e
63043

.D NURSING, Fifth Edition ISBN: 978-0-323-40170-8


**Notice**

best practice in this field are constantly changing. As new research and experience broaden
ng, changes in research methods, professional practices, or medical treatment may become

nd researchers must always rely on their own experience and knowledge in evaluating and
nation, methods, compounds, or experiments described herein. In using such information
should be mindful of their own safety and the safety of others, including parties for
a professional responsibility.
o any drug or pharmaceutical products identified, readers are advised to check the most
ion provided (i) on procedures featured or (ii) by the manufacturer of each product to be
verify the recommended dose or formula, the method and duration of administration,
tions. It is the responsibility of practitioners, relying on their own experience and
eir patients, to make diagnoses, to determine dosages and the best treatment for each
t, and to take all appropriate safety precautions.
extent of the law, neither the Publisher nor the authors, contributors, or editors, assume
ny injury and/or damage to persons or property as a matter of product liability,
nerwise, or from any use or operation of any methods, products, instructions, or ideas
material herein.

nal, Inc. *Nursing Diagnoses: Definitions & Classifications 2015-2017*, Tenth Edition. Edited by
an and Shigemi Kamitsuru. 2014 NANDA International, Inc. Published 2014 by John Wiley
panion website: www.wiley.com/go/nursingdiagnoses.

afe and effective judgments using NANDA-I nursing diagnoses, it is essential that nurses
ions and defining characteristics of the diagnoses listed in this work.

**ss Cataloging-in-Publication Data**
rsing/Emily Slone McKinney... [et al.].—Fifth ed.
phical references and index.
2775-3 (hardcover: alk. paper)
y Slone.
nal–Child Nursing—methods. 2. Pediatric Nursing—methods. WY 157.3]

*tegist:* Sandra Clark
*velopment Manager:* Laurie K. Gower
*ent Specialist:* Jennifer Wade
*Manager:* Jeff Patterson
*ager:* Anne Konopka
Ashley Miner

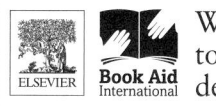



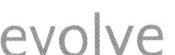

int number: 9 8 7 6 5 4 3 2 1

# Maternal–C
# Nursing

## Fifth Edition

Emily Slone McKinney, MSN, RN, C
(Deceased)
Nurse Educator and Consultant
Dallas, Texas

Susan Rowen James, PhD, RN
Professor Emerita
Curry College School of Nursing
Milton, Massachusetts

Sharon Smith Murray, MSN, RN
Professor Emerita
Health Professions
Golden West College
Huntington Beach, California

Kristine Ann Ne
Assistant Professor of
Tarrant County College
Trinity River East Camp
Professions
Fort Worth, Texas

Jean Weiler Ash
Assistant Dean
College of Nursing
University of Texas at A
Arlington, Texas

ELSEVIER

# SECTION EDITORS

## MATERNITY SECTION EDITORS


### Vanessa Flannery, DNP, PHCNS-BC, CNE
Associate Professor
Nursing Department
Morehead State University
Morehead, Kentucky

### Kari Mau, DNP, APRN-BC, RNFA, C-EFM
Instructor
College of Nursing
Medical University of South Carolina
Charleston, South Carolina;
Nurse Practitioner
The Breast Health Center
Bluffton, South Carolina

### Jennifer Rodriguez, RN, MSN
Nursing Instructor
Kellogg Community College
Battle Creek, Michigan

### Dawn Piacenza, MSN, BSN
Wesley Medical Center
Wichita, Kansas

### Karen Shaw Holub, RN, MS
Clinical Assistant Professor
Louise Herrington School of Nursing
Baylor University
Dallas, Texas

### Grace Moodt, DNP, MSN, RN
Associate Professor
School of Nursing
Austin Peay State University
Clarksville, Tennessee


## PEDIATRIC SECTION EDITOR


### Jacqueline Carroll, MSN, CPNP
Assistant Professor
School of Nursing
Curry College
Milton, Massachusetts

# CONTRIBUTORS

**Sheryl Cifrino, RN, DNP**
Associate Professor
Nursing Faculty
Curry College School of Nursing
Milton, Massachusetts

**Stephanie Clifford, MSN, ARNP, CPNP-AC/PC**
Pediatric Critical Care Nurse Practitioner
Department of Pediatrics
College of Medicine
University of Florida Health
Gainesville, Florida

**Cathleen C. Colleran, DNP, RN**
Professor of Nursing
Curry College, School of Nursing
Milton, Massachusetts

**Charlene Leonard, MSN**
Pediatric Critical Care Nurse Practitioner
University of Florida
Gainesville, Florida

**Karen Mehelich Lettre, MSN, RN, CEN, EMT**
Assistant Clinical Director
Emergency Center
Texas Children's Hospital Medical Center Campus
Dallas, Texas

**Michael A. Maymi DNP, ARNP, CPNP-AC, CCRN**
Cardiac Intensive Care Nurse Practitioner
Cardiology
Nemours Childrens Hospital
Orlando, Florida

**Eileen O'Connell PhD, PMHCNS-BC**
Professor
School of Nursing
Curry College
Milton, Massachusetts

## INSTRUCTOR AND STUDENT ANCILLARIES

**Jennifer T. Alderman, MSN, RNC-OB, CNL**
Assistant Professor
School of Nursing
University of North Carolina at Chapel Hill
Chapel Hill, North Carolina
*Study Guide*

**Martha Barry, MS, RN, APN, CNM**
Adjunct Clinical Instructor
College of Nursing
University of Illinois at Chicago
Chicago, Illinois
*Case Studies*

**Laura Bayless**
Bayless Editorial
Hazelwood, Missouri
*TEACH for Nurses*

**Meg Blair, PhD, MSN, RN, CEN**
Professor
Nursing Department
Nebraska Methodist College
Omaha, Nebraska
*Test Bank*

**Dusty Dix, MSN, RN**
Assistant Professor
School of Nursing
University of North Carolina at Chapel Hill
Chapel Hill, North Carolina
*Case Studies, Review Questions*

**Stephanie C. Evans, PhD, RN, CPNP-PC, CLC**
Assistant Professor
Harris College of Nursing and Health Sciences
Texas Christian University
Fort Worth, Texas
*Case Studies, Study Guide*

**Rhonda Lanning, RN, MSN, CNM, IBCLC**
Clinical Instructor
School of Nursing
University of North Carolina at Chapel Hill
Chapel Hill, North Carolina
*Case Studies*

**Karen Mehelich Lettre, MSN, RN, CEN, EMT**
Assistant Clinical Director
Emergency Center
Texas Children's Hospital Medical Center Campus
*Case Studies*

**Barbara Pascoe, RN, BA, MA**
Director—Maternity, Gynecology, and Pediatrics
Concord Hospital
Concord, New Hampshire
*PowerPoints*

**Kimberly Silvey, MSN, RN**
Assistant Professor
Department of Nursing
Morehead State University
Morehead, Kentucky
*Case Studies*

**Lynne L. Tier, MSN, RN**
Assistant Director of Simulation
Adventist University of Health Sciences
Orlando, Florida
*Review Questions*

# REVIEWERS

**Michael D. Aldridge, PhD, RN, CNE**
Assistant Professor of Nursing
Department of Pediatric Nursing
Concordia University Texas
Austin, Texas

**Brenda G. Alexander, MS, APRN-CNM**
Assistant Professor
Department of Nursing
St. Catharine College
St. Catharine, Kentucky

**Lilibeth Al-Kofahy, PhD, RN**
Sam Houston State University
The Woodlands, Texas

**Eryn Boyet, RN, MSN, WHNP-BC**
Faculty, Women's Health Nurse Practitioner
Nursing Department
North Central Texas College
Gainesville, Texas

**Shannon Smith Davis, MSN, BSN, RN**
Lead Faculty—Foundations of Nursing
School of Nursing
Jefferson Regional Medical Center
Pine Bluff, Arkansas

**Teresa Dawn Ferguson, RN, DNP, CNE**
Associate Professor of Nursing
Department of Nursing
Morehead State University
Morehead, Kentucky

**Cammie Fast, MS, RNC-OB**
Nursing Division Chair
Department of Nursing
Northern Oklahoma College
Tonkawa, Oklahoma

**Teresa L. Howell, DNP, RN, CNE**
Professor of Nursing
Department of Nursing
Morehead State University
Morehead, Kentucky

**Suzanne Miron, MSN, RN**
Associate Professor of Nursing
College of Health Sciences
Finlandia University
Hancock, Michigan

**Carolyn Morrisey, DNP, RN, CCRN**
Curriculum Coordinator, Instructor
Jefferson Regional Medical Center School of Nursing
Pine Bluff, Arkansas

**Jennifer Rodriguez, RN, MSN**
Nursing Instructor
Kellogg Community College
Battle Creek, Michigan

**Marilyn Murphy Shepherd PhD, RN, MBA, CAN, CDE, CWOCN, CNE**
Associate Professor
Blessing-Rieman College of Nursing and Health Sciences
Quincy University
Quincy, Illinois

**Madhu Soni, RN, MSN,MPsy,IBCLC, ICCE**
RN Educator/ Instructor
Nursing Department
Kaplan College
North Hollywood, California

**Melanie Stephens, MSN, RN, CNE**
Nursing Instructor
Department of Nursing
Fayetteville Technical Community College
Fayetteville, North Carolina

**Laura Williams, MSN, CNS, ONC, CCNS**
Orthopedic Clinical Nurse Specialist
Center for Nursing Research and Advanced Nursing Practice
Orlando Health
Orlando, Florida

# PREFACE

Children are a precious gift. Some of the most satisfying nursing roles involve helping families bring their children into the world, being a resource as they rear them, and supporting families during times of illness. In addition to providing care to young families as they bear and raise children, nurses play a crucial role in women's healthcare from the teen years through postmenopausal life. The fifth edition of *Maternal–Child Nursing* is written to provide a foundation for care of these individuals and their families and is intended to assist the nursing student or nurse entering maternity and women's health nursing or nursing of children from another area of nursing.

*Maternal–Child Nursing* builds on two successful texts to combine maternity, women's health, and nursing of children: *Nursing Care of Children: Principles and Practice,* fifth edition, by Susan Rowen James, Kristine Ann Nelson, and Jean Weiler Ashwill and *Foundations of Maternal-Newborn Nursing,* fifth edition, by Sharon Smith Murray and Emily Slone McKinney.

*Maternal–Child Nursing,* fifth edition, emphasizes evidence-based nursing care. The scientific base of maternal–newborn, women's health, and nursing care of children is demonstrated in the narrative and features in which the nursing process is applied. Physiologic and pathophysiologic processes are presented so the reader can understand why problems occur and the reasons underlying nursing care. Current references, many of them from Internet sources for best timeliness, provide the reader with the latest clinical information. National standards and guidelines, such as those from the Association of Women's Health, Obstetric and Neonatal Nurses (AWHONN); Society of Pediatric Nurses (SPN); and American Nurses Association (ANA), are used when applicable.

Maternal–newborn, women's health, and nursing of children may be practiced in a wide variety of settings. Where appropriate, our text discusses the care of patients in settings as diverse as acute and chronic care facilities, community, schools, and home. Methods to ease transition among facilities and improve continuity of care are highlighted when appropriate.

Legal and ethical issues add to the complexity of practice for today's nurse. A discussion of nurses' legal obligations when providing healthcare to women, newborns, and children optimizes care for all patients in each group. Legal topics include areas such as standards of care, informed consent, and refusal of treatment. Ethical principles and decision making are discussed in the first chapter of the text. Ethical issues, such as care of babies born at a very early gestation or nursing care at the end of life, are discussed in appropriate chapters.

Nursing students have time demands from work, family, and community activities in addition to their nursing education. For a significant number of nursing students and nurses, English is not their primary language. Considering those realities, we have written the text to effectively convey necessary information that focuses on critical elements and that is concise without the use of unnecessary complex language. Terms are defined throughout the chapter and are included with definitions in a glossary at the end of the book.

## CONCEPTS

Several conceptual threads are woven into our book. The *family* is a concept that is incorporated throughout our book as a vital part of maternal–child nursing care and nursing care of women. Family considerations appear in every step of the nursing process. A family may be the conventional mother–father–child arrangement or may be a single parent or multigenerational family. We consider several types of family styles as we present nursing care. We sometimes ask the reader to use critical thinking to examine personal assumptions and biases about families while studying.

Without *communication,* nursing care would be inadequate and sometimes unsafe. Teaching effective communication skills is incorporated into several features of the text as well as into the main narrative. Highlighted text within the narrative contains communication cues to give tips about verbal and nonverbal communication with patients and their families. Children are not little adults, and nowhere is this truer than when communicating with them. Therefore, communicating with children is presented in a separate chapter to supplement information given in other chapters on nursing of children.

*Health promotion* is obvious in chapters covering normal childbearing, child rearing, and women's health, but we also incorporate it into the chapters covering various disorders. Health promotion during illness may be as simple as reminding the reader that a technology-laden woman in labor is still having a baby, a usually normal process, and thus needs human contact. Sick children need activities to promote their normal growth and development as much as they need the technology and procedures that return them to physical wellness. This edition of *Maternal–Child Nursing* contains health promotion boxes in each of the developmental chapters. The goal of these boxes is to highlight anticipatory guidance appropriate for an infant's or child's developmental level according to the schedule of well visits recommended by the American Academy of Pediatrics (AAP).

*Teaching* is closely related to health promotion. Teaching is an expected part of nursing care to help patients and their families maintain health or return to health after illness or injury. Several features discussed later help the reader provide better teaching to patients in an understandable form.

*Cultural diversity* characterizes nursing practice today as the lines between individual nations become more blurred. The nurse must assess for unique cultural needs and incorporate them into care as much as possible to promote the acceptance of nursing care by the patient. Cultural influences are examined in many ways in our text, including critical thinking exercises to help the student "think outside the box" of his or her own culture.

*Growth and development* are concepts that appear throughout the book. We cover physical growth and development as the child is conceived and matures before birth and throughout childhood and as the woman matures through the childbearing years and into the climacteric. Specific chapters in the nursing of children section focus on growth and development issues, including anticipatory guidance, specific to each age group from infancy through adolescence.

*Advocacy* is emphasized in our text. Whether it is advocacy for a woman or family to be informed about their rights or advocacy for child and adult victims of violence, the concept is incorporated in the relevant places.

## FEATURES

Maternal–newborn and women's health nursing care differs from nursing care of children and their families in several important respects. Because of this fact, some features in the text appear in one part but not in the other, often with references to the chapter containing related content. Other features appear in both parts of the text.

Visual appeal characterizes many features in the text. Beautiful illustrations and photographs convey developmental or clinical information, capturing the essence of care for maternity, newborn, women's health, and child patients.

## OBJECTIVES

Objectives provide direction for the reader to understand what is important to glean from the chapter. Many objectives ask that the learner use critical thinking and apply the nursing process—two crucial components of professional nursing—to care for patients with the conditions discussed in that chapter. Other features within the chapters reinforce these two components of care.

## NURSING PROCESS

Several methods help the learner use the nursing process in the care of maternal–newborn, women's health, and child patients. The steps of the nursing process include performing assessment; formulating nursing diagnoses after analysis of the assessment data; planning care; providing nursing interventions; and evaluating the nursing interventions, expected outcomes, and appropriateness of nursing diagnoses as care proceeds. We address these steps in different ways in our book, often varying with whether the nursing process is discussed in the maternal–newborn, women's health, or nursing of children section. The varied approaches show the student that there is more than one way to communicate the nursing process. These different approaches to the nursing process also provide teaching tools to meet the needs of students' varied learning styles.

In the maternal–newborn and women's health section, the nursing process is presented in two ways. Nursing care is first presented as a *text discussion* that would apply to a typical patient with the condition. In addition, a *nursing care plan* that applies to a patient created in a specific scenario is constructed for many common conditions. This technique helps the student see individualization of nursing care. Many nursing care plans list *additional nursing diagnoses to consider* encouraging the reader to reflect on patient needs other than the obvious needs. The approach of scenario-based care plans is especially useful for showing learners how to apply the nursing process in dynamic conditions such as labor and birth.

In the nursing care of children section, the nursing process is applied to care for children with the most common childhood conditions by a blend of text discussion similar to the maternal–newborn and women's health section and a generic, rather than scenario-based, nursing care plan. The student thus has the benefit of seeing typical nursing diagnoses, expected outcomes, and interventions with their rationales discussed in a manner similar to care plans the learner may encounter in clinical facilities or be required to write in school. The evaluation step of the nursing process provides sample questions that the nurse would need to answer to determine whether the expected outcomes were achieved and whether further actions or revisions of nursing care are needed. The application of the nursing process in the nursing care of children provides a framework for the nursing instructor to help students individualize nursing care for their specific patients based on a generic plan of care. *Maternal–Child Nursing* demonstrates not only use of the nursing process when caring for acutely ill children but also emphasizes its application when providing care in the community setting. Community-based use of the nursing process applies to many nursing specialties, including those in both sections of this updated edition of *Maternal–Child Nursing.*

## CRITICAL THINKING EXERCISES

Critical thinking is encouraged in multiple ways in *Maternal–Child Nursing,* but specific Critical Thinking exercises present typical patient scenarios or other real-life situations and ask the reader to solve nursing care problems that are not always obvious. We use these exercises to help the student learn to identify the answer, choose the best interventions, or determine possible meanings or importance of signs and symptoms. Answers are provided on the Evolve Web site so that the student can check his or her solutions to these problems.

## EVIDENCE-BASED PRACTICE

As nursing care is grounded in evidence, the fifth edition of *Maternal–Child Nursing* continues to present timely evidence-based analyses in chapters where their topic is likely to be relevant to the patient care content. Reports of recent nursing research related to practice are summarized and give the reader a chance to identify possibilities to use the evidence in the clinical setting through questions at the end of each box.

## CRITICAL ALERTS

Students always want to know, "Will this be on the test?" The authors cannot answer that question, but consistent with Quality and Safety Education for Nurses (QSEN) terminology and the need to present critical and important information in a summative way, we have included both Safety Alerts and Nursing Quality Alerts that emphasize what is critical to remember when providing safe and optimal quality care.

## WANT TO KNOW

Because teaching is an essential part of nursing care, we give students teaching guidelines for common patient and family needs in terms that most lay people can understand. Both the Want to Know and the Patient-Centered Teaching boxes provide sample answers for questions that are most likely to be asked or topics that need to be taught, such as when to go to the birth center or methods of managing diet and insulin requirements for type 1 diabetes at home.

## HEALTH PROMOTION

Health Promotion boxes summarize needed information to perform a comprehensive assessment of well infants and children at various ages. Organized around the AAP-recommended schedule for well-child visits, examples are given of questions designed to elicit developmental and behavioral information from the parent and child. These boxes also include what the student might expect to see for health screening or immunizations and review specific topics for anticipatory guidance.

The topic of Health Maintenance is presented with the discussion of Women's Healthcare. Measures that may be taken for prevention of health problems or for early detection of specific diseases are often available to women.

## CLINICAL REFERENCE PAGES

Clinical Reference pages provide a resource for the reader when studying conditions that affect children. This feature provides the reader with basic information related to a group of disorders and includes a compact review of related anatomy and physiology; differences between children and adults in the system being studied; commonly used drugs, lab values, and diagnostic tests; and procedures that apply to the conditions discussed in that chapter.

## PATHOPHYSIOLOGY

Also present in many chapters in the nursing care of children are pathophysiology boxes. These boxes give the reader a brief overview of how the illness occurs. The boxes provide a scientific basis for understanding the therapeutic management of the illness and its nursing care.

## PROCEDURES

Clinical skills are presented in procedures throughout the text. Procedures related to maternal–newborn and women's health are presented in the chapters to which they apply. Because many procedures are common to the care of children with a variety of health conditions, they are covered in a chapter devoted to procedures, Chapter 37. Conditions such as asthma affect adults and children. The reader may find information about procedures that apply to both in a related pediatric chapter.

## DRUG GUIDES

Drug information may be presented in two ways: tables for related drugs used in the care of various conditions and drug guides for specific common drugs. Drug guides provide the nurse with greater detail for commonly encountered drugs in maternity and women's healthcare and in the care of children with specific pharmacologic needs.

## KEY CONCEPTS

Key concepts summarize important points of each chapter. They provide a general review for the material just presented to help the reader identify areas in which more study is needed.

Materials that complement *Maternal–Child Nursing* include the following:

### For Students

- *Evolve:* Evolve is an innovative Web site that provides a wealth of content, resources, and state-of-the-art information on maternity and pediatric nursing. Learning resources for students include Animations, Case Studies, Content Updates, Audio Glossary, Printable Key Points, Nursing Skills, and Review Questions.
- *Study Guide for Maternal–Child Nursing:* This student study aid provides learning exercises, supplemental classroom and clinical activities, and multiple-choice review questions to reinforce the material addressed in the text. An Answer Key is provided at the back of the book.
- *Virtual Clinical Excursions: Workbook and Online Companion* have been developed as a virtual clinical experience to expand student opportunities for critical thinking. This package guides the student through a computer-generated virtual clinical environment and helps the user apply textbook content to virtual patients in that environment. Case studies are presented that allow students to use this textbook as a reference to assess, diagnose, plan, implement, and evaluate "real" patients using clinical scenarios. The state-of-the-art technologies reflected in this CD demonstrate cutting-edge learning opportunities for students and facilitate knowledge retention of the information found in the textbook. The clinical simulations and workbook represent the next generation of research-based learning tools that promote critical thinking and meaningful learning.
- *Simulation Learning System:* The Simulation Learning System (SLS) is an online toolkit that effectively incorporates medium- to high-fidelity simulation into nursing curricula with scenarios that promote and enhance the clinical decision-making skills of students at all levels. The SLS offers a comprehensive package of resources including leveled patient scenarios, detailed instructions for preparation and implementation of the simulation experience, debriefing questions that encourage critical thinking, and learning resources to reinforce student comprehension.

### For Instructors

Evolve includes these teaching resources for instructors:

- *Electronic Test Bank in ExamView format* contains more than 1600 NCLEX-style test items including alternate format questions. An answer key with page references to the text, rationales, and NCLEX-style coding is included.
- *TEACH for Nurses* includes teaching strategies; in-class case studies; and links to animations, nursing skills, and nursing curriculum standards such as QSEN, concepts, and BSN Essentials.
- *Electronic Image Collection,* containing more than 600 full-color illustrations and photographs from the text, helps instructors develop presentations and explain key concepts.
- *PowerPoint Slides,* with lecture notes for each chapter of the text assist in presenting materials in the classroom. *Case Studies* and *Audience Response Questions* for iClickers are included.

# ACKNOWLEDGMENTS

Many people in addition to the authors made the fifth edition of *Maternal–Child Nursing* a reality. Thank you Sandra Clark, Senior Content Strategist; Laurie Gower, Senior Content Development Manager; Jennifer Wade, Content Development Specialist; Anne Konopka, Senior Project Manager; and Ashley Miner, Book Designer for your assistance throughout the publication process.

These acknowledgments would not be complete without thanking the current and past contributors to the nursing of children section. Their willingness and commitment to keeping current in their practice and sharing the benefit of their experience is most appreciated.

To Emily, Jean, Sharon, and Kris, with thanks for the many wonderful years of collaboration on this book, and to Jackie – I couldn't have asked for a better colleague. I would also like to express my love and gratitude to my family for their patience and support; I am truly blessed.

**Susan Rowen James**

# IN MEMORY OF EMILY S. MCKINNEY

Emily McKinney passed away in December 2013. It was my privilege to coauthor six editions of *Maternal-Newborn and Women's Health Nursing* and four editions of *Maternal-Child Nursing* with Emily. She also coauthored study guides for several other obstetric nursing textbooks. In 1999, she was awarded the honor of being included in the Dallas Fort Worth's Great 100 Nurses list. She was on the editorial staff of *JOGNN* (*Journal of Obstetric, Gynecologic, and Neonatal Nursing*) and was named Reviewer of the Year in 2006.

Emily was an excellent obstetric nurse and a talented nursing educator in the hospital as well as the classroom setting. She had an impressive knowledge of the science and the art of maternal-newborn nursing and was able to pass that knowledge on to her students an in easily digestible fashion.

It was Emily's idea to write a textbook that would be comprehensive yet easy to read. She realized that students often juggle several roles other than just being students. They are often parents and hold jobs to pay for their education and support their families. Emily used to say that simple words and short sentences could be just as effective as long, complicated words and sentences and much more easily absorbed by busy learners. When Trula Gorrie and I first met her in 1990, we knew that we shared Emily's vision and a wonderful partnership was formed.

Emily loved learning. She particularly looked forward to the yearly AWHONN (Association of Women's Health, Obstetric, and Neonatal Nursing) conventions. We met there each year and enjoyed hearing about the latest techniques and discoveries to advance obstetric nursing that were discussed. She was eager to find ways to apply new information to her clinical practice and teaching.

Throughout the years she was working on textbooks, Emily faced some difficult health problems. Yet she persevered in writing her chapters. She produced an amazing amount of quality work in short periods in spite of feeling ill. She was determined to do this as a way to advance nursing and nursing education.

Emily was also dedicated to her family. Her many interests included making clothes for her husband and two daughters as well as knitting hats for premature infants. Her daughters are following in her footsteps and are planning to go into nursing.

As an inspired nurse, Emily offered encouragement and practical help to her students and patients each day. Her passion for nursing was obvious to all. Emily is missed by everyone who knew her.

**Sharon S. Murray**

# CONTENTS

## UNIT III Pediatric Nursing Care

# 1

# Foundations of Maternity, Women's Health, and Child Health Nursing

http://evolve.elsevier.com/McKinney/mat-ch/

## LEARNING OBJECTIVES

*After studying this chapter, you should be able to:*

- Describe the historic background of maternity and child healthcare.
- Compare current settings for childbirth both within and outside a hospital setting.
- Identify trends that led to the development of family-centered maternity and pediatric care.
- Describe how issues, such as cost containment, outcomes management, home care, and technology, affect perinatal, a women's health, and child health nursing.
- Discuss trends in maternal, infant, and childhood mortality rates.
- Identify how poverty and violence on children and families affect nursing practice.
- Apply theories and principles of ethics to ethical dilemmas.
- Discuss ethical conflicts that the nurse may encounter in perinatal, women's health, and pediatric nursing practice.
- Relate how major social issues, such as poverty, homelessness, and access to healthcare, affect nursing practice.
- Describe the legal basis for nursing practice.
- Identify measures used to defend malpractice claims.
- Identify current trends in healthcare and their implications for nursing.

To better understand contemporary maternity nursing and nursing of children, the nurse needs to understand the history of these fields, trends, and issues that affect contemporary practice and the ethical and legal frameworks within which maternity and nursing care of children is provided.

## HISTORIC PERSPECTIVES

During the past several 100 years, both maternity nursing and nursing of children has changed dramatically in response to internal and external environmental factors. Expanding knowledge regarding the care of women, children, and families, as well as changes in the healthcare system markedly influenced these developments.

### Maternity Nursing

Major changes in maternity care occurred in the first half of the twentieth century as childbirth shifted from a home setting to a hospital setting. Rapid change continues as healthcare reforms attempt to control the increasing cost of care while advances in expensive technology accelerate. Despite changes, healthcare professionals attempt to maintain the quality of care.

### "Granny" Midwives

Before the twentieth century, childbirth usually occurred at home with the assistance of a "granny" or lay midwife whose training came through an apprenticeship with a more experienced midwife. Physicians were involved in childbirth only for serious problems.

Although many women and infants fared well when a lay midwife assisted with birth at home, maternal and infant death rates, resulting from childbearing, were high. The primary causes of maternal death were postpartum hemorrhage, postpartum infection also known as *puerperal sepsis* (or "childbed fever"), and hypertensive disorders of pregnancy. The primary causes of infant death were prematurity, dehydration from diarrhea, and contagious diseases.

### Emergence of Medical Management

In the late nineteenth century, technologic developments that were available to physicians but not to midwives led to a decline in home births and an increase in physician-assisted hospital births. Important discoveries that set the stage for a change in maternity care included the following:

- The discovery by Semmelweis that puerperal infection could be prevented by hygienic practices
- The development of forceps to facilitate birth
- The discovery of chloroform to control pain during childbirth
- The use of drugs to initiate labor or increase uterine contractions
- Advances in operative procedures such as cesarean birth

By 1960, 90% of births in the United States occurred in hospitals. Maternity care became highly regimented. All antepartum, intrapartum, and postpartum care were managed by physicians. Lay midwifery became illegal in many areas, and nurse–midwifery was not well established. The woman had a passive role in birth as the physician "delivered" her baby. Nurses' primary functions were to assist the physician and follow prescribed medical orders after childbirth. Teaching and counseling by the nurse were not valued at that time.

Unlike home births, early hospital births hindered the bonding between parents and infant. During labor, the woman often received medication, such as "twilight sleep," a combination of a narcotic and scopolamine, that provided pain relief but left the mother disoriented, confused, and heavily sedated. Birth became a delivery that was performed by a physician. Much of the importance of early contact between parents and child was lost as physician-attended hospital births became the norm. Mothers did not see their newborn for several hours after birth. Formula feeding was the expected method. The father was relegated to a waiting area and was not allowed to see the mother until sometime after birth and could only see his child through a window.

Despite the technologic advances and shift from home birth to hospital birth, maternal and infant mortality declined but slowly. The slow pace of this decline was caused primarily by preventable problems such as poor nutrition, infectious diseases, and inadequate prenatal care. These stubborn problems remained because of inequalities in healthcare delivery. Affluent families could afford comprehensive medical care that began early in the pregnancy, but poor families had very limited access to care or to information regarding childbearing. Two concurrent trends, federal involvement and consumer demands, led to additional changes in maternity care.

### Government Involvement in Maternal–Infant Care

The high rates of maternal and infant mortality among indigent women provided the impetus for federal involvement in maternity care. The Sheppard–Towner Act of 1921 provided funds for state-managed programs for mothers and children. Although this act was ruled unconstitutional in 1922, it set the stage for allocation of federal funds. Today, the federal government supports several programs to improve the health of mothers, infants, and young children (Table 1.1). Although projects supported by government funds partially solved the problem of maternal and infant mortality, the *distribution* of healthcare remained unequal. Most physicians practiced in urban or suburban areas where the affluent population could afford to pay for medical services, but women in rural or inner-city areas had difficulty obtaining care. The distribution of healthcare services is a problem that currently persists.

The ongoing problem of providing healthcare for poor women and children left the door open for nurses to expand their roles, and programs emerged to prepare nurses for advanced practice (see Chapter 2).

### Impact of Consumer Demands on Healthcare

In the early 1950s, consumers began to insist on their right to be involved in their healthcare. Pregnant women wanted a greater voice in their healthcare and wanted information regarding planning and spacing their children; moreover, they wanted to know what to expect during pregnancy. The father, siblings, and grandparents wanted to be part of the extraordinary events of pregnancy and childbirth. Parents began to insist on active participation in decisions concerning how their child would be born. Active participation of the patient is now expected in healthcare at all ages other than the very young or others who are unable to understand.

A growing consensus among child psychologists and nurse researchers indicated that the benefits of early, extended parent–newborn contact far outweighed the risk of infection. Parents began to insist that their infant remain with them, and the practice of separating the healthy infant from the family was abandoned.

### Development of Family-Centered Maternity Care

*Family-centered care* describes the safe, quality care that recognizes and adapts to both the physical and psychosocial needs of the family, including those of the newborn and older children (see also p. 5 for discussion of family-centered child care). The emphasis is on fostering family unity while maintaining physical safety.

Basic principles of family-centered maternity care are as follows:

- Childbirth is usually a normal, healthy event in the life of a family.
- Childbirth affects the entire family, and restructuring of family relationships is required.
- Families are capable of making decisions about care, provided that they are given adequate information and professional support.

Family-centered care increases the responsibilities of nurses. In addition to physical care and assisting the physician, nurses assume a major role in teaching, counseling, and supporting families in their decisions.

### Current Settings for Childbirth

As family-centered maternity care has emerged, the settings for childbirth have changed to meet the needs of new families.

**TABLE 1.1 Federal Projects for Maternal–Child Care**

| Program | Purpose |
|---|---|
| Title V of Social Security Act | Provides funds for maternal and child health programs |
| National Institute of Health and Human Development | Supports research and education of personnel needed for maternal and child health programs |
| Title V Amendment of Public Health Service Act | Established the Maternal and Infant Care (MIC) project to provide comprehensive prenatal and infant care in public clinics |
| Title XIX of Medicaid program | Provides funds to facilitate access to care by pregnant women and young children |
| Head Start program | Provides educational opportunities for low-income children of preschool age |
| National Center for Family Planning | A clearinghouse for contraceptive information |
| Special Supplemental Nutrition Program for Women, Infants, and Children (WIC) program | Provides supplemental food and nutrition information |
| Temporary Assistance to Needy Families (TANF) | Provides temporary money for basic living costs of poor children and their families, with eligibility requirements and time limits varying among states; tribal programs available for Native Americans<br>Replaces Aid to Families with Dependent Children (AFDC) |
| Healthy Start program | Enhances community development of culturally appropriate strategies designed to decrease infant mortality and causes of low birth weights |
| Individuals with Disabilities Education Act (PL 94-142) | Provides for free and appropriate education of all disabled children |
| National School Lunch/Breakfast program | Provides nutritionally appropriate free or reduced-price meals to students from low-income families |

### Traditional Hospital Setting

In the past, labor often took place in a functional hospital room, which was often occupied by several laboring women. When birth was imminent, the mother was moved to a delivery area similar to an operating room. After giving birth, the mother was transferred to a recovery area for 1 to 2 hours of observation and then taken to a standard hospital room in the postpartum unit. The infant was moved to the newborn nursery when the mother was transferred to the recovery area. Mother and infant were reunited when the mother was settled in her postpartum room. Beginning in the 1970s, the father or another significant support person could usually remain with the mother throughout labor, birth, and recovery, including cesarean birth.

Although birth in a traditional hospital setting was safe, the setting was impersonal and uncomfortable. Moving from room to room, particularly during late labor, was a major disadvantage. Each move was uncomfortable for the mother, disrupted the family's time together, and often separated the parents from the infant. Because of these disadvantages, hospitals began to devise settings that were more comfortable and included family participation.

*Labor, delivery, and recovery rooms.* Today most hospitals offer alternative settings for childbirth. The most common is the labor, delivery, and recovery (LDR) room. In an LDR room, labor, birth, and early recovery from childbirth occur in one setting. Furniture has a less institutional appearance but can be quickly converted into the setup required for birth. A typical LDR room is illustrated in Fig. 1.1.

During labor, significant others of the woman's preference may remain with her. The nurse often finds it necessary to regulate visitors in and out of the room to maintain safety and patient comfort. The mother typically remains in the LDR room for 1 to 2 hours after vaginal birth for recovery and is then transferred to the postpartum unit. The infant usually stays with the mother throughout her stay in the LDR room. The infant may be transferred to the nursery or may remain with the mother after her transfer to a postpartum room. Couplet care or the assignment of one nurse to the care of both mother and baby is common in today's postpartum units. The father or another primary support person is encouraged to stay with the mother and infant, and many facilities provide beds so they can stay through the night.

The major advantages of LDR rooms are that the setting is more comfortable and the family can remain with the mother. Disadvantages include the routine (rather than selective) use of technology such as electronic fetal monitoring and the administration of intravenous fluids.

*Labor, delivery, recovery, and postpartum rooms.* Some hospitals offer rooms that are similar to LDR rooms in layout and in function, but the mother is not transferred to a postpartum unit. She and the infant remain in the labor, delivery, recovery, and postpartum (LDRP) room until discharge. Frequent disadvantages of LDRP include a noisy environment and birthing beds that are less comfortable than standard hospital beds. Many hospitals have worked with the unit design so they have a group of beds in one area of the unit that are all postpartum.

### Birth Centers

Free-standing birth centers provide maternity care outside the acute-care setting to low-risk women during pregnancy, birth, and postpartum. Most provide gynecologic services such as annual checkups and contraceptive counseling. Both the mother and infant continue to receive follow-up care during the first 6 weeks. This may include help with breastfeeding, a postpartum examination at 4 to 6 weeks, family planning information, and examination of the newborn. Care is often provided by certified nurse-midwives (CNMs) who are registered nurses with advanced preparation in midwifery.

Birth centers are less expensive than acute-care hospitals that provide advanced technology that may be unnecessary for low-risk women. Women who want a safe, homelike birth in a familiar setting with staff they have known throughout their pregnancies express a high rate of satisfaction.

The major disadvantage is that most freestanding birth centers are not equipped for obstetric emergencies. Should unforeseen difficulties develop during labor, the woman must be transferred by ambulance to a nearby hospital to the care of a back-up physician who has agreed to perform this role. Some families do not feel that the very short stay after birth, often less than 12 hours, allows enough time to detect early complications in mother and infant.

### Home Births

In the United States only a small number of women have their babies at home. Because malpractice insurance for midwives attending home births is expensive and difficult to obtain, the number of midwives who offer this service has decreased greatly.

Home birth provides the advantages of keeping the family together in their own environment throughout the childbirth experience. Bonding with the infant is unimpeded by hospital routines, and breastfeeding is encouraged. Women and their support person have a sense of control because they actively plan and prepare for each detail of the birth.

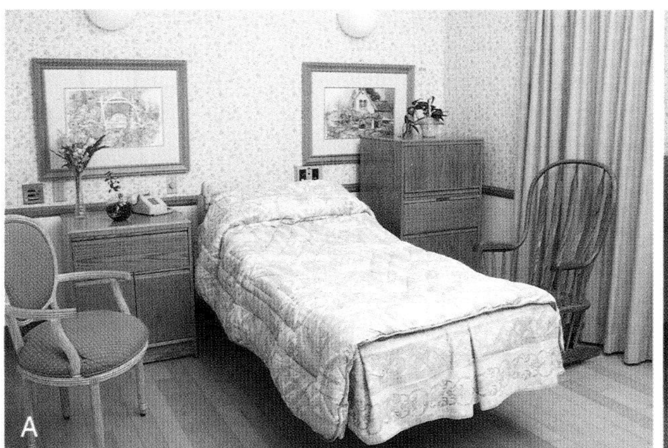


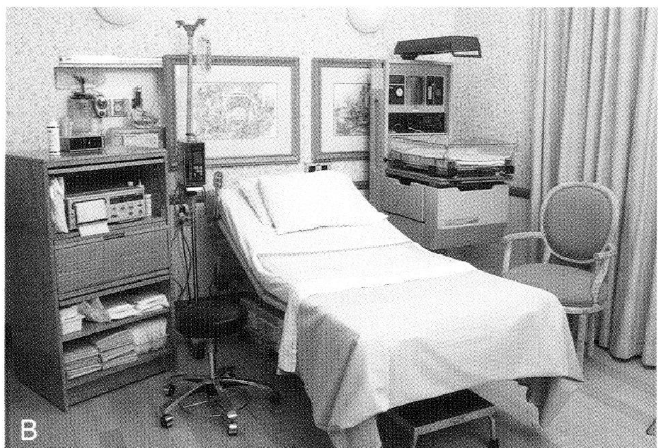


**FIG 1.1** A typical labor, delivery, and recovery room.Home-like furnishings **(A)** can be adapted quickly to reveal needed technical equipment **(B)**.

Giving birth at home also has disadvantages. The woman must be screened carefully to make sure that she has a very low risk for complications. If transfer to a nearby hospital becomes necessary, the time required may be too long in an emergency. Other problems of home birth may include the need for the parents to provide an adequate setting and supplies for the birth if the midwife does not provide supplies. The mother must care for herself and the infant without the professional help she would have in a hospital setting.

## Nursing of Children

To better understand contemporary child health nursing, the nurse needs to understand the history of this field, trends and issues affecting contemporary practice, and the ethical and legal frameworks within which pediatric nursing care is provided.

### Historic Perspectives

Nursing care for children has been influenced by multiple historic and social factors. Children have not always enjoyed the valued position that they hold in most families today. Historically, in times of economic or social instability, children have been viewed as expendable. In societies in which the struggle for survival is the central issue and only the strongest survive, the needs of children are secondary. The well-being of children in the past depended on the economic and cultural conditions of the society. At times, parents have viewed their children as property, and children have been bought and sold, beaten, and, in some cultures, sacrificed in religious ceremonies. In some societies, infanticide has been a routine practice. Conversely, in other instances, children have been highly valued and their birth considered a blessing. Viewed by society as miniature adults, children in the past received the same medical remedies as adults and, during illness, were cared for at home by family members, just as adults were.

### Societal Changes

As European settlements expanded on the North American continent during the seventeenth and eighteenth centuries, children were valued as assets to the community because of the desire to increase the population and share the work. Public schools were established, and the courts began to view children as minors and protect them accordingly. Devastating epidemics of smallpox, diphtheria, scarlet fever, and measles took their toll on children in the eighteenth century. Children often died of these virulent diseases within one day.

The high mortality rate in children led some physicians to examine common child-care practices. In 1748, William Cadogan's "Essay Upon Nursing" discouraged unhealthy child-care practices, such as swaddling infants in three or four layers of clothing and feeding them thin gruel within hours after birth. Instead, Cadogan urged mothers to breastfeed their infants and identified certain practices that were thought to contribute to childhood illness. Unfortunately, despite the efforts of Cadogan and others, child-care practices were slow to change. Later in the eighteenth century, the health of children improved with certain advances such as inoculation against smallpox.

With the flood of immigrants to eastern American cities in the nineteenth century, infectious diseases flourished as a result of crowded living conditions, inadequate and unsanitary food, and harsh working conditions for men, women, and children. Children frequently worked 12- to 14-hour days in factories, and their earnings were essential to the survival of the family. The most serious child health problems during the nineteenth century were caused by poverty and overcrowding. Infants were fed contaminated milk, sometimes from tuberculosis-infected cows. Milk was carried to the cities and purchased by mothers who had no means to refrigerate it. Infectious diarrhea was a common cause of infant death.

During the late nineteenth century, conditions began to improve for children and families. Lillian Wald initiated public health nursing at Henry Street Settlement House in New York City, where nurses taught mothers in their homes. In 1889, a milk distribution center opened in New York City to provide uncontaminated milk to sick infants.

### Hygiene and Hospitalization

The discoveries of scientists such as Pasteur, Lister, and Koch, who established that bacteria caused many diseases, supported the use of hygienic practices in hospitals and foundling homes. Hospitals began to require personnel to wear uniforms and limit contact between children in the wards. In an effort to prevent infection, hospital wards were closed to visitors. Because parental visits were noted to cause distress, particularly when parents had to leave, parental visitation was considered emotionally stressful to hospitalized children. In an effort to prevent such emotional distress and the spread of infection, parents were prohibited from visiting children in the hospital. Because hospital care focused on preventing disease transmission and curing physical diseases, the emotional health of hospitalized children received little attention.

During the twentieth century, as knowledge regarding nutrition, sanitation, bacteriology, pharmacology, medication, and psychology increased, dramatic changes in child health occurred. In the 1940s and 1950s, medications such as penicillin and corticosteroids and vaccines against many communicable diseases saved the lives of tens of thousands of children. Technologic advances in the 1970s and 1980s allowed more children to survive conditions that previously had been fatal (e.g., cystic fibrosis), thereby increasing the number of children living with chronic disabilities. An increase in societal concern for children brought about the development of federally supported programs designed to meet their needs, such as school lunch programs, the Special Supplemental Nutrition Program for Women, Infants, and Children (WIC), and Medicaid (see Table 1.1), under which the Early and Periodic Screening, Diagnosis, and Treatment program was implemented.

### Development of Family-Centered Child Care

Family-centered child healthcare developed from the recognition that the emotional needs of hospitalized children usually were unmet. Parents were not involved in the direct care of their children. Children were often unprepared for procedures and tests, and visiting was severely controlled and even discouraged.

Family-centered care is based on a philosophy that recognizes and respects the pivotal role of the family in the lives of both well and ill children. It strives to support families in their natural caregiving roles and promotes healthy patterns of living at home and in the community. Finally, parents and professionals are viewed as equals in a partnership committed to excellence at all levels of healthcare.

Most healthcare settings have a family-centered philosophy in which families are given choices, provide input, and are given information that is understandable by them. The family is respected, and its strengths are recognized.

The Association for the Care of Children's Health (ACCH), an international and interprofessional organization, was founded in 1965 to provide a forum for sharing experiences and common problems and to foster growth in children who must undergo hospitalization. Today the organization has broadened its focus on child healthcare to include the community and the home.

Through the efforts of ACCH and other organizations, increasing attention has been paid to the psychological and emotional effects of hospitalization during childhood. In response to greater knowledge about the emotional effects of illness and hospitalization, hospital policies and healthcare services for children have changed.

Twenty-four-hour parental and sibling visitation policies and home care services have become the norm. The psychological preparation of children for hospitalization and surgery has become standard nursing practice. Many hospitals have established child life programs to help children and their families cope with the stress of illness. Shorter hospital stays, home care, and day surgery also have helped minimize the emotional effects of hospitalization and illness on children.

## CURRENT TRENDS IN CHILD HEALTHCARE

During recent years, the government, insurance companies, hospitals, and healthcare providers have made a concerted effort to reform healthcare delivery in the United States and to control rising healthcare costs. This trend has involved changes in where and how money is spent. In the past, most of the healthcare budget was spent in acute care settings, where the facility charged for services after the services were provided. Because hospitals were paid for whatever materials and services they provided, they had no incentive to be efficient or cost conscious.

More recently, the focus has been on health promotion, the provision of care designed to keep people healthy and prevent illness. In late 2010, the USDHHS launched *Healthy People 2020,* a comprehensive, nationwide health promotion and disease-prevention agenda that builds on groundwork initiated 30 years ago. Developed with input from widely diverse constituencies, *Healthy People 2020* expands on goals and objectives developed for *Healthy People 2010,* and addresses "determinants of health," or those factors that contribute to keeping people healthy and achieving high quality of life (USDHHS, 2010). See http://www.healthypeople.gov to see and download objectives. Many of the national health objectives in *Healthy People 2020* are applicable to children and families. In fact, two objectives (Adolescent Health; Early and Middle Childhood) are specifically directed to the health of children and adolescents. National data for measuring progress toward these objectives are gathered from federal and state departments and from voluntary private, nongovernmental organizations. The mid-decade progress report states that more than 50% of leading health indicators have met goals or demonstrated progress toward achieving goals. For example, the infant mortality rate is approaching the target of 6.0 deaths per 1000 live births (USDHHS, 2014).

The focus of nursing care for children has changed as national attention to health promotion and disease prevention has increased. Even acutely ill children have only brief hospital stays because increased technology has facilitated parents' ability to care for children in the home or community setting. Most acute illnesses are managed in ambulatory settings, leaving hospital admission for the extremely acutely ill or children with complex medical needs. Nursing care for hospitalized children has become more specialized, and much nursing care is provided in community settings such as schools and outpatient clinics.

### Cost Containment

One way in which those paying for healthcare have attempted to control costs is by shifting to a *prospective* form of payment. In this arrangement, patients no longer pay whatever charges the hospital determines for services provided. Instead, a fixed amount of money is agreed upon in advance to cover necessary services for specifically diagnosed conditions. Several other strategies also have been used to contain the cost of services.

#### Diagnosis-Related Groups

Diagnosis-related groups (DRGs) are a method of classifying related medical diagnoses based on the amount of resources, severity of disease, and other patient characteristics. In some cases, DRG groupings articulate with the International Classification of Diseases (ICD) system. (Foley, 2015). This method of cost containment became a standard in 1987, when the federal government set the amount of money that would be paid by Medicare for each DRG. If the facility delivers more services or has greater costs than that covered by Medicare, the facility must absorb the excess cost. Conversely, if the facility delivers the care at lower cost than the payment for that DRG, the facility keeps the remaining money. Healthcare facilities working under this arrangement benefit financially if they can reduce the patient's length of stay, thereby decreasing the cost of services. Although the DRG system originally applied only to Medicare patients, most states have adopted the system for Medicaid payments, and most insurance companies use a similar system.

#### Managed Care

Health insurance companies also examined the cost of healthcare and instituted a healthcare delivery system that has been called *managed care*. Examples of managed care organizations are health maintenance organizations (HMOs), point of service plans (POSs), and preferred provider organizations (PPOs). HMOs provide relatively comprehensive health services for people enrolled in the organization for a set fee or premium. Similarly, PPOs are groups of healthcare providers who agree to provide health services to a specific group of patients at a discounted cost. When a patient needs medical treatment, managed care includes strategies such as payment arrangements and preadmission or pretreatment authorization to control costs.

Managed care, provided appropriately, can increase access to a full range of healthcare providers and services for women and children, but it must be closely monitored. Nurses serve as advocates in the areas of preventive, acute, and chronic care for women and children. The teaching timelines for preventive and home care have been shortened drastically, and the call to "begin teaching the moment the child or woman enters the healthcare system" has taken on a new meaning. Women, parents of the child, and other caregivers are being asked to do procedures at home that were once done by professionals in a hospital setting. Systems must be in place to monitor adherence, understanding, and the total care of a patient. Assessment and communication skills need to be keen, and the nurse must be able to work with specialists in other disciplines.

#### Capitated Care

Capitation may be incorporated into any type of managed care plan. In a pure capitated care plan, the employer (or government) pays a set amount of money each year to a network of primary care providers. This amount might be adjusted for the age and sex of the patient group. In exchange for access to a guaranteed patient base, the primary care providers agree to provide general healthcare and to pay for all aspects of the patient's care, including laboratory work, specialist visits, and hospital care.

Capitated plans are of interest to employers as well as the government because they allow a predictable amount of money to be budgeted for healthcare. Patients do not have unexpected financial burdens from illness. However, patients lose most of their freedom of choice regarding who will provide their care. Providers can lose money (1) if they refer too many patients to specialists, who may have no restrictions on their fees, (2) if they order too many diagnostic tests, or (3) if their administrative costs are too high. Some healthcare providers and consumers fear that cost constraints might affect treatment decisions.

### Effects of Cost Containment

Prospective payment plans have had major effects on maternal and infant care, primarily with respect to the length of stay. Mothers are typically discharged from the hospital at 48 hours after normal vaginal birth and 96 hours after cesarean birth, unless the woman and her healthcare provider choose an earlier discharge time. This leaves little time for nurses to adequately teach new parents about newborn care and to assess infants for subtle health issues. Nurses find that providing adequate information regarding infant care is particularly difficult when the mother is still recovering from childbirth. Problems with earlier discharge of mother and infant often require readmission and more expensive treatment than might have been required had the problem been identified early.

Despite efforts to contain costs related to the provision of healthcare in the United States, the percentage of the total government expenditures for services (gross domestic product [GDP]) allocated to healthcare was 17.4% in 2013 (National Center for Health Statistics [NCHS], 2014), markedly higher than many similar developed countries (Organization for Economic Co-operation and Development [OECD], 2015). This percentage has nearly doubled since 1980 but appears to be decreasing as new cost containment efforts increase. In March 2010, the *Patient Protection and Affordable Care Act* (ACA) was signed into the law. Designed to rein in healthcare costs while increasing access to the underserved, the provisions of this law have been phased in over several years (USDHHS, 2015). In general, improved access has occurred through the availability of affordable insurance coverage for all citizens. People who do not have access to insurance coverage through employer-provided insurance plans are able to purchase insurance through an insurance exchange, which was designed to offer various coverage options at competitive rates (USDHHS, 2015). In addition to increasing coverage, the ACA has had an effect on hospitalization and physicians' services, increasingly tying financial reimbursement to the quality of care and improved outcomes (USDHHS, 2015).

Several of the provisions of this law specifically address the needs of children and families and include the following (USDHHS, 2015):

- Prohibiting insurance companies from denying care based on pre-existing conditions for children younger than 19 years
- Keeping young adults on their family's health insurance plan until age 26 years
- Coordinated management for children and other individuals with chronic diseases
- Expanding the number of community health centers
- Increasing access to preventive healthcare
- Providing home visits to pregnant women and newborns
- Supporting states to expand Medicaid coverage
- Providing additional funding for the Children's Health Insurance Program (CHIP)

An additional provision of the ACA is the creation of accountable care organizations (ACOs). These are groups of hospitals, physicians' offices, community agencies, and any agency that provides healthcare to patients. Enhancing patient-centered care, the ACO collaborates on all aspects of coordination, safety, and quality for individuals within the organization. The ACO will reduce the duplication of services, decrease the fragmentation of care, and provide more control to patients and families (USDHHS, 2015).

Cost-containment measures have also altered traditional ways of providing patient-centered care, with increased focus on ensuring quality and safety through approaches such as case management, use of clinical practice guidelines and evidence-based nursing care, and outcomes management.

### Case Management

Case management is a practice model that uses a systematic approach to identify specific patients, determine eligibility for care, arrange access to appropriate resources and services, and provide continuity of care through a collaborative model (Lyon & Grow, 2011). In this model, a case manager or coordinator, who focuses on both quality of care and cost outcomes, coordinates the services required by the patient and family. Inherent to case management is the coordination of care by all members of the healthcare team. The guidelines established in 1995 by The Joint Commission require an interdisciplinary, collaborative approach to patient care. This concept is at the core of case management. Nurses who provide case management evaluate patient and family needs, establish needs documentation to support reimbursement, and may be part of a long-term care planning at home or a rehabilitation facility.

### Evidence-Based Nursing Care

The Agency for Healthcare Research and Quality (AHRQ), a branch of the U.S. Public Health Service, actively sponsors research in health issues that are faced by mothers and children. From research generated through this agency and others, high-quality evidence can be accumulated to guide the best and lowest cost clinical practices. The focus of research from AHRQ is primarily on accessing care for mothers, infants, children, and adolescents. This includes such topics as timeliness of care (care is provided as soon as necessary), patient centeredness (quality of communication with providers), coordination of care for children with chronic illnesses, access to a medical home, and affordability of care (AHRQ, 2015a). The effectiveness of healthcare also is a priority for research funding; this focus area includes recommendations for healthy living and preventive care in areas such as timely access to and provision of prenatal care, screening for mental health and developmental issues, immunizations, care of premature infants, and safety (AHRQ, 2015a). Clinical practice guidelines are an important tool in developing parameters for safe, effective, and evidence-based care for mothers, infants, children, and families. AHRQ has developed several guidelines related to adult and child care, as have other organizations and professional groups concerned with children's health. Important children's health issues, including quality and safety improvements, enhanced primary care, access to quality care, and specific illnesses, are addressed in the available practice guidelines. For detailed information, see the website at http://www.ahcpr.gov or http://www.guidelines.gov.

The Institute of Medicine (IOM, 2011) has published standards for developing practice guidelines to maximize consistency within and among guidelines, regardless of the guideline developers. The IOM recommends the inclusion of important information and process steps in every guideline. This includes ensuring the diversity of members of a clinical guideline group; full disclosure of conflict of interest; in-depth systematic reviews to inform recommendations; providing a rationale, quality of evidence, and strength of recommendation for each recommendation made by the guideline committee; and external review of recommendations for validity (IOM, 2011). The standardization of clinical practice guidelines will strengthen evidence-based care, particularly for guidelines developed by nurses or professional nursing organizations.

### Outcomes Management

The determination of lower healthcare costs while maintaining the quality of care has led to a clinical practice model called *outcomes management*. This is a systematic method to identify outcomes and to focus care on interventions that will accomplish the stated outcomes for children with specific issues, such as asthma.

***Nurse-sensitive indicators.*** In response to recent efforts to address both quality and safety issues in healthcare, various government and privately funded groups have sponsored research to identify patient care outcomes that are particularly dependent on the quality and quantity of nursing care provided. These outcomes, called *nurse-sensitive indicators*, are based on empirical data collected by such organizations as the AHRQ and the National Quality Forum (NQF), and represent outcomes that improve with optimal nursing care (American Nurses Association [ANA], 2011; Heslop, 2014). The following topics are in the process of development and delineation for pediatric nurses: adequate pain assessment, peripheral intravenous infiltration, pressure ulcer, catheter-related bloodstream infection, smoking cessation for adolescents, and obesity (ANA, 2011). Nurses need to use evidence-based intervention to improve these patient outcomes.

***Variances.*** Deviations or *variances* can occur in either the time line or in the expected outcomes. A variance is the difference between what was expected and what actually happened. A variance may be either positive or negative. A positive variance occurs when a child progresses faster than expected and is discharged sooner than planned. A negative variance occurs when progress is slower than expected, outcomes are not met within the designated time frame, and the length of stay is prolonged.

***Clinical pathways.*** One planning tool that is used by the healthcare team to identify and meet stated outcomes is the *clinical pathway*. Other names for clinical pathways include *critical* or *clinical paths, care paths, care maps, collaborative plans of care, anticipated recovery paths,* and *multidisciplinary action plans.* Clinical pathways are standardized, interdisciplinary plans of care that are devised for patients with a particular health problem. The purpose, as in managed care and case management, is to provide quality care while controlling costs. Clinical pathways identify patient outcomes, specify time lines to achieve those outcomes, direct appropriate interventions and sequencing of interventions, include interventions from various disciplines, promote collaboration, and involve a comprehensive approach to care. Home health agencies use clinical pathways that may be developed in collaboration with the hospital staff.

Clinical pathways may be used in various ways. For example, they may be used for change-of-shift reports to indicate information regarding the length of stay, individual needs, and priorities of the shift for each patient. They may also be used for documenting the person's nursing care plan and his or her progress in meeting the desired outcomes. The clinical pathway for a new mother may include care of her infant at term. Many pathways are particularly helpful in identifying families that require follow-up care.

## HOME CARE

Home nursing care has experienced dramatic growth since 1990. Advances in portable and wireless technology, such as infusion pumps for administering intravenous nutrition or subcutaneous medications, and monitoring devices such as telemonitors allow nurses and often patients or family to perform procedures and maintain equipment in the home. Consumers often prefer home care over hospitalization because this arrangement can be less stressful on the family when the patient is able to remain at home rather than be separated from the family support system because of the need for hospitalization. Optimal home care can also reduce readmission to the hospital for adults and children with chronic conditions.

Home care services may be provided in the form of telephone calls, home visits, information lines, developmental surveillance, and lactation consultations, among others. Online and wireless technology allows nurses to evaluate data transmitted from home. Infants with congenital anomalies, such as cleft palate, may require care that is adapted to their condition. Moreover, greater numbers of technology-dependent infants and children are now cared for at home, including those requiring ventilator assistance, total parenteral nutrition, intravenous medications, apnea monitoring, and other device-associated nursing care.

Nurses must be able to independently function within established protocols and must be confident of their clinical skills when providing home care. They should be proficient at interviewing, counseling, and teaching. They often assume a leadership role in coordinating all the services a family may require, and they frequently supervise the work of other care providers.

## COMMUNITY CARE

A model for community care of children is the school-based health center. These centers provide comprehensive primary healthcare services in the most accessible environment. Students can be evaluated, diagnosed, and treated on site. Services offered include primary preventive care (health assessments, anticipatory guidance, vision and hearing screenings, and immunizations), acute care, prescription services, and mental health and counseling services. Some school-based health centers are sponsored by hospitals, local health departments, and community health centers. Many are used in off hours to provide healthcare to uninsured adults and adolescents.

### Access to Care

Access to care is an important component when evaluating preventive care and prompt treatment of illness and injuries. Access to healthcare is strongly associated with having health insurance. The American Academy of Pediatrics states that all children through the age of 21 should have access to high quality healthcare that is comprehensive, takes place within the medical home, and incorporates new technologies (AAP, 2015). This care should be ensured through access to comprehensive health insurance that is designed to address the unique developmental and health needs of all children (AAP, 2015).

Having health insurance coverage, usually employer sponsored, often determines whether a person will seek care early in the course of a pregnancy or an illness. Many private health plans have restrictions such as prequalification for procedures and a set list of and services covered by the plan. People with employer-sponsored health insurance often find that they must change providers each year because the available plans change, a situation that may negatively affect the provider-patient relationship. The Affordable Care Act is designed to resolve some of these issues.

#### Public Health Insurance Programs

Improvements in federal and state programs that address children's health needs has resulted in a decrease of uninsured children in the United States. The percentage of children younger than age 17 years who lack health insurance is 6.6%, with 3.4% being uninsured for longer than 1 year. Although the overall percentage of uninsured children has decreased since 2009, this number has leveled off since 2012 (Cohen & Martinez, 2014). Health insurance coverage varies among children by poverty, age, race, and ethnic origin (Fig. 1.2). The proportion of children with health insurance is lowest among Hispanic children compared with white or black children and is lower among poor and near-poor children compared with those from higher-income families (Cohen & Martinez, 2014; Forum on Child and Family Statistics, 2015).

Children in poor and near-poor families are more likely to be uninsured (16.2%) (Cohen & Martinez, 2014), have unmet medical needs, receive delayed medical care, have no usual provider of healthcare, and have higher rates of emergency room service than those in families that are not poor. Approximately 4% of all children have no

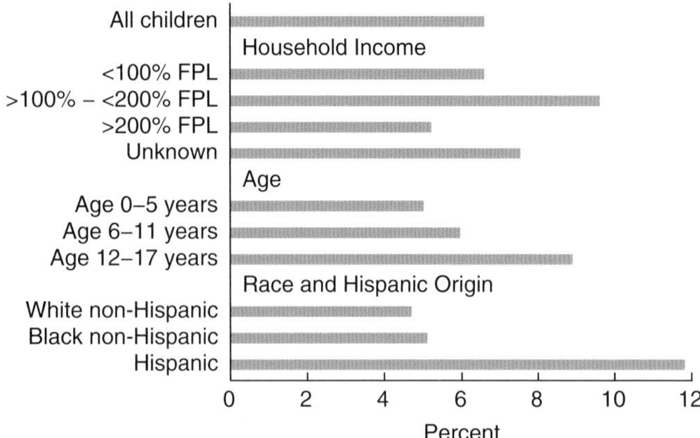


**FIG 1.2** Uninsured Children by Poverty Status, Household Income, Age, Race, and Hispanic Origin, 2014. FPL = Federal Poverty Level. (From: Cohen, R., & Martinez, M. (2014). *Health insurance coverage: Early release of estimates from the National Health Interview Survey, January to March, 2014.* Retrieved from http://www.cdc.gov/nchs; Federal Interagency Forum on Child and Family Statistics. (2015). *America's children: Key national indicators of well-being, 2015.* Retrieved from http://www.childstats.gov.)

usual place of healthcare, and this is more prevalent in children who are uninsured or underinsured (Federal Interagency Forum on Child and Family Statistics, 2015).

Public health insurance for children is provided primarily through Medicaid, a federal program that provides healthcare for certain populations of people living in poverty, or the CHIP (formerly the State Children's Health Insurance Program), a program that provides access for children not poor enough to be eligible for Medicaid but whose household income is less than 200% of poverty level. In 2009, funding was renewed for CHIP through the Children's Health Insurance Program Reauthorization Act (CHIPRA); in 2014, 8.1 million children nationwide were enrolled in CHIP (Centers for Medicare and Medicaid, 2015a).

Publicly sponsored health insurance covered 43% of children younger than age 18 years in 2013 (Cohen & Martinez, 2014). Medicaid provides healthcare for the poor, aged, and disabled, with pregnant women and young children especially targeted. Medicaid is funded by both the federal government and individual state governments. The states administer the program and determine which services are offered.

### Preventive Health

The oral health of children in the United States has become a topic of increasing focus as more is learned about the relationship between dental caries and overall health. Overall, 88% of children reported having seen a dentist within the previous year (Federal Interagency Forum on Child and Family Statistics, 2015). Services available through Medicaid are limited, and many dentists do not accept children who are insured by Medicaid. Economic, racial, and ethnic disparities exist in this area of health. Children living in poverty are far less likely to have seen a dentist over the past year than children from more affluent households. Furthermore, a high percentage of non-Hispanic black school-age children and Mexican-American children have untreated dental caries as compared to non-Hispanic white children (Federal Interagency Forum on Child and Family Statistics, 2015). In addition, maternal periodontal disease is emerging as a contributing factor to prematurity, with adverse effects on the child's long-term health.

Besides the obvious implication of not having health insurance—the inability to pay for healthcare during illness—uninsured children are less likely to receive immunizations and other preventive care, placing them at increased risk for preventable illnesses. Because practicing preventive healthcare is a learned behavior, these children are more likely to become adults who are less healthy.

## HEALTHCARE ASSISTANCE PROGRAMS

Many programs, some funded privately and others by the government, assist in the care of mothers, infants, and children. The WIC program, established in 1972, provides supplemental food supplies to low-income women who are pregnant or breastfeeding and to their children up to the age of 5 years. WIC has long been heralded as a cost-effective program that not only provides nutritional support but also links families with other services such as prenatal care and immunizations.

Medicaid's Early and Periodic Screening, Diagnosis, and Treatment (EPSDT) program was developed to provide comprehensive healthcare to Medicaid recipients from birth to 21 years of age. The goal of the program is to prevent health problems or identify them before they become severe. This program pays for well-child examinations and for the treatment of any medical problems diagnosed during such checkups.

Public Law 99-457 is part of the Individuals with Disabilities Education Act that provides financial incentives to states to establish comprehensive early intervention services for infants and toddlers with or at risk for developmental disabilities. Services include screening, identification, referral, and treatment. Although this is a federal law and entitlement, each state bases coverage on its own definition of developmental delay. Thus, coverage may vary from state to state. Some states provide care for at-risk children.

The Healthy Start program, begun in 1991, is a major initiative to reduce infant deaths in communities with disproportionately high infant mortality rates. Strategies used include reducing the number of high-risk pregnancies, reducing the number of low-birth-weight and preterm births, improving birth-weight–specific survival, and reducing specific causes of postneonatal mortality.

The March of Dimes, long an advocate for improving the health of infants and children, publishes an annual *Prematurity Report Card.* Designed to reduce the devastating toll that prematurity takes on the population, this organization emphasizes education, research, and advocacy. Prematurity often results in permanent health or developmental problems for survivors. The current percentage of babies born prematurely (less than 37 weeks) is nearly 10% in the United States (March of Dimes, 2015), with obvious regional differences; the lowest rate is in the northwest, while the highest rates are in the midwest and southeast. Racial and ethnic disparities continue to occur, with the highest rate of premature births occurring among Black and Native American populations (March of Dimes, 2015).

## STATISTICS ON MATERNAL, INFANT, AND CHILD HEALTH

Statistics are important sources of information about the health of groups of people. The newest statistics about maternal, infant, and child health for the United States can be obtained from the National Center for Health Statistics (http://www.cdc.gov/nchs).

### Maternal and Infant Mortality

Throughout history, women and infants have had high death rates, especially around the time of childbirth. Infant and maternal mortality rates began to decrease when the health of the general population improved, basic principles of sanitation were put into practice, and medical knowledge increased. A further large decrease resulted from the widespread availability of antibiotics, improvements in public health, and better prenatal care in the 1940s and 1950s. Today mothers seldom die in childbirth, and the infant mortality rate is decreasing, although the rate of change has slowed for both. Racial inequality in maternal and infant mortality rates continues, with nonwhite groups having higher mortality rates than white groups.

### Pregnancy-Related Mortality

In 2011, the pregnancy-related death ratio was 17.8 per 100,000 live births for all women in the United States. Black or African-American women are over three times more likely to die from pregnancy-related causes than white women (CDC, 2015). Although pregnancy-related deaths declined significantly over the past century, there has been a marked increase since 1987; the causes for this increase are unclear (CDC, 2015).

### Infant Mortality

The infant mortality rate (death before the age of 1 year per 1000 live births) has been decreasing since 2000. Most recent data report an infant mortality rate of 5.8, the lowest on record (Murphy, Kochanek, Xu, & Arias, 2015). The neonatal mortality rate (death before 28 days of life) dropped to 4.01 deaths per 1000 live births for the most recent reporting year (Murphy et al., 2015). Currently, the five leading causes of infant mortality are congenital malformations, deformations, and chromosome abnormalities; disorders related to low birthweight; newborn problems related to maternal complications; sudden infant death syndrome (SIDS); and unintentional injury.

The decrease in the infant mortality rate is attributed to better neonatal care and to public awareness campaigns, such as the Back to Sleep campaign to reduce the occurrence of sudden infant death syndrome. This campaign has contributed to more than a 50% decrease in the number of deaths attributed to SIDS in the United States since 1980 (Mathews & MacDorman, 2011; NCHS, 2011).

*Racial disparity for mortality.* Although infant mortality rates in the United States have declined overall, race-based differences remain. The 2012 mortality rate was 5.07 for white infants and 10.9 for African-American infants (NCHS, 2014). Fig. 1.3 compares the rates of infant mortality for all races and for whites and blacks or African-Americans since 1950. Much of the racial disparity in infant mortality is attributable to premature (born before 37 completed weeks) and low-birth-weight infants (less than 2500 g), both more common among Black infants. Premature and low-birth-weight infants have a greater risk of short- and long-term health problems, as well as death (March of Dimes, 2015).

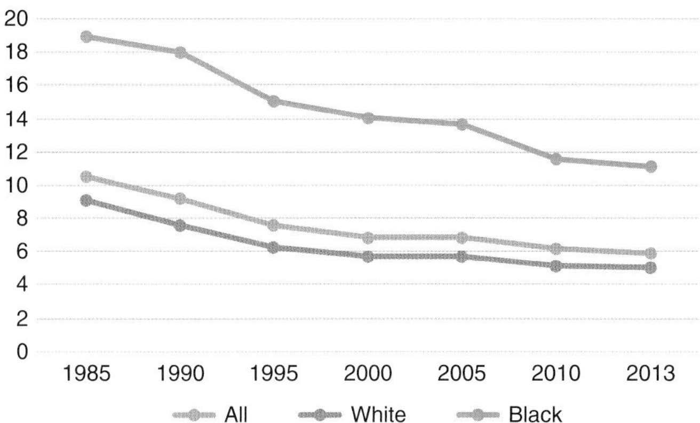


FIG 1.3 Infant Mortality Rates, 1985-2013. (From: *Infant mortality rates, 1950-2010.* Retrieved from http://www.infoplease.com; Mathews, T., MacDorman, M., & Thoma, M. (2015). Infant mortality statistics from the 2013 period linked birth/infant death data set. *National Vital Statistics Report, 64*(9). Retrieved from http://www.cdc.gov.)

Poverty is an important factor. Proportionally more nonwhites than whites are poor in the United States. Poor people are less likely to be in good health, to be well nourished, or to get the healthcare they need. Obtaining care becomes vital during pregnancy and infancy, and lack of care is reflected in the high mortality rates in all categories.

*International infant mortality.* One would expect that a nation such as the United States would have one of the lowest infant mortality rates when compared with other developed countries. However, data from 2010 (most current) places the United States 26th in the list of infant mortality rates of developed countries (Table 1.2) (MacDorman, Matthews, Mahangoo, & Zeitlin, 2014). International rankings are difficult to compare because countries differ in how they report live births. Preterm (<24 weeks) infant mortality is lower in the United States than many European countries, but the infant mortality rate for infants at 37 weeks in the United States is one of the highest (MacDorman et al., 2014).

### Adolescent Births

Teenage childbearing has been a long-standing concern in the United States. Young mothers are more likely to deliver low-birthweight (LBW) or preterm infants than older women. The babies of teen mothers have a greater risk of dying in infancy, and the public costs of teen births is estimated as $9.4 billion (Ventura, Hamilton, & Mathews, 2014). That adolescent birth rates in the United States have fallen to historic lows does not remove the health risks for mother and child.

Births to girls aged 15 to 19 years decreased from a 1991 peak of 61.8 births per 1000 girls to 26.5 births per 1000 girls. Births to girls

**TABLE 1.2 Infant Mortality Data for Selected Countries (Based on 2010 Data)**

| Country | Infant Mortality (Per 1000 Live Births) |
|---|---|
| Finland, Japan | 2.3 |
| Portugal, Sweden | 2.5 |
| Czech Republic | 2.7 |
| Norway | 2.8 |
| Spain | 3.2 |
| Denmark, Germany, Italy | 3.4 |
| Belgium, France | 3.6 |
| Greece, Ireland, Netherlands, Switzerland | 3.8 |
| Austria | 3.9 |
| Australia | 4.1 |
| United Kingdom | 4.2 |
| Poland | 5.0 |
| Hungary | 5.3 |
| New Zealand | 5.5 |
| Slovakia | 5.7 |
| United States | 6.1 |

From: MacDorman, M., Mathews, T. J., Mahangoo, A. D., & Zeitlin, J. (2014). International comparisons of infant mortality and related factors: United States and Europe, 2010. *National Vital Statistics Reports, 63*(5), Hyattsville, MD: National Center for Health Statistics.

in different age groups have had a 10% decrease from 2012-2013 (Martin, Hamilton, Osterman, Curtin, & Mathews, 2015):

- Teenagers 10 to 14 years: 0.3 per 1000; lowest ever reported
- Teenagers 15 to 17 years: decreased 13%, to 12.3 per 1000; record low
- Teenagers 18 to 19 years: decreased 8%, to 47.1 per 1000; record low

Among girls 15 to 19 years, births to non-Hispanic whites decreased 9%, non-Hispanic blacks and American Indian/Alaska natives decreased 11%, and Hispanics and Asian/Pacific Islanders decreased 10% (Martin et al., 2015).

### Childhood Mortality

Death rates for children have declined significantly over the past 20 years. Table 1.3 shows the leading causes of death in children. Although death rates attributed to unintentional injury also have dropped, they are still the leading cause of death in children aged 1 to 19 years. In all age groups except children 1 to 4 years, motor vehicle crashes lead the causes of death from unintentional injury; in children ages 1 to 4 years, drowning is the leading cause of unintentional death (Federal Interagency Forum on Child and Family Statistics, 2015). Homicide has become the third leading cause of death in children ages 1 to 4 years and is the fifth leading cause of death for children 5 to 14 years. Very concerning is that suicide has become the third leading cause of death for children ages 5 to 14 years and the second leading cause of death in adolescents (NCHS, 2014). Other common causes of death in children include congenital malformations, cancer, and cardiac and respiratory diseases. Self-inflicted firearm injury is a leading cause of death in the adolescent population (Forum on Child and Family Statistics, 2015).

### Morbidity

The morbidity rate is the ratio of sick people to well people in a population and is presented as the number of ill people per 1000 people.

**TABLE 1.3 Leading Causes of Death Among Children Ages 1 to 14 Years: Death Rates Per 100,000**

| | |
|---|---|
| **Ages 1 to 4 Years** | |
| Unintentional injury | 8.3 |
| Congenital malformations | 3.0 |
| Homicide | 2.1 |
| Cancer | 2.1 |
| Heart disease | 1.1 |
| **Ages 5 to 9 Years** | |
| Unintentional injury | 3.6 |
| Cancer | 2.2 |
| Congenital malformations | 0.9 |
| Homicide | 0.6 |
| Chronic lower respiratory diseases | 0.4 |
| **Ages 10 to 14 Years** | |
| Unintentional injury | 3.8 |
| Cancer | 2.2 |
| Suicide | 1.9 |
| Congenital malformations | 0.8 |
| Homicide | 0.7 |

From National Center for Health Statistics. (2013). *Deaths, percent of total death and death rates for the 15 leading causes of death in 5-year age groups by race and sex: United States 2013.* Retrieved from http://www.cdc.org/nchs.

This term is used in reference to acute and chronic illness as well as disability. Because morbidity statistics are collected and updated less frequently than mortality statistics, the presentation of current data in all areas of child health is difficult. The link between poverty and poorer health outcomes in children is well documented. Children in families with higher incomes and higher educational levels have a better chance of being born healthy and remaining healthy. Access to healthcare, the health behaviors of parents and siblings, and the exposure to environmental risks are among the factors contributing to this disparity in children's health (Federal Interagency Forum on Child and Family Statistics, 2015; NCHS, 2014).

Diseases of the respiratory system, including bronchitis or bronchiolitis, asthma, and pneumonia, are a major cause of physician visits and hospitalization for children younger than 18 years. A reported 8% of children in the United States currently have asthma; approximately 5% of these report having had one or more acute episodes during the previous year (Federal Interagency Forum on Child and Family Statistics, 2015). Obesity is a problem of significant concern. Over 10% of children between the ages of 2 and 5 years are considered to be obese; this percentage increases as children grow, and obesity affects more than 19% of adolescents (NCHS, 2014). Other issues of increasing concern include food allergies, attention deficit hyperactivity disorder (ADHD), and childhood and adolescent depression. Statistics regarding morbidity related to particular disorders are presented in this text as the disorders are discussed.

The Youth Risk Behavior Surveillance System conducts a national survey of students in grades 9 to 12 every 2 years in odd years. The CDC (2016) has identified the following health behaviors among youth in the United States that contribute to increased mortality, morbidity, and social problems: 1) behaviors that contribute to unintentional injuries and violence; 2) tobacco use; 3) alcohol and other drug use; 4) sexual behaviors related to unintended pregnancy and sexually transmitted infections (STIs), including HIV infection; 5) unhealthy dietary behaviors; and 6) physical inactivity. Many high school students engage in behaviors that place them at risk for the leading causes of morbidity and mortality. Since the earliest year of data collection, the prevalence of most health risk behaviors has decreased (e.g., riding with a driver who had been drinking alcohol, physical fighting, current cigarette use, current alcohol use, and current sexual activity), but the prevalence of other behaviors and health outcomes has not changed (e.g., suicide attempts treated by a doctor or nurse, smokeless tobacco use, having ever used marijuana, and attending physical education classes) or has increased (e.g., having not gone to school because of safety concerns, obesity, overweight, not eating vegetables, and not drinking milk). Monitoring emerging risk behaviors (e.g., texting and driving, bullying, and electronic vapor product use) is important to understand how they might vary over time (CDC, 2016).

## ETHICAL PERSPECTIVES ON MATERNITY, WOMEN'S HEALTH, AND CHILD NURSING

Maternal–child health nurses often struggle with ethical and social dilemmas that affect families. Nurses must know how to approach these issues in a knowledgeable and systematic manner.

### Ethics and Bioethics

*Ethics* involves determining the best course of action in a certain situation. Ethical reasoning is the analysis of what is right and reasonable. *Bioethics* is the application of ethics to healthcare. Ethical behavior or principle-based ethics for nurses is discussed in various codes, such as the ANA Code for Nurses. Ethical issues have become more complex as developing technology has allowed more options in healthcare.

### BOX 1.1 Ethical Principles

- *Beneficence.* One is required to do or promote good for others.
- *Nonmaleficence.* One must avoid risking or causing harm to others.
- *Autonomy.* People have the right to self-determination. This includes the right to respect, privacy, and the information necessary to make decisions.
- *Justice.* All people should be treated equally and fairly regardless of disease or social or economic status. Rendering to others what is due them.

These issues are controversial because of the lack of agreement over what is right or best and because moral support is possible for more than one course of action.

## Ethical Dilemmas

An *ethical dilemma* is a situation in which no solution appears completely satisfactory. Opposing courses of action may seem equally desirable, or all possible solutions may seem undesirable. Ethical dilemmas are among the most difficult situations in nursing practice. Finding solutions involves applying ethical theories and principles and determining the burdens and benefits of any course of action.

### Ethical Principles

Ethical principles are important in solving ethical dilemmas. Four of the most important principles are beneficence, nonmaleficence, autonomy, and justice (Box 1.1). Although principles guide decision making, in some situations, it may be impossible to apply one principle without encountering a conflict with another. In such cases, one principle may outweigh another in importance.

For example, treatments designed to be beneficial may also cause some harm. A cesarean birth may prevent permanent harm to a fetus in distress. However, the surgery that saves the fetus also harms the mother, causing pain, temporary disability, and possible financial hardship. Both mother and healthcare providers may decide that the principle of beneficence outweighs the principle of nonmaleficence. A third possibility is that if the mother does not want surgery, the principles of autonomy and justice must also be considered. Is the mother's right to determine what happens to her body more or less important than the right of the fetus to fair and equal treatment expected to be beneficial? Confidentiality is a cornerstone in healthcare relationships between multiple providers of care and is mandated by the Health Insurance Portability and Accountability Act (HIPAA). So does a woman's sexual partner have the right to know that she has been diagnosed with a sexually transmitted disease? What if the infection is HIV? What if the HIV infection has occurred in a 14-year-old girl? Can her parents be notified if she does not give consent (Stephenson, 2011)?

### Solving Ethical Dilemmas

Although using a specific approach does not guarantee a right decision, it provides a logical, systematic method for going through the steps of decision making.

Decision making in ethical dilemmas may appear straightforward, but it may not result in answers that are agreeable to everyone. Therefore, many agencies have bioethics committees to formulate policies for ethical situations, provide education, and help make decisions in specific cases. The committees include various professionals such as nurses, physicians, social workers, ethicists, and clergy members. If possible, the patient and family also participate. A satisfactory solution to ethical dilemmas is more likely to occur when people work together.

Ethical dilemmas may also have legal ramifications. For example, although the American Medical Association has stated that anencephalic organ donation is ethically permissible, it may be illegal. In many states, the legal criteria for death include cardiopulmonary and brain death.

## Ethical Concerns in Reproduction

Ethical issues often confront healthcare providers, families, and society at large. For example, conflicts between a woman and her fetus occur when the woman's requirements, behavior, or wishes may injure the fetus. Caregivers and society may respond to issues such as elective abortion, substance abuse, or a mother's refusal to follow advice of health professionals with anger rather than support. Pediatric ethical and legal issues may include the choice of treatments out of the mainstream or the refusal of medical treatment for a minor child in caregiver custody.

### Elective Pregnancy Termination

A woman's choice to electively have a pregnancy terminated or an *induced abortion* was a volatile legal, social, and political issue even before the *Roe vs. Wade* decision by the U.S. Supreme Court in 1973. Before that, states could prohibit induced abortion, making the procedure illegal. In *Roe vs. Wade,* the court stated that abortion was legal anywhere in the United States and that existing state laws prohibiting induced abortion were unconstitutional because they interfered with the mother's constitutional right to privacy. The Supreme Court's decision stipulated that (1) a woman could obtain an abortion at any time during the first trimester, (2) the state could regulate abortions during the second trimester only to protect the woman's health, and (3) the state could regulate or prohibit abortion during the third trimester, except when the mother's life might be jeopardized by continuing the pregnancy. Since 1973, many state laws have been upheld or struck down by the Supreme Court's decisions (Box 1.2).

Two conflicting major issues continue to be the belief that elective termination of pregnancy is a private choice and that this choice takes a life. Presidential candidates are confronted with the national abortion issue and their personal beliefs. Nurses also have personal beliefs concerning these two issues and those beliefs affect professional practice.

**Belief that induced abortion is a private choice.** At the heart of political action to keep induced abortion legal is the conviction that women have the right to make decisions concerning their reproductive function on the basis of their own ethical and moral beliefs and that the government has no place in these decisions. Advocates of the legal right point out that induced abortion, either legal or illegal, has always been a reality of life and will continue to be so, regardless of the legislation or judicial rulings. Advocates express concern about the unsafe conditions that accompany illegal abortion, citing the deaths that occurred as a result of illegal abortions that were performed before the *Roe v. Wade* decision.

**Belief that elective pregnancy termination is taking a life.** Many people believe that legalized abortion condones taking a life and feel morally bound to protect the lives of fetuses. People opposed to abortion have demonstrated their commitment by organizing to become a potent political force. They have been willingly arrested for civil disobedience when they attempted to prevent admissions to clinics where abortions are performed.

**Implications for nurses.** As healthcare professionals, nurses are involved in the conflict among differing beliefs about elective pregnancy termination. Nurses have their own beliefs about electively ending a pregnancy and respond in ways that illustrate the complexity of the issue and the ambivalence that it often produces. Nurses have several responsibilities that cannot be ignored. Nurses must

- Be informed about the induced abortion issue from a legal and ethical standpoint and should know the regulations and laws of their state.

**BOX 1.2 Supreme Court Decisions on Abortion Since *Roe V. Wade***

*1976:* States cannot give a husband veto power over his wife's decision to have an abortion.
*1977:* States do not have an obligation to pay for abortions as part of government-funded healthcare programs (considered by abortion rights advocates to be unfair discrimination against poor women who are unable to pay for an abortion).
*1979:* Physicians have broad discretion in determining fetal viability, and states have leeway to restrict abortions of viable fetuses.
*1979:* States may require parental consent for minors seeking abortions as long as an alternative, such as a minor getting a judge's approval, is also available.
*1989:* Upheld a Missouri law barring abortions performed in public hospitals and clinics or performed by public employees. Also required physicians to conduct tests for fetal viability at 20 weeks of gestation.
*1990:* States may require notification of both parents before a woman younger than 18 years has an abortion. A judge can authorize the abortion without parental consent.
*1992:* Validated Pennsylvania law imposing restrictions on abortions. The restrictions upheld include the following:
A woman must be told about fetal development and alternatives to abortion.
She must wait at least 24 hours after this explanation before having an abortion.
Unmarried women younger than 18 years must obtain consent from their parents or a judge.
Physicians must keep detailed records of each abortion, subject to public disclosure.
Struck down only one requirement of the Pennsylvania law: that a married woman must inform her husband before having an abortion.
*1993:* Rescinded the so-called *gag rule*, which restricted the counseling that healthcare professionals (with the exception of physicians) could provide at federally funded family planning clinics.
*1995:* Upheld a ruling that states cannot withhold state funds for abortions in case of pregnancies resulting from rape or incest or when the mother's life is in danger.
*2000:* Struck down a Nebraska law making late-term abortions illegal. The court held that the law placed undue burden on the pregnant woman because there was no provision for late abortion to protect the woman's health.

- Realize that abortion is an ethical dilemma that results in confusion, ambivalence, and personal distress for many.
- Recognize that the issue is not a dilemma for many but is a fundamental violation of personal or religious views that give meaning to their lives.
- Acknowledge the sincere convictions and the strong emotions of people on all sides of the issue.

The personal values of each nurse contribute to what nurses are willing to do if confronted by a woman's need for nursing care when having an elective abortion. For example, some nurses have no objection in participating in abortions. Others do not assist with elective pregnancy termination but may care for women after the procedure. Some nurses assist with a first trimester abortion but may object to later abortions. Many nurses are comfortable assisting in abortion if the fetus has severe anomalies but are uncomfortable in other circumstances. Some nurses believe that they could not provide care before, during, or after an abortion and that they are bound by conscience to try to dissuade a woman from the decision to abort.

Nurses have no obligation to support a position with which they disagree. Many states have laws that allow nurses to refuse to assist with the procedure if elective pregnancy terminations violate ethical, moral, or religious beliefs. However, nurses have an ethical obligation to disclose this information before becoming employed in an institution that performs abortions. For a nurse to withhold this information until being assigned to care for a woman having an abortion and then refusing to provide care would be unethical. The management must be informed by the nurse if he or she cannot provide compassionate care because of personal convictions so that appropriate care can be arranged (AWHONN, 2009b).

### Fetal Injury

The question of whether a mother should be restrained or prosecuted for actions that could cause injury to her fetus has both legal and ethical implications. Courts have issued jail sentences to women who have caused or who may cause fetal injury to prevent additional harm to the fetus. Women have been forced to undergo cesarean births against their will when physicians have testified that such a procedure was necessary to prevent fetal injury.

The state has an interest in protecting children, and the Supreme Court has ruled that a child has the right to begin life with a sound mind and body. Many states have laws requiring that evidence of prenatal drug exposure, which is considered child abuse, be reported. Women have been charged with negligence, involuntary manslaughter, delivering drugs to a minor, and child endangerment.

Yet forcing a woman to behave in a certain way because she is pregnant violates the principles of autonomy, self-determination of competent adults, bodily integrity, and personal freedom. Women are unlikely to seek prenatal care or treatment for substance abuse unless they feel safe from prosecution.

## Ethical Concerns in Child Health Nursing

Ethical concerns can arise in many areas of child healthcare. For example, disclosure of HIV status to HIV-positive children who are entering middle school is an issue that brings up ethical differences between pediatric providers and parents (see Chapter 42). Two additional important areas are withholding life-sustaining treatment and terminating life support.

### Withholding or Ceasing Life-Sustaining Treatment

An ongoing legal and ethical conflict has resulted from the case of Baby Doe and other potentially disabled infants, which occurred in the 1980s. This issue concerned an infant with Down syndrome who also was born with a tracheoesophageal fistula, normally treatable with surgery. The infant's parents refused surgery on the advice of the obstetrician, who was discouraging about the child's survival and subsequent quality of life (White, 2011). As a result of the parents' decision in this case and other similar cases in which infants died because of unrepaired defects, at the urging of the then Surgeon General, the Congress amended child abuse legislation to encompass the withholding of life-sustaining treatment from physically or intellectually disabled infants, essentially prohibiting discrimination because of their disability (White, 2011). The Baby Doe rules state that under circumstances where the physician's reasonable judgment would indicate that an acute medical issue could be resolved, treatment must be provided regardless of the child's disability. The only exceptions to this would be if the treatment prolonged the dying process in a child not expected to survive or if the child was in an irreversible coma (White, 2011). These rules, if applied, effectively remove the parent's or family's decision as to what is best for their child.

In 1994, the AAP Committee on Bioethics (1994/2012) issued a guideline that addresses the issue of withholding or ceasing life-sustaining treatments for all infants and children; since then, the guideline has been reaffirmed several times. The guideline recommends the use of the "best interests" standard–making recommendations for interventions to families based on what will benefit the child (improving the quality of remaining life, prolonging life so that the parent and child can have the best quality of relationship available until the child's death) versus what might harm the child (intractable pain and suffering, increased disability, prolonging life unnecessarily). This approach incorporates the consideration of the child's quality of life (AAP Committee on Bioethics, 1994/2012). Integral to the success of this approach is an honest and accurate communication between providers, the child, and the parents. Providers must convey realistic information about the likelihood of improvement, anticipated extent of pain, effect on the quality of life, and options for resuscitation. The goal is to assist the family with decisions that address both the *quality of life and the quality of dying* (Basu, 2013).

Similar to withholding treatment, the decision to cease treatment is an ethical situation that is always difficult and seems to be compounded when the patient is an infant or child. Children who would have died in the past can now have their lives extended through the use of life support. Parents must be involved in the decision-making process immediately and informed about available options. Laws in some states permit parents to provide advance directives for their minor children. When older children are involved, their views are considered.

### Terminating Life Support

Decisions to terminate life-support systems continue to present gut-wrenching ethical and legal situations to nurses, especially when an infant or child is involved. Contrary to the common belief that such decisions should be determined by *quality of life*, the legal system plays a major role in this area of healthcare.

Frequently parents become attached to a primary care nurse and request that the nurse participate in the decision as to whether to terminate life support for their child. A nurse might be faced with such a situation in the neonatal intensive care unit (NICU) with a teenage parent of a premature infant with a congenital defect or in a chronic care oncology unit with a terminally ill child.

In such instances, a team conference should be arranged with the parent, primary nurse, physician, clergy (if applicable), and a hospital staff attorney who is knowledgeable about applicable laws in that particular state. Problems may arise when there is a discrepancy among what families, physicians, and nurses think is best.

The issue of when first to discuss with adolescents the idea of cardiopulmonary resuscitation, mechanical ventilation, and do-not-resuscitate (DNR) orders is always sensitive. Adolescents who have reached majority age must give consent if they are of sound mind. In most states, minor status ends at the age of 18 years.

## SOCIAL ISSUES

Nurses are exposed to many social issues that influence healthcare and often have legal or ethical implications. Some of the issues that affect maternity and child healthcare include poverty, homelessness, access to care, and allocation of funds.

### Poverty

Poverty is an underlying factor in problems such as inadequate access to healthcare and homelessness and is a major predictor for unmet health needs in children and adults. The percentage of children in the United States who are living in poverty (22%) has increased steadily, exacerbated by the most recent downturn in the economy. Children younger than 5 years are more often found in families with incomes below the poverty line than are older children. Children in female-headed households and those with less than a high school education are more likely to be living in poverty; the poverty rate is nearly twice as high in black, Hispanic and Native American households than in white non-Hispanic households (National Center for Children in Poverty, 2015).

Poverty affects the ability to access healthcare for any age-group and decreases opportunities linked with health promotion. Nurses can play a role in helping to meet the healthcare needs of mothers and their infants and children by recognizing the adverse effect of poverty on health and identifying poverty as a practice concern. Several of the *Healthy People 2020* goals (USDHHS, 2010) have implications for maternal-child nurses:

- To reduce the infant mortality rate to no more than 6.0 per 1000 live births and the childhood mortality rate to 25.7 per 100,000 for children 1 to 4 years old and 12.3 per 100,000 for children 5 to 9 years old and to similarly reduce the rate of adolescent deaths
- To reduce the incidence of low birth weight to no more than 7.8% of live births and the incidence of very low birth weight to 1.4% of live births
- To ensure that 77.9 % of all pregnant women receive prenatal care in the first trimester of pregnancy
- To reduce preterm births to 8.1% of live births 34 to 36 weeks, 1.4% of live births 32 to 33 weeks, and 1.8% of live births at less than 32 weeks
- To achieve and maintain effective vaccination coverage levels for universally recommended vaccines in children aged 19 to 35 months and increase routine vaccination coverage for adolescents
- To reduce, eliminate, or maintain elimination of vaccine-preventable diseases
- To increase the fraction of people with health insurance to 100%

Poverty tends to breed poverty. Childbearing at an early age interferes with education and the ability to work. In low-income families, children may leave the educational system early, making them less likely to learn skills necessary to obtain good jobs. The cycle of poverty (Fig. 1.4) may continue from one generation to another as a result of hopelessness and apathy.

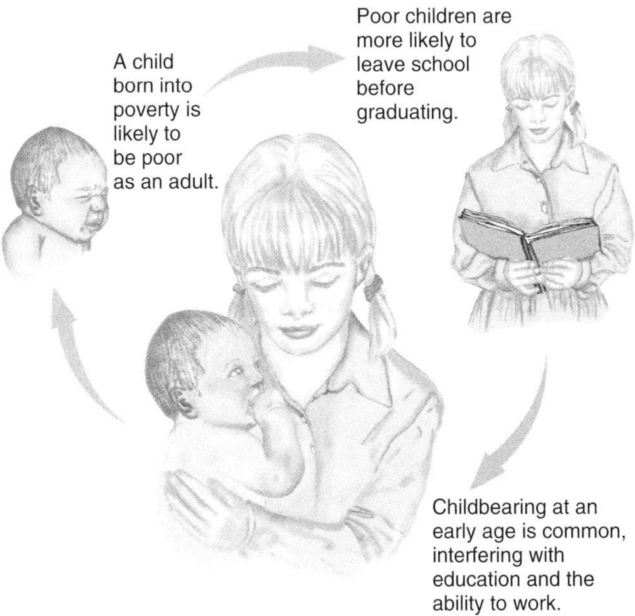

A child born into poverty is likely to be poor as an adult.
Poor children are more likely to leave school before graduating.
Childbearing at an early age is common, interfering with education and the ability to work.


**FIG 1.4** The cycle of poverty.

## Homelessness

Unemployment in the United States was 5% in late 2015, down considerably from its rate during the recent recession (Bureau of Labor Statistics, 2015). Unemployment can greatly increase the risk for or presence of homelessness to many families who were previously middle or low income because of its link to poverty (National Coalition for the Homeless, 2014a). Approximately 15% of the homeless population are families; most concerning is that homeless young people (younger than 24 years) comprise 33% of the homeless population (National Coalition for the Homeless, 2014a). In addition to poverty contributing to homelessness among women and their children, other factors include decreasing wages among the employed, lack of affordable housing, domestic violence, substance abuse, and mental illness. Homeless children are poorly nourished and are exposed to violence, experience school absences with subsequent learning difficulties, and are at risk for depression and other emotional consequences (National Coalition for the Homeless, 2011; National Coalition for the Homeless, 2014b; National Resource Center on Homelessness and Mental Illness, 2011).

Homeless women as well as their children can be poorly nourished and exposed to various infections. Rape and assault are problems, with a high rate of pregnancy among homeless girls. Infants born to homeless women are subject to low birth weight and have a greater likelihood of neonatal mortality. Pregnancy and birth, especially among teenagers, are important contributors to homelessness. Adolescent mothers are more likely to be single mothers, have incomplete education, and be poor. Pregnancy interferes with a woman's ability to work and may decrease her income to the point at which she loses her housing. Pregnancy among homeless youth is associated with longer periods of homelessness and may affect obtaining and keeping employment. In addition, homeless youth are more likely to have multiple sex partners and begin sexual intercourse at a young age. Children in families without money to pay for insurance or early healthcare have an increased chance of needing hospitalization (Begun, 2015).

Federal funding has provided assistance with shelter and healthcare for homeless people. The homeless, however, have the same difficulties in obtaining healthcare as other poor people because of lack of transportation, inconvenient hours, and lack of continuity of care.

## Prenatal Care in the United States

Prenatal care is widely accepted as an important element in improving the health of mothers and infants. For states using the more detailed updated birth certificate in 2008, almost three-quarters of mothers had prenatal care in the first trimester of pregnancy. Poor prenatal care often occurs because care is not easily available (NCHS, 2011; Osterman, Martin, Mathews & Hamilton, 2011). Preconception care is now recommended to provide the ideal circumstances in the mother from the earliest days of pregnancy. Goals for the woman to achieve before conception include adequate folic acid intake, updating immunizations as needed, and maintaining a healthy weight and healthy behaviors, such as avoiding smoking, alcohol, and the use of illegal and certain legal or therapeutic drugs (National Institute of Child Health and Human Development [NICHD], 2013).

Poor prenatal care access contributes to the infant mortality rate and the large number of low-birth-weight infants born each year in the United States. Because preterm infants form the largest category of those needing intensive care, millions of dollars could be saved each year by ensuring adequate prenatal care from the earliest weeks. Even a small improvement in an infant's birth weight decreases complications and hospital time.

In some situations, women can obtain prenatal care but choose not to. These women may not understand the importance of the care or may deny they are pregnant. Some have had such unsatisfactory experiences with the healthcare system that they avoid it as long as possible. Others want to hide substance use or other habits from disapproving healthcare workers. Language and cultural differences also play a part in whether a woman seeks prenatal care. Although these factors are not access issues as such, they must be addressed to improve healthcare.

## Government Programs for Healthcare: Medicaid

Having health insurance coverage (often employer sponsored) can determine whether a person will seek care early. Medicaid is a major government program that increases access to healthcare for those without private health insurance. Medicaid provides healthcare for the poor, aged, and disabled, with pregnant women and young children especially targeted. Medicaid is funded by the federal as well as state governments. The states administer the program and determine which services are offered. Although there is variation among states in just how poor one must be to qualify for assistance, all women at less than 133% of the current federal poverty level for income are eligible for perinatal care. Over 15% of the total population in the United States is insured by Medicaid (Irving & Loveless, 2015). Of this number, 27% are non-elderly adults and 48% are children younger than 21 years (Paradise, 2015).

Historically, qualifying for Medicaid has been a lengthy process; a woman not already enrolled at the beginning of her pregnancy is unlikely to finish the process in time to receive early prenatal care. The family must fill out lengthy, complicated forms, provide documentation of citizenship and income, and then wait for determination of eligibility. More recently, however, as a result of the Affordable Care Act expansion, many enrollees can be 'fast-tracked' through use of other computerized government program databases (Paradise, 2015). Facilitation of enrollment can ease the barriers related to program enrollment and retention.

Medicaid criteria may deny payment for some services that are routinely provided to those who hold private insurance. Some physicians and dentists are unwilling to care for Medicaid patients who are likely to be at high risk. Many are especially unwilling if reimbursement is slow and lower than that paid by other insurers. With their continual concern about malpractice suits, physicians may be less inclined to accept high-risk, lower-paying patients. Dental services for children are particularly limited.

Greater restrictions on private insurance are blurring the distinction between private and public health coverage. Many private health plans have restrictions such as prequalification for procedures, drugs the plan covers, and services that will be covered at all. Governmental actions related to healthcare and payment to providers are a current national issue in the United States.

## Allocation of Healthcare Resources

Expenditures for healthcare in the United States in 2014 totaled approximately $2.5 trillion. Healthcare expenditures are increasing on an annual basis. The average cost per person in 2014 was $7826 (NCHS, 2014). Although 48% of Medicaid recipients are children, they account for only 21% of Medicaid expenditures (Paradise, 2015). In 2014, 64.6% of non-elderly adults were insured by private insurance, many through the ACA health exchanges. Public insurance covered 24.2% and 13% remained uninsured (Cohen & Martinez, 2014).

Reforming healthcare delivery and financing is a complex area of national concern. How to provide care for the poor, the uninsured or underinsured, and those with long-term care needs must be addressed. In addition, major acute-care facilities often deal with greater financial burdens because of the growing numbers of uninsured patients who present for treatment with severe illness or injury. Escalating liability costs are another drain on healthcare dollars, leading some states to enact legislation that places a cap on awards for damages in malpractice cases.

### Care versus Cure

One problem to be addressed is whether the focus of healthcare should be on preventive and caring measures or on the cure of disease. Medicine has traditionally centered more on treatment and cure than on prevention and care. Yet prevention not only avoids suffering but is also less expensive than treating diseases once diagnosed.

The focus on cure has resulted in technologic advances that have enabled some people to live longer, healthier lives. Financial resources are limited, however, and the costs of expensive technology must be balanced against the benefits obtained. Indeed, the cost of one organ transplant would pay for the prenatal care of many low-income mothers, possibly preventing the births of many low-birth-weight infants who may suffer disability throughout life.

In addition, quality-of-life issues are important in regard to technology. Neonatal nurseries are able to keep very-low-birth-weight babies alive because of advances in knowledge. Some of these infants go on to lead normal or near-normal lives. Others gain time but not quality of life. Families and healthcare professionals face difficult decisions about when to treat, when to terminate treatment, and when suffering outweighs the benefits.

### Healthcare Rationing

Modern technology has had a large effect on healthcare rationing. Some might argue that such rationing does not exist, but it occurs when part of a population has no access to care and there is not enough money for all people to share equally in the technology available. Healthcare also is rationed when it is more freely given to those who have money to pay for it than to those who do not. The distance from the needed care facility may be another factor.

Many questions will need answers as the costs of healthcare increase faster than the funds available. Is healthcare a fundamental right? Should a certain level of care be guaranteed to all citizens? What is that basic level of care? Should the cost of treatment and its effectiveness be considered when one is deciding how much government or third-party payers will cover? Nurses will be instrumental in finding solutions to these vital questions.

### Violence

In today's society, women and children are the victims and sometimes the perpetrators of violence. Violence is not only a social problem but also a health problem. Acts of violence can include child abuse, domestic abuse, and murder. Children who live in an environment of violence feel helpless and ineffective. These children have difficulty sleeping and show increased anxiety and fearfulness. They may perpetuate the violence they see in their homes because they have known nothing else in family relationships.

Although violent crimes among children have decreased over the past decade, violence in schools continues to rise and is a daily stressor for many children. Bullying by other students, possibly without physical violence, has recently come to the forefront of public awareness because of the increased risk of suicide among adolescent victims. Experts in the field of education cite socioeconomic disparity, language barriers, diverse cultural upbringing, lack of supervision and behavioral feedback, domestic violence, and changes within the family as possible causes for this increased violence. Traditional approaches to aggressive behavior in the school, such as suspension, detention, and being sent to the principal's office, have been ineffective in changing behavior and only serve to exclude the student from education, leading to an increased dropout rate. Nurses need to educate themselves on the issue of violence and to work with schools and parents to combat the problem. In addition, they should not ignore the child who is afraid to go to school or is having other school-related problems.

Findings from a large body of recent research suggest that exposure to violence via the media is a contributing factor to the occurrence of violent acts by children and adolescents (AAP, 2013). Children and adolescents are exposed to violence via television, movies, video games, and youth-oriented music. The American Academy of Pediatrics (2013) encourages parents to monitor their children's media exposure and limit their children's screen time (TV, computer, video games) to no more than 1 to 2 hours per day. The AAP (2013) also recommends that parents remove televisions, computers and all other electronic devices (e.g., cell phones, tablets) from children's bedrooms, limit viewing of programs and video games that have sexual or violent content, monitor texting and access to websites and social media, view television programs with children and discuss these, and educate children and adolescents about media literacy.

The AAP (2013) suggests that clinicians ask parents and children about media exposure at every well visit. Providers also need to be concerned about adolescents who display aggressive or acting-out behaviors such as lying, stealing, temper outbursts, vandalism, excessive fighting, and destructiveness. It further recommends that healthcare providers promote the responsibility of every family to create a gun-safe home environment. The AAP recommendations include asking about the presence of guns in the home at every well visit and counseling children, parents, and relatives on the importance of firearm safety and the dangers of having a gun, especially a handgun.

Nurses working with children should ask them about violence in their school, home, or neighborhood and whether they have had any personal experience with violent behavior. In some cases it may be necessary to contact parents, human resource departments, police, or other authorities to protect children and adolescents who are in violent situations or at risk for violence.

## LEGAL ISSUES

The legal foundation for the practice of nursing provides safeguards for healthcare and sets standards by which nurses can be evaluated. Nurses need to understand how the law applies specifically to them. When nurses do not meet the standards expected, they may be held legally accountable.

### Safeguards for Healthcare

Three categories of safeguards determine how the law views nursing practice: (1) state nurse practice acts, (2) standards of care set by professional organizations, and (3) rules and policies set by the institution employing the nurse. Additional information regarding nursing responsibilities is presented in Chapter 2.

#### Nurse Practice Acts

Every state has a nurse practice act that determines the scope of practice for registered nurses in that state. Nurse practice acts define what a nurse is and is not allowed to do in caring for patients. Some parts of the law may be very specific, whereas others are stated broadly enough to permit flexibility in the role of the nurse. Nurse practice acts vary from state to state, and nurses must be knowledgeable about these laws wherever they practice.

In 2000, the National Council of State Boards of Nursing initiated a nurse licensure compact program. A nurse licensure compact allows a nurse who is licensed in one state to practice nursing in another participating state without having to be licensed in that state. Nurses must comply with the practice regulations in the state in which they practice. Since 1998, 25 states have become participants in the nurse licensure compact program (National Council of State Boards of Nursing, 2015). To learn the current status of this program, visit https://www.ncsbn.org.

Laws relating to nursing practice also delineate methods, called *standard procedures* or *protocols,* by which nurses may assume certain duties commonly considered part of healthcare practice. The procedures are written by committees of nurses, physicians, and administrators. They specify the nursing qualifications required for practicing the procedures, define the appropriate situations, and list the education required. Standard procedures allow for flexibility in the role of the nurse to meet changing needs of the community and to reflect expanding knowledge.

### Standards of Care

Courts have generally held that nurses must practice according to established standards and health agency policies, although these standards and policies do not have the force of law. Standards of care are set by professional associations and describe the level of care that can be expected from practitioners. For example, perinatal nurses are held to the specialty standards published by the Association of Women's Health, Obstetric, and Neonatal Nurses (http://www.awhonn.org). The Society of Pediatric Nurses is the primary specialty organization that sets standards for pediatric nurses (http://www.pedsnurses.org).

Other regulatory bodies, such as the Occupational Safety and Health Administration (OSHA), the U.S. Food and Drug Administration (FDA), and the Centers for Disease Control and Prevention (CDC) also provide guidelines for practice. Accrediting agencies, such as The Joint Commission (TJC) and the Community Health Accreditation Program, give their approval after visiting facilities and observing whether standards are being met in practice. Governmental programs such as Medicare, Medicaid, and state health departments require that their standards are met for the facility to receive reimbursement for services.

### Agency Policies

Each healthcare facility sets specific policies, procedures, and protocols that govern nursing care. All nurses should be familiar with those that apply in the facilities in which they work. Nurses are involved in writing nursing policies and procedures that apply to their practice and in reviewing or revising them regularly.

## Accountability

Nursing accountability involves knowledge of current laws. Accountability in child health nursing requires special consideration because the nurse must be accountable to the family as well as the child. For example, the Individuals with Disabilities Education Act (PL 94-142), which mandates free and appropriate education for all children with disabilities, provides for school nurses to be part of a team that develops an individual education plan for each child who is eligible for services. In school districts that are reluctant to involve the school nurse as part of the team, nurses may need to advocate for services for the child and family.

Federal as well as state legislative bodies have addressed the issue of child abuse. Considerable variation exists among state laws in the investigative authority and procedures granted to child protective workers. When child abuse is suspected, issues often arise as to whether a healthcare provider may investigate the home situation and obtain relevant records.

A recent issue pertaining to nursing accountability is inadequate hospital staffing as a result of budget cuts. A nurse has a duty to communicate concerns about staffing levels immediately through established channels. A nurse will not be excused from responsibility (e.g., late medication administration or injury resulting from inadequate supervision of a patient), just as a hospital will not be excused for insufficient staffing because of budget cuts.

Accountability also involves competency. If a nurse is not competent to perform a nursing task (e.g., to administer a new chemotherapeutic drug), or if a patient's status worsens to the point at which the care needs are beyond the nurse's competency level (e.g., a patient requiring hemodynamic monitoring), the nurse must immediately communicate this fact to the nursing supervisor or physician. Denial of a request for patient transfer to the intensive care unit (ICU) because the ICU is at full capacity is an insufficient defense in a charge of nursing negligence. In addition, the fact that a call was placed to a physician but there was no return call is no excuse for harm caused to a patient because of delayed treatment. The nurse has an obligation to pursue needed care through the established chain of command at the facility.

## Malpractice

*Negligence* is the failure to perform the way a reasonable, prudent person of similar background would act in a similar situation. Negligence may comprise doing something that should not be done or failing to do something that should be done.

*Malpractice* is the negligence by professionals, such as nurses or physicians, in performing their duties. Nurses may be accused of malpractice if they do not perform according to the established standards of care and in the manner of a reasonable, prudent nurse with similar education and experience. Four elements that must be present to prove negligence are duty, breach of duty, damage, and proximate cause (Guido, 2014).

**! NURSING QUALITY ALERT**

***Elements of Negligence***

*Duty.* The nurse must have a duty to act or give care to the patient. It must be part of the nurse's responsibility.

*Breach of Duty.* A violation of that duty must occur. The nurse fails to conform to established standards for performing that duty.

*Damage.* There must be actual injury or harm to the patient as a result of the nurse's breach of duty.

*Proximate Cause.* The nurse's breach of duty must be proved to be the cause of harm to the patient.

### Prevention of Malpractice Claims

Malpractice awards have escalated in both the number and amount of awards to plaintiffs, resulting in high malpractice insurance for all healthcare providers. In addition, more healthcare workers practice defensively, accumulating evidence that they are acting in the patient's best interest. For example, nurses must be careful to include detailed data when they document care. This responsibility is particularly important in perinatal nursing because this is the area in which most nursing lawsuits occur.

There are many reasons that perinatal nurses may become defendants in lawsuits. Complications are usually unexpected because parents view pregnancy and birth as normal. The birth of a child with a problem is a tragic surprise, and they may look for someone to blame. Although very small preterm infants now survive, some have long-term disabilities that require expensive care for the child's lifetime. Statutes of limitations vary in different states and with the cause for action, but plaintiffs may have more than 20 years to file lawsuits that involve a newborn.

The prevention of claims is sometimes referred to as *risk management* or *quality assurance.* Although it is not possible to prevent all malpractice lawsuits, nurses can help defend themselves against malpractice judgments by following guidelines for informed consent, refusal of care, and documentation; acting as a patient's advocate; working within accepted standards and the policies and procedures of the facility; and maintaining their level of expertise.

*Informed consent.* When adults receive adequate information, they are less likely to file malpractice suits. Informed consent is an ethical concept that has been incorporated in the law. Patients have the right to decide whether to accept or reject treatment options as part of their right to function autonomy. To make wise decisions, they need complete information regarding the treatments offered. Without proper informed consent, assault and battery charges can result.

The law mandates what procedures require informed consent and what to inform about as "risks" specific to each procedure. Nurses must be familiar with the procedures that require consent.

## ! NURSING QUALITY ALERT

### Requirements of Informed Consent

- Patient's competence to consent
- Full disclosure of information
- Patient's understanding of information
- Patient's voluntary consent

Competence. Certain requirements must be met before consent can be considered informed. The first requirement is that the patient be competent or able to think through a situation and make rational decisions. A patient who is comatose or severely developmentally disabled is incapable of making such decisions. Minors are not allowed to give consent. However, children should have procedures explained to them in age-appropriate terms. In most states, minor status for informed consent ends at the age of 18 years.

A patient who has received drugs that impair the ability to think is temporarily incompetent. In such cases, another person is appointed to make decisions for the patient if the patient has not specified that person in advance.

Most states allow some exceptions for parental consent in cases involving emancipated minors. An *emancipated minor* is a minor child who has the legal competency of an adult because of circumstances involving marriage, divorce, parenting of a child, living independently without parents, or enlistment in armed services. Legal counsel may be consulted to verify the status of the emancipated minor for consent purposes.

Most states allow minors to obtain treatment for drug or alcohol abuse or sexually transmitted diseases and to have access to birth control without parental consent. At present, the laws governing adolescent abortion widely vary from state to state.

Patient information about advance directives, such as a living will, durable power of attorney for healthcare, and an alternate decision maker for the person, must be assessed on admission to the healthcare facility. Hospitals are required to inform patients about advance directives, and this is often part of a nursing admission assessment. The person who has not made advance directives must be offered the opportunity to make these choices.

Full disclosure. The second requirement is that of full disclosure of information, including the treatment's purpose and expected results. The risks, side effects, and benefits as well as other treatment options must be explained to patients. The person must also be informed as to what would happen if no treatment were chosen.

For example, the National Childhood Vaccine Injury Act mandates that explanations about the risks of communicable diseases and the risks and benefits associated with immunizations should be provided to all parents to enable them in making informed decisions regarding their child's healthcare. Parents need to know the common side effects and what to do in case of emergency. Explanations should also be given to adults who receive these vaccines. The law stipulates that children injured by a vaccine must go through the administrative compensation system (funds from an excise tax levied on the vaccines) and reject an award before attempting to sue either the manufacturer or person who administered the vaccine in a civil suit. Furthermore, the law mandates certain record keeping and reporting requirements for nurses.

Understanding information. The patient, including the parent or legal guardian of a child, must comprehend information about the proposed treatment. Health professionals must explain the facts in terms the person can understand. Nurses must be patient advocates when they find that a person does not completely understand a treatment or has questions regarding it. If the nurse cannot explain it, she or he must inform the physician so that the patient's misunderstandings can be clarified.

During hospitalization and discharge preparations, considerations should be given to people who do not understand the prevailing language and to the hearing impaired. Foreign language and interpreters for the hearing impaired must be obtained when indicated. Provision for those who cannot read any language or adults with a low education level must also be considered.

*Voluntary consent.* Patients must be allowed to voluntarily make choices without undue influence or coercion from others. Although others can provide information, the patient alone or the parent or legal guardian of a child makes the decision. Patients should not feel pressured to choose in a certain manner or feel that their future care depends on their decision.

Children cannot legally consent for treatment or participation in research. However, they should be given the opportunity to give voluntary assent for research participation. Assent involves the principles of competence and full disclosure. Children should be provided information in a developmentally appropriate format. Patients 18 years and older must provide complete consent. When seeking assent from children, the nurse considers both the child's age and development. In general, when children have reached 14 years old, they are competent to understand the ramifications of a treatment or participation in a research; some children are competent at a somewhat younger age. Other factors to consider are the child's physical and emotional condition and behaviors, cognitive ability, history of family shared decision making, anxiety level, and disease context (Brothers, Lynch, Aufox, et al, 2014). In some states, the child's dissent to participate in research is legally binding; thus, nurses need to be aware of the legal issues in the states in which they practice. The Committee on Pediatric Emergency Medicine has issued a policy regarding consent for emergency medical services for children and adolescents. The policy recommends that every effort be made to secure consent from a parent or legal guardian, but emergency treatment should not be denied if there are problems in obtaining consent (American Academy of Pediatrics Committee on Pediatric Emergency Medicine, 2011).

### Refusal of Care

Sometimes patients decline treatment, including hospitalization, offered by healthcare workers. Patients may refuse treatment when they believe that the benefits of treatment do not outweigh its burdens or the quality of life they can expect after treatment. Patients have the right to refuse care, and they can withdraw their agreement to treatment at any time. When a person makes this decision, a number of steps should be taken.

First, the physician or nurse should establish that the patient understands the treatment and the results of refusal. The physician, if unaware of the person's decision, should be notified by the nurse. The nurse documents on the chart the refusal, the explanations given to the patient, and the notification of the physician. If the treatment is considered vital to the patient's well-being, the physician discusses the need with the patient and documents the discussion. Opinions by other physicians may also be offered to the patient.

Patients may be asked to sign a form wherein they indicate that they understand the possible consequences of rejecting treatment. This measure is to prevent a later lawsuit in which the person claims lack of knowledge of the possible outcomes of a decision. If there is no ethical dilemma, the patient's decision stands.

Refusal of care by a pregnant woman involves the life of the fetus, sometimes resulting in legal actions. One example is a woman's refusal to a cesarean birth, although her refusal is likely to cause grave harm to the fetus. The outcomes of legal actions have been divided, some upholding the mother's right to refuse treatment and others ordering a treatment despite the mother's objections. Court action is avoided if possible because it places the woman, family, and caregiver in adversarial positions. In addition, it invades the woman's privacy and interferes with her autonomy and right to informed consent.

When parents refuse to provide consent for what is deemed a necessary treatment of a child, the state may be petitioned to intervene. The court may place the child in the temporary custody of the government or a private agency. The nurse may be asked to witness such a transaction when physicians act in cases of emergencies, such as a lifesaving blood transfusion for a child despite parental objections based on religious beliefs.

### Adoption

Nurses may care for infants involved in adoptions. The nurse may need to consult with the birth parents, adoptive parents, social workers, obstetrician, or pediatrician to determine the various rights of the child, birth parents, and adoptive parents (e.g., in matters concerning visitation rights, informed consent, or discharge planning).

In open adoptions, the birth mother may opt to room in with the baby during hospitalization. The birth mother and adoptive parents typically have had contact before the delivery and have an informal agreement regarding shared responsibility for the baby. The birth parent may even participate in discharge planning because she may have extended rights to visit the child after adoption.

Issues may develop as to the state of mind of the birth mother at the time of relinquishing parental rights (which cannot occur until after birth, unlike the relinquishment of the birth father's rights). State laws vary as to the legal time period necessary (1 day to several weeks after the birth of the child) before a birth mother can lawfully relinquish her rights to the child.

Some state laws allow the birth mother to relinquish her rights immediately after birth. In such cases, the nurse has the responsibility of protecting the birth mother and child to ensure that the birth mother is not coerced into making a decision while under the effects of medication. Factual documentation of such circumstances may be requested if the birth mother later asserts her rights to the child, claiming "undue influence" or "coercion."

Birth fathers have the same rights as birth mothers. Unless the birth father relinquishes his legal rights to the child, he may later assert his rights to the child after attachment has occurred with the adoptive parents. This situation may occur if the birth mother denies knowledge of the father's identity.

### Documentation

Documentation, whether on paper or electronic media, is the best evidence that a standard of care has been maintained. All information recorded about a patient should reflect the standard of care at the time of occurrence. This information includes nurses' notes, electronic fetal monitoring records, flow sheets, and any other data in the patient record. In many instances, notations on hospital records, whether print or electronic, are the only proof that care was given. Expert witnesses, often registered nurses in the appropriate specialty, will search for evidence that the standard of care at the time of the incident was met. If not found in case documents, the expert witness must conclude that what should have been done was not done. When documentation is not present, juries tend to assume that care was not given. Although documentation is not listed as a step in the nursing process, it is in fact an integral part of the process.

Documentation must be specific and complete. Nurses are unlikely to be able to recall details of situations that happened years ago and must rely on their documentation to explain their care if sued. Documentation must show that the standards of care and facility policies and procedures in effect at the time of the incident were met. Documentation must demonstrate that appropriate patient assessment and continued monitoring, problem identification and provision of correct interventions, and changes in patient status were communicated to the primary care provider. If the nurse believes that the primary care provider has responded inappropriately, the nurse must refer the provider response through the appropriate chain of command for the facility and document the notification.

***Documenting discharge teaching.*** Discharge teaching is essential to ensure that new parents know how to take care of themselves and their newborn after their brief hospital stay. Nurses must document their teaching as well as the parents' degree of understanding of what was taught. The nurse should also note the need for reinforcement and how that reinforcement was provided. If follow-up home care is planned, teaching should be continued at home and documented by the home care nurse. Written documents of discharge teaching are signed by and provided to the patient.

***Documenting incidents.*** A type of documentation used in risk management is the *incident report,* often called a *quality assurance, occurrence,* or *variance report.* The nurse completes a report when something occurs that might result in legal action, such as in injury to a patient or a departure from the expectations in the situation. The report warns the agency's legal department that there may be a problem. It also helps identify whether changing processes within the system might reduce the risk for similar incidents in the future. Incident reports are not a part of the patient's chart and should not be referred to on the chart. Documentation of the incident on the chart should be restricted to the same type of factual information about the patient's condition that would be recorded in any other situation.

The analysis of medical error from a systems perspective is called a *root cause* analysis. The process involves identifying errors or near misses as soon as they occur, asking relevant questions about the factors that might have contributed to the error, analyzing the contributing causes, and developing interventions to prevent a similar error from occurring in the future. A root cause analysis is not intended to be punitive if an error was made. Instead, root cause analysis is used as a tool to prevent future errors or near misses.

### The Nurse as an Advocate

Malpractice suits may be brought if nurses fail in their role of patient advocate. Nurses are ethically and legally bound to act as the patient's advocate. This means that the nurse must act in the patient's best interests at all times. When nurses feel that the patient's best interests are not being served, they are obligated to seek help for the patient from appropriate sources. This usually involves taking the problem through the chain of command established at the facility. The nurse consults a supervisor and the patient's physician or that physician's supervisor. If the results are not satisfactory, the nurse continues through administrative channels to the director of nurses, hospital administrator, and chief of the medical staff, if necessary. All nurses should know the chain of command for their workplace.

In seeking help for patients, nurses must document their efforts. For example, if a postpartum woman experiences excessive bleeding, the nurse documents what was done to control the bleeding. The nurse also documents each time the physician was called regarding the problem, what information was given to the physician, and the response received. When nurses cannot contact the physician or do not receive adequate instructions, they should document their efforts to seek instruction from others, such as the nursing supervisor or chief of medical staff for the specialty. They should also complete an incident report. It is essential that they continue in their efforts until the patient receives the care needed.

Nurses also must be advocates for health promotion and illness prevention for vulnerable groups such as children. Nurses can participate in groups dedicated to the welfare of children and families, such as professional nursing societies, parent support groups, religious organizations, and voluntary organizations. Through involvement with healthcare planning on a political or legislative level and by working as consumer advocates, nurses can initiate changes for better quality healthcare.

### Maintaining Expertise

Maintaining expertise is another way for nurses and other health professionals to prevent malpractice liability. To ensure that nurses maintain their expertise to provide safe care, most states require proof of continuing education for renewal of nursing licenses. Nursing knowledge changes rapidly, and staying current is essential for all nurses. Incorporating new information learned by attending classes or conferences and reading nursing journals can help nurses perform as would a reasonably prudent peer. Journals provide information from nursing research that may be important in updating nursing practice. It is important for all nurses to analyze research articles to determine whether changes in patient care are indicated.

Employers often provide continuing education classes for their nurses. Many workshops and seminars are available on a wide variety of nursing topics. Membership in professional organizations such as state branches of the ANA or specialty organizations such as AWHONN and the Society of Pediatric Nurses gives nurses access to new information through publications as well as nursing conferences and other educational offerings.

Maintaining expertise may be a concern when nurses 'float' or are required to work with patients who have needs different from those of their usual patients. In these situations, the employer must provide orientation and education so that the nurse can perform care safely in new areas. Nurses who work outside their usual areas of expertise must assess their own skills and avoid performing tasks or taking on responsibilities in areas in which they are not competent. Many nurses learn to provide care in two or three different areas and are floated only to those areas. This system meets the need for flexible staffing while providing safe patient care.

## CURRENT TRENDS AND THEIR LEGAL AND ETHICAL IMPLICATIONS

Recent healthcare changes have affected the way nurses give care and may have legal and ethical implications as well. These changes result from efforts to lower healthcare costs. Two of special concern are the use of unlicensed assistive personnel and early discharge.

### Use of Unlicensed Assistive Personnel

In an effort to reduce healthcare costs, many agencies have increased the use of unlicensed assistive personnel to perform direct patient care and have decreased the number of nurses who supervise them. An unlicensed person may be trained to do everything from housekeeping tasks to drawing blood, performing diagnostic tests to giving medications, all in the same day. This practice raises grave concerns about the quality of care patients receive, as the nurse is responsible for the care of more patients but must rely on unlicensed personnel to perform much of the care formerly provided only by professionals. At the same time, use of an expert nurse for housekeeping and other mundane but necessary unit tasks is inefficient and detracts from available professional time for patient care. A balanced approach is needed when incorporating unlicensed assistive personnel into a unit's work.

Nurses must be aware of their legal responsibilities in these situations. They must know that the nurse is always responsible for patient assessments and must make the critical judgments necessary to ensuring patient safety. Nurses must know the capabilities of each unlicensed person caring for patients and must supervise them closely enough to ensure that they can perform their delegated tasks competently. More information about the use of unlicensed assistive personnel is available in a position statement from AWHONN (2015).

One area in which unlicensed assistive personnel may have greater responsibilities is in the school setting. Registered nurses who practice in schools are caring for children with more complex medical and nursing needs, responding to increased requirements for routine health screenings and dealing with budgetary cuts that result in a nurse caring for children in more than one school. These pressures have led to increased use of unlicensed assistive personnel to provide routine care to children with uncomplicated needs, including medication administration. If having a school nurse present at each school is not possible, then the school nurse can consider delegating certain responsibilities to properly trained, competent, unlicensed assistive personnel. Nurses who consider delegation must be familiar with their state's nurse practice act and appropriate professional standards (Shannon & Kubelka, 2013). Before delegating, the nurse needs to determine tasks that are appropriate and safe, the complexity of children's needs, and the school district policy (AAP, 2009b; Shannon & Kubelka, 2013). The nurse needs to work with the school administration to develop a comprehensive school-based policy (the nurse, not the administrator, decides what responsibilities will be delegated) before any responsibilities are delegated to others. The nurse is also responsible for educating and evaluating the competency of the unlicensed personnel; this includes requiring return demonstrations of procedures and regular onsite supervision (Shannon & Kubelka, 2013). Most important is that delegation does not relieve the nurse from regular assessment of the children's responses to all treatments and medications (National Association of School Nurses, 2012; Shannon & Kubelka, 2013).

### Concerns About Early Discharge

Patients are discharged from the hospital quickly, usually no later than 48 hours after vaginal birth and often with minimal recovery time after illness or surgery. Healthcare professionals are concerned about the ability of women to care for themselves or their infant or child when discharge occurs very early. Women may be exhausted from a long labor or complications and unable to take in all the information that nurses attempt to teach before discharge. Once home, many women must care for other children as well, often without family members or friends to help them.

While a patient is in the birth or acute-care facility, professionals may notice indications of complications that may not be apparent to lay people. Mothers at home may not recognize the developing signs of serious maternal or neonatal infection or jaundice, and care may be delayed until the illness is severe. There may be legal issues if a patient develops a complication after early discharge.

### Dealing With Early Discharge

Nurses must establish ways of helping patients who go home soon after birth or parents who must take their child home when only slightly less ill or very soon after surgery. New teaching tactics may be necessary, with more teaching taking place during pregnancy when the mother's physical needs do not interfere with her ability to assimilate new knowledge. Parent teaching can be done before actual admission of a child for surgery. If a child is admitted when acutely ill, parent teaching begins almost immediately after admission. Nurses can take advantage of any "teachable moment" to provide patients with the information they need to better care for themselves or their child.

Careful documentation and notification of the primary care provider are essential when abnormal findings develop so that patients are not discharged inappropriately. Methods of follow-up such as home visits, phone calls, or return visits by families to the birth facility for nursing assessments in the first 24 to 48 hours after discharge have become increasingly important. Nursing case managers are often involved to identify and advocate for the best avenues of care and to facilitate extension of stay if the patient's condition warrants.

## KEY CONCEPTS

- Maternity and child healthcare in the United States have changed because of technologic advances, increasing knowledge, government involvement, and consumer demands.
- Family-centered maternity and child healthcare, based on the principle that families can make decisions about healthcare if they have adequate information, have greatly increased the autonomy of families and the responsibilities of nurses.
- Prospective payment plans, such as PPOs or HMOs, control healthcare costs by negotiating reduced charges with providers, such as facilities and physicians, and by restricting patient access to a specific list of providers.
- Capitated plans are those in which a group of providers agrees to provide all services for a patient for a set annual fee. If the patient requires more costly care, the provider network pays those added charges. If the patient requires less care than the annual fee, the network keeps the remaining money.
- Case and outcome managements have resulted in new tools to reduce the length of stay for mothers and infants in the birth facility. The preparation for continuation of care at home begins as soon as the mother or child enters the healthcare system.
- Clinical pathways are interdisciplinary guidelines for assessments and interventions that are designed to accomplish the identified outcomes in the shortest time.
- Home care of patients has increased because of the need to control costs and because of the availability of portable technology. The number of uninsured adults and children continues to be excessive, reducing their chances of receiving preventive healthcare and increasing the costs of the late care they often seek.
- Infant and maternal mortality rates have dramatically declined in the past 50 years. However, the United States continues to rank well below other developed nations, and infant mortality rates still widely vary across ethnic groups. Unintentional injuries are the leading causes of death in children aged 1 to 19 years.
- Nurses must examine their beliefs and come to a personal decision about abortion before they are faced with the situation in their practice. Nurses are obligated to share objections related to abortion care with their employer before the need to provide that care arises.
- Punitive approaches to ethical and social problems may prevent patients from seeking care, particularly preventive care.
- Poverty is a major social issue that leads to questions about the allocation of healthcare resources, access to care, government programs to increase healthcare to indigent women and children, and healthcare rationing.
- To give informed consent, the patient must be competent, receive complete information, understand that information, and voluntarily consent. The parents usually give consent for a minor child, although adolescents may be able to consent to their own treatment related to sexually transmitted diseases, contraception, and alcohol and drug abuse.
- Nurses are accountable for their practice and must be acquainted with the laws, standards of care, and agency policies and procedures that affect their practice.
- Nurses can help defend malpractice claims by following the guidelines for informed consent, refusal of care, and documentation and by maintaining their level of expertise.
- Documentation is the best evidence that the standard of care was met in patient care. Therefore, nurses must ensure that their documentation accurately reflects the care given. The nurse is the professional who decides what tasks may safely be delegated to unlicensed assistive personnel. In making such decisions, the nurse is guided by the recommendations of the state licensing board, standards of care, and agency policy.

## REFERENCES AND READINGS

Agency for Healthcare Research and Quality. (2011). *AHRQ Publication No. 11-0005-2-EF: Child and adolescent health care: Selected findings from the 2010 National Healthcare Quality and Disparities Report.* Retrieved from http://www.ahrq.gov.

Agency for Healthcare Research and Quality. (2015a). *2014 National Healthcare Quality and Disparities Report.* Retrieved from www.ahrq.gov.

Agency for Healthcare Research and Quality. (2015b). *Depression screening. Rockville, MD: Author.* Retrieved from http://www.ahrq.gov/professionals/prevention-chronic-care/healthier-pregnancy/preventive/depression.html.

Alfaro-LeFevre, R. (2013). *Critical thinking and clinical judgment: A practical approach* (5th ed.). St. Louis: Saunders.

American Academy of Pediatrics. (2015). *AAP agenda for children 2014-2015: Finance.* Retrieved from http://www.aap.org.

American Academy of Pediatrics Committee on Pediatric Emergency Medicine. (2011). Consent for emergency medical services for children and adolescents. *Pediatrics, 126,* 427–433.

American Academy of Pediatrics, Council on Communications and the Media. (2013). Policy statement: Children, adolescents and the media. *Pediatrics, 132*(4), 958–961.

American Academy of Pediatrics, Council on School Health. (2009b). Policy statement: Guidelines for the administration of medication in school. *Pediatrics, 124,* 1244–1254.

American Academy of Pediatrics and American College of Obstetricians and Gynecologists. (2012). *Guidelines for perinatal care* (7th ed.). Elk Grove Village, IL and Washington, DC: Author.

American Academy of Pediatrics Committee on Bioethics. (1994, reaffirmed 2012). *AAP guidelines on foregoing life-sustaining medical treatment.* Retrieved from http://www.aap.org.

American Nurses Association. (2011). *Nursing sensitive indicators.* Retrieved from http://www.nursingworld.org.

Association of Women's Health, Obstetric, and Neonatal Nurses. (2009a). *Confidentiality in adolescent health care.* (Position statement). Retrieved from: (Position statement). Retrieved from http://www.awhonn.org.

Association of Women's Health, Obstetric, and Neonatal Nurses. (2009b). *Ethical decision making in the clinical setting: Nurses' rights and responsibilities.* (Position statement). Retrieved from http://www.awhonn.org.

Association of Women's Health, Obstetric, and Neonatal Nurses. (2015). *The role of unlicensed assistive personnel in the nursing care for women and newborns.* (Position statement). Retrieved from http://www.awhonn.org.

Basu, R. (2013). End-of-life care in pediatrics: Ethical controversies and optimizing the quality of death. *Pediatric Clinics of North America, 60*(3), 725–739.

Begun, S. (2015). The paradox of homeless youth pregnancy: A review of challenges and opportunities. *Social Work in Health Care, 54*(5), 444–460.

Brothers, K.B., Lynch, J.A., Aufox, S.A., et al. (2014). Practical guidance on informed consent for pediatric participants in a biorepository. *Mayo Clinic Proceedings, 89*(11), 1471–1480.

Bureau of Labor Statistics. (2015). *Labor force statistics from the current population survey.* Retrieved from http://www.labor.bls.gov.

Burston, S., Chaboyer, W., & Gillespie, B. (2014). Nurse-sensitive indicators suitable to reflect nursing care quality: a review and discussion of issues. *Journal of Clinical Nursing, 23*(13-14), 1785–1795.

Centers for Disease Control and Prevention. (2015). *Pregnancy mortality surveillance system.* Retrieved from http://www.cdc.gov/reproductivehealth/MaternalInfantHealth/PMSS.html.

Centers for Disease Control and Prevention. (2016). Youth Risk Behavior Surveillance System – 2015. *Morbidity and Mortality Weekly Reports, 65*(6), 1–180.

Centers for Disease Control and Prevention, National Center for Chronic Disease Prevention and Centers for Medicare and Medicaid. (2015a). *Children's health insurance program (CHIP).* Retrieved from http://www.medicaid.gov.

Centers for Medicare and Medicaid. (2015b). *NHE fact sheet.* Retrieved from http://www.cms.gov.

Cohen, R., & Martinez, M. (2014). *Health insurance coverage: Early release of estimates from the National Health Interview Survey, January–March 2014.* Retrieved from http://www.cdc.gov/nchs.

Foley, M. (2015). *DRG grouping and ICD-10-CM/PCS.* Retrieved from http://www.library.ahima.org.

Federal Interagency Forum on Child and Family Statistics. (2015). *America's children: Key national indicators of well-being, 2015.* Retrieved from http://www.childstats.gov.

Guido, G.W. (2014). *Legal and Ethical Issues in Nursing* (6th ed.). Upper Saddle River: Pearson.

Health Resources and Services Administration. (2014). *Adolescent childbearing.* Retrieved from http://www.hrsa.gov.

Heslop, L. (2014). Nursing-sensitive indicators: A concept analysis. *Journal of Advanced Nursing, 70*(11), 2469–2482.

Hobel, C.J., Lu, M.L., & Gambone, J.C. (2016). A life-course perspective for women's health care: Safe ethical and effective practice. In N.F. Hacker, J.C. Gambone, & C.J. Hobel (Eds.), *Hacker & Moore's essentials of obstetrics and gynecology* (6th ed., pp. 2–10). Philadelphia: Elsevier.

Institute of Medicine. (2011). *Clinical practice guidelines we can trust.* Retrieved from http://www.iom.edu/cpgstandards.

Irving, S., & Loveless, T. (2015). *Dynamics of economic well-being: Participation in government programs, 2009-2012: Who gets assistance?* Retrieved from http://www.census.gov.

Jiang, Y., Ekono, M., Skinner, C., & National Center for Children in Poverty. (2015). *Basic facts about low-income children.* Retrieved from http://www.nccp.org.

Lyon, F., & Grow, K. (2011). Case management. In M. Nies, & M. McEwen (Eds.), *Community/public health nursing: Promoting the health of populations* (5th ed., pp. 152–162). St. Louis: Saunders.

MacDorman, M., Matthews, T.J., Mahangoo, A.D., & Zeitlin, J. (2014). International comparisons of infant mortality and related factors: United States and Europe, 2010. *National Vital Statistics Reports, 63*(5), Hyattsville, MD: National Center for Health Statistics.

March of Dimes. (2014). *March of Dimes medical resources: Low birthweight.* Retrieved from http://www.marchofdimes.org.

March of Dimes. (2015). *2015 Premature birth report cards.* Retrieved from http://www.marchofdimes.org.

Martin, J.A., Hamilton, B.E., Osterman, J.K., Curtin, S.C., & Mathews, J. (2015). Births: Final Data for 2013. *National Vital Statistics Reports, 64*(1), Hyattsville, MD: Author.

Mathews, T.J., & MacDorman, M. (2011). Infant mortality statistics from the 2007 period. Linked birth/infant death data set. *National Vital Statistics Reports, 59*(6). National Vital Statistics System, National Center for Health Statistics. Retrieved from http://www.cdc.gov.

Murphy, S., Kochanek, K., Xu, Jiaquan, & Arias, E. (2015). *Mortality in the United States 2014.* National Center for Health Statistics Data Brief no.229. Hyattsville, MD: National Center for Health Statistics.

Murphy, S., Kochanek, K., Xu, J., & Heron, M. (2015). Deaths: Final data for 2012. *National Vital Statistics Reports, 63*(9), 11–13.

National Association of School Nurses. (2012). *Medication administration in the school setting.* Retrieved from http://www.nasn.org.

National Center for Health Statistics. (2011). *Health, United States, 2010 with special feature on death and dying.* Hyattsville, MD: Author.

National Center for Health Statistics. (2014). *Health, United States, 2014.* Hyattsville, MD: Author.

National Coalition for the Homeless. (2011). *Hunger and food insecurity.* Retrieved from http://www.nationalhomeless.org.

National Coalition for the Homeless. (2014a). *Homelessness in America.* Retrieved from http://www.nationalhomeless.org.

National Coalition for the Homeless. (2014b). *Senseless violence: A survey of hate crimes against the homeless.* Retrieved from http://nationalhomeless.org/wp-content/uploads/2014/01/Hate-Crimes-Report-2012.pdf.

National Council of State Boards of Nursing. (2015). *Nurse Licensure Compact.* Retrieved from https://www.ncsbn.org.

National Institute of Child Health & Human Development. (2013). *Preconception Care & Prenatal Care.* Retrieved from http://www.nichd.nih.gov.

National Resource Center on Homelessness and Mental Illness. (2011). *Current statistics on the prevalence and characteristics of people experiencing homelessness in the United States.* Retrieved from http://www.nrchmi.samhsa.gov.

Organization for Economic Cooperation and Development. (2015). *Health spending (excluding investment) as a share of GDP, OEO countries 2013.* Retrieved from http://www.oecd.org.

Osterman, M.J.K., Martin, J.A., Mathews, T.J., & Hamilton, B.E. (2011). Expanded data from new birth certificate 2008. *National Vital Statistics Reports, 59*(7), Hyattsville, MD: National Center for Health Statistics.

Paradise, J. (2015). *Medicaid moving forward.* Retrieved from http://www.kff.org.

Shannon, R.A., & Kubelka, S. (2013). Reducing risks of delegation…..use of procedure skills checklists for unlicensed assistive personnel in schools, part 2. *NASN School Nurse, 28*(5), 222–226.

Simpson, K.R. (2013). Perinatal patient safety and professional liability issues. In K.R. Simpson, & P.A. Creehan (Eds.), *AWHONN perinatal nursing* (4th ed., pp. 1–30). Philadelphia: Lippincott.

Stephenson, C. (2011). Ethics. In S. Mattson, & J.E. Smith (Eds.), *AWHONN core curriculum for maternal-newborn nursing* (4th ed., pp. 669–685). St. Louis: Saunders.

Sudia-Robinson, T. (2014). Legal and ethical issues in neonatal care. In C. Kenner, & J.W. Lott (Eds.), *Comprehensive neonatal nursing care: An interdisciplinary approach* (5th ed., pp.

863–868). New York: Springer Publishing Company.
Tilling, E. (2014). Effect of pregnancy on periodontal and oral health. *Dental Nursing, 10*(2), 72–75.
United States Department of Health and Human Services. (2010). *Healthy People 2020*. Retrieved from http://www.healthypeople.gov.
United States Department of Health and Human Services. (2011). *Accountable care organizations: Improving care coordination for people with Medicare*. Retrieved from http://www.healthcare.gov.
United States Department of Health and Human Services. (2014). *Healthy People 2020 leading health indicators: Progress update*. Retrieved from http://www.healthypeople.gov.
United States Department of Health and Human Services. (2015). *Key features of the Affordable Care Act by year*. Retrieved from http://www.healthcare.gov.
Ventura, S.J., Hamilton, B.E., & Matthews, T. (2014). National and state patterns of teenage births in the United States 1940-2013. *National Vital Statistics Reports, 63*(4), 1–33.
Wertz, R., & Wertz, D. (1992). *Lying-in: A history of childbirth in America* (2nd ed.). New Haven, CT: Yale University Press.
White, J. (2011). The end at the beginning. *The Ochsner Journal, 11*(4), 309–316.

2

# The Nurse's Role in Maternity, Women's Health, and Pediatric Nursing

http://evolve.elsevier.com/McKinney/mat-ch/

## LEARNING OBJECTIVES

*After studying this chapter, you should be able to:*

- Explain roles the nurse may assume in the practice of maternity nursing, women's health, and nursing of children.
- Explain the roles of nurses with advanced preparation in the practice of maternity nursing, women's health, and nursing of children.
- Explain the incorporation of critical thinking as a part of clinical judgment into nursing practice.
- Describe the steps of the nursing process and relate them to maternity, women's health, and nursing care of children.
- Explain issues surrounding the use of complementary and alternative therapies.
- Discuss the importance of nursing research and evidence-based care in clinical practice.

As care has changed from category-specific care for the woman, newborn, or child to family centered care, the fields of maternity, women's health, and nursing care of children have entered a new era of autonomy and independence. Women may have problems that are unique to women such as menstrual or menopausal issues. However, healthcare research shows that women may not respond to disorders such as cardiovascular disease as a man does; thus, women's healthcare has become a specialty. Nurses today must be able to effectively communicate with and teach people of many ages and levels of development and education. They must be able to critically think and use the nursing process to develop a plan of care that meets the unique needs of each person and their family. Nurses are expected to use current evidence to solve problems and to collaborate with other healthcare providers.

## THE ROLE OF THE PROFESSIONAL NURSE

The professional nurse has a responsibility to provide the highest quality of care to every patient. The American Nurses Association (ANA) Code of Ethics for Nurses (Box 2.1) provides guidelines for ethical and professional behavior. The code emphasizes a nurse's accountability to the person, community, and profession. The nurse should understand the implications of this code and strive to practice accordingly. Professional nurses have a legal obligation to know and understand the standard of care imposed on them. It is critical that nurses maintain competence and a current knowledge base in their areas of practice.

Standards of practice describe the level of performance expected of a professional nurse as determined by an authority in the practice. For example, perinatal nurses are held to the standards published by the Association of Women's Health, Obstetric, and Neonatal Nurses (AWHONN). The most recent edition of AWHONN *Standards for Professional Nursing Practice in the Care of Women and Newborns* and *Standards for Perinatal Nursing Practice and Certification in Canada* was published to guide nursing practice and shape institutional guidelines (AWHONN, 2009).

Nurses who care for children in all clinical settings can use the ANA/Society of Pediatric Nurses (SPN) Standards of Care and Standards of Professional Performance for Pediatric Nurses and the SPN/ANA Guide to Family Centered Care as guides for practice. Other standards of practice for specific clinical areas, such as pediatric oncology nursing and emergency nursing, are available from nursing specialty groups.

As healthcare continues to move toward family centered and community-based health services, all nurses should expect to care for children, adolescents, and their families at the point of contact. The Society of Pediatric Nurses has issued several position statements regarding the inclusion of pediatric nursing content when planning undergraduate nursing programs in response to these changes in settings of care. The statements address such important issues as social determinants of health, interdisciplinary collaboration in care, health promotion, accessibility to a full range of services, advocacy, and developmentally appropriate care (Friedman, 2014; SPN, 2015).

Nurses who provide care to women, children, and families function in various roles, including care provider, teacher, collaborator, researcher, advocate, and manager.

### Care Provider

The nurse provides direct patient-centered care to women, infants, children, and their families in times of childbearing, illness, injury, recovery, and wellness. Nursing care is based on the nursing process. The nurse obtains health histories, assesses patient needs, monitors growth and development, performs health-screening procedures, develops comprehensive plans of care, provides treatment and care, makes referrals, and evaluates the effects of care. Nursing of children is especially based on an understanding of the child's developmental stage and is aimed at meeting the child's physical and emotional needs at that level. Developing a therapeutic relationship with and providing support to patients and their families are essential components of nursing care. Maternity and pediatric nurses practice family centered care, embracing diversity in family structures and cultural

**BOX 2.1 ANA Code of Ethics for Nurses**

1. The nurse practices with compassion and respect for the inherent dignity, worth, and unique attributes of every person.
2. The nurse's primary commitment is to the patient, whether an individual, family, group, community, or population.
3. The nurse promotes, advocates for, and protects the rights, health, and safety of the patient.
4. The nurse has authority, accountability, and responsibility for nursing practice, makes decisions, and takes action consistent with the obligation to promote health and to provide optimal care.
5. The nurse owes the same duties to self as to others, including the responsibility to promote health and safety, preserve wholeness of character and integrity, maintain competence, and continue personal and professional growth.
6. The nurse, through individual and collective effort, establishes, maintains, and improves the ethical environment of the work setting and conditions of employment that are conducive to safe, quality healthcare.
7. The nurse, in all roles and settings, advances the profession through research and scholarly inquiry, professional standards development, and the generation of both nursing and health policy.
8. The nurse collaborates with other health professionals and the public to protect human rights, promote health diplomacy, and reduce health disparities.
9. The profession of nursing, collectively through its professional organizations, must articulate nursing values, maintain the integrity of the profession, and integrate principles of social justice into nursing and health policy.

From American Nurses' Association. *Code of ethics for nurses with interpretive statements.* (2015). ©2015 by American Nurses' Association. Reprinted with permission. All rights reserved.

backgrounds. These nurses strive to empower families, encouraging them to participate in self-care and the care of their child. Nurses who practice women's healthcare may need to coordinate care with pediatric nurses in families headed by grandparents rather than parents of the child.

## Teacher

Education is an essential role played by today's nurse. Teaching begins early—before and during a woman's prenatal care—and continues through her recovery from childbirth, learning to care for her newborn, and into her care in women's health (Fig. 2.1). Nurses who care for children prepare them for procedures, hospitalization, or surgery using knowledge of growth and development to teach at various levels of understanding. Families need information as well as emotional support so that they can cope with the anxiety and uncertainty of a child's illness. Nurses teach family members how to provide care, watch for important signs, and increase the child's comfort. They also work with new parents and parents of ill children so that the parents are prepared to assume responsibility for care at home after the child has been discharged from the hospital.

Education is essential to promoting health. The nurse applies principles of teaching and learning to change the behavior of family members. Nurses motivate women, children, and families to take charge of and make responsible decisions about their own health. Effective teaching must incorporate the family's values and health beliefs.

Nurses caring for children and families play an important role in preventing illness and injury through education and anticipatory guidance. Teaching about immunizations, safety, dental care, socialization, and discipline is a necessary component of care. Nurses offer guidance to parents with regard to child-rearing practices and preventing potential problems. They also answer questions about growth and development and assist families in understanding their children. Teaching often involves providing emotional support and counseling to children and families.

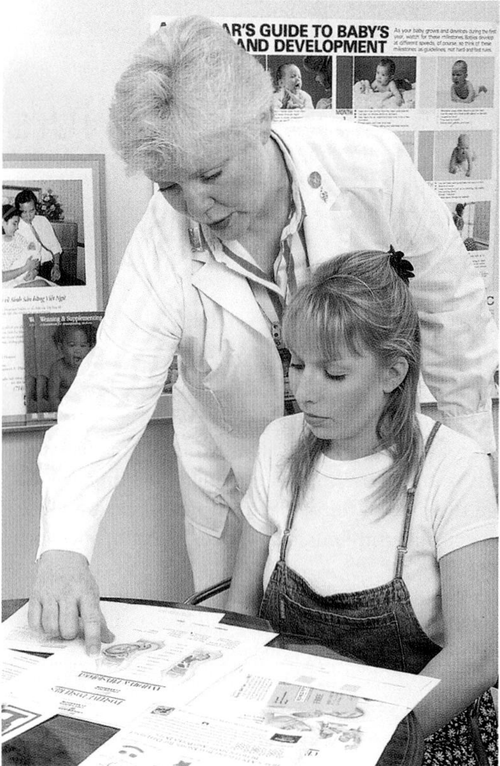

**FIG 2.1** In the prenatal clinic, the nurse teaches a woman one-on-one.

### Factors Influencing Learning

Numerous factors influence learning at any age. These include:

- *Developmental level.* Teenage parents often have very different concerns than older parents. Grandparents who assume long-term care for a child often need information that may not have been available when their own child was the same age. Developmental level also influences whether a person learns best by reading printed material, using computer-based materials, watching videos, participating in group discussions, play, or other means. Teaching must be adapted to the child's developmental level rather than the child's chronologic age.
- *Language.* Families for whom English is not the primary language may not understand idioms, nuances, slang terms, informal use of words, or medical words. An interpreter for the deaf may be necessary for the person who is hearing impaired.
- *Culture.* People tend to forget or disregard content with which they disagree. The nurse's teaching can be most effective if cultural considerations are weighed and incorporated into the education.
- *Previous experiences.* Parents who have other children may need less education about pregnancy care or infant and child care. However, they may have additional concerns about meeting the needs of several children and about sibling rivalry.

- *Physical environment.* The nurse must consider privacy when discussing sensitive issues such as adolescent sexuality or domestic violence, also called *intimate partner violence.* However, a group discussion may prompt participants to ask questions of concern to all members of the group, such as the experiences they can expect during labor.
- *Organization and skill of the teacher.* The teacher must determine the teaching objectives, develop a plan to meet those objectives, and gather all materials before teaching. The nurse must determine the best way to present the material for the intended audience. A summary of the information is helpful when concluding a teaching session.

### Principles of Teaching and Learning

- Applying the following principles will help nurses become effective teachers in the childbearing or childrearing setting:
- Real learning depends on the readiness of the family to learn and the relevance of the content.
- Active participation increases learning. Whenever possible, the learner should be involved in the educational process and not act as a passive listener or viewer. A discussion format in which all can participate stimulates more learning than a straight lecture.
- Repetition of a skill increases retention and promotes a feeling of competence.
- Praise and positive feedback are powerful motivators for learning. They are particularly important when the family is trying to master a frustrating task, such as breastfeeding an unresponsive infant or changing a wound dressing on a young child.
- Role modeling is an effective method for demonstrating behavior. Nurses must be aware that their behavior is scrutinized carefully at all times and that it may be copied later.
- Conflicts and frustration impede learning and should be recognized and resolved for learning to progress.
- Learning is enhanced when teaching is structured to present simple tasks before more complex material. For example, the nurse teaches how to care for the umbilical cord, which is simple, before teaching how to bathe and shampoo the newborn, which is more difficult for inexperienced parents.
- Various teaching methods are necessary to maintain interest and to illustrate concepts. Posters, videos, and printed materials supplement lectures and discussion. Models may be especially useful for teaching family planning or the process of labor or for teaching a child how to use a peak expiratory flow meter.
- Information is retained better when presented in small segments over a period of time. Short hospital stays do not support this practice, making follow-up care particularly important for some patients.

## Collaborator

Nurses collaborate with other members of the healthcare team, often coordinating and managing the patient's care. Care is improved by an interdisciplinary approach as nurses work together with dietitians, social workers, physicians, and others. Comprehensive and thorough interdisciplinary communication enhances the effectiveness of collaboration, promotes critical thinking skills and improves situation awareness (Cornell, Townsend Gervis, Yates & Vardaman, 2014). Such communication tools as Situation, Background, Assessment, and Recommendation (SBAR), hand-off reports, and closed loop communication (message sent, receiver acknowledges, receiver verifies with sender) facilitate the delivery of reliable and safe care (Cornell et al., 2014).

Managing the transition from a hospital or any other acute-care setting to the patient's home or another facility involves discharge planning and collaboration with other healthcare professionals. The trend toward home care makes collaboration increasingly important. The nurse must be knowledgeable about community resources, appropriate home care agencies for the type of patient or problem, and social work resources. Cooperation and communication are essential because patients, including parents of children, are encouraged to participate in their care.

## Researcher

Nurses contribute to their profession's knowledge base by systematically investigating theoretic or practice issues in nursing. Nursing does much more than simply "borrow" scientific knowledge from medicine and basic sciences. Nursing generates and answers its own questions based on evidence within its unique subject area. The responsibility to provide evidence-based, patient-centered care is not limited to nurses with graduate degrees. It is important that all nurses appraise and apply appropriate research findings to their practice rather than basing care decisions merely on intuition or tradition.

Evidence-based practice is no longer just an ideal but an expectation of nursing practice. Nurses can contribute to the body of professional knowledge by demonstrating an awareness of the value of nursing research and assisting in problem identification and data collection. Nurses should keep their knowledge current by networking and sharing research findings at conferences, by publishing, and by evaluating research journal articles.

## Advocate

An advocate is one who speaks on behalf of another. Care can become impersonal as the healthcare environment becomes more complex. The wishes and needs of children and families are sometimes discounted or ignored in the effort to treat and to cure. As the health professional who is closest to the patient, the nurse is in an ideal position to humanize care and to intercede on the patient's behalf. As an advocate, the nurse considers the family's wishes and preferences when planning and implementing care. The nurse informs families of treatments and procedures, ensuring that the families are involved directly in decisions and activities related to their care. The nurse must be sensitive to families' values, beliefs, and customs.

Nurses must be advocates for health promotion and healthcare access for vulnerable groups such as children, victims of domestic violence, and elders in the family. Nurses can promote the rights of children and families by participating in groups dedicated to their welfare, such as professional nursing societies, support groups, religious organizations, and voluntary organizations. Through involvement with healthcare planning on a political or legislative level and by working as consumer advocates, nurses can initiate changes for better quality healthcare. Nurses possess unique knowledge and skills and can make valuable contributions in developing healthcare strategies to ensure that all patients receive optimal care.

## Manager of Care

Because stays in acute-care facilities are short, nurses often are unable to provide total direct patient care. Instead they delegate concrete tasks, such as giving a bath or taking vital signs, to others. As a result, nurses spend more time teaching and supervising unlicensed assistive personnel, planning and coordinating care, and collaborating with other professionals and agencies. Nurses are expected to understand the financial effects of cost-containment strategies and to contribute to their institution's economic viability. At the same time, they must continue to act as patient advocates and to maintain a standard of care.

## ADVANCED PREPARATION FOR MATERNITY AND PEDIATRIC NURSES

The increasing complexity of care and a focus on cost containment have led to a greater need for nurses with advanced preparation. Advanced practice nurses may practice as certified nurse midwives (CNMs), nurse practitioners, clinical nurse specialists, or clinical nurse leaders (CNLs), among others. Advanced practice nurses also may work as nurse administrators, nurse educators, and nurse researchers. Preparation for advanced practice involves obtaining a master's or doctoral degree.

### Certified Nurse Midwives

CNMs are registered nurses who have completed an extensive program of study and clinical experience. They must pass a certification test administered by the American College of Nurse Midwives. CNMs are qualified to provide complete care during pregnancy, childbirth, and the postpartum period in uncomplicated pregnancies. They provide information about preventive measures and preparation for normal pregnancy and childbirth. They spend a great deal of time counseling and supporting the childbearing family. The CNM also provides gynecologic services as well as family planning and counseling.

Despite the proven effectiveness of nurse midwives, they were restricted in the scope and location of their practice for many years. However, many of these restrictions were lifted in 1970 when the American College of Obstetricians and Gynecologists, together with the Nurses Association of the American College of Obstetricians and Gynecologists (now known as the Association of Women's Health, Obstetric and Neonatal Nurses), issued a joint statement that admitted nurse midwives as part of the healthcare team. In 1981, Congress authorized Medicaid payments for the services of CNMs. This measure has greatly increased the use of nurse midwives, particularly by health maintenance organizations (HMOs), in birthing centers and in some hospitals.

### Nurse Practitioners

Nurse practitioners are advanced practice nurses who work according to protocols and provide many primary care services once provided only by physicians. Most nurse practitioners collaborate with a physician; depending on their scope of practice and their individual state's board of nursing mandates, they may work independently and prescribe medications. Nurse practitioners provide care for specific groups of patients in various settings (primary care facilities, schools, acute care facilities, rehabilitation centers). They may address occupational health, women's health, family health, and the health of the elderly or the very young.

*Women's health nurse practitioners* provide wellness-focused, primary, reproductive, and gynecologic care over the life span but do not usually manage care of women during pregnancy and birth. Common responsibilities include performing well-woman examinations, screening for sexually transmitted diseases, and providing family planning services. Some hospitals employ women's health nurse practitioners to assess and screen women who present to obstetric triage units, many of whom have nonobstetric problems.

*Family nurse practitioners* are prepared to provide care for people of all ages. They may care for women during uncomplicated pregnancies and provide follow-up care for the mother and infant after childbirth. Unlike certified nurse midwives, they do not assist with childbirth. They diagnose and treat patients holistically, with a strong emphasis on prevention.

*Pediatric nurse practitioners* use advanced skills to assess and treat well and ill children according to established protocols. The healthcare services they provide range from physical examinations and anticipatory guidance to the treatment of common illnesses and injuries. Staffing of newborn nurseries and children's hospital specialty units by neonatal or pediatric nurse practitioners is becoming more common.

*School nurse practitioners* receive education and training similar to that of pediatric nurse practitioners. However, because of the setting in which they practice, school nurse practitioners receive advanced education in managing chronic illness, disability, and mental health problems in a school setting and learn skills required to communicate effectively with students, teachers, school administrators, and community healthcare providers. School nurse practitioners expand the traditional role of the school nurse by providing on-site treatment of acute problems and providing extensive well-child examinations and services.

### Clinical Nurse Specialists

Clinical specialists are registered nurses who, through study and supervised practice at the graduate level (master's or doctorate), have become expert in the care of childbearing families or pediatric patients. Four major subroles have been identified for clinical nurse specialists: expert practitioner, educator, researcher, and consultant. These professionals often function as clinical leaders, role models, patient advocates, and change agents. Unlike nurse practitioners, clinical nurse specialists are not prepared to provide primary care.

### Clinical Nurse Leaders

The CNL is a master's-prepared nurse generalist whose focus is the quality, safety, and optimal patient outcomes at point of care, regardless of care setting (American Association of Colleges of Nursing [AACN], 2013). All CNLs receive the same basic preparation in a master's program, which includes advanced pathophysiology, pharmacology, and health assessment, along with other courses that prepare them to assume leadership roles within their specific practice setting. Extensive practicum experiences assist them with assessing quality and safety at the micro- and macro-systems level to improve direct patient care. A certification examination is available. CNLs work in various settings, some providing safe and optimal care to women, children, and families.

## IMPLICATIONS OF CHANGING ROLES FOR NURSES

As nursing care has changed, so also have the roles of maternity and pediatric nurses with both basic and advanced preparation. Nurses now work in various areas. Although they previously worked almost exclusively in the hospital setting, many now provide home care and community-based care. Some of the settings for care of maternity and pediatric patients include:

- Acute care settings: general hospital units, intensive care units, surgical units, postanesthesia care units, emergency care facilities, and onboard emergency transport craft
- Clinics and physicians' offices, including ambulatory care settings such as "minute clinics" that are often accessed by families with children
- Home health agencies
- Schools
- Rehabilitation centers and long-term care facilities
- Summer camps and daycare centers
- Hospice programs and respite care programs
- Psychiatric centers

### Therapeutic Communication

Therapeutic communication is a skill that nurses must have to carry out their many expected duties within the profession. Therapeutic

communication, unlike social communication, is purposeful, goal directed, and focused. Although it may seem simple, therapeutic communication requires conscious effort and considerable practice. Providing therapeutic communication often requires the nurse to be "present." Presence is a holistic model of communication where nurses connect with patients within an atmosphere of compassion and being "in the moment" with them (Fahlberg & Roush, 2016). When the nurse is truly present, the nurse is mindful of the patient's and family's needs and takes the time to listen, empathize, and "be" with them (Fahlberg & Roush, 2016).

### Guidelines for Therapeutic Communication

Therapeutic communication requires flexibility and cannot depend on a particular set of learned techniques. However, certain guidelines may prove helpful.

- A calm setting that provides privacy, reduces distractions, and minimizes interruptions is essential.
- Interactions should begin with introductions and clarification of the nurse's role. The nurse might say, "My name is Claudia Lyall. I am here to complete the discharge teaching that was started yesterday." This introduction describes the nurse's purpose and sets the stage for a discussion of the patient's concerns about what happens when the family is discharged from the hospital.
- Therapeutic communication should focus on meeting the needs expressed by the family. Beginning the interaction with an open-ended question such as "How do you feel about going home with your baby today?" is one method of focusing the interaction. Redirecting the conversation may also be necessary. For example, the nurse might say, "Thanks for showing me the beautiful pictures of the baby. I understand you are having a bit of trouble getting him to nurse."
- Nonverbal behaviors may communicate more powerful messages to the patient than the spoken word. For example, facial expressions and eye movements can confirm or contradict what is said. Repetitive hand gestures, such as tapping the fingers or twirling a lock of hair, may indicate frustration, irritation, or boredom. Body posture, stance, and gait can convey energy, depression, or discomfort. Voice tone, pitch, rate, and volume may indicate joy, anger, or fear. Communicating with a young child may require that the nurse sit or squat to get to the child's level (see Chapter 4). Personal grooming also conveys messages about the nurse's self-image.
- Active listening requires that the nurse attend to what is being said as well as to nonverbal clues. Attending behaviors that convey the nurse's interest and a sincere desire to understand include the following:
  - — Eye contact, which signals a readiness to interact.
  - — Relaxed posture, with the upper portion of the body inclined toward the person.
  - — Encouraging cues, such as nodding, leaning closer, and smiling. Verbal cues include "Uh huh, go on," "Tell me about that," or "Can you give me an example?"
  - — Touch, which can be a powerful response when words would break a mood or fail to convey the depth of feeling experienced between the woman and the nurse.
  - — Cultural differences influence communication. In some cultures, such as Chinese and Southeast Asian, prolonged eye contact is considered confrontational. People from Middle Eastern or Native American cultures are sometimes uncomfortable with touch and would be disturbed by unsolicited touching.
  - — Clarifying communication involves a unique process of the listener receiving the message as the sender intended. If the meaning of a statement is unclear, it may be necessary for the nurse to ask questions. For example, the nurse might say, "I'm not sure I understand."
  - — Emotions are part of communication, and nurses must often reflect feelings that are expressed verbally or nonverbally. The nurse might suggest, "You looked forward to delivery in a birth center and are disappointed that you needed a cesarean birth."

### Therapeutic Communication Techniques

Therapeutic communication involves responding as well as listening, and nurses must learn to use responses that facilitate rather than block communication. These facilitative responses, often called *communication techniques,* focus on both the content of the message and the feeling that accompanies the message. Communication techniques include clarifying, reflecting, being silent, questioning, and directing. A brief review of these and other communication techniques can be found in Box 2.2. In addition to being aware of effective communication techniques, nurses must be aware of behaviors that block communication, as listed with examples and alternatives in Table 2.1. More detailed methods of communicating with children and their families are described in Chapter 4.

## Critical Thinking

Optimal patient-centered care relies on the nurse's expertise in clinical judgment. Critical thinking, as a component of clinical judgment, underlies the nursing process steps (Gorton & Hayes, 2014).

### The Purpose of Critical Thinking

The critical thinking process begins when a nurse realizes that it is not enough to accumulate a fund of knowledge from texts and lectures. Nurses must also be able to *apply* the knowledge to specific clinical situations, and thus, to reach conclusions that provide the most effective care in each situation.

### Steps in Critical Thinking

A series of steps may help clarify how critical thinking is learned. These steps may be called the *ABCDEs* of critical thinking. They include recognition of assumptions, an examination of personal biases, analysis of how much pressure one has for closure, examination of how one collects and analyzes data, and evaluation of how emotions and environmental factors may interfere with one's ability to think critically.

***A. Recognizing assumptions.*** Assumptions are ideas, beliefs, or values that are taken for granted. Assumptions may lead to unexamined thoughts, unsound actions, or stereotyping.

***B. Examining biases.*** Biases are prejudices that sway an individual toward a particular conclusion or course of action on the basis of personal theories or stereotypes. Biases are based on unexamined beliefs, and many are widespread.

***C. Analyzing the need for closure.*** Many people look for immediate answers and experience anxiety until a solution is found for any problem. They have little tolerance for doubt or uncertainty, sometimes called ambiguity. As a result, they feel pressure to come to a decision, or to reach closure, as early as possible.

***D. Managing data.*** Expertise in collecting, organizing, and analyzing data involves developing an attitude of inquiry and learning to live with questions.

**Collecting data.** To obtain complete data, one must develop skill in verbal communication. Asking open-ended questions elicits more information than asking questions that require only a one-word

## BOX 2.2 Communication Techniques

| Definition | Examples |
|---|---|
| **Clarifying**<br>Clearing up or following up to understand both content and feelings expressed, to check the accuracy of how the nurse perceives the message | "I'm confused about your plans. Could you explain?"<br>"Tell me what you mean when you say you don't feel like yourself."<br>"Are you saying that ____________?"<br>"Can you tell me more about ____________?" |
| **Paraphrasing**<br>Restating in words other than those used by the patient, what the person seems to express; this is a form of clarification | **Example 1**<br>Patient: "My boyfriend won't even come into the room for the birth. I am furious with him."<br>Nurse: "You want him with you, and you are angry because he won't be here?"<br>**Example 2**<br>Patient: "My baby cries all of the time. We aren't getting any sleep."<br>Nurse: "You are feeling exhausted, and it seems like your baby cries a great deal? Can you tell me what a typical day is like?" |
| **Reflecting**<br>Verbalizing comprehension of what the patient said and what the person seems to be feeling. It is important to link content and feeling and to reflect the patient as a mirror reflects a person. The opinion, values, and personality of the nurse should not be in the reflected image. | **Example 1**<br>Patient: "I don't know what to do. My husband doesn't think a cesarean is needed, but the doctor says the baby is showing some stress."<br>Nurse: "You're confused and frightened because they don't agree?"<br>**Example 2**<br>Patient (woman in early labor): "It was my husband's idea for me to become pregnant. I wasn't too excited about it at first."<br>Nurse: "I'll bet the dad will be a pushover as a father." The nurse's statement reflects the nurse's opinion and fails to acknowledge the mother's statement.<br>A better response might be: "Your husband was more excited early in the pregnancy than you?" |
| **Silence**<br>Waiting and allowing time for the person to continue. Verbal communication need not be constant. | The nurse waits quietly for the person to continue. |
| **Structuring**<br>Creating guidelines or setting priorities | "You said you don't know how to take care of the baby and that you are afraid of getting pregnant again. What should we talk about first?" |
| **Pinpointing**<br>Calling attention to differences or inconsistencies in statements | Nurse talking to an 8-year-old child: "You said you didn't want your mother to spend the night with you, but you cry every night after she leaves. It can be scary being alone. I will sit with you, and we can talk about asking your mother to stay tomorrow night." |
| **Questioning**<br>Eliciting information directly; using open-ended questions to avoid yes or no answers and to prevent controlling the answers | "How do you feel about being pregnant?" instead of "Are you happy to be pregnant?"<br>"Will you tell me how you feel about your brother being very sick?" instead of "Are you frightened because your brother is very sick?" |
| **Directing**<br>Using nonverbal responses or succinct comments to encourage the patient to continue | Nodding. "Um mm." "You were saying." "Please go on." |
| **Summarizing**<br>Reviewing the main themes or issues that were discussed | "You had two major concerns today." "We have talked about breastfeeding and how to bathe the baby today." |

answer. Follow-up questions are often needed to clarify information or to pursue a particular train of thought.

**Validating data.** Information that is unclear or incomplete should be validated. This process may involve rechecking physical signs, collecting additional information, or determining whether a perception is accurate.

**Organizing and analyzing data.** Data are more useful when organized into patterns or clusters. The first step is to separate data that are relevant from data that may be interesting but that are not related to the current situation. The next step is to compare one's data with expected norms to determine what is within the expected range (normal) and what is not (abnormal).

**E. Evaluating *other factors*.** Various emotions and environmental factors can influence critical thinking, such as the hectic pace of the clinical area, time limitations, distractions, or fatigue that reduces one's ability to concentrate at the end of a 12-hour shift.

**TABLE 2.1 Behaviors That Block Communication**

| Behavior | Example | Alternative |
|---|---|---|
| Conveying lack of interest | Looking away, fidgeting | Attending behaviors such as eye contact, nodding |
| Conveying sense of haste | Checking the time, standing near the door | Sitting at bedside |
| Closed posture | Arms crossed over chest, holding clipboard in front of body | Leaning forward with arms relaxed |
| Interrupting, finishing sentences | Woman: "I'm not sure how ______." Nurse: "We will have a bath demonstration later." | "Go on ______." "You were saying ______." |
| Providing false reassurance | "You're going to be okay." | "I sense you are concerned about how to care for the baby. I will help you give the bath today." |
| Inappropriate self-disclosure | To woman in labor: "I was in labor 12 hours, then had a cesarean." | "What concerns you most about labor?" |
| Giving advice | "You should ______." "If I were you, I would ______." | "How do you feel about that?" "What do you think is most important?" |
| Failure to acknowledge comments or feelings | Mother: "Being a parent is hard work. I never have time for myself." Nurse: "It is going to get worse before it gets better. Parenting is hard work." | "Parenting is hard work. Let's talk about some ways that you might get a break." |

## THE NURSING PROCESS IN MATERNITY AND PEDIATRIC CARE

The nursing process is the foundation for all nursing. The nursing process consists of five distinct steps: (1) assessment, (2) nursing diagnosis, (3) planning, (4) implementation of the plan (interventions), and (5) evaluation. Despite the apparent complexity of the process, the nurse soon learns to use the steps of the nursing process in order when caring for patients (Box 2.3).

In maternal–newborn nursing, the nursing process must be adapted to a population that is generally healthy and is experiencing a life event that holds the potential for growth as well as for problems. Much maternal–newborn nursing activity is devoted to assessing and diagnosing patient strengths and healthy functioning and to supporting adaptive responses. This focus is similar to preventive care in both women's health and pediatric checkups and immunizations but differs somewhat from providing care for patients of any age who are ill.

Nursing of children, including care of a newborn, presents another challenge for many nursing students. While the nursing process when caring for adults may involve only the patient, in caring for infants and children it must involve the family as well. Therefore, it is common in planning and interventions to state what the parent is expected to do or to specify interventions (such as teaching a parent). The involvement of a third party (the family) may be new to the nursing student who has applied the nursing process only to care of adults in the past.

### Assessment

Nursing assessment is the systematic collection of relevant data to determine the patient's and family's current health status, coping patterns, needs, and problems. The data collected include not only physiologic data but also psychological, social, and cultural data relevant to life processes. Nurses must assess the belief systems, available support, perceptions, and plans of other family members in an effort to provide the best nursing care.

During the assessment phase, three activities take place: collecting data, grouping the findings, and writing the nursing diagnoses. Data can be collected through interview, physical examination, observation, review of records, and diagnostic reports, as well as through collaboration with other healthcare workers and the family. Two levels of nursing assessment are used to collect comprehensive data: (1) screening (database) assessment; and (2) focused assessment.

#### Screening Assessment

The screening, or database, assessment is usually performed during the initial contact with the person, whether in a well or inpatient setting. Its purpose is to gather information about all aspects of the adult's or child's health. This information, called **baseline data**, describes the individual's health status before interventions begin. Baseline data provide the basis for identifying both strengths and problems in the person's health. An example of baseline data would be information in a woman's prenatal record or the infant's birth information to begin his or her well-child checks.

Various methods can be used to organize the assessment. For example, information can be grouped according to body systems or functions. Assessment can also be organized around nursing models that are based on nursing theory, such as Roy's adaptation model, Gordon's functional health patterns, NANDA-International's (NANDA-I) human response patterns, or Orem's self-care deficit theory.

#### Focused Assessment

A focused assessment is used to gather information that is specifically related to an actual health problem or a problem that the patient or family is at risk for acquiring. A focused assessment is often performed at the beginning of a shift and centers on areas relevant to the patient's diagnosis and current status. For example, the nurse would perform a focused assessment of the respiratory system several times during the child's hospitalization for the child with acute asthma.

### Nursing Diagnosis

The data gathered during assessment must be analyzed to identify problems or potential problems. Data are validated and grouped in a process of critical thinking so that cues and **inferences** (drawing conclusions) can be determined. To reach a *nursing* diagnosis, the nurse identifies a person's responses to actual or potential health problems and to normal life processes. **Nursing diagnosis** provides a basis for nursing accountability for interventions and outcomes.

There are three types of nursing diagnoses. An *actual nursing diagnosis* describes a human response to a health condition or life process

## BOX 2.3 Developing Individualized Nursing Care Through the Nursing Process

Although the nursing process is the foundation for maternal-child nursing, its application in the clinical area is initially challenging, requiring proficiency in focused assessment of the patient as well as the ability to analyze data and plan nursing care for individual patients and families. It may be helpful to pose questions at each step of the nursing process.

**Assessment**

1. Were there data that were not within normal limits or expected parameters? For example, a woman states that she feels dizzy when she tries to ambulate.
2. If so, what else should be assessed? (What else should I look for? What might be related to this symptom?) For example, what are the blood pressure, pulse, skin color, temperature, and amount of lochia if the patient feels dizzy?
3. Did the assessment identify the cause of the abnormal data? What are the prepregnancy and current hemoglobin and hematocrit values? What was her estimated blood loss (EBL) during childbirth?
4. Are there other factors? What medication is the patient taking? How long has it been since she has eaten? Is the environment a related factor (crowded, warm, and unfamiliar)? Is she reluctant to ask for assistance?

**Analysis**

1. Are adequate data available to reach a conclusion? What else is needed? (What do you wish you had assessed? What would you look for next time?)
2. What is the major concern? (On the basis of the data, what are you worried about?) The woman who is dizzy may fall as she walks to the bathroom or she may drop her new baby. Or her dizziness may be a clue that a new complication is developing.
3. What might happen if no action is taken? (What might happen to the patient if you do nothing?) She may suffer an injury or a complication.
4. Is there a NANDA-I–approved diagnostic category that reflects your major concern? How is it defined? Suppose that during analysis you decide the major concern is that the patient will faint and suffer an injury. What diagnostic category most closely reflects this concern? Risk for Injury? Definition: "The state in which an individual is at risk for harm because of a perceptual or physiologic deficit, a lack of awareness of hazards, or maturational age."
5. Does this category and definition fit this patient? Is she at greater risk for a problem than others in a similar situation? Why? What are the additional risk factors?
6. Is this a problem that nurses can manage independently? Is collaboration with other health professionals needed?
7. If the problem can be managed by nurses, is it an actual nursing diagnosis (defining characteristics are present), a risk nursing diagnosis (risk factors are present), or possible problem (you have a hunch and some data, but not enough)?

**Planning**

1. What outcomes are desired? That the patient will remain free of injury during hospital stay? That she will demonstrate position changes that reduce the episodes of vertigo?
2. Would the outcomes be clear, specific, and measurable to anyone reading them?
3. What nursing interventions should be initiated and carried out to accomplish these goals or outcomes?
4. Are your written interventions specific and clear? Would another nurse know your planned interventions clearly enough to complete them after you leave? Are action verbs used *(assess, teach, assist)?* After you have written the interventions, look them over. Do they define exactly what is to be done (when, what, how far, how often)? Will they prevent the patient from suffering an injury?
5. Are the interventions based on sound rationale? For example, blood loss during birth may be excessive, resulting in hypotension that is aggravated when the woman stands suddenly.

**Implementing Nursing Interventions**

1. What are the expected effects of the prescribed intervention? Are there potential adverse effects? What are they?
2. Are the interventions acceptable to the patient and family?
3. Are the interventions clearly written so that they can be carefully followed?

**Evaluation**

1. What is the status of the patient right now?
2. What were the goals and outcomes? Are they specific? Can they be measured?
3. Compare the current status of the patient with the stated goals and outcomes.
4. What should be done now?

*NANDA-I,* North American Nursing Diagnosis Association–International.

affecting an individual, family, or community. Such a diagnosis is supported by defining characteristics (manifestations, signs, and symptoms) that can be clustered in patterns of related cues or inferences. A *risk nursing diagnosis* describes a human response to a health condition or life process that may develop in a vulnerable individual, family, or community. Such a diagnosis is supported by risk factors that contribute to increased vulnerability. A *wellness nursing diagnosis* describes a human response to levels of wellness in an individual, family, or community that has the potential for improvement.

Each nursing diagnosis is a concise term or phrase that represents a pattern of related cues or signs and symptoms. One problem that nurses often encounter is writing nursing diagnoses that nursing actions cannot address. For example, a medical diagnosis such as pyloric stenosis cannot be treated by a nurse. However, it is appropriate to say that there are nursing actions that can address the fluid volume deficit associated with pyloric stenosis.

An actual nursing diagnosis consists of two sections joined by the phrase "related to." The statement begins with the person's response to the current problem and then describes the causative factor or factors. An example is Interrupted Family Processes related to *the diagnosis of a child with cancer*. The causative factors can be physiologic, psychological, sociocultural, environmental, or spiritual. They assist the nurse in identifying nursing interventions as planning takes place.

## Planning

The nurse then makes plans to care for the problems identified during assessment and reflected in the actual nursing diagnoses. During this step, nurses set priorities, develop goals or outcomes that state what is to be accomplished by a certain time, and plan interventions to accomplish those goals. Goals cannot be achieved by nurse-prescribed actions in a risk nursing diagnosis but should reflect nursing responsibility in situations requiring physician-prescribed interventions.

### Setting Priorities

Setting priorities includes (1) determining what problems need immediate attention (i.e., life-threatening problems) and taking immediate action; (2) determining whether there are problems that call for a physician's orders for diagnosis, monitoring, or treatment; and

(3) identifying actual nursing diagnoses, which take precedence over at-risk diagnoses. For patients with many health and psychosocial problems, a realistic number of nursing diagnoses must be chosen.

### Establishing Goals and Expected Outcomes

Although the terms *goals* and *outcome criteria* are sometimes used interchangeably, they differ. Generally, broad goals do not state the specific outcome criteria and are less measurable than outcome statements. If broad goals are developed, they should be linked to more specific and measurable outcome criteria. For example, if the goal is that the parents will demonstrate effective parenting by discharge, *outcome criteria* that serve as evidence might be steps in that process such as prompt, consistent responses to infant signals and competence in bathing, feeding, and comforting the infant.

Certain rules should be followed when writing outcomes:

- Outcomes should be stated in patient terms. This wording identifies who is expected to achieve the goal (the woman, infant or child, or family).
- Measurable verbs must be used. For example, "identify," "demonstrate," "express," "walk," "relate," and "list" are verbs that are observable and measurable. Examples of verbs that are difficult to measure are "understand," "appreciate," "feel," "accept," "know," and "experience."
- A time frame is necessary. When is the person expected to perform the action? After teaching? Before discharge? By 1 day after hospitalization?
- Goals and outcomes must be realistic and attainable by nursing interventions only.
- Goals and outcomes are worked out in collaboration with a patient and family to ensure their participation in the plan of care.

### Implementation

Implementation is the action phase of the nursing process. Once the goals and desired outcomes are developed, it is necessary to select nursing interventions that will help the person meet the established outcomes. During this phase, the nurse is constantly evaluating and reassessing to determine that the interventions remain appropriate. As a patient's condition changes, so does the plan of care.

The type of nursing interventions implemented depends on whether the nursing diagnosis was an actual, risk, or wellness diagnosis and the setting in which the implementation is to occur. Nursing interventions for actual nursing diagnoses are aimed at reducing or eliminating the causes or related factors. Interventions for risk nursing diagnoses are aimed at (1) monitoring for onset of the problem, (2) reducing or eliminating risk factors, and (3) preventing the problem. For a wellness nursing diagnosis, interventions focus on supporting the individual's or family's coping mechanisms and promoting a higher level of wellness.

Nursing interventions in hospital care plans or protocols are most easily implemented if they are specific and spell out exactly what should be done. A well-written nursing intervention is specific: "Provide 200 mL of fluid [water or juice of choice] every 2 hours while the woman is awake." Vague interventions, such as "assist with breastfeeding," do not provide specific steps to follow.

### Evaluation

The evaluation determines how well the plan worked or how well the goals or outcomes were met. To evaluate, the nurse must assess the status of the patient and compare the current status with the goals or outcome criteria that were developed during the planning step. The nurse then judges how well the patient is progressing toward goal achievement and makes a decision. Should the plan be continued? Modified? Abandoned? Are the problems resolved or the causes diminished? Is another nursing diagnosis more relevant?

The nursing process is dynamic, and evaluation frequently results in expanded assessment and additional or modified nursing diagnoses and interventions. Nurses are cautioned not to view lack of goal achievement as a failure. Instead, it is simply time to reassess and begin the process anew.

## COMPLEMENTARY AND INTEGRATIVE HEALTH

Today's nurse will likely encounter individuals in many different care settings who use complementary health approaches (also referred to as complementary alternative medicine [CAM]). Terminology such as "complementary," "alternative," and "integrative" have been used interchangeably for many years; the field of complementary and integrative health is broad and constantly changing. The National Center for Complementary and Integrative Health (NCCIH, 2015) uses the term "complementary health approaches" when discussing practices and products of non-mainstream origin that are not generally considered part of conventional medicine (also called Western or allopathic medicine) as practiced by holders of medical doctor (M.D.) and doctor of osteopathy (D.O.) degrees and by allied health professionals such as physical therapists, psychologists, and registered nurses. However, the boundaries between complementary health approaches and conventional medicine are not absolute, and some complementary health approaches or practices may, over time, become widely accepted.

Complementary health approach therapies may be used instead of conventional medical therapy (alternative therapy) or in addition to it (complementary therapy). Integrative medicine combines conventional medical therapies with complementary health approach therapies that have substantial evidence as to their safety and effectiveness.

A major concern in the use of complementary health approaches is safety. People who use these techniques may delay needed care by a conventional healthcare provider, or they may take herbal remedies or other substances that are toxic when combined with conventional medications or when taken in excess. Adverse effects of complementary health approaches therapies may be unknown for the fetus (developing baby) or children. Safety and effectiveness of botanical or vitamin therapies are often unregulated. Thus, people may take in variable amounts of active ingredients from these substances. Some may not consider these therapies to be medicine and may not report them to their conventional healthcare provider, setting the stage for interactions between conventional medications and complementary health approaches therapies that have pharmacologic properties. Many people may not consider some of these therapies "alternative" at all because the therapy is mainstream in their culture.

Nurses may find that their professional values do not conflict with many of the complementary health approaches therapies. Nursing as a profession supports a self-care and preventive approach to healthcare in which the individual bears much of the responsibility for his or her health. Nursing practice has traditionally emphasized a holistic, or body-mind-spirit, model of health that fits with complementary health approaches. Nurses already practice complementary health approaches therapies such as therapeutic touch fairly often. The rising interest in complementary health approaches provides an opportunity for nurses to participate in research related to the legitimacy of these treatment modalities.

The National Center for Complementary and Integrative Health, a division of the National Institutes of Health, has a website (http://www.nccih.nih.gov) for information about and classification of the therapies.

## NURSING RESEARCH AND EVIDENCE-BASED PRACTICE

As nursing and the healthcare system changes, nurses will be challenged to demonstrate that what they do improves patient outcomes and is cost effective. To meet this challenge, nurses must participate in research and use evidence-based research to improve patient-centered care. With the establishment of the National Institute of Nursing Research (NINR) as a member of the National Institutes of Health (http://www.nih.gov/ninr), nurses now have an infrastructure in place to ensure that nursing research is supported and that a group of well-prepared nurse researchers will be educated. One way of doing this is through using the principles of evidence-based nursing practice.

Evidence-based practices to improve patient outcomes are a combination of the following: asking an appropriate clinical question; acquiring, appraising, and using the highest level of published research; clinical expertise; and patient values and preferences (Centre for Evidence-Based Medicine – Toronto, 2014; Melnyk & Fineout-Overholt, 2015). When considering a change in practice, nurses need to take into account both the level and quality (rigor, consistency, and sufficiency) of research to determine the strength of evidence (Melnyk & Fineout-Overholt, 2014). To accomplish this goal effectively, nurses need to be familiar with what constitutes the highest levels of evidence. The evidence level is based on the research design of a study or studies. There are several different approaches to categorizing levels of evidence for nursing, although all are very similar.

While the outcomes of research in nursing are expanding, few randomized controlled trials (RCTs) have been conducted and published by nurses. However, nurses can consider using high-quality evidence presented in integrative or systematic reviews (reviews of collected research on a particular health issue) conducted by various health professionals that includes nurses. One source of high-quality systematic reviews is the *Cochrane Database of Systematic Reviews;* another is the National Guideline Clearinghouse. Nurses should not exclude descriptive or qualitative studies from consideration of a practice change because these studies often provide more in-depth information about a particular clinical issue.

Finally, practice change should not be made without including the nurse's expertise and ability to assess what can or cannot be effective for patient outcomes. In some instances, it is not practical or cost effective to make a particular practice change. Nurses should also strongly consider whether a practice change will be acceptable to patients; if the change is not accepted, patients will not incorporate it into their self-care (Melnyk & Fineout-Overholt, 2014).

The amount of clinically based nursing research conducted is increasing rapidly as nurse researchers strive to develop an independent body of knowledge that demonstrates the value of nursing interventions. AWHONN has an ongoing commitment to develop and disseminate evidence-based practice guidelines through the association's research-based practice program. Implementation of evidence-based guidelines promotes application of the best available scientific evidence for nursing care rather than care based on tradition alone. The professional nurse is also expected to participate in research activities appropriate to her or his position, education, and practice environment (AWHONN, 2009). The Society of Pediatric Nurses (http://www.pedsnurses.org) also routinely publishes positions that address both clinical and educational issues related to nursing care of children and families. Although students and inexperienced nurses may not directly participate in research projects, they must learn how useful knowledge obtained by the research team is to their practice. Professional journals are the best sources of new information that can help nurses provide better care to specific patients. Searching for information can also identify unrecognized research needs to identify actions for a better practice.

## KEY CONCEPTS

- Maternal-newborn nurses, women's health nurses, and nurses who care for children and families function in various roles, including care provider, teacher, collaborator, researcher, advocate, and manager.
- The care settings in which maternity and pediatric nurses may practice include acute care settings, clinics, physicians' offices, home health agencies, schools, rehabilitation centers, summer camps, daycare centers, and hospices.
- Registered nurses with advanced education are prepared to provide primary care for women and children as certified nurse midwives and nurse practitioners.
- Clinical nurse specialists function as educators, researchers, and consultants to provide in-depth interventions for many problems encountered in maternity and pediatric care.
- Nurses must be adept at communicating and removing blocks to communication to meet their responsibilities as educators and counselors.
- A primary responsibility of nurses is to provide information to childbearing families and to children and their families; nurses must know the principles of teaching and learning to fulfill the role of educator.
- Nurses must learn to think critically by examining their own thought processes for flaws that can lead to inaccurate conclusions or poor clinical judgments.
- The nursing process begins with assessment and includes analysis of data that may result in nursing diagnoses. Nursing diagnoses are those problems that nurses are legally accountable for identifying and managing independently.
- Collaborative problems are usually physiologic complications that require both physician-prescribed and nurse-prescribed interventions.
- Nurses must consider the effect of complementary health approaches when assessing the patient and planning care.
- Competence in the collection and application of best evidence for specific care of common problems in nursing practice is now part of the role of every nurse. Relying on traditional care methods rather than determining whether evidence supports the methods is no longer sufficient.
- Risk nursing diagnoses are problems that require both physician-prescribed and nurse-prescribed interventions.

## REFERENCES AND READINGS


Ackley, B.J., & Ladwig, G.B. (2013). *Nursing diagnosis handbook: An evidence-based guide to planning care* (10th ed.). St. Louis: Mosby.

Alfaro-LeFevre, R. (2013). *Critical thinking and clinical judgment: A practical approach* (5th ed.). St. Louis: Elsevier Saunders.

American Association of Colleges of Nursing. (2013). *Competencies and curricular expectations for Clinical Nurse LeaderSM education and practice*. Retrieved from http://www.aacn.nche.edu.

American Nurses Association. (2015). *Code of ethics for nurses with interpretive statements. American Nurses Association*. Washington, DC. Retrieved from http://www.nursingworld.org.

Association of Women's Health, Obstetric, and Neonatal Nurses. (2009). *Standards for professional nursing practice in the care of women and newborns* (7th ed.). Washington, DC: Author.

Centre for Evidence-Based Medicine – Toronto. (2014). *Introduction to evidence-based nursing*. Retrieved from http://www.cebm.utoronto.ca/syllabi/nur/intro.htm.

Cornell, P., Townsend Gervis, M., Yates, L., & Vardaman, J.M. (2014). Impact of SBAR on nurse shift reports and staff rounding. *MEDSURG Nursing, 23*(5), 334–342.

Fahlberg, F., & Roush, T. (2016). Mindful presence: being "with" in our nursing care. *Nursing, 46*(3), 14–15.

Fontaine, K.L. (2014). *Complementary and alternative therapies for nursing practice* (4th ed.). Upper Saddle River: Prentice Hall.

Friedman, F. (2008/2014). *SPN Position statement: Position on family-centered care in the nursing curriculum*. Retrieved from http://www.pedsnurses.org.

Gorton, K.L., & Hayes, J. (2014). Challenges of assessing critical thinking and clinical judgment in nurse practitioner students. *Journal of Nursing Education, 53*(3S), S26–S29.

Melnyk, B., & Fineout-Overholt, E. (2015). *Evidence-based practice in nursing and healthcare* (3rd ed.). Philadelphia: Lippincott Williams & Wilkins.

Micozzi, M.S. (2015). Characteristics of complementary and integrative medicine. In M.S. Micozzi (Ed.), *Fundamentals of Complementary and Integrative Medicine* (5th ed., pp. 3–12). Philadelphia: Elsevier Saunders.

Micozzi, M.S., & Cassidy, C.M. (2015). Issues and challenges in integrative medicine. In M.S. Micozzi (Ed.), *Fundamentals of Complementary and Integrative Medicine* (5th ed., pp. 22–34). Philadelphia: Elsevier Saunders.

National Center for Complementary and Integrated Health. (2015). *Complementary, alternative, and integrative health: What's in a name?* Retrieved from http://www.nccih.nih.gov/health/integrative-health#term.

Riley, J.B. (2012). *Communication in nursing* (7th ed.). St. Louis: Elsevier Mosby.

Society of Pediatric Nurses. (2015). *Position statement: Child health content in the undergraduate nursing curriculum*. Retrieved from http://www.pedsnurses.org.

3

# The Childbearing and Child-Rearing Family

http://evolve.elsevier.com/McKinney/mat-ch/

## LEARNING OBJECTIVES

*After studying this chapter, you should be able to*

- Explain how important families are for the provision of effective nursing care to women, infants, and children.
- Describe different family structures and their effect on family functioning.
- Differentiate between healthy and dysfunctional families.
- List internal and external coping behaviors used by families when they face a crisis.
- Compare Western cultural values with those of other cultural groups.
- Describe the effect of cultural diversity on nursing practice.
- Describe common styles of parenting that nurses may encounter.
- Explain how variables in parents and children may affect their relationship.
- Discuss the use of discipline in a child's socialization.
- Evaluate the effects of an ill child on the family.

No factor influences a person as profoundly as the family. Families protect and promote a child's growth, development, health, and well-being until the child reaches maturity. A healthy family provides children and adults with love, affection, and a sense of belonging and nurtures feelings of self-esteem and self-worth. Children need stable families to grow into happy, functioning adults. Family relationships continue to be important during adulthood. Family relationships influence, positively or negatively, people's relationships with others. Family influence continues into the next generation as a person selects a mate, forms a new family, and often rears children.

For nurses in pediatric practice, the whole family is the patient. The nurse cares for the child in the context of a dynamic family system rather than caring for just an infant or a child. The nurse is responsible for supporting families and encouraging healthy coping patterns during the periods of normal growth and development or illness.

## FAMILY-CENTERED CARE

Family-centered maternity care and family-centered child care are integral for comprehensive care given by maternity and pediatric nurses. Family-centered care can be defined as an innovative approach to the planning, delivery, and evaluation of healthcare that is grounded in a mutually beneficial partnership between patients, families, and healthcare professionals (Schlucter, 2014). Some barriers to effective family-centered care are lack of skills in communication, role negotiation, and developing relationships. Other areas that interfere with the complete implementation of family-centered care are lack of time, fear of losing role, and lack of support from the healthcare system and from other healthcare disciplines (Harrison, 2010). One particular useful skill in family centered care is validation, which means accepting what the family member says or does as a valid expression of thoughts and feelings (Harvey & Ahmann, 2014). Clearly, there is a need for increased education in this area, based on evidence, to help nurses and other healthcare professionals implement this concept.

## FAMILY STRUCTURE

Family structures in the United States are changing. The number of families with children that are headed by a married couple has declined, and the number of single-parent families has increased. In addition, roles have changed within the family. While the role of the provider was once almost exclusively assigned to the father, both parents now may be providers, and many fathers are active in nurturing and disciplining their children.

### Types of Families

Families are sometimes categorized into three types: traditional, nontraditional, and high risk. Nontraditional and high-risk families often need care that differs from the care required by traditional families. Different family structures can produce varying stressors. For example, the single-parent family has as many demands placed on it for resources, such as time and money, as the two-parent family. However, only one parent is able to meet these demands.

#### Traditional Families

Traditional families (also called nuclear families) are headed by two parents who view parenting as the major priority in their lives and whose energies may not be depleted by stressful conditions such as poverty, illness, and substance abuse. Traditional families can be single-income or dual-income families. Generally, traditional families are motivated to learn all they can about pregnancy, childbirth, and parenting (Fig. 3.1). Today a family structure composed of two married parents and their children represents 69% of families with children. Twenty-four percent of children live with only their mother and 4% with no parents. The remaining percentage of children live with two parents who are not married (Federal Interagency Forum on Child and Family Statistics, 2015).

Single-income families in which one parent, usually the father, is the sole provider are a minority among households in the United

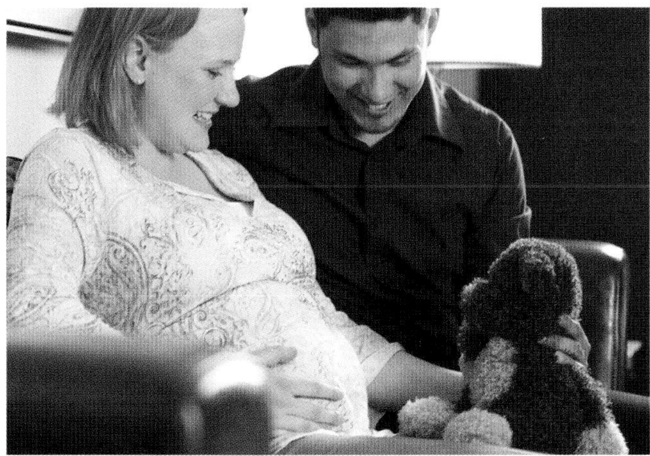

FIG 3.1 Traditional, two-parent families typically have the resources to prepare for childbirth and the needs of infants. (© 2012 Photos.com, a division of Getty Images. All rights reserved.)

States. Most two-parent families depend on two incomes, either to make ends meet or to provide nonessentials that they could not afford on one income. One or both parents may travel as a work responsibility. Dependence on two incomes has created a great deal of stress on parents, subjecting them to many of the same problems that single-parent families face. For example, reliable, competent child care is a major issue that has increased the stress experienced by traditional families. A high consumer debt load gives them less cushion for financial setbacks such as job loss. Having the time and flexibility to attend to the requirements of both their careers and their children may be difficult for parents in these families.

### Nontraditional Families

The growing number of nontraditional families, designated as "complex households" by the U.S. Census Bureau, includes single-parent families, blended families, adoptive families, unmarried couples with children, multigenerational families, and homosexual parent families (Fig. 3.2).

***Single-parent families.*** Millions of families are now headed by a single parent, most often the mother, who must function as homemaker and caregiver and is often the major provider for the family's financial needs. Factors contributing to this demographic include divorce, widowhood, and childbirth or adoption among unmarried women. Of the 28% of children who live with one parent, 24% live with their mothers (Federal Interagency Forum on Child and Family Statistics, 2015).

Single parents may feel overwhelmed by the prospect of assuming all child-rearing responsibilities and may be less prepared for illness or loss of a job than two-parent families.

***Blended families.*** Blended families are formed when single, divorced, or widowed parents bring children from a previous union into their new relationship. Many times the couple desires children with each other, creating a contemporary family structure commonly described as "yours, mine, and ours." These families must overcome differences in parenting styles and values to form a cohesive blended family. Differing expectations of children's behavior and development as well as differing beliefs about discipline often cause family conflict. Financial difficulties can result if one parent is obligated to pay child support from a previous relationship. Older children may resent the introduction of a stepmother or stepfather into the family system. This can cause tension between the biologic parent, the children, and the stepmother or stepfather.

***Adoptive families.*** People who adopt a child may have problems that biological parents do not face. Biological parents have the long period of gestation and the gradual changes of pregnancy to help them adjust emotionally and socially to the birth of a child. An adoptive family, both parents and siblings, is expected to make these same adjustments suddenly when the adopted child arrives. Adoptive parents may add pressure to themselves by having an unrealistically high standard for themselves as parents. Additional issues with adoptive families include possible lack of knowledge of the child's health history, the difficulty assimilating if the child is adopted from another country, and the question of when and how to tell the child about being adopted. Adoptive parents and biological parents need information, support, and guidance to prepare them to care for the infant or child and maintain their own relationships.

***Multigenerational families.*** The multigenerational or extended family consists of members from three or more generations living under one roof. Older adult parents may live with their adult children, or in some cases adult children return to their parents' home, either because they are unable to support themselves or because they want the additional support that the grandparents provide for the grandchildren. The latter arrangement has given rise to the term *boomerang* families. Extended families are vulnerable to generational conflicts and may need education and referral to counselors to prevent disintegration of the family unit.

Grandparents or other older family members now head a growing number of households with children because of the inability of the parents to care for their children. More than half of children who do not live with either parent live with a grandparent (Forum on Child and Family Statistics, 2015). The strain of raising children a second time may cause tremendous physical, financial, and emotional stress. These families might need multiple referrals for assistance for the child's care, such as Medicaid for health insurance, school lunch and breakfast programs, and psychological support.

***Same-sex–parent families.*** Families headed by same-sex parents have become increasingly more frequent in the United States. The children in such families may be the offspring of previous heterosexual unions, or they may be adopted children or children conceived by an artificial reproductive technique such as in vitro fertilization. The couple may face many challenges from a community that is unaccustomed to alternative lifestyles. The children's adaptation depends on the parents' psychological adjustment, the degree of participation and support from the absent biological parent, and the level of community support.

***Communal families.*** Communal families are groups of people who have chosen to live together as extended family groups. Their relationship to one another is motivated by social value or financial necessity rather than by kinship. Their values are often spiritually based and may be more liberal than those of the traditional family. Traditional family roles may not exist in a communal family.

## Characteristics of Healthy Families

In general, healthy families are able to adapt to changes that occur in the family unit. Pregnancy and parenthood create some of the most powerful changes that a family experiences.

Healthy families exhibit the following common characteristics, which provide a framework for assessing how all families function (Smith, 2013):

- Members of healthy families communicate openly with one another to express their concerns and needs.

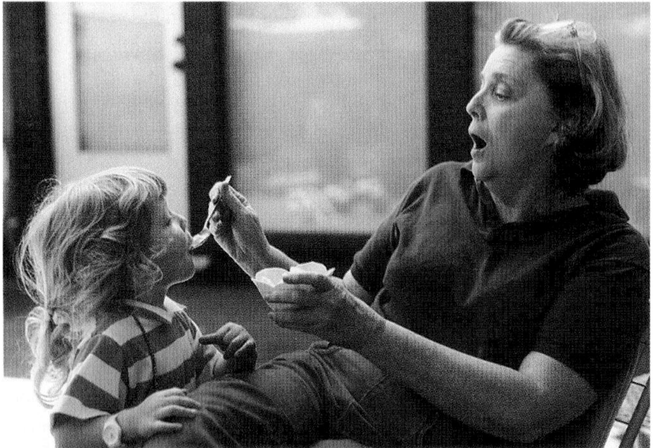

Busy parents may rely on grandparents for child care or for an additional measure of love and attention for their children. Some grandparents raise grandchildren because of their own children's inability to do so.

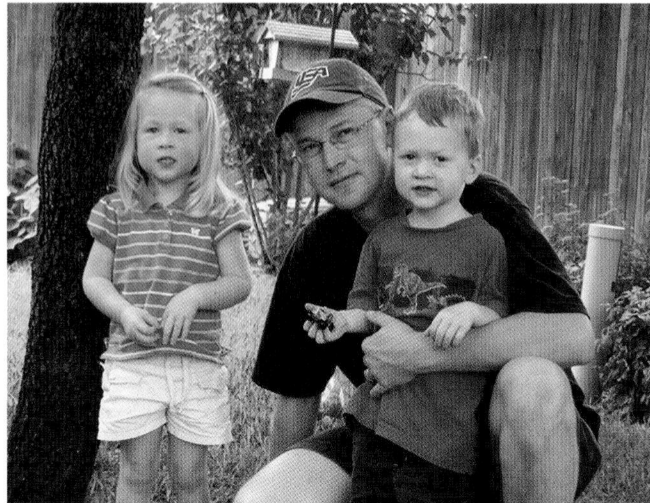

Fathers are the primary child-care providers in a growing number of families. Fathers who are not the primary caregivers often participate more actively in caring for their children than the fathers of previous generations.

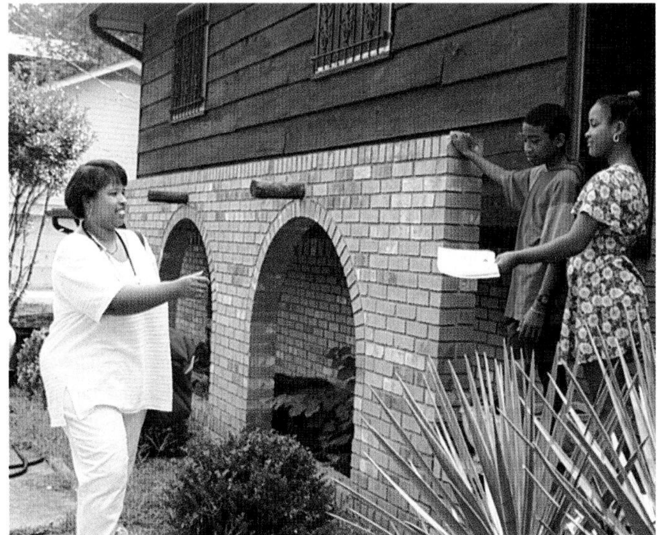

A single parent often experiences financial and time constraints. Children in single-parent families are often given more responsibility to care for themselves and younger siblings.

**FIG 3.2** A nurse caring for a child needs to know the child's family structure and the identity of the child's primary caregiver. This background becomes the context in which the nurse provides care. If family support is a concern, the nurse can provide information about local community resources. For example, in some communities, after-school programs and "warm lines" can help children with schoolwork and alleviate loneliness and fear.

- Healthy family members remain flexible in their roles, with roles changing to meet changing family needs.
- Adults in healthy families agree on the basic principles of parenting so that minimal discord exists about concepts such as discipline and sleep schedules.
- Healthy families are adaptable and are not overwhelmed by life changes.
- Members of healthy families volunteer assistance without waiting to be asked.
- Family members spend time together regularly but facilitate autonomy.
- Healthy families seek appropriate resources for support when needed.
- Healthy families transmit cultural values and expectations to children.

## FACTORS THAT INTERFERE WITH FAMILY FUNCTIONING

Factors that may interfere with the family's ability to provide for the needs of its members include lack of financial resources, absence of adequate family support, birth of an infant who needs specialized care, an ill child, unhealthy habits such as smoking and abuse of other substances, and inability to make mature decisions that are necessary to provide care for the children. Needs of aging members at the time children are going through adolescence or the expenses of college add pressure on middle-aged parents, often called the "sandwich generation."

### High-Risk Families

All families encounter stressors, but some factors add to the usual stress experienced by a family. The nurse needs to consider the additional needs of the family with a higher risk for being dysfunctional. Examples of high-risk families are those experiencing marital conflict and divorce, those with adolescent parents, those affected by violence against one or more of the family members, those involved with substance abuse, and those with a chronically ill child.

### Marital Conflict and Divorce

Although divorce is traumatic to children, research has shown that living in a home filled with conflict can also be detrimental both physically and emotionally (Kelly & El-Sheikh, 2011; Lindahl & Malik, 2011). Divorce can be the outcome of many years of unresolved family conflict. It can result in continuing conflict over child custody, visitation, and child support, changes in housing, lifestyle, cultural expectations, friends, and extended family relationships, diminished self-esteem, and changes in the physical, emotional, or spiritual health of children and other family members.

Divorce is loss that needs to be grieved. The conflict and divorce may affect children, and young children may be unable to verbalize their distress. Nurses can help children through the grieving process with age-appropriate activities such as therapeutic play (see Chapter 35). Principles of active listening (see Chapter 4) are valuable for adults as well as children to help them express their feelings. Nurses can also help newly divorced or separated parents through listening, encouragement, and referrals to support groups or counselors.

### Adolescent Parenting

The teenage birth rate in the United States fell to 26.5 per 1000 teen births in 2013, the lowest level ever reported in the seven decades for which a consistent series of rates is available (Martin, Hamilton, Osterman, Curtin, & Matthews, 2015). Adolescent birth rates vary by race; however, there has been a steady decline in teen birth rates for all racial and ethnic groups. The impact of strong pregnancy prevention messages directed to teenagers has been credited with the birth rate declines (National Center for Health Statistics, 2012).

Teenage parenting often has a negative effect on the health and social outcomes of the entire family. Adolescent girls are at increased risk for numerous pregnancy complications, such as preterm birth, low birth weight, and death during infancy (Ventura & Hamilton, 2011). Those who become parents during adolescence are unlikely to attain a high level of education and, as a result, are more likely to be poor and often homeless. An adolescent father often does not contribute to the economic or psychological support of his child. Moreover, the cycle of teen parenting and economic hardship is more likely to be continued because children of adolescent parents are themselves more likely to become teenage parents.

### Violence

Violence is a constant stressor in some families. Violence can occur in any family of any socioeconomic or educational status. Children endure the psychological pain of seeing the victimized parent experiencing violence from one who is supposed to provide love and care. Although women traditionally are more victimized by men (see Chapter 24), the reverse is not unlikely (Bureau of Justice Statistics, 2014). In addition, because of the role models they see in the adults, children in violent families may repeat the cycle of violence when they are adults and become abusers or victims of violence themselves.

Abuse of the child may be physical, sexual, or emotional or may take the form of neglect (see Chapter 53). Often one child in the family is the target of abuse or neglect, while others are given proper care. As in adult abuse, children who witness abuse are more likely to repeat that behavior when they are parents themselves, because they have not learned constructive ways to deal with stress or to discipline children.

### Substance Abuse

Parents who abuse drugs or alcohol may neglect their children because obtaining and using the substance(s) may have a stronger pull on the parents than does care of their children. Parental substance abuse interrupts a child's normal growth and development. The parent's ability to meet the needs of the child are severely compromised, increasing the child's risk for emotional and health problems (National Association for Children of Alcoholics Foundation, 2012).

The child may be the substance abuser in the home. The drug habit can lead a child into unhealthy friendships and may result in criminal activity to maintain the habit. School achievement is likely to plummet, and the older adolescent may drop out of school. Children, as well as adults, can die as a result of their drug activity, either directly from the drugs or from associated criminal activity or risk-taking behaviors.

### Child With Special Needs

When a child is born with a birth defect or has an illness that requires special care, the family is under additional stress (see Chapters 36 and 54). In most cases their initial reactions of shock and disbelief gradually resolve into acceptance of the child's limitations. However, the parents' grieving may be long term as they repeatedly see other children doing things that their child cannot and perhaps will not ever do.

These families often suffer financial hardship. Health insurance benefits may quickly reach their maximum. Even if the child has public assistance for healthcare costs, the family often experiences a decrease in income because one parent must remain home with the sick child rather than work outside the home.

Strains on the marriage and the parents' relationships with their other children are inevitable under these circumstances. Parents have little time or energy left to nurture their relationship with each other, and divorce may add yet another strain to the family. Siblings may resent the parental time and attention required for care of the ill child yet feel guilty if they express their resentment.

However, the outlook is not always pessimistic in these families. If the family learns skills to cope with the added demands imposed on it by this situation, the potential exists for growth in maturity, compassion, and strength of character.

## HEALTHY VERSUS DYSFUNCTIONAL FAMILIES

Family conflict is unavoidable. It is a natural result of a perceived unequal exchange or an imbalance in the use of resources by individual members. Conflict should not be viewed as bad or disruptive; the management of the conflict, not the conflict itself, may be problematic. Conflict can produce growth and improve family functioning if the outcome is resolution as opposed to dissolution or continued conflict. The following three ingredients are required to resolve conflict:

1. Open communication
2. Accurate perceptions about the nature and degree of conflict
3. Constructive efforts to resolve the conflict, such as willingness to consider the view of the other, consider alternate solutions, and compromise

Dysfunctional families have problems in any one or a combination of these areas. They tend to become trapped in patterns in which they maintain conflicts rather than resolve them. The conflicts create stress, and the family must cope with the resultant stress.

### Coping With Stress

If the family is considered a balanced system that has internal and external interrelationships, stressors are viewed as forces that change the balance in the system. Stressful events are neither positive nor negative, but rather neutral until they are interpreted by the individual. Positive as well as negative events can cause stress (Smith & Hamon, 2012). For example, the birth of a child is usually a joyful event, but it can also be stressful.

Some families are able to mobilize their strengths and resources, thus effectively adapting to the stressors. Other families fall apart. A *family crisis* is a state or period of disorganization that affects the foundation of the family (Smith & Hamon, 2012).

### Coping Strategies

Nurses can help families cope with stress by helping each family identify its strengths and resources. Friedman, Bowden, and Jones (2003) identified family coping strategies as internal and external. Box 3.1 identifies family coping strategies and further defines *internal strategies* as family relationship strategies, cognitive strategies, and communication strategies. *External strategies* focus on maintaining active community linkages and using social support systems and spiritual strategies. Some families adjust quickly to extreme crises, whereas other families become chaotic with relatively minor crises. Family functional patterns that existed before a crisis are probably the best indicators of how the family will respond to it.

**BOX 3.1 Coping Strategies of Families**

**Internal Coping Strategies**

***Relationship Strategies***

- Family group reliance
- Greater sharing together
- Role flexibility

***Cognitive Strategies***

- Normalizing
- Controlling the meaning of the problem by reframing and passive appraisal
- Joint problem solving
- Gaining of information and knowledge

**Communication Strategies**

- Being open and honest
- Use of humor and laughter

**External Coping Strategies**

***Community Strategy: Maintaining Active Linkages With the Community***

*Social Support Strategies*

- Extended family
- Friends
- Neighbors
- Self-help groups
- Formal social supports

*Spiritual Strategies*

- Seeking advice of clergy
- Becoming more involved in religious activities
- Having faith in God
- Prayer

From Friedman, M., Bowden, V., & Jones, E. (2003). *Family nursing: Theory, research, and practice* (5th ed.). Upper Saddle River, NJ: Prentice-Hall.

## CULTURAL INFLUENCES ON MATERNITY AND PEDIATRIC NURSING

Culture is the sum of the beliefs and values that are learned, shared, and transmitted from generation to generation by a particular group. Cultural values guide the thinking, decisions, and actions of the group, particularly regarding pivotal events such as birth, sexual maturity, illness, and death. Ethnicity is the condition of belonging to a particular group that shares race, language and dialect, religious faiths, traditions, values, and symbols as well as food preferences, literature, and folklore. Cultural beliefs and values vary between different groups and subgroups, and nurses must be aware that individuals often believe their cultural values and patterns of behavior are superior to those of other groups. This belief, termed ethnocentrism, forms the basis for many conflicts that occur when people from different cultural groups have frequent contact.

Nurses must be aware that culture is composed of visible and invisible layers that could be said to resemble an iceberg (Fig. 3.3). The observable behaviors can be compared with the visible tip of the iceberg. The history, traditions, beliefs, values, and religion are not necessarily observed but are the hidden foundation on which behaviors are based and can be likened to the large, submerged part of the iceberg. To comprehend cultural behavior fully, one must seek knowledge of the hidden beliefs that behaviors express. This knowledge comes from experiencing caring relationships with people of different cultures within the context of mutual respect and a sincere desire to understand the role of culture in another's "lived experiences" (Bearskin, 2011). One must also have the desire or motivation to engage in the process of becoming culturally competent to be effective in caring for diverse populations.

Nurses must first understand their own culture and recognize their biases before beginning to acquire the knowledge and understanding of other cultures. Applying the knowledge completes the process (Galanti, 2015).

Religious and spiritual beliefs often have a strong influence on families as they face the crisis of illness. Specific beliefs about the causes, treatment, and cure of illness are important for the nurse to know to empower the family as they deal with the immediate crisis. Table 3.1 describes how some religious beliefs affect healthcare.

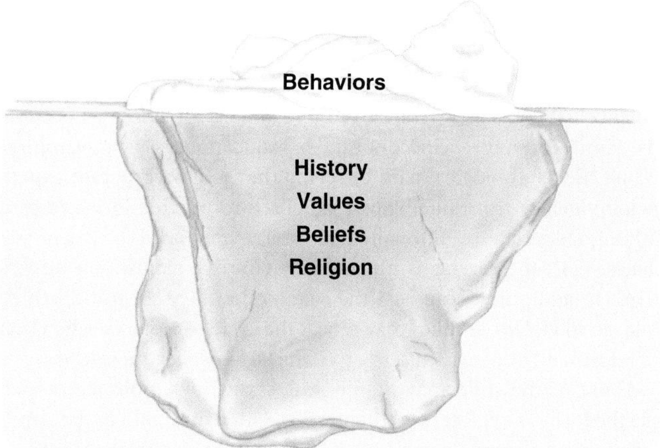


**FIG 3.3** Visible and hidden layers of culture are like the visible and submerged parts of an iceberg. Many cultural differences are hidden below the surface.

**TABLE 3.1 Religious Beliefs Affecting Healthcare**

| Religion and Basic Beliefs | Practices |
|---|---|
| **Christian** | |
| Christianity is generally accepted to be the largest religious group in the world. There are three major branches of Christianity and numerous religious traditions considered to be Christian. These traditions have much in common relative to beliefs and practices. Belief in Jesus Christ as the son of God and the Messiah comprises the central core of Christianity. Christians believe that it is through Jesus' death and resurrection that salvation can be attained. They also believe that they are expected to follow the example of Jesus in daily living. Study of biblical scripture; practicing faith, good works, and sacramental rites (e.g., baptism, communion, and others); and prayer are common among most Christian faiths. | |
| ***Christian Science*** | |
| Based on scientific system of healing. Beliefs derived from both the Bible and the book, Science, and Health with Key to the Scriptures. Prayer is the basis for spiritual, physical, emotional, and mental healing, as opposed to medical intervention (Christian Science, 2011). Healing is divinely natural, not miraculous. | Birth: Use physician or midwife during childbirth. No baptism ceremony. Dietary practices: Alcohol and tobacco are considered drugs and are not used. Coffee and tea also may be declined. Death: Autopsy and donation of organs are usually declined. Healthcare: May refuse medical treatment. View health in a spiritual framework. Seek exemption from immunizations but obey legal requirements. When Christian Science believer is hospitalized, parent or client may request that a Christian Science practitioner be notified. |
| ***Jehovah's Witness*** | |
| Expected to preach house to house about the good news of God. Bible is doctrinal authority. No distinction is made between clergy and laity. | Baptism: No infant baptism. Adult baptism by immersion. Dietary practices: Use of tobacco and alcohol discouraged. Death: Autopsy decided by persons involved. Burial and cremation acceptable. Birth control and abortion: Use of birth control is a personal decision. Abortion opposed on basis of Exodus 21 : 22-23.Healthcare: Blood transfusions not allowed. May accept alternatives to transfusions, such as use of non-blood plasma expanders, careful surgical technique to minimize blood loss, and use of autologous transfusions. Nurses should check an unconscious patient for identification that states that the person does not want a transfusion. Jehovah's Witnesses are prepared to die rather than break God's law. Respect the healthcare given by physicians, but look to God and His laws as the final authority for their decisions. |
| ***The Church of Jesus Christ of Latter-Day Saints (Mormon)*** | |
| Restorationism: True church of Christ ended with the first generation of apostles but was restored with the founding of Mormon Church. Articles of faith: Mormon doctrine states that individuals are saved if they are obedient to God's divine ordinances (faith, repentance, baptism by immersion and laying on of hands).Holy Communion: Hospitalized patient may desire to have a member of the church's clergy administer the sacrament. Scripture: Word of God can be found in the Bible, Book of Mormon, Doctrine and Covenants, Pearl of Great Price, and current revelations. Christ will return to rule in Zion, located in America. | Baptism: By immersion. Considered essential for the living and the dead. If a child older than 8 years is very ill, whether baptized or unbaptized, a member of the church's clergy should be called. Anointing of the sick: Mormons frequently are anointed and given a blessing before going to the hospital and after admission by laying on of hands. Dietary practices: Tobacco and caffeine are not used. Mormons eat meat (limited) but encourage the intake of fruits, grains, and herbs. Death: Prefer burial of the body. A church elder should be notified to assist the family. Birth control and abortion: Abortion is opposed unless the life of the mother is in danger. Only natural methods of birth control are recommended. Other means are used only when the physical or emotional health of the mother is at stake. Other practices: Believe in the healing power of laying on of hands. Cleanliness is important. Believe in healthy living and adhere to healthcare requirements. Families are of great importance, so visiting should be encouraged. The church maintains a welfare system to assist those in need. |
| ***Roman Catholic*** | |
| Belief that the Word of God is handed down to successive generations through scripture and tradition, and is interpreted by the magisterium (the Pope and bishops). Pope has final doctrinal authority for followers of the Catholic faith, which includes interpreting important doctrinal issues related to personal practice and healthcare. | Baptism: Infant baptism by affusion (sprinkling of water on head) or total immersion. Original sin is believed to be "washed away." If death is imminent or a fetus is aborted, anyone can perform the baptism by sprinkling water on the forehead, saying "I baptize you in the name of the Father, Son, and Holy Spirit." Anointing of the Sick: Encouraged for anyone who is ill or injured. Always done if prognosis is poor. Dietary practices: Fasting on Ash Wednesday and Good Friday required for all, except children, elders, and those who are ill. Avoidance of meat on Ash Wednesday and on Fridays during Lent required. Death: Organ donation permitted. |

*Continued*

**TABLE 3.1 Religious Beliefs Affecting Healthcare—cont'd**

| Religion and Basic Beliefs | Practices |
|---|---|
| ***Amish*** | |
| Christians who practice their religion and beliefs within the context of strong community ties. Focused on salvation and a happy life after death. Powerful bishops make healthcare decisions for the community. Problems solved with prayer and discussion. Primarily agrarian; eschew many modern conveniences. | Baptism: Late teen/early adult. Must marry within the church. Death: Do not normally use extraordinary measures to prolong life. Other practices: May have a language issue (modified German or Dutch) and need an interpreter. At increased risk for genetic disorders; refuse contraception or prenatal testing. May appear stoical or impassive—personally humble. Reject health insurance; rely on the Church and community to pay for healthcare needs. Use holistic and herbal remedies, but accept western medical approaches. |
| **Hindu** | |
| Belief in reincarnation and that the soul persists even though the body changes, dies, and is reborn. Salvation occurs when the cycle of death and reincarnation ends. Nonviolent approach to living. Congregation worship is not customary; worship is through private shrines in the home. Disease is viewed holistically, but Karma (cause and effect) may be blamed. | Circumcision is observed by ritual. Dietary practices: Dietary restrictions vary according to sect; vegetarianism is not uncommon. Death: Death rituals specify practices and who can touch corpse. Family must be consulted, as family members often provide ritualistic care. Other practices: May use ayurvedic medicine—an approach to restoring balance through herbal and other remedies. Same-sex health providers may be requested. |
| **Islam** | |
| Belief in one God that humans can approach directly in prayer. Based on the teachings of Muhammad. Five Pillars of Islam. Compulsory prayers are said at dawn, noon, afternoon, after sunset, and after nightfall. | Circumcision: Practiced<br>Dietary practices: Prohibit eating pork and other meat not slaughtered according to Islamic criteria. Alcohol is also prohibited. Fast during Ramadan (ninth month of Muslim year). Death: Oppose autopsy and organ donation. Death ritual prescribes the handling of corpse by only family and friends. Burial occurs as soon as possible. Same-sex health providers may be requested. |
| **Judaism** | |
| Beliefs are based on the Old Testament, the Torah, and the Talmud, the oral and written laws of faith. Belief in one God who is approached directly. Believe Messiah is still to come. Believe Jews are God's chosen people. | *Circumcision:* A symbol of God's covenant with Israel. Done on eighth day after birth. *Bar Mitzvah/Bat Mitzvah:* Ceremonial rite of passage for boys and girls into adulthood and taking personal responsibility for adherence to Jewish laws and rituals. *Dietary practices:* Some practice a Kosher diet, which requires food to be prepared in a Kosher kitchen; no pork or shellfish. *Healthcare:* May refuse to access healthcare on the Sabbath (from Friday at sundown to Saturday at sundown). *Death:* Remains are washed according to Jewish rite by members of a group called the Chevra Kadisha. This group of men and women prepare the body for burial and protect it until burial occurs. Burial occurs as soon as possible after death. |

Adapted from Carson, V.B. (1989). *Spiritual dimensions of nursing practice* (pp. 100–102). Philadelphia: Saunders; Betz, C.L., Hunsberger, M., & Wright, S. (1994). *Family-centered nursing care of children* (2nd ed., pp. 2230–2236). Philadelphia: Saunders; Graham, L., & Cates, J. (2006). Health care and sequestered cultures: A perspective from the old order Amish. *Journal of Nursing and Health, 12*(3), 60–66; Spector, R.E. (2012). *Cultural diversity in health and illness* (8th ed.). Upper Saddle River, NJ: Prentice-Hall; Davis, L., & Owens, C. (2013). *The impact of religion on health practices.* Retrieved from http://www.aacp.org.

## Implications of Cultural Diversity for Nurses

Many immigrants and refugees are relatively young, so nurses in most localities will provide care for families in culturally diverse circumstances. To provide effective care, nurses must be aware that culture is among the most significant factors that influence parenthood, health and illness, and aging. Nurses also need to be aware that there may be a dissonance in cultural beliefs and practices among generations, as the process of assimilation into a host environment occurs (Park, Chesla, Rehm, & Chun, 2011). Many healthcare workers' knowledge of other cultures and how to care for children and families in a culturally sensitive manner is limited (Johnson, Radesky, & Zuckerman, 2013). The following discussion summarizes the characteristics of family roles, healthcare beliefs and practices, and communication styles of some cultural groups. These descriptions are merely generalizations. Each family is unique and should be assessed and evaluated individually.

## Western Cultural Beliefs

Nursing practice in the United States is based largely on Western beliefs. Nurses need to recognize that these beliefs may differ significantly from those of other societies and that the differences have the potential to cause a great deal of conflict.

Leininger (1978) identified the following seven dominant Western cultural values; these values continue to greatly influence the thinking and action of nurses in the United States but may not be shared by their patients and families:

1. *Democracy* is a cultural value not shared by families who believe that elders or other higher authorities in the group make decisions. Fatalism, or a belief that events and results are predestined, may also affect healthcare decisions.
2. *Individualism* conflicts with the values of many cultural groups in which individual goals are subordinated to the greater good of the group.

3. *Cleanliness* is an American "obsession" viewed with amazement by many people of other cultures.
4. *Preoccupation with time,* which is measured by healthcare professionals in minutes and hours, is a major source of conflict with those who mark time by different standards, such as seasons or body needs.
5. *Reliance on machines and equipment* may intimidate families who are not comfortable with technology.
6. *The belief that optimal health is a right* is in direct conflict with beliefs in many cultures in the world in which health is not a major emphasis or even an expectation.
7. *Admiration of self-sufficiency and financial success* may conflict with the beliefs of other societies that place less value on wealth and more value on less tangible things such as spirituality.

Although Leininger recommended that nurses become culturally competent in care, newer views address the concept of cultural safety in care (Bearskin, 2011; Ulrich & Kear, 2014). In the practice of cultural safety, the nurse understands that the perspective of the patient and family, not the nurse, is central and forms the basis for the caring approach (Ulrich & Kear, 2014). In addition, if cultural beliefs and traditions in some way prevent access to or provision of optimal quality care, the available care is considered to be unsafe (Ramsden as cited in Bearskin, 2011). This approach demands a bidirectional and respectful sharing of cultural beliefs to enhance understanding and culturally appropriate care (Park et al., 2011). Additionally, it is the nurse's responsibility to recognize and address disparities in healthcare that are based on cultural perceptions, and to advocate for access to optimal healthcare for people of all cultures (American Academy of Pediatrics [AAP], 2013; Johnson et al., 2013).

## Cultural Influences on the Care of People From Specific Groups

To provide the best care for all patients, the nurse should know common cultural beliefs and practices that influence nursing care. Because communication is an essential component of nursing assessment and teaching, the nurse must understand cultural influences that may form barriers to communicating with people from another culture.

### Asians and Pacific Islanders

"Asian" refers to populations with origins in the Far East, Southeast Asia, and the Indian subcontinent, including Vietnam, China, Japan, and the Philippines. "Pacific Islander" refers to the original peoples of Hawaii, Guam, Samoa, and other Pacific islands. Their roots are in their ethnic viewpoint as well as their country of origin. They are not a homogeneous group, and differ in language, culture, and length of residence in the United States. Asians and Pacific Islanders constitute 5.5% of the U.S. population (United States Bureau of the Census, 2013).

In the Asian culture, the family is highly valued and often consists of many generations that remain close to one another. The elders of the family are highly respected. Self-sufficiency and self-control are highly valued. Asian-Americans place a high value on "face," or honor, and may be unwilling to do anything that causes another to "lose face." When medication or therapy is recommended, they seldom say no. They may accept the prescription or medication sample but not take the medicine, or they may agree to undergo a procedure but not keep the appointment. Stoicism may make pain assessment difficult. Herbal medicines and practices such as acupressure and music therapy may play an important part in healing for people of this culture.

In addition to the national languages of Vietnam, Cambodia, and Laos, numerous languages are spoken within subgroups in each country. People from Southeast Asia speak softly and avoid prolonged eye contact, which they consider rude. Even people who have been in the United States for many years often do not feel competent in English. The nurse should avoid "yes" or "no" questions and have the woman, parent, or child demonstrate an understanding of any teaching (Galanti, 2015). Special focus on education related to prevention of obesity, diabetes, and hypertension is needed for Pacific Islanders, as these conditions occur at a much higher rate than in other populations. The nurse needs to keep in mind that the English language is not native to these people and an interpreter might be necessary for health teaching (CMS Health Disparities Program, 2015).

### Hispanics

Hispanics, also called *Latinos,* include those whose origins are Mexico, Central and South America, Cuba, and Puerto Rico. They are a very diverse group that is growing rapidly in the United States, accounting for 17.1% of the total population in 2013 (United States Bureau of the Census, 2013).

Men are usually the head of household and considered strong (macho). Women are the homemakers. Hispanics usually have a close extended family and place a high value on children. Family is valued above work and other aspects of life.

Hispanics tend to be polite and gracious in conversation. Preliminary social interaction is particularly important, and Hispanics may be insulted if a problem is addressed directly without time first being taken for "small talk." This practice is counter to the value of "getting to the point" for many whites in the United States and may cause frustration for the patient as well as the healthcare worker.

Religion and health are strongly associated. The *curandero,* a folk healer, may be consulted for healthcare before an American healthcare worker is consulted. Hispanics have great respect for healthcare providers.

### African-Americans

African-Americans constitute 13.2% of the U.S. population (United States Bureau of the Census, 2013). African-Americans are often part of a close extended family, although many heads of household are single women. They have a sense of loyalty to their people and community, but sometimes distrust the majority group.

However, not all black people in the United States were born in this country. Natives of Africa and other countries are often found in both healthcare provider and patient populations within the United States.

The African-American minister is highly influential, and religious rituals, such as prayer, are frequently used. Illness may be seen as the will of God.

### American Indians and Alaska Natives

The terms *American Indian* and *Alaska Native* refer to people who have origins in any of the original peoples of North and South America and who maintain tribal affiliation or community attachment. This group makes up 0.12% of the total U.S. population (United States Bureau of the Census, 2013). Many who consider themselves Native Americans are of mixed race. The largest American Indian tribal groups are Cherokee, Navajo, Latin American Indian, Sioux, Chippewa, and Choctaw. The largest tribe among Alaska Natives are the Yupik (United States Census Bureau, 2011).

Native Americans may consider a willful child to be strong and a docile child to be weak. They have close family relationships, and respect for their elders is the norm. Although each American Indian nation or tribe has its own belief system regarding health, the overall traditional belief is that health reflects living in total harmony with nature, and disease is associated with the religious aspect of society, because supernatural powers are associated with the causing and curing of disease (Spector, 2012). Native Americans may highly respect a medicine man, whom they believe to be given power by supernatural forces. The use of herbs and rituals is part of the medicine man's curative practice.

#### Middle Easterners

Middle Eastern immigrants come from several countries, including Lebanon, Syria, Saudi Arabia, Egypt, Turkey, Iran, and Palestine. Islam is the dominant, and often the official, religion in these countries; its followers are known as *Muslims.* The man is typically the head of the household in Muslim families. Islam requires believers to kneel and pray five times a day, at dawn, noon, during the afternoon, after sunset, and after nightfall. Muslims do not eat pork or other meat not prepared according to Islamic law and do not use alcohol. Many are vegetarians. Other dietary standards vary according to the branch of Islam and may include standards such as how the acceptable animal is slaughtered for food.

Muslim women often prefer a female healthcare provider because of laws of modesty. Many Muslim women cover the head, arms to the wrists, and legs to the ankles, although there are many variations in the acceptable degree of coverage. Ritual cleansing before leaving the home or hospital room may be required before the woman dresses in her required modest apparel.

Communication in these countries is elaborate, and obtaining health information may be difficult because Islam dictates that family affairs be kept within the family. Personal information is shared only with friends, and the health assessment must be done gradually. When interpreters are used, they should be of the same country and religion, if possible, because of regional differences and hostilities. Because Islamic society tends to be paternalistic, asking the husband's permission or opinion when family members need healthcare is helpful.

### Cross-Cultural Health Beliefs

More than 100 different ethnocultural groups reside in the United States, and numerous traditional health beliefs are observed among these groups. For example, definitions of health are often culturally based. People of Asian origin may view health as the balance of yin and yang. Those of African or Haitian origin may define health as harmony with nature. Those from Mexico, Central and South America, and Puerto Rico often see health as a balance of hot and cold.

#### Traditional Methods of Preventing Illness

The traditional methods of preventing illness rest in a person's ability to understand the cause of a given illness in his or her culture. These causes may include the following:

- Agents such as hexes, spells, and the evil eye, which may strike a person (often a child) and cause injury, illness, or misfortune
- Phenomena such as soul loss and accidental provocation of envy, jealousy, or hate of a friend or acquaintance
- Environmental factors such as bad air, and natural events such as a solar eclipse

Practices to prevent illness have developed from beliefs about its cause. People must avoid those known to transmit hexes and spells. Elaborate methods are used to prevent inciting envy or jealousy of others and to avoid the evil eye. Protective or religious objects, such as amulets with magic powers or consecrated religious objects (talismans), are frequently worn or carried to prevent illness. Numerous food taboos and traditional combinations are prescribed in traditional belief systems to prevent illness. For example, people from many ethnic backgrounds eat raw garlic to prevent illness.

#### Traditional Practices to Maintain Health

Various traditional practices are used to maintain health. Mental and spiritual health is maintained by activities such as silence, meditation, and prayer. Many people view illness as punishment for breaking a religious code and adhere strictly to religious morals and practices to maintain health.

#### Traditional Practices to Restore Health

Traditional practices to restore health sometimes conflict with Western medical practice. Some of the most common practices include the use of natural substances, such as herbs and plants, to treat illness. Religious charms, holy words, or traditional healers may be tried before an individual seeks a medical opinion. Wearing religious medals, carrying prayer cards, and performing sacrifices are other practices used to treat illness.

Homeopathic care, often referred to as "complementary medicine" or "alternative medicine," is becoming more common in healthcare settings. Acupuncture, massage therapy, and chiropractic medicine are examples of homeopathic care (Spector, 2012).

Various substances may be ingested for the treatment of illnesses. The nurse should try to identify what the child or adult is taking and determine whether the active ingredient may alter the effects of prescribed medication.

Practices such as *dermabrasion,* the rubbing or irritation of the skin to relieve discomfort, are common among people of some cultures. The most frequently seen form is *coining,* in which an area is covered with an ointment, and the edge of a coin is rubbed over the area. All dermabrasion methods leave marks resembling bruises or burns on the skin and may be mistaken for signs of physical abuse.

***Cultural assessment.*** All healthcare professionals must develop skill in performing a cultural assessment so they can understand the meanings of health and illness to the cultural groups they encounter (AAP, 2013). When assessing a woman, child, or family from a cultural perspective, the nurse considers the following:

- Ethnic affiliation
- Major values, practices, customs, and beliefs related to pregnancy and birth, parenting, and aging
- Language barriers and communication styles
- Family, newborn, and child-rearing practices
- Religious and spiritual beliefs; changes or exemptions during illness, pregnancy, or after birth
- Nutrition and food patterns
- Ethnic healthcare practices, such as how time is marked, rituals to restore health or ease passage to the afterlife for a dying patient, and other views of life and death
- Health promotion practices
- How healthcare professionals can be most helpful

After such an assessment, plans for care should show respect for cultural differences and traditional healing practices. A guiding principle for nurses should be one of acceptance of nontraditional methods of healthcare as long as the practice does not cause harm. In some instances, cultural practices may actually cause unintentional harm; in these circumstances the nurse may need to consult other professionals familiar with the particular cultural practice to provide appropriate care and information for the family. Additional cultural information is presented throughout this book relating to specific areas in maternal and child healthcare.

## PARENTING

Parenting implies the commitment of an individual or individuals to provide for the physical and psychosocial needs of a child. Many believe that parenting is the most difficult and yet rewarding experience an individual can have. Many parents assume this important job with little education in parenting or child rearing. If the parents themselves have had parents that are positive role models, and if they seek appropriate resources for parenting, the transition to parenting is easier. Nurses are in a good position to provide parents with information on effective parenting skills through many venues, such as formal classes, anticipatory guidance at well-child checkups, and role modeling.

## Parenting Styles

Baumrind (1991) described three major parenting styles; these have been generally accepted by experts in child and family development. These include authoritarian, authoritative, and permissive. *Parenting style,* which is the general climate in which a parent socializes a child, differs from *parenting practices,* the specific behavioral guidance parents offer children across the age span. Although the characteristics of parenting styles are described in their general categories, many specialists in child development acknowledge that characteristics of several parenting styles may be present in parents. In addition, researchers recognize that parenting styles may work in different ways in different cultures.

*Authoritarian* parents have rules. They expect obedience from the child without any questioning about the reasons behind the rule. They also expect the child to accept the family beliefs and principles without question. Give and take is discouraged.

Children raised with this style of parenting can be shy and withdrawn because of a lack of self-confidence. If the parents are somewhat affectionate, the child may be sensitive, submissive, honest, and dependable. However, if affection has been withheld, the child may exhibit rebellious, antisocial behavior.

*Authoritative* parents tend to show respect for the opinions of each of their children by allowing them to be different. Although the household has rules, the parents permit discussion if the children do not understand or agree with the rules. The parents emphasize that even though they (the parents) are the ultimate authority, some negotiation and compromise may take place. This style of parenting tends to result in children who have high self-esteem and are independent, inquisitive, happy, assertive, and highly interactive.

*Permissive* parents have little or no control over the behavior of their children. If any rules exist in the home, they are inconsistent and unclear. Underlying reasons for rules may be given, but the children are generally allowed to decide whether they will follow the rules and to what extent. Limits are not set, and discipline is inconsistent. The children learn that they can get away with any behavior. Role reversal occurs: the children are more like the parents, and the parents are like the children.

Children who come from this type of home are typically disrespectful, disobedient, aggressive, irresponsible, and defiant. They tend to be insecure because of a lack of guidelines to direct their behavior. They are searching for true limits but not finding them. These children also tend to be creative and spontaneous.

Regardless of the primary parenting style, parenting is more effective when parents are able to adjust their parenting techniques according to each child's developmental level and when parents are involved and interested in their children's activities and friends.

## Parent–Child Relationship Factors

Relationships between parents and children are bidirectional, with the parents' behavior affecting the child and the child's behavior affecting the parenting. The parents' age, experience, and self-confidence affect the quality of the parent–child relationship, the stability of the marital relationship, and the interplay between the child's individualism and the parents' expectations of the child.

### Parental Characteristics

Parenting is multidimensional. Parenting goals include nurturing; facilitating the development of autonomy and self-sufficiency; providing comfort and support; conveying family knowledge, traditions, and values; socializing; and instilling confidence, among others. Parent personality type, personal history of parenting as a child, abilities and competencies, parental skills and expectations, personal health, quality of marital relationship, and relationship quality with others all play a part in determining how a person parents. Parenting behaviors that promote the development of social-emotional, cognitive, and language development include warmth, support, and vigilance without overprotection (Achtergarde, Postert, Wessing, Romer, & Muller, 2015).

In addition, parents who have had previous experience with children, whether through younger siblings, a career, or raising other children, bring an element of experience to the art of parenting. Self-confidence and age also can be factors in a person's ability to parent. How an individual was parented has a major effect on how he or she will assume the role. The strength of the parents' relationship also affects their parenting skills, as does the presence or absence of support systems. Support can come from the family or community. Peer groups can provide an arena for parents to share experiences and solve problems. Parents with more experience are often an important resource for new parents.

### Characteristics of the Child

Characteristics that may affect the parent-child relationship include the child's physical appearance, sex, and temperament. At birth, the infant's physical appearance may not meet the parents' expectations, or the infant may resemble a disliked relative. As a result, the parent may subconsciously reject the child. If the parents desired a baby of a particular sex, they may be disappointed or the disappointment may continue if the child's sex was identified during pregnancy. If parents are not given the opportunity to talk about this disappointment, they may reject the infant.

### Temperament and Parental Expectations

*Temperament* can be described as the way individuals behave or their behavioral style. Several researchers have studied temperament. Chess and Thomas (1996) developed the following three temperament categories, which are based on nine characteristics of temperament they identified in children (Box 3.2).

1. *Easy:* These children are even tempered, predictable, and regular in their habits. They react positively to new stimuli.
2. *Difficult:* These children are highly active, irritable, moody, and irregular in their habits. They adapt slowly to new stimuli and often express intense negative emotions.
3. *Slow to warm up:* These children are inactive, moody, and moderately irregular in their habits. They adapt slowly to new stimuli and express mildly intense negative emotions.

Some objection to the term *difficult* has been raised because it tends to have a negative connotation. However, that is the term established in temperament research, and parents should recognize that a "difficult" child is quite normal. As is true for other characteristics, such as appearance, the parent–child relationship is likely to have less conflict if the child's temperament meets the parents' expectations.

# DISCIPLINE

Children's behavior challenges most parents. The manner in which parents respond to a child's behavior has a profound effect on the

**BOX 3.2 Characteristics of Temperament in Children**

1. *Level of activity:* The intensity and frequency of motion during playing, eating, bathing, dressing, or sleeping
2. *Rhythmicity:* Regularity of biologic functions (e.g., sleep patterns, eating patterns, elimination patterns)
3. *Approach/withdrawal:* The initial response of a child to a new stimulus, such as an unfamiliar person, unfamiliar food, or new toys
4. *Adaptability:* Ease or difficulty in adjustment to a new stimulus
5. *Intensity of response:* The amount of energy with which the child responds to a new stimulus
6. *Threshold of responsiveness:* The amount or intensity of stimulation necessary to evoke a response
7. *Mood:* Frequency of cheerfulness, pleasantness, and friendly behavior versus unhappiness, unpleasantness, and unfriendly behavior
8. *Distractibility:* How easily the child's attention can be diverted from an activity by external stimuli
9. *Attention span/persistence:* How long the child pursues an activity and continues despite frustration and obstacles

Adapted from Chess, S., & Thomas, A. (1996). *Temperament: Theory and practice.* New York: Brunner-Mazel.

child's self-esteem and future interactions with others. Children learn to view themselves in the same way that the parent views them. Thus, if parents view their children as wild, the children begin to view themselves as wild, and soon their actions consistently reinforce their self-image. In this way, the children will not disappoint the parents. This pattern is called a *self-fulfilling prophecy* and is a cyclic process.

Discipline is designed to teach a child how to function effectively within society. It is the foundation for self-discipline. A parent's primary goal should be to help the child feel lovable and capable. This goal is best accomplished by the parent's setting limits to enhance a sense of security until the child can incorporate the family's values and is capable of self-discipline.

When a child is in the healthcare system, the nurse has the opportunity to aid in the socialization of the child to some degree. Although teaching principles of discipline are likely not practical when a child is ill or in the hospital, nurses can actively work with parents during well child visits. Through both formal instruction and informal role modeling, the nurse can help the parent learn how to discipline a child effectively. Box 3.3 lists ways in which a parent or nurse can facilitate children's socialization and increase their self-esteem.

**BOX 3.3 Effective Discipline for Positive Socialization and Self-Esteem**

- Attend promptly to an infant's and young child's needs.
- Provide structure and consistency for young children.
- Give positive attention for positive behavior; use praise when deserved.
- Listen.
- Set aside time every day for one-on-one attention.
- Demonstrate appreciation of the child's unique characteristics.
- Encourage choices and decision making, and allow the child to experience consequences of mistakes.
- Model respect for others.
- Provide unconditional love.

## Dealing With Misbehavior

A child's *misbehavior* may be defined as behavior outside the norms of acceptance within the family. Misbehavior stretches the limits of tolerance in all parents, even the most patient. A parent's response to the child's misbehavior can have minor consequences, such as short-term frustration, or major consequences such as child abuse. To prevent these negative consequences, the nurse can help teach parents various strategies for effective discipline. Whenever disciplinary strategies are used, the parent needs to consider the individual child's developmental level. In addition, discipline should be consistent, the parent should not "give in" to manipulation or tantrums, and the child's feelings should be acknowledged (AAP, 2011). The following are three essential components of effective discipline (AAP, 1998/2014):

1. Maintaining a positive, supportive, loving relationship between the parents and the child
2. Using positive reinforcement and encouragement to promote cooperation and desired behaviors
3. Removing reinforcement or applying punishment to reduce or eliminate undesired behaviors

Punishment is used to eliminate a behavior and can be in the form of a verbal reprimand or physical action to emphasize a point. The AAP discourages the use of spanking and other forms of physical punishment (AAP, 2011).

### Redirection

Redirection is a simple and effective method in which the parent removes the problem and distracts the child with an alternative activity or object. This method is helpful with infants through preadolescents.

### Reasoning

Reasoning involves explaining why a behavior is not permitted. Younger children lack the cognitive skills and developmental abilities to comprehend reasoning fully. For example, a 4-year-old may better understand the consequence that he will have to spend time in his room if he breaks his brother's toy than the concept of respecting the property of others.

When this technique is used with older children, the behavior should be the object of focus, not the child. The child should not be made to feel guilt and shame, because these feelings are counterproductive and can damage the child's self-esteem. The parent can focus on the behavior most effectively by using "I" rather than "you" messages.

A "you" message criticizes children and uses guilt in an attempt to get them to change their behavior. An example of a "you" message is "Don't take your little sister's toys away and make her cry. You're being a bad boy!" By contrast, an "I" message focuses on the misbehavior by explaining its effect on others. An example of an "I" message is, "Your little sister cries when you take her toys away because she doesn't know that you will give them back to her."

### Time-Out

Time-out is a method of removing the attention given to a child who is misbehaving. It involves placing the child in a nonstimulating environment where the parent can observe unobtrusively. For example, a chair could be placed facing a wall in a hall or nearby room. The child is told to sit on the chair for a predetermined time, usually 1 minute per year of age. If the child cries or fights, the timing is not begun until the child is quiet. The use of a kitchen timer with a bell is effective because the child knows when the time begins and when it has elapsed and the child can get up. After the child has calmed and the time is completed, discussion of the behavior that prompted the time-out at a level appropriate to the child's age may be helpful.

### Consequences

The consequences technique helps children learn the direct result of their misbehavior and can be used with toddlers through adolescents. If children must deal with the consequences of their behavior and the consequences are meaningful to them, they are less likely to repeat the behavior. Consequences fall into the following three categories:

1. *Natural:* Consequences that occur spontaneously. For example, a child loses a favorite toy after leaving it outside, and the parent does not replace it.
2. *Logical:* Consequences that are directly related to the misbehavior. For example, when two children are fighting over a toy, the parent removes the toy from both of them for a day.
3. *Unrelated:* Consequences that are purposely imposed. For example, a child comes in late for dinner and, as a consequence, is not allowed to watch TV that evening.

Some parents have difficulty allowing their children to face the consequences of their actions. When parents choose to deny their child this experience, the parent loses an important opportunity to teach responsibility for one's actions.

### Behavior Modification

The behavior modification technique of discipline rewards positive behavior and ignores negative behavior. This technique requires parents to choose selected behaviors, preferably only one at a time, that they desire to stop. They choose others that they want to encourage. The basic technique is useful for any age from toddlerhood through adolescence. For a young child, the selected positive behaviors are marked on a chart and explained to the child. For an older child, a contract can be written. The negative behaviors are kept in mind by the parents but are not recorded where the child can see them. A system of rewards is established. Stickers or stars on a chart for young children and tokens for older children are effective ways to record the behaviors. Children should receive a predetermined reward (e.g., a movie, book, or outing, but not food) after they successfully perform the behavior a set number of times. This system should continue for several months until the behavior becomes a habit for the child. Then the external reward should be gradually withdrawn. The child develops internal gratification for successful behavior rather than relying on external reinforcement. Children gain a sense of mastery and actually enjoy the process, often viewing it as a game.

**SAFETY ALERT**

***Avoiding the Use of Corporal Punishment as Discipline***

Corporal punishment can lead to child abuse if the disciplinarian loses control. It can also lead to false accusations of child abuse by either the child or other adults. Because of the high cost and low benefit of this form of punishment, parents should avoid its use.

Negative behaviors are simply ignored. If the parent refuses to give the child attention for the behavior, the child soon gives up that strategy. Consistency is the key to success for this technique, and many parents find this method difficult to enforce. Parents need to be warned that children frequently test the seriousness of this attempt by increasing their negative behavior soon after the parents begin ignoring it. If this technique is to be successful, the parents need to ignore the negative behavior every time.

### Corporal Punishment

Corporal punishment usually takes the form of spanking. It is highly controversial and should be discouraged. Corporal punishment has many undesirable results, which include physical aggression toward others and the belief that causing pain to others is acceptable (AAP, 2015). Adults who were spanked as children are more likely than those who were not spanked to experience depression, use substances, and commit domestic violence (AAP, 2015). Use of spanking as discipline can result in loss of control and child injury.

Because of the negative consequences of spanking and because it is no more effective than other methods of discipline, the AAP (2015) recommends that parents be encouraged and helped to develop methods of discipline other than spanking.

## NURSING PROCESS AND THE FAMILY

### Family Assessment

When assessing family health, the nurse first must determine the structure of the family. The structure is the actual physical composition of the family, the family's environment, and the occupations and education of its members. Diagrams can assist with this process. A *genogram,* (see Table 10.1) also known as a *pedigree,* which illustrates family relationships and health issues, looks like a family tree with three generations of family members represented. An *ecomap* is a pictorial representation of the family structure and relationships with factors in the external environment.

Next the nurse needs to determine how well the family is fulfilling its five major functions as described by Friedman et al. (2003):

1. *Affective function (personality maintenance function):* to meet the psychological needs of family members—trust, nurturing, intimacy, belonging, bonding, identity, separateness and connectedness, need–response patterns, and the therapeutic role of the individuals in the family.
2. *Socialization function (social placement):* to guide children to be productive members of society and transmit cultural beliefs to the next generation.
3. *Reproductive function:* to ensure family continuity and societal survival.
4. *Economic function:* to provide and effectively allocate economic resources.
5. *Healthcare function:* to provide the physical necessities of life (e.g., food, clothing, shelter, healthcare), to recognize illness in family members and provide care, and to foster a healthy lifestyle or environment based on preventive medical and dental health practices.

Health problems can arise from structural problems, such as too few or too many people sharing the same living quarters. If too few people are present, children may be left unattended; too many people may lead to overcrowding, stress, and the spread of communicable diseases. Environmental problems include impure drinking water, inadequate sewage facilities, damaged electric wiring and outlets, and inadequate sleeping conditions. Other environmental factors, such as rodents, crime, and noise, can affect health. Occupation and education can affect health through lack of adequate supervision of children; inability to purchase physical necessities, such as food; inability to purchase health insurance; and stress from employment dissatisfaction.

### Nursing Diagnosis and Planning

After using the various tools to assess the child's family completely, the nurse identifies the appropriate nursing diagnoses. These will differ according to the specific family assessment data. The following general nursing diagnoses can be used for families:

- Risk for Caregiver Role Strain
- Compromised Family Coping
- Interrupted Family Processes
- Impaired Parenting
- Risk for Impaired Parent-Infant Attachment
- Ineffective Family Therapeutic Regimen Management
- Social Isolation

Other diagnoses may also be appropriate. The expected outcomes for each diagnosis would be specifically tailored to the family's needs.

### Intervention and Evaluation

Interventions also are specific for the child and family, but most family interventions are directed toward enhancing positive coping strategies and directing the family to appropriate resources. The nurse adapts general family interventions to each family's unique needs but in particular helps the family to do the following:

- Identify and mobilize internal and external strengths
- Access appropriate resources in the extended family and community
- Recognize and enhance positive communication patterns
- Decide on a consistent discipline approach and access parenting programs if needed
- Maintain comforting cultural and religious traditions and sources of healing
- Engage in joint problem solving
- Acquire new knowledge by providing information about a specific health problem or issue
- Become empowered
- Allocate sufficient privacy, space, and time for leisure activities
- Promote health for all family members during times of crisis

Once families have participated in needed intervention, evaluation criteria are tailored to the specific intervention and individualized for the family.

### CRITICAL THINKING EXERCISE 3.1

Create a genogram of your family. Can you identify health issues and trends from looking at the genogram? What are the implications for nursing care?

## KEY CONCEPTS

- Traditional families may be single-income or dual-income families. Two-income families are much more common at present.
- Nontraditional family structures (single-parent, blended, adoptive, multigenerational [extended], and same-sex parent families) may require nursing care that differs from that required by traditional families.
- High-risk families have additional stressors that affect their functioning. Examples are families headed by adolescents, families affected by marital discord or divorce, violence, or substance abuse, and families with a severely or chronically ill member.
- All families experience stress; how the family deals with stress is the important factor.
- Identifying healthy versus dysfunctional family patterns can help the nurse implement effective strategies to care for the child and the family.
- During health and illness, women, children, and families are cared for within the framework of their families and their cultures.
- Traditional cultural beliefs may be used to prevent illness, maintain health, and restore health.
- Differing cultural beliefs and expectations between the healthcare provider and the family can create conflict.
- The nurse can help parents learn effective discipline methods by teaching and role modeling.
- Assessing the structure and function of the family is a basic part of caring for any child.

## REFERENCES AND READINGS

Achtergarde, S., Postert, C., Wessing, I., Romer, G., & Muller, J. (2015). Parenting and child mental health: Influences of parent personality, child temperament, and their interaction. *The Family Journal: Counseling Therapy for Couples and Family, 23*(2), 167–179.

American Academy of Pediatrics. (2011). *Disciplining your child*. Retrieved from http://www.healthychildren.org.

American Academy of Pediatrics. (2013).Policy statement: Enhancing pediatric workforce diversity and providing culturally effective pediatric care: Implications for practice, education, and policy making. *Pediatrics, 132*(4), e1105–e1116.

American Academy of Pediatrics. (2015). *Where we stand: Spanking*. Retrieved from http://www.healthychildren.org.

American Academy of Pediatrics Committee on Hospital Care. (2012). Family-centered care and the pediatrician's role. *Pediatrics, 129*(2), 394–404.

American Academy of Pediatrics Committee on Psychosocial Aspects of Child and Family Health. (1998). Guidance for effective discipline. *Pediatrics, 101*(4), 723–728, Policy reaffirmed in 2014.

Baumrind, D. (1991). Effective parenting during the early adolescent transition. In P. Cowan, & M. Hetherington (Eds.), *Family transitions* Hillsdale, NJ: Lawrence Erlbaum.

Bearskin, L.B. (2011). A critical lens on culture in nursing practice. *Nursing Ethics, 18*(4), 548–559.

Bureau of Justice Statistics. (2014). *National crime victimization survey*. Retrieved from http://www.bjs.gov.

Chess, S., & Thomas, A. (1996). *Temperament theory and practice*. New York: Brunner-Mazel.

Christian Science. (2011). *About Christian Science: Core beliefs*. Retrieved from http://www.christianscience.com.

CMS Health Disparities Program. (2015). *Native Hawaiians and Pacific Islanders*. Retrieved from http://www.cmspulse.org.

Davis, L., & Qwens, C. (2013). *The impact of religion on health practices*. Retrieved from http://www.aacp.org.

Dokken, D., Parent, K., & Ahmann, E. (2015). Family presence and participation: Pediatrics leading the way…and still evolving. *Pediatric Nursing, 41*(4), 204–206.

Federal Interagency Forum on Child and Family Statistics. (2015). *America's children: Key national indicators of well-being, 2015*. Washington, DC: U.S. Government Printing Office.

Friedman, M.M., Bowden, V.R., & Jones, E.G. (2003). *Family nursing: Theory, research and practice* (5th ed., pp. 593–594). Upper Saddle River, NJ: Prentice-Hall.

Galanti, G.A. (2015). *Caring for patients from different cultures.* (5th ed.). Philadelphia: University of Pennsylvania Press.

Harrison, T.M. (2010). Family-centered pediatric nursing care: State of the science. *Journal of Pediatric Nursing, 25,* 335–343.

Harvey, P. & Ahmann, E. (2014). Validation: a family-centered communication skill. *Pediatric Nursing, 40*(3), 143–147.

Johnson, L., Radesky, J., & Zuckerman, B. (2013). Cross-cultural parenting: Reflections on autonomy and interdependence. *Pediatrics, 131*(4), 631–633.

Kelly, R., & El-Sheikh, M. (2011). Marital conflict and children's sleep. *Journal of Family Psychology, 25*(3), 412–422.

Leininger, M. (1978). *Transcultural nursing: Concepts, theories, practices.* New York: Wiley.

Lindahl, L., & Malik, N. (2011). Marital conflict typology and children's appraisals: The moderating role of family cohesion. *Journal of Family Psychology, 25*(2), 194–201.

Martin, J.A., Hamilton, B.E., Osterman, J.K., Curtin, S.C. & Mathews, J. (2015). Births: Final Data for 2013. *National Vital Statistics Reports, 64*(1), Hyattsville, MD: Author.

National Association for Children of Alcoholics Foundation. (2012). *Healthy children and adolescents in families affected by substance abuse.* Retrieved from http://www.coaf.org.

National Center for Health Statistics. (2012). *Data Brief: Birth rates for U.S. teenagers reach historic lows for all age and ethnic groups.* Retrieved from http://www.cdc.gov/nchs/data/databriefs/db89.htm.

Park, M., Chesla, C., Rehm, R., & Chun, K.M. (2011). Working with culture: Culturally appropriate mental health care for Asian Americans. *Journal of Advanced Nursing, 67*(11), 2373–2382.

Schlucter, J. (2014). Patient-and family-centered transitions from pediatric to adult care. *Pediatric Nursing, 40*(6), 307–310.

Smith, C.M. (2013). A family perspective in community/public health nursing. In F. Maurer, & C. Smith (Eds.), *Community/public health nursing practice: Health for families and populations* (5th ed., pp. 335–337). St. Louis: Elsevier Saunders.

Smith, S.R., & Hamon, R.R. (2012). *Exploring family theories.* (3rd ed.). New York: Oxford University Press.

Spector, R.E. (2012). *Cultural diversity in health and illness* (8th ed.). Upper Saddle River, NJ: Prentice-Hall.

Tallon, M., Kendall, G., & Snider, P. (2015). Rethinking family-centred care for the child and family in hospital. *Journal of Clinical Nursing, 24,* 1426–1435.

Ulrich, B., & Kear, T. (2014). Patient safety and patient safety culture: Foundations of excellent health care delivery. *Nephrology Nursing Journal, 41*(5), 447–457.

United States Census Bureau. (2011). *2010 Census Briefs.* Retrieved from http://www.census.gov/prod/cen2010/briefs/c2010br-01.pdf.

United States Bureau of the Census. (2013). *Population Estimates Program (PEP).* Retrieved from http://www.census.gov.

Ventura, M.A., & Hamilton, B.E. (2011). *U.S. teenage birth rate resumes decline.* Retrieved from. : Centers for Disease Control and Prevention. NCHS Data Brief, Retrieved from http://www.cdc.gov/nchs/data/databriefs/db58.pdf

# 4

# Communicating With Children and Families

http://evolve.elsevier.com/McKinney/mat-ch/

## LEARNING OBJECTIVES

*After studying this chapter, you should be able to:*

- Describe the components of effective communication with children.
- Describe communication strategies that assist nurses in effectively working with children.
- Explain the importance of avoiding communication pitfalls in working with children.
- Describe effective family-centered communication strategies.
- Describe effective strategies for communicating with children with special needs. Describe warning signs of over and under involvement in child/family relationships.

To effectively work with children and their families, nurses need to develop keen communication skills. Because parents and other family members play a crucial role in the lives of children, nurses need to establish rapport with the family to identify mutual goals and facilitate positive outcomes. An awareness of body language, eye contact, and tone of voice must accompany good verbal communication skills when one is listening to children and their families. The same awareness helps nurses assess their own communication styles.

## COMPONENTS OF EFFECTIVE COMMUNICATION

Communication is much more than words going from one person's mouth to another person's ears. In addition to the words themselves, the tone and quality of voice, eye contact, physical proximity, visual cues, and overall body language convey messages. These nonverbal communications are often undervalued, yet comprise a significant portion of total communication. In choosing communication techniques to be used with children and families, the nurse considers cultural differences, particularly with regard to touch and personal space (see Chapter 3). Effective communication provides an important link between parents and providers that is based on honesty, caring, respect, and a direct approach (Fisher & Broome, 2011). It serves to ease stressful experiences for children and families, provide required information for the child's acute or preventive care, and it facilitates appropriate transitions from the hospital to home. Effective communication can empower children in situations where children are experiencing a loss of control and diminished autonomy (Lambert & McCarron, 2011; Livesley & Long, 2013).

### Touch

Touch can be a positive, supportive technique that is effective from birth through adulthood. Touch can convey warmth, comfort, reassurance, security, trust, caring, and support.

In infancy, the messages of love, security, and comfort are conveyed through holding, cuddling, gentle stroking, and patting. Infants do not have cognitive understanding of the words they hear, but they sense the emotional support, and they can feel, interpret, and respond to gentle, loving, supportive hands caring for them. Toddlers and preschoolers find it soothing and comforting to be held and rocked as well as gently stroked on the head, back, arms, and legs (Fig. 4.1).

School-age children and adolescents appreciate giving and receiving hugs and getting a reassuring pat on the back or a gentle hand on the hand. However, the nurse needs to request permission for any contact beyond a casual touch with these children.

### Physical Proximity and Environment

Children's familiarity and comfort with their physical surroundings affect communication. Normally, children are most at ease in their home environments. Once they enter a clinic, emergency department, or patient care unit, they are in an unfamiliar environment, and they experience increased anxiety. Hospital and clinic staff members have a tremendous advantage in knowing their clinic or unit as a familiar workplace. Nurses can gain a better picture of what a child is experiencing by trying to place themselves in the child's position and imagining the child's first impression of the triage desk, reception desk, admitting office, treatment room, and hospital room. A child's perspective is probably very different from an adult's. Creating a supportive, inviting environment for children includes the use of child-size furniture, colorful banners and posters, developmentally appropriate toys, and art displayed at a child's eye level.

Individuals have different comfort zones for physical distance. The nurse should be aware of differences and should cautiously move when meeting new children and families, respecting each individual's personal space. For example, standing over the child and family can be intimidating. Instead, the nurse should bring a chair and sit near the child and family. This action puts the nurse at eye level. If a chair is not accessible, the nurse may stoop or squat. The important part is to be at eye level while remaining at a comfortable distance for the child and family (Fig. 4.2).

The nurse should not overlook privacy or underestimate its importance. A room should be available for conducting private conversations away from roommates or family members and visitors. Privacy is particularly critical in working with adolescents, who typically will not discuss sensitive topics with parents present. The nurse's skill and ease

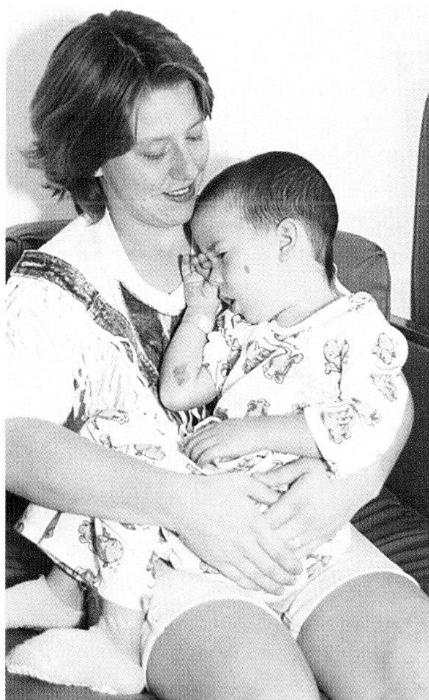

Touch is a powerful means of communicating. Toddlers and preschoolers often find touch in the form of cuddling and stroking to be soothing. Even older children who prize their independence find that a parent's hug or pat on the back helps them feel more secure.

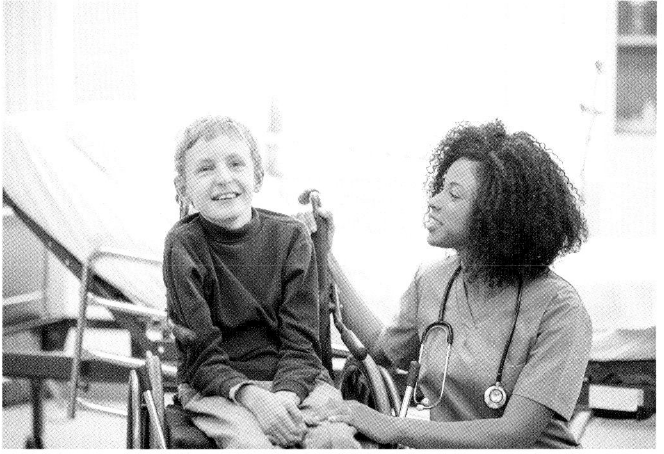

Communication with children is enhanced by touch and body language that conveys attentiveness and openness. (© 2016 Getty Images. All rights reserved.)

**FIG 4.1** Communication with children is enhanced by direct eye contact and by body language that conveys attentiveness and openness.

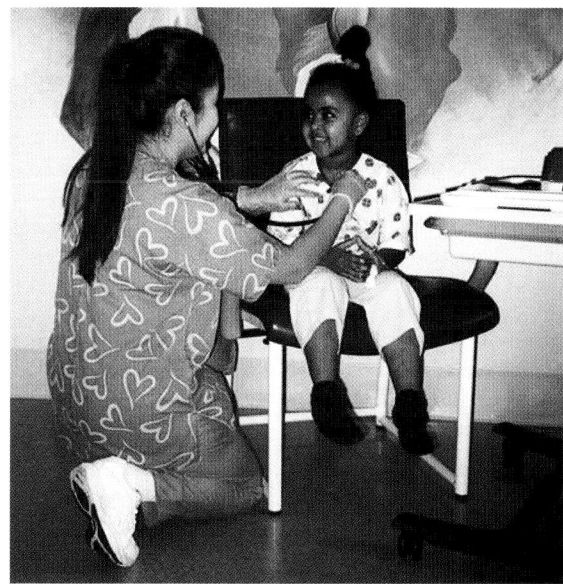

**FIG 4.2** For effective communication, the nurse needs to be at the child's eye level. (Courtesy Pat Spier, RN-C. In Leifer, G. [2011]. *Introduction to maternity & pediatric nursing.* [6th ed.]. St. Louis: Saunders.)

with parents of adolescents will increase the adolescents' trust in the nurse. Nurses need to avoid hallway conversations, particularly outside a child's room, because children and parents may overhear only some words or phrases and misinterpret the meaning. Overhearing may lead to unnecessary stress and mistrust between the healthcare providers and the child or family.

## Listening

Messages given must be received for communication to be complete. Therefore, listening is an essential component of the communication process. By practicing active listening skills, nurses can be effective listeners. Active listening skills are as follows:

### Attentiveness

The nurse should be intentional about giving the speaker undivided attention. Eliminating distractions whenever possible is important. For example, the nurse should maintain eye contact, close the room door, and eliminate potential distractions (e.g., television, computer, video games, smartphones, and tablets).

### Clarification Through Reflection

Using similar words, the nurse expresses to the speaker what was heard and understood about the content of the message. For example, when the child or family member says, "I hate the food that comes on my tray," a reflective response would be, "When you say you are unhappy with the food you've been given, what can we do to change that?" As the conversation progresses, the nurse can move the child through a dialogue that identifies those nutritional foods the child would eat.

### Empathy

The nurse identifies and acknowledges feelings expressed in the message. For example, if a child is crying after a procedure, the nurse might say, "I know it is uncomfortable to have this procedure. It is okay to cry. You did a great job holding still."

### Impartiality

To understand and avoid prejudicing what is heard with personal bias, the nurse listens with an open mind. For example, if a young adolescent shares that she is sexually active and is mainly concerned about sexually transmitted diseases, the nurse remains a supportive listener. The nurse can then provide her with educational materials and resources as well as discuss the possible outcomes of her actions in a manner that is open and not judgmental, regardless of the nurse's personal values and beliefs.

During shift handoff, descriptions of family must be shared objectively and impartially. Otherwise, perceptions of families may negatively affect how colleagues approach and interact with families.

To enhance the effectiveness of communication and maximize normal language patterns that contribute to language development, the nurse focuses on talking with children rather than to them and develops conversations with children.

The nurse needs to be prepared to listen with the eyes as well as the ears. Information will not always be audible, so the nurse must be alert to subtle cues in body language and physical closeness. Only then can one fully understand the messages of children. For example, when the nurse enters the room to complete an initial assessment of a 4-year-old child and observes the child turning away and beginning to suck her thumb, the child is communicating about her basic security and comfort level, although she has not said a word.

**! NURSING QUALITY ALERT**

***Tips to Enhance Listening and Communication Skills***

- Children understand more clearly than they can speak.
- To develop conversations with children, ask open-ended questions rather than questions requiring yes-or-no responses.
- Comprehension is increased when the nurse uses different methods to present and share information.
- Use "people-first" language (e.g., "Sally in 428 has cystic fibrosis" instead of "The CF patient in 428 is Sally").
- Encourage the child to be an active participant through creating a respectful listening environment where children can express concerns, ask questions, and participate in the development of a plan of care.

### Visual Communication

Eye contact is a communication connector. Making eye contact helps confirm attention and interest between the individuals communicating. For people in some cultures, direct eye contact may be uncomfortable; the nurse should be sensitive to responses when making eye contact.

Clothing, physical appearance, and objects being held are visual communicators. Children may react to an individual's presence on the basis of a white lab coat, a bushy beard, or a syringe or video game in the hand. The nurse needs to think ahead and anticipate visual stimuli a child may find startling and those that may be pleasing and to make appropriate adjustments when possible. For example, it is a routine practice for nurses to bring a medication in a syringe for insertion into an intravenous (IV) line. Unless the purpose of the syringe is immediately explained, children might quickly assume they are about to receive an injection.

Some children, and some adults, are visual learners. They learn best when they can see or read instructions, demonstrations, diagrams, or information. Using various methods of presenting and sharing information will increase comprehension for such children.

Concepts can be presented more vividly by using developmentally appropriate photographs, videos, dolls, computer programs, charts, or graphs than by using written or spoken words alone. The nurse needs to select teaching tools and materials that appropriately match the child's growth and developmental level.

### Tone of Voice

The spoken word comes to mind most often when communication is the topic. However, communication comprises not only what is said but also the way it is said. The tone and quality of voice often communicate more than the words themselves.

Because infants' cognitive understanding of words is limited, their understanding is based on tone and quality of voice. A soft, smooth voice is more comforting and soothing to infants than a loud, startling, harsh voice. Infants can sense from the tone of voice whether the caregiver is angry or happy, frustrated or calm. The nurse can assess how aware of and sensitive to these messages infants are by observing their body language. Infants are relaxed when they hear a calm, happy caregiver and tense and rigid when they hear an angry, frustrated caregiver.

Children can detect anger, frustration, joy, and other feelings that voices convey, even when the accompanying words are incongruent. This incongruity can be very confusing for children. The nurse should strive to make words and their intended meanings match.

Verbal communication extends beyond actual words. All audible sounds convey meaning. An infant's primary mode of audible communication is crying. Crying is a cue to check basic needs, including hunger, pain, discomfort (e.g., wet diaper), and temperature. Cooing and babbling, also heard during the first year of life, generally convey messages of comfort and contentment. As children develop and mature, they have larger vocabularies to express their ideas, thoughts, and feelings.

The choice of words is critical in verbal communication. The nurse needs to avoid talking down to children but should not expect them to understand adult words and phrases. Technical healthcare terms should be used selectively, and jargon should be avoided (see Table 4.4).

### Body Language

From the gentle caress of holding an infant to sitting and listening intently to an adolescent's story, body language is a factor in communication. An open body stance and positioning invite communication and interaction, whereas a closed body stance and positioning impede communication and interaction.

Using an open body posture improves the nurse's understanding of children and the children's understanding of the nurse. Nurses need to learn to read children's body language and should become more aware of their own body language. Table 4.1 compares open and closed body postures.

### Timing

Recognizing the appropriate time to communicate information is a developed skill. A distraught child whose parents have just left for work is not ready for a diabetes teaching session. The session will be much more productive and the information better understood if the child has a chance to make the transition. The convenience of meeting a schedule should be secondary to meeting a child's needs.

In the well or outpatient setting, scheduling teaching sessions that adapt to a parent's background and experiences, including work

**TABLE 4.1 Open and Closed Body Postures**

| Open | Closed |
|---|---|
| Leaning toward other person | Leaning away from other person |
| Arms loose at sides | Arms folded across chest |
| Frequent eye contact | No eye contact |
| Hands moving freely | Hands on hips |
| Soft stance, body swaying slightly | Rigid stance |
| Head up | Head bowed |
| Calm, slow movements | Constant motion, squirming |
| Smiling, friendly facial cues | Frowning, negative facial cues |
| Conversing at eye level | Conversing at a level that requires the child to move to listen |

schedule, can enhance child's or parent's understanding of information (Gallo, Campbell, Hoagwood, et al., 2016). For example, scheduling a teaching session during the late afternoon or early evening, or on a Saturday, at the parent's convenience assures increased attention because the parent is not distracted with needing to be at work or other demands on time.

## FAMILY-CENTERED COMMUNICATION

Any discussion about effective ways to communicate with children must also include a discussion of effective communication with families. Family-centered care emphasizes that the family is intimately involved in the care of the child. Parents need to be supported while sustaining their parental role during their child's hospitalization (Coyne, 2013). Family-centered care is achieved when healthcare professionals can create partnerships with families, recognizing that the family is essential to the child and that the family has the right to participate fully in planning, implementing, and evaluating the child's plan of care. It also means that families should have a choice in how much care they provide; overreliance on families to provide care can be detrimental to both the child and parent (Coyne, 2013).

Commitment to family-centered care means that the nurse respects the family's diversity. Children and parents live in various family structures. An expanded definition of family is required in the twenty-first century, because the term no longer refers to only the intact, nuclear family in which parents raise their biologic children. Contemporary family structures include adolescent parents, extended families with aunts, uncles, or cousins parenting, intergenerational families with grandparents parenting, blended families with stepparents and stepsiblings, gay or lesbian parents, foster parents, group homes, and homeless children. The nurse should be prepared to identify the foundational strengths in all family structures (see Chapter 3). Family-centered care also means that the nurse truly believes that the child's care and recovery are greatly enhanced when the family fully participates in the child's care (Fig. 4.3).

**! NURSING QUALITY ALERT**

***Communicating With Families***

- Include all involved family members. One essential step toward achieving a Family-centered care environment is to develop open lines of communication with the family.
- Encourage families to write down their questions.
- Remain nonjudgmental.
- Give families both verbal and nonverbal signals that send a message of availability and openness.
- Respect and encourage feedback from families.
- Recognize that families come in various shapes, sizes, colors, and generations.
- Avoid assumptions about core family beliefs and values.
- Respect family diversity.

### Establishing Rapport

Critical to establishing rapport with families is the nurse's ability to convey genuine respect and concern during the first encounter. A nonjudgmental approach and a willingness to assist family members in effectively caring for their child demonstrate the nurse's interest in their well-being.

### Availability and Openness to Questions

A nurse who does not take time to see how a child and family are doing—such as a nurse who leaves a room immediately after a treatment or administration of a medication—will not encourage or invite families to ask questions. Families want and need unrushed and uninterrupted time with the nurse. Sometimes this time can be made available only by purposefully scheduling it into the day. Encouraging families to write down their questions will enable them to take full advantage of their time with the nurse.

The nurse explains a child's test results to his mother and grandmother. Including all important family members in the child's healthcare reflects commitment to family-centered care. (Courtesy University of Texas at Arlington College of Nursing, Arlington, TX.)

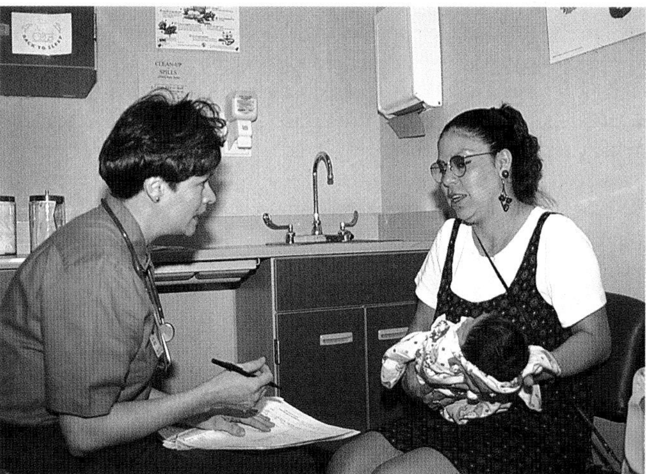

This nurse practitioner has learned Spanish to communicate better with her many Spanish-speaking patients. Speaking with family members in their own language encourages the family to remain in the healthcare system. The nurse is also using eye contact and has positioned herself at the mother's eye level. (Courtesy Parkland Health and Hospital System Community Oriented Primary Care Clinic, Dallas, TX.)

**FIG 4.3** The child's continuing healthcare, both preventive and during illness, is enhanced by participation of the family.

The nurse might encourage effective use of time by saying, "I know you have a lot of questions and are very anxious to learn more about your son's condition. I have another patient who has an immediate need, but I will be available in 10 minutes to meet with you. In the meantime, here is a parent handbook that gives general information about seizures. Please feel free to review it and write down any questions that we can discuss when I return."

### Family Education and Empowerment

Family empowerment occurs when the nurse and other health providers take the time to educate parents about their child's condition and the skills they need to participate, thus ensuring their continued involvement in planning and evaluating the plan of care. Families need support as they gain confidence in their skills, and they need guidance to assist them as they navigate through the healthcare experience. Communication is enhanced when families feel competent and confident in their abilities.

### Effective Management of Conflict

When conflict occurs, it needs to be addressed in an expedient manner to prevent further breakdown in communication. Box 4.1 suggests strategies for managing conflict, and Table 4.2 highlights the importance of choosing words carefully to make families feel welcome and to further facilitate family-centered care.

### Feedback From Children and Families

The nurse needs to be alert for both verbal and nonverbal cues. Routinely checking with family members about their experiences, satisfaction with communications, teaching sessions, and healthcare goals is an effective way to ensure that healthcare providers obtain appropriate feedback. To enhance the delivery of care, the nurse should explain how this feedback will be used. The nurse should listen and observe carefully to make sure that what family members are saying is truly what they are feeling.

The nurse should identify not only the child's primary caretaker but also other family members integral to the child's care. Support and physical care is often provided to the child by a family member other than a parent. Communicating with this important person will assist the nurse in providing comprehensive family-centered care.

For example, while one nurse was teaching the mother of a 2-year-old child who was recently diagnosed with type 1 diabetes mellitus, the mother reported that although she was her child's primary caregiver, the child's grandmother frequently cared for the child while the mother was at work. The nurse therefore notified the other team members and altered the teaching plan for diabetes care to include the child's grandmother.

### Spirituality

Children have rich spiritual lives, although they do not use the same vocabulary as adults to describe them. Spiritual care is a vital coping resource for many children. To provide holistic care to children, it is important to assess the child's beliefs and faith (Neuman, 2011). Supporting children's existing faith and spiritual practices is recommended. Children can be assisted in maintaining their rituals, whether they are bedtime prayers, songs, or blessings at meals. Nurses can provide spiritual care in ways that offer hope, encouragement, comfort, and respect. A resource to pursue in many hospital or healthcare settings is the pastoral care or chaplain's department.

### BOX 4.1 Strategies for Managing Conflict

- Understand the parents' perspective (walk in their shoes). Imagine yourself as the parent of a child in a hospital where your values and beliefs are exposed and scrutinized. Try to understand the parents' perspective better by encouraging them to share it.
- Determine a common goal and stay focused on it. Determine the agreed-on result, and work toward it. By staying focused on a common goal, the parties involved are more likely to find workable strategies to achieve the identified goal.
- Seek win-win solutions. Conflict should not be about who is right and who is wrong. Effective conflict management focuses on finding a solution whereby both parties "win." By establishing a common goal, both parties win when this goal is achieved.
- Listen actively. Critical to resolving situations of conflict is the ability to listen and understand what the other person is saying and feeling. In active listening, the receiver actively and empathically listens to gain a better understanding of the actual and the implied message.
- Openly express your feelings. Talking about feelings is much more constructive than acting them out. The nurse might say, "I am very concerned about Jamie's safety when you leave his side rails down."
- Avoid blaming. Each party owns part of the problem. Pointing fingers and blaming others will not solve the problem. Instead, identify the part of the problem that each party owns and work together to resolve it. Seek win–win solutions.
- Summarize the decision. At the end of any discussion, summarize what has been decided and identify who is responsible for follow-up. This process ensures that everyone is clear about the decision and facilitates accountability for implementing solutions.

### TABLE 4.2 Choosing Words Carefully

| Poor Words | Rationale | Better Words | Rationale |
|---|---|---|---|
| Policies allowed or not permitted | Convey attitude that hospital personnel have authority over parents in matters concerning their children | Guidelines, working together, welcome | Convey openness and appreciation for position and importance of families |
| Noncompliant, uncooperative, difficult (when referring to parents and other family members) | Imply that healthcare providers make decisions and give instructions that families must follow without input | Partners, colleagues, joint decision makers, experts about their child | Acknowledge that families bring important information and insight and that families and professionals form a team |
| Dysfunctional, in denial, overprotective, uninvolved, uncaring (labeling families) | Pronounce judgment that may not incorporate full understanding of family's situation, reactions, or perspective | Coping (describing family's reactions with care and respect) | Remain open to reaching a more complete and appreciative understanding of families over time |

## TRANSCULTURAL COMMUNICATION: BRIDGING THE GAP

Conflict can arise when the nurse comes from a cultural background that differs from that of the child and family. Such differences might influence the approach to care. As the demographics in the United States continue to change, healthcare professionals will be challenged to become more transcultural in their approach to patients if they want to remain effective in their relationships with children and families (American Academy of Pediatrics,[AAP], 2013). Healthcare professionals need to be aware of their own values and beliefs and to recognize how these influence their interactions with others. They also need to be aware of and respect the child's and family's values and beliefs. In working with children and families, the initial nursing assessment should address values, beliefs, and traditions. The nurse can then consider ways in which culture might affect communication style, methods of decision making, cultural adaptations for nursing intervention, and other behaviors related to healthcare practices.

During the initial interview, the nurse ascertains the following information related to the child and family:

*Decision-making practices:* Are decisions made by individuals or collectively as a group?

*Child-rearing practices:* Who are the primary caregivers? What are their disciplinary practices?

*Family support:* What is the family structure? To whom do the patient and family turn for support?

*Communication practices:* How is the information communicated to the rest of the family?

*Health and illness practices:* Do family members seek professional help or rely on other resources for treatment and advice?

Because language barriers can greatly affect the provision of healthcare, effective communication with a child or family for whom English is not the native language is an important challenge (AAP, 2013). The optimal approach to this issue is to access a trained interpreter or a family member or friend who is proficient in English. The AAP (2013) recommends not using a child to interpret.

The nurse can use the information obtained to individualize a treatment plan and approach suitable for the child's and family's needs. For example, if the parents of a child with an Orthodox Jewish religious background request a kosher diet, the nurse facilitates the routine delivery of kosher meals and communicates the family's wishes to the rest of the team members so that they can also respect the family's customs. If the family of a child who has a severe brain injury requests the services of a healer, the nurse enables the family to arrange the visit. Coordinating the child's daily schedule to provide an uninterrupted visit with the healer is one aspect of family-centered care. When the nurse communicates the family's cultural preferences to other members of the healthcare team, communication and holistic care are enhanced.

## THERAPEUTIC RELATIONSHIPS: DEVELOPING AND MAINTAINING TRUST

Trust is important in establishing and maintaining therapeutic relationships with families. Trust promotes a sense of partnership between nurses and families. Becoming overly involved with the child or family can inhibit a healthy relationship. Because nurses are caring, nurturing people and the profession demands that nurses sometimes become intimately involved in other people's lives, maintaining the balance between appropriate involvement and professional separation is quite challenging. Box 4.2 delineates behaviors that may indicate over involvement. Box 4.3 identifies behaviors that may indicate professional separation or under involvement. Whether nurses become too emotionally involved or find themselves at the other end of the spectrum, being under involved, they lose effectiveness as objective professional resources.

### BOX 4.2 Warning Signs of Over Involvement

- Buying gifts for individual children or families
- Giving out one's home phone number
- Competing with other staff for the child's or family's affection
- Inviting the child or family to social gatherings
- Accepting invitations to family gatherings (e.g., birthday parties, weddings)
- Visiting or spending time with the child or family during off-duty time
- Revealing personal information
- Lending or borrowing money
- Making decisions for the family about the child's care

### BOX 4.3 Warning Signs of Under Involvement

- Avoiding the child or family
- Calling in sick so as not to take assignment of a specific child
- Asking to trade assignments for a specific child
- Spending less time with a particular child

Family members may display feelings of incompetence, fear, and loss of control by expressing anger, withdrawal, or dissatisfaction. Most important in working with these families is to promote the parents' feelings of competence through education and empowerment. The nurse keeps parents well informed of the child's care through frequent phone calls and actively involves them in decision making. Teaching parents skills necessary to care for their child promotes confidence, enhances self-esteem, and fosters independence.

Nurses must be able to recognize their own personal and professional needs. Being aware of the motives for one's own actions will greatly enhance the nurse's ability to understand the needs of children and families and to give families the tools to manage care effectively.

### ! NURSING QUALITY ALERT

***Maintaining a Therapeutic Relationship***

Maintaining professional boundaries requires that the nurse constantly be aware of the fine line between empathy and over involvement.

## NURSING CARE

### Communicating With Children and Families

#### Assessment

A comprehensive needs assessment of the child and family elicits information about problem-solving skills, cultural needs, coping behaviors, and the child's routines. Any assessment requires the nurse to obtain information from the child and the family. It is important not to overlook the child's participation in providing information; many children want to provide input both to convey information and participate in their own care (Lambert, Geachen, & McCarron, 2011; Livesley & Long, 2013).

The nurse might say, "Mrs. Jiminez, I value your input as well as your child's. Hearing Ramon explain his understanding of his diabetic dietary restrictions in his own words will help us gain better insight into how best to manage his care. Let's take a few minutes to hear from Ramon, and then we can talk about your perspective."

Assessment enables the nurse to develop better insight by gathering information from multiple perspectives and facilitates the development of a more comprehensive plan of care. A thorough assessment of the child's communication skills presumes that the nurse understands developmental milestones and can relate comprehension and communication skills to the child's cognitive and emotional development and language abilities. During the initial assessment of the child and family, the nurse should also describe routines and provide information about what the child and family can expect during their visit.

The family's level of health literacy is an important component of a communication assessment. Because of language, educational, or other barriers, some family members may not understand medical or health terminology in ways nurses might expect. Miscommunication related to low health literacy has consequences for patients, such as not adhering to medication or recommended treatment routines or not being able to decipher medical forms (AAP, 2013; Kornburger et al., 2013). Assessment data that might suggest poor health literacy in family members include avoidance of reading or filling out hospital forms; giving rationales for not reading, such as saying they forgot their eye glasses at home; being unable to provide an appropriate health history; or waiting too long before seeking medical help (Lambert & Keogh, 2014). Providing instructions and explanations in language the caregiver understands as well as having the caregiver repeat or demonstrate back the instructions can increase understanding and adherence (Kornburger et al., 2013).

### Nursing Diagnosis and Planning

The nursing assessment may suggest diagnoses that affect communication but that arise from the child's encounter with the healthcare system. Other diagnoses are related to the child's and family's communication abilities.

- Anxiety related to potential or actual separation from parents (e.g., a 4-year-old girl who becomes withdrawn and unable to cooperate with an office hearing test when separated from her mother).

***Expected outcomes.*** The child verbalizes the cause of the anxiety and more readily communicates with the healthcare professional. The child exhibits posture, facial expressions, and gestures that reflect decreased distress.

- Fear related to a perceived threat to the child's well-being and inadequate understanding of procedures or treatments (e.g., a 7-year-old boy scheduled for tonsillectomy who wonders where his throat will be cut to remove his tonsils).

***Expected outcome.*** The child talks about fears and accurately describes the procedure or treatment.

- Hopelessness related to a deteriorating health status (e.g., an 11-year-old child in isolation with prolonged illness and uncertain prognosis).

***Expected outcomes.*** The child verbalizes feelings and participates in care. The child makes positive statements, maintains eye contact during interactions, and has appetite and sleep patterns that are appropriate for the child's age and physical health.

- Powerlessness related to limits to autonomy (e.g., a 3-year-old child with a C6 spinal fracture as a result of a motor vehicle trauma).

***Expected outcomes.*** The child expresses frustrations and anger and begins to make choices in areas that are controllable. The child asks appropriate questions about care and treatment.

- Impaired Verbal Communication related to physiologic barriers or cultural and language differences (e.g., a 17-year-old adolescent who has had her jaw wired subsequent to orthodontic surgery).

**Expected outcomes.** The adolescent effectively uses alternative communication methods. The child and family who speak and understand a different language appropriately communicate through an interpreter.

### CRITICAL THINKING EXERCISE 4.1

The nurse caring for an 8-year-old boy observes him lying in his bed with his back facing the door. He is crying, although he quickly wipes his eyes when he sees the nurse at the door. He has been hospitalized because of leukemia. He lives in a small community 350 miles from the hospital. His parents visit on the weekends.

1. Identify two things that might be upsetting the child.
2. What strategies could you use to encourage the child to talk about his feelings related to the problems you have identified?

### Interventions

Nurses working with children should determine the best communication approach for each child individually on the basis of the child's age and developmental abilities. Table 4.3 presents an overview of developmental milestones related to communication skills in children and some approaches to facilitate successful interactions. Other interventions that facilitate communication between the nurse and children include play, storytelling, and strategies for enhancing self-esteem.

***Play.*** Play can greatly facilitate communicating with children. Approaching children at their developmental level with familiar forms of play increases their comfort and allows the nurse to be seen in a more positive, less threatening role.

Because play is an everyday part of children's lives and a method they use to communicate, they are less likely to be inhibited when participating in play interactions. Through play, children may express thoughts and feelings they may be unable to verbalize (see Chapters 6 through 9 for normal play activities and Chapter 35 for therapeutic play).

Children's access to the World Wide Web and electronic social media sites has expanded the sources of health and illness information that children and families can obtain directly (Isaacs, 2014). Several sites appropriate for school age children's developmental level (e.g., http://www.kidshealth.org, http://www.medikidz.com) include informational interactive games, videos, and magazines that provide health information in an appealing format. Use of appropriate social networking sites is another vehicle for obtaining information and support for children. Nurses need to become familiar with some of these sites in order to evaluate them for appropriate and accurate information before recommending them to children and families.

***Storytelling.*** Storytelling is an innovative and creative communication strategy. It is also a skill that can be acquired and refined through practice. Familiarity with stories and frequent practice in storytelling increase a nurse's confidence and competence as a storyteller. Storytelling can be a routine part of a nurse's day. Its purposes range from establishing rapport to approaching uncomfortable topics, such as loss, death, fear, grief, and anger. In storytelling, there is a teller and a listener. In individual situations, the child may be the teller or the listener, although in a shared story, adult and child may each take a turn in both roles (Box 4.4).

***Explaining procedures and treatments.*** Preparation before a procedure, which includes explaining the reasons for the procedure and the expected sequence of events and outcomes, can greatly reduce a child's fears and anxieties (Copanitsanou & Valkeapaa, 2013). Preparation enables the child to experience some mastery over events, gives the child time to develop effective coping behaviors and fosters trust

**TABLE 4.3 Developmental Milestones and Their Relationship to Communication Approaches**

| Development | Language Development | Emotional Development | Cognitive Development | Suggested Communication Approach |
|---|---|---|---|---|
| **Infants (0-12 mo)** | | | | |
| Infants experience world through senses of hearing, seeing, smelling, tasting, and touching. | Crying, babbling, and cooing.<br>Single-word production.<br>Able to name some simple objects. | Dependent on others; high need for cuddling and security.<br>Responsive to environment (e.g., sounds, visual stimuli).<br>Distinguish between happy and angry voices and between familiar and strange voices.<br>Beginning to experience separation anxiety. | Interactions largely reflexive.<br>Beginning to see repetition of activities and movements.<br>Beginning to initiate interactions intentionally.<br>Short attention span (1-2 min). | Use calm, soft, soothing voice.<br>Be responsive to cries.<br>Engage in turn-taking vocalizations (adult imitates baby sounds).<br>Talk and read regularly to infants.<br>Prepare infant as you are about to perform care; talk to infant about what you are about to do.<br>Use slow approach and allow child time to get to know you. |
| **Toddlers (1-2 yr)** | | | | |
| Toddlers experience world through senses of hearing, seeing, smelling, tasting, and touching. | Two-word combinations emerge.<br>Participate in turn taking in communication (speaker/listener).<br>"No" becomes favorite word.<br>Able to use gestures and verbalize simple wants and needs. | Strong need for security objects.<br>Separation/stranger anxiety heightened.<br>Participate in parallel play.<br>Thrive on routines.<br>Beginning development of independence: "Want to do by self."<br>Still very dependent on significant adults. | Experiment with objects.<br>Participate in active exploration.<br>Begin to experiment with variations on activities.<br>Begin to identify cause-and-effect relationships.<br>Short attention span (3-5 min). | Learn toddler's words for common items, and use them in conversations.<br>Describe activities and procedures as they are about to be done.<br>Use picture books.<br>Use play for demonstrations.<br>Be responsive to child's receptivity toward you and approach cautiously.<br>Preparation should occur immediately before event. |
| **Preschool Children (3-5 yr)** | | | | |
| Preschool children use words they do not fully understand; they also do not accurately understand many words used by others. | Further development and expansion of word combination (able to speak in full sentences)<br>Growth in correct grammatical usage.<br>Use pronouns.<br>Clearer articulation of sounds.<br>Vocabulary rapidly expanding; may know words without understanding meaning. | Like to imitate activities and make choices.<br>Strive for independence but need adult support and encouragement.<br>Demonstrate purposeful attention-seeking behaviors.<br>Learn cooperation and turn taking in game playing.<br>Need clearly set limits and boundaries. | Begin developing concepts of time, space, and quantity.<br>Magical thinking prominent.<br>World seen only from child's perspective.<br>Short attention span (5-10 min). | Seek opportunities to offer choices.<br>Use play to explain procedures and activities.<br>Speak in simple sentences, and explore relative concepts.<br>Use picture and story books, puppets.<br>Describe activities and procedures as they are about to be done.<br>Be concise; limit length of explanations (5 min).<br>Engage in preparatory activities 1-3 h before the event. |
| **School-Age Children (6-11 yr)** | | | | |
| School-age children communicate thoughts and appreciate viewpoints of others.<br>Words with multiple meanings and words describing things they have not experienced are not thoroughly understood. | Expanding vocabulary enables child to describe concepts, thoughts, and feelings.<br>Development of conversational skills. | Interact well with others.<br>Understand rules to games.<br>Very interested in learning.<br>Build close friendships.<br>Beginning to accept responsibility for own actions.<br>Competition emerges.<br>Still dependent on adults to meet needs. | Able to grasp concepts of classification, conversation.<br>Concrete thinking emerges.<br>Become very oriented to "rules."<br>Able to process information in serial format.<br>Lengthened attention span (10-30 min). | Use photographs, books, diagrams, charts, videos to explain. Make explanations sequential.<br>Engage in conversations that encourage critical thinking.<br>Establish limits and set consequences.<br>Use medical play techniques.<br>Introduce preparatory materials 1-5 days in advance of the event. |

*Continued*

**TABLE 4.3 Developmental Milestones and Their Relationship to Communication Approaches—cont'd**

| Development | Language Development | Emotional Development | Cognitive Development | Suggested Communication Approach |
|---|---|---|---|---|
| **Adolescents (12 yr and older)** | | | | |
| Adolescents are able to create theories and generate many explanations for situations.<br>They are beginning to communicate like adults. | Able to verbalize and comprehend most adult concepts. | Beginning to accept responsibility for own actions.<br>Perception of "imaginary audiences" (see Chapter 9).<br>Need independence. Competitive drive.<br>Strong need for group identification.<br>Frequently have small group of very close friends.<br>Question authority. Strong need for privacy. | Able to think logically and abstractly.<br>Attention span up to 60 min. | Engage in conversations about adolescent's interests.<br>Use photographs, books, diagrams, charts, and videos to explain.<br>Use collaborative approach, and foster and support independence.<br>Introduce preparatory materials up to 1 wk in advance of the event.<br>Respect privacy needs. |

**BOX 4.4 Storytelling Strategies**

- Capture a story on paper or on video as told by a child or group of children.
- Tell a "yarn story" with two or more people. A long piece of yarn with knots tied at varied intervals is slid loosely through the hands of the teller until a knot is felt, at which time the yarn is passed to the next person, who continues the story.
- Initiate a game of sentence completion, either oral or written, with sentences beginning "If I were in charge of the hospital … ," "I wish … ," "When I get home I will … ," or "My family … "
- Read stories with themes related to issues a child is facing. The children's section of the local public library is an excellent resource.

in those caring for the child. Adequate preparation is the key to helping a child have a successful, positive healthcare experience.

In general, the younger the child, the closer in time to the event the child should be prepared for it. For example, a 3-year-old child will generally be very anxious and therefore should be prepared immediately before, whereas school age children and teenagers would benefit from a longer preparation time so that they can develop strategies for dealing with the situation. Table 4.3 gives age-related attention-span guidelines.

For nurses to adequately explain procedures and treatments to children and families, they themselves must first know what is involved. In this way, nurses can properly describe the sequence of events and collect the developmentally appropriate information and equipment needed to assist with the procedure or treatment explanation. Depending on the child's developmental level, the nurse provides **sensory information**, describing, step-by-step, what the child will see, hear, and feel; how long the procedure or treatment will last (e.g., as long as it takes to sing a favorite song or count slowly to ten), or how the equipment works. For example, in preparing a child for an IV line insertion, the nurse can show the child the catheter or explain the purpose of the tourniquet and allow the child to put it on or to put it on the arm of a doll, if the child so desires. The nurse should let the child smell an alcohol swab and feel its coolness when applied to the skin. Showing the child the place or room where procedures will occur may reduce some of the stress and anxiety associated with the unfamiliar environment. Often, this is done if the child will be experiencing a planned surgical procedure.

Teaching needs to be individualized to the specific child and the situation, with the child actively involved, if possible (Lambert et al., 2011). Kornburger and colleagues (2013) describe key elements for teaching children and families about procedures, treatments, and care of the child after discharge using the "teach back" method. The procedure is as follows (p. 284):

- *Assessing readiness.* The first step is to assess the child's or family's readiness to learn. Some children will prefer to be actively involved and interested in conveying opinions and feelings; other children might be passive participants (Lambert et al., 2011).
- *Providing information.* Once readiness has been established, the nurse begins to prepare the child using clear, descriptive language appropriate to the child's developmental level. Using words familiar to the child is important, and medical jargon is to be avoided. Consultation with the family will allow the nurse to learn specific words and terminology used by the child. Table 4.4 offers other concrete suggestions of appropriate language for nurses to use in working with children. Preparation should occur in an environment that is free from other distractions, so the child and/or family can focus on what is being said. The nurse should avoid information overload.
- *Verifying understanding.* When the teaching or preparation is complete, the nurse asks the child and family member to repeat in their own words the information provided; if teaching involves a procedure that the child or family member will perform, there should be a return demonstration of the skill. The nurse takes this opportunity to clarify any information that has been misinterpreted.
- *Asking* questions. The nurse will then solicit any questions from the family and answer them.

Open, honest communication about treatments and procedures and attentiveness to the learning needs of the child will greatly facilitate achievement of the treatment goals.

Because nonadherence to treatment protocols can be a problem in some families, it is essential that the nurse ensure that children and family members can describe the treatment plan. Using various written, verbal, interactive, and visual materials can improve comprehension and adherence. For psychomotor skill development, return demonstration is important. Reinforcement with written materials in the family's chosen language or at the family's assessed literacy level provides a ready reference for the family after the child's discharge (Lambert & Keogh, 2014).

***Strategies for enhancing self-esteem.*** Communication practices play an important role in the development of children's self-esteem and confidence. Nurses are in an excellent position to model communication practices that enhance self-esteem. Table 4.5 compares helpful and harmful communication practices.

The words adults choose, their tone of voice, and the place and timing of message delivery all influence the child's interpretation of the message. The interpretation may be positive, negative, or neutral. To enhance the child's self-esteem, adults should strive for positive language.

Allowing children to have a "voice" when care is provided increases their self-esteem and empowers them in situations where they feel out

**TABLE 4.4 Considerations in Choosing Language**

| Potentially Ambiguous | Possible Misinterpretation | Concrete Explanation |
|---|---|---|
| "The doctor will give you some dye." | To make me die? | "The doctor will put some medicine in the tube that will help her see your _______ more clearly." |
| Dressing, dressing change | Why are they going to undress me? Do I have to change my clothes? | Bandages; clean, new bandages. |
| Stool collection | Why do they want to collect little chairs? | Use child's familiar term, such as "poop," "BM," or "doody." |
| Urine | You're in? | Use child's familiar term, such as "pee." |
| Shot | When people get shot, they're really badly hurt. | Describe giving medicine through a (small, tiny) needle. |
| CAT scan | Will there be cats? | Describe in simple terms, and explain what the letters of the common name stand for. |
| PICU | Pick you? | Explain as above. |
| ICU | I see you? | Explain as above. |
| IV | Ivy? | Explain as above. |
| Stretcher | Stretch her? Stretch whom? | Bed on wheels. |
| Special; funny (words that are usually positive descriptors) | It doesn't look/feel special to me. | Odd, different, unusual, strange. |
| Gas, sleeping gas | Is someone going to pour gasoline into the mask? | "A medicine, called an anesthetic, is a kind of air you will breathe through a mask like this to help you sleep during your operation so you won't feel anything. It is a different kind of sleep." (Explain differences.) |
| "The doctor will put you to sleep." | Like my cat was put to sleep? It never came back. | "The doctor will give you medicine that will help you go into a very deep sleep. You won't feel anything until the operation is over. Then the doctor will stop giving you the medicine, so you can wake up." |
| "Move you to the floor." | Why are they going to put me on the ground? | Unit, ward. (Explain why the child is being transferred, and where.) |
| OR (or treatment room) table | People aren't supposed to get up on tables. | A narrow bed. |
| "Take a picture." | (X-ray, CT, and MRI machines are far larger than a familiar camera, move differently, and do not yield a familiar end product.) | "A picture of your insides." (Describe appearance, sounds, and movement of the equipment.) |
| "Flush your IV." | Flush it down the toilet? | Explain. |

Words can be experienced as "hard" or "soft" according to how much they increase the perceived threat of a situation. For example, consider the following word choices:

| Harder | Softer |
|---|---|
| "This part will hurt." | "It (you) may feel (or feel very) sore, achy, scratchy, tight, snug, full, or (other manageable, descriptive term)." |
| "The medicine will burn." | (Words such as scratch, poke, or sting might be familiar for some children and frightening to others.) |
| "The room will be very cold." | "Some children say they feel very warm." "Some children say they feel very cold." |
| "The medicine will taste (or smell) bad." | "The medicine may taste (or smell) different from anything you have tasted before. After you take it, will you tell me how it was for you?" |
| "Cut," "open you up," "slice," "make a hole." | "The doctor will make an opening." |
| "As big as _____" (e.g., size of an incision or of a catheter). | (Use concrete comparisons, such as "your little finger" or "a paper clip" if the opening will indeed be small.) "Smaller than _______." |
| "As long as _______" (e.g., for duration of a procedure). | "For less time than it takes you to _______." |
| "As much as _______." | "Less than _______." |
| (These are open-ended and "extending" expressions.) | (These expressions help confine, familiarize, and imply the manageability of an event or of equipment.) |

*Continued*

**TABLE 4.4 Considerations in Choosing Language—cont'd**

| The Unfamiliar Usage or Complexity of Some Common Medical Words or Expressions Can Be Confusing and Frightening. | |
|---|---|
| **Potentially Ambiguous** | **Concrete Explanation** |
| "Take your vitals" (or "your vital signs") | "Measure your temperature," "see how warm your body is," "see how fast and strongly your heart is working." (Nothing is "taken" from the child.) |
| Electrodes, leads | "Sticky like a Band-Aid, with a small wet spot in the center, and small strings that attach to the snap (monitor electrodes); paste like wet sand, with strings with tiny metal cups that stick to the paste (electroencephalogram [EEG] electrodes). The paste washes off easily afterward; the strings go into a box that will make a picture of how your heart (or brain) is working." (Show child electrodes and leads before using. Let child handle them and apply them to a doll or to self.) |
| "Hang your (IV) medication." | "We will bring in a new medicine in a bag and attach it to the little tube already in your arm. The needle goes into the tube, not into your arm, so you won't feel it." |
| NPO | "Nothing to eat. Your stomach needs to be empty." (Explain why.) "You can eat and drink again as soon as _______." (Explain with concrete descriptions.) |
| Anesthesia | "The doctor will give you medicine—you may hear it called 'anesthesia.' It will help you go into a very deep sleep. You will not feel anything at all. The doctor knows just the right amount of medicine to give you so you will stay asleep through your operation. When the operation is over, the doctor stops giving you that medicine and helps you wake up." |

*CT*, Computed tomography; *ICU*, intensive care unit; *IV*, intravenous; *MRI*, magnetic resonance imaging; *PICU*, pediatric intensive care unit.
Note: Words or phrases that are helpful to one child may be threatening for another. Health care providers must listen carefully and be sensitive to the child's use of and response to language.
Modified with permission from The Child Life Council, Inc., 11820 Parklawn Dr., Rockville, MD 20852-2529; from Gaynard, L., Wolfer, J., Goldberger, J., et al. (1998). *Psychosocial care of children in hospitals: A clinical practice manual from ACCH Child Life Research Project.* Rockville, MD: The Child Life Council, Inc.

**TABLE 4.5 Self-Esteem in Children: Communication Practices**

| Techniques to Enhance Self-Esteem | Practices That Harm Self-Esteem |
|---|---|
| Praise efforts and accomplishments. | Criticize efforts and accomplishments. |
| Use active listening skills. | Be too busy to listen. |
| Encourage expression of feelings. | Tell children how they should feel. |
| Acknowledge feelings. | Give no support for dealing with feelings. |
| Use developmentally based discipline. | Use physical punishment. |
| Use "I" statements. | Use "you" statements. |
| Be nonjudgmental. | Judge the child. |
| Set clearly defined limits, and reinforce them. | Set no known limits or boundaries. |
| Share quality time together. | Give time grudgingly. |
| Be honest. | Be dishonest. |
| Describe behaviors observed when praising and disciplining. | Use coercion and power as discipline. |
| Compliment the child. | Belittle, blame, or shame the child. |
| Smile. | Use sarcastic, caustic, or cruel "humor." |
| Touch and hug the child. | Avoid coming near the child, even when the child is open to touching, holding, or hugging. Touch and hold only when performing a task. |
| Rock the child. | Avoid comforting through rocking. |

of control (Lambert et al., 2011; Livesley & Long, 2013). Depending on the age and developmental level, children are competent to understand information about their condition and treatments and should be included in decision-making. Nurses need to be careful not to overlook children who appear reticent by excluding them from dialog. Depending on the particular situation, children might or might not want to participate in their care (Livesley & Long, 2013).

### Evaluation

While evaluation is traditionally considered as a closure activity, it should be a continuous activity throughout the nursing process. Keep expected outcomes visible, and evaluate whether they are being realized. Are the outcomes attainable? Could the wrong nursing diagnosis have been made? Adjust the plan of care as required.

## COMMUNICATING WITH CHILDREN WITH SPECIAL NEEDS

The opportunity to interact with children who have special communication needs presents an exciting challenge for nurses. It is essential for nurses to consider each child's particular routines and preferences when providing care (Oulton, Sell, Kerry, et al., 2015). Depending on the child's condition, communication strategies will differ. To ensure a consistent approach from all caregivers, the nurse might need to develop creative ways of conveying information to other health providers and family members (Oulton et al., 2015).

To identify successful alternative methods of communication, the nurse needs to learn particular techniques for working with children and families. Alternative methods of communicating are critical.

Children need to accurately express their wants and needs. Through adequate preparation and reassurance, the nurse can offer the child comfort and understanding. Successfully meeting this challenge is a rewarding experience for the nurse and a positive, supportive experience for the child and family.

### The Child With a Visual Impairment

For the child with a visual impairment, the nurse can do the following:

- Obtain a thorough assessment of the child's self-help skills and abilities (i.e., toileting, bathing, dressing, feeding, and mobility).
- Orient the child to the surroundings. Walk the child around the room and unit several times, indicating landmarks (e.g., doors, closets, bedside tables, and windows) while guiding the child by the hand or by the way the child prefers. Explain sounds that the child may frequently hear (e.g., monitors, alarms, and nurse call bells).
- Encourage a family member to stay with the child. This person can facilitate communication and greatly enhance the child's comfort in this unfamiliar environment.
- Keep furniture and other items consistently in the same place. Consistency aids in the child's orientation to the room, fosters independence, and promotes safety.
- Keep the nurse call bell in the same place and within the child's reach.
- Identify yourself when entering the room, and tell the child when you are departing.
- Carefully and fully explain all procedures.
- Allow the child to handle equipment as the procedure is explained.

**! NURSING QUALITY ALERT**

***Communicating With Children With Special Needs***

In working with children with special needs, the nurse must carefully assess each child's physical, mental, and developmental abilities and determine the most effective methods of communication.

## THE CHILD WITH A HEARING IMPAIRMENT

For the child with a hearing impairment, the nurse can do the following:

- Thoroughly assess the child's self-help skills and abilities.
- Identify the family's method of communication and, if possible, adopt it.
- Encourage a family member to stay with the child at all times to decrease the stress of hospitalization and facilitate communication.
- If sign language is used, learn the most frequently used signs and use them whenever able. Keep a chart of signs near the child's bed.
- Develop a communication board with pictures of most commonly used items or needs (e.g., television, cup, toothbrush, toilet, and shower).
- Determine whether the child uses a hearing aid. If so, make sure that the batteries are working and that the hearing aid is clean and intact.
- When entering the room, do so cautiously and gently touch the child before speaking.
- Always face the child when speaking. If the child is a lip reader, face-to-face visibility will greatly enhance the child's ability to understand.
- Do not shout or exaggerate speech. This behavior distorts the face and can be very confusing. Rather, speak in a normal tone and at a regular pace.
- Remember that nonverbal communication can speak as loudly as, if not louder than, speech (e.g., a frown or worried face can say more than words).
- When performing a procedure that requires standing behind the child, such as when giving an enema or assisting with a spinal tap, have another person stand in front of the child and explain the procedure as it is being performed.
- Whenever possible, use play strategies to help communicate and demonstrate procedures (see Table 4.3).

### The Child Who Speaks Another Language

For the child who speaks another language, the nurse can do the following:

- Thoroughly assess the child's abilities in speaking and understanding both languages.
- Identify an interpreter, perhaps another adult family member, friend of the family, or other individual with proficiency in both languages to be used for communication not related to healthcare. Other children should not be used as interpreters.
- Use an interpreter whenever possible but always when explaining procedures, determining understanding, teaching new skills, and assessing needs.
- Use a communication board with the names of items printed in both languages.
- Learn the words and names of commonly used items in the child's language, and use them whenever possible. Using the familiar language not only aids in communication but also demonstrates sincere interest in learning the language and respect for the culture.
- Learn as much about the child's culture as possible and develop plans of care that demonstrate respect for the culture. Sincere attempts to learn to communicate with the child and family demonstrate the nurse's concern for their well-being.
- Use play strategies whenever possible. Play seems to be a universal language.

### The Child With Other Communication Challenges

For the child who has more severe communication challenges, the nurse can do the following:

- Thoroughly assess the child's self-help skills and abilities. Determine the child's and family's methods of communicating and adopt them as much as possible.
- Encourage parents to stay with the child to decrease anxiety and foster communication.
- Determine whether the child uses sign language or augmented communication devices. Use a communication board if appropriate.
- Be attentive to and maximize the child's nonverbal communication. Facial grimaces, frowns, smiles, and nods are effective means of communicating responses and expressing likes and dislikes.
- If appropriate, encourage the child to use writing boards (dry erase or chalk; or pads of paper) to write needs, wants, questions, and concerns.

### The Child With a Profound Neurologic Impairment

Because hearing, vision, and language abilities are often hard to determine in the child who is profoundly neurologically impaired, the nurse should assume that the child can hear, see, and comprehend something of what is said. A friendly tone of voice that conveys warmth and respect should be used. For the child with a profound neurologic impairment, the nurse can do the following:

- Address the child when entering and exiting the room. Gently touch the child while saying the child's name.
- Speak softly, calmly, and slowly to allow the child time to process what you are saying.
- While in the room with the child, talk to the child. Do not talk as if the child is not there.

The nurse might say, "Jenny, I am going to wash your arm now," or "Jenny, now I am going to take your temperature by putting the thermometer under your arm." Identifying an assistant, the nurse might say, "Jenny, Kristi, another nurse, is here to help me lift you into your chair."

- Talk to the child about activities and objects in the room, things that the child might see, hear, smell, touch, taste, or sense.

For example, the nurse might say, "It is a sunny day today; can you feel the warm sun shining on you through the window?"

- When asking the child questions, allow the child adequate time to respond. Be careful to ask questions only of children who are capable of responding.
- Ascertain the child's ability to respond to simple questions. Some children can respond to yes-or-no questions by squeezing a hand or blinking their eyes (once for yes and twice for no).
- Be extremely attentive to any signs or gestures (e.g., facial grimaces, smiling, and eye movements) that may convey responses to likes or dislikes. Signs or gestures may be the child's only means of communicating.

As with all children with special communication needs, thoroughly document and communicate to others who interact with the child any special techniques that work. Providing information will greatly enhance continuity and more fully facilitate the child's ability to communicate.

## KEY CONCEPTS

- Components of effective communication involve verbal and nonverbal interactions that include touch, physical proximity, environment, listening, eye contact, visual cues, pace of speech, tone of voice, and overall body language.
- Touch is particularly important when communicating with infants, but positive and reassuring touch is valued by children of all ages. Nurses should always respect each person's sense of personal space.
- Creating and maintaining privacy facilitates communication, particularly for adolescents and families.
- The best communication approach for an individual child should be determined on the basis of the child's age, developmental abilities, and cultural preferences.
- Listening is an essential component of communication. Active listening skills include being attentive, clarification through reflection, empathy, and impartiality.
- The nurse also needs to be aware of the effects of visual communication, such as eye contact, body language, dress, and adverse visual stimuli.
- When communicating with families, it is essential for the nurse to first establish rapport and create a climate of trust.
- When the nurse is available and open to questions, the family feels empowered and more in control. Involving the family in the child's care and teaching them the skills needed to care for their child also is empowering.
- Conflict between families and the healthcare team is not unusual. The nurse can prevent conflict and facilitate conflict resolution by creating a welcoming climate and choosing words carefully when communicating with families.
- Communicating with families whose primary language is not English provides additional challenges; recognizing one's own cultural beliefs and attitudes and how they affect communication with others is important.
- For bridging the communication gap with families of different cultures, the nurse assesses child-rearing practices, family supports, who is the primary decision maker, communication practices and approaches to seeking healthcare.
- The nurse must be cautious about both over- and underinvolvement when caring for children and their families.
- Interventions that facilitate communication include such strategies as incorporating play and storytelling in care, and modeling communication practices that enhance self-esteem.
- Communication pitfalls, such as using jargon, talking down to children or beyond their developmental level, and avoiding or denying a problem, can lead to a breakdown in the relationship between the nurse and the child and family.
- Children with special communication needs include children who have a visual or hearing impairment, children who speak another language, children who have a communication disorder and children with profound neurologic impairment.
- In working with children with special needs, the nurse should carefully assess each child's personal routines and preferences as well as physical, mental, and developmental abilities and determine the most effective methods of communication.

## REFERENCES AND READINGS

American Academy of Pediatrics. (2013). Policy statement: Enhancing pediatric workforce diversity and providing culturally effective pediatric care: Implications for practice, education, and policy making. *Pediatrics, 132*(4), e1105–e1116.

Copanitsanou, P., & Valkeapaa, K. (2013). Effects of education of paediatric patients undergoing elective surgical procedures on their anxiety – a systematic review. *Journal of Clinical Nursing, 23,* 940–954.

Coyne, I. (2013). Families and health care professionals' perspectives and expectations for family-centred care: Hidden expectations and unclear roles. *Health Expectations, 18,* 796–808.

Crawford, D., Corkin, D., & Coad, J. (2013). Educating children's nurses for communicating bad news. *Nursing Children and Young People, 25*(8), 28–33.

Dion, X. (2015, February). Using social networking sites (namely Facebook) in health visiting practice – an account of five years experience. *Community Practitioner*, 28–31.

Fisher, M., & Broome, M. (2011). Parent-provider communication during hospitalization. *Journal of Pediatric Nursing, 26*, 58–69.

Gallo, K., Campbell, L., Hoagwood, K., et al. (2016). A narrative synthesis of the components of and evidence for patient- and family-centered care. *Clinical Pediatrics, 55*(4), 333–346.

Isaacs, D. (2014). Social media and communication. *Journal of Paediatrics and Child Health, 50*, 421–422.

Kornburger, C., Gibson, C., Sadowski, S., et al. (2013). Using "Teach-Back" for a safe transition from hospital to home: An evidence-based approach for improving the discharge process. *Journal of Pediatric Nursing, 28*,282–291.

Lambert, V., Glacken, M., & McCarron, M. (2011). Communication between children and health professionals in a child hospital setting: A Child Transition Communication Model. *Journal of Advanced Nursing, 67*(3), 569–582.

Lambert, V., & Keogh, D. (2014). Health literacy and its importance for effective communication Part 2. *Nursing Children and Young People, 26*(4), 32–36.

Livesley, J., & Long, T. (2013). Children's experience as hospital inpatients: Voice, competence, and work. Messages for nursing from a critical ethnographic study. *International Journal of Nursing Studies, 50*, 1292–1303.

Neuman, M. (2011). Addressing children's beliefs through Fowler's Stages of Faith. *Journal of Pediatric Nursing, 26*, 44–W50.

Olmstead, D., Scott, S, Mayan, M., et al. (2014). Influences in shaping nurses' use of distraction for children's procedural pain. *Journal for Specialists in Pediatric Nursing, 19*, 162–171.

Oulton, K., Sell, D., Kerry, S., et al. (2015). Individualizing hospital care for children and young people with learning disabilities: It's the little things that make the difference. *Journal of Pediatric Nursing, 30*(1), 78–86.

Ridgway, L., Mitchell, C., & Sheean, F. (2011). Information and communication technology use (ICT) in child and family nursing: What do we know and where to now? *Contemporary Nurse, 40*(1), 118–129.

5

# Health Promotion for the Developing Child

http://evolve.elsevier.com/McKinney/mat-ch/

## LEARNING OBJECTIVES

*After studying this chapter, you should be able to:*

- Define terms related to growth and development.
- Discuss principles of growth and development.
- Describe various factors that affect growth and development.
- Discuss the following theorists' ideas about growth and development: Piaget, Freud, Erikson, and Kohlberg.
- Discuss theories of language development.
- Identify methods used to assess growth and development.
- Describe the classifications and social aspects of play.
- Explain how play enhances growth and development.
- Identify health-promoting activities that are essential for the normal growth and development of infants and children.
- Discuss recommendations for scheduled vaccines.
- Discuss the components of a nutritional assessment.
- Discuss the etiology and prevention of childhood injuries.

Humans grow and change dramatically during childhood and adolescence. Normal growth and development proceed in an orderly, predictable pattern that establishes a basis for assessing an individual's abilities and potential. Nurses provide healthcare teaching and anticipatory guidance about the growth and development of children in many settings, such as newborn nurseries, emergency departments, community clinics and health centers, and pediatric inpatient units.

## OVERVIEW OF GROWTH AND DEVELOPMENT

Nurses are frequently the members of the healthcare team who parents approach. Parents are often concerned that their children are not progressing normally. Nurses can reassure parents about normal variations in development and can also identify problems early so that developmental delays can be addressed as soon as possible. Nurses who work with ill children must have a clear understanding of how children differ from adults and from each other at various stages. This awareness is essential to allow nurses to create developmentally appropriate plans of care to meet the needs of their young patients.

### Definition of Terms

Although the terms *growth* and *development* often are used together and interchangeably, they have distinct definitions and meanings. Growth generally refers to an increase in the physical size of a whole or any of its parts or an increase in the number and size of cells. Growth can be measured easily and accurately. For example, any observer can see that an infant grows rapidly during the first year of life. This growth can be measured readily by determining changes in weight and length. The difference in size between a newborn and a 12-month-old infant is an obvious sign of the remarkable growth that occurs during the first year of life.

Development is a more complex and subtle concept. Development is generally considered to be a continuous, orderly series of conditions leading to activities, new motives for activities, and patterns of behavior.

Another definition of development is an increase in function and complexity that occurs through growth, maturation, and learning—in other words, an increase in capabilities. The process of language acquisition provides an example of development. The use of language becomes increasingly complex as the child matures. At 10 to 12 months of age, a child uses single words to communicate simple desires and needs. By age 4 to 5 years, complete and complex sentences are used to relate elaborate tales. Language development can be measured by determining vocabulary, articulation skill, and word use.

Maturity and learning also affect development. *Maturation* is the physical change in the complexity of body structures that enable a child to function at increasingly higher levels. Maturity is programmed genetically and may occur as a result of several changes. For example, maturation of the central nervous system depends on changes that occur throughout the body, such as an increase in the number of neurons, myelinization of nerve fibers, lengthening of muscles, and overall weight gain.

Learning involves changes in behavior that occur as a result of both maturation and experience with the environment. Predictable patterns are observed in learning, and these patterns are sequential, orderly, and progressive. For example, when learning to walk, babies first learn to control their heads, then to roll over, next to sit, then to crawl, and finally to walk. The child's muscle mass and nervous system must grow and mature as well.

These examples show how complex and interrelated the processes of growth, development, maturation, and learning are. Children must be monitored carefully to ensure that these complicated events and activities unfold normally. Wide variations occur as children grow and develop. Each child has a unique rate and pattern of development, although parameters are used to identify abnormalities. Nurses must be familiar with normal parameters so that delays can be detected early. The earlier the delays are discovered and intervention initiated, the less dramatic their effect will be.

### Stages of Growth and Development

To simplify analysis and discussion of the complex processes and theories related to growth and development, researchers and theorists have identified stages or age-groupings. These stages serve as reference points in describing various features of growth and development

(Table 5.1). Chapters 6 through 9 discuss the physical growth and cognitive, emotional, language, and motor development specific to each stage.

**TABLE 5.1 Stages of Growth and Development**

***The Following Stages and Age-Groupings Refer to Stages of Childhood Growth and Development***

| Stage | Age |
|---|---|
| Newborn | Birth to 1 mo |
| Infancy | 1 mo-1 yr |
| Toddlerhood | 1-3 yr |
| Preschool age | 3-6 yr |
| School age | 6-11 or 12 yr |

### Parameters of Growth

Statistical data derived from research studies of large groups of children provide healthcare professionals with information about how children normally grow. Throughout infancy, childhood, and adolescence, growth occurs in bursts separated by periods when growth is stable or consistent.

Weight, length (or height), and head circumference are parameters that are used to monitor growth. They should be measured at regular intervals during infancy and childhood. The weight of the average term newborn infant is approximately 7½ lb (3.4 kg). Male infants are usually slightly heavier than female infants. The birth weight usually doubles by 6 months of age, triples by 1 year of age, and quadruples between 2 and 3 years of age. Slow, steady weight gain during childhood is followed by a growth spurt during adolescence.

The average newborn infant is approximately 20 inches (50 cm) long, with an average increase of approximately 1 inch (2.5 cm) per month for the first 6 months, followed by an increase of approximately ½ inch (1.2 cm) per month for the remainder of the first year. The child gains 3 inches (7.6 cm) per year from age 1 through 7 years and then 2 inches (5 cm) per year from age 8 through 15 years. Boys generally add more height during adolescence than do girls. Body proportion changes are shown in Fig. 5.1.

Head circumference indicates brain growth. The normal occipital-frontal circumference of the term newborn head is 13 to 15 inches (32 to 38 cm). Average head growth occurs according to the following pattern: 4.8 inches (12 cm) during the first year, 1 inch (2.54 cm) during the second year; ½ inch (1.27 cm) per year from 3 to 5 years, and ½ inch (1.2 cm) per year from 5 years until puberty. The average adult head circumference is approximately 21 inches (53 cm).

Dentition, the eruption of teeth, also follows a sequential pattern. Primary dentition usually begins to emerge at approximately 6 to 8 months. Most children have 20 teeth by age 2½ years. Permanent teeth, 32 in all, erupt beginning at approximately age 6 years, accompanied by the loss of primary teeth (see Chapter 33). Although some parents place importance on eruption of the teeth as a sign of maturation, dentition is not related to the level or rate of development.

## PRINCIPLES OF GROWTH AND DEVELOPMENT

### Patterns of Growth and Development

Growth and development are directional and follow predictable patterns (Boxes 5.1 and 5.2). The first direction of growth is cephalocaudal, or proceeding from head to tail (or toe). This means that structures

**BOX 5.1 Patterns of Growth and Development**

Although heredity determines each individual's growth rate, the normal pace of growth for all children falls into four distinct patterns:

1. A rapid pace from birth to 2 years
2. A slower pace from 2 years to puberty
3. A rapid pace from puberty to approximately 15 years
4. A sharp decline from 16 years to approximately 24 years, when full adult size is reached

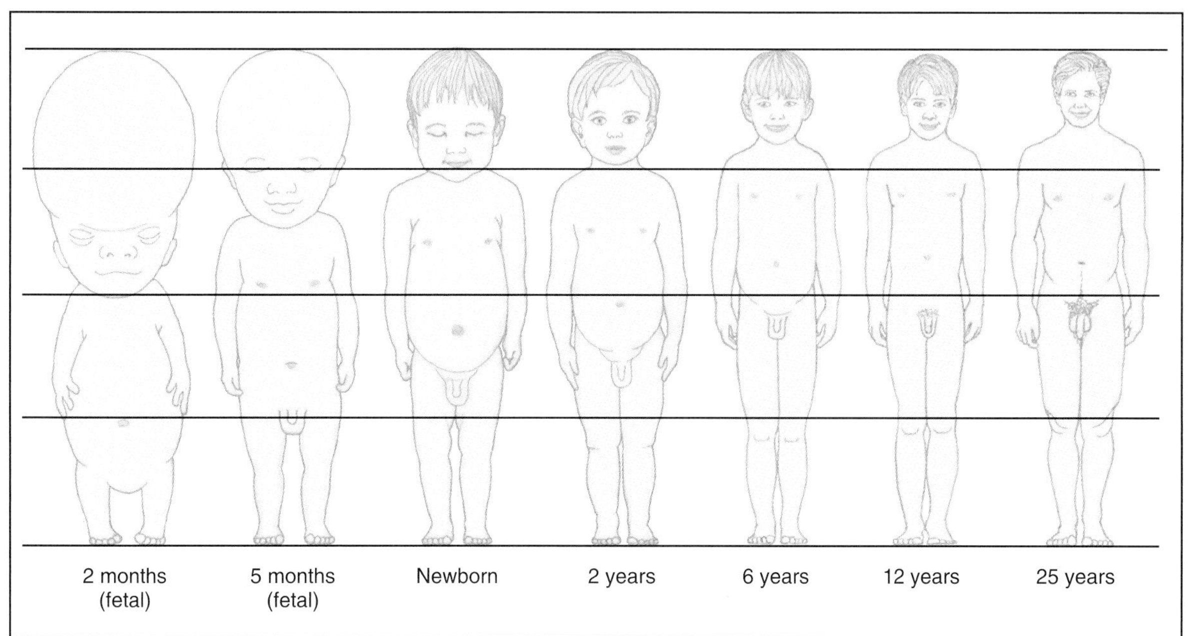


FIG 5.1 Changes in body proportions with growth.

## BOX 5.2 Directional Patterns of Growth and Development

**Cephalocaudal Pattern (Head to Toe)**

***Examples***

Head initially grows fastest (fetus), then trunk (infant), then legs (child).

Infant can raise the head before sitting and can sit before standing.

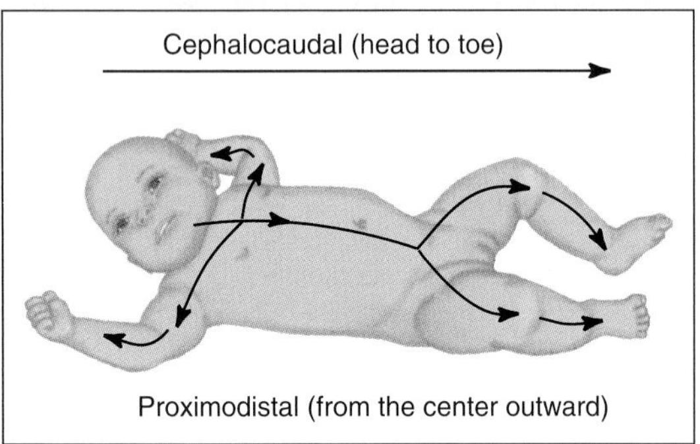


**Proximodistal Pattern (From the Center Outward)**

***Examples***

In the respiratory system, the trachea develops first in the embryo, followed by branching and growth outward of the bronchi, bronchioles, and alveoli in the fetus and infant.

Motor control of the arms comes before control of the hands, and hand control comes before finger control.

and functions originating in the head develop before those in the lower parts of the body. At birth the head is large, a full one fourth of the entire body length, the trunk is long, and the arms are longer than the legs. As the child matures, the body proportions gradually change; by adulthood, the legs have increased in size from approximately 38% to 50% of the total body length (see Fig. 5.1).

Directional growth and development are illustrated further by myelinization of the nerves, which begins in the brain and spreads downward as the child matures (see Box 5.1). Growth of the myelin sheath and other nerve structures contributes to cephalocaudal development, which is illustrated by an infant's ability to raise the head before being able to sit and to sit before being able to stand.

A second directional aspect of growth and development is **proximodistal**, which means progression from the center outward, or from the midline to the periphery. The growth and branching pattern of the respiratory tract illustrates this concept. The trachea, which is the central structure of the respiratory tree, forms in the embryo by 24 days of gestation. Branching and growth outward occur in the bronchi, bronchioles, and alveoli throughout fetal life and infancy. Alveoli, which are the most distal structures of the system, continue to grow and develop in number and function until middle childhood.

Growth and development follow patterns, one of which is general to specific. As a child matures, activities become less generalized and more focused. For example, a neonate's response to pain is usually a whole-body response, with flailing of the arms and legs even if the pain is in the abdomen. As the child matures, the pain response becomes more localized to the stimulus. An older child with abdominal pain guards the abdomen.

Another pattern is the progression of functions from simple to complex. This pattern is easily observed in language development. A toddler's first sentences are formed simply, using only a noun and a verb. By age 5 years, the child constructs detailed stories using many complex modifiers.

The rate of growth is not constant as the child matures. *Growth spurts,* alternating with periods of slow or stagnant growth, are observed throughout childhood. Spurts are frequently seen as the child prepares to master a significant developmental task, such as walking. An increase in growth around a child's first birthday may promote the neuromuscular maturation required for taking the first steps.

All facets of development (cognitive, motor, social/emotional, language) normally proceed according to these patterns. Knowledge of these concepts is useful when determining how a child's development is progressing and when comparing a child's development with normal patterns.

Mastery of developmental tasks is not static or permanent, and developmental stages do not always correlate with **chronologic age**. Children progress through developmental stages at varying rates within normal limits and may master developmental tasks only to regress to earlier levels when ill or stressed. Also, people can struggle repeatedly with particular developmental tasks throughout life, although they have achieved more advanced levels of development.

## Critical Periods

After birth, critical or sensitive periods exist for optimal growth and development. Similar to times during embryologic and fetal life, in which certain organs are formed and are particularly vulnerable to injury, critical periods are blocks of time during which children are ready to master specific developmental tasks. Children can master tasks outside these critical periods, but some tasks are learned more easily during particular periods.

Many factors affect a child's sensitive learning periods, such as injury, illness, and malnutrition. For example, the sensitive period for learning to walk seems to be during the latter part of the first year and the beginning of the second year. Children seem to be driven by an irresistible urge to practice walking and display great pride as they succeed. A child who is immobilized, for example, for the treatment of an orthopedic condition from age 10 months to 18 months, may have difficulty learning to walk. The child can learn to walk, but the task may be more difficult than for other children.

## Factors Influencing Growth and Development

### Genetics

One factor that greatly influences a child's growth and development is genetics. Genetic potential is affected by many factors. Environment influences how and to what extent particular genetic traits are manifested. See Chapter 10 for a discussion of genetics.

### Environment

The environment, both physical and psychosocial, is a significant determinant of growth and developmental outcomes before and after birth. Prenatal exposures, which include maternal smoking, alcohol intake, chemical exposures, infectious diseases, and diseases such as diabetes, can adversely affect the developing fetus. Socioeconomic status, mainly poverty, also has a significant effect on the developing child. Imported toys and other equipment for children can pose environmental hazards, particularly if they have multiple small pieces or components with high concentrations of lead or leaded paint.

Scientists suggest that factors in children's physical environment increasingly influence their health status (American Academy of Pediatrics [AAP] Council on Environmental Health, 2011). Children are vulnerable to environmental exposures for the following reasons (AAP Council on Environmental Health, 2011; Falck et al., 2015):

- Immature and rapidly developing tissue in multiple body systems, especially the neurologic system, increases the risk for injury from exposure to lower-level environmental toxins.
- Increased metabolic rate and growth, which necessitate a higher intake in relation to body mass of food and liquids, result in a higher concentration of ingested toxins.
- More rapid respirations increase inhalation of air pollutants.
- Larger body surface area enhances absorption through the skin.
- Developmental behaviors, such as mouthing or playing outdoors, increase the risk for hazardous ingestion from hand-to-mouth transfer.
- Decreased ability to metabolically clear ingested toxins.
- Environmental toxins can be passed to an infant through breast milk.

Nurses can assist parents in preventing environmental injury by teaching them how to avoid the most common sources of environmental exposure. Anticipatory guidance about avoiding sun exposure, secondhand smoke or other air pollutants, lead in the home environment and in toys, mercury in foods, use of pesticides in gardens and playground equipment, pet insecticides (e.g., flea and tick collars), and radon will provide parents with the information they need to reduce risk. As with communicable disease, teaching about the importance of hand hygiene is paramount.

During well visits, nurses can perform a brief or expanded environmental health screening. Fig. 5.2 provides an example of an environmental history. The AAP (Perrin, 2014) has expressed heightened concern that toxic chemicals in the environment are not being regulated to the extent required to protect children and pregnant women, and this position has been supported by the American Nurses' Association, the American Medical Association, and the American Public Health Association. The AAP (2011) recommends revisions to the Toxic Substances Control Act that would base decisions about toxic chemical exposures on a 'reasonable concern' for harm, especially their potential for harm to children and pregnant women (p. 988). Among other recommendations, the AAP (2011) recommends increased funding for evidence-based research to examine the effects of chemical exposures on children.

In addition to focusing substance exposure the AAP (Ahdoot & Council on Environmental Health, 2015; Perrin, 2014) has increased its focus on global climate change and its effects on children's health. Climate change affects air pollutants, water quality, environmental temperature, weather, and vector habitats. Adverse effects on children, especially the poor, could include increased respiratory conditions, illness from adverse effects on the food supply, and increased vector-borne illnesses (Ahdoot & Council on Environmental Health, 2015; Perrin, 2014). The AAP policy on global climate change recommends educating parents and politicians on its effects on children, advocating for decreased toxic emissions, reducing the carbon footprints of buildings and decreasing greenhouse gas emissions (Ahdoot & Council on Environmental Health, 2015).

Nurses can access and refer parents to several online resources, including the Environmental Protection Agency (http://www.epa.gov/children), Pediatric Environmental Health Specialty Units (PEHU) (http://www.aoec.org), Tools for Schools program (http://www.epa.gov/schools), and Tox Town (http://www.toxtown.nlm.nih.gov), among others. Nurses can advise parents to be aware of toy and equipment recalls and to suggest that parents examine toys carefully before purchasing them.

## Culture

Culture is the way of life of a people, including their habits, beliefs, language, and values. It is a significant factor influencing children as they grow toward adulthood.

When gathering data, nurses need to recognize how the common family structures and traditional values of various groups affect children's performance on assessment tests. The child's cultural and ethnic

Where does your child live and spend most of his/her time? ________

What are the age, condition, and location of your home? ________

Does anyone in the family smoke? ❑ Yes ❑ No ❑ Not sure

Do you have a carbon monoxide detector? ❑ Yes ❑ No ❑ Not sure

Do you have any indoor furry pets? ❑ Yes ❑ No ❑ Not sure

What type of heating/air system does your home have?
❑ Radiator ❑ Forced air ❑ Gas stove ❑ Wood stove ❑ Other________

What is the source of your drinking water?
❑ Well water ❑ City water ❑ Bottled water

Is your child protected from excessive sun exposure? ❑ Yes ❑ No ❑ Not sure

Is your child exposed to any toxic chemicals of which you are aware? ❑ Yes ❑ No ❑ Not sure

What are the occupations of all adults in the household? ________

Have you tested your home for radon? ❑ Yes ❑ No ❑ Not sure

Does your child watch TV, or use a computer or video game system more than two hours a day? ❑ Yes ❑ No ❑ Not sure

How many times a week does your child have unstructured, free play outside for at least 60 minutes? ________

Do you have any other questions or concerns about your child's home environment or symptoms that may be a result of his or her environment? ________

National Environmental Education Foundation
Knowledge to live by

Health & Environment

FIG 5.2 Pediatric environmental history (0 to 18 years of age). (Reprinted with permission from the National Environmental Education and Training Foundation at http://www.neefusa.org/pdf/PedEnvHistoryForm_complete.pdf.)

background must be considered when assessing growth and development. Standard growth curves and developmental tests do not necessarily reflect the normal growth and development of children of different cultural groups. Growth curves for children of various racial and cultural backgrounds are increasingly available. Nurse researchers and others conduct studies to determine the effectiveness of measurement tools for culturally diverse populations. In addition, culturally sensitive instruments are being developed to gather data to determine appropriate nursing interventions. To provide quality care to all children, nurses must consider the effect of culture on children and families (see Chapter 3).

### Nutrition

Because children are growing constantly and need a continuous supply of **nutrients**, nutrition plays an important role throughout childhood. Children need more nutritious food in proportion to size than adults do. Children's dietary and physical activity patterns can forecast the risk for later obesity. The Centers for Disease Control and Prevention (CDC) (2015b) list the major nutritional factors of concern: inappropriate food advertising directed toward children; decreased access to affordable foods, especially in inner city areas; ready availability of unhealthy sweetened beverages, including fruit drinks, which may be mistaken for 100% fruit juice; and, lack of breastfeeding support. Providing appropriate portion sizes is an important contributing factor as well, with many parents of preschool children unclear as to how much to feed them (Small et al., 2012). A complicating factor is that many parents cannot adequately control what their children are being fed because so many children eat at least one meal away from home.

### Health Status

Overall health status plays an important part in the growth and development of children. At the cellular level, inherited or acquired disease can affect the delivery of nutrients, hormones, or oxygen to organs and also can affect organ growth and function. Disease states that affect growth and development include digestive or malabsorptive disorders, respiratory illnesses, heart defects, and metabolic diseases.

### Family

A child is an inseparable part of a family. Family relationships and influences substantially determine how children grow and progress. Because of the special bond and influence of the family on the child, there can be no separation of a child from the family in the healthcare setting. For example, to diminish anxiety in a child, nurses sometimes attempt to reduce parental anxiety, which may then reduce the stress on the child. Nursing care of children involves nursing care of the whole family and requires skill in dealing with both adults and children.

Nurses might reduce parental anxiety about an ill child by saying, "Your child is in the best place possible here at the hospital. You brought him in at just the right time so that we can help him."

Family structures are in a constant state of change, and these dynamic states influence how children develop. Within the family, relationships change because of marriage, birth, divorce, death, and new roles and responsibilities. Societal forces outside the family, such as economics, population shifts, and migration, change how children are raised. These forces cause changes in family structures and the outcomes of child rearing, which must be considered when planning nursing care for children. The family is discussed in Chapter 3.

### Parental Attitudes

Parental attitudes affect growth and development. Growth and development continue throughout life, and parents have stage-related needs and tasks that affect their children. Superimposed on these developmental issues are other factors influencing parental attitudes: educational level, childhood experiences, financial pressures, marital status, and available support systems. Parental attitudes are also affected by the child's temperament or the child's unique way of relating to the world. Different temperaments affect parenting practices and have a bearing on whether a child's unique personality traits develop into assets or problems.

***Child-rearing philosophies.*** Child-rearing philosophies, shaped by myriad life events, influence how children grow and develop. For example, well-educated, well-read parents often provide their children with extra stimulation and opportunities for learning beginning at a young age. This enrichment includes extra parental attention and interaction—not necessarily expensive toys. Generally, development progresses best when children have access to enriched opportunities for learning.

Other parents may not recognize the value of providing a rich learning environment at home, may not have time, or may not appreciate this type of parenting. Children of these parents may not progress at the same rate as those raised in a more enriching atmosphere.

A significant point for parents to remember is that children must be ready to learn. If motor and neurologic structures are not mature, an overzealous approach for accomplishing a task related to those structures can be frustrating for both child and parent. For example, a child who is 6 months old will not be able to walk alone no matter how much time and effort the parent expends. However, at 12 to 14 months, a child usually is ready to begin walking and will do so with ease if given opportunities to practice.

## Theories of Growth and Development

Many theorists have attempted to organize and classify the complex phenomena of growth and development. No single theory can adequately explain the wondrous journey from infancy to adulthood. However, each theorist contributes a piece of the puzzle. Theories are not facts but merely attempts to explain human behavior. Table 5.2 compares and contrasts theories discussed in the text. The chapters on each age-group provide further discussion of these theories.

## Piaget's Theory of Cognitive Development

Jean Piaget (1896-1980), a Swiss theorist, made major contributions to the study of how children learn. His complex theory provides a framework for understanding how thinking during childhood progresses and differs from adult thinking. Like other developmental theorists, Piaget postulated that children pass through progressive stages as they develop intellectually (Piaget, 1962, 1967). The ages assigned to these periods are only averages. Piaget (1962, 1967) describes these stages as follows.

During the *sensorimotor* period of development, infant thinking seems to involve the entire body. Reflexive behavior is gradually replaced by more complex activities. The world becomes increasingly solid through the development of the concept of *object permanence,* which is the awareness that objects continue to exist even when they disappear from sight. By the end of this stage, the infant shows some evidence of reasoning.

During the *period of preoperational thought,* language becomes increasingly useful. Judgments are dominated by perception and are illogical, and thinking is characterized, especially during the early part of this stage, by egocentrism. In other words, children are unable to think about another person's viewpoint and believe that everyone perceives situations as they do. *Magical thinking* (the belief that events occur because of wishing) and *animism* (the perception that all objects have life and feeling) characterize this period.

## TABLE 5.2 Theories of Growth and Development

| | Piaget's Periods of Cognitive Development | Freud's Stages of Psychosexual Development | Erikson's Stages of Psychosocial Development | Kohlberg's Stages of Moral Development |
|---|---|---|---|---|
| ***Infancy*** | ***Period 1 (Birth-2 yr): Sensorimotor Period*** | ***Oral Stage*** | ***Trust vs. Mistrust*** | ***Premorality or Preconventional Morality, Stage 0 (0-2 yr): Naiveté and Egocentrism*** |
| | Reflexive behavior is used to adapt to the environment; egocentric view of the world; development of object permanence. | Mouth is a sensory organ; infant takes in and explores during oral passive substage (first half of infancy); infant strikes out with teeth during oral aggressive substage (latter half of infancy). | Development of a sense that the self is good and the world is good when consistent, predictable, reliable care is received; characterized by hope. | No moral sensitivity; decisions are made on the basis of what pleases the child; infants like or love what helps them and dislike what hurts them; no awareness of the effect of their actions on others. "Good is what I like and want." |
| ***Toddlerhood*** | ***Period 2 (2-7 yr): Preoperational Thought*** | ***Anal Stage*** | ***Autonomy vs. Shame and Doubt*** | ***Premorality or Preconventional Morality, Stage 1 (2-3 yr): Punishment–Obedience Orientation*** |
| | Thinking remains egocentric, becomes magical, and is dominated by perception. | Major focus of sexual interest is anus; control of body functions is major feature. | Development of sense of control over the self and body functions; exerts self; characterized by will. | Right or wrong is determined by physical consequences: "If I get caught and punished for doing it, it is wrong. If I am not caught or punished, then it must be right." |
| ***Preschool Age*** | ↓ | ***Phallic or Oedipal/ Electra Stage*** | ***Initiative vs. Guilt*** | ***Premorality or Preconventional Morality, Stage 2 (4-7 yr): Instrumental Hedonism and Concrete Reciprocity*** |
| | ↓ | Genitals become focus of sexual curiosity; superego (conscience) develops; feelings of guilt emerge. | Development of a can-do attitude about the self; behavior becomes goal-directed, competitive, and imaginative; initiation into gender role; characterized by purpose. | Child conforms to rules out of self-interest: "I'll do this for you if you do this for me"; behavior is guided by an "eye for an eye" orientation. "If you do something bad to me, then it's OK if I do something bad to you." |
| ***School Age*** | ***Period 3 (7-11 yr): Concrete Operations*** | ***Latency Stage*** | ***Industry vs. Inferiority*** | ***Morality of Conventional Role Conformity, Stage 3 (7-10 yr): Good-Boy or Good-Girl Orientation*** |
| | Thinking becomes more systematic and logical, but concrete objects and activities are needed. | Sexual feelings are firmly repressed by the superego; period of relative calm. | Mastering of useful skills and tools of the culture; learning how to play and work with peers; characterized by competence. | Morality is based on avoiding disapproval or disturbing the conscience; child is becoming socially sensitive. |
| | | | | Morality of Conventional Role Conformity, Stage 4 (begins at about 10-12 yr): Law and Order Orientation<br>Right takes on a religious or metaphysical quality. Child wants to show respect for authority, and maintain social order; obeys rules for their own sake. |

*Continued*

**TABLE 5.2 Theories of Growth and Development—cont'd**

| | Piaget's Periods of Cognitive Development | Freud's Stages of Psychosexual Development | Erikson's Stages of Psychosocial Development | Kohlberg's Stages of Moral Development |
|---|---|---|---|---|
| ***Adolescence*** | ***Period 4 (11 yr-Adulthood): Formal Operations*** | ***Puberty or Genital Stage*** | ***Identity vs. Role Confusion*** | ***Morality of Self-Accepted Moral Principles, Stage 5: Social Contract Orientation*** |
| | New ideas can be created; situations can be analyzed; use of abstract and futuristic thinking; understands logical consequences of behavior. | Stimulated by increasing hormone levels; sexual energy wells up in full force, resulting in personal and family turmoil. | Begins to develop a sense of "I"; this process is lifelong; peers become of paramount importance; child gains independence from parents; characterized by faith in self. | Right is determined by what is best for the majority; exceptions to rules can be made if a person's welfare is violated; the end no longer justifies the means; laws are for mutual good and mutual cooperation. |
| ***Adulthood*** | ↓ | ↓ | ***Intimacy vs. Isolation*** | |
| | | | Development of the ability to lose the self in genuine mutuality with another; characterized by love. | |
| | | | ***Generativity vs. Stagnation*** | ***Morality of Self-Accepted Moral Principles, Stage 6: Personal Principle Orientation*** |
| | | | Production of ideas and materials through work; creation of children; characterized by care. | Achieved only by the morally mature individual; few people reach this level; these people do what they think is right, regardless of others' opinions, legal sanctions, or personal sacrifice; actions are guided by internal standards; integrity is of utmost importance; may be willing to die for their beliefs. |
| | | | ***Ego Integrity vs. Despair*** | ***Morality of Self-Accepted Moral Principles, Stage 7: Universal Principle Orientation*** |
| | | | Realization that there is order and purpose to life; characterized by wisdom. | This stage is achieved by only a rare few; Mother Teresa, Gandhi, and Socrates are examples; these individuals transcend the teachings of organized religion and perceive themselves as part of the cosmic order, understand the reason for their existence, and live for their beliefs. |

At the end of the preoperational stage, the child shifts from egocentric thinking and begins to be able to look at the world from another person's view. This shifting enables the child to move into the *period of concrete operations,* where the child is no longer bound by perceptions and can distinguish fact from fantasy. The concept of time becomes increasingly clear during this stage, although far past and far future events remain obscure. Although reasoning powers increase rapidly during this stage, the child cannot deal with abstractions or with socialized thinking.

Adolescents normally progress to the *period of formal operations.* In this period the adolescent proceeds from concrete to abstract and symbolic and from self-centered to other centered. Adolescents can develop hypotheses and then systematically deduce the best strategies for solving a particular problem because they use a formal operations cognitive style. Newer theories of adolescent cognitive development suggest that appropriate adolescent decision-making is based on a combination of experiential and analytical thinking (Dansereau, Knight & Flynn, 2013). This theory may explain why some adolescents appear to have entered the period of formal operations and others have not, or why adolescent thinking and decision-making varies according to how they process their experiences at a given moment in time.

### Nursing Implications of Piaget's Theory

Although other developmental theorists have disputed Piaget's theories, especially the ages at which cognitive changes occur, his work provides a basis for learning about and understanding cognitive development. Piaget's theory is especially significant to nurses as they develop teaching plans of care for children.

Piaget believed that learning should be geared to the child's level of understanding and that the child should be an active participant in the learning process. For the child's optimal and active participation in learning about health or illness, nurses need to understand the different cognitive abilities of children at various ages. However, nurses should also assess each child's cognitive ability and readiness to learn, even if a child has not yet reached the expected age for a particular stage of cognitive development, because many children are capable of learning concepts more advanced than their age would suggest. Conversely, some children who might be expected to understand health issues might not have the literacy capabilities to do so (Lambert & Keogh, 2014). Nurses also need to know how to engage children in the learning process with developmentally appropriate activities. Because illness and hospitalization are often frightening to children, especially toddlers and preschoolers, nurses need to understand the cognitive basis of fears related to treatment and be able to intervene appropriately (see Chapter 35).

## Freud's Theory of Psychosexual Development

Sigmund Freud (1856-1939) developed theories to explain psychosexual development. His theories were in vogue for many years and provided a basis for other theories. Freud postulated that early childhood experiences provide unconscious motivation for actions later in life (Freud, 1960). According to Freudian theory, certain parts of the body assume psychological significance as foci of sexual energy. These areas shift from one part of the body to another as the child moves through different stages of development. Freud's work may help to explain normal behavior that parents may confuse with abnormal behavior, and it also may provide a good foundation for sex education.

Freud believed that during infancy, sexual behavior seems to focus around the mouth, the most erogenous area of the infant body (oral stage). Infants derive pleasure from sucking and exploring objects by placing them in their mouths. During early childhood, when toilet training becomes a major developmental task, sensations seem to shift away from the mouth and toward the anus (anal stage). Psychoanalysts see this period as a time of holding on and letting go. A sense of control or autonomy develops as the child masters body functions.

During the preschool years, interest in the genitalia begins (phallic stage). Children are curious about anatomic differences, childbirth, and sexuality. Children at this age often ask many questions, freely exhibit their own sexual organs, and want to peek at those of others. Children often masturbate, sometimes causing parents great concern. Although it is not universal, a phenomenon described by Freud as the Oedipus complex in boys and the Electra complex in girls is seen in preschool children. This possessiveness of the child for the opposite-sex parent, marked by aggressiveness toward the same-sex parent, is considered normal behavior, as is a heightened interest in sex. To resolve these disturbing sexual feelings, the preschooler identifies with or becomes more like the same-sex parent. The superego (an inner voice that reprimands and evokes guilt) also develops. The superego is similar to a conscience (Freud, 1960).

Freud describes the school-age period as the latency stage, when sexuality plays a less prominent role in the everyday life of the child. Best friends and same-sex peer groups are influential in the school-age child's life. Younger school-age children often refuse to play with children of the opposite sex, whereas prepubertal children begin to desire the companionship of opposite-sex friends.

During adolescence, interest in sex again flourishes as children search for identity (genital stage). Under the influence of fluctuating hormone levels, dramatic physical changes, and shifting social relationships, the adolescent develops a more adult view of sexuality. Cognitive skills, particularly in young adolescents, are not fully developed, however, and decisions are made often based on the adolescent's emotional state, rather than on critical reasoning (Dansereau et al., 2013). This can lead to questionable judgments about sexual matters and questions or confusion about sexual feelings and behaviors (A. Freud, 1974).

### Nursing Implications of Freud's Theory

Both children and parents may have questions and concerns about normal sexual development and sex education. Nurses need to understand normal sexual growth and development to help parents and children form healthy attitudes about sex and create an accepting climate in which adolescents may talk about sexual concerns.

## Erikson's Psychosocial Theory

Erik H. Erikson (1902-1994), inspired by the work of Sigmund Freud, proposed a popular theory about child development. He viewed development as a lifelong series of conflicts affected by social and cultural factors. Each conflict must be resolved for the child and adult to progress emotionally. How individuals address the conflicts varies widely. However, according to Erikson, unsuccessful resolution leaves the individual emotionally disabled (Erikson, 1963).

Each of eight stages of development has a specific central conflict or developmental task. These eight tasks are described in terms of a positive or negative resolution. The actual resolution of a specific conflict lies somewhere along a continuum between a perfect positive and a perfect negative.

Erikson (1963) describes the first developmental task as the establishment of trust. The basic quality of trust provides a foundation for the personality. If an infant's physical and emotional needs are met in a timely manner through warm and nurturing interactions with a consistent caregiver, the infant begins to sense that the world is trustworthy. The infant begins to develop trust in others and a sense of being worthy of love. Through successful achievement of a sense of trust, the infant can move on to subsequent developmental stages.

Erikson suggests that unsuccessful resolution of this first developmental task results in a sense of mistrust. If needs are consistently unmet, acute tension begins to appear in children. During infancy, signs of unmet needs include restlessness, fretfulness, whining, crying, clinging, physical tenseness, and physical dysfunctions such as vomiting, diarrhea, and sleep disturbances. All children exhibit these signs at times. However, if these behaviors become personality characteristics, unsuccessful resolution of this stage is suspected.

The toddler's developmental task is to acquire a sense of autonomy rather than a sense of shame and doubt. A positive resolution of this task is accomplished by the ability to control the body and body functions, especially elimination. Success at this stage does not mean that the toddler, even as an adult, will exhibit autonomous behavior in all life situations. In certain circumstances, feelings of shame and self-doubt are normal and may be adaptive.

Erikson's theory describes each developmental stage, with crises related to individual stages emerging at specific times and in a particular order. Likewise, each stage is built on the resolution of previous developmental tasks. However, during each conflict, the child spends some energy and time resolving earlier conflicts (Erikson, 1963).

### Nursing Implications of Erikson's Theory

In stressful situations, such as hospitalization, children, even those with healthy personalities, evoke defense mechanisms that protect them against undue anxiety. **Regression**, a behavior used frequently by children, is a reactivation of behavior more appropriate to an earlier stage of development. This defense mechanism is illustrated by a 6-year-old boy who reverts to sucking his thumb and wetting his pants under increased stress, such as illness or the birth of a sibling. Nurses can educate parents about regression and encourage them to offer their children support, not ridicule. They can provide constructive suggestions for stress management and reassure parents that regression normally subsides as anxiety decreases.

Erikson's main contribution to the study of human development lies in his outline of a universal sequence of phases of psychosocial development. His work is especially relevant to nursing because it provides a theoretic basis for much of the emotional care that is given to children. The stages are further discussed in the chapters on each age-group.

### Kohlberg's Theory of Moral Development

Lawrence Kohlberg (1927-1987), a psychologist and philosopher, described a stage theory of moral development that closely parallels Piaget's stages of cognitive development. He discussed moral development as a complicated process involving the acceptance of the values and rules of society in a way that shapes behavior. This cognitive-developmental theory postulates that, although knowing what behaviors are right and wrong is important, it is much less important than understanding and appreciating why the behaviors should or should not be exhibited (Kohlberg, 1964).

Guilt, an internal expression of self-criticism and a feeling of remorse, is an emotion closely tied to moral reasoning. Most children 12 years old or older react to misbehavior with guilt. Guilt helps them realize when their moral judgment fails.

Building on Piaget's work, Kohlberg studied boys and girls from middle- and lower-class families in the United States and other countries. He interviewed them by presenting scenarios with moral dilemmas and asking them to make a judgment. His focus was not on the answer but on the reasoning behind the judgment (Kohlberg, 1964). He then classified the responses into a series of levels and stages.

During the *Premorality* (preconventional morality) level, which has three substages (see Table 5.2), the child demonstrates acceptable behavior because of fear of punishment from a superior force, such as a parent. At this stage of cognitive and moral development, children cannot reason as mature members of society. They view the world in a selfish, egocentric way, with no real understanding of right or wrong. They view morality as external to themselves, and their behavior reflects what others tell them to do, rather than an internal drive to do what is right. In other words, they have an external locus of control. A child who thinks "I will not steal money from my sister because my mother will spank me" illustrates premorality.

During the *Morality of Conventional Role Conformity* (conventional morality) level, which is primarily during the school-age years, the child conforms to rules to please others. The child still has an external locus of control, but a concern for social order begins to emerge and replace the more egocentric thinking of the earlier stage. The child has an increased awareness of others' feelings. In the child's view, good behavior is that which those in authority will approve. If behavior is not acceptable, the child feels guilty.

Two stages, stage 3 and stage 4, characterize this level (see Table 5.2). This level of moral reasoning develops as the child shifts the focus of living from the family to peer groups and society as a whole. As the child's cognitive capacities increase, an internal sense of right and wrong emerges, and the individual is said to have developed an internal locus of control. Along with this internal locus of control comes the ability to consider circumstances when judging behavior.

Level 3, *Morality of Self-Accepted Moral Principles* (postconventional morality), begins in adolescence, when abstract thinking abilities develop. The person focuses on individual rights and principles of conscience during this stage. There is an internal locus of control. Concern about what is best for all is uppermost, and persons step back from their own viewpoint to consider what rights and values must be upheld for the good of all. Some individuals never reach this point. Within this level is stage 5, in which conformity occurs because individuals have basic rights and society needs to be improved. The adolescent in this stage gives as well as takes and does not expect to get something without paying for it. In stage 6, conformity is based on universal principles of justice and occurs to avoid self-condemnation (Colby, Kohlberg, & Kauffman, 1987; Kohlberg, 1964).

Only a few morally mature individuals achieve stage 6. These people, committed to a moral ideal, live and die for their principles.

Kohlberg believes that children proceed from one stage to the next in a sequence that does not vary, although some people may never reach the highest levels. Even though children are raised in different cultures and with different experiences, he believes that all children progress according to his description.

#### Nursing Implications of Kohlberg's Theory

To provide anticipatory guidance to parents about expectations and discipline of their children, nurses should be aware of how moral development progresses. Parents are often distraught because their young children apparently do not understand right and wrong. For example, a 6-year-old girl who takes money from her mother's purse does not show remorse or seem to recognize that stealing is wrong. In fact, she is more concerned about her punishment than about her misdeed. With an understanding of normal moral development, the nurse can reassure the concerned parents that the child is showing age-appropriate behavior.

## THEORIES OF LANGUAGE DEVELOPMENT

Human language has numerous characteristics that are not shared with other species of animals that communicate with each other. Human language has meaning, provides a mechanism for thought, and permits tremendous creativity.

Because language is such a complex process and involves such a vast number of neuromuscular structures, brain growth and differentiation must reach a certain level of maturity before a child can speak. Language development, which closely parallels cognitive development, is discussed by most cognitive theorists as they explain the maturation of thinking abilities. However, the process of how language develops remains a mystery.

Passive, or *receptive*, language is the ability to understand the spoken word. *Expressive* language is the ability to produce meaningful vocalizations. In most people, the areas in the brain responsible for expressive language are close to motor centers in the left cerebral area that control muscle movement of the mouth, tongue, and hands. Humans use various facial and hand movements as well as words to convey ideas.

Crying is the infant's first method of communication. These vocalizations quickly become distinct and individual and accurately convey such states as hunger, diaper discomfort, pain, loneliness, and boredom. Vowel sounds appear first, as early as 2 weeks of age, followed by consonants at approximately 5 months of age.

By age 2 years, children have a vocabulary of roughly 300 words and can construct simple sentences. By age 4 years, children have gained a sense of correct grammar and articulation, but several consonants, including "*l*" and "*r*," remain difficult to pronounce. For example, the sentence "The red and blue bird flew up to the tree" might be pronounced by the preschooler as "The wed and boo bud fwew up to the twee!"

The language of school-age children is less concrete and much more articulate than that of the preschooler. School-age children learn and understand language construction, use more sophisticated terminology, use varied meanings for words, and can write and express ideas in paragraphs and stories (Feigelman, 2016).

Infants learn much of their language from their parents. Children who are raised in homes where verbalization is encouraged and modeled tend to display advanced language skills. Also, in infancy, receptive ability (the understanding of language) is more developed than expressive skill (the actual articulation of words). This tendency, which persists throughout life, is important to realize when caring for children. In clinical situations, nurses must communicate what is happening to their young patients by use of simple, age-appropriate words, although the child may not verbalize understanding.

Nurses and other health providers need to assess for any concerns about a young child's language development at each well visit. Parent concern or positive family history of language problems can help identify children who may be at risk for disorders associated with altered expressive or receptive language and who might need a formal language evaluation (Siu & United States Preventive Services Task Force [USPSTF], 2015). Language development is discussed in more depth in chapters on each age-group and in Chapter 55.

## ASSESSMENT OF GROWTH

Because growth is an excellent indicator of physical well-being, accurate assessments must be made at regular intervals so that patterns of growth can be determined. Trained individuals using reliably calibrated equipment and proper techniques should perform growth measurement. Methods of obtaining accurate measurements in children are described in Chapter 33. To minimize the chance of error, data should be collected on children under consistent conditions on a routine basis, and values should be recorded and plotted on growth charts immediately.

Standardized growth charts allow an individual child's growth (length/height, weight, head circumference, body mass index [BMI]) to be compared with statistical norms. The most commonly used growth charts for boys and girls ages 2 years to 20 years are those developed by the National Center for Health Statistics. The World Health Organization growth charts are recommended for use for infants and children up to 2 years of age (available at http://www.cdc.gov/growthcharts).

Because height and weight are the best indicators of growth, these parameters are measured, plotted on growth charts, and monitored over time at each well visit. Brain growth can also be monitored by measuring infant frontal-occipital circumference at intervals and plotting the values on growth charts. It is important to relate head size to weight because larger babies have bigger heads. These measurements are routinely performed during the first 2 years of life.

BMI, which is a function of both height and weight, is an important measure of growth and overall nutritional status in children older than age 2 years. Because childhood overweight and obesity can contribute to health problems later in life, the American Academy of Pediatrics (Daniels, Hassink & Committee on Nutrition, 2015) recommends obesity prevention beginning during the prenatal period with appropriate management of maternal weight and weight gain during pregnancy. Infants and children younger than 2 years old can be screened for overweight using the weight-to-length measurement; concern is generated when that percentile exceeds the 95th. BMI charts are included in the most recent versions of charts available from the Centers for Disease Control and Prevention.

Growth rate is measured in percentiles. The area between any two percentiles is referred to as a *growth channel*. Childhood growth normally progresses according to a pattern along a particular growth channel. Deviations from normal growth patterns may suggest problems. Any change of more than two growth channels indicates a need for more in-depth assessment.

Recognition of abnormal growth patterns is an important nursing function. The earlier that growth disorders are detected, diagnosed, and treated, the better the long-term prognosis.

## ASSESSMENT OF DEVELOPMENT

Assessment of development is a more complex process than assessment of growth. To assess developmental progress accurately, nurses and health providers need to gather data from many sources, including observations and interviews, physical examinations, interactions with the child and parents, and various standardized assessment tools.

The AAP recommends that providers do a combination of developmental surveillance and developmental screening throughout a child's infancy and early childhood (Jenco, 2015). Developmental surveillance, which includes a combination of eliciting parent concerns, assessing for risks, and direct observation, is performed at every well visit during infancy and early childhood (AAP, 2016). If surveillance raises a concern, the provider refers the child for more formalized screening. In addition to developmental surveillance, formalized developmental screening with a sensitive and specific screening instrument occurs when the child is 9 months, 18 months, and 30 months of age (AAP, 2016). Using formalized screening in addition to routine surveillance can increase appropriate referrals for early intervention; however, the USPSTF (Siu & USPSTF, 2015) states there is insufficient evidence establishing benefits of routine screening of children whose parents or providers do not have developmental concerns.

Observation is a valuable method most often used to obtain information about a child's **developmental age** (level of functioning). By watching a child during daily activities, such as eating, playing, toileting, and dressing, nurses gather a great deal of assessment data. Observation of the child's problem-solving abilities, communication patterns, interaction skills, and emotional responses can yield valuable information about the child's level of development. Similarly, interviews and physical examinations can provide much information about how the child functions.

In addition to these sources of data, many standardized assessment tools are available for nurses and other healthcare professionals to use for developmental assessment. Standardized developmental tools should be both sensitive (accurately identifies developmental problems) and specific (accurately identifies those who do not have developmental problems). Additionally, they should be relatively easy to administer or to have the parent complete in a reasonable amount of time. General assessment screening instruments that meet these criteria include the Ages and Stages Questionnaire, the Infant Development Inventory, and the Parents' Evaluations of Developmental Status (PEDS), among others (Moodie et al., 2014). In general, screening tools are organized around major developmental areas (language, cognitive, social, behavioral, and motor). Many are given to parents to complete in the office setting or before the child's appointment. The Ages and Stages Questionnaire and the PEDS are considered to be reliable to administer to children with special needs; there is insufficient evidence to support reliability or validity in children whose primary language is other than English (Moodie et al., 2014).

Developmental assessment should be part of a newborn infant's assessment and of every well-child examination for several reasons. One reason is that parents want to know how their child compares with others and whether development is normal, especially if they had a difficult pregnancy or have other children who are developmentally delayed. Developmental assessment tends to allay fears. Probably the most important reason for assessment is that abnormal development must be discovered early to facilitate optimal outcomes through early intervention.

### Denver Developmental Screening Test II (DDST-II)

One, more in-depth, screening tool used for infants and young children is the Denver Developmental Screening Test II (DDST-II). The DDST-II provides a clinical impression of a child's overall development and alerts the user to potential developmental difficulties. It requires training to learn how to administer it properly.

The DDST-II, designed to be used with children between birth and 6 years of age, assesses development on the basis of performance of a series of age-appropriate tasks. There are 125 tasks or items arranged in four functional areas (Frankenburg & Dodds, 1992):

1. Personal-social (getting along with others, caring for personal needs)
2. Fine motor (eye-hand coordination, problem-solving skills)
3. Language (hearing, using, and understanding language)
4. Gross motor (sitting, jumping)

Items for rating the child's behavior are also included at the end of the test.

The test form is arranged with age scales across the top and bottom. After calculating the child's chronologic age (age in years), the test administrator draws an age line on the form. Each of the 125 tasks or items is arranged on a shaded bar depicting at which ages 25%, 50%, 75%, and 90% of the children in the research sample completed that particular item. The examiner assesses the child using the items clustered around the age line. The directions must be followed exactly during administration of the test. A score for performance on each item is recorded according to the following scale: pass *(P)*, fail *(F)*, no opportunity *(NO)*, and refusal *(R)*. At the completion of the test, the screener scores test behavior ratings (located at the bottom left of the form).

Interpretation of the test is based first on individual items and then on the test as a whole. Individual items are considered as "advanced, normal, caution, delayed, or no opportunity." Reliability and validity of the test can be altered if the child is not feeling well or is under the influence of medications. Parental presence and input as to whether the child is behaving as usual is desired (Frankenburg & Dodds, 1992).

The results of the test can be used to identify a child's developmental age and how a child compares with others of the same chronologic age. This information can be used to alert healthcare providers to potential problems. To ensure that the results are accurate, only individuals who are trained to administer the test in a standardized manner should perform testing. Training is obtained through study of the testing manual, review of the accompanying videotape, and supervised practice with children of various ages.

Although the DDST-II is widely used, it is a screening test only, not an intelligence quotient (IQ) test. It is not a definitive predictor of future abilities, and it should not be used to determine diagnostic labels. However, it is a useful tool for noting problems, validating hunches, monitoring development, and providing referrals.

## NURSE'S ROLE IN PROMOTING OPTIMAL GROWTH AND DEVELOPMENT

Nurses are particularly concerned with preventing disease and promoting health. One aspect of preventive care is providing anticipatory guidance or basic information for parents about normal growth and development as their child approaches different ages and developmental levels.

### Developmental Assessment

Nursing care for children is not complete without addressing the developmental issues that are unique to each child. Because children grow and change rapidly, the nurse must use knowledge of theories of growth and development to create plans of care for both healthy and ill children. Assessment data are collected from various sources, categorized, and analyzed with a theoretic knowledge base and clinical experience. A list of strengths and problems related to growth and development is generated. Nursing diagnoses are formulated with individualized goals, interventions, and evaluation to address specific problems that are related to, but differ from, physiologic and psychosocial needs.

#### Interview

During the initial interview, the nurse asks questions about the child's cognitive, language, motor, and emotional development. The parents' emotional state, level of education, and culture must be considered when information is gathered. For example, the nurse might use the following questions and statements when interviewing the parents of a 4-year-old child:

- What does your child like to do at home?
- Does your child know the days of the week?
- Describe your child's typical day.
- Does your child attend preschool? If so, how often?
- Can your child throw a ball, ride a tricycle, climb?
- Can your child draw pictures, color them?
- How effective is your child's use of language?
- How did your child's development progress during infancy and toddlerhood?

The nurse also assesses the child's ability to think through situations and to communicate verbally. In addition, how the child interacts with other children and adults can be a measure of cognitive abilities. The number, type, length, appropriateness, and correct use of words and sentences are also noted. Carefully observing the child in various situations, including play, provides valuable information about cognitive development.

A child's stage of emotional development can be assessed in numerous ways. From Erikson's theory, it is expected that a 4-year-old child's major conflict would be developing a sense of initiative rather than a sense of guilt. However, if the child is hospitalized, regressive behaviors might be exhibited if the anxiety of hospitalization becomes overwhelming. Questions directed to the parents, such as those that follow, could help validate inferences about the child's psychosocial development:

- What types of play activities does your child like best?
- How does your child get along with other children? With adults?
- How does your child usually handle stressful situations?
- What do you do to help your child cope with problems?
- How does your child's ability to cope compare with that of your other children?
- Is the behavior exhibited your child's usual behavior?

The nurse can also obtain valuable information from careful observation of a child who is hospitalized. The nurse should note how the child deals with pain, intrusive procedures, and separation from parents.

### Play

Although play is not work in the traditional sense, it is children's work. Play is those tasks, done to amuse oneself, that have behavioral, social, or psychomotor rewards. To adult observers, children's play may appear unorganized, meaningless, and even chaotic. However, anyone who watches carefully, quickly discovers that play is a rich activity, intricately woven with meaning and purpose. In adulthood, work is any activity during which one uses time and energy to create a product or achieve a goal. Play in childhood is similar to adult work in that it is undertaken by the child to accomplish developmental tasks and master the environment.

Play is also an important part of the developmental process. Play is how children learn about shape, color, cause and effect, and themselves. In addition to cognitive thinking, play helps the child learn social interaction and psychomotor skills. It is a way of communicating joy, fear, sorrow, and anxiety.

## Classifications of Play

Piaget (1962) described the following three types of play that relate to periods of sensorimotor, preoperational, and concrete operational functioning. These three types of play are overlapping and Piaget linked them to stages of cognitive development. Some, more current, researchers dispute the effects that play has on cognitive development; however, the complexity of variables that affect various types of play, suggest that, as a whole, play contributes positively to developmental outcomes in children (Weisberg, Hirsh-Pasek, & Golinkoff, 2013). It is also important to remember that demonstrations of play might differ according to a child's or family's culture.

*Sensorimotor*, which is also known as *functional play*, occurs when a child activates or manipulates an object and derives enjoyment from the result. The child will repeat the action for the pure fun involved. An example of this type of play is an infant throwing a spoon on the floor to see what happens, then repeats it after the parent has replaced it. This type of play is prominent during infancy, as infants begin to explore their world.

Symbolic play, which includes *pretend play*, occurs when a young child plays with an object or toy, but uses that object to represent another; for example, a pot and wooden spoon as a drum, or a cardboard box becomes a tent. The same object could become something else in a different play scenario. Pretend play also includes using objects or materials in pretend situations, such as when a child uses a toy cell phone to talk to a friend or dress-up clothes to be a policeman. There are no rules in symbolic play and the variety of play situations is only limited by the child's imagination. Symbolic play also can assist a child to adjust to a new or painful experience.

*Games* include rules and usually are played by more than one person, although some games can be played by oneself. For example, the card game solitaire is played by one person, as are many video games. Children younger than 4 years of age rarely play games with rules; games are most commonly seen in the school-age child (Piaget, 1962). Games continue throughout life as adults play board games, cards, and sports.

Through games, children learn to play by the rules and to take turns. Board games facilitate this accomplishment. Young children often make up games with unique sets of rules, which may change each time the game is played. Older children have games with specific rules; younger children tend to change the rules.

## Social Aspects of Play

As the child develops, increased interaction with people occurs. Certain types of play are associated with, but not limited to, social interaction in specific age-groups.

**Solitary play.** Solitary play is characterized by independent play (Fig. 5.3). The child plays alone with toys that are very different from those chosen by other children in the area. This type of play begins in infancy and is common in toddlers because of their limited social, cognitive, and physical skills. However, it is important for children in all age-groups to have some time to play by themselves.

**Parallel play.** Parallel play is usually associated with toddlers, although it can be found in any age-group. Children play side by side with similar toys, but there is a lack of interactive activity.

**Associative play.** Associative play is characterized by group play without group goals. Children in this type of play do not set group rules, and although they may all be playing with the same types of toys and may even trade toys, there is a lack of formal organization. This type of play can begin during toddlerhood and continue into the preschool age.

**Cooperative play.** Cooperative play begins in the late preschool years. This type of play is organized and has group goals. There is usually at least one leader, and children are definitely in or out of the group.

**Onlooker play.** Onlooker play is present when the child observes others playing. Although the child may ask questions of the players, the child does not attempt to join the play (see Fig. 5.3). Onlooker play is usually during the toddler years but can be observed at any age.

## Types of Play

**Dramatic play.** Dramatic play allows children to act out roles and experiences that may have happened to them, that they fear will happen, or that they have observed in others. This type of play can be spontaneous or guided, and it often includes medical or nursing equipment. It is especially valuable for children who have had or will have multiple procedures or hospitalizations.

Hospitals and clinics with child life specialists on staff usually have a medical play area as part of the activity room. Nurses may provide opportunities for spontaneous and guided dramatic play. The nurse may choose to observe spontaneous play or be an active participant with the child. Occasionally nurses will want to structure the dramatic play to review a specific treatment or procedure. In guided play situations, the nurse directs the focus of the play. Specialized play kits may be developed for specific procedures, such as central line care, casting, bone marrow aspirations, lumbar punctures, and surgery, using supplies related to the hospital or clinic setting.

**Familiarization play.** Familiarization play allows children to handle and explore healthcare materials in nonthreatening and fun ways (see Fig. 5.3). This type of play is especially helpful for but not limited to preparing children for procedures and the whole experience of hospitalization.

Examples of familiarization activities are as follows: using sponge mouth swabs as painting and gluing tools; making jewelry from bandages, tape, gauze, and lid tops; creating mobiles and collages with healthcare supplies; making finger puppets with plaster casting material; filling a basin with water and using tubing, syringes without needles, medicine cups, and bulb syringes for water play; decorating beds, wheelchairs, and intravenous poles with healthcare supplies; and using syringes for painting activities.

## Functions of Play

Play enhances the child's growth and development. Play contributes to physical, cognitive, emotional, and social development.

**Physical development and play.** Play aids in the development of both fine and gross motor activity. Children repeat certain body movements purely for pleasure, and these movements in turn aid in the development of body control. For example, an infant will first hit at a rattle, then will attempt to grasp it, and eventually will be able to pick up that same rattle. Next the infant will shake the rattle or perhaps bring it to the mouth.

The parent and child may make a game of repeating sounds such as "ma ma" or "da da," which increases the child's language ability. Repeating rhymes and songs can be a fun way for children to increase

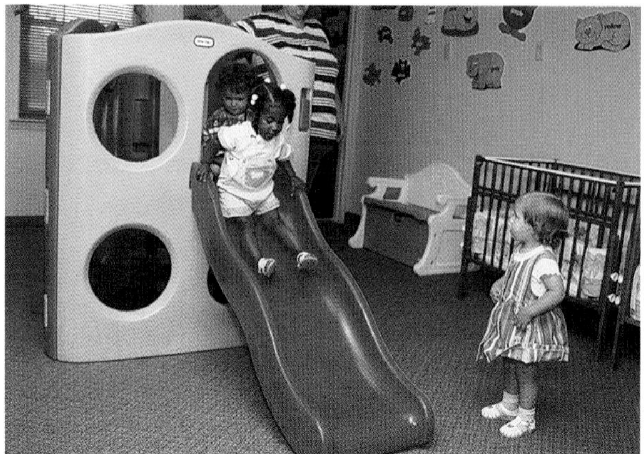

The little girl at right demonstrates onlooker play. She is interested in what is going on and observes another girl playing on the slide, but she makes no attempt to join the youngster on the slide.

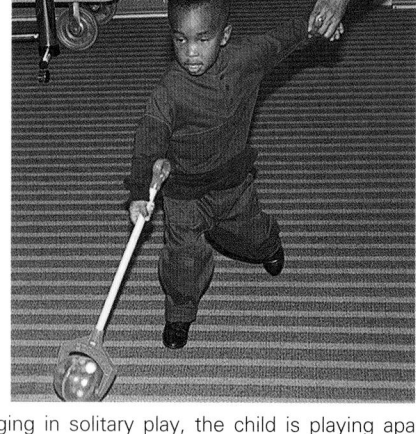

When engaging in solitary play, the child is playing apart from other children and with different types of toys. (Courtesy University of Texas at Arlington School of Nursing, Arlington, TX.)

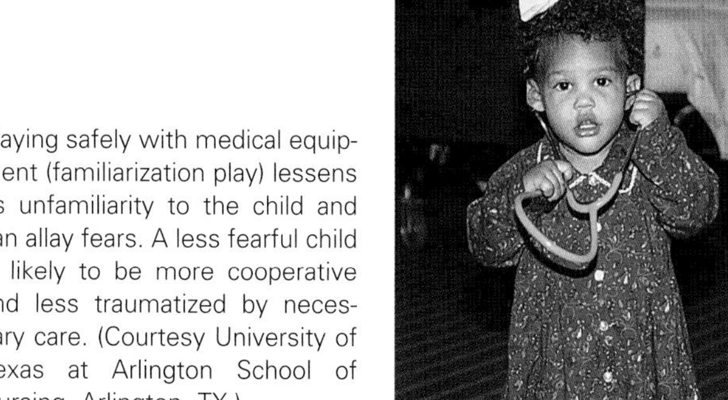

Playing safely with medical equipment (familiarization play) lessens its unfamiliarity to the child and can allay fears. A less fearful child is likely to be more cooperative and less traumatized by necessary care. (Courtesy University of Texas at Arlington School of Nursing, Arlington, TX.)

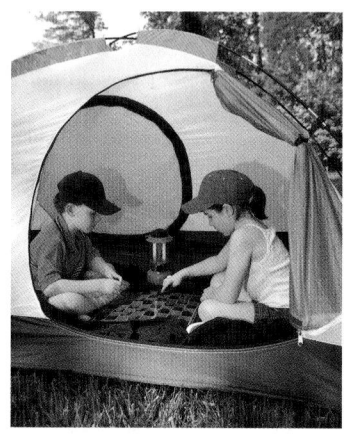

Games with rules, such as board games, help children learn boundaries, teamwork, taking turns, and competition. (©2012 Photos.com, a division of Getty Images. All rights reserved.)

**FIG 5.3** Types of play.

their vocabulary. Children love to color on a paper with a crayon and will scribble before being able to draw pictures and to color. This assists the child with eventually learning how to write letters and numerals.

***Play and cognitive development.*** Play is a key element in the cognitive development of children. Once a child has learned a general concept, further experiences with that concept expand from that beginning knowledge. Piaget gave the example of an infant learning to swing an object and then subsequently swinging other objects (Piaget, 1962). This could apply, for example, to things to be eaten, read, or ridden. Progression takes place as the child begins to have certain experiences, test beliefs, and understand the surrounding world.

Children can increase their problem-solving abilities through games and puzzles. Pretend play can stimulate several types of learning. Language abilities are strengthened as the child models significant others in role playing. The child must organize thoughts and be able to communicate with others involved in the play scenario. Children who play 'house' create elaborate details of what the characters do and say.

Children also increase their understanding of size, shape, and texture through play. They begin to understand relationships as they attempt to put a square peg into a round hole, for example. Books and videos increase a child's vocabulary while increasing understanding of the world.

***Play and emotional development.*** Children in an anxiety-producing situation are often helped by role playing. Play can be a way of coping with emotional conflict. Play can be a way to determine what is real and what is not. Children may escape through play into a world of fantasy and make-believe to make sense out of a sometimes senseless world. Play can also increase a child's self-awareness as an event or situation is explored through role playing or symbolic play.

As significant others in children's lives respond to their initiation of play, children begin to learn that they are important and cared for. Whether the child initiates the play or the adult does, when a significant person plays a board game with a child, shares a bike ride, plays baseball, or reads a story, the child gets the message, "You are more important than anything else at this time." This increases the child's self-esteem.

***Play and social development.*** The newborn infant cannot distinguish self from others, and thus, is narcissistic. As the infant begins to play with others and things, a realization of self and others begins to develop. The infant begins to experience the joy of interacting with others and soon initiates behavior that involves others. Infants discover that when they coo, their mothers coo back. Children will soon expect this response and make a game of playing with their mothers.

Playing make-believe allows the child to try on different roles. When children play "restaurant" or "hospital," they experiment with rules that govern these settings.

Of course, most games, from board games to sports, involve interaction with others. The child learns boundaries, taking turns, teamwork, and competition. Children also learn how to negotiate with different personalities and the feelings associated with winning and losing. They learn to share and to take turns (see Fig. 5.3).

*Play and moral development.* When children engage in play with their peers and their families, they begin to learn which behaviors are acceptable and which are not. Quickly they learn that taking turns is rewarded and cheating is not. Group play assists the child in recognizing the importance of teamwork, sharing, and being aware of the feelings of others.

## HEALTH PROMOTION

### Immunizations

Immunizations are effective in decreasing and, in some cases, eliminating childhood infectious diseases. Naturally occurring smallpox has been virtually eliminated, and the incidence of diphtheria, tetanus, measles, mumps, rubella, varicella, and poliomyelitis has greatly declined in the United States since vaccines against these diseases were introduced. In accordance with recommendations from the Centers for Disease Control and Prevention (CDC) and the AAP, children are immunized against 14 communicable diseases before they reach 2 years of age (CDC, 2016). In addition to those diseases mentioned previously, recommended vaccines have successfully provided protection against hepatitis A and B, *Haemophilus influenzae*, pneumococcal pneumonia, meningococcal disease, rotavirus, human papilloma virus (HPV), and pertussis (in older children and adolescents). Each year the Advisory Committee on Immunization Practices (ACIP) issues a recommended immunization schedule for children and adults in the United States; for the complete up-to-date schedule see http://www.cdc.gov. All states require immunizations for children enrolled in licensed child-care programs and school. Some states further require immunizations in the upper grades and at the time of college entrance. One group who may be overlooked includes children who receive home schooling. Therefore, it is of utmost importance that immunization records be traced and that vaccinations be given over the course of the fewest visits possible. Recommendations for some of the newer recommended vaccines follow (CDC, 2016):

- Hepatitis A vaccine is recommended for all children beginning at age 1 year (12 to 23 months). The two doses in the series should be administered at least 6 months apart. Children who are not vaccinated by age 2 years can be vaccinated at subsequent visits.
- Since the introduction of the hepatitis B vaccine, which is administered in a 3-dose series beginning shortly after birth, the childhood prevalence of hepatitis B in the United States has decreased. Much of this reduction is because of the decrease in perinatal and household transmission from adults to children. Subsequent doses of the vaccine usually are administered at 1-2 months and between 6 and 18 months of age. Four doses may be administered if the vaccine is given in combination with other vaccines given to infants.
- Diseases caused by *Haemophilus influenzae* type b (Hib), can cause meningitis in infants and young children. The World Health Organization (2011) reports that Hib infection is virtually nonexistent in industrialized nations, but is a leading cause of respiratory deaths in developing countries. Hib vaccine is administered in two or three primary doses (depending on vaccine manufacturer) followed by a booster dose at 12 to 15 months of age.
- Immunization with pneumococcal conjugate vaccine (PCV) introduced in 2000 has substantially reduced the number of cases of severe disease caused by the bacteria *Streptococcus pneumoniae*. PCV13 protects against 13 different strains of *Streptococcus pneumoniae*, and is routinely administered in four doses (at 2, 4, 6, and 12-15 months).
- Older children and adolescents can be susceptible to serious meningococcal infection, particularly those who are planning to reside in dormitories at college. Meningococcal conjugate vaccine should be administered routinely to all children at age 11 to 12 years with a booster dose at age 16 years. There are specific additional recommendations for children with health conditions that put them at increased risk (e.g., immunosuppressed, complement deficiency, asplenia).
- Rotavirus is one of the leading causes of gastrointestinal disease in infants and young children. Depending on the particular vaccine used, the dosage recommendation is for three doses given to infants at 2, 4, and 6 months of age, or two doses given at 2 and 4 months of age. Rotavirus vaccine is an oral vaccine and should not be given to children older than 8 months of age.
- Human papillomavirus (HPV) vaccine is available in various forms (2vHPV, 4vHPV, and 9vHPV). The vaccine prevents infection with certain strains of HPV that are known to be associated with later development of cervical cancer. Both boys (4vHPV or 9vHPV only) and girls receive the vaccine beginning at age 11 to 12 years. This is a 3-dose series, with the second dose administered one to two months after the first, and the third dose six months after the first dose.
- In response to an increasing incidence of pertussis (whooping cough), particularly among the adolescent population, an adult tetanus-diphtheria-pertussis (Tdap) vaccine is recommended as a booster. Pertussis can be a serious problem resulting in school absences and health consequences, including possible exposure of underimmunized infants. The dose is administered to 11- and 12-year-old children.
- Influenza vaccine is recommended annually prior to the beginning of the flu season for all healthy children beginning at 6-months of age. Household contacts of children in these groups, including siblings and caregivers, should also receive the vaccine. If not given previously, any child younger than 9 years needs to receive two doses initially, each dose being 1 month apart.

### Active and Passive Immunity

Immunizations are effective in preventing illness because of their activation of the body's immune response. *Active immunity* occurs when the body has been exposed to an antigen, either through illness or through immunization, and the immune system creates antibodies against the particular antigen. Active immunity generally confers long-term, and in some cases lifelong, protection against disease. A child acquires *passive immunity* when a serum that contains a disease-specific antibody is transferred to the child via parenteral administration (e.g., intravenous immune globulin) or, in some cases, through placental transfer from mother to infant. Protection from passive immunity is relatively short.

Live or *attenuated* vaccines have had their virulence (potency) diminished so as not to produce a full-blown clinical illness. In response to vaccination, the body produces antibodies and causes immunity to be established (e.g., measles vaccine). Killed or *inactivated* vaccines contain pathogens made inactive by either chemicals or heat. These vaccines also allow the body to produce antibodies but do not cause clinical disease. Inactivated vaccines tend to elicit a limited immune response from the body; therefore, several doses are required (e.g., polio and pertussis).

*Toxoids* are bacterial toxins that have been made inactive by either chemicals or heat. The toxins cause the body to produce antibodies (e.g., diphtheria and tetanus vaccines).

*Immune globulin* is made from the purified pooled plasma of many people. Large numbers of donors are used to ensure a broad spectrum of nonspecific antibodies. Disease-specific immune globulin vaccines are also available and are obtained from donors known to have high blood titers of the desired antibody (e.g., hepatitis B immune globulin [HBIG], rabies immune globulin [RIG]). The disadvantage of human immune globulin is that it offers only temporary passive immunity. Live vaccines must be given on the same day as immune globulin, or the two must be separated by 30 days to ensure appropriate immune response from both.

*Antitoxins* are made from the serum of animals and are used to stimulate production of antibodies in humans. Examples of antitoxins include rabies, snake bite, and spider bite. Animal serums have the disadvantage of being foreign substances, which may cause hypersensitivity reactions; thus, a history (including questions about asthma, allergic rhinitis, urticaria, and previous injections of animal serums), and skin sensitivity testing should always precede the administration of an antitoxin.

**SAFETY ALERT**

***Preventing Vaccine Reactions***

As all vaccines have the potential to cause anaphylaxis, it is imperative that the nurse ask about allergies and previous reactions before administering any vaccine.

### Obstacles to Immunizations

Major reasons identified for low immunization rates during healthcare visits are presented in Box 5.3. The media play an important part in the immunization status of children. News programs that highlight the side effects of vaccines, rather than their individual and collective protective effect, create fear and misunderstanding in the public. Healthcare providers need to address this issue when recommending various immunizations to parents. It is important for nurses to be aware of vaccine controversies and to know how to access appropriate, research-based information. The National Network for Immunization Information, an initiative of the Infectious Diseases Society of America, the Pediatric Infectious Diseases Society, the AAP, and the American Nurses Association, provides up-to-date information about immunization research. It can be accessed on-line at http://www.immunizationinfo.org.

### Informed Consent

The National Childhood Vaccine Injury Act of 1986 requires that the benefits and risks associated with immunizations be discussed with parents before immunizations. The act also requires that families receive vaccine information statements (VISs) before immunization.

All healthcare providers who administer immunizations are required by federal law to provide general information about immunizations to the child and parents, preferably in the family's native language. This information describes why the vaccine is being given, the benefits and risks, and common side effects. Before providers administer a vaccine, parents should read the federally required information about that vaccine (the VIS) and have the opportunity to ask questions (CDC, 2015d). It is necessary that the parents feel comfortable with the information and with the answers to any questions. VISs have been shown to increase the parents' knowledge level and to be beneficial. Providing the information before scheduled vaccinations allows parents the time to read all the information.

Providers are encouraged to obtain written informed consent for each vaccine administered. If signatures are not obtained, the patient's medical record should document that the vaccine information was reviewed. The CDC (2015d) recommends that providers check their state requirements for informed consent, before using the VIS as a consent form.

### Children With an Uncertain History of Immunization

When a lapse in immunization occurs, the entire series does not have to be restarted. Children's charts should be flagged to remind healthcare providers of these children's immunization status. For children of unknown or uncertain immunization status, appropriate immunization should be administered. Readministration of measles, mumps, and rubella (MMR) vaccine, Hib vaccine, or hepatitis B vaccine to someone who is immune has no harmful effects. For underimmunized children older than age seven years, one dose of the Tdap vaccine, rather than the DTaP vaccine, should be administered, followed by any necessary additional doses of Td vaccine (CDC, 2015a).

International adoptees, refugees, and exchange students should be immunized according to recommended schedules for healthy infants and children. If written records of prior immunization are not available, the child begins the schedule for children not immunized during infancy. This schedule is available through the CDC website (http://www.cdc.gov).

When taking an immunization history, the nurse should avoid asking the question, "Are your child's immunizations up to date?" This question will frequently be answered with "yes," but that does not give the nurse sufficient information. The nurse may gain more information by asking, "Can you tell me when and what was the last immunization your child had?"

### Administration of Vaccines

The manufacturer's packaging insert for each vaccine includes recommendations for handling, storage, administration site, dosage, and route. Nurses responsible for handling vaccines should be familiar with storage requirements to minimize the risk of vaccine failures. When multidose vials are used, sterile technique should be used to prevent contamination. To ensure safe administration, the vaccines should be given by the recommended route. The deltoid muscle can be used in children ages 18 months and older; for younger children and infants, the anterolateral thigh is used. Vaccines given intramuscularly need to be injected deep into the muscle mass to avoid irritation and possible necrosis.

More than one immunization may be administered at the same age or time. Some vaccines may be given as combined vaccine; several combination vaccines have been approved for use in the United States. When more than one injection is to be given, vaccines should be administered with separate syringes, not mixed into one, unless using

**BOX 5.3 Barriers to Immunization**

- *Complexity of the healthcare system,* which may lead to a delay in vaccinating children when parents become confused or frustrated with the healthcare system; special barriers include the following:
  - Appointment-only clinics
  - Excessively long waiting periods
  - Inconvenient scheduling
  - Inaccessible clinic sites
  - The need for formal referral from a primary healthcare provider
  - Language and cultural barriers
- *Expense* of immunization services
- *Parental misconceptions* about disease severity, vaccine efficiency and safety, complications, and contraindications
- *Inaccurate record keeping* by parents and healthcare workers
- *Reluctance of the healthcare worker* to give more than two vaccines during the same visit
- *Lack of public awareness* of the need for immunizations

a manufactured and approved combined vaccine. They should be given at different sites (preferably in different thighs), and the site used for each vaccine should be recorded to identify possible reactions. For infants and young children, to minimize the stress of vaccine administration, two nurses can give the vaccines simultaneously at different sites. The nurse should also record the lot number for each vaccine given. Box 5.4 lists nursing responsibilities associated with administering vaccines.

### Precautions and Contraindications

The main purpose of vaccination is to achieve immunity with the fewest possible side effects (Box 5.5). Most vaccines have no side effects; when side effects occur, they are usually mild. Fever and local irritation are not uncommon after administration of the DTaP vaccine, and fever and rash can occur 1 to 2 weeks after administration of a live-virus vaccine.

#### BOX 5.4 Nursing Responsibility in Administering Vaccines

- Know the recommended immunization schedule and the recommended alternative schedule for those with lapsed immunizations or unknown immunization history.
- Acquire up-to-date information because recommendations are revised frequently.
- Assess the family's beliefs and values to assist in the education of the family as to the rationale for immunizations, the risks and side effects, and the risks of nonimmunization.
- Take a careful history to determine possible contraindications or precautions and report any pertinent information to the practitioner. Educate the family as to the rationale for any contraindications.
- Some vaccines are combination vaccines (e.g., Pediarix—diphtheria, tetanus, pertussis, hepatitis B, and polio). Other vaccines should not be mixed. Check manufacturer's recommendations.
- Administer vaccines according to the manufacturer's recommended sites.
- Use hand hygiene before vaccine administration and between children.
- Review with the parents the common side effects and the signs of potentially severe reactions that warrant contacting the practitioner.
- Instruct the parents that they may administer age-appropriate doses of acetaminophen every 6 hours for 24 hours if the child has discomfort related to vaccine administration.
- For painful or red injection sites, advise the parents to apply cold compresses for the first 24 hours; then use warm or cold compresses as long as needed.
- Give multiple administrations in different sites and record those sites in the medical record.
- Document parental consent in the medical record. Documentation should also include the type of vaccine, date of administration, manufacturer and lot number, expiration date, administration site, any data pertinent to risks and side effects, and the signature and title of the person administering the immunization.

#### BOX 5.5 Common Misconceptions About Administration and Safety of Vaccines

The following conditions or circumstances are not contraindications to the administration of vaccines:

- Mild acute illness with low-grade fever or mild diarrhea in an otherwise healthy child.
- A reaction to a previous dose of diphtheria-tetanus-acellular pertussis (DTaP) vaccine with only soreness, redness, or swelling in the immediate vicinity of the injection site.

#### SAFETY ALERT

**_Special Considerations Related to Immunizations_**

- The preferred site for intramuscular administration of vaccines to infants and young children is the anterolateral thigh; the deltoid can be used in older children. Subcutaneous injections can be given in the thigh or upper arm.
- For intramuscular (IM) administration, use a needle of sufficient length to penetrate the muscle.
- When giving DTaP, Hib, and hepatitis B vaccines simultaneously, it is advisable to administer the most reactive vaccine (DTaP) in one leg and to inject the others, which cause less reaction, into the other leg.
- Live bacterial or virus vaccines should not be given to immunocompromised children, except under special circumstances.
- Live measles vaccine is produced by chick embryo cell culture, so there is a remote possibility of anaphylactic hypersensitivity in children with egg allergies. Most reactions from the MMR are reactions to other components of the vaccine, so MMR is not usually contraindicated for children with egg hypersensitivity (ACIP, 2011).
- Any immunization may cause an anaphylactic reaction. All offices and clinics must have epinephrine 1 : 1000 available.

However, some severe side effects have been reported. These events are usually not predictable. Because cases have been reported of development of paralytic polio in healthy children after administration of oral polio vaccine, the AAP and the CDC now recommend a full schedule of inactivated polio vaccine. Reactions to the MMR vaccine have included anaphylactic reactions, both in children with and in those without a history of egg allergy. This has prompted consideration of other possible causative agents. For example, the MMR vaccine contains neomycin, which may be the cause of the sensitivity.

Before a second dose of any vaccine is given, the nurse needs to ascertain and record whether any side effects or possible reactions occurred after the previous dose of that vaccine. The National Childhood Vaccine Injury Act of 1986 requires healthcare providers who administer vaccines to maintain permanent vaccination records and to report occurrences of certain adverse events stipulated in the act (Vaccine Adverse Event Reporting System [VAERS]). Anaphylaxis or anaphylactic shock and encephalopathy are examples of two reportable events associated with the tetanus and pertussis vaccines. Providers administering immunizations must be aware of reportable events and comply with the provisions of the act.

### Immunocompromised Children

In general, children who are immunologically compromised should not receive live bacterial or viral vaccines (e.g., MMR, varicella vaccine). There are some exceptions related to children with human immunodeficiency virus infection and in some specific instances of children in remission from cancer. Children with human immunodeficiency virus infection who are not severely compromised should receive MMR; varicella vaccine can be given, depending on the CD4+ count (see Chapter 42).

### Education

Immunization is a critical component of a child's healthcare. Knowledge of immunization schedules and an awareness of potential delays will aid the healthcare provider in identifying children who have not been fully immunized. Healthcare providers must provide parents with accurate information regarding immunizations because immunizations are the primary and safest means of managing preventable infectious diseases. All children in the United States should have access to appropriate immunization. The State Children's Health Insurance Program (see Chapter 1) and the Vaccines for Children program ensure that there are no financial barriers. Nevertheless, because access to healthcare may be difficult for certain populations, disparities in access to immunizations might result.

## Nutrition and Activity

To provide care for infants and children, the nurse needs to understand the body's nutritional needs. The body is nourished by food. Carbohydrates, fats, proteins, water, vitamins, and minerals are the basic *nutrients* in food. Carbohydrates, fats, and proteins provide energy, which is required by the cells of the body to transport all substances across the cell membrane, to synthesize substances within the cell, and to dispose of waste products.

### Carbohydrates

Carbohydrates provide most of the energy needed to maintain a healthy body. They exist in two forms, simple and complex. Complex carbohydrates should make up the majority of calories consumed. Most complex carbohydrates are found in starch from cereal grains, roots, vegetables, and legumes. The more mature the vegetable, the higher the starch content. Foods that are good sources of complex carbohydrates are relatively inexpensive and easily obtained. Insufficient calorie intake causes the body to break down protein and fat for energy and glucose production. Carbohydrates are a food source for many of the essential nutrients, including fiber, vitamins C and E, the majority of B vitamins, potassium, and the majority of trace elements.

### Fats

Fats serve as the secondary source of energy by providing 30% or less of daily calorie intake, with saturated fats comprising only 10% of total daily fat intake (United States Department of Agriculture [USDA] & United States Department of Health and Human Services [USDHHS], 2015). The Food and Drug Administration requires food manufacturers to list *trans* fat (i.e., *trans* fatty acids) on nutrition facts and some supplement facts panels. Trans fat, like saturated fat and dietary cholesterol, increases low-density lipoprotein cholesterol. Trans fat can be found in processed foods made with partially hydrogenated vegetable oils such as vegetable shortenings, some margarines, crackers, candies, cookies, snack foods, fried foods, and baked goods. Dietary fat allows the absorption of the fat-soluble vitamins (A, D, E, and K) and adds flavor to foods. The layer of fat beneath the skin plays a role in regulating body temperature. Fat is a component of cell membranes and acts as a protective padding for the internal organs. When excess calories are consumed, dietary fats are stored as excess body fat. The monounsaturated and polyunsaturated fats can increase high-density lipoprotein and decrease low-density lipoprotein cholesterol. For this reason, emphasis should be placed on replacing saturated fats with these fats whenever possible. Most whole grains, breads, pastas, and cereals are naturally low in fat. Families should be taught to choose lean meats, beans, and low-fat dairy products and to limit their intake of processed foods such as crackers, cookies, cakes, and higher-fat snacks.

### Proteins

Dietary *protein* is necessary for building and maintaining body tissues. Proteins are involved in homeostasis by working with other elements in the blood to maintain fluid balance. Many vitamins and minerals are bound to protein carriers for transport. Proteins, as antibodies, aid in the regulation of the body's immune system.

### Water

Water is essential for life. It transports nutrients to cells and waste products away from cells. It assists in the regulation of body temperature and in chemical reactions. Water lubricates joints and provides form and structure to the cells and the medium for body fluids. Water is found in most foods, including solids. Water requirements can be estimated by various methods. The child's activity level and ambient temperature influence the amount of water required.

### Vitamins and Minerals

*Vitamins* and *minerals* are necessary in the regulation of metabolic processes. They are present in a wide variety of foods. Vitamins and minerals are added to processed formulas and to other foods such as cereals. Except for vitamin D supplementation, it is generally not necessary for children to receive supplementation after infancy unless they are at nutritional risk (e.g., have anorexia or a chronic disease).

### Dietary Guidelines

The U.S. Department of Health and Human Services and the U.S. Department of Agriculture regularly publish and update dietary guidelines that are used as the basis for a federal nutrition policy. The guidelines recommend that various nutrient-dense foods and beverages within and among the basic food groups be consumed, but foods that contain saturated and trans fats, cholesterol, added sugars, salt, and alcohol should be limited (USDA & USDHHS, 2015) (Box 5.6).

The MyPlate system was developed to provide food-based guidance to help implement the recommendations of the guidelines (Fig. 5.4). The MyPlate image illustrates the recommended portion of daily nutrients in a way that children, as well as adults, can easily understand. MyPlate focuses on eating various foods to get the required nutrients and adequate energy. The dietary guidelines suggest consuming half of the daily requirements as fruits and vegetables, limiting saturated fats, sugars, and salt, using only lean meats, increasing other sources of

**BOX 5.6 Key Dietary Recommendations Specific to Children and Adolescents**

- Exclusively breastfeed infants for a minimum of 4 months and preferably 12 months; avoid introducing solid foods until 4 to 6 months of age.
- Consume whole-grain products often; at least half the grains should be whole grains.
- Children 1 to 8 years should consume 2 cups per day of milk; use fat-free or low-fat milk or equivalent milk products for children older than 2 years.
- Children 9 years of age and older should consume 3 cups per day of fat-free or low-fat milk or equivalent milk products.
- Limit juice to no more than 4 to 6 oz a day, but provide several servings of fruits and vegetables each day. Use 100% fruit juice and not juice drinks, which contain added sugar.
- Total daily fat intake should not exceed 30% to 35% of calories for children 2 to 3 years of age and 25% to 35% of calories for children and adolescents 4 to 18 years of age. Polyunsaturated and monounsaturated fatty acids, such as fish, nuts, and vegetable oils, should be the primary source of fats.
- Allow children to self-regulate food portions; do not force them to finish everything on their plate.
- Elementary school age children can be taught to read food labels.

Data from American Heart Association. (2015). *Dietary recommendations for healthy children.* Retrieved from http://www.heart.org.

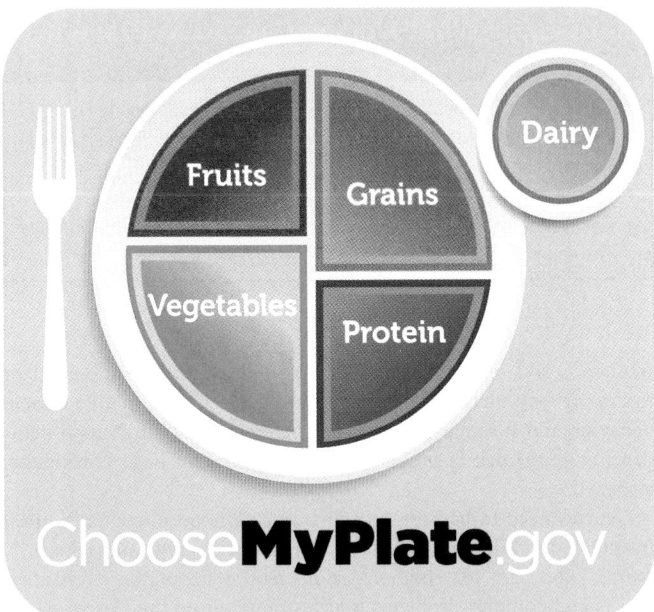


FIG 5.4 MyPlate. (Courtesy United States Department of Agriculture, Center for Nutrition Policy and Promotion. [2015]. *MyPlate*. Retrieved from http://www.choosemyplate.gov.)

protein, such as beans, and using low-fat or skim dairy products (USDA & USDHHS, 2015). Other web-based interactive tools and print materials can be accessed at http://www.choosemyplate.gov.

### Energy, Calories, and Servings

Energy is measured in calories. Energy or calorie needs depend on the person's age, sex, height, weight, and level of physical activity. Calorie needs vary during childhood. Infants need sufficient calories to support rapid growth; therefore, fat is not restricted in children younger than 2 years of age. Fat intake should be between 30% and 35% of calories for children 2 to 3 years of age and between 25% and 35% of calories for children and adolescents 4 to 18 years of age, with most fats coming from sources of polyunsaturated and monounsaturated fatty acids, such as fish, nuts, and vegetable oils (American Heart Association [AHA], 2015).

## Cultural and Religious Influences on Diet

Dietary intake is profoundly affected by both cultural and religious beliefs. An understanding of these patterns will assist the nurse in both the assessment and implementation of nutrition-related behaviors. Hospitalized children who become stressed by being in a new and strange environment do not need the added stress of unfamiliar foods. Information regarding a child's food preferences can be obtained during a dietary history.

A child's religious beliefs may also have an effect on the types of foods eaten and the way in which they are served. Within religious groups there may be various dietary observances. The nurse should assist and encourage the child and the child's family in communicating specific dietary needs.

## Assessment of Nutritional Status

A nutritional assessment is an essential component of the health examination of infants and children. This assessment should include anthropometric data, biochemical data, clinical examination, and dietary history. From these data, a plan of care can be developed. In addition, children at risk can be identified and areas of prevention pursued through teaching and further evaluation and follow-up.

### Anthropometric Data

Height and head circumference reflect past nutrition or chronic nutritional problems. Weight, midarm circumference, and BMI better reflect current nutritional status. The nurse should always be aware of the roles of birth weight and ethnic, familial, and environmental factors when evaluating anthropometric measurements. Infants and children should have anthropometric measurements done during each preventive healthcare visit.

### Clinical Evaluation

The clinical evaluation includes a physical examination and complete history. Special attention is paid to the areas where signs of nutritional deficiencies appear: the skin, hair, teeth, gums, lips, tongue, and eyes. Clinical symptoms usually are not by themselves diagnostic but may suggest conditions, which are then confirmed by biochemical tests and diet histories. More than one deficiency may be present.

### Dietary History

Obtaining an accurate history of dietary intake is difficult. The knowledge that what the child is eating is being recorded can influence what the parent feeds the child or what the child eats. Children often cannot remember what they have eaten. If the child or parent is not committed to the process, incomplete information may be obtained. However, it is still a useful assessment process and should be used. Patient teaching includes an understanding of the importance of recording the child's dietary intake and the need for accuracy. Common methods of assessing dietary intake include 24-hour recall, a food frequency questionnaire, and a food diary.

**Twenty-four-hour recall.** With the 24-hour recall method, the child or parent is asked to recall everything the child has eaten in the past 24 hours. A questionnaire may be used, or the nurse may conduct an interview asking the pertinent questions.

The child or parent may have difficulty remembering the kinds and amounts of food eaten, or the family may have had an atypical day on the previous day or may not feel comfortable relating what was eaten the day being evaluated. How the child or parents see the nurse may influence the response; they may say what they think the interviewer wants to hear. Asking for information in relation to meals eaten as opposed to food groups may increase the accuracy of the assessment.

**Food frequency questionnaire.** The food frequency questionnaire elicits information on the intake of particular foods or food groups on a daily, weekly, or monthly basis. This tool can be used to validate the 24-hour recall data. As for all methods of assessment, this requires the interviewer to be nonjudgmental and objective. Putting the information into a questionnaire may be less threatening to the child and family and will save time.

**Food diary.** When keeping a food diary, the child or parent records everything consumed during a specified period. Various sources recommend different lengths of time for keeping the diary; 3-day to 7-day records may be used. As in all nursing care, the nurse needs to evaluate what is a reasonable time to expect the family or child to keep the records. The time, place, and people present when the food was eaten may also be recorded. This provides the nurse with additional information, which may identify trends and other information related to the child's eating behaviors.

## Physical Activity

Over the past several decades, children of all ages have become less active and more sedentary. Along with dietary influences, the amount and frequency of physical activity affects a child's weight. The prevalence of overweight children ages 6 to 17 years in the United States more than tripled in the past 30 years, going from 6% in 1980 to 19%

in 2012; the rate among adolescents, ages 12 to 17 years, is 21% (Forum on Child and Family Statistics, 2015). Physical activity, dietary behavior, and genetics affect weight across all age-groups. Mexican-American children have the highest prevalence of obesity at 27% (Forum on Child and Family Statistics, 2015).

A person's BMI provides an indication of relative obesity, and this number (a function of weight and height) is being used more frequently to assess for obesity. For children, the BMI percentile for age is a more accurate measurement of overweight and obesity than the adult BMI measurement higher than 25. The CDC website (http://www.cdc.gov/growthcharts) contains information about the BMI for children of various ages.

Any health promotion counseling during childhood and adolescence needs to include an emphasis on increasing the child's and parents' daily physical activity. The USDA (2015) recommends at least 60 minutes a day of moderate to vigorous physical activity for children older than six years; at least three times a week, this activity should focus on muscle and bone-strengthening. Young children usually self-moderate activity, but need to be provided with opportunities for active play. Children particularly enjoy an activity if it is associated with fun and group involvement, and they are more likely to participate in physical exercise if they see their parents exercising as well.

When counseling parents and children about increasing physical activity, the nurse can emphasize the following points (CDC, 2015c):

- Children and adolescents should be physically active for at least 1 hour daily.
- Aerobic exercise should comprise the major component of children's daily exercise, but physical activity should also include muscle strengthening and bone strengthening activities.
- Make exercise fun and a habitual activity.
- Persuade schools to provide regular physical education classes, and encourage students to participate fully.
- Encourage parents to investigate their community's physical activity programs. City recreation centers, parks, and community YMCAs can provide fun places to engage in physical activities.

## Safety

Unintentional injury is the most significant but under recognized public health threat facing children today. Unintentional injury is the leading cause of death in children. Across age-groups, with the exception of children 1 to 4 years old, motor vehicle traffic injuries are the major causes of unintentional injury in children and adolescents; drowning is the leading cause of unintentional injury during early childhood (Federal Interagency Forum on Child and Family Statistics, 2015). (See Chapter 34 for a more detailed discussion of the causes of injury in childhood.)

The number of childhood deaths is staggering, but it is only a fraction of the number of children who are hospitalized and require emergency treatment and who have a permanent disability as a result of injury. The economic burden to society is equally astounding, reaching billions of dollars yearly. What cannot be quantified is the emotional loss, suffering, and pain the child and family must endure once an injury has occurred.

All children are at risk for injury because of their normal curiosity, impulsiveness, and impatience. Everywhere they venture, they are exposed to potentially hazardous situations.

### Injury Prevention

Injury prevention is a relatively new focus of health promotion. The term *accident,* with its implied meaning of random chance or lack of responsibility, has been replaced with *injury,* with its implication that injuries have causes that can be modified to prevent or lessen their frequency and severity. Safety education is a critical component of injury prevention. It increases awareness, it attempts to modify human behavior, and it reinforces changes implemented through legal mandates (e.g., seatbelt laws) or product modification (e.g., crib design, airbags).

Nurses need to become proactive in childhood injury prevention by increasing children's and adults' awareness of safety issues (Box 5.7). Nurses who care for children are acutely aware of the devastating effects and complex problems injuries cause. From their experiences, they become well-informed advocates for childhood safety.

**BOX 5.7 What Nurses Can Do to Prevent Childhood Injuries**

- Model safety practices in the home, workplace, and community.
- Educate parents and children through anticipatory safety guidance to help reduce needless injuries.
- Support legislative efforts that advocate prevention measures.
- Collaborate with other healthcare providers to promote safety and injury prevention.

### Anticipatory Guidance

To be most effective in providing anticipatory safety guidance, nurses must gear educational strategies to the child's level of growth and development. Knowledge of growth and development also helps the nurse understand the risks associated with each age-group and choose the educational strategy appropriate to a child's developmental level.

Early in their parenting experience, parents need to know how to provide a safe environment for their children and what behaviors they can expect at various developmental levels. Anticipatory guidance builds on the safety principles of the previous stage. Awareness of a child's changing capabilities allows the parent to be more alert and reactive to safety hazards that the child is likely to encounter. This awareness is especially important for first-time parents.

Simply telling parents to "watch your children" or to "child-proof" the home or telling a child to "be careful" has little educational impact. Educational efforts are much more likely to be effective if they focus on specific problems with specific solutions rather than providing broad or vague advice.

**SAFETY ALERT**

***Relationship Between Safety and Childhood Development***

Developmentally, children are vulnerable to injury for the following reasons:

- Children are naturally curious and enjoy exploring their surroundings.
- Children are driven to test and master new skills.
- Children frequently attempt activities before they have developed the cognitive and physical skills required to accomplish the task safely.
- Children often assert themselves and challenge rules.
- Children develop a strong desire for peer approval as they grow older.

### Teaching Strategies

Teaching can be formal or informal, simple or elaborate, as long as it provides relevant safety information and coincides with the child's or parents' cognitive abilities. For children younger than 5 or 6 years, it is advisable to incorporate the parents into the teaching process so that the parents can assist with reinforcement or questions the child later has about the safety issue. With younger children, who are easily distracted, the information should be presented in short sessions.

Many local and national organizations have safety information available for distribution. This information can be used to supplement the teaching process. Prepared materials range from pamphlets, booklets, posters, and audiovisual materials to entire teaching programs that can assist in providing injury prevention education to all age-groups. Some programs offer the materials free of cost. Internet information, such as that obtained at http://www.kidsafefoundation.org, can be extremely helpful to parents.

## KEY CONCEPTS

- Growth, development, maturation, and learning are complex, interrelated processes that produce complicated series of changes in individuals from conception to death.
- Growth and development proceed from simple to complex, from proximal to distal, and from head to lower extremities.
- As children grow and develop, wide variations within normal limits occur.
- Weight, height, and head circumference, common parameters used to monitor growth, should be measured and evaluated at regular intervals.
- The earlier that delays and deviations from normal are treated, the less severe the effect will be on growth and developmental outcomes.
- Numerous factors, including genetics, environment, culture, nutrition, health status, and family structure, affect how children grow and develop.
- Piaget's theory of cognitive development describes how children learn to deal with their environment through thinking and reasoning. Progress in learning during various periods is based on the child's ability to create patterns of understanding and behavior.
- Freud's psychosexual theory attempts to explain how humans struggle in both conscious and unconscious ways to become individual beings. During each stage of sexual development in children, a different area of the body is the focus of attention and pleasure.
- Erikson's theory of psychosocial development describes a series of crises emerging at specific times and in a particular order. These stages occur throughout life, and each must be resolved for an individual to progress emotionally.
- Kohlberg discusses moral development as a complex process involving progressive acceptance of the values and rules of society in a way that determines behavior. A maturing individual becomes less concerned with avoiding punishment and more interested in human rights and universal justice.
- Language development, a complex process involving extensive neuromuscular maturation, begins as undifferentiated crying at birth and proceeds throughout life to provide a vehicle for communication, thought, and creativity.
- Various screening tools are used by nurses to gain an overall picture of a child's developmental progress and to alert the nurse to potential developmental delays.
- Both developmental surveillance and formal screening at 9, 18, and 24 to 30 months improve health providers' assessment and identification of children with developmental delays.
- To provide high-quality, developmentally appropriate care to children and parents, nurses must be aware of normal patterns of growth and development.
- Piaget described three types of play, related to periods of sensorimotor, preoperational, and concrete operational functioning: practice play, symbolic play, and games.
- Play enhances the child's growth and development through physical, cognitive, emotional, social, and moral development.
- Personnel who administer and handle vaccines must be aware of recommendations for handling, storing, and administering the vaccines. Special attention should be given to the site of administration, dosage, and route.
- When a lapse in immunization occurs, the entire series does not have to be restarted.
- Children who are immunologically compromised generally should not receive live bacterial or viral vaccines.
- The six basic nutrients are carbohydrates, protein, fat, vitamins, minerals, and water.
- Components of a nutritional assessment are anthropometric data, biochemical data, clinical examination, and dietary history.
- Many childhood injuries and deaths are predictable and preventable.
- Understanding the developmental milestones of each age-group is important for promoting safety awareness for parents, caregivers, and children.

## REFERENCES AND READINGS


Advisory Committee for Immunization Practices. (2011). General recommendations on immunization: Recommendations of the Advisory Committee on Immunization Practices (ACIP). *Morbidity and Mortality Weekly Report*, *60*, 1–60.

Ahdoot, S. & Council on Environmental Health. (2015). Address causes of climate change to alleviate effects on children: AAP. *AAP News*. Retrieved from http://www.aappublications.org.

American Academy of Pediatrics. (2016). Recommendations for preventive pediatric health care. *Pediatrics*, *137*(1), 25–27.

American Academy of Pediatrics Council on Environmental Health. (2011). Policy statement: Chemical management policy, prioritizing children's health. *Pediatrics*, *127*, 983–990.

American Heart Association. (2015). *Dietary recommendations for healthy children*. Retrieved from http://www.heart.org.

Centers for Disease Control and Prevention. (2015a). *Catch-up immunization schedule for persons age 4 months through 18 years who start late or who are more than 1 month behind United States 2015*. Retrieved from http://www.cdc.gov

Centers for Disease Control and Prevention. (2015b). *Childhood obesity causes and consequences*. Retrieved from http://www.cdc.gov

Centers for Disease control and Prevention. (2015c). *Making physical activity part of a child's life*. Retrieved from http://www.cdc.gov.

Centers for Disease Control and Prevention. (2015d). *Vaccine information statements (VIS), Frequently asked questions*. Retrieved from http://www.cdc.gov.

Centers for Disease Control and Prevention. (2016). *Recommended immunization schedule for persons aged 0 through 18 years United States, 2016*. Retrieved from http://www.cdc.gov.

Colby, A., Kohlberg, L., & Kauffman, K. (1987). Theoretical introduction to the measurement of moral judgment. In A. Colby, & L. Kohlberg (Eds.), *The measurement of moral judgment* (Vol. 1). Cambridge, England: Cambridge University Press.

Daniels, S., Hassink, S., & Committee on Childhood Nutrition. (2015). The role of the pediatrician in primary prevention of obesity. *Pediatrics, 136*(1), e275–e292.

Dansereau, D., Knight, D., & Flynn, P. (2013). Improving adolescent judgment and decision-making. *Professional Psychology: Research and Practice, 44*(4), 274–282.

Erikson, E.H. (1963). *Childhood and society* (2nd ed.). New York: Norton.

Federal Interagency Forum on Child and Family Statistics. (2015). *America's children: Key national indicators of well-being, 2015.* Retrieved from http://www.childstats.gov

Feigelman, S. (2016). Middle childhood. In R. Kliegman, B. Stanton, J. St. Geme, & N. Schor (Eds.), *Nelson textbook of pediatrics* (20th ed., Chapter 13). Philadelphia: Elsevier.

Falck, A., Mooney, S., Kapoor, S., et al. (2015). Developmental exposure to environmental toxicants. *Pediatric Clinics of North America, 62*(5), 1173–1197.

Frankenburg, W.K., & Dodds, J.B. (1992). *Denver II screening manual.* Denver: Developmental Materials.

Freud, A. (1974). *Introduction to psychoanalysis.* New York: International Universities Press.

Freud, S. (1960). *The ego and the id (J. Riviere, Trans.).* New York: Norton, (Original work published 1923.).

Garvey, C. (1979). What is play? In P. Chance (Ed.), *Learning through play* New York: Gardner Press.

Jenco, M. (2015, July). Academy stands by its screening recommendations. *AAP News.* Retrieved from http://www.aapnews.org.

Kohlberg, L. (1964). Development of moral character. In M. Hoffman, & L. Hoffman (Eds.), *Review of child development research* (Vol. 1). New York: Russell Sage Foundation.

Kohlberg, L. (1984). *The psychology of moral development.* San Francisco: Harper & Row.

Lambert, V., & Keough, D. (2014). Health literacy and its importance for effective communication. Part 2. *Nursing of Children and Young People, 26*(4), 32–36.

Moodie, S., Daneri, P., Goldhagen, S., et al. (2014). *Early childhood developmental screening: A compendium of measures for children ages birth to five* (OPRE Report 201411). Washington, DC: Office of Planning, Research and Evaluation, Administration for Children and Families, U.S. Department of Health and Human Services

Perrin, J. (2014). Pediatric environmental health: Climate change and toxic exposures. *AAP News, 35*(10), 1.

Piaget, J. (1962). *Play, dreams and imitation childhood.* New York: Norton.

Piaget, J. (1967). *Six psychological studies.* New York: Random House.

Siu, A. & United States Preventive Services Task Force. (2015). Screening for speech and language delay and disorders in children aged 5 years or younger: United States Preventive Task Force recommendation statement. *Pediatrics, 136*(2), e474–e481.

Small, L., Bonds-McClain, D., Vaughan, L., et al. (2012). A parent-directed portion education intervention for young children: Be beary healthy. *Journal for Specialists in Pediatric Nursing, 17,* 312–320.

United States Department of Agriculture & United States Department of Health and Human Services. (2015). *Dietary guidelines for Americans, 2015-2020* (8th ed.). Retrieved from http://www.health.gov/dietaryguidelines/2015.

Weisberg, D., Hirsh-Pasek, K., & Golinkoff, R. (2013). Embracing complexity: Rethinking the relation between play and learning: Comment on Lillard et al. (2013). *Psychological Bulletin, 139*(1), 35–39.

World Health Organization. (2011). *Invasive Hib disease prevention.* Retrieved from http://www.who.int.

6

# Health Promotion for the Infant

http://evolve.elsevier.com/McKinney/mat-ch/

## LEARNING OBJECTIVES

*After studying this chapter, you should be able to:*

- Describe the physiologic changes that occur during infancy.
- Describe the infant's motor, psychosocial, language, and cognitive development.
- Discuss common problems of infancy such as separation anxiety, sleep problems, irritability, and colic.
- Discuss the importance of immunizations and recommended immunization schedules for infants.
- Provide parents with anticipatory guidance for common concerns during infancy, such as immunizations, nutrition, elimination, dental care, sleep, hygiene, safety, and play.

During no time after birth does a human being grow and change as dramatically as during infancy. Beginning with the newborn period and ending at 1 year, the infancy period, a child grows and develops from a tiny bundle of physiologic needs to a dynamo that is capable of locomotion and language and ready to embark on the adventures of the toddler years.

## GROWTH AND DEVELOPMENT OF THE INFANT

Although adults have historically considered infants unable to do much more than eat and sleep, it is now well documented that even young infants can organize their experiences in meaningful ways and adapt to changes in the environment. Evidence shows that infants form strong bonds with their caregivers, communicate their needs and wants, and socially interact. By the end of the first year of life, infants can independently move, elicit responses from adults, communicate through the use of rudimentary language, and solve simple problems.

Infancy is characterized by the need to establish harmony between the self and world. To achieve this harmony, the infant requires food, warmth, comfort, oral satisfaction, environmental stimulation, and opportunities for self-exploration and self-expression. Competent caregivers satisfy the needs of helpless infants, providing a warm, nurturing relationship so that the children have a sense of trust in the world and in themselves. These challenges make infancy an exciting yet demanding period for both child and parents.

Nurses play an important role in promoting and maintaining health in infants. Although the infant mortality rate in the United States has markedly declined over the past 30 years (see Chapter 1), many infants still die before the first birthday (nearly 6 per 1000 live births). The leading cause of death in infants younger than 1 year is congenital anomalies, followed by conditions related to prematurity or low birth weight (National Center for Health Statistics [NCHS], 2016). Sudden infant death syndrome (SIDS), which for a long time was the second leading cause of infant deaths, is now the fourth leading cause of death (NCHS, 2016), primarily because of international efforts, such as the *Back to Sleep* campaign. Unintentional injuries rank fifth in this age group and contribute to mortality and morbidity rates in the infant population (NCHS, 2016). Nurses provide anticipatory guidance for families with infants to reduce morbidity and mortality rates.

During the first year after birth, the infant's development is dramatic as he or she grows toward independence. Knowledge regarding developmental milestones helps caregivers determine whether the baby is growing and maturing as expected. The nurse needs to remember that these markers are averages and that healthy infants often vary. Some infants reach each milestone later than most. Knowledge of normal growth and development helps the nurse promote children's safety. Nurses teach parents to prepare for the child's safety before the child reaches each milestone.

Providing parents with information about immunizations, feeding, sleep, hygiene, safety, and other common concerns is an important nursing responsibility. Appropriate anticipatory guidance can assist with achieving some of the goals and objectives determined by the U.S. government to be important in improving the overall health of infants. Nurses are in a good position to offer anticipatory guidance on the basis of the infant's growth and achievement of developmental milestones. Table 6.1 summarizes growth and development during infancy.

### Physical Growth and Maturation of Body Systems

Growth is an excellent indicator of overall health during infancy. Although growth rates are variable, infants usually double their birth weight by 6 months and triple it by 1 year of age. From an average birth weight of 7½ to 8 lb (3.4 to 3.6 kg), neonates lose 10% of their body weight shortly after birth but regain birth weight by 2 weeks. During the first 5 to 6 months, the average weight gain is 1½ lb (0.68 kg) per month. Throughout the next 6 months, the weight increase is approximately 1 lb (0.45 kg) per month. Weight gain in formula-fed infants is slightly greater than in breastfed infants.

During the first 6 months, infants increase their birth length by approximately 1 inch (2.54 cm) per month, slowing to ½ inch (1.27 cm)/month over the next 6 months. By 1 year of age, most infants have increased their birth length by 50%.

The head circumference growth rate during the first year is approximately 5/10 inch (1.2 cm) per month. The posterior fontanel usually closes by 2 to 3 months of age, whereas the larger anterior fontanel

## HEALTH PROMOTION

### Healthy People 2020 *Objectives for Infants*

| | |
|---|---|
| MICH-20 | Increase the proportion of infants who are put to sleep on their back. |
| MICH-21 | Increase the percentage of infants who are breastfed, especially those exclusively breastfed. |
| MICH-29 | Increase the percentage of infants and children who are screened appropriately and referred for autism spectrum disorder and other developmental delays. |
| AHS-5 | Increase the percentage of infants and children who have an ongoing source of medical care. |
| EH-8 | Reduce blood lead levels in infants and children. |
| IID-7 | Achieve and maintain effective vaccination coverage levels for universally recommended vaccines among young children. |
| IVP-11 | Reduce deaths caused by unintentional injuries. |
| IVP-15 | Increase use of age-appropriate vehicle restraint systems. |
| ENT-VSL-1 | Increase the proportion of newborns who are screened for hearing loss by 1 month of age, have audiologic evaluation by age 3 months, and are enrolled in appropriate intervention services no later than age 6 months. |

Modified from U.S. Department of Health and Human Services. (2010). *Healthy People 2020.* Retrieved from http://www.healthypeople.gov.

may remain open until 18 months. Head circumference and fontanel measurements indicate brain growth and are obtained, along with height and weight, at each well-baby visit. Chapter 33 discusses growth-rate monitoring throughout infancy.

In addition to height and weight, organ systems grow and mature rapidly in the infant. Although body systems are developing rapidly, the infant's organs differ from those of older children and adults in both structure and function. These differences place the infant at risk for problems that might not be expected in older individuals. For example, the immature respiratory and immune systems place the infant at risk for various infections, and the immature renal system increases the risk of fluid and electrolyte imbalances. Knowledge of these differences provides the nurse with important rationales on which to base anticipatory guidance and specific nursing interventions.

### Neurologic System

Brain growth and differentiation occur rapidly during the first year of life, and they depend on nutrition and the function of the other organ systems. At birth, the brain accounts for approximately 10% to 12% of body weight. By 1 year of age, the brain has doubled its weight, with a major growth spurt occurring between 15 and 20 weeks of age and another between 30 weeks and 1 year of age. Increases in the number of synapses and expanded myelinization of nerves contribute to maturation of the neurologic system during infancy. Primitive reflexes disappear as the cerebral cortex thickens and motor areas of the brain

**TABLE 6.1 Summary of Growth and Development: the Infant**

| Physical | Motor | Psychosocial | Sensory/Cognitive | Language/ Communication |
|---|---|---|---|---|
| ***1-2 Mo*** | | | | |
| Fast growth; weight gain of 1½ lb (0.68 kg) per month and height gain of 1 in (2.54 cm) per month during first 6 mo.<br>Upper limbs and head grow faster.<br>Primitive reflexes present; strong suck and gag reflex.<br>Obligate nose breather.<br>Posterior fontanel closes by 2-3 mo. | **Gross**<br>May lift head when held against shoulder.<br>Head lag.<br>**Fine**<br>Palmar grasp. *1 mo:* Immediately drops object placed in hand.<br>Fist usually clenched (grasp reflex).<br>*2 mo:* Holds objects momentarily.<br>Hands often open (grasp reflex fading). | Erikson's stage of trust vs. mistrust.<br>Infant learns that world is good and "I am good."<br>This stage is the foundation for other stages.<br>Child is entirely dependent on parents and other caregivers.<br>Needs should be met in a timely fashion.<br>Touch is important. | Piaget's sensorimotor phase.<br>*1 mo:* Notes bright objects if in line of vision.<br>Vision 20/100.Reflexes dominate behavior.<br>*2 mo:* Begins to follow objects. | Strong cry.<br>Throaty sounds.<br>Responds to human faces.<br>*6-8 wk:* Begins to smile in response to stimuli. |
| ***3 Mo*** | | | | |
| Primitive reflexes fading. | **Gross**<br>Can get hand to mouth.<br>Can lift head off bed when in prone position.<br>Head lag still present but decreasing.<br>**Fine**<br>Holds objects placed in hands.<br>Grasp reflex absent. | Smiles in response to others.<br>Uses sucking to soothe self. | Follows an object with eyes.<br>Plays with fingers. | Babbles, coos.<br>Enjoys making sounds.<br>Responds to voices, watches speaker. |

**TABLE 6.1 Summary of Growth and Development: the Infant—cont'd**

| Physical | Motor | Psychosocial | Sensory/Cognitive | Language/ Communication |
|---|---|---|---|---|
| ***4-5 Mo*** | | | | |
| Can breathe when nose is obstructed.<br>Growth rate declines.<br>Drooling begins in preparation for teething.<br>Moro, tonic neck, and rooting reflexes have disappeared. | **Gross**<br>Plays with feet; puts foot in mouth.<br>Bears weight when held in a standing position.<br>Turns from abdomen to back.<br>**Fine**<br>Begins reaching and grasping with palm.<br>Hits at object, misses. | Mouth is a sensory organ used to explore environment.<br>Attachment is continuing process throughout infancy.<br>Has increased interest in parent, shows trust, knows parent.<br>Shows emotions of fear and anger. | *4 mo:* Brings hands together at midline. Vision 20/80.<br>Begins to play with objects.<br>Recognizes familiar faces.<br>Turns head to locate sounds.<br>Shows anticipation and excitement.<br>Memory span is 5-7 min.<br>Plays with favorite toys. | Crying becomes differentiated.<br>Babbling is common.<br>*4 mo:* Begins consonant sounds: *H, N, G, K, P, B.*<br>*5 mo:* Makes vowel sounds: *ee, ah, ooh.* |
| ***6-7 Mo*** | | | | |
| Weight gain slows to 1 lb (0.45 kg) per month.<br>Length gain of ½ in (1.27 cm)/month. Birth weight doubles; tooth eruption begins; chewing and biting occur.<br>Maternal iron stores are depleted. | **Gross**<br>Sits, leaning forward on both hands; when supine, lifts head off table.<br>Turns from back to abdomen.<br>**Fine**<br>Transfers objects from one hand to the other.<br>Picks up object well with the whole hand. | Smiles at self in mirror.<br>Plays peek-a-boo.<br>Begins to show stranger anxiety. | Can fixate on small objects.<br>Adjusts posture to see.<br>Responds to name.<br>Exhibits beginning sense of object permanence.<br>Recognizes parent in other clothes, places. Is alert for 1½-2 hr. | Produces vowel sounds and chained syllables.<br>Begins to imitate sounds.<br>Belly laughs.<br>Babbles (one syllable) with pleasure.<br>Calls for help.<br>"Talks" to toys and image in mirror. |
| ***8-9 Mo*** | | | | |
| Continues to gain weight, length.<br>Patterns of bladder and bowel elimination begin to become more regular. | **Gross**<br>Sits steadily unsupported.<br>Can crawl and pull up.<br>**Fine**<br>Pincer grasp develops.<br>Reaches for toys.<br>Rakes for objects and releases objects. | Stranger anxiety is at its height.<br>Separation anxiety is increasing.<br>Follows parent around the house. | Beginning development of depth perception.<br>Object permanence continues to develop.<br>Uses hands to learn concepts of in and out. | Stringing together of vowels and consonants begins.<br>First few words begin to have meaning (Mama, Dada, bye-bye, baby).<br>Begins to understand and obey simple commands, such as, "Wave bye-bye."<br>Responds to "No!"<br>Shouts for attention. |
| ***10-12 Mo*** | | | | |
| *12 mo:* Birth weight triples; birth length increases by 50%.<br>Head and chest circumference equal.<br>Babinski reflex disappears. | **Gross**<br>Can stand alone.<br>Can walk with one hand held but crawls to get places quickly.<br>**Fine**<br>Releases hold on cup.<br>*10 mo:* Finger-feeds self.<br>*12 mo:* Feeds self with spoon.<br>Holds crayon to mark on paper.<br>*12 mo:* Pincer grasp is complete. | Has mood changes.<br>Quiets self.<br>Is quieted by music.<br>Tenderly cuddles toy. | Vision 20/40.Searches for hidden toy.<br>Explores boxes, inserts objects in container.<br>Symbol recognition is developing (enjoys books). | Can say two or more words.<br>Says "Mama" or "Dada" specifically.<br>Waves bye-bye.<br>Begins to differentiate between words.<br>Enjoys jabbering.<br>Vocalization decreases when walking.<br>Knows own name. |

continue to develop, proceeding in a cephalocaudal pattern: arms first, then legs.

## Respiratory System

In the first year of life, the lungs increase to three times their weight and six times their volume at birth. In the newborn infant, alveoli number approximately 20 million, increasing to the adult number of 300 million by age 8 years. During infancy, the trachea remains small, supported only by soft cartilage.

The diameter and length of the trachea, bronchi, and bronchioles increase with age. However, these tiny, collapsible air passages leave infants vulnerable to respiratory difficulties caused by infection or foreign bodies. The eustachian tube is short and relatively horizontal, increasing the risk for middle ear infections.

### Cardiovascular System

The cardiovascular system undergoes dramatic changes in the transition from fetal to extrauterine circulation. Fetal shunts close, and pulmonary circulation increases drastically (see Chapter 46). During infancy, the heart doubles in size and weight, the heart rate gradually slows, and blood pressure increases.

**SAFETY ALERT**

***Risks Caused by the Infant's Immature Body Systems***

An immature respiratory system places the infant at risk for respiratory infection.
An immature immune system places the infant at risk for infection.
An immature renal system places the infant at risk for fluid and electrolyte imbalance.

### Immune System

Transplacental transfer of maternal antibodies supplements the infant's weak response to infection until approximately 3 to 4 months of age. Although the infant begins to produce immunoglobulins (Igs) soon after birth, by 1 year of age the infant has only approximately 60% of the adult IgG level, 75% of the adult IgM level, and 20% of the adult IgA level. Breast milk transmits additional IgA protection. The activity of T lymphocytes also increases after birth. Although the immune system matures during infancy, maximum protection against infection is not achieved until early childhood. This immaturity places the infant at risk for infection.

### Gastrointestinal System

The stomach capacity of a neonate is approximately 10 to 20 mL; with feedings, the capacity increases rapidly to approximately 200 mL at 1 year of age. In the gastrointestinal system, enzymes needed for the digestion and absorption of proteins, fats, and carbohydrates mature and increase in concentration. Although the newborn infant's gastrointestinal system is capable of digesting protein and lactose, the ability to digest and absorb fat does not reach adult levels until approximately 6 to 9 months of age.

### Renal System

Kidney mass increases threefold during the first year of life. Although the glomeruli enlarge considerably during the first few months, the glomerular filtration rate remains low. Thus, the kidney is not effective as a filtration organ or efficient in concentrating urine until after the first year of life. Because of the functional immaturity of the renal system, the infant is at great risk for fluid and electrolyte imbalance.

## Motor Development

During the first few months after birth, muscle growth and weight gain allow for increased control of reflexes and more purposeful movement. At 1 month, movement occurs in a random fashion, with the fists tightly clenched. Because the neck musculature is weak, and the head is large, infants can lift their heads only briefly. By 2 to 3 months, infants can lift their head 90 degrees from a prone position and can hold it steadily erect while in a sitting position. During this time, active grasping gradually replaces reflexive grasping and increases in frequency as eye-hand coordination improves (see Table 6.1).

The Moro, tonic neck, and rooting reflexes disappear at approximately 3 to 4 months. These primitive reflexes, which are controlled by the midbrain, probably disappear because they are suppressed by growing cortical layers. Head control steadily increases during the third month. By the fourth month, the head remains in a straight line with the body when the infant is pulled to a sitting position. Most infants play with their feet by 4 to 5 months, drawing them up to suck on their toes. Parents need anticipatory guidance about ways to prevent unintentional injury by "baby-proofing" their homes before each motor development milestone is reached.

The nurse might explain, for instance, "Infants grow and mature very rapidly, and you will be very busy with a new baby. Now is the time to 'baby-proof' your home before Mary turns over and begins crawling and reaching for objects. By doing this now, you can prevent later injuries and worries."

**PATIENT-CENTERED TEACHING**

***How to "Baby-Proof" the Home***

By the time babies reach 6 months of age, they begin to become much more active, curious, and mobile. Although your baby might not be creeping or crawling yet, it is difficult to predict when that will happen. For this reason, you need to be prepared by making sure your house and the toys with which the baby plays are safe. Babies learn through exploring and participating in many different types of experiences. By keeping the baby's environment safe, you can encourage these experiences for your baby.

Be sure to check the following:

- All small or sharp objects or dangerous substances should be out of the baby's reach. Get down to the baby's eye level to be sure. This includes plants and paint chips, which can be poisonous. Be sure to check that any bedside table near the baby's crib is kept clear of ointments, creams, pins, or any other small objects. Be sure to check that small pieces from older siblings' toys are put away. Keep money put away.
- Put plastic fillers in all plugs, and put cabinet and drawer locks on all cabinets and drawers. Doorknob covers are also available that prevent the infant from opening the door.
- Remove front knobs from the stove. Be sure to keep all pot and pan handles turned away from the edge of the stove.
- Remove from lower cabinets and lock away all dangerous or poisonous substances, including such items as pet food, household cleaning agents, cosmetic aids, pesticides, plant fertilizers, paints, matches, medicines, and plastic bags. Be sure to store these products in their original containers. Never give a small child a latex balloon.
- Place a gate on the top and bottom of stairways. Be sure the gate does not have openings that can trap the baby's head, hands, or fingers.
- Remove heavy containers from table tops covered with a tablecloth. Do not hold the baby on your lap while drinking or eating any kind of hot foods.
- Pad furniture with sharp edges. Be sure all windows have screens.
- Keep household hot water temperature at less than 120° F; always test water temperature before bathing the baby. **Never leave a baby unattended near water** (toilet, bathtub, swimming pool, hot tub). Keep water containers or tubs empty when not in use and toilet covers closed. Be sure there is no direct entrance to a backyard swimming pool through the house.
- Shorten all hanging cords (appliance, window cords, telephone) so they are out of the baby's reach. Be sure pull-toy cords are shorter than 12 inches.
- Have your house tested for sources of lead.
- Never leave your baby unattended or in the care of a young sibling.

During the fifth and sixth months, motor development accelerates rapidly. Infants of this age readily reach for and grasp objects. They can bear weight when held in a standing position and can turn from abdomen to back. By 5 months, some infants rock back and forth as a precursor to crawling.

Six-month-old infants can sit alone, leaning forward on their hands *(tripod sitting)*. This ability provides them with a wider view of the world and creates new ways to play. Infants of this age can roll from back to abdomen and can raise their heads from the table when supine. At 6 to 7 months, they transfer objects from one hand to the other. In addition, they can grab small objects with the whole hand and insert them into their mouths with lightning speed.

At 6 to 9 months, infants begin to explore the world by crawling. By 9 months, most infants have enough muscle strength and coordination to pull themselves up and cruise around furniture. These new methods of mobility enable the infant to follow a parent or caregiver around the house.

By 6 to 7 months, infants become increasingly adept at pointing to make their demands known. Six-month-old infants grasp objects with all their fingers in a raking motion, but 9-month-olds use their thumbs and forefingers in a fine motor skill called the *pincer grasp*. This grasp provides infants with a useful yet potentially dangerous ability to grab, hold, and insert tiny objects into their mouths.

Nine-month-old infants can wave bye-bye and clap their hands together. They can pick up objects but have difficulty releasing them on request. By 1 year of age, they can extend an object and release it into an offered hand. Most 1-year-old children can balance well enough to walk when holding another person's hand. However, they often resort to crawling as a more rapid and efficient way to move about.

An increased ability to move about, reach objects, and explore their world places infants at great risk for accidents and injury. Nurses provide information to parents about how quickly infant motor skills develop.

## Cognitive Development

Many factors contribute to the way in which infants learn about their world. Besides innate intellectual aptitude and motivation, infants' sensory capabilities, neuromuscular control, and perceptual skills all affect how their cognitive processes unfold during infancy and throughout life. In addition, variables such as the quality and quantity of parental interaction and environmental stimulation contribute to cognitive development.

Cognitive development during the first 2 years of life begins with a profound state of **egocentrism**. Egocentrism is the child's complete self-absorption and the inability to view the world from anyone else's vantage point (Piaget, 1952). As infants' cognitive capacities expand, they become increasingly aware of the outside world and their separateness from it. Gradually, with maturation and experience, they become capable of differentiating themselves from others and their surroundings.

According to Piaget's theory (1952), cognitive development occurs in stages or periods (see Chapter 5) as described in the following discussion. Infancy is included in the **sensorimotor** *stage* (birth to 2 years), during which infants experience the world through their senses and their attempts to control the environment. Learning activities progress from simple reflex behavior to trial-and-error experiments.

During the first month of life, infants are in the first substage, *reflex activity,* of the sensorimotor period. In this substage, behavior such as grasping, sucking, or looking is dominated by reflexes. Piaget believed that infants organize their activity, survive, and adapt to their world by the use of reflexes.

*Primary circular reactions* dominate the second substage, occurring from age 1 to 4 months. During this substage, reflexes become more organized, and new schemata are acquired, usually centering on the infant's body. Sensual activities such as sucking and kicking become less reflexive and more controlled and are repeated because of the stimulation they provide. The baby also begins to recognize objects, especially those that bring pleasure, such as the breast or bottle.

During the third substage, or the stage of *secondary circular reactions,* infants perform actions that are more oriented toward the world outside their own bodies. The 4- to 8-month-old infant in this substage begins to play with objects in the external environment, such as a rattle or stuffed toy. The infant's actions are labeled *secondary* because they are intentional (repeated because of the response that is elicited). For example, a baby in this substage intentionally shakes a rattle to hear the sound.

By age 8 to 12 months, infants in the fourth substage (*coordination of secondary schemata*) begin to relate to objects as if they realize that the objects exist even when they are out of sight. This awareness is referred to as **object permanence** and is illustrated by a 9-month-old infant seeking a toy after it is hidden under a pillow. In contrast, 6-month-olds can follow the path of a toy that is dropped in front of them; however, they will not look for the dropped toy or protest its disappearance until they are older and have developed the concept of object permanence.

Infants in the fourth substage solve problems differently from how they solve problems in earlier substages. Rather than randomly selecting approaches to problems, they choose actions that were successful in the past. This tendency suggests that they remember and can perform some mental processing. They seem to be able to identify simple causal relationships, and they show definite intentionality. For example, when an 11-month-old child sees a toy that is beyond reach, the child uses the blanket that it is resting on to pull it closer (Flavell, 1964; Piaget, 1952).

Cognitive development in the infant parallels motor development. Motor activity is necessary for cognitive development, and cognitive development is based on interaction with the environment, not simply maturation. Infant cognitive development lays the foundation for later cognitive functioning. Nurses can promote infants' cognitive development by encouraging parents to interact with their infants and to provide them with novel, interesting stimuli. At the same time, parents should maintain familiar, routine experiences through which their infants can develop a sense of security about the world. Within this type of environment, infants will thrive and learn.

**! NURSING QUALITY ALERT**

***Possible Signs of Developmental Delays***

Lack of eye muscle control after 4 to 6 months suggests a vision impairment and the need for further evaluation.

Lack of a social smile by 8 to 12 weeks requires further evaluation and close follow-up.

## Sensory Development

### Vision

The size of the eye at birth is approximately one half to three fourths the size of the adult eye. Growth of the eye, including its internal structures, is rapid during the first year. As infants grow and become more interested in the environment, their eyes remain open for longer periods. They show a preference for familiar faces and are increasingly able to fixate on objects. Visual acuity is estimated at approximately 20/100 to 20/150 at birth but improves rapidly during infancy and toddlerhood. Infants show a preference for high-contrast colors, such as black and white and primary colors. Pastel colors are not easily distinguished until approximately 6 months of age.

Young infants may lack coordination of eye movements and extraocular muscle alignment but should achieve proper coordination by age 4 to 6 months. A persistent lack of eye muscle control beyond age 4 to 6 months needs further evaluation. Depth perception appears to begin at approximately 7 to 9 months and contributes to the infant's new ability to move about independently (see Chapter 55).

### Hearing

Hearing seems to be relatively acute, even at birth, as shown by their reflexive, generalized reactions to noise. With myelination of the auditory nerve tracts during the first year, responses to sound become increasingly more specialized. By 4 months, infants should turn their eyes and head toward a sound coming from behind, and by 10 months they should respond to the sound of their name. However, an estimated 1 to 3/1000 newborns experience some degree of hearing impairment (American Academy of Audiology, 2011 The American Academy of Pediatrics (AAP) Joint Committee on Infant Hearing recommended in 2007 that all newborn infants be screened for hearing impairment either as neonates or before 1 month of age and that those infants who fail newborn screening have an audiologic examination to verify hearing impairment before age 3 months. The AAP also suggested that infants who demonstrate confirmed hearing loss be eligible for early intervention services and specialized hearing and language services as early as possible, but no later than 6 months of age (AAP, Joint Committee on Infant Hearing, 2007). These guidelines remain as recommended today (AAP Early Hearing Detection & Intervention Program [EHDI], 2015). Newborn hearing screening generally is done before hospital discharge. Rescreening of both ears within 1 month of discharge is recommended for those newborns with questionable results. Screening should be also available to those infants born at home or in an out-of-hospital birthing center (AAP, Joint Committee on Infant Hearing, 2007).

Health providers should assess risk for hearing deficits at every well visit (AAP, 2016). Risk factors include, but are not limited to, structural abnormalities of the ear, family history of hearing loss, pre- or postnatal infections known to contribute to hearing deficit, trauma, persistent otitis media, developmental delay, and parental concern (AAP Joint Committee on Infant Hearing, 2007; National Center on Birth Defects and Developmental Disabilities, 2015). Verification of referral or follow-up recommendations is important, as nearly 36% of infants who do not pass the newborn screening test are either rescreened or followed (AAP EHDI, 2015).

### Language Development

The acquisition of language has its roots in infancy as the child becomes increasingly intrigued with sound, begins to realize that words have meaning, and eventually uses simple sounds to communicate (Box 6.1). Although young infants probably understand tones and inflections of voice rather than words themselves, it is not long before repetition and practice of sounds enable them to understand and communicate with words. Infants can understand more than they can express.

The social smile develops early in the infant, usually by 3 to 5 weeks of age (Fig. 6.1). This powerful communication tool helps to foster attachment and demonstrates that the infant can differentiate between people and objects within the environment. The infant who does not display a social smile by 8 to 12 weeks of age needs further evaluation and close follow-up because of the possibility of developmental delay.

During infancy, connections form within the central nervous system, providing fine motor control of the numerous muscles required for speech. Maturation of the mouth, jaw, and larynx, bone growth, and development of the face help prepare the infant to speak.

Vocalization, or speech, does not appear to be reflexive but rather is a relatively high-level activity similar to conversation. The parents can usually elicit vocalization in their infant better than other adults can. Language includes understanding word meanings, how to combine words into meaningful sentences and phrases, and social use of conversation. The development of speech and language is intimately connected to adequate hearing. The development of both speech and language also can be influenced by sociodemographic factors, quality of communication in the environment, anatomic defects, neurologic disorders, developmental disorders, and family history (Crichton, 2013).

Although there is great variability, most children begin to make nonmeaningful sounds, such as "ma," "da," or "ah," by 4 to 6 months. The sounds become more meaningful and specific by 9 to 15 months, and by age 1 year the child usually has a vocabulary of several words, such as "mama," "dada," and "bye-bye." Infants who have older siblings

#### BOX 6.1 Language Development and Developmental Milestones in Infancy

**1 to 3 Months**
Reflexive smile at first, becoming more voluntary; sets up a reciprocal smiling cycle with parent. Cooing.

**3 to 4 Months**
Crying becomes more differentiated. Babbling is common.

**4 to 6 Months**
Plays with sound, repeating sounds to self. Can identify mother's voice. May squeal in excitement.

**6 to 8 Months**
Single-consonant babbling occurs. Increasing interest in sound.

**8 to 9 Months**
Stringing of vowels and consonants together begins. First few words begin to have meaning (mama, daddy, bye-bye, baby). Begins to understand and obey simple commands such as "Wave bye-bye."

**9 to 12 Months**
Vocabulary of two or three words. Gestures are used to communicate. Speech development may slow temporarily when walking begins.

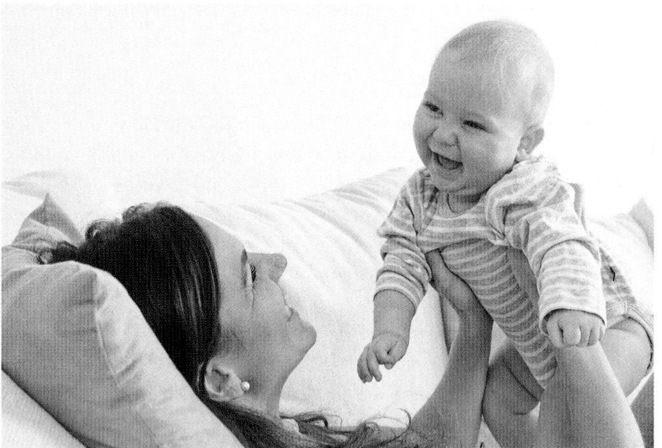

**FIG 6.1** This 6-month-old infant responds to her mother delightedly with a true social smile. Such interactive responses between parent and child promote communication and emotional development. (© 2016, Getty Images. Reprinted with permission.)

or who are raised in verbally rich environments sometimes meet these developmental milestones earlier than other infants.

## Psychosocial Development

Most experts agree that infancy is a crucial period during which children develop the foundation of their personalities and their sense of self. According to Erikson's theory of psychosocial development (1963), infants struggle to establish a sense of basic *trust* rather than a sense of basic mistrust in their world, their caregivers, and themselves. If provided with consistent, satisfying experiences delivered in a timely manner, infants come to rely on the fact that their needs will be met and that, in turn, they will be able to tolerate some degree of frustration and discomfort until those needs are met. This sense of confidence is an early form of trust and provides the foundation for a healthy personality.

Conversely, if infants' needs are ignored or met in a consistently haphazard, inadequate manner, they have no reason to believe that their needs will be met or that their environment is a safe, secure place. Erikson (1963) states that without consistent satisfaction of needs, the individual develops a basic sense of suspicion or mistrust.

Parallel to this viewpoint is Freudian theory, which regards infancy as the oral stage (Freud, 1974). The mouth is the major focus during this stage. Observation of infants for a few minutes shows that most of their behavior centers on their mouths. Sensory stimulation and pleasure, as well as nourishment, are experienced through their mouths. Sucking is an adaptive behavior that provides comfort and satisfaction while enabling infants to experience and explore their world. Later in infancy, as teething progresses, the mouth becomes an effective tool for aggressive behavior (see Chapter 7).

### Parent-Infant Attachment

One of the most important aspects of infant psychosocial development is parent–infant attachment. Attachment is a sense of belonging to or connection with each other. This significant bond between infant and parent is critical to normal development and even survival. Initiated immediately after birth, attachment is strengthened by many mutually satisfying interactions between the parents and the infant throughout the first months of life.

For example, noisy distress in infants signals a need, such as hunger. Parents respond by providing food. In turn, infants respond by quieting and accepting nourishment. The infants derive pleasure from having their hunger satiated and the parents from successfully caring for their children. A basic reciprocal cycle is set in motion in which parents learn to regulate infant feeding, sleep, and activity through a series of interactions. These interactions include rocking, touching, talking, smiling, and singing. The infants respond by quieting, eating, watching, smiling, or sleeping.

Conversely, continuing inability or unwillingness of parents to meet the dependency needs of their infants fosters insecurity and dissatisfaction in the infants. A cycle of dissatisfaction is established in which parents become frustrated as caregivers and have further difficulty providing for the infant's needs.

If parents can adapt to their infant, meet the infant's needs, and provide nurturance, attachment is secure. Psychosocial development can proceed on the basis of a strong foundation of attachment. Conversely, if parents' personalities and abilities to cope with infant care do not match their infant's needs, the relationship is considered at risk.

Although the establishment of trust depends heavily on the quality of the parental interaction, the infant also needs consistent, satisfying social interactions within a family structure. Family routines can help to provide this consistency. Touch is an important tool that can be used by all family members to convey a sense of caring.

### Stranger Anxiety

Another important aspect of psychosocial development is stranger anxiety. By 6 to 7 months, expanding cognitive capacities and strong feelings of attachment enable infants to differentiate between caregivers and strangers and to be wary of the latter. Infants display an obvious preference for parents over other caregivers and other unfamiliar people. Anxiety, demonstrated by crying, clinging, and turning away from the stranger, is manifested when separation occurs. This behavior peaks at approximately 7 to 9 months and again during toddlerhood, when separation may be difficult (see Chapter 7).

Although stressful for parents, stranger anxiety is a normal sign of healthy attachment and occurs because of cognitive development (object permanence). Nurses can reassure parents that although their infants seem distressed, leaving them for short periods does no harm. Separations should be accomplished swiftly, yet with care, love, and emphasis on the parents' return.

## HEALTH PROMOTION FOR THE INFANT AND FAMILY

Parents, particularly new parents, often need guidance in caring for their infant. Nurses can provide valuable information about health promotion for the infant. Specific guidance about everyday concerns, such as sleeping, crying, and feeding, can be offered, as well as anticipatory guidance about injury prevention. An important nursing responsibility is to provide parents with information about immunizations and dental care. Nurses can offer support to new parents by identifying strategies for coping with the first few months with an infant. The schedule of well visits corresponds with the schedule recommended by the AAP. At each well visit the nurse assesses development, administers appropriate immunizations, and provides anticipatory guidance. The nurse asks the parent a series of general assessment questions (Box 6.2) and then focuses the assessment on the individual infant.

### ? CRITICAL THINKING EXERCISE 6.1

Mary Brown and her 4-week-old daughter, Tonja, are being seen for a well-baby checkup. Tonja is Mrs. Brown's first child. Mrs. Brown looks very tired and begins to cry when you ask her how she is doing.

1. What are some of the possible causes the nurse should explore?
2. How will you approach exploring these possible causes?
3. What are some of the appropriate nursing measures?

### BOX 6.2 Continuing Assessment Questions

- Nutrition: How much is your child eating, how often, what kinds of foods?
- Elimination: How many wet diapers, stools? Consistency of stools?
- Safety: Use of car restraints? Gun violence? Smoking in the home?
- Hearing/vision: Any concerns?
- Can you tell me about the times you would feel it necessary to call your doctor?
- How is the family adjusting to the baby?
- Are you getting enough time alone and time together?
- Has there been any change in the household or family's lifestyle?
- Are there any financial concerns?
- Are there any other questions or concerns?

## Immunization

The importance of childhood immunization against disease cannot be overemphasized. Infants are especially vulnerable to infectious disease because their immune systems are immature. Term neonates are protected from certain infections by transplacental passive immunity from their mothers. Breastfed infants receive additional immunoglobulins against many types of viruses and bacteria. Transplacental immunity is effective only for approximately 3 months; however, for various reasons, many mothers choose not to breastfeed. In any case, this passive immunity does not cover all diseases, and infection in the infant can be devastating. Immunization offers protection that all infants need.

Nurses play an important role in health promotion and disease prevention related to immunization. Nursing responsibilities include assessing current immunization status, removing barriers to receiving immunizations, tracking immunization records, providing parent education, and recognizing contraindications to the receipt of vaccines. Chapter 5 provides detailed information regarding immunizations and their schedule.

## Feeding and Nutrition

Because infancy is a period of rapid growth, nutritional needs are of special significance. During infancy, eating progresses from a principally reflex activity to relatively sophisticated, yet messy, attempts at self-feeding. Because the infant's gastrointestinal system continues to mature throughout the first year, changes in diet, the introduction of new foods, and even upsets in routines can result in feeding problems.

Parents often have many questions and concerns about nutrition. They are influenced by various sources, including relatives and friends who may not be aware of current scientific practices regarding infant feeding. To provide anticipatory guidance, the nurse must have a clear understanding of gastrointestinal maturation and knowledge about breastfeeding and various infant formulas and foods. Families and cultures vary widely in food preferences and infant feeding practices. The nurse must remain cognizant of these differences when providing anticipatory guidance related to infant nutrition.

**! NURSING QUALITY ALERT**

***Essential Information for Infant Nutrition***

Breast milk or commercially prepared iron-fortified formula provides optimal nutrition throughout infancy.

Formula must be prepared according to instructions, and leftover formula should be stored or discarded according to the manufacturer's directions.

Some healthcare providers discourage the use of powdered formula until the infant is older than 6 weeks.

### Factors Influencing Choice of Feeding Method

The AAP (2012) and the American Heart Association (2015) strongly recommend exclusive breastfeeding for the first 4 to 6 months of life for all infants, including premature and sick newborns, with rare exceptions, and continuation of breastfeeding along with solid foods until the infant is 1 year old. Increasing the percentage of infants who are exclusively breastfed is a goal of *Healthy People 2020*. Although 79% of infants in the United States are breastfed at birth, only 49% of infants in the United States breastfeed for 6 months; this percentage drops to 27% at 1 year (Centers for Disease Control and Prevention [CDC], 2014). The percentage of infants who are breastfed exclusively at 6 months is only 19%.

***Breastfeeding.*** Breast milk provides complete nutrition for infants, and evidence suggests that breastfed infants are less likely to be at risk for overweight or obesity (Carling, Demment, Kjolhede, & Olson, 2015). Researchers also suggest that SIDS risk is decreased in infants who are breastfed (Goldstein, Trachtenberg, Sens, et al., 2016; Hauck, Thompson, Tanabe, et al., 2011).

Mothers who breastfeed need instruction and support as they begin. They are more likely to succeed if they are given practical information. Many facilities provide lactation consultants or home visits, or nursing staff may call to assess the mother's needs. Significant others are included in teaching to provide a support system for the mother. Breastfed infants need to receive vitamin D supplementation to prevent the occurrence of rickets. Breastfed infants may also need iron supplementation. In 2008, the AAP (CDC, 2015b; Greer, Sicherer, Burks, & the Committee on Nutrition and Section on Allergy and Immunology, 2008) recommended vitamin D supplementation of 400 IU/day for all breastfed and partially breastfed infants and for formula-fed infants who consume less than 1 L (33 oz) of vitamin-D–fortified formula a day. An in-depth discussion of breastfeeding can be found in Chapter 23.

***Formula feeding.*** Formula given by bottle is a choice selected by many women in the United States. This method is often easier for the mother who must return to work soon after her infant's birth, and it has the advantage of allowing other members of the family to participate in the infant's feeding. Infant formula does not have the immunologic properties and digestibility of human milk, but it does meet the energy and nutrient requirements of infants. If bottle feeding is chosen as the preferred feeding method, the formula should be iron fortified. The Infant Formula Act of 1980, which was revised in 1986, establishes the standards for infant formulas. It also requires that the label show the quantity of each nutrient contained in the formula. Special formulas are available for low-birth-weight infants, infants with congenital cardiac disease, and for infants allergic to cow's-milk–based formulas.

There are some physiologic reasons why some mothers choose to use formula. Infants with galactosemia or whose mothers use certain illegal drugs, are taking certain prescribed drugs (e.g., antiretrovirals, certain chemotherapeutic agents), or have untreated active tuberculosis should not be breastfed (AAP, 2012). In the United States and other developed countries where safe water is available, even if breastfeeding is culturally acceptable, women infected with HIV should avoid breastfeeding (AAP, 2012).

**Types of formula.** Formula can be purchased in three different forms: ready-to-use, concentrated liquid, and powdered. With the exception of the ready-to-use formula, all require the addition of water to obtain the appropriate concentration for feeding. Storage instructions differ, so nurses need to strongly encourage parents to carefully follow the storage directions for the specific type of formula they are using.

Although commercially prepared formulas have many similarities, there are also differences. Some commonly used brands are Enfamil, SMA, Similac, Gerber, and Good Start. There are formulas specifically designed for infants older than 6 months, but it is not necessary to change to a different formula when a child reaches that age. Some formulas are designed for feeding low-birth-weight or ill infants. Such formulas include high-calorie and predigested formulas (e.g., Pregestimil, Nutramigen).

**Cow's milk.** Cow's milk (whole, skim, 1%, 2%) is not recommended in the first 12 months. Cow's milk contains too little iron, and its high renal solute load and unmodified derivatives can put small infants at risk for dehydration. The tough, hard curd is difficult for infants to digest. In addition, skim milk and reduced-fat milk deprive the infant of needed calories and essential fatty acids. The incidences of allergy and iron deficiency anemia are higher in infants who are given cow's milk than in those who receive breast milk or formula.

**Formula feeding techniques.** Many different types of bottles and nipples are available for bottle feeding, including glass or plastic bottles or a plastic liner that fits into a rigid container. In response to concerns about environmental exposures, newly manufactured infant bottles in the United States are free of bisphenol A (BPA), a chemical found in some plastic bottles. Parents should be advised to purchase bottles labeled BPA-free, or if using older plastic bottles, to discard those having recycle #7 PC imprinted on the bottom (AAP, 2015a). Some nipples are designed to simulate the human nipple to promote jaw development. Selection of the type of bottles and nipples depends on individual preference.

It should not be assumed that parents know how to bottle-feed an infant. The nurse may need to teach them how often and how much to feed, how to hold and cuddle while feeding, when and how to burp, and how to prepare formula. See Chapter 23 for a more in-depth discussion of formula feeding.

### Weaning

Weaning is the replacement of breast or bottle feedings with drinking expressed breast milk or formula from a cup. Infants usually have a decreasing interest in the breast or bottle starting between ages 6 and 12 months. This varies from infant to infant, but if solids and a cup have been introduced, the infant will probably begin to indicate a readiness for the cup. Even young infants can be weaned to a regular plastic cup, although they will not be ready to hold the cup themselves until later. Some parents choose to use a sippy cup—a cup with a tight cover that prevents contents from spilling when dropped. When weaning is begun after age 18 months, the infant may resist because of increased attachment to the breast or bottle.

Behaviors that might indicate a readiness to begin weaning include the following:

- Throwing the bottle down
- Chewing on the nipple
- Taking only a few ounces of formula
- Refusing the breast or dawdling

Weaning should not take place during times of change or stress (e.g., illness, starting child care, the arrival of a new baby). Weaning is a gradual process and should start with the replacement of one bottle feeding or breastfeeding at a time. If breastfeeding must be terminated before age 6 months, it should be replaced with bottle feedings to meet the infant's sucking needs. The older infant who has learned to use a cup may not need to use a bottle.

The first bottle feeding or breastfeeding eliminated should be the one in which the infant is least interested. Initially the infant may accept the cup only after drinking some formula from the bottle or milk from the breast. The infant is next offered the cup before the feeding. After several days, another feeding can be eliminated if the infant is not resisting the change. The bedtime feeding is usually the last feeding to be eliminated.

During weaning, the child is giving up time that had been spent being held in the parent's arms. The parent needs to respond to the infant's continued need to be held and cuddled. Infants should not be encouraged to carry bottles or sippy cups around as toys, to take them to bed, or to use them as pacifiers.

### Juices

Once the infant takes fluids from a cup, the parent can introduce small amounts (no more than 4 to 6 oz/day) of fruit juice. Fruit juice lacks the fiber present in whole fruit, and for that reason, whole fruit is considered more nutritionally acceptable than fruit juice (American Heart Association, 2015). Fruit juice should be avoided in infants younger than 6 months of age and should not be given to infants at bedtime because it can contribute to tooth decay (American Academy of Pedodontics, 2012). Nurses need to be aware of the nutritional benefits and limitations of juice; advise parents to give children only 100% fruit juice and not juice drinks, which may contain added sugar.

In infants with a family history of allergies, orange and tomato juice should be delayed until age 1 year. Some prepared foods and dinners contain orange juice and tomato juice. Parents need to be taught to read labels. Juice is not warmed because heating destroys vitamin C. Juices should be kept in a covered container in the refrigerator to prevent the loss of the vitamin.

### Water

Sufficient water is provided in breast milk and in prepared formula during early infancy. When solid foods are introduced, it may be necessary to give a small amount of additional water because some foods (e.g., strained meats, high-meat dinners) have a high renal solute load. Additional fluid is necessary when intake is low or the infant has fluid loss because of illness (fever, respiratory disease). Young infants do not need fluoridated water.

### Solid Foods

The early introduction of solids may be detrimental to growth because the solids the infant eats cannot be adequately digested related to the immaturity of the gastrointestinal system. In addition, the nutrients in breast or formula milk will not be taken in because the infant's appetite has been satisfied with the less nutritious solids. Evidence suggests that early introduction of solid foods (before 4 months of age) in bottle-fed infants contributes to later overweight and obesity (Huh et al., 2011). However, nutrients supplied by solid foods in the older infant cannot be provided completely by formula or breast milk alone, so solid foods should be introduced beginning no earlier than 4 months and no later than 6 months of age (Greer et al., 2008).

The infant goes through a *transitional period* during which prepared foods are introduced and given together with human milk or formula. Each infant's growth and development vary, and milestones indicate the infant's readiness for solid foods (Box 6.3).

Solids should be introduced one at a time in small amounts (1 teaspoon to 2 tablespoons) for several days before introducing a new food. This is done to avoid confusion should a food intolerance be present. The order of introduction is not critical, but iron-fortified rice cereal is most often recommended as a first food because it is high in iron, is easily digested, and has a low allergenic probability. Other commercially available infant cereals include oatmeal, barley, mixed grain, and cereals with added fruit. When foods are first being introduced, mixed grains and cereals with added fruit should be avoided. Various meat, fish, poultry, and eggs can be introduced along with various fruits and vegetables. Foods should not be mixed with formula and fed

#### BOX 6.3 Readiness for Introduction of Solids

- Infant can sit.
- Birth weight has doubled and infant weighs at least 13 lb.
- Infant can reach for an object and maintain balance.
- Infant indicates a desire for food by opening mouth and leaning forward.
- Extrusion reflex has disappeared (4 to 5 months).
- Infant moves food to back of mouth and swallows during spoon feedings.

through a nipple with a large hole. This deprives the child of the chewing experience and changes the texture and taste of the food.

Several commercially prepared pureed fruits and vegetables are available. In addition, fruits and vegetables can easily be steamed or boiled and then pureed in a blender or food processor at home. It is usually necessary to add a small amount of water during the blending process. The parent should not give infants home-prepared orange or dark green leafy vegetables because of the elevated nitrate levels, which can cause methemoglobinemia. Elevated nitrates may also be present in well water; if using well water to mix formula, the well should be tested regularly for nitrate level. If the level exceeds 10 mg/L, it should not be used for infants (AAP, 2015c). As with cereals, mixed fruits should be avoided until the infant is older and has tolerated individual foods. The parent should avoid giving the infant mixed meats and vegetables as well; these baby foods may not contain enough meat.

Salt and sugar should not be added to commercial or home-prepared foods. Parents should avoid using canned foods or home-prepared foods that contain large amounts of sugar and salt. Feeding honey to infants under age 12 months has been associated with botulism, and thus, should be avoided.

***Finger foods.*** Between age 8 and 10 months the infant can be introduced to finger foods. At this time the pincer grasp is developing, and the infant can pick up foods. The infant will have a palmar grasp before this time; soft foods can be given, but the infant will mainly "play" with the food. This can be a positive experience that enables the infant to feel different textures and increase fine motor skills.

Finger foods should be bite-size pieces of soft food. Arrowroot biscuits, cheese sticks, slices of canned peaches or pears, cut pieces of bananas, and breads can be offered. As children's fine motor skills increase, they may enjoy eating some of the dry cereals, such as Cheerios. Be sure pieces of larger finger foods are not round and are small enough that they will not block the infant's airway, causing a choking hazard. The most common foods that represent a choking hazard to children ≤1 year of age include, liquids, biscuits (cookies), various fruits and vegetables (whole grapes, sliced bananas, raw carrots), seeds, or hard candy (Chapin et al., 2013). Hot dogs, while not usually given to infants, are the leading cause of choking episodes in children (Chapin et al., 2013). Nurses should advise parents not to give infants these foods without cutting them into small irregularly shaped pieces. Encourage parents to remain with an infant who is eating finger foods.

***Snacks.*** When the infant is on a three-meals-a-day schedule, small snacks are an appropriate addition to the nutritional intake. Because infants have small stomachs, they may not be content to wait until the next meal before eating. Snacks should be nutritious, and parents should resist the urge to give infants a bottle to satisfy their hunger. Some of the safe finger foods previously listed is nutritious snacks. If the infant is not hungry at mealtime, the snack should be given in a smaller portion or eliminated.

### Food Allergies

The early introduction (before 4 months of age) of solid foods may be associated with a higher incidence of food allergy in infants, especially those with a family history of allergy. However, recent evidence suggests that the introduction of various solid foods between 4 and 6 months of age, including foods suspected to be allergenic, does not increase the development of allergy in low risk infants (Grimshaw et al., 2015). In fact, early introduction of peanuts to an at-risk infant's diet may be protective against the development of peanut allergy (Fletcher et al., 2015). Furthermore, it is generally accepted that limiting allergenic foods during pregnancy and while breastfeeding also has no protective effect. Therefore, in general, a wide variety of culturally appropriate foods can be introduced, with a focus on foods that are high in iron, protein, and nutrient value. To identify foods to which an infant might react, the parent is taught to introduce one food at a time over 3 to 5 days before introducing another one and to read processed food labels for any allergenic components.

Some of the more common suspected allergens include cow's milk, egg, soy products, fish, peanuts, chocolate, corn, and wheat. Cow's milk protein intolerance is the most common food allergy during infancy, but this usually does not last past age 3 or 4 years.

Some of the common clinical manifestations of food allergies are abdominal pain, diarrhea, nasal congestion, cough, wheezing, vomiting, and rashes. Many children will outgrow their allergic response to certain foods.

### Dental Care

Eruption of the infant's first teeth is a developmental milestone that has great significance for many parents. Deciduous, or "baby," teeth usually erupt between 5 and 9 months of age. The first to appear are the lower central incisors, followed by the upper central incisors and then the upper lateral incisors. The next teeth to erupt are usually the lower lateral incisors, first primary molars, canines, and the second primary molars. The average child has six to eight teeth by the first birthday.

### Teething

Although sometimes asymptomatic, teething is often signaled by behavior such as night wakening, daytime restlessness, an increase in nonnutritive sucking, excess drooling, and temporary loss of appetite. Some degree of discomfort is normal, but a healthcare professional should further investigate elevated temperature, irritability, ear tugging, or diarrhea.

To help parents cope with teething, nurses can suggest that they provide cool liquids and hard foods (e.g., dry toast, Popsicles, frozen bagels) for chewing. Hard, cold teethers and ice wrapped in cloth may also provide comfort for inflamed gums. Nurses should explain to parents that over-the-counter topical medications for gum pain relief should be used only as directed. Home remedies, such as rubbing the gums with whiskey or aspirin, should be discouraged, but acetaminophen administered as directed for the child's age can relieve discomfort. Although these interventions can be helpful, parents should understand that absolute relief comes only with tooth eruption.

### Assessment of Dental Risk

The AAP (Clark & Slayton, 2014) and the United States Preventive Services Task Force (USPSTF) (Moyer, 2014) have issued recommendations about prevention and treatment of dental caries in infants and young children. The risk of tooth decay begins in infancy and is higher in families with a history of dental caries, children with special healthcare needs (especially those involving motor coordination), lower socioeconomic status, children with previous tooth decay, children who snack frequently on sugary foods (including 100% fruit juice), and those without a dentist (Clark & Slayton, 2014). Viewed as an infectious process, mothers with dental caries can transmit caries-causing bacteria to their infants. Taking a dental history from a mother can provide information about an infant's risk, and this should occur as early as the infant's teeth begin to erupt. The AAP (2011) has developed an oral health risk assessment tool available at http://www2.aap.org/oralhealth/RiskAssessmentTool.html. Infants with observable dental caries should be referred to a dentist as soon as these are observed by the healthcare provider.

The AAP (2016) recommends that pediatric providers assess infants' and children's oral caries risk periodically throughout infancy and childhood. This should occur along with dietary counseling on

## HEALTH PROMOTION

### *2-Week-Old to 1-Month-Old Infant*

**Focused Assessment**

- How have you been feeling? Have you made your postpartum checkup appointment?
- How have you and your partner been adjusting to the baby? Do you have other children? How are they adjusting?
- Have you discussed child-rearing philosophies?
- Does anyone in your household smoke cigarettes or use any substances?
- Have you recently been exposed to or had any sexually transmitted disease?
- Have you experienced any periods of sadness or feeling "down"?
- What concerns might you have about the costs of the baby's care?
- Do you feel that you and the baby are safe?

**Developmental Milestones**

- Personal/social: looks at parent's face; fixates, tracks, follows to midline; smiles responsively; prefers brightly colored objects
- Fine motor: newborn reflexes present
- Language/cognitive: prefers human female voice: responds to sounds; begins to vocalize
- Gross motor: equal movements; lifts head; lifts head and chin (by 1 month)

**Health Maintenance**

***Physical Measurements***

*Weight*: 7.5-8 lb (3.4-3.6 kg) average. Loses 10% of body weight after birth but gains it back by 2 weeks; gains on average ½ oz/day.

*Length*: Average 20 inches (50 cm). Gains 1 inch (2.5 cm)/month for the first several months.

*Head Circumference*: 13-15 inches (33-38 cm). Gains average of ½ inch (1.2 cm)/month until 6 months of age. Posterior fontanel closes by 2-3 months; anterior by 12-18 months.

***Immunizations***

Thimerosal-free hepatitis B #1 at birth and #2 at 1 to 2 months. Be sure to discuss side effects. Give the parent information about upcoming immunizations. If planning to use a combination vaccine that contains hepatitis B, wait until 2 months for second hepatitis B.

***Health Screening***

Verify that newborn metabolic and cystic fibrosis screening has been done
Verify that hearing screening has been done
Visual inspection for congenital defects

**Anticipatory Guidance**

***Nutrition***

Breast milk on demand at least every 2-3 hours
Iron-fortified formula 2-3 oz every 3-4 hours if not breastfeeding
Vitamin D supplement 400 IU/day for breastfed infants and for formula-fed babies consuming fewer than 1 liter (33 ounces) per day
Place on right side after feeding

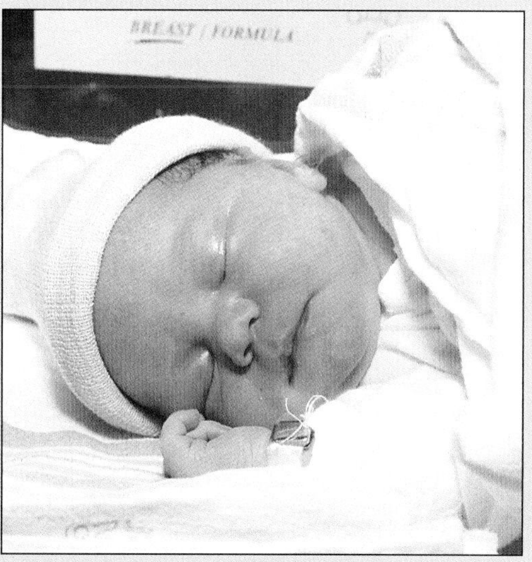

***Elimination***

6 wet diapers
Stools related to feeding method

***Dental***

Continue prenatal vitamins and calcium if breastfeeding

***Sleep***

**Place on back to sleep in parent's room in a separate crib/cradle/bassinet. Keep loose or soft bedding and toys out of the crib, offer pacifier for nap and bedtime if not breastfeeding or after breastfeeding is established.**
16 or more hours
By 1 month begin to establish nighttime routine

***Hygiene***

Bathe in warm water using mild soap and baby shampoo.
Keep diaper area clean and dry.

***Safety***

Be sure crib is safe: slats <2⅜ inches apart, firm mattress that fits the crib
Eliminate all environmental smoke
Rear-facing approved infant car seat
Fire prevention: smoke detectors, fire extinguishers
Water temperature <120° F
Cardiopulmonary resuscitation and first aid classes; emergency phone numbers
Violence: discuss shaking, guns in the home

avoiding food sources of sugar and provision of an appropriate dose of fluoride.

### Cleaning Teeth

Dental care must begin in infancy because the primary teeth are used for chewing until the permanent teeth erupt and because decay of the primary teeth often results in decay of the permanent teeth. The parent can use cotton swabs or a soft washcloth and water to clean the teeth with the infant positioned in the parent's lap or on a changing table; after age six months (to three years), the parent can smear the infant's erupting teeth with a rice-grain–sized amount of fluoridated toothpaste (Clark & Slayton, 2014). The teeth should be cleaned at least twice a day, and juice should be limited to no more than 4 to 6 oz a day given at meals.

## HEALTH PROMOTION

### *The 2-Month-Old Infant*

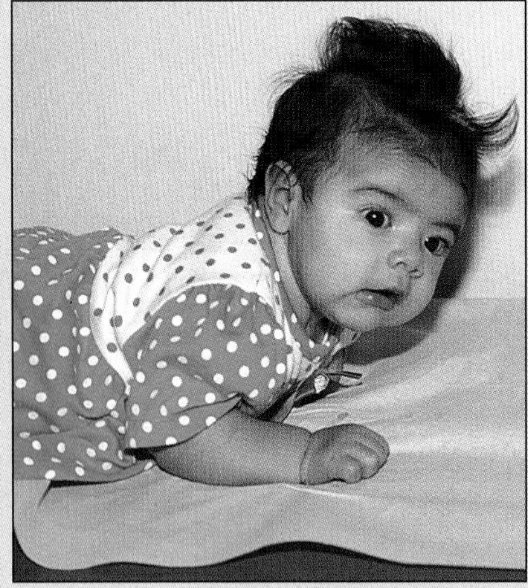

**Focused Assessment**

Ask the parent the following:

- How has your family adjusted to the baby?
- Are you able to plan time to give some individual attention to each of your other children?
- What opportunities do you have for continuing relationships and activities away from the baby?
- Will you describe your baby's behavior and general mood?
- Has your baby had any reaction to any immunizations? If so, what happened?

**Developmental Milestones**

*Personal/social:* Smiles spontaneously; enjoys interacting with others
*Fine motor:* Follows past midline; reflexes disappear
*Language/cognitive:* Vocalizes "ooh" and "ah" sounds; attends to voices
*Gross motor:* Beginning head control when upright; lifts head 45 degrees onto forearms

**Critical Milestones***

*Personal/social:* Smiles responsively; looks at faces
*Fine motor:* Follows to midline
*Language/cognitive:* Vocalizes making cooing or short vowel sounds; responds to a bell
*Gross motor:* Lifts head; equal movements

**Health Maintenance**

***Physical Measurements***

Measure length, weight, and head *circumference* and plot on appropriate growth charts

***Immunizations***

Diphtheria-tetanus-acellular pertussis (DTaP) #1; inactivated poliovirus (IPV) #1; *Haemophilus influenzae* type b (Hib) #1; pneumococcal #1; rotavirus #1 (combination *vaccines* are available for DTaP and IPV plus either Hepatitis B or Hib)
Discuss *potential* effects

***Health Screening***

Hearing screen if not done at birth; hearing risk assessment
Check eyes for strabismus
Assess ability to *follow* past midline

**Anticipatory Guidance**

***Nutrition***

Breastfeed on *demand* with increasing intervals
Formula, 4-6 oz *six* times per day
Vitamin D *supplementation* 400 IU/day for breastfeeding infants and for formula fed infants if taking less than 1 L (33 oz) of formula/day

***Elimination***

6 wet *diapers*
Stools related to *feeding* method; may decrease in number

***Dental***

Continue *prenatal* vitamins and calcium if breastfeeding
Do not prop *baby's* bottle

***Sleep***

**Place on back to sleep in parent's room in a separate crib/cradle/bassinet. Keep loose or soft bedding and toys out of the crib, offer pacifier for nap and bedtime. Continue nighttime routine**
Play with baby when awake

***Hygiene***

Bathe several *times* per week
Watch for diaper *rash* and seborrheic dermatitis

***Safety***

Review house and environmental safety and conditions for calling the doctor, posting of emergency numbers near the telephone, car safety, violence, avoidance of exposure to cigarette smoke
Discuss *preventing* falls; burns from hot liquids

***Play***

Imitate *vocalizations* and smile
Sing
Change infant's *environment*
Encourage *rolling* over

*Guided by Denver Developmental Screening Test II.

### Fluoride

To prevent tooth decay in developing teeth, supplemental oral fluoride has historically been prescribed for infants and children who live in areas where there is no community water fluoridation. The AAP (Clark & Slayton, 2014) recommends that oral fluoride supplementation begin in all children older than six months whose water supply contains less than 0.3 parts per million of fluoride. Additionally, topical fluoride varnish should be provided to all infants as soon as tooth eruption begins; this can be applied by pediatric providers during well visits every three to six months (AAP, 2016; Clark & Slayton, 2014; USPSTF, 2014).

### Bottle-Mouth Caries

Bottle-mouth caries, or nursing-bottle caries, is a well-described form of tooth decay that can develop in infants and children. The decay pattern usually involves the incisors initially and then spreads to other teeth. Decay may be so serious that tooth loss occurs prematurely. When the infant is allowed to fall asleep with a bottle containing milk or juice, the carbohydrate-rich solution bathes the teeth for a long period and may cause dental caries.

Nurses should discourage parents from giving bedtime bottles of milk or juice to infants. If a nighttime bottle is necessary, plain water is an acceptable substitute for carbohydrate-rich liquids. A pacifier is an acceptable alternative to a nighttime bottle, although the practice of dipping the pacifier in corn syrup or honey to encourage acceptance poses the same problem. An additional danger of the use of honey in infancy is botulism. Pacifier use after age 3 years can contribute to malocclusion.

## HEALTH PROMOTION

### *The 4-Month-Old Infant*

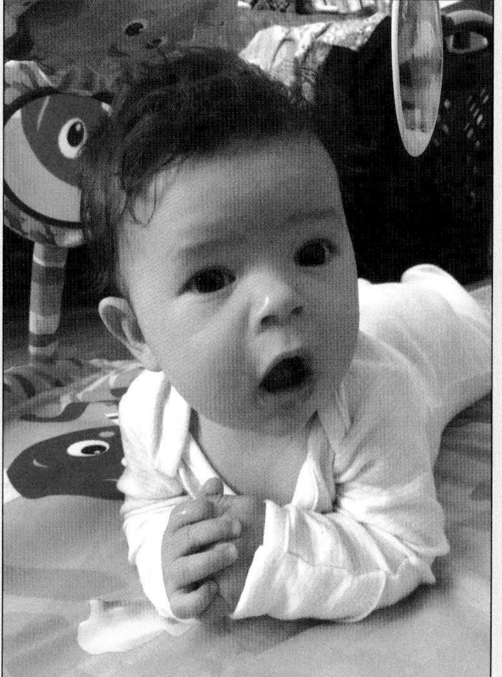

#### Focused Assessment

Ask the parent the following:

- What new activities is your baby doing?
- How well does your baby settle down to sleep without needing to be consoled?
- How are both parents included in the baby's care?
- Is the mother considering going back to work in the near future?

#### Developmental Milestones

*Personal/social:* Loves moving faces; knows parents' voices

*Fine motor:* Follows an object 180 degrees; binocular vision; bats objects; begins to hold own bottle

*Language/cognitive:* Initiates conversation by cooing; turns head to locate sounds

*Gross motor:* Supports weight on feet when standing; pulls to sit without head lag; begins to roll prone to supine

#### Critical Milestones*

*Personal/social:* Smiles responsively; smiles spontaneously; stares at own hand

*Fine motor:* Grasps a rattle; follows past midline; brings hands to middle of body

*Language/cognitive:* Laughs and squeals out loud; vocalizes; makes "ooh" sounds

*Gross motor:* Lifts head and chest 45 and 90 degrees when prone; head steady when sitting

#### Health Maintenance

##### *Physical Measurements*

Continue to measure and plot length, weight, and head circumference

Posterior fontanel closed

##### *Immunizations*

Diphtheria-tetanus-acellular pertussis (DTaP) #2, inactivated poliovirus (IPV) #2; *Haemophilus influenzae* type b (Hib) #2, (combination vaccines are available for DTaP and IPV plus either Hepatitis B or Hib), pneumococcal #2; rotavirus #2

Review side effects and ask about previous reactions

##### *Health Screening*

Assess for strabismus

Hearing risk assessment

No additional screening required

#### Anticipatory Guidance

##### *Nutrition*

Maintain breastfeeding schedule

Formula, 5-6 oz five or six times per day

Bottle supplement if breastfeeding mother has returned to work

Vitamin D supplementation 400 IU/day for breastfeeding infants and for formula-fed babies consuming fewer than 1 L (33 oz)/day

Begin iron supplementation for exclusively breastfed infants (1 mg/kg/day) (Greer, 2015)

##### *Elimination*

Similar to 2-month-old

##### *Dental*

May begin drooling in preparation for tooth eruption

##### *Sleep*

**Place on back to sleep in parent's room in a separate crib/cradle/bassinet. Keep loose or soft bedding and toys out of the crib; offer pacifier for nap and bedtime.**

Total sleep: 15-16 hour

Encourage self-consoling techniques

##### *Hygiene*

Continue daily routine of cleanliness

##### *Safety*

Review car safety and violence, exposure to cigarette smoke

Discuss choking hazards and management of choking; avoidance of walkers; playpen and swing safety; begin child-proofing

##### *Play*

Talk with the baby frequently and from different locations

Respond verbally and smile as infant does; cuddle

Sing; expose to different environmental sounds

Supervised water play

Provide bright rattles, tactile toys, mirror

*Guided by Denver Developmental Screening Test II.

## Sleep and Rest

Newborn infants may sleep as many as 17 to 20 hours per day. Sleep patterns vary widely, with some infants sleeping only 2 to 3 hours at a time. At approximately 3 to 4 months of age, most infants begin to sleep for longer periods during the night, although some children do not sleep through the night consistently until the second year.

Often one of the most difficult tasks for new parents is the regulation of their infant's sleep-wake cycles. Perception of sleep problems during infancy might result from parents' unrealistic expectations or lack of confidence in parenting. Parents need anticipatory guidance about what to expect regarding sleep and rest. Readiness for sleeping through the night begins when the infant is between six weeks and three months of age (Owens, 2016). Nurses advise parents that establishing a sleep routine is important for preventing later sleep problems. There are several different approaches to establishing and maintaining a sleep routine. Hauck, Hall, Dhaliwal, Bennett, and Wells (2011) describe active and passive settling techniques, as well as techniques that facilitate self-soothing. Using one or more of these techniques with which the parent is comfortable can assist the infant to establish a consistent sleep routine.

Some parents are distressed when an infant or child wakes in the middle of the night crying and are tempted to console by picking up the child. A certain amount of fussiness at bedtime is not unusual. Placing the infant in the crib or bassinet after cuddling, but before the infant is completely asleep, facilitates self-consoling behavior. Infants who do not learn to self-console when going to sleep expect the parents to console them should they awaken during the night. This can lead to a situation where neither the infant nor the parents are able to sleep through the night. Prevention is the best approach, but should the parents express concern about infant crying at night, the nurse can help with problem solving. The nurse assists the parent with learning how to interpret various infant crying behaviors. Other interventions include not picking up the child, but speaking softly and reassuringly to the infant until the infant becomes quiet, or playing soft music in the room (Hauck et al., 2011). It may take several nights of the infant crying and the parents consoling in this manner to mitigate the problem.

The sleep environment has become an important predictor in the prevalence of sudden unexpected infant death (SUID). The CDC (2015a) describes SUID as an unexpected infant death due to one of three causes: Sudden Infant Death Syndrome (SIDS), unknown cause, or death by suffocation or strangulation (accounts for 24% of SUID). The most current recommendations from the AAP (2011) for prevention of SIDS address primarily modifications in the infant's sleep environment; these strategies also address contributing factors to SUID. The policy includes the following recommendations for parents (AAP Task Force on Sudden Infant Death Syndrome, 2011):

- Put the infant to sleep in a supine position for the first year; if the infant can roll over both ways (supine to prone, prone to supine), the parent does not need to return the infant to a supine position.
- Put the infant to sleep for nap or night in the parent's room in a place other than the parent's bed (e.g., self-enclosed cradle, bassinet, crib); the crib or bassinet should not be near a window or other source of hanging cords or wires.
- Be sure to use the mattress that comes with the crib, that the mattress surface is firm and fits tightly; the mattress may be covered with a fitted sheet.
- There should be no soft or loose bedding (e.g., sheets, blankets, quilts) or toys in the crib.
- Young infants should not be put to sleep in car seats, infant carriers, or other equipment that keeps the infant in a sitting position; if using a sling or soft carrier, be sure that the infant's face is fully visible at all times.
- Avoid feeding infants while sitting on upholstered or soft furniture, especially if tired.
- Avoid exposing the infant to environmental smoke and avoid overheating the infant by dressing in clothes appropriate for the environmental temperature.
- Offer the infant a pacifier at nap and bedtime; be sure the pacifier is not attached to a string or other object.
- Do not use commercially marketed products that state they reduce the risk of SIDS.
- Breastfeed infants exclusively for at least the first 6 months, if possible, and be sure infants receive all recommended immunizations.
- Provide opportunities during awake time for "tummy" play.

Goldstein, Trachtenberg, Sens, et al. (2015) tracked the prevalence of sudden deaths in infants and compared it to infant deaths from other causes over the past 30 years. Their findings demonstrated that the rate of both SIDS and deaths from other causes have decreased markedly over the 30-year period and at a similar rate. The authors suggest that there may be intrinsic factors common to all major causes that have affected deaths over time, including decreased smoking during pregnancy, increase in exclusive breastfeeding, and increased access to care. They conclude that it may be as yet unidentified underlying system abnormalities that are the hallmark of SIDS (Goldstein et al., 2016). Additional information about SIDS is discussed in Chapter 45.

## Safety

The rapidly growing infant becomes mobile seemingly overnight. With newfound mobility comes the potential for unintentional injury. As the infant's musculature strengthens and coordination improves, the infant has an insatiable desire to explore. Without the cognitive skills needed to differentiate danger from safety, the rolling, crawling, toddling infant is at great risk for injury.

Infants are totally dependent on others for safety and protection. They are especially vulnerable to serious injury because of their relatively large head size. Motor development progresses to the point where infants quickly master new skills to learn more about their environment. They begin impulsively to reach out and move toward interesting objects around them.

Because of an infant's dependence, parents and caregivers are the primary recipients of anticipatory safety guidance. From the first day of life, safety must be considered and incorporated into the infant's world. Providing a safe environment for a rapidly growing infant is challenging. Potential safety hazards multiply as the baby learns to creep, crawl, climb, and explore. Some parents may not have a complete awareness of the safety issues that must be addressed to protect the infant from injury.

### Motor Vehicle Safety

Injuries associated with automobile crashes constitute the single greatest threat to an infant's life and health. Restraining seats are the only practical means of reducing this risk.

Infant safety in motor vehicles depends entirely on adults. Parents must be informed that they cannot protect their child from injury in a crash by cradling or holding the infant on their laps. Adults are neither strong enough nor quick enough to prevent the sudden forward motions or to overcome the inertial forces (external forces of motion caused by impact) exerted in a crash. An unrestrained adult is propelled forward, trapping and crushing the infant between the adult's body and the hard surfaces inside the car on impact. The only way to prevent injuries and death to an infant in a car is to use a car safety seat for each trip, no matter how short.

A lifelong practice begins with the newborn infant's first ride home. Getting a child accustomed to using a safety seat at a young age establishes a safety habit and may reduce resistance later (Fig. 6.2). All car safety seats should be placed in the rear seat of the vehicle, preferably in the center, away from the possibility of injury from a side crash (advise parents to consult their automobile operating manual for optimal seat positioning). Newborns and infants should be in a rear-facing seat with a three- or five-point harness until they are 2 years of age or have reached the upper parameters of the manufacturer's recommendation for the specific safety seat (AAP, 2014). Front-facing seats (Fig. 6.3) should be tethered to the tether anchor. LATCH (Lower Anchors and Tethers for Children) systems, which secure the seat without need for the seatbelt, keep the seat tightly anchored to the car. Both the car (those made after 2002) and seat must have the LATCH system for it to work without the seatbelt (AAP, 2014). Children should remain in an approved car safety seat or booster seat until they are approximately 4 feet 9 inches tall (between 8 and 12 years) (AAP, 2014). Nearly all states have passed laws regarding the age a child may use a regulation automobile seat belt; parents should be aware of the law in the state where they live or plan to travel (state regulations may be accessed through http://www.nhtsa.gov). Advise parents to check borrowed car seats to be sure they have not been in a previous crash, are not cracked or broken, and are not too old or without manufacturer directions (AAP, 2014).

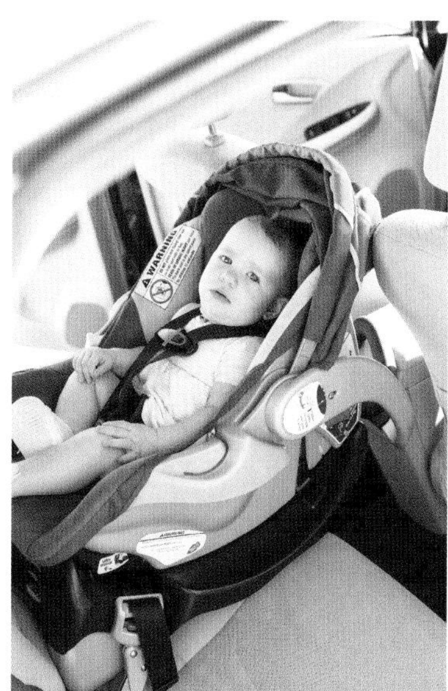

FIG 6.2 The infant rides facing the rear of the vehicle, ideally in the center of the back seat. The infant seat is secured to the vehicle with the seatbelt; straps on the car seat adjust to accommodate the growing baby. (© 2016, Getty Images. Reprinted with Permission.)

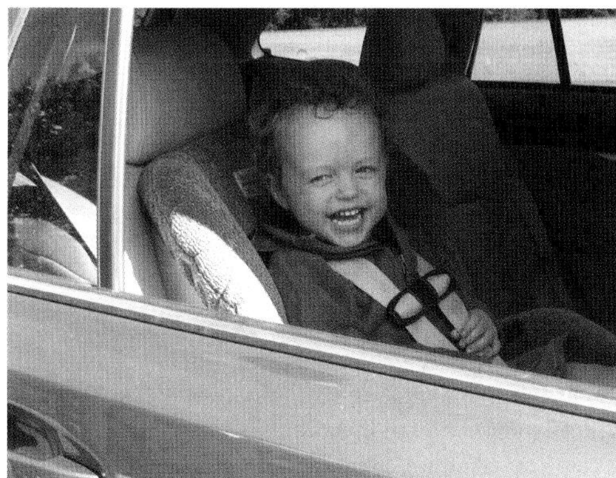

FIG 6.3 After the child reaches 2 years of age and has reached the manufacturer's height and weight recommendations for a rear-facing car seat, the child uses a forward-facing upright car safety seat. The safety straps should be adjusted to provide a snug fit, and the seat should be placed in the back seat of the car, ideally in the middle.

Some injuries and deaths have been associated with the deployment of airbags. Infants and children younger than 13 years should not be restrained in the front seat of cars equipped with airbags on the passenger side. When deployed, the airbag can severely jolt the car safety seat and harm the infant or child. Both the National Highway Traffic Safety Administration (NHTSA, 2015) and the AAP recommend placing all young children in the rear seat with the appropriate restraint.

### Providing a Safe Home Environment

During infancy and early childhood, when children are typically limited to the home environment, safety in and around the home is a top priority. With the exception of injuries and deaths related to motor vehicle crashes, most childhood injuries occur in the home. Major causes of unintentional injury that require visits to an emergency department include contact with sharp objects, bites and stings, cuts, and burns; however, the leading cause in infants and young children (younger than 9 years) is falls (CDC, 2013a). Besides motor vehicle crashes, unintentional suffocation (e.g., choking, strangulation), drowning, and fire and burn injury are the leading causes of death related to unintentional injury (CDC, 2013b). Parents must also consider safety as a factor when selecting daycare facilities for their child.

### Burn Prevention

Infants are especially vulnerable to inflicted burns, particularly scald burns. Infants' limited mobility makes it impossible for them to escape from immersion in hot water. Parents should be instructed to decrease the setting on water heaters to 120° F to prevent accidental scalds. Infant skin is thin, causing burns to occur faster at lower temperatures than in adults. With water temperature settings of 140° F, it takes only 3 seconds for the child to suffer serious burns. Lowering the temperature by 20° F causes the same degree of burn injury in 8 to 10 minutes of submersion. An adult should test the water temperature before the infant is submerged to decrease the risk of unintentional scald injuries.

Advise parents to avoid smoking, drinking hot liquids, or cooking while holding an infant. As infants begin to crawl around on the floor, open electrical sockets should be covered with appropriate socket protectors. Open stoves or fireplaces are especially intriguing to an exploring infant and should be outfitted with a guard or grid. Avoid use of a steam vaporizer to prevent scald injuries to a curious infant.

Burn injuries in infants can also be caused by various other sources. Exposure to sunlight can result in serious sunburn to their delicate skin. Young infants should not be exposed to sunlight, even for brief periods and on cloudy days; sunscreen should not be used on infants younger than 6 months old (AAP, 2015b; Balk & the Council on Environmental Health and Section on Dermatology, 2011). The best way to minimize the adverse effects of the sun is avoidance. If children are going to be in the sun, they should wear clothing to cover exposed areas of the skin, hat, and sunglasses. Parents should be encouraged to apply UVA and UVB sun blocks and sunscreens (minimum sun protection factor 15) liberally to older infants and children. Sunscreen should be applied 15 to 30 minutes in advance of exposure and be reapplied every

2 hours (AAP, 2015b; Balk & the Council on Environmental Health and Section on Dermatology, 2011).

### Safe Baby Furnishings

Baby furniture, although seemingly benign, can present lethal hazards to a growing infant. Parents should be aware of safety considerations when planning or decorating the infant's room. Parents need to be aware that older furniture that has been handed down may not meet current safety regulations. In older cribs, the gaps between slats may be large enough that infants could entrap their heads, or the paint may contain lead.

Hanging toys or mobiles placed over the crib should be positioned well out of the infant's reach to prevent entanglement and strangulation. Encourage the parent to avoid placing large toys in the crib because an older infant may use them as steps to climb over the side, resulting in a serious fall. Cribs should be positioned away from curtains or blinds to prevent accidental entanglement in dangling cords (see Patient-Centered Teaching box).

## PATIENT-CENTERED TEACHING

### *Crib Safety*

- The distance between slats must be no more than 2⅜ inches wide to prevent entrapment of the infant's head or body. Mesh-sided cribs should have mesh openings smaller than ¼ inch (6 mm).
- The interior of the crib must snugly accommodate a standard-size mattress so that the gap is minimal, less than the width of two adult fingers. Excessive space could allow the infant to become wedged, potentially suffocating.
- Decorative enhancements on the crib are not recommended because they can break apart and be aspirated by the infant. Design cutouts can trap an infant's arm or neck, causing death or serious injury.
- Corner posts or finials that rise above the end panels can snag garments and inadvertently strangle infants.
- The drop side must be impossible for an infant to release. Activating the drop side must take either a strong force (at least 10 lb) or a distinct action at each locking device. Never leave the drop side down when an infant is in the crib.
- Wood surfaces should be free of splinters, cracks, and lead-based paint.

### Preventing Falls

Infants are often placed on surfaces at heights that are convenient for the adult, such as on changing tables, counters, or furniture. These surfaces often have no restraining barriers. Infants begin to roll over as early as 2 months, and as they begin to scoot or crawl, fall injuries from these elevations are common. There must be constant adult supervision when infants are placed at such heights (Fig. 6.4). If the parent or nurse must move away from the infant, the adult should either take the infant or, if supplies are close, place a hand on the infant while reaching. At home, parents may choose to place their child on the floor for changing diapers or providing other care.

Falls from infant seats, out of highchairs, or out of strollers are common. Injuries can be prevented with supervision and the use of safety restraining straps to limit the mobility of the infant (see Fig. 6.4).

As infants begin to crawl, placing gates at the top and bottom of stairs can prevent falls. Infant walkers are dangerous and are not recommended. They allow infants mobility and the freedom to explore surroundings before they have developed the ability to interpret heights or protect themselves from falls.

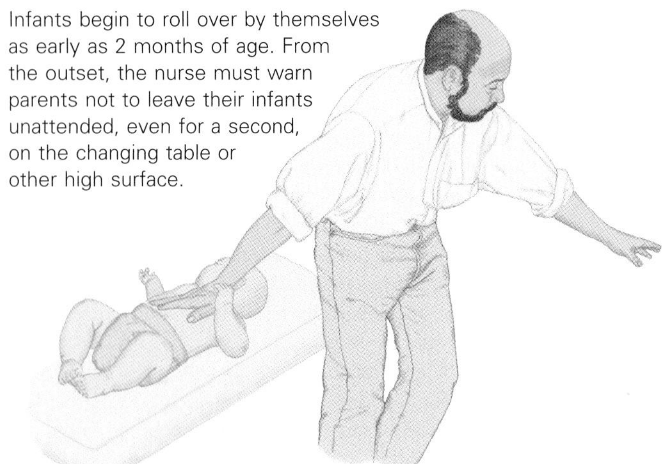

Infants begin to roll over by themselves as early as 2 months of age. From the outset, the nurse must warn parents not to leave their infants unattended, even for a second, on the changing table or other high surface.


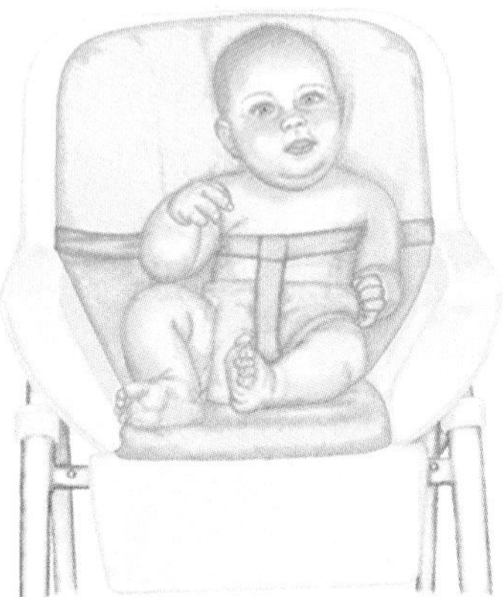

Close supervision and the use of restraining straps can prevent falls from highchairs, a common cause of injuries in children. After the straps are fastened, the highchair tray is secured to the front of the highchair.


**FIG 6.4** Safety education for parents of infants should emphasize the need for constant supervision and the use of restraining devices to prevent falls.

### Preventing Asphyxiation

**Asphyxiation** (suffocation) occurs when air cannot get into or out of the lungs and oxygen supplies are consequently depleted. Carbon dioxide levels then increase, causing life-threatening disruption of cardiac and cerebral functioning. Choking occurs when substances or objects are *aspirated* into the airway or into the branches of the lower airways, causing partial or complete obstruction of the lungs. Strangulation is typically thought of as a constriction of the neck, but it also includes blockage of the nose and mouth by airtight materials, such as plastic. This blockage prevents air exchange. Store all plastic bags or covers out of the infant's reach. Choking is a major concern in the first few months of an infant's life, when aspiration of feedings or vomit can occur easily because of the immature swallowing mechanism. Parents should be taught to position infants on their sides after feedings and to avoid placing small infants in bed with a bottle propped in their mouths.

As infants grow, they begin to explore the world around them by placing anything and everything in their mouths. Size, shape, and consistency are major determinants of whether a food or object is likely to be aspirated by an infant. Food that is round or similar to the size of the airway is especially dangerous. Dangerous foods include sliced hot dogs, hard candy, peanuts, grapes, raisins, and chewing gum, among others. These foods should be avoided until the child is able to chew thoroughly before swallowing. Food should be cut into small pieces, and the child should be supervised while eating. Advise parents

## HEALTH PROMOTION

### *The 6-Month-Old Infant*

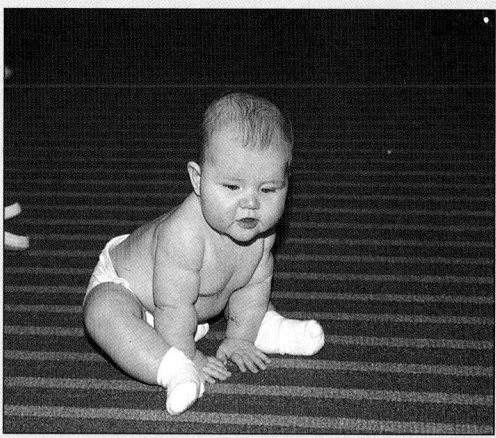

**Focused Assessment**

Ask the parent the following:

- What kind of new activities is your baby doing?
- If you have begun to give your baby solid foods, what solid foods have you introduced?
- How is any child care working out?
- What have you done about child-proofing your home?

**Developmental Milestones**

*Personal/social:* Interacts readily and noisily with parents and familiar people; may be cautious with strangers

*Fine motor:* Rakes objects with the whole hand; begins to transfer; mouths; can hold an object in each hand

*Language/cognitive:* Begins to imitate sounds (raspberries, clucking, kissing); babbles; says single sounds; beginning object permanence; awareness of time sequence

*Gross motor:* Tripod sitting unsupported; gets on hands and knees; bears full weight on legs; "swims" when prone

**Critical Milestones***

*Personal/social:* Reaches for toy out of reach; looks at hand; smiles spontaneously

*Fine motor:* Looks at raisin placed on contrasting surface; reaches out; follows completely side to side

*Language/cognitive:* Turns to rattle sound made out of vision on each side; squeals; laughs

*Gross motor:* Rolls over both directions; no head lag; lifts head and chest completely

**Health Maintenance**

***Physical Measurements***

Birth weight doubles

Continue to measure and plot length, weight, and head circumference

***Immunizations***

Diphtheria-tetanus-acellular pertussis (DTaP) #3 (may substitute combination vaccine); *Haemophilus influenzae* type b (Hib) #3 (depending on vaccine manufacturer); pneumococcal #3; rotavirus #3 (unless using the 2-dose vaccine); inactivated poliovirus (IPV) #3 (can be given between 6 and 18 months) and Hepatitis B #3 may be given between now and 18 months if not in combination vaccine

Influenza vaccine annually; two doses initially, separated by at least 4 weeks

Ask about previous reactions

Review side effects

***Health Screening***

Initial lead screening risk assessment (see Box 6.4)

Hearing risk assessment

**Anticipatory Guidance**

***Nutrition***

Begin introducing solid foods one at a time by spoon; use iron-fortified cereals

Hold or place in infant seat for feeding

Begin to offer a cup

Vitamin D supplementation 400 IU/day for breastfed infants and infants whose formula intake is less than 1 L (33 oz) per day

May discontinue iron supplementation for breastfeeding infants who are taking sufficient iron-rich solid foods

***Elimination***

Stools darken and become more formed as solids are increased

***Dental***

Tooth eruption begins with lower incisors

May have some pain and low-grade fever (<101° F)

May be fussy

Clean teeth and gums with wet cloth

Do not put to sleep with a bottle

Assess risk for tooth decay; begin fluoride supplementation for infants not receiving fluoridated water

Begin fluoride varnish application

***Sleep***

**Place on back to sleep (infant may roll over to prone position) in a separate crib. Keep loose or soft bedding and toys out of the crib; offer pacifier for nap and bedtime. Can move to a separate room**

Total sleep: 12-16 hour/day

Sleeps all night; two or three naps

Maintain sleep routine

***Hygiene***

Continue daily routine of cleanliness

Clean toys frequently

***Safety***

Review choking, walkers, violence, exposure to cigarette smoke

Discuss child-proofing, drowning prevention, poison prevention (see Chapter 34)

***Play***

Expose to different sounds and sights

Begin social games (pat-a-cake, peek-a-boo)

Provide bath toys, rattles, mirror, large ball, soft stuffed animals

Encourage to sit unsupported

Encourage to rock on hands and knees

*Guided by Denver Developmental Screening Test II.

to strongly discourage infants and young children from playing, singing, or other activities while eating, to avoid choking. Infants are equally endangered by rattles, pieces of toys, ribbons from stuffed animals, and common household objects such as coins, buttons, pins, or beads found on the floor or within their reach. Balloons should not be given to infants or young children or used where an infant or young child plays.

Anticipatory guidance for parents includes performing a thorough inspection of the infant's surroundings to remove all potential items that infants could grasp, place in their mouths, and choke on. Parents can be encouraged to crawl through the home to gain a better perspective of the infant's environment. Parents can then substitute safe objects for exploration.

Ornaments or toys with detachable parts are not recommended for infants because of the aspiration risk. The Consumer Product Safety Commission has a long-established toy standard to prevent choking hazards in nonfood products targeted for children younger than 3 years. Parents should take extra care to note the presence of small detachable parts on toys before allowing the infant to play with the items. Although the government regulates the size of parts on infants' toys, older children's toys are not regulated by the same standard. As the infant explores an older sibling's or a playmate's territory, adult supervision is important.

To prevent strangulation injuries, parents should not place a pacifier on a string or cord around the infant's neck, not put an infant to sleep with a bib in place, and not position a crib near blinds or curtain cords. Crib slats should comply with the $2\frac{3}{8}$-inch width requirement to prevent head entrapment.

In addition to inspecting and providing a safe environment for the infant, instruct parents in the appropriate action to take if the infant chokes (see Chapter 34 for a discussion of emergency procedures).

### Preventing Lead Exposure

Although lead poisoning in the United States has decreased markedly since the elimination of lead paint and solder used in homes and leaded gasoline, lead poisoning remains a significant risk, especially in cities where old housing predominates. In addition, paint from old homes can enter the soil and get on children's hands when they are playing. Children inhale lead dust as homes are being renovated. The lead risk assessment begins as the infant begins to be mobile (6 months of age). Risk should be assessed at every well visit beginning at the 6-month visit and education or treatment initiated as appropriate (Box 6.4) (see Chapter 34).

#### BOX 6.4 Lead Exposure Risk Assessment

Do you live in, or does your child spend time in, housing that was built before 1950 that has peeling paint or plaster or before 1978 that is being renovated?

Do you live near any sources of environmental lead, such as smelters or places that use leaded gasoline?

Does your child regularly come in contact with a household member who works with lead or lead solder (e.g., plumber, construction worker, stained glass artisan)?

Does your child have a sibling or any other household member who has tested positive for lead exposure or has had lead poisoning?

Has your child recently lived in a foreign country?

Has your infant or child been exposed to any other sources of lead: vinyl miniblinds, imported ceramics, toys, old baby furniture, leaded crystal, or foods that may have been stored in pottery from a foreign country?

Does your infant or child routinely put non-food items in his or her mouth?

If the infant has any risk factors, a capillary test for lead should be performed. Otherwise, a routine capillary lead screening should be done at the 9-month or 1-year visit.

## Concerns During Infancy

Parents, especially first-time parents have multiple concerns about their infants. Nurses can intervene to relieve parental anxiety and provide a realistic perspective about normal parental concerns.

### Patterns of Crying

Crying is a mode of communication for infants. It is especially challenging for new parents to learn and accurately interpret their individual infant's cry. Some infants respond readily to attempts to comfort them, sleep a great deal, and fit easily into their family's lifestyle. Other infants cry more readily and for longer periods and spend more time in a fretful, restless state than others. These infants often have more colic symptoms and sleep problems. This irritability may be caused by health problems, such as feeding difficulties, infection, or allergies, but often no clear cause emerges. In some cases, the infant's temperament may be the cause.

Nurses can suggest that parents, after ruling out physiologic causes for crying (e.g., hungry, soiled, gassy), console their infants when they cry by holding them, talking softly, or humming. Gently stroking an infant's head, back, and arms may also be soothing. Infant massage techniques and simply "centering" are easily accomplished by positioning the infant's arms and legs toward the midline of the body. Swaddling a new infant is a consoling technique that helps the infant to center.

Specific strategies to diminish infant irritability include activities such as taking the baby for a car ride, carrying the infant in a front pack close to the parent's chest, or swinging the baby in an infant swing. Vertical positioning and constant motion, such as that obtained when walking with the baby carried over the shoulder, are sometimes helpful. The football-carry position, with gentle patting on the back, can also be tried. Sometimes irritable infants need to be left alone to cry for brief periods. If parents choose this strategy, they must be cautioned to limit the crying time and to check the baby frequently.

Few interventions are consistently successful because infant responses may vary. However, providing parents with strategies helps decrease their anxiety and increase their feelings of control and competence. As infants grow and develop, they are better able to regulate their sleep-wake cycles. Generally, during the third or fourth month of life, sleep problems and irritability improve.

### The Infant With Colic

Colic usually refers to unexplained paroxysmal crying or fussing in infants, which may be characterized by infants pulling up their arms and legs. Periods of crying tend to occur at the same time of day, often in the late afternoon or evening. To be diagnosed with colic, an infant must have the symptoms several times daily for several days a week. Most infants outgrow symptoms of colic by 3 to 4 months of age.

***Etiology.*** The cause of colic is unknown, but several theories have been researched. The possibilities include but are not limited to allergy, cow's milk intolerance, maternal anxiety, familial stress, and too rapid feeding or overfeeding. It is highly likely that more than one factor may be involved. Colic is more common in infants with sensitive temperaments who seem to need increased attention.

## HEALTH PROMOTION

### *The 9-Month-Old Infant*

**Focused Assessment**

Ask the parent the following:

- What kind of new activities is your baby doing?
- How has your baby reacted to solid foods?
- Do you live in a house built before 1978 or an older home undergoing renovation?
- Do you live near sources of environmental lead?
- Does your baby regularly come in contact with someone who uses lead?
- Do you have a family member who has had lead poisoning?

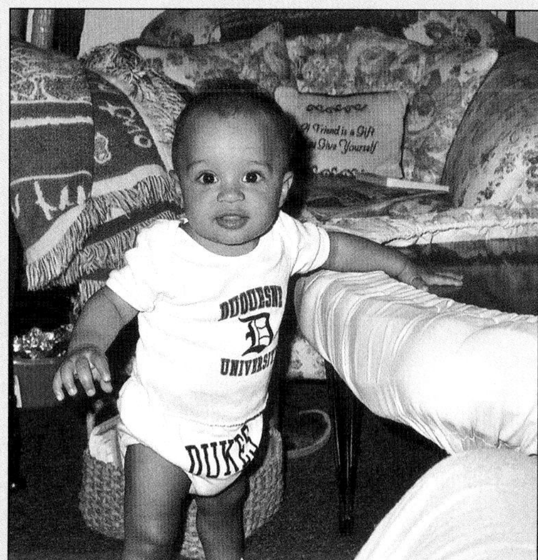

**Developmental Milestones**

*Personal/social:* Stranger wariness; waves bye-bye; plays social games; begins to indicate wants

*Fine motor:* Beginning pincer grasp; actively searches for out-of-sight objects; bangs toys together

*Language/cognitive:* Uses consonant and several vowel sounds; beginning to attach meaning to words; understands some symbolic language (blow a kiss); knows own name; says mama and dada specifically

*Gross motor:* Gets to a sitting position; pulls up to stand; creeps and crawls; walks holding on to furniture; may briefly stand alone

**Critical Milestones***

*Personal/social:* Feeds self finger foods; tries to get toys; looks at hands

*Fine motor:* Transfers; rakes a raisin or Cheerio; picks up and holds a small object in each hand

*Language/cognitive:* Imitates sounds; says single syllables; begins to put syllables together

*Gross motor:* No head lag; sits without support; stands holding onto furniture

**Health Maintenance**

Physical Measurements

Continue to measure and plot length, weight, and head circumference

***Immunizations***

Hepatitis B #3 (can give between 6 and 18 months); omit if combination vaccine has been used previously

Influenza vaccine annually

Provide information about upcoming measles-mumps-rubella (MMR), varicella, and Hepatitis A vaccines

***Health Screening***

Lead risk assessment (routine capillary lead screen at 9 or 12 months, usually in conjunction with hemoglobin and hematocrit)

Hemoglobin or hematocrit (screen at 9 or 12 months in conjunction with lead screen)

Formalized developmental screening

Hearing risk assessment

**Anticipatory Guidance**

***Nutrition***

Continue to breastfeed on established schedule

Formula, 16-32 oz/day

Vitamin D supplementation 400 IU/day if breastfed or taking less than 1 L (33 oz) of formula/day

Continue iron-fortified cereal

Begin to introduce various soft, mashed, or chopped table foods

Encourage cup rather than bottle

Avoid giving large pieces of food and foods known to be associated with choking

***Elimination***

Urinary and bowel patterns consistent

Appearance of undigested food in stools

***Dental***

Four teeth

Brush erupted teeth with soft toothbrush and water

Assess risk for dental caries

Fluoride varnish application

***Sleep***

Night waking diminishes if managed appropriately

***Hygiene***

More vigilant cleanliness of diaper area as bladder volume increases

Wash infant's hands and face frequently

Keep toys clean

***Safety***

Review child-proofing, violence, exposure to cigarette smoke

Discuss lowering crib mattress, household and plant poisons, burn prevention, sunscreen use, avoiding sources of lead

***Play***

Social games

Provide cloth, cardboard, or plastic books

Cuddle, rock, hug

Ball rolling

Pots and pans with wooden spoons

Plastic stacking or nesting containers

Hide-and-seek games with toys

*Guided by Denver Developmental Screening Test II.

## EVIDENCE-BASED PRACTICE

Inconsolable infant crying is one of the most distressing events for both new and experienced parents. Because infants do not talk, crying is their only means of communication, and there is nothing more frustrating to a parent than not being able to interpret their infant's communication signals. When the parent brings the infant to the provider and describes inconsolable crying, the provider tries to determine an underlying cause. If one is not discovered, the diagnosis is often infant colic. There is no way to accurately diagnose colic, other than to exclude other logical contributors to the crying symptoms.

Traditionally, colic has been described as inconsolable paroxysmal crying periods that occur on a daily basis for several days a week. Colic can last for several months and disappear spontaneously when the infant reaches approximately 3 to 4 months of age. It is difficult to manage, as there are few treatments available. Because nurses often assist parents to determine different types of crying behavior in their infants, it would be useful to know what symptoms are specific to a colicky infant that are usually not present in an infant without colic. To that purpose, Kvitvaer, Miller, and Newell (2012) conducted research to identify a collection of symptoms that would suggest an infant has colic, as opposed to another underlying cause of crying behavior. Of 1041 infants brought to a clinic with a complaint of unexplained crying, those for whom parental informed consent was provided were included in the study. Exclusions included those whose parent did not speak English and those who were ill or had a diagnosis that required referral. The final number was 186, or 17.8% of the crying infants, which the researchers say matches the estimated percentage of colicky infants in the infant population. Of the included infants, a group of 159 were described by their mothers as having colic, while 27 were not.

Mothers were given a survey that they completed when first bringing their infant to the clinic. The survey consisted of 45 descriptors previously validated to represent colic, along with seven other descriptors either known not be associated with colic or neutral. Using these descriptors, the researchers calculated the odds ratio of each for belonging to the colicky versus the noncolicky group. They used the significant descriptors to determine a constellation of symptoms that represent the likelihood of having or not having colic.

The results provided an interesting picture of a colicky infant. Characteristics that most predicted colic included the following: leg flexion, discomfort with bowel movements, irritability after feeding and when put to bed, appearance of being in pain, needing to be cuddled frequently, instantaneously going from happy to crying, and a family history of allergy or asthma. Following logistic regression analysis, the researchers suggested that infants with this constellation of symptoms have a 98% risk of having colic, while those without had a 3% risk.

Even though the study has limitations, an important one of which is the number discrepancy between groups, the results provide some insight as to what behavioral characteristics suggest colic as opposed to other causes of crying in infants. Knowing this information could help nurses reduce parental worry that their infant might have something seriously wrong as opposed to colic, which is relatively benign. Although the study does not address interventions for colicky infants, knowing the condition is not serious might, at the very least, reduce parental stress. Think about how you might use this information in providing anticipatory guidance.

Reference: Kvitvaer, B., Miller, J., & Newell, D. (2011). Improving our understanding of the colicky infant: A prospective observational study. *Journal of Clinical Nursing, 21,* 63–69.

***Management.*** The provider must determine whether, in fact, the infant is crying because of colic and not because of an acute condition such as intussusception, otitis media, or a fracture. Symptoms of milk allergy other than crying should be present before formula changes are made. Many practitioners avoid using medications to treat colic because of their limited success, lack of scientific data, and possible side effects. Perry, Hunt, and Ernst (2011) conducted a systematic review of randomized controlled trials of complementary therapies for the treatment of infant colic. They found that fennel extract and sucrose solution were the most effective treatments, and that the use of probiotics, such as *Lactobacillus reuteri,* and other therapies were not as effective. Herbal remedies should not be used without consulting a health provider first. If parents are using herbs such as chamomile, the nurse should be sure they know the appropriate dose, are aware of possible allergic reactions, and do not use so much as to interfere with adequate breast milk or formula intake.

***Nursing considerations.*** Because the etiology of colic and the care of an infant with colic are so individualized, it is very important that the nurse obtain a thorough history. The nurse should provide a concerned and caring atmosphere during the assessment and reassure the parents that colic is not related to bad parenting. It should be determined whether any other symptoms are associated with the crying. The infant's eating habits, including whether the infant is breastfed or bottle fed, should be discussed. The nurse should ask the parents whether commonalities are associated with the crying (time of day, associated activities, family members present) and ask what has been tried, what works, and what does not work. If the parents are unsure, they should keep a diary for 48 to 72 hours to determine patterns. The nurse should assess the parents' stress level and support system.

The nurse needs to educate the parents regarding the normal growth and development needs of infants related to sleep and awake times, feeding, soothing, and holding and listen to the parents with an empathic ear. Parents should be encouraged to soothe their infant by rocking and cuddling. Some infants will quiet when given a massage, pacifier, or warm bath. If the parent is busy, a swing may provide a soothing, rhythmic effect. Some of the same strategies for soothing infants may also be effective in quieting infants with colic.

Some infants seem most distressed during high-activity times when the family may be busy preparing meals, doing chores, gathering at the end of the day, and so forth. By assisting parents to see such trends, the nurse can help them establish alternative routines to decrease the infant's stimuli. The parent may choose to feed the infant away from all the activity or to have a later dinner. Each family will be unique, and the nurse's role is to facilitate problem solving.

All families need extra support after the birth of an infant. If the infant has colic, the need increases. During the first few months after the addition of a new baby, demanding work schedules, lack of recovery time from childbirth, the needs of other family members, physical exhaustion, and sleep deprivation can combine with the presence of a fretful infant to create stressful situations for the entire family. Sometimes infant temperament and parental coping styles are not compatible.

The nurse might, for example, explain to new parents, "Parenting is very much a challenge, even when parents care about their baby as much as you do. At first it is difficult to discern what Avery is telling you when she cries. But you will feel more and more comfortable, even recognizing that she has a different cry when she is hungry than when she is tired."

In validating the parents' feelings, the nurse recognizes that the infant's irritability or colic is real, not imagined, and that the infant is a challenge to handle. The nurse can reassure the parents that the infant is healthy, normal, and gaining weight and that the parents are competent in their nurturing role.

The emotional reserves of the parents can be restored through rest and pleasurable activities. Parents may need brief periods of relief from infant care responsibilities. Grandparents or other family members might be able to provide the parents with an evening out or a night of uninterrupted sleep. This direct support can help restore the parents' energy to cope with daily activities and feel more relaxed and confident in their parenting.

## HEALTH PROMOTION

### *The 12-Month-Old Infant*

**Focused Assessment**

Ask the parent the following:

- What approaches to discipline have you and your partner discussed and agreed on?
- Is your baby able to follow directions and carry out requests?
- Have you assessed your home and environment for sources of lead?

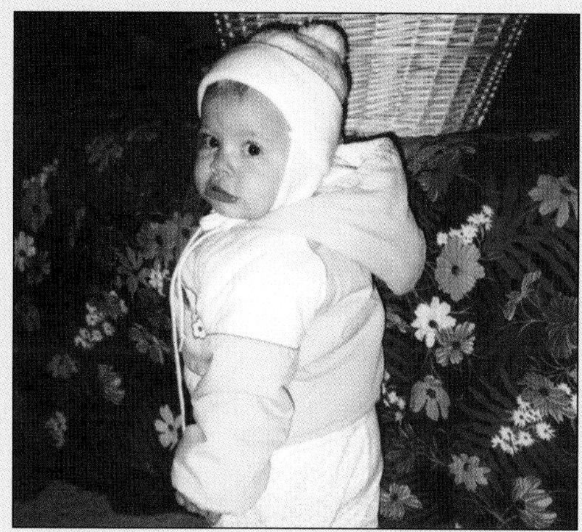

**Developmental Milestones**

*Personal/social:* Rolls or throws a ball with another person; explores; drinks from a cup; indicates wants without crying

*Fine motor:* Actively looks for hidden objects; puts blocks in containers; uses simple toys appropriately

*Language/cognitive:* Names the appropriate parent; begins to say one to three single words; understands simple requests

*Gross motor:* Stands alone for increasing lengths of time; stoops and recovers; walks holding onto a hand; may begin to walk alone and climb stairs (on knees)

**Critical Milestones***

*Personal/social:* Plays pat-a-cake; feeds self; works to get a toy

*Fine motor:* Developed pincer grasp; bangs objects together; picks up two cubes

*Language/cognitive:* Jabbers; combines syllables; mama/dada is nonspecific

*Gross motor:* Stands briefly without support; gets to sitting position; pulls to stand

**Health Maintenance**

***Physical Measurements***

Continue to measure and plot length, weight, and head circumference
Weight is usually triple birth weight
Length is 50% more than birth length

***Immunizations***

Measles-mumps-rubella (MMR) #1; varicella vaccine #1 (may use combination MMRV vaccine); Hepatitis A #1; pneumococcal and Hib boosters (if not scheduled to be given at 15 months); hepatitis B #3 (if not given previously)
Influenza vaccine annually
Hepatitis A #1

***Health Screening***

Hemoglobin/hematocrit if not done earlier
Lead screen if not done earlier
Hearing risk assessment
Tuberculosis (TB) screening if at risk

**Anticipatory Guidance**

***Nutrition***

May begin whole milk (2 or 3 cups daily)
Offer various table foods from different food groups
Vitamin D supplementation 400 IU/day if breastfed or taking less than 1 L (33 oz) of vitamin D fortified milk/day
Begins to use table utensils
Usually eats three meals and snacks
Avoid giving foods high in salt and sugar
Discuss highchair safety

***Elimination***

Remains dry for longer periods
Bowel movements decrease in number and become more regular

***Dental***

Eight teeth
Continue fluoride, if recommended, and brushing
Fluoride varnish application

***Sleep***

Sleeps through the night and has one or two naps

***Hygiene***

Continue as previously

***Safety***

Review poisons, burns, violence, exposure to cigarette smoke
Maintain the infant in a rear facing car safety seat
Discuss falls, water safety, toy and toy box safety, bike passenger helmet

***Play***

Beginning parallel play
Push-pull toys
Various-size balls
Picture books
Dolls and stuffed animals
"Busy" box
Sandbox – be sure to cover when not in use

*Guided by Denver Developmental Screening Test II.

## KEY CONCEPTS

- During the first year of life, the infant's organs grow and mature at a rapid rate, yet infants' organ systems remain very different from those of older children and adults.
- Weight gain and muscle growth during infancy allow the infant to have increased control of reflexes and increasingly coordinated movement.
- Sensory capabilities, neuromuscular control, perceptual skills, the quality and quantity of parental interaction, and environmental stimulation all affect cognitive development during infancy.
- Infants develop language first by listening to sounds of caregivers, then by realizing that certain sounds have special meaning, and eventually by using simple words to communicate.
- Infancy is the period during which children develop the foundation of their personalities, struggling to establish a sense of basic trust rather than mistrust.
- One of the most important features of psychosocial development during infancy is parent-infant attachment, or the sense of belonging with one another.
- Common problems during infancy, such as separation anxiety, sleep disorders, and fretfulness, cause parents concern and distress. Nurses should be available with information and support to provide anticipatory guidance.
- Nurses play an important role in health promotion and disease prevention related to immunizations.
- Because infancy is a period of very rapid growth and development, nutritional needs are of special significance. Parents frequently have many questions and concerns about nutrition.
- Breast milk or commercially prepared formulas provide the foundation of nutrition throughout infancy; exclusive breastfeeding for the first 6 months provides optimal nutritional benefit.
- Solid foods are usually introduced between 4 and 6 months of age in small amounts, one food at a time, on the basis of the infant's growth and development.
- Weaning usually begins between ages 6 and 12 months. It should never take place during stress, and the infant should receive breast milk or formula in the cup until age 12 months.
- Teething usually begins between 5 and 9 months of age. Some degree of discomfort is normal, and parents often need suggestions for coping with teething.
- Bottle-mouth caries is a form of tooth decay that can develop in infants and children as a result of prolonged breastfeeding or bottle feeding, especially at night, as well as frequent intake of sugary drinks.
- Improved motor development coupled with a keen desire to explore the environment places the infant at great risk for unintentional injury.
- Colic can be very stressful for parents. The cause of colic is unknown, and care of the infant must be individualized. Support of the parents is very important.

## REFERENCES AND READINGS


American Academy of Audiology. (2011). *American Academy of Audiology childhood hearing screening guidelines*. Retrieved from http://www.cdc.gov.

American Academy of Pediatrics. (2011). *Oral health risk assessment tool*. Retrieved from http://www.aap.org.

American Academy of Pediatrics. (2012). Breastfeeding and the use of human milk. *Pediatrics, 129*(3), e827–e841.

American Academy of Pediatrics. (2014). *Car safety seat checkup*. Retrieved from http://www.aap.org.

American Academy of Pediatrics. (2015a). *Baby bottles and bisphenol A (BPA)*. Retrieved from http://www.healthychildren.org.

American Academy of Pediatrics. (2015b). *Sun safety: Information for parents about sunburn and sunscreen*. Retrieved from http://www.healthychildren.org.

American Academy of Pediatrics. (2015c). *Where we stand: Testing of well water*. Retrieved from http://www.healthychildren.org.

American Academy of Pediatrics. (2016). Recommendations for preventive pediatric health care. *Pediatrics, 137*(1), 25–27.

American Academy of Pediatrics & Early Hearing Detection and Intervention Program. (2015). *Early Hearing Detection and Intervention*. Retrieved from http://www.aap.org.

American Academy of Pediatrics, Joint Committee on Infant Hearing. (2007). Year 2007 position statement: Principles and guidelines for early hearing detection and intervention programs. *Pediatrics, 120*, 898–920.

American Academy of Pediatrics, Task Force on Sudden Infant Death Syndrome. (2011). Policy statement SIDS and other sleep-related infant deaths: Expansion of recommendations for a safe infant sleeping environment. *Pediatrics, 128*(5), 1030–1039.

American Academy of Pedodontics. (2012). *Policy on dietary recommendations for infants, children, and adolescents*. Retrieved from http://www.aapd.org.

American Heart Association. (2015). *Dietary recommendations for healthy children*. Retrieved from http://www.heart.org.

Balk, S., & The Council on Environmental Health and Section on Dermatology. (2011). Technical report: Ultraviolet radiation, a hazard to children and adolescents. *Pediatrics, 127*(3), e791–e817.

Carling, S., Demment, M., Kjolhede, C. et al. (2015). Breastfeeding duration and weight gain trajectory in infancy. *Pediatrics, 135*(1), 111–119.

Centers for Disease Control and Prevention. (2013a). *National estimates of the 10 leading causes of nonfatal injuries treated in hospital emergency departments, United States—2013*. Retrieved from http://www.cdc.gov.

Centers for Disease Control and Prevention. (2013b). *10 leading causes of injury deaths by age group highlighting unintentional injury deaths, United States—2013*. Retrieved from http://www.cdc.gov.

Centers for Disease Control and Prevention. (2014). *Breastfeeding report card 2014*. Retrieved from http://www.cdc.gov.

Centers for Disease Control and Prevention. (2015a). *About SUID and SIDS*. Retrieved from http://www.cdc.gov.

Centers for Disease control and Prevention. (2015b). *Vitamin D supplementation*. Retrieved from http://www.cdc.gov.

Chapin, L., et al. (2013). Nonfatal choking on food among children 14 years or younger in the United States 2001-2009. *Pediatrics, 132*(2), 275–281.

Clark, M., & Slayton, R. (2014). Fluoride use in caries prevention in the primary care setting. *Pediatrics, 134*(3), 626–633.

Crichton, S. (2013). Understanding and supporting speech, language, and communication needs in children. *Community Practitioner, 86*(12), 44–48.

Erikson, E.H. (1963). *Childhood and society* (2nd ed.). New York: Norton.

Flavell, J.H. (1964). *The developmental psychology of Jean Piaget*. New York: Van Nostrand.

Fletcher, D., et al. (2015). Consensus communication on early peanut introduction and the prevention of peanut allergy in high risk infants. *Pediatrics, 136*(3), 600–604.

Freud, A. (1974). *Introduction to psychoanalysis.* New York: International Universities Press.

Goldstein, R., Trachtenberg, F., Sens, M., et al. (2016). Overall postneonatal morality and rates of SIDS. *Pediatrics, 137*(1), 1–10.

Greer, F. (2015). How much iron is needed for breastfeeding infants? *Current Pediatric Review, 11*(4), 298–304.

Greer, F., Sicherer, S., Burks, W., & The Committee on Nutrition and Section on Allergy and Immunology. (2008). Effects of early nutritional interventions on the development of atopic disease in infants and children: The role of maternal dietary restriction, breastfeeding, timing of introduction of complementary foods, and hydrolyzed formulas. *Pediatrics, 121*(1), 183–191.

Grimshaw, K., et al. (2015). Introduction of complementary foods and the relationship to food allergy. *Pediatrics, 132*(6), e1529-e1538.

Hauck, F., Thompson, J., Tanabe, K, et al. (2011). Breastfeeding and reduced risk of sudden infant death syndrome: A meta-analysis. *Pediatrics, 128*, 103–110.

Huh, S., Rifas-Shiman, S., & Taveras, E. (2011). Timing of solid food introduction and risk of obesity in preschool-aged children. *Pediatrics, 127*, e544–e551.

Moyer, V. (2014). Prevention of dental caries in children from birth through age 5 years: United States Preventive Services Task force recommendation statement. *Pediatrics, 133*(6), 1102–1111.

National Center on Birth Defects and Developmental Disabilities. (2015). *Hearing loss in infants and young children: Considerations for pediatric primary care providers.* Retrieved from http://www.cdc.gov.

National Center for Health Statistics. (2014). *Health, United States, 2014* (Table 21). Hyattsville, MD: Author.

National Center for Health Statistics. (2016). *Health, United States, 2015: With special features on racial and ethnic disparities.* Hyattsville, MD: Author.

National Highway Traffic Safety Administration. (2015). *Car seat by child's age and size.* Retrieved from http://www.safercar.gov.

Owens, J. (2016). Sleep medicine. In R. Kliegman, B. Stanton, J. St. Geme, N. Schor, & R. Behrman (Eds.), *Nelson textbook of pediatrics* (20th ed., Ch. 19). Philadelphia, PA: Saunders.

Perry, R., Hunt, K., & Ernst, E. (2011). Nutritional supplements and other complementary medicines for infantile colic: A systematic review. *Pediatrics, 127*, 720–733.

Piaget, J. (1952). *The origins of intelligence in children.* New York: International Universities Press.

United States Department of Health and Human Services. (2010). *Healthy People 2020.* Retrieved from http://www.healthypeople.gov.

United States Preventive Services Task Force. (2014). Prevention of dental caries in children from birth through age 5 years: United States Preventive Services Task Force recommendation statement. *Pediatrics, 133*(6), 626–633.

7

# Health Promotion During Early Childhood

http://evolve.elsevier.com/McKinney/mat-ch/

## LEARNING OBJECTIVES

*After studying this chapter, you should be able to:*

- Describe the physiologic changes and the motor, cognitive, language, and psychosocial developments of the toddler and preschooler.
- Provide parents with anticipatory guidance related to the toddler and preschooler.
- Discuss the causes of and identify interventions for common toddler behaviors: temper tantrums, negativism, and ritualism.
- Identify strategies to alleviate a preschool child's fears and sleep problems.
- Discuss strategies for disciplining a toddler and preschooler.
- Describe the signs of a toddler's readiness for toilet training and offer guidelines to parents.
- Offer parents suggestions for promoting school readiness in the preschool child.

The developmental changes that mark the transition from infancy to early childhood are dramatic. During the toddler years, ages 12 through 36 months, the child begins to venture out independently from a secure base of trust established during the first year. The preschool period, ages 3 through 5 years, is a time of relative tranquility after the tumultuous toddler period.

## GROWTH AND DEVELOPMENT DURING EARLY CHILDHOOD

The toddler years are characterized by a struggle for autonomy as the child develops a sense of self separate from the parent. Boundless energy and insatiable curiosity drive the toddler to explore the environment and master new skills (Fig. 7.1). The combination of increased motor skills, immaturity, and lack of experience places the toddler at risk for unintentional injury. Toddlers' egocentric and demanding behaviors, which are often marked by temper tantrums and negativism, have given this age the label the "terrible twos."

The preschooler becomes increasingly independent, mastering many self-care and motor skills and developing greater social and emotional maturity (Fig. 7.2). The preschooler is imaginative, creative, and curious. Many parents describe this period as their favorite age as they watch the dramatic transformation of a chubby toddler into an agile, articulate child who is ready to enter the world of peers and school.

The nurse's roles as healthcare provider, family counselor, and child advocate continue during the toddler and preschool years. Well-child checkups provide the nurse with opportunities for anticipatory guidance related to growth and development, safety, nutrition, and some of the common age-related concerns of parents. The American Academy of Pediatrics (AAP) (2016) recommends that pediatric providers conduct developmental surveillance (assessing developmental milestones and determining risk for developmental delay) at every routine well visit and that formal developmental screening, using a sensitive and specific screening test, be used at the 9-, 18-, and 30- (or 24-) month visits. In addition, an autism-specific screening should be performed at the 18- and 24-month visit (AAP, 2016). The United States Preventive Services Task Force (USPSTF) (2015a) issued a draft recommendation stating that evidence is lacking that universal screening for autism of asymptomatic young children improves outcomes; in addition, the USPSTF (2015b) issued a final recommendation stating similar conclusions for speech and language screening. Gabrielson, Farley, Speer, et al. (2015) conducted a research study to determine whether providers could recognize the signs of autism spectrum disorder (ASD) in young children within the approximately 10-minute window a provider has for assessment. Their findings indicated that children with ASD demonstrate more typical developmentally appropriate behaviors than atypical and that children without ASD frequently demonstrate atypical behaviors. This research makes a strong case for universal surveillance and follow-up for children whose parents express concerns regarding their development or providers notice a difference in their developmental progression (Gabrielson et al., 2015). Because parental concerns provide a reliable indicator of possible developmental delay, the nurse should elicit any concerns when taking a developmental history as part of every well visit.

### Physical Growth and Development

During early childhood, physical growth slows. The average weight gain is 2.25 kg (5 lb) per year. A child's birth weight has quadrupled by age 2 to 3 years. The rate of increase in height also slows, with the average toddler growing approximately 7.5 cm (3 inches) per year. Children attain half their adult height between ages 2 and 3 years. The brain grows at a slower rate during this period than during infancy. Head circumference reflects this growth, increasing approximately 3.7 cm (1½ inches) during the toddler years compared with the growth of 12 cm (4⅘ inches) in the first 12 months. By age 2 years, the head circumference has reached 90% of its adult size.

#### The Toddler

Immature abdominal musculature gives the toddler a potbellied appearance, with an exaggerated lumbar curve. The child's short legs may appear slightly bowed, and the feet seem flat because of a plantar fat pad that disappears around age 2 years. During the toddler years, muscle tissue gradually replaces much of the adipose tissue (baby fat)

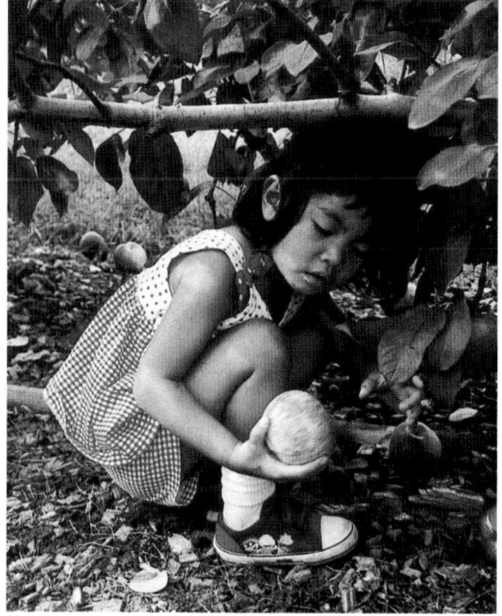

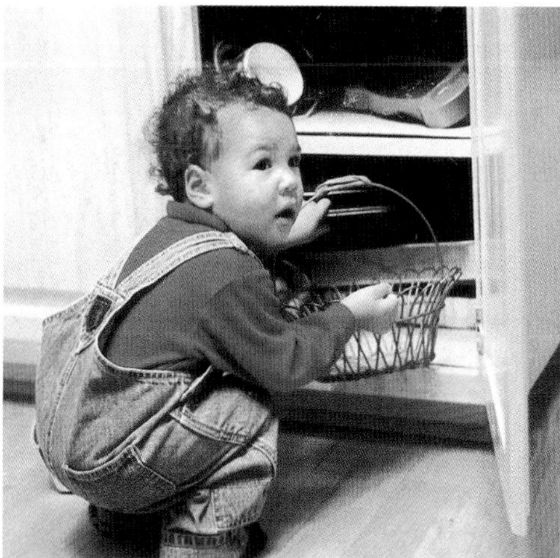

Pots and pans are popular toys for inquisitive toddlers. However, exploring cupboards can be a dangerous activity for toddlers. Toxic cleaning substances and other dangerous objects must be kept behind locked doors and out of reach.

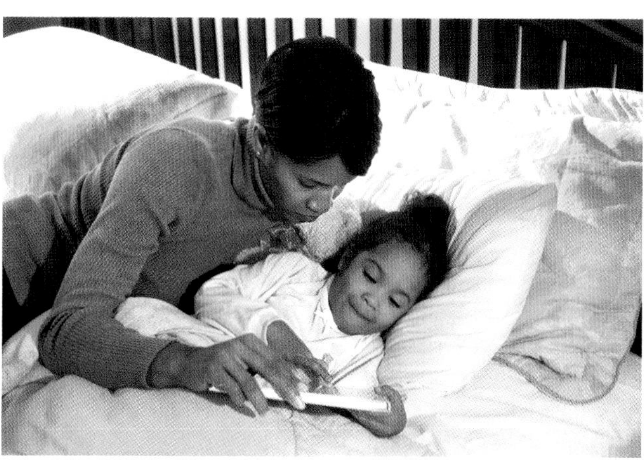

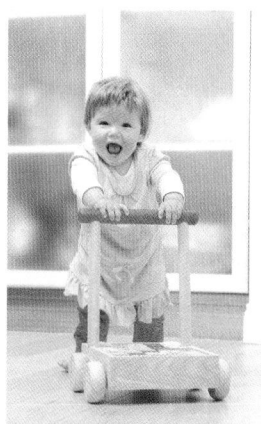

Toddlers enjoy push-pull toys. Toys should be strong and sturdy; wheeled toys should not tip over easily. (© 2016, Getty Images. Reprinted with Permission.)

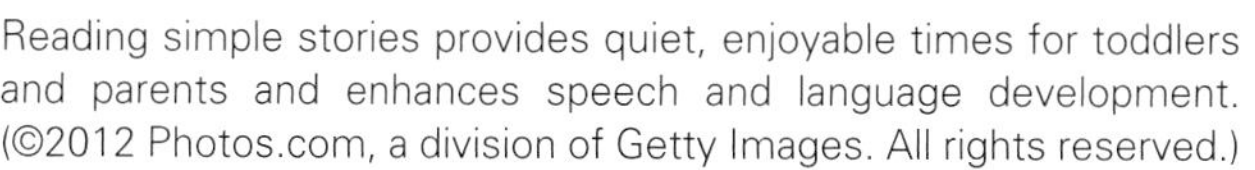

Reading simple stories provides quiet, enjoyable times for toddlers and parents and enhances speech and language development. (©2012 Photos.com, a division of Getty Images. All rights reserved.)

**FIG 7.1** Growth and development of the toddler.

present during infancy. As the musculoskeletal system matures and the child walks and runs more, the cherubic toddler disappears, and the child grows into a taller, leaner preschooler.

### The Preschooler

During the preschool years, growth occurs more rapidly in the legs than in the trunk, accumulation of adipose tissue declines, and the child's appetite decreases. As a result, the preschooler loses the potbellied appearance of the toddler, becoming slimmer and more agile. Muscles grow faster than bones during the preschool period. Muscle strength is influenced by nutrition, genetic makeup, and the opportunity to exercise and use the muscles. Knock-knees (see Chapter 50) are common in 3-year-olds and are often associated with occasional stumbling and falling. Maturation of the knee and hip joints usually corrects this problem by age 4 or 5 years.

As the lungs grow, the vital capacity increases, and the respiratory rate slows. Respirations remain primarily diaphragmatic until age 5 or 6 years. The heart rate decreases, and the blood pressure rises as the heart increases in size (see Chapter 33 for vital sign ranges). Cardiovascular maturation enables the preschooler to engage in more sustained and strenuous activity.

All 20 deciduous teeth are present by age 3 years. Deciduous teeth may begin to fall out at the end of the preschool period. The first permanent teeth to erupt, the back molars, usually appear in the early school-age years.

## Motor Development

### The Toddler

Learning to walk well is the crowning achievement of the toddler period. The child is in perpetual motion, seemingly compelled to pull up, take a few steps, fall, and repeat the process over and over, oblivious to bumps and bruises. The toddler will repeat this performance hundreds of times until the skill of walking has been perfected.

The age at which children learn to walk varies widely. Most children can walk alone by 15 months. By 18 months of age, toddlers walk well and try to run but fall often. At approximately 15 months of age, many toddlers become avid climbers. Chairs, tables, and bookcases present irresistible challenges and risks for injury. Parents may have difficulty

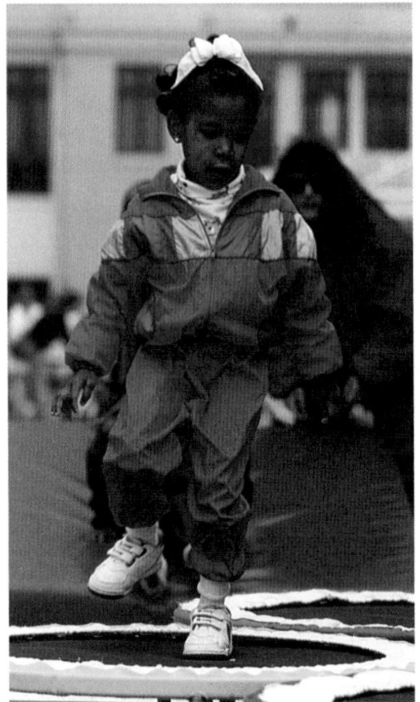

As the brain matures, the preschool child's motor development matures. Opportunities for practice contribute to the development of motor skills. (Courtesy Cook Children's Medical Center, Fort Worth, TX.)

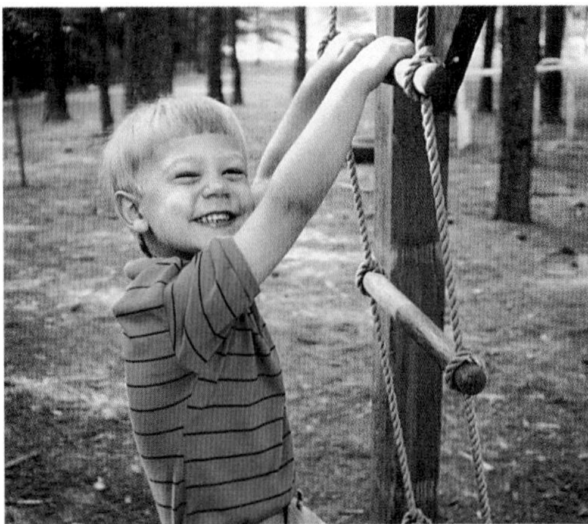

This 4-year-old's motor development has increased to the point that he can jump and climb well. A 4-year-old can also throw a ball overhand and cut on a curved line with scissors.

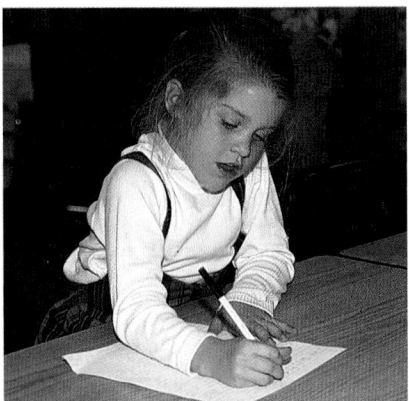

This 5-year-old is printing her name in readable letters. Children of this age can usually skip and can both throw and catch a ball. (Courtesy University of Texas at Arlington School of Nursing, Arlington, TX.)

**FIG 7.2** Growth and Development of the Preschooler.

## HEALTH PROMOTION

### Healthy People 2020 *Objectives for Toddlers and Preschoolers*

| | |
|---|---|
| EMC-2 | Increase the proportion of parents who use positive parenting and communicate with their doctors or other healthcare professionals about positive parenting. |
| IID-7 | Achieve and maintain effective vaccination coverage levels for universally recommended vaccines among young children (19 to 35 months). |
| IVP-9 | Prevent an increase in the rate of poisoning deaths. |
| IVP-16 | Increase age-appropriate vehicle restraint system use in children. |
| IVP-23 | Prevent an increase in the rate of fall-related deaths. |
| IVP-25 | Reduce drowning deaths. |
| NWS-11 | Prevent inappropriate weight gain in children ages 2 to 5 years. |
| TU-11 | Reduce the proportion of children ages 3 to 11 years exposed to secondhand smoke. |

Modified from U.S. Department of Health and https://Human Services. (2010). *Healthy People 2020.* Retrieved from http://www.healthypeople.gov.

keeping the toddler in a crib and may decide to move the child to a regular bed.

Toddlers are also engaged in perfecting fine motor skills. Hand-eye coordination improves with maturity and practice. Mealtimes are still messy. Although most 18-month-olds can hold a cup with both hands and drink from it without much spilling, eating with a spoon is difficult. Most of the food conveyed in a spoon is spilled. Children need a great deal of practice with a spoon before they can feed themselves without spilling. Most toddlers can feed themselves with a spoon by their second birthday if they have been allowed to practice.

At 18 months of age, the toddler enjoys removing clothing. By 24 months, the toddler can put on simple items of clothing but cannot differentiate front from back. Children at this age also can zip large zippers, put on shoes, and wash and dry their hands. Two-year-olds brush their teeth but need help in adequately removing plaque.

The toddler's increasing motor skills allow more independence in all areas of daily life. Feeding, dressing, and play provide opportunities for the child to develop autonomy. Motor development in this age-group is far ahead of development of judgment and perception. This difference in timing of the development of different skills increases the risk for injury.

### The Preschooler

Coordination and muscle strength increase rapidly between ages 3 and 5 years. Increases in brain size and nerve myelinization enable the child to perfect fine and gross motor skills.

Motor abilities vary widely among children. Although motor skill is less influenced by environment than other areas of development, such as language, opportunities to practice may contribute to better motor skills. For example, a 4-year-old who often plays catch with a sibling or parent generally finds playing Little League baseball as a 7-year-old easier than a child without a similar experience.

Handedness begins to emerge at approximately 3 years and is usually clearly established by 4 years. The nurse should encourage parents to provide left-handed children with appropriate tools, particularly left-handed scissors. Left-handed children should not be forced to use their right hands because coordination is usually better when they use the dominant side. Eye-hand coordination is usually good enough by age 5 years for a child to hit a nail on the head with a hammer. Increased coordination allows the child to perform many self-care skills and become more independent.

By age 4 or 5 years, the child is independent and can dress, eat, and go to the bathroom without help. Unlike the toddler, who must be restrained to avoid injury, the older preschooler can usually be trusted to heed verbal warnings of danger.

## Cognitive and Sensory Development

### The Toddler

Toddlers are consumed with curiosity. Their boundless energy and insatiable inquisitiveness provide them with resources for the tremendous cognitive growth that occurs during this period.

Toddlers between ages 12 and 18 months are in Piaget's sensorimotor period (Piaget, 1952) (see Chapter 5). Learning in this stage occurs mainly by trial and error. Toddlers spend most of a busy day experimenting to see what will happen as they dump, fill, empty, and explore every accessible area of their environment. Between 19 and 24 months, the child enters the final stage of the sensorimotor period. Object permanence is firmly established by this age. The child has a beginning ability to use symbols and words when referring to absent people or objects and begins to solve problems mentally rather than by repeating an action over and over. A toddler at this stage is often seen imitating the parent of the same sex performing household tasks (termed *domestic mimicry*). Late in this stage, the child displays *deferred imitation* (e.g., imitating the parent putting on makeup or shaving hours after that parent has left for work). The 18-month-old has a beginning ability to wait, as evidenced by an appropriate response of the toddler to a parent or caregiver who says "just a minute." However, the child's concept of time is still immature, and "a minute" may feel like an hour to the toddler.

Toddlers think in terms of the predictable routines of their daily schedule. When talking with the toddler, the nurse should use time orientation in relation to familiar activities. For example, a toddler understands "Your mother will be here after your nap" better than "Your mother will be here at 2 o'clock."

Many hours each day are spent putting objects into holes and smaller objects into each other as the child experiments with sizes, shapes, and spatial relations. Toddlers enjoy opening drawers and doors, exploring the contents of cabinets and closets, and generally wreaking havoc throughout the house, as well as exposing themselves to potential danger.

According to Piaget (1952), the preoperational stage of cognitive development characterizes the second half of early childhood (see Chapter 5). This stage is divided into two phases: the preconceptual phase (2 to 4 years) and the intuitive phase (4 to 7 years). During the preconceptual phase, the child is beginning to use symbolic thought—the ability to allow a mental image (words or ideas) to represent objects or ideas. Mental symbols allow the child to remember the past and describe events that happened in the past. At approximately 24 months, children enter the preconceptual phase, which ends at age 4 years. In this phase, children begin to think and reason at a primitive level. Two-year-olds have a beginning ability to retain mental images. This ability allows them to internalize what they see and experience. Symbols in the form of words can be used to represent ideas. Increasing amounts of play time are spent pretending. A box may become a spaceship or a hat; pebbles may be money or popcorn. The child's rapidly growing vocabulary enhances symbolic play. The toddler begins to think about alternative solutions to a problem and can even consider the consequences of an action without carrying it out (touching a hot stove, running too fast on a slippery sidewalk).

The toddler's thinking is immature, limited in its logic, and bound to the present. Egocentrism, animism, irreversibility, magical thinking, and centration characterize the preoperational thought of the toddler (Table 7.1). The predominant words in the toddler's language repertoire are "me," "I," and "mine."

**TABLE 7.1 Characteristics of Preoperational Thinking**

| Characteristic | Example |
|---|---|
| *Egocentrism:* Views everything in relation to self; is unable to consider another's point of view. | Toddler takes a toy away from another child and cannot understand that the other child also wants (or has a right to) the toy. |
| *Animism:* Believes that inert objects are alive and have wills of their own. | Toddler trips over a toy and scolds the toy for hurting her. She believes that the toy hurt her on purpose. |
| *Irreversibility:* Cannot see a process in reverse order. Cannot follow a line of reasoning back to its beginning. Cannot hold onto two or more sequential thoughts simultaneously. | If the child takes a toy apart, the child cannot remember the sequence for putting it back together. A child who is taken on a walk cannot retrace steps and find the way home. |
| *Magical thought:* Believes that magical thought is the cause of events and that wishing something will make it so. | Toddlers often feel extremely powerful and believe that their thoughts cause events to happen. |
| *Centration:* Tends to focus on only one aspect of an experience, ignoring other possible alternatives. Focuses on the dominant characteristic of an object, excluding other characteristics. | May have difficulty putting together a puzzle, concentrating on only one detail of a piece (e.g., shape) and ignoring other qualities (e.g., color, detail). Cannot follow more than one direction at a time. |

### The Preschooler

By age 3 years, maturation of the central nervous system contributes to the child's increasing cognitive abilities. The 3-year-old can retain a mental image of a loved one and can periodically "refuel" by thinking about that person. A photograph can help some children cope with separation by bridging the gap between physical presence and mental image. Preschoolers' ability to remember their parents and recognize that their needs can be met even though their parents are not present enhances their ability to tolerate separation.

Because preschoolers still engage in animism, they often endow inanimate objects with life-like qualities during play. A doll may become a crying baby, or a teddy bear may become a friend who listens sympathetically. Symbolic play is important for emotional development because it allows the child to work through distressing feelings. For this reason, allowing a child to play with medical equipment after a painful procedure can be therapeutic. Four-year-olds who have received injections may be found working out their feelings by giving their dolls "lots of shots."

During the preconceptual phase, reality may be distorted by transductive reasoning. The preschool child reasons from particular to particular rather than from particular to general and vice versa, as adults do. The child cannot understand that relationships exist and cannot view the whole with respect to its parts. The preschool child has difficulty in focusing on the important aspects of a situation. To a child, everything is important and interdependent. This type of thinking is called *field dependency.* For example, the preschooler may have difficulty falling asleep at night because the parent did not follow the usual bedtime routine. Objects, routine, and sameness are important to the preschool child. Rituals provide the preschool child with a feeling of control.

The second phase of Piaget's preoperational stage, the intuitive phase, is characterized by centration and the lack of reversibility. *Centration* is the tendency to center or focus on one part of a situation and ignore the other parts. The child cannot understand logical relationships and is unable to focus on more than one aspect of a

# HEALTH PROMOTION

## *The 15- to 18-Month-Old Child*

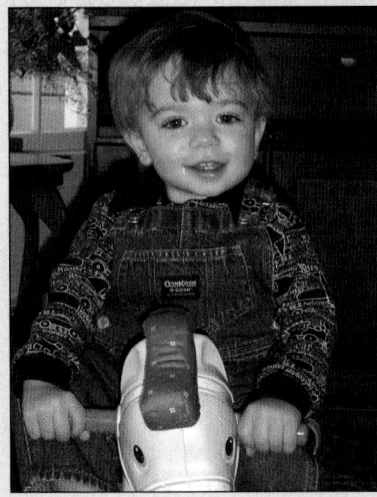

### Focused Assessment

Ask the parent the following:

- What new activities is your child doing?
- Can your child say single words? Put words together? Understand most of what you say? Communicate needs and wants?
- What kinds of foods does your child eat and how often? Do you have a concern that your child is eating items that are not food? Is your child able to eat with little assistance?
- Is your child walking well? Running? Jumping? Getting up and down the stairs?
- How does your child behave when frustrated? How do you and your partner handle this?
- What kinds of activities do you enjoy doing with your child?

### Developmental Milestones

*Personal/social:* May exhibit negativism, ritualism, and increasing tolerance of separation from parents; undresses; begins temper tantrums when frustrated; may have a transition object; begins to understand gender differences

*Fine motor:* Turns book pages; begins to imitate vertical and circular strokes; vision 20/50 by 18 months; drinks from a cup by holding it with two hands

*Language/cognitive:* Increasing receptive language; begins to understand and say "no"; may begin to put two words together; can point to familiar objects; begins to use memory; understands spatial and temporal relations and increased object permanence; has a basic moral understanding (reward and punishment); understands simple directions; by 18 months has a vocabulary of approximately 30 words; holographic speech (uses single words with gestures to express whole ideas)

*Gross motor:* Walks with increasing confidence and begins to run; climbs stairs first by creeping, then walking with hand held; jumps in place; begins to throw a ball overhand without falling

### Critical Milestones*

*Personal/social:* Begins to imitate; helps in the house; feeds self with increasing skill (still rotates the spoon, if used) and holds a cup

*Fine motor:* Builds a tower with increasing number of blocks; scribbles; able to put a block in a cup

*Language/cognitive:* Says 3 to 10 single words; can point to several body parts

*Gross motor:* Walks well forward and backward; stoops and recovers

### Health Maintenance

#### *Physical Measurements*

Continue to measure and plot length, weight, and head circumference

Anterior fontanel closed by 18 months

#### *Immunizations*

15 months: *Haemophilus influenzae* type b (Hib) #3 or #4 (depending on vaccine and if not given at 12 months); measles-mumps-rubella (MMR) #1 (if not given at 1 year); varicella (if not given at 1 year); pneumococcal (if not given at 1 year); hepatitis B #3 (if not given earlier)

18 months: diphtheria-tetanus-acellular pertussis (DTaP) #4; inactivated poliovirus (IPV) #3 (if not given earlier); hepatitis B #3 (if not given earlier)

Influenza vaccine annually

Hepatitis A #2 (6 months after first dose)

#### *Health Screening*

Standardized developmental screening

Autism-specific screening

Hearing risk assessment

### Anticipatory Guidance

#### *Nutrition*

Calorie, protein, and fluid requirements decrease slightly; offer various foods every 2 to 3 hours

Give 2 or 3 cups of whole milk daily for calcium

Vitamin D supplementation 400 IU/day if consuming less than 1 L (33 oz) per day of milk and vitamin D–fortified foods

Make mealtimes pleasant: use appropriate-size utensils and colorful dinnerware

Child may have fussy eating habits (physiologic anorexia)

Resist giving food as a comfort measure

Do not allow child to walk or play with food in the mouth

#### *Elimination*

Sphincters become physiologically under voluntary control, but child is usually not ready for toilet training; advise parents to wait but discuss signs of readiness

#### *Dental*

Continue to brush with a soft toothbrush twice daily (may use rice-sized amount of toothpaste); parent should floss the child's teeth

Maintain a diet low in sugar

Do not put the child to sleep with a bottle

Dental risk assessment (18 months); refer to dentist if not done earlier

Oral fluoride (0.25 mg) if water is not fluoridated

Fluoride varnish if no access to a dentist

#### *Sleep*

Sleep cycles decrease and the child has longer awake periods

Still naps one or two times per day

May resist going to bed; likes a bedtime routine

#### *Hygiene*

Begins to participate in self-care (washes face and hands with assistance)

#### *Safety*

Review car safety, violence, falls, water safety, toy and toy box safety, bicycle passenger helmet, and poisons

Discuss choking, toy safety, firearm access, burn prevention, and sun protection

#### *Play*

Provide push-pull toys with short strings

Noise-making toys

Dolls and stuffed animals (watch for small parts)

Musical toys

Art supplies: large crayons, finger paints, and clay

Large blocks and balls

*Guided by Denver Developmental Screening Test II.

## HEALTH PROMOTION

### *The 2-Year-Old Child*

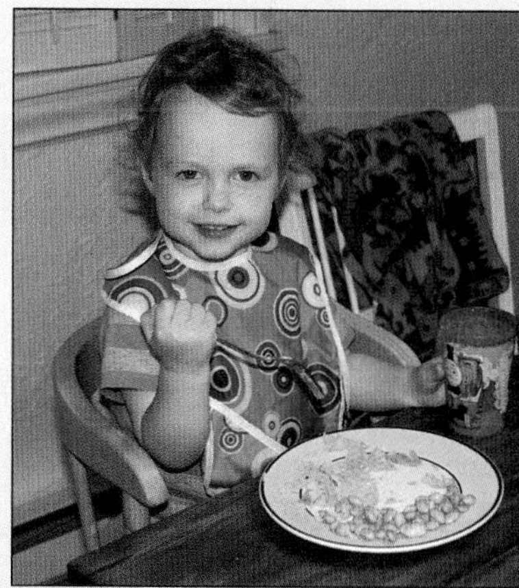

**Focused Assessment**

Ask the parent the following:

- How are you managing any discipline problems your child may be having?
- Do you have any concerns about any daycare arrangements you have?
- Does your child use a bottle or a cup?
- What do you do when your child has a temper tantrum? Do you feel confident about setting behavioral limits?
- How does your child communicate with others?
- What, if anything, have you done to begin toilet training your child?
- What activities do you enjoy doing together?

**Developmental Milestones**

*Personal/social:* Imitates household activities and begins to do helpful tasks; uses table utensils without much spilling; drinks from a lidless cup; removes a difficult article of clothing; begins developing sexual identity; is stubborn and negativistic: wants own way in everything; brushes teeth with help; is learning to walk; understands "soon"

*Fine motor:* Puts blocks into a cup after demonstration; builds tower of four to six blocks; able to imitate a horizontal and circular stroke with a crayon; turns a doorknob; turns book pages one at a time; can unzip and unbutton

*Language/cognition:* Has an approximately 300-word vocabulary, two-word sentences; points to six body parts and pictures of several familiar objects (e.g., bird, man, dog, plane); understands cause and effect, object permanence, sense of time; follows two-step directions; uses egocentric language (I, me, mine)

*Gross motor:* Stoops and recovers well; walks forward and backward; climbs stairs holding the railing; runs, jumps, kicks a ball

**Critical Milestones***

*Personal/social:* Removes one article of clothing; feeds a doll; uses a spoon or fork

*Fine motor:* Holds a pencil and spontaneously scribbles; dumps a raisin out of a bottle on command after demonstration; builds a two-block tower

*Language/cognitive:* Points to two pictures; says three to six words

*Gross motor:* Runs; walks up steps; kicks a ball forward

**Health Maintenance**

***Physical Measurements***

Gains approximately 2.25 kg (5 lb) per year

Length or height is approximately half eventual adult height

Grows approximately 7.5 cm (3 inches) per year

Compute and plot body mass index (BMI)

***Immunizations***

Administer any immunizations not given previously according to the recommended schedule

Influenza vaccine annually

***Health Screening***

Hemoglobin and lead screen

Standardized developmental screening (now or at 30 months)

Autism-specific screening

Fasting lipid screen for child with cardiovascular disease risk factors

Tuberculosis (TB) screening if at risk

**Anticipatory Guidance**

***Nutrition***

May begin low-fat milk

Daily diet: 2 or 3 cups of milk, two servings of protein, three small servings of vegetables, two servings of fruit, and six servings of bread

Modify diet for children with elevated cholesterol (no more than 200 mg cholesterol/day, no more than 30% calories from fat and 7% from saturated fat): egg substitute, low-fat cheeses and meats, added fiber

Decrease added fat and high-calorie, high-fat desserts; increase fruits, vegetables, and carbohydrates

Vitamin D supplementation 400 IU/day if consuming less than 1 L (33 oz) per day of milk and vitamin-D–fortified foods

***Elimination***

Bowel movements decrease in number and become more regular

Child remains dry for several hours

Begin to think about a positive approach to toilet training

***Dental***

Sixteen teeth; may use rice-size amount of fluoridated toothpaste, encourage not to swallow

Parent should floss the child's teeth

Schedule first dental visit if not done earlier

Oral fluoride as prescribed

Fluoride varnish application if no access to a dentist

***Sleep***

12 to 14 hours/day

Usually a long afternoon nap

Limit television viewing to no more than 1 hour/day

***Hygiene***

Girls are prone to vaginal irritation; advise to wipe from front to back; adding ¼ cup vinegar to bath water can relieve irritation

Boys' foreskin begins to retract; retract gently to clean; never force

***Safety***

Review toy safety, firearm safety, burn prevention, and other previously discussed subjects

May change to an approved forward-facing child safety seat

Discuss choking on food, street safety, water safety, outside poisons, playground safety, and sun protection

***Self-Esteem and Competence***

Discuss the following with parent:

- Modeling appropriate social behavior
- Encouraging the child to learn to make choices

*Continued*

## HEALTH PROMOTION—cont'd

### *The 2-Year-Old Child*

- Helping the child to appropriately express emotions
- Spending individual time with the child daily
- Providing consistent and loving limits to help the child learn self-discipline
- Beginning toilet training only when the child is ready (dry for 2 hours, able to pull pants down, can use appropriate toileting words, can indicate the need to use the toilet)

***Play***

Parallel play; play begins to become imitative and imaginative

Choose toys that are safe and durable: balls, picture books, puzzles with large pieces, sandbox toys, trucks, riding toys, household toys (e.g., broom, mop, carpet sweeper)

Limit screen time

*Guided by Denver Developmental Screening Test II.

situation at a time. For example, the child may not be able to follow a sequence of directions but will perform well if the directions are given one at a time.

The 4- or 5-year-old shows **irreversibility** in thought (Piaget, 1952). Children at this age cannot reverse a process or the order of events. They may be able to take a complex puzzle apart but have difficulty putting it back together. The 4- or 5-year-old also lacks reversibility for mathematical processes. The child may be able to add 3 and 1 and get 4 but reversing the problem ($4 - 1 = 3$) would be too difficult.

The preschool years are a period of rapid learning. The preschool child is curious and wants to know how things work. Preschoolers' thinking is still magical and egocentric (focused on the self). Children at this age tend to understand events only as these events affect them, believing that everyone else has had the same experience. Seeing their mother in distress, children may bring her a doll, assuming that it would comfort the mother as it does the child.

Preschool children often believe that their thoughts are powerful enough to cause things to happen. They may frighten themselves with some of their ideas, believing that they may become what they imagine they will be. Preschoolers may feel overwhelmed by guilt when a sibling is hospitalized because they believe that their hostile feelings caused the sibling's illness. Likewise, a child of this age may say, "I got sick because I was bad."

## Language Development

### The Toddler

The acquisition of language is one of the most dramatic developments of early childhood. Although the age at which children begin to talk widely varies, most can verbally communicate by their second birthday. The rate of language development depends on physical maturity and the amount of reinforcement that the child has received. Between 15 and 24 months of age, language ability rapidly develops. Toddlers understand many more words than they can say because receptive language (what the child understands) develops earlier and faster than speech. Sometime after 18 months, many children experience a sudden spurt in speech production and comprehension, resulting in a vocabulary of 300 or more words at 24 months. By 2 years of age, roughly 60% to 70% of toddlers' speech should be understandable. Because children age 24 to 30 months are less egocentric and are better able to consider another's point of view, they engage in more conversation with others and less monologue.

Despite variations in evidence relative to universal screening of children in early childhood (USPSTF, 2015b; Wallace et al., 2015), the AAP continues to recommend screening for speech and language delay at 18 and 24 (or 30) months (AAP, 2016). If language development is not progressing normally, parents should be advised to pursue follow-up care. Children of bilingual families, children who are twins, and children other than first-borns may have slower language development. Because language development depends on adequate hearing, delayed language can be seen in children who have had repeated ear infections or who have undiagnosed hearing loss (see Chapter 55).

Parents can promote language development by talking to their children and incorporating teaching into daily routines. Feeding, bathing, dressing, and going on outings to both new and familiar places offer opportunities for verbal interaction and the practice of growing language skills. The child should be encouraged to express needs rather than have the parent anticipate and provide what the child wants before the child asks for it. Reading simple, entertaining stories with colorful pictures provides quiet, enjoyable times for toddlers and parents and enhances speech and language development.

### The Preschooler

A dramatic increase in language skill in the preschool period promotes self-control and increases the child's ability to direct and be directed by others. Children at this age may be heard talking to themselves about things they have heard or been taught.

The preschooler's vocabulary increases rapidly, from 300 words at 2 years of age to more than 2100 words at 5 years. In less than 3 years, the child grows from a toddler who knows only a few words into a child who skillfully uses an extensive vocabulary to describe events, share feelings, and ask questions. Three-year-olds speak in short, telegraphic sentences. They may talk to themselves or to imaginary friends. A delightful characteristic of young preschoolers is the tendency to engage in lengthy monologues, regardless of whether anyone is listening or even present. Such self-talk provides the child with opportunities to practice speech and is often accompanied by symbolic play.

By 4 years old, children talk incessantly and tend to boast and exaggerate. They enjoy rhymes and silly ways to use similar words. Four-year-olds expect more detailed answers to their questions. They may use speech aggressively and may use profanity to gain attention. "Bad" language should be ignored, thus depriving the child of reinforcement of the behavior. When children feel that they gain power over their parents by using bad language, these verbalizations will continue.

Five-year-olds speak in sentences of adult length and use all parts of speech. They usually are proficient storytellers who produce elaborate tales for anyone who will listen. Their tendency to mix fantasy with reality may be perceived by adults as lying. The child of 5 years usually can recite the days of the week and can name the seasons.

Nurses can teach parents strategies to promote their child's language development. It is important for parents to talk with the child and respond to the child's attempts at communication. Reading to the child and making reading materials available can help build vocabulary and promote a lifelong love of reading. Watching educational programs or videos with their child may augment parents' communication skills with their child. Preschoolers spend a lot of time asking "how" and "why" questions, often taxing parents' patience. Short, simple, honest answers encourage vocabulary building and boost self-esteem.

## Psychosocial Development

### The Toddler

The toddler is developing a sense of autonomy, giving up the comfort of dependence enjoyed during infancy. If a basic sense of trust was established during the first year, the toddler can venture forward and separate from parents for short periods to explore and experience the world.

According to Erikson (1963), the toddler is struggling with the developmental task of acquiring a sense of autonomy while overcoming a sense of shame and doubt. Toddlers discover that they have a will of their own and that they can control others. However, asserting their will and insisting on their own way often lead to conflict with those they love, whereas submissive behavior is rewarded with affection and approval. Toddlers experience conflict because they want to assert their own will but do not want to risk losing the approval of loved ones. If the child continues to practice dependent behavior, doubt related to abilities develops. Toddlers may feel shame for independent impulses, particularly if frequent punishment is associated with their actions.

The toddler learns which behaviors gain approval and which result in censure and punishment. Two-year-olds do not have a conscience but avoid punishment by controlling their behavior. Right and wrong are determined by the consequences of actions.

At approximately 15 months, toddlers begin to demonstrate their developing autonomy with two almost universal behaviors: negativism and ritualism.

***Negativism.*** Negativism, one of the most dramatic expressions of independence, is shown in various ways. The toddler's favorite word seems to be "no." Unable to distinguish between requests and directives, the toddler seems to believe that saying "yes" would mean giving up free will. The child often seems to delight in this test of wills with the parent. Negativism may result in screaming, kicking, hitting, biting, or breath-holding. Parents often interpret the child's negative behavior as being bad or stubborn. Nurses can help parents understand their toddler's behavior as an important sign of the child's progress from dependence to autonomy and independence. The nurse should give support and encourage the parent to deal with the toddler's trying behavior with patience and a sense of humor. Although general permissiveness is not recommended, too much pressure and forceful methods of control often lead to defiance, tantrums, and prolonged negative behavior.

***Ritualism and the importance of routine.*** Ritualism helps the child venture out and away from the safety of the parents by ensuring uniformity and security. Ritualism allows the toddler to have a sense of control. The child feels more confident with a secure home base. The toddler insists on sameness. Milk may have to be poured into the same cup, parents may have to sit in the same chairs at dinnertime, and a specified routine may have to be followed countless times throughout the day. The child may be unable to go to sleep unless a bedtime ritual is followed exactly (e.g., a drink of water, two stories, prayers, and a teddy bear). The child may experience distress if this routine is not followed exactly the next night. Failure to recognize the importance of such rituals may increase stress and insecurity.

Events such as hospitalization, during which continuity of routine cannot be ensured, are difficult for the toddler. The nurse can decrease the stress of hospitalization by incorporating the child's usual rituals and routines from home into nursing care activities. Keeping hospital routines as similar to those of home as possible and recognizing ritualistic needs give the toddler some sense of control and security and reduce feelings of helplessness and fear. See Chapter 35 for further discussion of the hospitalized child.

***Separation anxiety.*** Separation anxiety peaks again in the toddler period. Although the concept of object permanence is fully developed in the toddler, children at this stage have difficulty differentiating their own feelings from those of their parents. Although the children experience a strong desire to be independent and leave their mothers, they fear that their mothers also want to leave them. A toddler may strike out independently across the room, only to rush back in tears to the mother, as if the child were frightened and angry with the mother for leaving. For a brief period, the parent may find talking on the telephone without interruption or even going into the bathroom without being followed virtually impossible. Leave-taking and brief separations are acceptable to a toddler if they are the toddler's idea, but the parent's departure may cause desperate clinging and crying. Games such as hide-and-seek help the child master fears of separation. Repeating separation under conditions the child can control helps the toddler overcome the anxiety associated with separation. The child learns from experience that loved ones will return after separation.

Being left with a stranger can be stressful. Toddlers should be told honestly and clearly about a separation shortly before it occurs. The parent or nurse should reassure the child that the parent is coming back. When the parent returns, the toddler often shows anger at being left by ignoring the parent or by pretending to be more interested in play than in going home. Parents of hospitalized toddlers are frequently distressed by such behavior when they visit their child (see Chapter 35).

Tolerating brief separations from parents is an important developmental task for the toddler. *Transition objects,* such as a favorite blanket or toy, provide comfort to the toddler in stressful situations, such as separation, illness, and even bedtime. Such objects help children make the transition from dependency to autonomy. Toddlers may become so attached to an object that they can hardly bear to part with it, even for a brief time while it is being laundered.

The nurse can offer support by explaining that the behavior is a normal growth and development milestone and telling the parents that plenty of affection and attention are needed to help the toddler cope with the stress of separation. The nurse counsels parents to leave a toddler only briefly at first and, if possible, to delay extended separations until the toddler can handle them better. The nurse who helps parents understand normal toddler behavior in response to separation helps parents cope with the frustrations of this transition.

***Play.*** Toddlers spend most of their time at play. Play is serious business to the toddler—it is the child's work. Many hours are spent each day in play, perfecting fine and gross motor skills, learning to control inner urges, and gaining self-esteem. Play during this period reflects the egocentric toddler's developmental level. The toddler engages in parallel play, in which children play alongside but not with other children (Fig. 7.3). Little regard is given to the feelings of others. Children engaged in this type of play frequently grab toys away from other children or may hit or fight to obtain a wanted toy. Because toddlers are egocentric, they do not realize that they are hurting the other child and feel no shame for aggressive actions.

Imitation and acting out scenes of everyday life are common as the toddler begins to try out roles and identify with adults. Active, large-muscle play helps the toddler vent frustrations and dissipate excess energy. The nurse can help parents understand the manner in which play enhances the toddler's development. The nurse should encourage parents to play with their toddler and provide opportunities for the toddler to play with other children. The nurse teaches parents about child proofing and checking the house on a daily basis. Toys must be strong, safe, and too large to swallow or place in the ear or nose.

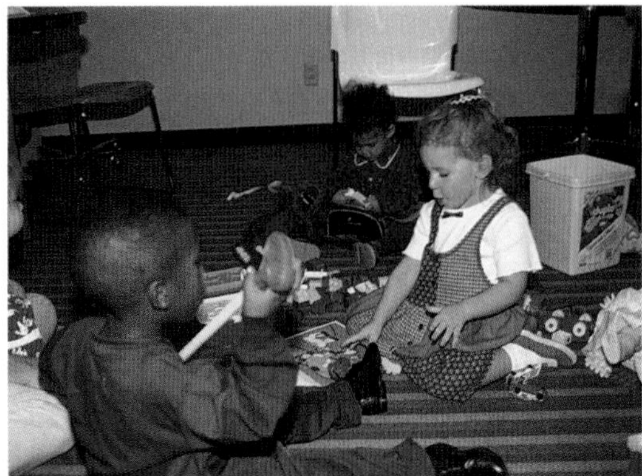

Parallel play occurs when children play side by side with similar toys but no organized group activity occurs. The children play *beside* one another but not *with* one another. (Courtesy University of Texas at Arlington School of Nursing, Arlington, TX.)

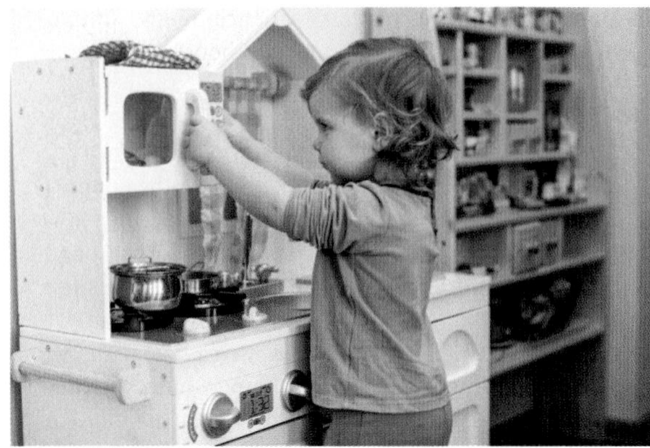

Symbolic play consists of activities that children use to express their perception of reality. This little girl is acting out a familiar adult scenario as she manipulates child-size toys that represent kitchen equipment. (© 2016, Getty Images. Reprinted with permission.)

**FIG 7.3** Types of play.

Toddlers need supervision at all times. Various play materials, which need not be expensive, and safe play environments enhance the toddler's development (Box 7.1).

***Psychosexual development.*** At approximately 18 months, toddlers enter the Freud's anal stage. Freud (1960) theorized that as children focus on the mastery of bowel and bladder functions, their attention is also directed to the genital area. Even before age 2 years, children are aware of their own gender and begin to develop a sense of gender identity. By 2½ or 3 years, toddlers can correctly identify anatomic pictures of boys and girls. Gender identity is not completely established until age 5 years, when the child understands gender as permanent (i.e., that gender does not change with the addition of a wig or a dress) (Kohlberg, 1966).

Children begin to be aware of expected gender role behaviors at an early age. By age 3 years most toddlers show an awareness of gender role stereotypes and tend to imitate the same-gender parent during play. Gender role identification continues throughout early childhood as the child incorporates the attitudes, roles, and values of the same-gender parent. Although gender role stereotypes have relaxed somewhat in recent years, children behave according to adult expectations. Children learn behavior by reinforcement and punishment, as well as by imitation. If a boy repeatedly hears that boys do not play with dolls, he will spurn such "girls' toys" and will play with toys that his parents consider masculine to gain their praise and approval. Nurses should be aware of their own biases about gender-typed behaviors and should support the parents in their choice of toys and activities for their child. The nurse can be most helpful by encouraging parents to make traditionally gender-typed toys available to both boys and girls if this approach is consistent with the parents' beliefs. Parents' expectations of appropriate gender role behavior differ according to their cultural backgrounds. In many cultures, boys and girls are differently treated, and thus, are taught "male" and "female" behaviors.

Parents are often concerned about their toddler's interest in and curiosity about gender differences. Sex play and masturbation are common among toddlers. Nurses can reassure parents that self-exploration or exploration of another toddler's body is normal behavior during early childhood. Parents should respect the child's curiosity as normal without judging the child as "bad." The child should be told that touching private parts is something that is done only in private. When parents discover children involved in sex play, casually telling them to dress and directing them to another activity can limit sex play without producing feelings of shame or anxiety. The nurse should explain to parents that positive attitudes toward sexuality are learned from parents who are comfortable with their own sexuality. As young children learn about their bodies and explore anatomic differences, they frequently ask questions about where babies come from or why "Brian looks different from Emily." Honest, straightforward answers

## BOX 7.1 Age-Related Activities and Toys for Toddlers and Preschoolers

### General Activities

***Toddler***

The toddler fills and empties containers, begins dramatic play, has increased use of motor skills, enjoys feeling different textures, explores the home environment, imitates orders, and likes to be read to and to look at books and television programs that are age-appropriate.

Toys should meet the child's need for activity and inquisitiveness.

The child also enjoys manipulating small objects such as toy people, cars, and animals.

***Preschooler***

Dramatic play is prominent.

The child likes to run, jump, hop, and, in general, improve motor skills.

The child likes to build and create things (e.g., sand castles and mud pies).

Play is simple and imaginative.

Simple collections begin.

### Toys and Specific Types of Play

***Toddler***

Continued exploring of the body parts of self and others; mechanical toys; objects of different textures such as clay, sand, finger paints, and bubbles; push-pull toys; large ball; sand and water play; blocks; painting; coloring with large crayons; nesting toys; large puzzles; trucks; dolls.

Therapeutic play can begin at this age.

***Preschooler***

Ride-on toys, materials for building such as sand and blocks, dolls, drawing materials, crayons, cars, puzzles, books, appropriate television and videos, nonsense rhymes, singing games, pretend play as something or somebody, dress-up, finger paints, clay, cutting, pasting, simple board and card games.

that use the correct terminology satisfy the toddler's curiosity and lay the foundation for healthy sexual attitudes.

## ! NURSING QUALITY ALERT

### *Important Tasks for the Toddler Period*

- Recognition of self as a separate person with own will
- Control of impulses and acquisition of socially acceptable ways to communicate wants and needs
- Control of elimination
- Toleration of separation from the parent

### The Preschooler

The preschool years are a critical period for the development of socialization. Children need opportunities to play with others to learn communication and social skills. They also need appropriate guidance to learn acceptable behavior.

According to Erikson (1963), the preschooler's developmental task is to achieve a sense of initiative. The preschooler is busy learning how to do things and takes great pride in new accomplishments. If the child acts inappropriately or is repeatedly criticized or punished for attempts to explore and learn, feelings of guilt, anxiety, shame, and fear may result. For example, an adult's comment, "That's nice, but it would look better if you did it this way," may cause the child to feel inferior. Such subtle criticism can make the child reluctant to try new activities. A feeling of inferiority also may develop if adults are always doing things for the child rather than encouraging independence. The child who does not achieve a sense of initiative will feel defeated, angry, and afraid of people and new situations. Nurses can promote healthy psychosocial development in preschoolers and help them gain a sense of initiative by teaching parents the importance of providing the child with opportunities to explore in a safe, stimulating environment. Adults should encourage the preschooler's imagination and creativity and should praise appropriate behavior.

*Play.* Learning to relate to age mates is another developmental task that is significant during the preschool period. Preschoolers need experience playing with other children to learn how to relate to other people. Three-year-olds are capable of sharing and are more likely to do so than toddlers. Four-year-olds tend to be more argumentative and less generous with playmates. Although this behavior may appear to be a step backward to parents, it is actually a sign of growth because 4-year-olds feel more secure in a group and are testing their roles and communication skills. The 5-year-old enjoys playing with other children and generally can play with another child for longer periods before arguments develop.

Children between ages 3 and 5 years enjoy parallel and associative play. Children also learn to share and cooperate (cooperative play) as they play in small groups. During play, preschoolers learn simple games and rules, language concepts, and social roles. Play is often imitative, dramatic, and creative. Various roles are explored through play as children imitate significant adults. Preschoolers enjoy dress-up clothes, housekeeping toys, doll houses, and other toys that encourage pretending (see Fig. 7.3). Tricycles and climbing toys help develop muscles and coordination. Preschoolers also enjoy materials for cutting, pasting, and painting. Such manipulative and creative materials stimulate imagination and fine motor development (see Box 7.1).

Imaginary friends are common near age 3 years. Boundaries between reality and fantasy are blurred at this age, and "pretend" can seem real, especially during play. Imaginary friends serve many purposes. They may take the blame when the child misbehaves, allowing the child to save face when feeling guilty about a certain behavior. Imaginary friends may be companions during lonely times. They may accomplish a task with which the child is struggling or allow the child to practice roles. For example, the child may scold an imaginary friend and administer punishment, just as a parent would. Imaginary friends seem to be more common in highly imaginative and intelligent children.

*Psychosexual development.* Sexual identity and body image are developing. Sexual curiosity and explorations are normal. Preschoolers are curious about anatomic differences and seek to investigate them. Preschoolers show interest in the differences between the sexes and often compare their bodies with those of others. Playing doctor and hiding with a friend to investigate anatomic differences are common activities during the preschool period. The nurse can reassure parents that the child is simply learning about his or her body and that the parents can direct the child to another activity. Preschoolers are interested in where they came from and how babies are made. Parents should be encouraged to assess what the child already knows about the subject and to determine why the child is asking the question. The parent should answer questions simply, honestly, and matter-of-factly. The child usually neither wants nor understands detailed explanations.

Parents greatly influence their children's sexual development. Positive signs of physical and emotional intimacy between parents send a positive signal to the child. A warm, accepting, matter-of-fact attitude toward sexual matters promotes a positive, healthy perspective in children. Parents can create an atmosphere of acceptance in the early preschool years when the first questions arise. A parental attitude of "You can ask me anything" can set the stage for healthy interaction from early childhood into adolescence, when parental guidance is so important.

Masturbation is common and may increase in frequency when the child is under stress. Parents often express concern about such behavior. The nurse can help parents handle these situations by explaining that such self-comforting behaviors are normal for this age. If the parent discovers the child masturbating, simple redirection of the child's attention without punishing, shaming, or reprimanding is best. Children should be taught that touching their genitals is not appropriate in public.

At this age, a sense of rivalry with the same-gender parent develops. Preschool boys commonly compete with their fathers for the attention of their mothers. A girl likewise may become "Daddy's girl," often cuddling and flirting with her father while excluding her mother from the relationship. This rivalry is usually resolved early in the school-age period as the child identifies strongly with the same-gender parent and same-gender peers. According to Freudian theory, the oedipal stage is resolved when the child strongly identifies with the parent of the same gender. By the end of the preschool period, the child identifies with and imitates the same-gender parent. In single-parent and nontraditional families, the child should have a friendly, stable relationship with an adult relative or friend of the same sex who can serve as a role model. By age 3 years, children know gender differences. They imitate masculine and feminine behaviors in play, and gender identity is well established by 6 years.

*Spiritual and moral development.* Learning the difference between right and wrong (the development of a conscience) is another important task of the preschool period. According to Kohlberg (1964), children between ages 4 and 7 years are in the second stage of the preconventional level of moral development. In this stage, children obey rules out of self-interest. They tend to believe that if the consequences of an action are personally advantageous, the action is right. An "eye-for-an-eye" orientation guides their behavior.

The preschooler begins to use self-control to resist temptation and tries to "be good" to avoid feelings of guilt. Preschoolers determine right from wrong by the consequences of disobeying their parents' rules. At this age, children have little understanding of the reason for a rule. For example, when asked why hitting another child is wrong, the preschooler might reply, "Because my mother says so." Preschoolers adhere to parents' rules dogmatically, deciding whether to break a rule on the basis of the resulting punishment.

Preschoolers often have difficulty applying rules in different situations. The child may know that hitting a sibling is wrong but may not understand that hitting another child at daycare is also wrong. Because the preschooler is egocentric, understanding another's viewpoint is difficult. The child begins to develop a conscience as a result of consistent rewards for good behavior and punishment for bad behavior.

The preschool child's concept of God is concrete. The family's religious beliefs and customs, such as bedtime prayers, mealtime grace, and Bible stories, are important to preschoolers. Such rituals, practiced in an atmosphere of love, can be deeply meaningful and comforting to children of this age.

## HEALTH PROMOTION DURING EARLY CHILDHOOD

When doing health promotion with parents of children in early childhood, the nurse inquires about areas discussed in Box 6.2 at every visit. These include nutrition (quantity and types of food), elimination, safety (car restraints, gun violence), hearing and vision, family adjustment, and any other concerns.

### Nutrition

The rate of growth slows during the toddler and preschool period, as does the child's appetite. This is sometimes referred to as physiologic anorexia. The child's food experiences during this period can have a lasting effect on how food and meals are viewed. The family is the primary influence at this time, although the media plays an important role. Children should be discouraged from eating while watching television, and family mealtimes should be encouraged.

#### Nutritional Requirements

The U.S. Department of Agriculture (USDA) and United States Department of Health and Human Services (USDHHS) (2015) have issued nutritional guidelines for the American public and have represented them graphically through the MyPlate icon (see Fig. 5.4). The MyPlate website (http://www.choosemyplate.gov) contains individualized eating plans for children of various ages and standardized weight and physical activity. The American Heart Association (2015) has also made recommendations for children (see Box 5.6). Children ages 2 to 8 years should consume 2 cups per day of fat-free or low-fat milk or equivalent milk products. Yogurt and cheese are other milk-group sources. Total fat intake should remain between 30% and 35% of calories for children ages 2 to 3 years and between 25% and 35% of calories for children ages 4 years and older. Most fats should come from sources of polyunsaturated and monounsaturated fatty acids, such as fish, nuts, and vegetable oils (American Heart Association, 2015). Poultry, fish, and lean meat are good sources of iron. Low-sugar breakfast cereals are sources of iron and vitamins. Snacks of fruits and vegetables assist in meeting the child's nutritional requirements (Box 7.2).

**BOX 7.2 Nutritious Snacks**

- Fresh fruit
- Celery sticks with cheese spread
- Yogurt
- Bagels
- Carrot sticks
- Graham crackers
- Pretzels
- Puddings

Many similarities exist in the nutritional needs of the toddler and the preschooler. Children this age who eat well-balanced diets should not experience iron deficiency. However, if milk remains the primary food, it will replace foods rich in iron, vitamins, and minerals, such as dark-green leafy vegetables, meats, and legumes. Although giving children a daily multivitamin is not harmful, in general the child who is healthy does not need vitamin supplementation. The exception to this is vitamin D. The AAP recommends vitamin D supplementation (400 IU daily) to children who consume fewer than 33 oz of milk or fortified dairy products a day (CDC, 2015; Greer, Sicherer, Burks, & the Committee on Nutrition and Section on Allergy and Immunology, 2008).

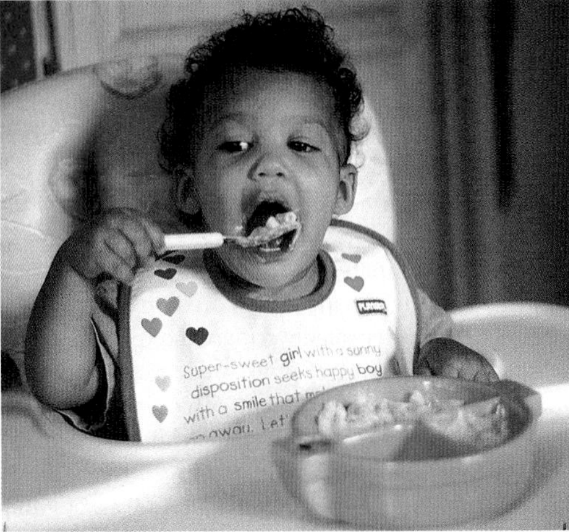


**FIG 7.4** By age 1 year, most children are eating the same foods as the rest of the family. Toddlers should be offered three meals and two healthy snacks each day. Most 2-year-olds can drink from a cup and use a spoon well if given the opportunity to practice.

#### Solid Foods

Children at this age are improving their proficiency in using a spoon and cup. By age 2 years, children can hold a cup in one hand and use a spoon well (Fig. 7.4). By age 12 months, most children are eating the same foods as the rest of the family. The child should be offered three meals and two snacks each day.

By age 3 to 4 years, the child begins to use a fork. The child continues to develop fine motor skills and by the end of the preschool period should begin to use a rounded knife for cutting.

One method to determine serving size for children is 1 tablespoon of solid food per year of age. Children may be more likely to try new foods and eat nutritious meals if smaller portions are served. Foods of different textures, colors, consistencies, tastes, and temperatures should be offered. The child should sit in a chair that allows easy access to the food; the dishes should be small, non-breakable and, when possible, steady enough to prevent spilling. Thick, short-handled spoons and forks and shallow bowls increase the toddler's ability to eat successfully.

Foods that could be aspirated should continue to be avoided during the toddler period. Soft drinks and candy need to be discouraged. Sugar is a source of calories and is naturally present in breast milk as lactose, in fruits as fructose, and in grain products as maltose. However, a diet with too much sugar can replace other, more nutritious foods and increase tooth decay. Artificial sweeteners and foods that contain artificial sweeteners are not recommended for children younger than 2 years.

### Age-Related Nutritional Challenges

*Food jags.* The volume of food the child eats may vary from day to day. The child may want the same food at every meal for several days and then suddenly reject the food completely. Children this age may refuse foods because of odor and temperature. They may not like mixing foods, and thus, may not eat casseroles. This dislike does not seem to apply to foods such as pizza, spaghetti, and macaroni and cheese. Many children prefer juices to milk and water. Too much milk is not good, but neither is too much juice, which can replace other foods and their nutrients. For toddlers and preschoolers, juices should be limited to no more than 4 to 6 oz/day (American Heart Association, 2015). Parents and older siblings can affect how a child views a food and should be careful about making negative comments about a certain food. Role modeling and making foods available assist children to develop tastes for new foods.

*Physiologic anorexia.* The nurse teaches parents appropriate ways to approach the child who is experiencing physiologic anorexia. Advise parents not to allow their child to fill up with snacks, milk, and juices. Small portions should be offered so that the child does not feel overwhelmed by the amount of food. Mealtimes should be pleasant and not times to discuss discipline problems or even the child's poor appetite. Being forced to sit at the table after the rest of the family has left only creates a negative association with mealtime. Parents need to maintain a balance between ignoring their child's nutritional intake and making it the focus of their parenting.

The nurse can encourage parents to focus more on their child's weekly nutritional intake, rather than on one day's intake. Frequently children are the best judges of what they need, and they may eat primarily fruit one day and peanut butter the next. Nutritional consumption tends to balance out over a week. Box 7.3 illustrates ways parents can increase their child's nutritional intake.

*Obesity risk.* The prevalence of obesity in the United States has risen dramatically among adults, but of particular concern is the prevalence of overweight and obese children. In *Healthy People 2020,* the United States Department of Health and Human Services (USDHHS) has specifically addressed the problem of obesity in young children, ages 2 to 5 years (USDHHS, 2010). Stating that 10.7% of 2- to 5-year-old children are identified as obese, objective NWS-10.1 is directed toward reducing obesity in children of this age-group. Strategies designed to approach this important issue include much of what has been discussed previously: increasing fruits and vegetables, increasing the percentage of whole grains, increasing calcium and iron intake, and decreasing solid fats, sodium, and sugar (USDHHS, 2010).

**BOX 7.3 Increasing Nutritional Intake**

- Limit to two nutritious snacks per day and give only at toddler's request.
- Limit to 4 to 6 oz of juice per day.
- Introduce to finger foods at age 8 to 10 months, and continue to make these types of food available.
- Limit to 16 to 24 oz of milk per day.
- Keep mealtimes pleasant.
- Do not force feed.
- Do not feed children who can feed themselves.

A report by Daniels, Hassink, & the Committee on Nutrition (2015) recommends screening children at risk for overweight and obesity beginning at age 2 years. This includes plotting a body mass index (BMI). Children with a family history of dyslipidemia or early cardiovascular disease development, and children whose BMI percentile exceeds the definition for overweight (>85th percentile) or who have high blood pressure, should have a fasting lipid screen (National Heart, Lung, and Blood Institute, 2013).

## Dental Care

Most toddlers have a complete set of 20 deciduous teeth by the time they are 30 months old. Although the exact time of eruption of teeth varies, an approximate rule of thumb to assess the number of teeth is the age of the toddler in months minus six. One tooth usually erupts for each month of age past 6 months up to 30 months of age.

Permanent teeth are calcifying during the toddler period, long before they are visible. Proper care of the deciduous teeth is crucial for the toddler's general health and for the health and alignment of the permanent teeth. Deciduous teeth play an important role in the growth and development of the jaw and face and in speech development. Premature loss of the deciduous teeth complicates eruption of the permanent teeth, often leading to malocclusion. Nurses need to be aware that some parents do not understand the value of preserving primary teeth.

Because toddlers do not have the manual dexterity to remove plaque adequately, parents must be responsible for cleaning their teeth. Children can be encouraged to brush their teeth after the teeth have been thoroughly cleaned by a parent. Because toddlers like to imitate, watching parents brush their teeth can be motivating. A small, soft, nylon-bristle brush works best. Optimal access and visibility are provided if the parent sits on the floor or bed with the child's head in the parent's lap and the child's body perpendicular to the parent's. This position also gives the parent some control of the child's head movement. In the young child (<3 years) the parent can smear a small amount of fluoride toothpaste onto the child's teeth; after age three, a pea-sized amount on the toothbrush is appropriate (AAP, 2014b). Ideally, teeth should be brushed after every meal and especially at bedtime. Flossing between teeth helps remove plaque and should be done daily by the parent after the toddler's teeth are brushed.

Fluoride makes tooth enamel resistant to acid attack, preventing decay. Recommendations currently state that pediatric providers should perform an oral risk assessment at regular intervals throughout childhood (AAP, 2016). Supplemental oral fluoride is prescribed for children without access to a community fluoridated water source. For these children, the dose of fluoride supplementation is as follows: 6 months to 3 years, 0.25 mg daily; 3 to 6 years, 0.5 mg daily (AAP, 2014b). Additionally, the AAP recommends an application of fluoride varnish every three to six months during early childhood if the child does not have access to a dentist (AAP, 2014b). A diet that is low in sweets and high in nutritious food promotes dental health. Sweets are most likely to cause caries if they are sticky or if they are eaten between meals rather than with meals. The nurse encourages the parent to offer nutritious snacks, such as fresh fruit, yogurt, or cheese, instead of candy, soda, or cookies.

All infants and children should have a source of dental care by age 1 year (AAP, 2016). Because bacterial organisms contribute to tooth decay, and children can acquire these organisms from their mother, primary preventive interventions need to be implemented as soon as possible in infancy. The AAP (2015c) suggests that the child should first see the dentist 6 months after the first primary tooth erupts and no later than age 12 months; this is especially important for infants and children at risk for tooth decay. The first appointment should

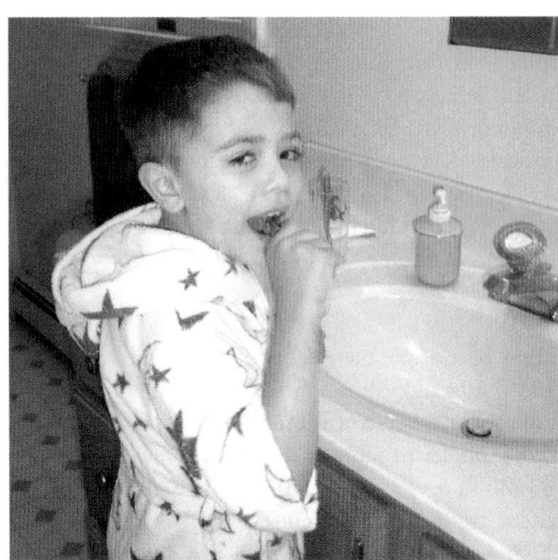

**FIG 7.5** Care of the deciduous teeth promotes healthy development of the permanent teeth. Some toddlers and preschoolers enjoy brushing their own teeth, but because toddlers and preschoolers lack the manual dexterity to remove plaque adequately, parents must assume this responsibility.

precede any needed dental work so that the visit is enjoyable and free from discomfort. This visit provides an opportunity for early assessment of the child's dental health as well as for teaching parents good preventive dental health practices, including not sharing eating or drinking utensils with the child.

Because the enamel on primary teeth is thinner than on permanent teeth, preschoolers' teeth are prone to destruction from decay. The distance from the tooth surface to the pulp is shorter also, so tooth abscesses from caries can occur rapidly. Untreated caries can lead to pain, abscess formation, and poor digestion because of ineffective chewing. Many parents do not realize that the deciduous teeth are important to protect the dental arch. If deciduous teeth are lost early (e.g., because of decay), the remaining teeth may drift out of position, blocking proper eruption of the permanent teeth and leading to malocclusion.

Nurses play an important role in the promotion of dental health by teaching proper tooth cleaning, including the removal of plaque, encouraging a balanced diet limited in sweets, and recommending twice-yearly visits to the dentist. Preschoolers can usually brush their own teeth (Fig. 7.5). Short back-and-forth or up-and-down strokes are easiest for the child to manage. Parents should monitor the child's toothbrushing and inspect the child's teeth to be sure that all plaque has been removed. Parents must help with flossing because it requires more manual dexterity than preschoolers have.

## Sleep and Rest

During the second year, children require approximately 12 to 14 hours of sleep each day. Most toddlers take one nap each day until the end of the second or third year, when many children give up the habit. Toddlers often resist going to bed, using dawdling or even temper tantrums to postpone separation from loved ones and the exciting events of the day. Firm, consistent limits are needed when toddlers try stalling tactics such as asking for one more drink of water.

Warning the child a few minutes before it is time for bed may reduce bedtime protests. Winding down with a quiet activity for 30 minutes before bedtime also helps toddlers prepare for sleep. Bedtime offers an opportunity for some snuggle time, when the parent and toddler can read a story and share the events of the day. Children of this age often have trouble relaxing and falling asleep. A warm bath before bedtime promotes relaxation. Bedtime rituals are important and should be followed consistently. Transition objects, such as a favorite blanket or stuffed animal, are often an important part of the child's bedtime routine.

Because preschoolers expend so much energy growing and learning, they need adequate rest. The preschooler needs an average of 10 to 12 hours of sleep in a 24-hour period. Some preschoolers do well without a nap during the day, but others still need a nap. Resistance to naps is common at this age. The child usually does not want to leave family or playmates, toys, and exciting activities to go into a darkened room to lie down and rest. A quiet time spent listening to music or looking at a favorite book may help the child relax and get some rest. Insufficient rest during the day may lead to irritability, decreased resistance to infection, and difficulty sleeping at night.

Sleep problems are more common during the preschool years than in any other period of childhood. Because of their active imaginations and immaturity, preschoolers often have nightmares and have trouble falling asleep at night. The boundaries between reality and fantasy are not well defined for children of this age, so monsters and scary creatures that lurk in the preschooler's imagination become real to the child after the light is turned off. Patience and repeated reassurance from a caring parent may be needed. Nightmares—frightening dreams that awaken the child from sleep—are common among preschoolers. A familiar environment and comfort with a hug and verbal reassurance from a parent usually enable the child to return to sleep. Night terrors differ from nightmares. Night terrors occur during deep sleep, and the child remains asleep even though the eyes may be open. The child does not awaken but moans, screams, or cries and does not recognize parents. Efforts to comfort the child may lead to agitation. The child does not remember the episode in the morning, even if awakened during the night terror. Parents should be instructed not to attempt to comfort or awaken the child during a night terror but should allow the child to sleep.

The nurse assesses sleep patterns during well-child visits and addresses parental concerns. The nurse can reassure parents that resistance to going to bed, fears, and nightmares are normal for children of this age. The nurse should assess the frequency of sleep problems and parents' reactions to them. If sleep problems occur often and are disruptive to the family, further investigation and intervention may be indicated.

Ritualistic techniques and transition objects that help decrease bedtime resistance in the toddler continue during the preschool period. Avoiding high-carbohydrate snacks and excitement before bedtime promotes relaxation. Children should not be forced to face their fears alone by sleeping in a completely dark room or with the door shut. Parents can search the room to reassure the preschooler that the room is safe. Progressive head-to-toe relaxation is an effective technique for helping preschoolers fall asleep. A set bedtime promotes security and healthy sleep habits.

A child who has slept for a long time at the babysitter's or at daycare may not be ready to sleep again. Communication with the child's daytime caretaker is important to determine whether the child is maintaining a balance of activity, rest, and sleep.

## Discipline

Effective discipline strategies should involve a comprehensive approach that protects children from harm and facilitates appropriate socialization (AAP, 1998/2014). How a parent uses discipline and the type of discipline used depends on various factors that include the maternal age and cultural background, experiences the parent had with

### CRITICAL THINKING EXERCISE 7.1

Mr. and Mrs. Thomas have brought 2-year-old Todd to the clinic for his annual physical examination. The parents report that bedtime is a major production almost every night. They state that he cries, comes out of his room, and displays various other behaviors that delay sleep. They wonder if he has a sleep disorder. They relate that, other than an occasional temper tantrum, they do not have any other concerns.

- What information do you need from the parents to assess the problem?
- After you have the above information, what advice should you give the Thomases?

discipline as a child, and the child's age (AAP, 1998/2014). When discipline is used in a positive manner, the child internalizes controls established by parental limits and begins to develop a conscience.

Toddlers need and want discipline to feel secure. They have little control over their behavior and need limits to learn how to behave and how to follow the rules and expectations of society. Toddlers' negativism, intense emotions, and curiosity put them at risk for injury. Because they are usually unaware of the consequences of their actions, vigilance and limits are needed for safety. Toddlers are frightened by a lack of limits and will deliberately test their parents until they are shown how far they can go. Firm discipline promotes the development of autonomy by giving the child a feeling of freedom within bounds.

Toddlers often repeat parental prohibitions to themselves while engaging in a forbidden activity. For example, a toddler may walk over to an electrical outlet, knowing that it is out of bounds, and mumble, "No, no, hurt!" while playing with the outlet. Although remembering the prohibition, the toddler lacks sufficient self-control to prevent the behavior.

Effective discipline techniques for children of this age include allowing natural and logical consequences, positive reinforcement for acceptable behavior, diversion and a time-out (1 minute per year of age) (AAP, 2015b). Teaching parents how to discipline their child helps avoid problems related to the incorrect use of discipline. Parents must be consistent. Physical punishment, such as spanking, is one of the least effective discipline techniques and is discouraged by the AAP (2011b) (see Chapter 3).

Preschoolers struggle to gain control over their strong inner impulses. To achieve this control, they need limits set on their behavior. When limits are set, the child feels more secure and can explore the environment and try new roles in an atmosphere of freedom and safety. Appropriate limit setting helps the child learn self-confidence, self-control, and moral values. The child must be consistently disciplined for acts that are destructive, socially unacceptable, or morally wrong. Limits must be clearly defined and consistently enforced to be effective. To prevent confusion and anxiety, the consequences of misbehavior should be spelled out in advance and carried out immediately after misbehavior occurs. When the child is disciplined for misbehavior, a simple, truthful explanation of why the behavior was unacceptable should be given.

The focus of the explanation should be on the behavior rather than on the child. For example, "Throwing toys could hurt someone. I don't like to see you doing that" is a better response than "I don't want to be around you when you act like that" or "You're a bad girl for doing that."

Discipline techniques that are effective with preschoolers include the following:

- Time-out (removing the child from a situation for a short period and offering an explanation for the punishment).
- Time-in (frequent, brief, nonverbal, physical contact when the child is acting appropriately). For example, the mother periodically strokes the child's hair or rubs his back when he is quietly playing on the floor near her while she talks on the telephone. The child who receives this type of reinforcement is more likely to continue what he is doing and much less likely to interrupt the mother.
- Offering restricted choices (e.g., "You may drink your juice in the kitchen or you may go into the living room without your juice.").
- Diversion (e.g., "You must stop marking on the wall with crayons. Here, mark on this paper instead.").

Consistent positive reinforcement for desired behavior is a powerful tool. If the parent does not care or is too busy to enforce rules consistently, the child will not internalize rules and will not feel guilty about breaking them. The child will be unruly and will be unable to follow the rules set by society.

Spending enjoyable time with their children is another way parents can model positive behaviors. Having good times with children increases their self-esteem and reinforces good behavior. Chapter 3 and the Parents Want to Know box, "Guidelines for Disciplining a Toddler," present additional discussions of discipline.

### PARENTS WANT TO KNOW

***Guidelines for Disciplining a Toddler***

- Discipline must be consistent. Inconsistency is confusing and counterproductive. Consistent follow-through every time is important.
- Discipline must be immediate. Consequences of behavior should occur as soon as possible after the behavior occurs. Threats such as "Just wait until your father gets home!" are confusing and ineffective for a child of this age.
- Discipline must be realistic and age appropriate. Toddlers should not be expected to act like "little ladies" or "little gentlemen."
- Discipline must be related to the incident. Consequences that are logical results of a behavior are most effective.
- Limits must be clearly explained to the child.
- Toddlers must be given time to respond to instructions.
- Withdrawal of love should never be used as punishment. Comforting the child after discipline promotes positive feelings. Love is the key to effective discipline.
- Arguments and extensive explanations should be avoided.
- Praise for good behavior should be used to build self-confidence and self-esteem.
- The toddler must be separated from the behavior: "I love you very much. Hitting your sister needs to stop."

## Toddler Safety

Understanding the developmental changes a toddler undergoes helps the nurse and parent appreciate why children are more injury prone in this stage of development than at any other time. Constant supervision is challenging for parents but is the most important factor in preventing injuries in this energetic age-group.

### Car Safety

Motor vehicle injuries are a significant threat to the toddler. Although toddlers begin to develop more independent behaviors, they are still wholly reliant on an adult for protection while traveling in a car. Toddlers should be secured in a rear-facing, approved car safety seat, placed in the middle of the rear seat until age 2 years or until the child has achieved the weight and height recommendations recommended by the car seat manufacturer (AAP, 2014a). Harness safety straps (used according to manufacturer weight and height guidelines) should be adjusted to provide a snug fit (AAP, 2014a). After age 2 years, toddlers are secured in an upright forward-facing safety seat with a three- or five-point harness (AAP, 2014a).

## SAFETY ALERT

### Car Safety

Toddlers should be restrained in an upright, forward-facing position in a car safety seat until they outgrow the manufacturer's weight or height recommendations.

Car doors should be locked while the car is in motion to prevent a curious toddler from opening a door.

Until passenger vehicles are equipped with airbags that are safe and effective for children, children younger than 13 years should not ride in a front passenger seat that is equipped with an airbag.

An approved booster seat (high-back seat preferred) may be used for a child who is older than 4 years or who has exceeded the height and weight recommended by the manufacturer for a forward-facing car safety seat. A booster seat raises the child to a level that accommodates the car's seatbelt system. Children usually use a booster seat until they are tall enough to properly wear the seat lap and shoulder belt (height 4 feet, 9 inches and 8 to 12 years old) (AAP, 2014a).

Because children begin to imitate their parents at an early age, the nurse encourages parents to model safe behavior by consistently wearing their seatbelts. As the toddler's cognitive and fine motor skills develop, some children wiggle free of the restraint system despite releases that are designed to be difficult for a child to operate. Parents must insist on adherence in spite of temper tantrums.

Because of the toddler's short physical stature, adults should visually inspect the area surrounding the automobile before placing it in gear. A toddler near the car may not be visible and can sustain serious crushing injuries if run over by the car or trapped between the car and a stationary object. Toddlers may also dart out on foot into oncoming traffic. Parents need to closely supervise play activities and remain physically close to the toddler to prevent these types of injuries.

Toddlers and infants should never be left unattended in a car, even for a moment. Exposure to extreme heat or cold is dangerous in this age-group. Injuries have occurred when parents have left a car running for various reasons and a curious toddler has disengaged the gears, causing the car to roll and collide with other objects.

### Airplane Safety

The Federal Aviation Administration (FAA) (2015) strongly suggest that infants and children younger than 4 years should be restrained during takeoff and landing, during turbulence, and as much as is feasible during flight. Children should be placed in properly secured age-appropriate safety seats, which have been government approved for both automobile and aircraft, in a similar manner as a car safety seat. The most desirable location of the safety seat is by a window (FAA, 2015). The FAA also has an approved harness restraint system (CARES) to be used for children weighing between 22 and 44 lb; parents need to request these restraint systems from the airline on which they are traveling (FAA, 2015). The FAA suggests that parents check with the airline to see if the airline will give a discount for the child who needs to be restrained.

### Fire and Burn Safety

Injuries related to fire and scalds are a significant cause of morbidity and mortality in children ages 1 to 4 years (CDC, 2013c). The CDC (2013a) has activated a national action plan to address the issue of preventing burns and scalds; the plan includes statistical surveillance, research, education, assessing healthcare infrastructure, modes of communication, and policy. Toddlers, with their increased mobility and developing fine motor skills, can reach hot water, open fires, or hot objects placed on counters and stoves above their eye level. A child at this age is at increased risk to reach up and pull a hot liquid off a surface or to grab or overturn a container of hot water onto himself or herself. Toddlers may pull objects off stoves, pull down cords attached to small appliances, open oven doors, and place electrical cords or frayed wires into their mouths. They may drink liquids that are dangerously hot. The nurse should emphasize to parents to remain in the kitchen when preparing a meal, use the back burners on the stove, and turn pot handles inward and toward the middle of the stove to reduce the toddler's risk of burn injuries. Dangling cords from irons or other small appliances should not be accessible to toddlers. Open fires and heaters are also inviting. Sturdy guards fixed to the wall prevent young children from getting too close to these burn hazards. In addition, curious toddlers are fascinated with matches and lighters, which must be kept out of reach.

Toddlers depend on adults for their protection in the event of a house fire. Anticipatory guidance emphasizes the importance of smoke detectors and escape plans.

### Preventing Falls

Toddlers move quickly and climb everywhere. Toddlers can fall from playground equipment, off tricycles, and out of windows. Falls are the leading cause of morbidity from unintentional injury during early childhood; 43% of all unintentional injuries during early childhood are related to falls (CDC, 2013c). Falls from above the first floor of a building can result in serious injury, particularly head injury. A chair next to a kitchen counter or table allows the toddler easy access to dangerously high places. Because climbing and exploration are normal aspects of the developmental process, safety education for the parent emphasizes constant supervision and some anticipatory planning, such as moving furniture, installing screen guards, and restricting access to potential climbing hazards.

### Water Safety

Toddlers love to play in water. Most drownings occur when a child is left alone in a bathtub or falls into a residential pool. Drowning has become the leading cause of death due to unintentional injury during early childhood (CDC, 2013b) and an increasing number of children are drowning in above-ground swimming pools (Shields, Pollack-Nelson, & Smith, 2011). Even when a child survives a submersion injury, the risk of permanent brain and lung damage is great (see Chapter 34).

Parents should not leave a child alone in or near a bathtub, pail of water, wading or swimming pool, or any other body of water, even for a moment; a competent swimmer should be within arm's reach when a child is near any swimming area (CDC, 2014). All swimming pools, whether in-ground or above ground require a "climb-resistant" fence (minimum height of 4 feet) that completely surrounds the pool and remains locked in a way that a young child cannot accidentally open it. Pool drains should be protected by covers that prevent children from being trapped or having long hair caught in the drain. Early swim instruction is one of the major drowning-prevention measures (CDC, 2014).

A toddler can drown in as little as 1 inch of water. Toilet lids need to remain closed. Toddlers can inadvertently fall headfirst into a toilet or bucket, and they lack the upper-body strength and coordination to remove themselves from submersion. Drowning prevention requires constant parental supervision of the toddler. Nurses need to be involved not only in individual counseling about drowning prevention, but also in advocacy at the community or state level for legislation that ensures pool safety.

### Preventing Poisoning

Children younger than 5 years are the most common victims of poisoning, with the majority being 1- to 3-year-olds (Majsak-Newman et al., 2014). Unintentional injury from poisoning affects more than 30,000 young children, and poisonings are the tenth leading cause of unintentional injury in the United States among children aged 1 to 4 years (CDC, 2013c). The home is the site of exposure in most cases, with causes being ingestions of medications, cleaning products, cosmetics or personal care products, plants, gardening products (e.g., pesticides) and alcohol (Majsak-Newman et al., 2014). The American Association of Poison Control Centers (AAPCC) (2016) reports concerns that new poisons are emerging; these include e-cigarette liquid, laundry detergent packets, energy drinks, and synthetic cannabis. With exploration, everything eventually finds its way to the child's mouth, even if it does not smell or taste good. Small children who are thirsty or hungry will ingest poisons that look or smell inviting.

## PATIENT-CENTERED TEACHING

### *Childhood Poison Prevention*

- Keep all poisons, medicines, cleaners, and toxic substances out of the reach of children. Never discard poisons in a wastebasket.
- Be familiar with poisons commonly found in or near the home, including detergents, drain cleaner, dishwashing soap, furniture polish, cleaning agents, window cleaners, all medicines, vitamins, children's medications, alcohol, sprays, powders, cosmetics, fingernail preparations, hair care products, sachets, mothballs, rodent poisons, fertilizers, gasoline, antifreeze, paints, glues, insecticides, cigarette butts, plants, and shrubs.
- Store poisons out of reach in areas that are secured with locks or protected by child-resistant safety latches.
- Medicines and all harmful substances should be purchased in child-resistant packages.
- Keep alcoholic beverages out of the reach of your children or locked in a separate cabinet. Do not give sips of alcohol to your children because small amounts can be toxic to young children.
- Children should not be allowed to chew on plants or shrubs.
- Keep ashtrays empty and out of the reach of small children.
- Handbags and overnight luggage of guests in the home often contain medicines or other toxic substances and should be kept out of a child's reach.
- Store poisons or harmful substances in the original container. Do not place toxic substances in food or beverage containers for storage.
- Teach your children to ask an adult before they touch a nonfood substance.
- Poison-proof all areas of the home, especially the kitchen, bathroom, pantry, bedroom, garage, basement, and work areas. Grandparents and other caregivers should be encouraged to do the same.
- Post the telephone number of the local poison control in an area that can be accessed immediately in the event of a poisoning. The American Association of Poison Control Centers' help line number (1-800-222-1222) will connect to the local poison control number, which is staffed 24 hours a day, 7 days a week. When contacting the poison control center, be able to provide the following information: the substance ingested (have the label on hand for prompt identification of toxic ingredients), time the substance was ingested, and the child's age and weight. Do not administer anything to your child without contacting the poison control center first.

Poisonings occur from a combination of factors that include not using safety equipment (e.g., child resistant medicine caps, gates, or putting poisons out of reach), hazards in the home (e.g., putting medications or other poisonous products in different containers than their original ones), and unsafe behaviors (e.g., leaving poisonous substances out after use) (Majsak-Newman et al., 2014). The nurse can help parents to poison-proof the home and teach them the appropriate action to take if an ingestion occurs (see Patient-Centered Teaching: Childhood Poison Prevention).

Calling the AAPCC help line (1-800-222-1222) needs to be the first action a parent takes if the child has ingested a poison; the professionals that staff the help line have experience in managing a wide variety of poisoning situations and can assist the parent to intervene immediately (AAPCC, 2011). In partnership with the AAPCC, pediatric health providers recommend this action, rather than having the parent call the emergency department or their health provider (AAPCC, 2011). If the child is unconscious, having a seizure, or not breathing, the parent should immediately call 911 or the local emergency number.

Medicine should not be called candy, and because young children often mimic their parents, adults should be discouraged from taking medicine in the child's presence. The nurse needs to advise parents to take the same precautions when small children go to a grandparent's home to visit. Childproof caps slow the child but are not an absolute barrier. Labels with characteristic symbols, such as the skull and crossbones or "Mr. Yuk," help provide visual cues to young children; however, labels are not absolute deterrents for a determined child. The best way to prevent toxic ingestions is by carefully storing all potential poisons in a place that is inaccessible to children. (See Chapters 5 and 34 for information about environmental poisonings.)

### Preschooler Safety

Preschoolers are active and inquisitive. They have greater self-control, but their understanding of danger is not fully developed. Safety becomes even more challenging for the parent because preschoolers are no longer content with their own backyards. Preschoolers are mesmerized by cartoons that depict make-believe situations. They see cartoon characters engaging in daring endeavors and walking away unharmed. Because of their magical thinking, preschoolers may believe that these feats are possible and may attempt them.

Safety education can now be directed toward the child as well as the parent. Children of this age have a strong sense of rhythm, and songs and rhymes about safety can enhance the learning process. Instruction should be simple, with one concept introduced at a time. Short stories, puppet shows, songs, coloring activities, and role-playing games are all suitable learning activities that help preschoolers learn safety-conscious behaviors.

### Car Safety

Preschoolers need to remain in an approved car safety seat until they are 4 years old or are too tall for the safety seat according to the manufacturer's recommendations (AAP, 2014a). Once a child has outgrown the child car safety seat, an approved booster seat, positioned high enough to safely use the lap and shoulder belt, is strongly recommended (Fig. 7.6). Although preferable to no restraints at all, standard seatbelts alone can contribute to injury because they fit poorly over the small frame of the preschooler. The standard shoulder harness often crosses the child's face or neck, and the lap belt is positioned across the midabdomen rather than across the bony structure of the pelvis. Booster seats are designed to raise the child high enough so that the restraining straps are correctly positioned over the child's smaller body frame.

Parents continue to have the primary responsibility for ensuring that a child is safely restrained before the vehicle is started and in

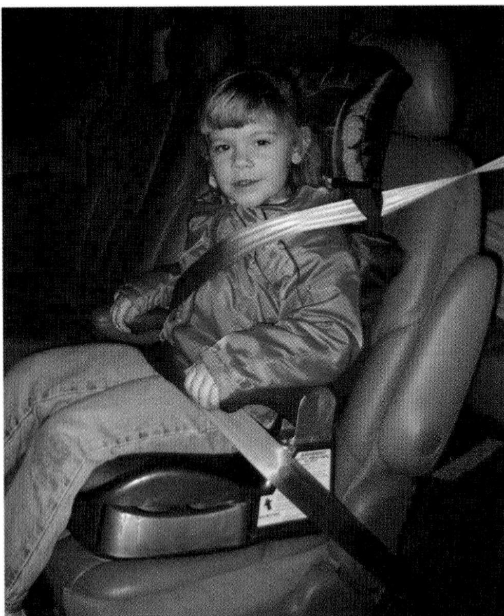

FIG 7.6 A high-back booster seat designed to properly hold a car lap and shoulder belt is strongly recommended for children who have outgrown a child safety seat. Booster seats raise the young child high enough to allow the car seatbelts to be correctly positioned over the child's chest and pelvis. (Courtesy M. Hayden, St. Louis, MO.)

motion. Parents must insist that children remain restrained at all times and that seatbelts be used correctly. Although riding in the open bed of a pickup truck or in the cargo area of a van or station wagon may seem fun and relatively harmless, it can be deadly in the event of a crash. Most states require children under a certain age to be restrained in an approved child safety seat at all times while riding in a vehicle.

### Fire and Burn Safety

Preschoolers imitate adults in all types of daily routines and activities. They may attempt household activities before they are able to manage an appliance safely (e.g., stove, iron, oven), increasing the risk of burn injuries. Matches and lighters continue to fascinate preschoolers. With their increased fine motor skills, preschoolers may be able to ignite a flame. Preschoolers should be taught that lighters and matches are adult tools and instructed to tell an adult immediately if they find these items. These actions can prevent burn injuries.

Children younger than 5 years are at the greatest risk for burn deaths in a house fire. They often panic and hide in closets or under beds rather than escape safely. Parents need to practice fire drills with their children to teach them what to do in the event of a house fire. Preschoolers should become familiar with the sounds emitted by smoke alarms and should be taught to crawl under smoke and to check doors for heat.

Preschoolers are at an ideal age to learn what to do if their clothing ignites in flames. Instruct preschoolers to stop immediately if their clothes catch on fire and to cover the face and mouth with the hands. They should then drop to the ground and roll to smother the flames. This simple command (stop, drop, and roll) can help prevent severe burn injuries. Teaching specific behaviors educates children to remain calm and not panic.

### Firearm Safety

Guns are often kept in the home loaded and readily accessible to young children. Parents should be encouraged to critically evaluate their need for a firearm in the home. Do the potentially devastating risks outweigh any benefits of keeping a weapon in the home? The nurse should talk to all parents about gun safety at every well visit because even though parents may not keep a gun in the house, children may visit friends whose parents do. Parents who choose to keep a gun in the home should receive anticipatory guidance about injury prevention. Guns kept in the home should always be unloaded, stored with trigger guards in place, securely locked in metal vaults, and inaccessible to all children. Ammunition should be stored in an inaccessible location separate from the gun.

### Personal Safety

Preschoolers have an interest in establishing relationships with others as they expand the boundaries of their world. With the child's increasing assertion of independence, parents are less able to provide the constant protection they once did.

Teaching children about personal safety encourages them to develop skills to detect danger and teaches appropriate ways to handle threatening situations. Strangers are often portrayed as evil characters, when in reality their appearance and approach may be nonthreatening and friendly. Distinguishing a stranger from a well-intentioned person is challenging and often difficult for the preschooler. Basic guidelines that a child needs to know about personal safety include saying no, getting away, and telling an adult.

Children need to know how to access emergency help if they need it. Parents should help their children learn to identify safety officials and how to dial 911 or other locally appropriate emergency numbers. Children need to respond to emergency operators with their full name, address, parent's name, and other appropriate information and should remain on the phone until help arrives. Parents can practice this safety skill with their children to ensure proper reactions in an emergency and help the child understand what constitutes an emergency situation.

### Sexual Abuse

Sexual abuse is another threat to personal safety. Preventing sexual abuse begins with teaching children the normal, healthy boundaries of their bodies and what constitutes inappropriate behavior. Often the perpetrators are known and trusted by the child. Abusers frequently intimidate the child into silence with threats of personal harm or suggestions that the child initiated the behavior. Children need to know that no matter how great the threat, if someone is touching their bodies in an inappropriate way, they should always tell an adult. If that adult cannot help them, they should tell as many adults as necessary until the inappropriate behavior is stopped (see Chapter 53).

## Selected Issues Related to the Toddler

### Toilet Training

Control of elimination is one of the major tasks of toddlerhood. Successful toilet training depends on both the child's and parent's readiness. The parent must be willing to spend the necessary time and emotional energy to encourage the child on a daily basis.

Toilet training is one of the most frustrating and time-consuming tasks that parents face. It can be so frustrating for some that researchers have linked toilet training accidents with many cases of child abuse. Parents who do not understand normal growth and development patterns often have unrealistic expectations and can become frustrated to the point of rage.

The nurse can assist parents by explaining developmental milestones and encouraging parents not to begin training until the child shows signs of readiness. Toilet training proceeds at different times in different cultures. Helping the parent recognize signs of readiness and

## HEALTH PROMOTION

### The 3-Year-Old Child

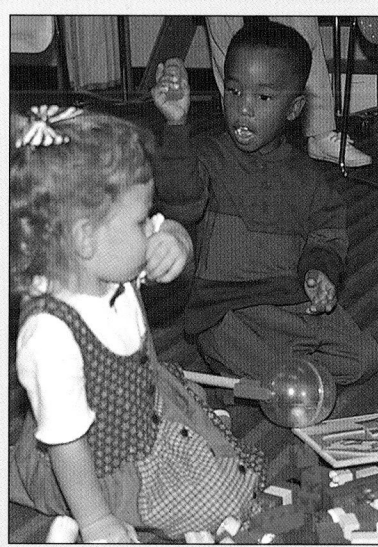

**Focused Assessment**

Ask the parent the following:

- How are you managing any discipline problems your child may be having?
- Have you been able to encourage your child to be independent? Does your child's developing independence create anxiety or conflict for you? Is your child in preschool or daycare? How many hours or days?
- How does your child get along with other children the same age?
- How well does your child communicate with others? Do you have any concerns about your child's speech?
- How well is your child doing with toilet training?
- What activities do you enjoy doing together?

**Developmental Milestones**

*Personal/social:* Puts on articles of clothing; brushes teeth with help; washes and dries hands using soap and water; notices gender differences and identifies with children of own gender; exhibits sexual curiosity, may begin to masturbate; knows own name and names one or more friends; increasing independence, may start preschool; ritualistic; understands taking turns and sharing but may not be ready to do so; begins to show fears (dark, shadows, animals)

*Fine motor:* Vision approaches 20/20; can build a tower of at least eight blocks; begins purposeful drawing, can imitate a circle and a cross and draw a person with three parts; feeds self well

*Language/cognition:* Increasing vocabulary with intelligible speech, although dysfluency is common (thinks faster than can talk); names four familiar objects and begins to describe qualities or actions of objects; knows meaning of common adjectives (sleepy, hungry, hot); begins color identification; uses symbolic language; still egocentric; increased concept of time, space, causality; constantly asks "how" and "why" questions; can count to three; can tell full name, age, and gender

*Gross motor:* Jumps with both feet up and down and over a short distance; throws a ball overhand; catches a large ball with both hands; balances on each foot for at least 2 seconds; begins to ride a tricycle

**Critical Milestones***

*Personal/social:* Brushes teeth with help, puts on clothing, feeds a doll

*Fine motor:* Builds a tower of at least four to six cubes

*Language/cognition:* Points to and names four familiar pictures (cat, horse, bird, dog, man); speech understandable 50% of the time

*Gross motor:* Throws a ball overhand; jumps; kicks a ball forward

**Health Maintenance**

***Physical Measurements***

Continue to plot height, weight, and body mass index (BMI)

Growth rate is similar to that of a 2-year-old

***Immunizations***

Administer any immunizations not given previously according to the recommended schedule

Influenza vaccine annually

***Health Screening***

Objective vision screening if cooperative (AAP, 2016) (see Chapter 33)

Objective hearing screening with age-appropriate audiometric equipment

Blood pressure measurement

Hemoglobin, hematocrit, and lead screening

Tuberculosis (TB) screening if at risk

Fasting lipid screen if at risk

**Anticipatory Guidance**

***Nutrition***

Similar to that of a 2-year-old

Vitamin D supplementation 400 IU/day if consuming less than 1 L (33 oz) per day of milk and vitamin-D–fortified foods

***Elimination***

Usually is toilet trained but not at night

***Dental***

Have the child brush with pea-sized amount of toothpaste

Parent should floss the child's teeth

Child should see the dentist every 6 months

Fluoride varnish if no access to a dentist

Change oral fluoride dose to 0.5 mg daily

***Sleep***

Similar to that of a 2-year-old

May relinquish the nap

Consider changing to a full bed if climbing out of the crib

May begin to experience night terrors

***Hygiene***

Similar to that of a 2-year-old

Remind the child about good handwashing, especially after toileting and before meals

***Safety***

Review choking on food, street safety, water safety, sun protection, outside poisons, playground safety

Discuss bicycle and tricycle safety, fire safety, car seats (child should be in an approved forward-facing car safety seat until the age of 4 years or until larger than the manufacturer's recommended size and weight for the particular model)

*Continued*

## HEALTH PROMOTION—cont'd

### The 3-Year-Old Child

**Self-Esteem and Competence**

Model appropriate social behavior
Encourage your child to learn to make choices
Help your child to express emotions appropriately
Spend individual time with your child daily, and encourage your child to talk about the day's events
Provide consistent and loving limits to help your child learn self-discipline

**Play**

Similar to that of a 2-year-old
Likes imitative toys, large building blocks, musical toys, and riding toys such as large trucks
Limit screen time

*Guided by Denver Developmental Screening Test II.

### BOX 7.4 Signs of Readiness for Toilet Training

**Physical Readiness**

Child can remove own clothing.
Child is willing to let go of a toy when asked.
Child is able to sit, squat, and walk well.
Child has been walking for 1 year.

**Psychological Readiness**

Child notices if diaper is wet.
Child may indicate that diaper needs to be changed by pulling on diaper, squatting, or repeating a word or phrase.
Child communicates need to go to the bathroom or can get there by self.
Child wants to please parent by staying dry.

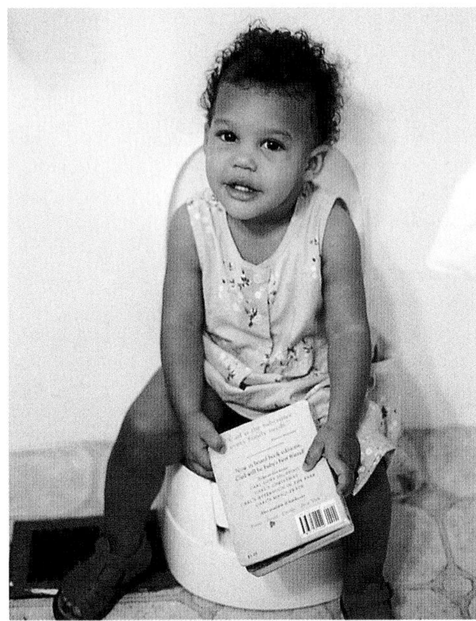

FIG 7.7 No set rules exist for toilet training. The nurse can help parents understand that both physical readiness and psychological readiness are necessary for success.

factors that interfere with toilet training, such as stress, can make the training easier (Box 7.4). The parent may not have the necessary reserves of patience and energy for toilet training during stressful times, such as near the birth of another child or while moving to a new house. Training may be easier if it is postponed until routines return to normal.

The nurse can assist parents with toilet training the toddler by explaining the importance of maturation to successful toilet training. Parents need to know that both physical readiness and psychological readiness are necessary for toilet training to be successful. Myelinization of the spinal cord, which usually occurs between 12 and 18 months, must be complete before the child can voluntarily control the bowel and bladder sphincters. The nurse can offer anticipatory guidance to parents by teaching them the signs that the toddler is ready for toilet training. The average toddler is not ready for toilet training to begin until 18 to 24 months of age. Waiting until the child is 24 to 30 months old makes the task considerably easier because toddlers of this age are less negative and usually are more willing to control their sphincters to please their parents. Nurses advise parents to try to be tuned in to their child's individual elimination patterns and responses to facilitate the ease of achieving control (AAP, 2015a).

There are no set rules or timetables for toilet training (Fig. 7.7). The age at which toilet training usually begins varies from culture to culture. If the child resists, training may be stopped for 30 to 60 days before it is begun again. Bowel control is usually achieved before bladder control. However, some children do achieve daytime bladder control before bowel control, which can be somewhat distressful for parents. Daytime bladder control occurs before nighttime bladder control. A relaxed, child-centered approach, with plenty of praise for each success, is most effective. Punishment and coercive techniques cause feelings of shame and lead to power struggles. The child should not be forced to sit on the toilet for long periods. Successful toilet training is a gradual process, and relapses must be expected. Toileting accidents often occur when children are too busy playing to notice a full bladder until too late. Many children cannot remain completely dry until age 3 years. Parents should respond to accidents with tolerance instead of scolding or shaming the child.

### Temper Tantrums

Temper tantrums are a common toddler response to anger and frustration and often result from thwarted attempts at mastery and autonomy. Tantrums may also occur as an emotional release of tension after a long, tiring day. Unable to express anger in more productive ways because of limited language and reasoning abilities, toddlers may react by screaming, kicking, throwing things, or even biting themselves or banging their heads. Tantrums occur more often when toddlers are tired, hungry, bored, or excessively stimulated.

The nurse can help parents by identifying strategies to decrease the frequency of tantrums. Limiting situations that are too much for the child to handle is helpful. Anticipating periods of fatigue, having a snack ready before the child gets too hungry, and offering the toddler choices when possible can minimize temper tantrums. Parental practices such as inconsistency, permissiveness, excessive strictness, and overprotectiveness increase the probability of tantrums.

Toddlers need appropriate and consistent limits. Letting the child know that temper tantrums will not be tolerated gives the child a sense of security. The intensity of a toddler's outburst almost seems to be a plea for someone to stop the behavior. Probably the most effective method for handling tantrums is to isolate the child safely and then ignore them. The child should learn that nothing is gained from a tantrum, not even attention. Giving in to the child's demands or scolding the child only increases the behavior. Toddlers stop using tantrums when they do not achieve their goals and as their verbal skills increase. Once the tantrum has subsided and the toddler has regained some self-control, the parent should offer comfort and let the child know that limits are necessary and that the child is loved. Acknowledging the child's angry feelings and rewarding more mature ways of expressing them assist the child in gaining self-control.

### Sibling Rivalry

Sharing parents' love and attention is difficult for most toddlers. Often toddlers have intense feelings of jealousy and envy toward a new infant sibling. Toddlers' egocentrism makes understanding that a parent can love more than one child at a time difficult.

Because the infant needs a great deal of time and attention, the toddler's routine is disrupted. The toddler has limited resources to cope with such stress and may react by treating the baby roughly, damaging property, or harming pets. The toddler may exhibit signs of regression by asking for a bottle or pacifier or by using baby talk.

Any changes, such as moving the toddler to a new bedroom or beginning daycare, should be made as far in advance as possible so that the toddler will not feel displaced by abrupt changes when the baby arrives. Many hospitals offer sibling preparation classes. When the mother and infant come home from the hospital, the mother's first concern should be greeting the older sibling. It is helpful if the father or another caregiver carries the newborn to allow the mother's arms to be free to hug the waiting toddler and express how much she missed her child. A toddler's jealous feelings can become intense when visitors lavish gifts and praise on the baby. Giving an inexpensive gift to the toddler each time the baby receives one can minimize these feelings. Visitors should be encouraged to pay attention to the older child as well as the baby. Parents should anticipate behavior changes, even if the toddler has been prepared for the arrival of a new baby. The parents should be present when the toddler is with the infant to prevent the toddler from inadvertently harming the newborn sibling.

#### PARENTS WANT TO KNOW

***Strategies to Decrease Sibling Rivalry***

- Include the toddler in preparations for the new baby.
- Explain to the toddler what new babies are like.
- Let the child feel the fetus move.
- Read picture books about new siblings.
- Talk about changes that the newborn might create.
- Acknowledge the older child's feelings about these changes.
- Refer to the baby as "ours."

Toddlers should be helped to recognize and identify negative feelings toward a new sibling. However, firm limits must be set if the toddler tries to harm the baby. The child may be told "It's okay to feel like you don't like the baby right now, but it's not okay to hurt the baby." Praise should be given for affectionate, cooperative behavior.

Planned, uninterrupted private time is important to maintain feelings of closeness between parent and toddler. Even 10 or 15 minutes each day while the baby is sleeping is valuable. Allowing the toddler to choose an activity for this time with the parent makes it even more special. This special time should be given to the child each day, regardless of the child's behavior.

## Selected Issues Related to the Preschooler

### Stuttering

Stuttering, or stammering, is a disturbance in the flow and time patterning of speech. It becomes apparent in children whose speech is normal until they reach early childhood (Reitzes, 2014). During the preschool years, children often have experiences they want to share but have difficulty putting the words together. Children this age commonly repeat whole words or phrases and interject "uh" and "um" in their speech. As children's communication skills develop, most grow out of their normal developmental dysfluency, but some might require a referral to a speech and language therapist (Krader, 2014). Dysfluency may be more frequent during times of excitement when formulating long and complex sentences, or when trying to think of a particular word.

Reactions from others can worsen the dysfluency. Indications for referral include the presence of speech difficulties occurring more often than not in conversation, facial tension or appearance of discomfort when talking, frustration or embarrassment, and parent concern (Krader, 2014).

Parents can help their child by focusing on the ideas the child is expressing, not on the way the child is speaking. Parents should not complete their child's sentences or draw attention to their child's speech. They should not criticize or correct the child's speech and should advise others to do the same (see Parents Want to Know: How to Help the Child Who Stutters).

#### PARENTS WANT TO KNOW

***How to Help the Child Who Stutters***

- Listen closely when your child speaks and refrain from interrupting.
- Speak slowly and clearly and pause frequently. Speak in short sentences. Doing so provides a model for the child and gives the child more time to understand what is being said and to formulate thoughts.
- Designate time every day to listen and talk individually with your child without distractions or competition from other family members. Let the child direct the content of the conversation.
- Restrict the number of questions you ask your child at one time. Do not ask a second question before the first question is answered. Be sure to listen attentively to the child's answer.
- Minimize stressful situations for your child.
- Recognize that certain environmental factors may have a negative effect on fluency: stress, competition to speak, excitement, time pressure, arguments, fatigue, new situations, unfamiliar listeners.
- Assist other family members to communicate with the child by modeling.
- Show your child love and acceptance and remain relaxed.

Data from Guitar, B., & Conture, E. (2015). *7 tips for talking with your child.* Retrieved from http://www.stutteringhelp.org.

### Preschool and Daycare Programs

A quality daycare program provides an environment in which the child can expand social and play skills as well as manipulate play materials unavailable at home. Working mothers often express guilt and concern about the effect of daycare on their children's emotional well-being and cognitive development. Some concerns about the effect of daycare on the child's development can be minimized by careful selection of the daycare facility.

The nurse is in an excellent position to advise parents about child care. Parents need specific advice about options that are affordable but will not compromise the child's health and development. Parents need to visit the provider or daycare center to evaluate the quality of the program. Areas to evaluate include the attitude and qualifications of the caregivers, as well as operating procedures, costs, child-care and disciplinary practices, meals, safety precautions, sanitary conditions, and the child-to-staff ratio. The parent should ask to see the center's health policy manual.

The child needs preparation before beginning daycare and information about what to expect in simple, concrete terms. Emphasizing the exciting parts of the experience will help the child view the experience positively. The parent should also explain the reason for separation. Imaginative preschoolers may believe that they are being "sent away" because of some misdeed.

## HEALTH PROMOTION

### The 4- and 5-Year-Old Child

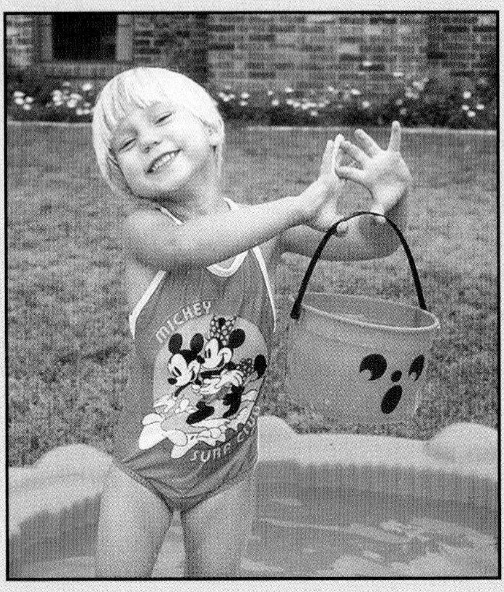


#### Focused Assessment

Ask the parent the following:

- Have you been able to encourage your child to be independent? Does your child's increasing independence create any anxiety or conflict for you?
- Is your child in preschool or daycare? How many hours or days?
- How does your child get along with other children the same age?
- How well does your child communicate with others? Do you have any concerns about your child's speech?
- Has your child's play become more imaginative? Does your child describe any fears?
- Can your child independently manage feeding, cleanliness, toileting, and dressing?
- Have you started giving your child small responsibilities or chores to do around the house?
- What activities do you enjoy doing together?

#### Developmental Milestones

*Personal/social:* Develops a sense of initiative; learns new skills and games; begins problem solving; develops a positive self-concept; develops a conscience: begins to learn right from wrong and good from bad (based on reward and punishment); learns to understand rules; identifies with parent of same gender, often closely imitating characteristics; aware of gender differences; independence in self-care; sociable and outgoing (might be aggressive or bossy); has an attention span of approximately 20 minutes

*Fine motor:* Proficient holding a crayon or pencil, draws purposefully; copies circle, cross, square, diamond, and triangle; draws a person with several body parts; drawings resemble familiar objects or people; may begin to write name or numbers; can tie shoelaces

*Language/cognitive:* Vocabulary of 1500 words; begins to understand concepts of size and time (related to familiar events such as meals and bedtime); understands two opposites (e.g., same/different, hot/cold, big/little); can follow several directions consecutively; uses four-word sentences with prepositions (e.g., on, under, behind); defines five words, counts to five, names four colors; begins to see others' viewpoints; uses magical thinking; very imaginative; can complete an 8- to 10-piece puzzle

*Gross motor:* Hops on one foot or alternate feet; walks heel to toe (front and back); balances on each foot for longer time; begins to ride bicycle with training wheels; throws and catches a ball; walks downstairs using alternate feet

#### Critical Milestones*

*Personal/social:* Puts on a T-shirt; washes and dries hands; names a friend

*Fine motor:* Imitates a vertical line; wiggles thumbs; builds a tower of eight cubes

*Language/cognitive:* Knows two adjectives (e.g., tired, hungry, cold); identifies one color; knows the use of two objects (e.g., cup, chair, pencil)

*Gross motor:* Balances on each foot for 1 second; jumps forward; throws a ball overhand

#### Health Maintenance

##### Physical Measurements

Weight increases 2.25 kg (5 lb) per year
Height increases approximately 7.5 cm (3 inches) per year
Compute and plot body mass index (BMI)

##### Immunizations

Diphtheria-tetanus-acellular pertussis (DTaP) #5; inactivated poliovirus (IPV) #4; measles-mumps-rubella (MMR) #2; varicella #2
Influenza vaccine annually

##### Health Screening

Hemoglobin and lead screen
Visual acuity screening (AAP, 2016) (see Chapter 33)Audiometry
Blood pressure
Fasting lipid screen if at risk
Tuberculosis (TB) screening if at risk

#### Anticipatory Guidance

Provide information and health teaching to the child as well as the parent

##### Nutrition

Continue as for a 3-year-old
Provide nutritious snacks (child too often in a hurry to eat at mealtime)
Begin to emphasize table manners
Vitamin D supplementation 400 IU/day if consuming less than 1 L (33 oz) per day of milk and vitamin-D–fortified foods

## HEALTH PROMOTION—cont'd

### *The 4- and 5-Year-Old Child*

***Elimination***

Bowel movements once or twice/day
Urinary output 1000 mL/day
Nighttime control achieved

***Dental***

Dental examinations every 6 months
Continue brushing and flossing
Child might begin to lose deciduous teeth
Fluoride varnish if no access to a dentist
Continue oral fluoride supplement

***Sleep***

10 to 12 hours, no nap
May experience night terrors or nightmares

***Safety***

Review bicycle safety, playground safety, fire safety, poisoning (outside plants), pedestrian safety, automobile safety, sun protection
May change to an approved booster seat if child has outgrown the forward-facing car safety seat
Discuss gun safety, stranger awareness, good touch versus bad touch

***Self-Esteem and Competence***

Discuss the following with the parent:
Modeling appropriate social behavior; begin to include participation in religious services
Encouraging the child to learn to make choices
Helping the child to express emotions appropriately
Spending individual time with the child daily and encouraging the child to talk about the day's events
Providing consistent and loving limits to help the child learn self-discipline
Encouraging curiosity, and providing formal learning experiences
Establishing opportunities for the child to do small household chores
Assessing the child's readiness for kindergarten entrance, and beginning to prepare the child for the school experience

***Play***

Peak of imaginative play: Misbehavior projected onto inanimate object or imaginary friend; participate in imaginary play; encourage curiosity and creativity
Teach songs and nursery rhymes
Read to the child frequently
Teach basic skills of sports and games
Provide playground equipment, household and garden tools, dress-up clothes, building and construction toys, art supplies, more sophisticated books and puzzles
Limit screen time

*Guided by Denver Developmental Screening Test II.

When parents must take their child to a babysitter or daycare center, they should give the child an explanation for the separation. A statement such as "I have to work so I can buy food and clothes for the family and toys for you" is not adequate. In response to this explanation, one 3-year-old boy wailed, "But I have enough toys!" More effective would be to explain the separation by saying, "We both have work to do. My work is at my office, and your work is at school."

The parent should reassure the child ("I'm really going to miss you today, and I wish you could be with me") and let the child know that separation is painful for the parent as well but is necessary. At the end of the day, when picking up the child, the parent should tell the child how happy the parent is to see the child. By responding to the child's feelings, parents can lessen the stress of separation.

Transition objects may help the child adjust to the new environment. Providing the staff with information about the child's interests, home routine, special terms, and names of pets and siblings helps the new caregiver make the child feel more comfortable. Parents should always assure the child that they will return to take the child home at the end of the day.

### Preparing the Child for School

Preparation for school begins long before the preschool period. The earliest interactions between parent and infant lay the foundation for school readiness. Probably the most important factor in the development of academic competency is the relationship between parent and child. Parents who are attuned to their child and who structure the environment to provide challenges as well as security facilitate the child's cognitive growth. An interesting environment, combined with parental encouragement and support, maximizes the child's potential.

Parents are the child's first and most important teachers. They structure the child's environment and offer opportunities for learning. Visiting a zoo, fire station, or museum and talking about the experience increase the child's general knowledge and vocabulary. Cooking together, playing simple games, or putting together puzzles also fosters intellectual development. Playing with clay, paint, and scissors promotes fine motor skills and provides opportunity for self-expression. Reading to the child is one of the most valuable activities for promoting school readiness. Listening to stories and discussing them can promote reading readiness. Dramatic play encourages reading readiness by providing opportunities for symbolic thinking and problem solving.

Preschool and daycare programs can supplement the developmental opportunities provided by parents at home. Opportunities to play with other children and learn how to share the attention of an adult are some benefits of a good preschool program. Head Start programs offer low-income children and their families opportunities for remedial and supportive activities. Kindergarten provides a transition between home and first grade through a structured learning environment. In kindergarten, children prepare for school by learning to cooperate with other children, developing listening skills, and forming a positive attitude toward school.

Nurses can provide parents with strategies designed to promote safety as part of preparation for school. Teaching children about street safety and dealing with strangers and ensuring that children know their home telephone numbers and addresses are important aspects of preparation for school.

Not every 5-year-old is ready for kindergarten. Both chronologic age and developmental maturity should be considered in the assessment of a child's readiness for school (Box 7.5). At this age, boys tend to lag behind girls developmentally by approximately 6 months.

**BOX 7.5 Checklist for School Readiness**

- Child is physically healthy and strong enough to enjoy the challenge of going to school and handle the increased stresses involved.
- Child attends to own toileting needs and washes hands independently.
- Child can separate from parent and spend several hours each day in an unfamiliar place with adults and children who are largely unknown at first.
- Child's attention span is long enough that child can sit for a fairly long period and concentrate on one thing at a time, gradually learning to enjoy the practicing and problem-solving activity involved.
- Child can listen to and follow two- or three-part instructions.
- Child can restrict talking to appropriate times.
- Child is able to tolerate the frustration of not receiving immediate attention from the teacher or others; can wait for and take turns.
- Child has some basic hand-eye skills necessary for learning to read and write.
- Child can hold a pencil properly and turn pages one at a time.
- Child knows the alphabet and can recognize some letters visually.
- Child can count to 10.
- Child can recognize the colors of the rainbow.

## KEY CONCEPTS

- The toddler's slower physical growth rate (compared with that of an infant) leads to a reduced demand for calories and decreased appetite (physiologic anorexia).
- The combination of increased motor skills, immaturity, and lack of experience places the toddler at risk for unintentional injury. Anticipatory guidance for the parents about child-proofing the home is an essential nursing role.
- Children's coordination and muscle strength increase rapidly between ages 3 and 5 years. Increases in brain size and nerve myelinization enable the child to perfect fine and gross motor skills. The preschool child has the skills needed to engage in activities such as running, riding a tricycle, cutting with scissors, and drawing.
- Toddlers' behavior is characterized by negativism, ritualism, and egocentrism.
- The preschool years are a critical period for the development of socialization. Children need opportunities to play with others to learn communication skills and ways to get along with others. Preschool children learn to share and cooperate as they play in small groups. Their play is often imitative, dramatic, and creative.
- Preschoolers' thinking is still magical and egocentric. They tend to understand events only as those events affect them, believing that everyone else has the same experience. Preschool children may be overwhelmed by guilt feelings if a loved one is injured or becomes ill because they believe their thoughts are powerful enough to cause events to happen.
- Toddlerhood is characterized by the struggle for autonomy as the child develops a sense of self as separate from the parent. Erikson (1963) defines the toddler's task as centered on autonomy versus shame and doubt.
- According to Erikson, the developmental task of the preschooler is to gain a sense of initiative. The preschooler is busy learning how to do things and takes great pride in new accomplishments.
- Gender identity and body image are developing in the preschool period. Sexual curiosity, anatomic explorations, and masturbation are common. The nurse should encourage parents to answer the preschooler's questions simply and honestly. Children should not be shamed or punished for self-comforting behaviors or for investigating gender differences.
- Food jags and physiologic anorexia are common occurrences in the young child.
- Toddlers need approximately 12 to 14 hours of sleep per day.
- The preschooler needs an average of 10 to 12 hours of sleep in a 24-hour period. Because of the preschooler's active imagination and immaturity, sleep problems are common.
- Firm, consistent discipline helps toddlers learn self-control. Effective discipline techniques include time-outs, diversion, and positive reinforcement.
- Preschool children need consistent discipline to learn acceptable behavior. Appropriate limit setting helps the child learn self-confidence, self-control, and moral values. Discipline techniques that are effective at this age include time-out, time-in, the use of restricted choices, and diversion.
- All 20 deciduous teeth are present by age 3 years. Proper care of deciduous teeth is crucial for the child's general health and for the health and alignment of permanent teeth. Nurses should teach parents the importance of good oral hygiene, adequate fluoride intake, good nutrition, and regular dental checkups.
- Nurses can help parents with toilet training by explaining the signs of physical and psychological readiness. Readiness depends on myelinization of the nerve pathways that enable the child to control the bowel and bladder sphincters.
- Sibling rivalry can be minimized with techniques such as including the toddler in preparations for the new baby, acknowledging the toddler's negative feelings while setting appropriate limits, and affirming the toddler as special and loved.
- The nurse plays an important role in helping parents prepare their children for school and in assessing children's readiness for school. Parents can help their child succeed in school by providing a stimulating environment and encouragement and support.
- Health promotion for the toddler or preschool child includes ensuring adequate sleep, optimal nutrition, dental care, immunizations, and prevention of injuries.

## REFERENCES AND READINGS

American Academy of Pediatrics. (1998, reaffirmed 2014). Guidance for effective discipline. *Pediatrics, 101*(4), 723–728.

American Academy of Pediatrics. (2011a). *Travel safety tips*. Retrieved from https://www.healthychildren.org.

American Academy of Pediatrics. (2011b). *What is the best way to discipline my child?* Retrieved from https://www.healthychildren.org.

American Academy of Pediatrics. (2014a). *Car safety seat checkup*. Retrieved from https://www.aap.org.

American Academy of Pediatrics. (2014b). Fluoride use in caries prevention. *Pediatrics, 134*(3), 626–633.

American Academy of Pediatrics. (2015a). *Creating a toilet training plan*. Retrieved from https://www.healthychildren.org.

American Academy of Pediatrics. (2015b). *Disciplining your child*. Retrieved from https://www.healthychildren.org.

American Academy of Pediatrics. (2015c). *How to prevent tooth decay in your baby*. Retrieved from https://www.healthychildren.org.

American Academy of Pediatrics. (2016). Recommendations for preventive pediatric health care. *Pediatrics, 137*(1), 25–27.

American Association of Poison Control Centers. (2011). *Health care providers and poison control centers: A partnership for patients*. Retrieved from http://www.aapc.org.

American Association of Poison Control Centers. (2016). *Alerts*. Retrieved from http://www.aapc.org.

American Heart Association. (2015). *Dietary recommendations for healthy children*. Retrieved from http://www.heart.org.

Centers for Disease Control and Prevention. (2013a). *A national plan for child injury prevention: Reducing fire and burn injuries*. Retrieved from http://www.cdc.gov.

Centers for Disease Control and Prevention. (2013b). *Ten leading causes of injury deaths by age group highlighting unintentional injury deaths: United States – 2013*. Retrieved from http://www.cdc.gov.

Centers for Disease Control and Prevention. (2013c). *Ten leading causes of non-fatal unintentional injuries: United States 2013, all races, both sexes, disposition all cases: Ages 1-4*. Retrieved from http://www.cdc.gov.

Centers for Disease Control and Prevention. (2014). *Unintentional drowning: Get the facts*. Retrieved from http://www.cdc.gov.

Centers for Disease Control and Prevention. (2015). *Vitamin D supplementation*. Retrieved from http://www.cdc.gov.

Centers for Disease Control and Prevention. (2016). *Recommended immunization schedule for persons aged 0 through 18 years – United States, 2016*. Retrieved from http://www.cdc.gov.

Daniels, S., Hassink, S., & the Committee on Nutrition. (2015). The role of the pediatrician in the primary prevention of obesity. *Pediatrics, 136*(1), e275–e292.

Erikson, E.H. (1963). *Childhood and society* (2nd ed.). New York: Norton.

Federal Aviation Administration. (2015). *Child safety: Keep your little one safe when you fly*. Retrieved from http://www.faa.gov.

Freud, S. (1960). *The ego and the id* (J. Riviere, Trans.). New York: Norton.

Gabrielson, T., et al. (2015). Identifying autism in a brief observation. *Pediatrics, 135*(2), e330–e338.

Greer, F., Sicherer, S., Burks, W., & The Committee on Nutrition and Section on Allergy and Immunology. (2008). Effects of early nutritional interventions on the development of atopic disease in infants and children: The role of maternal dietary restriction, breastfeeding, timing of introduction of complementary foods, and hydrolyzed formulas. *Pediatrics, 121*(1), 183–191.

Harris, V., Rochette, L., & Smith, G. (2011). *Pediatric injuries attributable to falls from windows in the United States in 1990-2008*. Retrieved from https://www.aap.org.

Jenco, M. (2015, August 4). Academy calls for continued autism screening despite the United States Preventive Services Task Force recommendation. *AAP News*. Retrieved from http://www.aapnews.org.

Kohlberg, L. (1964). Development of moral character. In M. Hoffman, & L. Hoffman (Eds.), *Review of child development research* (Vol. 1). New York: Russell Sage Foundation.

Kohlberg, L. (1966). A cognitive developmental analysis of children's sex-role concepts and attitudes. In E.E. Macoby (Ed.), *The development of sex differences*. Stanford, CA: Stanford University Press.

Krader, C. (2014). Empowering the stuttering child. *Contemporary Pediatrics, 31*(8), 23–31.

Majsak-Newman, G., et al. (2014). Keeping children safe at home: Protocol for a matched case-control study of modifiable risk factors for poisonings. *Injury Prevention, 20*, e10–e15.

National Heart, Lung, and Blood Institute. (2013). *Integrated guidelines for cardiac health and risk reduction in children and adolescents*. Retrieved from http://www.nhlbi.nih.gov.

Piaget, J. (1952). *The origins of intelligence in children*. New York: International Universities Press.

Reitzes, P. (2014). The powered up parent. *ASHA leader, 19*, 50–56.

Shields, B., Pollack-Nelson, C., & Smith, G. (2011). Pediatric submersion events in portable above-ground pools in the United States, 2001-2009. *Pediatrics, 128*(1), 45–52.

United States Department of Agriculture & United States Department of Health and Human Services. (2015). *Dietary guidelines for Americans, 2015-2020* (8th ed.). Retrieved from https://www.health.gov/dietaryguidelines/2015.

United States Department of Health and Human Services. (2010). *Healthy People 2020*. Retrieved from https://www.healthypeople.gov.

United States Preventive Services Task Force. (2014). *Prevention of dental caries in children from birth through age 5 years: US Preventive Services Task Force recommendation statement*. Retrieved from http://www.uspreventiveservicestaskforce.org.

United States Preventive Services Task Force. (2015a). *Draft recommendation statement: Autism spectrum disorder in children's screening*. Retrieved from http://www.uspreventiveservicestaskforce.org.

United States Preventive Services Task Force. (2015b). *Final recommendation statement: Speech and language delay and disorders in children age 5 and younger: Screening*. Retrieved from http://www.uspreventiveservicestaskforce.org.

Wallace, I., et al. (2015). Screening for speech and language delay in children 5 years old and younger: A systematic review. *Pediatrics, 136*(2), e448–e462.

# 8

# Health Promotion for the School-Age Child

ⓔ http://evolve.elsevier.com/McKinney/mat-ch/

## LEARNING OBJECTIVES

*After studying this chapter, you should be able to:*

- Describe the school-age child's normal growth and development and assess the child for normal developmental milestones.
- Describe the maturational changes that occur during the school-age period and discuss implications for healthcare.
- Identify the stages of moral development in the school-age child and discuss implications for effective parenting strategies.
- Discuss the effect school has on the child's development and implications for teachers and parents.
- Discuss anticipatory guidance related to various health and safety issues observed in the school-age child.
- Describe anticipatory guidance that the nurse can offer to decrease children's stress.

Middle childhood, ages 6 to 11 or 12 years, is probably one of the healthiest periods of life. Slow, steady physical growth and rapid cognitive and social development characterize this stage of life. During these years, the child's world expands from the tight circle of the family to include children and adults at school, at a worship community, and in the community at large. The child becomes increasingly independent. Peers become important as the child starts school and gradually moves away from the security of home. This period is a time for best friends, sharing, and exploring.

The school years are also a time that can be stressful for a child, and this stress can impede the child's successful achievement of developmental tasks. The Healthy People 2020 objectives that relate to school-age children include goals such as reducing obesity, improving nutrition, facilitating access to dental and mental healthcare, increasing physical activity, and preventing high-risk behaviors.

## GROWTH AND DEVELOPMENT OF THE SCHOOL-AGE CHILD

The child in middle childhood develops a sense of industry (Erikson, 1963) and learns the basic skills required to function in society. The child develops an appreciation of rules and a conscience. Cognitively, the child grows from the egocentrism of early childhood to a more mature thinking. The ability to solve problems and make independent judgments that are based on reason characterizes this new maturity. The child is invested in the task of middle childhood: learning to do things and do them well. Competence and self-esteem increase with each academic, social, and athletic achievement. The relative stability and security of the middle childhood period prepare the child to enter the emotional and physical changes of adolescence.

### Physical Growth and Development

Middle childhood is characterized by a slow and steady growth. The physical changes that occur during this period are gradual and subtle. Although growth rates vary among children, the average weight gain is 2.5 kg (5½ lb) per year, and the average increase in height is approximately 5.5 cm (2 inches) per year. During the early school-age period, boys are approximately 1 inch taller and 2 lb heavier than girls. At around age 10 or 11 years, girls begin to catch up in size as they undergo the preadolescent growth spurt. By 12 years, girls are 1 inch taller than boys and 2 lb heavier. Toward the end of middle childhood and into the beginning of adolescence, children of the same age can be of very different height (Fig. 8.1). A growth spurt, which signals the onset of puberty, usually occurs between ages 12 and 14 years and occurs 2 years later in boys than in girls.

#### Body Systems

School-age children appear thinner and more graceful than do preschoolers. Musculoskeletal growth leads to greater coordination and strength. The muscles are still immature, and thus, can be injured from overuse. Growth of the facial bones changes facial proportions. As the facial bones grow, the eustachian tube assumes a more downward and inward position, resulting in fewer ear infections than in the preschool years. Lymphatic tissues continue to grow until about age 9 years; immunoglobulin A and G (IgA, IgG) levels reach adult values at approximately 10 years. Enlarged tonsils and adenoids are common during these years and are not always an indication of illness. The frontal sinuses develop at age 7 years. Growth in brain size is complete by 10 years. The respiratory system also continues to mature. During the school-age years, the lungs and alveoli develop fully, and fewer respiratory infections occur.

#### Dentition

During the school-age years, all 20 primary (deciduous) teeth are lost and are replaced by 28 of the 32 permanent teeth. All permanent teeth, except the third molars, erupt during the school-age period. The order of eruption of permanent teeth and loss of primary teeth is shown in Fig. 33.7. The first teeth to be lost are usually the lower central incisors, at around age 6 years. Most first-graders are characterized by a snaggletooth appearance (see Fig. 8.1), and visits from the "tooth fairy" are important signs of growing up.

#### Sexual Development

Puberty is a time of dramatic physical change. It includes the growth spurt, development of primary and secondary sexual characteristics, and maturation of the sexual organs. The age at onset of puberty varies

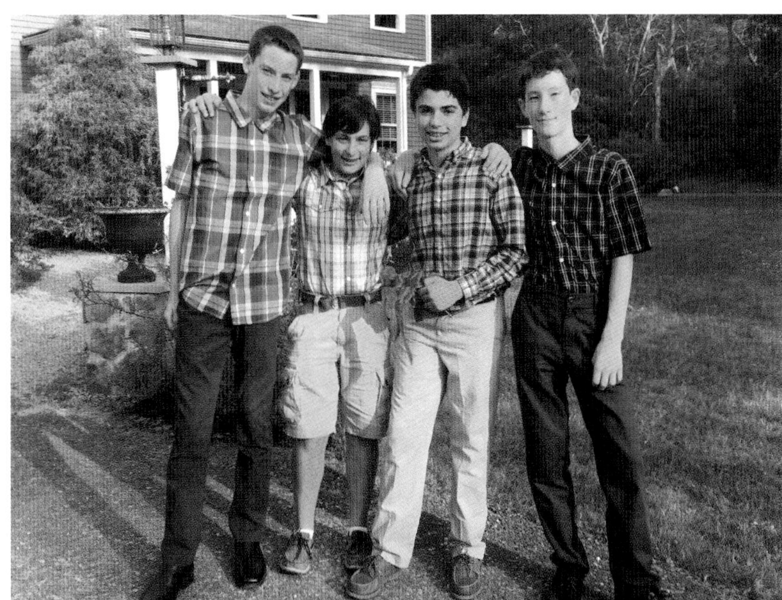

Children of the same age can vary significantly in height and physical development.

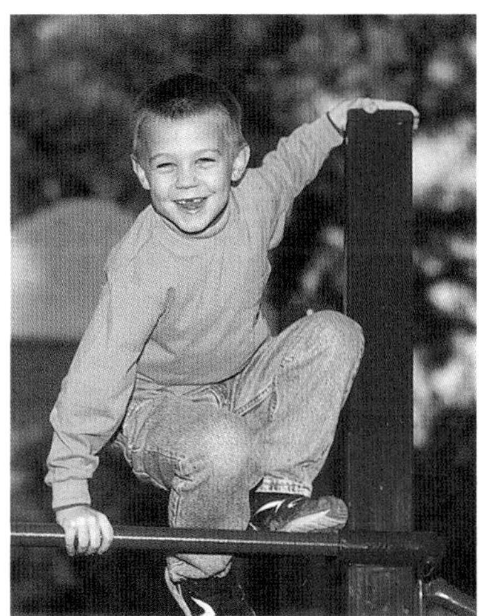

School-age children often have a snaggle-tooth appearance while they are losing their primary teeth.

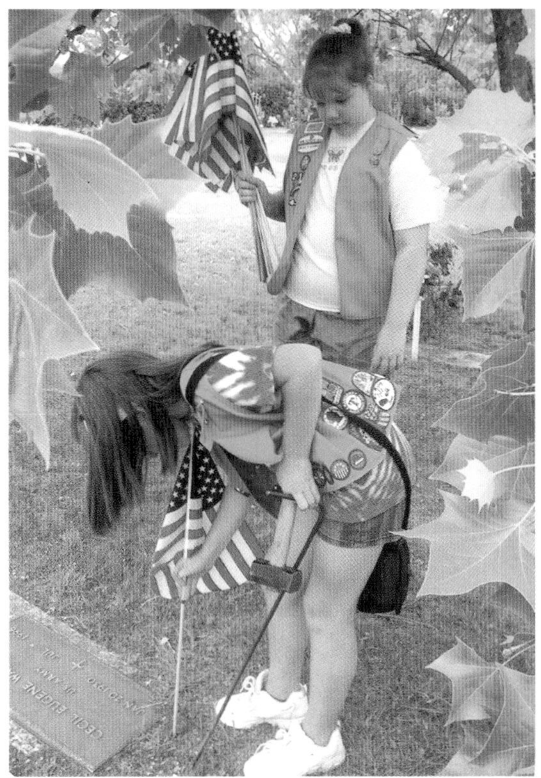

Organizations such as Girl Scouts help foster self-esteem and competence.

**FIG 8.1** Growth and development of the school-age child.

widely. Puberty is now occurring at a younger age than before (Kaplowitz, Bloch & AAP Section on Endocrinology, 2016), with its onset no longer unusual in girls who are 8 or 9 years old. On average, black girls begin puberty 1 year earlier than white girls (Kaplowitz, Bloch & AAP Section on Endocrinology, 2016). The reason for the earlier development among black girls is not known; however, recent research suggests that it may be related to food intake patterns. Puberty begins about 1½ to 2 years later in boys.

Menarche, the onset of menstruation, occurs at an average age of 12. However, with the decrease in the age of puberty onset, the age at menarche is also likely to decrease. Females who are significantly overweight tend to have earlier onset of puberty and menarche. Because puberty is occurring increasingly earlier, many 10- and 11-year-old girls have already had menarche. Wide variations in maturity at this age are a common cause of embarrassment because the school-age child does not want to appear different from peers. Children who mature either early or late may struggle with feelings of self-consciousness and inferiority. Table 9.1 describes the usual sequence of appearance of secondary sex characteristics during the school-age and adolescent periods.

## HEALTH PROMOTION

### Healthy People 2020 *Objectives for School-Age Children*

| | |
|---|---|
| ECBP-2 | Increase the proportion of elementary, middle, and senior high schools that provide comprehensive school health education to prevent health problems in the following areas: unintentional injury; violence; suicide; tobacco use and addiction; alcohol or other drug use; unintended pregnancy, HIV/AIDS, and sexually transmitted disease (STD); unhealthy dietary patterns; and inadequate physical activity. |
| ECBP-4 | Increase the proportion of elementary, middle, and senior high schools that provide school health education to promote personal health and wellness in the following areas: hand washing or hand hygiene; oral health; growth and development; sun safety and skin cancer prevention; benefits of rest and sleep; ways to prevent vision and hearing loss; and the importance of health screenings and checkups. |
| DH-14 | Increase the proportion of children and youth with disabilities who spend at least 80% of their time in regular education programs. |
| IVP-21 | Increase the number of States and the District of Columbia with laws requiring bicycle helmets for bicycle riders (especially for children younger than age 15 years). |
| MHMD-6 | Increase the proportion of children with mental health problems who receive treatment. |
| NWS-10 | Reduce the proportion of children and adolescents who are overweight or obese. |
| NWS-17—20 | Increase the contribution of number and variety of vegetables, fruits, and whole grains in the population ages 2 years and older; reduce consumption of solid fats (including saturated fats), added sugars, and sodium, and increase the consumption of calcium. |
| OH-1.2 | Reduce the proportion of children aged 6 to 9 years with dental caries experience in their primary and permanent teeth. |
| OH-9 and OH-12.2 | Increase the proportion of school-based health centers with an oral health component that includes dental sealants, dental care, and topical fluoride, and increase the proportion of children aged 6 to 9 years who have received dental sealants on one or more of their permanent first molar teeth. |
| PA-4 | Increase the proportion of the nation's public and private schools that require daily physical education for all students. |
| PA-8.2 | Increase the proportion of children and adolescents aged 2 years through 12th grade who view television, videos, or play video games for no more than 2 hours a day. |

Modified from United States Department of Health and Human Services. (2010). *Healthy People 2020.* Retrieved from https://www.healthypeople.gov.

## ! NURSING QUALITY ALERT

### *Components of Sex Education*

- Basic anatomy and physiology
- Body functions
- Expected changes related to puberty
- Menstruation, nocturnal emissions
- Reproduction
- Teenage pregnancy
- Human immunodeficiency virus (HIV) infection
- Sexually transmitted disease (STD)

Because of the earlier onset of puberty, sex education programs should be introduced in elementary school. Nurses are in an excellent position to serve as resource persons for parents and teachers who are responsible for sex education. Children's questions about sexuality and related issues should be answered honestly and in a matter-of-fact way. If sex education is presented within the context of learning about the human body, with its wonders and mysteries, children are less likely to feel embarrassed and anxious. Regardless of whether sex education is a part of a formal school curriculum, children need accurate information. Basic anatomy and physiology, information about body functions, and the expected changes of puberty should be introduced to children before the onset of puberty. Older school-age children need information about menstruation, nocturnal emissions, and reproduction. Sex education programs must also include information about responsible sexuality and related issues, such as teenage pregnancy, human immunodeficiency virus (HIV), and other sexually transmitted diseases (STDs).

## BOX 8.1 Age-Related Activities and Toys for the School-Age Child

**General Activities**

Play becomes organized with more direction.

Early school-age child continues dramatic play with increased creativity but loses some spontaneity.

Child is aware of rules when playing games.

Child begins to compete in sports.

**Toys and Specific Types of Play**

Collections, drawing, construction, dolls, pets, guessing games, complicated puzzles, board games, riddles, physical games, competitive play, reading, bicycle riding, hobbies, sewing, listening to the radio, watching television and videos, cooking

## Motor Development

### Development of Gross Motor Skills

During the school years, coordination improves. A developed sense of balance and rhythm allows children to ride a two-wheeled bicycle, dance, skip, jump rope, and participate in various sports. As puberty approaches in the late school-age period, children may become more awkward as their bodies grow faster than their ability to compensate.

### Importance of Active Play

School-age children spend much of their time in active play, practicing and refining motor skills. They seem to be constantly in motion. Children of this age enjoy active sports and games, as well as crafts and fine motor activities (Box 8.1). Activities requiring balance and strength, such as bicycle riding, tree climbing, and skating, are exciting and fun for the school-age child. Coordination and motor skills improve as the child is given an opportunity to practice.

Children should be encouraged to engage in physical activities. During the school-age years, children learn physical fitness skills that contribute to their health for the rest of their lives. Cardiovascular fitness, strength, and flexibility are improved by physical activity. Popular games such as tag, jump rope, and hide-and-seek provide a release of emotional tension and enhance the development of leader and follower skills.

Team sports, such as soccer and baseball, provide opportunities not only for exercise and refinement of motor skills but also for the development of sportsmanship and teamwork. Nurses should advise parents on ways to prevent sports injuries and how to assess a recreational sports program (see the Patient-Centered Teaching box: Assessing an Organized Recreational Sports Program). Sports activities should be well supervised, and protective gear (e.g., helmets for T-ball, shin guards for soccer) should be mandatory.

## PATIENT-CENTERED TEACHING

### *Assessing an Organized Recreational Sports Program*

Whenever your child begins playing in an organized recreational sports program, you need to consider the following:

- *Coaches' training:* Coaches not only need to understand how to play a sport and to teach it to young children but also should have undergone a training program in injury prevention, concussion management, and first aid. Check to see that the training emphasizes preventing overuse injuries and removal from play for children suspected of having a concussion.
- *Coaches' attitude:* Coaches should have a positive, encouraging manner with children—not critical and demeaning. Check whether the coach emphasizes skill development and plays all the children, regardless of whether required to. Be sure the coach is a good role model on the field and is courteous to referees, other coaches, and the children. Avoid coaches who have a "win at all costs" philosophy.
- *Safety:* Check to see that protective and athletic equipment is used correctly by all children participating in the sport. Facilities and equipment should be well maintained and safe. Be sure your child has enough fluids available and that the child stretches before playing. Children should be divided into teams according to size and maturation level rather than by age. Many sports programs require a preseason physical examination.
- *Enjoyment:* Sports programs can do wonderful things for your child's skill development, confidence, sense of cooperation, and self-esteem. Remember that it is your child playing the sport and not you. Be encouraging and positive, help the child when asked, and cheer the team on in an appropriate manner.

Obesity has become a major problem in children in the United States, with 18% of children ages 6 to 11 years being overweight; the percentage is higher (27%) in Mexican-American children (Forum on Child and Family Statistics, 2015). Time spent watching television, watching movies or playing computer games often diminishes a child's interest in active play outside. Nurses can help reverse this trend by advising parents to limit their children's screen time to 2 hours or less per day and to encourage them to engage in more active play. Parents need to provide adequate space for children to run, jump, and scuffle. Children should have enough free time to exercise and play. Parents also need to act as role models for both good nutrition and exercise.

### Preventing Fatigue and Dehydration

Because children enjoy active play and are so full of energy, they often do not recognize fatigue. Six-year-olds in particular will not stop an activity to rest. Parents must learn to recognize signs of fatigue or irritability and enforce rest periods before the child becomes exhausted. Because the child's metabolic rate is higher than an adult's and sweating ability is limited, extremes in temperature while exercising can be dangerous. Dehydration and overheating can pose threats to the child's health. Frequent rest periods and adequate hydration are essential for the child during physical exercise.

### Development of Fine Motor Skills

Increased myelinization of the central nervous system is shown by refinement of fine motor skills. Balance and hand-eye coordination improve with maturity and practice. School-age children take pride in activities that require dexterity and fine motor skill, such as model building, playing a musical instrument, and drawing.

## Cognitive Development

Thought processes undergo dramatic changes as the child moves from the intuitive thinking of the preschool years to the logical thinking processes of the school-age years. The school-age child gains new knowledge and develops more efficient problem-solving ability and greater flexibility of thinking. The 6- and 7-year-old remain in the intuitive thought stage (Piaget, 1962) characteristic of the older preschool child. By age 8 years, the child moves into the stage of concrete operations, followed by the stage of formal operations at around 12 years (Piaget, 1962). See Chapter 5 for a discussion of formal operations and Chapter 54 for a discussion of the child with cognitive deficits, including intellectual and developmental disabilities.

### Intuitive Thought Stage

In the intuitive thought stage (6 to 7 years), thinking is based on immediate perceptions of the environment and the child's own viewpoint (Piaget, 1962). Thinking is still characterized by egocentrism, animism, and centration (see Chapter 7). At 6 and 7 years old, children cannot understand another's viewpoint, form hypotheses, or deal with abstract concepts. The child in the intuitive thought stage has difficulty forming categories and often solves problems by random guessing.

### Concrete Operations Stage

By age 7 or 8 years, the child enters the stage of concrete operations. Children learn that their point of view is not the only one as they encounter different interpretations of reality and begin to differentiate their own viewpoints from those of peers and adults (Piaget, 1962). This newly developed freedom from egocentrism enables children to think more flexibly and to learn about the environment more accurately. Problem solving becomes more efficient and reliable as the child learns how to form hypotheses. The use of symbolism becomes more sophisticated, and children now can manipulate symbols for things in the way that they once manipulated the things themselves. The child learns the alphabet and how to read. Attention span increases as the child grows older, facilitating classroom learning.

**Reversibility.** Children in the concrete operations stage grasp the concept of *reversibility.* They can mentally retrace a process, a skill necessary for understanding mathematic problems ($5 + 3 = 8$ and $8 - 3 = 5$). The child can take a toy apart and put it back together or walk to school and find the way back home without getting lost. Reversibility also enables a child to anticipate the results of actions—a valuable tool for problem solving.

The understanding of time gradually develops during the early school-age years. Children can understand and use clock time at around age 8 years. Although 8- or 9-year-old children understand calendar time and memorize dates, they do not master historic time until later.

***Conservation.*** Gradually, the school-age child masters the concept of **conservation**. The child learns that certain properties of objects do not change simply because their order, form, or appearance has changed. For example, the child who has mastered conservation of mass recognizes that a lump of clay that has been pounded flat is still the same amount of clay as when it was rolled into a ball. The child understands conservation of weight when able to correctly answer the classic nonsense question, "Which weighs more, a pound of feathers or a pound of rocks?" The concept of conservation does not develop all at once. The simpler conservations, such as number and mass, are understood first, and more complex conservations are mastered later. An understanding of conservation of weight develops at 9 or 10 years old, and an understanding of volume is present at 11 or 12 years.

***Classification and logic.*** Older school-age children are able to classify objects according to characteristics they share, to place things in a logical order, and to recall similarities and differences. This ability is reflected in the school-age child's interest in collections. Children love to collect and classify stamps, stickers, sports cards, shells, dolls, rocks, or anything imaginable. School-age children understand relationships such as larger and smaller, lighter and darker. They can comprehend class inclusion—the concept that objects can belong to more than one classification. For example, a man can be a brother, a father, and a son at the same time.

School-age children move away from magical thinking as they discover that there are logical, physical explanations for most phenomena. The older school-age child is a skeptic, no longer believing in Santa Claus or the Easter Bunny.

***Humor.*** Children in the concrete operations stage have a delightful sense of humor. Around age 8 years, increased mastery of language and the beginning of logic enable children to appreciate a play on words. They laugh at incongruities and love silly jokes, riddles, and puns ("How do you keep a mad elephant from charging? You take away its credit cards!"). Riddle and joke books make ideal gifts for young school-age children. Evidence from multiple disciplines that address the needs of children suggests that children who have a good sense of humor may use it as a positive coping mechanism for stress associated with painful procedures and other situational life events.

## Sensory Development

### Vision

The eyes are fully developed by age 6 years. Visual acuity, ocular muscle control, peripheral vision, and color discrimination are fully developed by age 7 years. Just before puberty, some children's eyes undergo a growth spurt, resulting in myopia. Children with poor visual acuity usually do not complain of vision problems because the changes occur so gradually that they are difficult to notice. Usual behaviors that parents notice include squinting, moving closer to the television, or complaints of frequent headaches. The young child may never have had 20/20 vision and has nothing with which to compare the imperfect vision. For these reasons, yearly vision screening is important for children in middle childhood.

### Hearing

With maturation and growth of the eustachian tube, middle ear infections occur less frequently than in younger children. However, chronic middle ear infections are a problem for a few children and can result in hearing loss. Annual audiometric screening tests are important to detect hearing loss before unrecognized deficits lead to learning problems (see Chapter 55).

## Language Development

Language development continues at a rapid pace during the school-age years. Vocabulary expands, and sentence structure becomes more complex. By age 6 years, the child's vocabulary is approximately 8000 to 14,000 words. There is an increase in the use of culturally specific words at this age. Bilingual children may speak English at school and a different language at home.

Reading effectively improves language skills. Regular trips to the library, where the child can borrow books of special interest, can promote a love of reading and enhance school performance. School-age children enjoy being read to as well as reading on their own. Older children enjoy horror stories, mysteries, romances, and adventure stories.

School-age children often go through a period in which they experiment with profanity and "dirty" jokes. Children may imitate parents who use such words as part of their vocabulary.

## Psychosocial Development

### Development of a Sense of Industry

Erikson (1963) described the central task of the school-age years as the development of a sense of industry. Ideally, the child is prepared for this task with a secure sense of self as separate from loved ones in the family. The child should have learned to trust others and should have developed a sense of autonomy and initiative during the preceding years. The school-age child replaces fantasy play with "work" at school, crafts, chores, hobbies, and athletics. The child is rewarded with a sense of satisfaction from achieving a skill, as well as with external rewards, such as good grades, trophies, or an allowance. School-age children enjoy undertaking new tasks and carrying them through to completion. Whether it is baking a cake, hitting a home run, or scoring 100 on a math test, purposeful activity leads to a sense of worth and competence. Successful resolution of the task of industry depends on learning to do things and do them well. School-age children learn skills that they will need later to compete in the adult world. A person's fundamental attitude toward work is established during the school-age years.

### Fostering Self-Esteem

The negative component of this developmental stage is a sense of inferiority (Erikson, 1963). If a child cannot separate psychologically from the parent or if expectations are set too high for the child to achieve, feelings of inferiority develop. If a child believes that success is unattainable, confidence is lost, and the child will not take pleasure in attempting new experiences. Children who have this experience will then have a pervasive feeling of inferiority and incompetence that will affect all aspects of their lives. The child who lacks a sense of industry has a poor foundation for mastering the tasks of adolescence. The reality is that no one can master everything. Every child will feel deficient or inferior at something. The task of the caring parent or teacher is to identify areas in which a child is competent and to build on successful experiences to foster feelings of mastery and success. Nurses can suggest ways in which parents and teachers can promote a sense of self-esteem and competence in school-age children (see the Patient-Centered Teaching box: How to Promote Self-Esteem in School-Age Children).

At this age, the approval and esteem of those outside the family, especially peers, become important. Children learn that their parents are not infallible. As they begin to test parents' authority and knowledge, the influence of teachers and other adults is felt more and more. The peer group becomes the school-age child's major socializing influence. Although parents' love, praise, and support are needed, even craved during stressful times, the child begins to prefer activities with

## PATIENT-CENTERED TEACHING

### *How to Promote Self-Esteem in School-Age Children*

- Give your children household responsibilities according to their developmental level and capabilities. Set reasonable rules, and expect the child to follow them.
- Allow your child to solve problems and make responsible choices.
- Give praise for what is praiseworthy. Do not be afraid to encourage your child to do better. Refrain from being critical, but gently point out areas that could be improved.
- Allow your children to make mistakes and encourage them to take responsibility for the consequences of their mistakes.
- Emphasize your child's strengths and help improve weaknesses.
- Do not do your children's homework for them because this will make them think you do not trust them to do a good job; provide assistance and suggestions when asked and praise their best efforts.
- Model appropriate behavior toward others.
- Provide consistent and demonstrative love.

friends to activities with the family. As the child becomes more independent, increasing time is spent with friends and away from the family.

The concept of friendship changes as the child matures. At 6 and 7 years old, children form friendships merely on the basis of who lives nearby or who has toys that they enjoy. By the time children are 9 or 10 years old, friendships are based more on emotional bonds, warm feelings, and trust-building experiences. Children learn that friendship is more than just being together. Children at 11 and 12 years are loyal to their friends, often sharing problems and giving emotional support. School-age children tend to form friendships with peers of the same sex. Developing friendships and succeeding in social interactions lead to a sense of industry. Friendships are important for the emotional well-being of school-age children. Friends teach children skills they will use in future relationships.

Children learn a body of rules, sayings, and superstitions as they enter the culture of childhood. Rules are important to children because they provide predictability and offer security. Learning the sayings, jokes, and riddles is an important part of social interaction among peers. Sayings such as "Step on a crack and you'll break your mother's back" or "Finders, keepers; losers, weepers" have been part of childhood lore for generations.

Children become sensitive to the norms and values of the peer group because pressure to conform is great. Children often find that it is painful to be different. Peer approval is a strong motivating force and allows the child to risk disapproval from parents.

The school-age years are a time of formal and informal clubs. Informal clubs among 6-, 7-, and 8-year-olds are loosely organized, with fluid membership. Membership changes frequently, and it is based on mutual interests such as playing ball, riding bicycles, or playing with dolls. Children learn interpersonal skills, such as sharing, cooperation, and tolerance in these groups. Clubs among older school-age children tend to be more structured, often characterized by secret codes, rituals, and rigid rules. A club may be formed for the purpose of exclusion, in which children snub another child for some reason.

Formal groups organized by adults, such as Boy Scouts, Girl Scouts, Camp Fire USA, and 4-H, also foster self-esteem and competence as children earn ranks and merit badges (see Fig. 8.1). Transmission of societal values, such as service to others, duty to God, and good citizenship, is an important goal of these organizations.

## Spiritual and Moral Development

Middle childhood years are pivotal in the development of a conscience and the internalization of values. Tremendous strides are made in moral development during these 6 years. Several theorists have described the dramatic growth that occurs during this stage.

### Piaget

Piaget (1962) asserted that young school-age children obey rules because powerful, all-knowing adults hand them down. During this stage, children know the rules but not the reasons behind them. Rules are interpreted in a literal way, and the child is unable to adjust rules to fit differing circumstances. The perception of guilt changes as the child matures. Piaget stated that up to approximately age 8 years, children judge degrees of guilt by the amount of damage done. No distinction is made between accidental and intentional wrongdoing. For example, the child believes that a child who broke five china cups by accident is guiltier than a child who broke one cup on purpose. By age 10 years, children are able to consider the intent of the action. Older school-age children are more flexible in their decisions and can take into account extenuating circumstances.

### Kohlberg

Kohlberg (1964) described moral development in terms of three levels containing six stages (see Chapter 5). According to Kohlberg's theory, children 4 to 7 years old are in stage 2 of the preconventional level, in which right and wrong are determined by physical consequences. The child obeys because of fear of punishment. If the child is not caught or punished for an act, the child does not consider the act wrong. At this stage, children conform to rules out of self-interest or in terms of what others can do in return ("I'll do this for you if you'll do that for me."). Behavior is guided by an eye-for-an-eye philosophy.

Kohlberg describes children between ages 7 and 12 years as being in stage 3 of the conventional level. A "good-boy" or "good-girl" orientation characterizes this stage, in which the child conforms to rules to please others and avoid disapproval. This stage parallels the concrete operations stage of cognitive development. Around age 12 years, children enter stage 4 of the conventional level. There is an orientation toward respecting authority, obeying rules, and maintaining social order. Most religions place the age of accountability at approximately 12 years.

### Family Influence

Children manifest antisocial behaviors during middle childhood. Behaviors such as cheating, lying, and stealing are not uncommon. Often, children lie or cheat to get out of an embarrassing situation or to make themselves look more important to their peers. In most cases, these behaviors are minor; however, if they are severe or persistent, the child may need referral for counseling.

Parents and teachers profoundly influence moral development. Parents can teach children the difference between right and wrong most effectively by living according to their values. A father who lectures his child about the importance of honesty gives a mixed message when he brags about fooling his boss or cheating on his income tax return. The moral atmosphere in the home is a critical factor in the child's personality development.

Children learn self-discipline and internalization of values through obedience to external rules. School-age children are legalistic, and they feel loved and secure when they know that firm limits are set on their behavior. They want and expect discipline for wrongdoings.

For moral teaching to be effective, parents must be consistent in their expectations of their children and in administering rewards and punishment.

### Spirituality and Religion

Spiritually, school-age children become acquainted with the basic content of their faith. Children reared within a religious tradition feel a part of their religion. Although their thinking is still concrete, children begin to use abstract concepts to describe God and are able to comprehend God as a power greater than themselves or their parents. Because school-age children think literally, spiritual concepts take on materialistic and physical expression. Heaven and hell fascinate them. Concern for rules and a maturing conscience may cause a nagging sense of guilt and fear of going to hell. Younger school-age children still tend to associate accidents and illness with punishment for real or imagined wrong-doing. One 6-year-old child hospitalized for an appendectomy said, "God saw all the bad things I did, and He punished me." Reassurance that God does not punish children by making them sick reduces anxiety.

## HEALTH PROMOTION FOR THE SCHOOL-AGE CHILD AND FAMILY

It is recommended that during middle childhood, children should visit the healthcare provider at least every 2 years. Many school districts require documentation of a routine physical examination at least once during the elementary school years after the kindergarten visit. If children are participating in organized sports or attending camp, an annual physical examination might be required.

### Nutrition During Middle Childhood

#### Nutritional Requirements

Growth continues at a slow, regular pace, but the school-age child begins to have an increased appetite. Energy needs increase during the later school-age years. Children in this age-group tend to have few eating idiosyncrasies and generally enjoy eating to satisfy appetite and as a social function. Children who developed dislikes for certain foods during earlier periods may continue to refuse those foods. School-age children are influenced by family patterns and the limitations their activities put on them. They may rush through a meal to go out to play or watch a favorite program on television.

Children need to choose a variety of culturally appropriate foods and snacks daily. Dietary recommendations for school-age children include 2½ cups of a variety of vegetables; 1½ cups of a variety of fruits (slightly more for boys of fruits and vegetables); 5 oz grains (half of which should be whole grain); 5 oz protein (lean meat, poultry, fish, beans); and 3 cups of fortified nonfat milk or dairy products (American Heart Association [AHA], 2014a). They need to limit saturated fat intake and processed sugars to fewer than 10% of daily total calories (United States Department of Health and Human Services [USDHHS] & United States Department of Agriculture [USDA], 2015). Caloric and protein requirements begin to increase at about age 11 years because of the preadolescent growth spurt. The requirements for boys and girls also begin to vary at this age. A gradual increase in food intake will also occur. The nurse should ask children to describe specifically what they eat at meals and for snacks to develop a more comprehensive picture of their eating habits.

When children's nutritional status is assessed, it is important to also assess any body image concerns; be sure to ask children how they feel about the way they look. Eating disorders, although thought to be a problem of adolescence, can begin in the late elementary school years.

#### Age-Related Nutritional Challenges

During the school years, the child's schedule changes and more time is spent away from home. Most children eat lunch at school, and they usually have a choice of foods. Even if the parent packs a lunch for the child to take to school, there are no guarantees that the child will eat the lunch. Unless specifically prohibited by the school, children sometimes trade foods with other children or they may not eat a particular item. It is also during this period that the child becomes more active in clubs, sports, and other activities that interrupt the normal meal schedule.

The federal government funds the National School Lunch Program, which provides lunches free or at a reduced cost for low-income children. The school lunch program includes approximately one third of the recommended daily dietary allowances for a child. School lunch programs usually follow the dietary guidelines to meet recommended nutritional requirements; however, many school lunches are somewhat high in fat. Some schools also offer breakfast and milk programs. Many schools offer low-nutrient, high-calorie snacks as an add-on to the school lunch or in snack machines available in various locations throughout the school. In some cases, children use their lunch money to buy snacks. Advise parents to communicate with their children about appropriate lunch and snacks in school and to know what is being offered in the school cafeteria.

School-age children usually request a snack after school and in the evening. Encourage parents to provide their children with healthy choices for snacks. By not buying foods high in calories and low in nutrients, the parent can remove the temptation for the child to choose the less healthy foods.

Unpredictable schedules, advertising, easy access to fast food, and peer pressure all have an effect on the foods a child chooses. The child may begin to prefer 'junk foods,' which do not have much nutritional value. Most of these foods are high in fat and sugar. In addition, school-age children often skip breakfast. The family plays an important role in modeling good eating habits for the child. Schools also have a responsibility to provide nutritious meals for children.

### Dental Care

Although the incidence of dental caries (tooth decay) has declined in recent years, tooth decay remains a significant health problem among school-age children (American Academy of Pediatrics [AAP], 2014). Unfortunately, many parents and school-age children consider dental hygiene to be of minor importance. Some parents erroneously believe that dental care, even brushing, is not important for primary teeth because they will all fall out anyway. However, premature loss of these deciduous teeth can complicate eruption of permanent teeth and lead to malocclusion.

School-age children are able to assume responsibility for their own dental hygiene. Good oral health habits tend to be carried into the adult years, reducing cavity formation for a lifetime. Thorough brushing with fluoride toothpaste followed by flossing between the teeth should be done after meals and especially before bedtime. Proper brushing and flossing and a well-balanced diet promote healthy gums and prevent cavities. Sugary or sticky between-meal snacks should be limited. Candy that dissolves quickly, such as chocolate, is less cariogenic than sticky candy, which stays in contact with teeth longer. The AAP (Clark & Slayton, 2014) recommends an oral fluoride supplement for children ages 6 to 16 years who do not have access to fluoridated water; fluoride dose is 1 mg for children 6 years old or older.

### Malocclusion

Good *occlusion,* or alignment, of the teeth is important for tooth formation, speech development, and physical appearance. Many school-age children need orthodontic braces to correct malocclusion, a condition in which the teeth are crowded, crooked, or out of alignment. Factors such as heredity, cleft palate, premature loss of primary teeth, and mouth breathing lead to malocclusion. Pacifier use or thumb sucking is not believed to cause malocclusion unless it persists past age 2 to 4 years; because of the risk, children should stop using the pacifier before their permanent teeth erupt (AAP, 2015b). Malocclusion becomes particularly noticeable between ages 6 and 12 years, when the permanent teeth are erupting.

Children with braces are at increased risk for dental caries and must be scrupulous about their dental hygiene. School nurses can encourage children who wear braces to brush after every meal and snack, eat a nutritious diet, and visit the dentist at least once every 6 months. Use of a water flosser keeps gums healthy and helps remove food particles from around wires and bands.

Braces cause many children to feel self-conscious and may be difficult for a school-age child to accept. However, for some children, orthodontic appliances may be a status symbol. Parental support and encouragement are important to help the child adjust to orthodontic treatment.

### Preventing Dental Injuries

During the school-age years, injuries to the teeth can occur easily. Many injuries can be avoided by use of mouth protectors. These resilient shields protect against injuries by cushioning blows that might otherwise damage teeth or lead to jaw fractures (ADA, 2015). Children should wear a mouth protector when participating in contact and some non-contact sports, such as bicycle riding, gymnastics, or in-line skating. Custom-made mouth protectors constructed by the dentist are more expensive than stock mouth protectors purchased in stores, but their better fit makes them more comfortable and less likely to interfere with speech and breathing. If cost is an issue for a custom-made protector, a stock guard labeled with ADA/ANSI approved, is the next best option (ADA, 2015). Wearing a mouth protector is especially important for children with orthodontic braces; they protect against accidental disruption of the appliance as well as soft tissue injury that would occur from the contact between the orthodontic appliance and the interior of the lips and gums (ADA, 2015).

### Dental Health Education

Health education curricula need to be designed to foster attitudes and behaviors among children that promote good personal oral hygiene practices and awareness of the risks of dental disease. The school nurse is in an excellent position to educate children about dental health and to detect problems such as untreated caries, inflamed gums, or malocclusion. The nurse should look for signs of smokeless tobacco use (irritation of the gums at the tobacco placement site, gum recession, stained teeth) and should take this opportunity to explain to the child the risks of using tobacco. The use of snuff and chewing tobacco carries multiple dangers, including a greatly increased risk of oral cancer and heart disease.

## Sleep and Rest

The number of hours spent sleeping decreases as the child grows older. Children ages 6 and 7 years need about 12 hours of sleep per night. Some children also continue to need an afternoon quiet time or nap to restore energy levels. The 12-year-old needs about 9 to 10 hours of sleep at night. More sleep is needed when the child enters the preadolescent growth spurt. Adequate sleep is important for school performance and physical growth. Inadequate sleep can cause irritability, inability to concentrate, and poor school performance.

To promote rest and sleep, a period of quiet activity just before bedtime is helpful. A leisurely bedtime routine, with adequate time for the child to read, listen to the radio or MP3 player or just daydream, promotes relaxation. Keeping the room dark and quiet, without lights from computers, tablets, cell phones or television, is optimal for appropriate sleep (George, 2013). Children who do not obtain adequate rest often have difficulty getting up in the morning, creating a family disturbance as they rush to get ready for school, perhaps skipping breakfast or leaving the house in the heat of frustration. A set bedtime and waking time, consistently enforced, promote security and healthful sleep habits. Bedtime offers an ideal opportunity for parent and child to share important events of the day or give a kiss and a hug, unthinkable in front of peers earlier in the day.

Occasionally, school-age children have sleep problems, most commonly sleepwalking and sleep terrors (night terrors). Both conditions

## HEALTH PROMOTION

### *The 6- to 8-Year-Old Child*

**Focused Assessment**

Ask the child the following:

- Can you tell me how often and what foods you like to eat? How often do you eat at fast-food restaurants? How do you feel about how much you weigh? Do you think you need to gain or lose any weight?
- What types of physical activities do you like to do? How often and for how long do you do them? Do you have any quiet hobbies that interest you?
- How many hours each day do you watch television, movies, or use the computer, tablet or cell phone (including playing video games)? What is your favorite television program? Do you have a television in your room?
- How often do you brush your teeth, floss, and see the dentist?
- What time do you go to bed at night? What time do you get up in the morning? Do you have any trouble falling asleep, or do you wake up in the middle of the night?
- How often do you have a bowel movement? Are there any problems with urination? (Use the child's familiar terminology if known.) Do you wet the bed? If so, how often?
- What grade in school are you? Are you doing well in school or having any problems? Do you feel safe at school? Do you participate in any before- or after-school programs?
- What kinds of activities do you enjoy doing with your friends?
- How do you get along with other members of your family? Is there a special family member you could talk to if you are having a problem? If so, who?
- Do you do any or all of the following: use a seatbelt every time you get in a car; wear a helmet every time you ride a bicycle; wear a helmet and protective pads every time you skate or use a scooter; use sunscreen; swim with a buddy and only when an adult is present; always look both ways before crossing the street; use the right equipment when you play sports; know to avoid strangers and how to call for help if needed?
- Has anyone ever physically hurt you or touched you in a way that made you uncomfortable?

*Continued*

## HEALTH PROMOTION—cont'd

### *The 6- to 8-Year-Old Child*

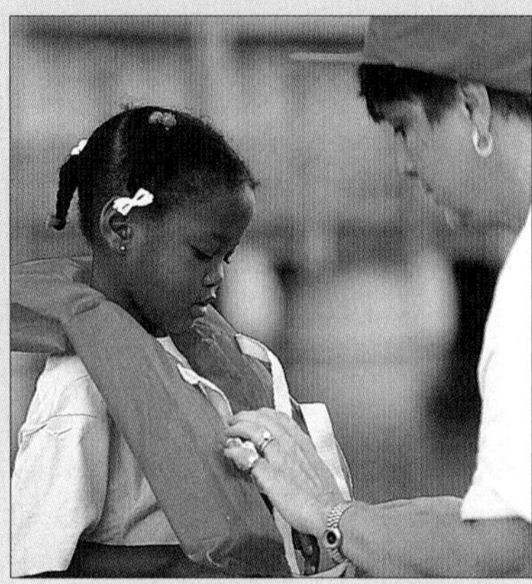

Ask the parent the following:

- Are there any concerns related to the child's nutrition, body image, physical activity, oral health, sleep, elimination, school, family interactions, self-esteem, and ability to practice safety precautions?
- Is there a gun in the home? If so, is it locked away and the ammunition stored locked in a separate place?
- Do you have a swimming pool? If so, is it fenced on all four sides and not directly accessible from the house?
- Do you have a fire escape plan that you practice regularly?
- Do you have any family history of heart problems or stroke; has anyone in your family had a heart attack or stroke at a young age?
- Is your child regularly exposed to second hand smoke?

#### Developmental Milestones

*Personal/social:* Develops positive self-esteem through skill acquisition and task completion; peer group becoming the primary socializing force; outgoing and boisterous, 'know-it-all,' but becomes more reflective and quiet by age 8 years; loves new ideas and places; has a good sense of humor, may tell crude jokes; may be argumentative and use tension-releasing behaviors such as nail biting, hair twisting, wriggling; likes to make things but often does not finish projects; loves family members but worries about them; has a strong sense of fairness and justice—uses rules to define cooperative relationships with others (sees rules as being imposed by others)

*Fine motor:* Ties shoelaces, buttons and zips clothes, dresses and undresses without help; can print, draw, color well, model clay, and cut with scissors; visual acuity is fully developed

*Language/cognitive:* Vocabulary expands; understands the different properties of language: play on words, puns, mnemonics, jokes; adapts well to changing physical properties of objects (e.g., conservation, reversibility, identity); improved long-term memory; organizes concepts and classifies in several ways; uses various memory strategies to improve schoolwork

*Gross motor:* Improved muscle mass and coordination allow for participation in various sports and games

#### Health Maintenance

##### *Physical Measurements*

Average weight gain is 2.5 kg (5½ lb) per year

Average increase in height is approximately 5.5 cm (2 inches) per year

Continue to plot height and weight

Plot body mass index (BMI) and percentile

Note any breast budding or signs of other secondary sex characteristics

##### *Immunizations*

If not given earlier, administer measles, mumps, and rubella (MMR) #2; varicella #2; diphtheria-tetanus-acellular pertussis (DTaP) #5 (if younger than 7 years; use Tdap if older than 7 years); and inactivated poliovirus (IPV) #4

Annual influenza vaccine

Administer other immunizations if not up to date

##### *Health Screening*

Objective hearing and vision screening

Speech assessment for fluency

Hemoglobin or hematocrit

Urine for sugar and protein

Blood pressure

Fasting lipid screen if at risk

Tuberculosis (TB) screening if at risk (see Chapter 45)

#### Anticipatory Guidance

Provide health teaching to the child as well as to the parent

##### *Nutrition*

Follow dietary guideline–recommended servings; teach the child how to keep track of servings and to give input into meal preparation

Advise to avoid fast foods and to eat a nutritious breakfast

Watch calcium and iron intake

Vitamin D supplementation 400 IU/day if consuming less than 1 L (33 oz) per day of milk and vitamin-D–fortified foods

##### *Elimination*

Regular bowel movements according to the child's pattern; treat constipation by increasing water intake and intake of fresh fruits and vegetables

Occasional bed-wetting is within the norm; refer for more serious problems (see Chapter 44)

##### *Dental*

Provide regular dental care every 6 months

Continue regular brushing with fluoride toothpaste and flossing (may need assistance with this)

May need dental sealants as permanent molars erupt

##### *Sleep*

Facilitate an individually appropriate sleep pattern; school-age children usually go to bed by 9 PM and are up by 7 AM

If the child is not tired, advise the parent to allow a quiet reading time in bed

##### *Safety*

Review gun safety; bicycle, skating, and scooter safety; playground safety; fire safety; automobile and pedestrian safety; water safety; sun protection; good touch versus bad touch, stranger awareness

Discuss exposure to contact allergens (poison ivy, oak, sumac), tick checks, sports safety, use of reflective clothing if out at night

##### *Play*

Encourage developing collections, playing complicated board and card games, crafts, electronic and science-related games

Advise limiting television watching to no more than 2 hours a day

Recommend increasing planned physical activity to at least 1 hour a day of moderate to vigorous exercise; incorporate age-appropriate activities to strengthen muscles and bones (Centers for Disease Control and Prevention [CDC], 2015c)

##### *Self-Esteem and Competence*

See Patient-Centered Teaching box (p. 135)

occur during deep sleep. Children with night terrors scream and appear excessively frightened; they may be difficult to console during the episode, but the episode is self-limiting, usually lasting less than 30 minutes. Children who walk in their sleep do not respond to their environment and are in danger of injuring themselves. Episodes of both sleep terrors and sleepwalking are frightening to parents, but the child is unlikely to remember the episode on awakening. The nurse can advise a parent to quietly soothe the child during an episode and protect the child from harm. Episodes may increase when the child is under stress.

### CRITICAL THINKING EXERCISE 8.1

Mrs. George states that Megan, 11 years old, has recently started to leave her belongings throughout the house and that her room is always a mess. Mrs. George states that she is frustrated and feels as if she is constantly asking Megan to pick up her things and clean her room.

- What assumptions might a nurse make on the basis of Mrs. George's report about her daughter's behavior?
- What other data does the nurse need to clarify to best help Mrs. George and Megan in this situation?
- What are some possible approaches the nurse might suggest to Mrs. George?

## Discipline

Because school-age children possess a strong sense of justice and believe in the importance of rules, they want and expect limits to be set on their behavior. Firm, consistent limits increase children's sense of security and reinforce the message that an adult cares about them. Realistic expectations, clearly defined rules, and logical consequences help children develop self-discipline and increased self-esteem. Some families have meetings where they discuss how responsibilities in the family will be shared. The child is made to feel more a part of the solution rather than the problem.

Responsibility can be developed in children through the use of natural and logical consequences related to actions. Children become accountable for their actions. If a child leaves a toy outside and it is damaged, the parent is empathetic but does not replace the toy. The parent does not get in a power struggle, nor does the parent verbally attack the child. The child begins to understand that there are consequences to actions. This type of discipline, correctly used, will allow the parent to separate the deed from the doer; not pass moral judgment; focus on the present, not the past; and show respect and firm kindness. In addition, the child will be given choices, and the consequence will relate to the logic of the situation.

Teachers' disciplinary efforts are often thwarted when parents do not support them or when they show no concern about their children's misbehavior in school. Teamwork between parents and teachers is essential for effective discipline. Regular parent-teacher conferences help make discipline effective.

## Safety

Unintentional injury is the leading cause of death in children of every age-group beyond 1 year of age (National Center for Health Statistics, 2016). Although the death rate from unintentional injury is lower in children ages 5 to 9 years than it is during early childhood, the patterns of injury differ. Aside from injury from falls, the leading causes of nonfatal unintentional injury in children of this age-group include being struck by or striking an object that resulted in injury, overexertion, lacerations, bites and stings, bicycle injury, and motor vehicle passenger, injuries (Centers for Disease Control and Prevention [CDC], 2013).

Approaches to safety education vary as the child grows older. Physically, middle childhood is a period of great activity, with the child moving back and forth between the home environment and the community. The school-age child has less fear when playing and frequently imitates adults by using tools and household items. Children in this age-group enjoy helping with adult routines and chores around the home. Anticipatory guidance related to safety is very important as children develop and try new projects that require use of more dangerous or sophisticated equipment.

Safety education is best accomplished by simply stating safety rules and providing reinforcement through short projects and immediate rewards. Role-playing activities and error-detection picture games are excellent ways to reinforce safety lessons. Children in this age-group are inquisitive and will frequently ask questions. The answers to their questions should contain concrete rationales. Group projects with safety topics help foster independent thinking while promoting interactions with the child's peer group.

### Car Safety

Once a child attains a height of 4 feet 9 inches and is between ages 8 and 12 years, he or she may be large enough to use the vehicle's three-point restraining system (AAP, 2014). The child needs to be tall enough that the shoulder belt crosses the middle of the chest and the lap belt rides low onto the thighs (AAP, 2014). Smaller and younger children can remain in an approved booster seat, which will position the belts properly in relation to the child (AAP, 2014). Parents should be aware of state laws regarding child automobile safety seats for school-age children where they reside and when they travel, as most states have specific ages at which a child may use the vehicle restraint system. Adherence often is determined by family values, with use or nonuse reflecting parental practices. Children should sit in a rear seat away from car passenger safety airbags.

### Water Safety

School-age children learn to swim well enough to keep their heads above water for a short time at about 8 years old. The length of time they can keep their heads above water and their swimming ability increase with age and experience. The incidence of drowning decreases in this age-group; however, drowning is the second leading cause of death after motor vehicle injury in the 5- to 9- and 10- to 14-year-old age-groups (CDC, 2014c). Adult supervision is still needed to prevent a water-related injury in children of these age-groups. School-age children often overestimate their swimming capabilities and endurance. As their swimming abilities improve, anticipatory guidance can include general swimming safety. Children should be taught to stay away from pools, canals and the fast-moving waters of creeks and rivers. Advise parents to teach children to wade into shallow water or to jump feet first into water of unknown depth to prevent neck injuries. Safety near the water includes never running, pushing, or jumping on others who are in the water.

### Fire and Burn Safety

Parents should continue to reinforce safety procedures associated with fire safety. Routine fire drills should be practiced in the home. Repetition of family drills helps ensure that the child will respond correctly and automatically to smoke alarms. Children of this age can better comprehend cause-and-effect relationships, so they can understand why they should not play with potentially flammable substances.

School-age children are eager to help parents with daily chores such as cooking or ironing. Parents need to invest the time to teach their children how to use tools and appliances properly and must

**SAFETY ALERT**

***Fire Safety Rules***

Know two specific escape routes from each area in the home.
Know how to dial 911.
Know how to crawl under the smoke to leave a burning house.
Have a predetermined meeting area outside the house.
Never return to a burning house.
Practice fire drills.

establish guidelines to avoid burn injuries as a result of the child's inexperience.

Fireworks create another burn hazard for children. Each summer, many children are seriously burned or permanently scarred by fireworks. To prevent serious burn injuries, the federal government, under the federal Hazardous Substances Act, prohibits the sale of the more dangerous fireworks to the general public. However, a degree of risk always is associated with any fireworks. There are no absolutely safe fireworks for children or adults. Fireworks are best left to the experts and viewed from a safe distance. Encourage families to enjoy the many community-sponsored fireworks displays.

### Bicycle, in-Line Skating, Scooter, and Skateboard Safety

Mastering the ability to ride a bicycle is a milestone in a child's life, leading to independence. The bicycle is typically considered a toy but is actually a vehicle that is capable of speedy transportation. Bicycle injuries are a leading cause of nonfatal injury in children 5 to 15 years old, with school age children and adolescents accounting for more than half of bicycle-related injuries (CDC, 2015a). For this reason, the public health community supports the mandatory use of bicycle helmets. Research has demonstrated that the use of a helmet can reduce the incidence of head injury, fractures, and traumatic brain injuries (McIntosh, Lai, & Schilter, 2012). Parents should choose a helmet that is the appropriate size for the child and meets the standards of the Consumer Product Safety Commission (AAP, 2015a). Bicycle safety practices actually begin when the child is a passenger in a bicycle seat on the back of a parent's bicycle. They continue as the child learns to ride a tricycle and progressively build as the child becomes more skilled and begins to ride a bicycle. A helmet and other safety accessories are essential for protection, but they are only an adjunct to the child's skill level and knowledge of the rules of the road. A young cyclist is unpredictable and may be preoccupied with managing the bicycle itself. For this reason, parents should set limits on where, when, and how far the child may ride until he or she can competently maneuver the bicycle. When parents on bicycles accompany children, it is essential that the parents wear helmets and follow the rules of the road to role model appropriate safety and emphasize the importance of the helmet and the rules.

In-line skating and skateboarding are recreational activities that are popular with school-age children. Balancing, stopping, and turning are challenging and require motor skills similar to those required for bicycling. As the child begins to learn these skills, falls are frequent, and protective gear is essential. Helmets and protective pads covering the knees and elbows help protect the most vulnerable areas of the child's body from serious injury. Key educational points and an overview of safety principles are described in the Patient-Centered Teaching box.

Unpowered scooters are very lightweight, small versions of an older, more stable type of scooter used by children in the 1950s. They are propelled by one foot and have a very narrow base and small wheels. Because of their portability, both adults and children use them, many times on crowded city sidewalks. Since the introduction of unpowered scooters in the late 1990s, scooter-related injuries have markedly increased, representing a significant number of children annually being seen in emergency departments for injuries related to unpowered scooter use. These injuries are mainly to the upper extremities and face (AAP Committee on Injury and Poison Prevention, 2002/2013). Recommendations for safe operation of scooters are similar to those for in-line skating, with the exception of wrist-pad use.

**PATIENT-CENTERED TEACHING**

***Bicycle, In-Line Skating, Scooter, and Skateboard Safety***

- Children should always wear a helmet when bicycle riding, in-line skating, or skateboarding. This safety practice should begin when the child begins to learn these activities.
- Helmets should fit properly and snugly on the head. Helmets need to be lightweight and ventilated and have reflective trim. Write your child's name and phone number in indelible ink on the inside of the helmet.
- Children should be taught not to ride at dusk or in the dark. They should always call home for a ride if it is after dark.
- Children should not ride two on a bicycle.
- Riding barefoot, in thongs, or in slippers is dangerous.
- Children need to avoid using audio headsets while riding a bicycle because headsets can diminish hearing capabilities.
- Encourage children to stay on sidewalks, paths, or driveways until they have mastered advanced bicycling skills and know the rules of the road.
- While bicycling or in-line skating, children should avoid uneven road surfaces, gravel, potholes, and bumps.
- Bicycles should be equipped with reflectors and lights. With their parents' help, encourage children to routinely inspect their own bicycles to ensure that they are functioning properly (e.g., brakes, tires, lights).
- Proper sizing is important when purchasing a bicycle for a child. Oversized bicycles are responsible for many injuries. The child should be able to place the balls of both feet on the ground when sitting on the seat with the hands on the handlebars.
- The child should be able to straddle the center bar with both feet flat on the ground. There should be about 1 inch of clearance between the crotch and the bar.
- The handlebars should be within easy reach for the child.
- Rules of the Road
- Children younger than 8 years old should ride only with adult supervision and not in the street. Limit in-line skating or skateboarding to areas where there is no car traffic.
- Children should not ride bicycles on roads with heavy traffic.
- A bicycle should be ridden on the right side of the road, with the traffic. Bicycle riders must obey all traffic laws, traffic signs, and lights.
- Children need to learn the appropriate hand signals and use them every time before turning.
- Bicycles should be walked across busy intersections, not ridden.
- Children need to learn to stop, look left, look right, and look left again before entering a street or leaving a driveway, alley, or parking lot.
- Children should stop at all intersections, marked and unmarked.
- Children riding bicycles should obey all stop signs and red lights.
- Children should look back and yield to traffic coming from behind before turning left at intersections.
- Basic bicycle safety rules apply to scooters, in-line skates, and skateboards.

### Pedestrian Safety

Children between ages 5 and 9 years are at great risk for automobile–pedestrian injuries (CDC, 2014a). The tremendous forces of impact and the lack of protection for the pedestrian can lead to severe injury. Children are commonly struck when they dart into traffic, especially where parked cars obscure the driver's view of the child (e.g., crossing the street in front of a school bus, playing near cars in driveways or yards). Several factors predispose this age-group to such injuries. Their smaller physical stature limits their visibility to drivers. In addition, children in this age-group have the misconception that if they can see the car, the driver must be able to see them and will be able to stop instantly. Focused on play activities, they often impulsively dart into the street, oblivious to boundaries and potential traffic dangers.

Children learn traffic safety by watching and doing. Exposure to traffic increases as the child begins to walk to and from school and friends' houses. Parents have the responsibility of practicing pedestrian safety hundreds of times before the child is allowed to venture across streets alone.

## Selected Issues Related to the School-Age Child

### Adjustment to School

Most children are eager to start school, particularly if they have older siblings. They even look forward to bringing home their books and doing "real" homework. However, this enthusiasm usually quickly fades. Most children adjust well to first grade, enjoying the opportunities it provides for peer interaction and stimulating experiences. First grade may be the child's first experience of being away from home. For these children, starting school may be a frightening experience. Even children who have attended preschool have some anxiety about beginning first grade. Adjustment to school depends on various factors, including the child's physical and emotional maturity, the child's experiences, and the parents' ability to support the child and accept the separation (see Chapter 7).

***Peer influence.*** School is often the first experience a child has with a large number of children of the same age. From peers children learn how to cooperate, compete, bargain, and follow rules. Peer approval is of major importance as children look to their friends for recognition and support. The influence of peers becomes stronger as the child grows older.

***Influence of teachers.*** Teachers have a significant influence on children's social and intellectual development. An effective teacher makes learning fun and capitalizes on the child's interests and talents. Teachers guide the child's learning by rewarding success and helping the child learn from and deal with failures. The teacher plays an important role in preventing feelings of inferiority in the child. By structuring the learning environment so that the child experiences success, the teacher bolsters feelings of industry.

## HEALTH PROMOTION

### *The 9- to 11-Year-Old Child*

**Focused Assessment**

Ask the child the following:

- Can you tell me how often and what foods you like to eat? How often do you eat at fast-food restaurants? How do you feel about how much you weigh? Do you think you need to gain or lose any weight?
- What types of physical activities do you like to do? How often and for how long do you do them? Do you have any quiet hobbies that interest you? How many hours each day do you watch television or movies, use the computer or tablet, or play video games? What is your favorite television program or computer game?
- How often do you brush your teeth, floss, and see the dentist? Do you take fluoride?
- What time do you go to bed at night? What time do you get up in the morning? Do you have any trouble falling asleep or do you wake up in the middle of the night?
- How often do you have a bowel movement? Are there any problems with urination? (Use the child's familiar terminology if known.) Do you wet the bed? If so, how often?
- What grade in school are you? Are you doing well in school or having any problems? Do you feel safe at school? In what before- or after-school programs do you participate?
- What kinds of activities do you enjoy doing with friends? Do you sometimes feel pressured to do things you don't want to do or know you shouldn't? Do you or your friends smoke or take any substances (alcohol, drugs)?
- How do you get along with other members of your family? Is there a special family member you could talk to if you are having a problem? If so, who?
- Do you do any or all of the following: use a seatbelt every time you get in a car; wear a helmet every time you ride a bicycle; wear a helmet and protective pads every time you skate or use a scooter; use sunscreen; swim with a buddy and only when an adult is present; always look both ways before crossing the street; use the right equipment when you play sports; know to avoid strangers and how to call for help if needed?

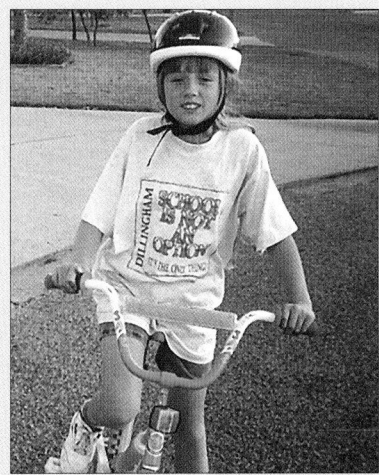


- Has anyone ever physically hurt you or touched you in a way that made you uncomfortable? Have you ever thought about hurting yourself?

Ask the parent the following:

- Are there any concerns related to the child's nutrition, body image, physical activity, oral health, sleep, elimination, school, family interactions, self-esteem, and ability to practice safety precautions?
- Is there a gun in the home? If so, is it locked away and the ammunition stored locked in a separate place?
- Do you have a fire escape plan that you practice regularly?
- Do you have any family history of heart problems or stroke; has anyone in your family had a heart attack or stroke at a young age?
- What types of information have you given to your child about puberty, sexual activity, and high-risk behaviors such as drug and alcohol use? Do you feel uncomfortable talking with your child about these issues?

*Continued*

## HEALTH PROMOTION—cont'd

### *The 9- to 11-Year-Old Child*

**Developmental Milestones**

*Personal/social:* Peers' opinions become more important than parents'; clubs, with secret codes and rituals, are at a peak; hero worship; fairly responsible, dependable, and polite to adults; boys tease girls, and girls may become "boy crazy"; may become angry but is learning to control it; critical of own work; rebelliousness may begin; ready for away-from-home experiences, such as camp

*Fine motor:* Hand-eye coordination fully developed; fine motor control approximates adults'

*Language/cognitive:* Reads more and enjoys comics and newspapers; understands fractions, conservation of volume and weight; likes to talk on the telephone; interested in how things work

*Gross motor:* May begin to be more awkward as growth spurt begins; may drop out of team sports to avoid embarrassment

**Health Maintenance**

***Physical Measurements***

Girls are 2.54 cm (1 inch) taller and 0.9 kg (2 lb) heavier on average than boys
About 90% of facial growth has been attained
Boys have greater physical strength
Girls may have rapid growth spurt and menarche
Compute and plot body mass index (BMI)

***Immunizations***

Review immunization records
Administer immunizations if not up to date; some children may need measles, mumps, and rubella (MMR) #2; varicella #2; hepatitis B series
Give tetanus-diphtheria-pertussis (Tdap) if child is 11 years old (unless received earlier as a catch up)
Meningococcal conjugate vaccine #1 at the age of 11 years
Consider immunizing against human papillomavirus (HPV) at the age of 11 years (see Chapters 5 and 9)
Annual influenza vaccine

***Health Screening***

Objective hearing and vision screening (may become myopic as growth spurt begins)
Hemoglobin or hematocrit
Urine for sugar and protein
Blood pressure
Baseline lipid screen (AAP, 2016)
Tuberculosis (TB) screening if at risk (see Chapter 45)
Scoliosis screening

***Anticipatory Guidance***

Provide health teaching to the child and the parent
Educate particularly about avoidance of smoke exposure and refer, if necessary, for tobacco cessation (AAP, 2011)

***Nutrition***

Follow recommended servings according to the dietary guidelines; teach the child how to keep track of servings, to read labels, and to give input into meal preparation
Advise to avoid fast foods and to eat a nutritious breakfast
Watch calcium and iron intake
Vitamin D supplementation 400 IU/day if consuming less than 1 L (33 oz) per day of milk and vitamin-D–fortified foods
Assess adequacy of diet and snacks

***Elimination***

Regular bowel movements according to the child's pattern

***Dental***

Provide regular dental care every 6 months
Continue regular brushing with fluoride toothpaste and flossing
Oral fluoride supplementation if no access to fluoridated water
May need dental sealants as permanent molars erupt
May need referral to orthodontist for malocclusion

***Sleep***

Facilitate an individually appropriate sleep pattern; school-age children usually go to bed by 9 PM and are up by 7 AM
If the child is not tired, advise the parent to allow a quiet reading time in bed
Limit sources of light in the room (e.g., computer, tablet, cell phone, television screens)

***Hygiene***

May resist baths and showers, may wear the same clothes every day, bedroom is usually messy
Early reluctance to keep clean may be followed by a period of overcleanliness (multiple showers daily, new outfit after each shower)

***Safety***

Review gun safety; bicycle, skating, and scooter safety; playground safety; fire safety; automobile and pedestrian safety; water safety; sun protection; exposure to outside allergens and ticks; sports safety; use of reflective clothing if out at night
Continue to have child belted in the back seat of the car away from airbags
Discuss not allowing others into the home if parent is not there; how to contact emergency services; not to open doors to strangers; avoiding listening to loud music through earphones

***Play***

Encourage reading age-appropriate fiction, developing collections, playing complicated board and card games, crafts, electronic and science-related games
Advise limiting television watching to no more than 2 hours a day
Recommend increasing planned physical activity to at least 1 hour a day of moderate to vigorous exercise (AAP, 2011)

***Self-Esteem and Competence***

See Patient-Centered Teaching box (p. 135)

The student-teacher relationship is a key factor in school success. Effective teachers motivate students by being warm and understanding, showing interest, and communicating at the child's level. Children value the opinion of such teachers and will work to gain their approval. Favorite teachers serve as role models and are often objects of hero worship by their students.

Even excellent teachers cannot do an effective job alone. They need the support of parents and school administrators to maximize children's learning potential.

***Parents' role.*** Parents play a key role in their children's academic success. By taking an active interest in children's progress and encouraging them to do their best, parents can foster learning. Positive reinforcement is given for honest efforts, not just good grades. Parents should enforce rules that encourage self-discipline and good study habits (e.g., no television until homework is finished). The child must create and adhere to a schedule for completing large assignments to prevent last-minute panic. If the child does not have a desk or another private place for homework, the kitchen table or another quiet, well-lighted area should be made available during study time. The television should be turned off during study time and distractions kept to a minimum. Adequate sleep is important for school performance. Parents may need to enforce bedtime rules to meet the child's needs. Rewarding children for meeting deadlines and for being organized encourages them to take responsibility for their learning and fosters skills that are important for success in jobs as adults.

Parents need to communicate with teachers and stay informed about their children's progress. Visiting the classroom and attending parent-teacher conferences and school activities are important. Showing respect and support for the teacher facilitates learning.

***School refusal.*** *School refusal* is considered to be one manifestation of a separation anxiety disorder that begins during middle childhood and can extend into adolescence (Rosenberg & Chiriboga, 2016). In the past, the term was used interchangeably with the terms *school phobia* and *school avoidance.* School refusal has been defined as the refusal to attend school, despite parental efforts to enforce attendance (Carless, Melvin, Tonge, et al., 2015). Some school-refusing children show specific fears that something "bad" will happen to parents while they are gone; older children often express anxiety that they will be embarrassed in some way (Rosenberg & Chiriboga, 2016). In some instances, school refusal might be related to underlying family dysfunction (Carless et al., 2015). Because some children with school-refusal behaviors have intense emotional distress related to school attendance, they are labeled *phobic.* The confusion over the use of these terms can make assessment and treatment of these children difficult. For an additional discussion of separation anxiety, see Chapter 53.

Children may go to school unwillingly or may refuse and have temper tantrums if the parents insist on taking the child to school. Younger children may complain of stomachaches, headaches, nausea, and vomiting. Older children may complain of palpitations and feeling faint. These symptoms typically resolve when the child returns home.

**Helping a child overcome school refusal.** In uncomplicated cases, the parent needs to calmly return the child to school as soon as possible. If symptoms are severe, a limited period of part-time or modified school attendance may be necessary. For example, part of the day may be spent in the counselor's or school nurse's office, with assignments obtained from the teacher. Communication and coordination of the treatment plan with school personnel is essential. The child should be gently questioned about factors at school that cause worry or fear. Specific causes, such as a bully or an overly critical teacher, should be dealt with immediately. Parents must support each other because the child may play one parent against the other to avoid school. Parents should be empathetic yet firm and consistent in their insistence that the child attend school. Parents should not pick the child up at school once the child is there. Positive reinforcement or reward for school attendance is essential. Encouraging and maintaining peer contacts and emphasizing the positive aspects of school are helpful. Family therapy might be required if the problem persists.

### Self-Care Children

The number of children who let themselves into their homes after school and are left alone continues to grow as the number of dual-income and single-parent families increases. These children are called **self-care children** or *home-alone children,* previously referred to as *latch-key children.* Ten percent of children ages 9 to 11 years and 33% of children 12 to 14 years care for themselves regularly; 2% of self-care children are between 5 and 8 years of age (Forum on Child and Family Statistics, 2015).

Parents often feel guilty about leaving children alone and may feel concern for their children's safety. Potential positive outcomes of this experience are learning to be independent and responsible. Because of time spent unsupervised at home, the risk of children engaging in problem behaviors (smoking, alcohol use, inappropriate eating) increases. The quality of the parent-child relationship and having parents who are emotionally supportive and establish firm rules play a role in moderating adverse effects on the child in self-care.

Nurses can help families by offering support and education to parents and children to reduce the risks for self-care children. Parents need to know when and how to prepare their children for self-care by teaching them specific strategies for staying safe at home alone. When considering whether a child is ready to stay home alone, parents should think about not only age, but maturity level. Parents can consider whether the child follows instructions well, exercises good decision-making, knows how to contact the parent and emergency personnel, and seems comfortable being alone (Child Welfare Information Gateway, 2013). An additional consideration includes the safety of the neighborhood and the home itself (Child Welfare Information Gateway, 2013). Nurses can serve as child advocates by working to develop expanded after-school child-care programs in the community. Numerous communities have established after-school telephone help lines to provide information, support, and assistance to self-care children. Nurses should also know the laws relating to self-care in their state of practice, as some states have established a minimum age at which children may be left home alone.

### Obesity

When intake of food exceeds expenditure, the excess is stored as fat. Obesity is an excessive accumulation of fat in the body and is assessed in children through a body mass index (BMI) that exceeds the 95th percentile for age.

Obesity can be a precursor of hyperlipidemia, sleep apnea, cholelithiasis (gallstones), orthopedic problems, hypertension, and diabetes. In addition, children who are obese can have psychosocial difficulties, particularly in the areas of self-esteem and body image, and are more likely to be teased by others (Feeg, Candelaria, Krenitsky, et al., 2014). Because the obese child develops increased numbers of fat cells, which are carried into adulthood, preventing obesity in childhood can reduce the risk of obesity in adulthood and plays a role in preventing disease.

Cultural, genetic, behavioral, environmental, and socioeconomic factors are linked to childhood obesity (Gahagan, 2016). Children with low metabolic rates and more fat cells tend to gain more weight, as do children whose parents are obese (Gahagan, 2016). Progress in obesity prevention has been made in preschool children. However, of the 17%

of children in the United States who are obese, the prevalence is highest in Hispanics (22.4%) and non-Hispanic blacks (20.2%), compared to 14% in non-Hispanic white children (CDC, 2015b). Both poverty and parental level of education affect the prevalence of obesity, with children in poor families and children whose parents did not complete high school at higher risk (CDC, 2015b). Environmental influences in the development of childhood obesity are extremely strong, with increased access to fast foods, decreased access to appropriate physical activity, and decreased sleep all having an impact (Daniels & Hassink, 2015; Gahagan, 2016). Obese children also are at risk for developing metabolic (insulin-resistance) syndrome (Gahagan, 2016). Features of this syndrome include obesity, elevated lipid levels, increased blood pressure, and elevated fasting blood sugar. Isolating factors that contribute to obesity is often difficult in a family in which the parents are obese. When a parent lacks nutritional knowledge, it is reflected in the meals and snacks provided in the home. The child is at risk for development of the same habits. Unstructured meals, 'meals on the run,' and meals at fast-food restaurants can lack proper nutrition and be high in calories. Lack of exercise also contributes to obesity. Youth Risk Behavior Surveillance demonstrates that as children get older, they are less likely to be involved in physical activity (Kann et al., 2014). The child who is given food for reward or punishment attaches more to eating than gaining nutrition. Some people still think that a fat baby is a healthy baby. This type of thinking leads to overfeeding.

Unfortunately, the long-term success rate for the elimination of childhood obesity is poor. Positive outcomes are increased when the child has a support system and understands the importance of diet and exercise.

***Assessing the scope of the problem.*** The child who is obese looks overweight. Experts define childhood overweight as a BMI between the 85th and 95th percentile for age and gender; BMI greater than or equal to the 95th percentile characterizes obesity.

Generally, obesity is caused by increased calorie intake combined with decreased physical activity. The amount of time spent watching television, at a computer, and playing video games takes away from time the child could be participating in active exercise. The possibility of disease as a contributing factor must be evaluated. Increased weight gain has been associated with central nervous system tumors, hypothyroidism, Cushing syndrome, and Turner syndrome.

***Prevention.*** Early identification of risk factors can target the child who needs special attention and support. All children should be taught healthy eating habits and the importance of regular exercise. School- and community-based interventions can, along with regular guidance from health providers, assist with obesity prevention. There is general agreement that an appropriate screening and counseling program throughout childhood can prevent or treat obesity (Aldrich, Gance-Cleveland, Schmiege, et al., 2014; Daniels & Hassink, 2015). The AAP (Daniels & Hassink, 2015) recommends regular assessment of obesity risk beginning in infancy, combined with counseling about appropriate dietary and physical activity requirements of childhood as obesity prevention measures.

***Interventions and anticipatory guidance.*** The approach to obesity prevention and treatment during middle childhood is multifaceted and addresses parenting and cultural practices, environmental modifications, children's personal behaviors and emotional state, and changes in lifestyle (Daniels & Hassink, 2015). Take a dietary history and evaluate the child's eating habits and patterns. The child or parents (or both) should keep a food diary for 1 week. The diary should include the time, place, and type and amount of food eaten and the reason for eating. The general dietary habits of the family should also be assessed. Additional strategies include watching portion size, avoiding having unhealthy foods or snacks available in the home, and parental role modeling (Daniels & Hassink, 2015). Parents may need support to increase their self-efficacy to prevent obesity (Grossklaus & Marvicsin, 2014).

One of the key elements of successful weight reduction in the child or adolescent is ownership by the child of whatever plan is proposed. Care should be taken to avoid a power struggle between the parent and child. Obviously the young child will need more parental involvement than the older child or adolescent. The family should be willing to support the child but should not take on the role of watchdog (see the Parents Want to Know box: How to Prevent and Manage Obesity).

## PARENTS WANT TO KNOW

### *How to Prevent and Manage Obesity*

You can help prevent and manage obesity in your child by doing the following:

- Do not use food as a reward.
- Establish consistent times for meals and snacks and discourage in-between eating.
- Offer only healthy food options (ask the child to choose between an apple or popcorn, not an apple or a cookie).
- Avoid keeping unhealthy food in the house and minimize trips to fast-food restaurants.
- Be a role model by improving your own eating habits and levels of activity.
- Encourage the child to do fun, physical activities with the family.
- Praise the child for making appropriate food choices and for increasing physical activity levels.

Caloric requirements vary depending on the age and gender of the child. By changing the obese child's lifestyle to include exercise and nutritious foods in smaller servings, the possibility of success is increased. Teach the family and child how to select and prepare foods that are tasty and how to restrict serving size. Reading labels assists with healthier food choices. The nurse should be mindful of considering cultural food preferences and traditions and including them in the child's daily meal plan, if possible. Teach family members how to assess culturally significant foods for nutritional value and how to modify them to be more nutritionally advantageous. The child's favorite foods should be identified and incorporated whenever possible. Because snacks are an important aspect in childhood nutrition, nutritious snacks should be identified. Involving the whole family will create family behaviors that support the child's new eating and activity behaviors.

The parent needs to limit television and computer game time. Children should be involved in regular physical exercise at school and at home. Children can be encouraged to ride their bicycles or to walk rather than ride in a car to a friend's house to play. Planned physical activities of at least 1 hour a day of moderate to vigorous exercise should be part of the child's after-school and weekend routine (AHA, 2014b).

Some older children and adolescents may find success in a support group, such as Weight Watchers or Overeaters Anonymous. Some centers have a special group for children. Other support groups may be associated with schools, summer camps, and children's hospitals in the community.

A team approach is often necessary for successful weight reduction. Psychological support may be essential for the child and family to be successful. A registered dietitian can provide expertise in the

## EVIDENCE-BASED PRACTICE

The increasing prevalence of overweight and obese children in America is of concern, and thus, is addressed as a priority in the *Healthy People 2020* goals. Statistics demonstrate that obesity is a particular problem for boys, poor children, and children from certain minority populations (CDC, 2015b). Although it is generally acknowledged that causes of obesity are multifactorial (e.g., genetic, environmental, cultural, and behavioral) and prevention is key for children, to be successful with prevention, parents need to have the confidence in their abilities to create an environment that is conducive to obesity prevention. Davies, Terhorst, & Nakonechny, et al (2014) wondered whether creating a health education website that could be used by a parent in a primary care setting would increase parental self-efficacy for obesity prevention.

In creating their website, Davies et al. (2014) conducted an extensive review of literature relating to both obesity prevention and parent self-efficacy. They looked at such obesity risk factors as family history, children's eating and physical activity habits, child temperament, sleep, and family and community environment. They wanted their website to be useful both in reading level and information presented. They used graduate nursing students in an informatics class to develop the website. They then pilot-tested the website with seven parents of preschoolers using a process called "think aloud," where the parents verbally expressed their thoughts while going through the website.

After perfecting the website usability, Davies et al. (2014) designed a study to measure parental self-efficacy related to obesity prevention before and after website use. They used a questionnaire that they developed from multiple published, reliable, and valid self-efficacy measures to measure parental self-efficacy related to obesity prevention. They then tested the website's influence on self-efficacy using the self-efficacy questionnaire, which they administered to a convenience sample of 13 mostly minority and low-income participants.

The results suggested that, in this population, self-efficacy improved in relation to some of the obesity risk factors after the parents viewed the website, most noticeably in the areas of family mealtime practices, child activities, and managing the child's temperament (Davies et al., 2014). The sample used in this study was very small, and results could not be generalized to the parenting population. However, the researchers suggest that viewing an educational website such as theirs might assist providers with identifying an individual child's risk, and providing targeted reinforcement of parenting confidence to manage these risks.

Think about informational websites you use regularly. Do you believe that this approach might be effective, both for educating children and parents about prevention of obesity? If you were to try to find such a website, how would you go about evaluating its usefulness?

Davies, M., Terhost, L., Nakonechny, A., et al. (2014). The development and effectiveness of a health information website designed to improve parents' self-efficacy in managing risk for obesity in preschoolers. *Journal for Specialists in Pediatric Nursing, 19,* 316–330.

identification and planning of foods that are not only nutritional but also items that the child likes.

The school nurse can assist children and families both by addressing individual needs and by advocating for healthy food practices within the school setting. Problems that need to be addressed include the availability of soda and other poor nutrient snacks and lack of regular daily physical education programs. Nurses can assist with developing wellness policies that address nutrition and physical exercise within the school setting.

### BOX 8.2 Manifestations of Stress in Children

How children perceive stress influences its effects. Whether the child has symptoms of stress is determined not only by the stress itself but also by how the child perceives and responds to the stress. Intervention is needed when a child shows the following signs of stress:

- Unhappiness, moodiness
- Irritability, increased aggressive behavior
- Fatigue, inability to concentrate
- Hyperactivity
- Changes in eating or sleeping habits
- Physical complaints (nausea, headaches, stomachaches)
- Bed-wetting
- Substance abuse
- Diminished school performance

### Stress

Today's children are subjected to stress as no generation has been before. Alarming increases in drug abuse, childhood suicide, child abduction and murder, and school failure attest to the overwhelming stress that children experience. Rapid, bewildering social change and ever-increasing demands for achievement often pressure children to grow up too quickly. Stressed children may not show serious symptoms during childhood but may develop patterns of emotional response that can lead to serious illness as adults (Box 8.2).

**Sources of stress in children.** Growing up is stressful, even for well-adjusted children with loving, supportive families. Children experience stress from societal change, family relationships, school, competitive athletics, rushed schedules, and the media.

Middle-class children in particular are pressured to grow up quickly. Achievement-oriented parents, focused on success and financial gain, often view children as extensions of themselves and unwittingly expect too much of their children. Pressure on children to succeed, to win, and to be the best and brightest is great, especially when parents value academic achievement. Children are often pressured into a frenzied schedule of music, dance, sports, and art lessons and may have little time for family meals or playing with friends. Self-esteem and peer relationships often suffer. Byrne, Thomas, & Burchell, et al. (2011) researched the primary daily stressors experienced by school-aged children. They found that stressors can be categorized into three main areas—family, peers, and school—and relate often to transitions in development. School-age children describe frequent stressors to include problems in relationships with friends (moodiness, arguments), impatient or upset parents, illness or injury of a family member, concerns about school work or homework, being victims of inappropriate touching, and not being listened to by others (Byrne et al., 2011). Additionally, Willard, Long, and Phipps (2016) describe stressful events considered to be traumatic, such as death of a family member or close friend, being in a car crash or other life-threatening situation, being a victim of a disaster, and witnessing violence. Their research also suggests it is the cumulative effect of stressful events, even those frequently encountered by children, that can result in psychological distress. Additionally, children who grow up in an environment where substance abuse exists experience significant stress (Charles et al., 2015). Economically deprived children must cope with an even greater burden of stress. Faced with the dangers of violence, drug and alcohol addiction, and gangs, these children must fight daily for survival. Children from lower-income families travel dangerous streets to and from school and suffer from the insecurity and uncertainty of poverty. Children who are homeless—as is increasingly common—have the added stress of living on the street or in shelters and having decreased access to appropriate nutritional, health, and educational resources.

**School pressures.** School can be a source of stress for children. Some children are unable to cope with the competitive, test-regulated curricula of school. They find it difficult to keep up with the unrelenting academic pressure. School imposes long-term stress on these children, and they tend to dislike school and stay home whenever they can. They are often tardy and may abuse alcohol and drugs. Eventually, they may drop out of school. These children rarely return to complete their education.

Other children, particularly those who are academically gifted, find school stressful because it is tedious or uninteresting. Boredom can be stressful. Meaningless, repetitive schoolwork can cause bright, talented children to become chronically fatigued, inattentive, and careless.

**Physical threats.** Children also face other types of stress at school. Violence and theft in schools are national problems. School-age children commonly voice fears of being beaten up or held up. The child who leaves a bicycle unlocked or a watch or jacket unattended quickly learns the hazards of such carelessness. Students who abuse drugs or participate in gang activity create a pervasive attitude of wariness and fear and are a real source of stress for children.

**Competitive sports.** Participation in competitive sports is stressful for some children. Fear of failure, especially in front of a cheering crowd, can be overwhelming. Some parents contribute to competitive stress by overemphasizing the importance of winning. Because of their own needs or interests, some parents push their children to participate in organized sports at an early age (Fig. 8.2).

**Tight schedules and adaptation overload.** As the number of single parents and working mothers increases, so does the stress on children who must adapt to parents' work schedules. Many children are rushed from home to school to carpool to daycare or a babysitter. Children must draw on their energy reserves to exercise self-control in these varying situations and may not be able to cope. Fatigue and exhaustion from such demands often result in behavioral problems and regression.

**Family pressures.** In today's mobile society, it is not unusual for families to move and for children to have to leave other family members and friends. Attending a new school, making new friends, and losing former support systems can be very stressful for children. This happens at a time when one or both parents are also making major adjustments

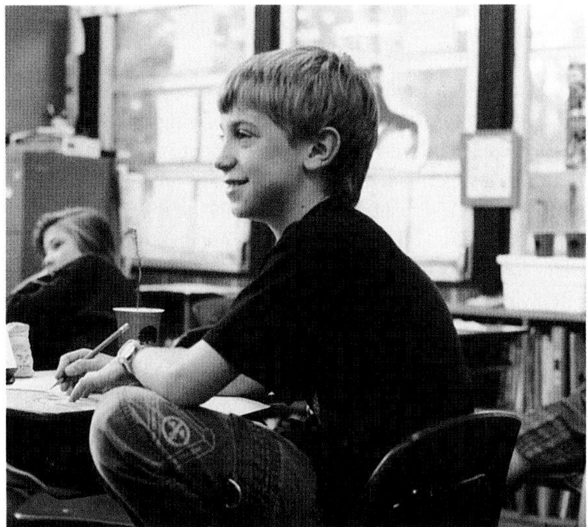

Attention span increases during the school-age years, facilitating classroom learning.

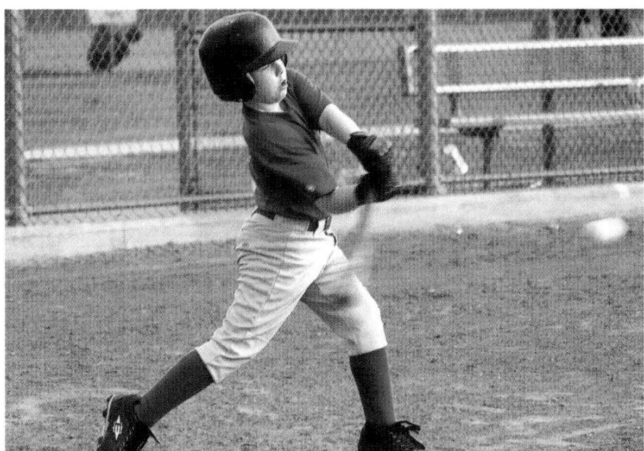

The nurse is in an excellent position to help parents and children identify factors that produce stress and to suggest ways to cope with its effects. Participation in competitive sports is stressful for some children, especially if parents push their child to play organized sports at an early age or overemphasize the importance of winning. Focusing on having fun and on the excitement of the game decreases competitive stress.

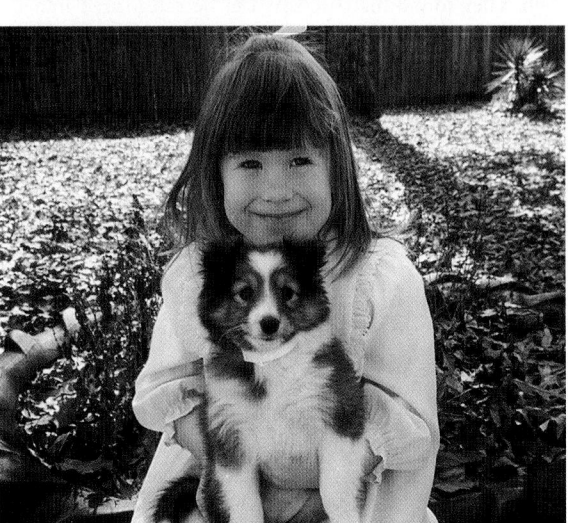

Spending time playing with and caring for pets can be fun and relaxing. Children who are given time and encouragement to play are better able to deal with the stresses of life.

**FIG 8.2** Health promotion for the school-age child and family.

in their lives, and they may not have the time and energy to meet all of the child's needs.

Overhearing parents quarrel produces anxiety and fear in children and erodes a child's sense of security. Some parents, although physically present, may be emotionally unavailable to children because of their own stresses. Divorce and separation are especially painful. Changes frequently caused by divorce, such as moving to a new house, attending a new school, and, usually the most stressful of all, separation from one of the parents, can cause great stress for children.

**Media influence.** The media are a common source of stress for today's children. Sexual and violent material portraying loss of control may frighten children because it suggests that they may not be able to master their own sexual and aggressive impulses. Television and violent video games expose children to vivid portrayals of the problems of today's society for many hours of their day. They also tend to isolate children from their parents and peers. Hours spent watching television or playing video games can limit children's participation in more creative play and contact and interaction with others.

Although many sociodemographic and psychologic factors influence whether an individual child turns to violence, there is a large body of epidemiologic research providing evidence that violence portrayed in the media has an adverse effect on developing children (Strasburger, Donnerstein, & Bushman, 2014). In response to this evidence, the AAP (2009) issued a policy statement on violent media exposure, which suggested that prolonged or frequent exposure to violence in the media can desensitize children to violence, lead to violent behavior toward others and emotional difficulties (irrational fears, nightmares) (p. 1495). Specific recommendations from the AAP include assessing media exposure at every well visit; encouraging parents to support the recommended daily limits for television and computer time; advising parents to be aware of potentially violent videos, programs, or computer games; and advocating for more positive media to be available for children along with an accurate rating system for various forms of media (AAP, 2009).

***Interventions and anticipatory guidance to reduce childhood stress.*** The nurse is in an ideal position to help parents and children identify factors that produce stress and to suggest ways to cope with its effects. Parents can meet basic psychological needs, influence self-esteem, shape values, control exposure to stressful events, and provide support. Parents may need guidance about realistic expectations from their children. Parents should watch for behavior changes in their children that may indicate signs of stress and offer appropriate reassurance. If significant tension is in the home, parents can try to resolve conflicts by negotiating rather than continuing to build an emotionally charged atmosphere. Parents should examine the child's schedule to make sure the child is not overburdened with school and extracurricular activities.

Close communication with teachers is important to prevent and deal with school-related stress. Becoming interested in and involved with the child's schoolwork conveys support and caring. Parents need to become active in parent-teacher associations and other community organizations to find solutions to the problems of violence and crime in the schools.

Children should be allowed to decide whether to participate in competitive athletics. It is important for parents to talk to coaches to determine what is expected of their children. Corrective instruction rather than punishment should be given for errors. A parent should serve as a role model for good sportsmanship.

Limiting the number of hours that children watch television and helping them select appropriate programs can decrease its negative effects. Watching television with children and discussing the content of programs are also helpful.

**! NURSING QUALITY ALERT**

***Sources of Stress for School-Age Children***

- Societal change
- School
- Competitive sports
- Tight schedules
- Family pressures
- Influence of the media
- Being bullied
- Fear of violence
- Chaotic living conditions

Children need to have time just to play. Parents should recognize that play is the child's work. Whether it is shooting baskets in the driveway, working on a collection, or building a model, play reduces stress for children. Toys and games that provide the greatest opportunity to use imagination are the best stress relievers. Most children love animals. Spending time playing with and caring for pets can be relaxing and fun. Children who are given the time and encouragement to play are better able to deal with the stresses of life (see Chapter 5). One of the most effective antidotes for childhood stress is a loving, attentive parent who takes the time to listen. A sympathetic adult who understands the stresses of childhood can offer valuable support. Discussion and modeling of ways to deal with the inevitable stresses of life can teach the child valuable lessons for living in today's society.

### Peer Victimization

Peer victimization, often called bullying, is becoming a significant problem for school-age children and adolescents in the United States. Although peer victimization is frequently found in the adolescent population, it is becoming more common during middle childhood. The United States Department of Education (2015) reports that nearly 28% of sixth grade students have been victims of bullying and 6% have been cyberbullied. Bullying occurs in students at all types of schools, public and private, urban and rural (U.S. Department of Education, 2015). The CDC defines bullying as aggression toward another in order to create a power imbalance. This aggression can be physical (pushing, shoving, tripping, fighting), verbal (teasing, name calling), social (spreading rumors, excluding from the group), or electronic (via cell phone or social media sites) (CDC, 2015d). Victimization can occur both in school and outside of school, with occurrences most often in a school hallway or outside on school property. The most frequent type of bullying in school age children is teasing, followed by spreading rumors (U.S. Department of Education, 2015). Peer victimization can cause extreme emotional distress in children and has been correlated with incidents of suicide (CDC, 2014b). Children can be bullies, victims, or both.

Signs that may indicate a child is being bullied are similar to signs of other types of stress and include nonspecific psychosomatic symptoms, loss of appetite, withdrawal, depression, school refusal, and decreased school performance (Perron, 2015; *Reducing the Impact*, 2015). Children may express fear of going to school or ask to be driven instead of riding the school bus. Some children spend inordinate amounts of time in the school nurse's office with vague complaints. Other children will have belongings that are missing or damaged for no known reason. Very often, children will not talk about what is happening to them.

It is important for nurses to emphasize to parents to be "tuned in" to their children to identify when there are problems with children being bullied or with possible bullying behavior by their child. Parents can be encouraged to talk with their children about bullying, empathize with the child who is being bullied, and provide reassurance that it is not the child's fault (USDHHS, 2011). A strategy that helps children deal with victimization includes role-playing actions to take when being bullied (speak up, walk away, don't retaliate, tell someone). It is most important for the parent to emphasize that no one should be bullied. Notifying the child's school can ensure that the child will be monitored in the school setting (USDHHS, 2011).

If parents think their child is bullying others, intervention is also warranted. Children who victimize other children can have long-term emotional consequences. Talking with the child, setting limits, stating that bullying is unacceptable, emphasizing the child's positive characteristics, and using appropriate discipline for misbehavior are all interventions to reduce bullying behavior (USDHHS, 2011).

Many school districts have introduced various anti-bullying programs; school nurses are often involved with planning and executing these programs. Additional information and resources are available through http://www.stopbullying.gov, a website maintained by the USDHHS.

## KEY CONCEPTS

- Slow, steady physical growth and rapid social and cognitive development characterize the school-age period, from 6 to 12 years. Average weight gain in the school-age child is 2.5 kg (5½ lb) per year, and the increase in height is approximately 5.5 cm (2 inches) per year. During the early school-age period, boys are approximately 2.54 cm (1 inch) taller and 0.9 kg (2 lb) heavier than girls.
- During the school-age years, children gradually move away from home and parents as a primary source of support, and they enter the wider world of peers and school.
- Physical changes include increased height and weight, increased muscle mass, maturation of body systems, and increased antibody production. During the school-age period, all 20 primary teeth are lost and are replaced by 28 of the 32 permanent teeth.
- The age at onset of puberty varies widely, but puberty is occurring at an earlier age than in the past. On average, black girls enter puberty approximately 1 year earlier than white girls.
- School-age children enjoy various activities. Cooperative play and team sports are typical of this age-group.
- According to Erikson, the developmental task of this period is the development of a sense of industry.
- The child develops a conscience and internalizes cultural and social values. The child is able to understand and obey rules.
- Thinking becomes less egocentric as children learn to consider viewpoints different from their own. School-age children can solve problems, form hypotheses, and make judgments based on reason.
- School-age children experience an increase in appetite, and older school-age children have increased energy needs as they approach puberty. Obesity is an important public health issue for which vigorous prevention approaches are necessary.
- Dental care is increasingly important as the primary teeth are replaced by permanent teeth. Malocclusion is not unusual in children of this age.
- Sources of stress for school-age children include societal change, school, competitive athletics, rushed schedules, fear of violence from bullies, chaotic living conditions if homeless, and the media. Teaching children coping strategies can reduce the effects of stress.
- Safety issues are related to the child moving more from the home environment to the community, less fear when playing, and the increased use of tools and household items. Important safety issues that impact school-age children include prevention of fire and burn injuries, pedestrian and motor vehicle injuries, pedestrian injury, and drowning.
- Peer victimization, or bullying, is becoming an important health issue for school-age children. It can occur within or outside the school setting and, without intervention, can cause long-term emotional problems for both the child being bullied and the child who bullies.

## REFERENCES AND READINGS

Aldrich, H., Gance-Cleveland, B., Schmiege, S., et al. (2014). School-based health center providers' treatment of overweight children. *Journal of Pediatric Nursing, 29*, 521–527.

American Academy of Pediatrics. (2009). Policy statement—Role of the pediatrician in youth violence prevention. *Pediatrics, 124*(1), 393–402.

American Academy of Pediatrics. (2011). Expert Panel on Integrated Guidelines for Cardiovascular Health and Risk Reduction in Children and Adolescents: Summary report. *Pediatrics,128*(5), S213–S256.

American Academy of Pediatrics. (2014). *Car safety seat checkup*. Retrieved from https://www.aap.org.

American Academy of Pediatrics. (2015a). *Bicycle helmets: What every parent should know*. Retrieved from https://www.healthychildren.org.

American Academy of Pediatrics. (2015b). *Pacifier and thumb sucking*. Retrieved from https://www.healthychildren.org.

American Academy of Pediatrics. (2016). Recommendations for preventive pediatric health care. *Pediatrics, 137*(1), 25–27.

American Academy of Pediatrics Committee on Injury and Poison Prevention. (2002, reaffirmed 2013). *Pediatrics, 133*(3), e799.

American Dental Association. (2015). *Mouthguards*. Retrieved from http://www.ada.org.

American Heart Association. (2014a). *Dietary guidelines for healthy children*. Retrieved from http://www.health.org.

American Heart Association. (2014b). *The AHA's recommendations for physical activity in children*. Retrieved from http://www.health.org.

Byrne, D., Thomas, K., & Burchell, J. (2011). Stressor experience in primary school-aged children: Development of a scale to assess profiles of exposure and effects on psychological well-being. *International Journal of Stress Management, 18*(1), 88–111.

Carless, B., Melvin, G., Tonge, B., et al. (2015). The role of parental self-efficacy in adolescent school refusal. *Journal of Family Psychology, 29*(2), 162–170.

Centers for Disease Control and Prevention. (2013). *10 leading causes of nonfatal unintentional injuries, United States – 2013, all races, both sexes, dispositions: All cases ages 6-14*. Retrieved from http://www.webappa.cdc.gov.

Centers for Disease Control and Prevention. (2014a). *Pedestrian safety*. Retrieved from http://www.cdc.gov.

Centers for Disease Control and Prevention. (2014b). *The relationship between bullying and suicide: What we know and what it means for schools*. Retrieved from http://www.cdc.gov.

Centers for Disease Control and Prevention. (2014c). *10 leading causes of injury deaths by age group highlighting unintentional injury deaths, United States—2013*. Retrieved from http://www.cdc.gov.

Centers for Disease Control and Prevention. (2015a). *Bicycle safety*. Retrieved from http://www.cdc.gov.

Centers for Disease Control and Prevention. (2015b). *Obesity facts.* Retrieved from http://www.cdc.gov.

Centers for Disease Control and Prevention. (2015c). *How much physical activity do children need?* Retrieved from http://www.cdc.gov.

Centers for Disease Control and Prevention. (2015d). *Understanding bullying: Fact sheet.* Retrieved from http://www.cdc.gov.

Centers for Disease Control and Prevention. (2016). *Recommended immunization schedule for persons aged 0 through 18 years United States, 2016.* Retrieved from http://www.cdc.gov

Charles, N. et al. (2015). Childhood stress exposure among preadolescents with and without family histories of substance use disorders. *Psychology of Addictive Behaviors, 29*(1), 192–200.

Child Welfare Information Gateway. (2013). *Leaving your child home alone.* Retrieved from https://www.childwelfare.gov.

Clark, M., & Slayton, R. (2014). Fluoride use in caries prevention in the primary care setting. *Pediatrics, 134*(3), 626–633.

Daniels, S., Hassink, S., & AAP Committee on Nutrition. (2015). The role of the pediatrician in primary prevention of obesity. *Pediatrics, 136*(1), e275–e292.

Erikson, E. (1963). *Childhood and society* (2nd ed.). New York: Norton.

Feeg, V., Candelaria, L., Krenitsky, S., et al. (2014). The relationship of obesity and weight gain to childhood teasing. *Journal of Pediatric Nursing, 29*(6), 511–520.

Forum on Child and Family Statistics. (2015). *America's children: Key national indicators of well-being, 2015.* Retrieved from http://www.childstats.gov.

Gahagan, S. (2016). Overweight and obesity. In R. Kliegman, B. Stanton, J. St. Geme, N. Schor, & R. Behrman (Eds.), *Nelson textbook of pediatrics* (20th ed., Chapter 47). Philadelphia: Elsevier.

George, N. (2013). Assessing sleep in adolescents through a better understanding of sleep physiology. *American Journal of Nursing, 113*(6), 26–31.

Grossklaus, H., & Marvicsin, D. (2014). Parenting efficacy and its relationship to the prevention of childhood obesity. *Pediatric Nursing, 40*(2), 69–86.

Kann, L., et al. (2014). Youth Risk Behavior Surveillance – United States 2013. *Morbidity and Mortality Weekly Report, 63*(4), 1–168.

Kaplowitz, P., Bloch, C., & American Academy of Pediatrics Section on Endocrinology. (2016). Evaluation and referral of children with signs of early puberty. *Pediatrics, 137*(1), 1–6.

Kohlberg, L. (1964). Development of moral character. In M. Hoffman & L. Hoffman (Eds.), *Review of child development research* (Vol. 1). New York: Russell Sage Foundation.

McIntosh, A., Lai, A., & Schilter, E. (2012). Bicycle helmets: Head impact dynamics in helmeted and unhelmeted oblique impact tests. *Traffic Injury Prevention, 14*, 501–508.

National Center for Health Statistics. (2016). *Health United States, 2015 with special feature on racial and ethnic health disparities.* Hyattsville, MD: Author.

Perron, T. (2015). Looking at the factors associated with bullying and visits to the school nurse, in the United States. *British Journal of School Nursing, 10*(6), 288–295.

Piaget, J. (1962). *Play, dreams, and imitation in childhood.* (C. Gattegno & F. M. Hodgson, Trans.). New York: Norton, (C. Gattegno & F.M. Hodgson, Trans.).

Reducing the impact of bullying: Useful resources and guidance. (2015). *British Journal of School Nursing, 10*(5), 248–249.

Rosenberg, D., & Chiriboga, J. (2016).Anxiety disorders. In R. Kliegman, B. Stanton, J. St. Geme, N. Schor, & R. Behrman (Eds.), *Nelson textbook of pediatrics* (20th ed., Ch. 25). Philadelphia, PA: Saunders.

Strasburger, V., Donnerstein, E., & Bushman, B. (2014). Why is it so hard to believe that media influence children and adolescents. *Pediatrics, 133*(4), 571–573.

United States Department of Education. (2015). *Student reports of bullying and cyberbullying: Results from the 2013 School Crime Supplement to the National Crime Victimization Survey.* Retrieved from http://www.nccs.ed.gov.

United States Department of Health and Human Services & United States Department of Agriculture. (2015). *Dietary guidelines for Americans, 2015-2020.* Retrieved from https://www.health.gov.

United States Department of Health and Human Services. (2011). *Bullying is a serious problem.* Retrieved from http://www.stopbullying.gov.

Willard, A., Long, A., & Phipps, S. (2016). Life stress versus traumatic stress: The impact of life events on psychological functioning in children with and without serious illness. *Psychological Trauma: Theory, Research, Practice & Policy, 8*(1), 63–71.

9

# Health Promotion for the Adolescent

http://evolve.elsevier.com/McKinney/mat-ch/

## LEARNING OBJECTIVES

*After studying this chapter, you should be able to:*

- Describe the adolescent's normal growth and development.
- Identify the sexual maturity rating and Tanner stages and recognize deviations from normal.
- Describe the developmental tasks of adolescence.
- Describe the concept of identity formation in relation to adolescent psychosocial development.
- Describe appropriate health-promoting behaviors for adolescents and young adults.
- Provide anticipatory guidance for adolescents and their families regarding risk-taking behaviors, nutrition, and safety.
- Discuss the prevalence of adolescent violence and strategies to deal with aggressive behavior.
- Discuss adolescent sexuality and related health risks.

Adolescence spans ages 11 to 21 years, although the developmental tasks of early adolescence, as well as the beginning stages of sexual maturation, may overlap with the school-age years. Adolescence is a time of change for teenagers and their families, a transition from childhood to adulthood. During this transition period, dramatic physical, cognitive, psychosocial, and psychosexual changes take place that are exciting and, at the same time, frightening.

*Healthy People 2020* (United States Department of Health and Human Services [USDHHS], 2010) objectives address many areas of adolescent health, some of which are contained in a new topic area specifically directed toward adolescents. These areas include access to comprehensive healthcare and education regarding appropriate reproductive health practices, violence reduction, and decreasing risk factors.

## ADOLESCENT GROWTH AND DEVELOPMENT

The adolescent tries out many new roles during this time as part of the important developmental task of identity formation. The peer group is of the utmost importance as adolescents experiment with new roles outside the confines of the family unit. When identity formation is complete, the young adult is emancipated from the family and establishes independence.

The rapid rate of physical growth during adolescence is second only to that of infancy. Adolescents come in many shapes and sizes, and the changes that take place during the teen years are obvious and dramatic. With physical changes come the development of secondary sexual characteristics and an intense interest in romantic relationships. In general, adolescents move from the same-sex friendships of childhood to the capacity for intimate, long-lasting relationships as young adults. Sexual orientation and gender identity are often recognized during adolescence as the teenager engages in exploration and self-discovery.

Both parents and adolescents need the nurse's support and guidance in understanding and facilitating health-promoting behaviors. Nurses can assist adolescents and their families in the areas of health promotion, disease prevention, and management of common problems by using effective communication strategies, knowledge of normal growth and development, anticipatory guidance, and early identification of potential problems.

### Physical Growth and Development

Physical development during the adolescent years is characterized by dramatic changes in size and appearance. Girls experience budding of the breasts followed by the appearance of pubic hair. Approximately 1 year after breast development, height increases rapidly until reaching its peak (peak height velocity [PHV]). Growth in height in girls typically ceases 2 to 2½ years after menarche.

Boys also experience physical changes, but those changes are not as obvious as in girls. Boys first experience testicular enlargement, followed in approximately 1 year by penile enlargement. Pubic hair usually precedes the growth of the penis. The growth spurt in boys occurs later than it does in girls, beginning between ages 10½ and 16 years and ending between 13½ and 17½ years. Growth continues at a much slower pace for several years after the spurt but usually ceases between 18 and 20 years of age.

Muscle mass increases in boys, and fat deposits increase in girls. Because of greater muscle mass, fully developed adolescent boys tend to be larger and stronger than adolescent girls.

### Psychosexual Development, Hormonal Changes, and Sexual Maturation

The physical development, hormonal changes, and sexual maturation that occur during adolescence correspond to Freud's final stage of psychosexual development, the genital stage (Freud, 1960) (see Chapter 5). The genital stage begins with the production of sex hormones and maturation of the reproductive system. Sexual tension and energy are manifested in the development of sexual relationships with others, and sexual gratification is sought. Freud's theory suggests that personality development is closely related to psychosexual development, with an emphasis on aggressive and sexual impulses as determining factors of personality. Freud's theories about male dominance, sexual repression, and the Oedipus and Electra complexes make the psychosexual theory of development highly controversial even today.

## HEALTH PROMOTION

### *Selected* Healthy People 2020 *Objectives for Adolescents*

| | |
|---|---|
| AH-1 | Increase the proportion of adolescents who have had a wellness checkup in the past 12 months. |
| AH-3 | Increase the proportion of adolescents who are connected to a parent or other positive adult caregiver. |
| AH-5.1 | Increase the proportion of students who graduate with a regular diploma 4 years after starting 9th grade. |
| AH-7 | Reduce the proportion of adolescents who have been offered, sold, or given an illegal drug on school property. |
| AH-11 | Reduce adolescent and young adult perpetration of, as well as victimization by, crimes. |
| ECBP-2 | Increase the proportion of senior high schools that provide comprehensive school health education to prevent health problems in the following areas: unintentional injury; violence; suicide; tobacco use and addiction; alcohol or other drug use; unintended pregnancy, HIV/AIDS, and sexually transmitted diseases (STDs); unhealthy dietary patterns; and inadequate physical activity. |
| FP-8 | Reduce pregnancies among adolescent females. |
| FP-9 | Increase the proportion of adolescents aged 17 years and younger who have never had sexual intercourse. |
| FP-10 & 11 | Increase the proportion of sexually active persons aged 15 to 19 years who use contraception to both effectively prevent pregnancy and provide barrier protection against disease. |
| FP-12 & 13 | Increase the proportion of adolescents who received formal instruction or talked to a parent about reproductive health topics including abstinence, birth control methods, HIV/AIDS prevention, sexually transmitted diseases (STDs) before they were 18 years old. |
| HIV-2, 3, & 4 | Reduce the rate of HIV/AIDS transmission and infection among adolescents. |
| IID-11 | Increase levels of routine vaccination coverage among adolescents. |
| IVP-29 | Reduce homicides. |
| IVP-34 | Reduce physical fighting among adolescents. |
| IVP-35 | Reduce bullying among adolescents. |
| IVP-36 | Reduce weapon carrying by adolescents on school property. |
| IVP-41 | Reduce nonfatal intentional self-harm injuries. |
| NWS-21 | Reduce iron deficiency among young children and females of childbearing age. |
| PA-3 | Increase the proportion of adolescents who meet current federal physical activity guidelines for aerobic physical activity and for muscle-strengthening activity. |
| SA-1 | Reduce the proportion of adolescents who report that they rode, during the previous 30 days, with a driver who had been drinking alcohol. |
| SA-2 & 3 | Increase the proportion of adolescents never using substances and who disapprove of substance use. |
| TU-2 & 3 | Reduce tobacco use by adolescents and reduce the initiation of tobacco use. |

Modified from United States Department of Health and Human Services. (2010). *Healthy People 2020.* Retrieved from https://www.healthypeople.gov.

Girls generally reach physical maturation before boys with the onset and establishment of menstruation (*menarche*). Menarche usually occurs between ages 9 and 15 years; however, recent evidence suggests that the initiation of pubertal development (Tanner 2) is occurring at a younger age than in previous times (Kaplowitz, Bloch, and the American Academy of Pediatrics [AAP] Section on Endocrinology, 2016). Statistical trending demonstrates that development in boys is also occurring earlier (Holland-Hall & Burstein, 2016). Racial and ethnic differences in pubertal onset occur, with black and Hispanic girls beginning puberty before white girls. Other environmental and personal factors, such as being overweight or obese, affect the timing of puberty (Holland-Hall & Burstein, 2016; Kaplowitz et al., 2016). Most young women achieve reproductive maturity 2 to 5 years after the start of menstruation. During the 2 to 5 years before reproductive maturity, the female sex hormones gradually increase, ovulation occurs more frequently, and menstrual periods become more regular.

Ultimately, diet, exercise, and hereditary factors influence adolescents' height, weight, and body build. The earlier onset of puberty has implications for the timing of sex education programs and anticipatory guidance. It also has implications for health issues, such as breast cancer, that have hormonal components.

The physical growth of boys and girls is directly related to sexual maturation and occurs in a relatively predictable sequence. The secretion of sex hormones—estrogen in girls and testosterone in boys—stimulates the development of breast tissue, pubic hair, and genitalia. Hormonal secretion at the time of puberty is the result of a complex regulatory process involving the environment, the central nervous system, the hypothalamus, the pituitary gland, the gonads, and the adrenal glands. Puberty is a biological process that brings about PHV, or the "growth spurt," the changes in body composition, and the development of primary and secondary sexual characteristics in both sexes. Although variable in both sexes, the PHV occurs at approximately age 10 to 11 years in girls and age 13½ years in boys. Table 9.1 describes five distinct stages in a sexual maturity rating (SMR) based on breast and pubic hair development in girls and genital and pubic hair development in boys and includes approximate age ranges for early, middle, and late puberty (Tanner, 1962). The beginning Tanner stages frequently occur in the school-age child, and Tanner stages 3 to 5 occur in adolescence.

In boys, puberty is considered delayed if testicular enlargement or pubic hair development has not occurred by age 14 years. Absence of breast budding or pubic hair development in girls by 13 years is reason for referral. Some of the more common causes of delayed puberty are chronic illnesses, malnutrition, extreme exercise, and hypothyroidism.

## ! NURSING QUALITY ALERT

### *Understanding Tanner Staging*

Knowledge of Tanner staging is essential for nurses to assess normal growth and development and provide adolescents and their parents with anticipatory guidance regarding sexual development. However, nurses must remember that sexual maturation and physical development are highly variable and that Tanner stages may overlap one another. A description of the adolescent's SMR provides greater information about the child's physical development than does chronologic age (age in years).

### Female Sexual Maturation

Sexual maturation in girls begins with the appearance of breast buds (thelarche), which is the first sign of ovarian function. Thelarche occurs at approximately age 8 to 11 years and is followed by the growth of pubic hair. The PHV is reached during thelarche, usually in Tanner stage 2 or 3. Linear growth slows, and menarche begins approximately 1 year after the PHV. As pubic hair increases in amount and becomes dark, coarse, and curly, the axillary hair develops. The apocrine sweat glands reach secretory capacity in Tanner stage 3 or 4. Frequent showers and deodorants become important to the adolescent. With increasing hormonal activity, girls develop a more adult body contour. As breasts mature, the nipples project more, and the pubic hair extends to the medial thighs; the young female is estimated to be at Tanner stage 5. Ovulation may be established, and conception can occur.

**TABLE 9.1 Sexual maturity rating (SMR): Tanner Stages of Adolescent Sexual Development**

**Boys**

| *Stage 1* | *Stage 2* | *Stage 3* | *Stage 4* | *Stage 5* |
|---|---|---|---|---|
| Pubic hair: none | Pubic hair: slight, long, straight, slightly pigmented at the base of the penis | Pubic hair: darker in color, starts to curl, small amount | Pubic hair: coarse, curly, similar to adult but less quantity | Pubic hair: adult distribution spread to inner thighs |
| Penis: preadolescent | Penis: slight enlargement | Penis: longer | Penis: larger, glans and breadth increase in size | Penis: adult in size and shape |
| Testes: preadolescent | Testes: enlarged scrotum, pink, slight alteration in texture | Testes: larger | Testes: larger, scrotum darker | Testes: adult |
| | *Early puberty:* Testes, 9½-13½ years; penis, 10½-14½ years; pubic hair, 12-12½ years | | | |
| | | *Middle puberty:* Testes, 13½-14½ years; penis, 13½-15 years; pubic hair, 12½-14½ years | | |
| | | | *Late puberty:* Testes, 13½-17 years; penis, 13½-16 years; pubic hair, 13½-16½ years | |

**Breast Development in Girls***

| *Stage 1* | *Stage 2* | *Stage 3* | *Stage 4* | *Stage 5* |
|---|---|---|---|---|
| Preadolescent | Breast bud stage (thelarche): breast and papilla elevated as small mound, areolar diameter increased | Breast and areola enlarged, no contour separation | Areola and papilla form secondary mound | Mature, nipple projects, areola part of general breast contour |
| | Early puberty: 9-13 years | | | |
| | | Middle puberty: 12-13 years | | |
| | | | Late puberty: 14-17 years* | |

**TABLE 9.1 Sexual maturity rating (SMR): Tanner Stages of Adolescent Sexual Development—cont'd**

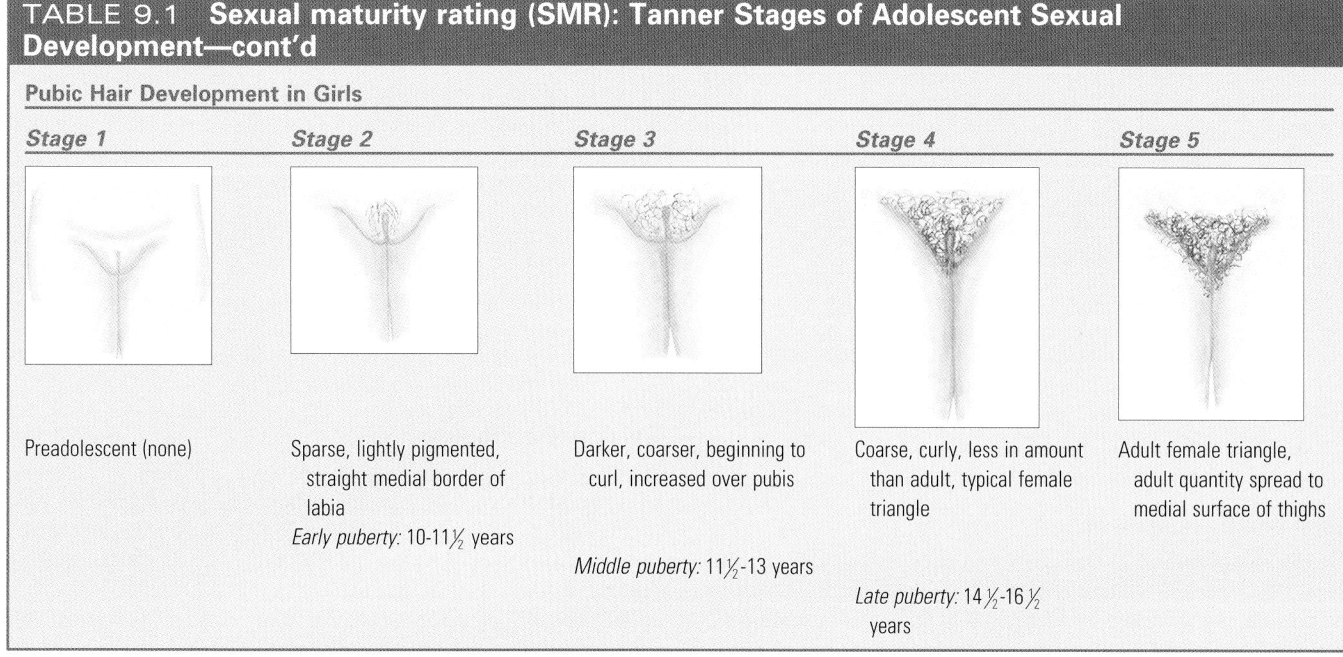

**Pubic Hair Development in Girls**

| *Stage 1* | *Stage 2* | *Stage 3* | *Stage 4* | *Stage 5* |
|---|---|---|---|---|
| Preadolescent (none) | Sparse, lightly pigmented, straight medial border of labia<br>*Early puberty:* 10-11½ years | Darker, coarser, beginning to curl, increased over pubis<br>*Middle puberty:* 11½-13 years | Coarse, curly, less in amount than adult, typical female triangle<br>*Late puberty:* 14½-16½ years | Adult female triangle, adult quantity spread to medial surface of thighs |

Modified from Tanner, J. M. (1962). *Growth at adolescence* (2nd ed.). Oxford: Blackwell Scientific Publications; Marshall, W. A., & Tanner, J. (1969). Variations in pattern of pubertal changes in girls. *Archives of Disease in Childhood, 44*(235), 291–303. Modified with permission from Blackwell Scientific Publications and the BMJ Publishing Group.

*Breast and pubic hair development may continue into late adolescence and may increase with pregnancy.

### Male Sexual Maturation

The first sign of pubertal changes in boys is testicular enlargement in response to testosterone secretion, which usually occurs in Tanner stage 2. Slight pubic hair is present, and the smooth skin texture of the scrotum is somewhat altered. As testosterone secretion increases, the penis, testes, and scrotum enlarge. The PHV usually occurs during Tanner stages 3 and 4, and the voice deepens and "cracks" as the cartilage in the larynx enlarges. Axillary hair develops, and the eccrine and apocrine sweat glands respond to stressful or emotional stimuli. Skin surface bacteria metabolize secretions from the apocrine glands, and body odor develops. *Gynecomastia* (male breast enlargement) occurs in approximately two thirds of young males during early adolescence and may be unilateral or bilateral (Ali & Donohoue, 2016). This phenomenon is often disturbing to boys, and they need considerable reassurance that the breast tissue will decrease over time. During Tanner stages 4 and 5, rising levels of testosterone cause sebaceous glands to enlarge, and excessive sebum may result in acne. The voice continues to deepen, facial hair appears at the corners of the upper lip and chin, and ejaculation may occur. Nurses need to provide anticipatory guidance to adolescent boys regarding involuntary nocturnal emissions of seminal fluid ("wet dreams") and assure them that this occurrence is normal. By Tanner stage 5, genital maturation is complete, spermatogenesis is well established, facial hair is present on the sides of the face, and the male physique is adultlike in appearance. Gynecomastia significantly decreases or disappears, much to the adolescent male's relief.

### Motor Development

Adolescents often engage in various forms of motor activity, from aerobic exercise to football. Motor activities such as sports and dancing provide an outlet for the adolescent's energy, as well as an opportunity for competition, teamwork, and social relationships. Large muscle mass increases in adolescents, and coordination of gross and fine muscle groups improves. With practice, adolescents become more adept at athletics and also at art, music, sewing, and other activities that require fine motor skills. The bones are not completely calcified until after puberty and are still fairly resistant to breaking in the young adolescent. Participants in sports activities should be grouped according to their size and sexual maturity rating rather than their chronologic age. A small, thin, late-maturing boy is less capable of competing with an early maturing, muscular classmate, and injuries are more likely to occur if they are grouped together.

**BOX 9.1 Nursing Goals for Preparticipation Sports Physical Examination**

- Assess the adolescent athlete's general health.
- Identify conditions that could limit participation or predispose to injury.
- Assess the adolescent athlete's physical and psychosocial maturity.
- Determine the athlete's fitness relative to performance requirements.
- Assess legal insurance requirements for participation.
- Provide wellness counseling and anticipatory guidance.

Nurses, particularly school nurses, may be helpful in assessing adolescents' growth and development and counseling them about sports activities in which they can succeed rather than those in which they will meet with physical and psychological failure. Adolescents should have a yearly physical examination and concussion screening if participating in high school athletics (Box 9.1); the school nurse keeps documentation of this matter. Because it is generally superficial, the school sports examination should not substitute for the recommended complete adolescent physical examination with counseling.

The development of the cardiovascular pump plays an essential role in the adolescent's participation in gross motor activities. Cardiopulmonary capacity increases during adolescence and is relatively mature

**SAFETY ALERT**

***The Adolescent Who Is Involved in Athletics***

Adolescents participating in athletics need the following:

- Adequate equipment
- Appropriate training schedules
- Frequent rest periods
- Adequate fluids to prevent injury, dehydration, and exhaustion
- Appropriate removal when concussion is suspected

in the late adolescent. The cardiovascular pump is not as efficient in young adolescents, whose lungs are smaller. Adolescents generally cannot run as fast or as long as young adults. The athlete's aerobic power, body composition, joint flexibility, and strength of skeletal muscles determine physical fitness.

## Cognitive Development

Cognitive development influences every aspect of adolescent psychosocial development. Cognition moves from concrete to abstract to analytical thinking during the three phases of adolescent development. According to Piaget (1969), formal operations, or abstract thinking, characterize the last stage of cognitive development. Early abstract thinking encompasses inductive and deductive reasoning, the ability to connect separate events, and the ability to understand later consequences. Abstract thinking in late adolescence is increasingly logical, and young adults are capable of using scientific reasoning, understanding complex concepts, and using analytic methods. Because of logical reasoning, adolescents are able to differentiate between others' perceptions and their own and to view social situations from a societal perspective.

In a review of adolescent cognitive development, Holland-Hall and Burnstein (2016) state that the brain is still maturing throughout adolescence and beyond, and this maturational process affects cognitive and emotional processing. Increased myelinization of neurons, along with neuromaturation (progressing anteriorly from the posterior to the prefrontal cortex) facilitates impulse control, decision-making skills, the ability to understand consequences of alternative actions, and prioritization (Holland-Hall & Burnstein, 2016). This change allows for increased organization and problem-solving skills, as well as critical thinking. Dansereau, Knight, & Flynn (2013) suggest that adolescent judgment and decision-making capabilities result from the interaction of cognitive maturation and life experiences, as well as analytical thinking and self-regulation. All of these factors, along with emotional influences, can affect adolescent stress and risk-taking behavior. The implications of this finding for nurses are especially relevant to health teaching. Adolescents think in different ways than adults. For example, sex education for ninth graders is quite different from that for college freshmen or adolescents with their first full-time jobs. The college freshman should be able to appreciate the later consequences of sexual behavior, whereas the young adolescent is focused on the here and now. For example, one should ask the ninth grader and the college freshman how an unwanted baby will affect their lives and compare their answers.

For various reasons (including, for example, poor comprehension, lack of education, and chronic substance abuse), some older adolescents remain concrete thinkers. Nurses and educators need to know their audiences and address them appropriately. Nurses may need to help parents learn how to communicate with their teens appropriately. Counseling a group of adolescent substance-abusers may be ineffective if the consequence of their behavior is tied to the future when their thinking is in the present. A professional approach to communicating with teens includes the following:

- Enjoy them.
- Be patient and flexible.
- Know adolescent development; consider how a teen will look to peers.
- Be open to their ideas and opinions and willing to negotiate choices.
- Listen nonjudgmentally, keeping criticism to a minimum.
- Encourage problem solving and mutual decision making.
- Maintain confidentiality.
- Be an advocate, but do not take sides against a parent.
- Explore feelings about healthcare choices, and allow for questions and analysis of healthcare options.

## Sensory Development

Adolescents' eyes and ears are fully developed, and with the exception of refractive errors and occasional minor infections of the eyes, ears, and sinuses, the sensory system remains quite healthy. Myopia occurs in early adolescence, between ages 11 and 13 years, often requiring frequent changes in corrective lenses.

Because of increased participation in competitive sports and outdoor activities, eye injuries are common in adolescence. Boys are more prone to eye injuries than are girls. Adolescents should always be required to wear safety or protective equipment when competing in sports or participating in any activity that may compromise eye safety.

## Language Development

With the acquisition of formal operational thought and adequate intellectual capacity, adolescents are able to understand abstract concepts, process complex thoughts, and express themselves verbally. Adolescents who read extensively are generally more articulate and have a larger vocabulary than those who do not. Social development and self-confidence play a significant role in how well adolescents express themselves verbally to others. Shy, introverted adolescents may have difficulty speaking to a group or members of the opposite sex but may write expressively. Conversely, extroverted, social adolescents who have no trouble with verbal expression may lack the reading and writing skills for effective written communication.

Computer technology has added to the adolescent's avenues for creative expression. Adolescents are capable of expressing ideas in symbols and abstract concepts, and many enjoy interpreting or even developing complex computer programs or applications for mobile phones and electronic devices. Teens may become more proficient with computer technology than their parents. In addition to teaching adolescents basic computer literacy, many high schools have computer clubs where students who excel in computer languages share ideas and knowledge of computer information systems.

Electronic and digital vehicles for communication have affected language communication as well. Social media websites, e-mail, telephone text messaging, instant messaging, blogs, and Twitter all contribute to abbreviated communication techniques, which eliminate not only grammar and sentence construction, but also word construction (e.g., using ur, for you are, or lol, for laughing out loud). Because of safety concerns with young adolescents using the internet and various social media and communication sites, parents need to monitor computer use and investigate whether parental controls, available through some Internet access companies, are appropriate for their child.

Communicating with adolescents sometimes presents a challenge to parents and other adults. Although adolescents are capable of verbal expression, they are also intensely private and may not wish to divulge their thoughts and feelings to others. Developmentally, the verbally expressive 12-year-old may turn into a relatively uncommunicative 14-year-old. Conflict with parents increases tension in communication (see Parents Want to Know box: Communicating with Adolescents).

Nurses who work with adolescents must develop communication skills that include assuring confidentiality, making no assumptions, remaining nonjudgmental, and posing open-ended questions. Questions such as "Tell me about your plans for the future" will glean more information than "Do you plan to go to college?" The question "Do you live with your parents?" makes an assumption about the living situation that could make the adolescent feel uncomfortable. "Describe where you live and who lives with you" gives the adolescent an opportunity to discuss the living situation.

## PARENTS WANT TO KNOW

### *Communicating With Adolescents*

Parents need encouragement to maintain open communication with their teenager while not appearing too intrusive. Inundating adolescents with questions or going through their belongings causes feelings of invasion and a lack of trust. Adolescents get more out of discussions in which they participate than they do out of lectures and are more likely to respond positively to adults who listen and appear interested in what they have to say.

## Psychosocial Development

Identity formation is the major developmental task of adolescence; other tasks include the formation of a sexual and vocational identity and the ability to emancipate oneself from the family or become independent (Fig. 9.1). Energy is focused within the self, and the younger adolescent is described as egocentric or self-absorbed. Frustrated parents often describe teenagers during this phase as self-centered, lazy, or irresponsible. In fact, they just need time to think, concentrate on themselves, and determine who they are going to be. Erikson (1968) described the conflict of this phase of psychosocial development as identity formation versus role confusion; this phase corresponds to Freud's genital stage of psychosexual development (see Chapter 5 for information on developmental theories).

In the transition period from childhood to adulthood, adolescents try new roles and experiment with the environment until they find a role that fits. The phase of experimentation has been termed the *moratorium*, meaning a period of delay granted to someone not yet ready to make more than a tentative commitment (Erikson, 1968). The adolescent's changing interests from year to year illustrate the lack of commitment. Parents may invest in expensive sports equipment or a musical instrument only to find it abandoned after a short time.

The peer group plays an essential role in adolescent identity formation. Teenagers take their cues on appearance, social behavior, and language from the peer group. The peer group serves as a safe haven as adolescents emotionally move away from the family and struggle to determine who they are. The peer group validates acceptable behavior, and teenagers feel secure in trying on new roles with peer-group approval. Teens frequently spend all day with friends in school and all evening rehashing the day's events over the phone or through postings on chat and social media websites (Box 9.2). Changes in the adolescent's body image, psychosocial development, and peer group acceptance are closely related. Early and middle adolescents are particularly audience conscious and feel that they are the focus of everyone's attention. A bad hair day or a blemish may throw the adolescent into despair. Clothing, hairstyles, and material possessions that are accepted by the group become the most important. Nurses counsel parents to negotiate choices with teens but always consider how peers will judge the child.

## ! NURSING QUALITY ALERT

### *The Adolescent and Erikson*

- Identity formation and establishment of autonomy
- Acquisition of abstract reasoning leading to the following:
- Analytic thinking
- Problem solving
- Planning for the future

Identity formation in adolescents of color may present special challenges. Brittian (2012) states that race and or ethnicity identification may complicate identity formation for these adolescents. Interactions with multiple aspects of the physical and social environment are critical for the development of positive or negative identity. Negative environmental attitudes, such as prejudice or discrimination, are risk factors for negative identity formation. Assisting adolescents of color with making connections with positive civil and community organizations or advocacy groups might facilitate positive identity formation in these adolescents (Brittian, 2012).

Early adolescence and middle adolescence are the periods when teens are prone to gang formation and activities. Peer modeling and peer acceptance, being of the utmost importance, lead some adolescents to form gangs that provide a collective identity and give them a sense of belonging. Peer pressure, companionship, and protection are the most frequently reported reasons for joining gangs, particularly those associated with violent or criminal acts.

Early and late adolescence have marked developmental differences. Each age-group has unique reactions to the developmental tasks, which are influenced by the adolescent's cognitive thinking. According to Piaget (1969), adolescent cognition is characterized by the transition from concrete operational thought to formal operational thought, the ability to think logically and use deductive and abstract reasoning (in addition to this chapter, see Chapters 5 through 8). The acquisition of formal operational thinking allows the adolescent to recall past experience and to apply knowledge to the future by drawing logical consequences from a set of observations. Adolescents are capable of using abstract symbols such as those derived from higher-order mathematics, making and testing hypotheses, and considering and arguing philosophic issues. Problem-solving and decision-making skills become more highly developed, although adolescents may still be conflicted about idealism versus reality.

### Early Adolescence

The early adolescent (11 to 14 years) has intense feelings about body image and the many physical changes taking place. Less confident with members of the opposite sex, early adolescents tend to group together and have best friends of the same sex. One has only to visit the local mall or a movie theater to see groups of young teens of the same sex, observing but rarely speaking to groups of the opposite sex.

The early adolescent is quite egocentric and may move from obedience to rebellion regarding parental authority. Parents are often shocked by the sudden turn of events and are hurt by the teen's rejection. Providing parents with anticipatory guidance regarding age-specific developmental changes is a primary nursing function. For example, the happy-go-lucky 11-year-old may turn into the shy, self-absorbed 12-year-old who seems comfortable only in the presence of

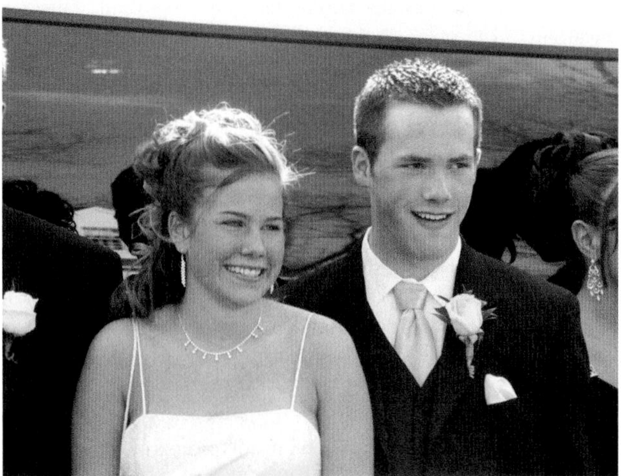

Relationships with the opposite sex are more mature by late adolescence. Late adolescents have more realistic expectations of both themselves and those who are important to them. They devote many hours and much anxious thought to making events, such as prom night, memorable for a lifetime. Some adolescents may be left out because they are unpopular or shy or do not have the financial resources to participate in these special events.

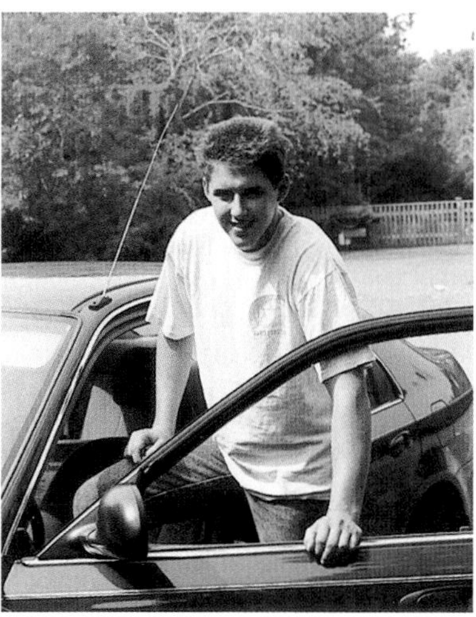

With the freedom driving brings to the adolescent comes responsibility. The adolescent's inexperience and risk-taking behaviors can be a lethal combination.

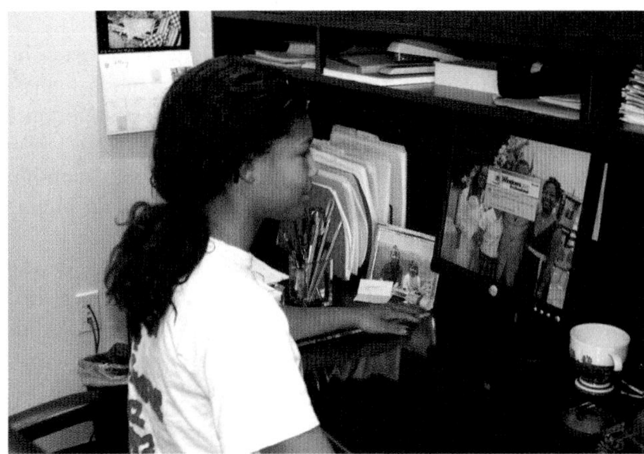

Computers in school and in many homes provide the adolescent with opportunities for learning, creative expression, communication, and entertainment. Adolescents often enjoy "surfing" the Internet, which can provide them with information not readily available locally. Parents must monitor their adolescent's computer connections; however, various social networking sites sometimes allow access to people and activities that conflict with family values.

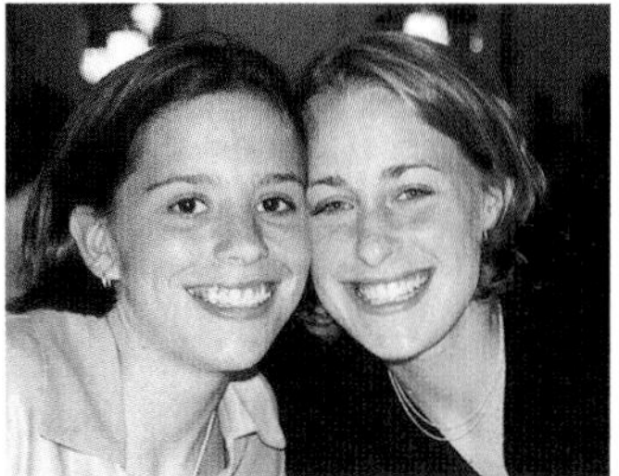

Although teens often have friends of both sexes, they are more comfortable sharing their hopes, dreams, secrets, and even embarrassing incidents with friends of the same sex.

**FIG 9.1** Adolescent Growth and Development.

## BOX 9.2 Age-Related Activities and Games for Adolescents

**General Activities**

Games and athletics are the most common forms of play.

Strict rules are in place.

Competition is important.

**Games and Special Types of Play**

Sports, videos, movies, reading, parties, hobbies, listening to favorite music, experimenting with makeup and hairstyles, talking on the telephone or cell phone, playing computer games, participating in social media discourse.

friends. Young teens, who are developmentally egocentric, fail to differentiate between how others see them and their own mental preoccupations, thinking everyone is as obsessed with them as they are with themselves. Elkind (1993) describes this phenomenon as a reaction to the imaginary audience. The belief in the imaginary audience is probably why young teens are so self-conscious; they believe everyone is critical of them, and indeed teens are quite critical of one another, especially those who are different. Self-conscious behavior may also be the result of the physical and emotional transition to middle adolescence. The early adolescent is losing the familiar role of the child but does not yet feel comfortable with the role of the adult. Ambivalence toward independence is common, and the teen who feels too grown up for a good-night kiss from a parent still falls asleep with a favorite teddy bear.

Elkind (1993) believes that because young teens are so audience conscious, they see themselves as unique and tell themselves a "personal fable" that supports feelings of invulnerability. They believe bad things will happen to others but not to them. Adolescent suicide attempts, for example, serve as a dramatic message to others, but young teens often do not realize the final consequences of their actions.

### Middle Adolescence

Middle adolescence (15 to 17 years) is often described by parents as the most frustrating period of adolescent development. The real audience gradually replaces the imaginary audience, and teens become even more introspective and narcissistic. Conformity to peer-group norms becomes even more important, and conflicts between teenagers and parents often escalate. Testing of limits, sulky withdrawal, and overt rebellion may occur over conflicts regarding curfews, friends, activities, appearance, cars, and money.

The adolescent may feel more secure by associating with or becoming a member of a gang (Box 9.3). Research suggests that youths, especially youths of color, who are gang members go through a transition between early and middle adolescence, where optimism and hope about achieving future goals can evolve into despair when faced with the reality of the consequences of gang membership (Morris & Fry-McComish, 2012). In some instances, gang members begin to accept the fact that what they want for themselves and their families may not be achievable without engagement in illegal activities (Morris & Fry-McComish, 2012). Additionally, adolescents who have been exposed to, or victims of, gang violence can exhibit mental health issues, such as anxiety or post-traumatic stress syndrome, secondary to fears for their safety (Kelly et al., 2012). When working with gang members, it is particularly important that nurses consider the risk for suicide (Morris & Fry-McComish, 2012).

In general, nurses who work with adolescents counsel parents to negotiate choices when possible and set limits that are perceived as reasonable by the adolescent. Consistent discipline and structure actually make adolescents feel more secure and assists them with decision making. With parental guidance, adolescents are able to make decisions that will result in desirable outcomes. However, adults must keep in mind that middle adolescents are impulsive and impatient. Parental concern may be seen as interference rather than guidance and may be met with resistance and resentment.

Feelings about self-image and social relationships are intense. Middle adolescence is generally a time of transition from same-sex friendships to an extreme interest in the opposite sex; it is also a time when adolescents may acknowledge homosexual feelings. The proportion of teens who are sexually experienced and sexually active has declined slightly, as has the teen birth rate (Centers for Disease Control and Prevention [CDC], 2015a; National Center for Health Statistics [NCHS], 2016). Nurses and other healthcare providers cannot become complacent in response to this change in trends. In a recent survey by the CDC (2016c), 3.9% of adolescents reported initiating sexual intercourse before age 13 years, and 41.2% of the ninth through twelfth graders surveyed had had sexual intercourse at least once. Of concern is the trend for early initiation of sexual intercourse.

Sexual activity is often related to peer pressure and self-esteem issues. Adolescents with low self-esteem are more vulnerable and are more apt to engage in negative risk-taking activities associated with sexuality. Decisions about sexual activity are often impulsive and made with little regard to later consequences or previous preparation. In fact, according to the 2015 Youth Risk Behavior Surveillance Survey (YRBSS) (CDC, 2016c), of the teenagers who reported being currently sexually active, 43.1% reported they did not use a condom at last intercourse.

Another concerning trend among adolescents is the participation in oral sex. Recent reports of national statistics suggest that the prevalence of oral sex among adolescents 15 to 19 years old is 45% in girls and 48% in boys (Copen & Chandra, 2012). Questions about oral sexual activity are not currently included in the YRBSS. Adolescents intend to have oral sex for various reasons, but primarily because they believe it is more socially acceptable than vaginal intercourse and does not carry the same risks (Copen & Chandra, 2012). Although many adolescents may know that various sexually transmitted diseases (STDs) can be contracted from engaging in oral sex, they, nevertheless, do not consider oral sex to be as risky as vaginal sex.

Nurses and other health professionals who assess adolescent health status need to be more specific when interviewing adolescents about sexual activity. The question of whether an adolescent is sexually active is no longer sufficient; questions should be directed toward assessing participation in various specific types of sexual activity as well as the method of barrier protection used. Nurses may help by providing accurate information to assist adolescents in making appropriate sexual choices. Parents need encouragement to maintain open communication and guide teenagers in sexual decision making. Providing parental guidance about sexual behavior is not easy during middle adolescence, when privacy is of extreme importance and communication with parents tends to decrease. In addition, some parents may find sexual behavior a difficult topic to discuss and often avoid talking with teens about sexual issues altogether.

***Vocational exploration.*** In the initial stages of establishing a vocational identity, adolescents are more likely to experience role confusion and have unrealistic expectations of themselves. Some adolescents identify a role that holds their interest, whereas others experiment with many roles, moving quickly from one role to another. Overidentification with glamorous roles takes precedence over reality and is enriched by daydreams and fantasy. A 15-year-old girl may spend time with her

#### BOX 9.3 Signs of Gang Involvement

- Associating with new friends while ignoring old friends. The adolescent usually will not talk about the new friends or what they do together.
- A change in hairstyle or clothing and associating with other youths with the same style. Usually some of the clothing, such as a hat or jacket, has the gang's colors, initials, or "street" name on it. Parents may note tattoos on the body.
- Unexplained source of money or possessions (e.g., stereos, jewelry, cars).
- Indications of drug, alcohol, or inhalant abuse (e.g., paint or correction fluid on the clothes, the smell of chemicals on the breath or clothes).
- Change in attitude toward activities such as sports, Scouting, or church. Discipline problems at school, in public, or at home. Youth no longer accepts parents' authority and challenges it frequently.
- Problems at school, such as failing classes, skipping school, and causing problems in class.
- Fear of the police.
- Unexplained signs of fighting, such as bruises, cuts, and reports of pain.
- Graffiti on or around residence or possessions.
- Threats from rival gang members. Sometimes a family member is a victim of a drive-by shooting before the family realizes the youth is involved in a gang.

**! NURSING QUALITY ALERT**

***Elements of Adolescent Care***

Nurses working with middle adolescents need to:
- Be approachable
- Maintain objectivity
- Encourage confidence
- Support parental authority
- Be a child advocate while not coming between adolescents and their parents
- Encourage the family to work as a mutually respectful unit

friends describing her future as a popular media star while failing to fold the laundry or do the dishes.

During middle adolescence, some teens acquire part-time jobs and identify various skills and interests. Part-time jobs are often a source of income for material possessions and activities not provided by parents. Such experiences help adolescents set realistic expectations about work, become more independent, and develop self-esteem. Those who are successful in the working world demonstrate a sense of responsibility and tend to have more positive social interactions. However, some adolescents may allow work to interfere with educational activity and have difficulty setting priorities. School nurses, in collaboration with parents and teachers, are in an excellent position to identify working students and assist them in setting realistic guidelines for both education and work.

### Late Adolescence (18 to 21 Years)

Late adolescence is characterized by the ability to think abstractly, conceptualize verbally, and express thoughts and feelings about various aspects of life. Late adolescents tend to be idealistic about love, social issues, ethics, and lifestyles until their experiences modify their beliefs. Conformity becomes less important as teens progress through late adolescence. With the development of a unique identity, self-esteem increases, and adolescents are able to resist group pressure if it is not in their best interest. Interactions with parents are less turbulent unless values clash, and relationships with both friends and family are maintained.

Emancipation (leaving home) is a major issue; late adolescents prepare themselves to meet this task through education or vocational training. Identifying realistic career goals is important, but many adolescents are not yet ready to make lifelong commitments. Changing career goals is not uncommon, but the nurse should watch for those adolescents who have set no career goals, who demonstrate apathy about the future, and who appear committed only to the present. Boredom and apathy are often symptoms of a greater problem: depression.

Social relationships are more mature, although partner selection often continues to fluctuate. Friendships developed in late adolescence may last a lifetime, and expectations of friends and loved ones become more realistic and less self-serving. The ability to consider others' needs increases, and recognition of societal needs is more apparent as the adolescent moves from adolescence to adulthood.

Failure to achieve identity formation may leave adolescents in role confusion and impede the successful mastery of the tasks of young adulthood. A positive ego identity depends on the adolescent's ability to accept the past, learn from experience, and become engaged in the future. Most adolescents move through the identity versus role confusion stage of development with minimal difficulty.

### Moral and Spiritual Development

Children develop moral reasoning in a sequential manner, as described by American psychologist Lawrence Kohlberg (1964). As adolescents move from concrete to analytic thinking, they advance to Kohlberg's stage 4 conventional level or Kohlberg's stage 5 postconventional level of moral development. Adolescents who remain concrete thinkers may never advance beyond Kohlberg's stage 3 of moral reasoning: conformity to please others and avoid punishment. The teenager's sense of justice is developed through interpersonal relationships with peers, family, and other adult role models. Behaviors that are modeled and rewarded, such as helping the less fortunate and showing loyalty to friends, contribute to the development of a conscience, which operates as a moral guide for subsequent behavior. For example, the middle to late teenager can appreciate that stealing from others is wrong regardless of whether one is caught and punished.

Adolescents and young adults develop a respect for law and order and a society-maintaining orientation (Kohlberg's stage 4). Young adults may even advance to the societal-perspective stage (Kohlberg's stage 5), which honors the moral rules of right and wrong, contractual agreements, majority opinion, and overall utility or the greatest good for the greatest number (see Chapter 5).

Older adolescents and young adults question the values of family and society and challenge existing moral codes before integrating their experiences and beliefs into a personal moral framework. Once the moral framework is developed, interpersonal relationships tend to be with those whose values and beliefs are similar.

Young adolescents in the stage of concrete operational thought are able to think logically. In this stage, children deal well with the observable but also begin to see other points of view and examine what they have learned. The young adolescent will accept religious teaching and examine how religious concepts relate to everyday life. Young adolescents are especially inclined to look to God for guidance when troubled.

Middle to late adolescents are capable of analytic thought and may begin to question the religious affiliation of the family, much as they question other family values. Older adolescents may explore different kinds of religion and share religious activities with the peer group.

Evidence suggests that spirituality has a positive effect on health-related quality of life and holistic wellness in adolescents (Spurr, Berry, & Walker, 2013; Wen, 2014). Spirituality may also be protective against engagement in high risk behaviors (Michaelson, Robinson, & Pickett, 2014). As part of providing holistic nursing care, nurses need to include an assessment of spiritual beliefs and values when working with adolescents and incorporate these values in nursing interventions.

## HEALTH PROMOTION FOR THE ADOLESCENT AND FAMILY

Adolescence is generally a period of wellness. Young people may seek healthcare for school or sports physicals, skin conditions (acne, contact dermatitis), acute minor illnesses (colds, flu), conditions related to sexuality (birth control, pregnancy, sexually transmitted diseases [STDs]), and the management of chronic illness (diabetes, epilepsy). Health promotion and disease prevention are achieved through adequate nutrition, rest, balanced exercise, and proper immunization against disease. It is important for adolescents to receive regular well care, as unmet health needs during adolescence can contribute to less than optimal health in adulthood (Hargreaves et al., 2015). Reasons that adolescents do not seek healthcare include concerns about confidentiality, not believing that preventive health is important, problems with access, belief that care is only necessary when ill, and cost (Aalsma, Gilbert, Xiao, et al, 2016; Hargreaves et al., 2015). Some adolescents may believe that their annual sports physical examination is sufficient.

During well visits for health promotion, adolescents confer privately with the nurse and the health provider; separately, parents are asked about any concerns they might have. Confidentiality is often an issue when adolescents are seen in the healthcare setting. Nurses should encourage adolescents to involve their parents, but adolescents frequently ask that communication be kept confidential. The adolescent must understand that the nurse will respect this confidentiality unless the information shared suggests a potentially life-threatening danger either to the adolescent or to others.

### CRITICAL THINKING EXERCISE 9.1

The nurse is caring for a 15-year-old girl, Heidi, who has been admitted to the hospital with dehydration. She is quiet and answers questions with a simple "yes" or "no." On the day Heidi is to be discharged, she says, "I'll tell you something, but you can't tell anyone else."

1. What factors must the nurse consider in this situation?
2. What would be the nurse's best response?

Adolescents need to be directly asked questions about their health. These include questions about diet and exercise, sexual risk behavior, substance use, preventive safety measures (e.g., seat belt, bicycle helmet, protective sports equipment), violence, peer and family relationships, and emotional health. The American Academy of Pediatrics [AAP] (2016) and the U.S. Preventive Services Task Force [USPSTF] (Siu & USPSTF, 2016) recommend routine screening for depression beginning at the age of 12 years. Both the Beck Depression Inventory and Patient Health Questionnaire for Adolescents can identify adolescents at risk for mental health problems (Siu & USPSTF, 2016). Some providers publically display their policy on confidentiality, always underlining the need to share information only if someone is in danger. Issues related to the time necessary for an adequate interview may arise in the current managed care environment. Nurses should be knowledgeable about communicating with adolescents and aware of when referral is warranted.

Access to regular quality healthcare for adolescents has become an issue of increasing concern because of its importance in preventing illness related to adolescent risk behavior. Regular health promotion visits to a provider during adolescence facilitates comprehensive health screening, preventive intervention, counseling, and referral. Many adolescents and their parents perceive the yearly sports physical as being sufficient. However, this physical, often performed by a school physician, is not comprehensive enough to identify subtle problems, nor is it likely to provide time for confidential communication of adolescent concerns to the provider (AAP Committee on Adolescence, 2008/2013). For this reason, the AAP Committee on Adolescence (2008/2013) recommends that access to comprehensive healthcare for adolescents be widely available in various venues that include school-based health clinics, physicians' offices, community or public health clinics, and hospitals. Recent evidence suggests that adolescents who are enrolled in a patient-centered medical home receive more comprehensive preventive services than those who access other models of care (Garcia-Huidobro, Shippee, DiCaprio, et al., 2016). In addition, the Committee on Adolescence recommends offering assurance of confidentiality, comprehensive services, care that is culturally and ethnically relevant, and health insurance coverage for all adolescents (AAP Committee on Adolescence, 2008/2013).

## Nutrition During Adolescence

The accelerated growth (in linear height, weight, and muscle mass) and sexual maturation during adolescence increase teenagers' nutritional needs, including that for protein, calories, zinc, calcium, and iron. Periods of intense growth require increased caloric intake, and the adolescent appears constantly hungry. Snacks and regular meals need to contain adequate nutrients to meet the body's anabolic needs. Adolescents are generally interested in nutrition and the effect food has on their bodies. Teenagers tend to be concerned about their weight, complexion, sexual development, and acceptance by their peers. These issues, together with the adolescent's growing independence, can have nutritional implications.

### Age-Related Nutritional Challenges

The adolescent's food habits are influenced by many factors (Box 9.4). Unfortunately, this happens at a time when the body has greater nutritional needs. Boys tend to have fewer nutritional deficiencies than girls because they take in more food and are less likely to be dieting. Soft drinks frequently replace milk. Fast foods and low-nutrient "junk foods" sometimes become the mainstay of the adolescent's diet. The social aspect of food consumption gains importance, and adolescents may prefer to eat meals with peers at social gatherings and restaurants of their choice. Parental supervision of meals declines as the adolescent spends more time away from home and engages in extracurricular activities with peers.

### Nutritional Guidance for the Adolescent

The nurse needs to understand growth and development to be successful in counseling adolescents and their parents about nutrition. Adolescents' increasing need to be independent and make their own choices should guide the nurse in teaching nutrition. The adolescent should always be involved in the planning.

The nurse should assess the adolescent's present diet and determine habits and eating patterns. The assessment should elicit how often the adolescent eats food from the different food groups and what foods the adolescent does not eat. Based on this information, nutritious foods for meals can be identified and a plan developed. Depending on physical activity level, the U.S. Department of Health and Human Services [USDHHS] and U.S. Department of Agriculture (USDA) (2015) recommend 1800 to 2000 calories/day for adolescent girls and 2000 to 2800 calories/day for adolescent boys, with foods coming from a variety of food groups—whole grains, fruits and vegetables, dairy, and protein (plant and animal). Adolescents should drink at least three cups of milk a day, limit fats to 25% to 35% of total daily calories consumed, and avoid added sugars (no more than 10% total daily calories. Adolescents need calcium and vitamin D to prevent future

### BOX 9.4 Factors Influencing the Adolescent's Diet

- Busy schedule (sports, activities, jobs)
- Body image concerns, which can lead to undereating
- Skipping breakfast
- Eating away from home
- Eating fast food frequently
- Beginning to buy and prepare own food
- Peer pressure
- Psychological and emotional problems

osteoporosis, and adolescent girls require adequate iron and folic acid (400 mcg/day from supplements or folic-acid–fortified foods) (USDHHS & USDA, 2015). Recently, the use of so-called energy drinks has increased in the adolescent population. These drinks contain large amounts of caffeine, along with glucose and other, non-regulated, substances. In addition to the danger from excessive caffeine and increased sugar intake, evidence suggests that regular consumption of energy drinks is related to increase risk-taking in the adolescent population (Arria, Bugbee, Caldeira, et al., 2014).

The nurse can also assist the adolescent by pointing out nutritious fast foods and snacks. An awareness of nutritious fast foods can also aid the adolescent in meal selection. Many fast-food chains have salads with nonfat or low-fat dressings, grilled chicken sandwiches, pasta, and nonfat yogurt. Fat and salt contents have been reduced, and vegetable fats have replaced animal fats at some restaurants. Adolescents should be guided to mix an occasional hamburger and fries with a regular selection of more nutritious foods. Permission should be given to eat foods that may be untraditional at a particular meal, such as pizza for breakfast.

Many adolescents decide to follow a vegetarian diet during their teen years. Several dietary organizations have suggested that a vegetarian diet, if correctly followed, is healthy for this population because the low-fat aspect of the diet can prevent future cardiovascular problems (Parks et al., 2016). If an adolescent wishes to follow a vegetarian diet, the nurse can assist with planning food choices that will provide sufficient calories and necessary nutrients. The focus is on obtaining sufficient calories for growth and energy through a variety of fruits and vegetables, whole grains, nuts, legumes, seeds, tofu, and soy milk; some vegetarians choose to eat eggs and dairy products as well. Vegetarian diets may be calcium- and Vitamin-D–deficient, so it is important to ensure intake of these nutrients through dark leafy vegetables and fortified drinks (Parks et al., 2016). As with any adolescent, nurses advise those who follow a vegetarian eating plan to avoid low-nutrient, high-fat foods.

Body image is of particular importance to adolescents. The media reinforce the belief that "thin is in." Adolescents hold themselves to standards set by the entertainment and advertising worlds, which emphasize fitness, glamour, and sexuality. Products that promise a quick weight loss or enhanced muscle mass with a lean physique are appealing to adolescents. Weight management techniques may include fasting, diet pills and laxatives, self-induced vomiting, and fad diets instead of low-fat, low-calorie, nutritionally sound diets and more aerobic exercise. Adolescents may not realize that unsound nutritional habits often follow them for a lifetime or that growth and development may be delayed or permanently impaired. School nurses are in an excellent position to identify adolescents who have nutritional problems or eating disorders and provide counseling or referral for adolescents and their families (see Chapter 53).

## Hygiene

Adolescents in general are meticulous about personal hygiene. However, a major concern is acne. Acne contributes to adolescent self-consciousness and, if severe, to decreased self-image. Nursing interventions to address acne are discussed in detail in Chapter 49.

## Dental Care

The incidence of dental caries decreases in adolescence, but dental hygiene remains important. Most permanent teeth have erupted, with the possible exception of the third molars (wisdom teeth), which erupt by late adolescence or remain impacted and may be removed surgically. The AAP (2014a) recommends continuing oral fluoride supplements until the adolescent reaches 16 years, if no access to fluoridated water. Several dental conditions are prevalent during the adolescent years: gingivitis, malocclusion, and dental trauma. Gingivitis is the inflammation and breakdown of the gingival epithelium; the gums appear pale and swollen and bleed easily. Increased hormonal activity at the time of puberty, diets high in sugar and simple carbohydrates, and the use of dental braces and appliances that make cleaning less effective are thought to contribute to the development of gingivitis.

Malocclusion (improper contact) occurs in approximately 50% of adolescents because of facial and mandibular bone growth and dental crowding. Treatment varies but generally entails dental devices such as braces to correct tooth position and redirect facial growth. Adolescents may be self-conscious if their peers are no longer in braces and may need reassurance that the condition is temporary. For economic reasons, some adolescents are unable to undergo correction of malocclusions and suffer the consequences indefinitely. Nurses can help by referring adolescents with no dental care to free clinics or agencies providing dental care at low cost. People with uncorrected malocclusions are at greater risk for dental trauma. Caring for the teeth and gums is critical to prevent dental caries associated with the orthodontic appliance. The child needs to floss and brush frequently; using a water flosser might be easier to manage than other flossing devices.

A tooth that has been completely knocked out of the mouth (avulsed) can sometimes be reimplanted. The sooner the reimplantation occurs, the greater is the likelihood of success. The prognosis is best if the injury is treated within 30 minutes. School and clinic nurses may be the first health professionals to see a child with a complete tooth avulsion and should be aware of the proper procedure (see Chapter 34). Parents should also know how to care for their child if such an incident occurs (see the Patient-Centered Teaching box: Caring for a Child with an Avulsed Tooth).

### PATIENT-CENTERED TEACHING

#### *Caring for a Child With an Avulsed Tooth*

If an avulsed tooth can be recovered, it should be touched only by the crown and placed in saline, milk, or a commercial tooth-preserving liquid. The tooth should not be scrubbed, and cleaning agents and disinfectants should be avoided. The child should be seen as soon as possible by a dentist or taken to the emergency department.

## Sleep and Rest

Along with increasingly independent activities, adolescents show a propensity for staying up late (particularly if working on a school project or attending a weekend party) and having difficulty waking up in the morning. Setting one's own bedtime and sleeping late on weekends are behaviors associated with gaining independence but may result in the adverse effects of decreased amounts of sleep. Hours of sleep may vary from 6 to 8 hours during the week to 12 hours on the weekends, but an overall average of 8 to 9 hours per night is recommended for adolescents and young adults. Nearly three quarters of adolescents report sleeping fewer than eight hours a night (CDC, 2016c). Babcock (2011) suggests that adolescents are more often than not in a state of sleep deprivation. Contributing factors include hectic after-school activities that postpone homework until late at night, electronic devices in the adolescent's bedroom, and the need to socialize late into the night. Effects of sleep deprivation include fatigue (including falling asleep in classes), distracted attention, poor school performance, and other physiologic and psychologic adverse effects (George & Davis, 2013).

Rapid physical growth and increased activities contribute to the adolescent's fatigue, and frustrated parents may complain that their teenager has energy for everything but household and family chores. Nurses can educate teens and their parents to set realistic schedules that allow time for adequate rest and relaxation. Some teens may find themselves so overscheduled that they develop sleep disturbances from excess fatigue and anxiety. Adult sleep cycles are formed during adolescence, and sleep disturbances continue into the adult years.

## HEALTH PROMOTION

### *The Adolescent*

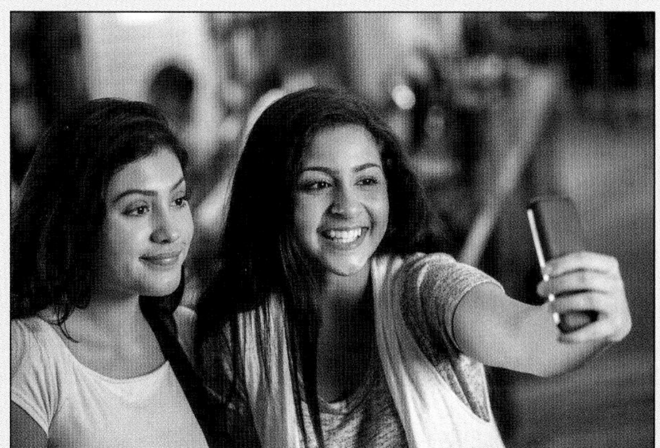

(© 2016, Getty Images. Reprinted with Permission.)

#### Focused Assessment

Ask the adolescent the following:

- Can you tell me how often and what foods you like to eat? How often do you eat at fast-food restaurants? How do you feel about how much you weigh and the shape of your body? Do you think you need to gain or lose any weight? Do you try to control your weight by making yourself vomit, by taking diet pills or laxatives, or by exercising too much?
- Can you describe how much physical activity and what kinds of physical activity you participate in daily?
- How often do you brush your teeth, floss, and see the dentist? What time do you go to bed at night? What time do you get up in the morning? Do you have any trouble falling asleep, or do you wake up in the middle of the night?
- How often do you have a bowel movement? Are there any problems with urination?
- What grade in school are you? How well do you think you are doing in school? Do any circumstances at school make you feel unsafe or threatened?
- Tell me about your friends. What types of enjoyable activities do you do together? Do your friends pressure you to do things you would rather not do? Do you or your friends smoke cigarettes or e-cigarettes, or take any substances (alcohol, drugs)?
- Tell me about your relationship with other members of your family. Do you have a special family member to talk to if you are having a problem? If so, whom?
- Do you do any or all of the following: use a seatbelt every time you get in a car; refuse to get into a car if the driver has been drinking or taking drugs; avoid talking on a cell phone or texting while driving; wear a helmet every time you ride a bicycle or motorcycle; wear a helmet and protective pads every time you skate; use sunscreen; swim with a buddy; protect yourself by not putting your personal information on social media websites (e.g., Twitter, Facebook, gaming sites) or reveal it to others in chat rooms or blogs?
- Has anyone ever physically harmed you or touched you in a way that made you uncomfortable? Have you ever thought about harming yourself? Do you or does anyone you know own a gun?
- Have you begun dating? Have you been or are you sexually active? (If sexually active, ask about condom use and birth control methods and any incidence of sexually transmitted diseases [STDs].) Do you have any questions or concerns about your sexual development (ask girls about the pattern and frequency of menstruation)?
- What kind of job do you have, if any? How many hours per week do you work?
- What kinds of things do you do to stay healthy? Do you regularly take any medications or dietary supplements? Do you regularly perform breast or testicular self-examinations? Do you have any concerns about any aspect of your health?

Ask the parent the following:

- Do you have any concerns related to your adolescent's nutrition, body image, physical activity, oral health, sleep, elimination, school, family interactions, self-esteem, or ability to practice safety precautions?
- Do you have any family history of heart problems or stroke; has anyone in your family had a heart attack or stroke at a young age (younger than 55 years for men or 65 years for women) (AAP, 2011)?
- Do you continue to stay involved in your child's life?
- What types of family rules do you consistently enforce?

#### Developmental Milestones

*Personal/social:* Experiences emotional and social turmoil associated with rapid changes in development and altered body image; is interested in opposite-sex relationships (some lead to a level of intimacy for which the adolescent is not ready); assumes varying roles to integrate social skills with new aspirations and to gain a sense of self; clarifies values and career directions; has more stable emotional control in later adolescence; may exhibit imaginary audience ("Everyone is staring at me") or personal fable ("It will never happen to me")

*Fine motor:* Adult fine motor control

*Language/cognitive:* Becomes future oriented; views the world in broad perspective; hypothesizes several alternatives to a problem; thinks and reasons abstractly; develops moral reasoning

*Gross motor:* Early growth-related awkwardness develops into coordinated muscle control

#### Health Maintenance

##### *Physical Measurements*

Girls achieve peak height velocity (PHV) approximately 2 years before boys

Average weight gain during growth spurt is 50% of adult weight, largely from body fat in girls and muscle mass in boys

Average height gain is 20% to 25% of adult height over a 2- to 3-year period (girls, 8.3 cm/year; boys, 9.4 cm/year)

Achieve Tanner stage 5 (see Table 9.1)

Compute and plot body mass index (BMI)

##### *Immunizations (CDC, 2016b)*

Review immunization records; administer immunizations if not up to date

Administer tetanus-diphtheria-pertussis (Tdap) at age 11 to 12 years.

Meningococcal conjugate vaccine at age 11 to 12 years. Administer a booster dose at age 16 years.

Human papillomavirus (HPV) vaccine—recommended at 11 to 12 years old for girls and boys (three doses—give second dose 2 months after the first; give third dose 6 months after the first)

Influenza vaccine annually

*Continued*

## HEALTH PROMOTION—cont'd

### *The Adolescent*

**Health Screening**

Objective hearing and vision screening (adolescent may become myopic as growth spurt begins)
Scoliosis screening
Hemoglobin or hematocrit
Urinalysis by dipstick
Blood pressure
Fasting lipid screen at 11 years and if at risk
Tuberculosis (TB) screening if at risk (see Chapter 45)
Sexually transmissible disease risk assessment with screening if applicable; HIV screening at 16 to 18 years (AAP, 2016)
Emotional and stress screening

**Anticipatory Guidance**

Provide anticipatory guidance and counseling to address concerns. Educate particularly about avoidance of smoke exposure and refer, if necessary, for tobacco cessation (AAP, 2011).

**Nutrition**

Follow recommended servings according to the USDA's Choose MyPlate website; teach the adolescent how to keep track of servings and give input into meal preparation
Advise to avoid fast foods and eat a nutritious breakfast; watch calcium and iron intake; assess adequacy of diet and snacks; recommend folic acid supplementation for adolescent girls
Vitamin D supplementation 400 IU/day if consuming less than 1 L (33 oz) per day of milk and vitamin-D–fortified foods
Teach principles of a vegetarian diet if applicable
Avoid caffeine-containing energy drinks

**Elimination**

Regular bowel movements according to individual pattern

**Dental**

Provide regular dental care every 6 months
Continue regular flossing and brushing with fluoride toothpaste
Supplemental fluoride until age 16 years if no access to fluoridated water
Discuss emergency care for fractured or avulsed teeth (see the Patient-Centered Teaching box: Caring for a Child with an Avulsed Tooth)

**Sleep and Activity**

Facilitate an individually appropriate sleep pattern; adolescent usually needs 8 hours
Recommend increasing planned physical activity to at least 1 hour a day of moderate to vigorous exercise and bone strengthening exercises three times a week

**Safety**

Review gun safety; automobile and motorized vehicle driver and passenger safety; water safety; sun protection; fire safety; avoiding listening to loud music through earphones
Discuss techniques to combat violence, particularly dating violence; wear protective equipment in the workplace; no drinking and driving; preventing STDs and pregnancy (if applicable); learn cardiopulmonary resuscitation (CPR)

**Emotional Health**

Tell another if concerned about a friend
Take every threat of suicide as real
Try to resist peer pressure
Learn stress-reduction techniques
Seek help if depressed or angry

Persistent difficulty in falling asleep, wakefulness during the night, and early waking may be signs of emotional problems associated with tension, anxiety, or depression and may warrant referral.

Several studies have suggested that adolescents' sleep patterns can interfere with their academic performance because the interaction between natural circadian sleep rhythm and social activities makes them less alert in the early morning (Carskadon, 2011). These findings have implications for schools in terms of scheduling start times and planning tests for high school students. School districts in various sections of the country are beginning to address this issue by looking at later start times.

Nurses can assist adolescents in obtaining sufficient sleep by providing information about sleep at each well visit. Encourage adolescents to maintain a routine bedtime and awakening schedule, avoid caffeine intake before bed, and shut down all electronic devices except for playing quiet music.

## Exercise and Activity

Although adolescents are often involved in many activities, these activities do not always promote physical fitness. One goal of *Healthy People 2020* is to increase physical activity in children of all ages. Surveys reveal that only 27.1% of adolescents meet the recommended levels of participation in regular exercise (60 minutes of mostly aerobic exercise daily), and 53.4% allocate three times a week for both muscle and bone-strengthening exercise (CDC, 2016c). Regular exercise enhances physical and emotional development and promotes healthy sleep patterns. Healthy diet and exercise habits formed during adolescence can follow into adulthood and significantly reduce the risk of cardiovascular disease.

Adolescence is an ideal time to initiate an exercise program, either as a team sport or as an individual activity. Exercise need not always involve an athletic activity but should provide for a program that gradually increases exercise over a 1- to 3-week period with a goal of vigorous exercise of at least 60 minutes daily to enhance cardiovascular fitness (USDHHS & USDA, 2015). Nurses can assist adolescents in designing an exercise program that allows gradual fitness and provides warm-up and cool-down sessions. Exercise programs are highly personal and should be structured for enjoyment, with consideration of physical capabilities and limitations.

## Safety

Injuries claim more lives during adolescence than all other causes of death combined. The predominance of injuries during adolescence results from a combination of factors: physical growth, psychomotor function, insufficient physical coordination for the task, energy, impulsivity, peer pressure, and inexperience. Impulsivity, inexperience, and peer pressure may place adolescents in unsafe situations. Feelings of invulnerability ("It can't happen to me") persist, and little thought may be given to the negative consequences of certain behaviors. Alcohol and other drugs that impair judgment are known to contribute to fatal injuries among adolescents, especially those involving firearms and motor vehicles (see Chapter 53 for a complete discussion of alcohol and substance abuse). The sad fact is that most serious or fatal injuries involving adolescents are preventable.

Nurses need to educate adolescents and their families about safety issues and injury prevention. Nurses in school and community action programs are increasingly focusing on preventing firearm and traumatic head injuries. Factual information with supportive explanations should be provided. Expressing a genuine interest in adolescents as individuals and listening in a nonjudgmental way are also important steps to gain confidence and trust. Helping the adolescent recognize choices when faced with difficult or potentially dangerous situations is an important component of safety promotion with this age-group.

The adolescent period is also a frightening time for parents because they are aware of the risks predisposing the adolescent to injury or death. Parents may request guidance from healthcare professionals in setting appropriate limits and establishing methods of effective enforcement. Parents should be encouraged to model the safe behaviors that they expect from the adolescent.

### Car Safety

Obtaining a driver's license signifies a passage into adulthood and provides the adolescent with the means to explore and experience the world more freely. Driving is a complex activity, and proficiency in it requires skill, judgment, and experience. The adolescent's lack of judgment, opposition to authority, and need to express independence often result in a disregard for sound defensive driving practices. Risk-taking behaviors appear to play a major role in the high incidence of car-related injuries and deaths among teenagers. The young, inexperienced driver tends to drive faster and take more chances while operating a car than does an older driver. The 2015 YRBSS of high school students found that 6.1% had rarely or never worn a seatbelt, a slight decline from the previous survey (CDC, 2016c). However, during the 30 days preceding the survey, 20% had ridden with a driver who had been drinking alcohol (CDC, 2016c).

The association between alcohol use and motor vehicle crashes by adolescents is alarming. Despite legal drinking age laws, alcohol is easily accessible to adolescents. The teenager's greater social activity combined with the availability of alcohol increases the incidence of impaired driving.

Distracted driving has gained importance as a contributing factor to motor vehicle crashes. With the explosion in the availability of electronic communication devices, especially cellular phones, texting and e-mailing on the go have become the standard for adolescents. This practice includes texting or e-mailing while driving, which has become a major factor in distracted driving for this population. Results from the YRBSS indicate that over 40% of adolescents surveyed admitted texting or e-mailing while driving, despite state laws that prohibit it (CDC, 2016c).

Nurses can promote car safety by supporting driver education programs for teenagers and the use of seatbelts and by discouraging teens from using a cell phone or texting while driving. In addition, many schools and community organizations have developed prevention programs that are helpful in presenting the facts about drinking and driving to adolescents. Nurses should encourage teens and their parents to set up a ride-home agreement to discourage any driving after drinking alcohol. Adolescents need to know that they have an option available to them if they find themselves in a situation in which the driver has been drinking. Dealing with the inconveniences of finding another ride home is much better than dealing with the injuries and damages of motor vehicle crashes.

### Water Safety

Drowning is a needless cause of death in teenagers, but it is the second leading cause of death from unintentional injury in the 10- to 14-year-old age-group and the third leading cause of unintentional injury death in the 15- to 24-year-old age-group (CDC, 2014). Most drowning deaths occur in lakes, rivers, and ponds, with the rest occurring in public or private swimming pools. Risk-taking behaviors contribute greatly to deaths from drowning and to the incidence of spinal cord injuries. Adolescents are able to travel to areas that are free of adult supervision. Frequently, alcohol and drugs are contributing factors. Given the combination of freedom and alcohol, adolescents may inadvertently place themselves at risk for injury by exceeding the limits for safe swimming and diving.

Safety promotion includes encouraging swimming lessons, water safety classes, and the completion of a course in cardiopulmonary resuscitation. Adolescents need to know how alcohol and drugs impair their ability to perform activities at which they are usually competent.

### Suicide

Intentional suicide is the third leading cause of death for children 5 to 14 years of age and the second leading cause of death in adolescents and young adults 15 to 24 years of age (NCHS, 2016). In a survey of adolescents, 17.7% had seriously considered committing suicide during the previous 12 months (CDC, 2016c). The identification of adolescents at risk for suicide is a priority. Depression is a common finding among suicidal youths; other risk factors are declining mental health, poor impulse control, poor school performance, family disorganization, conduct disorders, substance abuse, homosexuality, and recent stress. Nurses need to be involved in identifying high-risk adolescents. Adolescents identified as at risk for suicide and their families should be targeted for supportive guidance and counseling before a crisis situation. Nurses should counsel parents that all adolescent suicidal gestures should be taken very seriously. Suicidal gestures may appear minor to adults, but the actions may have serious intent (see Chapter 53).

With the increasing opioid epidemic nationwide, both illegal and prescription drugs are available to adolescents (CDC, 2013). Many adolescents do not know which types of drugs will actually harm them, and drug overdoses can lead to an unintentional poisoning death; poisoning is the second leading cause of unintentional death in adolescents aged 15 to 24 years (CDC, 2014). See Chapter 53 for discussion of drug use and abuse.

### Violence Toward Others

Violence continues to threaten the health and well-being of adolescents and society as a whole (see Chapter 1). Homicide is the fifth leading cause of death in children aged 5 to 14 years and the third leading cause of death in both teens and young adults aged 15 to 24 years and children aged 1 to 4 years (NCHS, 2016). Factors contributing to violence are multiple and complex (Box 9.5). A growing body of evidence suggests that exposure to violence at a young age contributes to later violent behavior. Exposure to violence in the family, community, and through various types of media (e.g., television, movies, video games, Internet) correlates with an increased likelihood that a child will use violent means to solve problematic relationships (Strasburger & Donnerstein, 2014). The behavior-related contributing factors provide the greatest opportunity for interventions initiated by healthcare professionals.

Nurses working with children, adolescents, and their families have the opportunity to include violence prevention as a component of anticipatory guidance. Ideally, prevention should begin when the child

**BOX 9.5 Factors Contributing to Adolescent Violence**

- Low socioeconomic status
- Crowded urban housing
- Single-parent family or limited parental supervision
- History of family violence or child abuse
- Access to guns
- Peer pressure or gang involvement
- Limited education
- Racism
- Drug or alcohol use or abuse
- Low self-esteem and hopelessness about the future
- Aggression

is young. Violence is a learned behavior. It is often reinforced by the actions of those closest to the child and by ever-increasing exposure to violence in the media. Assessing how a family deals with anger and resolves conflict provides insight into the way the child will likely react in similar situations. A family with violent tendencies should be referred to a counselor. Learning to react to anger or stress with non-violent actions through conflict resolution is the goal for the youth. Unfortunately, intervention cannot be a one-time educational session. Efforts must be reinforced in multiple facets of the adolescent's life, such as in school, youth organizations, and religious organizations, and at home.

Parents need to be aware of the amount and type of violence to which their children are exposed in the media. Parents cannot isolate their children from all media violence, but they can be encouraged to monitor and limit their children's television viewing and to co-view and discuss with their children the implications of violence shown.

The availability of firearms is related to violent acts. In a survey of students in grades 9 through 12 conducted by the CDC, 5.3% reported having carried a gun within the 30 days preceding the survey (CDC, 2016c). Carrying a weapon can establish a feeling of control or power, or it may be a response to fear of those with power. Regardless of the reasons, firearms in the hands of adolescents can be used impulsively, before the ramifications of such actions can be logically considered. A popular sport among adolescents, especially boys, is the use of so-called airsoft guns, which closely resemble real weapons but use ammunition that is some type of plastic pellet. Eye injuries have been reported from this type of weapon use, and it is imperative that adequate protection be used and the activity be appropriately supervised.

As society urgently seeks a solution to the growing problem of violence, healthcare professionals must become advocates of violence prevention. Opportunities for adolescents to discover and use less violent means to express themselves or resolve day-to-day issues should be taught and promoted. Peer mediation programs in schools have been successful in preventing violent behavior among teens. Given the tragic effects of violence on the safety and health of American children, nurses should participate in efforts to resolve the complex issues of violence in society.

## Selected Issues Related to the Adolescent

### Body Art

Body art encompasses both body piercing and tattooing. Many adolescents believe that such body art expresses their unique individuality or group identification (Armstrong et al., 2014). In some circumstances, body art correlates with an increase in other risk-taking behaviors (Dukes & Stein, 2014), especially as the number of piercings or tattoos increases (Armstrong et al., 2014). Although ear lobe piercing has been popular with teens for many years, piercings in other parts of the body, including the ear cartilage, tongue, lip, eyebrow, nose, navel, and nipple, are also common. Generally, body piercing is harmless, but nurses should caution teens about performing these procedures under unsterile conditions and should educate them about complications, such as bleeding, infection, keloid formation, and allergies to metal. There is a risk for contracting bloodborne diseases or infection from improperly sterilized needles, and most states carefully regulate places where piercings and tattoos can be obtained (American Academy of Dermatology [AAD], 2014). Qualified personnel using sterile needles and equipment should perform the piercing and tattooing procedures. Practices should include using single-use and disposable equipment and dyes and appropriately sterilizing reusable equipment (AAD, 2014).

Depending on the site of the piercing, healing time can take anywhere from 6 weeks up to a year. Important principles for caring for the piercing site include the following: refraining from touching the site or removing the jewelry until fully healed, appropriate hand hygiene, cleaning at least once each day (more often for a tongue piercing) with a recommended saline or antibacterial soap, protecting the site from friction stress, and teaching the adolescent to monitor for signs of infection (AAD, 2015). Tattooed skin may require application of a water-based lotion and avoidance of sun or other tanning exposure. Contacting a medical professional for any skin complication or infection from body art is essential to prevent complications (AAD, 2014).

Because of the invasiveness of the tattoo procedure, it should be considered a health-risk situation. Little oversight or regulatory compliance exists in the tattoo industry, and nurses should educate adolescents about the risks of bloodborne infections, skin infections, and allergic reactions to dyes used in the tattoo process. In addition, nurses need to be informed about tattoo removal to provide correct information to adolescents and their families (see Adolescents Want to Know: Tattooing box). Nurses need to caution adolescents with tattoos to notify health professionals of the tattoo if magnetic resonance imaging (MRI) is to be performed because many of the tattoo inks contain metal, such as iron. Additionally, in general, individuals must wait 12 months after receiving a tattoo before donating blood.

Nurses can provide education about body art during well visits, as well as at school. Because adolescents are not generally future-oriented, they may not adequately consider the consequences associated with body art acquisition. Nurses might need to initiate conversations about the topic, as adolescents might not think of body art as a health issue (Armstrong et al., 2014).

### Tanning

A "good" suntan does not exist. However, persuading adolescents that tanning is harmful to their skin and is a risk factor for developing skin cancer later in life is difficult. The media (advertising, movies, television) promote the image of beach glamour: young, well built, and tanned. Although most companies that manufacture tanning products promote the sun protection factor (SPF) in their products, the advertised image remains a bronzed, attractive, young person. Most exposure to ultraviolet radiation occurs during childhood and adolescence, and skin cancers care prevented with the appropriate and consistent use of sunscreens and sun blocks.

The estimated prevalence of indoor tanning salon use is approximately 13% of adolescents and 20% of adolescent girls in the United States (CDC, 2016a). An area of concern is that a fraction of the adolescents who use tanning salons do not use sun protection (either in the salon or when under natural sunlight) and are not aware of the

## ADOLESCENTS WANT TO KNOW

### Tattooing

- Carefully consider tattooing by talking with others about the process.
- Avoid making an impulsive decision about obtaining the tattoo, the location of the tattoo, or what the tattoo will represent.
- Understand that tattooing carries a risk for complications such as infection, allergic reaction to the dye, scarring or keloid formation, and bloodborne diseases such as hepatitis B and HIV; be sure you are immunized against hepatitis B. Tattoos are permanent, expensive, and painful to remove.
- Check the artist's technique; be sure that all equipment is sterile (e.g., ink and needles removed from the package and used just for you), the artist wears gloves and replaces them after touching anything else, and the artist displays a certificate of inspection by the health department.
- Be sure to obtain written instructions about caring for your skin after tattooing.

Data from American Academy of Dermatology. (2014). *Model regulations for body art establishments*. Retrieved from https://www.aad.org.

dangers of exposure to this type of ultraviolet light. Adverse effects from tanning beds include eye injury, premature aging of the skin, and increased risk of skin cancer of all types (CDC, 2016a). Evidence also suggests that regular use of a tanning salon is addictive for adolescents, and there is proposed legislation that no one younger than 18 years be permitted to use a tanning salon (Balk & the Council on Environmental Health, Section on Dermatology, 2011). Nurses who are doing anticipatory guidance with teens must address these issues along with teaching about the risks of tanning in natural sunlight.

Nurses need to educate teens about the benefits and side effects of different sun protection products and to encourage their use during water sports and all activities that involve sun exposure. Teens involved in athletic activities are often exposed to the sun for long periods without protection. Teenagers may be cognizant of body exposure at a beach but may forget about the exposure of body parts during a long tennis match or a baseball game, especially on a cloudy day, when up to 80% of the sun's radiation reaches the ground. Nurses should caution teens receiving any type of medication about the side effects related to sun exposure. Some medications may potentiate the sun's ultraviolet rays, resulting in quicker burning. The side effects of sunscreen products include itching, burning, and redness immediately or up to 24 hours after application. Some people are allergic or sensitive to the sunscreen agent (e.g., para-aminobenzoic acid [PABA], PABA esters, cinnamates, anthranilates, benzophenones) or other ingredients used, such as fragrances and preservatives. Sunscreen use should be discontinued if an allergic dermatitis is noted, and the teen should try another type of sunscreen. Various available products with different ingredients have protective capabilities. Sun damage can be prevented, and simple measures can minimize the effects of ultraviolet radiation on the skin. Many products are available over the counter or through professional salons that have the look of a tan when applied. Nurses can encourage adolescents to use these products rather than expose themselves to ultraviolet light.

### E-Cigarettes ("Vaping")

Used often by adults as a means of reducing cigarette smoking, e-cigarettes are being increasingly used by adolescents. The CDC (2015b) reports that e-cigarette use among youth tripled between 2013 and 2014. E-cigarettes, aerosol devices containing flavored nicotine in liquid form, create a vapor that is inhaled by the user, thus referred to as "vaping." Although the risks of inhalation of the by-products of cigarette smoke is reduced, nevertheless, the user receives a dose of nicotine, which can be harmful to the adolescents' developing brain (Duderstadt, 2015; Marynak, Holmes, King, et al., 2014). For the first time, the YRBSS (CDC, 2016c) asked adolescents about their e-cigarette use; 24.1% admitted to current vaping, as opposed to 10.8% smoking tobacco.

The sale and regulation of e-cigarettes remains under the states' control. Currently, 40 states have enacted regulations prohibiting the sale of these products to minors (younger than the age of 18 years). However, very few states have enacted regulations that limit use indoors and in public places, where they can expose others to the aerosolized nicotine (Marynak et al., 2014). Additionally, marketing strategies for e-cigarettes are increasingly directed toward attracting adolescents (Duderstadt, 2015).

During well visits, nurses need to ask adolescents about e-cigarette use. Emphasizing the risks to health is also important. Because there has been a reported increase in the number of toddlers and preschoolers who have been poisoned through access to the nicotine liquid (CDC, 2015b), it is imperative that nurses encourage users to keep these products out of reach, as with any other poison. Nurses can also advocate for stricter regulation of these products in states where they live.

### Sexual Activity

***Adolescent sexuality.*** *Adolescent sexuality* refers to the thoughts, feelings, and behaviors related to the adolescent's sexual identity. Middle adolescence typically marks the initial period of dating and experimentation with heterosexual and homosexual behaviors, although in some cultures sexual experimentation occurs much earlier. Initially, group dating may be popular, but this is quickly replaced by dating in couples, who might be sexual partners. Intimate relationships in middle adolescence are usually short lived as adolescents experiment with their sexual identity. Of greatest concern to parents during the adolescent's stage of sexual experimentation are unwanted pregnancies, STDs, and the teen's feelings of despair over failed relationships. Adolescents themselves are often impervious to the possibility of negative consequences of their sexual experimentation and believe that "It can't happen to me."

Although homosexual behavior in adolescence does not necessarily indicate that the adolescent will maintain a homosexual orientation, LGBT (lesbian, gay bisexual and transgender) adolescents face many challenges growing up in a society that is often unaccepting and discriminatory. Those adolescents who self-identify their sexual preference as LGBT during high school are at increased risk for suicide, victimization, risky sexual behaviors, homelessness, and multiple substance abuse (Lim, Brown, & Kim, 2014). Additionally, these adolescents often are victims of bullying, which exacerbates adverse emotions. Providing access to culturally appropriate preventive healthcare for LGBT adolescents is of primary importance because research has demonstrated that lack of appropriate primary care can contribute to adult health problems such as obesity, HIV infection, cancers, and depression.

***Sexual behaviors.*** Most very young teens have not had intercourse. However, the likelihood that teenagers will have vaginal intercourse increases with age. The 2015 YRBSS showed that 3.9% of the group had had sexual intercourse before the age of 13 years, a significant decrease from the prior survey (CDC, 2016c); 41.2% of all adolescents had been involved in sexual activity at some point during adolescence. The prevalence of sexual activity among adolescents is one reason the AAP (2016) is now recommending risk assessment for STDs during every adolescent visit, STD screening when appropriate, and HIV testing for all adolescents aged 16 to 18. At present, the

YRBSS does not ask questions about oral sex, although it is believed that a substantial percentage of teens engage in this behavior (Copen, Chandria, & Martinez, 2012). Adolescence is a period of risk taking, and many adolescents choose to be sexually active and to do so unprotected.

Early initiation of sexual activity correlates with increased risk for STDs and early pregnancy (Copen et al., 2012; Kao & Salerno, 2014). Sexual activity in adolescents is often associated with other risk behaviors, especially alcohol and other substance use, so nurses must approach the issue from multiple perspectives.

Some underlying themes influence whether an adolescent delays engaging in sexual activity. Adolescents who demonstrate high levels of self-esteem, who have goals for academic or other success, who are religious, and whose parents communicate about sexual expectations are more likely to delay sexual activity (Kao, & Salerno, 2014). The AAP (2014b) suggests that exposure to sexually explicit music, videos, movies, and television programs can contribute to early initiation of sexual activity in adolescents.

**Sexual behavior and the media.** A troublesome trend is that adolescents more frequently are obtaining information about sex and sexual relationships through social networking sites and information searches on the Internet (AAP Council on Communications and Media, 2013). An effect of this trend is that adolescents are being exposed to an environment where inappropriate sexuality and sexual behavior may be the norm. In addition, adolescents may be obtaining inaccurate information on which they base decisions about whether to engage in active sexual behavior.

Social media can facilitate adolescent sharing of personal information and inappropriate photographs (sexting). Studies show that there are various reasons adolescents engage in sexting behavior, such as peer pressure, low self-esteem, or to begin a romantic relationship (Ybarra, & Mitchell, 2014). Sometimes, adolescents do not recognize the possible consequences of such behavior. Inadvertent distribution to others can result in embarrassment and bullying, along with a potential adverse effect on the adolescent's reputation (Ouytsel, Walgrave, Ponnet & Heirman, 2015). Additionally, sexting is known to correlate with an increase not only in sexual risk behaviors but also in other high risk behaviors, such as substance and alcohol use (Ouytsel et al., 2015; Ybarra & Mitchell, 2014).

The AAP Council on Communications and Media (2013) suggests that the media could be used to send positive messages about sexuality and healthy relationships, but that this can only occur through advocacy and collaboration with the broadcast and entertainment industry. In addition, the Council recommends that parents limit their adolescents' exposure to sexually explicit media through monitoring adolescents' television viewing, use of social media websites, and access to R-rated movies.

**Relationship violence.** Results of the 2015 YRBSS (CDC, 2016c) indicate that approximately 10% of the adolescents who reported being sexually active experienced some form of relationship (dating) violence during the previous 12 months. Violence can be either sexual (being forced into some type of sexual activity) or physical (being hit or sustaining other physical injury). This violence can occur in any type of dating relationship—heterosexual or homosexual—and can be instigated by both boys and girls. The effects of dating violence can be severe and have lifelong physical and emotional effects, including unwanted pregnancy, contracting an STD, alcohol use, and depression (Lyons & Rabie, 2014). Nurses, especially school nurses, have an important responsibility to recognize signs of relationship abuse and refer victims appropriately for care. Additionally, school nurses who participate in health education can include discussions about relationship violence, and, more importantly, convey to adolescents that violence within the context of a dating relationship is never the norm nor acceptable (Lyons & Rabie, 2014).

***Pregnancy risk.*** The adolescent's limited cognitive abilities or lack of abstract thinking may influence contraceptive practices. Adolescents who feel invulnerable to pregnancy often cannot assimilate and apply to themselves information about sexual behavior, conception, and birth control. Lack of self-esteem and peer pressure also play a role in determining adolescents' sexual behavior. Teens may use sex to feel loved or desired, and they may fear abandonment by a partner if sex is refused. Some teens lack correct reproductive information and do not plan ahead for sexual encounters. Sexual activity is often impulsive, erratic, and unplanned because the relationships are relatively short term.

Nurses in schools and community clinics are in a position to identify teens at risk for pregnancy and provide guidance with appropriate information and referral in a confidential atmosphere. Nurses should strongly encourage adolescents to discuss sexuality, sexual behavior, and contraception with their parents whenever possible but must guarantee confidentiality of nurse-adolescent communication.

Sex education is best when it occurs within a positive parent-child relationship, where factual information dovetails with family values. School sex education programs have had varying success. Many are either abstinence based or protection based. A comprehensive program provides information about protection methods while emphasizing the benefits of abstinence, and may be more appropriate for adolescent development (Suleiman, Johnson, Shirtcliff, et al., 2015). Suleiman et al. (2015) describe the neurologic and hormonal influences that occur during early adolescent development, triggering romantic and sexual interests. Their research highlights goals for a sex education program that positively directs romantic and sexual interests while providing knowledge about sexual health.

The nurse's professional role is to ensure that adolescents have the knowledge, skills, and opportunities that enable them to make responsible decisions about sexual behavior. Education regarding sexuality and contraception should be oriented to the developmental level of the individual or group. The nurse uses primary preventive intervention by assisting adolescents to develop coping strategies to meet their needs in ways other than through sexual behavior.

## ! NURSING QUALITY ALERT

### *Factors to Consider in Selecting Adolescent Contraception*

- Cognitive development (concrete vs. abstract thinking)
- Understanding and acceptance of attitudes and values
- Sexual maturity rating
- Communication between partners
- Opportunity to counsel both partners
- Use of more than one method
- Frequency of intercourse
- Appropriate information (three messages per visit)
- Problem-solving abilities (appeal to logic and feelings of power over body)
- Communication with parents or other adults
- Physical and mental health
- Motivation of both partners
- Concrete, graphic instruction in all methods
- Number and gender of partners
- Encouragement that there is nothing wrong with abstinence

*Contraception.* Complete protection from pregnancy and STDs is achievable only through sexual abstinence. However, because approximately a third of adolescents aged 15 to 19 years are sexually active, nurses need to feel comfortable with managing health concerns related to sexuality. Comprehensive healthcare includes providing services for sexually active adolescents. Healthcare providers should provide screening for and management of STDs, contraceptive services, and psychosocial counseling.

The rate of all teen births in the United States has declined dramatically (42% since 2007) and continues to decline (Hamilton et al., 2015). Because teens might not seek contraception advice until it is too late, the AAP (2016) recommends assessing for sexual activity at every well visit during adolescence. When providing contraception and advice, providers need to routinely reassess for changes in sexual relationships, as well as determine adherence to the contraceptive recommendations (Ott, Sucato, & AAP Committee on Adolescence, 2014). Emphasizing use of condoms to prevent STDs as well as adhering to the chosen method of contraception is important. When the nurse is educating adolescents about birth control methods, consultation with the two partners together is ideal. Open communication between partners is essential, and decisions about contraception should be mutual. Both male and female adolescents need to assume responsibility for sexual behavior. Counseling teens about sexuality and contraception requires nurses who are open, forthright, and respectful of the decisions teens make about sexual activity. (See Chapter 5 for a discussion of media violence, Chapter 32 for information about contraception, and Chapter 41 for information about STDs.)

## Parenting Adolescents

Parenting adolescents is challenging at best. The wish of adolescents to be independent and autonomous often conflicts with the parents' desire to protect their children from harm. Parental monitoring and strong connections with schools have shown to be protective for adolescents engaging in high risk behaviors (CDC, 2015a). In addition to knowing the adolescent's friends and where they are going when they are out, monitoring their use of the Internet, social media sites, and texting is extremely important. However, overparenting can inhibit a healthy transition to adolescent independence. Research has shown that overparenting, defined as overinvolvement in the adolescent's day-to-day problem-solving strategies or physical and emotional well-being, can be counterproductive and inhibitory to positive emotional development (Segrin, Givertz, Swaitkowski, et al., 2015). Nurses can assist parents with striking a healthy balance between protection and overprotection, by advising parents to let their children make mistakes and problem-solve their own solutions; support, but not take over, school responsibilities, such as homework; require that adolescents keep parents informed about their whereabouts, but not use devices, such as phone trackers, to know where their child is every minute; and to gradually allow adolescents more freedom as they become more trustworthy.

## KEY CONCEPTS

- Adolescence is a period of transition from childhood to adulthood that is marked by important biological and psychological changes.
- Biological development during adolescence is variable. Primary and secondary sexual characteristics are acquired through the influence of reproductive hormones in males and females.
- Sexual maturity ratings (SMRs, or Tanner stages) are somewhat variable but predictable stages of sexual maturation that are based on the development of pubic hair and breasts in girls and pubic hair and genitals in boys.
- According to Erikson, the major developmental task in adolescence is the development of an identity and self-perception. Other developmental tasks are the development of a sexual identity, avocational/educational identity, and independence and autonomy.
- Early and middle adolescents are egocentric and concerned with themselves.
- Cognitive thinking during adolescence moves from concrete to abstract reasoning.
- According to Kohlberg, adolescents and young adults develop a respect for law and order and a society-maintaining orientation.
- Adolescents question the values of family and society before integrating their experiences and beliefs into a personal moral framework.
- Adolescents may be emotionally labile, with extreme highs and extreme lows.
- The pace of physical growth during adolescence is second only to the pace of growth during infancy.
- Poor eating habits and lack of aerobic exercise contribute to obesity and decreased overall physical fitness.
- Tanning, body piercing, tattooing, and use of e-cigarettes are behaviors associated with identity formation.
- Risk-taking behavior is considered part of normal growth and development.
- Safety issues related to sports activity, sexual activity, firearms, and the use of motor vehicles should be emphasized.
- Sexual maturation precipitates sexual activity; teen pregnancy and STDs are related issues.

## REFERENCES AND READINGS


Aalsma, M., Gilbert, A. Xiao, S., et al. (2016). Parent and adolescent views on barriers to adolescent preventive health care utilization. *Journal of Pediatrics, 169*, 140–145.

Ali, O., & Donohoue, P. (2016). Gynecomastia. In R. Kliegman, B. Stanton, J. St. Geme, N. Schor, & R. Behrman (Eds.), *Nelson textbook of pediatrics* (20th ed., Chapter 585). Philadelphia: Elsevier.

American Academy of Dermatology. (2014). *Model regulations for body art establishments.* Retrieved from https://www.aad.org.

American Academy of Dermatology. (2015). *Caring for pierced ears.* Retrieved from https://www.aad.org.

American Academy of Dermatology. (2016). *Caring for tattooed skin: Tips from dermatologists.* Retrieved from https://www.aad.org.

American Academy of Pediatrics. (2011). Expert Panel on Integrated Guidelines for Cardiovascular Health and Risk Reduction in Children and Adolescents: Summary report. *Pediatrics, 128*(S5), S213–S256.

American Academy of Pediatrics. (2014a). Fluoride use in caries prevention in the primary care setting. *Pediatrics, 134*(3), 626–633.

American Academy of Pediatrics. (2014b). *More sex and violence are creeping into movies as parents become less sensitive.* Retrieved from https://www.aap.org.

American Academy of Pediatrics. (2015). *Dental health and orthodontic problems.* Retrieved from https://www.healthychildren.org.

American Academy of Pediatrics. (2016). Recommendations for preventive pediatric health care. *Pediatrics, 137*(1), 25–27.

American Academy of Pediatrics Committee on Adolescence. (2008, Reaffirmed 2013). Achieving quality health services for adolescents. *Pediatrics, 121*(6), 1263–1270.

American Academy of Pediatrics Committee on Nutrition and the Council on Sports Medicine and Fitness. (2011). Sports drinks and energy drinks for children and adolescents: Are they appropriate? *Pediatrics, 127*(6), 1182–1189.

American Academy of Pediatrics Council on Communications and Media. (2013). Children, adolescents and the media. *Pediatrics, 132*(5), 958–961.

American Heart Association. (2014). *Dietary recommendations for healthy children*. Retrieved from http://www.heart.org.

Armstrong, M. Tustin, J., Owen, D., et al. (2014). Body art education, the earlier, the better. *Journal of School Nursing, 30*(1), 12–18.

Arria, A., Bugbee, B., Caldeira, M., et al. (2014). Evidence and knowledge gaps for the association between energy drink use and high risk behaviors among adolescents and young adults. *Nutrition Review, 72*(S1), 67–97.

Babcock, D. (2011). Evaluating sleep and sleep disorders in the pediatric primary care setting. *Pediatric Clinics of North America, 58*, 543–554.

Balk, S., & the Council on Environmental Health, Section on Dermatology. (2011). Technical report: Ultraviolet radiation: A hazard to children and adolescents. *Pediatrics, 127*(3), e791–e817.

Brittian, S. (2012). Adolescents' identity development: A relational developmental systems approach. *Journal of Black Psychology, 38*(2), 172–200.

Carskadon, M. (2011). Sleep in adolescents: The perfect storm. *Pediatric Clinics of North America, 58*, 637–647.

Centers for Disease Control and Prevention. (2013). *Addressing prescription drug abuse in the United States: Current activities and future opportunities.* Retrieved from http://www.cdc.gov.

Centers for Disease Control and Prevention. (2014). *10 leading causes of injury deaths by age group highlighting unintentional injury deaths, United States—2014*. Retrieved from http://www.cdc.gov.

Centers for Disease Control and Prevention. (2015a). *Adolescent and school health: Protective factors*. Retrieved from http://www.cdc.gov.

Centers for Disease Control and Prevention. (2015b). *E-cigarette study sparks national attention around e-cigarette and nicotine toxicity*. Retrieved from http://www.cdc.gov.

Centers for Disease Control and Prevention. (2015c). *Reproductive health: Teen pregnancy*. Retrieved from http://www.cdc.gov.

Centers for Disease Control and Prevention. (2016a). *Indoor tanning is not safe*. Retrieved from http://www.cdc.gov.

Centers for Disease Control and Prevention. (2016b). *Recommended immunization schedules for persons aged 0 through 18 years*. Retrieved from http://www.cdc.gov.

Centers for Disease Control and Prevention. (2016c). Youth Risk Behavior Surveillance—United States, 2015. *MMWR Morbidity & Mortality Weekly Report, 65*(6), 1–174.

Copen, C., Chandra, A., & Martinez, G. (2012). Prevalence and timing of oral sex with opposite sex partners among females and males aged 15-24 years: United States 2007-2010. *National Health Statistics Reports, 56*, 1–9.

Dansereau, D., Knight, D., & Flynn, P. (2013). Improving adolescent judgment and decision-making. *Professional Psychology: Research and Practice, 44*(4), 274–282.

Duderstadt, K. (2015). E-cigarettes: Youth and trends in vaping. *Journal of Pediatric Health Care, 29*(6), 555–557.

Dukes, R., & Stein, J. (2014). Evidence of anticipatory socialization among tattooed, wanabe, and non-tattooed adolescents: Differences in attitudes and behavior. *Sage Open*, 1–12.

Elkind, D. (1993). *Parenting your teenager*. New York: Ballantine Books.

Erikson, E. (1968). *Identity: Youth and crisis*. New York: Norton.

Freud, S. (1960). *The ego and the id*. (J. Riviere, Trans.). New York: Norton, (J. Riviere, Trans.).

George, N., & Davis, J. (2013). Assessing sleep in adolescents through a better understanding of sleep physiology. *AJN, 113*(6), 26–31.

Garcia-Huidobro, D., Shippee, N., DiCaprio, J., et al. (2016). Effect of patient-centered medical home on preventive services for adolescents and young adults. *Pediatrics, 137*(6), 1–9.

Hamilton, B., Martin, J., Osterman, M., et al. (2015). Births: Final data for 2014. *National Vital Statistics Reports, 64*(12), 1–64.

Hargreaves, D., Elliott, M., Viner, R., et al. (2015). Unmet health care need in United States adolescents and adult health outcomes. *Pediatrics, 136*(3), 513–570.

Holland-Hall, C., & Burstein, G. (2016). Adolescent development. In R. Kliegman, B. Stanton, J. St. Geme, N. Schor, & R. Behrman (Eds.), *Nelson Textbook of Pediatrics* (20th ed., Chapter 110). Philadelphia: Elsevier.

Husky, M., Miller, K., & McGuire, L. (2011). Mental health screening of adolescents in pediatric practices. *The Journal of Behavioral Health Services and Research, 38*(2), 159–169.

Kao, T., & Salerno, J. (2014). Keeping adolescents busy with extracurricular activities. *Journal of School Nursing, 30*(1), 57–67.

Kaplowitz, P., Bloch, C., & AAP Section on Endocrinology. (2016). Evaluation and referral of children with signs of early puberty. *Pediatrics, 137*(1), e20153732.

Kelly, S., Anderson, D., Hall, L., et al. (2012). The effects of exposure to gang violence on adolescent boys' mental health. *Issues in Mental Health Nursing, 33*, 80–88.

Kohlberg, L. (1964). Development of moral character. In M. Hoffman, & L. Hoffman (Eds.). *Review of child development research* (Vol. 1). New York: Russell Sage Foundation.

Lim, F., Brown, D., & Kim, S. (2014). Addressing disparities in the lesbian, gay, bisexual and transgender population: A review of best practices. *AJN, 114*(6), 24–34.

Lyons, J., & Rabie, G. (2014). Empowering adolescents and the wider community to recognize adolescent relationship abuse. *British Journal of School Nursing, 9*(3), 131–140.

Marshall, W.A., & Tanner, J. (1969). Variations in pattern of pubertal changes in girls. *Archives of Disease in Childhood, 44*(235), 291–303.

Marynak, K., Holmes, C., King, B. et al. (2014). State laws prohibiting sales to minors and indoor use of electronic nicotine delivery systems—United States 2014. *Morbidity and Mortality Weekly Reports, 63*(49), 1145–1150.

Mayer, J., Woodruff, S.I., Slymen, D.J., et al. (2011). Adolescents' use of tanning: A large-scale evaluation of psychosocial, environmental, and policy level correlates. *American Journal of Public Health, 101*(5), 930–938.

Michaelson, V., Robinson, P., & Pickett, W. (2014). Participation in church or religious groups and its association with health: A national study of young Canadians. *iJournal of Religion and Health, 53*, 1353–1373.

Morris, E., & Fry-McComish, L. (2012). Hope and despair: Diverse voices of hope from urban African-American adolescent gang members. *International Journal for Human Caring, 16*(4), 50–57.

National Center for Health Statistics. (2016). *Health, United States, 2015 with special feature on racial and ethnic disparities*. Hyattsville, MD: Author.

Ott, M., & Sucato, G., & AAP Committee on Adolescence. (2014). Contraception for adolescents. *Pediatrics, 134*(4), 1–15.

Ouytsel, J., Walrave, M., Ponnet, K., et al. (2015). The association between adolescent sexting, psychosocial difficulties and risk behavior: Integrative review. *Journal of School Nursing, 31*(1), 54–69.

Parks, E., Shaikhkhalil, A., Groleau, V., et al. (2016). Feeding healthy infants, children, and adolescents. In R. Kliegman, B. Stanton, J. St. Geme, N. Schor, & R. Behrman (Eds.), *Nelson textbook of pediatrics* (20th ed., Chapter 45). Philadelphia: Elsevier.

Piaget, J. (1969). *The theory of stages in cognitive development*. New York: McGraw-Hill.

Segrin, C., Givertz, M., Swaitkowski, P., et al. (2015). Overparenting is associated with child problems and a critical family environment. *Journal of Child and Family Studies, 24*, 470–479.

Siu, A., & U.S. Preventive Services Task Force. (2016). Clinical guideline screening for depression in children and adolescents: U.S. Preventive Services Task Force recommendation statement. *Annals of Internal Medicine, 164*, 360–366.

Spurr, S., Berry, L., & Walker, K. (2013). The meaning older adolescents attach to spirituality. *Journal for Specialists in Pediatric Nursing, 18*, 221–232.

Strasburger,V., & Donnerstein, E. (2014). The new media of violent video games. Yet same old media problems? *Clinical Pediatrics, 53*(9), 721–725.

Suleiman, A., Johnson, M. Shirtcliff, E., & Galvan, A. (2015). School based sex education and neuroscience: What we know about sex, romance, marriage and adolescent brain development. *Journal of School Health*, *85*(8), 567–574.

Tanner, J. (1962). *Growth at adolescence* (2nd ed.). Oxford: Blackwell Scientific Publications.

United States Department of Health and Human Services. (2010). *Healthy People 2020*. Retrieved from https://www.healthypeople.gov

United States Department of Health and Human Services and United States Department of Agriculture. (2015). *Dietary guidelines for Americans, 2015-2020*. Retrieved from https://www.health.gov.

Wen, M. (2014). Parental participation in religious services and parent and child well-being: Findings from the National Survey of America's Families. *Journal of Religion and Health*, *53*, 1539–1561.

Ybarra M., & Mitchell, K. (2014). "Sexting" and its relation to sexual activity and sexual risk behavior in a national survey of adolescents. *Journal of Adolescent Health*, *55*, 755–764.

10

# Hereditary and Environmental Influences on Development

http://evolve.elsevier.com/McKinney/mat-ch/

## LEARNING OBJECTIVES

*After studying this chapter, you should be able to:*

- Describe the structure and function of normal human genes and chromosomes.
- Give examples of ways in which genes and chromosomes are studied.
- Describe the transmission of single gene traits from parent to child.
- Relate chromosome abnormalities to spontaneous abortion and to birth defects in the infant.
- Describe the genetic components of selected disorders other than those related to reproduction.
- Explain the characteristics of multifactorial birth defects.
- Identify environmental factors that can interfere with prenatal development, and explain how their effects can be avoided or reduced.
- Describe the process of genetic counseling.
- Explain the role of the nurse in caring for individuals or families with concerns about birth defects.

Hereditary and environmental forces influence one's development from before conception until death. The nurse needs a basic knowledge of these forces to understand disorders evident at birth and those that develop later in life.

## HEREDITARY INFLUENCES

Hereditary influences on development result from the directions for cellular functions provided by genes located on the 46 chromosomes in every somatic cell. Abnormal structure or function results if too much or too little genetic material is present in the cells or if an abnormal gene provides incorrect directions. The disorders that result may be merely annoying or they may be devastating.

### Structure of Genes and Chromosomes

A review of the structure of genes and chromosomes aids in understanding how disorders occur. Chromosomes are composed of genes that in turn are composed of deoxyribonucleic acid (DNA) (Fig. 10.1).

#### DNA

DNA is the basic building block of genes and chromosomes. It has three units: (1) a sugar (deoxyribose), (2) a phosphate group, and (3) one of four nitrogen bases (adenine, thymine, guanine, and cytosine).

DNA resembles a spiral ladder, with a sugar and a phosphate group forming each side of the ladder and a pair of nitrogen bases forming each rung. The four bases of the DNA molecule pair with one another in a fixed way, allowing the accurate duplication of the DNA during each cell division.

- Adenine pairs with thymine.
- Guanine pairs with cytosine.

The sequence of base pairs within the DNA determines which amino acids are assembled to form a protein and the order in which they are assembled. Some of these proteins form the structure of body cells; others are enzymes that control metabolic processes within the cell. If the sequence of nitrogen bases in the DNA is incorrect or if some bases are missing or added, a defect in body structure or function may result.

#### Genes

A gene is a segment of DNA that directs the production of a specific product needed for body structure or function. Humans probably have approximately 21,000 genes in each cell (National Human Genome Research Institute [NHGRI], 2012).

Genes that code for the same trait often have two or more alternate forms (alleles). Many alleles are normal, such as those that code for a person's blood type. Normal alleles that are common in the population, or polymorphisms (alternate healthy forms of a gene), provide genetic variation and sometimes a biologic advantage. However, mutations often involve a change in a gene that alters or harms function, such as those that cause the production of abnormal hemoglobin in sickle cell disease, result in blood clotting disorders, or allow cells to grow in an uncontrolled way, causing cancer.

Genes are too small to be seen under a microscope, but through tissue analysis, many can be studied by:

- Measuring the protein product that the gene directs cells to produce
- Studying the DNA sequence of the gene directly
- Analyzing the association (linkage) of the gene with another gene that can be studied using one of the above methods

The Human Genome Project is an international effort begun in 1990 to identify all genes contained in the 46 human chromosomes. Sequencing of all human genes was completed in April, 2003 (NHGRI, 2015b). Information gained from this project may allow advances such as:

- Genetic testing to determine the risk for a disorder or the actual or probable presence of the disorder
- Basing reproductive decisions on more accurate and specific information than has been available
- Identifying genetic susceptibility to a disorder so that interventions to reduce risk can be instituted

- Using gene therapy to modify a defective gene
- Modifying therapy such as medication based on an individual's genetic code or the genetic makeup of tumor cells

The explosion of knowledge about the genetic basis for many diseases raises many legal and ethical issues. As our knowledge base grows, new issues are likely to emerge.

- Discovery of genetic information has implications for other family members, raising privacy issues.
- Identification of genetic problems could lead to poor self-esteem, guilt, and excessive caution, or, conversely, a reckless lifestyle.
- Presymptomatic identification of genetically influenced illness could be a source of long-term anxiety.
- Genetic knowledge could affect one's choice of a partner.
- Discrimination may occur, such as the imposition of high insurance rates, the denial of insurance coverage, or an employer's decision not to hire a qualified person who has a greater chance of genetically influenced illness.

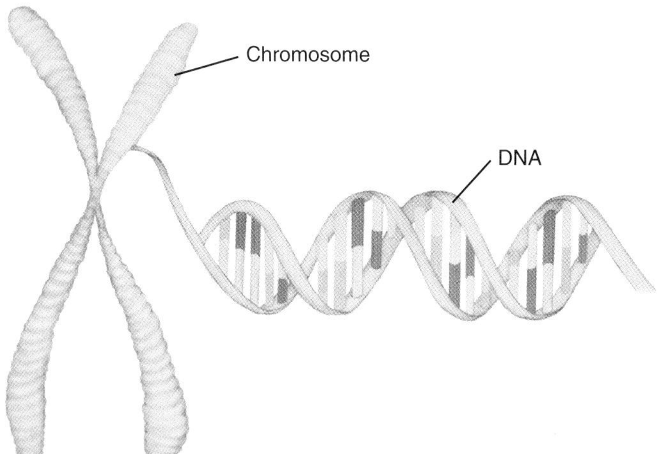

FIG 10.1 Diagrammatic representation of the deoxyribonucleic acid (DNA) helix, which is the building block of genes and chromosomes.

## Chromosomes

Genes are organized into 46 paired chromosomes in the nuclei of most somatic cells (non-sex body cells). Twenty-two chromosome pairs are autosomes (non-sex chromosomes), and the 23rd pair the sex chromosomes (XX in females, XY in males). Added or missing chromosomes or structurally abnormal chromosomes are usually harmful.

Mature gametes (reproductive cells) are called haploid because they have half the chromosomes (23) of other body cells. One chromosome from each pair is distributed randomly in the gametes, allowing variation of genetic traits among people. When the ovum and sperm unite at conception, the total is restored to 46 paired chromosomes, or diploid.

Cells used for full chromosome analysis must have a nucleus and must be living (Jorde, Carey, & Bamshad, 2010). Chromosomes can be studied using any of several types of live cells: white blood cells, skin fibroblasts, bone marrow cells, and fetal cells from the chorionic villi (finger-like projections of the placenta) or suspended in amniotic fluid.

Unlike genes, chromosomes can be seen under the microscope, but only during division of live cells. Specimens must be obtained and preserved carefully to provide enough living cells for chromosome analysis. Temperature extremes, clotting of blood, or adding improper preservatives can kill the cells and render them useless for analysis.

Chromosomes look jumbled when viewed under a microscope (Fig. 10.2). Photographing or using computer imaging allows paired chromosomes to be displayed in a karyotype from largest to smallest pairs (Fig. 10.3). The karyotype is then analyzed.

Finer analysis of chromosomes is possible using fluorescent in-situ hybridization (FISH), spectral karyotyping, and chromosome

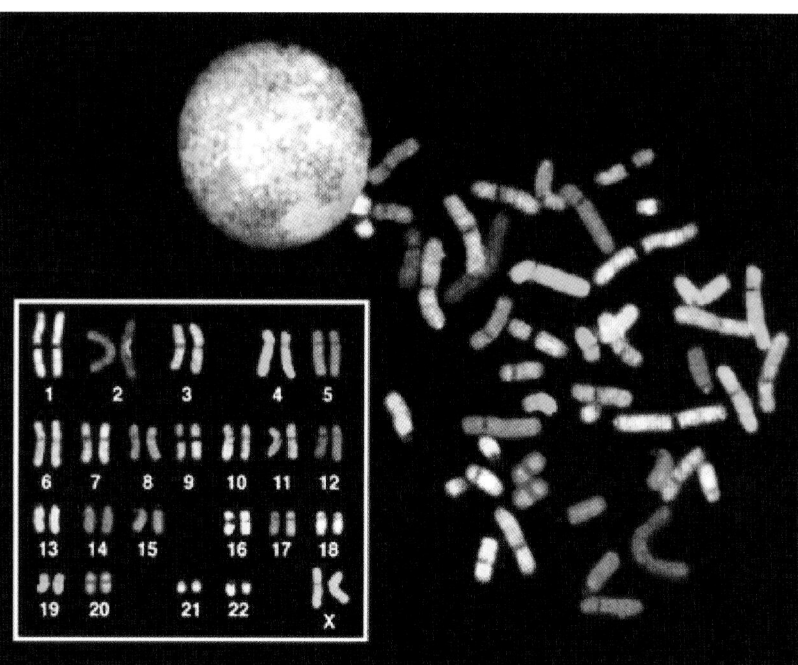

FIG 10.2 When viewed before karyotyping, chromosomes appear jumbled. The spectral karyotype (SKY) of a normal female is shown. (From National Human Genome Research Institute [2011]. Retrieved from http://www.genome.gov.)

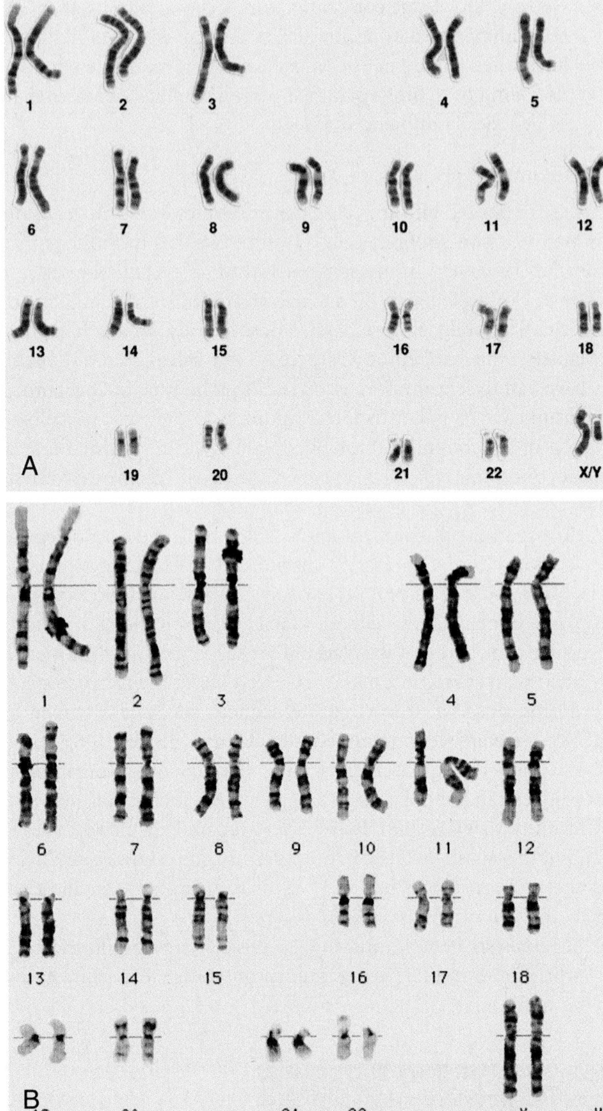


**FIG 10.3** Karyotypes comprising chromosomes that were stained, creating bands that distinguish each chromosome and can be used to identify missing or duplicated chromosome material. **A,** Normal male karyotype: 46, XY. **B,** Normal female karyotype 46, XX. (**A** from National Human Genome Research Institute [2013]. *Fact sheet: Karyotype.* Retrieved from http://www.genome.gov; **B** from Jorde, L.B., Carey, J.C., Bamshad, M.J., & White, R.L. [2003]. *Medical genetics* [3rd ed., pp. 108]. St. Louis: Mosby.)

microarray analysis (CMA). Spectral karyotyping (SKY) colors each chromosome differently to identify small rearrangements, losses, or gains of chromosome material (see Fig. 10.3). FISH and CMA use fluorescent-labeled DNA probes that attach to specific chromosomes and permits testing for added, missing, or rearranged chromosome material that otherwise may not be visible. FISH analysis does not require living cells, unlike other chromosome analyses (Jorde et al., 2010; NHGRI, 2015a).

## Transmission of Traits by Single Genes

Inherited characteristics are passed from parent to child by the genes in each chromosome. These traits are classified according to whether they are dominant (strong) or recessive (weak) and whether the gene is located on one of the autosome pairs or on the sex chromosomes. Both normal and abnormal hereditary characteristics are transmitted by these mechanisms.

### Alleles

Because humans have matched pairs of chromosomes (except the sex chromosomes in the male), they have two alleles for each gene—one on each member of the chromosome pair. The paired alleles may be identical (**homozygous**) or different (**heterozygous**).

Some alleles, both normal and abnormal, occur more frequently in certain groups than they do in the population as a whole. For example, the gene that causes Tay-Sachs disease is carried by approximately 1 of every 27 Ashkenazi Jews (of Eastern European origin) in the United States. A higher incidence of Tay-Sachs is found in non-Jewish French-Canadians, Louisiana Cajun people, and the Pennsylvania Amish. An estimated 1 of every 250 people outside this group, including non-Ashkenazi Jews, carries the gene (NHGRI, 2015a, b; National Tay-Sachs and Allied Diseases Association [NTSAD], 2015). Other disorders that are prevalent in certain ethnic groups are cystic fibrosis (primarily Whites of northern European descent) and sickle cell disease (primarily people of African, Mediterranean, Indian, or Middle Eastern descent).

A new trait (harmful, neutral, or sometimes beneficial) may emerge because of a change in the gene within the gamete. The DNA in the gamete is then different from that in the person's somatic cells. The offspring who receives the new version of the gene will have it in all somatic cells and can transmit it to future generations.

### Dominance

Dominance describes how one's genetic composition is translated into the **phenotype**, or observable characteristics. In the case of a dominant gene, one copy is enough to cause the trait to be expressed. For example, in the ABO blood system, genes for type A and type B are dominant. Therefore, a single copy of either of these genes is enough to be expressed in the person's blood type.

Two identical copies of a recessive gene are required for the trait to be expressed. The gene for blood group O is recessive. Laboratory testing will identify a person's blood group as O only if they carry the blood group O gene from both parents. If the person has the group O gene from one parent and the group A gene from the other parent, group A will be expressed in laboratory blood typing.

Other alleles are equally dominant. The person who receives a gene for blood group A from one parent and group B from the other will have type AB blood because both alleles are equally dominant and both are expressed in blood typing.

Dominance and recessiveness are not absolute for all genes. Some people with a single copy of an abnormal recessive gene (carriers) may have a slightly abnormal level of the gene product (e.g., an enzyme) that can be detected by laboratory methods. These people usually do not have the disease because the normal copy of the gene directs production of enough of the required product to allow normal or near-normal function.

### Chromosome Location

Genes located on autosomes are either autosomal dominant or autosomal recessive, depending on the number of identical copies of the gene needed to produce the trait. However, genes located on the X chromosome are paired only in females because males have one X and one Y chromosome.

A female with an abnormal recessive gene on one of her X chromosomes usually has a normal gene on the other X chromosome that compensates and maintains relatively normal function. However, the male is at a disadvantage if his only X chromosome has an abnormal gene. The male has no compensating normal gene because his other sex chromosome is a Y. The abnormal gene will be expressed in the male because it is unopposed by a normal gene.

## Patterns of Single-Gene Inheritance

Three important patterns of single-gene inheritance are (1) autosomal dominant, (2) autosomal recessive, and (3) X-linked. Box 10.1 summarizes the characteristics and transmission of each pattern. The inheritance patterns are graphically illustrated with a genogram, or pedigree, to represent a family's history and the relationships between family members.

The nurse may need to interpret the genogram for the patient. For example, when taking a genetic family history, the nurse might say, "I'm going to use several symbols to depict your family tree and its members' health histories. This diagram is often called a *genogram* or a *pedigree*."

Single-gene traits have mathematically predictable and fixed rates of occurrence. For example, if a couple has a child with an autosomal recessive disorder, the risk that future children from the same couple will have the disorder is one in four (25%) at every conception. The *risk* for the disorder is the same at every conception, regardless of how many of the couple's children are or are not affected.

**CRITICAL TO REMEMBER**

***Single-Gene Abnormalities***

- A person affected with an autosomal dominant disorder has a 50% chance of transmitting the disorder to each of his or her children.
- Two healthy parents who carry the same abnormal autosomal recessive gene have a 25% chance of having a child affected with the disorder caused by this gene.
- Parental consanguinity (blood relationship) increases the risk of having a child with an autosomal recessive disorder.
- One copy of an abnormal X-linked recessive gene is enough to produce the disorder in a male.
- Abnormal genes can arise as new mutations that are then transmitted to future generations.

### Autosomal Dominant Traits

An autosomal dominant trait is produced by a dominant gene on a non-sex chromosome. The expression of abnormal autosomal dominant genes may result in multiple and seemingly unrelated effects in the person. The gene's effects may vary substantially in severity, leading a family to think that a trait skips a generation. A careful physical examination may reveal subtle evidence of the trait in each generation. Some people may carry the dominant gene but may have no apparent expression of it in their physical makeup.

In some autosomal dominant disorders, such as Huntington's disease, the person having the gene will always have the disease if he or she lives long enough. In other disorders, only a portion of those carrying the gene will ever exhibit the disease. Achondroplasia, the most common type of dwarfism, is present at birth (congenital), while degeneration of the brain in Huntington's disease is not usually apparent until adulthood. See http://www.lpaonline.org and http://www.hdsa.org for support information for these disorders.

New mutations often account for the introduction of autosomal dominant traits into a family that has no previous history. Men who father children in their fifth decade or later are more likely to have offspring with a new autosomal dominant mutation.

The person who is affected with an autosomal dominant disorder is usually heterozygous for the gene; that is, the person has a normal gene on one chromosome and an abnormal gene on the other chromosome of the pair that overrides the influence of the normal gene. Occasionally a person receives two copies of the same abnormal autosomal dominant gene. Such an individual is usually much more severely affected than someone with only one copy.

### Autosomal Recessive Traits

An autosomal recessive trait occurs when a person receives two copies of a recessive gene carried on an autosome. Most people carry a few abnormal autosomal recessive genes without problems because a compensating normal gene produces enough of the gene's product for normal function. Because the probability that two unrelated people will share even one of the same abnormal genes is low, the incidence of autosomal recessive diseases is relatively low in the general population.

Situations that increase the likelihood that two parents will share the same abnormal autosomal recessive gene are:

- Consanguinity (blood relationship) of the parents
- Membership in groups that are isolated by culture, geography, religion, or other factors

Many autosomal recessive disorders are severe, such that affected people may not live long enough to reproduce. Two exceptions are phenylketonuria and cystic fibrosis. Improved care of people with these disorders has allowed them to live into their reproductive years. If one member of the couple has the autosomal recessive disorder, all of their children will be carriers. Their risk for having similarly affected children is higher as well, depending on the prevalence of the abnormal gene in the general population.

### X-Linked Traits

***X-linked recessive disorders.*** X-linked recessive traits are more common than X-linked dominant ones. Sex differences in the occurrence of X-linked recessive traits and the relationship of affected males to one another distinguish these disorders from autosomal dominant or recessive disorders. Males usually show full effects of an X-linked recessive disorder because their only X chromosome has the abnormal gene on it. Females can show the full disorder in two uncommon circumstances:

- When a female has a single X-chromosome (Turner syndrome, Fig. 10.4)
- When a female child is born to an affected father and a carrier mother

X-linked recessive disorders can be relatively mild, such as colorblindness, or severe, such as hemophilia. The severity of such diseases varies among those having the disorder.

## Chromosome Abnormalities

Chromosome abnormalities can be numerical or structural. They are quite common (50% or more) in the embryo or fetus that is spontaneously aborted, sometimes before pregnancy is recognized. Chromosome abnormalities often cause major defects because they involve many added or missing genes.

### Numerical Abnormalities

Numerical chromosome abnormalities are those involving added or missing single chromosomes and those with multiple sets of chromosomes. Trisomy and monosomy are numerical abnormalities of single chromosomes. Polyploidy describes abnormalities involving entire sets of chromosomes.

***Trisomy.*** A trisomy exists when each body cell contains an extra copy of one chromosome, bringing the total number to 47 (Fig. 10.5). Each chromosome is normal, but there is an extra one in every cell.

## BOX 10.1 Single-Gene Traits

### Genogram (Pedigree) Symbols

A genogram symbolically represents a family's medical history and the relationships of its members to one another. It can identify patterns of inheritance that may help distinguish one type of disorder from another.

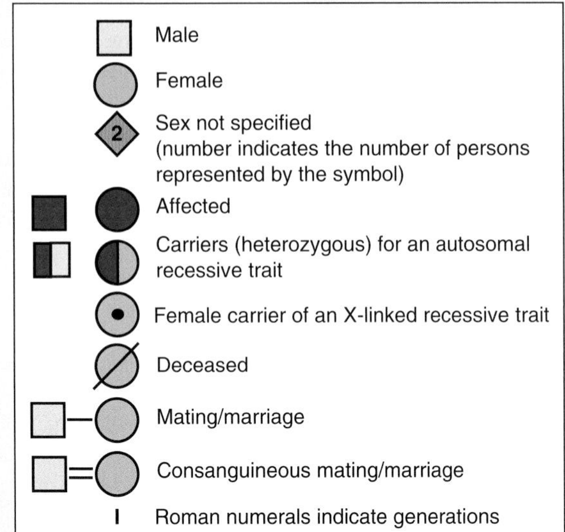


### Autosomal Recessive

#### *Characteristics*

Two autosomal recessive genes are required to produce the trait.
Males and females are equally likely to have the trait.
There is often no family history of the disorder before the first affected child.
If more than one family member is affected, they are usually full siblings.
Consanguinity (close blood relationship) of the parents increases the risk for the disorder.
Disorders are more likely to occur in groups isolated by geography, culture, religion, or other factors.
Some autosomal recessive disorders are more common in specific ethnic groups.

#### *Transmission of Trait From Parent to Child*

Unaffected parents are carriers of the abnormal autosomal recessive trait.
Children of carriers have a 25% (1 in 4) chance of receiving both copies of the defective gene, and thus, having the disorder.
Children of carriers have a 50% (1 in 2) chance of receiving one copy of the gene and being carriers like the parents.
Children of carriers have a 25% (1 in 4) chance of receiving both copies of the normal gene. They are neither carriers nor affected.

#### *Examples*

Normal traits: blood group O; Rh-negative blood factor.
Abnormal traits: Tay-Sachs disease; sickle cell disease; cystic fibrosis.

#### *Genogram*

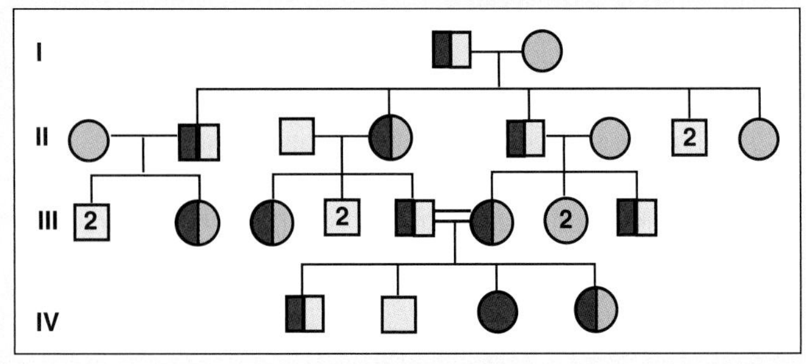


### Autosomal Dominant

#### *Characteristics*

A single copy of the gene is enough to produce the trait.
Males and females are equally likely to have the trait.
Often appears in every generation of a family, although family members having the trait may have widely varying manifestations of it.
May have multiple and seemingly unrelated effects on body structure and function.

#### *Transmission of Trait From Parent to Child*

A parent with the trait has a 50% (1 in 2) chance of passing the trait to the child.
The trait may arise as a new mutation from an unaffected parent. The child who receives the mutated gene can then transmit it to future generations.

#### *Examples*

Normal traits: blood groups A and B; Rh-positive blood factor.
Abnormal traits: Huntington disease; neurofibromatosis.

#### *Genogram*

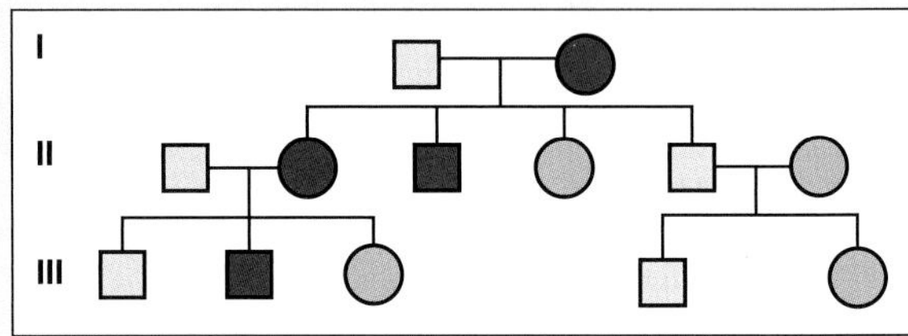


### X-Linked Recessive

#### *Characteristics*

Although recessive, only one copy of the gene is needed to cause the disorder in the male, who does not have a compensating X without the trait.
Males are affected, with rare exceptions.
Females are carriers of the trait but not usually adversely affected.
Affected males are related to one another through carrier females.
Affected males do not transmit the trait to their sons.

#### *Transmission of Trait From Parent to Child*

Males who have the disorder transmit the gene to 100% of their daughters and none of their sons.
Sons of carrier females have a 50% (1 in 2) chance of being affected. They also have a 50% chance of being unaffected.
Daughters of carrier females have a 50% (1 in 2) chance of being carriers like their mothers. They also have a 50% chance of being neither affected nor carriers.
A new X-linked recessive gene also may arise by mutation.

#### *Examples*

Colorblindness; Duchenne muscular dystrophy; hemophilia A

#### *Genogram*

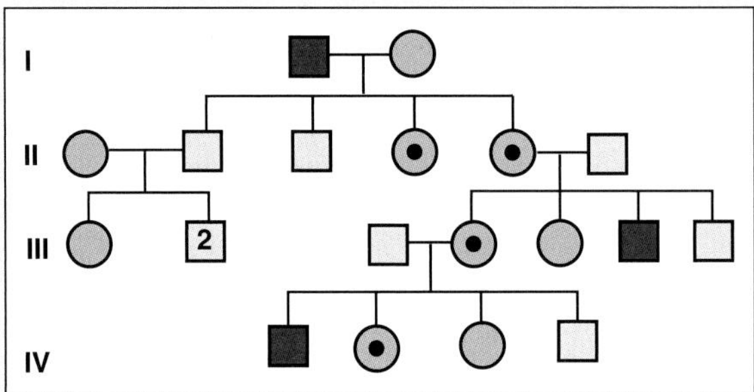

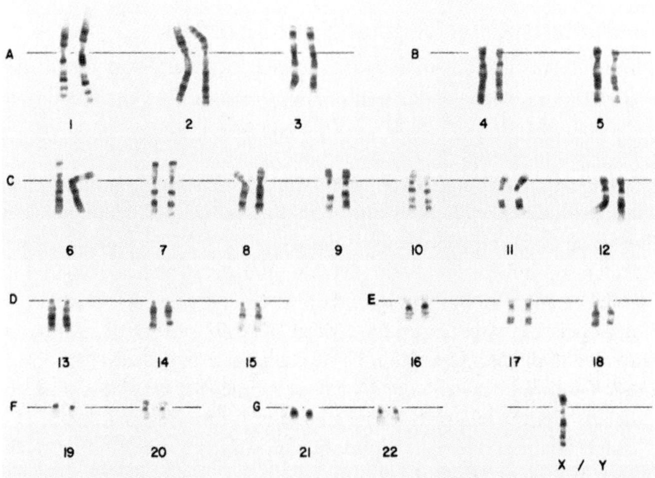


FIG 10.4 Karyotype of a female with monosomy X (Turner syndrome 45, X). (Courtesy Dr. Mary Jo Harrod, University of Texas Southwestern Medical Center, Dallas, TX.)

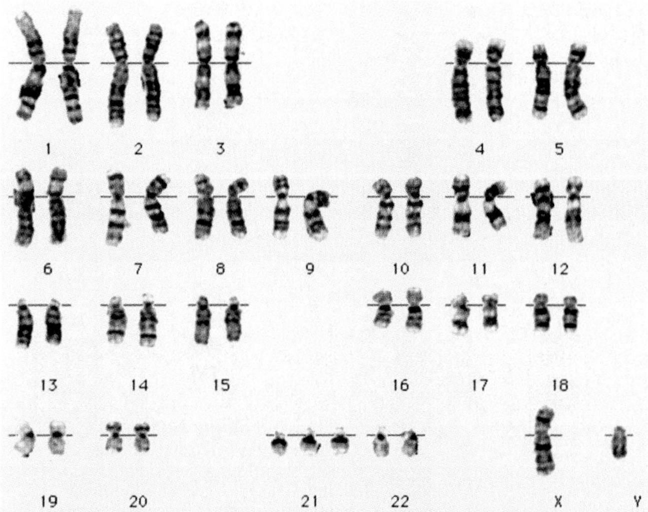

FIG 10.5 Karyotype of a male with trisomy 21 (Down syndrome: 47, XY, +21). (From Jorde, L.B., Carey, J.C., & Bamshad, M.J. [2010]. *Medical genetics* [4th ed., pp. 107]. St. Louis: Mosby.)

**CRITICAL TO REMEMBER**

***Chromosome Abnormalities***

Chromosome abnormalities are either numerical or structural.

**Numerical**

- Entire single chromosome added (**trisomy**)
- Entire single chromosome missing (**monosomy**)
- One or more added sets of chromosomes (**polyploidy**)

**Structural**

- Part of a chromosome missing or added
- Rearrangements of material within chromosome(s)
- Two chromosomes that adhere to each other
- Fragility of a specific site on the X chromosome

The most common trisomy is *Down syndrome*, or trisomy 21. In Down syndrome, each body cell has three copies of chromosome 21. Trisomies of chromosomes 13 and 18 are less common and have more severe effects. The incidence of trisomies increases with maternal age, so that most women who are 35 years old or older at conception are offered prenatal diagnosis to determine whether the fetus has Down syndrome or another trisomy. Noninvasive screening tests such as maternal serum alpha-fetoprotein or a quad-screen are offered to women who enter prenatal care during the first trimester of pregnancy. Additional testing is offered if the maternal serum tests are abnormal (see Chapter 15).

Infants with Down syndrome have characteristic features that are usually apparent at birth. Chromosome analysis of the neonate can be carried out to confirm the diagnosis and to determine whether Down syndrome is caused by trisomy 21 or a rarer anomaly involving a structural rather than a numerical addition of chromosome 21 material.

***Monosomy.*** A monosomy occurs when each body cell has a missing chromosome, with a total number of 45. The only monosomy that is compatible with extended postnatal life is *Turner syndrome*, or monosomy X (see Fig. 10.4). People with Turner syndrome have a single X chromosome and are female.

Liveborn infants with Turner syndrome have excess skin around the neck and edema that is most noticeable in the hands and feet. If Turner syndrome is not identified and treated during infancy or childhood, an affected girl will remain very short and will not have menstrual periods or develop secondary sex characteristics. Heart and aortic defects are common. Severe defects are surgically repaired. Children with Turner syndrome usually have normal intelligence, although they may have difficulty with spatial relationships or solving visual problems such as reading a map.

***Polyploidy.*** Polyploidy occurs when chromosome pairs do not separate during gamete formation or when two sperm fertilize an ovum simultaneously. The result is an embryo with one or more extra sets of chromosomes. The total number of chromosomes is a multiple of the haploid number of 23 (69 or 92 total chromosomes). Polyploidy usually results in an early spontaneous abortion but is occasionally seen in a liveborn infant.

### Structural Abnormalities

The structure of one or more chromosomes may be abnormal. Part of a chromosome may be missing or added, or DNA within the chromosome may be rearranged. Some of these rearrangements are harmless polymorphisms. However, others are harmful because important genetic material is lost or duplicated or the position of the genes in relation to other genes is altered, making normal gene function impossible.

Another structural abnormality occurs when all or part of a chromosome is attached to another (translocation). Many people with a translocation chromosome abnormality are clinically normal because the total of their genetic material is normal, or balanced (Fig. 10.6). If a parent has a balanced translocation, the offspring may have normal chromosomes or may have a balanced translocation like the parent. However, the offspring may receive too much or too little chromosome material at conception and may be spontaneously aborted or may have a birth defect (abnormality of structure, function, or body metabolism at birth that results in physical or mental disability or may be fatal). Either balanced or unbalanced chromosome translocations may occur spontaneously in the child of parents who have no translocation.

Fragile X syndrome is a structural chromosome abnormality that often causes intellectual disability in males. With this abnormality, a site on the X chromosome is more fragile than normal. Although

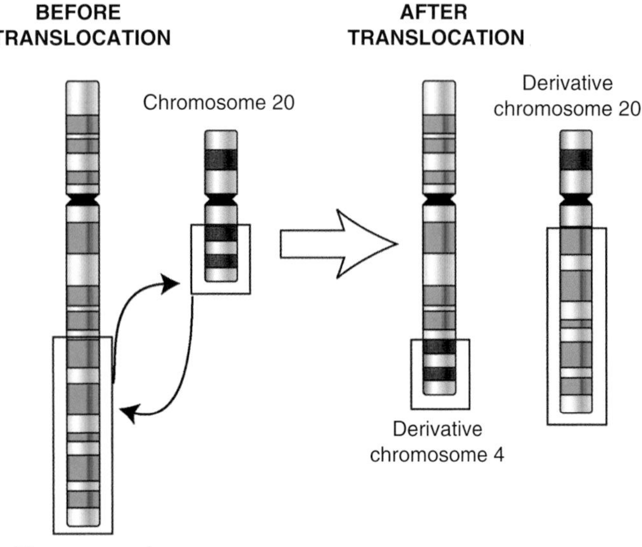


**FIG 10.6** Illustration of a translocation of chromosome material between chromosomes 4 and 20. (From National Human Genome Research Institute. [2010]. *Illustration: Translocation.* Retrieved from http://www.genome.gov.)

females can also be affected with fragile X syndrome, males are more severely affected because the female has a second X chromosome that is usually normal. The fragile X syndrome is inherited in an X-linked dominant pattern (ACOG, 2010; Jorde et al., 2010).

## MULTIFACTORIAL DISORDERS

Multifactorial disorders result from an interaction of genetic and environmental factors. The genetic tendency toward the disorder is modified by the environment. These interactions may influence prenatal and postnatal development either positively or negatively. For example, two embryos may have an equal genetic susceptibility for the development of a disorder such as spina bifida (open spine). However, the disorder will not occur unless an environment that favors its development, such as inadequate maternal intake of folic acid, also exists.

### CRITICAL TO REMEMBER

#### *Multifactorial Birth Defects*

- Multifactorial defects are some of the most common birth defects encountered in maternity and pediatric nursing practice.
- Multifactorial defects result from interaction between an individual's genetic susceptibility and environmental factors during prenatal development.
- Multifactorial defects are usually single, isolated defects, although the primary defect may cause secondary defects.
- Some occur more often in certain geographic areas.
- A greater risk of occurrence exists if:
  Several close relatives have the defect, whether mild or severe.
  One close relative has a severe form of the defect.
  The defect occurs in a child of the less frequently affected sex.
- Infants who have several major and/or minor defects that are not directly related probably do not have a multifactorial defect but have another syndrome, such as a chromosome abnormality.

### Characteristics of Multifactorial Disorders

Multifactorial disorders have two characteristics that distinguish them from other types of birth defects. They are typically (1) present and detectable at birth and (2) isolated defects rather than ones that occur with other unrelated abnormalities.

However, a multifactorial defect may *cause* a secondary defect. For example, infants with spina bifida often have hydrocephalus because abnormal development of the spine and spinal cord disrupts spinal fluid circulation, allowing it to build up within the brain's ventricular system.

The infant who has spina bifida plus one or more defects that are not associated with disrupted central nervous system development probably does *not* have a multifactorial disorder. In this case, the spina bifida is more likely to be part of a syndrome that may pose a much different risk for recurrence in the parents' future children.

Multifactorial disorders represent some of the most common birth defects that a maternal–child nurse encounters. Examples include:

- Many heart defects
- Neural tube defects such as anencephaly (absence of most of the brain and skull) and spina bifida
- Cleft lip and cleft palate
- Pyloric stenosis

### Risk of Occurrence

Unlike single-gene traits, multifactorial disorders are not associated with a fixed risk of occurrence or recurrence in a family. The risks are an average rather than a constant percentage. Factors that may affect the degree of risk are:

- Number of affected close relatives
- Severity of the disorder in affected family members
- Sex of affected person(s)
- Geographic location
- Seasonal variations

## ENVIRONMENTAL INFLUENCES

Environment may influence prenatal development positively, as when good nutrition supplies all necessary raw materials for fetal growth. However, some environmental influences are harmful such as teratogens or mechanical forces that disrupt development.

### Teratogens

Teratogens are agents in the fetal environment that either cause a birth defect or increase the likelihood that a birth defect will occur. People often ask whether a certain drug or other substance will harm the baby. Some drugs have been definitely established as either safe or harmful. However, for most agents, their potential for harming the fetus is not clear. Several factors make it difficult to establish the teratogenic potential of an agent:

- *Retrospective study.* Investigators must rely on the mother's memory about substances she ingested or was exposed to during pregnancy.
- *Timing of exposure.* Agents may be harmful at one stage of prenatal development but not at another.
- *Different susceptibility of organ systems.* Some agents affect only one fetal organ system, or they affect one system at one stage of prenatal development and another system if exposure occurs at a different stage of development.
- *Noncontrolled fetal exposure.* Exposures cannot be controlled to eliminate extraneous agents or to ensure a consistent dose.
- *Placental transfer.* Agents vary in their ability to cross the placenta.

- *Individual variations.* Fetuses show varying susceptibility to harmful agents.
- *Nontransferability of animal studies.* Results of animal studies cannot always be applied to humans.
- *Risk of damage from an uncontrolled maternal disorder.* Some maternal disorders, such as epilepsy or hypertension, may themselves cause fetal damage if not controlled, raising a question about whether the medication or the disorder caused the damage.

Teratogens typically cause more than one defect, which distinguishes teratogenic defects from multifactorial disorders. However, children affected by single-gene and chromosome defects are also likely to have multiple defects, often making diagnosis difficult.

Hundreds of individual agents are either known or suspected teratogens. Types of teratogens include:

- Maternal infectious agents (viruses or bacteria) that cross the placenta and damage the embryo or fetus
- Drugs and other substances used by the woman (therapeutic agents, illicit drugs, botanical preparations, tobacco, alcohol)
- Pollutants, chemicals, or other substances to which the mother is exposed in her daily life
- Ionizing radiation
- Maternal hyperthermia
- Maternal disorders, such as diabetes mellitus or phenylketonuria

It is theoretically possible to eliminate all or some of the risk to the developing fetus by avoiding exposure to the agent or changing the fetal environment in some way.

### Avoiding Fetal Exposure

Ideally, avoiding exposure to harmful influences begins before conception because major organ systems develop early in pregnancy, often before a woman realizes she is pregnant. To avoid some agents, such as alcohol or illicit drugs, pregnant women must be committed to make substantial lifestyle changes (Box 10.2).

**Infections.** Rubella immunization at least 4 weeks before pregnancy virtually eliminates the risk that the mother will contract this infection, which can damage the fetus severely. For infections that cannot be prevented by immunization, the nurse can counsel the woman to avoid situations in which acquiring the disease is more likely. Rubella immunization should be offered after birth with a waiting period of 4 weeks before conceiving again (American Academy of Pediatrics [AAP] & American College of Obstetricians and Gynecologists [ACOG], 2012; Centers for Disease Control and Prevention [CDC], 2014).

Zika virus infection during pregnancy is linked to birth defects. Fetal problems associated with Zika virus include microcephaly, defects of the eye, hearing deficits, and impaired growth. Zika virus is spread primarily via the bite of infected mosquitoes (*Aedes* species) but may also be spread through sexual contact with infected males. No vaccine is currently available, and pregnant women are encouraged to avoid traveling to areas with Zika virus (CDC, 2016).

**Drugs and other substances.** The U.S. Food and Drug Administration (FDA) has established pregnancy categories for therapeutic drugs based on their potential to harm the fetus. The categories range from A through D, and X. Class A drugs have no demonstrated fetal risk in well-controlled studies. At the opposite end, pregnancy category X drugs are well established as being harmful. For approximately 80% of therapeutic drugs, whether they are definitely safe or unsafe is unknown (See Appendix A on this book's Evolve website for a list of common drugs and other substances that may affect the fetus adversely.) In deciding whether to prescribe a drug, the physician must often balance the woman's need for the drug's therapeutic effects against the risk to the fetus. In addition, stopping a therapeutic drug may abrogate disease control in the mother, such as the reappearance of seizures or hypertension, which adversely affects the fetus.

**BOX 10.2 Selected Environmental Substances Known or Thought to Harm the Fetus***

Alcohol
Aminoglycosides
Anticonvulsant agents
Antihyperlipidemic agents (statins)
Antineoplastic agents
Antithyroid drugs
Cocaine
Diethylstilbestrol (DES)
Folic acid antagonists
Infections
- Cytomegalovirus
- Herpes simplex virus
- Human immunodeficiency virus
- Rubella
- Syphilis
- Toxoplasmosis
- Varicella
- Zika

Lithium
Mercury
Retinoic acid
Tetracycline
Tobacco
Warfarin

*The nurse should look for new information released about adverse fetal effects from these or other drugs that may be given during pregnancy.

Establishing whether an illicit drug can cause prenatal damage is especially difficult because women who abuse substances often have other problems that complicate the analysis of fetal effects. For example, these women may use multiple drugs and often have poor nutrition, untreated diseases, inadequate prenatal care, and a stressful life. In addition, illicit drugs are unlikely to be pure, and the substances used to dilute them may themselves be harmful.

Botanical preparations such as herbs may be used by many patients, including pregnant women. A woman might not consider these preparations to be potentially harmful, and thus, not make them known to her caregivers unless asked. Unlike therapeutic drugs, there is no FDA regulation of botanical products in terms of dose, effectiveness, or risk associated with use.

The best action for a pregnant woman is to eliminate use of nontherapeutic drugs and substances such as alcohol. If she takes therapeutic drugs, the physician may be able to prescribe an alternative drug with a lower risk to the fetus or may temporarily eliminate some therapeutic drugs.

**Ionizing radiation.** Nonurgent radiologic procedures may be done during the first 2 weeks after the menstrual period begins. This is usually before ovulation, and thus, before conception is possible. For urgent procedures, the lower abdomen should be shielded with a lead apron if possible. The radiation dose is kept as low as possible to reduce fetal exposure.

***Maternal hyperthermia.*** A mother's temperature may rise unavoidably during illness. Pregnant women should be cautioned to avoid or limit exposure to heat such as saunas or hot tubs.

#### Manipulating the Fetal Environment

Appropriate medical therapy can help a woman avoid fetal damage that could result from her illness. For example, a woman who has diabetes should try to keep her blood glucose levels normal and stable before and during pregnancy for the best possible fetal outcomes. A woman with phenylketonuria should closely adhere to a low-phenylalanine diet before conception to avoid buildup of toxic metabolic products in her body that may damage the fetus.

Occasionally, a pregnant woman is given a fetal therapy drug such as digoxin or propranolol for fetal cardiac dysrhythmias. In these cases, the fetus has the disorder, not the mother. The mother is the conduit for medicating the fetus to allow its normal development and function.

### Mechanical Disruptions to Fetal Development

Mechanical forces that interfere with normal prenatal development include oligohydramnios and fibrous amniotic bands.

*Oligohydramnios,* an abnormally small volume of amniotic fluid, reduces the cushion surrounding the fetus and may result in deformations such as clubfoot. Prolonged oligohydramnios interferes with fetal lung development because it does not allow normal development of the alveoli. Oligohydramnios may occur secondary to other fetal anomalies.

*Fibrous amniotic bands* may result from tears in the inner sac (amnion) of the fetal membranes and can result in fetal deformations or intrauterine limb amputation. Fibrous bands are usually sporadic and unlikely to recur. Because these bands can cause multiple defects, they may be confused with birth defects from other causes such as chromosome or single-gene abnormalities.

## GENETIC COUNSELING

Genetic counselors provide services to help people understand specific genetic disorders and the risk of occurrence in their family.

### Availability

Genetic counseling is often available through facilities that provide maternal–fetal medicine services. State departments of mental health and intellectual disability or rehabilitation services also may provide counseling services. Local chapters of the March of Dimes are an important source of information about birth defects and counseling sites. Fact sheets and other information about birth defects and their prevention or treatment are available online from the March of Dimes (http://www.modimes.com). Organizations that focus on specific birth defects provide valuable support and assistance in obtaining needed services for individuals and families affected by that disorder.

### Focus on the Family

Genetic counseling focuses on the family rather than on an individual. One family member may have a birth defect, but study of the entire family is often needed for accurate counseling. This study may involve obtaining medical records or performing physical examinations or laboratory studies on numerous family members. Counseling is impaired if family members are unwilling to provide their medical records or agree to examinations or laboratory studies. Moreover, those who seek counseling may be unwilling to request cooperation from other family members or to share genetic information they acquire. Very small families may be willing to provide information to the affected member, but there is less familial information (frequency of occurrence of the trait or condition) that can be obtained from so few.

### Process of Genetic Counseling

Genetic counseling is often a slow process that is not always straightforward. Several visits spread over months may be needed. In addition, some tests may be performed at only one or a few laboratories in the world, and several weeks may be needed to complete them. Despite a comprehensive evaluation, a diagnosis may never be established. An accurate diagnosis is crucial to provide families with the best information about the risks for a specific birth defect, the prognosis for the one affected, and options available to avoid or manage the disorder. Advances in knowledge about birth defects may allow a definite diagnosis later, and families are encouraged to contact the center for updates. Box 10.3 lists examples of procedures that may be used before conception, prenatally, and after birth to establish an accurate diagnosis related to birth defects.

A genetic evaluation may include many factors, such as:

- A complete medical history, including prenatal and perinatal history
- The medical history of other family members
- Laboratory, imaging, or other diagnostic studies
- Physical assessment of a child with the birth defect and other family members as needed
- Examination of photographs, particularly for family members who are deceased or unavailable
- Construction of a genogram, or pedigree, to identify relationships among family members and their relevant medical history

**BOX 10.3 Diagnostic Methods That May Be Used in Genetic Counseling**

**Preconception Screening**

- Family history to identify hereditary patterns of disease or birth defects
- Examination of family photographs
- Physical examination for obvious or subtle signs of birth defects
- Carrier testing
- People from ethnic groups with a higher incidence of some disorders
- People with a family history suggesting that they may carry a gene for a specific disorder
- Chromosome analysis
- Deoxyribonucleic acid (DNA) analysis

**Prenatal Diagnosis for Fetal Abnormalities**

- Maternal tests to screen for abnormalities
- Chorionic villus sampling
- Amniocentesis
- Ultrasonography
- Percutaneous umbilical blood sampling

**Postnatal Diagnosis for an Infant With a Birth Defect**

- Physical examination and measurements
- Imaging procedures (such as ultrasonography, radiography, echocardiography)
- Chromosome analysis
- DNA analysis
- Tests for metabolic disorders (phenylketonuria, cystic fibrosis)
- Hemoglobin analysis for disorders such as sickle cell disease
- Immunologic testing for infections
- Autopsy

If a diagnosis is established, genetic counseling educates the family about:

- What is known about the disorder and its cause
- The natural course of the disorder
- Options for care of an affected person
- The likelihood that the disorder will occur or recur
- The availability of prenatal diagnosis for the disorder
- How a couple may be able to avoid having an affected child
- The availability of treatment and services for the person with the disorder

Genetic counseling is nondirective; that is, the counselor does not tell the individual or parents what decision to make but educates them about options for dealing with the disorder. However, families often interpret the counseling subjectively. Some parents may regard a 50% risk of occurrence or recurrence as low, whereas others may think that a 1% risk is unacceptably high. The family's values and beliefs also influence whether they seek counseling and what they do with the information provided.

### Supplemental Services

Comprehensive genetic counseling includes services of professionals from many disciplines, such as biology, medicine, nursing, social work, and education. These professionals provide added support for families; they may offer referral to parent support groups, grief counseling, and intervention for problems that accompany the birth of a child with a birth defect, such as socioeconomic or family dysfunction.

## NURSING CARE FOR FAMILIES CONCERNED ABOUT BIRTH DEFECTS

Nurses have an important role in helping families who are concerned about birth defects. Some nurses work directly with family members who are undergoing genetic counseling. Many more nurses are generalists who bring knowledge about birth defects and their prevention to those they encounter in everyday practice.

### Nurses as Part of a Genetic Counseling Team

Genetic nursing may include:

- Providing counseling (after additional education)
- Guiding a woman or couple through prenatal diagnosis
- Supporting parents as they make decisions after receiving abnormal prenatal diagnostic results
- Helping the family deal with the emotional impact of a birth defect
- Assisting parents who have had a child with a birth defect locate needed services and support
- Coordinating services of other professionals, such as social workers, physical and occupational therapists, psychologists, and dietitians
- Helping families find appropriate support groups to help them cope with the daily stresses associated with a child who has a birth defect

(See also Chapter 54.)

### Nurses in General Practice

Nurses who work in women's healthcare and those who work in antepartum, intrapartum, newborn, or pediatric settings often encounter families who are concerned about birth defects. These families may include a member who has a birth defect. Other families may believe that they have an increased risk for having a child with a birth defect. Generalist nurses provide care and support that complements those of nurses who work on a genetic counseling team.

## PARENTS WANT TO KNOW

### *About Birth Defects*

**How Can This Birth Defect Be Genetic? No One Else in Our Family Has Ever Had Anything Like It.**
Autosomal recessive disorders are carried by parents who themselves are unaffected. The abnormal gene may have been passed down through many generations, with no risk of having an affected child until two carrier parents mate.

**Isn't There Only A One-In-A-Million Chance That This Birth Defect Will Happen to Another of Our Children?**
Autosomal recessive disorders have a 25% (1 in 4) chance of recurring in children of the same parents. Autosomal dominant disorders may pose a 50% risk of recurrence unless they resulted from a new mutation in the egg or sperm that created the baby.

**Isn't This Birth Defect Very Likely to Recur? We'd Better Not Have Any More Children.**
Some birth defects are associated with a relatively high risk of recurrence; others have a relatively low risk. How high a risk is perceived also varies among people. Prenatal diagnosis may offer parents a way to avoid having an affected child, and some disorders may be treated before birth.

**Because We've Already Had A Child With This Autosomal Recessive Birth Defect, Will The Next Three Be Normal?**
If both parents are carriers for an autosomal recessive disorder, there is a consistent 25% (1 in 4) risk for the birth defect to occur with each child conceived by the same parents. The chance is the same (1 in 4) that each child will not receive the gene from either parent and will be neither affected nor a carrier for the gene.

**If I Have Amniocentesis Or Other Prenatal Diagnostic Tests, Can The Test Detect All Birth Defects?**
Many but not all disorders can be prenatally diagnosed. Testing is offered for one or more specific disorders after a careful family history is taken to determine appropriate tests.

**If The Prenatal Test Is Normal, Will My Baby Be Normal?**
Normal results from prenatal testing exclude those disorders that were specifically tested for with varying accuracy. Every healthy couple has approximately a 5% risk of having a child with a birth defect, some of which are not obvious at birth. This baseline risk remains even if all prenatal test results are normal.

**Will I Have To Have An Abortion If My Prenatal Tests Show That My Baby Is Abnormal?**
Abortion may be an option for parents whose fetus has a birth defect. Most parents receive normal test results. If results are abnormal, some parents appreciate the time to prepare for a child with special needs. Better medical management can be planned for a newborn who is expected to have problems. Prenatal diagnosis gives many parents the confidence to have children despite their increased risk for having a child with a birth defect.

#### Women's Health Nurses

The ideal time to provide counseling is before conception so the childbearing couple has more options if problems are identified. As in antepartum care, the primary nursing role is to identify families who might benefit from counseling before conception. Personal and family histories are commonly taken at primary healthcare visits, and the nurse may identify a history that could affect a child that the couple might conceive.

### Antepartum Nurses

During the initial antepartum interview, the nurse may identify a pregnant woman or family who might benefit from genetic counseling. The antepartum nurse also assists families with decision making, teaching, and emotional support.

***Identifying families for referral.*** Nurses in antepartum settings often identify a woman or family who is appropriately referred for genetic counseling. The personal and family history of the woman and the father of her baby may reveal factors that increase their risks for having a child with a birth defect. In addition to the usual medical history about disorders such as hypertension or diabetes, the woman should be questioned about a family history of birth defects and intellectual or developmental disorders (often called mental retardation) that seem to "run in the family."

Some people are reluctant to disclose that they have a family member with delayed mental development or a birth defect. The nurse can gently probe for sensitive information by asking questions about whether there are family members who have learning problems or who are "slow." Using words that are lay-oriented often elicits more information than using harsh terms that are being phased out, such as *mental retardation.*

***Helping the woman decide about genetic counseling.*** If genetic counseling is appropriate, the physician or midwife usually discusses it with the woman and offers to refer her and her partner to an appropriate center if indicated. However, the final decision rests with the woman. The nurse can help the woman decide whether she wants genetic counseling at all and to weigh issues that are important to her and if she wants to include others in her decision.

Genetic counseling can raise issues that are uncomfortable, such as whether to undergo prenatal diagnosis, what to do if a condition cannot be prenatally diagnosed, and what options are acceptable if prenatal diagnosis shows abnormal results. Counseling may open family conflicts if information from other family members is needed or if family values differ on issues such as abortion of an abnormal fetus. In addition, the tests can show unexpected results (Boxes 10.4 and 10.5). The nurse must be careful not to allow personal values to influence the family's decision. It is the family members who must live with the decision they make.

***Teaching about lifestyle.*** Nurses can teach a pregnant woman about harmful factors in her lifestyle that can be modified to reduce the risk of defects to her offspring. The nurse can support the woman in making lifestyle changes that may be difficult, such as stopping alcohol consumption, reducing or eliminating smoking, or improving her diet. Liberal praise can motivate a woman to continue her efforts to promote an optimal outcome. A negative attitude from nurses or other professionals may make her feel like a failure, and she may abandon her efforts to create a healthier lifestyle.

***Providing emotional support.*** The time between prenatal testing and results sometimes spans several days or even weeks. Results are not always definite after several tests are done in an attempt to identify the fetal problem. In the meantime, the pregnancy is becoming more obvious and the woman may begin to feel fetal movement. Many women delay telling friends or family about their pregnancy until they know that prenatal test results are normal. They often delay investing emotionally in their pregnancy because it seems so tentative until test results are known. When results are abnormal, women face more difficult decisions about whether to terminate or continue the pregnancy.

***Helping the woman and family deal with abnormal results.*** Because prenatal diagnostic tests are performed to detect disorders involving serious physical and often mental effects, the woman or couple whose test results are abnormal must make painful decisions. For many of these disorders, no effective prenatal or postnatal treatment exists. In many cases there are only two choices: continue the pregnancy or terminate it. In addition, the decision to terminate a pregnancy must be made in a short time. Arriving at "no decision" is effectively a decision to continue the pregnancy. Although the physician or genetic counselor is the one who discusses abnormal results and available options, the nurse reinforces the information given to these anxious families.

When test results are abnormal, nurses can expect the couple to grieve. Even if a pregnancy was unplanned, the woman who reaches the time of prenatal diagnosis has already made the initial decision to continue the pregnancy. If results are abnormal, the woman must decide all over again about ending her pregnancy. Women who continue their pregnancies grieve over the expected normal infant. Indefinite conclusions about fetal health are likely to affect the woman and family until birth.

#### BOX 10.4 Reasons for Referral to a Genetic Counselor or Other Healthcare Specialist

- Pregnant women who will be 35 years of age or older when the infant is born
- Men who father children after the age of 40 years
- Members of a group with an increased incidence of a specific disorder
- Carriers of autosomal recessive disorders
- Women who are carriers of X-linked disorders
- Couples closely related by blood (consanguineous relationship)
- Family history of birth defect or intellectual disability
- Family history of unexplained stillbirth
- Women who experience multiple spontaneous abortions
- Pregnant women exposed to known or suspected teratogens or other harmful agents, either before or during pregnancy
- Pregnant women with abnormal prenatal screening results, such as triple- or quad-screen, or suspicious ultrasound findings

#### BOX 10.5 Problems Encountered in Genetic Counseling and Prenatal Diagnosis

- Inadequate medical records
  - Family members' refusal to share information
  - Records that are incomplete, vague, or uninformative
- Inconclusive testing
  - Too few family members available for family studies
  - Inadequate number of live fetal cells obtained during amniocentesis or chorionic villus sampling
  - Failure of cells for chromosome analysis to grow in culture
  - Ambiguous prenatal test results that are neither clearly normal nor clearly abnormal
- Unexpected results from prenatal diagnosis
  - Finding an abnormality other than the one tested for
  - Nonpaternity revealed
- Inability to determine the severity of a prenatally diagnosed disorder
- Inability to rule out all birth defects
- Patient misunderstanding of the mathematical risk as presented

### Intrapartum and Neonatal Nurses

Nurses working in intrapartum and neonatal settings encounter families who have given birth to an infant with a birth defect that often was unexpected. Stillborn infants sometimes have birth defects that contributed to their intrauterine death. Besides the loss of their baby, these parents face added pain because of the associated abnormality. An autopsy documents all anomalies and helps establish the most accurate diagnosis of the birth defect for counseling. Nursing care for families experiencing a perinatal loss, whether a result of the infant's death or the loss of the expected normal infant, is addressed in Chapter 24.

Nurses who care for these families in the intrapartum and neonatal settings will find the parents anxious, depressed, and sometimes hostile because of the unexpected event. The family's usual coping mechanisms may be inadequate for the situation. Various diagnostic studies are often recommended by neonatologists or other medical providers soon after the birth of an abnormal infant to establish a diagnosis and to give parents accurate information about the disorder and their options. However, a high anxiety level reduces a parent's ability to understand the often massive amount of information received. The nurse is in a position to evaluate the family's perception of the problem, help them understand the diagnostic tests, reinforce correct information, and correct misunderstandings. Moreover, the nurse is often most helpful by just being an available, active listener, helping to ease the family's pain over the event.

Nurses should encourage families to contact lay support groups. These groups are a significant source of support because they understand fully the daily problems encountered when caring for a child with a birth defect. They can help the parents deal with the stress and chronic grief associated with prolonged care of these children. Support groups also can help the parents see the positive aspects and victories when caring for their special-needs child.

### Pediatric Nurses

Children with birth defects typically have numerous recurrent medical problems. They usually are hospitalized more often and for longer periods than children without birth defects. They may have to travel to specialized hospitals for care, adding to the family's stress. Their families often have large expenses for medical care and equipment that are not covered by insurance or public assistance programs. There may be lost income because one parent, usually the mother, stops working to care for the child.

Family dysfunction is common, and the strain of having a child with a serious birth defect may lead to divorce. Siblings of the child often feel left out of their parents' attention because the needs of the sick child demand so much of the parents' time.

The pediatric nurse can reduce the family's stress by helping them locate appropriate support services. The nurse can contact social services departments to help the family find financial and other resources needed to care for the child. If parents have not connected with a lay support group, the pediatric nurse can encourage them to do so.

## KEY CONCEPTS

- The 46 human chromosomes are long strands of DNA, each containing up to several thousand different genes.
- With the exception of those genes located on the X and Y chromosomes in males, genes are inherited in pairs that may be identical or different. Some genes are dominant and some are recessive.
- Many genes can be analyzed by the products they produce, their DNA sequence, or their close association with another gene that is more easily analyzed.
- Specimens for chromosome analysis must be handled carefully to preserve cell viability.
- Chromosome abnormalities are either numerical, with the addition or deletion of an entire chromosome or chromosomes, or structural, with deletion, addition, rearrangement, or fragility of the chromosome material.
- Single-gene disorders are associated with a fixed risk of occurrence or recurrence. The type of single-gene abnormality (autosomal dominant, autosomal recessive, or X-linked) determines the level of risk.
- Multifactorial disorders are caused by a genetic predisposition combined with environmental factors.
- Of the many agents that can enter the fetal environment, the definitive teratogenicity or safety is known for only a few; environmental agents may differ with respect to the gestational age at which they are likely to be teratogenic.
- The purpose of genetic counseling is to educate individuals or families, providing them with accurate information so they can make informed decisions about reproduction and appropriate care for affected members.
- The nurse cares for people with concerns about birth defects by identifying those needing referral, teaching, coordinating services, and offering emotional support.

## REFERENCES AND READINGS


American Academy of Pediatrics and American College of Obstetricians and Gynecologists. (2012). *Guidelines for perinatal care* (7th ed.). Elk Grove Village, IL, and Washington, DC: Author.

American College of Obstetricians and Gynecologists. (2008; Reaffirmed 2014). *Ethical issues in genetic testing. (ACOG Committee Opinion No. 410)*. Washington, DC: Author, (ACOG Committee Opinion No. 410).

American College of Obstetricians and Gynecologists. (2009; Reaffirmed 2014). *Preconception and prenatal carrier screening for genetic diseases in individuals of Eastern European Jewish Descent. (ACOG Committee Opinion No. 442)*. Washington, DC: Author, (ACOG Committee Opinion No. 442).

American College of Obstetricians and Gynecologists. (2010). *Carrier screening for fragile X syndrome. (ACOG Committee Opinion No. 469)*. Washington, DC: Author, (ACOG Committee Opinion No. 469).

American College of Obstetricians and Gynecologists. (2011). *Update on carrier screening for cystic fibrosis. (ACOG Committee Opinion No. 486)*. Washington, DC: Author, (ACOG Committee Opinion No. 486).

American College of Obstetricians and Gynecologists. (2014). *Genetics and molecular diagnostic testing. (ACOG Technology Assessment No. 11)*. Washington, DC: Author, (ACOG Technology Assessment No. 11).

American College of Obstetricians and Gynecologists. (2015). *Cell-free DNA screening for fetal aneuploidy. (ACOG Committee Opinion No. 460)*. Washington, DC: Author, (ACOG Committee Opinion No. 460).

American College of Obstetricians and Gynecologists. (2015). *Identification and referral of maternal genetic conditions in pregnancy. (ACOG Committee Opinion No. 643)*.

Washington, DC: Author, (ACOG Committee Opinion No. 643).

American College of Obstetricians and Gynecologists. (2015). *Management of women with phenylketonuria. (ACOG Committee Opinion No. 636)*. Washington, DC: Author, (ACOG Committee Opinion No. 449).

Bacino, C.A., & Lee, B. (2011). Cytogenetics. In R.M. Kliegman, B.F. Stanton, J.W. St. Geme III, N.F. Schor, & R.E. Behrman (Eds.), *Nelson Textbook of Pediatrics* (19th ed., pp. 394–414). Philadelphia: Saunders.

Banasik, J.L. (2010). Genetic and developmental disorders. In L.C. Copstead, & J.L. Banasik (Eds.), *Pathophysiology* (4th ed., pp. 103–127). Philadelphia: Saunders.

Banasik, J.L. (2010). Molecular genetics and tissue differentiation. In L.C. Copstead, & J.L. Banasik (Eds.), *Pathophysiology* (4th ed., pp. 105–122). Philadelphia: Saunders.

Blackburn, S.T. (2013). *Maternal, fetal, and neonatal physiology: A clinical perspective* (4th ed.). St Louis: Saunders.

Callahan, L. (2016). Fetal and placental development and functioning. In S. Mattson, & J.E. Smith (Eds.), *AWHONN core curriculum for maternal-newborn nursing* (5th ed., pp. 37–62). St. Louis: Saunders.

Callahan, L. (2016). Genetics. In S. Mattson, & J.E. Smith (Eds.), *AWHONN core curriculum for maternal-newborn nursing* (5th ed., pp. 19–36). St. Louis: Saunders.

Centers for Disease Control and Prevention. (2014). *Guidelines for vaccinating pregnant women*. Retrieved from http://www.cdc.gov/vaccines.

Centers for Disease Control and Prevention. (2016). *Zika and Prenancy*. Retrieved from http://www.cdc.gov/Zika.

Hall, J.E. (2011). *Textbook of medical physiology* (12th ed.). Philadelphia: Saunders.

Jorde, L.B., Carey, J.C., & Bamshad, M.J. (2010). *Medical genetics* (4th ed.). St. Louis: Mosby.

Lee, B. (2011). Genetic counseling. In R.M. Kliegman, B.F. Stanton, J.W. St. Geme III, N.F. Schor, & R.E. Behrman (Eds.), *Nelson Textbook of Pediatrics* (19th ed., pp. 377–379). Philadelphia: Saunders.

National Genome Research Institute (2012). *National DNA Day Online Chatroom Transcript*. Retrieved from http://www.genome.gov.

National Human Genome Research Institute. (2015a). *FISH Fact Sheet*. Retrieved from http://www.genome.gov.

National Human Genome Research Institute. (2013). *SKY Fact Sheet*. Retrieved from: http://www.genome.gov.

National Human Genome Research Institute. (2015b). *All about the Human Genome Project*. Retrieved from http://www.genome.gov.

National Tay-Sachs and Allied Diseases Association. (2015). *What is Tay-Sachs disease?* Retrieved from http://www.ntsad.org.

Norton, M.E., Rose, N.C., & Benn, P. (2013). *Noninvasive Prenatal Testing for Fetal Aneuploidy*.

Scott, D.A., & Lee, B. (2011). Patterns of genetic transmission. In R.M. Kliegman, B.F. Stanton, J.W. St. Geme III, N.F. Schor, & R.E. Behrman (Eds.), *Nelson Textbook of Pediatrics* (19th ed., pp. 383–394). Philadelphia: Saunders.

11

# Reproductive Anatomy and Physiology

http://evolve.elsevier.com/McKinney/mat-ch/

## LEARNING OBJECTIVES

*After studying this chapter, you should be able to:*

- Explain the female and male sexual developments from prenatal life through sexual maturity.
- Describe the normal anatomy of the female and male reproductive systems.
- Explain the normal function of the female and male reproductive systems.
- Explain the normal structure and function of the female breast.

## SEXUAL DEVELOPMENT

Sexual development begins at conception when the union of an ovum and a sperm determines the genetic sex. During childhood, the sex organs are inactive.

### Prenatal Development

The mother's ovum carries a single X chromosome. Each of the father's spermatozoa carries either an X or Y chromosome. If an X-bearing sperm fertilizes the ovum, the offspring's genetic sex is female. If a Y-bearing sperm fertilizes the ovum, a male offspring results.

Although genetic sex is determined at conception, the reproductive systems of males and females are similar (sexually undifferentiated) for the first 6 weeks of prenatal life. During the 7th week, differences between males and females appear in the internal structures. The external genitalia look similar until the 9th week, when these outer structures begin to change. The differentiation of the external sexual organs is complete at approximately 12 weeks.

During fetal life, ovaries and testes secrete their primary hormones, estrogen and testosterone, respectively. Testosterone causes the development of male sex organs and external genitalia, and its absence results in female sex characteristics. Although the fetal ovary secretes estrogen, the hormone is not required to initiate the development of female sex structures. The trend for prenatal sexual development is to have female structures unless a Y chromosome is present. If a critical part of the Y chromosome is absent, a female rather than a male will develop from the XY genetic makeup.

### Childhood

The sex glands of girls and boys are inactive during infancy and childhood. At sexual maturity, the hypothalamus stimulates the anterior pituitary gland to produce hormones that will stimulate sex hormone production by the gonads (reproductive or sex glands).

### Sexual Maturation

Puberty refers to the time during which the reproductive organs become completely functional. Puberty is not a single event but a series of changes occurring over several years during late childhood and early adolescence.

#### Initiation of Sexual Maturation

Some factors that initiate sexual maturation remain unknown. Secretions of the hypothalamus, anterior pituitary, and gonads all play a part. The hypothalamus is capable of secreting gonadotropin-releasing hormone (GnRH) to initiate puberty during infancy and early childhood, but it does not do so in significant amounts until late childhood. Production of even tiny quantities of sex hormones by a young child's ovaries or testes inhibits secretions from the hypothalamus, preventing premature onset of puberty. Maturation of another unknown brain area probably triggers the hypothalamus to initiate puberty (Hall, 2011; Jones, 2009b).

The maturing child's hypothalamus gradually increases the production of GnRH beginning at 9 to 12 years of age (Blackburn, 2013; Hall, 2011; Jones, 2009b, 2009c). The level of GnRH slowly increases until reaching levels adequate to stimulate the anterior pituitary to increase its production of follicle-stimulating hormone (FSH) and luteinizing hormone (LH). The ovaries and testes increase their production of sex hormones and begin producing mature reproductive cells, or gametes, in response to the higher levels of FSH and LH. The sex hormones also induce the development of secondary sex characteristics (physical differences between mature males and females not directly related to reproduction). Table 11.1 presents the major hormones that play a role in reproduction.

There is individual variation in the age at which the changes of puberty begin and the time required to complete these changes. Research suggests that there is a direct correlation between obesity and

**TABLE 11.1 Major Hormones in Reproduction**

| Produced by | Target Organs | Action in Female | Action in Male |
|---|---|---|---|
| **Gonadotropin-Releasing Hormone (GNRH)** | | | |
| Hypothalamus | Anterior pituitary | Stimulates release of FSH and LH, initiating puberty and sustaining female reproductive cycles; release is pulsatile | Stimulates release of FSH and LH, initiating puberty; release is pulsatile |
| **Follicle-Stimulating Hormone (FSH)** | | | |
| Anterior pituitary | Ovaries (female)<br>Testes (male) | 1. Stimulates final maturation of follicle<br>2. Stimulates growth and maturation of Graafian follicles before ovulation | Stimulates Leydig cells of testes to secrete testosterone |
| **Luteinizing Hormone (LH)** | | | |
| Anterior pituitary | Ovaries (female)<br>Testes (male) | 1. Stimulates final maturation of follicle<br>2. Surge of LH approximately 14 days before next menstrual period causes ovulation<br>3. Stimulates transformation of Graafian follicle into corpus luteum, which continues secretion of estrogens and progesterone for approximately 12 days if ovum is not fertilized. If fertilization occurs, placenta gradually assumes this function. | Stimulates Leydig cells of testes to secrete testosterone |
| **Estrogen** | | | |
| 1. Ovaries and corpus luteum (female)<br>2. Placenta (pregnancy)<br>3. Formed in small quantities from testosterone in Sertoli cells of testes (male); other tissues, especially the liver, produce estrogen in the male | Internal and external reproductive organs<br>Breasts (female)<br>Testes (male) | 1. Reproductive organs<br>a. Maturation at puberty<br>b. Stimulation of endometrium before ovulation<br>2. Breasts: induce growth of glandular and ductal tissue; initiate deposition of fat at puberty<br>3. Stimulate growth of long bones, but cause closure of epiphyses, limiting mature height<br>4. Pregnancy: stimulate growth of uterus, breast tissue; inhibit active milk production; relax pelvic ligaments | Necessary for normal sperm formation |
| **Progesterone** | | | |
| Ovary, corpus luteum, placenta | Uterus, female breasts | 1. Stimulates secretion of endometrial glands; causes endometrial vessels to become dilated and tortuous in preparation for possible embryo implantation<br>2. Pregnancy: induces growth of cells of fallopian tubes and uterine lining to nourish embryo; decreases contractions of uterus; prepares breasts for lactation but inhibits prolactin secretion | Not applicable |
| **Prolactin** | | | |
| Anterior pituitary | Female breasts | Stimulates secretion of milk (lactogenesis); estrogen and progesterone from placenta have an inhibiting effect on milk production until after placenta is expelled at birth; sucking of newborn stimulates prolactin secretion to maintain milk production | Not applicable |
| **Oxytocin** | | | |
| Posterior pituitary | Uterus, female breasts | 1. Uterus: stimulates contractions during birth and stimulates postpartum contractions to compress uterine vessels and control bleeding<br>2. Stimulates letdown (milk-ejection reflex) during breastfeeding | Not applicable |
| **Testosterone** | | | |
| Adrenal glands (female)<br>Adrenal glands and Leydig cells in testes (male) | Sexual organs (male)<br>Male body conformation after puberty | Small quantities of androgenic (masculinizing) hormones from adrenal glands cause growth of pubic and axillary hair at puberty<br>Most androgens, such as testosterone, are converted to estrogen | 1. Induces development of male sex organs in fetus<br>2. Induces growth and division of the cells that mature sperm<br>3. Induces development of male secondary sex characteristics |

**TABLE 11.2 Comparison of Secondary Sex Characteristics in Females and Males**

| Females | Males |
|---|---|
| Development of glandular and ductal systems in the breast; deposition of fat selectively in the breast, buttocks, and thighs | Muscle mass 50% greater |
| Wide, round pelvis | Narrow, upright, and heavier pelvis |
| Pubic and axillary hair | Pubic and axillary hair; facial and chest hair; increased amount of hair on upper back in some males; male-pattern baldness, beginning on top of head |
| Soft, smooth skin texture | Coarser skin |
| Higher-pitched voice | Deeper voice |

early puberty in girls. Furthermore, girls who are underweight, with less body fat, typically experience a delay in puberty (Maron, 2015). Girls are approximately 6 months to 1 year younger than boys when hormonal changes of puberty begin. Changes of puberty occur in an orderly sequence in both sexes. Increases in height and weight are dramatic during puberty but slow after puberty until the mature height and weight are attained. Table 11.2 lists secondary sex characteristics of males and females. (See Chapter 9 for detailed information about the changes of puberty.)

### Female Puberty Changes

As a girl matures, the anterior pituitary gland secretes increasing amounts of FSH and LH in response to the hypothalamic secretion of GnRH. These pituitary hormones stimulate secretion of estrogens and progesterone by the ovary, resulting in the maturation of the reproductive organs and breasts and in the development of secondary sex characteristics such as axillary and pubic hair. The first noticeable changes of puberty begin at approximately 8 to 13 years in girls with the development of breast buds. The first menstrual period occurs 2 to 2½ years later, with an average age range from 9 to 16 years (Cromer, 2011).

**Breast changes.** The earliest outward changes of puberty occur in the breasts. First, the nipple enlarges and protrudes. The areola surrounding the nipple enlarges and becomes somewhat protuberant, although less so than the nipple. These changes are followed by growth of the glandular and ductal tissue. Fat is deposited in the breasts. During puberty, a girl's breasts may develop at different rates, resulting in a temporary lopsided appearance.

**Body contours.** The pelvis widens and assumes a rounded, basin-like shape that is favorable for passage of the fetus during childbirth. Fat is selectively deposited in the hips, giving them a rounder appearance than those of the male.

**Body hair.** Pubic hair appears downy at first but becomes thicker as puberty progresses. Axillary hair appears near the time of menarche (menstrual onset). The texture and quantity of pubic and axillary hair vary among women and in different ethnic groups. Women of African descent usually have body hair that is coarser and curlier than that of white women. Asian women often have sparser body hair than women of other racial groups.

**Skeletal growth.** In response to estrogen stimulation, girls grow taller for several years during early puberty. This growth spurt begins approximately 1 year after initial breast development. The other powerful effect of estrogen on the skeleton is to cause the epiphyses (growth areas of the bone) to unite with the shaft of the bones; this development eventually stops height growth.

**Reproductive organs.** The girl's external genitalia enlarge as fat is deposited in the mons pubis, labia majora, and labia minora. The vagina, uterus, fallopian tubes, and ovaries grow larger. The vaginal mucosa changes, becoming more resistant to trauma and infection in preparation for sexual activity. Changes in the reproductive organs occur during each female reproductive cycle.

**Menarche.** Early menstrual periods are often irregular and scant. Early menstrual cycles are not usually fertile because ovulation occurs inconsistently. Fertile reproductive cycles require preparation of the uterine lining precisely timed with ovulation. However, ovulation may occur during any female reproductive cycle, including the first. The sexually active girl can conceive even before her first menstrual period.

Delayed onset of menstruation is called *primary amenorrhea* if the girl's periods have not begun by the age of 16 years. Amenorrhea, or absence of menstruation, also may be considered primary if the girl is more than 1 year older than her mother or sisters were when their menarche occurred. *Secondary amenorrhea* describes absence of menstruation for at least three cycles after regular cycles have been established. Both primary and secondary amenorrhea are more common in females who are thin because they may have too little fat to produce enough sex hormones to stimulate ovulation and menstruation. Pregnancy is a common cause of secondary amenorrhea as well.

### Male Puberty Changes

Secretion of GnRH by the hypothalamus begins increasing as a boy enters puberty, stimulating secretion of LH and FSH from the anterior pituitary. LH and FSH then stimulate secretion of testosterone and eventually spermatogenesis, or formation of male gametes (sperm) in the testes. Testosterone stimulates development of a boy's reproductive organs and secondary sex characteristics.

**Growth of the testes and penis.** The first outward evidence of male sexual maturation is growth of the testes between approximately 9½ and 17 years. Growth in circumference and lengthening of the penis follow approximately a year after testicular growth begins. The skin of the scrotum thins and darkens.

**Nocturnal emissions.** Often called "wet dreams," nocturnal emissions are common during adolescence. The boy experiences a spontaneous ejaculation of seminal fluid during sleep, often accompanied by dreams with sexual content. Boys should be prepared for this normal occurrence so that they do not feel abnormal or ashamed.

**Body hair.** Pubic hair growth begins at the base of the penis. Gradually the hair coarsens and spreads upward and in the midline of the abdomen. Approximately 2 years later, axillary hair appears. Facial hair begins as a fine, downy mustache and progresses to the characteristic beard of the adult male. In most boys, chest hair develops, and some have hair on their upper backs. The amount and character of body hair varies between men of different racial groups, with Asian and Native American men often having less than white, black, or African-American men.

**Body composition.** Testosterone causes males to develop more muscle mass than females. At maturity, a man's muscle mass exceeds a woman's by 50%.

**Skeletal growth.** Testosterone causes boys to undergo a rapid growth spurt, especially in height. A boy's linear growth begins approximately a year later than a girl's and lasts for a longer time, resulting in the male's greater average height at maturity. Testosterone causes union of the epiphysis with the shaft of long bones, as does estrogen. The height-limiting effect of testosterone in the male is not as strong as that of estrogen in the female, so boys grow in stature for several years more than girls.

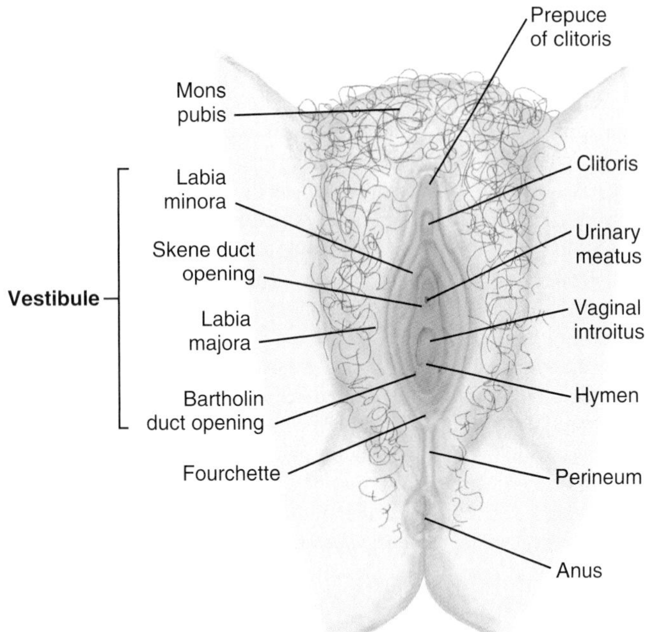


**FIG 11.1** External female reproductive structures.

A boy's shoulders broaden as his height increases. His pelvis assumes an upright shape, with a narrower diameter and heavier structure than the girl's.

***Voice changes.*** Hypertrophy of the laryngeal mucosa and enlargement of the larynx cause the male's voice to deepen. Before reaching the lower-pitched voice at maturity, many boys experience "cracking" or "squeaking" of their voices when they speak.

### Decline in Fertility

A woman's ability to reproduce decreases over a period of years involving physical and emotional changes, called the **climacteric**. In most women, the climacteric occurs between the ages of 45 and 50. At this time, maturation of ova and production of ovarian hormones decline. The external and internal reproductive organs atrophy somewhat as well. **Menopause** describes the final menstrual period. However, menopause and climacteric are often used interchangeably to describe the entire gradual process of change. **Perimenopause** is the time from the onset of symptoms associated with the climacteric until at least 1 year after the last menstrual period.

Males do not experience a marker event like menopause. Their production of testosterone and sperm gradually declines, but men in their 50s, 60s, and beyond may still be able to father children.

## FEMALE REPRODUCTIVE ANATOMY

### External Female Reproductive Organs

Collectively, the external female reproductive organs are called the *vulva* (Fig. 11.1).

#### Mons Pubis

The mons pubis is the rounded, fleshy prominence over the symphysis pubis that forms the anterior border of the external reproductive organs. It is covered with varying amounts of pubic hair.

#### Labia Majora and Labia Minora

The labia majora are two rounded, fleshy folds of tissue that extend from the mons pubis to the perineum. They have a slightly deeper pigmentation than surrounding skin and are covered with pubic hair. The labia majora protect the more fragile tissues of the external genitalia.

The labia minora run parallel to and within the labia majora. The labia minora extend from the clitoris anteriorly and merge posteriorly to form the fourchette, or posterior rim of the vaginal introitus. The labia minora do not have pubic hair. They are highly vascular and respond to stimulation by becoming engorged with blood.

#### Clitoris

The clitoris is a small projection at the anterior junction of the labia minora. The clitoris is composed of highly sensitive erectile tissue that is similar to tissue of the penis. The labia majora merge to form a prepuce over the clitoris.

#### Vestibule

The vestibule refers to structures enclosed by the labia minora. The urinary meatus, vaginal introitus, and ducts of Skene and Bartholin glands lie within the vestibule. Skene, or periurethral, glands provide lubrication for the urethra. Bartholin glands provide lubrication for the vaginal introitus, particularly during sexual arousal. The vaginal introitus is surrounded by erectile tissue. During sexual stimulation, blood flows into the erectile tissue, allowing the introitus to tighten around the penis. This process adds a massaging feeling that heightens the male's sexual sensations, encouraging release of semen.

The hymen is a thin fold of mucosa partially separating the vagina from the vestibule. The hymen may be broken with injury, with the use of tampons, during intercourse, or during childbirth. The intactness of the hymen, or lack thereof, is not a criterion of virginity.

#### Perineum

The perineum is the most posterior part of the external female reproductive organs. It extends from the fourchette anteriorly to the anus posteriorly and is composed of fibrous and muscular tissues that support pelvic structures.

### Internal Female Reproductive Organs

The internal reproductive structures are the vagina, uterus, fallopian tubes, and ovaries (Figs. 11.2 and 11.3).

#### Vagina

The vagina is a tube of muscular and membranous tissue approximately 8 to 10 cm (3 to 4 inches) long, lying between the bladder anteriorly and the rectum posteriorly. The vagina connects the uterus above with the vestibule below. The vaginal lining has multiple folds, or **rugae**, and a muscular layer that are capable of marked distention during childbirth. The vagina is lubricated by secretions of the cervix, the lowermost part of the uterus, and by the Bartholin glands.

The vagina does not end abruptly at the uterine opening but arches to form the vaginal **fornix**. Each fornix is described by its location: anterior, posterior, or lateral.

The three major functions of the vagina are:

- To allow discharge of the menstrual flow
- As the female organ of **coitus** (sexual union of male and female), to receive the male penis
- To allow passage of the fetus from the uterus

#### Uterus

The uterus is a hollow, thick-walled muscular organ that is shaped like a flattened upside-down pear. The uterus houses and nourishes the fetus until birth and then contracts rhythmically during labor to expel the fetus. Each month the uterus is prepared for a pregnancy, whether or not conception occurs.

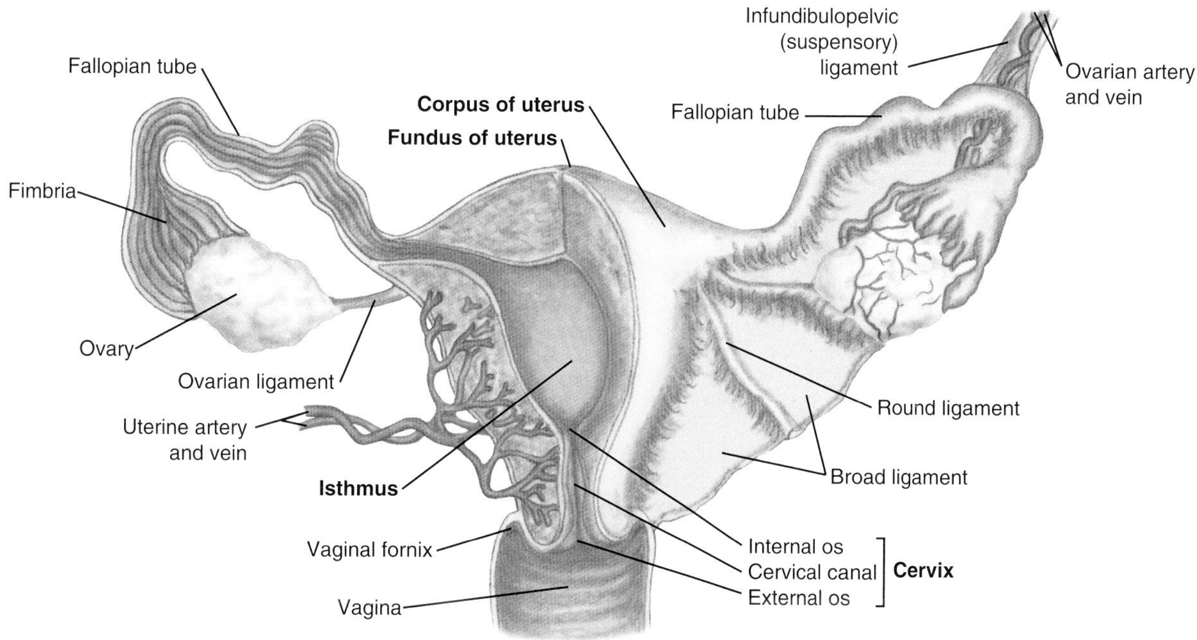


**FIG 11.2** Internal female reproductive structures, anterior view.

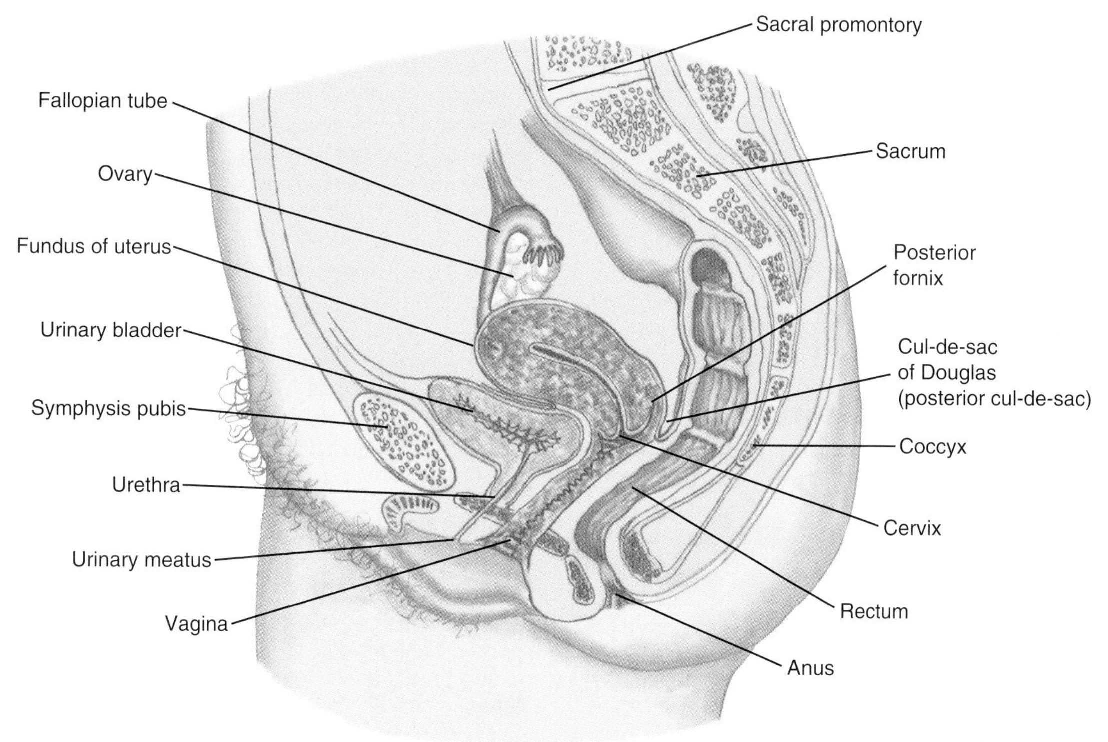


**FIG 11.3** Internal female reproductive structures, midsagittal view.

The uterus measures approximately 7.5 × 5 × 2.5 cm (3 × 2 × 1 inch) and is larger in a woman who has borne children than in one who has not. It is suspended above the bladder and is anterior to the rectum. Its normal position is anteverted (rotated forward) and slightly anteflexed (flexed forward).

***Divisions of the uterus.*** The uterus is divided into three parts.

**Corpus.** The upper part is the corpus, or body, of the uterus. The *fundus* of the uterus is the part of the corpus above the area where the fallopian tubes enter the uterus.

**Isthmus.** A narrower transition zone, the isthmus, is between the corpus of the uterus and the cervix. During late pregnancy the isthmus elongates and is known as the lower uterine segment.

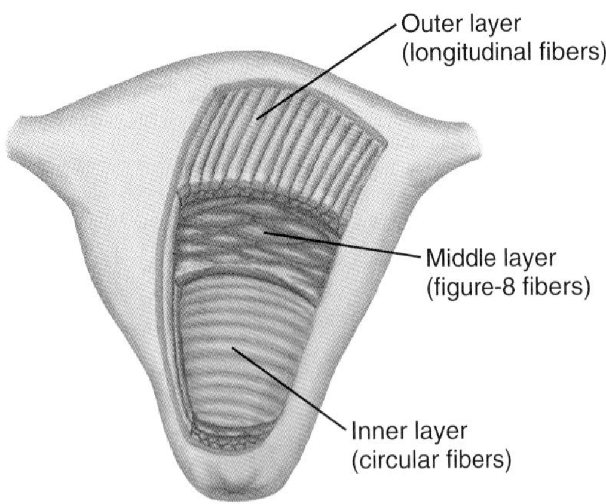


**FIG 11.4** Layers of the myometrium, showing the three types of smooth muscle fiber.

**Cervix.** The cervix is the tubular "neck" of the lower uterus and is approximately 2 to 3 cm (0.8 to 1 inch) long. The os is the opening in the cervix that runs between the uterus and the vagina. The upper part of the cervix is marked by the internal os, and the lower cervix is marked by the external os. The external os of a childless woman is round and smooth. After vaginal birth the external os has an irregular, slit-like shape and may have tags of scar tissue.

***Layers of the uterus.*** The uterus has three layers.

**Perimetrium.** The perimetrium is the outer peritoneal layer of serous membrane that covers most of the uterus. The perimetrium is continuous laterally with the broad ligaments on either side of the uterus.

**Myometrium.** The myometrium is the middle layer of thick muscle. Most of the muscle fibers are concentrated in the upper uterus, and their number diminishes progressively toward the cervix. The myometrium contains three types of smooth muscle fiber (Fig. 11.4). These types are:

- *Longitudinal fibers*, found mostly in the fundus and designed to expel the fetus efficiently toward the pelvic outlet during birth.
- *Interlacing figure-8 fibers*, which make up the middle layer. These fibers contract after birth to compress the blood vessels that pass between them to limit blood loss.
- *Circular fibers*, which form constrictions where the fallopian tubes enter the uterus and surround the internal cervical os. Circular fibers prevent reflux of menstrual blood and tissue into the fallopian tubes, promote normal implantation of the fertilized ovum by controlling its entry into the uterus, and retain the fetus until the appropriate time of birth.

**Endometrium.** The endometrium is the inner layer of the uterus. It is responsive to the cyclic variations of estrogen and progesterone during the female reproductive cycle (see p. 190). The endometrium has two layers:

- The *basal layer*, which is nearest the myometrium. This layer regenerates the functional layer of the endometrium after each menstrual period and after childbirth.
- The *functional layer*, which lies above the basal layer and contains the endometrial arteries, veins, and glands. This layer is shed during each menstrual period and after childbirth in the *lochia.*

### Fallopian Tubes

The fallopian tubes, also called *oviducts,* are 8 to 14 cm (3.2 to 5.6 inches) long and quite narrow (2 to 3 mm at their narrowest and 5 to 8 mm at their widest). The ovum travels from the ovary to the uterus through the fallopian tube. The fallopian tubes are lined with folded epithelium containing **cilia,** hair-like projections that move rhythmically toward the uterus to propel the ovum through the tube. Each fallopian tube enters the upper uterus at the *cornu,* or horn, of the uterus.

The fallopian has four divisions:

- The *interstitial* portion, which runs into the uterine cavity and lies within the uterine wall.
- The *isthmus,* the narrow part of the tube adjacent to the uterus.
- The *ampulla,* the wider area of the tube lateral to the isthmus where fertilization occurs.
- The *infundibulum,* the wide funnel-shaped terminal end of the tube. *Fimbriae* are finger-like processes surrounding the infundibulum.

The fallopian tubes are not directly connected to the ovary. At ovulation the ovum is expelled into the abdominal cavity. Wave-like motions of the fimbriae, which are very near the ovary, draw the ovum into the tube. However, the tubal isthmus remains contracted until 3 days after conception to allow the fertilized ovum to develop within the tube. Initial growth of the fertilized ovum within the fallopian tube promotes its normal implantation in the fundal portion of the uterine corpus. Implantation can occur within the tube, resulting in an ectopic pregnancy (see Chapter 25).

### Ovaries

The ovaries have two functions: to produce sex hormones and to develop an ovum to maturity during each reproductive cycle.

The ovaries secrete estrogen and progesterone in varying amounts during a woman's reproductive cycle to prepare the uterine lining for pregnancy. Ovarian hormone secretion gradually declines to very low levels during the climacteric.

At birth, the ovary contains all the ova that it will ever have: approximately 2 million immature ova. Many of these degenerate until 200,000 to 400,000 remain. Many ova begin the maturation process during each reproductive cycle but most never reach maturity. During the course of a woman's reproductive life, only approximately 400 of the ova ever mature enough to be released and fertilized. By the time a woman reaches the climacteric, almost all of her ova have been released during ovulation or have regressed. The few remaining ova are unresponsive to stimulating hormones and do not mature (Blackburn, 2013: Hall, 2011; Jones, 2009b; Moore & Persaud, 2008a, 2008b).

## Support Structures

The bony pelvis supports and protects the lower abdominal and internal reproductive organs. Muscles and ligaments provide added support for the internal organs of the pelvis against the downward force of gravity and the increases in intraabdominal pressure.

### Pelvis

The bony pelvis is a basin-shaped structure at the lower end of the spine. Its posterior wall is formed by the sacrum. The side and anterior pelvic walls are composed of three fused bones: the *ilium,* the *ischium,* and the *pubis.* Fig. 11.5 illustrates important anatomic landmarks on the pelvis.

The *linea terminalis,* also called the *pelvic brim* or *iliopectineal line,* is an imaginary line that divides the upper, or false, pelvis from the lower, or true, pelvis. The false pelvis provides support for the internal organs and the upper part of the body. The true pelvis is most important during childbirth, and its divisions and measurements are discussed in Chapter 16.

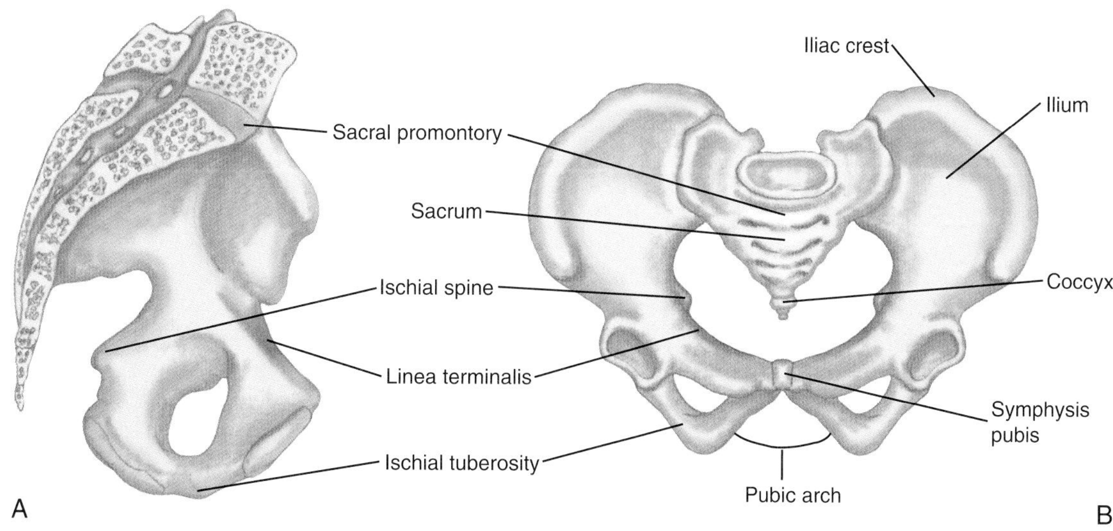


FIG 11.5 Structures of the bony pelvis, shown in lateral, **A,** and anterior, **B,** views.

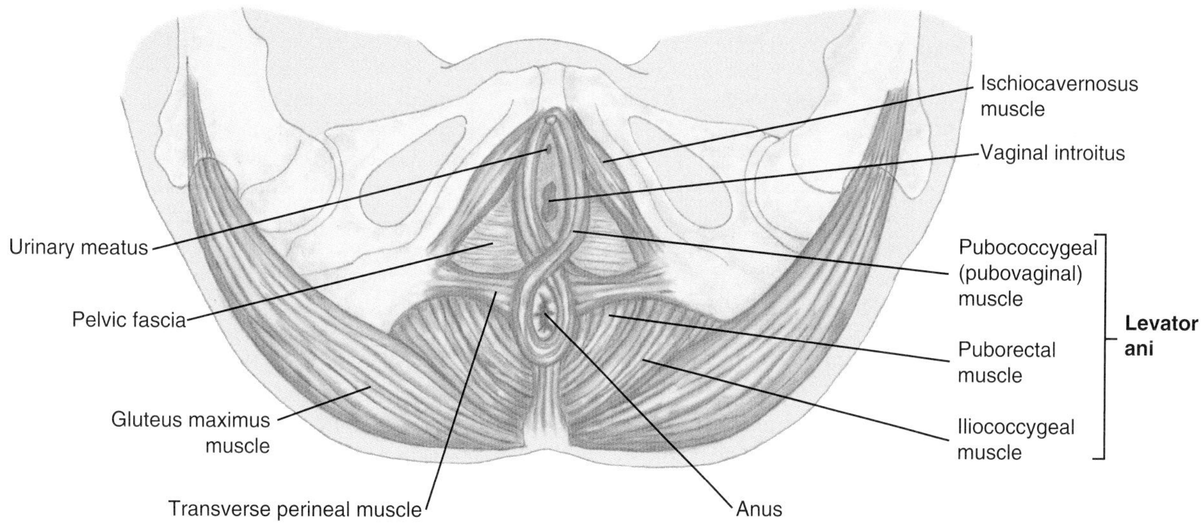


FIG 11.6 Muscles of the female pelvic floor.

## Muscles

Paired muscles enclose the lower pelvis and provide support for internal reproductive, urinary, and bowel structures (Fig. 11.6). A fibromuscular sheet, the *pelvic fascia,* also supports the pelvic organs. Vaginal and urethral openings are in the pelvic fascia.

The levator ani is a collection of three pairs of muscles: the *pubococcygeus,* which is also called the *pubovaginal muscle* in the female; the *puborectal;* and the *iliococcygeus.* These muscles support internal pelvic structures and resist increases in the intraabdominal pressure.

The *ischiocavernosus muscle* extends from the clitoris to the ischial tuberosities on each side of the lower bony pelvis. The two *transverse perineal muscles* extend from fibrous tissue of the perineum to the two ischial tuberosities, stabilizing the center of the perineum.

## Ligaments

Seven pairs of ligaments maintain the internal reproductive organs, with their nerve and blood supplies, in their proper positions within the pelvis (see Fig. 11.2).

**Lateral support.** Paired ligaments stabilize the uterus and ovaries laterally and keep them in the midline of the pelvis. The *broad ligament* is a sheet of tissue extending from each side of the uterus to the lateral pelvic wall. *The round ligament* and fallopian tube mark the upper border of the broad ligament; the lower edge is bounded by the uterine blood vessels. Within the two broad ligaments are the ovarian ligaments, blood vessels, and lymphatics.

The right and left *cardinal ligaments* provide support to the lower uterus and vagina. They extend from the lateral walls of the cervix and vagina to the sidewalls of the pelvis.

The *two ovarian ligaments* connect the ovaries to the lateral uterine walls. The *infundibulopelvic,* or *suspensory, ligaments* connect the lateral ovary and distal fallopian tubes to the pelvic sidewalls. The infundibulopelvic ligament also carries the blood vessel and nerve supply for the ovary.

**Anterior support.** Two pairs of ligaments provide anterior support for the internal reproductive organs. The *round ligaments* connect the upper uterus to the connective tissue of the labia majora. These ligaments maintain the uterus in its normal anteflexed position and help guide the fetal presenting part against the cervix during labor.

The *pubocervical ligaments* support the cervix anteriorly. They connect the cervix to the interior surface of the symphysis pubis.

**Posterior support.** The *uterosacral ligaments* provide posterior support, extending from the lower posterior uterus to the sacrum. These ligaments also contain sympathetic and parasympathetic nerves of the autonomic nervous system.

### Blood Supply

The uterine blood supply is carried by the *uterine arteries,* which are branches of the internal iliac artery. These vessels enter the uterus at the lower border of the broad ligament, near the isthmus of the uterus. The vessels branch downward to supply the cervix and vagina and upward to supply the uterus. The upper branch also supplies the ovaries and fallopian tubes. The vessels are coiled to allow for elongation as the uterus expands during pregnancy. Blood drains into the *uterine veins* and from there into the internal iliac veins.

Additional ovarian and tubal blood supply is carried by the *ovarian artery,* which arises from the abdominal aorta. The ovarian blood supply drains into the two *ovarian veins.*

### Nerve Supply

Most functions of the reproductive system are under involuntary, or unconscious, control. Nerves of the autonomic nervous system from the uterovaginal plexus and inferior hypogastric plexus control automatic functions of the reproductive system. Sensory and motor nerves that innervate the reproductive organs enter the spinal cord at the T12 through L2 levels. These nerves are important during childbearing for pain management.

## FEMALE REPRODUCTIVE CYCLE

The female reproductive cycle describes the regular and recurrent changes in the anterior pituitary secretions, ovaries, and uterine endometrium that are designed to prepare the body for pregnancy (Fig. 11.7). The female reproductive cycle is often called the *menstrual cycle* because menstruation provides a marker for each cycle's beginning and end if pregnancy does not occur.

The duration of the cycle is approximately 28 days, although it may range from 20 to 45 days (Hall, 2011; Jadack & Georges, 2010b; Jones, 2009a). Significant deviations from the 28-day cycle are associated with reduced fertility. The first day of the menstrual period is counted as day 1 of the woman's cycle. The female reproductive cycle is further divided into two cycles that reflect changes in the ovaries and uterine endometrium.

### Ovarian Cycle

In response to GnRH from the woman's hypothalamus, the anterior pituitary secretes FSH and LH. The FSH and LH stimulate the ovaries to mature an ovum, release it, and secrete other hormones that will prepare the endometrium for implantation of a fertilized ovum. The ovarian cycle consists of three phases: the follicular phase, the ovulatory phase, and the luteal phase.

#### Follicular Phase

The follicular phase is the period during which an ovum matures. It begins with the first day of menstruation and ends approximately 14 days later in a 28-day cycle. The length of this phase varies more among different women than do the lengths of the other two phases. The decrease in estrogen and progesterone secretion by the ovary just before menstruation stimulates secretion of FSH and LH by the anterior pituitary. As the FSH and LH levels rise, 6 to 12 Graafian follicles, each containing an oocyte (immature ovum), start growing faster. Each follicle secretes fluid containing high levels of estrogen, which accelerates maturation by making the follicle more sensitive to the effects of FSH. Eventually one follicle matures before the others. The mature follicle secretes large amounts of estrogen, which depresses FSH secretion. This brief dip in FSH secretion blocks further maturation of the less-developed follicles until after ovulation occurs. Occasionally more than one follicle matures and releases its ovum; this condition can lead to a multifetal pregnancy.

#### Ovulatory Phase

Near the middle of a 28-day reproductive cycle, approximately 2 days before ovulation, LH secretion rises markedly. Secretion of FSH also rises, but less than LH does. These surges in LH and FSH cause a slight fall in follicular estrogen production and a rise in progesterone secretion, stimulating final maturation of a single follicle and release of its mature ovum. Ovulation marks the beginning of the luteal phase of the female reproductive cycle and occurs approximately 14 days before the next menstrual period.

The mature follicle is a mass of cells with a fluid-filled chamber. A smaller mass of cells houses the ovum within this chamber. At ovulation, a blister-like projection, called a *stigma,* forms on the wall of the follicle, the follicle ruptures, and the ovum with its surrounding cells is released from the surface of the ovary. It is picked up by the fimbriated end of the fallopian tube for transport to the uterus.

#### Luteal Phase

After ovulation and under the influence of LH, the remaining cells of the old follicle persist for approximately 12 days as a *corpus luteum.* The corpus luteum secretes estrogen and large amounts of progesterone to prepare the endometrium for a fertilized ovum. Levels of FSH and LH decrease during this phase in response to higher levels of estrogen and progesterone. If the ovum is fertilized, it secretes human chorionic gonadotropin (hCG) that causes the corpus luteum to persist to maintain an early pregnancy. If the ovum is not fertilized, FSH and LH fall to low levels, and the corpus luteum regresses. Decline of estrogen and progesterone with the regression of the corpus luteum results in menstruation as the uterine lining breaks down.

The loss of estrogen and progesterone from the corpus luteum at the end of one cycle stimulates the anterior pituitary to increase secretion of FSH and LH, initiating a new cycle. The old corpus luteum is replaced by fibrous tissue called the *corpus albicans.*

### Endometrial Cycle

The uterine endometrium responds to ovarian hormone stimulation with cyclic changes. Three phases mark the changes in the endometrium: the proliferative phase, the secretory phase, and the menstrual phase.

#### Proliferative Phase

The proliferative phase takes place as the ovum matures and is released during the first half of the ovarian cycle. After completion of a menstrual period, the endometrium is very thin, with only the basal layer of cells remaining. These cells multiply to form new endometrial epithelium and endometrial glands under the stimulation of estrogen secreted by the maturing ovarian follicles. Endometrial spiral arteries and endometrial veins elongate to accompany thickening of the functional endometrial layer and to nourish the proliferating cells. As ovulation approaches, the endometrial glands secrete thin, stringy mucus that aids entry of sperm into the uterus.

#### Secretory Phase

The secretory phase occurs during the second half of the ovarian cycle as the uterus is prepared to receive a fertilized ovum. The endometrium continues to thicken under the influence of estrogen and progesterone

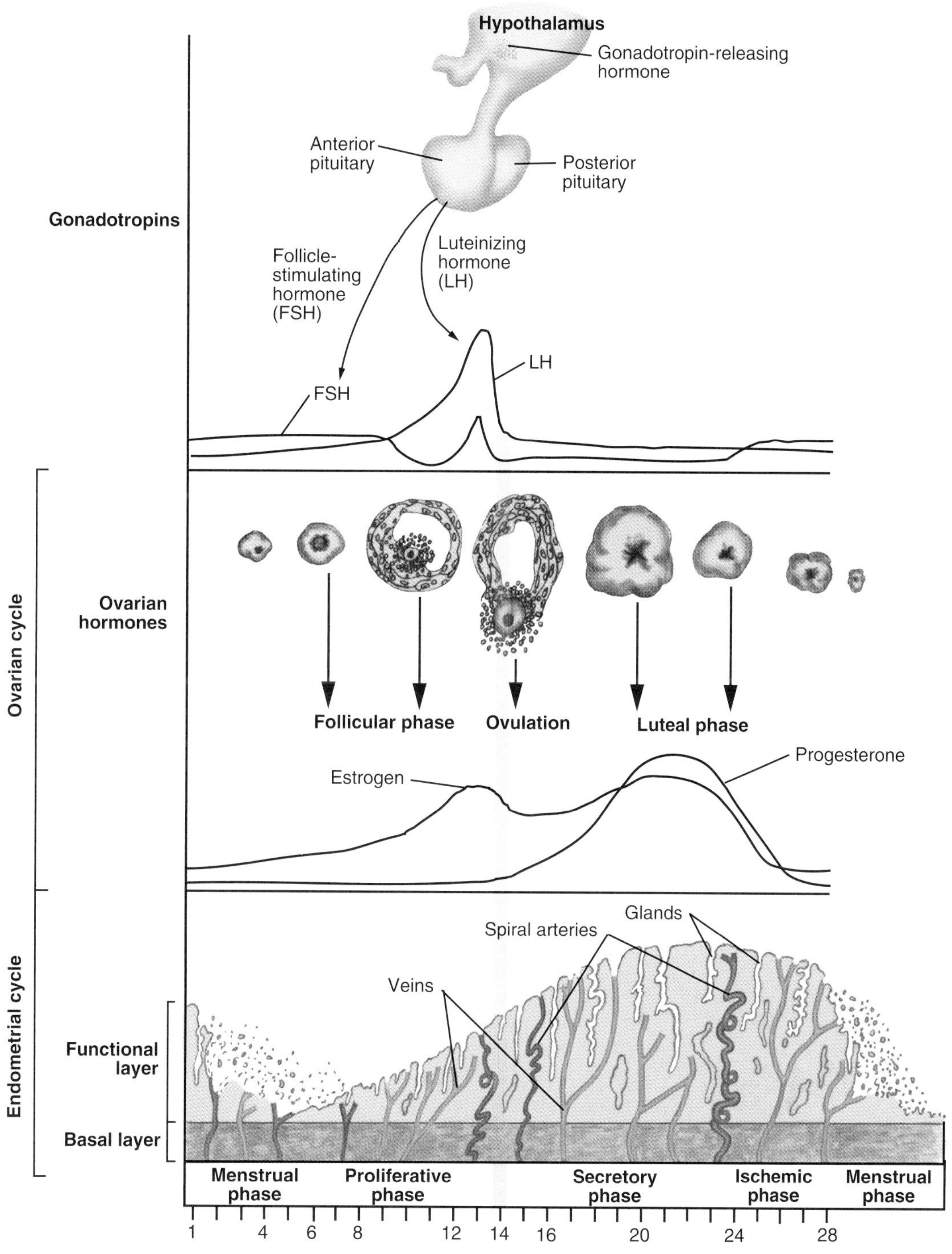


**FIG 11.7** The female reproductive cycle, showing the changes in hormone secretion from the anterior pituitary and interrelated changes in the ovary and uterine endometrium.

from the corpus luteum, reaching its maximum thickness of 5 to 6 mm. The blood vessels and endometrial glands become twisted and dilated.

Progesterone from the corpus luteum causes the thick endometrium to secrete substances that nourish a fertilized ovum. Large quantities of glycogen, proteins, lipids, and minerals are stored within the endometrium, awaiting arrival of the ovum.

## Menstrual Phase

If fertilization does not occur, the corpus luteum regresses, and its production of estrogen and progesterone fall. Approximately 2 days before the onset of the menses, vasospasm of the endometrial blood vessels causes the endometrium to become ischemic and necrotic. The necrotic areas of endometrium separate from the basal layers, resulting in menstrual flow. The average duration of the menstrual phase is approximately 5 days.

During a menstrual period, women lose approximately 40 mL of blood. Because of the recurrent loss of blood, many women are mildly anemic during their reproductive years, especially if their diets are low in iron.

### Changes in Cervical Mucus

During most of the female reproductive cycle, the mucus of the cervix is scant, thick, and sticky. Just before ovulation, cervical mucus becomes thin, clear, and elastic to promote passage of sperm into the uterus and fallopian tubes, where they can fertilize the ovum. Spinnbarkeit refers to the elasticity of cervical mucus (see Chapter 31). A woman may assess the elasticity of her cervical mucus to avoid or promote conception.

## THE FEMALE BREAST

### Structure

The breasts, or mammary glands, are not directly functional in reproduction, but they secrete milk after childbirth to nourish the infant. The small, raised nipple is at the center of each breast (Fig. 11.8). The nipple is composed of sensitive erectile tissue and can respond to sexual stimulation. Surrounding the nipple is a larger circular areola. Both the nipple and areola are darker than surrounding skin. Montgomery tubercles are sebaceous glands in the areola. They are inactive and not obvious except during pregnancy and lactation, when they enlarge and secrete a substance that keeps the nipple soft.

Within each breast are lobes of glandular tissue that secrete milk. These lobes are arranged like spokes of a wheel around the hub. Fifteen to twenty of these lobes are arranged around and behind the nipple and areola. Fibrous tissue and fat in the breast support the glandular tissue, blood vessels, lymphatics, and nerves.

Alveoli are small sacs that contain milk-secreting cells called *acini.* Acini extract substances needed from the mammary blood supply to manufacture milk when the breasts are properly stimulated by the anterior pituitary gland. Myoepithelial cells surround the alveoli to contract and eject the milk into the ductal system when signaled by secretion of the hormone *oxytocin* from the posterior pituitary gland.

The alveoli drain into lactiferous ducts that join to drain milk from all areas of the breast. The lactiferous ducts become wider under the areola and are called *lactiferous sinuses* in this area. The lactiferous sinuses narrow again as they open to the outside in the nipple.

### Function

The breasts are inactive until puberty, when rising estrogen levels stimulate growth of the glandular tissue. Fat is deposited in the breasts, resulting in the mature female contour. The amount of fat is the major determinant of breast size; the amount of glandular tissue is similar for all mature women. Therefore, breast size is unrelated to the amount of milk a woman can produce during lactation.

During pregnancy, high levels of estrogen and progesterone produced by the placenta stimulate growth of the alveoli and ductal system to prepare them for lactation. Prolactin secreted by the anterior pituitary gland stimulates milk production during pregnancy, but this effect is inhibited by estrogen and progesterone produced by the placenta. The inhibitory effects of estrogen and progesterone stop when the placenta is expelled after birth, and active milk production occurs in response to the infant's nursing.

## MALE REPRODUCTIVE ANATOMY AND PHYSIOLOGY

### External Male Reproductive Organs

The male has two external organs of reproduction: the penis and the scrotum (Fig. 11.9).

#### Penis

The penis has two functions. As part of the urinary tract, it carries urine from the bladder to the exterior during urination. As a reproductive organ, the penis carries semen into the female vagina during coitus.

The penis is composed mostly of erectile tissue, which is spongy tissue with many small spaces inside. There are three areas of erectile

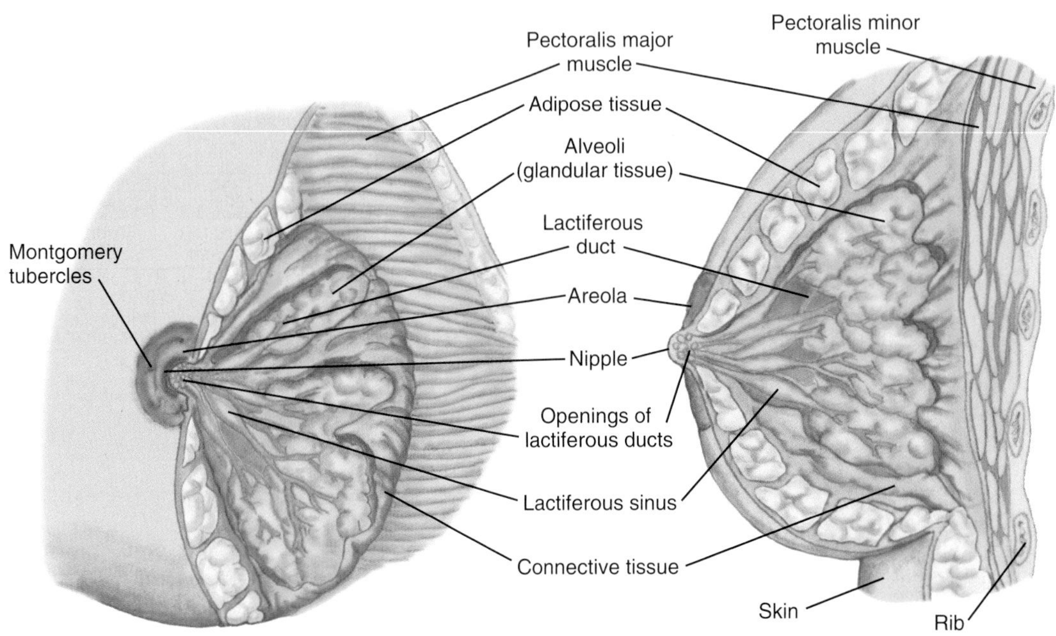


**FIG 11.8** Structures of the female breast.

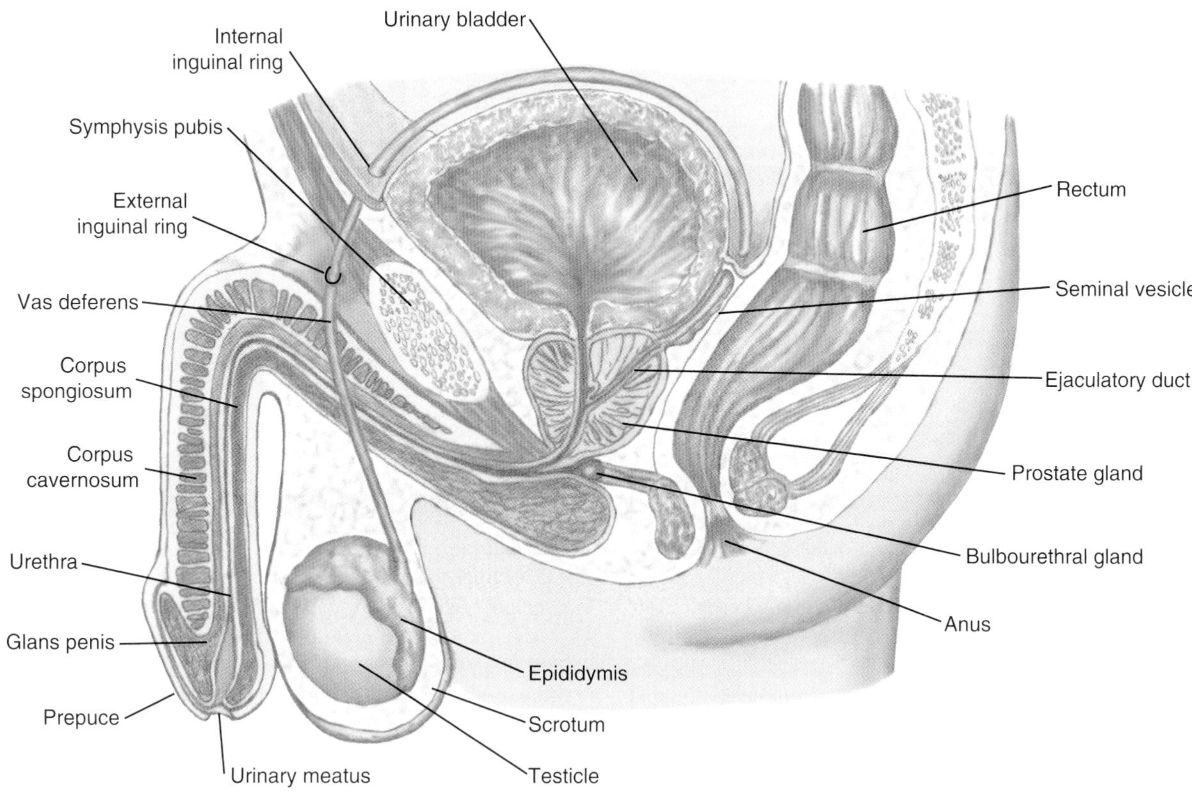


**FIG 11.9** Structures of the male reproductive system, midsagittal view.

tissue: the corpus spongiosum, which surrounds the urethra; and two columns of the corpus cavernosum, one on each side of the penis.

The penis is flaccid most of the time because small spaces within the erectile tissue are collapsed. During sexual stimulation, arteries within the penis dilate and veins are partly occluded, trapping blood in the spongy tissue. Entrapment of blood within the penis causes erection and enables the man to penetrate the vagina during sexual intercourse.

The glans is the distal end of the penis. The urinary meatus is centered in the end of the glans. Covering the glans is the loose skin of the prepuce, or foreskin. The prepuce may be removed by *circumcision*.

### Scrotum

The scrotum is a pouch of thin skin and muscle suspended behind the penis. The skin of the scrotum is darker than the surrounding skin and is covered with rugae. The scrotum is divided internally by a septum. One testicle is contained within each pocket of the scrotum.

The scrotum's main function is to keep the testes cooler than the core body temperature. Formation of normal sperm requires that the testes not be too warm. A cremaster muscle is attached to each testicle. This muscle can tighten, drawing the testes closer to the body and warming them, or it can relax, allowing the testes to fall away from the body and become cooler.

## Internal Male Reproductive Organs

### Testes

The male gonads, or testes, have two functions: they serve as endocrine glands and they produce male gametes, or sperm, also called *spermatozoa*. Androgens, the male sex hormones, are the primary endocrine secretions of the testes. Androgens are produced by Leydig cells of the testes. The primary androgen produced by the testes is testosterone.

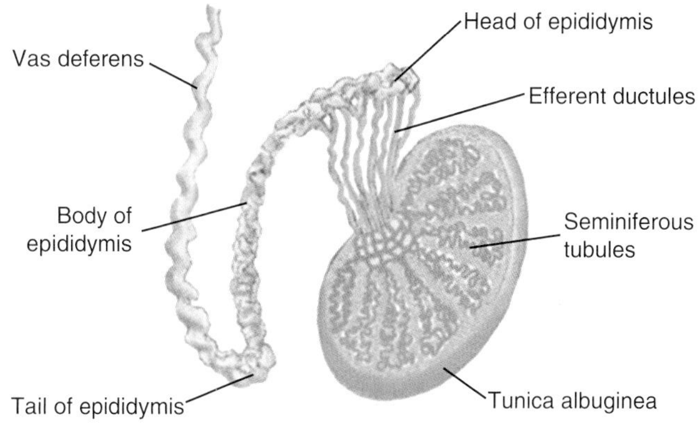


**FIG 11.10** Internal structures of the testis. Production of sperm begins within the tiny coiled seminiferous tubules. Immature sperm pass from the seminiferous tubules to the epididymis and then to the vas deferens. During their passage through these structures, the sperm mature and acquire the ability to propel themselves.

Unlike the female who experiences a cyclic pattern of hormone secretion, the male secretes testosterone in a relatively even pattern. A small amount of testosterone is converted to estrogen in the male and is necessary for sperm formation.

Spermatogenesis occurs within tiny, coiled tubes of the testes called the *seminiferous tubules* (Fig. 11.10). Leydig cells are interstitial cells that support the seminiferous tubules and secrete testosterone, a hormone necessary for forming new cells that will mature into sperm. Sertoli cells within the seminiferous tubules respond to FSH secretion by nourishing and supporting sperm as they mature. Unlike the female, who has a lifetime supply of ova in her gonads at birth, the male does not begin producing sperm until puberty. The normal male produces new sperm throughout life, although production declines with age.

At ejaculation, 35 to 200 million sperm are deposited in the vagina (Blackburn, 2013; Hall, 2011; Jones, 2009c). This large number is needed for normal fertility, although a single sperm fertilizes the ovum. Only a few sperm ever reach the fallopian tube, where an ovum may be available for fertilization.

### Accessory Ducts and Glands

From the seminiferous tubules, sperm pass into the epididymis within the scrotum for storage and final maturation. In the epididymis, sperm develop the ability to be motile. However, secretions within the epididymis inhibit actual motility until ejaculation occurs.

The epididymis empties into the vas deferens, where larger numbers of sperm are stored. The vas deferens leads upward into the pelvis and then back down toward the penis through the internal and external inguinal rings. Within the pelvis, the vas deferens joins the ejaculatory duct before connecting to the urethra.

Three glands—the *seminal vesicles,* the *prostate,* and the *bulbourethral glands*—secrete seminal fluids that carry sperm into the vagina during intercourse. The seminal fluid (1) nourishes the sperm, (2) protects the sperm from the acidic environment of the vagina, (3) enhances the motility of the sperm, and (4) washes the sperm out of the urethra so that the maximum number are deposited in the vagina.

## KEY CONCEPTS

- Initial prenatal development of the reproductive organs is similar for both males and females. If a critical part of the Y chromosome is not present at conception, female reproductive structures will develop.
- Puberty is the time when the reproductive organs become fully functional and secondary sex characteristics develop.
- Puberty begins approximately 6 months to 1 year earlier in girls than in boys, although a girl's early growth spurt makes it seem that she begins puberty much earlier than a boy.
- Girls are generally shorter than boys because they begin their growth spurt at an earlier age and complete it more quickly than boys.
- Girls often do not ovulate in early menstrual cycles, although it is possible for them to ovulate before the first one. A sexually active girl can become pregnant even before her first menstrual period.
- The onset of puberty is less obvious in boys than in girls and begins with growth of the testes and penis.
- Nocturnal emission of seminal fluids may be distressing to boys unless they are prepared for this normal event.
- At birth, a girl has all the ova she will ever have. New ova are not formed after birth, and most are depleted when a woman reaches the climacteric.
- The female reproductive cycle is often called the menstrual cycle. It includes changes in the anterior pituitary gland, ovaries, and uterine endometrium to prepare for a fertilized ovum. The character of cervical mucus also changes to encourage fertilization.
- Breast size is unrelated to glandular tissue or to the quantity or quality of milk a woman can produce for her infant after childbirth. Breast size is primarily related to the amount of fat present.
- For normal sperm to form, a man's testes must be cooler than his core body temperature.
- Seminal fluids secreted by the seminal vesicles, prostate, and bulbourethral glands nourish and protect the sperm, enhance their motility, and ensure that most sperm are deposited in the vagina during sexual intercourse.

## REFERENCES AND READINGS


Blackburn, S.T. (2013). *Maternal, fetal, and neonatal physiology: A clinical perspective* (4th ed.). St. Louis: Saunders.

Cromer, B. (2011). Adolescent physical and social development. In R.M. Kliegman, B.F. Stanton, J.W. St. Geme III, N.F. Schor, & R.E. Behrman (Eds.), *Nelson textbook of pediatrics* (19th ed., pp. 649–654). Philadelphia: Saunders.

Cunningham, F.G., Leveno, K.J., Bloom, S.L., et al. (2010). *Williams obstetrics* (23rd ed.). New York: McGraw-Hill.

Garibaldi, L., & Chemaitilly, W. (2011). Physiology of puberty. In R.M. Kliegman, B.F. Stanton, J.W. St. Geme III, N.F. Schor, & R.E. Behrman (Eds.), *Nelson textbook of pediatrics* (19th ed., pp. 1886). Philadelphia: Saunders.

Hall, J.C. (2011). *Guyton and Hall textbook of medical physiology* (12th ed.). Philadelphia: Saunders.

Jadack, R.M., & Georges, J.M. (2010a). Alterations in female genital and reproductive function. In L.C. Copstead, & J.L. Banasik (Eds.), *Pathophysiology: Biological and behavioral perspectives* (4th ed., pp. 769–789). Philadelphia: Saunders.

Jadack, R.M., & Georges, J.M. (2010b). Female genital and reproductive function. In L.C. Copstead, & J.L. Banasik (Eds.), *Pathophysiology: Biological and behavioral perspectives* (4th ed., pp. 751–768). Philadelphia: Saunders.

Jones, E.E. (2009a). Fertilization, pregnancy, and lactation. In W.F. Boron, & E.L. Boulpaep (Eds.), *Medical physiology* (2nd ed., pp. 1170–1192). Philadelphia: Saunders.

Jones, E.E. (2009b). The female reproductive system. In W.F. Boron, & E.L. Boulpaep (Eds.), *Medical physiology* (2nd ed., pp. 1146–1169). Philadelphia: Saunders.

Jones, E.E. (2009c). The male reproductive system. In W.F. Boron, & E.L. Boulpaep (Eds.), *Medical physiology* (2nd ed., pp. 1128–1145). Philadelphia: Saunders.

Maron, D.F. (2015). Why girls are starting puberty earlier. *Scientific American. 312*(5). 28-30.

Moore, K.L., & Persaud, T.V.N. (2008a). *Before we are born: Essentials of embryology and birth defects* (7th ed.). Philadelphia: Saunders.

Moore, K.L., & Persaud, T.V.N. (2008b). *The developing human: Clinically oriented embryology* (8th ed.). Philadelphia: Saunders.

Van Every, M., Mikkelson, D., & Cagle, C.S. (2010a). Alterations in male genital and reproductive function. In L.C. Copstead, & J.L. Banasik (Eds.), *Pathophysiology: Biological and behavioral perspectives* (4th ed., pp. 737–750). Philadelphia: Saunders.

Van Every, M., Mikkelson, D., & Cagle, C.S. (2010b). Male genital and reproductive function. In L.C. Copstead, & J.L. Banasik (Eds.), *Pathophysiology: Biological and behavioral perspectives* (4th ed., pp. 720–736). Philadelphia: Saunders.

12

# Conception and Prenatal Development

http://evolve.elsevier.com/McKinney/mat-ch/

## LEARNING OBJECTIVES

*After studying this chapter, you should be able to:*

- Describe the formation of the female and male gametes.
- Relate ovulation and ejaculation to the process of human conception.
- Explain the implantation and nourishment of the embryo before the development of the placenta.
- Describe normal prenatal development from conception through birth.
- Explain the structure and function of the placenta, umbilical cord, and fetal membranes.
- Describe how common deviations from usual conception and prenatal development occur.
- Describe prenatal circulation and the circulatory changes after birth.
- Explain mechanisms and trends in multifetal pregnancies.

A basic understanding of conception and prenatal development helps the nurse provide care to parents during normal childbearing and better understand problems such as infertility and birth defects. This chapter addresses the formation of the gametes, process of conception, prenatal development, and important auxiliary structures that support prenatal development. A short discussion of multifetal pregnancy is included.

## GAMETOGENESIS

To develop ova in females and spermatozoa in males, gametogenesis (creation of reproductive cells) requires a special reduction division called meiosis. Unlike mitosis, in which the diploid number of chromosomes (46) is retained in each new cell, meiosis halves the number of chromosomes (haploid number). Only one of each chromosome in a pair is directed to the gamete, yielding 22 autosomes and 1 sex chromosome. When the sperm and ovum unite at conception, the "halves" form a new cell and restore the chromosome number to 46 (Table 12.1).

### Oogenesis

Oogenesis (formation of ova or female gametes) begins during prenatal life when primitive ova (oogonia) multiply by mitosis, like other somatic (body) cells throughout life. Each oogonium contains 46 chromosomes (22 pairs of autosomes, or non-sex chromosomes, and a pair of X chromosomes), as do other body cells. Before birth, the oogonia enlarge to form primary oocytes with a layer of follicular cells surrounding each one (Fig. 12.1, *A*). These are called *primary follicles.* The primary oocyte begins its first meiotic division during fetal life but does not complete the process until puberty. The primary oocytes (still containing 46 chromosomes) remain dormant throughout childhood.

By the 30th week of gestation, the female fetus has all the ova she will ever have. Many of these ova regress during childhood (see Chapter 11). When reproductive cycles begin at puberty, some of the primary follicles that are present at birth begin maturing. The cyclic process of gamete maturation continues throughout a woman's reproductive years until the climacteric or menopause (Blackburn, 2013; Carlson, 2014; Jones, 2012a; Moore & Persaud, 2015, 2011).

When the oocyte matures, two meiotic divisions reduce the chromosome number from 46 paired to 23 unpaired chromosomes: 22 autosomes and an X chromosome. Shortly before ovulation, the primary oocyte completes its first meiotic division, which began during fetal life. A secondary oocyte, now containing 23 unpaired chromosomes, results. The cytoplasm in the primary oocyte is divided unequally with this division, with most retained by the secondary oocyte. The remainder of cytoplasm plus the other 23 chromosomes goes into a tiny, nonfunctional polar body that soon degenerates.

At ovulation, the secondary oocyte begins dividing again (second meiotic division) to form a mature ovum. The 23 chromosomes duplicate themselves in the second meiotic division, but half of the duplicated chromosomes will be discarded if fertilization occurs. The second meiotic division is prolonged, and the mature ovum remains suspended in metaphase, the middle part of cell division. If fertilization occurs, the second meiotic division is completed, resulting in a mature ovum containing 23 chromosomes and a second tiny polar body containing the 23 discarded chromosomes that degenerates. If the ovum is not fertilized, it does not complete the second meiotic division and degenerates. In oogenesis, one primary oocyte results in a single mature ovum.

When released from the ovary, two layers—the zona pellucida and the cells of the corona radiata—surround the mature ovum. These layers protect the ovum and prevent fertilization by more than one sperm. For fertilization to occur, the sperm must penetrate these two layers to reach the ovum's cell nucleus.

### Spermatogenesis

Spermatogenesis, or formation of sperm, begins during puberty in the male (Fig. 12.1, *B*). Primitive sperm cells *(spermatogonia)* develop during fetal life and begin multiplying by mitosis during puberty.

## TABLE 12.1 Comparison of Female and Male Gametogenesis

| | Oogenesis | Spermatogenesis |
|---|---|---|
| Time during which primary germ cells are produced | Fetal life. No others develop after approximately 30 wk of gestation. | Continuously after puberty |
| Hormones that control process | GnRH<br>FSH<br>LH<br>Estrogen | GnRH<br>FSH<br>LH<br>Testosterone<br>Estrogen (small amounts converted from testosterone)<br>Growth hormone |
| Number of mature germ cells that develop from each primary cell | One | Four |
| Quantity | One during each reproductive cycle of approximately 28 days | 35–200 million are released with each ejaculation. |
| Size | Large. Visible to naked eye. Abundant cytoplasm to nourish embryo until implantation | Tiny compared with ovum. Little cytoplasm. Head is almost all nuclear material (chromosomes). |
| Motility | Relatively nonmotile. Carried along by action of cilia and currents within fallopian tubes | Independently motile by means of whip-like tail. Mitochondria in middle piece provide energy for motility. |
| Chromosome complement | 23 total: 22 autosomes plus one X sex chromosome | 23 total: 22 autosomes, plus either an X or a Y sex chromosome |

*FSH,* Follicle-stimulating hormone; *GnRH,* gonadotropin-releasing hormone; *LH,* luteinizing hormone

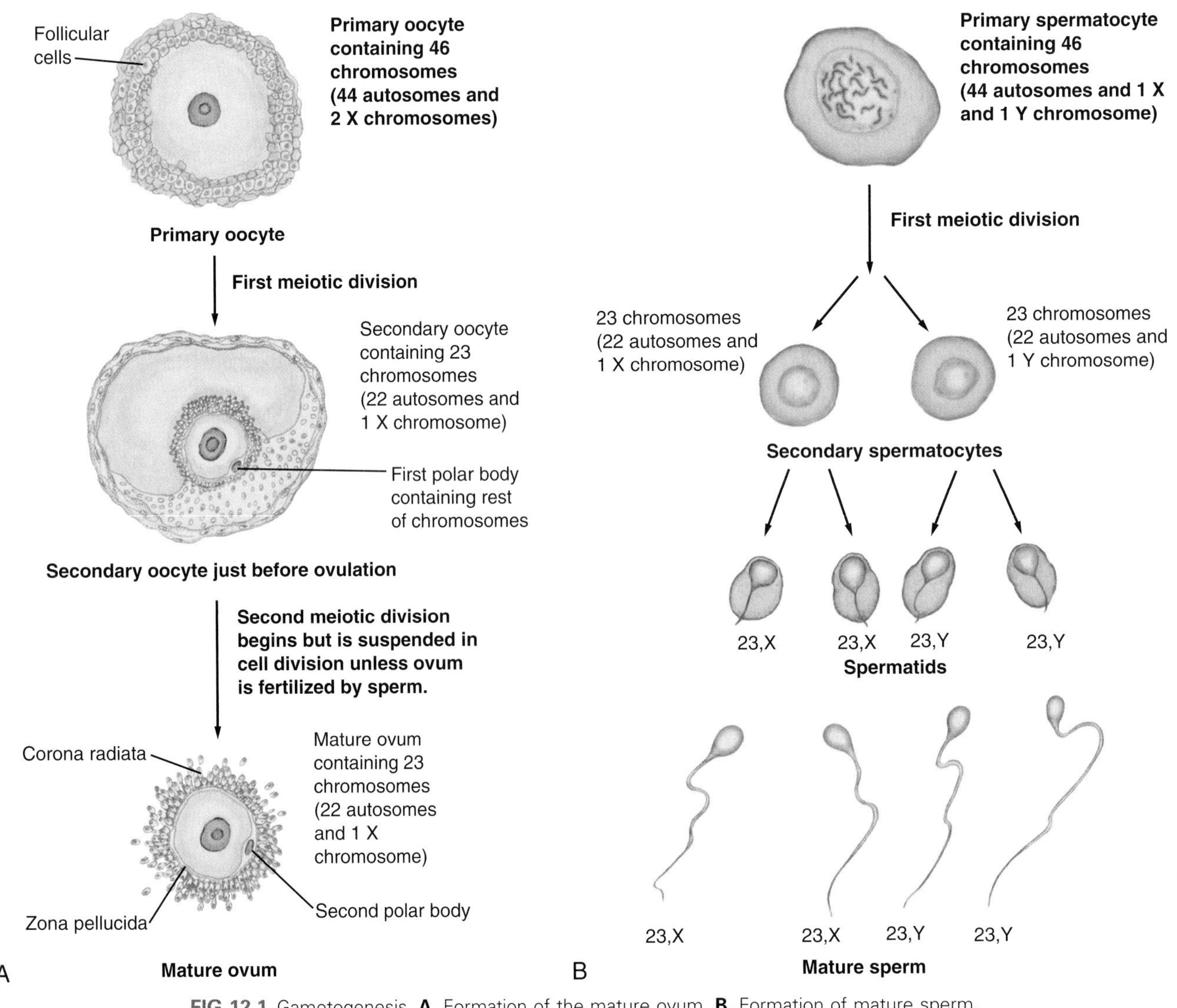


**FIG 12.1** Gametogenesis. **A,** Formation of the mature ovum. **B,** Formation of mature sperm.

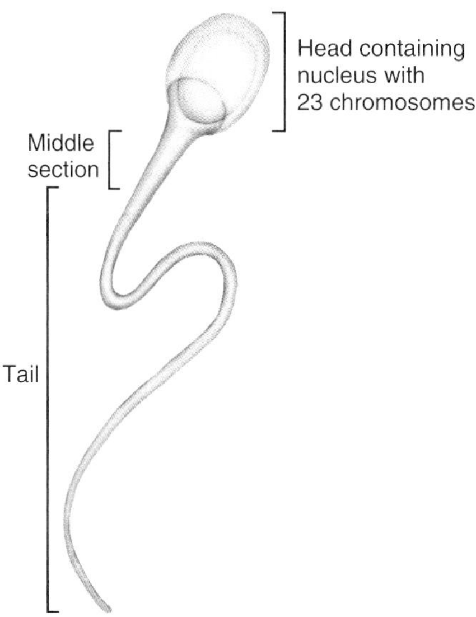


FIG 12.2 Mature sperm.

Unlike the female, the male produces new spermatogonia that can mature into sperm throughout his lifetime. Although male fertility gradually declines with age, men can father children in their 50s, 60s, and beyond.

Each spermatogonium contains 46-paired chromosomes, like other body cells. In the mature male, a spermatogonium enlarges to become a primary spermatocyte, still containing all 46 chromosomes. The first meiotic division forms two secondary spermatocytes and reduces the number to 23 unpaired chromosomes: 22 autosomes and 1 sex chromosome, either an X or a Y. Each secondary spermatocyte divides again in the second meiotic division to form two spermatids. Therefore, half of the four spermatids resulting from the two meiotic divisions of the spermatogonium carry an X chromosome and half carry a Y. The spermatids gradually mature into sperm.

The gamete from a male determines the sex of the new baby. If an X-bearing spermatozoon fertilizes the ovum, the baby is a girl. If a Y-bearing spermatozoon fertilizes the ovum, the baby is a boy.

The mature sperm has three sections: a head, a middle portion, and a tail (Fig. 12.2). The head is almost entirely the cell nucleus. The head contains the male chromosomes that will join the chromosomes of the ovum. The middle portion supplies energy for the tail's whip-like action. The movement of the tail propels the sperm toward the ovum.

## CONCEPTION

Conception requires correct timing between release of a mature ovum at ovulation and ejaculation of enough healthy, mature, motile sperm into the vagina. The ovum may have the capacity to be fertilized no longer than 24 hours after ovulation, although the exact duration of its viability is unknown. Most sperm survive no more than 1 to 2 days, although a few may remain fertile in the woman's reproductive tract up to 80 hours (Blackburn, 2013; Carlson, 2014).

### Female Preparation for Conception

Before ovulation, several oocytes begin to mature under the influence of follicle-stimulating hormone (FSH) and luteinizing hormone (LH) from the woman's anterior pituitary gland. Each maturing oocyte is contained in a sac within the ovary called the **Graafian** follicle, which produces estrogen and progesterone to prepare the **endometrium** (uterine lining) for a possible pregnancy. Eventually, one follicle outgrows the others. The less mature oocytes permanently regress.

### Release of the Ovum

**Ovulation**, or release of the ovum, occurs approximately 14 days before a woman's next menstrual period would begin. The follicle develops a thin spot on the surface of the ovary and ruptures, releasing the mature ovum with its surrounding cells on the surface of the ovary. There the collapsed follicle becomes the **corpus luteum**, which maintains the high estrogen and progesterone secretion necessary to make final preparation of the uterine lining for a fertilized ovum.

### Ovum Transport

Released on the surface of the ovary, the mature ovum is picked up by the fimbriated (fringed) ends of the fallopian tube near the surface of the ovary. Muscular action of the tube and movement of cilia within the tube transport the ovum through the tube. Fertilization normally occurs in the distal third of the fallopian tube, near the ovary. The ovum, fertilized or not, enters the uterus approximately 3 days after its release from the ovary.

### Male Preparation for Conception

Male preparation for fertilizing the ovum consists of ejaculation, movement of the sperm in the female reproductive tract, and preparation of the sperm for actual fertilization.

### Ejaculation

Expulsion of semen from the penis is **ejaculation**. When a male ejaculates during vaginal intercourse, 35 to 200 million sperm are deposited in the upper vagina and over the cervix (Blackburn, 2013; Hall, 2011; Jones, 2012b). The sperm are suspended in seminal fluid, which nourishes and protects them from the acidic vaginal environment. To hold the semen deeply in the vagina, the seminal fluid coagulates somewhat after ejaculation. The sperm are relatively immobile for approximately 15 to 30 minutes until other seminal enzymes dissolve the coagulated fluid and allow the sperm to begin moving upward through the cervix.

### Transport of Sperm in the Female Reproductive Tract

Whip-like movement of the tails of spermatozoa propels them through the cervix, uterus, and fallopian tubes. Uterine contractions induced by prostaglandins in the seminal fluid enhance movement of the sperm toward the ovum. Only sperm cells enter the cervix. The seminal fluid remains in the vagina.

Many sperm are lost along the way. Some are digested by vaginal enzymes and phagocytes in the female reproductive tract, whereas others move into the wrong tube or past the ovum and out into the peritoneal cavity. Only a few hundred reach the fallopian tube where the ovum waits.

### Preparation of Sperm for Fertilization

Sperm are not immediately ready to fertilize the ovum when they are ejaculated. While making the trip to the ovum, the sperm undergo changes *(capacitation)* that enable one to penetrate the protective layers surrounding the ovum. During capacitation, a glycoprotein coat and seminal proteins are removed from the acrosome (tip of the sperm head). After capacitation, the sperm look the same but are more active and can better penetrate the corona radiata and zona pellucida that surround the ovum.

The sperm that reach the ovum release an enzyme (hyaluronidase) to digest a pathway through the corona radiata and zona pellucida. Their tails beat harder to propel them toward the center of the ovum. Eventually, one spermatozoon penetrates the ovum.

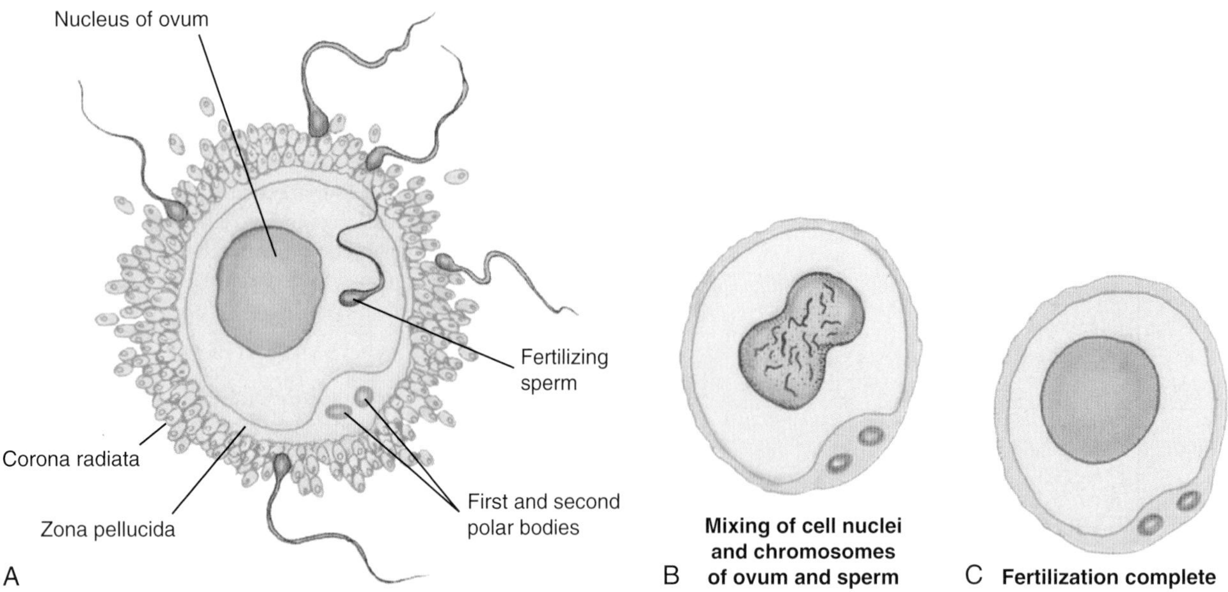


**FIG 12.3** Process of fertilization. **A,** A sperm enters the ovum. **B,** The 23 chromosomes from the sperm mingle with the 23 chromosomes from the ovum, restoring the diploid number to 46. **C,** The fertilized ovum, now called a *zygote*, is ready for the first mitotic cell division.

## Fertilization

Fertilization occurs when one spermatozoon enters the ovum and the two nuclei containing the parents' chromosomes merge (Fig. 12.3).

### Entry of One Spermatozoon Into the Ovum

Entry of a spermatozoon into the ovum has two consequences:

- Changes in the zona pellucida surrounding the ovum prevent other sperm from entering.
- The ovum, which has been suspended in the middle of its second meiotic division, completes meiosis.

The results are a nucleus with 23 chromosomes and expulsion of a second nonfunctional polar body. The mature ovum now contains 23 unpaired chromosomes, 22 autosomes, and 1 X chromosome in its nucleus.

### Fusion of the Nuclei of Sperm and Ovum

Fusion of the nuclei of the sperm and ovum begins when the sperm enters the ovum. The sperm head enlarges, and the tail degenerates. The nuclei of the gametes move toward the center of the ovum, where the membranes surrounding their nuclei touch and dissolve. The 23 chromosomes from the sperm mingle with the 23 from the ovum, restoring the diploid number to 46. Fertilization is complete within 24 hours, and cell division of the zygote can begin when the nuclei of the sperm and ovum unite.

## PRE-EMBRYONIC PERIOD

The pre-embryonic period is the first 2 weeks after conception. Fig. 12.4 illustrates the period from fertilization through implantation.

### Initiation of Cell Division

The zygote divides into two cells, then four, then eight cells while in the fallopian tube. Up to the 16-cell stage, the cells become smaller with each division, so they occupy approximately the same amount of space as the original ovum. When the conceptus (fertilized ovum) is a solid ball of 12 to 16 cells, it is called a *morula* because it resembles a mulberry.

The outer cells of the morula secrete fluid, creating a sac of cells (the *blastocyst*) that has an inner cell mass within the sac. The inner cell mass of the blastocyst develops into the fetus. Part of the outer layer of blastocyst cells develops into the placenta and fetal membranes.

### Entry of the Zygote Into the Uterus

The conceptus enters the uterus approximately 3 to 4 days after conception, when it contains approximately 100 cells. It lingers in the uterus another 2 to 4 days before beginning implantation. The endometrium, now called the *decidua,* is in the secretory phase of the reproductive cycle, 1½ weeks before the woman would begin her menstrual period. The endometrial glands are secreting at their maximum, providing rich fluids to nourish the conceptus before placental circulation is established. The endometrial spiral arteries are well developed in the secretory phase, providing easy access for developing the placental blood supply.

### Implantation in the Decidua

The conceptus carries a small supply of nutrients for early cell division, but implantation (nidation) at the proper time and location in the uterus is crucial for continued development. Complete implantation is a gradual process that occurs between the 6th and 10th days. Embryonic structures continue developing during implantation.

### Maintaining the Decidua

The implantation and survival of the conceptus are critically dependent on a continuing supply of estrogen and progesterone to maintain the decidua in the secretory phase. The zygote secretes human chorionic gonadotropin (hCG) to signal that a pregnancy has begun. With continued hCG production by the conceptus, the corpus luteum continues to secrete estrogen and progesterone rather than regressing.

### Location of Implantation

The conceptus must be in the right place at the right time for normal implantation to occur. The site of implantation is important because that is the place that the placenta develops. Normal implantation

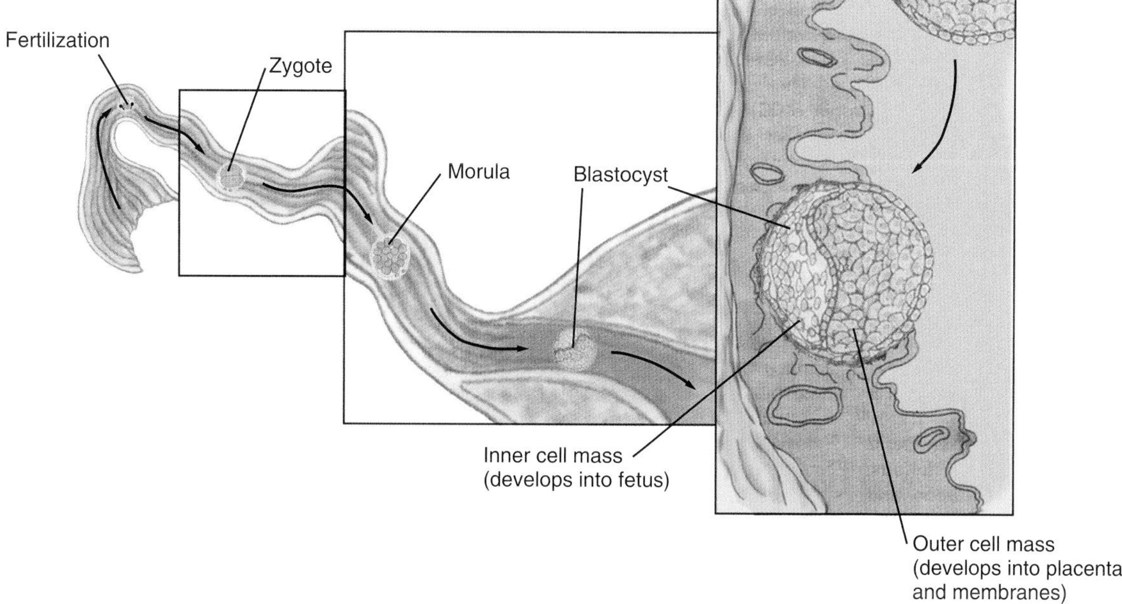


**FIG 12.4** Prenatal development from fertilization through the implantation of the blastocyst. Implantation gradually occurs from the 6th through the 10th days. Implantation is complete by the 10th day.

occurs in the upper uterus (fundus). The upper uterus is the best area for implantation and placental development for three reasons:

- The upper uterus is richly supplied with blood for optimal fetal gas exchange and nutrition.
- The uterine lining is thick in the upper uterus, preventing the placenta from attaching so deeply that it does not easily detach after birth.
- Implantation in the upper uterus limits blood loss after birth because strong interlacing muscle fibers in this area compress open vessels after the placenta detaches.

### Mechanism of Implantation

Enzymes produced by the conceptus erode the decidua, tapping maternal sources of nutrition. Primary chorionic villi are tiny projections on the surface of the conceptus. They extend into the decidua basalis that lies between the conceptus and the wall of the uterus. The chorionic villi eventually form the fetal side of the placenta; the decidua basalis forms the maternal side of the placenta (see Fig. 16.14).

At this early stage, nutritive fluid passes to the embryo by *diffusion* (passive movement across a cell membrane from an area of higher concentration to one of lower concentration) because no circulatory system is yet established. By 10 days, the conceptus is fully embedded within the mother's uterine decidua.

As the conceptus implants, usually near the time of the next expected menstrual period, a small amount of bleeding may occur at the site. The woman may think implantation bleeding is a normal menstrual period.

## EMBRYONIC PERIOD

The embryonic period of development extends from the beginning of the 3rd week through the 8th week after conception. Basic structures of all major body organs are completed during the embryonic period. Table 12.2 presents major developments in body systems during prenatal life. Fig. 12.5 illustrates the external appearance of the embryo from the 3rd through the 8th week after conception.

### Differentiation of Cells

The embryo progresses from having cells with identical functions (undifferentiated) to differentiated, or specialized, body cells. By the end of the 8th week, all major organ systems are in place, and many are functioning in a simple way.

Development of the specialized structures is controlled by three factors: (1) the genetic information in the chromosomes received from the parents, (2) interaction between adjacent tissues, and (3) timing. Although basic instructions are carried within the chromosomes, one tissue may induce change toward greater specialization in another but only if a signal between the two tissues occurs at a specific time during development. In this way, structures develop with appropriate size and relationships to each other.

During the embryonic period, organs are especially vulnerable to structural damage from teratogens, environmental agents that may cause damage, because they are developing rapidly. Normal development of one structure often requires normal and properly timed development of another. Unfortunately, a woman may not realize she is pregnant at this sensitive time. For this reason, the possibility of pregnancy should be explored with her before potentially harmful drugs or diagnostic procedures are prescribed. Some agents may be damaging at one time during pregnancy but not at another. Others may be damaging at any time during pregnancy. Appendix A contains information about substances that may cause prenatal damage.

Other teratogenic effects may occur because the mother does not take in a beneficial substance, either before or during pregnancy. One prominent example is inadequate maternal intake of folic acid, a substance that can reduce neural tube defects. Some mothers need standard amounts of folic acid, whereas those at higher risk for having an infant with a neural tube defect often needs several times the most frequently advised dose.

Prenatal growth and development proceed in patterns that continue after birth:

- Cephalocaudal direction (head-to-toe)
- Central-to-peripheral direction (from center outward)

**TABLE 12.2 Timetable of Prenatal Development Based on Fertilization Age***

| Nervous/Sensory System | Cardiorespiratory System | Digestive System | Genitourinary System | Musculoskeletal System | Integumentary System |
|---|---|---|---|---|---|
| ***3 Weeks: CRL, 1.5 mm*** | | | | | |
| Flat neural plate begins closing to form neural tube. Neural tube still open at each end. | Heart consists of two parallel tubes that fuse into a single tube. Contractions of heart tube begin. Chorionic villi of early placenta connect with heart. | Endoderm (inner germ layer) will become digestive tract. | | Paired, cube-shaped swellings (somites) appear and will form most of the head and trunk skeleton. Muscle, bone, and cartilage develop from mesoderm. | Epidermis (outer skin layer) will develop from ectoderm (outer germ layer). Dermis (deep skin layer) and connective tissue will develop from mesoderm (middle germ layer). |
| ***4 Weeks: CRL, 4 mm*** | | | | | |
| Neural tube closed at each end. Cranial end of neural tube will form brain; caudal end will form spinal cord. Eye development begins as an outgrowth of forebrain. Nose development begins as two pits. Inner ear begins developing from hindbrain. | Heart begins partitioning into four chambers and begins beating. Blood circulating through embryonic vessels and chorionic villi. Tracheal development begins as a bud on the upper gut and branches into two bronchial buds. | Development of primitive gut as embryo folds laterally. Stomach begins as a widening of the tube-shaped primitive gut. Liver, gallbladder, and biliary ducts begin as a bud from primitive gut. | Primordial germ (reproductive) cells are present on embryonic yolk sac. | Upper limb buds are present and look like flippers. Lower limb buds appear. | Mammary ridges that will develop into mammary glands appear. |
| ***6 Weeks: CRL, 13 mm*** | | | | | |
| Development of pituitary gland and cranial nerves. Head sharply flexed because of rapid brain growth. Eyelid development beginning. External ear development begins in neck region as six swellings. | Blood formation primarily in liver. Three right and two left lung lobes develop as outgrowths of the right and left bronchi. Partitioning of the heart into four chambers completed. | Most intestines are contained within the umbilical cord because the liver and kidneys occupy most of the abdominal cavity. Stomach nearing final form. Development of upper and lower jaws. | Kidneys are near bladder in the pelvis. Kidneys occupy much of the abdominal cavity. Primordial germ cells incorporated into developing gonads. Male and female gonads are identical in appearance. | Arms paddle shaped, fingers webbed. Feet and toes develop similarly, but a few days later than arms and hands. Bones cartilaginous, but ossification of skull begins. | Mammary glands begin development. Tooth buds for primary (deciduous) teeth begin developing. |
| ***8 Weeks: CRL, 30 mm*** | | | | | |
| Spinal cord stops at end of vertebral column. Taste buds begin developing. Eyelids fuse. Ears have final form but are low-set. | Heart partitioned into four chambers. Heartbeat detectable with ultrasound. Additional branching of bronchi. | Stomach has reached final form. Lips are fused. Intestines remain in umbilical cord. | Testes begin developing under influence of Y chromosome. Ovaries will develop if a Y chromosome is not present. External genitalia begin to differentiate but still appear quite similar. | Fingers and toes still webbed, but distinct by end of 8th wk. Bones begin to ossify. Joints resemble those of adults. | Auricles of ear low-set but beginning to assume final shape. |

| | | | | | |
|---|---|---|---|---|---|
| ***10 Weeks: CRL, 61 mm; Weight, 14 g*** | | | | | |
| Head flexion still present, but straighter. Eyelids closed and fused. Top of external ear slightly below eye level. | May be possible to detect heartbeat with Doppler transducer. Blood produced in spleen and lymphatic tissue. | Intestines contained within abdominal cavity as growth of this cavity catches up with digestive system development. Digestive tract patent from mouth to anus. | Kidneys in their adult position. Male and female external genitalia have different appearance but are still easily confused. | Toes distinct; soles face each other. | Fingernails begin developing. Tooth buds for permanent teeth begin developing below those for primary teeth. |
| ***12 Weeks: CRL, 87 mm; Weight, 45 g*** | | | | | |
| Surface of brain is smooth, without sulci (grooves) or gyri (convolutions). Nasal septum and palate complete development. | Heartbeat should be detected with Doppler transducer. | Sucking reflex present. Bile formed by liver. | Kidneys begin producing urine. Male and female external genitalia can be distinguished by appearance. | Limbs are long and thin. Involuntary muscles of viscera develop. | Downy lanugo begins developing at end of this week. |
| ***16 Weeks: CRL, 140 mm; Weight, 200 g*** | | | | | |
| Face appears human because eyes face forward rather than to side. | Pulmonary vascular system developing rapidly. | Fetus swallows amniotic fluid and produces meconium (bowel contents). | Urine excreted into amniotic fluid. | Lower limbs reach final relative length, longer than upper limbs. A woman who has been pregnant before may begin to feel fetal movements. | External ears have enough cartilage to stand away from head somewhat. Blood vessels easily visible through the delicate skin. Fingerprints developing. |
| ***20 Weeks: CRL, 160 mm; Weight, 460 g*** | | | | | |
| Myelination of nerves begins and continues through first year of postnatal life. | Heartbeat should be detectable with regular fetoscope. | Peristalsis well developed. | More than 40% of nephrons are mature and functioning. Testes contained in abdomen but begin descent toward scrotum. Primordial follicles of ovary reach peak of 5–7 million and then gradually decline. | Fetal movements felt by mother and may be palpable by an experienced examiner. | Skin is thin and covered with vernix caseosa. Brown fat production complete. Nipples begin development. |
| ***24 Weeks: CRL, 230 mm; Weight, 820 g*** | | | | | |
| Spinal cord ends at level of first sacral vertebra because of more rapid growth of vertebral canal. | Primitive thin-walled alveoli (air sacs) have developed and are surrounded by capillary network. Surfactant production begins in lungs. Respiration possible, but most fetuses die if born at this time. | | Testes descending toward inguinal rings. | Fetus is active. Fetal movements become progressively more noticeable to both mother and examiner. | Body appearance lean. Skin wrinkled and red. Fingerprints and footprints developed. Fingernails present. Eyebrows and lashes present. |

*Continued*

## TABLE 12.2 Timetable of Prenatal Development Based on Fertilization Age*—cont'd

| Nervous/Sensory System | Cardiorespiratory System | Digestive System | Genitourinary System | Musculoskeletal System | Integumentary System |
|---|---|---|---|---|---|
| ***28 Weeks: CRL, 270 mm; Weight, 1300 g*** | | | | | |
| Major sulci and gyri are present. Eyelids no longer fused after 26 weeks. Responds to bitter substances on tongue. | Erythrocyte formation completely in bone marrow. Sufficient alveoli, surfactant, and capillary network to allow respiratory function, although respiratory distress syndrome is common. Many infants born at this time survive with intensive care. | | Testes descended through inguinal canal into scrotum by end of 26th week. | | Skin slightly wrinkled but smoothing out as subcutaneous fat is deposited under it. |
| ***32 Weeks: CRL, 300 mm; Weight, 2100 g*** | | | | | |
| Maturation of parasympathetic nears that of sympathetic nervous system, resulting in fetal heart rate variability on electronic fetal monitor tracing. | Surfactant production nears mature levels. Respiratory distress still possible if born at 32 weeks. Fetal heart rate variability gradually increases toward full term. | | | | Skin smooth and pigmented. Large vessels visible beneath skin. Fingernails reach fingertips. Lanugo disappearing. |
| ***38 Weeks: CRL, 360 mm; Weight, 3400 g*** | | | | | |
| Sulci and gyri developed. Visual acuity approximately 20/600 at birth. | Newborn infant has approximately one eighth to one sixth the number of alveoli of an adult; well-developed ability to exchange gas. | | Both testes usually palpable in scrotum at birth. The newborn girl's ovaries contain approximately 1 million follicles. No new ones are formed after birth; their numbers continue to decline after birth. | | Fetus plump, and skin smooth. Vernix caseosa present in major body creases. Lanugo present on shoulders and upper back only. Fingernails extend beyond the fingertips. Ear cartilage firm. |

*Fertilization age is approximately 2 weeks less than gestational age.
*CRL,* Crown-rump length

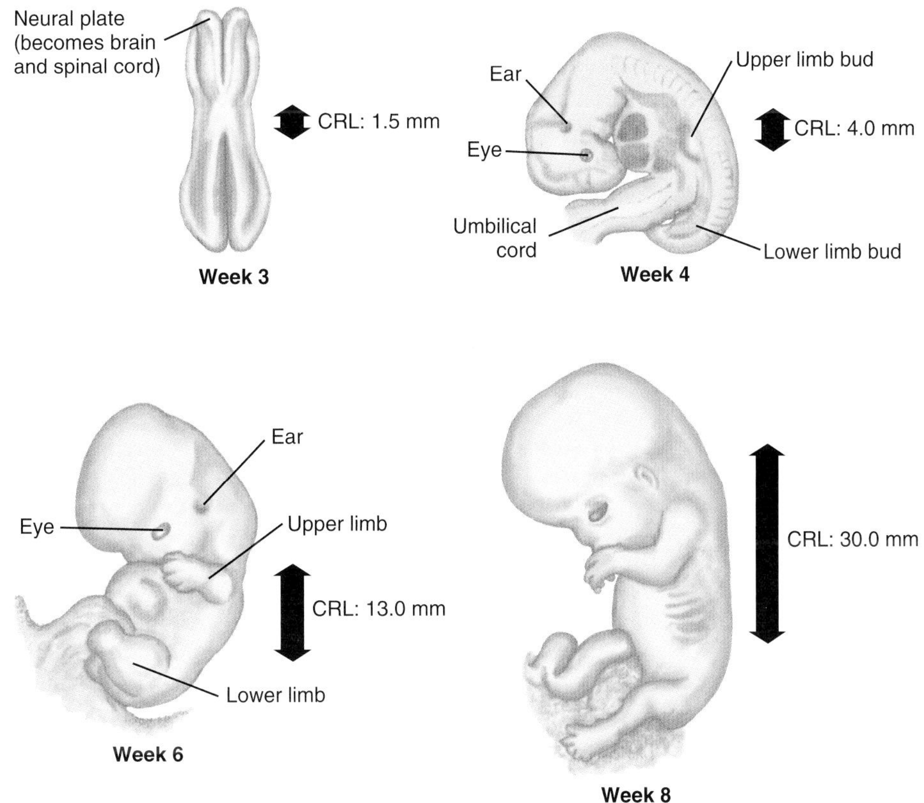


**FIG 12.5** Embryonic development from the 3rd week through the 8th week after fertilization. *CRL,* Crown-rump length.

- Simple-to-complex (early cells may become any cell of the body before they become specialized into specific structures with specific functions)
- General-to-specific (upper extremities begin as limb buds before detailed development of bones, joints, muscles, ligaments, and fingers)

See Box 5.2.

### Second Week

Implantation is complete by the end of the 2nd week. The most growth occurs in the outer cells *(trophoblast),* which eventually become the fetal part of the placenta. The inner cell mass that will develop into the baby becomes flattened into the *embryonic disk.* Cells that eventually form part of the fetal membranes develop.

### Third Week

Many women miss their first menstrual period during the 3rd week of pregnancy. The embryonic disk develops three layers *(germ layers)* that, in turn, give rise to the major organ systems of the body. The three germ layers are the ectoderm, the mesoderm, and the endoderm. Table 12.3 lists structures that develop from each germ layer.

The central nervous system begins developing during the 3rd week. A thickened, flat neural plate appears, extending toward the end of the embryonic disk that will become the head. The neural plate develops a longitudinal groove that folds to form the neural tube. At the end of the 3rd week, the neural tube is fused in the middle but is still open at each end.

**TABLE 12.3 Derivatives of the Three Germ Layers: Developing Structures**

| Ectoderm | Mesoderm | Endoderm |
|---|---|---|
| Brain and spinal cord | Cartilage | Lining of gastrointestinal and respiratory tracts |
| Peripheral nervous system | Bone | Tonsils |
| Pituitary gland | Connective tissue | Thyroid |
| Sensory epithelium of the eye, ear, and nose | Muscle tissue | Parathyroid |
| Epidermis | Heart | Thymus |
| Hair | Blood vessels | Liver |
| Nails | Blood cells | Pancreas |
| Subcutaneous glands | Lymphatic system | Lining of urinary bladder and urethra |
| Mammary glands | Spleen | Lining of ear canal |
| Tooth enamel | Kidneys | |
| | Adrenal cortex | |
| | Ovaries | |
| | Testes | |
| | Reproductive system | |
| | Lining membranes (pericardial, pleural, peritoneal) | |

Early heart development consists of a pair of parallel tubes that run longitudinally and join. The early heart begins beating at 21 to 22 days. Vessels developing in the chorionic villi and membranes join the heart tubes. Primitive blood cells arise from the endoderm lining the distal blood vessels.

### Fourth Week

The shape of the embryo is changing. It folds at the head and tail end laterally. The embryo resembles a C-shaped cylinder by the end of the 4th week. A "tail" is apparent during the embryonic period because the brain and spinal cord develop more rapidly than other systems.

The neural tube completes closure during the 4th week. If the neural tube does not close, defects such as anencephaly and spina bifida result.

The formation of the face and upper respiratory tract begins. Beginnings of the internal ear and the eye are apparent. The upper extremities appear as buds on the lateral body walls.

Because the embryo is sharply flexed anteriorly, the heart is near the embryo's mouth. Partitioning of the heart into four chambers begins during the 4th week and is completed by the end of the 6th week.

The lower respiratory tract begins growth as a branch of the upper digestive tract, which is tubular at this time. Gradually, the esophagus and trachea separate completely. The trachea branches to form the right and left bronchi. These bronchi in turn branch to form the three lobes of the right lung and two lobes of the left lung. Continued branching of the bronchi eventually forms the terminal air sacs *(alveoli)*. The alveoli proliferate and become surrounded near term by a rich capillary network that allows oxygen and carbon dioxide exchange at birth.

### Fifth Week

The head is very large because the brain grows rapidly during the 5th week. The heart is beating and developing four chambers. Upper limb buds are paddle shaped, with notches between the fingers. Lower limbs are also paddle shaped, but the area between the toes is less defined than the division between the fingers.

### Sixth Week

The head is prominent because of rapid development and is bent over the chest. The heart reaches its final four-chambered form. Upper and lower extremities continue to become more defined.

The eye continues to develop, and the beginning of the external ear is apparent as six small bumps near each side of the neck. Facial development begins with eyes, ears, and nasal pits widely separated, aligned with the body walls. Gradually the embryo grows so that the face comes together at the midline.

### Seventh Week

Growth and refinement of all systems occur. The face is now human looking. The eyelids begin to grow, and the extremities become longer and more defined. The trunk elongates and straightens, although a C-shaped spinal curve remains at birth.

During the embryonic period, the intestines grow faster than the abdominal cavity. The relatively large liver and kidneys also occupy much of the abdominal cavity. Therefore, most of the intestines are contained within the umbilical cord while the abdominal cavity grows to accommodate them. By 10 weeks, the abdomen is large enough to contain all its normal contents.

### Eighth Week

The embryo has a definite human form, and refinements to all systems continue. The ears are low-set but are approaching their final location. The eyes are pigmented but not fully covered by eyelids. Fingers and toes are stubby but well defined. The external genitalia begin to differentiate, but male and female characteristics are not distinct until after the 10th week.

## FETAL PERIOD

Beginning 9 weeks after conception and ending with birth, the rapidly dividing cells become a fetus. Dramatic growth and refinement in the structure and function of all organ systems occur during the fetal period. Teratogens may damage already formed structures but are less likely to cause major structural alterations. The central nervous system is vulnerable to damaging agents throughout the entire pregnancy. Fig. 12.6 illustrates growth and development during the fetal period.

### Weeks 9 Through 12

At the beginning of this period, the head is large, approximately half the total length of the fetus. The body begins growing faster than the head. The extremities approach their final relative lengths, although the legs remain proportionally shorter than the arms. The first fetal movements begin but are too slight for the mother to detect.

The face is broad, with a wide nose and widely spaced eyes. The eyes close at 9 weeks and reopen at 26 weeks after conception. The ears appear low-set because the mandible is still small.

The intestinal contents that were partly contained within the umbilical cord enter the abdomen as the capacity of the abdominal cavity catches up with their size. Blood formation occurs primarily in the liver during the 9th week but shifts to the spleen by the end of the 12th week. The fetus begins producing urine during this period, excreting it into the amniotic sac as part of amniotic fluid.

Internal differences in males and females become apparent in the 7th week. External genitalia look similar until the end of the 9th week. By the end of the 12th week, the fetal sex can often be determined by the appearance of the external genitalia on ultrasound.

### Weeks 13 Through 16

The fetus grows rapidly in length, so the head becomes smaller in proportion to the total length. Movements strengthen, and some women, particularly those who have been pregnant before, are able to detect them. Fetal movements produce the experience of *quickening*.

The face looks human because the eyes face forward. The external ears approach their final position, in line with the eyes.

### Weeks 17 Through 20

Fetal movements feel like fluttering, or "butterflies." Some women may not recognize these subtle sensations for what they are.

Changes in the skin and hair are evident. *Vernix caseosa*, a fatty, cheese-like secretion of the fetal sebaceous glands, covers the skin to protect it from constant exposure to amniotic fluid. *Lanugo* is fine, downy hair that covers the fetal body to help the vernix adhere to the skin. Both vernix and lanugo diminish as the fetus reaches term. Eyebrows and head hair appear.

*Brown fat* is heat-producing fat deposited on the back of the neck, behind the sternum, and around the kidneys. Brown fat helps the neonate maintain temperature stability after birth (see Fig. 21.3).

### Weeks 21 Through 24

The fetus continues growing and gaining weight but is thin and has little subcutaneous fat. The skin is translucent and looks red because the capillaries are close to its fragile surface.

The lungs begin to produce *surfactant*, a surface-active lipid that makes it easier for the baby to breathe after birth. Surfactant reduces surface tension in the lung alveoli and keeps them from collapsing with each breath.

The capillary network surrounding the alveoli is increasing but is still very immature, although some gas exchange is possible. If born

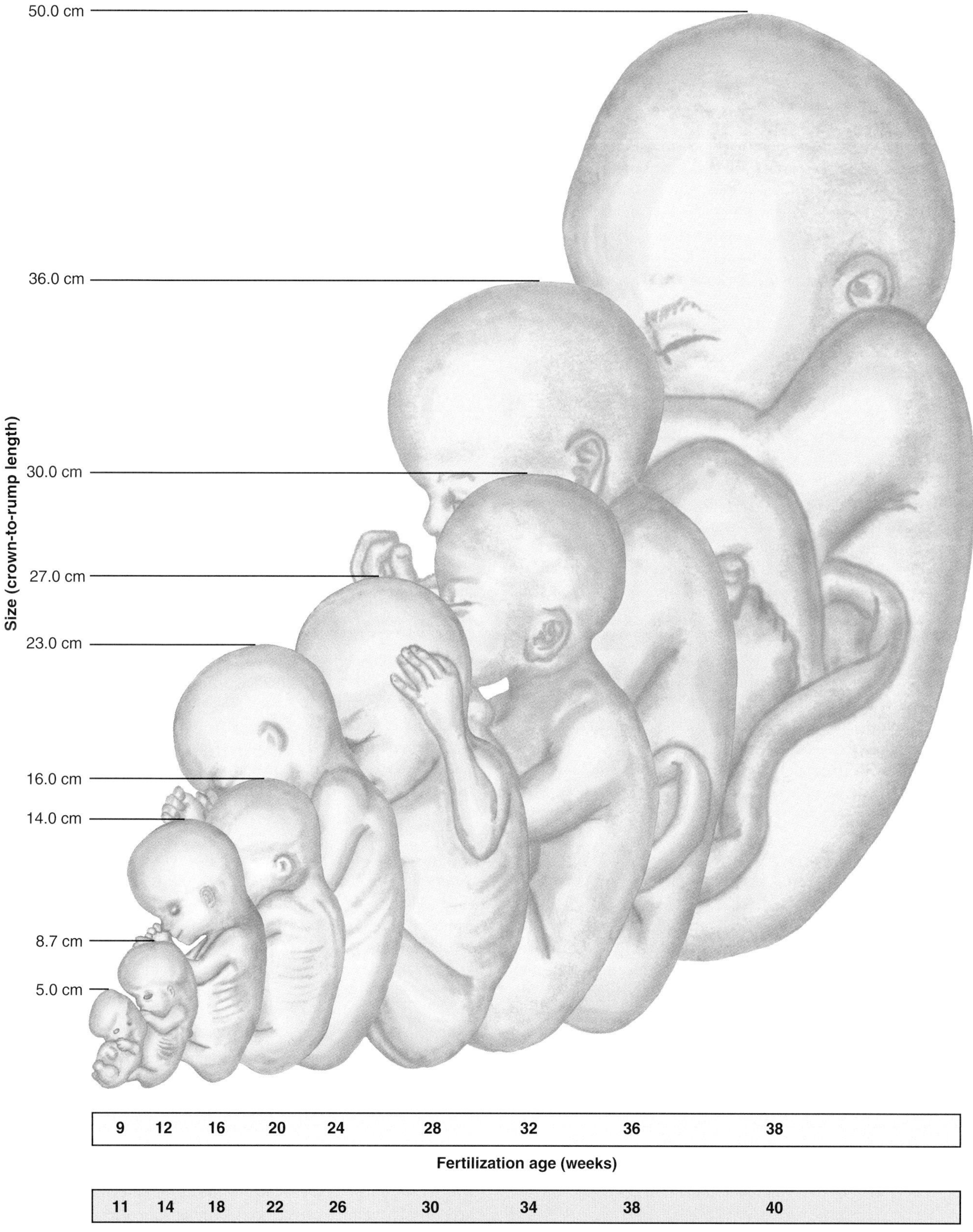


**FIG 12.6** Fetal development from 9 weeks of fertilization age through 38 weeks of fertilization age. Gestational age, measured from the first day of the last menstrual period, is approximately 2 weeks longer than the fertilization age.

at the end of this period, the baby may survive. However, multiple complications related to immaturity of all systems are likely, and the survivor has a high risk for permanent disability.

### Weeks 25 Through 28

With maturation of the lungs, pulmonary capillaries, and central nervous system, the fetus is more likely to survive if born after 24 weeks. The fetus becomes plumper and smoother skinned as subcutaneous fat is deposited under the skin. The skin becomes less red. The eyes, closed since 9 weeks, reopen. Head hair is abundant. Blood formation shifts from the spleen to the bone marrow.

During early pregnancy, the fetus floats freely within the amniotic sac. The fetus usually assumes a head-down position during this time for two reasons:

- The uterus is shaped like an inverted egg. The shape of the fetus in flexion is similar, with the head as the small pole of the egg shape, and with the buttocks, flexed legs, and feet as the larger pole.
- The fetal head is heavier than the feet, and gravity causes the head to drift downward in the pool of amniotic fluid.

### Weeks 29 Through 32

The skin is pigmented according to race and is smooth. Larger vessels are visible over the fetal abdomen, but small capillaries cannot be seen. Toenails are present, and fingernails extend to the fingertips. The fetus has more subcutaneous fat, rounding the body contours. If the fetus is born during this period, chances of survival are good with neonatal intensive care.

### Weeks 33 Through 38

Growth of all body systems continues until birth, but the rate of growth slows as full term approaches. The fetus is mainly gaining weight. The pulmonary system matures to enable efficient and unlabored breathing after birth.

The well-nourished term fetus is rotund, with abundant subcutaneous fat. Lanugo may be present over the forehead, upper back, and upper arms. Vernix may remain in major creases, such as the groin and axillae.

The testes are in the scrotum. Breasts of both male and female infants are enlarged, and breast tissue is palpable beneath the areola and nipple.

Full term ranges from 36 to 40 weeks of **fertilization age**, or 38 to 42 weeks of **gestational age**. Because conception occurs approximately 2 weeks after the first day of the last menstrual period, the fertilization age, used in this chapter, is approximately 2 weeks shorter than the gestational age. However, gestational age is most commonly used in practice because the last menstrual period provides a known marker, whereas most women do not know exactly when they conceived.

## AUXILIARY STRUCTURES

Three auxiliary structures develop simultaneously with fetal growth to sustain the pregnancy and permit normal prenatal development: the placenta, the umbilical cord, and the fetal membranes.

### Placenta

The placenta is a thick, disk-shaped organ (Fig. 12.7). Its major functions are (1) metabolic, (2) transfer of substances between mother and fetus, and (3) endocrine. The fetal side is smooth, with branching vessels covering the membrane covered surface. The maternal side is rough where it attaches to the uterus (see Fig. 16.14).

The umbilical cord is normally inserted on the fetal side of the placenta, near the center. However, it may insert off-center or even out on the fetal membranes. Fig. 12.8 illustrates the normal insertion and variations from normal.

The placenta is larger than the embryo or fetus during early pregnancy and appears to be low lying on ultrasound. The fetus grows faster than the placenta so that the placenta is approximately one sixth the weight of the fetus at the end of a term pregnancy and is implanted in the upper uterus (Benirschke, 2014b).

#### Maternal Component

***Development.*** When conception occurs, cells of the *endometrium* undergo changes that promote early nutrition of the embryo and enable most of the uterine lining to be shed after birth. These changes convert endometrial cells into the *decidua*. In addition to providing nourishment for the embryo, the decidua may protect the mother from uncontrolled invasion of fetal placental tissue into the uterine wall.

The three decidual layers are:

- The decidua basalis, which underlies the developing embryo and forms the maternal side of the placenta.
- The decidua capsularis, which overlies the embryo and bulges into the uterine cavity as the embryo and fetus grow.
- The decidua parietalis, which lines the rest of the uterine cavity. By approximately 22 weeks of gestation, the decidua capsularis fuses with the decidua parietalis, filling the uterine cavity.

***Circulation in the maternal side.*** Exchange of substances between mother and fetus occurs within the *intervillous space* of the placenta. While in the intervillous space, maternal blood is briefly outside her circulatory system. Approximately 150 mL of maternal blood is contained within the intervillous space, and it is changed approximately three or four times per minute.

Maternal blood enters the intervillous spaces through 80 to 100 spiral arteries in the decidua. After the oxygenated and nutrient-bearing maternal blood washes over the chorionic villi containing fetal capillaries, it returns to the maternal circulation through the endometrial veins for elimination of fetal waste products.

#### Fetal Component

***Development.*** The fetal side of the placenta develops from the outer cell layer (trophoblast) of the blastocyst at the same time that the inner cell mass develops into the embryo and fetus. The primary chorionic villi are the initial structures that eventually form the fetal side of the placenta.

***Circulation in the fetal side.*** Blood is circulated to and from the fetal side of the placenta by the fetal heart. The umbilical cord contains two umbilical arteries that spiral around one vein to transport blood between the fetus and placenta. The chorionic villi are bathed by oxygen-rich and nutrient-rich maternal blood in the maternal intervillous spaces. Each chorionic villus is supplied by a tiny fetal artery carrying deoxygenated blood and waste products from the fetus. The vein of the chorionic villus returns oxygenated blood and nutrients to the fetus.

Fetal capillaries in the chorionic villi are separated from direct contact with the mother's blood by the membranes of each villus. This arrangement allows contact close enough for exchange and avoids mixing of fetal and maternal blood, which may not be compatible.

#### Metabolic Functions

The placenta produces some nutrients needed for the embryo and for its own functions. Substances synthesized include glycogen, cholesterol, and fatty acids (Moore & Persaud, 2015).

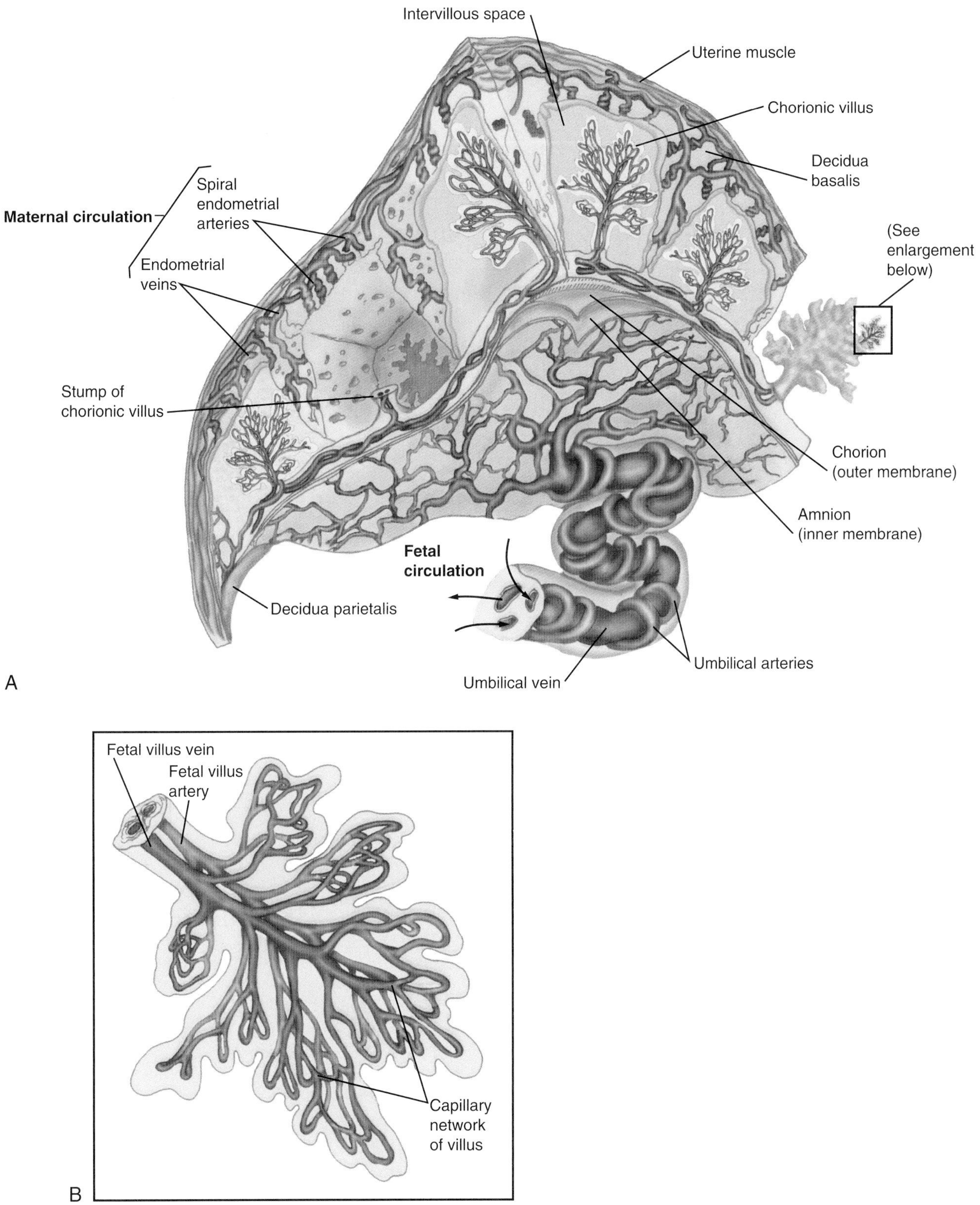

Intervillous space
Uterine muscle
Chorionic villus
Decidua basalis
(See enlargement below)
Maternal circulation
Spiral endometrial arteries
Endometrial veins
Stump of chorionic villus
Chorion (outer membrane)
Amnion (inner membrane)
Fetal circulation
Decidua parietalis
Umbilical arteries
Umbilical vein
A

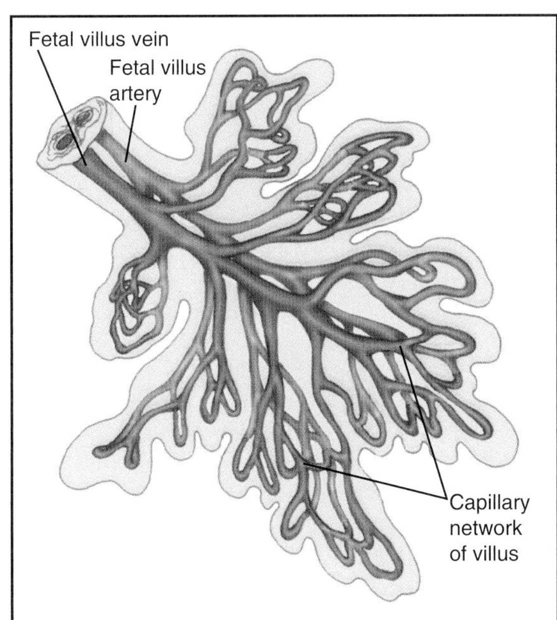


**FIG 12.7 A,** Placental structure, showing relationship of placenta, fetal membranes, and uterus. *Arrows* indicate the direction of blood flow between the fetus and placenta through the umbilical arteries and vein. Blood from the woman bathes the fetal chorionic villi within the intervillous spaces to allow exchange of oxygen, nutrients, and waste products without gross mixing of maternal and fetal blood. **B,** Structure of a chorionic villus, showing its fetal capillary network.

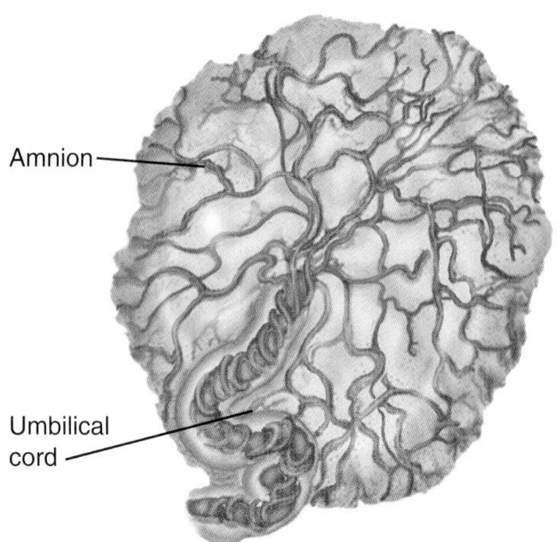
Amnion
Umbilical cord
Normal placenta, with insertion of umbilical cord near center and branching of fetal umbilical vessels over the surface

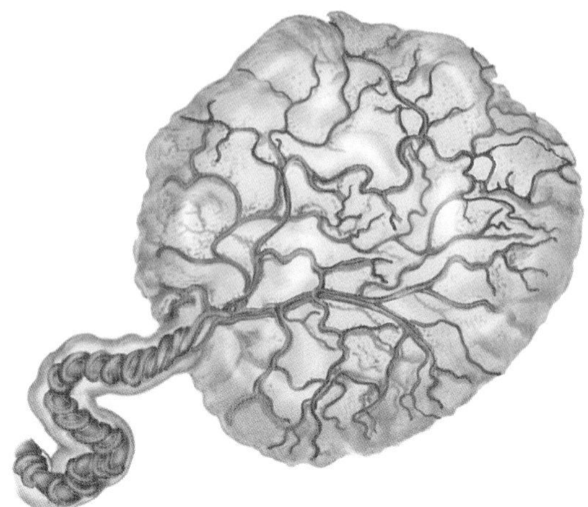
Placenta with cord inserted near margin of placenta

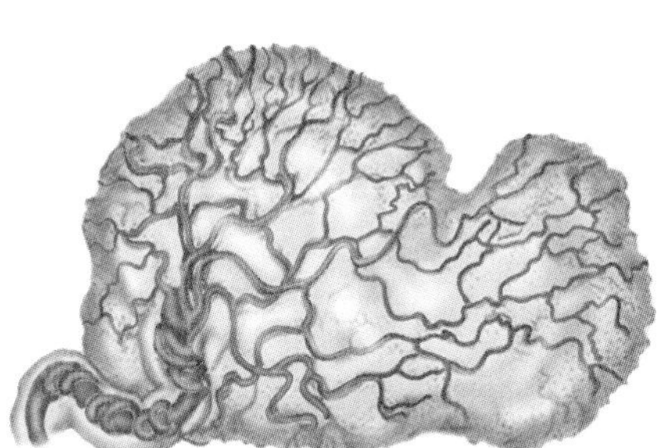
Placenta with a small accessory lobe

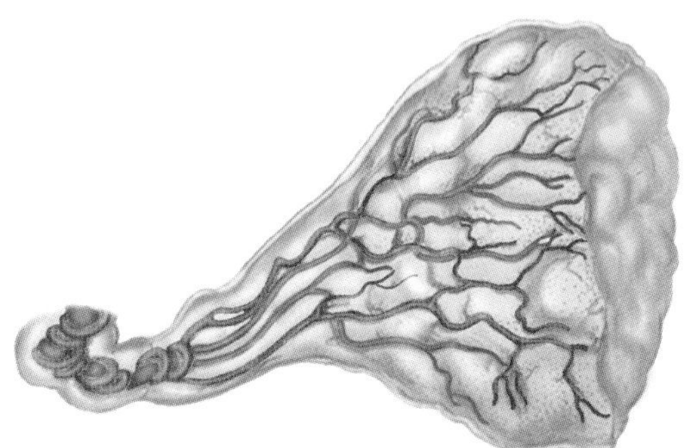
Velamentous insertion of umbilical cord.
Cord vessels branch far out on membranes.
When membranes rupture, fetal umbilical vessels may be torn, and the fetus can hemorrhage.

**FIG 12.8** Placental variations. Normal placenta, with insertion of umbilical cord near center and branching of fetal umbilical vessels over the surface Placenta with cord inserted near margin of placenta. Placenta with a small accessory lobe. Velamentous insertion of umbilical cord. Cord vessels branch far out on membranes. When membranes rupture, fetal umbilical vessels may be torn, and the fetus can hemorrhage.

### Transfer Functions

Exchange of oxygen, nutrients, and waste products across the chorionic villi occurs by several methods. Table 12.4 presents examples of substances transferred between the mother and the developing fetus.

Placental transfer of harmful substances also may occur. Most substances that enter the mother's bloodstream can enter the fetal circulation, and many agents enter it almost immediately.

***Gas exchange.*** A key function of the placenta is respiration. Oxygen and carbon dioxide pass through the placental membrane by simple diffusion. The average oxygen partial pressure ($Po_2$) of maternal blood in the intervillous space is 50 mm Hg. The average blood $Po_2$ in the umbilical vein (after oxygenation) is approximately 30 mm Hg (Hall, 2011). The fetus can thrive in this low-oxygen environment for three reasons:

- Fetal hemoglobin can carry 20% to 50% more oxygen than adult hemoglobin.
- The fetus has a higher oxygen-carrying capacity because of a higher average hemoglobin (15 to 24 g/dL) and hematocrit value (approximately 44% to 70%).
- Hemoglobin can carry more oxygen at low carbon dioxide partial pressure ($Pco_2$) levels than it can at high ones (Bohr effect). Blood entering the placenta from the fetus has a high $Pco_2$, but carbon dioxide diffuses quickly to the mother's blood, where the $Pco_2$ is lower, reversing the levels of carbon dioxide in maternal and fetal blood supplies. Therefore, the fetal blood becomes more alkaline and the maternal blood becomes more acidic. This difference allows the mother's blood to give up oxygen and the fetal blood to combine with oxygen readily.

***Nutrient transfer.*** The growing fetus requires a constant supply of nutrients from the mother. Glucose, fatty acids, electrolytes, and vitamins pass readily across the placenta.

***Waste removal.*** In addition to carbon dioxide, urea, uric acid, and bilirubin are readily transferred from the fetus to the mother for disposal.

***Antibody transfer.*** The immunoglobulin G (IgG) maternal antibodies are the primary ones transferred to the fetus by the placenta. Transfer of IgG antibodies to the fetus may provide temporary (passive) immunity against diseases such as rubella or tetanus if the mother is immune. The preterm or small-for-gestational-age infant has little disease protection because many maternal antibodies are not transferred until late pregnancy and are poorly transferred if placental function is inadequate.

**TABLE 12.4 Mechanisms of Placental Transfer**

| Mechanism | Description | Examples of Substances Transferred |
|---|---|---|
| Simple diffusion | Passive movement of substances across a cell membrane from an area of higher to lower concentration | Oxygen and carbon dioxide<br>Carbon monoxide<br>Water<br>Urea and uric acid<br>Most drugs and their metabolites |
| Facilitated diffusion | Passage of substances across a cell membrane by binding with carrier proteins that assist transfer | Glucose |
| Active transport | Transfer of substances across a cell membrane against a pressure or electrical gradient, or from an area of lower to higher concentration | Amino acids<br>Water-soluble vitamins<br>Minerals: calcium, iron, iodine |
| Pinocytosis | Movement of large molecules by ingestion within cells | Maternal IgG class antibodies<br>Some passage of maternal IgA antibodies |

*IgA*, Immunoglobulin A; *IgG*, immunoglobulin G

Passage of antibodies from mother to fetus also may be harmful. If maternal and fetal ABO blood types or Rh factors are not compatible, the mother may already have or may produce antibodies against fetal erythrocytes. The mother's antibodies can then destroy the fetal erythrocytes, causing fetal anemia or even fetal death.

***Transfer of maternal hormones.*** Most maternal protein hormones do not reach the fetus in amounts sufficient to cause abnormalities.

### Endocrine Functions

The placenta produces many hormones necessary for normal pregnancy. hCG causes the corpus luteum to persist and secrete estrogens and progesterone for the first 6 to 8 weeks. The placenta gradually takes over production of estrogens and progesterone, and the corpus luteum regresses after 20 weeks. When a Y chromosome is present in the male fetus, hCG also causes the fetal testes to secrete testosterone necessary for normal development of male reproductive structures.

Human chorionic somatomammotropin, formerly called human placental lactogen, promotes normal nutrition and growth of the fetus and maternal breast development for lactation. The hormone decreases maternal insulin sensitivity and utilization of glucose, making more glucose available for fetal growth.

Steroid hormones secreted by the placenta include estrogens and progesterone. Estrogens cause enlargement of the woman's uterus, enlargement of the breasts, growth of the ductal system of the breasts, and enlargement of the external genitalia. Estrogens enhance uterine activity, particularly as term approaches, playing a role as labor begins.

Progesterone causes the endometrium to change into the decidua, providing nourishment for the early conceptus. Progesterone reduces uterine contractions and suppresses maternal reactions to fetal antigens to prevent spontaneous abortion. Progesterone acts with estrogens and other hormones to cause growth of the breasts, budding of the alveoli that will secrete milk, and development of secretory characteristics in the alveolar cells.

Other hormones produced by the placenta include human chorionic thyrotropin and human chorionic adrenocorticotropin as well as many growth factors.

### Fetal Membranes and Amniotic Fluid

The two fetal membranes are the *amnion* (inner membrane) and the *chorion* (outer membrane). The two membranes are so close as to be one, although they can be separated. Together they are often called the *bag of waters*. If they rupture in labor, the amnion and chorion usually rupture together, releasing the amniotic fluid from within the sac.

The amnion is continuous with the surface of the umbilical cord, joining the epithelium of the fetus's abdominal skin. Chorionic villi proliferate over the entire surface of the gestational sac for the first 8 weeks after conception. A conceptus observed at this time looks like a shaggy sphere with the embryo suspended inside. As the embryo grows, it bulges into the uterine cavity. The villi on the outer surface gradually atrophy and form the smooth-surfaced chorion. The remaining villi continue to branch and enlarge to form the fetal side of the placenta.

Amniotic fluid protects the growing fetus and promotes normal prenatal development. Amniotic fluid protects the fetus by:

- Cushioning against an impact to the maternal abdomen
- Providing a stable temperature

Amniotic fluid promotes normal prenatal development by:

- Allowing symmetric development of the fetus as body surfaces fold toward the midline
- Keeping the membranes from adhering to developing fetal parts
- Providing room and buoyancy for fetal movement

Amniotic fluid is derived from two sources: fetal urine and fluid transported from the maternal blood across the amnion. Cast-off fetal epithelial cells and vernix are suspended in the amniotic fluid. The water of the amniotic fluid changes by absorption across the amnion, returning to the mother. Some fluid is absorbed by the fetal lungs with breathing movements. Additional amniotic fluid is swallowed and absorbed by the fetal digestive tract.

The volume of amniotic fluid increases during pregnancy until it is approximately 500 to 1000 mL at term, although the volume varies in the last trimester (Blackburn, 2013; Beall & Ross, 2014; Carlson, 2014; Hall, 2011). An abnormally small quantity of fluid (less than 50% of the amount expected for gestation, or less than 500 mL at term) is called *oligohydramnios* and is associated with poor fetal lung development and malformations that result from compression of fetal parts. Oligohydramnios may occur because the kidneys fail to develop, urine excretion is blocked, or placental blood flow is inadequate. *Hydramnios* (also called *polyhydramnios*) is the opposite situation, in which the quantity may exceed 2000 mL. Hydramnios may occur when the fetus has a severe malformation of the central nervous system or gastrointestinal tract that prevents normal ingestion of amniotic fluid.

### Fetal Circulation

The course of fetal blood circulation is from the fetal heart to the placenta, for exchange of oxygen and waste products, and back to the fetus for delivery to fetal tissues (Fig. 12.9, *A*).

### Umbilical Cord

The umbilical cord has two arteries that carry blood high in carbon dioxide and other waste products away from the fetus to the placenta, where these substances are transferred to the mother's circulation for elimination. The umbilical vein carries freshly oxygenated and nutrient-rich blood from the placenta back to the fetus. The umbilical arteries and vein are coiled within the cord to allow them to stretch and prevent obstruction of blood flow through them. The entire cord is cushioned by a soft substance called *Wharton's jelly* to prevent obstruction caused by pressure.

### Fetal Circulatory Circuit

Because the fetus does not breathe air or metabolize substances in the liver, several alterations of the postbirth circulatory route are needed. Three shunts—the ductus venosus, the foramen ovale, and the ductus arteriosus—divert most circulating blood away from the lungs and liver.

Oxygenated blood from the placenta enters the fetal body through the umbilical vein. Approximately half the oxygenated venous blood goes through the liver during early pregnancy and the rest bypasses the liver and enters the inferior vena cava through the first shunt, the *ductus venosus*. The blood then enters the right atrium. Most of the blood passes directly into the left atrium through the second shunt, the *foramen ovale,* where it mixes with the small amount of blood returning from the lungs. Blood is pumped from the left ventricle into the aorta to nourish the body. A small amount of blood from the right

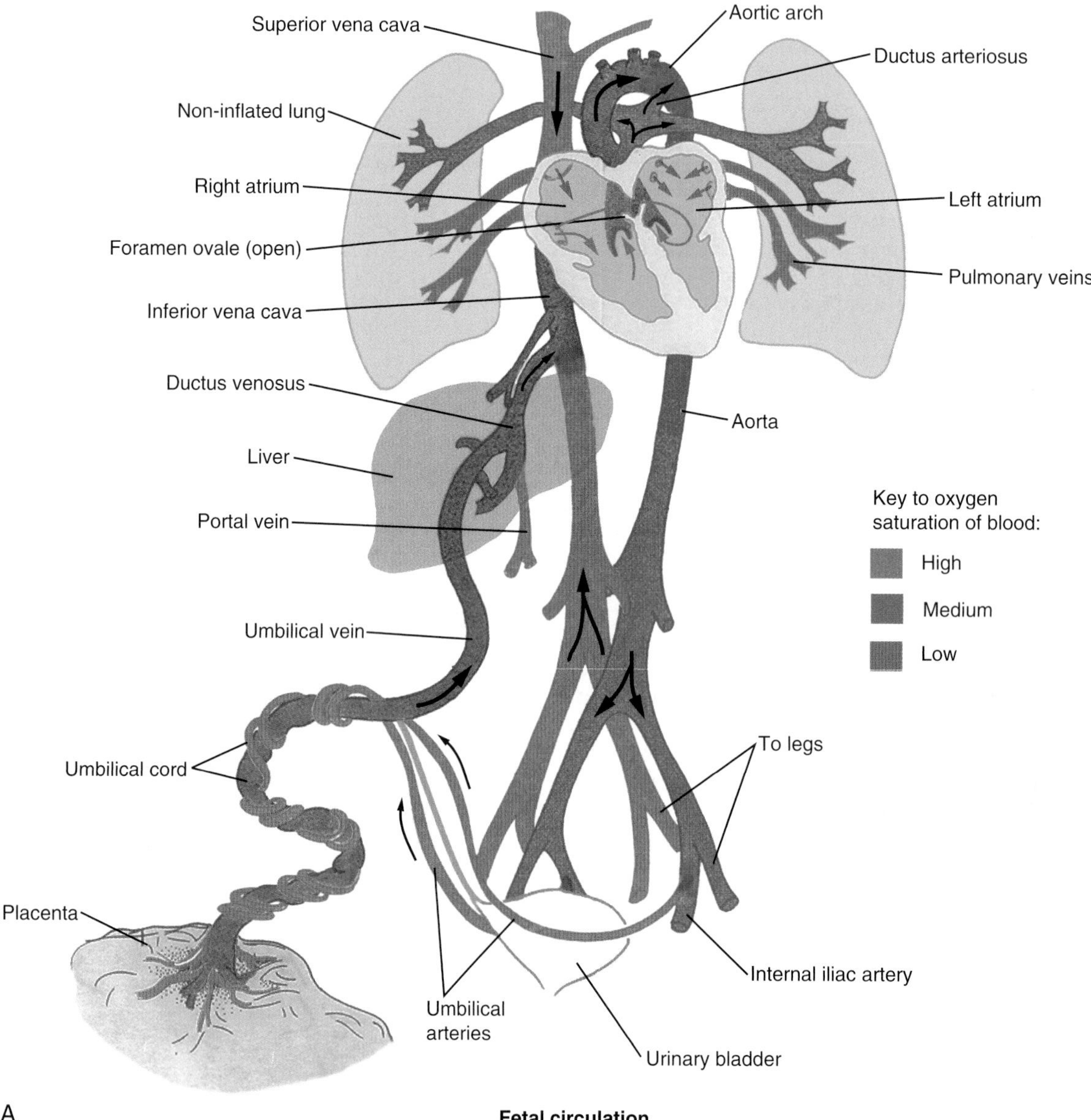


**FIG 12.9 A,** Fetal circulation. Three shunts—the ductus venosus, the ductus arteriosus, and the foramen ovale—allow most blood from the placenta to bypass the fetal lungs and liver.

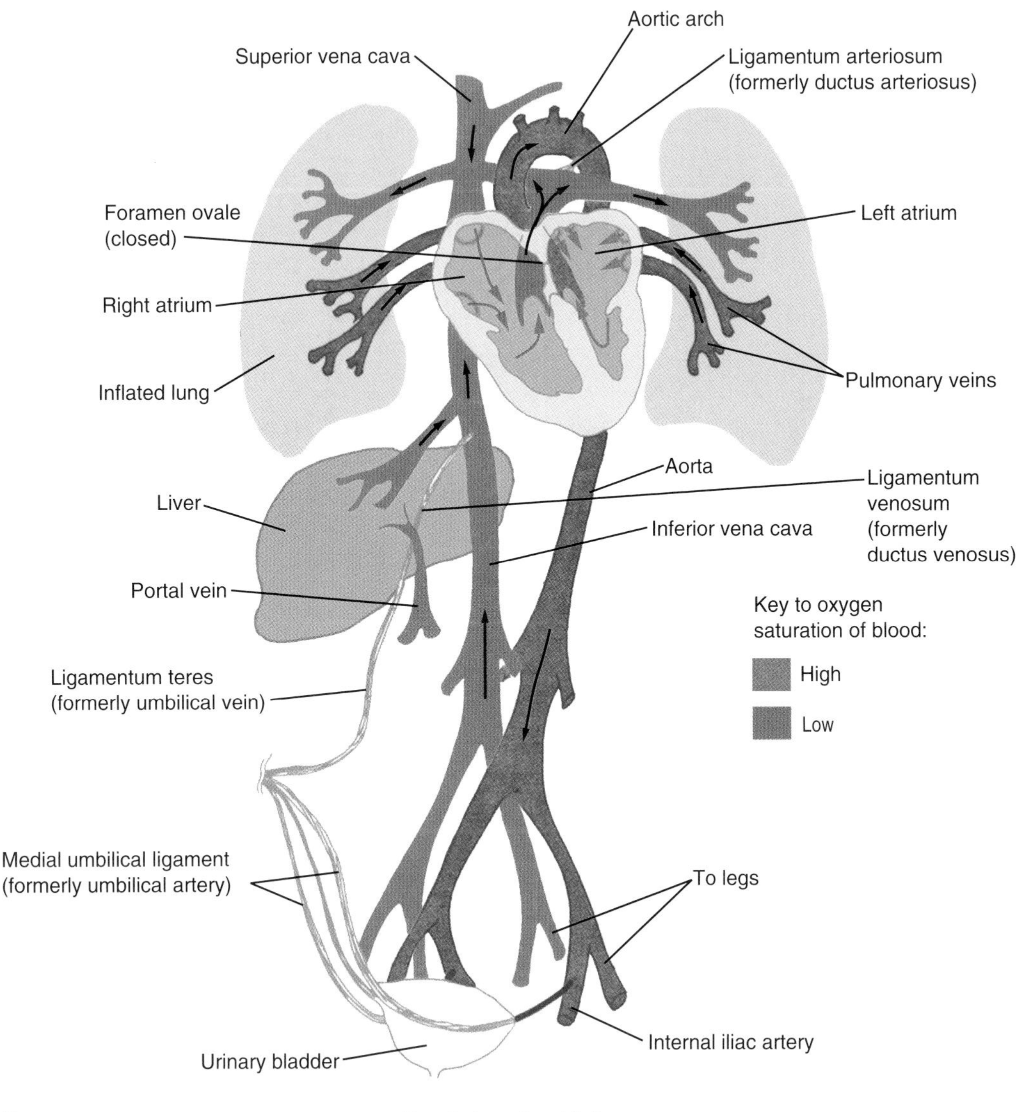


**FIG 12.9, cont'd B,** Circulation after birth. Note that the fetal shunts have closed. The umbilical vessels, the ductus venosus, and the ductus arteriosus have been converted to ligaments.

ventricle is circulated to the lungs to nourish the lung tissue. The rest of the blood from the right ventricle joins oxygenated blood in the aorta through the third shunt, the *ductus arteriosus*. The head and upper body receive the greatest amount of oxygenated blood. During late pregnancy, the liver receives 75% to 80% of the oxygenated venous blood (Blackburn, 2013; Fineman & Clyman, 2014; Jones, 2012b).

Resistance to blood flow through the uninflated lungs is high, causing the right ventricle to work harder and have a thicker wall than the left. After breathing is established, resistance to pulmonary blood flow falls and systemic resistance rises, causing the right ventricular wall to become thinner while the left becomes thicker.

### Changes in Blood Circulation After Birth

Fetal circulatory shunts are not needed after birth because the infant oxygenates blood in the lungs, metabolizes substances in the liver, and stops circulating blood to the placenta (see Fig. 12.9, *B*). As the infant breathes, blood flow to the lungs increases, pressure in the right heart falls, and the foramen ovale closes. Pressure in the aorta rises as pressure in the pulmonary artery falls, causing the direction of blood flow through the ductus arteriosus to reverse, from the aorta into the pulmonary artery. The ductus arteriosus constricts as the arterial oxygen level rises. The ductus venosus constricts when blood flow from the umbilical cord stops.

The foramen ovale and ductus venosus permanently close as tissue proliferates in these structures. The ductus venosus and ductus arteriosus become ligaments, as do the umbilical vein and arteries.

## MULTIFETAL PREGNANCY

Multifetal pregnancy is a deviation from the usual course of gestation. Twins occur *spontaneously* approximately once in 85 pregnancies, triplets approximately once in 8100 pregnancies, quadruplets once in 729,000 pregnancies, and quintuplets only once in more than 65 million pregnancies (Benirschke, 2014a; Moore & Persaud, 2015).

The twin birth rate has steadily increased each year since 1980. In 2013, the rate of twin births was up to 33.7 per 1000 births. Rates of

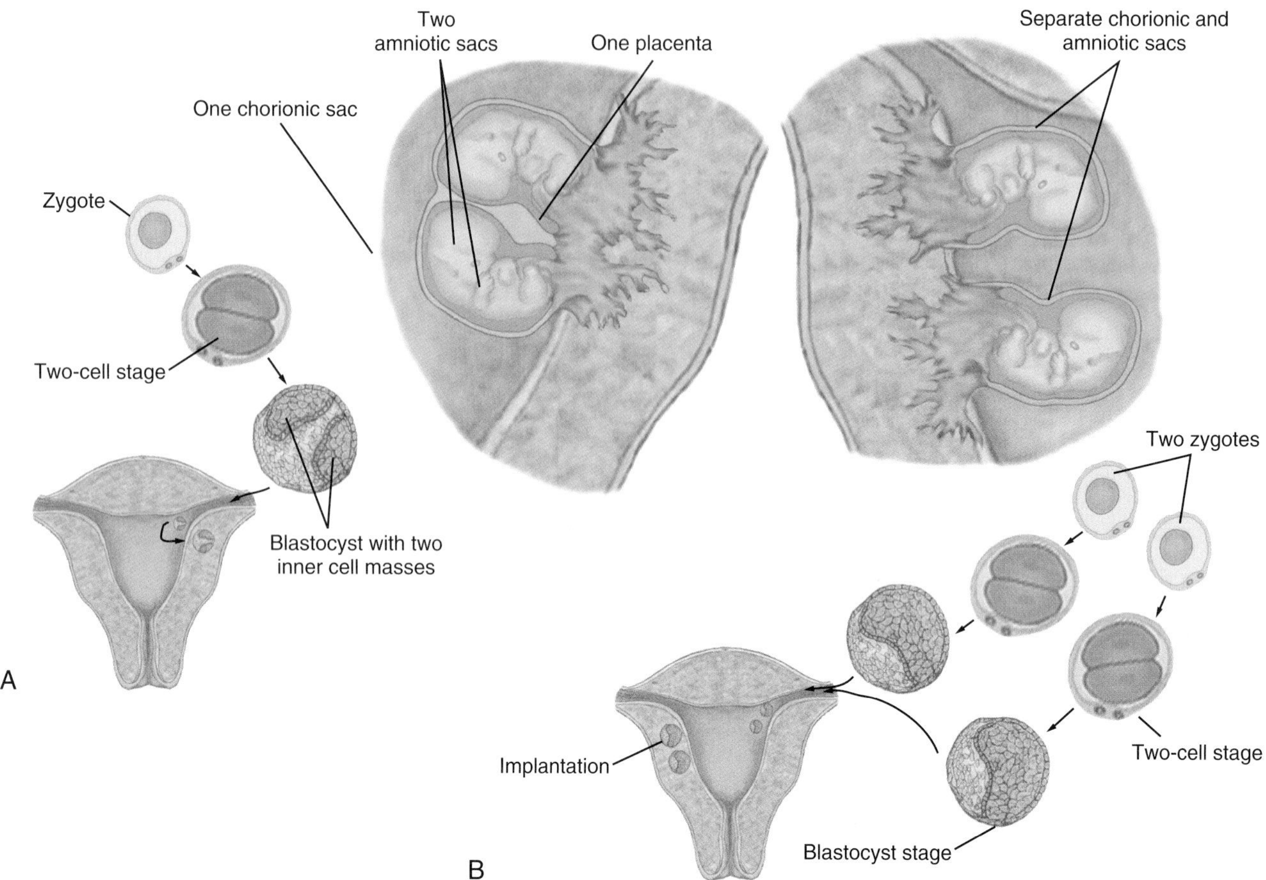


**FIG 12.10 A,** Monozygotic twinning. The single inner cell mass divides into two inner cell masses during the blastocyst stage. These twins have a single placenta and chorion, but each twin develops in its own amnion. **B,** Dizygotic twinning. Two ova are released during ovulation, and each is fertilized by a separate spermatozoon. The ova may implant near each other in the uterus, or they may be far apart.

high-order multiples (triplets or more) steadily increased between the mid-1990s, and 2003, when an all-time high of 187.4 per 100,000 births was recorded (Martin, Hamilton, Sutton, et al., 2010). However, these rates have since declined to 119.5 per 100,000 in 2013 (Martin, Hamilton, Osterman, et al., 2015). High-order multiple pregnancies pose greater hazards to the mother as well as the fetuses. The incidence of long-term handicaps is higher as the number of fetuses increases.

Twinning is the most common form of multifetal pregnancy. Processes that cause a twin pregnancy also may cause other multiple gestations. Twins are most accurately described by their genetic origin or by the number of ova and sperm involved. The two types of twins are monozygotic and dizygotic. Fig. 12.10 illustrates these two mechanisms of twinning (Benirschke, 2014a).

## Monozygotic Twinning

Monozygotic twins are conceived by the union of a single ovum and spermatozoon, with later division of the conceptus into two. Monozygotic twins have identical genetic complements and are of the same sex and are often called "identical" by laypeople; however, they do not always look exactly the same. Monozygotic twinning occurs at random and is unrelated to the use of assisted reproductive techniques (Blackburn, 2013; Moore & Persaud, 2015, 2011).

In monozygotic twinning, a single conceptus divides early in gestation. In most cases of monozygotic twins (65%), the formed *blastocyst* has two inner cell masses instead of one. With two inner cell masses, the fetuses have two amnions (inner membranes) but a single chorion (outer membrane).

If the conceptus divides earlier, two separate but identical morulas (and then blastocysts) develop and implant separately. These monozygotic twins have two amnions and two chorions. Although their placentas develop separately, they may fuse and appear as one at birth. Their chorions also may fuse during prenatal development. Therefore, examining the placenta and membranes after birth cannot always establish whether twins are monozygotic or dizygotic.

Late separation of the inner cell mass may result in twins with a single amnion and a single chorion. These twins often die if their umbilical cords become entangled. Incomplete separation of the inner cell mass may result in conjoined twins.

## Dizygotic Twinning

Dizygotic twins arise from two ova that are fertilized by different sperm. Because dizygotic twins are no more alike than siblings, laypeople often refer to them as "fraternal." Dizygotic twins may be the same or different sex, and they may or may not have similar physical traits. Infertility therapy and advancing maternal age are associated with the increased incidence of dizygotic twin births. See Chapter 31 for more information.

Dizygotic twinning may be hereditary in some families, presumably because of an inherited tendency of the women to release more than one ovum per cycle. Women of some races or country of origin are more likely to have dizygotic twins as well (Blackburn, 2013; Moore & Persaud, 2015, 2011):

- Africans: 1 in 20 births
- African-Americans: 1 in 70 births
- Whites: 1 in 125 births
- Asians: 1 in 500 births

The membranes and placentas of dizygotic twins are separate because they arise from two separate zygotes. The membranes, placentas, or both may fuse during development if they implant closely. Dizygotic twins are not conjoined because they do not involve division of a single cell mass into two.

## KEY CONCEPTS

- Gametogenesis produces ova and sperm that have half the full number of chromosomes, or 23 unpaired chromosomes. When an ovum and a sperm unite at conception, the number is restored to 46-paired chromosomes as in other body cells.
- No new ova are formed after 30 weeks of prenatal gestation.
- One primary oocyte results in one mature ovum that contains 23 unpaired chromosomes (22 autosomes and an X chromosome).
- A male can continuously produce new sperm from puberty through the rest of his life, although this production gradually declines with age.
- One primary spermatocyte results in production of four mature sperm. Two of the mature sperm have 22 autosomes and an X sex chromosome. Two have 22 autosomes and a Y sex chromosome.
- The male gamete determines the baby's sex because sperm carry either an X or a Y sex chromosome. The female contributes only an X chromosome to the baby.
- The basic structure of all organ systems is established during the first 8 weeks of pregnancy. Teratogens during this period may cause major structural and functional damage to the developing organs.
- The fetal period is one of growth and refinement of established organ systems.
- The placenta is an embryonic or fetal organ with metabolic, respiratory, and endocrine functions.
- Transfer of substances between mother and her developing baby occurs by four mechanisms: simple diffusion, facilitated diffusion, active transport, and pinocytosis.
- Most substances in the maternal blood can be transferred to the fetus.
- The fetal membranes contain the amniotic fluid, which cushions the fetus, allows normal prenatal development, and maintains a stable temperature.
- Two umbilical arteries carry deoxygenated blood and waste products to the placenta for transfer to the mother's blood. One umbilical vein carries oxygenated and nutrient-rich blood to the fetus. Coiling of the vessels and enclosure in Wharton's jelly reduce compression and torsion of the umbilical vessels.
- Three fetal circulatory shunts partially bypass the fetal liver and lungs: the ductus venosus, the foramen ovale, and the ductus arteriosus. These structures close functionally after birth but are not closed permanently until several weeks or months later.
- Multifetal pregnancy may be monozygotic or dizygotic. Twins are the most common form of multifetal pregnancy.
- Dizygotic twins are more likely to occur in certain families and racial groups, in older mothers, and in women who undergo infertility therapy.

## REFERENCES AND READINGS


Beall, M.H., & Ross, M.G. (2014). Amniotic fluid dynamics. In R.K. Creasy, R. Resnik, J.D. Iams, et al. (Eds.), *Creasy & Resnik's maternal-fetal medicine: Principles and practice* (7th ed., pp. 47–52). Philadelphia: Saunders.

Benirschke, K. (2014a). Multiple gestation: The biology of twinning. In R.K. Creasy, R. Resnik, J.D. Iams, et al. (Eds.), *Creasy & Resnik's maternal-fetal medicine: Principles and practice* (7th ed., pp. 53–65). Philadelphia: Saunders.

Benirschke, K. (2014b). Normal early development. In R.K. Creasy, R. Resnik, J.D. Iams, et al. (Eds.), *Creasy & Resnik's maternal-fetal medicine: Principles and practice* (7th ed., pp. 37–46). Philadelphia: Saunders.

Blackburn, S.T. (2013). *Maternal, fetal, and neonatal physiology: A clinical perspective* (4th ed.). St. Louis: Saunders.

Callahan, L. (2011). Fetal and placental development and functioning. In S. Mattson, & J.E. Smith (Eds.), *AWHONN core curriculum for maternal-newborn nursing* (4th ed., pp. 35–58). St. Louis: Saunders.

Carlson, B.M. (2014). *Human embryology and developmental biology* (5th ed.). Philadelphia: Mosby.

Fineman, J.R., & Clyman, R. (2014). Fetal cardiovascular physiology. In R.K. Creasy, R. Resnik, J.D. Iams, et al. (Eds.), *Creasy & Resnik's maternal-fetal medicine: Principles and practice* (7th ed., pp. 146–154). Philadelphia: Saunders.

Hall, J.C. (2011). *Guyton and Hall textbook of medical physiology* (12th ed.). Philadelphia: Saunders.

Jones, E.E. (2012a). Fertilization, pregnancy, and lactation. In W.F. Boron, & E.L. Boulpaep (Eds.), *Medical physiology* (2nd ed. Updated, pp. 1170–1192). Philadelphia: Saunders.

Jones, E.E. (2012b). Fetal and neonatal physiology. In W.F. Boron, & E.L. Boulpaep (Eds.), *Medical physiology* (2nd ed. Updated, pp. 1193–1210). Philadelphia: Saunders.

Lo, S.F. (2011). Laboratory medicine. In R.M. Kliegman, B.F. Stanton, & J.W. St. Geme III (Eds.), *Nelson textbook of pediatrics* (19th ed., pp. 2466). Philadelphia: Saunders, Retrieved from http://www.expertconsult.com.

Malone, F.D., & D'Alton, M.E. (2014). Multiple gestation: Clinical characteristics and management. In R.K. Creasy, R. Resnik, J.D. Iams, & C.J. Lockwood (Eds.), *Creasy & Resnik's maternal-fetal medicine: Principles and practice* (7th ed., pp. 578–598). Philadelphia: Saunders.

Martin, J.A., Hamilton, B.E., Sutton, P.D., et al. (2010). *Births: Final data for 2008. National Center for Health Statistics*. Hyattsville, MD: Author.

Martin, J.A., Hamilton, B.E., Osterman, M.J.K., et al. (2015). *Births: Final data for 2013. National Vital Statistics Reports: 64(1)*. National Center for Health Statistics: Hyattsville, MD.

Moore, K.L., & Persaud, T.V.N. (2015). *The developing human: Clinically oriented embryology* (10th ed.). Philadelphia: Saunders.

Moore, K.L., & Persaud, T.V.N. (2011). *Before we are born: Essentials of embryology and birth defects* (8th ed.). Philadelphia: Saunders.

# 13

# Adaptations to Pregnancy

http://evolve.elsevier.com/McKinney/mat-ch/

## LEARNING OBJECTIVES

*After studying this chapter, you should be able to:*

- Describe the physiologic and psychological changes that occur during pregnancy.
- Compute gravidity, parity, and estimated date of delivery.
- Describe preconception, initial, and subsequent antepartum assessments.
- Discuss maternal adaptations to multifetal pregnancy.
- Describe the common discomforts of pregnancy in terms of causes and measures to prevent or relieve them.
- Develop a plan of nursing care for common problems and discomforts of pregnancy.
- Identify the process of role transition.
- Explain the maternal tasks of pregnancy.
- Describe the developmental processes of the transition to the father role.
- Describe the responses of prospective grandparents and siblings to pregnancy.
- Discuss factors that influence psychosocial adaptation to pregnancy such as age, parity, social support, absence of a partner, socioeconomic status, and abnormal situations.
- Describe cultural influences on pregnancy and cultural assessment and negotiation.
- Describe the various types of education for childbearing families.

From the moment of conception, important changes occur in a pregnant woman's body. These changes are necessary to support and nourish the fetus and to prepare the woman for childbirth and lactation. Changes also occur in her psychological responses to the pregnancy. Nurses must understand not only the physiologic and psychological changes but also how these changes affect the daily lives of expectant mothers.

## PHYSIOLOGIC RESPONSES TO PREGNANCY

## CHANGES IN BODY SYSTEMS

Pregnancy challenges each body system to adapt to the increasing demands of the fetus.

### Reproductive System

#### Uterus

**Growth.** Before conception, the uterus is a small pear-shaped organ entirely contained in the pelvic cavity. It weighs up to 70 g (2.5 oz) and has a capacity of approximately 10 mL (one third of an ounce). By full term (the end of normal pregnancy) the uterus weighs approximately 1100 to 1200 g (2.4 to 2.6 lb) and has a capacity of approximately 5000 mL (Norwitz, Mahendroo & Lye, 2014). Uterine growth occurs as the result of hyperplasia and hypertrophy. Growth can be predicted for each trimester (one of three 13-week periods of pregnancy). During the first trimester, growth is mainly a result of hyperplasia caused by stimulation from estrogen and growth factors. During the second and third trimesters, uterine growth is caused by hyperplasia and hypertrophy as the muscle fibers stretch to accommodate the growing fetus. Fibrous tissue accumulates in the outer muscle layer of the uterus, and the amount of elastic tissue increases. These changes greatly increase the strength of the muscle wall (Cunningham, Leveno, Bloom, et al., 2010).

Muscle fibers in the myometrium increase in both length and width. By the third trimester, the uterine muscles are thin, and the fetus can be easily palpated through the abdominal wall. As the uterus expands into the abdominal cavity and rotates to the right, it displaces the intestines upward and laterally. Uterine rotation is caused by pressure from the rectosigmoid colon on the left side of the pelvis.

**Pattern of uterine growth.** The uterus enlarges in a predictable pattern that provides information about fetal growth and helps to confirm the estimated date of delivery (EDD), sometimes called the estimated date of birth (EDB) (Fig. 13.1). By 12 weeks of gestation, the fundus (top of the uterus) can be palpated above the symphysis pubis. At 16 weeks, the fundus reaches midway between the symphysis pubis and the umbilicus. It is located at the umbilicus by 20 weeks' gestation.

The fundus reaches its highest level at the xiphoid process at 36 weeks. Because it pushes against the diaphragm, many expectant mothers experience shortness of breath. By 40 weeks, the fetal head descends into the pelvic cavity and the uterus sinks to a lower level. This descent of the fetal head is called *lightening* because it reduces pressure on the diaphragm and makes breathing easier. Lightening is more pronounced in first pregnancies.

**Contractility.** Throughout pregnancy, the uterus undergoes irregular contractions called Braxton Hicks contractions. During the first two trimesters, contractions are infrequent and less noticeable. During the third trimester, contractions occur more frequently and may cause some discomfort. They are called false labor when they are mistaken for the onset of early labor.

**Uterine blood flow.** As the uterus increases in size, blood flow rises dramatically. In early pregnancy, when the uterus and placenta are relatively small, most of the blood flow is directed to the myometrium and endometrium. During late pregnancy, blood flow to the uterus and placenta reaches 1200 mL/min (Koos, Kahn, & Equils, 2010). Adequate perfusion of the placental intervillous spaces is essential for the

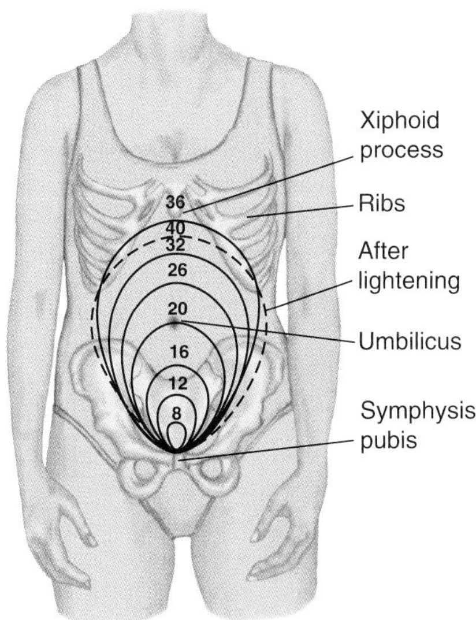


FIG 13.1 Uterine growth pattern during pregnancy.

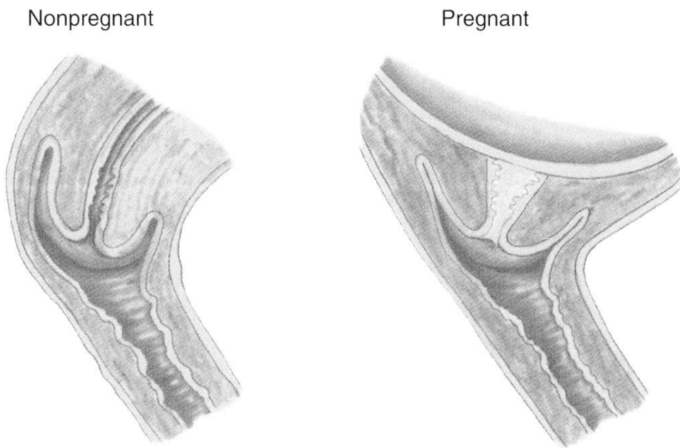


FIG 13.2 Cervical changes that occur during pregnancy. Note the thick mucous plug filling the cervical canal.

delivery of substances needed for fetal growth and the removal of metabolic wastes.

## Cervix

The most obvious cervical changes occur in color and consistency. Estrogen causes hyperemia (congestion with blood) of the cervix, resulting in the characteristic bluish purple color that extends to include the vagina and labia. This discoloration, referred to as Chadwick's sign, is one of the earliest signs of pregnancy.

Collagen fibers in the connective tissue of the cervix decrease, causing the cervix to soften. Before pregnancy, the cervix has a consistency similar to that of the tip of the nose. After conception, the cervix feels more like the lips or earlobe. The cervical softening is referred to as Goodell's sign.

The cervical glands proliferate during pregnancy, and the endocervical tissue resembles a honeycomb that fills with mucus. The mucus plugs the cervical canal and blocks the ascent of bacteria from the vagina into the uterus during pregnancy (Fig. 13.2). One of the earliest signs of labor may be "bloody show," which consists of the mucous plug plus a small amount of blood. This bleeding occurs from disruption of the cervical capillaries as the mucous plug is dislodged when the cervix begins to thin and dilate.

## Vagina and Vulva

Increased vascularity of the vagina causes the vaginal walls, as well as the cervix, to appear a bluish purple in color. Loosening of the abundant connective tissue allows the vagina to distend during childbirth. The vaginal mucosa thickens, and vaginal rugae (folds) become very prominent.

Vaginal cells contain increasing amounts of glycogen, which causes rapid sloughing and increased vaginal discharge. The pH of the vaginal discharge is acidic because of the increased production of lactic acid that results from the action of *Lactobacillus acidophilus* on glycogen in the vaginal epithelium (Cunningham et al., 2010). The acidic condition helps to prevent growth of harmful bacteria found in the vagina. However, the glycogen-rich environment favors the growth of *Candida albicans,* so that persistent yeast infections (candidiasis) are common during pregnancy.

Increased vascularity, edema, and connective tissue changes make the tissues of the vulva and perineum more pliable. Pelvic congestion during pregnancy can lead to heightened sexual interest and increased orgasmic experiences.

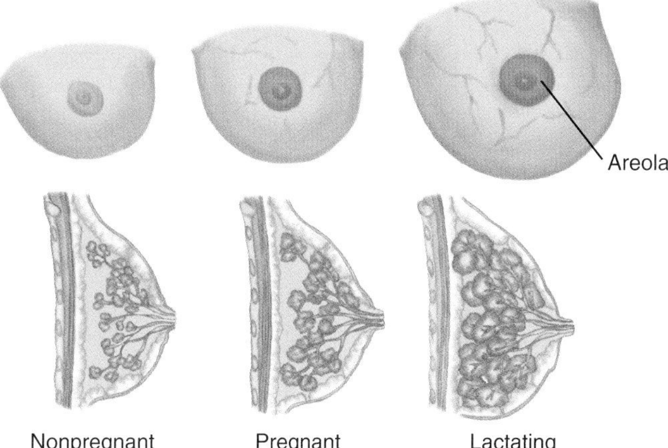


FIG 13.3 Breast changes that occur during pregnancy. The breasts increase in size and become more vascular, the areolae become darker, and the nipples become more erect.

**Ovaries.** After conception, the major function of the ovaries is to secrete progesterone from the corpus luteum for the first 6 to 7 weeks of pregnancy. Progesterone is called the hormone of pregnancy because adequate progesterone must be available from the earliest stages if the pregnancy is to be maintained. The corpus luteum secretes progesterone until the placenta is developed. Once developed, the placenta produces progesterone throughout pregnancy.

Ovulation ceases during pregnancy because the circulating levels of estrogen and progesterone are high, inhibiting the release of follicle-stimulating hormone (FSH) and luteinizing hormone (LH) necessary for ovulation.

**Breasts.** During pregnancy, the breasts change in size and appearance (Fig. 13.3). Estrogen stimulates the growth of mammary ductal tissue, and progesterone promotes the growth of lobes, lobules, and alveoli. The breasts become highly vascular, and a delicate network of veins is often visible. If the increase in breast size is extensive, lineal tears in the connective tissue (striae gravidarum or "stretch marks") may develop.

Characteristic changes in the nipples and areolae occur during pregnancy. The nipples increase in size and become darker and more erect, and the areolae become larger and more pigmented. Women with very light complexions exhibit less change in pigmentation than those with darker skin tones. Sebaceous glands, called *tubercles of Montgomery,* become more prominent during pregnancy and secrete a substance that lubricates the nipples. In addition, a thick, yellowish fluid (colostrum) is present beginning at 12 to 16 weeks of pregnancy and can readily be expressed from the breasts by the third trimester (Janke, 2014). Secretion of milk is suppressed during pregnancy by high levels of estrogen and progesterone.

## Cardiovascular System

### Heart

**Heart size and position.** Cardiac changes are relatively minor and reverse soon after childbirth. The muscles of the heart (myocardium) enlarge slightly because of an increased workload during pregnancy. The heart is pushed upward and toward the left as the uterus elevates the diaphragm during the third trimester. As a result of the change in position, the locations for auscultating heart sounds may be shifted upward and laterally in late pregnancy.

**Heart sounds.** During pregnancy, some heart sounds may be so altered that they would be considered abnormal in a nonpregnant state. The changes are first heard between 12 and 20 weeks and regress during the first week after childbirth. The most common variations in heart sounds include splitting of the first heart sound and a third heart sound. A systolic murmur is found in 95% of pregnant women. The murmur may persist beyond the 4th week for approximately 20% of postpartum women (Monga, 2014).

### Blood Volume

**Total volume.** Total blood volume is a combination of plasma and other components, such as red blood cells (RBCs, erythrocytes), white blood cells (WBCs, leukocytes), and platelets (thrombocytes). Total blood volume increases by as much as 45% (Jones, 2009).

**Plasma volume.** Plasma volume increases progressively from 6 to 8 weeks of gestation until approximately 32 weeks. This is an increase of 40% to 60% (1200 to 1600 mL) above nonpregnant values. Increases are greater in multifetal pregnancies. The increase may be related to vasodilation from nitric oxide and from estrogen and progesterone stimulation of the renin-angiotensin-aldosterone system, which stimulates sodium and water retention (Blackburn, 2013).

The increased volume is needed to: (1) transport nutrients and oxygen to the placenta, where they become available for the growing fetus; and (2) meet the demands of the expanded maternal tissue in the uterus and breasts. The greater volume also provides a reserve to protect the pregnant woman from the adverse effects of the blood loss that occurs during childbirth.

**Red blood cell mass.** RBC mass increases by 250 to 450 mL, approximately 20% to 30% above prepregnancy values (Blackburn, 2013). The increase in plasma volume is more pronounced and occurs earlier than the increase in RBC volume. The resulting dilution of RBC mass causes a decline in maternal hemoglobin and hematocrit. This condition is frequently called physiologic anemia or pseudoanemia of pregnancy because it reflects the dilution of RBCs in an expanded plasma volume rather than an actual decline in the number of RBCs. Therefore, it does not indicate true anemia.

Frequent laboratory examinations may be needed to distinguish physiologic anemia from true anemia. Generally, iron deficiency anemia occurs when the hemoglobin is less than 11 g/dL or the hematocrit is less than 33% in the first or third trimesters, or when the hemoglobin is less than 10.5 g/dL or the hematocrit is less than 32% in the second trimester (Johnson-Wimbley, Graham, 2011; Cunningham et al., 2010). Iron supplementation is often prescribed for pregnant women by the second trimester to prevent anemia.

Dilution of RBCs by plasma may also have a protective function. By decreasing blood viscosity, dilution may counter the tendency to form clots (thrombi) that can obstruct blood vessels and cause serious complications (see Chapter 28). Hemodilution may also increase intervillous perfusion (Monga, 2014).

### Cardiac Output

The expanded blood volume of pregnancy causes an increase in cardiac output—the amount of blood ejected from the heart each minute. It is based on stroke volume (the amount of blood pumped from the heart with each contraction) and heart rate (the number of times the heart beats each minute). Cardiac output rises up to 50%, with half of the rise occurring in the first 8 weeks of gestation (Beckmann, Ling, Barzansky, et al., 2010). The increase in cardiac output is caused primarily by a gain in stroke volume, but the heart rate also rises approximately 15 to 20 beats per minute (bpm) (Bond, 2011). Cardiac output is most efficient when the woman is lying in the lateral position and least efficient in the supine position.

### Systemic Vascular Resistance

Systemic vascular resistance diminishes during pregnancy. This change is likely the result of (1) vasodilation caused by the effects of progesterone and prostaglandins; (2) the addition of the uteroplacental unit, which provides low resistance and a greater area for circulation; (3) fetal, maternal, and placental heat production, which causes vasodilation; (4) decreased vascular sensitivity to angiotensin II; and (5) endothelial prostacyclin and endothelial-derived relaxant factors such as nitric oxide (Blackburn, 2013).

### Blood Pressure

As a result of decreased systemic vascular resistance, blood pressure (BP) changes little during pregnancy despite the increase in blood volume.

**Effect of position on blood pressure.** Arterial blood pressure is affected by the woman's position during pregnancy. With the woman in the sitting or standing position, the systolic pressure remains largely unchanged and diastolic pressure decreases (by approximately 10 mm Hg) by 24 weeks and then returns to prepregnancy levels by term. When the woman is lying in the left lateral position, systolic pressure decreases 5 to 10 mm Hg, and diastolic BP decreases 10 to 15 mm Hg (Monga, 2014).

**Supine hypotension.** When the pregnant woman is in the supine position, particularly during the second half of pregnancy, the weight of the gravid (pregnant) uterus partially occludes the vena cava and the aorta (Fig. 13.4). The occlusion may impede return of blood from the lower extremities and reduce cardiac return, cardiac output, and blood pressure. Collateral circulation developed in pregnancy generally allows blood flow from the legs and pelvis to return to the heart when the woman is in a supine position (Blackburn, 2013). However, some women develop supine hypotensive syndrome.

Symptoms include faintness, lightheadedness, dizziness, nausea, and agitation. Some may experience syncope, a brief lapse in consciousness. Blood flow through the placenta also decreases if the woman remains in the supine position for a prolonged period, which could cause fetal hypoxia.

Turning to a lateral recumbent position alleviates the pressure on the blood vessels and quickly corrects supine hypotension. Women should be advised to rest in a side-lying position to prevent supine hypotension. If they must lie in a supine position for any reason, a

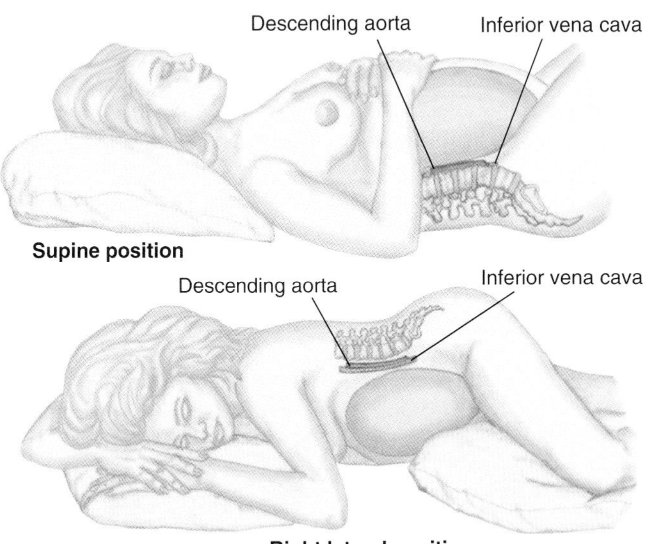


FIG 13.4 Supine hypotensive syndrome. When the pregnant woman is supine, the weight of the uterus partially occludes the vena cava and the descending aorta. A side-lying position corrects supine hypotension.

wedge or pillow under either hip is effective in decreasing supine hypotension.

### Blood Flow

Five major changes in blood flow occur during pregnancy (Koos et al., 2010):

- Blood flow is altered to include the uteroplacental unit.
- More blood must circulate through the maternal kidneys to remove the increased metabolic wastes generated by the mother and fetus.
- The woman's skin requires increased circulation to dissipate the heat generated by increased metabolism during pregnancy.
- Blood flow to the breasts increases resulting in engorgement and dilated veins with a feeling of heat and tingling.
- The weight of the expanding uterus on the inferior vena cava and iliac veins partially obstructs blood return from veins in the legs, causing stasis of blood and venous distention. Prolonged engorgement of the veins of the lower legs may result in varicose veins of the legs, vulva, or rectum (hemorrhoids).

### Blood Components

Although iron absorption and iron-binding power are increased during pregnancy, sufficient iron is not always supplied by diet. Iron supplementation is needed to promote hemoglobin synthesis and ensure that erythrocyte production is sufficient to prevent iron deficiency anemia (see Chapter 26). During pregnancy, erythrocyte production increases by 30% if the mother takes iron supplements and by 18% without supplementation (Gordon, 2012).

Leukocytes increase during pregnancy, ranging from 5000 to 12,000 cells/mm$^3$ to as high as 15,000 cells/mm$^3$ (Blackburn, 2013). Leukocytes increase further during labor and the early postpartum period, reaching 25,000 to 30,000 cells/mm$^3$ (Cunningham et al., 2010).

Pregnancy is a hypercoagulable state where the mother's blood clots more readily. This is because of an increase in factors that favor coagulation and a decrease in factors that inhibit coagulation. Fibrinogen (factor I) increases 50% and factors VII, VIII, IX, and X also rise (Beckmann et al., 2010). Fibrinolytic activity (to break down clots) decreases during pregnancy. Platelets may decrease slightly but remain within normal range (Blackburn, 2013). These changes offer some protection from hemorrhage during childbirth, but also increase the risk of thrombus formation. The risk is a particular concern if the woman must stand or sit for prolonged periods, causing stasis of blood in the veins of the legs. (Table 13.1 lists additional changes in blood components.)

**TABLE 13.1 Laboratory Values in Nonpregnant and Pregnant Women**

| Value | Nonpregnant | Pregnant |
|---|---|---|
| Red blood cell count | 4.2-5.4 million/mm$^3$ | 3.8-4.4 million/mm$^3$; Decreases slightly because of hemodilution |
| Hemoglobin | 12-16 g/dL | At least 11 g/dL during 1st and 3rd trimesters and at least 10.5 g/dL during 2nd trimester |
| Hematocrit, packed cell volume | 37%-47% | At least 33% during 1st and 3rd trimesters and at least 32% during 2nd trimester |
| White blood cell | 5000-10,000 /mm$^3$ | 5000-15,000 /mm$^3$ |
| Platelets | 150,000-400,000/mm$^3$ | Slight decrease but within normal range |
| Prothrombin time | 11-12.5 sec | Slight decrease |
| Activated partial thromboplastin | 30-40 sec | Slight decrease |
| D-dimer | Negative | Negative |
| Glucose, blood | | |
| Fasting | 70-110 mg/dL | 95 mg/dL or lower |
| Postprandial | <140 mg/dL | <140 mg/dL |
| Creatinine | 0.65 ± 0.14 mg/dL | 0.46 ± 0.13 mg/dL |
| Creatinine clearance, urine | 85-120 mL/min | 110-150 mL/min |
| Fibrinogen | 200-400 mg/dL | 300-600 g/dL |

Data from Blackburn, S.T. (2013). *Maternal, fetal, and neonatal physiology: A clinical perspective* (4th ed.). St. Louis: Saunders; Blackburn, S.T. (2014). Physiologic changes of pregnancy. In K.R. Simpson, & P.A. Creehan (Eds.), *AWHONN perinatal nursing* (4th ed., pp. 71–88). Philadelphia: Lippincott Williams & Wilkins; Cunningham, F.G., Leveno, K.J., Bloom, S.L., et al. (2010). *Williams obstetrics* (23rd ed.). New York: McGraw-Hill; Pagana, K.D., & Pagana, T.J. (2009). *Mosby's diagnostic and laboratory test reference* (9th ed.). St. Louis: Mosby.

### Respiratory System

***Oxygen consumption.*** Oxygen consumption increases by approximately 20% in pregnancy. Half the oxygen is used by the uterus, fetus, and placenta. The rest is consumed by the breast tissue, and increased cardiac, renal, and respiratory maternal demands (Beckmann et al., 2010). To compensate for the increased need for oxygen, the woman hyperventilates slightly by breathing more deeply, although her respiratory rate remains unchanged. This hyperventilation promotes the transfer of carbon dioxide from fetal to maternal circulation (Monga, 2014).

Hyperventilation also causes a tidal volume (the volume of gas moved into or out of the respiratory tract with each breath) increase of 30% to 40% causing an increase in the respiratory minute volume (the volume of air inspired or expired in 1 minute) (Beckmann et al.,

2010). As a result of the elevated minute volume, the partial pressure of carbon dioxide ($Pco_2$) is lowered. Renal excretion of bicarbonate from the kidneys compensates for the resulting respiratory alkalosis.

### Hormonal Factors

***Progesterone.*** Progesterone and prostaglandins play a role in decreasing airway resistance by relaxing smooth muscle in the respiratory tract. Progesterone is also believed to raise the sensitivity of the respiratory center (medulla oblongata) to carbon dioxide, thus stimulating the increase in minute ventilation. These two factors are responsible for the heightened awareness of the need to breathe experienced by many pregnant women.

***Estrogen.*** Estrogen causes increased vascularity of the mucous membranes of the upper respiratory tract. As the capillaries become engorged, edema and hyperemia develop within the nose, pharynx, larynx, and trachea. This congestion may result in nasal and sinus stuffiness, epistaxis (nosebleed), and deepening of the voice. Increased vascularity also causes edema of the eardrum and eustachian tubes, which may result in a sense of fullness in the ears or earaches.

### Physical Changes

Although the enlarging uterus lifts the diaphragm by approximately 4 cm (1.6 inches) by the third trimester, movement of the diaphragm is slightly increased. The total lung capacity is decreased 5% because of the elevated diaphragm (Callahan & Caughey, 2013). The ribs flare, the substernal angle widens, and the thoracic circumference increases by 5 to 7 cm (2 to 3 inches) (Bond, 2011). These changes result from relaxation of the ligaments around the ribs (Blackburn, 2013). Breathing becomes more thoracic than abdominal, adding to the dyspnea many women experience.

## Gastrointestinal System

### Mouth

Elevated levels of estrogen cause hyperemia of the tissues of the mouth and gums, which may lead to gingivitis and bleeding gums. Some women develop severe vascular hypertrophy of the gums, which appear reddened and swollen and bleed easily. The condition regresses spontaneously after childbirth.

Some women experience **ptyalism** (excessive salivation) that is unpleasant and embarrassing. The cause of ptyalism appears to be stimulation of the salivary glands by the ingestion of starch (Cunningham et al., 2010). Decreased swallowing during nausea and vomiting may also play a part (Bond, 2011). Small, frequent meals, gum chewing, and oral lozenges offer limited relief.

Some women believe pregnancy adversely affects tooth mineralization, but the teeth do not lose minerals to the fetus. However, existing periodontal disease may be exacerbated during pregnancy and dental care is important.

### Esophagus

The lower esophageal sphincter tone decreases during pregnancy, primarily because of the effect of progesterone on the smooth muscles. The relaxation of the esophageal sphincter and upward displacement of the stomach allow reflux of acidic stomach contents into the esophagus and produces heartburn (**pyrosis**).

### Stomach

Elevated levels of progesterone relax all smooth muscle, decreasing gastrointestinal tone and motility. The effect on gastric emptying time is unclear with some studies showing a decrease and others showing no change during pregnancy (Beckmann et al., 2010; Cunningham et al., 2010).

### Large and Small Intestine

The emptying time of the intestines is increased, allowing more time for nutrient absorption. Calcium, amino acids, iron, glucose, sodium, and chloride are better absorbed during pregnancy, but absorption of some of the B vitamins is reduced (Blackburn, 2013). Decreased motility in the large intestine allows time for more water to be absorbed, leading to constipation. Hemorrhoids may be caused or exacerbated by constipation if the expectant mother must strain to have bowel movements.

### Liver and Gallbladder

Progesterone causes functional changes of the liver and gallbladder. The gallbladder becomes hypotonic and emptying time is prolonged, resulting in thicker bile and predisposing to the development of gallstones. Reduced gallbladder tone also leads to a tendency to retain bile salts, which can cause itching (pruritus) (Cunningham, et al., 2010).

During the last trimester, the liver is pushed upward and backward by the enlarging uterus. Serum alkaline phosphatase rises to two to four times that of nonpregnant women, and levels of serum albumin and total protein fall (Williamson, Mackillop & Heneghan, 2014).

## Urinary System

### Bladder

The woman experiences frequency of urination throughout pregnancy. Although uterine expansion within the pelvis is one cause of these urinary changes, frequency begins before the uterus is big enough to exert pressure on the bladder. Hormonal influences, the increased blood volume, and changes in glomerular filtration rate (GFR) may play a significant role in urinary frequency (Blackburn, 2013). Many women experience stress or urge incontinence that begins at any time during pregnancy and continues until after delivery. Nocturia is also common.

The bladder, like all smooth muscle, relaxes in response to increasing levels of progesterone. The bladder mucosa becomes congested with blood, and the bladder walls become hypertrophied as a result of stimulation from estrogen. Decreased drainage of blood from the base of the bladder makes the tissues edematous and susceptible to trauma and infection during childbirth. The base of the bladder is pushed forward and upward near the end of pregnancy by pressure from the uterus.

### Kidneys and Ureters

***Changes in size and shape.*** During pregnancy, the kidneys change in both size and shape because of dilation of the renal pelves, calyces, and ureters above the pelvic brim. The dilation is caused by (1) the effect of progesterone, which causes the ureters to become elongated and more distensible; and (2) compression of the ureters between the enlarging uterus and the bony pelvic brim. The flow of urine through the ureters is partially obstructed, particularly on the right side, causing the ureters and renal pelvis to dilate. The resulting stasis of urine allows additional time for bacteria to multiply and increases the risk of urinary tract infection during pregnancy.

***Functional changes.*** Renal blood flow increases by 50% to 80% by the middle of pregnancy, then decreases as the pregnancy progresses to term (Blackburn, 2013). The rise is the result of increases in plasma volume and cardiac output. The GFR, the rate at which water and dissolved substances are filtered in the glomerulus, increases by 50% beginning in the second trimester (Cunningham et al., 2010). This increase is the result of the rise in renal blood flow and of decreased colloid osmotic pressure caused by a reduction in the concentration of plasma proteins.

The increases in renal plasma flow and GFR are necessary for excretion of additional metabolic waste from the mother and fetus, but they also affect the excretion of glucose, amino acids, electrolytes, and water-soluble vitamins. As the GFR increases, the filtered load of these substances exceeds the ability of the renal tubules to reabsorb them, and they spill into the urine (Blackburn, 2014). Therefore, glycosuria is common during pregnancy. Bacteria thrive in urine that is rich in nutrients, increasing the risk of urinary tract infections during pregnancy.

Mild proteinuria is common and does not necessarily indicate abnormal kidney function or preeclampsia (Blackburn, 2013). Urinary protein is monitored throughout pregnancy to identify increases that would indicate a problem. Tests of renal function may be misleading during pregnancy. As a result of increased GFR, blood urea nitrogen and serum creatinine normally decline (Blackburn, 2013).

## Integumentary System

### Skin

Circulation to the skin increases during pregnancy and encourages activity of the sweat and sebaceous glands. Pregnant women feel warmer and perspire more, particularly during the last trimester. Accelerated activity of the sebaceous glands fosters the development of acne. Additional changes include hyperpigmentation and vascular changes in the skin.

**Hyperpigmentation.** Increased pigmentation from elevated estrogen, progesterone, and melanocyte-stimulating hormone may begin as early as the 8th week. Women with dark hair or skin exhibit more hyperpigmentation than women with very light hair and skin.

Areas of pigmentation include brownish patches, called **melasma, chloasma**, or the **mask of pregnancy**, over the forehead, cheeks, and nose. Melasma may also occur in women taking oral contraceptives. It increases with exposure to sunlight, but use of sunscreen may reduce the severity.

The linea alba (the line that marks the longitudinal division of the midline of the abdomen) darkens to become the **linea nigra** (Fig. 13.5). The nipples, areolae, and preexisting moles (nevi) become darker as pregnancy progresses. Hyperpigmentation usually disappears after childbirth, when the levels of estrogen and progesterone decline, although melasma may persist in some women.

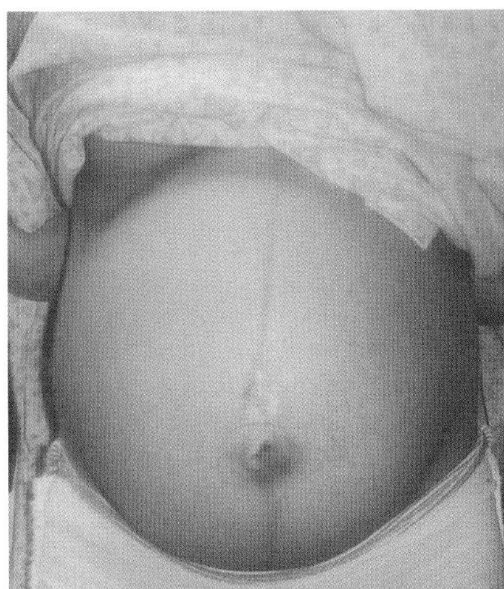

FIG 13.5 The linea nigra, a dark line of pigmentation from the fundus to the symphysis pubis, appears during pregnancy. (Courtesy Teresa Ortiz, Garden Grove, CA.)

**Cutaneous vascular changes.** Blood vessels dilate and proliferate during pregnancy, an effect of estrogen. Changes in surface blood vessels are obvious during pregnancy, especially in women with fair skin. These include spider angiomas that appear as tiny red elevations that branch in all directions. Redness of the palms or soles of the feet, known as palmar erythema, also occurs in many white women and in some black women. Vascular changes may be emotionally distressing for the expectant mother, but they are clinically insignificant and usually disappear shortly after childbirth.

### Connective Tissue

*Striae gravidarum* or "stretch marks" appear as slightly depressed pink to purple streaks on the abdomen, breasts, and buttocks. Striae fade to white or silvery lines but do not disappear after childbirth. Laser therapy is sometimes used after childbirth to reduce or eliminate severe striae. Many women believe that striae can be prevented by massage with oil, cocoa butter, or vitamin E, but no topical treatment has been found effective (Rapini, 2014). Lotions and antipruritic creams may be effective in controlling the itching that often occurs.

### Hair

Because fewer follicles are in the resting phase, hair grows more rapidly and less hair falls out during pregnancy. After childbirth, hair follicles return to normal activity. Many women become concerned about the rate of hair loss that begins 2 to 4 months postpartum. They need reassurance that more follicles have returned to the normal resting phase and that excessive hair loss will not continue. Hair growth returns to normal 6 to 12 months after delivery (Beckmann et al., 2010).

## Musculoskeletal System

### Calcium Storage

During pregnancy, fetal demands for calcium increase, especially in the third trimester. Absorption of calcium from the intestine is increased from the first trimester, and calcium is stored to meet the later needs of the fetus (Blackburn, 2013). The amount of calcium transferred to the fetus is small in comparison with maternal stores, and there is no loss of maternal bone density to supply fetal needs.

### Postural Changes

Musculoskeletal changes are progressive. They begin in the second trimester, when the hormones *estrogen* and *progesterone* initiate increased mobility of the pelvic ligaments. This facilitates passage of the fetus through the pelvis at the time of birth. At 28 to 30 weeks, the pelvic symphysis separates. Relaxation of the pelvic joints creates pelvic instability, and the woman may assume a wide stance and the waddling gait of pregnancy to compensate for a changing center of gravity.

During the third trimester, as the uterus increases in size, the expectant mother leans backward to maintain her balance. This posture creates a progressive *lordosis*, or curvature of the lower spine, and may lead to backache. Obesity or previous back problems increases the problem.

### Abdominal Wall

During the third trimester, the abdominal muscles may become so stretched that the rectus abdominis muscles separate (**diastasis recti**). The extent of the separation varies from slight, which is clinically insignificant, to severe, when a large portion of the uterine wall is covered only by peritoneum, fascia, and skin (see Fig. 20.4).

## Endocrine System

### Pituitary Gland

During pregnancy, prolactin from the anterior pituitary increases to prepare the breasts to produce milk. FSH and LH are suppressed because they are not needed to stimulate ovulation during pregnancy. The posterior pituitary produces oxytocin, which stimulates the milk-ejection reflex after childbirth. Oxytocin also stimulates contractions of the uterus, but during pregnancy, this action is inhibited by progesterone, which relaxes smooth muscle fibers of the uterus. After childbirth, progesterone levels decline when the placenta is removed, and oxytocin keeps the uterus contracted, preventing excessive bleeding at the placental site.

### Thyroid Gland

Hyperplasia and increased vascularity cause the thyroid gland to enlarge during pregnancy. Early in the first trimester, a rise in total serum thyroxine ($T_4$) and thyroxine-binding globulin occurs. The level of serum free (unbound) $T_4$ rises in early pregnancy and then returns to normal. Maternal thyroid hormones are important in the development of the fetal brain. The basal metabolic rate (BMR) increases up to 25% primarily because of the fetal metabolic activity (Cunningham et al., 2010).

### Parathyroid Glands

Parathyroid hormone, important for calcium homeostasis, decreases during the first trimester but then increases steadily throughout pregnancy (Cunningham et al., 2010). Calcium for transfer to the fetus is adequate.

### Pancreas

During pregnancy, alterations in maternal blood glucose and fluctuations in insulin production occur. Glucose levels are 10% to 20% lower than before pregnancy, and hypoglycemia may develop between meals and at night as the fetus draws glucose from the mother (Blackburn, 2013).

During the second half of pregnancy, maternal tissue sensitivity to insulin begins to decline because of the effects of human chorionic somatomammotropin, prolactin, progesterone, estrogen, and cortisol. The mother uses fat stores to meet her energy needs. The higher blood glucose level makes more glucose available for fetal energy needs and stimulates the pancreas of a healthy woman to produce additional insulin. Inadequate insulin production results in gestational diabetes (see Chapter 26).

### Adrenal Glands

During pregnancy, significant changes occur in two adrenal hormones: cortisol and aldosterone. Free (unbound) cortisol, the metabolically active form, is elevated. Cortisol regulates carbohydrate and protein metabolism. It stimulates gluconeogenesis (formation of glucose from noncarbohydrate sources such as amino or fatty acids) whenever the supply of glucose is inadequate to meet the mother's needs for energy.

Aldosterone regulates the absorption of sodium from the distal tubules of the kidneys. It increases during pregnancy to overcome the salt-wasting effects of progesterone to maintain the necessary level of sodium in the greatly expanded blood volume and to meet the needs of the fetus. Aldosterone is closely related to water metabolism.

### Changes Caused by Placental Hormones

**Human chorionic gonadotropin.** In early pregnancy, human chorionic gonadotropin (hCG) is produced by the trophoblastic cells that surround the developing embryo. The rapid increase of this hormone stimulates the corpus luteum to produce progesterone and estrogen until the placenta is sufficiently developed to assume that function at approximately 10 to 12 weeks after conception (Blackburn, 2014). It also causes a positive pregnancy test result.

**Estrogen.** In early pregnancy, estrogen is produced by the corpus luteum. It is produced primarily by the placenta for the remainder of pregnancy. Estrogen has numerous functions during pregnancy: (1) It stimulates uterine growth and increases blood supply to uterine vessels; (2) aids in developing the ductal system in the breasts in preparation for lactation; and (3) is associated with hyperpigmentation, vascular changes in the skin, increased activity of the salivary glands, and hyperemia of the gums and nasal mucous membranes.

**Progesterone.** Progesterone is produced first by the corpus luteum and then by the fully developed placenta. The major functions include:

- Maintaining the endometrial layer for implantation of the fertilized ovum
- Preventing spontaneous abortion by relaxing the smooth muscles of the uterus
- Preventing tissue rejection of the fetus
- Stimulating the development of the lobes and lobules in the breast in preparation for lactation
- Facilitating the deposit of maternal fat stores, which provide a reserve of energy for pregnancy and lactation
- Relaxing smooth muscle of the uterus and other areas (gastric sphincter, intestines, ureters, and bladder)
- Increasing respiratory sensitivity to carbon dioxide, stimulating ventilation
- Suppressing the immunologic response, preventing rejection of the fetus

**Human chorionic somatomammotropin (hCS).** Also called *human placental lactogen (hPL)* hCS increases the availability of glucose for the fetus. An insulin antagonist, hCS reduces the sensitivity of maternal cells to insulin. This decreases maternal metabolism of glucose, thereby freeing glucose for transport to the fetus. In addition, hCS promotes the mobilization and use of free fatty acids to provide energy for the pregnant woman.

**Relaxin.** Relaxin is produced by the corpus luteum, decidua, and placenta. Relaxin inhibits uterine activity, softens connective tissue in the cervix, and lengthens pubic ligaments (Cunningham et al., 2010).

### Changes in Metabolism

**Weight gain.** Because a correlation between small-for-gestational-age infants and inadequate weight gain in pregnancy has been found, women of normal prepregnancy weight are encouraged to gain 11.5 to 16 kg (25 to 35 lb during pregnancy [American College of Obstetricians and Gynecologists, 2013]) (See Table 14.1). The fetus, placenta, and amniotic fluid make up less than half the recommended weight gain. The remainder is found in the increased size of the uterus and breasts, increased blood volume, increased interstitial fluid, and maternal stores of subcutaneous fat (see Fig. 14.1).

**Water metabolism.** The requirement for water increases during pregnancy, and the kidneys must compensate for the many factors that influence fluid balance. Women accumulate water during pregnancy to allow for the added fluid needs of the fetus as well as those of the woman. Body water increases approximately 6.5 to 8.5 L during pregnancy (Gordon, 2012).

Atrial natriuretic factor, vasodilatory prostaglandins, and progesterone increase sodium excretion. However, increased concentrations of estrogen, deoxycorticosterone, hCS, and aldosterone all tend to promote the reabsorption of sodium. The net effect of the combined hormonal action is that appropriate sodium balance is maintained (Blackburn, 2013).

*Dependent edema.* Because of hemodilution, a slight decrease occurs in colloid osmotic pressure, which favors the development of edema during pregnancy. Edema increases further toward term, when the weight of the uterus compresses the veins of the pelvis. This process delays venous return, causing the veins of the legs to become distended, and increases venous pressure, resulting in additional fluid shifts from the vascular compartment to interstitial spaces.

As many as 70% of women have dependent edema during pregnancy. Water accumulation of edema varies from 1.5 to 5 L (Blackburn, 2013). Edema of the feet and ankles is obvious at the end of the day, particularly if a pregnant woman stands for prolonged periods. Dependent edema is clinically insignificant if no other abnormal signs are present.

*Carpal tunnel syndrome.* Fluid retention is also associated with carpal tunnel syndrome, believed to result when edema compresses the median nerve at the point where it passes through the carpal tunnel of the wrist. Symptoms include pain, burning, numbness, or tingling of the hand and wrist. Splinting of the wrist during the night may be necessary. The condition usually resolves by 3 months postpartum.

*Carbohydrate metabolism.* Carbohydrate metabolism changes markedly during pregnancy as more insulin is required as pregnancy progresses. Estrogen, progesterone, hCS, prolactin, and cortisol cause maternal tissue to be resistant to insulin. See the discussion under Pancreas, p. 241.

### Sensory Organs

#### Eye

During pregnancy, corneal edema causes thickening, which may result in discomfort for women who wear contact lenses. The problem resolves during the postpartum, so women should not get new prescriptions for lenses for several weeks after delivery. Intraocular pressure decreases, which may cause improvement in women with glaucoma (Blackburn, 2013; Cunningham et al., 2010).

#### Ear

Changes in the mucous membranes of the eustachian tube brought about by estrogen may cause women to have blocked ears and a mild temporary hearing loss.

### Immune System

Immune function is altered during pregnancy to allow the fetus, which is foreign tissue for the mother, to grow undisturbed without being rejected by the woman's body. Resistance to some infections is decreased for reasons that are not understood (Koos et al., 2010). Some autoimmune conditions such as rheumatoid arthritis improve during pregnancy (Cunningham et al., 2010).

## CONFIRMATION OF PREGNANCY

Although many women have an early ultrasound that proves they are pregnant, the diagnosis of pregnancy has traditionally been based on symptoms experienced by the woman as well as on signs observed by a physician, nurse-midwife, or nurse practitioner. Fig. 13.6 summarizes maternal changes that occur throughout pregnancy (see Chapter 12 for fetal growth and development).

These signs and symptoms are grouped into three classifications: presumptive, probable, and positive indications of pregnancy. A diagnosis of pregnancy cannot be made solely on the presumptive or probable signs. Table 13.2 lists other possible causes for these signs.

### Presumptive Indications of Pregnancy

Most, but not all, presumptive indications are subjective changes that the woman experiences. These changes are the least reliable indicators of pregnancy because they can be caused by conditions other than pregnancy.

#### Amenorrhea

**Amenorrhea** is the absence of menstruation. When it occurs in a sexually active woman who has menstruated regularly previously, conception is strongly suggested. Menses cease after conception because progesterone and estrogen, secreted by the corpus luteum, maintain the endometrial lining in preparation for implantation of the fertilized ovum. A small amount of bleeding from implantation of the blastocyst may cause the woman to think she is having a period.

#### Nausea and Vomiting

During pregnancy approximately 60% to 80% of women experience nausea and vomiting (Castro & Ogunyemi, 2010). Symptoms generally begin between 4 and 8 weeks of gestation (Beckmann et al., 2010). Nausea and vomiting are believed to be caused by the increase in hormones (hCG, estrogen) and decreased gastric motility (an effect of progesterone).

#### Fatigue

Fatigue and drowsiness during the first trimester are very common. The direct cause is unknown, but it may be related to progesterone.

#### Urinary Frequency

Urinary frequency begins in the first few weeks of pregnancy from hormonal and fluid volume changes and continues later when pressure is exerted on the bladder by the expanding uterus. Late in the third trimester, the fetus settles into the pelvic cavity and causes more frequency and urgency of urination as the uterus presses against the bladder.

#### Breast and Skin Changes

Breast changes begin at approximately the 4th to 6th week of pregnancy. The pregnant woman experiences breast tenderness, tingling, feelings of fullness, and increased size and pigmentation of the areolae. These changes are caused by estrogen and progesterone. Many women observe increased pigmentation of the skin (melasma, linea nigra) during pregnancy.

#### Vaginal and Cervical Color Changes

The labia, vagina, and cervix change from pink to a dark bluish purple. The color change, called Chadwick's sign, is another presumptive sign of pregnancy, (Bond, 2011; Cunningham et al., 2010; Gambone, 2010). It is caused by increased vascularity of the pelvic organs and is one of the earliest signs of pregnancy.

#### Fetal Movement

Unlike other presumptive indications of pregnancy, fetal movement is not perceived until the second trimester. Although some women feel movement sooner, most expectant mothers first notice subtle fetal movements (**quickening**) between 16 and 20 weeks. These movements gradually increase in intensity.

### Probable Indications of Pregnancy

Probable indications of pregnancy are objective findings that can be documented by an examiner. They are related primarily to physical changes in the reproductive organs. Although these signs are stronger

**Gestational age 5-8 weeks**

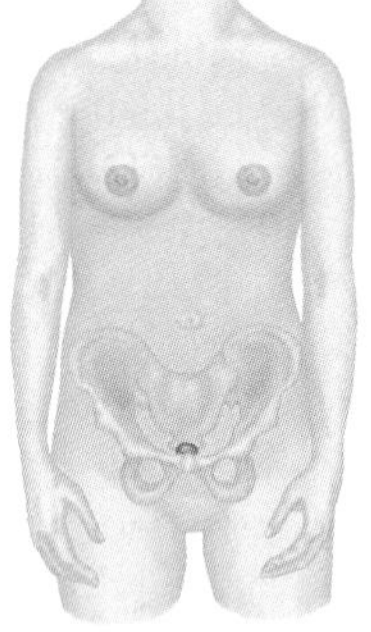

Woman misses menstrual period. Nausea; fatigue. Tingling of breasts. Uterus is size of a lemon; positive Chadwick's, Goodell's and Hegar's sign. Urinary frequency; increased vaginal discharge.

**Gestational age 9-12 weeks**

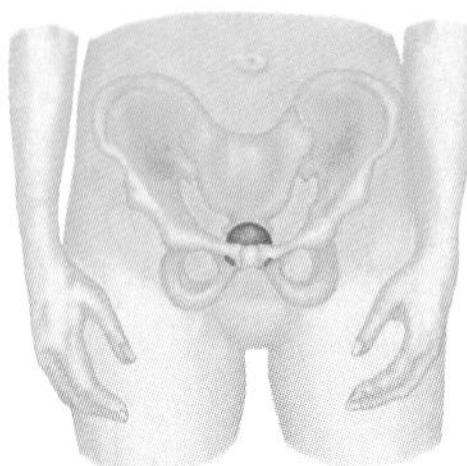

Nausea usually ends by 14 to 16 weeks. Uterus is size of an orange; palpable above symphysis pubis. Vulvar varicosities may appear.

**Gestational age 13-16 weeks**

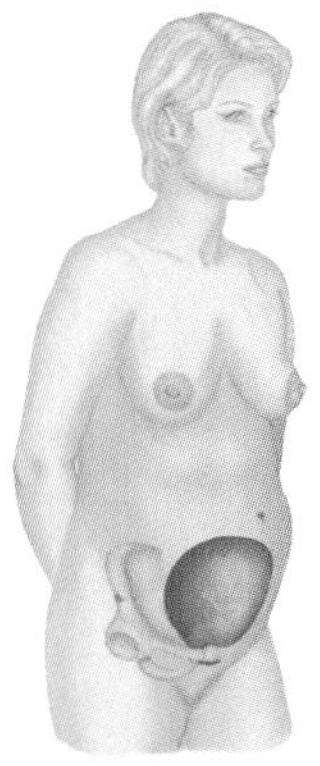

Fetal movements may be felt at about 16 weeks. Uterus has risen into the abdomen; fundus midway between symphysis pubis and umbilicus. Colostrum present; blood volume increases.

**Gestational age 17-20 weeks**

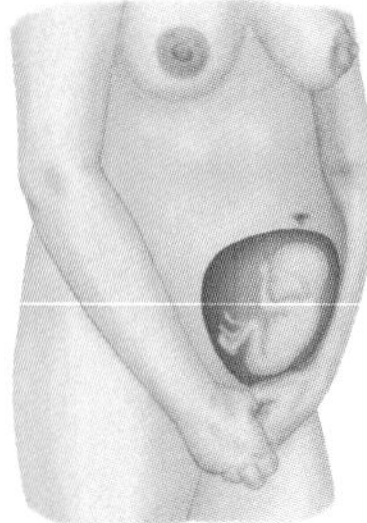

Fetal movements felt. Heartbeat can be heard with fetoscope or electronic device. Skin pigmentation increases: areolae darken; melasma and linea nigra may be obvious. Braxton Hicks contractions palpable. Fundus at level of umbilicus at about 20 weeks.

**Gestational age 21-24 weeks**

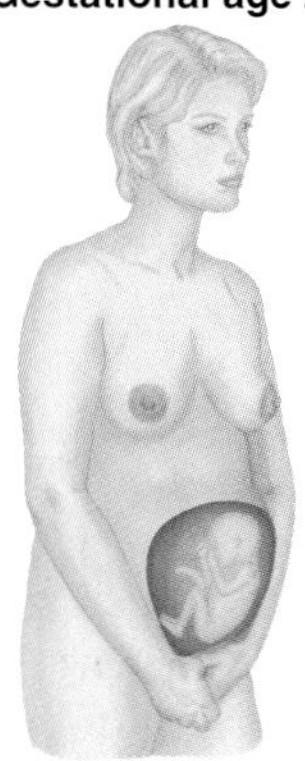

Relaxation of smooth muscles of veins and bladder increases the chance of varicose veins and urinary tract infections. Woman is more aware of fetal movements.

**Gestational age 25-28 weeks**

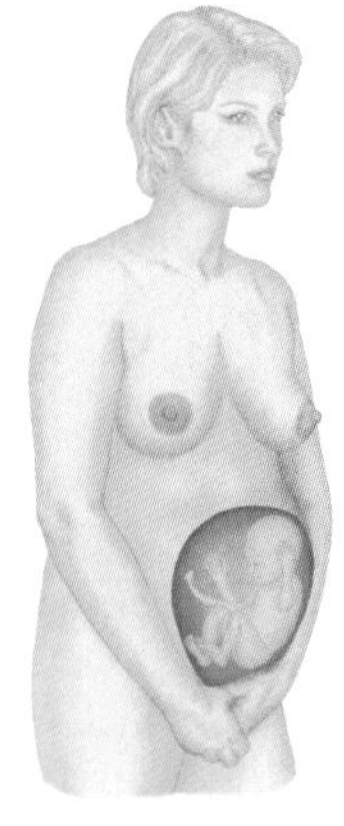

Period of greatest weight gain and lowest hemoglobin level begins. Lordosis may cause backache.

**Gestational age 29-32 weeks**

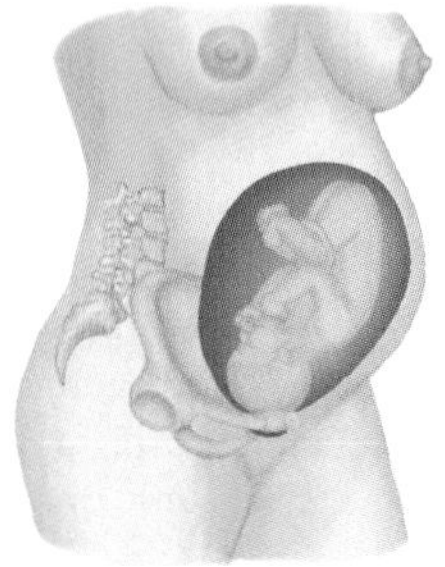

Heartburn common as uterus presses on diaphragm and displaces stomach. Braxton Hicks contractions more noticeable. Lordosis increases; waddling gait develops due to increased mobility of pelvic joints.

**Gestational age 33-36 weeks**

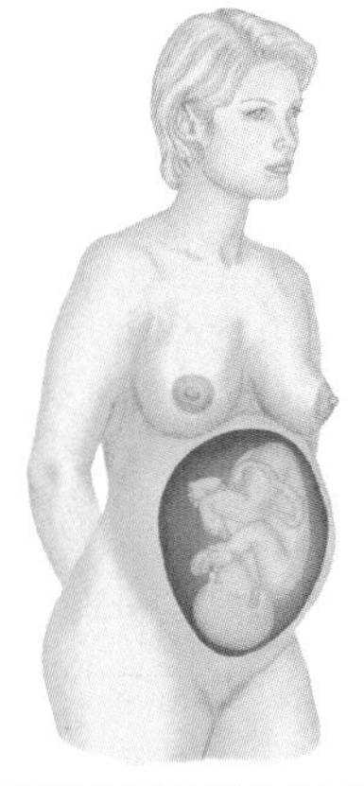

Shortness of breath caused by upward pressure on diaphragm; woman may have difficulty finding a comfortable position for sleep. Umbilicus protrudes. Varicosities more pronounced; pedal or ankle edema may be present. Urinary frequency noted following lightening when presenting part settles into pelvic cavity.

**Gestational age 37-40 weeks**

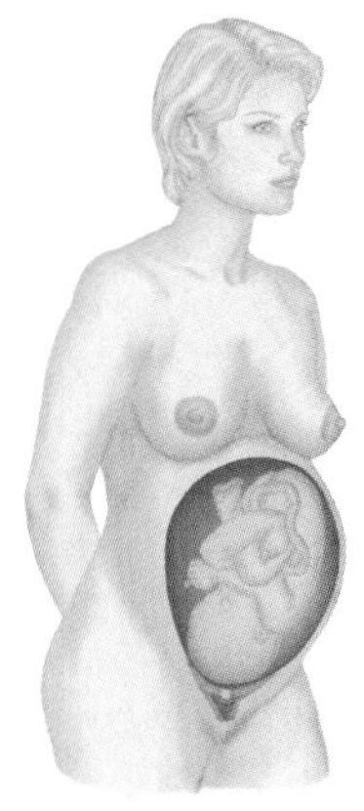

Woman is uncomfortable; looking forward to birth of baby. Cervix softens, begins to efface; mucous plug is often lost.

**FIG 13.6** Maternal changes based on the date of the last menstrual period.

**TABLE 13.2 Indications of Pregnancy and Other Possible Causes**

| Sign | Other Possible Causes |
|---|---|
| **Presumptive Indications** | |
| Amenorrhea | Emotional stress, strenuous physical exercise, endocrine problems, chronic disease, early menopause, low body weight |
| Nausea and vomiting | Gastrointestinal virus, food poisoning, emotional stress |
| Fatigue | Illness, stress, sudden changes in lifestyle |
| Urinary frequency | Urinary tract infections |
| Breast and skin changes | Premenstrual changes, use of oral contraceptives |
| Vaginal and cervical color changes (Chadwick's sign) | Infection or hormonal imbalance |
| Quickening | Intestinal gas, peristalsis, or pseudocyesis (false pregnancy) |
| **Probable Indications** | |
| Abdominal enlargement | Abdominal or uterine tumors |
| Cervical softening (Goodell's sign) | Hormonal imbalance, hormonal contraceptives |
| Ballottement | Uterine or cervical polyps |
| Braxton Hicks contractions | Intestinal gas |
| Palpation of fetal outline | Large leiomyomas (fibroids) (may feel like the fetal head); small, soft leiomyoma (may simulate small parts of the fetus) |
| Uterine souffle | Confusion with mother's pulse |
| Pregnancy tests | Incorrect procedure, testing too early, urine too dilute, certain medications, hematuria, proteinuria, or malignant tumors that produce human chorionic gonadotropins |
| **Positive Indications** | |
| Auscultation of fetal heart sounds | |
| Fetal movements felt by examiner | |
| Visualization of embryo or fetus | |

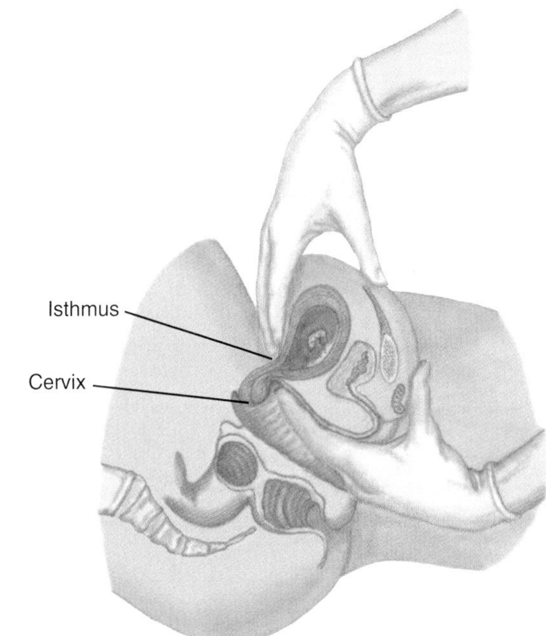


FIG 13.7 Hegar's sign—compressibility of the lower uterus—reflects softening of the isthmus of the cervix.

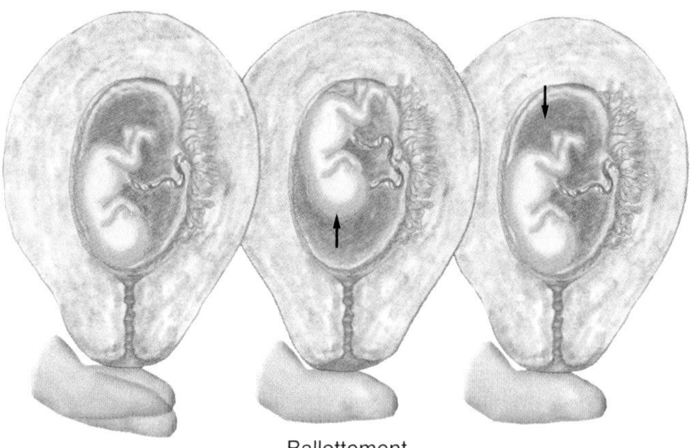


FIG 13.8 When the cervix is tapped, the fetus floats upward in the amniotic fluid. A rebound is felt by the examiner when the fetus falls back.

indicators of pregnancy, a positive diagnosis cannot be based on these findings because they may have other causes.

### Abdominal Enlargement

Enlargement of the abdomen during the childbearing years is a fairly reliable indication of pregnancy, particularly if it corresponds to a slow, gradual increase in uterine growth. Evidence of pregnancy is even more likely when uterine growth is accompanied by amenorrhea.

### Cervical Softening

Softening of the cervix *(Goodell's sign)* is noted by the examiner during pelvic examination. This is a result of pelvic vasocongestion.

### Changes in the Uterus

***Uterine consistency.*** At 6 to 8 weeks after the last menses, the lower uterine segment (the isthmus) is so soft that it can be compressed to the thinness of paper. This is called Hegar's sign (Fig. 13.7). Because of the softening, the uterus can be easily flexed against the cervix.

***Ballottement.*** Near midpregnancy, a sudden tap on the cervix during vaginal examination may cause the fetus to rise in the amniotic fluid and then rebound to its original position (ballottement) (Fig. 13.8). Ballottement is a strong indication of pregnancy, but may be caused by other factors such as uterine or cervical polyps.

***Braxton hicks contractions.*** Irregular, painless contractions occur throughout pregnancy, although many expectant mothers do not notice them until the third trimester. As the woman nears the end of pregnancy, the contractions become stronger and more frequent. Preterm labor may be mistaken for these *Braxton Hicks contractions*. Women who are unsure, have more than 5 or 6 regular contractions in an hour, or have other signs of early labor should check with their healthcare provider (Callahan & Caughey, 2013).

***Palpation of the fetal outline.*** Unless the woman is very obese, an experienced practitioner can palpate the outlines of the fetal body by the second half of pregnancy. Palpating the fetal outline becomes easier as the pregnancy progresses and the uterine walls become thinner.

***Uterine souffle.*** Late in pregnancy, the **uterine souffle**, a soft, blowing sound may be auscultated over the uterus. This is the sound of blood circulating through the dilated uterine vessels, and it corresponds to the maternal pulse. Therefore, to identify the uterine souffle, the rate of the maternal pulse must be checked simultaneously. Uterine souffle differs from **funic souffle**, the sharper whistling sound heard over the umbilical cord that corresponds to the fetal heart rate.

### Pregnancy Tests

Pregnancy tests detect hCG or the beta subunit of hCG, which is secreted by the placenta and present in maternal blood and urine shortly after conception.

***Agglutination inhibition test.*** This test uses antibodies to detect the beta subunit of hCG in blood or urine. The test is quick and ideal for early diagnosis of pregnancy. It can detect hCG in serum at very low concentrations and is positive as early as 3 to 7 days after conception (Pagana & Pagana, 2009). The tests may be performed in a laboratory or at home. For home testing, the woman places urine on a strip or wick and watches for a color change. Although the first morning void is most concentrated, samples from any time of day may be used with most kits.

***Radioreceptor assay.*** This test is accurate 6 to 8 days after conception. It is very sensitive and is used to detect very small amounts of hCG such as in ectopic pregnancies.

***Radioimmunoassay.*** Because radioimmunoassays use radioactively labeled markers to detect antibodies against beta subunit hCG in blood or urine, they must be performed in a laboratory. They are accurate before the first missed menstrual period but are currently seldom used (Pagana & Pagana, 2009).

***Inaccurate pregnancy test results.*** When pregnancy test results are reported as negative and the woman is in fact pregnant, the results are called *false-negative*. False-negative results may occur when the instructions are not followed properly, it is too early in the pregnancy, the urine is too dilute, or the woman is taking certain drugs such as diuretics. Hematuria or proteinuria may cause *false-positive* results, in which the test indicates a pregnancy when the woman is not pregnant. Some anticonvulsants, antiparkinsonian drugs, hypnotics, and tranquilizers cause a false-positive result (Pagana & Pagana, 2009). The woman should check with the manufacturer's instructions for a home pregnancy test if she is taking any drugs.

## Positive Indications of Pregnancy

Positive signs of pregnancy are those caused only by pregnancy.

### Auscultation of Fetal Heart Sounds

Fetal heart sounds can be heard with a stethoscope by 16 to 20 weeks of gestation. The electronic Doppler may detect heart motion and makes an audible sound as early as 9 weeks. The heartbeat can be seen on ultrasound as early as 8 weeks (Gambone, 2010).

It is important to distinguish the fetal heartbeat from the maternal pulse. The fetal heart rate ranges between 110 and 160 beats per minute (bpm) during the third trimester. It should be auscultated at the same time the examiner palpates the maternal radial pulse. The fetal heart rate is muffled by amniotic fluid, and the location changes because the fetus moves freely in the amniotic fluid.

### Fetal Movements Felt by Examiner

Fetal movements are considered a positive sign of pregnancy when felt by an experienced examiner who is not likely to be deceived by similar sensations produced by peristalsis in the large intestine.

### Visualization of the Fetus

Confirmation of pregnancy has become much simpler since the development of ultrasonography, which makes it possible to view the fetal outline and observe the fetal heartbeat very early in pregnancy. Positive confirmation of pregnancy is possible by transvaginal ultrasonography as early as 3 weeks of gestation (Katz, 2008).

# ANTEPARTUM ASSESSMENT AND CARE

Prenatal care includes assessment to identify potential problems as well as health education, counseling, and social support. Good antepartum care should begin before conception and continue in the first trimester and on a regular basis thereafter. Inadequate antepartum care is associated with low birth weight and a higher incidence of prematurity in neonates. These two complications lead to increased infant morbidity and mortality.

Some agencies use clinical pathways to provide guidelines and a time sequence for specific assessments and interventions during pregnancy. The pathways also alert the team when additional assessments or care may be needed.

## Preconception and Interconception Care

The early weeks of pregnancy are particularly important because fetal organs are forming and are especially sensitive to harm. Many women do not begin prenatal care until after this sensitive period and harm may already have occurred. Therefore, any visit to a healthcare professional by a woman of childbearing age should offer preconception or interconception care.

The purpose of such care is to identify any problems that might be harmful once pregnancy occurs and to teach health behaviors that will help achieve a healthy pregnancy. For women who have previously given birth, interconception care, a visit between pregnancies, identifies any new problems or provides a plan to manage previously known problems. Ideally, the woman has her first visit several months before conception.

At a preconception visit, the healthcare provider obtains a complete history and performs a physical examination. The woman is assessed for health problems (such as diabetes or hypertension), habits (such as use of alcohol or drugs), or social problems (such as intimate partner violence) that might unfavorably affect the pregnancy. If problems are discovered, treatment may begin before pregnancy.

If the woman is taking medications, their effect on pregnancy is reviewed and changes made, if needed. Women who are obese can obtain help to lose weight before conceiving. Referral to smoking cessation programs may be indicated. Smoking and use of alcohol or "recreational" drugs should end before the woman becomes pregnant. If not immune to rubella or varicella, vaccines can be given and the woman should be instructed to wait at least 1 month before conceiving. Hepatitis vaccine may be offered at the same time. Avoidance of common teratogens or other harmful substances is also discussed.

Previous recommendations have been for all women of childbearing age to consume 0.4 mg (400 mcg) folic acid daily to decrease the risk of neural tube defects. Updated recommendations are for an intake of 400 mcg to 800 mcg (0.4 mg to 0.8 mg) each day for all women capable of childbearing and at least one month before conception and 2 to 3 months after conception (U.S. Preventive Services Task Force,

2009). There has been no change to the recommendation of 0.6 mg (600 mcg) daily for the rest of pregnancy. Women who have given birth to an infant with a neural tube defect previously should take 4 mg of folic acid daily during the 4 weeks before pregnancy and throughout the first trimester (Gregory, Niebyl & Johnson 2012).

### Initial Visit

If the woman had a preconception visit, many of the initial prenatal assessments will have been completed. If not, the initial visit is a time for the nurse practitioner, nurse-midwife, or physician to establish rapport with the family and to perform a thorough assessment of the physiologic and psychosocial needs of the family. A thorough history and physical examination are included.

### History

***Obstetric history.*** The obstetric history provides essential information about prior pregnancies that may alert the healthcare provider to possible problems in the present pregnancy. Components of the obstetric history include:

- Gravidity, parity, abortions, and living children
- Weight of infants at birth, length of gestations
- Labor experiences, type of deliveries, locations of births, names of physicians or midwives
- Types of anesthesia and any difficulties with anesthesia during childbirth or previous surgeries
- Maternal complications, such as hypertension, diabetes, infection, or bleeding
- Infant complications
- Methods of infant feeding used in the past and currently planned
- Special concerns

**Gravida** refers to a woman who is or has been pregnant regardless of the duration of the pregnancy. A **primigravida** is a woman who is pregnant for the first time. A **multigravida** is a woman who has been pregnant more than once.

**Para** refers to the number of pregnancies that have ended at 20 or more weeks, regardless of whether the infant was born alive or was stillborn. A **nullipara** is a woman who has never completed a pregnancy beyond 20 weeks of gestation because she has never been pregnant or has had a spontaneous or elective abortion. A **primipara** is a woman who has delivered one pregnancy at 20 or more weeks of gestation. A **multipara** is a woman who has delivered two or more pregnancies at 20 or more weeks of gestation. The number of fetuses in a pregnancy does not change the para. Thus, a woman who gives birth to twins with her first pregnancy will be a gravida 1, para 1 if births occur at 20 or more weeks of gestation.

Use of the GTPAL acronym allows a more complete description of pregnancy outcomes than use of gravida and para alone. G stands for pregnancies or gravida; T, **term births** or pregnancies delivered between 38 and 42 weeks of gestation; P, **preterm births** (births between the 20th and 38th week of gestation); A, abortions; and L, living children. GTPAL is used by some authors to describe infants instead of pregnancies delivered. In this usage, (T) becomes term infants born and (P) becomes preterm infants born. Because the acronym is not used consistently, it can be confusing (Box 13.1).

Nurses must use caution when discussing gravida and para with the expectant mother in the presence of her family or significant other. Although the antepartum record may indicate a previous pregnancy or childbirth, she may not have shared this information with her family, and her right to privacy could be jeopardized by probing questions in their presence. The confidentiality of the pregnant woman must always be protected.

#### BOX 13.1 Calculation of Gravida and Para

A useful method for calculating gravida and para is to use the acronym GTPAL to describe pregnancies and their outcome: gravida (G), term (T), preterm (P), abortions (A), and living children (L).

To illustrate: A woman is 6 months pregnant. She previously had one spontaneous abortion and one elective abortion in the first trimester. She has a son who was born at 40 weeks of gestation and a daughter who was born at 34 weeks of gestation. She is gravida 5, para 2, and T = 1 (the son born at 40 weeks); P = 1 (the daughter born at 34 weeks); A = 2; L = 2. The two abortions are counted in the gravida but are not included in the para because they occurred before 20 weeks. Her GTPAL is 5-1-1-2-2.

***Menstrual history and estimated date of delivery.*** A complete menstrual history is necessary to establish the EDD. It is common practice to estimate the EDD on the basis of the first day of the last normal menstrual period (LNMP), although ovulation and conception occur approximately 2 weeks after the beginning of menstruation in a regular 28-day cycle. The average duration of pregnancy from the first day of the LNMP is 40 weeks, or 280 days. Nägele's rule is often used to establish EDD. The method involves subtracting 3 months from the first day of the LNMP, adding 7 days, and correcting the year, if appropriate.

*For example:* LNMP October 30, 2012
Subtract 3 months = July 30, 2012
Add 7 days and correct the year = August 6, 2013

Many healthcare providers also use a gestational calculator or wheel to calculate EDD quickly, although wheels are only accurate within plus or minus 5 days (Cunningham et al., 2010). A sonogram is often used to confirm the date. The EDD is also important to determine when to schedule certain tests commonly performed during pregnancy.

#### CRITICAL THINKING EXERCISE 13.1

Jenny gave birth to twin girls at 38 weeks of gestation 3 years ago. She had a spontaneous abortion last year at 12 weeks of gestation and thinks she may be pregnant now because she has missed a menstrual period and is nauseated in the mornings. Her last normal menstrual period (LNMP) began August 22.

1. If she is pregnant now, how would you record gravida and para?
2. Explain to Jenny why amenorrhea and morning sickness are not positive indications of pregnancy.
3. Use Nägele's rule to compute the expected date of delivery (EDD).

***Gynecologic and contraceptive history.*** Any previous gynecologic problems should be identified. Sexually transmitted diseases should be treated. Infertility problems with past or the present pregnancy should be discussed.

A detailed history of contraceptive methods is important. Although there has been some concern about congenital malformations when pregnant women inadvertently use hormonal contraceptives, studies have not shown the risk to be greater than for the general population (Nelson, 2011). Of course, any woman who suspects she might be pregnant should stop taking hormonal contraceptives and use another contraceptive until she has confirmation from a healthcare provider.

Although pregnancy with an intrauterine device (IUD) in place is unusual, it can cause complications such as spontaneous abortion and preterm delivery. The IUD should be removed promptly if the string is visible through the cervix. If the woman aborts during the second trimester, infection is likely to be present, and the woman should receive antibiotics and have her uterus evacuated (Cunningham et al., 2010).

***Medical and surgical history.*** Previous or current conditions can affect the outcome of the pregnancy and must be investigated. The history includes:

- Age, race, ethnic background (risk for specific genetic problems, such as sickle cell disease, thalassemia, cystic fibrosis, and Tay-Sachs disease)
- Childhood diseases and immunizations
- Chronic illnesses, such as asthma, heart disease, hypertension, diabetes, lupus, renal disease
- Previous illnesses, surgical procedures, injuries
- Previous infections such as hepatitis and tuberculosis
- History of anemia
- Bladder, bowel function (problems or changes)
- Amount of caffeine and alcohol consumed each day
- Tobacco use (number of years and number of packs per day)
- Prescription, over-the-counter, or illicit drugs
- Complementary or alternative therapies
- General nutrition, history of eating disorders
- Contact with pets, particularly cats (increased risk of infections such as toxoplasmosis)
- Allergies and drug sensitivities
- Occupation and related risk factors

***Family health history.*** A family history provides valuable information about the general health of the family, including chronic diseases such as diabetes and heart disease, and infections such as tuberculosis and hepatitis. Information about patterns of genetic or congenital anomalies also may be revealed.

***Partner's health history.*** The partner's history may include significant health problems such as genetic abnormalities, chronic diseases, and infections. The use of drugs such as cocaine or alcohol may affect the family's ability to cope with pregnancy and childbirth. Tobacco use by the father increases the risk of upper respiratory complications as a result of passive smoke to both the mother and infant. The father's blood type and Rh factor are important if the mother is Rh-negative because a blood incompatibility between the mother and the fetus is possible.

***Psychosocial history.*** The psychosocial history, which should be completed at the same time, is discussed on p. 248.

### Physical Examination

Many women have not had a recent physical examination before becoming pregnant. A thorough evaluation of all body systems is necessary to detect previously undiagnosed physical problems that may affect the pregnancy outcome. It also establishes baseline levels that will guide the treatment of the expectant mother and fetus throughout pregnancy.

***Vital signs***

**Blood pressure.** Position affects blood pressure in the pregnant woman. Blood pressure should be obtained with the woman seated and her arm supported in a horizontal position at the level of the heart. Documentation should include the position, arm used, pressure obtained, and type of sphygmomanometer used. Manual varieties are more accurate than automatic varieties.

All staff members should use the same Korotkoff's phase to measure blood pressure. Korotkoff's fifth phase (disappearance of sound) is most often used because the fourth phase (muffling) is not always identifiable. Blood pressures of 140/90 mm Hg and greater may indicate preeclampsia and require additional evaluation (see Chapter 25).

**Pulse.** The normal adult pulse rate is 60 to 90 bpm. Tachycardia is associated with anxiety, hyperthyroidism, and infection and should be investigated. The apical pulse should be assessed for at least 1 minute to determine the amplitude and regularity of the heartbeat and presence of murmurs. Pedal pulses should be strong, equal, and regular.

**Respiratory effort.** Respiratory rate during pregnancy is in the range of 16 to 24 breaths per minute. Tachypnea may indicate respiratory or cardiac disease. Breath sounds should be equal bilaterally, chest expansion should be symmetric, and lung fields should be free of abnormal breath sounds.

**Temperature.** Normal temperature during pregnancy is 36.6° C to 37.6° C (97.8° F to 99.6° F). Increased temperature suggests infection that may require medical management.

***Cardiovascular system***

**Venous congestion.** Additional assessment of the cardiovascular system includes observation for venous congestion, which can develop into varicosities. Venous congestion is most commonly noted in the legs and vulva (as varicosities), or rectum (as hemorrhoids).

**Edema.** Edema of the legs may be a benign condition that reflects pooling of blood in the extremities, which results in a shift of intravascular fluid into the interstitial spaces. When pressure exerted by a finger leaves a persistent depression, *pitting edema* is present.

***Musculoskeletal system***

**Posture and gait.** Body mechanics, as well as changes in posture and gait, should be addressed. Body mechanics during pregnancy may place strain on the muscles of the lower back and legs.

**Height and weight.** An initial weight is recorded to establish a baseline for evaluating weight gain throughout pregnancy (see Chapter 14). The body mass index should be calculated (see p. 279). Women who are underweight before pregnancy are at risk of having low-birth-weight infants. Obesity is associated with complications for the mother and newborn (see Chapter 14).

**Abdomen.** The contour, size, and muscle tone of the abdomen should be assessed. Fundal height should be measured if the fundus is palpable above the symphysis pubis (see p. 229). The fetal heart rate should be auscultated, counted, and recorded if the pregnancy is advanced enough so that it is audible.

***Neurologic system.*** A complete neurologic assessment is not necessary for women who are free of signs or symptoms that indicate a problem. However, deep tendon reflexes (DTRs) should be evaluated because hyperreflexia is associated with complications of pregnancy. (See Chapter 25, p. 541 for assessment of DTR.)

***Integumentary system.*** Skin color should be consistent with racial background. Pallor may indicate anemia. Jaundice may result from hepatic disease. Lesions, bruising, rashes, hyperpigmentation related to pregnancy (melasma, linea nigra), and stretch marks (striae), should be noted. Nail beds should be pink, with instant capillary return.

***Endocrine system.*** The thyroid enlarges slightly during the second trimester. However, gross enlargement or tenderness may indicate hyperthyroidism and requires further medical evaluation. Women with hypothyroidism should be treated during pregnancy to allow optimal development of the fetal central nervous system.

***Gastrointestinal system***

**Mouth.** The mucous membranes should be pink, smooth, glistening, and uniform. The lips should be free of ulcerations. The gums may be red, tender, edematous, and bleed more easily as a result of increased estrogen. The woman should be referred for regular dental care.

**Intestine.** Bowel sounds may be diminished because of the effects of progesterone on smooth muscle. Bowel sounds are often increased if a meal is overdue or if diarrhea is present. Constipation can be discussed at this time.

*Urinary system.* A clean-catch midstream urine sample is tested for signs of urinary tract infection and substances that may indicate a problem.

**Protein.** Although a trace amount of protein may be present in the urine, the amount should not increase. Its presence may indicate contamination by vaginal secretions, kidney disease, or preeclampsia.

**Glucose.** Small amounts of glucose may indicate physiologic "spilling" that occurs during normal pregnancy.

**Ketones.** Ketones may be found in the urine after heavy exercise or as a result of inadequate intake of food and fluid.

**Bacteria.** Increased bacteria in the urine is associated with urinary tract infection, which is common during pregnancy.

*Reproductive system*

**Breasts.** Breast size and symmetry, the condition of the nipples (erect, flat, inverted), and the presence of colostrum should be noted. Any lumps, dimpling of the skin, or asymmetry of the nipples requires further evaluation.

**External reproductive organs.** The skin and mucous membranes of the perineum, vulva, and anus are inspected for excoriations, growths, ulcerations, lesions, varicosities, warts, chancres, and perineal scars. Enlargement, tenderness, redness, or discharge from Bartholin's glands or Skene's glands may indicate gonorrheal or chlamydial infection. The examiner should obtain a specimen for culture of any discharge from lesions or inflamed glands to determine the causative organisms and to provide effective care.

**Internal reproductive organs.** A speculum inserted into the vagina permits the examiner to see the walls of the vagina and the cervix. Chadwick's sign and Goodell's sign are seen during pregnancy. The external cervical os is closed in *primigravidas* (women pregnant for the first time), but one fingertip may be admitted in multiparas. Routine cervical cultures for gonorrhea and chlamydial infection are generally obtained during the initial pregnancy examination. The examiner also collects a specimen for a Papanicolaou (Pap) test to screen for cervical cancer.

A bimanual examination involves using both hands, one on the abdomen and the other in the vagina, to palpate the internal genitalia. The examiner palpates the uterus for size, contour, tenderness, and position. The uterus should be movable between the two examining hands and should feel smooth. The ovaries, if palpable, should be about the shape and size of almonds and should not be tender.

**Pelvic measurements.** Pelvic measurements may be assessed at this time to determine if the bony pelvis is adequate to permit vaginal birth (see Fig. 16.4).

### Laboratory Data

Table 13.3 lists laboratory examinations commonly performed during pregnancy and the purpose and significance of each test. Table 13.1 shows laboratory values for pregnancy and nonpregnant women.

**TABLE 13.3 Common Laboratory Tests**

| Test | Purpose | Significance |
|---|---|---|
| Blood grouping with Rh factor and antibody screen | To determine blood type screen for possible maternal–fetal blood incompatibility | Identifies possible causes of maternal–fetal blood incompatibility. If father is Rh positive and mother is Rh negative and unsensitized, $Rh_0(D)$ immune globulin will be given during pregnancy and after birth |
| Complete blood count (CBC) | To identify infection, anemia, or cell abnormalities | More than 15,000/mm$^3$ white blood cells or decreased platelets require follow-up |
| Hemoglobin (Hgb) or hematocrit (Hct) | To detect anemia; often checked several times during pregnancy | Low Hgb or Hct may indicate a need for added iron supplementation |
| Venereal Disease Research Laboratory (VDRL) or rapid plasma reagin (RPR) | To screen for syphilis | Treat if positive. Retest if indicated. |
| Rubella titer | To determine immunity | If titer is 1:8 or less, mother is not immune Immunize postpartum if not immune |
| Tuberculin skin test | To screen for tuberculosis | If positive, refer for additional testing or therapy |
| Genetic testing (for sickle cell anemia, cystic fibrosis, Tay–Sachs disease, and other genetic conditions) | Offered if there is an increased risk for certain genetic conditions | If mother is positive, check partner Counseling appropriate to the results of testing |
| Hepatitis B | To detect presence of antigens in maternal blood | If present, infants should be given hepatitis immune globulin and vaccine soon after birth |
| Human immunodeficiency virus (HIV) screen | Voluntary test encouraged at first visit to detect HIV antibodies | Positive results require retesting, counseling, and treatment to lower infant infection |
| Urinalysis | To detect renal disease or infection | Requires further assessment if positive for more than trace protein (renal damage, preeclampsia), ketones (fasting or dehydration), or bacteria (infection) |
| Papanicolaou (Pap) test | To screen for cervical neoplasia | Treat and refer if abnormal cells are present |
| Cervical culture | To detect group B streptococci and sexually transmitted diseases | Treat and retest as necessary, treat group B streptococci during labor |
| Multiple marker screen: Maternal serum alpha-fetoprotein, human chorionic gonadotropin, and estriol. Inhibin A may also be measured. May be combined with ultrasound. | To screen for fetal anomalies | Abnormal results may indicate chromosomal abnormality (such as trisomy 18 or 21) or structural defects (such as neural tube defects) |
| Glucose challenge test | To screen for gestational diabetes | If elevated, a glucose tolerance test is recommended |

### Risk Assessment

Risk assessment begins at the initial visit, when the healthcare provider identifies factors that put the expectant mother or the fetus at risk for complications, and thus, in need of specialized care. Many women identified as high risk give birth to healthy term infants. Furthermore, risk factors change as pregnancy progresses, and risk assessment must be updated throughout pregnancy. Table 13.4 lists the major risk factors and their implications.

## Subsequent Assessments

Ongoing antepartum care is important to the successful outcome of pregnancy. The traditional schedule for prenatal assessment in a normal pregnancy follows.

Conception to 28 weeks: Every 4 weeks
29 to 36 weeks: Every 2 weeks
37 weeks to birth: Weekly

Although this is the usual model of prenatal care, there are other options. "Centering Pregnancy" is an example of an alternative method of care. The method involves ten 1.5- to 2-hour sessions with small groups of women and healthcare providers beginning at 12 to 16 weeks of pregnancy and ending in early postpartum. The women have an individual assessment before the first group session and during a small part of the subsequent group sessions. Women assess their own blood pressure and weight and participate in educational sessions appropriate for that point of pregnancy. The social support provided by the group is an important benefit (Herman, Rogers, & Ehrenthal, 2012). Women cared for in this way have been satisfied with the care and have had favorable pregnancy outcomes (Rotundo, 2011). Participants also receive more health promotion content and peer support than those receiving traditional care (Bell, 2012; Herman, Rogers, & Ehrenthal, 2012). More information is available at http://www.centeringpregnancy.org.

### Vital Signs

Significant deviations from baseline values for vital signs indicate the need for further assessment. The BP should be measured in the same arm with the woman in the same position each time.

### Weight

Weight should be recorded to document that the expected pattern of weight gain is occurring. A gain of 11.5 to 16 kg (25 to 35 lb) is recommended for the woman of normal prepregnancy weight. Inadequate weight gain may signify that the pregnancy is not as advanced as first thought or the fetus is not growing as expected. A sudden, rapid weight gain may indicate excessive fluid retention.

**TABLE 13.4 Summary of High-Risk Factors in Pregnancy**

| Factors | Implications |
|---|---|
| **Demographic Factors** | |
| Younger than 16 yr or older than 35 yr of age | Increased risk for preterm labor, preeclampsia, congenital anomalies, infant mortality |
| Low socioeconomic status or dependent on public assistance | Increased risk for preterm birth, low-birth-weight infants |
| Nonwhite race | Increased incidence of preterm birth and infant and maternal death for some groups |
| Multiparity | Higher parity increases risk for antepartum or postpartum hemorrhage, cesarean birth |
| **Social–Personal Factors** | |
| Low prepregnancy weight | Associated with low-birth-weight infants |
| Obesity | Increased risk for hypertension, prolonged labor, large-for-gestational-age infant, cesarean birth, wound infections, gestational diabetes, thromboembolic disorders, and postpartum hemorrhage |
| Height less than 152 cm (5 ft) | Increased incidence of cesarean birth because of cephalopelvic disproportion |
| Smoking | Associated with placenta previa, abruptio placentae, premature membrane rupture, spontaneous abortion, perinatal mortality, low-birth-weight, preterm birth, SIDS |
| Use of alcohol or unprescribed drugs | Increased risk for congenital anomalies, neonatal withdrawal, fetal alcohol syndrome |
| **Obstetric Factors** | |
| Birth of previous infant more than 4000 g (8.8 lb) | Increased need for cesarean birth; increased risk for infant birth injury, maternal gestational diabetes, neonatal hypoglycemia |
| Previous preterm birth | Increased incidence of repeated preterm birth |
| Previous fetal or neonatal death | Maternal psychological distress |
| Rh sensitization | Fetal anemia, erythroblastosis fetalis, kernicterus |
| **Existing Medical Conditions** | |
| Diabetes mellitus | Increased risk for preeclampsia, cesarean birth, preterm birth, infant small or large for gestational age, neonatal hypoglycemia, congenital anomalies |
| Hypothyroidism | Increased incidence of preeclampsia, abruptio placenta, low birthweight, preterm birth, and stillbirth |
| Hyperthyroidism | Maternal risk for preeclampsia, thyroid storm, or postpartum hemorrhage |
| Cardiac disease | Maternal risk for cardiac decompensation and death; increased risk for fetal and neonatal death |
| Renal disease | Maternal risk for renal failure and preterm delivery; fetal risk for intrauterine growth restriction |
| Concurrent infections | Increased incidence of spontaneous abortion or congenital anomalies (heart disease, blindness, deafness, bone lesions) if maternal disease occurred in the first trimester |

*SIDS*, Sudden infant death syndrome

### Urinalysis

Urine is tested at each visit for protein, glucose, and ketones. The urine may be checked for nitrates using a dipstick. A positive nitrate result indicates infection may be present, and a urine culture may be performed.

### Fundal Height

Measuring fundal height is an inexpensive and noninvasive method for evaluating fetal growth and confirming gestational age. The fundal height is measured at every visit once the fundus is able to be palpated in the woman's abdomen. The bladder must be empty to avoid elevation of the uterus by a full bladder. The woman lies on her back with her knees slightly flexed. The top of the fundus is palpated, and a tape measure is stretched from the top of the symphysis pubis, over the abdominal curve, to the top of the fundus (Fig. 13.9).

From 16 to 18 weeks until 36 weeks, the fundal height, measured in centimeters, is approximately equal to the gestational age of the fetus in weeks (Beckmann et al., 2010). If there is a discrepancy between fundal height and weeks of gestation, additional assessment is necessary. The EDD may be incorrect, and the pregnancy more or less advanced than thought. The number of fetuses present, fetal growth, the amount of amniotic fluid, presence of leiomyomata (fibroids), or gestational trophoblastic disease (hydatidiform mole) will affect the fundal height. Ultrasound may be performed to obtain further information.

### Leopold's Maneuvers

Leopold's maneuvers provide a systematic method for palpating the fetus through the abdominal wall during the later part of pregnancy. These maneuvers provide valuable information about the location and presentation of the fetus (see Chapter 16).

### Fetal Heart Rate

The fetal heart rate should be between 110 and 160 bpm. The location of the fetal heart sounds provides information that may help determine the position of the fetus. For example, a fetal heart rate heard in an upper quadrant of the abdomen suggests that the fetus is in a breech presentation.

### Fetal Activity

Usually first noticed by the expectant mother at 16 to 20 weeks of gestation, fetal movements gradually increase in frequency and strength. In the last trimester, the woman may be asked to count fetal movements. These are commonly called "kick counts." In general, fetal activity indicates the fetus is physically healthy.

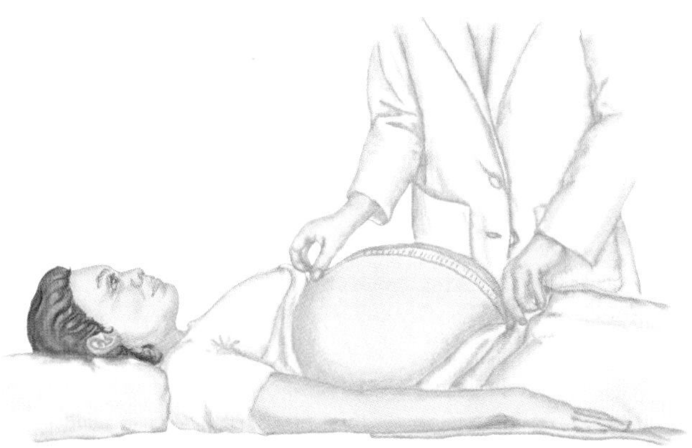

FIG 13.9 Measuring the uterus involves measuring from the upper border of the symphysis pubis to the top of the fundus.

### Signs of Labor

The woman should be asked about signs of labor at each visit. A discussion of contractions, bleeding, and rupture of membranes will help the woman know how to identify preterm labor. She should be cautioned to call her healthcare provider or go to the hospital if she thinks she might be in labor. During the third trimester, a discussion of the normal course of labor will help prepare the woman.

### Ultrasound Screen

Although an ultrasound examination is not necessary for all women, the test is often performed one or more times during pregnancy. Ultrasound helps determine gestational age and may show some fetal anomalies and determine the gender of the baby (see Chapter 15).

### Glucose Screen

Blood glucose is often screened at 24 to 28 weeks by a glucose challenge test. If the result is elevated, the woman has a glucose tolerance test to detect gestational diabetes (see Chapter 26). Glucose testing may not be necessary in women younger than 25 years and at low risk for developing gestational diabetes (Cunningham et al., 2010).

### Isoimmunization

Antibody tests may be repeated in the third trimester in women who are Rh negative if the father of the baby is Rh positive. If unsensitized, the woman should receive $Rh_o$ (D) immune globulin prophylactically at 28 weeks of gestation (see Chapter 25).

### Pelvic Examinations

During the last month of pregnancy the healthcare provider may perform a pelvic examination to determine cervical changes. The descent of the fetus and the presenting part also can be assessed at this time.

## Multifetal Pregnancy

A multifetal pregnancy is a pregnancy in which two or more embryos or fetuses are present simultaneously (see Chapter 12).

### Diagnosis

Women with multifetal pregnancies are larger than expected for the weeks of gestation, have more fetal movements, and gain more weight. More than one fetus should be suspected if the fundal height is 4 cm or more than expected based on gestational age (Beckmann et al., 2010).

Women who are older, black, have a personal or family history of twins, or have conceived using infertility therapy have an increased chance of multifetal pregnancies (Newman & Rittenberg, 2008). When more than one fetus seems likely, the diagnosis should be confirmed by sonography. Separate fetuses and heart activities may be seen as early as 6 weeks of gestation (Tarsa & Moore, 2010).

### Maternal Adaptation to Multifetal Pregnancy

Maternal physiologic changes are greater with multiple fetuses than with a single fetus. For example, with twins, blood volume increases 500 mL over that needed for a single fetus. This increases the workload of the heart and may contribute to fatigue and activity intolerance. The uterus may achieve a volume of 10 L or more and weigh more than 9 kg (20 lb) (Cunningham et al., 2010). Respiratory difficulty increases because the overdistended uterus causes greater elevation of the diaphragm.

The uterus also may cause more compression of the large vessels, resulting in more pronounced and earlier supine hypotension. Compression of the bowel makes constipation and hemorrhoids a persistent problem. Fatigue is greater than with a singleton pregnancy. Nausea and vomiting in early pregnancy may be greater than with single-fetus pregnancies.

### Antepartum Care in Multifetal Pregnancy

Prenatal visits to the healthcare provider increase with multifetal pregnancy because complications are more common. More frequent visits permit extra vigilance in the detection of complications such as spontaneous abortion, anemia, hypertension, preterm labor, gestational diabetes, and congenital anomalies (Mavridou, Norwitz, Robinson, et al., 2008). Ultrasound scanning may also be performed more frequently.

Education about diet and the necessity for increased rest is important. The need for calories, iron, vitamins, and folic acid increases. Women of normal pregestational weight carrying twins are advised to gain 17 to 25 kg (37 to 54 lb) or more (ACOG, 2013). Tests of fetal well-being are commonly performed twice a week in the third trimester. Preterm labor is more frequent, and the woman should be taught the signs and how to respond early in the pregnancy.

Concerns about the effect of more than one newborn on the family should be addressed. Referral for assistance with the financial burden of medical and hospital care during and after pregnancy for the mother and infants may be appropriate.

## Common Discomforts of Pregnancy

Many women experience discomforts of pregnancy that are not serious but detract from their feeling of well-being (see Patient-Centered Teaching box).

### Nausea and Vomiting

Nausea and vomiting during pregnancy are frequently called *morning sickness* because these symptoms are more acute on arising. However, they may occur at any time of day and are present in 70% to 80% of

## PATIENT-CENTERED TEACHING

### *How to Overcome the Common Discomforts of Pregnancy*

**Nausea and Vomiting**

- Eat dry crackers or toast before arising in the morning; then get out of bed slowly.
- Eat small amounts of carbohydrate and protein foods every 2 to 3 hours and a total of 5 or 6 small meals.
- Drink fluids separately from meals. Try small amounts of ice chips, water, and clear liquids like gelatin or Popsicles. Avoid coffee.
- Avoid fried, greasy, fatty, or spicy foods or those with strong odors. Instead try bland foods, which may be more easily tolerated.
- Try foods containing ginger or peppermint, or combine salty and tart foods like potato chips and lemonade.
- Increase protein intake and eat a protein snack before bedtime.
- Take prenatal vitamins at bedtime because they may increase nausea if taken in the morning.
- Rest more frequently and take naps, if possible.
- Use an acupressure band that applies pressure over a point approximately three fingerbreadths above the wrist crease on the inner arm.
- Ask your healthcare provider if vitamin $B_6$ (pyridoxine) would be helpful.
- Check with your primary caregiver before taking any herbal remedies.
- Notify your healthcare provider for severe nausea and vomiting or signs of dehydration (dry, cracked lips; elevated pulse; fever; concentrated urine).

**Heartburn**

- Eat small meals every 2 to 3 hours, and avoid fatty, acidic, or spicy foods.
- Eliminate or curtail smoking and drinking coffee and carbonated beverages, which stimulate acid formation in the stomach.
- Try chewing gum.
- Take a tablespoon of cream before meals if heartburn is not already present.
- Do not eat or drink just before bedtime, and sleep with an extra pillow.
- Walk or sit upright for 1 to 2 hours after meals to reduce reflux and relieve symptoms.
- Avoid bending over.
- Wear loose-fitting clothes.
- Take deep breaths and sip water to help relieve the burning sensation.
- Use only antacids suggested by your care provider, but avoid those that are high in sodium (Alka-Seltzer, baking soda), which cause fluid retention. Antacids high in calcium (Tums, Alka-Mints) provide relief but may cause rebound hyperacidity. Liquid antacids may be more effective.

**Backache**

- Maintain correct posture: head up, shoulders back.
- Do not gain excess weight.
- Avoid high-heeled shoes because they increase lordosis.
- To pick up objects, squat rather than bend at the waist.
- Do not lift heavy objects.
- When sitting, use foot supports, arm rests, and pillows behind the back.
- Perform exercises such as tailor sitting, shoulder circling, and pelvic rocking, which strengthen the back and prepare for labor.

**Round Ligament Pain**

- Use good body mechanics, and avoid strenuous exercise.
- Do not make sudden movements or position changes.
- Avoid stretching and twisting at the same time. When getting out of bed, turn to the side without twisting and then get up slowly.
- Bend toward the pain, squat, or bring the knees up to the chest to relieve pain by relaxing the ligament.
- Apply heat and lie on the right side to relieve the pain.

**Urinary Frequency**

- Decrease fluids in the evening but drink adequate amounts during the day.
- Avoid caffeine, which is a natural diuretic.
- Perform Kegel exercises to help maintain bladder control: Identify the muscles to be exercised by stopping the flow of urine midstream. Do not routinely perform the exercise while urinating because urinary retention may occur and increase the risk of urinary tract infection. Slowly contract the muscles around the vagina, and hold for 10 seconds. Relax at least 10 seconds. Repeat the contraction-relaxation cycle 30 times per day.

**Varicosities**

- Avoid constricting clothing and crossing the legs at the knees, which impedes blood return from the legs.
- Rest frequently with the legs elevated above the level of the hips.
- Wear support hose or elastic stockings that reach above the varicosities. Apply them before getting out of bed each morning.
- If working in one position for prolonged periods, walk around for a few minutes at least every 2 hours.

## PATIENT-CENTERED TEACHING—cont'd

### *How to Overcome the Common Discomforts of Pregnancy*

**Constipation**

- Use self-care measures that generally are as effective as using laxatives, but do not interfere with absorption of nutrients or lead to laxative dependency.
- Drink at least eight glasses of liquids including water, juice, or milk each day. These should not include coffee, tea, or carbonated drinks because of their diuretic effect. After drinking diuretic beverages, add a glass of water.
- Add foods high in fiber such as unpeeled fresh fruits and vegetables, whole-grain bread or cereals, bran muffins, oatmeal, baked potatoes with skins, dried beans, and fruit juices. Four pieces of fruit plus a large salad provide enough fiber for 1 day.
- Restrict cheese consumption, which causes constipation.
- Reduce intake of sweets, which increase bacterial growth in the intestine and can lead to flatulence.
- Do not discontinue taking iron supplements if they have been prescribed. If constipation persists, consult your healthcare provider for advice about stool softeners.
- Try swimming, riding a stationary bicycle, or taking a brisk walk of at least 1 mile per day to stimulate peristalsis and improve muscle tone.
- Establish a regular pattern by allowing a consistent time each day for elimination. One hour after meals is ideal to take advantage of the gastrocolic reflex (the peristaltic wave in the colon that is induced by taking food into the fasting stomach).
- Use a footrest or place your feet on a folded towel during elimination to provide comfort and decrease straining.

**Hemorrhoids**

- Avoid constipation to prevent straining that causes or worsens hemorrhoids. Drink plenty of water, eat foods rich in fiber, and exercise regularly.
- To relieve existing hemorrhoidal discomfort, take frequent, tepid baths. Apply cool witch hazel compresses or anesthetic ointments.
- Lie on your side with the hips elevated on a pillow.
- If pain persists or bleeding occurs, call your healthcare provider.

**Leg Cramps**

- To prevent cramps, elevate the legs often during the day to improve circulation.
- To relieve cramps, extend the affected leg, keeping the knee straight. Bend the foot toward the body, or ask someone to assist. If alone, stand and apply pressure on the affected leg with the knee straight.

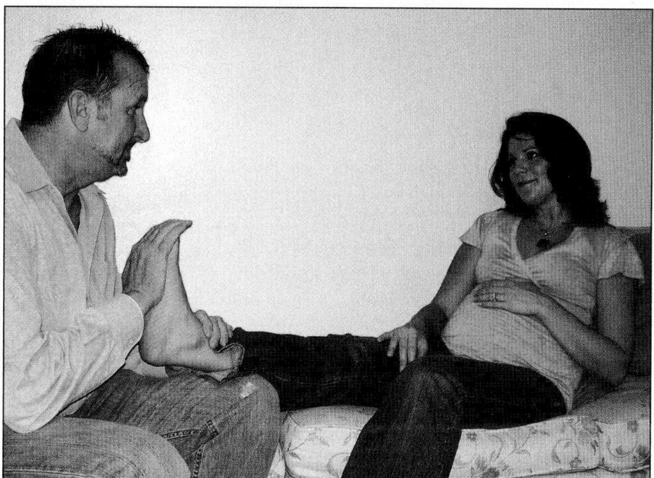

(Courtesy Steve and Michelle Henry, Tustin, CA.)

- Avoid excessive amounts of foods high in phosphorus. Check with your healthcare provider about taking additional calcium or magnesium.

pregnant women (Blackburn, 2014). Symptoms generally begin between 4 and 8 weeks of gestation and disappear by approximately 14 to 16 weeks (Beckmann et al., 2010). Women need reassurance that nausea and vomiting, however distressing, are common and that the condition is generally temporary. Morning sickness must be distinguished from hyperemesis gravidarum—severe vomiting accompanied by weight loss, dehydration, electrolyte imbalance, and ketosis (see Chapter 25).

Although the cause of nausea and vomiting is unknown, these symptoms are believed to be related to increased levels of hCG and estrogen, as well as periodic hypoglycemia. Symptoms may be aggravated by cooking odors, fatigue, and emotional stress. Vitamin $B_6$ and antihistamines may be prescribed for some women. Hypnosis and acupressure have also been found effective (Singh, Yoon, & Kuo, 2015).

### Heartburn

Heartburn is described as an acute burning sensation in the epigastric and sternal regions. It occurs in 70% of pregnant women when reverse peristaltic waves cause regurgitation of acidic stomach contents into the esophagus (Castro & Ogunyemi, 2010). The underlying causes are diminished gastric motility, displacement and compression of the stomach by the enlarging uterus, and relaxation of the lower esophageal sphincter. Improper diet and nervous tension may be precipitating factors.

### Backache

Backache is a common complaint during the third trimester. It is caused by the lordosis, relaxed ligaments, and muscle strain associated with pregnancy. A primary focus is to prevent backache by teaching correct posture (Fig. 13.10) and body mechanics (Fig. 13.11). Fig. 13.12 suggests exercises that relax the shoulders and thighs and help prevent backache.

### Round Ligament Pain

Round ligament pain is a sharp pain in the side or inguinal area, usually on the right side. It is caused by softening and stretching of the ligament from hormones and uterine growth. Because the uterus turns slightly to the right during pregnancy, the right round ligament is stretched more than the left one.

### Urinary Frequency

Although urinary frequency is a common complaint during pregnancy, the condition is temporary and is managed by most women without undue distress. Urinary incontinence may occur in the third

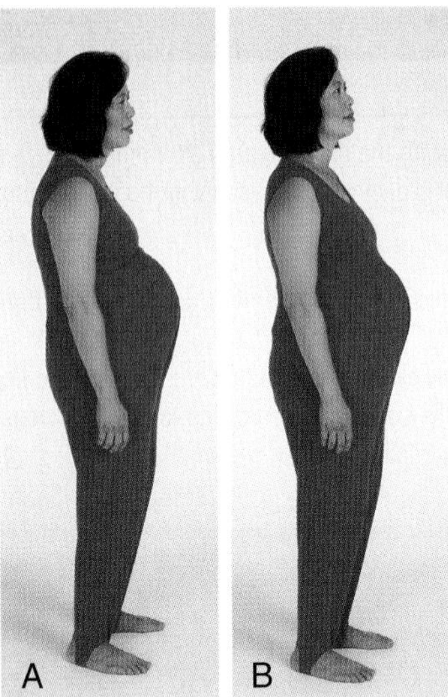


**FIG 13.10** Posture during pregnancy may cause or alleviate backache. **A,** Incorrect posture. The neck is jutting forward, the shoulders are slumping, and the back is sharply curved, creating back pain and discomfort. **B,** Correct posture. The neck and shoulders are straight, the back is flattened, and the pelvis is tucked under and slightly upward.

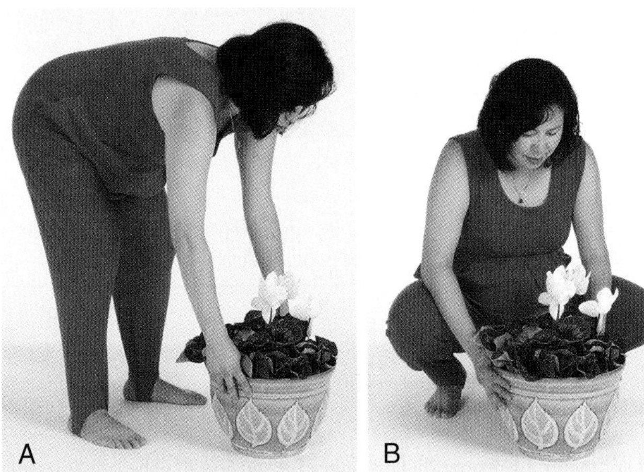


**FIG 13.11** Techniques for lifting. Squatting places less strain on the back. **A,** Incorrect technique. Stooping or bending places a great deal of strain on muscles of the lower back. **B,** Correct technique. Squatting and moving the object close permits the stronger muscles of the legs to do the lifting.

trimester. Kegel exercises are sometimes recommended to help maintain bladder control.

### Varicosities

Varicosities occur in 40% of pregnancies because the weight of the uterus partially compresses the veins that return blood from the legs and estrogen causes elastic tissue to become more fragile (Blackburn, 2013). The result is dilation of the vessels, which may become engorged, inflamed, and painful. The condition is usually confined to the legs but may involve the veins of the rectum (hemorrhoids) or vulva.

Varicosities occur most often in women who are obese, multiparas, or have a family history of varicose veins. The problem is exacerbated by prolonged standing, when the force of gravity makes blood return more difficult. There may be minimal discomfort at the end of each day or large, tortuous veins that produce severe discomfort with any activity.

### Constipation

Intestinal motility is reduced during pregnancy as a result of progesterone, pressure from the uterus, and decreased activity. These changes may cause hard, dry stools and decreased frequency of bowel movements. Iron supplementation often increases constipation.

### Hemorrhoids

Hemorrhoids are varicosities of the rectum that may be external (outside the anal sphincter) or internal (above the sphincter). Common causes include vascular engorgement of the pelvis, constipation, straining at stool, and prolonged sitting or standing. Pushing during the second stage of labor exacerbates the problem, which may continue into the postpartum. Hemorrhoids may continue into the postpartum period but often shrink and become less troublesome.

### Leg Cramps

Painful contraction of the muscles of the lower legs occurs most often during sleep, when the muscles are relaxed. Cramps may also occur when the woman stretches and extends her foot. Leg cramps are believed to be caused by an imbalance of serum calcium and phosphorus, but this has not been proven. Low magnesium levels also may be a cause (Erick, 2008). A 1 : 1 ratio of calcium to phosphorus is desired, but this ratio is difficult to achieve in pregnancy, when many women consume large amounts of dairy products high in calcium and phosphorus. Venous congestion in the legs during the third trimester also contributes to leg cramps.

## NURSING CARE

### Family Responses to Physical Changes of Pregnancy

The nursing process focuses on identifying each family's unique responses to the physiologic changes of pregnancy, determining factors that might interfere with the ability to adapt to changes, and finding solutions to identified problems.

#### Assessment

Assess the woman's responses to the physiologic processes of pregnancy and the family's preparation for the birth. Include structured interviews and informal discussions. Review the history and physical examination findings. Gather information from the expectant mother as well as from her partner and other significant family members, if appropriate.

#### Nursing Diagnosis and Planning

Most families express an intense desire to protect the health of the unborn child and the well-being of the mother. One of the most encompassing nursing diagnosis for the prenatal period is:

- Readiness for Enhanced Childbearing Process, prenatal health practices that provide optimal benefit to the fetus and mother.

***Expected outcomes.*** The woman and family will explain practices that promote the safety and well-being of the mother and fetus throughout pregnancy and will describe measures that provide relief from the common discomforts of pregnancy. During the first visit, the woman will describe a realistic plan to modify behaviors or habits that do not promote the health of herself or the fetus.

#### Interventions

***Teaching health behaviors.*** Teaching should be included in each visit and should focus on the mother's immediate questions and concerns.

**Shoulder circling**

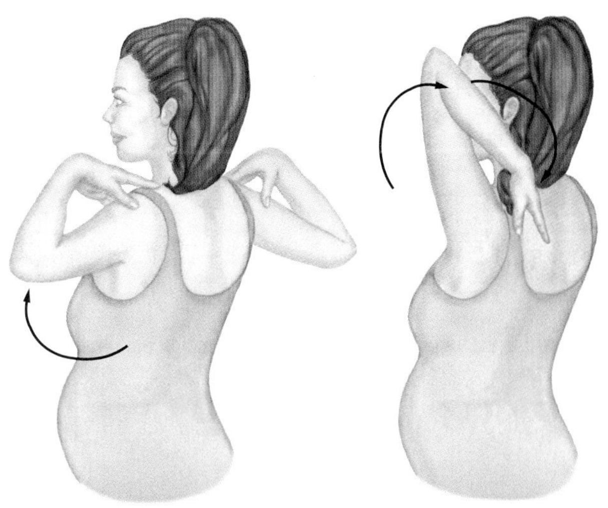

The fingertips are placed on the shoulders, then the elbows are brought forward and up during inhalation, back and down during exhalation. Repeat five times.

**Tailor sitting**

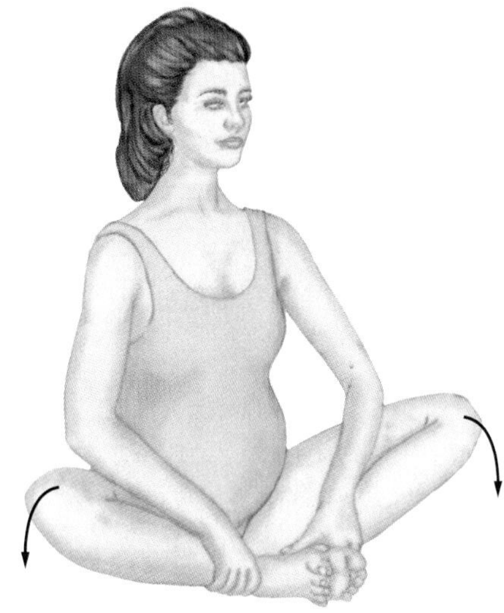

The woman uses her thigh muscles to press her knees to the floor. Keeping her back straight, she should remain in the position for 5 to 15 minutes.

**Pelvic tilt or pelvic rocking**

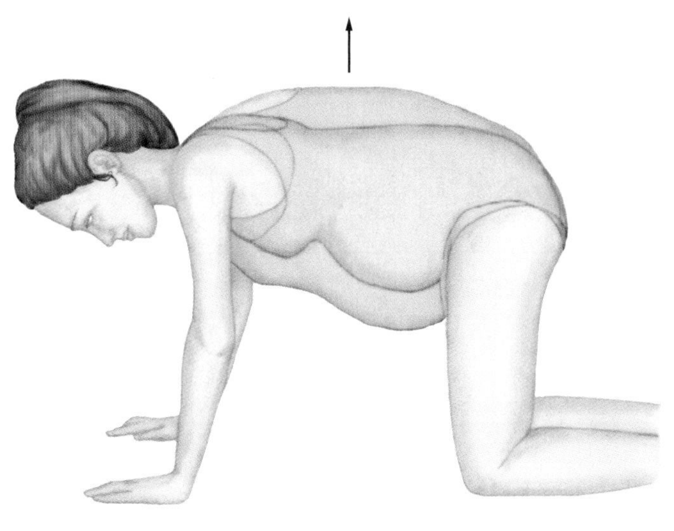

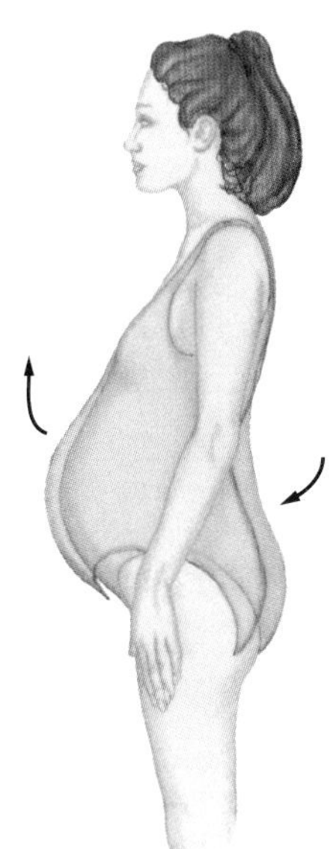

This exercise can be performed on hands and knees, with the hands directly under the shoulders and the knees under the hips. The back should be in a neutral position, not hollowed. The head and neck should be aligned with the straight back. The woman then presses up with the lower back and holds this position for a few seconds, then relaxes to a neutral position. Repeat 5 times. The exercise may also be performed in a standing position when the pelvis is rotated forward to flatten the lower back.

**FIG 13.12** Exercises to prevent backache.

**Bathing.** Bathing protects pregnant women from infection and promotes comfort by dissipating heat produced by increased metabolism. During the last trimester, when balance is altered by a changing center of gravity, caution the woman to use nonskid pads in the tub or shower.

**Hot tubs and saunas.** Instruct the woman to avoid activities that may cause maternal hyperthermia. Maternal hyperthermia, particularly during the first trimester, may be associated with fetal anomalies. A pregnant woman should not stay in a sauna for more than 15 minutes or a hot tub for more than 10 minutes and should keep her head, arms, and upper chest out of the water (American Academy of Pediatrics [AAP] & American College of Obstetricians and Gynecologists [ACOG], 2012; Beckmann et al., 2010).

**Douching.** Despite increased vaginal discharge in pregnancy, there is no need for douching during pregnancy or at any other time. Some women douche because they believe it increases cleanliness and prevents infection. However, infections such as bacterial vaginosis (BV) occur more often in women who douche (Cottrell, 2010). BV has been associated with preterm birth, premature rupture of membranes, and low birth weight (ACOG, 2014). Discuss the woman's reasons for douching, and explain the detrimental effects.

## NURSING CARE PLAN

### *Early Pregnancy Concerns*

**Focused Assessment**

Maria, a thin, 21-year-old primigravida who is 8 weeks pregnant, states she is often very tired during the day even though she is sleeping 8 to 10 hours at night. Fatigue concerns her because she is normally very energetic. Her job is demanding and requires that she concentrate and balance many factors at the same time. Her physical examination and laboratory tests are normal.

**Nursing Diagnosis**

Fatigue related to inadequate rest periods to accommodate the physiologic demands of pregnancy.

**Planning**

***Expected Outcomes***

Maria will:

1. Identify methods to cope with fatigue at home and at work.
2. Report increased energy by the second trimester.

**Interventions and *Rationales***

1. Acknowledge the fatigue and reassure Maria that it is self-limiting and occurs because of the change in hormone levels.
   *Reassurance helps alleviate the concern that fatigue indicates a problem with her pregnancy.*
2. Suggest she explore a flexible schedule or routine with her employer to allow rest periods at work. Advise a short nap after work before beginning other activities at home.
   *These changes are often all that is needed to continue to function effectively.*
3. Recommend that she lie down or sit comfortably with her legs elevated for a few minutes every 2 hours and consciously relax the muscles of the legs, abdomen, and shoulders.
   *Relaxation renews energy even when sleep is not possible.*
4. Suggest that she try deep breathing and visualizing a favorite location or pastime whenever possible. Progressive relaxation—conscious tensing and relaxing of groups of muscles beginning with those in the feet and working upward toward the head—may be helpful.
   *Such exercises relieve physical tension that adds to fatigue and also provide mental distraction.*
5. Recommend that Maria get as much sleep as she feels she needs when possible. Adequate rest may involve curtailing social activities and tasks that can be postponed.
   *Although recreation is important, the need for sleep is overwhelming for some women during early pregnancy.*
6. Recommend that she enlist the assistance of family, significant others, and friends to free her of all but the most essential home responsibilities.
   *This will allow her to rest more during this time.*
7. Explain that during the second trimester, Maria will probably have more energy, but it is normal to be tired again near the end of pregnancy.
   *If she knows the normal course of fatigue during pregnancy she can plan ahead for ways to cope with it.*

**Evaluation**

Maria was able to negotiate two short rest periods each day at work and rests after work. At 12 weeks of gestation, she continues to use learned techniques to renew energy. Maria reports increased energy at the third prenatal visit (16 weeks).

***Additional Nursing Diagnosis to Consider***

Activity Intolerance

**Breast care.** Instruct the expectant mother to avoid soap on her nipples because it removes the natural lubricant that forms there. Advise her to wear a supportive bra to help prevent loss of muscle tone as the breasts become heavier during pregnancy. Wide bra straps distribute the weight evenly across the shoulders and provide greater comfort. Explain that breast stimulation, which increases oxytocin secretion and may initiate uterine contractions, is unsafe if there has been a history of preterm labor or if signs of preterm labor are present.

**Clothing.** Recommend that all clothing be comfortable and nonconstricting. Tight jeans or pantyhose may constrict venous circulation and should be avoided or worn for short periods only. Explain that low heels do not interfere with balance, but high heels increase the lordosis prevalent during the last trimester.

**Exercise.** Teach women who have no medical or obstetric complications to exercise in moderation for 30 minutes or more each day (AAP & ACOG, 2012; Beckmann et al., 2010). Recreational sports can generally be continued if there is no risk for falling or abdominal trauma. Contact sports, exercise that requires balance or may cause injury, and exercise in the supine position after the first trimester are not safe. Moderate aerobic exercise may be prescribed for women who are overweight or obese with no other complications (ACOG, 2013).

Walking is an ideal exercise because it stimulates muscular activity of the entire body, gently increases respiratory and cardiovascular effort, and does not result in fatigue or strain. Swimming is an excellent exercise because the buoyancy of the water helps prevent injuries. Riding a stationary bike and yoga are also helpful. Exercise classes especially for pregnant women are often available and offer companionship with other women having similar experiences.

Instruct women not to *begin* strenuous exercise programs or intensify training during pregnancy. Women who have been exercising strenuously before pregnancy should consult their healthcare provider but may be able to continue some of their usual routine. As pregnancy progresses, it may be necessary to reduce the level of exercise to prevent physiologic stress or falls resulting from changes in the center of gravity.

Pregnant women must avoid becoming overheated because heat is transmitted to the fetus, causing an increase in fetal oxygen needs. Women should allow a cool-down period of mild activity after exercising. It is important to take liquids frequently while exercising to prevent dehydration. The woman should stop exercising and seek medical advice if she has chest or abdominal pain, dizziness, headache, vaginal bleeding, decreased fetal movement, or signs of labor while exercising.

**Sleep and rest.** Finding a comfortable position for rest becomes a problem in the third trimester. Suggest the woman use pillows to support the abdomen and back to enhance sleep (Fig. 13.13). Rest periods during the day also are beneficial.

**Nutrition.** A discussion of nutrition should be part of each visit. Assess the woman's use of prenatal vitamins and answer any questions she has (see Chapter 14).

**Employment.** Most women of childbearing age in the United States are employed outside the home, and most continue to work during pregnancy.

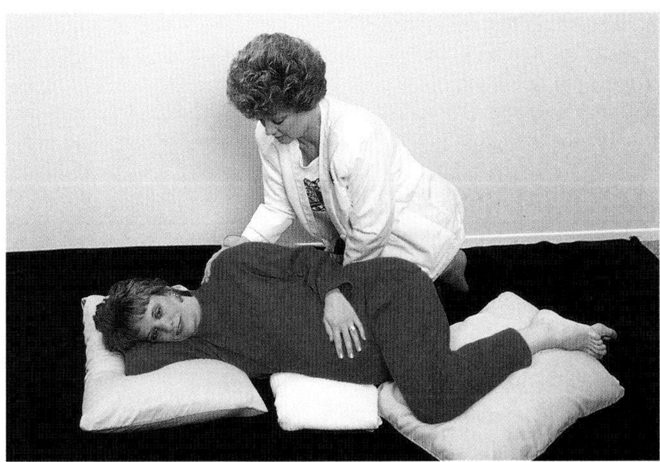

FIG 13.13 During the third trimester, pillows supporting the abdomen and back provide a comfortable position for rest.

***Maternal safety.*** Work leading to undue fatigue should be avoided. Frequent rest periods are essential. For jobs that require constant standing or sitting, suggest that the woman change positions frequently or walk briefly to stimulate circulation and reduce fatigue. Tasks that require balance may be hazardous because the uterus enlarges and the center of gravity shifts. Heavy lifting should be avoided.

Working women often have many home responsibilities that, for some, do not decrease during pregnancy. The fatigue and stress of the home and employment workload may be difficult during pregnancy. Recommend that the expectant mother adapt her home and employment workloads during pregnancy to reduce fatigue and stress if possible.

***Exposure to teratogens.*** Intrauterine exposure to toxic substances is of particular concern during the first trimester, the period of organogenesis. Advise women to investigate their own occupational hazards. For example, hairdressers are exposed to toxic substances in hair dyes and aerosol sprays and laundry, nail solon, and dry cleaning workers may be exposed to fetotoxic compounds. Nurses and hospital personnel may be exposed to infectious diseases, radiation, and anesthetic gases. Pesticides are another source of teratogen exposure. In addition, passive smoking is harmful to both mother and fetus.

**Travel.** Car travel is generally safe for uncomplicated pregnancies. Suggest the woman stop and walk for 10 minutes every 2 hours to decrease the chance of thrombosis which is more likely during pregnancy (Katz, 2008). Instruct the woman to fasten the seat belt snugly, with the lap belt under the abdomen and the shoulder belt in a diagonal position across her chest and above the bulge of the uterus. This position is uncomfortable for some women, and it causes concern about internal injuries should a collision occur. However, it is much safer to wear the belt than to leave it off and risk being ejected from the car during an accident.

Travel by plane is generally safe up to 36 weeks' gestation if there are no complications of the pregnancy (AAP & ACOG, 2012). Advise the woman to walk frequently to maintain adequate peripheral circulation. The woman should not travel to remote areas where medical care is unavailable. Suggest she take a copy of her medical records if traveling a long distance.

**Immunizations.** In general, immunizations with live virus vaccines (such as measles, mumps, rubella, varicella, and smallpox) are contraindicated during pregnancy because of possible teratogenic effects on the fetus. Inactivated vaccines such as those for tetanus, hepatitis B, and influenza are safe for women who have a risk for developing these diseases (Bruhn & Tillett, 2009). The CDC recommends that women who have not been previously vaccinated against pertussis receive the vaccine during the third or late second trimester (CDC, 2011). For current information, see the CDC website at http://www.cdc.gov/vaccines.

***Teaching necessary lifestyle changes.*** Many expectant parents are willing to make lifestyle changes to avoid adversely affecting the fetus.

**Prescription and over-the-counter drugs.** Advise the pregnant woman to consult with her healthcare provider before taking any drugs. This precaution is important for over-the-counter drugs as well as for prescription drugs. Some nonsteroidal antiinflammatory drugs such as aspirin should be avoided because they may increase bleeding. When prescription drugs are necessary, the healthcare provider must weigh the risks as opposed to the benefits to decide if a drug can safely be used or if changes are necessary. Drugs taken during the first trimester are of particular concern because of the risk to developing organs.

**Complementary and alternative therapies.** Some complementary and alternative therapies are very safe and helpful during pregnancy. However, some can be harmful. For example, herbs such as black or blue cohosh may cause contractions or harm the fetus if used in pregnancy (Skidmore-Roth, 2010). Ask about any complementary or alternative therapies used, and advise the woman to discuss them with her healthcare provider.

**Tobacco.** Approximately 16.4% of women in the United States smoke during pregnancy (Substance Abuse and Mental Health Services Administration, 2009). A *Healthy People 2020* objective is that the number of women who stop smoking during the first trimester and do not restart for the entire pregnancy increase to 30% from a baseline of 11.3% (U.S. Department of Health and Human Services, 2010).

Identify women who smoke, and explain the effects of smoking during pregnancy (see Chapter 14, p. 293). The Association of Women's Health, Obstetric and Neonatal Nurses (AWHONN) advocates that every nurse screen for tobacco use and refer women to smoking cessation programs as needed (2010). Make every effort to motivate the expectant mother to stop smoking and to avoid contact with others who smoke. Secondhand smoke exposure increases the risk of preterm birth, respiratory distress syndrome, neonatal intensive care unit (NICU) admission, and other complications (Ashford, Hahn, Hall, et al., 2010).

The "5 As" are tactics to encourage women to stop smoking. They include (1) *Asking* women about smoking and if they would like to quit, (2) *Advising* women about the importance of not smoking, (3) *Assessing* the woman's readiness to quit, (4) *Assisting* women in devising a plan, and (5) *Arranging* follow-up visits or phone calls for ongoing counseling (Barron, Petrilli, Strath, et al., 2014).

Although nonpharmacologic methods of smoking cessation such as counseling are best, nicotine replacement therapy (NRT) may be used if other methods are unsuccessful (Cunningham et al., 2010). Although NRT exposes women to nicotine, it may be safer than smoking, which exposes them to other harmful chemicals as well. More research is needed regarding the use of NRT (Forest, 2010). Women should consult their healthcare providers before using nicotine replacement products.

**Alcohol.** Alcohol is a known teratogen, and maternal alcohol use is a leading cause of intellectual disability in the United States. Alcohol may produce developmental anomalies known as *fetal alcohol spectrum disorders* (see Chapter 24, p. 508). Conclusive data about fetal effects of social or moderate drinking are not available, but no amount of alcohol during pregnancy is safe. Therefore, advise women who are pregnant or who plan to become pregnant to abstain from all alcohol use.

**Illegal drugs.** Use of so-called *street* or *recreational drugs,* such as cocaine, heroin, and methamphetamines, is harmful to the fetus. Assist the pregnant woman in obtaining help to discontinue all illicit drug use (see Chapter 24).

***Signs of possible complications.*** After the initial assessment, the woman is usually not seen by the healthcare provider for 4 weeks. Instruct her and her family about signs and symptoms of possible complications of pregnancy (see Safety Alert). She should be instructed to call her healthcare provider or go to the hospital immediately if she thinks she is experiencing complications.

**SAFETY ALERT**

***Signs of Possible Complications During Pregnancy***

| Sign of Possible Complication | Possible Causes |
|---|---|
| Vaginal bleeding with or without discomfort | Spontaneous abortion, placenta previa, abruptio placentae, lesions of the cervix or vagina, "bloody show" |
| Escape of fluid from the vagina | Rupture of membranes |
| Swelling of the fingers (rings become tight) or puffiness of the face or around the eyes | Excessive edema |
| Continuous pounding headache | Chronic hypertension or preeclampsia |
| Visual disturbances (such as blurred vision, dimness, flashing lights, spots before the eyes) | Worsening preeclampsia |
| Persistent or severe abdominal or epigastric pain | Ectopic pregnancy (if early), worsening preeclampsia, abruptio placentae |
| Convulsions | Eclampsia |
| Chills or fever | Infection |
| Painful urination | Urinary tract infection |
| Persistent vomiting | Hyperemesis gravidarum |
| Change in frequency or strength of fetal movements | Fetal compromise or death |
| Signs or symptoms of preterm labor: uterine contractions, cramps, constant or irregular low backache, pelvic pressure, watery vaginal discharge | Labor onset |

### Evaluation

- Do the woman and her family discuss plans to safeguard the mother and fetus?
- Can she discuss ways to obtain relief from the common discomforts of pregnancy?
- Can she explain how she will modify habits that do not promote health?

## PSYCHOLOGICAL RESPONSES TO PREGNANCY

Although each couple adapts to pregnancy in a unique manner, the psychological responses of prospective parents change as the pregnancy progresses. By the time the infant is born, the woman and her partner have completed certain developmental tasks, maturation steps that allow further development. These changes help them become parents in the true sense of the word. Both social and cultural factors influence their adjustment to pregnancy.

A woman's psychological response to pregnancy changes over time. Initially she may be uncertain or ambivalent about the pregnancy, and her primary focus is on herself. Her focus gradually shifts, and she becomes increasingly concerned about how she can protect and provide for the fetus.

## MATERNAL RESPONSES

### First Trimester

#### Uncertainty

During the early weeks, the woman is unsure if she is pregnant and tries to confirm it. She observes her body carefully for changes indicating pregnancy. She may use an over-the-counter pregnancy test kit for validation.

Reaction to the uncertainty of pregnancy depends on the individual. A woman may be eager to find confirming signs, or she may dread the possibility. Usually she seeks confirmation from a physician, nurse-midwife, or nurse practitioner during the first trimester of pregnancy.

#### Ambivalence

Because almost half of pregnancies are unintended, pregnancy is often unexpected. Once the pregnancy is confirmed, many women have conflicting feelings, or **ambivalence**, about being pregnant. Some feel that this is not the right time, even if the pregnancy is wanted. Women who had planned to become pregnant often say they thought it would take longer and that they feel unprepared for it. Many pregnancies are desired but unplanned, and these women may wish they had completed some goal before becoming pregnant.

Pregnancy results in permanent life changes for the woman, and she often begins to examine those changes and how she will cope with them. If it is a first pregnancy, the woman may worry about the added responsibility and feel unsure of her ability to be a good parent. A woman with other children may be apprehensive about how this pregnancy will affect her relationship with them or her partner.

#### The Self as Primary Focus

Throughout the first trimester, the woman's primary focus is on herself, not the fetus. Early physical responses to pregnancy, such as nausea or fatigue, confirm something is happening to her, but the fetus remains vague and unreal.

Physical changes and increased hormone levels may cause emotional lability (unstable moods). Her mood can change quickly from contentment to irritation or from optimistic planning to an overwhelming need for sleep. These changes may be confusing to her partner, who is accustomed to a more stable relationship.

Nurses should concentrate on the mother's physical and psychological needs during this period of maternal self-focus. Teaching should be aimed at the common early changes of pregnancy and their normality. Morning sickness and mood swings are important subjects to explore with the couple. The nurse should assess how they are managing these changes and explain that such changes are normal and generally do not indicate problems.

### Second Trimester

#### Physical Evidence of Pregnancy

During the second trimester, physical changes occur in the expectant mother that make the fetus "real." The uterus can be palpated in the abdomen, weight increases, and breast changes occur. Ultrasound examination allows her to see the fetus, and she may receive an ultrasound picture or video to share with her family. During this time she feels the fetus move *(quickening)*. This experience is important because it confirms the presence of the fetus with each movement. As a result, the mother no longer thinks of the fetus as simply a part of her body but now perceives it as separate, although entirely dependent on her (Fig. 13.14). This experience helps with early bonding, the development of strong emotional ties with the baby.

### The Fetus as Primary Focus

The woman's major focus during the second trimester becomes the fetus. Most pregnant women feel well because the discomforts of the first trimester have usually decreased. The woman is now concerned about producing a healthy infant. She often seeks information about diet and fetal development. She experiences a feeling of creative energy and satisfaction.

### Narcissism and Introversion

During this time many women become increasingly concerned about their ability to protect and provide for the fetus. This concern is often manifested as narcissism (undue preoccupation with oneself) and introversion (concentration on oneself and one's body). Selecting exactly the right foods to eat or the right clothes to wear may assume more importance than ever before. Some women may lose interest in their jobs because the work seems alien to the events taking place inside them. They may be less interested in current events as they focus on the pregnancy, or they may become fearful that world events threaten them and their fetus.

If she is a primigravida, the expectant mother wonders what the infant is like. She looks at baby pictures of herself and her partner and may want to hear stories about them as infants. Multiparas have concerns about how this child will be accepted by siblings and grandparents. Expectant mothers may also examine their relationships with others and how they will change after the birth.

### Body Image

Rapid and profound changes take place in the body during the second trimester. Changes in body size and contour are noticeable, with thickening of the waist, bulging of the abdomen, and enlargement of the breasts. The changes may be welcomed because they signify growth of the fetus and create pride in the woman and her partner. However, for some women, the change in body size and shape, coupled with hyperpigmentation of the skin and striae gravidarum, may contribute to a negative body image. Changes in body function, such as altered balance, less physical endurance, and discomfort in the pelvis and lower back areas also affect her body image (subjective image of herself).

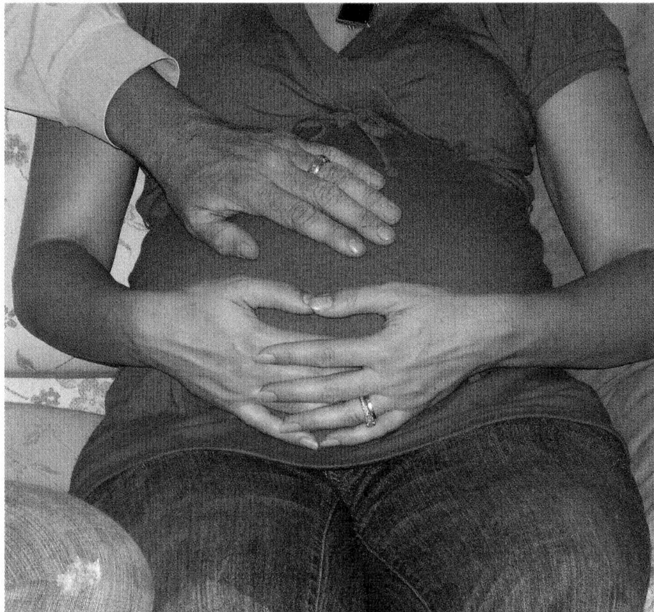

FIG 13.14 Fetal movement *(quickening)* confirms that a separate life is developing. (Courtesy Steve and Michelle Henry, Tustin, CA.)

### Changes in Sexuality

Sexual interest and activity of pregnant women and their partners are unpredictable: they may increase, decline, or remain unchanged. The culture of the couple is also important. Intercourse during pregnancy is allowed and encouraged in some cultures but strictly forbidden in others.

During the first trimester, freedom from worry about becoming pregnant or need for contraception may enhance sexuality for both partners. However, for some women, nausea, fatigue, and breast tenderness interfere with erotic feelings. Fear of miscarriage may cause couples to avoid intercourse, particularly if the woman has previously lost a pregnancy or has had infertility therapy. Nurses can help reassure the couple that there is no evidence that intercourse is related to pregnancy loss when no other complications are present.

In the second trimester, women experience increased sensitivity of the labia and clitoris and increased vaginal lubrication from pelvic vasocongestion. Nausea is generally no longer a problem by this time. A feeling of well-being and energy, coupled with not having to worry about getting pregnant, may increase sexual responsiveness. Orgasm may occur more frequently and with greater intensity during pregnancy because of these changes. Although orgasm causes temporary uterine contractions, they are not harmful if the pregnancy has been normal.

During the third trimester, the "missionary position" (male on top) may cause discomfort from abdominal pressure. Heartburn, indigestion, and supine hypotensive syndrome also may occur in this position. The nurse can suggest alternate positions such as side-to-side, female-superior, and vaginal entry from the back for intercourse. Fatigue, ligament pain, urinary frequency, and shortness of breath also may interfere with vaginal intercourse. Hugging, kissing, cuddling, and mutual massage or masturbation are expressions of affection that do not always lead to intercourse.

As they become larger, some women believe their bodies are ugly and worry about their partner's reaction to their increased size. Sexual response varies widely among men. Some men report heightened feelings of sexual interest, but other men perceive the woman's body in late pregnancy as unattractive. Moreover, fear of harming the fetus or causing discomfort may interfere with sexual activity.

The expectant couple should be made aware of the normal changes in sexual desire that occur during pregnancy and the importance of communicating their feelings openly with each other. Despite the need for information, many women are reluctant to ask questions about sexual activity. Health professionals often do not initiate such discussions because of discomfort with introducing the topic or concern about the patient's response.

Use of a broad opening statement to initiate discussion about sexual activity may be helpful. For example, "Sometimes couples are concerned about having sex during pregnancy." Such a statement provides a method of introducing the subject so that the woman feels comfortable to pursue it or let it drop.

Although not proven, some believe uterine contractions leading to labor may be initiated by nipple stimulation, orgasm, and semen. However, unless there are complications, intercourse is safe throughout pregnancy. Couples are advised to curtail sexual activity if the woman is at high risk for preterm labor. Intercourse should also be avoided if the woman has bleeding, placenta previa, ruptured membranes, or an

## NURSING CARE PLAN

### *Body Image During Pregnancy*

**Focused Assessment**

Ruth, a 34-year-old primigravida, is in the 26th week of pregnancy. Both she and her husband have been runners for several years. With her physician's permission, she continued running until 6 weeks ago when she began to find it uncomfortable. Ruth says she now walks "like other old ladies." She verbalizes concern about the brown discoloration on her face and her increasing size and says she feels "fat, awkward, and ugly." She states, "I hate the way I look. I can't wait to get back into shape."

**Nursing Diagnosis**

Disturbed Body Image related to changes in body size, contour, and function secondary to pregnancy.

**Planning**

***Expected Outcomes***

By the end of her next prenatal visit, Ruth will:

1. Make statements that indicate acceptance of expected body changes of pregnancy.
2. Express her feelings about body changes to her husband and the healthcare team.
3. Set realistic goals for weight loss and the resumption of a running program after childbirth.

**Interventions and *Rationales***

1. Acknowledge Ruth's feelings. "I can see you're disappointed at not being able to run, and concerned about how your body has changed as a result of pregnancy."
   *This will help her deal with the underlying causes.*
2. Clarify her concerns because she may fear changes of pregnancy will prevent her from participating in athletics. "You've always been an athlete.
   *Women often wonder if pregnancy will cause permanent body changes.*
3. Suggest that she share her feelings with her husband and seek his support.
   *She may assume that her partner understands when negative feelings exist, but this may not be true.*
4. Discuss types of low-impact, moderate exercise, such as walking or swimming, that would be beneficial for her.
   *Moderate daily exercise is encouraged during uncomplicated pregnancy.*
5. Describe the expected pattern of weight gain during the rest of the pregnancy and correlate this change with the growth and development of the fetus. Explain that adipose tissue provides a needed source of energy during birth and lactation.
   *Knowledge that weight gain shows normal pregnancy may allay unexpressed fears of excessive weight gain.*
6. Explain that the discoloration on her face (melasma) is normal and usually disappears after pregnancy. Suggest Ruth she limit exposure to the sun and use sunscreen to decrease the severity.
   *Knowledge of what is normal increases comfort with changes.*
7. Help Ruth make realistic plans to lose weight and regain strength after childbirth. *Many women are relieved to know that the added weight will be lost gradually.*
   a. Discuss the expected pattern of weight loss after birth.
   b. Demonstrate graduated exercises that increase muscle tone and strength.
   c. Discuss a diet that provides sufficient calories to meet her needs during breastfeeding.

**Evaluation**

At the next prenatal visit, Ruth speaks with pride about how big the baby is and makes other statements showing more acceptance of pregnancy body changes. She reports that she has discussed her feelings with her husband and that he is very supportive. She has explored other types of exercises and has found several she will use during the rest of her pregnancy. She also discusses realistic plans for diet and exercise after birth.

**Additional Nursing Diagnoses to Consider**

Risk for Situational Low Self-Esteem
Interrupted Family Processes

incompetent cervix. In addition, blowing into the vagina should be avoided because it may cause an air embolus (Coverston, 2011; Cunningham et al., 2010).

## Third Trimester

### Vulnerability

During the third trimester and particularly during the seventh month, pregnant women have increasing feelings of vulnerability (Coverston, 2011). They may worry that the precious baby may be lost or harmed if not protected at all times (Fig. 13.15). Many expectant mothers have fantasies or nightmares about harm coming to the infant and become very cautious as a result. They may avoid crowds because they feel unable to protect the infant from infectious diseases or physical dangers. They need reassurance that such dreams and fears are not unusual in pregnancy.

### Increasing Dependence

The expectant mother often becomes increasingly dependent on her partner in the last weeks of pregnancy. She may insist that the partner be readily available at all times and may call the partner's cell phone or place of work several times during the day. She may rely on her partner and others more at this time and seek their help in making decisions. Her need for love and attention from her partner is even more pronounced in late pregnancy. When she is assured of his concern and willingness to provide assistance, she feels more secure and able to cope.

Although the woman may not be able to explain the increasing dependence, she expects her partner to understand the feeling and may become angry if he is not sympathetic. Irritability may increase because of her fatigue at this time as well. The nurse can encourage couples to discuss fears and feelings openly so that misunderstandings can be avoided.

Some pregnant women have difficulty with tasks that require direct, sustained attention, particularly in the third trimester. Women may feel they have trouble concentrating or focusing on learning new material or skills at this time. Teaching should be clear and concise to help women learn most easily.

### Preparation for Birth

The feelings of vulnerability gradually decrease as the woman comes to terms with her situation. The fetus continues to grow, and fetal movements are no longer gentle. The woman's relationship with the

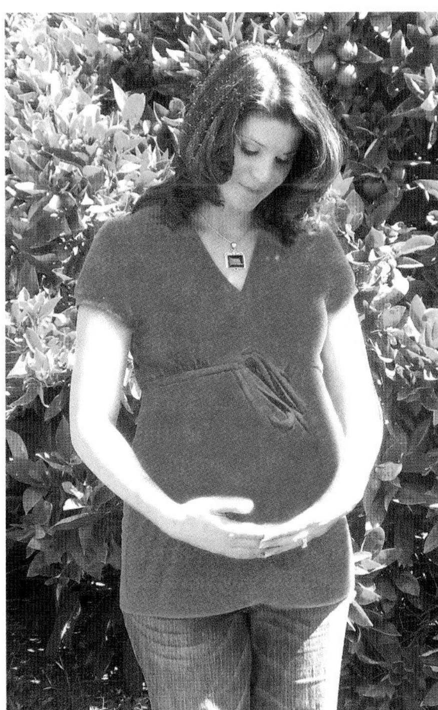

FIG 13.15 During the third trimester, the mother feels increasingly vulnerable. She cradles her fetus to signify her protectiveness. (Courtesy Steve and Michelle Henry, Tustin, CA.)

fetus changes as she acknowledges that although she and the fetus are interrelated, the baby is not a part of herself. Although she may not consciously acknowledge the increasing feelings of separateness, she longs to *see* the baby and to become acquainted with her child.

Most pregnant women are concerned with their ability to determine when they are in labor. They review the signs of labor and question friends and family members who have given birth. Many couples are concerned about how they will cope with labor and are worried that they will not get to the birth facility in time for the birth.

During the last few weeks, the woman becomes increasingly concerned with her due date and with the experience of labor and delivery. Some women fear labor and dread the due date, whereas others are so uncomfortable that they look forward to that day, anticipating it will be the exact day the birth will occur.

Women pregnant for the first time are more likely to fear childbirth than multiparas. Many women fear the pain of childbirth or that something will go wrong during labor. Multiparas who had a previous negative pregnancy or birth experience have increased concerns about the current pregnancy. Women may seek help for their fears by talking to members of their support system or by seeking information from health professionals, books, television, or the Internet. Women often watch TV shows that show pregnancy and childbirth to learn more about what their own experience might be like. However, information from websites or TV shows may not always be scientifically based.

During the third trimester, an expectant mother prepares for the infant, if that is appropriate in her culture. "Nesting" behavior includes obtaining clothing and arranging a place for the infant to sleep. Negotiation of how the couple will share household tasks also often occurs at this time. In addition, many couples complete childbirth education classes.

**TABLE 13.5 Progressive Changes in Maternal Responses to Pregnancy**

| First Trimester | Second Trimester | Third Trimester |
|---|---|---|
| **Emotional Response** | | |
| Uncertainty, ambivalence, focus on self | Wonder, increased narcissism, introversion, concern about changes in her body and sexuality | Vulnerability, increased dependence, acceptance that fetus is separate but totally dependent |
| **Physical Validation** | | |
| No obvious signs of fetal growth | Quickening, enlarging abdomen | Obvious fetal growth, discomfort, decreased maternal activity |
| **Role** | | |
| May begin to seek safe passage for self and fetus | Seeks acceptance of fetus and her role as mother | Prepares for birth |

Table 13.5 summarizes the progressive changes in maternal responses during pregnancy.

## MATERNAL ROLE TRANSITION

The transition into mothering begins during pregnancy and increases with gestational age. The woman must accept the pregnancy and the changes that will result. She develops a relationship with the unborn child, first as part of herself and then as a separate individual. Near the end of pregnancy she must prepare herself for the birth and for parenting the new baby (Ramer & Frank, 2001).

### Transitions Experienced Throughout Pregnancy

The woman undergoes transitions in relationships that continue throughout the pregnancy. She becomes more aware of herself and the changes occurring in her life. Her relationship with the father changes as they both prepare for parenthood. Her relationship with her own mother may change as the expectant mother develops a view of herself as a mother and what that role entails (Ramer & Frank, 2001).

### Steps in Adjusting to the Maternal Role

Rubin (1984), in her classic work, observed specific steps that provide a framework for understanding the process of maternal role taking: mimicry, role play, fantasy, the search for a role fit, and grief work.

#### Mimicry

**Mimicry** involves observing and copying the behaviors of other women who are pregnant or already mothers in an attempt to discover what the role is like. Mimicry often begins early, when the woman may wear maternity clothes before they are needed to see how women in more advanced pregnancy feel and to see how others react to her.

#### Role Play

Role play consists of acting out some aspects of what mothers actually do. The pregnant woman searches for opportunities to hold or care for infants in the presence of another person. Role playing gives her an opportunity to practice the expected role and to receive validation from an observer that she has functioned well. She is particularly sensitive to the responses of her partner and her own mother.

#### Fantasy

Fantasy allows the woman to explore a variety of possibilities and daydream or "try on" various behaviors. Fantasies often involve mental images of how the infant will look and what characteristics he or she will have. The woman may daydream about taking her child to the park or about holding the child and reading or playing music.

At times, fantasies are fearful. What if something is wrong with the infant? What if the baby cries and will not stop? Some women dream about a stranger entering their life. The stranger may represent the fetus (Driscoll, 2008). Fearful fantasies often provoke a pregnant woman to respond by seeking information or reassurance.

#### The Search for a Role Fit

Looking for a role fit occurs once the woman has built a set of role expectations for herself and has internalized a view of a "good" mother's behavior. She then observes various mothers and compares their behaviors with her own expectations of herself. She imagines herself acting in the same way and either rejects or accepts the behaviors, depending on how well they fit her sense of what is right. This process implies that the woman has explored the role of mother long enough to develop a sense of herself in the role and to be able to select behaviors that reaffirm her sense of herself fulfilling the role.

#### Grief Work

Grief work may seem incongruous with maternal role taking, but women often experience a sense of sadness when they realize that they must permanently give up certain aspects of their previous selves. A first-time mother will never again be a carefree woman without a child. She must relinquish some of her old patterns of behavior to take on the new identity of mother. Even simple things such as going shopping or to the movies will require planning to include the infant or find alternative care. Changes may be particularly difficult for the adolescent who is not used to planning ahead and who may have to give up or change school plans as well. A multipara will be unable to concentrate all her attention on other children.

### Maternal Tasks of Pregnancy

The psychological work of pregnancy has been grouped into four maternal tasks (Rubin, 1984):

1. Seeking safe passage for herself and the baby through pregnancy, labor, and childbirth
2. Securing acceptance of the baby and herself by her partner and family
3. Learning to give of herself
4. Developing attachment and interconnection with the unknown child

#### Seeking Safe Passage

Seeking safe passage for herself and her baby is the woman's priority task. If she cannot be assured of that safety, she cannot move on to the other tasks. Behaviors that ensure safe passage include seeking the care of a physician or nurse-midwife and following recommendations about diet, vitamins, rest, and subsequent visits for care. In addition to following the advice of healthcare professionals, the pregnant woman must adhere to cultural practices that ensure the safety of herself and the infant.

#### Securing Acceptance

Securing acceptance is a process that continues throughout pregnancy. It involves reworking relationships so that the important persons in the family accept the woman in the role of mother and welcome the baby into the family. In her first pregnancy, the woman and the father of the baby must give up their exclusive relationship and make a place in their lives for a child. When her partner expresses pride and joy in the pregnancy, the woman feels valued and comforted. This feeling is so important that many women retain a memory of the partner's reaction to the announcement of pregnancy for many years. Women with supportive partners are more likely to report the pregnancy is wanted.

Acceptance from her own mother is especially important. The pregnant woman gains energy and contentment when her mother freely offers acceptance and support. Many expectant mothers develop an increased closeness with their mothers during pregnancy.

Problems may occur if the family strongly desires a child with particular characteristics and the woman believes that the family may reject an infant who does not meet the criteria. For example, if family members wish for a boy, will they accept a girl?

#### Learning to Give of Herself

Giving is one of the most idealized components of motherhood but one that is essential. Learning to give to the coming infant begins in pregnancy when the woman allows her body to give space to the fetus. She tests her ability to derive pleasure from giving, often by providing food or care for her family. Their acceptance and enjoyment of the "gift" enhance her pleasure, and strengthen the role. She may also give small gifts to friends, especially those who are pregnant.

Pregnant women also learn to give by receiving. Gifts received at baby showers are more than needed items—they also confirm continued interest and commitment from friends and family and enhance the woman's ability to give. Intangible gifts from others, such as companionship, attention, and support, help increase her energy and affirm the importance of giving.

#### Committing Herself to the Unknown Child

Developing **attachment** (strong ties of affection) to the unborn baby begins in early pregnancy when the woman accepts the idea that she is pregnant, although the baby is not yet real to her. During the second trimester, the baby becomes real and feelings of love and attachment surge. This is especially true when quickening occurs or an ultrasound shows recognizable parts of the baby. Mothers report feedback from their unborn infants during the third trimester and describe unique characteristics of the fetus with regard to sleep-wake cycles, temperament, and communication. Love of the infant becomes possessive and leads to feelings of vulnerability. The woman integrates the role of mother into her image of herself. She becomes comfortable with the idea of herself as mother and finds pleasure in contemplating the new role (Mercer & Ferketich, 1994).

Some women delay attachment to the fetus until they feel sure the pregnancy is normal and will continue. This is especially true for women who have lost a pregnancy previously. They may begin to have feelings of attachment after they have passed a critical time that correlates to the time they lost a pregnancy before (Driscoll, 2008).

## PATERNAL ADAPTATION

Expectant fathers also must make major psychosocial changes to adapt to their new role. These changes may be more difficult because the male partner is often neglected by the healthcare team as well as by his peer group as attention is focused on the woman. His anxieties and concerns may remain unknown because of the lack of focus on him.

### Variations in Paternal Adaptation

Wide variations occur in paternal responses to pregnancy. Some men are emotionally invested and explore every aspect of pregnancy, childbirth, and parenting. Others are more task oriented and see themselves as managers. They may direct the woman's diet and act as coaches during childbirth but remain detached from the emotional aspects of the experience. Some men are more comfortable as observers and prefer not to participate. In some cultures, men are conditioned to view pregnancy and childbirth as "women's work," and may not express their true feelings about pregnancy and fatherhood.

Readiness for fatherhood is more likely if there is a stable relationship between the partners, financial security, and a desire for parenthood. Additional factors include the man's relationship with his own father, his previous experience with children, and his confidence in his ability to care for the infant.

Fathers have many concerns during a pregnancy. These include anxiety about the health of the mother and baby, financial concerns, and worry about his role during the birth and about the changes that will result from the birth of the baby. Financial concerns may be especially acute in a two-income family if the mother develops complications that prevent her from working as long as expected. A reduction in income coupled with an increase in expenses can result in added stress for both parents. Men may seek a second job or work overtime to prepare for the increased financial needs. Other concerns include the responsibility parenting will bring and whether he and his partner will be good parents.

## Developmental Processes

The developmental processes that an expectant father must work through include dealing with the reality of pregnancy and the new child, working to be recognized as a parent, and making an effort to be seen as relevant to childbearing (Jordan, 1990).

## Grappling With the Reality of Pregnancy and the Child

The pregnancy and the child must become real before a man can take on the identity of father. A man's initial reaction to the announcement of pregnancy may be pride and joy, but he often experiences the same ambivalence as his partner, particularly if he is unprepared for the added responsibility or commitment. Early pregnancy changes, such as the woman's nausea and fatigue, may be perceived by the father as symptoms of illness that have little to do with having a baby. Various experiences act as catalysts or "reality boosters" that make the child more real (Fig. 13.16). These include seeing the fetus on a sonogram, hearing the baby's heartbeat, and feeling the infant move.

Preparing room for the baby and accumulating supplies also reinforce the reality of the forthcoming child. These tasks often represent the first time that the expectant father has the opportunity to do something directly for the baby. The birth itself is the most powerful "reality booster," and the infant becomes real to the father when he has an opportunity to see and hold the infant.

### Struggling for Recognition as a Parent

Men are often perceived by others to be helpmates but not parents in their own right. Some men find it upsetting if their feelings are not validated because they want to be recognized as a parent as well as a helper. Support groups just for expectant fathers may be available. These groups allow a father-to-be to talk with other men about how changes resulting from the pregnancy have affected them. Knowing his experiences and feelings are shared by other men in the same situation is very helpful.

Expectant mothers play an important role in helping their partners gain recognition as parents. Women who openly share their physical sensations and emotions help expectant fathers feel that they are part of the process. These women often say "we" are pregnant and include their partners in all discussions and decisions.

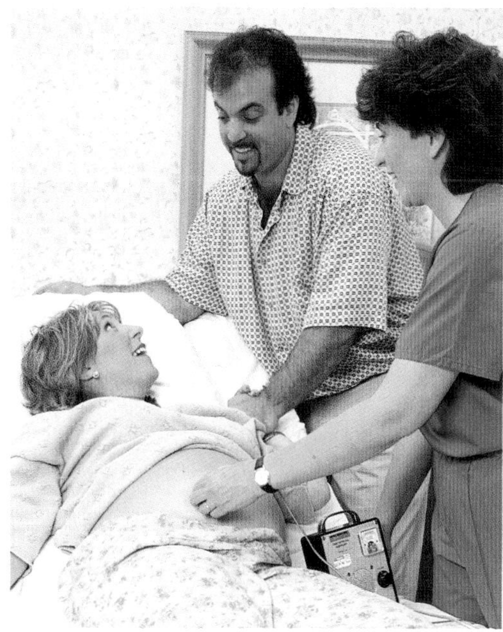

**FIG 13.16** Reality boosters such as hearing the sounds of the fetal heart make the fetus more real for the father.

Nurses must learn to view the mother, father, and infant as the patient and not focus exclusively on the mother and fetus. The nurse should encourage men to ask questions about the partner's pregnancy. These men are entitled to as much advice and reassurance as expectant women. The nurse can also guide the couple in discussing the role the father will play after the birth. Will he be involved in infant care from the start or wait until the baby is older? Will he change diapers and help with nighttime care, or does he see those tasks as belonging to the mother? The couple must consider each other's views and may need to negotiate to determine the roles each will play.

### Creating the Role of Involved Father

Men use various means to create a parenting role that is comfortable for them. They may seek closer ties with their fathers to reminisce about their own childhood. They also observe men who are already fathers and "try on" fathering behaviors to determine whether they are comfortable and fit their own concept of the father role. Some change their image of themselves and even change their appearance to fit their new image (Coverston, 2011).

***Parenting information.*** Many men assertively seek information about infant care and growth and development so that they will be prepared. Men who have sufficient information about pregnancy, birth, and newborn care are less likely to be psychologically stressed than those who feel they are lacking important information (Boyce, Condon, Barton, et al., 2007).

Although they may receive adequate information, some fathers may not gain enough parenting information to prepare them for care of their infants. This may be because the fathers are not ready to learn at the time information is provided. As a result, they may have unrealistic expectations of the newborn and may be unprepared to care for their infants. Nurses must review information about infant care and growth and development after the infant is born, when the information is immediately relevant.

***Couvade.*** The term couvade refers to pregnancy-related symptoms and behavior in expectant fathers. In primitive cultures, couvade took the form of rituals involving special dress, confinement, limitations of physical work, avoidance of certain foods, sexual restraint, and in some instances performance of "mock labor."

In modern practice, expectant fathers sometimes experience physical symptoms similar to those experienced by pregnant women: loss of appetite, nausea and vomiting, headache, fatigue, and weight gain. Symptoms are more likely to occur in early pregnancy and diminish as the pregnancy progresses. They may be caused by stress, anxiety, or empathy for the pregnant partner. They are usually harmless but may persist and result in nervousness, insomnia, restlessness, and irritability. Although the symptoms are rarely observed by the healthcare team, anticipatory guidance is beneficial for both partners.

## ADAPTATION OF GRANDPARENTS

The initial reaction of grandparents depends on a number of different factors.

### Age

Age is a major factor in determining the emotional responses of prospective grandparents. Older grandparents have usually dealt with their feelings about aging and react with joy when they find that they are to become grandparents. Younger grandparents may feel conflict and must resolve their self-image with the stereotype of grandparents as old people. They often have career responsibilities and may not be accessible because of the continuing demands of their own lives.

### Number and Spacing of Other Grandchildren

The number and spacing of other grandchildren also determine grandparents' reactions. A first grandchild may be an exciting event that creates great joy. However, if the grandparents have other grandchildren, the birth of another may be welcomed but with less excitement. The subdued reaction may be disappointing to the couple.

### Perceptions of the Role of Grandparents

Many grandparents see their relationships with grandchildren as second in importance only to the parent-child relationship. They want to be involved in the pregnancy and look forward to being intimately involved in child care. They offer to care for older children while the mother gives birth, and they assist during the first weeks after childbirth.

In the past, grandparents were often looked to for advice about childbearing and child rearing. Healthcare personnel have now become the "experts," and many grandparents have difficulty adjusting to this change. Special classes are often available for grandparents to bring them up to date with current childbearing practices.

Some contemporary grandparents hold different beliefs about the role of grandparents and plan much less participation in pregnancy or child care. This expectation often results in conflict with the parents, who may feel hurt by such an attitude. Parents and grandparents may need to negotiate how the grandparents can be involved without feeling that they must assume more care of the child than they desire.

## ADAPTATION OF SIBLINGS

Sibling adaptation to the birth of an infant depends largely on the child's age and developmental level.

### Toddlers

Children 2 years or younger are unaware of the maternal changes that occur during pregnancy and are unable to understand that a new brother or sister is going to be born. Because toddlers have little perception of time, many parents delay telling them that a baby is expected until shortly before the birth.

The nurse can make suggestions about helping prepare young children for the birth and what to expect from toddlers when the new baby comes home. Changes in sleeping arrangements should be made several weeks before the birth so the child does not feel displaced by the new baby. Parents need to realize that toddlers may have feelings of jealousy and resentment when they must share attention with a baby. Frequent reassurances of parental love and affection are of primary importance.

### Older Children

Children from 3 to 12 years are more aware of changes in the mother's body and may realize a baby is to be born. They may enjoy listening to the heartbeat or feeling the fetus move. Questions about how the fetus develops, how it started, and how it will get out of the abdomen are common. Younger children may expect that the infant will be a full-fledged playmate; however, they are shocked and disappointed when the infant is small and helpless. They also need preparation for the fact that the mother will go away for several days when the baby is born.

School-age children benefit from being included in preparations for the new baby. They are interested in preparing space and supplies for the infant. They should be encouraged to feel the fetus move, and many come close to the mother's abdomen and talk to the fetus. School-age children may wonder how the birth will affect their role in the family. Parents should address these concerns and reassure the children about their continued importance. Providing books about children's experiences after the birth of a sibling may be helpful.

Children as young as 3 years benefit from sibling classes. The classes provide an opportunity for them to discuss what newborns are like and what changes the new baby will bring to the family.

In some settings, siblings are permitted to be with the mother during childbirth. When they are to be present, children should attend a class that prepares them for the event. A familiar person who has no other role than to support and care for a younger child should be present at the birth to explain what is happening and to comfort or remove the child if events become overwhelming.

### Adolescents

The response of adolescents also depends on their developmental level. Some are embarrassed because the pregnancy confirms the continued sexuality of their parents. Others may be indifferent to the pregnancy unless it directly affects them or their activities. Some adolescents become very involved and want to help with preparations for the baby.

## FACTORS THAT INFLUENCE PSYCHOSOCIAL ADAPTATIONS

### Age

Pregnancy presents a challenge for teenagers, who must cope with the conflicting developmental tasks of pregnancy and adolescence at the same time. The pregnant woman older than age 35 may also have some concerns. Pregnancy may mean a major change in her life. She may have medical conditions that affect the pregnancy, as well. Concerns relating to the pregnant adolescent as well as the older woman are discussed further in Chapter 24.

### Multiparity

Pregnancy tasks are often much more complex for the multipara than for the primigravida. The multipara does not have time to take special care of herself as she did during the first pregnancy. She is likely to experience more fatigue and may have serious concerns about her other children. Mothers worry about finding time and energy for

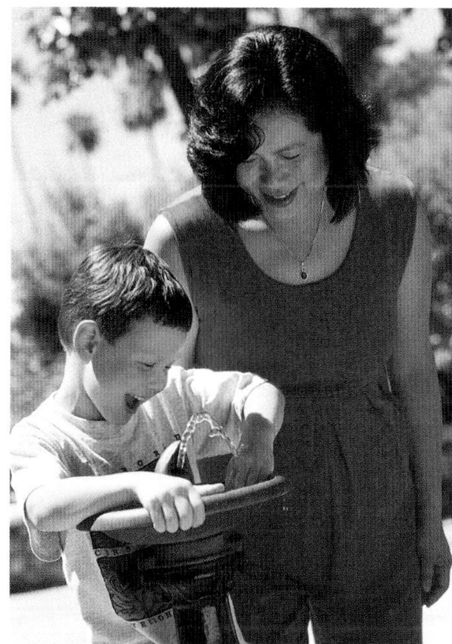
FIG 13.17 A pregnant woman spends time with her child to provide affection and a sense of security.

additional responsibilities. When seeking acceptance of the new baby, the multipara may find family members less excited than they were for the first child.

The woman spends a great deal of time working out a new relationship with the first child, who often becomes demanding. This behavior may foster feelings of guilt as she tries to expand her love to include the second child. Developing attachment for the coming baby is hampered by feelings of loss between herself and the first child. She senses that the child is growing up and away from her, and she may grieve for the loss of their special relationship (Fig. 13.17).

Nurses cannot assume that multiparas do not need information about labor, breastfeeding, and infant care. They also need special assistance in integrating an additional infant into the family structure.

### CRITICAL THINKING EXERCISE 13.2

Emma, a 24-year-old gravida 2, para 1 at 32 weeks of gestation appears apathetic and tired when she arrives at the prenatal clinic. She states that she is worried about how her 2-year-old son will accept the new baby and sometimes feels guilty that she is having this baby so soon.

1. How does multiparity affect the maternal tasks of pregnancy for Emma?
2. How should the nurse respond to her concerns?
3. Suggest measures Emma can take to prepare her son both before and after the new baby arrives.

### Social Support

Social support comes from the woman's partner, family, friends, and co-workers. Generally, support from the woman's partner and her mother is particularly important. Women who have social support as well as those enrolled in Medicaid or the Special Supplemental Nutrition Program for Women, Infants, and Children (WIC) are more likely to receive prenatal care (Potter, Pereya, Lamp, et al., 2009; Sunil, Spears, Hook, et al., 2010).

Depression may occur in women who have little support during pregnancy, and they are more likely to begin prenatal care late. The nurse should assess for signs of depression in all women and refer them for help when necessary. (See Chapter 28 for a discussion of postpartum depression that may have started during pregnancy.) When social support is inadequate, the nurse can help the woman explore potential sources such as support groups, childbearing education classes, church, work, or school.

### Absence of a Partner

Pregnant single women may have special concerns. Although some unmarried women have the emotional and financial support of a partner, others do not. They may experience more stress about how to tell their family and friends about the pregnancy. Enlisting social support to substitute for that of a partner may be important. They may also have legal concerns regarding the father's rights.

Many single women without partners live below the poverty level. They are more likely to delay prenatal care until the second or third trimester and are at increased risk for pregnancy complications and delivery of a low-birth-weight infant. Nurses must be prepared to offer special supportive care for single mothers. Needed social services may include Medicaid, WIC for food vouchers, and transportation to prenatal appointments.

Some women are single by choice. They may have been inseminated to achieve pregnancy or choose not to continue the relationship with the father. If the pregnancy was planned, these women may have fewer financial concerns.

### Socioeconomic Status

One of the greatest influences on childbearing practices is the socioeconomic status of the family (Table 13.6). Socioeconomic status refers to the resources available for the family to meet the needs for food, shelter, and healthcare. Socioeconomic status can be divided into affluent, middle class, working poor, and new poor.

### Abnormal Situations

Other factors influencing psychosocial adaptation during pregnancy include abnormal situations such as intimate partner violence and substance abuse (see Chapter 24). The nurse should assess all women for these risk factors during pregnancy so that appropriate referrals for help can be given.

## BARRIERS TO PRENATAL CARE

Women's access to prenatal care is limited by financial, systemic, and attitudinal barriers. Financial barriers are one of the most important factors that limit prenatal care. Many women have no insurance or not enough insurance to cover maternity care. Although Medicaid finances prenatal care for indigent women, the enrollment process is burdensome and lengthy. Some women may not know how to access this resource or do not qualify.

Systemic barriers include institutional practices that interfere with consistent care. For example, women must often wait weeks before being seen for their first visit. In one study, a researcher called 239 obstetric offices in one state and asked when a newly pregnant woman with insurance could be seen for her first prenatal visit. First visits were available at between 4 weeks of gestation and 10.6 weeks' gestation. The average appointment offered was at 6.37 weeks, and 25% of the appointments were for more than 8 weeks' gestation (Nettleman, Brewer, & Stafford, 2010).

Prenatal visits are usually scheduled during daytime hours, when some working women cannot attend. Taking time off from work often

**TABLE 13.6 Impact of Socioeconomic Factors on Family's Response to Pregnancy**

| Affluent | Middle Class | Working Poor and Unemployed | New Poor |
|---|---|---|---|
| **Resources** | | | |
| Is confident of ability, has financial reserves to protect from economic fluctuations, owns or rents home in a safe neighborhood, has health insurance or can pay for healthcare, able to provide enriched environment | Has relative security, but fewer reserves and more debt, owns or rents home in relatively safe neighborhood, depends on employment for health insurance | Lacks skills and bargaining power, is most vulnerable to economic fluctuations, struggles to meet basic needs | Was previously self-sufficient, but has lost previous resources; may have recently lost job and insurance; unfamiliar with public assistance |
| **Value Placed on Healthcare** | | | |
| Values preventive care | Values healthcare but must rely on health insurance related to employment | May value healthcare but often does not see a way to improve situation | Values healthcare but may no longer have finances to access it |
| **Time Orientation** | | | |
| Is future oriented and seeks prenatal care early, expects best possible care and education for children | Is future oriented and seeks early prenatal care, makes plans to provide best possible care and education for children | Priority is to meet needs of present, often seeks prenatal care late, uncertain future | Has middle-class time orientation but must meet present needs, may begin prenatal care late |

means loss of wages. Child care is rarely available at sites of care, and some women are unable to find it or it is too costly. Lack of transportation may also prevent women from getting prenatal care. In addition, interpreters may not be available for women who do not speak English.

An important barrier to healthcare results from the unsympathetic attitude of some healthcare workers toward those who are unable to pay for prenatal care. Women may experience long delays, hurried examinations, rudeness, and arrogance from some members of the healthcare team. Staff may be overworked and frustrated with the workloads they carry. Women may wait hours for an examination that lasts only a few minutes. Many never see the same healthcare provider more than once. These women may not keep clinic appointments because they do not see the importance of the hurried examinations.

Nurses must treat each family with respect and consideration and must insist that poor families who are unable to pay receive the same standard of care and respect as that received by families who can pay. Scheduling prenatal visits in the evening or on weekends, setting aside times for walk-in prenatal visits, and offering other services such as Medicaid and WIC applications might increase use of prenatal services.

Some women do not obtain early prenatal care because they do not realize they are pregnant, do not have the pregnancy confirmed, do not want anyone to know about the pregnancy, or are considering an abortion. Many women believe prenatal care is unimportant if they are healthy and having no problems.

## CULTURAL INFLUENCES ON CHILDBEARING

Many distinct cultural groups live in the United States. Each culture has its own health and healing belief system for major life events such as pregnancy and childbirth. The success of healthcare depends on how well it fits with the beliefs of those being served. Therefore, ignorance of culturally divergent beliefs may lead to failure of healthcare delivery.

### Differences Within Cultures

Wide variations of beliefs and practices exist within each culture, and nurses must recognize that people who share a culture may not have identical beliefs. Those who have lived in Western societies for years or even for generations often do not exhibit behaviors prescribed by their culture of origin. Nurses must be careful not to stereotype families or expect a certain set of behaviors from every person in a particular cultural group. Individual differences are as important as cultural variations.

A woman who does not normally follow certain beliefs of her culture may adhere to them during pregnancy. She may do this to show respect for family members to whom these beliefs are especially important during pregnancy, or she may fear that some part of the belief may be true after all and that she will harm her baby if she does not follow it.

### Cultural Differences That May Cause Conflict

Cultural differences that cause conflict between healthcare workers and families during pregnancy are observed most often in the areas of healthcare beliefs, communication, and time orientation. When health professionals violate cultural norms, patients are less likely to follow their advice.

#### Health Beliefs

***Health maintenance during pregnancy.*** The predominant U.S. culture treats pregnancy like an illness, with frequent visits to a physician, many laboratory tests, and hospitalization for delivery with various medical interventions. However, many other cultures see pregnancy as a natural condition that does not require medical care. Initial visits to a healthcare provider often occur later in pregnancy for them than U.S. culture dictates.

Different cultures have various requirements for maintaining health during pregnancy. Mexican women keep active to ensure a small baby and easy delivery. They may continue sexual intercourse to lubricate the birth canal (Dumonteil & Leon, 2008). Women from India avoid the sun and heat during pregnancy (Chatterjee, 2008). Prenatal care may not begin for Indonesian women until the second trimester, when the soul is believed to enter the fetus (Albright, 2008).

Puerto Rican women are often indulged by their families during pregnancy, and exercise is considered inappropriate at this time

## EVIDENCE-BASED PRACTICE

Prenatal care is recognized as important for helping to prevent complications in the mother and newborn. Yet some women have not had prenatal care at the time of delivery. Friedman, Heneghan, and Rosenthal studied a group of 211 such women to determine their characteristics and reasons for their lack of care. The reasons fell into six groups:

1. Substance Use Disorders

Thirty percent of the women had substance use problems. All were multiparas and most were older than age 30, unemployed, and had not completed high school. Some element of denial was seen in 28% of these women. Fear of losing custody or the child and legal prosecution were major issues.

2. Pregnancy Denial

This group of women (29%) had no substance use disorders but experienced denial of the pregnancy. They were either completely unaware they were pregnant or were aware but made no preparation and behaved as though they were not pregnant. Women who were younger than age 18 years and those who were students composed 25% of the group. Most had completed high school and many were employed. Pregnancy had occurred previously for 75% of the group.

3. Financial Problems

Eighteen percent of the women did not seek prenatal care because they had no insurance, had difficulty finding childcare, and did not want to take time off from work. Most were older than age 18 years, had not completed high school, and had previous pregnancies. The majority were unemployed.

4. Concealment of Pregnancy

Women who concealed the pregnancy (9%) were hiding it from parents, other family members, or friends. Another reason for concealment was fear of disapproval of their plan to place the infant for adoption. Most of the women were students and younger than age 29 years, with 40% less than 18 years.

5. Multiparity

This group of women (6%) did not seek prenatal care because they did not think it was necessary for this pregnancy. Although their general characteristics were similar to the group with financial problems, this group often had significant additional life stress.

6. Other/Unknown Reasons

Eight percent of the women had reasons that did not fit the categories, or the reasons were unknown.

Each of the women in the study was counseled regarding the importance of prenatal care for a future pregnancy and was referred to social services for help. The authors emphasized the need for identifying women who have not sought prenatal care and helping overcome difficulties that may be the cause.

Have you seen women who have not had prenatal care in your clinical practice?

What were reasons for their lack of prenatal care?

How would you counsel the women in each group?

### Barriers to Prenatal care for Teens

Early and continuous access to prenatal care and childbirth education are key factors in ensuring healthy outcomes for both mother and infant. Adolescents who are pregnant can be vulnerable to barriers to early prenatal care due to developmental needs, financial dependency, and unfinished formal education. Children born to teen mothers have higher rates of poverty, health problems and abuse and neglect.

Vanderbilt School of nursing targeted two high-volume, full-scope nurse midwifery group practices serving underserved areas and areas with a shortage of health professionals. The demographics of the OB patients included 94% low income, 14.5% teens, 42.4% Hispanic, 22.5% Black, 27.2% white, 2% Asian, 1% multiracial, 0.6% Native American/Alaskan, 4.5% unreported.

Healthy People 2010 goal was that 90% of all pregnant women should begin prenatal care in the first trimester. In Nashville, there were 1377 teen births in 2008; only 54% of teens 15-19 received prenatal care in the first trimester.

Vanderbilt's School of Nursing partnered with the Tennessee State Governor's Office of Children's Care Coordination, the two regional Medicaid Managed Care organizations and the local community health center of offer relationship care delivery model. This model addressed removal of transportation barriers, convenient scheduling, small incentives to keep appointments and make healthy lifestyle changes, and adherence to prescribed medication regimes. The results of this program after 18 months of operation demonstrated increased satisfaction and adherence to the program as reported by the participants.

Communicating the critical value of childbirth preparation in achieving healthy birth outcomes for baby and mother are some of the continued challenges of this innovative relationship based care model.

Reference: Friedman, S.H., Heneghan, A., & Rosenthal, M. (2009). Characteristics of women who do not seek prenatal care and implications for prevention. *Journal of Obstetric, Gynecologic, and Neonatal Nursing*, 38(2), 174–181.

Removing the Barriers to Prenatal Care and Education for Teens—Rock-a-Bye Teens: An Early SSTART Program. Pilon, Bonita; *International Journal of Childbirth Education,* Nov 2011; 26(4): 23–27.

(Torres, 2008). Korean women may practice Qi exercise that consists of physical postures, breathing techniques, and meditation. One study found women who practiced Qi exercise had less depression and physical discomfort and higher levels of interaction with the fetus (Ji & Han, 2010).

Some American Indian women may not tie knots or make braids during pregnancy to prevent complications involving the umbilical cord. Some Japanese women believe if they are happy during pregnancy, it will cause good fortune for the fetus, who is learning from the mother. Cambodian women may avoid standing in doorways to prevent the baby from becoming stuck in the birth canal. Eastern European women may avoid cutting or coloring their hair during pregnancy (Callister, 2014).

Avoidance of unclean objects and strong emotions like anger is believed necessary by some groups to prevent harm to the fetus or a difficult childbirth. Concentration, silence, prayer, and meditation to maintain mental and spiritual health are practiced by some. In many cultures, women must avoid contact with illness and death and may not attend funerals during pregnancy.

***Belief in fate.*** Some cultures (Southeast Asian, Middle Eastern) promote a strong belief in fate. Women often believe that the only way they can affect the outcome of pregnancy is by eating correctly and observing the taboos of their culture. Because of this belief, it may be difficult to convince women to seek early and regular prenatal care.

Advance preparation for the baby is also avoided in some cultures. Arabic Muslim women believe that preparing for the baby defies the will of Allah. Navajo families do not choose a name for the baby until after birth because they fear it will harm the infant (Callister, 2014). Some Jewish families select items needed for the new baby, but do not bring them home until after the birth (Kater, 2008). Russian women avoid being too optimistic about the pregnancy because it might bring bad luck. They also do not buy clothes or equipment until the baby is born well and healthy (Callister, 2014).

***Preventing illness.*** Practices that prevent illness include the use of protective religious objects or charms, such as amulets and talismans. Some women also believe that certain foods can prevent illness or provide a good pregnancy outcome. For example, those from many cultures eat raw garlic or onion or adhere to food taboos and prescribed combinations of foods. Strict adherence to religious codes, morals, and practices is also believed to prevent illness.

To be certain that all essential information about folk medicine is obtained, the nurse should inquire whether the patient is using folk remedies. "What do pregnant women take to protect themselves and the baby?" "Tell me about special foods and drinks that are important." "Are there any foods or drinks that you should not have when pregnant?"

***Restoring health.*** Traditional ways to restore health include natural folk medicine such as herbs and plants. Women may use charms, holy words, prescribed acts, and traditional healers before seeking other medical advice. Hispanics may consult *curanderas* for illness or a *partera* for care during pregnancy (Mann, Mannan, Quinones, et al., 2010).

***Modesty.*** Fear, modesty, and a desire to avoid examination by men may keep some women from seeking healthcare during pregnancy. In many cultures (Muslim, Hindu, Hispanic), exposure of the genitals to men is considered demeaning. The reputations of women from these cultures depend on their demonstrated modesty. If possible, female healthcare providers should perform examinations. If this is not possible, the woman should be carefully draped, with all areas of the body completely covered except for those being examined. A female nurse needs to remain with the woman at all times. It may be necessary to obtain permission from the husband before any examination or treatment can be performed.

***Female genital cutting.*** Female genital cutting (FGC) is also called *female circumcision* or *female genital mutilation*. The procedure is practiced in parts of Africa, Asia, and the Middle East and is usually performed at some time during childhood. Both Christian and Muslim women may have the procedure. Performing FGC is illegal in the United States for women younger than age 18 years (Hess, Weinland, & Saalinger, 2010).

FGC involves removal of part or all of the clitoris, labia minora, and labia majora (called infibulation). Urinary retention, incontinence, infection, and increased morbidity and mortality during childbirth may result from female genital cutting (AWHONN, 2008). The practice has been associated with premarital chastity and is a prerequisite for marriage in some cultures.

Women who have had the procedure and now live in North America need care from nurses and physicians who are knowledgeable about the custom and prepared for the abnormal appearance of the women's genitals. The nurse's own opinion of the practice should not cause the woman to be treated in a negative manner.

Nurses can assist the woman in locating a healthcare provider with whom she is comfortable, usually a woman. Pelvic examination is very painful because the introitus is so small and inelastic scar tissue makes the area especially sensitive. The examinations should be made as comfortable as possible by maintaining utmost privacy and draping the woman to provide maximum coverage. A pediatric speculum may be necessary because of the small vaginal opening. The woman may not give any verbal or nonverbal sign of pain, but this lack of response does not indicate an absence of pain.

### Communication Techniques

***Language.*** Language is a major barrier to healthcare. Trained female interpreters are ideal. Sometimes others may be used, but considerations of confidentiality, use of medical jargon, and the possible need to discuss sensitive issues indicate the need for professional interpreters. Interpreters are often available from a telephone service in the hospital.

Adults who came to the United States as children may speak English well and can interpret for their parents and grandparents. Other family members or friends, as well as clinic or hospital staff, may be helpful but not fluent. They may misunderstand instructions, particularly if medical jargon is used. Women may not want to discuss sensitive issues if the interpreter is a family member; is not appropriate to use children to discuss topics that might embarrass the parent or child.

***Communication style.*** Styles in communication differ between cultures. For example, among Asians, nodding and smiling may not mean agreement or even understanding but simply "Yes, I hear you." When presenting information, the nurse should validate the person's understanding by asking the listener to repeat the information: "Tell me what you understood" or "Show me what you learned."

Knowing the "rules" of communication helps the nurse avoid making errors. Hispanics are traditionally diplomatic and tactful. They frequently engage in small talk before bringing up questions about their care. Nurses can use small talk to establish rapport and help accomplish the goals of care. American Indians often converse in a low tone that may be difficult to hear in a noisy setting. They may consider note-taking taboo and expect the caregiver to remember what is said (Spector, 2009).

***Decision making.*** It is important to determine who makes decisions for the family. In some cultures, it is the husband or another family member. In those situations that person should be present when information is given or when the woman is asked to make decisions such as whether to have prenatal testing (Moore, Moos, & Callister, 2010).

***Eye contact.*** Many Americans and African-Americans consider eye contact important to communication. However, in some cultures respect is shown by avoiding eye contact (Spector, 2009). Eye contact between unmarried men and women may be considered seductive by those from Middle Eastern cultures.

***Touch.*** Touch is also an important component of communication. In some cultures (Hindu, Muslim), touch by a woman other than the wife is offensive to men. Hispanics are from a "high touch" culture and are more likely to appreciate touch, which may be viewed as a sign of sincerity. However, touch may not be appropriate with women if the nurse is male (Mann, Mannan, Quinones, et al., 2010). Nurses must remain sensitive to the response of the person being touched and should refrain from touching if the person indicates that touch is not welcomed.

### Time Orientation

Time orientation varies between cultures. Some American Indians, Middle Easterners, Hispanics, and American Eskimos tend to emphasize the moment rather than the future. This attitude causes conflicts in a healthcare setting in which appointments or tests are scheduled at particular times. If a woman does not place the same importance on keeping appointments, she may encounter anger and frustration in the healthcare setting that leaves her bewildered and ashamed.

## Culturally Competent Nursing Care

Culturally competent nursing care requires an awareness of, sensitivity to, and respect for the diversity of the patients served. It involves assessment of the family's culture and cultural negotiation when necessary.

### Cultural Assessment

Although nurses should be aware of the important aspects of the predominant cultures seen in their practice, they cannot know all the specific aspects of every culture. Some questions to help the nurse understand the family's beliefs about appropriate care during pregnancy include:

- How will you and your family prepare for the baby?
- What concerns do you have about the pregnancy?
- What would provide the greatest assistance?
- Where do you obtain most healthcare information?
- What foods are encouraged? Discouraged?

- Who will be with you during labor and birth?
- Who will help you at home?

### Cultural Negotiation

Cultural negotiation involves providing information while acknowledging that the family may hold different views. If the family indicates that the information would be helpful, it can be incorporated into the teaching plan.

If family members indicate that the information is not helpful or is harmful in their opinion, the conflict must be acknowledged openly and clarified. "I sense that you are unsure about this. Tell me your concerns about it." After allowing the family to express their beliefs, the nurse gives clear rationales for why the recommendation was made and works with the family to find a compromise satisfactory to all.

Cultural negotiation also involves being sensitive to specific concerns. For example, when caring for childbearing Muslim women, nurses must be aware of Islamic laws that require the woman to keep hair and body covered in the presence of men. In addition, a Muslim woman may be prohibited from being alone in the presence of a man other than a close relative. Female providers should be available to care for these women.

When talking to the woman's significant others, the nurse must call them by the right name. For example, a Vietnamese or Korean woman usually keeps her maiden name when she marries (Quach, Nguyen, & Nguyen, 2008; Yi, 2008a, 2008b). Therefore, the husband and wife will have different last names.

## NURSING CARE

### Psychosocial Concerns

#### Assessment

The purpose of a psychosocial assessment is to monitor the adaptation of the family to pregnancy, which some consider a maturational crisis that requires a major transition in role function and relationships. Some data such as age, gravida, para, and general health status, are obtained from the physical assessment. Table 13.7 identifies areas for psychosocial assessment, provides sample questions, and indicates nursing implications.

#### Nursing Diagnosis and Planning

Most families strive to maintain the health of the expectant mother and fetus and to complete developmental tasks needed for parenting. Perhaps the most encompassing nursing diagnosis is:

- Readiness for Enhanced Family Coping related to the desire to meet added family needs and assume parenting roles.

*Expected outcomes.* The expectant parents will verbalize emotional responses appropriate to each trimester and will describe methods that help them complete the developmental processes of pregnancy. The family will identify cultural factors that may produce conflicts and collaborate to reduce those conflicts.

#### Interventions

*Providing information.* Provide the expectant parents with information and anticipatory guidance about the emotional changes that

## NURSING CARE PLAN

### *Language Barrier During Pregnancy*

**Focused Assessment**

Diep, a young Vietnamese primigravida at 16 weeks of gestation speaks very little English. She listens quietly to the nurse's healthcare instructions, and although she appears confused, she asks no questions. Her husband speaks more English than Diep but has difficulty responding to questions about his wife's health. He frequently nods and smiles.

**Nursing Diagnosis**

Impaired Verbal Communication related to language barriers.

**Planning**

***Expected Outcomes***

Throughout the pregnancy, the family will demonstrate adequate understanding of instructions by:

1. Keeping scheduled appointments.
2. Following healthcare instructions.
3. Verbalizing basic needs and concerns at each prenatal visit.

**Interventions and *Rationales***

1. Assess the couple's ability to speak, read, and write in English and determine the languages in which each is fluent.
   *They may be able to read English better than they can speak it.*
2. Obtain the assistance of a fluent interpreter. Use the same interpreter whenever possible to enhance communication. Family or friends may be used if no professional interpreter is available but be aware of confidentiality issues and obtain the woman's permission first.
   *Asians do not always reveal they do not understand instructions.*
3. Use a translator to develop written materials in Vietnamese with common questions and answers printed in Vietnamese and English.
   *These help elicit basic information, reinforce information given verbally, and may answer unasked questions.*
4. Talk to Diep and her husband rather than to the interpreter *to show respect and concern.* Use a soft voice.
   *This will protect their privacy.*
5. Consider nonverbal factors when communicating.
   a. Speak slowly, and smile when appropriate.
   b. Keep an open posture. Avoid crossing the arms over the chest or turning away from the family.
   c. Attend carefully to what the family says. Nod, lean forward, or encourage continued talk with frequent "uh-huhs."
   d. Avoid fidgeting or watching a clock.
   e. Determine Diep's response to light touch on the arm, and use or avoid touch depending on her response.
   f. Do not expect prolonged eye contact.
   *This will show interest and respect for their culture.*
6. Locate prenatal classes in Vietnamese. Explain what is included in such classes, and encourage the couple to attend.
   *They will learn more easily in their own language and their cultural concerns will be addressed.*

**Evaluation**

Diep keeps all prenatal appointments, bringing an English-speaking family member with her to translate. She follows recommendations and asks appropriate questions at each visit.

***Additional Nursing Diagnoses to Consider***

Deficient Knowledge
Risk for Ineffective Health Maintenance

**TABLE 13.7 Psychosocial Assessment**

| Normal and Findings of Concern* | Sample Questions | Nursing Implications |
|---|---|---|
| **Psychological Response** | | |
| First trimester: uncertainty, ambivalence, mood changes, self as primary focus<br>Second trimester: wonder, joy, focus on fetus<br>Third trimester: vulnerability, preparing for birth (fear, anger, apathy, ambivalence, lack of preparation) | "How do you and your partner feel about being pregnant?" "How will the pregnancy change your lives?" "How do you feel about the changes in your body?" "What are you doing to get ready for the baby?" | Use active listening and reflection to establish a sense of trust. Reevaluate negative responses (fear, apathy, anger) in subsequent assessments. |
| **Availability of Resources** | | |
| Financial concerns (lack of funds or insurance)<br>Availability of grandparents, friends, family (family geographically or emotionally unavailable) | "What are your plans for prenatal care and birth?" "How do your parents feel about being grandparents?" "Who else can you depend on besides the family?" "Who helps you when there is a problem?" | Determine adequacy of financial means.<br>Refer to resources such as a public clinic for care, WIC for food.<br>Help the couple discover alternative resources if the family is unavailable.<br>Identify family conflicts early to allow time for resolution. |
| **Changes in Sexual Practices** | | |
| Mutual satisfaction with changes (excessive concern with comfort or safety, excessive conflict) | "How has your sexual relationship changed during the pregnancy?" "How do you cope with the changes?" "What concerns you most?" | Offer reassurance that intercourse is safe in normal pregnancy.<br>Suggest alternative positions and open communication. |
| **Educational Needs** | | |
| Many questions about pregnancy, childbirth, and infant care (no questions, absence of interest in educational programs) | "How do you feel about caring for an infant?" "What are your major concerns?" "Who do you ask for information?" | Respond to expressed needs. Refer couple to appropriate classes and reliable Internet sources of information. |
| **Cultural Influences** | | |
| Ability of either the woman or her family to speak English or availability of fluent interpreters<br>Cultural influences that support a healthy pregnancy and infant (harmful cultural beliefs or health practices) | "What foods and practices are recommended during pregnancy?" "What is forbidden?" "What is most important to you in your care?" "How do your religious beliefs affect pregnancy?" | Locate fluent interpreters if needed.<br>Avoid labeling beliefs as superstition.<br>Reinforce beliefs that promote a good pregnancy outcome.<br>Elicit help from accepted sources of information to overcome harmful practices. |

*WIC,* Special Supplemental Nutrition Program for Women, Infants, and Children
*Findings that require additional assessment or intervention are shown in parentheses.

occur during pregnancy, the developmental tasks of the mother and father, and role transition. Guidance is helpful to prepare prospective parents for the progressive changes that occur during pregnancy and to reassure them that their feelings and behaviors are normal. Such guidance also gives them an opportunity to ask questions and explore their feelings.

***Adapting nursing care to pregnancy progress.*** Adapt nursing care to the changes that occur in each trimester of pregnancy. During the first trimester, focus on the woman's acceptance of the pregnancy. Tailor teaching to her feelings (physical and psychological) because this is a period of self-focus. The second trimester is a time to concentrate more on the fetus and how the woman and her family will adapt to the changes the birth will bring. Ask about her fantasies regarding the baby and her relationships with significant others. The focus is on the woman's discomforts and readiness to give birth during the third trimester. Observe for signs the mother is having difficulty with any of the tasks or steps throughout pregnancy.

***Discussing resources.*** Help couples with limited financial resources or insurance coverage find the most convenient location for prenatal care. This concern is particularly important for the new poor, who have little idea of how to gain access to government-sponsored care.

Emotional resources include those that help the new family adjust to the demands of pregnancy and parenting. If family members who traditionally offer support in times of stress are unavailable, refer the prospective parents to community resources, such as childbirth education, sibling, breastfeeding, and new parenting classes and support groups.

***Helping the family prepare for the birth.*** During the last trimester, discuss lifestyle changes that will occur when the infant is born. Unanticipated changes that accompany this dramatic life event may add stress and disrupt family processes. Help the prospective parents make practical plans for the infant, such as obtaining clothing and equipment and choosing the method of feeding. Siblings should be prepared several weeks or months before the birth, depending on their ages. Older children often benefit from participating in planning for the baby.

Suggest that parents consider how they will work out the division of household and parenting tasks, as well as child care if the mother will return to work after childbirth. If these issues are not resolved, the couple can experience frustration and anger if one parent, usually the mother, assumes total care of the infant and attempts to complete all household tasks. Exhaustion and frustration can overwhelm the joys of parenting when one parent must provide all care.

*Modeling communication techniques.* When disagreements are evident, discuss and model therapeutic communication techniques that include all significant family members. Techniques that clarify, summarize, and reflect feelings can defuse negative feelings that might result in family disruption.

*Identifying cultural factors that can cause conflict.* Explore possible areas of conflict related to cultural beliefs and health practices that affect pregnancy.

Expectant mothers are reassured when nurses support beneficial health beliefs before confronting them with concerns about healthcare beliefs. For example, "It is so good for you and the baby when you eat so many vegetables. I was worried, though, when you missed your last appointment."

If there is conflict as a result of differences in time orientation, acknowledge the problem, convey understanding of the differences, and emphasize the importance of calling when appointments cannot be kept. Many families do not realize that when they miss their appointment, another family misses the opportunity for healthcare.

### Evaluation

- Does the family verbalize concerns and emotions at each visit?
- Do the partner and significant family members appear interested and involved?
- Are they making appropriate progress in meeting the tasks of pregnancy?
- Do the family members discuss compromises when cultural health practices are harmful?

## PERINATAL EDUCATION

Perinatal education helps couples learn about pregnancy, birth, and parenting. Classes focus not only on preparing for childbirth but also include information formerly received during a longer birth facility stay.

The goals of perinatal education are to help parents become knowledgeable consumers who make informed decisions, take an active role in maintaining health during pregnancy and birth, and learn coping techniques to deal with pregnancy, childbirth, and parenting.

### Providers of Education

Most perinatal education classes are taught by registered nurses, but some are taught by physical therapists or others with special preparation. Many instructors are certified by organizations such as the American Society for Psychoprophylaxis in Obstetrics (ASPO) or the International Childbirth Education Association (ICEA). Certification ensures that the instructors have received special preparation to provide sound education that adheres to the certifying organization's general philosophy.

### Class Participants

Participants in classes about childbearing have traditionally been middle-income couples who are older and better educated than those who do not take classes. Low-income women may not have money or transportation for classes. Although inexpensive or free classes are available in some areas, women with little or no prenatal care may not know about this form of education.

People take classes for various reasons. Many want to participate actively in all aspects of childbearing. Others are looking for coping strategies to deal with their fear of childbirth or pain. When women feel informed and believe that they have some control over what happens to them, they are more likely to expect birth to be satisfying and fulfilling and to experience it as such.

### Choices for Childbearing

One purpose of any perinatal education program is to help parents learn about available options so they can make appropriate choices. Parents learn that there are many ways of birthing and that none is the only "right" method. Knowledgeable parents can communicate assertively with their healthcare providers about their needs and desires.

Some women make a birth plan describing their preferences as they consider the various choices possible in childbirth. The plan may be very simple, such as the desire to keep the infant with the mother at all times, or it may be a list of very specific items to be included in the childbirth experience. Cultural preferences can be incorporated into the birth plan (Box 13.2). The birth plan is not always written. It may consist of the woman's beliefs about what she would like to have happen during her birth experience. Whether written or only in her mind, the woman should discuss her plans for birth with her healthcare provider during the pregnancy.

### Setting and Healthcare Provider

The woman and her partner must choose a birth setting and select a care provider who practices in that setting. Hospitals are the most common setting for birth in North America. They often have birthing suites that provide a home-like atmosphere. A freestanding birth center provides an atmosphere that is less institutional than that of the hospital. Home birth allows the woman to give birth in her own surroundings, with delivery managed by a midwife. The woman's insurance may limit her choice of setting for birth.

The woman must also choose a healthcare provider. The different roles of the physician, certified nurse-midwife, and nurse practitioner are discussed in Chapter 2.

### Support Person

During labor, the woman needs someone with her to help her through the experience. The support person is most often the father of her baby, but a relative or friend also may take this role (Fig. 13.18). Some women wish to share the birth experience with several relatives or close friends. Other women hire a **doula** to provide support during labor.

A doula is a trained labor support person who is employed by the mother to provide labor support. She gives physical support such as massage and help with relaxation and provides emotional support and advocacy throughout labor. Some doulas also help during the postpartum period.

**BOX 13.2 Birth Plan Considerations**

- Use of intermittent or continuous fetal monitoring
- Intravenous fluids: use, avoidance, saline lock
- Food and oral fluids allowed in labor
- Position and activity for labor, position for delivery
- Use of tubs, showers, birthing balls
- Episiotomy
- Methods of pain relief
- Support persons present during labor
- Medical interventions (such as induction of labor)
- Breastfeeding only, formula only, combination feeding
- Participation of siblings during/after birth
- Mother/baby couplet care
- Time of discharge

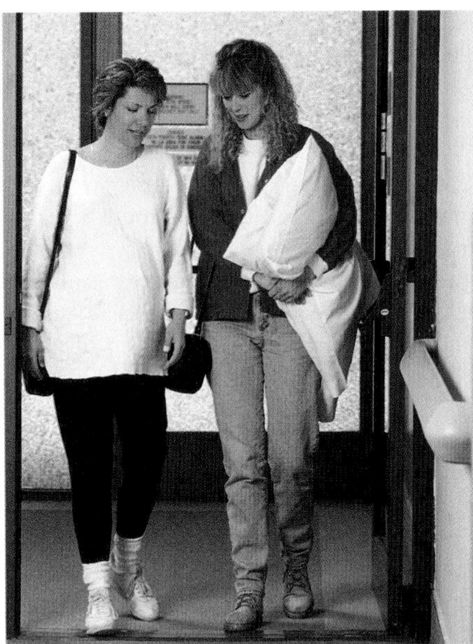

FIG 13.18 An expectant mother may ask a sister or close female friend to be her labor partner and to attend classes with her.

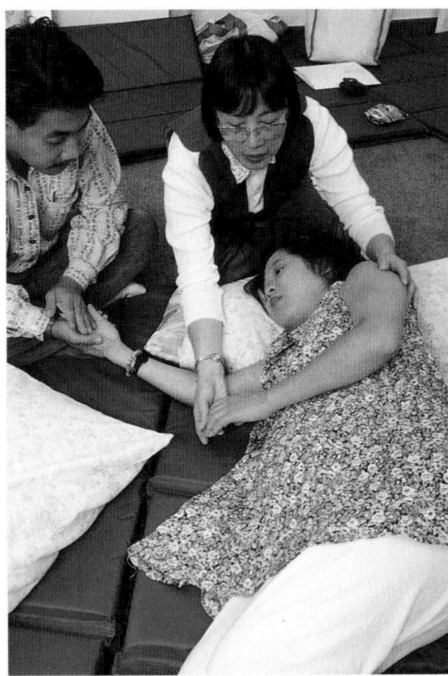

FIG 13.19 The nurse teaches the support person how to check for relaxation.

## Education

Expectant mothers must also decide on prenatal education classes. Their decisions are based on the classes available in the area, the costs, and the kinds of information they need. Some agencies offer many classes from which to choose. In others the selection is limited to childbirth preparation classes only. Classes in languages other than English often are available.

## Types of Classes Available

### Preconception Classes

Classes for couples who are thinking about having a baby are designed to help couples have a healthy pregnancy from the beginning. Information about nutrition before conception, healthy lifestyle, signs of pregnancy, and choosing a caregiver is presented. Preconception classes emphasize early and regular prenatal care and ways to reduce risk factors for poor pregnancy outcome.

### Early Pregnancy Classes

Early pregnancy classes focus on the first two trimesters. They cover information on adapting to pregnancy, dealing with early discomforts (such as morning sickness and fatigue), sexuality, and understanding what to expect in the months ahead. Emphasis is placed on obtaining prenatal care and avoiding hazards to the fetus.

Second-trimester classes focus on changes that occur during middle pregnancy, fetal development, and alterations in roles. Information on body mechanics, working during pregnancy, and what to expect during the third trimester is included. Teachers discuss childbirth choices and information to help students become more knowledgeable consumers.

### Exercise Classes

Exercise classes help women keep fit and healthy during pregnancy. Exercises should be low impact and preceded by warm-up routines. To prevent diversion of blood away from the uterus, women should avoid excessive heart rate elevation. Prenatal yoga classes may also be available.

### Childbirth Preparation Classes

In childbirth preparation classes, women and their support persons learn self-help measures and what to expect during labor and birth. Couples learn coping methods that help them approach childbirth in a positive manner. Teachers do not promise prevention of all pain in labor. The increased confidence and the techniques learned in prepared childbirth classes may help decrease pain perception and increase tolerance of pain during labor.

Classes include information about labor, pharmacologic and nonpharmacologic methods of pain relief (see Chapter 18), common complications, and a tour of the birth setting. Practice of relaxation, breathing techniques, and coping strategies is part of "labor rehearsals" (Fig. 13.19). DVDs assist women to develop a realistic picture of the birth process.

Many women plan to have epidural anesthesia during labor. However, having other techniques to help manage discomfort in labor is helpful until the epidural is administered.

Class series range from a 1-day class to four to eight meetings, depending on the content included. Women who have taken classes for a previous birth often take a refresher class for an update of current practices and review of techniques. These classes consist of supervised practice and discussion of role changes in the family and sibling adjustment.

Prepared childbirth classes based in birth facilities include detailed information on what to expect in that particular setting but may not cover options that are unavailable at that agency. Hospital classes have sometimes been criticized for teaching women to be "good," or compliant, patients. A woman may wish to talk to the instructor before taking a class to ask about class size and the teacher's philosophy, background, and teaching methods.

### Cesarean Birth Preparation Classes

Although cesarean birth is discussed in general childbirth classes, women planning a cesarean birth may take a separate class. Topics include indications, options, surgical procedure, and postoperative course. For those who had a cesarean birth previously, the class offers an opportunity to share experiences and feelings and to clarify misconceptions. Class discussion helps couples feel that they have some control over what happens and provides a basis for discussion with caregivers.

### Breastfeeding Classes

Prenatal breastfeeding classes help increase a woman's confidence in her ability to breastfeed successfully and provide her with resources if she encounters difficulties. Information includes physiology of lactation, feeding techniques, establishing a milk supply, and solutions to common problems. Partners who attend learn methods of providing support during breastfeeding. Classes may continue after the birth.

### Parenting Classes

Instruction on parenting and newborn care may be included in prepared childbirth classes or provided separately. Content typically includes general care and common concerns, such as the crying infant and advantages and disadvantages of circumcision. Baby equipment, such as various types of infant car seats, is often displayed. Practice with dolls also may be included. Classes sometimes continue after the birth of the infant.

### Classes for Fathers

Classes for fathers often focus on the male perspective of pregnancy, birth, and parenting. They provide an opportunity for men to meet other expectant fathers and ask questions they might not ask in classes that include expectant mothers. Some classes involve practicing infant care techniques such as diapering and bathing with dolls. Classes may be taught by a man to make the fathers feel more comfortable.

### Postpartum Classes

Although the postpartum period is covered in childbirth preparation classes, the mother can also attend classes after birth. Content includes the physiologic and psychological changes of the postpartum period, role transition, sexuality, and nutrition. Signs of postpartum depression often are discussed, with emphasis on when the woman should seek help. Some classes focus on exercise for the postpartum period.

## KEY CONCEPTS

- Pregnancy causes a predictable pattern of uterine growth. In general, the uterus can be palpated at the level of the umbilicus at 20 weeks of gestation and at the xiphoid process by 36 weeks.
- Thick mucus fills the cervical canal and protects the fetus from infection caused by bacteria ascending from the vagina.
- The plasma volume expands faster and to a greater extent than RBC volume, resulting in a dilution of hemoglobin concentration called physiologic (pseudo) anemia.
- Although blood volume increases, blood pressure is not elevated during normal pregnancy.
- The gravid uterus partially occludes the vena cava and aorta when the mother is supine. The occlusion causes supine hypotensive syndrome, which can be prevented or corrected by assuming a lateral position.
- Slight hyperventilation and decreased airway resistance allow increased oxygen needs to be met.
- The ribs flare, the substernal angle widens, and the chest circumference increases.
- Increased renal plasma flow results in an increased GFR, which often causes "spilling" of glucose and other nutrients into the urine.
- Hyperpigmentation during pregnancy includes melasma and linea nigra. Striae gravidarum occur from separation of connective tissue fibers.
- Increased hCG and estrogen levels and decreased gastric motility may cause nausea in early pregnancy.
- Increased progesterone causes relaxation of smooth muscles, resulting in stasis of urine and the risk of urinary tract infections and constipation.
- The expanding uterus results in progressive changes that can lead to muscle strain and backache may occur during the last trimester.
- Progesterone maintains the uterine lining, prevents uterine contractions, and helps prepare the breasts for lactation.
- Presumptive and probable signs of pregnancy may be caused by conditions other than pregnancy, and thus, cannot be considered positive or diagnostic signs. Positive signs can have no other cause.
- All women should have a preconception visit to the healthcare provider to ensure they are healthy before conceiving.
- The initial antepartum visit includes a complete history and physical examination to determine potential risks to the mother and fetus and to obtain baseline data so that a plan of care can be developed.
- Multifetal pregnancies impose greater physiologic changes than a single-fetus pregnancy and require extra vigilance to detect possible complications.
- Families need information on self-care and health promotion during pregnancy and ways to cope with the common discomforts of pregnancy that do not need or respond to medical management.
- Maternal psychological responses to pregnancy progress from uncertainty and ambivalence to feelings of vulnerability and preparation for the birth of the infant.
- As the fetus becomes real, usually in the second trimester, maternal focus shifts from self to the fetus, and the woman turns inward to concentrate on the processes going on in her body.
- Sexual activity varies between couples and may be culturally influenced. It is safe throughout pregnancy if there are no complications.
- Changes in the maternal body during pregnancy may result in a negative body image that affects sexual responses. This change may be especially troubling if the couple does not discuss emotions and concerns related to the changes in sexuality.
- Making the transition to the role of mother involves mimicking the behavior of other mothers, fantasizing about the baby, developing a sense of self as mother, and grieving the loss of previous roles.
- To complete the maternal tasks of pregnancy, the woman must seek safe passage for herself and the infant, gain acceptance of significant persons, give of herself, and form an attachment to the unknown child.
- Paternal responses depend on the ability to perceive the fetus as real, to gain recognition for the role of parent, and to create a role as involved father.
- The most powerful reality boosters for the expectant father during pregnancy are hearing the fetal heartbeat, feeling the fetus move, and viewing the infant on a sonogram.
- In primitive cultures, couvade refers to rituals performed by the man. In modern society, couvade often refers to a cluster of pregnancy-related signs and symptoms experienced by the man.

*Continued*

## KEY CONCEPTS—cont'd

- The response of grandparents to pregnancy depends on their age, the number and ages of other grandchildren, and their perception of the role of grandparents.
- The response of siblings to pregnancy depends on their ages and developmental levels.
- Completing the developmental tasks of pregnancy is more difficult for multiparas because they have less time, experience more fatigue, and must negotiate a new relationship with the older child or children.
- Socioeconomic status is a major factor in determining health practices during pregnancy. Low-income families have competing priorities for food and shelter and may seek prenatal care late in pregnancy.
- Cultural differences in language, time orientation, and health beliefs can create conflicts between expectant families and health-care workers.
- Education for childbearing helps couples become knowledgeable consumers and active participants in pregnancy and childbirth.
- Many classes are available for pregnant women and their families. Early pregnancy classes emphasize having a healthy pregnancy. Those conducted later in the pregnancy focus on preparing for childbirth, breastfeeding, and early parenting.

## REFERENCES AND READINGS


Albrecht, S.A. (2010). Smoking cessation in pregnancy. *Nursing for Women's Health, 3*(14), 177–179.

Albright, J.W. (2008). Indonesia. In C.E. D'Avanzo (Ed.), *Mosby's pocket guide to cultural health assessment* (4th ed., pp. 326–330). St. Louis: Mosby.

Alex, M.R. (2011). Occupational hazards for pregnant nurses. *American Journal of Nursing, 111*(1), 28–37.

American Academy of Pediatrics & American College of Obstetricians and Gynecologists. (2012). *Guidelines for perinatal care* (7th ed.). Elk Grove Village, IL. and Washington, DC: Author.

American College of Obstetricians and Gynecologists. (2015). *Nausea and vomiting of pregnancy, (ACOG Practice Bulletin #548).* Washington DC: Author.

American College of Obstetricians and Gynecologists. (2014). *Prediction and prevention of preterm birth, (ACOG Practice Bulletin #130).* Washington DC: Author.

American College of Obstetricians and Gynecologists. (2013). *Weight gain during pregnancy, (ACOG Committee Opinion #153).* Washington DC: Author.

Ashford, K.B., Hahn, E., Hall, L., Rayens, M.K., Noland, M. and Ferguson, J.E. (2010). The Effects of Prenatal Secondhand Smoke Exposure on Preterm Birth and Neonatal Outcomes. *Journal of Obstetric, Gynecologic, & Neonatal Nursing, 39*, 525–535. doi:10.1111/j.1552-6909.2010.01169.x

Association of Women's Health, Obstetric, and Neonatal Nurses. (2008). *Female genital cutting.* Washington, DC: Author.

Association of Women's Health, Obstetric, and Neonatal Nurses. (2009). *Standards for professional nursing practice in the care of women and newborns* (7th ed.). Washington, DC: Author.

Association of Women's Health, Obstetric, and Neonatal Nurses. (2010). *Smoking and women's health.* Washington, DC: Author.

Bailey, J.M., Crane, P., & Nugent, C.E. (2008). Childbirth education and birth plans. *Obstetrics and Gynecology Clinics of North America, 35*(3), 497–509.

Barron, M.L. (2014). Antenatal care. In K.R. Simpson, & P.A. Creehan (Eds.), *AWHONN perinatal nursing* (4th ed., pp. 89–121). Philadelphia: Lippincott Williams & Wilkins.

Beckmann, C.R.B., Ling, F.W., Herbert, W.N.P., et al. (2014). *Obstetrics and gynecology* (7th ed.). Philadelphia: Lippincott Williams & Wilkins.

Beddoe, A.E., Yang, C.P., Kennedy, H.P., et al. (2009). The effects of mindfulness-based yoga during pregnancy on maternal psychological and physical distress. *Journal of Obstetric, Gynecologic, and Neonatal Nursing, 38*(3), 310–319.

Bell, K.M. (2012). CenteringPregnancy: Changing the System, Empowering Women and Strengthening Families. *International Journal of Childbirth Education, 27*(1), 70–76 7p.

Blackburn, S.T. (2014). Physiologic changes of pregnancy. In K.R. Simpson, & P.A. Creehan (Eds.), *AWHONN perinatal nursing* (4th ed., pp. 71–88). Philadelphia: Lippincott Williams & Wilkins.

Blackburn, S.T. (2013). *Maternal, fetal, and neonatal physiology: A clinical perspective* (4th ed.). St. Louis: Saunders.

Boardman, L.A., & Kennedy, C.M. (2008). Benign vulvovaginal disorders. In R.S. Gibbs, B.Y. Karlan, A.F. Haney, et al. (Eds.), *Danforth's obstetrics & gynecology* (10th ed., pp. 625–647). Philadelphia: Lippincott Williams & Wilkins.

Bond, L. (2011). Physiology of pregnancy. In S. Mattson, & J.E. Smith (Eds.), *AWHONN core curriculum for maternal-newborn nursing* (4th ed., pp. 80–100). St. Louis: Saunders.

Boyce, P., Condon, J., Barton, J., et al. (2007). First-time fathers study: Psychological distress in expectant fathers during pregnancy. *Australian and New Zealand Journal of Psychiatry, 41*(9), 718–725.

Bruhn, K., & Tillett, J. (2009). Administration of vaccinations in pregnancy and postpartum. *MCN: The American Journal of Maternal/Child Nursing, 34*(2), 98–105.

Callahan, T.L., & Caughey, A.B. (2013). *Blueprints obstetrics & gynecology* (6th ed.). Philadelphia: Lippincott Williams & Wilkins.

Callister, L.C. (2014). Intergrating cultural beliefs and practices when caring for childbearing women and families. In K. R. Simpson, & P. A. Creehan (Eds.). *AWHONN perinatal nursing* (4th ed., pp. 41–70). Philadelphia: Lippincott Williams & Wilkins.

Castro, L.C., & Ogunyemi, D. (2010). Common medical and surgical conditions complicating pregnancy. In N.F. Hacker, J.C. Gambone, & C.J. Gobel (Eds.), *Essentials of obstetrics and gynecology* (5th ed., pp. 191–218). Philadelphia: Saunders.

Centers for Disease Control and Prevention. (2011). Updated recommendations for use of tetanus toxoid, reduced diphtheria tox-oid and acellular pertussis vaccine (Tdap) in pregnant women and persons who have or anticipate having close contact with an infant aged <12 months—Advisory Com-mittee on Immunization Practices, 2011. *MMWR Morbidity and Mortality Weekly Report, 60*(41), 1424–1426.

Centers for Disease Control and Prevention. (2015). *Vaccinating Pregnant Patients.* Retreived from http://www.cdc.gov/pertussis/pregnant/hcp/pregnant-patients.html.

Chalupka, S., & Chalupka, A.N. (2010). The impact of environmental and occupational exposures on reproductive health. *Journal of Obstetric, Gynecologic, and Neonatal Nursing, 39*(1), 84–102.

Chatterjee, S. (2008). India (Republic of). In C.E. D'Avanzo (Ed.), *Mosby's pocket guide to cultural health assessment* (4th ed., pp. 320–326). St. Louis: Mosby.

Cottrell, B.H. (2010). An updated review of evidence to discourage douching. *MCN: The American Journal of Maternal/Child Nursing, 35*(2), 102–107.

Coverston, C.R. (2011). Psychology of pregnancy. In S. Mattson, & J.E. Smith (Eds.), *AWHONN core curriculum for maternal-newborn nursing* (4th ed., pp. 101–114). St. Louis: Saunders.

Cunningham, F.G., Leveno, K.J., Bloom, S.L., et al. (2010). *William obstetrics* (23rd ed.) New York: McGraw-Hill.

Darby, S.B. (2007). Pre- and perinatal care of Hispanic families. *Nursing for Women's Health, 11*(2), 161–169.

Darby, S.B. (2009). Traditional Chinese medicine. *Nursing for Women's Health, 13*(3), 198–206.

Deane, R.A.K. (2010). Cultural competence: Nursing in a multicultural society. *Nursing for Women's Health, 14*(1), 50–59.

Driscoll, J.W. (2008). Psychosocial adaptation to pregnancy and postpartum. In K. R. Simpson, & P. A. Creehan (eds.), *AWHONN perinatal nursing* (3rd ed., pp. 78–87). Philadelphia: Lippincott Willians & Willkins.

Dumonteil, E., & Leon, M.R.G. (2008). Mexico (United Mexican States). In C. E. D'Avanzo (Ed.), *Mosby's pocket guide to cultural health assessment* (4th ed., pp. 477–481). St. Louis: Mosby.

Erick, M. (2008). Nutrition during pregnancy and lactation. In L. K. Mahan, S. Escott-Stump, & J. L. Raymond (Eds.), *Krause's food, nutrition, and diet therapy* (12th ed., pp. 159–198). St. Louis: Saunders.

Forest, S. (2010). Controversy and evidence about nicotine replacement therapy in pregnancy. *MCN: The American Journal of Maternal/Child Nursing, 35*(2), 89–95.

Freeman, L. (2009). *Mosby's complementary and alternative medicine: A research-based approach* (3rd ed.). St. Louis: Mosby.

Friedman, S.H., Heneghan, A., & Rosenthal, M. (2009). Characteristics of women who do not seek prenatal care and implications for prevention. *Journal of Obstetric, Gynecologic, and Neonatal Nursing, 38*(2), 174–181.

Galanti, G. (2008). *Caring for patients from different cultures* (4th ed.). Philadelphia: University of Pennsylvania Press.

Gambone, J.C. (2010). Clinical approach to the patient. In N. F. Hacker, J.C. Gambone, & C.J. Gobel (Eds.), *Essentials of obstetrics and gynecology* (5th ed., pp. 12–21). Philadelphia: Saunders.

Gilbert, E.S. (2011). *Manual of high risk pregnancy & delivery* (5th ed.). St. Louis: Mosby.

Gordon, M.C. (2012). Maternal physiology. In S.G. Gabbe, J.R. Niebyl, & J.L. Simpson (Eds.), *Obstetrics: Normal and problem pregnancies* (6th ed., pp. 42–65). New York: Churchill Livingstone.

Gregory, K.D., Niebyl, J.R., & Johnson, T.R. B., (2012). Preconception and prenatal care: Part of the continuum. In S.G. Gabbe, J.R. Niebyl, & J.L. Simpson (Eds.), *Obstetrics: Normal and problem pregnancies* (6th ed., pp. 101–124). Philadelphia: Churchill Livingstone.

Grewal, S.K., Bhagat, R., & Balneaves, L.G. (2008). Perinatal beliefs and practices of immigrant Punjabi women living in Canada. *Journal of Obstetric, Gynecologic, and Neonatal Nursing, 37*(3), 290–300.

Herman, J.W., Rogers, S., & Ehrenthal, D. (2012). Women's perceptions of CenteringPregnancy: A focus group study. *MCN The American Journal of Maternal/Child Nursing, 37*(1), 19–26.

Hess, R.F., Weinland, J., & Saalinger, N.M. (2010). Knowledge of female genital cutting and experience with women who are circumcised: A survey of nurse-midwives in the United States. *Journal of Midwifery & Women's Health, 55*(1), 46–54.

James, D.C., (2014). Psychosocial adaptation to the postpartum period. In K.R. Simpson, & P.A. Creehan (Eds.), *AWHONN perinatal nursing* (4th ed., pp. 570-572). Philadelphia: Lippincott Williams & Wilkins.

Janke, J. (2014). Newborn Nutrition. In K.R. Simpson, & P.A. Creehan (Eds.), *AWHONN perinatal nursing* (4th ed., pp. 626–661). Philadelphia: Lippincott Williams & Wilkins.

Ji, E.S., & Han, H. (2010). The effects of Qi exercise on maternal/fetal interaction and maternal well-being during pregnancy. *Journal of Obstetric, Gynecologic, and Neonatal Nursing, 39*(3), 310–318.

Johnson-Wimbley, T.D. & Graham, D.Y. (2011). Diagnosis and management of iron deficiency anemia in the 21st Century. *Therapeutic Advances in Gastroenterology, 4*(3), 177–184.

Jones, E.E. (2009). Fertilization, pregnancy, and lactation. In W.F. Boron, & E.L. Boulpaep (Eds.), *Medical physiology* (2nd ed., pp. 1170–1192). Philadelphia: Saunders.

Jordan, P. L. (1990). Laboring for relevance: Expectant and new fatherhood. *Nursing Research, 39*(1), 11–16.

Kater, V. (2008). Israel (State of). In C.E. D'Avanzo (Ed.), *Mosby's pocket guide to cultural health assessment* (4th ed., pp. 344–350). St. Louis: Mosby.

Katz, V.L. (2008). Prenatal care. In R.S. Gibbs, B.Y. Karlan, A.F. Haney, et al. (Eds.), *Danforth's obstetrics & gynecology* (10th ed., pp. 1–21). Philadelphia: Lippincott Williams & Wilkins.

Koos, B.J., Kahn, D.A., & Equils, O. (2010). Maternal physiologic and immunologic adaptation to pregnancy. In N.F. Hacker, J.C. Gambone, & C.J. Hobel (Eds.), *Essentials of obstetrics and gynecology* (5th ed., pp. 56–70). Philadelphia: Saunders.

Lu, M.C., Williams, J., & Hobel, C.J. (2010). Antepartum care: Preconception and prenatal care, genetic evaluation and teratology, and antenatal fetal assessment. In N.F. Hacker, J.C. Gambone, & C.J. Hobel (Eds.), *Essentials of obstetrics and gynecology* (5th ed., pp. 71–90). Philadelphia: Saunders.

Mandel, D. (2010). The lived experience of pregnancy complications in single older women. *MCN: The American Journal of Maternal/Child Nursing, 35*(6), 336–340.

Mann, J.R., Mannan, J., Quinones, L.A., et al. (2010). Religion, spirituality, social support and perceived stress in pregnant and postpartum Hispanic women. *Journal of Obstetric, Gynecologic, and Neonatal Nursing, 39*(6), 645–657.

Mathews, T.J., Minino, A.M., Osterman, M.J. K., et al. (2011). Annual summary of vital statistics: 2008. *Pediatrics, 127*(1), 146–157.

Mattson, S. (2011). Ethnocultural considerations in the childbearing period. In S. Mattson, & J.E. Smith (Eds.), *AWHONN core curriculum for maternal-newborn nursing* (4th ed., pp. 61–79). St. Louis: Saunders.

Mavridou, D., Norwitz, E.R., Robinson, J.N., et al. (2008). Management of multiple pregnancies. In E.F. Funai, E.I. Evans, & C.J. Lockwood (Eds.), *High risk obstetrics: The requisites in obstetrics and gynecology* (pp. 213–229). Philadelphia: Mosby.

Mercer, R.T., & Ferketich, S.L. (1994). Maternal-infant attachment of experienced and inexperienced mothers during infancy. *Nursing Research, 43*(6), 344–351.

Monga, M. (2014). Maternal cardiovascular, respiratory, and renal adaptation to pregnancy. In R.K. Creasy, R. Resnik, J.D. Iams, et al. (Eds.), *Maternal-fetal medicine: Principles and practice* (7th ed., pp. 93–99). Philadelphia: Saunders.

Moore, M. L., Moos, M., & Callister, L. C. (2010). *Cultural competence: An essential journey for perinatal nurses.* White Plains, NY: March of Dimes.

National Center for Health Statistics. (2009). *Health, United States, 2009 with special feature on medical technology.* Hyattsville, MD: Author.

Nelson, A.L. (2011). Combined oral contraceptives. In R.A. Hatcher, J. Trussell, A.L. Nelson, et al. (Eds.), *Contraceptive technology* (20th ed., pp. 249–341). New York: Ardent Media.

Nettleman, M.D., Brewer, J., & Stafford, M. (2010). Scheduling the first prenatal visit: Office-based delays. *American Journal of Obstetrics & Gynecology, 203*(207), e1–e3.

Newman, R.B., & Rittenberg, C. (2008). Multiple gestation. In R.S. Gibbs, B.Y. Karlan, A.F. Haney, et al. (Eds.), *Danforth's obstetrics & gynecology* (10th ed., pp. 220–245). Philadelphia: Lippincott Williams & Wilkins.

Norwitz, E.R., Mahendroo, M. & Lye, S.J. (2014). Biology of parturition. In R.K. Creasy, R. Resnik, J.D. Iams, et al. (Eds.), *Maternal-fetal medicine: Principles and practice* (7th ed., pp. 66-79). Philadelphia: Saunders.

Novick, G. (2009). Women's experience of prenatal care: An integrative review. *Journal of Midwifery & Women's Health, 54*(3), 226–237.

Pagana, K.D., & Pagana, T.J. (2009). *Mosby's diagnostic and laboratory test reference* (9th ed.). St. Louis: Mosby.

Potter, J.E., Pereyra, M., Lamp, M., et al. (2009). Factors associated with prenatal care use among peripartum women in the mother-infant rapid intervention at delivery study. *Journal of Obstetric, Gynecologic, and Neonatal Nursing, 38*(5), 534–543.

Quach, L., Nguyen, H.L., & Nguyen, H.T.N. (2008). Vietnam (Socialist Republic of). In C.E. D'Avanzo (Ed.), *Mosby's pocket guide to cultural health assessment* (4th ed., pp. 773–778). St. Louis: Mosby.

Ramer, L., & Frank, B. (2001). *Pregnancy: Psychosocial perspectives.* White Plains, NY: March of Dimes Birth Defects Foundation.

Rapini, R.P. (2014). The skin and pregnancy. In R.K. Creasy, R. Resnik, J.D. Iams, et al. (Eds.),

*Maternal-fetal medicine: Principles and practice* (7th ed., pp. 1146-1155). Philadelphia: Saunders.

Reid, J. (2007). CenteringPregnancy: A model for group prenatal care. *Nursing and Women's Health, 11*(4), 382–388.

Rotundo, G. (2011). CenteringPregnancy: The benefits of group prenatal care. *Nursing for Women's Health, 15*(6), 508–517.

Rubin, R. (1984). *Maternal identity and the maternal experience*. New York: Springer.

Russ, K. (2009). Health effects of personal care products: A review of the evidence. *Nursing for Women's Health, 13*(5), 392–401.

Sanders, L.B. (2009). Reproductive life plans: Initiating the dialogue with women. *MCN: The American Journal of Maternal/Child Nursing, 34*(6), 342–347.

Singh, P., Yoon, S.S., & Kuo, B. (2015). Nausea: a review of pathophysiology and therapeutics. *Therapeutic Advances in Gastroenterology. 9*(1), 98–112.

Skidmore-Roth, L. (2010). *Mosby's handbook of herbs & natural supplements* (4th ed.). St. Louis: Mosby.

Spector, R.E. (2009). *Cultural diversity in health and illness* (7th ed.). Upper Saddle River, NJ: Pearson Prentice Hall.

Substance Abuse and Mental Health Services Administration. (2009). *Results from the 2008 national survey on drug use and health: National findings*. (Office of Applied Studies, NSDUH Series H-36, HHS Publication No. SMA 09–4434). Rockville, MD. Retrieved from: (Office of Applied Studies, NSDUH Series H-36, HHS Publication No. SMA 09–4434). Rockville, MD. Retrieved from http://www.oas.samhsa.gov/nsduh/2k8nsduh/2k8Results.pdf.

Sunil, T.S., Spears, W.D., Hook, L., et al. (2010). Initiation of and barriers to prenatal care use among low-income women in San Antonio, Texas. *Maternal Child Journal, 14*(1), 133–140.

Tarsa, M., & Moore, T.R. (2010). Multifetal gestation and malpresentation. In N.F. Hacker, J.C. Gambone, & C.J. Gobel (Eds.), *Essentials of obstetrics and gynecology* (5th ed., pp. 160–172). Philadelphia: Saunders.

Torres, S. (2008). Puerto Rican Americans. In J.N. Giger, & R.E. Davidhizar (Eds.), *Transcultural nursing: Assessment and intervention* (5th ed., pp. 670–688). St. Louis: Mosby.

U.S. Department of Health and Human Services. (2000). *Healthy People 2010*. (Conference edition, in 2 volumes). Washington, DC: Author, (Conference edition, in 2 volumes).

U.S. Department of Health and Human Services. (2010). *Healthy People 2020*. Washington, DC: Author.

U.S. Preventive Services Task Force. (2009). *Folic Acid for the Prevention of Neural Tube Defects: U.S. Preventive Services Task Force Recommendation Statement*. AHRQ Publication No. 09-05132-EF-2, AHRQ Publication No. 09-05132-EF-2, Retrieved from http://www.uspreventiveservicestaskforce.org/uspstf09/folicacid/folicacidrs.htm.

Yi, M. (2008a). Korea, North (Republic of). In C.E. D'Avanzo (Ed.), *Mosby's pocket guide to cultural health assessment* (4th ed., pp. 384–387). St. Louis: Mosby.

Yi, M. (2008b). Korea, South (Republic of). In C.E. D'Avanzo (Ed.), *Mosby's pocket guide to cultural health assessment* (4th ed., pp. 387–391). St. Louis: Mosby.

Wallace, D.A., Dodd, M.M., McNeil, D.A., et al. (2009). A pregnancy wellness guide to enhance care through self-assessment, personal reflection, and self-referral. *Journal of Obstetric, Gynecologic, and Neonatal Nursing, 38*(2), 134–147.

Weiner, C.P., & Buhimschi, C. (2009). *Drugs for pregnant and lactating women* (2nd ed.). Philadelphia: Saunders.

Williamson, C., & Mackillop, L., & Heneghan, M.A. (2014). Diseases of the liver, biliary system, and pancreas. In R.K. Creasy, R. Resnik, J.D. Iams, et al. (Eds.), *Maternal-fetal medicine: Principles and practice* (7th ed., pp. 1075–1091). Philadelphia: Saunders.

14

# Nutrition for Childbearing

http://evolve.elsevier.com/McKinney/mat-ch/

## LEARNING OBJECTIVES

*After studying this chapter, you should be able to:*

- Explain the importance of adequate nutrition and weight gain during pregnancy.
- Compare the nutrient needs of pregnant and nonpregnant women.
- Describe common factors that influence a woman's nutritional status and choices.
- Describe how common nutritional risk factors affect nutritional requirements during pregnancy.
- Compare the nutritional needs of the postpartum woman who is breastfeeding with those of the woman who is not breastfeeding.
- Apply the nursing process to nutrition during pregnancy, postpartum, and lactation.

At no time in a woman's life is nutrition as important as it is during pregnancy and lactation when she must nourish her own body and that of her baby. Nurses have ongoing contact with women and can provide education about nutritional needs throughout this period. This is especially important because many women do not adequately understand the nutritional needs of pregnancy. Nutritional counseling can also be offered before conception to improve chances of a healthy pregnancy (American College of Obstetricians & Gynecologists [ACOG], 2005).

## WEIGHT GAIN DURING PREGNANCY

Weight gain during pregnancy, especially after the first trimester, is an important determinant of fetal growth. Insufficient weight gain during pregnancy has been associated with low birth weight (less than 2500 g, or 5.5 lb), small-for-gestational age infants, preterm birth, and failure to initiate breastfeeding. Poor maternal weight gain indicates not only lower caloric intake but also low intake of other important nutrients. Excessive weight gain is another problem and is associated with increased birth weight (macrosomia), cesarean birth, postpartum weight retention, low Apgar scores, hypoglycemia, and overweight in children (Luke, 2015; Robinson, Baird, & Godfrey, 2014; American College of Obstetricians and Gynecologists [ACOG], 2013b; American Dietetic Association [ADA], 2008).

### Recommendations for Total Weight Gain

Recommendations for weight gain in pregnancy are based on the woman's prepregnancy weight for her height or her body mass index (BMI). BMI is calculated by dividing the weight in kilograms by the height in meters squared. Another method is to divide the weight in pounds by the height in inches squared and multiply the result by 703 (Centers for Disease Control and Prevention [CDC], 2009). Tables are available that show the BMI for various weights and heights.

Suggested gains vary according to the woman's BMI (or weight for height) before pregnancy (Table 14.1). The recommended weight gain during pregnancy is 11.5 to 16 kg (25 to 35 lb) for women who begin pregnancy at normal BMI. The range allows for individual differences because no exact weight gain is appropriate for every woman (CDC, 2009).

Women who are underweight should gain more weight to meet the needs of pregnancy as well as meet their own need to gain weight. They should gain 12.5 to 18 kg (28 to 40 lb). The recommended gain for overweight women is 7 to 11.5 kg (15 to 25 lb).

Obesity is a growing problem. Obese women who become pregnant have an increased incidence of spontaneous abortion, gestational diabetes, gestational hypertension, preeclampsia, prolonged labor, cesarean birth, postpartum hemorrhage, wound complications, macrosomia, and congenital anomalies. Their children have an increased risk of childhood obesity. Overweight and obese women should be advised to lose weight before conception to achieve the best pregnancy outcomes (Cantor, Bougatsos, Dana, et al., 2015; Grieger, Grezeskowiak, & Clifton, 2014; Bond, 2011). The recommended weight gain for the obese woman is 5 to 9 kg (11 to 20 lb) to provide sufficient nutrients for the fetus (Flick & Artal, 2013; Bennett & McDonald-Mosley, 2011).

Lower weight gain or weight loss for obese women during pregnancy is not recommended at this time, as there is insufficient evidence about the effect on neurologic development of the infant. More research is needed in this area (Flick & Artal, 2013; Rasmussen, Abrams, Bodnar, et al., 2010).

In the past, women of small stature were advised to gain to the lower limits of the recommended range for their prepregnancy weight. Adolescents were advised to gain to the upper limits of their prepregnancy weight. However, evidence to support these guidelines has not been found. Therefore, these women should gain according to the recommendations for their BMI (ACOG, 2013b).

Infants of a multifetal pregnancy are often born before term and tend to weigh less than infants born of single pregnancies. A greater weight gain in the mother may help prevent low birth weight. The recommended gain for women of normal prepregnancy weight who are carrying twins is 17 to 25 kg (37 to 54 lb). When these women meet the recommended weight gain, they are less likely to deliver their twins before 32 weeks of gestation, and the infants are more likely to weigh more than 2500 gm (5.5 lb) (Luke, 2015).

**TABLE 14.1 Recommended Weight Gain During Pregnancy**

| Weight Before Pregnancy | Total Gain | Mean (Range) Weekly Gain (2nd and 3rd Trimesters)* |
|---|---|---|
| Normal weight (BMI 18.5-24.9) | 11.5-16 kg25-35 lb | 0.42 (0.35-0.5) kg1 (0.8-1) lb |
| Underweight (BMI <18.5) | 12.5-18 kg28-40 lb | 0.51 (0.44-0.58) kg1 (1-1.3) lb |
| Overweight (BMI 25-29.9) | 7-11.5 kg15-25 lb | 0.28 (0.23-0.33) kg0.6 (0.5-0.7) lb |
| Obese (BMI >30) | 5-9 kg11-20 lb | 0.22 (0.17-0.27) kg0.5 (0.4-0.6) lb |

*BMI,* Body mass index.
*Recommended weight gain during the first trimester is 0.5-2 kg (1.1-4.4 lb).
Data from Rasmussen, K.M., & Yaktine, A.L. (2009). (Eds.), *Weight gain during pregnancy: Reexamining the guidelines.* Washington, DC: National Academies Press.

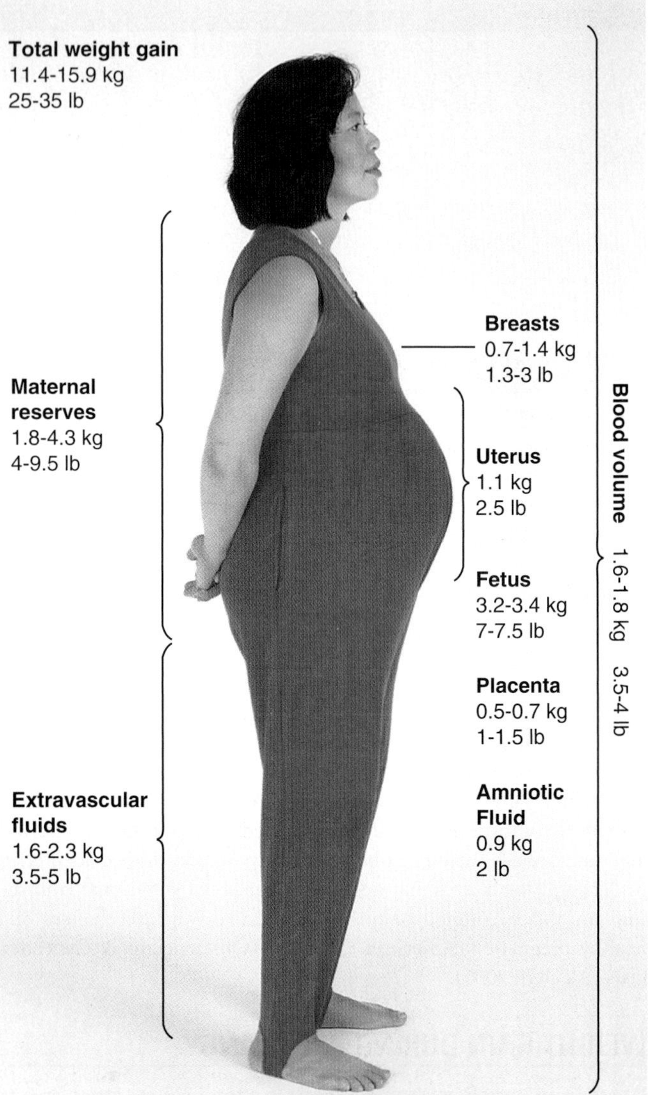


**FIG 14.1** Distribution of weight gain in pregnancy for women of normal prepregnancy weight. The numbers represent a general distribution because variation among women is great. Weight increases with the greatest fluctuation are those attributed to extravascular fluids (edema) and maternal reserves of fat.

### Pattern of Weight Gain

The pattern of weight gain is as important as the total increase. The general recommendation is for an increment of approximately 0.5 to 2 kg (1.1 to 4.4 lb) during the first trimester, when the mother may be nauseated and the fetus needs fewer nutrients for growth. During the rest of the pregnancy, the expected weekly weight gain for women of normal prepregnancy weight is 0.35 to 0.5 kg (0.8 to 1 lb) (ACOG, 2013b; Blackburn, 2013).

### Maternal and Fetal Distribution

Women often wonder why they should gain so much weight when the fetus weighs so little. Explaining the distribution of weight helps them understand this need (Fig. 14.1).

### Factors That Influence Weight Gain

Knowing about factors that may negatively influence nutrient intake and weight gain helps the nurse devise plans for improving nutrition. Women at risk for inadequate weight gain include those who are young, unmarried, low income, poorly educated, in poor general health, or receiving insufficient prenatal care. Multiparas are at higher risk for low weight gain than primiparas. Smoking or substance abuse may interfere with food intake and weight gain (Luke, 2015; Cardwell, 2013).

## NUTRITIONAL REQUIREMENTS DURING PREGNANCY

Nutrient needs increase during pregnancy to meet the demands of the mother and fetus. Usually the increases are not large and are relatively easy to obtain through the diet.

### Dietary Reference Intakes

In the United States, dietary reference intakes (DRIs) refer to terms that estimate nutrient needs. DRIs include four categories:

- Recommended dietary allowance (RDA), the amount of a nutrient that meets the needs of almost all (97% to 98%) healthy people in an age-group. The actual needs of individuals (particularly for calories and protein) may vary according to body size, previous nutritional status, and usual activity level.
- Adequate intake (AI), the nutrient intake assumed to be adequate when an RDA cannot be determined. It appears to sustain nutritional status.
- Tolerable upper intake level (UL), the highest amount of a nutrient that can be taken by most people without probable adverse health effects.
- Estimated average requirement (EAR), the amount of a nutrient estimated to meet the needs of half the healthy people in an age group.

Table 14.2 shows the current recommendations for DRIs for energy, carbohydrates, and protein for adult women.

### Energy

The energy provided by foods for body processes is calculated in kilocalories. Kilocalories (commonly called *calories,* the term used in this book) refers to a unit of heat used to show the energy value of foods.

**TABLE 14.2 Dietary Reference Intakes: Recommended Energy and Protein Intakes**

| Adult Female: Nonpregnant | Pregnancy | Lactation |
|---|---|---|
| **Energy** | | |
| Varies greatly according to body size, age, and physical activity level<br>*Example:*<br>Woman, 30 years, active, height 1.65 m (65 in), weight 50.4 kg (111 lb), body mass index (BMI) 18.5: 2267 kcal<br>Same woman, weight 68 kg (150 lb), BMI 24.99: 2477 kcal | Ages 14-50:First trimester: No change from nonpregnant needs<br>Second trimester: 340 kcal above nonpregnant needs<br>Third trimester: 452 kcal above nonpregnant needs | First 6 mo: 330 kcal above nonpregnant needs (with an additional 170 kcal drawn from maternal stores)<br>Second 6 mo: 400 kcal above nonpregnant needs |
| **Carbohydrate** | | |
| 130 g | 175 g | 210 g |
| **Protein** | | |
| 46 g | 71 g | 71 g |

Data from Institute of Medicine, Food, and Nutrition Board. (2002a). *Dietary reference intakes for energy, carbohydrates, fiber, fat, fatty acids, cholesterol, protein and amino acids (macronutrients)*. Washington, DC: National Academies Press.

Carbohydrates and proteins provide 4 calories/gram, and fats provide 9 calories/gram.

## Carbohydrates

Carbohydrates may be simple or complex. Simple carbohydrates include sucrose (table sugar, candy) and those found in fruits and vegetables. Complex carbohydrates are present in starchy foods such as cereals, pasta, and potatoes. They supply vitamins, minerals, and fiber. Because of their value in providing other nutrients, complex carbohydrates should be the major source of carbohydrates in the diet. Fiber, the indigestible carbohydrate in plant foods, is important because it produces bulk in the diet. Fiber absorbs water and stimulates peristalsis to help prevent constipation. It also slows gastric emptying, causing a sensation of fullness.

## Fats

Fats provide energy and fat-soluble vitamins. When reduction of calories is necessary, it is important to decrease but not eliminate carbohydrates and fats. If carbohydrate and fat intake provides insufficient calories, the body uses protein to meet energy needs. This use decreases the amount of protein available for building and repairing tissue.

Fat intake also is important because it provides essential fatty acids such as alpha linolenic acid and linoleic acid, which are needed for neurologic and visual development of the fetus. Docosahexaenoic acid (DHA) is also important for fetal visual and cognitive development. These fatty acids are found in canola, soybean, and walnut oil, as well as some seafood such as bass or salmon (Gunaratne, Makrides, & Collins, 2015; Ota, Tobe-Gai, Mori, et al., 2012).

## Calories

Approximately 80,000 additional calories are needed over the course of a pregnancy (Cunningham et al., 2010). These extra calories furnish energy for the production and maintenance of the fetus, placenta, added maternal tissues, and increased basal metabolic rate. Most pregnant women need a daily caloric intake of 2200 to 2900 calories depending on their age, activity level, and prepregnancy BMI (ADA, 2008).

During the first trimester of pregnancy, no added calories are needed. However, the daily caloric intake for pregnant women should increase by 340 calories during the second trimester and 452 calories during the third trimester (Institute of Medicine, Food, and Nutrition Board, 2002). This increase can be achieved relatively easily with various foods and only a small increase in food.

Nutrient density (quantity and quality of the various nutrients in each 100 calories of food) is an important consideration. Foods of high nutrient density have large amounts of quality nutrients per serving. During pregnancy, the increased need for most nutrients may not be met unless calories are selected carefully. The term empty *calories* refers to foods that are high in calories but low in other nutrients. Many snack foods contain excessive calories and low nutrient density and are high in fat and sodium. Increased calories should be "spent" on foods that provide the nutrients needed in increased amounts during pregnancy.

Women often use sugar substitutes to reduce their caloric intake. Saccharin (Sweet'N Low), sucralose (Splenda), and aspartame (Equal or NutraSweet) are considered safe for normal women during pregnancy. However, women with phenylketonuria lack the enzyme to metabolize aspartame and should never use it because it could lead to maternal and fetal brain damage (Smit, Lenters, Høyer, et al., 2012).

## Protein

Protein is necessary for metabolism, tissue synthesis, and tissue repair. The daily protein RDA for females is 46 g, depending on their age and size. During the second half of pregnancy, a protein intake of 71 g each day is recommended to expand the blood volume and support the growth of maternal and fetal tissues. This is an increase of 25 g of protein daily (Erick, 2012).

Protein is generally abundant in diets in most industrialized nations, but diets low in caloric intake may also be low in protein. If calories are low and protein is used to provide energy, fetal growth may be impaired.

The nurse should counsel women at risk for poor protein intake about how to determine protein intake and increase food sources. When a woman needs to increase her intake, she should eat more protein-rich foods rather than use high-protein powders or drinks. Protein substitutes lack the other nutrients provided by foods (Piccoli, Clari, Vigotti, et al., 2015).

## Vitamins

For most people, the daily intake of each vitamin is not always as high as recommended, but true deficiency states are uncommon in North America. Recommendations for vitamin intake and food sources are shown in Table 14.3.

The fat-soluble vitamins (A, D, E, and K) are stored in the liver. Deficiency states are not likely to occur, but fat-soluble vitamins can be toxic in excessive amounts. For example, too much vitamin A can cause fetal defects. The nurse should ask about vitamins and medications taken by pregnant women and alert them about the dangers of excess vitamins.

Water-soluble vitamins ($B_6$, $B_{12}$, and C, folic acid, thiamin, riboflavin, and niacin) are not stored in the body as well as fat-soluble vitamins. Therefore, they should be included in the daily diet. Because excess amounts are excreted in the urine, there is less chance of toxicity from excessive intake, but it can occur with megadoses. These vitamins

TABLE 14.3 **Dietary Reference Intakes: Recommendations for Vitamins and Minerals**

| Adult Females: Nonpregnant | Pregnancy and Lactation | Sources | Importance in Pregnancy |
|---|---|---|---|
| **Fat-Soluble Vitamins** | | | |
| ***Vitamin A*** | | | |
| Ages 14-50: 700 mcg (RDA) | *Pregnancy:*<br>Ages 14-18: 750 mcg<br>Ages 19-50: 770 mcg<br>*Lactation:*<br>Ages 14-18: 1200 mcg<br>Ages 19-50: 1300 mcg | Dark green, yellow, or orange vegetables; whole or fortified low-fat or nonfat milk; egg yolk; butter and fortified margarine | Fetal growth and cell differentiation<br>Excessive intake causes spontaneous abortions or serious fetal defects<br>Isotretinoin (Accutane), a vitamin A derivative for acne, should not be taken during pregnancy because it causes fetal defects |
| ***Vitamin D*** | | | |
| Ages 14-50: 400 IU (RDA) | Pregnancy and Lactation:600 IU | Fortified milk, margarine, and soy products; butter; egg yolks<br>Synthesized in skin exposed to sunlight<br>Vegans who are not exposed to sun and who do not eat fortified foods need supplements | Necessary for metabolism of calcium<br>Inadequate amounts may cause neonatal hypocalcemia, hypoplasia of tooth enamel<br>Excessive intake causes hypercalcemia and possible fetal deformities |
| ***Vitamin E*** | | | |
| Ages 14-50: 15 mg (RDA) | *Pregnancy:*<br>Ages 14-50: Same as nonpregnant needs<br>*Lactation:*<br>Ages 14-50: 19 mg (RDA) | Vegetable oils, whole grains, nuts, and dark green leafy vegetables | Antioxidant, important for tissue growth and integrity of cells, particularly red blood cell membranes |
| ***Vitamin K*** | | | |
| Ages 14-18: 75 mcg<br>Ages 19-50: 90 mcg (AI) | *Pregnancy and Lactation:*<br>Same as nonpregnant needs | Dark green leafy vegetables<br>Also produced by normal bacterial flora in small intestine | Necessary for blood clotting<br>Newborns are temporarily deficient and receive one dose by injection at birth to prevent hemorrhage |
| **Water-Soluble Vitamins** | | | |
| ***Vitamin $B_6$ (Pyridoxine)*** | | | |
| Ages 14-18: 1.2 mg<br>Ages 19-50: 1.3 mg (RDA) | Pregnancy:<br>Ages 14-50: 1.9 mg<br>Lactation:<br>Ages 14-50: 2 mg (RDA) | Chicken, fish, pork, eggs, peanuts, whole grains, cereals | Amino acid metabolism and in blood, hormone, and immune function |
| ***Vitamin $B_{12}$*** | | | |
| Ages 14-50: 2.4 mcg (RDA) | *Pregnancy:*<br>Ages 14-50: 2.6 mcg<br>*Lactation:*<br>Ages 14-50: 2.8 mcg (RDA) | Meat, fish, eggs, milk, fortified soy and cereal products | Cell division, protein synthesis, and formation of red blood cells<br>Prevents megaloblastic anemia |
| ***Folic Acid*** | | | |
| Ages 14-50: 400 mcg (RDA) | *Pregnancy:*<br>Ages 14-50: 600 mcg<br>*Lactation:*<br>Ages 14-50: 500 mcg (RDA) | Dark green leafy vegetables, legumes (beans, peanuts), orange juice, asparagus, spinach, and fortified cereal and pasta<br>May be lost in cooking | Cell replication and amino acid and hemoglobin synthesis<br>Deficiency in first weeks of pregnancy may cause cleft lip or palate, neural tube and cardiac defects |
| ***Thiamin*** | | | |
| Ages 14-18: 1 mg<br>Ages 19-50: 1.1 mg (RDA) | *Pregnancy and Lactation:*<br>Ages 14-50: 1.4 mg (RDA) | Lean pork, whole or enriched grain products, legumes, organ meats, seeds, nuts | Forms coenzymes necessary to release energy, aids in nerve and muscle functioning. Increased need in pregnancy due to greater intake of calories |
| ***Riboflavin*** | | | |
| Ages 14-18: 1 mg<br>Ages 19-50: 1.1 mg (RDA) | *Pregnancy:*<br>Ages 14-50: 1.4 mg<br>*Lactation:*<br>Ages 14-50: 1.6 mg (RDA) | Milk, meat, fish, poultry, eggs, enriched grain products, and dark green vegetables | Forms coenzymes necessary to release energy<br>Increased need in pregnancy due to greater intake of calories |

**TABLE 14.3 Dietary Reference Intakes: Recommendations for Vitamins and Minerals—cont'd**

| Adult Females: Nonpregnant | Pregnancy and Lactation | Sources | Importance in Pregnancy |
|---|---|---|---|
| ***Niacin*** | | | |
| Ages 14-50: 14 mg (RDA) | *Pregnancy:*<br>Ages 14-50: 18 mg<br>*Lactation:*<br>Ages 14-50: 17 mg (RDA) | Meats, fish, poultry, legumes, enriched grains, milk | Forms coenzymes necessary to release energy<br>Increased need in pregnancy due to greater intake of calories |
| ***Vitamin C*** | | | |
| Ages 14-18: 65 mg<br>Ages 19-50: 75 mg (RDA) | *Pregnancy:*<br>Ages 14-18: 80 mg<br>Ages 19-50: 85 mg<br>*Lactation:*<br>Ages 14-18: 115 mg<br>Ages 19-50: 120 mg (RDA) | Citrus fruit, peppers, strawberries, cantaloupe, green leafy vegetables, tomatoes, potatoes | Formation of fetal tissue, collagen formation, tissue integrity, healing, immune response, and metabolism |
| **Minerals** | | | |
| ***Iron*** | | | |
| Ages 14-18: 15 mg<br>Ages 19-50: 18 mg (RDA) | *Pregnancy:*<br>Ages 14–50: 27 mg<br>*Lactation:*<br>Ages 14–18: 10 mg<br>Ages 19–50: 9 mg (RDA) | Meats, dark green leafy vegetables, eggs, grain products, enriched bread and cereal, dried fruits, tofu, legumes, nuts, blackstrap molasses | Formation of hemoglobin and enzymes for metabolism<br>Expanded maternal blood volume, formation of fetal red blood cells, and storage in the fetal liver for use after birth |
| ***Calcium*** | | | |
| Ages 14-18: 1300 mg<br>Ages 19-50: 1000 mg (AI) | *Pregnancy and Lactation:*<br>Same as nonpregnant needs | Dairy products, salmon, sardines with bones, legumes, fortified juice, tofu, broccoli | Fetal bone and teeth formation, cell membrane permeability, coagulation, and neuromuscular function |
| ***Zinc*** | | | |
| Ages 14-18: 9 mg<br>Ages 19-50: 8 mg (RDA) | *Pregnancy:*<br>Ages 14-18: 12 mg<br>Ages 19-50: 11 mg<br>*Lactation:*<br>Ages 14-18: 13 mg<br>Ages 19-50: 12 mg (RDA) | Meat, poultry, seafood, eggs, nuts, seeds, legumes, wheat germ, whole grains, yogurt | Fetal and maternal tissue growth, cell differentiation and reproduction, DNA and RNA synthesis, metabolism, acid-base balance |
| ***Magnesium*** | | | |
| Ages 14-18: 360 mg<br>Ages 19-30: 310 mg<br>Ages 31-50: 320 mg (RDA) | *Pregnancy:*<br>Ages 14-18: 400 mg<br>Ages 19-30: 350 mg<br>Ages 31-50: 360 mg<br>*Lactation:*<br>Same as nonpregnant needs | Whole grains, nuts, legumes, dark green vegetables, small amounts in many foods | Cell growth and neuromuscular function; activates enzymes for metabolism of protein and energy |
| ***Iodine*** | | | |
| Ages 14-50: 150 mcg (RDA) | *Pregnancy:*<br>Ages 14-50: 220 mcg<br>*Lactation:*<br>Ages 14-50: 290 mcg (RDA) | Seafood, iodized salt | Important in thyroid function<br>Deficiency may cause abortion, stillbirth, congenital hypothyroidism, neurologic conditions |

*AI*, Adequate intake; *DNA*, deoxyribonucleic acid; *RDA*, recommended daily allowance; *RNA*, ribonucleic acid.
Dietary reference intakes are listed as RDA or AI.
Data from Institute of Medicine (IOM), Food and Nutrition Board (FNB). (1997). *Dietary reference intakes for calcium, phosphorus, magnesium, vitamin D, and fluoride*. Washington, DC: National Academies Press; IOM, FNB. (1998). *Dietary reference intakes for thiamin, riboflavin, niacin, vitamin $B_6$, folate, vitamin $B_{12}$, pantothenic acid, biotin, and choline*. Washington, DC: National Academies Press; IOM, FNB. (2000). *Dietary reference intakes for vitamin C, vitamin E, selenium, and carotenoids*. Washington, DC: National Academies Press; IOM, FNB. (2001). *Dietary reference intakes for vitamin A, vitamin K, arsenic, boron, chromium, copper, iodine, iron, manganese, molybdenum, nickel, silicon, vanadium, and zinc*. Washington, DC: National Academies Press; IOM, FNB. (2011). *Dietary reference intakes for calcium and vitamin D*. Washington, DC: National Academies Press.

are easily transferred from food to water in cooking. Foods should be steamed, microwaved, or prepared in only small amounts of water. The remaining water can be used in other dishes, such as soups.

## Folic Acid

Folic acid (also called *folate*) can decrease the occurrence of neural tube defects, such as spina bifida and anencephaly, in newborns. It may also help prevent cleft lip, cleft palate, and some heart defects (CDC, 2015; Peckenpaugh, 2010). Adequate intake of folic acid is especially important just before conception and during the first trimester of pregnancy. Because approximately half of pregnancies are unplanned, all women of childbearing age should consume adequate amounts of folic acid each day. A *Healthy People 2020* goal is for women of childbearing potential to take in at least 400 mcg of folic acid each day (U.S. Department of Health and Human Services, 2010).

In the past, the recommended amount of folic acid for women capable of childbearing has been 400 mcg (0.4 mg), but the U.S. Preventive Services Task Force (USPSTF) now recommends 400 mcg to 800 mcg (0.4 mg to 0.8 mg) each day. The dose should be taken for at least 1 month before and for 2 to 3 months after conception (USPSTF, 2009). There has been no change in the recommendation of 600 mcg (0.6 mg) of folic acid daily for the rest of pregnancy.

Women who are taking anticonvulsant drugs or who have previously had an infant born with a neural tube defect should take 4 mg daily before conception and during the first trimester (CDC, 2010; Johnson, Gregory, & Niebyl, 2007). This practice can decrease the risk of recurrence of neural tube defects by 80% (American Academy of Pediatrics [AAP] & American College of Obstetricians and Gynecologists [ACOG], 2013).

Women often do not realize the importance of folic acid in their diet before pregnancy begins, and many do not meet the recommended level, in spite of a national campaign to make the public more aware of this problem. One third of births occur to women aged 18 to 24 years, but women in this group have lower intake of supplements containing folic acid and less knowledge of the need for folic acid than older women (CDC, 2008). More education is necessary to increase folic acid use in women of childbearing age. Because of its importance, folic acid is added to all enriched cereal grain products.

## Minerals

Most minerals are supplied in adequate amounts in normal diets. However, dietary intake of iron and calcium may be below recommended levels in women of childbearing age (Grodner, Roth, & Walkingshaw, 2012). Recommendations for mineral intake and food sources are shown in Table 14.3.

### Iron

Approximately 1000 mg of absorbed iron is needed during pregnancy (Cunningham et al., 2010). This provides for the 20% to 30% increase in maternal red blood cells and for fetal iron storage and production of red blood cells. Infants use stored iron during the first 4 to 6 months, when their intake of iron is low. Iron is probably the only nutrient that cannot be supplied completely and easily from the diet during pregnancy. Table 14.4 lists common foods high in iron (Blackburn, 2013; Christian & Black, 2012).

Many adult women do not meet their daily nonpregnancy requirement for iron and begin pregnancy already anemic or with low iron stores (see Chapter 26). Women often have only 100 mg of nonhemoglobin iron stored at the beginning of pregnancy (Hall, 2015). Iron is transferred to the fetus even if the mother is anemic, so adequate intake is necessary to keep the mother's iron supply at normal levels (Cunningham et al., 2010).

**TABLE 14.4 Foods High in Iron**

| Food and Amount | Average Amounts of Iron Supplied (mg) |
|---|---|
| ***Meats and Fish (3 Oz)*** | |
| Beef, lean chuck | 3.1 |
| Beef, ground 15% fat | 2.2 |
| Chicken, dark meat | 1.3 |
| Tuna, light in water | 1.3 |
| ***Legumes (½ C)*** | |
| Kidney beans, dried and cooked | 2.6 |
| Lentils, dried, cooked | 3.3 |
| Chickpeas (garbanzo beans), canned | 1.6 |
| Soybeans, cooked | 4.4 |
| Tofu, firm ¼ block | 1.3 |
| ***Grains*** | |
| Bread, wheat (1 slice) | 0.9 |
| Rice, white enriched, cooked (1 c) | 3.2 |
| Total Raisin Bran cereal (¾ c) | 13.5 |
| ***Fruits*** | |
| Prune juice (8 oz) | 3 |
| Raisins (⅔ c) | 1.8 |
| ***Vegetables*** | |
| Potato, baked with skin, (1 med) | 2.2 |
| Sweet potatoes, canned, (1 c) | 2.8 |
| Tomatoes, canned and stewed (1 c) | 3.4 |
| Peas, green, cooked (1 c) | 2.4 |

The Recommended Dietary Allowance (RDA) for iron during pregnancy is 27 mg. Although many women take supplements because they do not eat enough iron-containing foods in their daily diet to meet this need, iron in foods is often better absorbed. Therefore, the nurse should suggest ways a woman can increase her dietary iron.
Data from United States Department of Agriculture. (2011). *USDA national nutrient database for standard reference.* Retrieved from http://www.ars.usda.gov/Services/docs.htm?docid=20958.

Iron is present in many foods, but in small amounts. Approximately 25% of iron from animal sources (called **heme iron**) is absorbed. Only approximately 5% of **nonheme iron** (iron from plant sources and fortified foods) is absorbed. Absorption of iron is affected by intake of other substances. Calcium and phosphorus in milk and tannin in tea decrease iron absorption from nonheme iron if they are consumed during the same meal. Coffee binds iron, preventing it from being fully absorbed. Antacids, phytates (in grains and vegetables), oxalic acid (in spinach), and ethylenediaminetetraacetic acid (EDTA, a food additive) also decrease absorption. Foods cooked in iron pans contain more iron. Foods containing ascorbic acid and meat, fish, or poultry eaten with nonheme-iron–containing foods may increase absorption (Rabel, Leitman, & Miller, 2015; Gallagher, 2012).

Because of the difficulty of obtaining enough iron in the diet, healthcare providers often prescribe iron supplements of 30 mg/day during pregnancy. Women who are anemic may need 60 to 120 mg/day. Women who take high doses of iron also need zinc and copper supplements because iron interferes with the absorption and use of these minerals. Supplementation may begin during the second trimester, when the need increases and morning sickness has usually ended (Cantor et al., 2015; Christian & Black, 2012; Ota et al., 2012).

Iron taken between meals is absorbed more completely, but many women find the side effects worse when iron is taken without food. Side effects occur more often with higher doses and include nausea, vomiting, heartburn, epigastric pain, constipation, diarrhea, and black stools. Taking iron at bedtime may make it easier to tolerate. For best absorption, it should be taken with water or juice but not with coffee, tea, or milk.

Women should be reminded to keep iron, like all other medicines, out of the reach of children. Accidental overdose with iron is a leading cause of childhood poisoning.

### Calcium

Calcium is transferred to the fetus, especially in the last trimester, and is important for mineralization of fetal bones and teeth. Although a small amount of calcium is removed from the mother's bones, it is insignificant and does not affect maternal bone mass. A common myth is that calcium is removed from the teeth during pregnancy, leading to excessive decay. Actually, calcium in the teeth is stable and is not affected by pregnancy.

Calcium absorption and retention increases during pregnancy and is stored for use in the third trimester when fetal needs are greatest. Women 18 years and younger need more calcium because their bone density is not complete. Calcium needs are unchanged during pregnancy and lactation.

The best source of calcium is dairy products. Whole, low-fat, and nonfat milk all contain the same amount of calcium and may be used interchangeably to increase or reduce calorie intake. However, women with **lactose intolerance** (lactase deficiency resulting in gastrointestinal problems when dairy products are consumed) need other sources of calcium (Box 14.1).

Although spinach and chard contain calcium, they also contain oxalates that decrease calcium availability and make them poor sources. Large amounts of fiber also interfere with calcium absorption. Caffeine increases the excretion of calcium.

Women who eat inadequate amounts of calcium-rich foods or avoid dairy products because of lactose intolerance, to avoid eating animal products, or for other reasons should take supplements. To ensure absorption of calcium, women should take supplements with meals, separately from iron supplements. Taking calcium with vitamin D also increases absorption (ACOG, 2011).

### Sodium

The need for sodium increases during pregnancy to provide for the expanded blood volume and the needs of the fetus. Although sodium is not restricted during pregnancy, excessive amounts should be avoided. Women are advised that a moderate intake of salt or the salting of foods to taste is acceptable, but that intake of high-sodium foods (Box 14.2) should be limited.

## Nutritional Supplementation

### Purpose

Food is the best source of nutrients. Although healthcare providers frequently prescribe prenatal vitamin-mineral supplements and many women expect to take them, supplementation may not be necessary during pregnancy if the diet is adequate. The exceptions are iron and folic acid, which may not be obtained in adequate amounts through normal food intake. Expectant mothers who are vegetarians, lactose intolerant, or have special problems in obtaining nutrients through diet alone may need supplements. Assessment of each woman's needs determines whether supplementation is appropriate (ADA, 2008).

### Disadvantages and Dangers of Nutritional Supplementation

The belief that supplements are a harmless way to improve their diets motivates some women to take large amounts without consulting a healthcare provider. No standardization or regulation of the amounts of ingredients contained in supplements is available at this time. Some supplements may not contain the amount of an ingredient listed on the label and may not fulfill the health claims made.

The use of supplements can increase the intake of some nutrients to doses much higher than recommended. Excessive amounts of some vitamins and minerals may be toxic to the fetus. Vitamin A can cause fetal anomalies when taken in high doses. Large amounts of vitamin A are taken by women using the drug isotretinoin (Accutane) for acne. In addition, high doses of some vitamins or minerals may interfere with the use of others. If women understand this, they are more likely not to exceed recommended doses (IOM, 2001; IOM, 2000; IOM, 1997).

#### BOX 14.1 Calcium Sources Approximately Equivalent to 1 Cup of Milk

- ¾ c yogurt, fruit, low fat
- 1½ oz cheddar cheese
- 1¼ c cottage cheese
- 4 oz almonds
- 3¾ c dried pinto beans, cooked
- 2 c cereal, Cheerios
- 3 packets instant oatmeal
- 3 English muffins
- 1 c collard greens, cooked
- 5 oz canned salmon with bones
- 3 oz canned sardines
- ½ block tofu made with calcium sulfate and magnesium chloride

This list can be used to counsel women who are vegans or lactose intolerant. Lactose-intolerant women can often eat small amounts of yogurt and cheese without distress. Although the amounts of some foods listed are more than would be likely to be eaten within a day, they serve for comparison.

Data from United States Department of Agriculture. (2011). *USDA national nutrient database for standard reference.* Retrieved from http://www.ars.usda.gov/Services/docs.htm?docid=20958.

#### BOX 14.2 Foods High in Sodium

- Products that contain the word "salt," "soda," or "sodium," such as table salt, seasoning salt, monosodium glutamate, bicarbonate of soda (baking soda)
- Foods that taste salty, including snack foods like popcorn, potato chips, pretzels, crackers
- Condiments and relishes, such as catsup, horseradish, mustard, soy sauce, bouillon, pickles, green and black olives
- Smoked, dried, or processed foods, such as ham, bacon, lunch meats, corned beef
- Canned soups, meats, and vegetables unless label states low in sodium
- Packaged mixes for sauces, gravies, cakes and other baked foods
- Canned tomato and vegetable juices

During pregnancy, foods high in sodium should be consumed in moderation. Expectant mothers should be taught to read labels and to avoid products in which sodium is listed among the first ingredients.

**TABLE 14.5 Food Plan for Pregnancy and Lactation**

| Food (Equivalent of 1 Oz or 1 Cup) | Recommended Intake for Pregnancy* | Recommended Intake for Lactation† |
|---|---|---|
| Whole grains (1 oz = 1 slice bread, ½ c rice or pasta) | 7-9 oz | 7 oz |
| Vegetables | 3-3½ c | 3 c |
| Fruits | 2 c | 2 c |
| Milk group (1 c milk or yogurt, 1½ oz cheese) | 3 c | 3 c |
| Meat/Beans (1 oz meat/poultry/fish, 1 egg, ¼ c dried beans [cooked], 1 tbsp peanut butter) | 6-6½ oz | 6 oz |

Data from http://www.choosemyplate.gov

*Example is for a woman 5 feet, 4 in tall and weighing 125 lb before pregnancy. Specific food plans for other women can be found at http://www.choosemyplate.gov.

†Amounts are for exclusive breastfeeding. If formula is also being used, 1 oz less of grains, ½ c less of vegetables, and ½ oz less of meat/beans is recommended.

**PATIENT-CENTERED TEACHING**

***Vitamins and Minerals***

Take only vitamin and mineral supplements prescribed by your healthcare provider. Ask your provider about over-the-counter supplements because they may not be formulated to meet your individual needs and could be harmful to you and your baby.

Take iron between meals, if possible. If you have nausea, heartburn, constipation, or diarrhea, try taking your iron at bedtime or with meals or a snack. Taking it with orange juice or another source of vitamin C may increase absorption. Do not take iron with calcium supplements, milk, tea, or coffee because these substances decrease its absorption.

Keep all vitamin and mineral supplements away from children because they may cause accidental poisoning.

### Water

Water is important during pregnancy for the expanded blood volume and as part of the increased maternal and fetal tissues. Women should drink approximately 8 to 10 cups of fluids each day, with water constituting most of the fluid intake. Fluids low in nutrients should be limited because they are filling and replace other, more nutritious, foods and drinks (Bond, 2011).

### Food Plan

The U.S. Department of Agriculture (USDA) has developed MyPlate, a food plan that provides a guide for healthy eating for adults and children. Guidelines for pregnancy and lactation are discussed below and are summarized in Table 14.5. Pregnant or lactating women can go to the website http://www.choosemyplate.gov to get an individualized diet plan specifically adapted for them and their needs during pregnancy.

#### Whole Grains

Breads, cereals, rice, and pastas provide complex carbohydrates, fiber, vitamins, and minerals. Whole grains provide more nutrients than do processed grain products. MyPlate recommendations are for 6 oz each day for adult women. Pregnant women should have 7 to 9 oz and lactating women should have 6 to 7 oz daily.

#### Vegetables and Fruits

The daily recommendation for vegetables in healthy adult women is 2.5 cups, 3 to 3½ cups for pregnancy, and 2½ to 3 cups for lactation. While 1.5 to 2 cups of fruits are recommended daily for adult women, those who are pregnant or lactating should have 2 cups daily. A wide range of fruits and vegetables provides the best nutrition. Dark green and orange or dark yellow vegetables are especially nutritious.

#### Dairy Group

The dairy group includes foods such as milk, yogurt, and cheese, which contain approximately the same nutrient values whether they are whole (4% fat), low fat (2% fat), or nonfat (skim); however, the calories and fat are less in the latter two forms. The milk group is an especially good source of calcium. Adult women and those who are pregnant or lactating need 3 cups or the equivalent from this group each day.

#### Protein Group

Many adults think of meat, poultry, fish, and eggs as the only sources of protein, but legumes (beans, peas, and lentils), nuts, and soybean products such as tofu also are good sources. Adult women should consume 5 to 5½ oz of foods from this group each day. Pregnant women need 6 to 6½ oz daily, and lactating women need 5½ to 6 oz daily. A typical serving of meat, fish, or poultry varies in size. A 3 oz portion is approximately the size of a deck of playing cards.

#### Other Elements

Fats, oils, and concentrated sugars should be eaten sparingly, as they provide calories for energy but few other nutrients. Adult women need 5 to 6 teaspoons of unsaturated fats daily, while pregnant women need 6 to 8 teaspoons and lactating women need 6 teaspoons daily. Foods containing saturated fats and *trans* fatty acids should be avoided.

## FOOD PRECAUTIONS

Although fish are an excellent source of protein and other nutrients, certain precautions should be taken. Large fish often have high levels of mercury, which can damage the fetal central nervous system. Pregnant and lactating women should not eat these fish. Certain fish have smaller amounts of mercury and can be eaten weekly. Raw fish may contain parasites or bacteria and should be avoided (Robinson, Baird, & Godfrey, 2014; Erick, 2012).

Some foods may be contaminated with *Listeria monocytogenes*, the agent that causes listeriosis. If contracted during pregnancy, listeriosis may result in abortion, premature labor, infant death, or severe illness in the newborn. Foods that are more likely to be contaminated include luncheon meats and hot dogs unless reheated until steaming hot. Other foods include soft cheeses, unpasteurized milk or milk products, and raw or undercooked meats and poultry (FDA, 2009b). (See Safety Alert.) More information about food safety during pregnancy can be obtained from the FDA website at http://www.fda.gov/Food/ResourcesForYou/HealthEducators/ucm081819.htm.

Eggs can be contaminated with harmful bacteria and should not be eaten unless fully cooked. Only eggs that have been pasteurized in the shell are safe to eat raw or partially cooked. Eating meat that is raw or undercooked or unwashed fruits or vegetables may cause toxoplasmosis, with severe consequences to the fetus. Toxoplasmosis may also be contracted by contact with cat feces.

## SAFETY ALERT

### *Food Safety During Pregnancy and Lactation*

- Do not eat shark, swordfish, king mackerel, or tilefish.
- Eat up to 6 oz canned albacore weekly.
- Eat up to 12 oz shrimp, canned light tuna, salmon, pollack, and catfish each week.
- Do not eat raw or undercooked fish, meat, poultry, or eggs.
- Avoid luncheon meats and hot dogs unless reheated until steaming hot.
- Avoid soft cheeses (brie, feta, blue cheese, Camembert, blue-veined cheeses, queso blanco, queso fresco, queso panela) unless made with pasteurized milk.
- Do not consume refrigerated pâté or meat spreads, refrigerated smoked seafood, raw or undercooked eggs or meat, or raw (unpasteurized) milk or milk products.

## FACTORS THAT INFLUENCE NUTRITION

The nurse must consider age, knowledge of nutrition, exercise, and cultural background when counseling women about their diets.

### Age

Age is an important consideration. The adolescent who is not fully mature needs nutritional support for her own growth. However, older women who are in good health have the same nutritional requirements as younger (nonadolescent) pregnant women (Black, 2013; Christian & Black, 2012).

### Nutritional Knowledge

Once pregnancy is confirmed, women often become interested in the relationship between what they eat and the effect on the fetus. Some lack basic understanding about nutrition and have misconceptions based on common food myths. They may seek information from books, magazines, television, and the Internet. They benefit from help from nurses in learning about nutrition.

### Exercise

Moderate daily exercise during pregnancy is encouraged. Women who exercise more strenuously or are athletes may need modifications of their diet to meet increased nutritional needs. Extra calories may be needed to make up for the energy used during exercise. A serving of fruit, yogurt, or pasta before and after exercise may be sufficient. Additional fluids should be taken during and after exercise as well (ACOG, 2002).

### Culture

Foods may have special cultural meanings during pregnancy or childbirth. Nurses need knowledge of the habits of various cultures so they can provide culturally appropriate nutrition counseling. Before making assumptions about the influence of a woman's culture on her diet, the nurse must assess each woman individually. Not all women follow food practices considered typical for their cultures (Callister, 2013; Galanti, 2008).

The nurse should assess the woman's age, how long she has lived in North America, and whether she has adopted any common American eating habits. Some women who usually follow an American diet may return to some aspects of their culture's traditional diet during pregnancy out of respect for elders or to "make sure" they do not harm the fetus (Callister, 2013; Galanti, 2008).

Nurses often use pamphlets as a part of teaching and may be able to obtain them in various languages.

The nurse should determine if the woman can read English or her own native language before giving her written materials. People who cannot read may not readily admit it to others. In addition, the reading level of the materials may be too complicated for the woman with little education. Having an interpreter discuss the material with the woman helps determine how well she can read and aids in other teaching.

People of many cultures believe that certain foods, conditions, and medicines are "hot" or "cold" and must be balanced to preserve health. Foods considered hot in one culture may not fit in that category in another culture, and the designation does not necessarily match the temperature or spiciness of the food. In the Chinese culture, this concept may be referred to as yin (cold) and yang (hot) and may influence what the mother eats during pregnancy and the postpartum period (Callister, 2013; Galanti, 2008).

Food taboos may determine what some women eat during the childbearing period. For example, Korean women may avoid eggs and duck because these foods are thought to have a harmful effect on the fetus. Samoan women do not eat octopus or raw fish during pregnancy. Haitian women believe eating white foods such as milk, white beans, and lobster after birth will increase the lochia. Special foods may be customary during pregnancy or after birth. A Korean family may bring the new mother a hot beef and seaweed soup to cleanse her body and increase breast milk production (Callister, 2013).

Great variety occurs in cultural preferences for foods. For example, some African-Americans may follow a diet similar to that of people living in the southeastern United States. Common foods include okra, collard greens, mustard greens, ham hocks, black-eyed peas, and hominy or grits. However, the diet of other African-Americans varies according to the geographic area in which they live. Lactose intolerance is common, resulting in lack of calcium if other sources are not present in the diet. Intake of high-sodium and fried foods may present health problems.

Some Jewish women follow a strict kosher diet. They avoid meat from animals with cloven hooves that do not chew their cud (no pork or pork products). Meat must be processed to remove all blood and cannot be eaten in the same meal as milk. Muslim women also do not eat pork and may fast on certain days. The religion exempts pregnant and nursing women from obligatory fasting, but women have to make up the fasting days at some other time. Some choose to fast for spiritual reasons or so they do not have to make up the days later (Callister, 2013).

The diet of Native American women may contain blue cornbread, potatoes, wild greens, legumes, nuts, tomatoes, and squash. Lactose intolerance is common, and milk and cheese are avoided. Meats may include wild game and poultry. Most foods are fried in lard or shortening (Callister, 2013).

Food preferences for two cultures, Southeast Asian and Hispanic, are explored further here to show the influence of culture on diet. Immigrants from Southeast Asia are likely to follow diets similar to those in their homelands. Hispanics are a large minority group in the United States, and nurses throughout the United States need information about food preferences prevalent in these groups.

#### Southeast Asian Dietary Practices

Southeast Asians include those from Cambodia, Laos, and Vietnam. Traditional cooking in these countries includes searing fresh vegetables quickly with small portions of meat, poultry, or fish in a little oil over high heat. Meals cooked in this manner are low in fat and retain vitamins. Most meals are accompanied by rice, which increases the intake of complex carbohydrates. A salty fish sauce called *nuoc mam* and fresh vegetables are also part of most meals (Stauffer, 2008). Tofu and fresh fruits are frequent additions.

Many Southeast Asians have added American foods to their diets. The addition of more eggs, beef, pork, and bread has increased nutrients but also fat to the diet. Coffee, candy, soft drinks, butter or margarine, and fast foods have been less favorable influences because they are low in nutrients but high in sugar or fat.

***Effect of culture on diet during childbearing.*** Pregnancy, especially the third trimester, is considered "hot," in Southeast Asian cultures; pregnant women eat "cold" foods to maintain a balance of hot and cold. Their diet includes sour foods, fruits, noodles, spinach, and mung beans but avoids fish, excessively salty or spicy foods, alcohol, and rice. The woman also avoids unfamiliar foods for fear that they may harm her or her fetus.

The postpartum period is considered "cold," partly because of the loss of blood, which is "hot." Mothers avoid losing more heat, which would have ill effects on their health. They stay warm physically and choose "hot" foods to eat, including rice with fish sauce, broth, salty meats, fish, chicken, and eggs. They may refuse cold drinks but welcome hot fluids, often requesting tea or plain hot water. Families frequently bring food to the mother while she is in the hospital because hospital food may not meet her preferences.

***Increasing nutrients with traditional foods.*** Milk products are not a large part of the traditional Southeast Asian diet, and lactose intolerance is common. Soy milk may be used instead. Some Vietnamese can tolerate dairy products in small amounts. However, increasing the intake of commonly used dark green leafy vegetables, such as mustard greens, bok choy, and broccoli, increases calcium, iron, magnesium, and folic acid intake. Tofu is a good source of calcium and iron. A broth made from pork or chicken bones soaked in vinegar (which removes calcium from the bones) is frequently served. If the mother avoids fortified milk, she may need vitamin D supplementation. Increasing the intake of meats and poultry elevates levels of vitamin $B_6$ and zinc.

### Hispanic Dietary Practices

Spanish-speaking people, such as Mexican-Americans, Puerto Ricans, and Cuban-Americans, are often referred to as *Hispanics* or *Latinos*. Like Asians, many Hispanics follow the theories of "hot" and "cold" foods and conditions. They also consider pregnancy to be "hot" and the postpartum period to be "cold" and adjust the diet accordingly. Hispanic women may not take prescribed prenatal vitamins or iron because they are considered "hot" or may take a "cold" food such as fruit juice to neutralize the effect (Callister, 2013).

Hispanic foods are often hot, spicy, and frequently fried. The diet is high in fiber and complex carbohydrates but may also be high in calories and fat. Dried beans (especially pinto beans) are a staple of the Mexican-American diet and are part of most meals, served alone, as refried beans, or mixed with other foods, such as rice. The major grain is corn, which is ground and made into a dough called *masa* to make corn tortillas, a good source of calcium. Corn or flour tortillas are eaten with most meals. Rice is also an important grain. Many Hispanics are lactose intolerant, but cheese is part of many dishes. Chili peppers and tomatoes are the most common vegetables used. Green leafy and yellow vegetables are seldom included.

Puerto Ricans and Cubans may add tropical fruits and vegetables common in the homeland, when available. *Viandas* (starchy fruits and vegetables such as plantain, green bananas, sweet potatoes, yams, and breadfruit) are common. They are sometimes cooked with codfish and onion. Guava, papaya, mango, and eggplant also are used when available.

## NUTRITIONAL RISK FACTORS

The nurse must identify risk factors that may interfere with a woman's ability to meet the nutritional needs of pregnancy.

### Socioeconomic Status

#### Poverty

Low-income women may have deficient diets because of lack of financial resources and education regarding nutrition. Carbohydrate-rich foods are often less expensive than others, resulting in a diet high in calories but low in vitamins and minerals. A referral to Temporary Assistance for Needy Families (TANF) or WIC may be helpful if the woman's food intake is inadequate because of lack of money. Vitamin and mineral supplementation may be important for the woman, especially if her diet is inconsistent.

#### Food Supplement Programs

The WIC program is administered by the USDA to provide nutritional assessment, counseling, and education to low-income women and children up to age 5 years who are at nutritional risk. The program also provides food vouchers for foods such as milk, cheese, eggs, tofu, whole grain bread (or brown rice or tortillas), whole grain cereal, fruit juice, dried or canned legumes, peanut butter, fruits, vegetables, and formula to qualified women and their children. Eligibility is based on an income of 185% of the federal poverty level or less. Women are eligible throughout pregnancy and for 6 months after birth if formula feeding or 1 year if breastfeeding. Children at risk for poor nutrition may be eligible until 5 years of age. Further information is available at http://www.fns.usda.gov/wic.

### Adolescence

Adolescent pregnancies are associated with higher risk for complications for both the expectant mother and the fetus (see Chapter 24). Pregnant adolescents who are the youngest in terms of gynecologic age (number of years since menarche) and those who are undernourished at conception have the greatest nutritional needs (Stang & Larson, 2012).

However, excessive weight gain during pregnancy should be avoided by adolescents as well as by adult women. Women who gain weight above the recommendations may have difficulty losing the weight and may become overweight or obese.

#### Nutrient Needs

The DRIs for nutrients needed by pregnant adolescents are the same as those for older women for most nutrients. They need more calcium, magnesium, phosphorus, and zinc to meet their own growth needs. Assessment of gynecologic age, nutritional status, and daily diet may indicate the need for added increases in some areas for individual adolescents.

#### Common Problems

The diets of teenagers before and during pregnancy are often low in vitamins A, $B_6$, and C, folic acid, calcium, iron, zinc, and magnesium. Supplements may be prescribed, but the adolescent may not take them regularly. This combination of poor intake and unreliable supplementation may further deplete nutrient stores and general nutritional status. Peer pressure is an important influence on nutritional status. Adolescents are often concerned about their body image (Stang & Larson, 2012). If weight is a major focus for a teenager and her peers, she may restrict calories to prevent weight gain during pregnancy. Teenagers tend to skip meals, especially breakfast. The fetus requires a steady supply of nutrients, and the

## NURSING CARE PLAN

### *Nutrition for the Pregnant Adolescent*

**Focused Assessment**

Patty, age 15, is 21 weeks pregnant and has gained 3.2 kg (7 lb). Her 24-hour diet history shows areas of deficiency and many food dislikes. She skips breakfast and eats from snack machines and fast-food restaurants for lunch and after school. She says she is disgusted with how heavy she is and wants to go on a diet to lose some weight. Her hemoglobin is 10.4 g/dL. She appears interested in nutrition, and her statements show concern about her baby's needs. Her weight was normal before her pregnancy, and a total weight gain of 11.5 to 16 kg (25-35 lb) is appropriate for her.

**Nursing Diagnosis**

Imbalanced Nutrition: Less Than Body Requirements related to concern about weight gain and diet choices inadequate to meet nutrient requirements of adolescent pregnancy.

**Planning**

***Expected Outcomes***

Patti will:

Explain the weight gain and amount of food from each food group recommended for pregnancy by the end of the visit.

Gain approximately 0.35 to 0.5 kg (0.8-1 lb) a week for the rest of her pregnancy and 11.5 to 16 kg (25-35 lb) by the end of pregnancy.

Attain a hemoglobin level of 11 g/dL or greater by the third trimester of pregnancy.

**Interventions and *Rationales***

1. Praise Patti for her interest in nutrition and her concern about gaining too much weight.
   *Praise helps foster rapport and may focus attention on learning.*
2. Discuss the reasons for appropriate weight gain during pregnancy and its effect on the fetus.
   *Adolescents may not understand how diet affects the fetus and themselves.*
3. Increase Patti's involvement in learning by helping her compare her food intake with that recommended from each food group. Point out areas of strength and praise her.
   *This will provide positive reinforcement.*
4. Ask Patti what problems she sees in her diet. Point out areas she may have missed. Explain the effect that lack of specific nutrients may have on the fetus.
   *Adolescents learn best when they see how the material applies to them.*
5. Discuss the high caloric intake of fast foods in relation to her present diet. Discuss "spending calories" to "buy" nutrients needed during pregnancy.
   *This increases understanding by relating concepts already understood to new information.*
6. From Patti's food preferences, determine foods suitable to meet her nutrient needs. Point out fruits and vegetables high in vitamins A and C yet low in calories.
   *Compliance is increased if the recommended diet is individualized to meet a woman's likes and dislikes.*
7. Suggest nutritional foods that Patti could choose at fast-food restaurants or from snack machines, and ask which ones are acceptable to her.
   *The ability to eat nutritious fast foods with her peers will help her remain a part of her group yet meet her nutritional needs.*
8. Discuss the importance of breakfast during pregnancy.
   *The fetus needs a steady supply of nutrients and needs food in the morning after the long fast during the night.*
9. Suggest that Patti eat foods not usually considered breakfast foods if she prefers. For example, cold pizza provides calcium and protein.
   *Nontraditional methods of meeting nutritional needs may be very effective.*
10. *Reinforce the importance of vitamin-mineral supplements. Adolescents may be inconsistent in taking them.*
11. Ask Patti to bring in another 24-hour diet history on her next visit.
    *This will allow new or continuing problems to be addressed.*
12. Ask Patti to share ways she has found to meet her diet needs that you could tell other teenagers. Ask for feedback on the methods discussed.
    *This will help Patti see that the nurse values her thoughts and ideas.*

**Evaluation**

Patti's 24-hour diet histories show that she is meeting the recommendations for each food group. She gains 1.8 to 2.7 kg (4-6 lb) per month throughout the rest of her pregnancy, for a total weight gain of 15 kg (33 lb). Her hemoglobin level rises to 11 g/dL. A healthy 3.4-kg (7½-lb) baby girl is born at term.

***Additional Nursing Diagnoses to Consider***

Disturbed Body Image

Situational Low Self-Esteem

expectant mother's stores may be used if intake is not sufficient to meet fetal needs.

Teenagers are often in a hurry, and they want foods that are fast and convenient. Meals may be irregular and often eaten away from home. Fast foods from restaurants or snack machines are a significant part of many teenagers' diets. These foods are often high in fat, sweeteners, and sodium and low in vitamins, minerals, and fiber. Choosing fast foods that do not make her appear different from her peers yet meet her added nutrient needs is important for the pregnant adolescent.

## Teaching the Adolescent

Teaching the adolescent about nutrition can be a challenge for nurses. It is essential to establish an accepting, relaxed atmosphere and show willingness to listen to the teenager's concerns. Her lifestyle, pattern of eating, and food likes and dislikes should be explored to determine if changes are needed in her diet.

The nurse should keep suggestions to a minimum, focusing on only those changes that are most important. Asking for the adolescent's input increases the likelihood that she will follow suggestions. When changes are necessary, the nurse should explain the reasons. A teenager, like other pregnant women, often makes changes for the sake of her unborn child that she would not consider for herself alone (see Nursing Care Plan).

The need to be like her peers is of major importance to the adolescent, especially when she is going through the changes of pregnancy. With education about what foods to choose, she can eat fast foods with her friends and still maintain a nourishing diet. Giving her plenty of examples of alternatives from which she can choose should be very helpful.

## Vegetarianism

**Vegetarians** eat a diet that contains wholly or mostly plant foods and avoid animal food-sources. Vegans avoid all animal products and may have the most difficulty meeting their nutrient needs. Their diet may be lacking in adequate calcium, iron, zinc, riboflavin, and vitamins D, $B_6$, and $B_{12}$ (Bond, 2011). Vegans may need to take supplements or foods fortified with these nutrients. Vegetarians whose diets include milk products (lactovegetarians), eggs (ovovegetarians), or milk products and eggs (lacto-ovovegetarians) can more easily meet their nutrient needs (Piccoli et al., 2015).

Although the knowledgeable vegetarian may eat a very nutritious diet, she is at higher risk during pregnancy. If she is new to vegetarian food practices, uninformed about pregnancy needs, or careless with her diet, she could fail to meet her nutrient needs. Vegetarians can follow the general guidelines during pregnancy by substituting plant sources for foods from animal sources.

### Meeting the Nutritional Requirements of the Pregnant Vegetarian

*Energy.* Vegetarian diets may be low in calories and fat and may not meet the energy needs of pregnancy. The diets are high in fiber and may cause a feeling of fullness before enough calories are eaten. A pregnant woman can increase caloric intake by eating snacks and higher-calorie foods. If carbohydrate and fat intakes are too low, her body may use protein for energy.

*Protein.* Although most vegetarians get enough protein, intake may be a concern in vegan diets. Complete proteins contain all the essential amino acids. Essential amino acids are those the body cannot synthesize from other sources. Animal and soy proteins are complete, but plant proteins (incomplete proteins) lack one or more of the essential amino acids. Even a diet with protein from plant sources only can meet the needs of pregnancy. Combining incomplete plant proteins with other plant foods that have complementary amino acids allows intake of all essential amino acids. Dishes that contain grains (wheat, rice, corn) and legumes (garbanzo, navy, kidney, pinto or soy beans; peas; and peanuts) are combinations that provide complete proteins. Complementary proteins do not have to be eaten at the same meal if they are consumed in a single day (Piccoli et al., 2015).

Incomplete proteins can also be combined with small amounts of complete protein foods like cheese to provide all amino acids. Therefore, women who include even small amounts of animal products meet their protein needs more easily.

Many vegetarians use tofu, made from soybeans, which provides protein as well as calcium and iron. Meat analogs that have a texture similar to meat but are made from vegetable protein are available. Some look and taste like hamburgers, bacon, lunch meats, chicken patties, and other commonly eaten foods. Meat analogs may be fortified with nutrients whose levels are often low in vegan diets (Piccoli et al., 2015).

*Calcium.* Vegetarians who include milk products in their diet may meet their pregnancy needs for calcium. Vegans obtain calcium from dark green vegetables and legumes, but their high-fiber diet may interfere with calcium absorption. Calcium-fortified juice or soy products, such as soy milk or tofu may meet the requirements. Calcium supplements may be necessary. Vitamin D supplementation is especially important if the woman drinks no milk and has little exposure to sunlight. Soy milks may be enriched with vitamin D.

*Iron.* Iron in the vegetarian diet is poorly absorbed because of the lack of heme iron from meats, poultry, and fish. Absorption is enhanced by eating a vitamin C source at the same meal as the nonheme iron. Iron supplementation is important for vegetarian women during pregnancy (Christian & Black, 2012).

*Zinc.* The best sources of zinc are meat and fish. Vegetarians may be deficient in this mineral and need supplements.

*Vitamin $B_{12}$.* Vitamin $B_{12}$ is obtained only from animal products. Because vegetarian diets contain large amounts of folic acid, anemia caused by inadequate intake of vitamin $B_{12}$ may not be apparent at first. Vegans may eat fortified foods such as cereal and some soy products or take $B_{12}$ supplements.

*Vitamin A.* Vitamin A is abundant in vegetarian diets. If the woman uses a daily multiple vitamin-mineral supplement, she may take in excessive amounts of vitamin A. Toxic effects include anorexia, irritability, hair loss, dry skin, and damage to the fetus. Supplementation should be individualized for each woman, based on her diet and her needs.

## Lactose Intolerance

Intolerance of lactose is caused by deficiency of the small intestine enzyme *lactase*, necessary for absorption of the milk sugar lactose. Some degree of lactose intolerance is normal for most of the world's population after early childhood. This includes many African-American, Hispanic, Asian, Pacific Islander, Native American, and Middle Eastern people. Although those with lactose intolerance may tolerate cultured or fermented milk products, such as aged cheese, buttermilk, and some brands of yogurt, symptoms may occur after drinking as little as a cup of milk. Symptoms include nausea, bloating, flatulence, diarrhea, and intestinal cramping (Zielinski, Searing, & Deibel, 2015).

Although the ability to tolerate lactose may increase during pregnancy, women who avoid dairy foods may not consume the recommended amounts of calcium. Most women tolerate small amounts (½ cup) of milk with meals, and they should increase their intake of other foods that provide calcium. Soy milk, low-lactose milk, and milk treated with lactase are available. The enzyme can be purchased to be added to milk or taken as a tablet. Calcium supplements may be necessary for some lactose-intolerant women.

## Pregnancy-Related Nausea and Vomiting

Many pregnant women experience morning sickness, and some also experience nausea at other times of day. Most women are able to manage frequent, small meals better than three large meals. Protein and complex carbohydrates are often tolerated best, but fatty foods increase nausea. Drinking liquids between meals instead of with meals often helps. At bedtime, a protein snack helps maintain glucose levels through the night. Eating a carbohydrate food such as dry toast or crackers before getting out of bed in the morning helps prevent nausea. Pregnancy-related nausea usually ends soon after the first trimester.

## Anemia

Anemia is a common concern during pregnancy. Hemoglobin values drop during the second trimester of pregnancy as a result of the dilution of the blood caused by plasma increases. This *physiological anemia* is normal (see Chapter 13). During the third trimester, hemoglobin levels generally return to prepregnant levels because of increased absorption of iron from the gastrointestinal tract, even though iron is transferred to the fetus primarily during this time. Fetal iron stores during the third trimester are generally sufficient to prevent anemia in the newborn for the first 4 to 6 months after birth.

The woman's iron stores may be measured by determining her serum ferritin level. A ferritin level less than 10 nanograms/100 mL indicates that the anemia is caused by iron deficiency. Generally, a woman is considered anemic if her hemoglobin is less than 11 g/dL or her hematocrit is less than 33% in the first or third trimesters or the hemoglobin is less than 10.5 g/dL or the hematocrit is less than 32% in the second trimester (Cunningham et al., 2010). Anemic women need iron supplements and help in choosing foods high in iron. Because high intake of iron inhibits the use of zinc and copper, anemic women may need to increase their intake of these minerals also (Cantor et al., 2015; Black, 2013; Christian & Black, 2012).

### Abnormal Prepregnancy Weight

In addition to teaching about dietary changes, the nurse should be alert for other problems associated with abnormal prepregnancy weight. The woman who is below normal weight may not have enough money for food or may have an eating disorder. Obese women may have other health problems, such as hypertension, that may affect the nurse's nutritional counseling plan.

### Eating Disorders

Eating disorders include anorexia nervosa (refusal to eat because of a distorted body image and feelings of obesity) and bulimia (overeating, followed by induced vomiting or use of laxatives or diuretics). These conditions are associated with electrolyte imbalance, low birth weight, and small-for-gestational-age infants. Many women with anorexia have amenorrhea and do not become pregnant; those with bulimia or subclinical anorexia are more likely to become pregnant (Cardwell, 2013; Cunningham et al., 2010).

All women should be asked about eating disorders, and nurses should watch for behaviors that may indicate disordered eating. Some women eat normally during pregnancy for the sake of the fetus, but others continue their previous eating patterns during pregnancy or in the early postpartum period if they do not lose weight immediately. Women with eating disorders need individual counseling to ensure that they meet the increased nutrient needs of pregnancy and understand normal postpartum weight loss (Cardwell, 2013).

### Food Cravings and Aversions

Women may have a strong preference or dislike for certain foods that is present only during pregnancy. Cravings for pickles, ice cream (not necessarily together), pizza, chocolate, cake, candy, spicy foods, and dairy products are common. Food aversions most often involve coffee, alcoholic beverages, highly seasoned or fried foods, and meat. The cause of cravings and aversions is not known, but they may be result from changes in the sense of taste and smell. They are generally not harmful, and some, like aversion to alcohol, may be beneficial.

### Pica

The practice of eating nonfood or some food components not considered part of a normal diet is called pica. Ice, clay, dirt, and laundry starch or cornstarch are the most common materials involved, but other items, such as chalk, baking soda, toothpaste, freezer frost, coffee grounds, and antacid tablets may be included. Pica is practiced by approximately 20% of pregnant women. Pica is more common in rural areas, inner cities, the southeastern United States, in African-Americans, women who live in poverty, those with poor nutrition, and in those with a childhood or family history of the practice. However, pica is not limited by socioeconomic group or geographic area. Pica may occur before pregnancy occurs (Miao, Young, & Golden, 2015; Lumish, Young, Lee, et al., 2014).

The cause of pica is unknown, although cultural values may be involved. Pica may be related to beliefs about the effect of the material eaten on labor or the baby. Iron deficiency is often associated with pica. Clay and dirt are not sources of iron and may decrease the absorption of iron and other nutrients. Zinc deficiency is also associated with pica. Studies about whether iron and zinc deficiencies are causes or results of pica are inconclusive (Miao, Young, & Golden, 2015; Christian & Black, 2012).

Pica can be harmful. The ingested substances may be contaminated with parasites, other organisms, or toxins such as lead. Clay and dirt may cause constipation or intestinal blockage. Eating large amounts of ice may cause dental problems. Another concern with pica is that it decreases the intake of foods, and thus, essential nutrients. Some women fear that their eating habits are harmful but are unable to ignore the cravings. They often keep their eating practices secret from caregivers who might disapprove (Miao, Young, & Golden, 2015).

#### CRITICAL THINKING EXERCISE 14.1

Joan, 6 months pregnant, very hesitantly confides that the reason she is not gaining much weight is that she eats large amounts of ice. She buys several bags of crushed ice daily. "I know I should be gaining more weight, but I'm just not hungry for anything besides ice," she says. How should the nurse handle this situation?

### Multiparity and Multifetal Pregnancy

The number and spacing of pregnancies, as well as the presence of more than one fetus, affects the mother's nutritional requirements. The woman who has had previous pregnancies may begin pregnancy with a nutritional deficit. In addition, she may be too busy meeting the needs of her family to be attentive to her own nutritional needs.

Closely spaced pregnancies may prevent a woman from making up any nutritional deficits from a previous pregnancy. Morning sickness from a new pregnancy may further interfere with an expectant mother's ability to eat an adequate diet. In addition, an interval of less than 6 months between pregnancies increases the risk of preterm and low-birth-weight infants as well as maternal morbidity and mortality (Luke, 2015; ACOG, 2005).

The woman with a multifetal pregnancy must provide enough nutrients to meet the needs of each fetus without depleting her own stores. The suggested weight gain for women of normal prepregnant weight who are pregnant with twins is 17 to 25 kg (37 to 54 lb), which is 5.5 to 9 kg (12 to 20 lb) more than for women with single pregnancies. The woman should consume an additional 300 calories per day for each fetus. Supplementation with calcium, iron, magnesium, zinc, and folic acid may also be necessary (Luke, 2015).

### Substance Use and Abuse

Substance abuse often accompanies a lifestyle that is unlikely to promote good eating habits. The expense of supporting a substance abuse habit may decrease the amount of money available to purchase food. Therefore, nutrition in pregnant women who abuse substances should be explored fully. Usually more than one substance is involved, and the effects of various combinations of substances on nutrition are not fully understood. The damaging effects of smoking, alcohol, and drug use on the fetus are further discussed in Chapter 24.

#### Smoking

Cigarette smoking increases the maternal metabolic rate and decreases appetite, which may result in a lower weight gain. Infant birth weight decreases in spite of adequate diet as the amount of smoking increases. Prematurity, spontaneous abortion, and other complications may also result. Smoking decreases the availability of some vitamins and minerals, making vitamin-mineral supplementation important during pregnancy (von Kobyletzki & Svensson, 2015). Counseling to help the woman stop smoking or at least decrease the number of cigarettes smoked during pregnancy is essential (see Chapter 13).

### Caffeine

Evidence regarding the effect of caffeine on nutrition during pregnancy is conflicting, and more research is needed. At this time, it appears that caffeine intake less than 200 mg/day is not a major contributing cause of miscarriage or preterm birth. Until more is known about its effects on nutrition and the fetus, caffeine intake should be limited during pregnancy to less than 200 mg/day (ACOG, 2010).

The nurse should discuss usual sources of caffeine. A 6 oz cup of brewed coffee contains approximately 103 mg; tea contains 36 mg/6 oz; cola beverages contain 35 to 50 mg/12 oz; and cocoa contains 4 mg/6 oz (ACOG, 2010). Some medications also contain caffeine. Caffeine changes the absorption or excretion of calcium, zinc, thiamine, and iron.

### Alcohol

Because of the association between drinking and fetal alcohol syndrome (see Chapter 24), women should avoid alcohol completely during pregnancy. Alcohol interferes with the absorption and use of vitamin $B_{12}$, folic acid, and magnesium, and often takes the place of food in the diet. Vitamin-mineral supplementation may be necessary for women whose intake of alcohol before pregnancy was large, because their nutrient stores may be depleted (Grieger, Grzeskowiak, & Clifton, 2014; Black, 2013; Erick, 2012).

### Drugs

The use of drugs other than those prescribed during pregnancy increases danger to the fetus and may interfere with nutrition. Marijuana increases appetite, but women may not satisfy their hunger with foods of good nutrient quality. Heroin use alters the metabolism and may cause the woman to be malnourished. Cocaine acts as an appetite suppressant, interfering with nutrient intake. Cocaine users tend to drink more beverages with alcohol or caffeine. Amphetamines and methamphetamines depress the appetite. Women who use amphetamines for dieting should be warned that these drugs should be discontinued during pregnancy (AAP & ACOG, 2013).

### Other Risk Factors

Women who follow food fads may not meet the nutritional requirements of pregnancy. Those who have followed a severely restricted diet may have depleted nutrient stores. The nurse can help them understand dietary changes needed during pregnancy. Women with complications of pregnancy, such as diabetes, heart disease, and preeclampsia, may need dietary alterations. Those with other medical conditions, such as extreme obesity, cystic fibrosis, and celiac disease, may need nutritional counseling from a dietitian (Black, 2013).

## NUTRITION AFTER BIRTH

Nutritional requirements after birth depend on whether the mother breastfeeds her infant or gives formula. The nurse should review the woman's nutritional knowledge as she returns to her prepregnancy diet and teach the breastfeeding mother how to adapt her diet to meet the needs of lactation.

### Nutrition for the Lactating Mother

The DRIs for lactating women are higher than those for nonpregnant adult women for many nutrients (see Tables 14.2 and 14.3).

### Energy

During the first 6 months of lactation, the estimated energy requirement (EER) is 330 calories each day in addition to normal needs for women according to age, weight, and height. In addition to the calories consumed, it is estimated that 170 calories per day are drawn from the woman's fat stores. This provides a total of 500 calories each day above prepregnancy requirements to meet the needs of lactation (Erick, 2012).

The EER for the second 6 months of lactation is 400 calories more than prepregnancy needs. Although the infant takes solids after 6 months and decreases milk intake, it is assumed that maternal energy stores have been used, and the calories should come from the woman's daily intake (Institute of Medicine, Food, and Nutrition Board, 2002). Women who were underweight before pregnancy or who had inadequate weight gain during pregnancy need more calories. Those who are overweight may need fewer calories than the EER. Milk volume is usually adequate even if a mother's diet is less than optimal, but the volume may be reduced and maternal stores of nutrients will be depleted with very low caloric intake (Erick, 2012).

### Protein

The recommended protein intake for pregnancy and lactation is 71 g/day. Although there is no change in protein needed for lactation, it is important for the woman to keep up her protein intake throughout the breastfeeding period.

### Fats

The long-chain polyunsaturated omega 3 and omega 6 fatty acids are present in human milk, and thus, should be included in the mother's diet during lactation.

### Vitamins and Minerals

The DRIs for lactating women are higher than those during pregnancy for vitamins A, $B_6$, $B_{12}$, C, and E and riboflavin, zinc, iodine, potassium, copper, and selenium. Lactating women who eat a well-balanced diet generally consume adequate amounts of essential nutrients to meet both the infant's and their own needs. The vitamin content of the milk may be lower than needed if the mother's diet is consistently low in vitamins. Lactating women with poor diets may have reduced milk levels of fatty acids, selenium, iodine, vitamin A, and some B vitamins (Erick, 2012). Vitamin D in the milk may be low if the mother has low intake, is not exposed to the sun, or has dark skin (Erick, 2012; ACOG, 2011). Mineral levels in the milk may remain constant because some minerals, such as calcium, are drawn from the mother's stores if her intake is poor. Routine vitamin-mineral supplements are unnecessary unless the diet is lacking in vitamins and minerals.

### Specific Nutritional Concerns

Some women are unlikely to consume the required nutrients, and they need special counseling.

***Dieting.*** Women who are concerned about losing weight after pregnancy need special consideration. After the initial losses in the first month, weight gradually decreases as maternal fat is used to meet a portion of the energy needs of lactation. However, breastfeeding does not necessarily result in weight loss, and some women maintain or even gain weight during lactation. This is more likely when weight gain during pregnancy was excessive.

Dieting should be postponed for at least 3 weeks after birth to allow the woman to recover fully from childbirth and establish her milk supply if she is breastfeeding. Gradual weight loss is preferable and should be accomplished by a combination of moderate exercise and a diet high in nutrients. Nursing mothers should avoid appetite suppressants, which may pass into the milk and harm the infant. Weight loss of approximately 0.45 to 0.68 kg (1 to 1.5 lb) a week is safe and will not affect milk supply or content (Bronner, 2014; IOM, 2009).

*Adolescence.* Problems associated with the adolescent diet continue to be of concern during lactation. The adolescent may be deficient in the same nutrients listed for other mothers during lactation, and she may be lacking in iron. If she avoids fruits and vegetables, her intake of vitamin A and C may be inadequate (Bronner, 2014; Lumish et al., 2014).

*Vegan diet.* The milk of the vegan mother may contain inadequate vitamin $B_{12}$ and D, and she and her infant may need supplements. The amounts of vitamin D in the diet also may be low. Vegans can meet their need for other nutrients during lactation by diet alone with careful planning. Those who are not knowledgeable about nutrition should take supplements.

*Avoidance of dairy products.* The recommendation for calcium remains the same for pregnancy and lactation, and the calcium content of breast milk is not affected by maternal intake. Less calcium is excreted in the urine during lactation. Women who do not eat dairy products should obtain calcium from other sources or take a calcium supplement.

*Inadequate diet.* Women with cultural or other food prohibitions may need help choosing a diet adequate for lactation. Low-income women may need referral to agencies such as WIC. If the mother must take medications that interfere with absorption of certain nutrients, her diet should be high in foods containing those nutrients.

*Alcohol.* Although it was once thought that the relaxing effect of alcohol would be helpful to the nursing mother, the deleterious effects of alcohol are too important to consider this suggestion appropriate today. An occasional single alcoholic beverage may not be harmful, but larger amounts may interfere with the milk-ejection reflex and be harmful to the infant. Alcohol in the milk peaks at 30 to 60 minutes if taken alone and 60 to 90 minutes after consumption with food. When mothers drink alcohol they should not breastfeed for at least 2 hours (Lawrence & Lawrence, 2011).

*Caffeine.* Foods high in caffeine should also be limited. The mother should restrict her caffeine intake to 2 cups of coffee or the equivalent each day. Caffeine in excessive amounts may make the infant irritable (ACOG, 2010).

### Fluids

Nursing mothers should drink fluids sufficient to relieve thirst, which often increases in the early breastfeeding period. Eight to 10 glasses of fluids, other than those containing caffeine, is adequate. Drinking large quantities of fluids is not necessary.

### Foods to Avoid

Lactating mothers are often concerned about whether they should avoid certain foods that might adversely affect the infant. Studies have shown that eliminating allergenic foods may be helpful for infants under 6 weeks of age with colic and when infants have a confirmed food allergy. However, there is insufficient evidence to recommend an elimination diet for other mothers during lactation. Infants at risk of developing allergies should be breastfed for at least 4 months (List & Vonderhaar, 2010).

## Nutrition for the Nonlactating Mother

The postpartum woman who is not breastfeeding can return to her prepregnancy diet if it meets the recommendations for adult women. Her diet should contain protein and vitamin C foods to promote healing. She may continue to take her prenatal vitamin-mineral supplements until her supply is finished to ensure adequate intake during the early weeks and help renew nutrient stores.

The nurse should assess the mother's understanding of the amount of food she needs from each food group. A review of important nutrient sources for calcium and iron may be relevant. If a woman was anemic during pregnancy, an iron supplement is important until her hemoglobin level returns to normal.

### Weight Loss

When her baby is born, a woman can expect to lose approximately 5.5 kg (12 lb) immediately. She loses approximately another 4 kg (9 lb) in the next 2 weeks and 2.5 kg (5.5 lb) by 6 months after delivery. If her weight gain during pregnancy has not been excessive, she will probably lose all but approximately 1.4 kg (3 lb) if she follows a well-balanced diet (Cunningham et al., 2010). She should decrease her caloric intake to her normal nonpregnant levels to avoid retaining weight.

Some women are impatient with slow weight loss. Because they need energy to meet the demands of infant care, new mothers should wait at least 3 weeks to start dieting to lose weight. Suggestions for sensible calorie reduction combined with exercise are appropriate.

Women who gain excess weight during pregnancy may have more difficulty losing it after birth and may need help from a dietitian in planning a weight loss program. Women who do not lose the weight gained during pregnancy risk beginning the next pregnancy overweight, and this may lead to further retention of weight after birth. Therefore, women need help with learning how to decrease their energy intake so they can return to their normal weight.

Mothers are sometimes so involved with the needs of the infant that they fail to eat properly. They may snack instead of planning meals for themselves, especially during the early weeks. The nurse should remind them that snacking often involves high-caloric intake without meeting nutritional needs. Meals and snacks should be high in nutrient content.

## NURSING CARE

### Nutrition for Childbearing

#### Assessment

*Interview.* The interview provides an opportunity to develop rapport and to identify any specific problems that affect dietary intake.

**Appetite.** Begin the interview by discussing the woman's appetite. How does it compare to her appetite before pregnancy? Morning sickness may decrease food intake during the first trimester. Determine the severity and duration of nausea and vomiting. Hyperemesis gravidarum is the most serious form of this problem and may require intravenous correction of fluid and electrolyte imbalance and parenteral nutrition (see Chapter 25).

**Eating habits.** Assess the usual pattern of meals to discover poor food habits, such as skipping breakfast or eating fast foods for most lunches. Determine who does the cooking for the family. If someone else does the cooking, discuss nutritional needs during pregnancy with that person.

**Food preferences.** Ask about the woman's food preferences and dislikes. During pregnancy, some women experience an aversion to certain foods, such as meats, that they do not have at other times. Determine whether she has food cravings or eats large amounts of any one particular food or group of foods. Discuss pica in a nonjudgmental, matter-of-fact manner to avoid giving an impression of disapproval.

In assessing for pica, the nurse might say, "Have you had any cravings for special things to eat during your pregnancy?" This can be followed by, "Women sometimes eat things like ice, clay, or starch during pregnancy. Have you tried these?" This provides an opening for a discussion of substitutes, such as nonfat dry milk powder for laundry starch, the woman may be willing to try.

**Identify potential problems.** Identify any obvious areas of potential deficiency. For example, the woman might eat little meat, avoid vegetables, be lactose intolerant, or follow a fad diet. Also determine her knowledge about nutritional needs during pregnancy. Ask about any cultural or religious practices that affect nutrition. Determine if these change during pregnancy and the effect on her nutrient intake.

Identify other factors that interfere with adequate nutrition. Women with low incomes may not know about sources of help. Ask the vegetarian how long she has followed the practice and assess her awareness of changes necessary during pregnancy. A woman's smoking habits, alcohol intake, and substance abuse may become obvious during the interview. Determine whether she takes medications that interfere with nutrient absorption.

Provide an opportunity for the woman to ask about special dietary concerns. This may bring out fears about weight gain, worry that specific foods could hurt the fetus, or other issues not yet addressed.

**Diet history.** Diet histories provide information about a woman's usual intake of nutrients. They form a basis for counseling about any changes required to meet pregnancy needs.

***Twenty-four-hour diet history.*** Ask the woman to recall what she ate at each meal and snack during the previous 24 hours. Use specific questions about the size of portions and ingredients used. Use models of food items and measuring utensils to help discuss portion sizes. Inquire about beverages and snacks. Ask whether this sample is typical of her usual daily food intake. If it is not, ask which foods are more representative. Analyze the diet to determine whether the woman has met the recommendations for specific food groups, calories, and protein. Detailed analysis of individual nutrients is unnecessary.

***Food intake records.*** Food intake records are used to report foods eaten over 1 or more days. Instruct the woman to list everything she eats throughout the day. The list is more accurate if she writes down each food immediately after eating.

***Food-frequency questionnaires.*** Food-frequency questionnaires contain lists of common foods and provide information about diet over a longer period. Ask the woman how often she eats each of the common foods listed. Analyze the list to determine whether foods from each food group are eaten in adequate amounts to meet pregnancy needs.

***Physical assessment.*** Information about nutritional status includes measurement of weight and examination for signs of nutritional deficiency.

**Weight at initial visit.** To get a baseline value for future comparison, weigh the woman at the first prenatal visit. Ask if this is her usual weight or if she has gained or lost weight. Measure her height without shoes. If her weight is low for height, nutritional reserves are marginal. If it is high, she may be overweight or obese.

## CRITICAL THINKING EXERCISE 14.2

Cheryl, age 22 years, has gained 4.5 kg (10 lb) more than recommended at 31 weeks of pregnancy. She asks the nurse for help because she is very worried about her weight gain and thinking of going on a severe weight loss diet. She started pregnancy at the upper end of the normal body mass index (BMI) and should gain 25 to 35 lb during the pregnancy. She has no apparent edema and no complications of pregnancy.

1. Why is Cheryl's weight gain a problem?
2. What suggestions should the nurse make to help Cheryl with her diet?

**Weight at subsequent visits.** Weigh the woman at each visit on the same scale with approximately the same amount of clothing. Record the weight on a weight chart at each visit throughout the pregnancy (Fig. 14.2). Use a chart that allows examination of the pattern as well as the total gain to date.

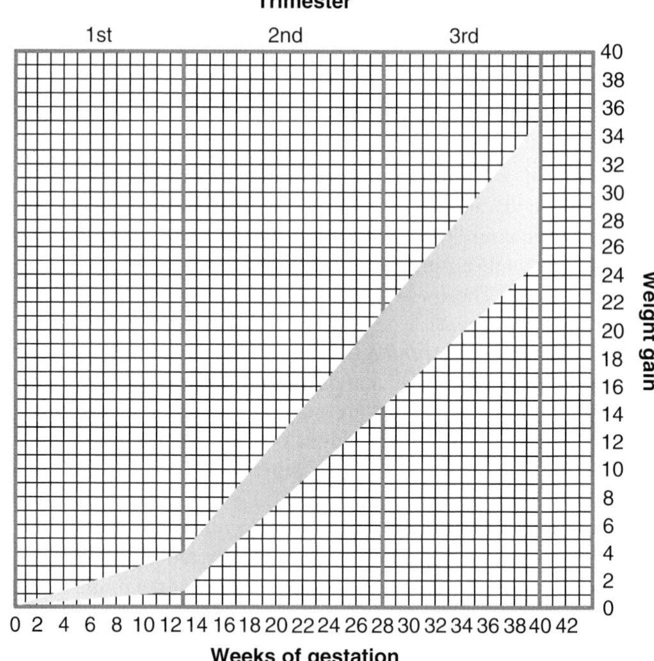


FIG 14.2 Weight gain for pregnancy. The range for weight gain in women of normal prepregnancy weight is 11.5 to 16 kg (25 to 35 lb). (From Rasmussen, K.M., & Yaktine, A.L. [2009]. [Eds.], *Weight gain during pregnancy: Reexamining the guidelines.* Washington, DC: National Academies Press.)

Be careful not to overemphasize weight gain. In some instances, a woman may be afraid that caregivers will be disapproving if she gains weight and consequently she may diet or fast a day or two before her prenatal visit.

**Signs of nutrient deficiency.** Observe for indications of nutritional status or signs of deficiency. For example, bleeding gums may indicate inadequate intake of vitamin C. However, actual deficiency states are not likely to occur in women in most industrialized countries. The exception is iron deficiency anemia, which is common in a mild form. Signs and symptoms include pallor, low hemoglobin level, fatigue, and increased susceptibility to infection.

***Laboratory tests.*** Laboratory tests for in-depth analysis of nutrient intake are generally impractical. Hemoglobin, hematocrit, and in some cases serum ferritin tests are used most often to detect anemia.

***Reassessing nutritional status at each visit.*** At each prenatal visit reassess the woman's dietary status. Ask about any difficulties with her diet. Check weight gain and evaluate hemoglobin and hematocrit levels, if appropriate. Explain what assessments are being made and why.

### Nursing Diagnosis and Planning

Although some women consume more calories than they need during pregnancy, the most common nursing diagnosis concerning nutrition is:

- Readiness for Enhanced Nutrition related to the desire to learn about the nutrient needs of pregnancy.

***Expected outcomes.*** The woman will eat a daily diet that includes the recommended amount of each food group for pregnancy. The woman with a normal BMI before pregnancy will gain approximately 0.5 to 2 kg (1.1 to 4.4 lb) during the first trimester and 0.35 to 0.5 kg (0.8 to1 lb) per week during the second and third trimesters for a total gain of 11.5 to 16 kg (25 to 35 lb).

### Interventions

***Explaining nutrient needs.*** Use the woman's diet history as a basis to introduce information about nutrition during pregnancy. Help the woman analyze her own diet for the amount of each food group included so she understands the process. Explain which important nutrients are provided in each food group and why they are necessary for her and the fetus.

Make a rough estimate of calories, protein, iron, folic acid, and calcium in the diet to help her determine if she eats enough of these foods on a regular basis. Compare the usual sources of these major nutrients with her diet history and favorite foods. Suggest ways she can increase her intake of nutrients she is lacking by increasing foods that are good sources.

***Providing reinforcement.*** Give frequent positive reinforcement when the woman is eating appropriately. Assist her in evaluating any weaknesses in her present diet and planning ways to remedy them (Fig. 14.3).

If the woman can read, give her written materials on nutrition during pregnancy and review them with her. A small pamphlet with pictures might be placed on the refrigerator to help her remember what foods she needs each day. Demonstrate portion sizes by showing her plastic models of common foods. These models are available for ethnic foods as well.

***Evaluating weight gain.*** Compare the woman's weight with a weight gain chart to ascertain whether she has gained the appropriate amount of weight for this point in her pregnancy. Discuss the importance and expected pattern of weight gain for her. Explain the concept of eating foods high in nutrient density when she is increasing calories.

For women of normal weight, a monthly gain of less than 1 kg (2.2 lb) should lead to a discussion of possible problems in food intake. A gain of more than 2.9 kg (6.5 lb) per month may signify edema. Errors in calculation of gestation may also reflect a pattern of weight gain different from that expected.

***Encouraging supplement intake.*** If vitamin-mineral supplements have been prescribed, determine whether the woman takes them regularly. If she forgets to take the supplements, suggest she take them with meals or at bedtime. If iron supplements are causing constipation, suggest increased intake of fluids or high-fiber foods. Let her know that black stools are a harmless side effect of iron supplements.

***Making referrals.*** Refer women with health problems such as diabetes, celiac disease, or extreme weight problems for a consultation with a dietitian and follow-up with the nurse. Refer women with inadequate financial resources to buy food to public assistance programs such as the WIC program. At the next visit, determine whether the woman obtained the help needed and whether other assistance is necessary.

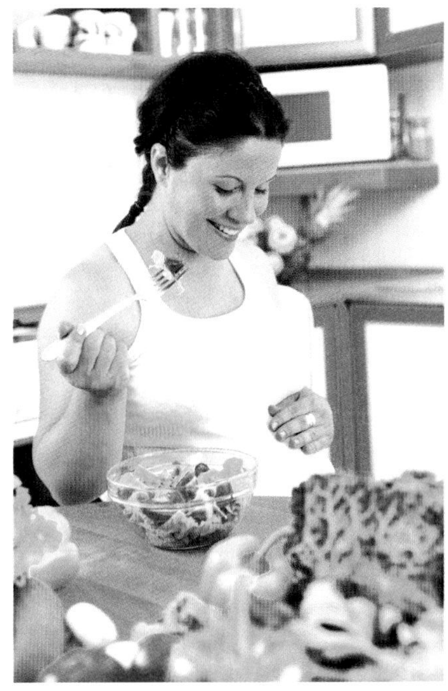

**FIG 14.3** Women often make changes in their diets for the good of their unborn children that they would not consider for themselves alone. (© 2016, Getty Images. Reprinted with permission.)

### Evaluation

- Does the woman report eating the recommended amount of each food group daily?
- Does the woman gain 0.5 to 2 kg (1.1 to 4.4 lb) during the first trimester and 0.35 to 0.5 kg (0.8 to 1 lb) per week during the second and third trimesters?
- Is her total pregnancy weight gain between 11.5 and 16 kg (25 and 35 lb)?

## KEY CONCEPTS

- Poor weight gain in pregnant women is associated with low-birth-weight infants and preterm birth. Excessive weight gain may lead to macrosomia and other complications.
- The recommended weight gain during pregnancy for women of normal prepregnancy weight is 11.5 to 16 kg (25 to 35 lb). The amount is greater for women who are underweight or who carry more than one fetus and less for overweight and obese women.
- The pattern of weight gain is important. The average woman should gain 0.5 to 2 kg (1.1 to 4.4 lb) during the first trimester and 0.35 to 0.5 kg (0.8 to 1 lb) per week thereafter.
- The recommended daily increase in energy intake during pregnancy is 340 calories in the second trimester and 452 calories in the third trimester.
- Protein should be increased to 71 g/day during pregnancy, an increase of 25 g/day over nonpregnancy needs.
- Women may not eat enough foods high in vitamins and minerals to meet recommendations.
- Fat-soluble vitamins (A, D, E, K) are stored in the liver. Excess consumption of fat-soluble vitamins (A, D, E, K) may result in toxic effects.
- Daily intake of water-soluble vitamins is necessary because excesses are not stored but excreted.
- Minerals most likely to be consumed in less-than-recommended amounts during pregnancy are iron and calcium. They are often added as a supplement.
- Vitamin-mineral supplements must be used carefully to prevent excessive intake and toxic effects. Increased intake of some nutrients interferes with the use of others.
- Pregnant women should drink approximately 8 of 10 cups of fluids each day. They should eat at least 7 to 9 oz of whole grains, 3 to 3½

*Continued*

## KEY CONCEPTS—cont'd

cups vegetables, 2 cups fruits, 3 cups milk products, and 6 to 8 oz of protein foods daily.

- Culture can influence diet during pregnancy. The nurse should assess whether a woman follows traditional cultural dietary practices and whether her food practices are consistent with good nutrition.
- Both Asian and Hispanic dietary practices include balancing yin and yang ("cold" and "hot") foods.
- Low-income women may not have enough money or knowledge to meet the nutrient needs of pregnancy. Nurses should refer them for financial assistance and nutritional counseling.
- Adolescents might skip meals and eat snacks and fast foods of low nutrient density. They are subject to peer pressure that may result in decreased nutritional intake.
- Pregnant vegetarians may need help choosing an adequate diet that includes nonanimal sources of needed nutrients.
- Lactose-intolerant women should increase calcium intake from foods other than milk, such as calcium-rich vegetables.
- Abnormal prepregnancy weight, anemia, eating disorders, pica, multiparity, substance abuse, closely spaced pregnancies, and multifetal pregnancies are all nutritional risk factors that warrant adaptations of diet during pregnancy.
- Compared to nonpregnant needs, a lactating woman should take in an added 330 calories daily during the first 6 months. An additional 170 calories is drawn from maternal stores. A daily intake of 400 calories over nonpregnant requirements are needed daily during the second 6 months.
- Lactating women should avoid alcohol and excess caffeine.
- The postpartum woman who does not breastfeed should resume her prepregnant calorie intake and eat a well-balanced diet to enhance recovery from childbirth. Weight loss should be accomplished slowly and sensibly.

## REFERENCES AND READINGS


American Academy of Pediatrics & American College of Obstetricians and Gynecologists. (2013). *Guidelines for perinatal care* (8th ed.). Elk Grove Village, IL, and Washington, DC: Author.

American Association of Nurse Practitioners. Retrieved from http://onlinelibrary.wiley.com/journal/10.1002/%28ISSN%292327-6924/earlyview?start=21&resultsPerPage=20.

American College of Obstetricians and Gynecologists. (2002). *Committee Opinion: Exercise during pregnancy and the postpartum period*. Washington DC: Author.

American College of Obstetricians and Gynecologists. (2005). Committee Opinion: The importance of preconception care in the continuum of women's health care. *Obstetrics & Gynecology*, 106(5), 665–666.

American College of Obstetricians and Gynecologists. (2010). *Committee opinion: Moderate caffeine consumption during pregnancy*. Washington DC: Author.

American College of Obstetricians and Gynecologists. (2011). ACOG Committee Opinion No. 495: Vitamin D: Screening and supplementation during pregnancy. *Obstetrics & Gynecology*, 118(1), 197.

American College of Obstetricians and Gynecologists. (2013b). Committee Opinion: Weight gain during pregnancy. *Obstetrics & Gynecology*, 121(1), 210–212.

American Dietetic Association [ADA]. (2008). Position of the American Dietetic Association: Nutrition and lifestyle for a healthy pregnancy outcome. *Journal of the American Dietetic Association*, 106(3), 553–561.

Bennett, W., & McDonald-Mosley, R. (2011). Management of severe obesity in pregnancy. *The Female Patient*, 36(7), 23–28.

Bhutta, Z., Das, J., Rizvi, A., et al. (2013). Evidence-based interventions for improvement of maternal and child nutrition: what can be done and at what cost? *The Lancet*, 382(9890), 452–77.

Blackburn, S.T. (2013). *Maternal, fetal, and neonatal physiology: A clinical perspective* (4th ed.). St. Louis: Saunders.

Bond, L. (2011). Physiology of pregnancy. In S. Mattson, & J.E. Smith (Eds.), *AWHONN Core curriculum for maternal-newborn nursing* (4th ed., pp. 80–100). St. Louis: Saunders.

Bronner, Y.L. (2014). Maternal nutrition during lactation. In J. Riordan, & K. Wambach (Eds.), *Breastfeeding and human lactation* (5th ed.). Sudbury, MA: Jones & Bartlett.

Callister, L.C. (2013). Integrating cultural beliefs and practices into the care of childbearing women. In K.R. Simpson, & P.A. Creehan (Eds.), *AWHONN perinatal nursing* (4th ed.). Philadelphia: Lippincott Williams & Wilkins.

Cantor, A., Bougatsos, C., Dana, T., et al. (2015). Routine iron supplementation and screening for iron deficiency anemia in pregnancy: a systematic review for the U.S. Preventive Services Task Force, *Annals of Internal Medicine*, 162(8), 566.

Cardwell, M.S. (2013). Eating disorders during pregnancy. *Obstetrics and Gynecology Survey*, 68(4), 312–323.

Centers for Disease Control and Prevention [CDC]. (2008). Use of supplements containing folic acid among women of childbearing age—United States, 2007. *MMWR Morbidity and Mortality Weekly Report*,57(01), 5–8.

Centers for Disease Control and Prevention [CDC]. (2009). *About BMI for adults*. Retrieved from http://www.cdc.gov/healthyweight/assessing/bmi/adult_bmi/index.html#Interpreted

Centers for Disease Control and Prevention [CDC]. (2015). *Folic acid: Questions and answers*. Retrieved from http://www.cdc.gov/ncbddd/folicacid/faqs.html.

Christian, P. & Black R. (2012). Food, micronutrients, and birth outcomes. *Journal of the American Medical Association*, 307(19), 2094.

Conrad, K, Russell, A., & Keister, K. (2011). Bariatric surgery and its impact on childbearing. *Nursing for Women's Health*, 15(3), 228–234.

Cunningham, F., Leveno, K., Bloom, S., et al. (2014). *Williams obstetrics* (24th ed.). New York: McGraw-Hill.

Cunningham, F.G., Leveno, K.J., Bloom, S.L., et al. (2010). *Williams obstetrics* (23th ed.). New York: McGraw-Hill.

Erick, M. (2012). Nutrition during pregnancy and lactation. In L.K. Mahan, S. Escott-Stump, & J.L. Raymond (Eds.), *Krause's food, nutrition, and diet therapy* (13th ed., pp. 340–374). St. Louis: Saunders.

Flick, A., & Artal, R. (2013). Obesity and weight gain in pregnancy. *Contemporary OB/GYN*, 58(7), 26–28.

Galanti, G. (2008). *Caring for patients from different cultures* (4th ed.). Philadelphia: University of Pennsylvania Press.

Gallagher, M.L. (2012). Intake: The nutrients and their metabolism. In L.K. Mahan, S. Escott-Stump, & J.L. Raymond (Eds.), *Krause's food, nutrition, and diet therapy* (13th ed., pp. 32–128). St. Louis: Saunders.

Grieger J.A., Grzeskowiak L.E., & Clifton V.L. (2014). Preconception dietary patterns in human pregnancies are associated with preterm delivery. *Journal of Nutrition*, 144(7), 1075–1080.

Grodner, M., Roth, S.L., & Walkingshaw, B.C. (2012). *Foundations and clinical applications of nutrition: A nursing approach* (5th ed.). St. Louis: Mosby.

Gunaratne, A., Makrides, M., & Collins, C. (2015). *Maternal prenatal and/or postnatal n-3 long chain polyunsaturated fatty acids (LCPUFA) supplementation for preventing allergies.* Retrieved from http://www.cochrane.org/

CD010085/PREG_fish-oil-n-3-or-omega-3-pregnant-mothers-or-breastfeeding-mothers-prevent-allergies-their-young

Hall, J.E. (2015). *Guyton and Hall textbook of medical physiology* (13th ed.). Philadelphia: Saunders.

Institute of Medicine. (2009). *Weight gain during pregnancy: Reexamining the guidelines.* Retrieved from http://iom.edu/Reports/2009/Weight-Gain-During-Pregnancy-Reexamining-the-Guidelines.aspx

Institute of Medicine, Food and Nutrition Board. (1991). *Nutrition during lactation.* Washington, DC: National Academies Press.

Institute of Medicine, Food and Nutrition Board. (1997). *Dietary reference intakes for calcium, phosphorus, magnesium, vitamin D, & fluoride.* Washington, DC: National Academies Press.

Institute of Medicine, Food and Nutrition Board. (1998). *Dietary reference intakes for thiamin, riboflavin, niacin, vitamin B6, folate, vitamin B12, pantothenic acid, biotin, & choline.* Washington, DC: National Academies Press.

Institute of Medicine, Food and Nutrition Board. (2000). *Dietary reference intakes for vitamin C, vitamin E, selenium, and carotenoids.* Washington, DC: National Academies Press.

Institute of Medicine, Food and Nutrition Board. (2001). *Dietary reference intakes for vitamin A, vitamin K, arsenic, boron, chromium, copper, iodine, iron, manganese, molybdenum, nickel, silicon, vanadium, and zinc.* Washington, DC: National Academies Press.

Institute of Medicine, Food and Nutrition Board. (2002). *Dietary reference intakes for energy, carbohydrates, fiber, protein and amino acids (macronutrients).* Washington, DC: National Academies Press.

Institute of Medicine, Food and Nutrition Board. (2010). *Dietary reference intakes for calcium and vitamin D.* Washington, DC: National Academies Press 623–633.

Johnson, T.R.B., Gregory, K.D., & Niebyl, J.R. (2007). Preconception and prenatal care: Part of the continuum. In S.G. Gabbe, J.R. Niebyl, & J.L. Simpson (Eds.), *Obstetrics: Normal and problem pregnancies* (5th ed., pp. 111–137). Philadelphia: Churchill Livingstone.

von Kobyletzki, L., & Svensson, Å. (2015). Prenatal and postnatal exposure to parental smoking increases odds allergic diseases during childhood and adolescence. *Evidence Based Medicine*, 20(3), 118.

Lawrence, R.A., & Lawrence, R.W. (2011). Medications, herbal preparations, and natural products in breast milk. In *Breastfeeding: A guide for the medical profession* (7th ed., pp. 364–405). Philadelphia: Mosby.

List, B.A., & Vonderhaar, K.J. (2010). Should breastfeeding mothers avoid allergenic foods? *MCN: The American Journal of Maternal/Child Nursing*, 35(6), 324–329.

Luke, B. (2015). Nutrition for multiples. *Clinical Obstetrics and Gynecology*, 58(3), 585–610.

Lumish, R., Young, S., Lee, S., et al. (2014). Gestational iron deficiency is associated with pica behaviors in adolescents. *Journal of Nutrition*, 144(10), 1533–1539.

Miao, D., Young, S., & Golden, C. (2015). A meta-analysis of pica and micronutrient status. *American Journal of Human Biology*, 27(1), 84–93.

Nix, S. (2009). *Williams' basic nutrition and diet therapy* (13th ed.). St. Louis: Mosby.

Ota, E., Tobe-Gai, R., Mori, R., et al. (2012). Antenatal dietary advice and supplementation to increase energy and protein intake. *Cochrane Database Systematic Review*, (9), CD000032.

Pagana, K.D., & Pagana, T.J. (2012). *Mosby's diagnostic and laboratory test reference* (10th ed.). St. Louis: Mosby.

Peckenpaugh, N.J. (2010). *Nutrition essentials and diet therapy* (11th ed.). St. Louis: Saunders.

Piccoli, G.B., Clari, R., et al. (2015). Vegan-vegetarian diets in pregnancy: danger or panacea? A systemic narrative review. *British Journal of Obstetrics and Gynecology*, 122(5), 623–633.

Piersma, A., Bonde, J., Toft, G., et al. (2015). Prenatal exposure to environmental chemical contaminants and asthma and eczema in school-age children. *Allergy*, 70(6), 653–660.

Rabel, A., Leitman, S., Miller, J. (2015). *Ask about ice, then consider iron.* Journal of the

Rasmussen, K.M., Abrams, B., Bodnar, L.M., et al. (2010). Recommendations for weight gain during pregnancy in the context of the obesity epidemic. *Obstetrics & Gynecology*, 116(5), 1191–1195.

Reinold, C., Dalenius, K., Smith, B., et al. (2009). *Pregnancy Nutrition Surveillance 2007 Report.* Atlanta: U.S. Department of Health and Human Services, Centers for Disease Control and Prevention.

Robinson, S., Baird, J., & Godfrey, K. (2014). Eating for two? The unresolved question of optimal diet in pregnancy. *American Journal of Clinical Nutrition*, 100(5), 1220–1.

Smit, L., Lenters, V., Høyer, B.B., et al. (2012). Nutrition in adolescence. In L.K. Mahan, S. Escott-Stump, & J.L. Raymond (Eds.), *Krause's food, nutrition, and diet therapy* (13th ed., pp. 410–430). St Louis: Saunders.

Stang, J., & Larson, N. (2012). Nutrition in adolescence. In L.K. Mahan, S. Escott-Stump, & J.L. Raymond (Eds.), *Krause's food, nutrition, and diet therapy* (13th ed., pp. 410–430). St Louis: Saunders.

Stauffer, R.Y. (2008). Vietnamese Americans. In J.N. Giger, & R.E. Davidhizar (Eds.), *Transcultural nursing: Assessment and intervention* (5th ed., pp. 494–536). St. Louis: Mosby.

U.S. Department of Agriculture. (2015). *Women, Infants, & Children [WIC] eligibility requirements.* Retrieved from http://www.fns.usda.gov/wic/wic-eligibility-requirements

U.S. Department of Health and Human Services. (2000). *Healthy People 2010.* (Conference edition, in 2 volumes). Washington, DC: Author, (Conference edition, in 2 volumes).

U.S. Department of Health and Human Services. (2010). *Healthy People 2020.* Washington DC: Author.

U.S. Food and Drug Administration. (2009b). While you're pregnant: Listeria. Washing-ton DC: *Author.*

U.S. Preventive Services Task Force. (2009). *Folic acid for the prevention of neural tube defects: U.S. Preventive Services Task Force Recommendation Statement.* AHRQ Publication No. 09-05132-EF-2. Retrieved from http://www.uspreventiveservicestaskforce.org/uspstf09/folicacid/folicacidrs.htm.

Zielinski, R., Searing, K., & Deibel, M. (2015). Gastrointestinal distress in pregnancy: Prevalence, assessment, and treatment of 5 minor discomforts. *Journal of Perinatal and Neonatal Nursing*, 29(1), 23–31.

# 15

# Prenatal Diagnostic Tests

http://evolve.elsevier.com/McKinney/mat-ch/

## LEARNING OBJECTIVES

*After studying this chapter, you should be able to:*

- Identify indications for fetal diagnostic procedures.
- Discuss the purpose, procedure, advantages, and risks of each diagnostic procedure presented in the chapter.
- Provide information in response to common questions parents have about procedures.

Methods to detect physical abnormalities in the fetus and to monitor the fetal condition in a high-risk pregnancy with greater accuracy are becoming common as knowledge regarding their usefulness accumulates. Many pregnant women now expect to know the sex of their baby before birth because of the routine use of technology such as ultrasound.

The ability to predict fetal outcome offers reassurance for most parents but not all. If the fetus is free of anomalies and is determined to be in good condition, the parents are relieved. However, testing may raise questions about fetal health rather than answer them, forcing parents to make decisions about having other tests or perhaps increasing their anxiety throughout the remainder of pregnancy. Decisions can create emotional conflict and raise ethical dilemmas that impose a great deal of stress on the family.

## INDICATIONS FOR PRENATAL DIAGNOSTIC TESTS

In general, fetal diagnostic and surveillance procedures are performed for the following three reasons: to detect congenital anomalies, to evaluate the condition of the fetus if the pregnancy is high risk and allow appropriate intervention, and to provide baseline information such as a more accurate gestational age. Procedures that were once done only if the pregnancy was high risk are currently routinely performed. Tests, such as ultrasound or maternal serum screening, are often offered to all pregnant women. Box 15.1 lists some risk factors for which prenatal diagnostic procedures are often recommended.

## ULTRASOUND

High-frequency sound waves aimed in a specific direction are deflected by objects in their path and return as echoes. The amount of energy returned as an echo depends on the density of the object that deflected the ultrasonic wave. In obstetrics, ultrasonic waves directed through the abdomen of a pregnant woman are deflected by deep tissues of the mother and fetus. The returning sound waves are converted into two- or three-dimensional images that show structures of different densities.

Ultrasound procedures in obstetrics use real-time scanning in which a rapid sequence of fixed images is displayed on the screen, showing movement in body tissues as it happens. This technique allows the observer to detect movement such as fetal heartbeat, fetal breathing activity, and fetal body movement. Still images are captured for purposes such as gestational age calculation using multiple measures (Fig. 15.1). Both still and video images may be captured for medical records as well as keepsakes for the parents. Three-dimensional images may be captured to reveal greater detail of the fetal body (Fig. 15.2).

### Emotional Responses

Some expectant mothers are excited and pleased and report feelings of love and protectiveness when they view the fetus. Others report increased feelings of vulnerability and anxiety about the fetus, fearing that something wrong will be found, and are thrilled if results are reassuring.

Expectant fathers are often fascinated by fetal movement and insist that the fetus "waved" at them or that they could see the facial expression as the fetus looked directly at them. Some couples wish to know the sex of the fetus, but others prefer to wait and "be surprised" even if the sex is obvious to the technician. Moreover, determining the fetal sex by ultrasound is sometimes not possible. Occasionally, a couple is surprised at birth if the infant's sex is not what they expected.

Although ultrasound is not yet a standard of care for all women, it is widely used because a great deal of information can be obtained with minimum risk to mother or fetus. Ultrasound may be used during any trimester, but the procedure and reasons for using it varies in each trimester.

### First Trimester

Transvaginal ultrasound is often used during the first trimester because the uterus, gestational sac, embryo, ovaries, and fallopian tubes are deep in the pelvis.

#### Procedure

The woman is placed in the lithotomy position for transvaginal ultrasound. A transvaginal probe that is encased in a disposable cover and coated with a gel that provides lubrication and promotes sound-wave conduction is inserted in the vagina. The woman may feel more comfortable if she inserts the probe herself.

## BOX 15.1 Indications for Fetal Diagnostic Procedures

**Medical Conditions**

Preexisting diabetes mellitus or gestational diabetes
Hypertension (chronic or preeclampsia)
Acute or nonacute infections (e.g., pyelonephritis)
Sexually transmitted diseases
Severe anemia
Parents carry or express a genetic disorder (e.g., sickle cell anemia, cystic fibrosis)

**Demographic Factors**

Maternal age <16 or >35 years
Poverty
Nonwhites (greater risk for prematurity and neonatal or infant death)
Inadequate prenatal care (initial visit after 20 weeks of gestation or fewer than five prenatal visits to physician or nurse-midwife)

**Obstetric Factors**

History of low-birth-weight (<2500 g [5 lb, 8 oz]) or preterm (<37 completed weeks of pregnancy) infant
Multifetal pregnancy
Malpresentation (breech, shoulder)
Previous fetal loss or birth of infant with congenital anomaly
Previous infant ≥4000 g (8 lb, 13 oz) at birth
Hydramnios (≥2000 mL at term; amniotic fluid index ≥24-25 cm [Cunningham et al., 2010])
Oligohydramnios (<500 mL at term; amniotic fluid index <5)
Decrease in or absence of fetal movements
Uncertainty about gestational age
Suspected intrauterine growth restriction
Discordant (unequal) fetal growth of twins
Postmaturity (>42 weeks)
Preterm labor (>20 weeks but <37 completed weeks of gestation)
Grand multiparity (>5 pregnancies)

**Concurrent Maternal Factors**

Prepregnancy body mass index (BMI) less than 18.5 kg/$m^2$
Prepregnancy BMI 25 kg/$m^2$ or higher
Inadequate weight gain or poor pattern of weight gain
Excessive weight gain
Use of drugs (legal, including prescribed, over-the-counter, and herbal; illegal), alcohol, tobacco

Reference: Cunningham, F.G., Leveno, K.J., Bloom, S.L., et al. (2010). *Williams obstetrics*. New York: McGraw-Hill.

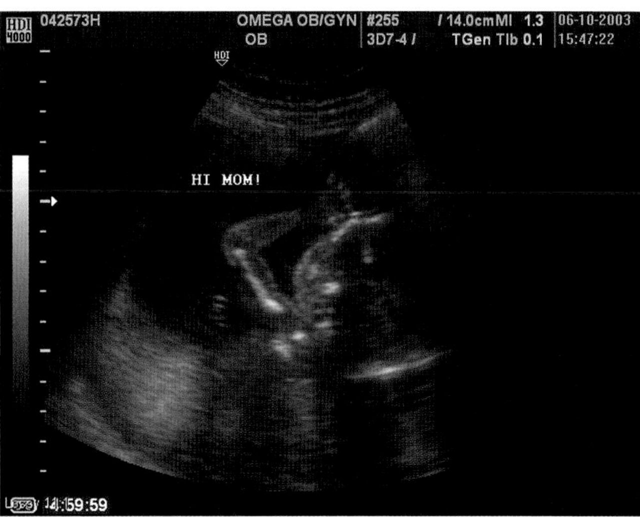


**FIG 15.1** Two-dimensional sonogram showing the fetal body profile and details of the fetal arm, hand, and fingers. (Courtesy Paul and Kerri Hamilton.)

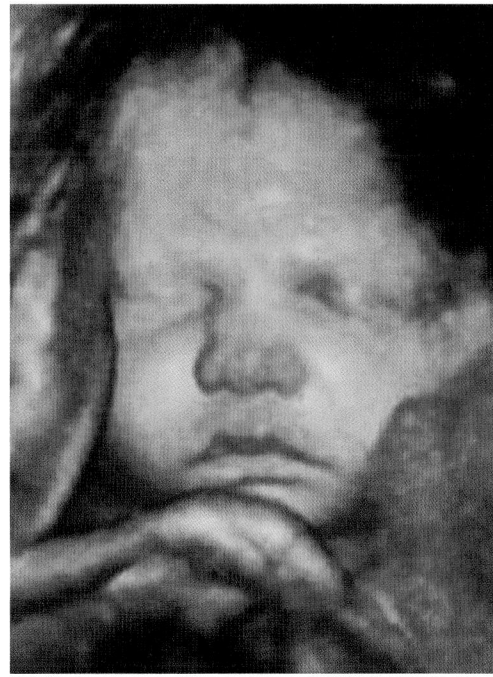

**FIG 15.2** Three-dimensional ultrasound image of a fetus in the third trimester, showing the detail of facial features. (From Benacerraf, B.R. [2008]. The role of three-dimensional ultrasound in the evaluation of the fetus. In P.W. Callen [Ed.], *Ultrasonography in obstetrics & gynecology* [5th ed.]. Philadelphia: Saunders.)

### Purposes

Transvaginal ultrasound is most common during the first trimester for:

- Determining the presence and location (intrauterine or elsewhere) of pregnancy
- Detecting multifetal gestations
- Estimating gestational age
- Confirming fetal viability
- Identifying the need for follow-up testing
- Identifying ultrasound characteristics that suggest fetal abnormality, such as chromosome defects
- As an adjunct for transcervical or transabdominal chorionic villus sampling

During the first trimester, the measurement of the crown-rump length of the embryo is the most reliable indicator of gestational age. Fetal viability is confirmed by the observation of the fetal heartbeat, which is visible when the embryo is at least 5 mm in length. Maternal structures and some abnormalities, such as uterine fibroids, ovarian cysts, and a bicornuate uterus, can also be seen (American College of Obstetricians and Gynecologists [ACOG], 2014).

### Second and Third Trimesters

Transabdominal ultrasound is common during the second and third trimesters because the uterus is out of the pelvis and accessible.

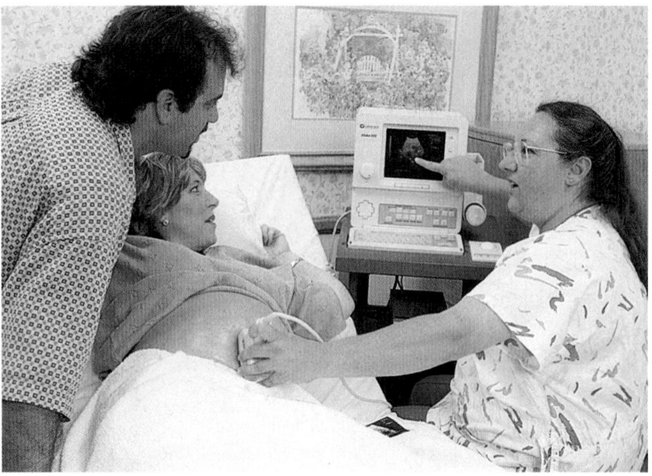

FIG 15.3 The sonographer provides information as she moves the transducer over the mother's abdomen to obtain an image.

Transvaginal ultrasound continues to be useful to evaluate the cervical and lower uterine areas.

### Procedure

The mother is positioned on her back with her head and knees supported by pillows. Her head should be elevated, and she should be turned slightly to one side with a wedge or rolled blanket under one hip to avoid supine hypotension (see p. 283). If she desires, the screen can be positioned so that she can see the images. Transmission gel is spread over her abdomen, and the sonographer, usually a physician or ultrasound technician, moves a transducer over the abdomen to obtain a picture (Fig. 15.3).

During the second trimester, a full bladder may be needed to displace the intestines and elevate the uterus for better visibility. If indicated, the woman should be instructed to drink several glasses of clear fluid an hour before the time of the examination and to delay urination until the examination is completed.

### Purposes

Ultrasound is used during the second and third trimesters for many reasons, including:

- Confirmation of fetal viability
- Evaluation of fetal anatomy
- Estimation of gestational age
- Assessment of fetal growth progress over a series of scans
- Comparison of fetal growth in multifetal gestation
- Evaluation of amniotic fluid volume (see also "Biophysical Profile," p. 283)
- Determination of the relative locations of the placenta and umbilical cord and the insertion of the cord into the fetal abdomen
- Determination of fetal presentation
- Guiding needle placement for procedures such as amniocentesis and percutaneous umbilical blood sampling

Several body measurements, including biparietal diameter, femur length, and abdominal circumference, are done to estimate gestational age during the last half of pregnancy. Sequential assessments of multiple fetal measurements will help date the pregnancy more accurately than a single measurement. Estimating fetal age by ultrasound after 32 weeks is subject to major error. At this time, the fetus can be evaluated for other signs of maturity and for signs of excessive or reduced growth rate (Copel, & Moore, 2014).

The true gestational age must be known if screening for the level of maternal serum **alpha-fetoprotein** (MSAFP), which changes with fetal age. Accurate gestational age is also important if intrauterine growth restriction is suspected or the expected date of delivery is uncertain.

A comprehensive ultrasound in the second trimester is used to evaluate the fetus when risk factors are present or the basic examination shows abnormal findings. Examples include previous birth of an infant with anomalies or abnormal clinical findings such as hydramnios (excessive amniotic fluid), oligohydramnios (insufficient amniotic fluid), or abnormal levels of MSAFP. Fetal anatomy is systematically examined to identify major system and organ structures. Anomalies that can be detected with comprehensive ultrasound include most open **neural tube defects** such as myelomeningocele and anencephaly (nonclosure of spinal cord); abdominal wall defects such as gastroschisis and omphalocele; malformed kidneys; hydrocephalus; obstruction in the fetal bowel or urinary system; cleft lip and palate; and limb abnormalities. Maternal obesity may limit the accuracy of ultrasound in pregnancy (Sharma, & Chervenak, 2011).

### Advantages

Ultrasound allows safe, clear visualization of the fetus and surrounding structures. Ultrasound is noninvasive and relatively comfortable, and the results are immediately available. Small portable scanners allow the machine to be moved easily for quick scans, as in the case of uncertain fetal presentation in a laboring woman.

### Disadvantages

Ultrasound and other prenatal diagnostic procedures cannot identify every fetal structural defect or defects that do not affect body structures, such as an inborn error of metabolism. In addition, women who do not have early prenatal care in the first trimester of pregnancy lose many benefits of early ultrasound examinations such as accurate estimation of gestational age. Cost may be a problem if the woman has no insurance coverage.

Ultrasound findings that are not normal but for which the implications are unknown may occur. The next step in the fetal diagnostic process may be uncertain, causing greater parental anxiety.

## DOPPLER ULTRASOUND BLOOD FLOW ASSESSMENT

When an ultrasound wave is directed at an acute angle to blood flowing through a vessel, the frequency of echoes changes as the cardiac cycle goes through systole and diastole. This change, referred to as the *Doppler shift*, indicates forward movement of blood within a vessel and resembles gentle hills and valleys that remain above the baseline.

### Purpose

Pregnancies complicated by hypertension or fetal growth restriction caused by placental insufficiency can be assessed using Doppler ultrasound of blood flow through the umbilical artery to identify abnormalities in the diastolic flow. The most common measurement is the systolic/diastolic (S/D) ratio, which normally decreases over the course of gestation. If fetal peripheral resistance rises, the diastolic flow falls, resulting in an increased S/D ratio. In severe cases of growth restriction caused by placental insufficiency, the diastolic flow may be absent or even reversed (American Academy of Pediatrics [AAP] & American College of Obstetricians and Gynecologists [ACOG], 2012; Kaimal, 2014).

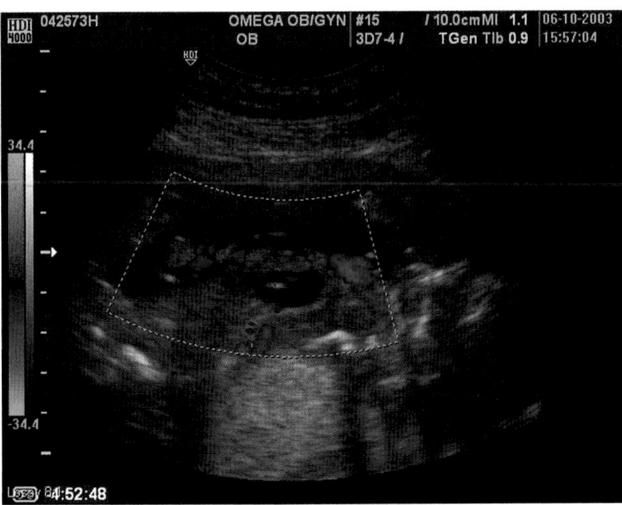


FIG 15.4 Color Doppler imaging of the umbilical vein and two arteries. Blood flow toward the transducer is typically shown as red whereas the flow away from the transducer is shown as blue. (Courtesy Paul and Kerry Hamilton.)

**BOX 15.2 Conditions Associated With Abnormal Maternal Serum Alpha-Fetoprotein Levels**

**Elevated Levels of Alpha-Fetoprotein (AFP)**

Open neural tube defects (anencephaly, spina bifida)
Esophageal obstruction
Abdominal wall defects (omphalocele, gastroschisis)
Increased amount leaked by fetal kidney (hydronephrosis)
Threatened abortion
Fetal demise
Normal fetus in conjunction with one or more of the following:
- Amniotic fluid contaminated with fetal blood during amniocentesis
- Underestimation of fetal age
- Multifetal gestation
- Incorrect maternal weight (lower than true weight)
- Maternal insulin-dependent diabetes

**Low Levels of AFP**

Chromosomal trisomies (e.g., Down syndrome)
Gestational trophoblastic disease
Normal fetuses in conjunction with the following:
- Overestimation of gestational age
- Incorrect maternal weight (higher than true weight)

## COLOR DOPPLER

Color Doppler imaging is useful for determining the relationships between body structures. Nondirectional color Doppler imaging uses a single color to identify structures, as in assessing the number of vessels in the umbilical cord. Directional color Doppler uses two or more colors to determine the direction and speed of blood flow and pulsations within cardiovascular structures (Fig. 15.4). This information can be used to determine whether the heart structure is normal and whether the relationships between the major vessels and the heart chambers are correct. Color Doppler imaging can determine blood flow and pulsations within umbilical cord vessels and other major vessels such as the cranial vessels.

## ALPHA-FETOPROTEIN SCREENING

Alpha-fetoprotein (AFP) is the main protein in fetal plasma. It diffuses from fetal plasma into fetal urine and is excreted into the amniotic fluid. Some AFP crosses placental membranes into the maternal circulation. Therefore, AFP can be measured both in maternal serum (i.e., MSAFP) and in amniotic fluid (i.e., amniotic fluid alpha-fetoprotein [AFAFP]). Abnormal concentrations of AFP are associated with serious fetal anomalies, requiring additional testing to determine the reason for the abnormal concentration.

The AFP concentration increases with advancing gestational age of the fetus and is higher in multifetal gestations because more than one fetus is producing the protein. Interpretation of MSAFP values must be corrected for maternal weight because AFP diffuses into a larger maternal compartment in heavier women.

### Purpose

Low levels of MSAFP are associated with chromosomal anomalies, such as trisomy 21 (Down syndrome). The most common cause of elevated AFP is failure of the embryonic neural tube or anterior body wall to close properly. In these conditions, neural or abdominal cavity tissues are exposed or covered with only a very thin layer of tissue, allowing high concentrations of AFP to seep into amniotic fluid and then enter maternal serum.

The most common open neural tube defects are anencephaly, in which the cranial vault is absent and most of the brain is undeveloped, and spina bifida, which varies widely in severity (see Chapter 52). Box 15.2 lists other conditions that are associated with abnormal MSAFP.

### Procedure

Pregnant women should be offered MSAFP screening, ideally between 16 and 18 weeks of gestation (AAP & ACOG, 2012). The mother is informed that MSAFP is a screening test rather than a diagnostic test. Further tests will be indicated to investigate abnormal concentrations. If MSAFP levels are abnormal, ultrasound is recommended initially to determine whether the abnormal concentration is caused by multifetal gestation, inaccurate gestational age, or fetal death.

### Advantages

MSAFP evaluation has several advantages:

- The procedure is simple and requires only a sample of maternal blood.
- It is the least invasive and most economical procedure to screen for an open body wall defect such as a neural tube defect or for chromosome abnormalities.
- Prenatal diagnosis allows parents time to examine their options or to prepare for the birth of an infant who will need special care.

### Limitations

MSAFP has several limitations:

- This screening tool must be viewed as the first step in a series of diagnostic procedures that are indicated if abnormal concentrations are found. Parents must decide about whether to proceed each time another diagnostic test is offered.
- Benign conditions, such as inaccurate estimation of gestational age, can result in apparently abnormal levels, causing the parents greater anxiety and expense if follow-up tests are indicated.

- Timing imposes limits. Evaluation is best performed between 16 and 18 weeks of pregnancy, but many women do not seek prenatal care until well after the 18th week, thus limiting their options.
- Because closed defects that are covered by skin do not produce elevated levels of AFP, a normal AFP level does not guarantee that the baby will be free of structural anomalies.

## MULTIPLE-MARKER SCREENING

Two other markers, human chorionic gonadotropin (hCG) and unconjugated estriol, have been added to routine MSAFP evaluation to screen for chromosomal abnormalities using maternal serum. This multiple-marker screening increases the detection of trisomy 18 and trisomy 21 (Cunningham, Leveno, Bloom, et al., 2010; Jorde, Carey, & Bamshad, 2010). Maternal serum samples are taken between 16 and 18 weeks of gestation, and the results are considered positive if MSAFP and estriol are low and if hCG is high. If the results are positive, the woman should be offered additional testing, such as amniocentesis (withdrawal of amniotic fluid through the abdomen) for karyotyping or additional ultrasound to look for physical characteristics associated with the chromosome defects.

A fourth marker, the placental hormone inhibin A, improves the accuracy of multiple-marker screening for identifying trisomy 21 in women younger than the age of 35 years. Added costs for more tests must be considered when considering their benefit to the woman.

## CHORIONIC VILLUS SAMPLING

Chorionic villi are microscopic projections from the outer membrane (chorion) that develop and burrow into endometrial tissue as the placenta is formed. The villi are composed of rapidly dividing cells of fetal origin that reflect the chromosomal and genetic makeup of the fetus. Chorionic villus cells can be used for diagnosis of fetal chromosomal, metabolic, or DNA abnormalities between 10 and 13 weeks of gestation.

### Purpose

Chorionic villus sampling (CVS) uses transcervical or transabdominal sampling to obtain villi to diagnose fetal chromosome or metabolic abnormalities. It cannot be used to diagnose anomalies for which amniotic fluid is essential, such as open neural tube or body wall defects, which require measuring AFP levels (AAP & ACOG, 2012) Cunningham et al., 2010; Wapner, 2014).

### Indications

CVS is usually performed between 10 and 13 weeks of gestation to diagnose fetal chromosomal, metabolic, or DNA abnormalities.

### Procedure

As with all diagnostic procedures, the woman should receive both counseling about the procedure itself and genetic counseling regarding the specific defect for which CVS is being performed. The benefits and limitations of the procedure should be carefully explained, and signed informed consent should be obtained.

CVS can be performed by a transcervical or transabdominal approach (AAP & ACOG, 2012; Cunningham et al., 2010; Wapner, 2014). In the transcervical technique, a flexible catheter is inserted through the cervix, and a sample of chorionic villi is aspirated (Fig. 15.5). In the transabdominal technique, a needle is inserted through the abdominal and uterine walls to collect chorionic tissue.

After the procedure, the woman is shown the fetal heart motion, and maternal vital signs are assessed. Heavy bleeding or the passage of amniotic fluid, clots, or tissue suggests possible miscarriage and should be reported. The woman should rest at home for several hours after the procedure.

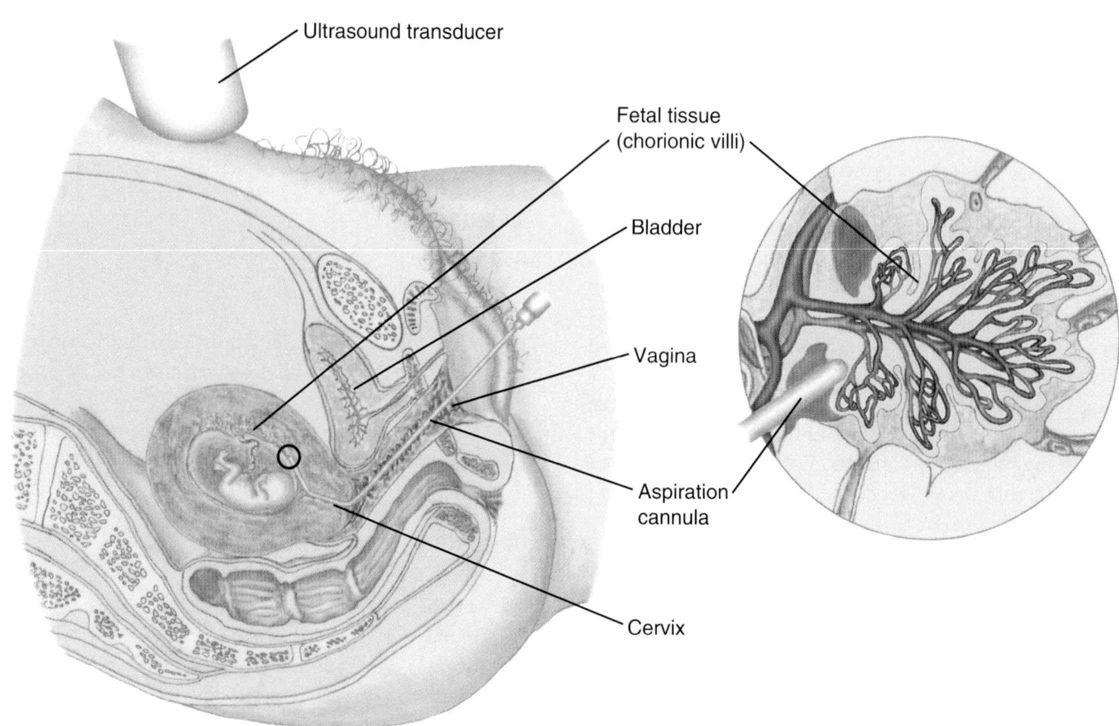


**FIG 15.5** Transcervical chorionic villus sampling. Tissue is aspirated to identify some genetic defects in the fetus. Transabdominal aspiration is an alternative method.

### Advantages

Fetal cells in the villi are actively dividing and results are usually available more quickly than amniocentesis. CVS is performed earlier in the pregnancy than is amniocentesis, offering an alternative to women who find later procedures unacceptable. Furthermore, if results are abnormal and the woman chooses abortion, she may consider the earlier abortion less physically and emotionally traumatic than a later procedure.

### Limitations

Although chorionic villus sampling is now considered a safe and effective technique for first-trimester prenatal diagnosis, there are limitations:

- The pregnancy loss rate is approximately 2.5% (Wapner 2014).
- Reports of a higher-than-expected rate of limb reduction defects is reported for CVS performed before 10 weeks. Although CVS is now performed at 10 to 13 weeks, families should be given information about reported problems before they choose the procedure.
- The risk of uterine infection is low, but it occurs occasionally. The presence of a cervical or vaginal infection is a contraindication for the transvaginal approach (Cunningham et al., 2010; Gilbert, 2011).
- Rh sensitization may occur as a result of entry of fetal Rh-positive blood cells into the circulation of an Rh-negative mother. $Rh_o$ (D) immune globulin (RhoGAM) should be administered to all unsensitized Rh-negative women following the procedure (see Chapter 26).
- CVS is labor intensive because maternal cells may be aspirated along with the fetal cells. Maternal cells must be removed from the sample before culture, adding to the procedure's cost.

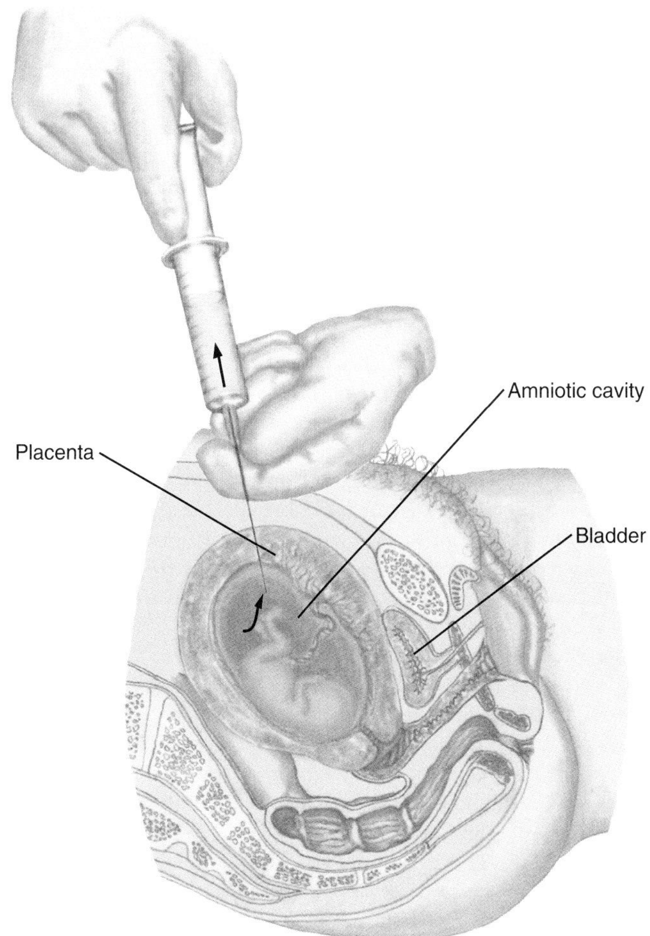


FIG 15.6 In amniocentesis, a needle is inserted through the mother's abdomen to aspirate fluid from the amniotic sac. The fluid can then be tested to detect chromosomal abnormalities in fetal cells or other problems and to determine fetal lung maturity.

## AMNIOCENTESIS

Amniocentesis is the aspiration of amniotic fluid from the amniotic sac for examination (Fig. 15.6). Amniocentesis may be performed during the second or third trimester of pregnancy, depending on the purpose. Second-trimester amniocentesis for fetal genetic abnormalities is best performed between 15 and 20 weeks because the amniotic fluid is of adequate volume and contains many viable fetal cells.

Early amniocentesis is possible between 11 and 14 weeks. Early amniocentesis is associated with a higher fetal loss rate than later amniocentesis. Fetal foot deformations are more likely to occur with removal of amniotic fluid at gestation earlier than 13 weeks (Cunningham et al., 2010).

### Purposes

#### Second-Trimester Amniocentesis

The primary purpose of midtrimester amniocentesis is to examine fetal cells present in amniotic fluid to identify chromosomal or biochemical abnormalities. Amniocentesis is also used to evaluate the fetal condition when the woman is sensitized to Rh-positive blood, to diagnose amnionitis (intrauterine infection), and to test the AFAFP for cases in which the MSAFP is abnormal and the cause cannot be determined by noninvasive tests (Box 15.3).

**BOX 15.3 Common Indications for Second-Trimester Amniocentesis**

- Maternal age 35 years or older
- Chromosomal abnormality in close family member
- Gender determination for maternal carrier of X-linked disorder (e.g., hemophilia, Duchenne muscular dystrophy)
- Birth of previous infant with chromosomal abnormality or a neural tube or body-wall defect
- Pregnancy after multiple spontaneous abortions
- Elevated levels of maternal serum alpha-fetoprotein that remain unexplained
- Maternal Rh sensitization of maternal Rh-negative blood to fetal Rh-positive blood

#### Third-Trimester Amniocentesis

During the third trimester, amniocentesis may be used to determine fetal lung maturity or to evaluate fetal hemolytic disease that is often caused by Rh incompatibility. Reduction amniocentesis is a variation in which excess amniotic fluid is removed and discarded when hydramnios occurs. Samples of the fluid removed in a reduction amniocentesis may be evaluated for the presence of infection or for substances that help evaluate the fetal condition.

***Tests to determine fetal lung maturity.*** A test for fetal lung maturity is recommended when non-emergency delivery is being considered before 38 weeks of gestation. This information can be used to reduce the risk of respiratory distress in the newborn. The lecithin/sphingomyelin (L/S) ratio is the best-known test for estimating fetal lung maturity. Lecithin and sphingomyelin are lipoproteins that make up surfactant, which is present in the pulmonary alveoli of term infants. Surfactant keeps the alveoli open by reducing surface tension on their inner walls. The decreased surface tension prevents collapse of the alveoli when the infant exhales, reducing the effort of breathing.

The proportion of lecithin to sphingomyelin is about equal until approximately the 30th week of gestation. At this time, the level of sphingomyelin plateaus, but lecithin continues to increase. An L/S ratio greater than 2 : 1 (twice as much lecithin as sphingomyelin) generally indicates that surfactant is adequate and the fetal lungs are mature. However, an L/S ratio of 2 : 1 does not ensure fetal lung maturity, particularly for the fetus of a woman who has diabetes. Therefore, amniotic fluid is also tested for the presence of phosphatidylglycerol (PG) and phosphatidylinositol (PI), other phospholipids that boost the properties of lecithin. Additional tests include the TDx fluorescence polarization immunoassay to determine the surfactant content in amniotic fluid. A foam stability index (FSI), often called the "shake test," may be used to determine fetal lung maturity (Mercer, 2014).

***Test for fetal hemolytic disease.*** Amniocentesis is used to obtain fluid for determining the fetal bilirubin concentration if the mother is Rh negative and is sensitized (i.e., has been exposed to the Rh antigen and has developed antibodies against Rh-positive erythrocytes). The level of bilirubin in amniotic fluid reflects the amount of fetal red blood cell destruction that occurs when maternal antibodies destroy Rh-positive fetal red blood cells, leaving the fetus vulnerable to erythroblastosis fetalis and hydrops fetalis (see Chapters 26 and 30).

### Procedure

The woman is placed in a supine position with a pillow or rolled towel under one buttock to shift the weight of the uterus off the major vessels. Maternal blood pressure and fetal heart rate (FHR) are assessed to establish baseline levels.

Ultrasound is used to locate the fetus and placenta, to identify the largest pockets of amniotic fluid that can safely be sampled, and to guide needle insertion. The skin is prepared with antiseptic solution. A small amount of local anesthetic is injected into the skin. The woman may experience the sensation of pressure as the needle is inserted and mild cramping as the needle enters the myometrium.

A 3- to 4-inch, 20- or 21-gauge needle is inserted into the pocket of fluid. The first 1 to 2 mL of fluid is discarded to avoid contamination of the fetal sample with maternal cells. Approximately 20 mL of fluid is removed for analysis. After fluid removal, the woman is shown the fetal heart beating and the fluid that remains (Cunningham et al., 2010). The fetus is monitored electronically for 30 to 60 minutes to identify continuing uterine contractions or nonreassuring fetal heart activity. The woman should avoid strenuous activity but may resume normal activities after 24 hours. She should report persistent uterine contractions, vaginal bleeding, leakage of amniotic fluid, or fever.

As with chorionic villus sampling, RhoGAM is administered to unsensitized Rh-negative women after amniocentesis to prevent sensitization.

### Advantages

Amniocentesis has several advantages, as it is:

- a simple, relatively safe procedure that permits the diagnosis of many fetal anomalies and confirms fetal lung maturity.
- a brief and relatively painless procedure.
- associated with few reported complications based on data from years of use. The fetal loss rate is <1% above the baseline risk for miscarriage during the midtrimester.

### Disadvantages

The major disadvantage of midtrimester amniocentesis for prenatal diagnosis is timing. The sample is taken at 15 to 20 weeks of gestation, and obtaining test results can take 2 or more weeks for less common tests. By this time, the pregnancy is obvious, the woman has felt fetal movement, and she may face an even more difficult decision about continuing the pregnancy if the results are abnormal.

Early amniocentesis avoids some of the timing disadvantages associated with later amniocentesis for prenatal diagnosis. However, early amniocentesis does carry a higher risk of fetal loss after the procedure, and smaller amounts of fluid can be withdrawn for analysis.

### Risks

Amniocentesis is a relatively safe prenatal diagnostic procedure. The risk of injury to the fetus or umbilical cord is minimal when ultrasound is used to guide needle insertion. The risk of infection is also minimal, because aseptic technique is used throughout the procedure. The risk of spontaneous abortion associated with amniocentesis during the second trimester is 0.5% or less (Cunningham et al., 2010).

As with all fetal diagnostic procedures, amniocentesis cannot guarantee the birth of a perfect infant. Parents must be counseled that not all defects are detectable by amniocentesis.

## PERCUTANEOUS UMBILICAL BLOOD SAMPLING

Percutaneous umbilical blood sampling (PUBS), also called *cordocentesis,* involves the aspiration of fetal blood from the umbilical cord near the placenta for prenatal diagnosis or therapy (Fig. 15.7). PUBS is infrequently needed to determine the karyotype (chromosome evaluation) because many tests can be done on fetal cells in amniotic fluid

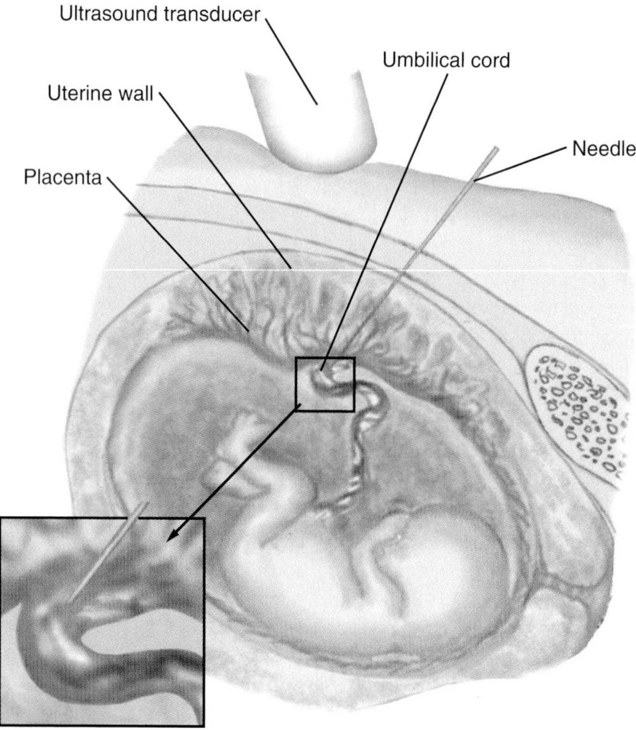


FIG 15.7 In percutaneous umbilical blood sampling, a needle is inserted through the mother's abdomen and into an umbilical vessel (vein or artery) to withdraw a sample of fetal blood.

using techniques such as fluorescent in-situ hybridization (FISH) or other DNA analysis (see Chapter 10). Major indications for PUBS include the diagnosis and intrauterine management of Rh disease, infections, or for diagnosing disorders that require fetal blood for testing (Cunningham et al., 2010; Kaimal, 2014; Wapner, 2014).

### Procedure

Ultrasound is used to locate the fetus, placenta, and umbilical cord. A needle is inserted through the abdomen and into the uterine cavity. The umbilical cord is punctured near the site where it meets the placenta to provide stability as blood is aspirated. The umbilical vein is targeted more commonly than one of the umbilical arteries because it is larger and less likely to constrict during the procedure. Which vessel is used (vein or artery) when sampling fetal blood is unimportant for genetic or coagulation studies but very important when testing fetal acid–base parameters. Blood from the umbilical vein contains oxygenated blood and has a lower carbon dioxide content than blood from an umbilical artery, leaving the fetus after circulation throughout the body.

### Risks

In addition to fetal loss, complications of PUBS include infection, fetal bradycardia, cord laceration, cord hematoma, thrombosis, thromboembolism, preterm labor, and premature rupture of membranes. RhoGAM is given to the unsensitized woman with Rh-negative blood (RhoGAM immune globulin drug guide in Chapter 26).

## ANTEPARTUM FETAL SURVEILLANCE

Antepartum fetal surveillance has three goals: to determine fetal health or compromise as accurately as possible, to guide intervention by the obstetric and neonatal teams, and to reduce perinatal morbidity and mortality. Three common methods of fetal surveillance are the nonstress test (NST), the contraction stress test (CST), and the biophysical profile (BPP).

### Nonstress Test

#### Purpose

The NST identifies whether an increase in the FHR occurs when the fetus moves, indicating adequate oxygenation, a healthy neural pathway from the fetal central nervous system to the fetal heart, and the ability of the fetal heart to respond to stimuli. FHR accelerations without fetal movement are also considered a reassuring sign of adequate fetal oxygenation. However, if the fetal heart does not accelerate with movement, fetal hypoxemia and acidosis are concerns. In such cases, an additional test such as the CST or BPP is necessary to evaluate the metabolic condition of the fetus. The NST is often included as part of the BPP.

#### Procedure

The nurse with training in fetal monitoring instructs the woman about the NST and explains why it is recommended. The test is termed "nonstress" because it consists of monitoring only. The fetus is not challenged or stressed by stimulated uterine contractions. A physician or midwife reviews and makes the final interpretation of the data.

The woman usually sits in a reclining chair or in bed in a semi-Fowler's position to prevent supine hypotension. Side lying or a lateral tilt is another positioning option. The nurse applies external electronic fetal monitoring (EFM) equipment to the woman's abdomen to detect the FHR and any contractions or fetal movement (Fig. 15.8). The woman may be given a remote event marker to press each time she senses movement. An accurate NST may be more difficult if a woman is obese because of her thick abdominal fat pad. (See Chapter 17 for more information about fetal monitoring.)

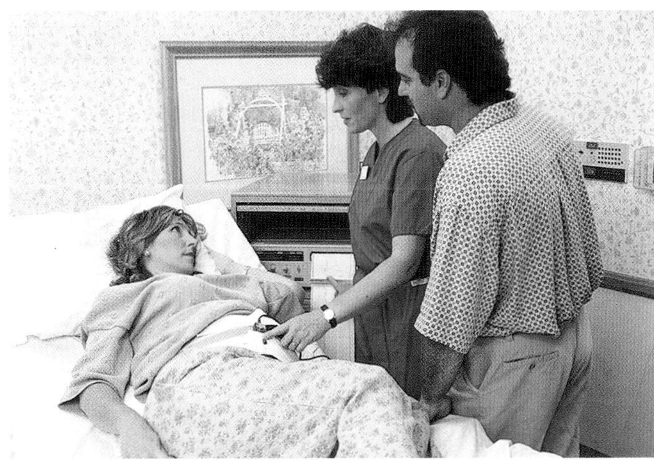

FIG 15.8 A nonstress test is a noninvasive test that measures the ability of the fetal heart to accelerate, often in response to fetal movements. Here, the nurse reassures the parents by pointing to fetal heart rate accelerations detected by the external fetal monitor.

#### Interpretation

Results are judged to be reactive (reassuring) or nonreactive (nonreassuring) (AAP & ACOG, 2012; ACOG, 2014; Cunningham et al., 2010; Kaimal, 2014) if the following characteristics are present:

- *Reactive (reassuring):* At least two FHR accelerations, with or without fetal movement, occurring within any 20-minute period and peaking at least 15 beats per minute (bpm) above the baseline and lasting 15 seconds ("15 by 15") from baseline to baseline (Fig. 15.9). Acoustic stimulation with a vibroacoustic stimulator of 1 second that elicits similar FHR accelerations is reassuring. Extending the testing time for 40 minutes or longer may be needed to allow for normal fetal sleep–wake cycles. Before 32 weeks, accelerations are acceptable at 10 bpm for 10 seconds ("10 by 10").

*Nonreactive (nonreassuring):* Tracing does not demonstrate the required characteristics of a reactive tracing within a 40-minute or longer period (AAP & ACOG, 2012; ACOG, 2014a; Cunningham et al., 2010; Kaimal, 2014).

#### Advantages

The NST is noninvasive, painless, and believed to be without risk to mother or fetus. For these reasons, it is the primary means of fetal surveillance in pregnancies that are at increased risk for uteroplacental insufficiency and consequent fetal hypoxia and acidosis. The NST is easy to administer and may be repeated weekly or even daily if necessary. Results are available immediately.

#### Disadvantages

A disadvantage is a false-positive test result that occurs in a well-oxygenated term fetus of 32 or more weeks gestation that does not have accelerations reaching a peak of 15 bpm or that last less than 15 seconds from baseline to baseline. Because of the high false-positive rate, women may undergo additional testing even though the fetus is actually healthy. Additional testing is usually a BPP or ultrasound examination.

Sleep is a common reason for lack of fetal movement. Fetal sleep cycles average 20 to 40 minutes, but other sleep cycles are longer. Vibroacoustic stimulation reduces many false-positive results.

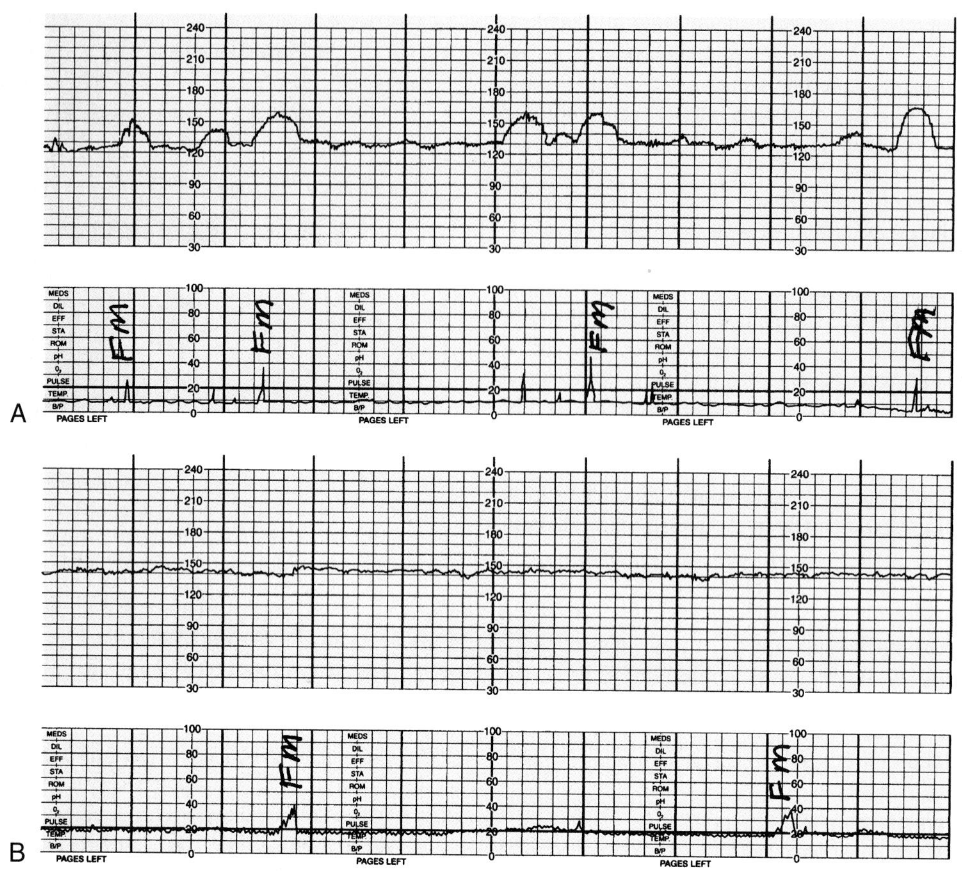


**FIG 15.9** **A,** Several accelerations have a duration of at least 15 seconds, reaching a peak of 25 to 30 beats per minute in this example of a reactive nonstress test. Comparable accelerations without fetal movement are also reassuring. **B,** In this recording of a nonreactive nonstress test, accelerations are absent after fetal movement. (Courtesy Graphic Controls, Buffalo, NY.)

## Vibroacoustic (Acoustic) Stimulation

### Purpose and Procedure

Vibroacoustic stimulation, also called VAS or acoustic stimulation, uses sound to confirm whether NST findings are reassuring and shorten the time to obtain quality NST data. Reactive test results obtained with a vibroacoustic stimulator, similar to an electronic larynx, appear to predict fetal well-being without interfering with the detection of a compromised fetus. VAS can be used in intrapartum monitoring to verify questionable findings (see Chapter 17).

A vibroacoustic stimulator is applied to the maternal abdomen over the area of the fetal head; stimulation with vibration and sound is given for up to 3 seconds. VAS can be repeated at 1-minute intervals up to three times.

### Fetal Responses

Brain responses to auditory stimulation appear between 26 and 28 weeks of gestation. The sound of VAS does not appear to damage hearing in the fetus. Fetuses near term show an increase in the number of gross (large and easily visible or felt) body movements to VAS, whereas healthy fetuses between 26 and 32 weeks of gestation may show no response, suggesting maturational changes to VAS (Harding, & Walker, 2014).

### Risks

VAS appears to be safe for the fetus in terms of hearing. The amniotic fluid and maternal tissues surrounding the fetus soften the sound of the VAS.

## Contraction Stress Test

### Purpose

A CST, or oxytocin challenge test (OCT) may be done if NST findings are nonreactive, although the next step is usually an ultrasound examination for a BPP. The concern is that if fetal oxygenation is only marginally adequate when the uterus is at rest, it will be decreased further during contractions generated by oxytocin infusion or nipple stimulation. Nipple stimulation by the woman to induce temporary contractions may be successful and eliminates the complexity of oxytocin infusion.

Uterine contractions compress the arteries supplying the placenta with oxygenated maternal blood, causing a recurrent decrease in fetal oxygen levels. The FHR pattern remains reassuring if the fetus has oxygen reserves adequate to tolerate the brief hypoxia during a contraction. However, if the fetus has inadequate reserves and if hypoxia has led to anaerobic metabolism, fetal acidosis may result. Fetal acidosis may be evidenced by late decelerations (slowing of the FHR after onset of a contraction that persists after the contraction ends) and loss of variability. (Chapter 17 reviews EFM and nonreassuring patterns.)

Because contractions are induced, the CST is contraindicated in some situations (AAP & ACOG, 2012; Cunningham et al., 2010):

- Preterm labor or women who have a high risk for preterm labor
- Preterm membrane rupture
- History of extensive uterine surgery or classic uterine incision for cesarean birth (see Chapters 19 and 27)
- Placenta previa (see Chapter 25)

### Procedure

The nurse places the woman in a supine position with her head comfortably elevated. A side-lying position or uterine displacement reduces uterine pressure on the woman's aorta and inferior vena cava. External EFM devices are applied to record both uterine activity and FHR. The FHR and patterns must be evaluated in relation to uterine contractions. Three contractions of at least 40 seconds each and occurring within a 10-minute period are required to interpret the CST. Two methods may be used to initiate uterine contractions if none are present:

1. *Breast self-stimulation* causes the release of oxytocin from the posterior pituitary, which then causes uterine contractions. The woman brushes her palm across one nipple through her clothing for 2 minutes, stopping if a contraction begins. The nipple stimulation is repeated after a 5-minute rest period if no contractions occur.
2. If nipple stimulation does not induce adequate uterine contractions, *intravenous infusion of low-dose oxytocin* is used. The nurse conducting the test inserts a primary intravenous line plus a piggyback line to administer the oxytocin solution. The administration of oxytocin is similar to that used to induce labor (see Chapter 19).

### Interpretation

Contraction stress test (CST) results are assigned one of five interpretations (ACOG, 2014 and Cunningham et al., 2010):

- *Negative (reassuring):* No late or significant variable decelerations.
- *Positive (nonreassuring):* Late decelerations follow 50% or more of contractions, even if fewer than three contractions occur in 10 minutes.
- *Equivocal-suspicious:* Intermittent late or significant variable decelerations.
- *Equivocal-tachysystole:* FHR decelerations occur in the presence of excessive contractions (more frequent than every 2 minutes or lasting longer than 90 seconds).
- *Unsatisfactory:* Fewer than three contractions within 10 minutes or a tracing that cannot be interpreted.

Figure 15.10 provides a summary of contraction stress test interpretations.

### Advantages

The availability of other tests that are more diagnostic of fetal well-being and placental function than the CST has decreased its original advantages. Reasons that CST may be chosen include:

- The test allows follow-up of a nonreactive NST result or BPP.
- If findings are negative, CST offers more than 99% reassurance that the uteroplacental unit is likely to support life for at least 1 more week (ACOG, 2012a).
- A positive CST result allows the physician to analyze available options and to make plans for the birth of an infant who may be compromised because of decreased placental functioning before or during labor.

### Disadvantages

The CST has three major disadvantages:

- The test is more time consuming than the NST.
- It requires precision, needing either the participation of the woman in breast self-stimulation or careful infusion of oxytocin by the nurse to obtain an adequate contraction pattern without causing tachysystole (6 contractions in a 10-minute period) of the uterus.
- The cost is higher than that of the NST, particularly if the oxytocin challenge test is used. The CST is usually performed in a hospital setting with a per-hour charge. Equipment and supplies such as intravenous lines, oxytocin, and infusion pumps add to the cost.

## Biophysical Profile

Predicting the condition of the fetus is more accurate if several parameters are evaluated. Unlike the NST and CST, which assess only fetal heart activity, the BPP assesses a total of five parameters of fetal well-being: the NST, fetal breathing movements, gross fetal movements (large trunk movements), fetal tone (small or fine body movements such as limb or hand extension and flexion or sucking movements), and amniotic fluid volume. The last four parameters require ultrasound evaluation. If all four ultrasound components are reassuring, the NST is not essential (AAP & ACOG, 2012; Cunningham et al., 2010; Kaimal, 2014).

### Purpose

The individual components of the examination are a combination of both acute and chronic markers of fetal well-being to improve the prognostic ability of the BPP. The acute markers are FHR reactivity, fetal breathing movements, gross body movements, and fetal tone. The major chronic or long-term marker is the volume of amniotic fluid. Normal values for each suggest adequate neurologic function and oxygenation.

The fetal central and autonomic nervous systems that control each parameter of the BPP react differently to hypoxemia. Control centers that develop later require higher oxygen levels than earlier-developing centers and are first to react when oxygen levels fall. Fetal activities that develop earliest in gestation are the last to disappear when fetal oxygenation is compromised. Thus, as hypoxemia begins, FHR reactivity will be less and then absent. Fetal breathing movements will slow, then cease. As hypoxemia progresses, characteristics that developed earlier in gestation, such as gross body movements and muscle tone, disappear as the fetus conserves energy and oxygen. Figure 15.11 illustrates the effects of gradual hypoxemia on the central nervous system of the fetus.

The amount of amniotic fluid provides important information about long-term hypoxia. During periods of hypoxemia, the fetus shunts blood from areas that are not critical to fetal life, such as the kidneys and lungs, toward the vital organs (heart, brain, and placenta). If the hypoxemia is prolonged, blood flow to the fetal kidneys and lungs, which produce most of the amniotic fluid, may virtually cease. Therefore, oligohydramnios indicates prolonged fetal hypoxia and strongly suggests fetal compromise.

### Procedure and Interpretation

FHR reactivity is measured and interpreted from an NST. The other four parameters are measured by real-time ultrasound. A scoring technique is used to quantify the data, with each of the five parameters contributing either 2 or 0 points out of 10 total points, or 8 total points if the NST is not done (Table 15.1). A score of 10 (8 for BPPs without the NST) is perfect; a score of 0 is the worst score. A total score of 8 to 10 out of 10 (expressed as "8/10" to "10/10") is reassuring; a score of 4 or less is nonreassuring. Oligohydramnios may indicate chronic fetal hypoxia and warrants more frequent BPP testing or consideration of delivery (AAP & ACOG, 2012; ACOG, 2014a).

The **amniotic fluid index** (AFI) is the sum of the maximum depth of amniotic fluid in four uterine quadrants and is used to evaluate amniotic fluid adequacy for gestational age. Established normal values for the AFI do not exist, but volume sums greater than 10 cm are

| | | |
|---|---|---|
| **Negative** | No late decelerations | Reassuring that the fetus can tolerate labor |
| **Positive** | Consistent late decelerations in ≥50% of the contractions, even if contraction frequency is less than 3 in 10 minutes | Indicates UPI and fetal compromise during contractions |
| **Equivocal-suspicious** | Intermittent late or significant variable decelerations | A second CST should be repeated within 24 hours |
| **Equivocal-tachysystole** | Late decelerations with excessive uterine activity (contractions closer than every 2 minutes or lasting longer than 90 seconds) | Repeat CST within 24 hours with careful monitoring of the situation |
| **Unsatisfactory** | Test cannot be interpreted; either not enough data or unsatisfactory tracing; fewer than three contractions in 10 minutes | Repeat CST with careful attention to maternal position, oxytocin infusion, and placement of tocotransducer |

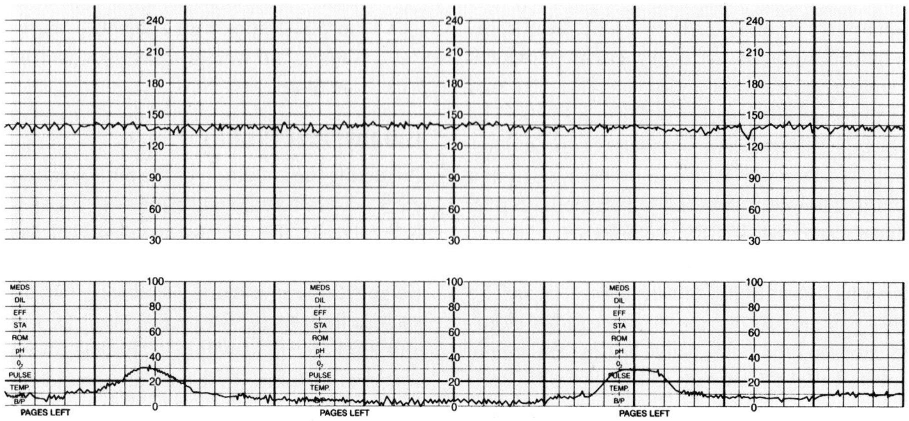

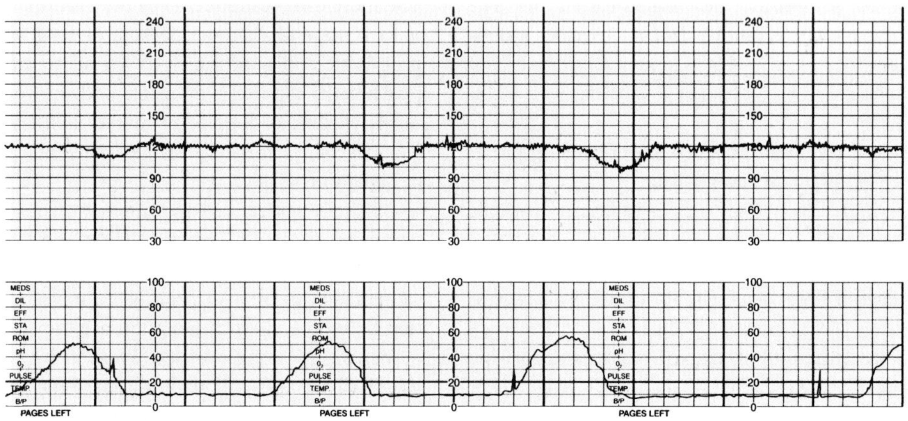

**FIG 15.10** Interpretation of contraction stress test (CST). *UPI,* Uteroplacental insufficiency. (Courtesy Graphic Controls, Buffalo, NY.)

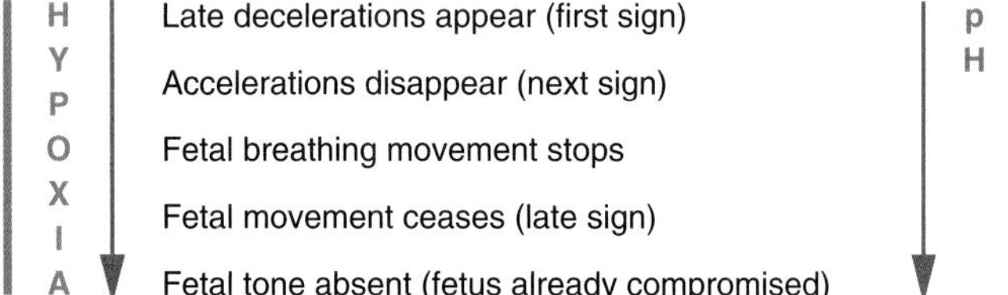


**FIG 15.11** Effects of gradual hypoxemia and worsening fetal acidosis.

considered reassuring, and less than 5 cm volume is considered oligohydramnios. An AFI higher than 24 to 25 cm suggests excess amniotic fluid volume, or hydramnios (Cunningham et al., 2010).

## Modified Biophysical Profile

Some physicians assess the fetus only by ultrasound and omit the NST if all ultrasound parameters are normal. Another modification includes only two parameters: an AFI and an NST (AAP & ACOG, 2012).

### Advantages

The BPP is noninvasive and is less costly than some tests because it can be done on an outpatient basis. Results are immediately available, and it may decrease the number of false-positive nonreactive NST findings. The evaluation allows conservative treatment of high-risk patients because delivery can be delayed if reassurance of fetal well-being exists.

### Disadvantages

Additional research is needed to refine interpretation of the test. For example, each variable is given equal weight, although some variables may be more important than others. The predictive accuracy of the BPP is best at the extremes, meaning that scores of 0 and 10 are highly predictive of the presence or absence of fetal acidosis, respectively. Scores toward the middle have less predictive accuracy.

Because perinatal asphyxia is a possible cause of cerebral palsy, antepartum surveillance techniques may allow fetal hypoxia to be identified and treated before it reaches critical levels. The BPP may be the

**TABLE 15.1 Scoring the Biophysical Profile for a Term Fetus**

| | Points | |
|---|---|---|
| *Criterion* | *Present (2 points)* | *Absent (0 points)* |
| Nonstress test (NST) (if used) | Reactive NST (at least 2 fetal heart rate [FHR] accelerations peaking at least 15 bpm above baseline for 15 sec within a 20-min period) | Nonreactive NST (absence of required characteristics for reactive test after 40 min of testing) |
| Fetal breathing movements (FBM) | ≥1 episode of rhythmic FBM of 30 sec or more within 30 min | Absent FBM or none that meet criterion for "present" |
| Gross body movements | ≥3 trunk movements in 30 min; limb and trunk movement is considered one movement | ≤2 trunk movements in 30 min |
| Fetal tone | ≥1 episode of fetal extremity extension with return to flexion; opening or closing of hand within 30 min | Extension with return to partial flexion; absence of flexion |
| Amniotic fluid volume | At least one pocket of fluid that measures at least 2 cm in two planes perpendicular to each other | Amniotic fluid volume that does not meet this criterion |

Adapted from American Academy of Pediatrics & American College of Obstetricians and Gynecologists. (2012). *Guidelines for perinatal care* (7th ed.). Elk Grove Village, IL, and Washington, DC: Author.

Interpretation: Normal (reassuring), 8 to 10 points; equivocal, 6 points; abnormal, ≤4 points and delivery may be considered. If oligohydramnios is present, more frequent testing is warranted and delivery may be considered.

main testing to identify problems before they result in permanent fetal injury, but other evaluations must often enter the diagnostic picture to best clarify fetal condition (Kaimal, 2014).

## MATERNAL ASSESSMENT OF FETAL MOVEMENT

Movements by the fetus, as assessed by the mother, are called "kick counts." Fetal movement is associated with fetal well-being, and a daily evaluation of these movements provides a low-tech way of evaluating the fetus. There is no consensus on exactly how the mother should be educated to perform a fetal kick count. Instructions range from there should be "5-10 movement in an hour" to there should be "at least 10 fetal movements within 12 hours". This is quite a range and can lead to inconsistency between care providers and confusion for pregnant women. Rather than having the mother focus on how many times the fetus moves, she should pay attention to patterns and changes from what she perceives as "normal movement" for her fetus and should be instructed to notify her care provider when deviation from her normal is noted. Maternal reporting of changes in fetal activity has shown to be as valid as formal counting and documentation of fetal movement (AAP & ACOG, 2012; ACOG, 2014a; Cunningham et al., 2010; Kaimal, 2014).

### Advantages

Counting fetal movements is one of the oldest methods for evaluating the condition of the fetus. Clear advantages include that it is:

- inexpensive.
- noninvasive.
- convenient for the patient and encourages her participation in care.

### Disadvantages

Many variables make interpretation of fetal movement counts difficult:

- Fetal resting state normally decreases movements.
- Maternal perception of fetal movement varies considerably, even in the same woman at different times.
- Time of day may affect fetal movement (fewer in the morning, more in the evening).
- Maternal use of drugs (sedative drugs, methadone, heroin, cocaine, alcohol, tobacco) may affect fetal activity.

## NURSING CARE

### The Patient Who Has Diagnostic Testing

#### Assessment

Nurses collect information important for conducting diagnostic tests or that is helpful to the physician for interpreting the results. Necessary information includes:

- Gravida, para, living children, gestation in weeks.
- Maternal health problems (hypertension, diabetes, heart disease).
- Current obstetric problems (vaginal bleeding, decreased fetal movement, multifetal gestation, intrauterine growth restriction, malpresentation, hydramnios, oligohydramnios, and preeclampsia).
- Previous obstetric problems (birth of stillborn infant or infant with congenital anomalies, birth of a low-birth-weight or large-for-gestational-age infant).
- History of substance abuse, including alcohol and tobacco.
- Knowledge of reasons for the test and the procedure to be performed. The nurse may ask, "What questions can I answer before we start the test?" Identify whether the woman needs added information from her healthcare provider who ordered the test.
- Patient knowledge of surveillance regimen if additional testing is necessary: "Will you tell me what you understand about the need to repeat the test every week?" "What changes in your baby's movement are important to report promptly?"
- Emotional response to the tests: "What are your major concerns?" "What can we do to make the tests easier for you?"
- The woman's or couple's expectations of the diagnostic tests. The risks and limitations of testing should be discussed as well as the indications. It also may be necessary to remind the couple that results from one test may indicate the need for another test. They must decide at each step whether to continue, with the mother making the final decision.

#### Nursing Diagnosis and Planning

The following nursing diagnosis is common when a woman requires fetal diagnostic testing:

- Anxiety related to lack of knowledge of diagnostic procedures and the uncertain condition of the fetus.

***Expected outcomes.*** The woman and her support person will verbalize knowledge of how, when, and why she is to be tested before testing procedures are initiated. The woman and her family will verbalize concerns and seek knowledge about the fetus.

### Interventions

***Providing information.*** Provide the woman and her family simple, clear explanations of what the test assesses and the purpose and frequency of any tests. Tell them how long the test takes, and describe the testing procedure to reduce anxiety caused by lack of knowledge. Some tests require teaching about follow-up care and events that the mother should report to the healthcare team.

Abnormal results from tests such as MSAFP usually result in anxiety for the woman. The nurse should remind the woman that other factors can cause abnormal results and that additional tests to clarify these results might be ordered. Because of parental anxiety, the nurse often reinforces physician explanations of the results and any additional tests needed.

***Providing support.*** Identify and respond to feelings expressed by parents when antepartum testing procedures are recommended or when fetal problems are confirmed. The woman often experiences frustration with the discomfort, limitations, and time-consuming demands of the pregnancy and the regimen of repeated fetal testing. Skill in therapeutic communication is never more important than when counseling about fetal diagnostic tests.

- Active listening conveys interest and concern.
- Paraphrasing allows for interpretation because it expresses in different words what concerns the family.
- Reflecting what is expressed about feelings helps the family "hear" their feelings.
- Clarifying helps prospective parents "see" the issues and what options are available.
- Comforting measures such as touch convey empathic concern and are especially important during difficult procedures.

Although nurses offer caring concern and careful reflection of feelings, they do not offer advice. The decisions must be made by the woman and her family, but nurses may help patients contact people to whom they turn in troubled times, such as a member of the clergy or a close relative.

**Helping patients set realistic goals.** Women benefit from understanding how prenatal diagnostic testing benefits the fetus. Although the repeated tests may seem tedious, they often offer the best chance for the fetus to be delivered at the best possible time. Explain that testing helps the perinatal team decide whether intervention is needed and choose the best possible intervention under the circumstances. The fetus has an improved chance of surviving and reaching maturity if test results remain reassuring.

If the woman is having testing to identify fetal abnormalities, help her understand that a **baseline risk** for abnormalities remains when tests show the fetus is normal. Even if it were possible for a woman to receive all diagnostic tests for birth defects, the background risk would remain.

**Supporting the woman's decision.** Prenatal genetic diagnosis sometimes leads a woman to choose pregnancy termination, often during the second trimester. The woman also has the right to indicated prenatal genetic diagnostic procedures even if she would not terminate her pregnancy for an abnormal fetus. Nurses must examine their own ethical beliefs before becoming involved in fetal diagnostic testing. They must be prepared to support whatever decision a family makes, even if it is not one they would make. A woman who decides to continue or terminate a pregnancy is entitled to compassionate care regardless of the nurse's personal views about her decision.

### Evaluation

- Did the woman (and her family) verbalize knowledge of why tests are recommended and express an idea of how and when they will be performed?
- Does she actively seek information about the fetal condition to relieve her anxiety?

## KEY CONCEPTS

- Ultrasound is used during pregnancy to determine a variety of fetal and placental conditions and to aid in the performance of other tests, such as amniocentesis.
- AFP assessment, a screening test performed on maternal serum or amniotic fluid, is used primarily to detect open body-wall defects and chromosomal abnormalities. Three other markers, hCG, estriol, and inhibin A, are often assessed with AFP to screen more precisely for chromosomal anomalies.
- CVS can be performed as early as 10 weeks of gestation to provide parents with information about many chromosomal defects in the first trimester of pregnancy.
- Amniocentesis is usually performed in the second trimester to identify fetal genetic anomalies and open defects such as neural tube defects. Amniocentensis can be performed during the third trimester to evaluate fetal lung maturity or Rh incompatibility problems.
- Percutaneous umbilical blood sampling involves aspirating blood from umbilical vessels to detect blood disorders, acid-base imbalance, infection, or fetal genetic disease.
- The NST evaluates FHR accelerations, with or without fetal movement. FHR reactivity with accelerations is a reassuring sign associated with adequate fetal oxygenation and intact neural pathway from the fetal brain to the heart. Reactivity in the fetus may not develop until 32 weeks.
- CSTs are used to determine how the fetal heart responds to uterine contractions that temporarily decrease placental blood flow. The CST cannot be done if stimulated uterine contractions are contraindicated.
- A BPP provides information on five parameters: the NST and ultrasound evaluation of fetal breathing movements, gross fetal movements, fetal tone, and amniotic fluid volume. The AFI is a method to quantify the amount of amniotic fluid visualized by ultrasound. The NST may be omitted.
- All perinatal nurses must be prepared to offer clear explanations of diagnostic procedures and to provide support for the family requiring fetal diagnostic tests.

## REFERENCES AND READINGS


American Academy of Pediatrics & American College of Obstetricians and Gynecologists. (2012). *Guidelines for perinatal care* (7th ed.). Elk Grove Village, IL, and Washington, DC: Author.

American College of Obstetricians and Gynecologists. (2013). *Screening for fetal chromosomal abnormalities (ACOG Practice Bulletin No. 77)*. Washington, DC: Author.

American College of Obstetricians and Gynecologists. (2014). *Antepartum fetal surveillance (ACOG Practice Bulletin No. 145)*. Washington, DC: Author.

American College of Obstetricians and Gynecologists. (2014). *Invasive prenatal testing for aneuploidy (ACOG Practice Bulletin No. 88)*. Washington, DC: Author.

American College of Obstetricians and Gynecologists. (2014). *Ultrasound in pregnancy (ACOG Practice Bulletin No. 101)*. Washington, DC: Author.

Blackburn, S. T. (2013). *Maternal, fetal, & neonatal physiology: A clinical perspective* (4th ed.). St. Louis: Saunders.

Copel, J.A., & Moore, T.R. (2014). Obstetrical Imaging. In R.K. Creasy, R. Resnik, J.D. Iams, et al. (Eds.), *Creasy & Resnik's maternal-fetal medicine: Principles and practice* (pp. 201–407). Philadelphia: Saunders.

Cunningham, F.G., Leveno, K.J., Bloom, S.L., et al. (2010). *Williams obstetrics* (23rd ed.). New York: McGraw-Hill.

Gilbert, E.S. (2011). *Manual of high risk pregnancy & delivery* (5th ed.). St. Louis: Mosby.

Harding, R., & Walker, D.W. (2014). Behavioral states in the fetus: relationship to fetal health and development. In R.K. Creasy, R. Resnik, J.D. Iams, et al. (Eds.), *Creasy & Resnik's maternal-fetal medicine: Principles and practice* (7th ed., pp. 155–162). Philadelphia: Saunders.

Jorde, L.B., Carey, J.C., & Bamshad, M.J. (2010). *Medical genetics* (4th ed.). St. Louis: Mosby.

Kaimal, A.J. (2014). Assessment of fetal health. In R.K. Creasy, R. Resnik, J.D. Iams, et al. (Eds.), *Creasy & Resnik's maternal-fetal medicine: Principles and practice* (7th ed., pp. 473–487). Philadelphia: Saunders.

Mercer, B.M. (2014). Assessment and induction of fetal pulmonary maturity. In R.K. Creasy, R. Resnik, J.D. Iams, et al. (Eds.), *Creasy & Resnik's maternal-fetal medicine: Principles and practice* (7th ed., pp. 507–515). Philadelphia: Saunders.

Mercer, B.M. (2014). Premature rupture of the membranes. In R.K. Creasy, R. Resnik, J.D. Iams, et al. (Eds.), *Creasy & Resnik's maternal-fetal medicine: Principles and practice* (7th ed., pp. 663–672). Philadelphia: Saunders.

Sharma, G., Chasen, S., & Chervenak, F. (2011). Routine use of obstetrical ultrasound. In Kurjak, A, & Chervenak, F. (Eds.), *Textbook of Ultrasound in Obstetrics and Gynecology* (3rd ed., pp. 35–55). New York: Jaypee Brothers Medical Publishers.

Wapner, R.J., (2014). Prenatal diagnosis of congenital disorders. In R.K. Cresy, R. Resnik, J.D. Imas, et al. (Eds.), *Cresey & Resnik's maternal-fetal medicine: Principles and practice* (7th ed., pp. 417–464). Philadelphia: Saunders.

# 16

# Giving Birth

http://evolve.elsevier.com/McKinney/mat-ch/

## LEARNING OBJECTIVES

*After studying this chapter, you should be able to:*

- Describe maternal and fetal responses to labor.
- Explain how components of the birth process affect the course of labor.
- Relate mechanisms of labor to the process of vaginal birth.
- Explain premonitory signs of labor.
- Compare true labor with false labor.
- Describe common differences in the labors of nulliparous and parous women.
- Compare the stages of labor and the phases within the first stage.
- Describe admission and continuing intrapartum nursing assessments.
- Identify nursing priorities when assisting the woman to give birth under emergency circumstances.
- Relate therapeutic communication skills to care of the intrapartum family.
- Apply the nursing process to care of the woman experiencing false labor.
- Apply the nursing process to care of the woman and her family during the intrapartum period.

Care of women and their families during labor and birth is a rewarding field of nursing. The birth of a baby is more than a physical event; it has deep personal and social significance for the family. Family roles and relationships are forever altered by this event.

## ISSUES FOR NEW NURSES

Common issues face new nurses and nursing students when caring for families during birth.

### Pain Associated With Birth

Working with people in pain is difficult, and most nurses feel compelled to relieve pain promptly. Yet pain is an expected part of labor and cannot be eliminated. Helping the woman *manage* the pain of birth is a crucial part of nursing care.

### Inexperience or Negative Experiences

The nurse who has never given birth may feel inadequate to care for laboring women, although she or he rarely feels it necessary to have experienced a fracture to care for someone with a broken bone. Nursing skills needed by the intrapartum nurse are basic: observation, critical thinking, problem solving, therapeutic communication, comfort promotion, empathy, and common sense.

Nurses also may be anxious because of their own difficult experiences during pregnancy or birth. They must be careful not to convey negative attitudes to the laboring woman and her partner.

### Unpredictability

Labor is a natural process that follows its own timetable. Some occurrences simply are not easily predicted or explained. Some nurses find the uncertain nature of intrapartum care troubling, whereas others find it exciting. Some days are busy from the start while others are uncannily quiet, only to erupt in adrenaline-charged action with no warning.

### Intimacy

The intimate nature of intrapartum care and its sexual overtones also make some nurses uncomfortable. They may feel that they are intruding on a private time.

The male nurse often finds this aspect of intrapartum care most anxiety provoking. Although he may have cared for other female clients, his care has not been this focused on the reproductive system. He often wonders how a woman's male partner will accept him as a care provider.

The best approach for both male and female nurses is to maintain professional conduct and take cues from the couple. If they want privacy, the nurse should intervene only as needed to assess the woman and fetus. In more advanced labor, both partners often welcome the presence of a competent, caring nurse of either sex.

## PHYSIOLOGIC EFFECTS OF THE BIRTH PROCESS

Labor and birth affect the physiologic systems of both the pregnant woman and her fetus. These effects are most striking in the maternal reproductive system and in relation to fetal and neonatal oxygenation.

### Maternal Response

Significant changes occur during labor in the woman's cardiovascular, respiratory, gastrointestinal, urinary, and hematopoietic systems as well as in her reproductive system.

#### Reproductive System

***Characteristics of contractions.*** Normal labor contractions are coordinated, involuntary, and intermittent.

**Coordinated contractions.** The uterus can contract and relax in a coordinated way, as can other smooth muscles such as the heart. As the woman approaches full term, contractions become organized and gradually assume a regular pattern of increasing frequency, duration, and intensity during labor. Coordinated labor contractions begin in

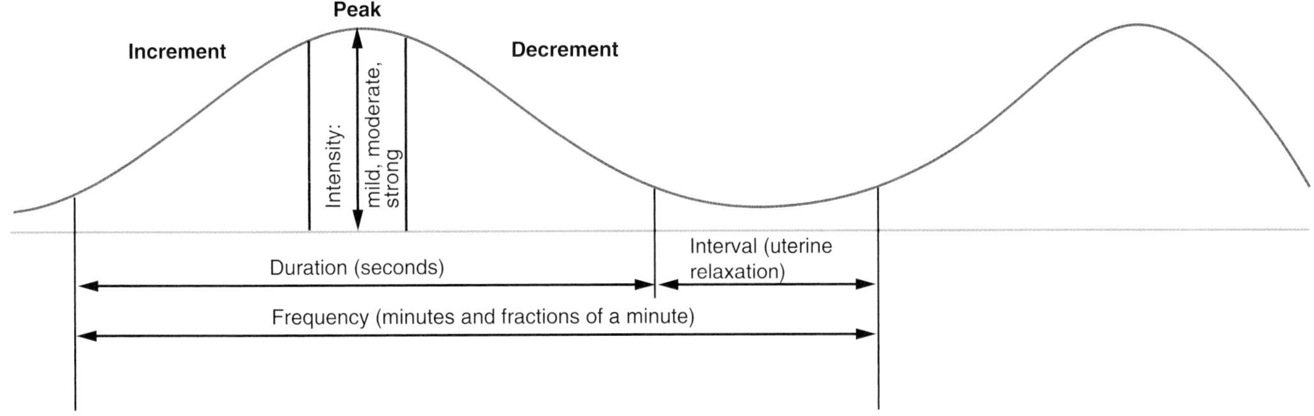


**FIG 16.1** Contraction cycle.

the uterine fundus and spread downward toward the cervix to propel the fetus through the pelvis.

**Involuntary contractions.** Uterine contractions are not under conscious control as are skeletal muscles. The mother cannot cause labor to start or stop by conscious effort. Walking or other activity may stimulate existing labor contractions. Anxiety and excessive stress can diminish them.

**Intermittent contractions.** Labor contractions are intermittent rather than sustained, allowing relaxation of the uterine smooth muscle and resumption of blood flow to and from the placenta to permit gas, nutrient, and waste exchange for the fetus.

***Contraction cycle.*** Each contraction consists of three phases (Fig. 16.1). The *increment* occurs as the contraction begins in the fundus and spreads throughout the uterus. The *peak,* or **acme**, is the period during which the contraction is most intense. The *decrement* is the period of decreasing intensity as the uterus relaxes.

The contraction cycle and the overall pattern of contractions are also described in terms of frequency, duration, and intensity. *Frequency* is the period from the beginning of one uterine contraction to the beginning of the next; it is usually expressed in minutes and fractions of minutes. For example, the nurse states, "Contractions are 3½ to 4 minutes apart."

*Duration* is the length of each contraction from beginning to end; it is usually expressed in seconds. For example, the nurse might report, "Her contractions last 55 to 65 seconds."

*Intensity* is the strength of the contractions. The terms "mild," "moderate," and "strong" are used to describe contraction intensity as palpated by the nurse. Mild contractions are often described as feeling like the tip of the nose, moderate contractions like the chin, and firm contractions like the forehead. Different descriptions of intensity may apply when the internal electronic fetal monitor is used to record contractions (see Chapter 17).

The *interval* is the period between the end of one contraction and the beginning of the next. The interval is the time when most fetal exchange of oxygen, nutrients, and waste products occurs. This is also called the resting tone.

***Uterine body.*** Uterine activity during labor is characterized by opposing features. The upper two thirds of the uterus contracts actively to push the fetus down. The lower one third of the uterus remains less active, allowing downward passage of the fetus. The cervix is similar to the lower uterine segment in that it is also passive. The net effect of labor contractions is enhanced because the downward push from the upper uterus is accompanied by reduced resistance to fetal descent in the lower uterus.

Myometrial (uterine muscle) cells in the upper uterus remain shorter at the end of each contraction rather than returning to their original length. In contrast, myometrial cells in the lower uterus become longer with each contraction. These two characteristics enable the upper uterus to maintain tension between contractions to preserve the cervical changes and downward fetal progress made with each contraction.

The opposing characteristics of myometrial contraction in the upper and lower uterine segments cause changes in the thickness of the uterine wall during labor. The upper uterus becomes thicker while the lower uterus becomes thinner and pulled upward during labor. The physiologic retraction ring marks the division between the upper and lower segments of the uterus (Fig. 16.2).

The opposing characteristics of contractions in the upper and lower uterine segments change the shape of the uterine cavity, which becomes more elongated and narrower as labor progresses. This change in uterine shape straightens the fetal body and efficiently directs it downward in the pelvis.

***Cervical changes.*** **Effacement** (thinning and shortening) and **dilation** (opening) are the major cervical changes during labor. Effacement and dilation occur together during labor but at different rates. The nullipara completes most cervical effacement early in the process of cervical dilation. In contrast, the parous woman's cervix is usually thicker than a nullipara's cervix at any point during labor.

**Effacement.** Before labor, the cervix is a cylindric structure, approximately 2 cm long, at the lower end of the uterus. Labor contractions push the fetus downward against the cervix as they pull the cervix upward. The cervix becomes shorter and thinner as it is drawn over the fetus and amniotic sac (Fig. 16.3). The cervix merges with the thinning lower uterus rather than remaining a distinct cylindric structure. Effacement is estimated as a percentage of the amount the cervix has thinned, so that a fully thinned cervix is 100% effaced. Effacement also may be recorded as cervical length, estimated in centimeters during vaginal examination.

**Dilation.** As the cervix is pulled upward and the fetus is pushed downward, the cervix dilates. Dilation is expressed in centimeters, with approximately 10 cm being full dilation, large enough to allow passage of the average-size term fetus. The action during effacement and dilation can be likened to pushing a tennis ball out the cuff of a sock.

### Cardiovascular System

During each uterine contraction, blood flow to the placenta gradually decreases, causing a relative increase in the woman's blood volume. This temporary change increases her blood pressure slightly and slows her pulse. Therefore, the mother's vital signs are best assessed during the interval between contractions.

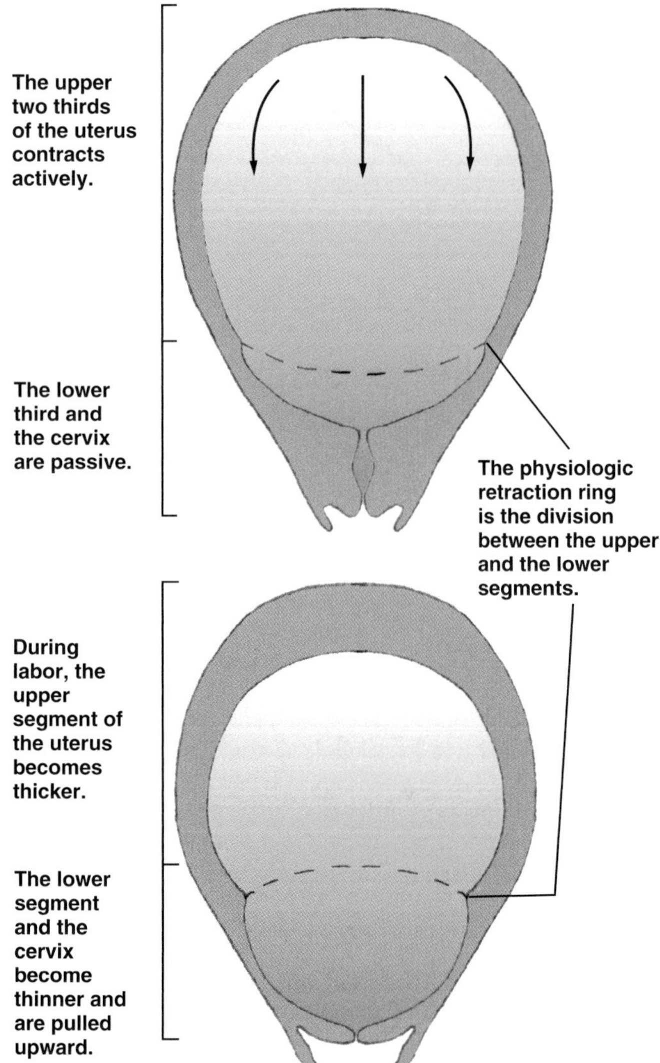
The upper two thirds of the uterus contracts actively.
The lower third and the cervix are passive.
The physiologic retraction ring is the division between the upper and the lower segments.
During labor, the upper segment of the uterus becomes thicker.
The lower segment and the cervix become thinner and are pulled upward.

**FIG 16.2** Opposing characteristics of uterine contraction in the upper and lower segments of the uterus.

Supine hypotension is most likely to occur during the antepartum period because the fetus has not yet started to descend but also may occur during labor if the mother lies on her back (see Fig. 13.4). *The mother should be encouraged to rest in positions other than the supine to promote blood return to her heart, and therefore, enhance blood flow to the placenta and promote fetal oxygenation.*

### Respiratory System

The depth and rate of respirations increase during labor, especially if the woman is anxious or in pain. A woman who breathes rapidly and deeply may experience symptoms of hyperventilation if she exhales too much carbon dioxide. She may feel tingling in her hands and feet, numbness, and dizziness. Helping her to slow her breathing and to breathe into a paper bag or her cupped hands can restore normal blood levels of carbon dioxide and relieve these symptoms.

### Gastrointestinal System

Gastric motility is reduced to varying degrees during labor. Ice chips are commonly provided, as are small amounts of other clear liquids or juices, Popsicles, or hard candy. Most women are not hungry but are often thirsty and have a dry mouth. However, recent research now supports allowing women to have a light meal during labor if wanted (American Society of Anesthesiologists, 2015). Providing women with the choice gives them a feeling of control and also provides them with extra calories to facilitate the work of labor and birth if they choose to eat.

### Urinary System

The most common change in the urinary system during labor is a decrease in sensing a full bladder. Because of intense contractions or the effects of regional pain management such as epidural, the woman may be unaware that her bladder is full. Yet a full bladder may contribute to general discomfort that remains after regional analgesia. A full bladder can also inhibit fetal descent because it occupies space in the pelvis.

After birth, the fluid retention that is normal during pregnancy is quickly reversed, and urine is excreted in large quantities. The bladder may fill rapidly during the first few days after birth.

### Hematopoietic System

Many authorities recognize 500 mL as a normal average blood loss during vaginal birth although women often lose and tolerate greater loss well because the blood volume increases during pregnancy by 1 to 2 L. Quantitative blood loss is often higher than estimated. A hemoglobin concentration of 11 g/dL and a hematocrit of 33% or higher give most women an adequate margin of safety for blood loss associated with normal birth. The leukocyte count averages 14,000 to 16,000/$mm^3$ but may be as high as 25,000/$mm^3$ or higher during labor, a level that might otherwise suggest infection (Blackburn, 2013; Cunningham, Leveno, Bloom, et al., 2010; Hall, 2011).

Levels of several clotting factors, especially fibrinogen, are elevated during pregnancy and continue to be higher during labor and after delivery. Fibrinolysis (clot breakdown) decreases during labor to promote coagulation at the placental site. Although the increase in clotting factors and decrease in fibrinolysis protect from hemorrhage, the combination also raises the mother's risk for venous thrombosis during pregnancy and after birth.

## Fetal Response

Fetal responses are most notable in the placental circulation, the cardiovascular system, and the pulmonary system.

### Placental Circulation

Exchange of oxygen, nutrients, and waste products between mother and fetus occurs in the intervillous spaces (see Chapter 12). During strong labor contractions, the maternal blood supply to the placenta stops intermittently as the spiral arteries supplying the intervillous spaces are compressed by the uterine muscle. Therefore, most placental exchange occurs during the interval between contractions.

The placental circulation usually has enough reserve over fetal basal needs to tolerate the intermittent interruption of blood flow. The fetus has protective mechanisms, such as fetal hemoglobin (which more readily takes on oxygen and releases carbon dioxide), a high hematocrit, and a high cardiac output. The fetus may not tolerate labor contractions well in conditions associated with reduced placental function, such as maternal diabetes or hypertension, or in conditions associated with reduced fetal oxygen–carrying capacity, such as fetal anemia.

### Cardiovascular System

The fetal cardiovascular system reacts quickly to events during labor. The fetal heart rate (FHR) is rapid, ranging from 110 to 160 beats per minute (bpm) at term (Lyndon, O'Brien-Abel, & Simpson, 2015). The preterm fetus may have a slightly higher heart rate than the term fetus, although persistent high FHRs at any gestation should be investigated

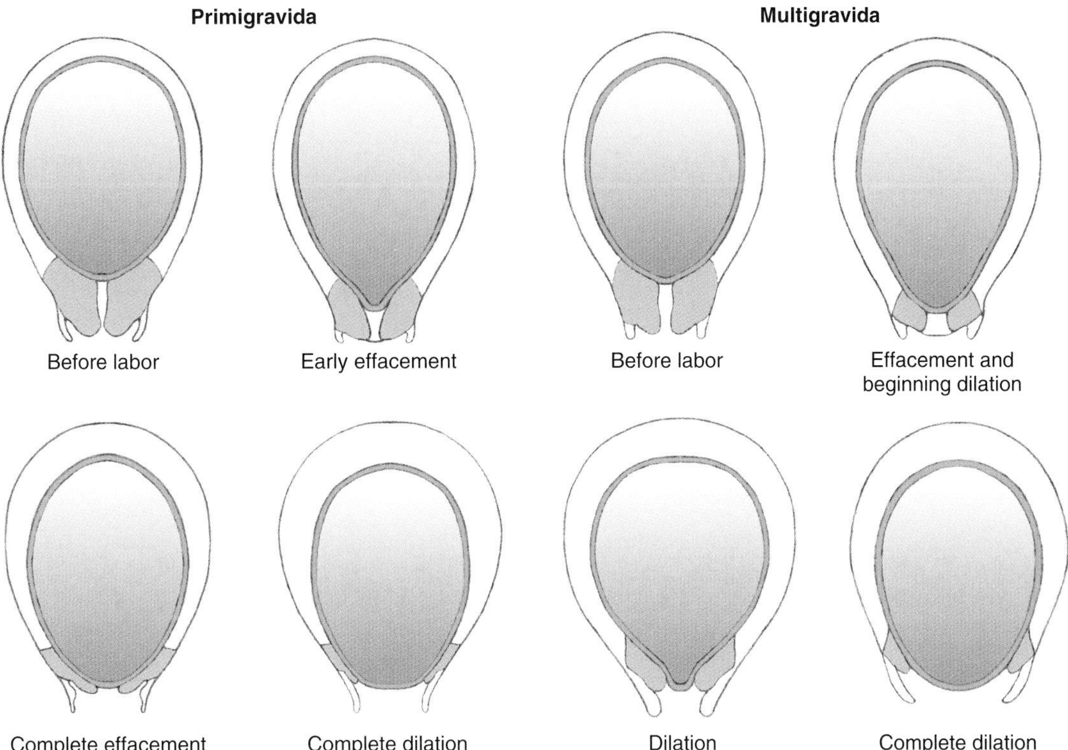


**FIG 16.3** Cervical dilation and effacement. During labor, the cervix of the multigravida remains thicker than that of the primigravida.

(see Chapter 17 for more discussion of FHR and responses during labor).

### Pulmonary System

Before birth, the fetal lungs are filled with fluid to allow normal development of the airways. This fluid must be cleared to allow air breathing. As term approaches, production of fetal lung fluid decreases and its absorption increases. Labor intensifies the absorption of lung fluid. Some fluid is expelled from the upper airways as the fetal head and thorax are compressed during passage through the birth canal. The remaining fluid is absorbed into the newborn's pulmonary and lymphatic circulations after birth. Chapter 21 contains added information about newborn transition.

## COMPONENTS OF THE BIRTH PROCESS

Four major factors, often called the "four Ps," interact during normal childbirth. They are the *p*owers, the *p*assage, the *p*assenger, and the *p*syche.

### Powers

The two powers of labor are uterine contractions and maternal pushing efforts.

#### Uterine Contractions

During the first stage of labor (onset through full cervical dilation), uterine contractions are the primary force moving the fetus through the maternal pelvis.

#### Maternal Pushing Efforts

At some point during the second stage of labor (full cervical dilation through birth of the baby), the woman adds her voluntary pushing efforts to the force of uterine contractions to propel the fetus through the pelvis.

### Passage

The passage for birth of the fetus consists of the maternal pelvis and its soft tissues. The bony pelvis is usually more important to the outcome of labor than the soft tissue because the bones and joints do not readily yield to the forces of labor. However, softening of the cartilage linking the pelvic bones increases as term approaches and the hormone *relaxin* increases.

The bony pelvis is divided by the linea terminalis (or pelvic brim) into the false pelvis above and the true pelvis below (see Chapter 11). The true pelvis is most important in childbirth. The true pelvis has three subdivisions: (1) the *inlet,* or upper pelvic opening; (2) the *midpelvis,* or pelvic cavity; and (3) the *outlet,* or lower pelvic opening. The true pelvis is like a curved cylinder with different dimensions at different levels. Fig. 16.4 (pp. 292-293) illustrates important pelvic measurements.

### Passenger

The passenger is the fetus plus the membranes and placenta.

#### Fetal Head

The fetus enters the birth canal in the cephalic presentation more than 96% of the time. The fetal shoulders are important because of their width, but they usually flex and adapt to the pelvis.

***Bones, sutures, and fontanels.*** The bones of the fetal head involved in birth are the two frontal bones on the forehead, the two parietal bones at the crown of the head, and the occipital bone at the back of the head (Fig. 16.5, p. 294). The five major bones are not fused but are connected by **sutures** composed of strong but flexible fibrous tissue. The **fontanels** are wider spaces at the intersections of the sutures.

**INLET**

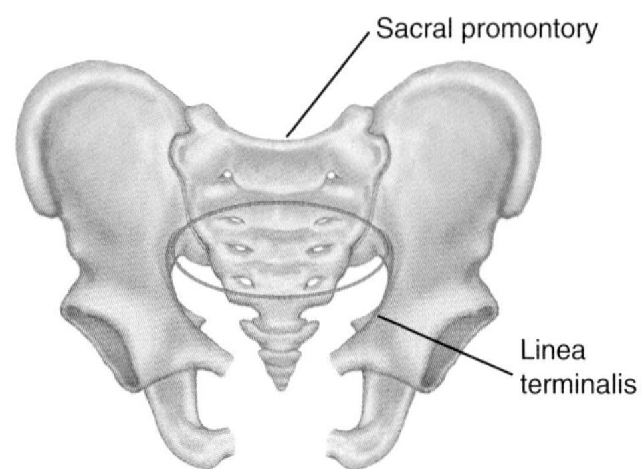


**Frontal view, cutaway**

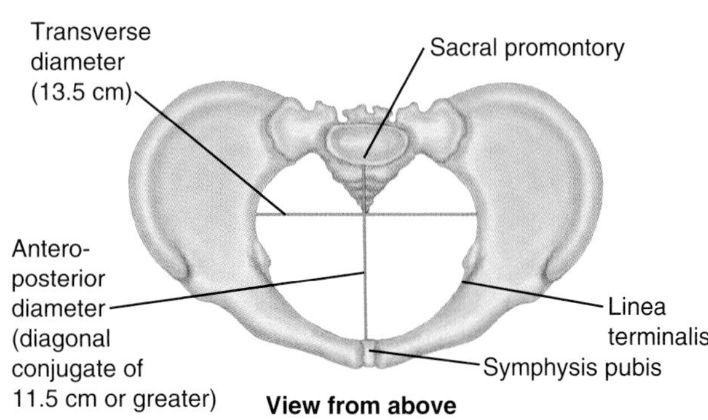


**View from above**

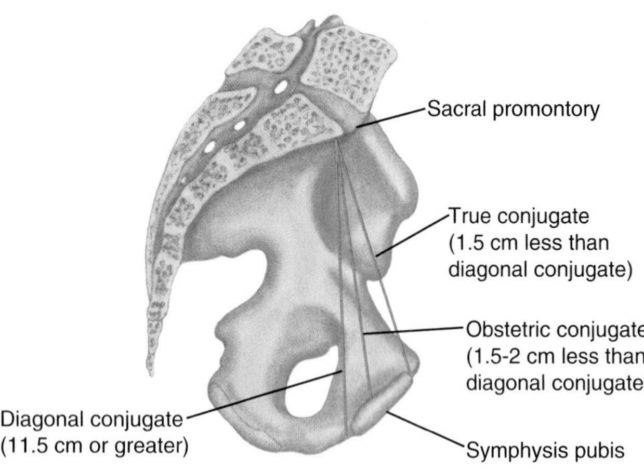


**Side view, cutaway**

**MIDPELVIS**

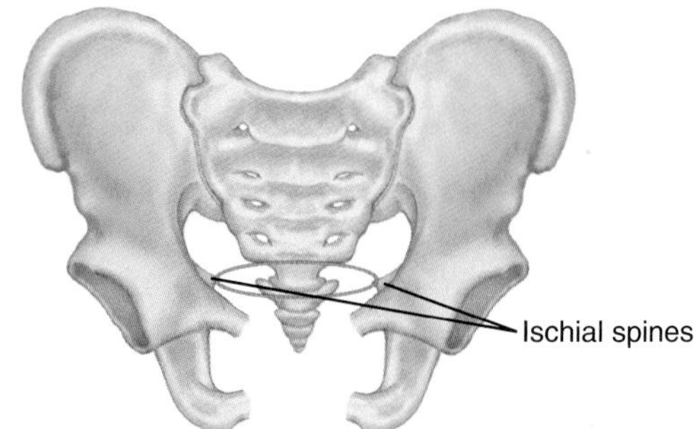


**Frontal view, cutaway**

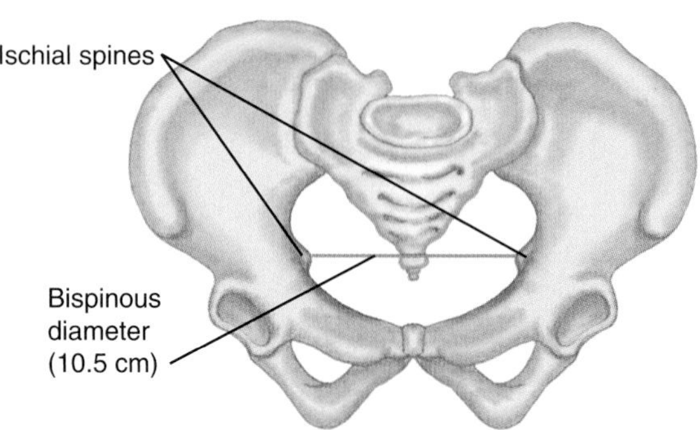


**View from above, with pelvis tilted anteriorly**

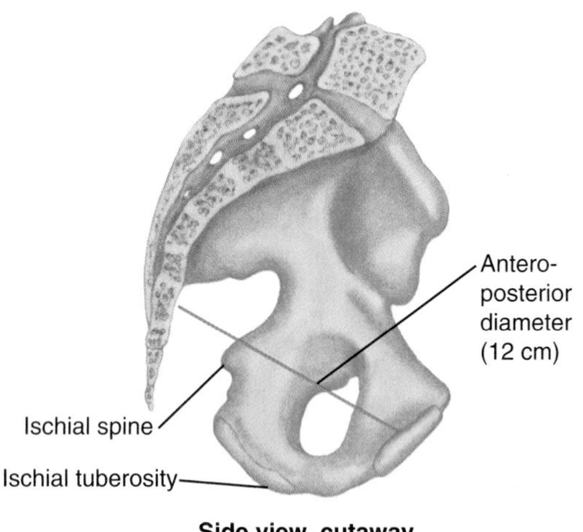


**Side view, cutaway**

The boundaries of the inlet are the symphysis pubis anteriorly, the sacral promontory posteriorly, and the linea terminalis on the sides. The inlet is slightly wider in its transverse diameter (13.5 cm) than in its anteroposterior (diagonal conjugate) diameter (11.5 cm or greater).

The diagonal conjugate is slightly larger than both the obstetric and true conjugates. The obstetric conjugate is the narrowest of the three conjugate diameters but cannot be measured directly. The obstetric conjugate is estimated by first measuring the diagonal conjugate and then subtracting 1.5 to 2 cm.

If the inlet is small, the fetal head may not be able to enter it. Because it is almost entirely surrounded by bone, except for cartilage at the sacroiliac joint and symphysis pubis, the inlet cannot enlarge much to accommodate the fetus. The bony measurements are essentially fixed.

The midpelvis, or pelvic cavity, is the narrowest part of the pelvis through which the fetus must pass during birth. Midpelvic diameters are measured at the level of the ischial spines. The anteroposterior diameter averages 12 cm.

The transverse diameter (bispinous or interspinous) averages 10.5 cm. Prominent ischial spines that project into the midpelvis can reduce the bispinous diameter.

**FIG 16.4** Pelvic divisions and measurements.

**OUTLET**

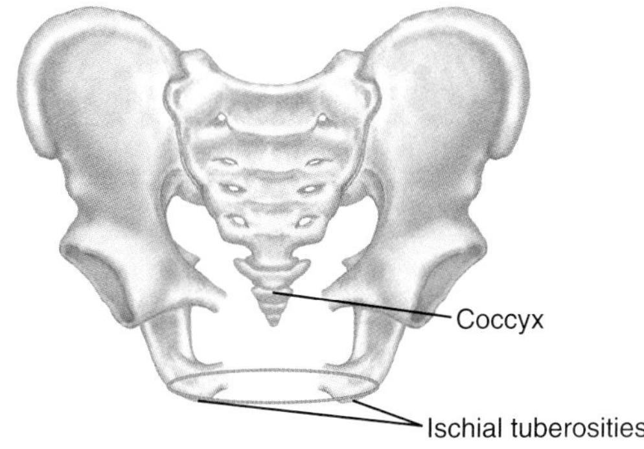


**Frontal view, cutaway**

Three important diameters of the pelvic outlet are (1) the anteroposterior, (2) the transverse (bi-ischial or intertuberous), and (3) the posterior sagittal. The angle of the pubic arch also is an important pelvic outlet measure.

The anteroposterior diameter ranges from 9.5 to 11.5 cm, varying with the curve between the sacrococcygeal joint and the tip of the coccyx. The anteroposterior diameter can increase if the coccyx is easily movable.

The transverse diameter is the bi-ischial, or intertuberous, diameter. This is the distance between the ischial tuberosities ("sit bones"), which averages 11 cm.

The posterior sagittal diameter measures the posterior pelvis—the distance from the sacrococcygeal joint to the middle of the transverse (bi-ischial) diameter.

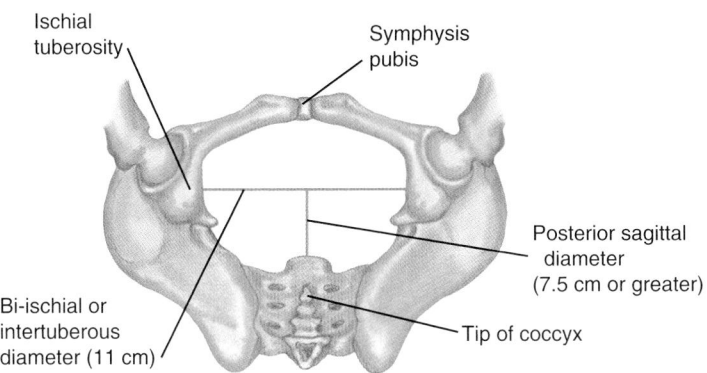

Ischial tuberosity
Symphysis pubis
Posterior sagittal diameter (7.5 cm or greater)
Bi-ischial or intertuberous diameter (11 cm)
Tip of coccyx

**View from below (woman is in lithotomy position)**

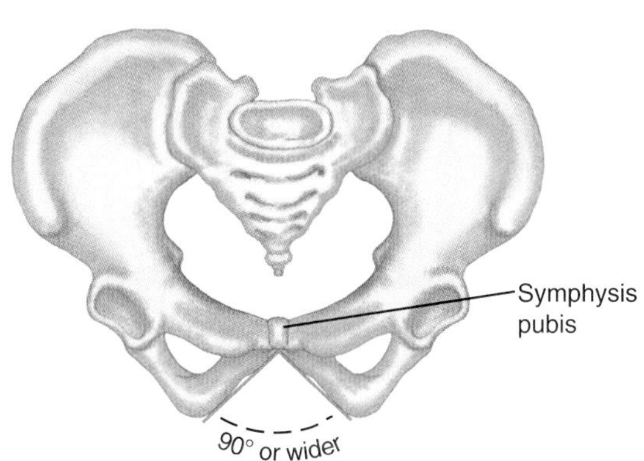


**Frontal view, with pelvis tilted anteriorly**

The angle of the pubic arch is important because it must be wide enough for the fetus to pass under it. The angle of the pubic arch should be at least 90 degrees. A narrow pubic arch displaces the fetus posteriorly toward the coccyx as it tries to pass under the arch.

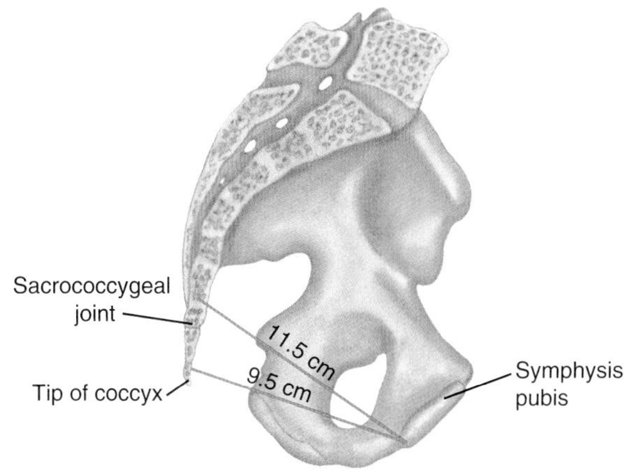


**Side view, cutaway**

**FIG 16.4, cont'd** Pelvic divisions and measurements.

The *anterior fontanel* is diamond shaped and formed by the intersection of four sutures: the two coronal, the frontal, and the sagittal, which connect the two frontal and the two parietal bones. The *posterior fontanel* has a triangular shape formed by the intersection of three sutures, one sagittal and two lambdoid, which connect the two parietal bones and the occipital bone. The posterior fontanel is very small, often more like a slight depression in the skull. The sutures and fontanels allow the bones to move slightly, changing the shape of the fetal head so that it can adapt to the size and shape of the pelvis by **molding**. The sutures and the different shapes of the fontanels provide landmarks to determine fetal position and head flexion during vaginal examination.

***Fetal head diameters.*** Although most fetuses enter the pelvis in the cephalic presentation, several variations are possible. The major transverse diameter of the fetal head is the biparietal, measured between the two parietal bones, which averages 9.5 cm in a term fetus.

The anteroposterior diameter of the head varies with the degree of flexion. In the most favorable situation, the head becomes fully flexed during labor and the anteroposterior diameter is the suboccipitobregmatic, averaging 9.5 cm. See Fig. 16.5, *B*, on p. 294, for anteroposterior head diameters in different degrees of head flexion and extension.

## Variations in the Passenger

***Fetal lie.*** The orientation of the long axis of the fetus to the long axis of the woman is the fetal lie (Fig. 16.6, p. 294). In more than 99% of pregnancies, the lie is longitudinal, or parallel to the long axis of the

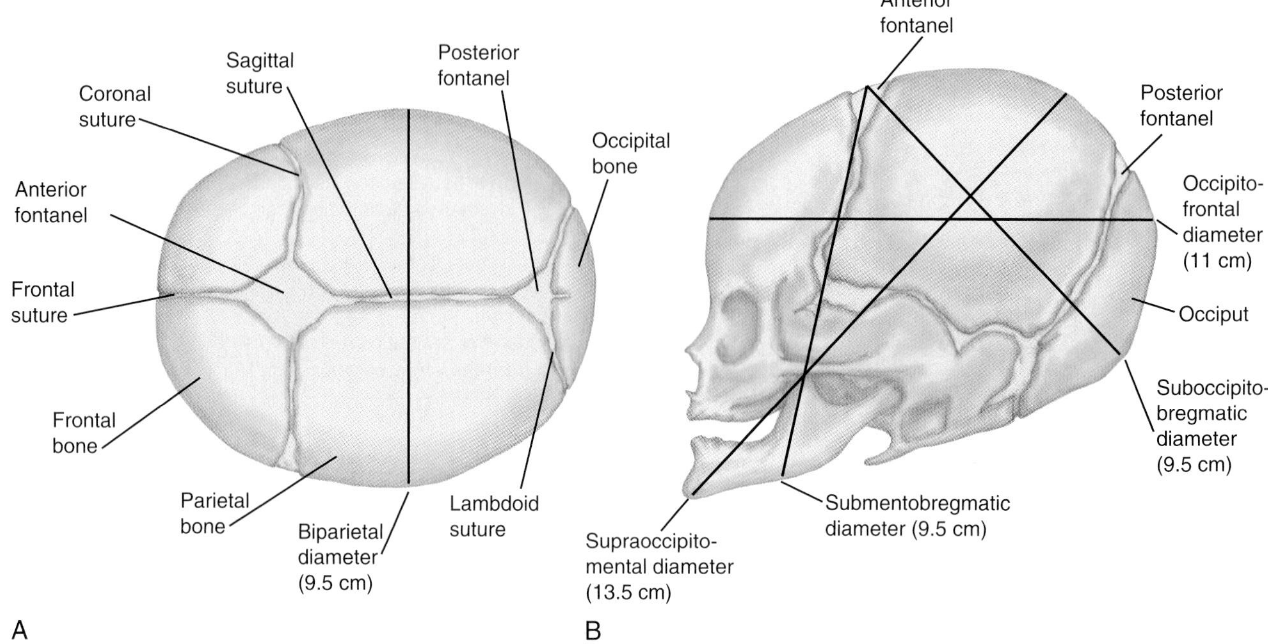


**FIG 16.5** **A,** Bones, sutures, and fontanels of the fetal head. Note that the anterior fontanel has a diamond shape, whereas the posterior fontanel is triangular. **B,** Lateral view of the fetal head. Anteroposterior diameters vary with the amount of flexion or extension.

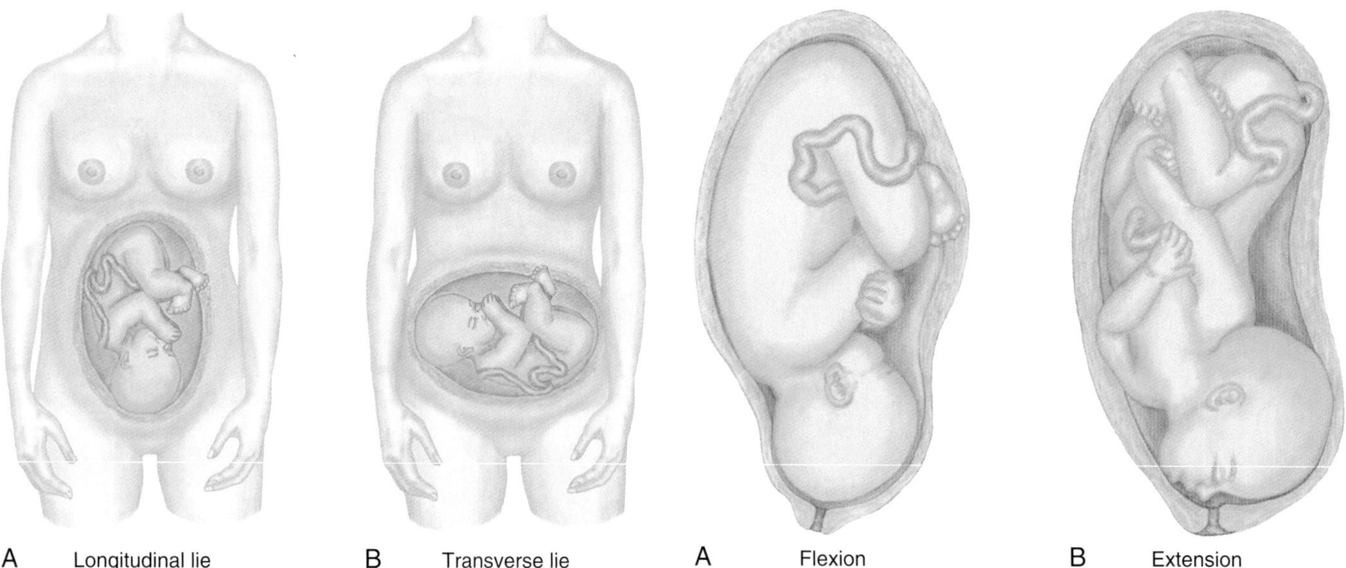


**FIG 16.6** Lie. **A,** Longitudinal lie: the long axis of the fetus is parallel to the long axis of the woman. **B,** Transverse lie: the long axis of the fetus is at right angles to the long axis of the mother. The woman's abdomen has a wide, short appearance.

**FIG 16.7** Attitude. **A,** The fetus is in the normal attitude of flexion, with the head, arms, and legs flexed tightly against the trunk. **B,** The fetus is in an abnormal attitude of extension. The head and the right arm are extended. A face presentation is illustrated.

woman. In the **longitudinal lie**, either the head or buttocks of the fetus enters the pelvis first. In a **transverse lie**, the long axis of the fetus is at right angles to the woman's long axis; this orientation occurs in less than 1% of pregnancies. A fetus in an **oblique lie** is at an angle between the longitudinal lie and the transverse lie.

***Attitude.*** The **attitude** of the fetus is the relation of fetal body parts to each other (Fig. 16.7, p. 294). The normal fetal attitude is one of flexion, with the head flexed toward the chest and the arms and legs flexed over the thorax. The back is curved in a convex C shape as labor starts.

***Presentation.*** The fetal part that enters the pelvis first is the presenting part. **Presentation** falls into three categories: (1) cephalic, (2) breech, and (3) shoulder. Cephalic presentation with the fetal head flexed is the most common (Fig. 16.8, p. 295). Other presentations are associated with prolonged labor or other problems and are more likely to require cesarean birth.

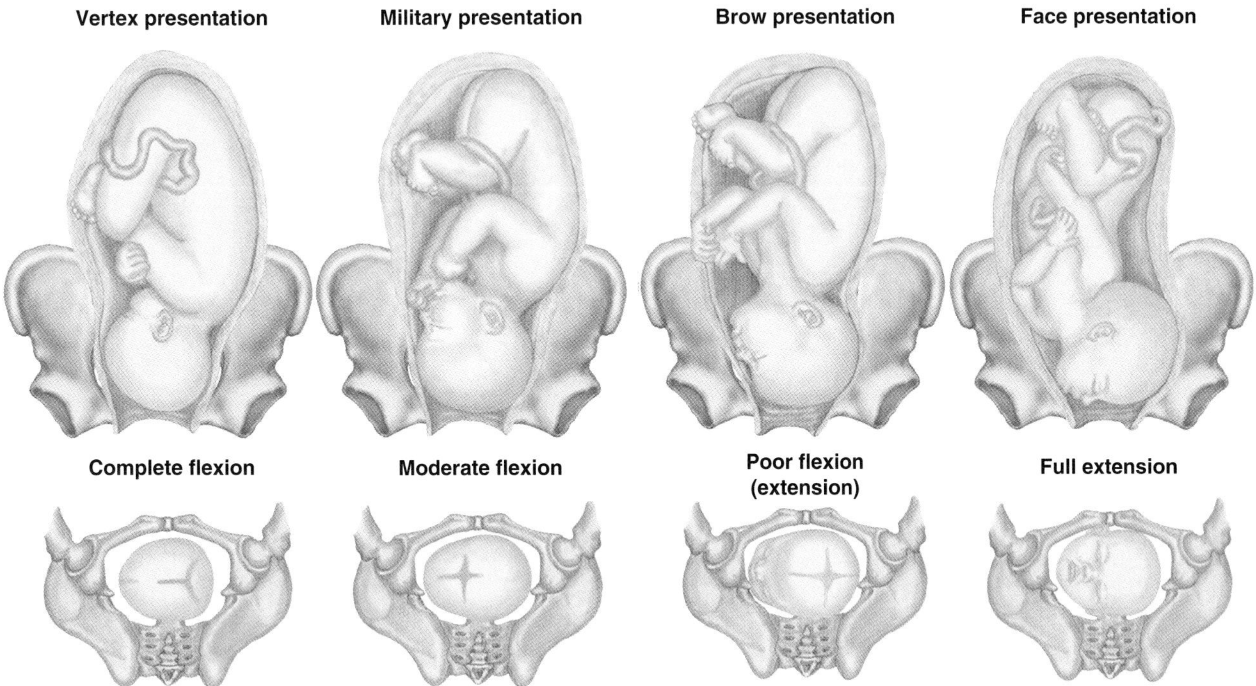


**FIG 16.8** Four types of cephalic presentation. The vertex presentation is normal. Note positional changes of the anterior and posterior fontanels in relation to the maternal pelvis.

**Cephalic presentation.** Cephalic presentation is more favorable than the others, for several reasons:

- The fetal head is the largest single fetal part. After the head is born, the smaller parts follow easily as the extremities unfold.
- During labor, the fetal head can gradually change shape to adapt to the size and shape of the maternal pelvis.
- The fetal head is smooth, round, and hard, making it an effective part to dilate the cervix, which is also round.

Cephalic presentation has four variations (see Fig. 16.8).

***Vertex.*** Vertex presentation is the most common. The fetal head is fully flexed. This presentation is the most favorable for a normal progression of labor because the smallest suboccipitobregmatic diameter is presenting.

***Military.*** In a military, or sinciput, presentation, the head is in a neutral position, neither flexed nor extended. The occipitofrontal diameter is presenting. This presentation is usually temporary and the head flexes into the vertex position or extends into the brow position.

***Brow.*** In a brow presentation the fetal head is partly extended. The longest supraoccipitomental diameter is presenting.

***Face.*** In a face presentation, the head is fully extended and the fetal occiput is near the fetal spine. The submentobregmatic diameter is presenting.

**Breech presentation.** A breech presentation occurs when the fetal buttocks or feet enter the pelvis first. They are common, occurring in approximately 3% of births (Cunningham et al., 2010; Tarsa & Moore, 2010). Breech presentations are associated with several disadvantages:

- The buttocks are not smooth and firm like the head and are less effective at dilating the cervix.
- The fetal head is the last part to be born. By the time the fetal head is deep in the pelvis, the umbilical cord is subject to compression between the baby's head and the maternal pelvis.
- Because the umbilical cord can be compressed after the fetal chest is born, the head must be delivered quickly to allow the infant to breathe. This necessary speed does not permit gradual molding of the fetal head as it passes through the pelvis.

The breech presentation has three variations, depending on the relationship of the legs to the body (Fig. 16.9).

***Frank breech.*** In the most common frank breech presentation the fetal legs are extended across the abdomen toward the shoulders.

***Full (or complete) breech.*** The full breech is a reversal of the usual cephalic presentation. The head is flexed, and the knees and hips are also flexed, but the buttocks are presenting.

***Footling breech.*** The footling breech occurs when one or both feet are presenting.

**Shoulder.** The shoulder presentation is a transverse lie and accounts for fewer than 1% of births, usually premature (Cunningham et al., 2010; Tarsa & Moore, 2010). A cesarean birth is necessary.

***Position.*** Fetal position describes the location of a fixed reference point on the presenting part in relation to the four quadrants of the maternal pelvis (Fig. 16.10): right and left anterior and right and left posterior. The fetal position is not fixed but rather changes during labor as the fetus moves downward and adapts to the pelvic contours. Abbreviations indicate the relationship between the fetal presenting part and the maternal pelvis.

**Right (R) or left (L).** The first letter of the abbreviation describes whether the fetal reference point is in the right or the left of the mother's pelvis. If the fetal point is neither to the right nor to the left of the pelvis, this letter is omitted.

**Occiput (O), mentum (M), or sacrum (S).** The second letter of the abbreviation refers to the fixed fetal reference point, which varies with the presentation. The occiput is used in a vertex presentation. The chin, or mentum, is the reference point in a face presentation. The sacrum is used for breech presentations. Letters may also designate the less common brow (F for fronto) and shoulder (Sc for scapula) presentations.

**Anterior (A), posterior (P), or transverse (T).** The third letter describes whether the fetal reference point is in the anterior or the posterior quadrant of the mother's pelvis. If the fetal reference point is in neither of these quadrants, it is described as transverse.

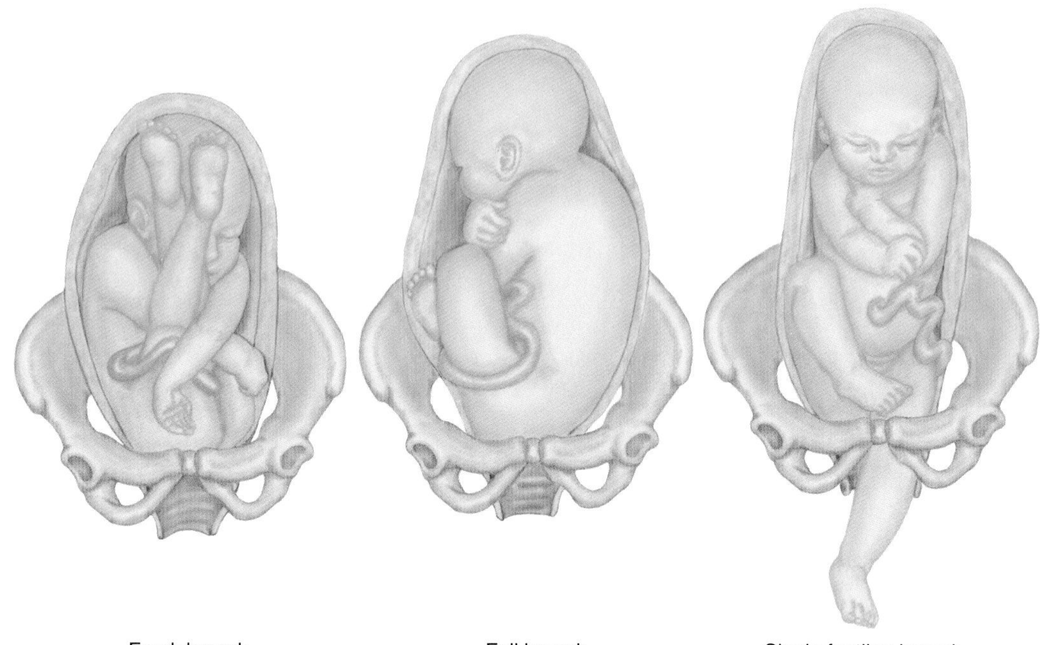


**FIG 16.9** Three variations of a breech presentation. Frank breech is the most common variation. Footling breeches may be single or double.

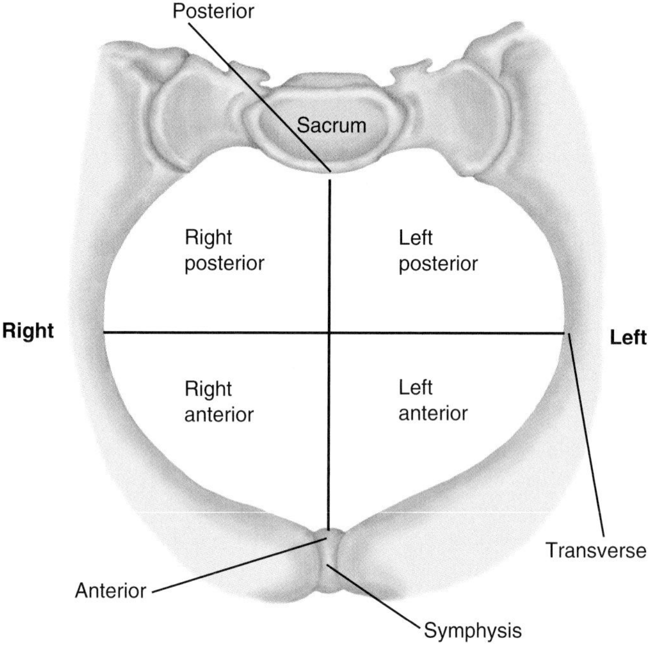


**FIG 16.10** The four quadrants of the maternal pelvis used to describe fetal position.

If the fetal occiput is located in the left anterior quadrant of the mother's pelvis, the position is described as left occiput anterior (LOA). If the occiput is in the mother's anterior pelvis, neither to the right nor to the left, it is described as occiput anterior (OA). If the fetal sacrum is located in the mother's right posterior pelvis, the description is R (right) S (sacrum) P (posterior). See Fig. 16.11 for different fetal presentations and positions.

## Psyche

The psyche is a crucial part of childbirth. Marked anxiety, fear, or fatigue decreases a woman's ability to cope with pain in labor. Maternal catecholamines secreted in response to anxiety or fear can inhibit uterine contractility and placental blood flow. However, relaxation augments the natural process of labor.

## Interrelationships Between the Components of Birth

The four Ps—the powers, passage, passenger, and psyche—are an interrelated whole. For example, a woman with a small pelvis (passage) and a large fetus (passenger) can have a normal labor and birth if the fetus is ideally positioned and the uterine contractions and maternal bearing-down efforts (powers) are vigorous. The nurse's supportive attitude strengthens positive psychologic elements (psyche) and enhances the processes of birth. The nurse can act as an advocate for the laboring woman and her family or partners to increase their sense of control and mastery of labor, often reducing anxiety and fear.

### Individual and Cultural Values

A family's culture affects its members' views of birth and the practices that surround it. Culture shapes the values that people hold, their expectations of the birth experience, and their responses to birth. A woman's culture gives her cues about how she should behave and react to labor and how she should interact with her newborn. If the woman, her family, and caregivers have similar views, little conflict in their values and expectations is likely. However, if these individuals hold markedly different views, they may be confused because each expects something different of the other (Callister, 2014).

Knowledge of the values and practices of cultural groups that the nurse encounters provides a framework to assess and care for the woman and her family, but within a culture, people are individuals. The nurse must assess the personal expectations and birth-related values of each woman and her family within this general framework. Aspects of cultural assessment for the intrapartum period might include:

- How long has the family been in the area? Are they recent immigrants, or have their relatives and friends lived in the area for generations?

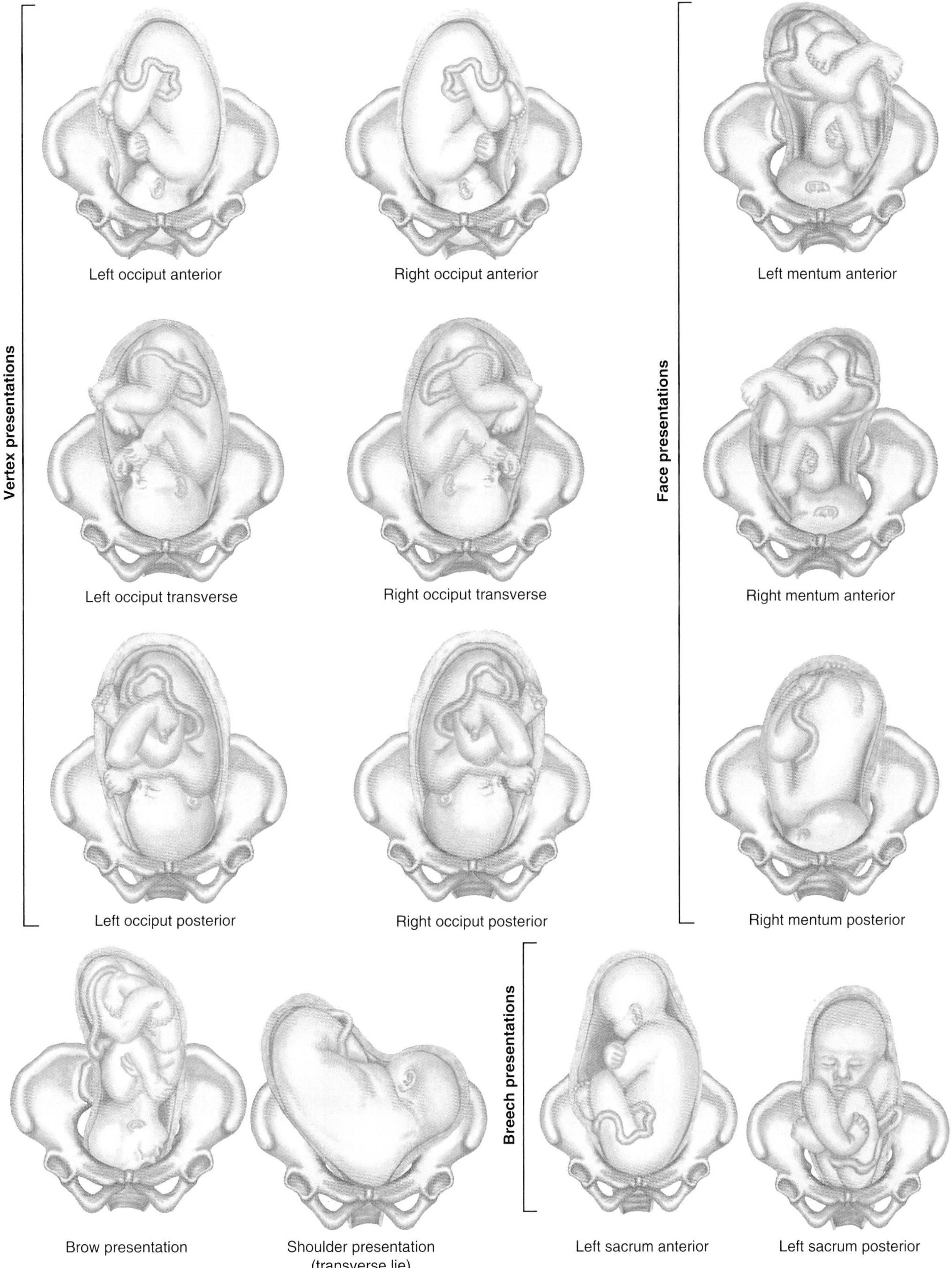


**FIG 16.11** Fetal presentations and positions.

- What is the family's primary language? Do the woman and her family speak the same language or does only one of them speak the dominant language? Is the dominant language not spoken by either the woman or her support person? Are they comfortable communicating in the nurse's language if the two are different? If an interpreter is needed, are there people the family considers unacceptable (e.g., a male or a member of certain religious groups)? How does a hearing-impaired woman communicate with people who hear?
- Who is the decision-maker in the family, or who must be consulted about important decisions?
- Will another relative (such as a grandmother) assume primary care for the infant?
- Is a caregiver of the same gender and cultural group essential?
- Who is the woman's primary support person for labor? What is that person's role? How extensively will that support person interact with the laboring woman? Who will be present at birth?
- What are the woman's feelings about touch? Is she comfortable telling the nurse when she does or does not welcome touch?
- Are specific symbols, practices, or ceremonies used during the birth period? Who will conduct any ceremonies?

### Birth as an Experience

Childbirth is a physical and emotional experience. It is also an irrevocable event that changes a woman and her family forever. Families describe the births of children as they describe other pivotal events in life: marriages, anniversaries, religious events, and even deaths. Women often have specific expectations about the experience of childbirth. The more realistic a woman's expectations about the birth are, the more likely she is to have a positive experience.

Nursing measures that increase a sense of control and mastery during birth help families perceive the birth as a positive event. Nursing measures to empower families include teaching them about their choices in childbirth in an unbiased way and supporting the choices they make.

## NORMAL LABOR

### Theories of Onset

Labor begins when forces favoring continuation of pregnancy are overcome by forces favoring its end. The body's preparation to give birth occurs gradually over the last few weeks of pregnancy. Although all reasons for initiation of labor are not known, factors that have a role in its onset include (Cunningham et al., 2010; Hall, 2011):

- Changes in the ratio of maternal estrogen to progesterone so that estrogen levels are higher than progesterone levels, reducing the relaxant effects of progesterone on the uterine muscle. Relatively higher estrogen levels near the onset of labor enhance uterine sensitivity to substances that stimulate uterine contractions: prostaglandins from the fetal membranes and oxytocin from the maternal posterior pituitary gland. Estrogens increase the number of gap junctions—connections that allow the individual uterine muscle cells to contract as a coordinated unit.
- Prostaglandins produced by the decidua and membranes may have a role in preparing the uterus for oxytocin stimulation at term. Prostaglandins are secreted from the lower area of the fetal membranes (forebag) during labor and may reflect inflammation caused by contact with microorganisms from the woman's vagina.
- Increased secretion of natural oxytocin appears to maintain labor once it has begun. Oxytocin alone does not appear to start labor but may play a part in labor's initiation in conjunction with other substances. Evidence of fetal oxytocin secretion also exists.
- Oxytocin receptors in the uterus increase markedly as labor begins, and the increase continues during labor and peaks at delivery. Oxytocin has little effect on the uterine muscle if the receptors have not developed.
- A fetal role in the initiation of labor appears likely. The fetal membranes release prostaglandin in high concentrations during labor. In addition to fetal oxytocin secretion, large quantities of cortisol are secreted by the fetal adrenal glands, possibly acting as a uterine stimulant.
- Stretching, pressure, and irritation of the uterus and cervix increase as the fetus reaches term size. During early pregnancy, the uterus has not reacted to stretching by contracting as smooth muscle normally does. A feedback loop is probably responsible for labor contractions at term: the fetal head stretches the cervix, causing the fundus of the uterus to contract, pushing the fetal head against the cervix, and causing more fundal contractions. Cervical stretching also causes secretion of oxytocin.

### Premonitory Signs

Before spontaneous labor begins, women usually notice one or more of the following premonitory, or warning, signs that labor is near:

- **Braxton Hicks contractions**, irregular mild contractions that occur throughout pregnancy increase in frequency and are sometimes painful. They may become regular at times, only to decrease spontaneously.
- **Lightening** ("dropping") occurs as the fetus descends toward the pelvic inlet. Lightening is most noticeable in nulliparas, occurring approximately 2 to 3 weeks before the onset of labor.
- Increased clear and nonirritating vaginal secretions occur as fetal pressure causes congestion of the vaginal mucosa.
- "**Bloody show**," a mixture of thick mucus and pink or dark brown blood, may occur as the cervix begins to soften, dilate, and efface slightly ("ripening").
- An energy spurt ("nesting").
- A small weight loss of 2.2 kg to 6.6 kg (1 to 3 lb) may occur because changing levels of estrogen and progesterone cause excretion of some of the extra fluid that accumulates during pregnancy.

### True Labor and False Labor

False labor, also called *prodromal labor,* is common because the time of spontaneous labor's onset is rarely known and the onset is usually gradual. False labor often causes women to be disappointed when their symptoms are not "the real thing." The term *false labor* may discourage a woman because she does not realize that these "false" contractions are simply preparation for the main event of true labor, rather than true labor itself.

Several characteristics distinguish true labor from false labor: contractions, discomfort, and cervical change. The best distinction between the two is that the contractions of true labor cause *progressive changes in the cervix*. Effacement and dilation occur with true labor contractions.

### Mechanisms of Labor

The mechanisms (cardinal movements) of labor occur as the fetus is moved through the pelvis during birth. The fetus undergoes several positional changes to adapt to the size and shape of the mother's pelvis at different levels (Fig. 16.12). Although the mechanisms of labor are

## PATIENT-CENTERED TEACHING

### *How to Know Whether Labor Is "Real"*

True labor differs from false labor in three categories.

| False Labor | True Labor |
|---|---|
| **Contractions** | |
| Inconsistent in frequency, duration, and intensity. | A consistent pattern of increasing frequency, duration, and intensity usually develops. |
| A change in activity, such as walking, does not alter contractions, or activity may decrease them. | Walking tends to increase frequency and strength of contractions. |
| **Discomfort** | |
| Felt in the abdomen and groin. | Begins in lower back and gradually sweeps around to the lower abdomen like a girdle. |
| May be more annoying than truly painful. | Back pain may persist in some women. Early labor often feels like menstrual cramps. |
| **Cervix** | |
| No significant change in effacement or dilation of the cervix after an observation period of 1 to 2 hours. | Effacement and/or dilation of cervix occurs. Progressive effacement and dilation of cervix are most important characteristics. |

described separately in Fig. 16.12, (pp. 300-301) some occur concurrently. In a vertex presentation, the mechanisms are:

- *Descent* of the fetal presenting part through the true pelvis.
- *Engagement* of the fetal presenting part as its widest diameter reaches the level of the ischial spines of the mother's pelvis.
- *Flexion* of the fetal head so that the smallest head diameter passes through the pelvis.
- *Internal rotation* to allow the largest fetal head diameter to match the largest maternal pelvic diameter.
- *Extension* of the fetal head as it passes beneath the mother's symphysis pubis.
- *External rotation* of the fetal head to allow the shoulders to rotate internally to fit the mother's pelvis.
- *Expulsion* of the fetal shoulders and fetal body.

The mechanisms of labor are different in presentations other than vertex, but the reason is the same: effective use of available space in the maternal pelvis.

## Stages and Phases of Labor

Each stage and phase of labor has qualities that set it apart from the others. Individual women vary in their labor patterns and responses to labor. Table 16.1 provides details of the characteristics of each stage of labor. Use of regional anesthetics, such as the epidural block, is likely to modify the typical maternal behaviors. Also, labor that is induced or augmented often differs from spontaneous labor.

### First Stage of Labor

Cervical effacement and dilation occur in the first stage of labor, or *stage of dilation*. It begins with the onset of true labor contractions and ends with complete dilation (10 cm) and effacement (100%) of the cervix. The first stage of labor is the longest for both nulliparous and parous women. Labor progress may be plotted on a graph, often called a *Friedman curve* (Fig. 16.13, p. 303). However, the Friedman curve cannot be the only measure of normal progress with today's technology. Current measures of maternal and fetal well-being, such as fetal monitoring, provide added information about whether a longer labor should be ended or allowed to continue.

First-stage labor differs from the other stages because it has three phases: latent (early), active, and transition. Each phase is characterized by typical maternal behaviors. These behaviors vary with the woman's preparation, use of coping skills, and analgesia.

**Latent phase.** The latent, or early, phase lasts from the beginning of labor until approximately 3 to 5 cm of cervical dilation. Its length varies among women. Despite being called *latent*, cervical effacement and subtle fetal position change occur during this phase, preparing for the more rapid changes of active labor. The woman is usually sociable and excited during this early phase of labor.

**Active phase.** The cervix dilates more rapidly as the woman enters the active phase, between approximately 4 cm and 6 cm. Research has demonstrated safety in a slower transition between latent and active labor than usually accepted in women in spontaneous labor (Zhang, Landry, Branch, et al., 2010). Effacement and dilation of the cervix are completed. Internal rotation occurs as the fetus descends in the pelvis during active labor. Discomfort usually increases as the pace of labor picks up. *Transition* may be used to describe the intense contractions of fetal descent and final cervical dilation, approximately 7 or 8 cm to complete.

Bloody show often increases with completion of cervical dilation. Transition is a short but intense phase, with very strong contractions. The woman may have an urge to push down during contractions as the fetal presenting part reaches her pelvic floor. Leg tremors, nausea, and vomiting are common as second stage nears.

The woman becomes more anxious and may feel irritable and helpless as the contractions intensify. The sociability of early labor is gone, replaced with a serious, inward focus. Her partner may be confused because actions that were helpful just a short time before now bother her.

### Second Stage of Labor

The second stage *(expulsion)* begins with complete (10 cm) dilation and full (100%) effacement of the cervix and ends with the birth of the baby. As the fetus descends, pressure of the presenting part on the rectum and the pelvic floor causes the mother to have an involuntary pushing response. She may say that she needs to have a bowel movement or "The baby's coming" or "I have to push." Her voluntary pushing efforts augment involuntary uterine contractions. As the fetus descends low in the pelvis and the vulva distends with crowning of the fetal head, she may feel a sensation of stretching or burning even if no trauma occurs.

Contractions are strong, but the woman may feel more in control because she is actively completing the process by pushing with them. "Labor" describes the second stage well. The woman exerts intense effort to push her baby out. Between contractions she may be oblivious to her surroundings and may appear asleep. She feels tremendous relief and excitement as the second stage ends with the birth of her baby.

### Third Stage of Labor

The third *(placental)* stage begins with the birth of the baby and ends with the expulsion of the placenta (Fig. 16.14). When the infant is born, the uterine cavity becomes much smaller. The reduced size decreases the size of the placental site, causing the placenta to separate from the uterine wall. Four signs suggest placenta separation:

- The uterus has a spherical shape.
- The uterus rises upward in the abdomen as the placenta descends into the vagina and pushes the fundus upward.
- The cord descends further from the vagina.

## DESCENT, ENGAGEMENT, AND FLEXION

*Descent*

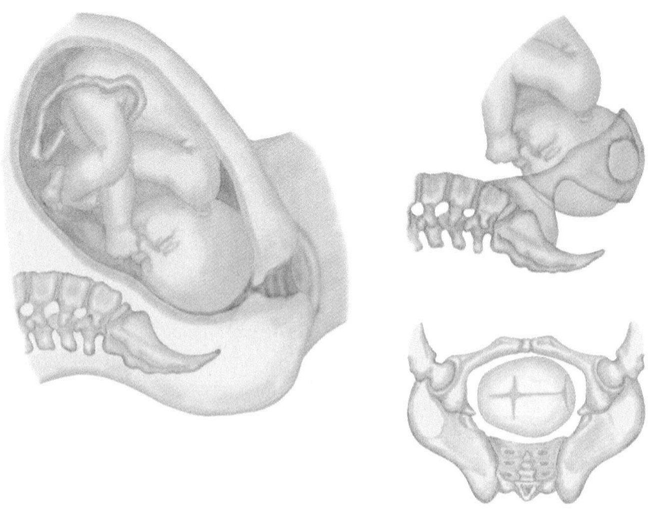

Descent of the fetus is a mechanism of labor that accompanies all the others. Without descent, none of the other mechanisms can proceed.

*Station*

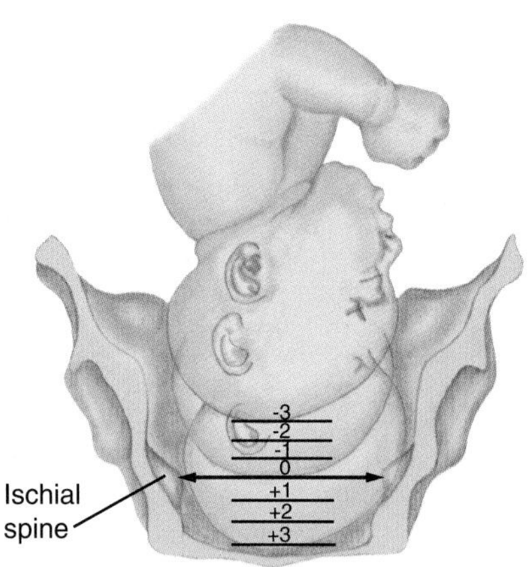


Station describes the descent of the fetal presenting part in relation to the level of the ischial spines. The level of the ischial spines is a zero station. Other stations are described with numbers representing the approximate number of centimeters above (negative numbers) or below (positive numbers) the ischial spines. As the fetus descends through the pelvis, the station changes from higher negative numbers (–3, –2, –1) to zero to higher positive numbers (+1, +2, +3, etc.). Sometimes the terms *floating* or *ballottable* may describe a fetal presenting part that is so high that it is easily displaced upward during abdominal or vaginal examination, similar to tossing a ball upward.

*Engagement*

Engagement occurs when the largest diameter of the fetal presenting part (normally the head) has passed the pelvic inlet and entered the pelvic cavity. Engagement is presumed to have occurred when the station of the presenting part is zero or lower. Engagement often takes place before onset of labor in nulliparous women. In many parous women and in some nulliparas, it does not occur until after labor begins.

*Flexion*

As the fetus descends, the fetal head is flexed farther as it meets resistance from the soft tissues of the pelvis. Head flexion presents the smallest anteroposterior diameter (suboccipitobregmatic) to the pelvis.

*Internal Rotation*

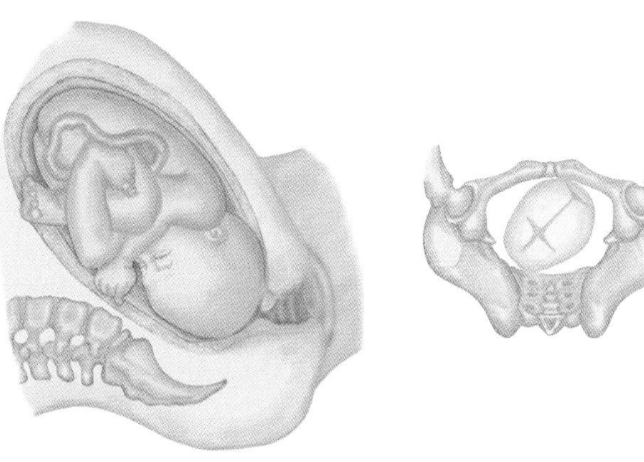

The fetus enters the pelvic inlet with the sagittal suture in a transverse or oblique orientation to the maternal pelvis because that is the widest inlet diameter. Internal rotation allows the longest fetal head diameter (the anteroposterior) to conform to the longest diameter of the maternal pelvis.

The longest pelvic outlet diameter is the anteroposterior. As the head descends to the level of the ischial spines, it gradually turns so that the fetal occiput is in the anterior of the pelvis (OA position, directly under the maternal symphysis pubis). When internal rotation is complete, the sagittal suture is oriented in the anteroposterior pelvic diameter (OA). Less commonly, the head may turn posteriorly so that the occiput is directed toward the mother's sacrum (OP).

**FIG 16.12** Mechanisms (cardinal movements) of labor.

## EXTENSION

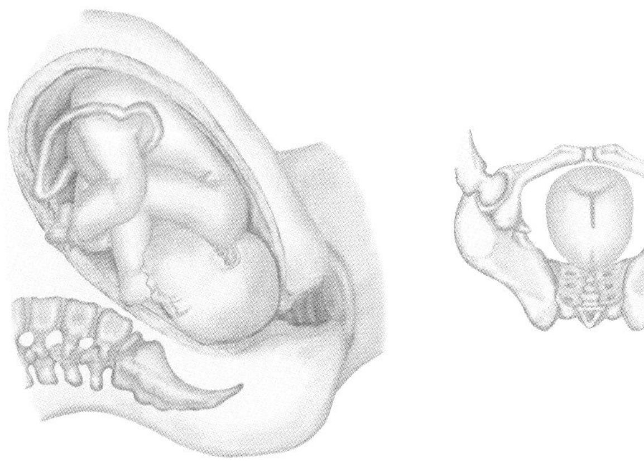

Extension beginning (internal rotation complete)

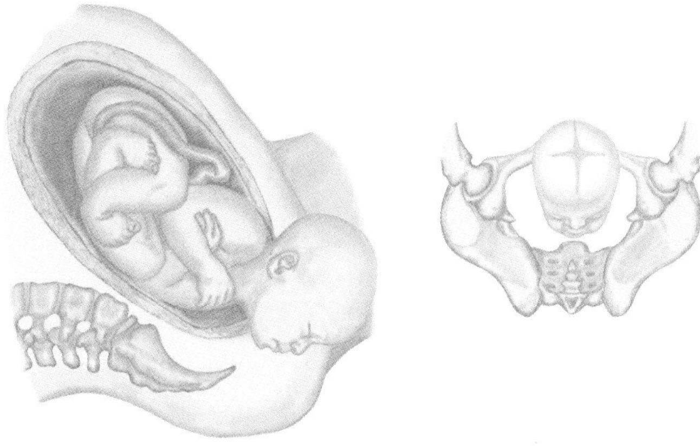

Extension complete

Because the true pelvis is shaped like a curved cylinder, the fetal head is directed posteriorly toward the rectum as it begins its descent. To negotiate the curve of the pelvis, the fetal head must change from an attitude of flexion to one of extension.

While still in flexion, the fetal head meets resistance from the tissues of the pelvic floor. At the same time, the fetal neck stops under the symphysis, which acts as a pivot. The combination of resistance from the pelvic floor and the pivoting action of the symphysis causes the fetal head to swing anteriorly, or extend, with each maternal pushing effort. The head is born in extension, with the occiput sliding under the symphysis and the face directed toward the rectum. The fetal brow, nose, and chin slide over the perineum as the head is born.

## EXTERNAL ROTATION

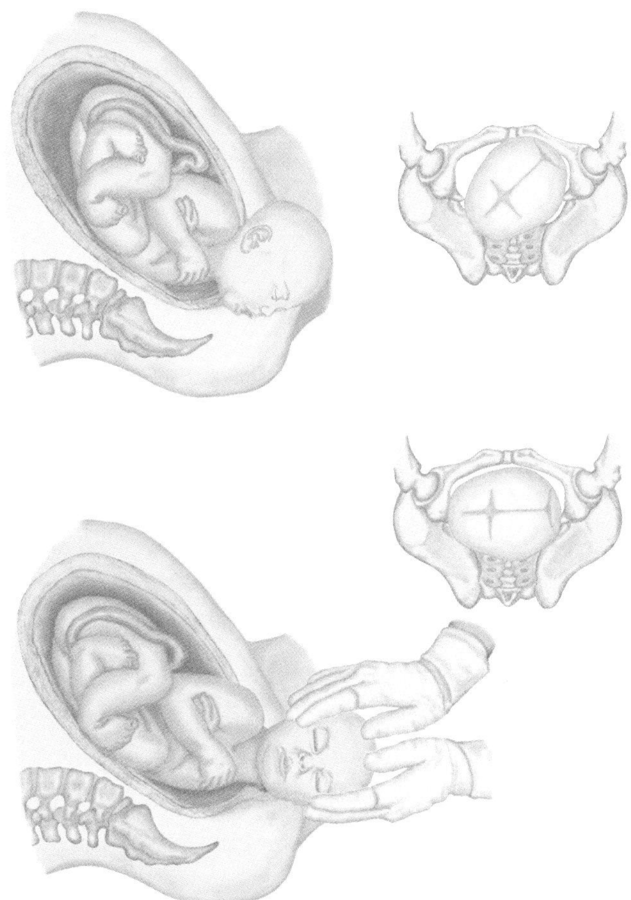

When the head is born with the occiput directed anteriorly, the shoulders must rotate internally so that they align with the anteroposterior diameter of the pelvis.

After the head is born, it spontaneously turns to the same side as it was in utero as it realigns with the shoulders and back (through a process called restitution). The head then turns farther to that side in external rotation as the shoulders internally rotate and are positioned with their transverse diameter in the anteroposterior diameter of the pelvic outlet. External rotation of the head accompanies internal rotation of the shoulders.

## EXPULSION

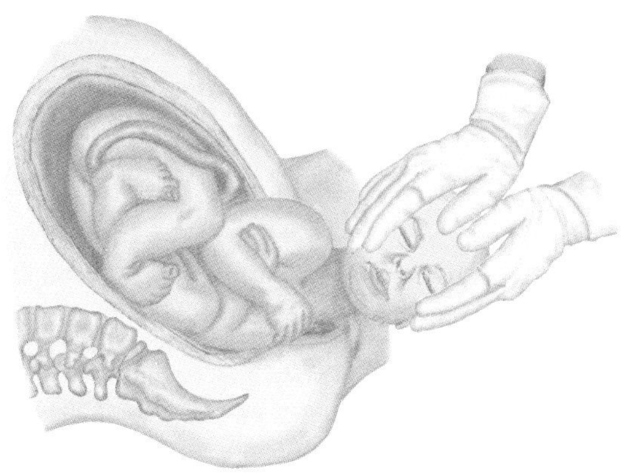

Expulsion occurs first as the anterior, then the posterior, shoulder passes under the symphysis. After the shoulders are born, the rest of body follows.

**FIG 16.12, cont'd** Mechanisms (cardinal movements) of labor.

**TABLE 16.1 Characteristics of Normal Labor**

| | First Stage | Second Stage | Third Stage | Fourth Stage |
|---|---|---|---|---|
| Work accomplished | Effacement and dilation of cervix | Expulsion of fetus | Separation of placenta | Physical recovery and bonding with newborn |
| Forces | Uterine contractions | Uterine contractions and voluntary bearing-down efforts | Uterine contractions | Uterine contraction to control bleeding from placental site |
| ***Average Duration*** | | | | |
| Nullipara | *Latent phase:* approximately 7.5-8.5 hr *Active phase:* 8-10 hr (range, 6-18 hr); dilation averages 1.2 cm/hr *Transition phase:* approximately 3.5 hr | Average, 50 min (range, 30 min-3 hr) | 5-10 min; up to 30 min is normal for unassisted placental separation | 1-4 hr after birth |
| Multipara | *Latent phase:* approximately 4-5.5 hr *Active phase:* 6-7 hr (range, 2-10 hr); dilation averages 1.5 cm/hr *Transition phase:* 0-30 min | Average, 20 min (range, 0-30 min) | Same as for nullipara | Same as for nullipara |
| Cervical dilation | *Latent phase:* 0-3 cm *Active phase:* 4-10 cm *Transition phase (if used):* final 8-10 cm | 10 cm (complete dilation) | Not applicable | Not applicable |
| Uterine contractions | *Latent phase:* Initially mild and infrequent; progress to moderate strength, every 5 min with a regular pattern; duration increases to 30-40 sec by end of latent phase *Active phase:* Increase in frequency, duration, and intensity until every 2-3 min, 40-60 sec, and moderate to strong intensity *Transition phase (if used):* Strong, every 1½-2 min, 60-90 sec | Strong, every 2-3 min, lasting 40-60 sec; may be slightly less intense than during transition phase of first stage; may pause briefly as second stage begins | Firmly contracted | Firmly contracted |
| Discomfort* | Often begins with a low backache and sensations similar to those of menstrual cramps; back discomfort gradually sweeps to lower abdomen in a girdle like fashion; discomfort intensifies as labor progresses | Urge to push or bear down with contractions, which becomes stronger as fetus descends; distention of vagina and vulva may cause a stretching or splitting sensation | Little discomfort; sometimes slight cramp is felt as placenta is passed | Discomfort varies; some women have afterpains, more common in multigravidas or those who have had a large baby; as anesthesia wears off, perineal discomfort may become noticeable |
| Maternal behaviors* | Sociable, excited, and somewhat anxious during early labor; becomes more inwardly focused as labor intensifies; may lose control during transition | Intense concentration on pushing with contractions; often oblivious to surroundings and appears to doze between contractions | Excited and relieved after baby's birth; usually very tired; often cries | Tired but may find it difficult to rest because of excitement; eager to become acquainted with her newborn |

*Maternal discomfort and behaviors often vary with pain-relief method chosen.
From Hobel, C.J., & Zakowski, M. (2010). Normal labor, delivery, and postpartum care. In N.F. Hacker, J.C. Gambone, & C.J. Hobel (Eds.), *Hacker & Moore's essentials of obstetrics and gynecology* (5th ed., pp. 91–118). Philadelphia: Saunders; Kilpatrick, S.J., & Laros, R.K. (1989). Characteristics of normal labor. *Obstetrics & Gynecology, 74*(1), 85–87; Simpson, K.R. (2014). Labor and birth. In K.R. Simpson, & P.A. Creehan (Eds.), *AWHONN's perinatal nursing* (4th ed., pp. 343–444). Philadelphia: Lippincott.

- A gush of blood appears as blood trapped behind the placenta is released.

The placenta may be expelled in one of two ways. In the more common *Schultze* mechanism, the placenta is expelled with the shiny, fetal side first (see Fig. 16.14, *A*). The *Duncan* mechanism is less common, with the rough maternal side presenting (see Fig. 16.14, *B*).

The uterus must contract firmly and remain contracted after the placenta is expelled to compress open vessels at the implantation site. Inadequate uterine contraction after birth may result in hemorrhage.

Pain during the third stage of labor results from uterine contractions and brief stretching of the cervix as the placenta passes through it.

### Fourth Stage of Labor

The fourth stage of labor is the *stage of physical recovery* for the mother and infant. It lasts from the delivery of the placenta through the first 1 to 4 hours after birth.

Immediately after birth, the firmly contracted uterus can be palpated through the abdominal wall as a firm, rounded mass approximately 10 to 15 cm (4 to 6 in) in diameter at or below the level of the umbilicus. The uterus is larger when the infant is large or the mother is a multipara. Uterine size is larger in the women who delivered twins or more at or near term.

The vaginal drainage during the fourth stage is **lochia rubra**, which consists mostly of blood. Small clots may also be present. See Chapter 20 for more information about lochia.

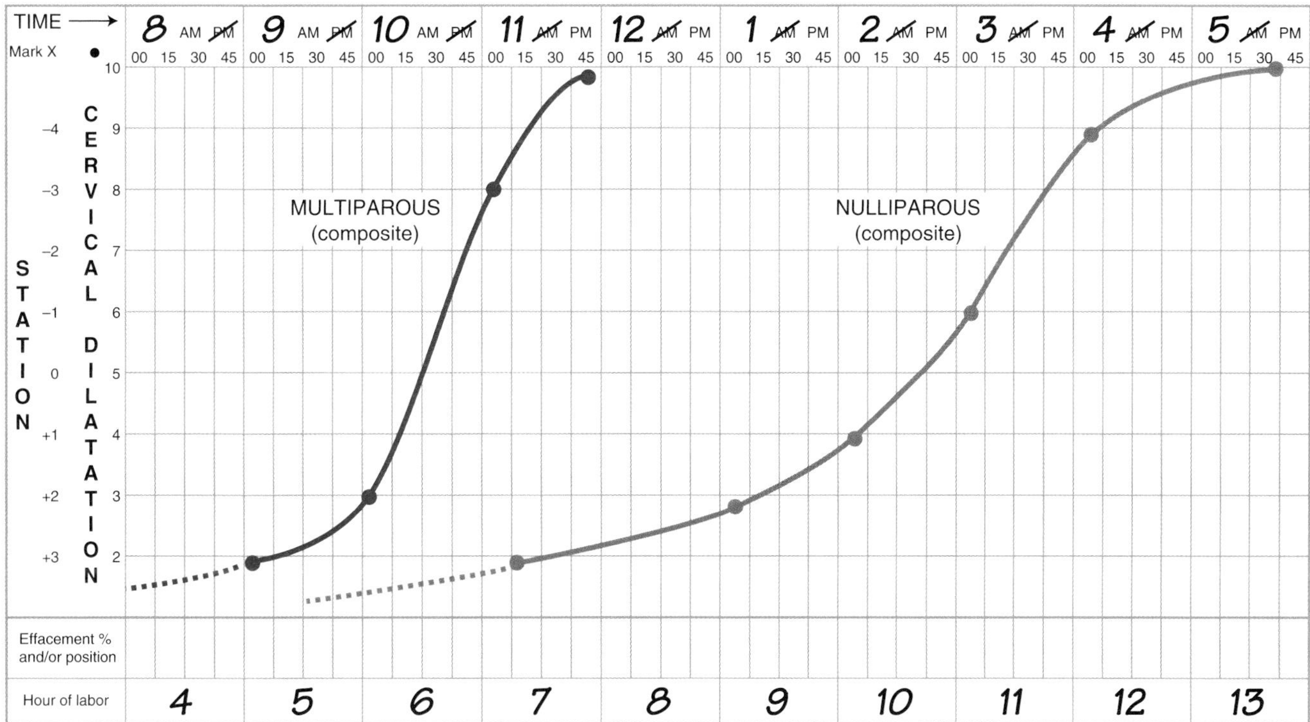


FIG 16.13 A labor curve, often called a *Friedman curve*, may be used to identify whether a woman's cervical dilation is progressing at the expected rate. Typical labor curves for a multiparous and a nulliparous woman are illustrated for comparison of patterns.

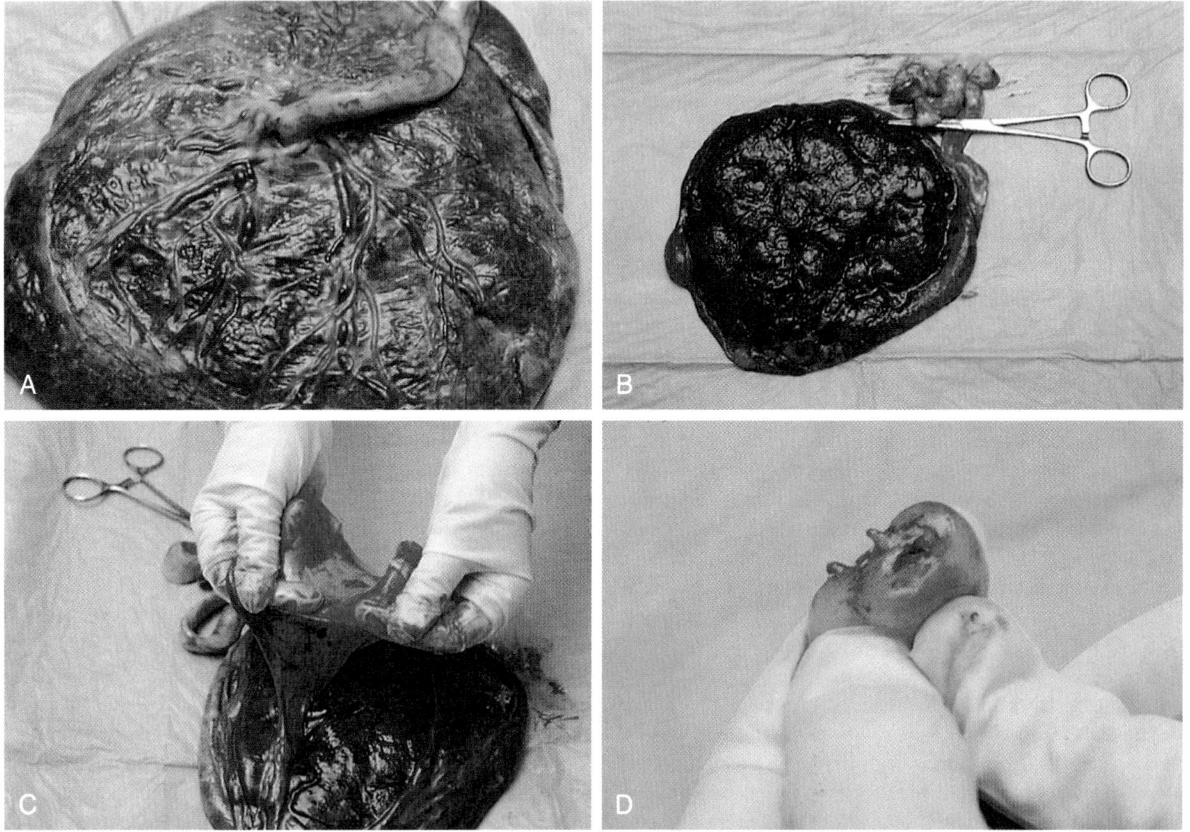


FIG 16.14 **A,** Fetal side of the placenta. **B,** Maternal side of the placenta. **C,** Separating membranes. **D,** Umbilical cord vessels—two arteries and one vein.

## EVIDENCE-BASED PRACTICE

Does delayed pushing versus immediate pushing during a woman's second stage have any physical advantages for her? What about her newborn? Two nursing research articles provide evidence that delaying pushing when a nullipara reaches second stage shortened the duration of pushing compared to the nulliparas in the immediate pushing group. However, the total length of second stage was longer in the delayed pushing group in each study, an expected finding. Primary outcome measures in both studies were the length of pushing during second stage, total length of second stage, and maternal fatigue.

Kelly, Johnson, Lee, et al. (2010) conducted a randomized clinical trial (RCT) including 44 nulliparas: immediate pushing for 28, delayed pushing for 16. Consent was obtained before full dilation and entry into the study. All women were receiving epidural anesthesia before reaching complete dilation. Labor was spontaneous or induced electively or was medically indicated. Fetal heart rate (FHR) at the time they entered the study was reassuring, and gestation was ≥38 weeks. Pain scores were ≥3 on a scale of 10 when they entered the study. This study delayed pushing up to 90 minutes, at which time pushing with contractions would be encouraged. The length of pushing time was 51% lower in the delayed pushing group (38.9 ± 6.9 minutes) than in the immediate pushing group (78.7 ± 7.9 min). The woman pushed sooner if she had a strong urge. The difference in actual pushing time was statistically significant. The duration of the second stage was approximately 30 minutes shorter in the immediate pushing group (87.1 ± 8.6 minutes) than in the delayed pushing group (117.6 ± 12.1 minutes), but not statistically significant. Maternal fatigue, measured with the visual analog scale (VAS) was similar in the two groups.

Gillesby, Burns, Dempsey, et al. (2010) had similar results with their group of 77 women, 39 in the immediate pushing group and 38 in the delayed pushing group. Their group was also nulliparas with epidural pain relief as they entered second stage. For the delayed pushing group, this RCT used 120 minutes as the maximum delay for pushing at which time pushing would be encouraged if the woman had no earlier urge. The duration of pushing time in the mothers with immediate pushing (94 ± 57 minutes) versus mothers with delayed pushing (68 ± 46 minutes) also differed significantly. Second stage labor duration averaged 107 ± 56 minutes in the immediate pushing group versus 163 ± 64 minutes in the delayed pushing group. Maternal fatigue scores were also similar between the two groups. The total second stage time was 59 minutes longer for the group who delayed pushing. Fatigue scores with the VAS were similar for the two groups.

These two studies support the benefit of delaying pushing without evidence of fetal compromise. Passive fetal descent and rotation is the likely reason why the second stage, while longer in total length, required a shorter period of pushing.

Above results confirmed by a two large meta analyses reported in 2014 by M. Kopas. Delayed pushing resulted in longer second stage, but less time spent actively pushing in the group of women who experienced delayed pushing (Kopas, 2014).

References: Gillesby, E., Burns, S., Dempsey, A., et al. (2010). Comparison of delayed versus immediate pushing during second stage of labor for nulliparous women with epidural anesthesia. *Journal of Obstetric, Gynecologic, and Neonatal Nursing, 39*(6), 635–644; Kelly, M., Johnson, E., Lee, V., et al. (2010). Delayed versus immediate pushing in second stage of labor. *MCN: The American Journal of Maternal-Child Nursing, 35*(2), 81–88; Kopas, M (2014). A Review of Evidence-Based Practices for Management of the Second Stage of Labor. *Journal of Midwifery and Wonem's Health*, 59(3), 264–276.

Many women have a chill after birth. The chill lasts for approximately 20 minutes and subsides spontaneously. A warm blanket, hot drink, or soup may help shorten the chill and make the woman more comfortable.

Discomfort during the fourth stage usually results from birth trauma or afterpains. Ice packs on the perineum limit discomfort and hematoma formation.

Afterpains are uterine contractions similar to menstrual cramps that occur after birth as the uterus begins its return to the prepregnancy state. The discomfort is similar to that of menstrual cramps. Afterpains are more intense in multiparas, in women who breastfeed, in women who have large babies or other causes of uterine over distention during pregnancy, or when something interferes with uterine contraction, such as a full bladder or a blood clot that remains in the uterus.

The mother is simultaneously excited and tired after birth. She may be exhausted but too full of nervous energy to rest. The fourth stage of labor is an ideal time for bonding of the new family because the interest of both parents and newborn is high. It is also the best time to start breastfeeding if no maternal or infant problems are present. The baby is alert and seeks to make eye contact with the new parents, giving powerful reinforcement for the parents' attachment to their newborn.

### Duration of Labor

The total duration of labor differs between women who have never given birth and those who have previously given birth vaginally. The parous woman usually delivers more quickly than does the nulliparous woman. However, women are individuals. Some nulliparas progress through labor quickly, whereas labor for some parous women resembles that of women who have never given birth. A woman who experienced a long labor with her first child may not have a long labor with every baby. However, if she has a history of rapid labor, later births are often rapid as well.

## NURSING CARE DURING LABOR AND BIRTH

### Admission to the Birth Center

During the last trimester, the woman needs to know when she should go to the hospital or birth center. Nurses teach women about the differences between false labor and true labor and offer guidelines for going to the birth center. Not everyone has a typical labor, so a woman should be encouraged to go to the birth center if she is uncertain or has other concerns.

### Nursing Responsibilities During Admission

The nurse has two priorities when the woman arrives at the birth center: (1) establishing a therapeutic relationship while (2) assessing the condition of the mother and fetus.

#### Establishing a Therapeutic Relationship

***Making the family feel welcome.*** A family's first impression influences how family members feel about the quality of the birth experience. Even if the unit is busy, the nurse should communicate interest, friendliness, caring, and competence. Families understand if the nurse is busy; they do not understand rudeness or insensitivity to their needs.

When caring for the woman who has not had prenatal care or childbirth classes, behaviors most nurses value, the nurse should avoid being judgmental in either words or actions. The woman's priorities and values may not be the same as those of the nurse, but she deserves the same respect, support, and care as the woman who made every preparation for her baby's birth.

## PATIENT-CENTERED TEACHING

### *When to Go to the Hospital or Birth Center*

These are guidelines for providing individualized instruction to women about when to enter the hospital or birth center.

**Contractions**

- A pattern of increasing regularity, frequency, duration, and intensity.
- Nullipara: Regular contractions, 5 minutes apart, for 1 hour.
- Multipara: Regular contractions, 10 minutes apart, for 1 hour.

**Ruptured Membranes**

A gush or trickle of fluid from the vagina should be evaluated, whether or not you have contractions, to determine if your membranes have ruptured ("water has broken").

**Bleeding**

Bright red bleeding that is not mixed with mucus should be evaluated promptly. Normal bloody show is thicker, pink or dark red, and mixed with mucus.

**Decreased Fetal Movement**

If you notice a decrease in the baby's movement, notify your physician or nurse-midwife or go to the labor unit.

**Other Concerns**

These guidelines cannot cover all situations. Go to the birth center for evaluation of any concerns or feelings that something may be wrong.

Nurses frequently encounter women who speak a language other than English. Arranging for a culturally acceptable interpreter who is fluent in the woman's language makes the woman and family feel more welcome and promotes safety because it enhances understanding among the woman, her family, and the nurse. Telephone interpreters may be available for languages encountered in a facility. Arrangements may be needed for sign language interpreters or other means for language translation between the hearing and the hearing impaired. See the National Institute on Deafness and Other Communication Disorders website at https://www.nidcd.nih.gov for more information.

## CRITICAL THINKING EXERCISE 16.1

A man phones you as you are working in the birth unit of your hospital one night. He says, "My wife's baby is almost due. She's been having some contractions off and on all day, and they are keeping her awake now. Should we come to the hospital?"

1. Do you need any other information? If so, what information do you need?
2. What should you tell her about her symptoms? What advice should you give her?

***Determining family expectations about birth.*** Regardless of how many children they have, women and their partners have expectations about the birth experience. The partners have often studied their options extensively and have planned a birth that best fits their ideals. Some may have a written birth plan filed with their prenatal records. Those who have not made specific plans also have expectations shaped by contact with relatives and friends or by previous birth experiences. Most women assume that their partner, usually the baby's father, will be present. Many want other close and trusted family or friends to be with them for all or part of labor and birth (Simpson & O'Brein-Abel, 2014).

Consider the different perspective implied by the phrases "give birth" and "be delivered." The woman who gives birth is an active and able participant; she is the principal action figure. However, when her baby is "delivered," the language implies that she is passive. The nurse might ask, "Who will attend you as you give birth?" or "Who is your doctor [or midwife]?" rather than, "Who will deliver your baby?"

***Conveying confidence.*** From the first encounter, the nurse should convey confidence in the woman's ability to give birth and her partner's ability to support her. Contractions and discomfort intensify as labor progresses. A woman having her first baby may find the power of normal labor contractions overwhelming. The nurse can reassure the woman that intense contractions are normal in active labor while helping her deal with them and watching for problems.

***Assigning a primary nurse.*** Birth, even if induced, does not fit neatly into nursing schedules. Thus, having one nurse give care during all of labor is unrealistic. However, the number of different caregivers should be limited as much as possible. The woman should know who each caregiver is and what to expect from each.

***Using touch for comfort.*** Touch can communicate acceptance and reassurance and can provide physical and emotional comfort to many laboring women. Women who do not usually welcome touch may appreciate it during labor. Cultural norms and personal history influence whether a woman is comfortable with touch from a stranger such as a nurse. One should not assume that the woman desires touch but should ask her if she wants it or benefits from it. As labor progresses, touch may become an irritant rather than a comfort measure during late labor.

***Respecting cultural values.*** Cultural beliefs and practices give structure and meaning to the birth experience. The nurse should incorporate a family's cultural practices into care as much as possible.

### Assessments at the Time of Admission

A paper or computer-based record of prenatal care is sent to the center where the woman plans to give birth before her due date and verified or updated on admission. Although prenatal records are becoming more accessible through computer networks, many factors may require paper records of care. Women who have not had prenatal care need a more extensive assessment by the nurse and physician or nurse-midwife. Table 16.2 lists intrapartum assessments, usual findings, significant findings, and appropriate nursing actions.

***Focused assessment.*** In the intrapartum unit, an initial focused assessment is done before the broader database assessment—opposite of the usual order. Assessment priorities are to determine the condition of the mother and fetus and whether birth is imminent.

**Fetal assessment.** Estimated gestational age should be determined by prenatal care records, previous ultrasound exams, or the mother's statement about her last menstrual period. Leopold's maneuvers (see Procedure on pp. 311-312) help identify the best place to assess the FHR. The rate, rhythm, and other characteristics should be assessed on admission and at intervals appropriate to the woman's risk status and labor. Fetal movement should be noted. If the membranes are ruptured, assess the color, odor, and clarity of leaking fluid. Chapter 17 provides detailed information about intrapartum fetal surveillance.

**Maternal vital signs.** Assess maternal vital signs primarily for signs of hypertension or infection. Hypertension during pregnancy is defined as a sustained blood pressure increase to 140 mm Hg systolic or higher or 90 mm Hg diastolic or higher (American Academy of Pediatrics [AAP] & American College of Obstetricians and Gynecologists [ACOG], 2012; Castro, 2010). A temperature of 38° C (100.4° F) or higher suggests infection.

*Text continued on p. 312*

**TABLE 16.2 Intrapartum Assessment Guide**

***Women Who Have Had Prenatal Care Have Much of This Information Available on Their Prenatal Record. The Nurse Need Only Verify It or Update It as Needed.***

| Assessment, Method (Selected Rationales) | Common Findings | Significant Findings, Nursing Action |
|---|---|---|
| ***Interview*** | | |
| *Purpose:* To obtain information about the woman's pregnancy, labor, and conditions that may affect her care. The interview is curtailed if she is in late labor. | | |
| *Introduction:* Introduce yourself and ask the woman how she wants to be addressed. Ask her if she wants her partner and/or family to remain during the interview and assessment. (Shows respect for the woman and gives her control over those she wants to remain with her) | Many women prefer to be addressed by their first names during labor. | The surname (family name) precedes the given name in some cultures. Clarify which name is used to properly address the woman and to properly identify both mother and newborn. Have the woman verify accuracy of identification bands before placing them on her and baby. |
| *Culture and language:* If she is from another culture, ask what her preferred language is and what language(s) she speaks, reads, or verbally understands. (Identifies the need for an interpreter and enables the most accurate data collection) | Common non-English languages of women in the United States are Spanish and some Asian languages. The most common non-English language varies with location. | Secure an interpreter fluent in the woman's primary language. Ask her if there are people who are not acceptable to her as interpreters (e.g., males or members of a group in conflict with her culture). Family members may not be the best interpreters because they may interpret selectively, adding or subtracting information as they see fit. Phone interpreters are available in many facilities. Hearing-impaired women may read lips well, or they may need sign-language interpreters or other assistance. |
| *Communication:* Ask the woman to tell you when she has a contraction, and pause during the interview and physical assessment. (Shows sensitivity to her comfort and allows her to concentrate more fully on the information the nurse requests.) | Women in active labor have difficulty answering questions or cooperating with a physical examination while they are having a contraction. Consider the stage and phase of labor to determine what information can wait. | If contractions are very frequent, assess the woman's labor status promptly rather than continuing the interview. Only ask questions related to vital information (see p. 336). |
| *Nonverbal cues:* Observe the woman's behaviors and interactions with her family and the nurse. (Permits estimation of her level of anxiety; identifies behaviors indicating that she should have a vaginal examination to determine whether birth is imminent) | *Latent phase:* Woman is sociable and mildly anxious. *Active phase:* Woman concentrates intently during contractions; often uses prepared childbirth techniques. | The unprepared or extremely anxious woman may breathe deeply and rapidly, displaying a tense facial and body posture during and between contractions. These behaviors suggest that birth is imminent:<br>1. Her statement that the baby is coming.<br>2. Grunting sounds (low-pitched, guttural sounds).<br>3. Bearing down with abdominal muscles.<br>4. Sitting on one buttock<br>Euphoria, combativeness, or sedation suggests recent illicit drug ingestion. |
| *Reason for admission:* "What brings you to the hospital/birth center today?" (Open-ended question promotes more complete answer) | Labor contractions at term, induction of labor, or observation for false labor are common reasons for admission. | Bleeding, preterm labor, pain other than labor contractions. Report these findings to the physician or nurse-midwife promptly. |
| *Prenatal care:* "Did you see a doctor or nurse-midwife during your pregnancy?" "Who is your doctor or nurse-midwife?" "How far along were you in your pregnancy when you saw the physician or nurse-midwife?" "Have you ever been admitted here before during this pregnancy?" (Enables location of prenatal record and previous visit records) | Early and regular prenatal care promotes maternal and fetal health. | No prenatal care or care that was irregular or begun in late pregnancy means that complications may not have been identified. |
| *Estimated date of delivery (EDD):* "When is your baby due?" (Determines if **gestation** is term.) "When did your last menstrual period begin?" (For estimation of EDD if woman did not have prenatal care) | *Term gestation:* 38-42 wk. The woman's gestation may have been confirmed or adjusted during pregnancy with an ultrasound or other clinical examination. | Gestations earlier than the beginning of the 38th wk (preterm) or later than the end of the 42nd wk (postterm) are associated with more fetal or neonatal problems. The physician may try to stop labor that occurs earlier than 36 wk if there are no contraindications for mother or fetus. |

**TABLE 16.2 Intrapartum Assessment Guide—cont'd**

***Women Who Have Had Prenatal Care Have Much of This Information Available on Their Prenatal Record. The Nurse Need Only Verify It or Update It as Needed.***

| Assessment, Method (Selected Rationales) | Common Findings | Significant Findings, Nursing Action |
|---|---|---|
| *Gravidity, parity, abortions:* "How many times have you been pregnant?" "How many babies have you had? Were they full term or premature?" "How many children are now living?" "Have you had any miscarriages or abortions?" "Were there any problems with your babies after they were born?" (Helps estimate probable speed of labor and anticipate neonatal problems) | Labor may be faster for the woman who has given birth before than for the nullipara. Miscarriage is used to describe a spontaneous abortion because many lay people associate the term abortion with only induced abortions. | Parity of 5 or more (grand multiparity) is associated with placenta previa (see Chapter 25) and postpartum hemorrhage (see Chapter 28). Women who have had several spontaneous abortions or who have given birth to infants with abnormalities may face a higher risk for an infant with a birth defect. |
| *Pregnancy history* (Identifies problems that may affect this birth) | | |
| Present pregnancy: "Have you had any problems during this pregnancy, such as high blood pressure, diabetes, infections, or bleeding?" | Complications are not expected. | Women who have diabetes or hypertension may have poor placental blood flow, possibly resulting in fetal compromise. Some complications of past pregnancies, such as gestational diabetes, may recur in another pregnancy. The woman who plans a VBAC may need more support and reassurance to give birth vaginally. |
| Past pregnancies: "Were there any problems with your other pregnancy (ies)?" "Were your other babies born vaginally or by cesarean birth?" | Women who had previous cesarean birth(s) may have a trial of labor and vaginal birth (VBAC). A woman who previously had a difficult labor or a cesarean birth may be more anxious than one who had an uncomplicated labor and birth. | Although the VBAC is less common, it may be chosen for various reasons. The nurse should be aware of the need for support and for complications that may be more likely in the current pregnancy. |
| Other: "Is there anything else you think we should know so that we can better care for you?" | This open-ended question gives the woman a chance to share information that may not be elicited by other questions. | |
| *Labor status:* "When did your contractions become regular?" "What time did you begin to think you might really be in labor?" (Facilitates a more accurate estimation of the time labor began.) | Varies among women. Many women go to the birth facility when contractions first begin. Others wait until they are reasonably sure that they are really in labor. | Women who say they have been "in labor" for an unusual length of time (e.g., "for 2 days") have probably had false (prodromal) labor. These women may be very tired from the annoying and apparently nonproductive contractions. |
| *Contractions:* "How often are your contractions coming?" "How long do they last?" "Are they getting stronger?" "Tell me if you have a contraction while we are talking." (Obtains the woman's subjective evaluation of her contractions; alerts the nurse to palpate contractions that occur during the interview) | Varies according to her stage and phase of labor. Labor contractions are usually regular and show a pattern of increasing frequency, duration, and intensity. | Irregular contractions or those that do not increase in frequency, duration, or intensity are more likely to represent false labor. Contractions that are too frequent or too long can reduce placental blood flow. Incomplete uterine relaxation between contractions also can reduce placental blood flow (see Chapter 17). |
| *Membrane status:* "Has your water broken?" "What time did it break?" "What did the fluid look like?" "Approximately how much fluid did you lose—was it a big gush or a trickle?" (Alerts the nurse to the need to verify whether the membranes have ruptured if it is not obvious. Identifies possible prolonged rupture of membranes or preterm rupture) | Most women go to the birth facility for evaluation soon after their membranes rupture. If a woman is not already in labor, contractions usually begin within a few hours after the membranes rupture at term. | If the woman's membranes have ruptured and she is not in labor or if she is not at term, a vaginal examination is often deferred. A speculum examination may be done by the physician or nurse-midwife to identify the woman's membrane status. Labor may be induced if she is at term with ruptured membranes. |
| *Allergies:* "Are you allergic to any foods, medicines, or other substances?" "Do you have an allergy to latex?" "What kind of reaction do you have?" "Have you ever had a problem with anesthesia when you have had dental work?" (Determines possible sensitivity to drugs that may be used) | Record any known allergies to food, medication, or other substances. As needed, describe how they affected the woman. | Allergy to seafood, iodized salt, or imaging contrast media may indicate iodine allergy. Because iodine is used in many "prep" solutions, alternatives should be used. Allergy to latex is more common. Allergy to dental anesthetics may indicate possible allergy to the drugs used for local or regional anesthesia. These drugs usually end in the suffix *-caine.* |

*Continued*

## TABLE 16.2 Intrapartum Assessment Guide—cont'd

***Women Who Have Had Prenatal Care Have Much of This Information Available on Their Prenatal Record. The Nurse Need Only Verify It or Update It as Needed.***

| Assessment, Method (Selected Rationales) | Common Findings | Significant Findings, Nursing Action |
|---|---|---|
| *Food intake:* "When was the last time you had something to eat or drink?" "What did you have?" (Provides information needed to most safely administer general anesthesia if required; identifies possible fluid or energy deficit) | Record the time of the woman's last food intake and what she ate. Include both liquids and solids. | If the woman says she has not had any intake for an unusual length of time, question her more closely: "Is there any food you may have forgotten, such as a snack or a drink of water or other liquid?" |
| *Recent illness:* "Have you been ill recently?" "What was the problem?" "What did you do for it?" "Have you been around anyone with a contagious illness recently?" | Most pregnant women are healthy. An occasional woman may have had a minor illness such as an upper respiratory tract infection. | Urinary tract infections are associated with preterm labor. The woman who has had contact with someone having a communicable disease may become ill and possibly infect others in the facility. |
| *Medications:* "What drugs do you take that your doctor or nurse-midwife has prescribed?" "Are there any over-the-counter or herbal drugs that you use?" "I know this may be uncomfortable to discuss, but we need to know about any illegal or abused substances that you use, to more safely care for you and your baby." (Permits evaluation of the woman's drug intake and encourages her to disclose nonprescribed use.) | Prenatal vitamins and iron are commonly prescribed. Record all drugs the woman takes, including time and amount of last ingestion. Women often do not consider botanical preparations as drugs. Women who use illegal substances often conceal or diminish the extent of their use because they fear reprisals. | Drugs may interact with other medications given during labor, especially analgesics and anesthetics. Substance abuse is associated with complications for the mother and infant (see Chapter 24). If the woman discloses that she uses illegal drugs, ask her what kind and the last time she ingested them (often referred to as "taking a hit"). A nonjudgmental approach in private is more likely to result in honest information. |
| *Tobacco or alcohol:* "Do you smoke or use tobacco in any other form? How many cigarettes a day?" "Do you use alcohol? How many drinks do you have each day (or week)?" (Evaluates use of these legal substances) | As in substance abuse, women may underreport the extent of their use of tobacco or alcohol. | Infants of heavy smokers are often smaller and may have reduced placental blood flow during labor. Infants of women who use alcohol may show fetal alcohol effects at birth or later (see Chapter 30). |
| *Birth plans* (shows respect for the woman and her family as individuals and promotes achievement of their expectations; enables more culturally appropriate care) | | |
| Coach or primary support person: "Who is the main person you want to be with you during labor?" Ask that person how he or she wants to be addressed, such as "Mr. Ramos" or "Carlos." | This is usually the woman's husband or the baby's father, but it may be her mother, her sister, or a friend, especially if she is single. | The woman who has little or no support from significant others probably needs more intense nursing support during labor and after the birth. These women are more likely to have problems with parent–infant attachment. |
| Other support: "Is there anyone else you would like to be present during labor?" | Women often want another support person present. | |
| Preparation for childbirth: "Did you attend prepared childbirth classes?" "Did someone go with you?" | Ideally, the woman and a partner have had some preparation in classes or self-study. Women who attended classes during previous pregnancies do not always repeat the classes during subsequent pregnancies. | The unprepared woman may need more support with simple relaxation and breathing techniques during labor. Her partner may need to learn techniques to assist her. |
| Preferences: "Are there any special plans you have for this birth?" "Is there anything you want to avoid?" "Do you plan to record the birth with pictures or video?" | Some women or couples have strong feelings regarding certain interventions. Common ones are (1) analgesia or anesthesia; (2) intravenous lines; (3) fetal monitoring; (4) use of episiotomy or forceps. | Conflict may arise if the woman has not previously discussed her preferences with her physician or nurse–midwife or if she is unaware of what services are available where she gives birth. |
| Cultural needs: "Are there any special cultural practices that you plan when you have your baby?" "How can we best help you to fulfill these practices?" | Women from Asian and Hispanic cultures may subscribe to the "hot-and-cold" theory of illness and want specific foods after birth, such as soft-boiled eggs. They may not want their water or other fluids iced. | Try to incorporate all positive or neutral cultural practices. If a practice is harmful, explain why and try to find a way to work around it if the family does not want to give it up. |

**TABLE 16.2 Intrapartum Assessment Guide—cont'd**

***Women Who Have Had Prenatal Care Have Much of This Information Available on Their Prenatal Record. The Nurse Need Only Verify It or Update It as Needed.***

| Assessment, Method (Selected Rationales) | Common Findings | Significant Findings, Nursing Action |
|---|---|---|
| ***Fetal Evaluation*** | | |
| *Purpose:* To determine if the fetus seems to be healthy and tolerating labor well. | | |
| *Fetal heart rate (FHR):* Assess by intermittent auscultation, or apply an external fetal monitor if that is the facility's policy (most common in the United States). Document FHR according to the stage of labor (see Chapter 17). Consider her risk status and facility policy. *Guidelines for assessment:* Active first stage, every 15-30 min; second stage, every 5-15 min (AWHONN) or every 5 min (ACOG) | Average rate at term is 110–160 bpm. Rate usually increases when the fetus moves. A reassuring response. | These signs may indicate fetal stress and should be reported to the physician or nurse–midwife:<br>1. Rate outside the normal limits<br>2. Slowing of the rate that persists after the contraction ends<br>3. No increase in rate when the fetus moves<br>4. Irregular rhythm<br>More frequent assessments should be made of the FHR and contractions if any finding is questionable. |
| ***Labor Status*** | | |
| *Purpose:* To identify whether the woman is in labor and if birth is imminent. If she displays signs of imminent birth, this assessment is done as soon as she is admitted. | | |
| *Contractions* (yields objective information about labor status): In addition to asking the woman about her contraction pattern, assess the contractions by palpation with the fingertips of one hand. Contractions should be assessed each time the FHR is assessed. | See Interview section earlier in table. | See Interview section earlier in table. Women who have intense contractions or who are making rapid progress should be assessed more frequently. |
| *Vaginal examination* (Determines cervical dilation and effacement; fetal presentation, position, and station; bloody show; and status of the membranes) | Varies according to the stage and phase of labor. It may not be possible to determine the fetal position by vaginal examination when membranes are intact and bulging over the presenting part. | A vaginal examination is not performed if the woman reports or has evidence of active bleeding (heavier and redder than bloody show) and may not be done if gestation is 36 wk or less and she does not seem to be in active labor. Report reasons for omitting a vaginal examination to the physician or nurse–midwife. |
| *Status of membranes:* During a vaginal examination a flow of fluid suggests ruptured membranes. A pH test and/or fern test may be done, often using a sterile speculum examination. (Test is not needed if it is obvious that the membranes have ruptured) | Amniotic fluid should be clear, possibly containing flecks of white vernix. Its odor is distinctive but not offensive. The pH test with a color change of blue-green to dark blue (pH > 6.5) suggests true rupture of the membranes but is not conclusive. The **fern test** is more diagnostic of true rupture of membranes because it is less likely to be affected by vaginal infections, recent intercourse, or other factors. | A greenish color indicates meconium staining, which may be associated with fetal compromise or postterm gestation. Thick meconium with heavy particulate matter ("pea soup") is most significant (see Chapter 30). Thick green-black meconium may be passed by the fetus in a breech presentation and is not necessarily associated with fetal compromise. Cloudy, yellowish, strong-smelling, or foul-smelling fluid suggests infection. Bloody fluid may indicate partial placental separation (see Chapter 25). |
| *Leopold's maneuvers:* Often done before assessing the FHR to locate the best place for assessment. (Identifies fetal presentation and position; most accurate when combined with information from vaginal examination) | A cephalic presentation with the head well flexed (vertex) is normal. The fetal head is often easily displaced upward ("floating") if the woman is not in labor. When the head is engaged, it cannot be displaced upward with Leopold's maneuvers. | A hard, round, freely movable object in the fundus suggests a fetal head, meaning the fetus is in a breech presentation. Less commonly, the fetus may be crosswise in the uterus: a transverse lie. |
| *Pain:* Note discomfort during and between contractions. Note tenderness when palpating contractions. (Distinguishes between normal labor pain and abnormal pain that may be associated with a complication) | There may be verbal or nonverbal evidence of pain with contractions, but the woman should be relatively comfortable between contractions. The skin around the umbilicus is often sensitive. | Constant pain or a tender, rigid uterus suggests a complication, such as abruptio placentae (separated placenta) (see Chapter 25) or, less commonly, uterine rupture (see Chapter 27). |

*Continued*

## TABLE 16.2 Intrapartum Assessment Guide—cont'd

***Women Who Have Had Prenatal Care Have Much of This Information Available on Their Prenatal Record. The Nurse Need Only Verify It or Update It as Needed.***

| Assessment, Method (Selected Rationales) | Common Findings | Significant Findings, Nursing Action |
|---|---|---|
| ***Physical Examination*** | | |
| *Purpose:* To evaluate the woman's general health and identify conditions that may affect her intrapartum and postpartum care. | | |
| *General appearance:* Observe skin color and texture, nutritional state, and appearance of rest or fatigue. Examine the woman's face, fingers, and lower extremities for edema. Ask her if she can take her rings off and put them on. | Women are often fatigued if their sleep has been interrupted by Braxton Hicks contractions, fetal activity, or frequent urination. Mild edema of the lower extremities is common in late pregnancy. | Pallor suggests anemia. Substantial edema of the face and fingers or extreme (pitting) edema of the lower extremities is associated with preeclampsia although it may occur in the absence of this hypertensive disorder (see Chapter 25). |
| *Vital signs:* Take the woman's temperature, pulse rate, respirations, and blood pressure. Reassess the temperature every 4 hr (every 2 hr after membranes rupture or if temperature is elevated); reassess blood pressure, pulse, and respirations every hour. | *Temperature:* 35.8-37.3° C (96.4-99.1° F)<br>*Pulse rate:* 60-100 bpm<br>*Respirations:* 12-20/min, even and unlabored Blood pressure near baseline levels established during pregnancy. Transient elevations in blood pressure are common when the woman is first admitted, but they return to baseline levels within approximately 30 min. | Report abnormalities to physician or nurse–midwife. Temperature of 38° C (100.4° F) or higher suggests infection. Pulse rate and respirations may also be elevated. Pulse rate and blood pressure may be elevated if the woman is extremely anxious or in pain. A blood pressure ≥140 mm Hg systolic or ≥90 mm Hg diastolic or higher is considered hypertensive. For women who did not have prenatal care, there is no baseline for comparison. |
| *Heart and lung sounds:* Auscultate all areas with a stethoscope. | Heart sounds should be clear with a distinct $S_1$ and $S_2$. A physiologic murmur is common because of the increased blood volume and cardiac output. Breath sounds should be clear, with respirations even and unlabored. | The woman who is breathing rapidly and deeply may have symptoms of hyperventilation: tingling and spasm of the fingers, numbness around the lips. |
| *Breasts:* Palpate for a dominant mass. | Breasts are full and nodular. Areola is darker, especially in dark-skinned women. Breasts may leak colostrum (clear, sticky, straw-colored fluid) during labor. | Report a dominant mass to the physician or nurse–midwife for later follow-up. |
| *Abdomen:* Observe for scars at the same time Leopold's maneuvers and the FHR are assessed. It is usually sufficient to assess the fundal height by observing its relation to the xiphoid process. | Striae (stretch marks) are common. If scars are noted, ask the woman what surgery she had and when. The fundus at term is usually slightly below the xiphoid process but varies with maternal height and fetal size and number. | Report a previous cesarean birth to the physician or nurse–midwife. Transverse uterine scars are the least likely to rupture during labor (see Chapter 27). Measure the fundal height (see p. 250) if the fetus seems small or if the gestation is questionable. |
| *Deep tendon reflexes (DTRs):* Assess patellar reflex (see Chapter 25). Upper extremity DTRs should also be evaluated at admission if epidural block analgesia is planned because they are normally not as strong as the patellar reflex. | A brisk jerk without spasm or sustained muscle contraction is normal. Some women normally have hypoactive reflexes, but at least a slight twitch is expected. Obese women may appear to have diminished reflexes because of the fat tissue over the tendon. | Report absent (uncommon unless the woman is receiving magnesium sulfate) or hyperactive reflexes. Hyperactive reflexes and clonus (repeated tapping when the foot is dorsiflexed) are associated with pregnancy-induced hypertension and often precede a seizure (see Chapter 25). |
| *Midstream urine specimen:* Assess protein and glucose levels using a dipstick. Follow instructions on the package for waiting times. Check for ketones if the woman has not eaten for a prolonged period or has been vomiting. Send a separate specimen for urinalysis if ordered. *Laboratory tests:* Women who have had prenatal care may not need as many admission tests. Common tests include:<br>1. Complete blood cell count (or hematocrit done on unit).<br>2. Blood type and Rh factor.<br>3. Serum tests for syphilis. Other routine admission tests may include serum HIV, vaginal gonorrhea and chlamydia, or vaginal group B streptococcus (GBS) tests. Routine drug screens are common for a woman who has not had prenatal care. | Negative or trace of protein; negative glucose and ketones.<br>1. Hemoglobin at least 10.5 g/dL; hematocrit at least 33%.<br>2. The woman who is Rh-negative and has had regular prenatal care receives Rh immune globulin at 28 wk of gestation to prevent formation of anti-Rh antibodies.<br>3. Negative on all. GBS screening may have been done recently during a prenatal visit late in pregnancy (see Chapter 13, Table 13.1, p. 238 for more information). | Proteinuria is associated with pregnancy-induced hypertension but may also be associated with urinary tract infections or a specimen that is contaminated with vaginal secretions. Glucosuria is associated with diabetes. Ketonuria is common in poorly controlled diabetes or if the woman does not eat adequate carbohydrates to meet her energy needs.<br>1. Values lower than these reduce maternal reserve for normal blood loss at birth.<br>2. Rh-negative mothers need Rh immune globulin after birth if the infant is Rh-positive.<br>3. A positive test indicates that the baby could be infected and needs treatment after birth. The mother should be treated if she has not been treated already. Maternal antibiotics are given for positive GBS to reduce newborn infection from organisms within the vagina. |

*ACOG,* American College of Obstetricians and Gynecologists; *AWHONN,* Association of Women's Health, Obstetric and Neonatal Nurses; *bpm,* beats per minute; *VBAC,* vaginal birth after cesarean

## PROCEDURE

### *Leopold's Maneuvers*

**Purposes**

To determine the presentation and position of the fetus and to aid in locating fetal heart sounds. Leopold's maneuvers are less likely to yield useful information if the woman has a thick abdominal fat pad, excessive amniotic fluid, or a very preterm fetus.

1. Explain the procedure, the reasons for the assessment, and what is found at each step to teach her and reassure her when the findings are normal.
2. Ask the woman to empty her bladder if she has not done so recently to reduce discomfort during palpation and make fetal parts easier to feel. Have her lie on her back with her knees flexed slightly or head slightly elevated to help her relax her abdominal muscles. Place a small pillow or folded towel under one hip to prevent supine hypotension.
3. Wash your hands with warm water to prevent transmission of microorganisms and to make your hands warmer when touching the woman. Wear gloves to avoid contact with the woman's secretions as indicated.
4. Stand beside the woman, facing her head, with your dominant hand nearest her, because the first three maneuvers are most easily performed in this position.

**First Maneuver**

5. Palpate the uterine fundus *to distinguish between a cephalic and breech presentation.* The breech (buttocks) is softer and more irregular in shape than the head. Moving the breech also moves the fetal trunk. The head is harder, with a round, uniform shape. The head can move without the entire fetal trunk moving.

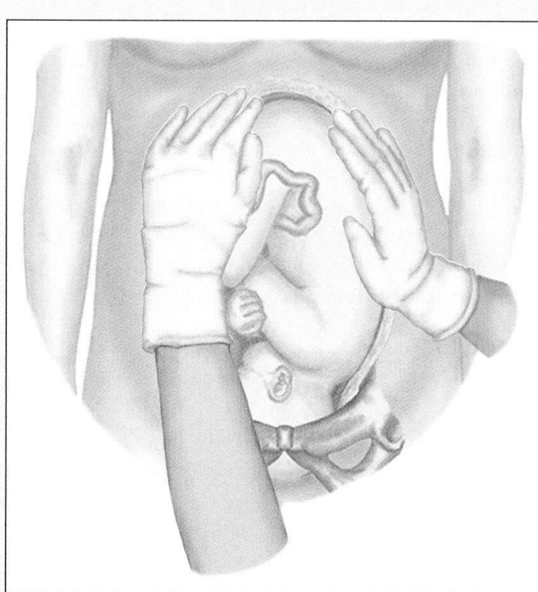

**Second Maneuver**

6. Hold your left hand steady on one side of the uterus while palpating the opposite side of the uterus with your right hand to determine which side the fetal back is on and which side the arms and legs ("small parts") are on. Then hold your right hand steady while palpating the opposite side of the uterus with your left hand. The fetal back is a smooth, convex surface. The fetal arms and legs feel nodular, and the fetus often moves them during palpation.

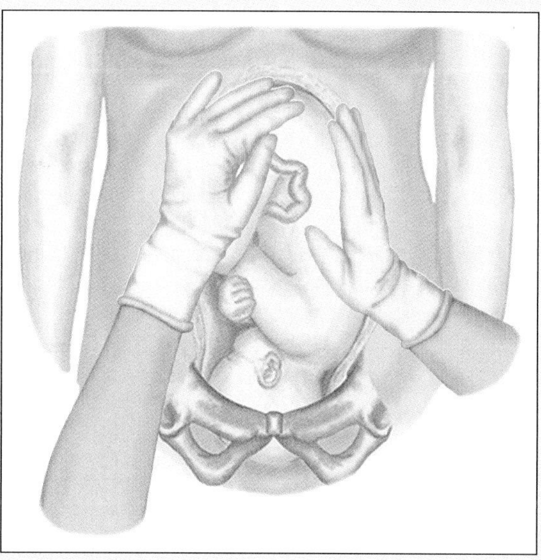

**Third Maneuver**

7. Palpate the suprapubic area to confirm the presentation felt in the first maneuver and to determine if the presenting part is engaged. If a breech was palpated in the fundus, expect a hard, rounded head in this area. Grasp the presenting part gently between the thumb and fingers. If the presenting part is not engaged, grasping with the fingers moves it upward in the uterus.
8. Omit the fourth maneuver if the fetus is in a breech presentation, because this maneuver is done only in cephalic presentations to determine if the fetal head is flexed.

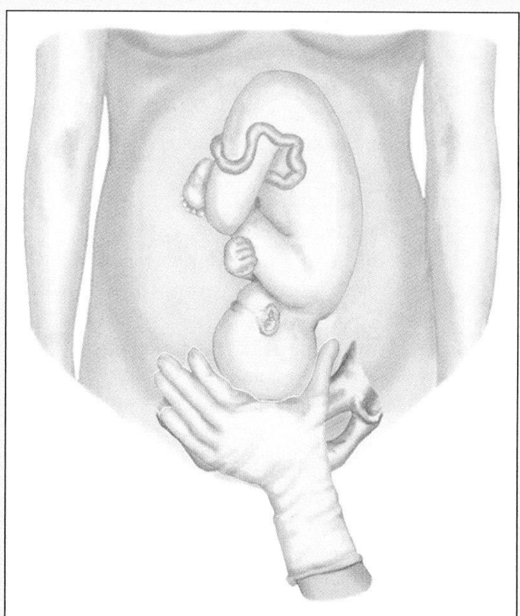

*Continued*

## PROCEDURE—cont'd

### *Leopold's Maneuvers*

9. To perform this maneuver most easily, turn so that you face the woman's feet.
10. Place your hands on each side of the uterus with your fingers pointed toward the pelvic inlet to determine whether the head is flexed (vertex) or extended (face). Slide your hands downward on each side of the uterus. On one side, your fingers easily slide to the upper edge of the symphysis. On the other side, your fingers meet an obstruction, the cephalic prominence. If the head is flexed, the cephalic prominence (the forehead in this case) is felt on the opposite side from the fetal back. If the head is extended, the cephalic prominence (the occiput in this case) is felt on the same side as the fetal back.

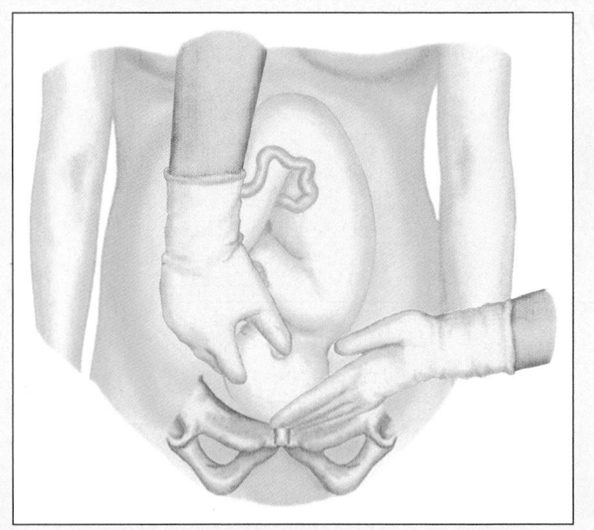

**Impending birth.** Occasionally a woman enters the intrapartum unit almost ready to give birth. Grunting sounds, bearing down, sitting on one buttock, or urgently saying something like "The baby's coming" suggests imminent birth. The nurse abbreviates the initial assessment and collects other information when possible.

Vital information to obtain if birth is imminent includes:

- Mother's name
- Support person's name
- Whether the woman had prenatal care
- Physician's or nurse-midwife's name
- Number of pregnancies and previous births, including whether vaginal or cesarean
- Status of membranes
- Estimated date of delivery (EDD)
- Any problems during this pregnancy
- Medications (see Database Assessment)
- Allergies
- Time and type of last oral intake
- Maternal vital signs and FHR
- Pain: location, intensity, intensifying or relieving factors, duration, whether it is constant or intermittent, acceptability to the woman

If focused assessments of mother and fetus are normal and birth is not imminent, complete the admission assessment. If the initial assessments are not normal or birth is near, notify the physician or nurse-midwife promptly.

***Database assessment.*** In addition to the focused assessment, assess the mother and fetus and available maternal support.

**Basic information.** Most intrapartum admission forms guide the nurse to ask for essential information. Prenatal records may be available to answer many of these questions if the woman had regular visits. Typical information includes:

- The woman's reason for coming to the hospital or birth center (e.g., contractions, rupture of membranes, bleeding)
- Prenatal care: when it began, most recent visit, name of physician or nurse-midwife
- EDD
- Number of pregnancies, births, spontaneous pregnancy losses (miscarriage), and abortions
- Allergies (medications, food, substances such as latex)
- Food intake: what food and when it was eaten
- Medical, surgical, and pregnancy history
- Recent illness, including treatment
- Medications, including prescription and over-the-counter drugs
- Complementary or alternative therapy; use of herbal and botanical preparations and their purpose
- Use of tobacco, alcohol, and substances of abuse
- The woman's subjective evaluation of her labor
- Birth plans, including expected pain management methods
- Support persons: who they are and the role of each
- Screening for domestic violence when the woman is alone (see Chapter 24)

Be careful when discussing previous pregnancies and births when a woman's family is present. She may have had an abortion or relinquished a baby for adoption, and her family may not know about it. Even if her partner knows about previous pregnancies, other family and friends may not.

**Fetal assessments.** Assess the fetal presentation and position and the FHR. Note the color of the amniotic fluid and the time of rupture if the membranes have ruptured.

**Labor status.** Determine the woman's labor status by:

- Assessing her contraction pattern
- Determining cervical dilation and effacement; and fetal station (measurement of fetal descent in the pelvis related to the ischial spines), presentation, and position
- Determining whether her membranes have ruptured

**Physical examination.** If birth is not imminent, perform a brief physical examination to evaluate the woman's overall health. Important general observations that relate to birth include the presence and location of edema, abdominal scars, and the height of the fundus.

### Admission Procedures

***Notifying the physician or midwife.*** After assessment, contact the woman's birth attendant to report on her status and obtain orders. Include the following data in the report:

- Gravidity, parity, abortions (spontaneous and elective), and term and preterm births
- EDD; fundal height

- Contraction pattern
- Fetal presentation and position
- Cervical dilation and effacement; fetal presentation and position; station of the presenting part
- FHR and pattern
- Maternal vital signs
- Any identified abnormalities or concerns about the maternal or fetal condition
- Pain, anxiety, or other reactions to labor

If the woman is admitted, any of several procedures may be done.

***Consent forms.*** The woman signs consent for care during labor, anesthesia, vaginal birth, cesarean birth, and blood transfusion. A separate consent for human immunodeficiency virus (HIV) is frequently required. Consent for newborn care is often completed as well. A separate consent for tubal ligation must be signed for women desiring permanent sterilization at delivery.

## CRITICAL THINKING EXERCISE 16.2

During a labor admission assessment, a woman quickly denies using drugs other than her prescribed prenatal vitamins. She becomes quiet, answering each of the nurse's questions tersely.

1. What might explain the woman's change in behavior?
2. Should the nurse alter the assessment interview? If so, why?

***Laboratory tests.*** A woman has routine admission laboratory tests plus other tests if indicated by her history and physical examination. Simple tests may be done on the unit, such as:

- Hematocrit
- Blood glucose levels
- Midstream urine specimen for dipstick evaluation of protein, glucose, and ketone levels. Urinalysis and culture and sensitivity may be ordered for possible urinary tract infection.

Other common routine tests done for every admitted perinatal patient include:

- Complete blood count
- Blood type and Rh factor
- Rapid plasma reagin (RPR) or other test for syphilis
- Hepatitis B surface antigen
- HIV testing, if the woman consents

***Intravenous access.*** If used, intravenous access is usually started with at least an 18-gauge catheter. A saline lock may be used, or the woman may receive continuous infusion of fluids. The lock facilitates walking during early labor and is less associated with illness, but it provides quick access if fluids or drugs are needed. Continuous fluid infusion helps prevent or relieve dehydration and is needed if epidural block analgesia is used. Isotonic electrolyte solutions, such as lactated Ringer's solution, are common.

### Assessments After Admission

After the admission assessment, the woman and her fetus need regular assessments based on their risk status and on whether interventions such as epidural analgesia are needed. General guidelines for continuing assessments are listed here.

The woman is usually observed if it is unclear after the initial assessment whether she is in true labor. After 1 or 2 hours, progressive cervical changes (effacement, dilation, or both) suggest true labor. Assess the woman and fetus during the observation period as if she were in early labor.

***Fetal assessments.*** Fetal assessments continue to identify signs of well-being and signs that suggest compromise. The principal fetal assessments include the FHR and patterns and the character of the amniotic fluid. Abnormalities revealed in these assessments may be associated with impaired fetal gas exchange or infection.

**FHR.** The FHR is usually assessed using electronic fetal monitoring. However, intermittent auscultation may be done with a Doppler transducer or a fetoscope (see Chapter 17).

**Amniotic fluid.** The membranes may rupture spontaneously (spontaneous rupture of membranes [SROM]), or **amniotomy** (artificial rupture of membranes [AROM]) may be performed. Assess the FHR for at least 1 minute after the membranes rupture. The umbilical cord could be displaced in a large fluid gush, resulting in compression and interruption of blood flow through it. Charting related to membrane rupture includes the time, FHR (which will appear on an electronic fetal monitor strip), and character of the fluid.

Amniotic fluid should be clear and may include bits of vernix, the creamy fetal skin lubricant. Cloudy, yellow, or foul-smelling amniotic fluid suggests infection. Green fluid indicates that the fetus has passed meconium before birth. Meconium passage may have been a response to transient hypoxia, although the cause may remain unknown. Meconium-stained fluid is not usually noted in the preterm infant, although it may be seen in the late preterm newborn born at 34 to 36 weeks of gestation.

Describe quantity in approximate terms. At term, a "large" amount is more than 1000 mL; a "moderate" amount is approximately 500 to 1000 mL; and "scant" amniotic fluid is only a trickle, barely enough to detect. If the fetus is well down into the pelvis when the membranes rupture, a small amount of fluid in front of the fetal head may be discharged (forewaters), with the rest lost at birth.

***Maternal assessments.*** Several maternal assessments, such as vital signs and contractions, also relate to the health of the fetus.

**Vital signs.** Guidelines for maternal vital signs assessment are listed in Table 16.2. Hypotension, hypertension, elevated pulse and respiratory rates, and elevated temperature should be reported, and repeat assessments should be done more frequently.

**Contractions.** Contractions can be assessed by palpation (see Procedure on p. 314) or with the electronic fetal monitor, using the guidelines in Table 17.1. With external monitoring, a combination of techniques is often used.

**Progress of labor.** Periodic vaginal examinations determine cervical dilation and effacement and fetal descent. The frequency of vaginal examinations depends on the woman's parity, the status of her membranes, and the overall speed of her labor. Vaginal examinations are limited to avoid introducing microorganisms from the perineal area into the uterus.

**Intake and output.** Oral and intravenous intakes are recorded. Each voiding is recorded. Labor or regional anesthesia reduces a woman's urge to void, so check her suprapubic area every 2 hours to identify bladder distention. Check more frequently if she has received large amounts of intravenous fluid.

Pressure of the fetal head on the rectum in late labor makes many women feel the need to defecate, even if they had epidural analgesia. Look at the woman's perineum for crowning of the fetal head if she abruptly expresses a need to defecate or says, "Something feels different" or a similar remark.

**Response to labor.** The woman's behavioral responses change as labor intensifies. She withdraws from interactions but needs more nursing presence and reassurance. She may become more anxious because of pain and fear of bodily injury, unknown outcome, loss of control, unresolved psychological issues that influence her readiness to give birth (e.g., sexual abuse, previous birth experiences), or unexpected occurrences during labor.

Women vary in the way they handle the pain of labor. The nurse must constantly assess whether added pain control measures are

## PROCEDURE

### Palpating Contractions

**Purpose**

To determine whether a contraction pattern is typical of true labor.

To identify abnormal contractions that may jeopardize the health of the mother or fetus or indicate another complication.

1. Assess contractions with each assessment of the fetal heart rate. Assess several contractions to evaluate average characteristics of the pattern. Palpate contractions periodically if an external fetal monitor is used because the monitor is less accurate for intensity as a result of variations in the thickness of the abdominal fat pad, maternal position, and fetal position.
2. Place the fingertips of one hand on the area where the contractions are best felt, usually the uterine fundus. The mother usually feels sensations in her lower abdomen and back. Use light pressure, and keep your fingertips relatively still rather than moving them over the uterus, because moving your hand over the uterus may stimulate contractions and give an inaccurate view of their true pattern. The fingertips are more sensitive to the first tightening of the uterus.
3. Note the time when each contraction begins and ends:
   a. Determine the frequency by noting the average time that elapses from the beginning of one contraction to the beginning of the next one.
   b. Determine the duration of contractions by noting the average time in seconds from the beginning to end of each contraction.
   c. Determine the interval between contractions by noting the average time between the end of one contraction and the beginning of the next one.
4. Estimate the average intensity of contractions by noting how easily the uterus can be indented during the peak of the contraction:
   a. Mild contractions are easily indented with the fingertips. They feel similar to the tip of the nose.
   b. Moderate contractions can be indented with more difficulty. They feel similar to the chin.
   c. Firm contractions feel "woody" and cannot be readily indented. They feel similar to the forehead.
5. Report hypertonic contractions that can reduce placental blood flow:
   a. Occurring less than 2 minutes apart and no more than 5 contractions in 10 minutes
   b. Durations longer than 90 to 120 seconds
   c. Intervals shorter than 30 seconds
   d. Incomplete relaxation of the uterus between contractions

**Hypertonic contractions** reduce placental blood flow by prolonged compression of vessels that supply the intervillous spaces. See Chapter 17 for details and interventions.

needed, because laboring women are often uncertain about when they are ready for added relief. Behaviors that suggest the woman needs help with pain management include:

- Expressing that nonpharmacologic measures are ineffective.
- Tensing her muscles or arching her back during contractions.
- Persistence of muscle tension between contractions.
- A tense facial expression; rolling in the bed.
- Expressions such as "I can't take it anymore."
- Specific requests for medication or other pain control such as epidural (see Chapter 18).

***The support person's response.*** Labor is stressful for the woman's support person, often the baby's father. He may become anxious, fearful, or tired. He feels a responsibility to protect and support the woman but may have limited resources for doing so. It is difficult for him to watch the woman he loves in pain, even if the pain is normal and she declines medication. He may respond to stress in many ways: by becoming quiet, suffering silently, pacing, expressing anger, or even vomiting. Some fathers respond by leaving the room frequently or for long periods, whereas others resist taking even short breaks that they need.

Nurses encourage and value the father's presence during labor and birth. However, this attitude may conflict with a couple's cultural norms, which may dictate that birth is a strictly female activity. The father may be pulled in two directions, wanting to be included but hesitant because men in his culture are not customarily involved in birth. The nurse should respect the values of each couple and their wishes about the father's involvement (Callister, 2014).

The support person also may be a parent or other relative, a friend of either sex, or a homosexual partner. The nurse must remember that anyone who assists the woman during labor may feel anxious or helpless at times. Reassurance and care for the labor partner strengthen that person's ability to support the woman and increase the likelihood that both will view the birth experience as positive.

## NURSING CARE

### The Woman With False or Early Labor

#### Assessment

After assessment it may be apparent that the woman is not in true labor. If findings are normal and her membranes are intact, she is usually discharged home. The woman who is in very early labor may be discharged to await active labor, especially if she is a nullipara and lives nearby.

#### Nursing Diagnosis and Planning

The woman may be frustrated because she cannot tell whether labor is real. She may resist returning to the birth center, possibly delaying care needlessly. A nursing diagnosis that applies to many women with false labor contractions is:

- Deficient Knowledge: Characteristics of true labor

***Expected outcomes.*** After the nurse teaches the woman and her support, they will restate the signs or symptoms for which she should return to the birth center.

#### Interventions

***Providing reassurance.*** A woman sent home after observation often feels foolish and frustrated. Reassure her that even professionals cannot always identify true labor and that false labor and early true labor have similar characteristics. Tell her that important preparation occurs during late pregnancy, such as cervical softening and fetal descent, even if objective progress like cervical dilation has not yet occurred.

**Teaching.** Review guidelines for returning to the birth center with her: regular contractions, leaking of amniotic fluid, active bleeding (more than bloody show and often not mixed with mucus), and decreased fetal movement. Explain that these are only guidelines and that she should call or return if she has any concerns. It is better for her to return with another false alarm than to arrive at the birth center in advanced labor or to develop complications at home.

### Evaluation

- Can the woman and her support person describe guidelines for returning to the birth center?

## NURSING CARE

### The Woman in True Labor

The admission assessment may confirm that the woman is in true labor, or true labor may be evident after observation. Nursing diagnoses and related care change during labor because the intrapartum period is an evolving process that involves two people who are connected: a mother and her fetus. Nursing care and medical or nurse-midwife care are also linked throughout. Care of mother and fetus before birth relates to fetal oxygenation, maternal discomfort, and maternal injury.

Nursing diagnoses are often interrelated during labor. For example, anxiety or fear can affect pain-relief measures. A maternal fluid volume deficit can alter fetal oxygenation because less blood is available to circulate to the placenta.

> **SAFETY ALERT**
>
> ***Conditions Associated With Fetal Compromise***
>
> - A fetal heart rate (FHR) outside the normal range of 110 to 160 beats per minute (bpm) for a term fetus.
> - Meconium-stained (greenish) thick amniotic fluid.
> - Cloudy, yellowish, or foul odor to the amniotic fluid (suggests infection).
> - Excessive frequency or duration of contractions.
> - Incomplete uterine relaxation.
> - Maternal hypotension (may divert blood flow away from the placenta to ensure adequate perfusion of the maternal brain and heart).
> - Maternal hypertension (may be associated with vasospasm in spiral arteries, which supply the intervillous spaces of the placenta).
> - Maternal fever (38° C [100.4° F] or higher).
>
> NOTE: Chapter 17 provides detailed fetal assessments and interpretation of data.

## FETAL OXYGENATION

### Assessment

Refer to assessments listed in Table 16.2 for intrapartum assessments. The main assessments related to fetal well-being are:

- FHR
- Contractions: frequency, duration, intensity, resting tone, interval
- Character of amniotic fluid, amount, and time of rupture
- Maternal vital signs

Chapter 17 contains detailed information about FHR and related observations.

### Nursing Diagnosis and Planning

Most fetuses tolerate labor well, but maternal conditions such as hypotension or hypertension, fever, excessive (tetanic) contractions, or fetal conditions that compress the umbilical cord can compromise fetal oxygenation. Nursing measures may restore good fetal oxygenation, or it may be necessary to notify the birth attendant for collaborative patient care. The nursing diagnosis for fetal observation throughout labor would be:

- Risk for Ineffective Peripheral Tissue Perfusion: Fetal, related to interruption in oxygen-rich blood flow through the placenta or through the umbilical cord.

**Expected outcome.** The FHR and contraction patterns are expected to remain reassuring throughout labor.

### Interventions

**Promoting placental function.** Maternal positioning is the most common measure to promote placental function during normal labor. The woman can choose any position other than supine to avoid aortocaval compression that would reduce blood flow to the placenta. If she must be in the supine position for a procedure such as catheterization, a small pillow or rolled towel or blanket wedged under one hip shifts her uterus to one side to maintain good placental blood flow.

**Observing for conditions associated with fetal compromise.** Determine whether any conditions associated with fetal compromise exist. If any are identified, assess the fetus more frequently and notify the birth attendant.

### Evaluation

A reassuring constant fetal evaluation includes a reassuring FHR pattern and ongoing maternal assessments within expected limits. Throughout labor, the nurse compares actual data with the norms for the mother and fetus. See Chapter 17 for integration of fetal assessments into intrapartum care planning.

## DISCOMFORT

### Assessment

See Table 16.2 for continuing assessments of the laboring woman.

### Nursing Diagnosis and Planning

Labor is painful. Women vary in their responses to pain and in the pain management methods they choose. Providing choices for pain management and supporting the woman's choice increase her sense of control over her birth experience. The woman who successfully masters the pain and other physical demands of labor is more likely to view her experience as positive. Her support person is likely to feel more satisfaction with the experience as well.

Pain and anxiety are related nursing diagnoses. Excess anxiety intensifies pain perception, and acute pain worsens anxiety. The nurse clusters assessment data and considers both pain and anxiety when determining the best approach to pain relief. Several cues may suggest that anxiety is a major contributor to labor pain that the woman might otherwise easily manage: a previous poor experience during birth or expressions of worry and concern. Therefore, the nursing diagnosis is:

- Pain related to effects of uterine contractions.

**Expected outcomes.** The woman will state that she is able to tolerate labor pain satisfactorily and will use breathing and relaxation techniques during labor. The woman's partner will express satisfaction with his or her ability to support her by discharge.

### Interventions

**Providing comfort measures.** Ordinary measures reduce irritating surroundings that impair a woman's ability to relax and use coping skills. Nurses must be creative when providing comfort to the laboring woman.

**Lighting.** Soft, indirect lighting is soothing, whereas a bright overhead light is an irritant. Bright lights imply a hospital ("sick") atmosphere rather than the normal life event that birth is. Use the overhead light only when needed. A small flashlight is handy if the woman wants her room truly dark.

**Temperature.** Labor is work. Women in labor are often hot and perspiring. Cool, damp washcloths on the woman's face and neck promote comfort. Keep an ample supply of damp washcloths available, and change them often to keep them cool. An electric fan circulates air in the labor room and directs a breeze on the woman. Be sure that the fan does not blow on the infant after birth, because cool air might cause hypothermia.

Have the woman wear socks if her feet are cold. She may shake, sometimes intensely, although her temperature is normal and she denies being cold.

**Cleanliness.** Bloody show and amniotic fluid leak from the woman's vagina during labor. Change the sheets and gown as needed to keep her dry and comfortable. Let her preferences be the guide, because she may not want to be disturbed during late labor. Change the under pad regularly to reduce microorganisms that may ascend into the vagina. A folded towel absorbs larger quantities of amniotic fluid than the pad alone. If using pillows near where fluid will leak, protect them with under pads.

**Mouth care.** Ice chips, Popsicles, or hard candy on a stick reduces the discomfort of a dry mouth. Avoid excess sugar intake that might contribute to neonatal hypoglycemia after birth. Oral intake restrictions among low-risk laboring women are a conflict among professional organizations in the United States and Canada. The American College of Nurse-Midwives advocates that the low-risk woman self-determine her oral intake. The World Health Organization does not promote interference with oral intake during labor (Sharts-Hopko, 2010).

If oral intake is contraindicated, brushing the teeth or simply rinsing the mouth helps. Many women appreciate a moist washcloth applied to their lips.

**Bladder.** A full bladder intensifies pain during labor and can delay fetal descent. Remind the woman to empty her bladder at least every 2 hours. Catheterization is often needed.

**Positioning.** Upright positions add the force of gravity to fetal descent. Women who labor upright often need less analgesia and have more effective contractions. Their infants often have improved pH and blood gases. The woman should avoid the supine position with no side tilt. Frequent changes reduce discomfort from constant pressure, help the fetus adapt to the pelvic contours, and promote fetal descent. Fig. 16.15 (pp. 317-321) illustrates various maternal positions for labor (Association of Women's Health, Obstetric and Neonatal Nurses [AWHONN], 2008).

The woman often has "back labor" if her fetus is in the occiput posterior position, because the fetal occiput presses on the mother's sacral promontory with each contraction. Positions that encourage the fetus to fall away from the sacral promontory, such as those in which the mother leans forward or uses the hands-and-knees position, promote comfort and enhance internal rotation to an occiput anterior position.

**Water.** Water in the form of a shower, tub, or whirlpool is relaxing and helps many women tolerate contractions of active labor. Nipple stimulation by water currents causes release of oxytocin by the posterior pituitary gland, which increases productive contractions that promote labor progression. If contractions become too strong, she simply removes her breasts from the water stream. Use of a bath in the latent phase may slow progress.

***Teaching.*** Teaching the woman in labor is a constant and changing task involving her support person.

**First stage of labor.** Many women become discouraged because several hours are needed to reach 4 or 5 cm of cervical dilation. They believe that the last 5 cm will take as long as the first 5 cm. It may help them to know that 5 cm is more like two thirds of the way to full dilation in time rather than half the way because the rate of dilation increases during the active phase.

The urge to push usually occurs when the woman's cervix is fully dilated and effaced and when the fetus descends deep into the pelvis and internally rotates. However, as she nears the second stage, her baby may descend enough to give her an urge to push before full cervical dilation. If her cervix, which is usually 8 or 9 cm dilated at this time, yields easily to downward pressure, pushing in response to her spontaneous urge rarely causes problems. Either of two problems may occur if she pushes against a cervix that does not easily open as the fetus applies pressure:

- The cervix may become edematous, which can block progress.
- The cervix may be lacerated.

Teach the woman to blow out in short breaths if she should not yet push.

**Second stage of labor.** The woman may need guidance to push effectively during second-stage labor. The support person should also be educated and supported to facilitate effective coaching.

***Laboring down.*** Two hours of intense pushing was once considered the upper limit for the duration of the second stage. It is now recognized that a second stage longer than 2 hours is safe if the mother and fetus show no signs of compromise. Nursing support is increasing and has resulted in inclusion of care based on solid evidence. Women push most effectively when they feel the reflex urge to do so. Closed-glottis pushing or the Valsalva maneuver can reduce fetal oxygenation. Nursing research has shown delayed pushing to result in significantly less time in active pushing and an insignificant increase in total second stage duration for nulliparous women with epidural analgesia (Gillesby, Burns, Dempsey, et al., 2010; Kelly, Johnson, Lee, et al., 2010).

***Positions.*** The mother may push in any position she prefers. Position changes promote her natural pushing efforts with fetal rotation and descent. Many women prefer semi-sitting and side-lying positions. Squatting enlarges the pelvic outlet slightly and adds the force of gravity to the mother's efforts, an advantage if her pelvis is small or the fetus is large. Some women push most effectively while sitting on the toilet because that is where they are accustomed to giving in to that sensation. The woman can also turn backward while sitting on the toilet, letting the tank (with a pillow on top) support her upper body. Several effective pushing positions are also valid if the woman has epidural analgesia.

Teach the mother to curve her body around her uterus in a C shape with her chin on her chest. To increase effectiveness, teach her to pull on her knees, hand-holds, or a squatting bar while pushing. Women often find that pulling on something from above is helpful to focus their pushing efforts.

***Method and breathing pattern.*** If she is pushing effectively and safely, do not interfere, but support the woman's spontaneous techniques. Prolonged breath-holding (>4 seconds per push) or pushing more than four times per contraction is discouraged. A deep breath helps her relax at the end of the contraction. The woman may grunt or groan when pushing and should be reassured that this is normal.

A woman who is modest or fears losing control may inhibit her best pushing efforts if she is instructed to push as if she were having a bowel movement, particularly if she is in a bed or chair. A more anatomically correct image is to teach the woman to push down and out under her symphysis ("pubic bone"), following the pelvic curve. Seeing a diagram of the pelvis helps her to visualize the curve.

***Labor support***

**Providing encouragement.** Success breeds success. Tell the woman when her labor is progressing. If she can see that her efforts are effective, she has more courage to continue. Help her touch or see the baby's head with a mirror as crowning occurs.

Praise the woman and her labor partner when they use breathing or other coping techniques effectively. This encouragement reinforces their actions, gives them a sense of control, and conveys the respect and support of the nurse. If one technique is not helpful after a reasonable trial (three to five contractions), encourage them to try other techniques.

**Giving of self.** The nurse's caring presence is a crucial element in labor support. Even women who are very independent may become dependent during labor and need human contact. Many times the woman simply needs reassurance that all is going well and that the nurse is there for her. The nurse's presence helps allay her fears of abandonment and conveys safety, acceptance, support, and comfort.

Although the woman and her support person may have prepared for childbirth, they often welcome suggestions and affirmation from the nurse. The nurse who is familiar with the techniques they are using can better support them and avoid contradicting what they have learned and practiced. The nurse's presence, gentle coaching, and encouragement help the laboring woman have confidence in her own body and her ability to give birth. See Chapter 18 for nonpharmacologic support and pain-relief measures.

**Offering pharmacologic measures.** Some women do not need pharmacologic pain relief during labor. Birth is usually a normal process, and the prepared woman and labor partner can deliver their infant without medication. However, most choose to have pharmacologic pain management. Inform the woman about medications available to her without pressuring her to take them. See Chapter 18 for additional information about pharmacologic measures.

A few women have a firm goal of avoiding all pain medication during labor. These women may then feel let down or guilty if they need medication. Other women may plan to use a specific pain-relief method, such as epidural analgesia. If something prevents use of their

***Standing***

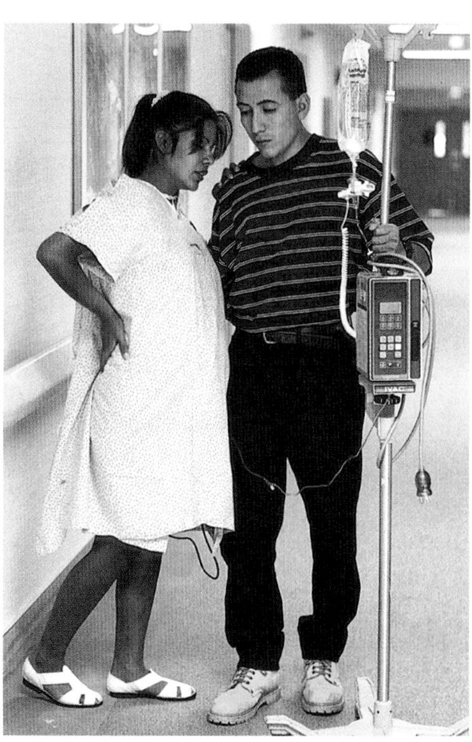

*Advantages*
Adds gravity to force of contractions to promote fetal descent.
Contractions are less uncomfortable and more efficient.
Variation: standing, leaning forward with support reduces back pain because fetus falls forward, away from the sacral promontory.
*Disadvantages*
Tiring over long periods.
Continuous electronic fetal monitoring is not possible without telemetry if woman is walking in the hall.
*Nursing Implications*
If the woman has intravenous fluid running, give her a rolling pole. Encourage her to alternate walking with other positions whenever she tires or desires to do so. Remind the woman and her partner when she should return to the labor area for evaluation of the fetal heart rate and her labor status.

***Sitting Upright***

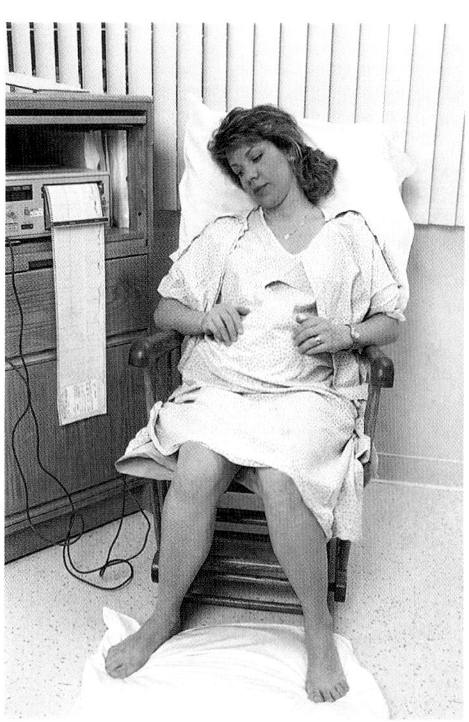

*Advantages*
Uses gravity to aid fetal descent.
Can be done when sitting on side of bed, in a chair, or on the toilet.
Can be used with continuous fetal monitoring.
Avoids supine hypotension.
*Disadvantages*
May increase suprapubic discomfort.
Contractions are the most efficient when the woman alternates sitting with other positions.
*Nursing Implications*
A rocking chair is soothing.
Place a pillow on a chair with a disposable underpad over the pillow to absorb secretions.
Use pillows or a footstool to keep a short woman's legs from dangling.
Encourage the woman to alternate positions periodically. For example, she can alternate walking with sitting or sitting with side-lying.

**FIG 16.15** Maternal positions for labor.

*Continued*

chosen method, they may be upset about this unexpected development in their birth experience. In either case, allow the woman to share her feelings about her experience. Although this development may not be what she wanted, expressing her feelings helps her put it into perspective.

**Caring for the birth partner.** The woman's support person is an integral part of her labor care. Her labor partner can provide care and comfort, which support the woman's ability to give birth. Do not expect too much of the partner or make assumptions about the desired type and amount of involvement.

Some partners are coaches in the true sense of the word, actively assisting the woman through labor. Others want the woman and nurse to lead them and tell them how to help. They are eager to do what they can but expect instructions about how and when to do it. Many couples see the partner's role as one of encouragement, moral support, and just being there for the woman.

To impose unrealistic expectations of leadership, care, and comfort on the partner makes the birth experience unnecessarily stressful. To ensure a positive experience for both people, accept whatever pattern of support the partner is able and willing to provide and whatever the couple finds comfortable. Without taking over or diminishing this role, provide support that the partner cannot.

Encourage the partner to conserve physical strength. The partner may have missed sleep during the hours of early labor or may need a break. The nurse may need to encourage the partner to eat or bring a snack. Remind the partner that support will be more effective if the partner's own needs are met. Support persons who do not eat for a long time are more likely to faint during the birth.

### Evaluation

- Is the woman satisfied with her pain control, whether it is nonpharmacologic or pharmacologic?
- Does the woman use the breathing and relaxation techniques that she was taught or that she creates for herself?
- Does her partner express satisfaction with his or her labor support?

As a nursing diagnosis, Pain and related goals for pain management are constantly re-evaluated during labor.

***Sitting, Leaning Forward with Support***

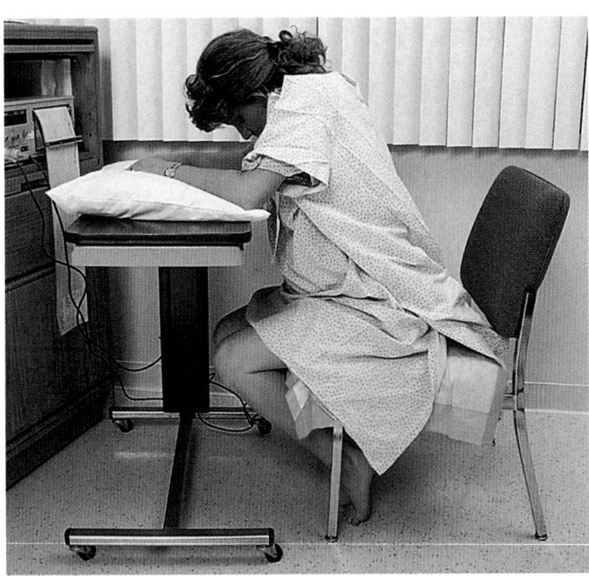

*Advantages*
Same as for sitting.
Reduces back pain because fetus falls forward, away from sacral promontory.
Partner or nurse can rub back or provide sacral pressure to relieve back pain.
*Disadvantages*
Same as for sitting.
*Nursing Implications*
Same as for sitting.

***Semi-Sitting***

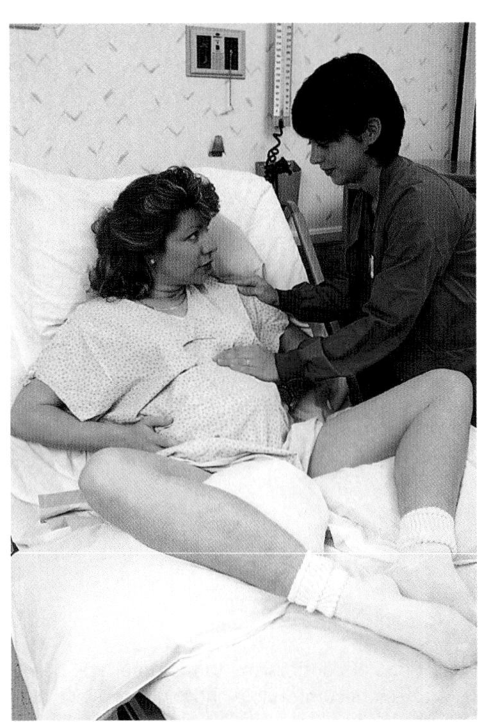

*Advantages*
Same as for sitting.
Aligns long axis of uterus with pelvic inlet, which applies contraction force in the most efficient direction through pelvis.
*Disadvantages*
Same as for sitting.
Does not reduce pain as well as the forward-leaning positions.
*Nursing Implications* Same as for sitting.
Raise bed to approximately a 30- to 45-degree angle.
Encourage the woman to use sitting (leaning forward) or side-lying position if she has back pain so that the caregiver can rub her back or apply sacral pressure.

**FIG 16.15, cont'd** Maternal positions for labor.

## PREVENTING INJURY

### Assessment

Nursing assessments of the mother and fetus continue as the woman nears birth. During the second stage of labor, observe the woman's perineum to determine when to make final birth preparations.

The exact time for final birth preparations varies according to the woman's parity, the overall speed of labor, the fetal station, and the distance of the physician or nurse-midwife from the labor and delivery unit. Final preparations are usually completed when crowning in the nullipara reaches a diameter of approximately 3 to 4 cm. The multipara is prepared sooner, when her cervix is fully dilated and the fetal head is well down in the pelvis but before much crowning has occurred.

### Nursing Diagnosis and Planning

The woman is vulnerable to injury immediately before and after birth for several reasons: (1) altered physical sensations, such as responses to intense pressure or medication; (2) positional changes for birth; and (3) unexpectedly rapid progress. Therefore, the nursing diagnosis selected for the laboring woman near the time of birth is:

- Risk for Maternal Injury related to altered sensations and positional or physical changes.

**Expected outcome.** The woman does not have an avoidable injury, such as muscle strains, thrombosis, or lacerations, during birth.

### Interventions

Transferring the woman to the delivery site or positioning her in the birthing bed is the first step in the sequence of events that culminates

***Side-Lying***

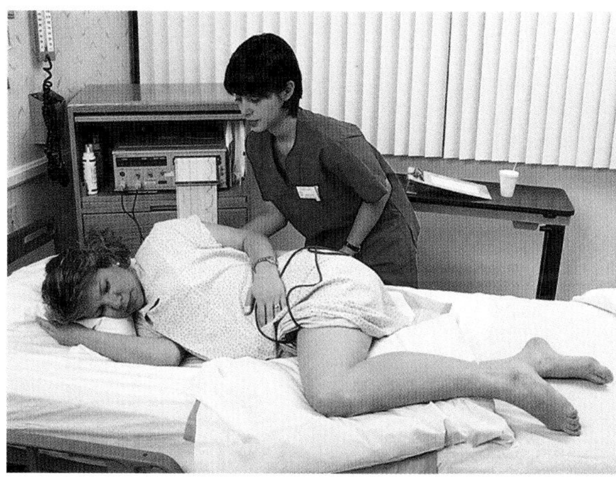

*Advantages*
It is a restful position.
Prevents supine hypotension and promotes placental blood flow.
Promotes efficient contractions, although they may be less frequent than with other positions.
Can be used with continuous fetal monitoring.
*Disadvantages*
Does not use gravity to aid fetal descent.
*Nursing Implications*
Teach the woman and her partner that although the contractions are less frequent, they are more effective.
This position offers a break from more tiring positions.
Use pillows for support and to prevent pressure: at her back, under her superior arm, and between her knees.
Use disposable underpads to protect the pillow between the woman's knees from secretions.
Some women like to put their superior leg on the bed rail. If the woman wants this variation, pad the bed rail with a blanket to prevent pressure.
If she wants to remain recumbent, she should use this position to promote placental blood flow.

***Kneeling, Leaning Forward with Support***

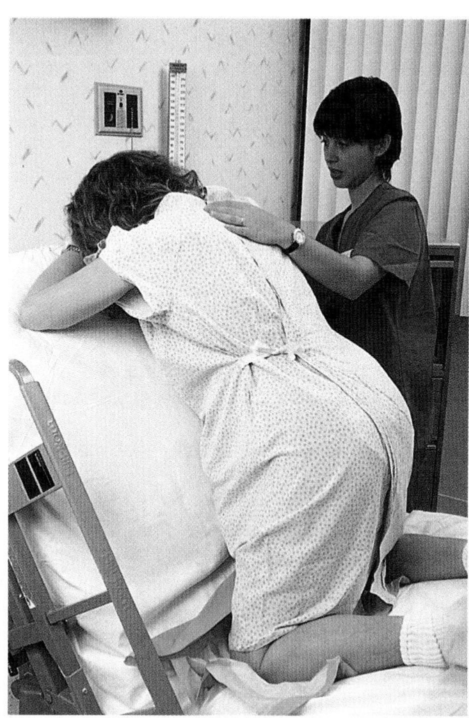

*Advantage*
Reduces back pain because fetus falls forward, away from sacral promontory.
Adds gravity to force of contractions to promote fetal descent.
Can be used with continuous fetal monitoring.
Caregivers can rub her back or apply sacral pressure.
Promotes normal mechanisms of birth.
*Disadvantages*
Knees may become tired or uncomfortable.
Tiring if used for long periods.
*Nursing Implications*
Raise the head of the bed, and have the woman face the head of the bed while she is on her knees.
Another method is for the partner to sit in a chair, with the woman kneeling in front, facing her partner, and leaning forward on him or her for support.
Use pillow under the knees and in front of the woman's chest, as needed, for comfort.
Encourage her to change positions if she becomes tired.

**FIG 16.15, cont'd** Maternal positions for labor.

*Continued*

in birth of the baby. During the period surrounding birth, the nurse reduces factors that contribute to maternal injuries.

***Transfer to a delivery room.*** Most vaginal births occur in a combination labor, delivery, and recovery room. With some patient conditions, such as a twin birth, the woman is transferred to a separate room for birth. Transfer her early enough to avoid rushed, last-minute preparations, which are stressful for all.

***Positioning for birth.*** To promote effective pushing and take advantage of gravity, raise the woman's back, shoulders, and head. Experimenting with the level of head elevation will probably be needed. Upright positions, such as squatting, promote vaginal birth but limit accessibility to the woman's perineum. Epidural block also limits birth positions.

***Hands and Knees***

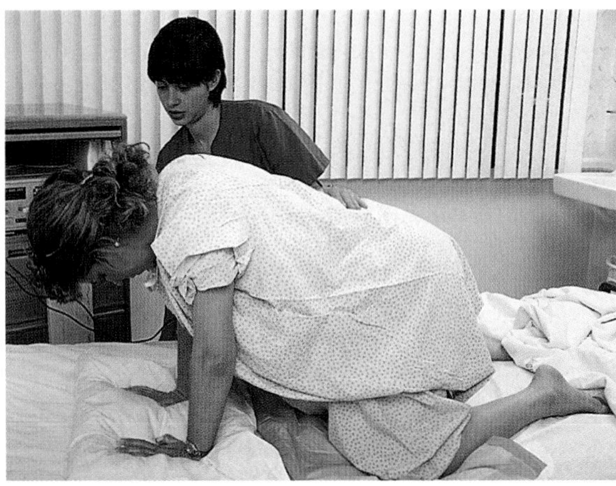

*Advantages*

Reduces back pain because the fetus falls forward, away from the sacral promontory.

Promotes normal mechanisms of birth.

The woman can use pelvic rocking to decrease back pain.

Caregivers can rub the woman's back or apply sacral pressure easily.

*Disadvantages*

The woman's hands (especially wrists) and knees can become uncomfortable.

Tiring when used for a long time.

Some women are embarrassed to use this position.

*Nursing Implications*

Encourage the woman to change to less tiring positions occasionally.

Ensure privacy when encouraging the reluctant woman to try this position if she has back pain.

A second hospital gown with the opening in front covers her back and hips but may be too warm.

***Positions for Pushing in Second Stage***

*Standing*

This position may be tiring, and access to the woman's perineum is difficult. Because the infant could fall to the ground if birth occurs rapidly, provide padding under the mother's feet. Gravity aids fetal descent.

*Hands and Knees*

Advantages and disadvantages are similar to those during first-stage labor. In addition, caregivers must reorient themselves because the landmarks are upside down from their usual perspective.

A variation is for the mother to kneel and lean forward against a beanbag or the side of the bed. This variation reduces some of the strain of wrists and hands.

***Squatting***

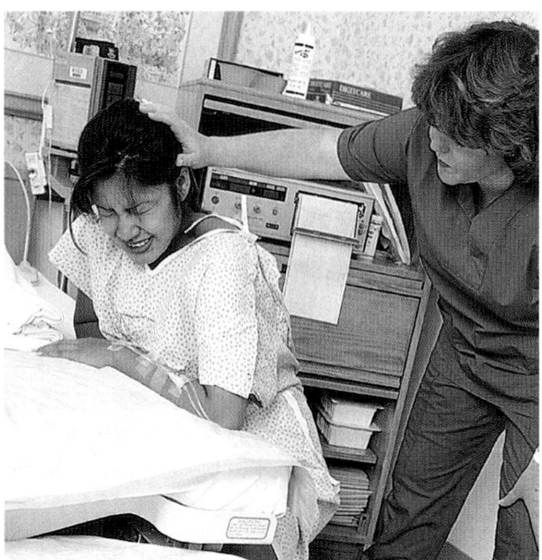

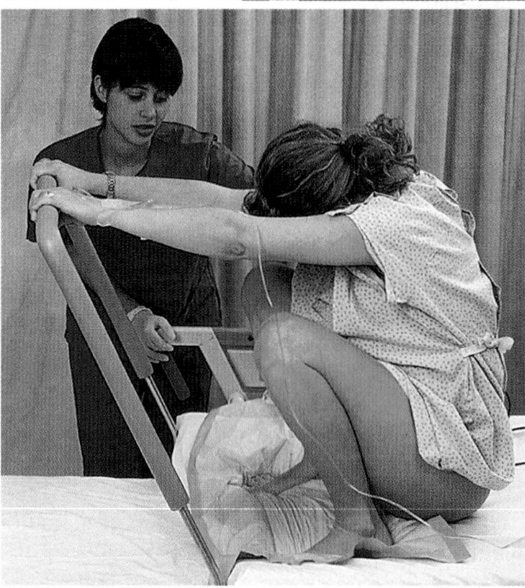

*Advantages*

Adds gravity to force of contractions to promote fetal descent.

Straightens the pelvic curve slightly for more direct fetal descent.

Increases dimensions of pelvis slightly.

Promotes effective pushing efforts in the second stage.

Caregivers can rub back or provide sacral pressure.

*Disadvantages*

Knees and hips may become uncomfortable because of prolonged flexion.

Tiring over a long time.

*Nursing Implications*

Provide support with a squat bar attached to the bed or by two people standing on each side of the woman.

If she becomes tired, or between contractions, she can lean back into the sitting position.

Variation: Have the woman squat beside the bed as she pushes.

**FIG 16.15, cont'd** Maternal positions for labor.

***Semi-Sitting***

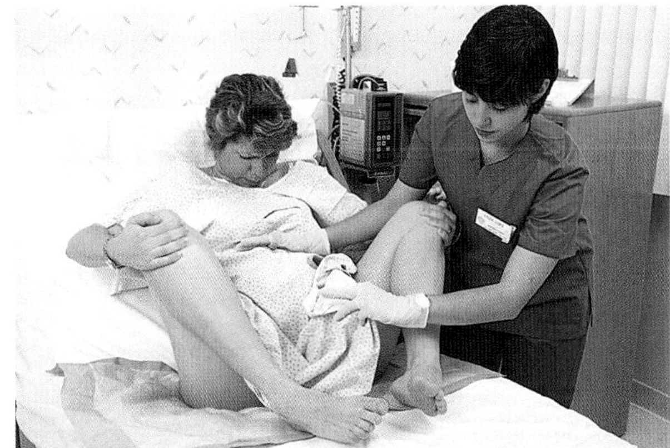

Many women prefer this because they have the security of a back rest; it is also familiar to caregivers and allows easy observation of the perineum. Elevate the woman's back at least 30 to 45 degrees so that gravity aids fetal descent. The woman pulls on her flexed knees (behind or in front of them) as she pushes. She should keep her head flexed and her sacrum flat on the bed to straighten the pelvic curve.

***Side-Lying***

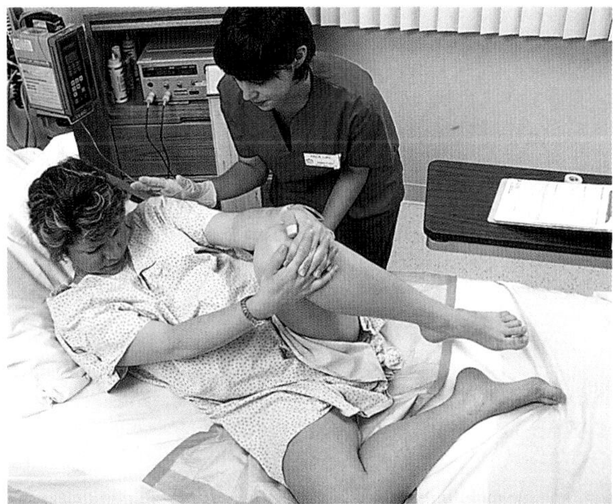

The woman flexes her chin on her chest and curls around her uterus as she pushes. She pulls on her flexed knees or the knee of the superior leg as she pushes.

**FIG 16.15, cont'd** Maternal positions for labor.

Padded stirrups or footrests support the woman's legs and feet and make her perineum more accessible. To reduce strain on muscles and ligaments, help her raise and lower her legs together and do not separate them too widely for her leg length. Surfaces that contact the popliteal space behind the knee should be padded to reduce pressure that can lead to thrombus formation. Do not leave her legs in stirrups for a prolonged time.

***Observing the perineum.*** The exact time at which a woman is ready to give birth is an educated guess. A woman who has been having a slow labor may suddenly make rapid progress. Birth is near when the fetal head swings anteriorly in extension as the occiput slips under the symphysis pubis. Observe the woman's perineum, especially during late second-stage labor.

*A classic sign of imminent birth is the mother's urgent cry, "The baby's coming!" Look at her perineum, and if the baby will be born before the physician or nurse-midwife arrives, remain calm and support the infant's head and body with gloved hands as it emerges* (Box 16.1).

### Evaluation

- During the postpartum period, does the woman show evidence of muscle strains or thrombus formation?

## NURSING CARE DURING THE LATE INTRAPARTUM PERIOD

### Responsibilities During Birth

The nurse has added responsibilities during the birth, although some may be assumed by other professionals. Nursing responsibilities may include:

- Preparation of a table with sterile gowns, gloves, drapes, solutions, and instruments, although the vagina is not sterile
- Perineal cleansing preparation
- Preparation for initial care and assessment of the newborn, including calling neonatal staff if indicated.
- Administration of medications such as oxytocin to contract the uterus and control blood loss (see Drug Guide: Oxytocin, in Chapter 19)

### BOX 16.1 Assisting With an Emergency Birth

The inexperienced nurse rarely must deliver a baby in the hospital or birth center but occasionally may help a more experienced nurse do so. Unplanned out-of-hospital births are not common, but they do occasionally occur.

**Nursing Priorities for an Emergency Birth in Any Setting**

- Prevent or reduce injury to the mother and infant.
- Maintain the infant's airway and temperature after birth.

**Preparing for an Emergency Birth in the Birth Facility**

- Study the delivery sequence in Figs. 16.17 and 16.18.
- Locate the emergency delivery tray ("precip" tray) on the unit.

**During the Birth**

- Remain with the woman to assist her in giving birth. Use the call bell, or ask her partner to call for help. Stay calm to reduce the couple's anxiety.
- Put on gloves to prevent contact with blood and other secretions. Sterile gloves reduce transmission of environmental organisms to the mother and infant. The nurse will be "catching" the infant in this situation. No invasive procedure is done.

**After the Birth**

- Observe the infant's color and respirations for distress. Suction excess secretions with a bulb syringe.
- Dry the infant, and place skin-to-skin with the mother and cover with warmed blankets to maintain warmth.
- Put the infant to the mother's breast and encourage suckling to promote uterine contraction, facilitating expulsion of the placenta and controlling bleeding.

Staff from the newborn or special care nursery and often a pediatrician, neonatologist, or neonatal nurse practitioner are usually present if the newborn is at risk for problems (e.g., preterm gestation) or has shown nonreassuring signs during labor. The nursery staff may routinely attend births in some facilities (Fig. 16.16, pp. 322-323).

***Transfer and Positioning for Birth***

*Action:* When the woman is almost ready to give birth, position the birthing bed. If birth will occur in a delivery room, such as for twins, transfer her to that location. The exact time varies with several factors (such as overall speed of labor and rate of fetal descent). *Rationale:* Rushed, last-moment preparations are anxiety-producing for the woman, her partner, and the nurse. Remaining in the birth position for a long time can be tiring.

*Action:* Continue observing her perineum while making final preparations for birth. *Rationale:* Birth may occur unexpectedly, and the nurse should be prepared to "catch" the infant if the attendant (physician or nurse-midwife) is not in the room.

*Action:* Continue observing the fetal heart rate (FHR) with continuous monitoring or intermittent auscultation. *Rationale:* Detects changes in fetal condition that may require interventions by the attendant to speed birth.

*Action:* Elevate the woman's back, shoulders, and head with a wedge (on a delivery table) or by raising the head of the birthing bed. *Rationale:* Allows more effective maternal pushing and uses gravity to aid fetal descent.

*Action:* Stirrups or footrests to support the woman's legs and feet may be used on a birthing bed. Pad the surface. *Rationale:* Padding reduces pressure, preventing venous stasis and possible thrombus formation.

*Action:* When placing the woman's legs in stirrups, elevate them and remove them simultaneously. Do not separate her legs widely. *Rationale:* Reduces strain on muscles and ligaments.

***Prepping and Draping***

*Action:* After the woman is in position, cleanse the perineal area with a standard prep solution unless the woman is allergic. *Rationale:* Removes secretions and feces from perineal area.

*Action:* With gloved hands, take a fresh sponge to begin each new area, and do not return to a clean area with a used sponge. Six sponges are needed. The proper order and motions are as follows:

1. Use a zigzag motion from clitoris to lower abdomen just above the pubic hairline.

2, 3. Use a zigzag motion on the inner thigh from the labia majora to approximately halfway between the hip and knee. Repeat for the other inner thigh.

4, 5. Apply a single stroke on one side from clitoris over labia, perineum, and anus. Repeat for the other side.

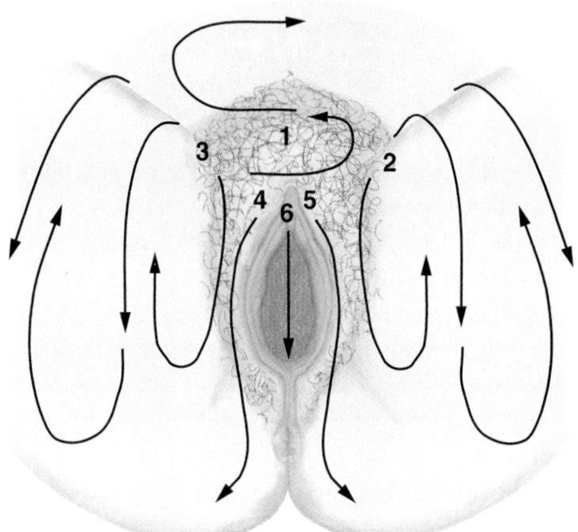


6. Use a single stroke in the middle from the clitoris over the vulva and perineum.

*Rationale:* Prevents cross-contamination or recontamination of an area that is already clean.

*Action:* The attendant may apply sterile drapes if desired. *Rationale:* A vaginal birth is a clean procedure rather than a sterile one because the vagina is not sterile. Sterile drapes are unnecessary, but some attendants may prefer to use them.

***Birth of the Head***

*Action:* If an episiotomy is needed, the attendant will perform it when the head is well crowned (see Chapter 19). *Rationale:* Minimizes blood loss from the episiotomy.

*Action:* As the vaginal orifice encircles the fetal head, the attendant applies gentle pressure to the woman's perineum with one hand while applying counter pressure to the fetal head with the other hand (Ritgen maneuver). The attendant may ask the mother to blow so that she avoids pushing, or to push gently. *Rationale:* Controls the exit of the fetal head so that it is born gradually rather than popping out; this minimizes trauma to the maternal tissues.

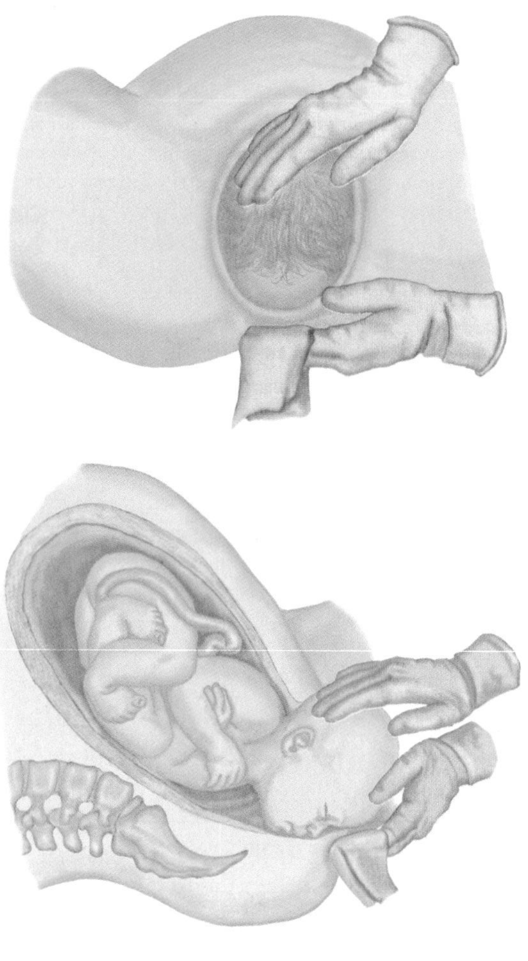

**FIG 16.16** Sequence of delivery.

*Action:* The attendant wipes secretions from the infant's face and suctions the nose and mouth with a bulb syringe. *Rationale:* Removes blood and secretions, preventing the infant from aspirating them with the first breaths.

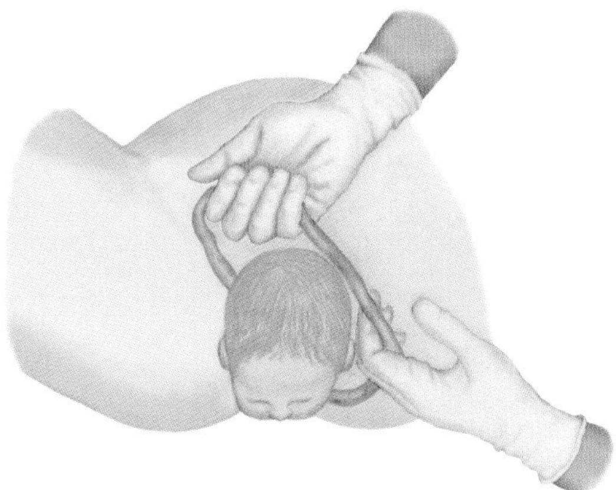

*Action:* The attendant feels for a cord around the fetal neck (nuchal cord). If it is loose, it is slipped over the head. If tight, it is clamped and cut between two clamps before the rest of the baby is born. *Rationale:* Allows the rest of the birth to occur and prevents stretching or tearing the cord.

***Birth of the Shoulders***

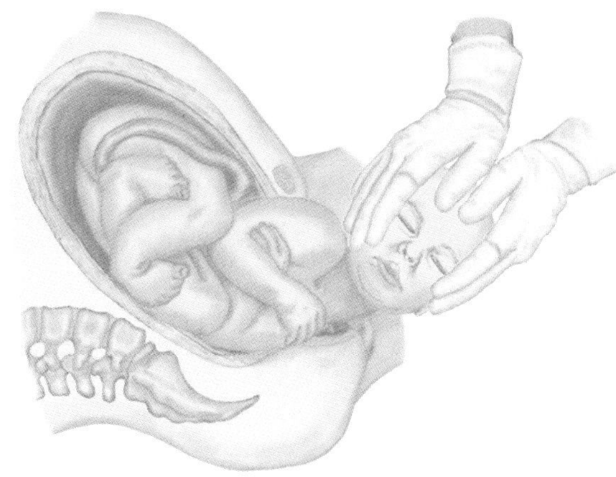

*Action:* After external rotation, the attendant applies gentle traction on the fetal head in the direction of the mother's perineum. *Rationale:* External rotation allows the shoulders to rotate internally and aligns their transverse diameter with the anteroposterior diameter of the mother's pelvic outlet. Traction on the head in the direction of her perineum allows the anterior fetal shoulder to slip under the symphysis pubis.

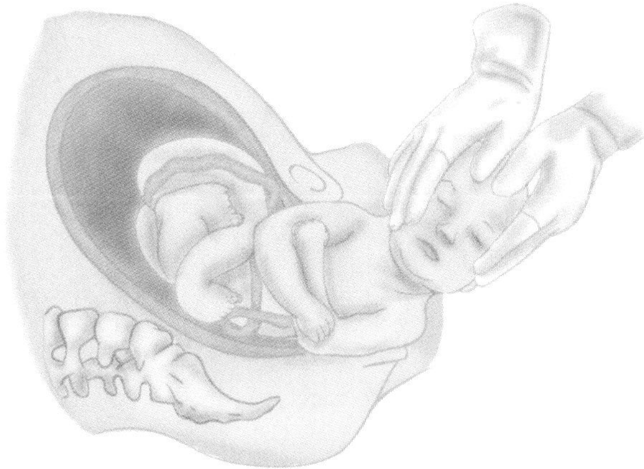

*Action:* The attendant then lifts the head toward the mother's symphysis pubis. *Rationale:* Permits the posterior fetal shoulder to be eased over the perineum, minimizing trauma to the maternal tissues.

***Clearing the Infant's Airway and Cutting the Cord***

*Action:* The rest of the infant's body is born quickly after the shoulders are born. The attendant maintains the infant in a slightly head-dependent position while suctioning excess secretions with a bulb syringe. The infant is often placed on the mother's abdomen. *Rationale:* Gravity aids spontaneous drainage of secretions and prevents aspiration of oral mucus and secretions.

*Action:* The attendant clamps the cord. Either the father or the attendant cuts the cord above the clamp. *Rationale:* Allows parents to interact more freely with their infant. Prevents flow of blood between placenta and infant, which might result in anemia (if infant is higher than placenta) or polycythemia (if infant is below the placenta).

***Delivery of the Placenta***

*Action:* After the placenta separates, it can usually be delivered if the mother bears down. The attendant may pull gently on the cord. *Rationale:* Excess traction on the cord may cause it to break, making the placenta harder to deliver.

*Action:* The attendant inspects both sides of the placenta. *Rationale:* Ensures that no fragments remain inside the uterus that might cause hemorrhage and infection.

After the infant and placenta are born, the attendant inspects the birth canal for injuries. If needed, any injuries and the episiotomy (if one was done) are repaired.

**FIG 16.16, cont'd** Sequence of delivery.

Standard precautions protect personnel from potentially infectious substances from mother or baby. At birth, the newborn is covered with blood, amniotic fluid, vernix, and other body substances (Fig. 16.17, pp. 324-325). To avoid contact with infectious secretions, personnel involved in infant contact should wear gloves and other protective equipment until after the first bath (Nursing Care Plan: Normal Labor and Birth [pp. 327-329] illustrates a normal labor and birth experience).

## Responsibilities After Birth

Intrapartum nursing care extends through the fourth stage of labor and includes care of the infant, the mother, and the family unit. See Chapters 20 through 23 for discussion of later postpartum care of the mother and infant.

### Care of the Infant

Immediate nursing care of the newborn includes supporting cardiopulmonary and thermoregulatory function and placing identifying bands on the infant and mother. In addition, the nurse assesses the infant for approximate gestational age and whether the infant is large or small for gestational age. Assessment of the blood glucose level is common for infants at increased risk for hypoglycemia such as those large or small for gestational age and infants of mothers with diabetes. Assessment for obvious anomalies or birth injuries and number of

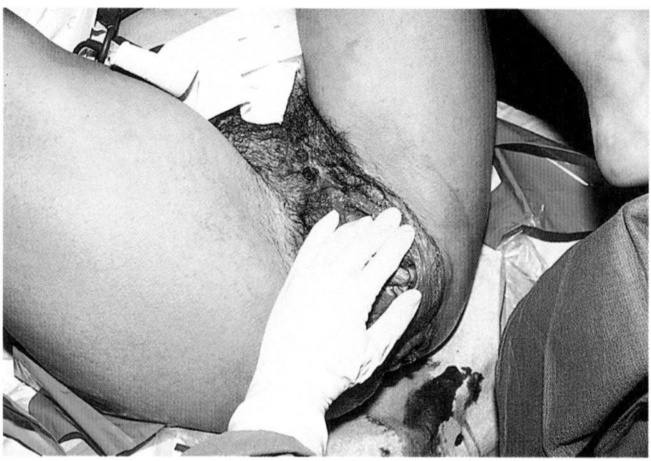

*A. Crowning*

The fetal head distends the labial and perineal tissues. The anus is stretched wide, and it is not unusual to see the woman's anterior rectal wall at this time. Any feces expelled are wiped posteriorly to avoid contaminating the vulva. The attendant (physician or nurse-midwife) is not holding the fetal head back but rather controlling its exit by using gentle pressure on the fetal occiput.

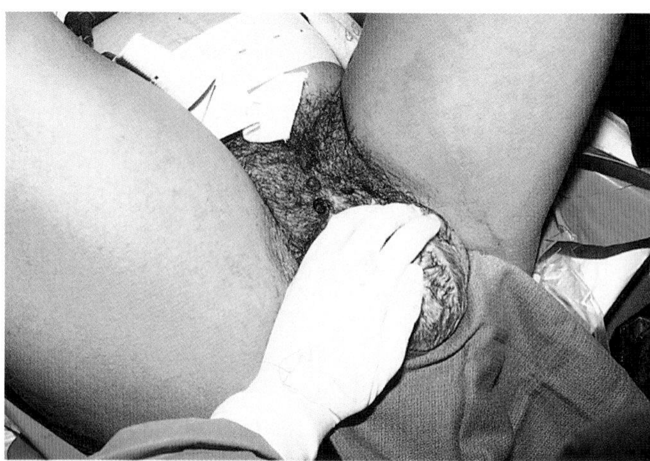

*B. Ritgen Maneuver*

Pressure is applied to the fetal chin through the perineum at the same time pressure is applied to the occiput of the fetal head. This action aids the mechanism of extension as the fetal head comes under the symphysis.

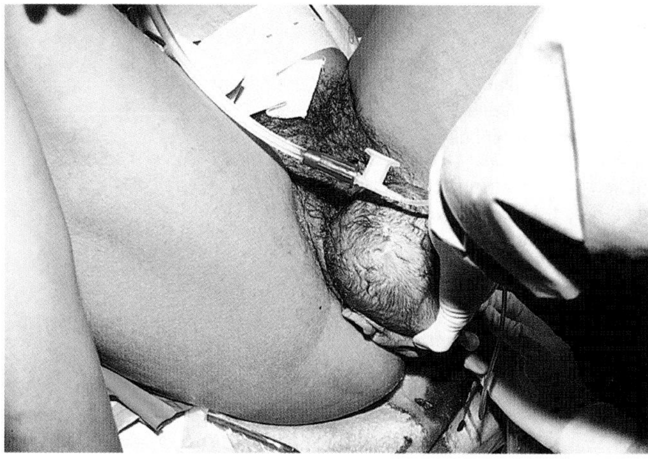

*C. Birth of the Head*

As the head emerges, the attendant prepares to suction the nose and mouth to avoid aspiration of secretions when the infant takes the first breath.

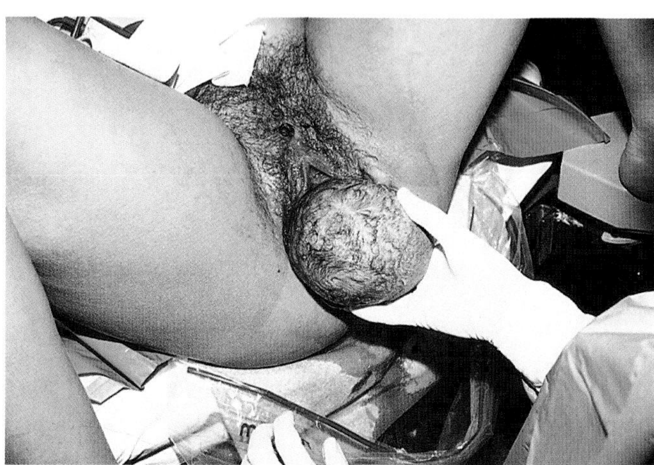

*D. Restitution and External Rotation*

After the head emerges, it realigns with the shoulders (restitution). External rotation occurs as the fetal shoulders internally rotate, aligning their transverse diameter with the anteroposterior diameter of the pelvic outlet.

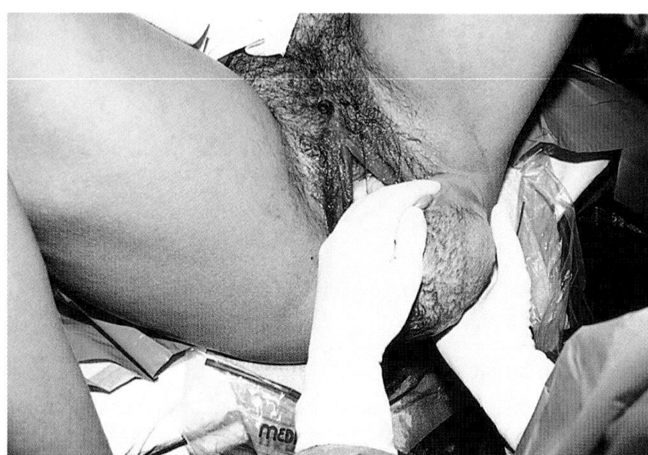

*E. Birth of the Anterior Shoulder*

The attendant gently pushes the fetal head toward the woman's perineum to allow the anterior shoulder to slip under her symphysis. The bluish skin color of the fetus is normal at this point; it becomes pink as the infant begins air breathing.

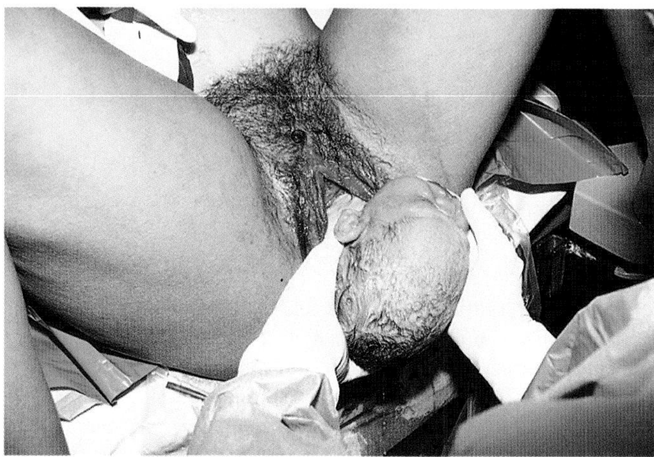

*F. Birth of the Posterior Shoulder*

The attendant now pushes the fetal head upward toward the woman's symphysis to allow the posterior shoulder to slip over her perineum

**FIG 16.17** Vaginal birth.

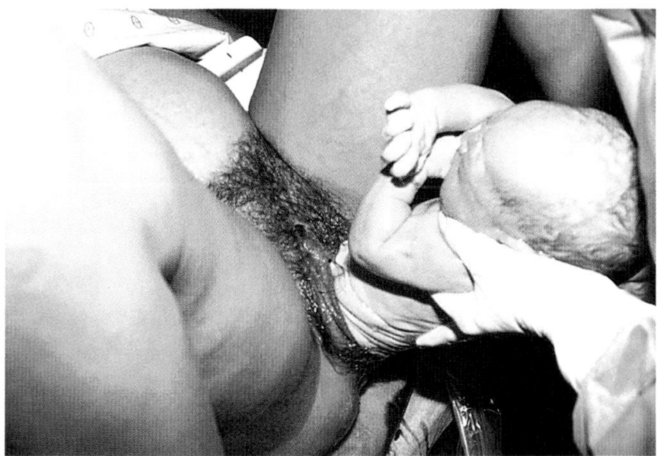

*G. Completion of the Birth*
The attendant supports the fetus during expulsion. Note that the fetus has excellent muscle tone, as evidenced by facial grimacing and flexion of the arms and hands.

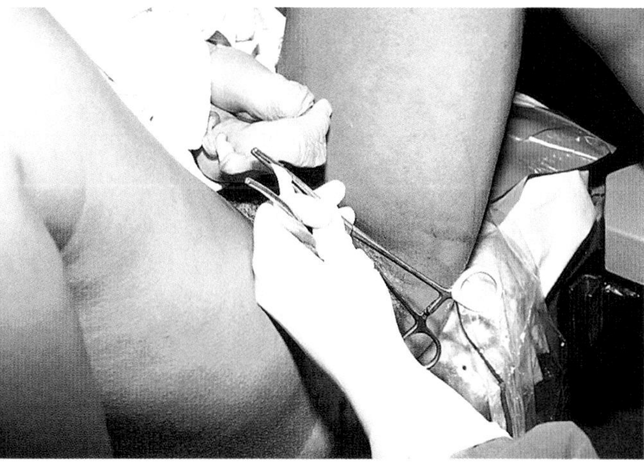

*H. Cord Clamping*
While the infant is in skin-to-skin contact on the mother's abdomen, the attendant doubly clamps the umbilical cord. The cord is then cut between the two clamps. Samples of cord blood are collected after it is cut.

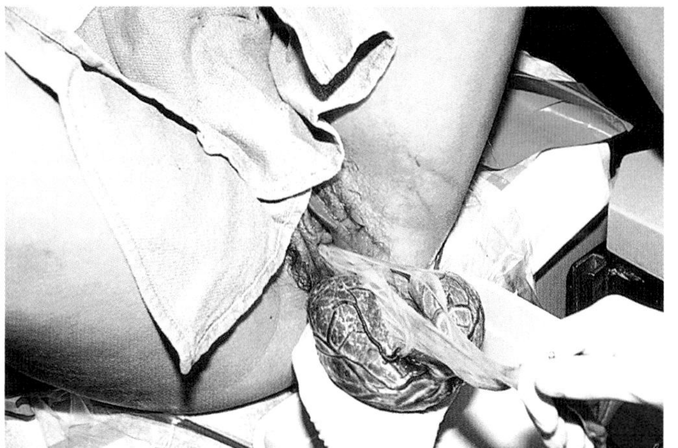

*I. Birth of the Placenta*
The attendant applies gentle traction on the cord to aid expulsion of the placenta. This placenta is expelled in the more common Schultze mechanism, with the shiny fetal surface and membranes emerging. Note the fetal membranes that surrounded the fetus and amniotic fluid during pregnancy. The chorionic vessels that branch from the umbilical cord are readily visible on the fetal surface of the placenta.

**FIG 16.17, cont'd** Vaginal birth.

cord vessels (see Fig. 16.14, *D*) should also be done. A stable newborn should be placed skin-to-skin with the mother immediately following delivery. A full admission assessment and bath can be done following an hour of skin-to-skin contact as long as the infant is stable.

***Maintaining cardiopulmonary function.*** Maintenance of the infant's cardiopulmonary function begins before birth by ensuring that equipment needed for neonatal resuscitation, such as suction equipment, oxygen, an appropriate-sized Ambu bag and mask, and intubation equipment, is ready. Ninety percent of infants need only gentle stimulation such as drying, but others need more vigorous resuscitation measures (Perlman, Wylie, Kattwinkel, et al., 2010).

Assess the infant's Apgar score (Table 16.3) at 1 and 5 minutes after birth for evaluation of early cardiopulmonary adaptation. If the Apgar score is 8 or higher, no intervention is needed other than supporting normal respiratory efforts. If the infant is obviously in distress (i.e., no or low heart rate and/or respirations, limp muscle tone, lack of response to stimulation, blue or pale color), interventions to correct the problem are instituted immediately rather than awaiting the 1-minute Apgar score.

Suction secretions from the infant's mouth and nose with a bulb syringe as needed. If deeper suction is needed for large amounts of fluid, use a neonatal suction apparatus with a mucus trap that is connected to regulated wall suction. Teach parents how to use the bulb syringe (see Chapter 22). Avoid keeping the infant in a head-dependent position without a specific indication, because the position limits diaphragm movement by upward pressure from the intestines.

***Supporting thermoregulation.*** To reduce evaporative heat loss, promptly dry the infant. Dry the head well, because substantial heat loss can occur from the head, which is approximately one fourth of the newborn's body surface area. Discard damp linens.

Place the infant in a prewarmed radiant warmer to limit heat loss while giving initial care. Skin-to-skin contact of the stable infant with a parent has the same effect, with the added benefit of promoting bonding. Avoid coming between the infant and the heat source. Wrap the infant in warm blankets when he or she is not in the warmer or making skin-to-skin contact. A stockinette cap further reduces heat loss if placed on the baby's *dry* head. A cap is not worn in the radiant warmer because the cap slows transfer of heat to the baby.

***Identifying the infant.*** Bands with matching imprinted numbers and identifying information are the primary means to ensure that the baby goes to the right mother after any separation (Fig. 16.18). Apply two bands on the infant, one on an arm and another on an ankle or one on each ankle to prevent facial scratching. Infant bands are applied more snugly than they would be if worn by an adult: leave

**TABLE 16.3 Apgar Score***

| Assessment | Points 0 | 1 | 2 |
|---|---|---|---|
| Heart rate | Absent | Below 100/min | 100/min or higher |
| Respiratory effort | No spontaneous respirations | Slow respirations or weak cry | Spontaneous respirations with a strong, lusty cry |
| Muscle tone | Limp | Minimal flexion of extremities; sluggish movement | Flexed body posture; spontaneous and vigorous movement |
| Reflex response | No response to suction or gentle slap on soles | Minimal response (grimace) to suction or gentle slap on soles | Responds promptly to suction or a gentle slap to the sole with cry or active movement |
| Color | Pallor or cyanosis | Bluish hands and feet only | Pink (light skinned) or absence of cyanosis (dark skinned); pink mucous membranes |

*The Apgar score is a method for rapid evaluation of the infant's cardiorespiratory adaptation after birth. The nurse scores the infant at 1 and 5 minutes after birth in each of five areas. The assessments are arranged from most important (heart rate) to least important (color). The infant is assigned a score of 0 to 2 in each of the five areas and the scores are totaled. Newborn resuscitation should not be delayed until the 1-minute score is obtained. However, general guidelines for the infant's care are based on three ranges of 1-minute scores:

| 0 1 2 3 | 4 5 6 | 7 8 9 10 |
|---|---|---|
| Infant needs resuscitation. | Gently stimulate by rubbing the infant's back while administering oxygen. Determine whether mother received narcotics that may have depressed the infant's respiration. | Provide no action other than support of the infant's spontaneous efforts and continue observation. |

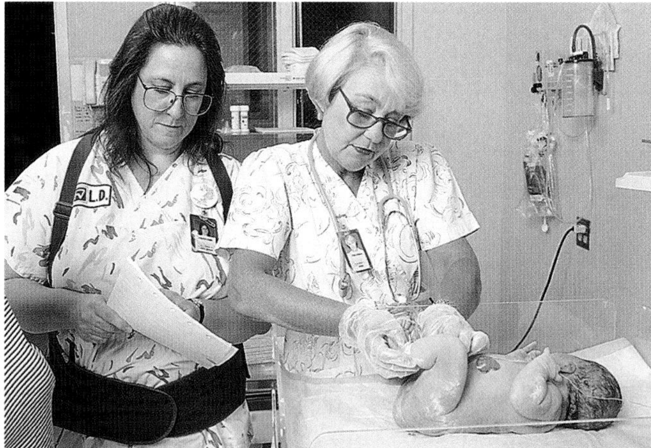

FIG 16.18 When the birthing room nurse turns over care of the newborn to the nursery nurse, both check the identification bands and medical record for the same information.

approximately one slender adult-finger-width of slack in the bands. Apply the larger band to the mother's wrist, similar to adult identification for any patient. A fourth band is provided to the father or other primary support person. Check that imprinted numbers and names are identical on each set of bands. A set is needed for each baby in a multiple birth. A digital photograph of the infant's face may be taken at birth for added visual identification.

## Care of the Mother

Nursing care of the mother during the fourth stage of labor focuses on observing for hemorrhage and relieving discomfort. Table 16.4 summarizes possible problems during the fourth stage of labor.

***Observing for hemorrhage.*** Important assessments related to hemorrhage are the woman's vital signs, uterine fundus, bladder, and lochia. For detailed information about these assessments, see Chapter 20.

***Vital signs.*** Assess the woman's temperature when recovery care begins and before transfer to a postpartum room. Added temperature checks will be needed for the woman who requires an extended recovery period. Assess her blood pressure, pulse, and respirations every 15 minutes during the first hour and every 30 minutes to 1 hour after the first hour, or as indicated by her condition. Evaluate her need for pain relief with vital signs. A rising pulse is an early sign of excessive blood loss because the heart contracts faster to compensate for reduced blood volume. The blood pressure may fall much later as the blood volume is severely reduced. A rising pulse rate also accompanies an elevated temperature.

If an indwelling catheter is in place, observe the urine output for adequacy. A low urine output (≤25 to 30 mL/hr) identifies water conservation by the kidneys in response to falling blood volume from any of several causes (e.g., dehydration, excess bleeding).

**Fundus.** The most common reason for excessive postpartum bleeding is that the uterus does not firmly contract and compress open vessels at the placental site. Assess the firmness, height, and positioning of the uterine fundus with each vital sign assessment. The fundus should be firm, in the midline, and at or below the umbilicus; it is approximately the size of a large grapefruit. If the fundus is firm, no massage is needed; if it is soft (boggy), massage it until it is firm (see Chapter 20). Nipple stimulation from the infant's suckling releases natural oxytocin from the mother's posterior pituitary to maintain firm uterine contraction. Oxytocin in the intravenous solution or given intramuscularly has the same effect.

**Bladder.** A full bladder interferes with contraction of the uterus and may lead to hemorrhage. Suspect a full bladder if the fundus is above the umbilicus or is displaced to one side, usually the right. If there is no contraindication, such as altered sensation, the mother can walk to the bathroom (with assistance the first time and as needed). Often, the first two or three voidings are measured until it is evident

**TABLE 16.4 Maternal Problems During the Fourth Stage of Labor**

| Sign | Potential Problem | Immediate Nursing Action |
|---|---|---|
| Rising maternal pulse rate and/or falling blood pressure; often accompanied by low or no urine output | An early sign of hypovolemia caused by excessive blood loss (visible or concealed) | Identify the probable cause of the blood loss, usually a poorly contracted uterus. Take steps to correct (see below) and notify birth attendant for further orders. Indwelling catheter may be inserted to observe urine output. |
| Soft (boggy) uterus | A poorly contracted uterus does not adequately compress large open vessels at the placental site, resulting in hemorrhage | With one hand securing the uterus just above the symphysis and the other on the fundus, massage the uterus until firm. Push downward on the firm uterus to expel any clots. Empty the woman's bladder (by voiding or catheterization) if fullness is contributing to uterine atony. |
| High uterine fundus, often displaced to one side | Suggests a full bladder, which can interfere with uterine contraction and result in hemorrhage | Massage the uterus if it is not firm. Help the woman urinate in the bathroom or in a bedpan. If she cannot void, catheterize her (usually a routine postpartum order). |
| Lochia exceeding one saturated perineal pad per hour during the fourth stage | Suggests hemorrhage; however, perineal pads vary in their absorbency, and this must be considered | Identify cause of hemorrhage; usually uterine atony, which is manifested by a soft uterus. Correct the cause. If lacerations are the suspected cause (excess bleeding with a firm fundus), notify the birth attendant. Keep the woman nothing by mouth (NPO) until the birth attendant evaluates her. |
| Intense perineal or vaginal pain, poorly relieved with analgesics | Hematoma, usually of vaginal wall or perineum; signs of hypovolemia may occur with substantial blood loss into tissues | If the hematoma is visible, apply cold packs to the area to slow bleeding into tissues. Notify the birth attendant, and anticipate possible surgical drainage. Keep the woman NPO. |

## NURSING CARE PLAN

### *Normal Labor and Birth*

**Focused Assessment**

Cathy, a 17-year-old gravida 1, para 0, is admitted in early labor. Her cervix is 3-cm dilated and completely effaced, and the fetus is at a zero station. Her membranes are intact. Her husband Tim is with her. They did not attend childbirth classes. She is holding Tim's hand tightly and breathing rapidly with each contraction. She says in a shaky voice, "I'm so scared. I've never been in a hospital before. I just don't know if I can do this."

**Nursing Diagnosis**

Anxiety related to unfamiliar environment and lack of birth preparation.

**Planning**

***Expected Outcomes***

Cathy will express being less anxious after admission procedures are completed, and have a relaxed facial expression and body posture between contractions.

**Interventions and *Rationales***

1. Maintain a calm and confident manner when caring for her. Express confidence in her ability to give birth.
   *The nurse's calm demeanor provides reassurance that labor is normal and that she has the resources within her to manage it.*
2. Use therapeutic communication when talking with Cathy. Adapt communication to the situation; simplifying explanations and directions as labor intensifies.
   *Clarity identifies dominant concerns so that they can be properly addressed. Intense physical sensations reduce the ability to comprehend complex information.*
3. Determine the couple's plans for birth, and work within them as much as possible.
   *This approach enhances their sense of control and helps them have a satisfying birth experience.*
4. Orient Cathy to the labor room, and explain procedures and equipment she will encounter.
   *This information will reduce fear of the unknown.*

**Evaluation**

Cathy relaxes a bit after talking with the nurse and slows her breathing. She says, "I feel a little better now. I hope I can have my baby before you go home." Tim also appears more relaxed.

**Focused Assessment**

Cathy's admission vital signs are all normal: temperature, 37.1°C (98.8°F); pulse, 88; respirations, 20 breaths per minute; and blood pressure, 112/70 mm Hg. The fetal heart rate averages 140 to 150 beats per minute (bpm). Her contractions occur every 4 minutes, last 50 seconds, and are of moderate intensity.

**Nursing Diagnosis**

Fetal observation throughout labor can be:

- Risk for Ineffective Tissue Perfusion: Fetal, related to interruption in oxygen-rich blood flow through the placenta or through the umbilical cord.

**Planning**

***Expected Outcome***

The fetal heart rate and contraction patterns are expected to remain reassuring throughout labor.

**Interventions and *Rationales***

1. Encourage her to use any position she desires except the supine. If she lies flat, a wedge should be placed under one hip to displace her uterus to one side. *The supine position can cause aortocaval compression, reducing blood flow to the placenta.*
   *Women in late pregnancy rarely want to be in the supine position because of this compression.*
2. Assess and document the fetal heart rate using the guidelines in Table 17.1. Report rates or patterns that are not reassuring. Assess the fetal heart rate more frequently if deviations from normal are identified. (Refer to Chapter 17 for detailed information.)
   *Observation allows prompt identification of changes in the rate or of abnormal rates. Fetal heart rate assessments that are outside expected limits need corrective action and should be reported for possible medical intervention.*

*Continued*

## NURSING CARE PLAN—cont'd

### *Normal Labor and Birth*

3. When the membranes rupture, observe the color, odor, and approximate amount of fluid, and note the time of rupture. Note the fetal heart rate after rupture.
   *This will help identify fetal conditions that should be promptly reported to Cathy's healthcare provider: meconium-stained fluid (possible fetal compromise); cloudy, yellow, or foul smelling (possible infection); prolonged membrane rupture (greater infection risk); low fetal heart rate (possible cord compression).*
4. Assess contractions when the fetal heart rate is assessed, at the interval between contractions.
   *This is when most placental exchange occurs.*
   Evaluate the interval between contractions to identify contractions that are too long (less than 30 seconds of full uterine relaxation), too strong, or longer than 90 to 120 seconds.
   *Contractions with an inadequate interval between them decrease the time available for the intervillous spaces of the placenta to eliminate wastes and refill with oxygenated blood and nutrients. Remember that the fetus with risk factors may not tolerate even less-than-normal labor contractions.*
5. Assess Cathy's blood pressure, pulse, and respirations every hour. Assess her temperature every 4 hours until her membranes rupture, then every 2 hours. If elevated, assess temperature every 2 hours or more frequently.
   *Maternal hypotension or hypertension can reduce blood flow to the placenta. Maternal fever increases the fetal temperature and metabolic rate, possibly raising fetal demand for oxygen beyond the mother's ability to supply it. A rising maternal pulse or fetal heart rate may precede the temperature elevation.*
6. See the Nursing Care Plan in Chapter 17, p. 381, for additional interventions.
   *This regular assessment is important if signs of fetal compromise occur.*

#### Evaluation

No nonreassuring fetal heart rate patterns appeared or persisted throughout labor.

#### Focused Assessment

In 1½ hours, Cathy's cervical dilation progresses to 5 cm, and the fetus descends to a +1 station. Her contractions occur every 3 minutes, last 60 seconds, and are of strong intensity. The fetal heart rate remains near its admission level. She is having difficulty relaxing between contractions and is complaining of back pain. She is relieved that her labor is progressing normally.

#### Nursing Diagnosis

Pain related to uterine contractions.

#### Planning

##### *Expected Outcome*

Cathy will express assurance that she can manage labor pain to her satisfaction.

#### Interventions and *Rationales*

1. Encourage Cathy to try positions such as standing/sitting and leaning forward, side-lying, leaning over the back of the bed, or on her hands and knees. Remind her to change positions approximately every half hour or when she feels the need for a change.
   *These positions shift the weight of the fetus away from the sacral promontory, reducing back pain. Alternating positions relieves strain and constant pressure and helps the fetus adapt to the pelvis.*
2. Teach Tim to rub or apply firm pressure to his wife's back. Ask her where the best place is and how hard to press.
   *Back rubs or firm pressure counteracts some of the back pain.*
3. Offer thermal pain management options:
   a. A warm blanket or warm pack applied to her back
   b. Cold packs applied to her back
   c. Alternating warm and cold packs, or use for 20 minutes on and 20 minutes off
   d. Warm water in a shower or whirlpool
   *Thermal stimulation interferes with transmission of pain impulses. Changing the thermal stimulation prevents habituation. Nipple stimulation in a shower or whirlpool causes release of oxytocin from the posterior pituitary and enhances contractions.*
4. Teach Cathy simple breathing and relaxation techniques (see Chapter 18). This will provide distraction and give her a sense of control and enhance her ability to manage pain in the normal labor process.
   *This will provide distraction and give her a sense of control and to enhance her ability to manage pain in the normal labor process.*
5. Observe the suprapubic area and palpate for a full bladder at least every 2 hours. Remind Cathy to void if she has not done so recently. A full bladder contributes to discomfort and can prolong labor by obstructing fetal descent.
   *A full bladder contributes to discomfort and can prolong labor by obstructing fetal descent.*
6. Tell Cathy about her progress in labor. Explain that she will probably begin to dilate faster now that she has entered active labor.
   *Encouragement and the knowledge that her efforts are having the desired results increase a woman's willingness to continue.*
7. Tell Cathy what pharmacologic pain-relief measures are available to her. *Knowing available options gives the woman a sense of control because she can choose whether she wants these measures.* (This action may be done during early labor to give a woman more time to consider her options.)

#### Evaluation

Cathy continues to have back pain that is 6 on a 0-to-10 scale but says that she is more comfortable sitting on the side of the bed with her head on a pillow on the over bed table. Her husband rubs her back during contractions. She says she is surprised to be able to manage the pain and does not want medication yet.

#### Focused Assessment

After another 2 hours, she is quite uncomfortable and requests pain medication. She is occasionally feeling an urge to push. She cries and says she is "losing it" and "can't take it anymore." Her husband asks anxiously, "What's wrong? Is she okay? Why is she acting this way?" The fetal heart rate remains near the admission range and shows no signs suggesting fetal compromise. Contractions occur every 2 minutes, last 70 seconds, and are strong. Her cervix is now 8 cm dilated and the station is +1. She asks for pain relief but does not want an epidural. Butorphanol (Stadol), 1 mg slow intravenous (IV) push, helps her regain control and work with her contractions. She avoids pushing by blowing out at the peak of each contraction. Cathy is fully dilated in 45 minutes, and the fetal station is +2. She pushes spontaneously several times with each contraction but tends to stiffen her back and push on the bed with her arms with each push. She pushes for approximately 10 seconds at a time, holding her breath each time. She prefers a semi-sitting position.

#### Nursing Diagnosis

Deficient knowledge related to effective pushing techniques.

#### Planning

##### *Expected Outcome*

Cathy will push more effectively after the nurse gives her instructions in good techniques.

## NURSING CARE PLAN—cont'd

### *Normal Labor and Birth*

**Interventions and *Rationales***

1. Observe Cathy's perineum for fetal crowning with each push. A woman having her first baby can still give birth rapidly. Observation permits the nurse to maintain her safety and that of the baby should rapid birth occur.
   *A woman having her first baby can still give birth rapidly. Observation permits the nurse to maintain her safety and that of the baby should rapid birth occur.*
2. Encourage her to exhale as she pushes strongly for approximately 4 to 6 seconds at a time.
   Prolonged pushing against a closed glottis reduces blood return to the heart and maternal oxygen saturation and decreases placental blood flow, especially if it is done with every contraction.
3. Teach her techniques:
   a. Instruct Cathy to flex her head with each push, directing each push downward into the pelvic cavity.
   b. Instruct her to pull against her flexed knees (or hand-holds on the bed) as she pushes, curving her body around her uterus. Encourage upright positions, including squatting. Pulling provides leverage to gain a more effective push from the abdominal muscles. Upright positions take advantage of gravity, and squatting enlarges the pelvic outlet slightly. Cathy has preferred upright positions throughout most of active labor.
   c. Have Cathy push toward the vaginal outlet because the vagina is the anatomically correct direction.
   d. Help Cathy relax her perineum as she pushes down reducing soft tissue resistance to fetal descent.
   e. Tell Cathy to keep her sacrum flattened against the bed when pushing in a semi-sitting position to straighten the pelvic curve somewhat. Similar to squatting. This position will make each push more effective.
4. Do not talk to her unnecessarily between contractions.
   *Silence allows Cathy to conserve energy for pushing efforts.*

**Evaluation**

Cathy pushes more effectively with the nurse coaching her during each contraction. In another hour she gives birth to a 3346 g (7 lb, 6 oz) boy. The baby's Apgar scores are 9 at both 1 and 5 minutes. Cathy has a small first-degree laceration that is sutured by her midwife using a local anesthetic. The new family gets acquainted during the recovery period. She expresses pride with her ability to "do it."

that the woman voids without difficulty and empties her bladder completely. Each void is usually at least 300 to 400 mL if she is emptying her bladder.

**Lochia.** Assess lochia with each vital sign and fundal assessment. The amount of lochia seems large to the inexperienced nurse and the new mother. Perineal pads vary in their absorbency, but *saturation* of one pad within the first hour is a guideline for the maximum normal lochia flow. Observe for lochia that pools under the mother's buttocks and back. Small clots are often present, but the presence of large clots is not normal, and the physician or nurse-midwife should be notified. A continuous trickle of bright red blood when the fundus is firm suggests a laceration in the birth canal. A hematoma causes bleeding into the tissues, but excess visible bleeding is unusual.

***Relieving discomfort.*** Uterine contractions (afterpains) and perineal trauma are common causes of pain after birth. A postpartum chill is often annoying. Pain is usually mild and readily relieved by simple measures. Pain that is intense or does not respond to common relief measures requires investigation, and the birth attendant should be notified.

**Ice packs.** To reduce edema and limit hematoma formation, apply a cold pack to the perineum promptly after vaginal birth. Small hematomas are common, but a rapidly enlarging hematoma suggests significant concealed blood loss and pain. Some perineal pads containing chemical cold packs vary in the amount of lochia they can absorb, which should be considered when estimating pad saturation. Many facilities use a diaper filled with ice because it is economical, more absorbent, and colder than the pads with cold packs.

**Analgesics.** Afterpains and perineal pain respond well to mild oral analgesics such as ibuprofen. Regular urination reduces the severity of afterpains because the uterus contracts effectively.

**Warmth.** A warm blanket is soothing and shortens the chill that is common after birth. A portable radiant warmer provides warmth to both the mother and infant. The mother may enjoy warm drinks or prefer cool ones.

#### Promoting Early Family Attachment

The first hour after birth is an ideal time for parent-infant attachment because the healthy neonate is alert and responsive. Provide privacy while unobtrusively observing the parents and infant. The infant can remain in the parent's arms while vital signs, minor suctioning of secretions, and many initial assessments are completed.

Assist the mother to nurse during the recovery period, if she desires. The infant is usually attentive and nurses briefly. Early nipple stimulation helps initiate milk production.

When the parents are ready, allow siblings, other family members, and friends to visit. Help siblings to see and touch their new brother or sister by putting a stool at the bedside or letting them sit on the bed. Preschool or school-age children may be fascinated by their new brother or sister. Adolescents may react in various ways to their parents' sexuality.

Observe for signs of early parent-infant attachment. Parent behaviors are tentative at first, progressing from fingertip touch to palm touch to enfolding of the infant. Expect parents to make eye contact with the infant and talk to a baby in higher-pitched, affectionate tones.

Cultural variations should be considered when assessing early attachment. The nurse should be knowledgeable about the typical practices of the populations commonly served. It is the nurse's responsibility to accept and accommodate the varying cultural traditions to meet the needs of all individuals, no matter their beliefs (Callister, 2014; Lewallen, 2011).

## KEY CONCEPTS

- Labor contractions are intermittent, allowing placental blood flow and exchange of oxygen, nutrients, and waste products between the maternal and fetal circulations during the interval.
- The upper uterus contracts actively during labor as it pushes the fetus down, maintaining tension to pull the more passive lower uterus and cervix over the fetal presenting part. These actions bring about cervical effacement and dilation.
- Fetal lung fluid production decreases and its absorption into lung tissue increases during late pregnancy and labor. Thoracic compression during labor aids in expulsion of additional fluid.
- Four interrelated components affecting the process of birth are the powers, the passage, the passenger, and the psyche. Presentation and position further describe the relation of the fetus (passenger) to the maternal pelvis.
- Natural mechanisms of labor favor efficient passage of the fetus through the mother's pelvis.
- As labor approaches, the woman may notice one or more premonitory signs that precede its onset: an increase in the frequency and intensity of Braxton Hicks contractions, lightening, increased vaginal secretions, bloody show, a spurt of energy, and weight loss.
- The conclusive difference between true labor and false labor is progressive effacement and dilation of the cervix.
- Some women do not have symptoms typical of true labor. They should enter the birth center for evaluation if they are uncertain or have concerns other than those listed in the guidelines.
- Four stages of labor are normal: Stage 1, cervical dilation and effacement; Stage 2, expulsion of the fetus; Stage 3, expulsion of the placenta; and Stage 4, maternal physiologic stabilization and parent-infant bonding.
- Normal labor is characterized by consistent progression of uterine contractions, cervical dilation and effacement, and fetal descent.
- Because of complete dependence on the mother's physiologic systems, the fetus is the more vulnerable of the maternal–fetal pair.
- The normal FHR at term averages 110 to 160 bpm. Other reassuring findings include the presence of variability in the electronically monitored term fetus, accelerations that peak at least 15 bpm above existing baseline with a total duration for the acceleration of at least 15 seconds, and absence of decelerations following contractions.
- Persistent contractions may reduce placental blood flow and fetal oxygen, nutrient, and waste exchange. The fetus with low reserves may be unable to cope with normal contractions. (See Chapter 17 for additional information about FHR and contraction patterns.)
- A maternal supine position can reduce placental blood flow because the uterus compresses the aorta and inferior vena cava.
- General comfort measures promote the woman's ability to relax and cope with labor.
- Regular changes in position during labor promote maternal comfort and help the fetus adapt to the pelvis.
- The nurse must be alert for signs of impending birth. The woman may urgently state, "The baby's coming," or she may make grunting sounds or bear down.
- The priority nursing care of the newborn immediately after birth is to promote normal respirations, maintain normal body temperature, and promote attachment.
- The priority nursing care of the mother after birth is to assess for hemorrhage, promote firm uterine contraction, and promote parent–infant attachment.

## REFERENCES AND READINGS

American Academy of Pediatrics & American College of Obstetricians and Gynecologists. (2012). *Guidelines for perinatal care* (7th ed.). Elk Grove Village, IL, and Washington, DC: Authors.

American Society of Anesthesiologist (2015). *Most healthy women would benefit from light meal during labor.* Retrieved from https://www.asahq.org/about-asa/newsroom/news-releases/2015/10/eating-a-light-meal-during-labor.

Association of Women's Health, Obstetric and Neonatal Nurses. (2008). *Nursing care and management of the second stage of labor (2nd ed.): Evidence-based clinical practice guidelines.* Washington, DC: Author.

Association of Women's Health, Obstetric, and Neonatal Nurses. (2009). *Standards for professional nursing practice in the care of women and newborns* (7th ed.). Washington, DC: Author.

Association of Women's Health, Obstetric, and Neonatal Nurses. (2015). *Fetal heart monitoring: Principles & practices* (5th ed.). Dubuque, IA: Kendall/Hunt.

Bernstein, D. (2011). The fetal to neonatal circulatory transition. In R. M. Kliegman, B. F. Stanton & J. W. St. Geme III (Eds.), *Nelson textbook of pediatrics* (19th ed., pp. 1529). Philadelphia: Saunders.

Blackburn, S.T. (2013). *Maternal, fetal, & neonatal physiology: A clinical perspective* (4th ed.). St. Louis: Saunders.

Burke, C. (2014). Pain in labor: Nonpharmacological and pharmacological management. In K.R. Simpson, & P.A. Creehan (Eds.), *AWHONN perinatal nursing* (4th ed., pp. 493–529). Philadelphia: Lippincott Williams & Wilkins.

Callister, L.C. (2014). Integrating cultural beliefs and practices when caring for childbearing women and families. In K.R. Simpson & P.A. Creehan (Eds.), *AWHONN perinatal nursing* (4th ed., pp. 41–70). Philadelphia: Lippincott Williams & Wilkins.

Castro, L.C. (2010). Hypertensive disorders of pregnancy. In N.F. Hacker, J.C. Gambone, & C. J. Hobel (Eds.), *Hacker & Moore's essentials of obstetrics and gynecology* (5th ed., pp. 173–182). Philadelphia: Saunders.

Cunningham, F.G., Leveno, K.J., Bloom, S.L., et al. (2010). *Williams obstetrics* (23rd ed.). New York: McGraw-Hill.

Gillesby, E., Burns, S., Dempsey, A., et al. (2010). Comparison of delayed versus immediate pushing during second stage of labor for nulliparous women with epidural anesthesia. *Journal of Obstetric, Gynecologic, and Neonatal Nursing, 39*(6), 635–644.

Hall, J.E. (2011). *Guyton and Hall: Textbook of medical physiology*. Philadelphia: Saunders.

Hobel, C.J., & Zakowski, M. (2010). Normal labor, delivery, and postpartum care. In N.F. Hacker, J.C. Gambone, & C.J. Hobel (Eds.), *Hacker & Moore's essentials of obstetrics and gynecology*, (5th ed., pp. 91–118). Philadelphia: Saunders.

Kelly, M., Johnson, E., Lee, V., et al. (2010). Delayed versus immediate pushing in second stage of labor. *MCN: The American Journal of Maternal-Child Nursing, 35*(2), 81–88.

Lewallen, L.P. (2011). The importance of culture in childbearing. *Journal of Obstetric Gynecologic & Neonatal Nursing, 40*(1), 4–8.

Lyndon, A., O'Brien-Abel, N., & Simpson, K.R. (2014). Fetal assessment during labor. In K.R. Simpson, & P.A. Creehan (Eds.), *AWHONN perinatal nursing* (4th ed., pp. 445–492), Philadelphia: Lippincott Williams & Wilkins.

Lyndon, A., O'Brien-Abel, N., & Simpson, K.R. (2015). Fetal heart rate interpretation. In A. Lyndon, & L. Usher (Eds.), *Association of Women's Health, Obstetric and Neonatal Nurses*

(AWHONN) *Fetal heart monitoring: Principles and practices* (5th ed., pp. 101–133). Washington, DC: Author.

Perlman, J.M., Wylie, J., Kattwinkel, J., et al. (2010). Special report—Neonatal resuscitation: 2010 International consensus on cardiopulmonary resuscitation and emergency cardiovascular care science with treatment recommendations. *Pediatrics, 126*(5), e1319–e1344.

Sharts-Hopko, N.C. (2010). Oral intake during labor: A review of the evidence. *MCN: The American Journal of Maternal-Child Nursing, 35*(4), 197–203.

Simpson, K.R., & O'Brien-Abel,N. (2014). Labor and birth. In K.R. Simpson & P.A. Creehan (Eds.), *AWHONN perinatal nursing* (4th ed., pp. 343–444). Philadelphia: Lippincott Williams & Wilkins.

Tarsa, M., & Moore, T.R. (2010). Multifetal gestation and malpresentation. In N.F. Hacker, J.C. Gambone, & C.J. Hobel (Eds.), *Hacker & Moore's essentials of obstetrics and gynecology* (5th ed., pp. 160–172). Philadelphia: Saunders.

Zhang, J., Landy, H., Branch, D.W., et al. (2010). Contemporary patterns of spontaneous labor with normal neonatal outcomes. *Obstetrics and Gynecology, 116*(6), 1281–1287.

# 17

# Intrapartum Fetal Surveillance

http://evolve.elsevier.com/McKinney/mat-ch/

## LEARNING OBJECTIVES

*After studying this chapter, you should be able to:*

- Identify the purposes of fetal surveillance before birth.
- Explain the normal and pathologic mechanisms that influence fetal heart rate (FHR).
- Identify the advantages and limitations of each method of fetal surveillance: auscultation and electronic monitoring.
- Explain the types of equipment used for electronic fetal monitoring (EFM) and the advantages and limitations of each.
- Describe the interpretation of EFM data. Explain the methods that may be used in addition to EFM to judge fetal well-being.
- Describe appropriate nursing responses to nonreassuring FHR patterns.
- Use the nursing process to plan care for a woman having electronic fetal monitoring.

Fetal surveillance uses any of the several methods to identify signs associated with well-being or with compromise. Accurate assessment of these signs promotes appropriate and timely care to reduce hazards to the fetus. Before birth, there are two patients: the mother and her fetus. The purposes of antepartum and intrapartum fetal surveillance are to evaluate the fetal condition during pregnancy and to identify possible hypoxic insult to the fetus during labor. Fetal surveillance cannot identify every compromised fetus. Although this chapter focuses on fetal surveillance of the woman during labor, many of these techniques and guidelines may be used in the care of a woman with an antepartum complication.

Two basic approaches are taken to intrapartum fetal surveillance—low- and high-tech approaches. Each has advantages and limitations. Neither is superior. The low-tech approach uses intermittent auscultation (IA) of the fetal heart rate (FHR) and palpation of the uterine activity. Electronic fetal monitoring (EFM) is the second approach for intrapartum fetal surveillance. Although EFM is dominant in U.S. hospital births, its routine use remains controversial because its benefits to the fetus are not always clear. Other data, such as assessment for fetal movement (see Chapter 15) or cord blood gases, may be added to FHR and contraction data to provide a balanced view of the fetal condition.

## FETAL OXYGENATION

Adequate fetal oxygenation requires five related factors:

- Normal maternal blood flow and volume to the placenta
- Normal oxygen saturation of maternal blood
- Adequate exchange of oxygen and carbon dioxide in the placenta
- An open circulatory path between the placenta and fetus through vessels in the umbilical cord
- Normal fetal circulatory and oxygen-carrying functions

Labor is stressful for a fetus, but several mechanisms compensate for these stresses. One must understand the dynamics of uteroplacental exchange and fetal circulation to understand fetal responses to labor. (See also Chapter 12 for a discussion of fetal circulation and placental functions.)

### Uteroplacental Exchange

Oxygen-rich and nutrient-rich blood from the mother enters the intervillous spaces of the placenta through the spiral arteries (see Fig. 12.7). Oxygen and nutrients in the maternal blood pass into the fetal blood that circulates in capillaries in the intervillous spaces. Carbon dioxide and other waste products pass from the fetal blood into the maternal blood at the same time. Maternal blood carrying fetal waste products drains from the intervillous spaces through endometrial veins and returns to the mother's circulation for elimination by her body. Substances pass back and forth between the mother and fetus without mixing the maternal and fetal blood if fetal capillaries remain intact.

During labor, contractions gradually compress the spiral arteries, temporarily stopping maternal blood flow into the intervillous spaces. During contractions, the fetus depends on the oxygen supply already present in the body cells, fetal erythrocytes, and intervillous spaces. The oxygen supply in these areas is enough for approximately 1 to 2 minutes. As each contraction relaxes, freshly oxygenated maternal blood re-enters the intervillous spaces and waste-laden blood drains out.

### Fetal Circulation

The fetal heart circulates oxygenated blood from the placenta throughout the body and returns deoxygenated blood to the placenta. The umbilical vein carries oxygenated blood to the fetus, and the two umbilical arteries carry deoxygenated blood from the fetus to the placenta (see Fig. 12.7).

### Fetal Heart Rate Regulation

Mechanisms that regulate FHR are balanced to maintain cardiac output at a level that keeps the fetal heart and brain oxygenated. Fetal cardiac output increase is primarily accomplished by an increase in the heart rate. Conversely, a marked decrease in FHR decreases the cardiac output.

Five fetal factors interact to regulate FHR:

- Autonomic nervous system
- Baroreceptors
- Chemoreceptors

- Adrenal glands
- Central nervous system

The balance among factors that increase and decrease the heart rate result in the characteristic fluctuations in FHR during late pregnancy.

### Autonomic Nervous System

The sympathetic and parasympathetic branches of the autonomic nervous system are balanced forces that regulate FHR. Sympathetic stimulation increases the heart rate and strengthens myocardial contractions through release of epinephrine and norepinephrine. The net result of sympathetic stimulation is an increase in cardiac output.

The parasympathetic nervous system, through stimulation of the vagus nerve, reduces FHR and maintains variability. The parasympathetic branch gradually exerts greater influence as the fetus matures, beginning between 28 and 32 weeks of gestation. Therefore, the average FHR is slightly lower in the term fetus than in the preterm fetus. However, variability in FHR near full term is often more dramatic than in a fetus just a few weeks younger than full term.

### Baroreceptors

Cells in the carotid arch and major arteries respond to stretching when the fetal blood pressure increases. These baroreceptors stimulate the vagus nerve to slow FHR and decrease the blood pressure, thus lowering cardiac output. As fetal blood pressure falls, the heart rate accelerates to maintain normal cardiac output.

### Chemoreceptors

Cells that respond to changes in oxygen, carbon dioxide, and pH are chemoreceptors found in the medulla oblongata and in the aortic and carotid bodies. Decreased oxygen content, increased carbon dioxide content, or a lower pH in the blood or cerebrospinal fluid triggers an increase in the heart rate. However, prolonged hypoxia (low oxygen), hypercapnia (excess carbon dioxide in blood [elevated carbon dioxide partial pressure {$Pco_2$}]), and acidosis (low pH from accumulation of acid [hydrogen ions] or depletion of base [bicarbonate ions]) depress FHR.

### Adrenal Glands

The adrenal medulla secretes epinephrine and norepinephrine in response to stress, causing a response from the sympathetic nervous system that accelerates FHR. The adrenal cortex responds to a decrease in the fetal blood pressure with release of aldosterone and retention of sodium and water, resulting in an increase in the circulating fetal blood volume.

### Central Nervous System

The fetal cerebral cortex causes the heart rate to increase during fetal movement and to decrease when the fetus sleeps. The hypothalamus coordinates the two branches of the autonomic nervous system. The medulla oblongata maintains the balance between stimuli that speed and stimuli that slow the heart rate.

## Pathologic Influences on Fetal Oxygenation

Fetal oxygenation may be compromised by alterations in the placenta, fetal factors, or the pregnant woman.

### Maternal Cardiopulmonary Alterations

Actual or relative reductions in the mother's circulating blood volume reduce perfusion of the intervillous spaces with oxygenated maternal blood. Hemorrhage causes an actual decrease in her blood volume. Relative reductions in maternal circulating volume result from altered distribution of the blood volume without blood loss. For example, epidural block analgesia may result in vasodilation, which increases the capacity of the maternal vascular bed. However, the amount of blood available to fill the vessels is unchanged. Hypotension can result, reducing placental blood flow.

Maternal hypertension may reduce blood flow to the placenta because of vasospasm and narrowing of the spiral arteries.

A lowered oxygen level in the mother's blood reduces the amount available to the fetus. Maternal acid–base alterations, which often accompany respiratory abnormalities or diabetic ketoacidosis, may also compromise exchange in the placenta. A lower maternal oxygen tension may result from respiratory disorders such as asthma or acute pulmonary infections or from smoking.

### Uterine Activity

Hypertonic contractions that are too long (≥90 to 120 seconds), too frequent (closer than every 2 minutes, or have an inadequate relaxation period (less than 30 seconds of complete relaxation) will not allow optimal uteroplacental exchange. Additional criteria may be specified when internal EFM is used. The uterus may never fully relax between contractions, applying continuous compression to the spiral arteries and reducing maternal-fetal exchange in the intervillous spaces. Excess uterine activity may occur with prostaglandin or oxytocin administration but can also occur in the absence of external stimulation. A fetus with good oxygen reserves may never show signs of compromise, even with excessive contractions. Likewise, the fetus with little reserve may show compromise, even with weak uterine activity.

### Placental Disruptions

Conditions such as abruptio placentae (separation of the placenta before birth) and infarcts (necrosis of varying amounts of placental tissue) reduce the placental surface area available for exchange. The amount and location of placental disruption relate to the degree of impairment in uteroplacental exchange.

### Interruptions in Umbilical Flow

The usual cause of interrupted blood flow through the umbilical cord is compression. Blood flow through the umbilical cord may be reduced by compression between the fetal presenting part and the pelvis, a nuchal cord (around the fetal neck), one that is wrapped around the fetal body, or a knot in the cord. Compression can occur with oligohydramnios because the amount of amniotic fluid is inadequate to cushion the cord. The umbilical cord may become tangled around fetal body parts. The fetus may compress the cord by grasping with the hand.

The thin-walled umbilical vein is compressed initially, reducing the flow of more highly oxygenated blood into the fetus. This compression results in initial hypoxia with hypotension. Baroreceptors and chemoreceptors respond by accelerating FHR. Flow from the fetus to the placenta through the firmer-walled umbilical arteries falls as cord compression continues, resulting in hypertension from increased fetal blood volume. Baroreceptors respond to hypertension by stimulating the vagus nerve, thus reducing fetal blood pressure and slowing the fetal heart. The FHR again accelerates as pressure on the arteries, and then the vein, is relieved.

### Fetal Alterations

Fetal tissues may be hypoxic despite an adequate oxygen supply from the mother and adequate exchange within the placenta. A low circulating fetal blood volume, fetal hypotension, or fetal anemia reduces the ability of fetal erythrocytes to deliver oxygen to body cells. Central nervous system or cardiac abnormalities may cause an abnormal rate

**BOX 17.1 Potential Maternal, Fetal, or Neonatal Risk Factors**

**Antepartum Period**

***Maternal History***

- Previous stillbirth (unexplained or possibly recurrent cause)
- Previous cesarean birth
- Poor nutrition, low prepregnancy weight, poor weight gain
- Multiple pregnancies, closely spaced
- Chronic diseases, such as cardiac disease, anemia, hypertension, diabetes, asthma, and autoimmune diseases
- Acute infections, such as urinary tract, pneumonia, gastrointestinal
- Hematologic problems, such as anemia, deep vein thrombosis
- Drug use (includes prescription, over-the-counter, herbal preparations, illegal drugs)
- Psychosocial stress, domestic violence

***Problems Identified During Pregnancy***

- Intrauterine growth restriction (IUGR)
- Gestation >42 wk
- Marked decrease in fetal movement
- Multifetal gestation
- Preeclampsia, eclampsia
- Gestational diabetes
- Placental abnormalities (placenta previa, abruptio placentae)
- Maternal severe anemia
- Maternal infection
- Maternal trauma

**Intrapartum Period**

***Maternal Problems***

- Hypotension or hypertension
- Hypertonic uterine contractions
- Abnormal labor: preterm or dysfunctional
- Prolonged rupture of membranes
- Chorioamnionitis
- Fever

***Fetal or Placental Problems***

- Fetal anemia
- Persistent abnormal or nonreassuring fetal heart rate or pattern
- Meconium-stained amniotic fluid
- Abnormal presentation or position
- Prolapsed cord
- Abruptio placentae

or rhythm. For example, a fetus with complete heart block may not respond to stimuli that would normally cause a rate increase.

Prolonged fetal bradycardia may be both a response to hypoxia and a contributing factor to hypoxia because fetal oxygenation is rate dependent. Prolonged tachycardia also can decrease cardiac output because the ventricles have less time to fill with oxygenated blood during diastole.

### Risk Factors for Fetal Compromise

When conditions associated with reduced fetal oxygenation are present (Box 17.1), surveillance by either IA and palpation or EFM should be carried out more often. No difference in perinatal outcome has been demonstrated between properly performed IA and EFM. However, EFM is used for most births in the United States (American Academy of Pediatrics [AAP] & American College of Obstetricians and Gynecologists [ACOG], 2012; American College of Nurse-Midwives [ACNM], 2010; ACOG, 2015b).

## AUSCULTATION AND PALPATION

The nurse may use IA of FHR and palpation of uterine activity for intrapartum fetal surveillance (Procedure: Auscultating the Fetal Heart Rate, p. 335). IA can be done using either the fetoscope or Doppler ultrasound (Fig. 17.1). Doppler auscultation is most common because of its ease of use, adjustable volume, and compact size. Many Doppler devices have a digital or paper display of the rate, and some may be used under water. The Doppler creates an electronic sound based on movements of the fetal heart and may be the only means of auscultation in women with a thick abdominal fat pad. However, the nonelectronic fetoscope is useful in cases of fetal cardiac dysrhythmias because its sound is that of actual opening and closing of heart valves, similar to the amplified sounds one hears with a stethoscope.

### Advantages

Mobility is the primary advantage of auscultation and palpation for intrapartum fetal monitoring of the fetus at low risk. The woman is

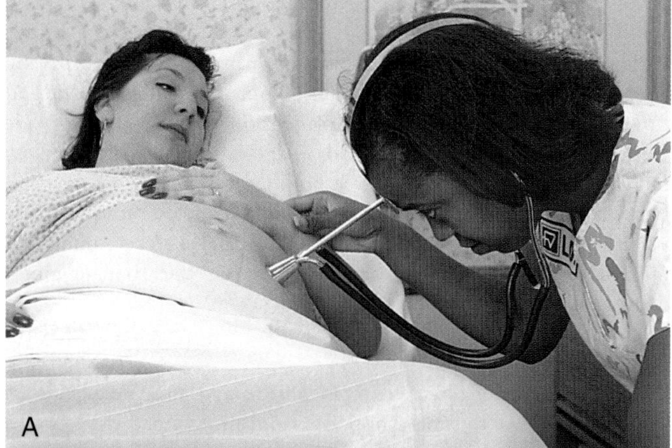


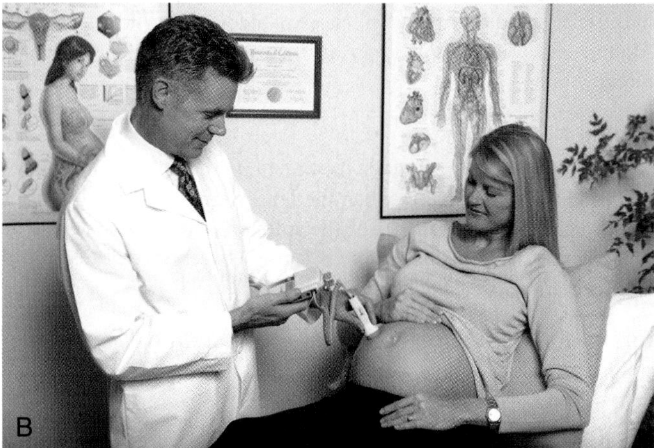


**FIG 17.1** Low intervention methods for evaluating fetal heart rate during labor. **A,** Fetoscope with head attachment to enhance conduction of faint fetal heart sounds. **B,** Doppler ultrasound transducer to sense the fetal heart rate electronically. (Courtesy Summit Doppler Systems, Inc., Golden, CO.)

## PROCEDURE

### *Auscultating the Fetal Heart Rate*

**Purpose**

To evaluate the fetal condition and tolerance of labor.

1. Explain the procedure to give information to the woman and her partner. Wash your hands with warm water to reduce the transmission of microorganisms and to make your hands warm when touching the woman's abdomen.
2. Use Leopold's maneuvers to identify the fetal back (see Chapter 16) because it usually is closest to the surface of the maternal abdomen, where fetal heart sounds are clearest. Illustrations show approximate locations of the fetal heart rate in different presentations and positions, whether assessing the fetus with auscultation or electronic fetal monitoring.
3. Assess the fetal heart rate (FHR) with a Doppler transducer or fetoscope. The external fetal monitor may be used for intermittent electronic fetal monitoring (short periods of electronic monitoring interspersed with periods with no fetal surveillance, such as maternal ambulation).
4. Doppler transducer (see Fig. 17.1, B): Place water-soluble conducting gel over the transducer to make an interface for clear signal transmission, and turn it on. Place the transducer over the fetal back and move it until you hear clear sounds that represent the fetal heart motion.
5. Fetoscope (see Fig. 17.1, A): Place the bell of the fetoscope over the fetal back. Part of the fetoscope, a head plate pressed against your forehead, may be attached to add bone conduction to the sound coming through the earpieces. Move the fetoscope until you locate where the sound is loudest.
6. With one hand, palpate the mother's radial pulse to verify that FHR is what is actually heard. If her pulse is synchronized with the sounds from the fetoscope or Doppler transducer, try another location for the fetal heart. Other sounds that may be represented by the Doppler are the funic souffle (blood flowing through the umbilical cord) or uterine souffle (blood flowing through the uterine vessels). The funic souffle is synchronized with the fetal heart and is the same rate; the uterine souffle is synchronized with the mother's pulse.
7. Count the baseline FHR for 30 to 60 seconds between contractions. Assessment during a contraction may clarify findings, but auscultation is difficult during contractions. Note accelerations or slowing of the rate. Other counting methods, such as counting for 6-second segments for a total of 1 minute, may be used.
8. Note reassuring signs that suggest the fetus is tolerating labor well:
   a. An average rate of 110 to 160 beats per minute (bpm)
   b. Regular rhythm
   c. Accelerations from the baseline rate
   d. No decrease in rate from the baseline rate
9. Note nonreassuring signs. An electronic fetal monitor is applied for continuous monitoring of FHR and more frequent assessments related to nonreassuring signs. Notify the physician or nurse-midwife for further evaluation if:
   e. Heart rate outside normal limits. Unexplained tachycardia or bradycardia for 10 minutes or longer
   f. Irregular rhythm
   g. Gradual or abrupt decrease in rate

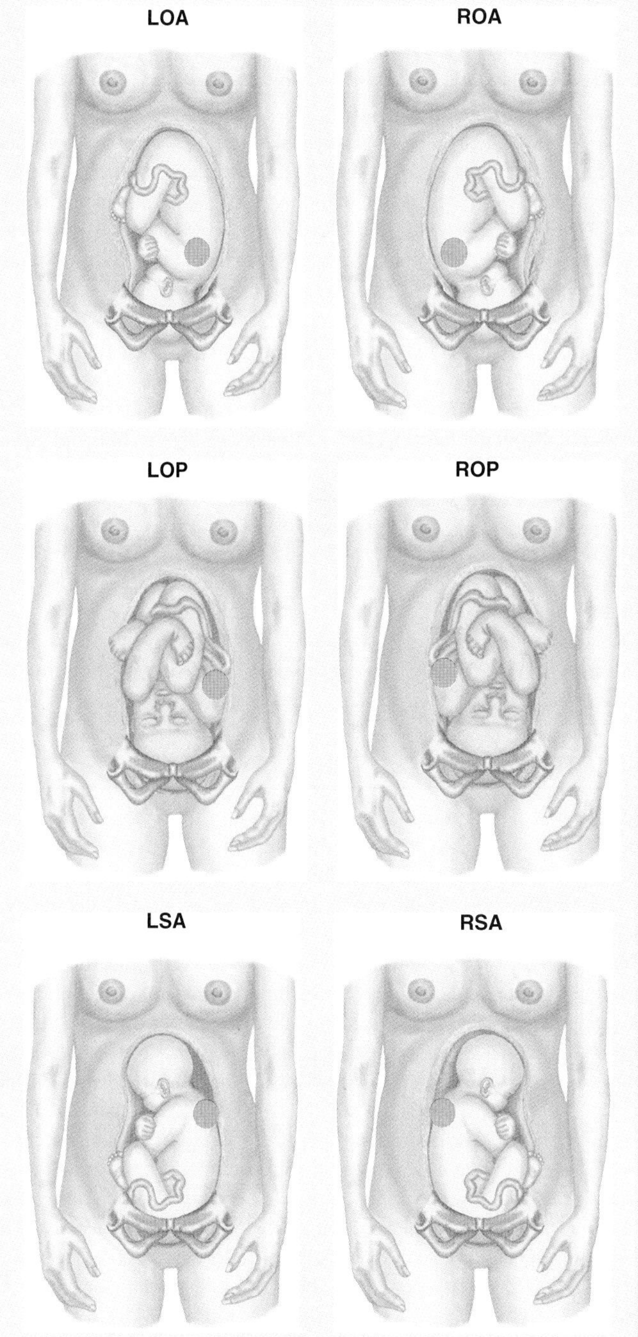


Modified from Feinstein, N. F., Sprague, A., & Trépanier, M. J. (Eds.), (2008). *Fetal heart rate auscultation* (2nd ed.). Washington, DC: Association of Women's Health, Obstetric and Neonatal Nurses; Simpson, K. R. (2008). Fetal assessment during labor. In K. R. Simpson & P. A. Creehan (Eds.), *AWHONN perinatal nursing* (3rd ed., pp. 339–442). Philadelphia: Lippincott Williams & Wilkins.

free to change position and walk, which is especially helpful during early labor or with a fetal occiput posterior position (see Chapter 16). She can use water-based methods of pain management, such as whirlpool baths or showers. The atmosphere is more natural than technologic, which is important to some families during their birth experience.

### Limitations

One disadvantage of IA and palpation as the primary method of fetal assessment is that FHR and uterine activity are assessed for a small part of the total labor. Labor contractions place stress on the fetus because of the normal decrease in blood flow to the placenta. Although FHR is assessed during some contractions, it is not recorded during every contraction. Continuous electronic or paper recording is not available on every Doppler to show the fetal response throughout labor or to identify subtle trends in the response.

Some women find that interruptions for auscultation are distracting. The pressure of the instrument on the abdomen is uncomfortable for some, and it may require several moves to locate the best place for auscultation with each assessment.

IA is staff intensive. Auscultation may not be a realistic option as the primary method of intrapartum fetal surveillance if the nurse-to-patient ratio must be greater than 1:1 for patients in normal labor. ACOG recommends continuous fetal monitoring in cases of high-risk conditions, such as diabetes or fetal growth restriction, in the woman or fetus (ACNM, 2010; ACOG, 2015b; Killion, 2015).

## EVALUATING AUSCULTATED FETAL HEART RATE DATA

Both the fetoscope and Doppler **transducer**, a device that translates one physical quantity into another, can be used to identify FHR baseline, rhythm, and changes from the baseline (see Table 17.1). Because the fetoscope detects actual fetal heart sounds, it is reliable for detecting fetal dysrhythmias. The Doppler transducer (and external fetal monitor if used for IA) also can be used to detect baseline, rhythm, and changes in the baseline. However, the Doppler transducer or external fetal monitor cannot be used to reliably detect fetal dysrhythmias. The fetoscope is rarely used in the United States, despite its reliability in evaluation of fetal dysrhythmias.

## ELECTRONIC FETAL MONITORING

EFM can be continuous, starting shortly after the woman is admitted, or **intermittent**, with a short recording made at regular intervals during labor, similar to auscultation.

The subjectivity of interpretation and use of varying descriptive terminology have made outcomes of research difficult to evaluate. A 2008 workshop was held to review and update definitions to describe EFM patterns and to make recommendations about a classification system for use in the United States. The most recent definitions are for visual interpretation of patterns, but the 2008 group recognized that computer programs for interpretation are being developed. Three categories, rather than the previous two categories, describe the fetus at that point in time and are not predictive of disorders such as cerebral palsy. Interventions may result in a change of the interpretation category (Macones, Hankins, Spong, et al., 2008). Guidelines from the Association of Women's Health, Obstetric and Neonatal Nurses (AWHONN) *Fetal Heart Monitoring: Principles and Practices* (Lyndon, O'Brien-Abel, & Simpson, 2015) and terminology from the National Institute of Child Health and Human Development (NICHD) workshops (2008) are used in a simplified form here.

### Advantages

The electronic monitor supplies more data about the fetus than auscultation and provides a permanent record that may be printed or stored electronically. Gradual trends in FHR and uterine activity are more apparent because the strip provides a graphic record for review. Continuous EFM shows the fetal response before, during, and after every contraction while it is in use rather than providing a sampling of fetal responses to contractions and between them. However, the many studies of IA versus EFM have found the two techniques equally valid for the low-risk fetus (ACOG, 2015a; Bashore & Koos, 2010).

The use of EFM is prevalent in U.S. births that occur in hospitals. Most women entering the hospital for birth expect electronic monitoring, even if their pregnancy has been low risk. The woman and support person may find the constant sound of the fetal heartbeat comforting. The coach can use the tracing of contractions on the monitor strip to help the woman anticipate the beginning and end of each contraction.

Electronic monitoring allows one nurse to observe two laboring women, primarily during uncomplicated early labor. A 1:1 nurse-to-patient ratio is needed during the second stage of labor or if high-risk conditions exist, regardless of the monitoring method used. Electronic monitoring gives the nurse more time for teaching and supporting the laboring woman with breathing and relaxation techniques if the nurse maintains the primary focus on the woman, not on the technology.

### Limitations

Reduced mobility is the major limitation of electronic fetal monitoring. Frequent maternal position changes or an active fetus may require constant adjustment of equipment to maintain a near-continuous trace. In addition, repositioning of the equipment is necessary as the baby moves downward in the pelvis during labor. The belts or stockinette used to keep sensors positioned properly for external monitoring are uncomfortable for some women, and obtaining a good trace is often difficult for the woman with a thick abdominal fat pad. A woman may concentrate on maintaining a good tracing rather than making herself comfortable or using a position to enhance fetal rotation and descent.

EFM and other procedures impart a technical air to the birth process and may be objectionable to a woman and her partner.

## ELECTRONIC FETAL MONITORING EQUIPMENT

EFM equipment consists of the bedside monitor unit and sensors for FHR and uterine activity. Sensors for each function may be either internal or external. Computer interfaces allow addition of chart annotations and admission and birth information and provide electronic storage of information. Models with **telemetry** (wireless transmission of data to the base for observation and storage) allow ambulation while monitoring.

Fetal monitor clocks should be synchronized throughout the unit, often by connection to an atomic clock. Using the fetal monitor clock to determine the birth time allows the most accurate reconstruction of the events of labor. In legal proceedings, the amount of time required to accomplish corrective interventions can make a difference in the defense of a lawsuit.

### Bedside Monitor Unit

The bedside fetal monitor unit uses the information from FHR and uterine activity sensors to provide a visual output in the form of a numeric display and a graphic strip. The strip may be printed by the monitor itself, similar to an electrocardiogram (ECG) strip, or viewed on a computer screen. The strip can be printed if electronic storage is not available in facilities that use a computer interface with the bedside monitor. Simultaneous monitoring of twins is possible for most fetal monitors.

### Paper Strip

Data regarding FHR and uterine activity can be displayed on paper using two horizontal grids—one for FHR and another for the uterine activity (Fig. 17.2). Each segment of paper between folds is numbered for identification and reassembly of a multipart strip. Time and date markers provide sequencing. Strips on computer screens have the same pattern.

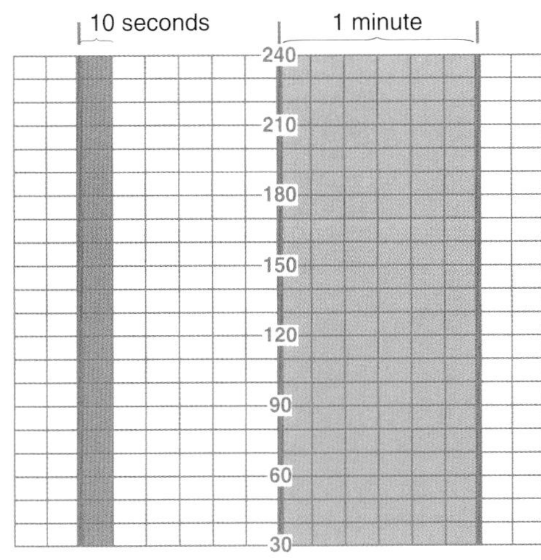


Upper grid for recording fetal heart rate. Vertically scaled in beats per minute (bpm)

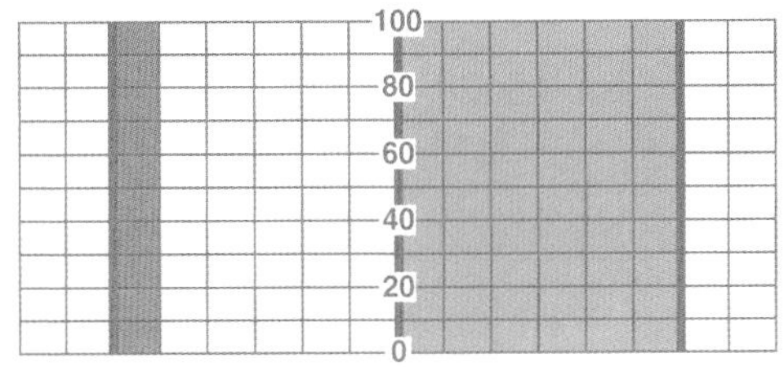


Lower grid for recording uterine activity. Vertically scaled in millimeters of mercury (mm Hg)

**FIG 17.2** Paper strip for recording electronic fetal monitoring data. Each dark vertical line represents 1 minute, and each lighter vertical line represents 10 seconds. Computerized displays that depict the fetal heart rate and uterine activity patterns have a similar appearance.

FHR is recorded on the upper grid. The range of recorded rates is from 30 to 240 beats per minute (bpm).

Uterine activity is recorded on the lower grid as bell-shaped curves with continuous smaller rises and falls that represent maternal breathing superimposed on the larger curve. Fetal movements, maternal coughing, vomiting, or position changes cause erratic curves or spikes on the uterine activity line. Contraction intensity and the degree of uterine muscle tension, or uterine resting tone (from 0 to 100 mm Hg), are recorded on the lower grid.

Vertical lines on both upper and lower grids are time divisions. At a paper speed of 3 cm per minute, dark vertical lines are 1 minute apart. Lighter lines subdivide the 1-minute divisions into six 10-second segments. The vertical lines are used to time the frequency and duration of contractions and to identify the fetal response to the contractions. The scroll speed of a screen display uses similar time divisions as a printed strip.

## Remote Surveillance

Many facilities have a display for each woman at central locations to allow surveillance when the nurse is not at the bedside. These units display the tracing on a screen and have settings for audible and visual alerts, such as an abnormal FHR or maternal blood pressure.

## Devices for External Fetal Monitoring

Both FHR and uterine activity can be monitored by external sensors (device that translates one physical quantity into another), or transducers. Transducers are secured on the mother's abdomen by elastic straps, a tube of wide stockinette, or an adhesive ring (Fig. 17.3). External devices are less accurate than internal ones but are noninvasive and suitable for most women in labor.

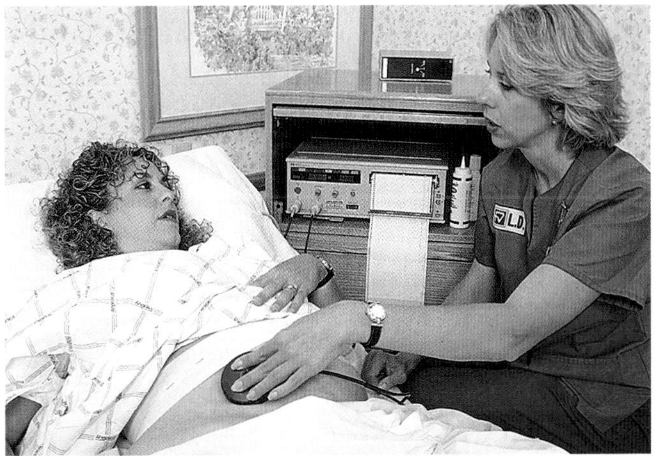

**FIG 17.3** The nurse applies the uterine activity transducer to the woman's upper abdomen, in the fundal area. The Doppler transducer for sensing the fetal heart rate is usually placed on her lower abdomen when the fetus is in the cephalic presentation.

### Fetal Heart Rate Monitoring With an Ultrasound Transducer

A Doppler ultrasound transducer detects fetal heart movement for rate calculation. It is similar to the hand-held Doppler unit. The transducer sends high-frequency sound waves into the uterus. The sound waves are reflected, and the monitor's computer continuously calculates FHR based on the movement sensed as the heart beats.

Fetal heart motion does not always correlate with electrical heart activity. Other movements, such as fetal or maternal activity or blood flow through the umbilical cord and the woman's aorta, also can be detected. Modern monitors ignore most of these extraneous sounds to provide a clean tracing.

The Doppler transducer produces a two-part sound with each heartbeat. Fetal or maternal activity produces a rough, erratic sound rather than the crisp, rhythmic sound characteristic of fetal heart motion. Fetal hiccups cause a "th-thump" sound at regular intervals that is superimposed on sounds created by heart activity. The volume can be adjusted or turned off.

### Monitoring Uterine Activity With a Tocotransducer

A tocotransducer ("toco") with a pressure sensor detects changes in abdominal contour to measure uterine activity. The uterus pushes outward against the mother's anterior abdominal wall with each contraction. The monitor calculates changes in this signal and prints them as bell- shaped curves on the lower grid of the strip.

Movement other than uterine activity also registers on the monitor. For example, maternal respirations superimpose a zigzag appearance on the uterine activity line. Other fetal or maternal movements appear as spikes on the uterine activity tracing.

Because uterine activity is sensed through the woman's abdomen, a tocotransducer is useful for observing the frequency and duration of contractions. It does not reliably measure internal contraction intensity and uterine resting tone. Factors that affect apparent intensity as printed on the strip include:

- *Fetal size.* A small fetus does not allow the uterus to push firmly against the abdominal wall with each contraction, making contractions appear less intense. In addition, an immature fetus floats in a relatively larger quantity of amniotic fluid than a term fetus if membranes are intact.
- *Abdominal fat thickness.* A thick layer of abdominal fat absorbs energy from uterine contractions, reducing their apparent

## PROCEDURE

### *External Fetal Monitor*

**Purposes**

To apply the electronic fetal monitor properly.

To perform a basic evaluation of the fetal heart rate (FHR) and uterine activity patterns to identify data needing further assessment by the experienced nurse, physician, or nurse-midwife.

1. Review agency policy for use of the electronic fetal monitor and how it interfaces with computer documentation.
2. Verify that the date and time for the monitor are accurate and consistent with computer documentation.
3. Perform a function test, following the manufacturer's instructions, to ensure that the bedside monitor unit is calibrated properly to give accurate data. Each manufacturer sets standards for indicators of proper function.
4. To decrease the woman's fear of the unknown, explain the basic procedure of electronic fetal monitoring to the woman and her partner or family. Teaching her that she can move with the monitor in place enhances her comfort and promotes normal labor. Vary instructions according to equipment used and hospital protocols. A sample is:
   a. Using the electronic fetal monitor does not mean that you or the baby has a problem. It is a common way we assess the baby's response to labor contractions.
   b. Two belts go around your abdomen—one for the fetal heart rate sensor and one for contractions (three belts are needed for most twin pregnancies).
   c. Feel free to move with the monitor on. If the tracing is poor, we can adjust the sensors.
5. Apply belts, an adhesive ring, or other method to secure the sensors:
   d. Slide both belts under the woman's back without the sensors attached. To enhance comfort, keep the belts smooth under her back.
   e. An additional belt that is tied in a knot rather than attached to the ultrasound transducer may apply pressure against the sensor to better maintain ideal tilt against the maternal abdomen. A folded or rolled washcloth, roll of tape, or other simple techniques may be used similarly to maintain the best tracing.
6. Use Leopold's maneuvers (see Chapter 16) to locate the fetus's back because the fetal heart rate is best detected through the back of the fetus.
7. Apply ultrasound gel to the Doppler ultrasound transducer because gel improves transmission and reception of the ultrasound waves to provide more accurate data. Place the transducer on the woman's abdomen at the approximate location of the fetal back. Move the transducer until a clear signal is heard, tilting the sensor slightly (without losing contact) if needed for a clear signal. Most bedside units have a flashing heart-shaped light or other indicator of a good signal. Continuously changing numbers indicate fluctuations of FHR.
8. Place the uterine activity sensor in the fundal area or the area where contractions feel the strongest when palpated because the external uterine activity monitor senses the change in the abdominal contour as the uterus rotates forward with each contraction. Contractions are usually strongest in the upper uterus. When the woman has a contraction, observe the tracing for the bell shape. The line for uterine activity is jagged because it also senses the rise and fall of the abdomen with breathing. Fetal or maternal movement causes a larger spike in the line. Observe through several contractions to verify correct placement, and improve placement if needed.
9. Observe the strip for baseline fetal heart rate, presence of variability, periodic changes, and uterine activity (contraction duration and frequency). Palpate contractions for intensity and relaxation between contractions to identify reassuring and nonreassuring fetal heart rate patterns (see Table 17.1). Contractions having a frequency greater than every 11/2 minutes (or 5 in 10 min), duration longer than 90 to 120 seconds, rest interval of less than 30 seconds, or incomplete uterine relaxation between contractions may reduce maternal blood flow into the intervillous spaces and impair exchange of oxygen and waste products. The external uterine activity sensor is useful for assessing contraction frequency and duration. It is not accurate for determining actual intensity or uterine resting tone.
10. Take corrective actions for nonreassuring patterns (p. 377). Notify the physician or nurse-midwife of nonreassuring patterns, corrective actions, and maternal and fetal responses. Document all calls, their content, and provider response.

intensity on the printed strip. Conversely, a thin woman whose uterus rotates sharply forward with each contraction may appear to have intense contractions when they are actually mild. Regular palpation of contractions should be done rather than relying only on the toco and contraction pattern.

- *Maternal position.* Different maternal positions may increase or decrease pressure against the transducer.
- *Location of the transducer.* Uterine activity is best detected where it is strongest and where the fetus lies close to the uterine wall. This location is usually over the upper uterus. Uterine contractions may not be detectable if the transducer is located elsewhere.

## Devices for Internal Fetal Monitoring

Accuracy is the main advantage of using internal devices for EFM, but their invasiveness slightly increases the risk of infection. Their use requires ruptured membranes and approximately 2 cm of cervical dilation.

### Fetal Heart Rate Monitoring With a Scalp Electrode

The fetal scalp electrode (FSE) detects electrical signals from the fetal heart (Fig. 17.4). Fetal or maternal movement interferes less with accuracy because the rate is calculated from electrical events in the fetal heart. The monitor unit generates a beeping sound with each fetal heartbeat, but the volume of the sound can be adjusted.

Areas to avoid for electrode application are the fetal face, fontanels, and genitals. The wire from the electrode protrudes from the mother's vagina and is attached to a leg plate to provide electrical grounding.

Because it barely penetrates the fetal skin (approximately 1 mm), the electrode is easily displaced. The tracing then becomes erratic or stops if the electrode is fully detached. Secure attachment of the electrode is often difficult if the fetus has thick hair. The electrode is removed by turning it counterclockwise approximately one and one half turns until it detaches.

### Uterine Activity Monitoring With an Intrauterine Pressure Catheter

Uterine activity, including contraction intensity and resting tone, can be measured using two types of intrauterine pressure catheters (IUPCs):

1. A solid catheter with a pressure transducer in its tip (Fig. 17.5) This catheter usually has an additional lumen for **amnioinfusion**, the infusion of sterile solution into the uterus (see p. 339).

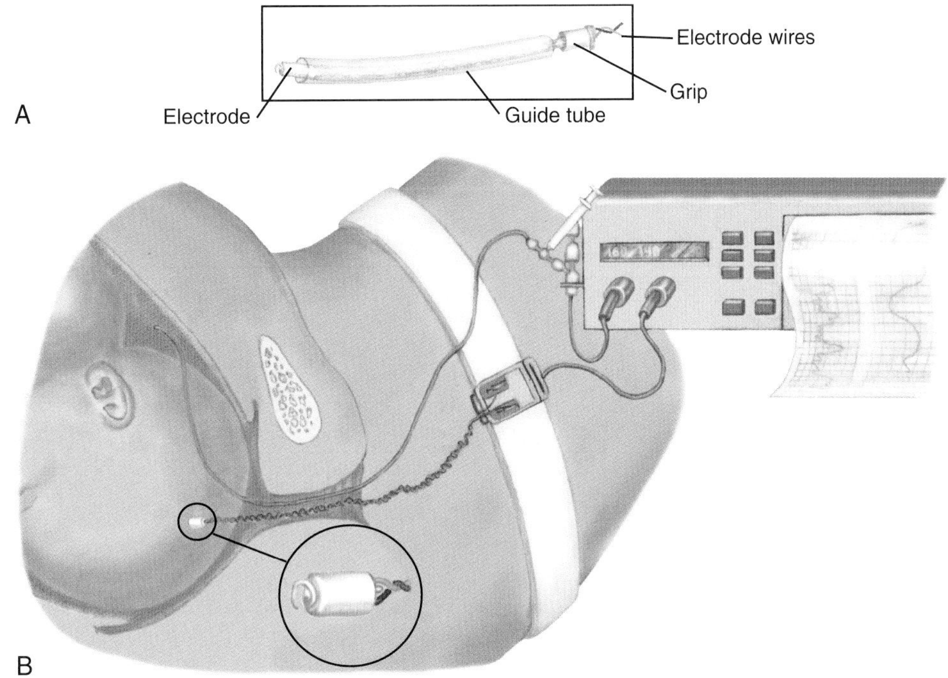


FIG 17.4 Fetal scalp electrode and intrauterine pressure catheter (IUPC). **A,** Parts of the fetal scalp electrode before it is applied. **B,** Fetal scalp electrode and IUPC in place and connected to the bedside monitor unit.

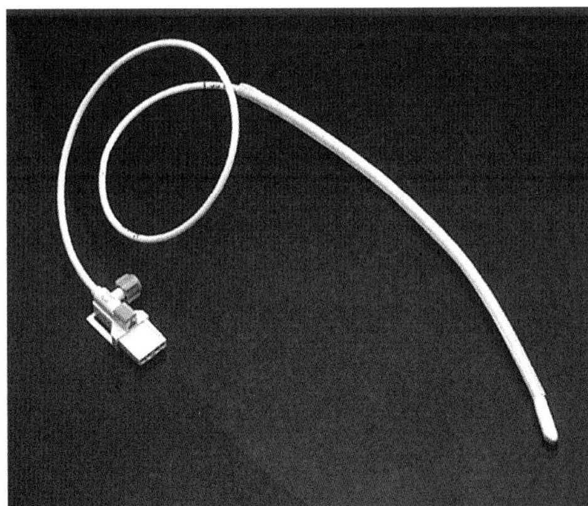

FIG 17.5 Intrauterine pressure catheter (IUPC) with transducer in its tip. This model has a lumen for amnioinfusion and is shown with its introducer over the catheter. The amnioinfusion port is on the side of the catheter connection and has a blue cap covering it when not in use. (Courtesy Utah Medical Products, Midvale, UT.)

2. A hollow, fluid-filled catheter that connects to a pressure transducer on the bedside monitor unit

Both types of IUPCs sense intrauterine pressure and increases in intraabdominal pressure, as with coughing or vomiting.

The solid catheter is not affected by height because its transducer is in the catheter. However, the sensor in its tip measures hydrostatic pressure from the amniotic fluid above the fetal presenting part as well as the pressure from uterine activity. Therefore, recorded intrauterine pressures from the solid catheter are higher than those from the fluid-filled catheter, and the nurse must consider this fact when assessing whether uterine activity is normal or hypertonic. The solid catheter is used more often than the fluid-filled catheter because it is simpler to use.

The tip of the fluid-filled catheter in the uterus should be at the level of the transducer on the outside for best accuracy. If the tip is lower than the transducer, the recorded pressure is lower than the actual intrauterine pressure. If the tip is higher, the recorded pressure may be artificially high. Changes in the mother's position may alter the height of the catheter tip, requiring adjustment of the transducer's height.

## EVALUATING ELECTRONIC FETAL MONITORING STRIPS

The nurse evaluates FHR tracing for baseline rate, variability, and any pattern of rate changes from the baseline. Uterine activity is evaluated by determining the frequency, duration, and intensity of contractions and by assessing uterine resting tone. FHR and uterine activity patterns must be evaluated together when assessing whether the fetal status is reassuring.

Other data relevant to strip interpretation are maternal vital signs; maternal position; drug, anesthetic, or oxygen administration; character of the amniotic fluid; labor status; and procedures performed. If paper charting is used, these are recorded on a paper strip as well as in the paper labor record. Computer systems that link charting and electronic FHR tracings reduce duplicate entries.

### Baseline Fetal Heart Rate

The FHR baseline is the average heart rate, rounded to 5 bpm, measured over 2 minutes of clear tracing within a 10-minute window. During this 2 or more minutes, the uterus must be at rest (Fig. 17.6), and episodes of significant increases or decreases in rate must not occur. The baseline also excludes periodic and nonperiodic changes (see Fig. 17.6) or segments of the baseline that differ by more than 25 bpm. The baseline rate is classified as follows (Lyndon, O'Brien-Abel, & Simpson, 2015; Macones et al., 2008):

- Normal—An average rate of 110 to 160 bpm. The preterm fetus at 26 to 28 weeks often has a rate at the upper end of this range

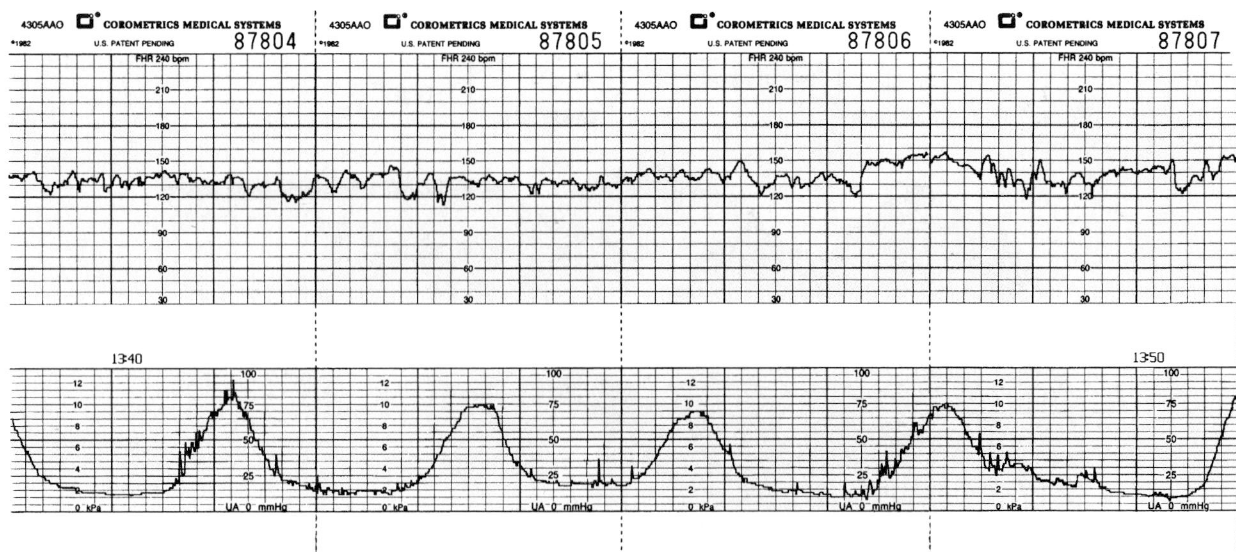


**FIG 17.6** Electronic fetal monitor strip showing a reassuring pattern of fetal heart rate and uterine activity. The baseline fetal heart rate averages 135 beats per minute (bpm), with a moderate variability of 10 bpm. An acceleration to 150 bpm is present. The contraction frequency is approximately every 2 to 3 minutes, duration is approximately 50 to 60 seconds, intensity is 75 to 90 mm Hg, and uterine resting tone is approximately 10 mm Hg. Fetal scalp electrode and intrauterine pressure catheter (IUPC) are being used. (Courtesy Corometrics Medical Systems, Inc., Wallingford, CT.)

because the parasympathetic nervous system, which slows the rate, is immature. Some healthy full-term fetuses have an average rate of 100 to 110 bpm.

- Bradycardia—Less than 110 bpm, persisting for at least 10 minutes.
- Tachycardia—More than 160 bpm, persisting for at least 10 minutes.

## Baseline FHR Variability

*Variability* describes fluctuations in the baseline FHR that cause the printed line to have an irregular wave-like appearance rather than a smooth, flat one (Fig. 17.7). Previous use of short-term (beat-to-beat) variability and long-term (broad fluctuations in rate over 1 minute) variability is no longer standard (Cunningham, Leveno, Bloom, et al., 2010; Macones et al., 2008).

Variability can be decreased by several nonpathologic and pathologic factors, such as (Cunningham et al., 2010; Killion, 2015):

- Fetal sleep
- Narcotics or other sedative drugs, such as magnesium sulfate, given to the woman
- Alcohol, illicit drugs
- Fetal tachycardia
- Gestation less than 28 weeks
- Fetal anomalies that affect central nervous system regulation of the heart rate, such as anencephaly
- Hypoxia that is severe enough to affect the central nervous system
- Abnormalities of the central nervous system, heart, or both
- Maternal acidemia (low blood pH) or hypoxemia (reduced oxygen in blood)

Variability occurs because multiple factors continuously speed and slow the fetal heart in a push-and-pull manner. Evaluation of variability helps clarify how a fetus is tolerating the stress of a pregnancy complication or labor, including factors that cause hypoxia. Variability is a significant component of FHR tracing on the electronic monitor, for two reasons:

Adequate oxygenation promotes normal function of the autonomic nervous system and helps the fetus adapt to the stress of labor.

Variability reflects the function of the fetal autonomic nervous system, especially the parasympathetic branch.

NICHD 2008 retains four categories of variability:

*Absent:* Undetectable
*Minimal:* Undetectable to ≤5 bpm
*Moderate:* 6 to 25 bpm
*Marked:* >25 bpm

## Periodic Patterns in FHR

Periodic patterns are temporary, recurrent changes from the baseline rate that are associated with uterine contractions. They include accelerations and decelerations. Periodic patterns are evaluated with respect to baseline characteristics (rate and variability).

### Accelerations

An acceleration is a temporary increase in FHR that peaks at least 15 bpm above the baseline and lasts at least 15 seconds (Fig. 17.8). Accelerations often occur with fetal movement. They may occur with vaginal examinations, uterine contractions, mild cord compression, and when the fetus is in a breech presentation. They may be nonperiodic (having no relation to contractions) as well as periodic. Accelerations are usually a reassuring sign, reflecting a fetus that has a responsive central nervous system and is not in acidosis.

The healthy preterm fetus may have shorter FHR accelerations less than 15 bpm. Before 32 weeks of gestation, an increase in FHR that peaks at least 10 bpm above the baseline and lasts at least 10 seconds is considered an acceleration. Variations in FHR in a fetus younger than 28 weeks may appear relatively flat because of autonomic nervous system immaturity.

Accelerations lasting longer than 2 minutes but less than 10 minutes are prolonged accelerations. Accelerations that last 10 minutes or longer are either a change in the baseline rate or a reflection of the merging of several accelerations that later return to the previous baseline.

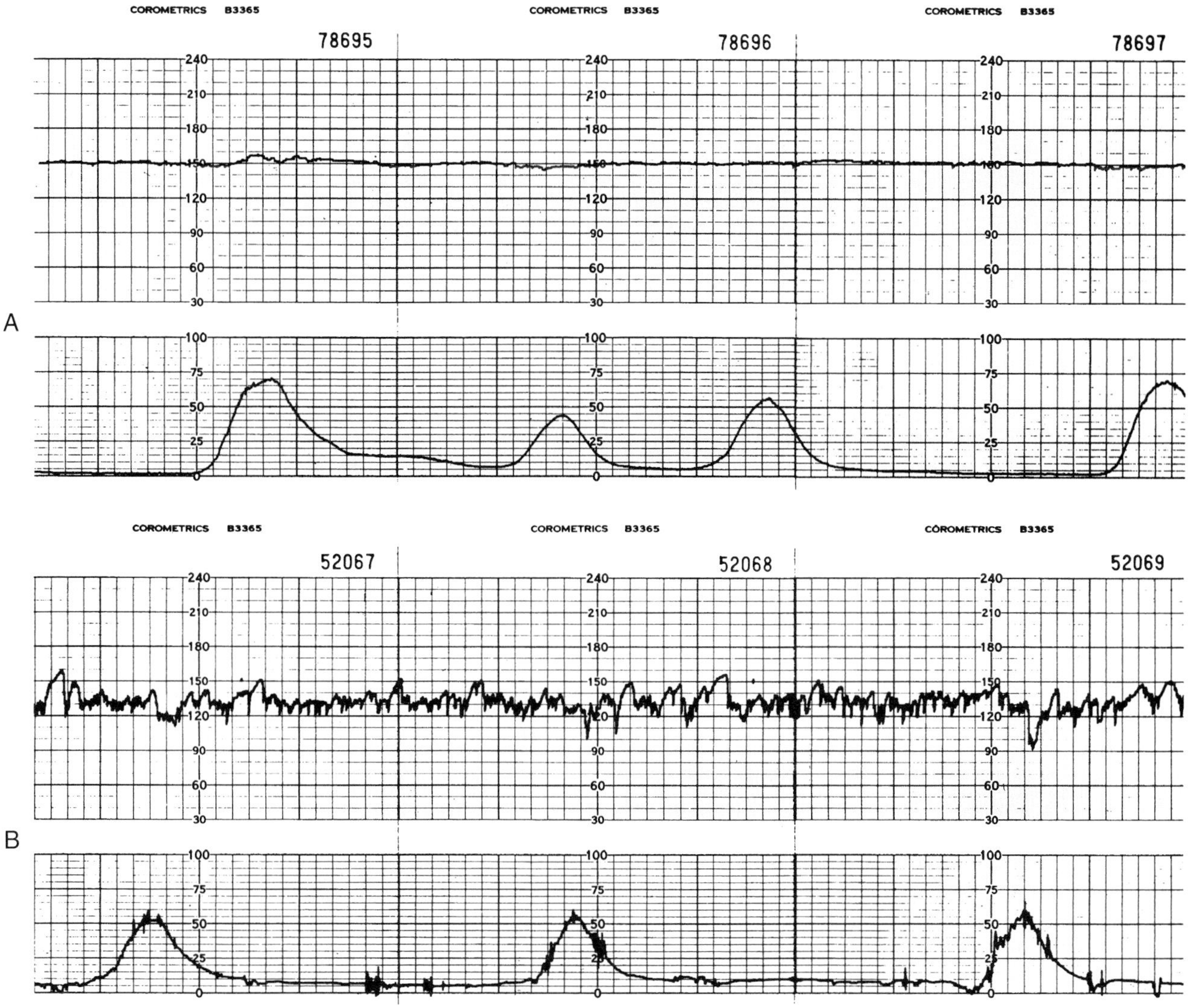

A

B

FIG 17.7 Contrasts in fetal heart rate variability. A fetal scalp electrode is being used. **A,** Minimal variability (less than 5 beats per minute [bpm]). Note the smooth, flat line in the *upper graph* for the fetal heart rate. **B,** Moderate variability (average 20 bpm variability). Note the zigzag appearance of the fetal heart rate line compared with the flat appearance in **A.** (Courtesy Corometrics Medical Systems, Inc., Wallingford, CT.)

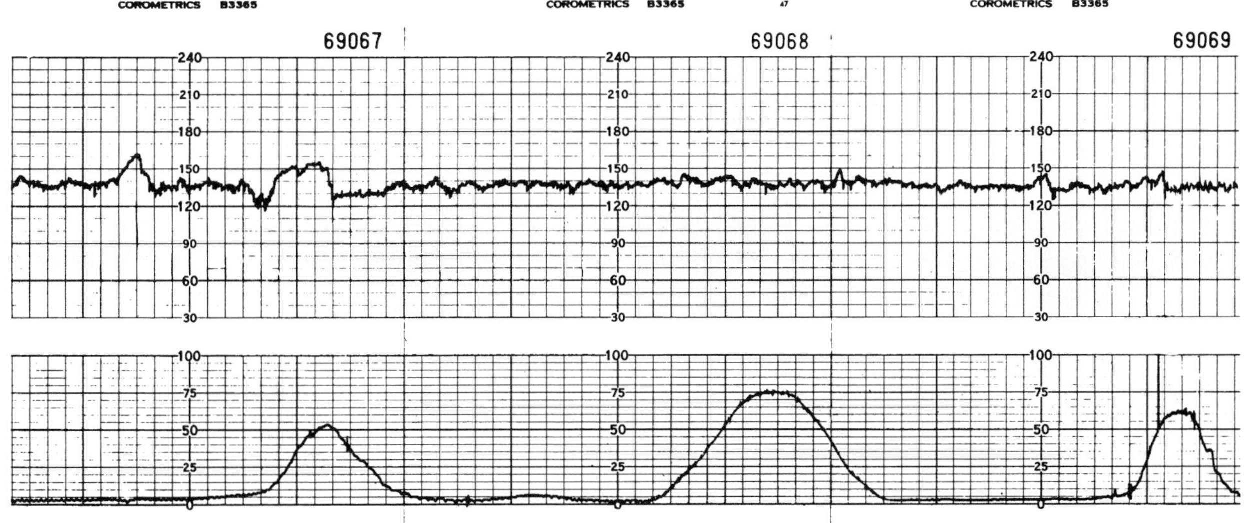


FIG 17.8 Accelerations in the fetal heart rate. (Courtesy Corometrics Medical Systems, Inc., Wallingford, CT.)

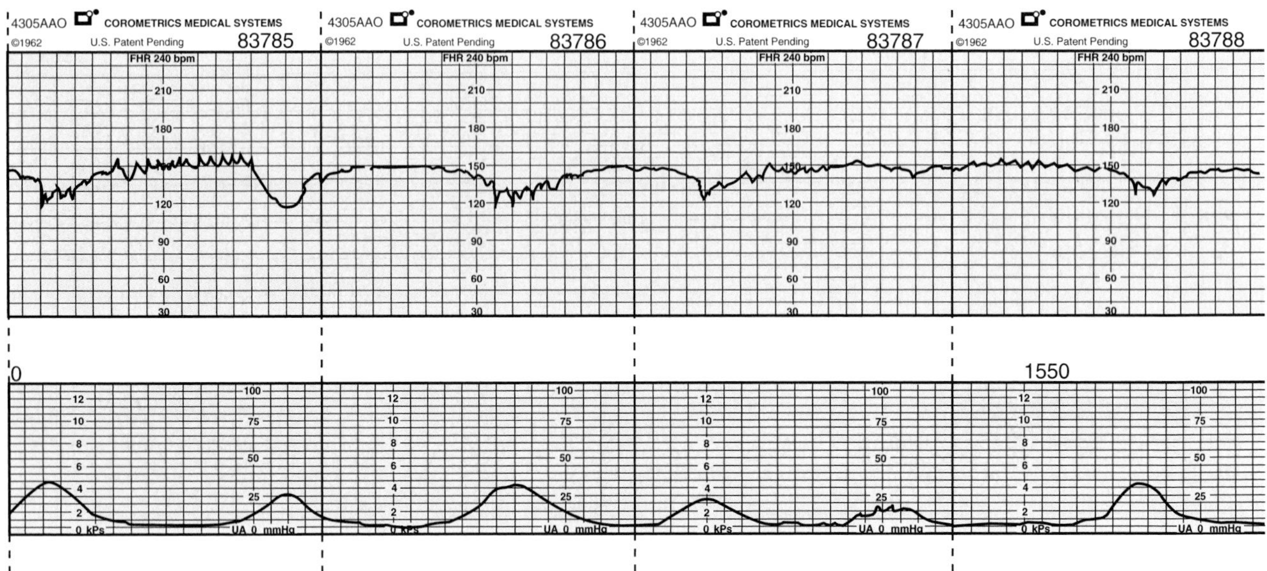

**FIG 17.9** Early decelerations. The slowing of the fetal heart rate is gradual, and the nadir of the deceleration occurs at the peak of the contraction. It returns to the baseline by the end of the contraction. Cause: fetal head compression. (Courtesy Corometrics Medical Systems, Inc., Wallingford, CT.)

### Decelerations

Periodic decelerations are classified into three types, based on their shape and relationship to uterine contractions.

***Early decelerations.*** Fetal head compression for any reason increases intracranial pressure, causing the vagus nerve to slow the heart rate. Early decelerations are not associated with fetal compromise and require no intervention. They occur during contractions as the fetal head is pressed against the woman's pelvis or soft tissues such as the cervix and are common during the second stage.

Early decelerations are consistent in appearance; they are uniform in that one early deceleration looks similar to others. They mirror the contraction, gradually falling from the baseline and gradually returning to the baseline by the end of the contraction (Fig. 17.9). The nadir (low point) of FHR occurs at the same time the contraction peaks. The rate at the nadir is usually no lower than 30 to 40 bpm from the baseline.

***Late decelerations.*** Impaired exchange of oxygen and waste products in the placenta (uteroplacental insufficiency) may result in a pattern of late (delayed) decelerations. Poor oxygen availability in the placenta requires a shift to anaerobic metabolism, resulting in acidemia that depresses cardiac function. The cause of uteroplacental insufficiency may be acute and transient, such as maternal hypotension or excessive uterine stimulation (tachysystole). It also may occur with chronic conditions that impair placental exchange, such as maternal hypertension or diabetes.

Although late decelerations are not reassuring, other signs can suggest whether the fetus is tolerating the uteroplacental insufficiency. A normal baseline rate with moderate variability and presence of accelerations suggests that the fetus is tolerating the conditions. However, the fetal reserves eventually will be depleted if the cause is not corrected, and reassuring signs will disappear.

Late decelerations look similar to early decelerations but are shifted to the right in relation to the contraction. They have a consistent and often subtle appearance in that one late deceleration looks similar to others. Late decelerations gradually fall from the baseline and gradually return *after* the contraction ends (Fig. 17.10). The FHR nadir occurs after the contraction peaks. The rate at the nadir is usually 5 to 30 bpm lower than the baseline rate and rarely lower than 40 bpm below baseline.

**SAFETY ALERT**

***Differences Between Early and Late Decelerations***

**Both Early and Late Decelerations**

- Decrease from the baseline fetal heart rate (FHR) and return to baseline gradually (onset to nadir of at least 30 sec)
- Occur with contractions
- Decrease at a rate rarely more than 30–40 beats per minute (bpm) below the baseline

**Early Decelerations**

- Are mirror images of the contraction (lowest point in FHR occurs with the peak of the contraction)
- Return to the baseline FHR by the end of the contraction
- Are usually unaffected with respect to pattern by maternal position changes
- Are associated with fetal head compression
- Are not associated with fetal compromise and require no added interventions

**Late Decelerations**

- Look similar to early decelerations but begin after the contraction begins (often near the peak).
- Are characterized by the occurrence of the nadir after the contraction peak.
- May remain in the normal range of deceleration and may not fall far from the baseline.
- Reflect possible impaired placental exchange (uteroplacental insufficiency).
- That are occasional, accompanied by moderate variability and accelerations, are not ominous.
- Should be addressed by nursing interventions to improve placental blood flow and fetal oxygen supply if persistent, especially with no accelerations and absent or minimal variability.

The FHR may remain in the normal range and may not fall much below its baseline level. The magnitude of the decrease in rate from baseline does not indicate the degree of uteroplacental insufficiency.

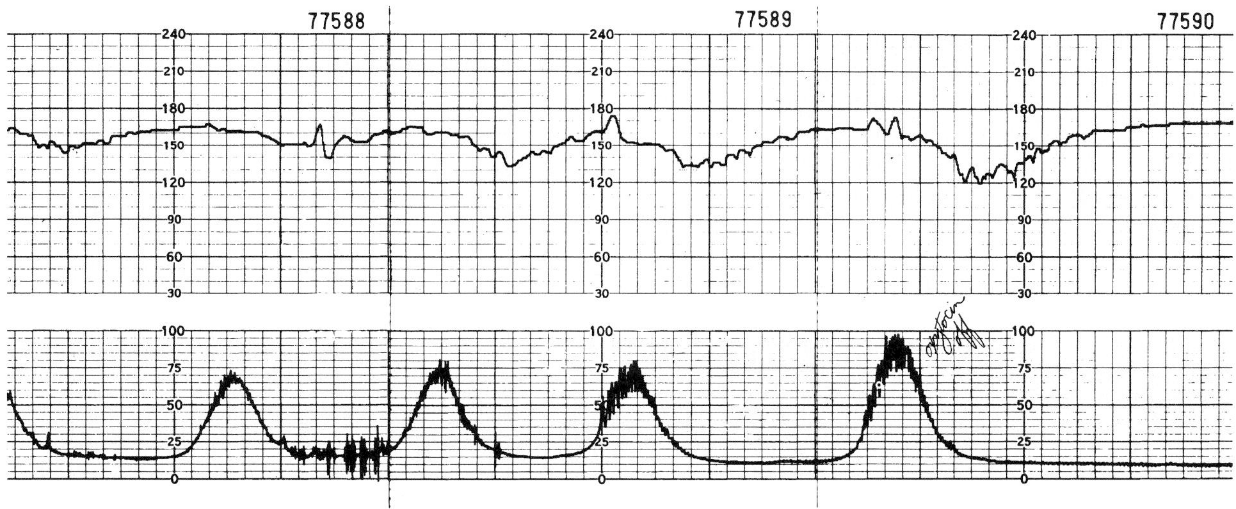


FIG 17.10 Late decelerations. Note that the decelerations look similar to early decelerations but are offset to the right. They begin at approximately the peak of the contraction, and the nadir occurs well after the peak of the contraction, often during the interval. Cause: uteroplacental insufficiency. (Courtesy Corometrics Medical Systems, Inc., Wallingford, CT.)

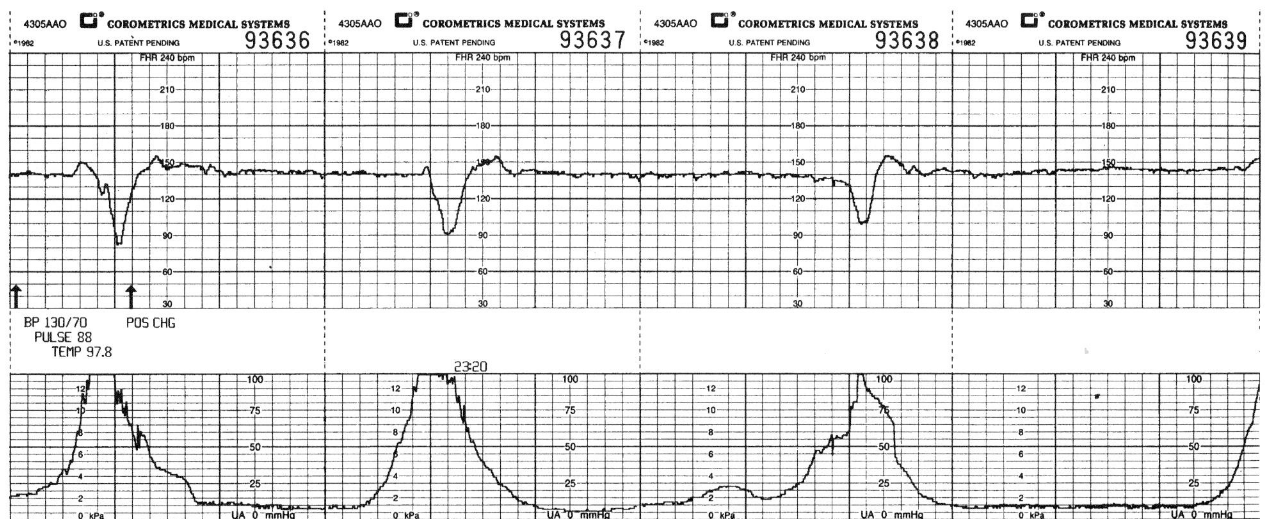


FIG 17.11 Variable decelerations. The decelerations are sharp in onset and offset. Note slight rate accelerations (shoulders) after each variable deceleration. These variable decelerations are periodic in that they occur during contractions. Cause: umbilical cord compression. (Courtesy Corometrics Medical Systems, Inc., Wallingford, CT.)

***Variable decelerations.*** Conditions that reduce flow through the umbilical cord result in variable decelerations. These decelerations do not have the uniform appearance of early and late decelerations. Their shape, duration, and degree of fall below baseline rate are variable. They fall and rise abruptly (within 30 seconds) with the onset and relief of cord compression, unlike the gradual fall and rise of early and late decelerations (Fig. 17.11). Variable decelerations also may be nonperiodic, occurring at times unrelated to contractions.

## Uterine Activity

Uterine activity is assessed using four components: frequency, duration, and intensity of the contractions; and uterine resting tone.

Palpation is used to estimate contraction intensity and uterine resting tone if uterine activity is monitored externally (see Procedure: External Fetal Monitor, p. 338). Contraction frequency and duration are measured with EFM as with palpation (beginning of one contraction to beginning of the next). Contraction intensity is described as *mild, moderate,* or *strong*. The uterus should relax between contractions for at least 30 seconds.

With the IUPC, the scale on the strip is used to describe intensity and resting tone. Contraction intensity changes as labor progresses. Average resting tone is 5 to 15 mm Hg. Contraction intensity with the IUPC is approximately 50 to 75 mm Hg during labor, although it may reach 110 mm Hg with pushing during the second stage.

Montevideo units (MVUs) may be used to describe contraction intensity (in mm Hg) when an IUPC is used. The MVU is calculated by noting the contraction intensity above the resting tone and multiplying by the number of contractions in 10 minutes. For example, if a woman has three contractions in 10 minutes, each of which has an intensity of 110 mm Hg and a resting tone of 15 mm Hg, the result in MVUs is 285. Excess uterine activity during labor would be 400 MVUs (Killion, 2015).

## SIGNIFICANCE OF FHR PATTERNS

The two previously used categories were reassuring and nonreassuring. The 2008 NICHD conference report has divided interpretations into the following three categories to guide needed interventions (Macones et al., 2008):

- Category I: Normal (reassuring)
- Category II: Indeterminate (often described as equivocal or ambiguous data)
- Category III: Abnormal (nonreassuring)

For category II patterns (equivocal or ambiguous patterns) or for questionable IA data, several methods may be used to further evaluate the fetal condition. Table 17.1 summarizes reassuring and nonreassuring patterns.

### Reassuring Patterns

Reassuring patterns, such as accelerations, often with fetal movement, are associated with fetal well-being. The nurse need only support optimal oxygenation because the patterns suggest that the fetus is tolerating intrapartum stressors.

### Indeterminate Patterns

Indeterminate patterns are those that do not clearly fall into reassuring or nonreassuring. Indeterminate patterns, often referred to as equivocal or ambiguous, have elements of reassuring characteristics but also data that may be nonreassuring. Examples include (Macones et al., 2008):

- Tachycardia
- Bradycardia with presence of variability
- Minimal or marked baseline variability
- Absent variability with no recurrent decelerations
- Absence of accelerations after fetal stimulation
- Periodic or episodic variations such as:
  - Recurrent variable decelerations accompanied by minimal or moderate baseline variability
  - Prolonged deceleration 2 minutes or longer but less than 10 minutes
  - Recurrent late decelerations with moderate baseline variability
  - Variable decelerations with other characteristics such as slow return to baseline and accelerations preceding or following ("overshoots," or "shoulders")

Numerous nurses, nurse-midwives, and physicians are seeking management guidelines for the many patterns described in category II (Parer & King, 2010).

### Nonreassuring Patterns

Category III includes nonreassuring patterns and those in which favorable signs are absent or signs associated with fetal hypoxia or acidosis are present. Nonreassuring patterns do not necessarily indicate that fetal hypoxia or acidosis has occurred. They indicate that steps should be taken to identify possible causes of the patterns and correct them.

Nonreassuring patterns are more significant if they occur together and are persistent. For example, bradycardia with variability of less than 5 bpm and late decelerations suggests greater physiologic stress than bradycardia with normal variability of the heart rate. The healthy fetus may demonstrate an occasional late deceleration, but a persistent pattern of late decelerations is more likely to represent compromise in a fetus. Nonreassuring patterns include but are not limited to:

- Absent baseline variability and
  - Recurrent late decelerations
  - Recurrent variable decelerations
  - Bradycardia
- Sinusoidal pattern, a visually undulating pattern (rare)

Hypertonic uterine activity (tachysystole), whether spontaneous or stimulated by drugs, may be a contributor to patterns that fall in the indeterminate or nonreassuring categories.

Nonreassuring patterns do not always indicate that labor should end immediately. Several interventions may be used to clarify the fetal condition and to determine the best course of action. Other interventions may increase fetal oxygenation, allowing the fetal heart patterns to return to normal.

**SAFETY ALERT**

***Nursing Responses to Nonreassuring Fetal Heart Rate Patterns***

1. Identify the cause of the nonreassuring pattern to plan appropriate interventions:
   - Evaluate characteristics of the pattern that are nonreassuring (late or variable decelerations, bradycardia or tachycardia, absent or minimal variability). Determine if combinations of nonreassuring characteristics are present (i.e., late decelerations with minimal variability).
   - Evaluate maternal vital signs to identify hypotension, hypertension, or fever that may contribute to the fetal response associated with a nonreassuring pattern.
   - If indicated, perform a vaginal examination to identify a prolapsed umbilical cord. Do not perform a vaginal examination if there is active vaginal bleeding, diagnosed placenta previa, preterm labor or preterm premature rupture of the membranes, or a high risk for infection.
2. Stop oxytocin or other uterine stimulants. A tocolytic such as terbutaline may be ordered.
3. Reposition the woman, avoiding the supine position, for patterns associated with cord compression. Repositioning often improves other nonreassuring patterns as well.
4. Increase the rate of infusion of a nonadditive intravenous fluid to expand the mother's blood volume and improve placental perfusion.
5. Administer oxygen by facemask at 8 to 10 L/min to increase maternal blood oxygen saturation, making more oxygen available to the fetus. Maternal pulse oximetry, available on many fetal monitors, allows ongoing assessment of maternal oxygen saturation and documentation on the strip if the information is crucial.
6. Consider starting continuous EFM with internal devices if no contraindication exists.
7. Notify the physician or nurse-midwife as soon as possible, or ask another nurse to notify. Report and document the following:
   - The pattern that was identified
   - Nursing interventions taken in response to the pattern
   - The fetal response after nursing interventions
   - The response of the physician or nurse-midwife (orders, other response)
8. If the nonreassuring pattern is severe, other staff members should be alerted to the possibility of immediate delivery (usually cesarean birth, unless operative vaginal birth is possible and quicker). Birth preparation should include staff prepared for neonatal resuscitation.

**TABLE 17.1 Reassuring (Normal) and Nonreassuring (Abnormal) Fetal Surveillance Assessments**

**REASSURING (NORMAL) ASSESSMENTS**

Baseline FHR: Stable, rate 110–160 bpm Moderate variability (6–25 bpm); Accelerations: Peaking at least 15 bpm above the baseline with a duration of 15 sec or more (10 bpm and 10 sec if gestation 32 weeks or less) Variable decelerations of less than 60 sec with rapid return to baseline, accompanied by normal baseline rate and moderate variability; *Uterine Activity:* Contraction frequency: No more frequent than every 1.5 min (or 5 within 10 min); Contraction duration: No longer than 90–120 sec; Interval between contractions: At least 30 sec; Uterine resting tone: Uterus relaxed between contractions (by palpation when intermittent auscultation or external fetal monitoring is used), uterine resting tone <20 mm Hg (with IUPC); Montevideo units <400

**NONREASSURING (ABNORMAL) ASSESSMENTS**

| Pattern and Description | Possible Cause or Causes |
|---|---|
| ***Tachycardia*** | |
| Baseline FHR >160 bpm for at least 10 min | Maternal fever (fetal tachycardia may precede fever or other signs of infection)<br>Maternal dehydration<br>Maternal or fetal hypoxia<br>Fetal acidosis<br>Maternal or fetal hypovolemia<br>Fetal cardiac dysrhythmias<br>Maternal severe anemia<br>Maternal hyperthyroidism<br>Drugs administered to mother (such as terbutaline, bronchodilators, decongestants, stimulant drugs) |
| ***Bradycardia*** | |
| Baseline FHR <110 bpm for at least 10 min<br>Baseline rates between 100 and 110 bpm are usually not associated with fetal compromise if there are no nonreassuring patterns | Fetal head compression<br>Fetal hypoxia, fetal acidosis, fetal heart block, umbilical cord compression, late second-stage labor with maternal pushing |
| ***Decreased or Absent Variability*** | |
| FHR baseline has a smooth, flat appearance | Fetal sleep episodes (usually 40 min or less; occasionally as long as 2 hr)<br>Fetal hypoxia with acidosis<br>Drug effects:<br>CNS depressants<br>Local anesthetic agents |
| ***Late Decelerations*** | |
| Gradual decelerations having a uniform appearance and a consistent relation to the contraction onset to nadir of 30 sec or longer<br>Nadir occurs after the peak of the contraction | Uteroplacental insufficiency, which may be secondary to:<br>Maternal hypotension or hypertension, excess uterine activity (spontaneous or stimulated)<br>Placental interruption, such as abruptio placentae or placenta previa<br>Maternal diabetes<br>Maternal severe anemia<br>Maternal cardiac disease |
| ***Variable Decelerations*** | |
| Sharp in onset and offset<br>May occur as a periodic or nonperiodic (random) pattern<br>Nonreassuring if:<br>Fall to less than 60 bpm for more than 60 sec<br>Return to baseline prolonged<br>Overshoots (exceeding baseline after deceleration) are present<br>Accompanied by tachycardia and/or loss of variability | Umbilical cord compression, which may be secondary to:<br>Prolapsed cord<br>Nuchal cord (around fetal neck)<br>Cord around fetal body parts<br>Oligohydramnios (abnormally small amount of amniotic fluid)<br>Cord between fetus and mother's uterus or pelvis, without obvious prolapse<br>Knot in cord |

*Bpm,* Beats per minute; *CNS,* central nervous system; *FHR,* fetal heart rate; *IUPC,* intrauterine pressure catheter

## Clarification of Data

Three methods may be used during the intrapartum period: fetal scalp stimulation, vibroacoustic stimulation (VAS), and fetal scalp blood sampling. A fourth method, analysis of umbilical cord blood gases and pH, is done immediately after birth. Fetal pulse oximetry was used a relatively short time but is described here.

***Fetal scalp stimulation.*** Scalp stimulation evaluates the fetus's response to tactile stimulation during labor (Fig. 17.12). This procedure may be performed by a nurse, physician, or nurse-midwife. The examiner applies pressure to the scalp (or other presenting part) with a gloved finger or fingers and sweeps the fingers in a circular motion. An acceleration in FHR of 15 bpm for at least 15 seconds is a reassuring response in the term fetus, suggesting normal oxygen

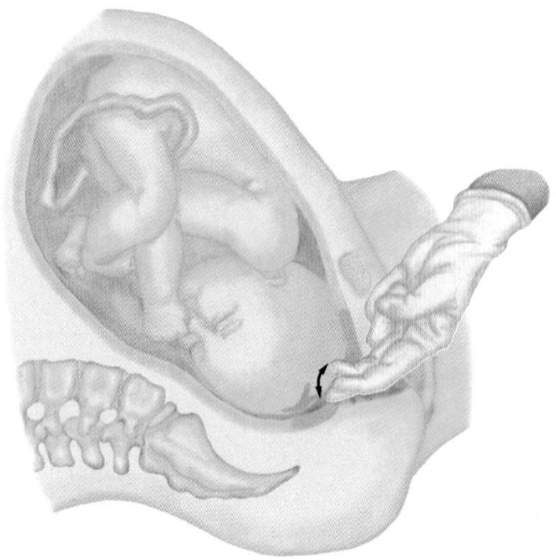

FIG 17.12 Fetal scalp stimulation assesses the fetal response to gentle massage. An acceleration in the fetal heart rate of 15 beats per minute for 15 seconds suggests that the fetus is in normal oxygen and acid–base balance. Accelerations often occur with vaginal examination unrelated to nonreassuring fetal heart rate patterns.

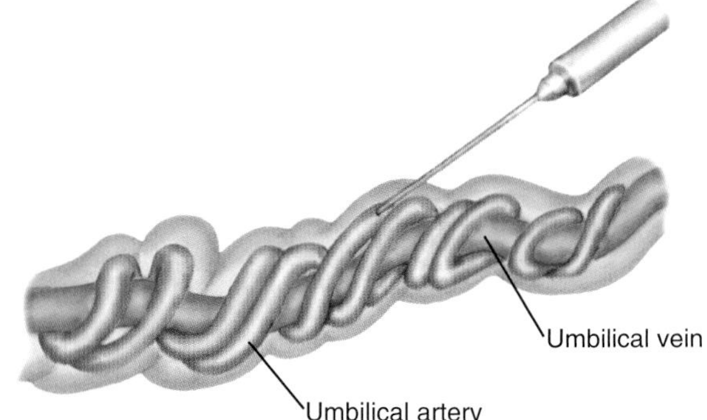


FIG 17.13 Obtaining a blood sample to determine umbilical cord blood gas values and pH. Samples are drawn from the umbilical artery and vein. Arterial samples most closely reflect fetal oxygen and acid–base status. The samples in capped syringes may be kept for up to 60 minutes at room temperature.

and acid–base balance. The acceleration may be delayed rather than immediate.

Fetal scalp stimulation is not done in some cases. These situations are similar to those in which vaginal examination should be restricted, such as:

- Preterm fetus (may cause or intensify contractions; may rupture intact membranes)
- Prolonged rupture of membranes (higher risk of infection)
- Chorioamnionitis (intrauterine infection)
- Placenta previa (may cause hemorrhage)
- Maternal fever of unknown origin (possibility of introducing microorganisms into the uterus)

***VAS.*** Acoustic stimulation, or VAS, may be used by the nurse, physician, or nurse-midwife to supplement fetal scalp stimulation or if scalp stimulation is contraindicated. Because of its simplicity and noninvasive nature, VAS is common.

A stimulator that uses a combination of sound and vibration is applied to the mother's lower abdomen and is turned on for up to 3 seconds. The reassuring response is the same as with fetal scalp stimulation: an acceleration in FHR of 15 bpm for 15 seconds or more. However, an absent response does not necessarily mean that the fetus is hypoxic or in acidosis.

***Fetal scalp blood sampling.*** This procedure is more complex than other intrapartum techniques and requires rupture of membranes. Normal scalp pH is 7.25 to 7.35. Acidosis is present if the pH is less than 7.20, and the clinician may hasten the birth by using forceps or cesarean delivery.

***Cord blood gases and pH.*** Umbilical cord blood analysis is used to assess the infant's acid-base balance immediately after birth rather than during labor. The samples are analyzed for pH, $PCO_2$, oxygen partial pressure ($PO_2$), and bicarbonate and for base deficit. This information helps identify whether acidosis exists and whether it is respiratory (short term), metabolic (prolonged), or mixed. Normal cord blood gases and pH can confirm that the fetus was adjusting normally to the stresses of labor, although the fetal monitoring pattern may have been nonreassuring or the 5-minute Apgar score low (see Table 16.3).

The cord is promptly double-clamped immediately after birth and cut to isolate a 10- to 30-cm (4- to 12-inch) segment. Arterial cord blood best reflects fetal oxygenation and acid-base status because this blood is leaving the fetus on its way to the placenta and should be drawn first. Blood is drawn into heparinized syringes to prevent coagulation; air is expelled, and the syringes are capped to avoid altering values by exposure to room air (Fig. 17.13). Venous blood is the second sample drawn. Samples should be carefully labeled as containing arterial or venous cord blood. Samples kept at room temperature are stable up to 60 minutes; they should be kept on ice if there is a delay beyond this time (AAP & ACOG, 2012; ACOG, 2015b; Cypher, 2015).

### Interventions for Nonreassuring Patterns

Any of several nursing and medical interventions may be indicated if a clearly nonreassuring (category III) FHR pattern is present. In addition, such interventions often are used for those of category II. All are directed toward identifying the cause of the nonreassuring pattern and improving fetal oxygenation.

***Identifying the cause of a nonreassuring pattern.*** Careful examination of the strip may suggest a cause for the nonreassuring FHR pattern and indicate direct interventions most likely to correct the presumed problem. For example, a pattern of recurrent late decelerations suggests uteroplacental insufficiency. However, uteroplacental insufficiency may be secondary to a number of conditions, such as maternal hypotension or excess uterine activity. Different causative conditions may require different corrective interventions. Checking the mother's vital signs may disclose hypotension, hypertension, or fever. Fetal tachycardia often precedes maternal fever. Maternal sedative medications may alter variability in a well-oxygenated fetus.

A vaginal examination may reveal a prolapsed cord, which can cause variable decelerations, bradycardia, or both, as it is compressed (see Chapter 27). A vaginal examination also evaluates the woman's labor status, which helps the birth attendant decide whether labor should continue or be ended with a cesarean birth.

***Increasing placental perfusion.*** The woman is positioned on her side to eliminate aortocaval compression, which reduces placental blood flow. Giving a bolus of isotonic intravenous fluid such as lactated Ringer's solution increases the maternal blood volume, which in turn improves perfusion of the placenta if hypotension develops secondary to regional block (see "Epidural Block," p. 362, in Chapter 18).

Uterine activity reduces blood flow into the intervillous spaces, and a fetus with little reserve for stress may be unable to tolerate even normal contractions. Persistent excess uterine activity may compromise a fetus with normal reserves. If a woman is receiving oxytocin, it is discontinued so that uterine activity is not stimulated. A tocolytic drug, such as terbutaline (0.125 to 0.25 mg intravenously or 0.25 mg subcutaneously), may be given to reduce uterine activity.

***Increasing maternal blood oxygen saturation.*** Administration of 100% oxygen at 8 to 10 L/min through a snug facemask makes more oxygen available for transfer to the fetus.

***Reducing cord compression.*** If cord compression is suspected, the woman is repositioned. She may be turned from side to side, or her hips may be elevated to shift the fetal presenting part toward her diaphragm. Several position changes may be required before the pattern improves or resolves. The fetal presenting part may be pushed upward slightly. See also Chapter 27 for information regarding umbilical cord prolapse, an intrapartum emergency.

Amnioinfusion, or infusion of sterile isotonic solution into the uterus, can be used to increase the fluid around the fetus and cushion the cord and reduce the likelihood of cesarean birth. Lactated Ringer's solution or normal saline is infused into the uterus through an IUPC. Amnioinfusion has been used to wash out or dilute fluid heavily stained with meconium, but evidence of its effectiveness for this purpose has been mixed (Bashore & Koos, 2010; Cunningham et al., 2010).

## NURSING CARE

### The Woman Having Intrapartum Fetal Monitoring

Either fetal heart auscultation with palpation or electronic monitoring is acceptable for low-risk women, but EFM is preferred for women with risk factors. The assessment frequency changes with risk status. The nurse may identify any of several problems if a woman has EFM. The woman or couple who prefer a nontechnical environment for birth may encounter a decision conflict because EFM may be needed for a problem. Anxiety is likely if the woman does not understand the electronic monitor or if problems develop. The complication of preterm rupture of membranes or preterm labor may heighten anxiety. Pain may be increased if mobility is restricted during labor.

Two nursing care needs related to intrapartum fetal monitoring are the woman's (or couple's) learning needs and an expansion of nursing care related to fetal oxygenation. Care related to fetal monitoring by either electronic means or auscultation should be combined with that for normal or complicated intrapartum nursing as needed.

## LEARNING NEEDS

### Assessment

Determine what the woman and her partner already know about fetal surveillance during labor. Does she believe that use of the electronic monitor (Fig. 17.14) indicates the development of a complication, or does she expect its use? Is the woman comfortable with intermittent FHR auscultation and palpation of contractions for fetal assessment? Which method is her preference?

Lack of knowledge contributes to anxiety. Note the anxiety level of the woman and her partner when the electronic monitor is used. For example, is the woman afraid to move because the fetal heart sounds and tracing skip at that time? Does she place the monitor's data above her own comfort? Note questions about the monitor and its data. Reassess after teaching to identify information that is still unclear or causing anxiety.

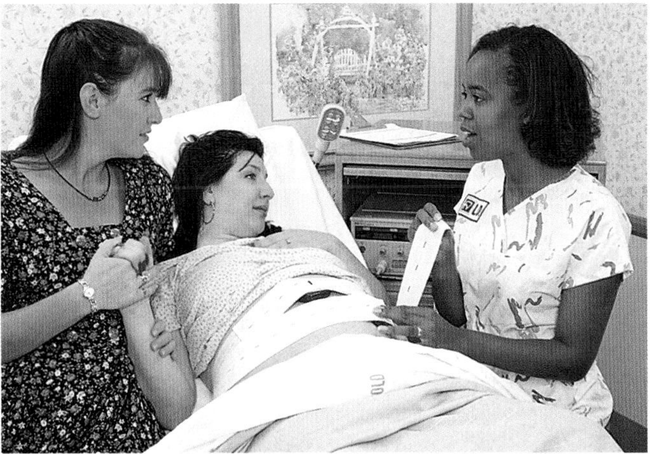

FIG 17.14 The nurse teaches the woman and her partner about electronic fetal monitoring to reduce anxiety and promote the woman's comfort during labor. Electronic fetal monitoring is only one method used to evaluate fetal well-being during labor.

### Nursing Diagnosis and Planning

Many women expect to have continuous EFM during labor and often have been informed of its use during prepared childbirth classes. Most women have additional questions; however, some women know little about this mode of fetal surveillance. The nursing diagnosis selected is:

- Deficient Knowledge of fetal monitoring.

***Expected outcome.*** After being taught about intrapartum fetal surveillance, the woman and her partner will express understanding of the equipment, procedures, limitations, and expected data.

### Interventions

***Explaining FHR auscultation with uterine palpation.*** Many women are surprised to know that auscultation and palpation are accepted modes of fetal surveillance during labor because they do not know of anyone who had this "low-tech" approach. Explain that the frequency of assessment by either method varies with risk status, procedures, and stage of labor. Also explain that the physician or nurse-midwife may recommend EFM for several reasons and that this does not necessarily indicate a complication.

***Explaining the electronic fetal monitor.*** Labor is a work in progress, and teaching needs vary as circumstances change. Explain the purposes of the monitor and the equipment to be used. A simple explanation entails telling the parents that the monitor is a tool to assess how the fetus reacts to labor, especially during contractions. If true, assure the woman that its use does not mean that something is wrong with her baby. Explain the reason for changes in the monitoring mode (external to internal). It may be helpful to explain that the physician or nurse-midwife evaluates many factors during labor and that the monitor strip is only one of those factors. If the woman will have intermittent monitoring, explain that, after a reassuring initial strip, she will be remonitored at regular intervals. Encourage her to walk around at this time.

***Addressing parents' safety concerns.*** Parents may be concerned about attachment of the scalp electrode to the fetal presenting part. Show them that the electrode is a very fine wire that penetrates the outer layer of skin only (approximately 1 mm, or the thickness of a dime). If she is concerned about the IUPC, tell her that it lies beside the fetus, next to the inner wall of the uterus.

***Coping with misleading data.*** Teach the woman that the monitor data sometimes suggest a problem when none exists. For example, FHR

## NURSING CARE PLAN

### *Intrapartum Fetal Compromise*

**Focused Assessment**

Glenda is a 30-year-old African-American woman, gravida 2, para 1, and has a 7-year-old son. She had early and regular prenatal care. She had a biophysical profile during her pregnancy because of a slight blood pressure elevation. Her labor is being induced with oxytocin (Pitocin) at $37\frac{5}{7}$ weeks of gestation because of hypertension during pregnancy (preeclampsia). Glenda's admission blood pressure was 148/94 mm Hg, and repeat assessments have been approximately the same level. Her baby will be monitored with electronic fetal monitoring. Glenda is accompanied by her husband Paul. They did not take classes because they felt that they remembered enough from their first birth. Chris is Glenda's nurse.

**Nursing Diagnosis**

Deficient Knowledge related to electronic fetal monitoring.

**Planning**

***Expected Outcome***

Glenda and Paul will state that they understand the reason for electronic monitoring, related equipment and procedures, and the data that are expected.

**Interventions and *Rationales***

1. Assess the parents' present knowledge about electronic fetal monitoring to build on existing accurate knowledge.
   *This will allow correction of misunderstandings.*
2. Explain information about the monitor to the parents, reinforcing that its use does not mean something is wrong with the woman or the baby.
   *This helps identify problems that develop so they can be corrected promptly.*
   a. Purpose: To record the fetal response to labor and guide interventions if nonreassuring patterns are identified.
      *This provides a realistic explanation of why the monitor is used.*
   b. Explain to the parents that monitoring sensors are electrically isolated from the wall current. The fetal scalp electrode (if used) penetrates the outer layer of skin, approximately a dime's thickness, less than the thickness of the fetal scalp. The intrauterine pressure catheter (IUPC) lies between the baby and the wall of the uterus.
      *This addresses possible safety concerns of the parents.*
   c. Encourage Glenda to call for assistance if she is concerned about anything related to the monitor, such as being unable to hear the fetal heartbeat because external and internal sensors are easily displaced.
      *The nurse will make needed adjustments.*
   d. Encourage Glenda to move about freely. Explain that she should urinate at least every 2 hours and that the nurse can help her roll the monitor to the bathroom door or temporarily disconnect the sensors. Remind Glenda to concentrate on coping with labor instead of maintaining monitor data.
      *Maternal movement and regular urination enhance normal labor*

**Evaluation**

Glenda and Paul say that they expected electronic fetal monitoring during labor and are familiar with the external monitor because it was used for her biophysical profile. Glenda agrees to have internal monitoring if needed, saying that she understands that greater accuracy is important because of her higher risk status.

**Focused Assessment**

Chris applies the electronic fetal monitor (EFM), which shows irregular spontaneous contractions. The fetal heart rate (FHR) baseline averages 125 to 135 beats per minute (bpm) with accelerations. Chris begins an oxytocin infusion to induce labor. Glenda's blood pressure is 160/96 mm Hg, pulse is 76 bpm, and respirations are 18 breaths per minute. Because of her continued hypertension, a magnesium sulfate infusion is started (see Chapter 25).

**Potential Complication**

Fetal Compromise

**Planning**

***Expected Outcomes***

Nurses manage fetal compromise with the woman's healthcare provider rather than independently, but care planning should reflect the following broad nursing actions to promote fetal well-being:

1. Compare FHR and uterine activity data with baseline levels before oxytocin induction.
2. Promote normal fetal oxygenation.
3. Take corrective actions for nonreassuring patterns.
4. Notify the physician or nurse-midwife if nonreassuring patterns develop.

**Interventions and *Rationales***

1. Identify relevant risk factors for fetal compromise.
   *Preeclampsia with magnesium sulfate therapy is a risk factor that requires increased frequency of fetal and maternal assessments.*
2. Encourage Glenda to assume any comfortable position other than the supine position. Encourage her to change positions regularly, approximately every half hour.
   *The supine position can reduce blood return to the heart by compressing the inferior vena cava and is often uncomfortable. Compression of the aorta and reduced cardiac output reduce placental perfusion. Regular changes of position promote normal labor progress and comfort.*
3. Evaluate and document the tracing and any nursing actions taken at the following times or according to facility policy:
   a. Every 15 to 30 minutes during active first stage labor and every 5 to 15 minutes during second stage or as directed by facility policy and medical provider orders related to Glenda's high risk condition.
   b. Before and after procedures such as amniotomy *(may result in cord compression)*, medications *(may alter rate or variability of FHR)*, epidural anesthesia *(possible hypotension that can reduce uteroplacental perfusion)*.
   c. With changes of activity, such as urination and repositioning, sensors may need adjustment.
      *Changes of activity could alter the uterine or umbilical cord blood flow.*
4. Use a systematic four-step approach to evaluate the fetal response to labor:
   a. Baseline FHR.
      *Tachycardia may be an early response to hypoxia. Bradycardia may occur in response to vagal stimulation or prolonged hypoxia.*
   b. Variability.
      *Normal variability suggests that the fetus is well oxygenated and not in acidosis.*
   c. Periodic changes: accelerations, a reassuring sign of fetal well-being, and decelerations. Note relationship of periodic changes to fetal movement, contractions, and Glenda's status and activity. Note nonperiodic (random) accelerations or variable decelerations. The nurse should attempt to identify cause of nonreassuring patterns, correct it if possible, and take steps to improve fetal oxygenation.
      *Early decelerations are a response to head compression. Late uteroplacental insufficiency and variable (umbilical cord compression) decelerations may be in the indeterminate patterns of category II or nonreassuring of category III.*

## NURSING CARE PLAN—cont'd

### *Intrapartum Fetal Compromise*

d. Uterine activity. (Evaluate frequency and duration using either external or internal devices. When external uterine activity monitoring is done, palpate three or more contractions. Note whether the uterus relaxes between contractions for at least 60 seconds. If an IUPC is used, read contraction intensity and uterine resting tone from scale on strip. Calculate Montevideo units [MVUs] if that is the facility's policy.)
*Contractions that are too long (more than 90 to 120 seconds in duration) or too frequent (closer than every 2 minutes), a resting interval of less than 30 seconds, or a baseline (resting) intrauterine pressure of more than 20 mm Hg reduces the time available for normal uteroplacental exchange. Because of Glenda's diabetes and hypertension, uteroplacental exchange may be reduced before labor begins. Oxytocin stimulates uterine activity and can add to risk.*

5. If nonreassuring patterns develop, take appropriate corrective actions such as discontinuing the oxytocin, increasing the rate of the nonadditive intravenous solution, repositioning the woman, and administering oxygen. The first priority is to identify the cause of the nonreassuring pattern and improve fetal oxygenation. Notify physician of the maternal-fetal status for needed medical orders or interventions as soon as possible. Document physician notification, response, and any orders.

#### Evaluation

Goals are not established for collaborative problems. Chris compared data from the fetal monitor and other nursing evaluations with the baseline data before oxytocin was started. For the first 4 hours of the oxytocin induction, FHR continued near its baseline of 125 to 135 bpm, with variability averaging 10 bpm. FHR accelerations continue. No nonreassuring patterns were noted.

#### Focused Assessment

The physician ruptures Glenda's membranes and inserts internal devices for FHR and uterine activity. Her blood pressure is 145/90 mm Hg, and her oxytocin and magnesium sulfate infusions continue. She is having contractions every 4 minutes of 50 seconds' duration and 50 mm Hg intensity, and she has a uterine resting tone of 10 mm Hg. One hour after Glenda's membranes are ruptured, the nurse notes that the baseline FHR has risen to approximately 145 to 150 bpm with variability averaging 3 bpm. A pattern of repeated late decelerations develops. Chris stops the oxytocin infusion and increases the rate of lactated Ringer's intravenous fluid, positions Glenda on her left side, and administers 100% oxygen at 10 L/min with a snug face mask. The physician is notified. Baseline variability improves to 5 bpm, but repeated late decelerations continue. Glenda is holding Paul's hand tightly and breathing rapidly. Her vital signs are blood pressure, 158/96 mm Hg; pulse, 90 bpm; respirations, 32 breaths per minute. Uterine activity is unchanged.

#### Nursing Diagnosis

Anxiety related to unexpected development of complications.

#### Planning

##### *Expected Outcomes*

Glenda will have a:

1. Reduced respiratory rate (12–20 breaths per minute) after interventions.
2. More relaxed face and body posture after interventions.

#### Interventions and *Rationales*

1. Maintain calm behavior while performing corrective actions and notifying the physician.
*This communicates competence to the parents in a nonverbal manner. Anxious behavior on the part of caregivers tends to increase the parents' anxiety.*
2. Use simple, concise language for all explanations.
*High anxiety or intense physical sensations impair a person's ability to comprehend explanations.*
3. Explain the following to the couple:
   a. The problem that was identified
   b. The usual cause of the problem
   c. Reasons for corrective actions
   d. Expected results
   e. That Glenda can talk with the oxygen mask on
*If the couple understands what is happening and why the corrective actions are taken, they are more likely to comply with the care. Knowledge decreases fear of the unknown. Assuring Glenda that she can talk with* the *oxygen mask on allows her to ask questions and express feelings to reduce anxiety and fear.*
4. Tell the couple if the pattern improves or is resolved to *decrease their anxiety about the fetal condition. For example, tell them when baseline variability improves.*
5. Allow Glenda and Paul to express their feelings about the labor and birth during the postpartum period. Explain any gaps in their understanding about what happened.
*This helps the couple accept and put unexpected occurrences in perspective. It decreases the possibility that one or both parents will feel like "a failure" if emergency intervention (cesarean birth) becomes necessary.*

#### Evaluation

The physician evaluates Glenda's condition and that of her baby. Over the next hour, FHR pattern gradually improves. The baseline rate slows (130 to 140 bpm), and late decelerations are sporadic. Variability improves to approximately 15 bpm. Glenda gradually relaxes her grip on her husband's hand and her body relaxes. Her respiratory rate slows to 20 breaths per minute. She requires a cesarean birth because her cervix does not dilate to greater than 7 cm, despite adequate contractions.

may suddenly fall to zero and the audible tone stop if the sensor (external or scalp electrode) is displaced. Tell her to call the nurse for adjustment or replacement of the sensor. Explain that normal labor progress and fetal movement may alter the best location for assessing FHR externally by either auscultation or external EFM.

The woman may be discouraged because the curves representing contractions on the electronic monitor do not look as strong on the strip as they feel to her. This situation is more likely if an external transducer is used. Explain the many factors that may cause the contraction curves to appear stronger or weaker than they really are. When an external tocotransducer is used, tell her that the strip is used mainly to assess the timing of contractions and the baby's reaction. Explain that an IUPC may be recommended if knowledge of intrauterine pressure is crucial. Explain also that data from the catheter may become inaccurate because of obstruction by amniotic fluid debris or pressure between the fetal head and pelvic structures during late labor.

Reassure the woman that her perception of her contractions and discomfort is important. Value the woman-generated data as well as

## PARENTS WANT TO KNOW

### *About Electronic Fetal Monitoring*

Women who have electronic fetal monitoring during labor often have questions that the nurse can answer. Here are some common questions and answers the nurse might provide.

**Can I Move Around With the Monitor?**

You can move freely with the monitor. If you notice that the machine isn't picking up the fetal heart sounds or contractions as well, call me and I'll readjust it. Make yourself comfortable; then we'll adjust the machine if necessary.

**What if I Need to Go to the Bathroom?**

If you need to go to the bathroom, we'll unplug the cords from the machine and you can walk in there or we can roll the monitor to the door of the bathroom. There may be some circumstances in which walking or discontinuation of the monitor is not recommended.

**Will the Monitor Shock Me? I Don't Know if I Want to Be Hooked to an Electrical Outlet, Especially Since My Water Has Broken**

Any monitor parts that are attached to you and your baby only transmit information into the machine for processing. The sensors on your body are isolated from electrical parts in the monitor.

**Why Is the Baby's Heart Beating so Fast?**

A baby's heart normally beats faster than an adult's, both before and after birth. The normal rate is approximately 110 to 160 beats per minute. A higher or lower rate does not necessarily mean that the baby has a problem, but we do look at the monitor strip closely to see how the baby is doing.

**Why Do Those Numbers for the Baby's Heart Rate Change All the Time?**

The heart rate of a healthy baby who is awake changes constantly. When the baby moves, the heart often speeds up, just as yours does. If the baby sleeps, the heart rate may change less.

**What Do Those Numbers for Contractions on the Machine (External Monitor) Mean? They Change All the Time.**

The numbers reflect a change in the pressure sensed by the monitor. The monitor senses many changes in pressure other than those from contractions, such as changes from breathing, coughing, or movement of you or the baby.

**My Contractions Don't Look Very Strong, but They Sure Seem Strong to Me! (External Uterine Activity Monitor Is Being Used.)**

The external monitor senses contractions indirectly rather than sensing the actual pressure inside the uterus. Their appearance on the tracing varies because of many factors, such as your position, the position of the sensor on your abdomen, and the thickness of your abdominal wall.

**Will the Internal Monitor Hurt My Baby?**

The spiral electrode attaches only to the outer layer of skin on the baby's head. We avoid sensitive areas on the head, such as the fontanels (soft spots) or the face. The uterine catheter or fetal pulse oximeter slides up beside the baby.

## CRITICAL THINKING EXERCISE 17.1

A woman is having her labor induced with oxytocin and is having internal electronic fetal monitoring. Contractions occur every 2 minutes, are 110 seconds in duration, and reach 75 mm Hg using an intrauterine pressure catheter (IUPC). The uterine resting tone between contractions is 20 mm Hg. The baseline fetal heart rate is 135 to 145 beats per minute (bpm), with approximately 15 bpm variability.

The nurse notes a pattern of uniform decelerations that begin at the peak of each contraction. The rate falls to 125 bpm before returning to the previous baseline approximately 30 seconds after the contraction ends.

1. What pattern do these findings describe? What is the probable cause?
2. What is the most appropriate nursing response? Why? If needed, are corrective actions urgent?

## CRITICAL THINKING EXERCISE 17.2

A woman in active labor is having external electronic fetal monitoring for fetal assessment. She has not had medication, and her labor has been normal so far. Her membranes ruptured approximately 1 hour ago, and the amniotic fluid was clear. Contractions occur every 3 minutes, are 60 seconds in duration, and are moderately intense. Her uterus fully relaxes between each contraction.

The nursing student who is helping to care for her notes abrupt slowing of the fetal heart rate to 90 beats per minute (bpm) during the next two contractions, each time lasting approximately 30 seconds.

1. What pattern do these findings describe? What is the probable cause?
2. Are any nursing actions needed? Why? If nursing actions are needed, what are they? What can the nursing student do? In what order should nursing actions be done?
3. When should the midwife or physician be contacted?

the machine-generated data. Palpate contractions at intervals and evaluate their appearance on the monitor strip.

It is natural for the nurse's attention to be drawn to the electronic fetal monitor when entering the room. Stay focused on the woman and her family rather than devoting excessive attention to the monitoring equipment. The woman, not the monitor, is giving birth to the baby.

***Including the labor partner.*** Tell the partner how to identify the onset and peak of contractions. During active labor, some women discover that contractions become intense before they can prepare for them. If this is the case, have the coach tell the woman when each contraction begins. The coach also can tell her when the peak has passed, to encourage her.

***Enhancing comfort.*** Auscultation and palpation allow intermittent fetal surveillance with minimal interruption of the woman's comfort measures for labor. However, the reassuring sounds generated by the electronic fetal monitor also may enhance emotional comfort.

Some women are reluctant to make themselves more comfortable when an electronic monitor is used. Nursing care involves finding ways to make the mother comfortable and the monitor as nonintrusive as possible. Teach her ways to improve comfort while still obtaining an adequate tracing.

Explain that staying in one position is uncomfortable and does not promote normal labor. The woman may assume any position other than supine unless a specific position is needed. Encourage her to find the position in which she is most comfortable; then adjust the external devices to best detect contractions and the fetal heartbeat. Internal devices may be an option if external devices cannot be adjusted to provide useful data.

If the woman finds the sound produced by the electronic fetal monitor distracting or inconsistent with the atmosphere she desires, lower the sound or turn it off. Remember that the auditory cues for rate accelerations and decelerations are absent.

If no other contraindications to walking exist, the woman may go to the bathroom when an electronic fetal monitor is used. Unplug the sensors at the machine and let her walk to the bathroom. Reconnect and adjust them when she returns. Alternatively, you may roll the machine to the door of the bathroom, keeping the cables connected. Sensors will need adjustment when she returns to bed, even if they were not disconnected. Document ambulation and other interruptions. If the fetus has a persistent nonreassuring pattern or internal sensors, it may be best not to interrupt the recording.

### Evaluation

The evaluation of parental knowledge is continual because most parents think of questions after initial explanations and as conditions change. Do the partners indicate their understanding after each explanation? Their understanding may be accompanied by a decrease in anxiety as well.

## FETAL OXYGENATION

### Assessment

Use a systematic approach to evaluate data from IA with palpation or a fetal monitoring strip. Assess FHR for baseline and for variability and periodic changes if using the electronic fetal monitor. Assess uterine activity for frequency, duration, and intensity of contractions and for uterine resting tone. Calculate MVUs for IUPC data if that is unit policy. Intervals for assessment and documentation are as follows (AAP & ACOG, 2012; ACNM, 2010):

- Active first stage labor, every 15 to 30 minutes shortly after a contraction
- Second stage labor, every 5 to 15 minutes

Box 17.2 provides additional guidelines for evaluating and documenting FHR. Guidelines for 2008 do not state different frequencies for the woman at higher risk.

Take the woman's temperature every 4 hours and then every 2 hours after the membranes rupture. Maternal fever increases the fetal temperature and fetal oxygen requirements. Assess the woman's pulse, respirations, and blood pressure at least hourly or with fetal assessments. Hypotension or hypertension may reduce maternal blood flow to the intervillous spaces.

Assessment of mother and fetus is continual during the dynamic process of labor. Compare data regarding FHR patterns, uterine activity, and maternal vital signs with baseline data and normal ranges. Observe for subtle trends in the data. Distinguish between patterns having similar appearances, such as early and late decelerations.

Vaginal examination (see Chapter 16) may be performed to evaluate specific FHR patterns—for example, to check for a prolapsed cord if a pattern of variable decelerations occurs.

### Nursing Diagnosis and Planning

The collaborative problem potential complication: fetal compromise is selected for nursing care related to fetal oxygenation when EFM is used.

Because the nurse cannot manage every instance of fetal distress independently, patient (fetal) goals are not made. The nurse's responsibility includes planning to:

- Promote adequate fetal oxygenation.
- Take corrective actions to increase fetal oxygenation if nonreassuring patterns are identified.
- Report nonreassuring patterns to the physician or nurse-midwife.
- Support the woman and her partner if a complication develops.
- Document assessments and care.

### BOX 17.2 Guidelines for Assessment and Documentation of Fetal Heart Rate Auscultation for Women at Low Risk

**Active First-Stage Labor**

Every 15–30 min, just after a contraction

**Second-Stage Labor**

Every 5–15 min

**Other Times to Document Fetal Heart Rate**

- Before artificial rupture of the membranes; after rupture of the membranes, either artificially or spontaneously
- Before and after ambulation
- If contractions become too frequent or last too long, or if there is an inadequate interval between them
- Before administration of oxytocin and when evaluating the dose for increase, maintenance, or decrease
- Before administration of cervical ripening agent-like misoprostol or cervidil.
- Before administration of sedative medications or central nervous system depressants and at time of peak action
- Before epidural analgesia is started and every 15 min for 1 hr thereafter

### Interventions

Measures to promote fetal oxygenation are discussed with the care of the woman in normal labor (see Chapter 16) and of the woman having an epidural or subarachnoid block (see Chapter 18).

***Taking corrective actions.*** If a nonreassuring pattern is noted, take actions to identify its cause and improve fetal oxygenation. Birth facilities have protocols for interventions if nonreassuring patterns develop. Nursing interventions may include both independent and delegated actions.

***Reassuring parents.*** Parents understandably become anxious when a nonreassuring fetal assessment occurs. Remain at the bedside and use a calm manner to avoid increasing their anxiety. Use the call bell to summon other nurses if needed to help with corrective actions and to notify the physician or nurse-midwife.

Explain the problem that was identified and the reason for corrective actions in simple, concise language. Severe anxiety reduces the parents' ability to understand information. Inform them if FHR returns to a reassuring pattern. Some corrective actions, such as oxygen administration and positioning, may continue after a reassuring pattern returns. Tell the woman that she may talk with the oxygen mask on.

***Reporting nonreassuring patterns.*** Notify the birth attendant of nonreassuring patterns as soon as possible after taking corrective actions. The priority of nursing care is to improve fetal oxygenation. Document the time and content of all consultations with the physician or nurse-midwife about the mother or fetus and document the birth attendant's response.

***Documenting assessments and care.*** Data related to fetal well-being in both the labor record and on the monitor strip are permanent records and should be complete. Box 17.3 shows guidelines for documentation on the monitor strip and labor record. Documentation can demonstrate good nursing care and show that the standard of care has been met.

Label a paper strip with the woman's name, the date, and the time when EFM begins. If a break in the strip occurs, such as to change

## BOX 17.3 Documenting Electronic Fetal Monitoring

**Documentation When Monitoring Is Initiated**

***Monitor Strip***

Woman's name and hospital or other permanent identifying number
Physician's or nurse-midwife's name
Date and time of admission
Date and time monitoring begins (verify accuracy of electronic monitor date and time)
Gravidity, parity, abortions, living children
Gestation in weeks
Presence of identified risk factors
Character of amniotic fluid (when membranes rupture)
Function test of monitor accuracy
Initial mode of monitoring (external or internal devices)

***Labor Record (if Paper-Only Documentation)***

Same information as on monitor strip
First panel number when a printed paper strip begins

**Continuing Documentation**

***Monitor Strip***

Maternal vital signs at appropriate intervals for stage of labor, membrane status, and interventions such as labor stimulation or pain management measures
Notations of strip review at intervals appropriate for risk factors and labor status (see Box 17.2)
Vaginal examinations, including cervical dilation, effacement, and fetal station
Rupture of membranes (spontaneously or artificially)
Color, quantity, and character (such as foul odor, cloudiness) of amniotic fluid
Maternal position changes
Maternal or fetal movement that affects tracing
Maternal vomiting, coughing, or other movement that affects tracing
Summaries while pushing in second stage
Equipment adjustments, problems maintaining continuous tracing (such as an active fetus)
Medication and anesthesia, including related interventions
Changes of equipment mode, such as external to internal device
Interventions for nonreassuring patterns and maternal-fetal response
Interruptions, such as the woman walking

***Labor Record***

Same information as on monitor strip
Periodic summary of maternal vital signs, baseline rate, variability, periodic changes, and uterine activity (frequency, duration, and intensity of contractions and uterine resting tone)
Nonreassuring maternal or fetal assessments, interventions, responses, provider notification, provider response
Actions taken in chain of command if the physician or nurse-midwife does not respond appropriately to the nurse's report of a problem

NOTE: Some of these actions may be entered automatically with electronic fetal monitoring (EFM) and computer interfaces.

paper, label the new strip with the woman's name, the date, and the time. Label each section of a multipart strip so that the entire paper record can be reassembled sequentially. Electronic "strips" include time for automatic and typed notations. Late entries also can be made as on a paper chart. Strips might not be automatically printed if they are stored electronically. Printing may be required if electronic storage is not functional at the time or if a printed view of a specific section of the strip is desired.

Continue documenting the heart rate and maternal observations until vaginal birth occurs. If a cesarean birth is needed, a minimum of one FHR assessment is done after arrival in the operating room, with additional assessments performed if surgery is delayed. Remove internal devices before securing the woman's legs to the operating table. Document the time of arrival in the operating room, all FHR and contraction assessments, the time of abdominal incision, and the time of birth. The unit should have a consistent method to document times, often using the electronic fetal monitor clock.

### Evaluation

Patient-centered goals are not formulated for a collaborative problem. The nurse compares data with established standards to determine whether they are within normal limits. If nonreassuring patterns are identified, the nurse:

- Takes measures to increase fetal oxygenation.
- Notifies the physician or nurse-midwife.
- Documents all relevant data.

## KEY CONCEPTS

- The purpose of intrapartum fetal surveillance is to identify fetal well-being and to identify the fetus who may be having hypoxic stress beyond the ability to compensate for it.
- The two approaches to intrapartum fetal monitoring are intermittent auscultation with palpation of uterine activity and electronic fetal monitoring. Each type has distinct advantages and limitations. EFM has not been shown to be superior to auscultation with palpation but is recommended for women with high-risk conditions.
- Fetal oxygenation depends on a normal flow of oxygenated maternal blood into the placenta, normal exchange within the placenta, patent umbilical cord vessels, and normal fetal circulatory and oxygen-carrying function.
- Stimulation of the sympathetic nervous system increases FHR and strengthens the heart contraction. Stimulation of the parasympathetic nervous system slows the heart rate. The push-pull action of speeding and slowing the heart rate is evidenced by the wavy appearance of the baseline in the fetus who is monitored electronically.
- IA and palpation allow the greatest amount of maternal movement but also require a 1:1 nurse-to-patient ratio for best surveillance.
- External EFM is less accurate for FHR and uterine activity patterns than internal monitoring, but it is noninvasive and does not require ruptured membranes.
- Greater accuracy is the main advantage of internal EFM devices, but these are invasive and require ruptured membranes.
- Nursing responsibilities related to intrapartum fetal surveillance by any mode include promoting fetal oxygenation, identifying and reporting nonreassuring findings, supporting parents, communicating with the physician or nurse-midwife, and documenting all care.

## REFERENCES AND READINGS


American Academy of Pediatrics & American College of Obstetricians and Gynecologists. (2012). *Guidelines for perinatal care* (7th ed.). Elk Grove Village, IL, and Washington, DC: Author.

American College of Nurse-Midwives. (2010). Intermittent auscultation for fetal heart rate surveillance. (Clinical Bulletin No. 11). *Journal of Midwifery & Women's Health*, *55*(4), 397–403.

American College of Obstetricians and Gynecologists. (2015a). *Intrapartum fetal heart rate monitoring: Nomenclature, interpretation, and general management principles (ACOG Practice Bulletin No. 106)*. Washington, DC: Author.

American College of Obstetricians and Gynecologists. (2015b). *Management of intrapartum fetal heart rate tracings (ACOG Practice Bulletin No.116)*. Washington, DC: Author.

Bashore, R. A., & Koos, B. J. (2010). Fetal surveillance during labor. In N. F. Hacker, J. C. Gambone & C. J. Hobel (Eds.). *Hacker & Moore's essentials of obstetrics and gynecology* (5th ed., pp. 119–127). Philadelphia: Saunders.

Blackburn, S. T. (2013). *Maternal, fetal, & neonatal physiology: A clinical perspective* (4th ed.). St. Louis: Saunders.

Cunningham, F. G., Leveno, K. J., Bloom, S. L., Hauth, J. C., Rouse, D. J., & Spong, C. Y. (2010). *Williams obstetrics* (23rd ed.). New York: McGraw-Hill.

Cypher, R. L. (2015). Assessment of fetal oxygenation and acid-base status. In A. Lyndon & L. Usher (Eds.). *AWHONN: Fetal heart monitoring: Principles and practices* (5th ed., pp. 148–169). Dubuque, IA: Kendall Hunt.

Feinstein, N. F., Sprague, A., & Trépanier, M. J. (2008). *Fetal heart rate auscultation* (2nd ed.). Washington, DC: Association of Women's Health, Obstetric, and Neonatal Nurses.

Grimes, D. A., & Peipert, J. F. (2010). Electronic fetal monitoring as a public health screening program: The arithmetic of failure. *Obstetrics and Gynecology*, *116*(6), 1397–1400.

Hall, J. E. (2011). *Guyton and Hall: Textbook of medical physiology* (12th ed.). Philadelphia: Saunders.

Killion, M.M. (2015). Techniques for fetal heart assessment. In A. Lyndon & L. Usher (Eds.), *AWHONN: Fetal heart monitoring: Principles and practices* (5th ed., pp. 65–98). Dubuque, IA: Kendall Hunt.

Lyndon, A., O'Brien-Abel, N., & Simpson, K. R. (2015). Fetal heart rate interpretation. In A. Lyndon & L. Usher (Eds.), *AWHONN: Fetal heart monitoring: Principles and practices* (5th ed., pp. 99-124). Dubuque, IA: Kendall Hunt.

Macones, G. A., Hankins, G. D. V., Spong, C. Y., Hauth, J., & Moore, T. (2008). The 2008 National Institute of Child Health and Human Development Workshop on electronic fetal monitoring: Update on definitions, interpretation, and research guidelines. (Copublished in Obstetrics & Gynecology, Vol. 112, No. 3, September 2008.) *Journal of Obstetric, Gynecologic, and Neonatal Nursing*, *37*(5), 510–515, (Copublished in Obstetrics & Gynecology, Vol. 112, No. 3, September 2008.).

Nageotte, M. P., (2014). Intrapartum fetal surveillance. In R. K. Creasy, R. Resnik, J. D. Iams, et al. (Eds.), *Creasy & Resnik's maternal-fetal medicine: Principles and practice* (7th ed., pp. 488–506). Philadelphia: Saunders.

National Institute of Child Health and Human Development [NICHD]. (2008). The 2008 National Institute of Child Health and Human Development Workshop Report on electronic fetal monitoring: Update on definitions, interpretation, and research guidelines. *Journal of Obstetric, Gynecologic, and Neonatal Nursing*, *37*(5), 510–515.

Parer, J. T., & King, T. L. (2010). Fetal heart rate monitoring: The next step? *American Journal of Obstetrics & Gynecology*, *203*(6), 520–521.

Lyndon, A., O'Brien-Abel, N., & Simpson, K. R. (2014). Fetal assessment during labor. In K.R. Simpson, & P.A. Creehan (Eds.), *AWHONN perinatal nursing* (4th ed., pp. 445–492). Philadelphia: Lippincott Williams & Wilkins.

Simpson, K. R. (2015). Physiologic interventions for fetal heart rate patterns. In A. Lyndon & L. Usher (Eds.), *AWHONN: Fetal heart monitoring: Principles and practices* (5th ed., pp. 125–147). Dubuque, IA: Kendall Hunt.

18

# Pain Management for Childbirth

http://evolve.elsevier.com/McKinney/mat-ch/

## LEARNING OBJECTIVES

*After studying this chapter, you should be able to:*

- Compare childbirth pain with other types of pain.
- Describe how excessive pain can affect the laboring woman and her fetus.
- Examine how physical and psychologic forces interact in the laboring woman's pain experience.
- Describe the use of nonpharmacologic pain management techniques in labor.
- Describe how medications may affect a pregnant woman and the fetus or neonate.
- Identify the benefits and risks of specific pharmacologic pain control methods.
- Explain nursing care related to different types of intrapartum pain management.

Each woman has unique expectations about birth, including expectations about pain and her ability to manage it. The woman who successfully handles the pain of labor is more likely to view her experience as a positive life event. A woman's experience with labor pain varies with several physical and psychologic elements, and each woman responds differently. Nonpharmacologic and pharmacologic methods give the nurse and laboring woman a selection of pain management techniques to choose from.

## UNIQUE NATURE OF PAIN DURING BIRTH

Pain involves two components:

- A physiologic component, which includes reception by sensory nerves and transmission to the central nervous system.
- A psychologic component, which involves recognizing the sensation, interpreting it as painful, and reacting to the interpretation.

However, childbirth pain differs from other pain in several important respects:

- Childbirth pain is part of a normal process, whereas other types of pain usually indicate an injury or illness. Pain may encourage the woman to assume different positions in labor, favoring rotation and descent of the fetus.
- The pregnant woman has several months to prepare for birth, including acquiring skills to help manage pain. Realistic preparation and knowledge about the birth process help her develop skills to cope with labor pain.
- Labor pain has a foreseeable end. A woman can expect her labor to end in hours, rather than days, weeks, or months.
- Labor pain is not constant but intermittent. A woman may describe little discomfort with contractions during early labor. Even during late labor, she may be relatively comfortable during the short rest periods between contractions.
- Labor ends with the birth of a baby. The emotional significance of her child's birth cannot be ignored when trying to understand a woman's response to pain. Concern about her fetus often motivates a woman to tolerate more pain during labor than she otherwise might be willing to endure.

## ADVERSE EFFECTS OF EXCESSIVE PAIN

Although expected during labor, pain that exceeds a woman's tolerance can have harmful effects on her and the fetus.

### Physiologic Effects

Labor increases a woman's metabolic rate and her demand for oxygen. Pain and anxiety escalate her already high metabolic rate by increasing the production of catecholamines or "fight or flight" hormones (epinephrine and norepinephrine), cortisol, and glucagon. In response to pain and the increase in sympathetic hormones, she may hyperventilate to obtain more oxygen, exhale too much carbon dioxide in the process, and have less oxygen to share with her fetus. Significant changes, more than those expected during labor, can occur in the woman's arterial oxygen pressure ($PaO_2$) and partial pressure of carbon dioxide in arterial blood ($PaCO_2$) and in her arterial pH. These maternal respiratory and metabolic changes alter the placental exchange of oxygen and waste products, even in the presence of normal placental circulation. The fetus has less oxygen available for uptake and decreased carbon dioxide exchange to the mother. The net result is that the fetus shifts to anaerobic metabolism, with the buildup of hydrogen ions (metabolic acidosis).

High catecholamine levels and excess stress hormones reduce blood flow to the uterus and placenta. The fetus is more likely to become hypoxic and eventually shift to an anaerobic metabolism if good placental blood flow is not restored.

Excessive catecholamine secretion inhibits the uterine response to oxytocin, secreted by the posterior pituitary. In addition, contractions become irritable, cramp like, and poorly effective, possibly resulting in dystocia and inhibiting labor progress, thus increasing pain further.

### Psychologic Effects

Poor pain control lessens the pleasure of this extraordinary life event for both partners. The mother may find it difficult to interact with her infant because she is depleted from a painful, exhausting labor. Unpleasant memories of the birth may affect her response to a sexual activity or another labor. Her partner may feel inadequate as a support person during birth.

## VARIABLES IN CHILDBIRTH PAIN

Physical and psychosocial factors contribute to a woman's response to the pain of labor.

### Physical Factors

Childbirth pain is of two types—visceral and somatic. Visceral pain, described as throbbing, is related initially to the contractions of the uterus and dilation and stretching of the cervix. Contractions cause ischemia of the arterioles in the uterine body. Later in labor, somatic pain, described as sharp and localized, is directly related to the stretching of the perineal tissue and adjacent structures.

#### Sources of Pain

Four potential sources of labor pain exist in most labors. Other physical factors may modify labor pain, increasing or decreasing it.

*Tissue ischemia.* The blood supply to the uterus decreases during contractions, leading to tissue hypoxia and anaerobic metabolism. Ischemic uterine pain has been likened to ischemic heart pain.

*Cervical dilation.* Dilation and stretching of the cervix and lower uterus are a major source of pain. Pain stimuli from cervical dilation travel through the hypogastric plexus, entering the spinal cord at the T10, T11, T12, and L1 levels (Fig. 18.1).

*Pressure and pulling on pelvic structures.* Some pain results from pressure and pulling on pelvic structures such as ligaments, pelvic bone, fallopian tubes, ovaries, bladder, and peritoneum. The pain is a visceral pain; a woman may feel it as referred pain in her back and legs.

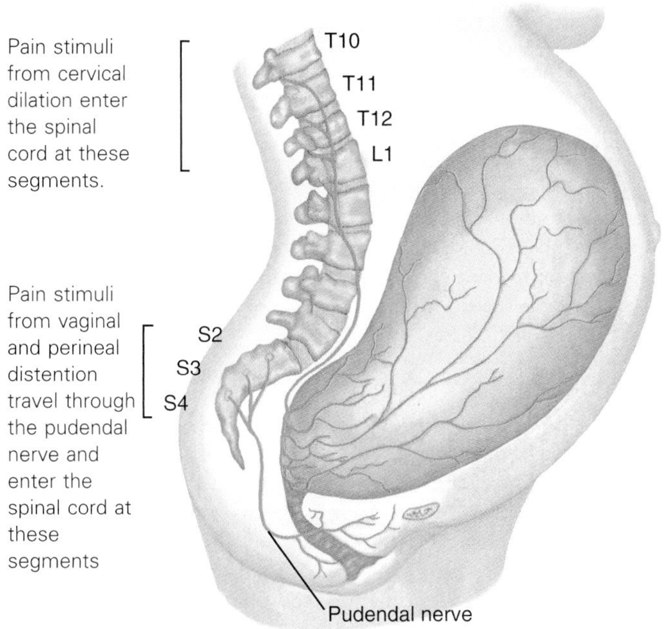

*Distention of the vagina and perineum.* Marked distention of the vagina and perineum occurs with fetal descent, especially during the second stage. The woman may describe a sensation of burning, tearing, or splitting (somatic pain). Pain from vaginal and perineal distention and pressure and pulling on adjacent structures enters the spinal cord at the S2, S3, and S4 levels (see Fig. 18.1).

Pain stimuli from cervical dilation enter the spinal cord at these segments.

T10

T11

T12

L1

Pain stimuli from vaginal and perineal distention travel through the pudendal nerve and enter the spinal cord at these segments

S2

S3

S4

Pudendal nerve

**FIG 18.1** Pathways of pain transmission during labor.

#### Factors Influencing the Perception or Tolerance of Pain

Although physiologic processes cause labor pain, a woman's tolerance of pain may be affected by other physical influences.

*Intensity of labor.* The woman who has a short, intense labor often complains of severe pain because each contraction does so much work (effacement, dilation, and fetal descent). A rapid labor may limit her options for pharmacologic pain relief as well.

Labor that is long or protracted can cause pain tolerance to decrease. If prelabor cervical changes (softening, with some dilation and effacement) are incomplete, the cervix does not open as easily. Ineffective contractions fail to achieve dilation and effacement, resulting in a longer labor and greater fatigue in the laboring woman.

*Fetal position and size.* The fetal position and presenting parts have an impact on labor progression and pain perception. Labor is likely to be longer and more uncomfortable when the fetus is in an unfavorable position. If the fetus is not well engaged, labor will be lengthened. An abnormal fetal position is a common variant seen in otherwise normal labors. The posterior occiput position can cause the woman to experience pain in between contractions, as the fetal structure presses on the sacrum. Macrosomic infants (>4000 g) cause increased pressure on pelvic structures and injury to perineal tissues.

*Characteristics of the pelvis.* The size and shape of a woman's pelvis influence the course and length of her labor. Abnormalities may cause a difficult and longer labor.

*Fatigue.* Fatigue reduces a woman's ability to tolerate pain and to use coping skills she has learned. She may be unable to focus on relaxation and breathing techniques that would otherwise help her tolerate labor.

Many women sleep poorly during the last weeks of pregnancy. Shortness of breath when lying down, frequent urination, and fetal activity interrupt sleep so that a woman often begins labor with a sleep deficit. If labor begins late in the evening, she may have been awake well over 24 hours by the time she gives birth. Even if a woman begins labor well rested, slow progress may exhaust her.

Prolonged, intense pushing during the second stage is exhausting as well. For this reason, promoting a physiologic second stage in which the woman delays pushing until she feels an urge to do so ("laboring down") is preferred.

*Intervention of caregivers.* Although needed for the well-being of a woman and fetus, some interventions add discomfort to the natural pain of labor. Intravenous (IV) lines cause pain when they are inserted and remain noticeable to many women during labor. Fetal monitoring equipment and the frequent need to adjust the sensors is uncomfortable to some women. Both can hamper a woman's mobility, decreasing her ability to assume a more comfortable position.

A woman whose labor is induced or augmented often reports more pain and increased difficulty coping with it because contractions reach peak intensity quickly rather than gradually over many hours. Vaginal examinations and internal fetal monitoring are uncomfortable because of vaginal and cervical stretching.

## Psychosocial Factors

Several psychosocial variables influence a woman's experience of pain.

### Culture

A woman's sociocultural roots influence how she perceives, interprets, and responds to pain during childbirth. Some cultures encourage loud and vigorous expression of pain, whereas others value self-control. However, women are individuals within their cultural groups. The experience of pain is personal, and one should not make assumptions about how a woman from a specific cultural or ethnic group will behave during labor.

Women should be encouraged to express themselves in any way they find comforting, and the diversity of their expressions must be respected. Accepting a woman's individual response to labor and pain promotes a therapeutic relationship.

The nurse should avoid praising some behaviors (e.g., stoicism) while belittling others (e.g., noisy expression). This restraint is difficult because noisy women are challenging to work with and may disturb others.

The unique nature of childbirth pain and women's diverse responses to it make nursing management complex. The nurse can miss important cues if the woman is either stoic, having little outward expression of pain, or expresses herself loudly and constantly. With either extreme, the nurse may not readily identify critical information such as impending birth or the symptoms of a complication.

### Anxiety and Fear

Extreme anxiety and fear magnify sensitivity to pain and impair a woman's ability to tolerate it. They consume energy she needs to cope with the birth process, including its painful aspects.

Anxiety and fear increase muscle tension, diverting oxygenated blood to the brain and skeletal muscles. Tension in pelvic muscles counters the expulsive forces of uterine contractions and the laboring woman's pushing efforts during the second stage. Prolonged tension results in general fatigue, increased pain perception, and reduced ability to use skills to cope with pain.

### Previous Experiences With Pain

Early in life, a child learns that pain is a symptom of bodily injury. Consequently, fear and withdrawal are a woman's natural reactions to pain during labor. Learning about the normal sensations of labor, including pain, helps a woman suppress her natural reactions of fear and withdrawal, allowing her body to do the work of birth.

A woman who has given birth previously has a different perspective. If she has had a vaginal delivery, she is probably aware of normal labor sensations and is less likely to associate them with injury or abnormality. Also, time has a way of blunting the memory of painful experiences.

A woman who had a child by cesarean birth may not have experienced labor and may be particularly anxious about pain. The experience of cesarean birth is known to her, whereas labor is often unknown. Subsequent babies are typically born by cesarean, but spontaneous labor may occur before the scheduled date of her surgery.

A woman who has previously had a long and difficult labor is more likely to be anxious about the outcome of the present one if a vaginal birth after cesarean (VBAC) is planned. If she had a cesarean birth following the difficult labor, she may doubt her ability to give birth vaginally. Her anxiety often intensifies when she reaches the point at which her previous labor ended with the cesarean birth.

Previous experiences do not always adversely affect a woman's ability to deal with pain. She may have learned ways to cope with pain during other episodes of pain or during other births and may use these skills adaptively during labor.

### Preparation for Childbirth

Preparation for childbirth does not ensure a pain-free labor. A woman should be prepared for pain realistically, including reasonable expectations about analgesia and **anesthesia** (loss of sensation with or without loss of consciousness). She may feel that her entire preparation is invalid if what she expects does not happen when she is in labor.

Preparation reduces anxiety and fear of the unknown. It allows a woman to rehearse for labor and learn a variety of skills to master pain as labor progresses. She and her partner learn about expected behavioral changes during labor, and their knowledge decreases their anxiety when those changes occur.

### Support System

An anxious partner or support person is less able to provide the encouragement and reassurance the woman needs during labor. In addition, anxiety in others can be contagious, and an anxious partner can increase the woman's anxiety. She may assume that if others are worried, something is probably wrong.

The birth experiences of a woman's family and friends cannot be ignored. Those individuals can be an important source of comfort and assistance if they convey realistic information about labor pain and its control. However, if they describe labor as simply intolerable with no relief steps taken, the woman may have needless distress. Equally detrimental is for her to hear that labor is painless. No two labors are alike, even for the same woman.

# STANDARDS FOR PAIN MANAGEMENT

The Joint Commission (http://www.jointcommission.org) has recognized that pain management is an essential part of care in all healthcare settings. Joint Commission standards require healthcare organizations to (The Joint Commission, 2015):

- Recognize the right of patients, residents, or clients to appropriate assessment and management of pain.
- Screen patients, residents or clients for pain during their initial assessment and, when clinically required, during ongoing, periodic re-assessments.
- Educate patients, residents, or clients suffering from pain, and their families, about pain management.

# NONPHARMACOLOGIC PAIN MANAGEMENT

The nurse who cares for women in labor and birth can offer nonpharmacologic and pharmacologic pain management methods. Education about nonpharmacologic pain management is the foundation of prepared childbirth classes. To be most helpful to women and their labor partners, the intrapartum nurse should know methods that are taught in local childbirth classes.

## Advantages

Nonpharmacologic methods have several advantages over pharmacologic methods if they produce adequate pain control. They do not slow labor and have no side effects, nor do they carry the risk of allergy or sedation.

Nonpharmacologic techniques are both an alternative and an adjunct to drugs. Most women use a combination of pharmacologic and nonpharmacologic techniques. The woman who chooses pharmacologic analgesia needs alternative pain management until the drug is given, usually after labor is established. Also, pharmacologic methods may not eliminate labor pain, and a woman may need nonpharmacologic methods to control the pain that remains. Nonpharmacologic techniques can help a person manage pain other than birth-related pain.

Nonpharmacologic methods may be the only realistic option for a woman who enters the hospital in advanced, rapid labor. In this case, there may not be time to obtain a good regional block or achieve analgesia from systemic drugs. Also, the newborn's respiration can be depressed by a systemic opioid narcotic that reaches its peak action near the time of birth.

### Limitations

Nonpharmacologic methods of pain control have limitations, especially if they are used as the sole method of pain control. Women do not always achieve their desired level of pain control using these methods alone. Because of the many variables in labor, even a well-prepared and highly-motivated woman may have a difficult labor and need pharmacologic analgesia or anesthesia.

## Preparation for Pain Management

The ideal time to learn nonpharmacologic pain control is before labor. During the last few weeks of pregnancy, the woman learns about labor, including its painful aspects, in childbirth classes. She can prepare to confront the pain, learning a variety of skills to use during labor. Her support person learns specific methods to encourage and support her. After admission, the nurse can review and reinforce what the partners learned in class.

The nurse can teach the unprepared woman and her support person nonpharmacologic techniques. The latent phase of labor is the best time for intrapartum teaching because the woman is usually anxious enough to be attentive and interested, yet comfortable enough to understand.

## Application of Nonpharmacologic Techniques

Methods for nonpharmacologic techniques in labor include relaxation, mind-body interventions, and breathing. Simple nursing interventions will improve the laboring patient's ability to relax and use the techniques.

### General Comfort

Comfortable surroundings support relaxation. The nurse can reduce irritants, such as bright lights, and can adjust the room temperature. Promoting the woman's personal comfort helps her focus on pain management during labor (Fig. 18.2). This includes actions to increase comfort and reduce the effect of irritants, such as a hot environment or wet bedding.

Assuming a comfortable position, changing positions as desired, and walking often improve a woman's ability to tolerate the discomforts of labor. Nurses can assist with the safe use of labor balls and other assistive devices during labor.

Music masks outside noise and provides a background for the use of imagery and breathing techniques. It will increase natural endorphin release to decrease pain perception. Music is a distraction that shifts the woman's attention from bodily sensations. Television may have the same effect for some women. Nurses should keep in mind that noise may also overstimulate the laboring woman and cause increased tension and anxiety.

### Reducing Anxiety and Fear

The nurse may reduce a woman's anxiety and increase her self-control by providing accurate information and focusing on the normality of birth. Hospitals are typically associated with illness or injury, situations that are anxiety provoking. Yet hospitals are the most common site for the normal event of birth in the United States.

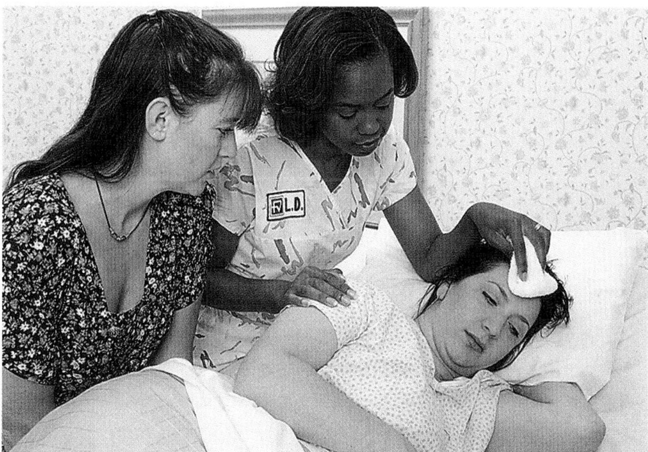


FIG 18.2 General comfort measures such as the nurse's reassuring presence or a cool, damp cloth applied to the face supplement other methods of nonpharmacologic and pharmacologic pain control.

Simple nursing actions keep the focus on the normality of childbirth, regardless of the setting. For example, referring to a woman as a *patient* reinforces the atmosphere of illness associated with being in a hospital, whereas calling her by name helps her to see birth as a normal process. Empowering the woman and her partner by giving them choices whenever possible helps them see themselves as competent people who can accomplish the task of giving birth.

### Relaxation

Promoting relaxation provides a base for all other methods, both nonpharmacologic and pharmacologic because relaxation does the following:

- Promotes uterine blood flow, thus improving fetal oxygenation
- Promotes efficient uterine contractions
- Reduces tension that increases **pain perception** (lowest level of stimulus that one perceives as painful) and decreases **pain tolerance** (maximum pain one is willing to endure)
- Reduces tension that can inhibit fetal descent

***Implementing specific relaxation techniques.*** Relaxation techniques work best if they are learned and practiced before labor. During practice sessions at home, couples may practice *progressive relaxation,* in which the woman contracts and then releases specific muscle groups until all muscles are relaxed. *Neuromuscular dissociation* helps the woman learn to relax all muscles except those that are working (the uterus or the abdominal muscles when pushing). The woman can learn *touch relaxation* in response to her partner's touch, and *relaxation against pain* as the partner deliberately causes mild pain and the woman learns to relax despite the pain.

Even if the woman did not practice these relaxation techniques at home, the nurse can teach her how to consciously relax as labor goes by. The partner can learn to watch for signs of tension, touch that area, and direct the woman to relax.

### Mind-Body Stimulation

Stimulation techniques have several variations that are often combined with each other or with other techniques.

***Self-massage.*** The woman may rub her abdomen, legs, or back in a self-massage called **effleurage** to counteract discomfort. Some women find abdominal touch irritating, especially near the umbilicus.

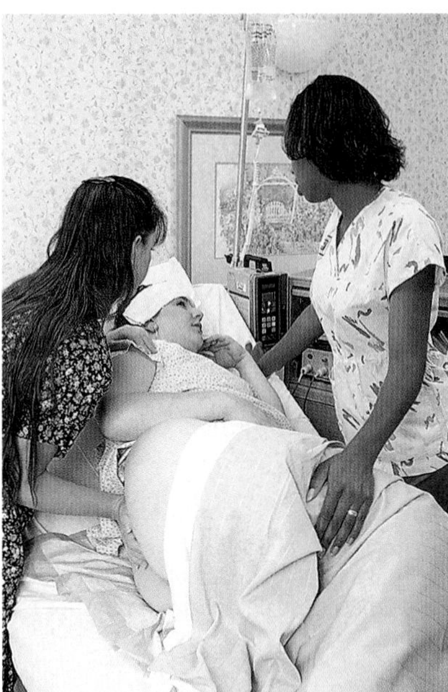

FIG 18.3 The coach applies sacral pressure to counter the back pain that is common during labor.

Women in labor may find firm stroking more helpful than very light stroking. They can trace figure eights or circles on the bed if touch irritates them.

Some women benefit from firm palm or sole stimulation during labor. They may like to have their palms rubbed vigorously by another, rub their hands or feet together, or bang their palms on, or grip, a cool surface. They may hold another person's hand tightly during a contraction. The nurse should determine if these actions indicate excess pain or if they are a woman's way of countering pain, and thus, useful.

***Massage by others.*** The partner or the nurse can rub the woman's back, shoulders, legs, or any area where she finds massage helpful. Sacral pressure is a variation that may help when the woman has back pain, which is usually most intense when the fetus is in an occiput posterior position. Sacral pressure may be applied using the palm of the hand, the fist or fists, or a firm object such as two tennis balls in a sock (Fig. 18.3).

Nonclinical touch by the nurse is a powerful tool if the woman does not object to it. Holding her hand, stroking her hair, or similar actions convey caring, comfort, affirmation, and reassurance at this vulnerable time.

***Thermal stimulation.*** Many women like to have warmth applied to their back, abdomen, or perineum during labor. A warm shower, tub bath, or whirlpool bath is relaxing and provides thermal stimulation. A sock filled with dry rice and microwaved provides gentle warmth and can be used to apply pressure to the sacral area.

Cool, damp washcloths may be comforting, especially if a woman is hot. She may put them on her head, throat, abdomen, or any place she wants. She also may want to put them in or over her mouth to relieve dryness (see Fig. 18.2).

***Acupressure.*** Acupressure is a directed form of massage in which the support person applies pressure to specific pressure points using hands, rollers, balls, or other equipment. Acupressure is related to its invasive counterpart, acupuncture, in which tiny needles are inserted into similar points. Data support the effectiveness of acupuncture and acupressure to relieve pregnancy-related nausea and vomiting, including "morning sickness." Few controlled studies have reported on their usefulness during birth. For updated, objective information on acupressure and other complementary and alternative medicine (CAM) techniques, visit the website for the National Center for Complementary and Alternative Medicine, one of the institutes of the National Institutes of Health (http://www.nncam.nih.gov).

### BOX 18.1 Use of Water Therapy During Labor

Use of water therapy has accompanied trends toward a low-intervention approach to intrapartum care. Water therapy can be delivered in several ways:

- Shower
- Standard tub
- Whirlpool

**Benefits**

- Associated with a more natural, home-like atmosphere.
- Gives a woman greater control over her labor.
- Upright position facilitates progress of labor.
- Faster labor progress if contractions are frequent when woman enters the tub.
- Buoyancy relieves tired muscles and reduces pressure.
- Facilitates fetal rotation from occiput posterior or transverse positions to the occiput anterior position. The woman can also assume different positions to aid rotation.
- Many women report a perception of less pain.
- Reduction in the mean arterial pressure, edema, and increased diuresis. This effect is especially helpful if the woman has pregnancy-induced hypertension.

**Disadvantages**

- Fetus must be assessed with intermittent auscultation rather than electronic fetal monitoring.

**Contraindications and Precautions**

- No specific contraindications if the woman can safely be out of bed.
- Thick meconium in the amniotic fluid is an indication for continuous electronic fetal monitoring in most birth facilities and would preclude the use of water therapy.
- Bleeding.
- Oxytocin induction or augmentation. The use of both oxytocin and water therapy could cause excess uterine activity. Oxytocin use is usually an indication for continuous fetal monitoring in a birth facility.

### Hydrotherapy

Water therapy (Box 18.1) in the form of a shower, tub bath, or whirlpool can supplement any relaxation technique. The buoyancy afforded by immersion supports the body, equalizes pressure, and aids muscle relaxation. In addition, fluid shifts from the extravascular space to the intravascular space, reducing edema as the excess fluid is excreted by the kidneys. Hydrotherapy for labor requires a supportive environment, adequate nursing policies and staffing, and collaborative relationships between nurses and other care providers. Systematic review of current research indicates there is little difference in neonatal outcomes between waterbirth and traditional birth. A decrease in the length of labor, labor pain, and degree of perineal tears with waterbirth was also found (Davies, Davis, Pearce, et al., 2014).

### Mental Stimulation

Mental techniques occupy the woman's mind and compete with pain stimuli. They also aid relaxation by providing a tranquil imaginary atmosphere.

*Imagery.* If the woman has not practiced a specific imagery technique, the nurse can help her create a relaxing mental scene. Most women find images of warmth, softness, security, and total relaxation most comforting.

Guided imagery can help the woman dissociate herself from the painful aspects of labor. For example, the nurse can help her visualize the work of labor: the cervix opening with each contraction or the fetus moving down toward the outlet each time she pushes. This technique is like visualizing success or movement toward a goal with each contraction.

*Focal point.* When using nonpharmacologic techniques, a woman may prefer to close her eyes or may want to concentrate on an external focal point. Keeping her eyes on a focal point may help the woman concentrate on something outside her body, and thus, away from the pain from contractions. She may bring a picture of a relaxing scene or an object to use as a focal point and to aid in the use of imagery. She can use any point in the room as a focal point.

### Breathing Techniques

Breathing techniques provide a different focus during contractions, interfering with pain sensory transmission (Fig. 18.4). Breathing techniques often supplement other nonpharmacologic and pharmacologic techniques. Techniques begin with simple breathing patterns and progress to more complex ones as needed. There is no single right time to begin using breathing techniques or to change patterns during labor. However, prolonged use of complex breathing techniques can be tiring.

*First-stage breathing.* Breathing in the first stage of labor consists of a cleansing breath and various breathing techniques known as *paced breathing*. The method begins with a very simple technique that is used as long as possible. When it is no longer effective, breathing that requires more concentration is added.

Cleansing breath. Each contraction in the first and second stages begins and ends with a deep inspiration and expiration known as the *cleansing breath*. Like a sigh, a cleansing breath helps the woman release tension. It provides oxygen to help prevent myometrial hypoxia, one cause of pain in labor. The cleansing breath also helps the woman clear her mind to focus on relaxing and signals her labor partner that the contraction is beginning or ending. The woman may inhale through the nose and exhale through the mouth or take her cleansing breath in any way comfortable for her.

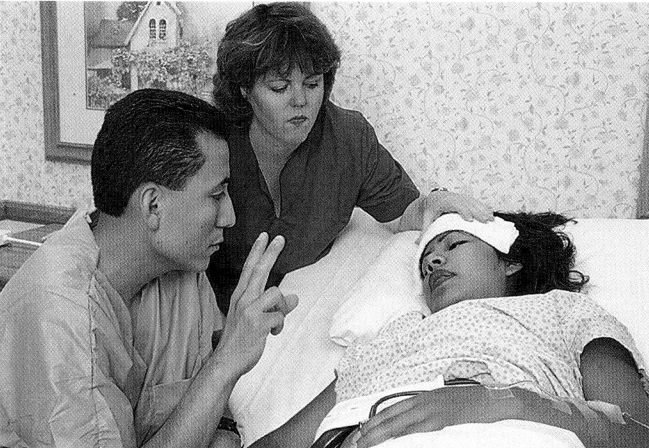

**FIG 18.4** A woman and her partner who are prepared for labor have learned a variety of skills to master pain as labor progresses. The coach uses hand signals to tell the woman how to change her pattern of paced breathing.

Slow-paced breathing. The first breathing is slow-paced breathing, a slow, deep breathing that increases relaxation (Fig. 18.5). The woman should concentrate on relaxing her body rather than on regulating the rate of her breathing. Relaxation naturally brings about slower breathing, similar to that which occurs during sleep. She can use nose, mouth, or combination breathing, depending on which is most comfortable.

The woman uses slow-paced breathing as long as possible during labor because it promotes relaxation and sufficient oxygenation. Slow-paced breathing is easy for the unprepared woman to learn between contractions and, with the support of the nurse, helps even a frightened woman become calm and able to work with her contractions.

### Modified-Paced Breathing

When the woman finds that slow-paced breathing is no longer effective, she begins modified-paced breathing (Fig. 18.6). This chest breathing at a faster rate matches the natural tendency to use more rapid breathing during stress or physical work, such as labor. Although modified-paced breathing is shallower than slow-paced breathing, the faster rate allows oxygen intake to remain about the same. As with slow-paced breathing, the focus is on release of tension rather than on the actual number of breaths taken.

Women can combine slow- and modified-paced breathing during the course of a contraction (Fig. 18.7). They begin slowly and use shallow, faster breathing at the peak of the contraction. Breathing should not interfere with relaxation but enhance it.

Pattern-paced breathing. Pattern-paced breathing (sometimes called "pant blow," "hee hoo," or "hee blow" breathing) involves focusing on a rhythmic pattern of breathing (Fig. 18.8). It is similar to modified-paced breathing. It differs in that after a certain number of breaths, the woman exhales with a slight emphasis or blow and then begins the modified-paced breathing again. The addition of a blow causes her to focus more on her breathing and reduces habituation. Some educators teach women to make a sound such as "hee" during this breathing and to blow through pursed lips with a "hoo" sound. Others avoid special sounds, which tighten the vocal cords and may decrease relaxation.

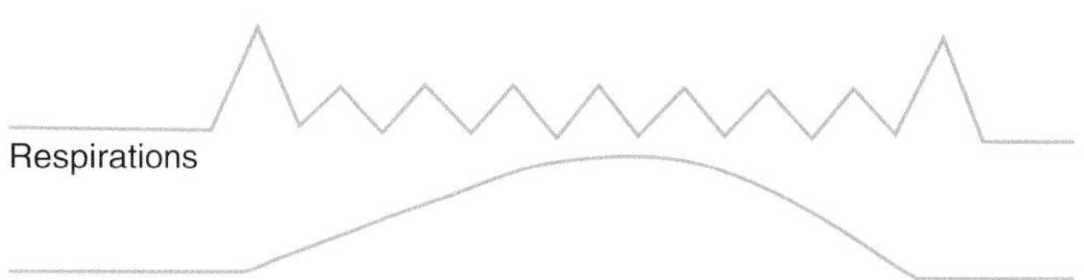


**FIG 18.5** Slow-paced breathing. Although a specific rate may or may not be taught, slow-paced breathing should be *no slower than half* the woman's usual respiratory rate to ensure adequate oxygenation. This pace is generally approximately six to nine breaths per minute.

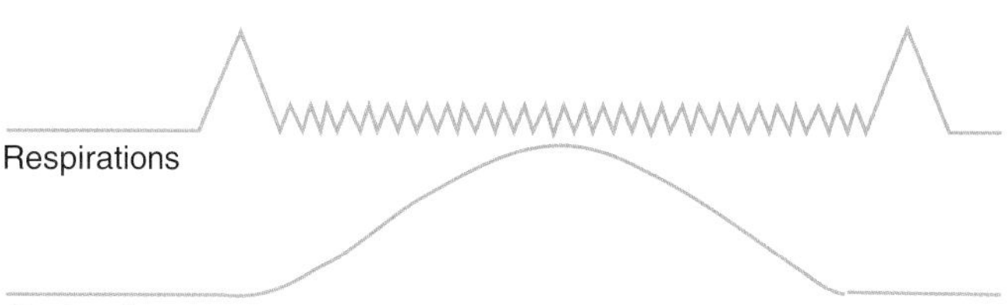


**FIG 18.6** Modified-paced breathing. The pattern for modified-paced breathing should be comfortable to the woman and *no faster than twice* her normal respiratory rate to prevent hyperventilation or interference with relaxation.

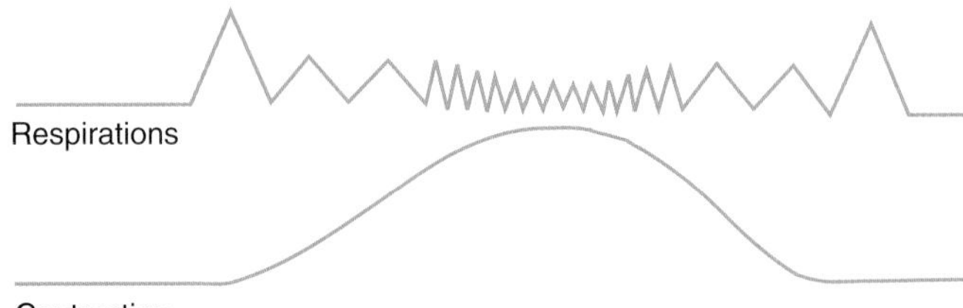


FIG 18.7 Combining breathing techniques during a contraction. Slow- and modified-paced breathing can be combined by using the slower breathing at the beginning and end of the contraction and the more rapid breathing over the peak of the contraction.

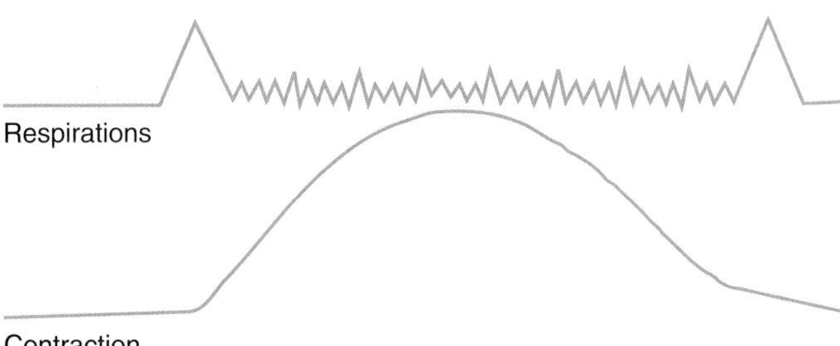


FIG 18.8 Pattern-paced breathing. Pattern-paced breathing adds a slight emphasis or "blow" on the exhalation in a pattern. The diagram shows the emphasis after every third inhalation.

The number of breaths before the blow may remain constant (usually between two and six) or may change in a pattern. Variations include a set pattern such as 3-1 or a stairstep pattern such as 6-1, 5-1, 4-1, 3-1. Some couples use a random pattern determined by the coach, who uses hand or verbal signals to show the number of breaths the woman should take before each blow.

**Controlling the urge to push.** If a woman pushes strenuously before the cervix is completely dilated, she risks injury to the cervix and reduced oxygenation of the fetus. Blowing prevents closure of the glottis and breath holding, which are a part of strenuous pushing. The woman blows repeatedly using short puffs when the urge to push is strong. The support person may learn to blow along with her to help the woman concentrate. Some women vary the blowing by using one short breath and one blow.

**Common problems.** Hyperventilation and mouth dryness may occur during breathing techniques. Hyperventilation is the result of rapid deep breathing that causes excessive loss of carbon dioxide, eventually resulting in respiratory alkalosis. The woman may feel dizzy or lightheaded and have impaired thinking. Vasoconstriction leads to tingling and numbness in fingers and lips. If hyperventilation continues, tetany caused by decreased calcium in tissues and blood may result in stiffness of the face and lips and carpopedal spasm.

The woman can slow her breathing between contractions or breathe in her own cupped hands if she feels dizzy. Rebreathing exhaled air in this way increases her blood carbon dioxide levels. Reassure the woman that these measures help restore her carbon dioxide level to normal and are relaxing.

Dryness of the mouth occurs when the woman uses prolonged mouth breathing. To avoid dryness, she can place her tongue gently against the roof of her mouth to moisturize entering air. The support person can offer ice, mouthwash, or liquids or encourage her to brush her teeth.

***Second-stage breathing.*** Care in the second stage of labor encourages a physiologic completion of labor, assisting the mother to respond to her urge to push rather than directing her to push as soon as her cervix is completely dilated even if she does not feel the urge. Lengthy pushing in second stage has been shown to result in greater maternal fatigue, more operative births and nonreassuring fetal heart rate (FHR) patterns, and does not significantly shorten the second stage.

With newer techniques of epidural block, women who choose this method of labor pain control often feel the urge to push, although not as strongly as unmedicated women. Using their natural urge to push, even if reduced, helps them push effectively with contractions. Delaying pushing for up to 1 to 2 hours after complete dilation has shown benefits similar to those of women who do not have epidural analgesia.

Research has shown that strenuous directed pushing increases risk for structural and neurogenic injury to a woman's pelvic floor. Closed-glottis pushing causes recurrent increases in intrathoracic pressure with a resulting fall in cardiac output and blood pressure. The woman's lower blood pressure then causes less blood to be delivered to the placenta, resulting in fetal hypoxia that is reflected in nonreassuring fetal heart patterns.

Promotion of a physiologic second stage uses spontaneous pushing. The woman makes her decision with the nurse about when it is time to start pushing. She may grunt, groan, sigh, or moan as she pushes, and the nurse should validate that these sounds are normal. Pushing three to four times for 6 to 8 seconds is likely to be effective in aiding descent and is safe for the baby. Allowing the mother to position for comfort is essential to improve fetal descent. Adjust the pushing process depending on the fetal status (AWHONN, 2014).

## PHARMACOLOGIC PAIN MANAGEMENT

Pharmacologic methods for pain management include systemic drugs, regional pain management, and general anesthesia.

### Special Considerations When Medicating a Pregnant Woman

Medicating a woman when she is pregnant is not straightforward for several reasons:

- Any drug taken by the woman may affect her fetus.
- Drugs may have effects in pregnancy that they do not have in a nonpregnant person.
- Drugs can affect the course and length of labor.
- Complications may limit the choice of pharmacologic pain management.
- Women who need other therapeutic drugs, use herbal or botanical preparations, or practice substance abuse may have fewer safe choices for labor pain relief.

#### Effects on the Fetus

Fetal effects of drugs given to the mother may be direct or indirect. Direct effects result from passage of the drug or its metabolites across the placenta to the fetus. An example of a direct effect on the fetus is decreased FHR variability after administration of an **analgesic** (systemic agent that relieves pain without causing loss of consciousness) to the woman. Indirect effects are secondary to drug effects on the mother. For example, a drug that causes maternal hypotension can reduce blood flow to the placenta. Fetal hypoxia and acidosis may result from major reductions in placental perfusion.

#### Maternal Physiologic Alterations

Normal pregnancy-related changes in four body systems have the greatest implications for pharmacologic pain management methods.

*Cardiovascular changes.* Cardiac output increases, which indirectly affects hepatic and renal blood flow. Decreased plasma binding increases the amount of free circulating medications. Plasma concentrations of free drug levels increase due to the decreased blood flow to lower extremities for women in supine positions.

*Respiratory changes.* A pregnant woman's full uterus reduces her respiratory capacity. To compensate, she breathes more rapidly and deeply. As a result, she is more vulnerable to reduced arterial oxygenation during induction of general anesthesia and is more sensitive to inhalational anesthetic agents.

*Gastrointestinal changes.* A pregnant woman's stomach is displaced upward by her large uterus; the stomach's interior also has a higher pressure. Progesterone slows peristalsis, reduces the tone of the sphincter at the junction of the stomach and esophagus, and decreases GI absorption of any oral medications. These changes make a pregnant woman more vulnerable to regurgitation and aspiration of acidic gastric contents during general anesthesia.

*Nervous system changes.* During pregnancy and labor, circulating levels of endorphins and enkephalins, morphine-like natural analgesics, are high. These substances modify pain perception and reduce requirements for analgesia and anesthesia medications.

The epidural and subarachnoid spaces (space between the arachnoid matter and the pia mater that contains the spinal fluid) are smaller during pregnancy, enhancing the spread of anesthetic agents used for epidural or subarachnoid blocks (SABs). The cerebrospinal fluid (CSF) pressure is higher, reaching a peak during the second stage of labor. Nerve fibers are more sensitive to local anesthetic agents, probably because of acid–base or hormonal alterations. High intraabdominal pressure causes engorgement of the epidural veins, increasing the risk for intravascular injection of anesthetic agents. The net result of these changes is that a smaller volume of the anesthetic agent may be needed to achieve satisfactory epidural or SAB.

### Effects on the Course of Labor

Caregivers must consider the adverse effects of excessive pain on labor's progress when helping a woman choose the method and timing of pain relief. Most analgesics are not given until labor is well established because they can slow progress if given too early. Regional anesthetics such as the epidural block reduce a woman's sensation of an urge to push, so she may need specific coaching when it is time to push.

### Pregnancy Complications

Patients with pregnancy complications may have limited choices regarding analgesia or anesthesia. Pregnancy complications also may require changes in how the medication is administered. For example, large volumes of IV fluids may be infused to prevent hypotension with regional anesthesia (anesthesia that blocks pain impulses in a localized area with no loss of consciousness). If a pregnant woman has heart disease, this fluid load could be detrimental. Yet without it, she is vulnerable to hypotension. Providers must exercise caution when considering pain management options.

### Interactions With Other Substances

A woman who ingests therapeutic or botanical agents may have fewer options that are also safe for the fetus because of interactions between these substances and analgesics or anesthetics. Women who have abused substances will have fewer options for pain management.

## Regional Pain Management Techniques

Regional pain control methods may be used for intrapartum analgesia, anesthesia, or both. These methods provide pain relief without loss of consciousness. Such methods include regional anesthesia such as pudendal and paracervical blocks. Neuraxial regional blocks include spinal, epidural, and combined spinal–epidural anesthesia.

The major advantage of regional pain management methods is that the woman can participate in birth yet still have good pain control. The woman usually feels some pressure and discomfort, although these sensations are greatly reduced. She can interact with her infant and partner and does not lose her protective airway reflexes, as can happen with general anesthesia. The disadvantages of regional pain control techniques depend on the specific technique used. The effect on the fetus depends on how the woman responds rather than on direct drug effects.

Epidural block analgesia or anesthesia provides pain control during much of labor and for the birth itself. Intrathecal opioids are used for pain control during labor; additional measures are needed during late labor and for the birth. Combined spinal–epidural (CSE) analgesia allows subarachnoid injection of opioids via a spinal needle followed by ongoing pain relief from anesthetics injected through the epidural catheter.

### Regional Anesthesia

Paracervical anesthesia provides comfort during the first stage of labor. The advantages of this method include its lack of effects on labor progress and on sensory or motor function. The major disadvantage is that is does not provide comfort in the second stage, so other analgesia must be considered. Pudendal nerve block is used in the second stage of labor immediately before delivery. It provides relief at delivery, but can be ineffective for repair of lacerations or episiotomy (Chestnut, 2014).

### Pudendal Block

A pudendal block anesthetizes the lower vagina and part of the perineum to provide anesthesia for an episiotomy and vaginal birth. A pudendal block does not block pain from uterine contractions, and the mother feels pressure. It is often used for repair of lacerations or episiotomy (Chestnut, 2014).

The physician or nurse-midwife injects the pudendal nerves near each ischial spine with local anesthetic (Fig. 18.9). The perineum is infiltrated with local anesthetic because the pudendal block does not fully anesthetize this area. As with local infiltration, a delay occurs

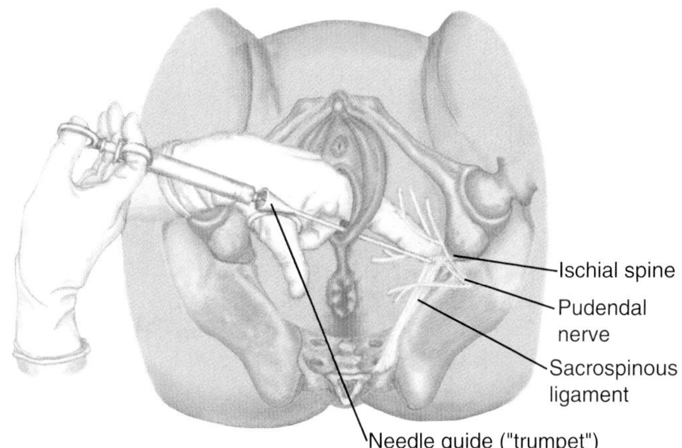


FIG 18.9 Pudendal block provides anesthesia for an episiotomy and the use of low forceps. A needle guide ("trumpet") protects the maternal and fetal tissues from the long needle needed to reach the pudendal nerve. Only approximately 1.25 cm (½ in) of the long needle protrudes from the guide.

between injection and the onset of numbness. Possible maternal complications include a toxic reaction to the anesthetic, rectal puncture, hematoma, and sciatic nerve block. If maternal toxicity is avoided, the fetus is usually not affected.

### Local Infiltration Anesthesia

Infiltration of the perineum with a local anesthetic is done by the physician or nurse-midwife just before performing an episiotomy or suturing a laceration (Fig. 18.10). Local infiltration does not alter pain from uterine contractions or distention of the vagina. The local agent provides anesthesia in the immediate area of the episiotomy or laceration. There is a short delay between anesthetic injection and the onset of numbness, and the drug burns before its anesthetic action begins. Local infiltration rarely has adverse effects on either mother or infant.

### Epidural Block

The epidural block is a popular and versatile regional block for relief of pain in labor and birth. It is useful for both vaginal and cesarean births.

The **epidural space** is outside the dura mater, between the dura and the spinal canal. It is loosely filled with fat, connective tissue, and epidural veins that are dilated during pregnancy (Fig. 18.11).

The epidural block is done by injecting local anesthetic into the tiny epidural space. Inclusion of opioids reduces the amount of local anesthetic needed for adequate pain relief, thus limiting loss of movement and sensation. Epidural analgesia provides substantial relief of pain from contractions and birth canal distention. The level of the epidural block can be extended upward to provide anesthesia for a cesarean birth or tubal ligation after birth. Higher concentrations of the anesthetic agent used for abdominal surgery result in loss of both motor and sensory function.

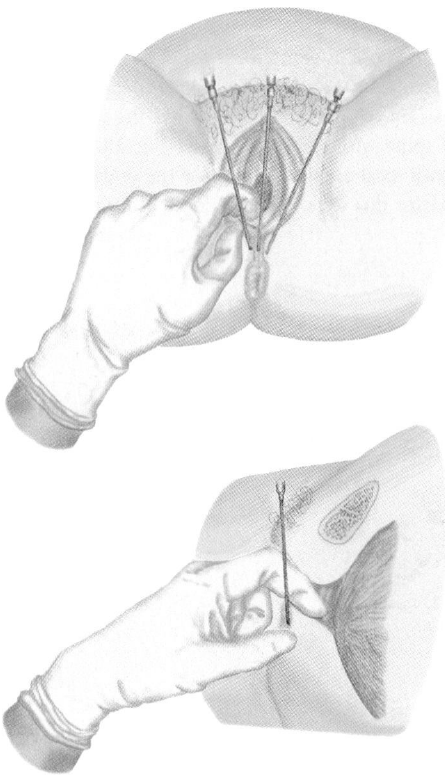

FIG 18.10 Local infiltration anesthesia numbs the perineum just before birth for an episiotomy or after birth for suturing of a laceration. The birth attendant protects the fetal head by placing a finger inside the vagina while injecting the perineum in a fan-like pattern or as needed.

***Technique.*** The epidural block is started after labor is established or just before a scheduled cesarean birth. The epidural space is entered at about the L3-L4 interspace (below the end of the spinal cord), and a catheter is passed through the needle into the epidural space (Fig. 18.12). The catheter allows continuous infusion or intermittent injection of medication to maintain pain relief during labor and vaginal or cesarean birth. Infusion of epidural medication can also be regulated by a patient-controlled epidural analgesia (PCEA) pump (American Society of Anesthesiologists (ASA), 2016; Wong, 2014).

A small (3 mL) test dose of local anesthetic may be injected before the full dose is given and before subsequent intermittent doses to verify catheter placement. Alternatively, the anesthesia provider may inject the total initial dose of the drug in small increments. If a large dose of anesthetic is injected into the subarachnoid space instead of the epidural space, the woman may experience rapid, intense motor and **sensory block** (loss of sensation). The test dose also can detect accidental intravascular injection. The woman has numbness of the tongue and lips, lightheadedness, dizziness, and tinnitus with intravascular injection. Epinephrine in the test dose produces tachycardia if injected intravascularly, helping distinguish tachycardia caused by labor pain from that caused by intravascular injection (ASA, 2016; Wong, 2014)

The local anesthetic drugs bupivacaine, levobupivacaine, and lidocaine are usually combined with a very small dose of an opioid analgesic such as fentanyl (Sublimaze), sufentanil (Sufenta), or morphine (Duramorph). All drugs injected into the epidural or subarachnoid spaces are preservative free. The drug combination provides rapid onset of relief and permits a lower total dose of local anesthetic with less **motor block**, or loss of voluntary movement (Wong, 2014). Epidural analgesics also are given after cesarean birth to provide long-acting pain relief with a low dose. The mother is comfortable enough to interact with her infant and family.

***Dural puncture.*** Because the tough dura and the fragile web-like arachnoid membranes lie close together, dural puncture also punctures the arachnoid. If the dura is unintentionally punctured with the needle used to introduce the catheter, substantial leakage of cerebrospinal fluid can occur, which may result in a spinal headache. Dural puncture and spinal headache also can occur without obvious cerebrospinal fluid leakage.

***Contraindications and precautions.*** An epidural block is suitable for most laboring women. Contraindications include the woman's refusal, coagulation defects, uncorrected hypovolemia, an infection in the area of insertion or a severe systemic infection, allergy, or a fetal condition that demands birth sooner than the block can become effective. Women who have had spinal surgery, as for scoliosis (spinal curvature), are evaluated individually. Compression of the aorta and inferior vena cava (aortocaval compression) by the uterus can also occur when a woman lies in the supine position. If placing a regional block or other procedure requires that the woman lie on her back, the uterus must be displaced to one side with the hands or with a small wedge placed under one hip. Operating room tables can often be tilted slightly to one side during a cesarean birth to provide a comparable safety measure.

***Adverse effects of epidural block.*** An epidural block can have adverse effects.

**Maternal hypotension.** Sympathetic nerves are blocked along with pain nerves, which may result in vasodilation and hypotension. Maternal hypotension with possible reduction in placental perfusion is most likely to occur within the first 15 minutes after epidural

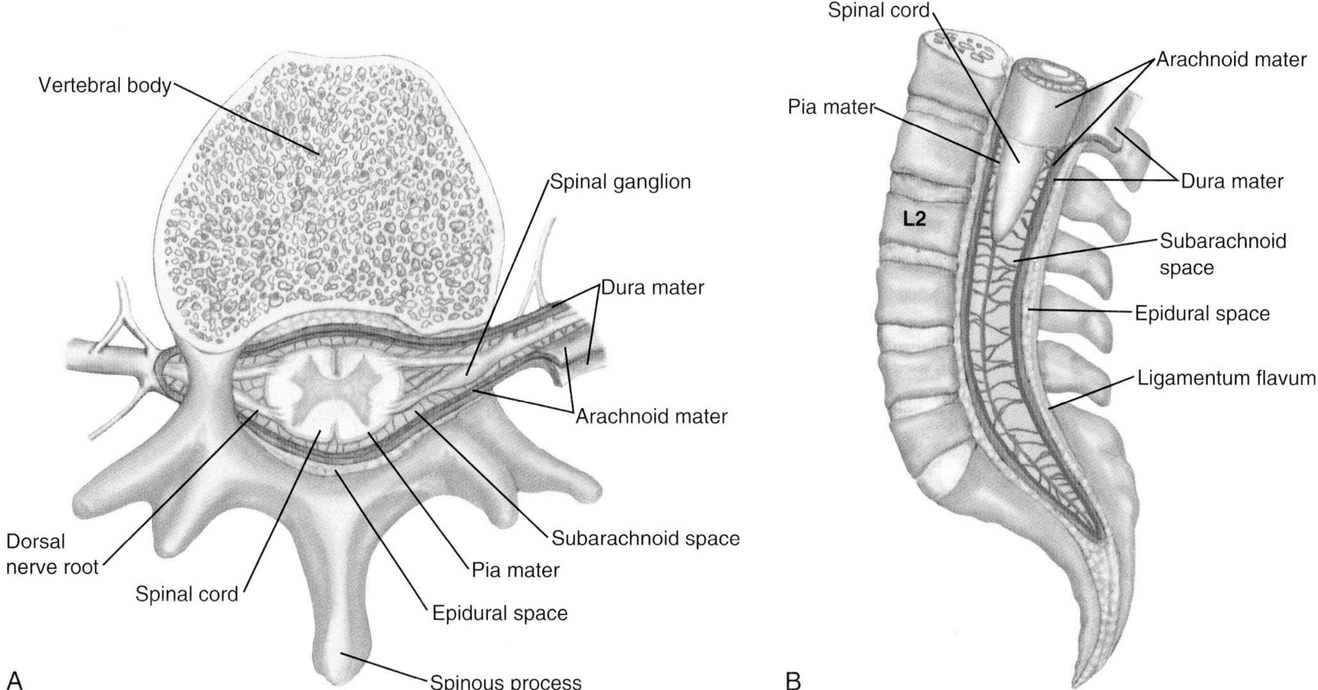


**FIG 18.11** **A,** Cross section of spinal cord, meninges, and protective vertebra. The dura and arachnoid lie close together. The pia mater is the innermost of the meninges and covers the brain and spinal cord. The subarachnoid space is between the arachnoid and pia mater. **B,** Sagittal section of spinal cord, meninges, and vertebrae. The epidural and subarachnoid spaces are illustrated. Note that the spinal cord ends at the L2 vertebra.

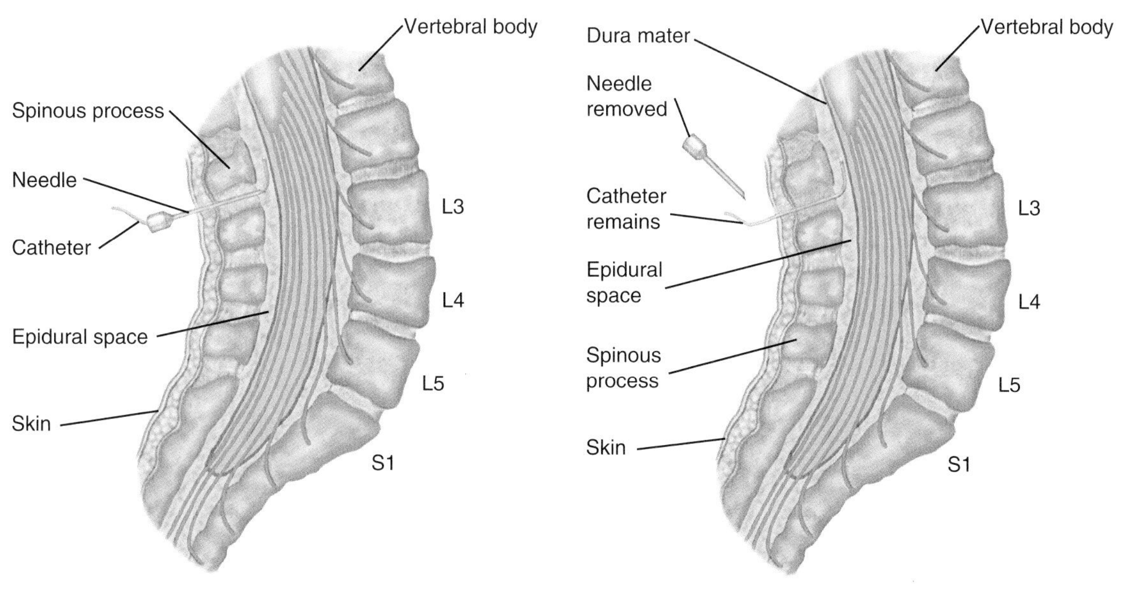


**FIG 18.12** Technique for epidural block.

initiation or injection of intermittent bolus doses to maintain pain relief. However, a significant percentage of women may have hypotension that occurs within 1 hour of initiation or repeat bolus doses (AWHONN, 2011; Cunningham, Leveno, Bloom, et al., 2014). In addition, if the mother has hypotension, the fetus is more likely to have nonreassuring fetal heart pattern on an electronic fetal monitor strip, such as a rising baseline, tachycardia, or late decelerations. However, nonreassuring fetal signs may also have other etiologies (see Chapter 17).

Rapid infusion of a nondextrose IV solution, often warmed, such as lactated Ringer's or normal saline, before initiation of the block fills the vascular system to offset vasodilation. Preload IV quantities are at least 500 to 1000 mL infused rapidly. If hypotension occurs, turn patient to left lateral side lying position, infuse intravenous crystalloid fluids, and IV ephedrine in 5- to 10-mg increments promotes vasoconstriction to raise the blood pressure. Additional maternal oxygen administration as needed.

**Bladder distention.** A woman's bladder fills quickly because of the large quantity of IV solution, yet her sensation to void is reduced. Continuous or intermittent bladder catheterization is usually required, increasing risk of infection.

**Prolonged second stage.** The urge to push is often less intense with reduced sensation. Forceps- or vacuum extractor-assisted births are more likely because of the reduced urge to push.

**Migration of the epidural catheter.** The catheter may move after accurate placement. A woman may then have symptoms of intravascular injection, an intense block, a block that is too high, absence of anesthesia, or a unilateral block.

**Fever.** Fever with no apparent infection may occur in a woman who has epidural analgesia, and its cause is not clear. The neonate's temperature may be elevated as well, possibly leading to unnecessary treatment for neonatal sepsis. Possible explanations for epidural-associated fever in the absence of infection include (AWHONN, 2011):

1. Decreased hyperventilation, sweating, and activity after onset of pain relief reduce heat dissipation.
2. Vasodilation redistributes heat from the core to the periphery of the body, where it is lost to the environment. The lower core temperature then signals the hypothalamus to increase heat production.
3. Shivering often occurs with sympathetic blockade accompanied by a dissociation between warm and cold sensations. In effect, the body believes that the temperature is lower than the true temperature and raises the "thermostat" to produce heat by shivering, thus increasing the core temperature.

***Adverse effects of epidural opioids.*** Adverse maternal effects associated with epidural opioids may include nausea and vomiting, pruritus (itching), and delayed respiratory depression.

**Nausea and vomiting.** As when opioids are given by other routes, nausea and vomiting may occur. Adjunctive drugs such as promethazine (Phenergan) reduce nausea and vomiting.

**Pruritus.** Itching of the face and neck is a harmless but annoying side effect of epidural opioids. Although she may not specifically complain of itching, a woman may rub or scratch her face and neck frequently. Diphenhydramine (Benadryl) or very small doses of naloxone (Narcan), nalbuphine (Nubain), or naltrexone (Trexan) may relieve bothersome pruritus (Wong, 2014) (Table 18.1).

**Respiratory depression.** The possibility of respiratory depression in the mother persists for up to 24 hours after the administration of an epidural opioid for cesarean pain relief, depending on the drug used.

***Nursing care***

**Nursing care for epidural placement.** Preparation for epidural anesthesia includes acquiring informed consent. Monitoring equipment for vital signs and fetal monitoring should be in place. The nurse should record baseline maternal vital signs and FHR and patterns for comparison with prenatal levels and those after the block. IV access is ensured, and the prescribed preload of 500 to 1000 mL fluid is given. The nurse supports the woman in lateral decubitus or sitting position and tells the anesthesia provider when the woman is having a contraction. The woman may feel a brief "electric shock" sensation as the catheter is passed. The nurse should assist her in remaining still while the block is completed. After the test dose medication is injected, the nurse observes for signs of subarachnoid puncture or intravascular injection.

Evidence-based practice guidelines from AWHONN (2011) state that evidence is insufficient to set firm guidelines for the frequency of maternal blood pressure and fetal heart monitoring during an epidural block. However, based on a literature review, the committee suggests assessing the blood pressure and FHR every 5 minutes during the first 15 minutes after initiation of the epidural or after any additional bolus doses. Repeat the blood pressure checks at 30 minutes and 1 hour after the epidural is started. Consider factors that may indicate more or less frequent monitoring for each patient.

The woman's bladder must be assessed frequently because of the large IV fluid load and her reduced sensation to void. Intermittent or indwelling catheterization is usual. Her temperature should be assessed for a rise with a possible rise in the baseline FHR before maternal fever.

The nurse should observe for signs associated with catheter migration from the epidural space and for adverse effects from epidural opioids, such as nausea, vomiting, and pruritus. Reassurance about the harmless and temporary nature of pruritus is often sufficient.

### Combined Spinal-Epidural Analgesia

Injection of an opioid analgesic into the intrathecal space provides labor pain management without sedation. The drug binds to opiate receptors in the subarachnoid space, allowing much smaller doses than systemic opioids. The woman can feel her contractions but not the pain. The CSE discussed earlier combines the epidural with the intrathecal opioid.

Advantages of intrathecal analgesics include:

- Rapid onset of pain relief without sedation
- No motor block, enabling the woman to ambulate during labor (unless she receives a concurrent epidural block)
- No sympathetic block, with its hypotensive effects

Disadvantages include:

- Dural puncture leads to potential for postdural headache

***Technique.*** The most common CSE technique is the needle-through-needle technique in the midlumbar spinous space. An epidural catheter is then placed for on-going analgesia and anesthesia for delivery or cesarean section.

The drug chosen depends on the expected duration of labor at the time of administration. Preservative-free drugs that can be used by this route include fentanyl, sufentanil, and morphine.

***Adverse effects of intrathecal opioids.*** As with epidural opioids, nausea, vomiting, and pruritus may occur. Delayed respiratory depression may occur, depending on the drug used.

***Nursing care.*** Vital signs and FHR are taken at the usual intervals for the woman's stage of labor. Side effects, such as nausea, vomiting, and pruritus, are reported and managed similarly to those occurring with the epidural block. Reduced effectiveness suggests that the drug's duration of action is ending or that the woman is in late labor. Other

**TABLE 18.1 Drugs Commonly Used for Intrapartum Pain Management**

| Drug/Dose | Comments |
|---|---|
| ***Opioid Analgesics*** | |
| Meperidine (Demerol) | Respiratory depression in the neonate at 3–5 hours |
| 12.5–50 mg every 2–4 hr IV; 50–100 mg every 204 hours IM | Long half-life for active metabolite normeperidine |
| Fentanyl (Sublimaze)<br>20–50 mcg IV; may be repeated every hour; may be given by PCA | Onset is quick (5 min for IV administration), but duration of action is short. Less nausea, vomiting, and respiratory depression occurs than with meperidine. Epidural use may cause pruritus. |
| Butorphanol (Stadol)<br>1–2 mg every 4 hr; IM or IV | Has some narcotic antagonist effects; should not be given to the opiate-dependent woman (may precipitate withdrawal) or after other narcotics such as meperidine (may reverse their analgesic effects); also a respiratory depressant. |
| Nalbuphine (Nubain)<br>10 mg every 3 hr IV or IM; | Opioid agonist/antagonist, lower neonatal neurobehavioral scores. Less nausea and vomiting, more sedation than meperidine. Low dose may decrease pruritus. |
| ***Adjunctive Drugs*** | |
| Metochlopramide (Reglan)<br>1–2 mg IV every 2–4 hours | Additive CNS depression with use of opioids, causes drowsiness. |
| Ondansetron (Zofran)<br>4 mg IV prior to anesthesia or after umbilical clamping, 0.15 mg/kg repeat every 4 hours, maximum dosage 16 mg | Prevention of nausea related to opioids should be adminstered prior to induction of anesthesia. |
| Diphenhydramine (Benadryl)<br>10–50 mg every 4–6 hr IV | Given to relieve pruritus from epidural narcotics. |
| ***Narcotic Antagonists*** | |
| Naloxone (Narcan)<br>Adult: | Action shorter than most narcotics it reverses; must observe for recurrent respiratory depression and be prepared to give additional doses. |
| To reduce respiratory depression induced by opioids: 0.4–2 mg IV<br>To reverse pruritus from epidural opioids:<br>0.04–0.2 mg IV or IV infusion 5–10 mcg/kg/hr | Small doses (0.04–0.08 mg) may be given to reduce pruritus from epidural opioids. |
| Neonatal resuscitation:<br>0.1 mg/kg IV (umbilical vein) or intratracheal | Neonatal resuscitation dose (see Chapter 30). |

*FHR,* Fetal heart rate; *IV,* intravenous; *PCA,* patient-controlled analgesia

References: Cunningham, F. G., Leveno, K. J., Bloom, S. L., Wong, C. Y., Dashe, J. S., Hoffman, B. L., ... & Sheffield, J. S. (2014). *Williams obstetrics* (24th ed.). New York: McGraw-Hill Medical; El-Wahab, N., & Fernando, R. (2014). Systemic analgesia: Parenteral and inhalation agents. In D. Chestnut, C. A. Wong, L. C. Tsen, D. N. K. Warwick, Y. Beilin, J. M. Mhyre & V. Naveen (Eds.), *Chestnut's Obstetric Anesthesia: Principles and practice* (5th ed) Philadelphia: Elsevier Saunders.

pain management methods may be needed for the remainder of labor and for birth.

Care of the woman having a CSE is the same as that for a noncombined block.

### Subarachnoid (Spinal) Block

A subarachnoid block (SAB) may be done when a quick cesarean birth is necessary and an epidural catheter is not in place. The typical SAB provides no pain relief during most of labor. Because of the popularity of epidurals for labor and the ability to give epidural opioids for long-lasting postoperative analgesia, the SAB is less common.

The anesthesia provider injects local anesthetic, often combined with an opioid such as fentanyl, into the subarachnoid space in a single dose. The woman loses both sensory and motor function below the level of the SAB, with complete relief of pain from contractions. A much lower dose of anesthetic agent is required because less absorption into surrounding tissues occurs than with the epidural block.

***Technique.*** A spinal needle is placed in the subarachnoid space. Appearance of cerebrospinal fluid at the needle hub assures correct placement, and the local anesthetic combination is injected (Fig. 18.13).

The level of anesthesia for both epidural blocks and SABs is determined by the volume, concentration, and density of the drug (Fig. 18.14).

***Contraindications and precautions.*** Contraindications and precautions are similar to those for epidural block: the woman's refusal, coagulation defects, uncorrected hypovolemia, infection in the area of insertion, systemic infection, allergy, and previous spinal surgery.

***Adverse effects of an SAB.*** Three adverse effects of an SAB are maternal hypotension, bladder distention, and spinal headache. Hypotension occurs because of sympathetic blockade as in epidural block but can be more severe. Treatment is the same, but a larger preload of IV fluid is common.

Postspinal headache may occur after SAB in some women because of cerebrospinal fluid leakage at the site of dural puncture. A spinal headache is postural; it is worse when a woman is upright and may disappear when she is lying flat. The incidence of spinal headache is lower if a small-gauge needle is used.

Bed rest with oral or IV hydration helps relieve the post-spinal headache. A blood patch often gives dramatic, definitive relief. Ten to 20 mL of the woman's blood (obtained using sterile technique) is injected by the anesthesia provider into the epidural space. The blood

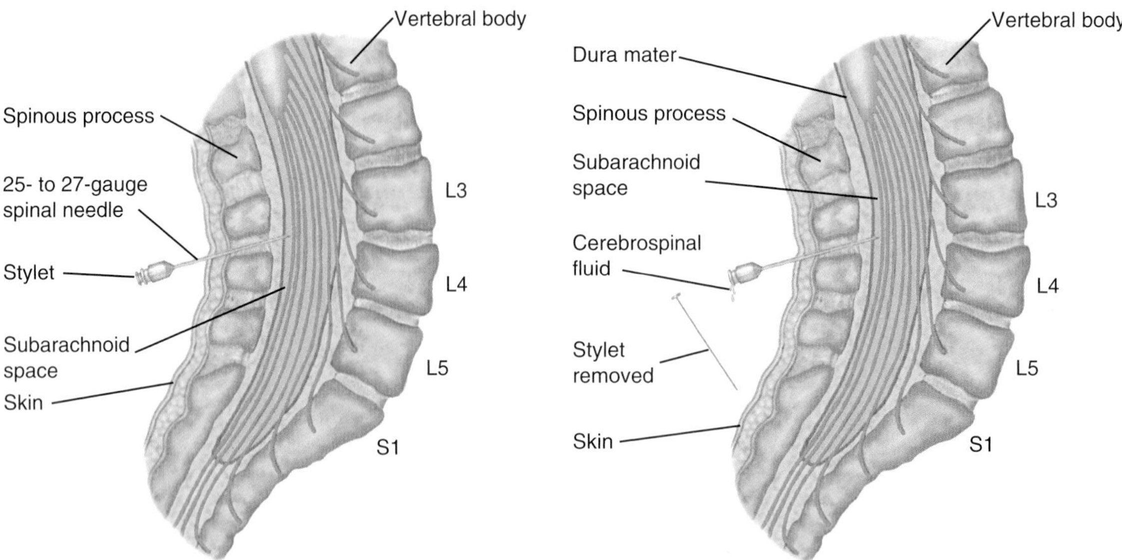


**FIG 18.13** Technique for subarachnoid block.

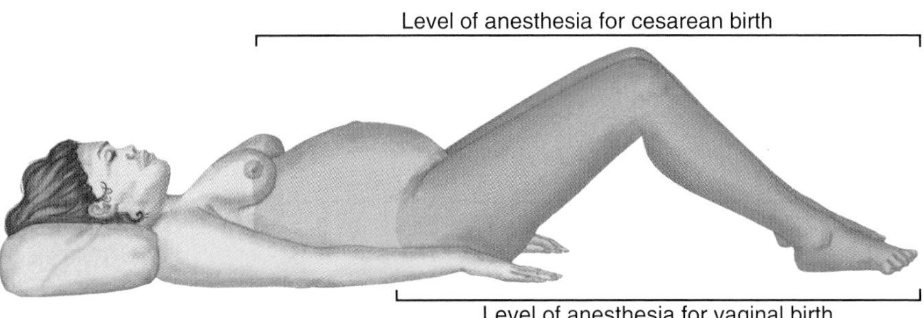


**FIG 18.14** Levels of anesthesia for epidural and subarachnoid blocks. A level of T10 through S5 is adequate for vaginal birth. A higher level, to T4-T6, is needed for cesarean birth.

forms a gelatinous seal over the hole in the dura, stopping spinal fluid leakage (Fig. 18.15). The blood patch can be repeated if needed.

## Systemic Drugs for Labor

Regional analgesia has become the preferred method of pain control during labor in the United States and Canada. However, a laboring woman may choose another method of pain control or she may have a contraindication to regional blocks. Systemic drugs have effects on multiple systems and on the neonate because they are distributed throughout the body and across the placenta. Systemic intrapartum drugs include inhalants, opioid analgesics, and adjunctive drugs. Agents used to induce general anesthesia are also systemic but are discussed separately because they are used only at birth.

### Inhalants

Globally, nitrous oxide is the most common inhalation agent used for labor management. Use in the United States as a safe method of pain control in labor has been increasing. Nitrous oxide is delivered by face mask in a 50% mixture with oxygen. The mask allows delivery of the medication on inhalation. The benefit of nitrous oxide is that it is cleared from the body through the lungs, so there is a minimal risk of

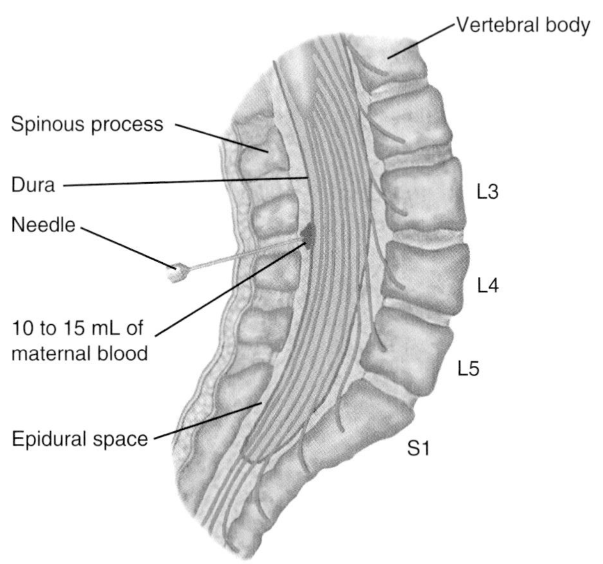


**FIG 18.15** Blood patch for relief of spinal headache. The woman's blood (10–15 mL) is injected into the epidural space to seal a dural puncture.

overdose. Major side effects include dizziness, nausea, vomiting, and dysphoria (Stewart & Collins, 2013).

### Nursing Considerations

Nitrous oxide must be self-administered with oxygen at a concentration no greater than 50%. The woman must be able to hold the mask herself without assistance, and the mask must have a demand valve so delivery stops when she is not inhaling.

### Opioid Analgesics

Opioid analgesics reduce the perception of pain without loss of consciousness. Injectable opioid analgesics are the systemic drugs of choice in labor. Analgesics that may be used in labor are meperidine (Demerol), fentanyl (Sublimaze), butorphanol (Stadol), and nalbuphine (Nubain). Table 15.1 summarizes common drugs used for intrapartum pain relief.

Meperidine is the most common narcotic analgesic used for intrapartum pain control. This drug can have a dysphoric, rather than analgesic, effect on the woman. She may be restless or irritable, have twitching, jerking, shaking, tremors, or even delirium. Of more concern is that meperidine produces a long-lasting active metabolite (normeperidine) that has a half-life of 3 to 6 hours in the woman but may affect newborn behavior for up to 24 hours. For this reason, meperidine is infrequently used for labor.

Fentanyl is a synthetic opioid with rapid onset, short duration of action, and no active metabolites. While fentanyl can be administered intramuscularly, it is commonly given intravenously, most frequently by a patient-controlled analgesia pump.

Opioid analgesics can cause respiratory depression, which is more likely to occur in the newborn than in the mother. An infant born at the peak of the drug's action is more likely to have respiratory depression than if born earlier or later. Prolonged action of active metabolites of drugs such as meperidine must also be considered in newborn care.

Meperidine and fentanyl are pure opioid agonists, a substance that causes a physiologic effect; butorphanol and nalbuphine have mixed opioid agonist and antagonist effects. Antagonists block the action of another substance. These agonist–antagonist drugs should not be given to a woman who is opiate dependent (on a drug such as heroin) to avoid withdrawal effects. These drugs also should not be given if she has already received a pure opioid agonist such as meperidine, because some analgesic effect of the first drug will be reversed.

Respiratory depression is limited with the mixed agonist–antagonist opioids, but pain relief also reaches a ceiling, making them poorly suited for intense pain as labor progresses.

During labor, opioid analgesics are usually given intravenously in small, frequent doses to provide a rapid onset of analgesia and a predictable duration of action. A woman benefits from rapid pain control, and there is less likelihood of neonatal respiratory depression. Starting the injection at the beginning of the contraction, when blood flow to the placenta is normally reduced, limits transfer to the fetus. When placental blood flow resumes, much of the drug is in maternal tissues (El-Wahab & Fernando, 2014).

### Opioid Antagonists

Naloxone (Narcan) reverses opioid-induced respiratory depression. Small doses may be given to the woman to reduce pruritus from epidural opioids. Naloxone does not reverse respiratory depression from other causes, such as barbiturates, anesthetics, nonopioid drugs, or pathologic conditions. Naloxone has a shorter duration of action than most of the opioids it reverses. In an opiate-dependent woman or newborn, naloxone may induce withdrawal symptoms. Naloxone for the infant is occasionally needed with neonatal resuscitation (see Chapter 30).

### Adjunctive Drugs

Adjunctive drugs during the intrapartum period include those with antiemetic and tranquilizing effects and sedatives. These drugs are given to reduce nausea and anxiety and to promote rest (see Table 18.1). They have no analgesic effects and do not potentiate analgesic drugs.

Promethazine (Phenergan) relieves the nausea and vomiting that may occur when opioid drugs are given. Promethazine is usually given intravenously but may be given by the intramuscular route. Promethazine must be diluted in normal saline and given slowly to reduce venous pain, inflammatory effects, and possible tissue necrosis.

### Sedatives

Sedatives such as barbiturates are not routinely given because they have prolonged depressant effects on the neonate. However, a small dose of a short-acting barbiturate may be given to promote rest if a woman is fatigued from false labor or a prolonged latent phase.

## General Anesthesia

General anesthesia is a systemic pain control that involves loss of consciousness. It is rarely used for vaginal births but still has a place in cesarean birth. Some women either refuse or are not good candidates for epidural block or SAB but require surgery. Occasionally, a planned epidural block or SAB proves inadequate for surgical anesthesia. In some cases, it may be necessary to perform a cesarean birth so quickly that no time is available to establish either type of regional block. General anesthesia may be required for emergency procedures at any stage of pregnancy, such as to repair injury that might result from an accident or domestic violence.

### Technique

To prepare for the induction of anesthesia, a woman breathes oxygen for 3 to 5 minutes, or four deep breaths, to increase her oxygen stores and those of her fetus for the short period of apnea during anesthesia induction. A wedge is placed under the woman's right side (or the operating table is tilted toward her left side) to displace the uterus from the aorta and inferior vena cava, promoting placental blood flow (Cunningham et al., 2014; Tsen, 2014). Medications are administered intravenously by the anesthesia provider to render the patient unconscious. The patient is intubated and monitored. The operation must begin immediately because of the decrease in uterine contractions and to reduce fetal exposure to medications.

### Adverse Effects of General Anesthesia

Major adverse effects are possible with the use of general anesthesia.

***Maternal aspiration of gastric contents.*** Regurgitation with aspiration of acidic gastric contents is a potentially fatal complication of general anesthesia. Aspiration of food particles may result in airway obstruction. Aspiration of acidic secretions results in chemical injury to the airways (aspiration pneumonitis). Infection may occur after the initial lung injury. For purposes of general anesthesia, anesthesia providers assume a pregnant woman has a full stomach.

***Respiratory depression.*** Respiratory depression may occur in either the mother or the infant but is more likely in the baby if delivery is delayed after starting anesthesia.

***Uterine relaxation.*** Some inhalational anesthetics may cause uterine relaxation. This characteristic is desirable for treating some complications, such as replacing an inverted uterus (see Chapter 27).

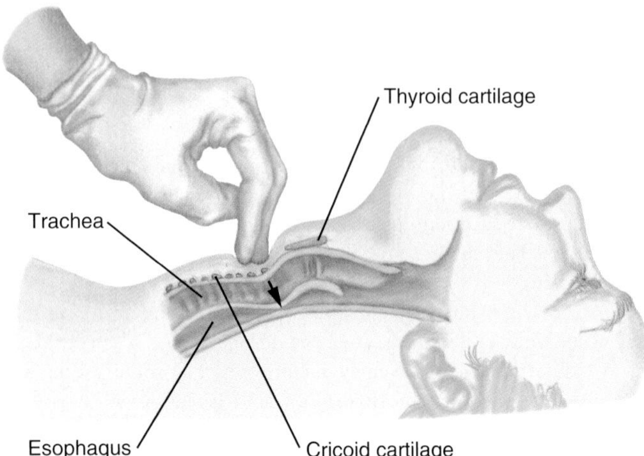


**FIG 18.16** Sellick maneuver to prevent vomitus from entering the woman's trachea while she is being intubated for general anesthesia. An assistant applies pressure to the cricoid cartilage to obstruct the esophagus. Once the woman is successfully intubated with a cuffed endotracheal tube, gastric secretions cannot enter the trachea.

However, postpartum hemorrhage may occur if the uterus relaxes after birth.

### Methods to Minimize Adverse Effects

Measures to reduce the risk of maternal aspiration (or of lung injury, if aspiration occurs) include:

- Restricting intake to clear fluids or maintaining nothing-by-mouth (NPO) status if surgery is expected, such as with a scheduled cesarean.
- Administering drugs to raise the gastric pH and make secretions less acidic, such as sodium citrate and citric acid (Bicitra), ranitidine (Zantac), cimetidine (Tagamet), or famotidine (Pepcid).
- Administering drugs to reduce secretions, such as glycopyrrolate (Robinul).
- Administering drugs to speed gastric emptying, such as metoclopramide (Reglan).
- Using cricoid pressure (Sellick maneuver) to block the esophagus by pressing the rigid trachea against it (Fig. 18.16).

Neonatal respiratory depression may be averted by:

- Reducing the time from induction of anesthesia until the umbilical cord is clamped.
- Minimizing the use of sedating drugs and anesthetics until the cord is clamped.

To reduce the time from induction of anesthesia to cord clamping, the woman is prepared and draped and the physicians are ready before anesthesia is begun. Before cord clamping, the anesthesia is so light that the woman may move on the operating table as the incision is made, but she rarely remembers the experience or does not recall it as painful. The anesthesia level is deepened after the cord is clamped.

## NURSING MANAGEMENT

### Pain Management

The nurse assists laboring women with both nonpharmacologic and pharmacologic methods of pain control as needed (see Nursing Care Plan: Intrapartum Pain Management). Nursing care related to pain management should be combined with that for normal labor, including care of the fetus, and any problems that arise. Two problems that commonly affect the woman are pain and her potential for respiratory compromise if she needs general anesthesia.

## PAIN

### Assessment

Pain assessment begins at admission and continues throughout labor. The assessments discussed in Table 16.1 guide the nurse to obtain data related to pain management. Pain-related assessments include:

- Preferences for pain management
- Previous surgeries, type of anesthesia, and any anesthesia-associated problems
- Maternal vital signs
- FHR and monitor patterns
- Allergies, focusing especially on allergy to opioid analgesics, dental anesthetics, and iodine (used in some prep solutions)
- Oral intake: time and type of last intake
- Evidence of pain: verbal evidence (verbal statement, requests for pain-relief measures, crying, moaning) and nonverbal evidence (tense, guarded posture or facial expression)

**Labor status.** In addition to these routine assessments, ask the woman if she needs help with pain management. A stoic woman may give little outward evidence of pain yet may say she wants medication or other pain control if asked.

When assessing pain, clarify the words a woman uses. When asked if she has "pain," the woman may deny it. Changing the word used to "discomfort," "aching," "pulling," "pressure," or other words to describe pain may bring a different response. Do not assume that everyone uses the same words to describe their pain. Just as pain is an individual experience, so also is the expression of pain, including verbal expression.

Asking a woman to rate her pain on a scale of 0 to 10 or a similar scale helps clarify her pain's intensity before and after relief measures. Zero represents no pain, whereas 10 is the worst possible pain (other scales that use drawings that range from smiling faces to crying are readily available). Ask the woman to rate her pain on this scale before and after pain-relief measures to evaluate their effectiveness. A surprising number of women have difficulty using a pain scale because they have little experience with pain. They may want to allow for an increase in the number later in labor, possibly underrating current pain, or they may say that they have no idea what the "worst pain imaginable" is, and thus, cannot guess what pain rated as 10 feels like. Document the woman's words and behavioral responses "when asked how bad" the pain is as well as the degree of relief at a reasonable time.

The woman who remains tense between contractions may be having difficulty coping with pain. Moaning, crying, thrashing, and an inability to use nonpharmacologic techniques suggest that she needs pharmacologic pain relief.

Assess the woman's labor status to help her choose the most appropriate method of pain control. If she has reached a point in labor at which she needs to decide for or against a specific pharmacologic method, inform her. This point does not occur at an exact time or with an exact amount of cervical dilation but is estimated according to when she is likely to give birth, the time needed to establish a specific method, and the pharmacology of the drug or drugs.

Avoid making assumptions about the amount of pain a woman is having based on her rate of labor progress, cervical dilation, or apparent intensity of contractions. It is tempting to assume that a woman whose cervix is 2 cm dilated has little pain and that a woman whose cervix is dilated 8 cm has intense pain. An obese woman's contractions may be strong, but they may seem mild if they are assessed by palpation or an external monitor because of her thick abdominal fat pad. *Labor*

## NURSING CARE PLAN

### Intrapartum Pain Management

#### Focused Assessment

Beth is a 28-year-old gravida 1, para 0, who was admitted 1 hour ago. Beth's cervix is 3 cm dilated and 100% effaced, the station is –2, and her membranes are intact. Contractions occur every 3 minutes, last 40 to 50 seconds, and are of moderate intensity. The fetal heart rate averages 135 to 145 beats per minute (bpm) and has no nonreassuring patterns. Beth says that back pain is most troubling. Beth and her husband Sam are using breathing techniques learned in childbirth classes.

#### Nursing Diagnosis

Pain related to effects of uterine contractions and pressure on pelvic structures.

#### Planning

*Expected Outcomes*

During labor Beth will:

1. Continue to use techniques she learned in prepared childbirth classes.
2. Have a relaxed facial and body posture between contractions.

#### *Interventions and Rationales*

1. Adjust the environment for comfort that is conducive to relaxation:
   a. Adjust room thermostat.
   b. Add warm blankets and socks for warmth.
   c. Offer small electric fan or hand fan if Beth is hot.
   *These interventions can help the woman use her coping skills to tolerate discomfort.*
2. Reduce distractions:
   a. Close door to reduce outside noise.
   b. Play music of Beth's choice to mask external noise.
   c. Do not stand in front of her focal point.
   d. Try to delay assessments or questions until after a contraction is over.
   *Distractions interfere with use of the skills for pain management taught in prepared childbirth classes.*
3. Reduce irritating stimulants:
   a. Keep sheets and underpads dry.
   b. Dim the lights as Beth desires. Use bright lights only when necessary.
   c. Do all procedures and nursing interventions as gently as possible.
   d. Avoid bumping the bed.
   e. Limit visitors as the couple wishes.
   *Irritating stimulants are distractions that decrease the woman's ability to use learned childbirth skills and add to her discomfort.*
4. Encourage Beth to assume the most comfortable positions and to change positions regularly (approximately every 30–60 min). If there is no contraindication, she may walk around or sit in a chair or on a birth ball at the bedside. A rolled pillow or blanket provides a wedge in a side-tilt position.
   *Frequent position changes favor fetal descent by encouraging the fetal head to adapt to the pelvic diameters most efficiently. Position changes also reduce muscle tension and unrelieved pressure:*
   a. Upright positions.
      *Reduces aortocaval compression with decreased placental perfusion.*
   b. If lying down, a side-lying or side-tilt position is more comfortable.
      *Enhance descent with gravity.*
5. Check for bladder distention hourly or more often if she has had large quantities of intravenous (IV) or oral fluid. Encourage voiding at least every 2 hours. With an order, catheterize her if her bladder is full and she cannot void.
   *A full bladder contributes to overall discomfort and may impede fetal descent and prolong labor.*
6. Give Beth small amounts of clear fluids such as ice chips. If oral intake is prohibited or she does not want fluids, moisten her mouth with a damp washcloth or have her rinse her mouth with water.
   *Women using relaxation or breathing techniques will use mouth breathing. This intervention diminishes the discomfort and promotes hydration. Clear liquids are often ordered because of the potential need for general anesthesia.*
7. Offer a back rub or firm, constant sacral pressure. Ask Beth where and how firm pressure should be applied. Use baby powder when rubbing her back. Have her tell caregivers if this technique becomes uncomfortable or if the location on her back needs to be changed. If Sam is rubbing her back, offer to relieve him occasionally and encourage him to take a break.
   *In early labor, back rubs can be beneficial; as labor progresses, they can become uncomfortable or even painful. The partner needs occasional breaks to conserve energy and help later in labor.*
8. Keep Beth and Sam informed about the progress of labor and their baby's condition.
   *Information reduces anxiety and fears. Anxiety and fear will increase pain perception and decrease pain tolerance.*

#### Evaluation

Beth concentrates on her breathing techniques with each contraction but has a relaxed body posture between them. She continues to use learned skills effectively for approximately 2 hours, when she begins to have more difficulty coping with her contractions.

#### Focused Assessment

Three hours after admission, Beth's cervix is 4 cm dilated and 100% effaced, and the fetal station is –1. Membranes have ruptured, and the amniotic fluid is clear. Contractions occur every 2 to 3 minutes, last 50 seconds, and are firm. Fetal heart rate and monitor patterns are reassuring. Back discomfort persists, and she is having difficulty relaxing between contractions and is discouraged that labor is not progressing as quickly as she expected. She is no longer able to use prepared childbirth techniques effectively and rates her labor pain as 8 on a 0 to 10 scale. Beth requests an epidural block, which will be given by continuous infusion.

**Critical Thinking:** *At this time, what are some advantages and disadvantages of having an epidural? Are added measures needed to safeguard the fetus because of an epidural?*

**Answer:** *an epidural may slow labor if performed earlier in labor, but labor progress may benefit from the pain relief and tension if done at this point or later. It is a disadvantage that Beth's activity will be limited, reducing her ability to enhance fetal descent and rotation in her pelvis.*

*To safeguard the fetus, the nurse should preload Beth with an IV of 500–1000 crystalloid fluid before the block is started. Continuous fetal monitoring is essential to identify any non-reassuring patterns that may occur. Beth should avoid a supine position to reduce compression of the aorta.*

The nurse gives Beth 500 mL of ordered IV solution before the block begins to offset hypotensive effects. Continuous electronic fetal monitoring is used to identify possible nonreassuring patterns.

#### Nursing Diagnosis

Risk for Injury related to altered sensation in her lower extremities.

#### Planning

*Expected Outcomes*

1. Beth will not fall or suffer injury while experiencing the effects of her epidural block.
2. Beth's baby will not be born in an uncontrolled manner.

#### *Interventions and Rationales*

1. Assist Beth to change positions regularly. Ambulation after birth should be delayed until movement and strength return, and assistance should be available until her legs have normal strength.

*Continued*

## NURSING CARE PLAN—cont'd

### *Intrapartum Pain Management*

*The epidural block causes a varying degree of motor block and weakness.*

2. Observe for signs of labor progress:
   a. Contractions increasing in frequency, duration, and intensity.
   b. Fetal heart rate changes such as early or variable decelerations that reflect head or cord compression.
   c. Increase in bloody show.
   d. Statement reflecting urge to push (not always present).

   *Rectal pressure associated with fetal descent may be reduced. To prevent the fetus from being born unattended, the nurse must observe for other signs that birth is near.*
3. Support Beth's pushing efforts. Teach her to avoid holding her breath while pushing and to push no longer than 6 to 8 seconds at a time. Explain to Beth and Sam that she may make grunting, moaning, or other sounds when pushing to avoid excessive breath-holding.

   *The urge to push may not be as strong, but it is usually felt when the fetus descends low in the pelvis.*

**Evaluation**

Beth is satisfied with her pain relief after the epidural block, rating her pain as 0 out of 10. She has little motor block. Her blood pressure and the fetal heart rate remain within expected limits. Cervical dilation progresses to 10 cm (complete) without injury to Beth or her fetus. However, despite her vigorous pushing efforts, the fetal station remains at 0. Beth has a cesarean birth, delivering an 8-lb, 10-oz girl (3912 g).

**Additional Nursing Diagnoses and Collaborative Problems to Consider:**

Anxiety
Risk of Aspiration
Powerlessness
Situational Low Self-esteem
Urinary Retention
Potential complication: Fetal Compromise

*progress or contraction intensity cannot be equated with a woman's pain perception or tolerance.*

A woman's need for pain relief should not be based on her outward expression alone. A quiet woman may need medication but may be reluctant to ask, whereas an expressive woman may be satisfied with nonpharmacologic measures. Women who do not speak the prevailing language or are hearing impaired may not know what is available; in such cases, seek an interpreter to communicate accurately.

## CRITICAL THINKING EXERCISE 18.1

Truc Pham is a Vietnamese-American in labor with her first baby. Her cervix is dilated 6 cm, effacement is 100%, and the fetus is at a +1 station. Truc's contractions occur every 3 minutes, last 50 to 60 seconds, and are of strong intensity. She smiles at the nurse each time the nurse talks to her but talks little. Truc stiffens her body during contractions and interacts little with her husband or the nurse at those times.

1. How should the nurse interpret these data?
2. Does the nurse need additional data?
3. What nursing actions are appropriate?

Observe for pain that is not typical of labor. Although labor pain is often intense, it should not be constant but should come and go with each contraction. The uterus should not be tender or board like between contractions. Report atypical pain to the physician or nurse-midwife.

### Nursing Diagnosis and Planning

Because pain is an expected part of normal childbirth, a common nursing diagnosis is:

- Pain related to effects of uterine contractions and fetal descent

***Expected outcomes.*** The woman will describe the pain-relief measures as satisfactory during labor and will use learned breathing and relaxation techniques during labor.

These two goals include both nonpharmacologic and pharmacologic measures.

### Interventions

Nursing care for intrapartum pain management is to reduce factors that hinder the woman's pain control and to enhance those that benefit it. Refer to Chapter 17 for nursing measures that should be included in the care of all laboring women, such as positioning, teaching, encouragement, and care of the partner. Although epidurals are very common in hospital births, do not assume that every woman will want one. Caring contact with a nurse enhances pain management and the overall experience of giving birth.

***Promoting relaxation.*** Simple attention to details promotes relaxation. Make the woman's environment more comfortable. If noise is a problem, suggest music or television to mask it. A warm blanket or a cool cloth provides tangible comfort and conveys the nurse's caring attitude. Change linens or underpads as needed to keep the woman reasonably clean and dry.

Offer the woman a warm shower or bath, especially if she is tense and there are no contraindications (see Box 18.1). In general, walking is good during early labor, and water therapy is better during active labor. The mild nipple stimulation that occurs in a whirlpool or shower may intensify contractions in a woman whose labor has slowed, because it causes her posterior pituitary gland to secrete oxytocin.

Reduce intrusions as much as possible. For example, wait until a contraction is over before asking questions or doing a procedure. Longer assessments and procedures may span several contractions, but try to stop during each contraction.

***Reducing outside sources of discomfort.*** Decrease the light and excessive noise in the room. Maintain a comfortable temperature for the woman. Anesthetize the site with lidocaine before inserting an IV catheter if the woman is not allergic and facility policy permits. Normal saline infiltration has a similar effect. Remind her to change position regularly to reduce tension and discomfort from constant pressure. Support her with pillows.

Observe the woman's bladder for distention hourly, and encourage her to void every 2 hours or more if she has received a large quantity of IV fluids. Catheterization is needed if she cannot void and her bladder is full.

***Reducing anxiety and fear.*** Accurate information reduces the negative psychologic impact of the unknown. Tell the woman about her labor and its progress. It is impossible to predict when she will give birth, but tell her if her labor progress is or is not on course. Sometimes she needs only the reassurance from an experienced nurse that her intense contractions are indeed normal. The woman may be willing to endure more discomfort than she otherwise would if she is making progress.

Be honest if problems do occur. A woman usually knows if there is a problem and is more anxious if she does not know what it is. Explain all measures taken to correct the problem, and keep her informed of the results.

**Helping the woman use nonpharmacologic techniques.** *If the nonpharmacologic method* is *safe for the woman and fetus and is effective, do not interfere with its use.* Try not to distract the woman from whatever technique she is using.

**Massage.** Fetal monitor belts hinder abdominal effleurage. Encourage the woman to do effleurage on uncovered areas of her abdomen or to stroke her thighs. Consider using intermittent fetal monitoring if this method is appropriate.

Powder reduces friction and skin irritation. The woman needs to tell the person who is providing sacral pressure or other massage how much pressure helps and the best location. Because this information may change during labor and massage may become uncomfortable rather than helpful, seek the woman's feedback regularly.

**Mental stimulation.** Use a low, soothing voice when helping a woman use imagery. It is often helpful to speak close to her ear when trying to create a tranquil imaginary scene or to calm her. Music can enhance mental stimulation techniques.

**Breathing.** Women learn a variety of breathing techniques in prepared childbirth classes and often modify them or invent some of their own during labor. Encourage the woman to change techniques when she needs to, avoiding complex techniques during early labor. If she has trouble maintaining her concentration, the nurse or her partner can make eye contact (if culturally appropriate) and breathe the pattern with her.

Symptoms of hyperventilation (dizziness, tingling and numbness of the fingers and lips, carpopedal spasm) are likely if a woman breathes fast and deep, whether or not she is using patterned breathing techniques. Breathing into her cupped hands, a paper bag, or a washcloth placed over her nose and mouth promotes rebreathing exhaled carbon dioxide to lessen the symptoms.

Teach breathing techniques to the unprepared woman when she is admitted. Review them when she seems to need a different method. Many women make up their own breathing techniques.

When teaching nonpharmacologic pain management techniques to the woman who is in advanced labor, follow these guidelines:

- Speak in a soft and calm tone.
- Teach one method at a time.
- Demonstrate the method between contractions.
- Use breathing techniques with the woman while maintaining eye contact.
- Allow her control over her labor: who is present, what technique she will use, and the like.

**Incorporating pharmacologic methods.** All pharmacologic methods require collaboration with medical personnel for orders. Soon after admission, tell the woman what medication is available if she needs it. This is not done to undermine her self-confidence but to allow her to better understand when she needs to make a choice about medication. Analgesia is most effective if it is given before pain is severe.

Tell her that her preferences about pain-relief methods will be honored if possible, but it is impossible to predict the course of her labor. Assure her that no pharmacologic method will be given without her understanding and consent.

If a woman finds some nonpharmacologic methods inadequate, try other nonpharmacologic methods or offer her available medication. When contacting the birth attendant for medication orders, report the fetal and maternal status and vital signs, labor status, and the woman's request for medication, including her pain rating on a scale. If she has a continuous epidural block, contact the person who inserted it if problems occur or added relief is needed. Observe special nursing considerations associated with the method used (Table 18.2).

## PARENTS WANT TO KNOW

### *How Will This Medicine Affect Our Baby?*

Women and their partners often ask whether pain medication or anesthesia will harm their baby. The nurse can help parents choose wisely from available options by providing honest information:

- Pain that you cannot tolerate is not good for you or your baby, and it reduces the joy of this special event.
- Some risk is associated with every type of pain medication or anesthesia, but careful selection and the use of preventive measures minimize this risk. If complications occur, corrective measures can reduce the risk to you and your baby.
- Some pain relievers can cause your baby to be slow to breathe at birth, but carefully controlling the timing and dose of the medication reduces the likelihood that this will occur. We can use another medication to reverse this effect if needed.
- Epidural or spinal anesthesia can cause your blood pressure to fall, which can reduce the blood flow to your baby. However, we give you lots of intravenous fluids to reduce this effect. We have other medications to increase your blood pressure if the fluids are not enough.
- General anesthesia can cause your baby to be slow to breathe at birth. To reduce this risk, the anesthesia will not be started until everything is ready for the surgery, and the doctors will clamp the baby's umbilical cord as quickly as possible.

### Evaluation

- Is the woman satisfied with her ability to manage her pain?
- Is she using coping skills somewhat consistently during labor?
- How did her pain scale rating change before and after the method (either nonpharmacologic or pharmacologic) was used? Is she satisfied with its relief?

## RESPIRATORY COMPROMISE

### Assessment

General anesthesia may be needed any time during birth, most often for cesarean birth. Document the type (solids or liquids) and time of the woman's last food intake. Question her closely if she reports an unusually long interval since her last oral intake. Anesthesia providers can anticipate and prevent problems better if they know the actual oral intake.

### Nursing Diagnosis and Planning

Nursing care of laboring women includes monitoring for the short-term risk of aspiration, because it is impossible to predict whether a woman will require general anesthesia. The nursing diagnosis is:

- Risk for Aspiration related to impaired protective laryngeal reflexes

**Expected outcome.** The woman will not aspirate gastric contents during the perioperative period.

**TABLE 18.2 Pharmacologic Methods of Intrapartum Pain Management**

| Method and Uses | Nursing Considerations |
|---|---|
| ***Opioid Analgesics*** | |
| Systemic analgesia during labor and for postoperative pain after cesarean birth. May be combined with an adjunctive drug such as promethazine to reduce the nausea and vomiting that sometimes occur with narcotic use and after surgery. | 1. Assess the woman for drug use at admission. Women who are opiate-dependent should not receive analgesics having mixed agonist and antagonist actions (butorphanol and nalbuphine).<br>2. Observe neonate for respiratory depression, especially if the mother had opioid narcotics within 4 hr of birth or at time of the drug's peak action or if the mother received multiple opioid doses during labor:<br>• Delay in initiating or sustaining normal depth and rate of respirations<br>• Respiratory rate <30 breaths per minute<br>• Poor muscle tone: limp, floppy<br>3. The use of adjunctive drugs for nausea, such as promethazine, enhances respiratory depressant effects.<br>4. Have naloxone available for infants exposed to opioids during labor. Respiratory and cardiac support precede drug administration in neonatal resuscitation. Observe for recurrent respiratory depression after administration of naloxone. |
| ***Epidural Opioids*** | |
| *Labor:* Mixed with a local anesthetic agent to give better pain relief with less motor block.<br>*Postoperatively:* Gives long-acting analgesia without sedation, allowing the mother and infant to interact more easily. | 1. Observe same nursing implications as with epidural block.<br>2. Do not give additional opioids or other CNS depressants except as ordered by the anesthesia provider. Nonsteroidal anti-inflammatory drugs or oral analgesics are often prescribed in routine orders.<br>3. Maternal respiratory depression may be delayed for up to 24 hr and varies with drug given. Observe respiratory rate, depth, oxygen saturation, and arousability hourly for 24 hr. Notify anesthesia provider for rate of <12 breaths per minute, persistent oxygen saturation of <95% on pulse oximetry, reduced respiratory effort, difficulty arousing, or as ordered by the provider. Cyanosis is a late sign of respiratory depression.<br>4. Have naloxone, 0.4 mg, an oral airway, and an Ambu bag and mask immediately available, such as on a "crash cart."<br>5. Observe for pruritus or rubbing of the face and neck. Routine postoperative orders to relieve pruritus are usually provided. Notify anesthesia provider if these are insufficient.<br>6. Urinary retention may occur after indwelling catheter removal. Observe for adequacy of voiding, as in all postpartum women.<br>7. Notify anesthesia provider for relief of nausea or vomiting.<br>8. Assess sensation and mobility before allowing ambulation. |
| ***Intrathecal Opioid Analgesics*** | |
| Provides analgesia for most of first-stage labor without maternal sedation. A very small dose of the drug is needed because it is injected very near the spinal cord where sensory fibers enter. Usually not adequate for late labor or the birth itself. Often combined with epidural block for the combined spinal-epidural (CSE) technique for labor. | 1. Observe for the common side effects of nausea, vomiting, and pruritus. Notify the anesthesia provider if these effects occur, and have an antagonist such as naloxone or naltrexone available.<br>2. Observe for delayed respiratory depression, depending on the drug given. Use a pulse oximeter as indicated.<br>3. Observe for nonreassuring fetal heart rate patterns that may be associated with reduced maternal oxygenation. |
| ***Local Infiltration Anesthesia*** | |
| Numbs perineum for episiotomy or repair of laceration at vaginal birth. No relief of labor pain. Not adequate for instrument-assisted birth (see Chapter 19). | 1. Assess for drug allergies, especially to dental anesthetics because they are related to those used in maternity care.<br>2. Apply ice to perineum after birth to reduce edema and hematoma formation and to increase comfort. |
| ***Pudendal Block*** | |
| Numbs the lower vagina and perineum for vaginal birth.<br>No relief of labor pain because it is done just before birth.<br>Provides adequate anesthesia for many instrument-assisted births. (See Chapter 19.) | 1. Use the same interventions as for local infiltration. A woman or her partner may be alarmed if she notices the long needle (about 6 in [15 cm]). Teach her that it must be long to reach the pudendal nerve through the vagina and that it will be inserted only about ½ inch (1.25 cm) near the location of the nerve. Tell her that a guide ("trumpet") will be used to avoid injuring her vaginal tissue or that of her baby. |

**TABLE 18.2 Pharmacologic Methods of Intrapartum Pain Management—cont'd**

| Method and Uses | Nursing Considerations |
|---|---|
| ***Epidural Block*** | |
| *Labor:* Insertion of catheter provides pain relief for labor and vaginal birth (T10–S5 levels).<br>*Cesarean birth:* If epidural was used during labor, level of block can be extended upward (T4–T6 level). Also used for cesarean birth. | 1. Prehydrate the woman with warmed nonglucose crystalloid solution such as Ringer's lactate or normal saline solution.<br>2. Displace uterus manually or with a wedge placed under the woman's side to enhance placental perfusion.<br>3. Assess for hypotension at least every 5 min for 15 min after block is begun and with each new dose until vital signs are stable. Report to anesthesia provider: systolic BP of <110 mm Hg or a fall of 20% or more from baseline levels, pallor, or diaphoresis. Facility procedures give further guidance.<br>4. Assess fetal heart rate for signs of impaired placental perfusion, and report to anesthesia provider and nurse-midwife: tachycardia (>160 bpm for 10 min) or bradycardia (<110 bpm for 10 min), late decelerations (see Table 18.1).<br>5. If hypotension or signs of impaired placental perfusion occur, increase the rate of infusion of nonadditive IV fluid, reposition the woman to her side, and administer oxygen by face mask (8–10 L/min). Have ephedrine available (usually included in epidural tray).<br>6. Observe for a full bladder, and catheterize as ordered.<br>7. Leg movement and strength vary after an epidural block. Transfer with help to avoid muscle strains to nurse or woman.<br>8. Ambulate only after sensation and movement have returned. Have another person's assistance with the first ambulation. |
| ***Subarachnoid Block*** | |
| *Cesarean birth:* Can be established slightly faster than epidural block.<br>May rarely be used for complicated vaginal birth.<br>Does not provide pain relief for labor because it is done just before birth.<br>May be combined with an epidural block in a combined spinal-epidural (CSE). See "Intrathecal Opioid Analgesics" for more information. | 1. See "Epidural Block" for these interventions:<br>• IV prehydration<br>• Uterine displacement<br>• Observation of blood pressure and fetal heart rate<br>• Care for hypotension or signs of impaired placental perfusion<br>• Observation and intervention for bladder distention<br>• Transfer and ambulation precautions<br>2. Observe for postspinal headache: a headache that is worse when the woman is upright and that may disappear when she is lying flat. Notify anesthesia provider if it occurs (a blood patch may be done).<br>3. Nursing interventions for postspinal headache: encourage bed rest, increase oral fluids if not contraindicated, give oral caffeine, and give analgesics as ordered. |
| ***General Anesthesia*** | |
| Cesarean birth if epidural or spinal block is not possible or if the woman refuses regional anesthesia. May be required for emergency procedures such as replacement of inverted uterus. | 1. Determine type and time of last food intake on admission.<br>2. Restrict oral intake to clear liquids or as ordered. Consult with physician or nurse-midwife if surgical intervention is likely.<br>3. Report to anesthesia provider: oral intake before and during labor, vomiting.<br>4. Displace uterus (see "Epidural Block").<br>5. Give ordered drugs such as sodium citrate and citric acid (Bicitra).<br>6. Maintain cricoid pressure (Sellick maneuver) during intubation.<br>7. The woman will remain intubated until protective (gag) reflexes have returned. Have oral airway and suction immediately available.<br>8. Interventions for postoperative respiratory depression: give positive-pressure oxygen by face mask; observe oxygen saturation with pulse oximetry until woman is awake and alert; have woman take several deep breaths if oxygen saturation falls below 95%. Notify anesthesia provider. |

*BP,* Blood pressure; *bpm,* beats per minute; *CNS,* central nervous system; *IV,* intravenous; *PCA,* patient-controlled analgesia

### Interventions

Nursing interventions relate to identifying factors that increase a woman's risk of aspiration, and to collaborative and nursing measures to reduce the risk of aspiration or lung injury.

***Identifying risk factors.*** Report oral intake both before and after admission to the anesthesia provider. Oral intake during labor is often restricted to medications, clear liquids, ice chips, Popsicles, or hard candies.

Vomiting is a common discomfort during normal labor, regardless of the mother's oral intake. If vomiting occurs, chart the time, quantity, and character (amount, color, presence of undigested food).

***Reducing risk of aspiration or lung injury.*** Nursing and medical personnel collaborate to reduce a woman's risk of pulmonary complications.

**Perioperative care.** Restrict oral intake as ordered if surgery is expected. Give ordered medications such as sodium citrate and citric acid (Bicitra). Either the nurse or anesthesia provider may give parenteral drugs, such as glycopyrrolate (Robinul), depending on when they are administered.

An experienced nurse or a trained anesthesia assistant provides cricoid pressure (Sellick maneuver) to block the esophagus until the woman is intubated and the cuff of the endotracheal tube is inflated. Successful intubation with the cuffed endotracheal tube blocks passage of any gastric contents into the trachea.

**Postoperative care.** Birth facility protocols guide postoperative care, including pre- and post-extubation care for the woman who had general anesthesia. The woman is extubated when her protective laryngeal reflexes have returned. Suction equipment and an Ambu bag with appropriate-size mask should be immediately available. Administer oxygen by mask or face tent for until the woman is awake and alert, because the agents used for general anesthesia are respiratory depressants. Monitor oxygen saturation with a pulse oximeter. If her oxygen saturation falls below 95%, have her take several deep breaths. Deep breathing helps her eliminate inhalational anesthetics and reduces stasis of pulmonary secretions.

Assess the woman's pulse, respiration, and blood pressure every 15 minutes for 1 hour or until stable; then continue according to policy. Observe her color for pallor or cyanosis, which suggests shock or hypoventilation.

### Evaluation

Interventions for this nursing diagnosis are preventive and short-term because it is a temporary high-risk situation. The goal is met if the woman does not aspirate gastric contents during the perioperative period.

See nursing care related to common pain management methods such as epidural analgesia (see Table 18.2).

## KEY CONCEPTS

- Childbirth pain is unique because it is normal and self-limiting, can be prepared for, and ends with a baby's birth.
- Excess or poorly relieved pain can be harmful to the mother and fetus.
- Pain is a complex physical and psychologic experience. It is subjective and personal.
- Four sources of pain, cervical dilation, uterine ischemia, pressure and pulling on pelvic structures, and vaginal and perineal distention, are present in most labors. Other physical and psychologic factors may alter the pain felt from these sources.
- Relaxation enhances other pain management techniques.
- Any drug that the expectant mother takes, whether therapeutic, herbal/botanical, or abused, may affect the fetus directly or indirectly.
- Cutaneous and mental stimulation techniques reduce pain perception. Techniques should be varied to prevent habituation.
- The purpose of breathing techniques is to increase relaxation.
- Physiologic alterations of pregnancy may affect a woman's response to medications.
- Major advantages of regional pain management methods are that the woman can participate in the birth and that she retains her protective airway reflexes.
- The nurse should observe for and take actions to prevent maternal hypotension with an epidural or SAB.
- The nurse should observe for FHR changes associated with impaired placental perfusion if the woman is at risk for hypotension, as with epidural or SABs.
- The main nursing observations of the woman who receives epidural or intrathecal opioids are for nausea and vomiting, pruritus, and delayed respiratory depression.
- The nurse should observe for respiratory depression, primarily in the newborn, when the mother has received opioid analgesics during labor.
- Regurgitation with aspiration of acidic gastric contents is the greatest risk for a woman who receives general anesthesia.

## REFERENCES AND READINGS


American College of Obstetricians and Gynecologists. (2010). *Obstetric analgesia and anesthesia (ACOG Practice Bulletin No. 36)*. Washington, DC: Author.

American Society of Anesthesiologists (2016) Practice guidelines for obstetric anesthesia: An updated report by the American Society of Anesthesiologists Task Force on Obstetric Anesthesia and the Society for Obstetric Anesthesia and Perinatology. *Anesthesiology, 124* (2), 270-300 doi: 10.1097/ALN.0000000000000935

Anderson, D. (2011) A review of systemic opioids commonly used for labor pain relief. *Journal of Midwifery and Women's Health, 56*, 222–239. doi:10.1111/j.1542-2011.2011.00061.x

Assessment of pain associated with childbirth: Women's perspectives, preferences and solutions. (2015). *Midwifery, 31*(7), 708–712. doi:10.1016/j.midw.2015.03.012

Association of Women's Health, Obstetric and Neonatal Nurses. (2011). *Evidence-based clinical practice guideline: Nursing care of the woman receiving regional analgesia/anesthesia in labor* (2nd ed.). Washington, DC: Author.

Association of Women's Health, Obstetric and Neonatal Nurses. (2014). Second stage of labor: Mother-initiated, spontaneous pushing. *Women's health and perinatal nursing care quality refined draft measures specifications.* Washington, DC: Author.

Blackburn, S. T. (2013). *Maternal, fetal, & neonatal physiology: A clinical perspective* (4th ed.). Amsterdam: Elsevier Saunders.

Chestnut, D. (2014) Alternative regional analgesic techniques for labor and vaginal delivery. In D. Chestnut, C. A. Wong, L. C. Tsen, D. N. K. Warwick, Y. Beilin, J. M. Mhyre, V. Naveen (Eds.), *Chestnut's Obstetric Anesthesia: Principles and practice* (5th ed) Philadelphia: Elsevier Saunders.

Chestnut, D., Wong, C. A., Tsen, L. C., Warwick, D. N. K, Beilin, Y, Mhyre, J. M., Naveen, V., (2014). *Chestnut's Obstetric Anesthesia: Principles and practice* (5th ed) Philadelphia: Elsevier Saunders.

Cunningham, F. G., Leveno, K. J., Bloom, S. L., Spong, C. Y., Dashe, J. S., Hoffman, B. L., … & Sheffield, J. S. (2014). *Williams obstetrics* (24th ed.). New York: McGraw-Hill Medical.

Davies, R., Davis, D., Pearce, M., & Wong, N. (2014) The effect of waterbirth on neonatal mortality and morbidity: A systematic review protocol. *Joanna Briggs Institute of Systematic Reviews and Implementation Reports. 12*(7) 1–8

DiFranco, J. T., & Curl, M. (2014) Healthy birth practice #5: Avoid giving birth on your back and follow your body's urge to push. *Journal of Perinatal Education, 23*(4) 207–210. doi:10.1891/1058-1243.23.4.207

Dozier, A., Howard, C., Brownell, E., Wissler, R., Glantz, J., Ternullo, S., … & Lawrence, R. (2013). Labor epidural anesthesia, obstetric factors and breastfeeding cessation. *Maternal & Child Health Journal, 17*(4), 689–698 10p. doi:10.1007/s10995-012-1045-4

El-Wahab, N., & Fernando, R. (2014). Systemic analgesia: Parenteral and inhalation agents. In D. Chestnut, C. A. Wong, L. C. Tsen, D. N. K. Warwick, Y. Beilin, J. M. Mhyre & V. Naveen (Eds.) *Chestnut's Obstetric Anesthesia: Principles and practice* (5th ed) Philadelphia: Elsevier Saunders.

Ramos-Torrecillas, J., & De Luna-Bertos, E. (2015). Retrospective study of the association between epidural analgesia during labour and complications for the newborn. *Midwifery, 31*(6), 613–616. doi:10.1016/j.midw.2015.02.013

Rooks, J. P. (2011). Safety and risks of nitrous oxide labor analgesia: A review. *Journal of Midwifery & Women's Health, 56*(6), 557–565 9p. doi:10.1111/j.1542-2011.2011.00122.x

Stewart, L. S., & Collins, M. (2013). Nitrous oxide as labor analgesia. *Nursing for Women's Health, 16*(5), 398–409. doi:10.1111/j.1751-486X.2012.01763.x

Sullivan, D. H., & McGuiness, C. (2015). Natural labor pain management. *International Journal of Childbirth Education, 30*(2), 20–25. Retrieved from Weatherspoon, D. (2011). Current practices in easing discomfort from labor and delivery: Alternative and medical practices. International Journal of Childbirth Education, 26(4), 44–48.

The Joint Commission. (2011). *Facts about pain management.* Retrieved from http://www.jointcommission.org.

Tsen, L. C. (2014) Anesthesia for cesarean delivery. In D. Chestnut, C. A. Wong, L. C. Tsen, D. N. K. Warwick, Y. Beilin, J. M. Mhyre & V. Naveen (Eds.) *Chestnut's Obstetric Anesthesia: Principles and practice* (5th ed) Philadelphia: Elsevier Saunders.

Wong, C. A. (2014) Epidural and spinal analgesia/anesthesia for labor and vaginal delivery. In D. Chestnut, C. A. Wong, L. C. Tsen, D. N. K. Warwick, Y. Beilin, J. M. Mhyre & V. Naveen (Eds.), *Chestnut's Obstetric Anesthesia: Principles and practice* (5th ed) Philadelphia: Elsevier Saunders.

# 19

# Nursing Care During Obstetric Procedures

http://evolve.elsevier.com/McKinney/mat-ch/

## LEARNING OBJECTIVES

*After studying this chapter, you should be able to:*

- Identify clinical situations in which specific obstetric procedures are appropriate.
- Explain risks, precautions, and contraindications for each procedure.
- Identify nursing considerations for each procedure.
- Identify methods to provide effective emotional support to the woman having an obstetric procedure.
- Apply the nursing process to plan care for the woman having a cesarean birth.

Although labor is a normal process, special procedures are sometimes needed to help the mother or fetus. A physician or nurse midwife performs these procedures while nurses provide supportive care. Descriptions of procedures and nursing considerations for each are addressed.

## AMNIOTOMY

### Indications

Amniotomy (artificial rupture of the amniotic sac) is often performed in conjunction with the induction or stimulation of labor or to permit internal electronic fetal monitoring (see Chapter 17). Although it is a common procedure, amniotomy implies a commitment to delivery (Cunningham, Leveno, Bloom, et al., 2014; Macones, Cahill, Stamilio, et al., 2012; Hobel & Zakowski, 2015).

### Risks

Amniotomy is seen by many professionals and expectant mothers as harmless, and it usually is, but the nurse must observe for three major associated risks and assist in any emergency procedures needed.

#### Prolapse of the Umbilical Cord

An immediate and continuing risk is that the umbilical cord will slip down in the gush of fluid. The cord can be compressed between the fetal presenting part and the woman's pelvis, obstructing blood flow to and from the placenta and reducing fetal gas exchange.

#### Infection

With the interruption of the membrane barrier, vaginal organisms have free access to the uterine cavity and may cause chorioamnionitis or infection of the amniotic sac. The risk is low at first but increases as the interval between membrane rupture and birth increases. Birth within 24 hours of amniotomy is desirable in the term pregnancy, although there is no absolute time when infection occurs.

#### Abruptio Placentae

Abruptio placentae (premature separation of a normally implanted placenta) may occur if the uterus is distended when the membranes rupture. The risk is greater if there is excessive amniotic fluid in the uterus (hydramnios) because of greater uterine distention. As the uterus collapses with discharge of the amniotic fluid, the area of placental attachment shrinks. The placenta then no longer fits its implantation site and partially separates. A large area of placental disruption reduces fetal oxygenation, nutrition, and waste disposal.

### Technique

A disposable plastic hook (Amnihook) is commonly used to perforate the amniotic sac (Fig. 19.1). The physician or nurse midwife performs a vaginal examination to determine cervical dilation and effacement, fetal station, and fetal presenting part. Amniotomy is deferred if the fetal presenting part is high in the pelvis or if the presentation is not cephalic. The risk for a prolapsed cord is greater in these situations because more room is available for the cord to slip down. In addition, a cesarean or surgical birth is usually performed for a noncephalic presentation.

The hook is passed through the cervix, and the membranes are snagged. The hole is enlarged with the finger, allowing fluid to drain.

### Nursing Considerations

#### Obtaining Baseline Information

The fetal heart rate (FHR) is assessed with auscultation or electronic monitoring to identify a reassuring rate and pattern before the amniotomy. A minimum of 20 to 30 minutes is needed for adequate fetal baseline evaluation and can be obtained with other admission information.

#### Assisting With Amniotomy

Before amniotomy, place underpads beneath the woman's buttocks to absorb the fluid. One or more folded bath towels under the buttocks absorb amniotic fluid well. Other supplies needed are a disposable plastic hook, a sterile glove or pair of gloves, and a packet of sterile lubricant.

#### Providing Care After Amniotomy

Nursing care after amniotomy is the same as that after spontaneous membrane rupture.

***Identifying complications.*** Assess the FHR for at least 1 full minute after membrane rupture, whether spontaneous or by amniotomy. A nonreassuring rate, other electronic fetal monitor patterns, or significant changes from previous assessments are reported promptly

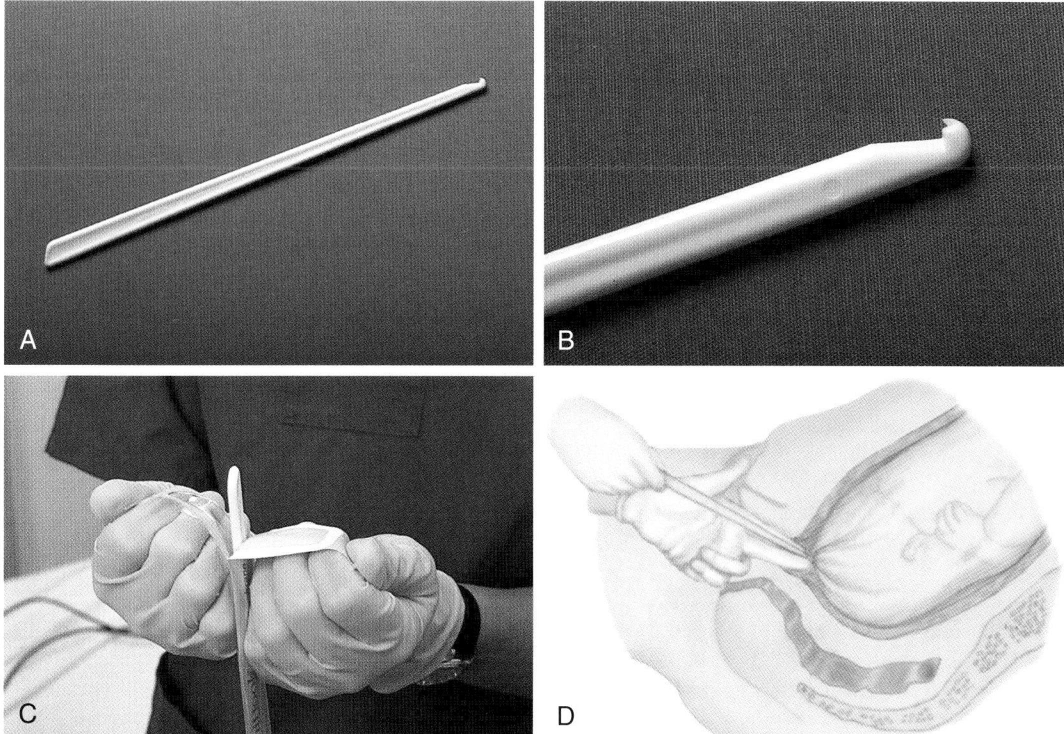

**FIG 19.1** **A,** Disposable plastic membrane perforator (Amnihook). **B,** Hook end of plastic membrane perforator. **C,** Correct method of opening the package. **D,** Technique for artificial rupture of membranes.

to the birth attendant. Cord compression is suspected if deep or prolonged variable decelerations occur during contractions or persistent bradycardia is present after contractions. Other nonreassuring FHR patterns also may occur (see Chapter 17).

Chart the quantity, color, and odor of the amniotic fluid. Refer to Chapter 16 for expected findings and signs of abnormality in the amniotic fluid.

Assess the woman's temperature every 2 hours after the membranes rupture. Report elevations greater than 38° C (100.4° F). Fetal tachycardia (sustained rate above 160 beats per minute [bpm]) often precedes maternal fever.

### CRITICAL THINKING EXERCISE 19.1

A physician performs an amniotomy on a laboring woman whose cervix is dilated to 5 cm. The amniotic fluid is pale yellow, moderate in amount, and has a strong odor. The fetal heart rate (FHR) averages 160 to170 beats per minute (bpm) and accelerates when the fetus moves. Maternal vital signs are temperature, 37.6° C (99.7° F); pulse, 92 bpm; respirations, 22 breaths per minute; and blood pressure, 116/80 mm Hg. Contractions are moderate to firm in intensity and occur every 3 to 4 minutes with a duration of 50 to 60 seconds and complete uterine relaxation between contractions.

1. Which of these observations should the nurse regard as normal? Which observations are abnormal?
2. Should the nurse modify routine labor care based on the postamniotomy assessments?

***Promoting comfort.*** Amniotic fluid leaks from the woman's vagina after membranes rupture. Change the underpads regularly for comfort and to reduce the moist environment that favors bacterial growth.

## INDUCTION AND AUGMENTATION OF LABOR

Induction and augmentation of labor use artificial methods to stimulate uterine contractions. Techniques and nursing care are similar for both induction and augmentation. After nearly 20 years of consecutive increases, the induction of labor for singleton births reached a high of 23.8% in 2010. Induction rates for late preterm births have declined since 2006, with the largest decrease at 38 weeks (iatrogenic, or the result of treatment) and the number of cesarean births has increased with the rise in labor inductions. A nullipara who has a cesarean after an unsuccessful induction usually has repeat cesareans for all other babies (American College of Obstetricians and Gynecologists [ACOG], 2015a; Wood & Ross, 2014; Hamilton, Martin, Osterman, et al., 2014; Martin, Hamilton, Osterman, et al., 2015). Few women who have regular prenatal care expect to deliver more than a few days past their due date.

### Indications

The induction of labor or artificial *initiation* of labor is considered when ending the pregnancy benefits the woman or fetus and when labor and vaginal birth are considered safe. Labor is not induced if the fetus must be delivered more quickly than the process permits; a cesarean birth would be performed instead. Examples of specific conditions that are indications for induction include (Simpson, 2008a):

- Fetal compromise (such as intrauterine growth restriction, maternal–fetal blood incompatibility)
- Spontaneous rupture of the membranes at or near term without onset of labor (premature rupture of the membranes or PROM)
- Postterm pregnancy

- Chorioamnionitis (inflammation of the amniotic sac)
- Hypertension associated with pregnancy or chronic hypertension, both of which are associated with reduced placental blood flow
- Abruptio placentae (large abruptions require immediate delivery) (see Chapter 27)
- Maternal medical conditions that are worsening with continuation of the pregnancy (such as diabetes, renal disease, pulmonary disease, and chronic hypertension)
- Fetal death

Elective induction for the convenience of the woman or her physician is not recommended, although it has become common. Factors such as a history of rapid labors and living a long distance from the hospital may be valid reasons for elective induction because of the possibility of birth under uncontrolled circumstances.

Prenatal testing may reveal a fetal anomaly for which specialized neonatal care at a distant facility will be needed. The mother may be transported to that facility for labor induction or cesarean birth, with the necessary equipment and specialists assembled to care for the newborn.

Augmentation of labor with oxytocin is considered when labor has begun spontaneously but progress has slowed or stopped because of poor contractions. The medical provider may use augmentation if progress is slower than expected, even if contractions seem to be adequate (ACOG, 2015a). The rate of oxytocin administration may be lower than that used for induction.

## Determining Whether Induction Is Indicated

The birth attendant evaluates whether labor and birth are safer for the woman or fetus than continuing the pregnancy. Labor is not induced if term gestation and/or fetal lung maturity are not established unless there is a compelling reason. Induction is more likely to be successful at term because prelabor cervical changes favor dilation.

The Bishop scoring system (Table 19.1) uses five factors to estimate cervical readiness for labor: cervical dilation, effacement, consistency, position, and fetal station. The Bishop score remains popular because of its ability to predict probable success of induction. The likelihood of vaginal birth is similar to that of spontaneous labor if the score is greater than 8 (ACOG, 2015a).

**TABLE 19.1 Bishop Scoring System to Evaluate the Cervix**

| | Score | | | |
|---|---|---|---|---|
| ***Factor*** | ***0*** | ***1*** | ***2*** | ***3*** |
| Dilation | 0 cm | 1-2 cm | 3-4 cm | 5-6 cm |
| Effacement | 0%-30% | 40%-50% | 60%-70% | ≥80% |
| Fetal station | −3 | −2 | −1 or 0 | +1 or +2 |
| Cervical consistency | Firm | Medium | Soft | |
| Cervical position | Posterior | Middle | Anterior | |

Modified from Bishop, E. H. (1964). Pelvic scoring for elective induction. *Obstetrics and Gynecology, 24*(2), 266–268.

NOTE: This system is used to estimate how easily a woman's labor can be induced. Higher scores are associated with a greater likelihood of successful induction because her cervix has undergone prelabor changes, often called *ripening*. A woman who has given birth before usually has a successful induction when her Bishop score is 5 or higher. Delivery in a woman who is having her first baby is most successfully induced if her score is 7 or higher.

## Contraindications

Any contraindication to labor and vaginal birth is a contraindication to induction or augmentation of labor. These conditions may include:

- Placenta previa (implantation in lower uterus), which can result in hemorrhage during labor
- Vasa previa, in which fetal umbilical cord vessels branch over the amniotic sac rather than inserting into the placenta; fetal hemorrhage is a possibility if the membranes rupture
- Abnormal presentation for which vaginal birth is often hazardous
- Umbilical cord prolapse (immediate birth by cesarean is indicated)
- Some uterine surgery, such as classic cesarean (see Fig. 19.2) and extensive surgery for uterine fibroids

Other maternal or fetal conditions are not contraindications to induction but require individual evaluation, such as the following:

- One or more previous low transverse cesarean births (see Fig. 19.2)
- Breech presentation (vaginal birth may be more hazardous; the fetus may turn to a normal position by the time spontaneous labor occurs)
- Maternal heart disease, which varies in severity
- Severe maternal hypertension
- Uterine over distention as occurs in multifetal pregnancy, especially triplets or higher, and hydramnios
- Fetal presenting part above the pelvic inlet, which may be associated with cephalopelvic disproportion (fetal head size that is too large to fit through maternal pelvis) or a preterm fetus
- Nonreassuring FHR patterns that do not yet mandate emergency delivery

## Risks

Induction and augmentation of labor are associated with the usual risks of spontaneous labor plus risks added by the procedure (Cunningham et al., 2014; Simpson, 2008a):

- Uterine tachysystole (hyperstimulation), which can reduce placental perfusion and fetal oxygenation caused by excessive frequency, duration, or intensity of contractions, or from poor uterine relaxation between contractions. Tachysystole may be accompanied by nonreassuring FHR patterns.
- Uterine rupture, more likely to occur with over distention.
- Maternal water intoxication caused by oxytocin's antidiuretic effects; more likely if hypotonic solutions are used to dilute the oxytocin.
- Greater risk for chorioamnionitis and cesarean birth.

## Technique

Surgical, medical, or mechanical methods can be used for labor induction or augmentation. Amniotomy is the surgical method of induction and augmentation, as rupturing membranes stimulates uterine contractions if the cervix is favorable (soft, some dilation and/or effacement). Medical methods for induction or augmentation involve the use of drugs such as prostaglandins, intravenous (IV) oxytocin (Pitocin), or both to stimulate contractions. Mechanical methods of induction use a variety of intracervical inserts to gradually stretch and soften the cervix.

### Cervical Ripening

Procedures to ripen (soften) the cervix, making it more likely to dilate with the forces of labor, are a common adjunct to induction. Cervical ripening may be done the morning of induction or possibly the day before.

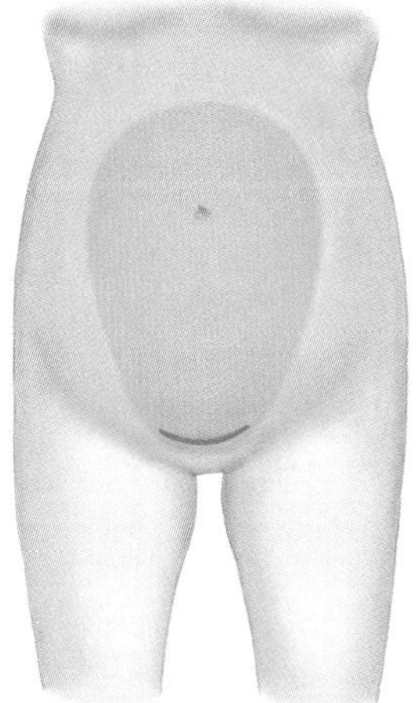


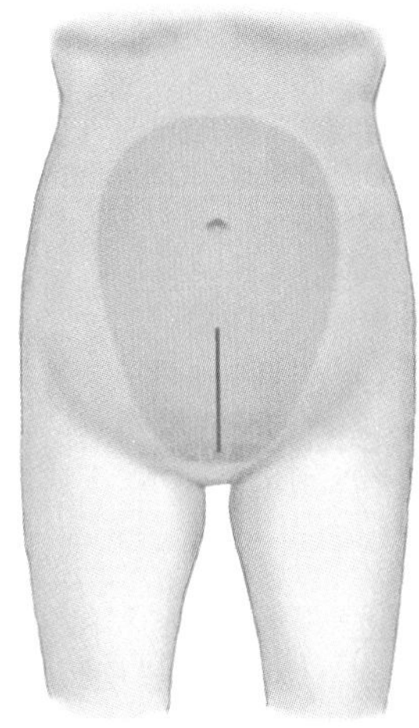


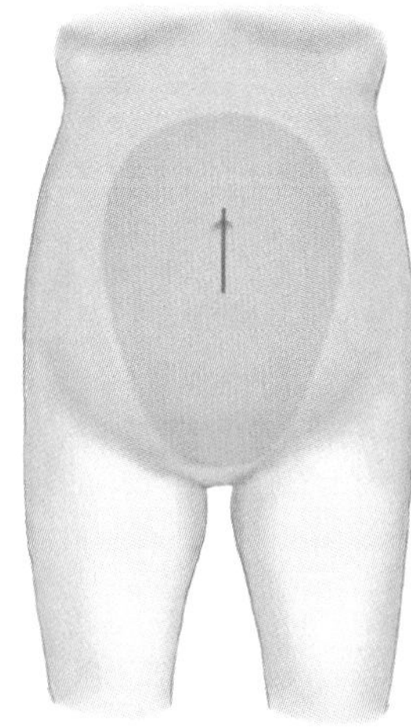


| Low Transverse | Low Vertical | Classic |
|---|---|---|
| *Advantages*<br>Unlikely to rupture during a subsequent birth<br>Makes VBAC possible for subsequent pregnancy<br>Less blood loss<br>Easier to repair<br>Less adhesion formation | *Advantage*<br>Can be extended upward to make a larger incision if needed | *Advantage*<br>May be the only choice in these situations:<br>Implantation of a placenta previa on the lower anterior uterine wall<br>Presence of dense adhesions from previous surgery<br>Transverse lie of a large fetus with the shoulder impacted in the mother's pelvis |
| *Disadvantage*<br>Limited ability to extend laterally to enlarge the incision | *Disadvantages*<br>Slightly more likely to rupture during a subsequent birth<br>A tear may extend the incision downward into the cervix | *Disadvantages*<br>Most likely of the uterine incisions to rupture during a subsequent birth<br>Eliminates VBAC as an option for birth of a subsequent infant |

**FIG 19.2** Uterine incisions for cesarean birth. The abdominal and uterine incisions do not always match. *VBAC*, Vaginal birth after cesarean.

***Medical methods.*** Preparations containing prostaglandin $E_2$ ($PGE_2$, or dinoprostone) can be used to facilitate cervical ripening. Prostaglandin is given as an intravaginal or intracervical gel or a timed-release vaginal insert (Table 19.2). It is administered in a setting in which fetal monitoring and emergency care, including immediate cesarean birth, are readily available.

Prostaglandin should be given cautiously to women who have asthma, glaucoma, ischemic heart disease, or pulmonary, hepatic, or renal disease. The major adverse reaction to prostaglandin for induction is tachysystole that can reduce placental blood flow and fetal oxygen exchange. The FHR and uterine activity should be monitored before prostaglandin insertion for a baseline and at least 30 minutes afterward for nonreassuring FHR patterns or excessive contractions.

Misoprostol (Cytotec) is popular for preinduction cervical ripening and labor induction because of its low cost, stability, and ease of use (see Table 19.2). Misoprostol is a synthetic prostaglandin tablet that is used for prevention of gastric ulcers. Its use for cervical ripening or labor induction remains an off-label use.

***Mechanical methods.*** Any of several techniques use mechanical means to ripen and begin dilation of the cervix:

- Transcervical catheter: Placement of a balloon-tipped Foley catheter in the cervix with possible saline infusion through the catheter into the space between the internal os and intact membranes (extra-amniotic saline infusion, or EASI).
- Placement of hydrophilic (moisture-attracting) inserts into the cervical canal, where they absorb water and expand, gradually dilating the cervix. Examples are:
  - Dilapan-S and Lamicel
  - Laminaria tents: sterile, cone-shaped preparations of dried seaweed; more than one can be placed in the vagina to absorb water and expand

## Oxytocin Administration

Oxytocin is a powerful drug, and it is impossible to predict a woman's response to it. Several precautions reduce the chance of adverse reactions in the mother and fetus:

- Oxytocin is diluted in an isotonic solution and given as a secondary (piggyback) infusion so that it can be stopped quickly if complications develop (Fig. 19.3). Oxytocin solutions are often premixed by the pharmacy.
- The oxytocin line is inserted into the primary (nonadditive, or maintenance) IV line as close as possible to the venipuncture site (the proximal port) to limit the amount of drug infused after changing to the nonadditive fluid.
- Primary nonadditive IV fluid is started first. Oxytocin is then started slowly, increased gradually, and regulated as the secondary line in the infusion pump.
- Uterine activity and the FHR and its patterns are monitored before induction, when oxytocin is started, and throughout labor.

The woman's uterus becomes more sensitive to oxytocin as labor progresses. Therefore, oxytocin administration is titrated to the uterine and fetal response. The rate of oxytocin infusion may be gradually reduced when the woman is in the active phase of labor, approximately

**TABLE 19.2 Prostaglandin Preparations for Cervical Ripening at Term**

| Prostaglandin Gel (Dinoprostone or Prepidil) | Vaginal Insert: Dinoprostone or Cervidil | Vaginal Insert: Misoprostol (Cytotec) |
|---|---|---|
| ***Dosage*** | | |
| 0.5 mg applied to cervix. May be repeated 6-12 hr later to a maximum of 1.5 mg (three applications) applied to the cervix; 2.5 mg vaginally. | 10 mg in a timed-release vaginal insert. Remove after 12 hr or at onset of active labor. | One quarter of 100-mcg tablet vaginally (approximately 25 mcg; see cautions below). Also used for labor induction by repeating 25-mcg dose every 3-6 hr. A 50-mcg dose is associated with hypertonic contractions. |
| ***Actions for Uterine Tachysystole, With or Without Nonreassuring Fetal Heart Rate Pattern*** | | |
| Place woman in side-lying position. Provide oxygen by facemask at 8-10 L/min.<br>Administer tocolytic drug such as terbutaline or magnesium sulfate.<br>Typically begins 1 hr after gel application.<br>Higher incidence with vaginal application. | Same as for dinoprostone gel.<br>Remove insert.<br>Hypertonic uterine activity may occur up to 9½ hr after insert placement. Greater incidence than with lower-dose intracervical dinoprostone gel. | Same as for dinoprostone gel. Higher doses or more frequent administration is more likely to cause excessive contractions, which may be accompanied by a nonreassuring FHR pattern. |
| ***When Oxytocin Induction Can Begin*** | | |
| Safe interval has not been established.<br>Delaying oxytocin administration for 6-12 hr after total intracervical dose of 1.5- or 2.5-mg vaginal dose recommended. | 30-60 min after removal of insert. | At least 4 hr after last dose. |
| ***Precautions and Comments*** | | |
| Limit dinoprostone gel to maximum of 1.5 mg dinoprostone gel in 24 hr.<br>Woman should remain recumbent with lateral uterine displacement for 15-30 min after application.<br>Has increased effect if combined with other oxytocics such as oxytocin (Pitocin). Increases hypertensive effect of the herb ephedra.<br>Use caution in women with asthma, hypertension, glaucoma, or severe renal or hepatic dysfunction, ischemic heart disease. | Remove after 12 hr or when active labor begins.<br>Adverse effects can be reduced within 15 min of removal.<br>Most expensive of the prostaglandin options. | Misoprostol is currently FDA approved only for treatment of peptic ulcers but is widely used for cervical ripening and the induction of labor. Manufacturer does not intend to seek approval, but American College of Obstetricians and Gynecologists supports its use for these purposes.<br>100-mcg tablet is not scored. Pharmacist should prepare the 25-mcg dose for best accuracy.<br>Cost is approximately 1%-2% that of other prostaglandin preparations.<br>Contraindicated in the woman with a previous cesarean or other uterine surgery. |

NOTE: Dosages can be higher in cases of fetal death.
*FDA,* U.S. Food and Drug Administration; *FHR,* fetal heart rate
From American Academy of Pediatrics. (2012). *Guidelines for perinatal care* (6th ed.). Elk Grove Village, IL, and Washington, DC: Author; American College of Obstetricians and Gynecologists. (2015c). *Induction of labor (ACOG Practice Bulletin No. 107).* Washington, DC: Author; Cunningham, F.G., Leveno, K.J., Bloom, S.L., et al. (2014). *Williams obstetrics* (24th ed.). New York: McGraw-Hill.

5 to 6 cm of cervical dilation. It may be stopped or reduced after her membranes rupture. If uterine tachysystole makes it necessary to stop oxytocin, the medical decision regarding whether to restart administration must be individualized. When labor is augmented with oxytocin, a lower total dose is usually needed to achieve adequate contractions.

## Nursing Considerations

In addition to basic intrapartum care, the nurse observes the woman and fetus for complications and takes corrective actions if abnormalities are noted. Nursing care is similar for the woman who has cervical ripening.

The nurse has a great responsibility when administering oxytocin or other uterine stimulants to a pregnant woman. The nurse must maintain safeguards to both mother and fetus when administering oxytocin and recognize when to start, change, or stop its infusion and when to notify the physician. Facility policies related to oxytocin must clearly support correct nursing and medical actions (Pearson, 2011).

### Observing the Fetal Response

Oxytocin stimulates uterine contractions, and they may become too strong (hypertonic). Hypertonic contractions can reduce placental blood flow, and thus, reduce exchange of fetal oxygen and waste products. Before induction or augmentation of labor, the nurse determines whether the FHR and patterns are reassuring. The FHR is charted in the labor record at least every 15 minutes during first-stage labor and every 5 minutes during the second stage (Simpson, 2013a).

The nurse remains alert for FHR patterns that suggest reduced placental exchange secondary to contractions that are too strong, too long, or do not relax at least 30 seconds (now termed *tachysystole*). Examples of these patterns are fetal bradycardia (<110 bpm at term), tachycardia (persistent rate >160 bpm at term), late decelerations (slowing after the peak of the contraction), and decreased FHR

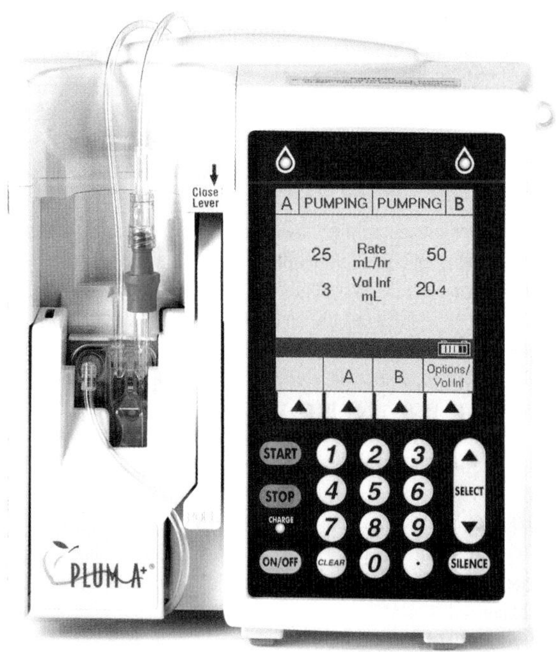


**FIG 19.3** Intravenous (IV) pump setup for infusion from two IV lines. Fluid in the primary line (nonadditive, or maintenance line) contains no medication but is regulated by the infusion pump to maintain the correct rate. Oxytocin solution is regulated in the secondary line in the same pump, giving the nurse options to change or discontinue the oxytocin infusion rate while maintaining the primary line infusion at the same rate. A single IV line at the lower part of the pump connects to the woman's infusion site. (Courtesy Hospira, Inc., Lake Forest, IL.)

variability (reduced rate fluctuations) that is not explained by medications or fetal sleep. Reduced placental exchange also may have causes other than excess uterine activity, such as maternal hypotension or maternal diabetes. The nurse must assess the woman and fetus carefully to identify the most likely cause of the problem and the indicated corrective actions.

If nonreassuring FHR patterns occur or if contractions are hypertonic, the nurse takes steps to reduce uterine activity and increase fetal oxygenation. These steps include:

1. Reducing or stopping the oxytocin infusion and increasing the rate of the primary nonadditive infusion.
2. Keeping the woman on her side to prevent aortocaval compression and increase placental blood flow.
3. Giving 100% oxygen by a snug facemask at a rate of 8 to 10 L/min to increase the woman's oxygen saturation, making more oxygen available for the fetus.

The physician may order a drug such as terbutaline (Brethine) or magnesium sulfate to reduce uterine activity. Terbutaline, 0.25 mg subcutaneously, can be given quickly to reduce uterine contractions.

## Observing the Mother's Response

Uterine activity must be assessed for tachysystole that can reduce fetal oxygenation and contribute to uterine rupture. Contractions are assessed for frequency, duration, and intensity, and uterine resting tone is assessed for relaxation of at least 30 seconds between contractions. Uterine activity observations are charted at the same intervals as the FHR patterns. Corrective actions for tachysystole are the same as those listed in the discussion of the fetal response. In addition, a tocolytic drug such as terbutaline may be given.

The woman's blood pressure and pulse are taken every 30 minutes or with each oxytocin dose change to identify changes from

## DRUG GUIDE

### *Oxytocin (Pitocin)*

**Classification:** Oxytocic

**Action:** Synthetic compound identical to the natural hormone from the posterior pituitary. Stimulates uterine smooth muscle, resulting in increased strength, duration, and frequency of uterine contractions. Uterine sensitivity to oxytocin increases gradually during gestation. Oxytocin has vasoactive and antidiuretic properties.

**Indications:** Induction or augmentation of labor at or near term. Maintenance of firm uterine contraction after birth to control postpartum bleeding. Management of inevitable or incomplete abortion.

#### Dosage and Route: Induction or Augmentation of Labor

1. *Intravenous infusion* via a secondary (piggyback) line. Oxytocin infusion is controlled with a pump. Various dilutions of oxytocin and balanced electrolyte solution may be used. Mixtures having 60 mU/mL are convenient because the mL/hr setting on the infusion pump is the same number as the mU/min infused, reducing the chance for errors. Common mixtures that provide 60 mU/mL of oxytocin include (1) 15 units of oxytocin (1.5 mL) plus 250 mL of solution; (2) 30 units (3 mL) of oxytocin plus 500 mL solution; (3) 60 units oxytocin plus 1000 mL solution. Lower concentrations, such as 10 to 20 units of oxytocin plus 1000 mL of solution, also may be used. The drug may be given in 10-minute pulsed infusions rather than continuously.
2. Guidelines for oxytocin administration from the American College of Obstetricians and Gynecologists* provide examples of low- and high-dose oxytocin labor-induction protocols. Depending on the protocol followed, the following recommendations are provided: (1) starting dosages of 0.5 to 6 mU/min, and (2) increasing dosage by 1 to 2 mU/min–increments every 15 to 40 minutes. High-dose protocols may increase the dose in increments of up to 6 mU/min. The actual oxytocin dose is based on the uterine response and absence of adverse effects. Higher starting doses, higher dose increases, and shorter intervals between dose increases are most likely to result in uterine hyperstimulation. A lower starting dose and lower rate-increase increments usually are required to augment labor.
3. After an adequate contraction pattern is established and the cervix is dilated 5 to 6 cm, the oxytocin may be reduced by similar increments.

***Control of Postpartum Bleeding:*** *Intravenous infusion:* Dilute 10 to 40 units in 1000 mL of intravenous solution. The rate of infusion must control uterine atony. Begin at a rate of 20 to 40 mU/min, increasing or decreasing the rate according to uterine response and the rate of postpartum bleeding. Correcting any identifiable cause of the hemorrhage should also be done. *Intramuscular injection:* Inject 10 units after delivery of the placenta (See Chapter 28 for other medications used to treat postpartum hemorrhage).

***Inevitable or Incomplete Abortion:*** Dilute 10 units in 500 mL of intravenous solution and infuse at a rate of 10 to 20 mU/min. Other dilutions are acceptable.

**Absorption:** Intravenous, immediate; intramuscular, 3 to 5 minutes.

**Excretion:** Liver and urine.

**Contraindications and Precautions:** Include, but are not limited to, placenta previa, vasa previa, nonreassuring fetal heart rate (FHR) patterns, abnormal fetal presentation, prolapsed umbilical cord, presenting part above the

*Continued*

## DRUG GUIDE—cont'd

### *Oxytocin (Pitocin)*

pelvic inlet, previous classic or other fundal uterine incision, active genital herpes infection, pelvic structural deformities, and invasive cervical carcinoma.

**Adverse Reactions:** Most result from drug hypersensitivity or excessive dosage. Adverse reactions include hypertonic uterine activity, impaired uterine blood flow, uterine rupture, and abruptio placentae. Uterine hypertonicity may result in fetal bradycardia, tachycardia, reduced FHR variability, and late decelerations. Fetal asphyxia may occur with diminished uterine blood flow. Fetal or maternal trauma, or both, may occur from rapid birth. Prolonged administration may cause maternal fluid retention, leading to water intoxication. Hypotension (seen with rapid intravenous injection), tachycardia, cardiac dysrhythmias, and subarachnoid hemorrhage are rare adverse reactions.

Drug interactions include vasopressors and the herb ephedra, causing hypertension.

**Nursing Considerations:** ***Intrapartum:*** Assess the FHR for at least 20 minutes before induction to identify reassuring or nonreassuring patterns. Perform Leopold's maneuvers, a vaginal examination, or both to verify a cephalic fetal presentation. If nonreassuring FHR patterns are identified or if fetal presentation is other than cephalic, notify the physician and do not begin induction until an ultrasound is done to ascertain fetal presentation.

Observe uterine activity for establishment of effective labor pattern: contraction frequency every 2 to 3 minutes, duration of 40 to 90 seconds, intensity of 50 to 80 mm Hg (measured with an intrauterine pressure catheter). Observe for hypertonic uterine activity (also known as tachysystole): contractions less than 2 minutes apart or more than 5 contractions within 10 minutes; rest interval shorter than 30 seconds, duration longer than 90 to 120 seconds, or an elevated resting tone greater than 20 mm Hg (measured with an intrauterine pressure catheter).

Observe FHR for nonreassuring patterns such as tachycardia, bradycardia, decreased variability, and late decelerations.

If uterine hypertonicity (tachysystole) or a nonreassuring FHR pattern occurs, intervene to reduce uterine activity and increase fetal oxygenation: stop the oxytocin infusion, increase the rate of nonadditive solution, position the woman in a side-lying position, and administer oxygen by snug facemask at 8 to 10 L/min. Notify the physician of adverse reactions, nursing interventions, and response to interventions. Record the maternal blood pressure, pulse, and respirations every 30 to 60 minutes and with each dosage increase. Record intake and output.

***Postpartum:*** Observe uterus for firmness, height, and deviation. Massage until firm if uterus is soft ("boggy"). Observe lochia for color, quantity, and presence of clots. Notify birth attendant if uterus fails to remain contracted or if lochia is bright red or contains large clots. Assess for cramping. Assess vital signs every 15 minutes or according to protocol. Monitor intake and output and breath sounds to identify fluid retention or bladder distention.

***Inevitable or Incomplete Abortion:*** Observe for cramping, vaginal bleeding, clots, and passage of products of conception. Observe maternal vital signs, intake, and output as noted under postpartum nursing implications.

*American College of Obstetricians and Gynecologists. (2009). *Induction of labor* (ACOG Practice Bulletin No. 107). Washington, DC: Author; American College of Obstetricians and Gynecologists. (2011). *Dystocia and augmentation of labor* (ACOG Practice Bulletin No. 49). Washington, DC: Author.

## CRITICAL THINKING EXERCISE 19.2

A woman is having term labor induced with oxytocin. Her cervix is 4 cm dilated and fully effaced, and the fetal head is at station 0. The nurse notes that the fetal heart rate (external monitor) is near its baseline of 120 to 130 beats per minute (bpm), with a variability of 10 bpm. Contractions are firm, occur every 2 minutes (every 120 seconds), and the duration is usually 100 seconds. The nurse must palpate contractions because the woman has thick abdominal fat. With palpation, the nurse notes that the woman's uterus does not fully relax before another contraction begins.

1. What is the correct interpretation of these assessments?
2. What are appropriate nursing actions in this situation, and why are they done?

her baseline. Her temperature is checked every 4 hours (every 2 hours after membrane rupture) to identify infection.

Recording intake and output identifies fluid retention, which precedes water intoxication. Signs and symptoms of water intoxication include headache, blurred vision, behavioral changes, increased blood pressure and respirations, decreased pulse, rales, wheezing, and coughing.

After birth, observe for postpartum hemorrhage caused by uterine relaxation. Postpartum uterine atony is more likely if the woman has received oxytocin for a long time because the uterine muscle becomes fatigued and does not contract effectively to compress vessels at the placental site. It is manifested by a soft uterine fundus and excess amounts of lochia, usually with large clots. Hypovolemic shock may occur with hemorrhage.

## SAFETY ALERT

### *Signs of Tachysystole*

- Contraction duration longer than 90-120 seconds.
- Contractions occurring less than 2 minutes apart or relaxation of less than 30 seconds between contractions.
- Uterine resting tone above 20 mm Hg or peak pressure higher than 90 mm Hg during first-stage labor (with intrauterine pressure catheter).
- Montevideo units greater than 400.
- An FHR pattern of late decelerations accompanying hypertonic uterine activity.

#### Nursing Actions for Tachysystole

- Reduce or stop the oxytocin infusion.
- Increase the rate of the primary nonadditive infusion.
- Keep the laboring woman in a lateral position.
- Give oxygen by snug facemask, 8 to 10 L/min.
- Notify the physician or nurse midwife.

## VERSION

Either of two methods may be used to change fetal presentation: external version or internal version. Each has different indications and a different technique. External version is much more common.

### Indications

#### External Cephalic Version

The fetus may be changed from a breech, shoulder (transverse lie), or oblique presentation to a cephalic presentation using external cephalic version (ECV) during late pregnancy. Successful version may allow the woman to avoid a cesarean birth. ECV to change the fetal presentation from breech to cephalic has shown a wide range of success given the many factors that affect the procedure. Some unsuccessful versions spontaneously change to cephalic before labor. Studies have shown mixed results regarding birth outcomes after ECV; some report that the cesarean rate is still higher than average after successful ECV, while others report no difference (ACOG, 2014; Cunningham et al., 2014).

### Internal Version

Malpresentation in twin gestations is usually managed by cesarean birth, but internal version may be used for vaginal birth of the second twin.

## Contraindications

Version is not done if a woman cannot or is unlikely to deliver vaginally. Maternal conditions that may contraindicate external version or reduce its success include:

- Uterine malformations that limit the room available to perform the version and may contribute to the abnormal fetal presentation.
- Previous cesarean birth, although some facilities offer version on an individualized basis.
- Disproportion between fetal size and maternal pelvic size.
- Fetal size 4000 g or larger.

Fetal conditions that may contraindicate version:

- Placenta previa. Manipulation of the fetus within the uterus may cause hemorrhage, endangering both mother and fetus. Placenta previa other than marginal is an indication itself for cesarean birth (see Chapter 25).
- Multifetal gestation, which reduces the available room to turn the fetus or fetuses. Internal version may be done after the first twin is born.
- Oligohydramnios (abnormally small amount of amniotic fluid), ruptured membranes, or a cord around the fetal body or neck (nuchal cord). These conditions limit the room in which to turn the fetus and may lead to cord compression and fetal hypoxia.
- Uteroplacental insufficiency. Uterine contractions occurring during the version or during labor may worsen the insufficiency and cause fetal compromise.
- Engagement of the fetal presenting part into the pelvis.

## Risks

There are few risks to the woman, and serious adverse effects on the fetus are rare. FHR changes are common during the procedure but usually return to normal after the procedure. The fetus may become entangled in or compress the umbilical cord, possibly resulting in transient or prolonged hypoxia. Abruptio placentae may occur if fetal manipulation disrupts the placental site. Mixing of fetal and maternal blood within small breaks in placental vessels may result in maternal sensitization to the fetal blood type. Cesarean birth may be needed for fetal compromise at the time of version or later if the fetus returns to an abnormal presentation.

## Technique

### External Version

A nonstress test or biophysical profile (see Chapter 15) is done before external version to evaluate fetal health and placental function. If the test is nonreactive or other nonreassuring signs are present, the procedure is not done. Version adds stress to the fetus already functioning with reduced physiologic reserve. An ultrasound examination confirms fetal gestational age and fetal presentation and demonstrates adequacy of amniotic fluid

External version is usually attempted at 37 or more weeks of gestation but before the woman is in labor, for the following reasons:

- As term nears, the fetus may spontaneously turn to assume a cephalic presentation.
- The fetus is more likely to return to an abnormal presentation if version is attempted before 37 weeks because of its smaller size.
- If fetal compromise or onset of labor occurs, the fetus will be at or near term at birth.

The woman may be given a tocolytic drug, such as terbutaline 0.25 mg subcutaneously, to relax the uterus while the version is performed.

An epidural block or other analgesic may be given to increase maternal comfort and relaxation.

Ultrasonography guides fetal manipulations during external version and helps monitor the FHR. The physician gently pushes the breech out of the pelvis in a forward or backward roll (Fig. 19.4).

If indicated, $Rh_o(D)$ immune globulin (RhoGAM) is given to the Rh-negative woman after external version to prevent Rh sensitization (Branch, Silver, & Aagaard-Tillery, 2008).

Labor may be induced immediately after a successful version, or the woman may be discharged to await spontaneous labor or a later induction.

### Internal Version

Internal version is an unexpected and urgent procedure. The physician reaches into the uterus with one hand and, with the other hand on the maternal abdomen, maneuvers the fetus into a longitudinal lie (cephalic or breech) to allow delivery.

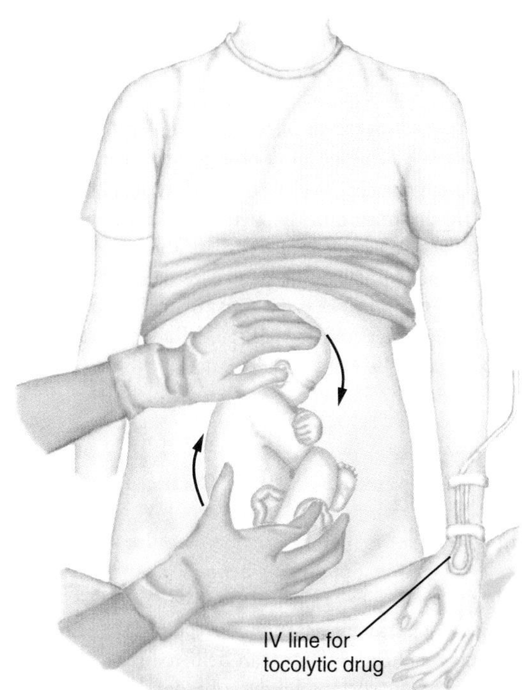


FIG 19.4 External version. Intravenous (IV) access is established in case of emergency or for some tocolytic drugs. If terbutaline is the tocolytic drug, it is given by subcutaneous injection.

### Nursing Considerations

When caring for the woman having external version, the nurse provides information, assesses the woman and fetus, and helps reduce her anxiety.

#### Providing Information

The physician explains the indications and risks for external version to the woman before she signs an informed consent form. The nurse verifies the woman's understanding of the purposes, risks, and limitations of version. Consent for cesarean birth is obtained. Also obtain consents if epidural or spinal anesthesia is planned.

The purposes and side effects of any tocolytic drug are reviewed. Tachycardia, flushing, headache, and tremors are common side effects of tocolytics such as terbutaline.

#### Promoting Maternal and Fetal Health

- Admission information is collected as if the woman were in labor or having a cesarean birth because the need for operative intervention may arise suddenly.
- Maternal vital signs are assessed for baseline value, and the initial nonstress test is administered. Abnormalities or nonreassuring FHR patterns should be reported promptly.
- An IV line is established for possible drug administration or fluid resuscitation if the FHR is nonreassuring.
- The nurse administers the tocolytic drug. Onset of action for terbutaline is 6 to 15 minutes after subcutaneous injection.
- Real-time ultrasound is used to guide the version and check the FHR periodically.
- After the version, the mother and fetus are observed for at least 1 hour. Reassuring fetal signs are a heart rate near the same range as baseline, resolution of bradycardia, and the presence of rate accelerations with fetal movement.
- Maternal tachycardia, flushing, or headache may be present for up to 4 hours if terbutaline was given to relax the uterus.
- Maternal vital signs are measured every 15 to 30 minutes until they return to near their baseline level. Maternal pulse should be no higher than 120 bpm.
- The presence of regular contractions suggests the onset of labor. Spontaneous rupture of membranes sometimes occurs.
- $Rh_o$(D) immune globulin is given to the Rh-negative woman.
- The woman usually has some discomfort during the version, but it should diminish quickly afterward. Persistent or continuous pain suggests a complication such as abruptio placentae.
- Because the woman undergoing external version is near term, the nurse should review the signs of true labor or membrane rupture with her and explain guidelines for returning to the hospital if she is not having induction immediately after the procedure (see Chapter 16).

#### Reducing Anxiety

The woman may be anxious before version because its success is not certain and complications may require rapid cesarean delivery. After successful version, she may still be anxious because the fetus can return to its previous position. Supporting her as she expresses her concerns and during the procedure can help reduce her anxiety.

Pointing out reassuring fetal monitor patterns, such as a normal heart rate and rate accelerations, can help reduce her anxiety about her baby. If problems such as bradycardia develop, the nurse should explain what has happened, what steps are being done to relieve it, and the result of these interventions. Explanations of tocolytic-associated side effects and when they should disappear should be provided.

## OPERATIVE VAGINAL BIRTH

An operative vaginal birth is one in which the physician applies traction to the fetal head during birth with a vacuum extractor or forceps to aid the woman's expulsive efforts. The use of forceps has decreased while use of vacuum extractors has increased. The number of births assisted by vacuum extraction is more than four times the number of forceps-assisted births. However, as the rate of cesarean births has risen, vaginal births assisted by either vacuum extractor or forceps have decreased since 1990 (Bofill & Martin, 2008; Martin et al., 2015).

Forceps are metal instruments having two curved blades with rounded edges that can be locked in the center. Many styles are available for different needs (Fig. 19.5). Disposable foam pads are available to cushion the fetal head. Forceps or a vacuum extractor also may be used during a cesarean birth to help pull the baby through the incision.

A vacuum extractor uses suction to grasp the fetal head as traction is applied (Figs. 19.6, p. 386, and 19.7, p. 386). This method is not used to deliver the fetus in a converted presentation, such as breech or face; otherwise, its use is similar to that for forceps. Three applications is the usual limit allowed by policy.

### Indications

Forceps or vacuum extraction is considered if shortening of the second stage is needed for the well-being of the woman, fetus, or both and if a vaginal birth can be accomplished quickly without undue trauma. Maternal indications may include exhaustion, inability to push effectively, cardiac or pulmonary disease, and intrapartum infection. Fetal indications may include cord compression, premature separation of the placenta, or nonreassuring FHR patterns.

### Contraindications

A cesarean birth is preferable if the maternal or fetal condition mandates a more rapid birth than can be accomplished with forceps or a vacuum extractor or if the procedure would be too traumatic. Examples of these conditions are severe fetal compromise or a high fetal station and acute maternal conditions such as pulmonary edema.

### Risks

Maternal risks include laceration or hematoma of the vagina, perineum, or periurethral area and a very large episiotomy. The infant may have ecchymoses, facial and scalp lacerations or abrasions, facial nerve injury, cephalhematoma, subgaleal hemorrhage, and other intracranial hemorrhage. A vacuum extractor creates circular scalp edema and redness or bruising called a **chignon** at the application area (see Fig. 19.6), which resolves quickly after birth.

### Technique

Preparation for forceps or vacuum extraction is the same as for any vaginal birth. The woman's bladder should be empty to limit bladder trauma. Membranes must be ruptured and the cervix completely dilated for forceps or vacuum-extraction birth. The woman needs adequate anesthesia, usually with a regional block such as an epidural.

Forceps- and vacuum extractor–assisted births are classified according to how far the fetal head has descended into the pelvis when these instruments are applied. Fewer teachers experienced in the more complex forceps deliveries and medical-legal concerns have reduced the number of practitioners skilled in midpelvis forceps (American Academy of Pediatrics [AAP] & American College of Obstetricians and Gynecologists [ACOG], 2012; ACOG, 2015d). The three classifications are outlet, low, and midpelvis (or mid-forceps):

- *Outlet operative vaginal delivery:* The fetal head is on the perineum, with the scalp visible at the vaginal opening without

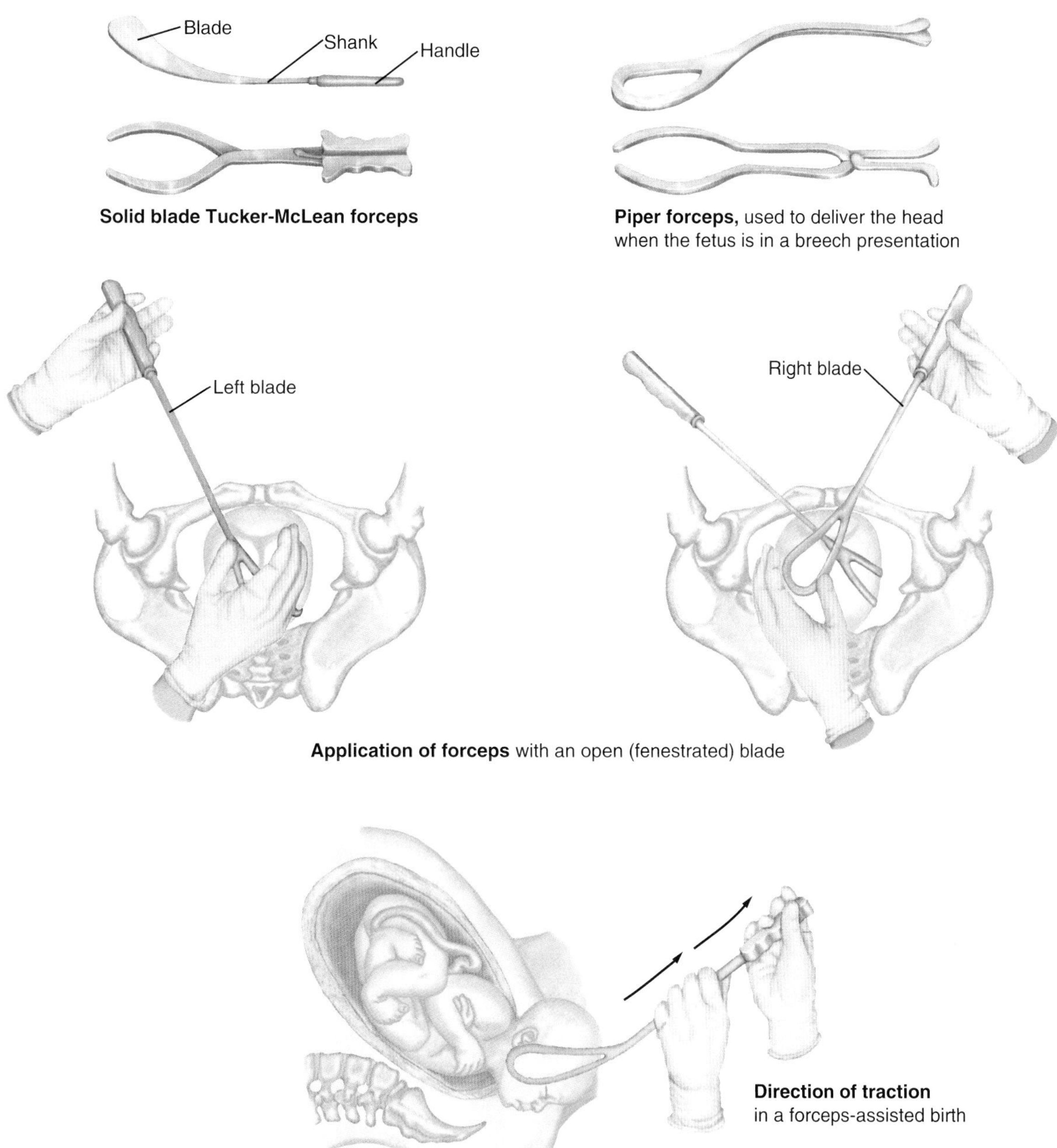


**FIG 19.5** Obstetric forceps and their application.

separating the labia. The position is occiput anterior or either right or left occiput anterior (ROA, LOA) or posterior (ROP, LOP).

- *Low operative vaginal delivery:* The leading edge of the fetal skull is at station +2 cm (approximately 4 cm below the level of the mother's ischial spines) or lower. Low operative vaginal birth is subdivided according to the amount of rotation of the fetal head needed. Births requiring 45 degrees or less of fetal head rotation are simpler.
- *Midpelvis operative vaginal delivery:* The station is above +2 cm, but the fetal head is engaged.

The physician determines the presentation, position, and station of the fetal head and the amount of cervical dilation. With correct application, the long axis of the forceps blades lies over the fetal cheeks and parietal bones. After checking for proper application, the physician locks the two blades in the center and pulls gently as the woman pushes, following the curve of the pelvis. The physician may keep the forceps on until the head is born or may remove the blades just before expulsion. The rest of the fetus is born in the usual way.

A hand pump is used to create suction to hold the vacuum cup on the fetal head in the midline of the occiput. The physician applies traction intermittently with the woman's push, as in a forceps-assisted birth. A vacuum release allows removal of the cup. The vacuum should go no higher than the green zone, indicated on the vacuum pump. A maximum of three pulls is the recommended limit.

## Nursing Considerations

The woman's bladder should be empty, usually by catheterization, before attempting an operative vaginal birth. The physician specifies

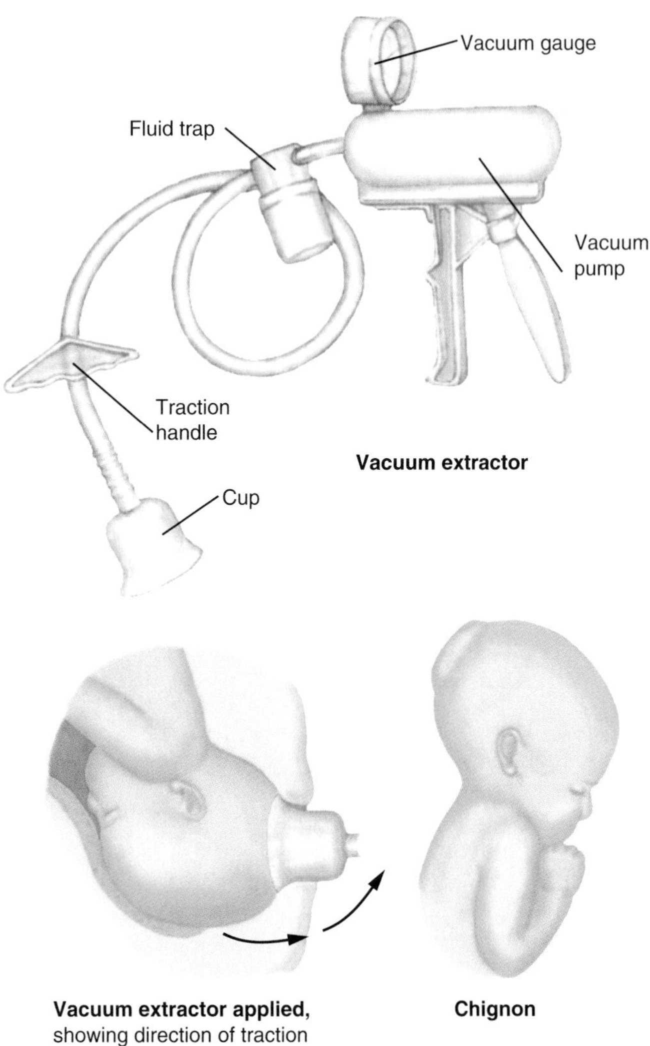


FIG 19.6 Birth assisted with a vacuum extractor. The chignon is scalp edema that often forms under the suction cup when the vacuum extractor is used.

the type of forceps or vacuum cup. The FHR should be assessed, and any rate less than 100 bpm should be reported.

After birth, the mother and infant are observed for trauma. The mother may have vaginal wall lacerations or hematoma (see Chapter 28). Cold applications for the first 12 hours reduce pain by numbing the area and limit bruising and edema of the tissues. Intermittent applications after 12 hours aid resolution of the edema and bruising. The fundus is usually firm unless uterine atony is present.

The infant often has reddening and mild bruising of the skin where the forceps were applied. Observe for skin breaks that allow entry of microorganisms; keep skin breaks clean. Facial asymmetry, most obvious when the infant cries, suggests facial nerve injury that is usually temporary. Neurologic abnormalities such as seizures suggest that the newborn has had an intracranial hemorrhage. However, seizures also may occur with neonatal hypoglycemia or sepsis. Scalp edema in the area of vacuum extractor cap is common.

After a forceps-assisted birth, a parent may ask why the baby's cheeks are reddened or bruised. A response is to explain that the pressure of the forceps on the baby's delicate skin may cause minor bruising that usually resolves without treatment. Parents of an infant born with assistance of a vacuum extractor may likewise be concerned about the edema on their baby's head. Reassure them that this edema will soon resolve. Point out improvement in the baby's cheeks or scalp during the postpartum stay.

## EPISIOTOMY

**Episiotomy**, or incision of the perineum just before birth, was once routine for vaginal births. The presumed maternal benefits of reducing pain, perineal tearing, and later pelvic relaxation with incontinence have not proven true. Data do not support liberal or routine episiotomy, and restrictive protocols are preferred. However, the birth attendant must decide if one is needed, and indications are not always clear (ACOG, 2015b; Cunningham et al., 2014; Lund & McManaman, 2008).

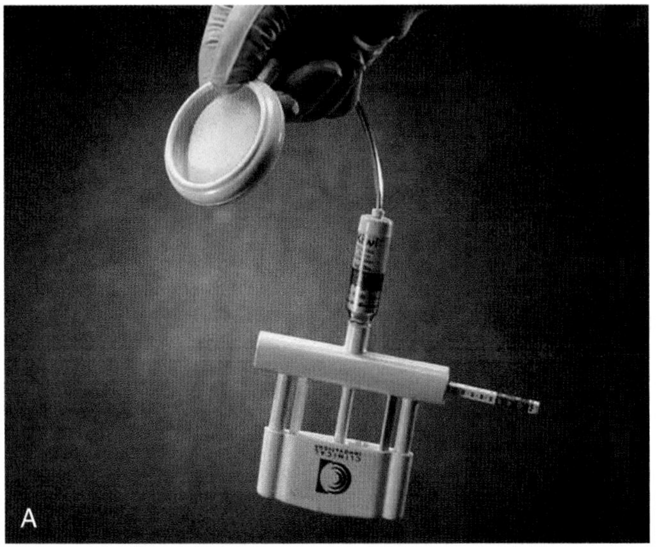


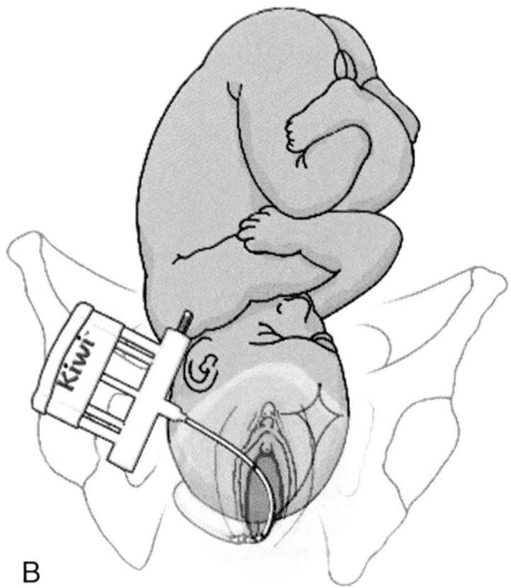


FIG 19.7 **A,** Vacuum extractor with a low-profile cup that can be used for occiput posterior fetal positions. Note the green band that denotes adequate suction and the red band that warns of excess suction. **B,** Application of the low-profile cup to the fetal head in an occiput posterior position. (Courtesy Clinical Innovations, Inc., Murray, UT.)

Examples of situations when the birth attendant may do an episiotomy include:

- Fetal shoulder dystocia, in which the shoulder of a fetus becomes lodged under the mother's symphysis during birth
- Forceps- or vacuum extractor–assisted births
- Birth with the fetus in an occiput posterior (face up) position

### Technique

An episiotomy is done when the fetal presenting part has crowned to a diameter of approximately 3 to 4 cm. The two types of episiotomies have different advantages and disadvantages: *median* or *midline;* and *mediolateral* (Fig. 19.8).

### Nursing Considerations

Gradual stretching of the perineum is the key to reducing the need for episiotomy. An upright position while pushing promotes gradual stretching of the woman's perineum. Laboring down, or delaying pushing until the urge is felt, also gradually distends the soft tissues of the pelvic floor. When the woman pushes, use of an open-glottis technique rather than prolonged breath-holding when pushing also promotes gradual perineal stretching.

Daily perineal massage and stretching by the woman from 36 weeks of gestation until birth has been shown to reduce the risk for perineal trauma during birth. Women older than 30 years of age, having their first baby, and adhering to the daily 10-minute perineal massage showed greatest benefit (Seehusen & Raleigh, 2014).

Nursing interventions during the recovery and postpartum periods are similar for all perineal trauma. Observe the perineum for hematoma and edema. Perineal cold applications are done for the first 12 hours, followed by intermittent perineal heat applications after at least 12 hours if needed.

## CESAREAN BIRTH

At one time, cesarean births made up only 5% of births; this number gradually rose to approximately 25% of births in the late 1980s. Efforts to reduce the number of cesarean births by use of vaginal birth after cesarean (VBAC) and reducing primary cesareans were successful until 1996, when the rates began to rise again. In 2013, the U.S. cesarean rate was 32.7% of deliveries (ACOG, 2015a; Martin et al., 2011).

Several factors contribute to the increasing U.S. cesarean birth rate (Cunningham et al., 2014; Scott & Porter, 2008; Thorp, 2013):

- Women are having fewer children, and those having their first baby are more likely to have a cesarean than those who have delivered vaginally in the past.
- Both medically indicated and elective inductions continue to rise, increasing the risk for cesarean, particularly for the nullipara having an induction.
- The high primary cesarean rate adds to the overall rate because more women will have repeat cesareans rather than attempting vaginal birth for their next children.
- Women are having children later, and cesareans are more common in the older pregnant woman.
- Obesity is prevalent, increasing the risk for pregnancy complications that result in cesarean.
- Use of assistance such as forceps or vacuum extractor for vaginal birth has decreased.
- Electronic fetal monitoring often prompts concerns about fetal oxygen and acid–base status or progress of labor.
- Most breech presentations are delivered by cesarean.
- There is fear of litigation if no tort reforms exist in the state of practice.

**Median or Midline**

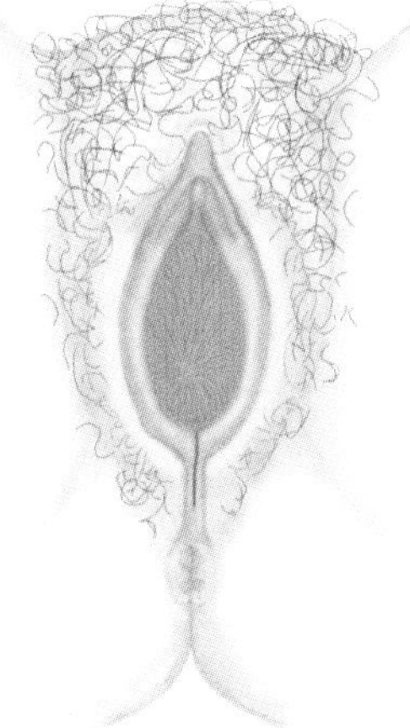

| ***Advantages*** | ***Disadvantages*** |
|---|---|
| Minimal blood loss<br>Neat healing with little scarring<br>Less postpartum pain than the mediolateral episiotomy | An added laceration may extend the median episiotomy into the anal sphincter<br>Limited enlargement of the vaginal opening because perineal length is limited by the anal sphincter |

**Mediolateral**

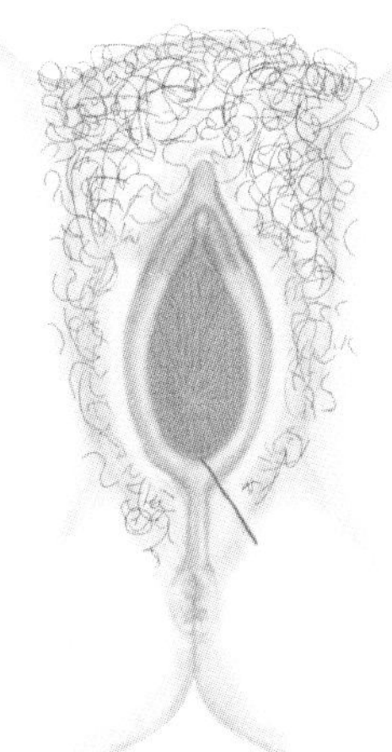

| ***Advantages*** | ***Disadvantages*** |
|---|---|
| More enlargement of the vaginal opening<br>Little risk that the episiotomy will extend into the anus | More blood loss<br>Increased postpartum pain<br>More scarring and irregularity in the healed scar<br>Prolonged dyspareunia (painful intercourse) |

**FIG 19.8** Types of episiotomies.

*Healthy People 2020* goals related to reducing cesarean birth rates show the increase since *Healthy People 2010* was released. More recent targets are to reduce the primary (first) cesarean rate to 23.9% and the repeat cesarean rate to no more than 81.7% for women at low risk for complications (https://www.healthypeople.gov). Promotion of vaginal birth after cesarean in women for whom it is appropriate is a major way to accomplish the goal. Other possibilities include more careful evaluation of **dystocia**, or prolonged labor, as a reason for cesarean and careful selection of women who are appropriate candidates for vaginal breech birth. External cephalic version (p. 382) is an option to attempt changing the presentation of a term or near-term to a cephalic presentation.

Experience with electronic fetal monitoring has improved knowledge of normal fetal responses to labor, promoting interventions for fetal benefit that may avoid cesarean delivery. Nurses and birth attendants increasingly recognize that simple interventions, such as upright positioning, often promote normal labor progress. Interventions, both nursing and medical, that reduce the primary cesarean birth rate also reduce the need for repeat (secondary) cesareans.

## VBAC

The decision about whether to have a VBAC has never been more difficult than now. The dictum "once a cesarean always a cesarean" was accepted without question and the only women who had VBACs were those who entered the hospital in such advanced labor that there was no time for a repeat cesarean.

As low transverse uterine incisions became the norm for most women having cesarean births, the safety of a trial of labor became established. VBAC gradually became an accepted way to lower the rise in cesarean births. Research continued on the safety of VBAC. AAP and ACOG, 2012 have affirmed their support for VBAC but have urged caution when considering a trial of labor after cesarean (TOL or TOLAC) because VBAC is associated with a small but significant risk of uterine rupture. For this and other reasons, many physicians are now conservative when discussing the option of VBAC with a woman. The risks and benefits of VBAC for each woman must be considered by her and her physician. For example, the risk of uterine rupture increases as the number of previous uterine incisions increases, and a woman who has had two cesarean deliveries might be reluctant to attempt VBAC for her third birth because of this added risk. In addition, the woman who tries VBAC and still needs a repeat cesarean birth incurs more costs because she has both labor and surgical expenses. She and her infant are more likely to have infections that further complicate their recovery and add to costs. The hospital also incurs greater costs for personnel and supplies.

When making the decision about whether to attempt VBAC, women need to know that surgical birth has risks, as do all surgeries. Besides risks common to any surgery, multiple cesarean births have a greater risk of placental abnormalities such as placenta previa (low-lying placenta) or placenta accreta (abnormal adherence of the placenta to the uterine wall, often along the previous incision area) (ACOG, 2015e). The woman and her physician must consider the risks and benefits of both methods.

Women may be anxious about attempting vaginal birth in a later pregnancy. A woman may know that she is a good candidate for VBAC but find it impossible to disregard even small risks. Scheduling a repeat cesarean may seem safer, simpler, and something on which she can count. The prospect of laboring and perhaps still needing a cesarean birth is worrisome as well.

The physician discusses VBAC during prenatal care if it is a reasonable option. The nurse reinforces these explanations and identifies misunderstandings. If the woman chooses VBAC, the nurse should reinforce the appropriateness of attempting VBAC and the advantages of a vaginal birth, such as fewer overall complications. VBAC should be presented in a positive way if it is a real option, yet the possibility of cesarean delivery should be acknowledged because the surgery can be needed unexpectedly in any birth (Box 19.1).

## Indications

Cesarean birth is performed when awaiting a vaginal birth would compromise the mother, the fetus, or both. Possible indications for cesarean birth include but are not limited to:

- Dystocia
- Cephalopelvic (fetopelvic) disproportion
- Hypertension, if prompt delivery is necessary
- Maternal diseases such as diabetes, heart disease, or cervical cancer, if labor is not advisable
- Active genital herpes at the time of birth
- Some previous uterine surgical procedures, such as a classic cesarean incision
- Persistent nonreassuring FHR patterns
- A prolapsed umbilical cord
- Fetal malpresentations, such as breech or transverse lie
- Hemorrhagic conditions, such as abruptio placentae or placenta previa

### BOX 19.1 Vaginal Birth After Cesarean Birth

Approximately 60% to 80% of women with one low transverse uterine incision from a previous cesarean birth have successful vaginal births.

Women who had their previous cesarean for a nonrecurring reason, such as breech presentation, are more likely to have a successful vaginal birth after cesarean (VBAC) birth than women who had their previous cesarean for dystocia.

Women who have had a vaginal birth before or since the previous cesarean birth are more likely to have successful VBAC.

Recommendations from the American College of Obstetricians and Gynecologists (ACOG) related to VBAC include:

- No more than two previous low transverse uterine incisions
- No other uterine scars (e.g., removal of fibroid tumors) or a previous uterine rupture
- A pelvis that is clinically adequate for the estimated fetal size
- Immediate availability of a physician during active labor if an emergency cesarean is needed
- Availability of anesthesia and personnel to perform an emergency cesarean
- Medical management of women who plan VBAC:
  - External cephalic version may be as successful for women having a previous cesarean as for women with an unscarred uterus.
  - Epidural analgesia and anesthesia may be used.
  - Labor can be induced or augmented with oxytocin. Misoprostol should not be used for cervical ripening.
  - Most authorities recommend electronic fetal monitoring.

Data from American Academy of Pediatrics & American College of Obstetricians and Gynecologists. (2007). *Guidelines for perinatal care* (6th ed.). Elk Grove Village, IL, and Washington, DC: Author; American College of Obstetricians and Gynecologists. (2009). *Induction of labor (ACOG Practice Bulletin No. 107).* Washington, DC: Author; American College of Obstetricians and Gynecologists. (2010). *Vaginal birth after previous cesarean delivery (ACOG Practice Bulletin No. 115).* Washington, DC: Author.

A previous cesarean birth alone is not an indication for another cesarean birth for most women. Many women will choose repeat cesarean rather than a trial of labor even if they are appropriate candidates for VBAC because of the small, but real, added risk of uterine rupture. Some choose elective (scheduled) repeat cesarean to avoid another unsuccessful experience or the pain of labor. For other women, trying to deliver their next baby vaginally—whether successful or not—is important.

### Contraindications

There are few absolute contraindications to cesarean birth, but there are conditions in which it is not desirable because the risks to the woman are too great when compared with the potential benefit to mother or fetus. These conditions include fetal death, a fetus that is too immature to survive, and maternal coagulation defects.

### Risks

Cesarean birth is one of the safest major surgical procedures, although it poses greater risk for the mother than does vaginal birth. Many maternal risks are those associated with any major abdominal surgery:

- Infection
- Hemorrhage and possibly transfusion
- Urinary tract trauma or infection
- Thrombophlebitis, thromboembolism
- Paralytic ileus
- Atelectasis
- Anesthesia complications

Cesarean delivery poses added risks to the infant, which may include:

- Inadvertent preterm birth
- Transient tachypnea of the newborn caused by delayed absorption of lung fluid (see Chapter 30)
- Persistent pulmonary hypertension of the newborn (see Chapter 30)
- Injury, such as laceration, bruising, fractures, or other trauma

Confirmation of fetal maturity is essential when a cesarean birth is planned. A gestational age of at least 39 weeks can be confirmed by (AAP, 2012 & ACOG, 2015a):

- Documentation of fetal heart sounds for 20 weeks by nonelectronic means or for 30 weeks by Doppler ultrasound
- An interval of 36 weeks since positive results for a serum or urine pregnancy test performed by a reliable laboratory
- An ultrasound examination between 6 and 11 weeks of pregnancy that supports a gestational age of 39 weeks or more
- Clinical history and later ultrasound examinations support a gestational age of 39 weeks or more

For women with questionable due dates, amniocentesis (see Chapter 15) can be used to establish fetal lung maturity if the cesarean is elective. Another alternative is to await the spontaneous onset of labor to perform the cesarean if VBAC is not planned.

## Technique

### Preparation

Routine laboratory studies vary with the mother's condition and type of anesthesia but may include a complete blood count, clotting studies such as prothrombin and partial thromboplastin times, and blood typing and screening. The physician may order one or more units of blood to be typed and screened or crossmatched to have available for transfusion if the woman's hemoglobin and hematocrit values are low or she has a high risk for hemorrhage, such as grand multiparity (five or more births) or abruptio placentae.

Epidural or combined spinal-epidural (CSE) block is typical for cesarean birth. General anesthesia may be required for either known or unexpected reasons. For emergency cesarean with no epidural in place, a general anesthetic may be chosen because it can be established most quickly. A drug such as famotidine (Pepcid) or sodium citrate with citric acid (Bicitra) is given to reduce gastric acidity before surgery. The woman does not receive routine premedication other than drugs to control gastric and respiratory secretions.

Additional preoperative care includes a "time-out" in which all members of the team validate the woman's identity, surgical site, and consents. Staff new to the woman identify themselves.

Fetal surveillance continues until just before the sterile abdominal skin prep (intermittent auscultation or external monitor) or just after the prep (internal monitor) (AAP, 2012 & ACOG, 2015a). A wedge placed under one hip prevents aortocaval compression and promotes placental blood flow.

A single IV dose of a prophylactic antibiotic such cephazolin is recommended preoperatively if she is not already on antibiotics. Additional antibiotic doses are ordered for added risks of infection (ACOG, 2011b).

If a Pfannenstiel (transverse or "bikini") skin incision is planned, the woman's lower abdominal hair is clipped from approximately 3 inches above the pubic hairline to the mons pubis, about where her legs come together. The fronts of the upper thighs are also clipped. For a vertical skin incision, the upper border of the abdominal hair clipping is near the umbilicus. Cordless electric clippers with disposable heads reduce skin nicks that provide an entry point for microorganisms.

An indwelling catheter inserted after the regional block is established but before the surgery keeps the bladder away from the operative area, reducing the risk for injury. The catheter may also be placed before the epidural. The catheter allows accurate observation of urine output during and after surgery, which helps evaluate circulatory status. The catheter also allows delay of ambulation to the restroom for urination until the woman can safely ambulate.

A grounding pad for the electrocautery is applied to an area with no bony prominences, usually the thigh. After application of the pad, the woman's legs are secured to the operating table with a wide, padded strap.

A sterile abdominal skin prep is done just before sterile draping and allowed to dry before sterile drapes are applied. As in other surgical skin preps, the direction of the scrub is generally circular, from the center of the operative area outward and from the pubic area downward on each upper thigh. The use of wide tape may be necessary to hold excess abdominal fat (the pannus, or "apron") upward, pulling it away from the skin incision area.

If a general anesthetic is required, preoperative preps are completed before anesthesia is begun to reduce newborn exposure to anesthesia. The team scrubs, dons gowns and gloves, and drapes the woman before general anesthesia is induced.

### Incisions

Two incisions are made: one in the abdominal wall (skin incision) and the other in the uterine wall. Either of two skin incisions is used: a midline vertical incision between the umbilicus and the symphysis or a Pfannenstiel incision just above the symphysis (Fig. 19.9).

Three types of uterine incisions are possible (Fig. 19.2): (1) low transverse; (2) low vertical; and (3) classic, a vertical incision into the upper uterus. The low transverse uterine incision is preferred unless a complication such as a very large fetus or placenta previa in the lower anterior uterus prevents its use. The uterine incision does not always match the skin incision. For example, a woman may have a vertical skin incision and a low transverse uterine incision, particularly if she is obese.

**Vertical**

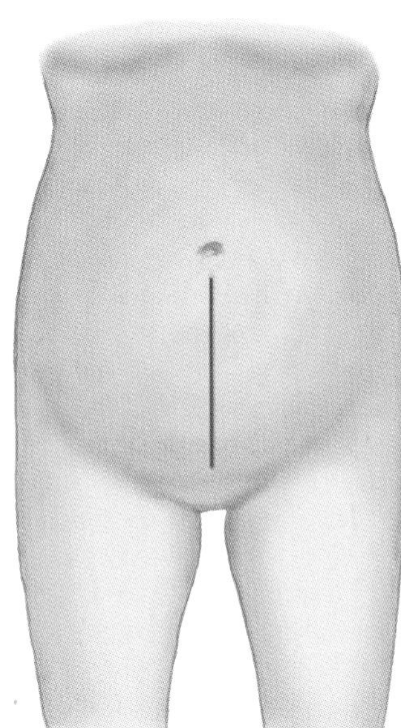

*Advantages*
Quicker to perform
Better visualization of the uterus
Can quickly extend upward for greater visualization if needed
Often more appropriate for obese women

*Disadvantages*
Easily visible when healed
Greater chance of dehiscence and hernia formation

**Pfannenstiel**

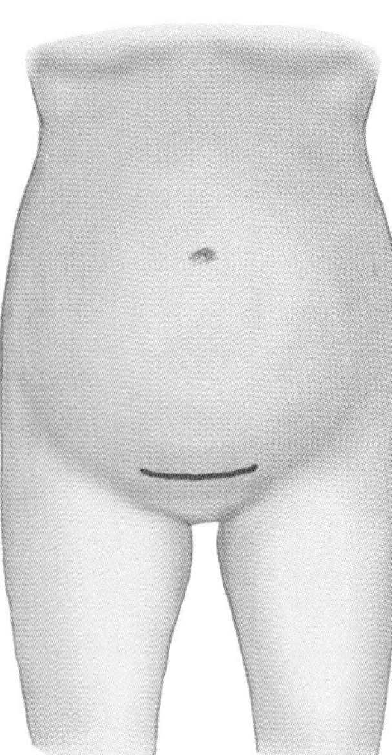

*Advantages*
Less visibility when healed and the pubic hair grows back
Less chance of dehiscence or formation of a hernia

*Disadvantages*
Less visualization of the uterus
Cannot be done as quickly, which may be important in an emergency cesarean birth
Cannot easily be extended to give greater operative exposure
Re-entry at a subsequent cesarean birth may require more time

**FIG 19.9** Skin (abdominal wall) incisions for cesarean birth.

## BOX 19.2 Nursing Care for a Woman Having a Cesarean Birth

**Before the Cesarean Birth**

1. Assess the time of last oral intake and what was eaten.
2. Assess for allergies. Include drug, food, and substance (e.g., latex or skin prep) allergies.
3. Determine medications taken and last dose. Include over-the-counter and herbal preparations.
4. Have the woman sign informed consents for surgery, anesthesia, and usually blood transfusion. Newborn care is usually signed at this time if not earlier.
5. Obtain ordered laboratory work.
6. Do preoperative teaching: what the woman can expect in the operating and recovery rooms, infant care, and who will be present.
7. Start ordered intravenous infusion and begin bolus dose for regional anesthetic at appropriate time (see "Epidural Block" in Chapter 18).
8. Clip abdominal hair using small scissors or an electric clipper.
9. Administer ordered medication to control gastric secretions if not done by anesthesiologist.
10. Insert a urinary indwelling catheter (or insert in operating room after regional block).
11. Assist woman to operating table, positioning her with a wedge under her hip to displace the uterus. Women having scheduled cesareans may walk to the operating room (OR).
12. Apply grounding pad for electrocautery.
13. Do sterile prep of abdomen.
14. Call infant care team if it is routine in the facility or for anticipated newborn complications.

**During the Recovery Period**

1. Begin anesthesia-related interventions: pulse oximeter, oxygen administration, cardiac monitor.
   a. Assess for return of sensation and movement if regional anesthesia was used.
   b. Assess level of consciousness if general anesthesia was used.
2. Do routine assessments every 15 min for the first hour, every 30 min during the second hour, and hourly thereafter until the woman is transferred to the postpartum unit. Assess:
   a. Vital signs; oxygen saturation.
   b. Electrocardiogram (ECG) pattern.
   c. Uterine fundus for firmness, height, and deviation (massage if poorly contracted).
   d. Lochia for color, quantity, and presence of large clots.
   e. Urine output for color, quantity, and patency of the catheter and tubing.
   f. Abdominal dressing for drainage.
   g. Return of lower body movement if regional block.
3. Assess need for analgesia, and administer as ordered.
4. Change position hourly if no contraindication exists. Have woman breathe deeply and cough at each routine assessment time. Provide a small pillow to support her incision when coughing or turning if sensation is present.

## Nursing Considerations

Nursing care for a woman who has a cesarean birth varies according to the situation (Box 19.2) (Nursing Care Plan: Cesarean Birth). She may be planning a cesarean birth, or a surgical birth may be unexpected. A planned cesarean may be her first, or she may have had a cesarean birth before. Her previous cesarean may have been planned or an emergency, and her feelings about the previous cesarean birth may be positive or negative.

Nursing care for all women having cesarean childbirth is similar, but the approach in each situation is different. For example, although preoperative teaching is important, it must be abbreviated or even omitted in a true emergency.

### Providing Emotional Support

Emotional support begins well before the birth and extends well after it. A mother who has had a previous cesarean birth may harbor

## NURSING CARE PLAN

### *Cesarean Birth*

**Focused Assessment**

Christina is 22 years old and expecting her first baby. Her due date is 2 weeks from today, and a cesarean was scheduled 1 week from today. Her baby remains in a complete (full) breech. Because her membranes ruptured this afternoon and she is in early labor, she will have her cesarean today. Epidural anesthesia is planned for her surgery. Although her physician has discussed cesarean birth with her, Christina is anxious and has many questions about what will happen to her and her baby. She says she is very nervous about the upcoming surgery. She has never been a patient in a hospital. Christina's mother and husband Bruce are with her.

**Nursing Diagnosis**

Anxiety related to unfamiliarity with the setting and procedures for cesarean birth.

**Planning**

***Expected Outcomes***

After interventions, Christina will:

1. State that she feels less apprehensive.
2. Verbalize understanding of preoperative and postoperative care.
3. Demonstrate postoperative techniques for coughing and deep breathing.

**Interventions and *Rationales***

1. Assess Christina's level of anxiety.
   *Assessment enables the nurse to approach her preoperative care in the most appropriate manner. Mild to moderate anxiety facilitates learning and is expected, but high levels impair learning.*
2. Remain with Christina as much as possible while completing preoperative procedures. Allow her to express her fears. Encourage her mother and Bruce to remain with her.
   *The presence of significant others and a caring nurse provide support. Expression of her fears enables the nurse to answer Christina's concerns specifically.*
3. Elicit Christina's feelings about surgery by using broad leads, such as, "What were your thoughts when you found out you might have your baby by cesarean?"
   *Identification of expectations of the birth experience allows actions to be taken to make it a positive one. If a woman's expected and actual experience closely match, she is likely to be more satisfied with it. Misunderstandings and possible feelings of inadequacy or anger are identified.*
4. Explain preoperative preparations using simple language, verifying Christina's understanding and giving her the opportunity to ask questions.
   *Knowledge decreases anxiety and fear of the unknown. Simple language facilitates understanding when a woman's attention is narrowed from anxiety. Explanations and the chance to ask questions show respect and give the woman a greater sense of control.*
5. Explain what to expect postoperatively, demonstrating as needed.
   *Knowledge reduces anxiety and fear of the unknown. The explanation promotes understanding and acceptance of care that will be painful while providing reassurance of pain control. Return demonstration verifies learning and identifies the need for additional teaching.*
6. Reduce unnecessary stimulation that can add to Christina's anxiety. Work efficiently but calmly.
   *Reducing anxiety emphasizes that Christina and Bruce are having a child and not just a surgical procedure.*

**Evaluation**

Christina agrees that a cesarean birth is best for her baby. She asks a few other questions and then states that she understands preoperative and postoperative care but that she is still "a little nervous." She demonstrates effective coughing and deep-breathing techniques.

**Focused Assessment**

She will have epidural anesthesia for her birth. Her vital signs are temperature, 37.2° C (99° F); pulse, 90 beats per minute (bpm); respirations, 22 breaths per minute; and blood pressure, 122/70 mm Hg. The fetal heart rate (FHR) is 130 to 140 bpm and accelerates with fetal movement. She walks to the operating room, and epidural anesthesia is begun.

**Nursing Diagnosis**

Risk for Injury related to altered sensation from epidural anesthesia and the use of electrical equipment during surgery.

**Planning**

***Expected Outcomes***

Christina will not have injury, such as pressure areas, muscle strains, and electrical injury, during the perioperative period.

**Interventions and *Rationales***

1. Pad bony prominences. Avoid obstructing her popliteal area. Place a wedge under her hip to tilt her uterus to one side. Padding reduces potential for tissue damage caused by pressure.
   *An unobstructed popliteal area reduces venous stasis and possible thrombus formation. Padding includes a uterine displacement wedge to avoid aortocaval compression.*
2. Transfer her from the operating table carefully after surgery, using enough staff members to keep her body in alignment. Brake the bed and operating table to keep them from separating. Be certain that the indwelling catheter tubing and intravenous (IV) line are free during the transfer.
   *Having adequate staff reduces the risk for a fall or muscle strains in both the woman and the staff.*
3. After anesthesia is in place, position her on the operating table and secure her legs with a safety strap.
   *The safety strap prevents falls or displacement of the woman's legs, which have lost sensation.*
4. Apply a grounding pad if electrocautery is to be used.
   *A grounding pad prevents electrical shock or burn.*

**Evaluation**

During surgery, her body was secured in proper alignment, with proper padding of all her bony prominences. The grounding pad ensured electrical safety when electrocautery was used. She gave birth to an appropriate-for-gestational-age baby, 3318 g (7 lb, 5 oz). She was transferred to postanesthesia care without incident. During recovery and postpartum, she showed no signs of pressure, electrical, or musculoskeletal injury.

***Additional Nursing Diagnoses to Consider***

Risk for Aspiration (general anesthesia)
Pain
Risk for Impaired Spontaneous Ventilation
Hypothermia
Readiness for Enhanced Family Coping

NOTE: Only nursing diagnoses related to the preoperative and intraoperative care of the woman are discussed here. See Chapter 17 for nursing care related to fetal oxygenation. See Chapter 18 for care related to anesthesia. See Chapters 16 and 20 for nursing care of the mother during the recovery and postpartum periods.

unresolved feelings of grief, guilt, or inadequacy because she perceives that she somehow failed in her expected birth experience.

The nurse in the prenatal setting can open the subject of a woman's previous cesarean or vaginal birth with a broad lead, such as, "Tell me about when you had your other baby."

Staff behavior can either reduce or increase the woman's anxiety. A calm and confident manner helps her feel that she is being cared for by competent professionals. A quiet, controlled voice is calming to the patient, her family, and the nurse and other staff.

The nurse and the woman's significant others are important sources of emotional support. Therapeutic communication with a caring nurse helps clarify her concerns, so explanations to reduce her fear of the unknown can be most effective.

The father or other support person should be encouraged to remain with her during surgery if she has regional anesthesia. In many hospitals the support person may come into the operating room (OR) after the woman is intubated for general anesthesia to foster attachment with the infant and help the mother integrate her birth experience.

Nurses also support a woman's birth partner and significant others during the cesarean birth. The partner may be as anxious as the woman but may be afraid to express it because the woman needs so much support. The partner may be physically exhausted after hours of labor coaching. Encourage breaks and snacks when appropriate. The staff should not expect more support from the partner than he or she can provide.

Although cesarean births are routine in the intrapartum unit, they are not routine to women who undergo them or to their families. Even a previous cesarean may have been unplanned. Avoid belittling their fears by telling women and their families not to worry or that everything will be all right, especially if an emergency occurs.

Talking with the mother and her family after birth allows the nurse to answer questions about the surgery and fill in any gaps in their understanding. This helps them understand the experience and promotes a positive perception of the birth.

### Teaching

Knowledge helps reduce fear of the unknown and increases a woman's sense of control over her infant's birth. The nurse cannot assume that a woman who had a previous cesarean birth already knows what will happen and why. If her previous surgery was done after a long labor or in an emergency, she may recall only part of it and may not understand what she does remember. Teaching should be done in simple language and should include her partner.

The nurse explains preoperative procedures and their purposes, such as labs, the abdominal skin prep, indwelling catheter, IV lines, medications, and dressings. The catheter and IV lines usually remain in place no longer than 24 hours after birth. Use of serial compression devices to reduce risks of venous thrombosis should be explained. The nurse may need to reinforce anesthetic information provided by the anesthesia clinician.

Women who have regional anesthesia, such as an epidural or subarachnoid block, often fear that they will feel pain during surgery. They do feel pressure and pulling, but these sensations do not mean that the anesthesia is wearing off. The nurse reassures her that her anesthesia clinician will regularly assess her needs for pain management.

If a woman is having general anesthesia, the nurse explains why operative preparations are completed before the woman is anesthetized. She should be reassured that her surgery will not begin until she is asleep and that she will not wake up during the procedure.

The nurse describes the OR and everyone who will be present to make it less intimidating to the woman. Staff she encounters in the OR before surgery should introduce themselves if possible. Explain that the room may seem cool, and the surgery table is narrow. Also explain that her room may be warm if a low-birth-weight or preterm infant is expected (see Chapter 29). Her labor nurse is often the circulating nurse during surgery, reassuring her with a familiar face and voice. Nursery staff is often the provider of newborn care in the OR.

The support person should be told when he or she can expect to come into the OR. If it is not already in place, an epidural block is often established after the woman goes to the OR. Bringing in the partner may be delayed until the regional block and other preparations, such as placement of the indwelling catheter, are complete. These preparations may take up to 30 to 45 minutes for a scheduled cesarean birth, varying with facility and provider practices. Assure the support person that he or she will not be forgotten. Estimating wait time helps reassure the partner that no problem has occurred during the preparation phase.

The nurse explains the postanesthesia care unit (PACU) and any equipment that will be used, such as a pulse oximeter, electrocardiogram (ECG) monitor, and automatic blood pressure cuff. Postoperative needs for routine assessments and interventions such as fundus and lochia checks, coughing, and deep breathing are explained. The woman is taught simple exercises to promote normal circulation in her legs when movement returns. The nurse reassures her that every effort will be made to promote her comfort with medication, positioning, and other interventions. She should be encouraged to ask for pain relief early, before it is severe, for best results.

The healthy newborn will often remain with parents in the PACU. Basic care is the same as that following vaginal birth. See Chapter 22 for early newborn nursing care.

### Promoting Safety

Although the need for general anesthesia during pregnancy occurs infrequently, the nurse must assume that it is possible. The woman's food intake is assessed for type and time upon admission. Oral intake and emesis during labor are recorded and reported to the anesthesia clinician. Usually the woman is on nothing per mouth (NPO) status, or only ice or clear liquids, if a cesarean birth is expected. Anesthesia-related drugs to control gastric and respiratory secretions are administered as ordered.

The woman is transferred and positioned carefully to prevent injury, especially if she has received regional anesthesia that reduces motor control and sensation. Her bony prominences are well padded. A safety strap placed across her thighs secures her on the narrow operating table. A wedge placed under one hip or tilting the operating table avoids aortocaval compression and reduced placental blood flow. During positioning, the drain tube of the indwelling catheter should be routed under her leg to promote drainage and keep the tube away from the operative area. The catheter bag is placed near the head of the table so that the anesthesia clinician can monitor urine output.

The nurse verifies proper function of machines such as suction devices, monitors, and electrocautery. Leads for the cardiac monitor and pulse oximeter are placed to observe heart and respiratory functions. A grounding pad permits safe use of the electrocautery. Infant care equipment should be readied for immediate use.

After the surgery, the incision area is cleansed with sterile water, and a sterile dressing is applied. Blood and amniotic fluid are cleaned from the woman's abdomen, buttocks, and back before she is transferred to a bed. Smooth transfers done by an adequate number of personnel reduce pain and hypotension.

### Providing Postoperative Care

Postoperative care for the mother who has had a cesarean birth is similar to that for one who has had a vaginal birth, with added interventions. Her temperature is assessed on admission to the PACU and according to protocol thereafter. If her condition is stable, other assessments are done on admission and every 15 minutes during the first 1 to 2 hours, progressing to every 30 minutes to 1 hour until transfer to her postpartum room. In addition to temperature, routine postoperative assessments include:

- Vital signs and character of respirations; oxygen saturation; ECG pattern (usually normal sinus rhythm)
- Return of motion and sensation (if a regional block was given)
- Level of consciousness (particularly if general anesthetic or sedating drugs were given)
- Abdominal dressing
- Uterine firmness and position (midline or deviated)
- Lochia (color, quantity, presence and size of any clots)
- Urine output (quantity, color, other characteristics)
- IV infusion
- Pain-relief needs

The nurse observes for return of motion and sensation if the woman had epidural or subarachnoid block anesthesia. The level of consciousness and respiratory status (skin or mucous membrane color; rate and quality of respirations; oxygen saturation) are important observations if she had general anesthesia. Detailed respiratory observations are essential for a longer period if the woman received epidural opioid narcotics, which can cause delayed respiratory depression. Have naloxone (Narcan) available to reverse opioid-induced respiratory depression (See Chapter 18 for more information about anesthesia and analgesia for cesarean birth).

The pulse, respirations, and blood pressure provide important clues to the woman's circulatory and respiratory status. If oxygen saturation falls below 95%, having her take several deep breaths usually raises it. Supplemental oxygen by nasal cannula, face tent, or mask is occasionally needed. A respiratory rate of less than 12 breaths per minute suggests respiratory depression. Deep breathing and coughing move secretions out of the lungs and promote full expansion. A small pillow to support her incision reduces pain when she coughs. Position changes every 2 hours improve ventilation and decrease discomfort from constant pressure.

As with a vaginal birth, the fundus is assessed for height, firmness, and position. To relax abdominal muscles, thus reducing pain from fundus checks if sensation has returned, she should flex her knees and take slow, deep breaths. The nurse gently "walks" his or her fingers toward the woman's fundus to determine uterine firmness. The woman who has a Pfannenstiel skin incision usually has less pain with fundus checks than the woman with a vertical skin incision. A firm fundus does not need massage. The dressing is checked for drainage with each fundus check.

The nurse assesses the lochia and urine output with other assessments. Lochia may pool under the mother's buttocks and lower back. Urine may be bloody temporarily if the cesarean birth occurred after a long labor or an attempted forceps or vacuum delivery. The urine drainage tube should be observed for gradual clearing of the blood. Urine should drain freely to prevent bladder distention, which worsens pain and increases the risk of postpartum hemorrhage. The nurse must remember that falling urine output is an early sign of hypovolemia, occurring well before the fall in blood pressure.

The woman's need for pain relief should be assessed with her vital signs. The woman who received an epidural analgesic may not need other analgesia during the early postpartum period. If she needs added pain relief while the epidural analgesic is still in effect, an oral analgesic often suffices. A nonsteroidal anti-inflammatory drug (NSAID) such as ibuprofen provides long-acting analgesia to supplement the epidural drug. A parenteral analgesic is usually given by a patient-controlled analgesia pump or occasionally by intermittent injections. Oral analgesics usually replace parenteral analgesics the day after surgery.

## KEY CONCEPTS

- Prolapse and compression of the umbilical cord are the primary risks of amniotomy. As the fluid gushes out, the cord can become compressed between the fetal presenting part and the woman's pelvis.
- The risk for infection is greater the longer membranes have been ruptured, especially if more than 24 hours has elapsed.
- Labor may be induced if continuing the pregnancy is more hazardous to the maternal or fetal health than is the induction. Induction is not done if a maternal or fetal contraindication exists to labor or vaginal birth.
- Oxytocin- or prostaglandin-stimulated uterine contractions may be hypertonic, decreasing placental perfusion.
- External version promotes vaginal birth by changing the fetal presentation from a breech or transverse lie to a cephalic lie. Internal version is sometimes used to change the presentation of the second twin after the birth of the first twin.
- Giving birth over an intact perineum results in less blood loss, less pain, and earlier resumption of comfortable intercourse postpartum. Therefore, episiotomy should be done selectively rather than routinely.
- Trauma to maternal and fetal tissue is the primary risk associated with use of forceps or a vacuum extractor. Possible trauma to the mother includes vaginal wall laceration and hematoma. Trauma to the infant may include ecchymoses, lacerations, abrasions, facial nerve injury, and intracranial hemorrhage.
- The low transverse uterine incision is that preferred for cesarean birth because it is least likely to rupture in a subsequent pregnancy. The skin incision does not always match the uterine incision and is unrelated to the risk of later uterine rupture.
- Some women have feelings of guilt or inadequacy if they have a cesarean birth. Therapeutic communication and sensitive family-centered care are essential to help them achieve a positive perception of their birth experience.
- The preferred uterine incision for cesarean birth is the low transverse incision because it is least likely to rupture in a subsequent pregnancy. The skin incision does not always match the uterine incision and is unrelated to the risk of later uterine rupture.

## REFERENCES AND READINGS


American Academy of Pediatrics & American College of Obstetricians and Gynecologists. (2012). *Guidelines for perinatal care* (7th ed.). Elk Grove Village, IL, and Washington, DC: Author.

American College of Obstetricians and Gynecologists. (2011a). *Dystocia and augmentation of labor (Practice Bulletin No. 49).* Washington, DC: Author.

American College of Obstetricians and Gynecologists. (2011b). *Use of prophylactic antibiotics in labor and delivery (ACOG Practice Bulletin No. 120).* Washington, DC: Author.

American College of Obstetricians and Gynecologists. (Reaffirmed 2015). *Cesarean delivery on maternal request (ACOG Committee Opinion No. 559).* Washington, DC: Author.

American College of Obstetricians and Gynecologists. (Reaffirmed 2015). *Episiotomy (ACOG Practice Bulletin No. 71).* Washington, DC: Author.

American College of Obstetricians and Gynecologists. (Reaffirmed 2015). *Induction of labor (ACOG Practice Bulletin No. 107).* Washington, DC: Author.

American College of Obstetricians and Gynecologists. (2015). *Operative vaginal delivery (ACOG Practice Bulletin No. 154).* Washington, DC: Author.

American College of Obstetricians and Gynecologists. (Reaffirmed 2015). *Vaginal birth after previous cesarean delivery (ACOG Practice Bulletin No. 115).* Washington, DC: Author.

American College of Obstetricians and Gynecologists. (Reaffirmed 2014). *External cephalic version (ACOG Practice Bulletin No. 13).* Washington, DC: Author.

Bishop, E.H. (1964). Pelvic scoring for elective induction. *Obstetrics and Gynecology, 24*(2), 266–268.

Bofill, J.A., & Martin, J.N. (2008). Operative vaginal delivery. In R.S. Gibbs, B.Y. Karlan, & A.F. Haney (Eds.), *Danforth's obstetrics and gynecology* (10th ed., pp. 462–490). Philadelphia: Lippincott Williams & Wilkins.

Branch, D.W., Silver, R.M., & Aagaard-Tillery, K. (2008). Immunologic disorders in pregnancy. In R.S. Gibbs, B.Y. Karlan, & A.F. Haney (Eds.), *Danforth's obstetrics and gynecology* (10th ed., pp. 313–339). Philadelphia: Lippincott Williams & Wilkins.

Cunningham, F.G., Leveno, K.J., Bloom, S.L., et al. (2014). *Williams obstetrics* (24th ed.). New York: McGraw-Hill.

Declercq, E.R., Sakala, C., & Corry, M.P. (2013). Executive summary in: *Listening to mothers III: Report of the Second National United States Survey of Women's Childbearing Experiences.* New York: Childbirth Connection.

Ehrenthal, D. B., Jiang, X., & Strobino, D. M. (2010). Labor induction and the risk of cesarean delivery among nulliparous women at term. *Obstetrics and Gynecology, 116*(1), 35–42.

Hamilton, B.E., Martin, J.A., Osterman, M., et al. (2014). *Births: Preliminary data for 2013. National Vital Statistics Reports, 63(2).* Hyattsville, MD: National Center for Health Statistics.

Hobel, C.J. (2015). Obstetric procedures. In N.F. Hacker, J.C. Gambone, & C.J. Hobel (Eds.), *Hacker & Moore's essentials of obstetrics and gynecology* (6th ed., pp. 224–235). Philadelphia: Saunders.

Hobel, C.J., & Zakowski, M. (2015). Normal labor, delivery, and postpartum care: Anatomic considerations, obstetric analgesia and anesthesia, and resuscitation of the newborn. In N.F. Hacker, J.C. Gambone, & C.J. Hobel (Eds.), *Hacker & Moore's essentials of obstetrics and gynecology* (6th ed., pp. 96–124). Philadelphia: Saunders.

Lund, K.J., & McManaman, J. (2008). Normal labor, delivery, newborn care, and puerperium. In R.S. Gibbs, B.Y. Karlan, & A.F. Haney (Eds.), *Danforth's obstetrics and gynecology* (10th ed.). Philadelphia: Lippincott Williams & Wilkins.

Macones, G., Cahill, A., Stamilio, D., et al. (2012). The efficacy of early amniotomy in nulliparous labor induction: a randomized controlled trial. *American Journal of Obstetrics & Gynecology, 207*(5), 403.e1–403.e5 1p. doi:10.1016/j.ajog.2012.08.032

Martin, J.A., Hamilton, B.E., Ventura, S.J., et al. (2011). *Births: Final data for 2009. National Vital Statistics Reports.* Hyattsville, MD: National Center for Health Statistics.

Martin, J.A., Hamilton, B.E., Osterman, M., et al. (2015). *Birth: Final Data for 2013. National Vital Statistics Report (64)1.* Hyattsville, MD: National Center for Health Statistics.

Menacker, F., & Hamilton, B.E. (2010). *Recent trends in cesarean delivery in the United States. National Center for Health Statistics Data Brief No. 35.* Hyattsville, MD: National Center for Health Statistics.

Pearson, N. (2011). Oxytocin safety: Legal implications for perinatal nurses. *Nursing for Women's Health, 15*(2), 110–117.

Scott, J.R., & Porter, T.F. (2008). Cesarean delivery. In R.S. Gibbs, B.Y. Karlan, & A.F. Haney (Eds.), *Danforth's obstetrics and gynecology* (10th ed., pp. 491–503). Philadelphia: Lippincott Williams & Wilkins.

Seehusen, D.A., & Raleigh, M. (2014). Antenatal perineal massage to prevent birth trauma. *American Family Physician, 89*(5), 335-336 2p.

Simpson, K.R. (2008a). *Cervical ripening and induction and augmentation of labor* (3rd ed.). Washington, DC: Association of Women's Health, Obstetric, and Neonatal Nurses.

Simpson, K.R. (2013a). Fetal assessment during labor. In K.R. Simpson, & P.A. Creehan (Eds.), *AWHONN perinatal nursing* (4th ed., pp. 445–487). Philadelphia: Lippincott.

Simpson, K.R. (2013). Labor and birth. In K.R. Simpson, & P.A. Creehan (Eds.), *AWHONN perinatal nursing* (4th ed., pp. 343–425). Philadelphia: Lippincott.

Thorp, J.M. (2013). Clinical aspects of normal and abnormal labor. In R.K. Creasy, R. Resnik, J.D. Iams, et al. (Eds.), *Creasy & Resnik's maternal-fetal medicine: Principles and practice* (7th ed., pp. 673–706). Philadelphia: Saunders.

Wood, S., Cooper, S., & Ross, S. (2014). Does induction of labour increase the risk of caesarean section? A systematic review and meta-analysis of trials in women with intact membranes. *BJOG: An International Journal of Obstetrics & Gynaecology, 121*(6), 674–685 12p. doi:10.1111/1471-0528.12328

# 20

# Postpartum Adaptations

http://evolve.elsevier.com/McKinney/mat-ch/

## LEARNING OBJECTIVES

*After studying this chapter, you should be able to:*

- Explain the physiologic changes that occur during the postpartum period.
- Describe nursing assessments and nursing care for postpartum physiologic and psychologic adaptations.
- Discuss the role of the nurse in health education and identify important areas of teaching.
- Compare nursing assessments and care for women who have undergone cesarean or vaginal births.
- Explain the process of bonding and attachment, including maternal touch and verbal interactions.
- Describe the progressive phases of maternal adaptation to childbirth and the stages of maternal role attainment.
- Identify maternal concerns and how they change over time.
- Discuss the cause, manifestations, and interventions for mild postpartum depression (blues).
- Describe the processes of family adaptation to the birth of a baby.
- Explain factors that affect family adaptation.
- Discuss cultural influences on family adaptation.
- Describe assessments and interventions for postpartum psychosocial adaptations.
- Describe criteria for discharge and available healthcare services.

The first 6 weeks after the birth of an infant are known as the *postpartum period* or **puerperium**. During this time, mothers experience numerous physiologic and psychosocial changes. Many postpartum physiologic changes are retrogressive—that is, changes that occurred in body systems during pregnancy are reversed as the body returns to the nonpregnant state. Progressive changes, such as the initiation of lactation, also occur.

## REPRODUCTIVE SYSTEM

### Involution of the Uterus

**Involution** refers to the changes the reproductive organs, particularly the uterus, undergo after childbirth to return to their nonpregnant size and condition. Uterine involution entails three processes: (1) contraction of muscle fibers, (2) **catabolism** (the process of breaking down cells into simpler compounds), and (3) regeneration of uterine epithelium. Involution begins immediately after the delivery of the placenta when the uterine muscle fibers contract firmly around maternal blood vessels at the area where the placenta was attached. This contraction controls bleeding from the area left denuded when the placenta separated. The uterus becomes smaller as the muscle fibers, which have been stretched for many months, contract and gradually regain their former contour and size.

The enlarged uterine muscle cells are affected by catabolic changes in protein cytoplasm that cause a reduction in individual cell size. The products of this catabolic process are absorbed by the bloodstream and excreted in the urine as nitrogenous waste.

Regeneration of the uterine epithelial lining begins soon after childbirth. The outer portion of the endometrial layer is expelled with the placenta. Within 2 to 3 days, the remaining **decidua** (endometrium during pregnancy) separates into two layers. The first layer is superficial and is shed in lochia. The basal layer provides the source of new endometrium. Regeneration of the endometrium, except at the site of placental attachment, occurs by 16 days after birth (Blackburn, 2013).

The placental site, which is approximately 8 to 10 cm (3 to 4 inches) in diameter, heals by a process of **exfoliation** (scaling off of dead tissue) (James, 2013). New endometrium is generated from glands and tissue that remain in the lower layer of the decidua after the separation of the placenta (Cunningham, Leveno, Bloom, et al., 2014). This process leaves the uterine lining free of scar tissue, which would interfere with the implantation of future pregnancies. Healing at the placental site takes approximately 6 weeks.

#### Descent of the Uterine Fundus

The location of the uterine **fundus** (top of the uterus above the openings of the fallopian tubes) helps determine whether involution is progressing normally. Immediately after delivery, the uterus is roughly the size of a large grapefruit and weighs approximately 1000 g (2.2 lb). The fundus can be palpated midway between the symphysis pubis and umbilicus and in the midline (middle) of the abdomen. Within 12 hours, the fundus rises to about the level of the umbilicus (Blackburn, 2013; James, 2013).

The fundus descends by roughly 1 cm or one fingerbreadth per day, so that by the 14th day, it is in the pelvic cavity and cannot be palpated abdominally (Blackburn, 2013) (Fig. 20.1). The fundus may be slightly higher in multiparas or in women who had an over distended uterus. When the process of involution does not occur properly, **subinvolution** occurs. Subinvolution can cause postpartum hemorrhage (see Chapter 28).

Descent is documented in relation to the umbilicus. For example, U − 1 or ↓ 1 indicates the fundus is palpable 1 cm or fingerbreadth below the umbilicus. Within a week, the weight of the uterus decreases to approximately 500 g (1 lb); at 4 weeks, the uterus weighs approximately 100 g (3.5 oz) or less (Cunningham et al., 2014).

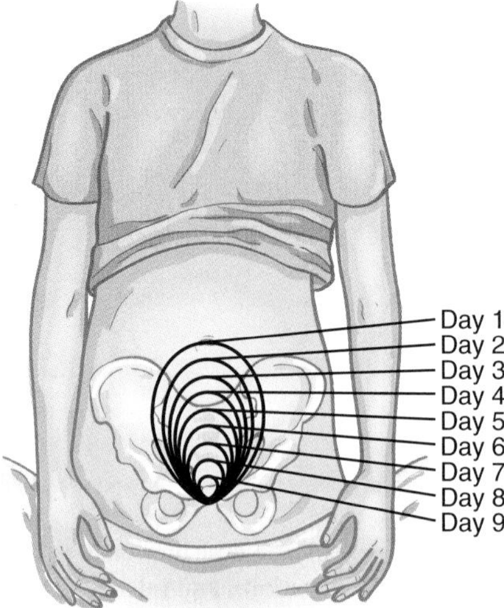


**FIG 20.1** Involution of the uterus. The height of the uterine fundus decreases by approximately 1 cm/day. The fundus is no longer palpable by 14 days.

### Afterpains

***Etiology.*** Intermittent contractions, known as *afterpains,* are a source of discomfort for many women. The discomfort is more acute for multiparas because repeated stretching of muscle fibers leads to the loss of muscle tone that causes alternate contraction and relaxation of the uterus. The uterus of a primipara tends to remain contracted, but she may also experience severe afterpains if her uterus has been overdistended by multifetal pregnancy, a large infant, polyhydramnios (excessive amniotic fluid), or if retained blood clots are present. Oxytocin released from the posterior pituitary during breastfeeding may cause strong contractions of the uterine muscles. Afterpains usually decrease to mild discomfort by the 3rd day postpartum (Cunningham et al., 2014).

***Nursing considerations.*** Analgesics are frequently used to lessen the discomfort of afterpains. Most commonly prescribed analgesics may be used for short-term pain relief without harm to the infant. The benefits of pain relief, such as comfort and relaxation, facilitate the milk ejection reflex or letdown reflex the release of milk from the alveoli into the ducts. These benefits usually outweigh the small effects of the medication on the infant.

Some mothers find that lying in the prone position with a small pillow or folded blanket under the abdomen helps keep the uterus contracted and provides relief. Afterpains are self-limited and decrease rapidly after 48 hours.

### Lochia

Changes in the color and amount of lochia also provide information about whether involution is progressing normally.

***Changes in color.*** For the first 3 days after childbirth, lochia consists almost entirely of blood, with small particles of decidua and mucus. Because of its reddish or red-brown color, it is called lochia rubra. The amount of blood decreases by approximately the 4th day, and the color of lochia changes from red to pink or brown-tinged (lochia serosa). Lochia serosa is composed of serous exudate, erythrocytes, leukocytes, and cervical mucus. By approximately the 11th day, the erythrocyte component decreases. The discharge becomes white, cream, or light yellow in color (lochia alba). Lochia alba contains leukocytes, decidual cells, epithelial cells, fat, cervical mucus, and bacteria. It is present in most women until the 3rd week after childbirth but may persist until the 6th week (Whitmer, 2011). Table 20.1 summarizes the characteristics of normal and abnormal lochia.

**TABLE 20.1 Characteristics of Lochia**

| Time and Type | Normal Discharge | Abnormal Discharge |
|---|---|---|
| Days 1–3: lochia rubra | Bloody; small clots; fleshy, earthy odor, red or red/brown | Large clots; saturated perineal pads; foul odor |
| Days 4–10: lochia serosa | Decreased amount; serosanguineous; pink or brown-tinged | Excessive amount; foul smell; continued or recurrent reddish color |
| Days 11–21: lochia alba (may last until 6th week postpartum) | Further decreased amounts; white, cream, or light yellow | Persistent lochia serosa; return to lochia rubra, foul odor; discharge continuing |

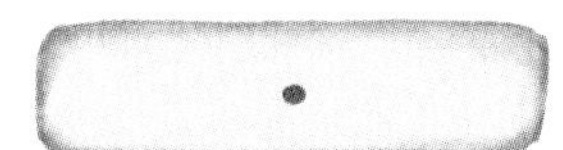

**Scant:** <2.5-cm (1-inch) stain

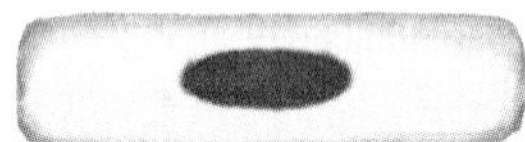

**Light:** 2.5- to 10-cm (1- to 4-inch) stain

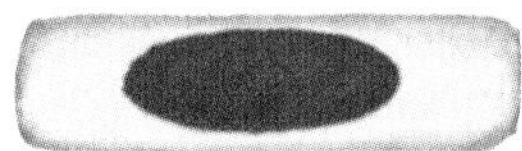

**Moderate:** 10- to 15-cm (4- to 6-inch) stain

**Heavy:** Saturated in 1 hour

**FIG 20.2** Guidelines for assessing the volume of lochia based on the amount of stain on a perineal pad in 1 hour.

***Amount.*** Because estimating the amount of lochia on a peripad (perineal pad) is difficult, nurses frequently record lochia in terms that are difficult to quantify, such as "scant," "moderate," and "heavy." One method for estimating the amount of lochia in 1 hour uses the following labels (Whitmer, 2011):

*Scant:* Less than a 2.5-cm (1-inch) stain on the perineal pad
*Light:* 2.5- to 10-cm (1- to 4-inch) stain
*Moderate:* 10- to 15-cm (4- to 6-inch) stain
*Heavy:* Saturated perineal pad
*Excessive:* Saturated peripad in 15 minutes

Determining the time the peripad has been in place is important in assessing lochia. What appears to be a light flow may actually be a moderate flow if the peripad has been in use less than an hour (Fig. 20.2).

Lochia may be less for women who had a cesarean birth because some of the endometrial lining is removed during surgery. The lochia will go through the same phases as that of the woman with a vaginal birth, but the amount may be less. Lochia is often heavier when the new mother first gets out of bed, because gravity allows blood that has pooled in the vagina during the hours of rest to flow freely when she stands.

### Cervix

Immediately after childbirth, the cervix is formless, flabby, and open wide. Small tears or lacerations may be present, and the cervix is often edematous. Healing occurs rapidly, and by the end of the 1st week the cervix feels firm, and the external os is dilated 1 cm (Whitmer, 2011). The internal os closes as before pregnancy, but the shape of the external os is permanently changed. It remains slightly open and appears slit-like rather than round, as in the nulliparous woman.

### Vagina

Soon after childbirth, the vaginal walls appear edematous, and multiple small lacerations may be present. Very few vaginal rugae (folds) are present. The hymen is permanently torn and heals with small, irregular tags of tissue visible at the vaginal introitus.

Although the rugae are regained by 3 to 4 weeks, it takes 6 to 10 weeks for the vagina to complete involution and to gain approximately the same size and contour it had before pregnancy. However, the vagina does not entirely regain its nulliparous size (Blackburn, 2013).

During the postpartum period, the vaginal mucosa becomes atrophic, and vaginal walls do not regain their thickness until estrogen production by the ovaries is reestablished. Because ovarian function, and thus, estrogen production, is not well established during lactation, breastfeeding mothers are likely to experience vaginal dryness and may experience dyspareunia (discomfort during intercourse).

### Perineum

Because of pressure from the fetal head, the muscles of the pelvic floor stretch and thin greatly during the second stage of labor. After childbirth, the perineum may be edematous and bruised. Some women have a surgical incision (episiotomy) of the perineal area to enlarge the opening for birth. Initial healing of the episiotomy site occurs in 2 to 3 weeks, but complete healing may take 4 to 6 months (Blackburn, 2013). Lacerations of the perineum also may occur during delivery. Lacerations and episiotomies are classified according to the tissue involved (Box 20.1). (See episiotomy discussion in Chapter 19, p. 386.)

#### Discomfort

Although the episiotomy is relatively small, the muscles of the perineum are involved in many activities (walking, sitting, stooping, squatting, bending, urinating, and defecating). An incision or laceration in this area can cause a great deal of discomfort. In addition, many pregnant women are affected by hemorrhoids (distended rectal veins) that are pushed out of the rectum during the second stage of labor.

#### Nursing Considerations

Hemorrhoids, as well as perineal trauma, episiotomy, or lacerations, can make physical activity or bowel elimination difficult during the postpartum period. Relief of perineal discomfort is a nursing priority and includes teaching self-care measures, such as applying ice, using topical anesthetics, and taking ordered analgesics.

### BOX 20.1 Lacerations of the Birth Canal

**Perineum**

Perineal lacerations are classified in degrees to describe the amount of tissue involved. Some physicians or nurse-midwives also use degrees to describe the extent of midline episiotomies.

- *First-degree:* Involves the superficial vaginal mucosa or perineal skin.
- *Second-degree:* Involves the vaginal mucosa, perineal skin, and deeper tissues, which may include fascia and muscles of the perineum.
- *Third-degree:* Same as second-degree lacerations but involves the anal sphincter.
- *Fourth-degree:* Extends through the anal sphincter into the rectal mucosa.

**Periurethral Area**

A laceration in the area of the urethra may cause women difficulty urinating after birth. An indwelling catheter may be necessary for a day or two.

**Vaginal Wall**

A laceration involving the mucosa of the vaginal wall.

**Cervix**

Tears in the cervix may be a source of significant bleeding after birth.

## CARDIOVASCULAR SYSTEM

Hypervolemia, which produces as much as a 45% increase in blood volume at term, allows the woman to tolerate a substantial blood loss during childbirth without ill effect (Jones, 2012). On the average, up to 500 mL of blood is lost in vaginal deliveries, and 1000 mL is lost in cesarean births (Blackburn, 2013).

### Cardiac Output

Despite the blood loss, a transient increase in maternal cardiac output occurs after childbirth. This increase is caused by (1) an increased flow of blood back to the heart when blood from the uteroplacental unit returns to the central circulation, (2) decreased pressure from the pregnant uterus on the vessels, and (3) the mobilization of excess extracellular fluid into the vascular compartment. The cardiac output returns to prelabor values within an hour after delivery. Gradually, cardiac output decreases and returns to prepregnancy levels by 6 to 12 weeks after childbirth (Blackburn, 2013).

### Plasma Volume

The body rids itself of the excess plasma volume needed during pregnancy by diuresis and diaphoresis:

- *Diuresis* (increased excretion of urine) is facilitated by a decline in the adrenal hormone aldosterone, which increases during pregnancy to counteract the salt-wasting effect of progesterone. As aldosterone production decreases, sodium retention declines and fluid excretion accelerates. A decrease in oxytocin, which promotes reabsorption of fluid, also contributes to diuresis. A urinary output of up to 3000 mL/day is common, especially on days 2 through 5 of the postpartum period (Blackburn, 2013).
- *Diaphoresis* (profuse perspiration) also rids the body of excess fluid, which can be uncomfortable and unsettling for the mother who is not prepared for it. Explanations of the cause and provision of comfort measures, such as showers and dry clothing, are generally sufficient.

### Blood Values

Several components of the blood change during the postpartum period. Marked leukocytosis occurs, with the white blood cell (WBC) count increasing to as high as 30,000/mm$^3$ during labor and the immediate postpartum period. The average range is 14,000 to 16,000/mm$^3$ (Cunningham et al., 2014). The WBC falls to normal values by 6 days after birth (Blackburn, 2013).

Maternal hemoglobin and hematocrit values are difficult to interpret during the first few days after birth because of the remobilization and rapid excretion of excess body fluid. The hematocrit is low when plasma increases and dilutes the concentration of blood cells and other substances carried by the plasma. As excess fluid is excreted, the dilution is gradually reduced. The hematocrit returns to normal values within 4 to 6 weeks unless excessive blood loss has occurred (Blackburn, 2013).

## Coagulation

During pregnancy, plasma fibrinogen and other factors necessary for coagulation increase. As a result, the mother's body has a greater ability to form clots, and thus, prevent excessive bleeding. Fibrinolytic activity (ability to break down clots) is decreased during pregnancy. Although fibrinolysis increases shortly after delivery, elevations in clotting factors continue for several days or longer, causing a continued risk for thrombus formation. It takes 4 to 6 weeks before the hemostasis returns to normal prepregnant levels (Blackburn, 2013).

Although the incidence of thrombophlebitis has declined greatly as a result of early postpartum ambulation, new mothers are still at increased risk (see Chapter 28). Women who have varicose veins, a history of thrombophlebitis, or a cesarean birth are at further risk, and the lower extremities should be monitored closely. Pneumatic compression devices should be applied before cesarean delivery for all women not already receiving anticoagulants (American College of Obstetricians, 2014). A national voluntary standard for perinatal care is that all women having a cesarean birth have prophylaxis with heparin or pneumatic compression devices (National Quality Forum, 2012).

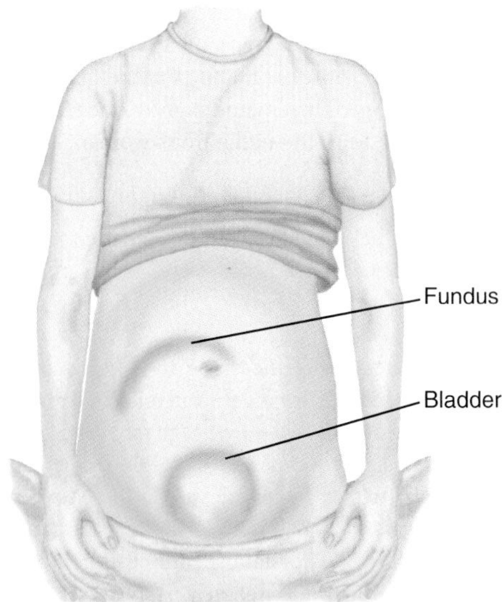


FIG 20.3 A full bladder displaces and prevents contraction of the uterus.

# GASTROINTESTINAL SYSTEM

Soon after childbirth, digestion begins to be active and the new mother is usually hungry because of the energy expended in labor. She is also thirsty because of the decreased intake during labor and the fluid loss from exertion, mouth breathing, and early diaphoresis. Nurses anticipate the mother's needs and provide food and fluids soon after childbirth.

Constipation is a common problem during the postpartum period for a variety of reasons. Bowel tone and intestinal motility, which were diminished during pregnancy as a result of progesterone, remain sluggish for several days. The abdominal musculature is relaxed. Decreased food and fluid intake during labor may result in small, hard stools. Perineal trauma, episiotomy, and hemorrhoids cause discomfort and interfere with effective bowel elimination. In addition, many women anticipate pain when they attempt to defecate and are unwilling to exert pressure on the perineum.

Temporary constipation is not harmful, although it can cause a feeling of abdominal fullness and flatulence. Stool softeners and laxatives are frequently prescribed to prevent or treat constipation. The first stool usually occurs within 2 to 3 days postpartum. Normal patterns of bowel elimination usually resume by 8 to 14 days after birth (Blackburn, 2013).

# URINARY SYSTEM

During childbirth, the urethra, bladder, and tissue around the urinary meatus may become edematous and traumatized as the fetal head passes beneath the bladder. This condition often results in diminished sensitivity to fluid pressure, and many new mothers have no sensation of needing to void even when the bladder is distended.

The bladder fills rapidly because of the diuresis that follows childbirth. As a consequence, the mother is at risk for overdistention of the bladder, incomplete emptying of the bladder, and retention of residual urine. Women who have received regional anesthesia are at particular risk for bladder distention and for difficulty voiding until feeling returns.

Urinary retention and overdistention of the bladder may cause urinary tract infection and increased postpartum bleeding. Urinary tract infection occurs when urinary stasis allows time for bacteria to multiply. Bleeding may increase because the uterine ligaments, which were stretched during pregnancy, allow the uterus to be displaced upward and laterally by the full bladder. The displacement results in decreased uterine muscle contraction (**uterine atony**), a primary cause of excessive bleeding (Fig. 20.3).

Stress incontinence may begin during pregnancy or the postpartum period. It usually improves within 3 months after birth (James, 2013). For some women, the problem resolves with pelvic floor exercises and time for healing. Others may have continued problems (see Chapter 32).

The dilation of the ureters and kidney pelvis improves by the end of the first week. The structures generally regain their nonpregnant state by 2 to 8 weeks after delivery (Cunningham et al., 2014). Both protein and acetone may be present in the urine in the first few postpartum days. Acetone suggests dehydration, which may occur during the exertion of labor. Mild proteinuria is usually the result of the catabolic processes involved in uterine involution.

# MUSCULOSKELETAL SYSTEM

## Muscles and Joints

In the first 1 to 2 days after childbirth, many women experience muscle fatigue and aches, particularly of the shoulders, neck, and arms, because of the effort of labor. Warmth and gentle massage increase circulation to the area and provide comfort and relaxation.

During the first few days, levels of the hormone relaxin gradually subside and the ligaments and cartilage of the pelvis begin to return to their prepregnancy positions. These changes can cause hip or joint pain that interferes with ambulation and exercise. The mother should be told that the discomfort is temporary and does not indicate a medical problem. Correct posture and good body mechanics are extremely important during this time to help prevent low back pain and injury to the joints (see Figs. 13.10 and 13.11).

## Abdominal Wall

During pregnancy, the abdominal walls stretch to accommodate the growing fetus, and muscle tone is diminished. Many women, expecting the abdominal muscles to return to the prepregnancy condition immediately after childbirth, are dismayed to find the abdominal muscles weak, soft, and flabby.

The longitudinal muscles of the abdomen may separate (diastasis recti) during pregnancy (Fig. 20.4). The separation may be minimal or severe. The mother may benefit from gentle exercises (Fig. 20.5) to strengthen the abdominal wall. The diastasis usually resolves within 6 weeks (Whitmer, 2011).

## INTEGUMENTARY SYSTEM

Many skin changes that occur during pregnancy are caused by an increase in hormones. When the hormone levels decline after childbirth, the skin gradually reverts to the nonpregnant state. For example, estrogen, progesterone, and melanocyte-stimulating hormone, which caused hyperpigmentation during pregnancy, decrease rapidly after childbirth and pigmentation begins to recede. This change is particularly noticeable when the melasma (mask of pregnancy) and linea nigra fade and disappear for most women.

The striae gravidarum (stretch marks), which develop during pregnancy when connective tissues in the abdomen and breasts are stretched, gradually fade to silvery lines but do not disappear.

The loss of hair may especially concern the woman. This is a normal response to the hormonal changes that caused decreased hair loss during pregnancy. Hair loss begins at 4 to 20 weeks after delivery and is regrown in 4 to 6 months for two thirds of women and by 15 months for the rest (Blackburn, 2013).

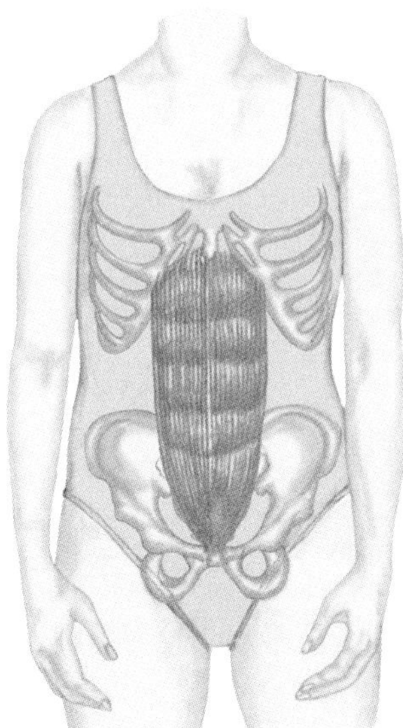

Normal location of rectus muscles of the abdomen

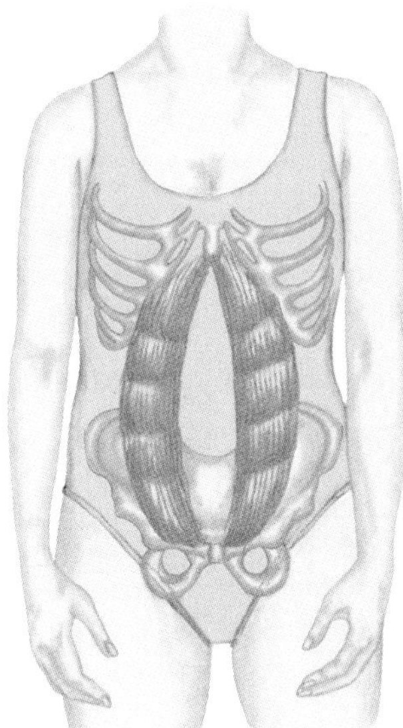

Diastasis recti: separation of the rectus muscles

FIG 20.4 Diastasis recti occurs when the longitudinal muscles of the abdomen separate during pregnancy.

## NEUROLOGIC SYSTEM

Many women experience discomfort and fatigue after childbirth. Afterpains, discomfort from episiotomy, lacerations, incisions, muscle aches, and breast engorgement (swelling from increased blood flow, edema, and presence of milk) may contribute to a woman's discomfort and inability to sleep. Anesthesia or analgesia may produce temporary neurologic changes such as lack of feeling in the legs and dizziness. During this time, prevention of injury that could occur as a result of falling is a priority.

Complaints of headache need careful assessment. Bilateral and frontal headaches are common in the first postpartum week and may result from changes in fluid and electrolyte balance (Blackburn, 2013). Although uncommon, spinal headaches after spinal anesthesia can occur. They may be most severe when the woman is in an upright position and relieved by a supine position. They should be reported to the appropriate healthcare provider, usually an anesthesiologist (see Chapter 18). Headache, proteinuria, blurred vision, photophobia, and abdominal pain may indicate development or worsening of preeclampsia (see Chapter 25).

Pain continues after discharge. Mothers report being surprised at the amount of pain they experienced when they went home. Some mothers feel that pain interferes with their ability to care for themselves and their infants (Eshkevari, Trout, & Damore, 2013).

## ENDOCRINE SYSTEM

After expulsion of the placenta, a fairly rapid decline occurs in placental hormones such as estrogen, progesterone, and human placental lactogen. Human chorionic gonadotropin is present for 3 to 4 weeks after birth. If the mother is not breastfeeding, the pituitary hormone prolactin, which stimulates milk secretion, returns to nonpregnant levels in 14 days (Lawrence & Lawrence, 2015).

### Resumption of Ovulation and Menstruation

Although the first few cycles for both lactating and non-lactating women are often anovulatory, ovulation may occur before the first menses (Whitmer, 2011). For some women, ovulation resumes as early as 3 weeks postpartum (Cunningham et al., 2014). Therefore, contraceptive measures are important considerations when sexual relations are resumed for both lactating and non-lactating women (see Chapter 31).

Approximately 40% to 45% of non-nursing mothers resume menstruation at 6 to 8 weeks after childbirth, 75% by 12 weeks, and all within 6 months. Menses while lactating may resume as early as 8 weeks or as late as 18 months (Whitmer, 2011). Frequent breastfeeding with no supplements is more likely to delay menses, but menses and ovulation are increasingly likely after the infant is 6 months old.

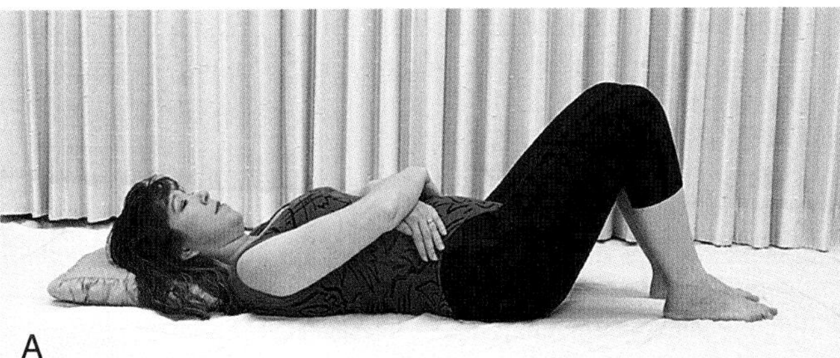

A

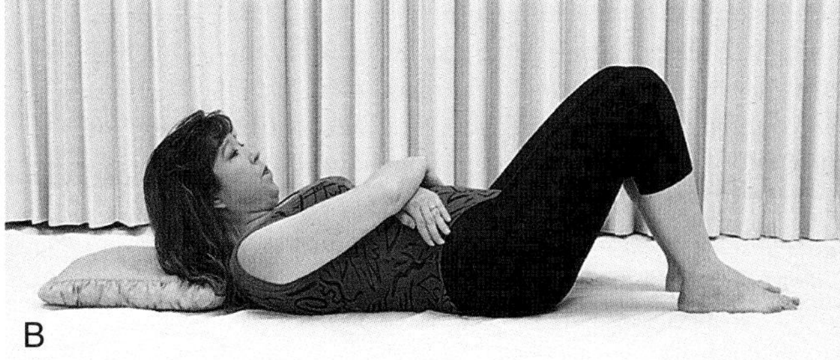

B

FIG 20.5 Abdominal exercises for diastasis recti. **A,** The woman inhales and supports the abdominal wall firmly with her hands. **B,** Exhaling, the woman raises her head as she pulls the abdominal muscles together.

### Lactation

During pregnancy, estrogen and progesterone prepare the breasts for lactation. Although prolactin also rises during pregnancy, lactation is inhibited at this time by the high levels of estrogen and progesterone. After expulsion of the placenta, estrogen and progesterone decline rapidly, and prolactin initiates milk production within 2 to 3 days after childbirth. Once milk production is established, it continues in response to frequent removal of milk from the breast.

Oxytocin is necessary for milk ejection, or "letdown." Oxytocin causes milk to be expressed from the alveoli into the lactiferous ducts during suckling (see Chapter 23).

### Weight Loss

Approximately 5.5 kg (12 lb) is lost during childbirth. This includes the weight of the fetus, placenta, amniotic fluid, and blood lost during the birth. An additional 4 kg (9 lb) over the next 2 weeks and another 2.5 kg (5.5 lb) are lost by 6 months after delivery (Cunningham et al., 2014). Adipose (fatty) tissue that was gained during pregnancy to meet the energy requirements of labor and breastfeeding is not lost initially, and the usual rate of loss is slow. Younger women with a lower pre-pregnancy weight and lower parity lose weight sooner and faster (Blackburn, 2013).

Many women do not lose all the weight gained and retain an average of 1 kg (2.2 lb) with each pregnancy (Blackburn, 2013). Women are often frustrated because they want to have an immediate return to prepregnancy weight. Nurses can provide information about diet and exercise that will produce an acceptable weight loss but does not deplete energy or impair the mother's health (see Chapter 14).

## POSTPARTUM ASSESSMENTS

Providing essential, cost-effective postpartum care to new families is a challenge for maternity nurses. Most women stay in the birth facility for 24-48 hours after a vaginal birth and 72-96 hours after a cesarean birth. However, some choose to go home earlier.

Although the length of stay is short, the family's need for care and information is extensive. This need causes nurses a great deal of concern for families who are discharged without adequate preparation or support.

### Clinical Pathways

Some institutions use clinical pathways (also called *critical pathways, care maps, care paths,* or *multidisciplinary action plans*) to guide necessary care while reducing the length of stay. Clinical pathways identify expected outcomes and establish time frames for specific assessments and interventions that prepare the mother and infant for discharge. The clinical pathway is a guideline and documentation tool.

### Initial Assessments

When caring for postpartum women, the nurse faces a high risk for contact with body fluids (colostrum, breast milk, and lochia from the mother as well as urine, stool, and blood from the infant). Therefore, the recommendations of the Centers for Disease Control and Prevention (CDC) for standard blood and body fluid precautions must be followed diligently. Postpartum assessments begin during the fourth stage of labor (the first 1 to 2 hours after childbirth). During this time, the mother is examined to determine whether she is physically stable. Initial assessments include:

- Vital signs
- Skin color
- Location and firmness of the fundus
- Amount and color of lochia
- Perineum (edema, episiotomy, lacerations, hematoma)
- Presence, degree, and location of pain
- Intravenous (IV) infusion (type of fluid; rate of administration; type and amount of added medications; patency of the IV line; and redness, pain, or edema of the site)
- Urinary output (time and amount of last void or catheterization, presence of a catheter, color and character of urine)
- Status of abdominal incision and dressing, if present
- Level of feeling and ability to move if regional anesthesia was administered

### Chart Review

When the initial assessments confirm the mother's physical condition is stable, nurses should review the chart to obtain pertinent information and determine if there are factors that increase the risk for complications during the postpartum period. Relevant information includes:

- Gravida, para
- Time and type of delivery (use of vacuum extractor, forceps)
- Presence and degree of episiotomy or lacerations
- Anesthesia or medications administered
- Significant medical and surgical history, such as diabetes, hypertension, or heart disease
- Medications given during labor and delivery or routinely taken and reasons for their use
- Food and drug allergies
- Chosen method of infant feeding
- Condition of the baby

Laboratory data are also examined. Of particular interest are the prenatal hemoglobin and hematocrit values, the blood type and Rh factor, hepatitis B surface antigen, rubella immune status, syphilis screen, and group B streptococcus status.

#### Need for $Rh_o$(D) Immune Globulin

Prenatal and neonatal records are checked to determine whether $Rh_o$(D) immune globulin should be administered. $Rh_o$(D) immune globulin may be necessary if the mother is Rh negative, the newborn is Rh positive, and the mother is not already sensitized. To prevent the development of maternal antibodies that would affect subsequent pregnancies, $Rh_o$(D) immune globulin should be administered within 72 hours after childbirth (see Chapter 25).

#### Need for Vaccines

**Rubella vaccine.** A prenatal rubella antibody screen is performed on each pregnant woman to determine if she is immune to rubella. If she is not immune, rubella vaccine is recommended after childbirth to prevent her from acquiring rubella during subsequent pregnancies, when it can cause serious fetal anomalies. Although there is no evidence of fetal damage in cases of inadvertent vaccination during pregnancy, there is a theoretical risk for defects because rubella vaccine contains live virus. Therefore, women are advised not to become pregnant for at least 28 days after receiving rubella vaccine (Atkinson, Wolfe, & Hamborsky, 2015).

Before administration, some agencies require that a woman sign a statement giving permission for vaccination and indicating that she understands the risks of becoming pregnant again too soon after the injection (see Drug Guide). If this statement is not required, the nurse should record in the chart that the risk has been explained and the woman has verbalized her understanding.

**Pertussis vaccine.** Recent outbreaks of pertussis have had serious effects in infants and young children. Although most adults have been

## DRUG GUIDE

### *Rubella Vaccine*

**Classification:** Attenuated live virus vaccine.

**Action:** Produces a modified rubella (German measles) infection that is not communicable, causing the formation of antibodies against rubella virus.

**Indications:** Administered at least 1 month before pregnancy or after childbirth or abortion to women whose antibody screen shows they are not immune to rubella. This vaccine prevents rubella infection and possible severe congenital defects in the fetus during a subsequent pregnancy.

**Dosage and Route:** 0.5 mL subcutaneously.

**Absorption:** Well absorbed.

**Contraindications and Precautions:** The vaccine is contraindicated in women who are immunosuppressed, pregnant, or sensitive to vaccine components, or have a moderate or severe illness. The attenuated virus may appear in breast milk and some infants may develop a rash but this is not a contraindication to vaccination of lactating women. Although it can be given near the time of $Rh_0$(D) immune globulin administration, women receiving the vaccine should be tested for immune status at 6 to 8 weeks to be sure they are immune (Atkinson, Wolfe, Hamborsky, et al., 2015).

**Adverse Reactions:** Transient stinging at site, fever, lymphadenopathy, arthralgia, and transient arthritis are most common.

**Nursing Implications:** Vials should be refrigerated. Reconstitute only with diluent supplied with the vial. Use immediately after reconstitution and discard if not used within 8 hours. Protect from light. Check with healthcare provider before giving near time of administration of $Rh_0$(D) immune globulin. Birth of infants with congenital rubella syndrome has not been documented when the vaccine has been given inadvertently during pregnancy, but women are advised to avoid pregnancy for at least 4 weeks after vaccination.

Reference: Atkinson, W., Wolfe, S., & Hamborsky, J. (Eds.). (2011). *Epidemiology and prevention of vaccine-preventable diseases* (12th ed.) Washington, DC: Public Health Foundation.

## SAFETY ALERT

### *Postpartum Risk Factors*

**Hemorrhage**

- Grand multiparity (five or more)
- Over distention of the uterus (large baby, twins, hydramnios)
- Rapid or prolonged labor
- Retained placenta
- Placenta previa or previous placenta accreta or abruptio placentae
- Drugs (tocolytics, magnesium sulfate, general anesthesia, prolonged use of oxytocin)
- Operative procedures (cesarean birth, vacuum extraction, forceps)
- Uterine fibroids
- History of postpartum hemorrhage
- Preeclampsia
- Coagulation defects

**Infection**

- Operative procedures (cesarean birth, vacuum extraction, forceps)
- Multiple cervical examinations
- Prolonged labor
- Prolonged rupture of membranes
- Manual extraction of placenta or retained fragments
- Diabetes
- Catheterization
- Bacterial colonization of lower genital tract

vaccinated as children, the effectiveness fades with time. Full protection of vaccinated infants does not occur until the entire series is completed.

The CDC (2010) recommends that all adults in contact with infants and young children get a booster dose of pertussis vaccine. The vaccine can be offered to women before hospital discharge after childbirth.

### Risk Factors for Hemorrhage and Infection

Nurses must be aware of conditions that increase the risk for hemorrhage and infection, the two most common complications of the puerperium.

## Focused Assessments After Vaginal Birth

Nurses perform postpartum assessments according to facility protocol. For example, a protocol might require assessment every 15 minutes for the first hour, every half hour for the next hour, every 4 hours for the first 24 hours, and every 8 hours thereafter. Of course, assessments are performed more frequently if findings are abnormal.

Although assessments vary according to particular problems presented, a focused assessment for a vaginal delivery generally includes the vital signs, fundus, lochia, perineum, bladder elimination, breasts, and lower extremities. The assessment for post-cesarean mothers is more extensive (see p. 405).

### Vital Signs

***Blood pressure.*** Blood pressure (BP) varies with position and the arm used. To obtain accurate results, the BP should be measured on the same arm with the mother in the same position each time. Postpartum BP should be compared with that of the predelivery period so that deviations from what is normal for the mother can be quickly identified. An increase from the baseline may be caused by pain or anxiety. If the BP is 140/90 mm Hg or higher, preeclampsia may be present. A decrease may indicate dehydration or hypovolemia resulting from excessive bleeding.

***Orthostatic hypotension.*** After birth, a rapid decrease in intraabdominal pressure results in dilation of blood vessels supplying the viscera. The resulting engorgement of abdominal blood vessels contributes to a rapid fall in BP of 15 to 20 mm Hg when the woman moves from a recumbent to a sitting position. This change causes mothers to feel dizzy or lightheaded or to faint when they stand. The nursing diagnosis Risk for Injury applies to women with orthostatic hypotension (see Nursing Care Plan: Postpartum Hypotension, Fatigue, and Pain, p. 408).

Hypotension may also indicate hypovolemia. Careful assessments for hemorrhage (location and firmness of the fundus, amount of lochia, pulse rate for tachycardia) should be made if the postpartum BP is significantly less than the prenatal baseline blood pressure.

***Pulse.*** Bradycardia, defined as a pulse rate of 40 to 50 beats per minute (bpm), may occur in some women (James, 2013). The lower pulse rate may reflect the large amount of blood that returns to the central circulation after delivery of the placenta. The increase in central circulation results in increased stroke volume and allows a slower heart rate to provide adequate maternal circulation.

Tachycardia may indicate pain, excitement, fatigue, dehydration, hypovolemia, anemia, or infection. If tachycardia is noted, additional assessments should include BP, location and firmness of the uterus, amount of lochia, estimated blood loss at delivery, and hemoglobin and hematocrit values. The objective of the additional assessments is to rule out excessive bleeding and to intervene at once if hemorrhage is suspected.

***Respirations.*** A normal respiratory rate of 12 to 20 breaths per minute should be maintained. Assessing breath sounds is especially important for mothers who have a cesarean birth, are smokers, have a history of frequent or recent upper respiratory infections or asthma, and for those receiving magnesium sulfate (see Chapter 25).

***Temperature.*** A temperature of up to 38° C (100.4° F) is common during the first 24 hours after childbirth and may be caused by dehydration or normal postpartum leukocytosis. If the elevated temperature persists for longer than 24 hours, if it exceeds 38° C (100.4° F), or if the woman shows other signs of infection, the nurse should report it to the physician or nurse-midwife (see Chapter 28).

***Pain.*** Pain, the fifth vital sign, should be assessed to determine the type, location, and severity on a pain scale. Nurses must remain alert to signs of afterpains, perineal discomfort, and breast tenderness. Nonspecific signs of discomfort include an inability to relax or sleep, a change in vital signs, restlessness, irritability, and facial grimacing. The nurse should encourage women to take prescribed medications as needed and should evaluate the effectiveness of pain-relief measures.

### Fundus

The fundus should be assessed for consistency and location. It should be firmly contracted and at or near the level of the umbilicus. If the uterus is above the expected level or shifted (usually to the right) from the middle of the abdomen (midline position), the bladder may be distended. The location of the fundus should be rechecked after the woman has emptied her bladder.

If the fundus is difficult to locate or is soft or "boggy," the nurse stimulates the uterine muscle to contract by gently massaging the uterus. The nondominant hand must support and anchor the lower uterine segment if it is necessary to massage an uncontracted uterus. Uterine massage is not necessary if the uterus is firmly contracted.

The uterus can contract only if it is free of intrauterine clots. To expel clots, the nurse must first massage the fundus until it is firmly contracted. The nurse then supports the lower uterine segment, as illustrated in the Procedure: Assessing the Uterine Fundus. This support prevents inversion of the uterus (turning inside out) when the nurse applies firm pressure downward toward the vagina to express clots that have collected in the uterus. Nurses should observe the perineum for the number and size of clots expelled. If lochia is excessive or large clots are present, they should be weighed to estimate the amount (see Chapter 28). Table 20.2 describes normal and abnormal findings of the uterine fundus and includes follow-up nursing actions for abnormal findings.

Drugs are sometimes needed to maintain contraction of the uterus, and thus, to prevent postpartum hemorrhage. The most commonly used drug is oxytocin (Pitocin) (see Drug Guide for oxytocin, Chapter 19, pp. 381-382).

### Lochia

Important assessments include the amount, color, and odor of lochia. Nurses observe the lochia on perineal pads and while checking the perineum. They also assess vaginal discharge while palpating or massaging the fundus to determine the amount of lochia and the number and size of any clots expressed during these procedures. Important guidelines include:

- A constant trickle, dribble, or oozing of lochia indicates excessive bleeding and requires immediate attention.
- Excessive lochia in the presence of a contracted uterus suggests lacerations of the birth canal. The healthcare provider must be notified so that lacerations can be located and repaired.

The odor of lochia is usually described as "fleshy," "earthy," or "musty." A foul odor suggests endometrial infection, and assessments should be made for additional signs of infection. These signs include maternal fever, tachycardia, uterine tenderness, and pain.

Absence of lochia, like the presence of a foul odor, may also indicate infection. If the birth was cesarean, lochia may be scant because some of the endometrial lining was removed. However, lochia should not be entirely absent.

**TABLE 20.2 Observations of the Uterine Fundus and Nursing Actions**

| Normal Findings | Abnormal Findings | Nursing Actions |
|---|---|---|
| Fundus firmly contracted. | Fundus soft, "boggy," uncontracted, or difficult to locate. | Support lower uterine segment. Massage until firm. |
| Fundus remains contracted when massage is discontinued. | Fundus becomes soft and uncontracted when massage is stopped. | Continue to support lower uterine segment. Massage fundus until firm, then apply pressure to express clots that may be accumulating in uterus. Notify healthcare provider and begin oxytocin administration, as prescribed, to maintain a firm fundus. |
| Fundus located at level of umbilicus and midline. | Fundus above umbilicus and/or displaced from midline. | Assess bladder elimination. Assist mother in urinating or catheterize, if necessary. Recheck the position and consistency of fundus after bladder is empty. |

### Perineum

The acronym REEDA is used as a reminder that the site of an episiotomy or a perineal laceration should be assessed for five signs: redness *(R)*, edema *(E)*, ecchymosis (bruising) *(E)*, discharge *(D)*, and approximation (the edges of the wound should be closed, as though stuck or glued together) *(A)*.

Redness of the wound may indicate the usual inflammatory response to injury. However, if accompanied by excessive pain or tenderness, it may indicate the beginning of localized infection. Ecchymosis or edema indicates soft tissue damage that can delay healing. There should be no discharge from the wound. Rapid healing requires that the edges of the wound be closely approximated (Procedure: Assessing the Perineum).

### Bladder Elimination

During the early postpartum period women may not experience the urge to void even if the bladder is full. Nurses must rely on physical assessment to determine whether the bladder is distended. Bladder distention often produces an obvious or palpable bulge that feels like a soft, movable mass above the symphysis pubis. Other signs include an upward and lateral displacement of the uterine fundus and increased lochia. Frequent voidings of less than 150 mL suggest urinary retention with overflow. Signs of an empty bladder include a firm fundus in the midline and a nonpalpable bladder.

Two or three voidings should be measured after birth or the removal of a catheter to determine if normal bladder function has returned. When the mother can void 300 to 400 mL, the bladder is usually empty. However, regardless of the amount voided, the fundus must be assessed after the woman voids to confirm that the bladder is empty. Subjective

## PROCEDURE

### Assessing the Uterine Fundus

**Purpose**

*To determine the location and firmness of the uterus.*

1. *To reduce anxiety and elicit cooperation,* explain the procedure and rationale before beginning the procedure.
2. Ask the mother to empty her bladder if she has not voided recently, *because a distended bladder displaces the uterus.*
3. Place the mother in a supine position with her knees flexed *to relax the abdominal muscles and permit accurate location of the fundus.*
4. Put on clean gloves. Lower the perineal pads *to observe lochia as the fundus is palpated.*
5. Place your nondominant hand above the woman's symphysis pubis *to support and anchor the lower uterine segment.*
6. Use the flat part of your fingers (not the fingertips) for palpation (see illustration), *because the larger surface provides more comfort.*
7. Begin palpation at the umbilicus, and palpate gently until the fundus is located. *This helps determine the firmness and location of the fundus.* It should be firm, in the midline, and approximately at the level of the umbilicus.
8. If the fundus is difficult to locate or is "boggy" (soft), keep the nondominant hand above the woman's symphysis pubis and massage the fundus with your dominant hand until the fundus is firm. *The nondominant hand anchors the lower segment of the uterus and prevents inversion while the uterus is massaged. The uterus contracts in response to tactile stimulation.*
9. After massaging a boggy fundus until it is firm, press firmly to expel clots. Do not attempt to expel clots before the fundus is firm *because this can increase the possibility of the uterus inverting.* Keep one hand pressed firmly just above the symphysis (over the lower uterine segment) throughout. *Removing clots allows the uterus to contract properly.*
10. If the fundus is above or below the umbilicus, use your fingers to determine the number of fingerbreadths between the fundus and the umbilicus. *Using the fingers to measure allows an approximation of the number of centimeters.*

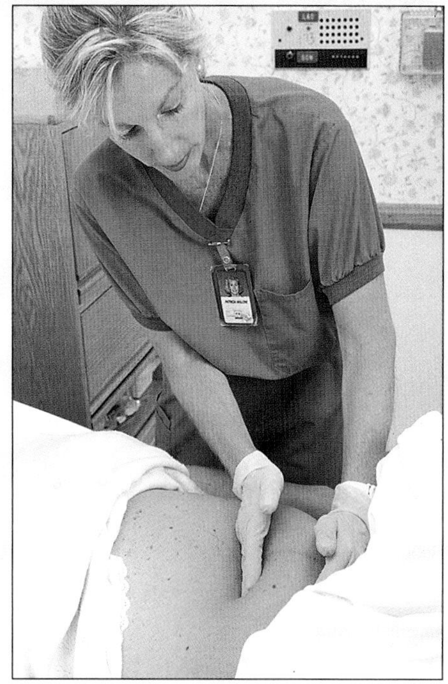

11. Document the consistency and location of the fundus *to promote accurate communication and identify deviations from expected findings.* Record consistency as "fundus firm," "firm with massage," or "boggy." Record fundal height in fingerbreadths above or below the umbilicus. For example, "fundus firm, midline, U ↓ 2" (two fingerbreadths or cm below umbilicus) or "fundus firm with light massage, U + 2, displaced to right."

## PROCEDURE

### Assessing the Perineum

**Purpose**

To observe perineal trauma and the state of healing.

1. Provide privacy, and explain the purpose of the procedure to elicit cooperation and reduce anxiety.
2. Put on clean gloves to implement standard precautions.
3. Ask the mother to assume a side-lying position and flex her upper leg. This allows visualization of the perineum and assessment of lochia that may be under the mother.
4. Lower the perineal pads and lift her superior buttocks to provide an unobstructed view of the perineum. If necessary, use a flashlight for better visibility during inspection of the perineal area.
5. Note the extent and location of edema or bruising. Extensive bruising or asymmetric edema may indicate formation of a hematoma (see Chapter 28).
6. Examine the episiotomy or laceration for redness, ecchymosis, edema, discharge, and approximation (REEDA), which may indicate infection or problems with healing.
7. Note the number and size of hemorrhoids. Swollen hemorrhoids interfere with activity and bowel elimination.

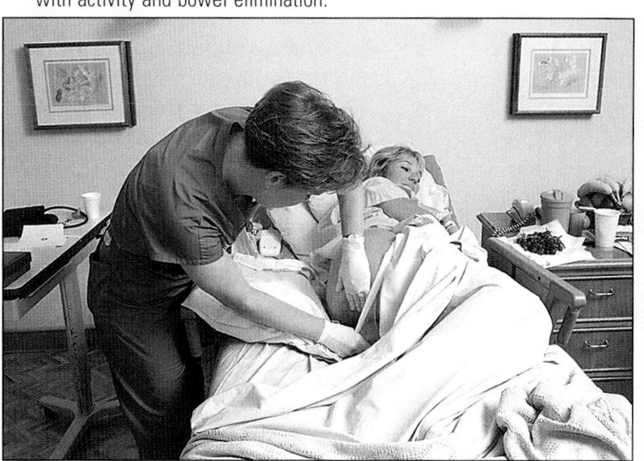

symptoms of urgency, frequency, or dysuria suggest urinary tract infection and should be reported to the healthcare provider.

**SAFETY ALERT**

### *Signs of a Distended Bladder*

- Location of fundus above baseline level
- Fundus displaced from midline
- Excessive lochia
- Bladder discomfort
- Bulge of bladder above symphysis
- Frequent voidings of less than 150 mL of urine, which may indicate urinary retention with overflow

### Breasts

For the first day or two after delivery, the breasts should be soft and nontender. After that, breast changes depend largely on whether the mother is breastfeeding. The breasts should be examined even if she chooses formula feeding because engorgement may occur. The size, symmetry, and shape of the breasts should be observed. The skin should be inspected for dimpling or thickening, which, although rare, can indicate a breast tumor.

The areola and nipple should be carefully examined for problems such as flat or retracted nipples, which may make breastfeeding more difficult. Signs of nipple trauma (redness, blisters, fissures) may be present during the first days of breastfeeding, especially if the mother needs assistance in positioning the infant correctly (see Chapter 23).

The breasts should be palpated for firmness and tenderness, which indicate increased vascular and lymphatic circulation that may precede milk production. The breasts may feel "lumpy" as various lobes begin to produce milk.

The breast assessment is an excellent opportunity to provide information or reassurance about breast care and breastfeeding techniques. The mother should be taught how to assess her own breasts so she can continue after discharge.

### Lower Extremities

The legs are examined for varicosities and signs or symptoms of thrombophlebitis. Indications of thrombophlebitis include localized areas of redness, heat, edema, and tenderness. Pedal pulses may be obstructed by thrombophlebitis and should be palpated with each assessment (see Chapter 28).

### Homans Sign

Discomfort in the calf with passive dorsiflexion of the foot is a positive Homans sign and may indicate deep vein thrombosis. A negative Homans sign is indicated by absence of discomfort. A positive Homans sign should be reported to the healthcare provider, along with redness, tenderness, or warmth of the leg. Assessment of Homans sign can be confusing because a deep venous thrombosis may not produce calf pain with dorsiflexion. In addition, women may report pain that is caused by strained muscles from positioning and pushing during delivery.

### Edema and Deep Tendon Reflexes

Pedal or pretibial edema may be present for the first few days, until excess interstitial fluid is remobilized and excreted. Diuresis is highest between the 2nd and 5th days after birth (Blackburn, 2013).

Deep tendon reflexes should be 1+ to 2+. Report brisker than average and hyperactive reflexes (3+ to 4+), which suggest preeclampsia. (See p. 541 for a description of assessing deep tendon reflexes.)

## CARE IN THE IMMEDIATE POSTPARTUM PERIOD

The postpartum period is often divided into three periods. The first 24 hours is the *immediate postpartum period;* the 1st week is the *early postpartum period;* and the 2nd week through the 6th week is the *late postpartum period.* Care of the mother during the immediate postpartum period focuses on physiologic safety, comfort measures, bladder elimination, and health education.

### Providing Comfort Measures

#### Ice Packs

Ice causes vasoconstriction and is most effective if applied soon after the birth to prevent edema and numb the perineum. Chemical ice packs and plastic bags or nonlatex gloves filled with ice may be used during the first 12 to 24 hours after a vaginal birth. The ice pack is wrapped in a washcloth or paper before it is applied to the perineum. It should be left in place until the ice melts. It is then removed for 10 minutes before a fresh pack is applied. Some peripads have cold packs in them. Condensation from ice may dilute lochia and make it appear heavier than it actually is.

#### Sitz Baths

Sitz baths are used in some agencies to cleanse and comfort the traumatized perineum. Cool water may be used during the first 24 hours to reduce pain from edema. Warm water increases circulation and promotes healing and may be most effective after 24 hours. Nurses must place the emergency bell within easy reach in case the mother feels faint during the sitz bath. The woman often takes the disposable sitz bath container home. She should clean it well between uses.

#### Perineal Care

Perineal care consists of squirting warm water over the perineum after each voiding or bowel movement. This is important for all postpartum women whether the birth was vaginal or by cesarean. The bottle should not touch the perineum. Perineal care cleanses, provides comfort, and prevents infection. The perineum is gently patted rather than wiped dry.

#### Topical Medications

Anesthetic sprays decrease surface discomfort and allow more comfortable ambulation. The mother is instructed to hold the nozzle of the spray 6 to 12 inches from her body and direct it toward the perineum. The spray should be used after perineal care and before clean pads are applied. Astringent compresses should be placed directly over the hemorrhoids to relieve pain. Hydrocortisone ointments may also be applied over the hemorrhoids to increase comfort.

#### Sitting Measures

The mother should be advised to squeeze her buttocks together before sitting and to lower her weight slowly onto her buttocks. This measure prevents stretching of the perineal tissue and avoids sharp impact on the traumatized area. Sitting slightly to the side is helpful to prevent the full weight from resting on the episiotomy site.

#### Analgesics

Mothers should be encouraged to take prescribed medications for afterpains and perineal discomfort. Many analgesics are combinations that include acetaminophen. The nurse should be careful that the woman receives no more than 4 g of acetaminophen in a 24-hour period. Nonsteroidal antiinflammatory drugs (NSAIDs), such as ibuprofen, are frequently prescribed for their antiinflammatory properties. They can be given along with other analgesics.

### Promoting Bladder Elimination

Many new mothers have difficulty voiding because of edema and trauma of the perineum and diminished sensitivity to fluid pressure in the bladder. As soon as they are able to ambulate safely, mothers should be assisted to the bathroom. It is important to provide privacy and to allow adequate time for the first voiding. Common measures to promote relaxation of the perineal muscles and to stimulate the sensation of needing to void include:

- Medicating the woman for perineal pain to help her relax
- Running water in the sink or shower, placing the mother's hands in warm water, and pouring water over the vulva
- Encouraging urination in the shower or sitz bath
- Providing hot tea or fluids of choice
- Asking the mother to blow bubbles through a straw

A nonpalpable bladder and firm fundus at or below the umbilicus and in the midline confirm that the bladder is empty and rule out urinary retention with overflow.

Because a distended bladder displaces the uterus, the uterus may not contract properly. The resulting uterine atony (loss of tone) permits excessive bleeding. Moreover, stasis of urine in the bladder predisposes the woman to urinary tract infection. Therefore, the mother must be catheterized if:

- She is unable to void.
- The amount voided is less than 150 mL and the bladder can be palpated.
- The fundus is elevated or displaced from the midline.

Repeated catheterizations increase the chance of urinary tract infection because bacteria may be pushed into the bladder despite scrupulous aseptic technique. In some situations, an indwelling catheter may be inserted for 24 hours if edema is excessive or catheterization is necessary more than once or twice.

 **CRITICAL THINKING EXERCISE 20.1**

Jenny, a 27-year-old gravida 4, para 4, was admitted from the labor, delivery, and recovery unit 2 hours after the birth of a 3628-g (8-lb) baby boy. Although all previous assessments were normal, her fundus is boggy, located three fingerbreadths above the umbilicus, and displaced to the right an hour after transfer. Her perineal pads, which were changed just before transfer, are saturated.

1. What do these data suggest? Why?
2. What nursing action should be taken first? What follow-up assessments are necessary?
3. Why is it necessary to remind and assist the woman to void?

### Providing Fluids and Food

Adequate fluids help restore the balance altered by fluid loss during labor and the birth process. Women should be encouraged to drink approximately 2500 mL of fluids each day. Offering ice water or cold drinks may be culturally inappropriate for some mothers. They may prefer hot or room-temperature water instead.

New mothers generally have a hearty appetite, and nurses should encourage healthy food choices with respect for the woman's ethnic background. Meals and snacks should be available at all times.

### Preventing Thrombophlebitis

The mother should be assisted to ambulate early after childbirth to prevent the development of thrombi. Frequent trips to the bathroom will help accomplish this goal.

## NURSING CARE AFTER CESAREAN BIRTH

In 2013, 32.7% of births were by cesarean (ACOG, 2015). These mothers must recover from childbirth as well as from major surgery and need special care. The usual length of stay after cesarean birth is 72 to 96 hours after surgery.

### Assessment

In addition to the usual postpartum evaluation, the postcesarean mother must be assessed like any other postoperative patient.

#### Pain Relief

Assessment of pain and the effectiveness of pain medication is an important part of nursing care for postcesarean women. Pain relief may be provided in various ways. Patient-controlled analgesia (PCA) is administered by continuous IV infusion of a low-concentration narcotic solution using a pump specifically designed for that purpose. If analgesia is insufficient, the woman can self-administer intermittent small doses of narcotic from the infusion pump. The machine limits the amount of narcotic available within a specific interval to prevent an overdose.

A single dose of opioid (often morphine or fentanyl) injected into the epidural or subarachnoid space immediately after the surgery provides 18 to 24 hours of postcesarean analgesia. If the woman has pain, oral analgesics usually suffice. Itching and nausea are common side effects. Side effects of both PCA and epidural narcotics include respiratory depression, itching (pruritus), nausea and vomiting, and urine retention.

#### Respirations

When mothers receive epidural narcotics for postoperative pain relief, respirations must be assessed frequently because narcotics depress the respiratory center. A pulse oximeter or an apnea monitor is used for 18 to 24 hours to detect decreased oxygen saturation from a decreased respiratory rate or depth. Capnography (end-tidal $CO_2$ monitoring) may also be used to detect opiate-related respiratory changes (Smith, 2015). These devices will emit an alarm if respirations decrease. The alarms should be loud enough to be heard easily by the nurse. Oxygen saturation or respiratory rate is documented hourly or according to facility policy.

In addition to observing respiratory rate and depth, the mother's breath sounds should be auscultated because depressed respirations as well as a longer period of immobility allow secretions to pool in the bronchioles.

#### Abdomen

Nurses assess gastrointestinal function by auscultating for bowel sounds until normal peristalsis is noted in all abdominal quadrants. Although paralytic ileus (lack of movement in the bowel) is rare after cesarean birth, nurses must be aware of the signs, which include abdominal distention, absent or decreased bowel sounds, and failure to pass flatus or stool.

If a surgical dressing is present, it should be observed for intactness and discharge. When the dressing is removed, nurses observe the incision, which should be approximated, and use the acronym REEDA to assess for signs of infection, such as redness and edema. A topical skin adhesive may be used instead of staples. Assessment of the wound is the same.

Assessment of the fundus is just as important after cesarean birth as after vaginal birth. However, palpation must be gentle because of increased discomfort caused by the uterine incision.

### Intake and Output

The IV should be monitored for patency, the rate of flow, and the condition of the site. Any signs of infiltration (edema or coolness at the site) and signs of infection (edema, redness, warmth, and pain) should be reported. Ice chips and clear fluids are usually allowed soon after cesarean birth. The amount, color, and clarity of urine should be monitored.

## Interventions

### The First 24 Hours

Nursing care for the mother who gave birth by cesarean is similar to that for other postoperative patients.

***Providing pain relief.*** The nurse should determine the need for pain relief on a regular basis. If the woman has a PCA, the nurse should check how often she is using it. The effectiveness of any type of medication must be observed. Pain relief aids ability to ambulate, which helps prevent thrombophlebitis and promotes healing.

The nurse should continue to assess the respiratory status in women who had epidural or spinal opioids. If the respiratory rate is less than 12 to 14 breaths per minute or the pulse oximeter shows persistent oxygen saturation less than 95%, the nurse should:

- Notify the anesthesiologist immediately.
- Elevate the head of the bed to facilitate lung expansion and ask the woman to breathe deeply.
- Administer oxygen, and apply a pulse oximeter (if not already in place) to measure oxygen saturation.
- Follow facility protocol to administer narcotic antagonists, such as naloxone hydrochloride (Narcan).
- Observe for recurrence of respiratory depression, because the effect of naloxone lasts as little as 30 minutes.
- Recognize that naloxone reduces the level of pain relief.

***Overcoming the effects of immobility.*** The new mother is on bed rest for the first 8 to 12 hours. To prevent pooling of secretions in the airways, she must be assisted to turn, cough, and expand the lungs by breathing deeply at least every 2 hours while she is awake. Splinting the abdomen with a small pillow reduces incisional discomfort when she coughs. An incentive spirometer may be used to help expand the lungs.

The woman should be encouraged to flex her knees and move her feet and legs frequently while she is in bed to improve peripheral circulation and prevent thrombi. Pneumatic compression devices may be used to prevent the pooling of blood in the lower extremities, especially for women who are obese or at a high risk for thrombus formation.

Her activity level will increase gradually. The woman needs assistance to sit and dangle her feet for the first few times before she gets out of bed. She should be assisted to walk within the first 24 hours to decrease the risk for thrombi. She will need help ambulating when the IV and catheter are still in place.

***Providing comfort.*** Placing a pillow behind her back and one between her knees prevents strain and discomfort when the woman is in a side-lying position. Excellent physical care (oral hygiene, perineal care, a sponge bath, and clean linen) comforts and refreshes her.

### After 24 Hours

***Resuming normal activities.*** After 24 hours, several normal functions return as postcesarean women are able to participate more actively in their own care:

- The indwelling catheter and the IV are usually discontinued.
- The dressing, if present, is usually removed in 24 hours, and staples (if used) may be removed before discharge. Staples may be removed after discharge by the physician if the woman is obese. Steri-Strips (small strips of adhesive), a small nonstick dressing, or a peripad may be placed over the incision to protect it from friction from clothing or adipose tissue, or the incision may be left open to air.
- Women are usually helped to ambulate on the 1st postpartum day and are comfortable sitting in a chair for brief periods. Nurses must encourage the mother to increase her activity and ambulation each postpartum day.
- Clear liquids are changed to a soft or regular diet once bowel sounds are audible or the woman is passing flatus. In some facilities, solids are given earlier.

***Assisting the mother with infant care.*** Pain after cesarean interferes with the mother's ability to breastfeed and care for her infant during the early days. Ensuring adequate pain relief is essential so the mother can focus on her infant. It is important to help the mother find a comfortable position for holding and feeding her infant. Some mothers prefer sitting with a pillow on the lap to protect the incisional area. A side-lying position or football hold may be most comfortable for breastfeeding because these positions avoid pressure on the incision. The side-lying position also allows the mother to rest while feeding (see Chapter 23). A support person or the nurse should be available to help the mother with infant care until she is able to take over herself.

***Preventing abdominal distention.*** Abdominal distention is a major source of discomfort. Measures to prevent or minimize it include:

- Early, frequent ambulation.
- Tightening and relaxing the abdominal muscles.
- Pelvic lifts. Lying supine with her knees bent, the woman lifts her pelvis from the bed and repeats the exercise up to 10 times, several times each day.
- Avoiding carbonated beverages which increase the accumulation of intestinal gas.
- Simethicone, as ordered, to help disperse upper gastrointestinal flatulence.
- Rectal suppositories, as ordered, to stimulate peristalsis and the passage of flatus.

## NURSING CARE

### Teaching After Birth

The first 12 weeks after birth are often called the **fourth trimester**. It is a time of transition for the parents and siblings. Nurses can do much to help during this adjustment period.

#### Assessment

Nurses are responsible for providing health education before the family is discharged from the birth facility. This is difficult because so much must be taught in a short time and women have not fully recovered from the birth process. Some women feel they have difficulty concentrating during the 1st week postpartum. They have much to think about with the many changes birth brings.

Before beginning teaching, determine the learning needs and the major concerns of the family. Multiparas remember some aspects of self-care but often benefit from a review. Primiparas may be anxious about self-care measures and all aspects of infant care. They may need more thorough teaching and more practice. Identify the effects of the most common barriers to learning: age and developmental level, cultural factors, and difficulty understanding the language.

#### Nursing Diagnosis and Planning

In general, mothers adapt well to the physiologic changes after childbirth, and most nursing care is wellness oriented. However, some new mothers lack knowledge of self-care and need education to prevent later problems. A nursing diagnosis that applies to these women is:

- Risk for Ineffective Health Maintenance related to insufficient knowledge of self-care, signs of complications, and preventive measures.

***Expected outcomes.*** The woman will verbalize or demonstrate understanding of self-care instructions by discharge and verbalize understanding of practices that promote maternal health by a specified date. By the day of discharge, the mother will describe plans for follow-up care and signs and symptoms that should be reported to the healthcare provider.

Additional diagnoses include Risk for Injury and Ineffective Sexuality Pattern, which are discussed in the Nursing Care Plan: Postpartum Hypotension, Fatigue, and Pain.

### Interventions

***Preparing for teaching.*** Before beginning teaching sessions, be sure the woman is comfortable. Give pain medication, if needed, to prevent her from being distracted by discomfort. Choose a time for teaching that does not interfere with meals, infant care needs, or visiting.

***Determining teaching topics.*** Discuss the teaching plan with the woman to include topics most important to her. Her perception of what is most important may differ from that of the nurse. Identifying the woman's educational needs ensures her interest and makes best use of the time available. Topics of less interest may require only a brief review.

***Teaching the process of involution.*** Provide the woman with basic information about involution, including how to assess lochia and how to locate and palpate the fundus. This information allows her to recognize abnormal signs, such as prolonged lochia, reappearance of bright-red lochia after lochia rubra has ended, or uterine tenderness, which should be reported to the healthcare provider. If the mother is a young adolescent, another family member may also need the information.

***Teaching self-care.***

**Handwashing.** Emphasize the importance of thorough handwashing before the woman touches the breasts, after diaper changes, after bladder and bowel elimination, before and after handling peripads, and always before handling the infant.

**Breast care for lactating mothers.** Instruct the breastfeeding mother to avoid using soap on her nipples because it will remove the natural lubrication secreted by the Montgomery's glands. Keeping the nipples dry between feedings helps prevent tissue damage, and wearing a good bra provides necessary support as breast size increases.

**Measures to suppress lactation.** If the mother chooses not to breastfeed, initiate measures to suppress lactation. Instruct the woman to wear a well-fitting bra or sports bra 24 hours a day until the breasts become soft.

Manage discomfort by applying ice, which reduces vasocongestion, and with analgesics. Advise the woman to refrain from stimulating milk production by pumping or massaging the breasts or allowing warm water to fall directly on the breasts during showers. Tenderness and engorgement should return to normal in 48 to 72 hours (Janke, 2013).

**Care of the cesarean incision.** If the birth was cesarean, the woman may have concerns about the care of the incision. If adhesive strips have been applied over the incision, teach her that she can shower with the strips in place and that they will gradually detach. If a topical skin adhesive was used, no dressing is necessary, and the woman is generally allowed to shower.

For each method, explain that the incision is closed and is unlikely to come apart. There should be little or no drainage from the incision. Instruct her to call her provider if the incision separates or drainage increases or has a foul smell.

**Perineal care.** Teach the woman how to clean the perineum. The most common method is to fill a squeeze bottle with warm water and spray the perineal area from the front toward the back. Remind the new mother not to separate the labia during this procedure to avoid allowing water to enter the vagina. The tip of the bottle should not touch the perineum during use.

Toilet paper or moist antiseptic towelettes are used in a patting motion to dry the perineum. Teach the mother to dry from front to back to prevent fecal contamination from the anal area to the vaginal introitus. She should perform perineal cleansing and change peripads after each voiding or defecation.

Some women do not use peripads for menstrual protection and must be taught how to use them correctly. Mesh panties and adhering pads are used in most facilities. Careful handling of the pads is important to prevent localized perineal infection:

- Thorough handwashing is a must before and after changing the pads.
- Unused pads should be stored inside their package.
- Pads should be applied without touching the side that comes into contact with the perineum.
- The pads should be applied and removed in a front-to-back direction to prevent contamination of the vagina and perineum.
- Used pads must be disposed of properly.

**Kegel exercises.** All women should become familiar with **Kegel exercises** (see Chapter 32). These movements strengthen the muscles that surround the vagina and urinary meatus. The exercise helps prevent the loss of muscle tone that can occur after childbirth and may decrease the risk for urinary incontinence.

The Kegel exercise involves contracting muscles around the vagina (as though stopping the flow of urine), holding tightly for 10 seconds, and then relaxing for 10 seconds. The woman should work up to 30 contraction-relaxation cycles or more each day.

***Promoting rest and sleep.*** Postpartum fatigue is common during the early days after birth and often continues for weeks or months. The extreme fatigue that mothers experience has a variety of contributing factors. Women are tired when they begin the postpartum period because they sleep poorly during the third trimester and are exhausted by the exertion of labor. Feelings of excitement and euphoria after childbirth interfere with rest. Numerous visitors and phone calls, hospital routines and noise, an unfamiliar environment, and physical discomfort all make it hard for the new mother to rest. Mothers often go home with a tremendous deficit in sleep and energy.

Screening women by a telephone call 2 weeks after they give birth may identify those with prolonged postpartum fatigue. Anemia, infection, and thyroid dysfunction may also be the cause of postpartum fatigue. Evaluation for these conditions should be considered in women at risk or suffering postpartum fatigue after the first 2 weeks (Giallo, Cooklin, Dunning, et al., 2014).

**Rest at the birth facility.** Frequent interruptions make rest difficult during the birth facility stay. Find ways to avoid interruptions and to increase mothers' opportunities for unbroken rest periods and relaxed time with their infants. Some agencies set aside a "quiet time" each afternoon where mothers are encouraged to rest without being disturbed. Group the assessments and care in a way that minimizes interruptions, and plan with the mother for a time for napping. Suggest that she restrict phone calls and visitors during these times. Encourage the use of the side-lying position for breastfeeding to allow her to rest during feedings.

## NURSING CARE PLAN

### *Postpartum Hypotension, Fatigue, and Pain*

**Focused Assessment**

Four hours after giving birth vaginally, Lani's vital signs are: blood pressure (BP), 126/80 mm Hg (baseline 124/78 mm Hg); pulse (P), 70 beats per minute (bpm); and respirations (R), 16 breaths per minute. Her fundus is firm, midline at the umbilicus, and her lochia is moderate rubra. Her hemoglobin at the end of pregnancy was 10.8 g/dL. When she attempts to ambulate the first time, she becomes weak and dizzy. Her gait is unsteady, and the nurse has to lower her back to bed to prevent her from fainting. Her color is pale and vital signs are: BP, 104/84 mm Hg; P, 86 bpm; and R, 20 breaths per minute.

**Nursing Diagnosis**

Risk for Injury related to physiologic effects of orthostatic hypotension.

**Planning**

***Expected Outcome***

Lani will remain free of injury caused by fainting or falling during the postpartum period.

**Interventions and *Rationales***

1. Obtain the assistance of a second staff person the next time ambulation is attempted until Lani is able to ambulate without feeling dizzy or faint.
   *This helps prevent injury to Lani or the staff if Lani should start to fall.*
2. Check her BP while she is in a supine position and in a sitting position before attempting to get her out of bed again.
   *This will determine if there has been a drop in BP, indicating orthostatic hypotension.* Use the same arm each time the BP is taken. *This procedure will improve accuracy.*
3. Elevate the head of the bed for a few minutes and then help Lani sit on the side of the bed for several minutes before standing. *This will allow her BP to stabilize before she stands.* Help her to stand slowly.
4. Instruct Lani to bend her knees and move her feet constantly when she first stands to increase venous return from the legs.
   *This helps maintain cardiac output and increases cerebral circulation.*
5. Suggest that she take brief, tepid (not hot) showers and that she bend her knees and "march" during the shower.
   *Hot water dilates peripheral blood vessels, allowing additional blood to remain in the vessels of the legs. Moving the feet and legs increases blood return from the legs.*
   Provide a chair in the shower for her to use if she feels weak or faint.
6. Initiate measures to prevent injuries that could occur if Lani were to faint:
   a. Stay with her when she ambulates, and be prepared to assist her in sitting down and lowering her head. *This will increase blood flow to the brain.* Gently lower her to the floor if she becomes faint.
   b. Call for additional assistance, if needed, before attempting to return her to bed. *Adequate assistance is needed to prevent injuries.*
   c. Remind Lani to call for assistance before trying to ambulate. Check to see that the call light is conveniently located. *This measure increases safety.*

**Evaluation**

Lani participates in self-care and has sustained no injury during her hospital stay.

**Focused Assessment**

On the second day after delivery, Lani expresses concern about her third-degree episiotomy and asks what she can do to prevent the pain she experienced during intercourse for several months after the birth of her first child, who is now 18 months old.

**Nursing Diagnosis**

Risk for Ineffective Sexuality Pattern related to fatigue and pain.

**Planning**

***Expected Outcomes***

Before discharge the couple will:

1. Verbalize measures to promote comfort during sexual activity.
2. Verbalize a plan to reduce fatigue, which interferes with interest in and energy for sexual activity by discharge.

**Interventions and *Rationales***

1. Recommend that the parents postpone vaginal intercourse until the perineum is well healed.
   *Such postponement will reduce pain or fear of pain during sexual activity.*
2. Suggest measures that may *lessen fatigue, which decreases interest in sexual activity after childbirth:*
   a. Recommend that each partner nap for 30 minutes sometime during the day or evening.
   b. Suggest that sexual activity occur in the morning or afternoon rather than at the end of a tiring day.
   c. Counsel the parents to rest when the infant has long periods of sleep and that they postpone additional home projects that will increase fatigue until the infant is older and is sleeping through the night.
3. Remind the mother to perform Kegel exercises until she can comfortably do 30 each day.
   *These exercises strengthen the muscles around the vagina and promote increased sexual satisfaction.*
4. Advise that the infant be breastfed just before the parents initiate sexual activity.
   *This will allow uninterrupted time while the infant sleeps. Breastfeeding also reduces the chance of leaking milk, which interferes with sexual pleasure for some couples.*
5. Remind parents that sexual arousal may be slower because of decreased hormone levels and fatigue. More stimulation may be necessary before the mother is sexually aroused.
   *This knowledge helps reduce the anxiety and tension that occur if the parents are unprepared.*
6. Recommend the use of a water-soluble vaginal lubricant (Lubrin, Replens, K-Y jelly).
   *This will increase comfort because breastfeeding decreases estrogen, causing vaginal dryness.*
7. Before vaginal intercourse, as part of foreplay, suggest that one finger be inserted into the vaginal introitus.
   *This will determine areas of tenderness or pain, gently stretch the perineal scar, and increase comfort.*
8. Advise that Lani assume the superior position during intercourse.
   *In this position, the woman controls the depth and location of penetration, which can help reduce her discomfort.*
9. Discuss the need for frank communication between partners regarding measures that reduce discomfort, as well as specific concerns and needs.
   *Communication facilitates understanding and fosters a feeling of closeness that can enhance sexual interest.*

**Evaluation**

Before discharge, the couple verbalizes a plan to reduce fatigue and provide rest for Lani. They express interest in trying measures to increase comfort during sexual activities.

***Additional Nursing Diagnoses to Consider***

Interrupted Family Processes
Ineffective Health Maintenance
Impaired Parenting
Disturbed Sleep Pattern

**Rest at home.** Help the mother understand the effect that her physical discomfort and the demands of the newborn and other family members will have on her energy when she returns home. If she understands that fatigue is normal and will continue for some time, she can plan ways to obtain extra help and conserve her energy. Start with the following suggestions:

- Maintain a relaxed, flexible routine that focuses on the care of the mother and infant.
- Nap or rest when the infant sleeps, if possible.
- Plan simple meals and flexible meal times.
- Limit visitors.
- Accept assistance with food shopping, meal preparation, laundry, and housework.
- Ask family or friends to care for the infant to provide nap times for the mother.
- Put off housework that is not absolutely necessary.
- Postpone major household projects.
- Involve friends and family to provide care for other children.

Explain to the mother that she should delay her return to employment, if possible, until the infant sleeps through the night (usually by 3 to 4 months) or later. It takes time to recover from the birth as well as to adjust to the changes that occur with a new baby.

Suggest relaxation exercises (lying quietly, alternately tightening and relaxing the muscles of the neck, shoulders, arms, legs, and feet) when a nap is not possible. Emphasize to the mother the importance of asking for help when she begins to feel exhausted or overwhelmed. Encourage her to share these feelings with her partner, family, friends, and other new mothers.

***Providing nutrition counseling***

**Food supply.** Families of low socioeconomic status may benefit from referral to government-sponsored programs, such as Temporary Assistance for Needy Families (TANF) or the Special Supplemental Nutrition Program for Women, Infants, and Children (WIC) to help them obtain adequate food. It also may be necessary to determine what facilities are available for cooking and storing food. Sometimes the new family may need referral to a social worker for solutions for their unique problems.

**Diet.** Although many women are unsatisfied with slow weight loss, they should avoid severe restriction of caloric intake. Explain the need to select foods that provide adequate calories to meet energy needs, taking into account the time and energy needed to care for a newborn (see Chapter 14). Strict dieting should be avoided.

***Promoting regular bowel elimination.*** Explain the role of progressive exercise, adequate fluid, and dietary fiber in preventing constipation. Walking is perhaps the best exercise, and the distance can be increased as strength and endurance increase. Drinking at least eight glasses of water daily helps maintain normal bowel elimination. Unpeeled fruits and vegetables are high in fiber and prunes act as a natural laxative. Additional fiber is found in whole-grain cereals, bread, and pasta.

A regular schedule of bowel elimination is important in overcoming constipation. For example, bowel elimination after breakfast allows the mother to take advantage of the gastrocolic reflex (stimulation of peristalsis induced in the colon when food is consumed on an empty stomach). Measures that reduce perineal and hemorrhoidal pain, such as witch hazel astringent compresses and hydrocortisone ointments, also facilitate bowel elimination.

***Promoting good body mechanics***

**Exercise.** Teach exercises in the early postpartum period to strengthen the abdominal muscles and firm the waist (Fig. 20.6, pp. 410-411). The exercises can be started soon after childbirth with five repetitions twice a day, at first. The number of exercises is gradually increased as the mother gains strength.

The nurse can reassure women seeking weight loss that moderate exercise will not interfere with lactation and will lead to more rapid weight reduction. Exercise classes that sometimes include the infant are often available for postpartum women. Common barriers to postpartum exercise are child care needs and lack of time. Walking is a common exercise, and women can take the infant with them on walks. Women who plan for exercise and do it with a friend are more likely to fit it into their schedules (Cochrum, 2015).

Instruct postcesarean mothers to follow the instructions of their healthcare provider. Less-vigorous exercise, such as walking, is appropriate at first. Women should not begin abdominal exercises for 4 weeks after cesarean birth (James, 2013).

**Preventing back strain.** Back strain often can be prevented if the mother and father find a location for infant care, such as a kitchen table or bathroom counter, that does not require bending or leaning forward. For lifting objects, teach parents to hold the back straight as they squat and use the legs rather than bending at the waist (see Fig. 13.11).

***Counseling about sexual activity.*** The couple may have concerns about resuming sexual intercourse and contraceptive choices. Fatigue, pain, concerns about the baby, and a feeling of unattractiveness may interfere with a woman's sexual desire. Couples can begin intercourse as early as 2 weeks after giving birth, if desire and comfort allow (Cunningham et al., 2014). A longer wait is needed if the woman is still sore. Breastfeeding women have low estrogen levels and may need to use a water-soluble lubricant to increase comfort. Some women have increased nipple sensitivity during lactation and do not want their breasts touched during love-making (Nobre, 2011). It is important that nurses provide such information to new mothers and their partners.

Many new parents are reluctant to ask about when to resume sexual activity and about potential changes in sexuality resulting from pregnancy and childbirth. If couples do not indicate such concerns, introduce the topic in a general, nonspecific manner, such as, "You have an episiotomy, which may cause some discomfort with intercourse until it has completely healed," or "Sometimes couples are not aware that some vaginal dryness occurs in breastfeeding women." Such broad opening statements permit the couple to pursue the topic as they desire (see Nursing Care Plan: Postpartum Hypotension, Fatigue, and Pain on p. 408).

Cultural or religious convictions may restrict the choice of contraceptive methods for some couples, and the availability of healthcare or limited finances may dictate the choice for others. Discuss previous experience with contraceptives and the satisfaction with those methods (see Chapter 31).

***Instructing about follow-up appointments.*** Remind the new mother to make an appointment with her physician or nurse-midwife for a postpartum examination at a time suggested by her provider (usually 4 to 6 weeks after childbirth after vaginal birth, 2 weeks after cesarean birth). Emphasize the importance of the postpartum examination because it allows early identification and treatment of problems that may develop. Instruct the woman to call her provider if problems occur before the appointment.

***Teaching about signs and symptoms that should be reported.*** Teach new mothers and at least one other family member which physical signs and symptoms should be reported to the healthcare provider immediately. These signs and symptoms include:

- Fever
- Localized area of redness, swelling, or pain in either breast
- Persistent abdominal tenderness
- Feelings of pelvic fullness or pressure
- Persistent perineal pain
- Frequency, urgency, or burning on urination

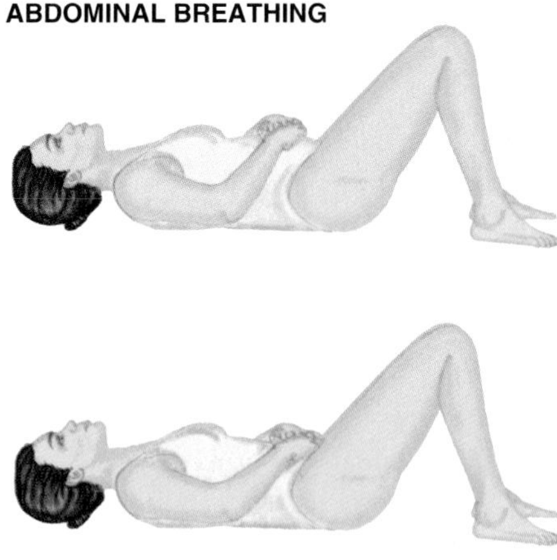


This is one of the simplest exercises and can be started on the first postpartum day. The woman assumes a supine position with knees bent. She inhales through the nose, keeps the rib cage as stationary as possible, and allows the abdomen to expand. She then contracts the abdominal muscles as she exhales slowly through the mouth.

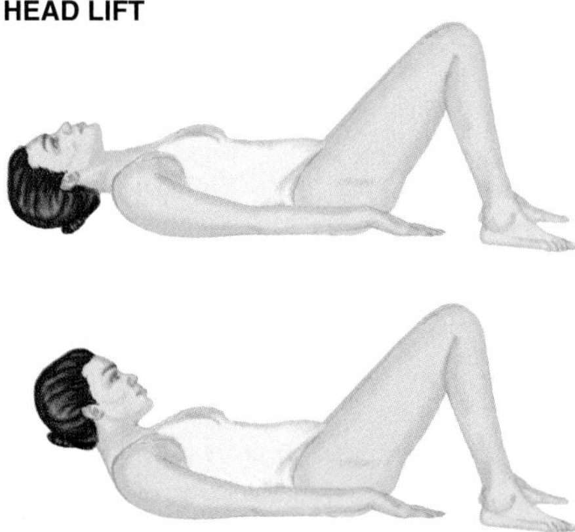


This exercise can be started within a few days after childbirth. The mother is supine with knees bent and arms outstretched at her side. She inhales deeply to begin, then exhales while lifting the head slowly; she holds the position for a few seconds and relaxes.

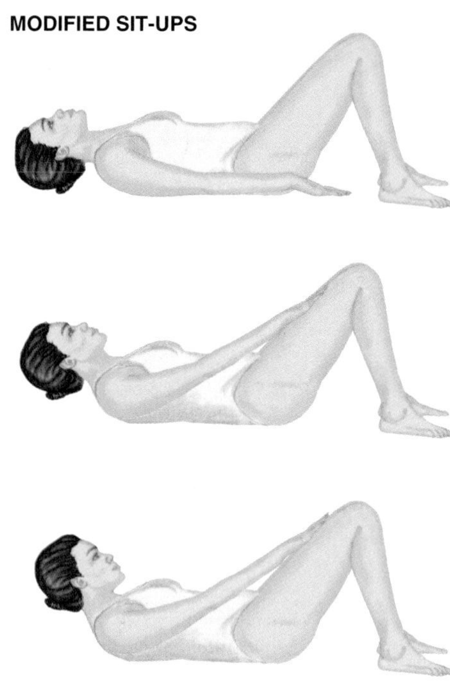


Head lifts may progress to modified sit-ups with the approval of the health care provider; the mother should follow the advice of the health care provider about the number of repetitions.

The exercise begins with the mother supine with arms outstretched and the knees bent. She raises her head and shoulders as her hands reach for her knees. She raises the shoulders only as far as the back will bend; her waist remains on the floor.

**FIG 20.6** Postpartum exercises.

- Abnormal change in character of lochia (increased amount, resumption of bright red color, passage of clots, foul odor)
- Localized tenderness, redness, edema, or warmth of the legs
- Redness, the separation of or foul drainage from an abdominal incision

***Ensuring that all elements have been taught.*** Streamline and organize information so it can be presented in the time available. Provide group instruction, such as infant care demonstrations and breastfeeding classes to use time for teaching efficiently. These provide an opportunity for mothers to ask questions pertaining to their own needs and concerns about their infants that watching videos or television shows do not. Innovations include conducting sensing sessions with patients, adding emergency information to discharge instructions, teleconferencing with a top decile hospital, adding questions related to leader rounding, adding a video to interactive woman education system, and adding a discharge pathway for postpartum patients (Fleischman, 2015). Individual teaching is necessary, in addition, to meet each woman's needs.

Although there are many subjects that must be discussed in parent teaching, avoid covering too much information at a time. Interspersing small segments of teaching throughout the day will help keep the woman from being overwhelmed and help her remember information better.

***Documenting teaching.*** Documentation is an important aspect of teaching, just as it is for other aspects of nursing care. Documentation that discharge teaching was performed and that the patient has indicated comprehension of teaching is required by accrediting agencies. To prevent omissions, many hospitals use teaching checklists to record the topics taught.

## Evaluation

- Does the mother demonstrate correct breast and perineal hygiene?
- Can the mother verbalize her plan to manage diet, rest, and exercise after discharge?
- Can she describe her plan for follow-up care and signs that indicate the need for immediate treatment?

**KNEE AND LEG ROLLS**

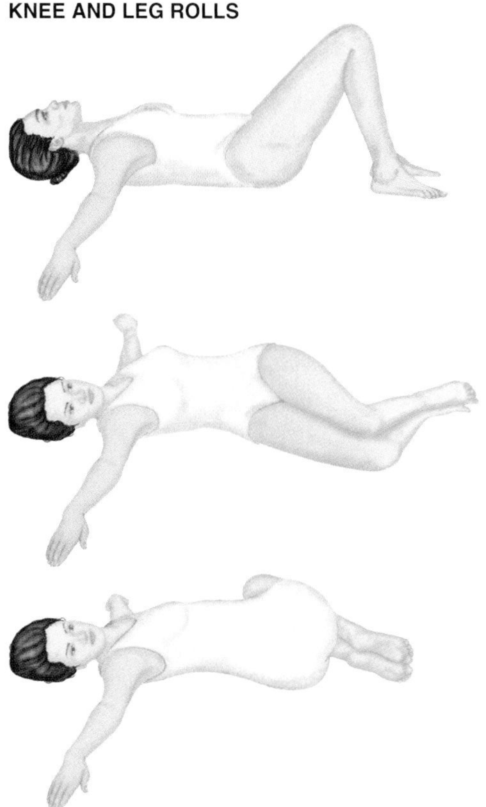

This is an excellent exercise to begin firming the waist. The mother lies flat on her back with knees bent and feet flat on the floor or bed; she keeps the shoulders and feet stationary and rolls the knees to touch first one side of the bed, then the other. She maintains a smooth motion as the exercise is repeated five times. Later, as flexibility increases, the exercise can be varied by the rolling of one knee only. The mother rolls her left knee to touch the right side of the bed, returns to center, and rolls the right knee to touch the left side of the bed.

**CHEST EXERCISES**

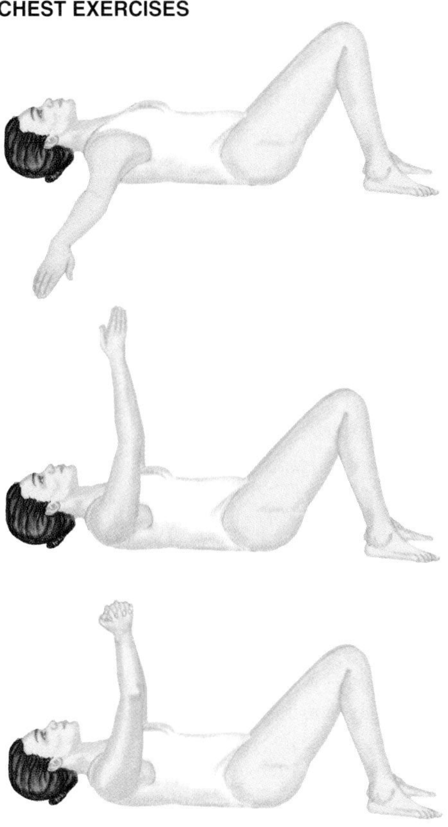

This is an excellent exercise to strengthen the chest muscles. The mother lies flat with arms extended straight out to the side; she brings the hands together above the chest while keeping the arms straight; she holds for a few seconds and returns to the starting position. She repeats the exercise five times initially and follows the advice of the health care provider for increasing the number of repetitions.

Isometric exercises also increase strength and tone; the mother bends her elbows, clasps her hands together above her chest, and presses her hands together for a few seconds. This is repeated at least five times.

**FIG 20.6, cont'd** Postpartum exercises.

## THE PROCESS OF BECOMING ACQUAINTED

Perhaps no other event requires such rapid change in family structure and function as the birth of a baby. The addition of a new baby requires that all family members adjust their roles.

The role of maternity nurses includes not only the care of the mother-infant dyad but the well-being of the entire family as well. Nurses are concerned about the family's adjustment to childbearing during the birth facility stay and the early weeks at home as new parents make the transition to parenthood.

Nursing literature has described how parents and newborns become acquainted and progress to develop feelings of love, concern, and deep devotion that last throughout life. The terms *bonding* and *attachment* are commonly used to describe the initial steps. Although the terms are sometimes used interchangeably, their meanings differ.

### Bonding

Bonding describes the initial attraction felt by parents for their infants. It is unidirectional, from parent to child, and is enhanced when parent and infant are permitted to touch and interact during the first 30 to 60 minutes after birth. During this time, the infant is in a quiet, alert state and seems to gaze directly at the parents (Fig. 20.7). Infants may be placed skin-to-skin on the mother's chest after delivery. Nurses frequently delay procedures such as instillation of prophylactic eye medications that can interfere with this time between parents and newborns so that parents can focus on their baby. When birth is by cesarean, mothers often hold their infants in the recovery room to enhance this process. Bonding can also occur later if parent-infant interaction does not occur immediately after birth.

### Attachment

Attachment is the process by which an enduring bond between a parent and child is developed through pleasurable, satisfying interaction. The process begins in pregnancy and extends for many months after childbirth. The infant receives warmth, food, and security from the parent. The parent (usually the mother) places the child's needs above her own for years to come. In return, she receives enjoyment and establishes her identity as a mother. Both benefit from the formation of irreplaceable links that continue long after the child ceases to be dependent.

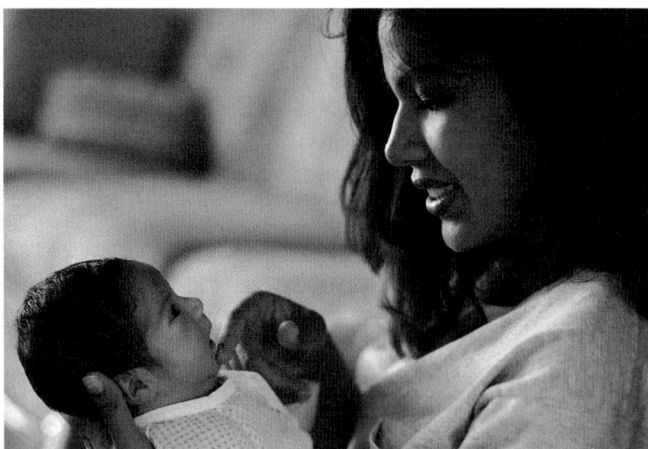

FIG 20.7 The infant is quiet and alert during the initial sensitive period. The newborn gazes at the mother and responds to her voice and touch. The mother touches only with her fingertips at first.

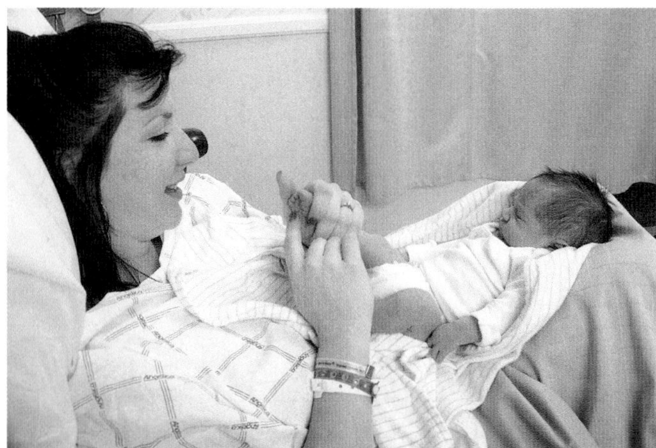

FIG 20.8 The mother begins to stroke her infant as she progresses in becoming acquainted.

Attachment follows a progressive course that changes over time. It is rarely instantaneous. Attachment occurs through mutually satisfying experiences. Therefore, if the newly delivered mother is in severe pain or is exhausted, she needs pain relief and assistance for her to enjoy the early experiences with the baby.

Unlike bonding, attachment is reciprocal—it occurs in both directions between parent and infant. Attachment is facilitated by positive feedback from the infant, either real or perceived. For example, an infant's grasp reflex around a parent's finger means "I love you" to the parent. Alert infants have a repertoire of responses called **reciprocal attachment behaviors** that promote early attachment. They are the infant's part in the process of early attachment that progresses to lifelong mutual devotion.

**! NURSING QUALITY ALERT**

***Reciprocal Attachment Behaviors***

Newborn infants have the ability to:

- Make eye contact and engage in prolonged, intense, mutual gazing
- Move their eyes and attempt to "track" the parent's face
- Grasp and hold the parent's finger
- Move synchronously in response to rhythms and patterns of the parent's voice (called **entrainment**)
- Root, latch on to the breast, and suckle
- Be comforted by the parent's voice or touch

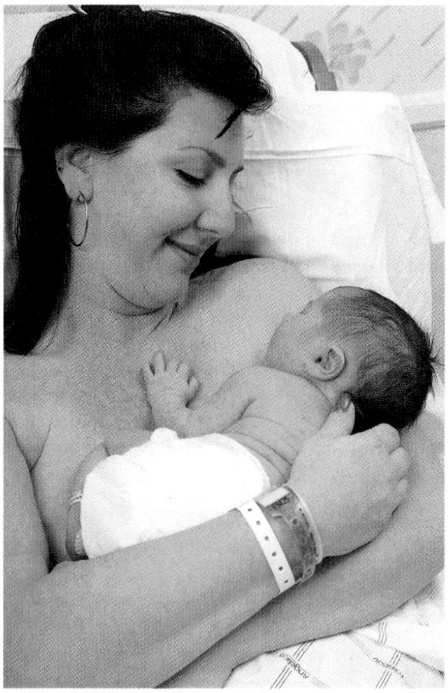

FIG 20.9 Mothers progress from exploratory touching to enfolding the infant. Their pleasure is enhanced by skin-to-skin contact.

## Maternal Touch

Maternal behavior, particularly maternal touch, changes rapidly as the mother progresses through a discovery phase with her infant. Initially the mother may not reach for the infant, but if the infant is placed in her arms, she holds the baby in an **en face** position, with the infant's face in the same vertical plane as her own so they can make eye contact. When the infant is awake, the two engage in prolonged mutual gazing (see Fig. 20.7).

**Fingertipping** is common during the early minutes as the mother gets acquainted with the tiny stranger. It describes the mother's first exploration of the infant's body. She may gently explore the infant's face, fingers, and toes with her fingertips only (see Fig. 20.7). She then begins to stroke the baby's chest and legs with her palm (Fig. 20.8). Next, the mother uses her entire hand to enfold the infant and to bring her baby close to her body. She strokes the baby's hair, presses her cheek against the infant's cheek, and finally feels comfortable enough to engage in a full range of consoling behaviors (Fig. 20.9).

The mother next begins to identify specific features of the newborn: "Look how bright his eyes are." Then she begins to relate features to family members. "He has his father's chin and nose" (Fig. 20.10). This identification process has been called *claiming* or *binding in* (Rubin, 1977).

## Verbal Behaviors

Verbal behaviors are also important indicators of maternal attachment. Most mothers speak to the infant in a high-pitched voice.

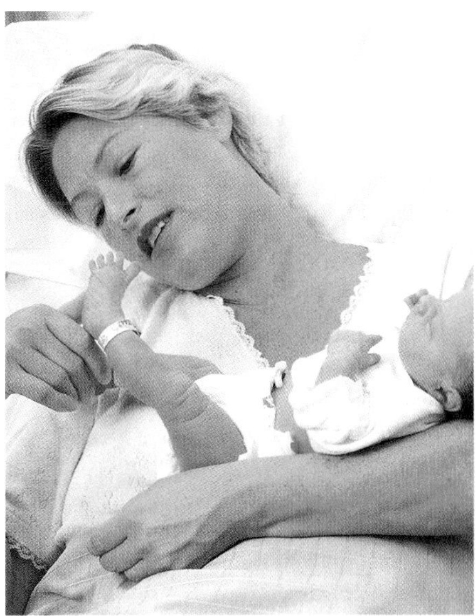

**FIG 20.10** The binding-in, or claiming, process includes the mother's identification of her baby's specific features, relating them to other family members. This mother states, "His long toes are exactly like mine."

Although many mothers have been calling the infant by name since seeing it on an ultrasound scan during pregnancy, some wait until after the birth to progress from calling the baby "it" to "he" or "she" and then to using the given name. Verbal behaviors may provide clues to a mother's early psychological relationship with her infant. Nurses observe the interactions of mothers and their infants and, if necessary, teach and model interactions that foster early attachment between them.

## THE PROCESS OF MATERNAL ROLE ADAPTATION

### Puerperal Phases

In the early 1960s, Rubin identified restorative phases that mothers go through to replenish the energy lost during labor and attain comfort in their new role. The puerperal phases are called *taking-in, taking-hold,* and *letting-go.* They provide one method of observing change in maternal behavior that can be helpful in anticipating maternal needs and in intervening to meet those needs.

#### Taking-in Phase

During the taking-in phase, the mother is focused primarily on her own need for fluid, food, and sleep. Inexperienced nurses may be puzzled by the mother's passive, dependent behavior as she takes in or receives attention and physical care. She also takes in every detail of the neonate, but she seems content to allow others to make decisions.

A major task for the mother during this time is to integrate her birth experience into reality. To do this she discusses her labor and delivery in detail with visitors or on the telephone. This process helps the mother realize that the pregnancy is over and the newborn is an individual separate from her.

Although Rubin (1961) believed that the taking-in phase lasted for approximately 2 days, it probably lasts a day or less today. The phase may be prolonged when a cesarean birth, especially in an emergency, has been necessary. These women may have difficulty assimilating the unfamiliar and intrusive procedures that occurred very rapidly and may have negative perceptions of the birth experience.

#### Taking-Hold Phase

The mother becomes more independent in the taking-hold phase. She exhibits concern about managing her own body functions and assumes responsibility for her own care. When she feels more comfortable and in control of her body, she shifts her attention to the behaviors of the infant. She welcomes information about the wide variety of behaviors exhibited by newborns.

During the taking-hold phase, the mother may verbalize anxiety about her competence as a mother. She may compare her caretaking skills unfavorably with those of the nurse.

The nurse must be careful not to take over the care of the infant. The mother should be encouraged to perform as much of the caretaking as possible as she assumes the mothering role. Fathers should also be encouraged to participate in caretaking as they take on a new role. The nurse should praise each attempt, even if the parents' early care is awkward.

The taking-hold phase, which extends over several days, has been called the "teachable, reachable, referable moment." Nurses who provide home or clinic care can take advantage of this ideal time to review previously taught material and provide additional instructions and demonstrations.

#### Letting-Go Phase

The letting-go phase is a time of relinquishment for the mother and often for the father. If this is a first child, the couple must give up their previous role as a childless couple and acknowledge the loss of their more carefree lifestyle. Many mothers must also give up idealized expectations of the birth experience. For example, they may have planned to have a vaginal birth with minimal or no anesthesia, but instead required a cesarean birth.

In addition, some mothers and fathers are disappointed by the size, gender, or characteristics of the infant who does not "match up" with the fantasy baby of pregnancy. They must relinquish the infant of their fantasies and accept the real infant. These losses often provoke feelings of grief that may be so subtle that they are unexamined or unacknowledged. However, both parents may benefit if given the opportunity to discuss unexpected feelings and to realize that these feelings are common. If the mother is very young or the pregnancy was unplanned, the feelings of loss and grief may be acute.

### Maternal Role Attainment

Role attainment is a process in which the mother achieves confidence in her ability to care for her infant and becomes comfortable with her identity as a mother. The process begins during pregnancy and continues for several months after childbirth. The transition to the maternal or paternal role follows four stages (Mercer, 1995b):

1. The anticipatory stage begins during the pregnancy when the pregnant woman chooses a physician or nurse-midwife. She may attend childbirth classes to prepare for the birth experience. She seeks out role models to learn the role of mother.
2. The formal stage begins with the birth of the infant and continues for approximately 4 to 6 weeks (Mercer, 1995a). During this stage, behaviors are mainly guided by others such as health professionals, close friends, or parents. A major task during this stage is for parents to become acquainted with their infants so that they can mesh their caregiving with infant cues.

### CRITICAL THINKING EXERCISE 20.2

Carol, a 35-year-old primipara, had a cesarean birth after failure to progress in labor. She is very tired, although she is relatively comfortable. On the day of delivery, Carol readily accepts attention and assistance with hygiene. She recounts the details of her labor to friends on the telephone. She examines her baby girl closely and touches the infant's face and hands gently with her fingertips. She remarks that she plans to breastfeed and is surprised that the infant sleeps so much.

Carol's husband is excited but expresses concern about discharge. He states he and Carol have little experience with infants and his job requires almost constant travel. He worries if she and the baby will be all right.

1. What are Carol's priority needs at this time?
2. What phase of recovery is she manifesting? Why does she "fingertip" the infant?

   On the first postoperative day, Carol's catheter is removed, and intravenous (IV) fluids are discontinued. She ambulates with minimal assistance and is pleased that she is able to urinate without difficulty. She asks about bowel function and requests the prescribed stool softener. She spends a great deal of time helping the baby breastfeed. She is very frustrated that the infant does not breastfeed well and asks for assistance from the lactation consultant.
3. What are Carol's priority needs now?
4. How have her behaviors changed?

   Before discharge, Carol is breastfeeding well. The infant latches on and nurses for 10 to 15 minutes on each breast, and Carol's nipples are free of tenderness or signs of trauma. She has no relatives in the area, and her husband is home for the weekend only. She states that she will just have to get along by herself after that.
5. What anticipatory guidance should Carol receive before discharge?
6. What further nursing interventions would be most helpful to her and the baby?

3. The informal stage may overlap the formal stage. It begins once the mother has learned appropriate responses to her infant's cues or signals. She begins to respond according to the unique needs of the infant rather than following textbook or health professionals' directives.
4. The personal stage is attained when the mother feels a sense of harmony in her role, sees the infant as a central person in her life, and has internalized the parental role. The mother accepts and feels comfortable with the role of parent.

Maternal role attainment implies an end point when the woman adjusts to motherhood. However, the process could better be called "becoming a mother" because it continues throughout motherhood. The mothering role grows and evolves as the mother responds to the challenges of her child's growth and development (Mercer, 2004). Most mothers do not feel competent and self-confident in the mothering role until approximately 4 months after childbirth (Mercer & Walker, 2006).

### Heading Toward a New Normal

Martell (2001) provides another view of early postpartum changes with *Heading Toward a New Normal* as the theme. This view also has three phases as the woman reorganizes her life as a mother. Although the phases have distinctive characteristics, they are continuous rather than separate.

***Appreciating the body.*** This phase centers on the way the woman feels physically as she copes with discomfort, fatigue, and changes in her body. The phase also involves dealing with emotional lability and changes in the way women think and retain information.

***Settling in.*** During settling in, mothers become more secure with their infants. They gradually gain in competence and confidence in their abilities to care for their infants without help from others. They adapt their needs and activities to meet the needs of the infant. Some find ways to integrate the infant into their usual activities with only minor changes.

***Becoming a new family.*** As women work toward becoming a new family, they modify relationships with their partners and other family members. They develop new routines to include the infant and enjoy spending time alone with their newly developed family.

### Redefining Roles

The mother is particularly concerned about redefining roles and focuses on maintaining a strong, adaptive relationship with her partner. She observes him carefully for any change in behavior and is acutely sensitive to his interaction with the infant. From the father's perspective, anxieties about succeeding in his new role put added pressure on the family. Conflicting demands between work and home, feelings of exclusion, and concerns about his relationship with his partner present additional challenges.

The new parents may need to agree on a division of tasks and responsibilities that was not necessary before the birth of the infant. This process is accomplished quickly and with very little discord in some families. Role assignment in other families is much less flexible, and any change can be a source of tension and frustration.

Although nurses are not actively involved in redefining family roles, they can use their skills in communication to assist the family in expressing their feelings and concerns so that the changes can be accomplished with minimal stress.

### Role Conflict

Role conflict occurs when one's perception of role responsibilities differs significantly from reality. For example, if the mother perceives that her responsibility is to provide most of the care and comfort for the infant but reality dictates that she must return to full-time employment, role conflict may occur. In the United States, nearly 64% of mothers with children younger than 6 years and more than 56.5% of mothers with infants younger than 1 year of age were employed in 2010 (U.S. Department of Labor, 2011).

Primiparas often do not realize how strong their attachment to the infant will be or how difficult it will be for them to leave the infant to return to work. Many women feel guilty and experience intense "separation grief" when they first leave the infant with a caregiver. Some report feeling jealous of the caregiver and fear that the caregiver will supplant them in the infant's affection.

The nurse can help by acknowledging these feelings and reassuring the mother that her emotions are normal. The mother needs to plan for time to reestablish feelings of closeness when she comes home from work. She should try to develop a schedule that allows maximum time with the infant when she is at home. She may have to negotiate with another family member to take over some of the household tasks until she feels more comfortable with the situation (Nursing Care Plan: Adaptation of the Working Mother).

## Major Maternal Concerns

As the woman gains confidence in her ability to care for the infant and her physical discomfort decreases, emotional concerns related to the self become more important. Body image and the experience of postpartum blues are particularly important.

## NURSING CARE PLAN

### *Adaptation of the Working Mother*

**Focused Assessment**

Rebecca, a 30-year-old single mother is ready to go home after giving birth to a baby boy by cesarean delivery 6 days ago. Breastfeeding is going well. During her visit to a nurse-managed postpartum clinic, Rebecca discusses her need to return to work as a sales executive in 6 weeks. She states that she hates the thought of leaving the baby with someone else while she works: "I've always wanted to stay home for at least 6 months when I had a baby, but it's just impossible. How can I be a mother and work full time?"

**Nursing Diagnosis**

Parental Role Conflict related to inability to perform the role of mother as she wishes secondary to the need to return to full-time employment.

**Planning**

***Expected Outcomes***

Rebecca will:

1. Describe her concerns and feelings about leaving her infant with a caregiver by the time of discharge.
2. Verbalize plans to achieve maximum satisfaction in her role as mother by the time of her postpartum checkup.

**Interventions and *Rationales***

1. Allow Rebecca to describe her perception of her role as mother and to express concerns about how employment will interfere with her ability to fulfill this role.
   *Venting helps her cope with the role conflict, stress, and grief she feels.*
2. Recommend free expression of feelings to significant others and to the care provider who is selected.
   *This may lead to a discussion of measures that will help to overcome her feelings of conflict.*
3. Acknowledge the feelings Rebecca expresses, and reassure her that the feelings are common.
   *This shows Rebecca that her feelings are not trivial and are experienced by others.*
4. Help her develop a schedule that allows her maximum time with the infant.
   *This will help alleviate feelings of stress and frustration.*
5. Recommend that she allow 30 to 45 minutes to hold the infant when she first gets home.
   *This will help make the transition from work to home.* Delay all other activities until this need is met. *This will help reestablish feelings of comfort and closeness.*
6. Suggest that Rebecca delay her return to employment, if possible, until the infant is at least 12 to 16 weeks old. Part-time work or work from home may also be a possibility for a time.
   *Most infants are sleeping long periods at night by 12 to 16 weeks of age. This reduces sleep deprivation in parents.*
7. Recommend that she investigate several daycare providers. She should check references, make unannounced visits, see required licenses and certification, discuss the number and ages of children cared for and the daily schedule, ask about the provider's philosophy of infant care and training in emergency measures, and know what emergency plans are in place.
   *This will increase her confidence in the competence of the caregiver she chooses.*
8. Suggest that she leave the infant with the chosen daycare provider for 2 or 3 days before resuming full-time employment.
   *This will help "practice separating" and make the transition less traumatic.*
9. Recommend that Rebecca pump her breasts and feed the infant by bottle at least once a day for a week or two before returning to work.
   *This will help her become proficient at pumping and help the infant adapt to bottle feeding during their separation.*

**Evaluation**

Rebecca expresses her feelings of guilt, anxiety, and concern about leaving her infant. She has a plan to investigate daycare in her area and verbalized plans to reorganize her work and social schedule so that she can spend as much time as possible with her son.

***Additional Nursing Diagnoses to Consider***

Deficient Diversional Activity
Grieving
Ineffective Role Performance

### Body Image

Women are very concerned about regaining their normal figures and may have unrealistic expectations about weight loss. Nurses must emphasize that weight loss should be gradual. Rigid restriction of calories can lead to depleted energy and decreased immunity. Appropriate exercise should also be discussed. Some birth facilities offer classes for postpartum mothers that include exercise and nutrition, as well as the opportunity to share concerns with other postpartum women.

### Smoking

Many women give up smoking during pregnancy to protect the health of the fetus. However, the majority of women resume smoking in the first 6 months postpartum. Factors that increase the likelihood of relapse include weight concerns and failure to breastfeed (Yang & Hall, 2014; Gyllstrom, Hellerstedt, & Hennrikus, 2012). Women who breastfeed their infants are less likely to resume smoking by 26 weeks postpartum (Oweis, 2012). Other factors that may cause relapse are depression, living with a smoker, stress, and planning to quit only during the pregnancy.

Nurses should discuss smoking with postpartum women to offer resources for those who stopped smoking prenatally and are at risk for relapse in the postpartum period. Explanations of the hazards to the infant from smoking may also be helpful because some mothers may believe the harmful effects occur only during pregnancy.

### Postpartum Blues

Mild depression, also known as postpartum blues, *baby blues,* or *maternity blues,* is a frequent concern. This mild, transient condition affects 70% to 80% of new mothers (Driscoll, 2014). The condition begins in the 1st week and usually lasts 2 to 10 days (Cunningham et al., 2014). It should last no longer than 2 weeks (Haskett, 2011). It is characterized by insomnia, irritability, fatigue, tearfulness, mood instability, and anxiety. The symptoms are usually unrelated to events, and the condition does not seriously affect the mother's ability to care for the infant.

Although the direct cause is unknown, postpartum blues may be caused by the mother's emotional letdown after birth, postpartum discomforts, fatigue, anxiety about her ability to care for the infant, and body image concerns (Cunningham et al., 2014). Hormonal fluctuations have not been proven to be a cause.

Although postpartum blues is self-limited, mothers benefit greatly when empathy and support are freely given by the family and the healthcare team. Nurses should prepare women for the occurrence of mild depressed or negative thoughts, let them know it is normal, and offer emotional support and encouragement.

Postpartum blues must be distinguished from postpartum depression and postpartum psychosis, which are disabling conditions and require therapeutic management for full recovery. Screening for risk factors and early signs is important during the birth facility stay (see Chapter 28). Nurses should teach the woman and her family to call the healthcare provider if the depression becomes severe, lasts longer than 2 weeks, or if the woman is unable to cope with daily life.

## THE PROCESS OF FAMILY ADAPTATION

The birth of an infant requires that family roles and relationships be reorganized. Each family member is affected.

### Fathers

The father's developing bond with his newborn is seen with engrossment. *Engrossment* is characterized by intense interest in how the infant looks and responds and a desire to touch and hold the baby. Many fathers comment on the baby's distinctive features. They experience strong attraction to the infant and elation after the baby's birth. The father's attachment behaviors increase when the infant is awake, makes eye contact, and responds to the father's voice (Fig. 20.11).

Many fathers eagerly look forward to co-parenting with their mate. However, they may lack confidence in providing infant care and are sensitive to being left out of instructions and demonstrations of infant care. They may feel that others expect them only to provide support to the mother. The nurse can assist the new father by involving him in child-care activities soon after birth to help him feel more confident and competent.

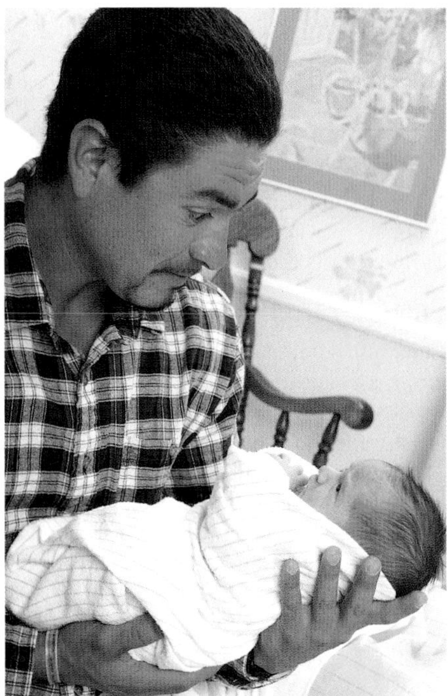

**FIG 20.11** Fathers' behaviors at initial contact with their infants often correspond to maternal behaviors. The intense fascination that fathers exhibit is called *engrossment*. Note the eye-to-eye contact between father and infant.

### Siblings

Sibling response to the birth of a new brother or sister depends on age and developmental level. Toddlers are usually not completely aware of the impending birth. Once the baby arrives, they may view the infant as competition or fear they will be replaced in the parents' affection. Negative behaviors such as sleep problems, an increase in attention-seeking efforts, and more infantile behaviors like renewed bed-wetting may surface. Some toddlers exhibit hostile behaviors toward the mother, particularly when she holds or feeds the newborn. Parents must find opportunities to affirm their continued love and affection for the very vulnerable sibling.

Preschool siblings may engage in more looking than touching. Most spend at least some time in proximity to the infant and talk to the mother about the infant (Fig. 20.12). A relaxed approach without time constraints may make it easier for young children to interact with the infant. Special care must be taken by the parents, visitors, and nurses to pay as much attention to the sibling as to the new baby.

### Grandparents

The involvement of grandparents with grandchildren depends on many factors. One of the most important factors is proximity. Grandparents who live near the child frequently develop a strong attachment. This evolves into unconditional love and a special relationship that brings joy to the grandparents and an added sense of security to the grandchildren (Fig. 20.13). Grandparents who live many miles from grandchildren must try to devise ways to foster a relationship with grandchildren they seldom see.

Grandparents are often a major part of the support system that new parents need. Grandmothers in particular provide assistance with household tasks and infant care to allow the mother to recover from childbirth and make the transition to parenthood.

### Factors Affecting Family Adaptation

Numerous factors influence the family's adjustment. Some, such as discomfort and fatigue, can be anticipated because they are so common. Unanticipated events, such as cesarean birth or birth of a preterm or ill infant, also affect the ease and speed with which the family adjusts.

#### Discomfort and Fatigue

Normally, discomfort associated with childbirth resolves within the first days after birth; nevertheless, such discomfort may diminish the mother's ability to focus on the newborn's needs. Fatigue often continues during the first few weeks and months, when the infant's schedule is erratic and uninterrupted sleep for parents is minimal. When the infant begins to sleep through the night (usually by 3 to 4 months), fatigue becomes less of a factor.

#### Knowledge of Infant Needs

First-time parents are often unsure about how to care for the newborn and may become very anxious if they are unable to console a crying infant. Moreover, many are concerned about feeding and specific procedures, such as the care of the umbilical cord or circumcision. Breastfeeding benefits both mother and infant, but may add to the stress that parents experience initially if they lack sufficient knowledge and support (see Chapter 23).

Some parents have concerns about spoiling the infant. They may believe that responding each time the infant cries causes the baby to cry to get attention. It may be necessary to teach parents that infants cry to indicate a need and to reassure the parents that responding to crying does not spoil the child. Suggesting a variety of methods to cope with crying may be helpful.

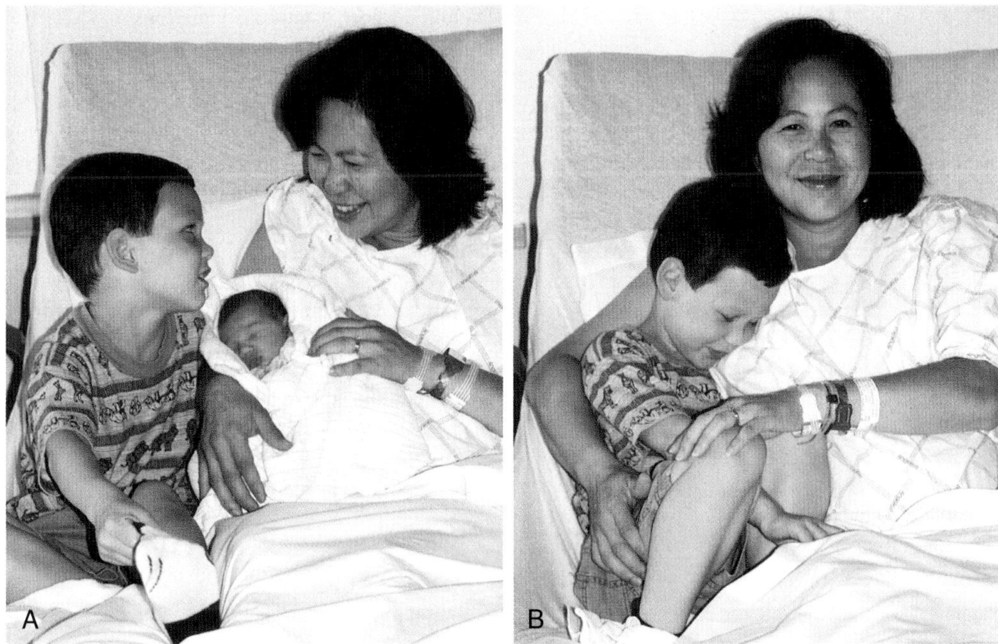


FIG 20.12 **A,** Although they may hesitate to touch the infant, children often want to be close. **B,** This boy's relief and joy are obvious as he reclaims a favorite spot.

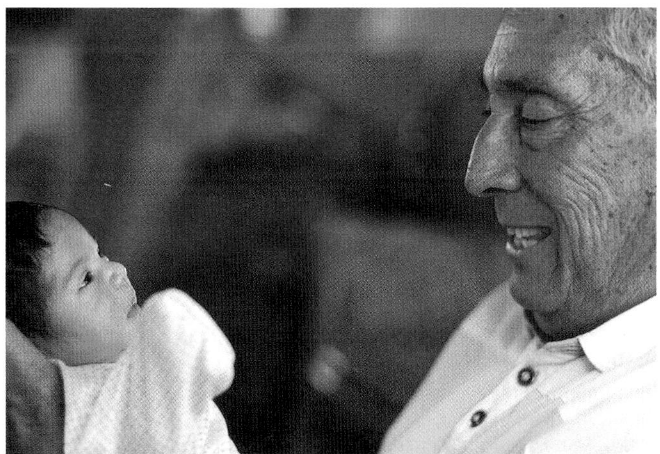

FIG 20.13 Grandparents may develop strong bonds with grandchildren.

### Previous Experience

Previous experience with newborns may also affect family adjustment. Multiparas are more comfortable with infants and exhibit attachment behaviors earlier than do primiparas. Mothers who have previously given birth to infants with anomalies or to infants who did not survive may need more time to feel comfortable with this infant.

### Expectations About the Newborn

Unrealistic expectations of the infant also may influence adjustment. Parents who have little experience with newborns may be surprised at the newborn's appearance. Some parents may be very disappointed in the gender of the child, or they may sense that their partners are disappointed. These feelings must be acknowledged and dealt with before attachment can take place.

Nurses must assist parents by teaching normal newborn characteristics such as molding or newborn rash. Some parents have misconceptions about newborn behavior and are in need of explanations. For example, the capacity of an infant's stomach is small and the infant must be fed frequently. Also, infants are neurologically unable to sleep through the night in the early weeks. Increasing the time the mother spends with the infant during the postpartum stay enhances opportunities for her to learn to care for the infant while a nurse is available to help her.

### Maternal Age

Adjustment to parenthood is a challenge for teenagers who have not achieved a strong sense of their own identity. The adolescent may talk less, respond less, and appear more passive or less affectionate with her infant than do adult parents. She needs special assistance to develop necessary parenting skills that promote optimal development of the infant (see Chapter 24).

### Maternal Temperament

Maternal personality traits also influence attachment. Mothers who are calm and secure in their ability to learn adjust more easily to the demands of motherhood. Conversely, mothers who are excitable, insecure, and anxious have more difficulty.

### Temperament of the Infant

The infant's temperament also affects maternal adjustment. Infants who are calm, easily consoled, and enjoy cuddling increase parental confidence and feelings of competence. In contrast, irritable infants who are difficult to console and do not respond to cuddling interfere with attachment.

### Availability of a Strong Support System

A strong, consistent support system is a major factor in the adjustment of the new mother. Friends and relatives who are parents can provide role modeling that is particularly important to first-time mothers. They also provide encouragement, praise, and reassurance that she is a good mother. In addition, the mother needs practical assistance with household tasks such as meal preparation, laundry, and shopping.

### Other Factors

***Cesarean birth.*** A cesarean birth, especially one that is not anticipated, may make parental adjustment more difficult. The surgical birth causes a longer recovery time, additional discomfort for the mother, and increased stress for the family. The mother's needs for both recovery and attachment with her infant must be considered in nursing care plans.

***Preterm or ill infant.*** Birth of a preterm or ill infant results in additional concern about the condition of the infant. Prolonged separation of parents and child may be necessary. Although attachment can occur in these situations, the separation may delay the process and create stress on the normally functioning family (see Chapter 29).

***Birth of multiple infants.*** Multiple birth often follows a high-risk pregnancy in which the woman was confined to restricted activity or bedrest. The infants may be preterm or have health problems. The birth of more than one infant may present problems of attachment. Parents attach to each infant separately as they get to know each infant's unique characteristics. Nurses must help the parents relate to each infant as an individual rather than as part of a unit by pointing out the individual responses and characteristics of each infant. Time alone with each infant is helpful. If infants are in a neonatal intensive care unit at first, frequent contacts should be arranged.

**! NURSING QUALITY ALERT**

***Factors That Affect Adaptation***

- Lingering discomfort or pain
- Chronic fatigue
- Knowledge of infant needs
- Available support system
- Expectations of the newborn
- Previous experience with infants
- Maternal temperament
- Infant characteristics
- Other factors: cesarean birth, preterm or ill infant, or birth of more than one infant

Mothers may be overwhelmed at the prospect of breastfeeding more than one infant. They need reassurance that they will produce an ample supply of milk for each infant because supply increases with demand.

## CULTURAL INFLUENCES ON ADAPTATION

A major goal of nursing practice in the postpartum period is to provide nursing care that fits the health beliefs, values, and practices of each woman. This provision can be difficult because of the wide ethnic diversity in countries such as the United States and Canada. A major challenge for nurses is to be aware of cultural beliefs and to acknowledge their importance in family adaptation. Postpartum is often thought to be a time of vulnerability for the woman and the infant (Mattson, 2011). Many cultural factors relevant to the postpartum period can be grouped into communication, dietary practices, and health beliefs.

### Communication

Verbal communication may be difficult because of the numerous dialects and languages spoken. An interpreter should be fluent in the language, of the same religion, and of the same country of origin if possible. This compatibility is particularly important for Middle Eastern families, whose religious orientations may vary widely and who come from countries with long histories of social and religious conflict.

Respecting the privacy and modesty of all people is important, but modesty is especially important to Hispanic, Middle Eastern, and Asian cultures. Laws of modesty require that Muslim women cover their hair, body, arms, and legs except when at home with family or in all female company (Giger, 2012).

Healthcare workers must remember that tactfulness and warmth are important. Direct communication can be distressing, particularly for some Hispanics and Native Americans, who approach a subject only after exchanging polite and gracious comments.

When the nurse and the family speak different primary languages, it is important to verify the family's understanding. Nodding or saying "Yes" may be a sign of courtesy rather than of understanding or agreement. To be certain the message has been received, the nurse should ask family members to explain in their own words what they have been told.

### Dietary Practices

Some dietary practices that must be considered center on the hot-cold theory of health and diet. This theory refers to the intrinsic properties and effects of certain foods rather than the temperature. Many cultures believe that postpartum is a cold time because heat is lost during delivery (Mattson, 2011; Moore, Moos, & Callister, 2010). Therefore, Southeast Asians (Cambodians, Vietnamese, Hmong, and Laotians) believe that after childbirth the woman should eat only "hot" foods. Some Chinese believe that a combination of yin and yang foods maintains balance. Food brought from home is a welcome sign of caring in many cultures. This is especially true if traditional foods are eaten after a woman gives birth. Nurses should encourage this practice and discuss any dietary restrictions with the family. (See Chapter 14 for more information about cultural dietary practices.)

### Health Beliefs

Cultural beliefs and practices provide a sense of security for new mothers. Provision of the care of the mother and baby by female relatives is a common thread among cultures. Women from parts of India return to the parents' home where the new mother is cared for by her mother for 16 weeks after birth (Katz, 2012).

For many Southeast Asians, the postpartum period is important to ensure health in later years. New mothers are expected to rest for 1 to 3 months while the grandmother or other female relatives take over the mother's usual responsibilities and care for her, the new baby, and other children. Korean women and their newborns are cared for by the husband's mother (Callister, 2013).

In India, a new mother and her baby are confined to their room for 40 days after childbirth to ward off any potential infection (Corbett & Callister, 2012). Native American women and their infants stay indoors and rest for 20 days or until the umbilical cord falls off (Callister, 2013). Chinese women believe in "doing the month" in which they rest, avoid exercise, and do not bathe for a month after giving birth. They believe that if they do not follow cultural proscriptions after giving birth, they will suffer problems such as aches, pains, arthritis, and other problems. African American women may also delay bathing and washing their hair until lochia ends. However, they will take a sponge bath (Galanti, 2014).

Southeast Asians and Hispanics believe that the mother should be kept warm to avoid upsetting the balance of hot and cold. These women drink hot water or other beverages to keep warm. Use of ice for perineal edema or breast engorgement may not be acceptable. Some women do not wish to take baths or wash their hair during the postpartum period. This practice is upsetting for some nurses who are

**TABLE 20.3 Assessing Maternal Adaptation**

| Assessments | Nursing Considerations |
|---|---|
| ***Progression Through Puerperal Phases*** | |
| Taking-in (passive, dependent); Taking-hold (autonomous, seeks information); Letting-go (relinquishes fantasy baby, begins to see self as mother) | Consider the mother's need for rest, her need to talk about the details of her labor and childbirth, and her readiness to learn infant care and assume control of her own care. |
| ***Maternal Mood*** | |
| Mood and energy level, eye contact, posture, comfort | Tense body posture, crying, or anxiety may indicate discomfort, fatigue, or beginning of postpartum blues. |
| ***Factors That Affect Maternal Adaptation*** | |
| Age of mother | May need additional support if adolescent. |
| Previous experience | Primiparas often progress through puerperal phases more slowly and may need more assistance. Multiparas have more experience with infant care. Birth of a child with anomalies or previous death of an infant may delay adaptation. |
| Maternal and infant temperaments | Mothers who are calm, secure, and free from anxiety need less assistance. Those with infants who are difficult to console need more assistance. |
| Other factors | Cesarean birth causes increased discomfort and longer recovery. The birth of a preterm or ill infant or more than one infant may create attachment problems. |
| ***Interaction With Infant*** | |
| Maternal touch | Progresses from fingertipping to enfolding and other comforting behaviors. |
| Verbal interaction | Mother may call infant "it" initially but progresses quickly to using given name and identifying specific characteristics. |
| Response to infant cues or signals | Prompt, gentle, consistent response indicates progressive adaptation to parenting role. |
| ***Preparation for Parenting*** | |
| Classes in breastfeeding, parenting, or infant care | Many mothers feel more prepared after completing classes and participate in care sooner. |

concerned about hygiene. Tact and sensitivity are needed to find a compromise. Although a shower or opportunity to wash should be offered to these women, whether to accept this care is the woman's choice.

## NURSING CARE

### Maternal Adaptation

#### Assessment

How the mother progresses through the puerperal phases, her mood, and interaction with the infant affect maternal adaptation to the birth (Table 20.3).

#### Nursing Diagnosis and Planning

Parenting may be difficult when maternal discomfort, fatigue, and lack of knowledge or confidence in infant care come into play. Therefore, a common nursing diagnosis is:

- Risk for Impaired Attachment related to multiple factors, such as fatigue, discomfort, and lack of knowledge of infant care.

***Expected outcomes.*** The mother will verbalize feelings of comfort and support as she progresses through the phases of recovery and will demonstrate progressive attachment behaviors by (specific date) and participate in the care of the newborn by (date).

#### Interventions

***Assisting the mother through recovery phases***

**"Mother" the mother.** The early taking-in phase is a time to "mother" the mother so that she can move on to more complex tasks of maternal adjustment. During the first few hours after childbirth, she has a great need for physical care and comfort. Provide ample fluids and favorite foods. Keep linens dry, tuck warm blankets around her until chilling has stopped, and use warm water for perineal care.

**Monitor and protect.** The new mother depends on nurses to monitor and protect her. Remind her of the need to void, and assist her to ambulate. Offer pain medication before discomfort is severe, at which time the analgesic is less effective. Encourage her not to delay requesting analgesia when needed. At the first signs of fatigue, encourage the mother to sleep.

**Listen to the birth experience.** Listen to details of the birth experience and offer sincere praise for her efforts during labor.

Many mothers spend so much time on the telephone that it is difficult to complete nursing care. When assessments and care are necessary for the mother's physical safety, the nurse might say, "Excuse me for a moment. I need to check you soon. I can do it now or come back in 10 minutes."

**Foster independence.** As the mother becomes more independent, allow her to schedule her care as much as possible. Collaborate with her to plan when care such as ambulating will be done. Encourage her to assume responsibility for self-care, and emphasize that the nurse's role at this point is to assist and teach.

**Promote bonding and attachment.** Early, unlimited contact between parents and infants is of primary importance to facilitate the attachment process. In most hospitals and birth centers, infants remain in the room with the parents unless complications intervene. This arrangement may be called *mother-baby care, couplet care,* or *dyad care.* One nurse cares for both the mother and the baby, providing education and help with bonding as part of ongoing nursing care. The nurse assists as the mother learns to care for her baby and gradually takes over all care as she is able (Fig. 20.14). This arrangement provides continuity of care and helps prepare for discharge.

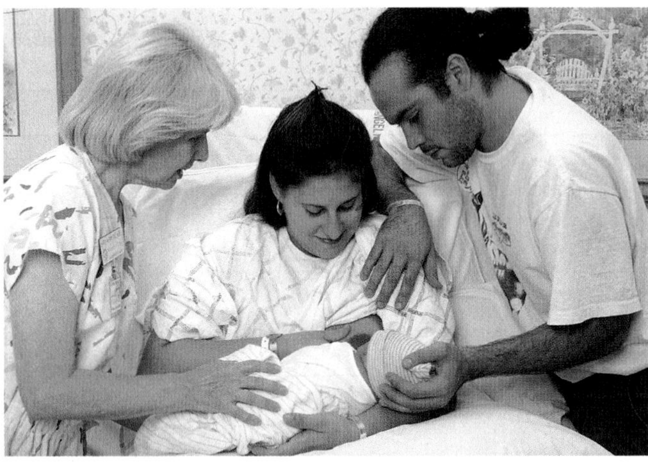

**FIG 20.14** By teaching about the newborn and family, the nurse helps parents develop confidence in their ability to provide care for the infant.

Prolonged contact between mothers and infants leads to more touching and caring for the infant, which enhances bonding. Specific nursing measures to promote bonding and attachment include to:

- Assist the parents in unwrapping the baby to inspect the fingers, toes, and body. This process allows the parents to become acquainted with the "real" baby that must replace the fantasy baby that was imagined during the pregnancy.
- Position the infant in an *en face* position because eye-to-eye contact is a first step in establishing mutual interaction between the infant and parent.
- Point out the reciprocal bonding activities of the infant: "Look how she holds your finger;" "He hasn't taken his eyes off you."
- Encourage the parents to spend time with the infant so they can progress at their own speed through the discovery or getting-acquainted phase.
- Assist the mother in feeding the infant, and answer her questions about feeding.
- Model behaviors by holding the infant close and speaking in high-pitched, soothing tones.
- Point out the infant's characteristics in a positive manner: "She has such pretty little hands and such fine hair."

**Involve parents in infant care.** Providing care for the infant fosters feelings of responsibility and nurturing and is an important component of attachment. In addition, it allows parents to develop confidence in their ability to care for their infant before they go home.

Help the parents take over the care of the infant gradually while providing assistance to enhance their self-confidence. Although teaching begins during pregnancy, review information and repeat demonstrations if time allows. It is important for the entire staff to agree on how to teach basic care. Mothers seek confirmation of information, and they become confused and lose faith in the credibility of the staff if information varies.

Offer parents repeated praise and encouragement because they become easily discouraged if they feel unsuccessful in early attempts to care for their infants.

Suggestions for care must be tactfully phrased to avoid the implication that the parents are inept: "You burped that baby like a professional. There are a couple of little hints I can share about diapering."

### Evaluation

- Does the mother verbalize comfort and support as she cares for her infant?
- Does she demonstrate attachment behaviors such as enfolding the infant, using the infant's name, and responding gently when the infant cries?
- Does she participate in infant care (diapering, feeding, and the care of the umbilical cord and circumcision)?

## NURSING CARE

### Family Adaptation

#### Assessment

***Fathers.*** The father's emotional status and interaction with the infant are particularly important because he usually serves as the mother's primary support person. The nurse should assess the father's interaction with the mother and infant and his knowledge about infants. Unrealistic expectations of the infant may lead to problems. In addition, if the father expects the mother to recover her energy and libido rapidly, he may become resentful if her recovery takes longer than anticipated.

***Siblings.*** Note the ages of siblings and their reactions to the newborn. Also assess the parents' reaction to sibling behaviors.

***Support system.*** Family members often provide a powerful support system, and their involvement is important to the adaptation of the family. Ask about who will assist the mother when she returns home.

***Nonverbal behavior.*** Nonverbal behavior is equally important. Are the parents' words congruent with their actions? For example, does the mother verbalize satisfaction with her infant's characteristics but respond slowly to infant signals? Table 20.4 summarizes the family assessment and briefly indicates nursing considerations.

#### Nursing Diagnosis and Planning

Sometimes a family who usually functions effectively is unable to cope because of a specific event, such as the birth of a baby. An appropriate nursing diagnosis is:

- Risk for Interrupted Family Processes related to lack of knowledge of infant needs and behaviors, stress during the early weeks at home, and sibling rivalry.

***Expected outcomes.*** By (specific date) the family will:

- Verbalize understanding of infant needs and behaviors.
- Identify methods for reducing stress during the early weeks at home.
- Describe measures to reduce sibling rivalry.
- Identify external resources and a support system.

#### Interventions

Teaching the family about the newborn.

***Infant needs.*** Provide parents with information about the infant's capabilities as well as the emotional and physical needs.

***Infant signals.*** Discuss the importance of responding promptly and gently to cues such as crying or fussing that indicate the infant needs attention. Reassure parents that responding to cues does not "spoil" their baby but helps the infant learn to trust that the world is a safe, secure place.

Help parents recognize signals that indicate when their infant has had enough interaction and needs to avoid further stimulation. These signals or *avoidance cues,* such as looking away, splaying the fingers, arching the back, and fussiness, indicate that the infant needs a quiet time.

***Helping the family adapt***

**Providing anticipatory guidance about stress reduction.** Help the family plan for the demands of the first weeks at home by

**TABLE 20.4 Assessing Family Adaptation**

| Assessments | Nursing Considerations |
|---|---|
| ***Characteristics of Infants That May Affect Family Adaptation*** | |
| Infant gender and size | Disappointment in the gender or concern about small size may interfere with bonding. |
| Unexpected characteristics (cephalhematoma, molding, jaundice, newborn rash) | Explain unexpected appearance or behavior in words parents can comprehend. |
| Illness or congenital anomalies | Explain the condition to parents and assist them during visits and while learning care. |
| Infant behavior (irritable, easily consoled, cuddles) | Infants who are easily managed make bonding and attachment easier. |
| ***Paternal Adaptation*** | |
| Response to mother and infant | The father often provides the most important support for the mother. His involvement with the infant indicates his acceptance of his parenting role. |
| Knowledge of infant care | The father's knowledge determines the teaching he needs. |
| Response to infant cues or signals (crying, fussing) | Many fathers feel awkward handling the infant but want to become proficient in infant care. |
| ***Ages and Developmental Ages of Siblings*** | |
| Reaction of siblings | Young children often fear that the newborn will replace them in the affection of parents. Parents may need anticipatory guidance about sibling rivalry. |
| ***Support System*** | |
| Interest and availability of family or friends to assist during early weeks | Families may need assistance to identify available support. |
| Plans for first few days at home | Review plans for support and rest. Provide resources such as postpartum clinics, "baby lines," or support groups. |
| Follow-up plans | Appointments at the clinic or healthcare provider for mother and infant should be scheduled. |
| ***Cultural Factors*** | |
| Cultural beliefs and practices that may affect nursing care | Culture-specific care can be planned for hygiene, dietary preferences, usual care of infants, and role of partner and family. |
| Expectations of the healthcare team | Expectations may vary between different cultures. |

providing anticipatory guidance. Fatigue is a common problem for both parents at this time of frequent interrupted sleep.

Emphasize that the priority during the first 4 to 6 weeks should be caring for the mother and baby. The mother should sleep when the infant sleeps and delay visits until she is rested. Suggest that the family establish a relaxed home atmosphere and a flexible meal schedule. Enlisting the aid of grandparents, other relatives, and friends to help with cooking, cleaning, and the care of the other children will provide the mother more time for rest.

Teach mothers breathing exercises and progressive relaxation to reduce stress and to energize, especially when a nap is not possible. To help them cope with stress, encourage parents to discuss their feelings openly. Remind them of the need for healthy nutrition and for recreation. Fatigue and tension can overwhelm the anticipated joys of parenting if no respite is available from constant care.

**Helping the father co-parent.** Help the father become involved with his infant by including him in teaching. Provide opportunities for him to participate in diapering, comforting activities, and feeding or helping the mother breastfeed. Offer frequent encouragement and praise.

**Providing ways to reduce sibling rivalry.** Suggest that parents plan time alone with older children and that they offer frequent expressions of love and affection. Suggest that visitors and family do not focus exclusively on the infant but include older children in gift giving and attention.

Emphasize the importance of responding calmly and with understanding when a sibling regresses to more infantile behaviors or expresses hostility toward the infant. Acknowledging the child's feelings and offering prompt reassurance of continued love are important.

**Identifying resources.** In many homes, women assume the major responsibilities of day-to-day homemaking. With the birth of an infant, this task becomes more difficult. A division of labor must be negotiated to prevent undue stress and fatigue. This division of labor is particularly important if there are other children who also need time, attention, and comfort.

The mother's primary support is often the father of the baby. Extended family members, particularly grandmothers and sisters, or friends also provide valuable support. Community resources such as daycare centers, parenting classes, and breastfeeding support groups are available in many areas. Remind the mother that resources are available when she begins to feel isolated and exhausted.

### Evaluation

- Do the parents discuss infant behaviors appropriately and respond to the infant's crying promptly and gently?
- Do the parents have a plan to reduce family stress and sibling anxiety?
- Are they able to describe family and community resources for support?

## POSTPARTUM HOME AND COMMUNITY CARE

### Criteria for Discharge

Most women leave the hospital when they are just beginning to recover from giving birth and starting to learn how to care for themselves and their infants. The American Academy of Pediatrics (2012) and the American College of Obstetricians and Gynecologists (2014) suggest the following criteria for discharge of mothers:

- The mother has no complications, and assessments (including vital signs, lochia, fundus, urinary output, incisions, ambulation, ability to eat and drink, and emotional status) are normal.
- Pertinent laboratory data including hemoglobin or hematocrit have been reviewed, and $Rh_o(D)$ immune globulin has been administered, if necessary.
- The mother has received instructions on self-care, deviations from normal, and proper response to danger signs and symptoms.
- The mother demonstrates knowledge, ability, and confidence to care for herself and her baby.
- The mother has received instructions on postpartum activity, exercises, and relief measures for common postpartum discomforts.
- Arrangements have been made for postpartum care.
- Family members or other sources of support are available to the mother for the first few days after discharge.

## COMMUNITY-BASED CARE

Many assessments and interventions of postpartum women occur in the clinic or outpatient setting. Mothers leave the birth facility when they are not fully recovered from the childbirth experience. New parents must be made aware of local community care services. Information lines, follow-up telephone calls from birth facility staff, nurse-managed postpartum outpatient clinics, and in some areas home visits provide information and guidance for postpartum families. Breastfeeding and parenting classes, "baby and me" walks or exercise sessions, and postpartum support groups may also be available. Comprehensive psychosocial support including telephone calls, home and clinic visits, and breastfeeding and parenting education have been shown to decrease the incidence of hospital readmission of normal newborns (Barilla, Marshak, Anderson, et al., 2010).

### EVIDENCE-BASED PRACTICE

Preparation for discharge from the hospital after the birth of a baby is essential to help mothers make the transition from hospital to home and to independent self and infant care. Weis and Lokken conducted a study of 141 postpartum mothers of healthy infants to identify predictors of maternal perception of readiness for discharge and the degree of difficulty they experienced after discharge. Data were taken from hospital records and during telephone interviews with the women 3 weeks after discharge. Additional outcome measures included post-discharge services as well as the Readiness for Hospital Discharge Scale and the Post-Discharge Coping Difficulty Scale, which has well-established validity and reliability.

Characteristics of the mothers and the type of delivery they experienced were not significant predictors for the mother's perceptions of readiness for discharge. Most mothers reported feeling ready for discharge on the day they went home. Overall, mothers stated they received high-quality teaching from nurses and more teaching than they needed. Mothers who felt most ready for discharge felt they received more information than they needed and more skillful teaching by the nurses than those mothers who felt less ready for discharge. Those who felt they received less skillful teaching covering less content than they needed felt less ready to go home when discharged. Mothers who felt unready for discharge were more likely to have difficulty coping in the first 3 weeks after they went home. They were more likely to ask for help from family and friends, and had more calls or visits to physicians after discharge.

Ask mothers in your facility how ready they feel for discharge on the day they go home. Also ask them what else could be done to help them feel more ready for discharge. If you have contact with postpartum mothers in a clinic, ask them about their early days at home and if they now feel less sure they were adequately prepared for discharge. Ask what else could be done to help them at home.

Reference: Weiss, M. E., & Lokken, L. (2009). Predictors and outcomes of postpartum mothers' perceptions of readiness for discharge after birth. *Journal of Obstetric, Gynecologic, & Neonatal Nursing, 38*(4), 406–417.

## KEY CONCEPTS

- After childbirth, the uterus returns to its nonpregnant size and condition by involution, which involves contraction of muscle fibers, catabolic processes, and regeneration of uterine epithelium.
- The site of placental attachment heals by a process of exfoliation, which leaves the endometrium smooth and without scars.
- Involution can be evaluated by measuring the descent of the fundus (approximately 1 cm/day). By the 14th day after childbirth, the fundus should no longer be palpable abdominally.
- Afterpains, or intermittent uterine contractions, cause discomfort for many women, particularly multiparas who breastfeed.
- Vaginal discharge (lochia) progresses from lochia rubra to lochia serosa to lochia alba in a predictable time frame. Lochia should be assessed for amount, type, and odor. Foul odor suggests endometrial infection.
- The vagina regains its nonpregnant size and contour in 6 to 10 weeks.
- Perineal trauma and hemorrhoids cause discomfort and can interfere with activity and bowel elimination.
- As blood from the uterus and placenta returns to the central circulation and extracellular fluid moves into the vascular compartment, the cardiac output increases and excess fluid is excreted by diuresis and diaphoresis.
- Increased clotting factors predispose the postpartum woman to clot formation. Early frequent ambulation helps prevent thrombi.
- Constipation may occur from decreased food and fluid intake during labor, reduced muscle and bowel tone, or fear of pain during defecation.
- Increased bladder capacity and decreased sensitivity to fluid pressure may result in urinary retention. Stasis of urine allows time for bacteria to grow and can lead to urinary tract infection.
- A distended bladder displaces the uterus and can interfere with uterine contraction and cause excessive bleeding.
- Exercises to strengthen the abdominal muscles, good posture, and body mechanics may reduce musculoskeletal discomfort.
- As hormone levels decline, the skin gradually returns to its nonpregnant state.

## KEY CONCEPTS—cont'd

- Breastfeeding may delay the return of ovulation and menstruation, but ovulation can occur before the first menses. All mothers need information about family planning.
- Breastfeeding mothers are more likely to experience dyspareunia as a result of vaginal dryness that results from inadequate estrogen.
- Lactation may be suppressed by wearing a sports bra and avoiding stimulation of the breasts.
- Orthostatic hypotension occurs when the mother goes from a supine to a standing position quickly.
- Tachycardia may be caused by pain, excitement, hypovolemia, fatigue, dehydration, anemia, or infection. Additional assessments are required to determine if excessive bleeding is the cause.
- The postpartum woman should be afebrile, but because of dehydration and leukocytosis, her temperature may be higher during the first 24 hours after delivery.
- The postcesarean woman requires postoperative as well as postpartum assessments and care. She may have problems associated with immobility and discomfort.
- The quick discharge from the hospital after childbirth challenges nurses to develop an effective plan for teaching self-care and infant care in a short period.
- Bonding and attachment are gradual processes that begin before childbirth and progress to feelings of love and deep devotion that last throughout life.
- Nurses foster bonding and attachment by providing early, unlimited contact between the parents and infant and by modeling attachment behaviors.
- Maternal touch changes over time as many mothers progress from exploratory fingertipping to enfolding, to demonstrating a full range of comforting behaviors.
- Verbal behaviors are important indicators of maternal attachment. Nurses often model how to speak to the infant and point out the infant's response to verbal stimulation.
- Maternal adjustment to parenthood is a gradual process that involves the phases of taking-in, taking-hold, and letting-go.
- Parents usually progress through four stages of role attainment (anticipatory, formal, informal, and personal) as they learn to structure their parenting behaviors to mesh with the infant's needs.
- Many women experience role conflict when they must leave the infant with a caregiver and return to work. Nurses can offer anticipatory guidance that makes the conflict less difficult.
- Postpartum blues is a temporary and self-limited period of tearfulness and mood instability. It should not last longer than 2 weeks.
- The birth of a baby requires reorganization of family structure and renegotiation of family responsibilities. Nurses can assist the father in co-parenting the infant and help the new parents identify family resources.
- Siblings may be jealous and fear that they will be replaced by the newborn in the affection of the parents. Nurses can help by providing information about how to reduce sibling rivalry.
- Attention to cultural concerns of postpartum families is important.

## REFERENCES AND READINGS


American Academy of Pediatrics & American College of Obstetricians and Gynecologists. (2012). *Guidelines for perinatal care* (7th ed.). Elk Grove Village, IL, and Washington, DC: Author.

American College of Obstetricians and Gynecologists. (Reaffirmed 2015). *Cesarean delivery on maternal request (ACOG Committee Opinion No. 559)*. Washington, DC: Author.

American College of Obstetricians and Gynecologists (ACOG). (2014). *Thromboembolism in pregnancy. (ACOG Practice Bulletin No. 123)*. Washington, DC: ACOG.

Association of Women's Health, Obstetric and Neonatal Nurses. (2009). *Standards for professional nursing practice in the care of women and newborns* (7th ed.). Washington, DC: Author.

Atkinson, W., Wolfe, S., & Hamborsky, J. (Eds.). (2015). *Epidemiology and prevention of vaccine-preventable diseases* (13th ed.). Washington, DC: Public Health Foundation.

Barilla, D., Marshak, H. H., Anderson, S. E., & Hopp, J. W. (2010). Postpartum follow-up: can psychosocial support reduce newborn readmissions? *MCN: The American Journal of Maternal/Child Nursing, 35*(1), 33–39.

Blackburn, S. T. (2013). *Maternal, fetal, and neonatal physiology: A clinical perspective* (4th ed.). St. Louis: Saunders.

Callister, L. C. (2013). Integrating cultural beliefs and practices when caring for childbearing women and families. In K. R. Simpson & P. A. Creehan (Eds.), *AWHONN perinatal nursing* (4th ed., pp. 41–64). Philadelphia: Lippincott Williams & Wilkins.

Centers for Disease Control and Prevention. (2010). *Pertussis—What you need to know.* Retrieved from http://www.cdc.gov/Features/Pertussis.

Cochrum, Robbie. (2015). Postpartum Weight Control and the Contribution of Exercise. *International Journal of Childbirth Education, 30*(1): 48–53.

Cunningham, F. G., Leveno, K. J., Bloom, S. L., Spong, C. Y., Dashe, J. S., Hoffman, B. L., … & Sheffield, J. S. (2014). *Williams obstetrics* (24th ed.). New York: McGraw-Hill.

Driscoll, J. W. (2014). Psychosocial adaptation to the postpartum period. In K. R. Simpson & P. A. Creehan (Eds.), *AWHONN perinatal nursing* (4th ed., pp. 570–571). Philadelphia: Lippincott Williams & Wilkins.

Eshkevari, L., Trout, K. K., & Damore, J. (2013). Management of Postpartum Pain. *Journal of Midwifery & Women's Health, 58*(6), 622–631. doi:10.1111/jmwh.12129

Fleischman, E. (2015). Improving Women's Readiness for Discharge Postpartum… Proceedings of the 2015 AWHONN Convention. *JOGNN: Journal of Obstetric, Gynecologic & Neonatal Nursing, 44*:S2–S2. doi:10.1111/1552-6909.12619

Galanti, G. (2014). *Caring for patients from different cultures* (5th ed.). Philadelphia: University of Pennsylvania Press.

Giallo, R., Cooklin, A., Dunning, M., & Seymour, M. (2014). The Efficacy of an Intervention for the Management of Postpartum Fatigue. *JOGNN: Journal of Obstetric, Gynecologic & Neonatal Nursing, 43*(5), 598–613. doi:10.1111/1552-6909.12489.

Giger, J. N. (2012). *Transcultural nursing: Assessment and intervention* (6th ed.). St. Louis: Mosby.

Gyllstrom, M., Hellerstedt, W., & Hennrikus, D. (2012). The Association of Maternal Mental Health with Prenatal Smoking Cessation and Postpartum Relapse in a Population-Based Sample. *Maternal & Child Health Journal, 16*(3), 685–693. doi:10.1007/s10995-011-0764-2.

Haskett, R. F. (2011). Psychiatric illness. In D. James, P. J. Steer, C. P. Weiner, et al. (Eds.), *High risk pregnancy: Management options* (2nd ed., pp. 997–1009). St. Louis: Saunders.

James, D. C. (2013). Postpartum care. In K. R. Simpson & P. A. Creehan (Eds.), *AWHONN perinatal nursing* (4th ed., pp. 530–577). Philadelphia: Lippincott Williams & Wilkins.

Janke, J. (2013). Newborn nutrition. In K. R. Simpson & P. A. Creehan (Eds.), *AWHONN perinatal nursing* (4th ed., pp. 626-655). Philadelphia: Lippincott Williams & Wilkins.

Jones, E. E. (2012). Fertilization, pregnancy, and lactation. In W. F. Boron & E. L. Boulpaep (Eds.), *Medical physiology* (2nd ed., pp. 1170–1192). Philadelphia: Saunders.

Katz, V. L. (2012). Postpartum care. In S. G. Gabbe, J. R. Niebyl, H. Galen, E. Jauniaux, M. Landon J. L. Simpson & D. Driscoll (Eds.), *Obstetrics: Normal and problem pregnancies* (6th ed., pp. 517–532). New York: Churchill Livingstone.

Lavender, T., Richens, Y., Milan, S., Smyth, R., & Dowswell, T. (2013). Telephone support for women during pregnancy and the first six weeks postpartum. *Cochrane Database of Systematic Reviews*, (7), N.PAG-N.PAG.

Lawrence, R. A., & Lawrence, R. M. (2015). *Breastfeeding: A guide for the medical profession* (8th ed.). Maryland Heights, MO: Mosby.

Levine, M. D., Marcus, M. D., Kalarchian, M. A., Houck, P. R., & Cheng, Y. (2010). Weight concerns, mood, and postpartum smoking relapse. *American Journal of Preventive Medicine*, *39*(4), 345–351.

Lund, K. J., & McManaman, J. (2008). Normal labor, delivery, newborn care, and puerperium. In R. S. Gibbs, B. Y. Karlan, A. F. Haney, et al. (Eds.), *Danforth's obstetrics and gynecology* (10th ed., pp. 22–42). Philadelphia: Lippincott Williams & Wilkins.

Mann, J. R., Mannan, J., Quinones, L. A., Palmer, A. A., & Torres, M. (2010). Religion, spirituality, social support, and perceived stress in pregnancy and postpartum women. *Journal of Obstetric, Gynecologic, & Neonatal Nursing*, *39*(6), 645–657.

Martell, L. K. (2001). Heading toward the new normal: A contemporary postpartum experience. *Journal of Obstetric, Gynecologic, & Neonatal Nursing*, *30*(5), 496–506.

Martin, J. A., Hamilton, B. E., Ventura, S. J., Osterman, M. J. K., Kirmeyer, S., Mathews, T. J., & Wilson, E. C. (2011). Births: Final data for 2009. Hyattsville, MD: National Center for Health Statistics. *National Vital Statistics Reports*, *60*(1), Hyattsville, MD: National Center for Health Statistics.

Mattson, S. (2011). Ethnocultural considerations in the childbearing period. In S. Mattson & J. E. Smith (Eds.), *AWHONN core curriculum for maternal-newborn nursing* (4th ed., pp. 61–79). St. Louis: Saunders.

Menacker, F., & Hamilton, B. E. (2010). *Recent trends in cesarean delivery in the United States. NCHS Data Brief, no 35*. Hyattsville, MD: National Center for Health Statistics.

Mercer, R. T. (1985). The process of maternal role attainment. *Nursing Research*, *34*(4), 198–204.

Mercer, R. T. (1990). *Parents at risk*. New York: Springer.

Mercer, R. T. (1995a). *Becoming a mother: Research on maternal identity from Rubin to the present*. New York: Springer.

Mercer, R. T. (1995b). Predictors of maternal role attainment. *Nursing Research*, *34*(4), 198–204.

Mercer, R. T. (2004). Becoming a mother versus maternal role attainment. *Journal of Nursing Scholarship*, *36*(3), 226–232.

Mercer, R. T., & Ferketich, S. L. (1994). Maternal-infant attachment of experienced and inexperienced mothers during infancy. *Nursing Research*, *43*(6), 344–351.

Mercer, R. T., & Walker, L. O. (2006). A review of interventions to foster becoming a mother. *Journal of Obstetric, Gynecologic, & Neonatal Nursing*, *35*(5), 568–582.

Moore, M. L., Moos, M., & Callister, L. C. (2010). *Cultural competence: An essential journey for perinatal nurses. White Plains*. NY: March of Dimes.

National Quality Forum. (2012). *Perinatal and Reproductive Health Endorsement Maintenance*. Washington, DC: Author.

Nobre, A. R. (2011). Breastfeeding and sexuality. *Nursing: Revista De Formacao Continua Em Enfermagem*, *23*(274), 8–16.

Oweis, A. (2012). TOWARD EVIDENCE-BASED PRACTICE. Smoking Behavior Before, During, and After Pregnancy: The Effect of Breastfeeding. *MCN: The American Journal Of Maternal Child Nursing*, *37*(6), 404–404.

Rubin, R. (1961). Puerperal change. *Nursing Outlook*, *9*(12), 743–755.

Rubin, R. (1977). Binding-in in the postpartum period. *MCN: The American Journal of Maternal/Child Nursing*, *6*(1), 65–75.

Rubin, R. (1984). *Maternal identity and the maternal experience*. New York: Springer.

Simpson, K. R. (2010). Quality measures for perinatal care. *MCN: The American Journal of Maternal/Child Nursing*, *35*(1), 64.

Smith, V. (2015). Oral analgesia for relieving post-caesarean pain. *Practising Midwife*, *18*(6), 34–36.

U.S. Department of Labor, Bureau of Labor Statistics. (2011). *Employment characteristics of families summary*. Retrieved from http://www.bls.gov/news.release/famee.nr0.htm.

Whitmer, T. (2011). Physical and psychological changes. In S. Mattson & J. E. Smith (Eds.), *AWHONN core curriculum for maternal-newborn nursing* (4th ed., pp. 301–314). St. Louis: Saunders.

Yang, I., & Hall, L. (2014). SMOKING CESSATION and Relapse Challenges Reported by Postpartum Women. *MCN: The American Journal of Maternal Child Nursing*, *39*(6), 375–380. doi:10.1097/NMC.0000000000000082.

21

# The Normal Newborn: Adaptation and Assessment

http://evolve.elsevier.com/McKinney/mat-ch/

## LEARNING OBJECTIVES

*After studying this chapter, you should be able to:*

- Explain the physiologic changes that occur in the respiratory and cardiovascular systems during the transition from fetal to neonatal life.
- Describe thermoregulation in the newborn.
- Compare gastrointestinal functioning in the newborn and adult.
- Explain the causes and effects of hypoglycemia.
- Describe the steps in normal bilirubin excretion and the development of physiologic, nonphysiologic, breastfeeding, and true breast milk jaundice.
- Describe kidney functioning in the newborn.
- Explain the functioning of the newborn's immune system.
- Describe the periods of reactivity and behavioral states of the newborn.
- Describe nursing assessments of the newborn.
- Explain the importance and components of gestational-age assessment.

At birth, neonates must make profound physiologic changes to adapt to extrauterine life and meet their own respiratory, digestive, and regulatory needs. During nursing assessments, nurses must be aware of those changes so they can identify behaviors signifying problems or abnormalities.

## INITIATION OF RESPIRATION

The first vital task in newborn adaptation is the initiation of respiration. Forces occurring throughout pregnancy and during birth bring about this change.

### Development of the Lungs

During fetal life, the alveoli produce fetal lung fluid that expands the alveoli and aids in lung development. As the fetus nears term, production of lung fluid decreases. During labor, the fluid begins to move into the interstitial spaces, where it is absorbed. Absorption is accelerated by the process of labor and may be delayed after cesarean birth that occurs without labor. This process continues throughout labor and during the early hours after birth. At birth, only about 35% of the original amount of fetal lung fluid remains (Blackburn, 2013).

Surfactant, a slippery detergent-like combination of lipoproteins, is detectable by 24 to 25 weeks of gestation (Blackburn, 2013). Surfactant reduces surface tension within the alveoli. Without surfactant, the alveoli collapse as the infant exhales and must be re-expanded with each breath, greatly increasing the work of breathing. Surfactant secretion increases during labor and immediately after birth to enhance the transition from fetal to neonatal life. Surfactant production is usually sufficient to prevent respiratory distress syndrome by 34 to 36 weeks of gestation (Gardner, Enzman-Hines, & Dickey, 2011).

Steroids may be given to women in preterm labor to help increase surfactant production and lung maturation. Complications such as hypertension, placental insufficiency, maternal infection, and rupture of membranes greater than 48 hours may cause accelerated lung maturity. Diabetes can delay surfactant production (Gardner et al., 2011).

### Causes of Respiration

The infant's first breath at birth must force the remaining fetal lung fluid out of the alveoli and into the interstitial spaces to allow air to enter the lungs, requiring a much larger negative pressure (suction) than subsequent breathing. Breathing is initiated by chemical, mechanical, thermal, and sensory factors that stimulate the respiratory center in the medulla of the brain and trigger respiration (Fig. 21.1).

#### Chemical Factors

Chemoreceptors in the carotid arteries and the aorta respond to changes in blood chemistry brought about by the hypoxia that occurs with normal birth. Decreases in the partial pressure of oxygen ($Po_2$) and pH and an increase in the partial pressure of carbon dioxide ($Pco_2$) in the blood cause stimulation of the respiratory center in the medulla. A forceful contraction of the diaphragm results, causing air to enter the lungs. However, stimulation of the respiratory center and breathing does not occur if prolonged hypoxia causes central nervous system depression.

#### Mechanical Factors

During a vaginal birth, the fetal chest is compressed by the narrow birth canal. Approximately one-third of the fetal lung fluid is forced out of the lungs into the upper air passages and expelled during birth. When the pressure against the chest is released at birth, recoil of the chest draws a small amount of air into the lungs. This reduces the amount of negative pressure needed for the first breath after birth.

#### Thermal Factors

The temperature change that occurs with birth also stimulates the initiation of respiration. Sensors in the skin respond to this sudden change in temperature by sending impulses that stimulate the respiratory center of the brain and breathing.

#### Sensory Factors

Tactile stimuli that occur during birth stimulate skin sensors. Nurses hold, dry, and place infants skin to skin with the mother or wrap them

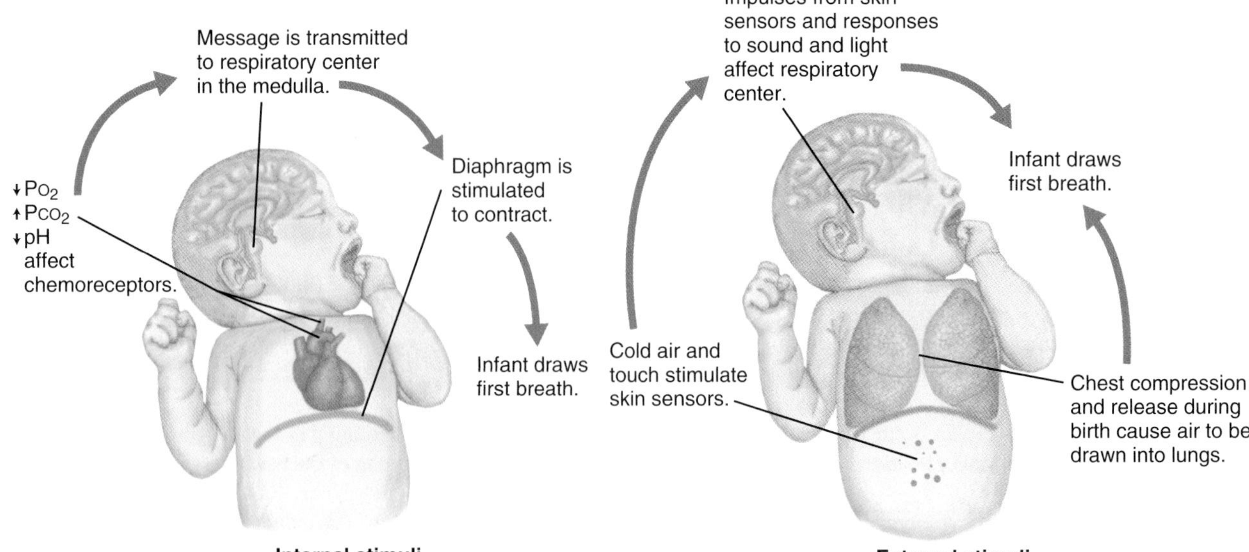


**FIG 21.1** Chemical changes that take place at birth are internal initiators of respiration. External initiators of respiration include thermal, sensory, and mechanical factors.

in blankets, providing further stimulation to skin sensors. Stimulation by sound, light, smell, and pain at delivery also may aid in initiating respiration.

### Continuation of Respiration

As the alveoli expand, surfactant allows them to remain partially open between respirations. Much of the air from the first breath remains in the lungs to establish the functional residual capacity. Subsequent breaths require less effort than the first one because the alveoli remain partly open.

As the infant cries, pressure within the lungs increases, causing the remaining fetal lung fluid to move into the interstitial spaces, where it is absorbed by the pulmonary circulatory and lymphatic systems. Although most fluid is absorbed within a few hours, complete absorption may take as long as 24 hours. Therefore, the lungs may sound moist when first auscultated but become clear a short time later.

## CARDIOVASCULAR ADAPTATION: TRANSITION FROM FETAL TO NEONATAL CIRCULATION

During fetal life, three shunts, the *ductus venosus, foramen ovale,* and *ductus arteriosus* carry much of the blood away from the lungs and some blood away from the liver. High pressure within the collapsed, fluid-filled lungs permits only a small amount of blood flow into the narrow pulmonary vessels.

### Ductus Venosus

Oxygenated blood from the placenta enters fetal circulation through the umbilical vein. About a third of the blood is directed away from the liver into the ductus venosus (DV), which connects to the inferior vena cava (IVC). The rest of the umbilical vein flow goes through the liver before entering the IVC. Near the end of pregnancy, the liver needs more perfusion, and 70% to 80% of the oxygenated blood from the umbilical vein flows through to the liver (Blackburn, 2013).

As blood from the DV or the portal system enters the IVC, it joins blood from the lower part of the body to travel to the heart in separate streams so that there is little mixing of the blood. When the blood enters the right atrium, the more highly oxygenated blood is directed across the atrium to the foramen ovale (Blackburn, 2013).

### Foramen Ovale

The foramen ovale is a flap in the septum between the right and left atria of the fetal heart. About 50% to 60% of the blood from the right atrium moves through the foramen ovale to the left atrium (Blackburn, 2013). The blood flows from the left atrium to the left ventricle and leaves through the ascending aorta. The majority of this better-oxygenated blood flows to the heart, brain, head, and upper body.

Blood that does not cross the foramen ovale moves to the right ventricle, but flow is restricted to the lungs by the narrow pulmonary artery and pulmonary blood vessels, elevating the pressure in the right side of the heart. Pressure is low on the left side of the heart because there is little resistance as blood leaves the left ventricle to travel to the rest of the body and into the widely dilated placental vessels. This difference in pressure between the right and left sides of the heart allows blood flow through the foramen ovale.

### Pulmonary Blood Vessels

Blood from the superior vena cava and the less oxygenated blood from the inferior vena cava flow into the right atrium, to the right ventricle, and into the pulmonary artery. Approximately 10% to 12% of the blood goes to the lungs; the rest passes through the ductus arteriosus to the aorta (Blackburn, 2013). Little blood is allowed into the lungs because the pulmonary artery and other blood vessels are constricted, causing high pulmonary vascular resistance. Blood perfusing the lungs returns to the left atrium via the pulmonary veins.

### Ductus Arteriosus

The ductus arteriosus connects the pulmonary artery and the aorta. Most of the blood that enters the pulmonary artery passes into the aorta through the widely dilated ductus arteriosus. Dilation of the ductus arteriosus is maintained by prostaglandins from the placenta and the low oxygen content of the blood.

## Changes at Birth

At birth, the shunts close and the pulmonary vessels dilate. These changes occur in response to increases in blood oxygen, shifts in pressure within the heart, pulmonary, and systemic circulations, as well as clamping of the umbilical cord. The changes necessary for transition from fetal to neonatal circulation occur simultaneously within the first few minutes after birth. They are discussed separately here (see Fig. 12.9).

As the newborn takes his or her first breaths at birth, the rise in the oxygen level of the blood causes the ductus arteriosus to constrict, preventing entry of blood from the pulmonary artery. The pulmonary blood vessels respond to the increased oxygenation by dilating. At the same time, fetal lung fluid begins to move into the interstitial spaces and is removed by blood and lymph vessels. These changes decrease pulmonary vascular resistance and allow more room for dilation of the pulmonary blood vessels. As a result, the pulmonary vessels can expand to hold the suddenly increased blood flow from the pulmonary artery.

At birth, pressures between the right and left sides of the heart are reversed. The sudden dilation of the vessels of the lungs allows blood to enter freely from the right ventricle and decreases pressure in the right side of the heart. Clamping of the umbilical cord further decreases pressure in the right side of the heart. Increased blood flow from the pulmonary veins into the left atrium causes pressure in the left side of the heart to build. Systemic resistance increases as blood flow to the placenta ends with clamping of the cord, further elevating pressure in the left heart.

Because the foramen ovale opens only from right to left, it closes when the pressure in the left atrium is higher than that in the right atrium. This change forces the blood from the right atrium into the right ventricle and pulmonary artery. Thus, blood flow through the heart and lungs changes from fetal to neonatal circulation and is similar to that in the normal adult.

The foramen ovale is functionally closed soon after birth because the unequal pressures between the atria prevent it from opening. Conditions such as asphyxia (insufficient oxygen and excess carbon dioxide in the blood and tissues) and persistent pulmonary hypertension, however, may reverse the pressures in the heart and cause the foramen ovale to reopen. The foramen ovale is permanently closed within several months (Kenney, Hoover, Williams, et al., 2011). The ductus arteriosus closes gradually as oxygenation improves and prostaglandins, which help keep it open, are metabolized. Functional closure occurs for most term infants at about 72 hours, and permanent closure occurs within 1 to 2 weeks (Kenney et al., 2011).

Until closure is complete, the blood that does flow through the ductus arteriosus usually reverses, moving from the aorta to the pulmonary artery and increasing blood flow to the lungs. This sequence occurs because pressure in the aorta is now higher than that in the pulmonary artery. A murmur may be heard as a result of blood flow through the partially open vessel.

Low levels of oxygen in the blood may cause the ductus arteriosus to dilate and the pulmonary vessels to constrict, increasing resistance to blood flow to the lungs. The result may be opening of the foramen ovale to allow a right-to-left shunt of blood and flow from the pulmonary artery through the ductus arteriosus and into the aorta. The ductus venosus closes shortly after birth. Permanent closure occurs by 1 to 2 weeks after birth (Kenney et al., 2011).

# NEUROLOGIC ADAPTATION: THERMOREGULATION

Although the fetus produces heat *in utero,* the consistently warm temperature of the amniotic fluid and the mother's body makes thermoregulation, the maintenance of body temperature, unnecessary. When

### CRITICAL THINKING EXERCISE 21.1

Understanding the changes that occur during the transition from fetal to neonatal circulation helps predict the effect on blood flow of various defects in the heart. What would be the effect on blood flow of an opening in the atrial septum of the heart?

the neonate moves from the warm uterus to the cooler outside environment, it must produce and maintain heat to prevent the serious effects of cold stress.

## Newborn Characteristics Leading to Heat Loss

Certain newborn characteristics predispose them to heat loss. The skin is thin, blood vessels are close to the surface, and there is little subcutaneous (white) fat to provide a barrier to loss of heat. Heat is readily transferred from the warmer internal areas of the body to the cooler skin surfaces and then to the surrounding air. Newborns have three times more surface area to body mass than the adult, and the rate of heat loss is four times greater than that of adults (Carlo, 2011a).

The flexed position of the healthy, full-term infant reduces the amount of skin surface exposed to the surrounding temperatures and decreases heat loss. Because of decreased muscle tone, the sick or preterm infant does not maintain a flexed position and is more susceptible to loss of heat.

## Methods of Heat Loss

The four methods of heat loss in the neonate are (Fig. 21.2):

- *Evaporation:* Evaporation is air-drying of the skin that results in cooling. Drying the infant immediately when wet helps prevent loss of heat by evaporation. Insensible water loss from the skin and respiratory tract increases heat loss from evaporation.
- *Conduction:* Movement of heat away from the body occurs when newborns come in direct contact with objects that are cooler than their skin. Contact with warm objects increases body heat by conduction. Warming objects that will touch the infant or placing the unclothed infant against the mother's skin ('skin to skin') helps prevent conductive heat loss.
- *Convection:* Transfer of heat from the infant to cooler surrounding air occurs through convection. When infants are in incubators, the circulating warm air helps keep them warm by convection. Providing a warm, draft-free environment avoids convective heat loss.
- *Radiation:* Radiation is the transfer of heat to cooler objects that are not in direct contact with the infant. Placing cribs and incubators away from windows and outside walls minimizes this type of heat loss. Use of a radiant warmer transfers heat from the warmer to the cooler infant.

## Nonshivering Thermogenesis

When newborns are cold, they become restless and cry, increasing flexion and activity to help maintain heat. Vasoconstriction occurs to decrease heat loss, and acrocyanosis (bluish discoloration of the hands and feet) may result. Body metabolism rises, increasing the need for oxygen and glucose (Blackburn, 2013). Adults shiver when they are cold, but shivering is rare in newborns. Shivering is seen only after prolonged exposure to cold and is not an important method of heat production. The primary method of heat production is nonshivering thermogenesis (NST), the metabolism of brown fat to produce heat. Newborns can increase heat production by 100% using NST (Blackburn, 2013).

Brown fat, also called *brown adipose tissue,* or *BAT,* is a specialized fat that provides heat when metabolized. It is located primarily around

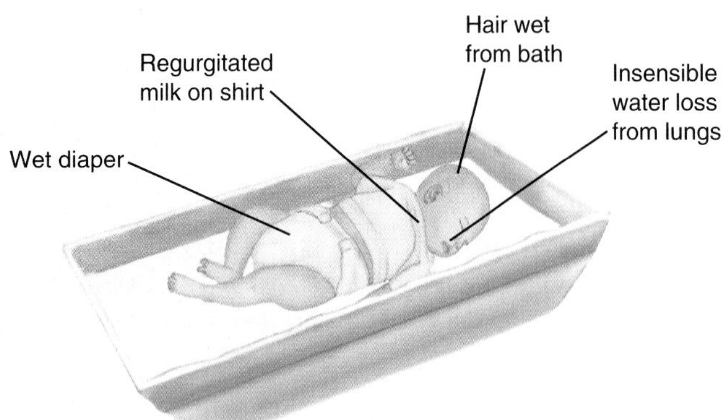


Evaporation can occur during birth or bathing from moisture on skin, as a result of wet linens or clothes, and from insensible water loss.

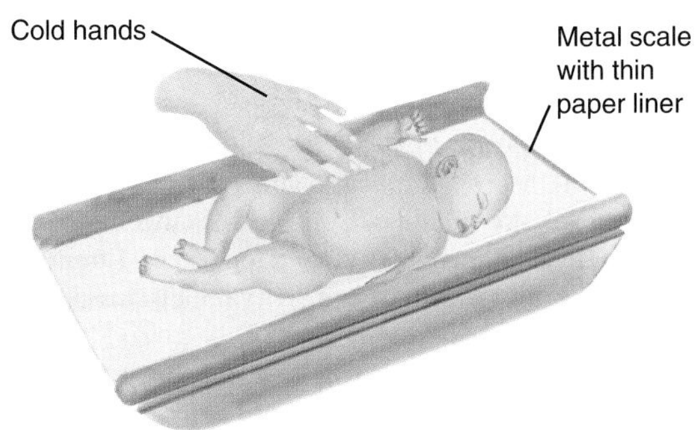


Conduction occurs when the infant comes in contact with cold objects or surfaces such as a scale, a circumcision restraint board, cold hands, or a stethoscope.

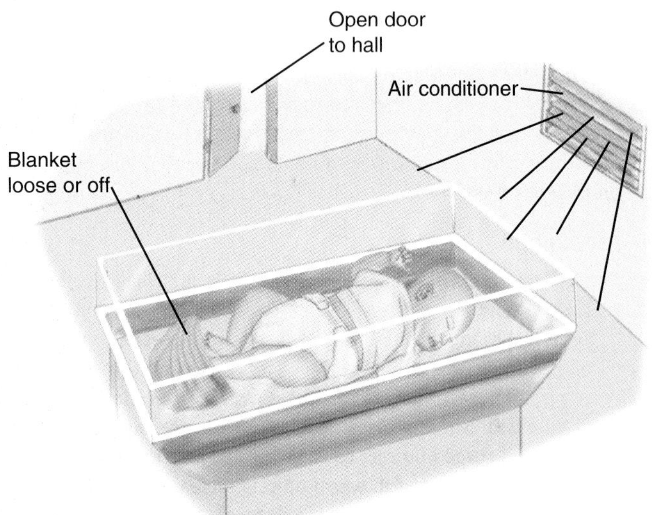


Convection occurs when drafts come from open doors, air conditioning, or even air currents created by people moving about.

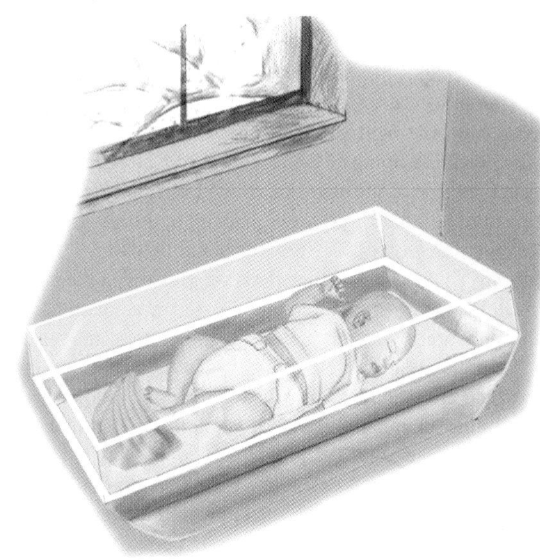

Heat is lost by radiation when the infant is near cold surfaces. Thus, heat is lost from the infant's body to the sides of the crib or incubator and to the outside walls and windows.

**FIG 21.2** Methods of heat loss.

the back of the neck, in the axillae, between the scapulae, along the abdominal aorta, and around the kidneys, adrenals, and sternum (Fig. 21.3). As brown fat is metabolized, it generates more heat than does white subcutaneous fat. Blood passing through brown fat is warmed and carries heat to the rest of the body.

NST begins when thermal receptors in the skin detect a drop in skin temperature. Thermal receptor stimulation causes the release of norepinephrine in brown fat, which initiates its metabolism. The process goes into effect even before a change occurs in the core or interior body temperature, as measured with a rectal thermometer. Therefore, NST may begin in an infant when skin temperature has been cooled, even though a temperature taken rectally shows a normal reading. A decrease in core temperature will not occur until NST is no longer effective.

Preterm infants and those with intrauterine growth restriction may have inadequate brown fat stores. Hypoxia, hypoglycemia, and acidosis may interfere with an infant's ability to generate heat. These infants are not able to raise their body temperature if subjected to cold stress, which can result in serious complications.

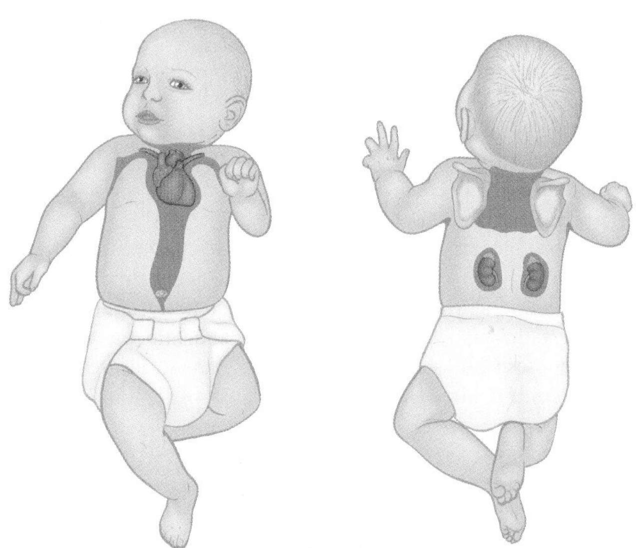

**FIG 21.3** Sites of brown fat in the neonate.

## Effects of Cold Stress

Cold stress causes many body changes (Fig. 21.4, Box 21.1). An increase in metabolic rate and metabolism of brown fat can lead to a significant rise in the need for oxygen. If an infant is having even mild respiratory distress, the problem can increase as oxygen is used for heat production. Cold stress also diminishes the production of surfactant, impeding lung expansion and leading to more respiratory distress.

More glucose is needed when the metabolic rate rises to produce heat. When glycogen stores are converted to glucose, they can be quickly depleted, causing hypoglycemia. Continued use of glucose for temperature maintenance leaves less glucose available for growth. Metabolism of glucose in the presence of insufficient oxygen increases the production of acids.

The metabolism of brown fat also releases fatty acids. This release can cause metabolic acidosis, which can be a life-threatening condition. Elevated fatty acids in the blood also interfere with the transport of **bilirubin** (unusable component of hemolyzed erythrocytes) to the liver, increasing the risk of **jaundice**, a yellow discoloration of the skin and sclera from excessive bilirubin in the blood.

**BOX 21.1 Hazards of Cold Stress**

- Increased oxygen need
- Decreased surfactant production
- Respiratory distress
- Hypoglycemia
- Metabolic acidosis
- Jaundice

As the infant's body attempts to conserve heat, vasoconstriction of the peripheral blood vessels occurs to reduce heat loss from the skin's surface. Decreased oxygen in the blood, however, can also cause vasoconstriction of the pulmonary vessels, leading to further respiratory distress.

## Neutral Thermal Environment

A **neutral thermal environment** is one in which the infant can maintain a stable body temperature with minimal oxygen need and without an increase in metabolic rate. The range of environmental temperature that allows this maintenance is called the *thermoneutral zone*. In healthy, unclothed full-term newborns, an environmental temperature of 32° C to 33.5° C (89.6° F to 92.3° F) provides a thermoneutral zone. When the infant is dressed, the thermoneutral range is 24° C to 27° C (75.2° F to 80.6° F) (Blackburn, 2013). The thermoneutral zone varies according to an infant's gestational age, size, and postnatal age.

## Hyperthermia

Infants also respond poorly to hyperthermia. With an elevated temperature, the metabolic rate rises, increasing the need for oxygen and glucose. In addition, peripheral vasodilation leads to increased insensible fluid losses. Sweating may occur but is often delayed because sweat glands are immature.

Newborns may be overheated by poorly regulated equipment designed to keep them warm. When radiant warmers, warming lights, or warmed incubators are used, the temperature mechanism must be set to vary the heat according to the infant's skin temperature

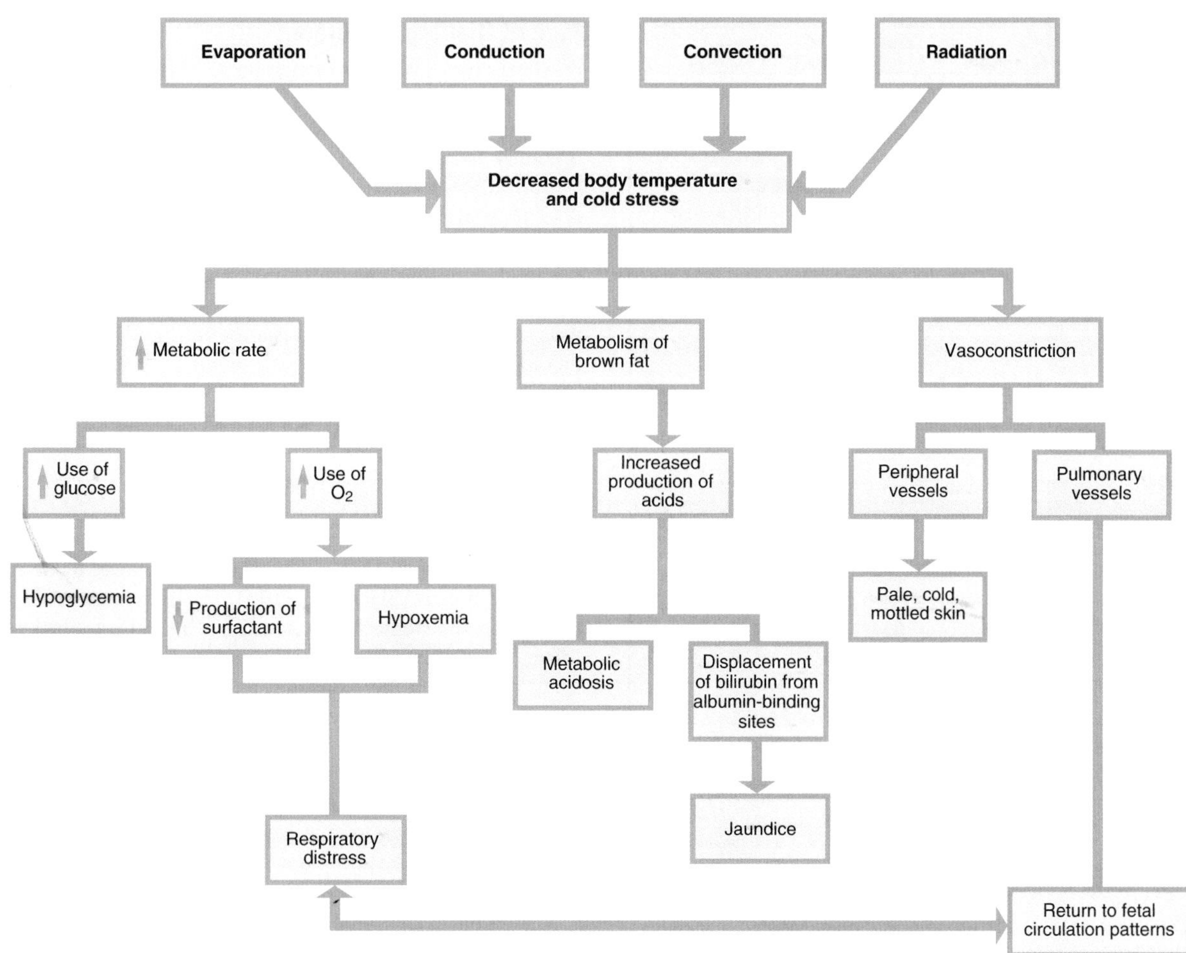

**FIG 21.4** Effects of cold stress.

and thus prevent heat that is too high or too low. Alarms to signal that the infant's temperature is too high or too low should be functioning properly.

## HEMATOLOGIC ADAPTATION

### Factors Affecting the Blood

The blood volume of the term newborn is 80 to 100 mL/kg, but this varies according to the time of cord clamping, the position of the infant when the cord is clamped, and the gestational age of the infant (Diehl-Jones & Askin, 2010). Preterm infants have a greater blood volume per kilogram than term infants.

Blood samples drawn from the heel, where the circulation is sluggish, show higher hemoglobin and hematocrit levels than samples taken from central areas. Venous blood samples are more accurate and are taken when precise measurement is essential. (Newborn values for common laboratory tests are listed in Table 21.1.)

### Blood Values

#### Erythrocytes and Hemoglobin

At birth, an infant has comparatively more erythrocytes (red blood cells [RBCs]) and higher hemoglobin and hematocrit levels than an adult. This difference is necessary because the partial pressure of oxygen of fetal blood is much lower than the normal adult level. The large number of erythrocytes (4.8 to 7.1 million/mm$^3$) and higher hemoglobin level (15 to 24 g/dL) enable the fetal cells to receive enough oxygen (Pagana & Pagana, 2011; Lo, 2011). In addition, fetal hemoglobin (hemoglobin F) has a greater affinity for oxygen than does adult hemoglobin (Verklan, 2011).

The newborn's erythrocytes have a shorter life span than those of the adult. Excess bilirubin caused by the hemolysis of large numbers of RBCs may lead to jaundice.

**TABLE 21.1 Laboratory Values in the Newborn**

| Test, Specimen, and Unit of Measurement | Age | Normal Range |
|---|---|---|
| Erythrocyte (red blood cell [RBC]) count, whole blood | Newborn | 4.8–7.1 (million/microliter) |
| Hemoglobin, whole blood | Newborn | 15–24 g/dL |
| Hematocrit, whole blood | Newborn | 44%–70% |
| Leukocytes, whole blood | Birth | 9.1–34 (thousand/mm$^3$) |
| Leukocyte differential count, whole blood | | |
| Myelocytes | | 0% |
| Neutrophils ("bands") | | 3%–5% |
| Neutrophils ("segs") | | 54%–62% |
| Lymphocytes | | 25%–33% |
| Monocytes | | 3%–7% |
| Eosinophils | | 1%–3% |
| Basophils | | 0%–0.75% |
| Platelet count, whole blood | Newborn | 84–478 (thousand/mm$^3$) |
| Glucose, serum | Cord | 45–96 mg/dL |
| | Newborn at 1 day | 40–60 mg/dL |
| | Newborn, >1 day | 50–90 mg/dL |
| Calcium, total serum | Cord | 9–11.5 mg/dL |
| | 3–24 hr | 9–10.6 mg/dL |
| | 24–48 hr | 7–12 mg/dL |
| | 4–7 days | 9–10.9 mg/dL |
| Magnesium, plasma | 0–6 days | 1.2–2.6 mg/dL |
| Bilirubin | Cord | <2 mg/dL |

Adapted from Lo, S. F. (2011). Reference intervals for laboratory tests and procedures. In R. M. Kliegman, B. E. Stanton, et al. (Eds.), *Nelson textbook of pediatrics* (19th ed., p. 2466). Philadelphia: Saunders; Pagana, K. D., & Pagana, T. J. (2011). *Mosby's diagnostic and laboratory test reference* (10th ed.). St. Louis: Mosby; Blackburn, S. T. (2013). *Maternal, fetal, and neonatal physiology: A clinical perspective* (4th ed.). St. Louis: Saunders.

#### Hematocrit

The hematocrit level in the normal newborn is 44% to 70% (Lo, 2011). A level above 65% from a central site indicates polycythemia, an abnormally high erythrocyte count (Luchtman-Jones & Wilson, 2011). Polycythemia increases the risk of jaundice and injury to the brain and other organs as a result of blood stasis. Respiratory distress and hypoglycemia are more common in these infants. Laboratory testing is performed if the infant has risk factors or signs of polycythemia or anemia.

#### Leukocytes

The leukocyte (white blood cell [WBC]) count at birth is 9,100 to 34,000/mm$^3$ (Lo, 2011). The WBC count falls to an average of 12,000/mm$^3$ by 4 to 5 days after birth (Blackburn, 2013). In newborns, an elevated WBC (leukocyte) count does not necessarily indicate infection. In fact, the WBC count may decrease in sepsis (Lott, 2010). Increased numbers of immature leukocytes are a sign of infection or sepsis. Platelets (thrombocytes) may decrease as a result of infections.

### Risk of Clotting Deficiency

Newborns have low levels of vitamin K, which is necessary to activate several of the clotting factors (factors II [prothrombin], VII, IX, and X). Vitamin K is synthesized in the intestines, but food and normal intestinal flora are necessary for this process (Luchtman-Jones & Wilson, 2011). To decrease the risk of hemorrhagic disease, vitamin K is administered intramuscularly to most newborns. Drugs such as phenytoin (Dilantin), phenobarbital, and antituberculosis drugs taken by the mother during pregnancy interfere with clotting ability in the infant after birth. Although the platelet counts in term newborns are near adult levels, the platelet response to stimuli is lower during the first few days of life.

## GASTROINTESTINAL SYSTEM

### Stomach

The newborn's stomach capacity is approximately 6 mL/kg at birth. Gastric emptying may be delayed at first. It is more rapid after ingestion of human milk than after formula and slower if the infant has swallowed mucus (Blackburn, 2013). The gastrocolic reflex is stimulated when the stomach fills, causing increased intestinal peristalsis. Infants frequently pass a stool during or after a feeding. The cardiac sphincter between the esophagus and the stomach is relaxed, which explains the tendency to regurgitate feedings easily.

### Intestines

The newborn's intestines are long in proportion to the infant's size and compared with those of the adult. The added length allows more surface area for absorption, but it also makes infants more prone to water loss should diarrhea develop. Air enters the gastrointestinal tract soon after birth, and bowel sounds are present within the first hour.

The digestive tract is sterile at birth. Once the infant is exposed to the external environment and begins to take in fluids, bacteria enter the gastrointestinal tract. Normal intestinal flora is established within the first few days of life.

### Digestive Enzymes

Maturation of the ability to digest and absorb occurs at different rates for various nutrients. Pancreatic amylase, needed to digest complex carbohydrates, is deficient for the first 4 to 6 months after birth (Blackburn, 2013). As a result, newborn digestion of complex carbohydrates such as those in cereals is limited. Amylase is also produced by the salivary glands, but in low amounts until about the third month of life. Amylase is present in breast milk.

The newborn is also deficient in pancreatic lipase, significantly limiting fat absorption. Lipase present in the mouth and stomach helps with some digestion of fat. Lipase is present in breast milk, which may make it more digestible for the newborn than formula. Protein and lactose, the major carbohydrate in the infant's milk diet, are both well digested.

### Stool

Meconium is the first stool excreted by the newborn. The components of meconium are particles from amniotic fluid such as vernix, skin cells, and hair, along with cells shed from the intestinal tract, bile, and other intestinal secretions. Meconium is greenish black with a thick, sticky, tarlike consistency. The first meconium stool is usually passed within 12 hours of birth, and 99% of newborns have the first stool within 48 hours (Carlo, 2011b). If meconium is not passed within that time, obstruction is suspected.

Meconium stools are followed by transitional stools, a combination of meconium and milk stools. Transitional stools are greenish brown and of a looser consistency than meconium. They are followed by milk stools characteristic of the type of feeding the infant receives.

The stools of infants fed with breast milk are seedy, with the color and consistency of mustard and a sweet-sour smell. The breastfed infant generally has more frequent stools than the infant who is formula fed. A stool may be passed with each feeding. Some older infants pass only one stool every 2 to 3 days. The normal breastfed newborn should have at least four or more stools daily (Lawrence & Lawrence, 2011).

The formula-fed infant excretes pale yellow to light brown stools. They are firmer in consistency than those of the breastfed infant. The infant may excrete several stools daily, or only one or two. The stools have the characteristic odor of feces.

## HEPATIC SYSTEM

Important liver functions include maintenance of blood glucose levels, conjugation of bilirubin, production of factors necessary for blood coagulation, storage of iron, and metabolism of drugs.

### Blood Glucose Maintenance

During the last trimester, glucose is stored in the fetal liver as glycogen for use after birth. Glucose is used rapidly by the newborn for energy during the stress of delivery and for breathing, heat production, movement against gravity, and activation of all the functions that the neonate must take on at birth.

Until newborn feedings are adequate to meet energy requirements, glucose present in the body is used, and stored glycogen is converted by the liver to glucose for use. In the term infant, glucose levels should be 40 to 60 mg/dL at day 1 and 50 to 90 mg/dL thereafter (Lo, 2011) but may be as low as 30 mg/dL for the first 1 to 2 hours after birth (Adamkin, 2011). While no general consensus has been established regarding the glucose level that defines hypoglycemia, less than 40 to 45 mg/dL in the term infant is often used as the lower limit of normal plasma glucose (Adamkin, 2011; McGowan, Rozance, Price-Douglas, et al, 2011).

Many newborns are at increased risk for hypoglycemia. In the preterm, late preterm (born between 340/7 and 366/7 weeks of gestation), and small-for-gestational-age infant, adequate stores of glycogen may not have accumulated. Stores may be depleted before birth in the postterm infant because of poor intrauterine nourishment from a deteriorating placenta. Large-for-gestational-age infants and those with diabetic mothers may produce excessive insulin that consumes available glucose quickly (see Chapters 29 and 30). Infants exposed to such stressors as asphyxia or infection may exhaust their stores of glycogen. Cold-stressed infants may deplete glycogen to increase metabolism and raise body temperature.

### Conjugation of Bilirubin

A major function of the liver is the conjugation of bilirubin (Fig. 21.5). The newborn's liver may not be mature enough to prevent jaundice during the first week of life. Jaundice results from **hyperbilirubinemia**, excessive bilirubin in the blood. Jaundice (or icterus) occurs in 60% of term newborns and 80% of preterm infants (Ambalavanan & Carlo, 2011).

#### Source and Effect of Bilirubin

The principal source of bilirubin is the hemolysis of erythrocytes. This process is normal after birth, when fewer erythrocytes are needed than during fetal life. Bilirubin is toxic to the body and must be excreted.

Bilirubin is released in an unconjugated form. Unconjugated bilirubin, also called *indirect bilirubin,* is not soluble in water. Before excretion can occur, the liver must change it to a water-soluble form by a process called *conjugation*. The bilirubin is then known as *conjugated* or *direct bilirubin*. Conjugated bilirubin is not toxic to the body and can be excreted.

Unconjugated bilirubin is fat soluble and can be absorbed by subcutaneous fat, causing the yellowish discoloration of the skin called *jaundice*. High levels of unconjugated bilirubin in the blood can lead to its accumulation in brain tissue, causing *acute* **bilirubin encephalopathy**, a neurologic condition resulting from bilirubin toxicity. If this condition becomes chronic, it is a permanent neurologic injury known as **kernicterus**. The level of bilirubin necessary to cause injury to the central nervous system is unknown and may differ among infants.

#### Normal Conjugation

When unconjugated bilirubin is released into the bloodstream, it attaches to binding sites on albumin in the plasma and is carried to the liver. If there are not enough albumin binding-sites, bilirubin circulates as unbound or free unconjugated bilirubin. Bilirubin can be displaced from albumin by some medications. Free fatty acids, acidosis, and infection also decrease the binding of bilirubin to albumin (Kamuth, Thilo, & Hernandez, 2011).

When albumin-bound bilirubin reaches the liver, it is changed to the conjugated form of bilirubin by the enzyme *uridine diphosphate glucuronosyltransferase (UDPGT)*. Conjugated bilirubin is excreted into the bile and then into the duodenum. In the intestines, the normal flora acts on bilirubin to reduce it to urobilinogen and stercobilin, which are excreted in the stool. A small amount of urobilinogen is excreted by the kidneys.

A small percentage of conjugated bilirubin may be deconjugated or converted back to the unconjugated state by the intestinal enzyme β-*glucuronidase*. This enzyme is important in fetal life because only unconjugated bilirubin can be cleared by the placenta for conjugation by the mother's liver. In the newborn, deconjugated bilirubin in the

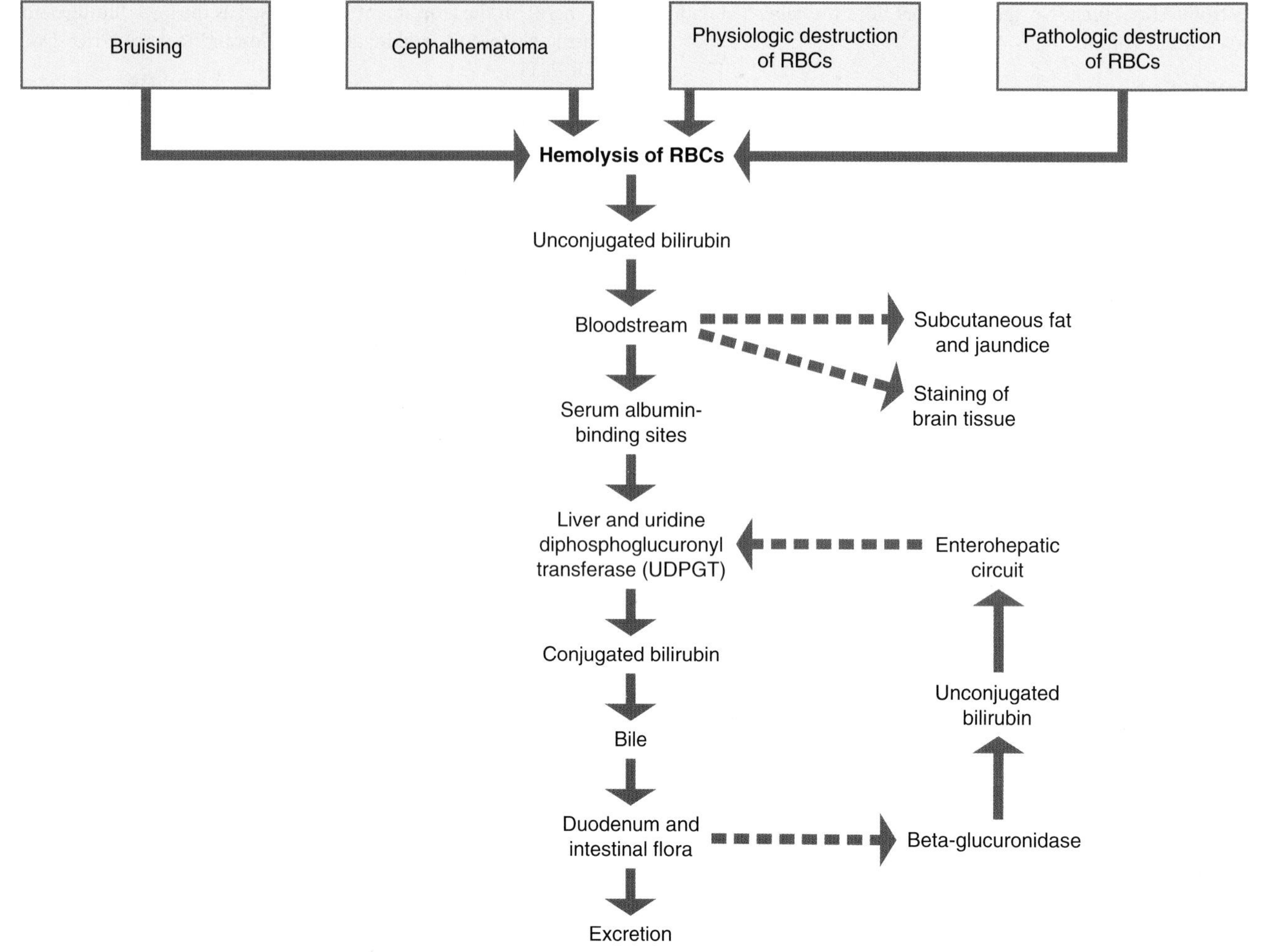


**FIG 21.5** Sources of bilirubin and how it is removed from the body.

intestines is absorbed into the portal circulation and carried back to the liver, where it again undergoes conjugation. This recirculation of bilirubin (the *enterohepatic circuit*) creates additional work for the liver. Blood tests for bilirubin measure total serum bilirubin (TSB) and direct (conjugated) bilirubin in the serum. TSB is a combination of indirect (unconjugated) and direct bilirubin.

### Risk Factors for Elevated Bilirubin

Factors that increase the risk for jaundice in the newborn include:

- *Excess production:* Twice as much bilirubin is produced in newborns as in adults. The rate of production remains higher in relation to their size for 3 to 6 weeks (Blackburn, 2013). Polycythemia further increases RBC breakdown.
- *Red blood cell life:* Fetal RBCs break down more quickly than do adult erythrocytes.
- *Albumin binding sites:* Newborns have fewer albumin binding-sites and decreased albumin binding capacity than do adults and older children (Kaplan, Wong, Sibley, et al., 2011).
- *Liver immaturity:* The newborn's immature liver may not produce adequate amounts of UDPGT and other substances during the first few days of life, limiting the amount of bilirubin that can be conjugated.
- *Blood incompatibility:* Rh, ABO, or others
- *Gestation:* Preterm and late preterm infants have immature conjugation abilities.
- *Intestinal factors:* Lack of adequate intestinal flora hinders excretion of conjugated bilirubin. High levels of the enzyme *β-glucuronidase* change bilirubin back to the unconjugated state. Intestinal motility is decreased, allowing more time for the enzyme to act.
- *Feeding:* When feedings are delayed or taken poorly, normal intestinal flora are not established, and passage of meconium, which is high in bilirubin, is delayed. Delayed passage of stools allows more time for conjugated bilirubin to be deconjugated by β-glucuronidase and reabsorbed. Meconium is especially high in bilirubin.
- *Trauma:* Trauma during birth (bruising, cephalhematoma [bleeding between the periosteum and skull from pressure during birth]) causes increased hemolysis of RBCs.
- *Fatty acids:* Fatty acids have a greater affinity than bilirubin for the binding sites on albumin and bind to albumin in place of bilirubin. Cold stress or asphyxia can increase circulating fatty acids.
- *Family background:* Increased risk in infants who are Asian, Native American, or Eskimo and in those with a sibling who had jaundice.
- *Other factors:* Birth to a diabetic mother, use of certain drugs, swallowing blood during birth, hypoglycemia, and infection also increase jaundice.

### Hyperbilirubinemia

Elevated levels of bilirubin in the newborn, or hyperbilirubinemia, results in jaundice that may be classified as physiologic or nonphysiologic, based on onset and severity.

### Physiologic Jaundice

Physiologic jaundice is also called nonpathologic or developmental jaundice. This condition is caused by transient hyperbilirubinemia and is considered normal. It is not present during the first 24 hours of life in term infants but appears on the second or third day after birth. Jaundice becomes visible when the serum bilirubin is 5 to 6 mg/dL (Blackburn, 2013).

Cord blood has an indirect bilirubin level of 1 to 3 mg/dL. In physiologic jaundice, the bilirubin peaks at 5 to 6 mg/dL between the second and fourth days of life. The bilirubin then begins to fall, declining to less than 2 mg/dL by 5 to 7 days (Ambalavanan & Carlo, 2011). Bilirubin normally rises higher and falls more slowly in Asian infants.

### Nonphysiologic (Pathologic) Jaundice

Normal jaundice must be differentiated from nonphysiologic, or pathologic, jaundice that requires further investigation. One of the most important differences is the time at which jaundice appears, as pathologic jaundice may occur during the first 24 hours. Bilirubin that rises more rapidly and to higher levels than is expected or stays elevated for longer than normal is more likely to lead to severe hyperbilirubinemia and may need earlier treatment.

Nonphysiologic jaundice is the result of abnormalities causing excessive destruction of RBCs or problems in bilirubin conjugation. These include incompatibilities between the mother's and infant's blood types (see Chapter 25), infection, and metabolic disorders. Nonphysiologic jaundice is often treated with phototherapy (discussed in Chapter 30).

Charts are available that show the rise and fall of bilirubin and the degree of risk for various levels of TSB according to the age of the infant in hours. For example, a full-term infant with no complications who is 24 hours old is considered at low risk if the TSB is 5 mg/dL or less and at high risk if the TSB is greater than 8 mg/dL. At 48 hours of age, that infant is at low risk if the TSB is 8.5 mg/dL but high risk if the TSB was that high before 48 hours. Infants who are preterm, late preterm, or who have other risk factors may receive treatment for hyperbilirubinemia at lower TSB levels than full-term infants.

### Jaundice Associated With Breastfeeding

The breastfed infant has a higher risk of developing jaundice, which may begin early or late after birth.

***Breastfeeding or early-onset jaundice.*** Bilirubin levels greater than 12 mg/dL develop in 13% of breastfed infants by 1 week of age (Ambalavanan & Carlo, 2011). The most common cause of jaundice in breastfed infants is insufficient intake. Jaundice begins within the first week of life, and serum bilirubin may rise above 12 mg/dL and reach dangerous levels if intake is not increased.

Infants who are sleepy, have a poor suck, or nurse infrequently may not receive enough colostrum, the substance that precedes true breast milk, to benefit from its normal laxative effect in eliminating bilirubin-rich meconium. Lack of adequate suckling depresses breast milk production, further increasing the problem. Helping the mother with breastfeeding to stimulate milk production and increase the infant's intake is essential. Supplementation with formula interferes with milk production. If breastfeeding is not adequate, weight loss is excessive, or the infant is dehydrated, supplementation with expressed breast milk or formula may be necessary. Glucose water will not decrease bilirubin levels and should be avoided.

***True breast-milk jaundice.*** True breast-milk jaundice, also called *late-onset breast-milk jaundice,* occurs after the first 3 to 5 days of life and lasts 3 weeks to as long as 3 months in some infants. The TSB usually peaks at 5 to 10 mg/dL and falls gradually over several months. In some infants, the TSB reaches levels of 20 to 30 mg/dL (Kaplan et al., 2011). The exact cause of true breast-milk jaundice is unknown. Substances in the breast milk may increase absorption of bilirubin from the intestine or interfere with conjugation. This condition may be a form of physiologic jaundice in breastfed infants. These infants have no signs of illness.

Treatment of breast milk jaundice includes close monitoring of TSB and at least 8 to 12 feedings each 24 hours. If bilirubin levels rise too high, phototherapy is begun while the mother continues frequent breastfeeding. Interruption of breastfeeding is not generally recommended. However, if the TSB levels are dangerously high, the health-care provider may order formula feeding for 1 to 3 days while the mother uses a breast pump to maintain her milk supply. Formula supplementation may be used instead. These measures should cause a rapid drop in bilirubin. If the level rises while breastfeeding is interrupted, jaundice from another cause should be investigated. The TSB may rise again when breastfeeding resumes, but the increase is usually not high enough to interfere with further breastfeeding.

### Blood Coagulation

Prothrombin and coagulation factors II, VII, IX, and X are produced by the liver and activated by vitamin K, which is deficient in the newborn.

### Iron Storage

Iron is stored in the fetal liver and spleen during the last months of pregnancy. Full-term infants who are breastfeeding usually do not need added iron until 4 to 6 months of age. At that time, they should begin consuming iron-containing foods or iron supplements. All infants who are not breastfeeding should be given iron-fortified formula (American Academy of Pediatrics [AAP] & American College of Obstetricians and Gynecologists [ACOG], 2012; Holt, Wooldridge, Story, et al., 2011).

### Drug Metabolism

The liver metabolizes drugs inefficiently in the newborn. Breastfeeding mothers should alert their physician or lactation consultant before taking medications, because harmful amounts of some drugs can be transferred to the infant through the breast milk.

## URINARY SYSTEM

### Kidney Development

Formation of the nephrons of the kidney is complete by 34 to 36 weeks of gestation (Frost, Fashaw, Hernandez, et al., 2011). Full kidney function, however, does not occur until after birth. Blood flow to the kidneys increases after birth because of decreased resistance in the renal vessels. The improved perfusion results in a steady improvement in kidney function during the first few days of life.

### Kidney Function

The newborn's kidney function is immature compared with that of the adult. The ability of the glomeruli to filter and the renal tubules to reabsorb is considerably less than in adults. The glomerular filtration rate doubles or triples during the first weeks after full-term birth but does not reach adult levels until 1 to 2 years of age (Frost et al., 2011). Therefore, infants have a decreased ability to remove waste products from the blood.

Small amounts of substances such as glucose and amino acids may escape into the urine of the neonate (Blackburn, 2013; Frost et al., 2011). Uric acid crystals may give a reddish color to the urine that is sometimes mistaken for blood.

**BOX 21.2 Intake and Output in the Newborn**

**First 3 to 5 Days of Life**
- Intake: 60–100 mL/kg (27–45 mL/lb) per day
- Output: At least 1 or 2 voids daily

**After the First 3 to 5 Days**
- Intake: 150–175 mL/kg (68–80 mL/lb) daily by 7 days
- Output: At least six voids daily by the 4th day

Voiding occurs within 12 hours for 50% of newborns; 92% void within 24 hours, and 99% void within 48 hours of life (Frost et al., 2011). The absence of kidneys or presence of abnormalities that interfere with urine excretion are usually discovered before birth because they cause low amniotic fluid volume. Only one or two voidings may occur during the first 2 days of life. The infant voids at least six times a day by the fourth day.

### Fluid Balance

Newborns have a lower tolerance for changes in total volume of body fluid than do older infants. In addition, the fluid turnover rate is greater than that in adults (Box 21.2). To maintain fluid balance, full-term infants need 60 to 100 mL/kg (27 to 45 mL/lb) per day during the first 3 to 5 days of life and 150 to 175 mL/kg (68 to 80 mL/lb) per day by 7 days of age (Halbardier, 2010).

#### Water Distribution

Water constitutes 75% of the newborn's body weight (Jones, Hayes, Starbuck, et al., 2011). Because infants have more fluid for their size than adults, with a larger proportion of the fluid located outside the cells, total body water is easily depleted. Conditions such as vomiting and diarrhea can quickly result in life-threatening dehydration. At birth, normal diuresis causes a 5% to 10% weight loss as excess extracellular water is lost (Halbardier, 2010; Jones et al., 2011).

#### Insensible Water Loss

Water lost from the skin and respiratory tract contributes to insensible water loss. The newborn's large body surface area and rapid respiratory rate cause increased insensible water loss. Fluid losses increase greatly when infants are placed under radiant warmers or phototherapy lights, which accelerate evaporation from the skin. An elevated respiratory rate or low humidity in the air surrounding the infant further raises insensible water loss.

#### Urine Dilution and Concentration

The ability of a newborn's kidneys to dilute urine is similar to that of adults, but they have only half the adult's ability to concentrate urine (Blackburn, 2013). Therefore, a newborn's kidneys cannot handle large increases in fluids, which results in fluid overload. This is most likely to happen if infants receive too much intravenous fluid. If abnormal conditions such as diarrhea cause excessive loss of fluid, the newborn's limited ability to conserve water leads to more rapid dehydration than in the older infant or child. The specific gravity of urine in the normal newborn is 1.002 to 1.01, and normal urine output is 2 to 5 mL/kg/hr (Jones et al., 2011).

### Acid-Base and Electrolyte Balance

The maintenance of acid-base and electrolyte balance is a primary function of the kidneys and may be precarious in neonates. In newborns, the tendency to lose bicarbonate at lower levels than adults and the lower ability to reabsorb it increases their risk for metabolic acidosis. In addition, the excretion of solutes is less efficient in newborns. Although newborns effectively conserve needed sodium, they are limited in sodium excretion, especially if the intake is excessive.

## IMMUNE SYSTEM

The neonate is less effective at fighting off infection than the older infant or child. Leukocytes are delayed in moving to the site of invasion and are inefficient in destroying the invader. The infant's decreased ability to localize infection leads to a tendency toward sepsis.

Fever and leukocytosis, which occur during infection in the older child, are often not present in the newborn with infection. This lack of response is the result of immaturity of the hypothalamus and the inflammatory response. Signs of infection in the neonate are nonspecific and include subtle changes in activity, tone, color, or feeding.

Because of their immature immune systems, infants are susceptible to pathogens that do not usually affect older children. Full-term newborns received antibodies from the mother during the last trimester of pregnancy. If the mother breastfeeds, the infant continues to receive antibodies in breast milk that provide passive immunity. Immunoglobulins (serum globulins with antibody activity) help protect the newborn from infection. The major immunoglobulins are IgG, IgM, and IgA.

### IgG

IgG, the only immunoglobulin that crosses the placenta, provides the fetus with passive temporary immunity to bacteria, bacterial toxins, and viruses to which the mother has immunity. Preterm infants have less IgG because transfer is greatest during the third trimester. Although the fetus makes some IgG, production at significant levels is delayed until after 6 months of age (Blackburn, 2013). The passive immunity from the mother gradually disappears over the first 6 to 8 months of life (Buckley, 2011).

### IgM

IgM helps protect against Gram-negative bacteria. Production increases rapidly a few days after birth as the infant is exposed to environmental antigens. IgM reaches adult levels at about 1 year of age (Buckley, 2011). If IgM is found in larger-than-normal amounts in the neonate, exposure to infection *in utero* is probable, as IgM does not cross the placenta.

### IgA

IgA also does not cross the placenta and must be produced by the infant. Because IgA is important for protecting the gastrointestinal and respiratory systems, newborns are particularly susceptible to infections of these systems. Immunoglobulin production begins at about 2 weeks of age. Secretory IgA is present in colostrum and breast milk (Kapur, Yoder, & Polin, 2011). Therefore, breastfed infants may receive protection that formula-fed infants do not.

## PSYCHOSOCIAL ADAPTATION

### Periods of Reactivity

In the early hours after birth, the infant goes through changes called *periods of reactivity*. The two periods of reactivity are separated by a period of sleep or decreased activity (Gardner & Hernandez, 2011).

#### First Period of Reactivity

The **first period of reactivity** begins at birth. Infants are wide awake, alert, and seem interested in their surroundings. Parents enjoy this phase, as the infant gazes directly at them when held in the *en face* (face-to-face) position. Infants move their arms and legs energetically, root, and appear hungry. If allowed to nurse, many infants latch on to the nipple and suck well. During this period, the temperature may be decreased, and the heart rate may be elevated to 180 beats per minute (bpm). Respiration may be as high as 80 breaths per minute. Rales, retractions, nasal flaring, and increased mucous secretions may be present. The pulse and respiration gradually slow, and the infant becomes sleepy.

#### Period of Sleep or Decreased Activity

After the first period of reactivity, infants fall into a deep sleep or exhibit greatly decreased activity. During this time, the pulse and respiration drop to the normal range.

#### Second Period of Reactivity

During the second period of reactivity, infants become interested in feeding and may pass meconium. The pulse, respiratory rate, and mucous secretions increase, and they may gag or regurgitate.

### Behavioral States

Six gradations in the infant's behavioral state, ranging from quiet sleep to crying, have been identified.

#### Deep or Quiet Sleep State

In the deep or quiet sleep state, the infant has no eye movements. Respirations are quiet, regular, and slower than in the other states. Although startles occur at intervals, the infant's body is still. Little or no response to noise or stimuli occurs, and the infant is difficult to arouse.

#### Light or Active Sleep State

In the light or active sleep state, infants move their extremities, stretch, change facial expressions, make sucking movements, and may fuss briefly. During this period, respiration tends to be more rapid and irregular, and rapid eye movements (REMs) occur. Infants are more likely to startle from noise or disturbances and may return to sleep or move to an awake state.

#### Drowsy State

The drowsy state is a transitional period between sleep and waking. The eyes may remain closed or, if open, appear glazed and unfocused. Infants startle and move their extremities slowly. They may go back to sleep or, with gentle stimulation, gradually awaken.

#### Quiet Alert State

The quiet alert state should be pointed out to parents because it is an excellent time to increase bonding. Infants focus on objects or people and seem bright and interested in their surroundings. They respond to stimuli and interaction with others. Body movements are minimal as they seem to concentrate on the environment. Full-term infants often are in this state shortly after birth.

#### Active Alert State

In the active alert state, infants are often fussy. They seem restless, have faster and more irregular respiration, may hiccup or regurgitate, and seem more aware of feelings of discomfort from hunger or cold. Although their eyes may be open, infants seem less focused on visual stimuli than during the quiet alert state.

#### Crying State

The crying state may quickly follow the active alert state if no intervention occurs to comfort the infant. The cries are continuous and lusty, and the infant does not respond positively to stimulation. A period of comforting may be required to move the infant to a state in which feeding or other activities can be accomplished.

## EARLY ASSESSMENTS

Immediately after birth, the infant is examined quickly for cardiorespiratory problems and obvious anomalies. The nurse determines whether resuscitation (see Chapter 30) or other immediate intervention is necessary. When the infant is stable and oxygenating well, a more thorough assessment can be performed. Table 21.2 summarizes newborn assessments.

**SAFETY ALERT**

***Protection From Bloodborne Infections***

When newborns are dried at birth, it is easy to forget that their skin is contaminated with blood and amniotic fluid. The nurse should wear gloves when handling newborns until they are bathed and all blood is removed from their skin and hair. This precaution helps protect the nurse from blood-borne infections.

### History

Information about the pregnancy, labor, and delivery is important in assessing the likelihood of problems at birth. The maternal age, health problems, and any complications during the pregnancy or birth may affect the neonate's adaptation at birth.

## ASSESSMENT OF CARDIORESPIRATORY STATUS

Assessments of respiratory and cardiovascular status are performed together because transitional changes take place in both systems simultaneously at birth.

### Airway

During birth, some fetal lung fluid is forced into the upper airway and expelled. Excessive fluid or mucus in the infant's respiratory passages may cause respiratory difficulty for several hours after birth.

#### Respiratory Rate

The nurse assesses respiration at least once every 30 minutes until the infant has been stable for 2 hours after birth (AAP & ACOG, 2012). If abnormalities are noted, respiration is assessed more often. The normal respiratory rate is 30 to 60 breaths per minute (Verklan, 2011). The average rate is 40 to 49 breaths per minute. The infant may breathe faster immediately after birth and during crying. Respiration should not be labored, and the chest movements should be symmetric.

Because the pattern and depth of respiration are irregular, they must be counted for a full minute for accuracy (see Procedure: Assessing Vital Signs in the Newborn). Periodic breathing, pauses in breathing lasting 5 to 10 seconds without other changes, followed by rapid respiration for 10 to 15 seconds may occur in some full-term infants during the first few days. Periodic breathing is more common in preterm infants. Apnea is any pause in breathing lasting 20 seconds or more, or any pause in breathing accompanied by cyanosis, pallor, bradycardia, or decreased muscle tone (Goodwin, 2010). Apnea is abnormal and requires prompt intervention.

#### Breath Sounds

The anterior and posterior lung fields are auscultated for breath sounds, which should be present equally throughout. Breath sounds should be clear over most areas. It is not unusual, however, to hear sounds of moisture in the lungs during the first hour or two after birth because fetal lung fluid has not been completely absorbed. Infants born by cesarean not preceded by labor may not experience the lung changes

*Text continued on p. 440*

## TABLE 21.2 Summary of Newborn Assessment

| Normal | Abnormal (Possible Causes) | Nursing Considerations |
|---|---|---|
| **Initial Assessment** | | |
| Assess for obvious problems first. If infant is stable and has no problems that require immediate attention, continue with complete assessment. | | |
| **Vital Signs** | | |
| ***Temperature*** | | |
| Axillary: 36.5° C–37.5° C (97.7° F–99.5° F).<br>Axilla is preferred site. | Decreased (cold environment, hypoglycemia, infection, CNS problem)<br>Increased (infection, environment too warm) | Decreased: Institute warming measures and check in 30 min. Check blood glucose.<br>Increased: Remove excessive clothing. Check for dehydration.<br>Decreased or increased: Look for signs of infection. Check radiant warmer or incubator temperature setting. Check thermometer for accuracy if skin is warm or cool to touch. Report abnormal temperatures to physician. |
| ***Pulses*** | | |
| Heart rate 120–160 bpm (100 sleeping, 180 crying).<br>Rhythm regular.<br>PMI at third to fourth intercostal space lateral to the midclavicular line.<br>Brachial, femoral, and pedal pulses present and equal bilaterally | Tachycardia (respiratory problems, anemia, infection, cardiac conditions)<br>Bradycardia (asphyxia, increased intracranial pressure)<br>PMI to right (dextrocardia, pneumothorax)<br>Murmurs (normal or congenital heart defects)<br>Dysrhythmias.<br>Absent or unequal pulses (coarctation of the aorta) | Note location of murmurs. Refer abnormal rates, rhythms and sounds, pulses. |
| ***Respiration*** | | |
| Rate 30–60 (average 40–49) breaths per min.<br>Respiration irregular, shallow, unlabored.<br>Chest movements symmetric.<br>Breath sounds present and clear bilaterally | Tachypnea, especially after the first hour (respiratory distress)<br>Slow respiration (maternal medications).<br>Nasal flaring (respiratory distress)<br>Grunting (respiratory distress syndrome)<br>Gasping (respiratory depression)<br>Periods of apnea more than 20 sec or with change in heart rate or color (respiratory depression, sepsis, cold stress)<br>Asymmetry or decreased chest expansion (pneumothorax)<br>Intercostal, xiphoid, or supraclavicular retractions or seesaw (paradoxical) respiration (respiratory distress)<br>Moist, coarse breath sounds (crackles, rhonchi) (fluid in lungs)<br>Bowel sounds in chest (diaphragmatic hernia) | Mild variations require continued monitoring and usually clear in early hours after birth.<br>If persistent or more than mild: suction, give oxygen, call physician, and initiate more intensive care. |
| ***Blood Pressure*** | | |
| Varies with age, weight, activity, and gestational age.<br>Average systolic, 65–95 mm Hg.<br>Average diastolic, 30–60 mm Hg | Hypotension (hypovolemia, shock, sepsis)<br>BP 20 mm Hg or more.<br>Higher in arms than legs (coarctation of the aorta) | Refer abnormal blood pressures.<br>Prepare for intensive care if very low. |
| **Measurements** | | |
| ***Weight*** | | |
| Weight 2500–4000 g (5 lb, 8 oz to 8 lb, 13 oz).<br>Weight loss up to 10% in early days. | High (LGA, maternal diabetes)<br>Low (SGA, preterm, multifetal pregnancy, medical conditions in mother that affected fetal growth)<br>Weight loss above 10% (dehydration, feeding problems) | Determine cause.<br>Monitor for complications common to cause. |
| ***Length*** | | |
| 48–53 cm (19–21 in). | Below normal (SGA, congenital dwarfism)<br>Above normal (LGA, maternal diabetes) | Determine cause.<br>Monitor for complications common to cause. |
| ***Head Circumference*** | | |
| 32–38 cm (12.5–15 in). Head and neck are approximately one-fourth of infant's body surface area. | Small (SGA, microcephaly, anencephaly)<br>Large (LGA, hydrocephalus, increased intracranial pressure) | Determine cause.<br>Monitor for complications common to cause. |
| ***Chest Circumference*** | | |
| 30–36 cm (12–14 in).<br>2 cm less than head circumference | Large (LGA)<br>Small (SGA) | Determine cause.<br>Monitor for complications common to cause. |

TABLE 21.2 **Summary of Newborn Assessment—cont'd**

| Normal | Abnormal (Possible Causes) | Nursing Considerations |
|---|---|---|
| ***Posture*** | | |
| Flexed extremities move freely, resist extension, return quickly to flexed state.<br>Hands usually clenched.<br>Movements symmetric.<br>Slight tremors on crying.<br>Extended, stiff legs if breech.<br>"Molds" body to caretaker's body when held.<br>Responds by quieting when needs met | Limp, flaccid, 'floppy,' or rigid extremities (preterm, hypoxia, medications, CNS trauma)<br>Hypertonic (neonatal abstinence syndrome, CNS injury)<br>Jitteriness or tremors (low glucose or calcium level)<br>Opisthotonos, seizures, stiff when held (CNS injury) | Seek cause, refer abnormalities. |
| **Cry** | | |
| Lusty, strong | High pitched (increased intracranial pressure)<br>Weak, absent, irritable, catlike 'mewing' (neurologic problems)<br>Hoarse or crowing (laryngeal irritation) | Observe for changes.<br>Report abnormalities. |
| **Skin** | | |
| Color pink or tan with acrocyanosis.<br>Vernix caseosa in creases.<br>Small amounts of lanugo over shoulders, sides of face, forehead, upper back.<br>Skin turgor good with quick recoil.<br>Some cracking and peeling of skin<br>**Normal Variations:** Milia, Skin tags,<br>Erythema toxicum ('flea bite' rash),<br>Puncture on scalp (from electrode),<br>Mongolian spots | **Color:** cyanosis of mouth and central areas (hypoxia).<br>Facial bruising (nuchal cord).<br>Pallor (anemia, hypoxia).<br>Gray (hypoxia, hypotension).<br>Red, sticky, transparent skin (very preterm).<br>Ruddy (polycythemia).<br>Greenish-brown discoloration of skin, nails, cord (possible fetal compromise, postterm).<br>Harlequin color (normal transient autonomic imbalance).<br>Mottling (normal or cold stress, hypovolemia, sepsis).<br>Jaundice (pathologic if first 24 hr).<br>Yellow vernix (blood incompatibilities).<br>Thick vernix (preterm)<br>**Delivery marks:** Bruises on body (pressure), scalp (vacuum extractor), or face (cord around neck).<br>Petechiae (pressure, low platelet count, infection).<br>Forceps marks<br>**Birthmarks:** Mongolian spots.<br>Nevus simplex (salmon patch, 'stork bite').<br>Nevus flammeus (port-wine stain).<br>Nevus vasculosus (strawberry hemangioma).<br>Café au lait spots (6 or more) larger than 0.5 cm in size (neurofibromatosis)<br>**Other:** Excessive lanugo (preterm).<br>Excessive peeling, cracking (postterm).<br>Pustules or other rashes (infection).<br>'Tenting' of skin (dehydration) | Differentiate facial bruising from cyanosis. Central cyanosis requires suction, oxygen, and further treatment.<br>Refer jaundice in first 24 hr or more extensive than expected for age.<br>Watch for respiratory problems in infants with meconium staining.<br>Look for signs and complications of preterm or postterm birth.<br>Record location, size, shape, color, type of rashes and marks. Differentiate mongolian spots from bruises.<br>Check for facial movement with forceps marks.<br>Watch for jaundice with bruising.<br>Point out and explain normal skin variations to parents. |
| **Head** | | |
| Sutures palpable with small separation between each.<br>Anterior fontanel diamond-shaped, 4-5 cm, soft, and flat.<br>May bulge slightly with crying.<br>Posterior fontanel triangular, 0.5–1 cm.<br>Hair silky and soft with individual hair strands<br>**Normal variations:** Overriding sutures (molding) Caput succedaneum or cephalhematoma (pressure during birth) | Head large (hydrocephalus, increased intracranial pressure) or small (microcephaly).<br>Widely separated sutures (hydrocephalus) or hard, ridged area at sutures (craniosynostosis).<br>Anterior fontanel depressed (dehydration, molding).<br>Full or bulging at rest (increased intracranial pressure).<br>Woolly, bunchy hair (preterm).<br>Unusual hair growth (genetic abnormalities). | Seek cause of variations.<br>Observe for signs of dehydration with depressed fontanel, increased intracranial pressure with bulging of fontanel and wide separation of sutures. Refer for treatment.<br>Differentiate caput succedaneum from cephalhematoma, and reassure parents of normal outcome. Observe for jaundice with cephalhematoma. |
| **Ears** | | |
| Ears well formed and complete.<br>Area where upper ear meets head even with imaginary line drawn from outer canthus of eye.<br>Startle response to loud noises.<br>Alerts to high-pitched voices | Low-set ears (chromosomal disorders).<br>Skin tags, preauricular sinuses, dimples (may be associated with kidney or other abnormalities).<br>No response to sound (deafness) | Check voiding if ears abnormal.<br>Look for signs of chromosomal abnormality if position abnormal.<br>Refer for evaluation if no response to sound. |

*Continued*

## TABLE 21.2 Summary of Newborn Assessment—cont'd

| Normal | Abnormal (Possible Causes) | Nursing Considerations |
|---|---|---|
| **Face** | | |
| Symmetric in appearance and movement.<br>Parts proportional and appropriately placed | Asymmetry (pressure and position *in utero*).<br>Drooping of mouth or one side of face, 'one-sided cry' (facial nerve injury).<br>Abnormal appearance (chromosomal abnormalities) | Seek cause of variations.<br>Check delivery history for possible cause of injury to facial nerve. |
| **Eyes** | | |
| Symmetrical.<br>Clear.<br>Transient strabismus.<br>Scant or absent tears.<br>Pupils equal, reactive to light.<br>Alerts to interesting sights.<br>Doll's-eye sign.<br>Red reflex present.<br>May have subconjunctival hemorrhage or edema of eyelids from pressure during birth. | Inflammation or drainage (chemical or infectious conjunctivitis).<br>Constant tearing (plugged lacrimal duct).<br>Unequal pupils.<br>Failure to follow objects (blindness).<br>White areas over pupils (cataracts).<br>Setting-sun sign (hydrocephalus).<br>Yellow sclera (jaundice).<br>Blue sclera (osteogenesis imperfecta) | Clean and monitor any drainage.<br>Seek cause. Reassure parents that subconjunctival hemorrhage and edema will clear. Refer other abnormalities. |
| **Nose** | | |
| Both nostrils open to air flow.<br>May have slight flattening from pressure during birth | Blockage of one or both nasal passages (choanal atresia).<br>Malformations (congenital conditions).<br>Flaring, mucus (respiratory distress) | Observe for respiratory distress.<br>Report malformations. |
| **Mouth** | | |
| Mouth, gums, tongue pink.<br>Tongue normal in size and movement.<br>Lips and palate intact.<br>Sucking pads.<br>Sucking, rooting, swallowing, gag reflexes present<br>**Normal variations:** Precocious teeth.<br>Epstein's pearls | Cyanosis (hypoxia).<br>White patches on cheeks or tongue (candidiasis).<br>Protruding tongue (Down syndrome).<br>Diminished movement of tongue, drooping mouth (facial nerve paralysis).<br>Cleft lip or palate, or both.<br>Absent or weak reflexes (preterm, neurologic problem).<br>Excessive drooling (tracheoesophageal fistula, esophageal atresia) | Administer oxygen for cyanosis.<br>Expect loose teeth to be removed.<br>Obtain order for antifungal medication for candidiasis.<br>Check mother for vaginal or breast infection.<br>Refer anomalies. |
| **Feeding** | | |
| Good suck/swallow coordination.<br>Retains feedings | Poorly coordinated suck and swallow (prematurity).<br>Duskiness or cyanosis during feeding (cardiac defects).<br>Choking, gagging, excessive drooling (tracheoesophageal fistula, esophageal atresia) | Feed slowly.<br>Stop frequently if difficulty occurs.<br>Suction and stimulate if necessary.<br>Refer infants with continued difficulty. |
| **Neck/Clavicles** | | |
| Short neck.<br>Turns head easily side to side.<br>Raises head when prone.<br>Clavicles intact | Weakness, contractures, or rigidity (muscle abnormalities).<br>Webbing of neck, large fat pad at back of neck (chromosomal disorders).<br>Crepitus, lump, or crying when clavicle or other bones palpated.<br>Diminished or absent arm movement (fractures) | Fracture of clavicle is more frequent in large infants with shoulder dystocia at birth.<br>Immobilize arm.<br>Look for other injuries.<br>Refer abnormalities. |
| **Chest** | | |
| Cylinder shape.<br>Xiphoid process may be prominent.<br>Symmetrical.<br>Nipples present and located properly.<br>May have engorgement, white nipple discharge (maternal hormone withdrawal) | Asymmetry (diaphragmatic hernia, pneumothorax).<br>Supernumerary nipples.<br>Redness (infection) | Report abnormalities. |
| **Abdomen** | | |
| Rounded, soft.<br>Bowel sounds present within first hour after birth.<br>Liver palpable 1-2 cm below right costal margin.<br>Skin intact.<br>Three vessels in cord.<br>Clamp tight and cord drying.<br>Meconium passed within 12–48 hr.<br>Urine generally passed within 12–24 hr<br>**Normal variation:** 'Brick dust' staining of diaper (uric acid crystals) | Sunken abdomen (diaphragmatic hernia).<br>Distended abdomen or loops of bowel visible (obstruction, infection, enlarged organs).<br>Absent bowel sounds after first hour (paralytic ileus).<br>Masses palpated (kidney tumors, distended bladder).<br>Enlarged liver (infection, heart failure, hemolytic disease).<br>Abdominal wall defects (umbilical or inguinal hernia, omphalocele, gastroschisis, exstrophy of bladder).<br>Two vessels in cord (other anomalies).<br>Bleeding (loose clamp).<br>Redness, drainage from cord (infection).<br>No passage of meconium (imperforate anus, obstruction).<br>Lack of urinary output (kidney anomalies) or inadequate amounts (dehydration) | Refer abnormalities.<br>Assess for other anomalies if only two vessels in cord.<br>Tighten or replace loose cord clamp.<br>If stool and urine output abnormal, look for missed recording, increase feedings, report. |

**TABLE 21.2 Summary of Newborn Assessment—cont'd**

| Normal | Abnormal (Possible Causes) | Nursing Considerations |
|---|---|---|
| **Genitals** | | |
| ***Female*** | | |
| Labia majora dark, covering clitoris and labia minora.<br>Small amount of white mucous vaginal discharge.<br>Urinary meatus and vagina present<br>**Normal variations:** Vaginal bleeding (pseudomenstruation).<br>Hymenal tags | Clitoris and labia minora larger than labia majora (preterm).<br>Large clitoris (ambiguous genitalia).<br>Edematous labia (breech birth) | Check gestational age for immature genitalia.<br>Refer anomalies. |
| ***Male*** | | |
| Testes within scrotal sac, rugae on scrotum, prepuce nonretractable.<br>Meatus at tip of penis | Testes in inguinal canal or abdomen (preterm, cryptorchidism).<br>Lack of rugae on scrotum (preterm).<br>Edema of scrotum (pressure in breech birth).<br>Enlarged scrotal sac (hydrocele).<br>Small penis, scrotum (preterm, ambiguous genitalia).<br>Empty scrotal sac (cryptorchidism).<br>Urinary meatus located on upper side of penis (epispadias), underside of penis (hypospadias), or perineum.<br>Ventral curvature of the penis (chordee) | Check gestational age for immature genitalia.<br>Refer anomalies.<br>Explain to parents why no circumcision can be performed with abnormal placement of meatus. |
| **Extremities** | | |
| ***Upper and Lower Extremities*** | | |
| Equal and bilateral movement of extremities.<br>Correct number and formation of fingers and toes.<br>Nails to ends of digits or slightly beyond.<br>Flexion, good muscle tone | Crepitus, redness, lumps, swelling (fracture).<br>Diminished or absent movement, especially during Moro reflex (fracture, nerve injury, paralysis).<br>Polydactyly (extra digits).<br>Syndactyly (webbing).<br>Fused or absent digits.<br>Poor muscle tone (preterm, neurologic injury, hypoglycemia, hypoxia) | Refer all anomalies.<br>Look for others. |
| ***Upper Extremities*** | | |
| Two transverse palm creases | Simian crease (normal or Down syndrome).<br>Diminished movement (injury).<br>Diminished movement of arm with extension and forearm prone (Erb-Duchenne paralysis) | Refer all anomalies.<br>Look for others. |
| ***Lower Extremities*** | | |
| Legs equal in length, abduct equally.<br>Gluteal and thigh creases and knee height equal.<br>No hip 'clunk'.<br>Normal position of feet. | Ortolani and Barlow tests abnormal, unequal leg length, unequal thigh or gluteal creases (developmental dysplasia of the hip).<br>Malposition of feet (position *in utero*, talipes equinovarus) | Refer all anomalies.<br>Look for others.<br>Check malpositioned feet to see if they can be gently manipulated back to normal position. |
| **Back** | | |
| No openings observed or felt in vertebral column.<br>Anus patent.<br>Sphincter tightly closed | Failure of one or more vertebrae to close (spina bifida), with or without sac with spinal fluid and meninges (meningocele) or spinal fluid, meninges, and cord (myelomeningocele) enclosed.<br>Tuft of hair over (spina bifida occulta).<br>Pilonidal dimple or sinus.<br>Imperforate anus | Refer abnormalities. Observe for movement below level of defect.<br>If sac is present, cover with sterile dressing and wet with sterile saline.<br>Protect from injury. |
| **Reflexes** | | |
| See Table 21.3. | Absent, asymmetric, or weak reflexes | Observe for signs of fracture, nerve injury, or CNS injury. |

*BP*, Blood pressure; *bpm*, beats per minute; *CNS*, central nervous system; *LGA*, large for gestational age; *PMI*, point of maximum impulse; *SGA*, small for gestational age

## PROCEDURE

### *Assessing Vital Signs in the Newborn*

**Purpose**

To obtain an accurate measurement of newborn vital signs.

**Temperature**

1. Place the thermometer vertically along the chest wall with the tip of the thermometer in the center of the axillary space. Hold the infant's arm firmly over the probe to *keep it positioned properly and avoid injury to the infant. If the thermometer is held horizontally, it may protrude behind the axilla and give an inaccurate reading.*
2. Read the thermometer at the proper time *to increase accuracy.* Electronic or digital: when the indicator sounds; other types: according to manufacturer's directions. Normal range: 36.5° C to 37.5° C (97.7° F to 99.5° F).

**Respiration**

1. Assess respiration when the infant is quiet or sleeping, if possible, *so that lung sounds can be heard more clearly.*
2. Observe, auscultate, or palpate the chest and abdomen. *Use of more than one method helps differentiate rapid, irregular respiration from other movements.*
3. Lift the infant's blanket and shirt *to see the chest and abdomen.* Observe the pattern of respiration before counting *to make it easier to count the rate.*
4. If desired, place a hand lightly to the side of the infant's chest or abdomen *to feel the movement.* Avoid covering the chest completely *so chest excursions can be watched as well as palpated.*
5. To auscultate respiration, place a stethoscope on the right side of the infant's chest *to decrease the sounds of the heart.* Then listen to breath sounds in all areas.
6. Count for a full minute *to increase accuracy, because respirations are normally irregular in the newborn.*
7. Offer a pacifier or gloved finger for sucking *to help quiet a crying infant.* If the infant continues to cry, count the respiration but make a note in the chart because the rate may be faster than when the infant is quiet. Recheck later when the infant is calm.
8. Expect the respiratory rate to be 30 to 60 breaths per minute with an average of 40 to 49 when the infant is at rest. Report signs of respiratory distress (tachypnea, retractions, flaring, cyanosis, grunting, seesawing, apneic periods, and asymmetry of chest movements) *to ensure follow-up care.*

**Apical Pulse**

1. If possible, listen to the apical pulse on a quiet or sleeping infant *so the sounds can be heard more clearly.*
2. Use a stethoscope equipped with a pediatric head, if available, to listen. *A small head allows better contact between the stethoscope and the chest wall and eliminates some of the sounds from the lungs and intestines.*
3. If the infant is crying, insert a pacifier or a gloved finger into the mouth *to quiet the infant.*
4. If the infant cannot be quieted, increase concentration and time spent listening *to focus on the heart sounds.*
5. Listen briefly before beginning to count. Tapping a finger in rhythm with the beat may be helpful. Count for a full minute to allow time *to identify abnormalities.* Expect the heart rate to be 120 to 160 beats per minute (bpm) at rest.
6. Move the stethoscope to listen over the entire heart area *to increase the chance of hearing abnormal sounds.* Refer any abnormal sounds (arrhythmias, murmurs) for follow-up.

that occur during labor and birth and are more likely to have coarse breath sounds for a short time. Continued abnormal or diminished sounds should always be reported to the primary care provider.

#### Signs of Respiratory Distress

The nurse must be alert for signs of respiratory distress, which may be present at birth or develop later.

***Tachypnea.*** **Tachypnea,** a respiratory rate of more than 60 breaths per minute, is the most common sign of respiratory distress. Tachypnea is not unusual during the first hour after birth and during periods of reactivity. Continued tachypnea, however, is abnormal.

***Retractions.*** Retractions result when the soft tissue around the bones of the chest is drawn in with the effort of pulling air into the lungs. Xiphoid (substernal) retractions occur when the area under the sternum retracts each time the infant inhales. When the muscles between the ribs are pulled in so that each rib is outlined, intercostal retractions are present. The muscles above the sternum and around the clavicles also may be used to aid in respiration (supraclavicular retractions). Occasional mild retractions are common immediately after birth but should not continue after the first hour.

***Flaring of the nares.*** A reflex widening of the nostrils occurs when the infant is receiving insufficient oxygen. Nasal flaring helps to decrease airway resistance and increase the amount of air entering the lungs. Intermittent flaring may occur in the first hour after birth. Continued flaring indicates a more serious respiratory problem.

***Cyanosis.*** Cyanosis is a purplish-blue discoloration that indicates the infant is not getting enough oxygen. It may be preceded by a dusky or gray hue to the skin. Central cyanosis involves the lips, tongue, mucous membranes, and trunk and shows true hypoxia. This sign indicates that not enough oxygen is reaching the vital organs, requiring

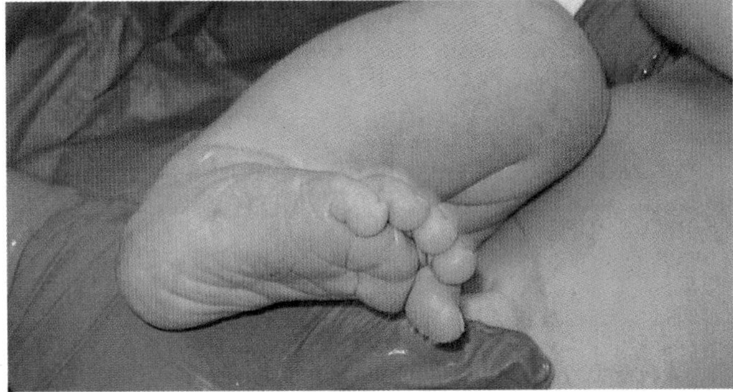

**FIG 21.6** Acrocyanosis. (Courtesy Todd Shiros, Santa Fe Springs, CA.)

immediate attention. To differentiate cyanosis from bruising, apply pressure to the area. A cyanotic area will blanch, but a bruised area remains blue. A pulse oximeter is used to determine oxygen saturation in infants with cyanosis.

Acrocyanosis is peripheral cyanosis involving just the extremities and is normal during the first day or when the infant is cold. Acrocyanosis is caused by poor perfusion of blood to the periphery of the body (Fig. 21.6).

***Grunting.*** In grunting, the infant first closes the glottis to keep air in the alveoli. Then the vocal cords are partially closed during expiration, producing the grunting sound (Carlo & DiFiore, 2011). Grunting may be very mild and heard only with a stethoscope, or it may be loud enough to hear unaided in an infant having severe respiratory difficulty. Persistent grunting is a common sign of respiratory distress syndrome and necessitates expanded assessment and referral for treatment.

*Seesaw or paradoxical respiration.* Normally, the chest and abdomen rise and fall together during respiration. In the infant with severe respiratory difficulty, the chest falls when the abdomen rises and the chest rises when the abdomen falls, causing a seesaw effect.

*Asymmetry.* Chest expansion should be equal on both sides. Asymmetry, or decreased movement on one side, may indicate the collapse of a lung (pneumothorax).

### Choanal Atresia

Choanal atresia is blockage or narrowing of one or both nasal passages by bone or tissue. Assessment for choanal atresia is important because newborns are preferential nose breathers for approximately the first 4 to 6 weeks of life (Sprecher & Arnold, 2011). They breathe mostly through the nose, except when crying. Bilateral choanal atresia causes severe respiratory distress and requires surgery. Blockage of one side puts the infant at risk for respiratory distress if the other side becomes occluded by mucus or edema.

The nurse can assess for choanal atresia by closing the infant's mouth and occluding one nostril at a time. The infant is observed for breathing, and breath sounds are auscultated while each nostril is occluded. Another method of assessment is to pass a small catheter through each nostril to check for patency. Infants with choanal atresia may become cyanotic when quiet but pink when crying.

### Color

In addition to cyanosis, the nurse assesses for pallor and ruddiness.

#### Pallor

Pallor can indicate that the infant is slightly hypoxic or anemic. A laboratory examination of hemoglobin and hematocrit or a complete blood count may be performed.

#### Ruddy Color

A ruddy or reddish skin color (plethora) may indicate polycythemia. Infants with elevated hematocrit levels are at increased risk for jaundice from the normal destruction of excessive red blood cells that occurs after birth.

### Heart Sounds

The heart is auscultated for rate, rhythm, and the presence of murmurs or abnormal sounds. The nurse should count the apical pulse for a full minute for accuracy and listen for abnormalities. The rate should range between 120 and 160 bpm with normal activity and can rise to 180 bpm during crying and drop as low as 100 bpm during deep sleep.

If no problems are present at birth, the heart rate should be recorded at least once every 30 minutes until the infant has been stable for 2 hours after birth (AAP & ACOG, 2012). Monitoring is more frequent if abnormalities are present. Once stable, the heart rate is checked once every 8 to 12 hours or according to agency policy, unless a reason for more frequent assessment develops.

The apex of the heart is located at the point of maximum impulse, where the pulse is most easily felt and the sound is loudest. This is at the third or fourth intercostal space, lateral to the midclavicular line (a line drawn from the middle of the left clavicle). Conditions that affect the position of the heart include pneumothorax and dextrocardia (in which the heart position is reversed from normal).

#### Rhythm and Murmurs

The rhythm of the heart should be regular, and the first and second sounds should be heard clearly. Abnormalities in rhythm and sounds such as murmurs should be noted. Murmurs are sounds of abnormal blood flow through the heart and may indicate openings in the septum of the heart or problems with blood flow through the valves. Most murmurs in the newborn are temporary, caused by incomplete transition from fetal to neonatal circulation. A murmur is common until the ductus arteriosus is functionally closed. Any abnormal sounds of the heart should be investigated further because they may be signs of cardiac defects.

### Brachial and Femoral Pulses

The brachial and femoral pulses should be present and equal bilaterally. The brachial pulse is located over the antecubital space, and the femoral pulse is located at the groin. Femoral pulses that are weaker than the brachial pulses may indicate impaired blood flow, as in coarctation of the aorta—a congenital heart defect (see Chapter 46).

### Blood Pressure

Measurement of blood pressure (BP) is not a necessary part of a routine assessment of the newborn. The BP is taken on all extremities, however, if the infant has unequal pulses, murmurs, or other signs of cardiac complications. Doppler ultrasonography or other electronic measurement is used. To ensure accurate measurement, the infant should be quiet during BP assessment because crying elevates the BP. The width of the BP cuff should be 40% to 50% of the circumference of the arm or leg or 25% to 55% wider than the diameter of the limb (Vargo, 2014).

BP varies according to the infant's age, weight, activity, and gestational age. The average BP for full-term newborns shortly after birth is 65 to 95 mm Hg systolic and 30 to 60 mm Hg diastolic (Gardner & Hernandez, 2011). A systolic blood pressure in the upper extremities that is more than 20 mm Hg higher than that of the lower extremities may indicate coarctation of the aorta (Vargo, 2014). Hypotension may occur in the sick infant.

### Capillary Refill

Capillary refill is assessed to help determine whether perfusion is adequate. Capillary refill is checked by depressing the skin over the chest, abdomen, or an extremity until the area blanches. The color should return within 3 to 4 seconds (Vargo, 2015).

## ASSESSMENT OF THERMOREGULATION

The neonate's temperature is assessed soon after birth while being held by the mother or in a radiant warmer using a skin probe attached to the abdomen. The probe allows the warmer to measure and display the infant's skin temperature continuously. The probe should not be attached over bony prominences or areas of brown fat. The temperature control is set to regulate the amount of heat produced according to the infant's skin temperature to avoid hyper- and hypothermia. The temperature should be assessed at least once every 30 minutes until it has been stable for 2 hours after birth (AAP & ACOG, 2012). The temperature is often checked again at 4 hours and then once every 8 hours or according to agency policy, as long as it remains stable (see Procedure: Assessing Vital Signs in the Newborn).

The most common method of taking the neonate's temperature is axillary measurement (Fig. 21.7). The normal range for axillary temperature is 36.5°C to 37.5°C (97.7°F to 99.5°F) (Brown & Landers, 2011). Axillary temperature measurement is safer than rectal temperature measurement because it avoids the possibility of irritation or injury to the rectum, which turns at a right angle approximately 3 cm (1.2 inches) from the anal sphincter (Brown & Landers, 2011). If a rectal temperature is necessary, the nurse should use great care because inserting the thermometer too far could result in fatal perforation of the intestinal wall. A thermometer should never be forced into the rectum because of the possibility of an imperforate (closed) anus.

Temperatures are usually measured with an electronic digital thermometer. Mercury thermometers are no longer used because of the

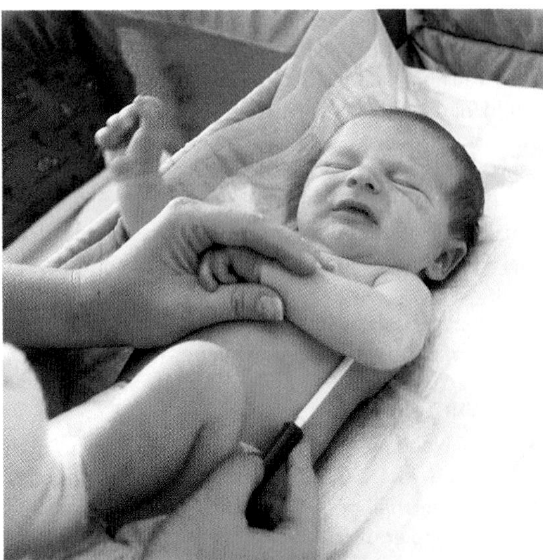

FIG 21.7 The infant is held securely to prevent injury and obtain an accurate reading when taking the temperature.

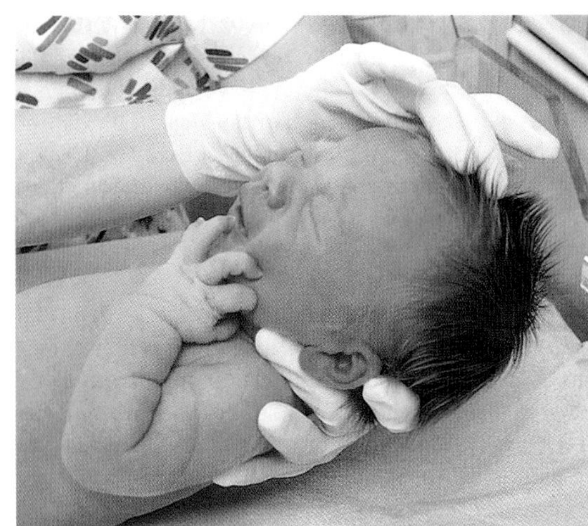

FIG 21.8 Palpation of the anterior fontanel. Note elevation of the head.

**BOX 21.3 Normal Vital Signs in the Newborn**

- Axillary Temperature: 36.5° C to 37.5° C (97.7° F to 99.5° F)
- Apical pulse: 120 to 160 beats per minute (bpm) (100 sleeping; 180 crying)
- Respiration: 30 to 60 breaths per minute

possibility of injury or contamination with mercury if the thermometer breaks. Inexpensive digital thermometers used while the infant is in the hospital may be given to the parents for home use. Disposable plastic strips that change color to indicate temperature readings are used less often than electronic models. Tympanic thermometers, used in some facilities for older infants and children, are not recommended for newborns at this time (Brown & Landers, 2011). (Box 21.3 lists normal temperature ranges for a newborn.)

## ASSESSING FOR ANOMALIES

### Head

The newborn's head is large in proportion to the rest of the body. The head and neck comprise 25% of the body surface area (Gardner & Hernandez, 2011). The head is palpated to assess the shape and to identify abnormalities. The degree of molding, size of the fontanels, and presence of caput succedaneum or later development of a cephalhematoma are noted.

The hair should be fine with a consistent pattern. Abnormal hair growth patterns may indicate genetic abnormalities. The nurse separates the hair, if necessary, to display bruises, rashes, or other marks on the scalp. A small red mark is present if a fetal monitor electrode was inserted into the skin of the scalp.

#### Molding

Molding refers to changes in the shape of the head from overriding of cranial bones at the sutures. Molding occurs most often in infants born vaginally because it allows the head to pass through the birth canal more easily. The condition usually resolves within a few days to a week after birth.

All sutures should be palpated. Separation may be the result of molding or, if it persists or widens, may indicate increased intracranial pressure. A hard, ridged area not resulting from molding may be caused by premature closure of the sutures, called *craniosynostosis*. This condition may impair brain growth and the shape of the head and necessitates surgery.

#### Fontanels

The nurse palpates the fontanels—the areas where the sutures of the head meet (Fig. 21.8). The infant's head is elevated during palpation for accurate assessment. The anterior fontanel is a diamond-shaped area where the frontal and parietal bones meet (see Fig. 16.5). It measures 4 to 5 cm from bone to bone, although this distance varies because of molding and individual differences. The fontanel closes by 18 months of age (Vargo, 2014).

The anterior fontanel should be soft and flat (even with the surrounding bones) or only slightly depressed. After molding resolves, a depressed fontanel may be a sign of dehydration. Vigorous crying may cause the fontanel to bulge. Fullness or bulging of the anterior fontanel of a quiet infant may indicate increased intracranial pressure. Abnormal signs are reported to the primary care provider.

The posterior fontanel is a triangular area where the occipital and parietal bones meet. Measuring 0.5 to 1 cm, the posterior fontanel is much smaller than the anterior fontanel. This fontanel closes by the time the infant is 2 to 4 months of age (Vargo, 2014).

#### Caput Succedaneum

A caput succedaneum is an area of localized edema that often appears over the vertex of the newborn's head as a result of pressure against the mother's cervix during labor (Fig. 21.9). The edematous area crosses suture lines, is soft, and varies in size. It resolves quickly and generally disappears within several days after birth (Vargo, 2014). Caput also can occur when a vacuum extractor is used to assist birth (see Chapter 19), with the lesion corresponding to the area where the extractor was placed on the skull. The amount of edema and presence of bruising are assessed.

#### Cephalhematoma

A cephalhematoma results from bleeding between the periosteum and the skull caused by pressure during birth (Fig. 21.10). It can occur on one or both sides of the head, usually over the parietal bones. The firm swelling is usually not present at birth but develops within the first 24 to 48 hours.

The nurse carefully palpates the area to differentiate cephalhematoma from caput succedaneum. A cephalhematoma has clear edges that end at the suture lines. Unlike caput succedaneum, it does not cross the suture lines because the bleeding is held between the bone and its covering, the periosteum. A cephalhematoma reabsorbs slowly and may take 2 weeks to 3 months to completely resolve (Mangurten & Puppala, 2011). Because of the breakdown of the red blood cells within the hematoma, affected infants are at greater risk for jaundice.

Both caput succedaneum and cephalhematoma may be frightening to parents. They need information, even if they do not ask, about the causes and how long it takes for the areas to resolve.

## Face

The face is examined for symmetry, positioning of the facial features, movement, and expression. A transient asymmetry from intrauterine pressure may be present, which lasts a few weeks or months. Drooping of the mouth appears as a one-sided cry and may be caused by facial nerve trauma. Irregularities in the facial features should be reported.

## Neck and Clavicles

The nurse assesses the infant's neck and notes the infant's ability to turn the head from side to side. The neck is very short. Webbing or an unusually large fat pad between the occiput and the shoulders may indicate a chromosomal anomaly. No masses should be present. When lying in a prone position, the term infant should be able to raise the head briefly and turn it to the other side.

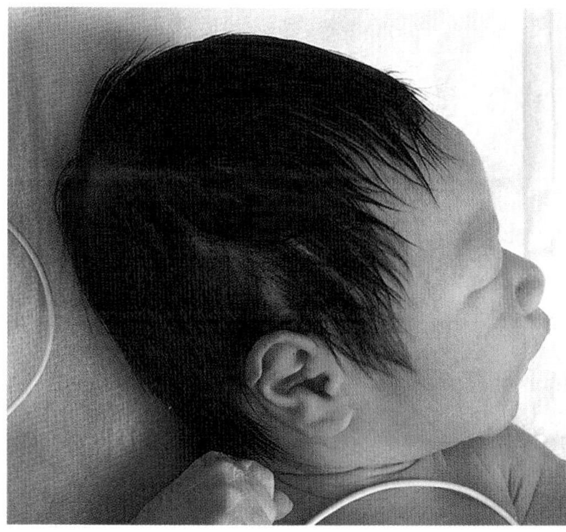

FIG 21.9 Caput succedaneum is an edematous area on the head from pressure against the cervix. It may cross suture lines.

Fractures of the clavicle are more likely to occur in large infants. A lump, swelling, or tenderness over the bone may occur. Crepitus (grating of the bone) or movement of the bone may be palpated if a fracture is present. Decreased movement of the affected arm is especially noticeable when the Moro reflex is elicited. Injury to the brachial plexus may cause paralysis of the arm on the side of the fracture. The arm is treated by immobilization.

## Cord

The umbilical cord should contain three vessels. The two arteries are small and may stand up at the cut end. The single vein is larger than the arteries and resembles a slit because its walls are more easily compressed. A two-vessel cord can be an isolated abnormality or associated with chromosomal and renal defects. The amount of Wharton's jelly in the cord is noted. If the cord appears thin, the infant may have been poorly nourished *in utero*. A yellow-brown or green tinge to the cord indicates that meconium was released before birth, perhaps as a result of fetal compromise. There should be no redness or discharge from the cord.

## Extremities

The infant should actively move the extremities equally in a random manner. The limbs of a term infant should remain sharply flexed and resist extension during examination. Poor muscle tone results in a limp or 'floppy' infant, which may occur from inadequate oxygen during birth but should resolve within a few minutes as oxygen intake increases. Continued poor muscle tone may be caused by prematurity or neurologic injury. Infants with previously good muscle tone may show decreased flexion if they become hypoglycemic or experience respiratory difficulty.

All extremities are examined for signs of fractures such as crepitus, redness, lumps, or swelling. Lack of independent movement of an extremity may indicate nerve injury. Brachial nerve plexus injury may result in Erb's palsy (Erb-Duchenne paralysis)—paralysis of the shoulder and arm muscles. The affected arm is extended at the infant's side with the forearm prone, and movement is diminished.

### Hands and Feet

The fingers and toes are examined for extra digits (polydactyly) and webbing between digits (syndactyly). Extra digits are often small and may not have bones. Tying the extra digits with sutures causes

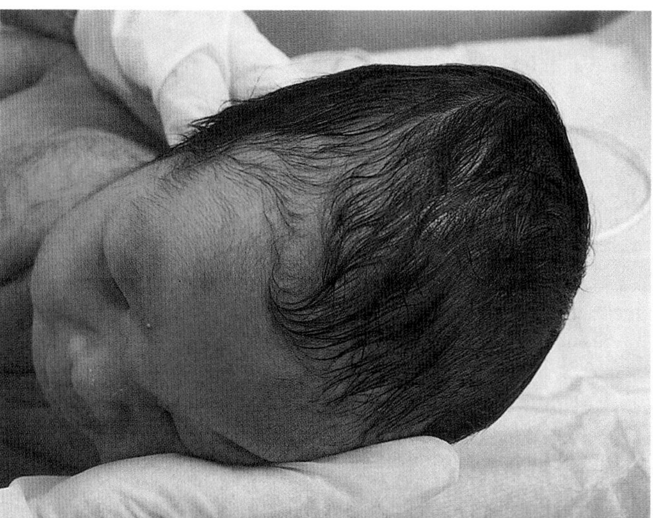

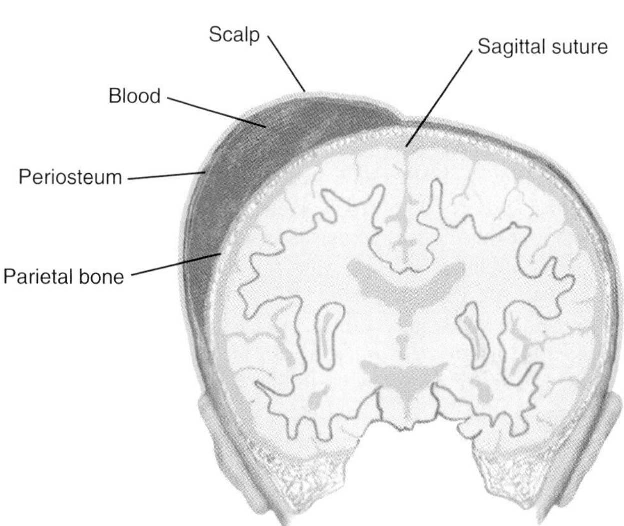


FIG 21.10 A cephalhematoma is characterized by bleeding between the bone and its covering, the periosteum. It can occur on one or both sides and does not cross suture lines.

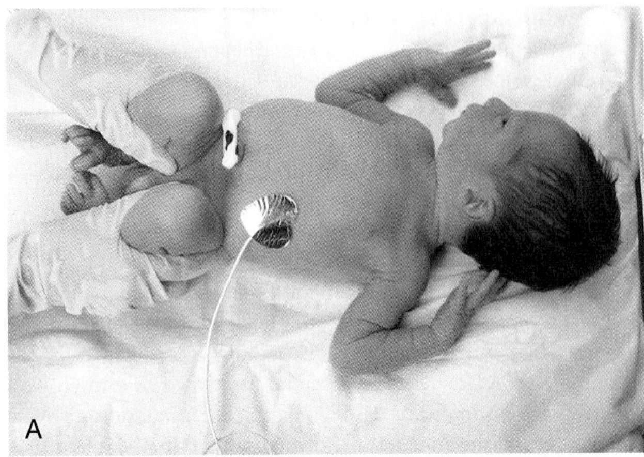


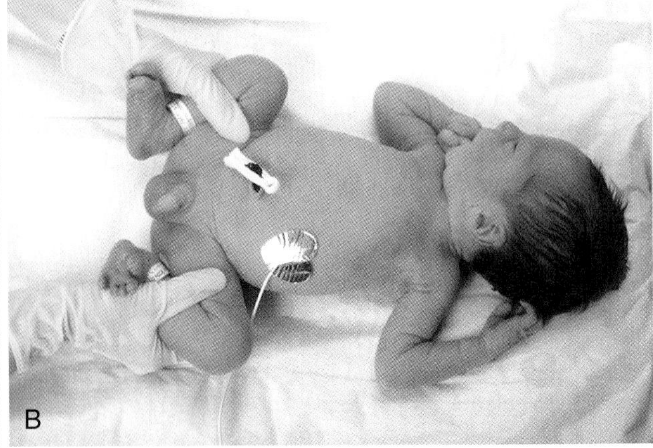


**FIG 21.11** Assessment of the hips. Place the fingers over the infant's greater trochanter and thumbs over the femur. Flex the knees and hips. **A,** Barlow test: adduct the hips, and apply gentle pressure down and back with the thumbs. In hip dysplasia, the examiner can feel the femoral head move out of the acetabulum. **B,** Ortolani test: abduct the thighs, and apply gentle pressure forward over the greater trochanter. A 'clunking' sensation indicates a dislocated femoral head moving into the acetabulum. A hip click is normal from ligament movement.

them to atrophy and fall off. Presence of a bone in the extra digit requires surgical removal. Webbed fingers or toes may be corrected by surgery. Nails in a term infant should extend to the end of the fingers or slightly beyond.

The hands are examined for a single, transverse palmar crease. Normally, two long transverse creases extend most of the way across the palm. A single crease parallel with the base of the fingers that crosses the palm without a break is referred to as a simian crease. This feature may be seen with incurving of the little finger and a low-set thumb in Down syndrome (trisomy 21). However, the simian crease alone is not diagnostic of Down syndrome, as it occurs in 4% of normal infants (Taperro, 2015).

The feet are assessed for talipes equinovarus, or clubfoot, a common malformation (see Chapter 50). If a foot looks abnormal, it should be gently manipulated. If it moves to a normal position, the abnormality is probably temporary, resulting from the position of the infant in the uterus. In true clubfoot, the foot turns inward and cannot be moved to a midline position.

### Hips

The hips are examined for developmental dysplasia (see Chapter 50). In this condition, instability of the hip joint occurs and the head of the femur can move in and out of the acetabulum. Partial dislocation and inadequate development of the acetabulum can occur.

Barlow and Ortolani tests are methods of assessing for hip instability in the newborn (Fig. 21.11). Both legs should abduct equally. Abduction of the affected hip may be more difficult. A hip click may be felt or heard but is usually normal and is different from the 'clunk' of hip dysplasia when the femoral head moves in the hip socket (Sankar, Horn, Wells, et al., 2011).

When the infant's legs are bent with the feet flat on the bed, the knee on the affected side is lower if the hip is dislocated. With the infant in a prone position, the legs are extended (Fig. 21.12). If the hip is dislocated, the leg on the affected side is shorter, and the creases are asymmetric. Because the hip may be unstable but not yet dislocated, these signs are not usually present at birth.

Treatment of developmental dysplasia of the hip involves immobilizing the leg in a flexed, abducted position, usually with a harness. Early identification and treatment are essential to prevent permanent injury to the joint.

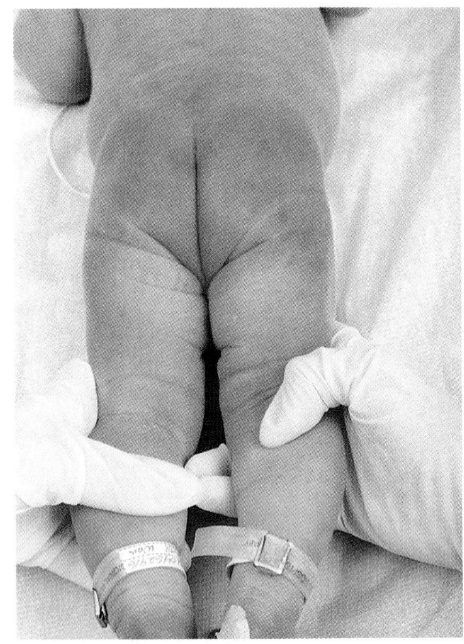

**FIG 21.12** Note the symmetry of gluteal and thigh creases.

### Vertebral Column

The nurse palpates the newborn's vertebral column to discover any defects in the vertebrae (see Chapter 52). An indentation, especially with a tuft of hair over it, is a sign of spina bifida occulta—failure of a vertebra to close completely. Other, more obvious neural tube defects include a meningocele (protrusion of spinal fluid and meninges) or myelomeningocele (protrusion of spinal fluid, meninges, and the spinal cord) through the defect in the vertebrae. These defects appear as a sack on the back that is sometimes covered by skin or only the meninges. A pilonidal dimple may be present at the base of the spine. It should be examined for a sinus and the depth noted.

### Measurements

Measurements provide information about the infant's growth *in utero*. The weight, length, and head and chest circumferences are compared with the norms for the infant's gestational age.

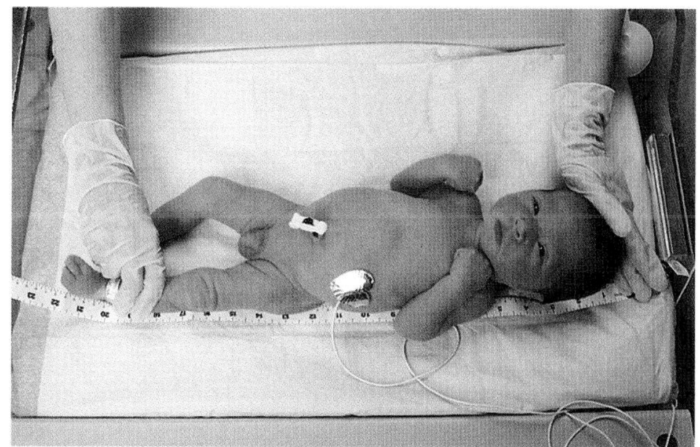

FIG 21.13 A tape is placed alongside the infant to measure the length. A mark can be made on the bed at the head and foot and the distance between the marks measured.

### Weight

The newborn's weight ranges between 2500 and 4000 g (5 lb, 8 oz and 8 lb, 13 oz) (Cheffer & Rannalli, 2016). The average weight of a full-term newborn is 3400 g (7 lb, 8 oz). Factors affecting weight include gestational age, placental functioning, genetic factors, and maternal diabetes, hypertension, and substance abuse.

Infants are weighed each day they are in the birth facility and at follow-up visits. They are expected to lose up to 10% of their birth weight during the first few days of life. This weight loss is caused by excretion of meconium from the bowel, normal loss of extracellular fluid, and inadequate intake of calories in the early days after birth. Infants normally regain or exceed their birth weight by 14 days of life. Thereafter, they gain approximately 20 to 30 g/day during the early months (Keane, 2011).

### Length

The infant's length is measured from the top of the head to the heel of the outstretched leg (Fig. 21.13). The normal length of a full-term newborn is 48 to 53 cm (19 to 21 inches) (Cheffer & Rannalli, 2016).

### Head and Chest Circumference

The diameter of the head is measured around the occiput and just above the eyebrows. The normal range of head circumference in the term newborn is 32 to 38 cm (12.5 to 14.5 inches) (Vargo, 2014). The measurement may be affected by molding of the skull during the birth process. If a large amount of molding occurred, the head is remeasured after regaining its normal shape. An abnormally small head may indicate poor brain growth and microcephaly. A very large head may be a sign of hydrocephalus.

The chest is measured at the level of the nipples and is usually 2 to 3 cm smaller than the head. The normal circumference of the chest is approximately 33 cm (13 inches) (Vargo, 2014). If molding of the head is present, the head and chest measurements may be equal at birth.

## ASSESSMENT OF BODY SYSTEMS

### Neurologic System

#### Reflexes

The nurse notes the presence and strength of the reflexes and whether both sides of the body respond symmetrically (Fig. 21.14). A diminished overall response occurs in preterm or ill infants. Absence of reflexes may indicate a serious neurologic problem. Asymmetric responses may indicate that trauma during birth caused nerve injury, paralysis, or fracture. Some of the newborn reflexes gradually weaken and disappear over a period of months (Table 21.3).

### CRITICAL THINKING EXERCISE 21.2

What might be the effect on normal development if reflexes are retained beyond the age when they should disappear?

### Sensory Assessment

**Ears.** The ears are assessed for placement, overall appearance, and maturity. An imaginary horizontal line drawn from the outer canthus of the eye should be even with the area where the ear joins the head (Fig. 21.15). Low-set ears may indicate chromosomal abnormalities. The nurse examines the ears for skin tags, preauricular sinuses, and dimples. Abnormalities of the ear may indicate chromosomal abnormalities, hearing problems, or kidney defects. The stiffness of the cartilage and degree of incurving of the pinna are checked as part of the gestational-age assessment.

Hearing is assessed by noting the infant's reaction to sudden loud noises, which should cause a startle response. The infant should respond to the sound of voices, particularly a high-pitched tone of voice, rhythmic sounds, or the mother's voice. Auditory testing is performed before discharge in most birth facilities (see Chapter 22).

**Eyes.** The eyes are examined for abnormalities and signs of inflammation. The eyes should be symmetric and equal in size. The usual slate gray–blue color of the eyes of infants with light skin tones gradually changes to the true color by about 6 months of age (Johnson, 2015; Vargo, 2014). Infants with dark skin may have dark brown eyes. Slanting epicanthal folds in a non-Asian infant may be a sign of Down syndrome. Edema of the eyelids and subconjunctival hemorrhages (reddened areas of the sclera) result from pressure on the head during birth and resolve within a week.

The sclera should be white or bluish white. A yellow color indicates jaundice. A blue color occurs in osteogenesis imperfecta—a congenital bone condition. Conjunctivitis may result from infection or a chemical reaction to medications. *Staphylococcus, Chlamydia,* and *Neisseria gonorrhoeae* are common organisms that cause infection. Maternal gonorrhea can infect the infant's eyes (ophthalmia neonatorum) and lead to blindness. All infants are treated prophylactically with antibiotics to the eyes to prevent this condition. Any discharge from the eyes is reported for possible culture and treatment.

Transient strabismus ('crossed eyes') is common in the newborn because they have poor control of their eye muscles. This condition should not last beyond 3 to 4 months after birth (Kaufman, Miller, & Gupta, 2011). The doll's-eye sign is a normal finding in the newborn. When the head is turned quickly to one side, the eyes move toward the other side. The setting-sun sign (the iris appears low in the eye and part of the sclera can be seen above the iris) may be an indication of hydrocephalus.

The pupils should be equal in size and react equally to light. Cataracts (opacities of the lens) appear as white areas over the pupils. They may develop in infants of mothers who had rubella or other infections during the pregnancy. When a light is directed into the eyes, the normal red reflex may not be seen if large cataracts are present. Tears are scant or absent for the first 4 to 6 months of life, when the lachrymal duct becomes fully patent (Vargo, 2014). Excessive tearing may indicate a plugged lacrimal duct, which is treated with massage or surgery.

Visual acuity is approximately 20/400 (Olitsky, Hug, Plummer, et al., 2011). The eyes cannot accommodate well, but newborns should show a visual response to the environment. They should make eye contact when held in a cradle position during a period of alertness. Although they focus best on objects that are 20 to 30 cm (8 to 12 inches) away, they can see objects to a distance of 76 cm (2.5 feet) (Blackburn, 2013). They should respond well to human faces and

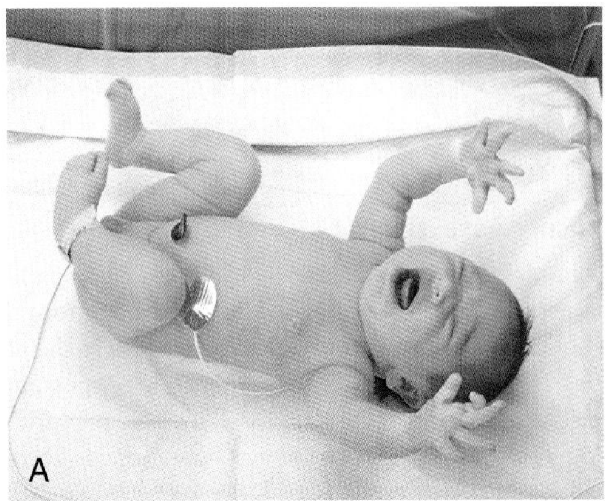


**Moro reflex**
The Moro reflex is the most dramatic reflex. It occurs when the infant's head and trunk are allowed to drop back 30 degrees when the infant is in a slightly raised position. The infant's arms and legs extend and abduct, with the fingers fanning open and thumbs and forefingers forming a C position. The arms then return to their normally flexed state with an embracing motion. The legs may also extend and then flex.

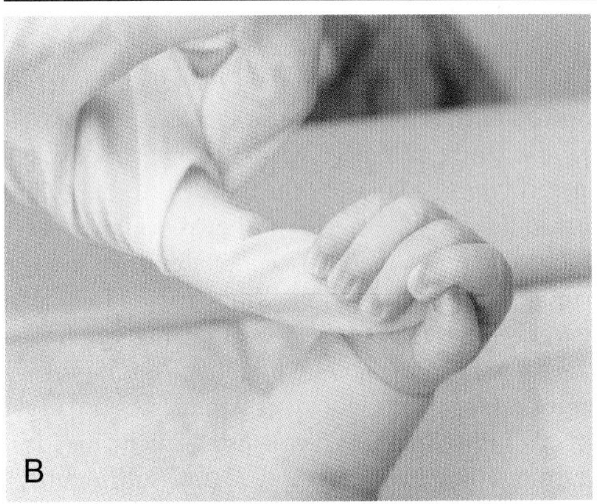


**Palmar grasp reflex**
The palmar grasp reflex occurs when the infant's palm is touched near the base of the fingers. The hand closes into a tight fist. The grasp reflex may be weak or absent if the infant has injury to the nerves of the arms.

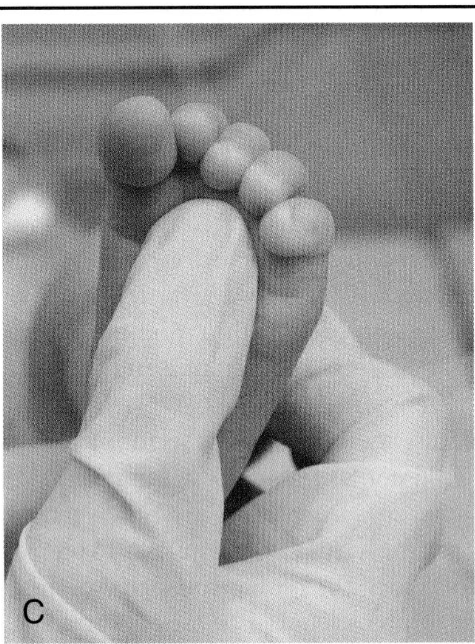


**Plantar grasp reflex**
The plantar grasp reflex is similar to the palmar grasp reflex. When the area below the toes is touched, the infant's toes curl over the nurse's finger.

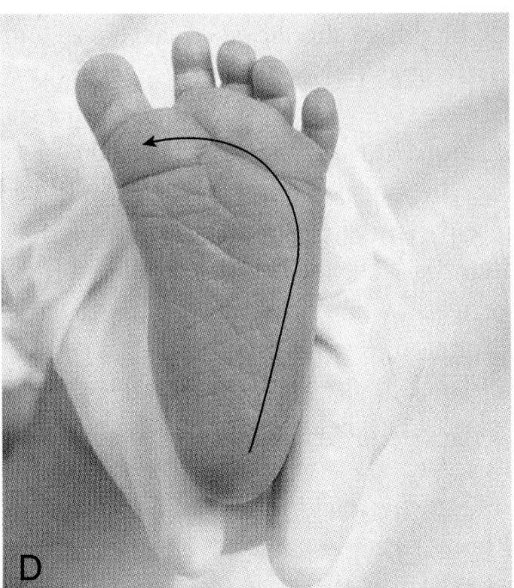


**Babinski reflex**
The Babinski reflex is elicited by stroking the lateral sole of the infant's foot from the heel forward and across the ball of the foot. This causes the toes to flare outward and the big toe to dorsiflex.

**FIG 21.14** Reflexes.

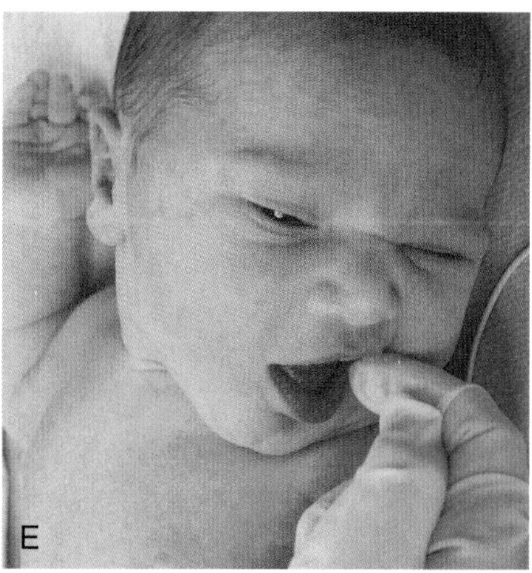


**Rooting reflex**
The rooting reflex is important in feeding and is most often demonstrated when the infant is hungry. When the infant's cheek is touched near the mouth, the head turns toward the side that has been stroked. This response helps the infant find the nipple for feeding. The reflex occurs when either side of the mouth is touched. Touching the cheeks on both sides at the same time confuses the infant.

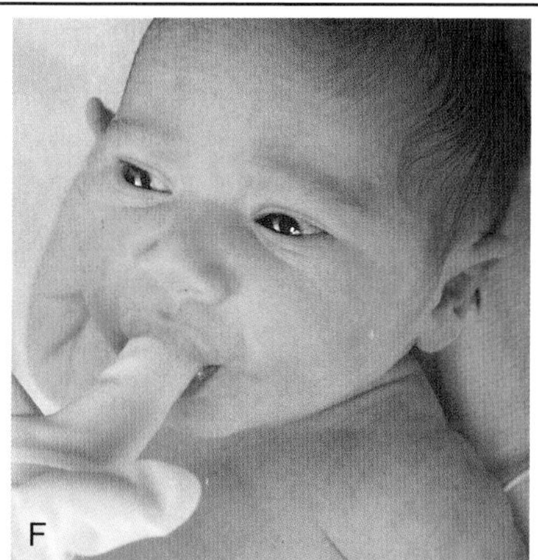


**Sucking reflex**
The sucking reflex is essential to normal life. When the mouth or palate is touched by the nipple or a finger, the infant begins to suck. The sucking reflex is assessed for its presence and strength. Feeding difficulties may be related to problems in the infant's ability to suck and to coordinate sucking with swallowing and breathing.

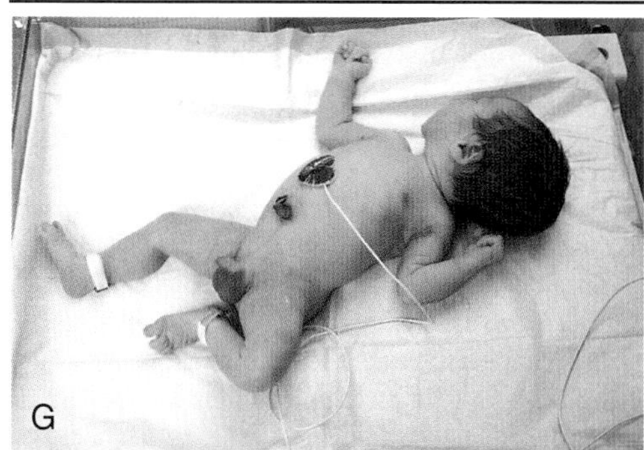


**Tonic neck reflex**
The tonic neck reflex refers to the posture assumed by newborns when in a supine position. The infant extends the arm and leg on the side to which the head is turned and flexes the extremities on the other side. This response is sometimes referred to as the "fencing reflex" because the infant's position is similar to that of a person engaged in a fencing match.

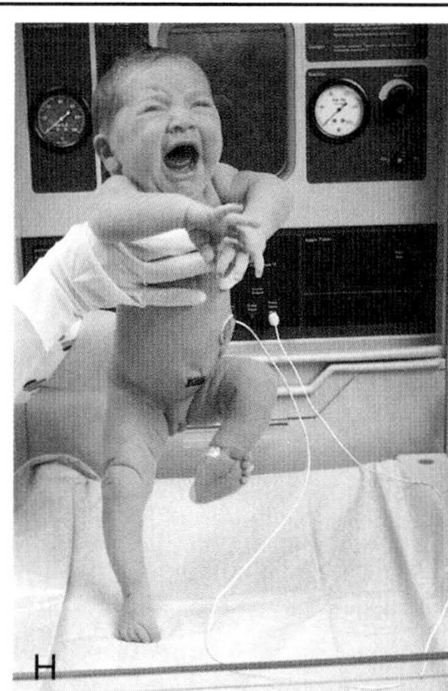


**Stepping reflex**
The stepping reflex occurs when infants are held upright with their feet touching a solid surface. They lift one foot and then the other, giving the appearance that they are trying to walk.

FIG 21.14, cont'd.

**TABLE 21.3 Summary of Neonatal Reflexes**

| Reflex | Method of Testing | Expected Response | Abnormal Response/Possible Cause | Time Reflex Disappears |
|---|---|---|---|---|
| Babinski | Stroke lateral sole of foot from heel to across base of toes. | Toes flare with dorsiflexion of the big toe. | No response: Bilateral, CNS deficit; Unilateral, local nerve injury | 8–9 mo |
| Gallant (trunk incurvation) | With infant prone, lightly stroke along the side of the vertebral column. | Entire trunk flexes toward stimulated side. | No response: CNS deficit | 4 mo |
| Grasp reflex (palmar and plantar) | Press finger against base of infant's fingers or toes. | Fingers curl tightly; toes curl forward. | Weak or absent: neurologic deficit or muscle injury | Palmar grasp: 2–3 mo<br>Plantar grasp: 8–9 mo |
| Moro | Let infant's head drop back approximately 30 degrees. | Sharp extension and abduction of arms followed by flexion and adduction to 'embrace' position. | Absent: CNS dysfunction; asymmetry: brachial plexus injury, paralysis, or fractured bone of extremity<br>Exaggerated: maternal drug use | 5–6 mo |
| Rooting | Touch or stroke from side of mouth toward cheek. | Infant turns head to side touched; difficult to elicit if infant is sleeping or just fed | Weak or absent: prematurity, neurologic deficit, depression from maternal drug use | 3–4 mo |
| Stepping | Hold infant so feet touch solid surface. | Infant lifts alternate feet as if walking | Asymmetry: fracture of extremity, neurologic deficit. | 3–4 mo |
| Sucking | Place nipple or gloved finger in mouth, rub against palate. | Infant begins to suck; may be weak if recently fed | Weak or absent: prematurity, neurologic deficit, maternal drug use. | 1 yr |
| Swallowing | Place fluid on the back of the tongue. | Infant swallows fluid; should be coordinated with sucking. | Coughing, gagging, choking, cyanosis: tracheoesophageal fistula, esophageal atresia, neurologic deficit | Present throughout life |
| Tonic neck reflex | Gently turn head to one side while infant is supine. | Infant extends extremities on side to which head is turned, with flexion on opposite side. | Prolonged period in position: neurologic deficit | May be weak at birth; disappears at 4 mo |

*CNS,* Central nervous system

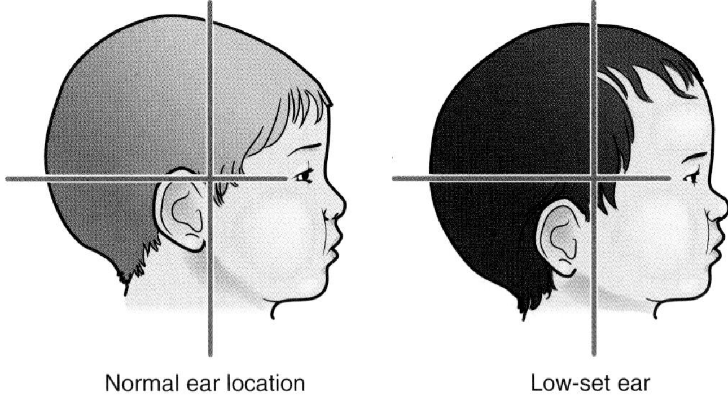


**FIG 21.15** An imaginary line is drawn from the outer canthus of the eye to the ear. The line should intersect the area where the upper ear joins the head.

geometric patterns of black and white or medium-bright colors, but they show little interest in pastel colors.

Newborns should blink or close their eyes in response to bright lights. Any infant who does not respond to visual stimuli should be reported to the physician or nurse practitioner for further investigation.

### Sense of Smell and Taste

The sense of smell allows newborns to recognize breast pads soaked with their mother's milk and differentiate them from pads soaked in water. The ability of infants to distinguish taste is shown by their preference for sweet tastes and aversion to sour and bitter tastes (Blackburn, 2013).

### Other Neurologic Signs

The newborn is assessed for tremors or jitteriness, which may be benign or caused by hypoglycemia, low calcium levels, or prenatal exposure to drugs. Tremors increase each time the infant is touched or moved but stop briefly if the extremity is flexed and held firmly.

Seizures indicate central nervous system or metabolic abnormality. To differentiate tremors from seizures, the infant's extremities are held in a flexed position. This position causes tremors to stop, but a seizure continues. Seizure activity may also include abnormal movements of the eyes or mouth and other subtle signs. Any infant thought to be having seizures is referred for further assessment and treatment (see Chapter 52).

The pitch of the cry is important. A shrill, high-pitched, hoarse, or catlike 'mewing' is abnormal. These cries may indicate a neurologic disorder or other problem.

Normal infants respond to holding and appear content when their needs are met. Rocking motions are often effective in quieting an irritable infant. Most infants 'mold' their bodies to that of the people holding them, making them easy to hold and cuddle. The neonate who stiffens the body, pulls away from contact, or arches the back when held may be showing signs of central nervous system injury. Infants should react to painful stimuli with crying and an increase in vital signs. Excessive irritability may also be a sign of nervous system injury or opioid withdrawal. All such abnormal signs are reported for further neurologic assessment.

## ASSESSMENT OF HEPATIC FUNCTION

The major early assessments of the hepatic system are related to blood glucose and bilirubin conjugation.

**BOX 21.4 Risk Factors for Hypoglycemia**

- Prematurity
- Postmaturity
- Late preterm birth
- Intrauterine growth restriction
- Large or small for gestational age
- Asphyxia
- Problems at birth
- Cold stress
- Maternal diabetes
- Maternal intake of terbutaline

## Blood Glucose

Observing for signs of hypoglycemia is necessary throughout routine assessment and care. Blood glucose screening is not necessary for normal-term infants (Adamkin, 2011). Those in risk categories (late preterm, large or small for gestational age, and infants of diabetic mothers) or showing signs of hypoglycemia should be screened (Box 21.4).

Neonatal blood glucose concentrations may be as low as 30 mg/dL during the first 1 to 2 hours after birth. Glucose levels usually stabilize above 45 mg/dL by 12 hours of age (AAP, 2011). Capillary blood is used in screening tests that are less accurate than laboratory tests using venous blood. Therefore, a laboratory analysis (per agency policy) should be used to verify low readings.

**SAFETY ALERT**

***Signs of Hypoglycemia***

- Jitteriness, tremors
- Poor muscle tone
- Diaphoresis (sweating)
- Poor suck
- Tachypnea
- Tachycardia
- Dyspnea
- Grunting
- Cyanosis
- Apnea
- Low temperature
- High-pitched cry
- Lethargy
- Irritability
- Seizures, coma
- No symptoms (some infants may be asymptomatic)

Avoiding injury to the infant's foot is important when taking blood from the heel. If the lancet goes into the calcaneus bone, osteomyelitis may result. Commercial devices for heel puncture are designed to puncture the foot to the proper depth and are available for both full- and pre-term infants. The site chosen must avoid the major nerves and arteries in the area (see Procedure: Obtaining Blood Samples from the Newborn by Heel Puncture).

**PROCEDURE**

***Obtaining Blood Samples From the Newborn by Heel Puncture***

**Purpose**

To obtain blood by heel puncture for various laboratory tests. (Instructions are given here for measuring the infant's blood glucose using a glucometer or reagent strips, but the same method applies to other testing.)

1. Wash the hands and gather supplies needed *to decrease contamination and increase organization.* Supplies vary with the test and equipment used but may include gloves, alcohol wipe, 2 × 2-inch gauze, glucometer, commercial lancing device, adhesive bandage, cotton balls, blood-collecting devices (glucose screening reagent strips, blotting paper for metabolic screening tests, capillary tubes, microtainers).
2. If the infant has not received a bath since birth, bathe the infant or wash the area before puncturing the skin *to avoid contamination of the puncture site with maternal blood on the infant's skin.*
3. Calibrate or program the glucometer and use quality-control measures according to manufacturer's guidelines *to ensure proper functioning of the machine.*
4. Warm the heel with a commercial heel warmer or a warm wet cloth according to agency policy. *Warming helps dilate the vessels.* Take care not to burn the infant.
5. Provide comforting measures such as swaddling, providing a pacifier, allowing the mother to hold or breastfeed, or giving oral sucrose (unless testing blood glucose and according to agency policy) *to help decrease the infant's pain.* Assess the infant's pain level before, during, and after the procedure using an infant pain scale according to agency policy *to determine the effectiveness of pain-relief methods* (see Evidence-Based Practice box).
6. Apply gloves *to prevent contamination of the hands with blood.*
7. Hold the heel in one hand. Locate the site. Palpate the bone of the heel *to avoid puncturing the calcaneus bone, which could result in infection.* Place the thumb or finger over the walking surface to avoid injury to area nerves and arteries. Choose a puncture site on the lateral heel that has not been used before, *to avoid infection or scarring.*
8. Clean the area with alcohol and dry with sterile gauze, or allow to air-dry *to prevent diluting the specimen with alcohol.*
9. Puncture the side of the heel with an automatic puncture device that penetrates to the appropriate depth *to avoid piercing the bone.* Place the device in a sharps container *to prevent injury to the infant and protect others from injury or unnecessary exposure to the infant's blood.*

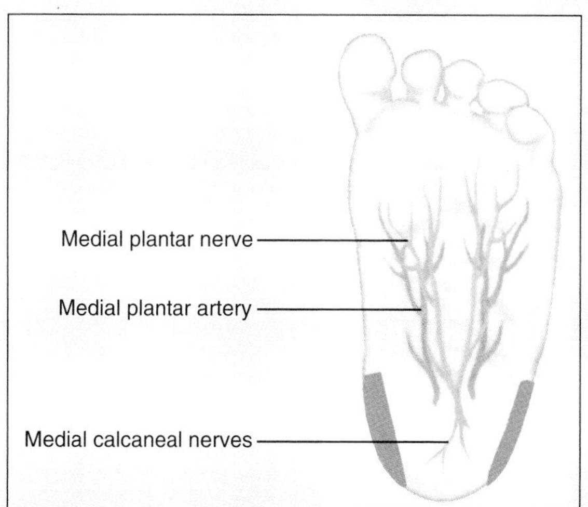


10. Wipe away the first drop of blood *to avoid contamination with tissue fluid or skin surface alcohol.*
11. Follow agency policy or manufacturer's directions for the type of test being performed regarding how to collect the sample, amount of blood to be collected, proper handling, and reading of results. *Following directions increases accuracy.*
12. Avoid excessive squeezing of the foot *because it dilutes the sample with tissue fluid and may cause bruising or hemolysis.*
13. Obtain blood sample. Apply pressure with gauze until the bleeding stops.
14. Document the procedure and record the results. Send specimens to the laboratory as appropriate. Report abnormal readings and follow-up according to agency policy. Confirm abnormal results by laboratory measurement according to agency policy. *This procedure ensures accuracy of testing and follow-up.*

Infants are often fed if the reading is 45 mg/dL or less to prevent further decreases in glucose, especially if the infant shows signs of hypoglycemia. Intravenous glucose may be necessary for persistent low glucose levels. Infants who are in the risk categories of small for gestational age or late-preterm are usually monitored for at least 24 hours after birth, while neonates who fall into the category of large-for-gestational-age or infants of diabetic mothers are screened for a minimum of 12 hours (Adamkin, 2011).

**EVIDENCE-BASED PRACTICE**

Healthy newborns endure painful procedures such as heel lancing (heel sticks) to obtain blood for various routine newborn tests. Morrow, Hidinger, and Wilkinson-Faulk compared differences in pain scores during heel lancing using swaddling and positioning. The Neonatal Inventory Pain Scale was used to measure pain before and just after the heel was lanced. Blood collection time was also measured. Forty-two infants were randomly assigned to a group for the study. In the experimental group, 22 infants were swaddled with one leg exposed and were held in an upright position. In the control group, 20 infants were lying on their backs and not swaddled during the procedure.

The results showed the infants in the experimental group had significantly lower pain scores than did those in the control group. The blood collection took an average of 30 seconds less time for the control group, but the difference was not significant. Swaddling and holding infants in an upright position for blood collections by heel lancing is a method of pain reduction that can be implemented easily. This study adds to current knowledge of various techniques for alleviating pain in neonates during painful procedures.

Reference: Morrow, C., Hidinger, A., & Wilkinson-Faulk, D. (2010). Reducing neonatal pain during routine heel lance procedures. *MCN: The American Journal of Maternal/Child Nursing, 35*(6), 346-354.

### Bilirubin

The nurse assesses for jaundice at least every 8 to 12 hours and is particularly watchful when infants have increased risk factors. Jaundice is identified by pressing the infant's skin over a firm surface, such as the end of the nose or the sternum. As the skin blanches, the yellow color can be seen. Jaundice begins at the head and moves down the body; the areas of the body involved should be documented. Jaundice becomes visible when serum bilirubin reaches 5 to 6 mg/dL (Blackburn, 2013). Box 21.5 lists risk factors for hyperbilirubinemia.

**BOX 21.5 Risk Factors for Hyperbilirubinemia**

- Premature or late preterm birth
- Cephalhematoma
- Bruising
- Delayed or poor intake
- Breastfeeding
- Cold stress
- Asphyxia
- Rh or ABO incompatibility or hemolytic anemia
- Infection
- Sibling with jaundice
- Male sex
- Polycythemia
- Infection
- Asian, Native American, Eskimo heritage
- Maternal diabetes or preeclampsia

Jaundice may not be physiologic if it appears before the second day of life. In many facilities, protocols allow the nurse to obtain transcutaneous bilirubin (TcB) measurements using a bilirubinometer or laboratory measurement of TSB without the order of a nurse practitioner or physician. Bilirubinometers are noninvasive devices for measuring bilirubin in the infant's skin, thus avoiding repeated skin punctures to obtain blood samples. The National Association of Neonatal Nurses (2010) recommends obtaining TSB or TcB measurements on every infant before discharge.

Abnormal TcB results should be confirmed by TSB. Charts are available to show the degree of risk for infants of different ages (in hours) by the level of the TSB. Commonly, all infants receive a TSB or TcB before discharge to determine if discharge should be delayed or early follow-up arranged. All abnormal results should be documented and reported to the nurse practitioner or physician. A plan of care for infants at risk for hyperbilirubinemia is included in Chapter 22, and phototherapy is discussed in Chapter 30.

## Gastrointestinal System

The initial assessment of the gastrointestinal tract occurs during the first hours after birth; the nurse visualizes the parts that can be seen while the infant takes the initial feeding.

### Mouth

The mouth is inspected visually and by palpation. Some infants are born with precocious teeth, usually lower incisors. If the teeth are loose, the physician usually removes them to prevent aspiration. Epstein's pearls may be noted on the hard palate or gums. These small, white, hard cysts are a form of milia and disappear without treatment within a few weeks.

The nurse examines the tongue for size and movement. A large, protruding tongue is present in hypothyroidism and some chromosomal disorders such as Down syndrome. Paralysis of the facial nerve causes unilateral drooping of the mouth, noticeable during crying or sucking, and affects the movement of the tongue.

Although candidiasis (thrush) is not apparent in the mouth immediately after birth, it may appear a day or two later. The lesions resemble milk curds on the tongue and cheeks and bleed if attempts are made to wipe them away. Newborns may become infected with Candida albicans during passage through the birth canal if the mother has a candidal vaginal infection. The infant is treated with antifungal medication such as nystatin suspension.

A cleft lip or palate results if the lip or palate fails to close (see Chapter 43). Cleft palate may involve the hard or the soft palate or both, and may appear alone or with a cleft lip. The palate is inspected when the infant cries. A gloved finger is inserted into the mouth to palpate both the hard and soft palate. A very small cleft of the soft palate may be missed if only a visual examination is done.

### Suck

The normal full-term infant should have a strong suck reflex that is elicited when the lips or palate are stimulated. The reflex is weaker in the neonate who is preterm, ill, or has just been fed. The newborn's cheeks have well-developed muscles and sucking pads that enhance the ability to suck. Blisters may be present on the newborn's hands or arms from strong sucking before birth.

### Initial Feeding

The initial feeding is an opportunity to assess the newborn further. If the mother is breastfeeding, the infant should nurse within the first hour, if possible. The nurse can observe the infant's response unobtrusively while assisting the mother to position the infant. To decrease regurgitation from overdistention of the stomach, an initial formula feeding should be no more than 1 ounce.

The nurse evaluates the infant's ability to suck, swallow, and breathe in a coordinated manner. Some newborns choke or gag during the first feeding. Others may become dusky or cyanotic because they become apneic while feeding. In either case, the nurse should stop the feeding immediately, suction if necessary, and stimulate the infant to cry by rubbing the back. Most full-term infants learn to coordinate sucking, swallowing, and breathing by the time the first feeding is finished.

Choking, coughing, and cyanosis may indicate a connection between the trachea and the esophagus, such as tracheoesophageal fistula (see Chapter 43). Infants with tracheoesophageal fistula or esophageal atresia also may have excessive secretions. Neonates who develop cyanosis during feedings may have a cardiac anomaly (see Chapter 46). Further assessment and referral are necessary.

### Abdomen

The abdomen should be soft, rounded, and protrude slightly, but should not be distended. A distended abdomen with stretched, shiny skin may indicate obstruction. Loops of bowel should not be visible through the abdominal wall. Visible bowel loops could indicate that air and meconium are not passing through the intestines normally.

A sunken or scaphoid appearance of the abdomen occurs in diaphragmatic hernia, in which the intestines are located in the chest cavity instead of the abdomen (see Chapter 43). The nurse listens over the abdomen for bowel sounds, which usually appear within the first hour after birth (Vargo, 2014). Bowel sounds heard in the chest may indicate diaphragmatic hernia.

An umbilical hernia occurs when the intestinal muscles fail to close around the umbilicus, allowing the intestines to protrude through the weak area. The condition is more common in low-birth-weight, male, and African-American infants. Often, the umbilical hernia disappears when the infant is walking well, although some hernias require surgical repair.

Palpating the abdomen is easiest when the infant is relaxed and quiet. The abdomen should feel soft because the muscles are not yet well developed. Masses may indicate tumors of the kidneys. Palpation of the liver is usually not part of routine nursing assessment of the abdomen but is performed by the primary care provider. The liver is normally 1 to 3 cm below the right costal margin. If the organ seems large, it should be reported to the physician or nurse practitioner because it may be a sign of congestive heart failure or congenital infection.

### Stools

Stools should be assessed for type, color, and consistency. There should never be a 'water ring' (a wet, stained area on the diaper where watery stool has been absorbed). There may be an area of more solid stool in the center. This indicates diarrhea. The nurse should be aware of the time that the infant's last stool occurred and whether any stools have been passed since birth. Newborns often pass the first meconium stool within 12 hours of birth and almost all within 48 hours.

## Genitourinary System

### Kidney Palpation

Palpation of the kidneys is not usually part of the routine nursing newborn assessment. The healthcare provider may palpate the kidneys just above the level of the umbilicus on each side of the abdomen during the first hours after birth. Abdominal masses may indicate enlargement or tumors of the kidneys. Anomalies of the kidney may accompany other defects because a problem early in fetal development may affect other organs being formed at the same time. For example, an infant with only one umbilical artery or defects involving the ears may have renal anomalies. The nurse should observe carefully for urinary output in these infants to determine if the kidneys are functioning adequately.

### Urine

The first void should be carefully noted on the chart. The newborn's bladder may empty as seldom as once or twice during the first 2 days, and the first void may be missed. Sometimes it occurs in the delivery room but goes unnoticed because attention is focused on the infant's overall condition. If there is no void in the expected time, the infant's fluid intake should be increased and the physician or nurse practitioner alerted. Each void is recorded in the infant's chart, including diapers the mother changes. The total number is correlated with what is appropriate for the age of the infant.

If a newborn is having feeding difficulties, it is especially important to note the number of wet diapers. Disposable diapers are very absorbent, and the pale color of the urine may not be noticed on the diaper. Wet diapers generally feel heavier than dry ones. A cotton ball or tissue placed in the diaper can be used to increase the visibility of small amounts of urine.

The newborn's urine may contain uric acid crystals that cause a reddish or pink stain on the diaper. This is known as 'brick dust staining' and may be frightening to parents, who may think the infant is bleeding. This condition does not continue beyond the first few days, as the kidneys mature.

### Genitalia

**Female.** In the full-term female infant, the labia majora should be large and completely cover the clitoris and labia minora. The labia may be darker than the surrounding skin from exposure to the mother's hormones before birth. Edema of the labia and white mucous vaginal discharge are normal. A small amount of vaginal bleeding, known as pseudomenstruation, may occur from the sudden withdrawal of the mother's hormones at birth. Hymenal or vaginal tags are small pieces of tissue at the vaginal orifice. These are normal and disappear in a few weeks. The urinary meatus and vagina should be present.

**Male.** The scrotum should be pendulous at term and may be dark brown from maternal hormones. Pressure during a breech delivery may cause it to be edematous. Rugae (creases in the scrotum) are deep and cover the entire scrotum in the full-term infant. Enlargement of one or both sides of the scrotum may be caused by a hydrocele—a collection of fluid around one or both testes, which usually resolves without treatment.

Palpation of the scrotum determines if the testes have descended (Fig. 21.16). Testes feel like small, round, movable objects that "slip" between the fingers. If the testes are not present in the scrotal sac, they may be felt in the inguinal canal. An empty scrotal sac appears smaller than one with testes. Undescended testis (cryptorchidism) can occur on one or both sides (see Chapter 44). They often descend by 6 months of age. If they do not descend by one year, surgery may be performed (Vargo, 2014).

The meatus should be at the tip of the glans penis. It may be abnormally located on the underside of the penis or on the perineum (hypospadias) or on the upper side (epispadias). The prepuce or foreskin of the penis covers the glans and is adherent to it. Attempts to retract it in the newborn are unnecessary and can cause injury. Abnormal

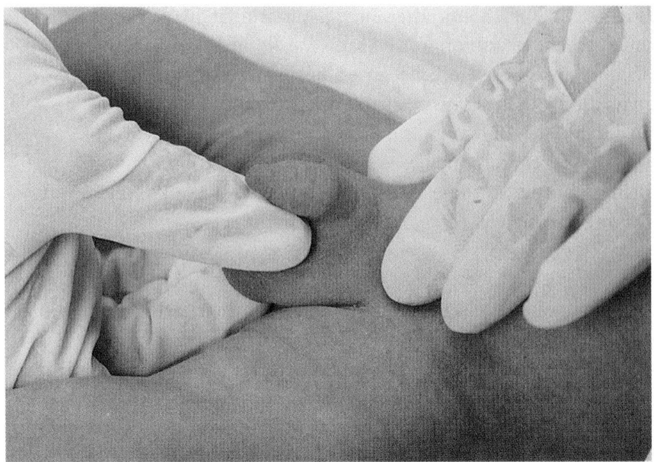

FIG 21.16 The testes are palpated from front to back with the thumb and forefinger. Placing a finger over the inguinal canal holds the testes in place for palpation.

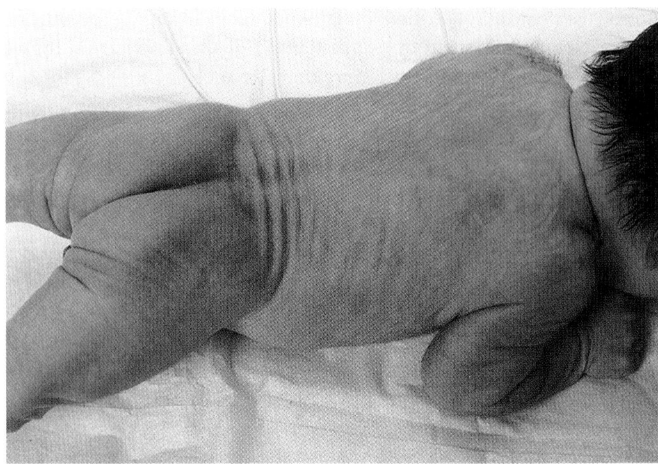

FIG 21.17 Lanugo is abundant on this slightly preterm infant.

placement of the meatus may not be visible because it is covered by the prepuce, but often the prepuce in these infants is incompletely formed. Hypospadias may be accompanied by chordee, a condition in which fibrotic tissue causes the penis to curve downward. These conditions can be corrected later by surgery (see Chapter 44).

Parents are very concerned about any abnormalities of the genitalia. If the meatus is abnormally positioned, they need an explanation of the condition and why the infant should not be circumcised. The foreskin may be needed for later plastic surgery to repair the defect.

## Integumentary System

### Skin

The newborn's skin is fragile, and reddened areas or rashes may develop during the early days of life. The nurse must carefully examine every inch of skin surface during the initial assessment and at the beginning of each shift.

***Color.*** The skin should be pink or tan. Red, thin skin occurs in preterm infants. Redness (ruddy color) in the full-term infant may indicate polycythemia. Acrocyanosis is common during the first day as a result of poor peripheral circulation. The infant's mouth and central body areas should not be cyanotic at any time. Blanching the skin over the nose or chest shows the presence of jaundice. Jaundice is abnormal during the first day of life but common during the first week.

A greenish-brown discoloration of the skin, nails, and cord results if meconium was passed before birth. This discoloration may indicate that the infant was compromised at some time before birth, and it is more common in the postterm infant. These infants must be watched for other complications, such as respiratory difficulty.

***Harlequin color change.*** A distinct color division with one side of the body deep pink or red and the other half of the body pale is called harlequin color change. This condition occurs more often in low–birth-weight infants, is transient, and benign. It is thought to be caused by an imbalance in the autonomic regulation of the vessels.

***Mottling.*** Mottling (cutis marmorata) is a lacy, red or blue marbling of the skin caused by vasomotor instability. This condition is seen when the infant is cold, stressed, or over-stimulated. Mottling is also seen in some chromosomal abnormalities.

***Vernix caseosa.*** Vernix, a thick white substance resembling cream cheese, provides a protective covering for the fetal skin in utero. The full-term infant has little vernix left on the body except small amounts in the creases. A thick covering of vernix may indicate a preterm infant.

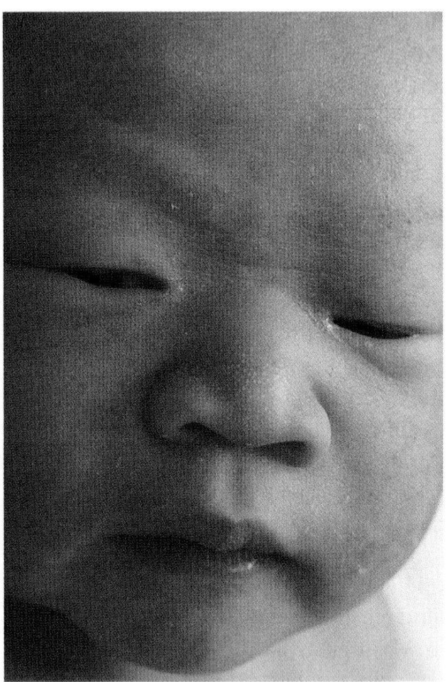

FIG 21.18 Milia.

Yellow-tinged vernix may indicate elevated bilirubin levels in utero and green-tinged vernix is caused by meconium staining.

***Lanugo.*** Lanugo is fine, soft hair that covers the fetus during intrauterine life (Fig. 21.17). The appearance of lanugo is used in gestational-age assessment.

***Milia.*** Milia are white cysts, 1 mm in size, caused by sebaceous gland secretions. They occur on the face over the forehead, nose, and cheeks and disappear within the first weeks without treatment (Fig. 21.18).

***Erythema toxicum.*** The nurse notes the presence of erythema toxicum, which are white or yellow papules or vesicles with a red base (Fig. 21.19). Commonly called "flea bite" rash or newborn rash, it resembles small bites or acne and occurs within 5 days of birth in approximately 50% of term newborns (Vargo, 2014). The rash usually appears during the first 24 to 48 hours after birth and up to 3 months of age. It occurs anywhere on the body except the palms and soles of the feet. The cause of erythema toxicum is unknown, and lesions disappear within hours or days.

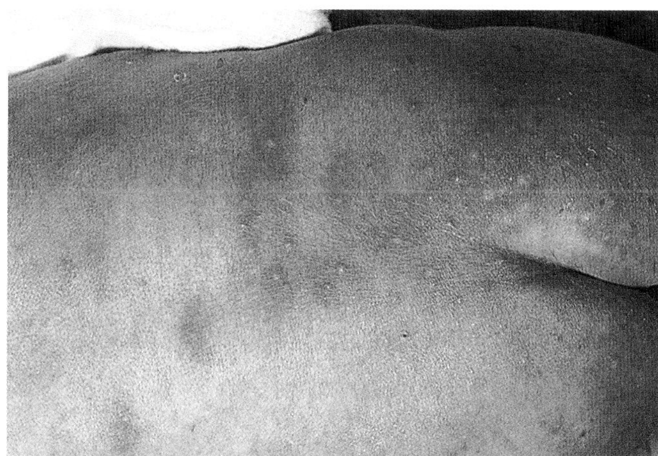

**FIG 21.19** Erythema toxicum. (From Hurwitz, S. [1993]. *Clinical pediatric dermatology* [2nd ed., p. 13]. Philadelphia: Saunders.)

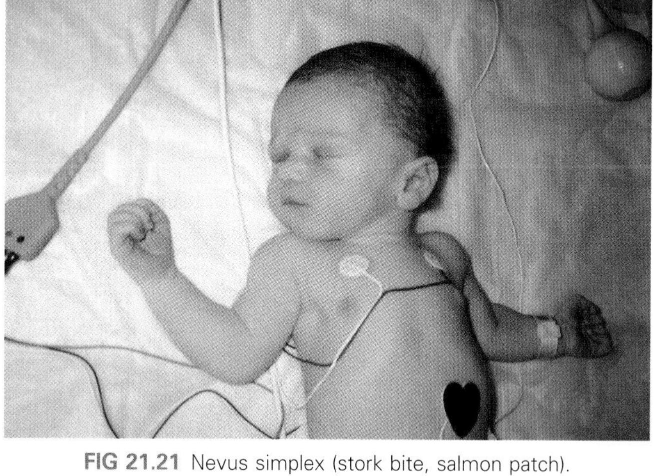

**FIG 21.21** Nevus simplex (stork bite, salmon patch).

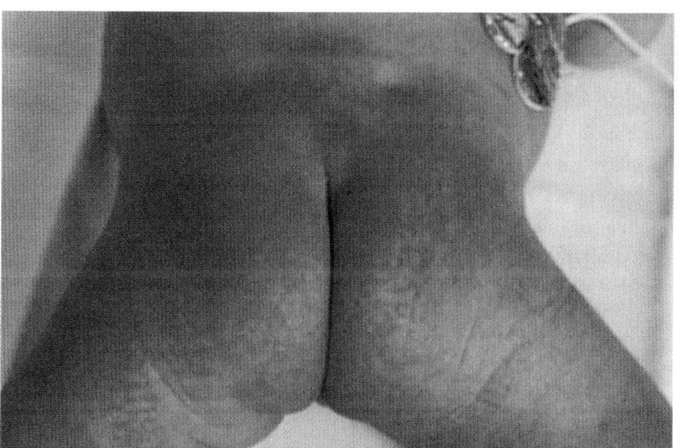

**FIG 21.20** Mongolian spots.

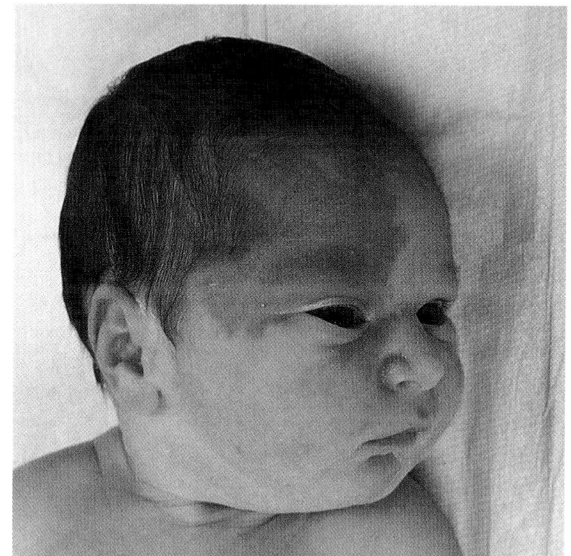

**FIG 21.22** Nevus flammeus (port-wine stain).

***Birthmarks.*** The size, location, color, elevation, and texture of all birthmarks should be carefully documented. Marks should be explained to parents, who are often concerned.

- **Mongolian** spots are bluish gray marks that resemble bruises on the sacrum, buttocks, arms, shoulders, or other areas (Fig. 21.20). They occur most frequently in newborns with dark skin and usually disappear after the first few years of life. Some continue into adulthood.
- A **nevus simplex** is also called a salmon patch or stork bite (Fig. 21.21). This flat, pink discoloration from dilated capillaries occurs on the eyelids, above the bridge of the nose, or at the nape of the neck. The color blanches when pressed and is more prominent during crying. Stork bites disappear by age 2 years, although those at the nape of the neck may persist.
- **Nevus flammeus (port-wine stain)** is a permanent, flat, pink to dark reddish-purple mark (Fig. 21.22). They vary in size and location and do not blanch with pressure. They can be removed by laser surgery. Some may occur as part of various syndromes.
- **Nevus vasculosus (strawberry hemangioma)** consists of enlarged capillaries in outer layers of the skin. They are dark red and raised, with a rough surface, giving a strawberry-like appearance. Such hemangiomas are usually located on the head. They may be present at birth or develop by 6 months of age. After growing larger for 5 to 6 months, they regress over several years. No treatment is necessary unless infection or ulceration occurs (Hoath & Narendran, 2011).
- **Café au lait spots** are permanent, light brown birthmarks that can occur anywhere on the body. Although they are harmless, the number and size are important. Six or more spots larger than 0.5 cm are associated with neurofibromatosis, a genetic condition of neural tissue.

***Marks from delivery.*** The nurse inspects the infant for marks that may have occurred from injury or pressure during labor or delivery.

- Bruises can occur on any part of the body where there was pressure during delivery. Bruising of the face may be present if the cord was wrapped around the neck during birth (nuchal cord). Bruising on the head may occur from use of a vacuum extractor.
- Petechiae, pinpoint bruises that resemble a rash, may appear on the back, face, and groin. They are caused by pressure during the birth process. Widespread or continued formation of petechiae may indicate infection or a low platelet count.
- A small puncture mark is present on the newborn's head if a fetal monitor scalp electrode was attached. The area should heal normally but is observed for signs of infection.
- Forceps marks occur over the cheeks and ears where the instruments were applied. Their size, color, and location are carefully documented. Lack of movement or symmetry of the face may indicate injury to a facial nerve.

***Other skin assessments.*** The nurse notes other aspects of the skin that may indicate abnormalities. Localized edema may be caused by trauma during delivery. Generalized edema indicates more serious conditions, such as heart failure. Peeling of the skin is normal in full-term newborns. Excessive amounts of peeling may indicate a postterm infant.

***Documentation.*** All marks or abnormalities of the skin must be recorded on the nurses' notes. The location, size, color, elevation, and texture of each mark should be described. Any changes that occur from previous assessments should also be documented.

### Breasts

The nurse notes the placement of the nipples and looks for extra (supernumerary) nipples, which may appear on the chest or in the axilla. Occasionally, the breasts become engorged and secrete a small amount of white fluid (sometimes called 'witch's milk'). This condition is caused by maternal hormones and resolves within a few weeks without treatment. Manipulation of the breasts could cause infection.

### Hair and Nails

The hair of the full-term infant should be silky and soft, whereas that of the preterm infant is woolly or fuzzy. The nails come to the end of the fingers or beyond. Very long nails may indicate a postterm infant. A green-brown staining of the nails may be a sign of passage of meconium from fetal distress.

## ASSESSMENT OF GESTATIONAL AGE

The gestational-age assessment is an examination of the newborn to determine the number of weeks from conception to birth. Such assessment is important because neonates born before or after term and those whose size is not appropriate for gestational age are at increased risk for complications.

### Assessment Tools

The New Ballard Score (Fig. 21.23) is frequently used to determine gestational age based on neuromuscular and physical characteristics. This score is accurate within 2 weeks of gestation (Furdon & Benjamin, 2010). A score is given for each assessment, and the total score is used to determine the gestational age of the infant.

### Neuromuscular Characteristics

#### Posture

The posture and degree of flexion of the extremities are scored before disturbing the quiet infant (Fig. 21.24). Preterm neonates with immature flexor muscles have extended, limp arms and legs. The limbs of full-term infants are sharply flexed. The legs should be flexed at the hips, knees, and ankles. The legs of infants who were in a frank breech position may be more extended than flexed even when they are full term.

#### Square Window

The 'square window' sign is elicited by flexing the hand at the wrist until the palm is as flat against the forearm as possible with gentle pressure (Fig. 21.25). The angle between the palm and the forearm is measured. The more mature the neonate, the smaller the angle, until the palm folds flat against the forearm at term.

#### Arm Recoil

To test for arm recoil, the nurse holds the neonate's arms fully flexed at the elbows for 5 seconds and then pulls the hands straight down to the sides (Fig. 21.26). The hands are quickly released, and the degree of flexion is measured as the arms return to their normally-flexed position. Preterm infants may move the arms slowly or not at all, whereas the full-term infant has a quick return to flexion.

#### Popliteal Angle

To measure the popliteal angle, the newborn's lower leg is folded against the thigh, with the thigh on the abdomen (Fig. 21.27). The lower leg is then straightened, just until resistance is met. Continued pressure causes the infant to extend the leg farther and results in an inaccurate score. The angle at the popliteal space is scored when resistance is first felt. The preterm infant extends the leg farther than the full-term infant.

#### Scarf Sign

To assess the scarf sign, the nurse grasps the infant's hand and brings the arm across the body to the opposite side, keeping the shoulder flat on the bed and the head in the middle of the body (Fig. 21.28). The position of the elbow in relation to the midline of the infant's body is noted. The full-term infant's elbow does not cross midline, but the preterm infant's arm extends farther toward the opposite side.

#### Heel to Ear

For the heel-to-ear assessment, the nurse grasps the infant's foot and pulls it straight up toward the ears while the hips remain flat on the surface of the bed (Fig. 21.29). When resistance is first felt, the position of the foot in relation to the head and the amount of flexion of the leg are compared with the diagrams. The more resistance and flexion, the more mature the infant.

### Physical Characteristics

#### Skin

The skin is assessed for color, visibility of veins, peeling, and cracking. The very preterm infant's skin is red, sticky, and fragile, with little subcutaneous fat and visible veins. In the mature newborn, the skin is thicker and the color is paler. Few veins are visible, and there is peeling and cracking. Peeling becomes even more apparent in the postterm infant and during the hours after birth as the skin loses moisture.

#### Lanugo

Lanugo appears by 20 weeks of gestation and increases in amount until 28 weeks (see Fig. 21.17), when it begins to disappear. Most is shed at 32 to 36 weeks (Gardner & Hernandez, 2011). At term, a small amount may remain over the upper back and shoulders, over the ears, or on the sides of the forehead. Infants with dark coloring may have more lanugo (which is dark and more easily noticed) than infants with fair skin and very light hair at the same gestational age. The infant receives a score based on the amount of lanugo present on the back.

#### Plantar Surface

Plantar creases (Fig. 21.30) begin to appear at 28 to 30 weeks of gestation and cover the entire sole by term (Trotter, 2015). The plantar creases must be assessed during the early hours after birth because as the infant's skin begins to dry, the creases appear more prominent. In very preterm infants, the foot length is measured.

#### Breasts

The nipples, areolae, and size of the breast buds are assessed and scored. To determine the size of the breast buds, the nurse places a finger on each side and measures the diameter (Fig. 21.31). Use of the thumb and forefinger may cause excess tissue to be drawn together, resulting in an inaccurate score.

## NEWBORN MATURITY RATING & CLASSIFICATION

ESTIMATION OF GESTATIONAL AGE BY MATURITY RATING
Symbols: X - 1st Exam 0 - 2nd Exam

NEUROMUSCULAR MATURITY

| | −1 | 0 | 1 | 2 | 3 | 4 | 5 |
|---|---|---|---|---|---|---|---|
| Posture | | | | | | | |
| Square window (wrist) | >90° | 90° | 60° | 45° | 30° | 0° | |
| Arm recoil | | 180° | 140°-180° | 110°-140° | 90°-110° | <90° | |
| Popliteal angle | 180° | 160° | 140° | 120° | 100° | 90° | <90° |
| Scarf sign | | | | | | | |
| Heel to ear | | | | | | | |

Gestation by Dates ________ wks

Birth Date ______ Hour ______ am pm

APGAR ______ 1 min ______ 5 min

MATURITY RATING

| score | weeks |
|---|---|
| −10 | 20 |
| −5 | 22 |
| 0 | 24 |
| 5 | 26 |
| 10 | 28 |
| 15 | 30 |
| 20 | 32 |
| 25 | 34 |
| 30 | 36 |
| 35 | 38 |
| 40 | 40 |
| 45 | 42 |
| 50 | 44 |

PHYSICAL MATURITY

| | | | | | | | |
|---|---|---|---|---|---|---|---|
| Skin | Sticky friable transparent | Gelatinous red, translucent | Smooth pink, visible veins | Superficial peeling &/or rash, few veins | Cracking pale areas rare veins | Parchment deep cracking no vessels | Leathery cracked wrinkled |
| Lanugo | None | Sparse | Abundant | Thinning | Bald areas | Mostly bald | |
| Plantar surface | Heel-toe 40-50 mm: −1 <40 mm: −2 | >50 mm no crease | Faint red marks | Anterior transverse crease only | Creases ant. 2/3 | Creases over entire sole | |
| Breast | Imperceptible | Barely perceptible | Flat areola no bud | Stippled areola 1-2 mm bud | Raised areola 3-4 mm bud | Full areola 5-10 mm bud | |
| Eye/Ear | Lids fused loosely: −1 tightly: −2 | Lids open pinna flat stays folded | Sl. curved pinna; soft; slow recoil | Well-curved pinna; soft but ready recoil | Formed & firm instant recoil | Thick cartilage ear stiff | |
| Genitals (male) | Scrotum flat, smooth | Scrotum empty faint rugae | Testes in upper canal rare rugae | Testes descending few rugae | Testes down good rugae | Testes pendulous deep rugae | |
| Genitals (female) | Clitoris prominent labia flat | Prominent clitoris small labia minora | Prominent clitoris enlarging minora | Majora & minora equally prominent | Majora large minora small | Majora cover clitoris & minora | |

SCORING SECTION

| | 1st Exam=X | 2nd Exam=O |
|---|---|---|
| Estimating Gest Age by Maturity Rating | ____ Weeks | ____ Weeks |
| Time of Exam | Date ____ Hour ____ am pm | Date ____ Hour ____ am pm |
| Age of Exam | ____ Hours | ____ Hours |
| Signature of Examiner | ____ M.D. | ____ M.D. |

**FIG 21.23** New Ballard Score. (Courtesy Bristol-Myers Company, Evansville, IN. From Ballard, J. L., Khoury, J. C., Wedig, K., et al. [1991]. New Ballard Score, expanded to include extremely premature infants. *Journal of Pediatrics, 19*[3], 417-423.)

### Eyes and Ears

The eyelids are fused until 26 to 28 weeks (Trotter, 2015). The incurving of the upper pinnae begins at the top and continues around the ear. In assessing the ear, the incurving and thickness of each pinna are rated (Fig. 21.32). The ear is folded to assess the resistance and the speed with which it returns to its original state. In infants less than 34 weeks of gestation, the ear has little cartilage to keep it stiff (Furdon & Benjamin, 2010). In the term neonate, the ear springs back to its original position immediately.

### Genitals

In the female infant, the relationship in size of the clitoris, labia minora, and labia majora is noted (Fig. 21.33). As the infant nears term, the

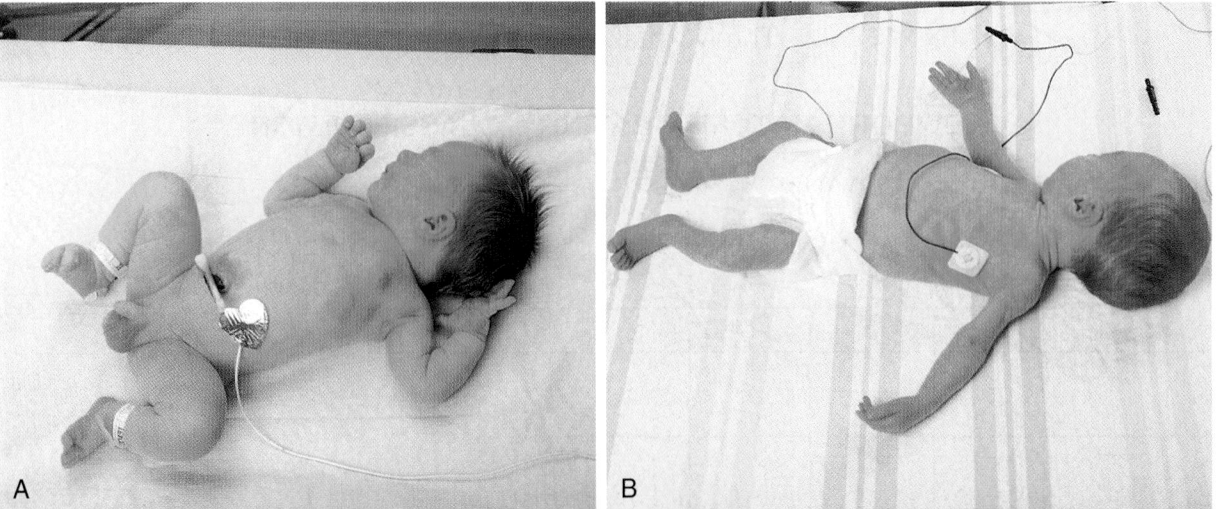

**FIG 21.24** Posture in newborns. **A,** The healthy, full-term infant remains in a strongly flexed position. **B,** The preterm infant's extremities are extended.

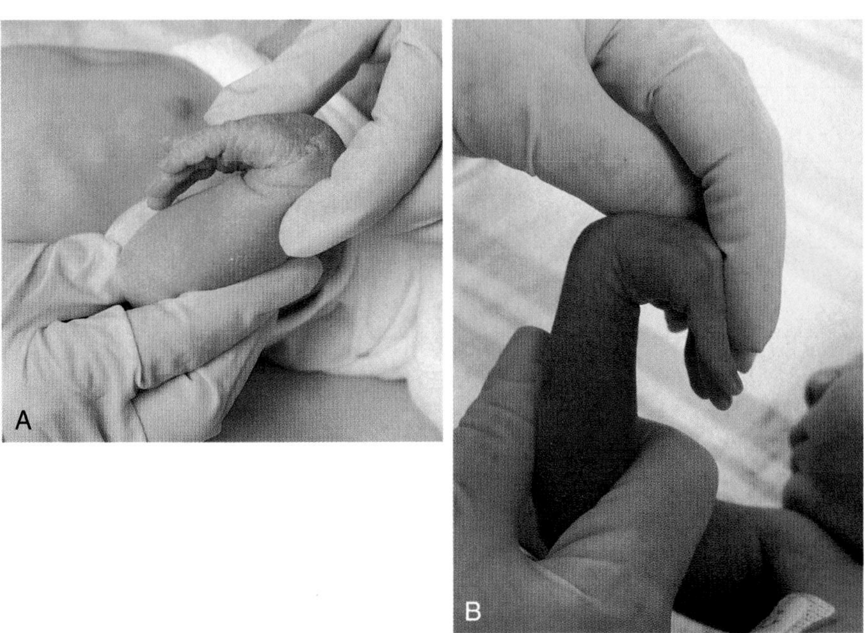

**FIG 21.25** The square window sign is performed on an arm without an identification bracelet. The nurse flexes the wrist and measures the angle. **A,** Infant near full term. **B,** Preterm infant.

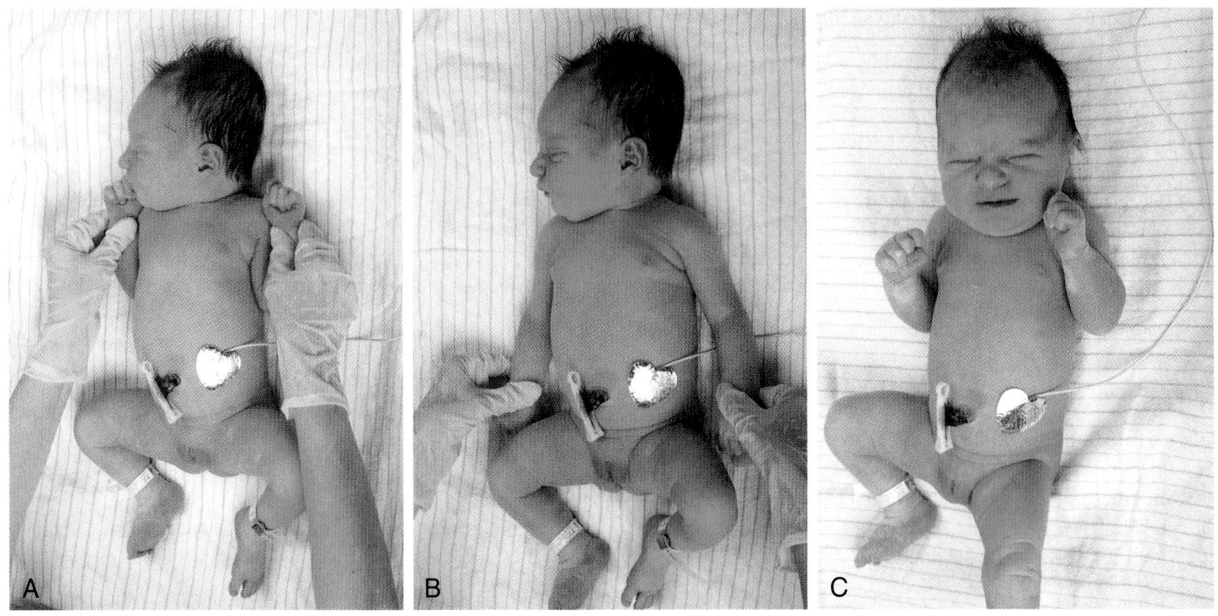

**FIG 21.26** Arm recoil. **A,** Arms flexed. **B,** Arms extended. **C,** Recoil for the full-term infant.

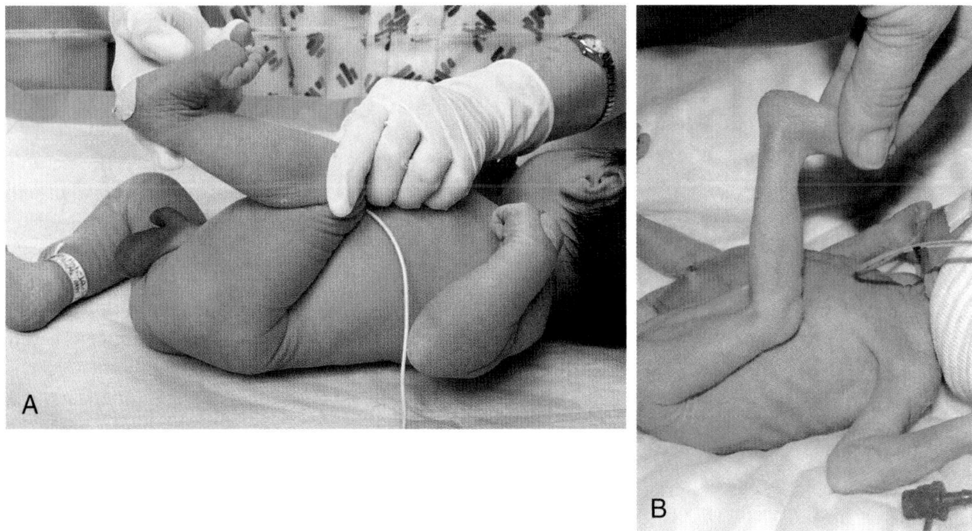

FIG 21.27 The popliteal angle is measured by flexing the thigh against the abdomen and extending the lower leg to the point of resistance. **A,** Full-term infant. **B,** Preterm infant.

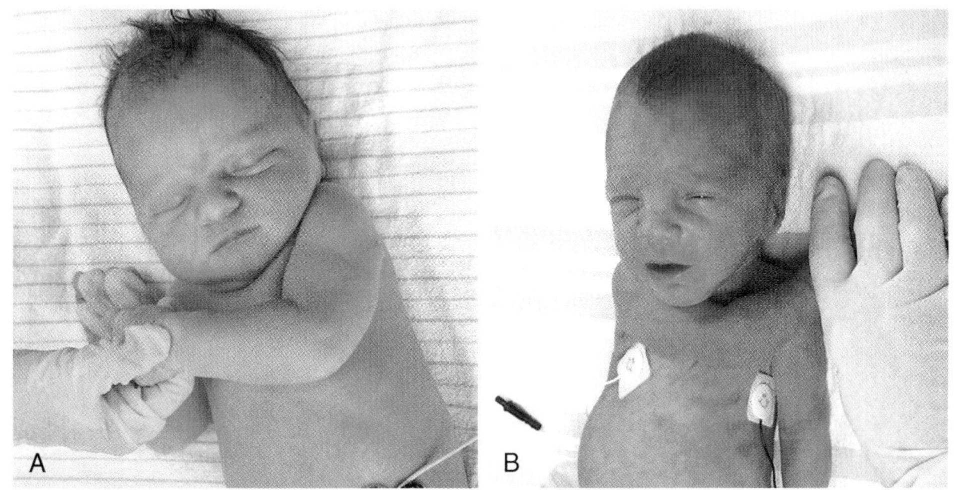

FIG 21.28 Scarf sign. The nurse determines how far the arm will move across the chest and observes the position of the elbow when resistance is felt. **A,** Full-term infant. **B,** Preterm infant. (Note the many visible veins in the preterm infant and the absence of visible veins in the full-term infant.)

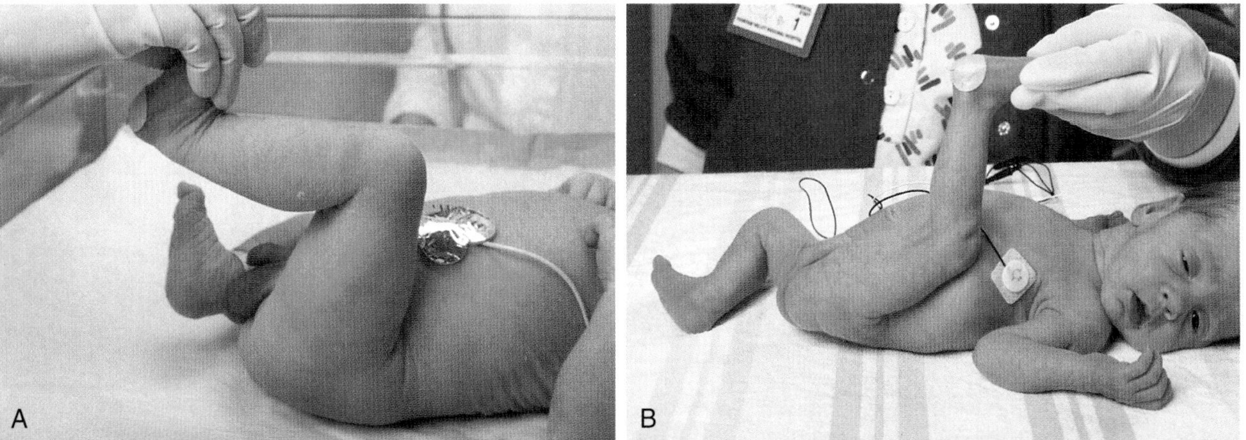

FIG 21.29 Heel to ear. The nurse grasps the foot and brings it up toward the ear. The score is recorded when resistance is felt. **A,** Full-term infant. **B,** Preterm infant.

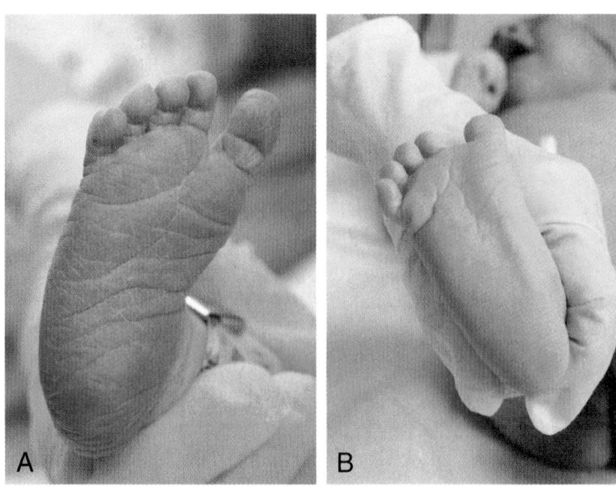

FIG 21.30 Plantar creases begin to develop at the base of the toes and extend to the heel. **A,** The postterm infant has deep creases. **B,** The preterm infant has few creases on the entire foot.

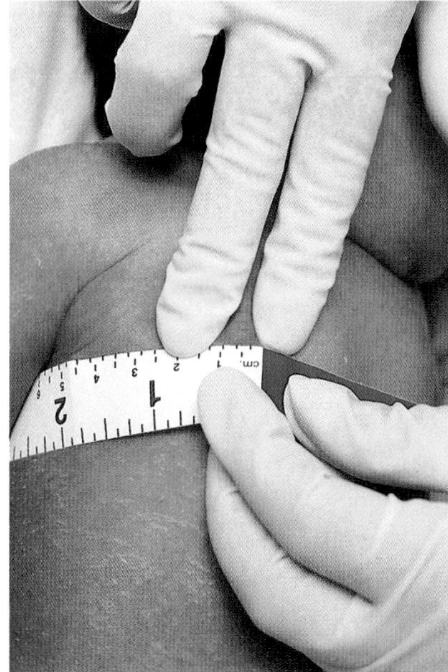

FIG 21.31 The nurse places a finger on either side of the breast bud and measures the size. In the full-term infant, the areola is raised and the nipple is easily distinguished from surrounding skin. (Note the peeling skin.)

labia majora enlarge until the clitoris and labia minora are completely covered.

In the male infant, the location of the testes and the rugae on the scrotum are assessed (Fig. 21.34). The testes originate in the abdominal cavity but have moved through the inguinal canal into the scrotum by term. Rugae forming on the surface of the scrotum cover the sac by 40 weeks. Once the testes are completely down into the scrotum, it appears large and pendulous.

## Scoring

As each part of the assessment is performed, the infant's response is matched with the diagrams and descriptions on the assessment tool (see Fig. 21.23). The total score is compared with the corresponding gestational age. It is important to understand that one or two characteristics alone are not enough to assign a gestational age. The total score of all assessed characteristics determines the gestational age.

## Gestational Age and Infant Size

The appropriateness of the neonate's size for gestational age is determined by plotting the gestational age, weight, length, and head circumference on a graph of intrauterine development. This score determines how well the infant has grown for the amount of time spent in the uterus. The infant whose size is appropriate for gestational age falls between the 10th and the 90th percentiles on the graph. The large-for-gestational-age (LGA) infant is above the 90th percentile, whereas the small-for-gestational-age (SGA) infant is below the 10th percentile.

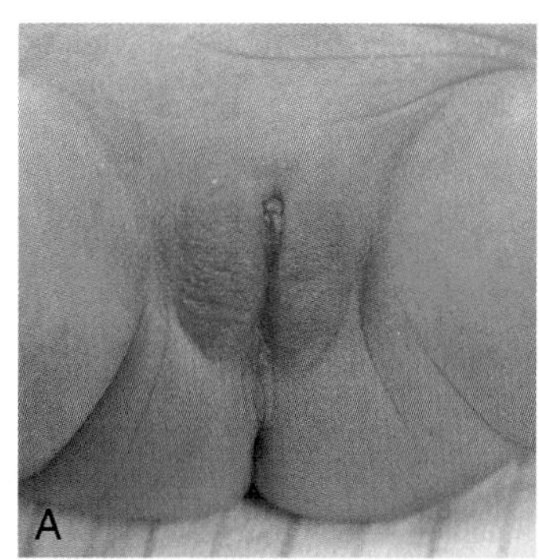

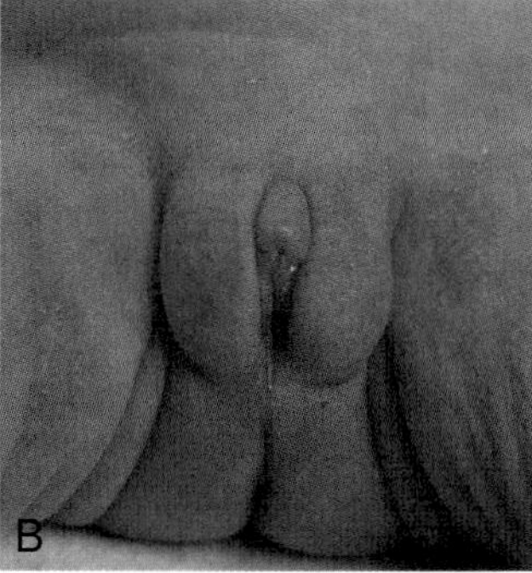

FIG 21.33 Female genitals. As the female fetus matures, the labia majora cover the labia minora and clitoris completely; in the preterm infant, these structures are not covered. **A,** Near-term infant. **B,** Preterm infant.

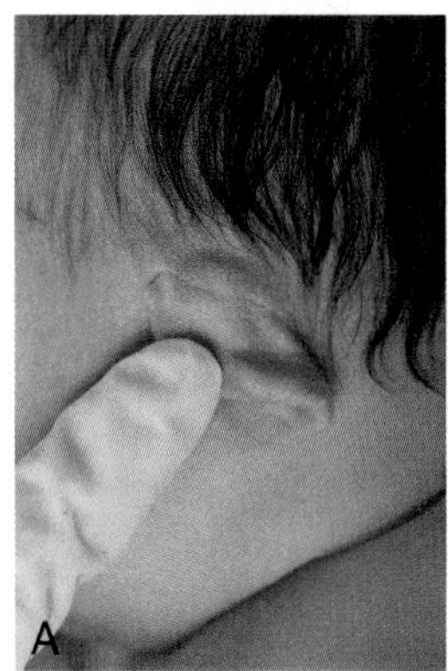

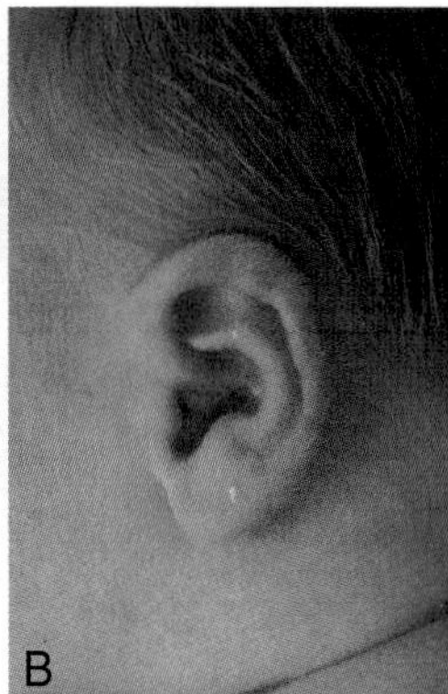

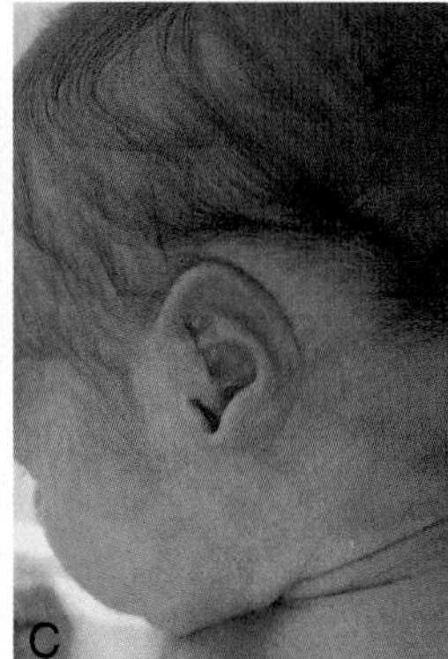

FIG 21.32 Ear maturation. **A,** The nurse folds the ears and notes how quickly they return to position. **B,** Ears in the full-term infant are well formed and have instant recoil. **C,** In the preterm infant, ears show less incurving of the pinna and recoil slowly or not at all.

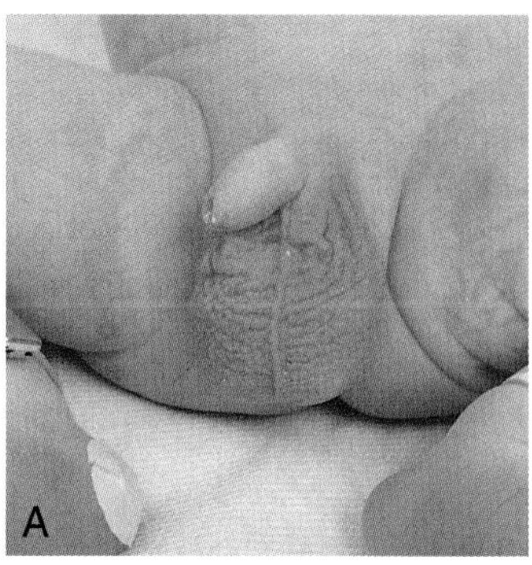

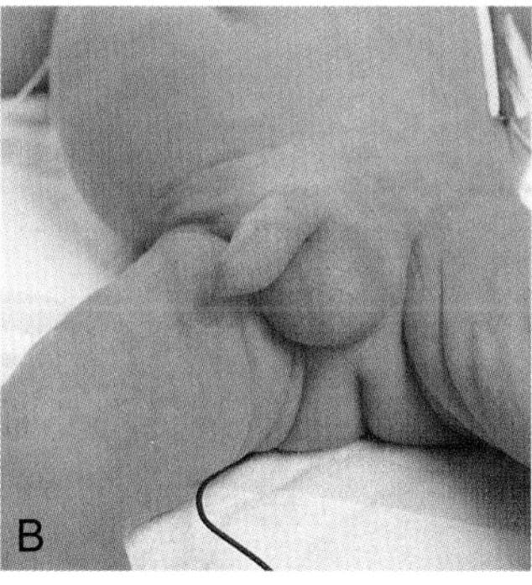


**FIG 21.34** Male genitals. **A,** The full-term infant has a pendulous scrotum with deep rugae. **B,** In the preterm infant, the testes may not be descended and rugae are few.

When an infant's gestational age or measurements fall outside the range expected, the nurse monitors for complications specific to the preterm, postterm, SGA, or LGA infant (see Chapter 29).

## ASSESSMENT OF BEHAVIOR

Assessment of the infant's behavior helps determine intactness of the central nervous system and provides information about ability to respond to caretaking activities.

### Periods of Reactivity

During the first and second periods of reactivity, newborns may have elevated pulse and respiratory rates, low temperatures, and excessive respiratory secretions. Careful observation is important at this time but can usually be done unobtrusively as parents hold the infant. During the sleep period between the first and second periods of reactivity, newborns cannot be awakened easily and are not interested in feeding.

### Behavioral Changes

Nurses assess the infant's behavior and alert the physician of abnormalities. Assessment includes the six different behavioral states: quiet sleep, active sleep, drowsy, quiet alert, active alert, and crying. Movement between states should be smooth, not abrupt.

The Brazelton Neonatal Behavioral Assessment Scale is often used when detailed knowledge about the infant is needed. In addition to assessing behavioral states, the scale analyzes other aspects of the newborn's behavior, such as orientation, habituation, self-consoling behaviors, and social behaviors.

#### Orientation

The nurse notes the infant's orientation (ability to pay attention) to interesting visual or auditory stimuli. It is most prominent during the quiet alert state. Infants focus their eyes and turn their heads toward a stimulus in an attempt to prolong contact with it.

#### Habituation

The infant's response to a visual, auditory, or tactile stimulus is assessed. Usually the first response of a healthy newborn to an interesting stimulus, such as a brightly colored object or a bell, is a period of alertness. If the stimulus is disturbing, like a bright light flashed in the eyes, the infant startles and attempts to escape by averting the eyes.

Infants gradually stop responding to continued unpleasant stimuli. This gradual habituation allows them to ignore the stimuli and save energy for physiologic needs. Newborns may go into a dull, drowsy state or fall into a deep sleep. Those who seem unresponsive in a bright, noisy environment may be in a state of habituation. The preterm infant or one with injury to the central nervous system may not be able to habituate.

#### Self-Consoling Activities

Normal newborns are able to console themselves for short periods. Self-consoling activities include attempting to bring their hands to the mouth and sucking on their fists. Infants who are ill, preterm, or exposed to drugs prenatally have less ability to console themselves.

#### Parents' Response

The parents' growing ability to respond to the infant's behavioral cues should be noted. To facilitate bonding and help the parents learn to interpret the infant's cues, the nurse can point out the infant's behavioral changes.

## KEY CONCEPTS

- Surfactant lines the alveoli and reduces surface tension to keep the alveoli open. Fetal lung fluid moves into the interstitial spaces before, during, and after birth and is absorbed by the lymphatic and vascular systems.
- Chemical, mechanical, thermal, and sensory factors combine to stimulate the respiratory center in the brain and initiate respiration at birth.
- Increases in blood oxygen levels, shifts in pressure in the heart and lungs, and closing of the umbilical vessels cause closure of the ductus arteriosus, foramen ovale, and ductus venosus at birth.
- Neonates must produce and maintain heat (thermogenesis) to prevent the effects of cold stress.
- Infants are predisposed to heat loss because they have thin skin with little subcutaneous (white) fat, blood vessels close to the surface, and a large skin surface area. They lose heat by evaporation, conduction, convection, and radiation.
- Heat is produced in newborns through increases in activity, flexion, metabolism by vasoconstriction and nonshivering thermogenesis. These factors increase oxygen and glucose consumption and may cause respiratory distress, hypoglycemia, acidosis, and jaundice.
- Laboratory values for erythrocytes, hemoglobin, and hematocrit are higher for newborns than for adults because less oxygen is available during fetal life than after birth.
- The stools progress from thick, greenish-black meconium to loose, greenish-brown transitional stools to milk stools. Stools of breastfed infants are frequent, seedy, and mustard colored, whereas those of formula-fed infants are pale yellow to light brown, firmer, and less frequent.
- The neonate uses glucose rapidly and is at risk for hypoglycemia. Infants at increased risk for hypoglycemia include those who are preterm, late preterm, small-for-gestational age, large-for-gestational age, born to diabetic mothers, or exposed to stressors.
- Physiologic, pathologic, breastfeeding, or breast-milk jaundice may occur in the neonate. Physiologic jaundice occurs in normal newborns after the first 24 hours of life as a result of hemolysis of red blood cells and immaturity of the liver. Pathologic jaundice begins

*Continued*

## KEY CONCEPTS—cont'd

in the first 24 hours and may require treatment with phototherapy. Breastfeeding jaundice is often caused by insufficient intake and requires assistance with breastfeeding techniques. True breast-milk jaundice begins later than physiologic jaundice and may be caused by substances in the milk.

- The ability of the newborn's kidneys to filter, reabsorb, and maintain fluid and electrolyte balance is less than that of the adult's kidneys. The newborn's body is composed of a greater percentage of water, with more located in the extracellular compartment, and fluid is more easily lost.
- Newborns usually pass the first stool within 12 hours of birth. The newborn's first void usually occurs within 24 hours. Absence of stool or urine for 48 hours may signify an abnormality.
- Newborns receive passive immunity when IgG crosses the placenta in utero. After birth, IgM, and IgA are produced to protect against infection.
- During the first and second periods of reactivity, newborns may have a low temperature, elevated pulse and respiratory rates, and excessive secretions.
- Newborns are active and alert and may be interested in feeding.
- Newborns progress through six behavioral states: deep or quiet sleep, light or active sleep, drowsy, quiet alert, active alert, and crying.
- Nurses assess newborns immediately after birth to detect serious abnormalities. If no problems are detected with a quick assessment, a more comprehensive examination is performed.
- Assessment of cardiorespiratory status includes history, airway, color, heart sounds, pulses, and may include blood pressure.
- Axillary temperatures are preferred over rectal temperatures because they are safer and provide accurate measurement.
- Molding of the head is normal during birth and may cause the head to appear misshapen. Caput succedaneum (localized swelling from pressure against the cervix) or a cephalhematoma (bleeding between the periosteum and the bone) may be present.
- Measurements are an important way to learn about growth before birth. Abnormal measurements alert the nurse that complications may occur.
- Reflexes are an indication of the health of the central nervous system. Asymmetry or retention of reflexes beyond the time when they should disappear is abnormal.
- Early signs of hypoglycemia include jitteriness, poor muscle tone, respiratory distress, sweating, low temperature, and poor suck.
- In performing heel sticks for blood samples, the nurse must choose the site carefully to avoid injury to the bone, nerves, or blood vessels of the heel.
- The initial feeding provides information about the neonate's ability to coordinate sucking and swallowing, with breathing as well as tolerance to feeding.
- Marks on the skin should be documented, including location, size, and a general description. Explain marks to parents, and offer emotional support if they are upset.
- The gestational-age assessment provides an estimate of the infant's age from conception. Gestational age alerts the nurse to possible complications of age and development.

## REFERENCES AND READINGS


Adamkin, D.H. Committee on fetus and newborn, American Academy of Pediatrics. (2011). Clinical report–Postnatal glucose homeostasis in late-preterm and term infants. *Pediatrics, 127*(3), 575–579.

Ambalavanan, N., & Carlo, W. (2011). Jaundice and hyperbilirubinemia in the newborn. In R.M. Kliegman, B.E. Stanton, J.W. St. Geme, et al. (Eds.). *Nelson textbook of pediatrics* (pp. 603–608). Philadelphia: Saunders.

American Academy of Pediatrics & American College of Obstetricians and Gynecologists. (2012). *Guidelines for perinatal care.* Elk Grove Village, IL, and Washington, DC: Author.

American Academy of Pediatrics, American Heart Association. (2011). *Textbook of neonatal resuscitation.* Elk Grove Village, IL: Author.

Association of Women's Health, Obstetric and Neonatal Nurses (2011). Position Statement: Newborn screening. *Journal of Obstetric, Gynecologic and Neonatal Nurses, 40*(1), 136–137.

Association of Women's Health, Obstetric and Neonatal Nurses (2015). Position Statement: Breastfeeding. *Journal of Obstetric, Gynecologic and Neonatal Nurses, 44*(1), 145–150.

Ballard, J.L., Khoury, J.C., Wedig, K., et al. (1991). New Ballard Score, expanded to include extremely premature infants. *Journal of Pediatrics, 19*(3), 417–423.

Blackburn, S.T. (2013). *Maternal, fetal, and neonatal physiology: A clinical perspective.* St. Louis: Saunders.

Brown, V.D., & Landers, S. (2011). Heat balance. In S.L. Gardner, B.S. Carter, M. Enzman-Hines, et al. (Eds.). *Merenstein & Gardner's handbook of neonatal intensive care* (pp. 113–133). St. Louis: Mosby.

Buckley, R.H. (2011). The T lymphocytes, B lymphocytes, and natural killer cells. In R.M. Kliegman, B.E. Stanton, J.W. St. Geme, et al. (Eds.). *Nelson textbook of pediatrics* (pp. 722). Philadelphia: Saunders.

Carlo, W.A. (2011a). Routine delivery room and initial care. In R.M. Kliegman, B.E. Stanton, J.W. St. Geme, et al. (Eds.). *Nelson textbook of pediatrics* (pp. 536–538). Philadelphia: Saunders.

Carlo, W.A. (2011b). Physical examination of the newborn infant. In R.M. Kliegman, B.E. Stanton, J.W. St. Geme, et al. (Eds.). *Nelson textbook of pediatrics* (pp. 532–536). Philadelphia: Saunders.

Carlo, W.A., & DiFiore, J.M. (2011). Assessment of pulmonary function. In R.J. Martin, A.A. Fanaroff, & M.C. Walsh (Eds.). *Fanaroff and Martin's neonatal-perinatal medicine: Diseases of the fetus and infant* (pp. 1092–1106). Philadelphia: Mosby.

Cheffer, N.D., & Rannalli, D.A. (2016). Transitional care of the newborn. In S. Mattson, & J.E. Smith (Eds.). *AWHONN core curriculum for maternal-newborn nursing* (pp. 345–362). St. Louis: Saunders.

Diehl-Jones, W., & Askin, D.F. (2010). Hematologic disorders. In M.T. Verklan, & M. Walden (Eds.). *Awhonn core curriculum for neonatal intensive care nursing* (pp. 666–693). St. Louis: Saunders.

Fraser, D. (2014). Newborn adaptation to extrauterine life. In K.R. Simpson, & P.A. Creehan (Eds.). *AWHONN perinatal nursing* (pp. 581-596). Philadelphia: Lippincott Williams & Wilkins.

Frost, M.S., Fashaw, L., Hernandez, J.A., et al. (2011). Neonatal nephrology. In S.L. Gardner, B.S. Carter, & M. Enzman-Hines (Eds.). *Merenstein & Gardner's handbook of neonatal intensive care* (pp. 717–747). Philadelphia: Mosby.

Furdon, S.A., & Benjamin, K. (2010). Physical assessment. In M.T. Verklan, & M. Walden (Eds.). *AWHONN core curriculum for neonatal intensive care nursing* (pp. 120–155). St. Louis: Saunders.

Gardner, S.L., Enzman-Hines, M., & Dickey, L.A. (2011). Respiratory diseases. In S.L. Gardner, B.S. Carter, M. Enzman-Hines, et al. (Eds.). *Merenstein & Gardner's handbook of neonatal intensive care* (pp. 581–677). St. Louis: Mosby.

Gardner, S.L., & Hernandez, J.A. (2011). Initial nursery care. In S.L. Gardner, B.S. Carter, M. Enzman-Hines, et al. (Eds.). *Merenstein & Gardner's handbook of neonatal intensive care* (pp. 78–112). St. Louis: Mosby.

Goodwin, M. (2010). Apnea. In M.T. Verklan, & M. Walden (Eds.). *Core curriculum for neonatal intensive care nursing* (pp. 484–493). St. Louis: Saunders.

Halbardier, B.H. (2010). Fluid and electrolyte management. In M.T. Verklan, & M. Walden (Eds.). *Core curriculum for neonatal intensive care nursing* (pp. 156-171). St. Louis: Saunders.

Hoath, S.B. & Narendran, V. (2011). The skin. In R.J. Martin, A.A. Fanaroff, & M.C. Walsh (Eds.). *Neonatal-Perinatal Medicine: Diseases of the Fetus and Newborn* (pp. 1705–1736). St. Louis: Elsevier.

Holt, K., Wooldridge, N., Story, M., et al. (2011). *Bright futures nutrition.* Elk Grove Village, IL: American Academy of Pediatrics.

Johnson, L., & Cochran, W.D. (2012). Assessment of the newborn history and physical examination of the newborn. In J.P. Cloherty, E.C. Eichenwald, A.R. Hansen, et al. (Eds.). *Manual of neonatal care* (pp. 91–102). Philadelphia: Lippincott Williams & Wilkins.

Johnson, P.J. (2015). Head, eyes, ears, nose, mouth, and neck assessment. In E.P. Tappero, & M.E. Honeyfield (Eds.). *Physical assessment of the newborn: A comprehensive approach to the art of physical examination* (pp. 61–78). Petaluma, CA: NICU Ink.

Jones, J.E., Hayes, R.D., Starbuck, A.L., et al. (2011). Fluid and electrolyte management. In S.L. Gardner, B.S. Carter, & M. Enzman-Hines (Eds.). *Merenstein & Gardner's handbook of neonatal intensive care* (pp. 333–352). St. Louis: Mosby.

Kamuth, B.D., Thilo, E.H., & Hernandez, J.A. (2011). Jaundice. In S.L. Gardner, B.S. Carter, M. Enzman-Hines, et al. (Eds.). *Merenstein & Gardner's handbook of neonatal intensive care* (pp. 531–552). St. Louis: Mosby.

Kaplan, M., Wong, R.J., Sibley, E., et al. (2011). Neonatal jaundice and liver disease. In R.J. Martin, A.A. Fanaroff, & M.C. Walsh (Eds.). *Fanaroff and Martin's neonatal-perinatal medicine: Diseases of the fetus and infant* (pp. 1443–1496). Philadelphia: Mosby.

Kapur, R., Yoder, M.C., & Polin, R.A. (2011). The immune system. In R.J. Martin, A.A. Fanaroff, & M.C. Walsh (Eds.). *Fanaroff and Martin's neonatal-perinatal medicine: Diseases of the fetus and infant* (pp. 761–885). Philadelphia: Mosby.

Kaufman, L.M., Miller, M.T., & Gupta, B.K. (2011). The eye: Examination and common problems. In R.J. Martin, A.A. Fanaroff, & M.C. Walsh (Eds.). *Fanaroff and Martin's neonatal-perinatal medicine: Diseases of the fetus and infant* (pp. 1737–1763). Philadelphia: Mosby.

Keane, V. (2011). Assessment of growth. In R.M. Kliegman, B.E. Stanton, J.W. St. Geme, et al. (Eds.). *Nelson textbook of pediatrics* (pp. 39). Philadelphia: Saunders.

Kenney, P.M., Hoover, D., Williams, L.C., et al. (2011). Cardiovascular diseases and surgical interventions. In S.L. Gardner, B.S. Carter, M. Enzman-Hines, et al. (Eds.). *Merenstein & Gardner's handbook of neonatal intensive care* (pp. 678-716). St. Louis: Mosby.

Lawrence, R.A., & Lawrence, R.M. (2011). *Breastfeeding: A guide for the medical profession.* Philadelphia: Mosby.

Lissauer, T., & Steer, P. (2013). Size and physical examination of the newborn infant. In A.A. Fanaroff & J.M. Fanaroff (Eds.). *Care of the High-Risk Neonate* (pp. 105–131.). Philadelphia: Saunders.

Lo, S.F. (2011). Reference intervals for laboratory tests and procedures. In R.M. Kliegman, B.E. Stanton, J.W. St. Geme, et al. (Eds.). *Nelson textbook of pediatrics* (pp. 2466). Philadelphia: Saunders.

Lott, J.W. (2010). Immunology and infectious disease. In M.T. Verklan, & M. Walden (Eds.). *AWHONN core curriculum for neonatal intensive care nursing* (pp. 694–723). St. Louis: Saunders.

Luchtman-Jones, L., & Wilson, D.B. (2011). The blood and hematopoietic system. In R.J. Martin, A.A. Fanaroff, & M.C. Walsh (Eds.). *Fanaroff and Martin's neonatal-perinatal medicine: Diseases of the fetus and infant* (pp. 1303–1373). Philadelphia: Mosby.

Mangurten, H.H., & Puppala, B.L. (2011). Birth injuries. In R.J. Martin, A.A. Fanaroff, & M.C. Walsh (Eds.). *Fanaroff and Martin's neonatal-perinatal medicine: Diseases of the fetus and infant* (501–529). Philadelphia: Mosby.

McGowan, J.E., Rozance, P.J., Price-Douglas, W., et al. (2011). Glucose homeostasis. In S.L. Gardner, B.S. Carter, & M. Enzman-Hines (Eds.). *Merenstein & Gardner's handbook of neonatal intensive care* (pp. 353–377). St. Louis: Mosby.

Morrow, C., Hidinger, A., & Wilkinson-Faulk, D. (2010). Reducing neonatal pain during routine heel lance procedures. *MCN: The American Journal of Maternal/Child Nursing, 35*(6), 346–354.

National Association of Neonatal Nurses. (2010). Position statement #3049: Prevention of acute bilirubin encephalopathy and kernicterus in newborns. *Advances in Neonatal Care, 10*(3), 112–118.

Olitsky, S.E., Hug, D., Plummer, L.S., et al. (2011). Disorders of the eye: Growth and development. In R.M. Kliegman, B.E. Stanton, & J.W. St. Geme (Eds.). *Nelson textbook of pediatrics* (pp. 2148). Philadelphia: Saunders.

Pagana, K.D., & Pagana, T.J. (2011). *Mosby's diagnostic and laboratory test reference.* St. Louis: Mosby.

Sankar, W.N., Horn, B.D., Wells, L., et al. (2011). Developmental dysplasia of the hip. In R.M. Kliegman, B.E. Stanton, & J.W. St. Geme (Eds.). *Nelson textbook of pediatrics* (2356–2360). Philadelphia: Saunders.

Smith, J.R. & Carley, A. (2014). Common neonatal complications. In K.R. Simpson, & P.A. Creehan (Eds.). *AWHONN perinatal nursing* (pp. 662–698). Philadelphia: Lippincott Williams & Wilkins.

Smith, V.C. (2012). The high-risk newborn: Anticipation, evaluation, management, and outcome. In J.P. Cloherty, E.C. Eichenwald, A.R. Hansen, et al. (Eds.). *Manual of neonatal care* (pp. 74–90). Philadelphia: Lippincott Williams & Wilkins.

Sprecher, R.C., & Arnold, J.E. (2011). Upper airway lesions. In R.J. Martin, A.A. Fanaroff, & M.C. Walsh (Eds.). *Fanaroff and Martin's neonatal-perinatal medicine: Diseases of the fetus and infant* (pp. 1170–1179). Philadelphia: Mosby.

Taperro, E.P. (2015). Musculoskeletal system assessment. In E.P. Tappero, & M.E. Honeyfield (Eds.). *Physical assessment of the newborn: A comprehensive approach to the art of physical examination* (5th ed., pp. 139–165). Petaluma, CA: NICU Ink.

Trotter, C.W. (2015). Gestational age assessment. In E.P. Tappero, & M.E. Honeyfield (Eds.). *Physical assessment of the newborn: A comprehensive approach to the art of physical examination* (pp. 23–43). Petaluma, CA: NICU Ink.

Vargo, L. (2015). Cardiovascular assessment. In E.P. Tappero, & M.E. Honeyfield (Eds.). *Physical assessment of the newborn: A comprehensive approach to the art of physical examination* (pp. 93–110). Petaluma, CA: NICU Ink.

Vargo, L. (2014). Newborn physical assessment. In K.R. Simpson, & P.A. Creehan (Eds.). *AWHONN perinatal nursing* (pp. 597–625). Philadelphia: Lippincott Williams & Wilkins.

Verklan, M.T. (2011). Adaptation to extrauterine life. In S. Mattson, & J.E. Smith (Eds.). *Awhonn core curriculum for maternal-newborn nursing* (pp. 72–90). St. Louis: Saunders.

Witt, C. (2015). Skin assessment. In E.P. Tappero, & M.E. Honeyfield (Eds.). *Physical assessment of the newborn: A comprehensive approach to the art of physical examination* (pp. 45–59). Petaluma, CA: NICU Ink.

22

# The Normal Newborn: Nursing Care

http://evolve.elsevier.com/McKinney/mat-ch/

## LEARNING OBJECTIVES

*After studying this chapter, you should be able to:*

- Describe the purpose and use of routine prophylactic medications for the normal newborn.
- Explain the nurse's responsibility in ongoing cardiorespiratory and thermoregulatory assessments and care.
- Describe collaborative interventions for hypoglycemia.
- Discuss prevention and parent teaching for jaundice.
- Explain the risks and benefits of circumcision.
- Describe the care of circumcised and uncircumcised male infants.
- Describe ongoing nursing assessments and care of the newborn.
- Describe methods to protect newborns by proper identification.
- Explain how nurses can help prevent infant abductions.
- Describe methods to prevent infections in newborns.
- Discuss important considerations in parent teaching.
- Explain the types and importance of newborn screening tests.
- Describe postdischarge nursing care included in home visits, clinic visits, and telephone follow-up.

The nurse's role in ongoing assessments and care of the newborn is to identify and respond to changes in their condition as they adapt to life outside the uterus, keep them safe, and teach parents how to provide care.

## EARLY CARE

Early care after birth involves assignment of Apgar scores, assessment, and stabilization of the infant as necessary. Immediate care is discussed in Chapter 16, and infant resuscitation is discussed in Chapter 30. Assessment is discussed in Chapter 21. Once the infant is stable, prophylactic medications are given.

The nurse wears gloves during all contact with the infant until the bath is completed to avoid contact with blood and amniotic fluid on the infant's skin from birth. After the bath, gloves are necessary only when contact with body fluids or stools will occur.

### Administering Vitamin K

Because infants cannot synthesize vitamin K in the intestines without bacterial flora, they are deficient in clotting factors (Luchtman-Jones & Wilson, 2011). Vitamin K should be given to the neonate to prevent vitamin K–deficiency bleeding. One dose of vitamin K intramuscularly within the first hour after birth, prevents bleeding problems until the infant is able to produce the vitamin independently. Although the injection is usually given within an hour, it can be delayed until the infant has finished breastfeeding in the delivery room (American Academy of Pediatrics [AAP] & American College of Obstetricians and Gynecologists [ACOG], 2012) (See Chapter 38 for administration of injections to infants).

### Providing Eye Treatment

Newborns also receive prophylactic eye treatment to help prevent ophthalmia neonatorum in case the mother is infected with gonorrhea. Erythromycin (0.5%) ophthalmic ointment (Fig. 22.1) is most commonly used. Tetracycline (1%) also may be used (AAP & ACOG, 2012). Because the ointment may temporarily blur the infant's vision, the treatment can be given near the end of the first hour to allow for bonding with the parents.

In some infants, a mild inflammation develops a few hours after prophylactic treatment. Any discharge from the eyes, especially if purulent, should alert the nurse to the possibility of infection. Drainage should be removed with sterile saline and cotton. If the mother is infected, the infant needs additional antibiotics because routine prophylactic treatment may not completely prevent infection.

## NURSING CARE

### Cardiorespiratory Status

Temporary problems in cardiorespiratory status can occur during the transition period in the early newborn.

#### Assessment

Assess the newborn for signs of a difficult transition. Note the rate and character of the heart rate, pulses, respirations, and breath sounds. Look for signs of respiratory distress, including tachypnea, retractions, flaring of the nares, pallor or cyanosis, grunting, seesaw respirations, and asymmetry of chest movements (see Chapter 21).

#### Nursing Diagnosis and Planning

Fluid from the lungs must be removed by absorption or drainage from the respiratory passages after birth. This process does not happen immediately and may cause a temporary problem during the early hours after birth. A common nursing diagnosis is:

- Ineffective Airway Clearance related to excessive secretions in the respiratory passages.

***Expected outcome.*** The newborn will maintain a patent airway as evidenced by a respiratory rate within the normal range of 30 to 60 breaths per minute and show no signs of respiratory distress.

## DRUG GUIDE

### *Vitamin $K_1$ (phytonadione)*

**Other Names:** AquaMEPHYTON, Konakion, Mephyton

**Classification:** Fat-soluble vitamin, antihemorrhagic

**Action:** Promotes the formation of factors II (prothrombin), VII, IX, and X by the liver for clotting. Provides vitamin K, which is not synthesized in the intestines until intestinal flora necessary for vitamin K production are established.

**Indication:** Prevention or treatment of vitamin K deficiency bleeding (hemorrhagic disease of the newborn)

**Neonatal Dosage and Route:** 0.5 to 1 mg (0.25 to 0.5 mL of solution containing 1 mg/0.5 mL) given once intramuscularly within 1 hour of birth for prophylaxis. May be delayed until after the first breastfeeding in the delivery room. May be repeated or higher doses used if the mother took anticonvulsants during pregnancy or the infant shows bleeding tendencies.

**Absorption:** Readily absorbed after intramuscular injection. Effective within 1 to 2 hours. Metabolized in the liver.

**Adverse Reactions:** Erythema, pain, and edema at injection site. Hemolysis or hyperbilirubinemia, especially in a preterm infant or when large doses are used.

**Nursing Considerations:** Protect the drug from light until just before administration because light causes decomposition and loss of potency. Observe all infants for signs of vitamin K deficiency: ecchymoses or bleeding from any site. Check to see that the infant had vitamin K before a circumcision is performed.

## DRUG GUIDE

### *Erythromycin Ophthalmic Ointment*

**Other Name:** Ilotycin ophthalmic ointment

**Classification:** Antibiotic

**Action:** Inhibits protein synthesis in bacteria; bacteriostatic or bactericidal (depending on organism)

**Indications:** Prophylaxis against the organism *Neisseria gonorrhoeae.* Prevents ophthalmia neonatorum in infants of mothers with gonorrhea. Prophylaxis against gonorrhea is required by law for all infants, regardless of whether the mother is known to be infected.

**Neonatal Dosage and Route:** A "ribbon" of 0.5% erythromycin ointment, 1 cm (0.4 in) long, is applied to the lower conjunctival sac of each eye within 1 hour after birth.

**Adverse Reactions:** Burning, itching. Irritation may result in chemical conjunctivitis, lasting 24 to 48 hours. Ointment may cause temporary blurred vision.

**Nursing Considerations:** Cleanse the infant's eyes as needed before application. Hold the tube in a horizontal rather than a vertical position to prevent injury to the eye from sudden movement. Administer from the inner canthus to the outer canthus. Do not touch the tip of the tube to any part of the eye because this may spread infectious material from one eye to the other. Do not rinse. Excess ointment may be wiped away after 1 minute. Observe for irritation. Use a new tube for each infant to prevent spread of infection.

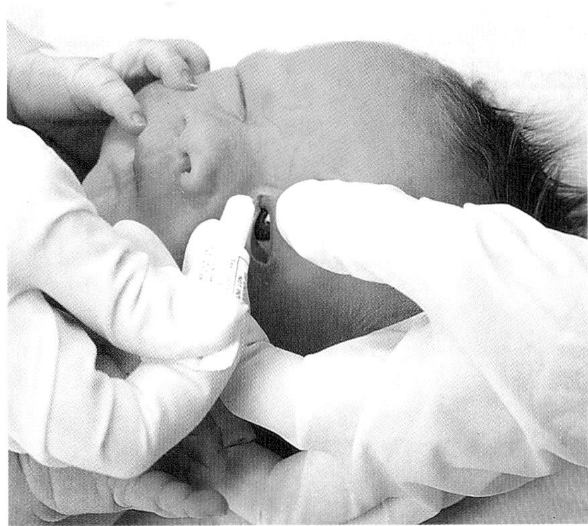

FIG 22.1 Administration of ophthalmic ointment. The nurse gently clears the eyes of blood or vernix, wiping from the inner to outer canthus. Then, placing a finger and thumb near the edge of each lid, the nurse gently presses against the periorbital ridges to open the eyes, avoiding pressure on the eye itself. A ribbon of ointment is squeezed into each conjunctival sac.

#### Interventions

***Positioning and suctioning.*** Position the infant on its back with the head in a neutral position or to the side. Use the bulb syringe as necessary to suction secretions as they drain into the infant's mouth or nose (see Procedure: Using a Bulb Syringe). Suction the mouth first because the infant may gasp and aspirate mouth fluids if the nose is suctioned first (Kattwinkel, 2011). Suction the nose gently and only if necessary because suctioning is traumatic to the tissues of the nose.

Keep the bulb syringe in the crib near the infant's head, where it is available if needed quickly. Teach both parents how to use the bulb syringe correctly. Send the syringe home with the infant so the parents can use it if the infant experiences a problem.

If mechanical suctioning is necessary to remove deeper secretions, choose a small catheter to avoid damaging the tissues of the respiratory tract. Suction for no more than 5 seconds at a time using minimal negative pressure to avoid trauma, laryngospasm, and bradycardia. Apply suction only when the catheter is being withdrawn.

***Providing continuing care.*** Continue monitoring the infant for problems throughout the birth facility stay. By the time of the second period of reactivity, the infant may be alone with the mother. Although nurses know that regurgitation, gagging, and brief episodes of cyanosis are normal during this time, they may be very frightening to the mother. Check in with her frequently to ask whether the infant is having difficulty and to provide needed instruction and assistance.

#### Evaluation

- Is the respiratory rate between 30 and 60 breaths per minute?
- Is the infant free of signs of respiratory distress?

## NURSING CARE

### Thermoregulation

Because any neonate can have difficulty with thermoregulation, the nurse must identify problems and intervene to prevent complications.

#### Assessment

Assess the newborn's temperature according to agency policy. The temperature is often assessed every half hour until it has been stable for 2 hours. It is generally checked again at 4 hours and then every 8 to 12 hours. Assess the temperature more often if it is abnormal.

## PROCEDURE

### *Using a Bulb Syringe*

**Purpose**

To maintain an open airway by removing secretions or regurgitated feeding from the infant's mouth and nose.

1. Position the infant's head to the side to allow fluids to pool in the lower cheek
2. Compress the bulb before inserting it into the mouth. Do not compress the bulb while it is in the infant's mouth or secretions in the bulb will be expelled back into the mouth.
3. Gently insert the syringe tip into the side of the infant's mouth. Avoid inserting it straight to the back of the throat, which could stimulate the gag reflex, causing regurgitation and stimulating a vagal response, resulting in bradycardia or apnea.
4. Release the bulb slowly to draw in the secretions from the mouth. Remove and empty the bulb by compressing it several times before using again to prevent inserting secretions back into the mouth.
5. Suction the nose, only if necessary, after the mouth is suctioned. Infants often gasp when the nose is suctioned and might aspirate secretions in the mouth if it is not cleared first.
6. Suction the nose gently because trauma could cause edema and obstruction of the nasal passages.

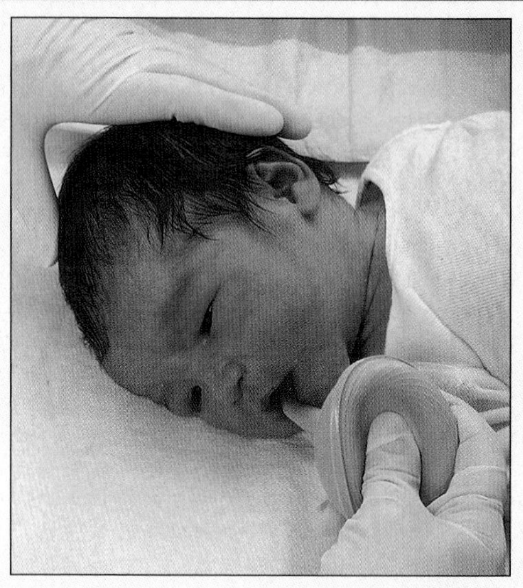

### Nursing Diagnosis and Planning

A common diagnosis is:

- Risk for Ineffective Thermoregulation related to immature compensation for changes in environmental temperature.

*Expected outcome.* The infant will maintain an axillary temperature within the normal range of 36.5°C to 37.5°C (97.7°F to 99.5°F).

### Interventions

#### *Preventing heat loss*

**Preparing the environment before birth.** Before the birth, prepare a thermal-neutral environment using a radiant warmer for use during initial assessments (Fig. 22.2). Check the radiant warmer to ensure it is functioning properly before the delivery. Turn it on early enough to warm the bed before the birth.

**Providing immediate care.** Immediately after birth, place the infant on the mother's abdomen to provide warmth from skin-to-skin contact or under the radiant warmer to counteract the cool temperature of the delivery room. Routine assessment and care can be performed while the infant is on the mother's abdomen; if the mother and infant are stable, breastfeeding can begin if the mother wishes.

Dry the wet infant quickly with warm towels to prevent heat loss by evaporation. Dry the hair well because the head has a large surface area, and damp hair increases heat loss. Remove towels or blankets as soon as they become wet, and replace them with dry, warmed linens. Cover the infant's head with a cap when the infant is not under a radiant warmer. Do not use a hat on an infant under the warmer because it prevents the transfer of heat to the head.

Attach a skin probe to the abdomen when the infant is placed under a radiant warmer. Set the skin temperature for servocontrol between 36°C and 36.5°C (96.8°F and 97.7°F) (Brown & Landers, 2011). This setting regulates the amount of heat produced by the warmer to maintain the infant's skin temperature at the normal level. Check frequently to see that the infant's skin temperature is increasing as expected.

**Providing ongoing prevention.** To avoid conduction of heat away from the body, objects that come into contact with the infant should be warmed. Add padding to cool surfaces such as scales before placing infants on them. Warm stethoscopes and clothing before using them. Before touching the infant, run warm water over your hands if they are cold.

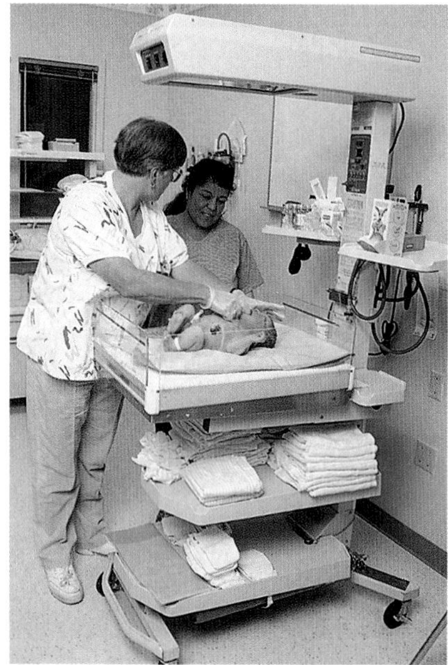

**FIG 22.2** Radiant warmers allow easy access to the infant without increasing heat loss caused by exposure. The nurse should be careful not to come between the infant and the overhead source of heat when giving care.

To prevent heat loss by radiation in cold weather, position the newborn's crib or incubator away from walls or windows that abut the outside of the building. When the objects and air around the infant seem warm, it is easy to overlook the fact that infants lose heat to objects not in close contact with them. Keep this possibility in mind when positioning cribs in mothers' rooms, which are often short of space. Place the crib between the beds (in a two-bed room) or near the head of the mother's bed and away from windows or doors, if possible. Avoid areas near hall doors or air conditioners, which may have drafts. Keep traffic low around radiant warmers because movement increases air currents.

When assessing or caring for newborns, avoid exposing more of their bodies than necessary. Remove clothing and blankets only from areas being assessed. Keep the upper part of the body covered when changing diapers. Wrap infants in blankets, and use a stockinette or insulated hat to prevent heat loss from the large surface area of the head.

***Restoring thermoregulation.*** If an infant with a previously normal temperature develops a low temperature, institute nursing measures to assist thermoregulation immediately. If the axillary temperature is low, some nurses check the rectal temperature to determine core temperature. However, the process of nonshivering thermogenesis begins before the core temperature becomes abnormal. Core temperature changes indicate that the infant's thermoregulatory resources are exhausted. Nurses must intervene before this happens.

Correct obvious causes first. The infant may be unwrapped or wearing wet clothing. The mother's room may be cold, or the crib may be placed near the air conditioner.

A small drop in temperature can be remedied by placing the infant, dressed in only a diaper and hat, next to the mother's bare skin. This skin-to-skin contact is very effective in using the mother's body to warm the infant. Place a warm blanket over both mother and infant.

If skin-to-skin contact is not possible, put a shirt on the infant upside down by placing the infant's legs in the sleeves for added warmth. Use two warmed blankets, each wrapped separately around the infant, to increase insulation of heat by trapping air between the layers. Place a hat on the infant's head and another blanket over the infant in the crib.

A greater drop in temperature or a temperature that has not improved within an hour using skin-to-skin contact requires additional measures. Place the infant under a radiant warmer for a short time. Observe the infant carefully during rewarming because it may cause apnea in some infants (Sedin, 2011).

***Performing expanded assessments.*** Expanded assessments are necessary whenever temperature is below normal in a newborn. Observe for signs of respiratory distress brought on by the additional oxygen requirement of nonshivering thermogenesis.

Because the cold infant uses more glucose to produce heat, test the blood glucose level when the temperature is abnormal. If the glucose is low, help the mother breastfeed or use formula. Warm colostrum or breast milk helps to warm the infant.

Notify the physician or nurse practitioner if the infant does not respond to these measures. Place the infant in a radiant warmer or incubator for close observation until the temperature stabilizes. Because low temperature may be a sign of infection, observe for other signs of infection (Sedin, 2011).

### Evaluation

- Is the temperature within normal range?
- Are there signs of complications from cold stress?

## NURSING CARE

### Hepatic Function

The major early assessments and care of the hepatic system are related to blood glucose levels and bilirubin conjugation.

### Blood Glucose

#### Assessment

Assess all infants for risk factors and signs of hypoglycemia (see Chapter 21, p. 445-449). Perform screening tests for blood glucose according to signs exhibited and agency policy.

#### Nursing Diagnosis and Planning

For infants who have glucose levels below 40 to 45 mg/dL (or value determined by agency policy), the collaborative problem Potential Complication: Hypoglycemia is appropriate. Patient-centered goals for hypoglycemia are not created because this problem requires collaboration between the nurse and the physician. Agency protocols usually allow the nurse to intervene for hypoglycemia and then notify the physician. Planning revolves around the nurse's role in:

- Assessing for signs of hypoglycemia
- Notifying the physician about signs of hypoglycemia, or following hospital protocol and then notifying the physician
- Intervening to minimize hypoglycemia

#### Interventions

***Maintaining safe glucose levels.*** Follow agency policy and physician orders regarding feeding infants with low glucose levels. A common practice is to feed infants if the glucose screening shows 40 to 45 mg/dL or less. Infants with severe hypoglycemia may need intravenous feedings to provide glucose rapidly. For most infants, breastfeeding or giving formula is sufficient. Glucose water alone is not recommended for newborns because the rapid rise in glucose results in increased insulin production, causing a further drop in blood glucose. Milk provides a longer-lasting supply of glucose.

Assist the breastfeeding mother with the first feeding. If she is unable to nurse the infant immediately (because of pain or exhaustion from delivery), feed the infant formula and help her breastfeed at the next feeding. Assist formula-feeding mothers to give the bottle. Explain the need for prompt feeding in infants with hypoglycemia.

***Repeating glucose tests.*** Until glucose levels are stable, closely observe newborns who have shown signs of hypoglycemia. Repeated glucose screenings may be performed according to agency policy. Keep the physician or nurse practitioner informed of the newborn's status. If the blood glucose does not remain at an adequate level, other causative factors are investigated. The infant may be transferred to an intensive care nursery for treatment, including intravenous feedings, until blood glucose is stabilized with oral feedings.

***Providing other care.*** Watch for signs of other complications. Infants who do not have enough glucose can experience a drop in temperature that could lead to respiratory distress, as oxygen is used for nonshivering thermogenesis. The parents will be distressed over the multiple heel sticks their infant must endure. Explain the importance of maintaining adequate blood glucose levels and why the tests and frequent feedings are necessary. Encourage parents to feed the newborn as instructed so that enough glucose is available to meet the infant's needs.

#### Evaluation

Evaluate the collaborative interventions for hypoglycemia by noting the infant's response to interventions and the presence or absence of continued signs of hypoglycemia.

### Bilirubin

Elevated bilirubin levels are common in newborns. Infants who need treatment for **hyperbilirubinemia** are discussed in Chapter 30. However, prevention is an important aspect of care.

## NURSING CARE PLAN

### The Normal Newborn

**Focused Assessment**

Nicholas, a full-term newborn, weighs 3402 g (7 lb, 8 oz) and is 50 cm (20 inches) long. He is the first baby for his mother, Vicki. He receives Apgar scores of 8 at 1 minute and 9 at 5 minutes. During the initial assessment he has an excessive amount of mucus. His respiratory rate is 62 breaths per minute, apical pulse is 156 beats per minute (bpm), and breath sounds are slightly moist. He has mild substernal retractions. His color is pink with acrocyanosis.

**Nursing Diagnosis**

Ineffective Airway Clearance related to excessive cheek secretions in airways.

**Planning**

***Expected Outcomes***

1. Nicholas will maintain a patent airway and show no signs of respiratory distress throughout the birth facility stay as demonstrated by respiratory rates of 30 to 60 breaths per minute, clear breath sounds, and no cyanosis, retractions, flaring, or grunting.
2. Before discharge, Vicki will demonstrate correct use of the bulb syringe and verbalize when it should be used.

**Interventions and *Rationales***

1. Position the infant's head to the side *to allow secretions to pool in the cheek and suction with a bulb syringe as needed.* If the nose also needs suctioning, suction it gently *because suctioning can traumatize the delicate nasal tissues.* Suction the mouth first *to avoid aspiration if the infant gasps when the nose is suctioned.*
2. Change the infant's position frequently.
   *Position changes promote expansion and drainage of all parts of the lungs.*
3. Provide reassurance for Vicki.
   *This will help allay her worry that something is wrong.*
4. Demonstrate and explain use of the bulb syringe. Observe Vicki's use of the bulb syringe and make suggestions as needed.
   *Demonstration and return demonstration help ensure that parents learn correct use.*
5. Continue to observe Nicholas for signs of respiratory distress. Count pulse and respirations every 30 minutes until they have been stable for 2 hours. Assess more often if there is any sign of abnormality. Continue to watch for other signs of ineffective airway clearance and respiratory difficulty such as cyanosis, retractions, flaring, and grunting.
   *Continued assessment must be based on the assessment results.*

**Evaluation**

Nicholas has clear breath sounds within 3 hours of birth, and his respiratory rate is 42 to 50 breaths per minute. He has no further signs of respiratory difficulty. Vicki uses the bulb syringe to suction the infant appropriately within 4 hours of the birth.

**Focused Assessment**

Nicholas's temperature is stable during the initial assessments, but later the axillary temperature is 36.2° C (97.2° F). His mother frequently removes his blankets to admire him and leaves him unwrapped after changing his diaper.

**Nursing Diagnosis**

Risk for Ineffective Thermoregulation related to parental lack of knowledge of newborn thermoregulation abilities and needs.

**Planning**

***Expected Outcomes***

1. Nicholas will maintain an axillary temperature within the normal range of 36.5° C to 37.5° C (97.7° F to 99.5° F) throughout his birth facility stay.
2. Vicki will verbalize and practice methods of preventing heat loss by the end of the first day.

**Interventions and *Rationales***

1. Explain to Vicki why newborns have problems with thermoregulation.
   If she understands the reasons behind precautions, she is more likely to practice them.
2. Place Nicholas, wearing only a diaper and a cap, next to Vicki's skin. Cover both of them with a warm blanket. Continue teaching her about thermoregulation while she holds the baby.
   *Skin-to-skin contact warms the infant. Vicki needs adequate education about maintaining thermoregulation.*
3. Teach Vicki to keep Nicholas wrapped as much as possible unless she is holding him skin to skin. Show her how to look at him and change his diaper while exposing only small areas of his body at a time.
   *This helps decrease heat loss by convection and radiation.*
4. Teach the mother to dry Nicholas promptly whenever he is wet, such as during bathing and when changing wet diapers or clothing.
   *This helps prevent heat loss from evaporation.*
5. Instruct Vicki to keep the infant's crib away from cold walls, windows, or drafts from air conditioners and open doors or windows.
   *This helps prevent heat loss from radiation and convection.*
6. Point out common objects that may be cold when they touch Nicholas. Explain the effect of this contact and suggest methods to warm them before use.
   *Heat can be gained or lost by conduction.*
7. Assess the infant's response to interventions by taking his axillary temperature every 30 minutes until it is once again stable for 2 hours.
   *Frequent assessment determines if further interventions are needed.*
8. If Nicholas becomes jittery or lethargic, check blood sugar according to birth facility routine.
   *Nonshivering thermogenesis may cause hypoglycemia.*
   If the blood sugar is low, help the mother breastfeed him or use formula.
   *Feeding provides calories for heat production. Contact with the mother's skin during breastfeeding helps warm the infant by conduction.*
9. Monitor for tachypnea or other signs of respiratory distress. Suction and apply oxygen if needed.
   *Cold stress increases oxygen need.*
10. If his temperature remains low or there are repeated episodes of low temperature, place Nicholas under a radiant warmer.
    *Radiant heat warms infants and can be adjusted according to their needs.*
    Alert the physician or nurse practitioner.
    *Temperature instability is one sign of infection in newborns.*
11. When Nicholas is ready to go back into an open crib, dress him in warmed clothes and blankets.
    *This will keep him warm by conduction.*
    Apply a stockinette or insulated hat to his head.
    *Covering the head decreases heat loss.*
12. Remove extra blankets according to the infant's temperature.
    *Overheating also increases oxygen and glucose consumption.*
13. After transfer to an open crib, assess Nicholas' temperature every 30 to 60 minutes until it is stable.
    *This promptly identifies any further problems that might develop.*
14. Teach Vicki how to take her son's axillary temperature at home.
    *This increases Vicki's ability to care for her son.*

**Evaluation**

The infant's axillary temperature rises to 37° C (98.6° F) and remains stable during his birth facility stay. Vicki is conscientious in using correct measures to keep the infant warm.

***Additional Nursing Diagnoses to Consider***

Risk for Infection
Risk for Ineffective Health Maintenance
Deficient Knowledge

### CRITICAL THINKING EXERCISE 22.1

You are caring for Callie and her first baby, Andy, who have both been doing well since the birth early this morning. As you enter the room after lunch, Callie says, "Andy's hands and feet are so cold! And his hands are so shaky. Is he all right?"

1. What are the nursing priorities in this situation?
2. What expanded assessments are necessary?
3. What interventions are necessary?
4. How will you respond to the mother?

#### Assessment

Assess for jaundice by blanching the infant's skin on the nose or sternum. Assess for jaundice every 8 to 12 hours along with vital signs. Determine how far down the body the jaundice extends. Because visual assessment of jaundice is unreliable for accurately determining the degree of hyperbilirubinemia, obtain transcutaneous bilirubin (TcB) or total serum bilirubin (TSB) measurements for any jaundiced infants. Compare the results to previous tests and to charts that show what is expected for the infant's age.

#### Nursing Diagnosis and Planning

Hyperbilirubinemia may not occur until after infants are at home, especially if discharge was early. A nursing diagnosis for this situation is:

- Risk for Injury related to lack of parental knowledge about hyperbilirubinemia.

*Expected outcomes.* Parents will identify methods of preventing or reducing jaundice when at home. Parents will identify and seek treatment for infants who develop jaundice or whose jaundice worsens when at home.

#### Interventions

Determine which infants are at increased risk for hyperbilirubinemia (see Chapter 21, p. 432). Pay particular attention to preterm and late preterm infants because parents may not realize the increased risk for jaundice.

Explain the significance of jaundice to parents, and show them how to assess for color changes in the skin. Answer parents' questions about bilirubin testing and care.

Discuss the importance of adequate feedings to stimulate passage of stools and help prevent high levels of bilirubin in the infant. When a newborn is feeding poorly, determine the reasons and intervene appropriately. Help mothers wake sleepy infants to feed, and encourage them to spend extra time with an infant with a poor suck. Explain that giving water to jaundiced infants does not stimulate stool excretion and should be avoided.

If the infant is breastfeeding, evaluate the infant's suck and the mother's understanding of positioning and other techniques. Instruct mothers to nurse at least 8 to 12 times every 24 hours for adequate lengths of time. Assist mothers having difficulty to ensure infants are feeding well before discharge.

Instruct parents to contact their care provider if they see an increase in jaundice after discharge or if the infant is not eating well, voiding at least six times a day by day 4, and is not producing stools appropriately (at least once daily for formula-fed infants; at least four stools daily for breastfed infants). Stress the importance of making and keeping follow-up appointments with the infant's healthcare provider. Offer written materials about jaundice for the parents to take home. Provide materials that are in the parents' language or use a translator for teaching to ensure understanding.

Continue to check the infant for jaundice during early clinic or home visits. Transcutaneous or serum bilirubin levels can be used to determine the degree of jaundice. Reinforce teaching about the identification of jaundice and importance of feedings and stooling. Answer questions that have occurred to parents since discharge from the birth facility.

If an infant develops true breast-milk jaundice, explain it to the parents. The mother who has been told she must discontinue breastfeeding for a day or two will be very concerned. Reassure her that her milk is adequate and not harmful to the infant. Help her maintain her milk supply by using a breast pump during the time the infant is taking formula.

#### Evaluation

- Are parents able to verbalize methods to prevent or reduce jaundice?
- Can parents describe what they will look for regarding jaundice and when to call the caregiver?

## ONGOING ASSESSMENTS AND CARE

A complete assessment is necessary every 8 hours or according to facility routine, but the nurse must always be alert for signs of change in the newborn's condition. Assessments are made more often if any are abnormal. The infant is weighed once daily, and weight loss or gain documented.

### Providing Skin Care

The skin is assessed for new marks or changes in old ones. To assess skin turgor, the nurse pinches a small area of skin over the chest or abdomen and notes how quickly it returns to its normal position. The return should be immediate in the normal newborn, with no "tenting." Skin that remains "tented" (raised in the pinched position) is an indication of dehydration.

#### Bathing

The infant receives a bath to remove blood and amniotic fluid as soon after birth as the temperature is stable. Removing all vernix is not necessary. Early bathing decreases exposure to maternal blood and possible bloodborne organisms on the infant's skin. The bath is given before invasive procedures such as injections or heel sticks to prevent drawing organisms on the skin into the infant's tissues. If the skin must be punctured before the bath is given, the area is washed well first.

Infants can be bathed by immersion in a tub. Tub bathing does not increase infection or decrease cord healing. Infants maintain their temperatures better during tub bathing than sponge bathing (Association of Women's Health, Obstetric, and Neonatal Nurses [AWHONN], 2013). Infants should be immersed in water that covers their shoulders to keep them warm. The water temperature should be approximately 38°C (100.4°F). A sponge bath under a radiant warmer also may be given.

While shampooing the hair, the nurse combs through it to remove dried blood. After the bath, the infant is thoroughly dried to prevent heat loss by evaporation. Combing the hair hastens drying. The infant remains under the radiant warmer until the hair is dry and the temperature returns to the previous level.

Bathing the infant in the presence of the parents allows the nurse to point out infant characteristics in addition to demonstrating the bath procedure and is also a good time to teach parents safety precautions.

After the initial bath, the infant may not receive another full bath during the birth facility stay. The skin is cleansed at diaper changes and to remove regurgitated milk. Clear water or a mild soap solution is used according to agency policy.

### Cleansing the Diaper Area

Because contact with body fluids is likely while changing diapers, it is important to wear clean gloves. Meconium is very thick and sticky and can be difficult to remove from the skin. Plain water or mild soap solutions may be used for cleaning the diaper area. If commercial diaper wipes are used, they should be free of detergent and alcohol (AWHONN, 2013).

## Providing Cord Care

The cord should be checked for bleeding or oozing during the early hours after birth. The cord clamp must be securely fastened with no skin caught in it. Purulent drainage, redness, or edema at the base indicates infection. The cord becomes brownish black within 2 to 3 days and falls off within approximately 10 to 14 days.

Evidence-based practice guidelines show that cleaning the cord with water when necessary and keeping it clean and dry is the best method of cord care. This natural treatment of cords may shorten the time to cord separation and does not lead to increased infections (AWHONN, 2013). The diaper is folded below the cord to keep it dry and free from contamination by urine.

The cord clamp is removed approximately 24 hours after birth if the end of the cord is dry (Fig. 22.3). Although the base of the cord is still moist, there is no danger of bleeding if the end is dry and crisp.

## Assisting With Feedings

The nurse must ensure that infants are eating well and that parents understand their chosen feeding method, which is particularly important for breastfeeding infants (see Chapter 23). A short period of observation at the start of feedings followed by checking back during the feedings will help the nurse identify any problems.

## Positioning the Infant

Teaching parents how to position infants properly is important. Placing infants in the prone position for sleep is associated with an increased risk of sudden infant death syndrome (SIDS) (see Chapter 45). AAP and ACOG recommend that mothers be taught to place infants on the back for sleep because this position is associated with the lowest rate of SIDS. The side position is not advised because of the possibility that the infant may roll to the prone position.

Parents should also be taught to use a firm sleep surface and to avoid loose or soft bedding that might interfere with breathing. Bumper pads are also not recommended. The infant should not sleep in a bed or couch with another person. However, placing the infant's bed in the parents' room is recommended. Giving a pacifier when putting the infant to sleep is also recommended, but this may be delayed for a month in breastfed infants to help establish breastfeeding. Overheating during sleep should be avoided (AAP, 2011; AAP & ACOG, 2012; Jana & Shu, 2015).

Infants who spend long periods in a supine position may develop flattening or asymmetry of the back of the head (positional **plagiocephaly**). This condition occurs because the bones are not fully developed and can be molded by positioning.

To prevent flattening of the head, infants should be placed on their abdomen while awake several times each day. This "tummy time" is an opportunity for play and interaction with the parents. The prone position helps the infant develop the neck, shoulder, and arm muscles. Toys placed in reach can help infants focus and begin to reach for objects. This position also helps the infant attain developmental milestones such as rolling over and crawling. It is essential that infants be supervised at all times when in the prone position, and they should be moved to a supine position if they fall asleep.

Infants tend to turn their heads toward the center of the room or the door. Therefore, they should be placed toward alternate ends of the crib when put down to sleep. Changing the position changes the side of the head that receives the most pressure. Infants who develop flattening should spend little time in infant seats, swings, or car seats because these put pressure on the back of the head. For bottle feeding, infants should be held on alternating sides for feedings to vary pressure points on the head.

## Protecting the Infant

Safeguarding the infant is a major role of the nurse. The primary ways in which nurses protect newborns include (1) ensuring that infants always go to the correct parents, (2) taking precautions to prevent infant abductions, and (3) preventing or recognizing early signs of infection.

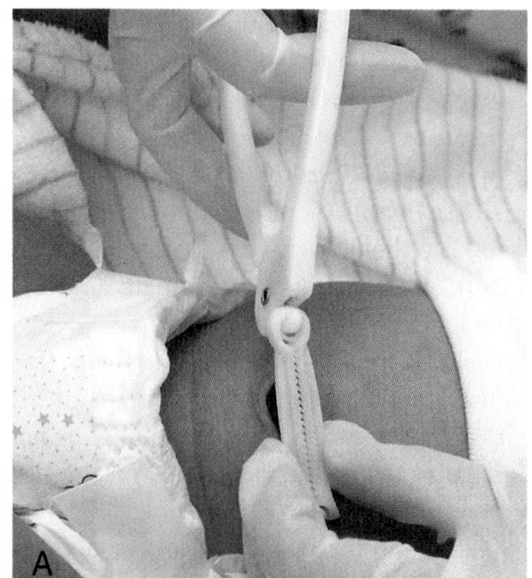


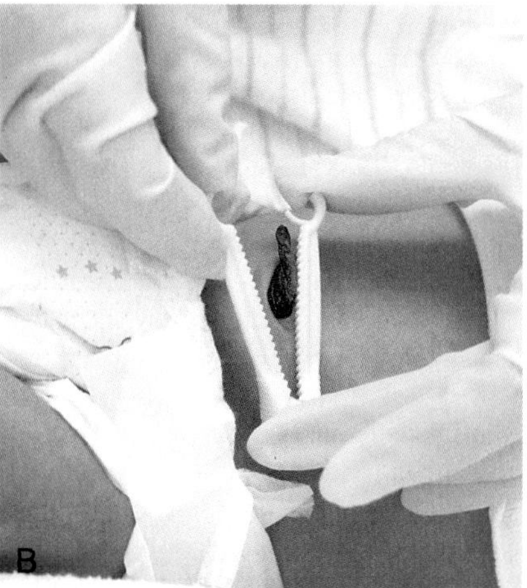


**FIG 22.3** The cord clamp is removed when the end of the cord is dry and crisp. The clamp is cut **(A)** and separated **(B)**.

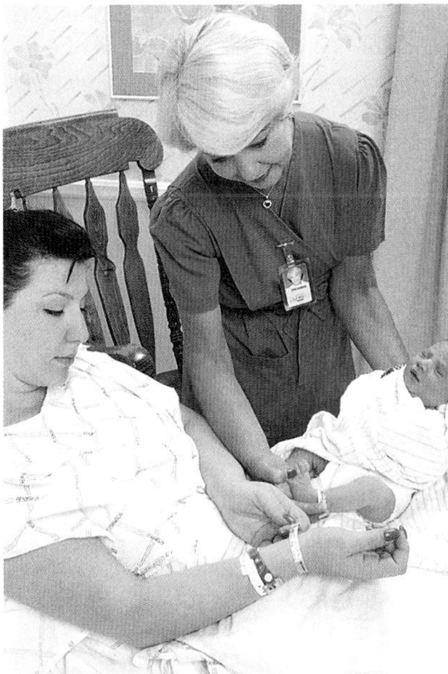

**FIG 22.4** The nurse unwraps the infant to compare the infant's identification band with the mother's band. The mother may be asked to read the identification number on her band as the nurse checks the infant's band or the nurse may look at both bands together.

### Identifying the Infant

Identification bands are placed on the mother, the infant, and the father or other support person at the infant's birth to ensure that an infant is never given to the wrong person. This type of mistake could result in interference with bonding, exposure to infections, lack of confidence in the staff, and lawsuits.

Information provided on each band includes the infant's gender, date and time of birth, delivering physician, mother's name and hospital number, and an imprinted number. Some bands also include a barcode. The imprinted number or barcode is used to identify the mother and the infant every time the infant is brought to the mother (or significant other) after a period of separation, however brief (Fig. 22.4). All staff must follow the facility protocol for identification of infants. In some facilities, electronic sensors are used to match the mother's band with that of the infant.

Other methods used to identify infants include taking footprints of the infant and a fingerprint of the mother or photographs of the infant. A notation of birthmarks or other distinguishing features is made on the nurses' notes. Cord blood can be used for DNA analysis if there is a later need for identification.

### Preventing Infant Abduction

An unfortunate but essential role of the nurse is protecting the infant from abduction (kidnapping). Between 1983 and 2015, 132 infants were abducted from healthcare facilities (National Center for Missing and Exploited Children, 2015).

Newborns are usually abducted by women who are familiar with the birth facility and its routines. They are of childbearing age, often overweight, and may live near the birth facility. They usually visit several agencies and learn the routines so they can impersonate birth facility staff to gain access to a newborn. They often know the layout of the facility and the locations of exits. The woman may have had a previous pregnancy loss or has been unable to have a child of her own. She may want an infant to solidify a relationship with her husband or boyfriend and may have pretended to be pregnant. Although the woman plans the kidnapping, she waits for an appropriate opportunity to take any infant. She may wear a uniform to impersonate hospital staff and tell parents she is taking the baby to have a test performed (Rabun, 2009).

Of the infants abducted from healthcare facility abductions, 58% were taken from the mother's room (National Center for Missing and Exploited Children, 2015). Therefore, it is important to include parents in safeguarding their infants. Precautions include teaching parents how to recognize the picture identification badge worn by birth facility personnel. There may be other identifying measures such as color-coded badges for maternity staff. Staff members who are working temporarily on the unit are assigned special identification badges that are carefully monitored so that none can be removed from the premises without alerting the regular staff. Parents receive written and verbal information and a picture of special identification badges worn by staff (Box 22.1).

Parents should be encouraged to ask for identification if they are unsure about anyone who asks to remove their infant for any reason. They must be cautioned never to give their infant to anyone who does not have proper identification and to call their primary nurse if they have questions.

#### BOX 22.1 Precautions to Prevent Infant Abductions

1. All personnel must wear picture identification that is easily visible at all times. No one without appropriate identification should handle or transport infants.
2. Enlist parents' help in preventing kidnapping. Teach them to allow only hospital staff with proper identification to take their infants from them.
3. Teach parents and staff to transport infants only in their cribs, never by carrying them. Question anyone carrying an infant outside the mother's room.
4. Question anyone with a newborn near an exit or in an unusual part of the facility.
5. Be suspicious of anyone who does not seem to be visiting a specific mother, asks detailed questions about infant or discharge routines, asks to hold infants, or behaves in an unusual manner.
6. Be suspicious of unknown people carrying large bags or packages that could contain an infant.
7. Respond immediately when an alarm signals that a remote exit has been opened or an infant has been taken into an unauthorized area.
8. Never leave infants unattended at any time. Teach parents that infants must be observed at all times. Infants may be taken into the bathroom with mothers, if necessary. Suggest that mothers have the nursing staff take over care of the infant if the mother wants to nap or feels unwell and no family members are present.
9. If infants need to be moved to another area, take one infant at a time. Never leave an infant in the hall unsupervised.
10. When infants are in mothers' rooms, place the cribs on the side of the mother's bed opposite the door to the hall.
11. Protect codes or card-keys that allow entrance to maternity units or nurseries so that unauthorized people cannot use them.
12. When a parent or family member comes to a nursery to take their infant, always match the infant and adult identification bracelet numbers. Never give an infant to anyone without the correct identification bracelet or other proper identification.
13. Alert hospital security immediately of any suspicious activity.
14. Suggest that parents do not place announcements in the paper or signs in their yard that might alert an abductor that a new baby is in the home.

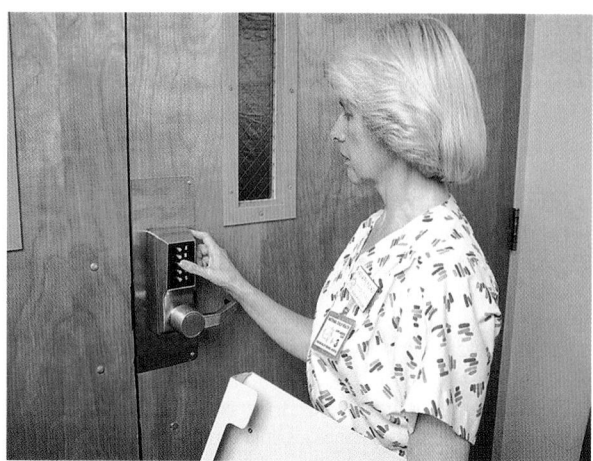

FIG 22.5 The nurse uses a code to open the door to maternity units.

Electronic security systems are used in some facilities. These systems use a sensing device attached to each infant by a bracelet or tag or on the cord clamp. The sensor activates an alarm if it goes near an exit or is cut or removed from the infant. With some systems, all exits lock automatically if an alarm is activated.

Entrances to the maternity unit should be observed at all times. Entrances should be locked so that visitors must press a call signal, and staff must use a card-key or a code to enter (Fig. 22.5). Visitors to maternity units may be required to check in with security guards or other staff members and wear special visitor identification tags.

Remote exits are locked and equipped with video cameras and alarms. Staff must respond quickly whenever an alarm sounds. Although alarms are usually triggered accidentally, it is always possible that a kidnapper is using a remote exit for a quick getaway.

Additional information about abduction is available for parents and professionals at the National Center for Missing and Exploited Children website, http://www.missingkids.com.

### Preventing Infection

Many nursing actions help prevent infection. Nurses wash their hands and arms at the beginning of their shift. Throughout the day, handwashing is important before and after touching any infant. It is essential not to handle one neonate and then another without again washing the hands. An infection that develops in one infant could quickly spread to others without these precautions. A special disinfectant for cleansing the hands may be used in place of handwashing when the hands are not visibly soiled. Dispensers may be placed in each mother's room and at other locations throughout the unit.

To avoid cross contamination, each infant's supplies should be kept separate from those used for other infants. Supplies in drawers or cupboards of each crib unit should be used only for that infant because they are likely to be touched by nurses giving care. Using them for another neonate could result in the transfer of infectious organisms.

The nurse should instruct parents and visitors to wash their hands before handling infants. Parents should be instructed to discourage visitors with colds or other infections from visiting the mother or newborn at the birth facility or during the early weeks at home.

When the mother has an infection, the healthcare provider decides whether it is safe for the newborn to remain with her. Although mothers and infants may well share the same organisms, the infant of a mother who is acutely ill may need to stay in the nursery until the mother is no longer contagious and feels able to perform infant care. Often the degree of the mother's fever is one of the determining factors.

Nurses must be vigilant for signs of infection during assessment and care of the infant (see Chapter 30). Instead of a fever, the infant's temperature may decrease. The infant may feed poorly, be lethargic, or have periods of apnea. Any change in behavior that is unexplained should be recorded and investigated.

## CIRCUMCISION

Circumcision is the most common surgical procedure performed on males in the United States (Swanson, 2009). Circumcision involves removal of the prepuce (foreskin), a fold of skin that covers the glans penis. Although the prepuce can be retracted easily for cleaning in the older child, it may not be fully retractable until 3 to 6 years of age (Smith, 2012). The prepuce should never be forcibly retracted in any infant because trauma and adhesions can result.

Circumcision is controversial, and parents may have questions about whether to have it performed. While the AAP and ACOG state that there are potential medical benefits as well as risks to circumcision, data presenting the benefits are not sufficient to recommend routine neonatal circumcision (AAP & ACOG, 2012).

### Reasons for Choosing Circumcision

Some conditions such as urinary tract infections, cancer of the penis, (which is uncommon), some sexually transmitted diseases (STDs), human immunodeficiency virus (HIV), and inflammation of the glans or prepuce occur more often in uncircumcised males. However, other factors, such as poor hygiene and risky behavior, can cause these conditions as well.

Some parents choose circumcision for religious, cultural, or social reasons. Jewish parents may have their infants circumcised on the eighth day after birth as part of a special ceremony. Muslim culture also includes circumcision. Some parents want their son to look like his circumcised father or peers. Others feel that circumcision is an expected part of newborn care, and some do not realize that they have a choice in the matter.

Parents may be concerned that when older, the uncircumcised child might develop phimosis, a tightening of the prepuce that prevents its retraction and requires circumcision. Although the number of such cases is small, surgery after the newborn period involves hospitalization and anesthesia and can be psychologically disturbing to the young child.

Lack of knowledge about the care of the prepuce leads to some circumcisions. Poor hygiene may increase the risk of infections and other problems. Teaching the parents and child proper care of the uncircumcised penis can prevent surgery and complications related to inadequate cleanliness.

### Reasons for Rejecting Circumcision

The reasons that parents decide against circumcision vary. Some parents believe that the incidence of conditions more common in uncircumcised males is too low to warrant the pain and risk of surgery. Others believe that having the infant circumcised to look like the father or peers is cosmetic surgery, and thus, unnecessary. These parents especially object to subjecting their sons to pain during and after surgery. Circumcision is less frequent among families from Asian, Hispanic, and Native American cultures. It is also less common in Europe, South and Central America, and Canada.

Parents may be concerned about removing the prepuce, which serves to protect the glans. The glans is more prone to irritation from constant exposure to urine and rubbing against diapers when unprotected by the prepuce. Many believe that circumcision decreases sexual pleasure later in life because the glans becomes less sensitive. Circumcision is not always covered by private insurance or

Medicaid. The lack of coverage may cause some parents to decide against the surgery.

Circumcision complications are unusual but most commonly include hemorrhage and infection. Removal of too much or too little of the prepuce and unsatisfactory cosmetic effect, urinary retention, stenosis or fistulas of the urethra, adhesions, necrosis, or other injury to the glans penis also may occur.

Only healthy newborns should undergo circumcision. The preterm or sick infant should not be circumcised until he is healthy enough to tolerate the procedure. Infants with blood dyscrasias may have excessive bleeding if circumcised. For the repair of anatomic abnormalities of the penis, such as hypospadias or epispadias, an intact prepuce may be needed for use in plastic surgery.

## Pain Relief

Circumcisions were once commonly performed without anesthesia because it was thought that newborns did not feel pain. It is now known that pain stimuli pass along fetal nerve pathways by the second and third trimesters of pregnancy. Pain responses include changes in vital signs, oxygen saturation levels, intracranial pressure, and catecholamine and cortisol levels. Infants may show irritability, altered sleep-wake states, and abnormal feeding patterns after a painful event (Gardner, Enzman-Hines, & Dickey, 2011).

A dorsal penile nerve block (injection of the dorsal penile nerves with anesthetic) is a safe method to eliminate pain during circumcision. Complications are uncommon but include hematomas and absorption of the medication into the bloodstream. A ring block (injection of anesthetic around the base of the penis) is also effective. Eutectic mixture of local anesthetic (EMLA) is a cream that can be applied to anesthetize the skin before the procedure, but it is less effective than anesthetic injection and requires a longer waiting period before it is effective.

Acetaminophen can be given just before the procedure or throughout the first day for postprocedure pain. Nonpharmacologic pain-relief methods include pacifiers, oral sucrose alone or on a pacifier, soothing music, recordings of intrauterine sounds, decreased lights, and talking softly to the infant. These methods are especially helpful at decreasing the stress of the procedure when combined with regional anesthesia. Pain and pain management in newborns is discussed further in Chapter 29.

## Methods

The Gomco (Yellen) clamp (Fig. 22.6) and the PlastiBell (Fig. 22.7) are two commonly used devices for performing circumcisions. In each method, the prepuce is first separated from the glans with a probe and incised to expose the glans. A Mogen clamp can also be used for circumcisions, especially in ritual circumcisions of Jewish infants.

## Nursing Considerations

### Assisting in Decision Making

Ideally, parents decide about circumcision early in pregnancy on the basis of careful consideration of the risks and benefits. However, this ideal is not always the case. Nurses may be called on to answer parents' questions or clarify misconceptions.

Although nurses generally teach parents of circumcised infants how to care for the penis, they may not think about educating parents who decide against circumcision. Proper care of the intact penis should be included in the teaching plan for these parents and also should be discussed with parents who are undecided about the procedure.

Nurses must be certain that their own biases about circumcision do not interfere with their ability to give objective information to parents. Once the parents come to a decision, the nurse should support it.

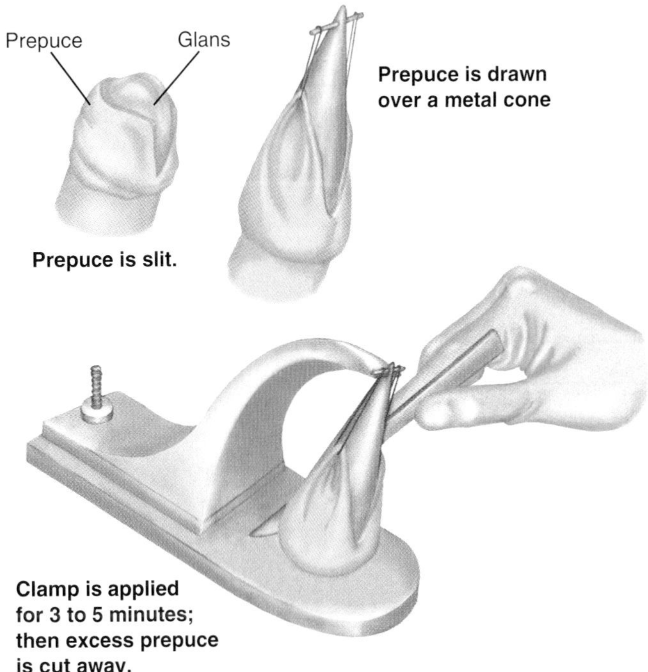
Prepuce
Glans
Prepuce is drawn over a metal cone
Prepuce is slit.
Clamp is applied for 3 to 5 minutes; then excess prepuce is cut away.

**FIG 22.6** Circumcision using the Gomco (Yellen) clamp. The physician pulls the prepuce over a cone-shaped device that rests against the glans. A clamp is placed around the cone and prepuce and is tightened to provide enough pressure to crush the blood vessels. This procedure prevents bleeding when the prepuce is removed after 3 to 5 minutes.

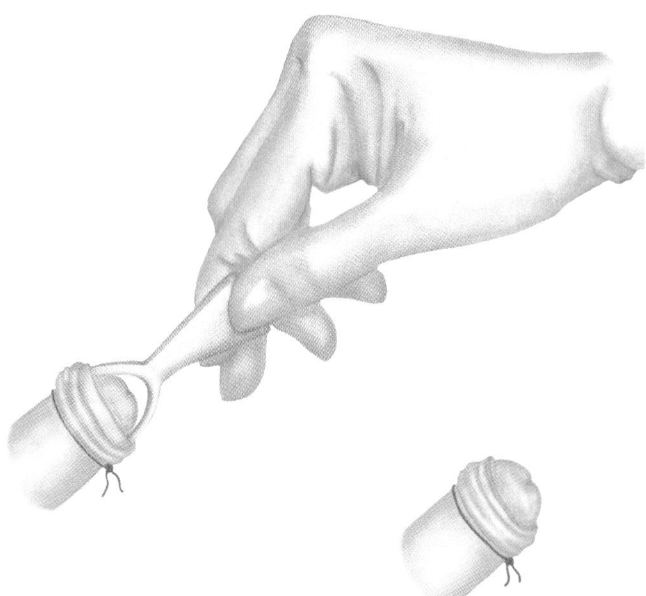

**FIG 22.7** Circumcision using the PlastiBell. The physician places the PlastiBell, a plastic ring, over the glans, draws the prepuce over it, and ties a suture around the prepuce and PlastiBell. This procedure prevents bleeding when the excess prepuce is removed. The handle is removed, leaving only the ring in place over the glans. The PlastiBell usually falls off in 7 to 14 days.

### Providing Care During Circumcision

As with any surgical procedure, informed consent from the parents is necessary before a circumcision. The nurse sees that the consent has been signed, the infant is stable, and that vitamin K has been given to prevent excessive bleeding. The physician is informed of any problems that might impair the infant's ability to withstand circumcision.

## PATIENT-CENTERED TEACHING

### How to Care for an Uncircumcised Penis

Wash your son's penis daily and when soiled diapers are changed. Do not retract the foreskin because it may not separate from the glans or end of the penis for 3 to 6 years after birth.

Occasionally, gently pull back on the foreskin to see how much separation has occurred. However, *never* force the foreskin to retract because it would be painful and might cause bleeding, infection, and adhesions. As your son gets older and takes over his own care, teach him to wash under the foreskin by gently pulling it back as far as it retracts, as part of his daily bath.

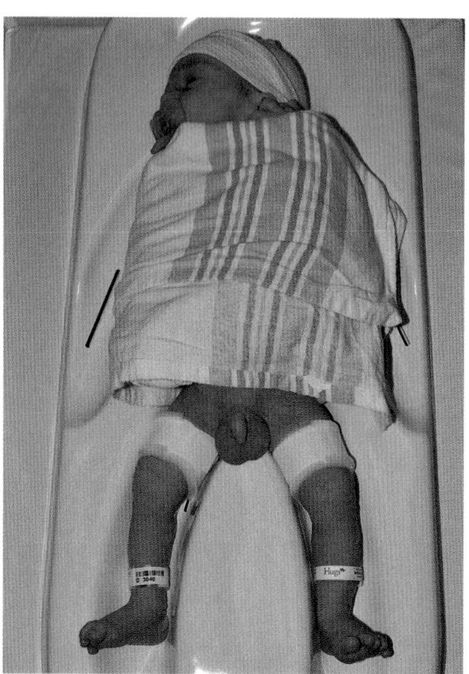

FIG 22.8 The infant is placed on the circumcision board just before the procedure is begun. (Courtesy Cheryl Briggs, RNC, Annapolis, MD.)

The nurse gathers equipment and supplies before the procedure. Feedings may be withheld for 2 to 4 hours before the procedure to prevent regurgitation and possible aspiration while the infant is restrained in a supine position. A bulb syringe should be placed nearby in case suction is necessary.

When the physician and equipment are ready, the infant is placed on a circumcision board and restrained (Fig. 22.8). A blanket is placed over the upper body, and a surgical drape provides warmth and maintains sterility. A heat lamp or radiant warmer helps prevent cold stress. During the procedure, the nurse provides comfort measures such as a pacifier and sucrose or talking to the infant.

### Evaluating Pain

Nurses should evaluate the infant's pain using one of the available pain scales for newborns. An example is Neonatal Inventory Pain Scale (NIPS) (Lawrence, Alcock, McGrath, et al., 1993). This scale measures facial expression, cry, breathing pattern, muscle tone of the extremities, and state of arousal. The infant's pain responses should be measured before, during, and after the procedure.

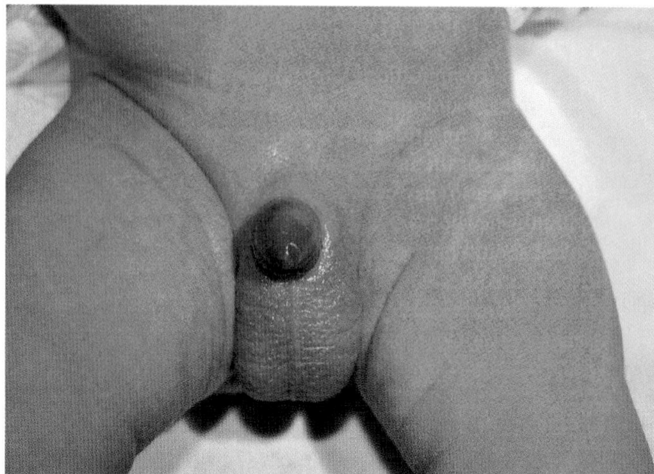

FIG 22.9 An infant with a newly circumcised penis. (Courtesy Cheryl Briggs, RNC, Annapolis, MD.)

### Providing Postprocedure Care

The infant should be removed from the restraints immediately after the circumcision is completed. If a Gomco clamp is used, the nurse squeezes petroleum jelly over the circumcision site to prevent the diaper from sticking to it. A small piece of gauze may be placed over the area. Petroleum jelly should not be used with a PlastiBell because it might displace the device. The diaper is attached loosely to prevent pressure. The infant should be comforted and returned to his mother, who may be anxious about her son.

The nurse watches carefully for signs of complications after the circumcision (Fig. 22.9). The wound is checked frequently for bleeding during the first few hours after the procedure. If the infant is to be discharged after the circumcision, he should be observed for at least 2 hours before release (AAP & ACOG, 2012).

If excessive bleeding occurs, pressure is applied to the site and the physician is notified. A small amount of blood loss may be significant in an infant, who has a small total blood volume. The physician may apply Gelfoam or epinephrine or suture the site.

Noting the first urination after circumcision is important because edema could cause an obstruction. If the infant goes home before voiding, the mother is instructed to call the physician if there is no urinary output within 6 to 8 hours.

## PATIENT-CENTERED TEACHING

### How to Care for a Circumcision Site

Observe the circumcision site at each diaper change. Call the physician if there are more than a few drops of blood with diaper changes during the first day or any bleeding after the first day. Continue to apply petroleum jelly to the penis with each diaper change for the first 4 to 7 days or as directed by your physician. If a PlastiBell was used, do not use petroleum jelly.

Squeeze warm water from a clean washcloth over the penis to wash it. Pat gently to dry the area. Fasten the diaper loosely to prevent rubbing or pressure on the incision site.

A yellow crust over the area is normal and should not be removed. If a PlastiBell was used, the plastic rim will fall off in 7 to 14 days. If it does not fall off by that time or falls off sooner, notify your physician. Watch for signs of infection such as fever or drainage that smells bad or has pus in it. *Call your physician if you suspect any abnormalities.* The area should be fully healed in approximately 10 days.

## PATIENT-CENTERED TEACHING

### *Techniques for Infant Care*

This guide is written in language that the nurse might use when teaching parents about infant care.

**Handling the Infant**

***Head Support***

An infant cannot support the heavy head when held in an upright position for the first few months of life. To help support the head, place one hand behind the head when you pick up or carry the baby.

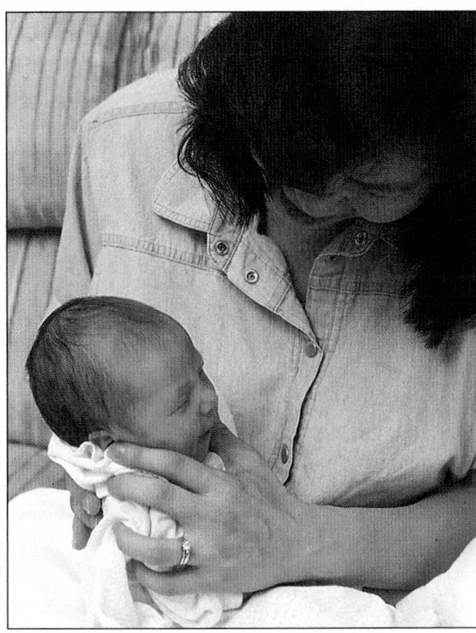

***Positioning***

Most mothers hold the infant in the cradle position. For the "football" position, support the baby's head in the palm of your hand with the body along your arm, supported against your side. This position allows one hand to be free when washing the baby's hair or breastfeeding.

The shoulder hold is good for burping the baby—or sit the baby on your lap and support the head and chest with one hand while gently patting or rubbing the infant's back with the other hand. This position allows you to see the baby's face in case of "spit-ups."

Always place your baby on the back for sleep. This position is recommended by the American Academy of Pediatrics because it helps prevent sudden infant death syndrome (SIDS), the sudden, unexplained death of an infant. The baby should sleep on a firm mattress and have no loose blankets or pillows in the bed. The baby should not sleep with anyone else. Use a pacifier when you put the baby down to sleep. If you are breastfeeding, you can wait a month to fully establish breastfeeding and then give the baby a pacifier.

Place your baby on the abdomen for play when the infant is awake and will be observed. This "tummy time" helps the infant develop muscles in the back and neck and prevents flattening of the back of the head. If the infant becomes sleepy, change the position to lying on the back for safety during sleep.

***Wrapping***

Young infants feel secure when wrapped firmly in a blanket. To swaddle the infant, turn down one corner of a blanket and position the baby's head over the edge. Fold one side of the blanket over the body and arm. Bring the lower corner up, and fold it over the chest. Then bring the other side around the infant and tuck it underneath.

**Normal Body Processes**

***Breathing***

Newborns normally breathe approximately 30 to 60 times a minute. Their breathing is irregular and may vary from loud to very soft.

***Using a Bulb Syringe***

Use the bulb syringe if the infant has excessive mucus in the mouth or nose or spits up milk. Be very gentle, and use the bulb only if necessary. Squeeze the bulb before you insert the tip into the side of the mouth. Do not aim it to the back. Do not suction the nose unless necessary. Extra mucus is common in the first days of life but is usually not a problem.

Clean the bulb with soap and water and dry well before using again. Call your physician if the baby's skin becomes blue or if the baby stops breathing for more than 15 seconds, has difficulty breathing, or has yellow or green drainage from the nose.

***Temperature***

Being cold can be dangerous for newborns because it causes them to use more calories and oxygen than when they are warm. Dress your baby as you would like to be dressed. Add a light receiving blanket, except in very hot weather.

***Using a Thermometer***

Check your baby's temperature during illness. Place the thermometer under the arm so it does not protrude behind the arm and hold the arm down firmly. Read the thermometer according to the manufacturer's directions. Call your doctor if the baby has a temperature higher than 100° F (37.8° C) or lower than 97.7° F (36.5° C).

***Urine Output***

Your baby will have at least one or two wet diapers a day during the first day or two and at least six wet diapers a day by the fourth day. Counting the number of wet diapers helps you know if the baby is getting enough milk. *Call your baby's doctor if the baby has no wet diapers for more than 12 hours.*

***Stool Output***

Breastfed infants pass at least four soft, seedy stools that have a sweet-sour odor and are mustard-yellow each day. Formula-fed infants pass one to several stools daily that are pale yellow to light brown and formed. Babies are not constipated when they turn red when passing a stool. Constipated infants pass small, hard stools that are fewer than usual.

***Diarrhea***

Babies with diarrhea pass more frequent stools that are greener and more liquid than usual. There may be a water ring—an area in the diaper where the liquid has absorbed, sometimes around an area of more solid stool. Call your physician if your baby has more than two diarrhea stools because serious dehydration can occur quickly.

***Skin Care***

A number of normal marks occur on the newborn's skin. The normal newborn rash resembles small insect bites or pimples. Small whiteheads disappear without treatment. Do not squeeze them or they may become infected. Newborns have very dry, peeling skin that will be soft after peeling. Lotions or creams are unnecessary and may cause irritation.

***Cord***

Clean the cord with plain water, if necessary, and keep it dry. Fold the diaper below the cord so that it is not wet by urine. The cord usually falls off by 10 to 14 days. Some healthcare providers suggest waiting for the cord to fall off

*Continued*

## Techniques for Infant Care

before tub bathing but others allow tub baths. Notify your physician if you see bleeding or signs of infection, such as redness, drainage, or a foul odor.

### *Diaper Area*

Clean the diaper area with each diaper change. For girls, separate the labia (folds) and remove all stool. Wipe the diaper area front to back. Wiping back and forth may move stool into the vagina or urethra, causing infection. For boys, wash under the scrotum to help prevent rashes. Changing the diaper frequently, avoiding commercial diaper wipes, and using absorbent diapers may help prevent diaper rash. If the diaper area becomes red, change the diaper more often. Leaving the diaper off to expose the area to air is also helpful. Petroleum jelly or a barrier-type zinc oxide ointment may be used. *If redness persists, ask your baby's doctor for suggestions.*

### *Bathing*

Because infants are washed as needed after regurgitation and with diaper changes, it is not necessary to give them a bath every day.

### *Sponge Baths*

Before the bath, gather all the supplies: a container or sink of warm water, washcloth, towel, baby shampoo, and clean clothes. Soap is not necessary for the young infant, but if used, it should be gentle and nonalkaline.

Give the bath in a room that is warm and free of drafts. Bathe the baby on a surface that is comfortable and safe. If you use a counter, pad it with blankets or towels.

*Never leave the infant alone on an unprotected surface, even for a minute.* Keep one hand on the infant at all times to prevent falls. Avoid answering the phone during baths so you are not distracted. If you must leave the room, take the baby along or place the baby in a crib.

Before undressing the baby, use the football position to shampoo the head. The fontanel, or "soft spot," is covered with a tough membrane and is not injured by washing. Pulse movements in the fontanel are normal. Dry the hair well to prevent heat loss.

Keep the baby warm by uncovering only the area you are washing. Wash the face with clear water. Use a separate clean area of the washcloth to wipe across each eyelid and around each eye. Clean in and around the ears, where regurgitated milk may accumulate. Do not use cotton-tipped swabs in the infant's ears or nose because injury may occur.

To clean the neck folds, put one hand under the baby's shoulders and lift slightly to cause the head to drop back enough that the creases in the neck can be washed. Clean the diaper area last.

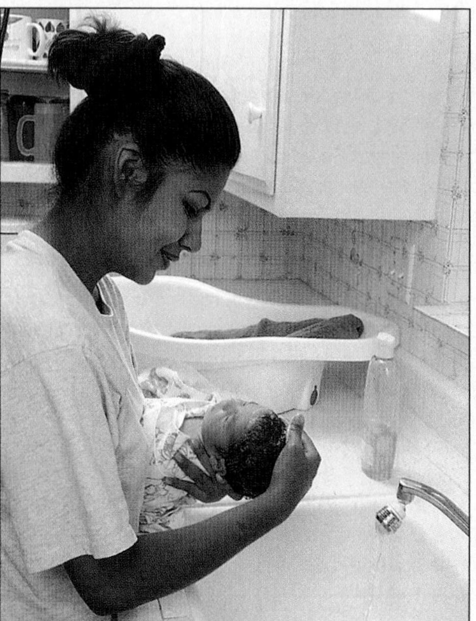

### *Tub Bath*

For a tub bath, use a plastic tub or a clean sink. Pad the bottom with a towel or foam pad. Place enough warm water in the tub to cover the infant's shoulders to prevent chilling. Wash the face and hair before placing the baby in the tub.

At first, it may be easier to lather the infant's body and then immerse the baby in the tub for rinsing. It is not unusual for young infants to be frightened when they are first put in water. To help the baby adjust, talk softly and calmly while holding your baby securely.

### Behavior

Knowing infants' different behavioral states helps you learn about your baby's individual characteristics.

### *Sleep Phases*

During quiet sleep the infant sleeps soundly with quiet breathing and little movement. Your baby will not be disturbed by noises from appliances or other children at this time. In active sleep, the baby moves or fusses while still asleep. During the drowsy state the baby is beginning to wake but may go back to sleep if not disturbed. However, if it is time for feeding or other activities, talk softly to help the baby awaken.

### *Awake Phases*

The quiet alert state is a good time for infant stimulation because the baby seems interested in objects and people. In the active alert, or "fussy," phase, infants signal hunger or discomfort. If you do not intervene, the baby soon moves to the crying state. The baby who cries too long may not respond at first to care activities. A few minutes of rocking and holding close may be necessary before the infant settles down.

### *Socialization*

Infants enjoy contact with people. Use an infant seat or an infant carrier to keep the baby near you and the rest of the family. Talking and holding the baby close provide social stimulation. Infants enjoy music that is not too loud. Because they focus their eyes best at a distance of 8 to 12 inches, items such as mobiles should be placed within this range. Infants especially like black-and-white geometric figures. Babies respond best to gentle stimulation during the quiet alert state. Too much stimulation can cause the baby to be irritable and have difficulty going to sleep.

### Teaching Parents

Each time the site is checked for bleeding, the nurse should show the parents the amount of blood on the diaper to help them understand how much to expect. The normal yellowish exudate that forms over the site should be described and differentiated from purulent drainage. Signs of complications should be discussed fully.

**SAFETY ALERT**

***Signs of Complications After Circumcision***

- Bleeding more than a few drops with first diaper changes
- Failure to urinate
- Signs of infection: fever or low temperature, purulent or foul-smelling drainage
- Displacement of the PlastiBell

## NURSING CARE

### Parents' Knowledge of Newborn Care

New mothers often feel anxious about taking over total care of their newborns. Therefore, the nurse must use every contact with the parents as an opportunity for further teaching.

#### Assessment

Assess parents' changing needs for learning throughout the birth facility stay. Consider the physical condition of the mother and infant and any special concerns that the mother may have.

Determine the learning needs of experienced mothers. They may be unaware of information that has changed since the birth of their last infant. Examples include current recommendations about positioning infants for sleep and immunization against hepatitis B. Experienced mothers may also be concerned about helping their other children adjust to the newborn.

Also assess the father's learning needs and his plans for involvement with infant care. Determine if there are cultural dictates about the father's participation in infant care.

#### Nursing Diagnosis and Planning

A common nursing diagnosis for the family with learning needs is:

- Readiness for Enhanced Parenting related to desire for information about infant care.

***Expected outcomes.*** Before discharge, the parents will seek assistance from nurses to meet their information needs, correctly demonstrate infant care, and express confidence in their ability to meet their infant's needs.

#### Interventions

***Determining who teaches.*** Because several different nurses care for mothers and infants during the birth facility stay, coordinate the teaching so that all concerns are addressed. Many facilities use a checklist to ensure that all important topics are covered.

***Setting priorities.*** With only a short time available for teaching, set priorities to determine what to teach. Make a teaching plan with the parents. Use a topic list to help them point out major concerns regarding infant care to ensure effective use of time. Begin by discussing their most pressing concerns to decrease anxiety. Then, as time allows, go on to other subjects.

***Using various teaching methods.*** Use a variety of teaching methods to increase effectiveness. Use verbal and written methods, as well as demonstrations and return demonstrations. Parents often learn best by seeing skills performed correctly and then practicing them while the nurse gives suggestions. To increase the likelihood that parents will follow instructions, explain the rationale for each point made during teaching sessions.

Discuss information with the mother alone or with her family members, roommate, or a group of mothers. Group teaching is a more efficient use of nursing time, but some mothers learn better with one-on-one teaching. Use audiovisual materials, including pamphlets, magazines, DVDs, television programs, and Internet sites. Internet sources such as the AAP website (https://www.healthychildren.org) provide reliable parent information. Highlight the most important areas taught, and clarify information as necessary to reinforce learning.

***Modeling behavior.*** Modeling by the nurse is an important teaching tool. Mothers watch closely when nurses handle infants. Nurses demonstrate mothering behavior by the way they hold, care for, and talk to infants. Point out different behavior states, how to console crying infants, and how to prepare infants for feedings. This guidance is particularly important for the mother with no experience in infant care.

***Teaching intermittently.*** Plan teaching in small segments that are interspersed with infant care. Check the parents' understanding often. Encourage them to take over tasks until they are performing all of the infant's routine care.

***Including the father.*** Identify fathers who would like to participate in care of their infants but hesitate because they lack experience. Offer them the same teaching given to the inexperienced mother. Give praise liberally to increase confidence when parents practice their new infant-care skills.

***Documenting teaching.*** Document all teaching performed and the parents' abilities to carry out infant care. This information helps other nurses know what teaching is still needed. It also provides legal proof that teaching was completed before discharge.

***Incorporating cultural considerations.*** When teaching, consider the family's cultural beliefs about child care. For example, some Southeast Asian, Hispanic, and Arab women are hesitant to breastfeed in the birth facility and want to wait until they are home and the milk comes in. Asian parents may be uneasy when caregivers are too complimentary about the baby or casually touch the infant's head. However, Hispanic parents may prefer that a person who compliments the infant touch the infant to ward off *mal ojo,* or the "evil eye."

Women from India may tie a black thread around the infant's wrist, ankle, or waist to ward of evil spirits (Grewal, Bhagat, & Balneaves, 2008). Amulets may be placed on the baby or in the room by parents from Israel, Italy, Kuwait, Iran, Iraq, Malaysia, and Greece (Spector, 2009). Naming of the baby can occur before the birth or as long as 30 days later, depending on the culture of the family (Watts & McDonald, 2007).

Care of the cord differs in various cultures too. Women from Mexico may strap a coin or marble, wiped with alcohol, to the umbilicus (D'Avanzo, 2008). Other women may use a binder or belly band or put a raisin or oil on the cord (Callister, 2013).

Teaching should include family members who will be caring for the infant. The people involved may vary according to the culture and the availability of the traditional caregiver. The woman's mother is often a major support person. However, in the Korean culture, the husband's mother is the primary caregiver for the infant and the mother in the early weeks (Callister, 2013).

If the new mother will not be the primary infant caregiver, she may appear uninterested in the nurse's teachings. Nurses must not assume the mother is not bonding with her infant because she is following the role prescribed by her culture. Asking the parents who will be helping them care for the infant helps determine which family members to include in the teaching.

Elicit questions during the discussions. However, be aware that women from some cultures will not ask questions. For many Native Americans, asking questions is considered rude. Other women may be too shy. When questions are not asked, discuss topics often brought up by other parents.

***Providing for follow-up care.*** If the mother and infant will be seen by a clinic or home visit nurse, provide information about unmet learning needs. Reinforcement can then be provided during outpatient care.

Give as much information as possible in written form so parents can then refer to it if they have concerns later. Also provide telephone numbers they can call for further help. Offer written information in the parents' primary language, if possible. Even if they speak English as a second language, parents may prefer to read in their own language.

### Evaluation

- Do the parents ask questions about the infant's care?
- Can they demonstrate correct infant care?
- Do they verbalize growing confidence in their caregiving abilities?

## IMMUNIZATION

Immunization for hepatitis B is now included with other routine childhood vaccinations. Newborns of mothers with acute or chronic hepatitis B infection (hepatitis B surface antigen [HBsAg] positive) can become infected from exposure to the mother's blood at birth. Infected infants have a very high chance for developing chronic infection, which can cause later cancer or other serious liver disease.

These infants should receive both the first dose of the vaccine and hepatitis B immune globulin (HBIG). HBIG provides passive immunity to hepatitis to protect infants until they develop their own antibodies and should be given within 12 hours of birth. The vaccine promotes antibody formation to protect infants from further exposure to the disease.

Newborns of uninfected mothers also receive the hepatitis B vaccine. It is often given during the birth facility stay or later at the pediatrician's office. A national voluntary standard for perinatal care is that all infants receive the appropriate hepatitis prophylaxis before discharge (National Quality Forum, 2009). Parents should be referred to their pediatrician for two more doses of the vaccine after discharge.

## NEWBORN SCREENING

Screening tests are used to identify infants who need more complex diagnostic testing for various conditions.

### Hearing Screening

In 2013, 97.2% of newborns were screened for hearing loss; of those screened, 9.8% were found to have impaired hearing (Centers for Disease Control and Prevention [CDC], 2013). This condition is the most common congenital abnormality in newborns (Cunningham & Sydlowski, 2009). Because early identification and treatment can prevent or reduce developmental delays and help the child communicate better, auditory screening of all newborns within the first month is recommended. Infants who do not pass the screening should be rescreened; if still not passing, they should have comprehensive audiologic evaluations by no later than 3 months of age (AAP, 2011). A goal of *Healthy People 2020* is to increase the proportion of newborns who are screened for hearing loss by age 1 month, have audiologic evaluation by age 3 months, and, if necessary, are enrolled in appropriate intervention services by age 6 months (U.S. Department of Health and Human Services [USDHHS], 2010).

To accomplish this goal, a screening test is usually given to infants before discharge from the birth facility, and referrals are made for further testing if the infant shows signs of hearing problems. Otoacoustic emissions and acoustic brainstem response tests are used for screening. The nurse ensures that infants receive screening and explains the tests to the parents. Infants who fail the first screening are often retested at the birth facility. Parents of infants referred for further testing after discharge need further explanations and emotional support (see Chapter 55).

### Other Screening Tests

Other screening tests are performed to detect conditions resulting from inborn errors of metabolism and other genetic conditions. In the United States, all states require newborn screening for metabolic disorders. Approximately 5000 infants with severe disorders are identified each year as a result of these tests (CDC, 2013). With early detection and treatment, infants with these conditions may avoid severe intellectual disability or other serious problems.

Although the conditions screened vary by state, common conditions often included are phenylketonuria (PKU) (see Chapters 30 and 51), hypothyroidism (see Chapter 51), galactosemia (see Chapter 51), and hemoglobinopathies such as sickle cell disease and thalassemia (see Chapter 47). Screening may be performed for congenital adrenal hyperplasia, maple syrup urine disease, biotinidase deficiency, homocystinuria, cystic fibrosis (see Chapter 45), and other conditions. In some situations, parents may ask that other tests be performed.

The tests are easy and inexpensive, and only one blood sample is needed for all tests. If any results are abnormal, further testing is necessary for confirmation. Testing is usually performed at 24 to 28 hours of age. If the blood specimens for testing are obtained before 24 hours after birth, the results may be inaccurate, and the tests should be repeated at 1 to 2 weeks of age (Mackie, 2015).

## DISCHARGE AND NEWBORN FOLLOW-UP CARE

### Discharge

Although state and federal legislation allows women and infants to stay in the birth facility for 48 hours after vaginal birth and 96 hours after cesarean birth, some women choose to go home earlier. The time of discharge varies according to the mother's wishes and the primary caregivers' assessments of their conditions.

Discharge is considered for term newborns who are appropriate for gestational age, have normal physical examination results, and show they are making the transition from fetal to neonatal life without difficulty. Infants should have normal vital signs, have fed successfully at least twice, passed urine and stool, and have had no excessive bleeding from the circumcision site for at least 2 hours. Newborn screening tests and evaluation for sepsis should have been completed. If infants have significant jaundice, plans should be made for follow-up after discharge or delay of the infant's discharge. The mother should have received teaching about infant care and should demonstrate the knowledge, ability, and confidence to provide adequate care of the newborn. An appropriate infant car seat should be used at discharge. The family should have an adequate support system and have plans for continued care from a healthcare provider (AAP, 2011; AAP & ACOG, 2012).

## Follow-Up Care

Care after discharge from the birth facility is very important. The AAP recommends that follow-up by a healthcare professional be provided within 48 hours of discharge to all newborns who go home from a birth facility less than 48 hours after birth. Care can be provided in the home, clinic, or office (AAP, 2011; AAP & ACOG, 2012). Any infant who is breastfeeding or has other risk factors should be seen within the first week and usually within 2 to 3 days of discharge (Sullivan & Dela Cruz-Rivera, 2009).

Nursing follow-up care can be provided by home visits, clinic visits, and telephone counseling.

### Home Visits

The home visit is ideally scheduled during the first 24 to 72 hours after discharge. This timing allows early assessment and intervention for problems with feedings, jaundice, newborn adaptation, and maternal–infant interaction. Visits usually are 60 to 90 minutes to allow enough time for assessment and teaching. Because home visits are expensive, they are not available in all areas.

*Content of the home visit.* The home visit includes a physical examination of the mother and infant and assessment of the support system and family adaptation. The nurse reinforces the teaching about self care and infant care that was begun at the birth facility. Blood may be obtained for metabolic screening if the infant went home too early for reliable testing.

*Identification of jaundice.* Home visits are especially valuable in recognizing jaundice and intervening before bilirubin levels become dangerously high. When jaundice is found, the nurse can discuss the implications and check the transcutaneous bilirubin level or draw blood for testing serum bilirubin levels. Appropriate care is discussed, as necessary, including hydration and phototherapy.

*Feeding concerns.* Mothers often have feeding questions, especially when they are breastfeeding. When the nurse observes a feeding and helps a woman deal with problems, the infant's intake may increase, preventing dehydration, hyperbilirubinemia, and possible hospital readmission.

*General considerations in home visits.* The nurse making a home visit is a guest of the family and must adapt nursing care to the home setting. The needs of other family members must also be considered. Examination of the infant may need to wait for a short time while the mother attends to her other small children.

Each visit is carefully planned to make the best use of the time available. The nurse calls to schedule the visit at a time convenient for the family and obtain directions to the home. The nurse must develop a rapport with family members quickly and work with them to meet shared goals. A brief social interaction may be beneficial at the beginning of the visit to develop a trusting relationship. The purpose of the visit should be explained and the family's expectations and desires discussed. Making suggestions in a positive manner is important.

The nurse should be aware of any cultural practices affecting the family's view of care. For example, in patriarchal cultures, the father is the head of the family and teaching should be performed through him. In some cultures, grandmothers are very important influences in the care of the mother and infant.

After the home visit, the nurse can provide the family with telephone numbers where they can receive further help if needed. The results of assessments, teaching, nursing care, referrals, and plans for follow-up should be recorded. Copies of the record are usually sent to the primary caregiver.

### Outpatient Visits

Outpatient visits may be provided by the pediatrician or by the birth facility in clinics often managed by nurses and included in the hospital maternity care charges. Assessment and care are essentially the same as those provided for home visits. The advantage of outpatient visits is that the nurse does not have to travel to the home and can see more patients each day, thereby reducing the cost of the service. The disadvantage is that the nurse does not have the opportunity to assess the home setting and family interaction. Clinic visits usually last 30 to 45 minutes.

### Telephone Counseling

Telephone counseling can occur during follow-up calls to discharged mothers or when parents call "warm lines" for help with problems or questions. Telephone calls are much less expensive than home or clinic visits. However, the nurse cannot perform an in-person assessment and must rely on the caller to present an accurate picture of the situation.

*Follow-up calls.* Follow-up calls are placed by nurses in the first few days after discharge. The nurse asks a series of questions to assess the physical condition of the mother and infant and to identify any needs or problems. Follow-up calls may be provided for all mothers or only for those considered at risk of problems. The nurse may schedule another call or a home visit, if available, or refer the woman to her primary care provider if problems are discovered.

*Warm lines.* Warm lines, also called 'help lines,' provide parents with an opportunity to ask a nurse questions about parenting. Warm lines are used for situations that cause parents concern but are not emergencies. The service should be available 24 hours per day. Parents often call about infant feeding, breastfeeding concerns, and basic care of the mother and infant. The nurse answers the caller's questions and assesses for other problems. The nurse may call back later to see if the situation has resolved.

*Telephone techniques.* Nurses caring for patients by telephone must understand telephone counseling techniques and triage. Open-ended questions such as, "How have you been getting along since you left the hospital?" or requests such as, "Tell me about any situations in which you weren't sure what to do" help the mother describe any problems in her own terms.

Telephone triage involves determining the presence of and solution to a serious problem. The nurse should help the caller describe the major concerns, which may not be those discussed first. "What worries you most?" may help focus on the most important problems. Although most problems discussed are concerns about normal infants, the nurse must be alert for serious situations needing immediate referral.

*Guidelines and documentation.* When nurses give care by telephone, they must have written protocols and policies to ensure that all who perform this service provide patients with similar information. A list of common questions can be compiled to help nurses give appropriate information to parents who call about a problem.

Parents should always be told when and how to seek more care if problems are not resolved. If the infant seems ill, referral to the pediatrician or hospital emergency department is most appropriate. The nurse's judgment, based on education, expertise, and experience, is the most important factor in how helpful the service is to patients.

All calls should be documented so that accurate legal records are available for future reference. The nurse may use a check-off form or a simple written description of the call. A copy of the information is sent to the primary caregiver to provide continuity of care.

## KEY CONCEPTS

- Prophylaxis against vitamin-K–deficiency bleeding (hemorrhagic disease of the newborn) and ophthalmia neonatorum is necessary shortly after birth, provided through vitamin K injection and erythromycin ophthalmic ointment, respectively.
- Newborns may need help in clearing the airway. Positioning, suction, and close observation may be necessary.
- Nurses can prevent heat loss in newborns by keeping them dry and covered, avoiding contact between them and cold objects or surfaces, and keeping them away from drafts and outside windows and walls.
- The nurse must identify actual or potential hypoglycemia and intervene appropriately.
- Important interventions for jaundice are to assess for its occurrence, to ensure the infant is feeding well, and to explain the condition to the parents.
- Parents should be taught to place infants supine for sleep to prevent SIDS. Infants should have supervised periods of lying prone each day.
- Parents and nurses must work together to prevent infant abductions. Parents must know how to identify hospital staff. Nurses should be alert for suspicious behavior.
- The identification band of the mother and the infant should be matched any time they have been separated to ensure the infant is given to the proper mother.
- Infection can best be prevented by scrupulous handwashing by staff and all who come into contact with newborns.
- Reasons parents may choose circumcision are to prevent certain conditions, for religious reasons, parental preference, or lack of knowledge about care of the foreskin.
- Parents reject circumcision because of the belief that uncommon risks do not necessitate surgery, pain caused to infants, and concerns about complications that can occur.
- Risks of circumcision include hemorrhage, infection, unsatisfactory cosmetic results, urinary retention, urethral stenosis or fistula, adhesions, necrosis, injury to the glans, and pain during and after the surgery.
- Infants who are circumcised should have pain relief provided. Dorsal penile nerve block or a ring block, along with nonpharmacologic methods of pain relief such as oral sucrose, are often used.
- Parents of circumcised infants should be taught signs of complications and how to care for the area.
- Parents with uncircumcised sons should be taught not to retract the foreskin until it becomes separate from the glans later in childhood.
- Every nursing contact with parents should be used as an opportunity to teach.
- Screening tests are commonly performed to rule out hearing loss, phenylketonuria, hypothyroidism, galactosemia, and hemoglobinopathies. Other tests commonly included vary.

## REFERENCES AND READINGS


American Academy of Pediatrics. (2007). Year 2007 position statement: Principles and guidelines for early hearing detection and intervention programs. *Pediatrics, 120*(4), 898–921.

American Academy of Pediatrics. (2011). Technical report—SIDS and other sleep-related infant deaths: Expansion of recommendations for a safe infant sleeping environment. *Pediatrics, 126*(5), e1–e27.

American Academy of Pediatrics. (2015). Policy statement—Hospital stay for healthy term newborns. *Pediatrics, 135*(5), 948–953.

American Academy of Pediatrics & American College of Obstetricians and Gynecologists. (2012). *Guidelines for perinatal care* (7th ed.). Elk Grove Village, IL, and Washington, DC: Author.

Association of Women's Health, Obstetric and Neonatal Nurses. (2013). *Evidence-based clinical practice guideline: Neonatal skin care* (3rd ed.). Washington, DC: Author.

Brown, V.D., & Landers, S. (2011). Heat balance. In S.L. Gardner, B.S. Carter, M. Enzman-Hines, et al. (Eds.), *Merenstein & Gardner's handbook of neonatal intensive care* (7th ed., pp. 113–133). St. Louis: Mosby.

Callister, L.C. (2013). Integrating cultural beliefs and practices into the care of childbearing women. In K.R. Simpson, & P.A. Creehan (Eds.), *AWHONN perinatal nursing* (4th ed., pp. 41–64). Philadelphia: Lippincott.

Centers for Disease Control and Prevention. (2013). *Summary of 2013 National CDC EHDI Data*. Retrieved from http://www.cdc.gov.

Centers for Disease Control and Prevention. (2014). *Laboratory Quality Assurance and Standardization Programs – Newborn Screening Quality Assurance Program*. Retrieved from http://www.cdc.gov.

Cunningham, D.R., & Sydlowski, S.A. (2009). Auditory screening. In T.K. McInery, H.M. Adam, D.E. Campbell, et al. (Eds.), *Textbook of pediatric care* (pp. 326–334). Elk Grove Village, IL: American Academy of Pediatrics.

D'Avanzo, C.E. (2008). *Mosby's pocket guide to cultural health assessment* (4th ed.). St. Louis: Mosby.

Fraser, D. (2014). Newborn adaptation to extrauterine life. In K.R. Simpson, & P.A. Creehan (Eds.). *AWHONN perinatal nursing* (4th ed., pp. 581–595). Philadelphia: Lippincott Williams & Wilkins.

Galuska, L. (2011). Prevention of in-hospital newborn falls. *Nursing for Women's Health, 15*(1), 59–61.

Gardner, S.L., Enzman-Hines, M., & Dickey, L.A. (2011). Pain and pain relief. In S.L. Gardner, B.S. Carter, M. Enzman-Hines, et al. (Eds.), *Merenstein & Gardner's handbook of neonatal intensive care* (7th ed., pp. 223–269). St. Louis: Mosby.

Grewal, S.K., Bhagat, R., & Balneaves, L.G. (2008). Perinatal beliefs and practices of immigrant Punjabi women living in Canada. *Journal of Obstetric, Gynecologic and Neonatal Nursing, 37*(3), 290–300.

Hatfield, L.A., Chang, K., Bittle, M., et al. (2011). The analgesic properties of intraoral sucrose: An integrative review. *Advances in Neonatal Care, 11*(2), 83–92.

Jana, L.A., & Shu, J. (2015). *Heading home with your newborn: From birth to reality* (3rd ed.). Elk Grove Village, IL: American Academy of Pediatrics.

Kattwinkel, J. (2011). *Neonatal resuscitation.* Elk Grove Village, IL: American Academy of Pediatricians and American Heart Association.

Lawrence, J., Alcock, D., McGrath, P., et al. (1993). The development of a tool to assess neonatal pain. *Neonatal Network, 14*(5), 59–62.

Lewallen, L.R. (2011). The importance of culture in childbearing. *Journal of Obstetric, Gynecologic, and Neonatal Nursing, 40*(1), 4–8.

Luchtman-Jones, L., & Wilson, D.B. (2011). The blood and hematopoietic system. In R.J. Martin, A.A. Fanaroff, & M.C. Walsh (Eds.), *Fanaroff & Martin's neonatal-perinatal medicine: Diseases of the fetus and infant* (Vol. 1, 8th ed., pp. 1303–1360). Philadelphia: Mosby.

Mackie, A. (2015). Expanded newborn blood spot screening. *British Journal of Midwifery*, *23*(2), 86 1p.

Mance, M.J. (2008). Keeping infants warm: Challenges of hypothermia. *Advances in Neonatal Care*, *8*(1), 6–11.

Mattson, S. (2011). Ethnocultural considerations in the childbearing period. In S. Mattson, & J.E. Smith (Eds.), *AWHONN core curriculum for maternal-newborn nursing* (4th ed., pp. 61–74). St. Louis: Saunders.

National Center for Missing and Exploited Children. (2015). *Newborn/infant abductions*. Retrieved from http://www.missingkids.com/en_US/documents/InfantAbductionStats.pdf.

National Quality Forum. (2009). *National voluntary consensus standards for perinatal care 2008: A consensus report*. Washington, DC: Author.

Rabun, J.B. (2009). *For healthcare professionals: Guidelines on prevention of and response to infant abductions* (9th ed.). Alexandria, VA: National Center for Missing and Exploited Children.

Sedin, C. (2011). The thermal environment. In R.J. Martin, A.A. Fanaroff, & M.C. Walsh (Eds.), *Fanaroff & Martin's neonatal-perinatal medicine: Diseases of the fetus and infant* (Vol. 1, 8th ed., pp. 555–576). Philadelphia: Mosby.

Shaefer, S.J.M., Herman, S.E., Frank, S.J., et al. (2010). Translating infant safe sleep evidence into nursing practice. *Journal of Obstetric, Gynecologic, and Neonatal Nursing*, *39*(6), 618–626.

Smith, L.M. (2012). Circumcision. In C.D. Berkowitz (Ed.), *Pediatrics: A primary care approach* (4th ed., pp. 121–124). Philadelphia: Saunders.

Spector, R.E. (2009). *Cultural diversity in health and illness* (7th ed.). Upper Saddle River, NJ: Pearson Prentice Hall.

Sullivan, C.K., & Dela Cruz-Rivera, S. (2009). Healthy newborn discharge. In T.K. McInery, H.M. Adam, D.E. Campbell, et al. (Eds.), *Textbook of pediatric care* (pp. 840–849). Elk Grove Village, IL: American Academy of Pediatrics.

Swanson, J.T. (2009). Circumcision. In T.K. McInery, H.M. Adam, D.E. Campbell, et al. (Eds.), *Textbook of pediatric care* (pp. 828–830). Elk Grove Village, IL: American Academy of Pediatrics.

U.S. Department of Health and Human Services. (2010). *Healthy People 2020*. Washington, DC: Author.

Vincent, J.L. (2009). Infant hospital abduction: Security measures to aid in prevention. *MCN: The American Journal of Maternal/Child Nursing*, *34*(3), 179–381.

Watts, N., & McDonald, C. (2007). The beginning of life (the perinatal period). In R.H. Srivastava (Ed.), *The healthcare professional's guide to clinical cultural competence* (pp. 203–226). Toronto: Mosby.

White, K.R., Forsman, I., Eichwald, J., et al. (2010). The evolution of early hearing detection and intervention programs in the United States. *Seminars in Perinatology*, *34*(2), 170–179.

# 23

# Newborn Feeding

http://evolve.elsevier.com/McKinney/mat-ch/

## LEARNING OBJECTIVES

*After studying this chapter, you should be able to:*

- Identify the nutritional and fluid needs of the infant.
- Compare the composition of breast milk with that of formula.
- Describe the benefits of breastfeeding for the mother and infant.
- Explain important factors in choosing a method of infant feeding.
- Explain the physiology of lactation.
- Describe nursing management of initial and continued breastfeeding.
- Explain nursing assessments and interventions for common problems in breastfeeding.
- Describe nursing assessments and interventions in formula feeding.

Helping women to choose and feel comfortable to use a feeding method are important nursing contributions that require knowledge of the newborn's nutritional needs and the techniques to meet those needs.

## NUTRITIONAL NEEDS OF THE NEWBORN

### Calories

The full-term newborn needs an average of 85 to 100 kcal/kg (39 to 45 kcal/lb) of body weight each day if breastfed and 100 to 110 kcal/kg (45 to 50 kcal/lb) if formula fed (Blackburn, 2013). Breast milk and formulas used for the normal newborn contain 20 kcal/oz.

During the early days after birth, infants may lose up to 10% of their birth weight because of the normal loss of extracellular water and the consumption of fewer calories than needed (Halbardier, 2010; Jones, Hayes, Starbuck, et al., 2011). Newborns have a small stomach capacity and may fall asleep before feeding adequately. Capacity increases rapidly so that many infants take 60 to 90 mL (2 to 3 oz) by the end of the first week.

Infants usually regain the lost weight by 2 weeks of age (Keane, 2011). They should be evaluated for feeding problems if weight loss exceeds 7% to 8%, if loss continues beyond 3 days of age, or if the birth weight is not regained by 2 weeks of age in the term infant (American Academy of Pediatrics [AAP] & American College of Obstetricians and Gynecologists [ACOG], 2012). This information should be explained to parents.

### Nutrients

The nutrients needed by the newborn are provided by carbohydrates, proteins, and fat in breast milk or formula. Full-term neonates digest simple carbohydrates and proteins well. Complex carbohydrates and fats are less well digested because of the lack of pancreatic amylase and lipase in the newborn. Vitamins and minerals are provided by both breast milk and formula.

### Water

Because newborns lose water easily from the skin, kidneys, and intestines, they must have adequate fluid intake each day. The normal full-term newborn needs approximately 60 to 100 mL/kg (27 to 45 mL/lb) during the first 3 to 5 days of life, which should gradually increase to 150 to 175 mL/kg (68 to 80 mL/lb) a day (Halbardier, 2010). Breast milk or formula supplies the infant's fluid needs. Additional water is unnecessary. Box 23.1 lists for daily calorie and fluid needs of the newborn.

## BREAST MILK AND FORMULA COMPOSITION

### Breast Milk

Breast milk is species specific (made for human infants) and offers many advantages over formula. The nutrients in breast milk are proportioned appropriately for the neonate and vary to meet the newborn's changing needs. Breast milk provides protection against infection and is easily digested. Maternal immunoglobulins, leukocytes, antioxidants, enzymes, and hormones important for growth are present in breast milk but not in formula.

#### Changes in Composition

The composition of breast milk changes in three phases: Lactogenesis (the production of milk) stages I, II, and III.

***Lactogenesis I.*** Lactogenesis I begins during pregnancy and continues through the early days after giving birth. At this time, the breast secretes colostrum—a thick, yellow substance. Colostrum has higher levels of protein and some vitamins and minerals than mature milk. It is lower in carbohydrates, fat, lactose, and some vitamins. Colostrum is rich in immunoglobulins, especially secretory IgA, which helps protect the infant's gastrointestinal tract from infection. Colostrum helps establish the normal flora in the intestines, and its laxative effect speeds the passage of meconium.

***Lactogenesis II.*** Lactogenesis II begins at 2 to 3 days after birth. Transitional milk, which gradually changes from colostrum to mature milk, appears over approximately 10 days (Lawrence & Lawrence, 2011). The amount of milk increases rapidly as it "comes in." Immunoglobulins and proteins decrease, and lactose, fat, and calories increase. The vitamin content is approximately the same as that of mature milk.

***Lactogenesis III.*** Mature milk replaces transitional milk during lactogenesis III. Because breast milk is bluish and not as thick as

**BOX 23.1 Daily Calorie and Fluid Needs of the Newborn**

- *Calories:* 85-100 kcal/kg (39-45 kcal/lb) if breastfed; 100-110 kcal/kg (45-50 kcal/lb) if formula fed
- *Fluid:* 60-100 mL/kg (27-45 mL/lb) for the first 3-5 days of life; gradually increasing to 150-175 mL/kg (68-80 mL/lb)

colostrum, some mothers think their milk is not "rich" enough for their infants. Nurses should explain the normal appearance of breast milk. Mature milk contains approximately 20 kcal/oz and nutrients sufficient to meet the infant's needs. It continues to provide immunoglobulins and other antibacterial components. Discussions of breast milk and its contents refer to mature milk unless otherwise stated.

### Nutrients

**Protein.** The concentrations of amino acids in breast milk are suited to the infant's needs and ability to metabolize them. Breast milk is high in taurine, which is important for bile conjugation and brain development. Breast milk is low in tyrosine and phenylalanine, corresponding to the infant's low levels of enzymes to digest them (Lawrence & Lawrence, 2011). The proteins produce a low solute load for the infant's immature kidneys.

Casein and whey are the proteins in milk. Casein forms a large, insoluble curd that is harder to digest than the curd from whey, which is very soft (Riordan, 2015). Breast milk is easily digested because it has a high ratio of whey to casein, especially in early lactation. Commercial formulas must be adapted to increase the amount of whey so the curd is more digestible. Infants use almost all of the protein in human milk but pass a large amount of protein from formulas in the stools (Eiger, 2016).

Allergy to cow's milk is the most common allergy in infants (Riordan, 2015). Because breast milk is made for the human infant, it is unlikely to cause allergies. Infants with a family history of allergies are less likely to develop them if they are breastfed (Lawrence & Lawrence, 2011). Although breast milk does not cause allergies, allergenic foods the mother has eaten may pass to her milk. If the infant reacts to the mother's diet, the offending food should be identified and eliminated. Foods in the mother's diet that may cause a problem for some infants include cow's milk or milk products, chocolate, cola, corn, citrus fruit, wheat, and peanuts (Bronner, 2015).

Studies have been inconclusive in determining whether avoiding common antigens in the mother's diet will protect against allergies in the infant. General recommendations are that the infant be exclusively breastfed for at least 4 months and that allergenic foods be avoided by the mother if her infant younger than 6 weeks of age has colic (Ribeiro, Leite, & deMorais, 2013).

**Carbohydrate.** Lactose is the major carbohydrate in breast milk. It improves absorption of calcium and provides energy for brain growth. Other carbohydrates in breast milk increase the intestinal acidity and impede the growth of pathogens (Riordan, 2015).

**Fat.** Fat provides half of the calories in breast milk (Kleinman & Greer, 2014). The amount of fat in breast milk varies during the feeding, between feedings, and on the same or different days. More fat is present in the **hindmilk**—the milk produced at the end of the feeding. Hindmilk helps the infant gain weight.

Triglycerides contribute the majority of the fat content. Cholesterol and essential fatty acids such as long-chain polyunsaturated fatty acids, docosahexaenoic acid (DHA), and arachidonic acid (ARA), important for vision and brain and nervous system development, are also present. The fat in breast milk is more easily digested by the newborn than that in cow's milk.

**Vitamins.** The content of vitamins A, E, and C is high in breast milk. The vitamin D content of breast milk is low, and daily supplementation with 400 IU is recommended within the first few days of life for all infants, whether breastfed or formula fed (Kleinman & Greer, 2014; Atisha, Ahmed, & Bim, 2010). Breastfeeding infants who are not exposed to the sun and those with dark skin are particularly at risk for insufficient vitamin D. The presence of water-soluble vitamins varies according to the mother's intake. The infant of a vegan mother may need supplementation with vitamin $B_{12}$.

**Minerals.** Although iron in breast milk is lower than that in formula, it is absorbed five times as well, and breastfed infants are rarely deficient in iron (Riordan, 2015). The full-term infant who is exclusively breastfed maintains iron stores for the first 6 months of life (Lawrence & Lawrence, 2011). Iron is normally added to the diet when the infant begins solids at 6 months. Preterm infants need iron supplements earlier. All formula-fed infants should receive formula fortified with iron (AAP & ACOG, 2012; Holt, Wooldridge, Story, et al., 2011).

As with iron, the content of calcium in breast milk is low, but it is better absorbed than that of cow's milk. Phosphorus is higher in cow's milk, but this may interfere with calcium absorption. Sodium, calcium, and phosphorus are higher in cow's milk than in human milk. Fluoride supplementation is unnecessary in infants younger than 6 months of age. After 6 months, fluoride may be given to formula-fed infants if water supplies do not contain sufficient fluoride (Kleinman & Greer, 2014).

### Enzymes

Breast milk contains enzymes that aid in digestion. Pancreatic amylase, necessary to digest carbohydrates, is low in the newborn but present in breast milk. Breast milk also contains lipase to increase fat digestion.

### Infection-Preventing Components

Substances in breast milk, such as bifidus factor, leukocytes, lysozymes, and lactoferrin, help prevent infection in the infant. Immunoglobulins are present in highest amounts in colostrum but are present throughout lactation. Secretory IgA produced in the breasts helps prevent viral and bacterial invasion of the intestinal mucosa, resulting in fewer intestinal infections. Infants who are breastfed have a decreased incidence of respiratory, gastrointestinal, and urinary tract infections, otitis media, asthma, diabetes, necrotizing enterocolitis, some cancers, obesity, sudden infant death syndrome, and infant mortality (Lawrence & Lawrence, 2011).

### Effect of Maternal Diet

Although the fatty acid content of breast milk is influenced by the mother's diet, malnourished mothers' milk has approximately the same amounts of total fat, protein, carbohydrates, and most minerals as milk from those who are well nourished. Levels of water-soluble vitamins in breast milk, however, are affected by the mother's intake and stores (Lawrence & Lawrence, 2011). It is important that breastfeeding women eat a well-balanced diet to maintain their own health and energy levels (see Nutrition for the Lactating Mother in Chapter 14, p. 268.)

## Formulas

Commercial formulas are produced to replace or supplement breast milk. They are sometimes called "breast milk substitutes" or "artificial breast milk" because manufacturers must adapt them to correspond to the components in breast milk as much as possible. However, an exact match is impossible. A variety of formulas that differ in price and ingredients is available.

### Cow's Milk

Unmodified cow's milk (whole, lowfat, or fat-free) is not recommended for infants younger than 12 months as it contains too much protein, potassium, chloride, and sodium; lacks sufficient fatty acids, iron, and vitamin E; and may cause gastrointestinal bleeding and anemia. It also causes the renal solute load to be too high (Kleinman & Greer, 2014).

Modified cow's milk is the source of most commercial formulas. Manufacturers specifically formulate it for infants by making changes in the protein and fat content and adding vitamins and other nutrients to simulate the contents of breast milk. Formula with added iron should be used for all infants receiving formula.

### Formulas for Infants With Special Needs

Infants with galactosemia, lactase deficiency, or those whose families are vegetarians can be fed soy formula. As many as half of infants allergic to cow's milk are also allergic to soy protein (Nguyen & Kerner, 2015). Protein hydrolysate formulas are better tolerated by infants with allergies. The protein in these formulas is treated to make it less allergenic. The formulas are also used for infants with malabsorption disorders. Amino acid formulas are used for allergic infants who do not thrive on extensively hydrolyzed protein formulas.

Lactose-free formula contains glucose instead of lactose for infants who do not tolerate lactose. Low-phenylalanine formulas are needed for infants with phenylketonuria, a deficiency in the enzyme that digests the phenylalanine found in standard formulas. The preterm infant may require a more concentrated formula, with more calories in less liquid. Modifications of other nutrients are also made. Human milk fortifiers can be added to breast milk to adapt it for preterm infants.

#### BOX 23.2 Benefits of Breastfeeding

**For the Infant**

- Allergies are less likely to develop.
- Immunologic properties help prevent infections. Decreased incidence of sepsis; meningitis; and respiratory, ear, gastrointestinal, and urinary tract infections.
- Decreased incidence of diabetes, asthma, obesity, some cancers, sudden infant death syndrome (SIDS), necrotizing enterocolitis, and infant mortality.
- Composition meets infant's specific nutritional needs.
- Nutritional and immunologic properties change according to infant's needs.
- Protein, fat, and carbohydrate in most suitable proportions.
- Easily digested; nutrients well absorbed.
- Less likely to result in overfeeding.
- Constipation less likely.
- No possibility of improper and potentially dangerous dilution.
- Unlikely to be contaminated; not affected by water supply.

**For the Mother**

- Oxytocin release enhances involution of uterus.
- Mother loses less blood because of delayed return of menses.
- Delays resumption of ovulation.
- May reduce the risk of some cancers.
- Mother more likely to rest while feeding.
- Mother likely to eat balanced diet that improves healing.
- Frequent, skin-to-skin contact enhances bonding.
- Convenient: always available, no bottles to wash or formula to buy, prepare, or heat.
- Economical: eliminates cost of formula and bottles and preparation time.
- Fewer costs associated with illness in the infant.
- Working mothers miss less work to care for sick infants.
- Traveling easier: no bottles to prepare, carry, refrigerate, or warm.

## CONSIDERATIONS IN CHOOSING A FEEDING METHOD

Many women decide on a feeding method well ahead of the birth. Nurses can help undecided parents choose a method and gain confidence in feeding their infants. For those who are undecided, nurses should explain the many benefits of breastfeeding for the mother and the infant.

However, nurses must be sensitive to mothers' feelings about feeding. Although nurses should encourage breastfeeding as the best method of feeding in most circumstances, they should be supportive of the mother's chosen method once the decision is made. The early days of parenting are a vulnerable time for new mothers, and the nurse's encouragement and teaching about the chosen feeding method are essential.

### Breastfeeding

Mothers choose breastfeeding because it offers many advantages for the mother and the infant (Box 23.2). The AAP recommends that infants receive only breast milk for approximately the first 6 months. Breastfeeding should continue until the infant is at least 12 months old with the addition of complementary foods (AAP, 2012; Kleinman & Greer, 2014). Breastfeeding and support to help mothers achieve it are also recommended by the American Dietetic Association (2015) and the U.S. Surgeon General (U.S. Department of Health and Human Services [USDHHS], 2011a).

A goal set by the USDHHS for 2020 is for 81.9% of all infants to be breastfed at some time, for at least 60.5% to be breastfeeding at 6 months, and 34.1% at 1 year. Additional goals are to increase the number of mothers who exclusively breastfeed their infants through 3 months to 44.3% and through 6 months to 23.7% (USDHHS, 2010).

The Centers for Disease Control and Prevention (CDC) reports that in 2011, 79% of infants were ever breastfed. The report also reveals that 49% of mothers breastfed their 6-month-old infants, and 27% of mothers continued breastfeeding their 12-month-old infants. Exclusive breastfeeding rates were 40.7% at 3 months and 18.8% at 6 months. These statistics show a gradual but steady increase over previous years, but continued improvement is needed (CDC, 2014).

In an effort to promote breastfeeding, the United Nations Children's Fund (UNICEF), the World Health Organization (WHO), and the U.S. Surgeon General advocate that birth facilities become certified as "baby-friendly" hospitals, with policies to actively encourage breastfeeding. Guidelines to becoming certified as a baby-friendly hospital emphasize the education of staff and parents about breastfeeding, early initiation of breastfeeding, demand feedings, avoidance of formula and pacifiers, and rooming-in. Unfortunately, less than 5% of U.S. hospitals are certified as baby-friendly (CDC, 2011a; USDHHS, 2011a). (More information is available at http://babyfriendlyusa.org.)

### Formula Feeding

Parents choose formula feeding for many reasons. Some women are embarrassed by breastfeeding, seeing the breasts only in a sexual context. Many mothers have little experience with family or friends who have breastfed infants. The woman's partner or mother may not be supportive of breastfeeding. Occasionally, a woman requires medications that might harm the infant. A frequent reason that mothers choose formula feeding instead of breastfeeding is a lack of understanding and education about the two methods.

## Combination Feeding

Some parents prefer a combination of breastfeeding and formula feeding. Unless medically indicated, it is best to delay giving formula until lactation has been well established at 3 to 4 weeks of age. Giving formula to breastfeeding infants leads to a decrease in breastfeeding frequency and milk production, making successful breastfeeding less likely (AAP & ACOG, 2012). However, if the mother chooses to feed both breast milk and formula, the nurse should educate and support her so the infant receives the benefits of breast milk at least part of the time.

A mother may give a bottle daily or only occasionally, such as when a baby-sitter is with the infant. Some mothers feel this allows them to be away from the infant for longer periods of time yet allows the closeness they enjoy with the infant, as well as the physical advantages of breastfeeding, to continue. Mothers may choose to use breast milk or formula for occasional bottle feedings.

## Factors Influencing Choice

Many factors influence a woman's choice of feeding method. These factors must be considered when educating women about their choices.

### Support From Others

The decision to breastfeed is strongly influenced by the woman's family and friends. She is likely to ask for advice from her partner first, followed by advice from her mother, family, and friends (USDHHS, 2011b). The woman with little support or with active discouragement from her family will probably have a more difficult time nursing. Advice from friends who have breastfed may also influence the mother's decision.

Involvement of the father in infant care is important for some families, and some may feel it is only possible with feedings. Nurses can suggest other infant care measures, such as holding, rocking, and bathing, which fathers can enjoy. Educating family members about the advantages of breastfeeding and how to deal with problems may lead to their encouragement and support.

Prenatal classes that include breastfeeding information may help a woman decide to breastfeed and may help her develop confidence that she will be successful. Educating fathers about the benefits of breastfeeding, as well as techniques for coping with any difficulties that might occur, is important. Fathers should also attend the classes so they can provide increased support based on their knowledge. Both prenatal classes and new-mother support groups led by lactation consultants are associated with higher breastfeeding rates at 6 months postpartum (Vital Signs, 2015).

Encouragement from the woman's healthcare provider can be a powerful influence in the woman choosing to breastfeed (Newton, 2012). The support the mother receives from the nursing staff plays a significant part in whether she feels comfortable with her chosen feeding method. Mothers who do not feel confident in their ability to breastfeed before they leave the birth facility are less likely to continue breastfeeding if they encounter difficulties at home.

Other support also can be important. Doulas, trained lay women who make home visits to assist women with breastfeeding after discharge, have been shown to increase the rate of breastfeeding at 6 weeks postpartum (Kozhimannil, Attanasio, Hardeman, & O'Brien, 2013). One study of African-American women found that breastfeeding self-efficacy, a woman's belief that she will be able to breastfeed successfully, was associated with a longer period of breastfeeding and more exclusive breastfeeding at 1 and 6 months postpartum (Robinson, 2010).

### Culture

Cultural influences may dictate decisions about how a mother feeds her infant. For example, many Mormon women believe that breastfeeding is an important part of motherhood. Muslim women often breastfeed for the first 2 years. Women who are most likely to breastfeed are Asian, Pacific Islander, or Hispanic. Those with the lowest breastfeeding rates include women who are non-Hispanic Black (USDHHS, 2011a).

Immigrants to the United States often would breastfeed infants if they were still in their own countries. For example, in Russia, women are expected to breastfeed, and formula is not available in birth houses (Gerbeda-Wilson & Powers, 2012). Hispanic women who are new immigrants are more likely to begin breastfeeding and continue for a longer period than more acculturated immigrants (Linares, Rayens, Gomez, Gokun & Dignan, 2015). Some of these women may think that formula is the preferred method of feeding in the United States because it is available in the hospital. Nurses must emphasize the superiority of breastfeeding and encourage these women to continue their cultural tradition of breastfeeding.

Nurses should be particularly watchful for ways to help mothers from other cultures who might wish to breastfeed but fail to do so because of lack of support. Some Asian and Latina mothers give their infants formula while in the birth facility and do not begin to breastfeed until at home. This practice may result from modesty regarding nursing in front of others in the birth facility, as well as lack of understanding about the value of colostrum. Women in some cultures believe that colostrum may be "spoiled" because it has been in the breasts for a long time. They may express colostrum and discard it before they begin to breastfeed the infant. Education by nurses can help mothers understand the importance of giving colostrum and that much of the milk is produced as the infant is **suckling** (feeding at the breast).

Rituals may be important in some cultures. In the Philippines, the ritual of *lihi,* stroking the mother's breasts with papaya leaves and sugar cane stalks ensures a good supply of rich milk (Riordan, 2015). Hispanic women may believe that they can transmit negative emotions to their breastfeeding infants. Navajo women believe they pass maternal attributes and model good behavior by breastfeeding (Kleinman & Greer, 2014).

### Employment

Women should be encouraged to continue breastfeeding when they return to work. Because of the decreased incidence of illness in breastfed infants, the mother is less likely to miss work to take care of a sick infant. This is an advantage for the employer as well as the breastfeeding family.

Unfortunately, returning to work or school is a major cause of discontinuation of breastfeeding. The mother may choose formula from the beginning, plan a short period of breastfeeding before weaning the infant to formula, or use a combination of breastfeeding and bottle feeding with breast milk or formula. Nurses who provide practical information about options, breastfeeding and working, breast pumps, and storage of breast milk help a mother continue breastfeeding for a longer period. Referral to a lactation consultant can provide a mother with continued education and support after she goes home.

### Staff Knowledge

It is important that all birth facility staff members are educated about how to help women breastfeed and do not provide inaccurate or conflicting information to new mothers. Educational programs are effective in helping to ensure that all staff have the same basic knowledge and skills to help breastfeeding mothers. Programs may involve formal classes, protocols, and self-paced learning modules (Bernaix, Beaman, Schmidt, et al., 2010; Mellin, Poplawski, & Gole, 2011).

### Other Factors

Other factors may also influence a woman's decision. Her knowledge and past experience with infant feeding are important. Lower breastfeeding rates are reported for women who receive assistance from the Special Supplemental Nutrition Program for Women, Infants, and Children (WIC), those with no college education, and those who live in the southeastern United States (USDHHS, 2011a). One study found that women were more likely to exclusively breastfeed in the hospital if they began prenatal care in the first trimester and had expressed an intention during pregnancy to breastfeed exclusively. Women who were overweight or obese were half as likely to exclusively breastfeed during the hospital stay (Tenfelde, Finnegan, & Hill, 2011).

## NORMAL BREASTFEEDING

### Breast Changes During Pregnancy

Breast changes begin early in pregnancy (see Chapters 11 and 13 and Figs. 11.8 and 13.3). The ducts, lobules, and alveoli develop in response to estrogen, progesterone, prolactin, and human chorionic somatomammotropin (hCs) (also called human placental lactogen). Prolactin levels are high, but milk production is prevented by estrogen, progesterone, and hCs, which inhibit the breast response to prolactin. Changes such as increased breast size indicate that the breasts are responding adequately to hormonal stimulation to prepare for lactation. Colostrum is present beginning at 12 to 16 weeks of pregnancy (Janke, 2014).

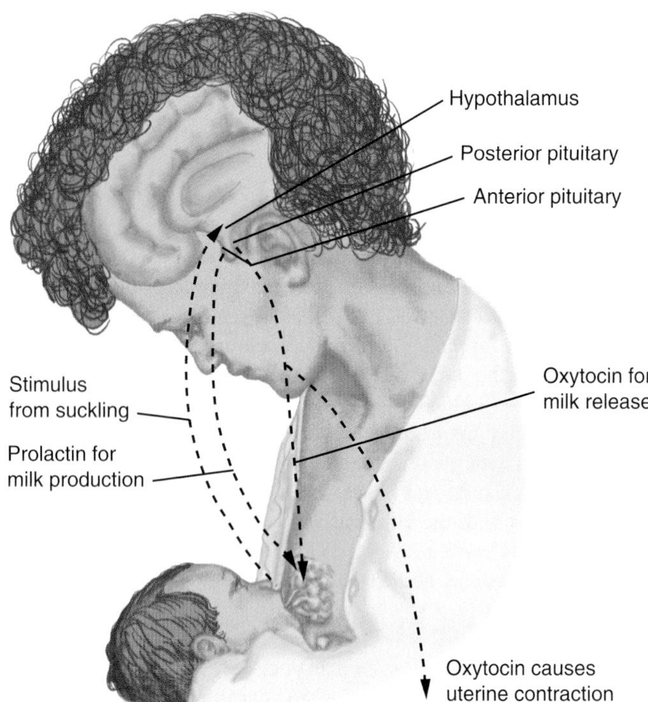


**FIG 23.1** Effect of prolactin and oxytocin on milk production. When the infant begins to suckle at the breast, nerve impulses travel to the hypothalamus and cause the anterior pituitary to secrete prolactin to increase milk production. Suckling causes the posterior pituitary to secrete oxytocin, producing the let-down reflex, which releases milk from the breast. Oxytocin also causes the uterus to contract, which aids in involution.

### Milk Production

Milk is produced in the alveoli of the breasts through a complex process by which materials from the mother's bloodstream are reformulated into breast milk. The milk is ejected from the secretory cells of the alveoli into the alveolar lumen by contraction of the myoepithelial cells. It travels through the lactiferous ducts to the nipple. The infant compresses the areola during nursing to eject a stream of milk through pores in the nipple. Although there is a small amount of milk in the breasts at the beginning of feedings, most of the milk is made during infant suckling (Brozanski & Bogen, 2012).

### Hormonal Changes at Birth

#### Prolactin

At birth, loss of placental hormones results in increased levels and effectiveness of prolactin to stimulate milk production. Suckling and the removal of colostrum or milk cause continued elevation of prolactin levels. Prolactin is secreted at highest levels with suckling and during the night (Lawrence & Lawrence, 2011). Levels are high during the early months and then gradually decrease until weaning.

#### Oxytocin

Oxytocin, the pituitary hormone, increases in response to nipple stimulation and causes the milk-ejection reflex, or let-down reflex, the release of milk from the alveoli into the ducts. The milk-ejection reflex occurs intermittently during each feeding. Mothers may have a tingling sensation of the breast when the let-down occurs.

When mothers see, hear, or think about their infants, they often have an increase in oxytocin, bringing about a let-down of milk. Pain or lack of relaxation can decrease oxytocin release. Oxytocin also causes the uterine contractions mothers may feel at the beginning of nursing sessions. These contractions are beneficial because they hasten involution of the uterus (Fig. 23.1).

### Continued Milk Production

The amount of milk produced depends primarily on adequate stimulation of the breast and removal of the milk. This "supply-and-demand" effect continues throughout lactation—that is, increased demand with more frequent and longer nursing results in more milk available.

If milk (or colostrum) is not removed from the breasts, components in the milk initiate feedback that decreases prolactin secretion and milk production. Milk in the ducts is eventually absorbed, the alveoli become smaller, the secretory cells return to a resting state, and milk production ends.

### Preparation of Breasts for Breastfeeding

Little preparation is needed during pregnancy for breastfeeding. The mother should avoid soap on her nipples to prevent removal of the natural protective oils from the Montgomery tubercles of the breasts. The use of creams and nipple rolling, pulling, and rubbing to "toughen" nipples does not decrease nipple pain after birth and may cause irritation or uterine contractions from the release of oxytocin.

The breasts should be assessed during pregnancy to identify flat or inverted nipples (Fig. 23.2). Normal nipples protrude. Flat nipples appear soft, like the areola, and do not stand erect unless stimulated by rolling them between the fingers. Inverted nipples are retracted into the breast tissue. Both conditions may make it difficult for infants to draw the nipples into the mouth. Some nipples appear normal but draw inward when the areola is compressed in the infant's mouth.

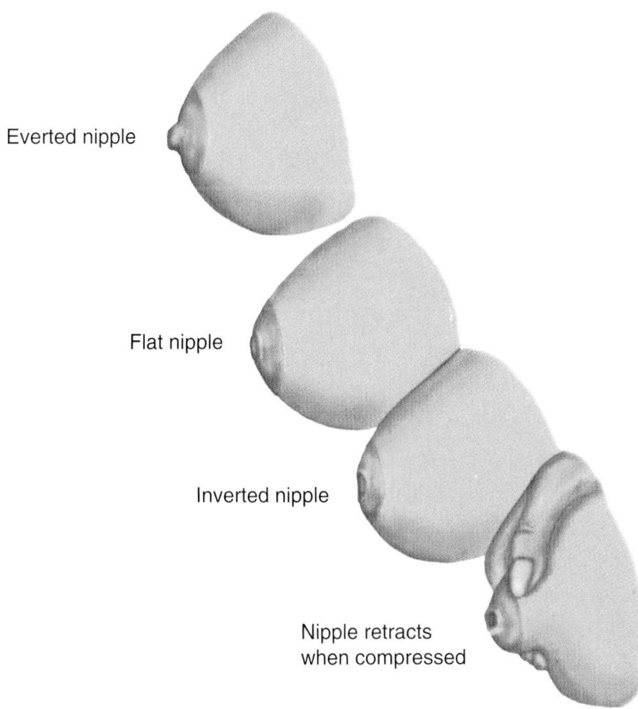


FIG 23.2 Normal everted nipple and other types of nipples that may cause the infant difficulty in latching on. Nipples shown after stimulation.

Compressing the areola between the thumb and forefinger determines whether the nipple projects normally or becomes inverted. Nipples that appear flat or inverted early in pregnancy may improve near term (Wambach & Riordan, 2015).

The helpfulness of breast shells for flat or inverted nipples is debated. Some authors find them helpful for some women, and others feel they decrease motivation to breastfeed and do not improve nipple eversion (Lawrence & Lawrence, 2011; Wambach & Riordan, 2015). These dome-shaped devices are worn during the last weeks of pregnancy and between feedings after birth. The shells are placed in the bra with the opening over the nipple. They exert slight pressure against the areola to help the nipples protrude. A breast pump used just before feedings to help bring the nipples out may be more effective.

## NURSING CARE

### Breastfeeding

#### Assessment

Assess the mother and the infant during the breastfeeding process.

***Maternal Assessment.***

**Breasts and nipples.** Assess the condition of the breasts and nipples and the mother's knowledge about breastfeeding to determine her need for assistance. Examine the breasts and nipples during late pregnancy to identify problems that might interfere with feeding. Assess the protrusion of the nipples to determine whether they are flat or inverted.

After birth, palpate the breasts with each postpartum assessment to see if they are soft, filling, or engorged. Soft breasts feel like a cheek. If milk is beginning to come in, the breasts may be slightly firmer, which is charted as "filling." **Engorgement** involves congestion and increased vascularity, edema from obstruction of drainage of the lymphatics, and accumulation of milk, as lactation is established. Engorged breasts may be hard and tender, with taut, shiny skin. Engorgement often is not seen until after discharge. Note any redness, tenderness, or lumps within the breasts. The nipples may be red, bruised, blistered, fissured, bleeding, or tender. Ask about nipple tenderness. Evaluate breastfeeding techniques if the mother is having problems with her nipples.

**Knowledge.** The mother breastfeeding for the first time may have many questions and may need substantial guidance during her first attempts. If she has nursed before, she may have a better understanding of breastfeeding but may have forgotten some aspects and have questions.

***Assessment of infant feeding behaviors.*** Before initiating a breastfeeding session, assess the infant's readiness for feeding (Box 23.3). The infant should be awake and alert. Sucking on the hands, rooting when the cheek or side of the mouth is touched, smacking the lips, and hand-to-mouth movements are hunger cues. Infants should be fed before they begin crying, which is a late sign of hunger. Crying infants must be calmed before they are ready to feed. Continue to assess for signs of problems throughout the feeding.

**BOX 23.3 Hunger Cues in Infants**

- Licking or sucking movements
- Lip smacking
- Rooting
- Hand-to-mouth movements
- Sucking on the hands
- Increased activity
- Crying (a late sign)

**LATCH scoring tool.** Assessing the infant's **latch** or attachment to the breast is important. The LATCH breastfeeding-assessment tool may be helpful (Jensen, Wallace, & Kelsay, 1994). The tool assigns a score of 0 to 2 in five areas. A score of 7 or less indicates the mother needs more assistance in feeding.

1. Latch: mouth positioned correctly for latch and rhythmic sucking, 2; repeated attempts needed, 1; no sustained latch, 0.
2. Swallow: spontaneous swallows, 2; a few swallows, 1; no audible swallowing, 0.
3. Nipples: everted, 2; flat, 1; inverted, 0.
4. Comfort: soft, nontender breasts, 3; redness, small blisters, or bruises with mild to moderate discomfort, 1; engorged breasts with cracked, bleeding, blistered, or bruised breasts or nipples, severe discomfort, 0.
5. Positioning: mother needs no assistance for correct positioning, 2; some assistance needed, 1; mother requires the staff to position the infant at the breast, 0.

#### Nursing Diagnosis and Planning

Women with and without experience often need information to have a successful breastfeeding experience. A woman's confidence in her ability to breastfeed may be an important determinant of her success. Therefore, nurses should help women increase their confidence and help prevent early weaning by using the nursing diagnosis:

- Risk for Ineffective Breastfeeding related to lack of understanding of breastfeeding techniques and confidence in using them.

***Expected outcomes.*** The infant will breastfeed using nutritive suckling for 10 to 15 minutes or more on each breast for most feedings before discharge. The mother will demonstrate breastfeeding techniques as taught and will verbalize satisfaction and confidence with the breastfeeding process before discharge.

***Interventions.*** Interventions are centered on teaching that nurses should provide to all breastfeeding mothers and their support persons. These techniques should be adapted as appropriate for mothers who have some knowledge of breastfeeding but need review or clarification.

***Assisting with the first feeding.*** The first feeding should take place within the first hour after birth if both mother and infant are in stable condition. Breastfeeding within the first hour is associated with a higher breastfeeding rate at 2 to 4 months after birth than later breastfeeding (Schanler, 2016). Early breastfeeding provides stimulation of milk production and improved suckling and may increase the duration of breastfeeding. The mother may need assistance in positioning herself and the infant and a demonstration of how to hold the breast. Stay with the mother during the first few feedings to help her with problems that may arise. After the first feedings, check back frequently to answer questions.

***Teaching feeding techniques***

**Position of the mother and infant.** Make the mother comfortable before beginning the feeding. Provide pain medications, if necessary. Provide privacy and prevent interruptions so she can concentrate. Breastfeeding mothers most often use the cradle, football or clutch, and cross-cradle holds and the side-lying position (Figs. 23.3 through 23.6). To increase her comfort, position pillows behind the mother's back, over an abdominal incision, or to support her arms. Her shoulders should be relaxed, and she should not be hunched over.

Use pillows or folded blankets to elevate the infant to the level of the nipple and prevent pulling and tension on the nipple. The infant's head and body should directly face the breast with the neck flexed, and the infant's nose, cheeks, and chin lightly touching the breast. If the infant must turn the head to reach the breast, swallowing is difficult. The infant's body should be aligned so that the ear, shoulder, and hips are in a straight line.

**Position of the mother's hands.** The mother's hand position is also important. In the palmar or C hand position, the mother holds her breast with her thumb on top and the fingers under the breast for support with the little finger against the chest wall (Fig. 23.7). Her fingers should be behind the areola, and her thumb should not press on the breast too deeply, or the infant will suck improperly, and the nipple may become sore.

Some women use the V hold, with their index and middle fingers supporting the breast. The fingers must be well behind the areola, or they may slip down the wet areola and interfere with the placement of the infant's mouth.

The mother should support her breast in place for the first few weeks if the weight of it makes it difficult for the infant to hold it in the mouth. As the infant becomes more adept at breastfeeding, the mother will not need to hold the breast.

Although mothers worry about the infant's ability to breathe while nursing, it is unnecessary to indent the breast tissue near the infant's nostrils. This might cause improper positioning of the nipple in the

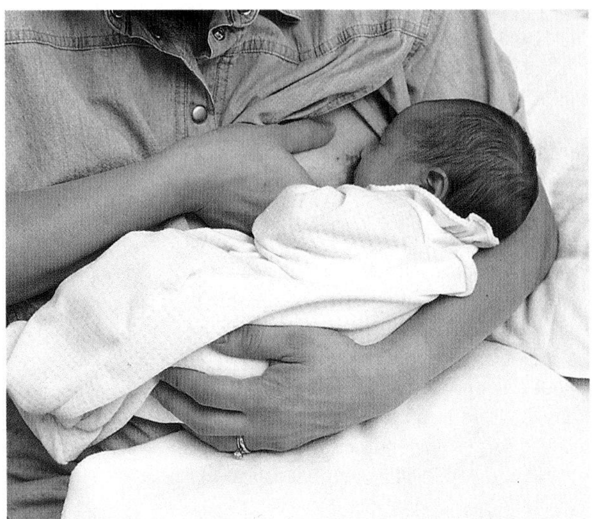

**FIG 23.3** For the cradle hold, the mother positions the infant's head at or near the antecubital space and level with her nipple, with her arm supporting the infant's body. Her other hand is free to hold the breast. Once the infant is positioned, pillows or blankets can be used to support the mother's arm, which may tire from holding the baby.

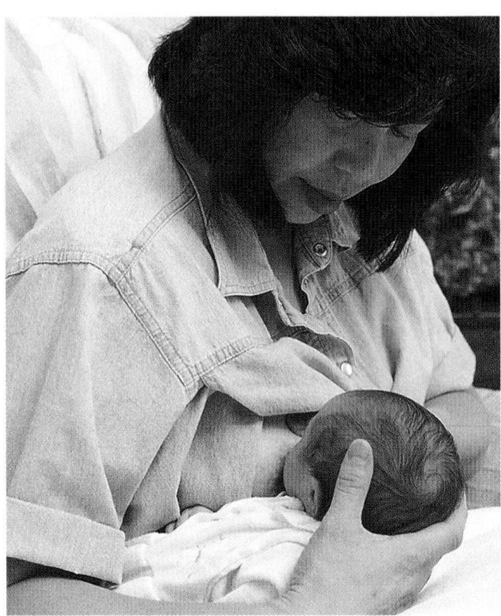

**FIG 23.4** For the football or clutch hold, the mother supports the infant's head in her hand, with the infant's body resting on pillows alongside her hip. This method allows the mother to see the position of the infant's mouth on the breast, helps her control the infant's head, and is especially helpful for mothers with heavy breasts. This hold also avoids pressure against an abdominal incision.

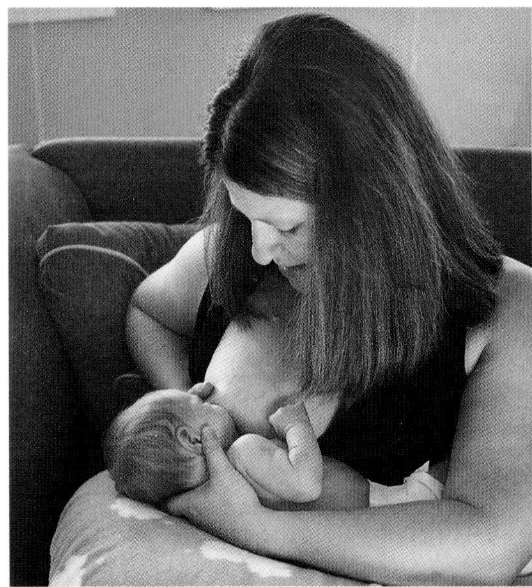

**FIG 23.5** The cross-cradle or modified cradle hold is helpful for infants who are preterm or have a fractured clavicle. The mother holds the infant's head in the hand opposite the side on which the infant will feed and supports the infant's body across her lap with her arm. The other hand holds the breast. The mother can guide the infant's head to the breast and see the mouth on the breast during the feeding.

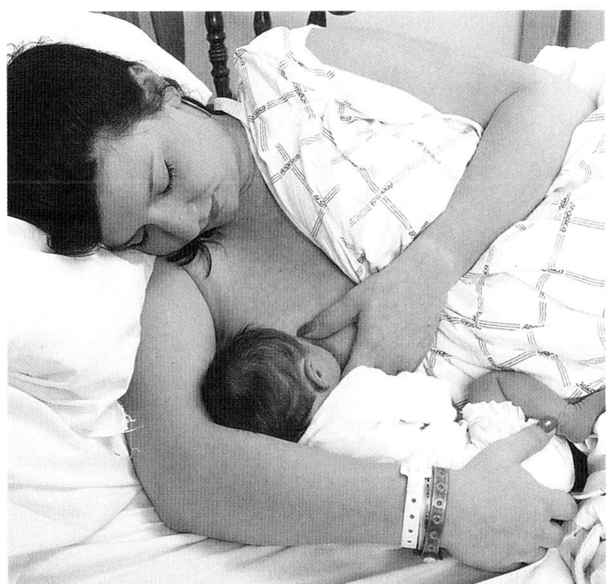

FIG 23.6 The side-lying position avoids pressure on episiotomy or abdominal incisions and allows the mother to rest while feeding. She lies on her side, with her lower arm supporting her head or placed around the infant. Pillows behind her back and between her legs provide comfort. Her upper hand and arm are used to position the infant on the side at nipple level and hold the breast. When the infant's mouth opens to nurse, the mother draws the infant to her to insert the nipple into the mouth.

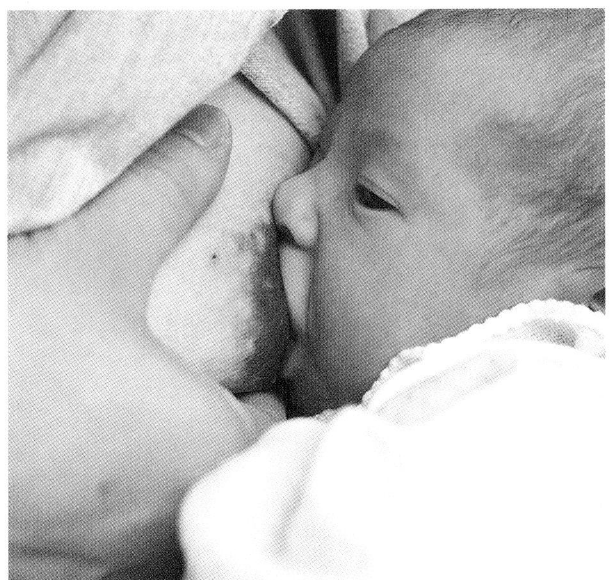

FIG 23.7 C position of hand on breast. The hand is positioned so the thumb is on top of the breast while the fingers support the breast from below. Note the flaring of the infant's lips.

infant's mouth, interfere with the grasp of the nipple, or impede milk flow. Bringing the infant's hips closer to the mother and lifting the body to a more horizontal position helps if there is concern about the infant's ability to breathe while nursing.

**Latch-on techniques.** Teach the mother techniques to help the infant latch on or attach to the breast.

**Eliciting latch-on.** After positioning the awake and hungry infant to face the breast, instruct the mother to hold her breast so the nipple

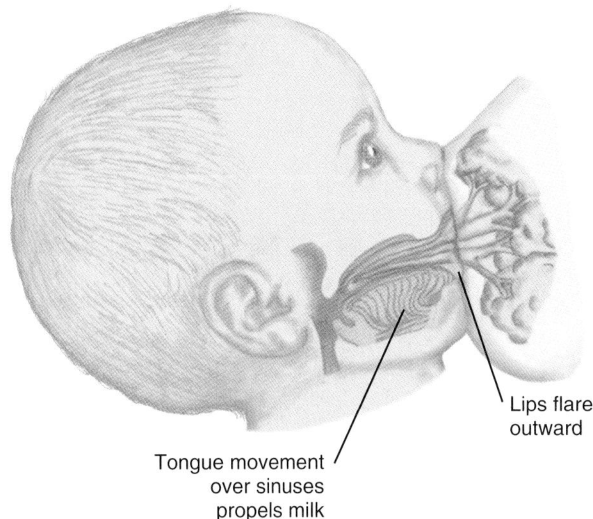
Lips flare outward
Tongue movement over sinuses propels milk

FIG 23.8 Position of infant's mouth while suckling. When the nipple and areola are properly positioned in the infant's mouth, the gums compress the areola instead of the nipple. The tongue is between the lower gum and the breast. The infant's lips are flared outward.

brushes against the infant's lips. A hungry infant will respond by opening the mouth, although up to a minute of stroking may be necessary. The breast should not be inserted until the infant's mouth is opened widely, or the infant will compress the end of the nipple, causing pain to the mother and little milk flow. When the mouth opens widely with the tongue down and over the gums, the mother should quickly bring the infant close to her so that the infant can latch on to the areola. The angle of the open mouth should be approximately 120 to 160 degrees (Smith & Riordan, 2015).

**Position of the mouth.** Assess the position of the infant's mouth on the breast (Fig. 23.8). The infant's lips should be positioned on the areola approximately 2.5 to 3.8 cm (1 to 1½ inches) from the base of the nipple to allow the nipple to be drawn toward the back of the mouth (Lawrence & Lawrence, 2011). This position prevents the infant from sucking on the nipple only and places the gums over the ducts so milk is released into the mouth as the gums compress the breast. The lips should be flared outward and the tongue cupped forward under the breast and over the gums.

**Suckling pattern.** Teach the mother about the infant's suckling pattern. During nutritive suckling, the infant sucks with smooth, continuous movements with occasional pauses to rest. Each suck may be followed by a swallow, or there may be several sucks before the swallow. Nonnutritive sucking is sucking during which little or no milk is obtained. It also refers to sucking on an object such as a pacifier. This type of sucking often occurs when the infant is falling asleep. A fluttery or choppy motion of the jaw with only occasional or no sounds of swallowing indicates nonnutritive sucking.

Mothers often wonder whether their infants are actually receiving milk from the breast. Point out the sound of swallowing when it occurs. A soft "ka" or "ah" sound indicates that the infant is swallowing colostrum or milk.

Explain that periodic short pauses between suckling periods are normal. Caution mothers not to jiggle the breast in the infant's mouth in an effort to start the suckling again. Moving the breast in the mouth may cause the infant to lose the grasp on the nipple and areola, resulting in "chewing" on the nipple and soreness. If necessary, she should take the infant off the breast to awaken the baby and then start again.

**Removal from the breast.** Teach the mother to remove the infant from the breast for burping midway in the feeding or if suckling becomes nonnutritive. Show her how to avoid trauma to the breast by inserting her finger into the corner of the infant's mouth between the gums to break the suction. She then removes the breast quickly before the infant begins to suck again.

**Frequency of feedings.** Breast milk moves through the stomach twice as fast as formula (Blackburn, 2013). Therefore, infants are breastfed every 1.5 to 3 hours, with 8 to 12 feedings every 24 hours (Schanler, 2016). Frequent feedings are especially important in the early days after birth, while lactation is being established and the stomach capacity is small. Explaining that the hormone *prolactin*, which is responsible for milk production, is released in increased amounts while the infant is suckling helps mothers understand the relationship of frequent feeding to milk supply.

During the early weeks of life, infants should be gently awakened every 3 hours for feeding to stimulate milk production (Association of Women's Health, Obstetric, and Neonatal Nurses [AWHONN], 2007). Long periods between feedings increase the likelihood of breast engorgement and decreased stimulation from prolactin.

Some infants vary the length of feedings and time between each feeding. Cluster feeding, when infants want to nurse several times close together, may occur on the second or third night at home or in later weeks when an appetite spurt occurs in the infant (Academy of Breastfeeding Medicine [ABM] Protocol Committee, 2009a). An infant's frequent need to nurse may cause the mother to think her milk supply is inadequate when it is actually normal. Strict scheduling of infant feedings is unnecessary and leads to frustration for both mother and infant. A mother should take her cues from her infant.

**Length of feedings.** Early feedings were once limited to only a few minutes per breast to prevent sore nipples; however, improper positioning, rather than time at breast, is the usual cause of nipple trauma. When feedings are too short, infants receive little or no colostrum or milk. The milk-ejection (let-down) reflex can take as long as 5 minutes to occur at first.

Generally, mothers can allow infants to set the length of feeding. Infants should suck vigorously for a period of time. When choppy, nonnutritive suckling without the sound of swallowing occurs, the mother should burp the infant and offer the other breast. When the infant is satisfied, the suckling pattern changes and the infant falls asleep.

Mothers who are uneasy without a specific length of time for feedings can be instructed to feed for a minimum of 10 to 15 minutes of effective suckling on each side, or longer if the infant continues to nurse vigorously (Orr, 2010). Although variations in the length of feedings occur, early feedings that last less than an average of 20 minutes and occur less than eight times in 24 hours may not be enough (Riordan & Hoover, 2015). Feeding time increases as needed by the infant over the next few days. Teach mothers that longer feedings do not cause sore nipples if the infant is positioned properly.

Explain the differences between **foremilk**, the watery first milk that quenches the infant's thirst, and hindmilk, which is richer in fat, is more satisfying, and leads to weight gain. Feeding for too short a time prevents the infant from getting the hindmilk and decreases weight gain.

Switching back and forth between breasts several times during a feeding increases the amount of foremilk the infant receives but decreases the amount of hindmilk. Therefore, the mother should continue feeding on the first side as long as the infant nurses vigorously, before burping and continuing on the other breast. For each feeding, the mother should alternate the breast offered first so that each breast is completely emptied.

***Preventing problems.*** Nurses can help prevent early problems in several ways.

**Teaching.** Intensive teaching during the short stay in the birth facility helps prevent problems after discharge, when the new mother may have no one to advise her. Check the woman frequently to answer her questions as she thinks of them.

Include suggestions about how to improve positioning and techniques. Discuss common problems that may occur after discharge and offer solutions. Pamphlets and DVDs provide another means of providing education. Review them before use, however, to ensure that the information is correct and that they contain no advertisements for formula. If the birth facility provides classes, telephone calls, home visits, or support groups, explain the service.

**Minimizing interruptions.** Once the mother is breastfeeding well, keep interruptions to a minimum. Ask her if she would like visitors to wait until she is through feeding. Hang a "Do Not Disturb" sign on the door to advise staff and visitors that the mother should not be interrupted. Tell the mother to use her call light to notify the nurse if she needs help or when she is ready for interruptions.

## EVIDENCE-BASED PRACTICE

Breastfeeding mothers are frequently interrupted during a breastfeeding session while in the birth facility. The reasons for interruptions vary but include need for assessments, laboratory tests, housekeeping, or other care needs. Because breastfeeding is a learned skill and having quiet, uninterrupted time together can increase breastfeeding success, Albert and Heinrichs-Breen conducted a small study to determine the effect of using a breastfeeding privacy sign during feeding sessions.

A convenience sample of 46 mother-infant dyads was used for the study. Twenty-three of the dyads (the control group) did not use the sign and received routine care. Mothers kept a feeding log (Study Feeding Diary) noting the date and time of feedings, wet diapers, stools, and number of interruptions during feeding sessions. Before discharge, they completed an Obstetric Research Study Questionnaire with questions pertaining to their feelings about the importance of alone time, feeling they had enough uninterrupted time, perception of the staff's concern for their privacy, perceptions of breastfeeding success, and additional comments. This questionnaire was completed before the study commenced.

The intervention group also consisted of 23 mother-infant dyads. They received routine hospital care but were given a privacy sign to be placed on their door at the beginning of breastfeeding sessions and removed at the end of each session. They were instructed to call the staff if they needed help at any time. The presence of anyone the mother wanted to have with her was not considered an interruption.

Intervention-group mothers kept a feeding log that had an additional column for recording whether or not they used the sign at each feeding. At discharge, they completed the study questionnaire, which had added questions regarding their use of the privacy sign and interruptions that occurred when they used the sign.

There were no differences between the groups in the number of feeding sessions, total minutes of breastfeeding, or day 2 percentage of infant weight loss. However, the intervention-group mothers reported they were interrupted during feeding sessions significantly less often than the control mothers. They also had significantly greater reporting that their breastfeeding sessions were successful. Fourteen of 23 control-group mothers made comments indicating that interruptions during feeding sessions were disturbing.

Are privacy measures for breastfeeding mothers in place at your facility? If not, what else besides a privacy sign could be used to help avoid interruptions during breastfeeding sessions? What effects of interruptions during breastfeeding have you seen in your patients?

Reference: Albert, J., & Heinrichs-Breen, J. (2011). An evaluation of a breastfeeding privacy sign to prevent interruptions and promote successful breastfeeding. *Journal of Obstetric, Gynecologic and Neonatal Nursing, 40*(3), 274–280.

**Formula gift packs.** Receiving a formula gift pack may be problematic in some situations. Having formula available may lead to an expectation for some parents that formula will be necessary. This message is contrary to the message nurses should give about breastfeeding. Gift packs that do not have formula are more appropriate for breastfeeding mothers.

**Formula supplements.** Avoid use of formula supplementation in the hospital unless there are medical indications. Supplements may lessen the success of breastfeeding because they decrease feeding from the breast and decrease milk production (AAP & ACOG, 2012; Schanler, 2016). A national goal is to reduce the proportion of breastfed newborns who receive formula in the first 2 days of life to no more than 15.6% (USDHHS, 2010). In 2011, nearly 19.4% of breastfed infants received formula before they were 2 days old (CDC, 2014).

Early initiation of breastfeeding is very important. The healthy newborn whose mother wishes to breastfeed should begin breastfeeding within the first hour after birth. Teach mothers that supplementing with formula will not lead to more sleep during the night.

**Insufficient milk supply.** One of the major reasons for early weaning to formula is parents' perception of insufficient milk supply. Women with positive attitudes toward breastfeeding and confidence that they will produce enough milk are less likely to wean early because of perceived lack of enough milk. Explain the normal course of breastfeeding and methods of handling problems to help mothers feel more confident in their abilities.

Teach the parents how to assess swallowing and nutritive suckling. Discuss ways to determine if the infant is receiving enough milk. Counting the number of wet and soiled diapers may be helpful. Infants should have at least three or four wet diapers and three or four stools a day by day 3 after birth (Janke, 2014). After that time, the normal breastfed infant should have at least four or more stools daily (Lawrence & Lawrence, 2011). There should be at least six wet diapers by day 4. Intake can also be gauged when weight gain is assessed. After the initial weight loss, infants generally gain approximately 20 to 30 g (0.7 to 1 oz) daily during the early months (Keane, 2011).

Common causes of decreased milk supply include ineffective suckling by the infant, feedings that are infrequent or too short, maternal fatigue, low maternal thyroid function, preterm or late preterm infants, and some medications including oral contraceptives containing estrogen. Intervene appropriately if any common causes are present.

Because the breasts are soft and the mother does not see large amounts of milk during the first few days, she may believe that little or none is present. This may lead her to give the infant formula before or after the feeding, decreasing milk production. Teach mothers who need to increase milk supply to feed more often and use a breast pump after feedings. If problems persist, refer the mother to a lactation consultant. These professionals are often available in the birth facility and in the community. They can help with the techniques of breastfeeding and special problems.

***Increasing confidence.*** Use every opportunity to offer praise and reinforcement of the woman's ability to breastfeed her infant. Point out the infant's positive response to the mother's handling and feeding. Mention the improvements she makes in recognizing hunger cues, positioning, latch-on, and other aspects of care. The nurse's support and encouragement will help the woman feel more confident with each feeding and may lead to longer duration of breastfeeding.

***Providing resources.*** Women who stop breastfeeding before they originally planned to stop may cite nipple pain, problems with latch-on, the belief that their milk supply was insufficient, and returning to work as their reasons. Giving them contact information for lactation consultants, support groups, the local La Leche League (http://www.llli.org), and other breastfeeding resources in their area may help them continue breastfeeding. Providing written material and Internet resources such as http://www.womenshealth.gov/breastfeeding is also helpful.

### Evaluation

- Does the infant nurse for 10 to 15 minutes or more per breast, with good latch-on and nutritive suckling?
- Does the mother use correct techniques for latch-on and positioning?
- Does the mother say she feels confident about the process?

### MOTHERS WANT TO KNOW

#### *Is My Baby Getting Enough Milk?*

Your baby is probably getting enough milk if:

- You hear the baby swallow frequently during feedings. It sounds like a soft "ka" or "ah" sound.
- You see nutritive suckling—a smooth series of sucking and swallowing with occasional rest periods. This pattern is different from short, choppy sucks that occur when the baby is falling asleep and not getting milk. After the first few days, you may feel a tingling of your nipples as a new let-down reflex occurs. This sensation is followed by more nutritive suckling as the infant swallows the increased milk available.
- Your breast is getting softer during the feeding. (However, your breasts do not have to be hard [engorged] for you to have enough milk.)
- You can see milk in the baby's mouth or dripping from your breast occasionally.
- You feed your baby 8 to 12 times every 24 hours. When you nurse often, you produce more milk.
- Your baby has at least one or two wet diapers daily by day 2 after birth, at least three wet diapers a day by day 3, and at least six wet diapers by day 4. If you are unsure if the diaper is wet, place a tissue or cotton ball inside it to show small amounts of urine. Urine should be light (not dark) yellow.
- By day 3, your baby passes at least three bowel movements and at least four stools a day after that time. The bowel movements are yellow by day 4.
- Your baby seems satisfied after feedings. Babies remain quietly awake or go to sleep for at least an hour after most feedings. (An occasional fussy time is not unusual and does not mean that the baby is not getting enough to eat.)
- Well-baby checks show that your baby is gaining weight.

## COMMON BREASTFEEDING CONCERNS

Because mothers may be discharged from the birth facility before problems arise, nurses should teach them how to prevent and treat common problems.

When the mother seeks help for problems, the nurse should ask the mother what has been done to try to solve the problem. It is important to ask about any complementary or alternative therapies the mother may have tried. The safety of any therapy should be determined.

Teas made from herbs such as orange spice, fenugreek, and raspberry are considered safe during lactation. However, no herbal tea should be consumed in large quantities (Lawrence & Lawrence, 2011; Skidmore-Roth, 2010). The mother may have used other herbs to encourage milk production. Because there has not been adequate research on the use of these therapies, she should be referred to the healthcare provider for information before using any substances, as some may be harmful.

Breastfeeding problems can be divided into those originating with the infant and those pertaining to the mother.

### Infant Problems

Infant problems require prompt attention to ensure successful breastfeeding.

**SAFETY ALERT**

***Infant Signs of Breastfeeding Problems***

- Falling asleep after feeding less than 5 minutes
- Refusal to breastfeed
- Tongue thrusting
- Smacking or clicking sounds
- Dimpling of the cheeks
- Failure to open mouth wide at latch-on
- Lower lip turned in
- Short, choppy motions of jaw
- No audible swallowing
- Use of formula

#### Sleepy Infant

During the first few days after birth, infants often sleep longer than expected or fall asleep at the breast after feeding for only a short time. They may be tired from the birth and may not respond appropriately to hunger. The nurse should show mothers how to arouse sleepy infants for breastfeeding. When infants fall asleep during feedings, the nurse should evaluate whether the infant has fed adequately, should be awakened to feed longer, or should be fed again sooner than usual. Irritating stimuli should not be used to awaken infants, because feedings should be associated with pleasurable feelings. Infants who continue to be excessively sleepy or to nurse poorly need further evaluation. Poor feeding may be an early sign of a complication such as sepsis (see Chapter 30).

#### Nipple Confusion

Nipple confusion (or nipple preference) can occur when an infant who has received bottle feedings confuses the tongue movements necessary for bottle feeding with the suckling of breastfeeding. Some infants may refuse to breastfeed or may use tongue movements that push the breast out of the mouth.

Movement of the mouth and tongue are different in breastfeeding and bottle feeding. In bottle feeding, infants must push their tongue over the latex nipple of a bottle to slow the flow of milk and prevent choking. The lips are relaxed because the infant does not need to hold the nipple in the mouth. If the infant uses the same thrusting tongue motion and relaxed lips while nursing, the breast can be pushed out of the mouth.

Nurses should discourage the use of formula in normal breastfeeding infants. It reduces breastfeeding time, which decreases prolactin secretion, and thus, milk supply. Formula takes longer to digest, and the infant is not hungry again for approximately 4 hours. The resulting decrease in breast stimulation can lead to engorgement.

Although some parents find pacifiers helpful, their use may be associated with suckling problems and an earlier weaning of infants from the breast. Some infants can use a pacifier without ensuing problems with breastfeeding, but their use should be discouraged at least until the infant is breastfeeding successfully. Although pacifiers are advised as one way to prevent sudden infant death syndrome, their use can be delayed for the first month to help establish breastfeeding (AAP, 2012).

#### Latch-on Problems

Suckling problems may occur when the nipple is poorly positioned in the mouth. Dimpling of the cheeks and smacking or clicking sounds may indicate that the infant is sucking on the tongue or nipple only. Some infants do not open their mouths widely and suck on the end of the nipple.

Inserting a gloved finger into the infant's mouth helps assess suckling. The motion of the tongue should be felt as the infant sucks. The infant who is thrusting the tongue may have become confused by the use of artificial nipples, which should be avoided until the problem is resolved. The tongue should be cupped under the breast and covering the lower gum. Helping the infant open the mouth widely before attachment may improve suckling. More complicated suckling problems may require assistance from a lactation consultant.

#### Infant Complications

Infant complications may be minor and cause minimal interference with breastfeeding or may prevent the infant from breastfeeding for a long period.

***Jaundice.*** Concern over adequate intake may be more prevalent in caring for the infant with jaundice. However, jaundice (hyperbilirubinemia) need not interfere with breastfeeding in most cases. Even when infants receive phototherapy, they can usually be removed from the lights for feedings. The mother should have help in giving frequent feedings with good latch to ensure optimum milk intake. Infants receiving phototherapy should not be given extra water because it may decrease the intake of breast milk. In addition, breastfeeding provides adequate intake of protein and fluid and increases the number of stools, decreasing intestinal reabsorption of bilirubin and aiding in its excretion. In some cases, supplementary formula may be necessary, but breastfeeding should continue.

***Prematurity.*** If the preterm infant cannot breastfeed immediately after birth, the mother needs encouragement and instruction on how to use a breast pump to establish and maintain her milk supply. Breast milk offers immunologic and nutritional benefits and is adapted to preterm needs. Breast milk can help to prevent or minimize the severity of necrotizing enterocolitis, a serious complication of prematurity. It also helps the mother feel she is providing care for her infant even if she cannot take the infant home with her. The woman can pump her milk and take it to the nursery for the infant's feedings. The nurse should provide sterile containers for the woman to take home and instruct her in special nursery requirements. The containers need to be labeled with the infant's name and the date and time the milk was pumped.

Some infants who are preterm or have other breastfeeding problems respond well to the use of supplementary feeding devices. These devices consist of a container of milk with a small plastic feeding tube attached to the breast. When the infant begins to breastfeed, milk is drawn from both the container and the breast. This system increases the infant's intake and motivation to continue suckling and provides stimulation to the breast. As the infant gains weight and its feeding ability increases, use of the device is gradually decreased until it can be discontinued completely.

Women who provide breast milk for their preterm infants may feel something is wrong with their milk when additions such as human milk fortifier are used. They should be reassured that their milk is very important in providing protection against infection and good nutrition but that the infant needs more of some nutrients during the period of very rapid growth.

***Late preterm infants.*** Infants born between the beginning of the 34th week of gestation and the end of the 36th week are called *late preterm infants.* Although they may look like full-term infants, they have many characteristics of preterm infants and often need extra help to breastfeed successfully. They may have poor coordination of sucking, swallowing, and breathing and may be sleepier than full-term infants.

## NURSING CARE PLAN

### *Breastfeeding an Infant With a Complication*

**Focused Assessment**

Ruth's son, David, is full term but develops complications at birth and is admitted to the neonatal intensive care unit. He will probably not be able to feed at the breast for a few days. His mother is disappointed and worried about whether she will be able to breastfeed at all.

**Nursing Diagnosis**

Interrupted Breastfeeding related to separation from infant secondary to illness.

**Planning**

**Expected Outcomes**

Within 2 days, Ruth will:

1. Verbalize the importance of breastfeeding her infant and her desire to maintain lactation.
2. Pump her breasts as taught.
3. Breastfeed her infant successfully (when it becomes possible).

**Interventions and *Rationales***

1. Explore Ruth's perception of the problem and her understanding of the cause for separation and the effect on breastfeeding.
   *This helps identify misconceptions and determines the type of teaching and support required.*
2. Use therapeutic communication to help her express her feelings of disappointment with the unexpected change in plans.
   *Expression of feelings may help her cope with the situation.*
3. Explain the value of breast milk for her infant.
   *This helps her understand the importance of breastfeeding.*
4. Teach her to use a breast pump. Instruct her to pump her breasts for approximately 15 to 20 minutes at least eight times in 24 hours.
   *Frequent use of a breast pump helps establish lactation by causing release of prolactin and oxytocin so that milk is produced and released from the breasts.*
5. Frequent pumping should prevent engorgement, but explain prevention and treatment of engorgement.
   *This will help prepare her for the possibility of engorgement.*
6. Teach Ruth how to store her milk and how to prepare it for use for her infant. Feed David breast milk if possible, whether by bottle or gavage.
   *Breast milk has properties that are especially valuable for the sick infant.*
7. Arrange for Ruth to spend as much time with her son as possible. Stay with her as she begins to breastfeed to answer her questions and provide support.
   *The nurse's presence provides support and an opportunity for teaching as needed.*
8. Offer praise and realistic encouragement frequently.
   *This will help increase her confidence.*
9. If she must go home before her son is ready for discharge, provide Ruth with information about purchase or rental of electric breast pumps.
   *Electric breast pumps are more effi cient than hand or battery pumps.*
   Give her containers to bring her milk into the nursery.

**Evaluation**

Ruth discusses her determination to provide breast milk for her son. She maintains lactation and brings breast milk to each visit. At 3 days of age, David is ready to begin breastfeeding. Ruth is very patient in helping her son learn to breastfeed with the nurses' help. David is able to nurse well at each feeding by the time of discharge.

They are at greater risk of difficulty with breastfeeding, jaundice, and the need for hospital readmission.

A lactation consultant should be involved in teaching the mother about her infant's special needs and in monitoring the effectiveness of feedings (AWHONN, 2010; Radke, 2011). Infants need to be positioned so that the head is supported, as with the football hold. Infants should be seen by a healthcare provider within 1 to 2 days after discharge to check the weight, adequacy of feeding, and jaundice. Frequent visits and weight checks should be made for any infants having feeding difficulties. Weekly weight checks should be performed until the infant reaches 40 weeks postconceptional age (ABM, 2011).

***Illness and congenital defects.*** Infant illness and congenital defects such as a cleft palate may cause breastfeeding problems. If the mother is unable to nurse, she will need assistance to maintain lactation until nursing is possible. Referral to support groups can be particularly helpful.

## Maternal Concerns

### SAFETY ALERT

### *Maternal Signs of Breastfeeding Problems*

- Hard, tender breasts
- Painful, red, cracked, blistered, or bleeding nipples
- Flat or inverted nipples
- Localized edema or pain in either breast
- Fever, generalized aching, or malaise

### Common Breast Problems

Early nursing intervention can help the mother overcome common breast problems.

***Engorgement.*** Many women have a temporary swelling or fullness of the breasts that begins on days 2 through 4 after birth, when the production of milk begins to increase or the milk "comes in." This normal, temporary engorgement should not interfere with breastfeeding.

Engorgement may become a problem if feedings are delayed or too short. The breasts become edematous, hard, and tender, making feeding or even movement painful. The areola may become so hard that the infant cannot compress it to nurse. The nipple can become flat, making it more difficult for the infant to draw it to the back of the mouth. Engorgement can lead to nipple trauma, mastitis (infection of the breasts), and even the discontinuation of breastfeeding.

***Nipple pain.*** Nipple pain lasting a minute or less at the beginning of feedings may occur during early breastfeeding as the infant stretches the tissue. Nipple pain usually peaks on days 3 to 6 after birth and resolves soon after (Smith & Riordan, 2015). Nipple trauma causes more sustained pain. Traumatized nipples appear red, cracked, blistered, or bleeding (Fig. 23.9). Minor nipple trauma can be treated by independent nursing interventions. Redness of breast tissue, purulent drainage, and fever indicate mastitis or breast abscess, requiring antibiotic treatment (see Chapter 28).

***Flat and inverted nipples.*** Nipple rolling just before feeding helps flat nipples become more erect so that the infant can grasp them more readily (Fig. 23.10, p. 492). A breast pump used for a few minutes just before feedings may help draw out inverted nipples.

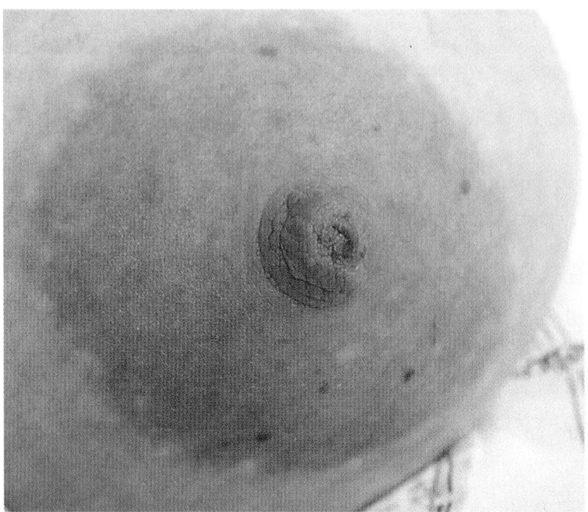

FIG 23.9 Note the cracked area on this nipple.

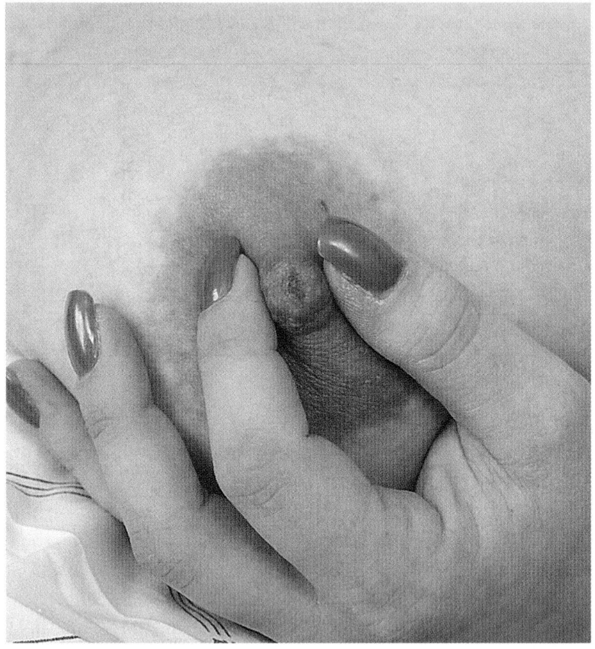

FIG 23.10 Rolling helps flat nipples become erect in preparation for latch-on.

*Plugged ducts.* Although the exact cause of occlusion of a lactiferous duct is unknown, engorgement, missed feedings, or a constricting bra may be involved. Localized edema and tenderness are present, and a hard area may be palpated. A tiny white area may be present on the nipple. Massage of the area (Fig. 23.11) followed by heat and continued breastfeeding using varied positions helps the duct to open. A plugged duct may progress to mastitis if not treated promptly. Mastitis involves localized pain accompanied by fever, generalized aching, and malaise.

### Illness in the Mother

It is seldom necessary for a mother to stop breastfeeding when she is ill. If breastfeeding must be temporarily stopped, the nurse should assist the mother in using a breast pump, if she wishes, until breastfeeding resumes. Abrupt weaning may lead to mastitis.

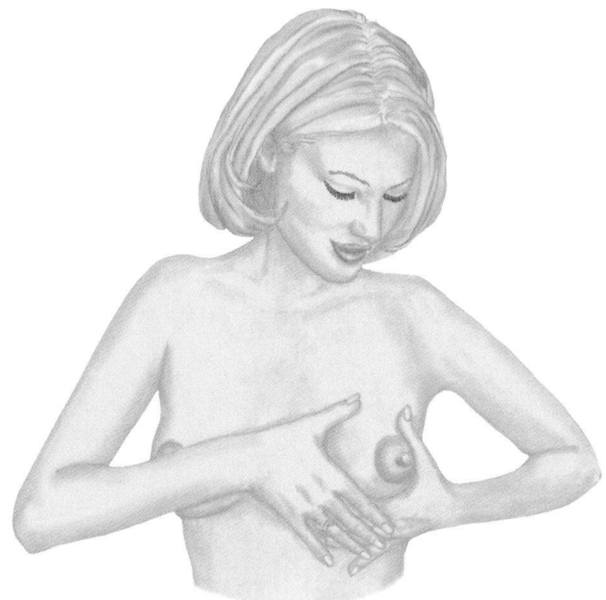

FIG 23.11 To massage the breasts, the mother places her hands against the chest wall with her fingers encircling the breasts. She gently slides her hands forward until the fingers overlap. The position of the hands is rotated to cover all breast tissue. Massaging with the fingertips in a circular motion over all areas of the breast also is helpful.

*Drug transfer to breast milk.* Most medications taken by the mother cross into the breast milk to some degree, but many pass in small amounts and are safe during lactation. Some drugs interfere with milk production. Use of both prescription and over-the-counter drugs should be approved by the healthcare provider. Another drug can often be substituted for one that adversely affects the infant. If a mother must take a drug that will be harmful to her infant, she should pump her breasts while she is taking the medication. Once the drug clears her bloodstream, she can resume breastfeeding (see Appendix B at http://evolve.elsevier.com/McKinney/mat-ch/). Some drugs may not reach the infant in harmful amounts if taken after a feeding or at night when there is a longer time between feedings. The U.S. National Library of Medicine has a website regarding the safety of drugs during lactation at http://toxnet.nlm.nih.gov.

*Conditions in which breastfeeding should be avoided.* In some situations, breastfeeding is contraindicated.

Examples are active untreated tuberculosis, human immunodeficiency virus (HIV) infection, galactosemia, maternal chemotherapy, and mothers who must take drugs that are unsafe for the infant. Maternal drug abuse is also usually a contraindication. Mothers with hepatitis A, B, or C may breastfeed. Infants of mothers with hepatitis B should receive hepatitis B vaccine and immune globulin. Mothers with herpes simplex may breastfeed if they have no lesions of their breasts and they use good handwashing (AAP & ACOG, 2012; Holt et al., 2011; Stettler, Bhatia, Parish, et al., 2011).

### Previous Breast Surgery

Women who have had surgery for breast reduction or augmentation may have difficulty with lactation. The type of surgical technique used and the amount of tissue involved determine breastfeeding ability. Surgery may disrupt the neural pathways, ducts, and blood supply. Some women can breastfeed without problem, and others may be able to do so by pumping or using a supplementation device to help build up milk supply if milk production is low.

## PATIENT-CENTERED TEACHING

### *Solutions to Common Breastfeeding Problems*

**Problem: Sleepy Infant**

Infant is sleepy at feeding time or falls asleep shortly after beginning feeding.

***Prevention***

- Unwrap the baby's blankets, and leave them off as you begin the feeding, keeping the baby skin-to-skin against your chest. Your body and a blanket added later will provide adequate warmth.
- If the infant continues to sleep, look for signs that he or she is ready to wake up, such as movement of the eyes through closed eyelids, small twitches or grimaces, sucking movements, or increased movements of the entire body.
- Gently awaken your baby when you see those signs. Talk, gently move the infant's arms and legs, and play with the infant for a short time before beginning the feeding.

***Solutions***

If your baby goes to sleep during the feeding and has fed less than 5 minutes, try the following:

- Remove the baby from the breast. Rub the infant's back to bring up bubbles of air and help awaken the baby.
- Change the diaper.
- Undress the baby except for the diaper and place the infant against your skin (if you have not done this already).
- Rub the baby's hair or cheeks gently, stroke around the mouth, or shift the baby's position slightly to see if the infant will wake up.
- Express a few drops of colostrum onto the nipple. The baby tastes the colostrum when the nipple is offered and often begins renewed suckling.
- Wipe the baby's face with a lukewarm washcloth to help wakening.
- If your baby cannot be aroused with a few of these gentle techniques, a longer sleep period may be needed. Let the infant sleep another half hour and then begin again. Watch for signs that the baby is in a lighter phase of sleep and can be awakened more easily.

**Problem: Nipple Confusion**

An infant who has taken bottles pushes the nipple out of the mouth and sucks poorly during breastfeeding. Infant is using sucking movements needed for bottle feeding.

***Prevention***

- Avoid all bottles and pacifiers unless necessary. If they are necessary, stop as soon as possible.
- Do not give the baby formula during the night.
- Avoid giving formula before or after breastfeeding because it is unnecessary for healthy newborns. It may cause the infant's stomach to become distended, resulting in more "spitting up." If the infant waits longer before nursing again, milk production will decrease.

***Solution***

Stop all bottle feeding and pacifier use so that the baby becomes accustomed to suckling from the breast instead of the bottle. Nurse more often to stimulate milk production and help the baby learn what to do.

**Problem: Latch-on Difficulty**

Infant sucks on the end of the nipple or fails to open the mouth widely enough.

***Prevention***

- Do not insert the breast into the infant's mouth until the infant opens the mouth wide with the tongue down and forward (like biting into a large sandwich). Then bring the baby to the breast.
- Pull down gently on the infant's chin to help the infant open the mouth wider if necessary.
- Be sure the nipple is at the back of the mouth and 1 to 1½ inches of the areola is in the mouth.

***Solution***

Stop the feeding and start again if the infant is sucking on the end of the nipple, if you see dimples in the infant's cheeks, or hear smacking or clicking sounds.

**Problem: Engorgement**

The mother's breasts are hard and tender from engorgement.

***Prevention***

- Breastfeed the infant every 2 to 3 hours day and night.
- Do not give bottles during the day or night.

***Solutions***

- To reduce edema and pain, apply cold packs to the breasts between feedings. Make inexpensive cold packs from frozen washcloths, a bag of frozen vegetables, or plastic bags filled with crushed ice. Cover cold packs with a washcloth before applying to the skin. A disposable diaper with ice placed between the layers can also be used.
- Some women find that application of cool cabbage leaves is helpful. Studies on their use report mixed results (Lawrence & Lawrence, 2011; Riordan & Hoover, 2015).
- Just before feedings, apply heat with compresses made with warm, wet washcloths or disposable diapers applied over each breast. Fasten the tabs to keep the diapers in place and prevent dripping. Or take a shower to stimulate milk flow.
- Massage the breasts before and during feedings to stimulate the let-down reflex.
- If the areolae are engorged, making it hard for your baby to latch on, express a little milk by hand or with a breast pump, or apply gentle pressure on the areola to move some swelling back into the breast and soften the areola to allow the infant to latch. As soon as the areolae are soft, begin to feed.
- Feed more often—every 1.5 to 2 hours.
- Wear a well-fitting bra for support during the day and at night for comfort.
- To help you feel more comfortable, take prescribed pain medication just before feedings.

**Problem: Nipple Pain**

Nipples are sore, cracked, blistered, or bleeding.

***Prevention***

- Position the baby at the breast with enough of the areola in the mouth that the nipple is not compressed between the baby's gums during nursing.
- Avoid engorgement by nursing frequently. Express enough milk to soften the areola if it becomes too hard for the infant to grasp.
- Vary the position of the baby to change the areas of pressure on the nipple.
- Do not use soap on the nipples because it removes the protective oils and causes drying.
- If you use breast pads for leaking milk, remove them when they become wet to prevent skin irritation. Avoid pads with plastic linings that retain moisture.

***Solutions***

- Use warm-water compresses or massage the breasts just before the feedings to help the milk flow more quickly.
- Apply warm water compresses between feedings to soothe nipples.

*Continued*

## PATIENT-CENTERED TEACHING—cont'd

### *Solutions to Common Breastfeeding Problems*

- Begin each feeding with the less sore side first. The let-down reflex causes milk to flow more quickly in the second breast.
- Massage the breast to encourage milk flow when the infant pauses in suckling.
- Vary the position of the infant during nursing. The area of the nipple directly in line with the infant's nose and chin is most stressed during the feeding.
- Nipple shields (artificial nipples that fit over your own nipples) may be helpful in some situations. A lactation consultant should help you to use them temporarily.
- Breast creams may cause sensitivity and irritation. If you choose to use lanolin for sore nipples, use only the purified form to protect against allergens and pesticides. Creams that must be removed before each feeding may increase soreness. Hydrogel may also be used to soothe nipples.
- Expose the nipples to air between feedings by lowering the flaps of your nursing bra, or use a breast shell to keep clothing from rubbing on the nipples.
- If you have burning, itching, or stabbing pain throughout your breast, look in the baby's mouth for the white patches of thrush, a yeast infection that can infect the nipples. Call your healthcare provider for medication to treat both you and your baby.
- Take prescribed pain medication just before feedings to help you relax.

**Problem: Flat or Inverted Nipples**

The baby has difficulty drawing flat or inverted nipples into the mouth.

***Prevention***

None.

***Solutions***

- Some women find that wearing breast shells in the bra helps the nipples to protrude.
- Just before beginning breastfeeding, roll the nipple between your thumb and forefinger to help it protrude (see Fig. 23.11).
- Use a breast pump just before feedings. Put the baby to your breast immediately after the pump causes the nipple to become erect. The normal suckling process usually causes the nipple to stay erect.
- A nipple shield may be used for a short time with the help of a lactation consultant to aid the infant in latching-on to inverted nipples correctly.

Reference: Lawrence, R.A., & Lawrence, R.M. (2011) *Breastfeeding: A guide for the medical profession* (7th ed.). Philadelphia: Mosby; Riordan, J., & Hoover, K. (2010). Perinatal and intrapartum care. In J. Riordan (Ed.), *Breastfeeding and human lactation* (4th ed., pp. 215–251). Boston: Jones & Bartlett.

### Employment

Although some women remain at home for 6 weeks or more after birth, others must return to work earlier. Breastfeeding offers many advantages for working women: mothers are less likely to miss work because of an ill infant, time and expense for formula preparation are unnecessary, and the mother can continue to provide nourishment for her infant. Breastfeeding can be combined very well with working if the woman does some advanced planning. Breastfeeding classes and support groups are often helpful in providing practical advice from nurses on how to merge employment with lactation.

The mother will need to purchase a breast pump. Breast pumps are covered under most insurance plans without a co-pay. A week or two before she returns to work, the mother can begin using a breast pump once or twice a day to practice pumping her breasts and to build up a small supply of frozen breast milk. Once breastfeeding has been well established, the woman can give the infant a bottle of breast milk occasionally to help the infant adjust more easily.

Most working mothers use a pump at work two or three times daily during lunch and breaks. The woman needs a clean, private place where she can pump. A national goal is to increase the proportion of employers that have worksite lactation support programs such as a specific place for mothers to pump (USDHHS, 2010). The milk should be refrigerated or placed in an insulated container with ice to be used by the caregiver for later feedings when the mother is at work. Breastfeeding just before the mother goes to work and when she returns home decreases the time between feedings. Frequent breastfeeding during the evenings and weekends will help to maintain her milk supply.

### Milk Expression and Storage

When milk expression is needed, the nurse teaches the mother to use hand expression (Fig. 23.12) or a breast pump (Fig. 23.13).

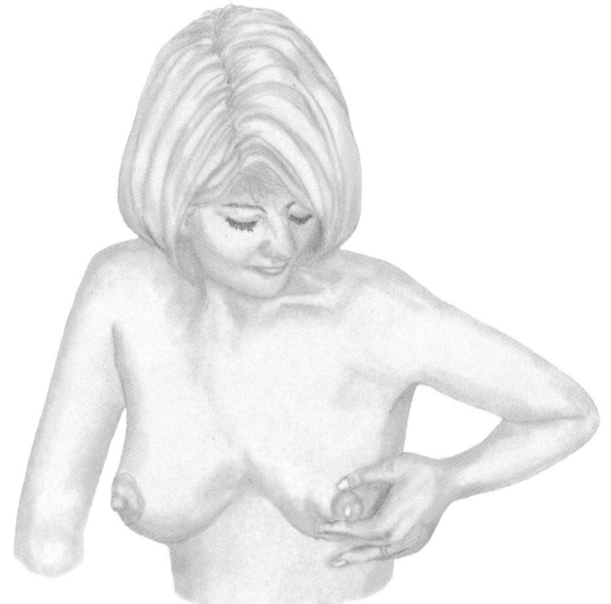

**FIG 23.12** To express milk from the breast, the mother places her hand just behind the areola, with the thumb on top and the fingers supporting the breast. The tissue is pressed back against the chest wall; then the fingers and thumb are brought together and toward the nipple to cause the milk to flow. The action is repeated to simulate the infant's suckling. Moving the hands around the areola allows compression of all areas and complete removal of milk from the breast. Compression should be gentle to avoid trauma.

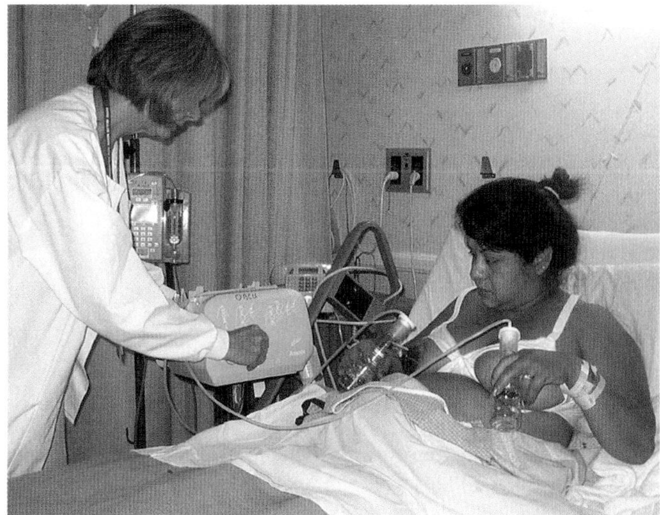

FIG 23.13 The nurse helps the mother to use an electric breast pump.

*Hand expression.* Hand expression can be done without other equipment but is usually not as effective as a breast pump. Hand expression or manual pumps are useful for the mother who wants to save breast milk for another feeding occasionally or whose areolae are so engorged that the infant cannot grasp them.

*Use of a breast pump.* The mother who plans to pump her milk for a prolonged period should use an electric breast pump. Battery-operated pumps are small, portable, and relatively inexpensive for short-term use. Large electric pumps can be rented for home use. Women who receive WIC services may also be able to borrow a breast pump from their local WIC facility. Electric pumps are more efficient than hand or battery pumps and are indicated when the mother must pump to maintain her milk supply for a long time. A double pump allows the mother to pump both breasts at once, saving time and increasing milk production.

Use of the breast pump should begin as soon as possible after birth if the woman cannot breastfeed her infant. She should pump her breasts approximately as often as her baby would nurse or at least eight times daily if she plans to breastfeed for a prolonged time. Sessions should last approximately 10 to 15 minutes (Hurst & Meier, 2015).

The mother should wash her hands before using the pump and before preparing pumped milk for storage or feeding. Use of massage and heat before pumping helps initiate milk flow. Massage during pumping may increase the volume of milk obtained.

The amount of pump suction should be set at a low level in the beginning and gradually increased, if necessary. Too much negative pressure traumatizes the breast. If the woman needs to increase her milk supply, pumping more often rather than for longer periods is most effective. The pump should be cleaned according to the manufacturer's instruction after each use.

*Milk storage.* Milk should be stored in clean glass or rigid polypropylene containers with a tight cap. The containers should be sterile if the infant is hospitalized. Plastic bags are more likely to spill or tear (Hurst & Meier, 2015). A nipple should not be used to cap the milk during storage because the hole allows passage of organisms.

Fresh, unrefrigerated breast milk should be used within 1 hour of pumping. Breast milk can be kept in a refrigerator for 48 hours. Milk that is fresh or has been refrigerated rather than frozen should be used as much as possible so that the leukocytes are available for the infant (Hurst & Meier, 2015).

If the milk is to be frozen, it should be placed in a freezer within 24 hours and kept at −18°C (0°F). It can be kept frozen in the back of a refrigerator freezer for 1 month and in a deep freeze for 6 months (Lawrence & Lawrence, 2011). Milk should be frozen in amounts that are likely to be used for one feeding. Containers should be marked with the date, and the oldest should be used first. Newly pumped milk should not be added to containers of previously pumped milk.

Breast milk should be thawed in a refrigerator or by holding the container under running water. It can be kept in a refrigerator for 24 hours after thawing, if necessary. Thawed breast milk can be warmed under warm running water or in a bowl of warm water rather than by heating it. It should not be refrozen or heated in a microwave. Thawed breast milk should be gently inverted a few times to mix the foremilk and the hindmilk. Milk that is not finished in one feeding should be discarded.

### Breastfeeding After Multiple Births

Mothers who have more than one newborn need help and support from nurses and family members. Explain to the mother that her milk supply adjusts to the demand and that she can make enough milk for her infants. Nursing every 2 to 3 hours to build up the milk supply is important. If the infants cannot breastfeed at first, the woman will need assistance in using a breast pump.

If the woman decides to feed two infants simultaneously, she will need help positioning them using the football (clutch) hold, cradle hold, or a combination of both. She should be encouraged to eat well, get enough rest, and ask for help from family and friends.

### Weaning

There is no one "right" time to wean the infant. Mothers choose to wean their infants for a variety of reasons. The nurse should provide information so that the mother can make an informed decision about weaning and should support the woman once her decision is made. Explaining that even a short period of breastfeeding offers her infant many advantages is reassuring.

Mothers may need help in planning a gradual weaning process to help avoid engorgement and allow the infant to get used to a bottle or cup slowly. Omitting one breastfeeding session a day and waiting several days or a week before omitting another will allow the mother and infant to adjust to the change more easily. Infants who are weaned before 12 months should be given iron-fortified formula instead of cow's milk (Holt et al., 2011).

### Home Care

Many infants have not breastfed well by the time of discharge from the birth facility, placing them at risk for failure to gain weight, dehydration, and hyperbilirubinemia. Problems with engorgement and sore nipples are more likely to occur after discharge. The infant should be seen by the physician or other healthcare provider 3 to 5 days after birth and again at 2 weeks of age to assess for any problems than might occur early after discharge (Noble, 2014).

The nurse can refer mothers to lactation consultants or organizations such as the La Leche League, a support group that gives assistance to breastfeeding mothers. La Leche League chapters are available in most communities and are listed in the telephone book. Support groups may also be provided by the birth facility.

### Other Concerns

Mothers may have questions about smoking, alcohol use, or foods they should avoid. See Chapter 14 for information about these concerns.

## FORMULA FEEDING

Formula feeding requires less knowledge and skill than breastfeeding, but the inexperienced parent often has many questions and may need assistance in learning to use formula correctly. Although breastfeeding is preferable in most situations, the nurse should support the woman who has decided to use formula.

## NURSING CARE

### Formula Feeding

#### Assessment

Assess the mother's knowledge of bottle feeding. Ask if she has fed an infant before, and elicit questions. Note how she holds the infant and bottle and evaluate her burping technique to identify problems. Point out infant feeding cues, which are the same for breast- and formula-fed infants.

#### Nursing Diagnosis and Planning

Because improper formula preparation and feeding techniques could harm the infant, an appropriate nursing diagnosis for the mother using formula feeding is:

- Risk for Ineffective Health Maintenance (infant) related to mother's lack of understanding of formula preparation and feeding techniques.

**Expected outcomes.** Before discharge, the mother will demonstrate correct techniques in holding the infant and bottle during feedings and will correctly describe how to prepare formula and the frequency of feedings.

#### Interventions

**Teaching about Formula.** The mother must learn about types of formula and how to prepare them.

**Types of formula.** Formula may be purchased in three different forms. All formula should be iron fortified.

**Ready-to-use.** Ready-to-use formula is available in bottles to which a nipple is added or in cans to be poured directly into a bottle. It should not be diluted. Although expensive, it is practical for traveling, when there is difficulty mixing the formula, or if water supply is in question. An open can should be refrigerated and used within 48 hours.

**Concentrated liquid.** Explain to the parents how to dilute concentrated liquid formula. Equal parts of concentrated liquid and water are mixed together in a bottle to provide the amount desired for each feeding. Opened cans should be stored in the refrigerator and used within 48 hours (Janke, 2014).

**Powdered formula.** Powdered formula is more economical and is particularly useful when a breastfeeding mother plans to give an occasional bottle of formula. Usually one level scoop of powder is added to each 2 oz of water in a bottle. Single-portion packets of powder are available for travel. Formula should be well mixed to dissolve the powder and make the solution uniform. New formula should be prepared for each feeding. Powdered formula is not sterile and may not be appropriate for preterm or immunocompromised infants.

**Equipment.** Many different types of bottles and nipples are available. Mothers may use glass or plastic bottles or a plastic liner that fits into a rigid container. Selection of the type of bottles and nipples depends on individual preference. Bottles and nipples should be free of bisphenol-A (BPA), which may be harmful to infants. Glass, polyethylene, and polypropylene bottles do not contain BPA (Morin, 2008).

**Preparation.** Teach the mother how to prepare formula correctly. Good handwashing is essential before beginning preparation. The top of the can and the can opener should be washed. Infection may occur if the milk or water used for preparation is contaminated. Emphasize the importance of following the directions on the label to mix the formula. Improper dilution of the formula may cause undernutrition or imbalances of sodium, which can be dangerous to the infant.

> **SAFETY ALERT**
>
> ***Formula Dilution***
>
> Formulas must be properly diluted to prevent serious illness and to promote weight gain and growth in the infant.
>
> - *Ready-to-use preparations:* use as is without dilution.
> - *Concentrated formulas:* dilute with equal parts of water.
> - *Powdered formulas:* mix 1 scoop of powder with 2 oz of water.

The mother can prepare a single bottle or a 24-hour supply. Although it is a good idea to sterilize equipment before the first time it is used, subsequent sterilization is not necessary if the water supply is safe. Bottles and nipples can be washed in a dishwasher or in hot, sudsy water using a brush to clean well and then rinsed.

Water mixed with formula should not contain any additives and should be boiled for 1 minute (Kleinman & Greer, 2014). If well water is used, it should be tested for high levels of nitrates. The formula and water are poured into the bottles, which are then capped. Prepared bottles should be used within 24 hours (Kleinman & Greer, 2014).

Explain that if the safety of the water supply is questionable, sterilization, by aseptic or terminal method, is necessary. In both methods, all equipment is washed and rinsed well before beginning.

In the aseptic method, the equipment needed for the procedure is boiled for 10 to 12 minutes in a sterilizer or deep pan (Nickols-Richardson, 2011). Water for diluting the formula is boiled separately. The bottles are then assembled, using sterilized tongs to avoid contamination by the hands. The formula and boiled water are added, and the bottles are capped and refrigerated until needed.

In the terminal sterilization method, the formula is placed in clean, loosely capped bottles. The bottles are then placed in the sterilizer or pan of water and boiled for 25 minutes (Eiger, 2016). After the bottles cool, the caps are tightened and the bottles refrigerated.

***Explaining feeding techniques***

**Positioning.** Show the parents how to position the infant in a semi-upright position such as the cradle hold. This allows them to hold the infant close with face-to-face contact. The bottle is held so that the nipple is kept full of formula to prevent excessive swallowing of air (Fig. 23.14). Place the infant in the opposite arm for each feeding to provide varied visual stimulation during feedings.

**Burping.** Burping or "bubbling" the infant after every ½ oz is important for the first few days. Gradually, the infant will be able to take more milk before burping and should be burped halfway through feedings. Show the parents how to place the infant over the shoulder or in a sitting position with the head supported while they pat and rub the infant's back.

**Frequency and amount.** Instruct the parents to feed the infant every 3 to 4 hours. The infant takes only ½ to 1 oz per feeding during the 1st day of life but increases to 2 to 3 oz per feeding within a week. An infant who is satisfied often goes to sleep.

**Cautions.** Explain that formula should not be heated in a microwave oven because the heating is uneven, resulting in some parts of the liquid being very hot, even when the outside of the bottle feels only warm. Formula can be heated by placing it in a container of hot water for 15 minutes. Suggest that the mother test the formula temperature by allowing a few drops from the bottle to fall on her inner arm.

Sometimes formula flow is too fast for infants. They may show this is happening by choking, gagging, sputtering, drooling, or biting the nipple. Some infants suck without stopping to breathe frequently

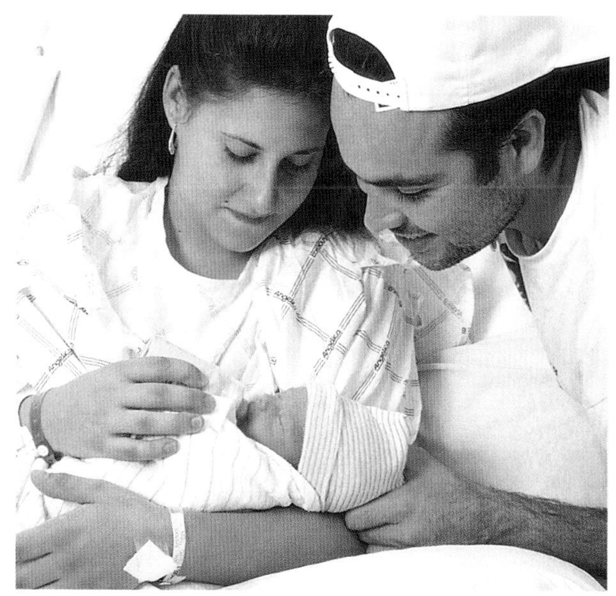

FIG 23.14 This mother holds her infant close during bottle feeding. The bottle is positioned so the nipple is filled with milk at all times. The father offers encouragement.

enough. To provide a rest period, the mother should tip the baby forward to stop the flow of milk

Caution parents not to prop the bottle. Propping increases the likelihood of choking if regurgitation occurs and eliminates the holding and cuddling that should accompany feeding. Infants who go to sleep with a bottle propped are at risk for aspiration. Pooled milk in the mouth leads to cavities once the teeth are in. Otitis media is more common in infants who sleep with a bottle or have a propped bottle.

The parents should not try to coax the infant to finish bottles because regurgitation and excessive weight gain could result. Discarding unused formula within an hour prevents feeding the infant formula contaminated by rapidly multiplying bacteria.

**Infant variations.** Although formula is usually given at room temperature, some infants take heated or cold formula better. The mother of a sleepy infant needs to use the same wake-up techniques discussed for the breastfeeding mother. Angling the tip of the nipple so that it rubs the palate triggers the suck reflex in most infants.

### Evaluation

- Does the mother position the infant and the bottle correctly?
- Does she feed the infant the right amount of formula with the right frequency?
- Can she explain how to prepare formula properly?

## KEY CONCEPTS

- Full-term breastfed infants need 85 to 100 kcal/kg (39 to 45 kcal/lb) daily. Formula-fed infants need 100 to 110 kcal/kg (45 to 50 kcal/lb) daily. They may lose weight in the first few days after birth as a result of insufficient intake and normal loss of extracellular fluid.
- Colostrum is rich in protein, vitamins, minerals, and immunoglobulins. Transitional milk appears between colostrum and mature milk. Mature milk follows transitional milk and continues to provide immunoglobulins and antibacterial components.
- Breast milk has nutrients in proportions needed by newborns and in an easily digested form. Most commercial formulas are cow's milk adapted to simulate human milk.
- Breast milk contains factors that help establish the normal intestinal flora and prevent infection. These include bifidus factor, leukocytes, lysozymes, lactoferrin, and immunoglobulins.
- A variety of commercial formulas is available, including modified cow's milk formula, soy-based or hydrolyzed formulas, and formulas for preterm infants and those with special problems.
- The AAP recommends exclusive breastfeeding for the first 6 months, with continued breastfeeding and the addition of complementary foods until the infant is at least 12 months of age.
- Factors that influence the mother's choice of feeding method include knowledge of each method, support from family and friends, cultural influences, and employment.
- Suckling at the breast causes the mother's posterior pituitary to release oxytocin, which triggers the let-down reflex. It also causes the anterior pituitary to release prolactin, which increases milk production.
- The principle of "supply and demand" applies to breastfeeding. Milk production increases when the infant feeds frequently. When breastfeeding ceases, prolactin secretion decreases, and eventually, the alveoli of the breasts stop producing milk.
- Flat and inverted nipples should be identified during pregnancy. Creams and methods to toughen the nipples are not necessary.
- The nurse should assess the mother's knowledge and the condition of her breasts and nipples. The LATCH score should be used to identify problems.
- The nurse can help the mother establish breastfeeding by initiating early feeding, assisting her to position the infant at the breast, and showing her how to position her hands. The nurse should teach the mother how to help the infant latch on to the breast, assess the position of the mouth on the breast, and remove the infant from the breast.
- The mother should feed the infant 8 to 12 times each day for an average of 10 to 15 minutes or more per side, nursing until the infant is satisfied.
- Wake-up techniques for sleepy infants include unwrapping the blankets, placing the infant skin to skin with the mother, talking to the infant, changing the diaper, and rubbing the infant's back.
- When infants suck from a bottle, they must push the tongue against the nipple to slow the flow of milk. When they suckle at the breast, they position the nipple far into the mouth so that the gums compress the areola.
- The nurse can help the woman with engorged breasts by encouraging her to nurse frequently, apply heat and cold, massage the breasts, and express milk to soften the areola if necessary.
- The nurse should help the mother with sore nipples to check the positioning of the infant at the breast. The mother should vary the position of the infant at the breast and apply warm-water compresses to the nipples. She should also expose the nipples to air.
- Teaching for the mother who plans to work and breastfeed includes expression of breast milk by hand or pump and proper storage of the milk.
- Mothers who use formula need information about the types of formula available, correct preparation, and feeding techniques.
- Formula should be diluted exactly according to directions to promote growth and avoid illness in the infant. It should not be heated in a microwave.

## REFERENCES AND READINGS


Academy of Breastfeeding Medicine. (2011). ABM clinical protocol no. 10: Breastfeeding the late preterm infant (34 0/7 to 36 6/7 weeks gestation) (First revision June 2011). *Breastfeeding Medicine*, *6*(3), 151–156.

Academy of Breastfeeding Medicine Protocol Committee. (2009a). ABM clinical protocol no. 3: Hospital guidelines for the use of supplementary feedings in the healthy term breastfed neonate, revised 2009. *Breastfeeding Medicine*, *4*(3), 175–283.

Academy of Breastfeeding Medicine Protocol Committee. (2009b). ABM clinical protocol no. 20: Engorgement. *Breastfeeding Medicine*, *4*(2), 111–113.

Academy of Breastfeeding Medicine Protocol Committee. (2010). ABM clinical protocol no. 22: Guidelines for management of jaundice in the breastfeeding infant. *Breastfeeding Medicine*, *5*(2), 175–182.

Albert, J., & Heinrichs-Breen, J. (2011). An evaluation of a breastfeeding privacy sign to prevent interruptions and promote successful breastfeeding. *Journal of Obstetric, Gynecologic and Neonatal Nursing*, *40*(3), 274–280.

American Academy of Pediatrics Section on Breastfeeding. (2012). Policy statement: Breastfeeding and the use of human milk. *Pediatrics*, *129*(3), e827–e841.

American Academy of Pediatrics & American College of Obstetricians and Gynecologists. (2012). *Guidelines for perinatal care* (7th ed.). Elk Grove Village, IL, and Washington, DC: Author.

American Dietetic Association. (2015). Position of the American Dietetic Association: Promoting and supporting breastfeeding. *Journal of the American Dietetic Association*, *115* (3), 444-449.

Association of Women's Health, Obstetric, and Neonatal Nurses. (2007). *Evidence-based clinical practice guideline: Breastfeeding support: Prenatal care through the first year* (2nd ed.). Washington, DC: Author.

Association of Women's Health, Obstetric, and Neonatal Nurses. (2010). *Assessment and care of the late preterm infant: Evidence-based clinical practice guideline: AWHONN late preterm infant initiative*. Washington, DC: Author.

Atisha, P., Ahmed, A., Nikila, P., & Bim, B. (2010). A case series of vitamin D deficiency in mothers affecting their infants. *Infant*, *6*(6), 196-201 6p.

Bernaix, L.W., Beaman, M.L., Schmidt, C.A., et al. (2010). Success of an educational intervention on maternal/newborn nurses' breastfeeding knowledge and attitudes. *Journal of Obstetric, Gynecologic, and Neonatal Nursing*, *39*(6), 658–666.

Blackburn, S.T. (2013). *Maternal, fetal, and neonatal physiology: A clinical perspective* (4th ed.). St. Louis: Saunders.

Bronner, Y.L. (2015). Maternal nutrition during lactation. In K. Wambach and J. Riordan (Eds.), *Breastfeeding and human lactation* (5th ed., pp. 497–518). Sudbury, MA: Jones & Bartlett.

Brozanski, B.S., Riley, M.M., & Bogen, D.L. (2012). Neonatology. In B.J. Zitelli, & H.W. Davis (Eds.), *Atlas of pediatric physical diagnosis* (6th ed., pp. 45–78). Philadelphia: Mosby.

Centers for Disease Control and Prevention. (2010). *Breastfeeding among U.S. children born 2000–2008, CDC national immunization survey*. Retrieved from http://www.cdc.gov/breastfeeding/data/NIS_data/index.htm.

Centers for Disease Control and Prevention. (2011a). *Breastfeeding report card–United States, 2011*. Retrieved from http://www.cdc.gov/breastfeeding/data/reportcard.htm.

Centers for Disease Control and Prevention. (2011). Vital signs: Hospital practices to support breastfeeding–United States, 2008 and 2009. *MMWR: Morbidity and Mortality Weekly Report*, *60*(30), 1020–1025.

Centers for Disease Control and Prevention. (2014). *Breastfeeding report card–United States, 2014*. Retrieved from http://www.cdc.gov/breastfeeding/data/reportcard.htm.

Dowling, D.A., & Tycon, L. (2010). Bottle/nipple systems: Helping parents make informed choices. *Nursing for Women's Health*, *14*(1), 61–66.

Eiger, M.S. (2016). Feeding of infants and children. In T.K. McInery, H.M. Adam, D.E. Campbell, et al. (Eds.), *Textbook of pediatric care* (2nd ed., pp. 212–219). Elk Grove Village, IL: American Academy of Pediatrics.

Gerbeda-Wilson, N., & Powers, N.G. (2012). Cultural practices and medical beliefs in pre-revolutionary Russia compared to modern textbook advice: Did Russian women breastfeed the "wrong" way? *Breastfeeding Medicine*, *7*(6): 514-520.

Halbardier, B. H. (2010). Fluid and electrolyte management. In M. T. Verklan, & M. Walden (Eds.), *AWHONN core curriculum for neonatal intensive care nursing* (4th ed., pp. 156–171). St. Louis: Saunders.

Halbardier, B.H. (2015). Fluid and electrolyte management. In M.T. Verklan, & M. Walden (Eds.), *AWHONN core curriculum for neonatal intensive care nursing* (5th ed., pp. 156–171). St. Louis: Saunders.

Hancock, M.E., & Brown, J. (2010). Formula feeding safety: What nurses need to teach parents who choose to formula feed. *Nursing for Women's Health*, *14*(4), 302–309.

Holt, K., Wooldridge, N., Story, M., et al. (Eds.), (2011). *Bright futures—nutrition* (3rd ed.). Elk Grove Village, IL: American Academy of Pediatrics.

Hurst, N.M., & Meier, P. (2015). Breastfeeding the preterm infant. In J. Riordan, & K. Wambach (Eds.), *Breastfeeding and human lactation* (5th ed., pp. 425–468). Sudbury, MA: Jones & Bartlett.

Linares, A., Rayens, M., Gomez, M., Gokun, Y., & Dignan, M. (2015). Intention to Breastfeed as a Predictor of Initiation of Exclusive Breastfeeding in Hispanic Women. *Journal Of Immigrant & Minority Health*, *17*(4), 1192–1198 7p. doi:10.1007/s10903-014-0049-0

Jana, L.A., & Shu, J. (2010). *Heading home with your newborn: From birth to reality* (2nd ed.). Elk Grove Village, IL: American Academy of Pediatrics.

Janke, J. (2014). Newborn nutrition. In K.R. Simpson, & P.A. Creehan (Eds.), *AWHONN perinatal nursing* (4th ed., pp. 626–655). Philadelphia: Lippincott Williams & Wilkins.

Jensen, D., Wallace, S., & Kelsay, P. (1994). LATCH: A breastfeeding charting system and documentation tool. *Journal of Obstetric, Gynecologic, and Neonatal Nursing*, *23*(1), 27–32.

Johnson, T.S., & Strube, K. (2011). Breast care during pregnancy. *Journal of Obstetric, Gynecologic and Neonatal Nursing*, *40*(2), 144–148.

Jones, J.E., Hayes, R.D., Starbuck, A.L., et al. (2011). Fluid and electrolyte management. In S.L. Gardner, B.S. Carter, & M. Enzman-Hines (Eds.), *Merenstein & Gardner's handbook of neonatal intensive care* (7th ed., pp. 333–352). St. Louis: Mosby.

Keane, V. (2011). Assessment of growth. In R.M. Kliegman, B.E. Stanton, J.W. St. Geme, et al. (Eds.), *Nelson textbook of pediatrics* (19th ed., pp. 39). Philadelphia: Saunders.

Kleinman, R.E., & Greer, F.R. (Ed.). (2014). *Pediatric nutrition handbook* (7th ed.). Elk Grove Village, IL: American Academy of Pediatrics.

Kozhimannil, K. B., Attanasio, L. B., Hardeman, R. R., & O'Brien, M. (2013). Doula Care Supports Near-Universal Breastfeeding Initiation among Diverse, Low-Income Women. *Journal Of Midwifery & Women's Health*, *58*(4), 378–382 5p. doi:10.1111/jmwh.12065.

Lawrence, R.A., & Lawrence, R.M. (2011). *Breastfeeding: A guide for the medical profession* (7th ed.). Philadelphia: Mosby.

Lewallen, L.P., & Street, D.J. (2010). Initiating and sustaining breastfeeding in African American women. *Journal of Obstetric, Gynecologic and Neonatal Nursing*, *39*(6), 667–674.

Mellin, P.S., Poplawski, D.T., & Gole, A. (2011). Impact of a formal breastfeeding education plan. *MCN: The American Journal of Maternal/Child Nursing*, *36*(2), 82–88.

Morin, K.H. (2008). Chemicals and infant nutrition. *MCN: The American Journal of Maternal/Child Nursing*, *33*(3), 189.

Morin, K.H. (2009). Preparing infant formula: Increasing caregiver knowledge. *MCN: The American Journal of Maternal/Child Nursing*, *34*(6), 387.

Newton, E.R. (2012). Breastfeeding. In S.G. Gabbe, J.R. Niebyl, & J.L. Simpson (Eds.), *Obstetrics: Normal and problem pregnancies* (6th ed., pp. 533–564). New York: Churchill Livingstone.

Nguyen, P.C., & Kerner, J.A. (2015). Gastrointestinal allergy. In T.K. McInery, H.M. Adam, D.E. Campbell, et al. (Eds.), *Textbook of pediatric care* (2nd ed., pp. 2064–2070). Elk Grove Village, IL: American Academy of Pediatrics.

Nickols-Richardson, S.M. (2011). Nutrition for normal growth and development. In E.D. Schlenker, & S. Long (Eds.), *Williams' essentials of nutrition and diet therapy* (10th ed., pp. 262–295). St. Louis: Mosby.

Noble, J.E. (2014). Breastfeeding. In C.D. Berkowitz (Ed.), *Pediatrics: A primary care approach* (5th ed., pp. 71–73). Elk Grove Village, IL: American Academy of Pediatrics.

Orr, S.S. (2010). Breastfeeding. In M.T. Verklan, & M. Walden (Eds.), *AWHONN core curriculum for neonatal intensive care nursing* (4th ed., pp. 315–334). St. Louis: Saunders.

Radke, J.V. (2011). The paradox of breastfeeding-associated morbidity among late preterm infants. *Journal of Obstetric, Gynecologic and Neonatal Nursing, 40*(1), 9–24.

Ribeiro, C. C., Leite Speridião, P. G., & de Morais, M. B. (2013). Knowledge and practice of physicians and nutritionists regarding the prevention of food allergy. *Clinical Nutrition, 32*(4), 624–629 6p. doi:10.1016/j.clnu.2012.10.014

Riordan, J. (2015). The biological specificity of breast milk. In K. Wambach, & J. Riordan (Eds.), *Breastfeeding and human lactation* (5th ed., pp. 117–160). Sudbury, MA: Jones & Bartlett.

Riordan, J., & Hoover, K. (2015). Perinatal and intrapartum care. In J. Riordan (Ed.), *Breastfeeding and human lactation* (5th ed., pp. 215–251). Boston: Jones & Bartlett.

Robinson, K. (2010). *African American women's infant feeding choices: Analyzing self-efficacy & narratives from a black feminist perspective.* African American Women's Infant Feeding Choices (pp. 187).

Schanler, R.J. (2016). Breastfeeding and the newborn. In T.K. McInery, H.M. Adam, D.E. Campbell, et al. (2nd ed.), *Textbook of pediatric care* (pp. 809–824). Elk Grove Village, IL: American Academy of Pediatrics.

Skidmore-Roth, L. (2010). *Mosby's handbook of herbs & natural supplements* (4th ed.). St. Louis: Mosby.

Smith, L.J., & Riordan, J. (2015). Postpartum care. In J. Riordan, & K. Wambach (Eds.), *Breastfeeding and human lactation* (5th ed., pp. 253–290). Boston: Jones & Bartlett.

Spatz, D.L. (2010). The critical role of nurses in lactation support. *Journal of Obstetric, Gynecologic and Neonatal Nursing, 39*(5), 499–500.

Stettler, N., Bhatia, J., Parish, A., et al. (2011). Feeding healthy infants, children, and adolescents. In R.M. Kliegman, B.E. Stanton, & J.W. St. Geme (Eds.), *Nelson textbook of pediatrics* (19th ed., pp. 160–170). Philadelphia: Saunders.

Tenfelde, S., Finnegan, L., & Hill, P.D. (2011). Predictors of breastfeeding exclusivity in a WIC sample. *Journal of Obstetric, Gynecologic and Neonatal Nursing, 40*(2), 179–189.

U.S. Department of Health and Human Services. (2010). *Healthy People 2020.* Washington, DC: Author.

U.S. Department of Health and Human Services. (2011a). *The Surgeon General's call to action to support breastfeeding.* Washington, DC: U.S. Department of Health and Human Services, Office of the Surgeon General.

U.S. Department of Health and Human Services. (2011). *Your guide to breastfeeding.* Washington, DC: Department of Health and Human Services, Office of Women's Health.

Vital Signs: Improvements in Maternity Care Policies and Practices That Support Breastfeeding - United States, 2007-2013. (2015). *MMWR: Morbidity & Mortality Weekly Report, 64*(39), 1112-1117 6p. doi:10.15585/mmwr.mm6439a5.

Wambach, K., & Riordan, J. (2015). Breast-related problems. In K. Wambach, & J. Riordan (Eds.), *Breastfeeding and human lactation* (5th ed., pp. 291–324). Sudbury, MA: Jones & Bartlett.

Weddig, J. (2011). Perspectives of hospital-based nurses on breastfeeding initiation best practices. *Journal of Obstetric, Gynecologic and Neonatal Nursing, 40*(2), 166–178.

# 24

# The Childbearing Family With Special Needs

http://evolve.elsevier.com/McKinney/mat-ch/

## LEARNING OBJECTIVES

*After studying this chapter, you should be able to:*

- Discuss the incidence and factors that contribute to teenage pregnancy.
- Identify the effects of pregnancy on the adolescent mother, her infant, and family.
- Describe the role of the nurse in the prevention and management of teenage pregnancy.
- Relate the major implications of delayed childbearing to maternal and fetal health.
- Describe the effects of substance abuse on the mother, fetus, and newborn.
- Identify nursing interventions to reduce or minimize the effects of substance abuse in the antepartum, intrapartum, and postpartum periods.
- Discuss parental responses when an infant is born with congenital anomalies, and identify nursing interventions to assist the parents.
- Describe parental responses to pregnancy loss, and identify nursing interventions to assist parents through the grieving process.
- Examine the role of the nurse when the mother places her infant for adoption.
- Identify the factors that promote violence against women, and describe the role of the nurse in its assessment, prevention, and interventions.

All families must make major changes as they adapt to pregnancy and childbirth. However, for some families, the changes are particularly difficult. These families have special needs related to the parents' age, substance abuse, birth of an infant with congenital abnormalities, perinatal loss, relinquishment, or intimate partner violence. Perinatal nurses have an opportunity to make a difference in the lives of these families.

## ADOLESCENT PREGNANCY

### Incidence of Teenage Pregnancy

In 2014, there were 24.2 births per 1,000 women aged 15 to 19 years in the United States, the lowest rate ever recorded. Approximately 250,000 teens gave birth. The birth rate for African-American teenagers was nearly twice as high as that for non-Hispanic white teens, while the rate for Hispanic teens was more than twice that for non-Hispanic white teenagers (Centers for Disease Control and Prevention [CDC], 2016). Asian/Pacific Islander adolescents have the lowest rate of teen pregnancy (Kochanek, Kirmeyer, Martin, et al., 2012).

Approximately 24 out of 1,000 girls in the United States become pregnant by the age of 20 years, and approximately 250,000 teen pregnancies occur each year (National Campaign to Prevent Teen and Unplanned Pregnancy [NCPTUP], 2014). The pregnancy and birth rates for teenagers in the United States are higher than those in other developed countries (U.S. Department of Health and Human Services [USDHHS], 2016). The Department of Health and Human Services' objectives for 2010 and 2020 include goals to reduce teen pregnancy (Levi & Dau, 2011). Between 1990 and 2014, the teen pregnancy rate declined from 116.9 to 24.2 pregnancies per 1,000 teen girls. This decline is attributed to an increase in the number of adolescents who are waiting to have sexual intercourse and the increased use of contraceptives by teens (CDC, 2016).

### Factors Associated With Teenage Pregnancy

Approximately 77% of teen pregnancies are unintended. Seventy percent of adolescents report that they have had sex by the age of 19 years (USDHHS, 2016). The high level of sexual activity and inconsistent or lack of contraceptive use among adolescents are directly related to the incidence of teenage pregnancies in the United States.

Adolescents often fail to recognize their vulnerability and believe that pregnancy cannot happen to them. Some risk pregnancy and parenthood as a means of gaining or maintaining a love relationship. They may see themselves as lacking power in their relationships and defer to their partner's wishes. Other teens see pregnancy as a means to gain independence (Box 24.1).

Adolescents who give birth are more likely to have a low income, which may mean they have less access to contraception and abortion. These teenagers may not believe that finishing their education and obtaining good jobs are possibilities for them and may see little reason to postpone pregnancy. Most pregnant adolescents are pregnant for the first time. However, 17% of pregnant adolescents have had one or more previous births (USDHHS, 2016) (Fig. 24.1).

### Sex Education

Sex education for teenagers should help them clarify their own values and beliefs about sexuality, understand how to set limits on sexual activity, and learn effective measures to prevent pregnancy and sexually transmitted infections (STIs) when they decide to become sexually active (see Chapter 31). Gonorrhea and chlamydial infection are particularly prevalent during these years, and these diseases can be transmitted to the infant and affect the eyes and lungs.

Learning how to set limits on sexual behavior is particularly important for younger teenagers, who may be pressured to become sexually

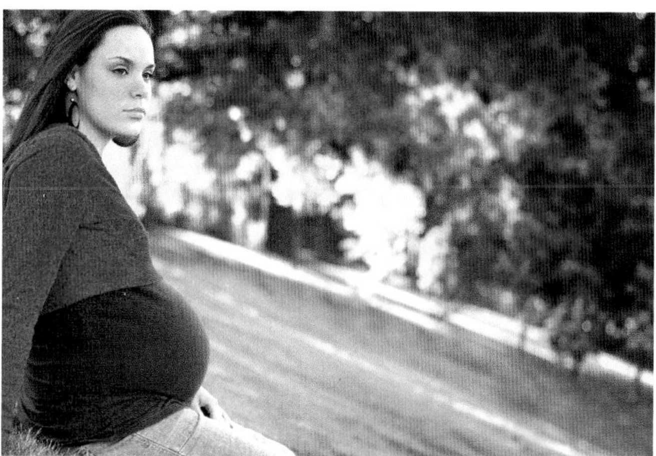

**FIG 24.1** Pregnant adolescent. Of teenage girls who become pregnant, approximately 1 in 5 has had a previous birth. (©2016 Getty Images. Reprinted with permission.)

**BOX 24.1 Factors That Contribute to Teenage Pregnancy**

- Peer pressure to begin sexual activity
- High rate of sexual activity
- Limited access to contraception
- Lack of accurate information about how to use contraceptives correctly
- Incorrect or lack of use of contraceptives
- Fear of reporting sexual activity to parents
- Ambivalence toward sexuality; intercourse not "planned"
- Feelings of invincibility
- Low self-esteem and consequent inability to set limits on sexual activity
- Desire to attain love or escape present situation
- Lack of appropriate role models

active before they have developed the maturity to responsibly deal with intercourse, contraception, or unplanned pregnancy. They need advice about how to handle pressure so that they can postpone sexual intercourse until they are emotionally and physically ready.

When providing sex education, nurses must keep in mind that adolescent males and females mature at different rates and may be more comfortable learning in separate groups. While talking to teenagers, nurses should use simple but correct language such as uterus, testicles, penis, and vagina.

## Preconception Counseling

Because adolescents are often seen by a healthcare provider for various reasons before they become pregnant, counseling to improve health for a future pregnancy should be offered to them during any healthcare visit. Smoking cessation, attaining optimum weight, folic acid intake, and screening for violence are all topics that should be discussed with all young women so that a future pregnancy has the most positive outcome (Heavey, 2010).

## Options When Pregnancy Occurs

An adolescent who becomes pregnant must choose one of three options: (1) terminate the pregnancy, (2) continue the pregnancy and place the infant for adoption, or (3) keep the infant. Some pregnant teens choose abortion, but this is not an acceptable option for others. Teenagers who might consider termination may not acknowledge the pregnancy or seek care until it is too late for abortion.

Approximately 1% of unmarried adolescents choose to relinquish their newborns for adoption (American Academy of Pediatrics [AAP], 2015). Those who choose adoption may have complicated feelings of grief, relief that a "bad" experience is over, and anger at parents who were unwilling to provide assistance, and thus, make adoption the only realistic option. For some pregnant adolescents, the autonomous decision to place the infant for adoption "for the child's good" may be an important step toward maturity.

Adolescents who choose abortion or adoption receive less assistance in dealing with their experience than those who keep their infants. They need help in coping with their feelings about their decision (see Adoption, p. 515).

## Socioeconomic Implications of Teenage Pregnancy

The medical expenses of adolescent pregnancy often are not covered by the family's health insurance, and public services become necessary. The public cost of teenage pregnancy in the United States is estimated at $9 to $10.9 billion each year (CDC, 2016, McCracken & Loveless, 2014). Costs include funds for Temporary Assistance for Needy Families (TANF), healthcare, Medicaid, food stamps, payment to care providers, loss of taxes, and administrative costs. Compared with older mothers, teenage mothers are more likely to be nonwhite, poor, less educated, unemployed, and unmarried, and many of the problems of early childbearing are related to these factors (McCracken & Loveless, 2014). They are more likely to have larger families at an earlier age, resulting in more children to feed and clothe on an already inadequate income.

Although the financial cost of teenage pregnancy is enormous, the cost in human terms is often tragic. The developmental tasks of adolescence, such as achieving independence from parents and establishing a lifestyle that is personally satisfying, may be interrupted. Instead of becoming independent, they often become more dependent on parents or a boyfriend as a result of pregnancy. Educational goals may be curtailed for some young mothers, limiting employment opportunities and resulting in reliance on the welfare system. Parenthood is a leading cause of school dropout among adolescent girls. Only 38% of teen mothers obtain a high school diploma, and less than 2% attain a college degree by the age of 30 years (National Campaign to Prevent Teen and Unplanned Pregnancy [NCPTUP], 2014).

Children born in these situations do not escape unscathed. They are at a higher risk for abuse and neglect (Ruedinger & Cox, 2012). They score lower on tests of cognitive ability, have inferior language skills, and may adjust poorly to the school environment. The negative cycle is often repeated: daughters of teenage mothers are three times more likely to become teen mothers than those of older mothers (NCPTUP, 2014). As a result, the children of adolescent parents are often among the poorest people in the United States.

However, for some adolescents, pregnancy motivates a desire to do well in school so that they can provide for their infants. Pregnancy and birth may have a stabilizing effect in adolescents who change past poor lifestyle choices and become more goal directed than they had previously been. They may become more determined to get an education to enable them to get jobs that allow them to provide for their children. Mothering may provide a new sense of purpose and reduced risk-taking that can enhance teen parenting abilities (Smith Battle, 2009).

## Implications for Maternal Health

Most pregnant teens have no medical complications during pregnancy. However, they are at an increased risk for anemia, labor dystocia, preeclampsia, and preterm birth. They also have an increased risk for being victims of violence during pregnancy. After birth, they are more likely to have infections and experience depression (Cunningham,

Leveno, Bloom, et al., 2010; Elfenbein & Felice, 2011). The high incidence of sexually transmitted diseases (STIs) among pregnant teenagers is another concern.

The reason for the higher incidence of complications among teenagers is uncertain but may be caused by inconsistent prenatal care and economic or sociocultural problems rather than age (Wildschut, 2011). Delayed prenatal care may result from denial of the pregnancy, lack of knowledge of how to get care, or a negative view of healthcare providers. Seven percent of pregnant adolescents have late or no prenatal care (Alan Guttmacher Institute, 2011).

### Implications for Fetal-Neonatal Health

Prematurity and low birth weight (less than 2500 g or 5.5 lb) are more likely to occur in infants born to adolescent mothers. These infants also have a higher infant mortality rate (Wildschut, 2011). Preterm infants are more likely to have a low birth weight and the added risks associated with immature organs. Low birth weights can also be caused by intrauterine growth restriction (IUGR), the failure of the fetus to grow as expected. This condition has various causes, including poor placental perfusion associated with preeclampsia, which is more common in adolescent pregnancy. Cigarette smoking is another cause of low birth weight. Teens are more likely to smoke during pregnancy than other maternal age groups (Grassley, 2011; McPeak et al., 2015).

### The Teenage Expectant Father

The majority of adolescent mothers have partners within 2 years of their age, but some have partners 6 or more years older. These men may accept the responsibility of the child, or they may become "phantom fathers," who are absent or rarely involved in raising the child.

Almost all adolescent expectant fathers indicate that they are not ready for fatherhood. Many are depressed as they grapple with the conflicting roles of adolescence and fatherhood. Although some express interest in learning about childbirth and child care, those who do not want to be fathers are less likely to be supportive. Some do not wish to be involved with the infant, leaving the pregnant girl to seek support elsewhere. Others are involved in some degree during the pregnancy and early years of the child's life but become less involved over time. Many adolescent mothers perceive that support from their partners is inadequate.

A disproportionate number of teenage expectant fathers are from environments of poverty and lack job skills or educational preparation. Many need job training before they can earn enough money to contribute to the support of their children.

### Impact of Teenage Pregnancy on Parenting

Adolescent mothers are at risk of becoming non-nurturing parents. Whether this risk results from adolescence per se, the higher incidence of premature births, the lower socioeconomic status, or the particular home environment is difficult to determine. Having to focus on an infant at a time when most teenagers are absorbed in their own thoughts and activities can make parenting difficult. Teens tend to respond in a less sensitive manner to their infants (Grassley, 2011; Chico & Gonzales, et al., 2015). Their own immature coping mechanisms may cause young adolescents experiencing stress (such as social isolation or inadequate financial resources) to use immature or punitive measures toward the infant.

Adolescent parents are likely to be surprised and dismayed at how difficult and time-consuming parenting can be. They may have little understanding of the expected growth and development of infants. For example, they may expect that the infant will sleep through the night, smile, or be toilet trained before it is possible for infants to do these things.

Preparing for parenthood is important. Although pregnant adolescents may want to be good mothers, they often do not actively seek information about infant care and development. The mother's relationship with the father of the baby may affect her parenting abilities. A close and satisfying relationship with the baby's father may increase attachment behaviors in the mother. Thus, the father should be included, when appropriate, in care of the mother and baby. However, many adolescent mothers do not have a good relationship with the father of their baby and will need support in coping.

## NURSING CARE

### The Pregnant Teenager

#### Assessment

***Physical assessment.*** Assessment of pregnant teenagers is similar to that of older women in many respects. At the initial visit, obtain a thorough health and family history to determine whether conditions such as diabetes or infectious diseases increase the risk for the mother and fetus. Monitor closely for signs of iron deficiency anemia, preeclampsia, or STIs. Attempt to identify behavioral risk factors such as poor nutrition, smoking, alcohol or drug use, or unprotected sex, which could harm the mother or fetus. Screen for physical or sexual abuse, which are more common in pregnant teenagers.

Structure the interview so that questions can be interspersed in a more general conversation that explores the teenager's likes and concerns. This approach helps to establish rapport and gain a better understanding of the teenager.

***Cognitive development.*** Determine the teenager's cognitive development and ability to absorb health counseling information. The three most important areas of cognitive development are:

1. *Egocentrism,* (interest centered on self) which involves the ability to defer personal satisfaction to respond to the needs of the infant: "What will you do when the baby is sick?"
2. *Present-future orientation,* which involves the ability to make long-term plans: "What are your plans for finishing high school?"
3. *Abstract thinking,* which involves identifying cause and effect: "Why is it important to keep clinic appointments?" "Why should condoms be used even though you are pregnant?"

***Knowledge of infant needs.*** Assess knowledge of infant needs and parenting skills. How does the teenager plan to feed the infant? What will she do when the infant cries? How will she know when the infant is ill and should be taken to a pediatrician? Does she know how much the infant should sleep? What plans have been made to provide for the safety needs of the infant?

***Family assessment.*** Begin assessment of the family unit by determining the degree of participation by the father of the infant. Fathers may plan to marry the expectant mother, participate in the pregnancy and rearing of the child without marriage, or be totally uninvolved.

It is important to assess the adolescent without her parents present, but it is also crucial to determine the availability and amount of family support. Families respond in various ways. A family member (usually the girl's mother) may take over the mothering role, or all infant care may be performed by the teenager. In other families, care and responsibilities are shared. This arrangement allows the adolescent to complete the developmental tasks of adolescence as well as learning the mother role.

The pregnant teenager's mother is particularly important when assessing the family. She may feel that she has "failed" as a mother, or she may resent the new cycle of child care in which the pregnancy involves her. Many pregnant adolescents live with their mothers, who provide various levels of support. If the family is unable or unwilling to provide care for an adolescent with an infant, what other social support can be located? In some situations, the family of the baby's father may be of assistance.

### Nursing Diagnosis and Planning

Many adolescents wait until the second or third trimester to seek prenatal care because they either do not realize that they are pregnant, continue to deny that they are pregnant, or want to hide the pregnancy. They may not know where to go for care and may fear the results of the pregnancy on their lives and relationships. Teenagers often have little information about physiologic demands, such as the increased need for nutrients that pregnancy imposes on their bodies. As a result, they may have a pattern of sporadic prenatal care and missed appointments (see Nursing Care Plan). One of the most relevant nursing diagnoses is:

- Risk for Ineffective Health Maintenance related to lack of knowledge of measures to promote health during pregnancy and increased family stress.

**Expected outcomes.** The expectant mother will keep scheduled prenatal appointments and follow healthcare instructions given throughout pregnancy. She will communicate her concerns throughout pregnancy. The family will verbalize emotions and concerns and maintain functional support of the expectant mother and her infant.

**Interventions**

**Eliminating barriers to healthcare.** Two major barriers to healthcare are scheduling conflicts and the negative attitudes of some healthcare workers. Help the adolescent locate the clinic closest to her that offers appointments when she (and her partner, if they wish) is available. Provide information about public transportation to that location, if necessary.

Pregnant women of all ages state that the negative attitude of some healthcare workers can discourage them from obtaining regular prenatal care. Nurses can be instrumental in finding ways to overcome these negative attitudes, thus encouraging pregnant women, including teenagers, to return for needed follow-up care. Nurses can acknowledge that frustration and staff burnout may occur when healthcare workers provide care for families with multiple problems. Allowing providers to see the same families consistently may help increase caring relationships and positive attitudes.

**Applying teaching or learning principles.** Arrange for the pregnant teenager to participate in small groups with common concerns. Being with peers may help her feel comfortable in asking

## NURSING CARE PLAN

### *An Adolescent's Responses to Pregnancy and Birth*

#### Focused Assessment

Ann, 16 years old, comes to the prenatal clinic during the 20th week of her pregnancy. She lives with her parents, who both work, and a younger sister. She sees her boyfriend sporadically but is unsure if he will be involved with the baby. She remains in school but discusses her concern about how she looks: "How much bigger am I going to get?" "Why is my face so blotchy?"

#### Nursing Diagnosis

Disturbed Body Image related to perceived negative effects of pregnancy, as evidenced by verbalized concern about appearance.

#### Planning

***Expected Outcomes***

Ann will:

1. Discuss her feelings about pregnancy and her perception of herself during each antepartum visit.
2. Make two positive statements about herself during the next antepartum visit.

#### Interventions and *Rationales*

1. Allow time at each prenatal visit for Ann to express concerns about weight gain and other physiologic changes of pregnancy, such as hyperpigmentation and stretch marks.
   *An adolescent is often ashamed and uncomfortable with her pregnant body. She feels more comfortable if she can share these feelings and be reassured they are a normal part of pregnancy.*
2. Initiate interaction about body changes by asking open-ended questions such as "How do you feel about your weight gain?"
   *Adolescents may be intimidated by healthcare professionals and may think their own feelings are not important enough to discuss.*
3. Provide anticipatory guidance about normal changes, such as the pattern of weight gain during pregnancy and weight loss after childbirth.
   *Most adolescents do not know what to expect during pregnancy. Anticipatory guidance reduces fear and provides needed information.*
4. Explain the reason for changes that are most troublesome at each prenatal visit (weight gain, hyperpigmentation, stretch marks, breast changes).
   *Knowing that some changes are temporary and that increasing weight indicates that the fetus is growing and developing is helpful. This may become a source of pride for the teenager.*
5. Involve Ann in scheduling prenatal appointments and classes and making plans for childbirth.
   *Participation in decision making promotes a positive sense of self.*
6. Promote a positive self-image by praising grooming, posture, and responsible behavior such as keeping prenatal appointments and following recommendations: "You have never missed an appointment, and your baby is growing very well."
   *Positive reinforcement is particularly important to help the adolescent meet the developmental tasks of developing a sense of identity and self-worth.*

#### Evaluation

Ann discusses her concerns about how she looks and begins to make positive statements about herself at each prenatal visit.

#### Focused Assessment

Ann reveals that her father says she has "shamed the family." She discusses her fears that her friends, none of whom have been pregnant, will reject her because she is pregnant. She tearfully confides that she will have to "drop out of everything" and feels guilty for "putting my family through this."

#### Nursing Diagnosis

Situational Low Self-Esteem related to feelings of rejection by family and friends, as manifested by statements indicating guilt and uncertainty about future support for herself and her infant.

#### Planning

***Expected Outcomes***

Ann will:

1. Identify at least two new measures to cope with anxiety by the end of the current antepartum visit.
2. Describe her implementation of these measures during subsequent antepartum visits.

*Continued*

## NURSING CARE PLAN—cont'd

### An Adolescent's Responses to Pregnancy and Birth

**Interventions and *Rationales***

1. Use therapeutic communication techniques to help her continue to express her feelings.
   *Listen to her to help Ann see her feelings as important and help the nurse prioritize interventions.*
2. Help Ann identify what she can do to overcome anxiety about rejection from her family and friends.
   a. Suggest that she talk to family members about her guilt for the unhappiness she is causing them and fear they will not assist her through the pregnancy and birth.
   *Although they seek independence, family values are important to adolescents. Rejection by the family would lead to great stress.*
   b. Role-play how she can initiate a conversation with her friends to discuss activities that they can continue to share.
   *Acceptance by the peer group is a major concern to the adolescent.*
   c. Recommend that she share her feelings with the father of the infant if she continues to see him.
   *He may be a source of emotional and financial support.*
3. Assist her in locating and joining the school-age mothers' program if available through her school district.
   *Teenagers in the same situation often replace the pregnant teenager's previous peer group.*
4. Encourage Ann to discuss her economic needs as well as her plans for continuing school when the infant is born.
   *Planning provides some sense of control and increases feelings of competency.*
5. Point out and praise any positive actions she takes, such as keeping prenatal appointments or eating a nutritious diet.
   *Sincere praise helps reinforce a positive self-image.*

**Evaluation**

Ann makes plans to talk with her family and at her next visit reports relationships are somewhat improved. She enters a school-age mothers' program and is very pleased. She states that her best friend has been very supportive.

**Focused Assessment**

Ann has a normal vaginal birth of a 6-lb, 3-oz girl at 38 weeks of gestation. She does not want to breastfeed because she feels uncomfortable with it. She will live at home, and her parents have agreed to pay for child care for the infant while she is in school. She seems unsure how to respond when the infant cries and handles her only during feedings.

**Nursing Diagnosis**

Risk for Impaired Parenting related to lack of knowledge of infant needs and little confidence in her ability to care for the infant, as evidenced by uncertain responses to the infant.

**Planning**

***Expected Outcomes***

Ann will:

1. Verbalize infant needs for gentle, prompt response to crying on the 1st postpartum day.
2. Demonstrate basic infant care (feeding, burping, bathing, swaddling) by discharge.
3. Demonstrate attachment behaviors (eye contact, gazing, holding, calling by name, and positive comments about the infant) before discharge.

**Interventions and *Rationales***

1. Demonstrate infant care on the 1st postpartum day. Obtain a return demonstration by the 2nd postpartum day.
   *This will help increase Ann's confidence in giving care.*
2. Demonstrate how to respond when the infant cries, and emphasize the importance of promptness and gentleness. Explain that infants develop a sense of trust when needs are met promptly and that crying does not indicate the infant is spoiled.
   *Modeling the way to respond to the infant helps Ann see what to do so she can respond in a like manner.*
3. Include the grandparents and the infant's father (if involved) in as many demonstrations as possible.
   *This will help promote consistency of care.*
4. Emphasize the importance of touch and verbal stimulation, and point out reciprocal bonding behaviors as in the infant following Ann with the eyes. Teach her the signs her infant is being overstimulated and needs a period of rest.
   *Newborns have many behaviors that stimulate attachment between parent and child. Recognition of overstimulation and the need for rest enhances caregiving ability.*
5. Instruct Ann in early growth and development of the infant (how often newborns need to eat, how much they sleep, behaviors to expect).
   *Anticipatory guidance helps parents have realistic perceptions of the infant.*
6. Encourage Ann to continue in the school-age mothers' program and to attend parenting classes along with other teenagers.
   *Learning along with her peers will help her increase her parenting skills and provides a continuing peer support group.*
7. Discuss Ann's future plans for her education and avoiding another pregnancy before she is ready. Provide information about contraceptives and refer her to her primary care provider.
   *Helping the teen make realistic plans for her future is important. Providing information about avoiding pregnancy may help her meet her goals.*

**Evaluation**

Ann responds quickly and gently when her infant cries. She gives basic care as taught and discusses what to expect in early growth and development of her baby. She makes frequent positive comments about her daughter.

***Additional Nursing Diagnoses to Consider***

Ineffective Coping
Interrupted Family Processes
Risk for Ineffective Health Maintenance
Risk for Delayed Growth and Development

questions and voicing concerns. Specific needs that might be addressed are the benefits of prenatal care or help in eliminating any unhealthy habits. Near the end of pregnancy, preparations for labor and delivery and infant care become the priorities.

Repetition is an important method of teaching and clarifying misinformation. Allow ample time for discussion. Although teenagers often do not read or benefit from printed materials to the same degree that older parents do, written materials prepared especially for adolescents may be helpful. Teens often respond well to audiovisual aids.

It is particularly important that the nurse does not sound like a parent when working with adolescents. Avoid using the words "should" or "ought," and do not make decisions for them.

**Counseling.** Allow time to counsel teenagers about their specific problems, such as nutrition, stress reduction, and infant care.

**Nutrition.** Counseling about nutrition is one way to help reduce the incidence of low-birth-weight infants. Determine the adolescent's general nutritional status, and assess for eating disorders that would reduce caloric intake and possibly affect fetal growth. Emphasize that because she is still growing, her intake must be adequate for her own growth as well as that of the fetus. Discuss nutrition during lactation, pointing out the advantages for both mother and baby. Tailor information to the individual adolescent's likes and peer group habits. Nutrition education must be socially and culturally appropriate (See Chapter 14 for suggestions on nutrition for adolescents).

Refer the teen to food stamp providers, the Special Supplemental Nutrition Program for Women, Infants, and Children (WIC), surplus food distributors, and food banks, if needed. Many teenagers have limited access to food and lack the ability to store or prepare it.

**Self-care.** Provide the same teaching about self-care that would be given to an older woman (see Chapter 13). In addition, emphasize prevention of STIs by using a condom even though she is pregnant. Counsel the adolescent about lifestyle changes, such as smoking or substance abuse cessation, that will benefit her and the fetus. Refer her to resources to help her with these problems.

**Stress reduction.** Identify the stressors in the adolescent's life. Stress may be related to basic needs such as food, shelter, and healthcare. Fear of labor and delivery and fear of being single, alone, and unsupported all create stress. Meeting the developmental tasks of adolescence while working on the developmental tasks of pregnancy is another stressor.

Various measures may be used to reduce stress, depending on the teenager's age, situation, and available support. Refer adolescents with chronic life stress to a social worker to achieve stability. If the girl is very young or if the pregnancy occurred as a result of rape or incest, social service and law enforcement agencies must become involved to provide protection and assistance.

The pregnant teenager often experiences stress because she has not told her parents or the father of the infant about the pregnancy. Role-play the encounter with her to help her work out a plan for breaking the news. Although there is strain on the relationship when the teen first tells her parents, her relationship with her parents may improve over time if her parents are supportive.

Teens who experience high levels of stress during pregnancy and postpartum display more negative parenting styles, resulting in poor behavioral, social-emotional, and cognitive outcomes for their children (Huang et al., 2014). Therefore, interventions to reduce stress in pregnant adolescents affect the infant as well as the mother.

Help the teen think ahead to how her life will change as a result of the pregnancy and what might interfere with the mother role. Help her identify possible solutions to the problems presented. Assistance with resolving conflict with support persons and identifying new sources of support are other important interventions.

**Attachment to the fetus.** Because attachment begins during pregnancy, helping the adolescent begin this process is important. Seeing the fetus move during an ultrasound often changes a pregnant woman's perceptions about the fetus. Hearing the fetal heartbeat and feeling the baby move may also increase attachment. Looking at illustrations of the fetus at different gestational ages increases the mother's interest. A heightened awareness of the fetus may make her more likely to follow suggestions that will enhance fetal well-being. Discussion of fetal changes month to month may lead to discussion of the capabilities and needs of the neonate.

**Breastfeeding.** Adolescents who decide to breastfeed their infants need much support in their endeavor. Adapt teaching to the mother's level of understanding. Encourage questions as they may have much misinformation. Privacy is important to adolescents, as they often feel embarrassed to breastfeed in front of others. Provide help with correct positioning and latching the infant. Show her how to drape a blanket to cover her breast and the nursing infant. Check on the mother frequently during feedings to identify any problems and intervene appropriately in a timely manner. Discuss problems that might occur, providing her with factual information so that she knows when and where to seek help, if necessary. Offer praise liberally. Success in latching the baby onto the breast and seeing the infant gain weight may be very rewarding for the mother.

**Promoting family support.** The pregnant teenager needs encouragement to include her family in her decision making and problem solving. Discuss topics such as who will care for the infant, whether the teenager will return to school, and what financial assistance is available from the family and the infant's father. Adolescent mothers who have adequate emotional support are more likely to learn appropriate parenting techniques.

However, if the family has problems such as substance abuse or domestic violence, involving family members may be inappropriate. The teenager should be encouraged to communicate with a family friend or other trusted adult instead.

**Providing support during labor.** The needs of the pregnant adolescent during labor are similar to those of the older woman. They need to feel respected and that the nurse cares about them. Help with pain management is particularly important. They also want to feel that their support persons are supported by the nurse. Younger teens respond to praise, while older teens may focus on receiving information from the nurse (Sauls, 2010).

**Providing referrals.** Make referrals to conveniently located community and national resources for pregnant adolescents. Include well-baby clinics offered by public health services, programs for school-age mothers offered by many school districts, TANF, and WIC. Church and community organizations may also provide needed assistance.

### Evaluation

- Does the pregnant adolescent keep prenatal appointments?
- Does she ask questions and follow the recommended plan of care?
- Is the family supportive, or have appropriate referrals been made?

## DELAYED PREGNANCY

An increasing number of women become pregnant relatively late in their reproductive lives. In 2014, the birth rate for women aged 40 to 44 years increased to 10.6 per 1000 women (Hamilton et al., 2015). Advances in contraception and improved infertility treatment allow women more options in childbearing.

### Maternal and Fetal Implications of Delayed Pregnancy

When the mature woman decides to conceive, she may experience a delay in becoming pregnant, particularly after the age of 35 years. This delay results from normal aging of the ovaries and the increased incidence of reproductive tract disorders with age. (See "Infertility" in Chapter 31.)

Although most pregnancies in mature women are normal, there is an increased risk of complications associated with pregnancy. The risks may be genetic, a result of preexisting medical conditions, or from obstetric complications. Advanced maternal age is associated with an increased risk for fetal chromosome abnormalities such as trisomy 21 (Down syndrome).

The most common examples of preexisting diseases that can cause maternal or fetal jeopardy are hypertension and diabetes mellitus.

Uterine myomas (fibroids) occur with greater frequency in women older than 35 years and may be associated with postpartum hemorrhage. The older woman is also at an increased risk for obstetric complications such as spontaneous abortion, gestational diabetes, cesarean birth, preterm delivery, preeclampsia, multifetal gestation, placenta previa, abruptio placentae, dysfunctional labor, and low-birth-weight infants (Bayrampour & Heaman, 2010; Cunningham et al., 2010; Lu, Williams, & Hobel, 2010; Von Kohler, 2016).

Most women who have delayed pregnancies have few problems and deliver healthy infants. Those who develop complications can often have a successful pregnancy with good medical and nursing care.

## Advantages of Delayed Childbearing

Mature primigravidas come to the parenting role with a range of personal resources: psychosocial maturity, self-confidence, and a sense of control over their lives. In addition, they are capable of solving complex problems and are often adept at maintaining interpersonal relationships. Many have made a conscious decision to wait until they are older to start their families. Because they are more likely to be financially secure, they can afford good care for their infants. They are experienced at setting priorities and developing plans. They are usually able to manage stress and will seek support and assistance when needed. They are often more accepting and feel less conflict in the parenting role (von Kohler, 2016) (Fig. 24.2).

## Disadvantages of Delayed Childbearing

Pregnancy complications that the woman did not expect may occur, requiring activity restrictions or missed work. After childbirth, mature primiparas need more time to recover and have less energy than their younger counterparts. They may find child care an exhausting experience for the first few weeks, particularly if they had a cesarean birth or pregnancy complications.

Peer support may be less available for mature primigravidas. Some older women have chosen to have a child without a partner and lack the support that women with partners have (Mandel, 2010). Many of their friends have teenage children and no longer relate to the concerns of a new mother. Younger mothers have some of the same concerns, but they often do not share the perspective of older mothers.

Family support may also be lacking for the older woman. Her parents are usually in their 60s or 70s and may not be able to assist with child care to the extent that younger grandparents can.

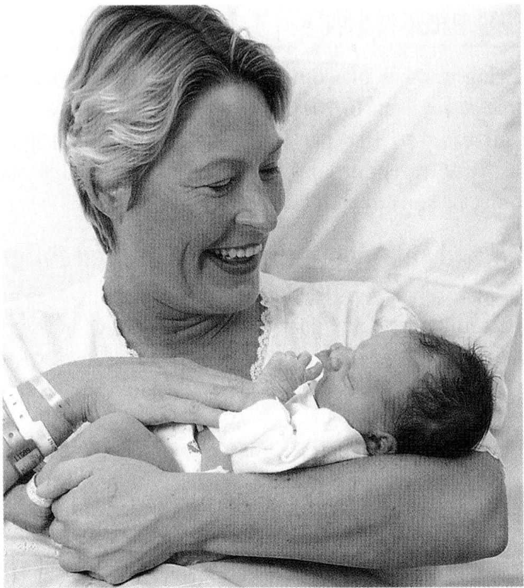

FIG 24.2 Older primigravidas bring maturity and problem-solving skills to the maternal role, but they are at somewhat increased risk for physiologic problems related to pregnancy and birth.

## Nursing Considerations

### Preconception Care

Preconception care is particularly important for the older woman planning to become pregnant. A visit to the nurse-midwife, nurse practitioner, or obstetrician can identify risk factors and correct them if possible. The preconception visit is essentially the same as for a younger woman but pays particular attention to any medical conditions more likely to occur in the older woman (see "Preconception Care" in Chapter 13).

### Reinforcing and Clarifying Information

Because the fetus of a mature woman is at an increased risk for chromosomal anomalies, information about available diagnostic tests will be provided (see Chapter 15). The tests most often recommended are multiple marker screening, chorionic villus sampling, amniocentesis, and ultrasonography. The family's beliefs and attitudes about abortion may determine whether the woman will have the recommended tests. The woman who would not consider abortion regardless of the condition of the fetus may refuse diagnostic studies or may choose to have them in preparation for problems that will occur at birth. Nurses must respect each woman's decision and acknowledge that it may have been difficult to make.

### Facilitating Expression of Emotions

Several days or weeks may pass between the performance of diagnostic studies and receipt of the results. This time is particularly difficult for many expectant parents, and nurses often assist the couple to express their concerns and emotions (see Chapter 15).

A broad statement such as, "Many couples find it difficult to wait for the results" will often elicit free expression of the parents' feelings. Follow-up questions such as, "What concerns you most?" may reveal anxiety about the procedure itself or about the possible effects of the procedure on the fetus. Simply acknowledging that it is a stressful time helps the couple cope with their emotions.

Mature gravidas also worry about complications that may affect the fetus or their own health. They are aware that they may not have another opportunity for pregnancy because of their age. They may also be concerned about their ability to balance their careers with increased family responsibilities.

### Providing Parenting Information

Nurses often help the mature primipara prepare for effective parenting. Anticipatory guidance about measures that will help conserve energy after childbirth is very useful. Such measures include meal planning and setting realistic housekeeping goals. In addition, many older mothers need to mobilize all available support so that they can reserve their energy for infant care.

During the first weeks after childbirth, the mother may experience feelings of social isolation, particularly if her friends have children who are much older. If she is accustomed to the mental stimulation of a job, she may miss it while staying at home. If she elects to return to work, she is likely to experience guilt and grief because she must leave her infant.

Older gravidas are more likely to seek out information they need from a variety of sources. First-time mothers older than 35 years are especially receptive to prenatal classes. Classes provide an opportunity to meet other older expectant parents with whom they have much in common. Women may have special concerns about the risks they face and may have many questions. They often adopt health-promoting activities such as improving nutrition and eliminating harmful substances. Printed materials that can be used to reinforce teaching are often helpful.

## SUBSTANCE ABUSE

The use of legal substances such as alcohol and tobacco, the use of illicit drugs, and prescription drug abuse increase the risk of medical complications in the mother and poor birth outcomes in the infant. Approximately 4.4% of pregnant women reported using illicit drugs during the preceding month in a government study (Wendell, 2013).

### Incidence

Although tobacco, alcohol, and marijuana are the most commonly abused substances, the use of opioids, cocaine, and amphetamines has had a major impact on healthcare for pregnant women and their offspring. A *Healthy People 2020* goal is to increase abstinence in pregnant women to 98.3% for alcohol, 98.6% for cigarette smoking, and 100% for use of illicit drugs (USDHHS, 2010).

### Maternal and Fetal Effects

When a pregnant woman uses drugs or alcohol, the fetus experiences the same systemic effects as the expectant mother but often more severely and for a longer time. A drug that causes intoxication in the woman causes it for prolonged periods in the fetus. The fetus cannot metabolize drugs efficiently and will experience the effects long after they have abated in the woman. The maternal, fetal, and neonatal effects of commonly abused substances are summarized in Table 24.1.

### Tobacco

Approximately 12.3% of women in the United States smoke during pregnancy (Tong, 2013). The active ingredients of cigarette smoke include nicotine, tar, and harmful gases, such as carbon monoxide and cyanide. Nicotine causes vasoconstriction and reduces placental blood circulation. Carbon monoxide inactivates fetal and maternal hemoglobin. Together, these effects reduce the amount of oxygen delivered to the fetus (Pitts, 2010). Cigarette smoking also decreases maternal appetite, resulting in inadequate intake of calories as well as decreased absorption of some nutrients. Suggestions for helping women to stop smoking are in Chapter 13.

Pregnant women who smoke have a higher rate of spontaneous abortion, low-birth-weight and -length infants, abruptio placentae, placenta previa, premature rupture of membranes, and perinatal mortality than women who do not smoke (Cunningham et al., 2010; Lu et al., 2010). Infants of smokers have a 30% higher chance of prematurity. Newborns born to smokers weigh approximately 200 g less than those born to nonsmokers and are 1.4 to 3 times more likely to die of sudden infant death syndrome (SIDS) (CDC, 2011). In addition, exposure to tobacco smoke before or after birth increases the odds of learning disabilities in children (Anderko, Braun, & Auinger, 2010). The

**TABLE 24.1 Maternal and Fetal or Neonatal Effects of Commonly Abused Substances**

| Substance | Maternal Effects | Fetal or Neonatal Effects |
|---|---|---|
| Caffeine (coffee, tea, cola, chocolate, cold remedies, analgesics) | Stimulates CNS and cardiac function, causes vasoconstriction and mild diuresis; half-life triples during pregnancy | Crosses placental barrier and stimulates fetus; teratogenic effects are undocumented |
| Tobacco | Decreased placental perfusion, abruptio placentae, anemia, PROM, preterm labor, spontaneous abortion | Prematurity, LBW, neurodevelopmental problems, increased incidence of SIDS |
| Alcohol (beer, wine, mixed drinks, after-dinner drinks) | Spontaneous abortion, abruptio placentae | Fetal demise, IUGR, fetal alcohol spectrum disorders, FAS (facial and cranial anomalies, developmental delay, intellectual impairment, short attention span) |
| Marijuana ("pot" or "grass") | Often used with other drugs: alcohol, cocaine, tobacco; exact effects undetermined | Unclear, more study needed, may be related to neurobehavioral problems; increased risk of anomalies or mortality unproven |
| Cocaine ("crack") | Hyperarousal state, euphoria, generalized vasoconstriction, hypertension, tachycardia, increased STIs, increased spontaneous abortion, abruptio placentae, preeclampsia, PROM, preterm labor, precipitous delivery | Tachycardia, stillbirth, prematurity, irritability, sleep followed by agitation, poor response to comforting or interaction, possible attention and language problems |
| Amphetamines and methamphetamines ("speed," "crystal," or "ice"; ecstasy) | Vasoconstriction, tachycardia, hypertension, spontaneous abortion, preterm labor, abruptio placentae, preeclampsia, and retroplacental hemorrhage | Increased risk for IUGR, prematurity, cleft palate, abnormal sleep patterns, agitation, poor feeding, vomiting |
| Antidepressants such as selective serotonin reuptake inhibitors | Relief of anxiety and depression, risk of anomalies with paroxetine, small risk of anomalies for other antidepressants | Transient respiratory distress, irritability, poor tone, persistent pulmonary hypertension |
| Opioids (heroin, methadone, morphine) | Malnutrition, anemia, increased incidence of STIs, HIV exposure, hepatitis, thrombosis, cardiac disease, spontaneous abortion, preterm labor | IUGR, LBW, perinatal asphyxia, meconium aspiration syndrome, neonatal abstinence syndrome, fetal or neonatal death, SIDS, child abuse and neglect, long-term developmental effects unclear |

*CNS,* Central nervous system; *FAS,* fetal alcohol syndrome; *FGR,* fetal growth restriction; *HIV,* human immunodeficiency virus; *LBW,* low birth weight; *PROM,* premature rupture of membranes; *SIDS,* sudden infant death syndrome; *STIs,* sexually transmitted diseases.

degree of fetal growth restriction varies with the number of cigarettes smoked daily. Women who stop smoking during pregnancy reduce the amount of growth restriction suffered by the fetus (Walker & Walker, 2011).Infants born too soon or too small are at an increased risk for adverse birth outcomes, and smoking may be a greater risk factor than illicit drugs (Bailey et al., 2012).

### Alcohol

Approximately 1 in 12 women reports drinking during pregnancy, and 1 in 30 pregnant women reports having five or more drinks on any one occasion during pregnancy. Alcohol passes easily across the placenta. During pregnancy, alcohol consumption can result in spontaneous abortion and abruptio placentae (Bandstra & Accornero, 2011). Alcohol is a teratogen, and its use during pregnancy can result in **fetal alcohol spectrum disorders,** conditions resulting in physical and mental abnormalities that range from mild to severe (CDC, 2014). The disorders include fetal alcohol syndrome (FAS), partial FAS, alcohol-related neurodevelopmental disorder, and alcohol-related birth defects. **Fetal alcohol syndrome,** a group of severe physical, behavioral, and mental abnormalities resulting from fetal exposure to alcohol, is the most severe of these disorders. Alcohol use during pregnancy is one of the top preventable causes of birth defects and developmental disabilities (Beckmann, Ling, Barzansky, et al., 2010). It is the leading cause of intellectual impairment and the only one that is preventable (Pitts, 2010).

The amount and timing of alcohol intake influence the specific effects on the fetus. During the first trimester, alcohol affects cell membranes and alters tissue organization, causing structural defects. Throughout pregnancy, alcohol interferes with the metabolism of nutrients, and thus, inhibits cell growth and division. Although binge drinking (four or more drinks on one occasion) is especially harmful, drinking in any amount and at any time can cause adverse fetal effects.

The teratogenic effects of alcohol include FAS, which is characterized by three clinical features: prenatal and postnatal growth restriction, central nervous system (CNS) impairment, and a recognizable combination of facial features. Growth restriction is noted in length, weight, and head circumference. CNS impairment includes intellectual impairment, learning disabilities, high activity level, short attention span, and poor short-term memory.

Common facial anomalies associated with FAS include microcephaly, short palpebral fissures (the openings between the eyelids), epicanthal folds, flat midface with a low nasal bridge, indistinct philtrum (groove between the nose and upper lip), and a thin upper lip.

Not every infant exposed to alcohol during pregnancy has all the characteristics of FAS. A range of defects may be exhibited. Because no safe level of alcohol consumption during pregnancy has been established, it is recommended that women abstain from drinking alcohol both when planning a pregnancy and throughout the pregnancy.

### Marijuana

Marijuana is the most commonly used illicit drug in the United States (Pitts, 2010). The active constituent of marijuana is tetrahydrocannabinol (THC), which crosses the placenta and accumulates in the fetus. Because it is often used with other drugs, such as cocaine and alcohol, its precise effects are difficult to determine. Studies are conflicting regarding the effects of marijuana use in pregnancy. Marijuana increases the carbon monoxide content of the mother's blood and can reduce the oxygen available to the fetus. Neurobehavioral problems may occur in the infant, including tremors and sleep disturbances. Research has not shown an increased risk of anomalies or infant mortality (Bandstra & Accornero, 2011).

### Cocaine

***Actions.*** Cocaine is a powerful, short-acting stimulant of the CNS. Cocaine blocks the reuptake of the neurotransmitters **norepinephrine** and **dopamine** at the nerve terminals, producing a hyperarousal state that results in euphoria, sexual excitement, increased alertness, and a heightened sense of well-being. The physical effects of cocaine use are related to cardiovascular stimulation and vasoconstriction. Hypertension, tachycardia, arrhythmias, tremors, anemia, and anorexia occur. Complications include myocardial infarction, convulsions, and death (Bandstra & Accornero, 2011; Pitts, 2010).

When the initial euphoria wears off, a period of irritability, exhaustion, lethargy, depression, and anxiety occurs. This state elicits a strong desire for additional cocaine so that the initial feelings can be recaptured.

***Maternal and fetal effects.*** Because many women who use cocaine also use additional drugs such as alcohol, tranquilizers, heroin, or marijuana to "come down" from the hyperarousal state that cocaine produces, it is difficult to determine the precise effects of cocaine on the fetus. Women who abuse cocaine are less likely to seek prenatal care or to eat a diet that contains adequate nutrition. Sex may be exchanged for drugs, so the woman is at an increased risk for STIs.

Because cocaine causes vasoconstriction of placental vessels, the incidence of abruptio placentae increases. Cocaine stimulates uterine contractions, resulting in an increased incidence of spontaneous abortion, premature rupture of membranes, preterm labor, and precipitous delivery. Additional complications include severe hypertension, pulmonary edema, fetal hypoxia, meconium staining, and stillbirth (Bandstra & Accornero, 2011; Pitts, 2010; Sullivan, 2016).

Clearance of the drug in the fetus requires a prolonged period of time. Fetal effects include hypoxia, tachycardia, hypertension, IUGR, and limb reduction syndrome (Oscar et al., 2014)

***Neonatal effects.*** Neonates exposed to cocaine *in utero* may exhibit central nervous system signs such as irritability followed by lethargy, alternating between sleep and agitation, and a poor response to interaction with others or comforting by caregivers (Pitts, 2010). Long-term effects are unclear but may include attention and language problems (Bandstra & Accornero, 2011).

### Amphetamines and Methamphetamines

These drugs are central nervous system stimulants that produce effects similar to cocaine but are longer acting. Common names include speed, crystal, ice, crank, and ecstasy.

***Maternal and fetal effects.*** Amphetamines and methamphetamines cause vasoconstriction, hypertension, and tachycardia. Effects on the mother and fetus appear similar to those of cocaine. Spontaneous abortion, IUGR, low birth weight, small-for-gestational-age, preterm labor, abruptio placentae, preeclampsia, and retroplacental hemorrhage may occur (ACOG, 2011; Pitts, 2010; Walker & Walker, 2011). Because these drugs are appetite depressants, the fetus may not receive required nutrients.

***Neonatal effects.*** Infants may have congenital defects such as cleft palate, abnormal sleep patterns, agitation, diaphoresis, poor feeding, and vomiting (Pitts, 2010; Walker & Walker, 2011).

### Antidepressants

Antidepressants such as selective serotonin reuptake inhibitors (SSRIs) are being prescribed more often in pregnancy for women with depression and anxiety. In some cases, the benefits of treatment outweigh any adverse effects known.

*Maternal and fetal effects.* Paroxetine (Paxil) is no longer recommended for use during pregnancy because of reports of congenital malformations. Further research is needed to determine the risks, but at this time, the risk of anomalies appears to be small (Buhimschi & Weiner, 2011).

*Neonatal effects.* Transient respiratory distress, irritability, poor tone, and persistent pulmonary hypertension have been reported (Buhimschi & Weiner, 2011). Long-term effects are unknown at this time.

### Opioids

Opioids include drugs such as morphine, heroin, methadone, meperidine, hydromorphone hydrochloride, propoxyphene, and oxycodone. Heroin is used here as an example of this class of drugs. Heroin, an illegal opiate derived from morphine, produces severe physical dependence. Like all opiates, heroin is a CNS depressant that produces mental dullness, drowsiness, and stupor. Dependence is present if discontinuation of the drug causes withdrawal symptoms (abstinence syndrome) that are quickly relieved by a dose of heroin.

Women who abuse heroin have poor general health, with multiple medical problems associated with their chemical dependence (physical and psychological dependence on a substance) and the associated lifestyle. Heroin is an appetite suppressant that also interferes with the absorption of nutrients, and many women who abuse heroin begin pregnancy malnourished and anemic. Additional problems include a high incidence of STIs, hepatitis, and exposure to human immunodeficiency virus (HIV) from sharing unclean needles. Spontaneous abortion, cardiac disease, and thrombosis can also occur (Pitts, 2010).

*Fetal effects.* The indirect effects of heroin use result from maternal malnutrition and fetal exposure to STIs. Because the woman's supply of heroin is usually not steady, episodes of maternal overdose alternate with periods of withdrawal. These episodes expose the fetus to intermittent hypoxia, which increases the risk of meconium aspiration syndrome. Fetal growth restriction, preterm labor, premature rupture of membranes, fetal distress, and stillbirth are other risks (Buhimschi & Weiner, 2011; Pitts, 2010; Walker & Walker, 2011).

*Neonatal effects.* Infants born to mothers dependent on opioids exhibit neonatal abstinence syndrome (NAS), physical signs that affect all organ systems. Most signs involve the neurologic and gastrointestinal systems. (See Chapter 30, p. 653 for withdrawal signs and management.) Infants are more likely to have low birth weight and an increased incidence of SIDS (Buhimschi & Weiner, 2011; Walker & Walker, 2011). Studies of long-term developmental and learning problems have produced conflicting results. The lifestyle of parents who are substance abusers is often associated with child neglect and abuse.

### Diagnosis and Management of Substance Abuse

In addition to toxicology screening, the pregnant woman who uses illicit drugs must be assessed throughout pregnancy for STIs, hepatitis, and exposure to HIV. Fetal diagnostic tests such as ultrasonography, nonstress tests, and biophysical profiles help identify problems. Nurses monitor weight and provide guidance in nutrition to prevent maternal anemia and inadequate weight gain.

Therapeutic management depends on the type of drug used and the problems presented. In the case of opioids, withdrawal during pregnancy has been associated with significant fetal stress, fetal seizures, and even fetal death. The pregnant woman who uses heroin is often prescribed an alternative drug, such as methadone, a synthetic opiate.

Methadone can be taken orally once daily and is long acting, providing consistent blood levels to decrease the adverse fetal effects of wide swings in blood level found with heroin use. At therapeutic levels, methadone does not produce the euphoria or sedation of heroin and allows the woman to live a relatively normal life. The woman in a drug-treatment program who receives a daily dose of methadone is more likely to receive prenatal care. However, the newborn must withdraw from methadone after birth. Some women taking methadone also use other illicit drugs such as cocaine or marijuana. Buprenorphine can be used instead of methadone, with less severe neonatal withdrawal (Walker & Walker, 2011).

Treatment is aimed at establishing abstinence and preventing relapse. Outpatient or residential treatment provides education, individual and group therapy sessions, and peer support groups (Narcotics Anonymous, Alcoholics Anonymous, or Cocaine Anonymous). Written contracts that focus on abstinence for one day at a time are often used to help the woman who has relapsed and experiences feelings of guilt and self-blame.

## NURSING CARE

### Maternal Substance Abuse

#### Antepartum Period

*Assessment.* Polydrug abuse appears to be the most common substance abuse problem among women. Because substance abuse occurs in all populations, the nurse must not make assumptions based on class, race, or economic status. All women must be screened at the first prenatal visit for tobacco, alcohol, and other drug use.

Certain behaviors are strongly associated with substance abuse: seeking prenatal care late in the pregnancy, failing to keep appointments, and following recommended regimens inconsistently. Poor grooming or inadequate weight gain may be signs of a lifestyle that includes substance abuse. Intravenous drug users may have needle punctures, thrombosed veins, or cellulitis.

Defensive or hostile behaviors may be overt signs of substance abuse. Women who use drugs have low self-esteem. They must cope with conflicting issues: the physical or psychological need for the substance and the guilt that they may be responsible for harming the fetus. Fear of prosecution for use of illegal drugs may keep the woman from seeking prenatal care, increasing the risk of harm to the woman and her fetus.

Many women with substance-abuse problems face discrimination and resentment from healthcare professionals who direct their frustration at the woman rather than at the problem. The nurse taking the health history must exhibit patience, empathy, and tolerance and must use a blend of approaches that reinforce concern for the woman and her infant. When women receive nonjudgmental, supportive care from knowledgeable healthcare workers, they are more likely to keep appointments for prenatal care (Lefebvre, Midmer, & Boyd, et al., 2010).

**CRITICAL TO REMEMBER**

***Behaviors Associated With Substance Abuse***

- Seeking prenatal care late in pregnancy
- Failure to keep prenatal appointments
- Inconsistent follow-through with recommended care
- Poor grooming, inadequate weight gain
- Needle punctures, thrombosed veins, cellulitis
- Defensive or hostile reactions
- Anger or apathy regarding pregnancy
- Severe mood swings

**Medical and obstetric history.** Determine whether the woman has medical conditions that are prevalent among those who use drugs, such as hepatitis, STIs, cellulitis, seizures, hypertension, depression, and suicide attempts. Evaluate for past and current pregnancy complications. Spontaneous abortions, premature deliveries, abruptio placentae, and stillbirths are associated with substance abuse. Current complications can include vaginal bleeding, an inactive or hyperactive fetus, and IUGR.

Identify emotional responses regarding the pregnancy. Anger or apathy is particularly significant during the latter half of the pregnancy, when normal feelings of ambivalence are usually resolved. Negative feelings toward the pregnancy may interfere with compliance with recommended care.

**History of substance abuse.** Obtaining an accurate history of substance abuse is difficult and depends in large part on the way the healthcare worker approaches the woman. A sincere, nonjudgmental, empathic approach promotes an open exchange of information.

Ask about all forms of drug use, including cigarettes (and e-cigarettes), over-the-counter drugs, prescribed medications, alcohol, and illicit drugs such as marijuana, amphetamines, cocaine, and heroin. Examine patterns of drug use, which can range from occasional recreational use to weekly binges to daily dependence on a particular drug or group of drugs.

***Nursing diagnosis and planning.*** Some women do not realize the adverse effects of the drugs they are using, and others are aware of the risks but are unable to stop. A nursing diagnosis that addresses both of these factors is:

- Ineffective Health Maintenance related to lack of knowledge of the effects of substance abuse on self and fetus and inability to manage stress without the use of drugs.

**Expected outcomes.** The woman will identify the harmful effects of substances on herself and her infant, will verbalize feelings related to continued use of harmful substances, and will identify personal strengths and accept resources offered by the healthcare delivery system to stop using drugs.

***Interventions.*** Effective interventions for substance abuse require that nurses realize that progress is slow and frustrating. The major priority is to protect the fetus and the expectant mother from the harmful effects of drugs.

**Examining attitudes.** When working with substance-abusing pregnant women, nurses must identify their own knowledge level, feelings, and prejudices. They may have limited knowledge about perinatal substance abuse and negative attitudes toward mothers who abuse substances. Maintaining feelings of empathy or concern without becoming judgmental or even unknowingly punitive to the pregnant woman may be difficult. Nurses may feel angry, helpless, and discouraged when the pregnant woman continues to abuse drugs despite the best efforts of the healthcare team. Inservice education, professional consultation, and peer support are all helpful when working with pregnant women who abuse drugs.

**Preventing substance abuse.** Participate in campaigns to prevent substance abuse throughout the community. Use posters, diagrams, pamphlets, and other visual aids to describe the effects of tobacco, alcohol, and other drugs on the fetus. Post visual aids in schools, supermarkets, shopping centers, and other areas where women of childbearing age will be exposed to them.

Focus on the benefits of remaining drug-free, which include a decrease in maternal and neonatal complications. For example, the effects of smoking tobacco are dose related and cumulative, and nurses need to encourage and support cessation at any point during pregnancy.

Women who use alcohol without other drugs during pregnancy may not realize the effect on the fetus. Social drinkers will often stop drinking once they know about the dangers of alcohol consumption during pregnancy. Those with heavy alcohol use need counseling and referral for further treatment.

**Communicating with the woman.** Ask the woman about stressors in her life that may be contributing to her substance abuse. These stressors may include inadequate housing, economic predicaments, intimate partner violence, and emotional or physical illness.

Be honest at all times, while displaying a patient, nonjudgmental attitude as well as genuine interest and concern. This demeanor is especially important when the woman relapses into substance-abusing patterns. Allow her to express guilt, and reassure her that abstinence is possible and that she can and must begin again.

**Helping the woman identify strengths.** Because she generally has a poor self-image, assist the substance-abusing pregnant woman in identifying personal strengths. Acknowledge her actions when she abstains from drugs or alcohol, even for a short time. Praise for maintaining adequate weight gain. Attending prenatal classes may increase her confidence and compliance with the recommended regimen of care.

**Providing ongoing care.** At each antepartum visit, consider the current status of substance use, social service needs, education needs, and compliance with treatment referrals. In particular, address current drug use because women may change their pattern of drug use during pregnancy. For example, they may stop using cocaine but increase their use of marijuana or alcohol.

Verify compliance with recommended treatment regimens such as antepartum clinics and chemical-dependence referral programs. Coordinate care among various service providers such as group therapy and prenatal classes.

Provide continuing prenatal education regarding the anatomy and physiology of pregnancy and consequences of prenatal substance abuse. Describe how the newborn benefits when the mother abstains from drugs, including tobacco and alcohol. Praise any attempts at abstinence, and encourage the expectant mother to try again if she relapses.

Assess maternal attachment to the fetus, because attachment may help her reduce or eliminate her substance use. Fetal movement often increases the woman's awareness of the fetus and may lead to a discussion about her plans for the infant and the changes that are occurring in her life.

***Evaluation***

- Can the expectant mother identify the effects of substance abuse on herself and her infant?
- Does she discuss her feelings about continued substance abuse?
- Does she identify her own strengths and work with the healthcare team to stop using drugs?

### Intrapartum Period

***Assessment.*** Nurses who work in labor and delivery units must become skilled at identifying drug-induced signs and symptoms.

**Cocaine.** Behaviors associated with frequent or recent use of cocaine include profuse sweating, hypertension, and irregular respirations, combined with a lethargic response to labor and apparent lack of interest in the necessary interventions. Additional signs include dilated pupils, increased body temperature, and sudden onset of severely painful contractions. Fetal signs often include tachycardia and excessive activity. Fetal bradycardia and late decelerations may occur.

Emotional signs of recent cocaine use include angry, caustic, or abusive reactions to those attempting to provide care. Emotional lability and paranoia are signs of cocaine intoxication.

**Heroin.** Typically, the pregnant woman with heroin dependence comes to the labor and delivery unit intoxicated from a recent drug administration. When the effects of the drug begin to wear off,

**CRITICAL TO REMEMBER**

***Signs and Symptoms of Recent Cocaine Use***

- Diaphoresis, hypertension, tachycardia, irregular respirations
- Dilated pupils, increased body temperature
- Sudden onset of severely painful contractions
- Fetal tachycardia
- Excessive fetal activity, late decelerations
- Angry, caustic, abusive reactions and paranoia

withdrawal symptoms may be observed. These include yawning, diaphoresis, rhinorrhea, restlessness, excessive tearing of the eyes, nausea, vomiting, and abdominal cramps.

***Nursing diagnosis and planning.*** One of the most relevant nursing diagnoses during the intrapartum period is:

- Risk for Injury related to physiologic and psychological effects of recent drug use.

**Expected outcome.** The woman and the fetus will remain free from injury during labor and childbirth.

***Interventions***

**Preventing injury.** When a laboring woman has recently used a substance such as cocaine, the nurse must intervene to meet the woman's needs for safety, oxygen, and comfort.

***Admitting procedure.*** Two nurses may be needed to admit the woman into the labor unit. One nurse helps the woman into bed, initiates electronic fetal monitoring, and begins administration of oxygen, as needed. The other nurse acts as communicator.

Because the woman who has recently used a drug may have difficulty following directions, only one nurse should tell her what to do. This nurse states firmly what is happening and exactly what the woman must do: "Lie on your left side," "This helps us watch how the baby is doing," "This gives you more oxygen." Maintain eye contact with the woman while giving her instructions.

***Setting limits.*** Setting limits is essential to protecting the safety of the mother and the fetus. For example, the mother cannot smoke when oxygen is in use. If she must remain in bed, she may become agitated. The nurse may say, "I know it's hard to stay in bed, but we can't take good care of the baby when you walk." If walking is safe for the woman, the nurse must set limits regarding where she can walk.

***Initiating seizure precautions.*** The laboring woman who has recently used cocaine is at risk for seizures. Take seizure precautions to protect her from injury in case of seizures. Keep the bed in a low, locked position. Pad the side rails and keep them up at all times. To prevent aspiration, make sure suction equipment functions properly. Reduce environmental stimuli (lights, noise) as much as possible.

**Maintaining effective communication.** Establishing a therapeutic pattern of communication is essential. Avoid confrontation. Instead, acknowledge feelings: "I know you hurt and you are frightened. I'll do everything I can to make you comfortable." If the woman is abusive, be careful not to take the abuse personally or react in a nontherapeutic manner.

Examine your own feelings when women are abusive, and acknowledge when anger is getting in the way of providing care. To allow some relief from unrelenting abusive comments, another nurse may need to assume care of the woman for a time.

**Providing pain control.** Pain control for women who are substance abusers poses a difficult problem because it is often impossible to determine the type or combination of drugs that were used before admission. If pain medication can be administered safely, do not withhold it under the false assumption that the woman does not need it or medication will contribute to her chemical dependence. Include nonpharmacologic comfort measures such as sacral pressure, back rubs, a cool cloth on the head, and continual support and encouragement as for any woman in labor.

**Preventing heroin withdrawal.** To prevent or stabilize heroin withdrawal during labor, give methadone or buprenorphine to the woman who usually takes it at a chemical-dependence center if she did not receive her daily dose. Administer methadone intramuscularly as ordered if the woman is nauseated or vomiting. Avoid narcotic agonists-antagonists such as butorphanol (Stadol) because they may cause acute withdrawal signs and symptoms in the woman and the fetus.

***Evaluation***

- Are the woman and her fetus free of injury during labor and childbirth?

### Postpartum Period

During the postpartum period, nursing care is focused on helping the mother with bonding, infant care, and planning to provide care for herself and the infant after discharge (see Chapter 30). Assess the mother-infant interaction so that bonding and attachment can be promoted. Encourage the woman to continue her efforts to stop taking substances. Women who stop or decrease use during pregnancy might return to using at previous levels after pregnancy and need support to continue abstinence. Referral to social services and child protective agencies may be necessary for follow-up care of the mother and infant.

## BIRTH OF AN INFANT WITH CONGENITAL ANOMALIES

Even when everything goes according to plan, childbirth is a time of stress for parents. When the infant is born with anomalies, the parents are often overwhelmed with shock and grief. Because nurses spend more time with the parents than the other members of the perinatal team, they have an opportunity to help the family adjust and cope with this situation.

### Factors Influencing Emotional Responses of Parents

#### Timing and Manner of Being Told

At one time, it was common practice to remove the infant from the delivery area before parents could see a congenital anomaly and tell them about it later instead. This practice changed when it was realized that parents experienced less stress if they were told at once and were permitted to hold their baby if the physical status of the infant allowed (Fig. 24.3). Physicians and nurses also became aware of the importance of helping the parents accept and bond with the newborn.

#### Previous Knowledge of the Defect

Although ultrasonography does not identify all fetal anomalies, many parents learn about fetal anomalies during ultrasound examinations performed during pregnancy. These parents may not experience the shock and disbelief at the birth seen in unprepared parents. Their reactions should not be interpreted as meaning that they do not experience grief. Instead, they have completed some of the early phases of grieving before the birth. Their grief is real and profound, even though it is expressed differently.

#### Type of Defect

Although any defect in a newborn produces extreme concern and anxiety, certain defects are associated with long-term parenting problems. Accepting an infant with facial or genital anomalies is particularly difficult for the family and the community. The face is visible to

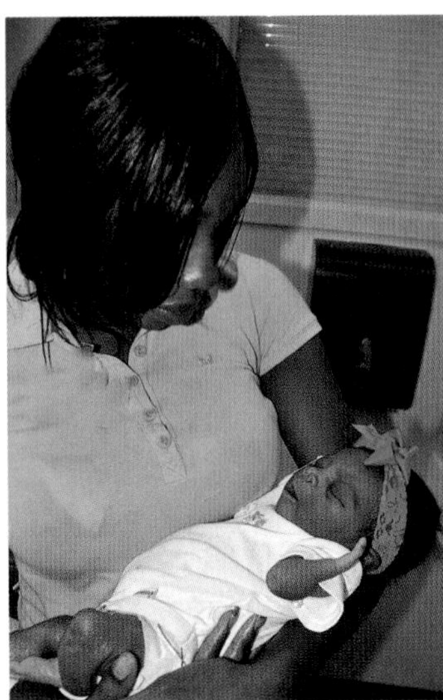

FIG 24.3 Touching and cuddling between parents and the infant with a congenital anomaly foster attachment and help resolve the grieving process. This infant has anomalies of the hand and arm. (Courtesy Cheryl Briggs, RNC, Annapolis, MD.)

everyone, and parents are fearful about whether their child will be accepted. If the defect is cleft lip and palate, the parents will be extremely concerned about surgical repair. Parents are often anxious about how grandparents and siblings will accept the child.

Gender is at the core of a person's identity, and any defect of the genitals arouses deep concern in both parents. Some anomalies, such as hypospadias (opening of the urethra on the underside of the penis), are repaired in early childhood. Other genital anomalies, such as ambiguous genitalia, when assignment of gender is in doubt, cause extreme concern in the family and affect such basic issues as what to name the infant, how to dress the infant, and how to respond to questions about the infant's gender.

### Irreparable Defect

Although the initial effect of any defect is deep disappointment and concern, irreparable defects cause the parents to grapple with the knowledge that their infant will have a lifelong disability. Examples of irreparable defects include Down syndrome, microcephaly, and amelia (absence of an entire extremity).

## Grief and Mourning

Grief describes the emotional response to loss. *Mourning* is the process of going through the phases of grief until the loss can be accepted and resolved. Birth of an infant with an anomaly evokes a grief response, and the family must mourn the loss of the perfect infant they imagined during the pregnancy. Detachment and mourning for the expected perfect infant must occur before the parents can attach to the actual infant (Gardner & Dickey, 2011). Early emotions include denial, anger, and guilt.

Denial and disbelief are the initial reactions of most parents to the discovery their infant has a congenital defect. Anger is often a pervasive response and may take the form of fault-finding or resentment. Anger may be directed toward the family, the medical personnel, or the self, but it is seldom directed toward the infant. Guilt may be expressed as a question of responsibility for the defect: "I shouldn't have worked so much while I was pregnant."

Other emotions include fear, which may be expressed as concern about what must be done in the immediate or distant future (surgical procedures, complicated care, the infant's potential for a normal life). Sadness and depression, manifested by crying, withdrawal from relationships, lack of energy, inability to sleep, and decreased appetite, may precede acceptance and resolution. Often after a prolonged period, feelings of sadness gradually abate and the family is able to adapt to the loss and resolve their grief.

## Nursing Considerations

### Assisting With the Grieving Process

If the condition is known before the birth, parents experience anticipatory grief. Both parents should be present when they are told about the infant's condition by the obstetrician or midwife. The nurse can use therapeutic communication techniques to help them express their feelings. They should receive as much information as possible about the condition and its effects. If the infant will go to the neonatal intensive care unit, a tour before the birth may increase their understanding of the care the infant will receive.

At birth, the parents experience the reality of the condition. They must continue to grieve the loss of the perfect infant they expected and begin to form an attachment to this newborn. Whether parents learned of the problem before or after the birth, it is helpful for the nurse to remain with them through the initial phase of shock and disbelief and maintain an atmosphere that encourages them to express their feelings.

Nurses must recognize that grief responses vary among individuals, and cultural and religious beliefs affect the expression of grief. Members of some groups express grief openly by crying, becoming angry, or seeking comfort from a support group. Those in other cultures (e.g., Chinese, Japanese, Native Americans) do not. They may appear stoic and may not reveal the depths of their grief. In some cultures (such as Latino), it is acceptable for women, but not for men, to grieve publicly.

The mother should be offered a private room, if possible. The infant should be examined in front of the parents so they can ask questions. Information about the normal needs of this newborn should be given at the same time as other information.

### Promoting Bonding and Attachment

A priority nursing intervention is to promote bonding and attachment, which may be disrupted when parents who expected a normal infant give birth to one with an abnormality. The process often begins when the nurse communicates acceptance of the infant.

To promote bonding, the nurse handles the newborn gently and presents the infant as someone precious. Parents are particularly sensitive to facial expressions of shock or distress. The infant should be called by name. Many nurses emphasize the normal aspects of the infant's body: "She's so alert, and she has beautiful eyes." Perhaps it is most important to help the parents hold their infant as soon as possible. Touching and cuddling are essential to caring.

### Providing Accurate Information

Nurses who work in perinatal settings are responsible for becoming informed about follow-up treatment and timing of surgical procedures for common anomalies so they can clarify and reinforce information provided by the physician. This process involves discussing the plan of care with the physician as well as researching the nursing care that will be required. Parents develop trust in the healthcare team when consistent information is presented clearly and explained fully.

If possible, one primary nurse or team should work with the family throughout the hospital stay. The nurse should expect to repeat information frequently because it may be difficult for the grieving parents to take in everything they are told at this time of intense emotions.

### Facilitating Communication

Nurses are sometimes fearful of being asked questions they cannot answer, or they fear that they will say the wrong thing.

The most helpful course of action is to answer questions as honestly as possible. If unsure of information, say so: "I'm not sure about that, but I'll find out for you." In addition to answers, parents need kindness, support, and genuine concern.

It is crucial that family members communicate with one another as well as with the health professionals. Information and empathy should be offered consistently to both parents. Fathers should be included in all discussions, demonstrations, and care of the infant. Without this attention, the father cannot be expected to support his partner, explain the infant's condition to relatives and friends, or begin to deal with his own shock and sadness.

The nurse should assess the mother for signs of postpartum depression (see Chapter 28). The support person should be made aware of the mother's increased risk for prolonged depression. The signs of depression and the differences between normal "baby blues," normal grieving, and postpartum depression should be explained.

### Participating in Infant Care

Parents should be involved in giving care to the infant as soon as possible to increase bonding and to help them feel that they can be real parents to their infant. Providing care for the infant also helps reduce parental anxiety as they get to know their baby (Klaus, Kennell, & Edwards, 2011).

### Planning for Discharge

Teach parents the special feeding, holding, and positioning techniques that their infant needs. Early participation in infant care fosters feelings of attachment and responsibility for the infant as well as increasing feelings of confidence.

Providing other anticipatory guidance may help prevent problems when the infant is discharged. The reaction and behavior of siblings depend on their ages and abilities to understand the needs of the infant. Young children, who are often jealous of the attention and care the infant requires, may regress to infantile behaviors such as bedwetting or thumb-sucking. Remind parents that this response indicates a need for attention rather than naughtiness.

Although grandparents can be a great source of strength and support, they may also have difficulty adjusting to the infant with an abnormality. When appropriate and if the parents are willing, include interested grandparents when teaching special care that the infant will need.

### Providing Referrals

Initiate referrals to national and community resources, if appropriate. Besides a referral to the social worker or grief counselor in the hospital, parents may also benefit from information about the Easter Seals Disability Services, the March of Dimes, or the disabled children's services of the public health department. In addition, organizations such as the Shriners provide funds for the care of children.

## PERINATAL LOSS

Perinatal death can occur at any time. Early spontaneous abortion, ectopic pregnancy, fetal demise at any point during pregnancy, stillbirth, or neonatal death when the infant survives for a few days or weeks can be equally devastating for the parents. The death may occur after a complicated pregnancy or after one in which all seemed well until the baby died.

Parents experiencing perinatal death often feel alone in their grief because many people do not consider perinatal loss to be on the same level as the loss of an older child or adult. In addition, friends and family members may be hesitant to discuss the loss for fear of saying the wrong thing.

### Early Pregnancy Loss

Early pregnancy loss from spontaneous abortion or ectopic pregnancy may precipitate intense grief in the parents. The parents may not have told family and friends about the pregnancy yet. Those who do know may minimize the grief that occurs at this time. Comments such as "You shouldn't have any problems getting pregnant again" discount the parents' feelings. When ectopic pregnancy is the reason for the loss, the woman must cope with the loss of the pregnancy as well as with the loss or damage of a fallopian tube.

### Concurrent Death and Survival in Multifetal Pregnancy

Parents experience conflicting and complex feelings of joy and grief when one or more infants in a multifetal pregnancy live while others in the same gestation die. Contrary to common belief, parents do not grieve less for the dead infant because of the joy they experience in the surviving infant.

For parents experiencing both survival and death of infants, the grieving process may be complicated. They may have fears about the health of the surviving infant, especially if the infant is preterm or ill. They may be unable to grieve for the dead child because of their concerns for the surviving child. They may also have problems with attachment to the surviving infant because of grieving and fear that they will lose that infant too. In addition, they may receive less support than parents who have lost the only child in a single gestation.

### Previous Pregnancy Loss

Women who have experienced previous pregnancy losses often have higher levels of anxiety than women who have not suffered such loss. They may also have symptoms of depression, which correlate with increased concern about the well-being of a healthy infant born after a previous loss (Côté-Arsenault et al., 2014).). Women find the entire pregnancy after a loss to be stressful but are most anxious in early pregnancy. They often tend to be pessimistic about the chance of a successful outcome near the beginning of pregnancy but gradually become more positive as the pregnancy progresses. They may delay telling family and friends about the pregnancy until they feel more confident about the outcome. They may be particularly fearful near the time in gestation when the previous loss occurred. Fathers may hide their worries about a new pregnancy in an effort to decrease worry in the mother.

Early prenatal care is especially important during a pregnancy following a loss. Both parents may be more comfortable if they can have frequent prenatal visits, which may need to be longer than usual. These parents require reassurance about the status of the fetus and emotional support throughout the pregnancy. Although mothers may request extra diagnostic testing to help relieve their anxiety, they may not always feel as reassured by normal test results as they had hoped. Nurses who provide them with an opportunity to express their distress and fears and make referrals to support groups or mental health providers may provide better relief of anxiety and a better use of health-care resources (Hutti, Armstrong, & Myers, 2011).

## NURSING CARE

### Pregnancy Loss

#### Assessment

Nursing assessment of the family that has experienced the loss of a fetus or infant requires great sensitivity. In the case of infant death, collect as much information as possible before meeting the woman and her family for the first time so that hurtful mistakes can be avoided. Knowing the child's gender, weight, length, gestational age, and whether any abnormalities were noted will help the nurse communicate effectively.

Many perinatal units design a sticker or symbol to place on the door, chart, and Kardex so that all staff who come in contact with the family, including auxiliary, housekeeping, and laboratory personnel, will be alerted that the infant has not survived. Designs include a fallen leaf, flower, teardrop, butterfly, or rainbow. This visual symbol diminishes the chance that an uninformed person will make inadvertent comments that cause the family pain.

Nurses are often unsure how to interact with a family that has experienced the loss of an infant. It is helpful to acknowledge the situation and to clarify the nurse's role at once: "I'm Dawn and I'll be your nurse today. I'm so sorry for your loss. What can I do today that would be most helpful to you?" This is not an appropriate time for self-disclosure or for false reassurance. Keep the focus on the family's response and their ability to support one another.

Nurses who provide home care or make follow-up telephone calls must be aware of subtle cues of grief, such as sighing, excessive sleeping, apathy, poor hygiene, or loss of appetite. These signs are especially important when assessing members of cultural groups who do not display grief publicly. In addition, nurses must observe for signs of anxiety or depression (Moore, Parrish & Black, 2011).

Evaluate the availability of a support system that includes family members or clergy. Ask whether a spiritual adviser would help the family cope with their grief, if appropriate. The family may want the infant baptized or blessed.

Assess the father's needs too, because they are sometimes perceived as needing less support than the mother, and they may not receive the support they need. Many fathers feel a need to appear strong so that they can support their partners. As a result, they often hold back their own feelings of grief and pain in an attempt to avoid increasing the mother's grief. In addition, each member of the couple may grieve differently and may be perceived as being unsupportive by others (Coverston, 2011). Mothers feel a sense of failure but often find it easier to express feelings of sadness. Some fathers feel that talking about feelings makes them appear weak. Fathers may express sadness as anger and may focus their attention on their work to help them cope with their grief.

#### Nursing Diagnosis and Planning

Because perinatal death affects the whole family, an appropriate nursing diagnosis for families is:

- Interrupted Family Processes related to grief over newborn (or fetal) death.

***Expected outcome.*** The parents will express the meaning of the loss, share their grief with significant others, and provide support to each family member.

#### Interventions

***Allowing expression of feelings.*** Stay with the parents as they express their feelings. Allow them to cry or respond as they wish. Parents may wish to have some time alone but may also appreciate having the nurse sit quietly nearby. When they are ready to talk, listen attentively.

***Acknowledging the infant.*** It was once believed that when an infant was stillborn or died shortly after birth, the parents would grieve less if the newborn was taken away quickly, before the parents could see it. Relatives often disposed of the clothes and infant equipment before the mother returned home. The parents were left with very few memories of the infant's birth.

The response to perinatal death changed as nurses discovered that the most helpful interventions for grieving parents were those that acknowledged the rights of the baby. These include the right to (Primeau & Lamb, 1995):

Be recognized as a person who was born and died.
Be named.
Be seen, touched, and held by the family.
Have end-of-life acknowledged.
Be put to rest with dignity.

**Presenting the infant to the parents.** The way in which the infant is presented to the parents is extremely important because these are the memories they will retain. If necessary, wash the infant and apply baby lotion or powder. Wrap the infant in a soft, warm blanket. Some parents wish to participate in bathing and dressing the baby.

If possible, bring the parents and infant together while the infant is still warm and soft. It may be necessary to keep the infant in a warmed incubator if some time elapses before the parents have contact with the infant. If this is not possible, tell the parents that the skin may feel cool. Call the infant by name, and allow the parents to keep the infant as long as they wish. Tell them to feel free to unwrap the infant.

When the stillborn infant has severe deformities, explain the defect briefly and gently. Wrap the infant to expose the most normal aspect. Use diapers to cover genital defects and booties and mittens to cover abnormalities of the hands and feet so the parents do not see those areas first. However, it is not advisable to try to hide the defects completely. Allow parents to progress at their own speed in inspecting the infant. Parents may look at the abnormality or choose to leave the infant wrapped.

Some parents provide infant care before their baby dies. If death is near, ventilators and other equipment may be removed so the parents can feel closer to the infant. They may hold the infant during the dying process. Many feel this is very helpful to them because it provides a chance to say goodbye and is the only opportunity they will have to parent their baby. Other family members may also be present at this time. Stay with the family, if they wish, to help them at this difficult time.

Allow as much privacy and time as the parents and other family members need to be together. Remain sensitive to cues that members of the family want to talk or prefer silence. A sympathetic smile and a promise to return in a specific time and then returning at that time are equally important. It is all right to ask, "Do you want to talk?" Then, listening quietly and reflecting the mother's or father's feelings are all that are required.

Although many parents want to spend time caring for or holding their baby before or after death, others may not. It is important not to make the parents feel guilty or that they should behave in a certain way. Nurses must accept that each family needs to go through this difficult experience in their own way (Limbo & Kobler, 2010).

**Preparing a memory box or packet.** Mourning requires memories. Nurses have explored measures that help the family create memories of the infant so that the existence of the child is confirmed and the parents can complete the grieving process.

Prepare a memory box or packet that includes items such as a photograph; the crib card with the infant's name, weight, and length;

identification band with the time and date of birth; blanket and cap used for the baby; and anything else used in care of the infant. Make paper handprints or soft modeling material impressions of the infant's hands and feet. If possible and with the parents' permission, cut a lock of hair from the nape of the neck, where it won't be noticeable. Some facilities offer commercial remembrance materials to give parents. The packets or boxes may contain clothing for the baby to wear or provide a place to keep baby items.

Take photographs of the infant to help the parents remember the baby's features and assist them in their grieving. Take photos of the infant dressed and undressed, wrapped and unwrapped, and of the parents and other family members with the infant. Professional photographs may be available from the Now I Lay Me Down To Sleep Foundation, a nonprofit organization that provides bereavement photos to families. A list of photographers and their locations is available at http://www.nowilaymedowntosleep.org. A website that offers help for caregivers who take pictures for the family is http://www.toddhochberg.com.

Keep the memory packet and photos on file if the parents do not want to take them home, because they may want them at a later time.

**Respecting cultural practices.** In some cultures, seeing or holding the baby after death is not acceptable. Cutting a lock of hair may not be permissible in some Muslim families. Certain Native American, Alaskan Native, Muslim, Hindu, and Amish groups do not want photographs taken of the infant because it is culturally unacceptable (Kavanaugh & Wheeler, 2007). Therefore, ask permission before taking pictures. Pictures taken before death occurs may be more acceptable. Discuss options with families about what they prefer, and don't make assumptions based on race.

Expression of grief may be loud and open or parents may appear stoic, depending on cultural expectations. The nurse must be accepting of the family's method of coping with their loss.

***Assisting with other needs.*** Help the parents plan how to tell other children about the death of the newborn. Provide the parents with written information about perinatal loss, grieving, and children's responses to death for later use. It is important that parents explain the cause of death in understandable terms because some children will believe they are to blame.

Offer to call clergy and discuss plans for a funeral or memorial service. Parents may wish to discuss this with their own clergy, or a hospital chaplain may assist them. Discuss the normal grieving process and explain that a considerable amount of time is involved. Describe common reactions that family members and friends may have and that grandparents will also experience grief because of the loss as well as the pain their children must endure.

Family members and friends often do not know how to help the grieving parents. Parents may find that friends and relatives expect them to recover quickly from perinatal loss and cannot understand their continued grief. Suggest they allow the parents to "tell the story" of the infant as often as they want because this helps them in the grief process. Suggest that they help the parents collect and talk about mementos to help establish memories of the infant.

Siblings are often expecting to be a "big brother" or "big sister" and need help understanding why that will not occur. Help the parents explore how they will tell their other children that the new baby will not be coming home. Explain that some young children think they have done something to cause the death and need reassurance. Young children may have questions (e.g., "Is the baby still dead?" or "Is the baby alive?") that should be answered simply but truthfully. See Chapter 36 for more on children's responses to a sibling's death.

***Providing referrals.*** Referrals to social services are important. Many hospitals provide bereavement programs or bereavement counselors to offer ongoing help to parents. Telephone calls may be made at specific intervals, and cards may be sent by agency staff to help parents cope with their grief. A list of resources that may be helpful may be included with a card.

The greatest help often comes from contact with people who have experienced a similar loss, and various support groups have been formed. Refer parents to resources at the birth facility or in the community that are designed to help parents cope with loss. Many Internet resources are available, for example, Share: Pregnancy & Infant Loss Support, Inc. at http://www.nationalshare.org/index.html; M.I.S.S. Foundation at http://www.misschildren.org; or Helping After Neonatal Death (HAND) at http://www.handonline.org.

### Evaluation

- Have the parents begun to acknowledge their grief and the meaning of the loss?
- Have they shared their grief with significant others?
- Are they able to be supportive of each other?

## ADOPTION

Some women carry their pregnancy to term and then relinquish the newborn to the care of another family for adoption. The decision to place the infant for adoption is a painful one that can produce long-lasting feelings of ambivalence and chronic sorrow. On the one hand, the expectant mother may be satisfied that the infant is going into a stable home where he or she is wanted and will receive excellent care. On the other hand, the social pressures against giving up one's child are often intense.

The relationship between the birth mother and the adoptive parents varies greatly. The adoptive parents may be unknown to the birth mother, or she may have chosen them after interviewing many candidates. Some adoptive mothers participate at the birth. The birth mother may never see the infant again or may keep in contact with and participate in the child's life.

Nurses are sometimes unsure of how to communicate with the woman who is placing her infant for adoption. First, the nursing staff who come into contact with the woman must be informed of her decision to place the infant for adoption. This information prevents inadvertent comments that could cause distress. Second, nurses must remember that adoption is *an act of love, not one of abandonment*, because the woman relinquishes the newborn to a family that is better able to provide financial and emotional support.

Nurses must also be prepared to respect any special wishes the mother may have about the birth. Most birth mothers plan ahead for the amount of involvement with the infant and adoptive parents they desire. Many want to know all about the infant. Encourage birth mothers to see and hold the newborn and give it a name. Many take photographs or save the crib card. Such actions provide memories of the infant and help the mother through the grieving process that accompanies relinquishment of a child.

The nurse should try to establish rapport and a trusting relationship with the birth mother. It is helpful to acknowledge the situation at the initial contact with the woman: "Hello, I'll be your nurse today. I understand the adoptive family is coming this morning. What can I do to help you get ready?" This approach is much more helpful than providing care without reference to an event that is of utmost concern to the mother. It also provides an opening for her to express feelings that may include attachment to the infant, ambivalence about her decision, and profound sadness.

Nurses also teach adoptive families how to care for the newborn and what to expect in growth and development. Teaching requires adequate time and a private place. The family benefits from all the teaching provided to other new parents. They may be anxious, and demonstrations as well as return demonstrations are appropriate.

## INTIMATE PARTNER VIOLENCE

Intimate partner violence (IPV) includes physical, sexual, emotional, social, and economic abuse. According to the CDC (2011) approximately 4.8 million acts of IPV occur annually to women in the United States. More than 25% of women report IPV at some time during their lives (Beckmann et al., 2010). Adolescents as well as older women are victims of IPV. Although some studies show an increased incidence in economically disadvantaged groups, IPV is seen at all educational levels, socioeconomic and ethnic groups, and in all areas of the country.

Physical violence occurs within the context of continuous mental abuse, threats, and coercion. Physical abuse may involve threats, slapping, or pushing. It may escalate to punching, kicking, and beating that results in internal injury, wounds from weapons, or death (Fig. 24.4). Sexual abuse, including rape, is often part of physical abuse, and many abused women report being forced into sex by their male partner. Reproductive coercion, such as interfering with a woman's use of contraception or threatening to leave her if she doesn't become pregnant, may also occur (Miller, Jordan, Levenson, et al., 2010).

Emotional abuse causes women to feel shame, loss of self-respect, and powerlessness. The abuser blames the victim for the abuse. Social abuse includes isolating the victim from friends and family and controlling where she can go. Economic abuse includes controlling the money and making the victim account for any money she spends. Such abuse can also involve interfering with the victim's ability to hold a job (Mattson & Smith, 2016).

Factors that are associated with violence include abuse of alcohol and other substances by the woman and her partner, depression, unwanted pregnancy, repeat pregnancy within 24 months, and frequent need for treatment for various problems including vague complaints, chronic pain, gynecologic problems, recurrent STIs, and inadequately explained injuries (Bacchus & Bewley, 2011; Ettinger & Gambone, 2010). Posttraumatic stress disorder and sleep and neuromuscular problems are also seen. Abused women often report that their partner is unwilling to use contraception or makes it difficult for them to use contraception, leading to unwanted pregnancies (Records, 2016).

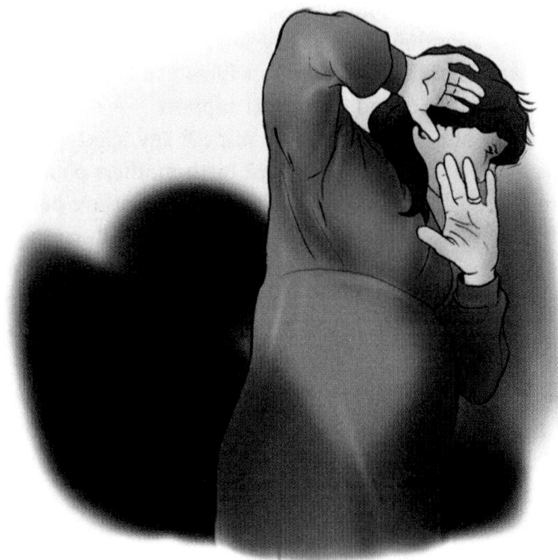

**FIG 24.4** The woman who is abused by her partner lives with an ever-present risk of violence. Because they may not seek help, all women should be asked about abuse whenever they receive healthcare.

### EVIDENCE-BASED PRACTICE

Intimate partner violence (IPV) affects women of all ethnic groups, but most of the related studies have included only white women. Liendo, Wardell, Engebretson, et al., conducted a study to learn more about the experience of women of Mexican descent who suffered IPV. Women were recruited from either a shelter for women who were victims of intimate partner violence or from an outreach agency for patients needing such services as legal support or safe haven. The sites were located near the Texas-Mexico border. Twenty-six women were interviewed in Spanish or English to discuss the effect of IPV on themselves and their families. Confidentiality was maintained for all women.

Eighteen of the women had suffered abuse as children or from more than one partner. Some described not allowing themselves to see what had been happening in the relationship because it was too painful. When they acknowledged the abuse, they wondered why they had stayed in the relationship so long. Women reported feeling dehumanized by the humiliation. Often they left the relationship because of the effects of seeing violence against their mother on their children. Some said they were also victimized by threats and blame by their partner's family. Those who were immigrants were threatened with deportation. The criminal justice and judicial systems were not always supportive.

Nurses and other healthcare and service providers should assess for abuse in women as a way to improve the lives of these women and their children. Education and prevention programs should be increased in community settings.

Reference: Liendo, N.M., Wardell, D.W., Engebretson, J., et al. (2011). Victimization and revictimization among women of Mexican descent. *Journal of Obstetric, Gynecologic, and Neonatal Nursing, 40*(2), 206–214.

### Effects of Intimate Partner Violence During Pregnancy

Up to 20% of women may be physically abused during pregnancy. Abuse is more common during pregnancy than is preeclampsia, diabetes, or other commonly screened pregnancy complications (Lu et al., 2010). IPV may begin or increase in frequency and severity during pregnancy and the period after birth. The greatest risk occurs during the postpartum period (Bacchus & Bewley, 2011).

Abuse during pregnancy is correlated with health problems for the mother and infant. Abused women are likely to have multiple injury sites, particularly of the face, arms, buttocks, abdomen, and breasts (Beckmann et al., 2010; Records, 2016). Abused women are more likely than nonabused women to start prenatal care late and to have health problems such as STIs. In addition, abused women have an increased risk of postpartum depression (Certain, Mueller, Jagodzinski, et al., 2010).

Infants born to abused mothers are more likely to have a low birth weight and be born preterm. Trauma to the abdomen can cause spontaneous abortion, abruptio placentae, premature rupture of membranes, preterm labor and birth, and fetal death (Bacchus & Bewley, 2011; Cunningham et al., 2010).

Abuse of the mother may be an indication of what life holds for the unborn child. Some men who batter women also batter the children, and some women who are victims of violence abuse their children. Child abuse occurs in 33% to 77% of homes where there is IPV. Approximately 27% of abused women abuse their children (AAP & ACOG, 2012).

Children who witness violence in their homes may have emotional, behavioral, developmental, and medical problems including anxiety, depression, aggressiveness, sleep problems, hyperactivity, and school difficulties (American Academy of Child and Adolescent Psychiatry [AACAP], 2013). Adults who abuse others were often abused as children.

### Factors That Promote Violence

Family violence occurs in cultures in which roles are based on gender and little value is placed on the woman's role. Men hold power, and women are viewed as less worthy of respect than men.

Women usually earn less than men in the job market, and they are often victimized by marriage. For example, women who hold full-time jobs still carry the major responsibilities for housekeeping and child care. They may remain in unhealthy relationships because they are financially dependent on their partners. If they divorce, women become single parents who often have a standard of living much lower than that of their former husbands.

Stereotyping males as powerful and females as weak and without value has a profound effect on the self-esteem of women. Many women internalize these messages and come to believe that they are less worthy than their partners and that they are the cause of their own punishment. They accept the implication from some members of society that when women are battered or raped, they "got what they deserved."

Although alcohol is often stated as a cause of violence against women, chemical dependence, and IPV are two separate problems. However, violence may become more severe or bizarre when alcohol or drugs are involved. Table 24.2 provides a summary of the myths and realities of violence against women.

**TABLE 24.2 Myths and Realities of Violence Against Women**

| Myths | Realities |
|---|---|
| The battered woman syndrome affects only a small percentage of the population. | Battering is the single major cause of injury to women. Approximately 4.8 million IPV-related physical assaults and rapes occur on women each year. |
| Violence against women occurs only in lower socioeconomic classes and minority groups. | Violence occurs in families from all social, economic, educational, racial, and religious backgrounds. |
| The problem is really "partner abuse," couples who assault each other. | Approximately 95% of serious assaults are male against female. Violence against women is about control and power. |
| Alcohol and drugs cause abusive behavior. | Substance abuse and violence against women are two separate problems. Substance abuse is a disease but violence is a learned behavior that can be unlearned. |
| The abuser is "out of control." | He is not out of control. He is making a decision, because he chooses who, when, and where he abuses. |
| The woman "got what she deserved." | No one deserves to be beaten. No one has the right to beat another person. Violent behavior is the responsibility of the violent person. |
| Women "like" it or they would leave. | Women are threatened with severe punishment or death if they attempt to leave. Many have no resources and are isolated, and they and their children are dependent on the abuser. |
| Couples counseling is a good recommendation for abusive relationships. | Couples counseling is ineffective for the couple and can be dangerous for the abused woman. |

*IPV,* intimate partner violence.

### Characteristics of the Abuser

Physical abuse concerns power and is only one of many tactics that abusive men use to control their partners. Other tactics include isolation, intimidation, and threats. Extreme jealousy and possessiveness are typical of the abuser. An abusive man often attempts to control all aspects of the woman's life, including where she goes and what she wears. He controls access to money and transportation and may force the woman to account for every moment spent away from him.

The abusive man often has a low tolerance for frustration and poor impulse control. He does not perceive his violent behavior as a problem and often blames the woman. Most abusive men come from homes where they witnessed the abuse of their mothers or were themselves abused as children.

### Cycle of Violence

Although IPV may be random, there is often a pattern. The violence occurs in a cycle that consists of three phases: (1) a tension-building phase, (2) a battering incident, and (3) a "honeymoon or calm phase." Being aware of the behaviors that accompany each phase will enable the nurse to counsel the woman (Fig. 24.5).

### Nurses' Role in Prevention of Abuse

Nurses can do a great deal to prevent physical abuse. First, they must examine their own beliefs to determine whether they accept the attitude that blames the victim: "Why does she stay with him?"

Second, nurses can consciously practice in ways that empower women. They should make it clear that the woman owns her body and has the right to decide how it should be treated. Nurses must use language that indicates the woman is an active partner in her care: "You understand your body; what do you think?"

During examinations, nurses can introduce aspects of care that increase the woman's control over the situation. For example, make sure that the woman meets the physician or nurse practitioner who is to examine her when she is seated and clothed rather than when she is unclothed and in a lithotomy position.

School nurses are in an excellent position to influence how teenagers define gender roles: "Real men don't beat up women." "Girls don't have to put up with verbal or physical abuse from anyone."

Nurses should be familiar with national resources that are designed to provide healthcare workers with technical assistance, training materials, posters, bibliographies, and relevant articles. The National Domestic Violence Hotline offers information on crisis assistance throughout the United States. They have interpreters for 170 different languages and are available 24 hours a day. The other sources listed below provide information but are not crisis lines.

Women who are being abused should be warned not to access Internet sources of information about abuse at home because their partners may be able to determine recently used Internet sites.

- National Domestic Violence Hotline, 1-800-799-SAFE (7233), http://www.thehotline.org
- National Coalition against Domestic Violence, 303-839-1852, http://www.ncadv.org
- National Resource Center on Domestic Violence, 1-800-537-2238, http://www.nrcdv.org

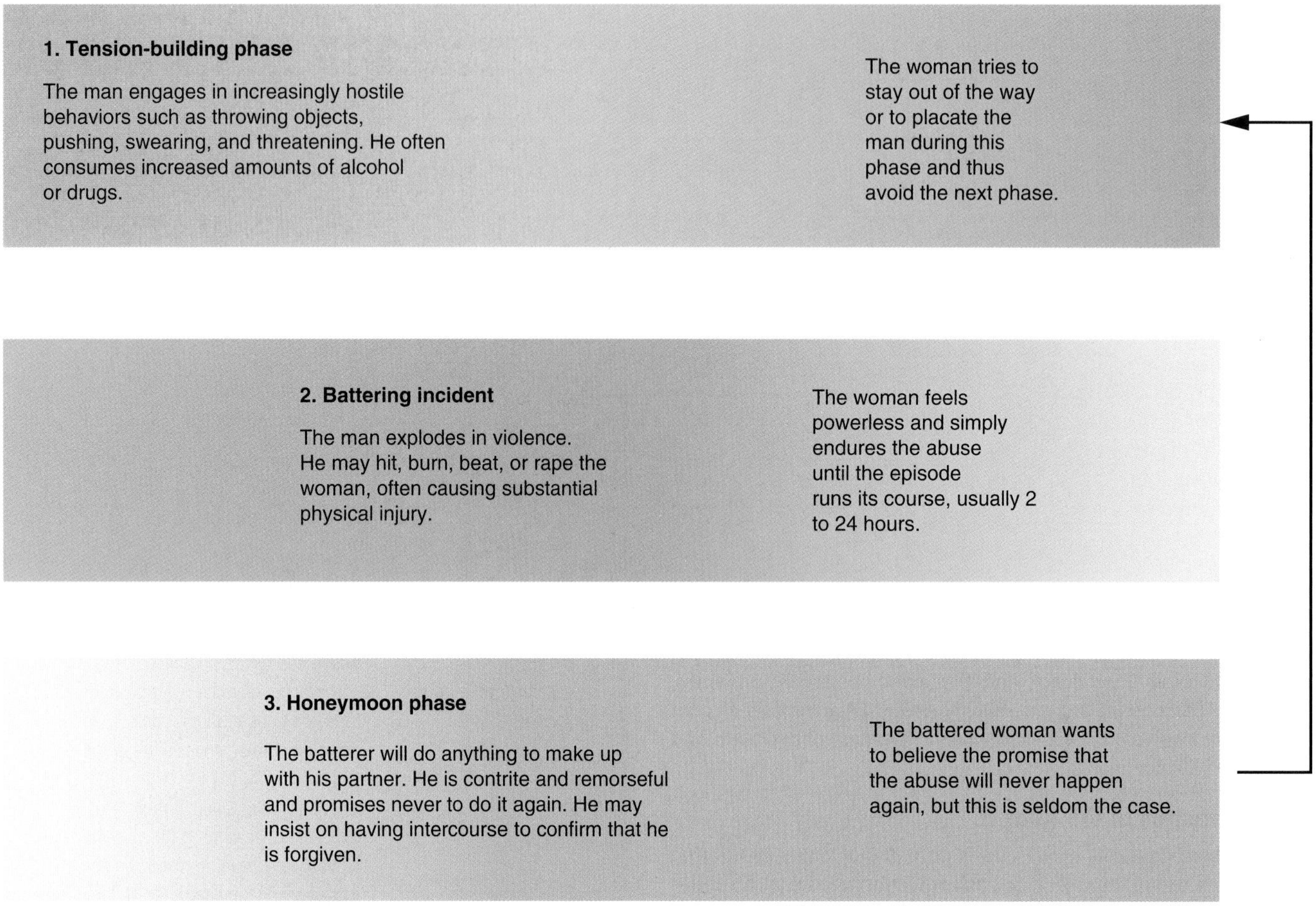

**1. Tension-building phase**

The man engages in increasingly hostile behaviors such as throwing objects, pushing, swearing, and threatening. He often consumes increased amounts of alcohol or drugs.

The woman tries to stay out of the way or to placate the man during this phase and thus avoid the next phase.

**2. Battering incident**

The man explodes in violence. He may hit, burn, beat, or rape the woman, often causing substantial physical injury.

The woman feels powerless and simply endures the abuse until the episode runs its course, usually 2 to 24 hours.

**3. Honeymoon phase**

The batterer will do anything to make up with his partner. He is contrite and remorseful and promises never to do it again. He may insist on having intercourse to confirm that he is forgiven.

The battered woman wants to believe the promise that the abuse will never happen again, but this is seldom the case.

**FIG 24.5** Types of behaviors evident in each step of the cycle of violence.

## NURSING CARE

### The Battered Woman

#### Assessment

During pregnancy, a woman is likely to have more frequent contact with healthcare providers than at any other time in her life. Because of the prevalence of IPV during pregnancy, it is recommended that all women be screened for physical abuse at each contact with the healthcare system. After pregnancy, opportunities for screening occur during visits to the pediatrician, which usually occur frequently during the infant's first year. The American Academy of Pediatrics (2010) recommends assessment for IPV during office visits as a means to prevent child abuse.

When first approached, women may deny that abuse has occurred. They may feel judged and stigmatized because they do not want to leave the relationship and are fearful that their children will be taken away if they reveal the situation. Asking, and especially asking more than once in a nonjudgmental way, may lead the woman to seek help at a later time. Leaving written information in women's restrooms also implies that discussion of violence is encouraged and safe.

Many nurses are unsure about how to approach the issue of suspected abuse. Women often seek care in the "honeymoon phase" of the violence cycle. During this phase the man is often overly solicitous ("hovering husband syndrome") and eager to explain any injuries that the woman exhibits. He often answers questions directed at the woman. *Introducing the subject of violence in the presence of the man who may be responsible for it places the woman in danger. It is essential to separate the woman from the man for the discussion of violence.* No other family members should be present for that part of the interview. Even children as young as 2 years may reveal to the partner or family members that abuse was discussed (Bacchus & Bewley, 2011; McFarlane, Parker, & Moran, 2007; Olshansky, 2014).

### CRITICAL THINKING EXERCISE 24.1

Claire, a 28-year-old primigravida, is admitted to the labor, delivery, and recovery unit in preterm labor at 30 weeks of gestation. The right side of her face is swollen. Old bruises that look like fingerprints are present on her upper arms, and a large bruised area is evident on her abdomen. She is accompanied by her husband, who is very solicitous. He verbalizes concern about her labor status and remains close beside her at all times. Claire appears lethargic and avoids eye contact with the nurse who is admitting her. She states that she fainted at home and hurt herself when she fell against the bathtub. The nurse accepts the explanation and asks no further questions.

1. What assumptions has the nurse made?
2. What should make the nurse examine her conclusion that the injuries resulted from falling?
3. Why did the nurse wait for time alone before asking questions?
4. How should the nurse respond? The nurse must guard against what bias?
5. How can Claire be protected?

A common concern about discussing IPV is having time with the woman without her partner. Sometimes the partner can be sent to another area to give insurance information. Telling the partner that the nurse plans to discuss "feminine hygiene" and needs privacy may also be a way to have time alone with the woman.

Other reasons nurses cite for not discussing IPV include lack of time, not knowing what to do if IPV is discovered, and language barrier. If language barriers are present, a family member or friend should never be used to translate. Instead, a professional interpreter is necessary.

When a private, secure place has been found, explain that many women experience abuse and that it is agency policy to ask every woman about abuse. Reassure her that her privacy will be protected and that confidentiality will be maintained. Commonly used questions to screen for violence include asking whether the woman has been threatened, hit, slapped, kicked, choked, or otherwise physically hurt or forced to have sexual relations by anyone during the past year and during the pregnancy and if she is afraid of anyone. A "yes" answer to these questions requires further assessment of the situation.

If trauma is apparent, appropriate questions include: "Did someone hurt you?" "Did you receive these injuries from being hit?" The abused woman often appears hesitant, embarrassed, or evasive. She may be unable to look the nurse in the eye and appears guilty, ashamed, jumpy, or frightened. She may initially deny abuse. Accept her answer without question to develop rapport and allow her to choose the time to disclose her situation.

Evaluate and document all signs of injury, both past and present. Such assessment includes areas of welts, bruising, swelling, lacerations, burns, and scars. Injuries are most commonly noted on the face, breasts, abdomen, and genitalia. Many women have new or old fractures of the face, nose, ribs, or arms. A photograph or a drawing can be used to show areas of injury. Such documentation may be important for future legal action. Record direct quotes of what the woman says about her experience. If there has been sexual abuse, a gynecologic examination is necessary because there is often trauma to the labia, vagina, cervix, or anus.

Be particularly alert for nonverbal cues indicating that abuse has occurred. Facial grimacing or a slow, unsteady gait may indicate pain. Vomiting or abdominal tenderness may indicate internal injury. A flat affect (absence of facial response) is indicative of women who mentally withdraw from the situation to protect themselves from the horror and humiliation they experience. Keep in mind that the woman may fear for her life because abusive episodes tend to escalate.

**CRITICAL TO REMEMBER**

### *Cues Indicating Violence Against Women*

- *Nonverbal:* Facial grimacing, slow and unsteady gait, vomiting, abdominal tenderness, absence of facial response
- *Injuries:* Welts, bruises, swelling, lacerations, burns, vaginal or rectal bleeding; evidence of old or new fractures of the nose, face, ribs, or arms
- *Vague somatic complaints:* Anxiety, depression, panic attacks, sleeplessness, anorexia
- *Discrepancy between history and type of injuries:* Wounds that do not match the woman's story, multiple bruises or lacerations in various stages of healing, bruising on the arms (which she may have raised to protect herself), old, untreated wounds

### Nursing Diagnosis and Planning

Nursing diagnosis depends on the data collected during the assessment. The most meaningful diagnosis may be:

- Fear related to possibility of severe injury to self and/or children during an unpredictable cycle of violence.

**Expected outcomes.** The woman will acknowledge the physical assaults, will develop a specific plan for when the cycle of abuse begins, and will identify community resources that provide protection for herself and her children.

The abused woman is often unwilling to leave the abusive situation, and nurses frequently must work with the woman to plan realistic short-term goals that will protect her from injury.

### Interventions

**Listening.** Use therapeutic communication techniques to listen and encourage the woman to share her feelings. Assure her that her situation is difficult and that she has been surviving as well as she can. Praise each positive step she takes to increase safety for herself and her children, no matter how small the step.

**Developing a personal safety plan.** Ask the woman what she does to decrease or avoid violence from her partner. If she hasn't already, help her make concrete plans to protect her safety as well as that of her children. Describe the cycle of behavior that culminates in physical abuse and instruct her about factors such as use of alcohol or other drugs that precipitate a violent episode. Discuss behaviors that indicate that the level of frustration and anger is increasing to the point where the danger is escalating. Assist her to:

- Locate the nearest shelter, safe house, or other safe place and make specific plans to go there once the cycle of violence begins.
- Identify the safest, quickest routes out of the home.
- Hide extra keys to the car and house, money, personal information (social security numbers, insurance policy information, birth certificates, driver's license, bank account numbers), medications, some clothes, and personal necessities. She should not hide them in the house but find another place such as with a friend or relative.
- Devise a code word, and prearrange with someone to call the police when the word is used.
- Memorize the telephone number of the shelter or hotline, because time is often a crucial element in the decision to leave. An easy number to remember is that for the National Domestic Violence Hotline (1-800-799-SAFE), which provides immediate crisis assistance in the caller's community.
- Review the safety plan frequently, because leaving the partner is one of the most dangerous times for her.

**Affirming that she is not to blame.** The abused woman often believes that she is responsible for the abuse. Let her know that no one deserves to be hurt for any reason. The one who hurt her is the person responsible. She did not provoke it or cause it and could not have prevented it. Nurses are often responsible for teaching that violence is not normal, is usually repeated, and usually escalates. She needs help to understand that battering is against the law and abused women have alternatives.

She also needs nonjudgmental acceptance and recognition of the difficulties involved in changing her situation. Praise her for any actions she takes, even if they are only minor steps toward making her life safer. Reassure her that she is doing the right thing for herself and her children when she seeks help and makes plans for escape.

**Providing education.** The pregnant woman is likely to worry about the effect of abuse on her pregnancy. Discuss the increased incidence of preterm labor with her and explain the signs. If she is using substances, explain the effects of smoking and alcohol and drug use and help her make plans to decrease or stop her use. Help her identify stressors and explore ways to reduce them wherever possible.

**Providing referrals.** Refer the family to community agencies such as the police department, legal services, community shelters, counseling services, and social service agencies as needed. Include mental health referrals, if necessary, for depression or counseling. Document that referrals were made and that the woman accepted them.

It is essential to accept the decisions of the battered woman and acknowledge that she is on her own timetable. She may not take any actions at the time they are recommended. Therefore, listening to her, believing her, and providing information about resources may be the only help the nurse can provide until the woman is ready to do more.

Do not become negative or pass judgment on the partner of an abused woman. She is often tied to the man by both economic and emotional bonds and may become defensive if her partner is criticized. Tell her that resources are available for her partner but that it is necessary for him to admit abuse and seek assistance before help can be offered. To initiate referrals for the partner before he asks for help will increase the danger to the woman if he believes he has been betrayed.

### Evaluation

- Does the woman acknowledge the violence?
- Has she made concrete plans to protect herself and her children from future injury?
- Does she make plans to use the community resources available to her?

## KEY CONCEPTS

- Teenage pregnancy is a major health problem in the United States. Adolescents need to receive accurate information about contraceptives and how to set limits on sexual behavior.
- Adolescent pregnancy poses serious physiologic risks that result in a higher incidence of complications for the mother and fetus.
- Teenage pregnancy interrupts the developmental tasks of adolescence and may result in childbirth before the parents are capable of providing a nurturing home for the infant without a great deal of assistance.
- The mature primigravida often has financial and emotional resources that younger women do not have. She may experience anxiety about recommended antepartum testing and about her ability to be an effective parent.
- Polydrug abuse is a widespread problem that can have devastating fetal and neonatal effects that can become long-term developmental problems for the child.
- The lifestyle associated with illicit drug abuse includes inadequate nutrition, inadequate prenatal care, and an increased incidence of STIs. Interdisciplinary interventions are required to prevent injury to the expectant mother and the fetus.
- The birth of an infant with congenital anomalies produces strong emotions of shock and grief in the family. A sensitive response from nurses can help the family grieve for the loss of the perfect or "fantasy" infant and to form an attachment to the newborn.
- Pregnancy loss at any stage produces grief that must be acknowledged and expressed. Nurses realize that mourning requires memories, and they intervene to arrange unlimited contact between the family and the stillborn infant and to prepare mementos for the family.
- Nursing care for the mother who is placing her infant for adoption is based on the knowledge that relinquishment for adoption is an act of love, not abandonment.
- Multiple factors are associated with intimate partner violence. It is deliberate, severe, and generally repeated in a predictable cycle that often causes severe physical harm (or death) to the woman.
- All perinatal nurses come into contact with abused women who require assistance to protect themselves and their children from serious injury.

## REFERENCES AND READINGS


Alan Guttmacher Institute. (2011). *Facts on American teens' sexual and reproductive health.* Retrieved from http://www.guttmacher.org/pubs/FB-ATSRH.html#18.

Albright, B.B., & Rayburn, W.F. (2009). Challenging issues in women's health care substance abuse among reproductive age women. *Obstetrics and Gynecology Clinics of North America, 36*(4), 891–906.

American Academy of Pediatrics. (2010). The role of the pediatrician in recognizing and intervening on behalf of abused women. *Pediatrics, 125*(5), 1094–1100.

American Academy of Pediatrics. (2015). *Choosing Adoption.* Retrieved from http://www.healthychildren.org.

American Academy of Child and Adolescent Psychiatry. (2013). *Facts for Families: Domestic violence and children.* Retrieved from http://www.aacap.org/AACAP/Families_and_Youth/Facts_for_Families/FFF-Guide/Helping-Children-Exposed-to-Domestic-Violence-109.aspx.

American Academy of Pediatrics & American College of Obstetricians and Gynecologists. (2012). *Guidelines for perinatal care* (7th ed.). Elk Grove Village, IL, and Washington, DC: Author.

American College of Obstetricians and Gynecologists. (2010). Committee Opinion 462: Moderate caffeine consumption during pregnancy. *Obstetrics & Gynecology, 116*(2), 467–468.

American College of Obstetricians and Gynecologists. (2011). Committee Opinion 479: Methamphetamine abuse in women of reproductive age. *Obstetrics & Gynecology, 117*(3), 751–755.

American College of Obstetricians and Gynecologists. (2012). Committee Opinion 518: Intimate Partner Violence. *Obstetrics & Gynecology, 119* (2), 412–417.

American Psychiatric Association. (2013). *Diagnostic and statistical manual of mental disorders* (5th ed.). Author, Washington, DC.

American Society of Addiction Medicine. (2011). *Public policy statement on women, alcohol and other drugs, and pregnancy.* Author, Chevy Chase, MD.

Anderko, L., Braun, J., & Auinger, P. (2010). Contribution of tobacco smoke exposure to learning disabilities. *Journal of Obstetric, Gynecologic and Neonatal Nursing, 39*(1), 111–117.

Association of Women's Health, Obstetric, and Neonatal Nurses. (2015). *Position Statement: Criminalization of pregnant women with substance use disorders.* Retrieved from http://www.AWHONN.org.

Bacchus, L., & Bewley, S. (2011). Domestic violence. In D.K. James, P.J. Steer, C.P. Weiner, et al. (Eds.), *High risk pregnancy: Management options* (4th ed., pp. 29–34). Philadelphia: Saunders.

Bailey, B.A., McCook, J.G., Hodge, A., & McGrady, L. (2012). Infant birth outcomes among substance using women: Why quitting smoking during pregnancy is just as important as quitting illicit drug use. *Maternal Child Health Journal, 16*(2), 414–422.

Bandstra, E.S., & Accornero, V.H. (2011). Infants of substance abusing mothers. In R.J. Martin, A.A. Fanaroff, & M.C. Walsh (Eds.), *Fanaroff & Martin's neonatal-perinatal medicine: Diseases of the fetus and infant* (9th ed., pp. 735–757). Philadelphia: Mosby.

Bayrampour, H., & Heaman, M. (2010). Advanced maternal age and the risk of cesarean birth: A systemic review. *Birth, 37*(3), 219–226.

Beckmann, C.R.B., Ling, F.W., Barzansky, B.M., et al. (2010). *Obstetrics and gynecology* (6th ed.). Philadelphia: Lippincott Williams & Wilkins.

Black, M.C., Basile, K.C., Breiding, M.J., Smith, S.G., Walters, M.L., Merrick, M.T., Stevens, M.R. (2011). *The National Intimate Partner and Sexual Violence Survey (NISVS): 2010 summary report.* National Center for Injury Prevention and Control, Centers for Disease Control and Prevention, Atlanta, GA.

Breiding, M.J., Smith, S.G., Basile, K.C., Walters, .L., Chen, J., & Merrick, M.T. (2014). *Prevalence and characteristics of sexual violence, stalking, and intimate partner violence victimization — National Intimate Partner and Sexual Violence Survey, United States. Surveillance Summaries.* Retrieved March 30, 2016 from http://www.cdc.gov/mmwr.

Broussard, A.B., & Broussard, B.S. (2010). Teaching pregnant teens: Lessons learned. *Nursing for Women's Health, 14*(2), 104–111.

Buhimschi, C.S., & Weiner, C.P. (2011). Medications. In D.K. James, P.J. Steer, C.P. Weiner, et al. (Eds.), *High risk pregnancy: Management options* (4th ed., pp. 579–597). Philadelphia: Saunders.

Burstein, G.R. (2011). Sexually transmitted infections. In R.M. Kliegman, B.F. Stanton, J.W. St. Geme, et al. (Eds.), *Nelson textbook of pediatrics* (19th ed., pp. 705–714). Philadelphia: Saunders.

Centers for Disease Control and Prevention. (2011). *Tobacco use and pregnancy.* Retrieved from http://www.cdc.gov/reproductivehealth/TobaccoUsePregnancy.

Centers for Disease Control and Prevention. (2011). *Understanding intimate partner violence: Fact sheet.* Retrieved from http://www.cdc.gov/violenceprevention/pdf/IPV_factsheet-a.pdf.

Centers for Disease Control and Prevention. (2011). Vital signs: Teen pregnancy—United States, 1991-2009. *MMWR: Morbidity and Mortality Weekly Report Early Release, 50*(13), 414–420.

Centers for Disease Control and Prevention (2014). *Fetal Alcohol Spectrum Disorders.* Retrieved from http://www.cdc.gov/Features/FASD/.

Centers for Disease Control and Prevention. (2016). *Teen Pregnancy in the United States.* Retrieved from http://cdc.gov/reproductivehealth/TeenPregnancy.

Certain, H.E., Mueller, M., Jagodzinski, T., & Fleming, M. (2010). Domestic abuse during the previous year in a sample of postpartum women. *Journal of Obstetric, Gynecologic and Neonatal Nursing, 37*(1), 35–41.

Chico, E. & Gonzalez, A., Ali, N., Steiner, M., & Fleming, A.S. (2015). Executive functioning and mothering: Challenges faced by teenage mothers. *Developmental Psychobiology, 56*(5), 1027–1035.

Cleveland, L., Gill, S. (2013). Try not to judge mothers of substance exposed infants. *American Journal of Maternal/Child Nursing, 38*(4), 200–205.

Côté-Arsenault, D., Schwartz, K, Krowchuk, H., & McCoy, T. (2014). Evidence-based intervention with women pregnant after perinatal loss. *The American Journal of Maternal/Child Nursing, 39*(3), 177–186.

Coverston, C.R. (2011). Psychology of pregnancy. In S. Mattson, & J.E. Smith (Eds.), *AWHONN core curriculum for maternal-newborn nursing* (4th ed., pp. 101–114). St. Louis: Saunders.

Cunningham, F.G., Leveno, K.J., Bloom, S.L., et al. (2010). *Williams obstetrics* (23th ed.). New York: McGraw-Hill.

Cunningham, F.G., Leveno, K.J., Bloom, S.L., et al. (2015). *Williams obstetrics* (24th ed.). New York: McGraw-Hill.

Discenza, D. (2010). When a baby dies: When families need you the most. *Neonatal Network, 29*(4), 259–261.

Dudgeon, A., Evanson, T. (2014). Intimate partner violence in rural U.S. areas: What every nurse should know. *American Journal of Nursing, 114*(5), 26–35.

Elfenbein, D.S., & Felice, M.E. (2011). Adolescent pregnancy. In R.M. Kliegman, B.F. Stanton, J.W. St. Geme, et al. (Eds.), *Nelson textbook of pediatrics* (19th ed., pp. 699–702). Philadelphia: Saunders.

Ettinger, B.B., & Gambone, J.C. (2010). Family and intimate partner violence and sexual assault. In N.F. Hacker, J.C. Gambone, & C.J. Hobel (Eds.), *Essentials of obstetrics and gynecology* (5th ed., pp. 322–325). Philadelphia: Saunders.

Fantasia, H.C., & Fontenot, H.B. (2011). The sexual safety of adolescents. *Journal of Obstetric, Gynecologic, and Neonatal Nursing, 40*(2), 217–224.

Gardner, S.L., & Dickey, L.A. (2011). Grief and perinatal loss. In S.L. Gardner, B.S. Carter, M. Enzman-Hines, et al. (Eds.), *Merenstein & Gardner's handbook of neonatal intensive care* (7th ed., pp. 898–937). St. Louis: Mosby.

Grassley, J.S. (2011). Adolescent mothers' breastfeeding social support needs. *Journal of Obstetric, Gynecologic, and Neonatal Nursing, 39*(6), 713–722.

Grassley, J.S. (2011). Promoting health among childbearing adolescents and their infants. *Journal of Obstetric, Gynecologic, and Neonatal Nursing, 39*(6), 694.

Hamilton, B.E., Martin, J.A., Osterman, M.J.K., Curtin, S.C., & Mathews, T.J. (2015). Births: Final data for 2014. *National Vital Statistics Reports, 64*(12), 1–64.

Heavey, E. (2010). Don't miss preconception care opportunities for adolescents. *MCN: The American Journal of Maternal/Child Nursing, 35*(4), 213–219.

Huang, C.Y., Costeines, J., Kaufman, J.S., & Ayala, C. (2014). Parenting stress, social support, and depression for ethnic minority adolescent mothers: Impact on child development. *Journal of Child and Family Studies, 23*(2), 255–262.

Hudak, M., & Tan, R. (2012). Neonatal drug withdrawal. *Pediatrics, 129*(2), e540–e560.

Hutti, M.H., Armstrong, D.S., & Myers, J. (2011). Healthcare utilization in the pregnancy following a perinatal loss. *MCN: The American Journal of Maternal/Child Nursing, 36*(2), 104–111.

Iverson, K.M., Wells, S.Y., Wiltsey-Stirman, S., Vaughn, R., & Gerber, M.R. (2013). VHA primary care providers' perspectives on screening female veterans for intimate partner violence: A preliminary assessment. *Journal of Family Violence, 28*(8), 823–831.

Kavanaugh, K., & Wheeler, S.R. (2007). When a baby dies: Caring for bereaved families. In C. Kenner, J.W. Lott, & A.A. Flandermeyer (Eds.), *Comprehensive neonatal nursing: An interdisciplinary approach* (4th ed., pp. 522–542). Philadelphia: Saunders.

Klaus, M.H., Kennell, J.H., & Edwards, W.H. (2011). Care of the mother, father, and infant. In R.J. Martin, A.A. Fanaroff, & M.C. Walsh (Eds.), *Fanaroff & Martin's neonatal-perinatal medicine: Diseases of the fetus and infant* (9th ed., pp. 615–627). Philadelphia: Mosby.

Kochanek, D.D., Kirmeyer, S.E., Martin, J.A., et al. (2012). Annual summary of vital statistics: 2009. *Pediatrics, 129*(2), 338–348.

Lefebvre, L., Midmer, D., Boyd, J.A., et al. (2010). Participant perception of an integrated program for substance abuse in pregnancy. *Journal of Obstetric, Gynecologic, and Neonatal Nursing, 39*(1), 46–52.

Lemacks, J., Fowles, K., Mateus, A., & Thomas, K. (2013). Insights from Parents about Caring for a Child with Birth Defects. *International Journal of Environmental Research and Public Health, 10*(8), 3465–3482.

Levi, A. & Dau, K.Q. (2011). Meeting the national health goal to reduce unintended pregnancy. *Journal of Obstetric, Gynecologic, and Neonatal Nursing, 40*(6), 775–781.

Liendo, N.M., Wardell, D.W., Engebretson, J., et al. (2011). Victimization and revictimization among women of Mexican descent. *Journal of Obstetric, Gynecologic and Neonatal Nursing, 40*(2), 206–214.

Limbo, R., & Kobler, K. (2010). The tie that binds: Relationships in perinatal bereavement. *MCN: The American Journal of Maternal/Child Nursing, 35*(6), 316–321.

Limbo, R., Kobler, K., & Levang, E. (2010). Respectful disposition in early pregnancy loss. *MCN The American Journal of Maternal/Child Nursing, 35*(5), 271–277.

Lu, M.C., Williams, J., & Hobel, C.J. (2010). Antepartum care: Preconception and prenatal care, genetic evaluation and teratology, and antenatal fetal assessment. In N.F. Hacker, J.C. Gambone, & C.J. Hobel (Eds.), *Essentials of obstetrics and gynecology* (5th ed., pp. 71–90). Philadelphia: Saunders.

Mandel, D. (2010). The lived experience of pregnancy complications in single older women. *MCN: The American Journal of Maternal/Child Nursing, 35*(6), 336–340.

March of Dimes. (2013). *A mommy after 35.* Retrieved from http://www.marchofdimes.com.

McCracken, K.A., & Loveless, M. (2014). Teen pregnancy: An update. *Current Opinion in Obstetrics and Gynecology, 26*(5), 355–359.

McFarlane, J., Parker, B., & Moran, B.A. (2007; reviewed 2014). *Abuse during pregnancy: A protocol for prevention and interventions* (3rd ed.). White Plains, NY: March of Dimes.

McPeak, K.E., Sandrock, D., Spector, N.D., & Patishall, A.E. (2015). Important determinants of newborn health: Postpartum depression, teen parenting, and breastfeeding. *Current Opinions in Pediatric, 27*(1)138–144.

Miller, E., Jordan, B., Levinson, R., et al. (2010). Reproductive coercion: Connecting the dots between partner violence and unintended pregnancy. *Contraception, 81*(6), 457–459.

Moats, C., Frederick, D., Edwards, M.D., & Files, J. (2014). More than meets the eye: The importance of screening for intimate partner violence. *Journal of Women's Health, 23*(3), 275–277.

Moore, M.L., Moos, M., & Callister, L.C. (2010). *Cultural competence: An essential journey for perinatal nurses.* White Plains, NY: March of Dimes.

Moore, R., Parrish, H., & Black, B.P. (2011). Interconception care for couples after perinatal loss: A comprehensive review of the literature. *The Journal of Perinatal and Neonatal Nursing, 25*(1), 44–51.

National Campaign to Prevent Teen and Unplanned Pregnancy. (2010). *Teen pregnancy and childbearing in the United States: Ten headlines.* Retrieved from http://www.TheNationalCampaign.org.

National Campaign to Prevent Teen and Unplanned Pregnancy. (2014). *Why it matters: Linking teen pregnancy prevention to other critical issues.* Retrieved from http://www.TheNationalCampaign.org.

National Institute on Drug Abuse, 2011. *Prenatal exposure to drugs of abuse.* Author, Bethesda, MD; 2011.

National Institute on Drug Abuse. (2009). *Treatment approaches for drug addiction.* Author, Bethesda, MD.

Olshansky, E. (2014). Assessment and health promotion. In Perry, S.E., Hockenberry, M.J., Lowdermilk, D.L., & Wilson, D. (Eds.), *Maternal child Nursing Care* (5th ed. Pp. 39–73). St. Louis, Missouri: Mosby.

Oscar, A.V., Soto, E.E., Bahado-Singh, R.O., Christensen, C.W., Chauhan, S.P, & Sibai, B.M. (2014). Fetal anomalies and long-term effects associated with substance abuse in pregnancy: A literature review. *American Journal of Perinatology, 32*(5), 405–415.

Patrick, S.W., Schumacher, R., Benneyworth, B., Krans, E.E., McAllister, J.M., & Davis, M.M. (2012). Neonatal Abstinence Syndrome and Associated Health Care Expenditures. *Journal of the American Medical Association, 307*(18),1934–1940.

Pitts, K. (2010). Perinatal substance abuse. In M.T. Verklan, & M. Walden (Eds.), *AWHONN core curriculum for neonatal intensive care nursing* (4th ed., pp. 41–71). St. Louis: Saunders.

Poole, J.H. (2014). Antenatal care. In K.R. Simpson, & P.A. Creehan (Eds.), *AWHONN perinatal nursing* (4th ed., pp. 89–121). Philadelphia: Lippincott Williams & Wilkins.

Porter, L.S., & Holness, N.A. (2011). Breaking the repeat pregnancy cycle. *Nursing for Women's Health, 15*(5), 368–381.

Primeau, M.R., & Lamb, J.M. (1995). When a baby dies: Rights of the baby and parents. *Journal of Obstetric, Gynecologic, and Neonatal Nursing, 24*(3), 206–208.

Records, K. (2016). Intimate partner violence. In S. Mattson, & J.E. Smith (Eds.), *AWHONN core curriculum for maternal-newborn nursing* (5th ed., pp. 417–434). St. Louis: Saunders.

Roark, S.V. (2010). Intimate partner violence: Screening and intervention in the health care setting. *Journal of Continuing Education in Nursing, 41*(11), 490–495.

Ruger, J.P., & Lazar, C.M. (2012). Economic evaluation of drug abuse treatment and HIV prevention programs in pregnant women: A systematic review. *Addictive Behaviors, 37*(1), 1–10.

Ruedinger, E., & Cox, J. E. (2012). Adolescent childbearing: consequences and interventions. *Current Opinion in Pediatrics, 24* (4), 446-452.

Sauls, D.J. (2010). Promoting a positive childbirth experience for adolescents. *Journal of Obstetric, Gynecologic and Neonatal Nursing, 39*(5), 703–712.

Shay-Zapien, G., & Bullock, L. (2010). Impact of intimate partner violence on maternal child health. *MCN: The American Journal of Maternal/Child Nursing, 35*(4), 206–212.

SmithBattle, L. (2009). Reframing the risks and losses of teen mothering. *MCN: American Journal of Maternal/Child Nursing, 34*(2), 122–128.

Substance Abuse and Mental Health Services Administration (2012). *Results from the 2012 national survey on drug use and health: summary of national findings.* Author, Rockville, MD.

Substance Abuse and Mental Health Services Administration. (2013). *Trends in substances of abuse among pregnant women and women of childbearing age in treatment.* Author, Rockville, MD.

Sullivan, C.J. (2016). Substance Abuse in Pregnancy. In S. Mattson, & J.E. Smith (Eds.), *AWHONN core curriculum for maternal-newborn nursing* (5th ed., pp. 417-434). St. Louis: Saunders.

Thackeray, J.D., Hibbard, R., & Dowd, D. (2010). Intimate partner violence: The role of the pediatrician. *Pediatrics, 125*(5), 1094–1100.

Tong, V.T., Dietz, P.M., Morrow, B., D'Angelo, D.V., Farr, S.L., Rockhill, K.M., & England, L.J. (2013). *Trends in Smoking Before, During, and After Pregnancy — Pregnancy Risk Assessment Monitoring System, United States, 40 Sites, 2000–2010.* Retrieved from http://www.cdc.gov/mmwr/preview/mmwrhtml/ss6206a1.htm.

U.S. Department of Health and Human Services. (2010). *Healthy People 2020.* Washington DC: Author.

U.S. Department of Health and Human Services. (2016). *Trends in Teen Pregnancy and Childbearing.* Retrieved March 28, 2016 from http://www.hhs.gov.

Von Köhler, C.S. (2016). Age-related concerns. In S. Mattson, & J.E. Smith (Eds.), *AWHONN core curriculum for maternal-newborn nursing* (5th ed., pp. 123–134). St. Louis: Saunders.

Walker, J.J., & Walker, A. (2011). Substance abuse. In D.K. James, P.J. Steer, C.P. Weiner, et al. (Eds.), *High risk pregnancy: Management options* (4th ed., pp. 565–578). Philadelphia: Saunders.

Wendell, A.D. (2013). Overview and epidemiology of substance abuse in pregnancy. *Clinical Obstetrics and Gynecology, 56*(1), 91–6.

Whitaker, C., Kavanaugh, K., & Klima, C. (2010). Perinatal grief in Latino parents. *MCN The American Journal of Maternal/Child Nursing, 35*(6), 341–345.

Wildschut, H.I.J. (2011). Constitutional and environmental factors leading to a high risk pregnancy. In D.K. James, P.J. Steer, C.P. Weiner, et al. (Eds.), *High risk pregnancy: Management options* (4th ed., pp. 11–28). Philadelphia: Saunders.

# 25

# Pregnancy-Related Complications

http://evolve.elsevier.com/McKinney/mat-ch/

## LEARNING OBJECTIVES

*After studying this chapter, you should be able to:*

- Describe the hemorrhagic conditions of early pregnancy, including spontaneous abortion, ectopic pregnancy, and gestational trophoblastic disease.
- Explain disorders of the placenta, such as placenta previa and abruptio placentae, that may result in hemorrhage during late pregnancy.
- Discuss the effects and management of hyperemesis gravidarum.
- Describe the development and management of hypertensive disorders of pregnancy.
- Compare Rh and ABO incompatibility in terms of etiology, fetal and neonatal complications, and management.

Complications during pregnancy sometimes threaten the well-being of the expectant mother, her fetus, or both. The most common pregnancy-related complications are hemorrhagic conditions that occur in early pregnancy, hemorrhagic complications of the placenta in late pregnancy, hyperemesis gravidarum, hypertensive disorders of pregnancy, and blood incompatibilities between the mother and fetus.

## HEMORRHAGIC CONDITIONS OF EARLY PREGNANCY

The three most common causes of hemorrhage during the first half of pregnancy are abortion, ectopic pregnancy, and gestational trophoblastic disease including hydatidiform mole.

### Abortion

**Abortion** is the loss of pregnancy before the fetus is viable, that is, before it is capable of living outside the uterus. The medical consensus today is that a fetus of less than 20 weeks of gestation or one weighing less than 500 g is not viable. Abortion may be either spontaneous or induced. Spontaneous abortion denotes termination of a pregnancy without action taken by the woman or any other person. *Miscarriage* is a term used by laypeople to denote an abortion that has occurred spontaneously as opposed to one that has been induced, and the term is becoming accepted by professionals as well. Elective termination of pregnancy, also called *induced abortion,* is described in Chapter 32.

#### Spontaneous Abortion

Determining the exact incidence of spontaneous abortion is difficult because many unrecognized losses occur in early pregnancy. The incidence of spontaneous abortion increases with parental age. The incidence is 12% for women younger than 20 years, rising to 26% for women older than 40 years. Increasing paternal age is also associated with rising spontaneous abortion rates, from 12% in men younger than 20 years to 20% in men older than 40 years. Most spontaneous abortions occur in the first 12 weeks of pregnancy, with the rate declining rapidly thereafter. Fetal death occurs before signs and symptoms appear (Cunningham, Leveno, Bloom, Spong, Dashe, Hoffman, Casey, & Sheffield, 2014).

The most common cause of spontaneous abortion is severe congenital abnormalities that are often incompatible with life. Chromosomal abnormalities account for approximately 50% to 60% of spontaneous abortions in the first trimester. Additional causes may include maternal infections and endocrine disorders such as hypothyroidism or insulin-dependent diabetes. Women who have repeated early pregnancy losses appear to have immunologic factors that play a role in their higher-than-expected spontaneous abortion incidence. Anatomic defects of the uterus or cervix can contribute to pregnancy loss at any gestational age (Cunningham et al., 2014).

Spontaneous abortion is divided into six subgroups: threatened, inevitable, incomplete, complete, missed, and recurrent. Fig. 25.1 illustrates threatened, inevitable, and incomplete abortion.

##### *Threatened abortion*

**Manifestations.** The first sign of threatened abortion is vaginal bleeding. Up to 25% of all women experience "spotting," or light bleeding, in early pregnancy, and approximately half of these pregnancies will not survive. Vaginal bleeding, which may be brief or last for weeks, may be followed by symptoms of uterine cramping, persistent backache, or feelings of pelvic pressure. The symptoms of pain and pressure are more likely to be associated with progression to loss of the pregnancy. When examined using a speculum, the cervix is closed. Laboratory tests show rising levels of beta–human chorionic gonadotropin (beta-hCG), and the uterine size increases with embryonic growth if the pregnancy remains viable (Cunningham et al., 2014).

**Therapeutic management.** Bleeding in the first half of pregnancy must be considered a threatened abortion, and women should be advised to notify their physician or nurse-midwife if they note vaginal bleeding. The nurse obtains a detailed history that includes length of gestation or time of last menstrual period and the onset, duration, and amount of vaginal bleeding. Accompanying discomfort, such as cramping, backache, abdominal pain, or pelvic pressure, is evaluated. Fever or uterine tenderness suggests infection.

Ultrasound (either transvaginal or abdominal) is performed to determine whether a fetus is present and, if so, whether it is alive. Beta-hCG levels may be assessed to determine whether they are appropriate for the gestation and if they are rising as the fetus grows.

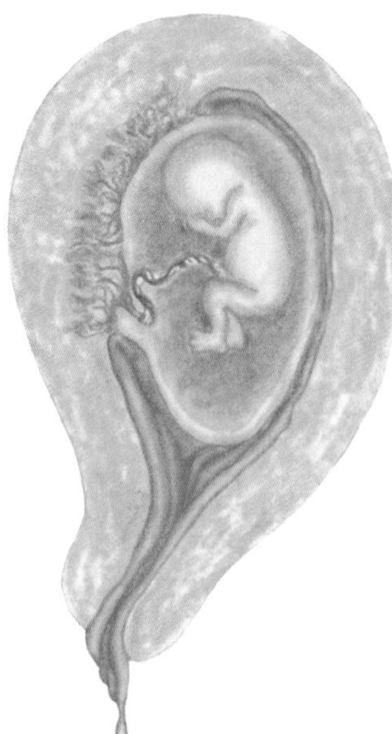

**Threatened abortion**
Vaginal bleeding occurs.

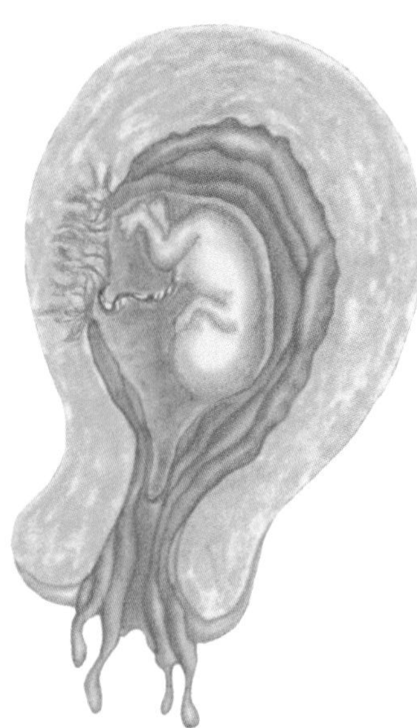

**Inevitable abortion**
Membranes rupture, and cervix dilates.

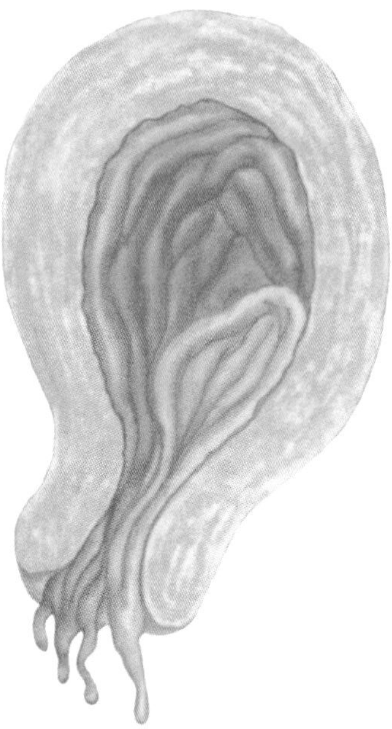

**Incomplete abortion**
Some products of conception have been expelled, but some remain.

**FIG 25.1** Three types of spontaneous abortion.

The woman may be advised to curtail sexual activity until bleeding has ceased. Bed rest or other restriction of physical activity has not been demonstrated to be effective in the treatment of threatened abortion. The woman is instructed to count the number of perineal pads (peripads) used and to note the quantity and color of blood on the pads. She should also look for tissue passage. Discharge with a foul odor suggests infection.

The woman often wonders whether her actions may have contributed to the situation and is anxious about her own condition as well as that of the fetus. The nurse should offer accurate information and avoid false reassurance, because the woman may lose the fetus despite every precaution. In addition, later complications, such as preterm birth or low birth weight may occur, even if the pregnancy progresses.

#### *Inevitable abortion*

**Manifestations.** Abortion is usually inevitable (i.e., it cannot be stopped) when the membranes rupture and the cervix dilates. Active bleeding may be present and heavy.

**Therapeutic management.** Natural expulsion of the uterine contents including fetal tissue is common, and no further treatment may be needed. This is often called products of conception. If tissue remains or if bleeding is excessive, the physician performs a dilation and vacuum curettage (D&C) **to clean the uterine walls and remove remaining uterine contents** while the woman is under intravenous (IV) sedation or anesthesia.

#### *Incomplete abortion*

**Manifestations.** Incomplete abortion occurs when some but not all of the products of conception are expelled from the uterus. The major manifestations are active uterine bleeding and severe abdominal cramping. The cervix is open, and fetal and placental tissue is passed. All products of conception may have been expelled from the uterus but remain in the vagina because of their small size, often no larger than a Ping-Pong ball if the gestation is very early.

**Therapeutic management.** Retained tissue prevents the uterus from contracting firmly, thus allowing profuse bleeding from uterine blood vessels. Initial treatment should focus on ensuring the woman's cardiovascular stability. Blood is drawn for a type and screen, and an IV line is inserted for fluid replacement and drug administration. A later pregnancy and a larger amount of fetal tissue may require greater cervical dilation and evacuation (D&E), followed by vacuum or surgical curettage. This procedure may be followed by IV administration of oxytocin (Pitocin) or intramuscular (IM) administration of methylergonovine (Methergine) to contract the uterus and control bleeding.

Because of the danger of excessive bleeding, curettage may not be performed if the pregnancy has advanced beyond 14 weeks. In this case, oxytocin or prostaglandin is administered to stimulate uterine contractions until all products of conception (fetus, membranes, placenta, and amniotic fluid) are expelled.

#### *Complete abortion*

**Manifestations.** Complete abortion occurs when all products of conception are expelled from the uterus. Uterine contractions and bleeding abate, and the cervix closes after all products of conception are passed.

**Therapeutic management.** Once complete abortion is confirmed, no additional intervention is required unless excessive bleeding or infection develops. The woman should be advised to rest and watch for further bleeding, pain, or fever. She should abstain from vaginal intercourse until after a follow-up visit with her healthcare provider. Contraception will be discussed at this visit if she wishes to avoid pregnancy.

#### *Missed abortion*

**Manifestations.** Missed abortion occurs when the fetus dies during the first half of pregnancy but is retained in the uterus. When the fetus dies, the early symptoms of pregnancy (nausea, breast tenderness, urinary frequency) disappear. The uterus stops growing and often decreases in size, reflecting the absorption of amniotic fluid and fetal maceration, or discoloration and softening of tissues, and eventual disintegration of the fetus.

**Therapeutic management.** In most cases, the pregnancy ends spontaneously after fetal death (Cunningham et al., 2010). If the fetus is not expelled, fetal death is confirmed by ultrasound examination. When fetal death is confirmed, the uterus may be evacuated by D&C. Prostaglandin $E_2$ or misoprostol (Cytotec) may be necessary to induce contractions and empty the uterus during the second trimester.

Two major complications of missed abortion are infection and disseminated intravascular coagulation (DIC). If there are signs of uterine infection, such as an elevated temperature, vaginal discharge with a foul odor, or abdominal pain, evacuation of the uterus is delayed until antibiotic therapy is initiated.

***Disseminated intravascular coagulation (consumptive coagulopathy).*** DIC is a defect in coagulation that may occur if the fetus is retained for a prolonged period. Although DIC may occur with other pregnancy complications, such as abruptio placentae (p. 531) or hypertension (p. 535), the coagulation defects may occur in the absence of pregnancy.

With DIC, anticoagulation and procoagulation factors are activated simultaneously. DIC develops when the clotting factor *thromboplastin* is released into the maternal bloodstream as a result of placental bleeding and consequent clot formation. The circulating thromboplastin may activate widespread clotting in small vessels throughout the body. This process consumes, or "uses up," other clotting factors such as fibrinogen and platelets. The condition is further complicated by activation of the fibrinolytic system to lyse, or destroy, clots. The result is a simultaneous decrease in clotting factors and increase in circulating anticoagulants, which leaves the circulating blood unable to clot. This situation allows bleeding to occur from any area, including IV sites, incisions, the gums or nose, as well as from expected sites such as the site of placental attachment during the postpartum period (Cunningham et al., 2014; Francois, 2012; Della Torre, Kilpatrick, Hibbard, Simonson, Scott, Koch, Gellar, 2011).

In DIC, fibrinogen and platelets are usually decreased, prothrombin and partial thromboplastin times may be prolonged, and fibrin degradation products, the most sensitive measurement, are increased. The D-dimer serum assay, which is normally negative, is a specific measurement of fibrin degradation activity.

The priority in treating DIC is delivery of the fetus and placenta to stop the production of thromboplastin, which is fueling the process. In addition, blood replacement products such as whole blood, packed red blood cells, and cryoprecipitate are administered to maintain the circulating volume and to transport oxygen to body cells (Francois, 2012).

### Recurrent Spontaneous Abortion

***Manifestations.*** Recurrent spontaneous abortion is sometimes referred to as habitual abortion; the current definition is three or more consecutive spontaneous abortions. The primary causes of recurrent abortion are believed to be genetic or chromosomal abnormalities or anomalies of the woman's reproductive tract, as in a bicornuate uterus, which has two horns, or incompetent cervix. The diagnosis of incompetent cervix or cervical insufficiency is considered when a patient experiences a second-trimester pregnancy loss as the result of painless cervical dilation.

Additional causes of habitual abortion include an inadequate luteal phase, with insufficient secretion of progesterone and immunologic factors involving increased sharing of human leukocyte antigens by the sperm and ovum of the man and woman who conceived. The theory is that because of this sharing, the woman's immunologic system is not stimulated to produce blocking antibodies that protect the embryo from maternal immune cells or other damaging antibodies. Systemic diseases, such as lupus erythematosus and diabetes mellitus, have been implicated in recurrent abortions. Reproductive infections and some sexually transmitted diseases are also associated with recurrent abortions.

***Therapeutic management.*** The first step in managing recurrent spontaneous abortion is a thorough examination of the woman's reproductive organs to determine whether anatomic defects, such as a bicornate uterus, are the cause. If her reproductive organs are normal, the woman is usually referred for genetic screening to identify genetic factors that would increase the possibility of recurrent abortions. Additional therapeutic management of recurrent pregnancy loss depends on the cause. For example, antimicrobials are prescribed for the woman with an infection, and hormone-related drugs may be prescribed if an imbalance preventing normal fetal implantation and support is found.

Recurrent spontaneous abortion may be caused by cervical incompetence, an anatomic defect that results in painless dilation of the cervix in the second trimester. In this case, the cervix can be sutured to keep it from opening (i.e., cerclage). Sutures are removed near term if vaginal delivery is expected, or they may be left in place if a cesarean birth is planned.

### Nursing Considerations

Spontaneous abortion may be accompanied by various amounts of bleeding. Prevention or identification and treatment of hypovolemic shock (rapid pulse, lightheadedness, syncope, falling blood pressure) are the nursing priorities when a woman is bleeding heavily. The nurse should observe for tachycardia (often the earliest sign of hypovolemia), falling blood pressure (late sign), pale skin and mucous membranes, confusion, restlessness, and cool and clammy skin. The nurse manages fluid and blood replacement as ordered.

Vaginal bleeding of any amount during pregnancy is frightening, and waiting and watching are difficult, although often the only reasonable treatment. Moreover, many families feel an acute sense of loss and grief with spontaneous abortion. Grief often includes feelings of guilt that may be expressed as wondering if the woman could have done something to prevent the loss. Nurses may be able to help by emphasizing that most spontaneous abortions occur because of factors or abnormalities that could not be avoided.

Anger, disappointment, and sadness are commonly experienced emotions, although the intensity of the feelings may vary. For many women, the fetus has not yet taken on specific physical characteristics, but they grieve for their fantasies of the lost child. The woman or couple may want to express their sadness but may feel that family, friends, and often health personnel are uncomfortable or diminish their loss. Nurses can determine whether their clinical facility offers options for disposing of fetal tissue and work to identify improvements (Limbo, Kobler, & Levang, 2010).

To recognize the meaning of the loss to each family, nurses must listen carefully to what the couples say and observe how the partners behave. Nurses must attempt to convey unconditional acceptance of the feelings expressed or demonstrated. The couple should be permitted to remain together as much as possible. Providing information and simple, brief explanations of what has occurred and what will be done facilitates the family's ability to grieve.

It is helpful for the family to realize that grief may last from 6 months to a year, or even longer. Grief may worsen at the time of the expected due date. Family support, knowledge of the grief process, spiritual counselors, and the support of other bereaved couples may provide needed assistance during this time.

## Ectopic Pregnancy

Ectopic pregnancy refers to implantation of a fertilized ovum in an area outside the uterine cavity. More than 95% of ectopic pregnancies are in the fallopian tube, usually in the ampulla (the middle part of the tube). Fig. 25.2 shows common sites of tubal implantation. Anything that slows the transport of the fertilized ovum through the tube

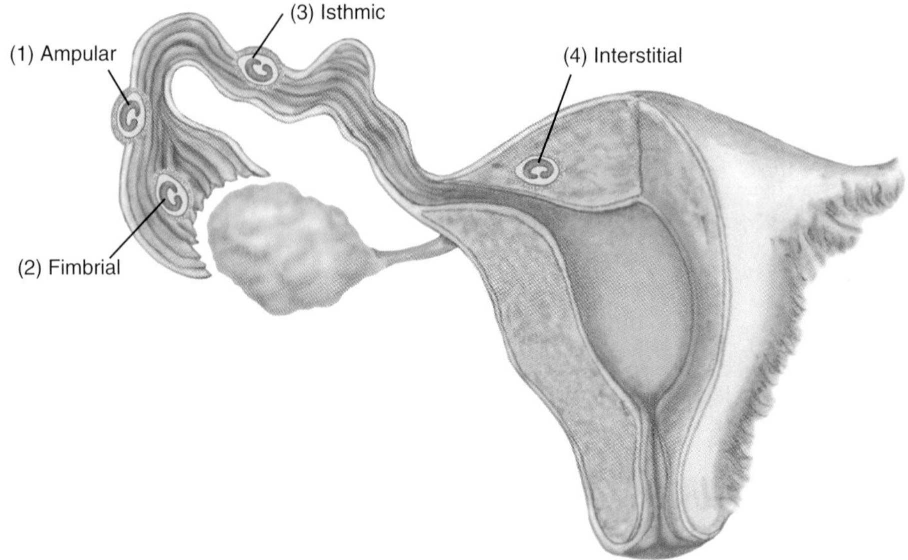


FIG 25.2 Sites of tubal ectopic pregnancy. Numbers indicate the order of prevalence. *(1) Ampular, (2) Fimbrial, (3) Isthmic, (4) Interstitial.*

**CRITICAL THINKING EXERCISE 25.1**

Alice, a 24-year-old primigravida, had an incomplete abortion at 12 weeks of gestation. When she was admitted to the hospital, IV fluids were administered, and blood was taken for blood typing and screen. A vacuum extraction with curettage was performed to remove retained placental tissue. She was discharged home after bleeding subsided. The nurse providing discharge instructions comments to the woman, "These things happen for the best, and you are so lucky it happened early." "You can have other children."

1. What assumptions has the nurse made? How might these comments affect the woman who suffered the spontaneous abortion or miscarriage?
2. Is the comment that the woman can have other children comforting? Why or why not?
3. If the nurse's response was not helpful, what responses from the nurse would be most helpful for Alice?

or causes it to implant too early increases the risk that implantation will occur in the tube rather than the uterus (American College of Obstetricians & Gynecologists [ACOG], 2010).

### Incidence and Etiology

The incidence of ectopic pregnancy has increased dramatically throughout the world since 1970, from 4.5 per 1000 pregnancies to 19.7 per 1000 pregnancies. Ectopic pregnancy rates are higher in nonwhite women and older women. The highest rate is seen in nonwhite women older than 35 years (Cunningham et al., 2014; ACOG, 2010c). The rapid increase in incidence is attributed to the growing number of women of childbearing age who experience scarring of the fallopian tubes caused by pelvic infection, inflammation, or surgery. Pelvic infection or inflammation (pelvic inflammatory disease [PID]) is often the result of sexually transmitted diseases such as *Chlamydia* or *Neisseria gonorrhoeae*. Pelvic infection also can occur after induced abortion or childbirth. Women who require assisted reproductive techniques to conceive also have a greater risk, probably resulting from the underlying pathology that caused infertility (Box 25.1).

**BOX 25.1 Risk Factors for Ectopic Pregnancy**

- History of sexually transmitted diseases (gonorrhea, chlamydial infection)
- History of pelvic inflammatory disease
- History of previous ectopic pregnancies
- Failed tubal ligation
- Intrauterine device
- Multiple induced abortions
- Maternal age older than 35 years
- Some assisted reproductive techniques, such as gamete intrafallopian transfer (GIFT)

Additional risk factors for ectopic pregnancy include:

- Use of the intrauterine device (IUD) for contraception
- Anatomic or functional defects in the fallopian tubes
- Cigarette smoking
- Vaginal douching

### Manifestations

Early signs and symptoms of ectopic pregnancy are:

- Missed menstrual period
- Abdominal and pelvic pain
- Vaginal "spotting" or light bleeding
- May have positive urine pregnancy test

More subtle signs and symptoms depend on the site of implantation. If implantation occurs in the distal end of the fallopian tube, which can accommodate a larger embryo, the woman may at first exhibit the usual early signs of pregnancy. Several weeks into the pregnancy, intermittent abdominal pain and small amounts of vaginal bleeding occur. These early manifestations are easily mistaken for those of threatened abortion.

If implantation has occurred in the proximal end of the fallopian tube, rupture of the tube may occur within 2 to 3 weeks of the missed period. Symptoms include sudden, severe pain in one of the lower quadrants of the abdomen as the tube tears open and the embryo is expelled into the pelvic cavity. Pain is often accompanied by intraabdominal hemorrhage. Irritation of the diaphragm, manifested by shoulder or neck pain that is worse on inspiration, occurs in approximately half of women (Cunningham et al., 2014). Signs of hypovolemic shock may develop with no or minimal external bleeding. Identification of risk factors for bleeding is important.

### Diagnostic Evaluation

The combined use of transvaginal ultrasound examination (see Chapter 15) and determination of the beta-hCG level usually results in early detection of ectopic pregnancy. An abnormal pregnancy is suspected if beta-hCG is present but at lower levels than expected. If a gestational sac cannot be visualized when beta-hCG is present, a diagnosis of ectopic pregnancy can be made with great accuracy. Visualization of an intrauterine pregnancy, however, does not absolutely rule out an ectopic pregnancy, as a woman can have an intrauterine pregnancy concurrent with an ectopic pregnancy.

The use of sensitive pregnancy tests, maternal serum progesterone levels, and high-resolution transvaginal ultrasound has largely eliminated invasive tests for ectopic pregnancy. Laparoscopy (examination of the peritoneal cavity by means of a laparoscope) occasionally may be necessary to diagnose rupture of an ectopic pregnancy. A characteristic bluish swelling within the tube is the most common finding.

### Therapeutic Management

The management of tubal pregnancy depends on whether the tube is intact or ruptured. Medical management may allow preservation of the tube, thus improving the chance of future fertility. Medical management is most successful if the tube is intact, the pregnancy is early, the size of the pregnancy is less than 3.5 cm, and the fetus is not living. The cytotoxic drug methotrexate (a folic acid antagonist that interferes with cell reproduction) inhibits cell division in the embryo. Single-dose methotrexate therapy has shown a higher failure rate and two-dose or fixed multidose therapy is more often used. Laboratory evaluation of beta-hCG levels are repeated as needed to evaluate success of drug therapy. Surgical treatment may be needed if methotrexate treatment fails or if the woman shows a high suspicion of tubal rupture (Cunningham et al., 2014; ACOG, 2010c).

Surgical management of an unruptured tubal pregnancy may involve a linear salpingostomy to salvage the tube for future pregnancies. The tube is opened with a fine linear incision, the products of conception are removed, and to reduce scarring, the tubal incision is left to heal without suturing. Linear salpingostomy also can be attempted if the fallopian tube is minimally ruptured and a slightly greater tubal opening is needed for removal of tubal pregnancy material.

When ectopic pregnancy results in rupture of the fallopian tube, the goal of therapeutic management is to control the bleeding and prevent hypovolemic shock. When the woman's cardiovascular status is stable, a salpingectomy is performed to remove the affected tube and ligate bleeding vessels. Future pregnancies can still occur when only one tube is present, although fertility decreases. In addition, the same conditions that caused the ectopic pregnancy in the tube that was removed may exist in the other tube.

### Nursing Considerations

Nursing care focuses on preventing or identifying hypovolemic shock, controlling pain, and providing psychological support for the woman who experiences an ectopic pregnancy. If methotrexate is used, the nurse must explain temporary side effects (e.g., nausea and vomiting) and the importance of communicating to the healthcare team bothersome drug effects or worsening symptoms that suggest rupture (e.g., pelvic, shoulder, or neck pain; dizziness or faintness; increased vaginal bleeding). The woman must be instructed to refrain from drinking alcohol or ingesting vitamins that contain folic acid, which would reduce the drug's effectiveness. She should not have sexual intercourse until beta-hCG levels are undetectable (Cunningham et al., 2010). The importance of keeping follow-up appointments should be emphasized because medical treatment is not always successful, and surgical intervention may be needed.

The woman and her family often need support to resolve emotions, which may include anger, grief, guilt, and self-blame. The woman may also be anxious about her ability to become pregnant in the future. Although the pregnancy is unsuccessful very early, the nurse should be aware that these women may feel an acute sense of loss similar to that of women suffering miscarriage. Nurses may need to clarify the physician's explanation and to use therapeutic communication techniques that help the woman to deal with her anxiety and grief.

## Gestational Trophoblastic Disease (Hydatidiform Mole)

Gestational trophoblastic diseases are a spectrum of diseases that include benign hydatidiform mole and gestational trophoblastic tumors, such as invasive moles and choriocarcinoma. Hydatidiform mole (molar pregnancy) occurs when the trophoblasts (peripheral cells that attach the fertilized ovum to the uterine wall) develop abnormally. As a result of the abnormal growth, the placenta, but not the fetus, develops. Hydatidiform mole is characterized by proliferation and edema of the chorionic villi. The fluid-filled villi form grape-like vesicles that can grow large enough to fill the uterus to the size of an advanced pregnancy if not diagnosed and treated (Fig. 25.3). The mole may be *complete*, with no fetus present, or *partial*, in which fetal tissue or membranes are present. Malignant change and proliferation of residual trophoblastic tissue (gestational trophoblastic neoplasm, or choriocarcinoma) is a life-threatening complication. Acute respiratory distress may occur if vesicles of the hydatidiform mole enter the woman's circulation and embolize to her lungs (Osborn & Dodge, 2012).

### Incidence and Etiology

In the United States and Europe, the incidence of gestational trophoblastic disease is 1 in every 1000 to 1500 pregnancies. Age is a factor,

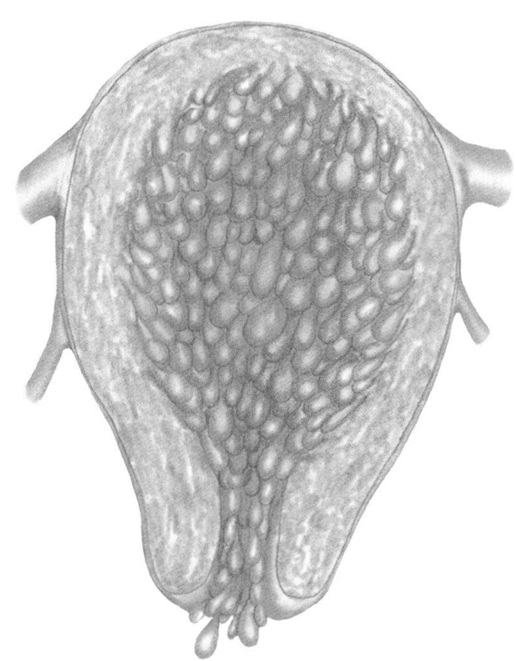

**FIG 25.3** Hydatidiform mole.

with the frequency of molar pregnancies highest at both ends of reproductive life. Women who have had one molar pregnancy are at greater risk for another (Cunningham et al., 2014)

A *complete mole* is believed to occur when the ovum is fertilized by a sperm that duplicates its own chromosomes while the chromosomes of the ovum are inactivated. In a *partial mole,* the maternal contribution is usually present, but the paternal contribution is double, and thus the karyotype is triploid (69,XXY or 69,XYY). Anomalies are present in an accompanying fetus.

Persistent gestational trophoblastic disease may undergo malignant change (choriocarcinoma), with possible rapid spread to distant sites such as the vagina, lung, liver, kidney, and brain. (Osborn & Dodge, 2012).

### Manifestations

Most molar pregnancies are diagnosed early by ultrasound that reveals the vesicles and no fetal gestational sac or cardiac action. Levels of beta-hCG are high because of the rapidly proliferating abnormal villi. Other signs and symptoms of a complete molar pregnancy vary with gestation, but may include:

- Vaginal bleeding, which varies from dark brown spotting to profuse hemorrhage
- A uterus larger than expected for the duration of the pregnancy
- Excessive nausea and vomiting, possibly related to high beta-hCG levels
- Early development (before 24 weeks) of preeclampsia

### Diagnostic Evaluation

Ultrasound examination allows a differential diagnosis to be made between two types of molar pregnancies. A complete mole shows multiple small cystic structures but no fetus. Current diagnostic techniques allow early identification and treatment of a molar pregnancy rather than later, when it ends spontaneously and is more likely to be accompanied by hemorrhage.

### Therapeutic Management

Management includes (1) evacuation of the mole and (2) follow-up to detect any malignant changes in any remaining trophoblastic tissue. Before evacuation, chest imaging studies, metabolic and blood chemistry tests, and a baseline serum beta-hCG level are done. A complete blood count, laboratory assessment of clotting factors, and blood typing and crossmatching are performed in case a transfusion is needed. Treatment for hypertension or hyperemesis may be needed if these added complications have occurred (Cunningham et al., 2014).

Vacuum aspiration is usually used to extract the mole. After tissue has been removed, IV oxytocin (Pitocin) is used to contract the uterus. Misoprostol (Cytotec) may also be used for uterine contraction. It is important to avoid uterine stimulation with these medications before evacuation. Uterine contractions can cause trophoblastic tissue to be drawn into the venous circulation, resulting in embolization of the vesicles. Curettage with a sharp curette follows the evacuation to remove all remaining molar tissue, and the tissue obtained is sent for laboratory evaluation to identify malignant changes. Diagnosis is confirmed from the pathologic findings of the products of conception after the evacuation of the pregnancy.

Follow-up is critical to assess for choriocarcinoma. The follow-up protocol involves evaluation of serum beta-hCG levels every 1 to 2 weeks until three normal prepregnancy levels are attained. The test is repeated every 1 to 2 months for up to a year and following any subsequent pregnancies (Cunningham et al., 2010). Pregnancy, which normally raises beta-hCG levels, must be avoided during follow-up because evidence of choriocarcinoma would be obscured.

Malignant transformation of any remaining tissue is suspected if the beta-hCG levels do not fall or if they rise after an initial fall. Chemotherapy is the primary treatment for gestational trophoblastic neoplasm (choriocarcinoma) and has a high cure rate (Osborn & Dodge, 2012).

### Nursing Considerations

Women who have had a hydatidiform mole experience many of the same emotions as those who have had any other type of pregnancy loss. In addition, they may be anxious about the possibility of malignancy and the need to delay pregnancy.

## NURSING CARE

### The Woman With a Hemorrhagic Condition of Early Pregnancy

Nurses play a vital role in the management of early pregnancy bleeding, regardless of its cause. Nurses monitor the condition of the pregnant woman and collaborate with the physician to provide treatment.

#### Assessment

Confirmation of pregnancy and length of gestation is an important initial step. Physical assessment priorities are to determine the amount and character of bleeding and the description, location, and severity of pain. Estimate the amount of vaginal bleeding by examining linen and peripads. If necessary, make a more accurate estimation by weighing the linen and peripads (1 g weight equals 1 mL volume).

When asking a woman how much blood she lost at home, ask her to compare the amount lost with a common measure, such as a tablespoon or a cup. Ask how many pads she has used in the past hour. Ask how long the bleeding episode lasted and what she has done to control the bleeding.

Bleeding may be accompanied by pain. Uterine cramping usually accompanies spontaneous abortion; deep, severe pelvic pain is associated with ectopic pregnancy. Remember that in ruptured ectopic pregnancy, bleeding may be concealed within the abdomen and pain may be the only symptom.

Assess the woman's vital signs and urine output to evaluate her cardiovascular status. Check laboratory values for complete blood count (CBC) including hemoglobin and hematocrit, and report abnormal values to the physician. Determine the Rh factor so that all women who are Rh-negative can receive $Rh_o$(D) immune globulin (RhoGAM) (see p. 545).

Because any spontaneous abortion can be associated with infection, assess the woman for signs and symptoms of fever, malaise, and prolonged or malodorous vaginal discharge. Teach her to continue these observations. Determine the family's knowledge of needed follow-up care and how to prevent complications such as infection.

#### Nursing Diagnosis and Planning

The potential complications *prenatal bleeding* and *infection* are collaborative problems that should be considered in the woman with a bleeding complication in early pregnancy. Because current diagnostic techniques allow early diagnosis before hemorrhage, a nursing diagnosis that is more often encountered that applies to early bleeding disorders is:

- Deficient Knowledge related to diagnostic and therapeutic procedures, signs and symptoms of additional complications, dietary measures to prevent infection or improve hemoglobin level, and importance of follow-up care.

***Expected outcomes.*** The woman will verbalize understanding of diagnostic and therapeutic procedures, signs, and symptoms of additional complications, and measures to reduce the risk of infection. The woman will develop a plan for obtaining follow-up care, including signs or symptoms that should be reported.

### Interventions

***Providing information about tests and procedures.*** Women and their families experience less anxiety if they understand what is happening. Explain necessary diagnostic procedures, such as transvaginal or abdominal ultrasound. Include the purpose of the tests, their duration, and whether the procedures cause discomfort. If surgical intervention is necessary, reinforce the explanations of the physicians who will perform the surgery and administer anesthesia. Briefly describe the reasons for blood tests, such as determination of beta-hCG, hemoglobin, or hematocrit values, coagulation factors, blood type, and screen. Explain that diagnostic and therapeutic measures are performed quickly at times to reduce blood loss.

***Teaching measures to prevent infection.*** The risk of infection is greatest during the first 72 hours after spontaneous abortion or operative procedures, but most women are discharged within a few hours of uterine evacuation. To prevent infection, peripads should be used instead of tampons until bleeding has stopped. Teach the woman to wash her hands before and after changing peripads. She should consult with the healthcare provider before resuming sexual intercourse.

***Providing dietary information.*** Nutrition and adequate fluid intake help maintain the body's defense against infection and help correct anemia. The woman needs foods high in iron to increase hemoglobin and hematocrit values. These foods include liver, red meat, spinach, egg yolks, carrots, and raisins. In addition, the woman needs foods high in vitamin C (citrus fruits, broccoli, strawberries, cantaloupe, cabbage, and green peppers), which may increase the utilization of iron (Erick, 2012).

Iron supplementation is often prescribed, and the woman may require information about how to reduce the gastrointestinal upset that is often experienced with oral iron. Less gastric upset is experienced when iron is taken with meals. Iron supplements with a slow release may also be better tolerated. A diet high in fiber and fluid helps prevent the commonly associated constipation.

***Teaching signs of infection to report.*** Tell the woman where she can buy a thermometer if she does not have one, and instruct her to take her temperature every 8 hours for the first 3 days at home. Tell her to seek medical help if her temperature goes above 37.8° C (100° F) or as instructed by her physician. She should also report to the physician additional signs of infection, such as vaginal discharge with foul odor, pelvic tenderness, or general malaise.

***Emphasizing the importance of follow-up care.*** A variety of follow-up procedures such as repeat ultrasound examinations or repeated determinations of serum beta-hCG levels may be necessary, depending on the pregnancy disorder. The couple who experiences recurrent abortions may become involved in complex investigations of immunologic or genetic abnormalities. Teaching about contraceptive use may be needed before discharge.

The nurse should acknowledge the couple's grief, which often manifests as anger. Many women have guilt feelings that must be recognized. They often need repeated reassurance that the loss was not caused by anything they did or by anything they neglected. Older mothers are often more concerned about pregnancy loss or the need to delay pregnancy after gestational trophoblastic disease because their age imposes limits for successful subsequent pregnancy. A woman also may be anxious about the possible development of choriocarcinoma.

### Evaluation

- Did the woman verbalize comprehension of diagnostic and therapeutic procedures, signs and symptoms of additional complications, and hygienic and dietary measures to support the body's healing and reduce the risk of infection?
- Did the woman develop and follow the plan of care suggested for her complication?

## HEMORRHAGIC CONDITIONS OF LATE PREGNANCY

After 20 weeks of pregnancy, the two major causes of hemorrhage are disorders of the placenta called *placenta previa* and *abruptio placentae.* Abruptio placentae may be further complicated by DIC.

### Placenta Previa

Placenta previa is an implantation of the placenta in the lower uterus, near the fetal presenting part. Use of both abdominal and transvaginal ultrasound allows measurement of the distance between the internal cervical os and the lower border of the placenta to classify placenta previa as follows (Fig. 25.4):

- *Marginal* (sometimes called *low-lying*): Placenta is implanted in the lower uterus, but its lower border is more than 3 cm from the internal cervical os.
- *Partial:* Lower border of the placenta is within 3 cm of the internal cervical os but does not completely cover the os.
- *Total:* Placenta completely covers internal cervical os.

Marginal placenta previa is common in early ultrasound examinations and often appears to "move" upward and away from the internal cervical os. The growing placenta does not move, however, but is drawn upward as the myometrium beneath it develops with pregnancy progression.

#### Incidence and Etiology

Placenta previa occurs in approximately 1 in 200 to 300 pregnancies in the United States. It is more common in older women, multiparas, women who have had cesarean births, and women who have had suction curettage for induced or spontaneous abortion. Placenta previa is also more likely to recur in a future pregnancy. Women of Asian or African ethnicity have an increased risk. Smoking and cocaine use are also associated with placenta previa. Placenta previa is also more likely to occur if the fetus is male (Cunningham et al., 2014).

#### Manifestations

The classic sign of placenta previa is the sudden onset of painless uterine bleeding in the latter half of pregnancy. However, many cases of placenta previa are diagnosed by ultrasound examination before the onset of bleeding. Bleeding occurs when the placental villi are torn from the uterine wall, resulting in hemorrhage from the uterine vessels. Bleeding is typically painless because it does not occur in a closed cavity and therefore does not cause pressure on adjacent tissue. Bleeding may be scanty or profuse, and it may cease spontaneously, only to recur later.

Bleeding may not occur until labor starts, when cervical changes disrupt placental attachment. The admitting nurse may be unsure whether the bleeding represents heavy "bloody show" or is a sign of a placenta previa. The woman may have pain associated with the bleeding because of active labor contractions.

Digital examination of the cervical os when placenta previa is present can cause additional placental separation or can tear the

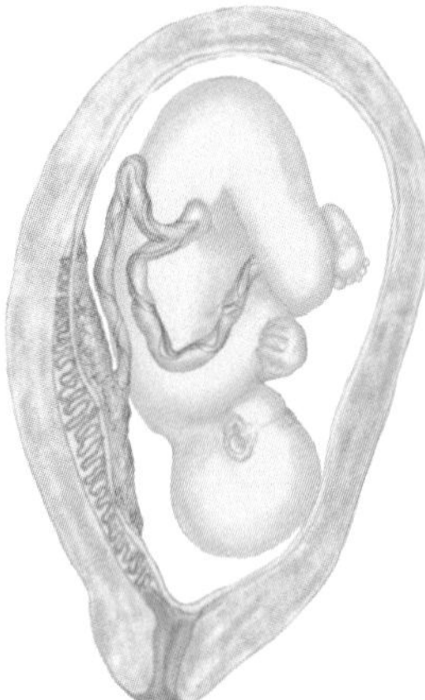


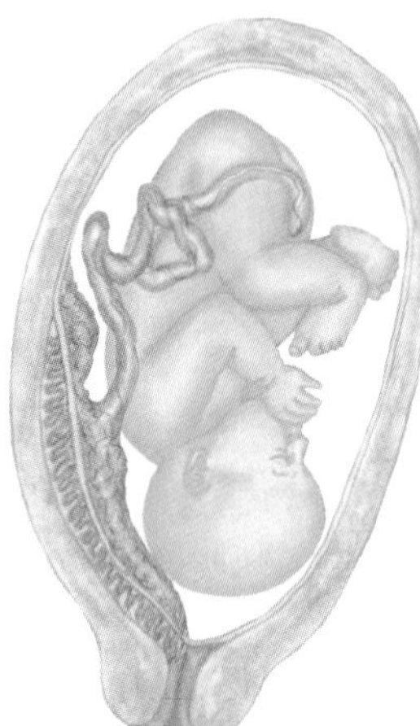

Partial
Lower border of placenta is within 3 cm of internal cervical os but does not fully cover it.


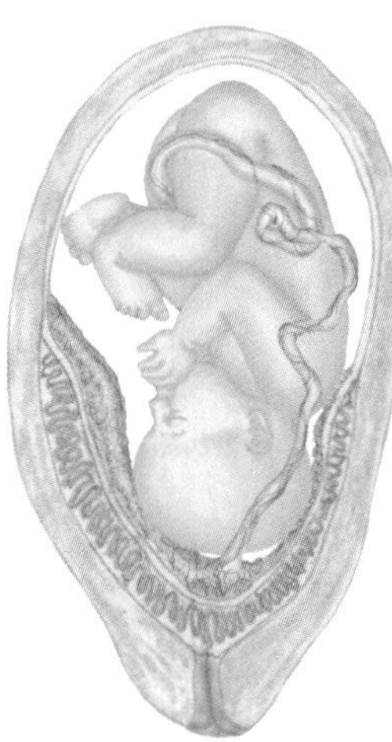


**FIG 25.4** The three classifications of placenta previa.

placenta itself, causing severe maternal and fetal bleeding. *Until the location and position of the placenta are verified by ultrasound to determine the cause of excessive vaginal bleeding, manual examinations and administration of oxytocin to stimulate labor should be avoided. Manual vaginal examination or contraction stimulation can interrupt connections between maternal and placental vessels if the placenta is attached low in the uterus.*

### Therapeutic Management

When the diagnosis of placenta previa is confirmed, medical interventions are based on the condition of the mother and fetus. The woman is evaluated carefully to determine the amount of hemorrhage, and external electronic fetal monitoring is initiated to determine whether the patterns are reassuring (see Chapter 17). A third consideration is the fetal gestational age.

Options for management include conservative, expectant management if the mother's cardiovascular status is stable and the fetus is immature and has a reassuring status according to monitoring and ultrasound examination. Delaying birth may increase birth weight and maturity and allow administration of corticosteroids to the mother to speed maturation of the fetal lungs. Conservative management can take place in the home or hospital (Cunningham et al., 2014).

### Nursing Considerations

Nursing care can be provided in the home or the hospital if conservative management is chosen by the caregivers.

**Home care.** Criteria for outpatient management include:

- The woman is clinically stable, with no evidence of active bleeding.
- The woman can maintain bed rest at home.
- Home is within a reasonable distance from the hospital.
- Emergency transportation is available 24 hours a day.
- The woman can verbalize understanding of the risks associated with placenta previa and how to manage her care.

Nurses help the family develop a plan of care that includes bed rest as ordered, the presence of a responsible adult at all times, and ready transportation to the hospital. Nurses must teach the mother and the family what to monitor and emphasize the importance of (1) assessing vaginal discharge or bleeding after each urination or bowel movement or more often as needed; (2) counting fetal movements daily (see Chapter 15); (3) assessing uterine activity daily; and (4) omitting sexual intercourse to prevent disruption of the placenta. Spontaneous membrane rupture can occur at any time and with varying amounts of fluid loss, so the woman and her family should be instructed to return to the hospital for evaluation. Home care nurses may provide assessments of uterine activity (cramping; regular or sporadic contractions), bleeding, fetal activity, and adherence to the prescribed treatment plan with regular phone contact. In addition, nurses can make regular home visits for maternal–fetal assessments such as nonstress tests with portable equipment. The family is instructed to report decreased fetal movements, uterine contractions, or increased vaginal bleeding immediately.

Nurses should also provide specific, accurate information about the condition of the fetus. For example, parents are reassured when they hear that the fetal heart rate and daily 'kick counts' are within the expected range, indicating fetal well-being. Moreover, it may be necessary for nurses to help the family understand the physician's plan of care, such as a cesarean delivery with possible blood transfusion.

**Inpatient care.** Hospitalization is needed if the woman does not meet the criteria for home care. Nursing assessments in the hospital are similar to those done at home and are focused on observing the presence and character of bleeding and looking for signs of preterm labor. Periodic nonstress tests and biophysical profile ultrasounds provide added information about the fetal condition. A significant change in fetal heart activity, an episode of increased vaginal bleeding, or signs of preterm labor should be reported immediately to the physician. Rupture of membranes should be reported, whether at home or in the hospital.

Conservative management is not always an option. For example, delivery by cesarean birth is often scheduled if the fetus is greater than 36 weeks of gestation and the lungs are mature as determined by fetal lung studies from amniocentesis. Immediate delivery of an immature fetus may be necessary if bleeding is excessive and does not stop, the woman's cardiovascular status is unstable, or there are signs of fetal compromise.

Nurses prepare the woman for surgery whenever cesarean birth becomes necessary (see Chapter 19). Signed consents for cesarean birth, blood transfusion, and anesthesia should be kept current for women with late-pregnancy bleeding because surgery may be required suddenly. IV access can be maintained with a saline lock in women with late-pregnancy bleeding for whom immediate delivery is not necessary. Crossmatched blood may be kept on hold. When many emergency preparations occur at once, the nurse should constantly provide appropriate reassurance to reduce the woman's anxiety and that of her family.

## Abruptio Placentae

Separation of a normally implanted placenta before the fetus is born (called *abruptio placentae, placental abruption;* or *premature separation of the placenta*) occurs when there is bleeding and formation of a hematoma on the maternal side of the placenta. As the clot expands, further separation occurs. The severity of the complication depends on the amount of bleeding and the size of the hematoma. The hematoma can expand and thus obliterate intervillous spaces where fetal gas and nutrient exchange occurs. Moreover, fetal vessels will be disrupted as placental separation occurs, resulting in fetal as well as maternal bleeding. Small abruptions may, however, be self-limiting (Cunningham et al., 2010).

The major danger for the woman is hemorrhage and consequent hypovolemic shock and clotting abnormalities such as DIC (see p. 525). The major dangers for the fetus are related to anoxia, blood loss, and preterm birth.

### Incidence and Etiology

Abruptio placentae occurs in approximately 0.5% to 1% of pregnancies but accounts for 10% to 15% of perinatal deaths. The cause of abruptio placentae is unknown, but risk factors include hypertension, smoking, multigravida status, abdominal trauma from a motor vehicle accident or domestic violence, and a history of a previous premature separation of the placenta. Maternal use of cocaine, which causes vasoconstriction (narrowing of the vessel lumen) of the endometrial arteries is a leading cause of abruptio placentae (Cunningham et al., 2014).

Autoimmune factors have been identified recently as associated with abruptio placentae. These factors include anticardiolipin antibodies and lupus anticoagulant. Other coagulopathies may be genetic in origin, as with the factor V Leiden mutation. Women who have these coagulopathies tend to form clots in the placenta. Hypertension, a frequent companion of abruptio placentae, also occurs more frequently in women with certain autoimmune disorders.

### Manifestations

The five classic signs and symptoms of abruptio placentae are:

- Vaginal bleeding (which may not reflect the true amount of blood loss)
- Abdominal and low back pain, often described as aching or dull
- Uterine irritability with frequent low-intensity contractions
- High uterine resting tone, as determined using an intrauterine pressure catheter
- Uterine tenderness that may be localized to the site of the abruption

Additional signs include back pain, nonreassuring fetal heart rate patterns, signs of hypovolemic shock, and fetal death. The woman may feel pain if an epidural analgesia is in place.

Hemorrhage from abruptio placentae can be either concealed or apparent. In either type, the placental abruption may be complete or partial. Concealed hemorrhage is bleeding that occurs behind the placenta while the margins remain intact. The hemorrhage is apparent when bleeding separates or dissects the membranes from the endometrium and blood flows out through the vagina. The amniotic fluid often has a classic "port-wine" color. Fig. 25.5 illustrates variations of abruptio placentae with external and concealed bleeding. The actual amount of blood lost can be greater than the visible bleeding. Signs of

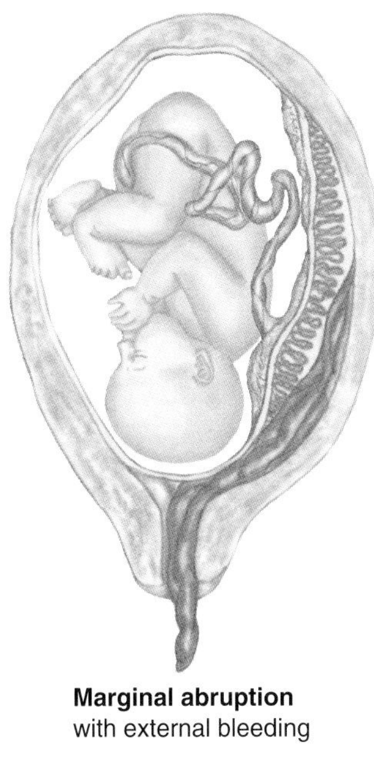

**Marginal abruption**
with external bleeding

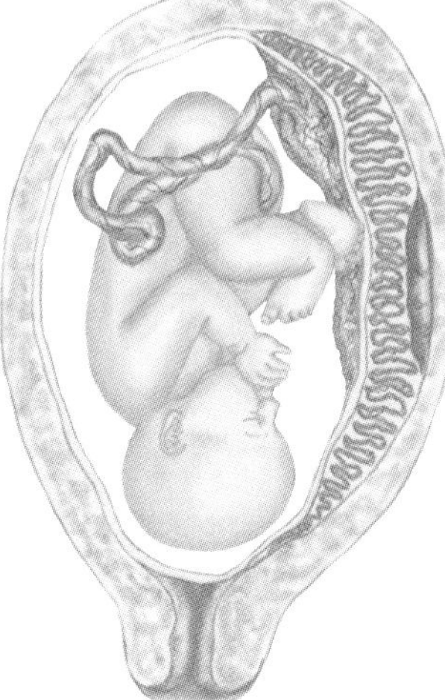

**Partial abruption**
with concealed bleeding

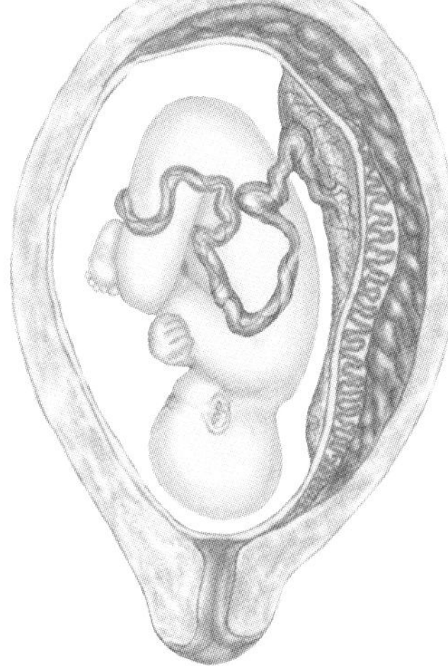

**Complete abruption**
with concealed bleeding

**FIG 25.5** Types of abruptio placentae.

maternal hypovolemia may be present when there is little or no external bleeding.

Abdominal pain is also related to the type of separation. It can be sudden and severe when there is bleeding into the myometrium (uterine muscle) or intermittent and difficult to distinguish from labor contractions. The abdomen may become exceedingly firm (board like) and tender, making palpation of the fetus difficult. Ultrasound examination is helpful to rule out placenta previa as the cause of bleeding, but it cannot be used to diagnose abruptio placentae because placental separation and bleeding look similar on ultrasound images.

### Therapeutic Management

A woman who exhibits signs of abruptio placentae should be hospitalized and evaluated immediately. Evaluation focuses on the condition of the fetus and the cardiovascular status of the mother.

**SAFETY ALERT**

***Signs and Symptoms Suggesting Concealed Hemorrhage in Abruptio Placentae***

- Increase in fundal height
- Hard, board-like abdomen
- High uterine baseline tone on electronic monitoring strip
- Persistent abdominal pain
- Systemic signs of early hemorrhage (tachycardia [maternal and fetal], falling blood pressure, restlessness)
- Persistent late deceleration in fetal heart rate or decreasing baseline variability
- Vaginal bleeding can be slight or absent

Expectant, conservative management in an inpatient setting can be initiated if the abruption is mild and the fetus is less than 34 weeks of gestation, shows no signs of distress, and if bleeding is minimal. Measures include bed rest and may include administration of tocolytic medications to decrease uterine activity. Serial Kleihauer–Betke (K-B) tests determine whether fetal bleeding is worsening. For the Rh-negative woman, RhoGAM is ordered to prevent maternal Rh sensitization.

Women may be observed for 24 hours after significant abdominal trauma such as a motor vehicle collision or domestic violence, because abruptio placentae can take this amount of time to become evident. If there are no contractions after the trauma and the fetal heart rate pattern and laboratory studies are reassuring, monitoring for 4 to 6 hours may be sufficient.

If signs of fetal compromise are present or the woman or her fetus exhibit signs of excessive bleeding, either obvious or concealed, prompt delivery of the fetus is necessary. Intensive monitoring of both the woman and the fetus is essential because rapid deterioration of either can occur. One or more large-gauge IV lines should be placed for replacement of fluid and blood.

**CRITICAL THINKING EXERCISE 25.2**

All women who have experienced prenatal bleeding and invasive procedures are at increased risk of infection. What common assumptions do nurses make about those who are at risk for developing infections?

### Nursing Considerations

If immediate cesarean delivery is necessary, the woman may feel frightened and powerless as the healthcare team hurriedly prepares her for surgery. She may be experiencing severe pain and be aware of the risks to her baby and herself. If at all possible, nurses should explain the anticipated procedures to the woman and her family to reduce their feelings of fear and anxiety.

Excessive bleeding and fetal hypoxia are always major concerns with abruptio placentae. Nurses are responsible for continuous monitoring of both the expectant mother and the fetus so that problems can be detected early, before the condition of either deteriorates.

## NURSING CARE

## The Woman With a Hemorrhagic Condition of Late Pregnancy

### Assessment

For hemorrhagic conditions of late pregnancy, medical and nursing assessments are concurrent. Some assessments are delayed or omitted if the maternal or fetal condition is not reassuring. The priority assessments are:

- *Amount and nature of bleeding:* Time of onset, estimated blood loss before admission to hospital, and description of tissue or clots passed. Peripads and underpads should be saved so that blood loss can be estimated more accurately.
- *Pain:* Type (constant, intermittent, sharp, dull, severe), onset (sudden, gradual), and location (generalized over abdomen, localized). Is the uterus tender or irritable when palpated gently?
- *Maternal vital signs:* To identify hypertension, hypotension, or tachycardia that occurs with hypovolemia. A normal blood pressure can be misleading in a woman with abruptio placentae because she may have been hypertensive before the blood loss caused her blood pressure to fall to normal or hypotensive levels. An indwelling catheter helps to identify reduced urine output that can occur before hypotension is evident.
- *Condition of the fetus:* Application of an electronic monitor to identify trends and patterns in fetal heart rate, baseline variability, and fetal response to uterine activity (late decelerations or loss of baseline variability are of particular concern).
- *Uterine contractions:* An external uterine contraction monitor is used. If the membranes are ruptured, placement of an intrauterine pressure catheter allows more precise evaluation of baseline pressure and contraction intensity. Inadequate uterine relaxation, uterine irritability, and high baseline pressures (greater than 20 mm Hg) are common.
- *Obstetric history:* Gravida, para, previous abortions, preterm infants, previous pregnancy outcomes. History of abruptio placenta.
- *Length of gestation:* Date of last menstrual period, fundal height, correlation of fundal height with estimated gestation, results of ultrasound examinations performed during pregnancy. With bleeding into the myometrium, the fundus enlarges rapidly as bleeding progresses.
- *Laboratory data:* Laboratory studies include a complete blood count and blood typing and screening. Blood crossmatching is done if transfusion is likely. Type and Rh factor identify the possible need for RhoGAM. Other tests may be done serially to identify whether the abruption is stable or worsening. The K-B test detects fetal blood cells in the maternal circulation. Coagulation studies include fibrinogen, fibrin split products (FSPs), prothrombin and partial thromboplastin times (PT/PTTs), and D-dimer to identify fibrin degradation fragments. A drug screen is done if illegal drug use is suspected or if the woman had no prenatal care.
- Referrals may include a neonatology and perinatology consult.

Despite the emphasis on physical assessment, the emotional response of the mother as well as her partner must be addressed (Nursing Care Plan: Antepartum Bleeding). They will most likely be anxious, fearful, confused, and overwhelmed by the activity. They may have very little knowledge of expected medical management and may not realize that the fetus must be delivered as quickly as possible and that a surgical procedure is necessary. Moreover, they may fear for the life of the woman and the fetus. Also, the baby may be dead when the mother is admitted, adding shock and grief to their anxiety.

### Nursing Diagnosis and Planning

The most dangerous potential complication is *hypovolemia,* which jeopardizes the life of the mother as well as the fetus. The nurse cannot independently manage this collaborative problem but must confer with physicians for medical orders for treatment. Planning should therefore reflect the nurse's responsibility to:

## NURSING CARE PLAN

### *Antepartum Bleeding*

#### Focused Assessment

Beth is a 28-year-old gravida 2, para 1, admitted at 32 weeks of gestation after an episode of vaginal bleeding caused by total placenta previa. Vital signs are stable, and the fetal heart rate is 140 to 150 beats per minute with no nonreassuring signs. She and her husband Bob appear anxious about the condition of the fetus and the plan of care. Both are worried about their 5-year-old son, who is now staying with a neighbor. Jenny is their nurse.

#### Nursing Diagnosis

Anxiety related to unknown effects of bleeding and lack of knowledge of predicted course of management.

#### Planning

***Expected Outcomes***

The couple will:

1. Verbalize expected routines and projected management by the end of the first day after admission.
2. Express less anxiety after teaching.

#### Interventions and *Rationales*

1. Remain with the couple and acknowledge the emotions that they exhibit: "I know this is unexpected, and you must have many questions. Perhaps I can answer some of them."
   *Jenny's presence and empathic understanding prepare the family to cope with the unexpected situation. Even if Beth knew that bleeding might occur with the previa, she might not have truly expected an episode.*
2. Determine the couple's level of understanding of the situation and the projected management: "Tell me what you've been told to expect."
   *Assessing understanding allows reinforcement of earlier explanations and identifies if additional explanations are necessary.*
3. Provide Beth and Bob with factual information about projected management.
   *This information will prevent and/or reduce their anxiety and fear.*
   Examples of potential teaching topics:
   a. Hospitalization that may be necessary to closely watch her condition and that of the fetus, allowing rapid intervention if needed.
   b. The necessity for a cesarean birth this time even though she delivered vaginally before.
   c. Information about hospital routines (meals, visitors [including their son]) and monitoring techniques that will be used (electronic fetal monitoring, nonstress tests, biophysical profiles, and testing for fetal lung maturity).
4. Explain the corticosteroid therapy ordered to hasten fetal lung maturity if preterm birth is necessary. Include explanations of any maternal side effects that may occur.
   *Knowing the benefits of corticosteroids in hastening fetal lung maturity may reduce Beth's anxiety if a preterm birth occurs.*
5. Ask Beth if she would like to talk with a nurse from the special care nursery in case preterm birth occurs. Include Bob and other family in the teaching, as Beth wishes.
   *Continued bleeding or nonreassuring fetal factors are likely to result in a preterm birth.*
6. Encourage Beth and her family to participate in the routine as much as possible.
   *This involvement will reduce the sense of powerlessness that many high-risk antepartum patients experience.*
   Schedule procedures around times when her husband and son can visit.
   *Such inclusion promotes family involvement with Beth and the expected newborn.*
7. Refer Beth to online support groups if available.

#### Evaluation

The interventions are considered successful if Beth and Bob demonstrate knowledge of the projected management and why it is necessary and verbalize decreased anxiety by the end of the first day.

#### Focused Assessment

Although Beth has no more episodes of vaginal bleeding, she cries frequently. She tells the nurse, "I miss my son so much. He just started kindergarten, and he is so shy. I feel useless, and he really needs me now. It's hard on my husband, too. He has to do everything."

#### Nursing Diagnosis

Situational Low Self-Esteem related to temporary inability to provide care for family.

#### Planning

***Expected Outcomes***

Beth will:

1. Identify positive aspects of self during hospitalization.
2. Identify ways of providing comfort and affection for her son during the hospital stay.

#### Interventions and *Rationales*

1. Encourage Beth to express her concerns about the need for hospitalization: "What bothers you most about being away from home?"
   *Major concerns may not be identified or may be misunderstood unless she clarifies them.*
2. After acknowledging Beth's feelings, encourage her to examine the need for hospitalization and its consequences—It provides time for her baby to mature. Remind her of what she learned from the nurse in the special care nursery if that meeting occurred.
   *Careful consideration identifies positive aspects of her important role in maturing her fetus.*
3. Ask Beth if she feels the benefit of various therapies available in the facility with a physician's order, such as physical, occupational, and recreational therapy. Explore the availability of complementary therapies such as aromatherapy or music therapy.
   *These therapies can help Beth maintain better physical condition and may also help her interact with other women hospitalized for a long period. Physician orders for therapy make them more likely to be covered by insurance.*
4. Explore Beth's self-appraisal ("I feel useless") by helping her to investigate ways to provide nurturing care for her son while she is hospitalized.
   *Daily involvement with her child may reduce Beth's feelings of isolation and failure to meet family obligations.*
5. Assist Beth to involve her son in plans for the newborn. He might benefit from sibling classes or play time with his mother that involves caring for dolls.
   *Involving "big brother" combines family interaction that may increase Beth's feeling of self-worth. Young boys often benefit from understanding that they can be beneficial to their new sibling's life.*

#### Evaluation

Beth makes positive comments about the importance of rest to the health of the baby, and she initiates numerous activities that permit her to continue close, comforting contact with her child during the period of hospitalization. She enjoys the return to needlework that she has not done for several years.

#### *Additional Nursing Diagnoses to Consider*

Interrupted Family Processes
Deficient Diversional Activity
Fear

- Observe for signs of hypovolemic shock.
- Consult the physician if signs of hypovolemic shock are observed.
- Perform actions to minimize the effects of hypovolemic shock.

#### Interventions

***Monitoring for signs of hypovolemic shock.*** Observe for any sign of developing hypovolemic shock. The body attempts to compensate for decreased blood volume and to maintain oxygenation of essential organs by increasing the rate and effort of the heart and lungs and by shunting blood from less essential organs. This compensatory mechanism results in the following early signs and symptoms of hypovolemic shock before birth:

- Fetal tachycardia (often the first sign of either maternal or fetal hypovolemia)
- Maternal tachycardia, weak peripheral pulses
- Normal or slightly decreased maternal blood pressure
- Increased respiratory rate
- Low oxygen saturation
- Cool, pale skin and mucous membranes

The compensatory mechanism fails if hypovolemic shock progresses and blood volume is insufficient to perfuse the brain, heart, and kidneys. Later signs of hypovolemic shock include:

- Falling blood pressure and oxygen saturation levels
- Pallor of skin and mucous membranes; cold, clammy skin
- Urine output less than 30 mL/hr
- Restlessness, agitation, decreased mentation

**SAFETY ALERT**

***Signs and Symptoms of Impending Hypovolemic Shock Caused by Blood Loss***

- Increased pulse rate, falling blood pressure, increased respiratory rate
- Weak, diminished, or "thready" peripheral pulses
- Cool, moist skin; pallor; or cyanosis (late sign)
- Decreased urinary output (<30 mL/hr)
- Decreased hemoglobin, hematocrit levels
- Change in mental status (restlessness, agitation, difficulty concentrating)

***Monitoring the fetus.*** Initiate continuous electronic fetal monitoring to identify nonreassuring signs that can occur as the placental surface area for gas exchange is disrupted, such as decreasing baseline variability or late decelerations (see Chapter 17). Notify the physician if nonreassuring patterns are noted, because these may occur before maternal signs of hypovolemia are obvious. The physician should be given a report on new laboratory data that suggest increasing placental abruption.

***Promoting tissue oxygenation.*** To promote oxygenation of tissues:

- Place the woman in a lateral position, with the head of the bed flat to increase cardiac return and thereby increase circulation and oxygenation of the placenta and other vital organs.
- Restrict maternal movements and activity to decrease the tissue demand for oxygen.
- Provide simple explanations, reassurance, and emotional support to the woman to help reduce anxiety, which increases the metabolic demand for oxygen.

***Collaborating with the physician for fluid replacement.*** To maintain circulating maternal blood volume:

- Insert IV lines, often two large-gauge catheters or a central line, to allow rapid blood replacement.
- Obtain an order for blood typing and screening or crossmatching so that blood is available for replacement if necessary.
- Administer replacement IV crystalloids such as normal saline and lactated Ringers as directed by the physician to maintain a urinary output of at least 30 mL/hr.

***Providing emotional support.*** Explain to the woman the cause of her discomfort, and reassure her that pain-relief measures will be initiated as soon as possible without causing harm to the fetus. While it is unwise to offer false reassurance about the condition of the fetus, provide accurate and timely information to the woman and her family.

***Care related to surgery.*** Quick preparation of the woman for cesarean birth may be necessary (Care for the woman having a cesarean birth is discussed fully in Chapter 19). Remain with the woman and her family as much as possible to provide information.

After birth, assess bleeding from the vagina and from any surgical sites or puncture wounds (epidural, IV sites). Report uncontrolled bleeding or bleeding from unexpected sites, which may indicate DIC. Perform all routine postpartum assessments as well as those related to surgery and to the hemorrhagic complication.

#### Evaluation

Although patient-centered goals are not developed for collaborative problems, the nurse collects and compares data with established norms and judges whether the data are within normal limits. The desired outcome is that the maternal vital signs remain within normal limits and the fetal heart rate demonstrates no signs of compromise, such as late decelerations or decreasing baseline variability.

## HYPEREMESIS GRAVIDARUM

Hyperemesis gravidarum (HEG) is persistent, uncontrollable vomiting that begins in the first weeks of pregnancy and may continue throughout pregnancy. Hyperemesis is associated with loss of 5% or more of prepregnancy weight, dehydration, acidosis from starvation, elevated blood and urine ketones, alkalosis from loss of hydrochloric acid in the gastric fluids, and hypokalemia. Short-term hepatic dysfunction with elevated liver enzymes can occur. Deficiency of vitamin K may cause coagulation disorders, and deficiency of thiamine can cause encephalopathy.

### Etiology

The cause of HEG is not known. This condition is more common among unmarried white women, during first pregnancies, and in multifetal pregnancies. Possible causes include allergy to fetal proteins. Elevated levels of pregnancy-related hormones, such as estrogen and beta-hCG, are considered a possible cause, as is maternal thyroid dysfunction. Persistent hyperemesis may result in low pregnancy weight gain and a newborn with low birth weight. More recently, an association with the organism that causes peptic ulcer disease, *Helicobacter pylori (H. pylori)*, has been associated with hyperemesis. Psychological factors may interact with the nausea and vomiting that occur during early pregnancy to worsen it (ACOG, 2011; Cunningham et al., 2010; Williamson & Girling, 2011).

### Therapeutic Management

The physician will exclude other causes for persistent nausea and vomiting, such as cholecystitis or peptic ulcer disease, before diagnosing and treating hyperemesis. Laboratory studies include determining the hemoglobin and hematocrit, which may be elevated as a result of dehydration. Electrolyte studies may reveal low sodium, potassium, and chloride. Elevated creatinine levels indicate renal dysfunction.

Treatment often occurs in the home, where the woman attempts to control the nausea by methods used for morning sickness (see Chapter 13). Pyridoxine (vitamin $B_6$) and vitamin $B_6$ plus doxylamine have consistent evidence of benefits. Ginger has shown some benefit in reducing the episodes of vomiting. Antiemetics such as promethazine (Phenergan) provide some short-term relief. Drugs that act on the central nervous system, such as ondansetron (Zofran) or metoclopramide (Reglan), may be used. The steroid *methylprednisolone* has recently been found to reduce the nausea and vomiting (ACOG, 2011).

If methods to relieve nausea and vomiting are unsuccessful and weight loss or electrolyte imbalance persists, IV fluid and electrolyte replacement or total parenteral nutrition (TPN) may be necessary and often relieves nausea quickly. Enteral nutrition via a feeding tube also has been used successfully (ACOG, 2011; Cunningham et al., 2014).

### Nursing Considerations

Physical assessment begins with determining the woman's intake and output. Intake includes IV fluids and parenteral nutrition as well as oral fluids and nutrition, which is allowed once vomiting is controlled. A description of the output includes the amount and character of emesis and urinary output. As a rule of thumb, the normal urinary output is approximately 1 mL/kg (2.2 lb)/hr. A record of bowel elimination also provides significant information about oral nutrition because bowel movements will be decreased and hard with dehydration. Findings associated with dehydration include decreased fluid intake (less than 2000 mL/day), decreased urinary output, increased urine specific gravity (more than 1.025), dry skin or dry mucous membranes, and nonelastic skin turgor.

The woman should be weighed daily during acute illness and her urine tested for ketones. Weight loss and the presence of ketones in the urine suggest that fat stores and protein are being metabolized to meet energy needs. Consultation with a dietitian is indicated. Nursing interventions focus on reducing nausea and vomiting, maintaining nutrition and fluid balance, and providing emotional support.

#### Reducing Nausea and Vomiting

Food portions should be small so that the amount does not appear overwhelming. Present foods attractively, and eliminate foods with strong odors because nausea is often associated with food smells. Lowfat foods and easily digested carbohydrates, such as fruit, breads, cereals, rice, and pasta, provide important nutrients and help prevent low blood sugar, which can cause nausea. Soups and other liquids should be taken between meals so as not to overly distend the stomach and trigger vomiting. Sitting upright after meals reduces gastric reflux. Pharmacologic therapy may also be prescribed.

#### Maintaining Nutrition and Fluid Balance

Women with nausea and vomiting should eat every 2 to 3 hours. Salting food helps replace chloride lost when hydrochloric acid is vomited. Potassium- and magnesium-rich foods should be encouraged because these nutrients are likely to be depleted, and magnesium deficiency can worsen nausea (see Chapter 14).

IV fluids and TPN are administered as directed by the physician. Small oral feedings of clear liquids are started when nausea and vomiting begin to subside. When oral fluids are tolerated, parenteral fluids and nutrition are gradually discontinued. Any inability to tolerate oral feedings or continued episodes of vomiting should be reported to the physician so that continued parenteral fluids and nutrition can be prescribed.

#### Providing Emotional Support

The persistence and severity of HEG has a significant effect on the woman's daily life as she tries to assume her role as mother. Rather than pregnancy being a pleasant time overall, HEG interferes with her common activities and relationships. The unpredictability of nausea and vomiting may cause her to decrease contact with others, even avoiding getting out of bed each morning. Setting up the nursery or preparing for birth may not hold the pleasure she anticipated (Meighan & Wood, 2005).

The woman with HEG needs the opportunity to express how it feels to be pregnant and to live with ever-present nausea, but these women often experience a curious lack of sympathy and support. This attitude may stem from reports that the cause of HEG is always psychological. Observation of the woman and her family can provide clues about family dynamics that may be contributing to her response to pregnancy-related nausea. Nurses must use critical thinking to examine personal beliefs and biases so that they can provide comfort and support.

## HYPERTENSION DURING PREGNANCY

The terminology used to describe hypertension in pregnancy is often nonuniform and confusing. To standardize classifications of pregnancy-related hypertension and identify the best management, the National Heart, Lung, and Blood Institute assembled a working group to update older recommendations (Table 25.1; ACOG, 2010a, 2010b; National Institutes of Health: National Heart, Lung, and Blood Institute [NHLBI], 2001).

**TABLE 25.1 Classifications of Hypertension in Pregnancy**

| Classification | Comments |
|---|---|
| Gestational hypertension (replaces term pregnancy-induced hypertension [PIH]) | Systolic blood pressure ≥140 mm Hg or diastolic blood pressure ≥90 mm Hg that develops after 20 wk of pregnancy but returns to normal within 6 wk postpartum. Proteinuria (negative or trace on random urine dipstick) is not present. |
| Preeclampsia | Systolic blood pressure ≥140 mm Hg or diastolic blood pressure ≥90 mm Hg that develops after 20 wk of pregnancy and is accompanied by proteinuria ≥0.3 g in 24-hr urine collection (random urine dipstick is usually ≥1+). |
| Eclampsia | Progression of preeclampsia to generalized seizures that cannot be attributed to other causes. |
| Chronic hypertension | Systolic blood pressure ≥140 mm Hg or diastolic blood pressure ≥90 mm Hg that was known to exist before pregnancy or develops before 20 wk of gestation. Also diagnosed if the hypertension does not resolve during the postpartum period. |
| Preeclampsia superimposed on chronic hypertension | Development of new-onset proteinuria ≥0.3 g in 24-hr urine collection in a woman who has chronic hypertension. In women who had proteinuria before 20 wk, preeclampsia should be suspected if woman has a sudden increase in proteinuria from her baseline levels or a sudden increase in blood pressure that had been well controlled previously, development of thrombocytopenia (platelets <100,000/mm$^3$), or abnormal elevation of liver enzymes (AST or ALT). |

*ALT*, Alanine aminotransferase (formerly SGPT); *AST*, aspartate aminotransferase (formerly SGOT).

Four categories of hypertensive disorders occurring during pregnancy were identified by the group working within the NHLBI of the National Institutes of Health for the United States and remain current at this revision:

- *Gestational hypertension:* Blood pressure elevation after 20 weeks of pregnancy that is not accompanied by proteinuria. Gestational hypertension must be considered a working diagnosis because it can progress to preeclampsia. If gestational hypertension persists more than 6 weeks after birth, chronic hypertension is diagnosed.
- *Preeclampsia:* A systolic blood pressure ≥140 mm Hg or diastolic blood pressure ≥90 mm Hg occurring after 20 weeks of pregnancy that is accompanied by significant proteinuria (>0.3 g in a 24-hour urine collection, which usually correlates to a random urine dipstick evaluation ≥1+). Edema, although common in preeclampsia, is now considered to be nonspecific because it occurs in many pregnancies not complicated by hypertension.
- *Eclampsia:* Progression of preeclampsia to generalized seizures that cannot be attributed to other causes. Seizures can occur postpartum.
- *Chronic hypertension (pre-existing):* The elevated blood pressure was known to be present before pregnancy. Unrecognized chronic hypertension may not be diagnosed until after the end of pregnancy during a postpartum visit.

**BOX 25.2 Risk Factors for Pregnancy-Related Hypertension**

- First pregnancy
- First pregnancy for father of baby
- Men who have fathered one preeclamptic pregnancy
- Age >35 years
- Anemia
- Family or personal history of preeclampsia
- Chronic hypertension or preexisting vascular disease
- Chronic renal disease
- Obesity
- Diabetes mellitus
- Antiphospholipid syndrome
- Multifetal pregnancy
- Pregnancy from assisted reproductive techniques

From Bowers, N.A., Curran, C.A., Freda, M.C., et al. (2008). High-risk pregnancy. In K.R. Simpson, & P.A. Creehan (Eds.), *AWHONN's perinatal nursing* (3rd ed., pp. 125–299). Philadelphia: Lippincott; Cunningham, F.G., Leveno, K.J., Bloom, S.L., et al. (2010). *Williams obstetrics* (23rd ed.). New York: McGraw-Hill; Dekker, G. (2011). Hypertension. In D.K. James, P.J. Steer, C.P. Weiner, et al. (Eds.), *High risk pregnancy: Management options* (4th ed., pp. 599–626). Philadelphia: Saunders; Roberts, J.M., & Funai, E.M. (2009). Pregnancy-related hypertension. In R.K. Creasy, R. Resnik, & J.D. Iams, et al. (Eds.), *Creasy and Resnik's maternal-fetal medicine* (6th ed., pp. 651–688). Philadelphia: Saunders.

## Preeclampsia

Preeclampsia affects approximately 5% to 8% of U.S. pregnancies each year, although its incidence varies. It is a major cause of perinatal death and is often associated with intrauterine growth restriction (IUGR). Recurrent preeclampsia is associated with more severe maternal and fetal problems (Sibai, 2012).

### Risk Factors

Although the cause of preeclampsia is unknown, several factors increase a woman's risk that the condition will develop, and many risk factors are interrelated. Box 25.2 lists common risk factors.

Preeclampsia is most likely to occur in a first pregnancy, in women at the extremes of maternal age, and in multifetal pregnancies. Chronic hypertension increases the risk for preeclampsia. Being overweight or obese also increases a woman's risk. Maternal diabetes, often present with chronic hypertension, adds to maternal risk if preeclampsia is superimposed. Black Americans, those with a positive family history, and in those with chronic hypertension or renal disease also have a higher risk for preeclampsia. Immunologic and genetic disorders, such as lupus and clotting disorders, add to the risk for preeclampsia that is often severe. Women who had previous pregnancies without hypertension are more likely to have preeclampsia if the father is a new partner who previously fathered a pregnancy in another woman that was complicated by the disorder (Sibai, 2012; ACOG, 2010b).

### Pathophysiology

Preeclampsia is the result of generalized vasospasm. The underlying cause of the vasospasm remains a mystery, but some of the physiologic processes are known. In a normal pregnancy, vascular volume is significantly increased, and cardiac output is increased. Despite these factors, blood pressure does not rise in a normal pregnancy, probably because pregnant women develop resistance to the effects of vasoconstrictors such as angiotensin II. Moreover, a decrease in peripheral vascular resistance occurs from the effects of certain vasodilators, such as prostacyclin ($PGI_2$), prostaglandin $E_2$ ($PGE_2$), and endothelium-derived relaxing factor (EDRF).

In preeclampsia, however, peripheral vascular resistance increases because of the sensitivity of some women to angiotensin II and a decrease in vasodilators. For example, the ratio of thromboxane $A_2$ to $PGI_2$ increases. Thromboxane, produced by kidney and trophoblastic tissue, causes vasoconstriction and platelet aggregation (clumping). $PGI_2$, produced by placental tissue and endothelial cells, causes vasodilation and inhibits platelet aggregation.

Vasospasm reduces the diameter of blood vessels, resulting in endothelial cell damage and decreased EDRF. Vasospasm also results in impeded blood flow and elevated blood pressure. As a result, circulation to all body organs, including the kidneys, liver, brain, and placenta, decreases. The following changes are most significant:

- Decreased renal perfusion reduces the glomerular filtration rate. Consequently, blood urea nitrogen, creatinine, and uric acid levels rise.
- Glomerular damage secondary to reduced renal blood flow allows protein to leak across the glomerular membrane.
- Loss of protein from the kidneys reduces colloid osmotic pressure and allows fluid to shift to interstitial spaces. This fluid shift may result in relative hypovolemia, which causes increased viscosity of the blood and a rise in hematocrit. Generalized edema often occurs.
- In response to hypovolemia, additional angiotensin II and aldosterone are secreted to trigger the retention of both sodium and water. The pathologic processes spiral: additional angiotensin II results in further vasospasm and hypertension; aldosterone increases fluid retention, and edema worsens.
- Decreased circulation to the liver impairs liver function and leads to hepatic edema and subcapsular hemorrhage, which can result in hemorrhagic necrosis. This process is manifested by elevated liver enzyme levels in maternal serum. Liver dysfunction can manifest as epigastric pain.
- Vasoconstriction of cerebral vessels leads to pressure-induced rupture of thin-walled capillaries, resulting in small cerebral

hemorrhages. Signs and symptoms of arterial vasospasm include headache and visual disturbances, such as blurred vision and "spots" before the eyes, as well as hyperreflexia.

- Decreased colloid oncotic pressure can lead to pulmonary capillary leaks that result in pulmonary edema. Dyspnea is the primary symptom.
- Decreased placental circulation results in infarctions that increase the risk for abruptio placentae and HELLP (which stands for hemolysis, elevated liver enzymes, and low platelets) syndrome (see p. 544). In addition, the fetus may experience IUGR and persistent fetal hypoxemia.

### Preventive Measures

Although it does not prevent preeclampsia, early and regular prenatal care with attention to the pattern of weight gain, as well as careful monitoring of blood pressure and urinary protein, can minimize maternal and fetal morbidity and mortality.

Attempts at prevention in women at high risk for recurrence have included low-dose aspirin, calcium and magnesium supplements, and fish oil supplements. Low-dose aspirin of 81 mg/day appears to have a modest preventive effect in women at high risk but little effect in low-risk women. Women on medications for chronic hypertension continued to have a greater risk of preeclampsia. In Europe, calcium supplementation reduced the risk of preeclampsia only in women with low calcium levels. No consensus on measures to reliably prevent preeclampsia in high-risk women exists at this time (Cunningham et al., 2010); National Institutes of Health: NHLBI, 2001).

### Manifestations

*Classic signs.* The first indication of preeclampsia is usually hypertension. Blood pressure measurements vary with the woman's position, so it should be measured uniformly at each office visit. Blood pressure should be measured with the woman seated and her arm supported, using an appropriately-sized cuff. The diastolic pressure should be recorded at Korotkoff's phase V, disappearance of sound (ACOG, 2010b; National Institutes of Health: NHLBI, 2001). Hospitalizing the woman for serial blood pressure observations of her can distinguish true elevations from those induced by anxiety.

Proteinuria can be identified using a clean-catch specimen to prevent contamination of the specimen by vaginal secretions or blood. Women with a urinary tract infection often have erythrocytes and leukocytes in the urine, which would elevate urine protein in the absence of preeclampsia. Because the degree of proteinuria varies during the day, a 24-hour urine specimen is often ordered to provide greater accuracy than a single specimen.

*Additional signs.* When the retina is examined, vascular constriction and narrowing of the small arteries are obvious in most women with preeclampsia. The vasoconstriction visible in the retina is occurring throughout the body. Deep tendon reflexes (DTRs) may be very brisk (hyperreflexia), suggesting cerebral irritability secondary to decreased circulation and edema. Upper extremity reflexes should be assessed if the woman has epidural analgesia in place because lower extremity reflexes may be depressed by the epidural medication. Edema may impede ideal DTR assessment.

Laboratory studies may identify liver, renal, and hepatic dysfunction if preeclampsia is severe. Coagulation may be impaired as evidenced by a fall in platelets, which are often in the high-normal range in a pregnant woman without preeclampsia.

Although generalized edema is a nonspecific sign that may have many causes, it often occurs with preeclampsia and can be severe. Edema may first present as a rapid weight gain caused by fluid retention. Edema may be present in the lower legs, which is common in pregnancy, and in the hands and face (Fig. 25.6; Table 25.2). Edema may be so massive that the woman's appearance is distorted. However, edema is not present in all women who develop preeclampsia, and it can

**TABLE 25.2 Assessment of Edema**

| Characteristics | Grade |
|---|---|
| Minimal edema of lower extremities | +1 |
| Marked edema of lower extremities | +2 |
| Edema of lower extremities, face, hands, and sacral area | +3 |
| Generalized massive edema that includes ascites (accumulation of fluid in peritoneal cavity) | +4 |

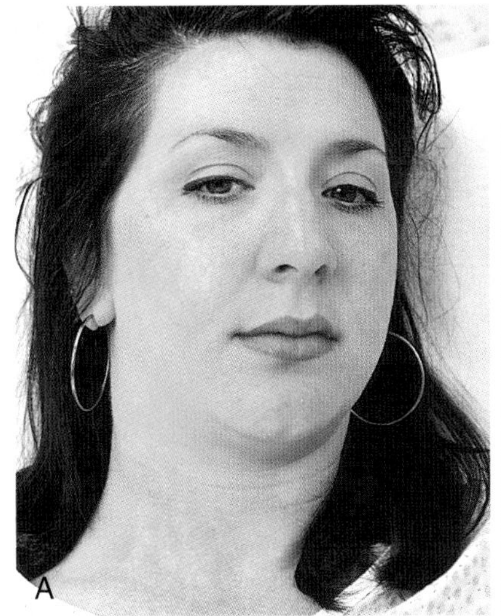


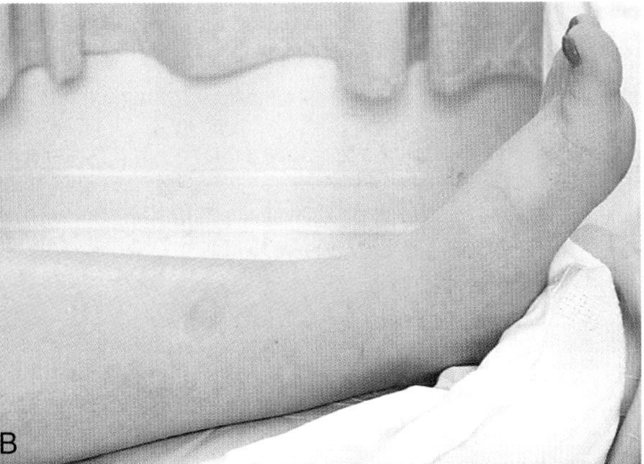


**FIG 25.6** Generalized edema is a possible sign identified with preeclampsia, although it may occur in both normal pregnancy or in a pregnancy complicated by another disorder. **A,** Facial edema may be subtle. **B,** Pitting edema of the lower leg.

be severe in women who do not have the disorder. Pulmonary edema is also more common in women with massive edema from any cause, including drug therapy given to stop preterm labor (see Chapter 27).

*Symptoms.* Preeclampsia is dangerous for the expectant mother and fetus for two reasons: (1) it can develop and progress rapidly; and (2) the early symptoms often go unnoticed by the woman or may be attributed to other causes. By the time she experiences symptoms, the disease has often progressed to an advanced state, and valuable treatment time has been lost.

Certain symptoms, such as continuous headache, drowsiness, or mental confusion, indicate poor cerebral perfusion and may be precursors of generalized seizures. Visual disturbances, such as blurred or double vision or spots before the eyes, indicate arterial spasms and edema in the retina. Some symptoms, such as epigastric pain or "upset stomach," are particularly ominous because they indicate distention of the hepatic capsule and often warn that a seizure is imminent. Decreased urinary output indicates poor perfusion of the kidneys and may precede acute renal failure.

### Therapeutic Management

Preeclampsia is categorized as either mild or severe, depending on the frequency and intensity of presenting signs and symptoms (Table 25.3). Because the disease can progress rapidly, an apparently mild condition can become severe in a very short time, or it may progress to eclampsia from mild disease. Delivery is the only definitive treatment but may not be ideal if preeclampsia is mild and the fetus is immature.

If the fetus is less than 34 weeks of gestation, steroids to accelerate fetal lung maturity will be given and an attempt made to delay birth for 48 hours. However, if the maternal or fetal condition deteriorates, the woman will be delivered, regardless of fetal age or administration of steroids. Vaginal birth is preferred because of the multisystem impairments.

*Home care for mild preeclampsia.* Initial evaluation of the severity of preeclampsia will be done in the hospital. Home management is possible if preeclampsia is mild. The woman and fetus must be in stable condition, and she must be willing to adhere to the treatment plan and make follow-up visits every 3 or 4 days. The woman on home care and her family should be taught blood pressure assessment and the signs of worsening preeclampsia, such as visual disturbances, severe headache, or epigastric pain. She must also be taught the signs that suggest nonreassuring fetal status, such as diminished movements (see Chapter 15) and signs and symptoms that suggest onset of labor (see Chapter 16). If any of these occur, she should return to the hospital or clinic. Frequent prenatal care office visits are often implemented.

**Activity restrictions.** Activity is usually restricted, although full bed rest is not required. The woman will most likely need to stop working for the duration of home management, although computer-based work may be possible. Lying down for at least 1.5 hours per day in a side-lying position maximizes placental blood flow.

**Fetal activity.** The woman often keeps a record of fetal movements, also called a "kick count" (see Chapter 15). She should report a significant decrease in movements or absence of movement during a 4-hour period.

**Blood pressure.** The family must be taught to use electronic blood pressure equipment, readily available at grocery and discount stores and pharmacies. Blood pressure should be checked two to four times per day on the same arm and with the woman in the same position.

**Weight.** The woman should weigh herself each morning, preferably on the same scale and in similar clothing.

**Urinalysis.** A urine dipstick test for protein, using the first voided midstream specimen, should be performed daily. The physician may request that the woman test at other times also.

**Diet.** A regular diet without salt or fluid restriction is usually prescribed. Women who also have chronic hypertension or diabetes

**TABLE 25.3 Mild vs Severe Preeclampsia**

| Parameter Evaluated | Mild | Severe |
|---|---|---|
| Systolic blood pressure | ≥140 but <160 mm Hg | ≥160 mm Hg (two readings, 6-hr apart, while on bed rest) |
| Diastolic blood pressure | ≥90 but <110 mm Hg | ≥110 mm Hg |
| Proteinuria (24-hr specimen is preferred to eliminate hour-to-hour variations) | ≥0.3 g but <2 g in 24-hr specimen (1+ or higher on random dipstick) | ≥5 g in 24-hr specimen (3+ or higher on random dipstick samples) |
| Creatinine, serum (renal function) | Normal | Elevated (>1.2 mg/dL) |
| Platelets | Normal | Decreased (<100,000 cells/mm$^3$) |
| Liver enzymes (alanine aminotransferase [ALT] or aspartate aminotransferase [AST]) | Normal or minimal increase in levels | Elevated levels |
| Urine output | Normal | Oliguria common, often <500 mL/day |
| Severe, unrelenting headache not attributable to other cause; mental confusion (cerebral edema) | Absent | Often present |
| Persistent right upper quadrant or epigastric pain or pain penetrating to the back (distention of the liver capsule); nausea and vomiting | Absent | May be present and often precedes seizure |
| Visual disturbances (spots or "sparkles"; temporary blindness; photophobia) | Absent to minimal | Common |
| Pulmonary edema; heart failure; cyanosis | Absent | May be present |
| Fetal growth restriction | Normal growth | Growth restriction; reduced amniotic fluid volume |

From American Academy of Pediatrics & American College of Obstetricians and Gynecologists. (2007). *Guidelines for perinatal care* (6th ed.). Elk Grove Village, IL: Author; American College of Obstetricians and Gynecologists. (2008). *Diagnosis and management of preeclampsia and eclampsia* (ACOG Practice Bulletin No. 33). Washington, DC: Author; National High Blood Pressure Education Program Working Group on High Blood Pressure in Pregnancy. National Institutes of Health: National Heart, Lung, and Blood Institute. (2001). *Report of the national high blood pressure education program working group on high blood pressure in pregnancy.* Retrieved from http://www.nhlbi.nih.gov.

should have diet management appropriate to these disorders, whether they are inpatient or outpatient.

**Fetal assessment.** Fetal surveillance includes sonography for fetal growth and quantity of amniotic fluid or as part of a biophysical profile (BPP). A diminishing amount of amniotic fluid suggests placental impairment. Corticosteroids can be given to accelerate fetal lung maturity if the pregnancy is less than 34 completed weeks. Amniocentesis can be performed to evaluate fetal lung maturity before labor induction. Referrals to specialists including perinatology and neonatology may be ordered.

***Inpatient management for severe preeclampsia.*** Preeclampsia is severe if the systolic blood pressure is ≥160 mm Hg or the diastolic blood pressure is ≥110 mm Hg or if evidence of multisystem involvement is present (see Table 25.3). Delivery may be necessary, even if the gestation is less than 34 weeks, because of disease severity.

**Antepartum management.** The woman will be hospitalized for assessment and management. The goals of management are to prevent seizures and to maintain the pregnancy until it is safe to deliver the fetus.

***Bed rest.*** The hospitalized woman is kept on bed rest, and her environment is kept quiet. External stimuli (lights, noise) that might precipitate a seizure should be reduced.

***Anticonvulsant medications.*** Magnesium sulfate is the drug most commonly used in the management of preeclampsia. Magnesium acts as a central nervous system (CNS) depressant by blocking neuromuscular transmission and decreasing the amount of acetylcholine liberated. Magnesium is not an antihypertensive medication, but it relaxes smooth muscle, including the uterus, and thus reduces vasoconstriction, possibly resulting in modest blood pressure reduction. Decreased vasoconstriction promotes circulation to maternal vital organs and increases placental circulation. Increased circulation to the maternal kidneys improves diuresis, as interstitial fluid is shifted into the vascular compartment and excreted.

Although magnesium sulfate is not risk free, it has the major advantage of a long safety record for mother and baby while preventing maternal seizures. Fetal magnesium levels are nearly identical to those of the mother. As a result, the fetal monitor tracing may show decreased fetal heart rate variability. No cumulative effect occurs, however, because the fetal kidneys excrete magnesium effectively.

The therapeutic serum level for magnesium is 4 to 8 mg/dL or as set by the healthcare facility. Adverse reactions to magnesium sulfate usually occur if the serum level becomes too high. The most important is CNS depression, including depression of the respiratory center. Magnesium is excreted solely by the kidneys, and the reduced urine output that often occurs in preeclampsia allows magnesium to accumulate to toxic levels in the woman. Frequent assessment of serum levels, DTRs (see Procedure), respiratory rate, and oxygen saturation can identify CNS depression before it progresses to respiratory depression or cardiac dysfunction. Monitoring urine output identifies oliguria that could allow magnesium to accumulate and reach excessive serum levels.

***Antihypertensive medications.*** If the woman's systolic blood pressure is ≥160 mm Hg or her diastolic blood pressure is ≥110 mm Hg, the risk for stroke or congestive heart failure is higher. Hydralazine (Apresoline) is commonly used because of its record of safety. The major advantage of hydralazine over other antihypertensives is its vasodilator activity that increases cardiac output and blood flow to the placenta. Other antihypertensive medications such as nifedipine (a calcium channel blocker) and labetalol (a beta-adrenergic blocker) are often used.

**Intrapartum management.** Most seizures occur during labor and the postpartum period. During labor, the woman must be monitored continuously to detect signs of imminent seizures. She should be kept in a lateral position to promote circulation through the placenta, and pain that may cause agitation and precipitate seizures should be controlled. Narcotic analgesics or epidural analgesia can be administered to reduce pain that could precipitate a seizure and lower blood pressure.

Labor is induced by IV oxytocin if the maternal or fetal condition deteriorates. Vaginal birth is usually the first choice because depression of coagulation factors and other multisystem involvement adds to the surgical risk for cesarean birth. Oxytocin to stimulate uterine contractions and magnesium sulfate to prevent generalized seizures are often administered simultaneously during labor. The woman will have two secondary infusions in addition to her primary infusion: one for oxytocin and one for magnesium sulfate.

Continuous electronic fetal monitoring identifies fetal heart rate patterns that suggest compromise. If nonreassuring patterns occur, the corrective actions depend on the pattern identified (see Chapter 17). Late decelerations (associated with reduced placental perfusion) and decreased variability (associated with reduced placental perfusion or magnesium use) are most common, but any other nonreassuring pattern can occur as well.

## DRUG GUIDE

### *Magnesium Sulfate*

**Classification:** Electrolyte.

**Action:** Decreases acetylcholine released by motor nerve impulses, thereby blocking neuromuscular transmission. Depresses the central nervous system (CNS) to act as an anticonvulsant; also decreases frequency and intensity of uterine contractions. Produces flushing and sweating as a result of decreased peripheral blood pressure.

**Indications:** Prevention and control of seizures in severe preeclampsia. Prevention of uterine contractions in preterm labor.

**Dosage and Route:** A common intravenous (IV) administration protocol for preeclampsia includes a loading dose and a continuous infusion. The loading dose is 4 to 6 g magnesium sulfate administered in 100 mL IV fluid over 15 to 20 minutes. The continuing infusion to maintain control is commonly 2 g/hr. Doses are individualized as needed. Deep intramuscular (IM) injection is acceptable but painful.

Magnesium sulfate can also be administered in a similar dose profile to stop preterm labor contractions because of its relaxant effects on smooth muscle.

**Absorption:** Immediate onset following IV administration.

**Excretion:** Excreted by the kidneys.

**Contraindications and Precautions:** Contraindicated in persons with myocardial damage, heart block, myasthenia gravis, or impaired renal function. Magnesium toxicity, possibly related to incomplete renal drug excretion, may be evidenced by thirst, mental confusion, or decreased reflexes.

**Adverse Reactions:** Result from magnesium overdose and include flushing, sweating, hypotension, depressed deep tendon reflexes, and CNS depression, including respiratory depression.

**Nursing Implications:** Monitor blood pressure closely during administration. Assess woman for respiratory rate of at least 12 breaths per minute, oxygen saturation of 95% or higher; presence of deep tendon reflexes, and urinary output greater than 30 mL/hr before administering magnesium. Place resuscitation equipment (suction, oxygen) in the room. Keep calcium gluconate, which acts as an antidote to magnesium, in the room along with syringes and needles.

Magnesium is usually administered by intravenous infusion, which allows for immediate onset of action and does not cause the discomfort associated with IM administration. Intravenous magnesium is administered via a secondary ("piggyback") line so that the medication can be discontinued at any time while the primary line remains functional.

A pediatrician, neonatologist, or neonatal nurse practitioner should be available to care for the newborn at birth.

**Postpartum management.** After birth, careful assessment of the mother's blood loss and signs of shock is essential because the hypovolemia caused by preeclampsia can be aggravated by blood loss during the birth. Assessments for signs and symptoms of preeclampsia must be continued for at least 48 hours, and magnesium may be continued to prevent seizures.

Signs that the woman is recovering from preeclampsia are:

- Urinary output of 4 to 6 L/day, which causes a rapid reduction in edema and rapid weight loss
- Decreased protein in the urine
- Gradual improvement in serum laboratory values (Table 25.4)
- Return of blood pressure to normal, usually within 2 weeks

**TABLE 25.4 Nursing Assessments for Preeclampsia and Magnesium Toxicity**

| Assessment | Implications |
|---|---|
| Daily weight | Provides estimate of fluid retention. |
| Blood pressure | To determine worsening condition, response to treatment, or both. |
| Respiratory rate, pulse oximeter readings | Drug therapy (magnesium sulfate) causes respiratory depression, and drug should be withheld and the physician notified if respiratory rate is 12 breaths/min or as specified by hospital policy. Pulse oximeter readings 95% or greater. |
| Breath sounds | To identify sounds of excess moisture in lungs associated with pulmonary edema. |
| Deep tendon reflexes | Hyperreflexia indicates increased cerebral irritability and edema; hyporeflexia is associated with magnesium excess. |
| Edema | For estimation of interstitial fluid. |
| Urinary output | Output of at least 30 mL/hr indicates adequate perfusion of the kidneys (25 mL/hr is used by some authorities). Magnesium levels may become toxic if urinary output is inadequate. |
| Urine protein | Normal protein in a random dipstick urine sample is negative or trace. Higher protein levels suggest greater leaking of protein secondary to glomerular damage with worsening preeclampsia. A 24-hr urine sample is most accurate for quantitative urine protein level. |
| Level of consciousness | Drowsiness or dulled sensorium indicates therapeutic effects of magnesium; lack of responsive behavior and muscle weakness are associated with magnesium excess. |
| Headache, epigastric pain, visual problems | These symptoms indicate increasing severity of the condition caused by cerebral edema, vasospasm of cerebral vessels, and liver edema. Eclampsia may develop quickly. |
| Fetal heart rate and baseline variability | Rate should be between 110 and 160 beats per minute in a term fetus. Decreasing baseline variability may be caused by therapeutic magnesium level or by inadequate placental perfusion. |
| Laboratory data | Elevated serum creatinine, elevated liver enzymes, and decreased platelets (thrombocytopenia) are significant signs of increasing severity of disease. Serum magnesium levels should be in the therapeutic range designated by the physician. |

Recent evidence shows that hypertension is more likely to recur well after preeclampsia, however, and may be a risk factor for both the woman and her baby in the pregnancy with preeclampsia. Cardiovascular disease is now the number one killer of women, and more research is needed to determine whether there is a true association between a pregnancy complication that is usually in young adulthood and a medical problem in middle or old age (Arslanian-Engoren, 2011; Fedorka & Heasley, 2008). See also Chapters 26 and 32.

### Therapeutic Management of Eclampsia

Eclampsia is a potentially preventable extension of severe preeclampsia marked by the onset of one or more generalized seizures. Early identification of preeclampsia in a pregnant woman allows intervention before the condition reaches the seizure stage in most cases. Generalized seizures usually start with facial twitching, followed by rigidity of the body. Tonic-clonic movements then begin and last for approximately 1 minute. Breathing stops during a seizure but resumes with a long, noisy inhalation. The woman is temporarily in a coma and is unlikely to remember the seizure when she resumes consciousness. Transient fetal heart rate patterns may be nonreassuring, such as bradycardia, loss of variability, or late decelerations. Fetal tachycardia may occur as the fetus compensates for the period of maternal apnea during the seizures. Eclampsia can occur during pregnancy or in the intrapartum or postpartum period.

Magnesium sulfate is administered as part of the treatment for eclampsia. Other anticonvulsants or sedatives are not routinely given.

The woman's blood volume is usually severely contracted in eclampsia, increasing the risk for poor placental perfusion. Fluid shifts from her intravascular space to the interstitial space, including the lungs, causing pulmonary edema and possibly heart failure as forward blood flow is impeded. Renal blood flow is severely reduced, with oliguria (less than 30 mL/hr urine output) and possible renal failure. Cerebral hemorrhage may accompany eclampsia because of the high blood pressure and coagulation deficits. The woman's lungs should be auscultated at regular intervals, usually hourly. A pulse oximeter provides continuous readings of oxygen saturation. Furosemide (Lasix) may be administered if pulmonary edema develops. Oxygen by facemask at 8 to 10 L/min improves maternal and fetal oxygenation. Digitalis may be needed to strengthen contraction of the heart if circulatory failure results. Urine output should be assessed hourly; if output drops below 30 mL/hr, renal failure should be suspected.

Because eclampsia stimulates uterine irritability, the woman should be monitored carefully for ruptured membranes, signs of labor, or abruptio placentae. While the woman is unresponsive, she should be kept on her side to prevent aspiration and to improve placental circulation. The side rails should be padded and raised to prevent injury from a fall. When maternal and fetal vital signs have stabilized, delivery of the fetus should be considered.

Aspiration of gastric contents is a leading cause of maternal morbidity after an eclamptic seizure. After initial stabilization, the nurse should anticipate orders for chest radiography and arterial blood gas determination to identify aspiration.

## NURSING CARE

### The Woman With Preeclampsia

#### Assessment

The frequency of assessments will vary according to the severity of the woman's preeclampsia. Weigh her on admission and then daily. Check vital signs every 4 hours, and auscultate the chest for moist breath sounds that suggest pulmonary edema. Assess the location and severity of edema at least every 4 hours. Table 25.2 on p. 537 describes a useful

## PROCEDURE

### *Assessing Deep Tendon Reflexes*

**Purpose**

To identify exaggerated reflexes (hyperreflexia) or diminished reflexes (hyporeflexia).

1. You will need a reflex hammer to best assess the brachial and the patellar reflexes. The patellar reflex is less reliable if the woman has had epidural analgesia, and upper extremity reflexes should be assessed.
2. Support the woman's arm and instruct her to let it go limp while it is being held so that the arm is totally relaxed and slightly flexed as you assess the brachial reflex. If you have difficulty identifying the correct tendon to tap, have the woman flex and extend her arm until you can feel it moving beneath your thumb. Have her fully relax her arm after you identify the tendon.
3. Place your thumb over the woman's tendon, as illustrated, to allow you to feel as well as see the tendon response when it is tapped. Strike your thumb with the small end of the reflex hammer. The normal response is slight flexion of the forearm.

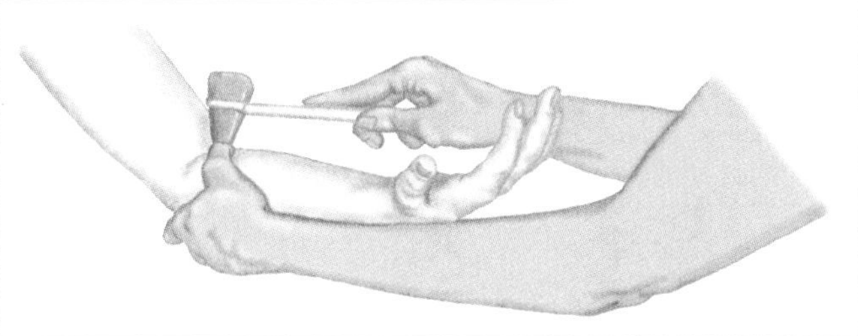

4. The patellar, or "knee-jerk," reflex can be assessed with the woman in two positions, sitting or lying. When the woman is sitting, allow her lower legs to dangle freely to flex the knee and stretch the tendons. If her patellar tendon is difficult to identify, have her flex and extend her lower legs slightly until you palpate the tendon. Strike the tendon directly with the reflex hammer, just below the patella.

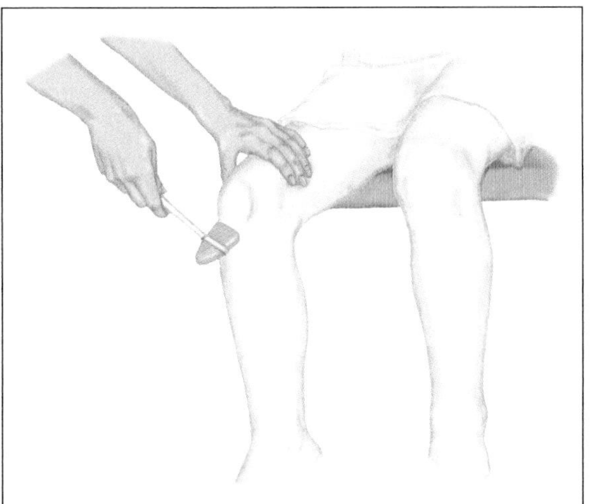

5. When the woman is supine, the weight of her leg must be supported to flex the knee and stretch the tendons. An accurate response requires that the limb be relaxed and the tendon partially stretched. Strike the partially stretched tendons just below the patella. Slight extension of the leg or a brief twitch of the quadriceps muscle of the thigh is the expected response.

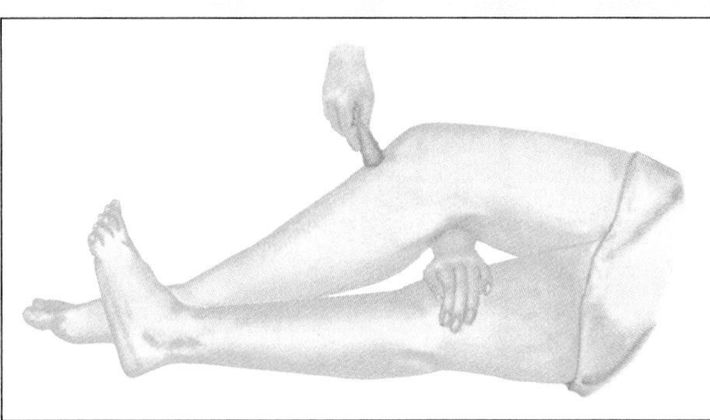

6. To assess clonus, the woman's lower leg should be supported, as illustrated, and the foot well dorsiflexed to stretch the tendon. Hold the flexion. If no clonus is present, no movement will be felt. When clonus (indicating hyperreflexia) is present, rapid rhythmic tapping motions of the foot are present.

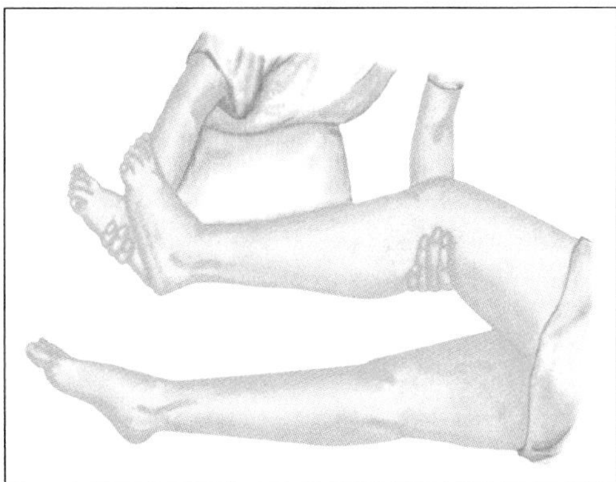

**Deep Tendon Reflex Rating Scale**

0: Reflex absent
+1: Reflex present, hypoactive
+2: Normal reflex
+3: Brisker than average reflex
+4: Hyperactive reflex; clonus may also be present.

*Note:* The rating scales of some facilities may omit the plus signs.

method for describing edema. Measure urine output hourly. An indwelling catheter is often ordered. Check the urine for protein every 4 hours. Apply an electronic fetal monitor to identify changes in fetal heart rate or variability, which suggest poor placental perfusion or other problems.

Check brachial, radial, and patellar reflexes for hyperreflexia, which indicates cerebral irritability. Clonus (rapidly alternating muscle contraction and relaxation) may be present when reflexes are hyperactive. Procedure 25.1 details how to assess and rate DTRs.

Question the woman carefully about symptoms she may be experiencing, such as headache, visual disturbances, epigastric pain, nausea or vomiting, or a sudden increase in edema.

An open-ended question such as "How do you feel?" may not be adequate. Ask targeted questions, such as "Do you have a headache?

Describe it for me." "Do you have any pain in the abdomen? Show me where it is, and describe it." "Have you had an upset stomach or vomiting?" "Do you see spots before your eyes? Flashes of light? Double vision?" "Is your vision blurred?" "Does light bother your eyes?" "Have you had an increase in swelling? Where is it located? When did you notice it?"

**Assessments for magnesium toxicity.** Obstetrical units have protocols that address routine assessments when magnesium is being administered and their frequency. Serum magnesium levels provide numerical data for blood levels of the drug. However, direct assessment provides detailed evaluation of the drug's true effects on the woman at any time. Hypotonic or absent reflexes indicate CNS depression that precedes respiratory depression. Determining the respiratory rate, lung sounds, and oxygen saturations by pulse oximetry identifies the adequacy of maternal respirations. Checking urine output identifies oliguria (less than 30 mL/hr) that may result in magnesium toxicity as the drug accumulates. Assess the woman's level of consciousness (alert, drowsy [expected], confused, oriented or disoriented). Table 25.4 summarizes nursing assessments and their implications.

**Psychosocial assessment.** The development of preeclampsia places a great deal of stress on the childbearing family. The woman may be on bed rest at home or hospitalized for some time. Preeclampsia also can require abrupt hospitalization. Whether care can be provided at home or requires hospitalization, the situation creates anxiety and mixed emotions about the condition of the fetus as well as that of the expectant mother. The family may not understand the seriousness of the disease because the woman feels well initially.

## NURSING CARE PLAN

### *Preeclampsia*

**Focused Assessment**

Julie is a 16-year-old primigravida seen in the prenatal clinic at 30 weeks of gestation. Julie's mother accompanies her. Julie's blood pressure is 136/90 mm Hg, and there is slight edema of the lower legs and trace proteinuria in a single voided specimen. Julie and her mother are given instructions about home care for gestational hypertension. The regimen includes rest; frequent monitoring of blood pressure, weight, and urine; and doing fetal "kick counts." She is told that she must return to the clinic in a week. She states that she feels fine and doesn't want to miss school. She says that she doesn't see the reason for "constant rest" and "doing nothing."

**Nursing Diagnosis**

Impaired Adjustment related to lack of knowledge of health status and the need for a change in lifestyle.

**Planning**

**Expected Outcomes**

Julie will:

1. Verbalize the benefits of the recommended regimen by the end of the first prenatal appointment.
2. Comply with the recommended care for the next week.
3. Keep prenatal appointments.

**Interventions and *Rationales***

1. Encourage Julie to verbalize her feelings about the recommended regimen: "What concerns you most about missing school?"
   *Acknowledge her feelings as important to reduce Julie's anxiety so that teaching and learning can begin.*
2. Identify family support that will permit compliance with the recommended regimen of rest and home care. Contact social worker for additional assistance needed, such as homebound teaching.
   *Compliance with the regimen is impossible without family assistance, which includes assistance with activities of daily living and necessary assessments. Homebound classes alleviate her concern that she is falling behind with schoolwork.*
3. Describe in general terms the pathophysiologic processes that affect Julie and her baby.
   *Expectant mothers are usually motivated to comply with a therapeutic management that will benefit the fetus. Julie's support from friends and family can strengthen her motivation and compliance.*
4. Tell Julie that she may feel well even though the condition worsens and that she must be observed for signs and symptoms at home and at the clinic.
   *A woman does not physically notice hypertension and proteinuria. Edema is not always present in hypertensive complications during pregnancy, and women may not be aware that it can be associated with other problems.*
5. Instruct Julie and her mother or other primary home caregiver to call the clinic or go to the hospital for evaluation if she notices headache, double vision, or spots before her eyes.
   *These signs suggest rapid progression of the disease and that additional management is promptly needed. Such an agreement will allow a schedule to provide peer support but allow for prolonged periods of quiet.*
6. Collaborate with Julie to arrange contact with her boyfriend and/or selected friends and to arrange for ongoing home-bound classes as needed.
   *Such an agreement will allow a schedule to provide peer support but allow for prolonged periods of quiet rest.*

**Evaluation**

Despite following the recommended regimen of rest with the help of her mother and sister and keeping prenatal appointments, Julie's condition worsens; preeclampsia is her updated medical diagnosis. She develops a rise in blood pressure and rapid weight gain, indicating generalized edema.

**Focused Assessment**

Julie is admitted to the hospital at 32 weeks of gestation with a blood pressure of 160/110 mm Hg, heart rate of 92 beats per minute, and respiratory rate of 22 breaths per minute. There is 2+ proteinuria and marked edema of the hands and face as well as her lower extremities. The fetal heart rate is 136 beats per minute with average variability. An intravenous infusion of magnesium sulfate is started, seizure precautions are initiated, and environmental stimuli are reduced. Julie is agitated and verbalizes concern that the procedures are going to hurt her or the fetus. She frequently asks, "How sick am I?" "Is the baby going to be okay?" Her hands are perspiring, and they shake when she reaches for a tissue.

**Nursing Diagnosis**

Anxiety related to hospitalization and concern about her health and the health of the fetus.

**Planning**

**Expected Outcomes**

Julie will:

1. Verbalize her concerns and describe the benefits of treatment while her family is present.
2. Manifest less anxiety (agitation, physiologic signs such as tremors, tachycardia, and perspiration).

## NURSING CARE PLAN—cont'd

### *Preeclampsia*

**Interventions and *Rationales***

1. *Because anxiety is an ominous feeling of tension resulting from a physical or emotional threat to the self and a global, often unnamed sense of doom, it needs to be ventilated and then addressed by conveying that the person is not alone and will be protected.* Julie expresses a feeling of helplessness, isolation, and insecurity when she must enter the hospital after following all prescribed measures at home. Nursing measures that may reduce her anxiety include the following:
   a. Reassure Julie that a solution for anxiety can be found: "I can see you are really worried, and I will try to answer all your questions."
   b. Allow Julie to cry, get angry, or express any feeling that is present.
   c. Encourage a discussion of feelings: "Tell me more about how you feel."
   d. Reflect observations: "I see you wringing your hands; do you want to talk about it?"
   e. Convey empathy and positive regard; use nonverbal behavior, including touch, when appropriate.
2. *Perception is somewhat narrowed with high anxiety. Knowledge of what to expect in the hospital gives Julie a sense of control that can reduce her anxiety and help her regain a sense of control. Provide brief information about hospital routines and procedures when Julie's anxiety has diminished enough for learning to take place:*
   a. Be very specific about procedures, such as fetal monitoring, assessment of deep tendon reflexes, taking of vital signs, and care specific for magnesium sulfate therapy. Explain the reasons for these procedures, who will perform them, and how long they will be continued after birth.
   b. Focus on Julie's present concerns; she is not able to be future-oriented at this time.
   c. Speak slowly and calmly, give very short directions, and do not ask Julie to make decisions: "Turn on your side." "Breathe slowly."
   d. Allow a friend or family member to remain with Julie, and instruct the person about the need for a low-stimulus environment.

**Evaluation**

Julie discusses her feelings with the nurse and with her sister. She feels in control of anxiety, as manifested by fewer signs of agitation and fewer physiologic signs (tachycardia, tachypnea) and by the ability to use relaxation techniques that she learned earlier.

**Potential Complications to Consider**

1. Magnesium Toxicity
2. Seizures

Investigate how the family will function while the woman is hospitalized or on bed rest at home. Determine how the woman is adapting to the "sick role" and the necessity of depending on others instead of functioning in her primary role. Ask how much support is available and who is willing to participate. Finally, determine the major concerns of the family (Sittner, DeFrain, & Hudson, 2005).

## Nursing Diagnosis and Planning

Analysis of the data collected can lead to nursing diagnoses (Nursing Care Plan: Preeclampsia) as well as collaborative problems or potential complications. Potential complications require nurses to monitor for the onset of new problems or changes in status. Physician-prescribed and nurse-prescribed interventions are used to minimize the complications. Potential medical complications for the woman with preeclampsia are *eclamptic seizures* and *magnesium toxicity*.

Potential complications of eclamptic seizures and magnesium toxicity are not appropriate for independent nursing management. The nurse must confer with physicians and use established protocols for treatment. For seizures, planning should reflect the nurse's responsibility to:

- Perform actions that reduce the risk of seizures and prevent maternal or fetal injury if seizures do occur.
- Monitor for signs of impending seizures.
- Support the family of the woman with eclampsia.

For magnesium toxicity, planning should reflect these nursing responsibilities:

- Monitor for signs of magnesium toxicity.
- Consult with the physician if signs of magnesium toxicity are observed.
- Perform actions that will minimize the possibility of magnesium toxicity.

## Interventions

### *Interventions for seizures*

**Initiating preventive measures.** In the presence of cerebral irritability, seizures may be precipitated by excessive visual or auditory stimuli. Nurses should reduce external stimuli by:

- Admitting the woman to a room in the quietest section of the unit and keeping the door to the room closed. The need for intense nursing observation and care exists regardless of the room location.
- Reducing noise when the door must be opened and closed.
- Keeping lights low and noise to a minimum; this may include blocking incoming telephone calls or visitors.
- Grouping nursing assessments and care to allow the woman periods of undisturbed quiet.
- Moving carefully and calmly around the room and avoiding bumping into the bed or startling the woman.
- Collaborating with the woman and her family to restrict visitors.

**Monitoring for signs of impending seizures.** Maternal findings that may precede seizures include:

- Hyperreflexia, the presence of clonus, or both
- Increasing signs of cerebral irritability (headache, visual disturbances)
- Epigastric or right upper quadrant pain, nausea, or vomiting

None of these signs is a predictor of imminent seizure in any woman. Nurses must be alert for subtle changes and be prepared for seizures in all women with preeclampsia.

**Preventing seizure-related injury.** Hard side rails should be padded and the bed kept in the lowest position with the wheels locked to prevent trauma during a seizure.

Oxygen and suction equipment should be assembled and ready to use to remove secretions and to provide oxygen if it is not already being administered. Check equipment and connections when the woman arrives and at the beginning of each shift for use readiness. Common emergency supplies include a medium plastic airway, an Ambu bag with mask, endotracheal tubes in assorted sizes, an ophthalmoscope, a tourniquet, a reflex hammer, syringes, and needles. Calcium gluconate should be immediately available to reverse the effects of excess magnesium sulfate.

**Protecting the woman and fetus during a seizure.** The nurse's primary responsibilities to protect the woman and the fetus during a generalized seizure are to:

- Remain with the woman and press the emergency bell for assistance.
- Attempt to turn the woman onto her side when the tonic phase begins. A side-lying position permits greater circulation through the placenta and can help prevent aspiration.
- Note the time and occurrences during the seizure.
- Insert an airway after the seizure, and suction the woman's mouth and nose to clear secretions and prevent aspiration. Provide oxygen by mask at 8 to 10 L/min to increase oxygenation of the placenta and all maternal body organs.
- Observe fetal monitor patterns for nonreassuring signs, such as bradycardia, tachycardia, or decreased variability. These may resolve within a few minutes as maternal oxygenation is restored.
- Notify, or have another nurse notify, the physician that a seizure has occurred. Administer medications and prepare for additional medical interventions as directed by the physician.

**Providing information and support for the family.** Explain to the family what has happened without minimizing the seriousness of the situation. A seizure is frightening for anyone who witnesses it, and the family is often reassured when the nurse explains that the seizure lasts only a few minutes and that the woman may not be alert for some time afterward. Acknowledge that the seizure indicates worsening of the condition and that it will be necessary for the physician to determine future management, which may include delivery of the infant as soon as possible. Vaginal birth is preferred if the maternal and fetal conditions permit because of the abnormalities in coagulation and other body systems.

***Interventions for magnesium toxicity***

**Monitoring for signs of magnesium toxicity.** Magnesium excess depresses the entire central nervous system, including the brainstem, which controls respiration and cardiac function, and the cerebrum, which controls memory, mental processes, and speech. Carbon dioxide accumulates if the respiratory rate or depth is inadequate, leading to respiratory acidosis and further CNS depression, which could end in respiratory arrest.

Signs of magnesium toxicity include:

- Respiratory rate less than 14 breaths per minute (hospital protocols may specify a respiratory rate of less than 12 breaths per minute)
- Maternal pulse oximeter reading lower than 95%
- Absence of DTRs
- Sweating, flushing
- Altered sensorium (confusion, lethargy, slurring of speech, drowsiness, disorientation)
- Hypotension
- A serum magnesium concentration greater than the therapeutic range of 4 to 8 mg/dL

**Responding to signs of magnesium toxicity.** Discontinue magnesium and notify the physician for signs of magnesium toxicity. Magnesium is excreted by the kidneys, and the physician should be notified if the urinary output falls below 30 mL/hr.

Calcium opposes the effects of magnesium at the neuromuscular junction. Magnesium toxicity can be reversed by slow IV administration of 1 g calcium gluconate (10 mL of 10%) at 1 mL/min.

### Evaluation

Collect and compare data with established norms and then judge whether the data are within normal limits. For seizures, interventions are judged to be successful if:

- DTRs remain within normal limits (+1 to +3).
- The woman is free of visual disturbances, severe headache, and epigastric or right upper quadrant pain.
- The woman remains free of seizures or free of preventable injury if a seizure occurs.
- For magnesium toxicity, determine whether respiratory rates remain at least 12 breaths per minute, DTRs are present, and maternal serum levels of magnesium do not exceed the therapeutic range.

## HELLP SYNDROME

The acronym HELLP describes a life-threatening occurrence that complicates approximately 10% of pregnancies in women with severe hypertension. As in preeclampsia, HELLP syndrome can occur during the postpartum period (Dekker, 2011).

Hemolysis is believed to occur as a result of the fragmentation and distortion of erythrocytes during passage through small, damaged blood vessels. Liver enzyme levels increase when hepatic blood flow is obstructed by fibrin deposits. Hyperbilirubinemia and jaundice can occur as a result of liver impairment. Low platelet levels are caused by vascular damage resulting from vasospasm; platelets aggregate at sites of damage, resulting in systemic thrombocytopenia (Dekker, 2011).

The prominent symptom of the HELLP syndrome is pain in the right upper quadrant, the lower chest, or epigastric area. There may also be tenderness because of liver distention. Additional signs and symptoms include nausea, vomiting, and severe edema. It is important to avoid traumatizing the liver by abdominal palpation and to use care in transporting the woman. A sudden increase in intraabdominal pressure, including a seizure, could lead to rupture of a subcapsular hematoma, resulting in internal bleeding and hypovolemic shock.

Women with the HELLP syndrome should be managed in a setting with full intensive care facilities available. Their treatment includes that which is appropriate for preeclampsia or eclampsia. After delivery, most women begin recovering within 72 hours.

## CHRONIC HYPERTENSION

A diagnosis of chronic hypertension is made whenever evidence suggests that hypertension preceded the pregnancy or when a woman is hypertensive before 20 weeks of gestation. Chronic hypertension is seen most often in older women, in those who are obese, and in those with diabetes. Heredity, including race, plays a role in the development of chronic hypertension, which is more common in Black-Americans at any age than in other races (Centers for Disease Control and Prevention [CDC], 2011). Late childbearing and rising obesity rates will no doubt fuel an increase in hypertension. Chronic hypertension is usually essential, or primary. However, it may be secondary to another problem, such as diabetes, renal disease, or an autoimmune disorder.

The most common maternal hazard is the development of preeclampsia in chronic hypertension. New-onset proteinuria or a significant rise in preexisting proteinuria identifies the development of superimposed preeclampsia. The rise in blood pressure with preeclampsia is likely to be greater in these women (Cunningham et al., 2010; Dekker, 2011)

A dietitian should be consulted about the appropriate diet and weight gain, because many of these pregnant women are obese, and they often have diabetes. Adequate intake of protein helps counteract the protein lost in urine. Prenatal visits will be needed more frequently. Regular fetal surveillance by biophysical profile and kick counts (see Chapter 15) is usual to identify poor growth patterns or signs that are nonreassuring, such as a falling volume of amniotic fluid.

Antihypertensive medications must be chosen carefully because they may reduce placental blood flow. Antihypertensive medication should be initiated if the diastolic pressure is consistently higher than 100 mm Hg in early pregnancy. Methyldopa (Aldomet) is the drug of choice because of its record of safety and effectiveness in pregnancy. Beta blockers and calcium channel blockers also can be used if methyldopa is not effective, but their record of safety in pregnancy is not as well established. Angiotensin-converting enzyme (ACE) inhibitors are contraindicated in pregnancy but can be used in the postpartum period. Hydralazine is a vasodilator reserved for hypertensive crisis. Diuretics are avoided, if possible, in superimposed preeclampsia because they can further shrink the blood volume.

## INCOMPATIBILITY BETWEEN MATERNAL AND FETAL BLOOD

### Rh Incompatibility

Rhesus (Rh) factor incompatibility during pregnancy is possible only when two specific circumstances coexist: (1) the expectant mother is Rh-negative; and (2) the fetus is Rh-positive. For such a circumstance to occur, the father of the fetus must have an Rh-positive blood type. Rh incompatibility is a problem that affects the fetus; it causes no harm to the expectant mother during pregnancy (Tidblad, Wesgren, Pasupathy, Karlsson, & Wikman, 2013).

Rh-negative blood is a recessive trait; therefore a person must inherit the same gene from both parents to be Rh-negative. Approximately 15% of the white population in the United States is Rh-negative. The incidence is lower in Black Americans and Asians.

#### Pathophysiology

People who are Rh-positive have the Rh antigen on their red blood cells, whereas people who are Rh-negative do not. When blood from a person who is Rh-positive enters the bloodstream of a person who is Rh-negative, the body reacts as it would to any foreign substance: It develops antibodies to destroy the invading antigen. To destroy the Rh antigen, which is part of the red blood cell, the entire red blood cell must be destroyed.

Theoretically, no mixing of fetal and maternal blood occurs during pregnancy. But in reality, small placental accidents can allow a drop or two of fetal blood to enter the maternal circulation and initiate the production of antibodies to destroy the Rh-positive blood cells (isoimmunization). Sensitization can also occur during a spontaneous or elective abortion or during antepartum procedures such as amniocentesis and chorionic villus sampling. Fig. 25.7 illustrates the process of maternal sensitization.

Most exposure of maternal blood to fetal blood occurs during the third stage of labor, when active exchange of fetal and maternal blood can occur as the placenta separates. The woman's first Rh-positive child is usually unaffected because maternal antibodies are formed after the birth of the infant. Subsequent Rh-positive fetuses can be affected, however, unless the mother receives RhoGAM to prevent antibody formation after the birth of each Rh-positive infant. The use of

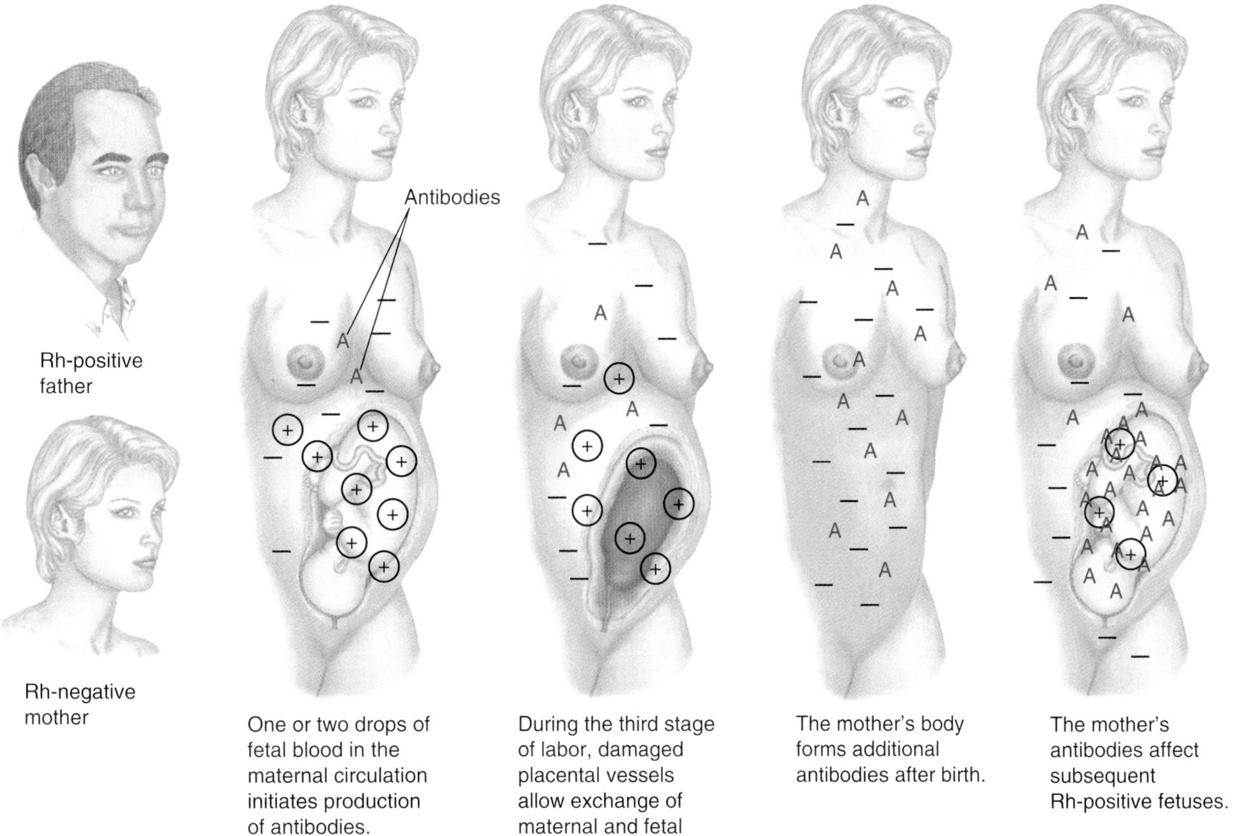

Rh-positive father
Rh-negative mother
Antibodies
One or two drops of fetal blood in the maternal circulation initiates production of antibodies.
During the third stage of labor, damaged placental vessels allow exchange of maternal and fetal blood.
The mother's body forms additional antibodies after birth.
The mother's antibodies affect subsequent Rh-positive fetuses.


**FIG 25.7** The process of maternal sensitization to the Rh factor.

RhoGAM has greatly reduced the fetal and neonatal complications of Rh incompatibility. The complication does still occur, however, and can be fatal to the fetus.

### Fetal and Neonatal Implications

If antibodies to the Rh factor are present in the mother's blood, they cross the placental barrier and destroy Rh-positive fetal red blood cells. The fetus becomes deficient in red blood cells, which are needed to transport oxygen to fetal tissue. As fetal red blood cells are destroyed, fetal bilirubin levels increase *(icterus gravis)*, which can lead to severe neurologic disease (bilirubin encephalopathy or **kernicterus**) with staining of the brain tissue. This hemolytic process results in the rapid production of erythroblasts (immature red blood cells) that cannot carry oxygen. The entire syndrome is termed **erythroblastosis fetalis**. The fetus may become so anemic that generalized edema (hydrops fetalis) results and can end in fetal congestive heart failure. Management of the infant born with erythroblastosis fetalis is discussed in Chapter 30.

## PARENTS WANT TO KNOW

### *About Rh Incompatibility*

**What does it mean to be Rh-negative?**
Those who are Rh-negative lack a substance that is present on the red blood cells of those who are Rh-positive.

**How can the expectant mother be Rh-negative and the fetus be Rh-positive?**
The fetus can inherit the Rh-positive factor from the father.

**What does sensitization mean?**
Sensitization means that the expectant mother has been exposed to Rh-positive blood and has developed antibodies against the Rh factor.

**Do the antibodies harm the expectant mother?**
No. The mother is unaffected because she does not have the Rh factor.

**Do Rh-positive men always father Rh-positive children?**
No. Rh-positive men who have an Rh-positive gene and an Rh-negative gene can also father Rh-negative children.

**Why is $Rh_0$(D) immune globulin (RhoGAM) necessary during pregnancy and following childbirth?**
RhoGAM prevents maternal development of Rh antibodies, which might be harmful to the current Rh-positive fetus as well as subsequent fetuses. The fetus is presumed Rh-positive.

**Why will the next fetus be jeopardized if RhoGAM is not administered?**
Although the degree of risk varies, if RhoGAM is not administered to the mother when the newborn is Rh-positive, she may develop antibodies to fetal Rh-positive blood. These antibodies can cross the placenta and destroy the erythrocytes of the next Rh-positive fetus.

### Prenatal Assessment and Management

All pregnant women should have a blood test to determine their blood type and Rh factor at the initial prenatal visit. Rh-negative women should have an antibody titer (indirect Coombs test) to determine whether they are sensitized (have developed antibodies) as a result of previous exposure to Rh-positive blood. If the indirect Coombs test is negative, it is repeated at 28 weeks of gestation to identify cases of later sensitization. A negative indirect Coombs test result accurately determines that the fetus is not at risk for hemolytic disease of the newborn at that time.

As a preventive measure, the fetus is considered Rh positive, and RhoGAM is administered to the unsensitized, Rh-negative woman at 28 weeks of gestation. RhoGAM is a commercial preparation of passive antibodies against Rh factor. It effectively prevents the formation of active antibodies if a small amount of fetal Rh-positive blood enters the circulation of an Rh-negative mother during the remainder of the pregnancy. RhoGAM is repeated after birth if the woman delivers an Rh-positive infant (Moise & Argoti, 2012).

A positive indirect Coombs test result indicates maternal sensitization and the presence of antibodies against Rh-positive erythrocytes. The indirect Coombs test is repeated at frequent intervals throughout the pregnancy to determine whether the antibody titer is rising, which indicates that the process is continuing. The fetus will be in jeopardy because fetal erythrocytes are being attacked by maternal anti-Rh antibodies.

Amniocentesis can be performed to evaluate changes in the optical density (delta [Δ] OD 450) of amniotic fluid. This measure reflects the amount of bilirubin (residue of red blood cell destruction) present in the amniotic fluid. If the fluid OD remains low, it indicates that the fetus is either Rh-negative or is in no jeopardy if Rh-positive. If the OD is elevated, the fetus is in jeopardy.

Ultrasound examination is used to noninvasively evaluate the condition of the fetus. Doppler studies allow evaluation of cardiac

## DRUG GUIDE

### *$Rh_0$(D) Immune Globulin (RhoGAM, HypRho-D, Gamulin Rh)*

**Classification:** Concentrated immunoglobulins directed toward the red blood cell antigen $Rh_0$(D).

**Action:** Prevents production of anti-$Rh_0$(D) antibodies in Rh-negative women who have been exposed to Rh-positive blood by suppressing the immune reaction of the Rh-negative woman to the antigen in Rh-positive blood. Prevents antibody production, which subsequently prevents hemolytic disease of the newborn in future pregnancies of women who have conceived an Rh-positive fetus.

**Indications:** Administered to Rh-negative women who have been exposed to Rh-positive blood through:
- Delivering an Rh-positive infant
- Aborting an Rh-positive fetus
- Having chorionic villus sampling, amniocentesis, or intraabdominal trauma while carrying an Rh-positive fetus
- Accidental transfusion of Rh-positive blood to an Rh-negative woman

**Dosage and Route:** One *standard dose* administered intramuscularly:
- At 28 weeks of pregnancy and within 72 hours of delivery
- Within 72 hours following the termination of a pregnancy of 13 weeks gestation or more

One *microdose* within 72 hours following the termination of a pregnancy of less than 13 weeks gestation.

After accidental transfusion with Rh-positive blood, dosage is calculated based on the volume of blood erroneously administered.

**Absorption:** Well absorbed from intramuscular sites.

**Excretion:** Metabolism and excretion unknown.

**Contraindications and Precautions:** Women who are Rh-positive or women previously sensitized to $Rh_0$(D) should not receive $Rh_0$(D) immune globulin. Used cautiously for women with previous hypersensitivity reactions to immune globulins.

**Adverse Reactions:** Local pain at intramuscular site, fever, or both.

**Nursing Implications:** Type and screen of mother's blood and cord blood of the newborn must be performed to determine the need for the medication. The mother must be Rh-negative and negative for Rh antibodies; the newborn must be Rh-positive. If there is doubt regarding the fetal blood type following spontaneous or elective abortion, the medication should be administered. The drug is administered to the mother, not the infant. The deltoid muscle is recommended for intramuscular administration.

function and blood flow in fetal vessels. Generalized fetal edema, ascites, an enlarged heart, or hydramnios occurs when the fetus is very anemic. Percutaneous umbilical blood sampling (PUBS) or cordocentesis (see Chapter 15), allows invasive sampling of fetal blood from cord vessels to determine the degree of erythrocyte destruction. Because it is invasive, PUBS is reserved for use in the fetus thought to be significantly affected (Papantoniou, Sifakis, & Antsaklis, 2013; Weiner, 2011).

### Postpartum Management

If the mother is Rh-negative, umbilical cord blood is taken at delivery to determine the baby's blood type, Rh factor, and antibody titer (direct Coombs test). Rh-negative, unsensitized mothers who give birth to Rh-positive infants are given an IM injection of RhoGAM within 72 hours after delivery. As a result, the fetal Rh antigens present in her circulation are destroyed, and she does not form natural, permanent antibodies.

If the infant is Rh-negative, there is no antibody formation, and RhoGAM is not necessary. RhoGAM is also administered when fetal-to-maternal transfusion is possible after abortion, chorionic villus sampling, and amniocentesis and the fetal blood type is unknown and at 28 weeks of gestation if the mother is Rh-negative and unsensitized. The drug may also be given after trauma if fetal-to-maternal hemorrhage is detected. More than the single 300-μg dose may be needed for large fetal hemorrhages.

Families are often very concerned about the fetus. Nurses must be sensitive to clues and signals that indicate that the family is anxious and must be able to offer honest reassurance. These skills are especially important if the pregnant woman is sensitized and fetal testing is necessary throughout pregnancy.

At birth, the physician or nurse should collect cord blood to determine the blood type and Rh factor of the newborn. During the postpartum period, nurses are responsible for follow-up to determine whether RhoGAM is necessary and to administer the injection within the prescribed time.

## ABO Incompatibility

ABO incompatibility occurs when the expectant mother is blood type O and the fetus is blood type A, B, or AB. Blood types A, B, and AB contain a protein component (antigen) that is not present in type O blood. Neonatal morbidity can range from uncomplicated hyperbilirubinemia to more severe anemia (Greenberg, Narendran, Schibler, et al., 2009).

People with type O blood develop anti-A or anti-B antibodies naturally as a result of exposure to antigens in the foods that they eat or to infection by gram-negative bacteria. As a result, some women with type O blood have developed high serum anti-A and anti-B antibody titers before pregnancy. The antibodies, or immune globulins, can be either IgG or IgM. When the woman becomes pregnant, the IgG antibodies cross the placental barrier and cause hemolysis of fetal red blood cells. Although the first fetus can be affected, ABO incompatibility is less severe than Rh incompatibility because the primary antibodies of the ABO system are IgM, which do not cross the placenta.

No specific prenatal care is needed, but the nurse must be aware of the possibility of ABO incompatibility. At birth, cord blood is taken to determine the blood type of the newborn and the antibody titer (direct Coombs test). The newborn is carefully screened for jaundice, which indicates hyperbilirubinemia. See Chapter 30 for medical and nursing management of hyperbilirubinemia in newborns.

## KEY CONCEPTS

- Spontaneous abortion is a leading cause of pregnancy loss. Treatment focuses on preventing complications, such as hypovolemic shock and infection, and providing emotional support for grief.
- The incidence of ectopic pregnancy in the United States is increasing as a result of pelvic inflammation associated with sexually transmitted diseases. The goals of therapeutic management are to prevent severe hemorrhage and to preserve the fallopian tube so that future fertility is retained.
- Management of hydatidiform mole involves two phases: (1) evacuation of the molar pregnancy, and (2) regular follow-up for 1 year to detect malignant changes.
- A woman with placenta previa typically presents with painless vaginal bleeding during the last half of pregnancy. Bleeding from abruptio placentae can be visible or concealed and is likely to be accompanied by pain, uterine tenderness, and uterine hyperactivity.
- DIC is a life-threatening complication of missed abortion, abruptio placentae, and preeclampsia, in which procoagulation and anticoagulation factors are simultaneously activated.
- The goals of HEG management are to prevent dehydration, malnutrition, and electrolyte imbalance. Emotional support is a most important therapy and a responsibility of nurses.
- Generalized vasospasm, which occurs with preeclampsia, decreases circulation to all organs of the body, including the placenta. Major maternal organs affected include the liver, kidneys, and brain.
- The treatment of preeclampsia includes bed rest, reducing environmental stimuli, and administering anticonvulsants.
- Magnesium sulfate is used to prevent seizures in preeclampsia. Its most serious adverse effect is central nervous system depression, which includes depression of the respiratory center. Hyporeflexia precedes respiratory depression.
- Nurses monitor the woman with preeclampsia to determine the effectiveness of medical therapy and to identify signs that the condition is worsening, such as greater hyperreflexia. Nurses also control external stimuli and initiate measures to protect the woman in case of eclamptic seizures.
- Women who have chronic hypertension are at increased risk for preeclampsia and should be monitored closely for proteinuria and generalized edema. Antihypertensive medication should be continued or initiated if diastolic blood pressure is consistently higher than 100 mm Hg.
- Rh incompatibility can occur when an Rh-negative woman conceives a child who is Rh-positive. Maternal antibodies may then develop after exposure to fetal Rh-positive blood and cause hemolysis of fetal Rh-positive red blood cells in subsequent pregnancies. Administration of RhoGAM prevents production of anti-Rh antibodies, thus preventing destruction of Rh-positive red blood cells in subsequent pregnancies.
- ABO incompatibility usually occurs when the mother has type O blood and has naturally-occurring anti-A and anti-B antibodies, which cause hemolysis if the fetal blood is not type O. ABO incompatibility may result in hyperbilirubinemia of the infant, but this condition is usually mild.

## REFERENCES AND READINGS


Abalos, E., Duley, L., & Steyn, D. (2014). Antihypertensive drug therapy for mild to moderate hypertension during pregnancy. *Cochrane Database Systemic Review*. Retrieved from http://onlinelibrary.wiley.com/enhanced/doi/10.1002/14651858.CD002252.pub3.

American Academy of Pediatrics & American College of Obstetricians and Gynecologists. (2013). *Guidelines for perinatal care* (8th ed.). Elk Grove Village, IL, and Washington, DC: Author.

American College of Obstetricians and Gynecologists. (2010). Emergent therapy for acute-onset, severe hypertension during pregnancy and the postpartum period (Committee opinion No. 623). *Obstetrics & Gynecology, 125*(2), 521–525.

American College of Obstetricians and Gynecologists. (2010a). *Chronic hypertension in pregnancy (ACOG Practice Bulletin No. 29)*. Washington, DC: Author.

American College of Obstetricians and Gynecologists. (2010b). *Diagnosis and management of preeclampsia and eclampsia (ACOG Practice Bulletin No. 33)*. Washington, DC: Author.

American College of Obstetricians and Gynecologists. (2010c). *Medical management of ectopic pregnancy (ACOG Practice Bulletin No. 94)*. Washington, DC: Author.

American College of Obstetricians and Gynecologists. (2011). *Nausea and vomiting of pregnancy (ACOG Practice Bulletin No. 52)*. Washington, DC: Author.

American College of Obstetricians and Gynecologists (2013). Hypertension in pregnancy: Report of the American College of Obstetricians and Gynecologists' Task Force. *Obstetrics & Gynecology, 122*(5), 1122–31.

American College of Obstetricians and Gynecologists. (2013). *Medically indicated late-preterm and early-term deliveries. (ACOG Practice Bulletin No. 560)*. Washington, DC: Author.

Arslanian-Engoren, C. (2011). Women's risk factors and screening for coronary heart disease. *Journal of Obstetric, Gynecologic, and Neonatal Nursing, 40*(3), 337–347.

Blackburn, S.T. (2013). *Maternal, fetal, and neonatal physiology: A clinical perspective* (4th ed.). St. Louis: Saunders.

Bobrowski, R.A. (2011). Trauma. In D. James, P. Steer, & P. Weiner (Eds.), *High risk pregnancy: Management options* (4th ed., pp. 973–995). Philadelphia: Saunders.

Centers for Disease Control and Prevention. (2011). *Hypertension: High blood pressure facts*. Retrieved from http://www.cdc.gov.

Cunningham, F.G., Leveno, K.J., Bloom, S.L., et al. (2010). *Williams obstetrics* (23rd ed.). New York: McGraw-Hill.

Cunningham, F.G., Leveno, K.J., Bloom, S.L., Spong, C.Y., Dashe, J.S., Hoffman, B.L., Casey, B.M., & Sheffield, J.S. (2014). *Williams obstetrics* (24th ed.). New York: McGraw-Hill.

Della Torre, M., Kilpatrick, S.J., Hibbard, J.U., Simonson, L., Scott, S., Koch, A., & Geller, S.E. (2011). Assessing preventability for obstetric hemorrhage. *American Journal of Perinatology, 28*(10), 753–760.

Dekker, G. (2011). Hypertension. In D.K. James, P.J. Steer, & C.P. Weiner (Eds.), *High risk pregnancy: Management options* (4th ed., pp. 599–626). Philadelphia: Saunders.

Erick, M. (2012). Nutrition during pregnancy and lactation. In L.K. Mahan, & S. Escott-Stump (Eds.), *Krause's food & nutrition therapy* (13th ed., pp. 340–374). Philadelphia: Saunders.

Fedorka, P.D., & Heasley, S.W. (2008). Preeclampsia: The little known truth. *American Nurse Today, 3*(2), 9–11.

Francois, K. (2012). Antepartum and postpartum Hemorrhage. In M. Foley, T. Strong, & T. Garite (Eds.), *Obstetrics: Normal and Problem Pregnancies* (6th ed.). Saunders: Philadelphia.

Gilbert, E.S. (2011). *Manual of high risk pregnancy & delivery* (5th ed.). St. Louis: Mosby.

Greenberg, J.M., Narendran, V., Schibler, K.B., et al. (2009). Neonatal morbidities of prenatal and perinatal origin. In R.K. Creasy, R. Resnik, & J.D. Iams (Eds.), *Creasy & Resnik's maternal-fetal medicine: Principles and practice* (6th ed., pp. 1197–1227). Philadelphia: Saunders.

Hutti, M.H., Armstrong, D.S., & Myers, J. (2011). Healthcare utilization in the pregnancy following a perinatal loss. *MCN: American Journal of Maternal-Child Nursing, 36*(2), 104–111.

Kavak, S., Atilgan, R., Demirel, I., Celik, E., Ilhan, R., & Sapmaz, E. (2013). Endouterine hemostatic square suture vs. Bakri balloon tamponade for intractable hemorrhage due to complete placenta previa. *Journal of Perinatal Medicine, 41*(6), 705–9.

Limbo, R., Kobler, K., & Levang, E. (2010). Respectful disposition in early pregnancy loss. *MCN: American Journal of Maternal-Child Nursing, 35*(5), 271–277.

Lisonkova, S., & Joseph, K. (2013). Incidence of preeclampsia: risk factors and outcomes associated with early- versus late-onset disease. *American Journal of Obstetrics & Gynecology, 209*(6), 544.

Magee, L., Helewa, M., Moutquin, J., & von Dadelszen, P. (2014). Diagnosis, evaluation, and management of the hypertensive disorders of pregnancy. *Journal of Obstetrics and Gynaecology Canada, 36*(5), 416–438.

Meighan, M., & Wood, A.F. (2005). The impact of hyperemesis gravidarum on maternal role assumption. *Journal of Obstetric, Gynecologic, and Neonatal Nursing, 34*(2), 172–179.

Moise, K., & Arogti, P. (2012). Management and prevention of red cell alloimmunization in pregnancy: a systematic review. *Obstetrics & Gynecology, 120*(5), 1132–9.

National Institutes of Health: National Heart, Lung, and Blood Institute. (2001). *Report of the working group on research on hypertension during pregnancy*. Retrieved from http://www.nhlbi.nih.gov.

Osborn, R., & Dodge, J. (2012). Gestational trophoblastic neoplasia. *Obstetrics Gynecology Clinics of North America, 39*(2), 195–212.

Sittner, B.J., DeFrain, J., & Hudson, D.B. (2005). Effects of high-risk pregnancies on families. *MCN: The American Journal of Maternal/Child Nursing, 30*(2), 121–126.

Papantoniou, N., Sifakis, S., & Antsaklis, A. (2013). Therapeutic management of fetal anemia: a review of standard practice and alternative treatment options. *Journal of Perinatal Medicine, 41*(1), 71–82.

Sibai, B. (2012). Etiology and management of postpartum hypertension-preeclampsia. *American Journal of Obstetrics and Gynecology, 206*(6), 470–475.

Tiblad, E., Wesgren, M., Pasupathy, D., Karlsson, A., & Wikman, A. (2013). Consequences of being Rhesus D immunized during pregnancy and how to optimize new prevention strategies. *Acta Obstetricia et Gynecologica Scandinavica, 92*(9), 1079–1085.

Tikkanen, M., Luukkaala, T., Gissler, M., Ritvanen, A., Ylikorkala, O., Paavonen, J., Nuutila, M, Andersson, S., Metsäranta M. (2013). Decreasing perinatal mortality in placental abruption. *Acta Obstetricia et Gynecologica Scandinavica, 92*(3), 298–305.

Weiner, C.P. (2011). Fetal hemolytic disease. In D.K. James, P.J. Steer, & C.P. Weiner (Eds.), *High risk pregnancy: Management options* (4th ed., pp. 209–227). Philadelphia: Saunders.

Williamson, C., & Girling, J. (2011). Hepatic and gastrointestinal disease. In D.K. James, P.J. Steer, & C.P. Weiner (Eds.), *High risk pregnancy: Management options* (4th ed., pp. 839–860). Philadelphia: Saunders.

Yoong, W., Ridout, A., Memtsa, M., Stavroulis, A., Aref-Adib, M., Ramsay-Marcelle, Z., & Fakokunde, A. (2012). Application of uterine compression suture in association with intrauterine balloon tamponade ('uterine sandwich') for postpartum hemorrhage. *Acta Obstetricia et Gynecologica Scandinavica, 91*(1), 147–151.

26

# Concurrent Disorders During Pregnancy

http://evolve.elsevier.com/McKinney/mat-ch/

## LEARNING OBJECTIVES

*After studying this chapter, you should be able to:*

- Describe the effects of pregnancy on glucose metabolism.
- Discuss the effects and management of preexisting diabetes mellitus during pregnancy.
- Explain the effects and management of gestational diabetes mellitus.
- Describe the management of the pregnant and postpartum woman who has a heart disease.
- Explain the maternal and fetal effects of specific hematologic disorders and the required management during pregnancy.
- Identify the effects, management, and nursing considerations of specific preexisting conditions discussed in this chapter.
- Discuss the maternal, fetal, and neonatal effects of the most common infections that can occur during pregnancy.

Pregnancy can alter the course of a concurrent disease, or a disease and its treatment may have unwanted effects on the pregnancy. As a result, the usual antepartum care must be adapted to include increased surveillance of the mother and fetus. Moreover, some disorders that are mild or even subclinical in the pregnant woman can cause massive damage to a fetus.

## DIABETES MELLITUS

### Pathophysiology

#### Etiology

Preexisting, or type 1, diabetes mellitus is a complex disorder of carbohydrate metabolism caused primarily by a partial or complete lack of insulin secretion by the beta cells of the pancreas. Some cells, such as those in skeletal and cardiac muscles and in adipose tissue, require insulin to carry glucose across their membranes. Without insulin, glucose accumulates in the blood, resulting in hyperglycemia. The body attempts to dilute the glucose load by any means possible. The first strategy is to increase thirst *(polydipsia)*, one of the classic symptoms of diabetes mellitus. Next, the fluid from the intracellular spaces is drawn into the vascular bed, resulting in dehydration at the cellular level but fluid volume excess in the vascular compartment. The kidneys attempt to excrete large volumes of this fluid plus the heavy solute load of glucose (osmotic diuresis). This excretion produces the second sign of diabetes, polyuria, and *glycosuria* (glucose in the urine). Without glucose, the cells starve, so weight loss occurs, although the person ingests large amounts of food (polyphagia).

If the body cannot metabolize glucose, it begins to metabolize protein and fat (lipogenesis) to meet energy needs. The metabolism of protein produces a negative nitrogen balance, and the metabolism of fat results in the accumulation of ketone bodies (e.g., acetone, acetoacetic acid, or beta-hydroxybutyric acid) or ketosis (accumulation of ketone bodies or acids) in the body.

If the disease is not well controlled, serious complications can occur. Hypoglycemia or hyperglycemia can result if the amount of insulin does not match the diet. Moreover, fluctuating periods of hyperglycemia and hypoglycemia damage small blood vessels throughout the body. This damage can cause serious impairment, especially in the kidneys, eyes, and heart.

### Effect of Pregnancy on Fuel Metabolism

Pregnancy has a profound impact on metabolism and is known as an insulin-resistant state. To understand the relationship between diabetes mellitus and pregnancy, knowledge of how pregnancy and diabetes alter food metabolism is necessary.

***Early pregnancy.*** Metabolic changes can be divided into those that occur early in pregnancy (from 1 to 20 weeks of gestation) and those that occur late in pregnancy (from the end of 20 weeks of gestation until birth). During early pregnancy, maternal metabolic rates and energy needs change little. However, during this time, insulin release in response to serum glucose levels increases. Significant hypoglycemia may result, particularly in women who experience the nausea, vomiting, and anorexia that often occur during the first weeks of pregnancy.

In an uncomplicated pregnancy, the availability of glucose and insulin favors the development and storage of fat during the first half of pregnancy. The accumulation of fat prepares the mother for the increase in energy use by the growing fetus during the second half of pregnancy.

***Late pregnancy.*** During the second half of pregnancy, when fetal growth accelerates, levels of placental hormones rise sharply. These hormones, particularly estrogen, progesterone, and human placental lactogen, create resistance to insulin in maternal cells to provide an abundant supply of glucose for the fetus. The hormones have a diabetogenic effect, or a condition that produces the effects of diabetes mellitus. These effects may leave the woman with insufficient insulin and episodes of hyperglycemia.

For most women, insulin resistance is not a problem. The pancreas responds by simply increasing the production of insulin. However, if the pancreas is unable to respond, the woman will experience periods of hyperglycemia.

During late pregnancy, the fetus continuously withdraws nutrients, such as glucose and amino acids, from maternal blood. The result is an earlier-than-normal switch from carbohydrate metabolism to gluconeogenesis (formation of glycogen from noncarbohydrate sources such as proteins and fat). Because the fetus uses many of the amino acids, the process becomes predominantly one of fat utilization. This process produces high levels of free fatty acids that further inhibit the uptake and oxidation of glucose, and thus, preserve glucose for use by the central nervous system (CNS) and fetus. These metabolic changes are similar to those that occur during "accelerated starvation," when fat is metabolized to meet the body's energy needs.

## Classification

Diabetes is classified as type 1 (insulin deficient) or type 2 (insulin resistant, with a relative deficiency of insulin to metabolize carbohydrate) according to whether the person requires the administration of insulin to prevent ketoacidosis. A third type, *gestational diabetes mellitus* (GDM), is one in which any degree of glucose intolerance has its onset or first recognition during pregnancy (Box 26.1).

An additional classification of diabetes can be used for descriptive purposes. The White classification describes the age at onset of diabetes, its duration based on the woman's current age, and vascular complications, such as retinopathy, that are present. GDM descriptions in White's classification also include $A_1$ (diet controlled) or $A_2$ (diet and insulin controlled) (Cunningham, Leveno, Bloom, Spong, & Dash, 2014; Berggren, Boggess, Stuebe, & Funk, 2011).

## Incidence

Diabetes mellitus is a medical condition that can adversely affect pregnancy, and its frequency is increasing along with obesity and abnormal lipid profiles. Approximately 90% to 95% of diagnoses in the total population are type 2, whereas type 1 accounts for only 5% to 10% of those diagnosed. Diabetes during pregnancy can be the result of preexisting diabetes (type 1 or type 2) or the development of GDM during the course of the pregnancy. A pregnant woman may have had undiagnosed type 2 diabetes that is discovered during pregnancy screening for GDM or her postpartum visit at 6 to 12 weeks (American College of Obstetricians and Gynecologists [ACOG], 2015, American Diabetes Association [ADA], 2015).

Approximately 7% of all pregnancies are affected by GDM, but the range varies from 1% to 14% among different ethnic groups, with higher rates in African-Americans, Latinas, American Indians, some Asian-Americans, and Pacific Islanders. Women who have GDM have a 35% to 60% likelihood of developing diabetes in the following 10 to 20 years (ACOG, 2015; ADA, 2015).

### BOX 26.1 Classification of Diabetes Mellitus

- *Type 1:* Insulin dependent. Onset in childhood or young adulthood. Involves autoimmune destruction of pancreatic beta cells. Prone to ketosis.
- *Type 2:* Can be diet controlled or require insulin, depending on the level of insulin resistance. Usual onset after age 40 years. Associated with obesity that often occurs in young adults or children. Ketosis less likely to occur than in type 1 diabetes mellitus.
- *Gestational (GDM):* Onset of glucose intolerance first diagnosed during pregnancy. Two subgroups are GDM $A_1$ (diet control) and GDM $A_2$ (insulin control with diet).

Data from American Diabetes Association. (2011). Diagnosis and classification of diabetes mellitus. *Diabetes Care, 34*(1), S62–S69, January 2011.

## Pathology

The root cause of type 2 diabetes is insulin resistance, in which body cells do not use glucose properly. The need for insulin rises, and the pancreas gradually loses the ability to supply enough of the hormone needed to metabolize glucose. Type 2 diabetes may be controlled by diet, exercise, and weight reduction, or it may require oral agents or insulin to control high glucose levels.

## Preexisting Diabetes Mellitus

### Maternal Effects

Preeclampsia occurs more often in women with diabetes than in the unaffected population (ACOG, 2014; Cunningham et al., 2014). The development of ketoacidosis is a threat to women who require insulin to properly control their diabetes. Ketoacidosis is often precipitated by infection or missed insulin doses, particularly in the woman with type 1 diabetes. Moreover, during pregnancy, ketoacidosis can develop at lower thresholds of hyperglycemia. Untreated ketoacidosis can progress to fetal and maternal death.

Urinary tract infections are more common, possibly because glucose-rich urine provides a good medium for bacterial growth. Other effects include hydramnios (excess volume of amniotic fluid), resulting from fetal hyperglycemia and consequent fetal diuresis. Premature rupture of membranes can also occur, caused by overdistention of the uterus by hydramnios or a large fetus. A difficult labor, shoulder dystocia (delayed or difficult birth of fetal shoulders after the head is born), and injury to the birth canal are more likely if the fetus is large. Large fetal size also increases the likelihood that a cesarean birth will be necessary and increases the risk for postpartum hemorrhage (Cunningham et al., 2014; Gilbert, 2011).

Production of excess amniotic fluid (hydramnios) can occur if maternal insulin control is not optimal. The excess fluid distends the uterus, possibly leading to early rupture of membranes, prolapsed cord (see Chapter 27), abnormal labor, and postpartum hemorrhage caused by failure of the uterus to contract effectively.

### Fetal Effects

The fetal and neonatal effects of preexisting diabetes depend on the timing and severity of maternal hyperglycemia and the degree of maternal vascular impairment. During the first trimester, when major fetal organs develop, the effects of the abnormal metabolic environment (hypoglycemia, hyperglycemia, or ketosis) increase the incidence of spontaneous abortion and major fetal malformations.

***Congenital malformation.*** The most common major congenital malformations associated with preexisting diabetes are neural tube defects, caudal regression syndrome (failure of the sacrum, lumbar spine, and lower extremities to develop), and cardiac defects. Women who are hyperglycemic during the first trimester have three to four times the risk of having an infant with a structural anomaly compared to women with normal serum glucose. Fewer malformations occur in women who have good glycemic control during the formation of major body structures. Maternal glycemic control reduces the risk of childhood obesity (Cunningham et al., 2014; Simpson, 2011).

The occurrence of maternal and fetal–neonatal complications can be greatly diminished if the mother maintains normal and stable blood glucose levels before and throughout pregnancy. The objective of the team providing treatment is to devise a plan that allows the woman to maintain blood glucose levels as close to normal as possible (see Nursing Care Plan).

***Variations in fetal size.*** Fetal growth is related to maternal vascular integrity. In women without vascular impairment, glucose and oxygen are easily transported to the fetus; if the woman is

## NURSING CARE PLAN

### *Pregnancy and Diabetes Mellitus*

#### Focused Nursing Assessment

Kathy is a 24-year-old primigravida at 9 weeks of gestation. She was diagnosed with type 1 diabetes mellitus 6 years ago. She has been on a daily regimen of insulin and is comfortable with insulin administration and blood glucose monitoring. She is experiencing daily nausea and occasional vomiting. She states that she is concerned because she is not eating as much as before becoming pregnant. She also reveals that she had sometimes "binged" on food before becoming pregnant and didn't always monitor blood glucose as often as directed. She does not see why her blood glucose must be watched so carefully when pregnant.

#### Nursing Diagnosis

Risk for Ineffective Health Maintenance related to deficient knowledge of the effects of pregnancy on diabetes control.

#### Planning

##### *Expected Outcomes*

Kathy will:

1. Describe predicted changes in insulin needs throughout pregnancy.
2. Follow prescribed schedule of blood glucose monitoring, insulin administration, diet, and exercise.
3. Describe the importance of frequent fetal surveillance and follow the prescribed schedule.

#### Interventions and *Rationales*

1. *Motivation and readiness to learn are essential for permanent learning to occur. Kathy will learn only if she sees the value of the information. To accomplish this result, the nurse should reduce barriers to Kathy's learning.* Possible nursing actions are to:
   a. Allow Kathy to express emotions and concerns before teaching.
   b. Examine with Kathy her beliefs and past experiences related to diabetes.
   c. Assess Kathy's readiness to learn based on interest, attention, and participation in scheduled learning sessions.
2. Instruct Kathy about the predicted changes in diabetes management during pregnancy.
   *Understanding how insulin needs change throughout pregnancy, labor, and the postpartum period increases the likelihood that Kathy will follow the recommended regimen:*
   a. Explain the importance of blood glucose testing; she will need less insulin because of the nausea and vomiting occurring in the first trimester.
   b. Emphasize that she will probably need more insulin as the second and third trimesters progress because of the effects of the placental hormones. Insulin requirements usually fall immediately after birth but will achieve longer-term levels after the immediate postbirth period.
   c. Describe the importance of following the prescribed diet and exercise regimen to maintain normal blood glucose levels.
3. Inform Kathy about specific fetal surveillance techniques often recommended (serial nonstress tests, biophysical profiles). Explain the importance of the tests because *some frequently-ordered tests are time-consuming and expensive. Kathy is more likely to comply if she understands the importance of monitoring her baby's condition at frequent intervals.*
4. Allow time for Kathy to focus on her feelings and concerns at each teaching session; offer praise and encouragement for her adherence to the prescribed regimen.
   *Motivation to comply with the regimen is strengthened by praise and the awareness that her feelings are important.*
5. Explain in simple, positive terms the advantages to the fetus of maintaining a normal maternal blood glucose level. Advantages include an optimal pattern of growth, the increased likelihood that the baby will be born at or near term, and have fewer prematurity associated complications.
   *Understanding that her baby benefits when maternal glucose levels are normal reduces anxiety and increases the likelihood that Kathy will comply with recommended treatment that may frequently change.*
6. Review the recommended plan for diet and exercise during pregnancy, and determine whether Kathy knows the importance of these factors in her care.
   *Maintaining a normal blood glucose depends on coordinating the amount of food, insulin, and exercise. If any of these factors is altered, the others must also be altered to prevent hypoglycemia or hyperglycemia.*

#### Evaluation

Kathy verbalizes her understanding of the changing insulin needs during pregnancy and the importance of glucose monitoring. She states that she feels in better control of the diabetes and plans to comply with the recommended schedule of fetal surveillance, diet, and exercise.

#### Focused Assessment

At 32 weeks of gestation, Kathy's blood glucose is consistently above the desired level, and twice-weekly nonstress tests and fetal ultrasounds for biophysical profiles are prescribed. The tests are reactive, and ultrasounds show appropriate fetal growth, movements, and amniotic fluid quantities, indicating no fetal compromise. However, Kathy verbalizes anxiety about the condition of the fetus and asks when it will be safe for the baby to be born.

#### Nursing Diagnosis

Anxiety related to perceived threat to the health of the fetus, including the expected gestation when born.

#### Planning

##### *Expected Outcomes*

Kathy will:

1. Relate her perception of the condition of the fetus and the significance of the fetal surveillance as the tests are performed.
2. Describe her concerns about the timing of the delivery at the conclusion of the nonstress test and fetal ultrasound.

#### Interventions and *Rationales*

1. Ask Kathy to describe her concern about the fetus and to clarify her feelings.
   *Her concerns must be identified and clarified so that misconceptions do not occur in nurse-patient communication.*
2. Explain that it is a reassuring sign that the fetus is not in immediate jeopardy if the nonstress test is reactive and accelerates whenever the baby moves. Frequency of fetal surveillance will be changed if a need is identified.
   *Reassurance that the tests will usually detect early signs of a problem may reduce Kathy's anxiety about her baby's well-being.*
3. Ask Kathy how she feels about her labor and delivery. Determine whether she is taking childbirth education classes and whether she has selected her coach.
   *It is normal for women to become concerned about the birth process and how they will cope with labor during the last few weeks of pregnancy. Medical professionals should not neglect the need for normal pregnancy care for women with high-risk pregnancies.*
4. Assist Kathy in investigating a childbirth education class if she has not done so previously, and suggest that she and her coach begin classes.
   *Knowledge learned at childbirth classes may reduce anxiety about the birth processes. Birth units usually have referral locations for classes.*
5. Acknowledge that the prospect of labor and delivery causes many women some anxiety, even when the condition of the infant is not at risk.
   *Kathy's understanding that her feelings are common to most women may provide some relief from anxiety.*

#### Evaluation

Kathy says she is reassured by explanations regarding the reactive nonstress test and the ultrasound photos of her baby. However, she is concerned about how she will do in labor. She plans to attend a childbirth education class with her sister as the coach.

##### *Additional Nursing Diagnoses to Consider*

Readiness for Enhanced Family Coping
Risk for Injury

hyperglycemic, so is the fetus. Although maternal insulin does not cross the placental barrier, the fetus produces insulin by the 10th week of gestation. Fetal macrosomia (large fetal size, ≥4000 g at term) results when elevated levels of blood glucose stimulate excessive production of fetal insulin, which acts as a powerful growth hormone.

Conversely, placental perfusion can decrease with vascular impairment. Vascular impairment can be caused by complications of the diabetes or by vasoconstriction that occurs in preeclampsia, a common added complication for all women with diabetes. With impaired placental perfusion, the supply of glucose as well as oxygen decreases. If placental perfusion is impaired for a prolonged period, the infant is likely to experience fetal growth restriction (FGR).

### Neonatal Effects

The four major complications of maternal diabetes for the newborn are hypoglycemia, hypocalcemia, hyperbilirubinemia, and respiratory distress syndrome. All can be minimized by stabilizing and maintaining maternal glucose levels near normal, particularly in the last weeks of pregnancy and during labor.

Newborns of a woman with poorly controlled diabetes and no vascular impairment are more likely to be very large, often weighing well over 4500 g (9 lb, 15 oz). Approximately 30% of these newborns have an enlarged heart (cardiomegaly), and 5% to 10% require care for congestive heart failure.

*Hypoglycemia.* The neonate is at higher risk for hypoglycemia because fetal insulin production was accelerated during pregnancy to metabolize excessive glucose received from the expectant mother. The constant stimulation of hyperglycemia leads to hyperplasia and hypertrophy of the islets of Langerhans in the pancreas. At birth, when the maternal glucose supply is withdrawn, the level of neonatal insulin exceeds the available glucose, and hypoglycemia develops rapidly.

*Hypocalcemia.* Hypocalcemia, defined as a calcium concentration of less than 7 mg/dL, usually occurs within 72 hours of birth. The risk for hypocalcemia is less if the maternal glucose level is controlled.

*Hyperbilirubinemia.* The fetus who experiences recurrent hypoxia caused by maternal vascular impairment compensates by producing additional erythrocytes to carry oxygen supplied by the mother, resulting in polycythemia. After birth, the excess erythrocytes are broken down, releasing large amounts of bilirubin into the neonate's circulation.

*Respiratory distress syndrome.* Fetal hyperinsulinemia retards cortisol production, which is necessary for synthesis of surfactant, thereby increasing the risk of respiratory distress syndrome in the newborn. Reduced lung fluid clearance and delayed thinning of lung connective tissue may also play a part, although other authorities believe that gestational age is the primary determinant of whether an infant will have respiratory distress syndrome (Cunningham et al., 2014). (See Chapter 29 for additional information about neonatal complications.)

### Maternal Assessment

The initial prenatal assessment for the woman with preexisting diabetes includes a history, physical examination, and laboratory tests.

*History.* A detailed history should include the onset and management of the diabetic condition. How long has the woman had the disease? How does she maintain normal blood glucose levels? Can she monitor her blood glucose level and self-administer insulin? The degree of glycemic control before pregnancy is of particular interest. Effective management depends on the woman's adherence to a plan of care. Therefore, her knowledge of how diabetes and pregnancy interact must be determined. Her support person's knowledge also must be assessed, and specific learning needs should be identified. In addition, the woman's emotional status should be assessed to determine how well she is coping with pregnancy superimposed on preexisting diabetes.

All women with diabetes should be seen by a qualified nurse educator for an individualized assessment to ensure that they can monitor blood glucose accurately. Accurate readings depend on performing the test correctly and as often as recommended by the healthcare team. Most pregnant women who need a hypoglycemic agent take insulin rather than an oral agent, although an occasional woman refuses to take injectable medication for blood glucose control. The nurse, who is often a diabetes educator, must confirm the woman's skill in mixing and administering insulin, using a sliding scale for added insulin, or using an insulin pump if needed. A woman who has taken insulin before pregnancy often needs more information about why very tight control is needed during pregnancy and why the need for progressively more insulin is common in the later weeks of pregnancy.

*Physical examination.* In addition to routine prenatal examination (see Chapter 13), specific efforts should be made to assess the effects of diabetes. A baseline electrocardiogram (ECG) determines cardiovascular status. Evaluation for retinopathy should be performed, with referral to an ophthalmologist if necessary. The woman's weight and blood pressure must be monitored carefully because of the increased risk for the development of preeclampsia. The fundal height should be measured, noting any abnormal increase in size that could indicate macrosomia or hydramnios. Reduced growth in fundal height suggests FGR associated with maternal vascular impairment. Ultrasonography is indicated to determine true gestational age and to identify any abnormal fetal growth or amount of fluid (Cunningham et al., 2014).

*Laboratory tests.* In addition to routine prenatal laboratory examinations, baseline renal function should be assessed using a 24-hour urine collection for total protein excretion and creatinine clearance. A random midstream urine sample should be checked at each prenatal visit for possible urinary tract infections and for the presence of protein, glucose, and ketones. Thyroid function tests should be performed because of the risk for coexisting thyroid disease (Cunningham et al., 2014).

Glycemic control should be evaluated on the basis of *glycosylated hemoglobin,* or $HbA_{1c}$. Prolonged hyperglycemia causes some of the hemoglobin in erythrocytes to remain saturated with glucose for the life of the red blood cell. Unlike tests that reflect the amount of glucose in the plasma at that moment, the $HbA_{1c}$ assay is not affected by recent intake or restriction of food.

### Fetal Surveillance

Because of greater risk for congenital anomalies or fetal death, surveillance should begin early for women with preexisting diabetes. Testing for anomalies includes multiple marker screening to identify possible neural tube or other open defects and chromosome abnormalities. Testing also includes ultrasonography and fetal echocardiography at 20 to 22 weeks to determine the integrity of the fetal body and cardiac structure (Cunningham et al., 2014).

During the third trimester, the care goal is to identify markers that suggest a worsening intrauterine environment with a higher probability of fetal death. Surveillance may include maternal perception of fetal movement, biophysical profiles, and nonstress or contraction stress tests. Ultrasound is also used to document fetal growth rates and estimate amniotic fluid volume. Doppler velocimetry can be used to detect vascular complications and hypertension. See Chapter 15 for a description of fetal surveillance methods.

### Therapeutic Management

The goals of therapeutic management for a pregnant woman with diabetes are to (1) normalize and maintain maternal blood glucose levels as near normal as possible, (2) increase the likelihood that the baby will be born healthy, and (3) avoid accelerated impairment of maternal blood vessels and other major organs. Pregnant women with diabetes are cared for by a team that can include a diabetologist, who assists in regulation of maternal blood glucose; an obstetrician, who monitors the mother and fetus and determines the optimal time for birth; a registered dietitian (RD) or registered dietary technician (DTR), who provides a balanced meal plan that considers the woman's individual needs; and a diabetes educator, often a nurse, who provides ongoing education and support as the therapy changes during pregnancy. The team is completed by a neonatologist, who will care for the newborn, and the family physician and the pediatrician, who will provide ongoing care for the infant and mother after birth. A maternal–fetal medicine specialist and support staff may be added if multiple fetal evaluation procedures are needed.

*Preconception care.* Ideally, care should begin before conception. Both prospective parents should participate in care sessions to learn more about the following issues if diabetes exists before pregnancy:

- Establishing the optimal time to undertake pregnancy (based on maintenance of normal maternal blood glucose levels) to reduce the risk for major fetal malformations.
- Determining whether diabetes complications are affecting other organ systems.
- Determining the degree of glycemic control based on patient records or laboratory studies.
- Instructing a woman about the use of a glucometer to monitor blood glucose levels and having the woman demonstrate a correct technique.
- Taking a daily prenatal vitamin that contains 400 μg (0.4 mg) of folic acid. A dose of 4 mg per day is recommended for the woman who has had a previous child with a neural tube defect.

*Diet.* Diet recommendations are individualized during a diabetic pregnancy. The average recommended caloric intake for the pregnant diabetic woman of normal weight is 30 kcal/kg/day. Approximately 40% to 45% of the calories should be from carbohydrates, 12% to 20% from protein (approximately 60 g), and up to 40% from fat. Caloric intake should be distributed among three meals and two or more snacks. The bedtime snack should include a complex carbohydrate and protein. Women who are overweight or underweight usually have lower or higher caloric goals (Franz, 2012).

*Self-monitoring of blood glucose (SMBG).* The optimal frequency for SMBG has not yet been established. One common testing regimen requires obtaining fasting and 2-hour postprandial levels. Another includes testing six times per day: a fasting capillary glucose, 1 to 2 hours after breakfast, before and after lunch, before dinner, and at bedtime. One study found that the postprandial levels were most effective at predicting fetal macrosomia and other adverse outcomes (Moore & Catalano, 2009). In addition to regular monitoring, the woman should also perform a glucose test whenever she experiences symptoms of hypoglycemia. She should record all test results to a log for review by the healthcare provider at each visit. Most glucometers for SMBG have a memory to provide accurate recall of times and glucose levels and to verify accuracy of log book entries.

*Insulin therapy.* Maintaining rigorous control of maternal metabolism during pregnancy requires more frequent doses of insulin than usual. Most treatment regimens rely on three daily injections, with a combination of short-acting (regular) insulin and intermediate-acting (neutral protein Hagedorn [NPH]) insulin given before breakfast, regular insulin before dinner, and NPH insulin at bedtime. Lispro and aspart (Humalog and NovoLog, respectively) insulins act rapidly and should be injected just before a meal. The rapid-acting insulins have been shown to control postprandial hyperglycemia with less between-meal hypoglycemia. Because placental hormones cause insulin needs to change throughout pregnancy, adjustment of insulin coverage will be needed as pregnancy progresses.

First trimester. Insulin needs generally decline during the first trimester because the secretion of placental hormones that are antagonistic to insulin remains low during this time. The woman may also experience nausea, vomiting, and anorexia, resulting in reduced food intake, and thus, may need less insulin. Moreover, the fetus receives its share of glucose, which reduces maternal plasma glucose levels and decreases the need for maternal insulin.

Second and third trimesters. Insulin needs increase markedly during the second and third trimesters, when placental hormones reach their peak and cause greater maternal resistance to the effects of insulin. The nausea of early pregnancy usually resolves, and the woman needs additional calories per day to meet the increased metabolic demands of pregnancy.

During labor. Maintenance of tight maternal glucose control during birth is desirable to reduce neonatal hypoglycemia. Continuous infusion of a regular insulin solution combined with a separate intravenous solution containing glucose, such as 5% dextrose in Ringer's lactate, allows titration to maintain blood glucose levels between 80 and 110 mg/dL. The insulin infusion rate is raised, lowered, or discontinued to maintain euglycemia based on hourly capillary blood glucose levels. If blood glucose levels remain too high, the insulin infusion is adjusted, and the primary infusion is changed to one without glucose.

Women with type 2 or GDM that has been controlled by diet during pregnancy can usually maintain normal glucose levels during labor if intravenous solutions containing glucose are avoided (Cunningham et al., 2014).

Postpartum. Insulin needs should fall rapidly after delivery of the placenta and the abrupt cessation of placental hormones. However, blood glucose levels should be monitored at least four times daily so that the insulin dose can be adjusted to meet individual needs. However, up to one third of women who had GDM will have diabetes or impaired glucose metabolism that requires either lifestyle modifications or medication. Postpartum screening at 6 to 12 weeks is recommended to identify long-term health-promotion needs for these women. Women who had GDM have a 35% to 60% chance of developing diabetes during the 10 to 20 years following birth.

*Timing of delivery.* If possible, the pregnancy should be allowed to progress to 39 weeks or later to allow fetal lungs to mature, reducing the risk for neonatal respiratory distress syndrome. With evidence of fetal compromise, such as nonreassuring biophysical profile or reduced amniotic fluid, prompt delivery may be needed. Amniocentesis is usually done if delivery is considered for non-emergency reasons before completion of 38 weeks because fetal lung maturation can be slower than in nondiabetic pregnancies.

## Gestational Diabetes Mellitus

### Risk Factors

GDM is a carbohydrate intolerance of variable severity that develops or is first recognized during pregnancy. Some women diagnosed with GDM may actually have unrecognized type 2 diabetes. Factors associated with a higher risk for GDM are similar to those for type 2 diabetes (ACOG, 2015; ADA, 2015).

- Overweight (body mass index [BMI] 25 to 25.9 kg/m$^2$), obese (BMI 30 to 39.9 kg/m$^2$), or morbidly obese (BMI ≥40 kg/m$^2$)
- Maternal age older than 25 years
- Previous birth outcome often associated with GDM (neonatal macrosomia, maternal hypertension, infant with unexplained congenital anomalies, previous fetal death)
- GDM in previous pregnancy
- History of abnormal glucose tolerance
- History of diabetes in a close (first-degree) relative
- Member of a high-risk ethnic group (Hispanic, African, Native American, South or East Asian, or Pacific Islands ancestry)

### Identifying Gestational Diabetes Mellitus

All pregnant women should be screened by identification of a history or risk factors that are consistent with GDM or by blood glucose testing. A common prenatal screening test is the glucose challenge test (GCT) administered between 24 and 28 weeks. An oral glucose tolerance test may be used as the initial test if a woman is at high risk for GDM but is more likely to be used as a diagnostic test when abnormally high GCT results occur. Women with a fasting glucose level greater than 126 mg/dL or a nonfasting level of more than 200 mg/dL meet the criteria for GDM, and no added testing is needed (ACOG, 2015; ADA, 2015; Cunningham et al., 2014).

***Glucose challenge test.*** Fasting is not necessary for a GCT, and the woman is not required to follow any pretest dietary instructions. The woman should ingest 50 g of oral glucose solution; 1 hour later, a blood sample is taken. If the blood glucose concentration is 140 mg/dL or greater, a 3-hour oral glucose tolerance test (OGTT) is recommended. Some practitioners use a lower cutoff of 130 or 135 mg/dL to identify more women at risk (ACOG, 2015; ADA, 2015; Cunningham et al., 2014).

***Oral glucose tolerance test.*** The OGTT is the gold standard for diagnosing diabetes, but this test is more complicated. After the fasting plasma glucose level is determined, the woman should ingest 100 g of oral glucose solution. Plasma glucose levels are then determined at 1, 2, and 3 hours. GDM is the diagnosis if the fasting blood glucose level is abnormal or if two or more of the following values occur on the OGTT (Berggren et al., 2011).

- Fasting, greater than 95 mg/dL
- 1 hour, greater than 180 mg/dL
- 2 hours, greater than 155 mg/dL
- 3 hours, greater than 140 mg/dL

### Maternal, Fetal, and Neonatal Effects

With a few important exceptions, the effects of GDM are similar to those associated with preexisting type 2 diabetes. Because GDM develops after the first trimester, which is the critical period for major fetal organ development (organogenesis), it is not associated with an increased incidence of major congenital abnormalities. Nevertheless, poorly controlled GDM, with maternal hyperglycemia during the third trimester, is associated with fetal macrosomia and neonatal hypoglycemia. Hypocalcemia, hyperbilirubinemia, and respiratory distress also can occur. Table 26.1 summarizes the maternal, fetal, and neonatal effects of diabetes mellitus and their probable causes.

**TABLE 26.1 Major Effects of Diabetes Mellitus on Pregnancy**

| Effect | Probable Cause |
|---|---|
| **Increased Maternal Risks** | |
| Hypertension; preeclampsia | Unknown but increased even without renal or vascular impairment |
| Urinary tract infections | Increased bacterial growth in nutrient-rich urine |
| Ketoacidosis (risk for mother and fetus) | Uncontrolled hyperglycemia or infection; most common in women with type 1 diabetes |
| Labor dystocia; cesarean birth; uterine atony with hemorrhage after birth | Hydramnios secondary to fetal osmotic diuresis caused by hyperglycemia; uterus is overstretched |
| Birth injury to maternal tissues (hematoma, lacerations) | Fetal macrosomia causing difficult birth |
| **Increased Fetal and Neonatal Risks** | |
| Congenital anomalies | Maternal hyperglycemia during organ formation in first trimester |
| Perinatal death | Poor placental perfusion because of maternal vascular impairment, primarily in woman with type 1 diabetes |
| Macrosomia (>4000 g) | Fetal hyperglycemia stimulating production of insulin to metabolize carbohydrates; excess nutrients transported to fetus |
| Intrauterine fetal growth restriction | Maternal vascular impairment |
| Preterm labor; premature rupture of membranes; preterm birth | Overdistention of uterus caused by hydramnios and large fetal size at preterm gestation |
| Birth injury | Large fetal size; shoulder dystocia or other difficult delivery |
| Hypoglycemia | Neonatal hyperinsulinemia after birth when maternal glucose is no longer available but newborn insulin production remains high |
| Polycythemia | Fetal hypoxemia stimulating erythrocyte production |
| Hyperbilirubinemia | Breakdown of excessive red blood cells after birth |
| Hypocalcemia | Transfer of calcium abruptly stopped at birth; reduced fetal parathyroid function |
| Respiratory distress syndrome | Delayed maturation of fetal lungs; inadequate production of pulmonary surfactant; slowed absorption of fetal lung fluid |

### Therapeutic Management

***Diet.*** Ideally, an RD, RDT, or diabetes educator determines the dietary needs of the woman with GDM. The diet should provide the calories and nutrients needed for maternal and fetal health, result in euglycemia, avoid ketosis, and promote appropriate weight gain. Calories should be distributed similarly to that for preexisting diabetes. Simple sugars found in concentrated sweets should be eliminated from the diet. The obese woman can be prescribed a diet with a smaller percentage of carbohydrates than the woman of normal weight. Carbohydrates should be adequate to prevent ketosis in all women. Calories should be divided between three meals and at least three snacks (ACOG, 2015; Franz, 2012).

***Exercise.*** Exercise plays a significant role in managing blood glucose levels in women who develop GDM and in women with type 2 diabetes who become pregnant. The exercise regimen should be recommended by a physician who takes into account each woman's risk factors and risks to the fetus. Regular exercise improves glucose metabolism, offers cardiorespiratory benefits, and aids in weight control.

***Glucose level monitoring.*** As in care of the woman with preexisting diabetes, SMBG levels help guide diet and insulin therapy (see p. 555). A common method is measurement of fasting glucose (no food for the previous 4 hours) and 2-hour postprandial blood glucose levels (2 hours after each meal). If blood glucose levels repeatedly exceed 95 mg/dL or postprandial values exceed 120 mg/dL, insulin administration is started. Additional checks for glucose levels may be performed if needed.

***Fetal surveillance.*** Antepartum surveillance to identify fetal compromise (see Chapter 15) may begin as early as 28 weeks of gestation if the woman has poor glycemic control or by 34 weeks in lower-risk women with GDM. Surveillance testing may include maternal "kick counts," ultrasound assessment of fetal growth and amniotic fluid volume, biophysical profile, nonstress or contraction stress tests, or amniocentesis for fetal lung maturity.

### Nursing Considerations

The care of a pregnant woman with diabetes mellitus focuses primarily on helping her maintain normal blood glucose levels and an optimum fetal condition. Some women respond calmly to the intense medical supervision. Other women respond with anxiety, fear, denial, or anger and may feel unable to control the diabetes to the degree expected by the healthcare team. Still others fear for their own or their baby's health, especially when the diagnosis is a new one.

*Increasing effective communication.* Nurses must ask specifically about the feelings and concerns the woman and her family have about the pregnancy to help the woman avoid unnecessary guilt, anxiety, or frustration, and thus, promote her active participation in her plan of care.

Broad opening questions, such as "What are your major concerns?" and "How do you feel about the plan of care?" help identify the woman's greatest concerns. These should be followed by more specific questions, such as "How do you feel about the fetal testing?" and "What would you like to change about your diet?"

The nurse must be an active listener and allow time for the woman and her family to express concerns and feelings. The nurse must convey acceptance of feelings that are expressed, whether they are negative or positive. Sharing emotions may help promote positive feelings about her ability to participate successfully in her plan of care.

*Providing opportunities for control.* Providing ways for the woman to make decisions increases her sense of control. For example, she can select foods from the exchange list that provide the necessary nutrients but still give choices. A dietitian should be consulted if the list does not include food the woman likes or that suits her ethnic or cultural preferences. The woman should be assisted to develop a regular schedule of exercise and sleep that helps maintain good blood glucose control. Nurses should allow as much flexibility as possible when scheduling stressful events such as fetal monitoring tests and amniocentesis.

*Providing normal pregnancy care.* A woman with diabetes also needs to know about the normal aspects of pregnancy. The nurse caring for a woman with diabetes should provide education and counseling regarding normal pregnancy changes and discomforts.

## NURSING CARE

### The Pregnant Woman With Diabetes Mellitus

#### Assessment

Determine how well the woman understands the prescribed management and how she plans to carry out the recommended regimen. She may be newly diagnosed, with no experience in the necessary skills and procedures, or she may be skilled in monitoring glucose levels and administering insulin but has no knowledge of the effects of diabetes on pregnancy or the effects of pregnancy on diabetes management. If she has used an oral hypoglycemic to manage her glucose, she may be unfamiliar with the use of insulin for that purpose.

To determine whether her techniques are accurate, ask the pregnant woman to demonstrate how she monitors her blood glucose level and observe how she mixes and injects insulin. Verify that she and her family are aware of the need to select appropriate sites and injection techniques.

Although diet is often prescribed individually, it is necessary to assess how well the family understands the diet. Determine whether there are special problems with food preferences or the availability of recommended foods. Diet recommendations include a target number of calories, plus targets for grams of carbohydrate, protein, and fat to meet calorie needs. Any of several methods to count and exchange foods can be used. One method uses exchange lists, in which the listed foods all have about the same grams of carbohydrate, protein, and fat. Thus, one food from the list can be substituted, or exchanged, for another in the same list. Another method uses carbohydrate counting, in which foods on the starch, fruit, or milk list supply approximately 15 g of carbohydrate, or one carbohydrate choice. The diet plan would prescribe the number of carbohydrate choices for each meal and snack. Insulin is often adjusted according to the carbohydrate count for each meal or snack.

Identify the woman's knowledge of potential complications, such as hypoglycemia and hyperglycemia, so that she and her family can be provided with pertinent information to avoid and treat it.

Explain why greater fetal surveillance is often ordered. Some women are highly motivated to continue the treatment regimen when test results indicate the fetus is thriving. Other women find the frequent testing stressful and inconvenient.

#### Nursing Diagnosis and Planning

One of the most common nursing diagnoses is:

- Risk for or Actual Ineffective Health Maintenance related to knowledge deficit of specific measures to: maintain normal blood glucose levels; signs, symptoms, and management of hypoglycemia and hyperglycemia; and recommended fetal surveillance procedures.

*Expected outcomes*

- Demonstrate competence in SMBG and administration of insulin before home management is initiated.
- Describe a plan for meeting dietary recommendations that fits family lifestyle and food preferences.
- Identify signs and symptoms of hypoglycemia and hyperglycemia and the management required for each.
- Verbalize knowledge of fetal surveillance procedures and keep scheduled appointments for testing.

#### Interventions

Although management of diabetes mellitus during pregnancy is a team effort, a nursing responsibility is to provide accurate information about the recommended therapeutic regimen and to offer consistent support for the woman's efforts to comply with the recommendations. It may be necessary to demonstrate specific skills that the woman and her support person must master and to review and reinforce information that comes from other members of the healthcare team.

*Teaching self-care skills.* Demonstration and return demonstration are effective ways to teach and evaluate psychomotor skills. The woman (and her family) must learn to use a meter and obtain a small sample of blood to determine glucose levels and to correctly mix and inject insulin. Both procedures are invasive and cause mild discomfort, which may make the woman reluctant to start. Mixing insulins accurately or using a sliding scale may be intimidating at first. Using food exchanges is often unfamiliar to the woman who is newly diagnosed, but it is critical to glucose control. Acknowledge these feelings before teaching begins. As needed, reinforce skills taught. Also give positive reinforcement when the woman demonstrates these skills successfully.

**Self-monitoring of blood glucose.** Spring-loaded lancets make home blood-glucose–monitoring easier. The side of the fingertip is less sensitive than the pad and may be less uncomfortable. Teach her to cleanse the area with warm water before obtaining a sample to prevent infection. The first drop of blood is wiped away, and the second drop is used to place blood on the meter's strip. Each home monitoring kit contains specific instructions for use of the meter. Teach her how to record glucose values in a handwritten log. Teach her that glucometers have a memory option for retrieval of previous glucose readings.

**Insulin administration.** The woman is often prescribed a combination of short- and intermediate-acting insulins. Teach the woman the difference in onset, peak, and duration of action of each type of insulin. She also needs to learn how to mix the two insulins in the same syringe. If she will use a sliding scale to keep glucose levels close to normal, she will need teaching about how to determine the additional dose of insulin if she has never used sliding scale insulin administration.

Insulin is administered subcutaneously. Common sites include the upper thighs, abdomen, and upper arms. Because the pregnant woman is injecting insulin frequently, emphasize these precautions:

- To prevent hypoglycemia, a meal should be taken 30 minutes after regular insulin is injected. Because of its 10-minute onset of action, lispro (Humalog) insulin is injected just before eating.
- Unless the woman is very thin in the injection site, insulin should be injected with the short needle inserted at a 90-degree angle so that the tip of the needle reaches the fatty tissue layer.
- The needle should be inserted quickly to minimize discomfort.
- The tissue pinch, if used, is released after inserting the needle and before injecting insulin because pressure from the pinch can promote insulin leakage from the subcutaneous tissue.
- Aspirating when injecting into subcutaneous tissue is not necessary.
- Insulin is injected slowly (over 2 to 4 seconds) to allow tissue expansion and minimize pressure, which can cause insulin leakage.
- The needle is withdrawn quickly to minimize the formation of a track, which might permit insulin to leak out.

Emphasize the importance of administering the correct dosage at the correct time. Teach the woman and her family the function of insulin and the importance of following the directions of her physician in regard to coordinating meals with the administration of insulin.

**Continuous subcutaneous insulin infusion.** Many women who have preexisting diabetes use continuous subcutaneous insulin infusion and wish to continue this method during pregnancy. The programmable insulin infusion pump allows tailoring of insulin administration to the woman's individual lifestyle. Prompt emergency counseling and assistance must be available 24/7 to deal with unexpected problems such as pump malfunction.

***Teaching dietary management.*** A dietitian prescribes the recommended diet, and the nurse must be aware of the general requirements and be sensitive to the expectant mother's dietary habits and preferences. Often, Reviewing and clarifying how exchange lists are used to plan meals and snacks is often needed. Encourage the woman to avoid simple sugars (candy, cake, cookies, juice), which raise the blood glucose levels quickly but can result in wide swings between high and low levels.

It may be necessary to help the woman select foods high in nutrients but low in cost or to meet cultural or religious constraints. Animal protein is especially expensive, and alternative sources of protein (beans, peas, corn, grains) can be substituted to meet some of the protein needs as well as provide high-quality carbohydrate and fiber.

***Recognizing and correcting hypoglycemia and hyperglycemia.*** Every woman and her family must be aware of the signs and symptoms that indicate abnormal blood glucose levels. If they are not identified and corrected quickly, hypoglycemia and hyperglycemia pose a threat to mother and fetus.

**Hypoglycemia.** Treat hypoglycemia at once to prevent damage to the brain, which depends on glucose. The woman should take 15 g of carbohydrate if she can swallow. Retest after 15 minutes. If the level is less than 70 mg/dL, repeat carbohydrate intake and retest every 15 minutes until the blood glucose level returns to normal (Franz, 2012). Examples of foods containing 15 g of carbohydrate include:

- Three glucose tablets, depending on their carbohydrate content; oral glucose gel
- 4 to 6 ounces fruit juice or regular soft drink
- Six saltine crackers
- 1 tablespoon of syrup or honey

Family members should read instructions on commercial glucose preparations. Teach family members to inject glucagon if the woman cannot retain oral glucose or food and to notify the physician at once. Intravenous glucose will be given if the woman is hospitalized. If untreated, hypoglycemia can progress to seizures and death.

To prevent episodes of hypoglycemia, instruct the woman to have meals at a fixed time each day and to plan snacks at the recommended times. Suggest that she carry glucose tablets or dry crackers whenever possible.

## SAFETY ALERT

### *Signs and Symptoms of Maternal Hypoglycemia*

- Shakiness (tremors)
- Sweating
- Pallor; cold, clammy skin
- Disorientation, irritability
- Headache
- Hunger
- Blurred vision

**Hyperglycemia.** Because infection is the most common cause of hyperglycemia in a woman with preexisting diabetes, pregnant women must be instructed to notify the physician whenever they have an infection of any type.

Untreated hyperglycemia can lead to ketoacidosis, coma, and maternal and fetal death. If signs and symptoms occur, notify the physician at once so that treatment can be initiated for hyperglycemia and any underlying infection. Hospitalization is necessary for monitoring blood glucose levels and intravenous administration of insulin and antibiotics if needed.

## SAFETY ALERT

### *Signs and Symptoms of Maternal Hyperglycemia*

- Fatigue
- Flushed, hot skin
- Dry mouth, excessive thirst
- Frequent urination
- Rapid, deep respirations; odor of acetone on the breath
- Drowsiness, headache
- Depressed reflexes

***Explaining procedures, tests, and plan of care.*** Explain the schedule and the reasons for frequent checkups and tests. Encourage the woman and her family to ask questions if any part of the schedule is confusing. Pregnant women and their families need to know why frequent antepartum surveillance tests are necessary. They should know that their diabetic care will take more time and effort than it did before pregnancy but that this care greatly improves the likelihood that they will have healthy infants.

### Evaluation

After the procedures, tests, and plan of care have been explained, the family should be evaluated.

- Can the woman and one support person demonstrate competence in blood glucose monitoring and administration of insulin?
- Can the woman describe a plan for meeting individual dietary requirements?
- Can the woman and one support person list the signs and symptoms of hypoglycemia and hyperglycemia and describe their initial management?
- Can the woman verbalize knowledge of the reason for fetal surveillance procedures and keep appointments for tests?

## CARDIAC DISEASE

Cardiovascular function changes during pregnancy to meet additional maternal metabolic demands and the needs of the fetus. Plasma volume, venous return, and cardiac output all increase. Heart rate and stroke volume, the two components of cardiac output, increase during pregnancy. The heart rate gradually rises above baseline during the third trimester, but an increase in stroke volume is primarily responsible for the overall rise in cardiac output during early pregnancy. For additional information about cardiac disease and the woman who is not pregnant, see Chapter 32.

A normal heart adapts to the changes so that the woman tolerates pregnancy and birth without difficulty. However, with the underlying heart disease, the changes can impose an additional burden on an already compromised heart, and cardiac decompensation and **congestive heart failure** (failure of heart to maintain adequate circulation) can result.

**SAFETY ALERT**

***Signs and Symptoms of Congestive Heart Failure***

- Cough (frequent, productive, hemoptysis)
- Progressive dyspnea with exertion
- Orthopnea
- Pitting edema of legs and feet or generalized edema of face, hands, or sacral area
- Heart palpitations
- Progressive fatigue or syncope with exertion
- Moist rales in lower lobes, indicating pulmonary edema

### Incidence and Classification

Successful treatment of congenital cardiac anomalies or mitral stenosis resulting from rheumatic heart disease now allows many girls to reach childbearing age and bear children. Rheumatic heart disease, a complication of streptococcal infection, is not common in the United States but may be found in recent immigrants. The growing incidence of obesity in the general population may result in unexpected cardiovascular complications during pregnancy such as myocardial infarction. Congestive heart failure may be secondary to underlying heart disease or damage or may occur secondary to treatment for other conditions.

### Rheumatic Heart Disease

Rheumatic heart disease is a complication that sometimes follows a streptococcal pharyngitis infection (strep throat). Even one bout of rheumatic fever can cause scarring of the heart valves, resulting in stenosis (narrowing) of the openings between the chambers of the heart. Early diagnosis and treatment of the streptococcal infection has resulted in a near-eradication of rheumatic fever in North America and Europe.

The mitral valve is the most common site of stenosis. Mitral stenosis obstructs free flow of blood from the left atrium to the left ventricle. The left atrium becomes dilated. As a result, pressure in the left atrium, the pulmonary veins, and pulmonary capillaries is chronically elevated. This elevation can lead to pulmonary hypertension, pulmonary edema, or congestive heart failure. The first warnings of heart failure include persistent rales at the base of the lungs, dyspnea on exertion, cough, and hemoptysis. Progressive edema and tachycardia are additional signs of heart failure.

### Congenital Heart Disease

Congenital heart defects can be grouped into those that cause a left-to-right shunt and those that result in a right-to-left shunt. Defects that produce left-to-right shunting include atrial and ventricular septal defects and patent ductus arteriosus (PDA). Right-to-left shunting occurs with a cyanotic heart defect, such as tetralogy of Fallot. However, right-to-left shunting can also occur through a septal defect or a PDA when pulmonary vascular resistance exceeds peripheral vascular resistance, leading to pulmonary hypertension (Eisenmenger syndrome).

The risk to the fetus varies with the severity of disease in the mother. The risk for a congenital heart defect in the fetus is also higher and varies with the number of affected relatives. See Chapter 46 for information about congenital heart defects in children.

#### *Left-to-right shunt*

**Atrial septal defect.** Atrial septal defect (ASD) is often first discovered in women of childbearing age because symptoms are absent or vague. This defect produces a left-to-right shunt because pressure in the left side of the heart is higher than that in the right side. Pregnancy is well tolerated by women with no complications. Bacterial endocarditis is rare, and prophylactic antibiotics are not required. ASDs are not associated with heart failure; therefore, digitalis, diuretics, and extreme limitation of intravenous infusions are not indicated. However, left-to-right shunting increases the chance of pulmonary hypertension because the additional blood that moves to the right side of the heart is transported to the lungs via the pulmonary artery (Cunningham et al., 2014).

**Ventricular septal defect.** Although ventricular septal defects (VSDs) are more common at birth than ASDs, VSDs are usually detected and corrected before children reach childbearing age. Most women with uncorrected defects who become pregnant are asymptomatic, but occasionally fatigue or symptoms of pulmonary hypertension become evident with the hemodynamic changes of pregnancy.

How pregnancy is tolerated is directly related to the size of the defect. Small defects are unlikely to cause pulmonary hypertension and heart failure. If heart failure or dysrhythmias occur, they are managed as in nonpregnant women. Bacterial endocarditis is common with unrepaired defects, and antibacterial prophylaxis is usual.

**Patent ductus arteriosus.** The communicating shunt between the pulmonary artery and aorta is usually discovered and treated in childhood. If untreated, the physiologic effects are related to size. If

## EVIDENCE-BASED PRACTICE

Despite the fears of breast cancer, coronary heart disease (CHD) remains the greatest killer of American women. Medical advances have improved survival in women age 25 to 64 years with better secondary prevention, revascularization, treatment of initial myocardial infarction (MI), heart failure treatment, and reduction of risk factors (total cholesterol, systolic blood pressure, smoking, and physical inactivity). However, other risk factors are increasing as a group: obesity and the prevalence of diabetes mellitus (DM), leading to greater CHD death rates. Black women have a higher CHD mortality. The author, Cynthia Arslaneum-Engoren, concludes that data suggest modifying lifestyle behaviors can have a favorable effect on reducing future CHD events in women.

Demographic variables include age, race, and low socioeconomic status. Women's risk of dying from CHD rises with age and is the number one risk for women 65 years and older. Although mortality has been higher for the older woman, it has also been rising for younger women age 35 to 44 years. Black women have been most affected overall, with the highest overall mortality rates, out-of-hospital death rates, and highest premature death rates. Compared to white women, they have a 28% higher age-adjusted death rate. Women of all races with a low socioeconomic status are at greater risk for MI, coronary insufficiency, and coronary death.

*Co-morbid* risk factors include hypertension (HTN), DM, hypercholesterinemia and hyperlipidemia, and obesity, and all have a chance for improvement. Hypertension is defined as systolic blood pressure (SBP) ≥140 mm Hg and diastolic blood pressure (DBP) ≥90 mm Hg. Hypertension occurs in approximately 31% of non-Hispanic white women, 31% of Mexican-American women, and 45% of Black women, with 75% of Black women older than 75 years having hypertension. DM now affects 11.5 million women who have the added risk of developing gestational diabetes and glucose intolerance during pregnancy. Glucose intolerance has a 40% to 60% chance of developing into DM within 5 to 10 years of diagnosis. In addition, approximately 55 million women have cholesterol levels ≥200 mg/dL despite treatment goals to bring those levels down.

Lifestyle behaviors can be modified. White women are more likely to smoke than Black or Hispanic women. Lowest rates of smoking are among women with graduate degrees and women age 65 and older. Smoking causes 2 million years potential life lost and costs $32.6 billion yearly in lost productivity. Two guidelines mentioned in the article from American Heart Association and American College of Sports Medicine to modify physical activity are to do 30 minutes of moderate-intensity exercise 5 days a week or 150 minutes per week of vigorous-intensity aerobic physical activity. Physical inactivity and a high–saturated-fat diet are likely to increase obesity (body mass index ≥30 kg/m$^2$).

Sex hormones (estrogen and progesterone) decrease with increasing age and are associated with CHD as women age. Although estrogen and progesterone were replaced in the Women's Health Initiative (WHI) to provide cardiac protection, continuation of the study revealed that these hormones increased CHD significantly, and that arm of the study was discontinued. A secondary analysis of the data from that study found that women who were started on hormone therapy had no increased risk for CHD.

Preeclampsia was identified as an independent risk factor for later CHD in women younger than 66 years in one study that Arslaneum-Engoren used. Another study found that women who had preeclampsia or eclampsia had a twofold higher risk of ischemic heart disease after 11.7 years and are 1.5 times more likely to die 14.5 years after preeclampsia or eclampsia.

Nontraditional risk factors will not be detailed here.

### U.S. Preventive Services Task Force (USPSTF) CHD Screening Recommendations

Arslaneum-Engoren brings many facts together with the specific work for routine screening of CHD, citing the grading system for best screening among women. Task force recommendations include:

- Hypertension: Screen all women age 18 and older to identify a SBP ≥140 mm Hg or DBP ≥90 mm Hg (grade A, high certainty of benefit). The Joint Commission also recommends BP screening every 2 years for women with SBP <120 mm Hg and DBP <80 mm Hg, and annually for women with SBP of 120 to 139 mm Hg or DBP of 80 to 90 mm Hg.
- DM: The task force recommends (grade B, moderate net benefit) that women who have a sustained BP >135/80 mm Hg be screened for DM, but the task force stated insufficient screening for asymptomatic adults with BP <135/80 mm Hg (inconclusive [I]).
- Tobacco use: The task force recommends that all women be screened for tobacco use, and women who use tobacco be provided with tobacco cessation interventions, including pregnancy-tailored counseling (grade A, high certainty of benefit).

The USPSTF does not recommend that low-risk women have routine screening for coronary artery stenosis, electrocardiography, exercise treadmill test, or electron beam computer tomography. There is also insufficient evidence for nontraditional risk factors reviewed in the article.

### Implications for Nursing Practice

A nurse needs to use counseling skills that are based on trust and communication to help a woman alter her risks with protective behaviors such as exercise, lowfat diet, and smoking cessation. A qualitative study by Arslaneum-Engoren found that women associated CHD risk with obese men who smoked and led a stressful life, a misperception of women's risk for the problem. Education strategies should alter a woman's perception of her risk and promote her heart health. Lifestyle behavior change is lifelong, and the nurse must encourage and reinforce patient behaviors so that patients progress toward their goals. Lifestyle changes involving customs, food patterns, and living space as well as a woman's caregiver and family can also affect her cardiac health and incorporation of health recommendations.

Arslaneum-Engoren concludes that preventive screening for women based on demographic characteristics, co-morbid conditions, lifestyle behaviors, and risk factors should be performed routinely based on USPSTF recommendations to reduce their risk for CHD.

Reference: Arslaneum-Engoren, C. (2011). Women's risk factors and screening for coronary heart disease. *Journal of Obstetric, Gynecologic, and Neonatal Nursing, 40*(3), 337–347.

small, this lesion, like septal defects, may be well tolerated during pregnancy unless complicated by pulmonary hypertension. The PDA tends to become infected, so antibiotic prophylaxis is recommended during labor.

***Right-to-left shunt***

**Tetralogy of Fallot.** The primary cause of right-to-left shunting is tetralogy of Fallot, a combination of four defects (VSD, pulmonary valve stenosis, right ventricular hypertrophy, and displacement of the aorta so that it overrides part of the right ventricle). Untreated patients with tetralogy of Fallot have obvious symptoms of heart disease that include (1) cyanosis, (2) clubbing of the fingers, indicating proliferation of capillaries to transport blood to the extremities, and (3) inability to tolerate activity.

Women who have undergone repair often do well during pregnancy. Uncorrected tetralogy of Fallot places a woman at high risk for morbidity or mortality (Cunningham et al., 2014).

**Eisenmenger syndrome.** Eisenmenger syndrome is a left-to-right shunt resulting from an uncorrected VSD, ASD, or PDA. Pulmonary resistance equals or exceeds systemic resistance to blood flow and a shunt reversal develops, resulting in a right-to-left shunt and cyanosis. Operative closure of the shunt should be done before pregnancy. Pregnancy that extends past the first trimester carries a 40% maternal mortality risk, usually from right ventricular failure. If the maternal arterial oxygen saturation ($SaO_2$) is less than 85%, the fetus is likely to die before reaching a viable gestation. Preterm delivery is likely for 85% of fetuses, and their survival is near 90%.

**Mitral valve prolapse.** The leaflets of the mitral valve prolapse into the left atrium during ventricular contraction in mitral valve prolapse (MVP). Most women with MVP are asymptomatic. Some experience dysrhythmias or chest pain, but most women with MVP tolerate pregnancy well. The condition is considered by some to be a significant risk factor for bacterial endocarditis, and some physicians administer prophylactic antibiotics before and during labor and delivery. Beta blockers such as atenolol or metoprolol may be given for chest pain or dysrhythmias. The incidence of MVP among otherwise healthy young women is approximately 1% (Cunningham et al., 2014).

### Peripartum and Postpartum Cardiomyopathy

Cardiomyopathy in the peripartum or postpartum period is a rare condition exclusively associated with pregnancy after exclusion of other causes. Women with the condition have no underlying heart disease, but symptoms of cardiac decompensation appear during the last weeks of pregnancy or from 2 to 20 weeks postpartum. The symptoms are those of congestive heart failure: dyspnea, edema, weakness, chest pain, and heart palpitations. Cardiomyopathy can appear suddenly in a woman who has been healthy. An abrupt downhill course in which the woman can be saved only with cardiac transplantation occurs in approximately 20% of women. Approximately 50% of other women with cardiomyopathy have a partial recovery, with persistent congestive heart failure or other cardiac dysfunction. The remaining women show recovery. Peripartum cardiomyopathy often recurs with subsequent pregnancies, particularly in women who did not have complete recovery of left ventricular function. The woman should be informed of this risk (Cirillo & Cohn, 2015; Cunningham et al., 2014).

Anticoagulation with low-molecular-weight heparin is typical to prevent clot formation during pregnancy when coagulation factors are higher than normal. Other medical therapy includes fluid restriction to reduce pulmonary edema and treatment of congestive heart failure and other pathologies associated with cardiomyopathy.

## Diagnostic Evaluation of Cardiac Disease

Early recognition of underlying heart disease is essential, and careful assessment for specific signs and symptoms of heart disease is part of every preconception or initial prenatal visit. Signs and symptoms include dyspnea, syncope (fainting) with exertion, hemoptysis, paroxysmal nocturnal dyspnea, and chest pain with exertion. Additional signs that confirm the diagnosis are (1) diastolic, presystolic, or continuous heart murmur; (2) cardiac enlargement; (3) a loud, harsh systolic murmur associated with a palpable thrill; or (4) serious dysrhythmias.

The diagnosis of heart disease is made from clinical signs and symptoms and physical examination. It is confirmed by tests such as chest imaging, electrocardiography, and echocardiography.

Once the diagnosis is made, the severity of the disease can be determined by the woman's ability to endure physical activity. A clinical classification based on the effect of exercise on the heart has been developed by the New York Heart Association (Box 26.2).

**BOX 26.2 New York Heart Association Functional Classification of Heart Disease**

- Class I: Uncompromised. No limitation of physical activity. Asymptomatic with ordinary activity.
- Class II: Slightly requiring slight limitation of physical activity. Comfortable at rest, but ordinary physical activity causes fatigue, dyspnea, palpitations, or anginal pain.
- Class III: Marked limitation of physical activity. Comfortable at rest, but less than ordinary activity causes excessive fatigue, palpitation, dyspnea, or anginal pain. Markedly compromised.
- Class IV: Inability to perform any physical activity without discomfort. Symptoms of cardiac insufficiency even at rest. Compromised.

In general, maternal and fetal risks with classes I and II disease are small but are greatly increased with classes III and IV.

## Therapeutic Management

### Class I and Class II Heart Disease

Because demands on the pregnant woman's heart are higher, a woman with heart disease should do the following (Cunningham et al., 2014):

- Limit physical activity so that cardiac demand does not exceed the functional capacity of the heart. The woman should remain free of symptoms of cardiac stress, such as dyspnea, chest pain, or tachycardia.
- Avoid excessive weight gain, which adds to demands on the heart. A diet adequate in protein, calories, and sodium is necessary. A low-sodium diet may be advised to avoid congestive heart failure.
- Prevent anemia, which decreases the oxygen-carrying capacity of the blood and results in a compensatory increase in heart rate that a diseased heart may be unable to tolerate. Most anemia is prevented by administration of iron and folic acid.
- Prevent infection such as upper respiratory infections. Immunizations for influenza and pneumonia are available. Prophylactic antibiotics may be included. Avoid contact with those who may be ill during times when upper respiratory infections are prevalent, such as winter months.
- Undergo careful assessment for the development of congestive heart failure, pulmonary edema, or cardiac dysrhythmias. Characteristics of heart failure may include persistent basilar rales, often accompanied by a cough during the night as the woman tries to sleep, sudden inability to carry out usual activities, dyspnea, hemoptysis, increasing edema, and tachycardia (Cirillo & Cohn, 2015; Cunningham et al., 2014).

### Class III and Class IV Heart Disease

The primary goal of management is to prevent cardiac decompensation and the development of congestive heart failure. Moreover, every effort is also made to protect the fetus from hypoxia and FGR, which can occur if placental perfusion is inadequate. In addition to the precautions listed for classes I and II heart disease, the woman may require bed rest, especially during the last trimester because she has little reserve to tolerate rising metabolic demands. Reduced activity increases the risk for thrombus formation and will require prophylaxis such as elastic compression stockings or a serial or boot compression device. Prophylactic anticoagulation may be needed.

### Drug Therapy

Drug therapy for maternal cardiac disorders can extend from the prenatal period through postpartum. Drugs that were part of a woman's treatment before pregnancy may require a change during pregnancy if the mother tolerates the change. The medical team must consider risks and benefits when treating the pregnant woman with cardiac disease.

***Anticoagulants.*** During pregnancy, clotting factors normally increase and thrombolytic activity decreases. These changes predispose the pregnant woman to thrombus formation. Superimposed cardiac problems such as mitral valve stenosis may require anticoagulant therapy during pregnancy because they add to the tendency to form thrombi. Warfarin (Coumadin) is associated with fetal malformations and should be avoided throughout pregnancy. Subcutaneous heparin, which does not cross the placental barrier, is an effective alternative anticoagulant for most women. Careful monitoring of the partial thromboplastin time, activated partial thromboplastin time, and platelet count is essential to achieve effective, safe anticoagulation. Enoxaparin (Lovenox) can be used instead of heparin because it requires less-frequent monitoring for bleeding complications. Enoxaparin and heparin are not interchangeable. Both are given subcutaneously. Use of enoxaparin should be changed to heparin at 36 weeks of gestation because regional anesthesia is contraindicated within 24 hours of the last enoxaparin dose.

***Antidysrhythmics.*** Use of medications for heart disease during pregnancy must balance benefits to the mother against possible harm to the fetus. Another consideration is that maternal heart failure itself is harmful to the fetus. Digoxin, adenosine, and calcium channel blockers appear to be safe. Beta blockers have been associated with neonatal respiratory depression, sustained bradycardia, and hypoglycemia when administered late in pregnancy or just before delivery but may be needed in selected cases (Cunningham et al., 2014).

***Antiinfectives.*** Antiinfective agents for endocarditis are chosen based on the infecting agent and the woman's individual risk. Dental procedures are considered high risk for blood-borne infections. Gram-positive staphylococcus infections are common in intravenous drug users (IDUs), and the mortality is high. Maternal gonorrhea infection can cause acute, rapidly developing endocarditis. A woman with an increased risk for bacterial endocarditis can receive prophylactic antibiotics at delivery, such as amoxicillin, penicillin, ampicillin, and gentamicin. Ceftriaxone or vancomycin also can be given for acute endocarditis.

***Drugs for heart failure.*** Diuretics may be needed when congestive heart failure is uncontrolled by restriction of activity and sodium intake. Careful monitoring of electrolytes and water balance is necessary to avoid excessively reducing maternal blood volume with resulting adverse effects on the fetus. Experience is greatest with furosemide and thiazide diuretics. FGR has been associated with furosemide; neonatal jaundice, thrombocytopenia, anemia, and hypoglycemia have been associated with thiazide diuretics. Beta blockers, angiotensin-converting enzyme (ACE) inhibitors, angiotensin receptor blockers, and digoxin also can be used if beneficial for treatment of pregnancy-associated heart failure. These drugs cross the placental barrier and are often category D (known fetal risk), particularly during the second and third trimesters of pregnancy. However, maternal heart failure is also a known fetal risk.

### Intrapartum Management

Every effort is made to minimize the effects of labor on the cardiovascular system. With every contraction, 300 to 500 mL of blood is shifted from the uterus and placenta into the central circulation. The fluid shift causes a sharp rise in cardiac workload. Therefore, careful management of intravenous fluid administration is essential to prevent fluid overload. The woman should be positioned on her side, with her head and shoulders elevated. Oxygen is administered to increase the blood oxygen saturation, which is monitored by pulse oximetry. Discomfort should be reduced as much as possible, but the use of epidural block should be monitored closely because of its hemodynamic effects (see Chapter 18). The environment is kept as quiet and calm as possible to decrease anxiety, which can cause tachycardia (Cunningham et al., 2014).

The fetus is monitored electronically, and signs of fetal compromise, as well as maternal signs of cardiac decompensation (tachycardia, rapid respirations, moist rales, exhaustion), should be reported immediately to the physician. Maternal pulse oximetry is usually ongoing throughout labor and post anesthesia.

A vaginal delivery is recommended for a woman with heart disease unless there are specific indications for cesarean birth, which can be hazardous. Vacuum extraction or outlet forceps are often used to minimize pushing during the second stage (Cunningham et al., 2014).

The fourth stage of labor is associated with special risks. After delivery of the placenta, approximately 500 mL of blood returns to the maternal intravascular volume. To minimize the risks of overloading the heart, abrupt positional changes should be avoided. Moreover, the uterus should not be massaged to expedite separation of the placenta. Careful assessment for signs of circulatory overload, such as a bounding pulse, distended neck and peripheral veins, and moist rales in the lungs, is performed throughout labor and postpartum.

### Postpartum Management

Women who have shown no evidence of cardiac distress during pregnancy, labor, or childbirth can still decompensate during the postpartum period. They must be observed closely for signs of infection, hemorrhage, or thromboembolism. These conditions can act together to precipitate postpartum heart failure in women with underlying heart disease.

## Nursing Considerations

To plan care better, the nurse should determine what functional classification the physician has assigned the woman. Assess for changes in vital signs such as tachycardia. Note increasing fatigue or other signs of congestive heart failure at office visits. Review the chart to identify other factors that can increase the woman's cardiac workload, such as anemia, infections, anxiety, or inadequate support to manage the activities of daily living.

During pregnancy, nursing care focuses on helping the woman and her family understand factors that increase the workload of the heart and measures they can take to help the woman maintain any needed activity restrictions. Explain how gaining excessive weight during pregnancy or any other time increases the burden on the heart. Anemia causes the heart to pump faster to circulate available erythrocytes to the tissues. A well-balanced diet that yields approximately 2200 kcal/day is recommended, with adequate high-quality protein. Emphasize the importance of taking iron and folic acid supplements to prevent anemia.

Identify modifications to allow the woman to live within her cardiac reserve. Explain how she can take rest periods during the day and for an hour after meals. Instruct her to sit rather than stand, if possible, when performing activities. If she performs an activity that increases her heart rate, teach her to rest every few minutes to allow the heart to recover. She should stop the activity if she experiences dyspnea, chest pain, or tachycardia. Chapter 27 contains suggestions for coping with bed rest if it is required.

The woman should avoid extremes of temperature when possible. Instruct her to dress for the cold in layers and to avoid exertion during hot and humid weather.

Emotional stress increases cardiac demand. Discuss methods for stress management, such as meditation, progressive relaxation, and biofeedback. Teach that cigarette smoking and the use of illicit drugs, such as cocaine and amphetamines, greatly increase stress to her heart and are associated with hypertension.

The woman is vulnerable postpartum, as interstitial fluid is mobilized into the vascular space for elimination. Continue to observe for signs of congestive heart failure. Observe urine output, because inadequate urine output may reflect the heart's inability to circulate blood adequately to the kidneys. If the mother cannot assume care of her infant, nurses should make every effort to promote contact between the mother, her significant others, and the infant. Breastfeeding imposes extra demands on the mother's heart, and whether it is advised is individualized.

The mother and new family may need help at home. Consult physicians and make any needed referrals for follow-up care, which may include home visits by a nurse or nursing assistant. Before the woman is discharged, review the signs and symptoms of cardiac complications and note the times when she should contact the physician.

## ANEMIAS

Anemia is a condition in which a decline in circulating red blood cell mass reduces the capacity to carry oxygen to the vital organs of the mother or fetus. Significant maternal anemia is associated with preterm birth and low birth weight. A woman is usually considered anemic if her hemoglobin is lower than 11 g/dL in the first and third trimesters or lower than 10.5 g/dL in the second trimester (Cunningham et al., 2014).

Anemia is one of the most common problems of pregnancy worldwide. The incidence varies according to geographic location and socioeconomic group, being a major problem in developing nations. Anemia is caused by various factors, including poor nutrition, hemolysis, and blood loss. Anemias that are often seen in a pregnant woman include iron deficiency anemia, folic acid deficiency anemia, the anemia associated with sickle cell disease, and thalassemia (ACOG, 2015; Cunningham et al., 2014).

### Iron Deficiency Anemia

Iron deficiency causes 75% of anemias in pregnancy. Meeting pregnancy needs for iron through the diet alone is difficult, although iron is present in many foods. The primary sources are meat, fish, chicken, and green leafy vegetables.

#### Maternal Effects

Signs and symptoms of iron deficiency anemia are often minimal but may include pallor, fatigue, lethargy, and headache. Clinical findings also can include inflammation of the lips and tongue. Pica (consuming nonfood substances such as clay, dirt, ice, or starch) is another sign of iron-deficiency anemia. Laboratory findings include red blood cells that are *microcytic* (small) and *hypochromic* (pale). The plasma iron and serum ferritin concentrations are low, and the total iron-binding capacity rises. Women who have multifetal pregnancies or bleeding complications are more likely to be anemic during pregnancy (Cunningham et al., 2014).

#### Fetal and Neonatal Effects

Even with significant maternal iron deficiency, the fetus will usually receive adequate iron at a cost to the mother. However, if the mother is severely anemic, the fetus can have reduced red blood cell volume, hemoglobin, and iron stores. Poor iron stores at birth can result in anemia during the first year, when the infant's oral iron intake is poor.

#### Therapeutic Management

Prenatal vitamins that contain iron are part of routine care. However, routine supplemental iron therapy rather than therapy based on an indication of anemia is controversial. Ferrous sulfate (325 mg, one to three times per day) is a common supplement. Many women experience less gastrointestinal discomfort if iron is taken with meals. Taking iron with 500 mg of vitamin C may enhance the iron absorption. Therapy is often continued for approximately 6 months after the anemia has been corrected. Parenteral therapy may be necessary for the woman who cannot or will not take oral iron and is significantly anemic (ACOG, 2015).

### Folic Acid Deficiency (Megaloblastic) Anemia

Folic acid is essential for cell duplication and for fetal and placental growth. It is also an essential nutrient for the formation of red blood cells.

#### Maternal Effects

Maternal needs for folic acid double during pregnancy in response to the demand for greater production of erythrocytes and for fetal and placental growth. A deficiency in folic acid results in a reduction in the rate of deoxyribonucleic acid (DNA) synthesis and mitotic activity of individual cells, resulting in the presence of *large, immature erythrocytes (megaloblasts)*. Folate deficiency is the primary cause of megaloblastic anemia during pregnancy.

Non-nutritional factors that contribute to folic acid deficiency include hemolytic anemias with increased red blood cell turnover; some medications, such as anticonvulsants; and malabsorption entities. Folic acid deficiency is often present in association with iron deficiency anemia.

#### Fetal and Neonatal Effects

Folate deficiency is associated with an increased risk for spontaneous abortion, abruptio placentae, and fetal anomalies, especially neural tube defects such as spina bifida and anencephaly.

#### Therapeutic Management

The recommended daily allowance for folic acid doubles during pregnancy, and some women have difficulty ingesting the amount needed, even though folic acid occurs widely in foods. The best sources of folic acid are kidney beans, lima beans, and fresh, dark green leafy vegetables. Because the demand for this vitamin increases during pregnancy, supplementation with folic acid (400 μg [0.4 mg]/day) is recommended for all women of childbearing age, and 600 μg (0.6 mg) is recommended when pregnancy is confirmed. Treatment is 1 mg folic acid daily and usually corrects megaloblastic anemia within a week. Women who have had a previous child with a neural tube defect should take 4 mg of folic acid for 1 month before and during the first trimester of pregnancy (American Academy of Pediatrics [AAP] & American College of Obstetricians and Gynecologists [ACOG], 2013; Cunningham et al., 2014).

### Sickle Cell Disease

Sickle cell disease is an autosomal recessive genetic disorder that causes anemia because an abnormal hemoglobin results in distortion and destruction of erythrocytes. It occurs when the gene for the production of hemoglobin S is inherited from both parents. The abnormal hemoglobin in the erythrocytes responds to hypoxia, acidosis, or dehydration by changing its shape to become a long, rigid rod. The change of hemoglobin S into rigid molecules distorts erythrocytes into a crescent, or sickle, shape. After erythrocytes lose their round, smooth, concave shape, they tend to clump together and occlude the smaller blood vessels.

The disease is characterized by chronic anemia, increased susceptibility to infection, and periodic crises when the abnormally shaped erythrocytes obstruct blood vessels. Sickle cell disease occurs most often in people who have ancestors from Africa, southern Europe, Near and Middle Eastern nations, South or Central America, Saudi Arabia, and India. Approximately 1 in 500 African-American and 1 in 1000 to 1400 Hispanic births in the United States will result in an infant with sickle cell anemia. Sickle cell anemia affects approximately 70,000 persons in the United States. More than 2 million Americans are carriers of the sickle cell gene and can pass it on to their children even though they are not affected (National Institutes of Health {NIH}, 2014).

### Maternal Effects

The physiologic anemia, increased coagulation factors, and venous stasis that are normal in pregnancy may bring on *sickle cell crisis,* sometimes for the first time. Any of several conditions can result, including temporary cessation of bone marrow function, hemolytic crisis with massive erythrocyte destruction resulting in jaundice, and severe pain caused by infarctions in the joints and other major organs. A sickle cell crisis can damage multiple organ systems. Women with sickle cell trait and sickle cell disease have higher risks for urinary tract infections during pregnancy (Cunningham et al., 2014).

### Fetal and Neonatal Effects

In the absence of maternal sickle cell crisis, the fetus usually does well, although complications such as prematurity and FGR are more common. The incidence of fetal loss is high if sickle cell crisis occurs because of placental infarctions with loss of exchange surface on the placenta.

### Therapeutic Management

Most treatment of sickle cell anemia during pregnancy is symptomatic and directed toward avoiding sickle cell crisis. Evaluations of hemoglobin, complete blood count, serum iron, total iron-binding capacity, and serum folate determine the degree of anemia and iron and folic acid stores. Folic acid 4 mg per day is recommended because of the continual turnover of red blood cells. Testing is carried out to detect infections such as hepatitis, human immunodeficiency virus (HIV), tuberculosis, and sexually transmitted diseases. Hepatitis B vaccine may be given to the noninfected woman. Urinalysis identifies clinical, as well as subclinical, infections that should be treated. Fetal surveillance studies (ultrasonography, nonstress tests, biophysical profiles) assess fetal growth and development and placental function. Exchange transfusions or prophylactic transfusions may be used to increase the amount of normal hemoglobin in the circulation and to reduce severe anemia (Cunningham et al., 2014).

The goal of nursing management is to help the pregnant woman maintain a healthy status and avoid hospitalization. Women must be encouraged to keep all prenatal care appointments, usually every other week. Topics in prenatal education include (1) the need to maintain adequate hydration to prevent sickling, (2) the need for adequate nutrition to meet metabolic needs, (3) the need for folic acid supplementation for erythrocyte production, (4) the need for rest periods throughout the day, (5) good hygiene practices and the avoidance of people with infectious illnesses, and (6) the need for prompt treatment of fever or other signs of infection that could precipitate a crisis. Additional medications may be prescribed based on the individual.

Nurses must be alert for signs of sickle cell crisis in an affected woman. The most common indications are pain in the abdomen, chest, vertebrae, joints, or extremities; pallor; and signs of cardiac failure. Nurses must also provide comfort measures such as repositioning, good skin care, assisting with ambulation and movement in bed, and assisting the woman to splint the abdomen with a pillow when she must cough or breathe deeply.

Intrapartum care focuses on preventing development of sickle cell crisis. Oxygen is administered continuously, and fluids should be administered to prevent dehydration because hypoxemia and dehydration as well as exertion, infection, and acidosis stimulate the sickling process. Packed red blood cells (PRBCs) can be administered to women who have a hemoglobin concentration less than 8 g/dL or hematocrit less than 20%.

## Thalassemias

Like sickle cell disease, thalassemia is a genetic disorder that involves the abnormal synthesis of alpha or beta chains of hemoglobin. This mutation leads to alterations in the red blood cell membrane and a decreased life span of red blood cells. Thalassemia is named and classified by the type of chain that is inadequately produced. Beta-thalassemia is most frequently encountered in the United States. Beta-thalassemia minor refers to the heterozygous form that results from the inheritance of one abnormal gene from either parent. Beta-thalassemia major refers to inheritance of the gene from both parents. Newborns with beta-thalassemia major (Cooley's anemia) are usually healthy at birth but the fetal hemoglobin F falls, leading to severe anemia and failure to thrive. Pregnancy was once rare in women with Cooley's anemia but may possibly be successful today. Pregnancy is only recommended if there is adequate cardiac function and maintenance of a hemoglobin value of 10 g/dL. Beta-thalassemia is most often found in those of Mediterranean or Asian (particularly Chinese) origin (Cunningham et al., 2014; ACOG, 2013).

### Maternal Effects

Women with beta-thalassemia minor are often mildly anemic but otherwise healthy. Laboratory values normally associated with beta-thalassemia minor indicate a mild hypochromic and microcytic anemia. Beta-thalassemia major is often known before pregnancy. Fertility is usually low. Avoidance of iron overload requiring the chelating drug is ideal during pregnancy because of unknown fetal effects.

### Fetal and Neonatal Effects

Whether the disorders are associated with increased fetal or neonatal morbidity remains unknown because of the many variants of thalassemia. There appears to be no increase in the rate of prematurity, low-birth-weight infants, or abnormal size for gestation. Fetal anemia can be serious if inadequate fetal hemoglobin is produced. The fetus can inherit the serious problem of beta-thalassemia major if both parents have beta-thalassemia minor.

### Therapeutic Management

There is no specific therapy for beta-thalassemia minor during pregnancy. Most often, the outcomes for the mother and fetus are satisfactory. Infections, which depress production of red blood cells and accelerate erythrocyte destruction, should be identified and treated promptly (Cunningham et al., 2014; ACOG, 2013).

# IMMUNE COMPLEX DISEASES

## Systemic Lupus Erythematosus

Systemic lupus erythematosus (SLE) is a chronic, inflammatory autoimmune disease that can affect any organ or system in the body.

Although the cause is unknown, an imbalance appears to develop between immune response and tolerance of specific antigens, so that the body produces antibodies to its own cells and tissue. Signs and symptoms result from inflammation of multiple organ systems, especially the joints, skin, kidneys, and nervous system. The most common signs or symptoms are joint pain, photosensitivity, thrombocytopenia, and a "butterfly" rash on the face that is easily confused with normal pigmentation changes of pregnancy. Fatigue is a common symptom. Remissions occur periodically, during which no symptoms are present.

The disease tends to affect young women, but it may occur in any age group. The exact incidence is unknown. It is more common in women of African or Hispanic ancestry (National Institutes of Health: National Institute of Arthritis and Musculoskeletal and Skin Diseases [NIAMS], 2015). For more information on SLE, see http://www.lupus.org.

SLE is associated with an increased incidence of miscarriage and fetal death during the first trimester. There is an increased risk for later pregnancy loss or premature birth because of hypertension, renal complications, and preterm rupture of membranes. Preeclampsia may be early and severe for the woman who has SLE.

An infrequent *neonatal lupus syndrome* can occur, including a transient photosensitive rash, thrombocytopenia, hepatitis, and hemolytic anemia. Congenital heart block may be recognized in pregnancy and require a pacemaker.

Because pregnancy can worsen previously well-controlled SLE, the woman must be carefully observed for signs that the disease has progressed. Renal complications pose a special risk. Women with a history of kidney problems should be advised to seek the advice of a physician before becoming pregnant. Pregnancy is most likely to have a favorable outcome in the woman whose disease is under good control at the beginning and who does not have renal involvement.

### Antiphospholipid Syndrome

Antiphospholipid syndrome (APS) is an autoimmune condition characterized by the production of antiphospholipid antibodies, combined with certain clinical features. The most specific clinical features include thrombosis, decreased platelets, and pregnancy loss. Pregnancy complications that are more common with APS include fetal loss, early onset preeclampsia, IUGR, and preterm birth. Stroke related to arterial thrombosis may occur.

Although the syndrome occurs most often in women with other underlying autoimmune diseases, such as SLE, it is also diagnosed in women with no other recognizable autoimmune disease.

Women with APS should be informed of the potential maternal and obstetric problems, ideally before conception. They should be assessed for evidence of anemia, thrombocytopenia, and underlying renal disease. Low-dose aspirin and prophylactic heparin or enoxaparin are currently recommended for pregnant women with APS. Research for the best treatments continues (ACOG, 2015; Cunningham et al., 2014).

### Hashimoto's Thyroiditis

Hashimoto's thyroiditis, also known as chronic lymphocytic thyroiditis, is an autoimmune disorder and the cause of most cases of hypothyroidism in women. Many women with Hashimoto's thyroiditis are euthyroid but later become hypothyroid. Untreated maternal hypothyroidism during pregnancy can adversely affect the child's mental development. Thyroid-stimulating hormone should be tested before or in early pregnancy and hypothyroidism corrected within the first trimester (Cunningham et al., 2014).

## SEIZURE DISORDERS: EPILEPSY

Generalized seizures are the most common form of epilepsy, which is a recurrent disorder of cerebral function. Seizure disorders affect approximately 1% of the general population. Other types of seizures are partial (simple and complex) and nonepileptic. Status epilepticus, or continuous seizures, are a medical emergency (see also Chapter 52). Pregnancy can affect frequency and management of seizures, and the seizure disorder can affect the course of pregnancy. The frequency of seizures can increase, decrease, or remain the same. Antiseizure drug levels often decrease in the pregnant woman and may or may not alter her previous frequency. In general, the longer the woman has been seizure-free before pregnancy, the less likely she is to develop seizures during pregnancy. Those with partial seizures are more likely to have an increased frequency. Vomiting, reduced gastric motility, use of gastrointestinal medications, and weight gain of pregnancy affect the absorption and distribution of anticonvulsant drugs. Serum levels of anticonvulsants may rise, fall, or remain the same during pregnancy.

A major concern is the teratogenic effects of anticonvulsant drugs possibly related to folate deficiency. One specific syndrome is *fetal hydantoin syndrome,* which includes craniofacial abnormalities, neural tube defects, limb reduction defects, growth restriction, intellectual disability, and cardiac anomalies. Newer anticonvulsants such as oxcarbazepine have less data available related to fetal effects (Cunningham et al., 2014).

Preconception management by an obstetrician and a neurologist is ideal for seizure control with minimal anticonvulsant drug doses. Treatment goals are to prevent generalized seizures and to reduce the adverse effects of anticonvulsant medications on the fetus. The woman and her family must be made aware of the risks involved with specific anticonvulsants that they should continue during pregnancy. Treatment is not expected to be stopped unless the woman has been seizure free for 2 years. The decision to discontinue anticonvulsants will be made by the physicians. Generalized seizures result in fetal hypoxia and acidosis, and thus, pose a serious problem for the fetus (Cunningham et al., 2014).

## INFECTIONS DURING PREGNANCY

Infections can harm the woman, the fetus, or both. A mild infection in the adult may have devastating effects on the developing fetus. Table 26.2 presents nursing considerations in relation to sexually transmitted diseases and vaginal and urinary tract infections.

### Viral Infections

Viral infections are often mild or even asymptomatic in adults, but they can have catastrophic fetal or neonatal consequences. Maternal infections with cytomegalovirus, rubella, varicella-zoster virus, herpes simplex, hepatitis B, and HIV have the greatest potential for harming the fetus or neonate.

#### Cytomegalovirus

Cytomegalovirus (CMV), a member of the herpesvirus group, is widespread and eventually infects most humans. Although CMV is widespread, the most serious effects occur in the fetus and immunocompromised people. CMV has been isolated from urine, saliva, blood, cervical mucus, semen, breast milk, and feces. Young children who have close contact with infected playmates are the most likely reservoirs for transmission to adults, including pregnant women. Many infections are asymptomatic or produce minimal symptoms, so they may not be suspected or diagnosed (ACOG, 2015).

**TABLE 26.2 Infections That Impact Pregnancy: Sexually Transmitted Diseases, Vaginal and Urinary Tract Infections**

| Maternal, Fetal, and Neonatal Effects | Nursing Considerations |
|---|---|
| **Sexually Transmitted Diseases** | |
| ***Syphilis (Causative Organism: Spirochete* Treponema pallidum*)*** | |
| If untreated, the organism can cross the placenta to the fetus, resulting in spontaneous abortion, a stillborn infant, premature labor and birth, or congenital syphilis. Major signs of congenital syphilis are enlarged liver and spleen, skin lesions, rashes, osteitis, pneumonia, and hepatitis. | Penicillin G is the primary treatment to cure the disease in both the woman and fetus. Women who are allergic are desensitized and then treated.*‡ |
| ***Gonorrhea (Causative Organism: Bacterium* Neisseria gonorrhoeae*)*** | |
| Not transmitted via the placenta; vertical transmission from mother to newborn during birth can cause ophthalmia neonatorum. Endocervicitis and weakness of the fetal membranes increase the risk for premature rupture of membranes and preterm labor. *Chlamydia* infection is likely to accompany gonorrhea infection. | Cephalosporins such as cefixime or ceftriaxone (pregnancy category B) are recommended for gonorrhea during pregnancy.* Because 20% to 50% of women with gonorrhea also have chlamydial infection, azithromycin or amoxicillin (pregnancy category B) is recommended to accompany gonorrhea treatment.*† The partner must also be treated to prevent reinfection. Infants are treated with an ophthalmic antibiotic such as ceftriaxone at birth to prevent ophthalmia neonatorum. |
| ***Chlamydial Infection (Causative Organism: Bacterium* Chlamydia trachomatis*)*** | |
| Chlamydial infection is the most common sexually transmitted disease in the United States. The fetus can be infected during birth and suffer neonatal conjunctivitis or pneumonitis. Conjunctivitis is prevented by erythromycin ophthalmic ointment. *Chlamydia* can cause premature rupture of membranes, premature labor, and chorioamnionitis. | Education is particularly important because infection is usually asymptomatic. Both partners should be treated to prevent recurrent infection. As with all sexually transmitted diseases, the use of condoms decreases the risk for infection. Azithromycin, amoxicillin, or clindamycin are recommended treatments.*† |
| ***Trichomoniasis (Causative Organism: Protozoan* Trichomonas vaginalis*)*** | |
| Common cause of vaginitis in 10% to 50% of pregnant women and in the prostatic fluid of up to 70% of their sexual contacts. Organism can also infect urethra, periurethral glands, and bladder. Associated with premature rupture of membranes, preterm birth, and postpartum endometritis.*† | Metronidazole (Flagyl), pregnancy category B, may be given to the pregnant woman as a 2-g single oral dose. Tinidazole (Tindamax), pregnancy category C, may be chosen in a 2-g single oral dose. Consistent association between fetal abnormalities or injury and metronidazole use has not been upheld.*† |
| ***Condyloma Acuminatum (Causative Organism: Human Papillomavirus [HPV])*** | |
| Transmission of condyloma acuminatum, also called *venereal* or *genital warts*, can occur during vaginal birth and is associated with the development of epithelial tumors of the mucous membranes of the larynx in children. Pregnancy can cause proliferation of lesions, which are associated with cervical dysplasia and cancer. | The common choices for nonpregnant therapy (podophyllin, podofilox, imiquimod) are not recommended during pregnancy. Maternal lesions can be excised using cryotherapy or cautery.<br>*†Immunization of girls and women age 11 through 26 and boys and men age 9 through 26 is now recommended to combat HPV virus. Full immunization is three doses. See also Chapter 32. |
| ***Vaginal Infections*** | |
| ***Candidiasis (Causative Organism: Yeast* Candida albicans*)*** | |
| Oral candidiasis (thrush) can develop in newborns if infection is present at birth. Thrush is treated with application of nystatin (Mycostatin) over the surfaces of the oral cavity four times a day for several days. Characteristic "cottage cheese" vaginal discharge with vulvar pruritus, burning, and dyspareunia. Vulva may be red, tender, and edematous. | Candidiasis (sometimes called *Monilia vaginitis*) is a persistent problem for many women during pregnancy. Examples of maternal treatment choices include topical miconazole, clotrimazole, and oral or intravenous fluconazole for 7 days.*†‡ |
| ***Bacterial Vaginosis§ (Causative Organism:* Gardnerella vaginalis*)*** | |
| Adverse pregnancy outcomes include preterm rupture of membranes, preterm labor and birth, intraamniotic infection, and postpartum endometritis. Marked by a major shift in vaginal flora from the normal predominance of lactobacilli to a predominance of anaerobic bacteria. Causes profuse, malodorous, "fishy" vaginal discharge, itching, and burning.*‡ | Metronidazole or clindamycin oral therapy for 7 days is recommended during pregnancy. Clinical trials have shown that women at high risk for preterm birth may benefit from this medication regimen.*‡ |
| ***Urinary Tract Infections*** | |
| ***Asymptomatic Bacteriuria (Causative Organisms:* Escherichia coli, Klebsiella, Proteus*)*** | |
| Ascending bacterial infection can result in cystitis or pyelonephritis in later pregnancy if condition remains untreated. | Recovery of a urinary pathogen from a midstream, clean-catch urine specimen is defined as 100,000 colony-forming units (CFUs) per mL of urine. Urine dipsticks can identify nitrites that suggest but do not diagnose possible bacteriuria. |

**TABLE 26.2 Infections That Impact Pregnancy: Sexually Transmitted Diseases, Vaginal and Urinary Tract Infections—cont'd**

| Maternal, Fetal, and Neonatal Effects | Nursing Considerations |
|---|---|
| ***Cystitis (Causative Organisms:* E. coli, Klebsiella, Proteus*)*** | |
| Signs and symptoms include dysuria, frequency, urgency, and suprapubic tenderness. Ascending infection can lead to pyelonephritis. | Antibiotics used for both asymptomatic bacteriuria and cystitis include amoxicillin, ampicillin, trimethoprim-sulfamethoxazole, nitrofurantoin, or a third-generation cephalosporin such as ceftriaxone. Emphasize importance of reporting signs of urinary tract infection. Stress the importance of taking all the medication prescribed in the 7-day course, even if symptoms abate. Provide information about hygiene measures such as front-to-back perineal care after urination or bowel movements. A test of cure may be performed after completion of treatment.[‡] |
| ***Acute Pyelonephritis (Causative Organisms:* E. coli, Klebsiella, Proteus*)*** | |
| Increased risk for preterm labor and premature delivery. Maternal complications include a high fever, septic shock, and adult respiratory distress syndrome. Pregnant women often require hospitalization for acute care. | Inform women with asymptomatic bacteriuria or cystitis of signs and symptoms, such as sudden onset of fever (often higher than 39° C [102.2° F]), chills, flank pain or tenderness, nausea, and vomiting, so that treatment can begin promptly. Blood culture may be required to diagnose pyelonephritis if antibiotics have been started for asymptomatic bacteriuria or cystitis. Skin cooling may be used to lower the woman's temperature below 38° C (100.4° F), reducing possible compromise of fetal oxygen level. Intravenous (IV) antibiotics are used for at least 48 hr followed by oral medications. Common combinations include ampicillin or a cephalosporin plus an aminoglycoside. Serum levels of aminoglycosides are often determined to ensure an adequate dose without reaching a toxic level.[‡] |

*Centers for Disease Control and Prevention. (2010). Sexually transmitted diseases treatment guidelines, 2010. *MMWR: Morbidity and Mortality Weekly Report, 59*(RR-12).

[†]Duff, P., Sweet, R.L., & Edwards, R.K. (2009). Maternal and fetal infections. In R.K. Creasy, R. Resnik, J.D. Iams, et al. (Eds.), *Creasy & Resnik's Maternal-fetal medicine: Principles and practice* (6th ed., pp. 739–795). Philadelphia: Saunders.

[‡]Yudin, M.H. (2011). Other infectious conditions. In D.K. James, P. J. Steer, C.P. Weiner, et al. (Eds.), *High risk pregnancy: Management options* (4th ed., pp. 521–542). Philadelphia: Saunders.

[§]Roos, T., & Baker, D.A. (2011). Cytomegalovirus, herpes simplex virus, adenovirus, coxsackievirus, and human papillomavirus. In D.K. James, P.J. Steer, C.P. Weiner, et al. (Eds.), *High risk pregnancy: Management options* (4th ed., pp. 503–520). Philadelphia: Saunders.

After primary (first) infection, the virus becomes latent, but like other herpesviruses, CMV may produce periodic reactivation and shedding of the virus. Primary CMV infection is the most dangerous to the fetus. Determining the viral load in the fetus or newborn may be done by polymerase chain reaction (PCR) in amniotic fluid, newborn dry blood spot, or tissue.

***Fetal and neonatal effects.*** The most severe neonatal infection usually occurs if a woman develops a primary CMV infection during pregnancy. Mortality is as high as 20% to 30% at birth, with 90% of survivors having late complications. Possible newborn problems include enlarged spleen and liver, CNS abnormalities, jaundice, chorioretinitis, and growth restriction. Newborns may become infected during the first 6 months because of transmission from the mother at birth or breastfeeding. CMV is the leading cause of hearing loss in children, and routine newborn hearing screens help identify the loss early.

***Therapeutic management.*** No effective therapy is currently available for the treatment of congenital infection. Ultrasound scanning may identify manifestations of the infection, such as cranial abnormalities or growth restriction. Antiviral agents, such as ganciclovir and foscarnet, may be used for severe infections, but these drugs are toxic and only temporarily suppress shedding of the virus. Primary prevention, such as emphasizing handwashing, especially to women who care for small children, warning of the risks imposed by having several sexual partners, and transfusing only CMV-free blood, is most effective (Cunningham et al., 2014).

## Rubella

Rubella is caused by a virus transmitted by droplets or through direct contact with articles contaminated with nasopharyngeal secretions. Rubella is a mild disease; major symptoms are fever, general malaise, and a characteristic maculopapular rash that begins on the face and spreads over the body. Although the overall incidence has declined since rubella vaccine became available, many young adults remain at risk, and outbreaks have occurred. One outbreak in the United States had an incidence of almost 90% in women born in Latin America. Rubella immunization campaigns in Latin America and Mexico have reduced the incidence of congenital rubella syndrome (CRS).

***Fetal and neonatal effects.*** Rubella remains a serious concern because the virus crosses the placental barrier and can infect the fetus. The greatest risk to the fetus occurs during the first trimester, when fetal organs are developing. If maternal infection occurs during this time, approximately 90% of fetuses will have CRS. Hearing loss, intellectual disability, cataracts, cardiac defects, growth restriction, and microcephaly are common fetal complications. Infants born to mothers who had rubella during pregnancy shed the virus for many months, and thus, pose a threat to other infants as well as to susceptible children and adults who come into contact with them (Cunningham et al., 2014).

***Therapeutic management.*** Prevention is the only effective protection for the fetus. Active international immunization against rubella is aimed at eliminating the infection and CRS. Women who are immune do not become infected, so it is critical to determine the immune status of all women of childbearing age. A rubella titer of 1:8 or greater provides evidence of immunity. Women who are not immune should be vaccinated before they become pregnant, and they should be advised not to become pregnant for 4 weeks after vaccination because the live-virus vaccine poses a possible risk to the fetus. However, the risk of the vaccine to the fetus appears to be very low and may not exist. Nonimmune women are usually vaccinated during the postpartum period so that they will be immune before becoming pregnant again.

### Varicella-Zoster Virus

Varicella infection (chickenpox) is caused by varicella-zoster virus, a herpesvirus that is transmitted by direct contact or via the respiratory tract. The varicella virus can become latent in nerve ganglia. When the virus is reactivated, herpes zoster (shingles) results. Adults have usually acquired immunity by the time they reach childbearing age.

**Fetal and neonatal effects.** Fetal and neonatal effects depend on the time of maternal infection. If the infection occurs during the first trimester, the fetus has a small risk for congenital varicella syndrome (0.4% to 2%). The greatest risk for the development of congenital varicella syndrome occurs from 13 to 20 weeks of pregnancy, and the risk is low (2%). Clinical findings include limb hypoplasia, cutaneous scars, chorioretinitis, cataracts, microcephaly, and FGR. In later pregnancy, transplacental passage of maternal antibodies usually protects the fetus. However, if the woman develops varicella within 2 weeks of birth, newborn varicella may occur because the mother has not had time to develop antibodies to the virus. Varicella-zoster immune globulin (VZIG) will be given to a newborn during this time period. Infants born earlier than 28 weeks or who weigh 1000 g are given VZIG because maternal antibodies to varicella earlier in pregnancy have not yet crossed the placenta, reducing natural passive immunity (ACOG, 2015).

**Therapeutic management.** A live attenuated varicella vaccine (Varivax) is available, and children and susceptible adults can receive the vaccine if they live in the same household as a susceptible pregnant woman. VZIG should be administered within 96 hours to provide passive (temporary) immunity to pregnant women who have been exposed and are susceptible. A nonimmune postpartum woman should receive her first immunization before discharge and her second one 4 weeks postpartum. Pregnancy should be avoided for 1 month after each dose.

A pregnant woman should be told to promptly report pulmonary symptoms such as shortness of breath or cough. Hospitalization, fetal surveillance, full respiratory support, and hemodynamic monitoring should be available for women diagnosed with varicella pneumonia. Women and infants with varicella should be placed in airborne and contact isolation. Only staff members known to be immune to varicella should come into contact with these patients. Pregnant women with shingles should be in contact isolation.

### Herpesvirus Serotypes 1 and 2

Genital herpes is one of the most common sexually transmitted diseases. It is caused by herpesvirus serotype 1 or serotype 2, but most episodes of genital herpes are caused by type 2. Infection occurs as a result of direct contact of the skin or mucous membrane with an active lesion. Lesions form at the site of contact and begin as a group of painful papules that progress rapidly to become vesicles, shallow ulcers, pustules, and crusts. The woman sheds the virus until the lesions are completely healed. The virus then migrates along the sensory nerves to reside in the sensory ganglion, and the disease enters a latent phase. It can be reactivated later as a recurrent infection, usually less severe, but with viral shedding.

*Vertical transmission* (from mother to infant) occurs in two ways: (1) after rupture of membranes, when the active virus ascends from active lesions; and (2) during birth, when the fetus comes into contact with infectious genital secretions. The risk for neonatal infection is highest if the infant is exposed during the mother's primary (first) infection.

A reliable diagnosis for herpes simplex virus (HSV) requires viral cell culture from a lesion or PCR assays of the viral DNA.

**Fetal and neonatal effects.** Complications during pregnancy from a recurrent maternal infection are rare. Neonatal herpes infection acquired during vaginal birth is the major perinatal problem, particularly if the maternal infection is primary. Severity of neonatal HSV infection may be local infection of the skin, mouth, or eyes; encephalitis; or disseminated disease. Encephalitis or disseminated HSV infection has a high mortality rate and most survivors are not normal. Viral culture is the only reliable method of diagnosis.

**Therapeutic management.** To reduce symptoms and shorten the duration of lesions, acyclovir, famciclovir, or valacyclovir may be given orally during pregnancy. Some specialists recommend treatment with these drugs during late pregnancy for women who have recurrent lesions to reduce the likelihood of active lesions at term (ACOG, 2014).

For women with a history of genital herpes, vaginal delivery is planned if there are no genital lesions at the time of labor. For women with recurrent or primary active lesions at the time of labor, cesarean birth is recommended. Use of fetal scalp electrodes, which cause a break in the skin, should be limited in the woman with active lesions but is acceptable if there are no active lesions.

After delivery, isolation of the mother from her infant is not necessary as long as direct contact with lesions is avoided and mothers use careful handwashing techniques. Mothers may breastfeed if there are no lesions on the breasts. The infant is observed carefully for signs of infection, including temperature instability, lethargy, poor sucking reflex, jaundice, seizures, and herpetic lesions. Acyclovir therapy is prescribed for neonatal infection.

Expectant mothers need information regarding effective ways to deal with the emotional as well as the physical effects of herpes. Many women are concerned about privacy and do not want family members to know why cesarean birth is necessary. Such women must be assured that their wishes will be respected. Many women need an opportunity to discuss their feelings of shame, anger, or anxiety about the disease.

### Parvovirus B19

Erythema infectiosum, also called *fifth disease*, is caused by human parvovirus B19. This acute, communicable disease is characterized by a distinctive "lace like" rash. The rash starts on the face with a "slapped-cheeks" appearance, followed by a generalized maculopapular rash. Other symptoms include fever, malaise, and joint pain. Erythema infectiosum is more common among children and often occurs in community epidemics. The disease is most contagious the week before the rash appears. The prognosis is usually excellent. However, if the disease occurs in pregnancy, there are possible fetal and neonatal effects. Maternal antibody titers or PCR analysis of viral DNA can be done to identify in utero infection risk.

**Fetal and neonatal effects.** When infection occurs during pregnancy, fetal death can result, usually from failure of fetal red blood cell production, followed by severe fetal anemia, hydrops (generalized edema), and heart failure. Serial ultrasonography can be performed to detect hydrops. Intrauterine transfusion is an option to treat severe fetal anemia if it does not resolve spontaneously. The risk to the fetus is greatest when the mother is infected in the first 20 weeks of pregnancy, although this risk is approximately 10%, and risk of loss after 20 weeks is less than 1%. The affected newborn is examined for any defect, and the child is assessed regularly for several years to identify delayed complications.

*Therapeutic management.* Infection with parvovirus B19 has no specific treatment. Starch baths may help reduce pruritus, and analgesics may be necessary to relieve mild joint pain.

### Hepatitis B

Six types of hepatitis virus subtypes have been identified: A, B, C, D, E, and G. Type B in the perinatal period is the focus in this chapter. Hepatitis A virus (HAV) accounts for approximately one-third of hepatitis cases in the United States. Hepatitis A is mostly transmitted by contaminated food or water. Supportive care is usually sufficient. Immune globulin to neonates born to mothers with recent HAV may be given.

The incidence of hepatitis B virus (HBV) has fallen significantly with screening and immunization of at-risk people, including healthcare providers. Goals to eliminate HBV in the United States include:

- Universal newborn vaccination
- Routine screening of all pregnant women and provision of immunoprophylaxis to infants born to infected mothers or women with unknown infection status
- Routine vaccination to unvaccinated children and adolescents
- Vaccination of adults at increased risk of infection, including healthcare workers, those with sexually transmitted diseases (STDs), household contacts or sex partners with those having chronic HBV infection, multiple sex partners, recipients of certain blood products, or dialysis patients (ACOG, 2014).

Hepatitis C may go undiagnosed until the woman develops chronic liver disease that often requires liver transplantation. Hepatitis C is often associated with intravenous drug use, HIV infection, and frequent transfusions, although transfusion-acquired hepatitis C is now very rare.

HBV is caused by a virus that is transmitted through blood, saliva, vaginal secretions, semen, or breast milk and readily crosses the placental barrier. The disease is prevalent in certain population groups, including immigrants from central and Southeast Asia, the Middle East, and Africa, and in Native Americans, Eskimos, and intravenous drug users. Symptoms may include vomiting, abdominal pain, jaundice, fever, rash, and painful joints. Fortunately, most infected adolescents and adults recover within 6 months and acquire long-lasting immunity. However, chronic infection can result in liver failure with possible carcinoma.

*Fetal and neonatal effects.* HBV infection in pregnancy is associated with an increased incidence of prematurity, low birth weight, and neonatal death. Infants born to mothers who had HBV during pregnancy or who are chronic carriers of hepatitis B surface antigen (HBsAg) are at risk for the development of acute infection at birth. The younger the age when exposed to HBV, the more likely that chronic carrier status will develop (ACOG, 2014).

*Therapeutic management.* HBV infection is preventable. Simple hygiene measures such as handwashing, standard precautions with body fluids, and safe sex with condom use provide primary prevention. HBV vaccine is now recommended for newborns, and the first dose may be given before discharge or at the infant's first visit to the pediatrician. The second dose is given at 2 months and third dose at 6 to 18 months. HBV vaccines are available as a series of three intramuscular injections into the deltoid for adults, with the second and third doses given at least 1 and 4 months after the first. A combination of vaccines against HVA and HBV (Twinrix) is given in three doses, with the second and third doses given 1 month and 6 months after the first. Vaccination is recommended for any population at risk, including nurses who frequently come into contact with infectious body fluids. See http://www.cdc.gov for the most current adult and pediatric immunization schedules and alternate dosing (CDC, 2015).

All pregnant women should be screened for HBsAg, and those having risk factors should be offered the vaccine. Household members and sexual contacts should be tested and offered vaccination if they are not immune. No specific treatment exists for acute HBV. Recommended supportive treatment includes bed rest and a high-protein, low-fat diet.

Chronic infection of a newborn whose mother is known to be HBsAg-positive can usually be prevented by administration of hepatitis B immune globulin (HBIG, Hep-B-Gammagee) and HBV vaccine (Recombivax-HB, Engerix-B) within 12 hours of birth. The priority within 12 hours is the HBIG. To prevent infection from contamination of the infant's skin with maternal blood, the newborn's skin should be cleaned well before injections or heel sticks. The infant is tested 1 to 3 months after completing the HBV immunization schedule to identify presence of chronic infection. Breastfeeding is considered safe as long as the newborn has been vaccinated.

### Human Immunodeficiency Virus (HIV)

Acquired immunodeficiency syndrome (AIDS) is a failure of immune function caused by the retrovirus HIV. HIV infection is most often transmitted to women or infants in one of three ways: (1) heterosexual transmission from an infected person, (2) parenteral exposure to infected blood or tissue, or (3) from an infected mother to an infant (vertical transmission) perinatally. Perinatal transmission has fallen with routine prenatal HIV testing for most women, antiviral therapy to the infected pregnant woman and to her newborn. Although there is still no cure, better control of opportunistic infections has greatly extended life for those with HIV.

Approximately one-half of HIV infections in 2009 occurred in women, and almost one-fourth of new infections were in women. In 2009, HIV infections among black women in the United States were 57%, 21% in white women, and 16% in Hispanic/Latinas. Transmission in women is usually related to high-risk heterosexual contact and intravenous drug use (Cunningham et al., 2014).

*Pathophysiology.* Like other retroviruses, HIV can integrate its viral genetic makeup into the genetic makeup of the cell when infecting it. This process produces a cell that cannot perform its functions properly. At the same time, this abnormal cell replicates and produces more viruses that invade more cells. The disease worsens as more and more cells cease to function, and at the same time, a greater number of viruses are produced. The principal mechanism whereby HIV leads to immunodeficiency is through its effect on helper (CD4) lymphocytes. These cells play a key role in organizing the body's immune response.

As the number of CD4 cells declines, the immune response becomes inadequate, and opportunistic infections are able to overwhelm the person who is HIV-positive. Antiretroviral therapy is usually started when the CD4 count is less than 500 to 600 cells/mm$^3$; almost half of infected people will show evidence of AIDS with a CD4 count of 100 cells/mm$^3$ or less.

The clinical course of HIV infection follows four fairly predictable stages:

- Stage 1: An early, or acute, stage occurs several weeks after HIV exposure. Flu-like symptoms may develop and last a few weeks. Antibodies to HIV (seroconversion) generally appear within a few months but occasionally can be delayed for more than a year.
- Stage 2: A middle, or asymptomatic, period of minor or no clinical problems occurs. This period is characterized by continuous low-level viral replication and CD4 cell loss. The latent

period from infection to AIDS is approximately 11 years but varies with the decision to accept or deny treatment.

- Stage 3: There is a transitional period of symptomatic disease, characterized by immune dysfunction.
- Stage 4: A late, or crisis, period of symptomatic disease can last months or years. This period is characterized by infections and cancers that occur principally in people with immune system compromise.

During stages 1 and 2, the infected person is said to be HIV-positive; during stages 3 and 4, the immune system no longer offers adequate protection and opportunistic diseases occur. The person is then said to have AIDS.

***Fetal and neonatal effects.*** Because of new antiretroviral drugs, the prognosis for HIV-infected women and their infants has improved. Antiretroviral therapy should be done even though the woman is not yet on the drugs when not pregnant to reduce perinatal transmission to the infant. Therapy should include three drugs, with the primary antiretroviral being zidovudine (ZDV, also abbreviated AZT). Antiretroviral drugs will be delayed until 10 to 12 weeks' gestation if the woman has a low enough viral load for her safety. Three drug combinations of antiretrovirals have reduced perinatal transmission, with zidovudine being the principal drug. Mothers who receive no or minimal HIV care during the prenatal period have higher rates of infected infants. Infant infection can occur during pregnancy, labor, and birth, or after birth if the infant is breastfed. Maternal therapy will stop after birth unless the mother continues to need therapy. Zidovudine therapy for the infant should begin 6 to 12 hours after birth. Zidovudine syrup 2 mg/kg every 6 hours continues for 6 weeks after birth.

Infant HIV tests can remain positive for up to 18 months after birth because of passive maternal antibodies. An infected newborn is typically asymptomatic at birth, but signs and symptoms may become obvious during the first year of life. Early signs include enlargement of the liver and spleen, lymphadenopathy, failure to thrive, persistent thrush, and extensive seborrheic dermatitis (cradle cap). Infected infants often have bacterial infections such as meningitis, pneumonia, osteomyelitis, septic arthritis, and septicemia. Prompt treatment of the HIV-infected infant with appropriate antiretroviral medications and other prophylactic therapy can slow the infection's progress. See Chapter 42 for more information about HIV infection and its treatment in infants and children.

***Prevention.*** Prevention remains the only way to avoid HIV infection. Sexual transmission can be avoided by several methods. Abstinence would render a person safe from all STDs, including HIV, but most are not willing to practice lifelong total abstinence. Sexual transmission of HIV can also be prevented if infected individuals do not have intercourse with susceptible persons. Consistent condom use reduces but does not eliminate HIV transmission.

Intravenous drug users who refuse rehabilitative treatment should be taught to wash the equipment with water, soap, and bleach before each use to prevent transmission of the virus from one person to another via a soiled needle.

***Therapeutic management.*** Multiple antiretroviral drugs from different classes are beneficial in extending the woman's life after infection. Guidelines for the latest treatments from the National Institutes of Health for pregnant as well as nonpregnant patients may be found at http://www.aidsinfo.nih.gov.

Maternal ZDV therapy to reduce infant HIV infection must consider many situations such as:

- If the mother has had any antiretroviral therapy during pregnancy, including ZDV, and when it began
- If the mother had any prenatal care and when she started
- Fetal gestational age
- If the membranes have ruptured, how long they have been ruptured

See Box 26.3 for measures to reduce infection in the infant.

### BOX 26.3 Recommendations for Prevention of Perinatal Human Immunodeficiency Virus Infection of the Infant

- Pregnancy: Zidovudine (ZDV), 100 mg orally five times per day initiated between 14 and 34 weeks of gestation. Alternative adult dose regimens for oral ZDV are 200 mg three times per day or 300 mg twice daily.
- Labor: Intravenous zidovudine with a 1-hour loading dose of 2 mg/kg, followed by continuous infusion of 1 mg/kg/hr until delivery.
- Newborn: Oral ZDV syrup, dose of 2 mg/kg every 6 hours for 6 weeks, beginning 8 to 12 hours after birth.

A cesarean delivery at 38 weeks of pregnancy, before the onset of labor and rupture of membranes, is usual to reduce maternal transmission of human immunodeficiency virus (HIV) to the fetus. HIV-infected mothers are advised not to breastfeed because of the presence of the virus in their milk.

Data from American Academy of Pediatrics & American College of Obstetricians and Gynecologists. (2007). *Guidelines for perinatal care* (6th ed.). Elk Grove Village, IL, and Washington, DC: Author; Cunningham, F.G., Leveno, K.J., Bloom, S.L., et al. (2010). *Williams obstetrics* (23rd ed.). New York: McGraw-Hill; Watts, D.H. (2011). Human immunodeficiency virus. In D.K. James, P.J. Steer, C.P. Weiner, et al. (Eds.), *High risk pregnancy: Management options* (4th ed., pp. 479–491). Philadelphia: Saunders.

Additional actions to prevent infant infection include cesarean birth before the onset of labor or membrane rupture, at 38 weeks of gestation. Breastfeeding is not recommended because of possible viral transmission through the milk.

***Nursing considerations.*** Testing for HIV with other laboratory studies is routine at an early prenatal visit, but the woman does have the right to opt out of this test. It is essential for the nurse to document the woman's decision to opt out. Learning of HIV infection during pregnancy can have a devastating and immobilizing effect on the entire family. Even though appropriate antiretroviral drug treatment and birth interventions can reduce risk of transmission to the infant, grief in the family is a real possibility. Anticipatory Grieving, a nursing diagnosis related to possible deaths of the mother and infant at some time in the future, should be considered. Crisis intervention may be necessary to help the family cope with a serious and unexpected diagnosis during pregnancy.

Nurses must often determine what the family perceives as the most pressing needs and worries. Some of the most common fears are loss of control, loss of support and love, social isolation, and loss of privacy. The nurse's response may involve finding ways for the woman to retain control while she is physically able and to assist her in selecting those in her family who will provide continued love and emotional support. Above all, it is necessary to reassure the woman that her right to privacy will not be violated.

Nurses can help the woman maintain the highest level of wellness possible. Adequate, high-quality nutrition decreases the risk for opportunistic infections and promotes vitality. A daily regimen should include sufficient rest and activity. It is important to avoid large crowds, traveling to areas with poor sanitation, and exposure to those with other infections. Meticulous skin care is essential, especially during recurrent herpes infections that often occur.

The woman should know that breastfeeding is contraindicated but that she can provide all other care for her infant. She will almost certainly experience a great deal of anxiety about whether the infant will be infected with HIV. Nurses need to respond honestly that testing will be required but that many infants do not get the virus if their medication regimen is followed. Moreover, nurses must reinforce information about antiretrovirals that slow maternal disease and reduce the rate of vertical transmission to the infant.

Frequently updated information for patients and professionals may be found at http://aidsinfo.nih.gov.

## Nonviral Infections

### Toxoplasmosis

Toxoplasmosis is a protozoal infection caused by *Toxoplasma gondii*. Infection is transmitted through organisms in raw or undercooked meat, through contact with infected cat feces, or across the placental barrier to the fetus if the expectant mother acquires the infection during pregnancy.

Toxoplasmosis is often subclinical; the woman may experience a few days of fatigue, muscle pains, and swollen glands but may be unaware of the disease. If infection is suspected, diagnosis can be confirmed by positive serologic test results, amplification of specific DNA sequences with PCR, identification of the parasite or its antigens, or isolation of the organism (Cunningham et al., 2014).

***Fetal and neonatal effects.*** The severity of fetal and neonatal effects secondary to toxoplasmosis varies with timing during pregnancy. Transmission of maternal infection to the fetus is highest during the third trimester. However, severe infant effects are more likely when acute infection occurs in the first trimester. Severe infant complications include chorioretinitis, hydrocephaly, microcephaly, and calcifications within the cranium.

***Therapeutic management.*** Women should be advised to use these precautions to avoid infection at any time:

- Cook meat thoroughly to an internal temperature of at least 160° F or as high as 180° F for large poultry such as whole chickens and turkeys.
- Avoid touching mucous membranes of the mouth or eyes while handling raw meat.
- Wash all kitchen surfaces that come into contact with uncooked meat.
- Do not use the same utensils or cutting board for raw meat and raw produce.
- Wash the hands thoroughly after handling raw meat.
- Avoid uncooked eggs and unpasteurized milk.
- Wash fruits and vegetables before eating.
- Do not feed house cats raw or undercooked meat.
- Avoid contact with materials that are possibly contaminated with cat feces when pregnant (cat litter boxes, sandboxes, garden soil). Wash hands well after working with soil or handling animals.

Maternal treatment of toxoplasmosis during pregnancy is essential to reduce the risk for congenital infection. Spiramycin is successfully used in Europe, Canada, and Mexico for maternal toxoplasmosis and can be used under specific guidelines from the CDC within the United States. Pyrimethamine and sulfadiazine can be added after the first trimester to reduce teratogenic effects.

### Group B Streptococcus Infection

Group B streptococcus (GBS) is a leading cause of life-threatening perinatal infections in the United States. The gram-positive bacterium colonizes the rectum, vagina, cervix, and urethra of pregnant and nonpregnant women. Approximately 10% to 30% of pregnant women are colonized with GBS in the vaginal or rectal area, but isolating the organism may be possible only intermittently. Symptomatic maternal infections such as urinary tract infection, chorioamnionitis, and endometritis can occur during pregnancy. GBS is associated with preterm rupture of membranes and preterm birth. Transmission to the newborn can result in the most serious infection (Cunningham et al., 2014).

***Fetal and neonatal effects.*** Early onset newborn GBS infection occurs during the first week after birth, often within 48 hours. Women who have GBS in the rectovaginal area at the time of birth have a 60% chance of transmitting the organism to their newborn, and approximately 1% to 2% of these infants will develop early onset GBS disease. Sepsis, pneumonia, and meningitis are the primary infections in early onset GBS disease. Late onset occurs after the first week of life through 3 months, and meningitis is the most common manifestation (Cunningham et al., 2014).

***Therapeutic management.*** Identifying women who are asymptomatic carriers of GBS is difficult because the duration of carrier status varies. Optimal identification of the GBS carrier status is obtained by vaginal-rectal culture between 35 and 37 weeks of gestation. Penicillin is the first-line agent for antibiotic treatment of the infected woman during birth if she is not allergic. Ampicillin, cefazolin, clindamycin, or erythromycin are possible alternatives.

Guidelines for testing and management are:

- GBS testing for all pregnant women at 35 to 37 weeks gestation
- Intrapartum antibiotic prophylaxis treatment for GBS infection is not required for a woman who:
- Will have a planned cesarean birth in the absence of labor or membrane rupture
- Had a positive culture in a previous pregnancy, but the current pregnancy is GBS negative
- Has a negative GBS culture in later gestation
- Intrapartum antibiotic prophylaxis is indicated for GBS if
- Previous infant had GBS infection
- GBS bacteriuria this pregnancy
- Positive GBS screening current pregnancy unless woman with planned cesarean has labor or membrane rupture
- Unknown GBS status and delivery at 37 weeks or less of gestation; membrane rupture at 18 hours or later; or intrapartum temperature at 100.4° F (38° C) or higher

### Tuberculosis

Tuberculosis (TB) results from infection by *Mycobacterium tuberculosis*. It is transmitted by aerosolized droplets of liquid containing the bacterium that are inhaled by a noninfected individual and taken into the lungs. Initially, most individuals are asymptomatic until a critical number of organisms replicates in the lungs. Women obtaining prenatal care should be screened for TB. This screening involves an intradermal injection of mycobacterial protein (purified protein derivative [PPD]). If the reaction is positive, the woman's abdomen should be protected by a lead shield while a radiograph is taken of her chest. The diagnosis is confirmed by isolating and identifying the bacterium in the sputum.

Symptomatic individuals have general malaise, fatigue, loss of appetite, weight loss, and fever. These symptoms occur in the late afternoon and evening and are accompanied by night sweats. As the disease progresses, a chronic cough develops and mucopurulent sputum is produced.

Pregnant women from high-frequency areas of Asia, Africa, Mexico, and Central America have an increased frequency of TB. Women with HIV have a greater likelihood of a positive tuberculin test (Cunningham et al., 2014).

***Fetal and neonatal effects.*** Although perinatal infection is rare, it can be acquired as the fetus aspirates infected amniotic fluid or is exposed through the umbilical vein. The diagnosis is made by finding the bacilli in a gastric aspirate of the neonate or in placental tissue. Signs of congenital TB include failure to thrive, lethargy, respiratory distress, fever, and enlargement of the spleen, liver, and lymph nodes. If the mother remains untreated, the newborn is at high risk for acquiring TB by inhalation of infectious respiratory droplets from the mother (see Box 26.3) (Cunningham et al., 2014).

***Therapeutic management.*** Multidrug therapy is used to protect the woman and her fetus. Drug management for the woman with latent TB is isoniazid and pyridoxine during pregnancy and postpartum. Active disease should be treated more aggressively with a combination of isoniazid, rifampin, and ethambutol during pregnancy. Streptomycin should not be used during pregnancy because of adverse fetal effects. Women with active TB should be on respiratory isolation.

Management of the infant born to a mother with TB involves preventing the disease or treating early infection. Breastfeeding is not contraindicated. Prevention focuses on teaching family members how the disease is transmitted so that they can protect the infant from airborne organisms. The infant should be skin tested at birth and may be started on preventive isoniazid therapy. Skin testing should be repeated at 3 to 4 months. Isoniazid is usually continued for at least 9 months. Infant TB medication may stop if the mother and family members are well treated and show no additional disease. If the skin test result converts to positive, a full course of drug therapy should be given.

For additional information regarding medical conditions and their effect on pregnancy, see Table 26.3.

**TABLE 26.3 Medical Conditions and Their Effect on Pregnancy**

| Condition | Maternal-Fetal Effects | Nursing Considerations |
|---|---|---|
| **Appendicitis** | | |
| Inflammation of the appendix, often with fever. The most common nongynecologic surgical emergency during pregnancy. | Difficult to diagnose during pregnancy. Early symptoms mimic common conditions of pregnancy. Ultrasonography may help rule out other diagnoses such as ectopic pregnancy. | When reasonable doubt exists that the patient has appendicitis, the appendix should be removed to prevent rupture and consequent complications. The location often is altered by the growing uterus. |
| **Asthma** | | |
| An obstructive lung disease caused by airway inflammation. Characterized by dyspnea, cough, wheezing. Course in pregnancy is variable. | Effective therapy and avoidance of severe attacks are associated with a good pregnancy outcome. Medications used are well tolerated in pregnancy and appear to be safe for the fetus. Breastfeeding is safe for the newborn and can reduce the risk for allergies. | Early use of antiinflammatory agents such as inhaled corticosteroids, such as beclomethasone, can prevent severe attacks. Cromolyn sodium and nedocromil sodium are effective but require more time to become effective than inhaled corticosteroids. Bronchodilators such as theophylline and inhaled beta-agonists may be required. |
| **Glucose-6-Phosphate Dehydrogenase Deficiency** | | |
| Female-linked genetic disorder that predisposes to lysis of red blood cells when exposed to oxidizing drugs (salicylates, acetaminophen, phenacetin, and some sulfa drugs) and ingestion of fava beans in some people. | Not affected by pregnancy unless complicated by anemia. Iron and folic acid supplementation is recommended. Newborn males have a higher incidence of severe jaundice. | Advise woman of risks and suggest she consult with her healthcare provider for recommended list of drugs for minor discomforts. |
| **Hyperthyroidism** | | |
| An overactive, enlarged thyroid gland. Difficult to diagnose and manage during pregnancy because the normal changes of pregnancy increase the metabolic rate and mimic hyperthyroidism. Graves' disease is the most common cause during pregnancy. Treatment ideally begins before pregnancy. | Increased incidence of hypertension such as preeclampsia and postpartum hemorrhage if not well controlled during pregnancy. Treatment is complicated by the presence of the fetus, which may be jeopardized by surgery or antithyroid medications. Propylthiouracil has limited placental transfer and is widely used during pregnancy to control thyroid function. Additional drugs such as iodides and beta blockers may be needed, particularly in a thyroid crisis. | Be aware of the major signs that should be reported. These include a resting pulse rate greater than 100 bpm, loss of weight or failure to gain weight in spite of normal intake of food, heat intolerance, and abnormal protrusion of the eyes (exophthalmos). |
| **Hypothyroidism** | | |
| Characterized by inadequate thyroid secretion; confirmed by an elevated level of thyroid-stimulating hormone and low levels of triiodothyronine and thyroxine. | Women with hypothyroidism have a higher incidence of preeclampsia, abruptio placentae, and low-birth-weight or stillborn infants. If the pregnant woman is untreated, there is an increased risk of neonatal goiter and congenital hypothyroidism; severity of symptoms depends on time of onset and severity of the deprivation but can include neurologic deficits. Treatment is with levothyroxine. | Suspect neonatal hypothyroidism when the infant is large for gestational age, with respiratory and feeding difficulties, rough and dry skin, and an umbilical hernia. |

**TABLE 26.3 Medical Conditions and Their Effect on Pregnancy—cont'd**

| Condition | Maternal-Fetal Effects | Nursing Considerations |
|---|---|---|
| **Maternal Phenylketonuria (PKU)** | | |
| Inherited single-gene recessive defect leading to an inability to metabolize essential amino acid phenylalanine, resulting in high serum levels of phenylalanine. Irreparable intellectual disability of the fetus occurs if the pregnant woman is not treated early with a diet that provides adequate protein but restricts phenylalanine. | The woman must be on a low-phenylalanine diet before conception and pregnancy. If not, the fetal risk for microcephaly, intellectual disability, heart defects, and intrauterine growth restriction increases. | The child either will be a carrier of the gene or inherit the disease, depending on the presence of the gene in the father of the child. Special low-phenylalanine foods are expensive, but they may be obtained through the state's Supplemental Food program for Women, Infants, and Children (WIC) or Medicaid, or may be covered by insurance. |

*bpm,* beats per minute

## KEY CONCEPTS

- Episodes of hypoglycemia may occur during the first 20 weeks of pregnancy with increased insulin release. Levels of placental hormones rise sharply after 20 weeks and create resistance to insulin in maternal cells and changes in maternal insulin needs throughout pregnancy.
- Women with type 1 diabetes mellitus have a greater risk for preeclampsia, urinary tract infections, and ketosis.
- Because maternal hyperglycemia during the first trimester increases the risk for congenital anomalies in the fetus, a major goal of management is to establish normal blood glucose levels before conception.
- Fetal growth depends on the condition of maternal blood vessels and blood glucose levels. With no vascular impairment and adequate placental perfusion, the infant is likely to be of normal size with normal maternal glucose levels or large (i.e., having macrosomia) with high maternal glucose levels. With high maternal glucose levels and vascular impairment, placental perfusion may be compromised, and the fetus may be growth restricted.
- In addition to congenital anomalies, the infant of a diabetic mother is at increased risk for hypoglycemia, hypocalcemia, hyperbilirubinemia, and respiratory distress syndrome.
- The maternal effects of GDM include increased risks for urinary tract infections, hydramnios, premature rupture of membranes, and the development of preeclampsia.
- GDM is responsible for two major complications for the fetus or neonate—fetal macrosomia and neonatal hypoglycemia.
- GDM can usually be treated by diet and exercise. Insulin may be started if blood glucose remains high.
- Cardiovascular changes that occur in normal pregnancy impose an additional burden that may result in cardiac decompensation if the expectant mother has preexisting heart disease.
- The primary goal of pregnancy management of heart disease is to prevent the development of congestive heart failure. Limiting the woman's activity, weight gain, and preventing anemia and infection helps keep cardiac demand below cardiac reserves.
- Intrapartum and postpartum management of heart disease focuses on preventing fluid overload, which can cause a sharp rise in cardiac effort.
- Iron supplementation is needed during pregnancy because most women do not have sufficient iron stores to meet the demands of pregnancy.
- Folic acid deficiency is associated with an increased risk for spontaneous abortion, abruptio placentae, and fetal anomalies, such as neural tube defects. A folic acid supplement may be necessary to prevent maternal and fetal effects.
- Sickle cell disease is worsened by pregnancy changes, and a primary goal is to prevent sickle cell crisis during pregnancy.
- Laboratory values for thalassemia are similar to those of iron deficiency, but administration of iron is risky because increased iron absorption and storage make the woman susceptible to iron overload.
- Although women with SLE can have a normal pregnancy and give birth to a normal newborn, the pregnancy must be treated as high risk because of the increased incidence of abortion, fetal death during the first trimester, and possible exacerbation of the disease.
- APS is a cluster of clinical entities and is associated with an increased risk for thrombosis, fetal loss, and low platelets. Preeclampsia has a higher incidence in the woman with APS.
- The management of epilepsy is complicated by the teratogenic effects of anticonvulsant medications. Alterations in epilepsy therapy may be possible to reduce teratogenic effects on the fetus.
- Viral infections that occur during pregnancy can be transmitted to the fetus in two ways: across the placenta or by exposure to organisms during birth. Although they are mild or even subclinical in the mother, viral infections can have serious effects for the fetus.
- HIV is a retrovirus that gradually causes a decrease in the effectiveness of the maternal immunity, often over many years in the treated woman. Maternal treatment with ZDV and other antiretroviral medications can substantially reduce the risk of fetal infection with HIV.
- The newborn should be started on ZDV 6 to 12 hours after birth. The mother will be continued on previous antiretroviral therapy, or maternal therapy may be delayed until her CD4 levels decline to less than 500 to 600 cells/mm$^3$.
- Specific pregnancy and postbirth treatment of nonviral infections such as toxoplasmosis, group B streptococcus infection, and TB reduce long-term maternal and newborn complications.

## REFERENCES AND READINGS


AIDSinfo/National Institutes of Health (2012). *HIV and pregnancy*. Retrieved from http://www.aidsinfo.nih.gov.

AIDSinfo/National Institutes of Health (2015). *Recommendations for use of antiretroviral drugs in pregnant HIV-1-infected women for maternal health and interventions to reduce perinatal HIV transmission in the United States*. Retrieved from http://www.aidsinfo.nih.gov.

American Academy of Pediatrics & American College of Obstetricians and Gynecologists. (2013). *Guidelines for perinatal care* (8th ed.). Elk Grove Village, IL, and Washington, DC: Author.

American College of Obstetricians and Gynecologists. (2013). *Inherited thrombophilias in pregnancy. (ACOG Practice Bulletin No. 138)*. Washington, DC: Author.

American College of Obstetricians and Gynecologists. (2014). *Management of herpes in pregnancy (ACOG Practice Bulletin No. 82)*. Washington, DC: Author.

American College of Obstetricians and Gynecologists. (2014). *Viral hepatitis in pregnancy (ACOG Practice Bulletin No. 86)*. Washington, DC: Author.

American College of Obstetricians and Gynecologists. (2014). *Pregestational diabetes (ACOG Practice Bulletin No. 60)*. Washington, DC: Author.

American College of Obstetricians and Gynecologists. (2015). *Nausea and vomiting of pregnancy (ACOG Practice Bulletin No. 153)*. Washington, DC: Author.

American College of Obstetricians and Gynecologists. (2015). *Anemia in pregnancy. (ACOG Practice Bulletin No. 95)*. Washington, DC: Author.

American College of Obstetricians and Gynecologists. (2015). *Gestational diabetes mellitus (ACOG Practice Bulletin No. 137)*. Washington, DC: Author.

American College of Obstetricians and Gynecologists. (2015). *Cytomegalovirus, parvovirus B19, varicella zoster, and toxoplasmosis in pregnancy. (ACOG Practice Bulletin No. 151)*. Washington, DC: Author.

American College of Obstetricians and Gynecologists. (2015). *Antiphospholipid syndrome. (ACOG Practice Bulletin No. 132)*. Washington, DC: Author.

American Diabetes Association (2015). Management of diabetes in pregnancy. *Diabetes Care, 38*(1), S77–79.

Andrews, J.I. (2011). Hepatitis viral infections. In D.K. James, P.J. Steer, & C.P. Weiner (Eds.), *High risk pregnancy: Management options* (4th ed., pp. 469–477). Philadelphia: Saunders.

Arslaneum-Engoren, C. (2011). Women's risk factors and screening for coronary heart disease. *Journal of Obstetric, Gynecologic, and Neonatal Nursing, 40*(3), 337–347.

Berggren, E.K., Boggess, K.A., Stuebe, A.M., Funk, M.J. (2011). National Diabetes Data Group versus Carpenter-Coustan Criteria to Diagnose Gestational Diabetes. *The American Journal of Obstetrics and Gynecology, 205*(3), 253.e1–253.e7.

Centers for Disease Control and Prevention. (2012). Prevention of perinatal group B streptococcal disease: Revised guidelines from CDC, 2010. Retrieved from *MMWR: Morbidity and Mortality Weekly Report, 59*(RR-10) http://www.cdc.gov/mmwr.

Centers for Disease Control and Prevention. (2014). *Vaccines for pregnant women*. Retrieved from http://www.cdc.gov.

Centers for Disease Control and Prevention. (2015). *Sexually transmitted diseases treatment guidelines, 2015*. Retrieved from http://www.cdc.gov/mmwr.

Centers for Disease Control and Prevention. (2015). *HIV among women*. Retrieved from http://www.cdc.gov/hiv.

Centers for Disease Control and Prevention. (2015). *Recommended adult immunization schedule—United States, 2015*. Retrieved from http://www.cdc.gov/vaccines/schedules/dowloads/adult/adult-schedule.pdf.

Cirillo, P.M., & Cohn, B.A. (2015). Pregnancy complications and cardiovascular disease death: 50-year follow-up of the Child Health and Development Studies pregnancy cohort. *Circulation, 132*(13), 1234–1242.

Cunningham, F., Leveno, K., Bloom, S., Spong, C., & Dash, L. (2014). *Williams obstetrics* (24th ed.). New York: McGraw-Hill.

DeVon, H.A., Saban, K.L., & Garrett, D.K. (2011). Recognizing and responding to symptoms of acute coronary syndromes and stroke in women. *Journal of Obstetric, Gynecologic, and Neonatal Nursing, 40*(3), 372–382.

Erick, M. (2012). Nutrition during pregnancy and lactation. In L.K. Mahan, & S. Escott-Stump (Eds.), *Krause's food, nutrition, and diet therapy* (13th ed., pp. 340–374). Philadelphia: Saunders.

Franz, M. (2012). Medical nutrition therapy for diabetes mellitus and hypoglycemia of nondiabetic origin. In L.K. Mahan, & S. Escott-Stump (Eds.), *Krause's food, nutrition, and diet therapy* (13th ed., pp. 675–710). Philadelphia: Saunders.

Gilbert, E.S. (2011). *Manual of high risk pregnancy & delivery* (5th ed.). St. Louis: Mosby.

Hartling, L., Dryden, D.M., Guthrie, A., Muise, M., Vandermeer, B., Donovan, L. (2014). Benefits and harms of treating gestational diabetes mellitus: a systematic review and meta-analysis for the U.S. Preventive Services Task Force and the National Institutes of Health Office of Medical Applications of Research. *Annals of Internal Medicine, 159*(2), 123–9.

McSweeney, J.C., Pettey, C.M., & Souder, E. (2011). Disparities in women's cardiovascular health. *Journal of Obstetric, Gynecologic, and Neonatal Nursing, 40*(3), 362–371.

Moore, T. R., & Catalano, P. (2009). Diabetes in pregnancy. In R. K. Creasy, R. Resnik, J. D. Iams, et al. (Eds.), *Creasy & Resnik's maternal-fetal medicine: Principles and practice* (6th ed., pp. 953–993). Philadelphia: Saunders.

National Institutes of Health: National Heart, Lung, and Blood Institute. (2001). *Report of the working group on research on hypertension during pregnancy*. Retrieved from http://www.nhlbi.nih.gov.

National Institutes of Health: National Heart, Lung, and Blood Institute. (2014). *Evidence-based management of sickle cell disease: Expert panel report, 2014*. Retrieved from http://www.nhlbi.nih.gov.

National Institutes of Health: National Institute of Arthritis and Musculoskeletal and Skin Diseases. (2015). *Handout on health: Systemic lupus erythematosus*. Retrieved from http://www.nhlbi.nih.gov.

Pagana, K.D., & Pagana, T.J. (2011). *Mosby's diagnostic and laboratory test reference* (10th ed.). St. Louis: Mosby.

Savitz, D.A., Danilack, V.A., Elston, B., & Lipkind, H.S. (2014). Pregnancy-induced hypertension and diabetes and the risk of cardiovascular disease, stroke, and diabetes hospitalization in the year following delivery. *American Journal of Epidemiology, 180*(1), 41–44.

Scifres, C., Feghali, M., Althouse, A.D., Caritis, S., & Catov, J. (2015). Adverse Outcomes and Potential Targets for Intervention in Gestational Diabetes and Obesity. *Obstetrics & Gynecology, 126*(2), 316–325.

Simpson, K.R. (2011). Diabetes in pregnancy: To screen or not to screen. *MCN: The American Journal of Maternal/Child Nursing, 36*(1), 72.

Viana, L.V., Gross, J.L., & Azevedo, M.J. (2014). Dietary intervention in patients with gestational diabetes mellitus: a systematic review and meta-analysis of randomized clinical trials on maternal and newborn outcomes. *Diabetes Care, 37*(12), 3345–3355.

27

# The Woman With an Intrapartum Complication

http://evolve.elsevier.com/McKinney/mat-ch/

## LEARNING OBJECTIVES

*After studying this chapter, you should be able to:*

- Explain abnormalities that may result in dysfunctional labor.
- Describe maternal and fetal risks associated with the premature rupture of the membranes.
- Analyze factors that increase a woman's risk for preterm labor.
- Explain maternal and fetal problems that may occur if pregnancy persists beyond 42 weeks.
- Describe common intrapartum emergencies.
- Explain the therapeutic management of each intrapartum complication.
- Apply the nursing process to the care of women with intrapartum complications and to their families.

Birth is usually free of major complications. However, sometimes complications make childbearing hazardous for the woman or her baby. The nurse's challenge is to identify and manage the complications promptly and to provide effective care for these mothers while supporting the entire family at this significant time in their lives.

## DYSFUNCTIONAL LABOR

Normal labor is characterized by progress. Dysfunctional labor is one that does not result in the normal progress of cervical effacement, dilation, and fetal descent. Dystocia is a general term that describes any difficult labor or birth. A dysfunctional labor results from problems with the powers of labor, the passenger, the passage, the psyche, or a combination of these. Dysfunctional labor is often prolonged but may be unusually short and intense. Combined medical and nursing care is indicated for the care of the woman having dysfunctional labor (Cunningham et al., 2014; ACOG, 2010; Simpson & Obrien-Abel, 2013).

An operative birth (vacuum extractor- or forceps-assisted or cesarean) may be needed if dysfunctional labor does not resolve or if fetal or maternal compromise occurs. Signs that indicate the need for an operative birth include persistent nonreassuring fetal heart rate (FHR) patterns (see Chapter 17), fetal acidosis, and meconium passage. Maternal exhaustion or infection can occur, especially during long labors (Cunningham et al., 2014).

### Problems of the Powers

The powers of labor may not be adequate to expel the fetus because of ineffective contractions or ineffective maternal pushing efforts.

#### Ineffective Contractions

Effective uterine activity is characterized by coordinated contractions that are strong and numerous enough to propel the fetus past the resistance of the woman's bony pelvis and soft tissues. It is not possible to say how frequent, long, or strong labor contractions must be. One woman's labor may progress with contractions that would be inadequate for another woman. Possible causes of ineffective contractions include:

- Maternal fatigue
- Maternal inactivity
- Fluid and electrolyte imbalance
- Hypoglycemia
- Excessive analgesia or anesthesia
- Maternal catecholamines secreted in response to stress or pain
- Disproportion between the maternal pelvis and the fetal presenting part
- Uterine overdistention, as with multiple gestation or hydramnios (excess amniotic fluid; also called *polyhydramnios*)

Two patterns of ineffective uterine contractions are hypotonic and hypertonic dysfunction (Table 27.1). Hypotonic dysfunction is more common than hypertonic. Characteristics and management of each are different, but the result—poor labor progress—is the same if they persist.

***Hypotonic labor dysfunction.*** Hypotonic contractions are coordinated but too weak to be effective. They are infrequent and brief, and the abdomen can be easily indented with fingertip pressure at the peak.

Hypotonic dysfunction or secondary arrest usually occurs during the active phase of labor, when progress normally quickens. Uterine overdistention is associated with hypotonic dysfunction because the stretched uterine muscle contracts poorly.

The woman may be fairly comfortable because her contractions are weak. However, persistent hypotonic dysfunction is fatiguing and frustrating for the mother. Fetal hypoxia is not usually seen with hypotonic labor.

Management depends on the cause. Providing intravenous (IV) or oral fluids corrects maternal fluid and electrolyte imbalances or hypoglycemia. Maternal position changes, particularly upright positions, including walking or showering, favor fetal descent and promote effective contractions. The woman who moves about actively typically has better labor progress and is more comfortable than one who remains in one position. Pain management techniques such as epidural block can have outcomes that reduce contraction effectiveness, requiring interventions specific to that factor. On the other hand, effective pain management can improve the progress of labor.

The nurse should use therapeutic communication to help the woman identify anxieties or beliefs about labor and its progress.

**TABLE 27.1 Patterns of Labor Dysfunction**

| Hypotonic Dysfunction | Hypertonic Dysfunction |
|---|---|
| **Contractions** | |
| Coordinated but weak.<br>Become less frequent and shorter in duration.<br>Easily indented at peak.<br>Woman may have minimal discomfort because the contractions are weak. | Uncoordinated, irregular.<br>Short and poor intensity, but painful and cramp like. |
| **Uterine Resting Tone** | |
| Not elevated. | Higher than normal. Important to distinguish from abruptio placentae, which has similar characteristics (see p. 531). |
| **Phase of Labor** | |
| Active. Typically occurs after 4 cm dilation.<br>More common than hypertonic dysfunction. | Latent. Usually occurs before 4 cm dilation.<br>Less common than hypotonic dysfunction. |
| **Therapeutic Management** | |
| Amniotomy (increases the risk of infection).<br>Oxytocin augmentation.<br>Cesarean birth if no progress. | Correct cause if it can be identified.<br>Light sedation to promote rest.<br>Hydration.<br>Tocolytics to reduce high uterine tone and promote placental perfusion. |
| **Nursing Care** | |
| Interventions related to amniotomy and oxytocin augmentation.<br>Encourage position changes. An abdominal binder may help direct the fetus toward the mother's pelvis if her abdominal wall is very lax.<br>Ambulation if no contraindication and if acceptable to the woman.<br>Emotional support: Allow her to express feelings of discouragement. Explain measures taken to increase effectiveness of contractions. Include her partner or family in emotional support measures because they may have anxiety that will heighten the woman's anxiety. | Promote uterine blood flow: side-lying position.<br>Promote rest, general comfort, and relaxation.<br>Pain relief.<br>Emotional support: Accept the reality of the woman's pain and frustration. Reassure her that she is not being childish. Explain reason for measures to break abnormal labor patterns and their goal or expected results. Allow her to ventilate her feelings during and after labor. Include partner or family (see Hypotonic Labor Dysfunction). |

Helping her to get her anxieties out in the open is the first step to managing them effectively so that the stress response does not slow her labor (Simpson & Obrien-Abel, 2013).

Some women need measures such as amniotomy or oxytocin infusion to promote labor progress. The birth attendant evaluates the woman's labor to confirm that she is having hypotonic active labor rather than a long latent phase (approximately the first 3 cm of dilation) of labor. The maternal pelvis and fetal presentation and position are assessed to identify problems.

Amniotomy or oxytocin augmentation (see Chapter 19) can be used to stimulate a labor that slows after it is established. Reduced placental perfusion caused by excessive uterine contractions is the most common risk of oxytocin labor augmentation (Cunningham et al., 2014).

***Hypertonic labor dysfunction.*** Hypertonic dysfunction of labor is less common than hypotonic. Contractions are uncoordinated and erratic in their frequency, duration, and intensity. The contractions are painful but ineffective. Hypertonic dysfunction usually occurs during the latent phase of labor.

The uterine resting tone between contractions is high, reducing uterine blood flow. This ischemia decreases fetal oxygen supply and causes the woman to have almost constant cramping pain. Because high resting tone and constant pain are also seen in abruptio placentae (premature separation of the normally implanted placenta), this complication should be considered as well.

The mother becomes very tired because of long yet nonproductive discomfort. She may lose confidence in her ability to cope with labor and give birth. Frustration and anxiety further reduce her pain tolerance and interfere with normal processes of labor. The nurse should accept her frustration and discomfort. It is important not to equate cervical dilation with the amount of pain a woman "should" experience (Simpson & Obrien-Abel, 2013).

Management of hypertonic labor depends on the cause. Relief of pain is the primary intervention to promote a normal labor pattern. Warm showers or baths promote relaxation and rest, often allowing a normal labor pattern to ensue. Systemic analgesics for therapeutic rest or epidural analgesia may be needed to achieve this goal.

Oxytocin is not usually given because it can intensify the already high uterine resting tone. However, administration of a very low dose of oxytocin sometimes promotes the coordination of uterine contractions. Amniotomy may be performed if the hypertonic contractions occur in active labor. Tocolytic drugs (inhibit uterine contractions) can reduce uterine resting tone and improve placental blood flow (Cunningham et al., 2014).

### Ineffective Maternal Pushing

A reflex urge to push with contractions usually occurs as the fetal presenting part reaches the pelvic floor during second-stage labor. Ineffective pushing can result from:

- Use of incorrect pushing techniques or inefficient pushing positions
- Fear of injury because of pain and tearing sensations felt by the mother when she pushes
- Minimal or absent urge to push

- Maternal exhaustion
- Regional block analgesia that may suppress the woman's urge to push
- Psychological unreadiness to "let go" of her baby

Management focuses on correcting the causes contributing to ineffective pushing. If maternal and fetal vital signs are normal, there is no maximum allowable duration for the second stage. Each woman is evaluated individually by her birth attendant to determine whether labor should be ended with an operative delivery or can continue safely (see Chapter 16). Nursing care to promote effective pushing helps the mother make each effort productive. Upright positions such as squatting add the force of gravity to her efforts. Semi-sitting, side-lying, and pushing while sitting on the toilet are other options. Regional analgesia methods can restrict possible maternal positions and alter a woman's spontaneous urge to push. On the other hand, women who have regional pain management often feel an adequate urge to push that is not complicated by excess pain (Graseck, Tuuli, Roehl, et al., 2014).

The woman who fears injury because of the sensations she feels when she pushes may respond to accurate information about the process of fetal descent. If she understands that sensations of tearing often accompany fetal descent but that her tissues can expand to accommodate the baby, she may be more willing to push with contractions.

The woman who is exhausted may push more effectively if she is encouraged to rest until she feels the urge. Encouraging her to push with intermittent contractions, such as every other contraction, also allows her to maintain adequate pushing effort. Oral or IV fluids provide energy for the strenuous work of second-stage labor. Reassuring the woman if there is no apparent fetal or maternal harm to a prolonged second stage may encourage her. Remind her that there is progress as the baby moves down through the pelvis even if the mother is not pushing for a period of time (Graseck et al., 2014).

## Problems With the Passenger

Fetal problems associated with dysfunctional labor are those related to:

- Fetal size
- Fetal presentation or position
- Multifetal pregnancy
- Fetal anomalies

These variations can cause mechanical problems and contribute to ineffective contractions.

### Fetal Size

**Macrosomia.** The macrosomic infant weighs more than 4000 g (8 lb, 13 oz) at birth, although some authorities define it as a weight of 4500 g (9 lb, 15 oz) or greater. The head or shoulders may not be able to adapt to the pelvis, known as *cephalopelvic,* or fetopelvic, *disproportion* (CPD). In addition, distention of the uterus by the large fetus reduces the strength of contractions both during and after birth.

However, size is relative. The woman with a small pelvis or one that is abnormally shaped may not be able to deliver an average-size or small infant. A woman with a large pelvis may easily give birth to an infant heavier than 4000 g. Fetal position as the baby descends through the pelvis is another important factor in terms of fetal size and maternal pelvic size (Dennedy & Dunne, 2013).

**Shoulder dystocia.** Delayed or difficult birth of the shoulders can occur as they become impacted above the maternal symphysis pubis. As soon as the head is born, it retracts against the perineum, much like a turtle's head drawing into its shell ("turtle sign"). Failure of the shoulders to complete external rotation is another sign (see Fig. 16.12). Nursing interventions to help rotate the fetal head and promote descent also can help prevent shoulder dystocia (Simpson & Obrien-Abel, 2013).

Shoulder dystocia is unpredictable and can occur in a baby of any weight. This complication requires urgent intervention by available physicians, midwives, nurses, anesthesia personnel, and neonatology staff because the umbilical cord is compressed, and chest compression within the vagina prevents respirations. Any of several methods can be used to relieve the impacted fetal shoulders quickly (Fig. 27.1). The infant's clavicles should be checked for crepitus, deformity, or bruising, each of which suggests fracture. Nerve injury to the brachial plexus, or Erb's palsy, can cause flaccid muscle tone on the affected side. Most cases of Erb's palsy resolve in a few weeks, but exercises and physical therapy can be started in the immediate postbirth period (Cunningham et al., 2014; Graseck et al., 2014).

### Abnormal Fetal Presentation or Position

An unfavorable fetal presentation or position can interfere with cervical dilation or fetal descent.

**Rotation abnormalities.** Persistence of the fetus in the occiput posterior (OP) or occiput transverse (OT) position can contribute to dysfunctional labor and possible shoulder dystocia. These positions delay fetal descent and other mechanisms of labor (cardinal movements). Most fetuses in an OP position during early labor rotate spontaneously to an occiput anterior position while descending through the pelvis, promoting normal extension and expulsion of the head. Some women with a large pelvis relative to the fetal size may be able to deliver their fetus in the OP position.

Labor is usually longer and more uncomfortable when the fetus is in the OP or OT position. Intense back or leg pain that is poorly relieved with analgesics makes it difficult for the woman to cope with labor. "Back labor" aptly describes the sensations a woman feels when her fetus is in the OP position (Cunningham et al., 2014; Graseck et al., 2014).

Maternal position changes promote fetal head rotation to an occiput anterior position and fetal descent (see Chapter 16). Examples are:

- Hands and knees. Rocking the pelvis back and forth while on hands and knees encourages rotation.
- Side-lying (on her left side if the fetus is in a right OP position and on her right side for a left OP position).
- The lunge, in which the mother places one foot on a chair with her foot and knee pointed to that side. She lunges sideways repeatedly during a contraction for 5 seconds at a time. This action can also be performed in a kneeling position.
- Squatting (for second-stage labor).
- Sitting, kneeling, or standing while leaning forward.

Using a birthing ball—a large plastic ball capable of supporting an adult's weight—helps support the woman when in the hands-and-knees position. She can also sit on it, providing many of the benefits of squatting. In addition, the woman tends to move her hips back and forth, favoring fetal descent.

### CRITICAL THINKING EXERCISE 27.1

A woman having her first baby has been in labor for several hours. Her nurse-midwife performs a vaginal examination and says that the cervix is dilated 6 cm and completely effaced, with the fetus in the right occiput posterior position. The mother is having persistent back pain that worsens during contractions.

1. How should the nurse interpret this information?
2. Should the nurse take any specific action based on the examination?

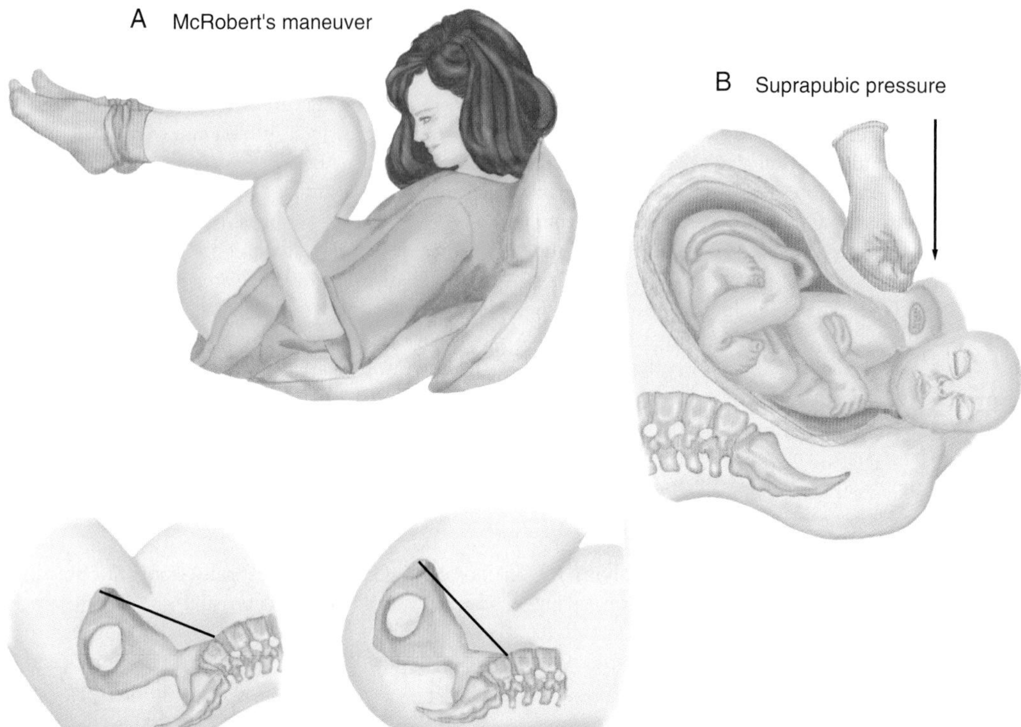


**FIG 27.1** Methods used to relieve shoulder dystocia. **A,** McRoberts maneuver. The woman flexes her thighs sharply against her abdomen, which straightens the pelvic curve. A supported squat has a similar effect and adds gravity to her pushing efforts. **B,** Suprapubic pressure by an assistant pushes the fetal anterior shoulder downward to displace it from above the mother's symphysis pubis. Fundal pressure should not be used because it will push the anterior shoulder more firmly against the mother's symphysis.

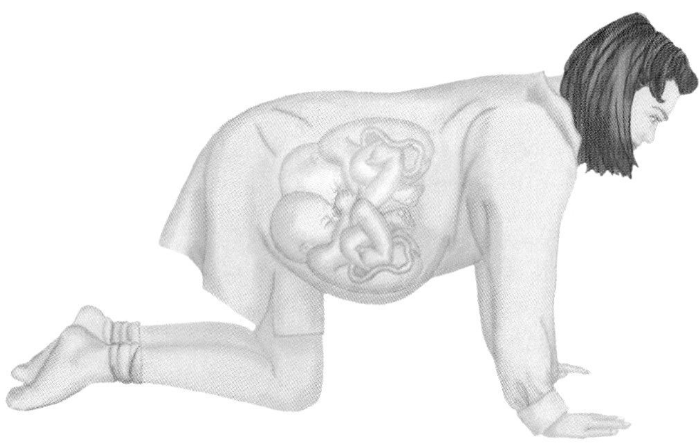

**FIG 27.2** A hands-and-knees position helps the fetus rotate from a left occiput posterior (LOP) position to an occiput anterior position.

Upright maternal positions promote descent, which is usually accompanied by fetal head rotation. The hands-and-knees and the side-lying positions promote rotation because the mother's abdomen is dependent in relation to her spine. The convex surface of the fetal back tends to rotate toward the convex anterior uterus, similar to nesting two spoons together (Fig. 27.2). Moreover, these positions decrease the mother's discomfort by reducing fetal head pressure on her sacrum. A side-lying position has a similar effect.

The lunge widens the side of the pelvis toward which the woman lunges. If the fetal position is known, she lunges toward the side where the occiput is located (Fig. 27.3). If the fetal position is not known, the woman can lunge toward the side that gives her greater comfort.

All variations of the squatting position aid rotation and fetal descent by straightening the pelvic curve and enlarging the pelvic outlet. They also add gravity to the force of maternal pushing.

If spontaneous rotation does not occur, the physician may assist rotation and descent of the head with a vacuum extractor or forceps. Some types of vacuum extractors cannot be applied to the fetal head when it remains in an OP position. Cesarean birth may be needed if forceps or vacuum extractor use is not successful.

***Deflexion abnormalities.*** The poorly flexed fetal head presents a larger diameter to the pelvis than if flexed with the chin on the chest (see Fig. 16.8). In the *face presentation,* the head diameter is similar to that of the vertex presentation, but the maternal pelvis can be traversed only if the fetal chin (mentum) is anterior.

***Breech presentation.*** Cervical dilation and effacement are often slower when the fetus is in a breech presentation because the buttocks or feet do not form a smooth, round dilating wedge like the head. The greatest fetal risk is that the head—the largest fetal part—is last to be born. By the time the lower body is born, the umbilical cord is well into the pelvis and may be compressed. The shoulders, arms, and head must be delivered quickly so that the infant can breathe.

A breech presentation is common well before term, but only 3% to 4% of term fetuses remain in this presentation. Most breech births in North America are by cesarean, but a surgical birth does not eliminate all problems associated with breech birth, which may include:

- Fetal injury, particularly with a difficult vaginal birth
- Prolapsed umbilical cord

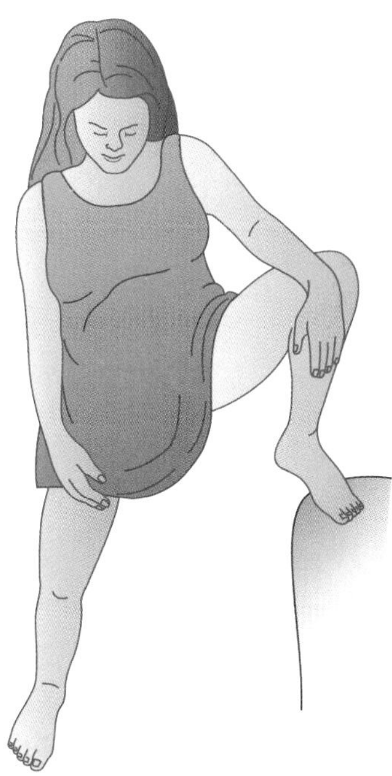

FIG 27.3 The "lunge" to one side promotes rotation of the fetal occiput from a posterior position to an anterior one.

- Low birth weight as a result of preterm gestation, multifetal pregnancy, or intrauterine growth restriction
- Fetal anomalies contributing to the breech presentation, such as hydrocephalus
- Complications secondary to placenta previa (implantation of the placenta in the lower uterus, at or very near the cervical os) or cesarean birth

*External cephalic version (ECV)* may be attempted to change the fetus in a breech presentation or transverse lie to a cephalic presentation (see Chapter 19). If the fetus remains in the abnormal presentation, cesarean birth is recommended to avoid complications of a difficult vaginal birth if the woman is not in active labor. A woman who first enters the labor unit in advanced active labor may have a fetus remaining in a breech presentation and perhaps a very immature fetus. In such cases, ECV is not always possible, and vaginal birth may be necessary simply because labor ends very quickly (Cunningham et al., 2014)).

### Multifetal Pregnancy

Multifetal pregnancy, also known as multiple gestation, can result in dysfunctional labor because of uterine overdistention, which contributes to hypotonic dysfunction, and abnormal presentation of one or both fetuses (Fig. 27.4). In addition, the potential for fetal hypoxia during labor is greater. The risk of postpartum hemorrhage resulting from uterine atony because of uterine overdistention is greater (ACOG, 2014).

Because of these problems, birth for a woman with a twin pregnancy is often cesarean, although vaginal birth is common also. Pregnancies with more than two fetuses are most often delivered by cesarean if the gestation is viable. The physician considers fetal presentations, maternal pelvic size, and the presence of other complications, such as hypertension, as well as the multiple fetuses (ACOG, 2014).

During labor, each twin's FHR is monitored separately. When in bed, the woman should remain in a lateral position to promote adequate placental blood flow. After vaginal birth of the first twin, assessment of the second twin's FHR continues until birth. The nurse observes for signs of hypotonic dysfunction throughout labor and for uterine atony, often related to the overdistended uterus, after birth.

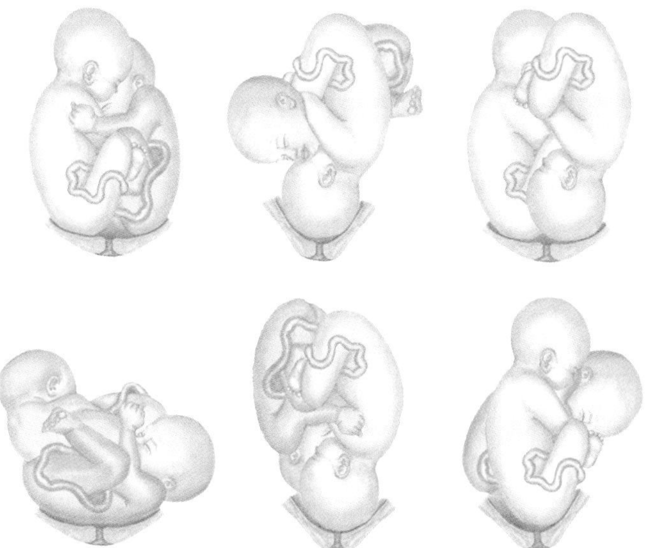

FIG 27.4 Twins can present in any combination of presentations and positions.

Whether the birth is vaginal or cesarean, the intrapartum staff must be prepared for the care and possible resuscitation of multiple infants as with the birth of a single infant. Cord clamps, bulb syringes, radiant warmers, and resuscitation equipment must be prepared for each infant. A team of neonatal care providers including neonatal nurses, a neonatal nurse practitioner, and a pediatrician or a neonatologist should be available to care for each infant. Another nurse should be free to care for the mother.

### Fetal Anomalies

Fetal anomalies such as hydrocephalus or a large fetal tumor can prevent normal descent of the fetus. Abnormal presentations such as breech or transverse lie are also associated with fetal anomalies. These abnormalities may be discovered by ultrasound examination before labor. A cesarean birth is scheduled if vaginal birth is not possible or if it is inadvisable.

## Problems of the Passage

Dysfunctional labor can occur because of variations in the maternal bony pelvis or soft tissue problems that inhibit fetal descent.

### Pelvis

A small (contracted) or abnormally shaped pelvis can retard labor and obstruct fetal passage. The woman may experience poor contractions, slow dilation, slow fetal descent, and a long labor. The danger of uterine rupture (tear in the uterine wall) is greater with thinning of the lower uterine segment, especially if contractions remain strong.

There are four basic pelvic shapes, each with different implications for labor and birth (Fig. 27.5). Most women have mixed characteristics of two or more types.

### Maternal Soft-Tissue Obstructions

During labor, a full bladder is a common soft-tissue obstruction. Bladder distention reduces available space in the pelvis and intensifies maternal discomfort. The woman should be assessed for bladder distention regularly and encouraged to void every 1 to 2 hours.

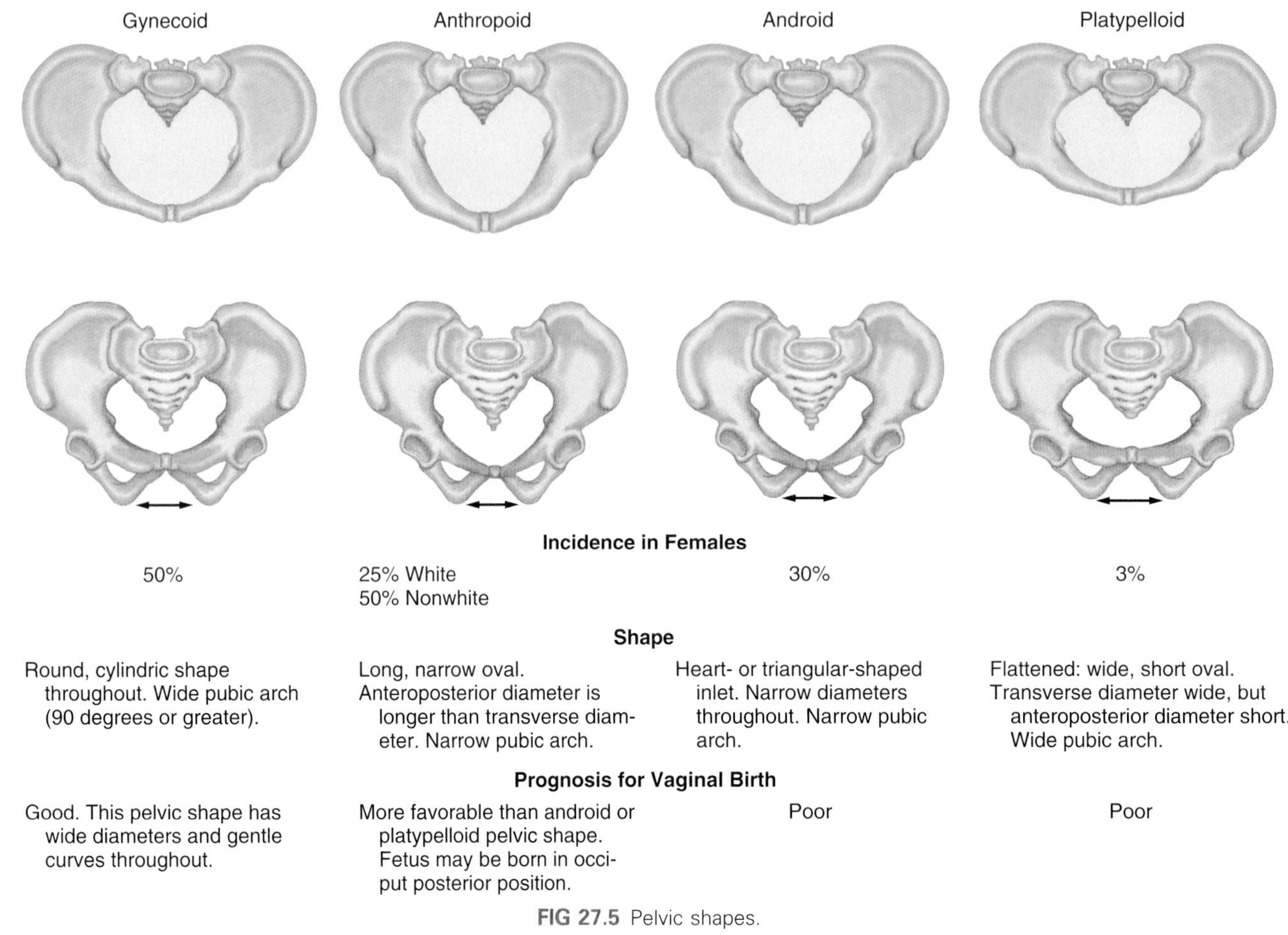


| | Gynecoid | Anthropoid | Android | Platypelloid |
|---|---|---|---|---|
| **Incidence in Females** | 50% | 25% White<br>50% Nonwhite | 30% | 3% |
| **Shape** | Round, cylindric shape throughout. Wide pubic arch (90 degrees or greater). | Long, narrow oval. Anteroposterior diameter is longer than transverse diameter. Narrow pubic arch. | Heart- or triangular-shaped inlet. Narrow diameters throughout. Narrow pubic arch. | Flattened: wide, short oval. Transverse diameter wide, but anteroposterior diameter short. Wide pubic arch. |
| **Prognosis for Vaginal Birth** | Good. This pelvic shape has wide diameters and gentle curves throughout. | More favorable than android or platypelloid pelvic shape. Fetus may be born in occiput posterior position. | Poor | Poor |

**FIG 27.5** Pelvic shapes.

Catheterization may be needed if she cannot urinate or if she receives regional block analgesia (see Chapter 18).

## Problems of the Psyche

A perceived threat caused by pain, fear, nonsupport, or personal circumstance can result in great maternal stress and interfere with normal labor progress. The woman's perception of stress is more important than the actual existence of a threat.

The body responds to stress, preparing itself for fight or flight. Responses to excessive or prolonged stress interfere with labor in several ways:

- Increased glucose consumption reduces the energy supply available to the contracting uterus.
- Maternal catecholamines can impair labor by interfering with adequate uterine contractility. Maternal blood supply to the placenta may be reduced.
- Labor contractions and maternal pushing efforts are less effective because these powers are working against the resistance of tense abdominal and pelvic muscles.
- Pain perception is increased and pain tolerance is decreased, further increasing maternal anxiety and stress.

Helping the woman relax helps her body work more effectively with the forces of labor and promotes normal progress. General nursing measures involve:

- Establishing a trusting relationship with the woman and her family
- Making the environment comfortable by adjusting temperature and light
- Promoting physical comfort, such as cleanliness
- Providing accurate information
- Implementing nonpharmacologic and pharmacologic pain management

Chapters 16 and 18 describe additional methods to encourage relaxation and promote comfort, including individual and family cultural values that are part of childbirth.

## Abnormal Labor Duration

An unusually long or short labor can result in maternal, fetal, or neonatal problems.

### Prolonged Labor

Prolonged labor is a type of dysfunctional labor that results from problems with any of the factors in the birth process. After the woman reaches the active phase of labor, cervical dilation should proceed at a minimum rate of 1.2 cm per hour in the nullipara and 1.5 cm per hour in the parous woman. Descent of the fetal presenting part is expected to occur at a minimum rate of 1 cm per hour in the nullipara and 2 cm per hour in the parous woman (Cunningham et al., 2014). If all previous births were by cesarean before much cervical dilation occurred, the criteria that apply to a nullipara may be applied.

Potential maternal and fetal problems related to prolonged labor include:

- Maternal infection, intrapartum or postpartum
- Neonatal infection, which can be severe or fatal
- Maternal exhaustion
- Higher levels of anxiety and fear during a subsequent labor

Maternal and neonatal infections are more likely if the membranes have been ruptured for a prolonged time, because organisms ascend from the vagina. The mother is more likely to have an intrapartum infection, a postpartum infection, or both (ACOG, 2016c; Belfort & Dildy, 2011).

Nursing measures for the woman who has prolonged labor include promotion of comfort, conservation of energy, emotional support, position changes that favor normal progress, and assessment for infection. Nursing care for the fetus includes observation for signs of intrauterine infection and for compromised fetal oxygenation (see Chapter 17).

### Precipitate Labor

Precipitate labor is a rapid birth that occurs within 3 hours of labor onset. There is often an abrupt onset of intense contractions rather than the more gradual increase in frequency, duration, and intensity that typifies most spontaneous labors. The mother or her fetus or newborn may be affected by several conditions that can be associated with the precipitate labor. These conditions may include abruptio placentae, fetal meconium, maternal cocaine use (also may be associated with abruptio placentae in any labor), postpartum hemorrhage, or low Apgar scores for the infant (Cunningham et al., 2014).

Precipitate labor is not the same as precipitate birth. A precipitate birth occurs after a labor of any length, in or out of the hospital or birth center, when a trained attendant is not present to assist. A woman in precipitate labor can also have a precipitate birth. The nurse should simply wear gloves while supporting the baby as it emerges. The mother's legs should not be forced together or the fetal head held back to delay birth. Such actions can result in fetal hypoxia or other injury.

If the maternal pelvis is adequate and the soft tissues yield easily to fetal descent, little maternal injury is likely. However, trauma such as uterine rupture, cervical lacerations, or hematoma of the vagina or vulva can occur.

The fetus may suffer direct trauma, such as intracranial hemorrhage or nerve damage, during a precipitate labor. The fetus may become hypoxic because intense contractions with a short relaxation period reduce time available for gas exchange in the placenta.

Priority nursing care of the woman in precipitate labor includes promotion of fetal oxygenation and maternal comfort. The woman should remain in a side-lying position to enhance placental blood flow and reduce the effects of aortocaval compression. An added benefit of the side-lying position is to slow the rapid fetal descent and minimize perineal tears. Additional measures to enhance fetal oxygenation include administering oxygen to the mother and maintaining adequate blood volume with nonadditive IV fluids. If oxytocin is being used, it should be stopped. A tocolytic drug is often ordered.

Promoting comfort is difficult in a precipitate labor because intense contractions give the woman little time to prepare and to use coping skills such as breathing techniques. Pharmacologic measures (opioid analgesia or regional block) are not useful if rapid labor progression does not allow time for them to become effective. In addition, possible newborn respiratory depression must be considered when opioids are given near birth. The nurse helps the woman focus on techniques to cope with pain one contraction at a time. The nurse must remain with her, to provide support and to assist with an emergency birth if it occurs.

## NURSING CARE

### The Woman in Dysfunctional Labor

Several nursing diagnoses and collaborative problems may be appropriate in dysfunctional labor. Observing for fetal compromise should be part of all intrapartum management (see Chapter 17). Pain management is often more difficult, and the woman may find that practiced coping skills are inadequate if labor is not normal. Anxiety or fear is often higher with abnormal labor, which also can reduce the effectiveness of pharmacologic or regional block (e.g., epidural block) pain control methods. Maternal or newborn injury sometimes becomes apparent after the birth (Cunningham et al., 2014; Gee, 2011).

In addition to these problems, nursing care in this section is directed toward two other concerns: possible intrauterine infection and maternal exhaustion.

#### Intrauterine Infection

***Assessment.*** Infection can occur with both normal and dysfunctional labors. Assess the FHR and maternal vital signs for evidence of infection:

- FHR: persistent fetal tachycardia (more than 160 beats per minute [bpm] for more than 10 minutes) is often an early sign of intrauterine infection and often occurs with maternal fever.
- Maternal temperature: assess every 2 to 4 hours in normal labor and every 2 hours after membranes rupture; assess hourly if elevated (≥38° C [100.4° F]) or if other signs of infection are present.
- Maternal pulse, respirations, and blood pressure: assess at least hourly to identify tachycardia or tachypnea, which often accompany temperature elevation. Maternal vital signs are usually added to the fetal monitor tracing.

Assess amniotic fluid for normal clear color and mild odor. Small flecks of white vernix are normal. Yellow or cloudy fluid or fluid with a foul or strong odor suggests infection, and vernix may be stained by discolored fluid. The strong odor may be noted before birth or afterward on the infant's skin.

***Nursing diagnosis and planning.*** For the woman without signs of infection but with risk factors, the nursing diagnosis selected is:

- Risk of Infection related to presence of favorable conditions (specify) for development.

**Expected outcomes.** Maternal temperature will remain less than 38° C (100.4° F). The electronic fetal monitoring (EFM) pattern will maintain a reassuring pattern near the baseline and below 160 bpm. The amniotic fluid will remain clear and without a foul or strong odor.

***Interventions***

**Reducing the risk of infection.** Nurses should wash their hands before and after each contact with the woman and her infant to reduce transmission of organisms. Use gloves and other protective wear to prevent contact with potentially infectious secretions.

Limit vaginal examinations to reduce transmission of vaginal organisms into the uterine cavity, and maintain aseptic technique during essential vaginal examinations. Keep underpads as dry as possible to reduce the moist, warm environment that favors bacterial growth. Periodically clean excessive secretions from the vaginal area in a front-to-back motion to limit fecal contamination and promote the mother's comfort.

**Identifying infection.** Assess the woman and fetus for signs of infection. Increase the frequency of assessments if labor is prolonged. If signs of infection are noted, report them to the birth attendant for definitive treatment. Note the time at which the membranes ruptured to identify prolonged rupture, which adds to the risk of infection.

The birth attendant may collect specimens after birth from the uterine cavity or placenta for culture to identify infectious organisms and determine antibiotic sensitivity. Both aerobic and anaerobic culture specimens may be collected. Transport specimens to the laboratory promptly because living organisms are required for culture and sensitivity study.

Inform the newborn staff if maternal risk factors for infection exist and if signs of infection are noted. If available, specialized caregivers such as neonatal nurse practitioners should be notified of an increased risk for newborn infection and resuscitation. Specimens of infants' secretions may be obtained for testing after birth. Prophylactic antibiotics to prevent neonatal sepsis are often given. See Chapter 30 for additional information about neonatal infection.

*Evaluation*

- Did the woman's temperature remain below 38° C (100.4° F)?
- Did the amniotic fluid have normal characteristics?
- Did the EFM tracing have a reassuring pattern, without tachycardia?

The woman remains at higher risk for postpartum infection and should continue to be observed for signs and symptoms of infection.

**SAFETY ALERT**

***Signs Associated With Intrapartum Infection***

- Fetal tachycardia (>160 beats per minute [bpm])
- Maternal fever (≥38° C [100.4° F])
- Foul- or strong-smelling amniotic fluid
- Cloudy or yellow amniotic fluid

### Maternal Exhaustion

*Assessment.* Many women begin labor with a sleep deficit because of fetal movement, frequent urination, and shortness of breath associated with advanced pregnancy. As labor drags on, the mother's reserves are further depleted.

Assess the mother for signs and symptoms of exhaustion:

- Verbal expression of tiredness, fatigue, or exhaustion
- Verbal expression of frustration with a prolonged, unproductive labor ("I can't go on any longer. Why doesn't the doctor just take the baby?")
- Ineffectiveness of or inability to use coping techniques (e.g., patterned breathing) that she previously used effectively
- Changes in her pulse, respiration, and blood pressure (increased or decreased)

*Nursing diagnosis and planning.* The intense energy demands of a dysfunctional labor can exceed a woman's physical and psychological ability to meet them. For this reason, an appropriate nursing diagnosis is:

- Activity Intolerance related to depletion of maternal energy reserves.

**Expected outcomes.** The woman will rest between contractions with her muscles relaxed. She will use coping skills such as breathing and relaxation techniques.

*Interventions*

**Conserving maternal energy.** Reduce factors that interfere with the woman's ability to relax. Lower the light level and turn off overhead lights. Reduce noise by closing the door or masking it with soft music or other comforting sounds. Silence the EFM if she prefers. Maintain a comfortable maternal temperature with blankets or a fan. If there is no contraindication, a warm shower or bath is soothing.

Position the woman to encourage comfort, promote fetal descent, and enhance fetal oxygenation. Support her with pillows to reduce muscle strain and added fatigue. Help her change positions regularly (approximately every 30 minutes) to reduce muscle tension from constant pressure. Regular position changes also promote maternal comfort by maintaining an even distribution of regional analgesia such as epidural block.

Even though epidural block is a common pain relief for birth, a woman may become tense in the upper body areas that are not affected by epidural effects, such as the shoulders and upper or middle back. Several pain management methods are options for women regardless of whether they choose any medical pain relief for labor. A soothing back rub can reduce muscle tension that increases fatigue. Firm sacral pressure or assuming positions that are helpful for fetal OP positions can reduce back pain. Use of the birthing ball can relax and support the woman in some positions. Warmth to her back can reduce back pain. However, the mother's skin sensation of warm applications may be reduced by a regional block, and they should be avoided in those areas. Warm applications to areas unaffected by the block may be comforting. Maintain IV fluids at the rate ordered to provide fluid and electrolytes, and occasionally glucose. Assess intake and output to identify dehydration, which can accompany prolonged labor and cause maternal fever, often preceded by fetal tachycardia. If there is no contraindication, provide juice, lollipops, Popsicles, or other liquids to moisten the woman's mouth and replenish her energy.

**Promoting coping skills.** When medical therapy or position changes are used to enhance labor, explain their purpose and expected benefits. Encourage the woman to visualize her baby passing downward smoothly through her pelvis as a result of her efforts. Provide her with mental images that allow her to "see" herself giving birth.

Generous praise and encouragement of the woman's use of skills such as breathing techniques motivate her to continue them even when she is discouraged. As with any laboring woman, tell her when she is making progress. Tell her that FHRs and patterns are reassuring if this is true. Knowing that her efforts are having the desired results and that her fetus is doing well gives the woman courage to continue.

*Evaluation*

- Does the woman rest and relax between contractions? If she cannot relax, discuss analgesia options with her. Inability to relax between contractions is associated with pain beyond the woman's tolerance.
- Does the woman continue to demonstrate adequate use of learned skills to cope with labor?

## PREMATURE RUPTURE OF THE MEMBRANES

Rupture of the amniotic sac before the onset of true labor, regardless of length of gestation, is called *premature rupture of the membranes* (PROM). A related term, *preterm premature rupture of the membranes* (often abbreviated PPROM or pPROM), describes membranes ruptured earlier than the end of the 37th week of gestation, with or without contractions. PROM may be a normal occurrence that precedes term birth at 38 weeks or later, even if labor induction is needed to initiate labor. However, PPROM is often associated with preterm labor (PTL), with the greatest risk of preterm birth occurring before completing 34 weeks of gestation (ACOG, 2016b). However, brief delays of an inevitable preterm birth from PPROM can enable interventions to reduce these risks.

### Etiology

Several conditions can cause early membrane rupture, but the exact cause is not always identified. Most cases of PPROM have no identifiable cause. Possible causes include (ACOG, 2016c):

- Infections, possibly asymptomatic, of the vagina or cervix by agents such as *Neisseria gonorrhoeae, Chlamydia trachomatis, Trichomonas vaginalis,* group B streptococcus (GBS), or *Gardnerella vaginalis* (bacterial vaginosis)
- Amniotic sac with a weak structure

- Chorioamnionitis (intraamniotic infection) associated with GBS, *N. gonorrhoeae, Listeria monocytogenes*, or species of *Mycoplasma, Bacteroides*, and *Ureaplasma* in the amniotic fluid
- Previous preterm birth, especially if preceded by PPROM
- Fetal abnormalities or malpresentation
- Incompetent cervix or a short cervical length (≤25 mm)
- Overdistention of the uterus
- Maternal hormonal changes
- Recent vaginal intercourse
- Maternal stress or low socioeconomic status
- Maternal nutritional deficiencies

## Complications

Both mother and newborn are at risk for infection during the intrapartum and postpartum periods. Intraamniotic infection (chorioamnionitis) can be either the cause or result of PPROM. The mother is at higher risk for postpartum infection. The newborn is at greater risk for sepsis after birth, with the most immature preterm infants having the greatest risk for systemic infection.

Chorioamnionitis, characterized by maternal fever and uterine tenderness, is most likely to precede preterm birth in the infant born before 34 weeks of gestation. Preterm infants with the lowest maturity (e.g., 23 weeks of gestation) are at greater risk for infection than those who are even a few weeks more mature. The exact time at which infection occurs cannot be predicted for either term or preterm infants.

Membranes ruptured well before term can form a seal, stopping the fluid leak and allowing the amniotic fluid cushion to become reestablished. However, membranes can continue to leak, prolonging the loss of the amniotic fluid cushion (oligohydramnios) for the fetus. Umbilical cord compression, reduced lung volume, and deformities resulting from compression can result, particularly in the fetus affected early in gestation.

## Therapeutic Management

Management of PROM depends on the gestation and whether there is evidence of infection or other fetal or maternal compromise. If infection is present, further management also depends on the type of infection. For a woman at term, PROM may herald the imminent onset of true labor. Usually, the cervix is soft with some dilation and effacement, and the fetal head is at or near zero station. Labor induction or cesarean birth may be reasonable if the fetus is 34 to 36 weeks of gestation or more because the negative effects of an active infection may be greater than a late preterm birth. Studies to determine fetal lung maturity are often performed.

If the pregnancy is earlier than 34 weeks of gestation, therapeutic management is more complex. The risk of infection or preterm birth is weighed against the hazards of actively promoting birth, whether vaginally or by cesarean. Accurate gestational age and evaluation of fetal lung maturity are important and may not be well defined in women with little or no prenatal care.

### Determining True Membrane Rupture

The first step is to determine whether the membranes are truly ruptured. Urinary incontinence, increased vaginal discharge, or loss of the mucous plug can cause a woman to believe her membranes have ruptured when they have not. A vaginal examination is avoided if the gestation is preterm and there is no evidence of labor. Instead, the physician or nurse-midwife performs a sterile speculum examination to look for a pool of fluid near the cervix and to estimate cervical dilation and effacement. A pH test or fern test (see Chapter 16) can verify whether the vaginal fluid is amniotic, although blood, semen, or vaginal infections may alter test results. Tests to assess fetal lung maturity and identify infection may be performed. Transvaginal ultrasound can be used to measure cervical length to identify a short cervix (≤25 mm), which is more likely to continue effacement and dilation (ACOG, 2016a; Cunningham et al., 2014).

### Gestation Near Term

If labor does not begin spontaneously, the woman's pregnancy is at or near term, and her cervix is favorable, labor may be induced (see Chapter 19). If the cervix is not favorable and no infection is present, induction may be delayed 24 hours or longer to allow cervical softening and administration of drugs to combat infection associated with early membrane rupture. If induction is unsuccessful or if infection or other complications develop, a cesarean birth is most common. However, the nurse should remember that cesarean birth also increases the risk of infection for any mother.

### Preterm Gestation

If the fetus is less than 34 weeks of gestation, the physician weighs the risks of infection against the infant's risk for complications of prematurity. Cesarean birth is more common if delivery at the earlier gestation is needed. The physician considers factors such as gestational age, amount of amniotic fluid remaining, and fetal lung maturity in addition to possible infection of mother and infant.

## Maternal Antibiotics

Maternal antibiotics may stop the infection that caused or will occur with the rupture, thus delaying the onset of labor and allowing the fetus to mature. Drugs used to stop infection if early membrane rupture occurs include ampicillin, erythromycin, amoxicillin, and azithromycin. The current recommendation to treat or prevent PPROM-associated infections is the administration of IV antibiotics for 48 hours, followed by 5 days of oral antibiotics. GBS is also treated if indicated (see Chapter 26) (ACOG, 2016b; ACOG, 2011).

## Nursing Considerations

The woman will either remain hospitalized until birth or return home after a few days of hospital observation and 48 hours of treatment with IV antibiotics. If she is hospitalized, the nurse observes for signs of infection. Preparation for home management includes teaching the woman to:

- Avoid sexual intercourse, orgasm, or insertion of anything into the vagina, as these increase the risk of infection caused by ascending organisms and can stimulate contractions.
- Avoid breast stimulation if the gestation is preterm because it can cause release of oxytocin from the posterior pituitary, thereby stimulating contractions.
- Take her temperature at least four times a day, reporting any temperature greater than 37.8° C (100° F).
- Maintain any activity restrictions.
- Note and report uterine contractions or vaginal drainage with a foul odor.

# PRETERM LABOR

Preterm labor (PTL) is that beginning after the 20th week but before the end of the 37th week of pregnancy. The physical risks to the mother are no greater than labor at term unless complications such as infection, hemorrhage, or the need for a cesarean delivery are also present. However, PTL can result in the birth of an infant who is ill-equipped for extrauterine life, particularly if earlier than 32 weeks of gestation. (ACOG, 2016a; Cunningham et al., 2014).

## Associated Factors

As the triggers of labor onset at full term are unknown, the causes of PTL are also unclear. Many factors are associated with PTL:

- Maternal medical conditions such as infections of the urinary tract, reproductive organs, or systemic organs; preexisting or gestational diabetes; connective tissue disorders; chronic hypertension; and drug abuse
- Maternal obesity, with difficult evaluation of the need for early delivery of the possibly macrosomic fetus (Jorgensen, 2008a)
- Chronic health disorders, often associated with older mothers (Jorgensen, 2008a)
- Conceptions achieved by assisted reproductive technology, including those resulting in a single fetal gestation
- Present and past obstetric conditions such as short cervical length (≤25 mm), previous preterm birth, multifetal gestation, preterm membrane rupture, preeclampsia, and bleeding disorders that involve the woman, fetus, or placental implantation area
- Fetal conditions such as growth restriction, inadequate amniotic fluid volume, and chromosomal or other birth defects
- Social and environmental factors such as inadequate or absent prenatal or dental care, maternal domestic violence episodes, maternal smoking, and housing deficiency such as homelessness
- Demographic factors such as race and age of the parents, financial stability, and the number and birth intervals of the woman's other children

However, many women who have PTL and preterm birth do not have known risk factors. Other women may reach full term despite having many risk factors. Table 27.2 lists more details about possible risk factors.

### SAFETY ALERT

**_Late Preterm Is Not Term_**

Term birth occurs after at least 37 to 41 weeks of gestation.
Late preterm infants are born at 34 to 36 completed weeks.
Late preterm infants may appear to be full term at birth.
Infant appearance is deceiving.
Mortality for late preterm infants is three times higher than that of term infants.

## Manifestations

Signs and symptoms near the beginning of a PTL episode are subtle and often occur in normal pregnancies as well. Prenatal visits and routine ultrasounds may reveal evidence of cervical changes that have been occurring over several weeks during the second and third

### EVIDENCE-BASED PRACTICE

This study examines possible reasons why a large inner-city public hospital had fewer preterm births, defined as less than 37 weeks, from 1995 to 2002 compared to the total U.S. preterm birth rates for that same period. The "inner city" is Dallas, Texas, and the facility is Parkland Memorial Hospital. Hispanic women, mostly from Mexico, were the largest minority in the Parkland study sample of women who had preterm births (70%). African-American women were the second largest minority at 20%, and white women constituted 8%. The U.S. sample for preterm birth rates was 61% white women, 19% Hispanic, and 14% African-American. Parkland Hospital had data from 1988 to 2006 and continues to gather data on births, racial differences, disparities between women's races, and other data. Parkland Hospital is using the period from 1995 to 2002 to compare the hospital preterm birth statistics to national data for those years. The staff participating in this study and providing care to the women and their babies in the healthcare system described included:

- Faculty physicians from the Departments of Obstetrics and Gynecology and Pediatrics at University of Texas Southwestern Medical School
- Residents (house officers) in each specialty at Parkland Hospital
- Nurses who gather data and provide antepartum care at outpatient clinics and inpatient perinatal care at Parkland Hospital

Adverse pregnancy outcomes are related to poverty and poor access to care. Policy makers at Parkland focused their efforts to improve birth outcomes by improving access to care. During the early 1990s, Parkland Hospital, in conjunction with University of Texas Southwestern Medical School, developed a neighborhood-based, administratively and medically integrated public healthcare system. Prenatal clinics in this system were located with comprehensive medical and pediatric clinics. The inner-city pregnant women that this system was designed to serve often have no other resources, and the aim of Parkland Hospital's system was to provide access to the available care so that they would be more likely to take advantage it. The aim of this system was to make that care seamless from the clinic system to the hospital setting.

Prenatal protocols are used by nurse-practitioners at all clinic sites to provide homogenous care. Standardized referrals are made to the hospital centralized clinic system for women with high-risk pregnancies. The high-risk pregnancy clinics provide prenatal care for women with previous preterm birth, gestational diabetes, infectious diseases, multiple gestations, and hypertensive disorders. Maternal–fetal medicine faculty staff these specialty clinics. Prenatal care in the Parkland system is "considered one component of a comprehensive and orchestrated public healthcare system that is community based" (Leveno, McIntire, Bloom, et al., 2009).

The Parkland study was prompted by a 2006 Institute of Medicine report, *Preterm Birth: Causes, Consequences, and Prevention.* The purpose of this study was to compare preterm births among African-American and Hispanic women served at Parkland with national data in the 1995 to 2002 period. One general finding was that the preterm birth rate (<37 weeks gestation) at Parkland decreased from 1988 to 2006, from 10.4% to 4.9%, while the U.S. total preterm birth rate increased during the 1995 to 2002 period, from 9.4% to 10.1%. Preterm births before 37 weeks of gestation were lower in the Parkland cohort than the U.S. group for African-American and Hispanic women. Except for 1 year, white women in the Parkland group had a preterm birth rate just slightly lower than the U.S. group of white women. Disparity between the preterm birth rates for white, African-American, and Hispanic women narrowed in the Parkland group when compared to the U.S. group.

Parkland researchers did not expect the results of this study to show that their preterm birth rate was significantly lower than that of the nation for this 8-year period. The staff cannot definitively conclude whether the neighborhood access to prenatal care in a system providing care for problem pregnancies is what made Parkland Hospital's preterm birth rate lower than that of the U.S. from 1995 to 2002. An additional finding from Parkland's data was that women who did not have prenatal care did not show this decrease in preterm births.

Reference: Leveno, K.J., McIntire, D.D., Bloom, S.L., et al. (2009). Decreased preterm births in an inner-city public hospital. *Obstetrics and Gynecology, 113*(3), 578–584.

**TABLE 27.2 Maternal Risk Factors for Preterm Labor**

| Medical History | Obstetric History | Present Pregnancy | Lifestyle and Demographics |
|---|---|---|---|
| Low weight for height<br>Obesity<br>Uterine or cervical anomalies, uterine fibroids<br>History of cone biopsy<br>Diethylstilbestrol (DES) exposure as a fetus<br>Chronic illness (e.g., cardiac, renal, diabetes, clotting disorders, anemia, hypertension) | Previous preterm labor<br>Previous preterm birth<br>Previous first-trimester spontaneous abortion (>2)<br>Previous second-trimester spontaneous abortion<br>History of previous pregnancy losses (≥2)<br>Incompetent cervix<br>Cervical length ≤25 mm (2.5 cm [1 in]) at midtrimester of pregnancy<br>Number of embryos implanted (assisted reproductive techniques [ARTs]) | Uterine distention (e.g., multifetal pregnancy, hydramnios)<br>Abdominal surgery during pregnancy<br>Uterine irritability<br>Uterine bleeding<br>Dehydration<br>Infection<br>Anemia<br>Incompetent cervix<br>Preeclampsia<br>Preterm premature rupture of membranes (PPROM)<br>Fetal or placental abnormalities | Little or no prenatal care<br>Poor nutrition<br>Age <18 yr or >40 yr<br>Low educational level<br>Low socioeconomic status<br>Smoking >10 cigarettes daily<br>Nonwhite<br>Employment with long hours and/or long standing<br>Chronic physical or psychological stress<br>Domestic violence<br>Substance abuse |

trimesters. The woman may be vaguely aware that something seems different, or she may not detect that anything is amiss. Only when PTL reaches the active phase is it more typical of labor at term. Signs and symptoms that a woman may experience when PTL begins include:

- Uterine contractions that may or may not be painful; contractions may not be felt by the woman at all
- A sensation that the baby is frequently "balling up"
- Cramps similar to menstrual cramps
- Constant low backache; intermittent or irregular mild low back pain
- Sensation of pelvic pressure or a feeling that the baby is pushing down or is heavier
- Pain, discomfort, or pressure in the vulva or thighs
- Change or increase in vaginal discharge (increased, watery, bloody)
- Abdominal cramps with or without diarrhea
- A sense of "just feeling bad" or "coming down with something"

## Preventing Preterm Birth

### Community Education

Preterm birth can impose substantial physical, emotional, and financial burdens on the child, family, and society. Ideally, nursing strategies to prevent preterm birth begin before conception, through community education. Programs often include teaching related to the:

- Role of early and regular prenatal care in preventing preterm birth
- Duration of normal pregnancy
- Conditions that increase a woman's risk for preterm birth
- Signs and symptoms that PTL may be occurring
- Consequences of preterm birth for mother and baby

Women who are aware of the consequences of preterm birth may be more likely to take action to prevent it. If they recognize that they have risk factors, they may seek prenatal care earlier in gestation.

### During Pregnancy

During pregnancy, measures to prevent preterm birth include:

- Reducing barriers and improving access to early and regular prenatal care for all women
- Assessing for risk factors to promote changes in those that can be reduced
- Promoting adequate nutrition
- Promoting maternal smoking cessation
- Teaching women and their partners about characteristics of early PTL that are often subtle and how these differ from normal pregnancy changes
- Empowering women and their partners to take an active approach in seeking care if they have signs and symptoms of PTL

*Improving access to care.* To improve access to prenatal care, the community setting must be considered. Difficult access is a serious problem for women who rely on public clinics for their care. Women who live in a rural area may find access difficult whether they seek public or private prenatal care. Long waits to see the provider for just a few minutes, fragmented care, language or cultural barriers, and insensitivity of caregivers may discourage women from seeking care. Expanding the number of caregivers by using nurses with advanced education, such as certified nurse-midwives and nurse practitioners, can reduce waits for care and enhance the communication process between professionals and the pregnant woman and her family. Nurses can help coordinate various aspects of care to limit the number of appointments a woman must obtain to complete care.

*Identifying risk factors.* Women who have risk factors for preterm birth can benefit from programs to reduce the risk and identify PTL early. These women benefit from frequent prenatal care appointments, reinforcement of the symptoms of PTL, telephone contacts, and assessments of fetal growth and health.

Some risk factors can be reduced or eliminated if the woman changes her lifestyle. Despite the difficulty involved, many women have stopped smoking or using drugs to benefit their babies. While getting more rest or to stopping work would be beneficial for some women, such change can be difficult or impossible. Nurses can work with the woman to help reduce her risks as much as possible by helping her identify sources of support.

Infections of the urinary and reproductive tracts are associated with PPROM and PTL. Screening for abnormal microorganisms in the urine, vagina, and cervix identifies women who might benefit from antibiotic therapy.

*Progesterone supplementation.* Progesterone (17 alpha-hydroxyprogesterone caproate, or 17P, formerly under the trade name sDelalutin) was used in the past to prevent spontaneous abortion. The drug proved to be ineffective for that purpose and was pulled from the market. However, it continues to be studied for decreasing the incidence of preterm birth in women with a previous preterm birth or a high risk for singleton birth earlier than 34 weeks. 17P was not found to prevent preterm birth or newborn morbidity in multiple pregnancies (ACOG, 2016c; Cunningham et al., 2014). Studies are ongoing, and nurses might encounter a woman who has taken 17P weekly by intramuscular injection or daily by vaginal suppository.

***Promoting adequate nutrition.*** An adequate maternal diet contributes positively to the length of gestation and the infant's weight. Every pregnant woman should be offered culturally appropriate diet counseling that considers her means. The Special Supplemental Nutrition Program for Women, Infants, and Children (WIC) is available to supplement the diet of some low-income women. Anemia can be corrected by appropriate supplementation. Women carrying more than one fetus need additional food intake.

***Educating women and their partners about preterm labor.*** *All pregnant women and their partners should be taught about symptoms of PTL, because most preterm births occur in women who have no identified risk factors.* Language barriers can be reduced by using fluent interpreters and printed materials in the woman's primary language. Diagrams should supplement the words of any language because some women have limited reading skills. Respecting cultural norms of the woman and her family is also an essential part of prenatal care.

The vague signs and symptoms of early PTL should be reinforced regularly as part of prenatal care. Women who often have uterine irritability may be given guidelines to observe at home before they must go to the hospital. PTL often causes only vague sensations if the cervix dilates minimally, so any home-care guidelines are individualized according to the woman's risk for a preterm birth, the gestation and prenatal status, and the likelihood that specific interventions are beneficial to mother and baby. In addition, women should enter the hospital for evaluation if they are not sure about the seriousness of their sensations. Examples of home care guidelines include:

- Drinking adequate amounts of water to improve hydration or reduce bladder irritation that can accompany a urinary tract infection.
- Emptying the bladder frequently, because a full bladder is associated with uterine irritability and contractions.
- Lying down in a side-lying position to promote uterine blood flow. Limiting physical activity can increase diuresis. Prolonged limitation of physical activity is not usually beneficial or safe for prevention of premature labor, although it may be required for serious maternal disorders such as cardiac disease.
- Palpating contractions for 1 hour daily or as instructed because of the duration of any previous labor. However, the woman should notify her birth attendant or go directly to the labor unit for assessment if contractions increase in frequency, duration, or sensitivity.

The nurse should verify the woman's understanding by seeking feedback, such as having her restate the signs and symptoms of PTL and the appropriate responses to them.

***Empowering women and their partners.*** Delaying birth when PTL occurs depends on its early identification. Women should be taught to report to the labor unit promptly for assessment if contractions or other discomfort intensifies. They should be encouraged to communicate their concerns when they arrive at the clinic or hospital to avoid long waits to be seen. It is equally important not to make the woman feel foolish if she reports signs and symptoms but is not in labor; otherwise she may not seek care for recurrent episodes when she truly is in labor, possibly losing the opportunity to stop it.

The nurse might suggest that a woman who is seeking care for possible PTL say, "I'm not due for 8 more weeks, but I think I may be in labor. I need to be seen right away, or I might have a premature baby."

## Therapeutic Management

Management focuses on predicting those at risk for preterm birth, identifying PTL early, delaying birth, and accelerating fetal lung maturity if preterm birth is likely.

### Predicting Preterm Birth

Because treatment for PTL has been less than satisfactory at preventing preterm birth, research has focused on identifying women who are most likely to deliver early. The key is to identify those who are truly at risk for preterm birth and to treat them intensively while continuing regular prenatal care for those experiencing PTL symptoms as a variant of normal pregnancy. An inexpensive, noninvasive screening test giving quick results to predict preterm birth risk is not presently available. For this reason, various evaluations are used in an attempt to determine the best medical management.

A major preterm prediction study looked at multiple factors and found that their relevance to preterm birth was interrelated. The factors most strongly associated with predicting preterm birth included:

- A short cervical length of ≤25 mm (1 inch)
- A previous preterm birth
- A positive fetal fibronectin (fFN) result after 22 weeks of gestation

***Cervical length.*** A short cervix (≤25 mm), measured by transvaginal ultrasound during the second trimester, may allow vaginal organisms easier access to the uterus, where they weaken the membranes and cause premature rupture. Alternatively, the shortened cervix may reflect structural changes caused by an intrauterine infection or uterine contractions. The woman may have no symptoms of infection or pressure against the cervix (Cunningham et al., 2014).

***Fetal fibronectin.*** Fetal fibronectin (fFN) is a protein present in fetal tissues that is normally found in the cervical and vaginal secretions until 16 to 20 weeks of gestation and again at or near term. Early appearance suggests that labor might begin early, similar to the rise in cardiac enzyme levels in the person with a myocardial infarction. A positive fFN test during midpregnancy can identify the woman at risk for PTL, possibly because this result is associated with maternal or fetal infection. The test must be collected before significant vaginal manipulation from examination to reduce false positives. Cervical examination, recent sexual intercourse, and vaginal bleeding can result in a false-positive test. Combining cervical length measurement with an accurate fFN test may provide more accurate prediction of PTL (Cunningham et al., 2014).

***Infections.*** Infections often increase the risk for preterm membrane rupture or birth, even if the woman does not initially have clinical signs or symptoms. A urinary tract infection is common with PTL, so catheterized or midstream urine is often obtained for urinalysis and for culture and sensitivity testing. Tests for other infections associated with preterm birth risk include those often found upon premature membrane rupture (see Premature Rupture of the Membranes, p. 580).

Blood peak and trough levels of indicated antibiotics, such as gentamicin, ensure that the woman is receiving a therapeutic level (peak) of the drug. Determining whether the blood drug level is excessive just before the next dose (a high trough level) is important to prevent possible damage to mother or baby. Testing for peak and trough drug levels allows the dose to be adjusted appropriately.

A woman with an infection that is not always related to pregnancy may present for care. Relevant testing may relate to acute gastrointestinal or respiratory infections. More serious maternal infections may require cultures of maternal blood, respiratory, or other secretions to determine the ideal treatment. Although rare during pregnancy, maternal pneumonia increases the risk of fetal and maternal death as well as the risk that the woman will give birth to a preterm infant. Other poor health conditions during pregnancy, including crowded living conditions and a chronic condition such as asthma, increase a woman's risk of pneumonia as well.

### Identifying Preterm Labor

The best way for caregivers to identify PTL is more frequent patient contact to identify risk for preterm birth or to identify PTL early, possibly delaying birth and promoting further fetal maturation.

Women at risk for preterm birth should have more frequent prenatal visits, at which time they are checked for evidence of PTL and their ability to follow preventive therapy, in addition to their regular prenatal checkup. They should be assessed for development of new risk factors with each visit. Gentle cervical examinations, usually with a sterile speculum, are done if indicated. A transvaginal ultrasound may identify the shortened, thinned cervix that often precedes onset of labor in the asymptomatic woman. Infections can be identified and treated promptly before rupture of membranes or onset of labor occurs (ACOG, 2016a).

### Stopping Preterm Labor

Once diagnosis of PTL is made, management focuses on stopping uterine activity before the point of no return, usually after approximately 3 cm dilation. Preterm delivery may be inevitable, but steroid therapy promotes earlier fetal lung maturation. Particularly for very early gestations, such as 25 weeks, treatment may buy enough time for the steroids to be on board. Even one more day of fetal maturation may improve the outcome for the very premature infant.

***Initial measures.*** The physician initially determines whether any maternal or fetal conditions contraindicate continuing the pregnancy. Examples of these conditions are:

- Preeclampsia or eclampsia; persistent hypertension from any cause
- Significant or prolonged maternal alterations, such as hypovolemia, hypoxemia, or acid-base imbalance
- Serious infection, including chorioamnionitis or maternal infection such as maternal pyelonephritis
- Fetal heart rate monitoring data showing inability to correct signs that are nonreassuring for the gestation of the fetus

Initial measures to stop PTL include identifying and treating infections, identifying other causes of PTL that may be treatable, and reducing activity. Hydration with IV fluids may be chosen if maternal dehydration is a factor. Excess fluid hydration increases the risk for pulmonary edema if some drugs also are used to stop PTL.

***Identifying and treating infections.*** Infection, both systemic and local, has a strong association with preterm birth and PROM. However, it may be unclear whether various microorganisms found at diagnosis of PTL are significant if the membranes remain intact. Blood studies identify signs of infection and conditions, such as anemia, that are associated with PTL or affect its management. Common studies include a complete blood count with differential white blood cell analysis and cultures for GBS, chlamydia, gonorrhea, or other suspected infections. Amniocentesis may be done to obtain amniotic fluid for culture if chorioamnionitis is suspected because this infection would contraindicate stopping PTL. Fetal lung maturity testing (see Chapter 15) may be done on an amniotic fluid specimen. Urinalysis with culture and sensitivity may be done to determine if treatment is indicated.

Culture results require at least 24 to 48 hours to complete, so anti-infectives that are usually effective against the probable organisms are started as soon as the specimen is obtained. Prompt treatment of acute infections such as pyelonephritis, improves maternal and fetal outcomes. Broad-spectrum antibiotics such as ampicillin, penicillin, and an aminoglycoside such as gentamicin, that are effective against many organisms, may be chosen for possible chorioamnionitis. Anaerobic organisms may also cause infection for a woman who requires a cesarean birth, and medications such as clindamycin or metronidazole may be prescribed (ACOG, 2016a).

***Identifying other causes for preterm contractions.*** The woman with polyhydramnios, identified by ultrasonography, may have more contractions because her uterus is stretched more than normal. A therapeutic amniocentesis to remove some amniotic fluid can reduce uterine irritability. Multifetal gestations can be identified by ultrasonography if not previously diagnosed. These mothers may benefit from improved nutrition, stress reduction, assistance with household care, and other interventions.

***Limiting activity.*** Activity limits, usually by relaxing in a side-lying or semi-sitting position, increase placental blood flow and reduce fetal pressure on the cervix. However, lengthy and substantial activity restriction (e.g., complete bed rest) has not been shown to prolong pregnancy significantly. As in other individuals, activity restriction is associated with serious maternal side effects, some of which develop within as few as 24 hours. Adverse effects of substantial activity restriction during pregnancy may include:

- Muscle weakness, including aching; muscle atrophy; and bone loss
- Diuresis as the body tries to reduce the normally higher fluid level of pregnancy
- Poor nutrition as a result of appetite loss, lower intake, and increased indigestion; weight loss, or inadequate weight gain
- Orthostatic hypotension caused by the change in blood pressure regulation by baroreceptors
- Psychological effects, such as increased stress on the woman about separation from her family, anxiety about the pregnancy's outcome, depression, boredom from a decreased activity level and less contact with other people, and concerns about finances if the woman's job is essential to her family
- Sleep changes as depression increases or usual activities that direct the woman's sleep-wake cycles are not present

Because of problems and lack of benefits for most women, limited and individualized activity reductions are now prescribed if preterm birth risk is higher. Changes may be relatively simple, such as a change in work hours or duties or finding ways to help the woman meet the needs for her other children, such as transportation to school or other activities. Several rest periods may be prescribed for home care when the woman's risk status is lower. Positions for rest may include a semi-sitting position with the feet and legs elevated. If lying down for rest, a mother's frequent change of the side-lying position reduces discomfort from the pressure of remaining on one side for a prolonged time. Frequent position changes are also beneficial to women who require hospitalization for their PTL.

Women hospitalized for the care of PTL may have a greater activity restriction. Because of IV hydration and drug therapy, bed rest is common during initial care. Ambulating to the bathroom may be contraindicated because of maternal sedative effects from a drug that depresses uterine activity, such as magnesium sulfate (also given for preeclampsia; see Chapter 25). The woman may have an indwelling catheter for precise urine output assessment with administration of magnesium, although these women usually have normal output. If PTL stops and the sedating drug is discontinued, the woman may usually walk to the restroom for showers, voiding, and bowel movements. If she remains hospitalized for longer-term care, she may sit in a chair periodically or take occasional short trips to another area in a wheelchair that her family or friends push.

Although preterm birth may occur, the severity of infant effects may be less if even a few days are gained in the duration of pregnancy. Whether the woman is expected to be hospitalized briefly or for a longer time, the following services may improve her adherence to care:

- Physical therapy to help maintain muscle strength and coordination, and to reduce muscle aching, fatigue, and bone loss
- Recreational therapy to identify appropriate activities to relieve boredom
- Occupational therapy to help the woman cope physically with lifestyle changes, particularly if discharge home is anticipated
- Complementary therapy to reduce stressors and enhance physical care measures
- Social work to identify how needs such as financial and child care can be met
- Consultation with a psychologist to help the woman and family cope with the added stressors

***Hydrating the woman.*** Hydration to stop preterm contractions has not been shown to be beneficial for all women. High-volume IV infusions may cause maternal respiratory distress if a drug, such as magnesium sulfate, to decrease uterine contractions is being administered because the drug may also reduce the respiratory rate, even if a woman has a normal blood pressure level.

However, dehydration may contribute to uterine irritability for some women. This condition is often the case in those who have had an illness such as acute gastrointestinal infection in which loss of fluid through diarrhea exceeds the nauseated woman's ability to drink water or other fluids. Infections with maternal fever (≥38° C [100.4° F]) can also decrease the woman's fluid intake. IV fluids are ordered according to their expected benefit, such as magnesium sulfate drug therapy to stop PTL or initiation of an antibiotic. Adequate fluid intake also promotes urination to reduce the risk of infection.

## Tocolytics

The benefits of tocolytic therapy to delay preterm birth are not clear. Tocolysis may be ordered if labor occurs before the 34th week of gestation because the infant's risk for respiratory and other complications of prematurity is high if born during this time. Delay of preterm birth with tocolysis may provide time to give maternal corticosteroids to reduce respiratory distress in the newborn or time to transfer the mother to a facility with an appropriate neonatal intensive care unit. Delay of birth until full term is not expected.

Current tocolytic drugs are used primarily for conditions other than PTL, and thus, have effects on body systems other than the reproductive system. Risks and possible benefits of the drug chosen must be considered and communicated clearly to the woman. The lowest possible dose that inhibits contractions is used. Four types of drugs are used for tocolysis: (1) magnesium sulfate, (2) calcium antagonists, (3) prostaglandin synthesis inhibitors, and (4) beta-adrenergics. (Table 27.3 summarizes doses and routes of administration for each of these drugs.)

***Magnesium sulfate.*** Magnesium sulfate is used in management of pregnancy-associated hypertension to prevent seizures (see the Drug Guide on p. 539 in Chapter 25). It often is used to inhibit PTL because of the additional effect of quieting uterine activity. Although the evidence to support magnesium sulfate as a tocolytic is weak, it is a common choice for the initial suppression of PTL because the physician is familiar with use of the drug. Magnesium sulfate for tocolysis is given intravenously using a similar protocol to that for hypertension during pregnancy. The loading dose (4 to 6 g) is given over 30 minutes. The maintenance dose ranges from 1 to 4 g/hr to stop PTL. The magnesium sulfate infusion is continued until 12 hours after contractions have stopped or until contractions are no more than one in 10 minutes (six or fewer per hour). Magnesium sulfate therapy can be continued for a total of 48 hours so the mother can receive the full course of corticosteroids to speed fetal lung maturation. When magnesium sulfate is discontinued, the physician may start another tocolytic or discontinue tocolysis.

Common hospital criteria to continue magnesium sulfate therapy include the following:

- Urine output of at least 30 mL/hr
- Presence of deep tendon reflexes
- At least 12 respirations per minute

In addition, the nurse should check heart and lung sounds with hourly vital signs because fluid overload and electrolyte imbalances can lead to pulmonary edema or cardiac dysrhythmias. Oxygen saturations are included with the hourly vital signs and other assessments. Bowel sounds are checked when therapy begins and every 4 to 8 hours because the smooth muscle in the intestinal tract can relax as with the uterus. Serum magnesium level measurements guide maintenance of therapeutic levels. EFM identifies drug effects on the fetus, such as reduced variability, that are common in PTL and with magnesium sulfate therapy.

Calcium gluconate (10%) should be available to reverse magnesium toxicity and prevent respiratory arrest if serum levels become high. Excess serum levels of magnesium are less likely when the drug is given for PTL because the woman's renal function is usually normal. However, the nurse must remain alert for this complication.

An unexpected finding in research investigating the effectiveness of magnesium to stop PTL is an apparent neuroprotective effect, with a lower incidence of cerebral palsy in the child (Cunningham et al., 2014).

***Calcium antagonists.*** Nifedipine (Adalat, Procardia) is a calcium channel blocker usually given for hypertension. Calcium is essential for the contraction of smooth muscle such as the uterus, so blocking calcium reduces muscle contraction. Flushing of the skin, headache, and a transient increase in the maternal and fetal heart rates are common side effects. Because nifedipine is a vasodilator, the woman can develop orthostatic hypotension.

The nurse should observe for side effects of nifedipine and report a maternal pulse greater than 120 bpm. The woman should be given information about possible dizziness or faintness with nifedipine's hypotensive effects. She should sit or stand slowly and call for assistance if needed (see Chapter 20, p. 408).

***Prostaglandin synthesis inhibitors.*** Because prostaglandins stimulate uterine contractions, drugs can be used to inhibit their synthesis. Indomethacin (Indocin) is the drug in this class most often used for tocolysis.

The main fetal and neonatal side effects are constriction of the ductus arteriosus, pulmonary hypertension, and oligohydramnios. These effects are unlikely if treatment is no longer than 48 to 72 hours and the gestation is less than 32 weeks. The effect of reducing the amount of amniotic fluid makes indomethacin useful for normalizing the volume in hydramnios. The amniotic fluid volume usually returns to its previous level when indomethacin treatment is discontinued. Regular ultrasound examinations and fetal echocardiography are used to determine whether indomethacin is having adverse effects on the fetus. Assessment of the infant after birth for other complications, such as pulmonary hypertension or intracranial hemorrhage, may be done related to the duration of maternal indomethacin intake, gestation, and the probability that delivery will occur less than 24 hours after the drug is discontinued (Cunningham et al., 2014).

The nurse should observe the woman for side effects such as nausea, heartburn, vomiting, and rash. Because indomethacin can prolong bleeding time, the nurse observes for abnormalities such as prolonged

TABLE 27.3 **Drugs Used in Preterm Labor**

| Drug and Purpose | Common Dose Regimens* | Side or Adverse Effects |
|---|---|---|
| Magnesium sulfate (use as tocolytic) | *IV:* Loading dose, 4-6 g over 30 min.<br>Maintenance dose for tocolysis, 1-4 g/hr.<br>When contraction frequency is no higher than 1 per 10 min (≤6 per hr), maintain infusion rate for 12 hr; then discontinue drug.<br>An oral tocolytic can be ordered to continue tocolysis after magnesium sulfate is stopped. | Side and adverse effects are dose-related, occurring at higher maternal serum levels<br>Depression of deep tendon reflexes, which should be present, although less active<br>Respiratory or cardiac depression if serum levels are high; greatest risk is in woman with poor urinary elimination of drug<br>Less serious side effects: lethargy, weakness, visual blurring, headache, sensation of heat, nausea, vomiting, constipation<br>Fetal–neonatal effects: reduced fetal heart rate (FHR) variability, hypotonia |
| Nifedipine (Procardia); nicardipine (Cardene) (calcium channel blockers for tocolysis) | Oral loading dose of 10-20 mg.<br>Continued oral therapy: 10-20 mg every 3-6 hr until contractions are rare followed by long-acting formulations of 30-60 mg every 8-12 hr until antepartum steroids have been administered. | Maternal flushing, dizziness, headache, nausea<br>Transient maternal tachycardia<br>Mild hypotension<br>Modest blood glucose level increases |
| Indomethacin (Indocin); sulindac (Clinoril) (prostaglandin synthesis inhibitors) | Limit use to preterm labor before 32 wk of gestation.<br>Use indomethacin for no longer than 48-72 consecutive hr.<br>Loading dose: 50 mg (oral).<br>Maintenance dose: 25 mg orally every 6 hr for 48 hr.<br>Ultrasound examinations and fetal echocardiography help determine if maternal indomethacin has adverse effects on fetus. | Epigastric pain, nausea, gastrointestinal bleeding.<br>Asthma in aspirin-sensitive woman.<br>Increased blood pressure in hypertensive woman.<br>Fetus: adverse fetal effects include constriction of ductus arteriosus, particularly if mother receives indomethacin for more than 48-72 hr and gestation is later than 32 wk; impairs fetal renal function, which can decrease amniotic fluid volume, possibly resulting in cord compression. |
| Terbutaline (beta-adrenergic for tocolysis) | IV infusion: Begin at ordered rate of approximately 0.01 to 0.05 mg/min. Increase rate by 0.01 mg/min at 10- to 30-min intervals until contractions or the maximum dose of 0.08 mg/min is reached. Maintain this dose for 1 hr, then reduce the rate at 20-min intervals to reach the minimum maintenance dose when contractions stop. Continue maintenance dose for 12 hr or as ordered.<br>Subcutaneous (most common parenteral route): Intermittent injections, 0.25 mg, every 4 hr. By subcutaneous infusion pump: low-dose continuous (baseline) drug infusion plus intermittent bolus doses. A subcutaneous pump is typically placed, and its programming for continuous and bolus doses is verified before removing the IV infusion line for terbutaline or magnesium sulfate.<br>Oral: 2.5 to 5 mg every 2-4 hr.<br>When changing from IV to oral therapy, give oral dose 30 min before discontinuing IV infusion. | Terbutaline is not approved by the U.S. Food and Drug Administration (FDA) for inhibiting uterine activity and now carries a new *Boxed Warning and contraindications* ("black box") against use as a tocolytic rather than its intended use as a bronchodilator.<br>Infusion rate is not increased and can be decreased if maternal pulse rate exceeds 120 bpm or systolic BP falls below 80 to 90 mm Hg.<br>Adverse reactions:<br>1. Cardiovascular: Maternal and fetal tachycardia, palpitations, cardiac dysrhythmias, chest pain, wide pulse pressure<br>2. Respiratory: Dyspnea, chest discomfort<br>3. Central nervous system: Tremors, restlessness, weakness, dizziness, headache<br>4. Metabolic: Hypokalemia, hyperglycemia<br>5. Gastrointestinal: Nausea, vomiting, reduced bowel motility<br>6. Skin: Flushing, diaphoresis |
| Corticosteroids (betamethasone and dexamethasone) | See Drug Guide: Betamethasone, Dexamethasone (p. 588) | |
| 17 Alpha-hydroxyprogesterone caproate (17P) (currently in clinical research trials) | Women in studies currently receive 17P in daily vaginal suppositories or weekly IM injections. Drug must be prepared by a compounding pharmacist. 17P is discontinued if woman reaches 37 wk of gestation. | 17P is now being studied to evaluate effectiveness for prevention of preterm birth in women who had previous preterm birth(s); side effects also being evaluated.<br>Previously known as diethylstilbestrol (DES, or Delalutin); withdrawn from market because of ineffectiveness for stopping spontaneous abortion |

*Doses and frequency of administration are examples; actual protocols may vary.

Data from American Academy of Pediatrics & American College of Obstetricians and Gynecologists. (2007). *Guidelines for perinatal care* (6th ed.). Elk Grove Village, IL, and Washington, DC: Author; Iams, J.D., Romero, R., & Creasy, R.K. (2009). Preterm labor and birth. In R.K. Creasy, R. Resnik, J.D. Iams, et al. (Eds.), *Creasy & Resnik's maternal-fetal medicine: Principles and practice* (6th ed., pp. 545–582). Philadelphia: Saunders; Svigos, J.M., Dodd, J.M., Robinson, J.S. (2011). Threatened and actual preterm labor including mode of delivery. In D.K. James, P.J. Steer, C.P. Weiner, et al. (Eds.), *High risk pregnancy: Management options* (4th ed., pp. 1065–1074). Philadelphia: Saunders.

bleeding from injections and bruising with no apparent cause. The antiinflammatory effect of indomethacin can mask infection because fever may not be present. Checking the height of the fundus at the beginning of therapy and daily thereafter helps identify reduced amniotic fluid volume. Ultrasound calculation of the amniotic fluid index (AFI) is a more precise volume measurement. Decreased fetal movements and absent FHR accelerations with fetal movement can occur if the fetal condition deteriorates.

**Beta-adrenergic drugs.** Although ritodrine (Yutopar) is the only beta-adrenergic currently approved by the FDA for tocolysis, it is used infrequently because of significant side effects and only minimal increases in the length of pregnancy, similar to other tocolytics. Terbutaline (Brethine) is prescribed to treat bronchospasm. However, terbutaline is used off-label for its tocolytic activity to stop PTL. Terbutaline has been widely used for tocolysis because it is less expensive, has a longer duration of action between doses, and can be administered promptly by the subcutaneous rather than the oral route if needed (AAP & ACOG, 2007; ACOG, 2011a; Agency for Healthcare Research and Quality [AHRQ], 2010).

The main side effects of beta-adrenergic drugs, including terbutaline, involve the cardiorespiratory system. Maternal and fetal tachycardia are common. Other potential maternal side effects include decreased blood pressure, wide pulse pressure, dysrhythmias, myocardial ischemia, chest pain, and pulmonary edema. Metabolic changes include hyperglycemia and hypokalemia. Headaches, tremors, and restlessness are other side effects, with headaches often becoming less severe as the woman becomes accustomed to the drug. Propranolol (Inderal), an agent that blocks beta-adrenergic drugs, should be readily available to reverse severe adverse effects.

Because of reported cardiovascular events, terbutaline now carries a *Boxed warning and Contraindications* ("black box") against parenteral use longer than 48 to 72 hours or prolonged treatment with oral terbutaline (FDA, 2011). A beta-adrenergic such as terbutaline can be given by the IV, subcutaneous, or oral route. See http://www.fda.gov for the FDA drug safety report.

The nurse should assess a woman's apical heart rate and lung sounds before administering each intermittent dose of terbutaline for PTL. Addition of these maternal assessments to scheduled maternal vital signs and FHR is often adequate when a woman receives terbutaline by subcutaneous infusion pump. However, infusion pump therapy may not be insured. Drug toxicity necessitating discontinuation of terbutaline is suggested by a maternal heart rate greater than 120 bpm or respiratory findings such as "wet" lung sounds and a more rapid rate, possibly accompanied by shortness of breath. Nonreassuring maternal or fetal assessments should be reported promptly to the physician.

## DRUG GUIDE

### *Betamethasone, Dexamethasone*

**Classification:** Corticosteroids.

**Indications:** Acceleration of fetal lung maturity to reduce the incidence and severity of respiratory distress syndrome (RDS). Studies suggest that antenatal steroids can reduce the incidence of intraventricular hemorrhage (IVH) and neonatal death in the preterm infant. Greatest benefits accrue if at least 24 hours elapse between the initial dose and birth of the preterm infant, but the drug is indicated if birth is not imminent.

**Dosage and Route:** Betamethasone: 12 mg intramuscular (IM) for two doses, 24 hours apart. Dexamethasone: 6 mg IM every 12 hours for four doses.

**Absorption:** Rapid and complete after IM administration.

**Excretion:** Metabolized in the liver. Excreted in urine.

**Contraindications:** Active infection, such as chorioamnionitis, is a relative contraindication, although further study is needed. The National Institutes of Health (NIH) recommend use of corticosteroids for the woman who has preterm rupture of the membranes (24 to 34 weeks of gestation). The American Academy of Pediatrics (AAP) and American College of Obstetricians and Gynecologists (ACOG) agree with the NIH recommendation but recommend that the time period for administration be 24 to 32 weeks and that 32 and 33 weeks might be beneficial; however, evidence supporting this recommendation is unclear.

**Precautions:** Possible infection. Pregnancies complicated by diabetes.

**Adverse Reactions:** Few, owing to the short-term use of the drug. Pulmonary edema is possible secondary to sodium and fluid retention.

**Nursing Considerations:** Explain to the woman the potential benefits of corticosteroid administration to the preterm neonate. Explain that the drug cannot prevent or lessen the severity of all complications of prematurity. If the woman has diabetes, explain that more frequent blood glucose determinations are common because these levels are often elevated while taking either of the corticosteroids. A temporary rise in platelet and white blood cell (WBC) levels can last 72 hours. WBC levels greater than 20,000/mm$^3$ can indicate infection. Assess lung sounds. Report chest pain or heaviness or dyspnea.

Reference: American Academy of Pediatrics & American College of Obstetricians and Gynecologists. (2007). *Guidelines for perinatal care* (6th ed.). Elk Grove Village, IL, and Washington, DC: Author.

## Accelerating Fetal Lung Maturation

Corticosteroids are often administered to speed fetal lung maturation if birth before 34 weeks seems inevitable. Steroid therapy can reduce the incidence and severity of respiratory distress syndrome (RDS) and intraventricular hemorrhage (IVH) in the preterm infant. Steroid administration as late as 37 weeks gestation may be chosen if fetal lung maturity studies demonstrate immature lungs after 34 weeks gestation. Betamethasone or dexamethasone can be used for this purpose (see Drug Guide: Betamethasone, Dexamethasone for corticosteroids used to accelerate fetal lung maturation).

Corticosteroids are indicated if the woman is between 24 and 34 weeks of gestation because of the high incidence of problems, including RDS, that affect an infant of this age. Delaying preterm birth for at least 24 hours after a woman begins corticosteroid therapy provides the greatest benefit in reducing critical problems associated with prematurity. Evidence shows that even a fetus born sooner than 24 hours after the mother begins taking the corticosteroid can have some lung maturation benefits. Thus, one benefit of tocolytic drugs is to prolong labor enough that the fetus can benefit from the corticosteroid drug given. Benefits of corticosteroids to the preterm infant are known to last for 7 days after the drug is initiated, although they may last longer. Repeating the corticosteroid therapy process 7 days after the initial dose is not recommended (AAP & ACOG, 2013; Cunningham et al., 2014).

A temporary increase in leukocytes or glucose intolerance can occur with betamethasone or dexamethasone therapy. An increase in the insulin dose may be required for the woman with gestational diabetes or preexisting diabetes during steroid therapy. The nurse should tell the woman about common but temporary side effects of nervousness and insomnia when receiving steroids.

Vital signs should be assessed to identify fever and elevated pulse that can indicate infection associated with steroid administration. Lung sounds should be assessed with vital signs because corticosteroids can cause sodium retention with accompanying fluid retention and pulmonary edema. The nurse should observe for and teach the woman about signs of pulmonary edema. The woman is taught to report any chest pain or heaviness or any difficulty breathing, because these symptoms could indicate pulmonary edema or pneumonia. Pain and burning with urination are symptoms of urinary tract infection that is common in pregnancy, even when steroids are not given.

## NURSING CARE

### The Woman in Preterm Labor

Nursing care for the woman with PTL can include interventions related to tocolytic, corticosteroid, or antibiotic drug therapy. If labor cannot be stopped, care is similar to that for other laboring women, with additional care to prepare for a preterm infant's needs at birth. Support for anticipatory grieving may be needed if the infant is very immature and not expected to live.

Care for the family expecting an extremely preterm infant (approximately 20 through 24 weeks of gestation) can be heavily laden with ethical and legal issues. For example, what is the true accuracy of the gestational age? Has a corticosteroid been administered to accelerate fetal lung maturity and when was the last dose? If labor cannot be halted, is fetal monitoring beneficial? Nonreassuring fetal monitoring patterns in the very immature fetus can distress parents and caregivers alike. On the other hand, knowledge of the fetal response to labor helps the neonatologist make better decisions about how to treat the infant. In addition, ultrasound estimates of gestational age have considerable variation at present. A fetus presumed to be 23 weeks of gestation before birth may be assessed as 25 weeks or older after birth and suited to more intense treatment than planned, especially if the woman had no prenatal care before entering the hospital (ACOG, 2016a).

General nursing care for a woman having PTL often applies to women with other high-risk pregnancies. Women may need multiple hospitalizations, with admission occurring in the middle of the night, disrupting sleep and family routines. These women often have some activity restriction and may have to stop working. This section focuses on the family's psychosocial concerns, management of home care, and the woman's boredom that may result from restrictions.

#### Psychosocial Concerns

***Assessment.*** The entire family is affected by stressors associated with a complicated pregnancy. Assess how the woman and her family usually cope with crisis situations and how they are coping with this one. To set priorities for care, identify their greatest concerns.

The woman or her family members may have physical, emotional, and cognitive ailments because of the unexpected problems. Physical signs of emotional distress, such as trembling, palpitations, and restlessness, are also side effects of beta-adrenergic drugs or corticosteroids. The woman may express fear, helplessness, or disbelief. She may be irritable and tearful. Her ability to concentrate may be impaired at a time when she needs to absorb new information.

Her partner often feels at loose ends. He struggles to keep the household running if she must be inactive. Young children pick up on their parents' anxiety and may misbehave or regress.

The family may be under financial strain. The woman must often curtail or stop working. If she does not have sick time or other benefits, the family suffers an abrupt drop in income at a time when medical expenses are mounting. A woman may be admitted to a distant hospital that has the better capacity to care for her and her preterm baby. A distant transfer to a higher-level maternity care facility removes the woman from familiar friends, family, and support groups.

Overlaid on the sudden change in lifestyle is the family's concern for the well-being of the fetus. A woman may feel pulled in opposite directions by the needs of all her children—those already born and the fetus she is trying to mature. She may be concerned about the effects of drug therapy and their side effects on the fetus and on her own body.

***Nursing diagnosis and planning.*** The outcome of any pregnancy is never certain, and this is especially true when the pregnancy is high risk for any reason. The unexpected development of complications during pregnancy can prevent a woman and her family from using their normal coping mechanisms. Goals focus on the family's ability to cope with the crisis of PTL. The nursing diagnosis is:

- Anxiety related to uncertain outcome of the pregnancy, disruption of family relationships, and financial concerns.

**Expected outcome.** The woman and family will identify methods to cope with the temporary disruption in their lives.

***Interventions***

**Providing information.** Knowledge decreases anxiety and fear related to the unknown. Include appropriate family members so that they are more likely to be supportive. Determine what the woman knows about preterm birth and about the specific recommended therapy. Determine what information the parents need regarding the problems that her preterm infant may face. Use this opportunity to correct misinformation and reinforce accurate information.

Initially, the woman for whom activity restriction is prescribed may be highly motivated to maintain the recommended activity level. Because her contractions often diminish, even if only for a short time, she may become restless from minor restrictions. She may feel that there is now no need for a restrictions regarding, for example, how far she should ambulate. Help her understand the purpose of activity restrictions and that these restrictions may diminish as the condition of her pregnancy stabilizes.

**Promoting expression of concerns.** Encourage the woman and her family to express their concerns. Begin by exploring common concerns of women with problem pregnancies. For example, say, "Most women are worried when they need to stop working. How has this affected your family?" An open question gives them a chance to ventilate their feelings so that they can take the next step: identifying constructive methods to cope with the situation. Collaboration with a social worker may identify financial or other community resources available. Offering to refer a chaplain to the woman may help her talk about her concerns associated with care related to her pregnancy, the pregnancy outcome, or her personal life. Referral to a psychologist may be indicated.

**Teaching what may occur during a preterm birth.** Because preterm birth may occur despite all interventions, a pregnant woman and her partner should be prepared for that possibility. If the hospital has a neonatal intensive care unit, a nurse often visits the parents to explain what might occur there if their baby is born early. One or both parents tour the unit to see the equipment and care infants receive there. A tour of the intensive care nursery may motivate the woman to maintain the recommended therapy as she tries to "buy time" for the baby to mature.

In hospitals with neonatal intensive care units, one or more neonatal nurses, a neonatal nurse practitioner, a neonatologist, or a combination of these professionals is present at birth to care for the infant. The woman who planned to give birth in a hospital that does not have a neonatal intensive care unit or has one of a lower level of critical care may be transferred before the birth to an appropriate facility. Such a move will allow immediate care and stabilization of her newborn. The infant may also be transferred after birth if there is no time to transfer the woman before birth or if the infant has more problems than anticipated. Hospitalization of the mother, infant, or both at a distant location adds to the stress on the family. However, the pregnancy and fetal maturity also may progress after the early complications, allowing the woman to return to care in a familiar environment.

*Evaluation*

- Can the woman and her family identify constructive methods to deal with their anxiety?

If a high-risk pregnancy situation is prolonged or if the family has difficulty adapting constructively to the situation, a nursing diagnosis of Interrupted Family Processes may be more appropriate. (Also see Nursing Care Plan: Preterm Labor for other nursing diagnoses.)

### Management of Home Care

*Assessment.* The care of women with high-risk pregnancies, including risk of preterm birth, often occurs in their homes if the gestation is sufficiently advanced and the signs and symptoms of PTL and birth have diminished significantly. Many daily household activities are managed by the woman, even if only by her directions to others. However, when the PTL complication becomes greater, family roles are again disrupted because of the changed relationships between family members.

Clarify the level of activity prescribed by the physician, and identify the role of each family member. A good way to do this is to have the woman describe a usual day before any limitations were recommended. Determine the number and ages of children in the home.

Evaluate the home itself, either by visual inspection or by questioning the family. Does the home or apartment have more than one level? Determine whether a telephone is available for emergency contact.

Evaluate the family's resources and their willingness to use them. Ask whether family members and friends in the area are available to help. Explore local support groups such as churches or mother-to-mother networks that the family might contact for assistance. Determine financial reimbursements that might be available through insurance coverage.

*Nursing Diagnosis and planning.* The nursing diagnosis is:

- Impaired Home Maintenance related to change in usual roles and responsibilities.

**Expected outcomes.** Two outcomes are often appropriate for the woman and family faced with a preterm birth that will occur at an unknown time:

- Short term: The family will identify methods for managing daily household routines.
- Long term: The woman will be able to maintain the prescribed level of activity and drug therapy.

*Interventions.* The pregnancy threatened by PTL or other complications is a self-limiting situation, making temporary adjustments somewhat easier. Needed changes in home routines may be brief but sometimes unexpectedly extend over several weeks.

**Caring for children.** The concerns of a woman who has children differ from those of a woman who does not. Knowledge of growth and development helps the nurse identify the most appropriate way to ensure adequate care for the children and strengthen family relationships.

Toddlers and preschoolers rarely understand why their mother does not play with them as usual. If they are already in daycare, this arrangement can continue if the family can afford it. They might live with a relative or friend temporarily. Toddlers may feel that their parents have abandoned them if they are sent away, although this might be the only realistic solution if no one besides the mother is available to supervise them.

School-age children usually understand the situation better and are often quite helpful. They can assist with the care of other children, but they should not be put into the role of an adult. They may resent responsibility that is excessive for their age. School-age children often enjoy learning new facts about their mother's pregnancy and tests the baby may need.

Adolescents may welcome the trust their parents have in them, but they also may resent the intrusion on independent activities with their peers. Teenagers who drive safely can be helpful in taking younger siblings to school and other activities. They can be enlisted for grocery shopping and meal preparation. If resentment flares, the parents and nurse can remind teenagers that the situation is temporary and that they are making valuable contributions to the health of the new baby.

**Maintaining the household.** The first step to home maintenance during this time may be for the woman to lower her standards of housekeeping. Things may not be as clean or as organized as she would like. The partner may take over many household tasks, but these could compete with responsibilities outside the home.

Advise the woman to have a list of tasks ready when friends and family ask, "Can I do anything to help?" If they offer to bring a meal or do laundry, encourage her to accept. Remind her that people who offer to help mean it and that she may be able to return the favor to someone else. Homemaker services may be an option to help the family deal with the woman's temporary disability.

Transportation of school-age children may be a concern. If no family or friends are available, the school nurse or Parent-Teacher Association (PTA) may help find someone willing to take the children to school each day.

*Evaluation.* Short-term expected outcomes help the nurse and patient (often including the family) to identify resolution of their immediate needs. Longer-term outcomes can be evaluated over a series of days or weeks as the prescribed therapy for the complicated pregnancy changes.

- Short term: Does the family identify how to manage minimal household care?
- Long term: Can the woman maintain the prescribed therapy until birth?

### Boredom

*Assessment.* If activity is to be restricted, determine what skills the woman has for coping with boredom. An occupational or recreational therapist may help the woman identify activities that are possible within prescribed restrictions. Although the use of bed rest to prolong gestation is usually brief, some reduction in activity is prescribed. The nurse should consider helping the woman choose appropriate activities, whether hospitalized or managing her care at home.

To identify activities that are still appropriate within the restrictions prescribed, ask about a usual day. Ask about hobbies, present and past. What type of leisure activities does the woman enjoy? Which activities are available or possible? Does she have more than one resting place to give her a change of scenery and surrounding activity?

Assess her personality. Is she calm and composed, taking whatever comes with serenity, or does she need to be busy most of the time? No matter how motivated, the woman who finds inactivity tiresome will find even limited activity restrictions difficult to maintain.

*Nursing diagnosis and planning.* A possible nursing diagnosis is:

- Deficient Diversional Activity related to lack of knowledge about appropriate activities for her pregnancy restrictions.

**Expected outcome.** The woman will pursue (with the help of others) appropriate activities to relieve boredom while maintaining recommended activity limits.

*Interventions*

**Identifying appropriate activities.** Determine the woman's understanding about needed activity restrictions to identify misunderstandings. The type and amount of ideal physical activities may vary with complications and the progression of pregnancy. Reinforce which of her usual activities are permitted and which are not and why. If the

## NURSING CARE PLAN

### *Preterm Labor*

**Focused Assessment**

Rhonda, a 28-year-old woman, is a gravida 4, para 3. Her children were born at 40 weeks, 28 weeks, and 32 weeks of gestation. Her children are 7 and 4 years and 18 months old. She has mild cramping and pelvic pressure at 28 weeks and comes to the hospital right away. Her cervix is dilated 1 to 2 cm and is beginning to efface. She responds to intravenous (IV) magnesium sulfate to stop her contractions. The physician also orders two doses of betamethasone 12 mg intramuscular (IM), 24 hours apart. After her contractions stop, she is started on oral terbutaline to maintain tocolysis and will be discharged home in 48 hours if no recurrent symptoms develop. Terbutaline will probably be discontinued before discharge.

**Nursing Diagnosis**

Possible Impaired Home Maintenance related to activity restrictions and family demands.

**Planning**

***Expected Outcome***

By hospital discharge, Rhonda will:

Relate ways that she can maintain prescribed activity restrictions.

**Interventions and *Rationales***

1. Assess what support systems are available and financially feasible to help Rhonda with child care and transportation, such as daycare, "mother's day out" programs at churches, family, and friends.
   *Responsibilities for other children may impede maintaining activity limits. Coordination among several resources helps provide all-day coverage for child care.*
2. Encourage Rhonda to lower her standards for home management temporarily and reallocate some of her usual roles. Alternate arrangements increase the chance to maintain therapy:
   a. Eat nourishing take-out or fast food.
   b. Set priorities regarding household tasks that must be done.
   c. Let her children do tasks that are within their abilities.
   d. Make lists of tasks for different people who ask to help her. Encourage her to consider the talents, resources, and obligations of volunteers.
   *Considering the strengths and personal obligations of those who volunteer to help her will increase the satisfaction of both Rhonda and her family as well as the satisfaction of those who help.*
3. Encourage Rhonda to accept help from others. Remind her that this situation is temporary and that she may be able to help someone else at another time.
   *If a woman feels that she may be able to help others at a later time, she may be more willing to accept help when she needs it.*

**Evaluation**

Rhonda identifies three friends in addition to her mother-in-law who may be able to help with child care. She says she cannot afford to continue sending her children to their daycare center if she is not working. She feels that if her children are cared for, her husband can handle the other home management needs.

**Focused Assessment**

At 31 weeks of gestation, Rhonda again experiences preterm labor and goes to the hospital. Her cervix is dilated 2 to 3 cm and is 75% effaced (approximately 0.5 cm long). Her contractions occur every 6 to 7 minutes, and last approximately 20 to 30 seconds each. The physician again orders a magnesium sulfate infusion. The physician explains that preterm birth may be delayed but will probably occur within the next 24 to 48 hours. Rhonda begins crying and says, "I did what I was supposed to do and now I'm still going to have another preemie! It will be weeks before I can be a real mother!"

**Nursing Diagnosis**

Grieving related to loss of expected term birth experience.

**Planning**

***Expected Outcome***

Rhonda will:

Express her feelings about the loss of her expected birth at term.

**Interventions and *Rationales***

1. Sit down and spend time with Rhonda. Use therapeutic communication to encourage her to express her feelings.
   *Unhurried time allows expression of feelings, which is the first step in dealing with the anticipated loss.*
2. When she has expressed her frustration about this development in her pregnancy, explain that much remains unknown about why labor begins, whether at term, preterm, or postterm.
   *If a woman knows that professionals do not have all the answers but must make recommendations based on what is known or appears to work for an individual woman, Rhonda may be more accepting of the inevitability of preterm birth.*
3. Tell Rhonda that her efforts have paid off because she has gained 3 valuable weeks of gestation for her baby. In addition, the drug betamethasone can reduce the chance that her preterm newborn will have the usual degree of common respiratory problems if born at this time.
   *Knowing that her self-care has benefits, although not the hoped-for term birth, reduces the sense of failure that Rhonda may feel.*

**Evaluation**

Rhonda cries and expresses her frustration about the developments in her pregnancy. She says that she knew she was more likely to have another preterm infant but hoped that this time would be different. As the day goes by, she gradually begins expressing feelings that she did do something positive for this baby. Because contractions have not diminished but have become more intense, she plans to deal with the probable preterm birth within 24 hours.

**Additional Nursing Diagnoses to Consider**

Readiness for Enhanced Self-Health Management
Interrupted Family Processes
Ineffective Health Maintenance
Ineffective Coping (Individual and/or Family)
Readiness for Enhanced Family Processes

woman understands the rationale, she may be more willing to comply with restrictions.

Some women continue work activities such as paperwork or phone calls that can be accomplished with minimal physical exertion. Work that can be done online may relieve boredom and reduce anxiety about unfinished deadlines. Workplace deadlines can increase stress, even if the woman works at home. However, the feeling of usefulness gained by such activities may be beneficial if it means she is willing to maintain activity restrictions. Moreover, work-related activities can reduce some of the family's financial concerns.

Online support organizations such as Sidelines National Support Network (http://www.sidelines.org) provide online support for women with high-risk pregnancies. Pregnancy complications other than PTL are included on the website.

Suggest activities to help the woman keep busy and productive. These may include household activities that can be done at rest, volunteering for activities such as phone calls, and leisure activities such as puzzles, home movies, games, and needlework. Help her identify someone who can obtain the necessary supplies for her. This might be a good time to reactivate an old (quiet) hobby.

The woman can participate in many activities with her children while she rests. She can read to them and play board or card games. Encourage her to help the children with their homework and stimulate their development with thought-provoking discussions. Working with children on video games may help them learn during their playtime.

**Changing the physical surroundings.** Encourage the woman to identify at least two locations where she can maintain her prescribed rest periods. A change of location increases the woman's willingness to reduce her activities because she can still take part in family activities. Each area should include pillows, blankets, and a clipboard with writing materials. A laptop computer can be taken from place to place by another person. Small rolling carts made of plastic help keep small things organized and together. The carts can be used after the baby is born for household needs. Ideally, the telephone is within reach and is cordless or she has effective use of a cell phone. Either programming or writing important phone numbers of family and friends, physicians, and emergency numbers helps assure the family that phone contacts are easily available for emergency as well as social needs.

***Evaluation***

- Does the woman accurately identify appropriate and inappropriate activities that she pursues?

## PROLONGED PREGNANCY

A prolonged pregnancy is defined as one that lasts longer than 42 weeks. Many apparent cases of prolonged pregnancy are only a miscalculation of the estimated date of delivery (EDD) because the woman has had irregular menstrual periods or has forgotten the date of her last period. Late or no prenatal care limits the use of clinical methods such as ultrasonography that are most useful for pinpointing the EDD and avoiding potential problems associated with a prolonged gestation.

### Complications

The main physical risk in prolonged pregnancy is to the fetus or newborn. Insufficiency of the placental function secondary to aging can occur if pregnancy is truly postterm. Infarctions of small areas reduce the transfer of oxygen and nutrients to the fetus and removal of carbon dioxide and other wastes. Because the fetus with placental insufficiency has less reserve to tolerate uterine contractions, signs of fetal compromise, such as late decelerations and decreased variability, can develop during labor. In addition, the reduced amniotic fluid volume (oligohydramnios) that often accompanies placental insufficiency can result in umbilical cord compression. Meconium in the amniotic fluid can cause respiratory distress in the newborn if it is aspirated before or during birth. The infant may have growth restriction and appear to have lost weight.

Many postterm fetuses do not suffer from placental insufficiency and continue growing. The woman and fetus can have complications related to dysfunctional labor or injury if the birth is traumatic. The woman's postpartum uterine contractions may be inadequate to control bleeding. However, some women and their postterm fetus have an uneventful labor and birth.

Psychologically, the woman often feels as if her pregnancy will never end. She may fear induction of labor, a possible cesarean birth, and problems with her baby. The added fatigue imposed by prolonged pregnancy diminishes her resources for tolerating the added stress and anxiety.

### Therapeutic Management

Therapeutic management begins with determination of the most accurate gestational age. If a woman did not have early prenatal care, several markers used to pinpoint gestation, such as ultrasonography, fundal height measurements, and dates of quickening and first auscultation of the fetal heart tones with a nonamplified fetoscope, may be lost. Also, the woman may have forgotten the date of her last menstrual period or have irregular periods.

Fetal condition is another factor in management decisions. If antepartum tests such as the biophysical profile (BPP) indicate that the fetus is doing well but other tests do not yet verify a term gestation, the birth attendant often takes a more conservative approach than if the fetus is suffering from reduced placental function.

If the gestation appears to be truly postterm and there is no fetal urgency to deliver quickly, management depends on whether the cervix is favorable for induction of labor. If the cervix is favorable, induction is often started. If the cervix is not favorable, the physician may take a "wait-and-see" approach, repeating fetal surveillance tests as needed. The woman can undergo a cervical ripening procedure (see Chapter 19) to make the cervix more favorable for induction.

### Nursing Considerations

Nursing care for the woman with a prolonged pregnancy is tied to the management chosen. The nurse's role may include:

- Teaching about procedures such as antepartum testing or induction of labor
- Support for the woman's psychological and physical fatigue
- Nursing care related to specific procedures such as induction of labor

## INTRAPARTUM EMERGENCIES

### Placental Abnormalities

Women with placental abnormalities (see Chapter 25) can experience hemorrhage during the antepartum or intrapartum period. Placenta previa or previous cesarean birth is often associated with an abnormally adherent placenta (**placenta accreta**). Placenta accreta can cause immediate or delayed hemorrhage immediately after birth because the placenta does not separate cleanly, often leaving small fragments that prevent full uterine contraction. More extreme degrees of abnormal adherence occur when the placenta penetrates the uterine muscle itself (**placenta increta**) or even all the way through the uterus (**placenta percreta**). Prenatal ultrasound images help identify the placental abnormality before birth, and a cesarean hysterectomy is often planned. However, massive hemorrhage can occur unexpectedly. Methotrexate (see Chapter 32) can be used to speed degeneration of the remaining placental tissue (Belfort & Dildy, 2011; Cunningham et al., 2014).

### Prolapsed Umbilical Cord

A prolapsed umbilical cord slips down after the membranes rupture, subjecting it to compression between the fetus and pelvis (Fig. 27.6). It may slip down immediately with the fluid gush or long after the membranes rupture. Interruption in blood flow through the cord interferes with fetal oxygenation and is potentially fatal.

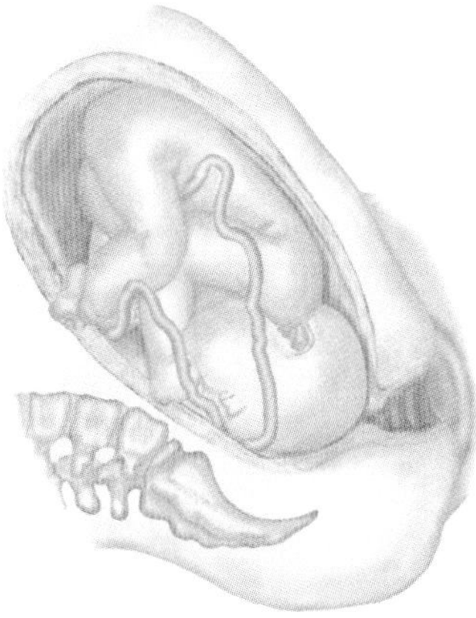

**Occult (hidden) prolapse**

The cord is compressed between the fetal presenting part and pelvis but cannot be seen or felt during vaginal examination.

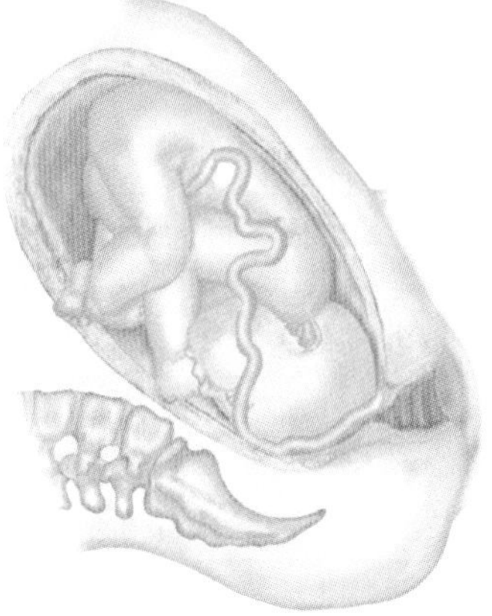

**Cord prolapsed in front of the fetal head**

The cord cannot be seen but can probably be felt as a pulsating mass during vaginal examination.

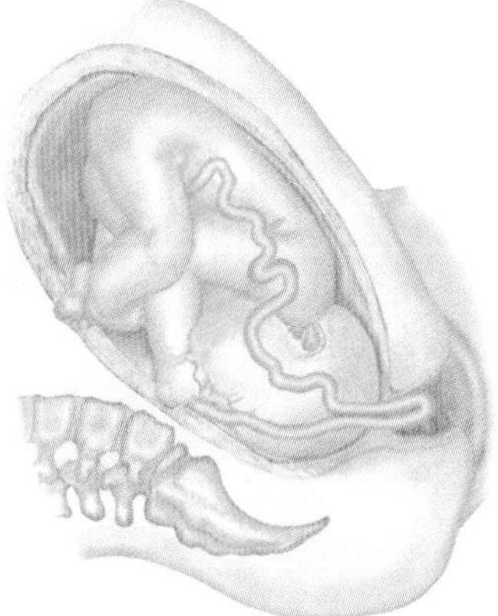

**Complete cord prolapse**

The cord can be seen protruding from the vagina.

FIG 27.6 Variations of prolapsed umbilical cord.

### Etiology

Prolapse of the umbilical cord (displacement of the umbilical cord in front of or beside the fetus) is more likely when the fit is poor between the fetal presenting part and the maternal pelvis when membranes rupture. When the fit is good, the presenting part fills the pelvic opening, leaving little room for the cord to slip down. Cord prolapse is more likely if any of the following conditions are present:

- A fetus that remains at a high station
- A very small fetus
- Breech presentation (the footling breech is more likely to be complicated by a prolapsed cord because the feet and legs are small and do not fill the pelvis well)
- Transverse lie
- Hydramnios (often associated with abnormal presentations; also, the unusually large amount of fluid exerts more pressure to push the cord out)

### Manifestations

Prolapse can be complete, with the cord visible at the vaginal opening. A prolapsed cord may not be visible but may be palpated on vaginal examination as it pulsates synchronously with the fetal heart. A speculum may allow visualization of the cord. An occult prolapse of the cord is one in which the cord slips alongside the fetal head or shoulders. The prolapse cannot be palpated or seen but is suspected because of changes in the FHR, such as bradycardia or variable decelerations.

### Therapeutic Management

Medical and nursing management overlap, as they do in many emergency situations. The nurse or birth attendant may be the first to discover cord prolapse. Birth is almost always cesarean unless vaginal delivery can be accomplished more quickly and less traumatically. If fetal death has already occurred, the care of the mother is the focus.

The priority is to relieve pressure on the cord to restore blood flow after cord prolapse occurs. None of these interventions should delay the promptest possible delivery. Push the call light to summon help. Others should call the physician and prepare for birth. Notify neonatal nurses and the pediatrician or neonatologist to prepare for neonatal resuscitation.

**SAFETY ALERT**

***Factors That Increase a Woman's Risk for a Prolapsed Umbilical Cord***

Ruptured membranes *and:*

- The fetal presenting part at a high station
- A fetus that poorly fits the pelvic inlet because of small size or abnormal presentation
- Excessive volume of amniotic fluid (hydramnios)

Prompt actions are taken to relieve cord compression and increase fetal oxygenation:

1. Position the woman's hips higher than her head to shift the fetal presenting part toward her diaphragm. Methods (Fig. 27.7) include:
   a. Knee-chest position
   b. Trendelenburg position
   c. Hips elevated with pillows, with side-lying position maintained
2. If elevation of the maternal hips does not result in an upward shift of the fetus to relieve cord compression, vaginal elevation of the presenting part using a sterile gloved hand may be required. Maintain this position until the physician orders it stopped, usually just before cesarean delivery, while minimizing added cord compression from the hand.
3. Avoid or minimize manual palpation or handling of the cord because vasospasm or trauma of cord vessels can further reduce umbilical blood flow to and from the fetus.
4. Ultrasound examination can be used to confirm presence of fetal heart activity before cesarean delivery.

Give oxygen at 8 to 10 L/min by facemask to increase maternal blood oxygen saturation, making more oxygen available to the fetus.

Umbilical cord prolapse occurs with varying degrees of severity, and other options may be ordered by the physician. However, prompt delivery of the viable fetus remains the priority. A tocolytic drug with a rapid onset of action, such as subcutaneous terbutaline, may be ordered to inhibit contractions, increasing placental blood flow and reducing intermittent pressure of the fetus against the pelvis and cord.

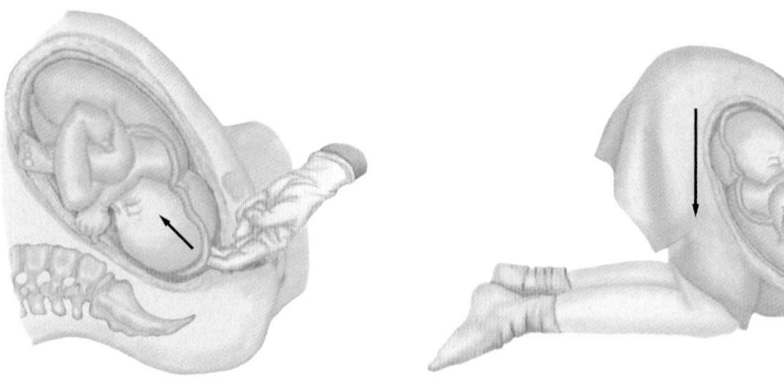

A gloved hand in the vagina pushes the fetus upward and off the cord.

Knee-chest position uses gravity to shift the fetus out of the pelvis. The woman's thighs should be at right angles to the bed and her chest flat on the bed.

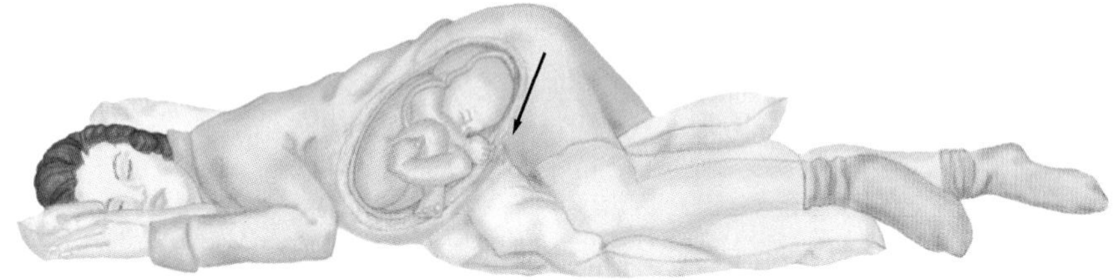

The woman's hips are elevated with two pillows; this is often combined with the Trendelenburg (head down) position.

**FIG 27.7** Measures to relieve pressure on a prolapsed umbilical cord until delivery can take place.

Warm, saline-moistened towels retard cooling and drying of the cord that protrudes from the vagina if any delay in cesarean delivery is required. Cooling causes vasospasm within the cord.

Prognosis for the woman is usually good because additional risks of umbilical cord prolapse are those associated with cesarean birth. Prognosis for the infant depends on how long and how severely blood flow through the cord has been impaired and on the gestational age. With prompt recognition and corrective actions, the infant usually does well (ACOG, 2010).

### Nursing Considerations

In addition to prompt corrective actions, the nurse must consider the woman's anxiety. The nurse must remain calm during this time and acknowledge the woman's anxiety. Explanations must be simple because anxiety interferes with the woman's ability to comprehend them. Her partner and family should be included as much as possible.

## Uterine Rupture

Sometimes a tear in the wall of the uterus occurs because the uterus cannot withstand the pressure against it (Fig. 27.8). The three variations of uterine rupture are as follows:

- *Complete rupture* is a direct communication between the uterine and peritoneal cavities.
- *Incomplete rupture* is rupture into the peritoneum covering the uterus or into the broad ligament but not into the peritoneal cavity.
- *Dehiscence* is a partial separation of an old uterine scar. There may be little or no bleeding. There may be no signs or symptoms, and the rupture ("window") may be found incidentally during a subsequent cesarean birth or other abdominal surgery.

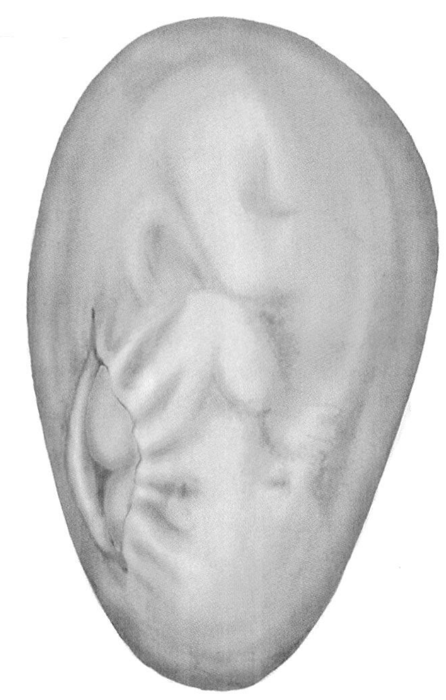

**FIG 27.8** Uterine rupture in the lower uterine segment.

### Etiology

Although uterine rupture is rare, dehiscence is not unusual. Uterine rupture is associated with previous uterine surgery, such as cesarean birth or surgery to remove fibroids. The risk of rupture in a woman who has had a prior cesarean birth depends on the type of uterine incision. The risk for rupture is greater in women with a classic incision (vertical into the upper uterine segment) than in women with a low transverse incision. For this reason, vaginal birth after cesarean (VBAC) is not recommended for women who have had a previous birth through a classic cesarean incision (see Fig. 19.9 [types of uterine incisions]). The decision regarding VBAC is made by the woman and her physician with consideration of the benefits and potential problems associated with vaginal birth that follows a previous cesarean.

Rupture of the unscarred uterus is more likely for women of high parity with a thin uterine wall, women sustaining blunt abdominal trauma, and women with intense contractions, especially if fetopelvic disproportion is present. Excessively strong (hypertonic) contractions can cause the intrauterine pressure to exceed the tensile strength of the uterine wall. If the fetus cannot be expelled downward through the pelvis, contractions may push it through the lower uterine segment. Intense contractions are more likely to occur when oxytocin or misoprostol are administered to stimulate labor, but uterine rupture can occur spontaneously (Belfort & Dildy, 2011; Cunningham et al., 2014).

### Manifestations

Dehiscence does not produce symptoms initially and may not interfere with labor or vaginal delivery if the area is small. However, labor progress may stop because the open area prevents efficient expulsion of the fetus. The intrauterine pressure may change little during contractions. A larger area of dehiscence may cause abdominal pain that persists despite analgesic.

Manifestations of uterine rupture vary with the degree of rupture and can mimic other complications. Possible signs and symptoms of uterine rupture include:

- Abdominal pain and tenderness. The pain may not be severe; it can occur suddenly at the peak of a contraction. The woman may describe a feeling that something "ripped" or "gave way."
- Chest pain, pain in the shoulder area, between the scapulae, or pain on inspiration. Pain occurs because of the irritation of blood below the woman's diaphragm.
- Hypovolemic shock caused by hemorrhage: tachycardia, tachypnea, falling blood pressure, pallor, cool and clammy skin, anxiety. Signs of hypovolemia may not occur until after birth, and the fall in blood pressure is often a late sign of the hemorrhage.
- Signs associated with impaired fetal oxygenation, such as late decelerations, reduced variability, tachycardia, and bradycardia.
- Absent fetal heart sounds with a large disruption of the placenta.
- Cessation of uterine contractions.
- Palpation of the fetus outside the uterus (usually occurs only with a large, complete rupture). The fetus is often dead if the placenta is involved.

If the rupture is incomplete, blood loss is slower and signs of shock, chest pain, or shoulder pain may be delayed. Complete rupture results in massive blood loss. Signs of shock and pain develop quickly. External bleeding may not be impressive because most of the blood is lost into the peritoneal cavity.

### Therapeutic Management

Initial management is to stabilize the woman and fetus and to perform cesarean delivery. If the rupture is small and the woman wants other children, the uterus may be repaired. A woman with a large uterine rupture requires hysterectomy. Blood products are replaced if needed.

### Nursing Considerations

The nurse must be aware if the woman is at increased risk for uterine rupture and must stay alert for the signs and symptoms. Administer oxytocin cautiously to reduce the likelihood of excessive contractions. Keep in mind that hypertonic contractions can occur in either a stimulated or unstimulated labor, and monitor for their presence. Notify the birth attendant if hypertonic contractions occur.

Uterine rupture may not be detected before birth. If postpartum bleeding is excessive and the fundus is firm after vaginal birth, injury to the birth canal, including uterine rupture, is possible. Bleeding may be concealed if the ruptured area bleeds into the broad ligament. In this case, signs of hypovolemic shock are likely to develop quickly.

## Uterine Inversion

An inversion occurs when the uterus completely or partly turns inside out, usually during the third stage of labor. Such an event is uncommon but potentially fatal.

### Etiology

Often no single cause is identified. Predisposing factors include:

- Pulling on the umbilical cord before the placenta detaches from the uterine wall
- Fundal pressure during birth
- Fundal pressure on an incompletely contracted uterus after birth
- Increased intraabdominal pressure
- An abnormally adherent placenta
- Weakness of the uterine wall
- Fundal placenta implantation

### Manifestations

The birth attendant notes that the uterus is either absent from the abdomen or a depression in the fundal area is present. The interior of the uterus may be seen through the cervix or protruding into the vagina. Massive hemorrhage, shock, and pain quickly become evident. The woman has severe pelvic pain.

### Therapeutic Management

Quick action by nursing and medical personnel is essential to prevent maternal morbidity and mortality. The physician tries to replace the uterus through the vagina into a normal position. If that is not possible, laparotomy with replacement is done. Hysterectomy may be required, and several units of blood are usually ordered immediately (Belfort & Dildy, 2011; Cunningham et al., 2014).

Two IV lines are established to allow rapid fluid and blood replacement. An arterial line is often placed for oxygen saturation monitoring. General anesthesia or a tocolytic drug is often needed to relax the uterus enough to replace it. After the uterus is replaced, oxytocin or a prostaglandin, such as carboprost, is given to contract the uterus and control blood loss. *Uterine contraction is stimulated until the uterus is repositioned to avoid trapping the inverted fundus in the cervix.*

### Nursing Considerations

Nursing care during the emergency will supplement that of other staff members. Postpartum nursing care is directed toward observing and maintaining maternal blood volume and correcting shock. The woman may be transferred to the intensive care unit.

Assess the uterine fundus for firmness, height, and deviation from the midline. Initially, frequent maternal vital signs and oxygen saturation checks maintain observation of hemodynamic factors. After postbirth outcomes stabilize, the assessment frequency of the woman's hemodynamic status is gradually reduced to a standard recovery room frequency while continuing observation for other complications that may be less obvious. Observe for tachycardia and a falling blood pressure and falling urine output, which are associated with hypovolemic shock. Cardiac dysrhythmias can occur because of severe hypovolemia and the secondary effects from drugs used to manage the complications. Laboratory studies of blood count and clotting factors are frequent.

An indwelling catheter allows observation of fluid balance and keeps the bladder empty so that the uterus can contract well. Assess the catheter for patency, and record intake and output. Urine output should be at least 30 mL/hr. A fall in urine output may indicate hypovolemia or an obstructed catheter.

The woman is allowed nothing by mouth until her condition stabilizes. She can usually receive fluids and progress to solid foods quickly if uterine inversion does not recur. It may recur in a future pregnancy if conditions favor its development.

### Anaphylactoid Syndrome

Pregnancy-related anaphylactoid syndrome, often called *amniotic fluid embolism (AFE),* occurs when amniotic fluid is drawn into the maternal circulation and carried to the woman's lungs. Fetal particulate matter (skin cells, vernix, hair, meconium) in the fluid obstructs pulmonary vessels. Failure of the right ventricle occurs early and can lead to hypoxemia. Left ventricular failure follows. Abrupt respiratory distress, depressed cardiac function, and circulatory collapse can occur rapidly. Disseminated intravascular coagulation (DIC) (see Chapter 25) is likely because thromboplastin-rich amniotic fluid interferes with normal blood clotting. This infrequent disorder is often fatal, and survivors may have neurologic deficits.

Entry of amniotic fluid containing fetal cells and other matter, such as vernix, is more likely if labor is very strong. High intrauterine pressure forces amniotic fluid into open uterine or cervical veins. The meconium that often accompanies a stressed fetus in such a labor adds to the particulate matter forced into the woman's circulation.

Although this disorder has been called amniotic fluid embolism, the newer name *anaphylactoid syndrome* is preferred because of findings related to other complications. Other maternal conditions that are not characterized by leaking of amniotic fluids into the woman's circulation include septic shock, preeclampsia, and cardiac disease. Other complications may be associated with this disorder but are not fully known. Fetal cells are often found in the blood samples of women who never developed this often fatal complication (Robbins, Martin, & Wilson, 2014).

Rapid therapeutic management of pregnancy-related anaphylactoid syndrome is primarily medical and includes:

- Cardiopulmonary resuscitation and support
- Oxygen with mechanical ventilation
- Correction of hypotension
- Blood component therapy (e.g., fibrinogen, packed red blood cells, platelets, fresh frozen plasma) to correct coagulation defects

If the pregnant mother is in cardiac arrest, immediate cesarean delivery is likely to improve survival odds for the baby (Cunningham et al., 2014).

## TRAUMA

Most major trauma during pregnancy occurs because of motor vehicle accidents, assault, or suicide. Battering is a significant cause of maternal–fetal trauma during pregnancy. (Social and emotional issues of battering, or interpersonal violence, are addressed in Chapter 24.) Trauma may be blunt, such as that sustained in an automobile accident, or penetrating, as in gunshot and knife wounds. Burns and electrical injuries also can occur.

Although injury may not be fatal, infant neurologic deficits may be found after birth. Direct fetal trauma, such as skull fracture or intracranial hemorrhage, can occur from maternal pelvic fracture, penetrating wounds, or blunt trauma. Indirect causes of fetal injury or death include abruptio placentae and disruption of the placental blood flow secondary to maternal hypovolemia or uterine rupture. The most common cause of fetal death is death of the mother.

The anatomic and physiologic changes of pregnancy make trauma care unique. During early pregnancy, the uterus is surrounded by the pelvis and is well protected from direct damage. As the uterus grows, it protrudes and becomes a large target for trauma. At the same time, it acts as a shield for some maternal organs such as the kidneys, often protecting them from direct trauma. The growing uterus pushes abdominal organs such as the liver, kidney, stomach, and intestines upward and outward, moving them out of their nonpregnant locations. Obesity often alters where organs will be found.

Normal alterations of pregnancy can affect the maternal and fetal outcomes after traumatic injury and can affect the interpretation of diagnostic studies. Pregnant women have a greater blood volume than nonpregnant women, which gives them a cushion against blood loss. However, the fetus may suffer if the woman hemorrhages because maternal blood is diverted from the placenta to increase her blood volume. Fetal hypoxia, acidosis, and death may then occur.

Maternal fibrinogen levels are higher during pregnancy (300 to 600 mg/dL). A decrease to lower levels is associated with abruptio placentae and suggests DIC.

### Therapeutic Management

The care of the pregnant trauma victim will vary with the extent of her injuries. The initial response of the trauma team should be to treat injuries that threaten the woman's life, using the basic ABCs of resuscitation. The mnemonic stands for airway, breathing, circulation. Priorities include:

- Maintenance of maternal cardiopulmonary function
- Evaluation and stabilization of maternal injuries

Placing a wedge along the woman's right or left side or assuming a lateral tilt allows lateral uterine displacement to reduce compression of the large blood vessels by the heavy uterus. Venous access is often by central line, and maternal hemodynamic status can be monitored using an arterial line. Laboratory studies often include complete blood count, blood type and screen or crossmatch, clotting studies, Kleihauer–Betke (K-B) test, urinalysis, and others. Blood alcohol and urine drug tests may be performed.

Evaluation continues after stabilization for fractures, bleeding, and internal injuries. The uterus and fetus are part of this further evaluation. Management of the fetus depends on whether the fetus is living and a viable gestation. The fetus may be delivered by cesarean birth if it is mature enough to survive and if the maternal or fetal condition is likely to be improved by prompt delivery. The fetus that is dead or too immature to survive is not usually delivered unless delivery will improve the mother's outcome.

Fetal heart tones are assessed by Doppler or continuous electronic monitoring after 24 weeks. A K-B test may be ordered at intervals to identify placental disruptions that allow fetal blood to leak into the circulation. The baby should be monitored at least 4 to 6 hours before discharge, even if the mother has no significant trauma (Mendez-Figueroa, Dahlke, Vrees, et al., 2013).

### Nursing Considerations

Nonuse or incorrect use of automobile restraints such as seat belts or air bags can result in greater trauma or fatality in the mother and fetus. The pregnant woman should buckle the lap belt under her belly and over her hips with the shoulder restraint comfortably between her breasts. Driving a short distance with an unbuckled belt is unsafe for a pregnant woman, as it is for any other person. Remind a woman that her baby will need a car carrier so that she can consider what to look for early. Visit the website for the National Highway Traffic Safety Administration for up-to-date information on correct use of seatbelts and airbags during pregnancy and on choosing the correct infant or child restraint (http://www.nhtsa.dot.gov).

Continued nursing focuses on maintaining maternal and fetal stability. Vital signs are taken as needed, based on the woman's condition. Vital signs and urine output (at least 30 mL/hr) provide information about the adequacy of her blood volume. Bloody urine suggests bladder or renal damage. Other nursing care is directed toward specific injuries and implementation of medical care.

Signs suggesting abruptio placentae (vaginal bleeding with uterine pain and tenderness) should be reported because this complication can occur with abdominal trauma, and its signs are not always immediate. The fundal height may increase as the uterus fills with blood. Maternal tachycardia usually precedes a fall in blood pressure. Fetal tachycardia or cessation of the FHR is likely to occur in more extensive uterine trauma or maternal hemorrhage. Fetal hemorrhage can occur with trauma to the placenta or the umbilical cord.

Once the woman's condition is stable, nursing care intensifies for the fetus. External monitoring is appropriate if the fetus has reached a viable gestational age. PTL may occur but may not be recognized if the woman is unconscious or if pain from injuries overshadows discomfort from contractions. Recurrent restlessness or moaning may accompany contractions. *The nurse should palpate the woman's uterus for contractions periodically because they may not be evident on the fetal monitor, especially if the fetus is small.*

Although the nurse is usually anxious in an emergency situation, it is important to keep a calm attitude. The woman and her family quickly pick up on the staff's anxiety, and theirs consequently escalates. To reduce fears of abandonment, the nurse should remain with the woman and, if possible, hold her hand. The nurse should speak in a low, calm voice.

## KEY CONCEPTS

- Dysfunctional labor is caused by abnormalities in the powers, the passenger, the passage, or the psyche. Combinations of abnormalities are common.
- Nursing care in dysfunctional labor focuses on prevention or prompt identification and action to correct additional complications: fetal hypoxia, infection, injury to the mother or fetus, and postpartum hemorrhage.
- PROM is associated with infection as both a cause and an effect.
- The early indications of PTL are often vague. Prompt identification of PTL enables the most effective therapy to delay preterm birth.
- Nursing care for the woman at risk for a very early preterm birth focuses on helping her delay birth long enough to promote fetal lung maturation with corticosteroids, allow transfer to a facility with an appropriate level of neonatal intensive care, or reach a gestation at which the infant's problems with immaturity are minimal.
- The main risk in prolonged pregnancy is reduced placental function, which can compromise the fetus during labor and result in meconium aspiration in the neonate. Dysfunctional labor can occur as a fetus continues growing during the prolonged pregnancy.
- The key intervention for umbilical cord prolapse is to relieve pressure on the cord without compressing its blood vessels and to expedite delivery.
- Be aware of women at risk for uterine rupture, and observe for signs and symptoms: signs of shock, abdominal pain, a sense of tearing, chest pain, pain in the shoulder area, abnormal FHR patterns, cessation of contractions, and palpation of the fetus outside the uterus.
- Uterine inversion is often accompanied by massive blood loss and shock. Recovery care promotes uterine contraction and maintenance of adequate circulating volume.
- Anaphylactoid syndrome is more likely to occur when labor contractions are intense, forcing particulate matter into the mother's circulation. Once thought to result only from amniotic fluid entering the maternal circulation, this critical complication is also associated with other complications such as maternal sepsis, preeclampsia, and cardiac disease.
- Automobile accidents are the major cause of blunt force trauma in pregnant women and can result in premature separation of the placenta, hemorrhage, fractures, and internal injuries. Penetrating injuries caused by knives or bullets are particularly dangerous for the fetus.
- The treatment of trauma during pregnancy is similar to that in a nonpregnant person. Providing cardiopulmonary support and controlling bleeding are the priorities. Careful evaluation of the uterus and fetus is also essential.

## REFERENCES AND READINGS


Agency for Healthcare Research and Quality. (2010). *Evidence-based practice center systematic review protocol: Project title: Comparative effectiveness of terbutaline pump for the prevention of preterm birth*. Retrieved from http://www.effectivehealthcare.ahrq.gov.

American Academy of Pediatrics & American College of Obstetricians and Gynecologists. (2007). *Guidelines for perinatal care* (6th ed.). Elk Grove Village, IL, and Washington, DC: Author.

American Academy of Pediatrics & American College of Obstetricians and Gynecologists. (2013). *Guidelines for perinatal care* (8th ed.). Elk Grove Village, IL, and Washington, DC: Author.

American College of Obstetricians and Gynecologists. (2010). *Preparing for clinical emergencies in obstetrics & gynecology (ACOG Practice Bulletin No. 487)*. Washington, DC: Author.

American College of Obstetricians and Gynecologists. (2011). *Prevention of early-onset group B streptococcal disease in newborns. (ACOG Committee Opinion No. 487)*. Washington, DC: Author.

American College of Obstetricians and Gynecologists. (2011a). *Dystocia and the augmentation of labor (ACOG Practice Bulletin No. 49)*. Washington, DC: Author.

American College of Obstetricians and Gynecologists. (2014). *Multifetal gestations* (ACOG Practice Bulletin No. 144). Washington, DC: Author.

American College of Obstetricians and Gynecologists. (2016a). *Management of preterm labor (ACOG Practice Bulletin No. 159)*. Washington, DC: Author.

American College of Obstetricians and Gynecologists. (2016b). *Premature rupture of membranes (ACOG Practice Bulletin No. 139)*. Washington, DC: Author.

American College of Obstetricians and Gynecologists. (2016c). *Critical care in pregnancy (ACOG Practice Bulletin No. 158)*. Washington, DC: Author.

Balchin, I., & Steer, P.J. (2011). Prolonged pregnancy. In D.K. James, P.J. Steer, & C.P. Weiner (Eds.), *High risk pregnancy: Management options* (4th ed., pp. 1139–1143). Philadelphia: Saunders.

Belfort, M.A., & Dildy, G.A., III. (2011). Postpartum hemorrhage and other problems of the third stage. In D.K. James, P.J. Steer, & C.P. Weiner (Eds.), *High risk pregnancy: Management options* (4th ed., pp. 1283–1311). Philadelphia: Saunders.

Bobrowski, R.A. (2011). Trauma. In D.K. James, P.J. Steer, & C.P. Weiner (Eds.), *High risk pregnancy: Management options* (4th ed., pp. 973–995). Philadelphia: Saunders.

Cheng, Y.W., Shaffer, B.L. Nicholson, J.M., et al. (2014). Second stage of labor and epidural use: a larger effect than previously suggested. *Obstetrics & Gynecology, 123*(3), 527–535.

Cunningham, F., Leveno, K., Bloom, S., et al. (2014). *Williams obstetrics* (24th ed.). New York: McGraw-Hill.

Dennedy, M., & Dunne, F. (2013). Macrosomia: defining the problem worldwide. *Lancet, 381*(9865), 435–436.

Forsythe, E.S., & Allen, P.J. (2013). Health risks associated with late-preterm infants. *Pediatric Nursing, 39*(4), 197–201.

Gee, H. (2011). Dysfunctional labor. In D.K. James, P.J. Steer, & C.P. Weiner (Eds.), *High risk pregnancy: Management options* (4th ed., pp. 1169–1183). Philadelphia: Saunders.

Gherman, R.B. (2011). Shoulder dystocia. In D.K. James, P.J. Steer, & C.P. Weiner (Eds.), *High risk pregnancy: Management options* (4th ed., pp. 1169–1183). Philadelphia: Saunders.

Gibson, P.S., & Powrie, R.O. (2011). Respiratory disease. In D.K. James, P.J. Steer, & C.P. Weiner (Eds.), *High risk pregnancy: Management options* (4th ed., pp. 657–682). Philadelphia: Saunders.

Gilbert, E.S. (2011). *Manual of high risk pregnancy & delivery* (5th ed.). St. Louis: Mosby.

Graseck, A., Tuuli, M., Roehl, K., et al. (2014). Fetal descent in labor. *Obstetrics & Gynecology, 123*(3), 521–526.

Jorgensen, A.M. (2008a). Late preterm birth: A rising trend. *Nursing for Women's Health, 12*(4), 308–314.

Leveno, K.J., McIntire, D.D., & Bloom, S.L. (2009). Decreased preterm births in an inner-city public hospital. *Obstetrics and Gynecology, 113*(3), 578–584.

Lim, A.D., Schuit, E., Bloemenkamp, K., et al. (2011). 17-Alpha-hydroxyprogesterone caproate for the prevention of adverse neonatal outcome in multiple pregnancies. *Obstetrics and Gynecology, 118*(3), 513–520.

Malone, F.D., & D'Alton, M.E. (2014). Multiple gestation: Clinical characteristics and management. In R.K. Creasy, R. Resnik, J.D. Iams, C. Lockwood, T. Moore, & M. Greene. (Eds.), *Creasy & Resnik's maternal-fetal medicine: Principles and practice* (7th ed.). Philadelphia: Saunders.

March of Dimes. (2011). *Preterm labor: Progesterone treatment to reduce preterm birth.* Retrieved from http://www.marchofdimes.com.

Martin, J.A., Hamilton, B.E., Osterman, M.J., et al. (2015). Births: Final data for 2013. National Center for Health Statistics. *National Vital Statistics Reports, 64*(1), 1–13.

Mendez-Figueroa, H., Dahlke, J., Vrees, R., et al. (2013). Trauma in pregnancy: An updated systematic review. *American Journal of Obstetrics & Gynecology, 209*(1), 1–10.

Mercer, B.M. (2014). Assessment and induction of fetal pulmonary maturity. In R.K. Creasy, R. Resnik, J.D. Iams, C. Lockwood, T. Moore, & M. Greene. (Eds.), *Creasy & Resnik's maternal-fetal medicine: Principles and practice* (7th ed.). Philadelphia: Saunders.

Mercer, B.M. (2014). Premature rupture of the membranes. In R.K. Creasy, R. Resnik, J.D. Iams, C. Lockwood, T. Moore, & M. Greene. (Eds.), *Creasy & Resnik's maternal-fetal medicine: Principles and practice* (7th ed.). Philadelphia: Saunders.

Ogle, R., Hyett, J., & Marren, A.J. (2011). Screening for spontaneous preterm labor and delivery. In D.K. James, P.J. Steer, & C.P. Weiner (Eds.), *High risk pregnancy: Management options* (4th ed., pp. 1065–1074). Philadelphia: Saunders.

Robbins, K.S., Martin, S.R., & Wilson, W.C. (2014). Intensive care considerations for the critically ill parturient. In R.K. Creasy, R. Resnik, J.D. Iams, C. Lockwood, T. Moore, & M. Greene. (Eds.), *Creasy & Resnik's maternal-fetal medicine: Principles and practice* (7th ed.). Philadelphia: Saunders.

Simhan, H., Berghella, V., & Iams, J. (2014) Preterm labor and birth. In R.K. Creasy, R. Resnik, J.D. Iams, C. Lockwood, T. Moore, & M. Greene. (Eds.), *Creasy & Resnik's maternal-fetal medicine: Principles and practice* (7th ed.). Philadelphia: Saunders.

Simpson, K.R. & O'Brien-Abel, N. (2013). Labor and birth. In K.R. Simpson, & P.A. Creehan (Eds.), *AWHONN perinatal nursing* (4th ed.). Philadelphia: Lippincott Williams & Wilkins.

Svigos, J.M., Dodd, J.M., & Robinson, J.S. (2011). Prelabor rupture of membranes. In D.K. James, P.J. Steer, & C.P. Weiner (Eds.), *High risk pregnancy: Management options* (4th ed.). Philadelphia: Saunders.

Svigos, J.M., Dodd, J.M., & Robinson, J.S. (2011). Threatened and actual preterm labor including mode of delivery. In D.K. James, P.J. Steer, & C.P. Weiner (Eds.), *High risk pregnancy: Management options* (4th ed.). Philadelphia: Saunders.

Thorp, J.M. & Laughon, S.K. (2014). Clinical aspects of normal and abnormal labor. In R.K. Creasy, R. Resnik, J.D. Iams, C. Lockwood, T. Moore, & M. Greene. (Eds.), *Creasy & Resnik's maternal-fetal medicine: Principles and practice* (7th ed.). Philadelphia: Saunders.

U.S. Food and Drug Administration (FDA). (2011). *FDA drug safety communication: New warnings against use of terbutaline to treat preterm labor.* Retrieved from http://www.fda.gov.

# The Woman With a Postpartum Complication

http://evolve.elsevier.com/McKinney/mat-ch/

## LEARNING OBJECTIVES

*After studying this chapter, you should be able to:*

- Describe postpartum hemorrhage in terms of predisposing factors, causes, signs, and therapeutic management.
- Explain major causes, signs, and therapeutic management of subinvolution.
- Describe three major thromboembolic disorders (superficial venous thrombosis, deep vein thrombosis, pulmonary embolism) and their predisposing factors, causes, signs, and therapeutic management.
- Discuss puerperal infection in terms of location, predisposing factors, causes, signs and symptoms, and therapeutic management.
- Describe the major mood disorders (peripartum depression, postpartum psychosis, and bipolar II disorder) and anxiety disorders (panic disorder, postpartum obsessive-compulsive disorder, and posttraumatic stress disorder).
- Describe the role of the nurse in the management of women who have a postpartum complication.

Complications that occur during the postpartum period are uncommon but life threatening. Nurses must be aware of problems that may occur and their effects on the family. The most common physiologic complications are hemorrhage, thromboembolic disorders, and infection. Complications that are psychogenic in origin include mood and anxiety disorders.

## POSTPARTUM HEMORRHAGE

Postpartum hemorrhage is a major cause of maternal death and morbidity in the United States and the world (Abdul-Kadir, McLintock, Ducloy, et al., 2014; Main, Goffman, Scavone, et al., 2015; Callaghan, Creanga, & Kuklina, 2012). Traditionally, postpartum hemorrhage was defined as blood loss greater than 500 mL for a vaginal birth and greater than 1000 mL for a Cesarean birth (Cunningham, Leveno, Bloom, et al., 2014; Main et al., 2015). However, the nomenclature consensus conference of the American College of Obstetricians and Gynecologists revised the definition of early postpartum hemorrhage as, "Cumulative blood loss of ≥1000 mL or blood loss accompanied by sign/symptoms of hypovolemia within 24 hours following the birth process (includes intrapartum loss)." (American College of Obstetricians and Gynecologists, 2014). Blood loss is frequently underestimated, reporting only approximately half the actual loss (Cunningham et al., 2014). Therefore, blood loss should be quantified by weighing or measuring, and records of cumulative loss should be maintained. (Association of Women's Health, Obstetric and Neonatal Nurses, 2015a; Main et al., 2015). Hemorrhage in the first 24 hours after childbirth is called *early postpartum hemorrhage.* Hemorrhage after 24 hours for up to 12 weeks after birth is called *late postpartum hemorrhage.* Hemorrhage is a leading cause of maternal morbidity and mortality (Creanga, Berg, Syverson, et al., 2015).

### Early Postpartum Hemorrhage

Early postpartum hemorrhage usually occurs during the first hour after birth and is most often caused by uterine atony (Cunningham et al., 2014; ACOG, 2015). Atony refers to lack of muscle tone that results in failure of the uterine muscle fibers to contract firmly around blood vessels when the placenta separates. Trauma to the birth canal during labor and birth, hematomas (localized collections of blood in a space or tissue), retention of placental fragments, and abnormalities of coagulation are other causes. Hemorrhage from disseminated intravascular coagulation and placenta previa are discussed in Chapter 25. Placenta accreta (abnormal adherence of the placenta to the uterine wall) and inversion of the uterus are other causes that are described in Chapter 27.

#### Uterine Atony

With uterine atony, the relaxed muscles allow rapid bleeding from the endometrial arteries at the placental site. Bleeding continues until the uterine muscle fibers contract to stop the flow of blood. Fig. 28.1 illustrates the effect of uterine contraction on the size of the placental site and the amount of bleeding that occurs.

***Predisposing factors.*** Knowledge of factors that increase the risk of uterine atony helps the nurse anticipate and reduce excessive bleeding. Over distention of the uterus from any cause, including conditions such as multiple gestation, a large infant, and hydramnios, makes it more difficult for the uterus to contract with enough firmness to prevent excessive bleeding. Multiparity results in muscle fibers that have been stretched repeatedly, and these flaccid muscle fibers may not remain contracted after birth. Obesity increases the risk of postpartum hemorrhage (Cunningham et al., 2014). Intrapartum factors include minimally effective contractions, resulting in prolonged labor and excessively vigorous contractions resulting in precipitate labor. Labor that was induced or augmented with oxytocin is more likely to be followed by post-birth uterine atony and hemorrhage. Retention of a segment of the placenta does not allow the uterus to contract firmly, and thus, can result in uterine atony. Box 28.1 summarizes predisposing factors for postpartum hemorrhage.

***Manifestations.*** Major signs of uterine atony include:

- A uterine fundus that is difficult to locate
- A soft or "boggy" feel when the fundus is located

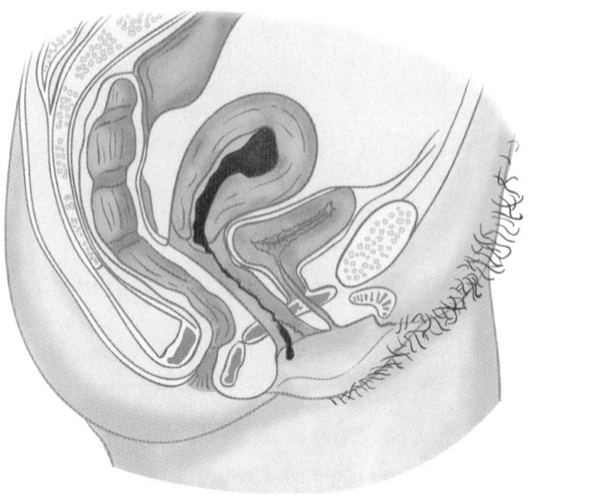

A Contracted uterus

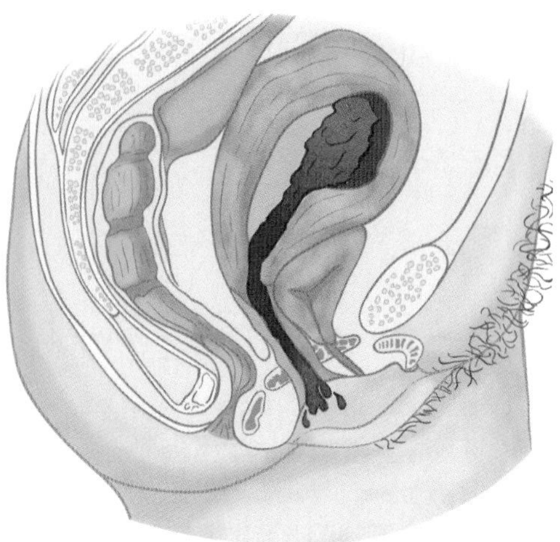

B **Uterine atony**
Uterus remains inadequately contracted

FIG 28.1 **A,** When the uterus remains contracted, the placental site is smaller, so bleeding is minimal. **B,** If uterine muscles fail to contract around the endometrial arteries at the placental site, hemorrhage occurs.

- A uterus that becomes firm as it is massaged but loses its tone when massage is stopped
- A fundus that is located above the expected level
- Excessive lochia, especially if it is bright red
- Excessive clots expelled

For the first 24 hours after childbirth, the uterus should feel like a firmly contracted ball roughly the size of a large grapefruit. It should be easily located at about the level of the umbilicus. Lochia should be dark red and scant to moderate in amount. Saturation of one peripad in 15 minutes indicates excessive blood loss (Whitmer, 2016). The nurse must realize that although bleeding may be profuse and dramatic, a constant steady trickle, dribble, or slow seeping is just as dangerous (see Chapter 20 for assessment of the uterus and lochia).

***Therapeutic management.*** Early administration of oxytocin is recommended for all births as a prophylaxis against postpartum hemorrhage (Abdul-Kadir et al., 2014; Main, et al., 2015; AWHONN, 2015b). Intravenous (IV) infusion of dilute oxytocin (not IV Push) should be given during the third stage of labor. Oxytocin may also be administered intramuscularly. (AWHONN, 2015b) (see Drug Guide: Oxytocin, p. 382). Nurses are with the mother during the hours after childbirth and are responsible for assessments and initial management of uterine atony. If the uterus is not firmly contracted despite preventative measures, the first intervention is to massage the fundus until it is firm and to express clots that may have accumulated in the uterus. One hand is placed just above the symphysis pubis to support the lower uterine segment while the other hand gently but firmly massages the fundus in a circular motion (Fig. 28.2) Clots that may have accumulated in the uterine cavity interfere with the ability of the uterus to contract effectively. They are expressed by applying firm but gentle pressure on the fundus in the direction of the vagina. It is critical that the uterus is contracted firmly before attempting to express clots. *Pushing on a uterus that is not contracted could invert the uterus and cause massive hemorrhage and rapid shock* (see Chapter 27).

If the uterus does not remain contracted as a result of uterine massage or if the fundus is displaced, the problem may be a distended bladder. A full bladder lifts the uterus, moving it up and to the side, preventing effective contraction of the uterine muscles. If atony persists despite prophylactic oxytocin and uterine massage, further pharmacologic measures may be necessary. Initially, additional oxytocin may be ordered. Methylergonovine (Methergine) is a common second drug of choice when oxytocin is not effective. Methergine elevates blood pressure and should not be given to a woman who is hypertensive. The usual route of administration is IM. (see Drug Guide: Methylergonovine). Misoprostol (Cytotec), a synthetic prostaglandin E1 given orally or sublingually may also be used to control bleeding. (California Maternal Quality Care Collaborative, 2015, Cunningham et al., 2014). Analogs of prostaglandin F2-alpha ($PGF_2\alpha$; carboprost tromethamine [Hemabate; Prostin/15M]) are also effective

### BOX 28.1 Common Predisposing Factors for Postpartum Hemorrhage

- Over distention of the uterus (multiple gestation, large infant, hydramnios)
- Multiparity (five or more)
- Precipitate labor or birth
- Prolonged labor
- Use of forceps or vacuum extractor
- Cesarean birth
- Manual removal of the placenta
- Uterine inversion
- Placenta previa, placenta accreta, or low implantation
- Drugs: oxytocin, prostaglandins, tocolytics, or magnesium sulfate
- General anesthesia
- Chorioamnionitis
- Clotting disorders
- Previous postpartum hemorrhage or uterine surgery
- Disseminated intravascular coagulation
- Uterine leiomyomas (fibroids)

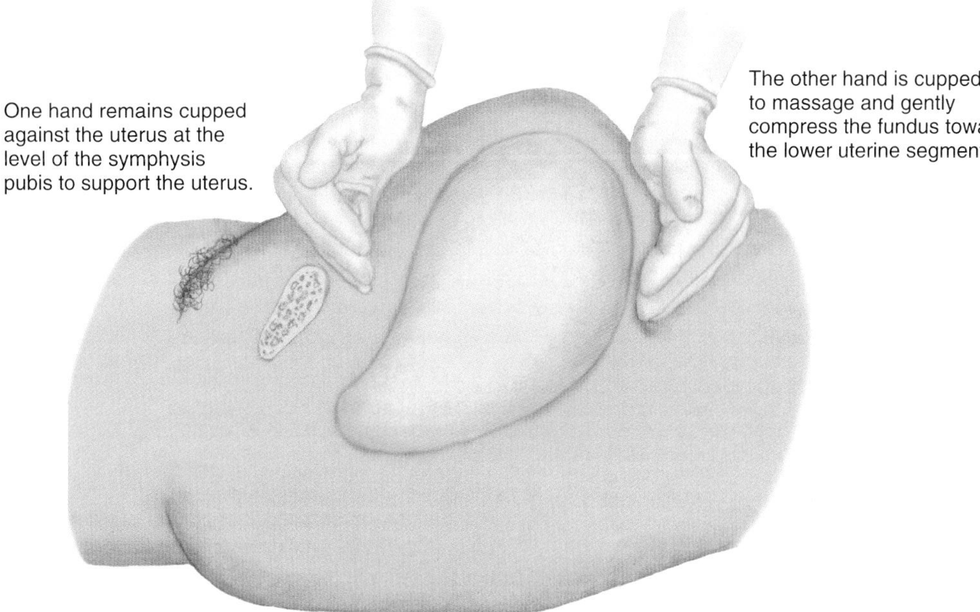
One hand remains cupped against the uterus at the level of the symphysis pubis to support the uterus.
The other hand is cupped to massage and gently compress the fundus toward the lower uterine segment.

**FIG 28.2** Technique for fundal massage.

## DRUG GUIDE

### *Methylergonovine (Methergine)*

**Classification:** Ergot alkaloid, uterine stimulant

**Action:** Stimulates sustained contraction of the uterus and causes arterial vasoconstriction.

**Indications:** Used for the prevention and treatment of postpartum or post abortion hemorrhage caused by uterine atony or subinvolution.

**Dosage and Route:** Usual dosage is 0.2 mg intramuscularly (IM) every 2 to 4 hours for a maximum of five doses. Change to the oral route 0.2 mg every 6 to 8 hours for a maximum of 7 days. Intravenous use not recommended; use in life-threatening emergency only and give over at least 60 seconds with close monitoring of blood pressure (BP) and pulse; may cause severe hypertension.

**Absorption:** Well absorbed after oral or IM route.

**Excretion:** Metabolized by the liver; excreted in the feces and urine.

**Contraindications and Precautions:** Methylergonovine should never be used during pregnancy or to induce labor. Do not use if the mother is hypersensitive to ergot. Contraindicated for women with hypertension, severe hepatic or renal disease, thrombophlebitis, coronary artery disease, peripheral vascular disease, hypocalcemia, sepsis, or before the fourth stage of labor.

**Adverse Reactions:** Nausea, vomiting, uterine cramping, hypertension, dizziness, headache, dyspnea, chest pain, palpitations, peripheral ischemia, seizure, and uterine and gastrointestinal cramping.

**Nursing Considerations:** Before administering the medication, assess the blood pressure. Follow facility protocol to determine at what BP level medication must be withheld. Caution the mother to avoid smoking, because nicotine constricts blood vessels. Remind her to report any adverse reactions.

## DRUG GUIDE

### *Carboprost Tromethamine (Hemabate, Prostin/15M)*

**Classification:** Prostaglandin, oxytocic.

**Action:** Stimulates contraction of the uterus.

**Indications:** Used for the treatment of postpartum hemorrhage caused by uterine atony. Also used for abortion.

**Dosage and Route:** Postpartum hemorrhage: 250 mcg intramuscularly. May repeat at 15- to 90-minute intervals. Maximum total dose, 2 mg.

**Absorption:** Metabolized by the liver and by enzymes in the lungs.

**Excretion:** Primarily excreted in urine.

**Contraindications and Precautions:** Contraindicated for women with hypersensitivity to carboprost or other prostaglandins; acute pelvic inflammatory disease; cardiac, pulmonary, renal, or hepatic disease. Use caution if the woman has a history of asthma, hypotension or hypertension, anemia, jaundice, diabetes, epilepsy, or previous uterine surgery.

**Adverse Reactions and Side Effects:** Excessive dose may cause tetanic contraction and laceration or uterine rupture. May cause uterine hypertonus if used with oxytocin. Nausea, vomiting, diarrhea (frequent), fever, chills, facial flushing, headache, hypertension or hypotension, tachycardia, pulmonary edema.

**Nursing Considerations:** Should be refrigerated. Give via deep intramuscular (IM) injection. Rotate sites if repeated. Monitor vital signs. Administer antiemetics and antidiarrheals as ordered.

when given IM or into the uterine muscle (CMQCC, 2015) (See Drug Guide: Carboprost Tromethamine).

If uterine massage and pharmacologic measures are ineffective in stopping uterine bleeding, the healthcare provider may use bimanual compression of the uterus. In this procedure, one hand is inserted into the vagina, and the other compresses the uterus through the abdominal wall (Fig. 28.3). A balloon may be inserted into the uterus to apply pressure against the uterine surface to stop bleeding (Cekmez et al., 2015; Martin et al., 2015). Uterine packing may also be used. It may be necessary to return the woman to the birthing area for exploration of the uterine cavity and removal of placental fragments that interfere with uterine contraction.

A laparotomy may be necessary to identify the source of the bleeding. Uterine compression sutures may be placed to stop severe

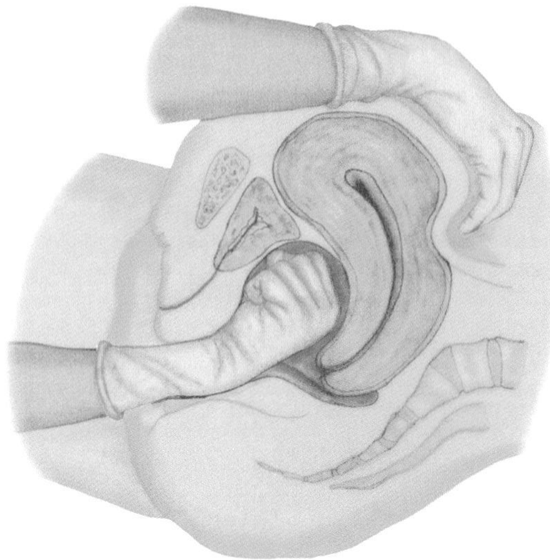

**FIG 28.3** Bimanual compression. One hand is inserted in the vagina, and the other compresses the uterus through the abdominal wall.

bleeding. Ligation of the uterine or hypogastric artery or embolization (occlusion) of pelvic arteries may be required if other measures are not effective. Hysterectomy is a last resort to save the life of a woman with uncontrollable postpartum hemorrhage.

Hemorrhage requires prompt replacement of intravascular fluid volume. Lactated Ringer's solution, whole blood, packed red blood cells, normal saline, or other plasma extenders are used. Enough fluid should be given to maintain a urine flow of at least 30 mL/hr (Cunningham et al., 2014). Typically, the nurse is responsible for obtaining properly typed and cross-matched blood and inserting large-bore IV lines that are capable of carrying whole blood.

### Trauma

Trauma to the birth canal is the second-most common cause of early postpartum hemorrhage. Such trauma includes vaginal, cervical, and perineal lacerations as well as hematomas.

***Predisposing factors.*** Many of the same factors that increase the risk of uterine atony increase the risk of soft tissue trauma during childbirth. For example, trauma to the birth canal is more likely to occur if the infant is large or if labor and birth occur rapidly. Induction and augmentation of labor and the use of assistive devices such as a vacuum extractor or forceps increase the risk of tissue trauma.

***Lacerations.*** The perineum, vagina, cervix, and the area around the urethral meatus are the most common sites for lacerations. Small cervical lacerations occur frequently and generally do not require repairs. Lacerations of the vagina, perineum, and periurethral area usually occur during the second stage of labor with rapid descent of the fetal head or the use of assistive devices in birth such as a vacuum extractor or forceps.

Lacerations of the birth canal should always be suspected if excessive uterine bleeding continues when the fundus is contracted firmly and is at the expected location. Bleeding from lacerations of the genital tract often is bright red, in contrast to the darker red color of lochia. Bleeding can be heavy or appear to be minor, with a steady trickle of blood.

***Hematomas.*** Hematomas occur when blood enters loose connective tissue occurs while the overlying tissue remains intact. Hematomas develop as a result of blood vessel injury in spontaneous deliveries and deliveries in which vacuum extractors or forceps are used. Hematomas may be found in vulvar, vaginal, and retroperitoneal areas.

The rapid bleeding into soft tissue can cause a visible vulvar hematoma, a discolored bulging mass that is sensitive to touch. Hematomas in the vagina or retroperitoneal areas cannot be seen. Hematomas produce deep, severe, unrelieved pain and feelings of pressure that are not relieved by usual measures. Formation of a hematoma should be suspected if the mother demonstrates systemic signs of concealed blood loss, such as tachycardia or decreasing blood pressure, when the fundus is firm and lochia is within normal limits.

***Therapeutic management.*** When postpartum hemorrhage is caused by trauma to the birth canal, surgical repair is often necessary. Because lacerations of the vagina or cervix are difficult to see, it is necessary to return the mother to the birthing area, where surgical lights are available. She is placed in a lithotomy position and carefully draped. Surgical asepsis is required while the laceration is being examined and repaired.

Small hematomas usually reabsorb naturally. Large hematomas may require incision, evacuation of the clots, and location and ligation of the bleeding vessel.

## Late Postpartum Hemorrhage

Late postpartum hemorrhage, also called *secondary postpartum hemorrhage,* is defined as hemorrhage occurring between 24 hours and 12 weeks after birth (ACOG, 2015). The most common causes of late postpartum hemorrhage are **subinvolution** (delayed return of the uterus to its nonpregnant size and consistency) and retained placental fragments. (Cunningham et al., 2014; Doussou, Debost-Legrand, Dechelotte, et al., 2015) Clots form around the retained fragments, and excessive bleeding can occur when the clots slough away several days after birth. Infection of the uterus can also be a cause. Subinvolution is discussed on p. 605.

Late postpartum hemorrhage caused by retained placental fragments is generally preventable. When the placenta is delivered, the healthcare provider carefully inspects it to determine whether it is intact. If a portion of the placenta is missing, the provider manually explores the uterus, locates the missing fragments, and removes them.

Because late postpartum hemorrhage frequently happens after discharge and can be dangerous for the unsuspecting mother, women must be taught how to assess the fundus and normal characteristics and duration of lochia flow. They should be instructed to notify their provider if bleeding persists or becomes unusually heavy.

### Predisposing Factors

Attempts to deliver the placenta before it separates from the uterine wall, manual removal of the placenta, placenta accreta (see Chapter 27), previous cesarean birth, and uterine leiomyomas are primary predisposing factors for retention of placental fragments. Debost-Legrand et al. (2015) found that early postpartum hemorrhage and advanced maternal age (≥ 35 years) were also risk factors.

### Therapeutic Management

Initial treatment for late postpartum hemorrhage is directed toward control of the excessive bleeding. Oxytocin, methylergonovine, and prostaglandins are the most commonly used pharmacologic measures. Placental fragments can be dislodged and swept out of the uterus by the bleeding, and if the bleeding subsides when oxytocin is administered, no other treatment is necessary. Sonography may identify placental fragments that remain in the uterus. If bleeding continues or recurs, dilation and curettage (stretching of the cervical os to permit suctioning or scraping of the walls of the uterus) may be necessary to remove fragments. Broad-spectrum antibiotics can be given if postpartum infection is suspected because of uterine tenderness, foul-smelling lochia, or fever.

## HYPOVOLEMIC SHOCK

During and after giving birth, the woman can tolerate blood loss that approaches the volume of blood added during pregnancy (approximately 1500 to 2000 mL). The amount of blood lost can be estimated by comparing the hematocrit values before and after birth. If the hematocrit is lower after birth, the woman lost the amount of blood added during pregnancy plus an additional 500 mL for each 3% drop in the hematocrit value (Cunningham et al., 2014)

When blood loss is excessive, hypovolemic shock (acute peripheral circulatory failure resulting from loss of circulating blood volume) can ensue. Hypovolemia, abnormally decreased volume of circulating fluid in the body, endangers vital organs by depriving them of oxygen. The brain, heart, and kidneys are especially vulnerable to hypoxia and can suffer damage in a short time.

### Pathophysiology

Recognition of hypovolemic shock may be delayed because the body activates compensatory mechanisms that mask the severity of the problem. Baroreceptors are stimulated to constrict peripheral blood vessels, shunting blood into the central circulation and away from less essential organs such as the skin and extremities. The skin becomes pale and cold, but cardiac output and perfusion of vital organs are maintained.

The adrenal glands release catecholamines, which compensate for decreased blood volume by promoting vasoconstriction in nonessential organs, increasing the heart rate, and raising the blood pressure. As a result, blood pressure remains normal initially, although a decrease in pulse pressure (difference between systolic and diastolic blood pressures) may be noted. The tachycardia that develops is an early sign of compensation for excessive blood loss.

As shock worsens, the compensatory mechanisms fail, and physiologic insults spiral. Inadequate organ perfusion and decreased cellular oxygen for metabolism result in a buildup of lactic acid and the development of metabolic acidosis. Acidosis results in vasodilation, which further increases bleeding. Eventually, circulating volume becomes insufficient to perfuse cardiac and brain tissue. Cellular death occurs as a result of anoxia, and the mother dies.

### Manifestations

Early signs of blood loss such as mild tachycardia or hypotension may not appear until 25% to 30% of the woman's blood volume has been lost (Robbins, Martin, & Wilson, 2014). Tachycardia is one of the earliest signs of hypovolemic shock; even gradual increases in the pulse rate should be noted. A decrease in blood pressure and narrowing of pulse pressure occur when the circulating volume of blood is sufficiently decreased. The respiratory rate increases as the woman becomes more anxious and attempts to take in more oxygen to overcome the deficit created by the lack of hemoglobin.

Skin changes also provide early clues. Vasoconstriction in the skin causes it to become pale and cool to the touch. As hemorrhage worsens, the skin changes become more obvious; pallor increases, and the skin becomes cold and clammy.

As shock progresses, changes occur in the central nervous system. The mother becomes anxious, then confused, and finally lethargic as blood loss increases. Urine output decreases and eventually stops.

### Therapeutic Management

The goals of therapy are to control bleeding and prevent hypovolemic shock from becoming irreversible. A second IV line should be inserted with a large-bore (14- to 18-gauge) catheter capable of carrying whole blood. A central IV catheter may be placed. Sufficient fluid volume is infused to produce a urinary output of at least 30 mL/hr. Vasopressors may be needed for low blood pressure. The healthcare team makes every effort to locate the source of bleeding and to stop the loss of blood.

### Nursing Considerations

#### Immediate Care

Multidisciplinary work groups of the National Partnership for Maternal Safety under the guidance of the Council on Patient Safety in Women's Health Care outlined critical clinical practices called safety bundles that should be implemented in every maternity unit to address obstetric hemorrhage. These practices fall into four categories: *Readiness* (immediate access to supplies and medications, identification of a response team and the method for immediate communication, protocols for emergency blood transfusions, staff education with regular drills), *Recognition and Prevention* (risk assessment at multiple times during the antepartum, intrapartum and postpartum periods, quantification of blood loss, early postpartum administration of oxytocin), *Response* (an emergency management plan for obstetric hemorrhage, support programs for patient, families and staff) and *Reporting and System Learning* (culture of safety, including huddles and debriefs, multidisciplinary quality reviews of hemorrhages with ongoing monitoring of outcomes and practice changes). (Council on Patient Safety in Women' Health, 2015; Main et al., 2015). These practices should be used to facilitate implementation of evidenced based practices to decrease severe maternal morbidity and mortality.

When postpartum hemorrhage is identified, the response team should be notified. One person should be assigned to evaluate and record vital signs. Blood pressure and pulse should be assessed every 3 to 5 minutes. The location and consistency of the fundus, amount of lochia, skin temperature and color, and capillary return are assessed. Oxygen can be administered by tight face mask at 8 to 10 L/min to increase the saturation of the remaining red blood cells. Oxygen saturation levels are carefully monitored. Nurses often follow protocols that allow them to draw blood for hemoglobin, hematocrit, clotting studies, and type and cross match. Nurses are responsible for administering fluids, whole blood, and medications as directed and for reporting their effectiveness. A urinary catheter is inserted to measure hourly urinary output, which should be at least 30 mL/hr. The catheter is also necessary if a surgical procedure is required. In addition, nurses must make every effort to provide information and emotional support to the woman and her family.

**SAFETY ALERT**

***Signs of Postpartum Hemorrhage***

- A uterus that does not contract or does not remain contracted
- Large gush or slow, steady trickle, ooze, or dribble of blood from the vagina
- Saturation of one peripad per 15 minutes
- Severe, unrelieved perineal or rectal pain
- Tachycardia

## NURSING CARE

### The Woman With Excessive Bleeding

#### Assessment

The initial postpartum assessment includes a chart review to determine whether risk factors for hemorrhage are present. This alerts the nurse to women at increased risk for hemorrhage.

***Uterine atony.*** Priority assessments for uterine atony include the fundus, bladder, lochia, vital signs, skin temperature, and color. Assess the consistency and the location of the uterine fundus. The fundus should be firmly contracted at or near the level of the umbilicus and midline. If the fundus is above the level of the umbilicus and displaced, a full bladder may be the cause of excessive bleeding. Assist the mother to urinate, or obtain an order and catheterize her to correct uterine atony caused by bladder distention. Note urine output, and then reassess the uterus.

An accumulation of clots also expands the uterus, making contraction difficult and promoting continued bleeding. (See Procedure: Assessing the Uterine Fundus on p. 403 for fundal assessment.)

Obese women have an increased risk for uterine atony with subsequent postpartum hemorrhage (Blomberg, 2011); however, assessment of the fundus is difficult in this population. Monitor these women frequently for other signs of uterine atony and attempt to assess the uterine fundus while watching for increased lochia flow or clots to be expelled.

Remember to check under the woman's legs, buttocks, and back for lochia drainage by asking her to turn on her side. While bleeding can be profuse and dramatic, a continuing small but steady trickle can also lead to significant blood loss that becomes increasingly life threatening.

Estimation of the lochia volume by visual examination of peripads is difficult. More accurate information is obtained by weighing peripads, linen savers, and bed linens before and after use and determining the difference. One gram (weight) equals approximately 1 mL (volume).

Measure vital signs at least every 15 minutes or more often if necessary. Apply a pulse oximeter to determine oxygen saturation levels. Because the body initially compensates for excessive bleeding by constricting the peripheral blood vessels and shunting blood to vital organs, the vital signs may remain normal at first, even though the woman is becoming hypovolemic. The skin should be warm and dry, mucous membranes of the lips and mouth should be pink, and capillary return should occur within 3 seconds when the nails are blanched. These signs confirm adequate circulating volume to perfuse the peripheral tissue.

***Trauma.*** If the fundus is firm but bleeding is excessive, the cause may be lacerations of the cervix or birth canal. Inspect the perineum to determine whether a laceration is visible. Lacerations of the cervix or vagina are not visible, but bleeding in the presence of a firmly contracted uterus suggests a laceration. This suspicion warrants examination of the vaginal walls and cervix by the healthcare provider.

Assess comfort level. If the mother complains of deep, severe pelvic or rectal pain, or if vital signs or skin changes suggest hemorrhage but excessive bleeding is not obvious, the cause may be concealed bleeding and hematoma formation. Examine the vulva for bulging masses or discoloration. However, a hematoma developing in the vagina or in the retroperitoneal area will not be obvious when the vulva is examined. Table 28.1 summarizes assessments, abnormal signs and symptoms, and nursing implications.

#### Nursing Diagnosis and Planning

Postpartum hemorrhage is a complication that requires the efforts of all members of the healthcare team to control the hemorrhage and prevent further complications. Patient-centered goals are inappropriate for this potential complication because the nurse cannot manage postpartum hemorrhage independently but must use orders from healthcare providers to treat the condition. Planning should reflect the nurse's responsibility to:

- Monitor for signs of postpartum hemorrhage.
- Perform actions that minimize postpartum hemorrhage and prevent hypovolemic shock.
- Notify the healthcare provider if signs of excessive blood loss are observed or if the woman does not respond as desired.

#### Interventions

***Preventing hemorrhage.*** The key to successful management of early postpartum hemorrhage is early recognition and response. All postpartum women are at risk for hemorrhage. However, be aware of factors that further increase this risk and be particularly vigilant in

**TABLE 28.1 Nursing Assessments for Postpartum Hemorrhage**

| Assessments | Abnormal Signs and Symptoms | Nursing Implications |
|---|---|---|
| Chart review | Presence of predisposing factors | Perform more frequent evaluations. |
| Fundus | Soft, boggy, displaced | Massage, express clots, and assist to void or catheterize; notify primary healthcare provider if measures are ineffective. |
| Lochia | Bleeding (steady trickle, dribble, oozing, seeping, or profuse flow); heavy, saturation of 1 pad/hr; excessive, 1 pad/15 min | Assess for trauma; save and weigh pads, linen savers, and bed linens so estimation of blood loss will be more accurate. Notify healthcare provider. |
| Vital signs | Tachycardia, decreasing pulse pressure, falling blood pressure, decreasing oxygen saturation level | Report signs of excessive blood loss. |
| Urine output | Decreased urine output<br>Should be at least 30 mL/hr | Report decrease in output. |
| Comfort level | Severe pelvic or rectal pain | Assess for signs of hematoma, usually perineal or vaginal; examine vulva for masses or discoloration; report findings. |
| Skin | Cool, damp, pale | Look for signs of hypovolemia; vigilant assessment and management by entire healthcare team are necessary. |

monitoring these women so that excessive bleeding can be anticipated and minimized.

When predisposing factors are present, initiate frequent assessments. Many hospitals and birth centers have a protocol that calls for assessments every 15 minutes during the first hour after birth, every 30 minutes for the next 2 hours, and hourly for the next 4 hours. This plan may not be adequate for the woman at known risk for postpartum hemorrhage. A delay in assessment could result in excessive blood loss.

***Collaborating with the healthcare provider.*** When excessive bleeding is suspected and the fundus is boggy, begin uterine massage. Check the woman's bladder for distention and have her empty it if necessary. If she is not able to void, and the bladder is distended, obtain an order and catheterize the woman. Weigh blood-soaked pads, linen savers, and linens to accurately determine the amount of blood lost. If massage is not effective in controlling bleeding promptly, notify the healthcare provider. Save any tissue or clots passed.

Follow facility protocols to initiate specific laboratory studies such as determining hemoglobin and hematocrit levels and typing and cross matching blood so that blood is available should transfusions become necessary. Coagulation studies that may be ordered include fibrinogen, prothrombin time, partial thromboplastin time, fibrin split products, fibrin degradation products, platelets, D dimer, and blood chemistry. Many protocols also allow the nurse to increase the flow rate of an existing IV or insert a large-bore catheter to start IV fluids while the healthcare provider is being informed of the mother's condition. These actions do not substitute for notifying the healthcare provider, but they do allow nurses to make initial interventions quickly.

Keep the woman on bed rest to increase venous return and maintain cardiac output. The full Trendelenburg's position may interfere with cardiac and pulmonary function and is not advised. A modified Trendelenburg position can be used with the legs elevated 10 to 30 degrees to increase blood return from the legs, the trunk horizontal, and the head slightly elevated. Continue assessments, call for assistance, and save all blood-soaked materials so that an accurate estimation of blood loss can be made. Assistance is necessary; one nurse must continue to massage the uterus and perform and record assessments while another notifies the provider of the mother's condition and gathers medications and supplies needed.

Administer medications, fluids, and treatments as ordered by the healthcare provider or as stated in the facility's protocol. Evaluate the effects and relay the information to the provider. Physicians and nurse-midwives depend on the nurse for accurate information, on which they base medical management.

Because of oxytocin's antidiuretic effect, listen to breath sounds to identify signs of pulmonary edema from fluid overload if large amounts of oxytocin are given. Document blood pressure if methylergonovine is given. If measures fail to control bleeding, notify the healthcare provider so that additional procedures can be initiated. These may include preparation for operative intervention.

***Providing support for the family.*** The unusual activity of the hospital staff may make the mother and her family anxious. Be alert to their nonverbal cues, and when they appear frightened acknowledge their feelings. Keeping the family informed is one of the most effective ways of reducing anxiety.

Acknowledge the anxiety and provide simple, appropriate explanations of the activity. "I know all this activity must be frightening. She is bleeding a little more than we would like and we are doing several things at once."

***Posthemorrhage care.*** After the hemorrhage is controlled, continue to assess the woman frequently for a resumption of bleeding. The woman may be anemic and fatigued. Allow rest periods and organize work to help her conserve energy. Because the woman may experience orthostatic hypotension, assist her in getting out of bed after dangling her legs and assessing for dizziness and low blood pressure. Encourage intake of fluids and of foods high in iron. She may need assistance feeding her newborn.

***Home care.*** Nurses who work in home care or nurse-managed postpartum clinics must be aware that women who have had postpartum hemorrhage are subject to various complications. In general, they are exhausted, and it can take weeks for them to feel well again. Anemia often results, and a course of iron therapy may be prescribed to restore hemoglobin level. Activity may be restricted until strength returns. Some women need extra assistance with housework and care of the new infant. Fatigue may interfere with attachment. Because extensive blood loss increases the risk of postpartum infection, the woman must be taught to observe for specific signs and symptoms.

## CRITICAL THINKING EXERCISE 28.1

Dawn, a 26-year-old gravida 5, para 4, is admitted to the hospital. She has a rapid labor and delivers a baby boy weighing 4000 g (8 lb., 13 oz.). Two hours later, she is transferred to the postpartum unit. At the initial postpartum assessment, Dawn's fundus is firm, at the level of the umbilicus. Lochia is heavy, with occasional small clots expressed. Vital signs are unchanged from prenatal norms.

1. Do any "red flags" suggest a potential problem or complication? What actions should the nurse take?
2. At the next assessment, the nurse observes that the fundus is soft and lochia is excessive. What are the priority interventions? Why?
3. Within an hour, the fundus becomes "boggy" again and is located 3 cm above the umbilicus and displaced to the right. What is the priority nursing action? Why?
4. Dawn voids 500 mL. However, the fundus is difficult to locate, and lochia is excessive. What is the next nursing action? Why?

### Evaluation

Although patient-centered goals are not developed for potential complications (collaborative problems), the nurse collects and compares data with established norms and judges whether the data are within normal limits. If problems arise, the nurse acts to minimize hemorrhage and notifies the healthcare provider.

## SUBINVOLUTION OF THE UTERUS

Subinvolution refers to a slower-than-expected return of the uterus to its nonpregnant size after childbirth. Normally, the uterus descends at the rate of approximately 1 cm (one fingerbreadth) per day. By 14 days, it is no longer palpable above the symphysis pubis. The endometrial lining has sloughed off as part of the lochia, and the site of placental attachment is well healed by 6 weeks after childbirth if involution progresses as expected.

The most common causes of subinvolution are retained placental fragments and pelvic infection. Signs of subinvolution include prolonged discharge of lochia, irregular or excessive uterine bleeding, and sometimes profuse hemorrhage. Pelvic pain or feelings of pelvic heaviness, backache, fatigue, and persistent malaise are reported by many women. On bimanual examination, the uterus feels larger and softer than normal for that time of the puerperium.

### Therapeutic Management

Treatment is tailored to correct the cause of subinvolution. Methylergonovine given orally provides long, sustained contraction of the uterus. Infection responds to antimicrobial therapy.

### Nursing Considerations

In most cases, subinvolution is not obvious until the mother has returned home after childbirth; nurses must teach the mother and her family how to recognize its occurrence.

The mother is taught how to locate and palpate the fundus and how to estimate fundal height in relation to the umbilicus. The uterus should become smaller each day (by approximately one fingerbreadth) Explain the progressive changes from lochia rubra to lochia serosa to lochia alba (see Chapter 20).

The mother is instructed to report any deviation from the expected pattern or duration of lochia. A foul odor often indicates uterine infection, for which treatment is necessary. Additional signs include pelvic or fundal pain, backache, and feelings of pelvic pressure or fullness. The mother should be able to verbalize the warning signs before leaving the facility.

## THROMBOEMBOLIC DISORDERS

A **thrombus** is a collection of blood factors (primarily platelets and fibrin) on a vessel wall. **Thrombophlebitis** occurs when the vessel wall develops an inflammatory response to the thrombus. This inflammation further occludes the vessel. An **embolus** is a mass, possibly composed of a thrombus or amniotic fluid released into the bloodstream, that obstructs the capillary beds in another part of the body, frequently the lungs. A **pulmonary embolus** is a potentially fatal complication that occurs when the pulmonary artery is obstructed by an embolism. The three most common thromboembolisms encountered during pregnancy and the postpartum period are superficial venous thrombophlebitis (SVT), deep vein thrombosis (DVT), and, occasionally, pulmonary embolism (PE). SVT generally involves the saphenous venous system and is confined to the lower leg. DVT can involve veins from the foot to the iliofemoral region. It is a major concern because it predisposes to PE.

### Incidence and Etiology

Approximately 1 per 1000 pregnancies is complicated by thromboembolic events (Cunningham et al., 2014). Thrombi can form whenever the flow of blood is impeded. Once started, the thrombus can enlarge through successive layering of platelets, fibrin, and blood cells as the blood flows past the clot. Thrombus formation is often associated with thrombophlebitis.

The three major causes of thrombosis are venous stasis, hypercoagulable blood, and injury to the endothelial surface (the innermost layer) of the blood vessel. (Pettker & Lockwood, 2012) Two of these conditions—venous stasis and hypercoagulable blood—are present in all pregnancies, and the third, blood vessel injury, is likely to occur during birth.

#### Venous Stasis

During pregnancy, compression of the large vessels of the legs and pelvis by the enlarging uterus causes venous stasis. Stasis is most pronounced when the pregnant woman stands for prolonged periods of time. It results in dilated vessels that increase the potential for continued pooling of blood postpartum. Relative inactivity and activity restriction caused by complications during pregnancy lead to venous pooling and stasis of blood in the lower extremities. Prolonged time in stirrups for birth and repair of an episiotomy can also promote venous stasis and increase the risk of thrombus formation.

#### Hypercoagulation

Pregnancy is characterized by changes in the coagulation and fibrinolytic systems that persist into the postpartum period. During pregnancy, the levels of many coagulation factors are elevated. In addition, the fibrinolytic system, which causes clots to disintegrate (lyse), is suppressed. The result is that factors that promote clot formation are increased, and factors that prevent clot formation are decreased to prevent maternal hemorrhage, resulting in a higher risk for thrombus formation during pregnancy and the postpartum period.

**BOX 28.2 Factors That Increase the Risk of Thrombosis**

- Inactivity
- Prolonged bed rest
- Obesity
- Cesarean birth
- Sepsis
- Smoking
- History of previous thrombosis
- Varicose veins
- Diabetes mellitus
- Trauma
- Prolonged labor
- Prolonged time in stirrups in second stage of labor
- Maternal age older than 35 years
- Increased parity
- Dehydration
- First-degree relative with thrombosis
- Use of forceps
- Antiphospholipid antibody syndrome
- Inherited thrombophilias
- Air travel

#### Blood Vessel Injury

Vascular damage is possible during pregnancy, especially at birth. Lower extremity trauma, operative birth, and prolonged labor can cause vascular damage (Rhode, 2016). Cesarean birth significantly increases the risk for thromboembolic disease (Leung & Lockwood, 2014).

#### Additional Predisposing Factors

Women with varicose veins, obesity, a history of thrombophlebitis, and smoking are at additional risk for thromboembolic disease (Box 28.2). An age greater than 35 years doubles the risk (Leung & Lockwood, 2014).

### Superficial Venous Thrombosis

#### Manifestations

SVT is most often associated with varicose veins and limited to the calf area. It can also occur in the arms as a result of IV therapy. Signs and symptoms include swelling of the involved extremity as well as redness, tenderness, and warmth. Palpation of an enlarged, hardened, cord-like vein may be possible. The woman may experience pain when she walks, but some women have no signs at all.

#### Therapeutic Management

Treatment includes analgesics, rest, and elastic support. Elevation of the lower extremity improves venous return. Warm packs can be applied to the affected area. Anticoagulants are not usually needed, but anti-inflammatory medications may be used. After a period of bed rest with the leg elevated, the woman may ambulate gradually if symptoms have disappeared. She should avoid standing for long periods and should continue to wear support hose to help prevent venous stasis and a subsequent episode of superficial thrombosis. There is little chance of PE if the thrombosis remains in the superficial veins of the lower leg.

## Deep Venous Thrombosis

Signs and symptoms of DVT or PE are absent in most women affected (Leung & Lockwood, 2014). When present, they may be attributed to normal benign changes of pregnancy (Farquharson & Greaves, 2011). Those that occur are caused by an inflammatory process and obstruction of venous return. The woman may report pain in the leg, or groin (Rhode, 2016). Swelling of the leg, erythema, heat, and tenderness over the affected area are the most common signs. Homan's sign is not a reliable or valid test. Reflex arterial spasms can cause the leg to become pale and cool to the touch, with decreased peripheral pulses. Additional symptoms include pain on ambulation, chills, general malaise, and stiffness of the affected leg.

### Diagnostic Evaluation

Venous ultrasonography with vein compression and Doppler flow analysis of the deep veins of the upper legs are most commonly used to detect alterations in blood flow that are diagnostic of DVT. Noncontrast magnetic resonance imaging (MRI) is considered very sensitive and accurate in diagnosing pelvic and leg thrombosis (Leung and Lockwood, 2014). D-Dimer tests may be performed, but the results are normally higher during pregnancy and postpartum, and the test may not be as accurate as at other times. (Cunningham et.al, 2014; Leung & Lockwood, 2014).

### Therapeutic Management

***Preventing thrombus formation.*** Women who have had a previous DVT or PE are at risk for another. These women and others at high risk may receive prophylactic heparin, which does not cross the placenta. Either standard unfractionated heparin (UH) or a low-molecular-weight heparin (LMWH), such as enoxaparin (Lovenox) or tinzaparin (Innohep), can be used. Women receiving LMWH during pregnancy are changed to UH at approximately 36 weeks of gestation. The change is necessary because UH has a shorter half-life, and epidural anesthesia, which may be needed in labor, is contraindicated within 24 hours of the last dose of LMWH. Heparin is discontinued during labor and birth and resumed approximately 6 to 12 hours after uncomplicated birth and 12 hours after the epidural catheter is removed (ACOG, 2014).

If stirrups must be used during the birth, they should be padded to prevent prolonged pressure against the popliteal angle. If possible, the time in stirrups should be no more than 1 hour.

To prevent thrombus formation after childbirth, all new mothers are encouraged to ambulate frequently and as early as possible. Ambulation prevents stasis of blood in the legs and decreases the likelihood of thrombus formation. If the woman is unable to ambulate, range-of-motion and gentle leg exercises, such as flexing and straightening the knee and raising one leg at a time, should begin within 8 hours after childbirth. The mother should not use pillows under her knees or the knee gatch on the bed. These devices can cause sharp flexion at the knees and pressure against the popliteal space, leading to pooling of blood in the lower extremities.

Graduated compression stockings or sequential compression devices are used for mothers with varicose veins, a history of thrombosis, or a cesarean birth. Sequential compression devices should be applied preoperatively for a woman undergoing a cesarean birth who is not on anticoagulant therapy and should be continued until she begins to ambulate postpartum (ACOG, 2014). Compression stockings should be applied before the mother gets out of bed to prevent venous congestion, which begins as soon as she stands. It is important that she understands the correct way to put on the stockings. Improperly applied stockings can roll or bunch and slow venous return from the legs.

***Initial treatment.*** Anticoagulant therapy is started to prevent extension of the thrombus. Clotting studies should be monitored to ensure safe but therapeutic levels. The woman is placed on bed rest, with the affected leg elevated to decrease interstitial swelling and to promote venous return from the leg. She is allowed to ambulate when symptoms have disappeared. Analgesics may be prescribed to control pain, and antibiotics will be used as necessary to prevent or control infection. Moist heat provides relief of pain and increases circulation.

***Subsequent treatment.*** The long-term management of DVT depends on whether the woman is pregnant or in the postpartum period. The pregnant woman with a DVT receives anticoagulation therapy until labor begins. It is resumed 6 to 12 hours after birth and continued for 6 weeks to 6 months after birth (ACOG, 2014). Warfarin (Coumadin) is contraindicated during pregnancy because of teratogenic effects and the risk of fetal hemorrhage. Therefore, pregnant women are given UH or LMWH, which do not cross the placenta.

During the postpartum period, warfarin is started before heparin is stopped to provide continuous anticoagulation. Warfarin therapy is continued for at least 6 weeks postpartum (Ambrose & Repke, 2011). Warfarin is safe for use during lactation. Longer use of warfarin is necessary in some women with continuing risk factors. The INR is used to monitor coagulation time when warfarin is used.

Before discharge from the birth facility, the mother should be taught about lifestyle changes that can improve peripheral circulation. Clothing that is constricting around the legs and prolonged sitting should be avoided. If sitting for long periods is necessary, walking for a short time hourly or moving her feet and legs frequently will help prevent circulatory stasis.

## NURSING CARE

### The Mother With Deep Venous Thrombosis

#### Assessment

Assessment focuses on determining the status of the venous thrombosis. Inspect both legs at the same time so that the affected leg can be compared with the unaffected leg. DVT is most often unilateral, usually affecting the woman's left side (Leung and Lockwood, 2014). Warmth or redness indicates inflammation; coolness or cyanosis indicates venous obstruction. Palpate the pedal pulses, comparing the strength of the right and left. Measure the affected and unaffected leg, comparing the circumferences. Record the measurements for ongoing assessment. It may be helpful to mark the woman's legs at the location of the measurement for consistency in assessments. Ask the woman about the degree of her discomfort. Pain is caused by tissue hypoxia, and increasing pain indicates progressive obstruction.

Evaluate the laboratory reports of clotting studies. Thrombocytopenia is a concern when heparin is administered for a prolonged time.

#### Nursing Diagnosis and Planning

The treatment of DVT includes the administration of anticoagulants for a prolonged time. An appropriate nursing diagnosis for this situation is "Risk for Bleeding related to lack of understanding of anticoagulant therapy precautions."

***Expected outcomes.*** The woman will remain free of bleeding from anticoagulant therapy. She will discuss precautions needed when taking anticoagulants and verbalize her plan for changes necessary as a result of anticoagulant therapy.

#### Interventions

***Monitoring for signs of bleeding.*** At least twice a day, inspect the mother for the appearance of bruising or petechiae. Instruct her to

## WOMEN WANT TO KNOW

### How Do I Prevent Thrombosis (Blood Clots)?

Methods to improve peripheral circulation will help prevent the occurrence of thrombophlebitis:

- Improve your circulation with a regular schedule of activity, preferably walking.
- Avoid prolonged standing or sitting in one position.
- When sitting, elevate your legs and avoid crossing them. This will increase the return of venous blood from the legs.
- Maintain a daily fluid intake of 12 or more 8-oz glasses to prevent dehydration and consequent sluggish circulation.
- Stop smoking. Smoking is a risk factor for thrombosis and can cause respiratory problems in you and your newborn.

report any signs of bleeding: bruises, bloody nose, blood in urine or stools, bleeding gums, or increased vaginal bleeding. Be alert for signs of hemorrhage, such as tachycardia, falling blood pressure, or other signs that may indicate internal bleeding.

Observe for excessive or bright red lochia. If the uterus is boggy, the cause is uterine atony. Massage the uterus and express clots. If the fundus is firm, bleeding may be from trauma or anticoagulant therapy. In either case the provider should be notified.

Unless frank hemorrhage is present, the usual treatment for excessive anticoagulation is temporary discontinuation of the anticoagulant. Protamine sulfate, which is the antidote for UH and is partially effective against LMWH, should be available. The antidote for warfarin is vitamin K.

*Explaining continued therapy.* Teach the woman how to prevent excessive anticoagulation. Carefully explain the treatment regimen, including the schedule of medication. Help the woman develop a method for remembering to take the medication as directed, for example, marking a calendar each time the drug is taken. Caution her not to "double up" if a dose is missed. If necessary, teach her and another family member how to inject heparin or enoxaparin. Explain the need for repeated laboratory testing to regulate the dose of the anticoagulant. Emphasize the importance of careful attention to dosage changes to keep the medication at the appropriate blood levels.

Because oral anticoagulants are associated with many clinically significant drug interactions, emphasize the importance of keeping the healthcare provider informed about any medications the woman takes. Caution her that common over-the-counter medications, such as aspirin and other nonsteroidal anti-inflammatory drugs, increase the risk of hemorrhage.

Instruct the woman taking warfarin that eating large amounts of vitamin K–containing foods can interfere with anticoagulation. These foods include broccoli, cabbage, lettuce, spinach, and lentils. The woman should use effective contraception as long as she is taking warfarin because the drug can cause fetal defects.

Suggest that the mother use a soft toothbrush and floss her teeth gently to prevent bleeding from the gums. An electric toothbrush may be too vigorous, causing bleeding. The woman should postpone dental appointments until the therapy is completed. Using a depilatory or waxing product or shaving with an electric razor to remove unwanted hair is safer than using a blade razor during anticoagulant therapy.

Remind the mother not to go barefoot and to avoid activities that could cause injury. Caution her against drinking alcohol, which inhibits the metabolism of oral anticoagulants. Also emphasize the importance of reporting unusual bleeding. Explain that many herbs affect the potency of anticoagulants, and the woman should check with her healthcare provider before using any herbs or dietary supplements.

*Helping the family adapt to home care.* Nurses often assist the family to adapt to home care. Assess the family structure and function to determine how prepared the family is to cope with the mother's illness. Determine the ages of any children and availability of family members or friends to help while the mother is confined to bed or on limited activity. Although the health of the mother is of primary importance, care must be taken that the attachment process between her and the infant progresses normally.

### Evaluation

- Does the woman maintain therapeutic levels of her anticoagulant?
- Is she free from signs of unusual bleeding or other side effects of the medication?
- Can she explain how she will keep safe while on anticoagulation medication?

## PULMONARY EMBOLISM

### Pathophysiology

PE is a serious complication of DVT that can lead to maternal mortality. PE occurs when fragments of a blood clot dislodge and are carried to the lungs. An embolus can also consist of amniotic fluid and its debris, a condition called *anaphylactoid syndrome* (see Chapter 27). The embolus lodges in a vessel and partially or completely obstructs the flow of blood into the lungs. If pulmonary circulation is severely compromised, death can occur within a few minutes. If the embolus is small, adequate pulmonary circulation can be maintained until treatment can be initiated.

### Manifestations

Clinical signs and symptoms depend on how much the flow of blood is obstructed. Dyspnea, chest pain, tachycardia, tachypnea, and hemoptysis are the most common signs (Rhode, 2016). Syncope is uncommon and may indicate massive emboli (Leung and Lockwood, 2014). Pulmonary rales, cough, abdominal pain, and low-grade fever can also occur. Pulse oximetry shows decreased oxygen saturation. Arterial blood gas determinations show decreased partial pressure of oxygen, and chest radiography reveals areas of atelectasis and pleural effusion. Other possible diagnostic tests include computed tomographic pulmonary angiography (CPTA) and ventilation-perfusion (V/Q) scan. A venous ultrasound can also be performed to identify a DVT (Leung and Lockwood, 2014).

### Therapeutic Management

Treatment of PE is aimed at dissolving the clot and maintaining pulmonary circulation. Oxygen is used to decrease hypoxia, and narcotic analgesics are given to reduce pain and apprehension. Bed rest with the head of the bed elevated is used to help reduce dyspnea. The level of care, including support of ventilation, depends on the woman's pulmonary status. Pulse oximetry and arterial blood gases are evaluated. Heparin therapy is initiated and is continued throughout pregnancy if the embolism occurs before birth. Warfarin therapy can be continued for months after birth to prevent further emboli.

### Nursing Considerations

#### Monitoring for Signs

When caring for a woman with DVT, nurses must be aware of the danger of PE and focus the assessment on early signs and symptoms. Such measures include frequent assessment of respiratory rate as well as thorough and frequent auscultation of breath sounds. Abnormalities such as diminished or unequal breath sounds or coughing should be reported immediately to the healthcare provider. Additional signs that require immediate attention include air hunger, dyspnea, tachycardia, pallor, and cyanosis.

### Facilitating Oxygenation

Oxygen should be administered at 8 to 10 L/min by tight face mask. The nurse should remain with the mother to allay fear and apprehension. The head of the bed should be raised to facilitate breathing. Narcotic analgesics such as morphine can be used to relieve pain. Sedatives can be given to help control anxiety.

### Seeking Assistance

The woman's condition is precarious until the clot is lysed or until it adheres to the pulmonary artery wall and is reabsorbed. The primary nurse should call for assistance to initiate interventions, including continuous assessment of vital signs and administration of IV heparin and emergency drugs that may be needed. The woman who has PE requires critical care nursing skills and is usually transferred to an intensive care unit.

## PUERPERAL INFECTION

**Puerperal infection** is a term used to describe bacterial infections after childbirth. Until the advent of antibiotics, puerperal infection often resulted in death and remains a cause of maternal death, especially in developing nations. The most common postpartum infections are **endometritis**, wound infections, urinary tract infections, **mastitis** (infection of the breast), and septic pelvic thrombophlebitis. **Endomyometritis** is an infection of the muscle and inner lining of the uterus. If the surrounding tissues are also involved, **endoparametritis** is present. **Metritis** is an infection of the decidua, myometrium, and parametrial tissues of the uterus.

### Definition

The definition of puerperal infection is a temperature of 38° C (100.4° F) or higher after the first 24 hours and occurring on at least 2 of the first 10 days following childbirth (Adair, 1935). Although a slight elevation in temperature can occur during the first 24 hours because of dehydration or the exertion of labor, any mother with fever should be assessed for other signs of infection.

### Pathophysiology

To understand the serious nature of infection of the reproductive tract, consider the anatomy of the region. Every part of the reproductive tract is connected to every other part, and organisms can move from the vagina, through the cervix, into the uterus, and through the fallopian tubes to infect the ovaries and the peritoneal cavity. The entire reproductive tract is particularly well supplied with blood vessels during pregnancy and after childbirth. Bacteria that invade or are picked up by the blood vessels or lymphatics can carry the infection to the rest of the body, which can result in life-threatening septicemia.

The normal physiologic changes of childbirth increase the risk of infection. During labor and birth, the acidity of the vagina is reduced by the amniotic fluid, blood, and lochia, which are alkaline. An alkaline environment encourages bacterial growth.

Necrosis of the endometrial lining and the presence of lochia provide a favorable environment for the growth of anaerobic bacteria. Many small lacerations, some microscopic in size, occur in the endometrium, cervix, and vagina during birth and allow bacteria to enter the tissue. Although the uterine interior is not sterile until 3 to 4 weeks after childbirth, infection does not develop in most women, partly because granulocytes in the lochia and endometrium help prevent infection. Scrupulous aseptic technique during labor and birth and careful hand washing during the postpartum period are also major preventive factors.

### Etiology

Other factors can predispose a woman to infection (Table 28.2). Cesarean birth is a major predisposing factor (Mackeen, Packard, Ota, et al., 2015) because of the tissue trauma that occurs in surgery, the incision that provides an entrance for bacteria, the possibility of contamination during surgery, and foreign bodies, such as sutures, that can promote infection. In addition, women who have a surgical birth because of a problem that develops during labor can have other risk factors (e.g., prolonged labor) that raise the chances of infection. Colonization of the vagina with organisms also predisposes the woman to the development of infection after childbirth.

Any trauma to maternal tissues increases the hazard of infection. Trauma during vaginal birth can occur with rapid birth, birth of a large

**TABLE 28.2 Risk Factors for Puerperal Infection**

| Risk Factor | Reason |
|---|---|
| History of previous infections (urinary tract infection, mastitis, thrombophlebitis) | May be more vulnerable to infection |
| Colonization of lower genital tract by pathogenic organisms | Infections usually caused by several microbes that have ascended to uterus from lower genital tract |
| Cesarean birth | Provides increased portals of entry for bacteria |
| Trauma | Provides entrance for bacteria and makes tissues more susceptible |
| Prolonged rupture of membranes | Removes barrier of amniotic membranes and allows access by organisms to interior of uterus |
| Prolonged labor | Increases number of vaginal examinations; allows time for bacteria to multiply |
| Catheterization | Could introduce organisms into bladder |
| Excessive number of vaginal examinations | Increases chance that organisms from vagina or outside source are carried into uterus |
| Retained placental fragments | Provides growth medium for bacteria and may interfere with flow of lochia |
| Hemorrhage | Results in loss of infection-fighting components of blood |
| Poor general health (excessive fatigue, anemia, frequent minor illnesses) | Increases vulnerability to infections and complications of labor |
| Poor nutrition (decreased protein, vitamin C) | Less able to repair tissue and defend against infection |
| Poor hygiene | Increases exposure to pathogens |
| Medical conditions such as diabetes mellitus | Decreases ability to defend against infections of any kind; diabetes increases glucose level in urine |
| Low socioeconomic status | More likely to have poor nutrition and inadequate prenatal care |

infant, use of a vacuum extractor or forceps, manual delivery of the placenta, or lacerations and episiotomies. Catheterization during labor increases the chance of introducing organisms into the bladder and adds to the urinary tract trauma that occurs during normal childbirth.

When prolonged rupture of membranes occurs during labor, organisms from the vagina are more likely to ascend into the uterine cavity. A long labor or many vaginal examinations during labor increases the danger of infection. Each vaginal examination increases the possibility of contamination from organisms in the vagina that are carried through the open cervix. Use of a fetal scalp electrode or intrauterine pressure catheter has the same effect. If part of the placenta remains inside the uterus after birth, the tissue becomes necrotic and provides a good place for bacteria to grow.

Additional factors include postpartum hemorrhage, which causes loss of infection-fighting components of the blood, such as leukocytes, and leaves the mother in a weakened condition. Prenatal conditions (poor nutrition, anemia) interfere with the mother's ability to resist infection. Lack of knowledge of hygiene or lack of access to facilities that permit adequate hygiene increase the risk of postpartum infection.

## Specific Infections

### Endometritis

Endometritis occurs in 1% to 3% of women following vaginal birth and 5% to 15% of women having scheduled cesarean birth. If extended labor and rupture of membranes precede cesarean birth, infection occurs in 30% to 35% of women who have no prophylactic antibiotics and 10% or less of those who receive prophylactic antibiotics (Cunningham et al., 2014; Duff, 2014).

***Etiology.*** Endometritis is usually caused by organisms that are normal inhabitants of the vagina and cervix. Most infections are polymicrobial, with both aerobic and anaerobic organisms involved. Organisms most often found include aerobic and anaerobic streptococci, *Escherichia coli, Klebsiella pneumoniae, Proteus, Bacteroides*, and *Gardnerella*. (Dickinson, 2011). *Chlamydia trachomatis* is most often associated with late-onset infections, 2 or more weeks after birth (Rhode, 2016).

***Manifestations.*** The mother with severe endometritis looks sick. She presents a different picture from the typical happy new mother. The major signs and symptoms are temperature of 38° C (100.4° F) or higher; chills; malaise; anorexia; abdominal pain and cramping; uterine tenderness; and purulent, foul-smelling lochia. Additional signs include tachycardia and subinvolution. In most cases, the signs and symptoms occur within 36 hours after birth (Duff 2014).

Laboratory data can confirm the diagnosis. The results of a complete blood count typically shows an elevation in the number of leukocytes (15,000/mm$^3$ to 30,000/mm$^3$). Leukocyte levels are normally elevated to as high as 30,000/mm$^3$ during the early postpartum time (Blackburn, 2013). However, leukocytosis that is not decreasing should prompt further evaluation. A blood culture and catheterized urine specimen may be obtained. Cultures of the vagina or endometrium are not usually helpful.

***Therapeutic management.*** Administration of IV antibiotics is the initial treatment for endometritis. The goal is to confine the infection to the uterus and to prevent its spread throughout the body. Broad-spectrum antibiotics such as the cephalosporins, clindamycin plus gentamicin, or ampicillin plus aminoglycosides are often used. Metronidazole with penicillin also can be given. Antibiotics are continued until the woman has been afebrile and asymptomatic for 24 hours (Duff, 2014).

To decrease the incidence of endometritis and wound infections, a single prophylactic IV dose of an antibiotic before skin incision should be given to any woman who is having a cesarean birth (Duff, 2014). Other medications include antipyretics for fever and oxytocics such as methylergonovine to increase drainage of lochia and promote involution.

***Complications.*** If the infection spreads outside the uterine cavity, it can affect the fallopian tubes (salpingitis) or the ovaries (oophoritis), possibly resulting in sterility. Peritonitis (inflammation of the membrane lining the walls of the abdominal and pelvic cavities) can occur and lead to pelvic abscess formation. In addition, the risk of pelvic thrombophlebitis is increased when pathogenic bacteria enter the bloodstream during episodes of endometritis.

Signs and symptoms that the infection is spreading are similar to those of endometritis but more severe. Fever and abdominal pain will be particularly pronounced. Peritonitis can result in paralytic ileus and abdominal distention with absent bowel sounds.

***Nursing considerations.*** The woman with endometritis should be placed in a Fowler's position to promote drainage of lochia. She should be medicated as needed for abdominal pain or cramping, which can be severe. Monitor the woman's response to treatment and note signs of improvement or of continued infection (nausea and vomiting, abdominal distention, absent bowel sounds, and severe abdominal pain). Assess vital signs every 2 hours while fever is present and every 4 hours afterward. Comfort measures include warm blankets, cool compresses, cold or warm drinks, or use of a heating pad. Foods high in vitamin C and protein to aid healing are encouraged, along with oral fluids to maintain hydration.

Teaching should include signs and symptoms of worsening condition, side effects of therapy, and the importance of adhering to the treatment plan and follow-up care. If the woman is so sick that she must be separated from her infant or the infant is discharged before the mother, a nursing diagnosis of "Risk for Impaired Attachment related to separation from infant" should be considered. If the mother is breastfeeding, she will need help pumping her breasts to establish and maintain lactation.

### Wound Infection

Wound infections are common types of puerperal infection because any break in the skin or mucous membrane provides a portal of entry for organisms. The most common sites are cesarean surgical incisions, episiotomies, and lacerations. Infection of the incision occurs along with endometritis in 3% to 5% of women after cesarean (Duff 2014). Risk factors include obesity, diabetes, hemorrhage, anemia, chorioamnionitis, corticosteroid therapy, and multiple vaginal examinations.

***Manifestations.*** Signs of wound infection are edema, warmth, redness, tenderness, and pain. The edges of the wound may pull apart, with seropurulent drainage present. If the wound remains untreated, generalized signs of infection, such as fever and malaise, can develop as well. As with other puerperal infections, cultures may reveal mixed aerobic and anaerobic bacteria. Necrotizing fasciitis is a rare infection that can occur at any incision site. The necrosis can spread, and the condition can be fatal.

***Therapeutic management.*** Incision and drainage of the affected area may be necessary. The wound exudate is cultured, and broad-spectrum antibiotics are ordered until a report of the organism is returned. Analgesics are often necessary, and warm compresses or sitz baths provide comfort and promote healing by increasing circulation to the area. Surgical debridement is performed for necrotizing fasciitis.

***Nursing considerations.*** Despite their small size, wound infections are painful and annoying to the mother. Perineal infections cause discomfort during many activities, including walking, sitting, and defecating and are particularly troublesome because they are not expected by the new mother.

Wound infections may require readmission to the hospital or home healthcare visits. The woman requires reassurance and supportive care. Comfort measures include sitz baths, warm compresses, and frequent perineal care. She should be taught to wipe from front to back and to change perineal pads frequently. Good hand washing techniques are emphasized. Adequate fluid intake and a healthy diet are important. Activity may be modified depending on the site, severity, and treatment of the wound infection.

The infant is not routinely isolated from the mother with a wound infection, but the woman must be advised about how to protect her infant from contact with contaminated articles such as dressings. Anticipatory guidance should include teaching regarding the side effects of medications, signs of worsening condition, self-care measures, and the importance of hand washing.

### Urinary Tract Infections

***Etiology.*** During childbirth the bladder and urethra are traumatized by pressure from the descending fetus. Catheter insertion, with its risk of infection, may also be performed during labor. After childbirth, the bladder and urethra are hypotonic, with urinary stasis and retention as common problems. Residual urine and reflux of urine can occur during voiding.

Women who had bacteria in the urine during pregnancy, often without symptoms, are at increased risk for cystitis and pyelonephritis, which can result in preterm labor. Asymptomatic bacteriuria are discovered during urine screens in 2% to 11% of pregnant women (Duff, 2014). Urinary tract infections are most often caused by coliform bacteria such as *E. coli*. Other organisms include *K. pneumoniae* and *Proteus* species (Ambrose & Repke, 2011).

***Manifestations.*** Symptoms typically begin on the 1st or 2nd postpartum day. They include dysuria (a burning pain on urination), urgency, frequency, and suprapubic pain. Hematuria can also occur. A low-grade fever is sometimes the only sign. In some women, an upper urinary tract infection, such as pyelonephritis, may develop the 3rd or 4th postpartum day, with chills, spiking fever, costovertebral angle tenderness, flank pain, nausea, and vomiting. This infection of the kidney pelvis can cause permanent damage to the kidney if not promptly treated.

***Therapeutic management.*** Most urinary tract infections can be treated with antibiotics on an outpatient basis. Asymptomatic bacteriuria during pregnancy increases the risk of pyelonephritis 20 to 30 times. Treatment reduces the incidence of pyelonephritis significantly (Duff, 2014). Pyelonephritis during pregnancy may require hydration and IV administration of broad-spectrum antibiotics. In addition, the woman should be observed for signs of preterm labor. If the postpartum woman is only mildly ill, she can be treated with oral antibiotics at home. Urinary analgesics, such as phenazopyridine (Pyridium), may also be prescribed. Antibiotics that are safe for use during lactation are given if the mother is breastfeeding.

***Nursing considerations.*** The woman with a urinary tract infection must be instructed to take the medication for the entire time it is prescribed and not to stop when symptoms abate. In addition, she must drink at least 2500 to 3000 mL of fluid each day to help dilute the bacterial count and flush the infection from the bladder. Acidification of the urine inhibits multiplication of bacteria, and drinks that acidify urine, such as apricot, plum, prune, and cranberry juices, are frequently recommended. Grapefruit and carbonated drinks should be avoided because they increase urine alkalinity. Teaching should also include measures to prevent urinary tract infections, such as using proper perineal care, increasing fluid intake, and urinating frequently.

### Mastitis

Mastitis, an infection of the breast, occurs most often 2 to 4 weeks after childbirth, although it can develop at any time during breastfeeding. Approximately 5% to 10% of lactating women are affected (Duff, 2014). It usually affects only one breast.

***Etiology.*** Mastitis is often caused by *Staphylococcus aureus*, including methicillin-resistant staphylococcus aureus (MRSA), *E. coli*, and *Streptococci* (Lawrence & Lawrence, 2016). The bacteria are most often carried on the skin of the mother or in the mouth or nose of the newborn. The organism can enter through an injured area of the nipple, such as a crack or blister, even though no obvious signs of injury is apparent. Soreness and pain of a nipple may result in insufficient emptying of the breast during breastfeeding.

Mastitis is often preceded by engorgement and stasis of milk, which can occur when a feeding is skipped, when the infant begins to sleep through the night, or when breastfeeding is suddenly stopped. Constriction of the breasts by a bra that is too tight can interfere with duct emptying, leading to infection. The mother who is fatigued or stressed or who has other health problems that might suppress her immune system is also at increased risk for mastitis.

***Manifestations.*** Initial symptoms may be flu like, with fatigue and aching muscles. Symptoms progress to include a temperature of 39° C (102.2° F) or higher, chills, malaise, and headache. Mastitis is characterized by a localized lump or wedge-shaped area of pain, redness, heat, inflammation, and enlarged axillary lymph nodes. A hard, tender area is palpable (Fig. 28.4). Untreated mastitis can progress to breast abscess.

***Therapeutic management.*** Antibiotic therapy and continued emptying of the breast by breastfeeding or breast pump constitute the first line of treatment. With early antibiotic treatment, mastitis usually resolves within 24 to 48 hours. Antibiotics should be continued for 7 to 10 days (Duff, 2014). Women who develop a breast abscess are treated with surgical drainage and antibiotics. Approximately 10% of women with mastitis develop a breast abscess (Ambrose & Repke, 2011).

Supportive measures include application of moist heat or ice packs, breast support, bed rest, and analgesics. The mother should continue to breastfeed from both breasts. If the affected breast is too sore, she can use a breast pump. Regular emptying of the breast is important in preventing abscess formation. If an abscess forms and is surgically drained, breastfeeding can be continued as long as the incision is not near the areola and the mother is comfortable. If an abscess ruptures into the milk ducts, breastfeeding on that side should be discontinued temporarily and a breast pump used to empty the breast (Lawrence & Lawrence, 2016).

***Nursing considerations.*** Because mastitis rarely occurs before discharge from the birth facility, the nurse must provide adequate information for prevention. Measures to prevent mastitis include positioning the infant correctly and avoiding nipple trauma and milk stasis. The mother should breastfeed every 2 to 3 hours and should avoid formula supplements. Nursing pads should not have a plastic layer and should be changed as soon as they are wet. The mother should also avoid continuous pressure on the breasts from tight bras or infant carriers.

Once mastitis occurs, nursing measures are aimed at increasing comfort and helping the mother maintain lactation. Moist heat promotes comfort and increases circulation. A disposable diaper wet with warm water and placed over the breast is an easy way to apply heat. The thickness helps to maintain the temperature, and the plastic cover prevents dripping. A shower or hot packs should be used before feeding or pumping the breasts. The woman should complete the entire course of antibiotics to prevent recurrence or a breast abscess.

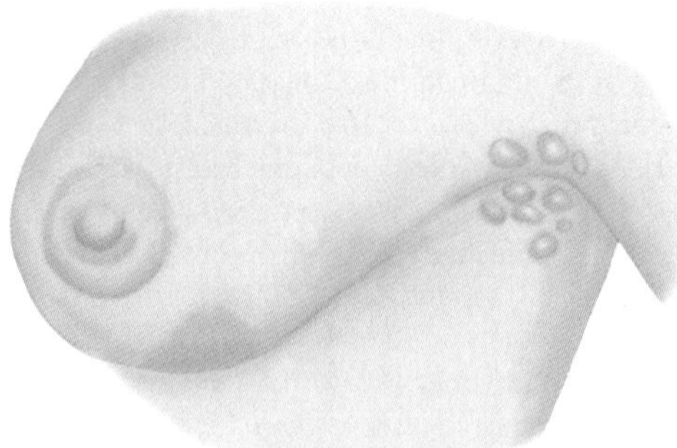


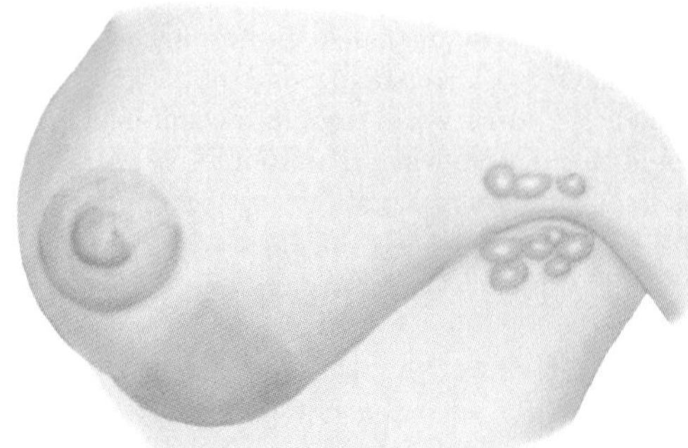


**FIG 28.4** Mastitis typically occurs in the breast of a woman who breastfeeds after 2 to 3 weeks following birth.

The breast should be completely emptied at each feeding to prevent stasis of milk, which can result in an abscess. If the mother is too sore to breastfeed on the affected side, she should be shown how to express the milk or use a pump to empty the breasts.

Breastfeeding or pumping every 1.5 to 2 hours makes the mother more comfortable and prevents stasis. Starting the feeding on the unaffected side causes the milk-ejection reflex to occur in both breasts, making milk available in the painful breast as soon as the infant begins to nurse on that side. Massage over the affected area before and during the feeding helps to ensure complete emptying. The mother should stay in bed during the acute phase of her illness. Her fluid intake should be 2500 to 3000 mL per day. Analgesics may be required to relieve discomfort.

The mother with mastitis is likely to be very discouraged. Some mothers decide to stop breastfeeding because of the discomfort involved. Weaning during an episode of mastitis can increase engorgement and stasis, leading to abscess formation or recurrent infection. The mother may need much encouragement, and she will need help in arranging care for other children or with other responsibilities so that she can rest. The nursing diagnosis "Interrupted Breastfeeding related to discomfort, infectious process, or effects of therapy" may be appropriate.

### Septic Pelvic Thrombophlebitis

Septic pelvic thrombophlebitis is the least common of the puerperal infections, occurring in 1 of 2000 pregnancies (Duff, 2014). This condition usually is not seen until 2 to 4 days after childbirth. It occurs when infection spreads along the pelvic venous system and thrombophlebitis develops.

***Manifestations.*** The primary symptom is pain in the groin, abdomen, or flank. Spiking fever, tachycardia, gastrointestinal distress, and decreased bowel sounds may be present. The only sign may be fever that does not respond to antibiotic therapy. Laboratory data can be used to exclude other diagnoses and usually include a complete blood count with differential, blood chemistries, coagulation studies, and cultures. Pelvic ultrasound, computed tomography, or MRI may be performed.

***Therapeutic management.*** Readmission to the hospital is usually necessary. Primary treatment includes anticoagulation therapy with IV heparin and IV antibiotics. Warfarin may be given when heparin is discontinued. Supportive care is similar to that for DVT and includes monitoring for safe levels of anticoagulation therapy and for signs and symptoms of PE.

## NURSING CARE

### The Woman With an Infection

#### Assessment

Although all women are observed for indications of infection as part of routine nursing assessments, the nurse must practice increased vigilance for mothers who are at increased risk of infection.

Pay particular attention to signs that may be expected in infection, such as fever, tachycardia, pain, or unusual amount, color, or odor of lochia. Generalized symptoms of malaise and muscle aching may also be significant. Examine all wounds each shift for signs of localized infection such as redness, edema, tenderness, discharge, or pulling apart of incisions or sutured lacerations. Ask the mother if she has difficulty emptying her bladder or discomfort related to urination.

Assess the mother's knowledge of hygiene practices that prevent infections, such as proper handwashing, perineal care, and handling of perineal pads. Evaluate her knowledge of breastfeeding and any problems that might result in breast engorgement and stasis of milk in the ducts. Examine the nipples for signs of injury that might provide a portal of entry for organisms.

#### SAFETY ALERT

***Signs and Symptoms of Postpartum Infection***

- Fever, chills
- Pain or redness of wounds
- Purulent wound drainage or wound edges not approximated
- Tachycardia
- Uterine subinvolution
- Abnormal duration of lochia, foul odor
- Elevated white blood cell count
- Frequency or urgency of urination, dysuria, or hematuria
- Suprapubic pain
- Localized area of warmth, redness, or tenderness in the breasts
- Body aches, general malaise

#### Nursing Diagnosis and Planning

Because all women are at risk for infection after childbirth, most facilities have developed standards of practice that protect postpartum women from infection. However, when predisposing factors increase the likelihood of infection, routine assessments and care must be modified and preventive measures intensified. In this case, the most relevant nursing diagnosis is "Risk for Infection related to the presence of significant risk factors."

*Expected outcome.* See the Nursing Care Plan: Risk for Postpartum Infection, which develops expected outcomes and interventions for this nursing diagnosis.

## AFFECTIVE DISORDERS

Childbearing is a major life stressor that can provoke or aggravate affective disorders including mood disorders (prenatal and postpartum depression, postpartum psychoses, and bipolar disorders) and anxiety disorders (obsessive-compulsive disorder, generalized anxiety disorder, panic disorder, social anxiety disorder, specific phobias, and posttraumatic stress disorder) (AWHONN, 2015c).

### Mood Disorders

Mood disorders are disturbances in function, affect, or thought processes that can affect the family after childbirth as severely as physiologic problems. Postpartum blues ("baby blues") is a transient, self-limiting mood disorder (discussed in Chapter 20). Depression, postpartum psychosis, and bipolar disorder are more serious disorders that disrupt the family and require intervention.

### Peripartum Depression

Peripartum depression is a term used to describe the onset of a depressive disorder during pregnancy or postpartum. This disorder is designated 'peripartum' rather than 'postpartum' depression because fifty percent of depressive episodes occurring during the perinatal period first present during the antepartum period. Peripartum depression involves at least a 2-week period of depressed mood or loss of interest in almost all activities accompanied by at least four of the following: changes in appetite or weight, sleep, and psychomotor activity; decreased energy; feelings of worthlessness or guilt; difficulty thinking, concentrating, or making decisions; or recurrent thoughts of death or plans or attempts of suicide that occur during pregnancy or the first 4 weeks after birth (American Psychiatric Association, 2013). Most

## NURSING CARE PLAN

### *Risk for Postpartum Infection*

**Assessment**

Patty, a thin, 26-year-old primipara, is admitted to the postpartum unit after a cesarean birth. She was in labor for 16 hours, and her membranes were ruptured for 14 hours before the birth. She was catheterized twice during labor, with insertion of an indwelling catheter shortly before her surgery. She plans to breastfeed her infant.

**Nursing Diagnosis**

Risk for Infection related to presence of favorable conditions for infections.

**Planning**

***Expected Outcomes***

Patty will:

1. Remain free of signs of infection during the postpartum period.
2. Verbalize methods of prevention of infection by discharge.
3. List signs of infection that should be reported to her healthcare provider.

**Interventions and *Rationales***

1. Assess vital signs every 4 hours.
   *Temperature above 38° C (100.4° F) or tachycardia suggests an infectious process and should be reported.*
2. Observe the surgical incision for redness, tenderness, edema, drainage, and approximation, and note the odor of lochia every 4 hours. Determine character of urine and whether Patty experiences frequency, urgency, or pain with urination after the catheter is removed.
   *Redness, pain, or edema of the incision suggests wound infection. Drainage could be bleeding or a sign of infection. Separation also can indicate infection. Foul odor of lochia suggests endometrial infection. Frequency, urgency, or painful urination may indicate urinary tract infection.*
3. Instruct Patty in hygienic practices to prevent infection:
   a. Careful handwashing before and after perineal care
   b. Perineal cleansing after elimination
   c. Changing peripads frequently
   d. Wiping the perineum from front to back
   *Good hygiene helps prevent infection. Handwashing is the most important defense against infection and its spread. Perineal cleansing helps prevent growth of bacteria. Frequent pad changes remove accumulated lochia, an excellent culture medium for bacteria. Wiping from front to back prevents fecal contamination of the vagina.*
4. Initiate measures to reduce the risk of urinary tract infection.
   a. Provide fluids of Patty's choice when she is able to take them, and emphasize the importance of drinking 2500 to 3000 mL/day.
   b. Monitor bladder distention to prevent overfilling. Teach her the importance of emptying her bladder every 2 to 3 hours during the first days after childbirth.
   c. Use methods to promote bladder emptying such as running water in the shower or sink, pouring warm water over the perineum, and providing pain medication as needed.
   *Adequate hydration and frequent emptying of the bladder help prevent stasis of urine, which increases the risk of urinary tract infection. The sound of running water may stimulate the urge to void. Relief of pain may allow the mother to relax enough to void.*
5. Assist her with breastfeeding. Explain the reasons for proper positioning and frequent, adequate feedings.
   *Poor positioning and short, infrequent feedings may cause nipple trauma, engorgement, and incomplete emptying of the breasts, leading to mastitis.*
6. Offer and encourage Patty to eat well-balanced meals when she progresses to a regular diet. Emphasize the importance of a diet high in protein and vitamin C.
   *Adequate protein and vitamin C are necessary for healing damaged tissues.*
7. Organize nursing care to allow periods of rest.
   *Rest is important to help the body heal and fight infection.*
8. Teach her signs of infection that she should report to her healthcare provider. Include fever, chills, dysuria, increased incisional tenderness or drainage, lochia with a foul odor, or pain and redness of the breast.
   *Prompt recognition and reporting of signs of infection ensures early treatment and reduces further complications*

**Evaluation**

Patty is free of signs and symptoms of infection throughout her hospital stay and at her postpartum checkup. She verbalizes measures she will take to reduce her risk of infection when she is discharged from the hospital and signs of infection she will report to her healthcare provider, if necessary.

***Additional Nursing Diagnoses to Consider***

Activity Intolerance
Pain
Interrupted Breastfeeding
Risk for Impaired Parenting

experts in postpartum depression extend the time to the first 12 months since birth (Beck, 2014; Stuart-Parrigon & Stuart, 2014).

### Incidence and Etiology

Peripartum depression occurs in up to 20% of women during pregnancy or the first three months postpartum. (O'Hara et al., 2014). The cause of peripartum depression is unknown. Most of the research available has focused on postpartum depression (PPD). Theories include interactions between biochemical, genetic, psychosocial factors, and life stress (Beck, 2014). The relationships between sleep, fatigue, and physical health to postpartum depression are topics of recent research (Bhati & Richards, 2015; Giallo et al., 2015, Woolhouse et al., 2014). Risk factors include depressive symptoms during pregnancy or previous PPD (strong predictors), first pregnancy, personal or family history of depression, mental illness, or alcoholism, personality characteristics such as immaturity and low self-esteem, medical problems during pregnancy or after birth (preeclampsia, preexisting diabetes mellitus, anemia, or postpartum thyroid dysfunction), child care stress (infant with health problems, including preterm and low birth weight, anomalies, or a difficult temperament), inadequate social support, fatigue and lack of sleep, financial worries, and chronic stressors.

### Manifestations

While PPD can occur at any time during the first 12 months after the birth of the baby, the most likely time is during the first three months postpartum (Beck, 2014). The woman experiencing PPD shows a depressed mood with loss of interest in her usual activities and a loss of her usual emotional response toward her family. These are not mood swings but a persistent depressed state. Even though she cares for the infant, she is unable to feel pleasure or love. She sees the infant as demanding and herself as inept at mothering.

The woman may have intense feelings of anxiety, unworthiness, guilt, agitation, and shame, and she often expresses a sense of loss of self. Generalized fatigue, irritability, complaints of ill health, and difficulty concentrating and making decisions are also present. She often has little interest in food, may have weight changes, and experiences sleep disturbances (insomnia or excessive sleeping). Most of the symptoms are intensely and consistently present for at least a 2-week period and tend to become worse over time.

### Impact on the Family

PPD creates strain on the family's usual methods of coping and often causes difficulties in relationships. Stressors tend to be magnified, and as a result, family members may decrease their interactions with the depressed mother at a time when she needs support the most. Communication is impaired because she gradually withdraws from contact with others. The decreased libido commonly associated with depression can also affect her relationship with her significant other.

Partners of depressed women report a sense of loss of the partner and the relationship they had known previously. They express feelings of loss of control, anger, frustration, and embarrassment. Fathers may take on household chores and child care duties that the depressed mother is unable to manage. The father may also suffer from depression. Researchers are beginning to examine postpartum depression in new fathers. Findings suggest that PPD in the mother is the most significant risk factor for depression in the father during the first year after the birth of a baby (Stadtlander, 2015).

Depressed mothers interact differently with their infants than do women who are not depressed. They appear tense, are more irritable, and feel less competent as mothers. They may not notice the infant's cues or smiles, and thus, may fail to meet the infant's needs and to enjoy the positive feedback. They are less likely to provide healthy feeding and sleep practices or positive enrichment activities with their infants. Maternal PPD creates a home environment that can have a negative effect on the development of the infant's physical and psychosocial development, especially if her depressive symptoms continue after the postpartum period (Newland & Parade, 2016; Agnafors, Sydsjö, deKeyser, et al., 2013).

### Therapeutic Management

Depression responds best to a combination of psychotherapy, social support, and medication. Psychotherapy may be helpful to assist the woman to cope with changes in her life. The woman's partner and immediate family must be included in counseling sessions so they can develop an understanding of what the woman feels and needs. If psychotherapy alone is not effective, it should be combined with medication. Selective serotonin reuptake inhibitors and tricyclic antidepressants are the most commonly prescribed medications (Beck, 2014).

Whether the woman is still pregnant or is breastfeeding must be considered when drugs are prescribed, as some are safer than others for use in pregnancy and lactation. Women who discontinue medications for depression during pregnancy are more likely to have a relapse during pregnancy or postpartum (Cunningham et al., 2014). Electroconvulsive therapy may be necessary for mothers who are suicidal. It is used when the woman has not improved with other treatment.

## Postpartum Psychosis (PPP)

**Psychosis** is a mental state in which a person's ability to recognize reality, communicate, and relate to others is impaired. This rare condition affects 1 or 2 women per 1000 births (Kendall, Chalmers & Platz, 1987). It can occur as early as 2 days after birth and is a psychiatric emergency that usually requires hospitalization. Manifestations include agitation, irritability, rapidly shifting moods, disorientation, and disorganized behavior. Some mothers also have delusions about the baby and experience hallucinations (Beck, 2014). Women who have a personal or family history of PPP are at an increased risk. Management requires hospitalization, pharmacologic treatment, and psychiatric care (Cunningham et al., 2014).

Assessment and management of postpartum psychosis are beyond the scope of maternity nurses, and mothers who experience this condition must be referred to specialists for comprehensive therapy. Women with signs of postpartum psychosis need immediate medical attention, and hospitalization is usually necessary to prevent suicide or infanticide.

## Bipolar II Disorder

Women with bipolar disorder suffer from periods of irritability, hyperactivity, euphoria, and grandiosity. They exhibit little need for sleep and are seldom aware they have a problem. The poor judgment and confusion they experience make self-care and infant care impossible and can be life-threatening for the mother and infant.

The depressions of the bipolar disorder and major depression are similar and are characterized by tearfulness, preoccupation with guilt, feelings of worthlessness, sleep and appetite disturbances, and an inordinate concern with the baby's health. Delusions about the infant being dead or defective are common. Hallucinations may also be present. Women who have depressive symptoms must be assessed for risk of suicide or harming the infant and should be treated according to the severity of the threat.

## Postpartum Anxiety Disorders

The most common postpartum anxiety disorders include panic disorder, postpartum obsessive-compulsive disorder (OCD), and posttraumatic stress disorder. Panic disorder manifests as episodes of tachycardia, palpations, shortness of breath, chest pain, and fear of dying or of "going crazy." Episodes are repetitive and interfere with the woman's daily life. Antianxiety and antidepressant medications and counseling are the treatment for this condition.

Postpartum OCD is a condition in which the woman has consuming thoughts that she might harm the baby and fears being alone with the baby. Anxiety and depression occur, and the woman may perform compulsive behaviors to avoid acting on her thoughts. Some mothers avoid their infants while others obsessively check on the infant. Treatment includes cognitive-behavioral therapy and, if necessary, pharmacotherapy (Beck, 2014).

In posttraumatic stress disorder, women perceive childbirth as a traumatic event. They have nightmares and flashbacks about the event, anxiety, and avoidance of reminders of the traumatic event; some have depression after giving birth. Feeling a lack of caring or communication or having a birth very different from what they expected can contribute to this disorder. Women need to talk about their experiences and how they perceived them and often search for answers about their experiences. They may feel isolated from their infants and have prolonged difficulty feeling close to them. Celebrating the child's birthdays may be distressing, as they are anniversaries of the trauma experienced when the child was born (Beck, 2014).

## NURSING CARE

### Postpartum Affective Disorders

#### Assessment

Early identification and treatment of peripartum mood and anxiety disorders is a significant factor in appropriate management of these conditions (AWHONN, 2015c). Assess all women for depression during pregnancy, at the birth facility, and during follow-up visits after birth. If follow-up phone calls are made from the birth facility, questions about depression should be included in the assessment. The woman should be reassessed at each contact with healthcare providers. Women whose infants are in a neonatal intensive care unit should be assessed for PPD during visits to their infants. Pediatricians and pediatric nurse practitioners are also in a position to identify PPD. New mothers take their infants to the pediatrician's office frequently during the early months after childbirth. These are ideal settings in which to assess the new mother's emotional state and provide referrals if necessary Assessment tools such as the Postpartum Depression Predictors Inventory-Revised may be helpful. This inventory identifies prenatal depression, life stress, social support, prenatal anxiety, satisfaction with marital relationship, history of depression, self-esteem, unwanted or unplanned pregnancy, marital status, socioeconomic status, child care stress, infant temperament, and maternity blues as factors that can predict the likelihood of a woman developing PPD (Beck, Records, & Rice, 2006). In addition, screening for excessive fatigue in the first 2 weeks after childbirth may help identify women who will later develop PPD and enable them to get early treatment. Other screening tools include the Edinburgh Postnatal Depression Scale (Cox, Holden, & Sagovsky, 1987) and the Postpartum Depression Screening Scale (Beck & Gable, 2002). Ask the woman if she is often sad or depressed, or if she has felt a loss of pleasure or interest in things she once enjoyed. These questions may enable early identification and treatment of depression, reducing its duration and severity. Asking shows interest and acceptance of expressions of feelings and opens the door for further discussion. Inform the mother that many women feel depressed after childbirth and that help is available.

Observe for subjective symptoms, such as apathy, lack of interest or energy, anorexia, or sleeplessness. The mother's verbalizations of failure, sadness, loneliness, anxiety, or vague confusion are important cues. Focus on the frequency, duration, and intensity of the woman's feelings to determine their severity.

Assess for objective data such as crying, sleeplessness, poor personal hygiene, or inability to follow directions or concentrate. Determine what support, if any, is available. Single mothers or mothers with an absent or unavailable support system can feel increasingly isolated, leading to stress that they are unable to manage. Inappropriate expressions of blame or anger toward the partner and unmet expectations of the baby or the parenting role are sometimes present.

**SAFETY ALERT**

***Signs and Symptoms of Postpartum Depression***

- Feelings of sadness, crying
- Loss of pleasure in usual activities
- Anxiety, agitation or irritability
- Feelings of guilt
- Fatigue, sleep disturbances
- Difficulty concentrating or making decisions
- Depression (may not be present at first)
- Suicidal thoughts

#### Nursing Diagnosis and Planning

A likely nursing diagnosis is: Risk for Ineffective Coping related to depression secondary to stressors associated with childbirth and parenting.

***Expected outcomes.*** The new mother will demonstrate effective coping by verbalizing her feelings with the healthcare provider and the significant other throughout the postpartum period and by identifying strengths and resources that are available during her postpartum period.

#### Interventions

***Providing anticipatory guidance.*** Because of short hospital stays for new mothers together with timing of the usual onset of affective disorders, most incidences of PPD (and postpartum psychosis) occur after the woman has gone home. Anticipatory guidance of the mother and her family is the most critical nursing intervention. Success of treatment is largely affected by early diagnosis. All pregnant and postpartum women should be screened for affective disorders (AWHONN, 2015c). During the prenatal period, initiate a discussion with all new mothers and their partners regarding perinatal mood and anxiety disorders. Explain the signs of disorders and the importance of seeking early help to decrease the length of time the condition lasts.

Discuss the need for frequent contact with other adults so that the mother does not become isolated. Emphasize the importance of continued communication with the partner or a close friend who can provide support when loneliness or anxiety becomes a problem. Explain that adequate rest and nutrition can help the mother maintain energy and a feeling of health and well-being. Teach mothers and their support persons the signs of PPD and other peripartum psychological disorders, including when they should seek help.

***Demonstrating caring.*** Conveying a caring attitude is an important nursing strategy to help mothers decrease their emotional distress and guide them in regaining their well-being during the postpartum period. Acknowledge that something is wrong and that the woman seems depressed. Spend time with her and reassure her that the condition is not her fault. It is an illness that can be treated, and it will end.

## EVIDENCE-BASED PRACTICE

Post Partum Depression (PPD) is a common disorder that causes significant functional impairment and increases risk of poor mother-infant bonding and delays in infant development. Kayton et al studied 3039 women receiving prenatal care and delivering at the University of Washington. Of these women 1515 were excluded due to lack of post partum assessment. The participants of this study were screened at four months or eight months of pregnancy (or both) and then again at six weeks post partum.

This study found that younger age, unemployment, antenatal depressive symptoms, taking anti depressants, psychosocial stressors, prepregnancy chronic physical illnesses (diabetes, and neurologic conditions), and smoking were independent predictors of development of PPD.

With knowledge of risk factors for PPD, what can the maternity do to initiate dialogue with new mothers and their families about post partum mood disorders? What screening tools are appropriate for use prior to discharge from the facility? What should be included in discharge teaching about PPD. What resources are available?

Katon, W., Ruso, J., & Gavin, A. (2014). Predictors of Postpartum Depression, *Journal of Women's Health* (15409996), 23(9), 753-759 7p.

Explain to the woman that what she is feeling is a common experience after childbirth. Encourage her to talk about her feelings and reassure her that help is available for her.

***Helping the mother verbalize feelings.*** Because women are expected to be happy after giving birth, many women do not discuss their negative feelings with others. They may feel ashamed and believe there is a social stigma to admitting to depression at any time and especially after giving birth. They may fear that their infants will be taken away from them if they disclose their problem. If they do discuss their feelings, their friends or even healthcare workers may trivialize the problem by making comments such as, "You'll get over it. After all, you have a beautiful baby." Women and their families minimize depression because they cannot identify the exact cause.

Recommend that although some of her feelings may seem "unreasonable" (anger, guilt, shame), the woman should acknowledge negative feelings to herself and insist that others recognize them too. Discuss the realities of parenting and the fact that it is often exhausting. It may be helpful to rehearse some of the situations that can occur, such as a fussy baby or being home alone and feeling lonely, as a means to develop perspective and to find solutions before the situation arises.

***Increasing sensitivity to infant cues.*** Point out infant cues and explain their meaning. Model behavior to show the mother how to respond to the infant's cues. Suggest measures that may increase her sensitivity to cues. Kangaroo care (skin-to-skin) can also help increase attachment and may help the woman feel better about herself and her ability to care for the infant. Measures to help the mother relax can help improve her mood and her response to her infant.

Assess the infant's growth and development. Depressed mothers may not give the care and nurturing needed. Determine the infant's weight gain or loss and observe the mother's response to the infant's crying. If the mother is breastfeeding, make suggestions to help her continue, as it may increase her feelings of closeness to the infant. If she is taking medication, be sure it is recommended for use during lactation.

***Helping family members.*** Include the father in discussions about depression, before and after the birth. Acknowledge his feelings as well as those of the mother. Stress his role in helping his partner and other family members. Offer practical suggestions of ways he can help manage the changes in their lives. Discuss ways to help, such as arranging for the mother to get more sleep and to eat better, which may help decrease her irritability and anxiety. Explain the impact of PPD on each family member. Emphasize the importance of the mother taking medications as ordered. Discuss signs that the mother is getting worse and when to call the healthcare provider. Because depressed mothers do not interact with their infants well, emphasize the importance of other family members holding and interacting with the infant.

***Discussing options and resources.*** Ask the mother about stressors in her life that may be contributing to her depression. Help her plan ways to reduce common areas of stress. Assist the mother and her partner to identify people who are available to provide support. In addition, provide telephone numbers for local PPD support groups. Internet sources are another place to find help. Examples are Postpartum Support International (http://www.postpartum.net), Depression After Delivery (http://www.depressionafterdelivery.com), and the National Women's Health Information Center (http://www.womenshealth.gov).

### Evaluation

- Can the mother verbalize her feelings with others?
- Does she identify personal strengths?
- Can she name community and family resources and describe how she will use them?

## CRITICAL THINKING EXERCISE 28.2

Aricella, a 23-year-old multipara, gave birth 5 days ago to her second baby. It is clear to the nurse making a telephone follow-up call after discharge that Aricella is crying. She says, "I don't know what's wrong with me! I can barely get out of bed in the morning, and I'm worn out just trying to take care of the kids." The nurse responds, "Oh, that's just the 'baby blues.' Just look at that beautiful baby and you'll feel better."

1. What assumptions has the nurse made?
2. Is the nurse's response helpful for Aricella? Why or why not?
3. What would be a more therapeutic response?
4. What additional action should the nurse take?

## KEY CONCEPTS

- Postpartum hemorrhage can sometimes be prevented by careful examination of factors that predispose to excessive bleeding.
- Overstretching of the muscle fibers during pregnancy and repeated stretching during past pregnancies predispose to uterine atony and excessive uterine bleeding.
- Initial management of uterine atony focuses on measures to contract the uterus and provide fluid replacement.
- Soft tissue trauma (lacerations, hematomas) can cause rapid loss of blood even when the uterus is firmly contracted. Management involves repairing the trauma before excessive blood loss occurs.
- Compensatory mechanisms maintain the blood pressure so that vital organs receive adequate oxygen. When these mechanisms fail, hypovolemic shock follows.

## KEY CONCEPTS—cont'd

- The process of uterine involution may be delayed (subinvolution) when placental fragments are retained or when the uterus is infected.
- Subinvolution of the uterus develops after the mother goes home. The nurse teaches the family the process of normal involution and the signs and symptoms that should be reported to the healthcare provider.
- Venous stasis that occurs during pregnancy, increased levels of coagulation factors, and decreased levels of thrombolytic factors that persist into the postpartum period increase the risk of thrombus formation during the puerperium.
- Treatment for deep venous thrombosis includes anticoagulants, analgesics, and bed rest with the affected leg elevated.
- Nurses who administer anticoagulant therapy assess the mother to determine whether her laboratory tests are within the recommended therapeutic range so that overmedication with anticoagulants does not result in unexpected bleeding.
- Pulmonary embolism occurs when a clot is dislodged from the vein, or amniotic fluid debris is carried by the blood to a pulmonary vessel, which may be completely or partially occluded.
- The risk of infection is increased with childbearing because there is open access to bacteria from the vagina through the fallopian tubes and into the peritoneal cavity. Increased blood supply to the pelvis and the alkalinization of the vagina by the amniotic fluid further increase the risk of infection.
- Any break in the skin or mucous membranes during childbirth provides a portal of entry for pathogenic organisms and increases the risk of puerperal infection. Nurses should assess women with an incision or laceration for signs of localized wound infections.
- Urinary stasis and trauma to the urinary tract increase the risk of urinary tract infection. Nurses should initiate measures to prevent urinary stasis.
- Nurses should provide information about the importance of completely emptying the breasts at each feeding and about measures to avoid nipple trauma to prevent mastitis.
- Mood disorders include postpartum blues, postpartum depression, and postpartum psychosis.
- Postpartum depression is a disabling affective disorder that affects the entire family. Nurses help the woman acknowledge her feelings and assist her in identifying measures that will help her cope with the condition.
- Anxiety disorders include panic disorder, postpartum obsessive compulsive disorder, and posttraumatic stress disorder.

## REFERENCES AND READINGS


Abdul-Kadir, R., McLintock, C., Ducloy, A., et al. (2014). Evaluation and management of postpartum hemorrhage: consensus from an international expert panel. *Transfusion, 54*, 1756–1768.

Adair, F.L. (1935). The American Committee of Maternal Welfare, Inc: Chairman's Address. *American Journal of Obstetrics and Gynecology, 30*(6):868–871.

Agnafors, S., Sydsjö, G., deKeyser, L., et al. (2013). Symptoms of Depression Postpartum and 12 years Later-Associations to Child Mental Health at 12 years of Age. *Maternal & Child Health Journal, 17*(3), 405–414 10p. doi:10.1007/s10995-012-0985-z.

Ambrose, A., & Repke, J. (2011). Puerperal problems. In D.K. James, P.J. Steer, C.P. Weiner, et al. (Eds.), *High risk pregnancy: Management options* (4th ed., pp. 1313–1329). Philadelphia: Saunders.

American College of Obstetricians and Gynecologists. (2011). Practice bulletin no. 123: Thromboembolism in pregnancy. *Obstetrics and Gynecology, 118*(3), 718–729.

American College of Obstetricians and Gynecologists. (2014). *Obstetric data definitions (version 1.0)*. Retrieved from http://www.acog.org/-/media/Departments/Patient-Safety-and-Quality-Improvement/2014reVITALizeObstetricDataDefinitionsV10.pdf.

American College of Obstetricians and Gynecologists (2015). *Postpartum hemorrhage. Practice Bulletin No. 76, October 2006, Reaffirmed 2015.* Retrieved from http://www.acog.org/-/media/Practice-Bulletins/Committee-on-Practice-Bulletins----Obstetrics/Public/pb076.pdf?dmc=1&ts=20160227T1325017755.

American Psychiatric Association. (2013). *Diagnostic and Statistical Manual of Mental Disorders.* 5th ed. DSM-5. Arlington, VA. Author.

Association of Women's Health, Obstetric and Neonatal Nurses. (2015a). Quantification of Blood Loss: AWHONN Practice Brief Number 1. *JOGNN: Journal of Obstetric, Gynecologic & Neonatal Nursing, 44*(1), 158-160. doi: 10.1111/1552-6909.12519.

Association of Women's Health, Obstetric and Neonatal Nurses. (2015b). Guidelines for Oxytocin Administration after Birth: AWHONN Practice Brief Number 2. *JOGNN: Journal of Obstetric, Gynecologic & Neonatal Nursing, 44*(1), 161-163 3p. doi:10.1111/1552–6909.12528.

Association of Women's Health, Obstetric and Neonatal Nurses. (2015c). AWHONN Position Statement. Mood and Anxiety Disorders in Pregnant and Postpartum Women. *JOGNN, 44*(5), 687–689. doi: 10.1111/1552-6909.12734

Beck, C.T. (2014). *Postpartum mood and anxiety disorders: Case studies, research, and nursing care,* 3rd ed. Washington, DC: Association of Women's Health, Obstetric, and Neonatal Nurses.

Beck, C.T., & Gable, R.K. (2002). *Postpartum depression screening scale manual.* Los Angeles, CA: Western Psychological Services.

Beck, C.T., Records, K., & Rice, M. (2006). Further development of the postpartum depression predictors inventory—Revised. *JOGNN: Journal of Obstetric, Gynecologic & Neonatal Nursing, 35*(6), 735–745.

Bhati, S., & Richards, K. (2015). A Systematic Review of the Relationship Between Postpartum Sleep Disturbance and Postpartum Depression. *JOGNN: Journal of Obstetric, Gynecologic & Neonatal Nursing, 44*(3), 350-357 8p. doi:10.1111/1552-6909.12562

Blackburn, S.T. (2013). *Maternal, fetal, and neonatal physiology: A clinical perspective* (4th ed.). St. Louis: Saunders.

Blomberg, M. (2011). Maternal obesity and risk of postpartum hemorrhage. *Obstetrics and Gynecology, 118*(3), 561–568.

California Maternal Quality Care Collaborative. (2015). *Obstetric hemorrhage toolkit version 2.0. Stanford, CA: California Department of Public Health.* Retrieved from http://www.cmqcc.org/ob_hemorrhage

Callaghan, W.M., Creanga, A.A., Kuklina, E.V. (2012). Severe Maternal Morbidity among delivery and postpartum hospitalizations in the United States. *Obstetrics& Gynecology, 120*(5), 1029–1036.

Cekmez, Y., Ozkaya, E., Ocal, F., et al. (2015). Experience with different techniques for the management of postpartum hemorrhage due to uterine atony: compression sutures, artery ligation and Bakri balloon. *Irish Journal of Medical Science [serial online]. 184*(2):399–402. Available from: MEDLINE, Ipswich, MA.

Council on Patient Safety in Women' Health (2015). *Obstetric Hemorrhage Bundle.* Retrieved from http://www.safehealthcareforeverywoman.org/national-partnership.php.

Cox, J.L., Holden, J.M., & Sagovsky, R. (1987). Detection of postnatal depression. Development of the 10-item Edinburgh Postnatal Depression Scale. *British Journal of Psychiatry, 150*, 782–786.

Creanga, A.A., Berg, C.J., Syverson, C., et al. (2015). Pregnancy-Related Mortality in the United States, 2006-2010. *Obstetrics & Gynecology, 125*(1), 5–12.

Cunningham, F.G., Leveno, K.J., Bloom, S.L., et al. (Eds.), (2014). *Williams Obstetrics* (24th ed.). New York: McGraw-Hill.

Debost-Legrand, A., Riviere, O., Dossou, M., et al. (2015). Risk Factors for Severe Secondary Postpartum Hemorrhages: A Historical Cohort Study, *Birth (Berkeley, Calif.), 42*(3), 235–241. doi: 10.1111/birt.12175.

Dickinson, J.E. (2011). Cesarean section. In D.K. James, P.J. Steer, C.P. Weiner, et al. (Eds.), *High risk pregnancy: Management options* (4th ed., pp. 1269–1280). Philadelphia: Saunders.

Doussou, M., Debost-Legrand, A., Dechelotte, P., et al. (2015). Severe secondary postpartum hemorrhage: a historical cohort. *Birth (Berkeley, Calif.), 42*(2), 149-155. doi: 10.1111/birt.12164.

Duff, P. (2014). Maternal and fetal infections. In R.K. Creasy, R. Resnik, J.D. Iams, et al. (Eds.), *Creasy & Resnik's maternal-fetal medicine: Principles and practice* (7th ed., pp. 802–851). Philadelphia: Saunders.

Farquharson, R.G., & Greaves, M. (2011). Thromboembolic disease. In D.K. James, P.J. Steer, C.P. Weiner, et al. (Eds.), *High risk pregnancy: Management options* (4th ed., pp. 753–762). Philadelphia: Saunders.

Giallo, R., Gartland, D., Woolhouse, H., et al. (2015). Differentiating maternal fatigue and depressive symptoms and six months and four years post partum: Considerations for assessment, diagnosis and intervention. *Midwifery, 31*, 316–322.

Kendall, R.E., Chalmers, J.C., & Platz, C. (1987). Epidemiology of puerperal psychoses. *The British Journal of Psychiatry: The Journal OF Mental Science, 150*: 662–673.

Lawrence, R.A., & Lawrence, R.M. (2016). *Breastfeeding: A guide for the medical profession* (8th ed.). Philadelphia: Mosby.

Leung, A.N., & Lockwood, C.J. (2014). Thromboembolic disease in pregnancy. In R.K. Creasy, R. Resnik, J.D. Iams, C.J. Lockwood, T.R., Moore & M.F. Greene (Eds.), *Creasy & Resnik's maternal-fetal medicine: Principles and practice* (7th ed., pp. 906–917). Philadelphia: Saunders.

Mackeen, A.D., Packard, R.E., Ota, E., et al. (2015). Antibiotic regimens for postpartum endometritis. *The Cochrane Database of Systemic Reviews*, 2CD001067. doi: 10.1002/14651858.CD001067.pub3.

Main, E.K., Goffman, D., Scavone, B.M., et al. (2015). National Partnership for Maternal Safety: Consensus Bundle on Obstetric Hemorrhage. *Obstetrics and Gynecology, 126*(1), 155–162. doi: 10.1097/AOG.0000000000000869.

Martin, E., Legendre, G., Bouet, P., et al. (2015). Maternal outcomes after uterine balloon tamponade for postpartum hemorrhage. *Acta Obstetricia Et Gynecologica Scandinavica, 94*(4), 399–404. doi: 10.1111/aogs.12591.

Negron, R., Martin, A., Almog, M., et al. (2013). Social support during the postpartum period: Mothers' views on needs, expectations, and mobilization of support. *Maternal Child Health Journal, 17*, 616–623. doi: 10.1007/s10995-02-1037-4.

Newland, R.P., & Parade, S.H. (2016). Screening and treatment of postpartum depression: Impact on children and families. *Brown University Child & Adolescent Behavior Letter, 32*(1), 1–6 3p. doi:10.1002/cbl.30092.

O'Hara, M.W., Wisner, K.L., Asher, N., et al. (2014). Perinatal mental illness: Definition, description and aetiology. *Best Practice & Research, Clinical Obstetrics & Gynaecology, 28*(1), 3–12. doi: 10.1016/i.bpobgyn.2013.09.002.

Pettker, C.M., & Lockwood, C.J. (2012). Thromboembolic disorders. In S.G. Gabbe, J.R. Niebyl, J.L., Simpson, M.B. Landon, H.L. Galan, E.R.M. Jauniaux, & D.A. Drisdoll (Eds.), *Obstetrics: Normal and problem pregnancies* (6th ed., pp 980–993). Philadelphia: Elsevier.

Rhode, M.A. (2016). Postpartum complications. In S. Mattson, & J.E. Smith (Eds.), *Core curriculum for maternal-newborn nursing* (5th ed., pp. 645-661). St. Louis: Elsevier.

Robbins, K.S., Martin, S.R., & Wilson, W.C. (2014). Intensive care considerations for the critically ill parturient. In R.K. Creasy, R. Resnik, J.D. Iams, et al. (Eds.), *Creasy & Resnik's maternal-fetal medicine: Principles and practice* (7th ed., pp. 1182–1211). St. Louis: Elsevier.

Stadtlander, L. (2015). Paternal Postpartum Depression. *International Journal of Childbirth Education, 30*(2), 11–13.

Stuart-Parrigon, K., & Stuart, S. (2014). Perinatal Depression: An update and overview. *Current Psychiatry Reports, 16*, 468–476. doi: 10.1007/s11920-014-0468-6

Swanson, L.M., Pickett, S.M., Flynn, H., et al. (2011). Relationships among depression, anxiety, and insomnia symptoms in perinatal women seeking mental health treatment. *Journal of Women's Health, 20*(4), 553–558.

Whitmer, T. (2016). Physical and psychologic changes after birth. In S. Mattson, & J.E. Smith (Eds.), *Core curriculum for maternal-newborn nursing* (5th ed., pp. 297–313). St. Louis: Elsevier.

Woolhouse, H., Gartland, D., Perlen, S., et al. (2014). Physical health after childbirth and maternal depression the first 12 months post partum: Results of an Australian nulliparous pregnancy cohort study. *Midwifery, 30*, 378–384.

29

# The High-Risk Newborn: Problems Related to Gestational Age and Development

http://evolve.elsevier.com/McKinney/mat-ch/

## LEARNING OBJECTIVES

*After studying this chapter, you should be able to:*

- Describe the implications of late preterm birth.
- Explain the special problems of the preterm infant. Flourish
- Identify common nursing diagnoses for preterm infants and explain the nursing care for each.
- Explain the complications that may result from premature birth.
- Describe the characteristics and problems of the infant with postmaturity syndrome.
- Explain the effects of fetal growth restriction.
- Compare the problems of the large-for-gestational-age infant with those of the small-for-gestational-age infant.

Maternity nurses identify and begin care for the immediate needs of neonates with gestational complications until neonatal intensive care unit (NICU) nurses assume care. Nurses from both areas also provide information and emotional care for parents. Neonatal intensive care is a nursing specialty that requires additional education and experience to prepare for this role.

## CARE OF HIGH-RISK NEWBORNS

Nurses care for minor illness in the mother-baby unit or the normal newborn nursery, but more serious problems require care in NICUs, nurseries designed for that purpose (Fig. 29.1). Approximately 9% of all newborns are sick enough at birth to require special or intensive care (Carlo & Amalavanan, 2015).

## LATE PRETERM INFANTS

Infants born between 34-0/7 and 36-6/7 weeks of gestation are called **late preterm infants** (LPIs) because they have many needs that are similar to those of **preterm infants**. In the past, LPIs often received care similar to full-term infants because they are more stable than infants of lower gestational age. However, they are physiologically and metabolically immature and have higher mortality and morbidity rates than full-term infants (Phillips et al., 2013).

### Incidence and Etiology

Late preterm births accounted for 8.66% of all births in 2009 and more than 70% of all preterm births. Contributing factors in late preterm birth include difficulty in accurately estimating gestational age before delivery, multifetal pregnancies, obesity, assisted reproductive technology, elective and medically indicated inductions and cesarean deliveries, advanced maternal age, and all the causes of preterm birth.

### Characteristics of Late Preterm Infants

Because LPIs often look like full-term infants, they may not be recognized as being preterm. They are at risk for respiratory disorders, problems with temperature maintenance, hypoglycemia, hyperbilirubinemia, feeding difficulties, acidosis, and sepsis because of their immaturity. They are also at risk for long-term neurodevelopmental disorders as well as cognitive and behavioral problems. They are more likely to be admitted to the NICU after birth and are at increased risk for rehospitalization after discharge.

### Therapeutic Management

Therapeutic management varies according to the problems presented. Many interventions are similar to those for preterm infants discussed in this chapter.

### Nursing Considerations

#### Assessment and Care of Common Problems

LPIs need closer monitoring for complications during the hospital stay than do full-term infants. Nursing care is similar to that for preterm infants in many aspects.

***Thermoregulation.*** Once stable, normal newborns usually have their temperature checked only once per shift. To prevent unrecognized cold stress, the temperature of the LPI should be checked every 3 to 4 hours, depending on need and agency policy. **Kangaroo care (KC)**, (a method of providing skin-to-skin contact between infants and their parents [see p. 632]), a radiant warmer, or an incubator may be used if the infant cannot maintain normal temperature (Boundy, Dastjerdi, Spiegelman, et al., 2016; Hardy, 2011b).

***Feedings.*** LPIs can have immature suck and swallow reflexes, shorter awake periods, and fall asleep during feedings before they have fed adequately, or they may sleep through feedings (Cleveland, 2010). They may have difficulty with latch when breastfeeding. Their low tone and weak suck can limit the amount of milk they obtain. They have an increased caloric need and should be fed every 2 to 3 hours.

Feeding problems are common, and nurses should assess feeding sessions to ensure swallowing is occurring. Urine and stool output are monitored as indications of adequate intake. Breastfeeding mothers need special help to ensure infants are feeding well. Because LPIs are at greater risk for breastfeeding-associated rehospitalization than term infants, lactation consultants should be involved in their care. Use of the football and cross-cradle holds is helpful in positioning these

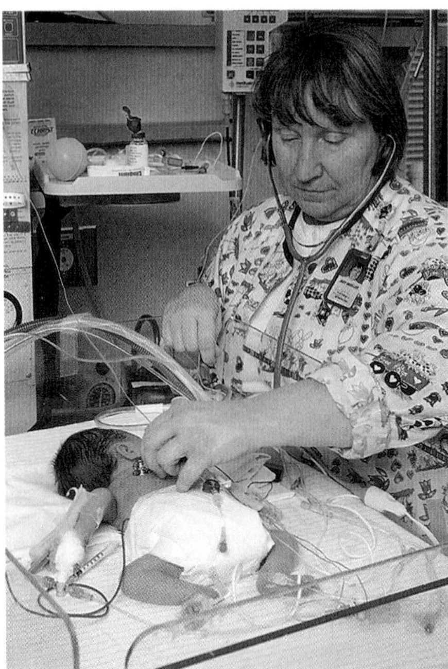

**FIG 29.1** The infant in a neonatal intensive care unit (NICU) is cared for by nurses with highly specialized skills.

infants at the breast. Breastfeeding should be evaluated at least twice daily. Supplemental feedings by bottle, gavage, or use of a supplemental nursing system may be necessary.

LPIs are at risk for hypoglycemia. Therefore, blood glucose level measurements should be performed according to hospital protocol, especially during the first 24 hours.

***Discharge.*** In addition to the usual discharge criteria for term infants, other considerations apply for the LPI. Infants should not be discharged before 48 hours of age. Nurses should ensure that infants have fed successfully and have had normal vital signs for at least 24 hours before discharge. Bilirubin levels should also be assessed before discharge.

Parents should be taught signs of common complications such as jaundice or dehydration and what to do if they occur. A follow-up visit with the healthcare provider should be arranged for 24 to 72 hours after discharge.

Teaching should include the need for keeping the infant warm. The infant should be kept away from drafts and dressed with one more layer than an adult would wear. A car seat challenge should be conducted before discharge to ensure the infant can tolerate sitting in a car seat without bradycardia, apnea, or decreased oxygen saturation.

LPIs are subject to overstimulation. This can occur when parents take the baby home to an environment with many different stimuli. The nurse should teach signs of overstimulation and how to minimize them.

## PRETERM INFANTS

**Preterm infants** (also called *premature infants*) are born before the beginning of the 38th week of gestation. The word *preterm* is sometimes confused with the term **low birth weight** (LBW), which refers to infants weighing 2500 g (5 lb, 8 oz) or less at birth. **Very-low-birth-weight** (VLBW) infants weigh 1500 g (3 lb, 5 oz) or less at birth. **Extremely low-birth-weight** (ELBW) infants weigh 1000 g (2 lb, 3 oz) or less at birth. Although most of these infants are preterm, others are full term and have failed to grow normally while in the uterus, a condition called fetal growth restriction (FGR).

### Incidence and Etiology

#### Scope of the Problem

Advances in technology have resulted in infant survival at much lower birth weights than ever. Although the incidence of preterm births was increasing, the rate in 2009 decreased for the third year in a row to 12.18% of all births. A *Healthy People 2020* goal is to reduce preterm births to not more than 11.4% of live births (U.S. Department of Health and Human Services, 2010). Disorders related to short gestation and low birth weight are the second leading cause of infant mortality, surpassed only by those from congenital anomalies.

#### Causes

The exact causes of preterm birth are not known, but all risk factors in pregnancy are potential causes (see Chapters 13 and 27).

#### Prevention

Preventing preterm birth is best accomplished by providing adequate prenatal care for every pregnant woman to identify and treat risk factors as early as possible. Teaching women to recognize signs of preterm labor will help them seek care early enough that stopping labor is still a possibility (see Chapter 27).

### Characteristics of Preterm Infants

Preterm infant characteristics vary by gestational age. For example, the appearance and problems of infants born at 33 weeks of gestation are different from those of infants born at 26 weeks of gestation. However, some characteristics are common to all preterm infants.

#### Appearance

Preterm infants often appear frail and weak, and they have less developed flexor muscles and muscle tone compared to full-term infants. Their extremities are limp, and infants typically lie in an extended position (see Fig. 21.24). The infant's head appears large in comparison with the rest of the body.

Preterm infants lack subcutaneous or white fat, which makes their thin skin appear red and translucent, with blood vessels clearly visible. The nipples and areola may be barely perceptible, but vernix caseosa and lanugo may be abundant. Plantar creases are absent in infants of less than 32 weeks of gestation (see Fig. 21.30).

The pinna of the ear is soft, flat, and contains little cartilage (see Fig. 21.32). In the female infant, the clitoris and labia minora appear large and are not covered by the small, separated labia majora. The male infant may have undescended testes, with a small, smooth scrotal sac (see Figs. 21.33 and 21.34).

#### Behavior

Behavior varies according to gestational age. In general, preterm infants have little excess energy for maintaining muscle tone. They are easily exhausted from noise and routine activities. Their responses are varied, including lowered oxygenation levels and stress-related behavior changes. The cry may be feeble.

### Assessment and Care of Common Problems

Preterm infants are prone to problems that affect all systems and body processes.

### Problems With Respiration

Problems of the respiratory system are a major concern because preterm newborns have immature lungs. The presence of surfactant in adequate amounts is of primary importance. Surfactant reduces surface tension in the alveoli and prevents their collapse with expiration. It allows the lungs to inflate with lower negative pressure, decreasing the work of breathing. Infants born before surfactant production is adequate develop respiratory distress syndrome (RDS) (see p. 634). In addition, preterm infants have a poorly developed cough reflex and narrow respiratory passages, which increase the risk of respiratory difficulty.

***Assessment.*** The infant's respiratory status must be observed constantly. The lungs are assessed for adventitious breath sounds or areas of absent breath sounds.

The nurse differentiates periodic breathing from apneic spells. Periodic breathing is the cessation of breathing for 5 to 10 seconds without other changes. It may be followed by rapid respirations for 10 to 15 seconds. Apneic spells are a lack of breathing lasting more than 20 seconds or accompanied by cyanosis, pallor, bradycardia, or hypotonia (Goodwin, 2010). Apneic spells are common in preterm infants, increasing in incidence with lower gestational age. Apnea without an identified cause in a preterm infant is called *idiopathic apnea* or *apnea of prematurity* and generally improves as the infant matures. The infant may require gentle tactile stimulation, medications, or continuous positive airway pressure (CPAP).

The nurse observes the effort required for breathing and the location and severity of retractions. Retractions are particularly noticeable in preterm infants, whose weak chest wall is drawn in with each inspiration. The excessive compliance (elasticity) of the chest cage during retractions can interfere with full expansion of the lungs.

Grunting may be an early sign of RDS. It closes the glottis and increases the pressure within the alveoli, keeping the alveoli partially open during expiration and increasing the amount of oxygen absorbed.

***Nursing interventions.*** Interventions focus on collaborating with other team members, such as the respiratory therapist, to manage technical equipment and facilitate removal of secretions.

**Working with respiratory equipment.** An oxygen hood is often used for infants who can breathe alone but need extra oxygen. The hood is a plastic dome that fits over the infant's head or head and upper body. The infant breathes the higher levels of oxygen within the hood, and the device does not interfere with access to the rest of the infant's body for care (Fig. 29.2).

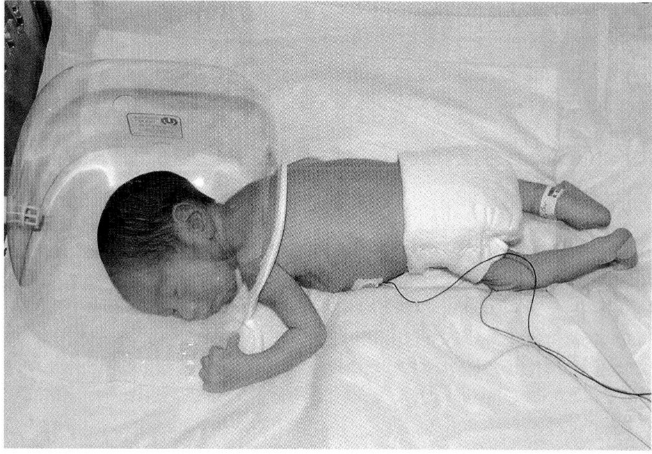

FIG 29.2 The oxygen hood is one way of delivering oxygen to an infant who can breathe unassisted. (Courtesy Cheryl Briggs, RNC, Annapolis, MD.)

Oxygen also can be given by nasal cannula to the infant who breathes well alone. After discharge, many preterm infants continue to receive oxygen via nasal cannula at home. Oxygen must be humidified to prevent insensible water loss and drying of the delicate mucous membranes. It is warmed to maintain body temperature.

CPAP may be necessary to keep the alveoli open and improve expansion of the lungs. It can be delivered with nasal prongs, a mask, or an endotracheal tube. The infant may need conventional mechanical ventilation when respiratory failure, severe apnea or bradycardia, or other conditions are present. High-frequency ventilation can be used to provide very fast, frequent respirations with less pressure and volume, which helps decrease lung injury from pressure (barotrauma) and volume (volutrauma).

When oxygen is administered, it should be warmed and humidified. Because both too little and too much oxygen can cause problems, the level of oxygen in the infant's blood must be monitored. Arterial blood is drawn for testing oxygen levels. Pulse oximetry is also used. It is less invasive than blood testing and provides continuous information about oxygen partial pressure ($Po_2$) levels through sensors attached to the skin. Nurses and respiratory therapists titrate oxygen based on the pulse oximetry or arterial oxygen levels according to agency policy.

The nurse must observe the infant's increasing or decreasing dependence on breathing assistance and need for oxygen. Handling, feeding, and linen changes can increase oxygen need. Changes in settings on equipment may be needed during such activities.

**Positioning the infant.** The side-lying and prone positions facilitate drainage of respiratory secretions and regurgitated feedings. These positions are not recommended for normal newborn infants because they are associated with an increased incidence of sudden infant death syndrome (SIDS). However, in the preterm infant, the prone position increases oxygenation and enhances respiratory control, improves lung mechanics and volume, and reduces energy expenditure.

Supine positioning for sleep is begun when the infant can tolerate it and before discharge so the infant can become accustomed to sleeping on the back before going home. Before discharge, parents should be taught the importance of the supine position for sleep to prevent SIDS. It is important for nurses to model SIDS prevention by placing infants in the supine position as soon as they are able; parents are more likely to position infants as they saw them positioned in the hospital.

**Suctioning secretions.** The nurse checks suction equipment at the beginning of each shift to ensure it is available and functioning properly at all times. The infant is suctioned only as necessary when the need becomes apparent. Suction should be gentle to avoid traumatizing the delicate mucous membranes. Trauma could cause edema, decreasing the size of the air passages and leading to more respiratory difficulty.

Suctioning also provides an entry for organisms and decreases oxygenation during the procedure. The procedure causes changes in heart rate, blood pressure, and cerebral blood flow. Suction should be applied for only 5 to 10 seconds at a time, and increased oxygen should be provided before and after each suction attempt. The mouth is suctioned before the nose because stimulation of the nares causes reflex inspiration that could cause aspiration of fluids in the infant's mouth. Rest periods should be provided after suctioning.

**Maintaining hydration.** Adequate hydration is essential to keep secretions thin so that they can be removed by drainage or suction. If infants become dehydrated, secretions will become thick and viscous and could obstruct tiny air passages. Fluid intake should be increased, as ordered by the physician, if secretions seem to indicate minimal dehydration.

### Problems With Thermoregulation

Although heat loss can be a problem for full-term infants, it is even more significant for preterm infants. They have thin skin with blood vessels near the surface and little subcutaneous (white) fat for insulation. Less brown fat is present for nonshivering thermogenesis. Preterm infants' body surface area in proportion to their body mass is five times that of adults (Blackburn, 2013). Their extended extremities increase exposure to the air for heat loss. The temperature control center of the brain of preterm infants is less mature and may be further impaired by asphyxia. These conditions all contribute to heat loss.

Complications of heat loss are more likely in the preterm infant than in the full-term infant. They include hypoglycemia, metabolic acidosis, pulmonary vasoconstriction, impaired surfactant production, and hyperbilirubinemia. In addition, calories used for heat production are unavailable for growth and weight gain.

*Assessment.* The infant's temperature is monitored continuously by a skin probe on the infant's abdomen, which is attached to the heat control mechanism of the radiant warmer or incubator. The abdominal skin temperature is usually maintained at 36° C to 36.5° C (96.8° F to 97.7° F). The infant's temperature should be recorded every 30 to 60 minutes initially and every 1 to 3 hours when the infant is stable. The axillary temperature should be compared with the heat control reading to ensure that the equipment is functioning properly.

The axillary temperature for a preterm infant should remain between 36.3° C and 36.9° C (97.3° F and 98.4° F), slightly lower than the temperature of a full-term infant (Brown & Landers, 2011). If the infant has accumulated brown fat, an axillary temperature reading may be misleading. A normal axillary temperature when the skin temperature is decreased can indicate that heat from brown fat in the axillary space is being used to maintain the infant's core temperature.

Indications of inadequate thermoregulation include poor feeding or intolerance to feedings in an infant who previously had little difficulty, lethargy, irritability, poor muscle tone, cool skin temperature, and mottled skin (Fig. 29.3). Hypoglycemia and respiratory distress may be the first signs that the infant's temperature is low. Because temperature instability may be an early sign of infection, the nurse should assess for other evidence of infection.

**SAFETY ALERT**

***Signs of Inadequate Thermoregulation***

- Axillary temperature <36.3° C to >36.9° C (<97.3° F to >98.4° F)
- Abdominal skin temperature <36° C to >36.5° C (<96.8° F to >97.7° F)
- Poor feeding or feeding intolerance
- Irritability followed by lethargy
- Weak cry or suck
- Decreased muscle tone
- Skin pale, cool to touch, mottled or acrocyanotic
- Hypoglycemia
- Respiratory distress
- Poor weight gain if chronic

*Nursing interventions.* Maintenance of heat in preterm infants involves the same basic nursing care principles as for the full-term infant (see Chapter 22). However, these principles must be adapted to meet the needs of the preterm infant (Premji, Young, Rogers, et al., 2012).

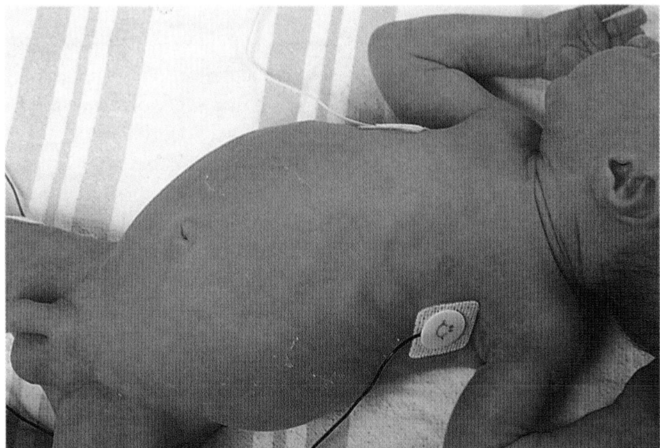

**FIG 29.3** This preterm infant has mildly mottled skin and slight abdominal distention and retractions.

**Maintaining a neutral thermal environment.** A neutral thermal environment is especially important to prevent the need for increased oxygen to maintain body temperature. The delivery room should be warm to decrease heat loss at birth. Immediately after birth, the infant is dried and placed on the mother's abdomen or a prewarmed radiant warmer for care. Infants less than 29 weeks of gestation should be placed in a polyethylene bag or wrap that covers the body from the shoulders down before the infant is dried. This prevents heat loss by evaporation during initial care and transfer to the NICU and is used until the infant is stabilized. It also decreases insensible water loss.

Because they produce heat less effectively and lose more heat than larger or older infants, smaller, less mature infants need more warmth to maintain body heat. Radiant warmers or incubators are used until infants can maintain normal body temperature alone. Some devices convert from a radiant warmer to an incubator and back again to eliminate the need to move the infant from one device to another.

Infants needing many procedures are usually placed under an open radiant warmer to make it easier to see them and work with equipment. However, air currents around an unclothed infant can cause heat loss by convection despite the heat generated by the warmer. Doors near the warmer should be closed and traffic kept to a minimum to decrease convective heat loss. The infant should receive only warmed oxygen, because thermal receptors in the face are very sensitive to cold. Cold oxygen could quickly lead to cold stress.

Equipment or caregivers should not come between the infant and the heat source, thus preventing heat from reaching the infant. A transparent plastic blanket over the infant allows heat from the warmer to pass across to the infant and decreases exposure to drafts and insensible water loss while maintaining visibility of the infant's body.

Incubators are used for infants who do not need to be under radiant warmers. They have double walls to minimize radiant heat loss to the cooler outer walls. Warmed air circulating inside the incubator provides heat. Humidity may be added to decrease evaporative heat loss and insensible water loss, especially in very preterm infants. Incubators should be placed away from air conditioning ducts or windows that could affect the temperature.

When infants are in incubators, nurses should keep portholes and doors closed as much as possible. A significant amount of heat is lost every time the incubator is opened, and it takes time to build up again. When removed from the incubator for procedures or holding, the infant should be wrapped in heated blankets and a hat applied. The incubator doors should be closed while the infant is outside to maintain heat inside.

Although temperature loss is the most common concern, overheating also is a problem for preterm infants. Overheating can occur when heating devices such as radiant warmers are set too high or a skin probe is accidentally removed. Overheating leads to an increase in the metabolic rate, with increased oxygen and glucose needs, and insensible water losses. Alarms to detect high and low temperature should be turned on at all times.

Temperature regulation in preterm infants is usually provided in incubators until infants can maintain their own temperature, but warmth can also be provided when parents hold them. Adequate temperature is maintained in stable infants during KC.

**Weaning to an open crib.** Preparation of infants for moving to open cribs should begin early. When stable, infants can wear a shirt, diaper, and hat while in the incubator. Clothing conserves heat and helps infants adjust to a different temperature on the face than the rest of the body. Infants who weigh approximately 1500 g (3 lb, 5 oz), have a consistent weight gain for 5 days, have no medical complications, and are tolerating **enteral feedings** (feedings into the gastrointestinal tract orally or by feeding tube) can begin gradual weaning from external heat.

Each NICU has its own protocol for the weaning process. The incubator temperature is usually decreased gradually and increased if the infant's temperature falls below the desired range. If the temperature remains stable, the process can continue.

When the infant is ready for transfer to an open crib, double-wrapping with warm blankets at first helps insulate body heat. The temperature is assessed at gradually increasing intervals until the infant is on a routine schedule. A blanket is added for a low temperature, but if the temperature does not rise to normal, the infant is returned to the incubator. Nurses should observe infants carefully during the first few days after transfer to an open crib.

### Problems With Fluid and Electrolyte Balance

Preterm infants lose fluid very easily. The rapid respiratory rate and use of oxygen increase fluid loss from the lungs. Their thin skin has little protective subcutaneous white fat and is more permeable than the skin of term infants. The large surface area in proportion to body weight and lack of flexion further increase transepidermal water losses. Radiant warmers heighten insensible water losses by 40% to 50% compared with water loss in an incubator. Heat from phototherapy lights causes more fluid loss through the skin.

The ability of the kidneys to concentrate or dilute urine is poor, causing a fragile balance between dehydration and overhydration. The fluid needs of preterm infants vary according to size, gestational age, insensible water loss, and medical needs. Normal urinary output is 2 to 5 mL/kg/hr for preterm infants. After 24 hours of life, output less than 0.5 mL/kg/hr is oliguria (Blackburn, 2013).

Insufficient electrolyte regulation by the kidneys is also a problem. Preterm infants need higher intakes of sodium because the kidneys do not reabsorb it well. However, if they receive too much sodium, they may be unable to increase sodium excretion adequately and are susceptible to sodium overload.

***Assessment.*** Monitoring intake and output of fluids is important in determining fluid balance. The infant's intake and output by all routes are carefully calculated. The measured intake comprises fluids administered parenterally, by feeding tube, and orally, including medications. Output from regurgitation, drainage tubes, stools, and urine should be measured. The nurse must also keep track of the amount of blood taken for laboratory tests because the loss can be substantial.

**Urinary output.** Several methods are used for measuring urinary output. Plastic bags that adhere to the perineum are not suitable for the preterm infant because they can damage the fragile skin. Weighing diapers is less invasive. The weight of dry diapers is subtracted from the weight of wet diapers to determine the weight of urine excreted. One gram is equivalent to 1 mL of urine. Humidification can add moisture to the diaper, and a radiant warmer can cause evaporation of urine from the diaper. When precise measurement is essential, diapers can be fastened instead of placing them open under the infant.

Specific gravity should be checked to determine if urine is more concentrated or dilute than expected. Urine is collected by placing cotton balls at the perineum. The specific gravity should range between 1.002 and 1.01.

**Weight.** Changes in the infant's weight can give an indication of fluid gain or loss, especially if the changes are sudden and greater than would be expected. The undressed infant should be weighed at the same time each day with the same scale. Very small infants are often placed in a bed with a scale so that they are not disturbed for daily weighing. They can be weighed two or three times a day to monitor fluid status more closely.

**Signs of dehydration or overhydration.** The nurse should observe for signs indicating that the infant has received too little or too much fluid. Early signs of dehydration include decreased urine output (less than 2 mL/kg/hr) and increased specific gravity. Weight loss may exceed that expected for the infant's age and general condition. Dry skin or mucous membranes, sunken anterior fontanel, and poor tissue turgor are late signs. Changes in the blood include increased sodium, protein, and hematocrit levels resulting from decreased plasma volume.

Signs of overhydration include increased urine output (more than 5 mL/kg/hr) with a below-normal specific gravity. Edema and weight gain occur from retention of fluids. Bulging fontanels, moist breath sounds, and decreased blood sodium, protein, and hematocrit levels also are present. Complications of excess fluid may include patent ductus arteriosus and congestive heart failure.

**SAFETY ALERT**

***Signs of Fluid Imbalance in the Newborn***

**Dehydration**

- Urine output <2 mL/kg/hr
- Urine specific gravity >1.01
- Weight loss greater than expected
- Dry skin and mucous membranes
- Sunken anterior fontanel
- Poor tissue turgor
- Blood: elevated sodium, protein, and hematocrit levels

**Overhydration**

- Urine output >5 mL/kg/hr
- Urine specific gravity <1.002
- Edema
- Weight gain greater than expected
- Bulging fontanels
- Moist breath sounds
- Difficulty breathing
- Blood: decreased sodium, protein, and hematocrit levels

*Nursing interventions.* The nurse must carefully monitor intravenous (IV) fluids using infusion control devices that administer fluid with a precision of 0.1 mL/hr to help prevent fluid volume overload. IV medications should be diluted in as little fluid as is consistent with safe administration of the drug and should be included when measuring intake. Starting IV lines on infants with poor veins is a lengthy, difficult procedure. Infants must be restrained as necessary to prevent infiltration. Some solutions cause extensive damage if infiltrated as a result of tissue sloughing.

IV sites should be assessed at least every hour for signs of infiltration. Many infants have central venous catheters or umbilical lines, which must be assessed for infection and position changes. Small blood transfusions may be necessary to replace blood drawn for frequent laboratory tests.

### Problems With the Skin

Preterm infants have fragile, permeable, easily damaged skin. They often have endotracheal tubes, IV lines, electrodes, and other equipment that must be maintained in place, but standard adhesive tape can be very damaging to the skin, especially during removal. Preparations used to disinfect the skin before invasive procedures can be harmful to fragile skin and may be absorbed.

*Assessment.* The nurse should frequently assess the condition of the infant's skin and record any changes. The infant's response to products used for cleansing and disinfection should be noted.

*Nursing interventions.* Adhesives should be used as little as possible. Commercial devices are available to secure tubes and catheters. Skin damage can be minimized by backing tape with cotton, waiting more than 24 hours to remove it, and using gauze wraps instead of tape. Pectin or hydrocolloid barriers, transparent semipermeable dressings, hydrogel or silicone-based adhesive products, and barrier films are less traumatic to the skin and can be used to attach devices. Hydrogel and hydrocolloid dressings can be used if skin breakdown or wounds occur. These substances promote moist healing and need no adhesive (Lund & Durand, 2015).

All disinfectants have potential risks when used on neonates. Aqueous chlorhexidine gluconate solutions are commonly used at this time. Povidone-iodine can injure the skin and exert toxic effects on the thyroid in premature infants. All disinfectants should be removed with sterile water or saline. Alcohol should not be used (Lund & Durand, 2011).

Cleansers with a pH of 5.5 to 7 can be used for bathing infants. Infants should not be bathed more often than every other day. Warm water without soap should be used for infants less than 32 weeks of gestational age for the first week after birth. Sterile water is not necessary unless there are concerns about the safety of tap water or there is a break in skin integrity. Stable preterm infants without umbilical IV lines can be immersed in water that covers the shoulders for bathing if there are no contraindications. Emollients can help reduce fissures in dry skin and transepidermal water loss. They are safe to use under radiant warmers and during phototherapy.

Infants and their equipment should be positioned to avoid undue pressure on the skin. Frequent position changes are important but should be based on the infant's ability to tolerate changes.

### Problems With Infection

The incidence of infection in preterm LBW infants is 3 to 10 times greater than that in full-term, normal-birth-weight newborns. Many preterm infants have one or more episodes of sepsis during their hospital stays. Factors contributing to the high rate of infection include exposure to maternal infection, lack of transfer of immunoglobulin G (IgG) from the mother during the third trimester, and immature immune response to infection.

Preterm infants are often exposed to situations that promote infection. They are subject to many invasive procedures such as insertion of IV lines, leading to catheter-related bloodstream infections. A prolonged stay in the hospital increases the likelihood of acquiring an infection from multiple exposures to organisms.

*Assessment.* The nurse should be alert for signs of sepsis at all times (see Chapter 30, p. 648).

*Nursing interventions.* Hand hygiene is the most important factor in preventing nosocomial infections. Nursing care involves scrupulous cleanliness and maintaining the infant's skin integrity. Even the normal flora on the hands of caretakers can cause sepsis. Therefore, parents and staff members should thoroughly wash their hands and arms before handling infants. Exposure to family or staff members who have contagious diseases should be prevented.

Early signs of infections should be identified and reported so that treatment can begin immediately. The nurse carefully notes the infant's response to treatment because some organisms become resistant to antibiotics. Other nursing care for infections is discussed in Chapter 30.

### Problems With Pain

Infants in the NICU undergo many painful procedures each day. Caregivers once thought that newborns, particularly preterm infants, were neurologically too immature to feel pain. It is now recognized that preterm infants do feel pain, and pain stimuli cause physiologic and behavioral changes in infants.

Pain can have numerous untoward effects. For example, increases in intracranial pressure resulting from pain can elevate the risk for intraventricular hemorrhage. Other risks include hypoxia, changes in metabolic rate, and adverse effects on growth and wound healing. Stress and pain in the newborn can alter pain thresholds and cause permanent changes in neural pathways (Blackburn, 2013). The long-term effects of pain in the neonate are not yet fully understood. The American Academy of Pediatrics and the American College of Obstetricians (AAP & ACOG, 2013) recommend that pain be routinely assessed, painful procedures be minimized, and environmental and pharmacologic interventions be used to prevent, reduce, or eliminate pain in neonates.

*Assessment.* The nurse performs pain assessment whenever vital signs are taken. In addition, the nurse must assess the infant's response to painful stimuli and to pharmacologic and nonpharmacologic interventions. Assessment tools are available to evaluate physiologic and behavioral responses to pain in term and preterm infants. One example is the Premature Infant Pain Profile (PIPP), designed for use with term or preterm infants. The tool assesses gestational age and behavior states, heart rate, oxygen saturation, brow bulge, eye squeeze, and nasolabial furrow (lines from the edge of the nose to beyond the corners of the mouth) to assign a pain score.

Physiologic changes are unpredictable and cannot be used alone to assess pain. Behavioral responses must also be assessed (see Nursing Quality Alert: Common Signs of Pain in Infants). Behavioral changes include high-pitched, intense, harsh crying. Infants who are intubated or too weak to cry have a "cry face," a facial expression of crying without the sound of a cry. Less than half of preterm infants experiencing painful stimuli respond with crying. Infants who have been exposed to prolonged or repeated pain may no longer be able to show behavioral changes even though they are experiencing pain. Critically ill or very immature infants may not show the same pain responses as older, less sick infants. Therefore, a lack of response to a painful situation should not be interpreted as an absence of pain. Because parents often spend many hours with their infants, the nurse should involve them in helping to assess their infant's pain.

## ! NURSING QUALITY ALERT

### *Common Signs of Pain in Infants*

- Increased or decreased heart rate and respirations, apnea
- Decreased oxygen saturation
- Increased blood pressure
- High-pitched, intense, harsh cry
- Whimpering, moaning
- "Cry face"
- Eyes squeezed shut
- Grimacing
- Bulging or furrowing of the brow
- Tense, rigid muscles or flaccid muscle tone
- Rigidity or flailing of extremities
- Sleep-wake pattern changes

*Nursing interventions.* Nurses should prepare infants for potentially painful procedures by waking them slowly and gently and using containment. **Containment** simulates the enclosed space of the uterus and is comforting to infants. It involves keeping the extremities in a flexed position and midline by swaddling, positioning devices, or the nurse's hands. At least one of the infant's hands should be near the mouth for sucking. Containment is also called facilitated tucking (Fernandes, Campbell-Yeo, & Johnston, 2011). KC and breastfeeding are also used to reduce pain.

The infant should be allowed to rest before and after procedures. The infant is often hypersensitive after a painful stimulus and may perceive other activities as painful. Comfort measures help the infant cope with short-term, mild pain and reduce agitation. They include using a pacifier for nonnutritive sucking. Sucrose placed on the pacifier or given by mouth 2 to 3 minutes before a painful stimulus increases pain relief. However, sucrose may not be appropriate for very young preterm infants. Talking softly, holding, rocking, and prone positioning are other methods of pain relief that can be used alone or with sucrose. Measures should be adapted according to infants' responses. Methods can be combined (e.g., skin-to-skin contact with a sucrose-dipped pacifier).

Comfort measures alone are not enough for moderate to severe pain. The nurse should discuss the infant's pain with the primary care provider to ensure that medications are available when necessary. Opioids such as morphine and fentanyl, can be tolerated by preterm infants. Nonnarcotic analgesics such as acetaminophen can also be used. Topical anesthesia can be used to reduce pain during some procedures. Sedatives are effective for agitation, but they are not effective for pain. Regional or general anesthesia is used during surgery.

The nurse gives ordered medications before painful procedures and when the infant demonstrates signs of pain. The infant's response is assessed frequently to determine the need to increase or decrease the dosage. Analgesics can be given continuously or on an as-needed basis.

## NURSING CARE

### The Preterm Infant

Preterm infants commonly have difficulty with environmental stress and obtaining adequate nutrition. Their parents may have difficulty with bonding.

## EVIDENCE-BASED PRACTICE

Managing pain in the preterm infant is of concern to both nurses and parents. Herrington and Chiodo conducted a study on gentle human touch (GHT) and the reduction of pain responses in patients in the neonatal intensive care unit (NICU). Eleven premature infants were randomly assigned to control and experimental groups. GHT was provided to infants in the experimental group during a heelstick. Infants who did not receive GHT experienced increased heart rate and cry times and decreased respiratory rates. Conversely, the group who received the GHT experienced none of these changes. This study presented evidence that GHT reduces pain in patients in the NICU. GHT is an effective and feasible intervention that bedside nurses can perform to improve patient outcomes.

Herrington, C.J., & Chiodo, L.M. (2014). Human touch effectively and safely reduces pain in the newborn intensive care unit. *Pain Management Nursing, 15*(1), 107–115.

#### Environmentally Caused Stress

Recognition of the effects of environmental factors on the preterm infant has led to the use of developmentally supportive care. Developmental care keeps stressors in the environment to a minimum based on the infant's physiologic and behavioral responses.

In the past, preterm infants were often exposed to bright lights and a noisy environment without understanding their effect on infants. Improvements have been made, but noise continues to be a problem. Although the recommended noise level in NICUs is below 45 decibels, levels range between 38 and 90 decibels or higher. Noise levels tend to be highest during report and caregiver rounds and in areas where staff congregate such as entrances, sinks, and computer areas. The sounds of alarms, ventilators, incubators, doors, and people create a noise level that increases the risk of hearing loss and other complications. In addition, stimulation of any kind can cause increased energy expenditure by the preterm infant. Noise and even routine handling and nursing interventions are often accompanied by changes in heart rate, oxygen saturation levels, and behavior states.

Preterm infants undergo multiple assessments, procedures, and treatments that cause frequent interruptions of sleep and can interfere with the development of normal sleep–wake cycles. Sleep disruption alters neuronal maturation and growth hormone secretion and interferes with growth and development. The energy used to cope with an overstimulating and stressful environment may be unavailable for normal growth and development.

Although touch is generally thought to be comforting to infants, it is often associated with painful events for preterm infants. This association can cause infants to develop touch aversion, a negative response to touch of any kind. They may cry, squirm, and recoil when touched, expecting that touch will lead to pain.

*Assessment.* Assess the amount of noise to which the infant is exposed. Determine how often interruptions occur and how the infant responds to different types of care. Assess the infant's ability to tolerate activity and noise. Overstimulation results in changes in oxygenation and behavior.

*Nursing diagnosis and planning.* A nursing diagnosis appropriate for preterm infants having difficulty enduring the multiple stimuli in their environment is:

- Risk for Disorganized Infant Behavior related to stress from an overstimulating environment.

**Expected outcomes.** The infant will show decreasing signs of overstimulation during routine activity, as evidenced by fewer respiratory and behavioral changes during handling and increased periods of relaxed behavior or sleep.

## SAFETY ALERT

### Signs of Overstimulation in Preterm Infants

**Oxygenation Changes**

- Blood pressure, pulse, and respiratory instability
- Cyanosis, pallor, or mottling
- Flaring nares
- Decreased oxygen saturation levels
- Sneezing, coughing

**Behavior Changes**

- Stiff, extended arms and legs
- Fisting of the hands or splaying (spreading wide apart) of the fingers
- Arching
- Alert, worried expression
- Turning away from eye contact (gaze aversion)
- Regurgitation, gagging, hiccupping
- Yawning
- Fatigue signs

***Interventions.*** Interventions are focused on providing developmentally supportive nursing care that meets the preterm infant's ability to tolerate stimulation.

**Scheduling care.** Schedule periods of undisturbed rest to allow the infant to recover from treatments. Avoid waking the infant during the short, quiet sleep phase. If the infant must be awakened for care, try to wait until the infant is in an active sleep phase and more easily aroused with quiet talking and gentle touch. Arrange routine care to correspond with the infant's awake periods and avoid disturbing rest.

Coordinate diagnostic tests and care given by other healthcare workers to ensure the infant is not stressed. Decrease the frequency of taking vital signs and performing other routine care as soon as possible. Even the handling involved in routine sponge bathing may cause stress in small infants. Routine daily baths are unnecessary and should be avoided. Bathing every fourth day does not lead to increased skin flora or pathogen counts. Bathing should be postponed until infants are physiologically stable.

Arrange group care activities so that several tasks are performed at one time to allow for more rest between care activities. Keep clustered care short and be alert to the infant's signs of stress. Too many activities may be more than the infant can tolerate. Clustered care may not be appropriate for preterms less than 28 weeks of gestational age.

Provide short rest periods within grouped activities or during long or painful procedures. Do not include painful procedures in a cluster of other care activities. Rest is needed before and after painful procedures.

**Reducing stimuli.** Keep noise near the infant as low as possible. Place incubators away from traffic and congestion areas, and avoid talking near the incubator. Use incubator covers to help lower sound inside the incubator. Set alarm volumes on low, and respond quickly when they sound. Open and close incubator portholes and doors and cupboards quietly. Do not place objects on top of the incubator or use it as a writing surface because it increases the noise inside. Teach parents and others to avoid tapping on the incubator. Soft classical music is sometimes used to help promote rest.

Lights that are on 24 hours a day in the nursery may interfere with the development of sleep cycles. Position the incubator so the infant is not facing bright lights, and drape blankets or incubator covers over the back and ends to decrease light as well as noise. Use dimmer switches to vary the intensity of lights as needed. Reduce lighting at night to as low as possible to help promote rest and conserve energy for growth.

Some NICUs have single rooms for each infant. This arrangement reduces noise and allows environmental stimuli to be adapted to each infant's individual needs. It also provides more privacy for visiting family members and can reduce nosocomial infections.

**Promoting rest.** When possible, schedule "quiet times" when lights and noise in the unit are kept to a minimum to promote rest. Only emergency procedures should take place during rest times. Rest periods should be at least an hour long to allow preterm infants to complete a sleep cycle.

Scheduled naps when infants are disturbed as little as possible can help decrease waking and lead to longer uninterrupted sleep. Naps also help the infant begin to differentiate day and night sleeping patterns. Lowering lights at night helps the infant to develop circadian rhythms.

Contain the infant's arms and legs to promote flexion of the joints and reduce energy loss from flailing extremities. Containment is used to promote quieting, enhance physiologic stability, and reduce stress (Gardner & Goldson, 2011). Provide boundaries with rolled blankets or commercial positioning devices placed around the infant.

Stroking and gentle massage may be calming for stable preterm infants. It can help increase weight gain and improve development. It also involves parents in the care of their infant. However, it may not be appropriate for smaller, more fragile infants.

**Promoting motor development.** Preterm infants can have musculoskeletal and developmental problems from prolonged immobilization and the effects of gravity on their immature neuromuscular system. Because the extensor muscles mature before the flexor muscles, the infant tends to remain in an extended, "frog-leg" position. Shoulder retraction, abduction and external rotation of the lower extremities, lateral flexion of the arms, neck hyperextension, and flattening of the sides of the head can be prevented with correct positioning.

Reposition the infant every 2 to 3 hours or when other care is provided. Change the position slowly, as repositioning may be stressful. When possible, position the infant with the extremities flexed and the hands positioned in midline and near the mouth to allow the infant to suck the hands for comfort. Use swaddling, blanket rolls, or commercial positioning devices to maintain flexion.

**Individualizing care.** When possible, the same nurse or several nurses should be assigned care for an infant to provide consistency in care and handling techniques. This model of care allows the nurse to learn the infant's unique responses and to individualize nursing care. It is also very helpful to parents to relate to a small number of nurses who know their infant well.

The ability to tolerate stress varies with each infant. Adapt general care according to the infant's ability to tolerate it. Even positive stimuli, such as soft music or soft talking, can overstimulate some infants.

Infants often require extra energy to adjust to changes in care. Observe how well they tolerate changes such as moving from assisted to more independent breathing or introduction of new feeding methods. Increase rest periods during these times.

**Communicating infants' needs.** Use the nursing care plan, Kardex, and shift reports to inform other caregivers of techniques that are especially effective for certain infants. Tape notes at the bedside as reminders of each infant's needs. Explain all techniques to parents so they can participate in care appropriately.

***Evaluation***

- Does the infant display signs of overstimulation less often?
- Are periods of relaxed behavior and sleep increased?

### Nutrition

Preterm infants are born before they are able to accumulate stores of nutrients, and their digestive systems are immature. Full-term newborns have reservoirs of calcium, iron, and other nutrients, but these are lacking in preterm infants. Fat stores are minimal or absent, and glucose reserves are used soon after birth. Low blood glucose develops very rapidly and must be prevented or treated quickly.

Preterm infants receiving enteral feedings need approximately 105 to 130 kcal/kg/day. This amount varies according to activity, illness, and other factors. These infants also need more protein, iron, calcium, phosphorus, and magnesium. The average healthy preterm infant should gain approximately 15 to 20 g/kg/day.

#### *Assessment*

**Feeding tolerance.** Assess how well the infant tolerates enteral feedings, whether by gavage or nipple. Aspirate the stomach contents to measure the residual amount of feeding in the stomach before intermittent gavage feedings or every 2 to 4 hours or according to hospital policy for continuous feedings. This procedure helps determine whether the stomach is emptying and prevents over distention. If the residual measures more than half the previous feeding or more than 2 to 4 mL/kg or a 1-hour volume for continuous feedings, report it to the physician. Excessive residuals indicate that the amount, type, or formula flow rate needs to be changed or that complications such as **necrotizing enterocolitis** (NEC) (a serious inflammatory condition of the intestines) are occurring.

Unless they are bloody, have large amounts of mucus, or are otherwise abnormal, gastric residuals are often replaced to prevent loss of electrolytes. Abnormal residuals are reported to the physician, and the feeding is held. The next feeding may be reduced by the amount of the residual. If residuals are not replaced, observe carefully for signs of electrolyte imbalance.

Vomiting or frequent regurgitation may indicate that the feedings are too large. Vomitus or residuals containing bile are be a sign of intestinal obstruction. Diarrhea can be caused by too rapid advancement of the feeding or intolerance to the type of formula.

Observe for signs of intestinal complications. Obtain objective data about abdominal distention using a tape to measure abdominal girth at the level of the umbilicus every 4 to 8 hours. Stools may be tested for reducing substances (which indicate malabsorption of carbohydrates) or occult blood if feeding intolerance is suspected. Report signs to the healthcare provider because they may be early indications of complications such as ileus, sepsis, intestinal obstruction, or NEC.

**Readiness for nipple feeding.** During gavage feedings, watch for signs that nipple feeding will soon be possible. Such signs include rooting, a respiratory rate below 60 breaths per minute, and an increasing ability to tolerate holding and handling. Although sucking on the gavage tube, a finger, or a pacifier may be a sign of readiness, it is not enough. Infants must also have an intact gag reflex; otherwise, they are more likely to aspirate feedings. Note whether the infant gags on the catheter or a gloved finger inserted into the mouth.

When the infant begins to feed by nipple, assess coordination of suck, swallow, and breathing, and observe for aspiration. Frequent choking, gagging, or cyanosis during feedings indicate that the infant cannot coordinate sucking, swallowing, and breathing well enough for nipple feeding. Some infants are so weak that the usual signs of aspiration are minimal or absent.

Assess the respiratory rate before and during feedings. When the respiratory rate is more than 60 breaths per minute before feedings, gavage feed to prevent aspiration. Observe for signs that the effort of nipple feeding requires too much energy and oxygen for the infant.

> **! NURSING QUALITY ALERT**
>
> ***Advancing to Nipple Feeding***
>
> **Signs of Readiness for Nipple Feedings**
> - Rooting
> - Sucking on gavage tube, finger, or pacifier
> - Able to tolerate holding
> - Respiratory rate <60 breaths per minute
> - Presence of gag reflex
>
> **Signs of Nonreadiness for Nipple Feedings**
> - Respiratory rate >60 breaths per minute
> - No rooting or sucking
> - Absence of gag reflex
> - Excessive gastric residuals
>
> **Adverse Signs During Nipple Feedings**
> - Increased or decreased heart rate
> - Increased or decreased respiratory rate
> - Markedly decreased oxygen saturation level
> - Apnea
> - Cyanosis, pallor
> - Coughing, choking
> - Gagging, spitting up
> - Drooling, gulping
> - Falling asleep early in the feeding
> - Feeding time more than 20 to 30 minutes

***Nursing diagnosis and planning.*** The nursing diagnosis that addresses the nutritional problems of the preterm infant is:

- Risk for Imbalanced Nutrition: Less Than Body Requirements related to uncoordinated suck and swallow and fatigue during feedings.

**Expected outcomes.** The infant will take in adequate amounts of breast milk or formula to meet nutrient needs for age and weight and will gain 15 to 20 g/kg/day. The actual amount of feedings and weight gain vary according to the infant's gestational age and other conditions. Discuss what is appropriate for a particular infant with the physician or nurse practitioner.

#### *Interventions*

**Administering parenteral nutrition.** The nurse manages the administration of total parenteral nutrition, which may be necessary for very immature infants because of respiratory problems, limited gastric capacity, surgery, or reduced peristalsis. **Total parenteral nutrition** is the IV infusion of solutions containing the major nutrients needed for metabolism and growth. It provides calories, amino acids, fatty acids, vitamins, and minerals in amounts adapted to the needs of infants. Total parenteral nutrition is continued in decreasing amounts until the infant is able to tolerate full enteral feedings.

**Administering enteral feedings.** Enteral feedings (feeding into the gastrointestinal tract, orally or by feeding tube) are usually begun within the first few days using **minimal enteral feedings** (also called trophic feedings). Given by gavage, they contain only a few milliliters of breast milk or formula. Trophic feedings promote maturation of the intestinal tract, intestinal motility, and gastric hormone production. Feeding tolerance and weight gain are improved, and infants achieve full enteral feedings earlier if they are given trophic feedings. Human milk is preferred if it is available. Colostrum is especially high in immune agents to help prevent infection. Feedings are gradually increased according to the infant's tolerance.

Preterm infants need special formulas or fortified breast milk. Such formulas are adapted to meet the need for easily digestible, concentrated nutrients in a smaller volume of fluid. Preterm infants may need 24 kcal/oz (instead of 20 kcal/oz used for the full-term infant) to meet their requirements. Preterm formulas contain added calories, protein, vitamins, minerals, and complex fatty acids. Additional components are added to formulas to meet the needs of individual infants. Breast milk fortifiers add needed nutrients to breast milk.

**Administering gavage feedings.** Gavage feedings are usually started before oral feedings for preterm infants (see Procedures on page 935 and on page 937). A small, soft catheter is inserted through the nose or mouth to provide intermittent or continuous feedings.

Intermittent bolus feedings provide a more normal feeding pattern, with periodic stimulation of gastric hormones and enzymes. They should be given slowly over 30 to 60 minutes. Continuous feedings may be better for infants with short bowel syndrome, congenital heart disease, intolerance to bolus feedings, or those recovering from NEC. However, continuous feedings have a higher risk of aspiration because the infant is not attended at all times during the feeding. In addition, bacterial counts in the milk or formula may become too high, and fats tend to adhere to the tubing during continuous feeding.

Pacifiers are often used during gavage feedings. Preterm infants have been exposed to noxious stimulation around the mouth, such as intubation and suctioning. As a result, they may react negatively to any additional oral stimulation, thus interfering with feedings. Providing a pacifier during gavage feedings gives positive oral stimulation and helps associate the comfortable feeling of fullness with sucking. Nonnutritive sucking also increases later success in oral feedings.

**Administering oral feedings.** The ability to feed orally and weight gain are important milestones. Most infants are ready for oral feedings when they reach what would be 34 to 35 weeks of gestation, and some are ready by 30 to 34 weeks (Gardner & Goldson, 2011). Infants must have a functional gag reflex and the ability to coordinate sucking and swallowing with breathing.

The first nipple feedings may be only a few milliliters once a day, completed by gavage. Feedings are based on infant cues showing readiness for oral feeding such as rooting, hand-to-mouth movements, and sucking on a pacifier. The feedings are gradually increased in amount and frequency until the infant feeds by breast or bottle once every 8 hours, then every second or third feeding, and eventually, every feeding (Fig. 29.4).

Oral feedings should be cue-based (begun when the infant shows signs of physiologic and behavioral readiness to feed) rather than on a time schedule. Crying is a late hunger sign and can cause the infant to be too tired to eat. Cue-based feedings help infants to develop sleep-wake cycles and to begin to self-regulate.

***Preparing for feedings.*** Provide for heat maintenance during feedings. When infants have stable temperature maintenance, wrap them in warm blankets, and hold them for feedings.

Nipple feedings involve a greater expenditure of energy by the infant than do gavage feedings. Provide a period of rest before and after feedings. Use a pacifier before feedings to help bring the infant to an alert state to improve feeding success.

***Giving bottle feedings.*** A variety of nipples are available for neonates taking bottle feedings. Soft nipples require less energy for sucking but may deliver milk too rapidly. Standard nipples deliver milk more slowly and are better for some infants. Nursing interventions for bottle feeding the preterm infant are presented in the Nursing Care Plan.

**Facilitating breastfeeding.** Breast milk is best for most infants and especially for preterm infants.

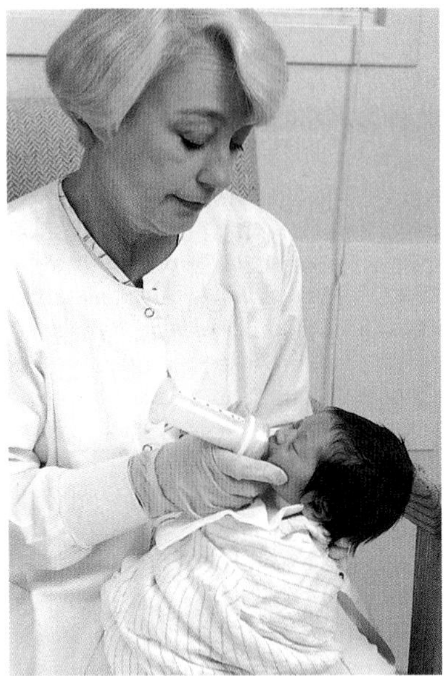

**FIG 29.4** The nurse feeds a preterm infant.

### CRITICAL THINKING EXERCISE 29.1

What are the major differences between formula feeding a preterm infant and a full-term infant?

Explain to parents that the immunologic benefits of breast milk are particularly important to the preterm infant who did not receive passive immunity during fetal life. Human milk provides protection against infections and decreases the incidence of NEC. Breast milk stimulates the immune system and gastrointestinal maturation. It is well tolerated, and nutrients are more available than those in cow's-milk formulas. Nutrients in breast milk are more easily digested, and it provides antimicrobial components, enzymes, hormones, and growth factors important for the preterm infant.

In addition, breastfeeding may be less stressful than bottle feeding for preterm infants. Oxygenation levels are often higher during breastfeeding because the infant can regulate breathing and suckling better than with bottle feeding (Hurst & Meier, 2010).

Offer support and encouragement to mothers who would like to breastfeed. Contributing her milk helps the mother realize she has something important to offer at a time when she may feel that she can do little to help her baby.

The mother who plans to breastfeed needs help in maintaining lactation until the infant is mature enough to nurse. Help her begin to use a breast pump as soon as possible after birth and instruct her to pump at least eight times daily for 10 to 15 minutes. Give her sterile containers to store her milk. Show her how to label her milk and where to take it when she brings it to the NICU. When she goes home, tell her to place the milk in a refrigerator if the infant will receive it within 24 hours or in a freezer if it will be more than 24 hours.

Although milk from mothers of preterm infants has many components necessary for these infants, it is usually necessary to add fortifiers to meet total nutrient needs. If fortifiers will be added to the milk, explain the higher needs of the preterm infant so the mother does not think something is wrong with her milk.

In some facilities, healthy preterm infants progress to breastfeeding from gavage feedings without using the bottle at all. This progression

## NURSING CARE PLAN

### *The Preterm Infant*

#### Focused Assessment

Giovanni was born at 31 weeks of gestation and now weighs 1800 g (4 lb). He breathes on his own with oxygen by hood. He needs many treatments throughout the day. Giovanni becomes pale and has an increased respiratory rate when tired. Noises often cause a drop in oxygen saturation. When held or disturbed for care, he may stiffen and extend his arms with the fingers splayed. He sleeps most of the time when he is undisturbed.

#### Nursing Diagnosis

Activity Intolerance related to weakness, fatigue, and possible overstimulation.

#### Planning

***Expected Outcomes***

Giovanni will:

1. Show fewer signs of overstimulation (increased respirations, pallor, decreased oxygen saturation level, stiffening of arms and legs, splaying of fingers) as a result of normal activity.
2. Increase tolerance to activity gradually, as demonstrated by fewer signs of fatigue or stress.

#### Interventions and *Rationales*

1. Whenever possible, arrange routine care to correspond with Giovanni's natural awake periods.
   *Preterm infants need undisturbed sleep to promote growth.*
2. Schedule periods of uninterrupted rest, especially before and after energy-draining activities.
   *Infants tolerate activities best when they begin in a rested state and are allowed to recover before other activities are necessary.*
3. Experiment with clustering care to determine the number and combination of activities that he tolerates best.
   *Clustering allows for longer rest periods between tasks but too many activities may be too fatiguing.*
4. Assess Giovanni's stress signs before beginning care activities, during each period of care, and after care.
   *Careful assessment helps the nurse individualize nursing care to meet the changing needs of the infant.*
5. Determine which activities bring about signs of overstimulation and fatigue. Stop activities and allow Giovanni to rest, if possible.
   *Careful assessment allows the nurse to be sensitive to the infant's ability to tolerate care.*
6. Reduce the noise level around the infant. Avoid unnecessary talking; open and close doors softly; keep alarm volumes low.
   *Noise may be overstimulating and cause increased oxygen need.*
7. Place Giovanni facing away from bright lights. Partially cover the incubator to keep out light but allow visibility of the infant. Schedule regular nap times when lights are turned down.
   *These changes in lighting will increase rest.*
8. Use positioning devices to form "boundaries" around him and keep his extremities flexed.
   *Enclosed space promotes rest and comfort.*
9. Collaborate with parents and other nurses. Tape signs on the bed to provide this information to parents and others.
   *Determine what works best to provide consistent care and decrease Giovanni's fatigue.*
10. Explain the infant's needs for rest and low stimulation to his parents. Suggest ways they can interact appropriately to meet his needs, and point out signs that he is receiving too much stimulation. For example, splayed fingers are a "stop sign." Ask for their input.
    *Informed parents can care for the infant appropriately and feel that they are members of the team.*

#### Evaluation

Giovanni gradually shows a greater ability to tolerate progressive activity and has fewer episodes of overstimulation. His respirations and oxygen saturation levels remain stable. He shows fewer signs of overstimulation during handling and has increased periods of sleep.

#### Focused Assessment

Several times a day Giovanni receives feedings by nipple supplemented by gavage when he becomes too tired. The feeding plan is for him to receive 120 kcal/kg/day to meet his needs. He has occasional episodes of increased respirations or short cyanotic spells when fed. He sometimes takes only half the feeding before falling asleep and must receive the rest by gavage. Giovanni's mother has decided to formula feed.

#### Nursing Diagnosis

Ineffective Infant Feeding Pattern related to muscle weakness and fatigue during feedings.

#### Planning

***Expected Outcomes***

Giovanni will:

1. Take 120 kcal/day to meet his needs at a weight of 1800 g.
2. Gain 27 to 36 g (15 to 20 g/kg) daily.
3. Complete nipple feedings without signs of excessive fatigue (e.g., increased respiratory rate, falling asleep during feeding).

#### Interventions and *Rationales*

1. Schedule rest periods before and after nipple feedings. Feed Giovanni when he begins to show hunger cues and before he begins to cry with hunger.
   *Rest helps avoid excessive fatigue that might prevent the infant from completing the feeding. Crying increases energy use.*
2. Use a pacifier before feedings.
   *Nonnutritive sucking helps alert the infant to prepare him for feeding.*
3. Use a feeding container on which each milliliter is marked.
   *This allows the intake to be measured accurately.*
4. Determine the type of nipple that prevents Giovanni from receiving too much or too little milk at a time.
   *If milk flows too fast, choking may occur. If the flow is too slow, frustration and fatigue may result.*
5. Wrap Giovanni in warmed blankets with his extremities flexed and midline. Place a hat on his head to keep him warm. Use a quiet area and avoid distractions or interruptions during feedings.
   *Quiet and comfort will enhance feedings.*
6. Position him at a 45- to 60-degree angle. Support his head and neck in a neutral position.
   *A flexed, upright position helps the infant control the flow of formula.*
7. Feed slowly, and allow the infant to rest when he stops sucking to avoid fatigue. Remove the nipple from his mouth if he has signs of stress or long sucking bursts without pausing to breathe.
   *Preterm infants have difficulty regulating their breathing while feeding.*
8. Do not move the nipple around in his mouth to force him to resume feeding. Burp frequently.
   *Moving the nipple interferes with the infant's ability to pace the feeding. Preterm infants may swallow more air than full-term infants because sucking is less efficient.*
9. Observe for coughing, gagging, cyanosis, apnea, and changes in heart rate, respirations, or oxygen saturation. Stop feeding, and evaluate the infant's ability to continue. Provide or increase oxygen if needed.
   *These signs show difficulty coordinating sucking, swallowing, and breathing, and possible aspiration. Feeding requires more oxygen intake.*

*Continued*

## NURSING CARE PLAN—cont'd

### *The Preterm Infant*

10. Assess for signs of overfatigue: falling asleep during feedings, feedings lasting more than 20 to 30 minutes, increased respirations, decreased oxygen saturation.
    *Feedings may require more energy than the infant has available. Infants who are overfatigued are more likely to aspirate. Calories may be used for feeding instead of for growth.*
11. Finish feeding by gavage if necessary.
    *This method will conserve energy, prevent aspiration, and ensure the infant receives the desired nutrient intake.*
12. Involve parents in giving feedings as soon as possible. Teach them to assess feeding cues and Giovanni's response to feedings. Help them learn the infant's usual pattern of sucking, swallowing, and breathing and to watch for changes such as milk dribbling out of his mouth or breathing irregularities that indicate a need to stop the feeding temporarily.
    *Feeding allows parents to participate in the infant's care. Their comfort with feedings and learning about the infant's responses will help them prepare for discharge.*

**Evaluation**

- Giovanni consumes approximately 110 to 130 kcal daily and does not show excessive fatigue during feedings. He gains 28 to 32 g each day.

***Additional Nursing Diagnoses to Consider***

- Ineffective Thermoregulation
- Ineffective Airway Clearance
- Interrupted Family Processes
- Risk for Caregiver Role Strain
- Risk for Impaired Parenting
- Risk for Infection
- Acute Pain

should be encouraged for eligible infants and mothers who want to breastfeed. If the amount of breast milk obtained at a feeding is of concern, the infant can be weighed before and after the feeding. The difference between the weights in grams equals the volume (in mL) taken in.

Ongoing support for the mother is important. Encourage her efforts in feeding, which may be difficult at first. Remind her that even full-term infants must learn to breastfeed. Mothers who have not breastfed previously have to learn the basic techniques and also how to adapt them for the preterm infant. Provide as much privacy as possible, using a separate room or screens. Help the mother feel comfortable holding the tiny infant and any attached equipment. The presence of a lactation consultant during initial breastfeeding sessions is very helpful.

Adapt breastfeeding teaching to the needs of a very small infant. Show the mother how to use the football and cross-cradle holds (see Figs. 23.4 and 23.5), which allow her to see the infant's face well during latching-on and throughout the feeding. A supplemental nursing system, a device that holds expressed breast milk in a bag with a small tube attached to the mother's nipple, helps infants receive more milk with less effort during early feedings. Feedings should begin gradually and progress as with initial bottle feedings.

Make the same observations of the infant during breastfeeding as for bottle feeding. Signs of fatigue, bradycardia, tachypnea, or apnea may show lack of readiness for breastfeeding. Be sure that the infant stays warm. The mother's body heat will help maintain the infant's temperature during feedings.

**Making ongoing assessments.** Continually assess the infant's responses to all feeding methods. Watch for signs of distress, especially when feedings are first initiated. Record the amount of breast milk or formula the infant takes by gavage or bottle and compare it to the amount needed to meet nutrient needs for the infant's age and weight. Infants can be weighed on an electronic scale before and after breastfeeding to determine intake. The weight allows supplementary gavage-feeding amounts to be calculated based on the infant's oral intake of breast milk.

Weigh the infant daily at the same time with the same scale. Record the length and head circumference each week. Plot measurements on a growth chart for preterm infants and compare results with expected ranges. Weight increase not accompanied by increased length can be caused by edema and may be a sign of a complication such as congestive heart failure.

Observe changes in the infant's ability to take feedings. As the infant becomes more mature, less energy should be expended during the feeding sessions. The infant will take the feedings more quickly and show fewer signs of fatigue, such as falling asleep during feedings.

***Evaluation***

- Does the infant consume adequate amounts of formula or breast milk to meet nutrient needs for age and weight?
- Is the pattern of weight gain approximately 15 to 20 g/kg/day?

### Parenting

The extended hospitalization of a preterm infant causes separation of the parents from their newborn, produces emotional trauma, and disrupts family life. The inability of parents to assume the parenting role they had expected is stressful for them, and they may state that they do not feel like parents during this time. Although attachment begins during pregnancy, premature birth and prolonged hospitalization interfere with the process of attachment after birth.

Preterm infants often look and behave very differently from those who are full term. When NICU care is required, many parents are unable to participate fully in infant care for a prolonged period. This hampers their ability to learn their baby's unique characteristics such as how they respond to stress and the consolation methods that work best. Separation and inability to assume the parenting role delay the development of the parent-infant relationship and can impair bonding. Nurses must evaluate the progress of attachment to help parents feel important in caring for their infant (Boykova & Kenner, 2012).

***Assessment.*** Assess for signs of parental attachment on the first and subsequent visits to the NICU nursery. Expect parents to be fearful at first but more able to focus on the infant as they recover from the initial shock of preterm birth. Assess for common behaviors that show normal progression of attachment. These include talking about the infant in positive terms, making eye contact, pointing out physical characteristics, naming the infant, and calling the infant by name. When they can hold and participate in the care of the infant, observe for gradual increase in comfort and skill. The parents should smile and talk to the infant and verbalize increasing confidence in their caretaking abilities.

Watch for signs that bonding is not occurring as expected. These include failure to show usual attachment behaviors or a decrease in behaviors that were previously present. Determine if there are other stressors in the parents' lives that could interfere with their ability to visit and attach to the infant. The financial need to return to work, lack of transportation, long distances to travel, or the need to care for other children can prevent parents from visiting as often as they wish.

## ! NURSING QUALITY ALERT

### *Signs of Delayed Bonding*

- Using negative terms to describe the infant
- Discussing the infant in impersonal or technical terms
- Failing to give the infant a name or to use the name
- Visiting or calling infrequently or not at all
- Decreasing the number and length of visits
- Showing equal interest in other infants and their own
- Refusing offers to hold and learn to care for the infant
- Showing a decrease in or lack of eye contact
- Spending less time talking to or smiling at the infant

After the critical period in the early days after birth, healthy preterm infants become more stable. They still require specialized nursing care and hospitalization but gradually need fewer technologic interventions. They are sometimes called "growers" at this time. This is a time when parental participation in the infant's care should increase in preparation for discharge.

***Nursing diagnosis and planning.*** For most parents of preterm infants, an important nursing diagnosis is:

- Risk for Impaired Attachment related to separation of parents from infant and lack of understanding about the preterm infant's condition and characteristics.

**Expected outcomes.** The parents will demonstrate bonding behaviors, including visiting or calling frequently and interacting as appropriate for the infant's condition throughout the hospital stay. The parents will verbalize understanding of the preterm infant's condition and characteristics within 2 days and will express gradually increasing comfort with their participation in infant care throughout the hospital stay.

***Interventions***

**Making advance preparations.** Preparing for threatening situations such as preterm birth helps parents cope with the actual event. Parents at higher risk for a preterm birth should visit the NICU before delivery. If the mother is confined to bed, arrange for a nurse from the NICU to visit her. The father or another support person should tour the nursery so that he can discuss the nursery environment with the mother. Encourage the parents to ask questions about how the infant will be cared for if it is born early.

**Assisting parents at birth.** After the birth, allow the parents to see and touch the newborn in the delivery room so that they have a realistic idea of the infant's appearance and condition. If possible, allow the father or primary support person to watch the initial care in the NICU. Explain what is happening and why. This attention allows him to see the intensive efforts made on behalf of his infant, increases confidence in the staff, and enables him to give the mother a full description later. Support the father as well as the mother by using therapeutic communication during this difficult time.

If the infant must be transported to another facility, ask the transport team to visit the parents before leaving, if possible. The visit helps them feel connected to their infant and to the staff providing care. Leaving photographs with the mother is another way of helping her bond even though the infant is not with her.

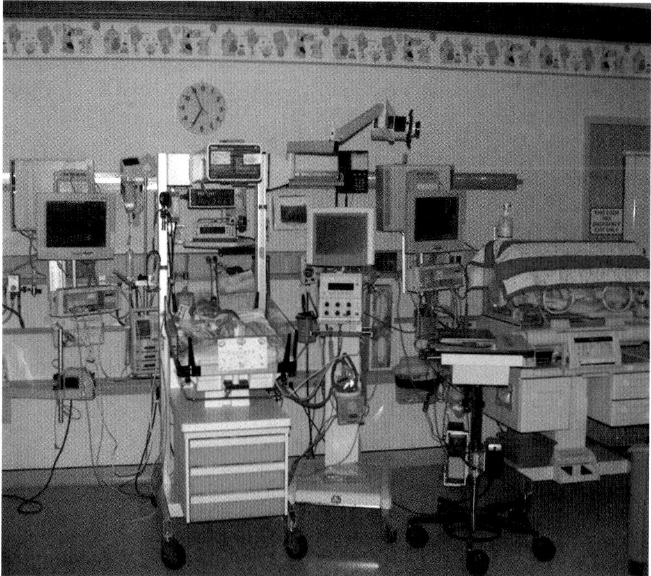

**FIG 29.5** An infant in the NICU is surrounded by highly technologic equipment. This can be very frightening to parents at first. Preparing parents before they visit is an important nursing responsibility. (Courtesy Cheryl Briggs, RNC, Annapolis, MD.)

**Supporting parents during early visits.** Take the parents to the NICU as soon as possible. If the mother is too sick to be with her infant, give her photographs. Prepare parents before the first visit. Describe the equipment and its purposes, the various attachments to the infant, and the sounds of alarms (Fig. 29.5). Explain how the infant will look and behave. Box 29.1 provides specific steps that the nurse can follow to help parents become familiar with the NICU setting.

At first, stay with the parents during their time in the NICU. When they are comfortable, allow them time alone with the infant so that they can interact in private. Answer questions and explain changes in the infant's condition and treatment. Expect to repeat explanations because stressed parents may not understand or remember what was said at first. Parents may not know what questions to ask at first or may be too overwhelmed to ask questions. In this situation, discuss questions that are common when parents first visit the NICU. Use therapeutic communication as the parents cope with their grief, guilt, and emotional turmoil.

Parents should touch the infant as soon as possible because touching helps promote attachment. They may be hesitant initially for fear that they will interfere with equipment. Some parents hesitate to touch because they are afraid of becoming attached to an infant whom they might lose. They need sensitive support from the nurse until they are ready to progress in their relationship with the infant.

Show parents how to touch in ways appropriate for the infant, such as holding the infant's hand through the portholes of the incubator. Explain that handling is kept to a minimum for physiologically unstable infants because it is too stressful for them. When the infant is ready, show parents which forms of touch work best for their infant.

Help the parents to hold the baby as soon as possible. Holding the baby is particularly important to parents who interpret it as a very positive sign of the infant's condition. Yet it may be frightening too, especially if the infant is attached to various equipment. Help the

**BOX 29.1 Introducing Parents to the Neonatal Intensive Care Unit Setting**

**Before Parents Visit the Neonatal Intensive Care Unit (NICU)**

- If possible, provide parents with a tour of the NICU before the birth.
- If a tour is not possible, describe the NICU environment. Include alarm noise, staff activity, and the number of people and sick infants.
- Describe the equipment. Include ventilators, intravenous (IV) lines, feeding tubes, and monitors. Describe how they look and how they are attached to the infant. Keep explanations simple, without technical details.
- Show parents photographs of the infant. Photos help prepare them but are not as overwhelming as seeing the infant in person.
- Describe the infant. Include the size, lack of fat, breathing, and weak cry. Explain that no sound of crying can be heard if the infant is intubated. Include some personal aspects: "He's a real fighter" or "She makes the funniest faces during her feedings."

**When Parents Visit the NICU**

- Help parents perform thorough handwashing while explaining its importance.
- Stay with the parents during their visit. Having a familiar person nearby will help them feel more comfortable while they adjust to this unfamiliar environment.
- Introduce them to the infant's nurse. Ask the nurse to explain some of the care being provided for the infant.
- Give parents written information about the NICU so that they can take it home to read later. This list should include visiting hours, telephone updates, available classes on preterm infant care, and support groups.
- Tell the parents that they will receive instruction on how to care for their infant in time. Encourage them to visit the infant as much as they can. Emphasize how important they are to their infant.
- Offer realistic encouragement based on the infant's condition.
- Provide an opportunity for the parents to express their concerns and feelings and to ask questions.

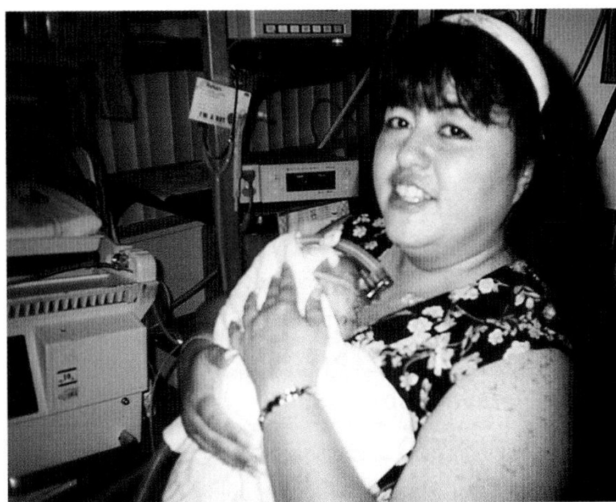

**FIG 29.6** This mother holds her 27-week-gestation infant under her clothes against her skin as she gives kangaroo care.

parents find a comfortable position for themselves and the infant, and point out positive responses from the infant.

Nurses often focus on the mother in providing support. However, fathers also need support in learning about their infant and how to parent a preterm infant. One study showed fathers of NICU infants had elevated levels of stress and symptoms of depression throughout the 7 weeks of the study. They may be less comfortable in the NICU setting because they have work and other family responsibilities. Encourage them to participate in hands-on care whenever possible. Complement each parent as they care for the infant so they are encouraged to participate even more.

**Providing information.** An important role of the nurse is providing information to parents. Allow parents to express their concerns before beginning to teach. Encourage them to ask questions about all aspects of their infant's condition and care. Although some mothers are not hesitant to ask questions, others avoid asking for explanations or advocating for their need to care for their infants because they are afraid that they might be seen as difficult or demanding. Give information about common concerns of parents if the parents do not ask questions.

Explain the equipment used to care for the infant. Interpret the information obtained from monitors and the meaning of alarms. Clarify all nursing care, its purpose, and the expected response. Point out how preterm infants are similar to and different from full-term infants to help parents develop an understanding of the infant's capabilities.

Offer realistic reassurance about the infant's condition, emphasizing positive aspects while being truthful. If parents have misconceptions or did not understand a physician's explanations, clarify or ask the physician to go over specific information again. Translate medical terms into words the parents can understand. Repeat explanations, especially at first. Because of their emotional distress, parents are often unable to comprehend fully or remember what is said to them.

Use an interpreter if the parents do not understand English. Offer written information in the parents' language about NICU policies and procedures. Explanations about visiting hours, who can visit, routines for handwashing, and the role of parents can be reinforced in writing and be available for later reading by overwhelmed parents.

**Instituting kangaroo care (KC).** Begin KC as soon as possible, if the parents are interested. KC is a method of providing skin-to-skin contact between preterm infants and their parents. During KC, the infant, wearing only a diaper and hat, is placed upright under the mother's clothes between her breasts. A blanket is placed over them both (Fig. 29.6). Mothers can breastfeed if they wish and if the infant is able. Fathers are encouraged to participate in KC also. The infant is monitored for changes in vital signs and behavior.

Explain the advantages of KC to parents, and elicit their participation. This method of care has been found safe for stable infants, even if intubated. It provides an opportunity for parents to participate in the very important developmental care of their preterm infant. KC is associated with more stable vital signs, increased weight gain, shorter length of stay, more quiet sleep, and less crying. It also promotes thermoregulation, bonding, and helps relieve pain (Boundy et al., 2016; Hardy, 2011a).

The upright position of the infant against the parent's chest makes the infant's breathing easier. The containment of the extremities decreases purposeless movements that use needed oxygen and calories. Breastfeeding is facilitated, and the infant has more alert periods and increased deep sleep. Contact with the parent's skin maintains the infant's body temperature. In addition, KC enhances early and long-term maternal–infant interaction and maternal confidence and competence.

Provide privacy for parents interested in KC. Assist them in transferring the infant from the bed, managing attachments, and making the infant comfortable. Explain that infants often set off alarms because of changes in vital signs or oxygenation during the transfer process, but that they become stable again once settled. KC should be provided daily if the infant remains stable and should last at least an hour to improve the infant's sleep.

**Facilitating interaction.** Preterm infants often have little facial expression and seldom make eye contact. Parents may feel rejected by the infant's lack of response or negative responses during interactions. Explain that the type of interaction that is effective with full-term infants may be too stimulating for very young or sick preterm infants. Suggest forms of touch and interaction based on the individual infant's capacity. Quiet holding may be better until the infant can tolerate more stimulation.

Help parents understand the infant's behavior and cues. Teach them signs of overstimulation, and explain that these signs show that the infant needs a quiet rest period without stimulation. Help them adapt their interactions to meet the infant's needs. Discuss methods to avoid too much stimulation and ways to calm the infant. If several types of simultaneous stimulation (e.g., rocking, eye contact, and talking) cause signs of distress, suggest they stop one or more activities until the infant has had a rest period.

Teach parents how to soothe infants when they show stress signs. Explain containment and demonstrate how to do it. Placing the palm of the hand over the infant's chest or holding the infant's arms on the chest may help quiet the infant. Show them how to position the infant with the hands near the mouth so the infant can suck on them as a self-comforting measure. When the infant is ready for more interaction, suggest appropriate types of stimulation.

Point out small signs of improvement and even minor strengths. Talk about normal preterm characteristics and emphasize individual traits that make this infant different from all others. The way the infant eats, reacts to sounds, or seems to get tangled in the monitor leads may help parents feel closer to their newborn.

Involve the parents in care of the infant as soon as possible to help them feel a sense of control (Fig. 29.7). Plan to change the linens in the incubator or radiant warmer when the parents are there so that they can hold their infant. Save baths and other routine caregiving for times when parents can be present so they can participate. As the infant's condition improves, parents can develop skill in caring for the tiny infant by changing diapers, feeding, and bathing.

Include other family members by allowing them to visit with the parents. Involve family members in learning how to feed and care for the infant if they will be helping the parents after discharge.

**Increasing parental decision making.** Parents should be considered essential parts of the healthcare team rather than visitors. Give parents the information they need to take an active part in decisions made about the infant's treatment plan, even if the decisions seem insignificant to the staff. Such participation will increase their feelings of control over a situation in which many parents feel they have little power. Although parents often feel like outsiders when first visiting the NICU, they will move into the role of partners with the NICU staff in caring for the infant in time. Look for opportunities to praise parenting abilities. Point out positive ways the infant responds to the parents' touch and caregiving. As parents become more knowledgeable and participate more in caregiving, seek their input about how the infant is progressing and practices that seem to work best. Demonstrate respect for their concerns and suggestions and incorporate their preferences into the plan of care when possible.

**Alleviating concerns.** Invite parents to call the NICU at any time for information about their infant. Phone calls are especially beneficial for parents who cannot visit the infant because of distance or other reasons.

Put them in touch with parents of other preterm infants, and refer them to support groups, parent-to-parent groups with veteran NICU parents, telephone support, educational offerings, or counseling sessions. Internet sources of support are also available such as http://www.preemiecare.org. Talking with others who have faced the same problems can be very comforting as parents compare notes and get practical suggestions from an experienced parent's point of view. Taking language and culture into consideration is important during this process.

Cultural practices should be incorporated into the care of the infant. Determine who in the family will make the decisions and who will be managing the infant's care. In some cultures, the father makes decisions, and the grandmother is the major caregiver (Fig. 29.8). In these cases, it is essential that the right persons be included in teaching. In many cultures, the mother is expected to stay at home to recover after giving birth. This arrangement interferes with her ability to spend

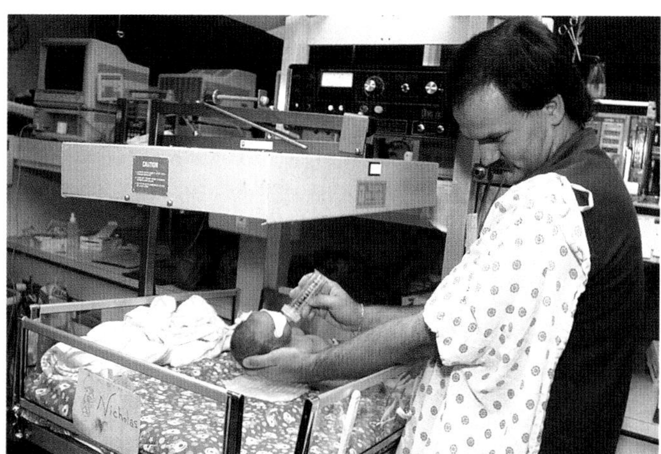


FIG 29.7 To promote family bonding with the infant, parents are involved as much as possible in the care of their infant. This father bottle feeds his infant in a radiant warmer.

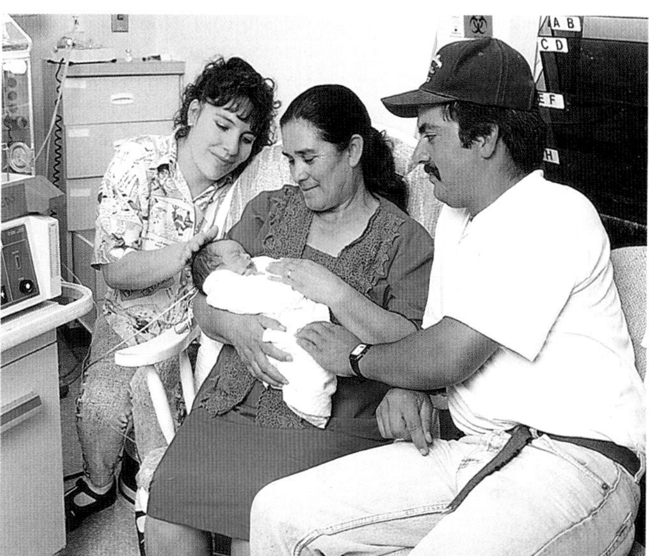

FIG 29.8 The parents look on while the grandmother holds the infant in the NICU.

time in the NICU. Another family member may be enlisted to be with the infant in these cases.

**Helping with ongoing problems.** Parents may be unprepared for the inconsistent progress infants often make after surviving the risks of the early days. They expect steady progress once the infant can breathe alone and take feedings. However, complications such as NEC or sepsis can cause major setbacks at this time. To cope with a new crisis, parents need extensive support from the nurse. Use therapeutic communication techniques such as reflecting feelings to help them express and cope with their extreme disappointment. Give information about the infant's changing condition and what to expect in the days ahead.

Having a hospitalized child can be exhausting for the parents. Remind the parents to take breaks away from the infant, whether to go to the cafeteria for a meal or to go home and rest. As the infant's condition improves parents may take more time away as they begin to prepare for the infant's discharge. Encourage them to do this, while at the same time making sure they feel welcome to stay with the infant as much as they want. Mothers with LBW infants in the NICU may have problems with sleep disturbances and depressive symptoms. Fatigue and having an ill infant are factors that can lead to postpartum depression (see Chapter 28).

**Preparing for discharge.** Because infants go home very early in their development, it is important that the parents understand the expected hospital course. If a clinical pathway is being used for the infant, give them a copy. They can chart the infant's achievement of major milestones in development and changes in care as the infant moves toward discharge.

Begin early to teach parents and other caregivers any special procedures, treatments, and medications that the infant will need after discharge. Observe the parents performing care until they are comfortable and can do it safely. Praise their efforts and provide hints to make care easier. Help them learn what is normal for their infant and how to recognize and respond to abnormal signs. Some hospitals have parents spend a night or two in a special "parent room," where they take over full 24-hour care of the infant yet still have help available if problems arise. This arrangement helps increase parents' confidence that they can care for the infant alone. It also allows staff to confirm the parents' abilities to care for the infant.

Help the parents determine what adaptations they will need to make at home before discharge. Utility companies should be notified if the infant is considered medically fragile to ensure the family receives priority service in case of power failure. Arrange home nursing services, purchase of supplies, and delivery of special equipment before discharge.

Discuss what to expect in providing care for the infant after discharge. Infants may require oxygen, cardiorespiratory monitoring, suctioning, tube feedings, or other treatments that parents will have to learn to perform. Many infants need feedings every 3 hours, day and night, to help them gain weight adequately. Feedings may be time consuming, and parental fatigue resulting from sleep interruptions may be greater than they expected.

Explore with parents what kind of help they will need to meet the everyday requirements of the infant and the rest of the family. Help them identify where they might find assistance from family and friends. Reassure them that friends and family often welcome opportunities to help.

AAP and ACOG (2007) recommend the following in determining the time of discharge:

- Signs of readiness for discharge include a sustained pattern of weight gain, adequate maintenance of body temperature in an open bed, feeding without cardiorespiratory compromise, and stable cardiorespiratory function.
- Appropriate immunizations should have been given, metabolic screening performed, assessment of hearing, the eyes, hematologic status, and nutritional risks performed, and appropriate treatment plans completed before discharge.
- The family and home should have been evaluated. The family must have at least two members who demonstrate the ability to feed and provide all needed care, perform cardiopulmonary resuscitation, give medications, operate equipment, and show understanding of signs of problems and what to do about them.
- A primary care physician and other appropriate follow-up care have been arranged.

Help parents form realistic expectations of the infant. For example, they should know that the infant will accomplish developmental tasks, such as crawling and walking, later than full-term infants. Parents should base expectations on the infant's developmental or **corrected age** (the age the infant would be if still in utero or born at full term) rather than chronologic age. Developmental or corrected age is the chronologic age minus the number of weeks the infant was born early.

Assist the parents to plan for integrating the new infant into the family. Meeting the needs of their other children in addition to the new responsibilities of caring for the preterm infant is a major source of worry. Listen to their concerns about other children and encourage siblings who do not have infections to visit the NICU. Help the parents prepare siblings for what they will see and do while visiting. Siblings should touch or hold the infant, if possible, to help them bond. Put them in touch with support groups for parents after discharge.

Before discharge, infants are evaluated for apnea or bradycardia in the car seat the parents will use. Proper positioning with blanket rolls may be necessary because infants may slump over, interfering with chest expansion. Some infants need car beds to allow them to ride in a recumbent position. Car seats or beds should always be placed in the backseat of the car. Airbags in the area the infant is placed should be disconnected because they can cause injury if inflated.

#### *Evaluation*

- Do the parents demonstrate common bonding behaviors?
- Do they verbalize understanding of the preterm infant's special needs and treatments?
- How active are the parents in caring for the infant?

## COMMON COMPLICATIONS OF PRETERM INFANTS

Complications of prematurity increase as the infant's gestational age and birth weight decrease. Some complications, such as hyperbilirubinemia, are common to full-term and preterm infants and are discussed in Chapter 30. Complications most common in prematurity are discussed here.

### Respiratory Distress Syndrome (RDS)

Respiratory distress syndrome (RDS) is a condition caused by insufficient surfactant in the lungs. It occurs most frequently in preterm infants and increases as gestational age decreases. It also occurs when there has been asphyxia, cesarean delivery, multiple births, male infants, cold stress, and maternal diabetes, because these conditions interfere with surfactant production. It occurs less often, however, when chronic fetal stress, such as heroin addiction, maternal hypertension, prolonged rupture of membranes, or antenatal corticosteroids, cause the lungs to mature more quickly.

#### Pathophysiology

RDS is caused by insufficient production of surfactant, a phospholipid that lines the alveoli. Surfactant production is usually sufficient beginning at 34 to 36 weeks of gestation to prevent RDS.

Surfactant decreases surface tension, allowing the alveoli to remain open when air is exhaled. It must be continuously produced. With too little surfactant, the alveoli collapse each time the infant exhales. The lungs and thorax become noncompliant or "stiff," and resist expansion. Noncompliant lungs require a much higher negative pressure to allow opening of the alveoli each time the infant inhales. The effort required to exert such pressure results in severe retractions with each breath, because the chest wall is very compliant and the weak muscles of the chest wall are drawn inward. The resulting pressure on the lungs further interferes with expansion.

As fewer alveoli expand, atelectasis, hypoxia, and hypercapnia (increased carbon dioxide) occur. This condition causes pulmonary vasoconstriction and decreased blood flow to the lungs because of the high resistance within the pulmonary blood vessels. Persistent pulmonary hypertension (see Chapter 30) can result in a return to fetal circulation patterns, with opening of the ductus arteriosus. Acidosis and alveolar ischemic injury interfere with surfactant synthesis.

Lecithin, sphingomyelin, phosphatidylglycerol, and phosphatidylinositol are components of surfactant that can be detected by tests of amniotic fluid. These tests can predict whether the fetal lungs are mature enough for survival outside the uterus (see Chapter 15). The incidence and severity of RDS is decreased by giving the mother corticosteroids before birth of an infant less than 32 weeks of gestation.

#### Manifestations

Signs of RDS begin during the first hours after birth and include tachypnea, nasal flaring, retractions, and cyanosis. Grunting on expiration is characteristic and signifies physiologic efforts to maintain lung expansion. Breath sounds may be decreased, and rales may be present. Acidosis develops as a result of hypoxemia. Blood gases show increased carbon dioxide levels and decreased oxygen. Chest radiographs show the "ground glass" reticulogranular appearance of the lungs that is characteristic of RDS. Signs become worse and peak within 3 days, then begin to improve gradually.

#### Therapeutic Management

Surfactant replacement therapy can be instilled into the infant's trachea immediately after birth or as soon as signs of RDS become apparent. Doses are repeated if necessary. Infants treated with surfactant have higher survival rates, but it does not reduce other complications of prematurity such as bronchopulmonary dysplasia.

Other supportive treatment includes oxygen, CPAP or mechanical ventilation, inhaled nitric oxide therapy, correction of the acidosis, IV fluids, and care of other complications. Maintenance of thermoregulation is essential.

#### Nursing Considerations

The nurse observes for signs of developing RDS at birth and during the early hours after birth. Changes in the infant's condition are constantly assessed. Changes in ventilator settings may be necessary as the infant's ability to oxygenate increases. Observation for signs of common complications, such as patent ductus arteriosus and bronchopulmonary dysplasia, is important. The nurse must monitor the results of laboratory tests for abnormalities in blood gases and acid-base balance. Early signs of sepsis must be identified and reported. Other care is similar to general care for the preterm infant.

### Bronchopulmonary Dysplasia (Chronic Lung Disease)

Bronchopulmonary dysplasia (BPD), also known as chronic lung disease, is a chronic condition occurring most often in infants weighing less than 1000 g born at 28 weeks of gestation or less (Carlo & Ambalavanan, 2011). This condition is discussed in detail in Chapter 45.

### Intraventricular Hemorrhage

Intraventricular hemorrhage (IVH), also called periventricular-intraventricular hemorrhage or germinal matrix hemorrhage, is bleeding around and into the ventricles of the brain. Approximately 30% of preterm infants weighing less than 1500 g develop IVH (Carlo & Amalavanan, 2015). The first few days of life are the most common times for hemorrhage to occur. This condition can also occur in term infants from asphyxia or trauma.

#### Pathophysiology

IVH results from rupture of the fragile blood vessels in the germinal matrix, located around the ventricles of the brain. It is associated with increased or decreased blood pressure, asphyxia or respiratory distress requiring mechanical ventilation, and increased or fluctuating cerebral blood flow. Rapid blood volume expansion, hypercarbia, acidosis, and hypoglycemia are other causes.

Hemorrhage is graded 1 through 3, according to the amount of bleeding. Grade 1 is a very small bleed at the germinal matrix, producing few if any clinical changes. Grade 2 hemorrhage extends into the lateral ventricles, and grade 3 causes distention of the ventricles. The condition is diagnosed using cranial ultrasound.

#### Manifestations

Signs of IVH correspond to the severity of the hemorrhage. Infants may have no signs or may show lethargy, poor muscle tone, deterioration of respiratory status with cyanosis or apnea, drop in hematocrit level, acidosis, hyperglycemia, decreased reflexes, tense fontanel, and seizures. Mild aberrations of eye position or movement may occur. Signs may be few and subtle.

#### Therapeutic Management

Because most hemorrhages occur during the first week, ultrasonography is often performed at 7 days of age on preterm infants at risk. Serial ultrasonography can be used to assess progression of the problem.

Treatment is supportive and focuses on maintaining respiratory function and dealing with other complications. Hydrocephalus can develop from blockage of cerebrospinal fluid flow. A ventriculoperitoneal shunt (catheter leading from the ventricles of the brain to the peritoneal cavity) may be necessary to drain the fluid.

#### Nursing Considerations

Many aspects of care can cause increases in cerebral blood flow and blood pressure. These include mechanical ventilation, suctioning, and excessive handling. Even crying can produce changes in cerebral blood flow. Therefore, the nurse must prevent situations that increase the risk of IVH and be alert for early signs. Nursing care includes daily measurement of the head circumference and observation for changes in neurologic status, which may be subtle. Pain and stress should be as low as possible.

Parents need assistance to cope with the diagnosis and their concerns regarding long-term implications. They should learn how to assess for signs of increasing intracranial pressure from hydrocephalus and understand that follow-up care may include periodic ultrasound examinations.

### Retinopathy of Prematurity

Retinopathy of prematurity (ROP) can result in visual impairment or blindness in preterm infants. It occurs most often in those weighing less than 1000 g and less than 29 weeks of gestational age.

### Pathophysiology

ROP results from injury to retinal blood vessels. The exact cause is unknown, but one risk factor is high levels of oxygen. However, ROP develops in some infants who never received supplementary oxygen. Prolonged ventilation, acidosis, sepsis, shock, IVH, hyperglycemia, and fluctuating blood oxygen levels have all been reported as associated with ROP.

In ROP, immature blood vessels in the eye constrict and are obliterated. New vessels proliferate throughout the retina and into the vitreous humor in some infants. Fluid leakage and hemorrhage can cause scarring, traction on the retina, and retinal detachment. However, the pathologic progress stops in more than 90% of infants, with little or no visual loss.

### Therapeutic Management

Infants born at 30 weeks of gestation or less, those weighing 1500 g or less at birth, and those with a birthweight of 1500 to 2000 g who were unstable should be screened for changes in the eyes 4 weeks after birth or at 31 weeks gestational age. Laser surgery to destroy abnormal blood vessels is the current treatment of choice. Cryosurgery or reattachment of a detached retina also may be necessary.

### Nursing Considerations

The nurse should check the pulse oximetry readings frequently for any infant receiving oxygen. Parents should be informed about ophthalmologic tests and receive an explanation of the results. Eye examinations can be very stressful to the infant, and swaddling and rest periods should be provided as appropriate. If surgery is performed, the eye is assessed for drainage, and pain medication should be given. Support for parents is essential throughout the examinations and especially if eye injury is found.

## Necrotizing Enterocolitis (NEC)

NEC is a serious inflammatory condition of the intestinal tract that can lead to necrosis of the intestinal mucosa. It occurs in 1% to 5% of infants admitted to NICUs and 6% to 10% of infants with birthweights under 1500 g. Ninety percent of infants with NEC are preterm (Bradshaw, 2015). The mortality rate is 10% to 30%. The ileum and proximal colon are the areas most often affected.

### Pathophysiology

Although the exact causes are unknown, immaturity of the intestines is a major factor. The rate of NEC increases with decreasing gestational age. Previous ischemia of the intestines is another cause. Most infants with NEC have received feedings. Although minimal enteric feedings are thought to increase maturation of the intestines, feedings that are too early or increased too fast increase the risk. Bacterial colonization with pathologic organisms can be present. Eventually, necrosis, perforation, and peritonitis can occur. Breast milk, which contains immunoglobulins, leukocytes, and antibacterial agents, may have a preventive effect on the development of NEC.

### Manifestations

Signs include feeding intolerance, increased abdominal girth caused by distention, increased gastric residuals, decreased bowel sounds, visible loops of bowel, vomiting, abdominal tenderness, erythema of the intestinal wall, blood in the stools, and signs of infection. Respiratory difficulty can occur because of pressure from the distended abdomen on the diaphragm. Apnea, bradycardia, temperature instability, lethargy, hypotension, and shock also may be present. Thrombocytopenia, increased or decreased leukocytes, and metabolic acidosis can occur. The presence of air within the intestinal wall on a radiograph is diagnostic of the condition. Free air in the peritoneum indicates that perforation has occurred, although perforation can occur without this sign.

### Therapeutic Management

Use of probiotics is under study as a means of establishing normal intestinal flora and preventing NEC, but further research is necessary. Treatment of NEC includes antibiotics, discontinuation of oral feedings, gastric suction, IV fluids, and use of parenteral nutrition to rest the intestines. Peritoneal drainage may be performed. Surgery is necessary for perforation or continued lack of improvement. The necrotic area is removed, and an ostomy is performed. Infants who have had large areas of bowel removed can develop short-bowel syndrome, with malabsorption and malnutrition (see Chapter 43).

### Nursing Considerations

Nurses should encourage interested mothers to provide breast milk for their infants because NEC is less likely to occur in breastfed infants. Because nurses are constantly observing the infant, they often are able to detect the early, subtle signs that lead to prompt diagnosis. If one or more signs are noted, the nurse withholds the next feeding and notifies the physician.

Abdominal girth is measured, and IV fluids and parenteral nutrition must be managed. Intake and output are important, as third-space fluid loss occurs when fluid moves from the intravascular spaces to the extracellular spaces. The infant should be positioned on the side to minimize the effects of pressure on the diaphragm from the distended intestines. During recovery, the nurse must manage pain. Observation for signs of feeding intolerance when feedings are resumed is important. Scar tissue may cause partial or complete bowel obstruction.

# POSTTERM INFANTS

**Postterm infants** are those born after the 42nd week of gestation. Their longer-than-normal gestation places them at risk for a number of complications.

## Scope of the Problem

In some cases, the postterm fetus continues to be well supported by the placenta. Infants are usually of normal size or large for gestational age. Some grow to more than 4000 g (8 lb, 13 oz), placing them at risk for birth injuries or cesarean birth.

In other cases, placental functioning decreases when pregnancy is prolonged (see Chapter 27). If placental insufficiency is present, decreased amniotic fluid volume (oligohydramnios) and umbilical cord compression can occur. The fetus may not receive the appropriate amount of oxygen and nutrients and may be small for gestational age. This condition results in hypoxia and malnourishment in the fetus and is called ***postmaturity syndrome*** or *dysmaturity syndrome*. Postmaturity syndrome occurs in approximately 20% of postterm pregnancies.

When labor begins, poor oxygen reserves can cause fetal compromise. The fetus may pass meconium as a result of hypoxia before or during labor, increasing the risk of meconium aspiration (see Chapter 30). Postterm infants have a higher perinatal mortality rate than infants born at term.

## Assessment

The infant with postmaturity syndrome may have an apprehensive look associated with hypoxia. The infant may be thin, with loose skin and little subcutaneous fat. There is little or no vernix caseosa, but the infant generally has abundant hair on the head and long nails. The skin

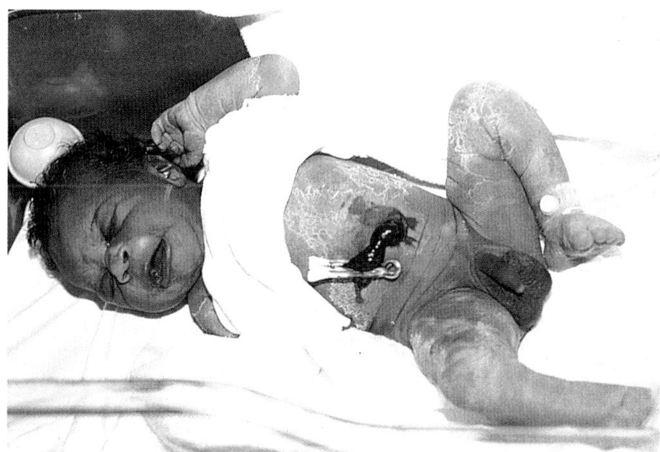

FIG 29.9 The postmature infant has dry, cracked, peeling skin and no vernix.

is wrinkled, cracked, and peeling (Fig. 29.9). If meconium was present in the amniotic fluid for some time, the cord, skin, and nails may be stained. Postterm infants should be assessed for hypoglycemia because of rapid use of glycogen stores. If loss of subcutaneous fat has occurred, the infant may have a low temperature.

### Therapeutic Management

Therapeutic management focuses on prevention and symptomatic treatment. Labor is induced if signs of placental deterioration are present during fetal diagnostic testing. In cases of asphyxia or meconium aspiration, respiratory support is needed at birth (see Chapter 30).

### Nursing Considerations

Signs of postmaturity syndrome in infants are noted during the initial assessment. Respiratory problems may necessitate continued assessment and care. Infants with any indications of postmaturity should be tested for hypoglycemia soon after birth and again an hour later or according to hospital policy. They need early and more frequent feedings to help compensate for the period of poor nutrition before birth.

Temperature regulation can be poor because fat stores were used for nourishment before birth. Extra blankets, frequent temperature assessment, and teaching parents about prevention of cold stress are important. Polycythemia from hypoxia before birth increases the risk of hyperbilirubinemia.

## SMALL-FOR-GESTATIONAL-AGE INFANTS

Small-for-gestational-age (SGA) infants are those who fall below the 10th percentile in size on growth charts. They have failed to grow in the uterus as expected, which is called fetal growth restriction (FGR). The terms SGA and FGR are often used interchangeably, although not all infants who have had some growth restriction are SGA.

SGA infants can be preterm, full-term, or postterm. Infant mortality and morbidity increase steadily as growth restriction increases. Approximately 30% of LBW infants born in the United States after 37 weeks of gestation have FGR.

### Etiology

The many risk factors associated with SGA include congenital malformations, chromosomal anomalies, genetic factors, and fetal infections. Poor placental function resulting from aging, small size, separation, or malformation can interfere with fetal growth. Illness in the expectant mother such as preeclampsia or severe diabetes restricts uteroplacental blood flow and decreases fetal growth. Smoking, drug or alcohol abuse, and severe maternal malnutrition also impair fetal growth.

### Scope of the Problem

Infants affected with FGR have perinatal morbidity and a mortality rates that are 10 to 20 times higher those of infants who are not growth restricted. Death can occur from asphyxia before or during labor or from complications, congenital anomalies, or prematurity.

Full-term SGA infants are subject to many of the same complications as those who are preterm or postterm, depending on the cause and degree of growth restriction. Problems tend to be greatest in infants who are preterm in addition to being SGA.

Low Apgar scores, meconium aspiration, and polycythemia are more frequent in SGA infants. Hypoglycemia is common because of inadequate storage of glycogen in the liver. Infants are prone to inadequate thermoregulation because subcutaneous white fat and brown fat stores have been used to survive *in utero*.

### Characteristics of Small-for-Gestational-Age (SGA) Infants

The appearance of the SGA infant varies according to whether the cause of growth restriction began early or late in the pregnancy. Variation occurs because growth restriction affects the weight first. If it continues, the length and then the head size will eventually be affected.

*Symmetric* growth restriction involves the whole body and is caused by congenital anomalies, genetic disorders, exposure to infections or drugs early in pregnancy, or normal genetic predisposition. Although the infant's weight, length, and head circumference are all below the 10th percentile, the body is proportionate and appears normally developed for size. The total number of cells is decreased, and the infant may have long-term complications. These infants are often small throughout their lives. Approximately 20% of SGA infants have symmetric growth restriction.

*Asymmetric* growth restriction is caused by conditions that begin in the third trimester that interfere with uteroplacental function or nutrition. In asymmetric restriction, the head is normal in size but seems large for the rest of the body. The length is normal, but the weight is below the 10th percentile for gestational age. Brain growth is normal, but the liver, spleen, thymus, adrenals, and placenta are smaller than normal. Infants generally catch up in growth if they are adequately nourished after birth.

The infant appears thin and wasted. The dry, loose skin has longitudinal thigh creases from loss of subcutaneous fat and a sunken abdomen. The infant has a thin cord and the facial appearance of being elderly. The anterior fontanel may be large with wide or overlapping cranial sutures.

### Therapeutic Management

Therapeutic management focuses on prevention through good prenatal care and to identify and treat problems early. When growth restriction cannot be prevented, ultrasound examination assists in early discovery of the condition. Serial nonstress tests and biophysical profiles help determine whether the infant should be delivered early, and preparation can be made for the expected complications at birth. Common problems include asphyxia, meconium aspiration, temperature instability, hypoglycemia, and polycythemia.

### Nursing Considerations

Because the causes of growth restriction are so varied, care of the SGA infant must be adapted to meet the specific problems demonstrated.

When signs of growth restriction are present, the nurse must observe for complications that commonly accompany it. The general appearance and measurements give an indication of the type of growth restriction that has occurred. Measurements of the head, chest, length, and weight are below normal in the infant with symmetric growth restriction. If the restriction is asymmetric, the head circumference and length are normal, while the abdominal circumference and weight are low.

The nurse should assess for hypoglycemia, especially in asymmetric growth-restricted infants. The brain of the infant is normal and needs large amounts of glucose, but the liver is small and has inadequate stores of glycogen. Caloric needs are greater than for a normal infant, making early and more frequent feedings important. Temperature regulation and respiratory support are added nursing concerns. Observation for jaundice is important in infants with polycythemia because a large amount of bilirubin is released when the red blood cells break down.

## LARGE-FOR-GESTATIONAL-AGE INFANTS

Large-for-gestational-age (LGA) infants are those with a weight above the 90th percentile for gestational age on intrauterine growth charts. They may have macrosomia (weigh more than 4000 g [8 lb, 13 oz]) and are usually born at term, although they may be preterm or postterm. The preterm LGA infant can be mistaken for full term but has the same problems as other preterm infants.

### Etiology

LGA infants are born to multiparas, large parents, mothers who are obese, and members of certain ethnic groups known to have large infants. Diabetes in the mother can also cause increased size, as can erythroblastosis fetalis (see Chapter 30).

### Scope of the Problem

The LGA infant is more likely to go through a longer labor, have injury during birth, or need a cesarean birth. Shoulder dystocia can occur if the shoulders are too large to fit through the pelvis. Fractures of the clavicle or skull, damage to the brachial plexus or facial nerve, cephalhematoma, and bruising occur more often in these infants than in those of normal size. Congenital heart defects are more common, and the mortality rate is higher.

### Therapeutic Management

Therapeutic management is based on identification of increased size during pregnancy by measurements of fundal height and ultrasound examination. Delivery problems can lead to the use of vacuum extraction, forceps, or cesarean birth. Specific treatment involves identification and treatment of birth injuries and complications as they arise.

### Nursing Considerations

The nurse assists in a difficult delivery or cesarean birth resulting from dystocia when the infant is LGA. After birth, the infant is carefully assessed for injuries or other complications such as hypoglycemia (p. 448), polycythemia (p. 653), or being born to a diabetic mother (p. 652). Nursing care is geared to problems presented.

## KEY CONCEPTS

- Late preterm infants, born between 34 and 36-6/7 weeks, are at risk for respiratory, thermoregulation, and feeding problems, as well as hypoglycemia, hyperbilirubinemia, acidosis, and sepsis.
- Preterm infants differ in appearance from full-term infants. Some differences include small size, unflexed posture, red skin, abundant vernix and lanugo, and immature ears and genitals.
- The lungs of preterm infants may lack adequate surfactant, which interferes with lung expansion, increasing the amount of energy necessary for breathing and leading to atelectasis.
- Other factors that increase respiratory problems are poor cough reflex, narrow respiratory passages, and weak muscles.
- The prone position is used for preterm infants because it decreases breathing effort and increases oxygenation. The supine position is used as soon as possible.
- Preterm infants are subject to cold stress because they have thin skin with blood vessels near the surface, little subcutaneous white fat or brown fat, a large surface area, a limp position, and an immature temperature control center.
- It is important to maintain a neutral thermal environment at all times for infants. The nurse should prevent drafts, use warmed oxygen, and keep incubator doors and portholes closed. When taken out of heating devices, the infant should be wrapped in warmed blankets and wear a hat.
- Preterm infants are subject to increased insensible water losses and have difficulty maintaining fluid balance. Their kidneys do not concentrate or dilute urine as well as those of full-term infants. Intake and output must be carefully measured.
- The fragile skin of a preterm infant is easily damaged. Adhesives or chemicals that could injure the skin should be avoided. Special products designed to prevent injury to the skin should be used.
- Preterm infants are subject to infections because they lack passive antibodies from the mother, have an immature immune system, have fragile skin, and are subjected to many invasive procedures.
- The nurse must watch carefully for signs of pain and use comfort measures, containment, pacifiers, sucrose, breastfeeding, kangaroo care, and medications to alleviate it.
- Infants demonstrate that they are receiving too much stimulation through changes in oxygenation and behavior. The nurse should schedule care to allow rest periods, keep noise to a minimum, and teach parents how to interact with the infant appropriately.
- Preterm infants lack nutrient stores and need more nutrients. They lack coordination in sucking and swallowing and fatigue easily.
- Signs indicating an infant may be ready for nipple feeding include rooting, sucking on a gavage catheter or pacifier, presence of gag reflex, and a respiratory rate less than 60 breaths per minute.
- The nurse can help mothers who wish to breastfeed their preterm infants by teaching them how to use a breast pump and store milk. Nurses provide privacy, give support, explain the infant's behavior, and answer questions about breastfeeding.
- Nurses can increase parents' comfort with their preterm infant by providing information about the infant's condition and characteristics, the NICU, equipment, and infant care. Spending time with parents during visits, offering therapeutic communication and realistic encouragement, and involving parents in care of the infant also help with bonding.
- Preparation for discharge should be started early in the infant's hospital stay. This allows parents to learn gradually and take on increasing responsibility in the care of the infant until they are comfortable with complete care.

## KEY CONCEPTS—cont'd

- Common complications of preterm birth are respiratory distress syndrome, bronchopulmonary dysplasia, intraventricular hemorrhage, retinopathy of prematurity, and necrotizing enterocolitis.
- Infants with postmaturity syndrome may appear thin, with loose skinfolds, cracked and peeling skin, and meconium staining. They can have respiratory difficulties at birth and suffer from hypoglycemia and inadequate temperature regulation.
- Infants with fetal growth restriction may be small-for-gestational-age at birth. In symmetric growth restriction, the infant is proportionately small; in asymmetric growth restriction, the head and length are normal and the body is thin.
- Large-for-gestational-age infants can incur birth injuries such as fractures, nerve damage, or bruising as a result of their size. They may have hypoglycemia or polycythemia.

## REFERENCES AND READINGS


American Academy of Pediatrics & American College of Obstetricians and Gynecologists. (2007). *Guidelines for perinatal care* (6th ed.). Elk Grove Village, IL, and Washington, DC: Author.

American Academy of Pediatrics. (2012). Breastfeeding and the Use of Human Milk. *Pediatrics, 129*(3).

American Academy of Pediatrics & American College of Obstetricians and Gynecologists. (2013). *Guidelines for perinatal care* (8th ed.). Elk Grove Village, IL, and Washington, DC: Author.

Association of Women's Health, Obstetric and Neonatal Nurses. (2015). Breastfeeding. *Journal of Obstetric, Gynecologic, and Neonatal Nursing, 44*(1), 145–150.

Blackburn, S.T. (2013). *Maternal, fetal, and neonatal physiology: A clinical perspective* (4th ed.). St. Louis: Saunders.

Boucher, C.A., Brazal, P.M., Graham-Certosini, C., et al. (2011). Mothers' breastfeeding experiences in the NICU. *Neonatal Network, 30*(1), 21–28.

Boundy, E., Dastjerdi, R., Spiegelman, D., et al. (2016). Kangaroo mother care and neonatal outcomes: a Meta-analysis. *Pediatrics, 137*(1), 1–16.

Boykova, M., & Kenner, C. (2012). Transition from hospital to home for parents of preterm infants. *Journal of Perinatal and Neonatal Nursing, 26*(1), 81–87.

Bradshaw, W.T. (2015). Gastrointestinal disorders. In M.T. Verklan, & M. Walden (Eds.), *AWHONN Core curriculum for neonatal intensive care nursing* (5th ed.). St. Louis: Mosby.

Brown, L., Hendrickson, K., Evans, R., et al. (2015). Enteral nutrition. In S.L. Gardner, B.S. Carter, M. Enzman-Hines, & J. Hernandez (Eds.), *Merenstein & Gardner's handbook of neonatal intensive care* (8th ed.). St. Louis: Mosby.

Cardner, S., & Hernandez, J. (2015). Heat balance. In S.L. Gardner, B.S. Carter, M. Enzman-Hines, & J. Hernandez (Eds.), *Merenstein & Gardner's handbook of neonatal intensive care* (8th ed.). St. Louis: Mosby.

Carlo, W., & Ambalavanan, N. (2011). Respiratory distress syndrome (hyaline membrane disease). In R.M. Kliegman, B.E. Stanton, J.W. St. Geme, et al. (Eds.), *Nelson textbook of pediatrics* (19th ed., pp. 555–564). Philadelphia: Saunders.

Carlo, W. & Ambalavanan, N. (2015). Intracranial-intraventricular hemorrhage and periventricular leukomalacia. In R.M. Kliegman & B.E. Stanton (Eds.) *Nelson textbook of pediatrics* (20th ed., pp. 835-877). Philadelphia: Elsevier.

Centers for Disease Control and Prevention (2013). Progress in increasing breastfeeding and reducing racial/ethnic differences- United States, 2000-2008. *Morbidity & Mortality Weekly Report, 62*, 77–80.

Cleveland, K. (2010). Feeding challenges in the late preterm infant. *Neonatal Network, 29*(1), 37–41.

Ditzenberger, G.R. (2014). Nutritional management. In M.T. Verklan, & M. Walden (Eds.), *AWHONN core curriculum for neonatal intensive care nursing* (5th ed.). St. Louis: Saunders.

Ellard, D., & Anderson, D.M. (2011). Nutrition. In J.P. Cloherty, E.C. Eichenwald, A.R. Hansen, et al. (Eds.), *Manual of neonatal care* (7th ed., pp. 230–262). Philadelphia: Lippincott Williams & Wilkins.

Fernandes, A., Campbell-Yeo, M., & Johnston, C.C. (2011). Procedural pain management for neonates using nonpharmacological strategies. *Advances in Neonatal Care, 11*(4), 235–241.

Gardner, S.L., Enzman-Hines, M., & Argawal, R. (2015). Pain and pain relief. In S.L. Gardner, B.S. Carter, M. Enzman-Hines, & J. Hernandez (Eds.), *Merenstein & Gardner's handbook of neonatal intensive care* (8th ed.). St. Louis: Mosby.

Gardner, S.L., Enzman-Hines, M., & Nip, M. (2015). Respiratory diseases. In S.L. Gardner, B.S. Carter, M. Enzman-Hines, & J. Hernandez (Eds.), *Merenstein & Gardner's handbook of neonatal intensive care* (8th ed.). St. Louis: Mosby.

Gardner, S.L., Goldson, E., & Hernandez, J. (2015). The neonate and the environment: Impact on development. In S.L. Gardner, B.S. Carter, M. Enzman-Hines, & J. Hernandez (Eds.), *Merenstein & Gardner's handbook of neonatal intensive care* (8th ed.). St. Louis: Mosby.

Goodwin, M. (2010). Apnea. In M. T. Verklan, & M. Walden (Eds.), *AWHONN core curriculum for neonatal intensive care nursing* (4th ed., pp. 484–493). St. Louis: Saunders.

Hardy, W. (2011a). Facilitating pain management. *Advances in Neonatal Care, 11*(4), 279–281.

Hardy, W. (2011b). Integration of kangaroo care into routine caregiving in the NICU. *Advances in Neonatal Care, 11*(2), 119–121.

Herrington, C.J., & Chiodo, L.M. (2014). Human touch effectively and safely reduces pain in the newborn intensive care unit. *Pain Management Nursing, 15*(1), 107–115.

Hurst, N.M., & Meier, P. (2010). Breastfeeding the preterm infant. In J. Riordan, & K. Wambach (Eds.), *Breastfeeding and human lactation* (4th ed., pp. 425–468). Sudbury, MA: Jones & Bartlett.

Jana, L.A., & Shu, J. (2011). *Heading home with your newborn: From birth to reality* (2nd ed.). Elk Grove Village, IL: American Academy of Pediatrics.

Kattwinkel, J. (Ed.). (2011). *Textbook of neonatal resuscitation* (6th ed.). Elk Grove Village, IL: American Academy of Pediatrics and American Heart Association.

Kochanek, D.D., Kirmeyer, S.E., Martin, J.A., et al. (2012). Annual summary of vital statistics: 2009. *Pediatrics, 129*(2), 338–348.

Lessen, G.S. (2011). Effect of the premature infant oral motor intervention on feeding progression and length of stay in preterm infants. *Advances in Neonatal Care, 11*(2), 129–139.

Lund, C.H., & Durand, D.J. (2015). Skin and skin care. In S.L. Gardner, B.S. Carter, M. Enzman-Hines, & J. Hernandez (Eds.), *Merenstein & Gardner's handbook of neonatal intensive care* (8th ed.). St. Louis: Mosby.

Lutsive, O., Giglia, L., Pullenayegum, E., et al. (2013). A population-based cohort study of breastfeeding according to gestational age at term delivery. *Journal of Pediatrics, 163*(5), 1283–8.

Maheshwari, A., & Carlo, W.A. (2011). Neonatal necrotizing enterocolitis. In R.M. Kliegman, B.E. Stanton, J.W. St. Geme, et al. (Eds.), *Nelson textbook of pediatrics* (19th ed., pp. 601–603). Philadelphia: Saunders.

Martin, J.A., Hamilton, B.E., Osterman, M.J., et al. (2015). *Births: Final data for 2013.* National vital statistics reports. Retrieved from http://www.cdc.gov.

Munson, M., Saatkamp, R., & West, C. (2011). Late preterm infants: Steps to success. *Neonatal Network, 30*(4), 267–270.

National Association of Neonatal Nurses (2011). *The use of human milk and breastfeeding in the neonatal intensive care unit*. (Position Statement No.3052.). Glenview, IL: Author, (Position Statement No.3052.).

Nightlinger, K. (2011). Developmentally supportive care in the neonatal intensive care unit: An occupational therapist's role. *Neonatal Network, 30*(4), 243–248.

Nyp, M., Brunkhorst, J., Reavey, D., et al. (2015). Fluid and electrolyte management. In S.L. Gardner, B.S. Carter, M. Enzman-Hines, & J. Hernandez (Eds.), *Merenstein & Gardner's handbook of neonatal intensive care* (8th ed.). St. Louis: Mosby.

Pappas, B.E., & Robey, D. (2014). Care of the late preterm infant. In M.T. Verklan, & M. Walden (Eds.), *AWHONN core curriculum for neonatal intensive care nursing* (5th ed.). St. Louis: Saunders.

Parsons, J., Seay, A., & Jacobson, M. (2015). Neurologic disorders. In S.L. Gardner, B.S. Carter, M. Enzman-Hines, & J. Hernandez (Eds.), *Merenstein & Gardner's handbook of neonatal intensive care* (8th ed.). St. Louis: Mosby.

Phillips, R.M., Goldstein, M., Hougland, K., et al. (2013). Multidisciplinary guidelines for the care of late preterm infants. *Journal of Perinatology, 33*(Suppl), S5–S22.

Premji, S., Young, M., Rogers, C., et al. (2012). Transitions in the early-life of late preterm infants: Vulnerabilities and implications for postpartum care. *Journal of Perinatal and Neonatal Nursing, 26*(1), 57–68.

Radtke, J.V. (2011). The paradox of breastfeeding-associated morbidity among late preterm infants. *Journal of Obstetric, Gynecologic and Neonatal Nursing, 40*(1), 9–24.

Sprull, C.T. (2014). Developmental support. In M.T. Verklan, & M. Walden (Eds.), *AWHONN core curriculum for neonatal intensive care nursing* (5th ed.) St. Louis: Saunders.

U.S. Department of Health and Human Services (2010). *Healthy People 2020*. Washington DC: Author.

30

# The High-Risk Newborn: Acquired and Congenital Conditions

http://evolve.elsevier.com/McKinney/mat-ch/

## LEARNING OBJECTIVES

*After studying this chapter, you should be able to:*

- Describe the steps involved in neonatal resuscitation.
- Explain common respiratory problems in the newborn.
- Explain the causes and significance of nonphysiologic jaundice.
- Describe the nursing care of the infant with nonphysiologic jaundice.
- Describe causes of neonatal infections and nursing care for infants with infections.
- Explain the effect of maternal diabetes on the newborn and implications for nursing care.
- Explain hypocalcemia and phenylketonuria and the nursing considerations of each.
- Describe the effect of maternal substance abuse on the newborn and the nursing care.

In addition to the high-risk conditions related to gestational age discussed in Chapter 29, the newborn at risk can have acquired or congenital complications. Acquired conditions are associated with prenatal complications or occur at birth or shortly thereafter.

## RESPIRATORY COMPLICATIONS

Respiratory distress is one of the most common problems of the neonate. It is caused by asphyxia before or during birth, disease of the respiratory system, and other conditions that affect the infant's ability to breathe. The nurse is responsible for evaluation of respiratory status at birth and throughout the hospital stay.

### Asphyxia

Asphyxia is a lack of oxygen and increase of carbon dioxide in the blood. This condition can occur *in utero,* at birth, or later. When asphyxia occurs at birth, it is either the continuation of asphyxia that began before birth or the result of other factors, such as preterm lungs with insufficient surfactant to function adequately.

Lack of oxygen transported to the cells leads to anaerobic metabolism and the production of lactic acid. Metabolic acidosis develops when not enough bicarbonate is available to buffer the accumulating acids. Respiratory acidosis occurs as carbon dioxide accumulates. The partial pressure of carbon dioxide increases in arterial blood ($Paco_2$), and the partial pressure of oxygen ($Po_2$), pH, and bicarbonate levels decrease.

Vasoconstriction caused by low oxygen decreases blood flow to all organs except the brain, myocardium, and adrenal glands. Under such conditions, the ductus arteriosus and foramen ovale can remain open because of the low oxygen in the blood, high resistance to blood flow through constricted pulmonary vessels, and elevated pressure on the right side of the heart. Thus, even circulating blood remains low in oxygen. Progression toward brain injury and death is rapid unless intervention is prompt.

#### Manifestations

If asphyxia occurs after birth, rapid respirations are followed by cessation of respirations (primary apnea) and a rapid fall in heart rate. Stimulation alone or with oxygen can restart respirations. If asphyxia continues without intervention, gasping respirations may resume weakly until the infant enters a period of secondary apnea. In secondary apnea, the oxygen levels in the blood continue to decrease, the infant loses consciousness, and stimulation is ineffective. Resuscitative measures must be initiated immediately to prevent permanent injury to the brain or death. Asphyxia seen at birth may be a continuation of asphyxia that began before or during birth. Therefore it is essential to begin resuscitation without delay.

#### Infants at Risk

Complications during pregnancy, labor, or birth increase the infant's risk for asphyxia. In addition, if the expectant mother receives narcotics shortly before birth, the infant may be too depressed at birth to breathe well spontaneously. Naloxone (Narcan; see Drug Guide) can be given to these infants if they have a normal color and heart rate with depressed respirations and the mother received opiates within 4 hours of the birth.

#### Neonatal Resuscitation

Although 90% of newborns have no difficulty with breathing at birth, approximately 10% require some help to begin respirations, and 1% require extensive resuscitative measures (Kattwinkel, 2011). Therefore, all personnel involved in deliveries should know how to perform resuscitative measures (see Procedure: Performing Resuscitation in Newborns). Equipment should be readily available and functioning properly at all times so there is no delay in starting resuscitation. Nurses begin resuscitation as necessary and assist the physician or nurse practitioner with intubation, insertion of umbilical vein catheters, and administration of medications.

## DRUG GUIDE

### *Naloxone Hydrochloride (Narcan)*

**Classification:** Opiate antagonist.

**Action:** Reverses central nervous system and respiratory depression caused by narcotics (opiates). Competes with narcotics at receptor sites.

**Indications:** Severe respiratory depression in the newborn when the mother has received narcotics within 4 hours of birth.

**Dosage and Route:** Available in 0.2 mg/mL, 0.4 mg/mL, and 1 mg/mL. Dosage for neonates is 0.1 mg/kg. Given via intravenous (IV), intramuscular (IM), subcutaneous, or into an endotracheal tube. IV route is preferred during neonatal resuscitation; IM is acceptable, but action may be delayed. There are no studies of the efficacy of endotracheal tube administration (Kattwinkel, 2011).

**Absorption:** Well absorbed by all routes. Onset of action is 1 to 2 minutes if given via IV.

**Excretion:** Metabolized by the liver and excreted by kidneys.

**Contraindications and Precautions:** Duration of effect is 20 to 60 minutes. The dose may need to be repeated because the opiate may have a longer half-life than naloxone. If given to the infant of a mother addicted to opiates, it will cause withdrawal and can cause seizures. Resuscitative measures should be used as necessary.

**Nursing Considerations:** Note the strength of the medication available when calculating the dose. When depression from opiates is expected, prepare the syringe before birth by drawing up more than is needed. After birth, the excess is removed from the syringe and the amount is given according to the estimate of the infant's weight. Monitor for response, and be prepared to give repeated doses if necessary.

Reference: Kattwinkel, J. (2011). *Textbook of neonatal resuscitation* (6th ed.). Elk Grove Village, IL: American Academy of Pediatrics and American Heart Association.

Maintaining thermoregulation is very important throughout care. A warming pad placed under linens in the radiant warmer provides extra heat. Infants less than 29 weeks of gestation can be placed in a polyethylene bag up to the neck before drying to reduce heat loss from evaporation. The bag also reduces stress from handling during drying. Prevention of hyperthermia is also important (Kattwinkel, 2011).

Some infants develop hypoxic-ischemic encephalopathy after asphyxia. Therapeutic hypothermia has been used to improve neurologic outcomes for these infants. Infants must be 36 or more weeks of gestation, have evidence of an acute perinatal hypoxic-ischemic event, and be in a facility where the treatment can be initiated within 6 hours of birth (Kattwinkel, 2011).

Once the infant is stabilized, the nurse continues to assess for changes. Infants with asphyxia often have other complications such as hypoglycemia, feeding and thermoregulation problems, seizures, hypotension, pulmonary hypertension, metabolic acidosis, renal problems, and fluid and electrolyte imbalances. They need close monitoring and often need intensive nursing care. Communication with the parents is a vital nursing function. Parents need explanations, realistic reassurance, and continued support after the crisis.

## Transient Tachypnea of the Newborn

Infants with **transient tachypnea of the newborn** (TTN) develop rapid respirations soon after birth when inadequate absorption of fetal lung fluid occurs. The condition resolves within 24 to 72 hours. Risk factors include cesarean birth without labor, precipitous delivery, male gender, perinatal asphyxia, and maternal diabetes or asthma. Infants are usually term or late preterm, although some may be preterm.

### Etiology

Although the exact cause of TTN is unknown, it is thought to result from a delay in absorption of fetal lung fluid by the pulmonary capillaries and lymph vessels. This condition causes decreased lung compliance and air trapping and produces signs similar to respiratory distress syndrome (RDS).

### Manifestations

In TTN, respirations of 60 to 120 breaths per minute develop within hours of birth. Retractions, nasal flaring, grunting, and mild cyanosis are present. Chest radiography shows hyperinflation, perihilar streaking showing interstitial fluid along the bronchovascular spaces, and fluid in the fissures between the lobes of the lungs.

### Therapeutic Management

Treatment is supportive and may include oxygen for cyanosis and gavage feedings while the respiratory rate is high to prevent aspiration and conserve energy. Because the signs are similar to those of RDS and sepsis, the infant is observed for those complications. Antibiotics may be given until sepsis is ruled out.

### Nursing Considerations

After identifying signs, the nurse notifies the provider and carries out treatment. General nursing care is similar to that of the respiratory care of the preterm infant (see Chapter 29).

## Meconium Aspiration Syndrome

Meconium-stained amniotic fluid occurs in 10% to 15% of births. **Meconium aspiration syndrome** (MAS), a condition in which there is obstruction, air trapping, and chemical pneumonitis caused by meconium in the infant's lungs, develops in 5% of those infants (Ambalavanan & Carlo, 2011). The condition occurs most often in infants who are postterm, small for gestational age (SGA), and compromised before birth by placental insufficiency or cord compression (Abu-Shaweesh, 2011).

### Etiology

Although the normal fetus can pass meconium, MAS most often occurs when hypoxia causes increased peristalsis of the intestines and relaxation of the anal sphincter before or during labor. MAS develops when meconium in the amniotic fluid enters the lungs during fetal life or at birth. It is drawn into the lungs if gasping movements occur *in utero* as a result of asphyxia and acidosis. When the infant takes the first breaths after birth, meconium in the upper airways can be pulled deep into the respiratory passages.

Obstruction of the airways can be complete or partial. Atelectasis can result if small airways are completely obstructed. In partial obstruction, air can enter but not escape from the alveoli. During inhalation, the bronchioles expand slightly as air flows into them past the meconium. During exhalation, the passages constrict, and meconium blocks movement of air out of the lungs. This ball-valve mechanism results in air trapping. The overdistended alveoli can develop an air leak, with escape of air into the pleural cavity (pneumothorax) or mediastinum (pneumomediastinum). Surfactant production may be inhibited, increasing the respiratory distress. In addition, meconium is irritating to lung tissue and causes an inflammatory reaction and chemical pneumonitis.

Severe MAS develops in only a small number of newborns with meconium below the vocal cords. The addition of meconium to lungs damaged by asphyxia can increase the severity of the condition. Injury from asphyxia interferes with clearing of lung fluid and production of

## PROCEDURE

### *Performing Resuscitation in Newborns*

**Purpose**

To ensure adequate oxygenation of the neonate with asphyxia.

Note: Although this procedure is listed by steps, resuscitation is performed as an integrated process rather than individual steps. Because two or more people often are working together, several steps can be performed at once.

1. Place the infant under a preheated radiant warmer immediately. *Prevention of cold stress is important to prevent increased oxygen need.*
2. Position the infant with the neck slightly extended ("sniffing") position. Place a small rolled blanket under the shoulders to help maintain an open airway. Avoid hyperextension or flexion of the neck. *Proper positioning helps maintain an open airway. Hyperextension or flexion can obstruct the airway.*

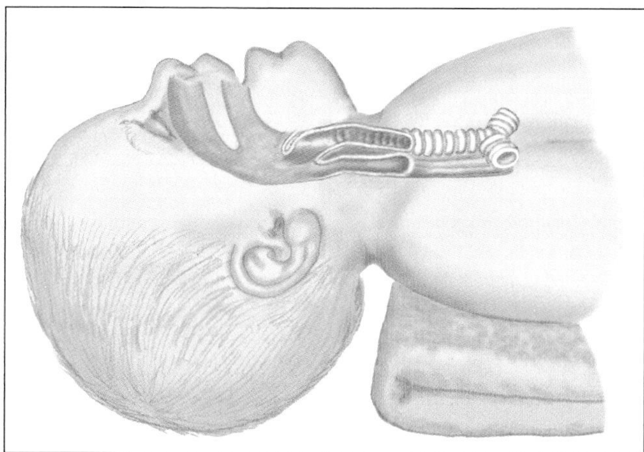

3. Suction the mouth and then the nose. If meconium is present and the infant is vigorous (showing strong respiratory effort, good muscle tone, and heart rate greater than 100 beats per minute [bpm]), suction the mouth and nose, and continue with usual care. If the infant is not vigorous, an endotracheal tube can be used for suction. After suctioning, the endotracheal tube is inserted or placed later, if necessary, to provide an open airway. *Infants often gasp when the nose is suctioned and can aspirate secretions from the mouth into the lungs. Tracheal suctioning removes more meconium in the infant who is not vigorous.*
4. Dry the infant. Remove and replace wet linens. Stimulate the infant if necessary by gently rubbing the back, body, or extremities, or flicking or slapping the soles of the feet. If two people are present, one can dry the infant while the other positions and suctions. Reposition the head as necessary. Positioning, clearing the airway, drying, and stimulation should take no more than 30 seconds. *Drying helps prevent cold stress and increased oxygen need. Removal of wet linens prevents heat loss. The tactile stimulation of drying and suctioning the infant can cause spontaneous respirations. Repositioning may be necessary because the infant has been moved.*
5. If no response occurs after stimulating once or twice, stop and evaluate need for immediate resuscitation. Do not delay resuscitation to continue stimulating or until the Apgar scores are given. *Resuscitation becomes more difficult the longer it is delayed. Apgar scores can be determined without interrupting the resuscitation process.* Also assess scores at 10, 15, and 20 minutes if the score is under 7 at 5 minutes.
6. Evaluate the respirations, heart rate, and color. Count the heart rate by feeling the pulsations at the base of the umbilical cord or using a stethoscope. Count for 6 seconds and multiply by 10 for a quick estimate of the heart rate. *Evaluation helps determine the next steps.*
7. If central cyanosis is present, the infant is breathing, and the heart rate is more than 100 bpm, give supplemental oxygen. Hold a mask or oxygen tubing close to the infant's nose (called "blow by" or "free flow" oxygen) to provide oxygen mixed with room air. Attach a pulse oximeter probe to the infant's right palm or wrist; then, connect the probe to the pulse oximeter. If the infant becomes pink with oxygen, and oximeter readings are 85% to 90%, the oxygen can be gradually removed. *Oxygen will help relieve cyanosis and prevent damage to vital tissues. An oximeter measures oxygen saturation in the blood and helps determine whether the infant is receiving the right amount of oxygen. It is more accurate than assessment of color.*
8. If the term infant fails to breathe spontaneously with initial stimulation, has gasping respirations, a heart rate less than 100 bpm when respirations have begun, or remains cyanotic and has low oxygen saturation with supplemental oxygen, begin positive-pressure ventilation (PPV) with an appropriate-size bag and mask and 21% oxygen (room air). If the infant is preterm, a higher oxygen content may be necessary. The amount of oxygen used is varied as necessary according to the oximeter reading. The mask should rest on the chin and cover the mouth and nose but not the eyes. *PPV ensures oxygen entry into the lungs. An oxygen blender is used to vary the percent of oxygen used. An appropriately-sized mask allows a seal to prevent oxygen from escaping around the sides.*
9. Place the mask snugly over the infant's nose and mouth. Squeeze the bag gently to force air into the infant's lungs. Use a bag with a pressure gauge and a pressure-release valve. Start with a pressure of 20 cm $H_2O$. *A pressure gauge shows the amount of pressure being used. A pressure-release valve opens if the pressure is high enough to cause lung injury.*
10. Ventilate the infant at a rate of 40 to 60 breaths per minute until the infant is breathing spontaneously and the heart rate is above 100 bpm. At that point, PPV is gradually discontinued and free-flow oxygen given. *PPV is adjusted according to the infant's response.*
11. If the heart rate and oxygen saturation do not improve, breath sounds are not heard, and the chest does not move, reposition the mask and the head, and suction secretions. If necessary, gradually increase the pressure until chest movement and bilateral breath sounds are present. If chest expansion is not adequate, an endotracheal tube should be inserted. *The airway must not be occluded by positioning or secretions. Pressure must be high enough to inflate the lungs without causing injury from overinflation. More pressure is needed for the first breaths and for diseased lungs.*
12. If PPV with a mask is necessary for more than a few minutes, insert an 8 Fr feeding tube through the mouth to the stomach. Suction the stomach contents and leave the tube in place and open. *The feeding tube allows air that enters the stomach to escape.*
13. Assess the heart rate, color, muscle tone, and presence of spontaneous breathing. If the heart rate is above 60 bpm after 30 seconds, continue PPV and assess as above every 30 seconds. If the heart rate is less than 60 bpm after 30 seconds of effective assisted ventilation, a second person should begin chest compressions while the first continues to ventilate the infant. An endotracheal tube can be inserted if it has not been placed previously. Increase oxygen to 100%. *Adequate ventilation causes improvement of bradycardia in most infants. Evaluation of the infant's status determines whether ventilation can be discontinued or chest compressions must be added for the infant to survive. The oximeter may not be accurate if the heart rate is below 60 bpm.*

*Continued*

## PROCEDURE—cotn'd

### *Performing Resuscitation in Newborns*

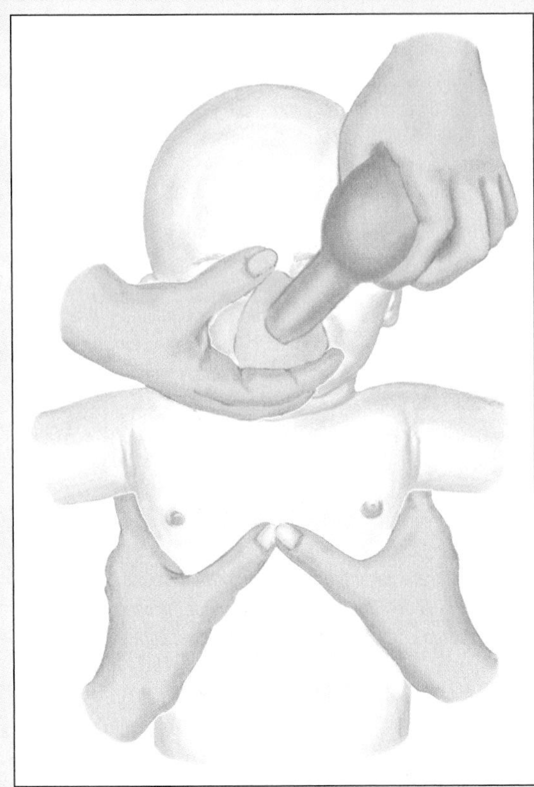

14. Compress the chest by placing the hands around the infant's chest with the fingers under the back to provide support and the thumbs over the lower third of the sternum (below an imaginary line drawn between the nipples and above the xiphoid process). *This method is preferred because it gives more consistent pressure and depth control.* An alternate method is to use two fingers of one hand to compress the chest with the other hand under the back to provide support. *Correct hand position compresses the heart but avoids or minimizes injury to the liver, fractures of the ribs, and pneumothorax. The alternate method may be necessary to allow access to umbilical vessels or for people with small hands.*
15. Compress the sternum to a depth of approximately one third of the anterior-posterior diameter of the chest. Release the pressure between compressions but do not remove the fingers from the chest. The size of the infant determines the depth of compressions. Keep the fingers in contact with the chest at all times *so they do not have to be repositioned each time.*
16. Use three compressions followed by one ventilation for a combined rate of 120 compressions and ventilations each minute. This provides 90 compressions and 30 ventilations each minute. Pause after every third compression (during "breathe-and") for ventilation. Counting "one-and-two-and-three-and-breathe-and-one- ..." may be helpful. *Simultaneous compression and ventilation can interfere with efficacy. The short pause allows air to enter the lungs.*
17. Check the heart rate after at least 45 to 60 seconds of coordinated compressions and ventilation. If it is 60 bpm or more, discontinue compressions but increase PPV to a faster rate of 40 to 60 bpm until the heart rate is more than 100 bpm and spontaneous breathing begins. Then, discontinue PPV slowly. *Periodic evaluation is necessary to ensure that treatment is appropriate to the infant's status.*
18. If the heart rate is less than 60 bpm, an endotracheal tube should be inserted (if not done previously). Recheck to see that ventilation and compressions are being given correctly and 100% oxygen is being used for PPV. *Endotracheal intubation may be necessary to ensure an adequate airway.*
19. An umbilical catheter should be inserted, and epinephrine should be given if the heart rate remains below 60. If necessary, it can be given through an endotracheal tube until intravenous (IV) access is established. IV volume expanders, such as normal saline, Ringer's lactate, or type O Rh-negative packed red blood cells (if severe fetal anemia is expected) can be given. *Epinephrine stimulates the heart. The endotracheal route results in less predictable epinephrine levels. Volume expanders are given for hypovolemic shock from fluid or blood loss.*
20. Naloxone can be given via IV to infants who have normal heart rate and color but continued depressed respirations. It is used only if the mother received opiates within 4 hours of delivery. The intramuscular route is acceptable if necessary but has a delayed onset. *Naloxone counteracts effects of opiates given the mother.*

Data from Kattwinkel, J. (2011). *Textbook of neonatal resuscitation* (6th ed.). Elk Grove Village, IL: American Academy of Pediatrics and American Heart Association.

surfactant and causes pulmonary vasoconstriction that can result in return to fetal circulation patterns. Persistent pulmonary hypertension of the newborn occurs in one-third of infants with MAS (Burris, 2012).

#### Manifestations

Signs of mild to severe respiratory distress are present at birth, with tachypnea, cyanosis, retractions, nasal flaring, grunting, rales, and in severe cases, a barrel-shaped chest from hyperinflation. The infant's nails, skin, and cord may be stained with meconium. Radiography shows atelectasis, consolidation, and hyperexpansion from air trapping.

#### Therapeutic Management

Suctioning the infant as soon as the head is born has not been found to reduce the incidence of MAS. The vigorous infant (good respirations and muscle tone; heart rate above 100 bpm) does not need special suctioning at birth. In infants with depressed respirations and insufficient muscle tone or a heart rate below 100 beats per minute (bpm), an endotracheal tube is used to remove as much meconium as possible (Kattwinkel, 2011).

Some infants only need warmed, humidified oxygen, while others require extensive respiratory support with mechanical ventilation. High-frequency ventilation may be used. Surfactant lavage has been used in severe cases but is controversial (Abu-Shaweesh, 2011). Supportive care is given to meet the problems presented. Infants with severe MAS who do not respond to conventional treatment may benefit from extracorporeal membrane oxygenation (ECMO). ECMO, which is available in some hospitals, oxygenates the blood while bypassing the lungs to allow the infant's lungs to rest temporarily and recover.

#### Nursing Considerations

When meconium is noted in the amniotic fluid during labor, the nurse notifies the primary caregiver so that delivery care can be adapted as necessary. Nurses from the neonatal intensive care unit (NICU) and a neonatologist may be present for the delivery. The nurse ensures that equipment for oxygenation and suction is functioning properly and assists with care at delivery. After the infant's birth, nursing care is adapted as needed. Although meconium is sterile, lung injury promotes the growth of bacteria, and infants should be closely observed for infection. Nursing attention to thermoregulation and decreased stimulation is important.

## Persistent Pulmonary Hypertension of the Newborn

Persistent pulmonary hypertension of the newborn (PPHN) is a condition in which vasoconstriction of pulmonary vessels prevents the normal decrease in vascular resistance of the lungs after birth, impairing the changes in neonatal circulation that should occur. For this reason, the condition is also called *persistent fetal circulation*.

### Etiology

PPHN occurs in infants who are late preterm, preterm, or term. The cause can be abnormal lung development, maternal use of nonsteroidal antiinflammatory drugs or selective serotonin reuptake inhibitors, or unknown. This condition is often associated with hypoxemia and acidosis from asphyxia, meconium aspiration, sepsis, polycythemia, diaphragmatic hernia, and RDS (Ambalavanan & Carlo, 2011).

Inadequate oxygenation results in vasoconstriction, instead of the normal dilation, of the pulmonary artery and small pulmonary vessels, increasing resistance in the lungs. The elevated pulmonary vascular resistance causes a rise in pressure on the right side of the heart. This results in a right-to-left shunt of unoxygenated blood that flows through the foramen ovale. In addition, unoxygenated blood from the pulmonary artery flows through the ductus arteriosus to the aorta. Thus, blood bypasses the lungs, as occurs during fetal circulation. Metabolic acidosis causes more pulmonary vasoconstriction, further worsening the condition.

### Manifestations

Infants with PPHN develop signs within the first 24 hours after birth. Tachypnea, respiratory distress, and progressive cyanosis often become worse with handling. Oxygen saturation and partial pressure of oxygen in arterial blood ($Pao_2$) are decreased, $Paco_2$ is increased, and acidosis is present. Other signs may result from associated conditions. An echocardiogram demonstrates shunting.

### Therapeutic Management

Management involves treating the underlying cause and relieving pulmonary vasoconstriction. Arterial pH can be increased with respiratory and drug therapy to cause pulmonary vasodilation. Sedation, high-frequency ventilation, surfactant therapy, and inhaled nitric oxide (which dilates pulmonary vessels) may be necessary. If other therapies fail, ECMO can be helpful.

### Nursing Considerations

Nursing care is similar to care of other infants with severe respiratory disease. Because infants with PPHN become hypoxic with activity and other stimuli, handling and noise are kept to a minimum. Attention to thermoregulation and assessment for hypoglycemia, hypocalcemia, anemia, and metabolic acidosis is important.

# HYPERBILIRUBINEMIA

Jaundice is a common concern in caring for neonates. Conjugation of bilirubin and physiologic jaundice are discussed in Chapter 21. Nonphysiologic or pathologic jaundice is discussed here.

Jaundice becomes visible when the total serum bilirubin (TSB) reaches 5 to 6 mg/dL (Blackburn, 2013). Jaundice is considered abnormal or nonphysiologic when TSB rises more rapidly and to higher levels than is expected or stays elevated for longer than normal. Charts showing the expected rise and fall of bilirubin according to infant age in hours are used to identify infants who need treatment for rising TSB.

Nonphysiologic jaundice may be seen in the first 24 hours of life. This condition is a concern because it can lead to bilirubin encephalopathy, a condition caused by bilirubin toxicity. Chronic and permanent effects of bilirubin toxicity (kernicterus) can occur. In kernicterus, bilirubin deposits cause yellowish staining of the brain, especially the basal ganglia, cerebellum, hippocampus, and brainstem.

Although bilirubin encephalopathy and kernicterus are rare today because of improved treatment measures, the mortality and morbidity rate of affected infants is high. Those who survive may have cerebral palsy, intellectual impairment, hearing loss, or more subtle long-term neurologic and developmental problems. The exact level at which bilirubin encephalopathy develops is unknown. The toxic level may not be the same for all infants. It occurs at lower TSB levels and is more severe in infants who have complications or are preterm, late preterm, or low birth weight than in healthy, full-term infants.

### Etiology

The most common cause of pathologic jaundice is hemolytic disease of the newborn resulting from incompatibility between the blood of the mother and that of the fetus. The best known cause is Rh incompatibility, in which the Rh-negative mother forms antibodies when Rh-positive blood from the fetus enters her circulation (see Chapter 25). Antibodies develop during a previous pregnancy or after injury, abortion, amniocentesis, or a transfusion of Rh-positive blood. The antibodies cross the placenta and destroy fetal red blood cells. Excessive hemolysis causes erythroblastosis fetalis, a condition involving agglutination and hemolysis of fetal erythrocytes from incompatibility between fetal and maternal blood types.

Infants with erythroblastosis fetalis are anemic from destruction of red blood cells. Severely affected infants can develop hydrops fetalis, a severe anemia that results in heart failure and generalized edema. Intrauterine fetal transfusions can be given. After birth, phototherapy and exchange transfusions are used to prevent kernicterus (Gruslin & Moore, 2011). Use of $Rh_o(D)$ immune globulin, such as RhoGAM, to prevent the mother from forming antibodies against Rh-positive blood has greatly decreased the incidence of erythroblastosis fetalis.

ABO incompatibility also causes pathologic jaundice. Mothers with type O blood have natural antibodies to types A and B blood. The antibodies cross the placenta and cause hemolysis of fetal red blood cells. However, the destruction is much less severe than with Rh incompatibility and causes milder signs.

Other causes of nonphysiologic jaundice include infection, hypothyroidism, glucuronyl transferase deficiency, polycythemia, glucose-6-phosphate dehydrogenase deficiency, and biliary atresia. Infants of diabetic mothers are more likely to develop nonphysiologic jaundice, especially if they have macrosomia. Any condition that causes destruction of erythrocytes or impairment of the liver can result in elevated bilirubin levels.

### Therapeutic Management

The focus of therapeutic management is prevention of bilirubin encephalopathy and kernicterus. The cause is determined by history and diagnostic tests to identify infections or blood abnormalities. During pregnancy, an Rh-negative expectant mother will have an indirect Coombs test to identify the presence of antibodies against fetal blood. If the test is positive, amniocentesis can determine the fetal Rh factor and the degree of hyperbilirubinemia (see Chapter 25).

When infants are jaundiced, the cord blood is used in a direct Coombs test to determine the infant's blood type. A positive Coombs test indicates that antibodies from the mother have attached to the infant's red blood cells. TSB levels are followed closely to detect changes indicating that treatment should be initiated or changed.

Nurses often assess infants for changes in jaundice. However, visual inspection for jaundice is not an accurate way to determine the true bilirubin level. Other tests can be used to reduce the number of blood draws the infant must have. Transcutaneous bilirubinometers are hand-held devices that measure skin color to determine transcutaneous bilirubin (TcB) levels. These noninvasive tests allow frequent checks of jaundice with no discomfort to the infant. However, they may not be accurate in preterm infants, infants receiving phototherapy, or if TSB levels are above 15 mg/dL (Grabenhenrich, Grabenhenrich, Bührer, et al, 2014).

### Phototherapy

Phototherapy is the most common treatment of jaundice and involves placing the infant under special lights. During phototherapy, bilirubin in the skin absorbs the light and changes into water-soluble products, the most important of which is lumirubin. These products do not require conjugation by the liver and can be excreted in the bile and urine. Because preterm infants are more vulnerable to bilirubin toxicity, phototherapy is begun at lower TSB levels than for full-term infants.

Phototherapy can be delivered in several ways. A bank of fluorescent lamps or "bili lights" can be placed above the infant, whether in an incubator, under a radiant warmer to maintain heat, or in an open crib. The infant wears only a diaper to ensure maximal exposure of the skin. The diaper is removed if the TSB is becoming dangerously high. The eyes are closed and patches placed over them to prevent injury. More than one bank of lights can be used if the bilirubin level is high.

Other options for phototherapy include light-emitting diodes (LEDs), halogen lamps, and fiberoptic phototherapy blankets. The LED device is placed above the infant as with fluorescent lights. The LED is long lasting and does not generate excessive heat. The halogen spotlight is used alone or with other lamps. The infant can be swaddled with a fiberoptic phototherapy blanket against the skin; such treatment does not require patches over the eyes. With the blanket, the mother can hold the infant without interfering with therapy. The blanket can be combined with phototherapy lights.

Side effects of phototherapy include frequent loose green stools resulting from increased bile flow and peristalsis. The stools can injure the skin and cause fluid loss. Insensible water loss is increased as well. A 25% increase in fluid intake is needed during phototherapy (Kaplan, Wong, Sibley, et al., 2011). Bronze baby syndrome, a grayish brown discoloration of the skin and urine, occurs in some infants with cholestatic jaundice. A macular skin rash can occur. The color changes and rash disappear gradually when phototherapy is completed.

TSB determinations are performed frequently to show the effectiveness of treatment and when it can be discontinued. When phototherapy is discontinued, TSB should be monitored for 24 hours to ensure further phototherapy is not necessary. Explain to parents that the infants often have an elevation in bilirubin after phototherapy ends and that the healthcare provider may order additional blood tests after discharge.

### Exchange Transfusions

Exchange transfusions are seldom necessary but are performed when phototherapy cannot reduce dangerously high bilirubin levels quickly enough. This treatment removes sensitized red blood cells, maternal antibodies, and unconjugated bilirubin and corrects severe anemia.

***Procedure.*** During the exchange transfusion, small portions of blood are removed and replaced with an equal amount of donor blood. The total volume administered is double the infant's blood volume. When an immediate transfusion is needed for Rh incompatibility, type O, Rh-negative blood cross-matched against the mother and infant is used. In ABO incompatibility, type O, Rh-negative (or Rh-compatible with the mother and infant) packed red blood cells with type AB plasma are used so that there are no anti-A or anti-B antibodies present (Gregory, Martin, & Cloherty, 2012).

At the end of the transfusion, approximately 85% of the infant's red blood cells have been replaced, and the bilirubin level is reduced by 50% (Kaplan et al., 2011). When the level in the blood decreases, bilirubin from the tissues moves into the plasma. This rebound elevation of bilirubin may necessitate repeat transfusions, but phototherapy is generally adequate to resolve it.

***Complications.*** Complications of exchange transfusions include electrolyte and acid-base imbalance, hypocalcemia, infection, hypoglycemia, necrotizing enterocolitis, cardiac dysrhythmias, hemorrhage, thrombosis, and thrombocytopenia. Samples of the blood are analyzed for complete blood count (CBC), bilirubin and calcium levels, and other tests as needed.

***Role of the nurse.*** The nurse's role during exchange transfusion is to prepare equipment, assess the infant during and after the procedure, and keep accurate records. A cardiac monitor is attached to the infant, and a radiant heater provides warmth. The nurse must clarify any misunderstandings that the parents may have about the treatment and help allay their anxiety.

## NURSING CARE

### The Infant With Hyperbilirubinemia

Although collaborative care of the infant with jaundice is an important part of the nurse's role, several nursing diagnoses are appropriate. Risk for Injury is discussed in this section. The nursing diagnosis Risk for Deficient Fluid Volume is discussed in the Nursing Care Plan: The Infant with Jaundice.

#### Assessment

Assess the level of jaundice at least every 8 hours by pressing the skin over a bony prominence and noting the color in the area before the blood returns. Assess the skin with phototherapy lights turned off because they distort the skin color. In infants with dark skin, assess the color of the conjunctivae of the eyes, palate, and oral mucous membranes. Determine the areas of the body affected by the jaundice, and document carefully for comparison during future assessments. Jaundice begins at the head and moves down the body as the bilirubin levels rise. Keep in mind that visual assessment is not an accurate method of assessing true bilirubin levels. Monitor TcB and laboratory TSB levels for change.

Assess for risk factors that might further increase bilirubin levels. Note temperature fluctuations, hypoglycemia, and infection. Determine the infant's oral intake and number of stools.

#### Nursing Diagnosis and Planning

Nurses can do many things to prevent situations that might cause further rises in bilirubin. They must also protect the infant from injury from the light during phototherapy. The nursing diagnosis is:

- Risk for Injury related to preventable causes of further elevation of bilirubin or injury to the eyes secondary to phototherapy.

## NURSING CARE PLAN

### *The Infant With Jaundice*

**Focused Assessment**

Holly, a 2-day-old full-term infant born by cesarean is jaundiced secondary to ABO incompatibility and is receiving phototherapy. She weighs 3.2 kg (7 lb, 1 oz), and her mucous membranes appear slightly dry. Skin turgor is good with quick recoil, and the anterior fontanel is flat. Urine appears slightly dark. She had three loose green stools with no water ring on this shift. She is a sleepy infant who takes formula poorly. Valerie, her mother, appears tired and frustrated with her infant's slow eating behavior.

**Nursing Diagnosis**

Risk for Deficient Fluid Volume related to inadequate oral intake to meet needs of increased insensible water loss and frequent loose stools.

**Planning**

***Expected Outcomes***

Within 24 hours, Holly will:

1. Take at least 191 to 320 mL of fluid per day 60 to 100 mL/kg (27 to 45 mL/lb) to meet normal needs.
2. Show adequate hydration (moist mucous membranes, elastic skin turgor, flat fontanels, pale yellow urine, and at least three wet diapers daily).

**Interventions and *Rationales***

1. Instruct Valerie to feed her infant every 2 to 3 hours. Feed Holly in the nursery at night or when Valerie needs rest, if she prefers.
   *Adequate intake of breast milk or formula is needed to meet the infant's nutrient and fluid needs and ensure excretion of bilirubin in the stools. The mother's needs for rest must be met without interfering with the infant's needs.*
2. Explain to Valerie that Holly needs frequent feedings to help her pass stools that contain the bilirubin that causes her jaundice.
   *The mother's understanding of the reasons will increase her willingness to work with the infant.*
3. Observe Valerie feeding Holly and offer suggestions as needed. Show her how to awaken the infant by unwrapping and gentle stimulation. Try warming the formula slightly. Use a pacifier or insert a gloved finger into the infant's mouth to elicit the suck reflex before feedings.
   *Observation of feedings may identify problems. A wide-awake infant is more likely to feed well. Some infants prefer warm milk. Nonnutritive sucking may help the infant suck effectively during feedings.*
4. Tell the parents about the need for frequent feeding to provide added fluid, protein, and other nutrients.
   *Infants receiving phototherapy have an increased insensible water loss. Albumin (protein) is necessary to carry bilirubin to the liver for conjugation. Heightened intestinal motility decreases absorption of nutrients.*
5. Avoid offering water or dextrose water. Use breast milk or formula instead.
   *Water supplements can decrease milk intake. Milk increases excretion of bilirubin in stools, but water does not have the same effect.*
6. If water loss appears excessive, weigh the diapers and check the specific gravity of the urine. Urine output should be 2 to 5 mL/kg/hr, which is a total of 154 to 384 mL/day for Holly. Specific gravity should be 1.002 to 1.01 for full-term infants.
   *Weighing the diapers and checking specific gravity will identify inadequate output and dehydration early. The wet diaper weight in grams minus the weight of a dry diaper equals the milliliters of urine.*
7. Use therapeutic communication techniques to help Valerie vent her frustrations. Offer praise for her attempts to feed her infant.
   *Helping the mother cope with her feelings helps her meet the infant's needs. Praise increases her concept of herself as a "good mother."*
8. Before discharge, teach the parents to call the physician if the infant has increasing jaundice, fewer than six wet diapers daily, poor feeding, is lethargic or irritable, or has other changes in behavior.
   *Increases in bilirubin may occur after discharge, and the parents should know when to call the physician.*

**Evaluation**

Holly drinks a total of 224 mL (7.5 oz) of formula during 24 hours. Valerie is able to wake the infant, who begins to suck more vigorously. Her mucous membranes are moist, and there are eight diapers with pale yellow urine during the 24 hours.

***Additional Nursing Diagnoses to Consider***

Impaired Skin Integrity
Anxiety
Impaired Parenting
Ineffective Thermoregulation

***Expected outcomes.*** The infant will avoid injury resulting from increased bilirubin or exposure of the skin or eyes secondary to the use of phototherapy lights.

### Interventions

***Maintaining a neutral thermal environment.*** Prevent situations such as cold stress or hypoglycemia that could result in increased fatty acids in the blood caused by acidosis. Increased fatty acids decrease the availability of albumin-binding sites for unconjugated bilirubin. Prevent cold stress at birth and during all care by maintaining the infant in a neutral thermal environment. Check the infant's axillary temperature every 2 to 4 hours to identify an early decrease before it becomes a problem. Dress the infant in warmed clothes and blankets on removal from phototherapy lights.

Prevent elevation of the infant's temperature from exposure to the heat of the "bili lights." Position the lights according to the manufacturer's guidelines to prevent overheating the infant. Use a skin probe when the infant is in an incubator or radiant warmer to maintain the appropriate settings for the infant's needs.

***Providing optimal nutrition.*** Ensure that the infant receives feedings every 2 to 3 hours, whether by breast or bottle. Breastfeeding should not be stopped because the infant is receiving phototherapy. Provide extra support for breastfeeding mothers. Frequent feedings prevent hypoglycemia, provide protein to maintain the albumin level in the blood, and promote gastrointestinal motility and prompt removal of bilirubin in the stools.

Avoid offering water, because the infant may decrease intake of milk, which is more effective in removing bilirubin from the intestines. If breastfeeding must be supplemented, use formula instead of water. Weigh the infant twice a day and monitor intake and output to identify dehydration early and intervene appropriately.

***Protecting the eyes.*** Provide patches to protect the eyes from retinal injury from the phototherapy lights (Fig. 30.1). To avoid abrasions to the cornea, close the infant's eyes before placing the patches.

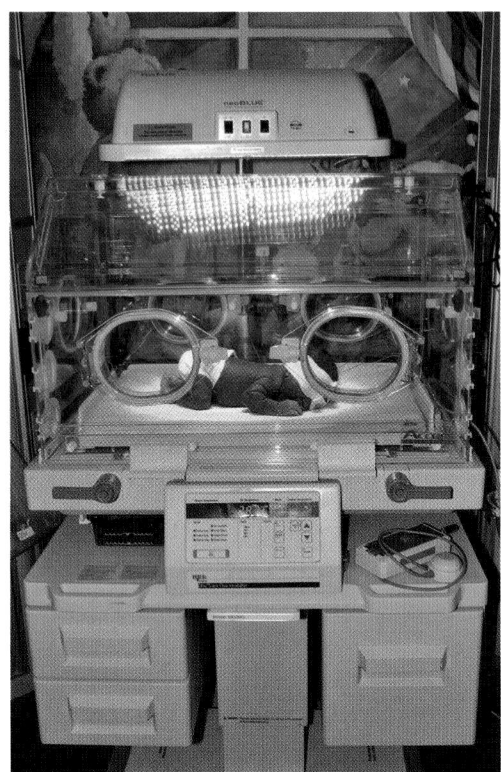

FIG 30.1 The infant receiving phototherapy is wearing eye patches to protect the eyes. (Courtesy Cheryl Briggs, RNC, Annapolis, MD.)

Check the position of the patches at least every hour. Infants can dislodge the patches so that they do not cover the eyes, press too hard on the eyes, or compress the nose and interfere with breathing. Turn off the lights and remove the patches to assess for skin irritation around and under the patches at least every 4 hours.

*Enhancing response to therapy.* Position the lights the proper distance away from the infant. Lights that are too close risk burning the skin. Lights too far away from the infant will not be effective in reducing jaundice. Halogen lights must be placed farther away from the infant than other lights to prevent burning. Follow the manufacturer's instructions regarding light placement. Although phototherapy increases insensible water loss from the skin, avoid the use of creams or lotions on the infant's skin because they might cause burning.

Use a light meter to check the level of irradiance (energy output) to be sure the apparatus is functioning properly and to determine whether the bulbs need replacement. Check laboratory reports of TSB levels to determine the effectiveness of treatment and when it can be discontinued.

Expose as much skin as possible to the light. Remove all clothing except a diaper. Turn the infant every 2 hours to expose all areas evenly and prevent skin irritation. If a fiberoptic blanket is used, check the position frequently. Infants sometimes need to be repositioned to keep the blanket in contact with the skin.

*Detecting complications.* Observe for other complications. Although bilirubin encephalopathy is rare today, monitor for signs that indicate its presence. Signs include lethargy, increased or poor muscle tone, poor feeding, decreased or absent Moro reflex, high-pitched cry, opisthotonos, and seizures.

*Teaching parents.* Explain care to parents, who may be frightened to see their infant in an incubator with the eyes covered. Explaining the causes of jaundice and the purpose of phototherapy will decrease their worry. Removing the infant from phototherapy for feeding and interaction with the parents for periods up to an hour at a time does not decrease the effectiveness of phototherapy (Kaplan et al., 2011). Explain the importance of minimizing further interruptions to phototherapy.

Note the presence of rashes or changes in the color of the skin, and inform parents that they are not harmful and will disappear when phototherapy is discontinued.

When the infant is discharged, explain the need for follow-up laboratory work and visits to the healthcare provider. Teach parents how to assess for further jaundice and signs of complications and when to call the healthcare provider. Explain that most infants have no further problem with jaundice.

#### Evaluation

- Is the infant free of signs of injury?
- Are the eyes protected from injury from the phototherapy lights?

### CRITICAL THINKING EXERCISE 30.1

Why is it important to remove the patches from the eyes each time the infant is taken from the phototherapy lights for feeding or when parents visit?

## INFECTION

Nurses must be constantly alert for signs of infection in neonates. Up to 10% of infants develop infections in the first month of life (Stoll, 2011).

### Transmission of Infection

Newborns can acquire infections before, during, or after birth. Vertical infection is acquired from the mother before or during birth. Organisms, such as those causing rubella, cytomegalovirus, syphilis, human immunodeficiency virus (HIV), and toxoplasmosis, can pass across the placenta and cause infection during pregnancy. During labor and birth, organisms in the vagina, such as group B streptococci (GBS), herpes, and hepatitis, can enter the uterus after rupture of membranes or infect the infant during passage through the birth canal. Horizontal infection occurs after birth from contact with hospital staff members, contaminated equipment (health-care associated or nosocomial infections), or from family members or visitors. An example is staphylococcal infection.

Some of the most common infections and their effects on the neonate are listed in Table 30.1. Other infections are discussed in Chapter 26.

### Sepsis Neonatorum

Infection that occurs during or after birth can cause sepsis neonatorum, a systemic infection from bacteria in the bloodstream. Newborns are particularly susceptible to sepsis because their immune systems are immature and they react more slowly to invasion by organisms. Newborns and especially preterm infants have fewer antibodies and are unable to localize infection as well as older children. This inability allows the infection to spread easily from one organ to another. In addition, the blood-brain barrier is less effective in keeping out organisms, and central nervous system infection can result.

#### Etiology

Common causative agents of neonatal sepsis include GBS, *Escherichia coli,* coagulase negative *Staphylococcus, Staphylococcus aureus, Haemophilus influenzae,* and *Candida albicans* (Wilson & Tyner, 2014;

**TABLE 30.1 Common Infections in the Newborn**

| Transmission | Effect on Newborn | Nursing Considerations |
|---|---|---|
| **Viral Infections** | | |
| ***Cytomegalovirus*** | | |
| Transplacental, during birth, in breast milk. | Most asymptomatic at birth. SGA, FGR, enlarged liver, jaundice, CNS abnormalities, learning impairment, hearing loss, purpura, chorioretinitis, thrombocytopenia, microcephaly, seizures. Can have no signs for months or years. | Diagnosed by pharyngeal or urine culture. Can shed virus in saliva and urine for years. Antiviral drug therapy is used but has toxic effects and is not recommended routinely. Treatment supportive. |
| ***Hepatitis B*** | | |
| Usually during birth through contact with maternal blood. Also transplacental; in breast milk. | Asymptomatic at birth. LBW, prematurity. Most of those infected become chronic carriers. Risk of later liver cancer. | Wash well to remove all maternal blood before infant's skin is punctured for any reason. After cleaning, administer hepatitis B immune globulin (HBIG) and hepatitis B vaccine to prevent infection. May breastfeed if infant receives vaccine and HBIG. |
| ***Herpes*** | | |
| Usually during birth through infected vagina or ascending infection after rupture of membranes. Transplacental rarely. Transmission highest with primary infection. | Clusters of vesicles, temperature instability, lethargy, poor suck, seizures, encephalitis, jaundice, purpura. Death or severe neurologic impairment is likely with disseminated infection.<br>High mortality and morbidity if untreated. | Contact precautions. Obtain specimens of lesions for culture. Antiviral drugs given to mother during pregnancy. Acyclovir given to treat infant after birth. Breastfeeding OK if no lesions on the breasts. |
| ***Human Immunodeficiency Virus or Acquired Immunodeficiency Syndrome*** | | |
| Transplacental, during birth from infected blood and secretions, or from breast milk. Transmission rate is much lower if mother takes antiretroviral drugs during pregnancy and if birth is by cesarean before rupture of membranes. | Asymptomatic at birth, signs usually apparent at 12–24 months: enlarged liver and spleen, lymphadenopathy, failure to thrive, pneumonia, persistent *Candida* and bacterial infections, diarrhea, meningitis, septic joints. | Diagnosis can be delayed because of maternal antibodies. Some early tests available. Wash early to remove blood before infant's skin is punctured. Treat with zidovudine, other antiretroviral drugs, and prophylaxis against other infections. Advise against breastfeeding. |
| ***Rubella*** | | |
| Transplacental. | Spontaneous abortion, asymptomatic or FGR, cataracts, cardiac defects, deafness, microcephaly, intellectual impairment, jaundice. Injury greatest if infected in first trimester. | Contact precautions. Infant can shed virus for 1 year after birth. Diagnosed by presence of antibody and virus. Treatment supportive. |
| ***Varicella-Zoster Virus (Chickenpox, Shingles)*** | | |
| Transplacental. | Congenital varicella syndrome (skin scarring, limb hypoplasia, CNS and eye abnormalities, severe intellectual impairment, death). Highest incidence if between 13th and 20th wk of gestation. Severe effects with maternal infection between 5 days before and 2 days after birth. | Varicella immune globulin for pregnant women exposed in pregnancy or for infants of mothers infected just before or after delivery. It modifies but does not prevent infection. Acyclovir to treat. Strict isolation precautions for mothers and infants with lesions. |
| **Other Infections** | | |
| ***Group B Streptococcal Infection*** | | |
| During birth or ascending after rupture of membranes. | Sudden onset of respiratory distress in infant usually well at birth, temperature instability, pneumonia, meningitis, shock. May have early or late onset. | Early identification essential to prevent death. Treatment of infected mothers during labor has decreased neonatal infection. IV antibiotics given to infected infants. |
| ***Gonorrhea*** | | |
| Usually during birth. | Conjunctivitis (ophthalmia neonatorum), with red, edematous lids and purulent eye drainage. May result in blindness if untreated. | All infants receive prophylactic treatment. Erythromycin eye ointment is most common. Infected infants are treated with IV antibiotics. |

*Continued*

TABLE 30.1 **Common Infections in the Newborn—cont'd**

| Transmission | Effect on Newborn | Nursing Considerations |
|---|---|---|
| ***Chlamydial Infection*** | | |
| During birth. | Conjunctivitis 1-2 wk after birth, pneumonia 4-11 wk after birth, otitis media, bronchiolitis. | Erythromycin eye ointment given to all infants minimizes conjunctivitis but does not affect pneumonia. Pneumonia treated with oral erythromycin. Ophthalmic erythromycin for conjunctivitis. |
| ***Candidiasis*** | | |
| During vaginal birth. | White patches in mouth (thrush) that bleed if removed. Rash on perineum. Can be systemic in preterm or LBW. | Administer nystatin drops or cream, and teach parents how to administer them. Assess mother for vaginal or breast infection. IV antifungal drugs for systemic infection. |
| ***Toxoplasmosis*** | | |
| Transplacental. | Asymptomatic or LBW, preterm, FGR, thrombocytopenia, enlarged liver and spleen, jaundice, cerebral calcifications, encephalitis, seizures, microcephaly, hydrocephalus, chorioretinitis. Signs may not develop for years. | Consider in infants with FGR. Confirmed by serum tests. Treatment: spiramycin during pregnancy. Pyrimethamine, sulfadiazine, and folinic acid for 1 year for the infant. |
| ***Syphilis*** | | |
| Transplacental. | Spontaneous abortion, stillbirth, asymptomatic or enlarged liver and spleen, jaundice, hepatitis, anemia, rhinitis, pink or copper-colored peeling rash, pneumonitis, periostitis, osteochondritis, CNS involvement. | Diagnosed by blood and cerebrospinal fluid testing. Treated with penicillin. |

NOTE: Standard Precautions for infection control apply to all patients and are not listed in this table.
*CNS,* Central nervous system; *FGR,* fetal growth restriction; *IV,* intravenous; *LBW,* low birth weight; *SGA,* small for gestational age.

Edwards, 2011). Sepsis is categorized as early or late onset according to when the signs of disease begin.

Early onset sepsis is acquired during birth, often from complications of labor such as prolonged rupture of membranes, prolonged labor, or chorioamnionitis. Onset is usually in the first 72 hours but can be as late as 7 days after birth. This rapidly developing, multisystem illness has high mortality and morbidity rates. Pneumonia and meningitis are commonly seen.

Late-onset sepsis generally develops after the first week of life. It is acquired during or after birth, before or after hospital discharge. Infection is localized, as with meningitis, and serious long-term effects are common.

### Therapeutic Management

***Diagnostic testing.*** Neonatal sepsis can be confused with other illnesses. For example, group B streptococcal pneumonia has the same initial symptoms as RDS. Diagnostic testing helps identify sepsis and the organisms responsible. For sepsis, a CBC with differential will show decreased total neutrophils, increased bands (immature neutrophils), an increased ratio of immature neutrophils to total neutrophils, and decreased platelets. While newborns normally have a higher leukocyte level than older infants or children, a sudden rise or fall in leukocyte levels is abnormal.

The presence of elevated immunoglobulin M (IgM) levels in cord blood or in the neonate shortly after birth indicates that infection was acquired *in utero,* because this immunoglobulin does not cross the placenta. IgM elevation often indicates transplacental infection.

C-reactive protein (CRP) levels may be elevated, a sign of an inflammatory process. Serial tests of CRP are often performed to check for rise and then fall as infection improves. Cultures of the blood, urine, cerebrospinal fluid, or any skin lesions may be obtained. Cultures of the nasopharynx, the cord, and gastric aspirate usually show colonization with organisms but not infection. Chest radiography helps differentiate between RDS and sepsis. Blood glucose levels should be checked because they can be unstable (high or low) in sepsis.

Infants who appear well, are at least 37 weeks of gestation, and had amniotic membranes ruptured less than 18 hours before birth are observed for 48 hours or more after birth if their mothers received treatment during labor for GBS. Infants of mothers who did not receive antibiotics during labor yet who seem well but are less than 37 weeks of gestation or with membranes ruptured over 18 hours receive a blood culture, CBC, and observation only.

***Treatment.*** Broad-spectrum antibiotics are given intravenously until culture and sensitivity results are available. Continued antibiotic therapy is based on culture results. Commonly used antibiotics include ampicillin, aminoglycosides, and cephalosporins. Vancomycin is used also. Intravenous (IV) immunoglobulins are being studied for use in preterm infants.

Other care is supportive to meet the infant's specific needs. Infants sometimes require oxygen and mechanical ventilation. They may need treatment for shock, hypoglycemia or hyperglycemia, electrolyte and acid-base imbalances, and problems in temperature regulation.

### Nursing Considerations

#### *Assessment*

**Risk factors.** The nurse should identify infants at risk for infection. Prematurity and low birth weight are important risk factors.

Preterm infants of less than 32 weeks of gestation have a 4 to 25 times greater risk of infection (Wilson & Tyner, 2014).

Infants of mothers who have rupture of membranes longer than 18 hours have an increased risk of infection (Venkatesh, Adams, & Weisman, 2011). Other risk factors for sepsis include prolonged or precipitous labor, signs of maternal infection before or during labor, and chorioamnionitis. The nurse needs to identify women known to have GBS and those who show signs of infection so they can be treated with antibiotics during labor to reduce risk to the infant.

Any infant in the NICU is at risk for healthcare–associated infections. These infants have complications, such as prematurity, that make them more susceptible to infection. The risk of infection increases with decreasing gestational age and birth weight. Preterm infants have not received maternal antibodies to help protect them from infection. In addition, they sometimes spend prolonged periods in the NICU, where they are exposed to many invasive procedures (e.g., the use of IV catheters and endotracheal tubes) that increase their risk of infection. Catheter-related blood stream infections are a significant problem in NICUs.

**Signs of infection.** In the newborn, early signs of infection are often subtle and could indicate other conditions. There may be temperature instability, respiratory problems, and changes in feeding habits or behavior. Other than the parents, the nurse is the only person who spends significant time with the infant, and thus, is able to identify early subtle changes in behavior that can indicate sepsis. Experienced nurses may have a feeling that the infant is not doing well even before specific signs of infection are present. When this occurs, the nurse expands the assessment and watches carefully for the development of other signs. Early identification and treatment are important because infants can develop septic shock with little warning.

*Nursing interventions*

**Preventing infection.** Although it is not always possible to prevent infection, every effort should be made to do so. Careful and frequent handwashing is the most important aspect of infection prevention. The nurse should practice and teach parents to use good handwashing or hospital-provided hand disinfectants before and after touching infants. Equipment must be disinfected according to hospital protocols. Meticulous sterile technique must be used during invasive procedures. Invasive procedures should be kept to the lowest number possible.

The skin is delicate in the newborn and particularly so in preterm infants. Handling and trauma to the skin should be minimized as much as possible to prevent skin breakdown and infection.

Transmission of infection to other infants in the nursery is prevented by handwashing, separation of infants' supplies, and Standard Precautions for infection control. Placing the infant in an incubator provides a physical separation between infected and well infants, similar to placing adults in isolation in private rooms.

**Providing antibiotics.** Because signs of infection are nonspecific and the disease can be fatal, physicians may order antibiotics before an actual diagnosis is made for infants who are at high risk or show early signs. Broad-spectrum IV antibiotics are given after samples for culture are obtained and before the results are known. Continued antibiotic therapy is based on the organisms found in cultures. The nurse must be knowledgeable about the specific antibiotics used and possible side effects.

The nurse starts the IV fluids and ensures that medications are administered on time. If more than one antibiotic is ordered, the timing of administration must be coordinated to increase effectiveness. Laboratory analysis of peak and trough levels indicate blood levels of medications at the times when they are expected to be the highest and lowest. Changes in dosage are based on the results of the laboratory tests. Antibiotics are usually continued for 10 to 14 days for sepsis and 21 days for meningitis (Wilson & Tyner, 2014).

**Providing other supportive care.** Critically ill infants need intensive nursing care. Care involves the use of oxygen or other respiratory support as needed. Fluid balance maintenance, monitoring of vital signs, and hourly urine output measurements are important. IV or gavage feeding is necessary if the infant cannot take oral feedings. The nurse must be constantly alert for signs of other complications such as disseminated intravascular coagulopathy.

**Supporting parents.** The infant with sepsis often appears healthy at birth but suddenly becomes critically ill. Parents experience feelings of shock, fear, and disappointment when their apparently healthy newborn is suddenly moved to the intensive care nursery. The preterm infant parents thought was making good progress might suddenly develop a life-threatening illness. Parents benefit from a chance to talk about their feelings with an understanding nurse who can explain the infant's treatment and care. Keeping the parents informed about the

## SAFETY ALERT

***Signs of Sepsis in the Newborn***

**General Signs**
Temperature instability
Nurse's feeling that infant is not doing well

**Respiratory Signs**
Tachypnea
Respiratory distress—nasal flaring, retractions, grunting
Apnea

**Cardiovascular Signs**
Color changes—cyanosis, pallor
Tachycardia
Hypotension
Decreased peripheral perfusion
Edema

**Gastrointestinal Signs**
Poor feeding
Vomiting
Increased gastric residuals
Diarrhea
Abdominal distention
Hypoglycemia or hyperglycemia

**Central Nervous System Signs**
Decreased or increased muscle tone
Lethargy
Irritability
Full fontanel
High-pitched cry

**Signs That Indicate Advanced Infection**
Jaundice
Evidence of hemorrhage—petechiae, purpura, pulmonary bleeding
Anemia
Enlarged liver and spleen
Respiratory failure
Shock
Seizures

infant's treatments and changes in condition and involving them in care are essential.

## INFANT OF A DIABETIC MOTHER

### Scope of the Problem

The infant of a diabetic mother (IDM) faces many risks. The neonatal mortality rate is five times that of infants born to nondiabetic mothers (Carlo, 2011a). Cardiac, urinary tract, gastrointestinal, and neural tube anomalies and sacral agenesis are most frequent. Cardiomegaly is common and can lead to heart failure. The incidence of anomalies in infants of insulin-dependent mothers is two to three times that of normal women but is not increased in infants of women with gestational diabetes. Congenital anomalies are less frequent with good control of diabetes before conception and in the early weeks of gestation when fetal organs are forming (Kalhan & Devaskar, 2011).

Insulin acts as a growth hormone. Protein synthesis is accelerated and fat and glycogen are deposited in fetal tissues, resulting in macrosomia (Fig. 30.2). Macrosomic infants are at risk for trauma during birth, including fractures of the clavicles from shoulder dystocia, cephalhematoma, and facial nerve and brachial plexus injury. Strict control of maternal blood glucose levels, especially in the third trimester, reduces the risk of macrosomia (Blackburn, 2013).

When the mother is hyperglycemic, large amounts of amino acids, free fatty acids, and glucose are transferred to the fetus. Insulin does not cross the placenta because the molecules are too large. The excessive glucose received by the fetus causes the fetal pancreas to secrete large amounts of insulin and leads to hypertrophy of the islet cells. Hypoglycemia can occur after birth, when the maternal supply of glucose is no longer available but the infant's high insulin production continues.

Infants of mothers with long-term diabetes and vascular changes may have fetal growth restriction instead of macrosomia because of decreased placental blood flow. Hypertension occurs more often in diabetic women and further compromises uteroplacental blood flow.

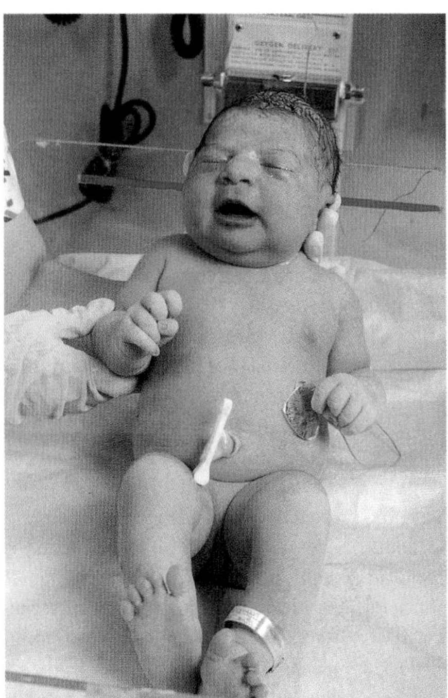

**FIG 30.2** Macrosomia is common in infants of diabetic mothers.

The IDM has a higher risk of asphyxia and RDS. RDS occurs because high levels of insulin block the effect of cortisol on surfactant production (Lee-Parritz & Cloherty, 2012). Hypocalcemia (p. 653) can result from decreased parathyroid hormone production. Magnesium levels also can be low. Polycythemia, a response to chronic hypoxia *in utero,* can cause hyperbilirubinemia as the large number of red blood cells break down after birth.

### Characteristics of Infants of Diabetic Mothers

The macrosomic IDM has hypertrophy of the liver, spleen, and heart. All organs except the brain and possibly the kidneys are larger than normal (Kalhan & Devaskar, 2011). The length and head size are generally within the normal range for gestational age. These infants have a characteristic appearance. The face is round, the body is obese, and the skin may be red (plethoric). The infant has poor muscle tone at rest but becomes irritable and may have tremors when disturbed. The SGA IDM is similar to infants who are SGA from other causes but is more likely to have congenital anomalies.

### Therapeutic Management

Therapeutic management includes controlling the mother's diabetes throughout pregnancy to decrease complications in the fetus and newborn (see Chapter 26). If the infant is large, shoulder dystocia or cephalopelvic disproportion can occur, and a cesarean birth may be required. Immediate care of respiratory problems and continued observation for complications determine treatment of the infant.

### Nursing Considerations

#### Assessment

The IDM is assessed for signs of complications, trauma, and congenital anomalies at delivery and during the early hours after birth. Respiratory problems can be apparent at birth or develop later. The initial assessment may reveal injuries. For example, an infant who cries when an arm is moved or fails to move an arm may have a fractured clavicle or nerve injury.

Hypoglycemia occurs in 25% to 50% of infants of mothers with pregestational diabetes and 15% to 25% of those with gestational diabetes (Carlo, 2011a). The most common sign of low blood glucose is jitteriness or tremors, but some infants show no signs at all. Diaphoresis is uncommon in newborns but can occur with hypoglycemia. Rapid respirations, low temperature, and poor muscle tone are common (see Chapter 21, p. 449). These signs also occur in other conditions, and the nurse must be alert for other complications if the signs continue after feeding.

#### Nursing Interventions

The nurse assesses blood glucose level according to hospital policy. Glucose levels below 40 to 45 mg/dL as measured with a bedside glucometer should be reported and verified by laboratory analysis.

Infants should be fed early to prevent hypoglycemia and immediately if low blood glucose occurs. Breast milk or formula is used. IDMs are often poor feeders. Gavage feeding may be necessary if the infant does not suck well or if the respirations are rapid. Infants whose condition does not allow enteral feedings or those whose glucose levels are very low or are not maintained with feedings need IV glucose.

The nurse must be alert for signs of other complications that occur in IDMs. Signs of RDS or other respiratory complications may develop. Cold stress increases the need for oxygen and glucose, increasing hypoglycemia and respiratory problems. Infants with polycythemia need adequate hydration to prevent sluggish blood flow and ischemia in vital organs. Hypocalcemia should be suspected if tremors continue and the blood glucose is normal.

Providing support to parents is important. They may not understand why their infant, who appears fat and healthy to them, needs close observation and frequent blood tests. The mother who had a difficult pregnancy might feel guilty, even if she followed a program of good diabetic control. Ample opportunity to discuss feelings, as well as information about the infant's care, is important.

## POLYCYTHEMIA

Infants with polycythemia have a hematocrit above 65% and hemoglobin level higher than 22 g/dL (Luchtman-Jones & Wilson, 2011). The resulting increased blood viscosity causes resistance in blood vessels and decreases blood flow. Thromboemboli, stroke, congestive heart failure, hypoglycemia, renal vein thrombosis, PPHN, and necrotizing enterocolitis can follow. Hyperbilirubinemia can occur from the excessive red blood cell breakdown after birth.

### Causes

Polycythemia occurs when the fetus produces more erythrocytes than normal to compensate for poor intrauterine oxygenation. This condition is more common in infants with postmaturity, large for gestational age (LGA), SGA, or maternal hypertension, diabetes, or smoking. Delayed clamping of the cord or a transfusion from one twin to another also can cause this condition.

### Manifestations

Most infants have minimal or no signs of polycythemia. Symptomatic infants often exhibit a plethoric color, lethargy, irritability, poor tone, and tremors. Abdominal distention, decreased bowel sounds, poor feeding, hypoglycemia, and respiratory distress also can be present. Hyperbilirubinemia occurs as red cells are broken down.

### Therapeutic Management

Treatment is primarily supportive. Nonsymptomatic infants with hematocrits of 70% or less are observed with attention to adequate hydration. Symptomatic infants or those with a hematocrit above 70% may receive a partial exchange transfusion, wherein blood is replaced with crystalloid solutions. Phototherapy is used to treat hyperbilirubinemia.

### Nursing Considerations

Bilirubin levels should be monitored to determine whether treatment for jaundice is necessary. Infants must be hydrated adequately to prevent dehydration that would slow already-sluggish blood flow and increase ischemia to vital organs. If a partial exchange transfusion is performed, the nurse assists and watches for complications.

## HYPOCALCEMIA

Hypocalcemia is a total serum calcium concentration below 7 mg/dL. This condition is classified as *early onset* (in the first 72 hours of age) or *late onset* (after 1 week of age) (Jones, Hayes, Starbuck, et al., 2011).

### Etiology

Early onset hypocalcemia occurs most often in IDMs and infants with asphyxia, prematurity, and fetal growth restriction. Late onset hypocalcemia is caused by low magnesium levels, maternal hyperparathyroidism or congenital hypoparathyroidism, and high-phosphate formula.

### Manifestations

Signs of hypocalcemia include jitteriness, irritability, muscle twitching, poor feeding, high-pitched cry, and seizures, although it is often asymptomatic.

### Therapeutic Management

Laboratory testing of serum calcium identifies the problem. Enteral or IV calcium gluconate is given if feeding alone does not raise the calcium level. A cardiac monitor is necessary when IV calcium is given, because bradycardia can occur.

### Nursing Considerations

Oral calcium should be given with feedings to prevent gastric irritation. IV calcium should be administered slowly and stopped immediately if bradycardia or dysrhythmia develops. The IV site should be assessed frequently because infiltration can cause necrosis.

## PRENATAL DRUG EXPOSURE

Substance abuse affects the fetus at any time during pregnancy. Most drugs readily cross the placenta and cause a variety of problems. The effects of substance abuse on pregnancy, the fetus, and the neonate are discussed in Chapter 24. Neonatal abstinence syndrome (NAS), a disorder in which neonates demonstrate signs of drug withdrawal from *in utero* exposure to maternal drugs, is discussed here.

**EVIDENCE-BASED PRACTICE**

Neonatal Abstinence Syndrome (NAS) is a growing concern in nursing care. As the use and abuse of addictive substances increases in pregnant mothers, so will the incidence of NAS. Care of the drug-addicted mothers and their drug-dependent newborns brings many challenges to health care personnel.

Most infants born to drug-dependent mothers will undergo NAS and will require pharmacotherapy for withdrawal symptoms. According to the findings of the 2009 National Survey on Drug Use and Health (W.S. Department of Health and Human Services, (2010), nurses are in a unique position to assess pregnant drug-addicted mothers and to observe for signs and symptoms of withdrawal in their newborns (Nelson, 2013).

Since symptoms begin within 8-48 hours of life the nurses in the newborn nursery may be the first to observe withdrawal symptoms in these newborns.

After screening these infants may require transfer to the NICU for specialized withdrawal care. The nurse will be responsible to assess, feed, and comfort the infant while in withdrawal. These infants need to be rocked, and have a quiet and calm atmosphere. Many times the mothers of these infants are not present to provide care.

Nelson concluded that NAD is a growing nursing, medical, social, and psychological issues. Further research is needed for best practices of care for these infants and nursing has the opportunity to lead the research in nursing interventions and best practices for the care of the infant with NAS (Nelson, 2013).

Nelson, M. M. (2013). Neonatal Abstinence Syndrome: The Nurse's Role. *International Journal Of Childbirth Education, 28*(1), 38-42 5p.

### Identification of Drug-Exposed Infants

Maternal substance abuse may be identified before an infant is born, or it may be unknown to health professionals. A history of minimal or no prenatal care or the mother's behavior during labor can alert nurses to suspect substance abuse. When there is any reason to suspect drug use, the infant is observed closely for signs of prenatal drug exposure.

NAS occurs in infants who have suffered prenatal opiate exposure sufficient to cause withdrawal signs after birth. Women who use heroin are generally switched to methadone during pregnancy to decrease wide variations in the drug dose, which is harmful to the fetus. These women usually receive better prenatal care, but their infants must undergo withdrawal after birth.

Withdrawal syndromes are also seen in infants exposed to other drugs such as codeine, hydroxyzine, amphetamine, and antidepressants (Carlo, 2011b). Neonates exposed to cocaine exhibit central nervous system signs such as irritability followed by lethargy, tremors, and increased tone. They respond poorly to comforting and become distressed easily. These effects are thought to be caused by the drug rather than withdrawal.

Selective serotonin reuptake inhibitors and other antidepressants taken during pregnancy can result in some behaviors similar to NAS, but the effect is usually milder (Carlo, 2011b). Methamphetamine exposure results in lethargy, irritability, high-pitched cry, and hypertonicity in infants (Altshul, 2012).

Signs of drug exposure usually begin during the first 24 to 72 hours after birth but may not occur for up to 4 weeks, depending on the specific drug and the time of the mother's last use (Bandstra & Accornero, 2011). Use near the time of delivery causes a later onset but more severe signs of withdrawal in the newborn. Some signs can continue for 4 to 6 months (Weiner & Finnegan, 2011). Polydrug use is common, and signs vary according to the drug or combination of drugs used but often include neurologic and gastrointestinal abnormalities. Some infants with prenatal drug exposure show no abnormal signs at all.

Infants with NAS may be irritable and have hyperactive muscle tone and a high-pitched cry. Tremors may be present, but the blood glucose level is normal. Infants appear hungry and suck vigorously on their fists but have poor coordination of suck and swallow. Frequent regurgitation, vomiting, and diarrhea are common. The infant's excessive activity, coupled with poor feeding ability, results in failure to gain weight.

Various scoring systems are available to determine the number, frequency, and severity of behaviors that indicate NAS. The score is helpful in determining the necessity of drug therapy to alleviate withdrawal. Behaviors are generally scored every 2 to 4 hours until low scores are obtained consistently.

Congenital anomalies and other effects of prenatal drug exposure may be apparent at birth. Fetal growth restriction and prematurity are common. Infants are more likely to have respiratory distress at birth, jaundice, or sudden infant death syndrome (SIDS). Infants with fetal alcohol syndrome have a characteristic appearance.

When drug exposure is suspected, a urine specimen is collected from the infant for analysis (see the procedure on page 929). Drugs or their metabolites are present in the newborn's urine for various lengths of time after the mother has used them. Some drugs last several days because of the infant's difficulty in excreting them, whereas others disappear very soon. Therefore, it is important to obtain the first urine output from the infant, if possible. Meconium may also be tested for drugs because the drug is present for a longer period. A segment of the umbilical cord is tested in some facilities.

## Therapeutic Management

Therapeutic management includes dealing with the complications common to drug-exposed infants during and after birth. Respiratory problems and those related to prematurity are treated as for other infants. Drug therapy may be necessary for approximately 50% to 60% of these infants if they have high scores on abstinence scales (Weiner & Finnegan, 2011).

Medications commonly used include diluted tincture of opium, oral morphine, methadone, and phenobarbital. The dosage is gradually tapered until the infant no longer needs it. Although these drugs help relieve the signs of withdrawal, all have undesirable side effects.

Gavage or IV feeding may be required because the infant's suck and swallow are uncoordinated. Some infants need more than the normal caloric requirements because of their excessive activity. Involvement of social services is important to deal with the long-term effects of the drugs, placement of the infant after hospitalization, and follow-up with the mother or other caretaker to help provide for the infant's needs.

> **SAFETY ALERT**
>
> ***Signs of Intrauterine Drug Exposure***
>
> **Behavioral Signs**
> Irritability
> Jitteriness, tremors, seizures
> Muscular rigidity, increased muscle tone
> Restless, excessive activity
> Exaggerated Moro reflex
> Prolonged high-pitched cry
> Difficult to console
> Poor sleeping patterns
> Yawning
>
> **Signs Relating to Feeding**
> Excessive sucking
> Uncoordinated sucking and swallowing
> Frequent regurgitation or vomiting
> Diarrhea
> Weight loss
>
> **Respiratory Signs**
> Nasal stuffiness, sneezing
> Tachypnea, apnea
> Retractions
>
> **Other Signs**
> Fever
> Diaphoresis
> Excoriation
> Mottling
>
> NOTE: Some infants with prenatal drug exposure have no abnormal signs at all, or signs may be delayed.

## Nursing Considerations

The infant who has been exposed to drugs prenatally needs special care to cope with drug withdrawal. Care is focused on feeding, rest, and, if possible, enhancing parental attachment (Nursing Care Plan: The Drug-Exposed Infant).

### Feeding

Feeding can be difficult and time consuming. The poor suck and swallow coordination of drug-exposed infants interferes with caloric intake, yet their excessive activity increases caloric needs.

***Assessment.*** The nurse should assess the infant's ability to coordinate sucking and swallowing with respirations. Changes in the frequency and amount of regurgitation or vomiting or the length of time it takes infants to finish feedings should be noted.

*Nursing interventions.* Gavage feedings may be necessary to conserve the infant's energy and prevent aspiration if the infant is excessively agitated, cannot suck and swallow adequately, or has rapid respirations. Formula with 24 kcal/oz increases calorie intake. More frequent feedings may be needed. Infants should be swaddled during feedings to prevent excessive movement. Other types of stimulation such as rocking or talking should be minimized during feedings.

### Rest

The excessive activity and poor sleep patterns of drug-exposed neonates interfere with their ability to rest.

*Assessment.* The infant's muscle tone, tremors, and tendency for excessive activity with and without being disturbed should be assessed. The degree of tremors and stimuli that increase or decrease irritability are important. The nurse also keeps track of the number of hours the infant sleeps after each feeding.

*Nursing interventions.* Keep stimulation of the drug-exposed infant to a minimum by reducing noise and bright lights as much as possible. Organize nursing care to reduce handling and disturbances. A calm approach and slow, smooth movements during care help avoid startling the infant. If signs of overstimulation occur, all activity should be stopped, if possible, and a rest period provided.

Swaddling the infant in a flexed position helps prevent startling and agitation. A pacifier for nonnutritive sucking also helps quiet the infant. Skin excoriations from excessive activity or diarrhea can increase discomfort and agitation. They should be prevented if possible and treated promptly if they occur. Covering the infant's hands with mittens or the end of the shirtsleeves helps prevent scratches to the face. Placing the infant in a prone position promotes better sleep for some infants, but supine positioning should be used as soon as possible.

### Bonding

When infants test positive for drugs, child protective services becomes involved. The infant may not be released to the mother until her ability to care for her infant safely has been assessed by social services or a court. Some mothers are required to enter a drug rehabilitation program before they can obtain custody of the infant. After hospital discharge, the infant may receive care by family members approved by the court, in a foster home, or in an institution. However, the mother will most likely gain custody of the infant eventually if she complies with court-ordered treatment, and attachment to the infant should be encouraged.

*Assessment.* The frequency of the mother's visits and her response to the infant may give an indication of her apparent interest in the infant. Bonding behaviors such as calling the infant by name and smiling at the infant should be noted.

*Nursing interventions.* Child neglect or abuse and failure to respond appropriately to the infant are associated with alcohol and drug abuse. Because the mother might become the infant's primary caretaker, it is vital that nurses do whatever they can to enhance mother-infant bonding. Helping the mother feel welcome when she visits the infant provides a challenge. It can be difficult for the nurse to be accepting of a mother whose behavior has harmed her infant. Yet a friendly approach will make the mother more likely to visit the infant and accept teaching from the nurse.

Promote bonding by encouraging mothers to participate actively in infant care during visits. If the mother feels that the nurses trust her to care for the infant, her confidence may grow. Increased confidence can encourage the mother's effort to go through recovery to regain custody of her newborn.

The mother's participation also provides a chance for the nurse to assess her infant care skills and areas in which further discussion of the newborn's needs will be helpful. In addition, it gives the nurse an opportunity to demonstrate parenting skills. Many mothers who use drugs have not had good parenting role models and do not know how to care for an infant. Frequent positive feedback about the mother's participation is important.

Offer the mother the same teaching given to all new parents, as well as special techniques necessary to meet the needs of drug-exposed infants. Point out the newborn's special characteristics and help her take on more of the infant's care as she demonstrates readiness.

The mother may feel rejected when the infant doesn't respond to her care as other infants do. Explain that infants are easily overstimulated and demonstrate how to comfort them. In addition, these infants cannot tolerate more than brief periods of interaction. They may not make eye contact, or they may avert their eyes after 30 to 60 seconds of social interaction. The nurse should teach the mother that the infant responds poorly to everyone so that she does not think that only she is being rejected.

Cocaine, amphetamines, heroin, and other drugs pass into breast milk. Breastfeeding an infant with poorly developed feeding skills may be too much stress for the mother who is trying to recover from addiction. Mothers likely to continue drug use after delivery should be discouraged from breastfeeding. Women receiving methadone maintenance may be allowed to breastfeed if they are not taking other drugs that are contraindicated (Altshul, 2012). If the woman has a strong desire to breastfeed, the nurse should consult the healthcare provider.

The nurse can provide information and referral to any special programs available to help parents learn stimulation techniques appropriate for drug-exposed infants. If the mother cannot care for the newborn, the same interventions can be used to help the infant's caregiver on hospital discharge.

## PHENYLKETONURIA

Phenylketonuria (PKU) is a genetic disorder that causes central nervous system injury from toxic levels of the amino acid phenylalanine in the blood. Severe intellectual impairment occurs in untreated infants and children. In the United States, all newborns are screened for this condition before or shortly after discharge from the birth facility. Positive screening tests are followed by other testing.

### Etiology

PKU is caused by a deficiency of the enzyme phenylalanine hydrolase, which is necessary to convert phenylalanine to tyrosine for use. This disorder is autosomal recessive.

### Manifestations

Signs of untreated disease begin with digestive problems and vomiting and later progress to seizures, musty odor to the urine, and intellectual impairment. Older children have eczema, **hypertonia, hyperactive behavior, and hypopigmentation of the hair, skin, and irises**.

### Therapeutic Management

Treatment is a low-phenylalanine diet. Small amounts of phenylalanine are allowed because it is a necessary amino acid. Early and continued treatment throughout life is necessary to prevent intellectual

## NURSING CARE PLAN

### The Drug-Exposed Infant

Beth was born at 39 weeks of gestation to Gloria, who was on a methadone maintenance program. During labor, Gloria admitted to using heroin several times during the last weeks of pregnancy.

#### Focused Assessment

Beth sleeps less than an hour after feedings. When she awakens, her high-pitched cry and agitation begin immediately. Her activity elicits the Moro reflex, which leads to more agitation. She is irritable and does not respond to caretaking activities as quickly as other infants.

#### Nursing Diagnosis

Disturbed Sleep Pattern related to agitation from own activity and irritability.

#### Planning

***Expected Outcomes***

The infant will:

1. Sleep for periods of 2 hours or more after feedings within 3 days.
2. Decrease crying by at least 1 hour a day within the first week after birth.

#### Interventions and *Rationales*

1. Place Beth's crib in the quietest corner of the nursery. Place a sign nearby to remind others of the need for quiet in that area.
   *Drug-exposed infants are easily overstimulated by noise and activity.*
2. Keep lights turned down as much as possible. Partially cover the crib with a blanket to decrease light.
   *Lowered lighting provides a more restful environment.*
3. Keep Beth swaddled in a flexed position during sleep and feedings.
   *The drug-exposed infant's own movements can cause startling, awakening, and agitation.*
4. Use a pacifier, and position her hands near her mouth.
   *Nonnutritive sucking may have a calming effect on the infant. Positioning the hands near the mouth allows the infant to self-comfort by sucking.*
5. Organize nursing care so that Beth is not disturbed unnecessarily, especially when sleeping.
   *Drug-exposed infants may have difficulty going back to sleep if awakened.*
6. Stop all activity if she shows signs of increased stress.
   *Providing a time-out in response to stress allows the infant to rest.*

#### Evaluation

The infant gradually lengthens her sleep periods to 2 hours and decreases crying episodes within the first week after birth.

#### Focused Assessment

Gloria visits her infant sporadically. She seems hesitant when she comes into the nursery and afraid to touch or care for her infant. She asks, "Why does she cry so much?" When the nurse helps her hold her infant, Gloria says, "I don't think she likes me."

#### Nursing Diagnosis

Impaired Parenting related to lack of understanding of the infant's characteristics and how to relate to an irritable infant.

#### Planning

***Expected Outcomes***

Within 1 week Gloria will:

1. Visit at least every other day.
2. Participate in Beth's care by holding and feeding her.
3. Make positive statements about her daughter.

#### Interventions and *Rationales*

1. Show acceptance of Gloria when she comes to visit her infant. Greet her, and provide her with an update on her infant's progress.
   *A mother is more likely to visit her infant if she feels accepted by staff. The more she visits, the more she is likely to learn about parenting her infant.*
2. Assist Gloria to hold and feed Beth. Explain nursing actions such as placing the crib in a secluded area. Offer kangaroo care.
   *Participating in care of the infant helps the mother get to know her infant and gain comfort in providing infant care. Kangaroo care can help Gloria feel closer to her infant.*
3. Demonstrate comfort measures such as swaddling. Show her how to place a rolled blanket or positioning device around the infant to provide a feeling of security.
   *When the mother learns ways to comfort her infant, the positive response from the infant may increase bonding.*
4. Explain common behaviors in drug-exposed infants and that Beth's stiff body posture and excessive activity are normal at this time. Point out signs such as gaze aversion that show the infant is overstimulated.
   *Understanding that Beth's behavior is part of the infant's problem and is not caused by Gloria's handling of her is reassuring to the mother.*
5. Model ways of interacting with Beth and calming her. Point out signs that she is ready to interact. Suggest only one stimulus at a time, such as talking softly without rocking.
   *Gloria will learn appropriate interaction when she sees it performed by the nurse. Decreasing multiple stimuli may be effective in calming Beth.*
6. Point out positive points about Beth, such as her long eyelashes or delicate fingers. Discuss signs that show that she is making progress.
   *Gloria needs help to focus on positive aspects of the infant as well as the problems.*
7. Explain the routine care of a newborn. Spread teaching out over visits.
   *Gloria needs to learn the usual care of any newborn as well as the infant's special needs.*
8. Give praise and encouragement frequently as Gloria works with her infant.
   *The mother needs positive reinforcement and help to feel that she is capable of mothering her infant.*
9. Use therapeutic communication techniques to help Gloria discuss her feelings as she cares for Beth.
   *Mothers often find it frustrating to care for the drug-exposed infant. Helping them vent their feelings may increase their ability to cope with the infant's needs.*
10. Discuss sources of support from family members or friends. Refer Gloria to support groups in the community.
    *Ongoing support is necessary for the woman with addiction problems. Support for Gloria will help her care more effectively for her infant.*
11. If Gloria will have custody of her infant, help her make plans for discharge. Discuss ongoing problems and concerns such as sudden infant death syndrome (SIDS). Explain that some withdrawal behaviors can last as long as 6 months.
    *Infants have ongoing problems that will continue in the home setting. Infants exposed to heroin have an increased incidence of SIDS.*

#### Evaluation

Gloria begins to visit more often, coming three or four times a week. She participates in care, begins to talk about her "pretty little girl," and discusses plans for taking her infant home with her.

***Additional Nursing Diagnoses to Consider***

Imbalanced Nutrition: Less Than Body Requirements
Ineffective Infant Feeding Pattern
Ineffective Coping
Impaired Skin Integrity
Disorganized Infant Behavior

impairment. Women who are not following the diet closely need to return to it before conception and throughout pregnancy to avoid abnormalities in the fetus (Rezvani & Melvin, 2011).

### Nursing Considerations

The nurse should see that all newborns are screened for PKU at the appropriate time in the hospital. Screening performed before 24 hours of age should be repeated because the infant's protein intake may be too low for the test to be accurate.

The nurse assists parents in regulating the diet. Parents can be reassured that good control helps avoid long-term neurologic problems. However, subtle intellectual and behavioral problems may occur (see Chapter 51).

## KEY CONCEPTS

- Asphyxia before or during birth can cause apnea, acidosis, pulmonary hypertension, and possible death. Neonatal resuscitation must be initiated immediately.
- Nurses must identify conditions that increase the risk of asphyxia, begin resuscitation promptly, and assist other members of the team during treatment. Continued follow-up of the infant and parental support are important.
- In transient tachypnea of the newborn, respiratory difficulty in full-term or preterm infants is caused by failure of fetal lung fluid to be absorbed completely. It usually resolves spontaneously with supportive care.
- In meconium aspiration syndrome, meconium in amniotic fluid enters the lungs before birth or during the first breaths after birth. It causes obstruction, air trapping, and inflammation.
- Persistent pulmonary hypertension is a condition in which pulmonary vascular resistance remains high after birth and right to left shunting of blood occurs causing severe respiratory difficulty.
- Nonphysiologic jaundice appears in the first 24 hours of life, and bilirubin rises faster and to higher levels than physiologic jaundice. If untreated, it can result in injury to the brain.
- The nurse's role in phototherapy is to decrease situations such as cold stress or hypoglycemia that can further elevate bilirubin levels, protect the eyes, ensure that lights are used properly, observe for excessive fluid loss or skin impairment, ensure adequate oral intake, and teach parents.
- Infection can be transmitted to the neonate from the mother during pregnancy or birth or from the mother, family members, visitors, or agency staff after birth.
- Infants of diabetic mothers can have congenital anomalies, can be large or small for gestational age, and can have respiratory distress syndrome, hypoglycemia, hypocalcemia, and polycythemia.
- Nursing responsibilities in caring for IDMs include early identification and follow-up of complications, monitoring blood glucose levels, ensuring early and adequate feedings, and supporting parents.
- Infants with polycythemia have increased blood viscosity that can cause thromboemboli, stroke, hyperbilirubinemia, and other complications.
- Hypocalcemia is treated with oral or IV calcium.
- Infants with prenatal exposure to drugs can have behavioral and feeding abnormalities. They may have difficulty relating to others and fail to gain weight.
- Nursing care for infants with neonatal abstinence syndrome includes decreasing stimuli from lights, noise, or handling; increasing feeding abilities; and fostering the mother's attachment to and ability to care for her infant.
- Infants with phenylketonuria must be on a low phenylalanine diet to prevent severe intellectual impairment.

## REFERENCES AND READINGS


Abu-Shaweesh, J.M. (2011). Respiratory disorders of preterm and term infants. In R.J. Martin, A.A. Fanaroff, & M.C. Walsh (Eds.), *Fanaroff and Martin's neonatal-perinatal medicine: Diseases of the fetus and infant* (9th ed., vol. 2, pp. 1141–1168). Philadelphia: Mosby.

Altshul, K.W. (2012). Maternal drug abuse, exposure, and withdrawal. In J.P. Cloherty, E.C. Eichenwald, A.R. Hansen, et al. (Eds.), *Manual of neonatal care* (7th ed., pp. 134–165). Philadelphia: Lippincott Williams & Wilkins.

Ambalavanan, N., & Carlo, W. (2011a). Meconium aspiration. In R.M. Kliegman, B.E. Stanton, J.W. St. Geme, et al. (Eds.), *Nelson textbook of pediatrics* (19th ed., pp. 590–592). Philadelphia: Saunders.

Ambalavanan, N., & Carlo, W. (2011b). Persistent pulmonary hypertension of the newborn (persistent fetal circulation). In R.M. Kliegman, B.E. Stanton, J.W. St. Geme, et al. (Eds.), *Nelson textbook of pediatrics* (19th ed., pp. 592–594). Philadelphia: Saunders.

American Academy of Pediatrics & American College of Obstetricians and Gynecologists. (2013). *Guidelines for perinatal care* (8th ed.). Elk Grove Village, IL, and Washington, DC: Author.

American Academy of Pediatrics Subcommitee on Fetus and Newborn (2014). Respiratory support in preterm infants at birth. *Pediatrics, 133*(1), 171–174.

American Academy of Pediatrics Subcommittee on Hyperbilirubinemia. (2004). Management of hyperbilirubinemia in the newborn infant 35 or more weeks of gestation (Clinical Practice Guideline). *Pediatrics, 114*(1), 297–316.

Anadkat, J.S., Kuzniewicz, M.W., Chaudhari, B.P., et al. (2012). Increased risk for respiratory distress among white, male, late preterm and term infants. *Journal of Perinatology, 32*(10), 780–5.

Anderson, B.L., & Gonik, B. (2011). Perinatal infections. In R.J. Martin, A.A. Fanaroff, & M.C. Walsh (Eds.), *Fanaroff and Martin's neonatal-perinatal medicine: Diseases of the fetus and infant* (9th ed., vol. 1, pp. 399–422). Philadelphia: Mosby.

Bandstra, E.S., & Accornero, V.H. (2011). Infants of substance-abusing mothers. In R.J. Martin, A.A. Fanaroff, & M.C. Walsh (Eds.), *Fanaroff and Martin's neonatal-perinatal medicine: Diseases of the fetus and infant* (9th ed., vol. 1, pp. 735–757). Philadelphia: Mosby.

Bhutani, V.K. (2011). Phototherapy to prevent severe neonatal hyperbilirubinemia in the newborn infant 35 or more weeks of gestation: Technical report. *Pediatrics, 128*, e1046–e1052.

Blackburn, S.T. (2013). *Maternal, fetal, and neonatal physiology: A clinical perspective* (4th ed.). St. Louis: Saunders.

Burris, H.H. (2012). Meconium aspiration. In J.P. Cloherty, E.C. Eichenwald, A.R. Hansen, et al. (Eds.), *Manual of neonatal care* (7th ed., pp. 429–434). Philadelphia: Lippincott Williams & Wilkins.

Carlo, W.A. (2011a). Infants of diabetic mothers. In R.M. Kliegman, B.E. Stanton, J.W. St. Geme, et al. (Eds.), *Nelson textbook of pediatrics* (19th ed., pp. 627–629). Philadelphia: Saunders.

Carlo, W.A. (2011b). Metabolic disturbances. In R.M. Kliegman, B.E. Stanton, J.W. St. Geme, et al. (Eds.), *Nelson textbook of pediatrics* (19th ed., pp. 622–626). Philadelphia: Saunders.

Cunningham, F., Leveno, K., Bloom, S., et al. (2014). *Williams obstetrics* (24th ed.). New York: McGraw-Hill.

Dhillon, R. (2012). The management of neonatal pulmonary hypertension. *Archives of Disease in Childhood, 97*(3), F223–F228.

Edwards, M.S. (2011). Postnatal bacterial infections. In R.J. Martin, A.A. Fanaroff, & M.C. Walsh (Eds.), *Fanaroff and Martin's neonatal-perinatal medicine: Diseases of the fetus and infant* (9th ed., vol. 2, pp. 793–830). Philadelphia: Mosby.

Gardner, S.L., Enzman-Hines, M., & Dickey, L.A. (2011). Respiratory diseases. In S.L. Gardner, B.S. Carter, M. Enzman-Hines, et al. (Eds.), *Merenstein & Gardner's handbook of neonatal intensive care* (7th ed., pp. 581–677). St. Louis: Mosby.

Grabenhenrich, J., Grabenhenrich, L., Bührer, C., et al. (2014). Transcutaneous bilirubin after phototherapy in term and preterm infants. *Pediatrics, 134*(5), e1324–e1329.

Gregory, M.L. P., Martin, C.R., & Cloherty, J.P. (2012). Neonatal hyperbilirubinemia. In J.P. Cloherty, E.C. Eichenwald, A.R. Hansen, et al. (Eds.), *Manual of neonatal care* (7th ed., pp. 304–339). Philadelphia: Lippincott Williams & Wilkins.

Gruslin, A.M., & Moore, T.R. (2011). Erythroblastosis fetalis. In R.J. Martin, A.A. Fanaroff, & M.C. Walsh (Eds.), *Fanaroff and Martin's neonatal-perinatal medicine: Diseases of the fetus and infant* (9th ed., vol. 1, pp. 357–375). Philadelphia: Mosby.

Hatfield, L., Schwoebel, A., & Lynyak, C. (2011). Caring for the infant of a diabetic mother. *MCN: The American Journal of Maternal/Child Nursing, 36*(1), 10–16.

Jones, J.E., Hayes, R.D., Starbuck, A.L., et al. (2011). Fluid and electrolyte management. In S.L. Gardner, B.S. Carter, M. Enzman-Hines, et al. (Eds.), *Merenstein & Gardner's handbook of neonatal intensive care* (7th ed., pp. 333–352). St. Louis: Mosby.

Kalhan, S.C., & Devaskar, S.U. (2011). Disorders of carbohydrate metabolism. In R.J. Martin, A.A. Fanaroff, & M.C. Walsh (Eds.), *Fanaroff and Martin's neonatal-perinatal medicine: Diseases of the fetus and infant* (9th ed., vol. 2, pp. 1497–1523). Philadelphia: Mosby.

Kaplan, M., Wong, M.J., Sibley, E., et al. (2011). Neonatal jaundice and liver disease. In R.J. Martin, A.A. Fanaroff, & M.C. Walsh (Eds.), *Fanaroff and Martin's neonatal-perinatal medicine: Diseases of the fetus and infant* (9th ed., vol. 2, pp. 1443–1496). Philadelphia: Mosby.

Kattwinkel, J. (Ed.). (2011). *Textbook of neonatal resuscitation* (6th ed.). Elk Grove Village, IL: American Academy of Pediatrics and American Heart Association.

Lee-Parritz, A., & Cloherty, J.P. (2012). Diabetes mellitus. In J.P. Cloherty, E.C. Eichenwald, A.R. Hansen, et al. (Eds.), *Manual of neonatal care* (7th ed., pp. 11–23). Philadelphia: Lippincott Williams & Wilkins.

Luchtman-Jones, L., & Wilson, D.B. (2011). Hematologic problems in the fetus and neonate. In R.J. Martin, A.A. Fanaroff, & M.C. Walsh (Eds.), *Fanaroff and Martin's neonatal-perinatal medicine: Diseases of the fetus and infant* (9th ed., vol. 2, pp. 1303–1360). Philadelphia: Mosby.

McGowan, J.E., Rozance, P.J., Price-Douglas, W., et al. (2011). Glucose homeostasis. In S.L. Gardner, B.S. Carter, M. Enzman-Hines, et al. (Eds.), *Merenstein & Gardner's handbook of neonatal intensive care* (7th ed., pp. 353–377). St. Louis: Mosby.

Miller, M.Q., & Morris, L.A. (2011). Developmental considerations in working with newborn infants of mothers with diabetes. *Neonatal Network, 30*(1), 37–45.

More, K., Sakhuja, P, & Shah, P.S. (2014). Minimally invasive surfactant administration in preterm infants: a meta-analysis review. *Journal of the American Medical Association, 168*(10), 901–908.

Patrick, S.W., Dudley, J., Martin, P.R., et al. (2015). Prescription opioid epidemic and infant outcomes. *Pediatrics, 135*(5), 842–50.

Perlman, J.M., Wyllie, J., Kattwinkel, J., et al. (2010). Neonatal resuscitation: 2010 international consensus on cardiopulmonary resuscitation and emergency cardiovascular care science with treatment recommendations. *Pediatrics, 126*(5), e1319–e1344.

Polin, R.A., & Carlo, W.A. (2014). Surfactant replacement therapy for preterm and term neonates with respiratory distress. *Pediatrics, 133*(1), 156–163.

Reynolds, R., & Talmage, S. (2011). "Caution! Contents should be cold": Developing a whole-body hypothermia program. *Neonatal Network, 30*(4), 225–230.

Rezvani, I., & Melvin, J.J. (2011). Phenylalanine. In R.M. Kliegman, B.E. Stanton, J.W. St. Geme, et al. (Eds.), *Nelson textbook of pediatrics* (19th ed., pp. 418–422). Philadelphia: Saunders.

Spain, J.E., Tuuli, M.G., Macones, G.A., et al. (2015). Risk factors for serious morbidity in term nonanomalous neonates. *American Journal of Obstetrics & Gynecology, 212*(6), e1–e7.

Stokowski, L.A. (2011). Fundamentals of phototherapy for neonatal jaundice. *Advances in Neonatal Care, 11*(5S), S10–S21.

Stoll, B.J. (2011). Infections of the neonatal infant. In R.M. Kliegman, B.E. Stanton, J.W. St. Geme, et al. (Eds.), *Nelson textbook of pediatrics* (19th ed., pp. 629–648). Philadelphia: Saunders.

Stroustrup, A., Trasande, A., & Holzman, I.R. (2012). Randomized controlled trial of restrictive fluid management in transient tachypnea of the newborn. *Journal of Pediatrics, 160*(1), 38–43.

Tolia, V.N., Patrick, S.W., Bennett, M.M., et al. (2015). Increasing incidence of the neonatal abstinence syndrome in U.S. neonatal ICUs. *New England Journal of Medicine, 372*(22), 2118–2126.

Venkatesh, M.P., Adams, K.M., & Weisman, L.E. (2011). Infection in the neonate. In S.L. Gardner, B.S. Carter, M. Enzman-Hines, et al. (Eds.), *Merenstein & Gardner's handbook of neonatal intensive care* (7th ed., pp. 553–580). St. Louis: Mosby.

Walker, J.J., & Walker, A. (2011). Substance abuse. In D.K. James, P.J. Steer, C.P. Weiner, et al. (Eds.), *High risk pregnancy: Management options* (4th ed., pp. 565–578). Philadelphia: Saunders.

Weiner, S.M., & Finnegan, L.P. (2011). Drug withdrawal in the neonate. In S.L. Gardner, B.S. Carter, M. Enzman-Hines, et al. (Eds.), *Merenstein & Gardner's handbook of neonatal intensive care* (7th ed., pp. 201–222). St. Louis: Mosby.

Wilson, D.J., & Tyner, C.I. (2014). Immunology and infectious disease. In M.T. Verklan, & M. Walden (Eds.), *AWHONN core curriculum for neonatal intensive care nursing* (5th ed., pp. 689–719). St. Louis: Saunders.

Wynn, J.L., Wong, H.R., Shanley, T.P, et al. (2014). Time for a neonatal-specific consensus definition for sepsis. *Pediatric Critical Care Medicine, 15*(6), 523–528.

31

# Management of Fertility and Infertility

http://evolve.elsevier.com/McKinney/mat-ch/

## LEARNING OBJECTIVES

*After studying this chapter, you should be able to:*

- Describe the role of the nurse in helping couples choose contraceptive methods.
- Describe important considerations when choosing a contraceptive method.
- Explain why informed consent is important for contraception.
- Compare and contrast contraceptive needs of adolescent and perimenopausal women.
- Explain the mechanism of action, advantages, disadvantages, side effects, and teaching needed for methods of family planning.
- Discuss the nurse's role in contraceptive counseling and education.
- Explain factors that can impair a couple's ability to conceive.
- Describe factors that can cause repeated pregnancy losses.
- Specify evaluations performed when a couple seeks help for infertility.
- Explain the use of procedures and treatments that may aid a couple's ability to conceive and carry the fetus to viability.
- Discuss the nurse's role for families needing care related to fertility or infertility.

Family planning involves choosing the time to have children. It includes contraception—the prevention of pregnancy—as well as methods to achieve pregnancy. This chapter discusses preventing pregnancy with contraception as well as helping couples with infertility or difficulty achieving pregnancy.

## CONTRACEPTION

Approximately 90% of sexually active women who do not use contraception will conceive within 1 year if both partners are fertile (Cunningham, Leveno, Bloom, et al., 2014). Therefore, those who wish to control the timing of pregnancies cannot leave contraception to chance.

Approximately 43 million women in the United States are sexually active and could become pregnant but do not want a pregnancy at this time. Of those women, 62% are practicing contraception. However, they may not be using contraception consistently. Eighteen percent of women use contraception inconsistently or incorrectly, which accounts for 41% of all unintended pregnancies (Alan Guttmacher Institute [AGI], 2015b).

Unintended pregnancies are those that are unwanted or that occur in women who want to become pregnant at some time in the future but not at the time their pregnancy occurs. These pregnancies can result in economic hardship, health problems, interference with educational or career plans, and other disruptions in the lives of women and their families. Pregnancies that are spaced less than 6 months apart result in a higher risk for maternal mortality and morbidity, preterm birth, and low birthweight infants (AGI, 2015b).

Over three million unintended pregnancies occur each year in the United States (AGI, 2015b). A *Healthy People 2020* goal is to increase the number of pregnancies that are intended to 56% from a baseline of 51% (U.S. Department of Health and Human Services [USDHHS], 2010).

## ROLE OF THE NURSE

The nurse's role in family planning is that of counselor and educator. To fulfill this role, nurses need current, correct information about contraceptive methods and need to share this information with the women they see in their practice.

Women who do not plan to become pregnant may have gaps in contraceptive use when there are changes in their relationships or when they are planning to change contraceptive methods. Approximately 40% of unintended pregnancies occur in women who used their contraceptive method incorrectly or inconsistently (AGI, 2015b). Such errors might occur less often if women had adequate ongoing education about their chosen method. Nurses can increase the likelihood of a woman using contraception by providing contraceptive counseling that is directed to the woman's specific needs. Therefore, the nurse must provide individualized family planning information to women in every situation for which it is appropriate.

Nurses must be comfortable discussing contraception and be sensitive to the woman's concerns and feelings. It is important that nurses do not introduce their own biases for or against specific methods. The nurse's personal experiences and choices regarding contraception are not pertinent. Counseling must be focused on the needs, feelings, and preferences of the woman and her partner (Fig. 31.1). For example, nurses working in maternity settings should discuss family planning with postpartum women to provide an opportunity to clarify misinformation and answer questions. Then the woman will be ready to discuss contraception further with her primary caregiver, if necessary.

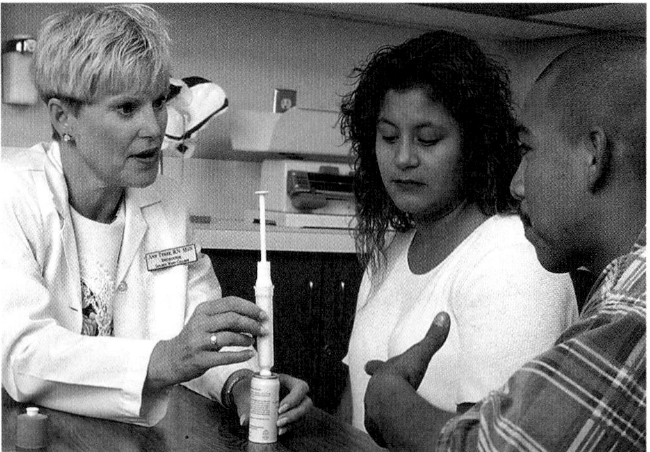

FIG 31.1 Successful contraception is more likely when both the woman and her partner are involved in discussions. The nurse demonstrates filling a foam applicator.

## CONSIDERATIONS WHEN CHOOSING A CONTRACEPTIVE METHOD

No contraceptive method is perfect. Each has advantages and disadvantages (Table 31.1). Sexually active women who do not want to become pregnant will need to use contraceptives for more than 30 years and are likely to change their contraceptive choices over that time. Women change contraceptive methods as circumstances in their lives change and in response to dissatisfaction with side effects or other features of contraceptives. Careful consideration of all factors can help women choose methods that best meet their needs and they will use consistently.

The most popular methods of contraception in the United States are **oral contraceptives (OCs)**, female sterilization, and male **condoms** (AGI, 2015a). However, the most popular methods are not right for every woman. Nurses can help women weigh factors involved in choosing a family planning method.

**TABLE 31.1 Advantages and Disadvantages of Most Common Contraceptive Methods**

| Method | Advantages | Disadvantages |
|---|---|---|
| Sterilization | Ends concern about contraception<br>Tubal sterilization performed during or right after childbirth or between pregnancies<br>Vasectomy performed in the physician's office with local anesthesia<br>Low long-term cost | No protection against STDs<br>Reversal is difficult, expensive, and can be unsuccessful<br>Potential complications of any surgery<br>Vasectomy requires another contraceptive method until semen is free of sperm<br>Expensive initially |
| Intrauterine devices or intrauterine system | Unrelated to coitus<br>In place at all times<br>Low long-term cost<br>Effective for 5-10 years<br>Decreases dysmenorrhea and menstrual blood loss<br>Some become amenorrheic<br>Copper IUD can also be used for EC | No protection against STDs<br>High initial cost<br>Can be expelled without the woman's knowledge—must check for strings<br>Potential side effects or complications: menorrhagia, infection near time of insertion, perforation, ectopic pregnancy or spontaneous abortion if pregnancy occurs |
| Progestin implant | Unrelated to coitus<br>Provides 3-year protection<br>Safe during lactation<br>Body weight has no effect<br>Low long-term cost | No protection against STDs<br>Minor surgical procedure to insert and remove<br>Major side effect is irregular bleeding |
| Progestin injections (Depo-Provera) | Unrelated to coitus<br>Avoids need for daily use<br>May cause amenorrhea with continued use<br>Requires use only every 12 wk | No protection against STDs<br>Must remember to repeat every 12 wk<br>Cause temporary decrease in bone density. Long-term effects unknown.<br>Side effects similar to other progestin contraceptives |
| Oral contraceptives | Taken at time unrelated to coitus (see Box 31.1) | No protection against STDs<br>Must be taken daily at or near same time<br>Can have side effects and complications (see Box 31.1) |
| Emergency contraception (EC) | Helps prevent pregnancy after unprotected coitus<br>Some available over the counter to patients 17 years and older | No protection against STDs<br>Oral EC must be taken within 120 hr of unprotected intercourse<br>May cause nausea |
| Transdermal contraceptive patch | Unrelated to coitus<br>Requires only weekly application<br>Regulates menstrual cycles | No protection against STDs<br>Must remember to apply on the right day<br>May be less effective for women over 90 kg (198 lb)<br>May cause skin irritation<br>Other side effects similar to OCs<br>May have higher risk of clot formation |
| Vaginal contraceptive ring | Unrelated to coitus<br>In place for 3 wk at a time<br>No fitting required | No protection against STDs<br>Must remember when to remove and when to insert<br>Side effects include expulsion, vaginal discomfort or discharge, and others similar to OCs |

**TABLE 31.1 Advantages and Disadvantages of Most Common Contraceptive Methods—cont'd**

| Method | Advantages | Disadvantages |
|---|---|---|
| **Barrier** | | |
| All methods | Avoid use of systemic hormones<br>Some offer some protection against STDs | Most coitus-related (must be used shortly before coitus)<br>May interfere with sensation<br>Contraindicated for allergies to components of spermicide or latex |
| Spermicides | Quick and easy<br>No prescription needed<br>Inexpensive per single use<br>Provide lubrication | Films and suppositories must melt to be effective<br>Effective time varies from less than 1-8 hr<br>No douching for 6 hr<br>May cause irritation<br>Can be messy<br>New application needed for repeated intercourse |
| Condoms | Quick and easy<br>No prescription needed<br>Best protection available for STDs<br>Inexpensive per single use<br>Can be carried discreetly<br>Vaginal condoms increase women's control over contraceptive use and protection from STDs | Interferes with spontaneity<br>Must be checked for expiration date and holes<br>Can break or slip off<br>Can be used only once<br>Female condoms may seem unattractive |
| Sponge | Available over the counter<br>Can be inserted several hours before coitus<br>Effective for repeated intercourse<br>No prescription needed | No protection against STDs<br>Must remain in place for 6 hr after last intercourse but no more than 30 hr total<br>May cause irritation<br>Risk of toxic shock syndrome if used too long or during menstruation |
| Diaphragm | Can be inserted several hours before coitus<br>Provides some protection from STDs<br>Can remain in place up to 24 hr | Initially expensive; requires healthcare provider to fit<br>Requires education on proper use<br>Difficult to insert or remove for some women<br>Added spermicide necessary for repeat coitus<br>Possibility of toxic shock syndrome or bladder infection<br>Must remain in place at least 6 hr after coitus |
| Cervical cap | Smaller than a diaphragm and may fit women who cannot wear a diaphragm<br>No pressure against bladder<br>Less noticeable than a diaphragm<br>Can remain in place 48 hr<br>Requires less spermicide<br>Provides some protection against STDs | Initially expensive<br>Requires healthcare provider to fit<br>Requires education on proper use<br>Added spermicide necessary for repeat coitus<br>Possibility of toxic shock syndrome<br>Must remain in place at least 6 hr after coitus |
| **Natural Family Planning** | | |
| All methods | Inexpensive<br>No drugs or hormones<br>Help a woman learn about her body<br>Can be combined with barrier methods to increase effectiveness<br>Acceptable to most religions<br>May be used to help achieve pregnancy | No protection against STDs<br>Requires high level of motivation and extensive education<br>Requires abstinence for large part of each cycle<br>High risk of pregnancy from error<br>Many factors may change ovulation time |

*IUD*, Intrauterine device; *OCs*, oral contraceptives; *STDs*, sexually transmitted diseases.

### Safety

The safety of the method is a primary consideration. Medical conditions make some methods unsafe for certain women. For example, women who have had thrombophlebitis or stroke should not use OCs because the hormones increase the risk for these conditions to recur.

### Protection From Sexually Transmitted Diseases

No contraceptive (other than total abstinence) is 100% effective in preventing sexually transmitted diseases (STDs). The risk of exposure to STDs should be discussed when counseling women about contraceptive choices. The male condom is inexpensive and offers the best protection available. It should be used whenever there is a risk that one partner has an STD, even when another form of contraception is practiced or the woman is pregnant.

### Effectiveness

The importance of avoiding pregnancy must be considered when choosing a contraceptive method. Effectiveness is determined by how often the method prevents pregnancy. Effectiveness rates reflect two different types of contraceptive failure: that of the method itself and that related to the user. The ideal, perfect, or theoretical effectiveness

**TABLE 31.2 Usa Pregnancy Rates for Common Types of Contraception**

| Method | Pregnancy Rate: Actual or Typical Use (%) |
|---|---|
| Sterilization | |
| Vasectomy | 0.15 |
| Tubal sterilization | 0.5 |
| Intrauterine devices | |
| LNG-IUS (Mirena) | 0.2 |
| Copper T 380A (ParaGard) | 0.8 |
| Contraceptive Implant | 0.05 |
| Injectable (Depo-Provera) | 6 |
| Oral contraceptives | 9 |
| Transdermal contraceptive patch (Evra) | 9 |
| Vaginal contraceptive ring (NuvaRing) | 9 |
| Spermicides, gel, foam, films, suppositories (used alone) | 28 |
| Condoms | |
| Male | 18 |
| Female | 21 |
| Sponge | |
| Nulliparous women | 12 |
| Parous women | 24 |
| Diaphragm with spermicide | 12 |
| Cervical cap | |
| Nulliparous women | 16 |
| Parous women | 32 |
| Natural family planning (all types) | 24 |
| Coitus interruptus (withdrawal) | 22 |
| No contraceptive use | 85 |

Data from Trussell, J. (2011). Contraceptive failure in the United States. *Contraception, 83*(15), 307–404; Speroff, L., & Darney, P.D. (2011). *A clinical guide for contraception* (5th ed.). Philadelphia: Lippincott Williams & Wilkins.

rate refers to perfect use of the method with every act of intercourse. The typical, actual, or user effectiveness rate is most useful because it refers to the actual occurrence of pregnancy in people using the method (Table 31.2).

Effectiveness drops greatly when the user does not understand how to use the method. The failure rate commonly decreases after the first year of use because experience with a method leads to more accurate use. Combining two less reliable methods, such as a condom and a spermicide, increases effectiveness.

### Acceptability

The effectiveness of a method must be balanced against its acceptability to the couple. For example, a spermicide may be considered unacceptable because it seems "messy" to the woman. Teenagers who are not comfortable with their bodies are unlikely to accept methods that require insertion of a device into the vagina. Although sterilization is very effective, it is not chosen by those who want to have more children. Side effects cause some women to choose less effective methods. The woman or her partner may be concerned about certain contraceptives because of potential effects such as weight gain.

### Convenience

Convenience is another important factor in choosing a contraceptive method. If the woman perceives her contraceptive as difficult to use, time-consuming, or too much "bother," she is less likely to use it consistently. Methods that can be used monthly or weekly instead of daily or with each intercourse are more convenient and likely to lead to better compliance. Spotting or bleeding between periods, common with some methods, can be viewed as very inconvenient.

The desire to avoid monthly menstruation should also be considered. Some women prefer extended cycles with several months between menses, and others want to avoid menstrual periods altogether. Extended or continuous use of OCs, the patch, and the ring can be used. Hormone implants or injections and intrauterine devices (IUDs) can also lead to amenorrhea in some women.

### Education Needed

Some women fail to use contraception because they do not understand their risk for pregnancy. They may be unfamiliar with the variety of methods available or the risks and benefits of the different types. Some methods, such as condoms, involve very little education, whereas others are more complicated. Women using natural family planning methods need extensive education to practice these methods successfully. Women knowledgeable about a contraceptive technique are less likely to feel that the contraceptive is difficult to use.

### Benefits

Some methods have special benefits that should be discussed with women. OCs have many beneficial side effects such as improvement of acne, decreased bleeding with periods, or prolonged amenorrhea. Natural family planning methods offer freedom from exposure to hormones. Condoms provide better protection against human immunodeficiency virus (HIV).

### Side Effects

Many methods of contraception have bothersome side effects that should be explained. When women know what to expect, they are often more willing to tolerate side effects, especially if they know they do not indicate a health risk.

### Effect on Spontaneity

Contraceptive methods related to coitus (sexual intercourse), such as spermicides and some barrier methods, must be readily available and used just before sexual intercourse. They interrupt love making, increasing the chance that the method will not be used. Some couples remedy this problem by making placement of the contraceptive device a part of foreplay. Others prefer methods such as OCs or IUDs that do not interrupt sexual activity.

### Availability

Condoms and spermicides are readily available without prescriptions. They can be purchased anonymously, at any time. Their availability may be important to an adolescent who wants to hide her sexual activity or to women who are embarrassed to discuss contraception with a healthcare provider.

### Expense

The cost of family planning methods is important. Less expensive contraceptives are chosen by some couples to save money. Less expensive methods are often less effective, and thus, more likely to result in pregnancy, which costs more than the yearly expense of any contraceptive.

The "per use" cost of a contraceptive can be compared with long-term expense. The price of condoms and spermicides is relatively low, but frequent use makes them expensive over a period of years. Methods that depend on periodic visits to a healthcare provider are more costly than over-the-counter methods. However, these visits provide an opportunity for teaching about correct use that improves the contraceptive effectiveness. The visits also provide the woman an opportunity to discuss other health concerns. Long-term contraceptives such as IUDs are very cost-effective over a 5- or 10-year period because they prevent pregnancy so well.

Publicly funded clinics may provide free or low-cost contraceptives. However, many require a long wait, and the woman is likely to see a different healthcare provider at each visit. Twenty-eight states have laws in place that insurance companies must cover prescription medications, including contraceptive drugs and devices. These laws are is important, as millions of women rely on insurance coverage to help them afford contraception (AGI, 2015a).

### Preference

The woman usually makes the final decision about her contraceptive method. Consistent use of any method depends on whether it meets the needs of the woman and her partner. If the woman feels pressured to choose a certain method or if a chosen method fails to live up to her expectations, use is more likely to be inconsistent. The opinion of the woman's partner and her friends can also influence what method she chooses.

### Religious and Personal Beliefs

Religious or other personal beliefs also affect the choice of contraceptives. Ninety-nine percent of Protestants and Catholics have used contraception at some time in their lives. Two percent of Catholics rely on natural family planning (AGI, 2015a).

### Culture

Another potential influence is the woman's culture. Some cultures place a high value on large families and especially on sons. A woman may have more pregnancies in an effort to have sons. Asian and Hispanic women are often very modest and do not talk about sexuality with others. They need to feel very comfortable with the nurse before talking about sexual matters. Taking time to establish rapport before discussing intimate subjects is important.

Some cultures restrict a woman's activities during menses. Methods that have increased bleeding or break-through bleeding as a side effect may not be acceptable to these couples. Some African-American women believe that menses removes dirty or excess blood. These women may not want to use contraception that increases or decreases bleeding.

### Other Considerations

Women also consider other factors when choosing a contraceptive. The length of time before another pregnancy is desired will determine if a long-acting contraceptive is appropriate. Breastfeeding women must choose a method that will not harm the baby or reduce milk production. A woman at risk for acquiring or transmitting an STD should use condoms either alone or with another, more effective, method of preventing pregnancy.

Obese women using combined OCs have a higher risk of thromboembolic disorders than nonobese women. However, the risk is less than that of pregnancy. Evidence is inconsistent as to whether the effectiveness of OCs is less for obese women (Robinson & Burke, 2013).

## INFORMED CONSENT

Because some methods have potentially dangerous side effects, it is necessary for the woman choosing surgical sterilization, hormone injections, implants, and IUDs to sign an informed consent form. Of course, whether or not a consent form is used, every woman should receive information about the chosen contraceptive method and its proper use, risks and benefits, and alternative methods available.

## ADOLESCENTS

In a national survey of high school students, 46% reported ever having sexual intercourse, and 38.9% of currently sexually active students reported they had not used a condom at last sexual intercourse. Although the rate of adolescent pregnancies has diminished in recent years, adolescent pregnancy is still a major problem. Because of the serious effect of pregnancy on the teenager, finding methods to increase contraception use among adolescents is extremely important. (See Chapter 24 for more about adolescent pregnancy.)

The U.S. *Healthy People 2020* goals include:

- Increasing the number of adolescents ages 15 to 17 years who have never had sexual intercourse to 79.3% of females and 78.3% of males
- Increasing condom use at first intercourse to 73.6% of adolescent females and 88.6% of males
- Increasing the number of sexually active adolescents ages 15 to 17 years who used a condom and hormonal or intrauterine contraception at first and last intercourse (USDHHS, 2010)

### Adolescent Knowledge

Many adolescents have little knowledge about their own anatomy and physiology, including how and when conception occurs. They are likely to learn about contraception from other teenagers, who often pass on incorrect information. Contraceptive failure is twice as likely in teenagers as in women age 30 years or older (Speroff & Darney, 2011).

#### Misinformation

Misinformation and erroneous beliefs cause adolescents to use ineffective methods of contraception or no method at all. Even adolescent mothers are more likely to be inconsistent in contraceptive use or use ineffective methods. Some teenagers think they cannot become pregnant the first time they have intercourse. Others assume they must have an orgasm or must have been menstruating a certain length of time to become pregnant. However, conception can result from any intercourse near ovulation. Although many adolescents have anovulatory menstrual cycles during the early months after menarche, they cannot depend on failure to ovulate to prevent pregnancy because some will ovulate before their first menses.

Teenagers and older women may douche (insert a solution into the vagina) after intercourse to prevent pregnancy. However, douching is ineffective because sperm enter the cervix very soon after ejaculation. **Coitus interruptus** (withdrawal of the penis before ejaculation) is another unreliable method used by teenagers. It requires more control over timing of ejaculation than most adolescent boys have. In addition, **semen** (sperm and fluid discharged during ejaculation) spilled near the vagina can enter and cause pregnancy even without penetration by the penis.

#### Risk-Taking Behavior

Adolescents are more likely than adults to take risks in sexual activity because they believe their chances of becoming pregnant are low. Because of their immaturity and feelings of invincibility, teenagers often do not plan intercourse and are not prepared with contraceptives. They are more likely to engage in risk-taking behavior than older women, and this can lead to STDs and pregnancy. Some teenagers wait months after becoming sexually active to begin contraception.

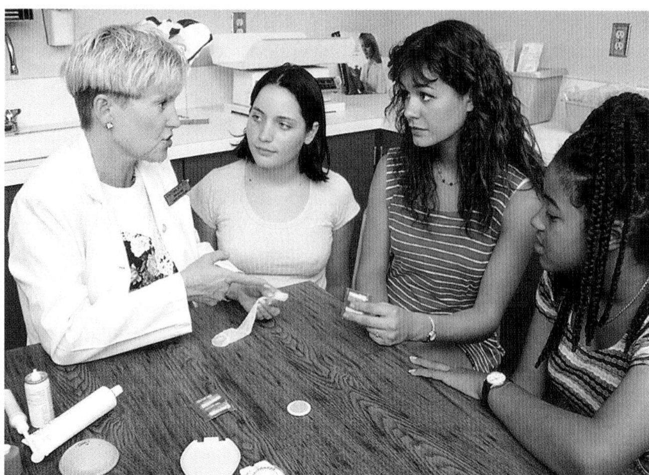

**FIG 31.2** Although many adolescents choose oral contraceptives, the nurse emphasizes the need to use condoms for protection against sexually transmitted diseases. Demonstrating with actual contraceptives increases understanding.

### Counseling Adolescents

Nurses who counsel adolescents about sexuality must be sensitive to their feelings, concerns, and needs (Fig. 31.2). They must be accepting of the teenager regardless of personal feelings about adolescent sexuality. Teenagers may not ask about contraception because they do not want anyone to know they are sexually active. Their need for secrecy may cause them to miss family planning appointments. The nurse must reassure teenagers that their visits are confidential.

Visits to a healthcare provider for checkups, minor illnesses, or pregnancy testing can provide unplanned opportunities for the nurse or other healthcare provider to discuss contraception. After a negative pregnancy test, a teenager may be particularly interested in learning about contraception.

Although nurses should encourage adolescents to discuss contraception with their parents, many teenagers will forego contraception rather than talk to their parents about it. Therefore, they need other reliable sources of information. Many schools provide information about sexuality. Discussions include information about contraception as well as abstinence. Encouragement to delay sexual activity and discussion regarding the effect of pregnancy on the adolescent are often included. Family planning clinics that are open after school and in the evenings are also a source of contraception education and supplies.

The pelvic examination, greatly dreaded by many women, is not necessary for a prescription for OCs and can be delayed until a later healthcare visit. The American Cancer Society (ACS) recommends that yearly Papanicolaou (Pap) tests should begin at age 21. During the first contraceptive visit, the teenager receives information about contraceptive methods. Taking the time to explain the different methods helps to dispel misinformation and allay common concerns.

Because of her youth and possible lack of knowledge about anatomy and physiology, the adolescent often needs more extensive teaching than the older woman. Liberal use of audiovisual materials, such as pictures, anatomic models, and samples of various methods, helps the teenage girl understand the information more easily. Giving her a patch, vaginal ring, and condom to manipulate or showing her the packet of pills she will be using are important aids.

Using understandable terminology is especially important when teaching adolescents. The nurse must know street terms for body parts and sexual intercourse because they may be the only terms the teenager knows.

Adolescents have most success when they choose contraceptive methods that are easy to use and that seem unrelated to coitus. The most popular contraceptives for adolescents are OCs and condoms (Speroff & Darney, 2011). Teenagers choose OCs because they are safe, have few contraindications for teenagers, seem unrelated to sex, and are not difficult or messy. In addition, they increase bone density, regulate periods, may decrease acne, and reduce menstrual flow and cramping (Cunningham et al., 2014; Speroff & Darney, 2011).

However, adolescent girls may be inconsistent in taking pills every day. They are more likely than older women to discontinue any method for side effects such as spotting. Their concerns should be taken seriously and attempts made to alleviate side effects so they will continue using the method. Methods that do not have to be used every day may be more appropriate for teens who tend to forget their pills or do not like the side effects of OCs.

Adolescents may use condoms alone to prevent pregnancy and STDs, especially at the beginning of a relationship or with casual partners. With long-term partners, they may switch from condoms to hormonal methods. Increased use of hormonal methods is associated with decreased use of condoms for many adolescents. Some seldom use condoms except if they have casual partners or if they are very concerned about pregnancy and STDs. Many young women are uneasy about asking a partner to use a condom. Discussions about how to negotiate condom use with a partner are helpful. Using a condom and an OC provides highly efficient contraception along with protection from STDs and should be encouraged.

#### CRITICAL THINKING EXERCISE 31.1

A 15-year-old girl approaches a nurse with questions about contraception. She says she does not want to become pregnant, but her boyfriend does not want to use condoms, and she is too embarrassed to go to see a physician for other contraceptive methods. How should the nurse handle the situation?

## PERIMENOPAUSAL WOMEN

Pregnancy is uncommon after age 50. However, perimenopausal women may continue to ovulate as long as they have regular menstrual periods, and some ovulate even when indications of menopause are present. Fertility begins to decline when women reach 35 to 40 years, but they are still at risk for an unintended pregnancy (Nelson, 2011). In fact, more than 30% of pregnancies in women older than age 35 years are unintended (Godfrey, Chin, Fielding, et al., 2011). Therefore, the nurse must offer these women contraceptive counseling whenever possible. To avoid pregnancy, effective contraception should be used until 1 year after a woman's last menses (Barry, 2011).

The most common method used by women in the United States who are older than 30 years is sterilization (AGI, 2015a). Low-dose OCs can be used by nonsmokers to prevent contraception and help regulate the irregular bleeding that often occurs during perimenopause. However, women older than age 35 years who smoke or have significant cardiac risk factors should not use combined hormonal contraceptives. Barrier methods or contraceptives that contain only **progestin** (any form of progesterone), such as the progestin IUD (Mirena), Depo-Provera, or progestin only OCs, are also good choices for the older woman. Perimenopausal women should have regular physical examinations to identify any conditions that would require a change in contraceptive method.

# METHODS OF CONTRACEPTION

## Sterilization

Sterilization (male and female combined) is one of the most widely used methods of contraception in the United States (AGI, 2015b). Approximately one in three married couples uses this method. Although it is expensive at the time of surgery, sterilization ends all further contraceptive costs. It should always be considered a permanent end to fertility because reversal surgery is difficult, expensive, not always successful, and often not covered by insurance.

Couples considering sterilization need counseling to ensure that they understand all aspects of the procedure. When surgery is planned for immediately after childbirth, the decision should be made well before labor begins. Future marriage, divorce, or death of a child can cause couples to regret their decision. Although pregnancy is rare after sterilization, the risk of failure should be discussed. Pregnancies that occur after tubal sterilization are more likely to be ectopic.

### Tubal Sterilization

Tubal sterilization (also called tubal ligation) is widely used throughout the world. It involves cutting or occluding the fallopian tubes to prevent fertilization. The surgery is easiest during abdominal surgery such as cesarean birth when a woman is sure that she wants the procedure regardless of the outcome of the birth. During the first 48 hours after vaginal birth, the fundus is located near the umbilicus, and the fallopian tubes are directly below the abdominal wall, making this a good time for tubal sterilization. Interval tubal sterilization, not associated with childbirth, is often performed as outpatient surgery. General anesthesia is most common, but regional or local anesthesia can be used.

Several surgical methods are used for tubal sterilization. One uses a minilaparotomy incision near the umbilicus during the postpartum period or just above the symphysis pubis at other times. Another is performed through a laparoscope inserted through a small incision. In each method, the surgeon blocks the tubes with clips, bands, or rings, removes a piece of the tubes, and either ties the ends or uses electrocoagulation to destroy a portion of the tubes.

Two nonsurgical methods of sterilization are available. Essure involves the insertion of a small coil through the vagina and uterus into each fallopian tube. The Adiana system uses radiofrequency energy to remove a thin layer of tissue and a silicone implant is inserted into each tube. The procedures can be performed in the physician's office. The tubes become permanently blocked over the next 3 months as tissue grows in and around the inserts. During this time, another contraceptive method is necessary. A hysterosalpingogram is performed at the end of 3 months. The American College of Obstetricians and Gynecologists (ACOG) (2013a,b) emphasizes the importance of the hysterosalpingogram at 3 months to ensure the tubes are completely blocked.

### Vasectomy

Vasectomy, the male sterilization procedure, involves making a small incision or puncture in the scrotum to cut, tie, cauterize, or remove a section of the vas deferens, which carries sperm from the testes to the penis. After vasectomy, sperm no longer pass into the semen.

Vasectomy is safer, easier, less expensive, and has a lower failure rate than tubal sterilization (Speroff & Darney, 2011). It can be performed in a physician's office under local anesthesia and is less expensive. After surgery, the man rests and wears a scrotal support for 2 days. He applies ice to the area for 4 hours and takes a mild analgesic if needed. Strenuous activity should be avoided for 1 week (Roncari & Hou, 2011).

Sperm may be present in the ductal system, distal to the ligation of the vas deferens when the surgery is performed. The couple should understand that the man may be able to impregnate a woman until sperm are no longer present in the semen, which may be 3 months or more. He should submit semen specimens for analysis until two specimens show no sperm present.

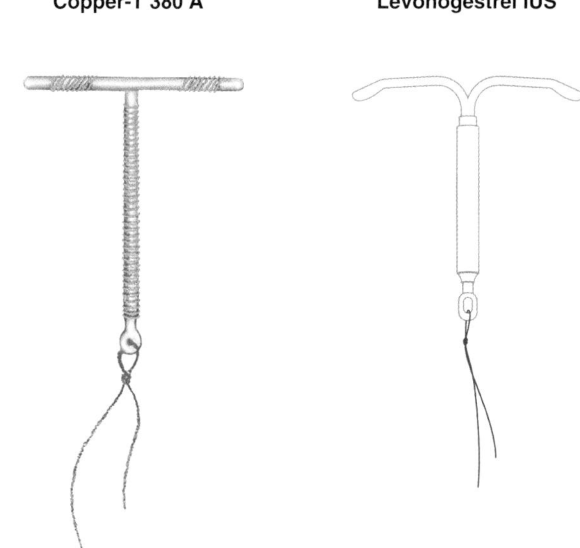


**FIG 31.3** The Copper T 380A (ParaGard) intrauterine device (IUD) and the levonorgestrel intrauterine system (LNG-IUS or Mirena). Currently, the IUD is considered a very safe method for preventing pregnancy.

## Intrauterine Devices (IUDs)

An IUD is inserted into the uterus to provide continuous pregnancy prevention. The Copper T 380A (ParaGard) and the levonorgestrel intrauterine system (LNG-IUS or Mirena) are shaped like the letter T (Fig. 31.3). ParaGard is effective for 10 years and Mirena for 5 years. Fertility returns when the device is removed. Increasing the use of IUDs is recommended by ACOG as a long-term, cost-effective means of lowering unintended pregnancy (ACOG, 2011).

Many women have misperceptions regarding the safety and effectiveness of IUDs (Hladky, Allsworth, Madden, et al., 2011). Although there was concern about safety with early models, IUDs are considered very safe at this time. More education about IUDs is necessary to increase their use. IUDs provide contraception without the need to take pills, have injections, or perform other tasks just before intercourse. They can be inserted immediately postpartum or after an abortion, although expulsion is higher in the immediate postpartum period (ACOG, 2011).

IUDs can be used by some women who cannot use hormonal contraception. They are safe for adolescents and women who have never had a baby. There is a slight risk of infection during the first 20 days after insertion, but there is no increased risk of pelvic inflammatory disease or infertility in women who use IUDs or when couples are not mutually monogamous if condoms are used (ACOG, 2011). Women at high risk for STDs should use another method.

### Action

IUDs cause a sterile inflammatory response that results in a spermicidal intrauterine environment. They do not cause abortion (Speroff & Darney, 2011). Progestin is continuously released from the LNG-IUS, Mirena. The progestin causes decreased sperm and ova viability, thickening of the cervical mucus (barring sperm penetration), inhibits sperm motility, prevents ovulation some of the time, and makes the endometrium hostile to implantation.

### Side Effects

Side effects include cramping and bleeding with insertion. Menorrhagia (increased bleeding during menstruation) and dysmenorrhea (painful menstruation) are common reasons for removal of the copper device. Ibuprofen may relieve cramping and reduce bleeding. Irregular bleeding or spotting may occur during the early months with the LNG-IUS, but bleeding is less than with the copper IUD and may be followed by amenorrhea. The LNG-IUS can be used by women who had amenorrhea before using an IUD.

Complications include expulsion of the IUD and perforation of the uterus. Although pregnancy with an IUD is rare, ectopic pregnancy or spontaneous abortion is more likely if pregnancy does occur. Infection can occur in the first few weeks after insertion because of contamination at the time of insertion. Women with recent or recurrent pelvic infections, a history of ectopic pregnancy, bleeding disorders, or abnormalities of the uterus should choose another contraceptive method.

### Teaching

Teaching the woman about side effects and to check for the presence of the plastic strings, or "tail," extending from the IUD into the vagina is important. The woman should feel for the strings once a week during the first 4 weeks, then monthly after menses, and if she has signs of expulsion (cramping or unexpected bleeding). If the strings are longer or shorter than they were previously, she should see her physician, nurse-midwife, or nurse practitioner. The healthcare provider should be informed about signs of infection, such as unusual vaginal discharge, pain or itching, low pelvic pain, and fever. Any signs of pregnancy should be reported to rule out ectopic pregnancy and remove the device if pregnancy has occurred.

## Hormonal Contraceptives

Hormonal contraceptives alter the normal hormone fluctuations of the menstrual cycle. Hormones are delivered by implant, injection, patch, or vaginal ring, or can be taken orally.

### Hormone Implants

The progestin implant, Implanon (or Nexplanon), a single rod implant, is inserted subcutaneously into the upper inner arm. Implanon is 2 mm thick and 4 cm (1.6 in) long and releases progestin continuously to provide 3 years of contraception. Like other progestin-only contraceptives, it inhibits ovulation, thickens cervical mucus to prevent sperm penetrability, and makes the endometrium unfavorable for implantation. Increasing the use of hormone implants is recommended by ACOG as a means of offering effective long acting reversible contraception (ACOG, 2011).

Side effects include irregular menstrual bleeding. The woman should be taught that bleeding is expected and not a sign of abnormality. Amenorrhea can occur with longer use. Implanon is safe during lactation; body weight does not affect its effectiveness, and fertility returns within a few weeks after the implant is removed. If it is inserted within 7 days of the start of menses, no back-up method is needed. If it is inserted later, a back-up contraceptive should be used for at least 3 days (Speroff & Darney, 2011).

### Hormone Injections

Medroxyprogesterone acetate, or DMPA (Depo-Provera), is an injectable progestin that is available for intramuscular (IM) and subcutaneous (Sub Q) administration. It is convenient, has no estrogen, and prevents ovulation for 14 weeks, although injections should be scheduled every 12 weeks. Action and side effects are similar to those of other progestin contraceptives. Women who should not use other hormone contraceptives should avoid Depo-Provera as well.

The IM form of Depo-Provera is given by deep intramuscular injection. The Sub Q form is given in the anterior thigh or abdomen. The site should not be massaged after injection because massage accelerates absorption and decreases the period of effectiveness. A back-up method of contraception should be used for the first 7 days unless the injection is given within 5 days after a menstrual period starts. Back-up contraception is also recommended if the woman is more than 2 weeks late in returning for subsequent injections, and a pregnancy test may be performed.

Menstrual irregularity is the major reason for discontinuation. Although spotting and break-through bleeding are common, amenorrhea occurs in 80% of women using the IM form at 5 years and in 55% of women using the Sub Q form at 1 year (Speroff & Darney, 2011). Other side effects include breast tenderness, weight gain, headaches, depression, and decreased bone density.

Because of the loss of bone density that occurs with prolonged use, the prescribing information states that Depo-Provera should not be used for more than 2 years unless no other contraceptive is suitable. Although bone density losses reverse after the drug is discontinued, it is not known if the bone loss is fully reversible. Bone loss could be a bigger problem for women who begin Depo-Provera during adolescence or in the perimenopausal period. Women who use Depo-Provera should get adequate amounts of calcium and vitamin D and should increase weight-bearing exercises.

Depo-Provera can be started in the immediate postpartum period. It increases the quantity of milk in lactating women, and its effectiveness is not affected by a woman's weight. After the drug is discontinued, there is a delay in return to fertility. Approximately 59% of women resume menses in 6 months, and 25% do not resume menses for a year or more.

### Oral Contraceptives

Oral contraceptives are widely used in the United States. They are available as combination OCs containing both estrogen and progestin or as minipills that contain only progestin. Both types have much lower hormone levels than the original OCs, thus decreasing the risk of long-term side effects.

***Progestin only.*** Progestin-only pills (POPs) are less effective at inhibiting ovulation but avoid the use of estrogen, which cannot be used by some women. POPs cause thickening of the cervical mucus to prevent penetration by sperm, and they make the endometrial lining unfavorable for implantation. The woman should start POPs during the first 5 days of her menstrual cycle and take one pill at the same time of day continuously. She can start the pills on another day if she is sure she is not pregnant. If she misses any pills or does not take them at the same time each day, the chance of pregnancy increases. The woman should use a back-up method of contraception for 2 days when the pills are first started, if she is more than 3 hours late in taking a pill, or has vomiting or diarrhea within 4 hours of taking a pill (Raymond, 2011). Break-through bleeding and greater chances of error have made these OCs less popular than the combination OCs.

***Combination.*** Combined OCs (COCs) containing estrogen and progestin are the most common OCs. COCs suppress estrogen and luteinizing hormone (LH), inhibiting maturation of the follicle and ovulation. They cause thickening of the cervical mucus, preventing sperm from entering the fallopian tubes. In addition, tubal motility is slowed, and the endometrium becomes less hospitable to implantation.

Monophasic or multiphasic dosages are available. The estrogen and progestin content of monophasic pills remains constant throughout the cycle. With multiphasic pills, the estrogen and progestin doses vary at different times of the cycle to help reduce side effects. Because of the changes in dose over the course of the menstrual cycle, women must take the pills in the proper order.

Many COCs are available in packets of 21 or 28 tablets. With 21-tablet packets, the woman takes 1 pill daily for 3 weeks and then stops for a week, during which the menses occur. Packets of 28 tablets include 21 active tablets and 7 tablets made of an inert substance that the woman takes during the fourth week. These extra pills avoid disrupting the everyday routine of taking pills. Some formulations contain 24 active tablets with 4 inactive tablets. Women using these pills have shorter, lighter withdrawal bleeding.

Some women prefer extended cycles in which the menses are delayed for a few days for special occasions or for a longer time. These women take two or more pill packs without taking the placebo pills for several packs or indefinitely. A COC designed to provide 84 days of active pills and seven placebo pills or seven pills with a small amount of estrogen allows women to have menses only four times a year. The added estrogen is given to decrease breakthrough bleeding and give a shorter withdrawal bleed. Another formulation is taken every day without stopping to suspend menstrual periods indefinitely. Breakthrough bleeding and spotting are a common problem with extended or continuous use, but they usually lessen with time. A disadvantage is that a woman might not recognize a pregnancy early.

***Benefits, risks, and cautions.*** When choosing OCs, the balance between the benefits and risks must be weighed for each individual (Box 31.1). Women often believe the risks of OCs are higher than they actually are, yet taking OCs is safer for most women than pregnancy (Beckmann et al., 2010). In addition to safe, reliable contraception, OCs result in regular menses and decreases in flow, premenstrual syndrome, and dysmenorrhea, reduced acne, and improved bone density.

OCs should not be used by women who have certain medical complications (see Safety Alert: Cautions in Using Oral Contraceptives). Smoking significantly increases complications for women of all ages. Women older than age 35 who smoke should not use OCs. Women who have previously smoked must abstain from all sources of nicotine for at least 6 to 12 months to be considered a nonsmoker (Speroff & Darney, 2011).

Obese women have a higher risk of thromboembolic problems, but this is not considered a contraindication to OC use. Evidence is inconsistent regarding the effect of body weight on OC effectiveness. OCs provide no protection against STDs and may increase susceptibility to chlamydia. A woman should be advised to use a condom and spermicide if her partner could be infected or the relationship is not monogamous.

***Side effects.*** Approximately 33% of women who do not wish to become pregnant discontinue OC use within a year, (Trussell, 2011) usually because of side effects. Most side effects are minor. Using formulations with less estrogen helps relieve nausea and breast tenderness. Break-through bleeding occurs most often in the first 3 months and then usually subsides. Some women complain of weight gain while taking OCs, but studies have not shown it to be caused by the pills. Other side effects include fluid retention, amenorrhea, and melasma (brownish pigmentation of the face).

***Teaching.*** Many unintended pregnancies result from failure to take OCs correctly. However, education about proper use greatly increases

**BOX 31.1 Potential Benefits, Disadvantages, and Risks of Oral Contraceptives**

| Benefits | Disadvantages | Risks* |
|---|---|---|
| Unrelated to coitus | Must be taken every day at or near same time, especially progestin-only pills | No protection against STDs |
| Highly effective contraception | Side effects may include: | May increase risk of cervical cancer |
| Regulate menstrual cycles and reduce dysmenorrhea, menstrual blood loss, and associated anemia | Break-through bleeding | Increased incidence of: |
| Amenorrhea (may be seen as a disadvantage) | Nausea | Deep and superficial vein thrombosis |
| Fertility returns within 3 mo usually | Headache | Pulmonary embolism |
| Decreased incidence of: | Breast tenderness | Myocardial infarction |
| Premenstrual dysphoric disorder symptoms | Chloasma | Stroke (in smokers) |
| Benign breast disease | Amenorrhea (may be seen as an advantage) | Hypertension |
| Pelvic inflammatory disease | | Chlamydial infection |
| Salpingitis | | Gallbladder disease |
| Ectopic pregnancy | | |
| Ovarian cancer | | |
| Endometrial cancer | | |
| Colorectal cancer | | |
| Improves: | | |
| Acne | | |
| Endometriosis | | |
| Many premenstrual symptoms | | |
| Dysmenorrhea | | |
| Bleeding from fibroids | | |
| Bone mass (combined OCs only) | | |
| Hirsutism (excessive hair growth) | | |
| Rheumatoid arthritis | | |

*OCs,* Oral contraceptives; *STDs,* sexually transmitted diseases

*Incidence of many risks is significantly reduced with low-dose OCs presently used. Avoiding OC use in women who smoke or have other risk factors significantly lowers risk of cardiovascular disease.

**SAFETY ALERT**

***Cautions in Using Oral Contraceptives***

Combined oral contraceptives (OCs) should not be used by women with a history of any of the following:

- Thrombophlebitis and thromboembolic disorders
- Cerebrovascular or cardiovascular diseases
- Any estrogen-dependent cancer or breast cancer
- Benign or malignant liver tumors
- Hypertension
- Migraines with aura or women older than 35 years of age having migraines without aura
- Diabetes longer than 20 years duration or with vascular or other organ involvement

Combined OCs should not be used by women who have any of the following:

- Any of the above conditions
- Impaired liver function
- Suspected or known pregnancy
- Undiagnosed vaginal bleeding
- Age older than 35 years and any smoking
- Major surgery requiring prolonged immobilization

effectiveness. Because the instructions can be complicated, the woman should receive written as well as verbal instructions in her own language if she can read.

Teaching about when to start taking OCs is especially important. The woman will be told to start taking her pills either on the day they are prescribed (if it is reasonably sure she is not pregnant [Quick Start method]), on the first day of the next menstrual period, or on the first Sunday after her next menses begins. The Quick Start method provides immediate protection. A Sunday start prevents the woman from having periods on weekends. Unless she begins her pills on the first day of her menses, the woman is usually told to use a back-up contraceptive for the first week.

One study showed that women who did not fully understand the advantages of OCs and had low confidence in their ability to use them were less likely to continue use at 6 months (Dempsey, Johnson, & Westhoff, 2011). The nurse should listen carefully to women's concerns about side effects and help them find methods of relief. Teaching about temporary side effects may help the women endure them until they are no longer present.

When women discontinue OCs because they are unhappy with the side effects, they might not use another contraceptive or use one that is less effective, becoming pregnant as a result. Women should be instructed to keep a back-up contraceptive method readily available should they decide to stop taking their OCs.

***Blood hormone levels.*** Maintaining a constant blood hormone level is important for effectiveness, especially with POPs. The woman must take the pills close to the same time each day. Many women take the pills as a part of their morning or bedtime routine. The pills can be taken with a meal to avoid nausea. Illness can affect the blood hormone levels. A woman who experiences vomiting or diarrhea should use a back-up method of contraception for 7 days because the hormones may not have been properly absorbed.

**Missed doses.** The woman should follow instructions from her provider if she misses one or more doses of her OC. Instructions vary according to the type of OC she uses, the number of doses missed, and the time in the cycle when the OC is missed.

Instructions for missed OCs commonly include (Speroff & Darney, 2011):

- One missed dose: Take the pill as soon as remembered. Take the next dose at the usual time. No back-up contraception is necessary.
- Two missed doses in the first 2 weeks: Take two pills for 2 days, and then take one tablet each day. Use back-up contraception for the next 7 days.
- Two missed doses in the third week or more than two active pills missed at any time: If using the Sunday start schedule, take one active pill each day until Sunday. On Sunday, start a new package. If on a different schedule, start a new package immediately. Use another form of contraception for 7 days.
- Missing inactive tablets will not increase the risk of pregnancy. Discard the tablets missed.

If a woman misses a period and thinks she may be pregnant because she missed one or more doses, she should stop taking the pills and get a sensitive pregnancy test immediately. It is essential that she use another contraceptive method during this time. Although an association with significant fetal anomalies has not been established, continued use of OCs during pregnancy is not advisable.

**Postpartum and lactation.** Women have an increased risk of thrombosis after giving birth. They are usually advised to wait 3 to 4 weeks to begin COCs (Nelson & Cwiak, 2011). COCs reduce milk production in lactating women, and small amounts are transferred to the milk. POPs are a better choice because they do not decrease milk production; in fact, they can increase it. POPs can be started immediately after delivery (Speroff & Darney, 2011).

**Other medications.** OCs can interact with other medications. Drugs that stimulate metabolism in the liver, such as St. John's wort and some anticonvulsants, can alter the effectiveness of OCs. Most broad-spectrum antibiotics and antifungals do not decrease OC effectiveness. The woman should always tell her healthcare providers and her pharmacist about other drugs she is taking.

**Follow-up.** The only essential follow-up for women who take OCs is yearly blood pressure measurement. Yearly pelvic examinations, Pap tests, and breast examinations are not necessary to receive prescriptions for OCs. Women should follow the same recommendations for these examinations as women who do not take OCs.

The woman's ability to remember to take a pill every day should be evaluated, and other methods should be discussed if this requirement is a problem. Return of fertility usually occurs within 3 months after the pills are discontinued in women who were ovulating before pill use (Cunningham et al., 2014). Any signs of adverse reaction should be reported immediately. Use of the word ACHES may help the woman remember the signs that indicate complications (Table 31.3).

### Emergency Contraception

Emergency contraception (EC; also called the "morning-after pill") prevents pregnancy after unprotected intercourse. This method can be used after contraceptive failure, such as condom breaking during intercourse, after rape, or after contraceptives were used incorrectly or not at all.

Two types of EC (Plan B One-Step and Next Choice) contain the progestin levonorgestrel. Both are available at pharmacies without a prescription for women who are 17 years of age and older with picture identification for proof of age. Those under 17 need a prescription. Another type of EC is ulipristal acetate (Ella), which requires a prescription for all ages (Levy, Jager, Kapp, et al., 2014; Glasier, 2013).

The progestin ECs delay or inhibit ovulation and interfere with corpus luteum function. They are effective if ovulation has not already occurred. The treatment is ineffective if implantation has already

**TABLE 31.3 ACHES***

***Warning Signs of Oral Contraceptive Complications***

| | Warning Sign | Possible Complication |
|---|---|---|
| A | Abdominal pain (severe) | Mesenteric or pelvic vein thrombosis, benign liver tumor, gallbladder disease |
| C | Chest pain, dyspnea, hemoptysis, cough | Pulmonary embolism or myocardial infarction |
| H | Severe headache, weakness or numbness of extremities, hypertension | Stroke, migraine |
| E | Eye problems (complete or partial loss of vision, headache) | Stroke, migraine, retinal vein thrombosis |
| S | Severe pain or swelling, heat, or redness of calf or thigh | Deep vein thrombosis |

*The acronym ACHES can be used to help women remember warning signs that indicate complications of oral contraceptives. Other signs include jaundice, a breast lump, and depression. The woman should contact her healthcare provider if any of these signs develop.

Data from Nelson, A.L., & Cwiak, C. (2011). Combined oral contraceptives (COCs). In R.A. Hatcher, J. Trussell, A.L. Nelson, et al. *Contraceptive technology* (20th ed., pp. 249–341). New York: Ardent Media.

occurred. It does not harm a developing fetus (Speroff & Darney, 2011; Trussell & Schwarz, 2011). Ulipristal acetate (Ella) acts to delay or block the luteinizing surge and ovulation. It also inhibits implantation. Pregnancy should be excluded before Ella is taken because it can interfere with an existing pregnancy.

EC involves taking one or two tablets (taken together) that contain a high dose of progestin. Treatment reduces the risk of pregnancy by approximately 85% (Speroff & Darney, 2011). Combined OCs in larger-than-usual doses can also be used for this purpose. The dose varies with the brand and may require taking a large number of tablets. EC is most effective if used as soon as possible within 72 hours of intercourse but can be used with lessened effectiveness within 120 hours. Ulipristal acetate (Ella) can be taken within 5 days of unprotected intercourse. EC will not prevent pregnancy if unprotected intercourse occurs after EC is used.

Insertion of the copper IUD within 5 days of intercourse is up to 99% effective in preventing pregnancy (Trussell & Schwarz, 2011). Mifepristone is also used for EC. The drug inhibits ovulation and prevents endometrial development. However, mifepristone will disrupt an existing pregnancy. Because it is also used for medically induced abortion, some women will prefer to use another method.

Many women are unaware of the availability of EC. One survey found that although most female college students had heard of EC, many had inaccurate knowledge about the action, side effects, and how to obtain it. Information about its use and how to obtain it should be included any time education about contraception is offered. Women who need EC should receive counseling about their regular contraceptive method. They may not understand how to use their method correctly or may want information about other, more effective options. Because of the short time during which EC is effective, some health providers give women prescriptions to use at a later date, if needed. Women who use EC are not more likely to have risky sex, future unplanned pregnancies, or STDs (Levy et al., 2014; Glasier, 2013).

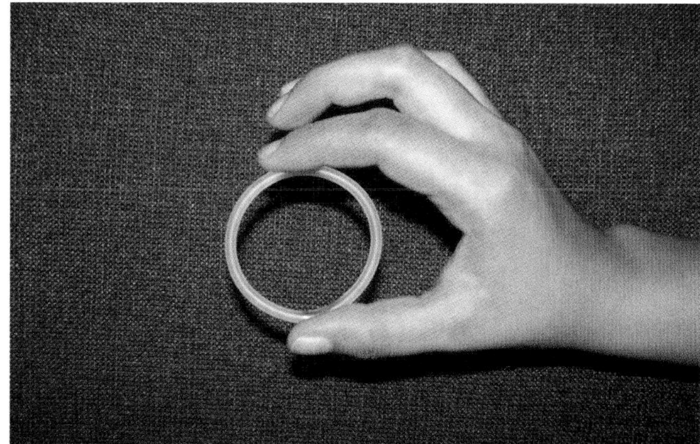

**FIG 31.4** The vaginal contraceptive ring (NuvaRing) is 5 cm (2 in) across and 4 mm thick.

### Transdermal Contraceptive Patch

The ethinyl estradiol and norelgestromin transdermal contraceptive patch (Ortho Evra) releases small amounts of estrogen and progestin that are absorbed through the skin to suppress ovulation and make cervical mucus thick. It also regulates menstrual cycles. A nonhormonal contraceptive should also be used during the first week of use unless the patch is started on the first day of the menstrual period.

The patch is applied to clean, dry, nonirritated skin of the abdomen, buttock, upper torso (excluding the breasts), or upper outer arm. It should not be placed over areas where lotions or oils have been used or where the patch would be rubbed by clothing. A new patch is applied to a different site on the same day of the week each week for 3 weeks and worn continuously for 7 days. No patch is worn during the fourth week. During the patch-free week, the woman has a period. After 7 patch-free days, she applies a new patch and begins the cycle again. Women can have extended cycles without menses by using patches for several cycles or continuously. Patches should not be cut or altered, and no more than one patch should be worn at a time.

The patch usually adheres to the skin even in the shower or when exercising or swimming. However, approximately 5% of patches detach (Speroff & Darney, 2011). A patch should be replaced with a new patch if it cannot be reattached. Extra patches are available by prescription. The day the patch is changed does not change even if a replacement for a detached patch is necessary. If a patch is detached for more than 24 hours or there is a delay of more than 2 days within the cycle, a new patch is applied to start a new cycle. The patch change day will be the day of the week the new patch is applied. Back-up contraception is necessary for 1 week of the first cycle (Speroff & Darney, 2011).

Side effects include spotting, especially during the first two cycles, breast tenderness, and skin reactions. Other side effects and risks are similar to combination OCs. The patch may be less effective in women who weigh more than 90 kg (198 lb) (Nandra, 2011). The risk of venous thromboembolism may be higher with patch use than with OC use because the estrogen exposure is 60% higher over time when patches are used. However, studies report conflicting results (Cunningham et al., 2014). Women with risk factors for thromboembolic conditions should discuss the risks and benefits of patch use with their healthcare provider.

### Contraceptive Vaginal Ring

Women using the ethinyl estradiol contraceptive ring (NuvaRing) insert a soft, flexible ring into the vagina and leave it in place for 3 weeks (Fig. 31.4). The ring releases small amounts of progestin and estrogen continuously to prevent ovulation. The woman removes the ring at the end of the third week, and bleeding occurs. A new ring is inserted to begin the next cycle a week after the old ring was removed. Although a prescription is required, no fitting or particular placement in the vagina is necessary. Unless the ring is inserted on the first day of menses, a back-up contraceptive should be used during the first 7 days of the first cycle.

Side effects such as break-through bleeding are less common than with OCs. Some women experience expulsion, vaginal discharge, or discomfort because they feel the ring in the vagina. Although some couples can feel the ring during intercourse, it is not generally a problem. The ring can be removed for short periods. However, if more than 3 hours elapse, a back-up method of contraception is needed until the ring has been used continuously for the next 7 days. If the woman desires extended cycles, she can insert a new ring at the end of the third week and avoid withdrawal bleeding.

## Barrier Methods

The barrier methods of contraception involve chemicals or devices that prevent sperm from entering the cervix. All of the barrier methods are coitus-related and may interfere with spontaneity. They avoid the use of systemic hormones and provide some protection from STDs.

### Chemical Barriers

The chemicals that kill sperm, called *spermicides,* come in many forms. Creams and gels are generally used with mechanical barriers such as the diaphragm or cervical cap. Foams, foaming tablets, suppositories, and vaginal film are used alone or with another contraceptive. They are inserted deep into the vagina approximately 30 minutes before sexual intercourse. Spermicides are effective for less than an hour to as long as 8 hours, depending on the type used and should be reapplied before repeated intercourse (Speroff & Darney, 2011). Women should not douche for at least 6 hours after intercourse.

Spermicides are readily available without a prescription, are inexpensive per use, and are easy to use. They can be used with condoms to enhance lubrication, decreasing the risk of condom breakage. They may be helpful during lactation or in the menopausal woman when vaginal secretions are diminished.

Spermicides do not protect against STDs. Frequent use or sensitivity to the products can cause genital irritation, which increases susceptibility to infection. Some women and their partners think that spermicides are messy and interfere with sensation during intercourse. Effectiveness is increased when spermicides are used with a mechanical barrier method.

### Mechanical Barriers

Mechanical barriers are devices placed over the penis or cervix to prevent sperm from entering the uterus. They include the condom, sponge, diaphragm, and cervical cap.

***Male condom.*** Condoms, one of the most popular contraceptive methods in the United States, cover the penis to prevent sperm from entering the vagina. They are most often made of latex. Latex condoms provide the best protection available (other than abstinence) against STDs, including HIV. Condoms should be used during any possible exposure to an STD, even if another contraceptive technique is used or if the woman is pregnant.

People allergic to latex should avoid the use of latex condoms because severe reactions are possible. Polyurethane, other synthetic materials, and natural membrane condoms are also available. Polyurethane condoms are thinner than latex but can require lubrication to avoid breakage and are more likely to slip off. Natural membrane condoms do not prevent passage of organisms that cause STDs.

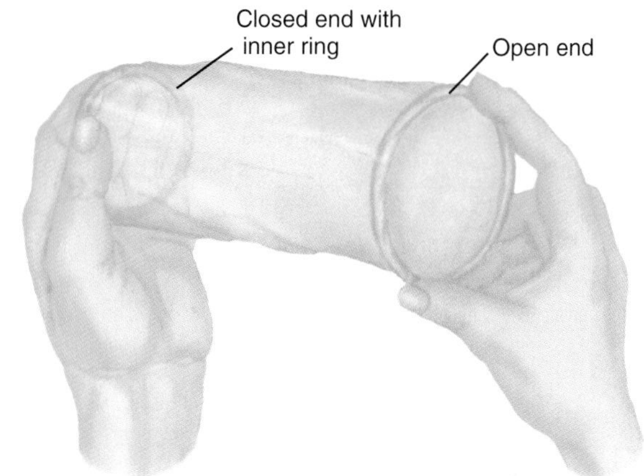


**FIG 31.5** The female condom. A woman can protect herself from sexually transmitted diseases without relying on use of the male condom.

Condoms are readily available, inexpensive, and can be carried inconspicuously by a man or a woman. The effectiveness can be increased by combining condom use with another contraceptive method. Reservoir tips and water-based lubricants help prevent breakage. The slippage and breakage rate is approximately 5% to 8%. Some couples reject condoms because they interfere with spontaneity or sensation. Condoms are affected by some vaginal medications and should not be used concurrently.

***Female condom.*** The female condom (also called a *vaginal pouch*) is a polyurethane or nitrile sheath inserted into the vagina. A flexible ring inside the closed end of the condom fits over the cervix like a diaphragm. Another ring extends outside the vagina to partially cover the perineum (Fig. 31.5).

The female condom is the first contraceptive device that allows a woman some protection from STDs without relying on the male condom. Male and female condoms should not be used together because they may adhere to each other.

***Sponge.*** The contraceptive sponge is made of soft polyurethane that traps and absorbs semen. It contains the spermicide nonoxynol-9. It does not require a prescription, contains no hormones, is easy to use, and can be inserted just before intercourse or hours ahead of time. It provides contraception for 24 hours.

To use the sponge, the woman should wash her hands and wet the sponge with approximately 2 tablespoons of water, squeezing it until it becomes sudsy. She folds the sponge with the concave ("dimple") area inside and the loop on the outside of the fold and inserts it into the vagina. When the sponge is released, the "dimple" covers the cervix. Repeated intercourse does not require added spermicide or a new sponge. It should remain in place for at least 6 hours after the last intercourse, but should not remain in the vagina longer than 30 hours total. It is removed by inserting a finger into the loop and pulling slowly.

Use during menstruation increases the risk of toxic shock syndrome (see Chapter 32). The sponge should not be used by women with a history of toxic shock syndrome and does not protect against STDs. It can cause irritation or be difficult to remove for some women.

***Diaphragm.*** The diaphragm is a latex dome surrounded by a spring or coil. The woman places spermicidal cream or gel into the dome and around the rim and then inserts it over the cervix. The diaphragm prevents passage of sperm into the cervix while holding spermicide for additional protection. It must be fitted by a healthcare provider. Weight

## COUPLES WANT TO KNOW

### *What Is the Proper Way to Use Condoms?*

Although condoms are easy to use, proper use increases their effectiveness.

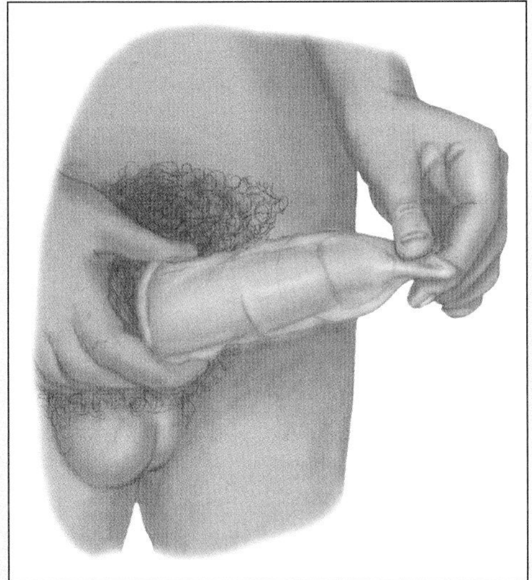

Condoms are available in a variety of colors, textures, and materials, but those made of latex are most effective. Others may help protect against pregnancy but not against sexually transmitted diseases.

Check the expiration dates on packages because condoms can deteriorate after 5 years. Open the package carefully and check the condom to see that it is not damaged.

Lubrication may increase comfort for the woman and reduce the risk of breakage. Use a water-soluble lubricant because oil-based products (such as petroleum jelly or baby oil) deteriorate latex condoms.

Always apply the condom before there is any contact of the penis with the vagina.

Squeeze the air out of the tip of the condom, and leave ½ inch of space at the tip as the condom is unrolled onto the erect penis. This space allows a place for sperm to collect, which helps prevent breakage.

While holding the condom at the base, withdraw the penis from the vagina while it is still erect so the condom does not slip off and spill semen into the vagina.

Use a new condom each time intercourse is repeated.

changes or vaginal delivery can affect the fit of the diaphragm. The woman should be checked for size changes after a gain or loss of 10 lb or more and after a pregnancy (Cates & Harwood, 2011).

Pressure on the urethra can cause irritation and urinary tract infections. Voiding after intercourse helps to prevent infections. An allergy to latex or a history of toxic shock syndrome precludes use. The diaphragm can be damaged by oil-based lubricants and some medications used for vaginal infections.

***Cervical cap.*** The cervical cap is similar to the diaphragm but smaller. It is fitted by a healthcare provider. The flexible silicone cap fits over the cervix and remains in place by suction. The cap causes no pressure on the bladder and can stay in place for 48 hours. Spermicide is placed on both sides of the cap before insertion; if intercourse is repeated, more spermicide is inserted into the vagina without removing the cap. The nurse should teach the woman to feel her cervix to check placement before and after intercourse, because the cap can be dislodged. The cap should not be removed for 6 hours after the last intercourse. It should not be used during menses or in women with a history of toxic shock syndrome (see Chapter 32).

***Lea's Shield.*** Lea's Shield is a silicone device that fits over the cervix. It has a central valve to allow drainage of cervical secretions and a loop for easy removal. It is used with spermicide like the diaphragm or cervical cap. The shield is obtained by prescription but does not require fitting by a healthcare provider. It should remain in place for 8 hours after last intercourse but not longer than 48 hours. It should not be used during menses.

### Natural Family Planning Methods

Natural family planning methods, also called *fertility awareness* or *periodic abstinence* methods, use physiologic cues to predict ovulation and avoid coitus when conditions are favorable for fertilization. These methods can also help women who want to become pregnant. The methods are based on knowledge that the ovum may be fertilized for approximately 24 hours and that most sperm live only 48 hours in the female genital tract, but some may live up to 80 hours (Blackburn, 2013).

Natural family planning helps women learn about how their bodies change throughout the menstrual cycle. This method is acceptable to most religious groups and avoids the use of drugs, chemicals, and devices. However, couples must be highly motivated because they must abstain from intercourse during as much as half the menstrual cycle. Although the methods are very effective if used perfectly, the overall failure rate for typical use is 24% (Table 31.4). The methods are very unforgiving, and errors in predicting ovulation can lead to pregnancy from having intercourse during the fertile time. Women often combine the various fertility awareness methods to improve effectiveness. Some women use the methods to determine when they are fertile and use another contraceptive at that time. For additional information about fertility awareness, see the Planned Parenthood website (http://www.plannedparenthood.org).

#### Calendar or Rhythm Method

The calendar or rhythm method is based on the timing of ovulation, approximately 14 days before the onset of menses. The couple must abstain or use another method during the days calculated to be fertile. This method is unreliable because many factors, such as illness or stress, can affect the time of ovulation.

#### Standard Days Method

This method uses a string of color-coded beads to help keep track of the fertile and infertile days of each cycle. It can be used by women with cycles that range from 26 to 32 days in length but is ineffective for other women. Days 8 through 19 are considered fertile days.

#### Cervical Mucus and Two-Day Method

Also called the "Ovulation" or *Billings* method, the cervical mucus technique is based on changes in cervical mucus that is assessed by wiping it from the vaginal orifice with tissue each day. There is no mucus for the first 3 to 4 days after menses; thick, sticky mucus then begins to appear. As estrogen increases, the mucus changes to clear, slippery, and stretchy, like egg white (a quality known as spinnbarkeit). After ovulation, mucus decreases in amount and becomes thick and sticky again.

To prevent pregnancy, couples must avoid intercourse from the time mucus is first present after menses until 4 days after the end of the slippery mucus. Intercourse is allowed only every other day when there is little or no mucus, because semen interferes with mucus assessment.

## WOMEN WANT TO KNOW

### *How to Use a Diaphragm*

Follow instructions carefully when using your diaphragm. Skill at insertion and removal increases with practice.

Plan to insert the diaphragm up to 6 hours before intercourse. Empty your bladder before insertion.

Spread about a tablespoon of spermicidal cream or gel inside the dome and around the rim.

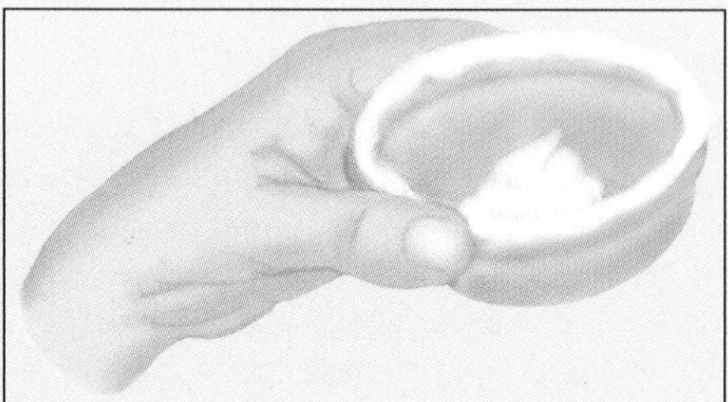

Insert it into the vagina with the spermicide toward the cervix. A squatting position or placing one foot on the tub or toilet seat makes insertion and removal easier.

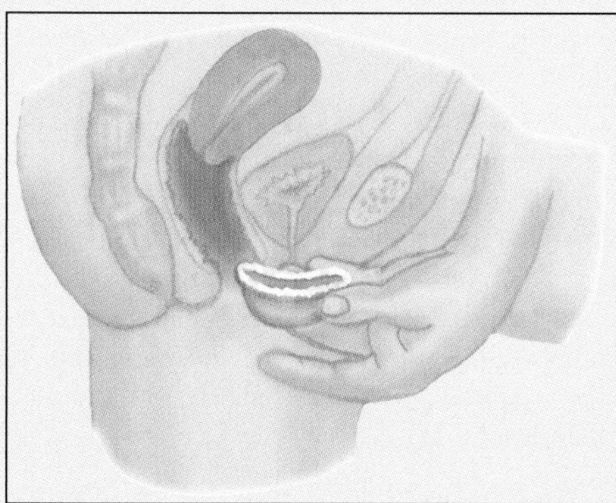

Be sure that the front rim fits behind your pubic bone and that you can feel the cervix through the center of the diaphragm.

If more than 6 hours elapse between insertion and intercourse or if you have intercourse again, insert more spermicide into the vagina without removing the diaphragm.

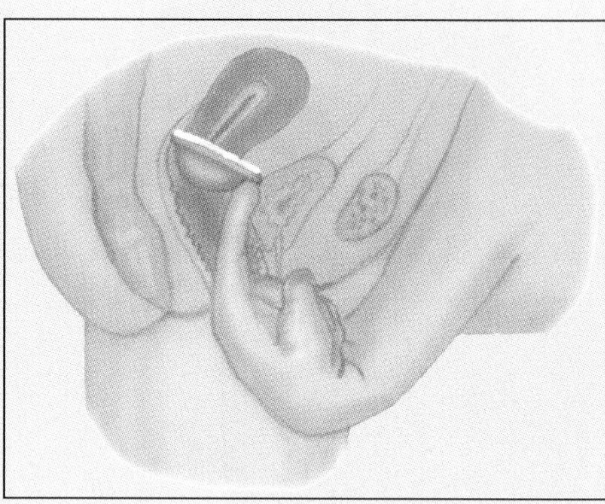

Leave the diaphragm in place for at least 6 hours after the last intercourse. To reduce risk of infection, remove it by 24 hours after insertion.

Douching with the diaphragm in place is unnecessary and will lessen its effectiveness.

To remove the diaphragm, assume a squatting position and bear down. Hook a finger around the front rim to break the suction, and pull down.

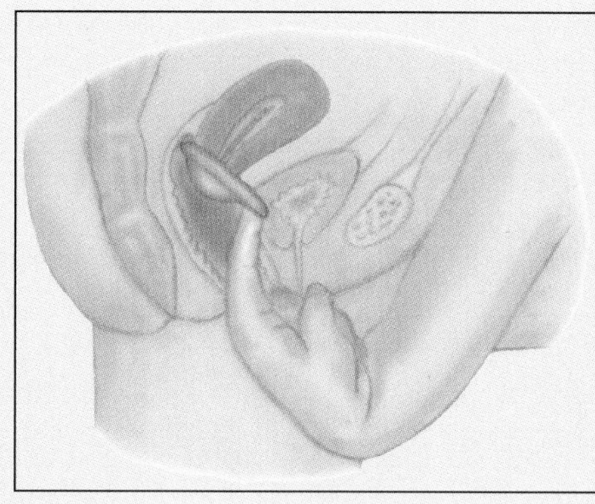

Wash the diaphragm with mild soap and dry well after each use. Inspect it for holes by holding it up to a light or filling it with water. If you find a hole, use another contraceptive method and go to your healthcare provider for a new diaphragm.

## TABLE 31.4 Natural Family Planning Methods

| Method | Application | Comments |
|---|---|---|
| Calendar | Record length of six cycles. Subtract 18 days from shortest cycle and 11 days from longest cycle to determine fertile period. | Example: cycle length, 28-32 days fertile days, 10-21 |
| Standard days method | Intercourse is allowed only on days 1-7 and 20 to the end of the cycle. Fertile days are days 8-19. | Ineffective if the cycle length is shorter than 26 days or longer than 32 days. |
| Cervical mucus (Ovulation or Billings) Two-Day method | Assess mucus at vaginal orifice daily. Avoid intercourse during menses and from the time mucus appears until 4 days after the clear, slippery, stretchy mucus ends. Fertility is determined by presence of cervical mucus today or yesterday. | Intercourse is allowed only every other day, as semen interferes with assessment of mucus. Intercourse is avoided if the woman notices any secretions at all. |
| Symptothermal | Combines cervical mucus and basal body temperature. May also assess weight gain, libido, bloating, and mittelschmerz. | Requires much education and motivation. |

Data from Speroff, L., & Darney, P.D. (2011). *A clinical guide for contraception* (5th ed.). Philadelphia: Lippincott Williams & Wilkins.

## COUPLES WANT TO KNOW

### *How to Assess Cervical Mucus and Basal Body Temperature*

**Cervical Mucus Assessment**

Your cervical mucus normally changes throughout your menstrual cycle. If you check the mucus each day, you can estimate when ovulation occurs. Before and after ovulation, the mucus is scant, thick, sticky, and whitish. It stretches less than 6 cm (2.3 inches). Just before and for 2 to 3 days after ovulation, the cervical mucus is thin, slippery, and clear—similar to raw egg white. It stretches 6 cm (2.3 inches) or more. When this mucus is present, you have probably ovulated and could become pregnant.

Use a tissue to obtain a small sample of mucus each day from just inside your vagina. Note the following:

- The general sensation of wetness (around ovulation) or dryness (not near ovulation) on your labia
- The appearance and consistency of the mucus: thick, sticky, and whitish; or thin, slippery, and clear or watery
- The distance the mucus will stretch between your fingers

Your cervical mucus may be thicker if you take antihistamines. Vaginal infections, contraceptive foams or jellies, sexual arousal, and semen can make the mucus thinner even if ovulation has not occurred. Keep a daily record of the type of mucus present and anything that might affect it.

To use cervical mucus assessment as a method of contraception, avoid intercourse from the time secretions first occur until 4 days after the slippery mucus ends. Intercourse is allowed only every other day when there is no mucus because semen interferes with mucus assessment.

As a method to enhance conception, you should have intercourse on each of the 2 days during the period of ovulatory mucus. Ovulation predictors available over the counter provide added information that is helpful if you are trying to conceive.

**Basal Body Temperature (BBT)**

BBT is the lowest, or resting, temperature of the body. It is assessed to detect the slight elevation in temperature that occurs near the time of ovulation. Your temperature is lower during the first half of the menstrual cycle than during the second half of the cycle. The BBT may drop slightly just before ovulation. Not all women experience this fall in temperature.

Progesterone is secreted during the second half of the cycle, rising just after ovulation. Progesterone causes an increase in BBT. The BBT rises near ovulation and remains higher during the second half of the cycle. However, some women do not have a temperature rise even when they ovulate. The BBT remains higher if conception occurs and falls approximately 2 to 4 days before menstruation if conception does not occur.

An electronic thermometer digitally displays temperature in tenths of a degree. You should place the thermometer under your tongue as soon as you awaken each morning and before any activity. It should remain in place until the electronic signal sounds. Record your BBT on a chart.

Also note relevant events that may alter your BBT, such as menstrual periods, intercourse, illness, or other occurrences. The BBT can be altered by illness, restless or inadequate sleep (fewer than 6 hours), waking later than usual, traveling across time zones (jet lag), alcohol intake the evening before, sleeping under an electric blanket, or performing any activity before taking the temperature.

As a method to avoid pregnancy, you should not have intercourse from the onset of your menstrual period until the night of the third day of elevated temperature. This method has limited value for increasing the chances of conception because the rise in temperature indicates that ovulation has already occurred. It is helpful as a screening method to identify whether the woman is likely to be ovulating and if progesterone is secreted to prepare the endometrium for implantation.

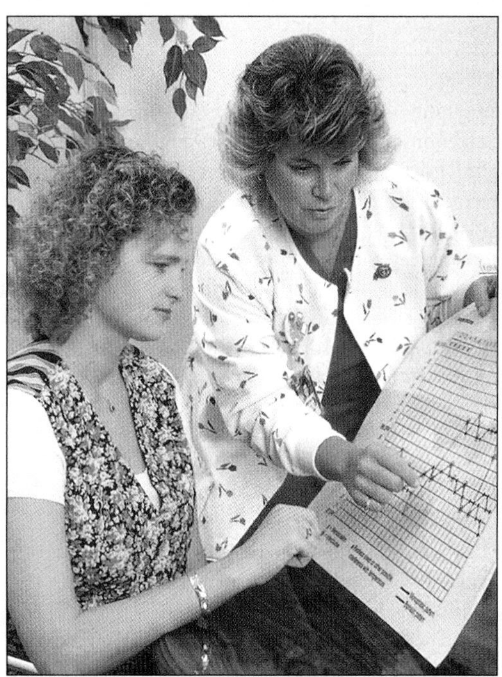

The Two-Day method is a simpler form of this method. The woman assesses cervical secretions daily. If she notices vaginal secretions of any kind today or yesterday, she considers herself fertile. If there were no secretions either day, she considers herself infertile (Jennings & Burke, 2011).

### Symptothermal Method

The symptothermal method combines assessment of basal body temperature (BBT; body temperature at rest) and cervical mucus daily. (See Couples Want to Know: How to Assess Cervical Mucus and Basal Body Temperature.) In addition, symptoms that occur near ovulation, such as weight gain, abdominal bloating, mittelschmerz (pain on ovulation), or increased libido (sexual desire), are noted.

Some women also use an electronic hormonal fertility monitor. The monitor is designed for women trying to become pregnant but can also be used to avoid pregnancy by identifying fertile times in the cycle.

### Abstinence

Abstinence is avoidance of sexual intercourse and any activity that allows sperm to enter the vagina. Although it is the only completely effective method of preventing pregnancy and STDs, abstinence requires perfect use to be effective. Depending on the time within the menstrual cycle it occurs, intercourse without the use of a contraceptive has up to an 85% chance of resulting in pregnancy.

Most women are not abstinent all of their reproductive lives but many practice abstinence at various intervals. Some women practice abstinence part of the time but have other methods available to use if they decide to become sexually active. Periodic abstinence is also practiced by women using the natural family planning methods.

Sex education programs in schools often include information on ways to maintain abstinence. Abstinence-only education programs have not been successful in reducing teen pregnancy (Speroff & Darney, 2011). Adolescents who choose abstinence need help to learn practical methods to reach their goal. They need to think through just what abstinence entails and should role-play situations they might encounter so they know what to say and do before it becomes necessary. Women who choose abstinence should know where to get information and contraception if they later decide to become sexually active.

## Least Reliable Methods of Contraception

The following methods of contraception are not considered reliable but they are used by women who lack information about their risks, lack other options, or do not want to use other methods for medical or personal reasons. The nurse needs to be familiar with these methods to help women understand the risks involved.

### Breastfeeding

Breastfeeding inhibits ovulation because suckling and prolactin interfere with secretion of gonadotropin-releasing hormone and LH. The frequency, intensity, and duration of suckling are very important in inhibiting ovulation.

Women who breastfeed completely (day and night with no supplementary feedings) may avoid ovulation and resumption of the menstrual cycle. Use of formula or solid foods decreases breastfeeding frequency and can lead to ovulation. Ovulation generally occurs before menses, making it difficult to know when the menstrual cycle is resuming. Ovulation usually occurs by 6 months, even in women fully breastfeeding. Another method of contraception should be used by that time or earlier if menses has resumed or if supplementary feedings are used.

### Coitus Interruptus

Also called *withdrawal,* coitus interruptus is the removal of the penis from the vagina before ejaculation. The method requires great control by the man and may be unsatisfying for both partners. Sperm spilled on the vulva can enter the vagina and cause pregnancy.

## NURSING CARE

### Choosing a Contraceptive Method

#### Assessment

Perform the assessment in a quiet area where interruptions are unlikely. Assure the woman that her confidentiality will be maintained. Keep voices low to increase the woman's comfort.

***Introducing the subject.*** In the postpartum setting, introduce the subject by asking the woman if she plans to have more children. Most women indicate a desire to wait a period of time before the next pregnancy. Ask the woman what contraceptive method she is planning to use or how she liked methods she has used before. Introduce the subject during well-woman checks by asking about the woman's current contraceptive and how satisfied she is with it. These questions will help identify problems and questions that the woman may have about contraception.

***Determining the woman's understanding.*** Determine the woman's understanding of her contraceptive technique. For example, ask where she places her patch or if it is hard for her to remember to take her OC each day. The woman should know how to use her technique effectively and what to do in special circumstances, such as missing an OC pill. Explore any misinformation, concerns, or problems that she may have in regard to effectiveness, technique, or common side effects of the method.

***Assessing the woman's satisfaction.*** Assess the woman's satisfaction with her contraceptive. Women may be unsure about their method in the early months until they gain comfort from repetitive use. Side effects also affect satisfaction. They can be severe enough to cause the woman to consider another method, or they may be relieved by simple techniques. Discussing side effects helps differentiate them from serious complications and leads to a discussion of relief methods.

***Assessing appropriate choices.*** If the woman is considering a change in contraceptive method, assess factors to help determine the best method for her. Include a history of medical conditions, childbearing history, cultural and religious beliefs, and intensity of her desire to prevent pregnancy. The woman's ability to understand and follow complicated directions is important as well.

The relationship of the couple is important. If intercourse is frequent, the woman may wish to have a method that is always in place, such as an IUD or hormone implant. In a mutually monogamous relationship, there is no risk of STDs if neither partner is infected. If either of the couple has more than one partner, condom use to protect against STDs is essential, even if the woman uses another contraceptive method.

#### Nursing Diagnosis and Planning

Lack of knowledge about family planning is common. A nursing diagnosis that addresses this problem is:

- Risk for Ineffective Health Maintenance related to lack of understanding about contraceptive methods chosen and available.

***Expected outcomes.*** By the end of the visit, the woman will:

- Correctly describe how to use her contraceptive method, including solving common problems
- Describe common side effects, indications of complications, and correct follow-up
- Report that she and her partner are satisfied with their contraceptive method or will explore another method

#### Interventions

***Increasing understanding of the chosen method.*** Fill in gaps in the woman's knowledge about how her contraceptive method works, its effectiveness, advantages and disadvantages, common side effects and complications, and when to seek help. Use demonstrations (such as applying a patch or inserting a vaginal ring) and return demonstrations for using the method. Give suggestions for managing side effects and common problems. Understanding common side effects and the ability to manage them helps women continue to use a method.

***Teaching about other methods.*** Provide information about other forms of contraceptives, if the woman wishes. Discuss characteristics of other methods that are most important to the woman and her lifestyle. Compare various methods to the one she is currently using. Include benefits, disadvantages, and risks so she can make an informed choice. If a prescription or fitting is needed, discuss what will happen during the visit. Provide written information she can take home to discuss with her partner, if she wishes, before making a final decision.

***Protecting against sexually transmitted diseases.*** Address defense against STDs, particularly if the woman is using a method that does not provide protection. This is a delicate subject. A way to approach it might be to say, "The method you are using is very effective against pregnancy but does not protect you against diseases such as HIV that you might catch from a partner. If there is any chance that you or your partner might have sex with someone other than each other or that your partner might have an infection, you should protect yourself by using condoms with your regular contraceptive."

***Including the woman's partner.*** Invite the woman to include her partner in discussions, if possible. If the partner understands the proper method of use, he may be more cooperative and willing to help ensure contraceptive success.

***Ongoing teaching.*** Instruct the woman to call if she has any questions or difficulties. If she chooses a new method, suggest she visit again in 1 to 2 months to discuss her satisfaction with it. Make a note to talk about contraception with her again at the next visit, even if it is for another reason.

### Evaluation

- Can the woman explain the proper use of her contraceptive technique?
- Can she describe side effects, complications, and how to solve common problems?
- Do she and her partner report satisfaction with their chosen method?
- Has she discussed other methods and chosen one if she is unhappy with her present contraceptive?

## ROLE OF THE NURSE IN INFERTILITY CARE

Although infertility care is a specialty, many general practice nurses meet people who are seeking help for infertility or who have had infertility treatment in varied settings, such as perioperative and maternity settings. The nurse could be one of those people who seeks treatment. Achieving parenthood with infertility therapy is not always easy, and nurses who work in pediatric or psychosocial settings may counsel families needing help with parenting and changes in their personal relationships. Menopause after perhaps many attempts at childbearing may have a different perspective for a woman.

### Extent of Infertility

The extent of infertility depends on how the problem is defined. Infertility is not an absolute condition but instead a reduced ability to conceive. Infertility is strictly defined as the inability to conceive after 1 year of unprotected regular sexual intercourse. A more workable definition does not specify a time limit but recognizes that infertility is any involuntary inability to conceive at the time desired. The definition is commonly expanded to include couples who conceive but repeatedly lose a pregnancy (pregnancy wastage) before the fetus is old enough to survive. Couples with primary infertility have never conceived. Couples with secondary infertility may have conceived before but are unable to conceive again.

From 6% to 15% of U.S. women cannot have a baby when they desire (Centers for Disease Control & Prevention [CDC], 2015). Some couples delay childbearing until their mid to late 30s, when a natural decline in fertility begins. As improved diagnostic and treatment options become available, couples who might have accepted childlessness may now choose to enter infertility therapy or resume therapy they had abandoned. Women who want to have a child without a male partner are served by infertility services.

### Factors Contributing to Infertility

The ability to conceive depends not only on normal reproductive function in each partner but also on a sensitive interaction between the partners. For some couples, identification and treatment of infertility are simple; for other couples, complex evaluation and treatment are required. Because many factors contributing to infertility remain unknown, treatment of an identified problem does not always lead to a successful pregnancy.

#### Factors in the Man

The test of a man's fertility is his ability to initiate pregnancy in a fertile woman. Few absolute criteria distinguish normal from abnormal male fertility, although an adequate number of sperm having normal structure and function must be deposited near the woman's cervix. Problems can occur with the sperm, with erection or ejaculation, or with the seminal fluid (semen) that carries the sperm into the woman's reproductive tract.

***Abnormalities of the sperm.*** Many factors can impair the number, structure, or function of sperm. Some conditions, such as an acute illness, are temporary. Other conditions, such as a genetic disorder, are permanent. A single finding or several findings may be abnormal. Normal daily variations in semen further complicate the evaluation of a man's fertility.

Evaluation of the semen can reveal azoospermia (absence of sperm in semen) or oligospermia (low number of sperm in semen). The average number of sperm released at ejaculation is 35 to 200 million. Twenty million sperm per milliliter of semen is considered the minimum number adequate for unassisted fertilization.

A sufficient number of normal sperm must move in a purposeful direction to reach the ovum in the fallopian tube. Abnormal sperm structure or movement reduces fertility, regardless of the actual number of sperm. Inflammatory processes in the man's reproductive organs can cause the sperm to clump, inhibiting their motility and fertilizing ability. Other sperm look normal but are unable to penetrate the ovum.

Many factors can impair the number and function of the sperm, including:

- Abnormal hormonal stimulation of sperm production
- Acute or chronic illness such as mumps, cirrhosis, or renal failure
- Infections of the genital tract
- Anatomic abnormalities, such as a varicocele or obstruction of the ducts that carry sperm to the penis
- Exposure to toxins, such as lead, pesticides, or other chemicals
- Therapeutic treatments, such as antihypertensives or antineoplastic drugs or radiation for cancer
- Excessive alcohol intake
- Use of illicit drugs, such as marijuana or cocaine
- An elevated scrotal temperature resulting from febrile illness, repeated use of saunas or hot tubs, or sitting for prolonged periods
- Immunologic factors produced by the man against his own sperm (autoantibodies) or by the woman, causing the sperm to clump or be unable to penetrate the ovum

***Abnormal erections.*** Abnormal erections reduce the man's ability to deposit sperm-bearing seminal fluid in the woman's upper vagina near her cervix. Erections are influenced by both physical and psychological factors. Central nervous system dysfunction, which can be caused by drugs, psychiatric disturbance, or chronic illness, can interfere with erections. Spinal cord disorders and disorders or surgery affecting the autonomic nervous system also can disrupt normal erections. Peripheral vascular disease reduces the amount of blood entering the penis, and thus, reduces the ability to maintain an erection. Drugs such as antihypertensives can decrease the erection size or shorten its duration.

***Abnormal ejaculation.*** Abnormal ejaculation prevents deposition of the sperm in the ideal place to achieve pregnancy. Retrograde ejaculation (discharge of semen into the bladder) can occur in the man who has diabetes or neurologic disorders, has had surgery that impairs function of the sympathetic nerves, or takes drugs such as antihypertensives or psychotropics. Men who have suffered spinal cord injury may retain the ability to ejaculate, depending on the level of cord damage.

Anatomic abnormalities, such as hypospadias (urethral opening on the underside of the penis), cause deposition of semen near the vaginal outlet rather than near the cervix.

Excessive alcohol intake and the use of some therapeutic or illicit drugs can adversely affect ejaculation, as well as sperm number and function. Ejaculation can be slow, absent, or retrograde if a man takes drugs that affect the neurologic coordination of this event. Premature ejaculation can be related to psychological disorders such as performance anxiety or unresolved conflicts. Erectile dysfunction (consistent inability to achieve or maintain an erection that is sufficiently rigid and sustained for vaginal intercourse) makes it difficult for the man to furnish semen for study or fertilization on demand.

***Abnormalities of seminal fluid.*** The seminal fluid nourishes, protects, and carries sperm into the vagina until they enter the cervix. Only sperm enter the uterus. Most seminal fluid remains in the vagina because it contains prostaglandins that would cause intense uterine contractions if large amounts enter the uterus. Semen coagulates immediately after ejaculation but should liquefy within 60 minutes to permit forward movement of sperm. Seminal fluid that remains thick traps the sperm, impeding their movement into the cervix. The pH of seminal fluid is slightly alkaline to protect the sperm from the acidic secretions of the vagina. Adequate fructose, citric acid, and other nutrients must be present to provide energy for the sperm to move forward in the woman's reproductive tract. Seminal fluid that is abnormal in amount, consistency, or chemical composition suggests obstruction, inflammation, or infection. The presence of large numbers of leukocytes suggests infection.

### Factors in the Woman

A woman's fertility depends on:

- Regular production of normal ova
- An open path from her cervix to the fallopian tube to permit fertilization and movement of the embryo into the uterus for implantation
- A uterine endometrium that supports the pregnancy after implantation

***Disorders of ovulation.*** Normal ovulation depends on delicately timed and balanced secretions from the hypothalamus and pituitary and an ovarian response to mature and release an ovum. At puberty, the hypothalamus secretes GnRH in regular pulses. In turn, GnRH causes the pituitary to release follicle-stimulating hormone (FSH) and LH. FSH stimulates maturation of several follicles in the ovary. As the follicles mature, the ovary secretes estrogen to thicken the endometrium. Approximately 24 to 36 hours before ovulation, LH surges markedly, stimulating the final maturation and release of one ovum from its follicle. The collapsed follicle from which the ovum was released, now called a *corpus luteum,* produces progesterone and estrogen, which further prepare the endometrium for implantation and nourishment of the fertilized ovum (see Chapter 12) (Jones, 2009a).

Ovulation can be disrupted by:

- Dysfunction in the hypothalamus or pituitary gland that alters the secretion of GnRH, FSH, and LH
- Failure of the ovaries to respond to FSH and LH stimulation, preventing maturation and release of the ovum

Disruption of hormone secretion or of the ovarian or endometrial responses to hormone secretion can be caused by many factors, including cranial tumors, stress, obesity, anorexia, systemic disease, and abnormalities in the ovaries or other endocrine glands. Infertility may be the presenting problem for women with polycystic ovary syndrome (PCO or PCOS). Obesity, amenorrhea, other menstrual abnormalities, and high androgen levels are common PCOS characteristics. A few women have premature ovarian failure, also known as *early menopause.*

As a woman approaches the end of her reproductive life, responses to reproductive hormones become irregular. Ovulation and menstruation are more erratic as the pool of ova diminishes and fewer are available for fertilization. Oocytes are produced only during prenatal life and are vulnerable to cumulative toxic effects of therapeutic drugs, abused substances, and environmental agents. In addition to normal aging of oocytes, factors that impair normal ovulation include cancer chemotherapeutic agents, excessive alcohol intake, and cigarette smoking.

Women with ovulation disorders often have abnormal menses because hormone levels do not permit normal development and shedding of the endometrium. Some women have absent, scant, or heavy menstrual periods, but others have no menstrual disorders. Inability to conceive may be a woman's only complaint.

***Abnormalities of the fallopian tubes.*** At least one open fallopian tube is needed for normal conception and implantation. Tubal obstruction can be the result of scarring and adhesions following reproductive tract infections. STDs such as chlamydia and gonorrhea are responsible for many cases of infertility from tubal obstruction.

Endometriosis (growth of uterine lining tissue outside the uterine cavity) can cause tubal adhesions, painful menstrual periods, and painful intercourse. Small lesions are unlikely to affect tubal patency, but large lesions can distort tubal anatomy and lead to infertility.

Tubal obstruction can occur if adhesions develop after pelvic surgery, ruptured appendix, peritonitis, or ovarian cysts. In addition, the fallopian tubes and other reproductive organs can be affected by congenital anomalies that disrupt normal function.

The conditions that cause obstruction can interfere with normal motility within the fallopian tube. Poor movement of the fimbriated (distal) end of the tube prevents the pickup of the ovum from the ovarian surface after ovulation. Abnormal action of the cilia within the tube prevents normal transport of the ovum toward the uterine cavity.

Depending on the extent and location of the blockage, fallopian tube obstructions can prevent fertilization of the ovum or lead to an ectopic pregnancy. Complete tubal occlusion prevents sperm from reaching the ovum, and the woman will be sterile without the use of advanced techniques such as *in vitro* fertilization (IVF). Because sperm can reach the ovum to fertilize it but the embryo cannot reach the uterine cavity to implant, partial obstruction can result in a tubal pregnancy.

***Abnormalities of the cervix.*** Estrogen levels from the ovary peak twice during the menstrual cycle—once before ovulation and again approximately 1 week after ovulation. The first peak occurs approximately 2 days before ovulation and causes the woman's cervix to dilate slightly and produce the clear, thin, slippery mucus described on p. 671. This mucus facilitates sperm passage into the uterus and prepares them for fertilization. Low estrogen levels prevent development of this mucus and are usually associated with anovulation.

Polyps or scarring from past infections or surgical procedures can obstruct the woman's cervix. Abnormal cervical mucus caused by estrogen deficiency, surgical destruction of the mucus-secreting glands, and cervical damage secondary to infection or other factors prevents normal capacitation and movement of the sperm into the uterus and fallopian tubes for fertilization.

## Repeated Pregnancy Loss

Couples who repeatedly lose pregnancies have the same result as those unable to conceive: no living child. Recurrent losses can result from

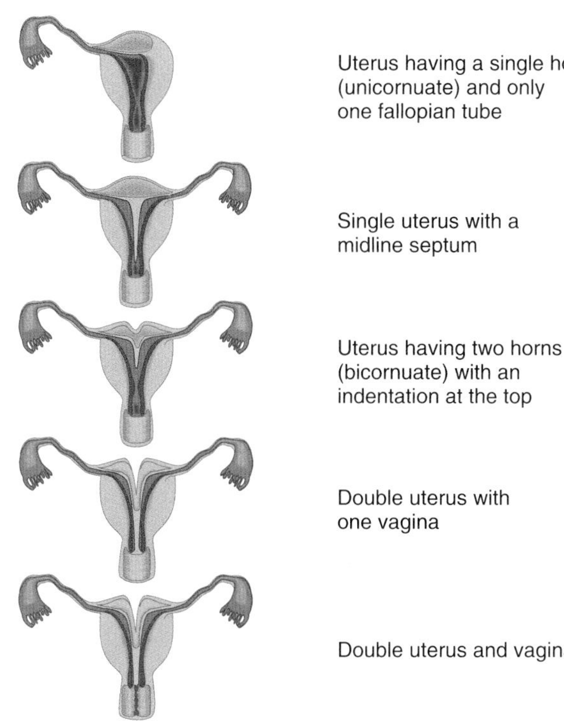


FIG 31.6 Types of uterine malformations that can cause infertility or repeated pregnancy loss.

abnormalities in the fetus or placenta or from maternal factors such as structural abnormalities or autoimmune disease.

### Abnormalities of the Fetal Chromosomes

Errors in the fetal chromosomes can result in spontaneous abortion, usually in the first trimester. Chromosome abnormalities often severely disrupt development, and the embryo or fetus cannot survive to live birth. Maternal-age–associated chromosome abnormalities in the ova increase spontaneous abortions and decrease live births in older women who conceive.

### Abnormalities of the Cervix or Uterus

Stenosis or congenital malformations of the cervix or uterine cavity can cause repeated loss of a normal embryo or fetus (Fig. 31.6). These malformations prevent normal implantation of a fertilized ovum that is ready to implant.

Cervical or uterine abnormalities and possibly hysterectomy also can occur after surgery or trauma from a previous birth. Painless and premature cervical dilation, often early in the second trimester, is characteristic in women with an incompetent cervix. Although the woman can conceive, she is unable to carry the pregnancy long enough for the fetus to survive if born.

Uterine myomas, or fibroids (benign tumors of the uterine muscle), and adhesions inside the uterine cavity can cause repeated fetal loss. These lesions alter the blood supply to the developing fetus or cause uterine irritability that leads to preterm labor and birth.

### Endocrine Abnormalities

Inadequate progesterone secretion by the corpus luteum (luteal phase defect) prevents normal thickening of the endometrium for implantation and establishment of the placenta (see Chapter 12). The embryo does not implant, or it implants poorly. In other cases, the corpus luteum develops and functions properly, but the woman's endometrium does not respond to its secreted progesterone.

Infertility related to menstrual irregularities and anovulation can lead the woman with PCOS to seek care. Obesity is often a contributing factor to infertility. Androgen excess, increased LH, and reduced FSH impair ovum maturation. Endocrine abnormalities in the woman with PCOS who conceives and delivers successfully prevent her from producing adequate milk for infant needs.

Hypothyroidism and hyperthyroidism are associated with the inability to conceive and with recurrent pregnancy loss. Because of its effects on maternal blood glucose levels and the vascular system, poorly controlled diabetes can result in repeated pregnancy loss as well as many other complications of pregnancy.

### Immunologic Factors

Immunologic factors are implicated in some cases of recurrent pregnancy loss, although not all are established conclusively. The embryo has antigens that differ from those of the mother and ordinarily would be rejected as would any other foreign tissue. However, the mother's body normally blocks this rejection response and tolerates the developing baby. Some women's bodies respond inappropriately to the embryo, rejecting it. These women often have recurrent spontaneous abortions.

Women with autoimmune disease such as systemic lupus erythematosus (SLE) are more likely to experience spontaneous abortion. Pregnancy loss in these women appears to be related to thrombosis or other damage in placental blood vessels, perhaps related to a genetic cause for abnormal clotting. Women with SLE can have other complications during pregnancy, such as exacerbation of their symptoms, fetal heart block, fetal distress, and stillbirth (see Chapter 26).

### Environmental Agents

Some environmental agents have a well-established relationship to impaired fertility and pregnancy loss. In addition to diethylstilbestrol (DES), other common toxic agents include ionizing radiation, alcohol, and isotretinoin (Accutane). Suspected toxins are numerous; among them are cigarette smoke, anesthetic gas, organic solvents, pesticides, lead, and mercury. Some of these agents are directly toxic to the embryo or fetus, causing its death, while others interfere with the normal placental function necessary to sustain the pregnancy.

### Infections

Infections of the reproductive tract are associated with poor pregnancy outcomes in general, and may be related to early pregnancy losses as well (see Chapter 26). These infections are often asymptomatic, making their link to pregnancy loss difficult to establish.

## Evaluation of Infertility

Infertility is defined as 1 year of unprotected intercourse without conceiving. Eighty-five percent of couples conceive within 1 year. The rate of conception in the first cycle of treatment for infertility is 15% to 25%, falling as the months pass. Only 3% of couples conceive in the 12th cycle. Couples are often in a hurry for definitive therapy before the end of the woman's reproductive years, but a thorough assessment of their problem is essential for effective and financially sound treatment. Some tests, such as semen evaluation, are repeated sequentially for better accuracy. Usefulness and well-accepted normal values are not yet established for all tests, and newer diagnostic tests are investigational. Despite many examinations and tests, infertility remains unexplained in 10% to 20% of couples who seek care.

Numerous professionals can be involved in evaluation and care of infertile couples: nurses, physicians specializing in reproductive medicine, gynecologists, radiologists, endocrinologists, urologists, microsurgeons, biologists, embryologists, laboratory technical workers, and ultrasonographers. In addition, general and specialized laboratory facilities often provide diagnostic services to enhance treatment. Nurses working in infertility clinics often coordinate communication among the many providers and help the couple negotiate the maze of evaluation and treatment.

### Preconception Counseling

Couples are usually offered preconception counseling to help them evaluate their risk for birth defects and perhaps reduce their risk for bearing a child with a serious birth defect. Many women seeking infertility care are older than 35 years, an age at which having an infant with a chromosome defect increases (see Chapter 10). A thorough history and physical examination of both members of the couple, including their family histories, can identify an increased risk for having a child with a single-gene defect. Counseling can help the woman understand *before conception* the importance of an adequate diet and avoidance of teratogens that can harm the developing fetus before she knows she is pregnant.

### History and Physical Examination

A thorough history and physical examination of each partner can help identify the appropriate diagnostic tests and therapy and identify risks for birth defects in the couple's offspring.

***History***

- The woman's age at menarche and menstrual characteristics (frequency, regularity, duration, amount of flow, presence of pain)
- Any pregnancies, complications, and their outcomes
- Contraceptive methods, past and present
- Previous fertility of the man or woman with other partners
- Previous surgeries, infections (including childhood infections), pelvic inflammatory disease, STDs, abnormal Pap tests and treatments, serious illness
- Pattern of intercourse in relation to the woman's cycles
- Length of time the couple has had intercourse without contraception
- Exposure to possible toxins, prescribed and over-the-counter medications
- Family history of multiple pregnancy losses, birth defects, intellectual disabilities
- Any home tests the couple has used, such as over-the-counter ovulation predictor kits

The detailed personal and family histories of each partner help determine what specific tests to do first. The pattern of a couple's intercourse related to ovulation can improve or impair conception.

***Physical examination.*** Couples who seek help for infertility are usually healthy. However, a thorough physical examination of each partner can identify endocrine disturbances, cranial tumors, or undiagnosed chronic disease. Examination of the reproductive organs can reveal structural defects, infection, cysts, or other abnormalities. Chromosomal analysis and maternal blood clotting studies are often conducted for couples experiencing repeated pregnancy losses.

**Diagnostic tests.** Each couple's evaluation is individualized, but testing generally proceeds from the simple and less expensive to the more complex and expensive diagnostics. Simple evaluations are done simultaneously, but more complex tests are delayed until the need for them is established. Two methods of identifying ovulation, BBT and assessment of cervical mucus, can be used as contraceptive measures in addition to their use in infertility care.

## INFERTILE COUPLES WANT TO KNOW

### *What Is Infertility Treatment Like?*

**General**

Both members of the couple are evaluated systematically to identify the most time- and cost-effective therapy.

Simpler evaluations and therapies are done before more complex efforts are undertaken.

A complete medical history and physical examination is done for each partner.

The ages of the partners, particularly the woman's, are considered. Evaluations and therapy proceed more quickly if the woman is in her mid-30s or older.

Costs may be partially covered by insurance; check to see what your insurance covers.

Difficult decisions may be required at different times during evaluation and treatment. Decisions might include whether to proceed to more complex and expensive tests and therapies, whether to take a break from treatment, or whether to abandon treatment altogether.

Infertility treatment can be stressful, can occupy many hours per week, and requires a substantial commitment to self-care.

Infertility remains unexplained in as many as 20% of couples.

Internet resources for information on infertility include the Centers for Disease Control and Prevention (http://www.cdc.gov), American Society for Reproductive Medicine (http://www.asrm.org), and Resolve (http://www.resolve.org).

**Men**

Semen analysis is often the first test. Several semen specimens are obtained over a period of weeks to obtain the best evaluation.

Depending on your medical history, physical examination, and semen analysis, other diagnostic tests might be done (hormone assay, an ultrasound of your reproductive organs, a biopsy of your testicles, and specialized tests of sperm function).

Potential corrective measures include medications, surgery, and methods to reduce the scrotal temperature.

**Women**

The first evaluation is usually to determine whether you are ovulating each month. An ovulation predictor kit is most often used for this purpose. Self-assessment of your basal body temperature, or temperature immediately on awakening each morning, and cervical mucus may also be taught (see p. 673). These assessments are often done at the same time as other tests.

Other common evaluations include an ultrasound examination of your reproductive organs, and imaging your uterus and fallopian tubes with dye (hysterosalpingogram).

For some tests and therapies, an operative procedure is required (e.g., hysteroscopy, laparoscopy, laser surgery, microsurgery).

Typically, infertility evaluations and treatments require more of the woman's time, energy, physical discomfort, and risk than the man's.

Corrective measures depend on the problem identified. Examples include medications, surgery, and advanced reproductive techniques, such as *in vitro* fertilization.

Several basic tests are common in early infertility evaluation, and others may be used as indicated:

- BBT (see Couples Want to Know How to Assess Cervical Mucus and Basal Body Temperature, p. 673) or, more commonly, ovulation monitoring kits to identify if ovulation has occurred
- Evaluation of the cervical mucus to identify changes that occur with ovulation
- Hormone evaluations such as estrogen, progesterone, LH, FSH, thyroid function
- Ultrasound imaging of internal reproductive organs
- Radiographic imaging to visualize the uterine cavity and fallopian tubes
- Semen analysis
- Testicular biopsy

Table 31.5 describes selected diagnostic tests that may be offered to the infertile couple and the nursing care associated with each.

## Therapies to Facilitate Pregnancy

Evaluation of the couple identifies what therapy would best improve their chance of conceiving and completing a pregnancy. A variety of procedures are available, depending on the couple's initial and ongoing evaluations and their personal choices. Some therapy is simple, like timing intercourse to better coincide with ovulation. Other procedures involve considerable expense, discomfort, or unpleasant side effects. Many couples need a combination of treatments to improve their chances of conception.

Determination of the appropriate infertility therapy is not always straightforward. Many factors must be considered by care providers and the couple, including their personal and family history, medical evaluations, financial resources, maternal age and other time constraints, and religious and cultural values.

### Medications

Medications are used to improve semen quality, reduce endometriosis, induce ovulation, prepare the uterine endometrium, and support the pregnancy once established. Table 31.6 summarizes the medications used in infertility therapy.

Medications to induce ovulation are prescribed for the woman who does not ovulate or who ovulates erratically. Such medications are also given to produce multiple ova in women who plan undergo assisted reproductions. Progesterone vaginal suppositories and clomiphene citrate (Clomid) are often used to stimulate follicle development. Human chorionic gonadotropin (hCG) can then be given to induce the release of several ova. Human menopausal gonadotropin (hMG) can be injected in small, regular pulses for pituitary insufficiency of LH and FSH, similar to delivery by an insulin pump.

Ovulation induction, also known as *superovulation,* increases the risk of multiple births because several ova can be released and fertilized. Another serious complication is *ovarian hyperstimulation syndrome,* which involves marked ovarian enlargement with exudation of fluid and protein into the woman's peritoneal and pleural cavities. Adjustment of medication dosage and serial ultrasound examinations to determine the number of mature follicles reduces the occurrence of high-order multifetal pregnancy (triplets or more) and ovarian hyperstimulation syndrome.

### Surgical Procedures

Endoscopic procedures are used to correct obstructions, with minimal invasiveness, in either the man or the woman. The woman may need a laparotomy to relieve pelvic adhesions and obstructions caused by endometriosis, infection, or previous surgical procedures if these cannot be corrected via laparoscopy. Adhesions are often removed using laser surgery techniques because they are minimally invasive, precise, and less likely to cause new adhesions. Correction of a varicocele by ligating or embolizing the dilated vein can improve sperm quality and quantity, although there is no consensus on its usefulness. Microsurgical techniques are used to correct obstructions in the fallopian tubes and male tubal structures.

Transcervical balloon tuboplasty is a minimally invasive procedure used to unblock the fallopian tubes. A thin catheter is threaded through the cervix and uterus into the fallopian tube. The balloon is then inflated to clear the blockage.

### Therapeutic Insemination

Therapeutic insemination uses either the partner's semen or that of a donor to overcome a low sperm count. Donor insemination also can be used if the man carries a genetic defect or if a woman wants a biological child without having a relationship with a male partner. Intrauterine insemination (IUI) is a variation that allows the sperm to bypass cervical mucus and reduces immunologic incompatibilities by injecting prepared sperm directly into the uterus.

Sperm used for therapeutic insemination or IUI are obtained from semen collected by masturbation. The sperm are washed in laboratory solutions to remove prostaglandins that cause uterine cramping and then concentrated before insemination. Washing also removes many of the antibodies that interfere with sperm motility and ability to penetrate the ovum. If the man has retrograde ejaculation, he can take sodium bicarbonate 2 hours before obtaining the semen to render the urine alkaline. The urine is collected in a sterile container and washed with a medium to separate sperm from urine. Sperm can be aspirated from epididymal fluid to overcome some types of male factor infertility.

Men who donate semen for insemination are screened to reduce the risk of transmitting diseases or genetic defects. They are questioned about their personal and family health histories, including genetic disorders or birth defects. Questions about their social habits and personality can disclose high-risk behaviors and give recipient parents information about traits their child might have. Physical and laboratory examinations are performed to evaluate the man's general health, determine his blood type and Rh factor, and screen for infections such as STDs or HIV. Carrier testing for specific genetic defects such as sickle cell anemia and Tay-Sachs disease reduces the risk of passing on these disorders. To reduce the risk of transmitting diseases that are not yet apparent at the initial screening, donor semen is frozen and held for 6 months before use. The man is retested for diseases such as HIV several times during the 6 months.

Inadvertent consanguinity (blood relationship) is a possibility with donor sperm insemination because half-siblings from different families may not know they were conceived with donor gametes. They could later conceive a child who shares a larger number of genes, both normal and abnormal, than the general population. For this reason, the number of donations from a single donor may be limited.

### Egg Donation

Use of donor eggs (oocytes) is an option for some women who do not produce ova because of premature ovarian failure, who do not respond to ovarian stimulation, whose ova are not successfully fertilized despite apparently normal sperm, or following radiation or chemotherapy. Younger fertile women are usually the donors, and the success rate of IVF is higher (approximately 40%). Eggs from a single donor are limited to avoid inadvertent consanguinity. The donor is more likely to be known to the recipient and may be a family member, increasing the possibility of attachment to the child. Egg donation has donor risks from the medications used to stimulate ovulation, ovarian

**TABLE 31.5 Selected Diagnostic Tests in Infertility**

| Test and Purpose | Nursing Implications |
|---|---|
| **Male** | |
| ***Semen Analysis*** | |
| Evaluates structure and function of sperm and composition of seminal fluid.<br>Semen volume: 2 mL or more<br>pH: 7.2-7.8<br>Sperm concentration: ≥20 million/mL<br>Motility: 50% or more with normal forms<br>Morphology: 30% or more with normal forms<br>Viability: 50% or more live<br>Liquefaction: within 60 min<br>Leukocytes (white blood cells): <1 million/mL | Explain purpose of semen analysis: three or more specimens are usually collected over several weeks' time for improved accuracy.<br>Explain to the man that he should collect the specimen by masturbation after a 3-day abstinence; semen may be collected in a condom if masturbation is unacceptable.<br>Teach him to note the time the specimen was obtained so the laboratory can evaluate liquefaction of the semen. To maintain warmth, the specimen should be transported near the body and should arrive in the laboratory within 1 hr. |
| ***Endocrine Tests*** | |
| Evaluate function of hypothalamus, pituitary gland, and the response of the testicles. Assays are made to determine testosterone, luteinizing hormone (LH), and follicle-stimulating hormone (FSH) levels.<br>Additional tests may be done based on history, physical findings, and results of other tests. | Teach the man about the relationship between hypothalamic and pituitary function and sperm formation; LH stimulates testosterone production by Leydig cells of the testes, and FSH stimulates Sertoli cells of the testes to produce sperm. |
| ***Ultrasonography*** | |
| Evaluates structure of prostate gland, seminal vesicles, and ejaculatory ducts by use of a transrectal probe. | Teach the man that ultrasonography uses sound waves to evaluate these structures; no radiation is involved. |
| ***Testicular Biopsy*** | |
| An invasive test for obtaining a sample of testicular tissue; identifies pathology and obstructions. | Explain the purpose of the test; a local anesthetic is used, and there should be little discomfort. Ask the man questions to confirm that he understands the test. |
| ***Sperm Penetration Assay*** | |
| Evaluates fertilizing ability of sperm; assesses ability of sperm to undergo changes that allow penetration of a hamster ovum from which the zona pellucida has been removed. | Explain the purpose of the test and that abnormal penetration of the hamster ovum does not necessarily mean that the sperm cannot fertilize a human ovum. |
| **Female** | |
| ***Ovulation Prediction*** | |
| Identifies the surge of LH that precedes ovulation by 24-36 hr; improves ability to time intercourse to coincide with ovulation, and identifies the absence of ovulation.<br>Common prediction methods include commercial ovulation predictor kits and cervical mucus assessment (see Patient-Centered Teaching: Couples Want to Know How to Assess Cervical Mucus and Basal Body Temperature, p. 673). Basal body temperature (BBT) can be used to determine whether ovulation has occurred and the timing of intercourse in relation to probable ovulation. | Explain the purpose of the assessments.<br>Teach the woman to follow the instructions on commercial ovulation predictor.<br>Teach her how to do the BBT and cervical mucus assessment if that is used.<br>Teach her to indicate days on which she and her partner had intercourse to determine the frequency during the menstrual cycle and intercourse near ovulation. |
| ***Ultrasonography*** | |
| Evaluates structure of pelvic organs.<br>Evaluates cyclic endometrial changes.<br>Identifies ovarian follicles and release of ova at ovulation.<br>Evaluates for presence of ectopic or multifetal pregnancy. | Teach the woman that ultrasonography uses sound waves to evaluate these structures; no radiation is involved. Explain preparations needed for specific evaluations. |
| ***Hysterosalpingogram*** | |
| Evaluates patency of uterus and fallopian tubes by injection of contrast medium into the cervix while imaging the pelvis to visualize passage of the dye. | Review purposes of the imaging test to determine if the woman understands the procedure. |
| ***Postcoital Test*** | |
| Evaluates characteristics of cervical mucus and sperm function within that mucus at time of ovulation.<br>Ultrasonography ensures proper timing for test. | Explain that the test is performed 6-12 hr after intercourse; the woman may have to rearrange her personal or work commitments each time this test is done. Use is infrequent because of stress on the woman and her partner. |

**TABLE 31.6 Selected Medications for Infertility Therapy**

| Drug | Primary Use |
|---|---|
| Bromocriptine (Parlodel); cabergoline (Dostinex) | Corrects excess prolactin secretion by anterior pituitary, improving gonadotropin-releasing hormone (GnRH) secretion, in turn normalizing release of follicle-stimulating hormone (FSH) and luteinizing hormone (LH). These drug actions increase ovulation and support early pregnancy by stimulating progesterone secretion by the corpus luteum. |
| Chorionic gonadotropin, human (hCG; [Novarel, Pregnyl]); recombinant deoxyribonucleic acid (DNA) origin (r-hCG; [Ovidrel]) | Used in conjunction with gonadotropins to stimulate ovulation in the female or sperm formation in the male. Stimulates progesterone production by corpus luteum. |
| Clomiphene citrate (Clomid) Letrozole (Femara) | Induction of ovulation in women who have specific types of ovulatory dysfunction. The drug increases frequency of GnRH secretion from the hypothalamus, thus increasing FSH and LH release, maturing the ovarian follicle, and causing release of the ovum. |
| FSH, recombinant DNA origin (follitropin alfa [Gonal-F]) | Stimulation of ovarian follicle growth; ovulation-induction gonadotropin. |
| GnRH antagonists (e.g., cetrorelix [Cetrotide], ganirelix [Antagon]) | Reduces endometriosis; adjunct to drugs given to stimulate ovulation by suppressing LH and FSH, reducing ovarian hyperstimulation. |
| GnRH agonists (goserelin [Zoladex], leuprolide [Lupron], nafarelin [Synarel]) | Stimulates release of FSH and LH from the pituitary gland in men and women who have deficient GnRH secretion by their hypothalamus. FSH and LH, in turn, stimulate ovulation in the female and stimulate testosterone production and spermatogenesis in the male. |
| Gonadotropins (urofollitropin [Bravelle], menotropins [Humegon, Pergonal, Repronex]) | Induction of ovulation with human-derived FSH and LH; brands may differ in the proportions of FSH to LH; recombinant DNA preparations are becoming more common because of their greater purity. |
| LH, recombinant DNA origin | Replacement of LH via subcutaneous pump; promotes ability of mature ovarian follicle to rupture and luteinize when hCG is secreted. |
| Progesterone (parenteral or vaginal preparations) | Luteal phase support; prepares uterine lining and promotes implantation of embryo. |
| Metformin (Glucophage) | Adjunct treatment for ovulation induction in women with polycystic ovary syndrome. |
| Erectile agents (sildenafil [Viagra], tadalafil [Cialis], vardenafil [Levitra]) | Increase blood flow to the penis, improving erectile function. |

hyperstimulation, bleeding, cramping, and infection. Other medications prepare the recipient to receive the conceptus. Legal and ethical issues involve disclosure of the donor to the recipient and her partner and possible later disclosure to the child. The egg donor must receive information regarding the risks of donating.

### Surrogate Parenting

A surrogate mother may enter the picture if the woman is infertile because she does not have a uterus or if she has been unable to carry a healthy fetus to live birth. Surrogacy is different from therapeutic insemination or egg donation because it is not anonymous. In addition, the woman who carries the child inevitably forms bonds with the fetus during the months of pregnancy. For these and many other reasons, extensive interviewing and counseling of both the infertile couple and the surrogate mother are required.

Custody issues are clearer when the birth mother is a gestational surrogate than when she also donates her ovum to the child. Courts have more often recognized the genetic parents as the legal parents and upheld the contracts between them and the gestational surrogate.

## Assisted Reproductive Techniques

Assisted reproductive technology (ART) uses medical, surgical, laboratory, or micromanipulation techniques to handle the ovum and sperm. ART includes several techniques to bypass natural obstacles to conception and place gametes together to promote fertilization. The success rates for ART in 2008 showed that the use of these techniques doubled over the previous decade, with over 1% of infants born in the United States conceived using ART. However, couples eager to conceive should know all the facts and risks before choosing any ART method.

IVF places the conceptus into the uterus. Procedures that place the conceptus into the fallopian tube at varying times after fertilization include gamete intrafallopian transfer (GIFT), zygote intrafallopian transfer (ZIFT), tubal embryo transfer (TET), a variation of ZIFT. Intracytoplasmic sperm injection (ICSI) has had good results related to male infertility.

Couples with concerns about a specific genetic defect in the family may be offered preimplantation genetic testing of their fertilized ova. As in other types of prenatal screening, genetic testing of the fertilized ovum cannot rule out every potential abnormality in the offspring. Rather, the testing allows parents to make informed decisions about whether to implant a fertilized ovum into the uterus.

### In Vitro Fertilization (IVF)

IVF, the most commonly used ART method, bypasses blocked or absent fallopian tubes (Fig. 31.7). The physician removes the ova by ultrasound-guided transvaginal retrieval or occasionally by laparoscopy and mixes them with prepared sperm from the woman's partner or a donor. Ova are examined for successful fertilization approximately 18 hours later and then either returned to the uterus or cultured for 48 to 96 more hours, allowing 5 days of cell division (see Fig. 31.7). The number of fertilized ova returned is individualized but is approximately two or three based on the prognosis for success balanced against the woman's risks of multifetal pregnancy. Older women often receive more ova than younger women to improve their chances of pregnancy without greatly increasing the risk of having a triplet or higher pregnancy. Pregnancy complications in the single older woman are more likely, and she might lack the needed support in her pregnancy.

Supplemental progesterone is given to the woman to promote implantation and support the early pregnancy (luteal phase support). Because of the supplemental progesterone, the woman will not have a menstrual period even if she is not pregnant. Transvaginal ultrasounds

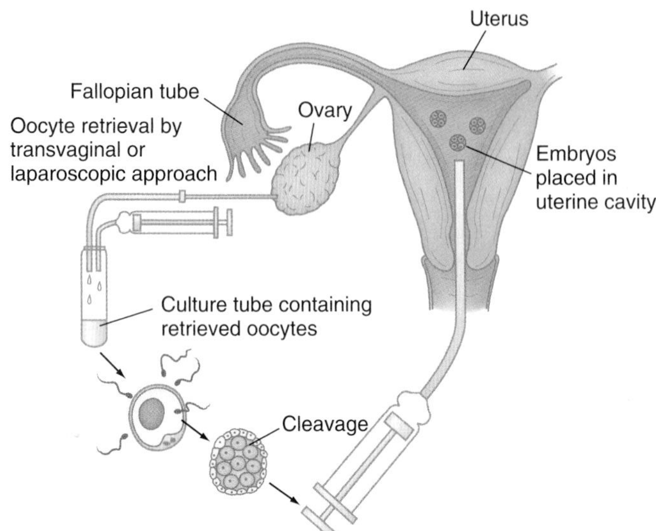


**FIG 31.7** *In vitro* fertilization (IVF). Multiple oocytes are obtained using a transvaginal or laparoscopic approach. The retrieved oocytes are mixed with prepared sperm, incubated approximately 18 hours, and then evaluated for cell division. Embryos are then transferred to the uterus immediately or after 48 to 96 hours to allow 5 days of further cell division before implantation.

are used to identify whether one or more gestational sacs have implanted with IVF and to determine whether a tubal (ectopic) pregnancy occurred after methods such as IUI, GIFT, or ZIFT (see Chapter 25).

### Gamete Intrafallopian Transfer (GIFT)

The woman must have at least one patent fallopian tube for GIFT to be an option. The procedure begins in a manner similar to that of IVF, using multiple retrieved ova and washed sperm. The ova are drawn into a catheter that also carries prepared sperm. Sperm and up to two ova per tube are injected into each fallopian tube through a laparoscope. Additional prepared sperm may be injected into the uterus through the cervix to improve the chance of successful fertilization. Progesterone is given as in IVF.

### Zygote Intrafallopian Transfer (ZIFT)

ZIFT, often called TET, is a hybrid of IVF and GIFT. The woman's ova are fertilized outside her body as in IVF, but the resulting fertilized ova are placed into the distal fallopian tube and enter the uterus naturally for implantation. The woman must have at least one patent fallopian tube.

### Comparison of In Vitro Fertilization, Gamete Intrafallopian Transfer, and Zygote Intrafallopian Transfer

One advantage of GIFT is that some people and religious groups find these procedures more acceptable than IVF or ZIFT because ova and sperm are placed directly into the woman's body. With IVF and ZIFT, there is evidence of fertilization before placement in the uterus or tubes, which reassures other people.

### Intracytoplasmic Sperm Injection (ICSI)

Microsurgical techniques are related to IVF but are considerably more complex. These techniques now help couples conceive despite severe male factor infertility when standard IVF, GIFT, and ZIFT are unlikely to be successful.

Men who have obstructions to or absence of the epididymis may be able to father children with the use of percutaneous or microsurgical sperm aspiration. The sperm are retrieved from the epididymis by percutaneous aspiration using a small-gauge needle. Alternatively, a microsurgical incision can be made to aspirate the sperm if the percutaneous approach cannot be used. The sperm obtained are then used to fertilize ova by ICSI.

All ARTs have some degree of invasiveness for the woman and possibly the man. To obtain more ova and increase the likelihood of pregnancy with a procedure, a woman may undergo controlled ovarian hyperstimulation (COH). Placement of gametes or fertilized ova in the distal fallopian tube requires a laparoscopy, whereas IVF can be achieved transcervically, making it the most common procedure. Tubal pregnancy may result if embryos cannot reach the uterine cavity to implant. IVF is used approximately 99% of the time because it is less invasive. Higher rates of prematurity and low- or very-low-birth-weight infants have been linked to more frequent multiple births associated with ART.

## Responses to Infertility

The desire for children is strong in many couples. If a couple does not achieve pregnancy or produce a living child as expected, the man and woman often experience psychological distress and a threat to their self-images. Either or both partners may feel like failures. Their marital and family relationships can be stressed, and they may withdraw from relationships that they previously found satisfying.

### Assumption of Fertility

Many couples use contraception before they decide to have a baby. When they want a child, they discontinue contraception and assume that pregnancy will occur within a few months at most.

Either or both partners may experiment with the role of parent as they anticipate pregnancy. They develop a heightened awareness of children and parenting. Being with others who are expecting or who already have children is exciting because they plan to join their ranks shortly. Many discuss issues such as full-time parenting by one partner, child care, and future lifestyle changes. They may begin acquiring the toys and furnishings a child will need and perhaps move to a larger home. Both partners can develop a fantasy child or a concept of what their baby will be like.

### Growing Awareness of a Problem

As the months pass, the couple gradually becomes concerned about the inability to conceive. If the woman is older, they feel the urgency of the limited time before her reproductive years end. Repeated loss of a pregnancy causes repeated grief after the thrill of conceiving.

The couple begins to feel uneasy with child-related activities. Now they are not so sure when they will be parents. Events such as baby showers or christenings can become melancholic rather than joyful occasions. Family members and friends who are having children may feel guilty at their good fortune when they are around the couple that cannot conceive.

The potential grandparents may feel that their children are waiting too long to start a family or even that they are selfish. If they are aware that the couple is trying to conceive, they become even more worried as the months pass without the longed-for announcement of a pregnancy. They are twice saddened by the lack of a grandchild and by the hurt their adult children are enduring.

### Seeking Help for Infertility

Eventually, couples must decide whether to seek help to conceive. They may reach this point after only a few menstrual cycles or, at the opposite extreme, never seek help. Many factors enter into their decision. These include their ages (especially the woman's), how long they have been unable to conceive, how much they want a biological child, how they regard adoption, and how they feel about a child-free life.

*Identifying the importance of having a baby.* Each partner may place a different priority on having a baby. Conflicts can arise when one partner wants help to conceive sooner than the other. In addition, cultural or religious beliefs influence how each feels about procreation and whether options such as assisted reproductive procedures or adoption are acceptable. How the couple resolves these differences is crucial to the stability of the relationship.

Men and women often differ in their reactions to infertility. Women may want to talk about their feelings and frustrations, but men often internalize their feelings or feel that they must be strong for their partner. The man may worry silently that he is the one with the problem. The woman may interpret her partner's reluctance to express his feelings and his stoicism as disinterest or lack of concern and care for her. Either or both partners may feel guilty about earlier decisions to postpone having a family.

*Sharing intimate information.* Although the infertility specialist will ask only necessary questions, evaluation and treatment for infertility require that both partners reveal intimate information about their sexual relationship, such as the frequency and timing of intercourse. In addition, infertile couples may feel that the evaluation calls their sexual adequacy into question.

*Considering financial resources.* Financial concerns enter into the couple's decision about whether to seek treatment and how far to carry it. Ovulation predictors and records of BBT are inexpensive ways to identify whether ovulation occurs and if they have intercourse at an ideal time. But complex problems will require more detailed testing of the couple. Advanced techniques such as IVF are expensive, and success varies based on multiple factors. Health insurance may not cover infertility care at all or may not cover all tests and procedures because the problem does not directly threaten the health of either partner. Investigational treatments are often not covered. The drugs that must be taken to achieve pregnancy are often quite expensive. Expense and restricted coverage limit treatment choices for many couples.

*Ethical issues.* Ethical issues enter infertility care as well (see Chapter 1). Those who seek and pursue infertility treatment usually have greater financial resources than those who do not, creating a disparity in availability to pursue parenthood. Money paid to a woman who donates ova or a surrogate mother can raise issues of baby selling. Participation by professionals in arranging surrogacy even may be illegal in some states. Could a poor but fertile woman feel compelled to provide her body for a more well-to-do couple? Yet not compensating a woman for the real physical and emotional risks of this undertaking can be construed as exploitive as well. Not implanting live embryos that have a genetic defect or reducing the number of fetuses in a high multiple pregnancy is viewed as abortion by many people.

*Committing to involvement in care.* Infertility evaluation and treatment require commitment of the couple's time, energy, and money. Couples participate on a day-to-day basis as they do home assessments, take medications, and keep detailed records. For infertility diagnosis and therapy to be most effective, couples must consider their ability and desire to be directly involved in the process over what may be a long time. Age of the woman affects decisions repeatedly.

### Reactions During Evaluation and Treatment

Couples undergoing infertility evaluation and treatment have different reactions to the process. In addition, their reactions can change as infertility care progresses.

#### Influences on Decision Making

If evaluations show that a treatment or procedure may enable them to conceive, the couple must then decide whether to proceed. The decision-making process begins early and must be repeated during therapy if pregnancy does not occur. A complex array of factors enters into their decisions about beginning and continuing treatment or whether to end their pursuit of pregnancy. These factors interact dynamically as the couple makes each decision. As part of an interdisciplinary team, the nurse helps both partners examine each factor and arrive at a decision that is best for them.

*Social, cultural, and religious values.* Not all medically appropriate options are acceptable to every couple. Surrogate parenting, IVF, and therapeutic insemination (especially with donor sperm) are inconsistent with the personal or religious beliefs of many people. If a procedure offers the partners hope for a child but is incompatible with their beliefs, they have two choices: use the technology despite their beliefs, or accept childlessness. Adoption is a third alternative for some couples if the desire for a biological child is not absolute. Placement of a remaining embryo into the uterus of the adoptive mother may be possible. As in other decisions, couples must work out conflicting personal values to decide which therapy is acceptable.

*Difficulty of treatment.* The couple must consider how difficult, risky, and uncomfortable therapy will be. The level of difficulty involves physical, psychological, geographic, and time factors. Employment constraints often affect treatment decisions as well.

Several infertility treatments involve invasive procedures or surgery. Medications to induce ovulation of multiple ova cause wide mood swings and physical discomfort. The person who undergoes the procedure must be the one who ultimately decides whether to do it. That person alone can decide whether the hope of a child is worth the risks and discomfort of the procedure.

Infertility treatment is stressful. Often the partners are willing to tolerate different levels of stress. To reduce the stress, they may abandon treatment completely or take a several-month vacation from the constant preoccupation with conceiving. Women nearing or in their 40s often feel that they do not have the luxury of skipping a treatment cycle.

Some couples encounter geographic difficulties if they must travel a long distance for therapy. Time stresses are substantial. The partners, particularly the woman, feel that achieving pregnancy is their new career. One or both partners may spend many hours every week in pursuit of pregnancy.

Employment constraints can be a barrier to infertility therapy because of the time required for treatment. The impact of time is usually greatest on the woman. Time away from work can burden the employer or coworkers. Stopping work may not be an option because the family needs the money and often needs the insurance coverage that comes with employment. Job loss may be a realistic fear for either partner.

*Probability of success.* Couples often have a biased interpretation of their statistical probability of success, especially when they begin treatment with a new procedure. For example, if a procedure has a 20% likelihood of success in any given cycle, they may expect that they will be in the successful group rather than in the 80% who do not conceive. However, as time goes by, they must weigh the likelihood of success of any therapy against financial concerns and their own willingness to accept the discomfort and difficulty associated with it. The fact that a couple with no infertility problems has only a 20% chance of conceiving in any given month is little comfort to those investing so much time, money, and effort.

*Financial concerns.* Couples who have ample resources and a strong desire for a biological child can pursue expensive treatments and continue them longer than those of more limited means. They may do so despite a low probability of success. Couples with financial limitations find that they must abandon treatment sooner than they want. Other couples go heavily into debt, adding financial strain to the other stresses of treatment in their quest for a biological child.

### Psychological Reactions

A couple's initial reaction to infertility is often one of shock because the partners are usually healthy and do not expect to have problems conceiving. Their reactions vary according to how easily their infertility is alleviated, their personalities and self-images, and the strength of their relationship.

*Guilt.* A partner having the only identified problem might feel that he or she is depriving the other of children. This feeling can be compounded if the "normal" partner has children from another relationship. It may be difficult for this person to understand that not all factors affecting fertility can be detected and that what seems like the one partner's problem is often the couple's problem.

Guilty about past choices that now affect fertility can be felt by either partner. A woman with adhesions resulting from a sexually acquired infection may regret her past choices. The man who wanted to delay pregnancy longer than the woman may feel guilty if her age is now limiting the time she has for conceiving.

*Isolation.* Infertile couples often feel different from friends and relatives who do not have difficulty conceiving. To insulate themselves from painful reminders of their infertility, they may withdraw from these relationships. Some couples develop supportive relationships with others who are also infertile, which somewhat diminishes their sense of isolation but may increase it if one of those couples conceives.

*Depression.* One or both partners may experience depression as their sense of competence and control over their bodies is challenged, especially if therapy is not successful quickly. They often feel as if they are on a roller coaster of hope alternating with despair when the woman has her menstrual period each month. In an attempt to insulate themselves from disappointment, couples with long-term infertility try not to expect too much with each cycle.

The couple may feel envious of those who conceive easily. They may become judgmental and angry when they see those who seem to "have no business having a baby," such as an adolescent, a woman who abuses drugs, or a woman who cannot support an added child.

*Stress on the relationship.* Because infertility can challenge one's identity and self-esteem, the partners may find less satisfaction in their relationship. They may feel unlovable or unappealing to their mates.

The man may find it difficult to perform on demand for examinations that require him to ejaculate, feeling that others will judge his sexual function. The fact that semen samples are best obtained by masturbation is unacceptable to some men. Both partners are stressed when intercourse must be scheduled to coincide with specific evaluations or with ovulation. Intercourse can become a chore or a medical procedure more than an expression of love. It may come to be associated with failure rather than fulfillment.

If sperm from an anonymous donor is used for therapeutic insemination or other techniques, the man may feel that his masculinity is further threatened. He may have difficulty distinguishing fatherhood as a biological achievement from fatherhood as a relationship with his child.

The partners find their relationship strained if they disagree on which treatments are appropriate and how long they should be pursued. One partner may want to keep trying "One more month," and the other may want to abandon treatment. If they are considering adoption, their relationship may be strained if they differ on whether to adopt and what kind of child they are willing to accept.

## Outcomes After Infertility Therapy

After infertility therapy, three outcomes are possible. Pregnancy can be achieved and then lost, causing mixed emotions of optimism and grief. The couple can become parents, either biologically or through adoption. The couple also may decide to remain childless after unsuccessful infertility therapy.

### Pregnancy Loss After Infertility Therapy

Couples who suffer pregnancy loss after infertility therapy may interpret the experience with mixed feelings of loss and gain. Couples undergoing infertility evaluation and treatment are often aware of a pregnancy much earlier than fertile couples. They want to hope yet expect to be disappointed again. If a miscarriage or birth before fetal viability occurs, they may grieve profoundly for what they achieved and then lost.

Yet despite their grief about the pregnancy loss, the partners may be encouraged because they have proved that they can achieve a pregnancy. They may feel that if they succeeded once, they can do it again.

### Parenthood After Infertility Therapy

Women or couples who conceive experience varied emotions. Pregnancy after infertility therapy is emotionally tentative for many infertile couples, especially those who have been trying to conceive for a long time or have lost a pregnancy. They may distance themselves from the pregnancy until late in gestation, emotionally "holding their breath" until the baby is born. The woman has grown accustomed to sensing and reporting every symptom and may interpret normal physiologic changes and discomforts of pregnancy as threatening.

The previously infertile couple may find little sympathy from those who do not understand why they are tentative about the pregnancy. Friends or family may be annoyed because they expect the couple to be overjoyed at a successful and apparently normal pregnancy. Outsiders may feel that the partners are self-centered and cannot decide what they want. Other infertile couples, who were previously a source of mutual support, may withdraw from the expectant couple.

The parents' anxiety can be heightened during labor. They are afraid that something will go wrong at the last moment. Even after the birth of a healthy term infant, some parents have difficulty relaxing and enjoying their baby.

These new parents often need much nursing support as they gain experience with their child. Infertile couples who eventually have biological or adopted children may have unrealistic expectations about parenting. After investing so much financial, physical, and emotional resources into having a child, they may be reluctant to express any unhappiness or frustration over the realities of raising children (Rockliff, Lightman, Rhidian, et al., 2014).

### Choosing to Adopt

Couples who consider adoption must confront their personal preferences, limitations, and biases. As much as they want a child, couples may not be willing to adopt any child. Most couples prefer to adopt a newborn or an infant of their race. Some prefer an infant but are also willing to adopt an older child, one with special needs, one of a mixed or different race, or a pair or group of siblings. Other couples, for a variety of reasons, will not consider adopting these children. Couples, particularly older ones, may turn to foreign adoption because they are considered too old to be adoptive parents by most U.S. agencies. Adoption of children from abroad usually requires multiple trips to the nation to complete documents and multiple interactions with the child they hope to adopt. Adopting children from orphanages in foreign countries carries the risk of having a developmentally delayed child because of the limited interactions with adults or other children.

Some couples fear adopting a child because the woman might become pregnant. Although pregnancy has been the goal for a long time, they may worry that they would love their adopted child differently from their biological child.

Couples who decide to adopt face further scrutiny of their personal lives. Agencies investigate their home, financial means (which may be drained), and fitness as parents. Once again, they may feel that their personal competence is questioned. Their age also may limit their options.

The couple that decides on adoption can have emotions similar to those who achieve a pregnancy. They may be slow to invest in the process emotionally because they expect disappointment. In addition, the adopted child often comes to them suddenly and unexpectedly. Although they may have been waiting months for this happy event, they have little time to adjust to the reality that they are becoming parents.

### Menopause After Infertility

A woman or couple may decide when to stop unsuccessful infertility treatment, or natural aging may make that decision for her in menopause. After many attempts to conceive and carry a child to term, the biological clock that she was watching closely is running out quickly. A woman may find a new sense of self as her body changes are not related to infertility therapy.

## NURSING CARE

### The Infertile Couple

Nursing care of the infertile couple is challenging but can be most satisfying. Regardless of the clinical setting where the nurse encounters infertile couples, meeting the emotional needs associated with infertility evaluation, treatment, and outcomes of therapy is an important part of their care.

#### Assessment

Most infertile couples previously had a positive self-image and feelings of competence. The diagnosis of infertility shakes their positive view. The nurse should be aware that these feelings may underlie their physical concerns.

Determine at what point the couple is in their infertility treatment. Couples who have just discovered their infertility may be shocked yet optimistic that therapy will result in a baby for them. Couples with long-standing infertility may have a deeper sense of failure and a pessimistic outlook. Listen for remarks that are negative, expressing guilt or helplessness.

Evaluate how infertility has affected the partners' relationship. Are there conflicts or differences in their values? Observing their body language, such as eye contact, can provide clues about differences in their commitment to diagnosis and treatment. Ask them how their relationship has changed. Are they more or less satisfied with their relationship than they were before they had problems conceiving?

Ask about support systems. Couples suffering from infertility often withdraw from old relationships but do not form new, supportive ones. Do others who are significant in the partners' lives know that they are trying to conceive? Are family members and friends nearby, and are they supportive? Have they encountered assumptions that infertility is the "fault" of one partner or the other? Are they subjected to questions that invade their privacy, such as, "When are you two going to have a baby of your own?" What unique issues must the single woman face as menopause draws closer with no expected father of the baby she wants?

Determine how the couple's culture, religion, or personal values view infertility and the effect of these values on treatment. Are any therapies unacceptable to one or both partners?

Determine how the couple is coping with the stresses of treatment. How much has infertility cost them in time, money, and discomfort? Identify the successes and failures they have experienced. Their ages, especially the woman's, add another unavoidable stressor.

If the woman is pregnant or has given birth recently or if the couple has adopted a child recently, observe for high levels of anxiety in either or both parents. Assess them for negative behaviors and comments, such as reluctance to feel joy or a sense that they will "fail" again.

#### Nursing Diagnosis and Planning

A nursing diagnosis commonly encountered is the risk for or actual:
- Situational Low Self-Esteem related to perception of reproductive inadequacy.

***Expected outcomes.*** The person(s) will express feelings about infertility and its evaluation and treatment, will explore ways to increase control within the situation of infertility, and will identify aspects of self that are positive. Expected outcomes can apply to the man, the woman, or both.

#### Interventions

***Assisting communication.*** Use a variety of communication techniques, such as active listening and exploration, to encourage the partners to express their feelings honestly, both as a couple and individually. Provide privacy and acceptance of their feelings.

Encourage the partners to accept their feelings, both positive and negative. For example, the couple that has finally achieved pregnancy may be living a lie to some extent. They might act elated because they believe they should feel happy yet inside feel cautious and hesitant to become attached to their baby. Explain that feelings are neither right nor wrong. It may be helpful to open the subject of negative feelings (fear of attachment) within a successful situation (pregnancy or birth) to reinforce the normality of their mixed emotions. This technique gives them the opportunity to talk about emotional reactions that they or others feel are inappropriate and might otherwise be reluctant to discuss.

Discuss possible differences in ways the man and woman communicate. For example, explain that the woman may feel more comfortable than the man in talking about their problem and concerns about treatment. Explain that these differences in communication style can cause misunderstandings because one partner believes that the other does not care as much about their problem. Encourage them to be open with each other for the best mutual support.

***Increasing the couple's sense of control.*** Explore how the couple has dealt with stressors and how these techniques might be applied to their present crisis. Reinforce positive coping skills such as learning more about infertility and the proposed therapy for it (Frederiksen, Farver-Vestergaard, Skovgård, et al., 2015).

Some couples experiencing undue stress benefit from relaxation techniques such as visualization and moderate exercise. Frequent strenuous exercise can reduce the woman's ability to ovulate. Although a hot tub is relaxing for many people, it should be avoided because the high temperatures inhibit spermatogenesis. The woman also could become pregnant, and high body temperature in early pregnancy is associated with fetal anomalies.

Discuss behaviors that enhance the ability to handle stress and provide a good environment for pregnancy. Reinforce healthy choices such as good nutrition and a balance between exercise and rest. Teach the couple ways to increase general health if deficiencies are identified.

Explain any procedures and their purpose in language that the couple can understand. Reinforce medical explanations they have been given. Clarify information they have obtained from outside sources such as the Internet. Encourage questions so that the couple is fully informed. Have the partners review teaching to reduce misunderstandings.

Help the couple explore options at each decision point. No one else can decide the best course of action, but the nurse can help identify pros and cons of each choice so the partners can arrive at a decision appropriate for them. Be nondirective so that the choices are theirs and do not reflect the biases of the nurse or other caregivers.

***Reducing isolation.*** Because couples often avoid friends and family relationships that they find painful, they may distance themselves from those who want to be supportive. Refer them to available support groups to provide emotional outlets, a sense of belonging, and a source of information for them and their affected friends and family. Help the couple identify ways they can improve communication with family and friends who want to support them. Remind them that they have undergone significant shifts in self-image that have also affected those around them.

***Promoting a positive self-image.*** Explore areas of competence and activities with the couple that make them feel good about themselves. Reinforce positive attitudes and self-evaluations. Encourage them to maintain activities such as hobbies, sports, or volunteer work. The career of either partner can be a source of stress that needs relief, or it may be an avenue that fosters a positive self-perception.

### Evaluation

- Did the partners express their feelings about their situation over a period of time?
- Did the partners explore ways to increase personal control over their lives and express diminished feelings of helplessness and dependence?
- Did the partners identify one or more aspects of self-perceived as positive and identify areas of competence?

## KEY CONCEPTS

- The nurse plays an important role in educating women about contraceptive techniques and their correct use.
- Important issues in choosing contraceptives include safety, protection from STDs, effectiveness, acceptability, convenience, education needed, benefits, side effects, effect on spontaneity, availability, expense, preference, religious beliefs, and culture.
- Written informed consent may be necessary for some contraceptive choices.
- Adolescents often have erroneous beliefs and incorrect information about contraception that increase their risk of pregnancy and STDs.
- Adolescents feel more comfortable talking about contraception with a nurse who has an accepting attitude, provides extra time for education, and uses understandable terms and audiovisual materials.
- Women older than 35 years who smoke or have cardiac risk factors should not use combined oral contraceptives (OCs).
- Tubal sterilization can be performed soon after childbirth or at any time. Vasectomy is less expensive and can be performed in a physician's office under local anesthesia. Although surgery to reverse sterilization is possible, it is expensive and not always successful.
- Intrauterine devices (IUDs) are very effective and safe. Women must check for the IUD strings and know when to seek medical treatment.
- Hormonal contraceptives include hormone implants, injections, OCs, patches, or vaginal rings. Hormonal contraceptives inhibit ovulation and make the cervical mucus unreceptive to sperm. Side effects and complications make these unsuitable for some women.
- OCs, the patch, and the ring are used on a monthly basis, for extended cycles, or indefinitely to decrease menstrual periods.
- Emergency contraception (EC) protects against pregnancy if taken within 3 to 5 days after unprotected intercourse.
- Barrier methods are chemical or mechanical. They kill sperm or prevent sperm from entering the cervix and provide some protection against STDs.
- Natural family planning methods involve avoidance of coitus when physiologic cues suggest that ovulation is likely. They involve extensive education and high motivation and have a high risk of pregnancy should error occur.
- Because of the many unknown factors in reproduction, identification and correction of problems in one or both partners will not necessarily resolve their infertility.
- A variety of structural and functional abnormalities can contribute to a couple's infertility. The man may have abnormalities of the sperm or of the seminal fluid or with ejaculation. The woman may have ovulation disorders, anatomic problems such as fallopian tube occlusion, or physiologic disorders such as hormone imbalances.
- A systematic evaluation of both partners, proceeding from simple to complex, identifies therapy most likely to be successful and cost-effective. The couple may decide to stop evaluation or therapy at any point.
- Infertility is a crisis for the couple and often for the extended family. Either or both partners may feel that the inability to conceive represents a personal failure.
- Infertile couples must make choices at many points before and during evaluation and therapy. Some major factors that enter into their decisions involve social, cultural, and religious values; difficulty of treatment; probability of success; financial resources; and age, particularly the woman's.
- The possible outcomes of infertility therapy present new challenges to the partners and their families: unsuccessful therapy and the choice of whether to pursue adoption, pregnancy loss after infertility, and parenthood after infertility. Stopping infertility therapy and remaining childless is another options.

## REFERENCES AND READINGS


Alan Guttmacher Institute (AGI). (2014). *Facts on American teens' sexual and reproductive health.* Retrieved from http://www.guttmacher.org/fact-sheet/american-teens-sexual-and-reproductive-health#18.

Alan Guttmacher Institute (AGI). (2015a). *Fact sheet: Unintended pregnancy in the United States.* Retrieved from http://www.guttmacher.org/pubs/FB-Unintended-Pregnancy-US.html?gclid=CjwKEAiAoIK1BRCRiMqphvnlwlwSJAAOebPMS5YcPku00IMOQLOA_N9rccCT92CwzdvXYhSw9mCcTBoC_xHw_wcB

Alan Guttmacher Institute (AGI). (2015b). *Facts on contraceptive use in the United States.* Retrieved from http://www.guttmacher.org/fact-sheet/contraceptive-use-united-states.

Alkema, L., Kantorova, V., Menozzi, C., et al. (2013). National, regional, and global rates and trends in contraceptive prevalence and unmet need for family planning between 1990 and 2015: a systematic and comprehensive analysis. *Lancet, 381*(9878), 1642–1652.

Allen, R.H., Cwiak, C.A., & Kaunitz, A.M. (2013). Contraception in women over 40 years of age. *Canadian Medical Association Journal, 185*(7), 565–573.

American Cancer Society. (2014). *Cervical cancer: Prevention and early detection.* Retrieved from http://www.cancer.org/acs/groups/cid/documents/webcontent/003167-pdf.pdf.

American College of Obstetricians and Gynecologists (ACOG). (2010). *Noncontraceptive uses of hormonal contraceptives (Practice Bulletin No. 110).* Washington, DC: Author.

American College of Obstetricians and Gynecologists (ACOG). (2011). *Long-acting Reversible Contraception: Implants and intrauterine devices (ACOG Practice Bulletin No. 121).* Washington, DC: Author.

American College of Obstetricians and Gynecologists. (2012). *Adoption (ACOG Committee Opinion No. 528).* Washington, DC: Author.

American College of Obstetricians and Gynecologists (ACOG). (2013a). *Benefits and risks of sterilization (ACOG Practice Bulletin No. 133).* Washington, DC: Author.

American College of Obstetricians and Gynecologists. (2013b). *Multifetal pregnancy reduction (ACOG Committee Opinion No. 553).* Washington, DC: Author.

American College of Obstetricians and Gynecologists (ACOG). (2015). *Emergency contraception (Practice Bulletin No. 112).* Washington, DC: Author.

American College of Obstetricians and Gynecologists. (2015). *Polycystic ovary syndrome (ACOG Practice Bulletin No. 108).* Washington, DC: Author.

American Society for Reproductive Medicine. (2006). *Patient's fact sheet: Ovulation detection.* Retrieved from http://www.reproductivefacts.org/uploadedFiles/ASRM_Content/Resources/Patient_Resources/Fact_Sheets_and_Info_Booklets/ovulation_detection.pdf.

Barry, M. (2011). Preconception care at the edges of the reproductive life span. *Nursing for Women's Health, 15*(1), 68–74.

Beckmann, C.R.B., Ling, F.W., Barzansky, B.M., et al. (2010). *Obstetrics and gynecology* (6th ed.). Philadelphia: Walters Kluwer Lippincott Williams & Wilkins.

Blackburn, S.T. (2013). *Maternal, fetal, & neonatal physiology: A clinical perspective* (4th ed.). St. Louis: Saunders.

Cates, W., & Harwood, B. (2011). Vaginal barriers and spermicides. In R.A. Hatcher, J. Trussell, A.L. Nelson, et al. (Eds.), *Contraceptive technology* (20th ed., pp. 391–408). New York: Ardent Media.

Centers for Disease Control & Prevention [CDC]. (2015). *Infertility FAQs.* Retrieved from http://www.cdc.gov/reproductivehealth/infertility/.

Cunningham, F., Leveno, K., Bloom, S., et al. (2014). *Williams obstetrics* (24th ed.). New York: McGraw-Hill.

Dempsey, A.R., Johnson, S.S., & Westoff, C.L. (2011). Predicting oral contraceptive continuation using the transtheoretical model of health behavior change. *Perspectives on Sexual and Reproductive Health, 43*(1), 23–29.

Frederiksen, Y., Farver-Vestergaard, I., Skovgård, N.G., et al. (2015). Efficacy of psychosocial interventions for psychological and pregnancy outcomes in infertile women and men: a systematic review and meta-analysis. *British Medical Journal, 5*(1), e006592.

Glasier, A. (2013). Emergency contraception: clinical outcomes. *Contraception 2013, 87*(3), 309–313.

Godfrey, E.M., Chin, N.P., Fielding, S.L., et al. (2011). Contraceptive methods and use by women aged 35 and over: A qualitative study of perspectives. *BMC Women's Health, 11*, 5.

Hall, J.E. (2011). *Guyton and Hall's textbook of medical physiology* (12th ed.). Philadelphia: Saunders.

Hershberger, P.E., Schoenfeld, C., & Tur-Kaspa, I. (2011). Unraveling preimplantation genetic diagnosis for high-risk couples: Implications for nurses at the front line of care. *Nursing for Women's Health, 15*(1), 36–45.

Hladky, K.J., Allsworth, J.E., Madden, T., et al. (2011). Women's knowledge about intrauterine contraception. *Obstetrics & Gynecology, 117*(1), 48–54.

Jennings, V.H., & Burke, A.E. (2011). Fertility awareness-based methods. In R.A. Hatcher, J. Trussell, A.L. Nelson, et al. (Eds.), *Contraceptive technology* (20th ed., pp. 417–434). New York: Ardent Media.

Jones, E.E. (2009a). The female reproductive system. In W.F. Boron, & E.L. Boulpaep, (Eds.), *Medical physiology: A cellular and molecular approach* (2nd ed., pp. 1146–1169). Philadelphia: Saunders.

Kochanek, D.D., Kirmeyer, S.E., Martin, J.A., et al. (2012). Annual summary of vital statistics: 2009. *Pediatrics, 129*(2), 338–348.

Lee, K.C. (2011). Fertility treatments and the cost of a healthy baby. *Nursing for Women's Health, 15*(1), 15–18.

Levy, D.P., Jager, M., Kapp, N., et al. (2014). Ulipristal acetate for emergency contraception: postmarketing experience after use by more than 1 million women. *Contraception 2014, 89*(5) 431–433.

Link, D.G. (2011). Contraception. In S. Mattson, & J.E. Smith (Eds.), *AWHONN Core curriculum for maternal-newborn nursing* (4th ed., pp. 335–342). St. Louis: Saunders.

Nandra, K. (2011). Contraceptive patch and vaginal contraceptive ring. In R.A. Hatcher, J. Trussell, A.L. Nelson, et al. (Eds.), *Contraceptive technology* (20th ed., pp. 343–369). New York: Ardent Media.

Nelson, A.L. (2011). Perimenopause, menopause, and postmenopause: Health promotion strategies. In R.A. Hatcher, J. Trussell, A.L. Nelson, et al. (Eds.), *Contraceptive technology* (20th ed., pp. 737–777). New York: Ardent Media.

Nelson, A.L., & Cwiak, C. (2011). Combined oral contraceptives (COCs). In R.A. Hatcher, J. Trussell, A.L. Nelson, et al. (Eds.), *Contraceptive technology* (20th ed., pp. 249–341). New York: Ardent Media.

Practice Committee of the American Society for Reproductive Medicine, Practice Committee of the Society for Assisted Reproductive Technology, Practice Committee of the Society of Reproductive Biology and Technology. (2014). Revised minimum standards for practices offering assisted reproductive technologies: a committee opinion. *Fertility and Sterility, 102*(3), 682–686.

Raymond, E.G. (2011). Progestin-only pills. In R.A. Hatcher, J. Trussell, A. Nelson, et al. (Eds.). *Contraceptive technology* (20th ed., pp. 237–247). New York: Ardent Media.

Robinson, J.A., & Burke, A.E. (2013). Obesity and hormonal contraception efficacy. *Women's Health, 9*(5), 453–466.

Rockliff, H.E., Lightman, S.L., Rhidian, E., et al. (2014). A systematic review of psychosocial factors associated with emotional adjustment in in vitro fertilization patients. *Human Reproduction Update, 20*(4), 594–613.

Roncari, D., & Hou, M.Y. (2011). Female and male sterilization. In R.A. Hatcher, J. Trussell, A.L. Nelson, et al. (Eds.), *Contraceptive technology* (20th ed., pp. 435–482). New York: Ardent Media.

Slama, R, Hansen O.K., Ducot, B., et al. (2012). Estimation of the frequency of involuntary infertility on a nation-wide basis. *Human Reproduction, 12*(5), 1489–1498.

Speroff, L., & Darney, P.D. (2011). *A clinical guide for contraception* (5th ed.). Philadelphia: Lippincott Williams & Wilkins.

Tepper, N.K., Curtis, K.M., Steenland, M.W., et al. (2013). Physical examination prior to initiating hormonal contraception: a systematic review. *Contraception 2013, 87*(5), 650–654.

Trussell, J. (2011). Contraceptive failure in the United States. *Contraception, 83*(5), 307–404.

Trussell, J., & Schwarz, E.B. (2011). Emergency contraception. In R.A. Hatcher, J. Trussell, A.L. Nelson, et al. (Eds.), *Contraceptive technology* (20th ed., pp. 113–145). New York: Ardent Media.

Wise, L.A., Mikkelsen, E.M., Sørensen, H.T., et al. (2015). Prospective study of time to pregnancy and adverse birth outcomes. *Fertility & Sterility, 103*(4), 1065–1073.

U.S. Department of Health & Human Services. (2010). *Healthy People 2020.* Washington D.C.: Author.

# 32

# Women's Healthcare

http://evolve.elsevier.com/McKinney/mat-ch/

## LEARNING OBJECTIVES

*After studying this chapter, you should be able to:*

- Explain examinations and screening procedures that are recommended to maintain the health of women.
- Explain benign disorders of the breast, relate them to the common age of onset, and describe the diagnostic procedures used to rule out breast cancer.
- Describe the incidence, risks, pathophysiology, management, and nursing considerations of malignant breast tumors.
- Discuss cardiovascular disease in women, including risk factors, signs and symptoms, and measures to reduce risk.
- Discuss the four most common menstrual cycle disorders. Explain management options for premenstrual syndrome (PMS) and premenstrual dysphoric disorder (PMDD) and nursing considerations.
- Discuss procedures, possible complications, and follow-up care related to elective termination of pregnancy, also called induced abortion.
- Describe physical and psychological changes associated with menopause and options to alleviate uncomfortable changes.
- Discuss osteoporosis and measures to reduce severity.
- Discuss the major disorders associated with pelvic relaxation in terms of causes, treatments, and nursing considerations.
- Discuss the signs and symptoms, management, and nursing considerations for the most common benign and malignant disorders of the reproductive tract.
- Describe the care of a woman with an infectious disorder of the reproductive tract, including sexually transmitted diseases, pelvic inflammatory disease, and toxic shock syndrome.

Women are not pregnant the majority of their lives, and some are never pregnant. However, they often consider their primary care provider for their unique preventive healthcare to be the same person they saw for obstetrics or annual Papanicolaou (Pap) tests. Many obstetricians continue to provide gynecology care after retiring from obstetrics. Certified nurse-midwives usually provide preventive healthcare to nonpregnant women. The advanced practice women's health nurse practitioner (WHNP) provides basic reproductive system care to women in many settings. Therefore, the provider that a woman sees for her well-woman examination (WWE) must be prepared to examine her for nonreproductive problems to determine referrals that she may need. A nurse in the outpatient setting plays varied roles in routine assessments, screening procedures, and management of the woman's specific health concerns, acting as educator and advocate for the woman. Nurses explain screening and diagnostic procedures, clarify options so that women can make informed decisions about care, and provide support to women when they experience disruptions in their health.

## WOMEN'S HEALTH INITIATIVE

The Women's Health Initiative (WHI) began in 1991 by the National Heart, Lung, and Blood Institute of the National Institutes of Health (NHLBI) as a 15-year national study focusing on the best prevention for four diseases that have a major effect on postmenopausal women of all races and socioeconomic backgrounds. The study was extended to 2010 adding research findings for these diseases:

- Cardiovascular disease
- Breast cancer
- Colorectal cancer
- Osteoporosis

Breast cancer, cardiovascular disease, and osteoporosis are covered in this chapter. For additional nursing information about these three diseases and about cardiovascular disease and colorectal cancer, refer to a medical-surgical nursing text.

Information about clinical trials, observational studies, and community prevention measures that are now completed can be found at http://www.nhlbi.nih.gov/whi/.

## HEALTHY PEOPLE 2020

*Healthy People 2020* has now been released with a total of 13 new topics with objectives. Several goals in *Healthy People 2020* that are relevant to women's health include:

- Increase the proportion of adults aged 20 and older who were at a healthy weight from 2005 to 2008 from 30.8% to 33.9%.
- Reduce female breast cancer deaths from 22.9 per 100,000 in 2007 to 20.6 per 100,000.
- Increase proportion from 73.7% to 81.1% of women aged 50 to 74 years who received a breast cancer screening based on the most recent guidelines.
- Reduce deaths from cancer of the cervix from 2.4 per 100,000 to no more than 2.2 per 100,000; increase the number of women aged 21 to 65 years who receive screening for cervical cancer according to current guidelines from 84.5% in 2008 to 93%.
- Increase the percentage of adults aged 50 to 75 years who undergo a colorectal cancer screening according to current guidelines from 54.2% to 70.5%.
- Reduce the proportion of adults aged 50 and older with osteoporosis from 5.9% to 5.3% or less. Reduce the number of women aged 65 and older hospitalized with hip fractures from 823.5 per 100,000 to 741.2 per 100,000.

- Increase the number of sexually active females enrolled in Medicaid screened for *Chlamydia trachomatis* from 52.7% to 74.4% (aged 16 to 20 years) and 59.4% to 80% (aged 21 to 24 years).
- Increase the number of sexually active females enrolled in commercial insurance screened for *C. trachomatis* from 40.1% to 65.9% (aged 16 to 20 years) and 43.5% to 78.3% (aged 21 to 24 years).
- Reduce the gonorrhea rates in females aged 15 to 44 years from 285 new cases per 100,000 to 257 per 100,000.
- Reduce the number of females aged 15 to 44 years who have required treatment for pelvic inflammatory disease (PID) from 3.99% to 3.59%.

Information on many other topics and updates as they occur can be found at http://www.healthypeople.gov.

## HEALTH MAINTENANCE

*Health maintenance* refers to measures that can be taken for prevention or early detection of specific diseases. Unfortunately, many women do not practice recommended health maintenance procedures. Some seek care only when they have a problem. For others, the only healthcare they receive comes from a gynecologist or nurse practitioner, often with their annual checkup. Therefore, it is important that those who provide healthcare for women are familiar with principles of screening and counseling in areas that are not traditionally associated with gynecology, such as assessing risk factors for colon cancer and heart disease.

### Health History

The health history is most important in determining risk factors for a variety of conditions. The woman's health history can also help her identify what she does that improves her health. The focus of a health history depends on the woman's age, but some topics need to be discussed with all women. Box 32.1 provides a summary of information that should be obtained.

Family history is essential to assess risk profiles for identifying risks that cannot be modified. Family and/or personal history of hyperlipidemia, diabetes mellitus, heart disease, osteoporosis, and thyroid disease suggests screening tests, and examinations are needed. A list of family members who have had cancer, its type, and their ages at diagnosis provides important information about the risk of cancer, particularly of the breast and colon.

Drug use (prescribed, over-the-counter (OTC), and illicit) should be discussed, including the use of any complementary and alternative medicines (CAM) that many people do not think are medical therapy.

### Physical Assessment

A thorough physical examination is necessary to detect general health problems. Vital signs and weight are measured at each visit. Height is taken at the initial examination and yearly thereafter. Loss of height and abnormal curvature of the vertebral column (dorsal kyphosis or scoliosis) are important observations in evaluating osteoporosis.

The heart is auscultated at the initial visit to determine whether the rate and rhythm are normal and to detect heart murmurs. The extremities are observed for varicosities or edema, and pedal pulses are palpated. Palpation of the abdomen for tenderness, masses, or distention is an important part of the physical examination.

Additional assessments are necessary if the woman is at higher risk of disease. For example, if the woman has a family history of diabetes mellitus, an oral glucose tolerance test or glycosylated hemoglobin ($HbA_{1c}$) may be indicated. If she has a history of multiple sexual partners or a sexual partner with multiple contacts, she should be tested for sexually transmitted diseases (STDs) and human immunodeficiency virus (HIV).

**BOX 32.1 Health History**

**Personal History**

Demographic data (name, age, marital status or whether living with a partner of either gender)
Reason for seeking medical care (chief complaint)
Current and past state of health, previous surgeries
Height, weight, vital signs
Allergies (drugs, food, environmental allergens)
Medications, usual and reason for taking (over-the-counter; prescribed; illicit)
Use of complementary or alternative therapies, such as herbal or botanical preparations, acupressure; chiropractic treatment
Habits (smoking, use of alcohol, drugs)
Appetite, usual dietary intake
Exercise pattern (type, frequency, duration)
Patterns of elimination (current or chronic problems)
Sleep and rest patterns
Degree of stress and stress management techniques

**Menstrual History**

Age of menarche
Regularity, duration of menstrual cycle
Menstrual discomfort (time during cycles, intensity, relief measures)
Age at menopause, if applicable

**Obstetric History**

Gravida, para, length of gestation, weight of infant at birth
Labor experience, medical interventions, and method of delivery

**Sexual History**

Sexual activity (one partner, multiple partners, age when first sexually active)
Method of contraception (satisfaction with method, adverse reactions, accuracy of use)
Previous sexually transmitted disease and treatment
Knowledge or practice of measures to protect self from sexually transmitted diseases

**Family History**

Cardiovascular problems (anemia, hypertension, clotting disorders, stroke, heart attacks)
Cancer (breast, uterine, ovarian, bowel, lung, other)
Osteoporosis

**Psychosocial History**

Primary language, additional languages spoken or understood, ability to read
Marital status, employment, occupation, education (relevant to determine financial, social, and emotional support)
Evaluation for possible domestic violence

### Preventive Counseling

Physical examination provides an excellent opportunity to counsel women about preventive care. Major preventable problems are obesity, inactivity, and smoking. Approximately two-thirds of adults in the United States were overweight and approximately one-third were obese in 2011-2012. Obesity often begins in childhood, and almost one in five children 5 years of age or older was obese according to the 2011-2012 statistics. A normal adult body mass index (BMI) is from 18.5 to 24.9 kg/m$^2$. BMI of 25.0 to 29.9 kg/m$^2$ is overweight, 30.0 to 34.9 kg/m$^2$ is obese, while grade 2 obesity is a BMI of 35.0 kg/m$^2$ or higher, and grade 3 is a BMI of 40.0 kg/m$^2$ or higher. A BMI greater than 30.0 kg/m$^2$ correlates with higher mortality in women. Obesity in women has continued to increase from 25% in 1988 to 36.4% in 2012. The percentage of obese women in the 2012 population varied by race and ethnicity (National Center for Health Statistics [NCHS], 2013):

| | |
|---|---|
| Whites | 33.1% |
| Non-Hispanic Blacks | 58% |
| Mexican origin | 44% |

Obesity is associated with diabetes, hypertension, and other chronic diseases, including breast, endometrial, and colon cancers. Inactivity associated with obesity brings other problems such as osteoporosis, osteoarthritis, **dyslipidemia** (abnormal amount of cholesterol and other fats in the blood), stroke, and coronary artery disease (CAD). Gynecologic conditions include abnormal menses and infertility (Centers for Disease Control and Prevention [CDC], 2015a).

Infections, often STDs, are a source of many health problems that should be reinforced in the nursing care of women. Chlamydia and gonorrhea are the two most frequently reported STDs. Use of latex condoms provides some protection against the transmission of HIV and human papillomavirus (HPV), a risk factor for cervical cancer (American Cancer Society [ACS], 2010; CDC, 2015a).

The history or physical examination can indicate other areas for which counseling or screening should be provided. These include the dangers of malignant melanoma with repeated exposure to ultraviolet rays of the sun. In addition, the health risks associated with alcohol and other substance abuse is particularly important for some women. Domestic violence may be discovered, requiring counseling for the woman to deal with this complex social problem.

## Screening Procedures

Screening procedures are important because early diagnosis allows early therapy while the pathologic process is still treatable. A variety of screening procedures are recommended for all women, including three screening procedures for early detection of breast cancer as well as vulvar self-examination and screening for cervical cancer. Other procedures are based on the woman's age and risk status. Table 32.1 summarizes purposes for common screening procedures for women.

### Breast Self-Examination

Most breast cancers are discovered by the woman herself; yet only approximately half of all women examine their breasts each month.

**TABLE 32.1 Screening Procedures**

| Procedure | Purpose |
|---|---|
| Breast self-examination (BSE) | To assess monthly for breast changes or masses that might indicate breast tumors |
| Clinical breast examination (CBE) | To detect masses that women might miss |
| Mammography with additional imaging such as ultrasonography as needed 40 years or older (routine screening mammography) | To detect breast lumps before they become palpable, promoting long-term survival. Diagnostic mammograms and other imaging may be started at a younger age for women having a higher risk for breast cancer or previous breast cancer or other disorders |
| Cholesterol test | To detect blood levels that raise risk of heart disease; usually combined with additional tests for high-quality screening (lipid profile) such as triglyceride level, high-density (HDL), and low-density (LDL) lipoprotein (see Box 32.3) |
| Vulvar self-examination | To detect signs of precancerous conditions or infection |
| Pelvic examination | To confirm that no disease exists, or for early detection if disease does exist |
| Pap test | To detect abnormal cervical cytology as early as possible |
| Rectal examination | To check for hemorrhoids and lesions and to evaluate sphincter control |
| Fecal occult blood test (FOBT) | To detect blood in stool, an early sign of colon cancer |
| Urinalysis | To screen for diabetes and urinary tract infections |
| **ADDITIONAL PROCEDURES MAY BE BASED ON RISK FACTORS** | |
| **Procedure** | **Risk Factors** |
| Bone density ≥2 years starting at 65 years. Begin bone density screening earlier than 65 years for high-risk women | Family history, fracture history, estrogen deficiency, fall history, physically inactive, underweight, poor nutrition, tobacco or alcohol abuse, chronic steroid use, dementia, European or Asian ancestry |
| Sexually transmitted disease (STD) testing; human immunodeficiency virus (HIV) testing | Multiple sexual partners of the woman or her partner, history of STDs; seeking treatment for STDs, injection drug use, sexual partner who is HIV-positive or bisexual or injects drugs, recurrent or persistent episodes of STDs such as candidiasis and herpes |
| Lipid profile | Diabetes, smoking, no estrogen use after menopause, family history of high cholesterol or coronary artery disease |
| Fasting glucose test | Overweight, history of gestational diabetes, family history of diabetes |
| Rubella antibodies | To determine immunity to rubella |
| Thyroid-stimulating hormone (TSH) | Signs or strong family history of thyroid disease |
| Blood tests to evaluate genetic risk for reproductive cancers (see Box 32.5) | To determine the degree of higher risk influenced by genetic alterations, improving options for therapy |
| Transvaginal ultrasound examination | Family history of ovarian cancer |
| Sigmoidoscopy (every 5 years) or colonoscopy (every 10 years) | Family history of bowel cancer or older than 50 years |
| Tuberculosis testing | To determine infection in a person at higher risk for tuberculosis |

*American Cancer Society. (2014b). *Breast cancer: Early detection.* Retrieved from http://www.cancer.org.

## WOMEN WANT TO KNOW

### *How to Perform Breast Self-Examination (BSE)*

- Lie down. Flatten your right breast by placing a pillow under your right shoulder. If your breasts are large, use your right hand to hold your right breast while you do the examination with your left hand.
- Use the sensitive pads of the middle three fingers on your left hand and a massaging motion to feel for lumps or changes in the breast tissue.
- Press firmly enough to distinguish different breast textures: light pressure to feel tissues near the skin, medium pressure to feel slightly deeper, and firm pressure to feel tissues near the chest and ribs.
- Completely palpate or feel all parts of the breast and chest area. Examine breast tissue extending from the ribs under the arm to the center of the sternum or chest bone. Examine breast tissue that extends from the lower ribs up to the neck or collarbone. The amount of time required to completely palpate all the breast tissue depends on the size of the breast. Women with small breasts need at least 2 minutes to examine each breast. Larger breasts take longer.

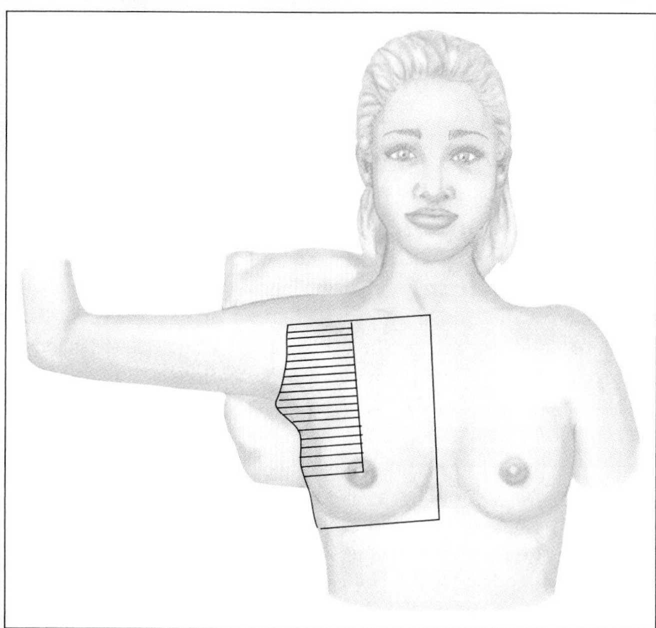

- Use the same routine or pattern to feel every part of the breast tissue. Any of three patterns can help you make sure you have covered your entire breast: the vertical strip, the circular pattern, and the wedge. Choose the method you find easiest. Evidence suggests the up-and-down pattern is the most effective to avoid missing breast tissue.

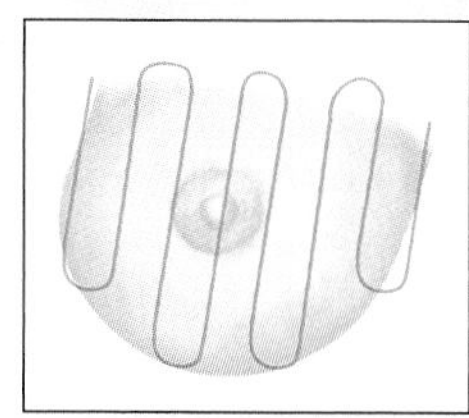

- When you have completely examined your right breast, examine the left breast with your right hand using the same method. Compare what you feel in one breast with the other.
- You may also want to examine your breasts while bathing, when the skin is wet and lumps may be more easily palpated.
- You can check your breasts in a mirror by raising your arms and looking for an unusual shape, dimpling of the skin, and any changes in the nipple.

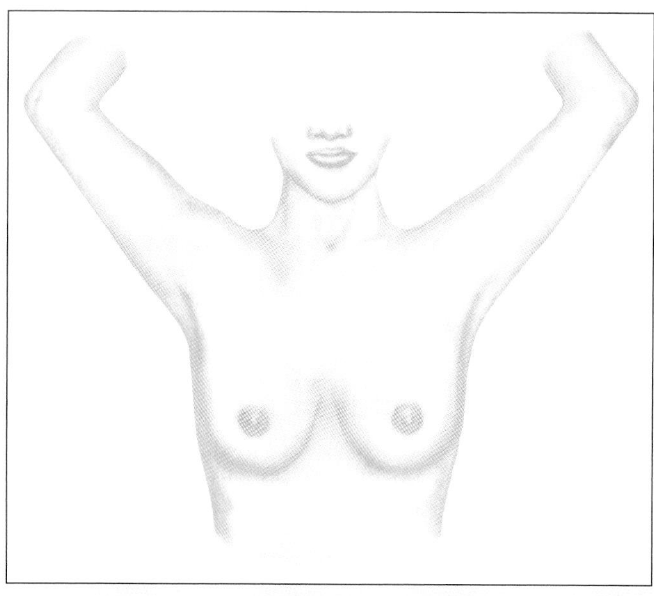

- Examine each underarm, either when sitting or standing, by raising your arm slightly to better feel the area. Raising your arm high will tighten tissues in the area, reducing what you can feel.

Modified from the American Cancer Society. (2011). *Breast cancer: Early detection.* Retrieved from http://www.cancer.org.

Breast self-examination (BSE) is ideally done monthly by a woman starting at 20 years of age. A good time is approximately 1 week after the onset of menses, when hormonal influences on the breasts are at a low level. If the woman no longer menstruates, perform her monthly BSE on a day that is easy to remember is ideal. An example is the first day of the month.

### Clinical Breast Examination

Clinical breast examination (CBE) performed by a healthcare professional can detect questionable areas that the woman misses during BSE. CBE should be routinely performed every 3 years for women aged 20 to 39 years and yearly for those 40 years or older. Some conditions need more frequent examinations because they are associated with a higher risk for breast cancer than the general population. The examination includes inspection and palpation.

***Inspection.*** Follow these steps for breast inspection:

1. While the woman is in an upright position, the examiner inspects the breasts for size, symmetry, color, and skin changes. The nipples and areola are inspected for differences in size and color, unilateral retraction of a nipple, and asymmetric nipple direction, which can indicate an underlying tumor.
2. The woman raises her hands above her head, and the examiner inspects the sides and underneath portions of the breast for asymmetry and differences in color.
3. The woman places her hands on her hips and presses down to reveal skin dimpling or masses.

***Palpation.*** Follow these steps for breast palpation:

1. With the woman in an upright position and while the arm is at the side and relaxed, each axilla is carefully palpated for enlarged or tender lymph nodes.

2. The woman lies in a supine position for palpation of the breasts. A small pillow or folded towel is placed under the shoulder, and the arm is placed at a 90-degree angle to stretch the tissue, and thus, flatten the breast. The examiner uses the flat part of the first three fingers to palpate the breast, rotating the fingers against the chest wall. Tissue that extends into the axilla, **the tail of Spence**, or **axillary tail**, should also be palpated. The procedure is repeated on the opposite side. Normal breast tissue is described as firm, lumpy, nodular, tender, and thickened. Abnormal breast tissue is often likened to a raisin, watermelon seed, or grape. If a suspicious area is found, follow-up by mammography, often with related ultrasonography, is recommended.
3. The nipples are compressed to detect the presence of discharge. A sample of any discharge should be collected for culture and examination of cells.

### Mammography

Mammography is used either to screen for cancer or assist in the diagnosis of a palpable mass in the breast. Mammography is the primary screening tool that can detect breast lumps long before they are large enough to be palpated. This procedure, often accompanied by ultrasound studies, allows early diagnosis and treatment, thus increasing the chance of long-term survival.

ACS (2014b) recommends yearly mammography to screen for breast cancer in women starting at the age of 40 years. Women at higher risk for breast cancer or with a suspicious growth in the breast may need mammography and other diagnostic studies at a younger age. Despite the value of screening mammography, many women have never had a **mammogram** (study of breast tissue using very-low-dose-radiography). Reasons include expense, fear that x-ray exposure will cause cancer, fear of pain, and reluctance to hear "bad news."

Nurses provide information and reassurance to help the woman overcome her objections to the use of this valuable screening tool. Although mammography is relatively expensive, the cost is often covered by health insurance, Medicaid, and Medicare, and screening mammograms are frequently offered by the community at low cost. It is important to acknowledge that some discomfort occurs when the breast is compressed between two plates while the radiograph is taken. One measure that reduces discomfort is scheduling the mammography after a menstrual period, when the breasts are less tender. Knowledge that the risk of mammography is minimal to nonexistent because of the very-low-dose x-rays used may help women overcome some of their fear. Digital mammography, although more expensive, can provide clearer images. Ultrasound images or magnetic resonance imaging (MRI) can also be used if needed.

No screening test is 100% accurate. Therefore, nurses must emphasize that the mammogram should be performed *in conjunction with* a monthly BSE and the recommended frequency of CBEs.

### Vulvar Self-Examination

Vulvar self-examination should be performed monthly by all women older than 18 years and by those younger than 18 years who are sexually active. Chronic HPV is a risk factor for vulvar cancer and can spread to other parts of the body. Vulvar self-examination involves visual inspection and palpation of the female external genitalia to detect signs of precancerous conditions or infections (ACS, 2014g).

The woman should sit in a well-lighted area and use a hand-held mirror to see her external genitalia. She is taught to examine the vulva in a systematic manner, starting at the mons pubis and progressing to the clitoris, labia minora, labia majora, perineum, and anus. Palpation of the vulvar area should accompany visual inspection. The woman should report new moles, warts or growths of any kind, ulcers, sores, changes in skin color, or areas of inflammation or itching to her health-care provider as soon as possible.

### Pelvic Examination

The gynecologic assessment includes a pelvic examination. The woman is advised to schedule the examination approximately 2 weeks after her menstrual period and not to douche or have sexual intercourse for at least 48 hours before the examination. She is advised to avoid vaginal medications, douches, sprays, or deodorants that can interfere with a Pap test or other specimens obtained during the examination.

Before the examination, the procedure is carefully explained, and the woman empties her bladder. She is placed in the lithotomy position, with a pillow under her head. If she wishes, she may assume a semi-sitting position and use a hand mirror so that she can observe the external genitalia and the examination. She is draped so that only the parts being examined are exposed.

Equipment needed for the pelvic examination includes gloves, a speculum of appropriate size, plus equipment to obtain test specimens needed, including a Pap test (also called a *Pap smear*). Additional equipment for collecting tissue specimens for the Pap test may include slides, cotton swabs, a fixative agent, and a cytobrush and spatula. Newer equipment for the Pap test transfers cervical cells to a liquid preservative. A stool specimen may be obtained by the examiner during the rectal examination, and a slide for this specimen should also be available. Equipment to obtain specimens for suspected infection should also be available.

***External organs.*** The pelvic examination is conducted systematically and gently. The external organs are scrutinized for the degree of development or atrophy of the labia, the distribution of hair, and the character of the hymen. Any cysts, tumors, or inflammation of Bartholin's glands are noted. The urinary meatus and Skene's glands are inspected for purulent discharge. Perineal scarring caused by childbirth is noted.

***Speculum examination.*** A bivalve speculum of the appropriate size is used to inspect the vagina and cervix. If a metal speculum is used, it is usually warmed with tap water or a low-temperature electric warmer (heating pad) to reduce chilling and is gently inserted into the vagina. To avoid interference with test accuracy, vaginal lubrication with a water-based lubricant may be delayed until specimens for the Pap test or cultures are obtained. The size, shape, and color of the cervix are noted. A sample is taken for the Pap test. In addition, a sample of any unusual discharge is obtained for microscopic examination or culture.

***Bimanual examination.*** The bimanual examination provides information about the uterus, fallopian tubes, and ovaries. The labia are separated, and the gloved, lubricated index finger and middle finger of the examiner's hand are inserted into the vaginal introitus.

The cervix is palpated for consistency, size, and tenderness to motion. The uterus is evaluated by placing the other hand on the abdomen with the fingers pressing gently just above the symphysis pubis so that the uterus can be felt between the examining fingers of both hands. The size, configuration, consistency, and motility of the uterus are evaluated (Fig. 32.1).

The ovaries are palpated between the fingers of both hands. Because ovaries atrophy after **menopause** (permanent cessation of menstruation), it is often impossible to palpate the ovaries of a postmenopausal woman.

### Pap Test

***Purpose.*** Changes occur in cells of the cervix before cervical cancer develops. Cervical cytology, or the Pap test, is the most useful procedure for detecting precancerous and cancerous cells that are shed by the cervix. Because infection with HPV contributes to cervical neoplasms, testing for this virus is usually done during the pelvic examination.

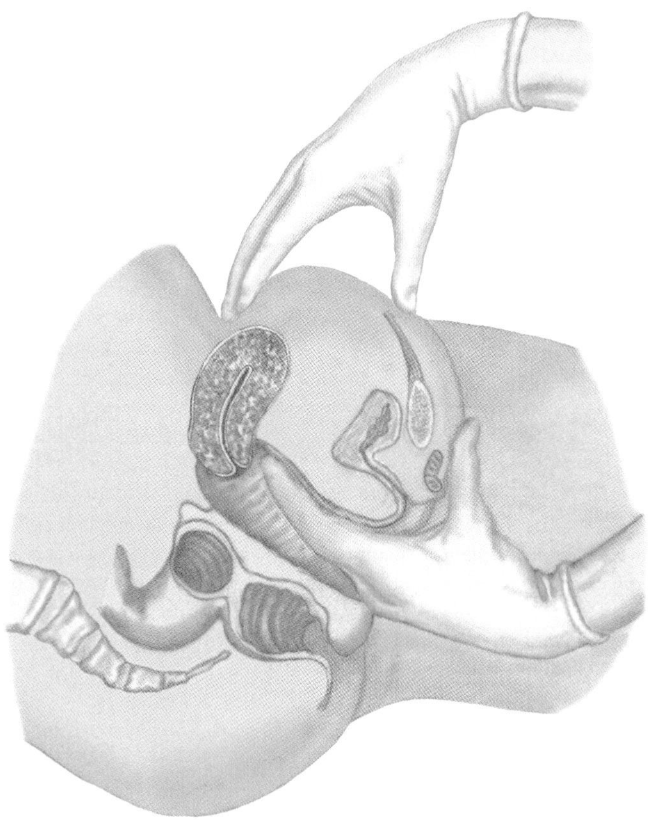

**FIG 32.1** Bimanual palpation provides information about the uterus, fallopian tubes, and ovaries.

***Procedure.*** With the speculum blades open and the cervix in view, samples of the superficial layers of the cervix and endocervix are obtained. Samples are best obtained with a spatula and a cytobrush or with a broom-type sampling device. A sample is taken where most lesions develop, at the squamocolumnar junction (the border where developing squamous tissue meets the immature columnar epithelium).

Cervical tissue is placed on slides that are then sprayed with or immersed in a fixative solution before being sent to the laboratory for analysis (if the older Pap test technique is used). Specimens obtained with the broom-type device as used in the liquid-based Thin-Prep or AutoCyte tests, are rotated in a liquid that preserves the cells for analysis. The liquid-based tests use image processing to select the slides that need additional reading by a technician for best analysis.

***Classification of cervical cytology.*** The widely used Bethesda system describes standard terminology for results of both the conventional Pap test and the liquid preparation. The most recent (2001) Bethesda system reports three elements: (1) a statement of specimen adequacy, (2) a general descriptive category (normal or abnormal), and (3) a descriptive diagnosis for abnormal cytology, whether results suggest malignancy or another disorder.

Categories for epithelial cell abnormalities include:

- Squamous cells:
  1. Atypical squamous cells of undetermined significance (ASCUS).
  2. Squamous intraepithelial lesion (SIL), which is subdivided into (a) low-grade, or LSIL (including cellular changes of HPV); and (b) high-grade, or HSIL (previously categorized as carcinoma in situ). HSIL is more likely to become cancerous without definitive treatment.
  3. Squamous cell cancer that is likely to be invasive.
- Glandular cells:
  4. Atypical glandular cells of uncertain significance (AGCUS).
  5. Adenocarcinoma.

The woman's follow-up depends on the nature of the abnormality and whether it is persistent. Pap tests that have persistent abnormal findings after a 3- to 6-month interval usually are evaluated by a colposcopy (examination of vaginal and cervical tissue with a colposcope for cell magnification), and biopsy is conducted on suspicious lesions.

DNA testing is now available for the types of HPV most likely to cause cervical cancer. The sample of cervical cells is collected in the same way as the Pap test. HPV cell types most strongly associated with cancers are HPV 16, HPV 18, HPV 31, HPV 33, and HPV 45. Approximately two-thirds of cervical cancers are caused by HPV 16 and 18 (ACS, 2014d).

### Rectal Examination

The anus is inspected for hemorrhoids, inflammation, and lesions. The lubricated index finger is gently inserted, and sphincter tone is noted. A slide may be prepared to test for the presence of occult blood in stool.

Fecal occult blood testing (FOBT) is a useful screening measure for colorectal cancer. Special instructions are necessary to prevent false test results when materials for FOBT are sent home with the woman. She should be instructed to:

- Avoid aspirin and nonsteroidal antiinflammatory drugs (NSAIDs), such as ibuprofen or naproxen, for at least 7 days before collecting the specimen.
- Avoid red meat, raw fruits and vegetables, horseradish, and vitamin C for 72 hours before testing.
- Collect a specimen from three consecutive stools.
- Return slides as directed within 4 to 6 days after the specimens are collected.

## BREAST DISORDERS

### Benign Disorders of the Breast

There are four relatively common benign disorders of the breast. The risk of each disorder is age-specific.

#### Fibrocystic Breast Changes

Fibrocystic breast changes commonly occur during the reproductive years. Fibrosis, or thickening of the normal breast tissue, occurs in the early stages. Cysts may form in the later stages and are felt as multiple, smooth, well-delineated nodules that have a tender, movable character. The lumpy, rubbery, or rope-like nodules often vary in size, from less than 1 cm to several centimeters. Fibrocystic changes are not cancerous, although atypical hyperplasia of the terminal breast ducts or lobules is associated with a greater risk for breast cancer. For women at higher risk for breast cancer, tissue specimens can be obtained to identify malignant changes (ACS, 2014b; Gemignani, 2008).

Pain and tenderness (mastalgia) as the breasts respond to hormonal variations during the menstrual cycle are common. The pain is often bilateral and most apparent during the premenstrual phase of the normal cycle. Women with large pendulous breasts may have pain associated with stretching of breast ligaments.

Treatment for fibrocystic breast changes is based on the woman's symptoms. NSAIDs may provide adequate pain relief. Some women find that reducing their intake of caffeine and stimulants known as *methylxanthines* (present in coffee, tea, chocolate, and many soft drinks) helps. Other women may need oral contraceptives to reduce painful fibrocystic changes (ACS, 2014b; Gemignani, 2008).

#### Fibroadenoma

Fibroadenomas are the most common benign tumors of the breast, usually occurring during the teenage years and the 20s. Fibroadenomas are composed of both fibrous and glandular tissue. They are firm, rubbery, freely mobile nodules that may or may not be tender when palpated. The nodules are usually located in the upper, outer quadrant of the breast, and more than one may be present.

Treatment can involve careful observation for a few months. Persistent symptoms require mammogram and ultrasound. Because the woman's risk for breast cancer is increased with fibroadenomas, fine needle aspiration (FNA) or a core biopsy may be used to obtain cells for analysis, particularly if the mass continues to enlarge. The aspiration of cells sometimes collapses a cystic mass. A woman may prefer to have the mass surgically excised (ACS, 2014b; Gemignani, 2008).

### Ductal Ectasia

Ductal ectasia usually occurs as a woman approaches menopause. It is characterized by dilation of the collecting ducts, which become distended and filled with cellular debris, initiating an inflammatory process that results in:

- A mass that feels firm and irregular
- Enlarged axillary node
- Nipple retraction, pain, and discharge

These signs and symptoms are similar to those of breast cancer, and accurate diagnosis through biopsy is vital. Although ductal ectasia is benign, the ducts may be excised to prevent further discharge or to remove an abscess that results from infection.

### Intraductal Papilloma

Intraductal papilloma develops most often just before or during menopause. It occurs when papillomas (small elevations or protuberances) develop in the epithelium of the ducts of the breasts, often under the areola. As a papilloma grows, it causes trauma and erosion within the ducts that result in serous or serosanguineous discharge from the nipple. Treatment consists of excision of the mass and ductal area, plus analysis of nipple discharge to rule out a malignant tumor. Regular follow-up after the excision is essential to identify any subsequent malignancy early (ACS, 2010, 2014b; Gemignani, 2008).

### Diagnostic Evaluation

When a lesion or lump is discovered in the breast, the physician must determine whether it is benign or malignant. *Mammography* is used to locate and visualize suspicious areas of the breasts. However, mammography is not as effective a screening technique for breasts that are dense, as in younger women or because of changes associated with a disorder. *Digital mammograms* are becoming more widely available and can be adjusted in size and clarity to help the reader better evaluate images. *Ultrasound* imaging differentiates fluid-filled cysts from solid tissue that is more likely to be malignant. For this reason, mammography and ultrasound examinations are often done together for improved diagnostic imaging. MRI also can be used. Variations of these imaging techniques are used to guide biopsy and excision of some small masses.

Options for biopsy vary with the type of lesion. FNA can be performed to remove fluid or small tissue fragments for analysis of cells. *Core needle biopsy* uses a larger needle to obtain a cylinder of tissue from an area of abnormal breast tissue. *Open,* or *surgical, biopsy* is performed to obtain tissue for analysis and to remove all or part of the lump of breast tissue. Other types of biopsy may be needed to obtain the most accurate tissue sample with minimal trauma. Examples of conditions that may require a biopsy include:

- Suspicious mass that persists through a menstrual cycle
- Bloody fluid aspirated from a cyst
- Failure of a mass to disappear completely after fluid aspiration
- Recurrence of a cyst after one or two aspirations
- Solid dominant mass not diagnosed as fibroadenoma
- Serous or serosanguineous nipple discharge
- Nipple ulceration or persistent crusting
- Skin edema and erythema suggesting inflammatory breast carcinoma
- Suspicious findings on mammography or other imaging studies
- Known or possible genetic abnormality that increases a woman's risk for breast cancer

### Nursing Considerations

All women feel anxiety when a breast disorder is discovered. The apprehension continues for most women while they await a final diagnosis after biopsy. Some women may find it helpful to learn that most breast disorders are benign. However, as discussed, some benign disorders do increase the risk for later occurrence of cancer. For others, the most helpful intervention is to encourage them to express their concerns such as a genetic risk factor that increases their likelihood of developing cancer.

The nurse should reinforce medical explanations of procedures that are planned to diagnose the woman's breast disorder, such as ultrasound examination, mammography, needle biopsy, or surgical biopsy. Explanations should include what the procedures entail and how long the woman will have to wait for the results.

## Malignant Tumors of the Breast

### Incidence

The risk of a woman developing invasive breast cancer at some time in her life is slightly under one in eight. Fewer than 1% of men develop breast cancer. The American Cancer Society estimates that in the United States in 2015, approximately 246,660 new cases of invasive breast cancer will be diagnosed in women. The incidence of invasive breast cancer before the age of 45 years is 1 in 8, but 2 of 3 women aged 55 years or older are likely to have invasive breast cancer when screened. White women have a higher incidence than Black women, but African-American women have a higher risk of dying from breast cancer because they are more likely to have fast-growing tumors and be diagnosed at a more advanced stage. Asian-American, Hispanic, and Native Indian or Alaska Native women have a lower risk for developing cancer than white or Black women (ACS, 2014b; Gemignani, 2008).

### Predisposing Factors

Although the actual cause of breast cancer remains unknown, several factors are known to increase the risk of developing breast and ovarian cancer and other diseases (see p. 695 [see Box 32.2] and p. 710 [see Box 32.5]). Mutations in two genes (*BRCA1* and *BRCA2*) thought to be responsible for most cases of familial breast cancer have been identified. Mutation of the *CHEK-2* gene increases the risk of breast cancer in both women and men. Studies of genetic links to many types of cancers are ongoing. Because research has linked these and other genes to an increased risk of breast or other cancers, testing is offered to the woman at higher risk or who has developed cancer at a younger age than expected.

Knowledge of risk factors is important to guide breast cancer screening and treatment processes so that a cancer is diagnosed at the earliest stage possible. It is also important for nurses to convey to women that many breast cancers develop in those with no known risk factors, while others with one or more risk factors do not develop breast cancer.

### Pathophysiology

Approximately 65% to 80% of cases of breast cancer are infiltrating (invasive) ductal carcinoma, which originates in the epithelial lining of the mammary ducts. A cancer tumor becomes invasive when it is

**BOX 32.2 Risk Factors for Breast Cancer**

- Female
- Age: 1 in 8 invasive breast cancers in women younger than 45 years; invasive breast cancers found in 2 of 3 women aged 55 years or older
- Race: White women are more likely to develop breast cancer, but Black women are more likely to die because they tend to have a more aggressive form. Asian, Hispanic, and Native American women have a lower risk of developing and dying from breast cancer.
- Early menarche (<12 years), late menopause (>55 years)
- Nulliparity or first pregnancy after 30 years
- Personal history of breast cancer
- Genetic risk factors
  - Family history in first-degree relatives (mother, sister, daughter)
  - Family history of other cancer
  - Mutations in the *BRCA1* and *BRCA2* genes
  - Mutations in other genes: *CHEK-2* gene, *ATM* (ataxia-telangiectasia mutated) gene, *PTEN* gene, p53, CDH1, STK11
- Previous irradiation of the chest area as a child or young woman as treatment for another cancer (such as Hodgkin's disease or non-Hodgkin's lymphoma)
- Previous abnormal breast biopsy results:
  - Atypical hyperplasia increases the risk four to five times
  - Fibrocystic changes without proliferative changes does not change breast cancer risk
- Long-term hormone replacement therapy with estrogen and progesterone
- Excessive alcohol consumption
- Overweight or obesity
- Physical inactivity

Data from American Cancer Society. (2011). *Breast cancer: Early detection*. Retrieved from http://www.cancer.org.

no longer confined to the duct and spreads to surrounding breast tissue. Another 10% of breast cancers are infiltrating lobular cancer, originating in the milk-secreting pockets of breast tissue. Uncommon inflammatory cancers account for only 1% to 3% of breast cancers, but these cancers grow rapidly and are highly malignant. Tumors of the common types of breast cancer grow in irregular patterns and invade the lymphatic channels, eventually causing lymphatic edema and the dimpling of the skin that resembles an orange peel (peau d'orange) (ACS, 2014b; Gemignani, 2008).

Cancer cells are carried by the lymph channels to the lymph nodes, and 40% to 50% of patients have involvement of axillary lymph nodes at the time of diagnosis. By the time a patient consults a physician, breast cancer may be a systemic disease rather than confined to local tissue. Metastasis occurs when malignant cells are spread by blood and lymph systems to distant organs. The most common sites of metastasis are the brain, lungs, liver, and bones.

### Manifestations

When breast cancer becomes palpable, the woman or caregiver feels a breast lump, thickening, or distortion. Dimpling, nipple retraction, or changes in the skin or shape of the breast may occur. Most breast pain is benign. Changes on the mammogram or ultrasound images may occur before the cancer is palpable.

### Staging

Although confirmation of malignancy is the first step in evaluating the woman with cancer, staging is necessary to understand the severity of the cancer. Staging is generally based on the tumor, node, and metastasis (TNM) system used to describe the cancer's anatomic extent. Stages of breast cancer progress from stage 1, indicating a small tumor without lymphatic involvement or metastases, to stage 4, which indicates spread to lymph nodes and metastases to other organs. The stages are often used to determine treatment, and they are useful guides to prognosis. The type of cancer cell, the presence of hormone receptors, and the proliferative rate of the breast cancer cells are also important factors in the rate of recurrence.

### Therapeutic Management

The woman with breast cancer must choose from a variety of treatments with involvement of multiple medical specialties. A combination of surgical excision and adjuvant therapy (additional treatment that increases or enhances the action of the primary treatment) is often recommended. Radiation therapy of the breast minimizes chances of recurrence or spread of the cancer.

**Surgical treatment.** The surgical procedure depends on the type, stage, and location of the disease. The most common surgeries are as follows (ACS, 2014b; Gemignani, 2008):

- *Breast conservation surgery* involves wide local excision (lumpectomy) of the malignant tissue to reach microscopically clear margins of healthy tissue surrounding the tumor. The excision can be performed without major cosmetic deformity. Varying numbers of axillary lymph nodes are usually removed to identify the stage of the woman's breast cancer.
- *Quadrantectomy* is a more extensive surgery for a breast tumor, removing a quadrant of tissue. Removal of the tumor involves resection of the skin and other tissue in the area to reach a microscopically clear margin of healthy tissue. Analysis of lymph nodes removed during the quadrantectomy allows staging of the cancer.
- *Simple mastectomy* is removal of the entire breast but not all axillary lymph nodes. However, some lymph nodes may be removed for cancer staging. Simple mastectomy is recommended for some women in whom prophylactic removal of the opposite breast is considered. It is also performed for older adult women who are poor operative risks and in whom no axillary involvement or distant disease is present.
- *Modified radical mastectomy* involves removal of breast tissue, axillary nodes, and some chest muscles. However, the pectoralis major and minor muscles are preserved. This surgical procedure is recommended when a large primary lesion is found in a relatively small breast, radiation therapy is contraindicated, or a higher genetic risk for breast cancer exists. Breast reconstruction, ultimately the woman's choice, may be offered at the time of mastectomy. Timing of reconstruction is individualized by anticipated postoperative therapy and by the woman's choice.

*Sentinel lymph node (SLN) biopsy* is a technique used to remove a small number of key lymph nodes for evaluating cancer spread rather than removing most nodes in the area (axillary dissection). A radioactive suspension or a dye and often both materials are injected near the tumor site. The dye flows by the lymphatics toward the axillary nodes and is trapped by the first one or two lymph nodes, or the "sentinel" nodes, which are then removed for examination. Sentinel node biopsy can reduce the number of lymph nodes removed, decreasing problems caused by lymphedema (see p. 696).

**Adjuvant therapy.** Adjuvant therapy is supportive or additional therapy that follows a surgical procedure. Radiation therapy, chemotherapy, hormonal therapy, and immunotherapy are often recommended. The decision about whether to use adjuvant therapy is based on the woman's age, the stage of the disease, the woman's preference, and the hormone receptor status of the lesion. Radiation and chemotherapy are known to improve the chance of long-term survival after surgery for many cancers. Research is ongoing within many centers to determine the best uses for these adjuvant therapies for each individual woman when treating breast cancer. The oncology nurse must keep up with broad changes in adjuvant therapy as well as changes for each patient.

***Radiation therapy.*** Radiation therapy uses high-energy rays to destroy cancer cells that remain in the breast, chest wall, and the underarm area after surgery. The effects on skin in the treated area are similar to sunburn. Lymphedema is more likely to occur if the axillary nodes are treated. Intensity-modulated radiation therapy (IMRT) is a newer technology used to deliver precise doses of radiation to the tumor or within the tumor to limit the adverse effects of radiation on normal tissue.

***Chemotherapy.*** Chemotherapy uses a combination of drugs designed to kill proliferating cancer cells. Normal body cells, especially rapidly dividing cells such as those in the mouth, are also killed by chemotherapy but will regenerate. The drugs, doses, and schedule of administration are individualized for each woman based on factors such as type of cancer cells, age, hormone receptor status of malignant cells, and medications needed for nonmalignant disorders. Temporary loss of head and body hair is a side effect of many chemotherapeutics. Nausea, anemia, reduced clotting factors, and reduced immunity are other common side effects of many drugs.

***Hormonal therapy.*** Estrogen-blocking medications are prescribed because many breast tumors are estrogen-receptor positive, meaning that their growth is stimulated by estrogen. Estrogen-receptor–positive tumors occur in premenopausal as well as postmenopausal women. Risks and benefits of proposed estrogen-blocking medications are discussed with the oncologist, particularly in women who have not reached menopause. Osteoporosis is a greater risk with estrogen-blocking medications.

Tamoxifen (Nolvadex) blocks estrogen by binding to estrogen receptors, thereby suppressing tumor growth by reducing the effects of estrogen. Hot flashes, vaginal dryness or an increased vaginal discharge, nausea, or anorexia can occur with tamoxifen therapy. Anastrozole (Arimidex), exemestane (Aromasin), and letrozole (Femara) are aromatase inhibitors with estrogen-blocking capabilities, as they block conversion of androgens to estrogen.

The Study of Tamoxifen and Raloxifene (STAR) was conducted by the National Cancer Institute to compare the effectiveness of tamoxifen and raloxifene (a drug to reduce osteoporosis) in preventing breast cancer in high-risk women. Results of the STAR research, completed in 2006, showed these drugs to be equally effective in preventing invasive breast cancer in postmenopausal women. Those on raloxifene had a lower incidence of uterine cancer and less likelihood of developing blood clots than those on tamoxifen. See http://www.cancer.gov/clinicaltrials for more information about drug trials for cancer therapy.

***Immunotherapy.*** This biologically based therapy targets specific cell pathways that promote cancer growth. Approximately 25% of women with breast cancer have tumors that overexpress HER2/neu, a protein that promotes the growth of breast cancer cells. Trastuzumab (Herceptin) is a monoclonal antibody given to reduce overexpression of this protein. Others being studied at the time of this text revision are lapatinib (Tykerb), pertuzumab, and neratinib.

### Breast Reconstruction

***Timing.*** Breast reconstruction to normalize the body's appearance is often an option after breast cancer treatment. Reconstruction options are discussed with the woman during treatment planning. Immediate reconstruction appeals to many women because it quickly restores their breast contour and often makes them feel normal again. However, breast cancer treatment can involve factors for which later breast reconstruction is best. Some women prefer later reconstruction, even if not required, because it allows more time to learn about options for reconstruction surgery and other methods to restore their appearance. The woman is able to physically heal from the mastectomy and to consider her personal values and desires regarding the added surgery.

***Methods.*** Several methods of breast reconstruction are available. The *tissue expansion method* uses an empty silicone implant fitted with a valve that can be accessed by percutaneous needle puncture. The bag is filled with saline in small increments to slowly expand the tissue. When the desired volume is attained, the incision is reopened, the device is removed, and the expander is exchanged for the appropriate implant. In some models, only the valve must be removed and the expander serves as the permanent implant (ACS, 2009).

*Tissue flap procedures* move autogenous tissue from the back, abdomen, or buttocks to create a breast mound. Although these procedures do not always involve implants of a foreign substance as the tissue expansion method does, they involve at least two incisions: one at the breast and one at the site of the donor tissue. Not all women are suitable for muscle flap grafts, particularly those with diabetes, connective tissue disorders, and smokers, because these procedures involve altering the blood supply to the transplanted tissue with the possibility of poor wound healing. Thin women may not have sufficient tissue for transplant to the breast (ACS, 2009).

Types of tissue flap procedures include:

- Transverse rectus abdominis muscle (TRAM) flap, which uses extra abdominal tissue in either of two ways. A *pedicle flap* allows the tissue to remain attached to its original blood supply while it is tunneled under the skin to its site for breast reconstruction. The *free flap* involves removal of the tissue from its original site for attachment to the breast site. Because blood vessels are disconnected in free flap removal, microsurgery is required to reconnect the vessels and tissue, preserving blood flow in the graft.
- Deep inferior epigastric artery perforator (DIEP) flap detaches skin and fat tissue from the lower abdominal area but does not use muscle in creating the new breast. Microsurgery is also required to connect blood vessels.
- Latissimus dorsi flap moves muscle and skin tissue from the upper back under the skin to the site of breast reconstruction. Weakness of the back, shoulder, or arm may persist after the surgery.
- Gluteal free flap uses surgical transfer of skin, fat, muscle, and blood vessels from the gluteal area to re-create the breast.

*Nipple/areola reconstruction* improves the natural appearance in the reconstructed breast through a small skin graft. Tissue is taken from the opposite nipple, from skin that covers the prosthesis mound, or from other body tissue. After the nipple has been reconstructed, tattooing promotes natural coloring to the nipple and areola (ACS, 2009).

### Psychosocial Consequences of Breast Cancer

The time from discovery to treatment of breast cancer is the most stressful for many women. Factors that contribute to presurgery distress include a sense of uncertainty, inadequate information, the need to make difficult treatment decisions, and scheduling problems. Treatment usually involves consultations with multiple specialists, including a surgeon, a radiotherapist, a plastic surgeon, and a medical oncologist. When there are scheduling difficulties or conflicting opinions expressed by the healthcare team, the woman feels frustrated and confused.

Concerns frequently expressed during breast cancer treatment include fear of recurrence and death, uncertainty about the quality of life, changes in body image, the effect on sexuality, and side effects of therapy. For many women, the knowledge that they will lose their hair as a result of chemotherapy creates one of the most difficult situations in therapy.

Breast cancer can have psychological consequences not only for women but also for their significant others. Difficulties reported include sleep disturbances, eating disorders, and problems with work responsibilities. The marital relationship may be strained, primarily in the areas of sexual relations and communication about matters related to the illness. Women and their partners sometimes differ regarding how much they want to discuss the illness. Some women have a great need to discuss their diagnosis, treatment, and fears of recurrence. Other women and many men view discussion of such fears as negative thinking that delays adjustment.

### Nursing Considerations

The woman who is diagnosed with breast cancer depends on nurses for emotional support and accurate information. The nurse must allow time for the woman to express her feelings and must convey a sense of empathic understanding by quiet presence, touch, and close attention to the woman's concerns. Many women feel that they have lost control and that their lives have been taken over by cancer and the recommended treatments. They may have concerns about family relationships and how their sexual partner will respond. Each woman should be allowed to express her fears and worries. Use of communication techniques such as clarifying, paraphrasing, and reflecting feelings helps the woman participate in her care.

The anxiety that most women experience is reduced when procedures and care are clearly understood. Preoperative teaching should include significant others to increase their ability to support the woman. Teaching should include the length of the hospital stay and what will happen during that time. The nurse should describe the dressings, drainage tubes, and appearance of incisions for the breast procedure or procedures being planned (lumpectomy, mastectomy, reconstruction). Lymphedema of the arm on the side of the mastectomy is possible because of blocked lymphatic vessels, but it may not appear in the immediate postoperative period. Specific exercises such as arm lifts and pulley exercises may be necessary to promote flexibility in surgical areas.

Discharge teaching focuses on follow-up care and treatment. Some areas of concern are how to minimize the risk of wound infection, side effects of adjuvant therapy, and signs and symptoms that should be reported to the physician. Most women also benefit from support groups such as American Cancer Society's Reach to Recovery (http://www.cancer.org) and community support groups often found in healthcare centers and churches. Survivors may find satisfaction in giving back to support others with breast cancer through these organizations.

Using nursing diagnoses to plan and implement care could ensure that care is complete. Relevant diagnoses might include:

- Fear related to uncertain outcome
- Disturbed Body Image related to loss of breast and temporary loss of hair during chemotherapy
- Interrupted Family Processes related to the woman's illness, changes in work and home activity, or inadequate information about the course of the disease
- Ineffective Sexuality Patterns related to concern about altered body structure

## CARDIOVASCULAR DISEASE

Heart disease is the leading cause of death for women in the United States, killing 292,188 women in 2009, 1 in every 4 female deaths (CDC, 2015d). Cardiovascular diseases include disorders of the heart and blood vessels, such as myocardial infarction (MI), congenital abnormalities, and stroke. Those discussed here primarily relate to diseases of the blood vessels, particularly CAD. The topic is extensive, and only an overview will be presented in this text. A medical-surgical text should be consulted for more extensive information.

Most women fear dying from cancer, often breast cancer, but cardiovascular disease is the leading cause of death in both women and men in the United States. Almost twice as many American women die of heart disease and stroke as from all forms of cancer, including breast cancer. Most people tend to think of heart and other blood vessel diseases as a male problem that does not affect many women, particularly not women before menopause.

### Recognition of Coronary Artery Disease (CAD)

Women are more likely to die from MI than men. Women are usually older when it occurs and may have other complicating diseases, contributing to their higher death rate. In addition, MI tends to present with atypical, vague symptoms in women that can delay recognition and treatment. The classic crushing or stabbing chest pain or pressure in the chest is not the usual presentation in women as it is with men. Women may report having some vague symptoms such as fatigue for several weeks before seeking care for an imminent acute MI or one that has already occurred. The symptoms of CAD in women include the following (DeVon, Saban, & Garrett, 2011; Keresztes & Weisel, 2009):

- Fatigue, weakness
- Angina (chest pain with exertion) or pain at rest
- Dyspnea, sometimes paroxysmal nocturnal dyspnea
- Dizziness, faintness, lightheadedness
- Upper abdominal pain, heartburn, loss of appetite
- Nausea, vomiting, sweating
- Pain in the upper body, other than the chest (arm, neck, upper back, jaw, throat, teeth)

Because the pain may be subtle or different from what she associates with a heart attack, the woman may not consider MI as a possibility. Caregivers must be aware that the woman's symptoms could be cardiac related. For example, a dentist must consider that a woman with a toothache but no apparent tooth disease could have cardiac ischemia and an MI.

### Risk Factors

While many factors increase the risk of cardiovascular disease, the most common include hypertension, inadequate physical activity, overweight and obesity, and a diet of poor nutritional quality. These and other risk factors often contribute to the development of other problems, such as type 2 diabetes and high cholesterol, that further increase the risk of cardiovascular disease (CDC, 2015b). Each risk factor may add to the risk for developing another of the problems listed here.

Risk factors can be fixed, unmodifiable, or changeable. Aging is a major risk factor because the woman loses the protection that estrogen, secreted before menopause, exerts on the blood vessels. Estrogen's protective effect delays the onset of cardiovascular disease, making most women older at the disease onset than men. However, cardiovascular disease remains the number one killer of women, not breast cancer as many women believe. Other risk factors are listed in Box 32.3 and are similar to those for men. Several risk factors deserve added discussion.

The leading preventable cause of CAD and other diseases in women and men is smoking. Cigarette smoking adds to the burden of heart, blood vessel, respiratory, cancers, and other diseases in females. Smoking is often more attractive to a woman if others in her family and friends smoke, if she feels that smoking helps control her weight, or she feels that smoking reduces her anxiety.

Both systolic and diastolic blood pressure elevations are associated with CAD and other vascular disorders. Adequate control of hypertension reduces death and disability from MI, stroke, and other blood vessel disorders. A woman with hypertension may not notice the problem because symptoms are not always present. Smoking,

## EVIDENCE-BASED PRACTICE

Too many women believe that cancer is their number one killer, while it is not. Cardiovascular disease (CVD) is actually their number one killer. The four most common types of CVD are coronary heart disease, ischemic stroke, hypertension, and heart failure. Cardiovascular disease and ischemic stroke and their effects on women are discussed in this article.

Stroke is the third leading cause of death for women, and kills twice as many women as breast cancer. Risk factors for stroke include family history, high blood pressure, high cholesterol, diabetes, smoking lack of exercise, and being overweight. Women face unique risk factors which include:

- Oral contraceptives
- Pregnancy: Stroke risk increases during a normal pregnancy due to changes such as increased blood pressure and stress on the heart.
- Hormone Replacement Therapy: Combined hormone therapy of progestin and estrogen, to relieve menopausal symptoms
- Suffering from migraine headaches with aura: Migraines can increase a woman's stroke risk two and a half times and most people in the U.S. suffer migraines are women.

Only approximately 54% of women are aware that CVD is the leading cause of death in women. Black (43%), Hispanic (44%), and Asian (34%) women were less aware than white (60%) women of the CVD mortality. Another study found that fewer than 20% of physicians knew that more women than men die each year from CVD. Lower risk awareness among women and clinicians results in less risk reduction, poor response to symptoms by clinicians, and less likelihood that the woman will seek treatment. Despite the need to improve symptom awareness, deaths from CVD declined 22% from 1996 to 2006.

Stroke can be ischemic if a cerebral artery is blocked or hemorrhagic if a cerebral artery ruptures. Almost 90% of strokes are ischemic. Women aged 45 to 74 years have a lower mortality rate than men in this age group. However, women older than 85 years have a higher stroke mortality rate than men in their age group. Metabolic syndrome (abdominal obesity, dyslipidemia, hypertension, and hyperglycemia) doubles the stroke risk in women but does not affect the stroke risk in men. Migraine, particularly with an aura, was found to double the risk of stroke in women younger than 45 and has also been associated with increased CVD risk. Another study found that stroke risk was tripled with use of oral contraceptives.

DeVon, Saban, and Garrett present two case studies using pseudonyms to illustrate two women's risk perception. Ruth Nolan has a CVD event over a week but does not promptly respond to symptoms that are more common in women than men: severe pain in her upper back, unusual fatigue, and loss of appetite over the week. During the week, Ruth helped her daughter pack to move and cared for three young grandchildren, ignoring the symptoms. On arrival in the emergency department, she was nauseated and sweaty and stated that she had "stomach flu." Ruth was diagnosed with acute coronary syndrome (ACS) with an ST-elevation myocardial infarction (MI), also known as STEMI. Non-ST-elevation MI (NSTEMI) and unstable angina (UA) are the other two terms under ACS. She was sent immediately for cardiac catheterization for angioplasty and stent placement.

The other case study presented Tom Finnegan (pseudonym) and his wife (no pseudonym for her) and demonstrated his response to her stroke-like symptoms while they were watching fireworks on July 4. He saw that she was having difficulty speaking and seemed confused but unconcerned as she watched. He knew that she had a history of hypertension. As her symptoms worsened, he knew she needed professional help and walked to concessions, where bystanders called 911. Following a computerized tomography (CT) in the emergency department (ED), and reperfusion interventions, her symptoms subsided. Mrs. Finnegan eventually made a full recovery.

These two case studies illustrate the benefit of quick response to symptoms that may not seem "bad." Ms. Nolan did not seek treatment for a week despite persistent symptoms of fatigue and loss of appetite, and now severe upper back pain and nausea. The case study demonstrates how a woman's significant delay in seeking care reduces the effectiveness of fibrinolytics, angioplasty, or stent placement in reperfusion. Ms. Nolan arrived too late for reperfusion therapy that might have prevented the actual MI. However, Ms. Finnegan illustrates the benefits of quick and accurate response by her full recovery. Her husband's prompt recognition of her worsening symptoms and action to get her to ED made it possible for reperfusion therapy to be effective and give her a full recovery from her ischemic stroke.

Research has found that women often experience symptoms with MI that are atypical of men: unusual fatigue, upper back pain, nausea and/or vomiting, loss of appetite, dizziness, palpitations, jaw pain, and neck pain. Two tables summarizing appropriate responses to ACS and stroke help the nurse educate patients on ACS and ischemic stroke, encouraging prompt response to either rather than delaying care. Inclusion of family provides added information about responses to significant symptoms. The nurse should emphasize when teaching patients that these life-saving therapies are time dependent.

Symptoms of ischemic stroke appear to have few sex differences. "Traditional" symptoms include arm and/or leg weakness and speech disturbance. Less common symptoms include facial weakness, loss of sensation in arm and/or leg, headache, and nonorthostatic dizziness. Other researchers reported mental status changes, lightheadedness, and face or other pain on one side of the body as "nontraditional." Four groups have investigated sex differences and reported inconsistent findings.

Authors list some reasons why women often ignore symptoms and delay or miss effective treatment: lack of awareness of their risk, tendency to be more passive than men, failure to recognize symptoms of MI, attribution of their symptoms as being "old age," and barriers to self-care, often putting others' needs before their own. Authors also list possible areas for future research.

Nurses should maintain awareness to identify possible risk factors in the women they encounter in care so appropriate teaching and referrals can be made if needed. The nurse often has the chance to raise a woman's awareness of her risks in the obstetrics and gynecologic setting, which helps her respond appropriately to get the care she needs. The nurse should also share knowledge about risk factors and symptoms of CVD with the healthcare provider so referrals to specialists or appropriate laboratory tests are carried out. An environment of collaborative and participatory care may help women adopt health-promoting behaviors and receive specialized care when needed. In addition it may help women achieve better health with weight control and exercise.

References: DeVon, H.A., Saban, K.L., & Garrett, D. K. (2011). Recognizing and responding to symptoms of acute coronary syndromes and stroke in women. *Journal of Obstetric, Gynecologic, and Neonatal Nursing, 40*(3), 372–382.
American Heart Association: 2015 Guidelines Stroke.org (2016)

being overweight, and diabetes further contribute to hypertension. Hypertension is more prevalent in Blacks than in Whites.

Inadequate exercise contributes to many of the risk factors listed. Overweight and obesity are more likely when a person is sedentary, and these weight problems increase the likelihood that diabetes and hypertension will occur. Dyslipidemia (abnormal levels of cholesterol and fat in the blood) is more likely in women, as well as men, who do not get adequate exercise, adding to their risk.

### Prevention

Prevention is the key to reducing death and illness from all cardiovascular diseases among women. The promise of estrogen replacement

**BOX 32.3 Risk Factors for Coronary Artery Disease in Women**

Cigarette smoking
Hypertension (including isolated systolic hypertension)
Serum lipids (dyslipidemia):
Elevated total cholesterol (normal: ≤199 mg/dL; borderline: 200-239 mg/dL; high: ≥240 mg/dL)
Low levels of high-density lipoprotein (HDL) cholesterol: <35 mg/dL (<40 mg/dL men; <50 mg/dL women [American Heart Association])
Cholesterol ratio: The ratio of cholesterol to HDL cholesterol is often used instead of total blood cholesterol. The goal is to keep the ratio lower than 5 (total cholesterol) to 1 (HDL cholesterol), with an optimum ratio of 3.5 : 1.
Triglyceride levels: >150 mg/dL
Diabetes mellitus
Overweight and obesity
Sedentary lifestyle
Poor nutrition, especially a diet high in saturated fat and cholesterol but low in fiber and fruit
Age older than 60 years
Postmenopause status
Family history of coronary artery disease

Sources: American Heart Association. (2011). *What your cholesterol levels mean.* Retrieved from http://www.heart.org; Crowder, B. (2009). Assessment of the cardiovascular system. In J.M. Black, & J.H. Hawks (Eds.), *Medical-surgical nursing: Clinical management for positive outcomes* (8th ed). St. Louis: Saunders; Pagana, K.D., & Pagana, T.J. (2011). *Mosby's diagnostic and laboratory test reference* (10th ed.). St. Louis: Mosby.

therapy to reduce a woman's risk for cardiovascular disease after menopause has not proven true (see p. 705).

### Hypertension

People may be unaware of current definitions for the desired blood pressure and do not seek the help needed to bring it under control before it causes subtle damage over a long period of time. Current standards that define hypertension are lower than what most people expect (CDC, 2015b):

- Normal: systolic, lower than 120 mm Hg; diastolic, lower than 80 mm Hg
- Prehypertension: systolic, 120 to 139 mm Hg; diastolic, 80 to 89 mm Hg
- Hypertension: systolic, 140 mm Hg or higher; diastolic, 90 mm Hg or higher

Lowering the incidence of hypertension, including isolated prehypertension in women, reduces the risk of CAD and stroke. Medication should be considered if regular aerobic exercise, weight reduction, improved nutrition, and stress management do not lower the blood pressure adequately (DeMartinis, 2009). The Dietary Approaches to Stop Hypertension (DASH) diet plan from the NHLBI is often recommended for people to maintain good control. Updated DASH dietary guidelines including recipes can be obtained from http://www.nhlbi.nih.gov.

### Smoking Cessation

Stopping smoking can cause a woman to gain weight, particularly if she increases food calories or reduces her activity. However, smoking cessation has a positive effect on reducing angina and stopping the progression of CAD. Stopping smoking also reduces the risk of lung cancer, the number one cancer in women. Improvement in other respiratory conditions is likely as well. Medication patches prescribed to gradually reduce nicotine are helpful for some women.

### Diet and Glucose Control

Women with diabetes have a relatively greater risk for CAD than do men, so maintaining weight and glucose within normal limits is especially important. Diet is the primary means to control the lipid profile. Diet recommendations should be individualized, but general guidelines are that fat intake should be a maximum of 25% to 35% of daily calories, and saturated fat (found in foods like meat, butter, cream, and cheese) make up less than 7% of daily calories. Cholesterol intake maintained below 200 mg/day is ideal. Increasing evidence shows that fish, especially fatty fish, confers cardiovascular benefits, and at least two servings per week are recommended. A diet high in vegetables, fruits, and low-fat dairy products and limiting sodium intake to 1500 mg/day and alcohol to a maximum of one drink per day for women has shown to be beneficial for reducing blood pressure (Raymond & Couch, 2012).

### Increased Activity

Aerobic exercise helps control weight, blood pressure, the lipid profile, and glucose. It reduces body fat while increasing muscle mass and improving muscle tone. The Surgeon General has recommended at least 30 minutes of daily moderate physical activity such as a brisk walk or stair climbing. Low- to moderate-intensity exercises also have some benefits.

### Aspirin

Daily low-dose aspirin therapy (81 mg or "baby aspirin") is beneficial for inhibiting the platelet aggregation that increases clot formation and leads to CAD. Acute chest pain should be treated with a single adult-dose tablet (325 mg, equivalent to four baby aspirin tablets) as soon as MI is suspected to reduce clot formation and increase the chances of full recovery. For those unable to tolerate aspirin or who have recent gastrointestinal bleeding, prescription drugs such as clopidogrel (Plavix) may be prescribed. Individual needs are based on age, risk factors, and history.

## MENSTRUAL CYCLE DISORDERS

Although most menstrual cycle disorders are benign, all require comprehensive gynecologic assessment. Nurses must be knowledgeable about underlying processes, diagnostic procedures, and expected treatment so they can provide patient advocacy, education, and supportive counseling.

### Amenorrhea

Amenorrhea (absence of menstruation) is normal before menarche (onset of menstruation), during pregnancy, during the puerperium and lactation, and after menopause. Amenorrhea at other times is abnormal, and it is called either *primary* or *secondary amenorrhea,* depending on when it occurs.

#### Primary Amenorrhea

Primary amenorrhea occurs if the girl passes the age by which menstruation has normally started, from 9 to 15 years. Ninety percent of girls have started menstruating if they have completed the sexual maturity rating 4 (SMR 4) (see Chapter 9). Primary amenorrhea is considered if onset of menstrual periods has not occurred, particularly if associated sexual changes have not taken place. Primary amenorrhea may be suspected if the girl is more than 1 year older than the age at which her mother and sisters had menarche (Cohen, 2008; Cromer, 2011).

*Etiology.* The most common cause for primary amenorrhea associated with absence of breast or pubic hair development is Turner syndrome. This syndrome occurs when girls have only one normal X chromosome. Primary amenorrhea in the woman with secondary sex characteristics can result from incomplete development of the uterus, ovaries, or fallopian tubes. Intrauterine exposure to diethylstilbestrol is associated with abnormal development of the uterus. Other causes include hormonal imbalances, systemic disease, and hypothalamic-pituitary abnormalities that result in inadequate secretion of gonadotropins. Primary amenorrhea also results from excessive exercise, malnutrition, and eating disorders such as anorexia nervosa and bulimia, which cause a decrease in ovarian hormones because of inadequate body fat.

*Therapeutic management.* The success of medical management depends on the cause. Counseling for eating disorders and reducing excessive exercise may prove helpful. Hormone therapy can establish normal menses if the cause is a hormone imbalance. Some conditions cannot be successfully treated. For example, if the cause is reproductive tract or congenital anomalies, normal menses and fertility may not be possible, and psychological support becomes the most important therapy.

### Secondary Amenorrhea

Secondary amenorrhea is the cessation of menstruation for 6 months or more in a woman who has established a pattern of menstruation or absence for the duration of three normal cycles. In addition to pregnancy, there are a variety of causes, including systemic diseases such as diabetes mellitus, tuberculosis, hypothyroidism, and central nervous system lesions. Hormone imbalances, strenuous aerobic exercise, poor nutrition, use of hormonal contraceptives, and ovarian tumors can also cause secondary amenorrhea. Events such as divorce, the death of a close friend or family member, moving, or a job change often result in stress that is associated with secondary amenorrhea.

Assessment includes a thorough medical and obstetric history and laboratory testing of hormone levels, as well as questions about stressors, eating habits, history of dieting, and current exercise pattern. Women are also questioned about their use of drugs, such as hormonal contraceptives, phenothiazines, and antihypertensives, which can cause secondary amenorrhea.

Medical treatment aims at identifying and correcting the underlying cause and will vary. Pregnancy testing is done for a sexually active woman, and medications that are potentially teratogenic must be withheld until pregnancy is ruled out. Other treatment may include testing levels of hormones related to the menstrual cycle, therapy to improve timing of the cycle, treatment of anovulation, and identification of other abnormalities that may be related to the disorder. Excess androgen levels may be linked to polycystic ovary syndrome (PCOS), characterized by acne, excess weight and body hair, as well as the anovulation that results in amenorrhea.

### Nursing Considerations

Amenorrhea causes a great deal of concern for the young woman and her family, who may worry that it indicates a serious disease. Moreover, menstruation is a unique function of women, and absence of menstruation may provoke concerns about femininity and the ability to have children.

Teaching includes the importance of adequate nutrition and discouragement of rigorous dieting. The nurse should explain that although exercise is beneficial, strenuous workouts or aerobic training can cause amenorrhea. Effective weight control can reduce factors related to PCOS. The nurse also provides emotional support and explanation of the proposed treatment.

## Abnormal Uterine Bleeding

Abnormal uterine bleeding is that which occurs with abnormal frequency, lasts an abnormal length of time, occurs irregularly, or is excessive in amount. Most abnormal bleeding occurs in cycles without ovulation, often near puberty and perimenopause. Complications of an unrecognized pregnancy, such as spontaneous abortion, must be considered when making the diagnosis. Uterine cancer must be considered in the woman with postmenopausal vaginal bleeding.

### Etiology

Common causes of abnormal uterine bleeding fall into five basic categories:

1. Pregnancy complications, such as spontaneous abortion
2. Anatomic lesions, either benign or malignant, of the vagina, cervix, or uterus
3. Drug-induced bleeding, such as "breakthrough" bleeding that occurs in some women who are taking hormonal contraceptives
4. Systemic disorders such as diabetes mellitus, uterine myomas (fibroids), hypothyroidism, or blood coagulation disorders
5. Failure to ovulate

### Management

Evaluation of abnormal uterine bleeding may include a sensitive pregnancy test, coagulation studies, and tests to determine whether ovulation is occurring. Hormone and liver function tests plus tests to determine if the woman is anemic will often be done. Ultrasonography or hysteroscopy may be used to look for polyps and check the uterine lining.

A common hormone treatment is progestin-estrogen combination oral contraceptives that suppress ovulation and allow a more stable endometrial lining to form. Surgical therapies include **laparoscopy** (view of abdominal contents through illuminated tube to locate bleeding or perform surgical procedures) and possibly dilation and curettage (D&C) to remove polyps or to diagnose **endometrial hyperplasia** (proliferation of normal cells of the uterine lining, possibly due to estrogen during the postmenopausal period). Hysterectomy may be performed if the uterus is enlarged as a result of fibroids oradenomyosis (benign invasive growth of the endometrium into the muscular layer of the uterus) and if the woman does not want more children. Laser ablation can be used to permanently remove the endometrial lining without hysterectomy. Excessive uterine bleeding from any cause may warrant treatment for iron deficiency anemia (Goldstein, 2008).

### Nursing Considerations

Nurses are often responsible for encouraging women to seek medical attention promptly when irregular or prolonged bleeding occurs. Nurses also help the woman keep a record of the bleeding episodes and the amount of blood lost, instructing her to keep a calendar and note any vaginal bleeding (spotting, menses) that occurs as well as the number of pads and tampons saturated each day.

A nurse teaches the importance of adequate nutrition and discourages rigorous dieting. For women who are concerned about amenorrhea, the nurse should explain that although exercise is beneficial, excess workouts or aerobic training can cause amenorrhea. In addition, the nurse explores methods to reduce stress and promote relaxation with the woman. Finally, nurses must provide support for women who fear that irregular bleeding indicates a serious disease, such as cancer. Offering false reassurance is unwise, but information about diagnostic procedures, such as pelvic examinations, Pap test, and other tests is helpful.

## Pain Associated With the Menstrual Cycle

Cyclic pelvic pain must be distinguished from acute pelvic pain. Acute pelvic pain is sudden in onset and is not experienced with each menstrual cycle. It can indicate a serious disorder such as ectopic pregnancy or appendicitis. Cyclic pelvic pain occurs repetitively and predictably in a specific phase of the menstrual cycle. The most common causes of cyclic pelvic pain are mittelschmerz, dysmenorrhea, and endometriosis.

Cyclic pelvic pain can be primary dysmenorrhea, with no definite known cause, or secondary dysmenorrhea associated with pelvic pathologic changes. Primary dysmenorrhea is cramping pain with the onset of menses, whereas secondary dysmenorrhea may not be cyclic.

### Mittelschmerz

Mittelschmerz ("middle pain") refers to unilateral pelvic pain that occurs midway between menstrual periods at the time of ovulation. The pain is caused by growth of the dominant follicle in the ovary or rupture of the follicle and subsequent spillage of follicular fluid and blood into the peritoneal space. The pain is fairly sharp and usually lasts from a few hours to 2 days, and slight vaginal bleeding may accompany the discomfort. Usually, explanation of the cause of the discomfort or mild analgesics are sufficient treatments.

### Primary Dysmenorrhea

Primary dysmenorrhea refers to menstrual pain without an identified pathologic process. Commonly called *cramps,* primary dysmenorrhea affects many women. Women often have mothers or sisters with primary dysmenorrhea (Davis, 2008).

***Manifestations.*** The pain of dysmenorrhea begins within hours of the onset of menses and is spasmodic or colicky in nature. It is felt in the lower abdomen but often radiates to the lower back or down the legs. The pain gradually resolves over 48 to 72 hours. Primary dysmenorrhea occurs in ovulatory cycles and is most common in young, nulliparous women. Pelvic examination is usually normal.

***Etiology.*** One of the most confusing aspects of primary dysmenorrhea is that it is experienced by some but not all women. Some women produce excessive endometrial prostaglandins during the late luteal phase of the menstrual cycle. The prostaglandins (particularly $E_2$) diffuse into the endometrial tissue, causing abnormal uterine muscle contractions, uterine ischemia, and hypoxia. This process accounts for the cramping uterine pain as well as symptoms that often accompany it, such as diarrhea, nausea, and vomiting.

***Therapeutic management.*** Oral contraceptives and NSAIDs, such as ibuprofen (Advil, Motrin) and naproxen (Naprosyn, Anaprox), provide effective dysmenorrhea relief by reducing prostaglandin secretion in endometrial tissue. For best pain management using NSAIDs, the drug should be taken around the clock for 48 to 72 hours, starting at the onset of menstrual flow. Rest in a comfortable position and application of warmth may provide added relief.

### Endometriosis

Endometriosis occurs when endometrial tissue is present outside the uterus. The incidence of endometriosis is estimated as approximately 10%. Endometriosis is often associated with secondary dysmenorrhea, chronic pelvic pain, and infertility (Psaroudakis, Hirsch, & Davis, 2014; Schenken, 2008).

***Etiology.*** The cause of endometriosis remains unknown. One theory is that retrograde menstruation (reflux of menstrual flow through the fallopian tubes) causes endometrial cells to attach to adnexa, nearby structures such as fallopian tubes and ovaries, and proliferate, creating spots of endometrial tissue. Other possible causes include genetic predisposition, immunologic changes, and hormonal changes. Endometriosis is often diagnosed when a woman is in her 20s to 30s. It remains mild in some women and increases in severity in others. Because the misplaced tissue is hormone responsive, endometriosis is most often found during the reproductive years (Psaroudakis et al., 2014; Schenken, 2008).

***Pathophysiology.*** Endometrial tissue outside the uterus responds to stimulation from estrogen and progesterone in the same manner that tissue inside the uterus responds. That is, it grows and proliferates during the follicular and luteal phases of the cycle and then sloughs during menstruation.

However, the menstruation from endometriosis lesions occurs in a closed cavity, which can cause pressure and pain on adjacent tissue. In addition, prostaglandins secreted by the endometriosis lesions irritate nerve endings and stimulate uterine contractions that further increase pain. Moreover, cyclic bleeding into the pelvic cavity initiates chronic inflammation that can cause scarring and adhesions that make conception and implantation difficult. The most common sites of endometriosis lesions are illustrated in Fig. 32.2.

***Manifestations.*** The two major symptoms of endometriosis are cyclic pain and infertility. The pain of endometriosis differs from that of primary dysmenorrhea. Endometriosis pain may be deep, unilateral or bilateral, and either sharp or dull. Secondary dysmenorrhea of endometriosis is constant as opposed to the spasmodic or colicky pain of primary dysmenorrhea and often begins 36 to 48 hours before menses. Dyspareunia (painful intercourse) is typical, particularly with deep penetration. Rectal pain is common, especially during defecation. Diarrhea, constipation, and sensations of rectal pressure or urgency are other common symptoms of endometriosis. Vaginal examination near menstrual onset may identify large and tender masses of endometrial tissue. Although the cause of infertility remains unknown, pelvic adhesions and tubal disease caused by chronic inflammatory changes are likely contributing factors (Psaroudakis et al., 2014).

***Therapeutic management.*** Treatment is either medical or surgical, and the therapy chosen must weigh the need for pain relief and the desire to maintain fertility against the side effects that accompany many treatment regimens. Growth of endometrial tissue depends on adequate production of ovarian hormones during the menstrual cycle.

Continuous oral contraceptives suppress endometrial tissue proliferation. This choice is particularly suited to a woman who desires pregnancy within 6 to 12 months after endometriosis treatment is

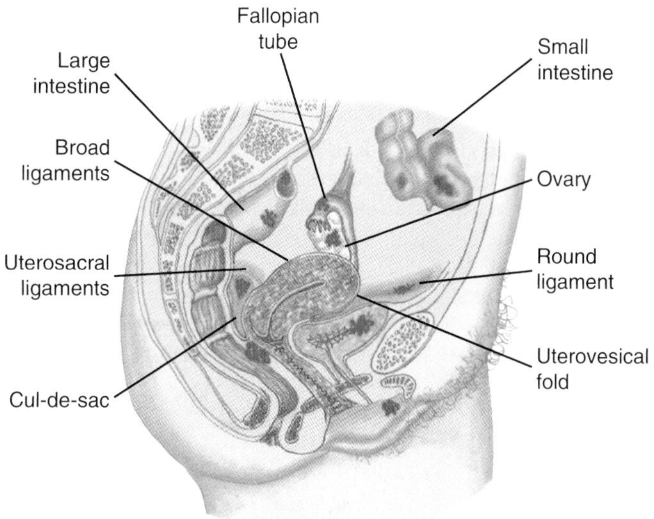


**FIG 32.2** Common sites of endometriosis.

complete. Progestins such as medroxyprogesterone acetate (Depo-Provera) and norethindrone (Micronor) directly inhibit growth of the excessive endometrial tissue (Schenken, 2008).

Both the testosterone derivative danazol (Danocrine) and gonadotropin-releasing hormone (GnRH) agonists such as leuprolide acetate (Lupron) and nafarelin (Synarel) interfere with hormones needed for ovulation and the menstrual cycle, creating a "pseudomenopause" while taken. The woman may have hot flashes, vaginal dryness, insomnia, decreased libido, and reduced bone density. In addition, danazol can produce masculinizing effects such as deepening of the voice, facial and body hair, and weight gain. A woman takes the drug for a period of time that varies, often between 3 and 6 months, depending on the drug and the degree of her endometriosis (Schenken, 2008).

Aromatase inhibitors are a different approach to inhibiting estrogen production in endometrial tissue and have been used successfully combined with daily progesterone or norethindrone. One limitation to long-term use of aromatase inhibitors is bone loss. Two common aromatase inhibitors prescribed for endometriosis are anastrazole (Arimidex) and letrozole (Femara) (Schenken, 2008).

Surgical treatment options for endometriosis differ depending on the size, number, and location of lesions, the age of the affected woman, and whether endometriosis contributes to her infertility. Laparoscopy can be performed for lysis of adhesions and laser vaporization of the lesions. This procedure is used especially when infertility is a problem. For women with severe pain who no longer wish to have children, a hysterectomy, sometimes including bilateral salpingo-oophorectomy to remove both fallopian tubes and ovaries, and excision of all lesions offer relief. Removal of both ovaries causes loss of their hormone production, resulting in an early menopause. Postoperative hormone replacement therapy may be recommended if endometriosis lesions are removed. Any remaining endometrial tissue may respond to hormone replacement after hysterectomy, so this factor must be considered in making treatment decisions.

***Nursing considerations.*** Dysmenorrhea varies from mild "menstrual awareness" to incapacitating pain that affects the quality of life for many days each month. Too often the pain is belittled (e.g., "It's just cramps."). One of the most important nursing actions is to acknowledge the pain in a supportive manner.

The nurse should suggest nonpharmacologic pain relief measures, such as frequent rest periods, application of heat to the lower abdomen, moderate exercise, and a well-balanced diet. The woman should avoid scheduling stress-provoking situations during the menstrual period if possible. The nurse should counsel the woman about the expected effects of OTC or prescribed medications. The woman should also be instructed about side or adverse effects specific to the medications recommended that should be reported.

The nurse should allow time for the woman to express her concerns about the therapy. She should be taught expected effects for drugs given for endometriosis and about the drug's precautions and any side or adverse effects. Some women benefit from information about measures that promote sleep and relaxation, and, most important, from the knowledge that someone is available to provide support and guidance when needed. A woman may demonstrate emotional distress if she has not had all the children she desires but must decide whether to have a hysterectomy to reduce physical pain that simpler measures have not relieved.

### Premenstrual Syndrome (PMS)

Premenstrual syndrome, or PMS, is a group of symptoms that occur during the second half of the menstrual cycle and cause varied types and severity of problems in a woman's work and relationships with others (Box 32.4). As many as 85% of women are affected with PMS. Of these, approximately 8% have more severe symptoms known as *premenstrual dysphoric disorder* (PMDD) (American College of Obstetricians and Gynecologists [ACOG], 2010; Reid, 2008). Once thought to be trivial problems, PMS and PMDD can significantly impair a woman's work productivity and her social interactions. Severe anger, aggression, anxiety, and depression are serious psychiatric effects that occur with PMDD and can have an effect on the welfare of the woman or those affected by her behaviors.

#### BOX 32.4 Symptoms of Premenstrual Syndrome (PMS)

**Physical Symptoms**
- Headache, dizziness
- Abdominal bloating or swelling; swelling of extremities
- Weight gain
- Breast tenderness
- Hot flashes
- Abdominal cramps
- Generalized muscle and joint pain
- Fatigue
- Appetite changes: binge eating, food craving
- Sleep changes: excessive or insomnia
- Reduced sexual interest

**Behavioral Symptoms**
- Depression or sadness
- Feelings of hopelessness
- Marked anxiety
- Confusion, forgetfulness, poor concentration
- Accident prone
- Irritability and anger
- Emotional lability: tearfulness or crying easily, loneliness, mood instability
- Reduced interest in normal daily activities
- Social avoidance
- Lethargic or energetic

***Etiology.*** The cause of PMS is unknown. Theories include an imbalance between estrogen and progesterone, low levels of beta-endorphins, low serotonin levels, and abnormal production of prostaglandins.

Manifestations

- Signs and symptoms must be cyclic and recur during the luteal phase (after ovulation) of the menstrual cycle.
- The woman should be symptom-free during the follicular phase (before ovulation) of the menstrual cycle, and the cycle must include 7 symptom-free days.
- Symptoms must be severe enough to affect the woman's work, lifestyle, and personal relationships.
- Diagnosis should be based on *prospective* symptom recording by the woman, meaning that symptoms are recorded as they occur rather than recalling symptoms that occurred in the past.

Fig. 32.3 illustrates one type of calendar or diary the woman can use to record her PMS/PMDD symptoms and their severity. Other records may include additional factors such as appetite and food cravings, life events, how the symptoms affect her lifestyle, and her psychosocial reactions. Other PMS records are available on the Internet.

PMS puts a regular strain on family relationships because major symptoms recur monthly. Clinical descriptions of severe family disruptions include increased family conflict, disrupted communication, and decreased family cohesion. Of particular concern is the group of women who report symptoms of loss of control, child battering, self-injury, and increased accidents.

## WOMEN WANT TO KNOW

### *How to Relieve Symptoms of Premenstrual Syndrome (PMS)*

**Diet**

- Reduce consumption of caffeine (coffee, tea, colas, chocolate), which increases irritability, insomnia, anxiety, and nervousness.
- Avoid simple sugars (cake, candy) to prevent elevations in blood glucose followed by a rapid decline and a period of low blood glucose (hypoglycemia).
- Decrease intake of salty foods to reduce fluid retention.
- Drink at least 2000 mL (2 quarts) of water per day, and do not include other beverages in this total.
- Eat six small meals a day to prevent hypoglycemia. Plan well-balanced meals with emphasis on fresh fruits and vegetables, complex carbohydrates, and nonfat milk products.
- Avoid alcohol, which aggravates depression.

**Exercise**

- Increase physical exercise to relieve tension and to decrease depression. Aerobic activity, such as jogging or walking, several times a week is recommended.

**Stress Management**

- During the time when there are no symptoms of PMS, acknowledge the effect of PMS on daily life and make plans to avoid stressful situations during the premenstrual period when symptoms are acute.
- Use guided imagery, conscious relaxation techniques, warm baths, and massage to reduce stress.

**Sleep and Rest**

To reduce fatigue and combat insomnia:

- Adhere to a regular schedule for sleep.
- Drink a glass of milk, which is high in tryptophan and known to promote sleep, before bedtime.
- Schedule exercise in the morning or early afternoon rather than late afternoon.
- Engage in relaxing activities, such as reading, before bedtime, and avoid excitement at this time.

*Therapeutic management.* Treatment of PMS is based on the symptom profile of each woman after ruling out other problems, especially psychiatric diagnoses such as depression. Fluoxetine (Prozac) and sertraline (Zoloft) have shown effectiveness in treating PMS. Alprazolam (Xanax) has been useful in some women for anxiety treatment. Oral contraceptives have improved physical symptoms of PMS.

Varied dietary measures may provide relief. Carbohydrate-rich foods and beverages may improve moods and food cravings for some women. Vitamin $B_6$, 100 mg/day, is considered safe, but the woman should be cautioned that excessive doses of vitamin $B_6$ can cause peripheral neuropathy. Other trials have shown that calcium supplements (1200 mg/day) have some effectiveness, and magnesium (200 to 400 mg/day) is minimally effective. Reducing caffeine and taking vitamin E (400 International Units/day) during the luteal phase of the cycle may reduce breast pain (mastalgia) in some women (ACOG, 2010; Reid, 2008).

Women with physical, emotional, and cognitive symptoms may be prescribed antidepressant medications, oral contraceptives to suppress ovulation, or both. Danazol taken in low doses relieves mastalgia, but higher doses may be required for the drug to relieve other PMS symptoms. Preferred antidepressants are selective serotonin reuptake inhibitors (SSRIs) such as fluoxetine (Sarafem), sertraline (Zoloft), and paroxetine (Paxil), although tricyclic antidepressants also may be useful. Short-acting drugs to reduce anxiety, such as alprazolam (Xanax) or buspirone (BuSpar), have shown benefit (ACOG, 2010; Reid, 2008).

*Nursing considerations.* Many women experience some of the symptoms and diagnose themselves as having PMS. Nurses must discourage this practice because serious systemic disease can be missed if the criteria for diagnosis are ignored. A nurse should recommend that the woman consult with her healthcare provider so that a complete history and physical examination can be performed to rule out other causes.

Once the diagnosis of PMS is confirmed, nurses can educate the family about lifestyle changes that may help. Nurses should acknowledge that dietary changes are particularly difficult because many women crave salty or sweet foods, which should be limited. Women also benefit from education about expected cyclic changes. As they learn to predict the pattern of symptoms and gain a sense of control over them, the symptoms often diminish.

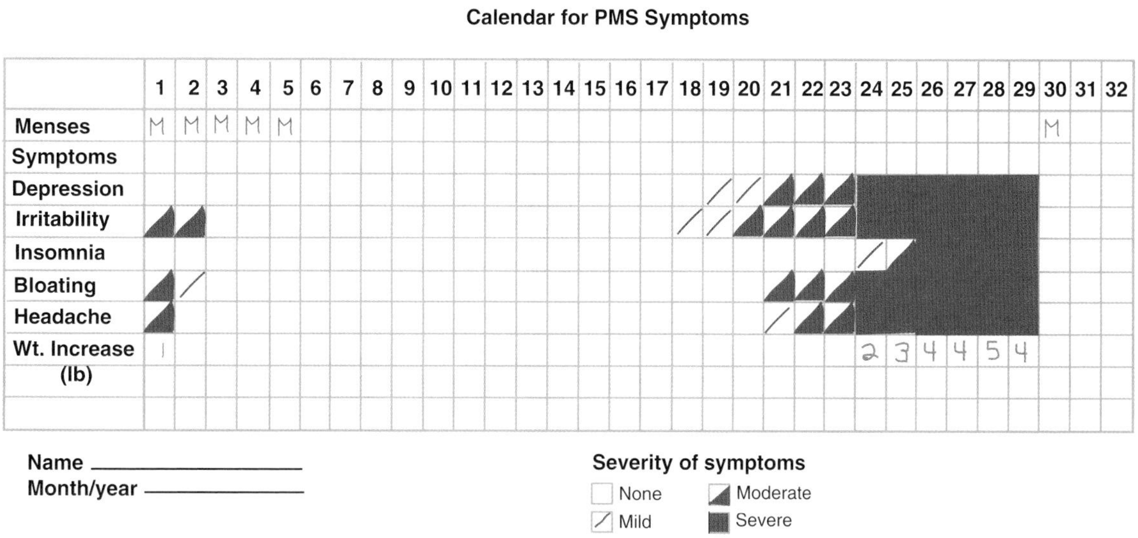

**Calendar for PMS Symptoms**

| | 1 | 2 | 3 | 4 | 5 | 6 | 7 | 8 | 9 | 10 | 11 | 12 | 13 | 14 | 15 | 16 | 17 | 18 | 19 | 20 | 21 | 22 | 23 | 24 | 25 | 26 | 27 | 28 | 29 | 30 | 31 | 32 |
|---|---|---|---|---|---|---|---|---|---|---|---|---|---|---|---|---|---|---|---|---|---|---|---|---|---|---|---|---|---|---|---|---|
| **Menses** | M | M | M | M | M | | | | | | | | | | | | | | | | | | | | | | | | | M | | |
| **Symptoms** | | | | | | | | | | | | | | | | | | | | | | | | | | | | | | | | |
| **Depression** | | | | | | | | | | | | | | | | | | | | | | | | | | | | | | | | |
| **Irritability** | | | | | | | | | | | | | | | | | | | | | | | | | | | | | | | | |
| **Insomnia** | | | | | | | | | | | | | | | | | | | | | | | | | | | | | | | | |
| **Bloating** | | | | | | | | | | | | | | | | | | | | | | | | | | | | | | | | |
| **Headache** | | | | | | | | | | | | | | | | | | | | | | | | | | | | | | | | |
| **Wt. Increase (lb)** | 1 | | | | | | | | | | | | | | | | | | | | | | | 2 | 3 | 4 | 4 | 5 | 4 | | | |
| | | | | | | | | | | | | | | | | | | | | | | | | | | | | | | | | |

**Name** ____________________

**Month/year** ____________________

**Severity of symptoms**

None; Moderate; Mild; Severe

FIG 32.3 The woman uses a calendar to record occurrence and severity of premenstrual symptoms.

Education and support must be expanded to include the family. When the woman exhibits symptoms of PMS, family members often respond by withdrawing or confronting her. Family members should also be encouraged to express their feelings so that anger and resentment within the family can be diminished.

The nurse must help the woman make concrete arrangements to obtain relief when she feels she is losing control or when she fears that she may harm herself or a child. A neighbor, friend, or family member should be identified to provide immediate relief, without questions or explanations, when the woman feels she is losing control.

## ELECTIVE TERMINATION OF PREGNANCY

Elective termination of pregnancy, also called *induced abortion,* is a voluntary method of ending a pregnancy at the request of the woman but not for reasons of impaired maternal health or fetal disease. Therapeutic termination is usually performed to preserve the health of the mother, to prevent the birth of an infant with severe birth defects, or to end a pregnancy caused by rape or incest. A woman may choose elective termination for a variety of reasons, possibly economic or social. Therapeutic and elective terminations involve many social and ethical issues (see Chapter 1). In 2010, the induced abortion rate was 14.6 per 1000 women ages 15 to 44 years, a slight decrease from the number in 2007 (Pazol, Creanga, Burley, et al., 2013).

### WOMEN WANT TO KNOW

#### *Guidelines for Self-Care After Elective Termination of Pregnancy*

- Normal activities can be resumed, but strenuous work or exercise should be avoided for a few days.
- Bleeding or cramping may occur for a week or two. If either becomes severe, medical advice should be sought. Light "spotting" may occur for approximately a month.
- Sanitary pads should be used instead of tampons for the first week after the abortion to avoid possible infection.
- To prevent infection, douching should be avoided for at least 1 week. Ask the healthcare provider for advice about whether douching should be continued at all.
- Intercourse should be curtailed for 1 week after the abortion because of the possibility of infection until the uterine lining heals.
- Birth control measures should be used if sex is resumed before menstruation begins because it is possible to become pregnant during this time. Menstruation usually resumes in 4 to 6 weeks.
- Temperature should be taken twice a day to detect possible infection; a temperature above 37.8° C (100° F) should be reported to the healthcare provider.
- Attending the follow-up appointment in 2 weeks is important.

### Methods of Induced Abortion

The technique used to terminate a pregnancy depends on the length of gestation. Medication-based abortion techniques are options within 7 weeks of the woman's last menstrual period. Inducing uterine contractions with specific medications to end pregnancy early makes the process more private, eliminates risks such as uterine trauma or perforation, and does not require anesthesia. Medications used include:

- Mifepristone (Mifeprex, or RU-486), an antiprogesterone drug, followed by misoprostol (Cytotec), a prostaglandin drug commonly used to reduce gastric acid secretion. Oral or vaginal use of misoprostol in medical abortion is unlabeled by the manufacturer. The woman receives an initial dose of 600 mg mifepristone orally. Oral or vaginal misoprostol (400 μg) follows in 48 hours to promote expulsion if pregnancy has not ended. The woman usually expels the early pregnancy within 14 days of her first visit. Newer regimens use a combination of mifepristone 200 mg followed by a patient-administered dose of vaginal misoprostol (800 μg) and can be prescribed up to 9 weeks of gestation (ACOG, 2009; Holmquist & Gilliam, 2008).
- Methotrexate (Folex, Mexate) is an antimetabolite also used to treat certain types of cancer. Although not U.S. Food and Drug Administration (FDA) approved for medical abortion, individualized doses have been successfully used for medical pregnancy termination. Misoprostol may be prescribed to enhance expulsion of the uterine contents (ACOG, 2009; Holmquist & Gilliam, 2008).

Surgical abortion techniques are needed if the woman has been pregnant for more than 7 weeks or if her medical abortion failed and she still desires pregnancy termination. Through 12 weeks of gestation, vacuum aspiration with curettage is the method of choice. The cervix is dilated after locally injecting anesthetic in the area, and a plastic cannula is inserted into the uterine cavity. The contents are aspirated with negative pressure, and the uterine cavity may be scraped with a curet to ensure that the uterus is empty. Cramping may last 20 to 30 minutes after the procedure is completed. Complications include uterine perforation, hemorrhage, cervical lacerations, and adverse reactions to the anesthetic agent.

For second-trimester abortions, *dilation with removal of the fetus and placenta,* also known as *dilation and evacuation,* or *D & E,* is generally performed. The procedure is similar to vacuum curettage but requires greater cervical dilation and a larger aspirator because the products of conception have grown in size and must be removed gradually. Laminaria are rounded, cone-shaped materials made of dry seaweed that absorb water. They are inserted into the cervix approximately 24 hours before the procedure to allow expansion and cervical dilation. If needed before aspiration and removal of the products of pregnancy, additional cervical dilation is performed.

Medical methods are available for abortion in the second trimester, but these involve labor. Retention of the placenta often occurs, requiring a D&C to fully clean the uterus. Laminaria are inserted approximately 12 hours before the procedure to start cervical dilation. Prostaglandin $E_2$, which stimulates contractions, may be given via vaginal suppository or intraamniotic infusion. Oxytocin is not effective at starting labor because of the early gestation, but it may shorten labor after it has been established by other methods. Similar methods may be required if fetal death occurs in the second trimester. Because of the emotional distress caused by the longer procedure and the increased risks involved, elective termination of pregnancy is not often chosen in the second trimester.

### Nursing Considerations Related to Elective Pregnancy Termination

The nurse's role in caring for women seeking induced abortion is to provide physical and emotional support and information. The nurse may take a history and collect specimens for laboratory testing. Counseling and emotional support are nursing responsibilities. Nurses should reinforce instructions about returning to the clinic and provide information for self-care. They should teach women signs of complications such as excessive bleeding or infection (temperature >37.8° C [100° F], foul-smelling vaginal drainage). Nurses may teach the use of a recommended contraceptive method after the pregnancy has ended. Rh-negative women should receive $Rh_o(D)$ immune globulin (RhoGAM) if they do not have a preexisting sensitivity to Rh-positive blood.

## MENOPAUSE

*Menopause* simply means "the end of menstruation," usually 2 consecutive months without menses. However, many people use the term to indicate all changes that occur at the end of the reproductive period. The entire process, frequently called the *change of life,* is correctly termed the climacteric to include endocrine, body, and psychological changes that occur at the end of a woman's reproductive cycles. *Premenopause* refers to the early part of the climacteric, before menstruation ceases but after the woman experiences some of the climacteric symptoms, such as irregular menses. Perimenopause includes premenopause, menopause, and at least 1 year after menopause. *Postmenopause* refers to the phase after menopause, when menstrual periods have ceased altogether.

Once a woman is postmenopausal, *unplanned vaginal bleeding should always be investigated as soon as possible* because it is highly suggestive of endometrial cancer. Women who take estrogen and progesterone sequentially have planned bleeding when they stop taking the drugs, usually once a month. This allows the uterine lining to be sloughed and prevents endometrial hyperplasia.

### Age at Menopause

The woman's reproductive function falls during the climacteric, from approximately 45 to 50 years of age, as the ovarian hormones decline and then cease. Menopause occurs at the time of the woman's final period during the climacteric. If therapeutic, menopause can be created artificially at any age, through surgical removal of the ovaries or their destruction by radiation therapy, often related to treatment for cancer. Young women who experience artificial menopause often have more symptoms associated with menopause than do women who go through the natural process gradually.

Women can now expect to live another 30 years after menopause at the expected age. During this period, they must deal with physical, psychological, and social changes that often require a reevaluation of their primary roles and restructuring of personal goals.

### Physiologic Changes

During premenopause, the ovaries are less responsive to gonadotropins. Although increased amounts of follicle-stimulating hormone are secreted, ovulation is sporadic, and menstrual periods are irregular. With progressive aging, the ovaries become unresponsive, even to high levels of gonadotropins, and ovulation, menstruation, and the secretion of ovarian hormones (estrogen and progesterone) cease. Menstrual periods become less frequent as menopause approaches.

When estrogen levels decline, the organs of reproduction undergo regression. The labia become thin and pale. The vaginal mucosa atrophies, and vaginal tissue loses its lubrication and is easily traumatized. Dyspareunia is not uncommon, and bacterial invasion of the epithelium may lead to frequent vaginal infections. This process is called *atrophic vaginitis*. Breasts become smaller, and atrophy of the uterus and ovaries occurs. A concurrent benefit is that uterine myomas (fibroids) and endometriosis lesions also atrophy. Estrogen deficit can also result in atrophic changes in the bladder and urethra that give rise to loss of urethral tone and frequent atrophic cystitis.

In addition, absence of estrogen is associated with an adverse change in serum lipids. Low-density lipoproteins (LDLs), which carry cholesterol to blood vessels, increase. High-density lipoproteins (HDLs), which carry cholesterol to the liver and protect against the development of CAD, decrease.

Many menopausal women experience hot flashes or flushes, which are the result of vasomotor instability. The cause of vasomotor instability is unknown, but it is closely associated with increased secretion of gonadotropins. Hot flashes are characterized by a sudden feeling of heat or burning of the skin, followed by perspiration. They occur more frequently during the night, causing fatigue from interrupted sleep.

### Psychological Responses

Psychological and social changes accompany menopause, and individual responses vary widely. Many women are relieved that their childbearing and child-rearing tasks are coming to an end. Other women grieve that the possibility of childbearing is past, especially if they are childless. "Boomers" born from 1946 to 1964 entering menopause are likely to change many of society's ideas about menopause because of the sheer size of their group. As they have grown up and matured, boomers have changed the social fabric of the United States dramatically.

Some symptoms do not have a physiologic explanation, but they are no less real to women who experience them. Depression, mood swings, irritability, and agitation are common climacteric complaints. Insomnia and fatigue are frequently mentioned as major problems.

One of the most puzzling aspects of menopause is the wide variation in physical and psychological symptoms. For some women, the only changes are mild, infrequent hot flashes and amenorrhea. Others experience severe, debilitating hot flashes, atrophic vaginitis, and multiple psychological symptoms such as irritability and prolonged depression.

### Therapy for Menopause

Although many women comfortably undergo the age-associated changes of menopause, others seek assistance for their individual discomforts such as hot flashes, interrupted sleep, or vaginal dryness. The belief that increasing reproductive hormones would slow the aging process and promote a more youthful appearance increased the use of replacement therapy during the climacteric. Additional beneficial effects were once thought to be a reduction in cardiovascular disease, colorectal cancer, breast cancer, and osteoporosis as well as other medical-surgical conditions associated with aging.

As greater research results emerged, including that of the WHI, additional risk factors, as well as benefits, of hormone therapy became evident. Two groups of perimenopausal women were included in the hormone studies of the WHI research:

- Estrogen and progesterone were given to women with a uterus. Combining progesterone with estrogen therapy prevented uterine hyperplasia, a precursor to uterine cancer, in this group.
- Estrogen therapy alone was given to women who had had a hysterectomy, because uterine hyperplasia was not a risk.

*Menopause hormone therapy* (MHT) is an umbrella term used to describe several hormone preparations. Estrogen alone can only be used in women who no longer have a uterus; estrogen plus progesterone is needed if the woman has a uterus, and thus, an endometrium. Another common abbreviation for the combination of estrogen and progesterone replacement is *hormone replacement therapy,* or *HRT,* whereas the estrogen-only replacement therapy may be called *ERT* (National Institutes of Health: Institute on Aging, 2012).

Although once routinely prescribed to reduce the annoying changes of menopause for many women, the decision regarding hormone therapy is complex because both the associated benefits and risks for each woman must be considered. In addition, complementary therapy often is more useful for women having mild menopausal changes.

Some women do not qualify for hormone therapy, such as those who have breast cancer or blood coagulation disorders. Women who had breast cancer before the climacteric often should not take hormone therapy because their risk of cancer recurrence is higher than that of the general population. Smoking, hypertension, diabetes, cardiovascular disease, and renal or liver disease are often contraindications for hormone therapy, whether it includes estrogen and progesterone or estrogen alone.

## Nursing Considerations Related to Menopause

Nursing care focuses on helping women understand the physical and psychological changes that occur during perimenopause. If the woman chooses hormone therapy, nurses must reinforce both the prescribed regimen as well as the risks and benefits of the therapy. For example, women should be told that although MHT effectively treats atrophic vaginitis and reduces dyspareunia, it may not correct the loss of libido that some women experience.

If MHT is contraindicated or not chosen by the woman, nurses often provide information about measures to reduce problems and promote comfort:

- Using water-soluble lubricants, such as K-Y Liquid, Lubrin, Replens, or K-Y Silk-E to relieve vaginal dryness and dyspareunia. Oil-based lubricants should not be used because they adhere to the mucous membrane for long periods and provide a medium for bacterial growth.
- Discussing alternatives to estrogen, such as botanical preparations, if the woman does not want estrogen replacement therapy. The woman should discuss these with her healthcare provider because some have side or adverse effects or interactions with other drugs.
- Doing Kegel exercises to increase muscle tone around the vagina and urinary meatus to counteract the effects of genital atrophy.
- Drinking at least eight glasses of water a day to decrease the concentration of urine, to flush urine from the bladder, and to reduce bacterial growth, thereby preventing atrophic cystitis.
- Wiping from front to back after urination and defecation to reduce the transfer of bacteria from the anus to the urinary meatus and to help prevent cystitis at any age.

## Osteoporosis

**Osteoporosis** (increased spaces in bone; increases after menopause) is one of the greatest hazards of the postmenopausal years, yet bone loss begins well before menopause. The decrease in estrogen at menopause accelerates bone loss and slows bone regeneration. Osteoporosis is characterized by reduced bone density, leaving the bones porous, fragile, and susceptible to fractures. The vertebrae and hips are the most common sites of fractures, with wrists, forearms, feet, and toes also susceptible. In the United States, 1.5 million osteoporosis-related fractures occur yearly, with women having the highest risk. More osteoporosis-related fractures are expected as the age of the U.S. population rises (National Institutes of Health: National Institute of Arthritis and Musculoskeletal and Skin Diseases [NIAMS], 2011).

### Predisposing Factors

The combination of peak bone density and the rate of bone loss influences the severity of osteoporosis. Small-boned, fair-skinned white women of northern European extraction and Asian women are at greatest risk for osteoporosis, but Black and Hispanic women also are at risk. Other risk factors may include a family history of the disease, late menarche, early menopause, and a sedentary lifestyle. Women who smoke, drink alcohol, or consume excessive amounts of caffeine have an increased risk for osteoporosis. Drug intake such as corticosteroids, some anticonvulsants, and aromatase inhibitors for breast cancer can reduce bone density. Inadequate lifetime intake of calcium or vitamin D is a risk factor because reaching one's peak bone mass near the age of 30 does not occur.

### Manifestations

Osteoporosis has been called the "silent thief" because it takes place gradually over the course of many years without symptoms. The first noticeable signs are loss of height and back pain that occurs when the vertebrae collapse. Later signs include the "dowager's hump," which occurs when the vertebrae can no longer support the upper body in an upright position. Secondary to this, the waistline disappears and the abdomen protrudes because the rib cage moves closer to the pelvis. Depending on the number of fractures, several inches of height may be lost. Fig. 32.4 illustrates progressive changes in posture associated with osteoporosis.

Diagnosis of osteoporosis depends on history and physical examination. Bone mineral analysis may be performed if results will influence the decision to use hormone replacement therapy. Conventional radiography is of little help because more than 30% of the bone mass must be lost before changes are apparent. Dual-energy x-ray absorptiometry (DEXA) is a highly accurate, fast diagnostic method that involves low exposure to radiation.

### Prevention and Therapeutic Management

The major goal of treatment is to prevent or slow osteoporosis and to stabilize remaining bone mass. Although research has upheld estrogen therapy to reduce osteoporosis by inhibition of bone resorption, fewer women are choosing the hormone because of its potential adverse effects.

***Drug therapy.*** Other drug categories to reduce osteoporosis include:

- Calcitonin (Calcitonin, Miacalcin, Fortical), a calcium regulator usually prescribed as a daily nasal spray.
- Bisphosphonates, which inhibit osteoclasts (cells that break down bone), reducing bone turnover. Alendronate (Fosamax), risedronate (Actonel), and ibandronate (Boniva) are used to prevent and

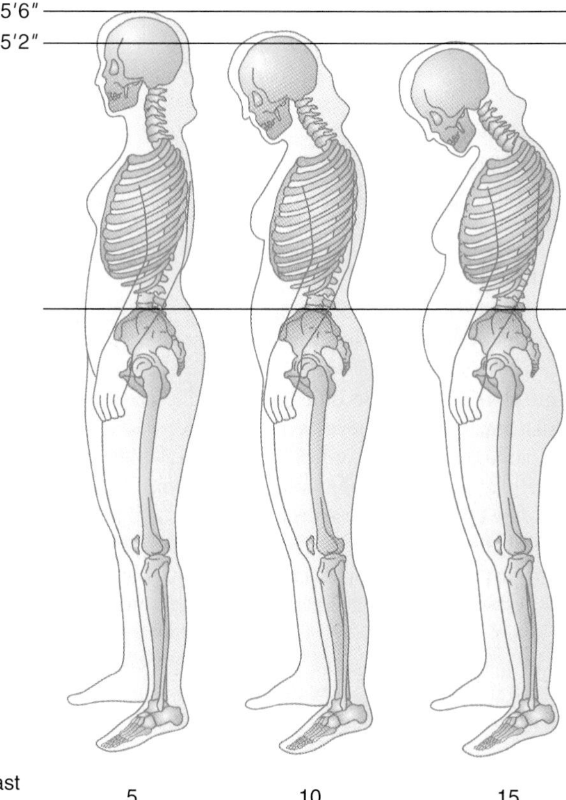


**FIG 32.4** With progression of osteoporosis, the vertebral column collapses, causing loss of height and back pain. Dowager's hump is the term used for this curvature of the upper back.

treat postmenopausal osteoporosis. Oral bisphosphonates may be contraindicated for women with ulcers or an inflammatory gastrointestinal disease such as dysphagia or esophagitis. Alendronate and risedronate are also approved to treat bone loss that results from glucocorticoids and to treat men with osteoporosis. Zoledronic acid (Reclast) is approved for treatment of postmenopausal osteoporosis and is given by intravenous (IV) infusion yearly. Headache or flu-like pain in muscles or joints may occur for 2 or 3 days after zoledronic acid infusion (NIAMS, 2011; Wilton, 2011).
- Raloxifene (Evista), a selective estrogen receptor modulator, or SERM, that binds to estrogen receptors to reduce bone loss. Because of the combined estrogen agonist and estrogen antagonist effects of SERMs, raloxifene is being studied to see if its effects also improve cardiac health without raising breast or uterine cancer risks (NIAMS, 2011).
- Teriparatide (Forteo), an injectable parathyroid hormone approved for postmenopausal women and men at high risk of fracture. Current approved duration of use is a maximum of 24 months. Teriparatide stimulates new bone formation, reducing the risk of both vertebral and nonvertebral fractures. Nausea, dizziness, and leg cramps are side effects (NIAMS, 2011).
- Denosumab (Prolia) is a recently approved receptor activator of nuclear factor-kappa B (RANK) ligand (RANKL) inhibitor that inhibits osteoclasts. Increased RANKL in postmenopausal women results in greater bone resorption by the osteoclasts. Denosumab reduces bone loss by inhibiting osteoclasts produced by higher RANKL levels (NIAMS, 2011; Wilton, 2011).

***Calcium and vitamin D.*** Although calcium does not prevent bone loss, other therapies cannot be effective if calcium is deficient. A woman older than 50 years needs 1200 mg of calcium daily. Daily calcium supplements are recommended because it is difficult to ingest these quantities through food intake only. Vitamin D is necessary for calcium to be absorbed from the intestine. Supplemental vitamin D, 600 International Units (IU) per day, is recommended for adults up to 70 years and 800 IU daily after the age of 70 (ACOG, 2014c; NIAMS, 2011). Foods high in calcium are dairy products, dark green, leafy vegetables, and foods fortified with calcium such as breads, orange juice, and cereals.

***Exercise.*** Weight-bearing and resistance exercises have been shown to increase bone density and build muscle mass in women. Walking, hiking, stair climbing, and dancing are examples of weight-bearing exercises. Use of free weights or weight machines build muscle mass and increase bone strength. High-impact exercises should be avoided if vertebrae are fragile. At least 30 minutes of daily therapeutic exercise is needed. Other exercises, such as swimming or water-based exercises, often improve cardiovascular and respiratory fitness while managing weight, although their primary use is not to limit bone loss.

### Nursing Considerations

Nurses often counsel women about lifestyle factors that contribute to bone loss, such as cigarette smoking, excessive alcohol or caffeine intake, and the importance of following the recommended medical regimen. Adolescents and young women should be counseled about factors that impair, as well as promote, achievement of their ideal peak bone density. Nurses are also concerned about how to prevent falls, thereby reducing the risk of fractures. Suggestions to increase safety in the home include adequate lighting and avoiding objects that might increase falls, such as loose electrical cords or rugs without nonskid backing.

### Nursing Diagnoses

A variety of nursing diagnoses are relevant for the woman with osteoporosis. Examples are:

- Activity Intolerance related to discomfort, lack of appropriate exercise, or fear of falling
- Chronic Pain related to pressure and inflammation of nerves that exit the spinal column
- Disturbed Body Image related to altered posture and functional limitations
- Self-Care Deficit (specify) related to physical limitations and depression

## PELVIC FLOOR DYSFUNCTION

Pelvic floor dysfunction occurs when muscles, ligaments, and fascia that support the pelvic organs become damaged or weakened. This relaxation of pelvic support allows the pelvic organs to prolapse into, and sometimes out of, the vagina. Urinary incontinence may accompany pelvic floor dysfunction. Pelvic disorders usually occur in the perimenopausal period. Some are a delayed result of vaginal childbirth.

### Vaginal Wall Prolapse

The vagina may prolapse, or herniate, at either the anterior or posterior wall. Anterior wall prolapse involves the bladder and urethra and is called *cystocele*. Prolapse of the posterior wall produces *enterocele* or *rectocele*. A woman can have both anterior and posterior vaginal wall prolapse. Combinations of these pelvic organ prolapses, which require surgical repair, can occur.

#### Cystocele

When the weakened upper anterior wall of the vagina is no longer able to support the weight of urine in the bladder, cystocele develops (Fig. 32.5, *A*). The bladder protrudes downward into the vagina, resulting in incomplete emptying of the bladder and consequent cystitis. Urethral displacement occurs when the bladder bulges into the lower anterior vaginal wall, producing stress incontinence. Stress incontinence is the loss of urine that occurs with a sudden increase in intraabdominal pressure from sneezing, coughing, lifting, or other sudden, jarring motions.

#### Enterocele

Enterocele refers to prolapse of the upper posterior vaginal wall between the vagina and rectum. This condition is almost always associated with herniation of the pouch of Douglas (a fold of peritoneum that dips down between the rectum and the uterus) and may contain loops of bowel (see Fig. 32.5, *B*). Enterocele often accompanies uterine prolapse.

#### Rectocele

Rectocele occurs when the posterior wall of the vagina becomes weakened and thin. When the woman strains at defecation, feces are pushed against the thin wall, causing further stretching, until finally the rectum protrudes into the vagina (see Fig. 32.5, *C*). Many rectoceles are small and produce few symptoms. If the rectocele is large, the woman may have difficulty emptying the rectum. Some women facilitate bowel elimination by applying digital pressure on the posterior vaginal wall to keep the rectocele from protruding during a bowel movement.

### Uterine Prolapse

Uterine prolapse occurs when the cardinal ligaments that support the uterus and vagina are stretched during pregnancy and do not return to normal after childbirth. As the ligaments stretch, the uterus sags backward and downward into the vagina. Fig. 32.6 illustrates three levels of uterine prolapse, from first degree, in which the uterus remains

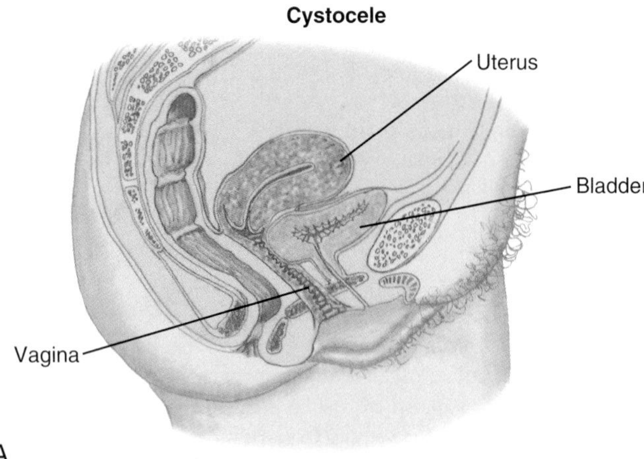


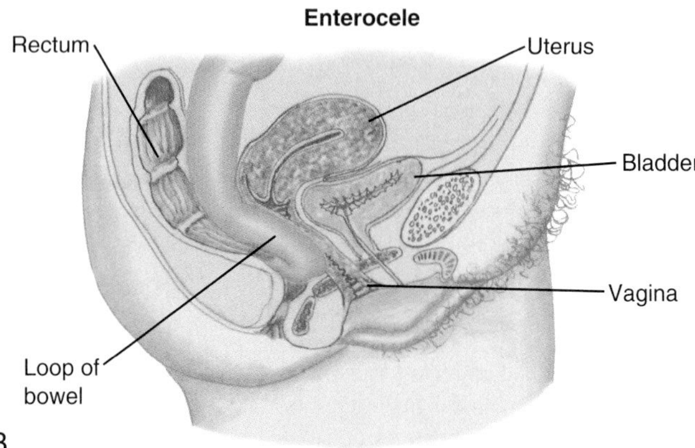


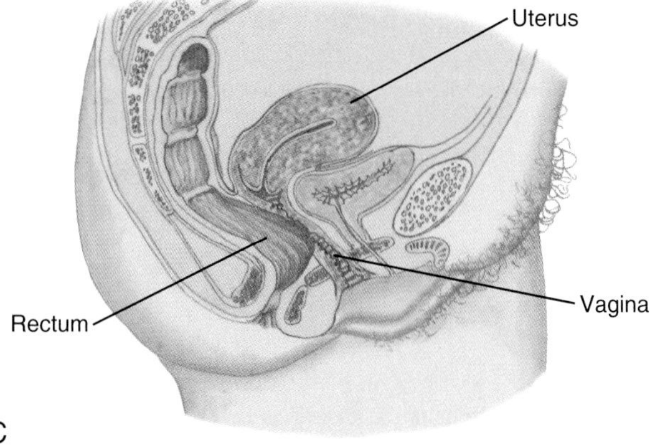


**FIG 32.5** Three types of vaginal wall prolapse. **A,** Note bulging of bladder into the vagina. **B,** Note loop of bowel between rectum and uterus. **C,** Note bulging of rectum into vagina. More than one type of vaginal wall prolapse can be present in the same woman.

in the vagina, to third degree, in which the cervix protrudes through from the vagina (DeLancy, 2008).

### Manifestations

Symptoms usually become obvious during the menopausal period, when decreased estrogen causes atrophic changes in the supporting

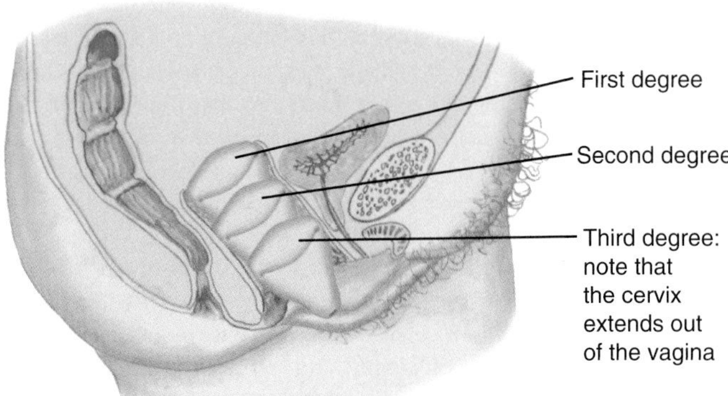


**FIG 32.6** Three degrees of uterine prolapse.

structures. Symptoms include feelings of pelvic fullness, a dragging sensation, pelvic pressure, and fatigue. Low backache and a feeling that "everything is falling out" are sometimes described.

Symptoms relate to the affected area and the level at which support has decreased. For example, urinary frequency, urgency, and incontinence often occur in women with cystocele because the support of their urethra and lower vaginal wall has decreased. Constipation, flatulence, and difficulty defecating are major symptoms of rectocele. Regardless of the structures involved, symptoms become worse after prolonged standing and are relieved by lying down. Symptoms of uterine prolapse are produced by the weight of the descending pelvic structures and include pelvic pressure, backache, and fatigue. Cervical ulceration and bleeding occur if the cervix protrudes from the vaginal introitus. Some women fear their symptoms are caused by cancer in the affected structures.

### Therapeutic Management

Treatment of disorders related to pelvic floor dysfunction depends on the woman's age, physical condition, sexual activity, and degree of prolapse. American Urological Association set some clinical guidelines in 2011 to guide management in a risk-benefit order depending on invasiveness. First-line treatments are most conservative, such as relaxation, stress management, and self-care. Second-line therapies are more invasive and have potential risk, while third- through sixth-line treatments involve progressively greater risk (Gish, 2011).

Maintaining adequate fluid intake and best pain control requires experimentation. Elimination of bladder irritants from the diet will require teaching about common irritants that the woman might eliminate or decrease. Interventions for most effective pain relief require guidance from the healthcare team and feedback from the woman.

Surgical procedures provide the most satisfactory therapy for women who have significant discomfort. The most common procedures are the anterior and posterior colporrhaphy. The anterior colporrhaphy, performed for a cystocele, involves suturing the pubocervical fascia to support the bladder and urethra. For a rectocele, a posterior colporrhaphy (suturing the fascia and perineal muscles that support the perineum and rectum) is performed. Combined procedures may be required.

Surgical treatment for prolapse of the uterus is individualized to best correct both the degree and location of uterine prolapse. An anterior and posterior colporrhaphy may be effective for a first-degree prolapse. Treatment for more severe prolapse may include vaginal hysterectomy, in which the uterus is removed through the vaginal canal rather than through an abdominal incision. Vaginal hysterectomy may be combined with anterior and posterior colporrhaphy to improve vaginal support for the bladder or rectum.

If surgery is contraindicated, a pessary (a device to support pelvic structures) may be inserted into the vagina. The pessary must be inspected and changed as needed by a physician or nurse practitioner to prevent vaginal discharge, ulceration, or infection. Teaching the woman to insert the pessary and remove it nightly reduces discharge. Topical or systemic estrogen treatment may be indicated (Gish, 2011; National Institutes of Health: National Institute of Diabetes and Digestive and Kidney Diseases [NIDDKD], 2013; Nygaard, 2008).

### Nursing Considerations

**Pelvic exercises.** Kegel exercises strengthen the pubococcygeus muscle, which surrounds the urethra, vagina, and rectum and provides partial support for the pelvic floor. Kegel exercises cannot relieve all muscle relaxation that is part of pelvic floor dysfunction. When teaching Kegel exercises, the nurse should ask the woman to contract the pubococcygeus muscle as if she were trying to pick up a marble with her vagina. The nurse should teach a woman how she should perform the Kegels as recommended but not while urinating.

Kegel exercises involve conscious contracting and relaxing of the pubococcygeus muscle. Muscles of the abdomen, thighs, and buttocks should *not* tighten. Women should be taught to exhale and keep the mouth open to avoid bearing down when contracting the pelvic muscles for at least 3 seconds, building to a maximum hold of 10 seconds, and then gradually relaxing the muscle contraction. A minimum of 10 seconds of muscle relaxation should follow the pelvic muscle contractions. The reported optimal number of repetitions varies, but 30 to 80 daily repetitions are beneficial. To maintain pubococcygeal muscle tone, the woman should continue Kegel exercises for the rest of her life (NIDDKD, 2013).

Measures that help reduce the symptoms of pelvic relaxation may prove helpful. These include lying down with the legs elevated or assuming a knee-chest position for a short time several times a day. Additional teaching includes measures to prevent constipation.

**Urinary incontinence.** Nurses must acknowledge the reluctance many women feel about discussing incontinence and help them overcome these feelings and seek medical intervention.

Women of any age may be reluctant to admit problems with urinary incontinence. Direct questions such as, "Do you have trouble with your bladder?" or "Do you ever unexpectedly lose urine?" may encourage women to discuss urine control problems.

Evaluation of the characteristics of a woman's urinary incontinence guides treatment. Three major patterns are (NIDDKD, 2013; Norton, 2008):

- *Stress incontinence,* with urine leakage occurring as the woman increases her intraabdominal pressure. Examples of situations in which intraabdominal pressure increases sufficiently include coughing, sneezing, laughing, or physical exertion such as picking up a full shopping bag or heavy load.
- *Urge incontinence,* characterized by urine leakage that accompanies a woman's strong need to void promptly.
- *Mixed incontinence,* in which a woman's urine leakage has associated factors from both the stress and urge incontinence patterns.

Overactive bladder (OAB) can occur with both urge and mixed incontinence. OAB is characterized by frequent sensations of urgency and nocturia and accompanies many neurologic, anatomic, and structural disorders.

Several evaluations may be carried out to best determine the type of urinary incontinence and choose the best corrective actions. In addition to physical examination, the woman may be asked to keep a daily record of her urinary pattern and sensations. Additional tests may include those that identify leakage patterns and specialized testing of urinary tract functions.

Continence may be enhanced by teaching health promotion activities such as Kegel exercises and bladder training. Kegel exercises are designed to improve the strength of the pelvic floor as described earlier and also to help the woman intentionally contract the pubococcygeus muscles to control urine leaking. Bladder training helps the woman decrease the frequency of urination during waking and sleeping hours. Women may benefit from biofeedback, electrical stimulation, or physical therapy. Surgery may be necessary to reposition or stabilize the bladder neck and proximal urethra (NIDDKD, 2013; Nager & Kane, 2008).

Women often benefit from knowing about some of the commercial products that protect the skin and prevent odor. These products are made of material that traps urine and prevents constant contact with the skin.

Women often restrict fluids, believing that this will decrease urinary incontinence. Restricting fluids may actually make the condition worse because the bladder does not fill to its normal capacity. Furthermore, decreased fluid intake can lead to highly concentrated urine that irritates bladder mucous membranes and increase the urge to void. Alcohol and caffeine can irritate the bladder and worsen incontinence.

Obesity is associated with urinary incontinence, increasing the benefits for a woman to achieve her ideal weight range.

Drug treatment can enhance bladder control. Drugs that may be prescribed include (Amir & Bent, 2008):

- Vaginal estrogen administered as a cream, tablet, or vaginal ring to reduce atrophy of the urinary and vaginal areas.
- Anticholinergic drugs, including their long-acting versions, such as oxybutynin or tolterodine.
- Research continues to identify drugs that improve bladder control.

## DISORDERS OF THE REPRODUCTIVE TRACT

### Benign Disorders

The most common benign conditions of the reproductive tract include cervical polyps, uterine leiomyomas (fibroids), and ovarian cysts.

#### Cervical Polyps

Polyps are small tumors, usually only a few millimeters in diameter, that are usually on a pedicle (a stem-like structure). They are caused by proliferation of the cervical mucosa and often cause intermittent vaginal bleeding.

Cervical polyps are surgically removed in an outpatient setting, and the specimen is sent for pathologic examination to rule out malignancy. Endometrial polyps are found in some women with abnormal uterine bleeding.

#### Uterine Leiomyomas

Uterine leiomyomas (fibroids) are the most common gynecologic tumors. Although the cause is unknown, uterine fibroids develop from smooth muscle cells and are estrogen dependent. As a result, they grow rapidly during the childbearing years and may be very apparent when the uterus is palpated during late pregnancy. During menopause, they begin to atrophy, although estrogen replacement therapy can cause the benign tumors to persist. Fibroids can occur throughout the muscular layer of the uterus and can have different forms. Fibroids near the endometrium are more often associated with heavy menstrual bleeding than are those in outer levels of the uterus.

Uterine fibroids usually produce no symptoms, but increased uterine size, pelvic pain, or excessive menstrual bleeding may occur. Excessive bleeding can result in anemia, weakness, and fatigue. Additional symptoms include feelings of pelvic pressure, bloating, and urinary frequency that occurs when the tumor applies pressure on the bladder.

Treatment depends on multiple factors, including the size, number, and location of the fibroids, the symptoms experienced, whether future childbearing is desired, and how near the woman is to natural menopause. In the absence of symptoms, treatment may involve observation only. If abnormal bleeding is a problem, surgical intervention might be necessary. Hysterectomy may be appropriate for the woman who does not want to become pregnant. Myomectomy, or removal of the fibroid from uterine muscle, is an option for the woman who wants children in the future. Uterine artery embolization (UAE) is a procedure done under fluoroscopic guidance in the interventional radiology department that focuses on reducing the fibroid size by obstructing the arteries that supply the fibroid. The woman may want to retain childbearing potential, but amenorrhea can occur despite functional ovaries. Pregnancy after UAE is more likely to involve intrauterine growth restriction or preterm birth (Goldstein, 2008; Haney, 2008).

Medical treatment with progesterone-only or estrogen–progesterone oral contraceptives can reduce heavy menstrual flow. Short courses of GnRH agonists can decrease the size of myomas and lessen symptoms before surgical removal of the tumor. However, GnRH agonists induce menopausal changes that many women find less tolerable, and prolonged use of the drug can decrease bone density. Mifepristone (RU-486) is being studied as a drug to reduce fibroid size without loss of bone density.

### Ovarian Cysts

Ovarian cysts are either follicular or luteal. A follicular cyst can develop if the ovarian follicle fails to rupture during ovulation. These cysts are usually asymptomatic, and they usually regress during the next menstrual cycle. A lutein cyst can develop if the corpus luteum becomes cystic and fails to regress. A lutein cyst is more likely to cause pain and some delay in the next menstrual cycle. Occasionally, an ovarian cyst ruptures or twists on its pedicle and becomes infarcted, causing pelvic pain and tenderness.

Treatment depends on differentiating a cyst from a solid ovarian tumor. If the woman is in her childbearing years, when the risk of ovarian cancer is less, the physician may wait until after the next menstrual cycle and examine the woman again. Transvaginal ultrasound examination is useful to determine if it is a fluid-filled cyst or a solid tumor. Laparoscopy (insertion of illuminated tube into abdomen to see contents, locate bleeding, and perform surgical procedures) or laparotomy (incision through abdominal wall to examine organs) can be performed to remove the cyst from the ovary for examination by a pathologist.

**SAFETY ALERT**

***Signs and Symptoms That Should Always Be Investigated***

- Irregular vaginal bleeding
- Unexplained postmenopausal bleeding
- Unusual vaginal discharge
- Dyspareunia
- Persistent vulvar or vaginal itching
- Elevated or discolored lesions of the vulva
- Persistent abdominal bloating or constipation
- Persistent anorexia or vomiting
- Blood in stools

## Malignant Disorders

The primary sites for cancer in the female reproductive organs are the cervix, uterus, and ovaries. Although cancer can occur at any age, the incidence increases with age. Risk factors associated with cancer of the reproductive area are summarized in Box 32.5.

### Manifestations

Cancer of the reproductive organs may not be diagnosed until it is advanced because few symptoms are experienced in the early stages. When symptoms occur, they are often nonspecific and could be caused by other conditions. Cancer of the ovaries is particularly difficult to diagnose early because the condition may remain "silent" until far advanced, when the chance of long-term survival is reduced.

### Diagnostic Evaluation

A variety of screening and diagnostic procedures are useful for early detection, which improves long-term survival among women with a reproductive cancer. Screening tests include periodic pelvic examinations, Pap tests, and ultrasonography. Serum tests for tumor markers such as CA-125 determine whether ovarian or other cancers have spread beyond their primary site. Women carrying genes such as *BRCA1* and *BRCA2* (see p. 694) that are linked to other cancers may undergo more diagnostic procedures than those without this genetic risk. Specific strains of the HPV are a risk factor for cervical cancer, even if the original infection has healed. Diagnostic procedures include

**BOX 32.5 Risk Factors for Cancer of the Reproductive Organs**

**Uterus**

- Blacks: higher risk for leiomyosarcoma
- Obesity
- Nulliparity
- Middle-aged and older adults
- Late menopause (>52 years)
- Diabetes mellitus
- Breast, colon, or ovarian cancer
- Estrogen replacement therapy

**Cervix**

- Human papillomavirus (HPV) infection
- Sexual risks: young age at start of intercourse (<20 years), multiple sexual partners, uncircumcised male partners
- Many pregnancies
- Obesity
- Diet low in fruits and vegetables
- Smoking
- Lower socioeconomic status (may be related to infrequent gynecologic examinations)
- History of STDs, such as chlamydia or HIV infection

**Ovaries**

- Menses started at <12 years
- No child or first child after 30 years of age
- Late menopause (>55 years)
- Infertility; infertility drugs
- Family history of ovarian, breast, or colorectal cancer
- Personal history of breast cancer

*HIV*, Human immunodeficiency virus; *STDs*, Sexually transmitted diseases

endometrial sampling and colposcopy (examination of vaginal and cervical tissue with a colposcope to magnify cells), which can identify patterns of abnormality near the cervical os, where most cancers of the cervix develop.

### Therapeutic Management

Treatment of cervical, endometrial, and ovarian cancer is based on the location and extent of the disease and the woman's desire to bear more children. The extent of surgical treatment for these cancers varies with the tumor's size, degree of malignancy, and spread beyond the primary site of the tumor. Chemotherapy and radiation oncology therapy supplement treatment for many invasive cancers. Drugs such as anastrozole (Arimidex) and exemestane (Aromasin), aromatase inhibitors, reduce estrogen secretion that increases cancer growth in most breast and reproductive organs.

***Cervical cancer.*** A lesion of early cervical cancer is usually SIL. HPV is associated with most cervical cancers. Early treatment of cervical cancer often involves cryosurgery, destruction of abnormal tissue by laser, loop electrosurgical excision procedure (LEEP), or surgical conization to remove the central cervix. Regular surveillance following cervical cancer therapy is recommended to identify recurrence, particularly in the woman who had an HSIL because her risk for repeated cervical cancer is greater.

Treatment for advanced cervical cancer usually consists of a total abdominal hysterectomy as well as bilateral salpingo-oophorectomy. Removal of the uterus and ovaries and SLN biopsy can be achieved laparoscopically. Adjuvant therapy with radiation and chemotherapy is likely (ACS, 2014d; Giuntoli & Bristow, 2008; McCormish, 2011).

***Endometrial cancer.*** Endometrial cancer is the fourth most common cancer in women following lung, breast, and colon cancers. Abnormal vaginal bleeding near or after menopause is the primary symptom. Spread into the deeper uterine tissues and to tissue outside the uterus can occur. Older women are likely to have a higher grade of malignancy than younger women. The highest cure rate is with surgery (hysterectomy and salpingo-oophorectomy), but poor surgical candidates can be treated using chemotherapy or radiation therapy (ACS, 2014d; Mutch, 2008).

***Ovarian cancer.*** Surgery involving removal of the healthy ovary as well as the affected ovary is an essential part of therapy and can be curative for women in the earliest stages of ovarian cancer. Surgery for more advanced ovarian cancer improves diagnostic information, allows more accurate staging, and permits surgical reduction of the cancer. Chemotherapy is required after surgery for all but the very early cancers. The 5-year survival rate varies with the stage at diagnosis and response to chemotherapy (ACS, 2014a; Cass & Karlan, 2008).

## INFECTIOUS DISORDERS OF THE REPRODUCTIVE TRACT

### Candidiasis

Candidiasis, also known as *moniliasis* and *yeast infection,* is the most common form of vaginitis. Changes in the vaginal pH allow accelerated growth of *Candida albicans,* a yeast-like fungus commonly found in the digestive tract and on the skin. Some conditions, such as pregnancy, diabetes mellitus, oral contraceptive use, and systemic antibiotic therapy cause changes in the vaginal pH and flora that favor accelerated growth of *C. albicans*. Although not considered an STD, recurrent candidiasis in sexually active women can occur. A small number of exposed male partners develop erythema and itching of the glans penis (balanitis).

The main symptoms of candidiasis are vaginal and perineal itching. Vulvar and vaginal tissues are inflamed, causing burning on urination. Vaginal discharge is white with a typical "cottage cheese" appearance. Diagnosis is made by identifying the spores of *C. albicans.*

Treatment involves nonprescription or prescription medications. Medications available without prescription include butoconazole, miconazole, clotrimazole, terconazole, and tioconazole by vaginal application. The duration for most of the nonprescription medications for candidiasis ranges from 3 to 7 days, depending on the specific medication. Women should be advised to seek medical attention with the first infection or if the infection persists or recurs frequently. Prescription vaginal medications include nystatin and higher doses of butoconazole and terconazole. Oral fluconazole is a prescription medication for candidiasis. Recurrent yeast infections that resist treatment are associated with diabetes mellitus and HIV infection.

### Sexually Transmitted Diseases (STDs)

STDs, also called *sexually transmitted infections,* are transmitted through sexual activity. For some diseases, such as gonorrhea and chlamydial infection, sexual activity is almost the only method of transmission. For other diseases, such as bacterial vaginosis, sexual activity may or may not be the mode of transmission. A woman can have more than one STD at a time. Recommended regimens for treatment are listed here, but alternative regimens are listed in the *Sexually Transmitted Diseases Treatment Guidelines, 2010,* available at http://www.cdc.gov. Updates to treatment recommendations appear on the same website. Treatment is varied for infection sites other than the reproductive tract.

#### Incidence

STDs are most frequent among adolescents and young adults. Because the vagina and microscopic tears in mucosa from intercourse provide favorable conditions for infection, women are twice as likely as men to contract an STD (CDC, 2015c; Eschenbach, 2008).

Methods of contraception have a significant effect on the risk for STDs. The best protection is the use of condoms. Barrier methods, such as the diaphragm and cervical cap, are less effective than the condom in preventing STDs, but they provide some protection for the upper genital tract. Other methods can prevent pregnancy but do not prevent exposure to STDs.

Major concerns include:

- The vulnerability of women to STDs
- The resistance of some organisms to antibiotics
- The relationship between HIV infection and other STDs
- Failure of asymptomatic people to seek treatment when their sexual partner is infected

See Chapter 26 for the effect of some STDs on pregnancy and the fetus.

### Types of Sexually Transmitted Diseases (STDs)

#### Trichomoniasis

Trichomoniasis is caused by *Trichomonas vaginalis,* a protozoon that thrives in an alkaline environment. The presenting symptoms include a purulent vaginal discharge that is thin or frothy, malodorous, and yellow-green or brownish gray. The pH of the vaginal discharge is usually greater than 4.5, higher than the normal acidic pH of the vagina (3.8 to 4.5). Vulvar itching, edema, and redness may be present. The diagnosis is made by identifying the organism in a wet-mount preparation.

Treatments of choice are metronidazole (Flagyl) (2 g) or tinidazole (Tindamax) (2 g) in a single oral dose. Alcohol ingestion when taking metronidazole can result in a disulfiram-like (Antabuse) reaction. Women should be advised to avoid using alcohol during treatment and for 24 hours (metronidazole) or 72 hours (tinidazole) after treatment is complete.

Sexual partners should refrain from intercourse until a cure is established. Reinfection can result if the woman's partner is not treated. In particular, emphasize that all sexual partners should be treated and that condoms should be used with a new partner.

### Bacterial Vaginosis

This infection, previously referred to as *nonspecific vaginitis,* is associated with organisms that replace normal lactobacilli with *Gardnerella vaginalis* or *Mycoplasma hominis* or with anaerobic bacteria, such as *Prevotella, Mobiluncus, Ureaplasma,* or *Mycoplasma.* Causes of the bacterial proliferation are not known, although tissue trauma and vaginal intercourse have been identified as contributing factors. Multiple partners, douching, and lack of vaginal lactobacilli are associated with bacterial vaginosis.

Chief signs and symptoms are a thin, grayish white vaginal discharge that typically exudes a fishy odor. The diagnosis is made by preparing a saline wet mount and identifying characteristic clue cells (epithelial cells with numerous bacilli clinging to their surface).

Treatment with metronidazole or clindamycin is directed toward reestablishing the balance of flora in the vagina. The woman should refrain from sexual intercourse until cured, or her partner should use a condom. Treatment of her male partner has not been shown to be beneficial (CDC, 2015c).

### Chlamydial Infection

The incidence of infection by the gram-negative bacterium *Chlamydia trachomatis* is particularly high in the sexually active teen and young adult populations. Chlamydial infection is often asymptomatic in men and women, which makes diagnosis and control of the disease difficult. The woman exhibits symptoms similar to those of gonorrhea, such as a yellowish vaginal discharge and painful urination. Gonorrhea and chlamydial infections often coexist.

Left untreated, chlamydial infection ascends from the cervix to involve the fallopian tubes and is one of the chief causes of tubal scarring that results in PID, infertility, or ectopic pregnancy. Treatment is usually directed to eradicate both chlamydia and gonorrhea. Treatment options include azithromycin or doxycycline. Ofloxacin, levofloxacin, or erythromycin is also commonly ordered. Treatment of all sexual partners is essential to prevent recurrence and further spread. Use of condoms until a cure is established is essential as well. A test for cure may be done, particularly if there is doubt about whether a woman would take the ordered treatment.

### Gonorrhea

Gonorrhea is an infection of the genitourinary tract that is caused by the gonococcus *Neisseria gonorrhoeae.* Gonorrhea is often asymptomatic in women, but symptoms that do occur include purulent discharge, dysuria (pain with urination), and painful intercourse. Diagnosis is based on a positive culture for the gonococcus. As with chlamydia, gonorrhea is associated with PID, which increases the risk of tubal scarring and can result in infertility or ectopic pregnancy.

Dual treatment of gonorrhea and chlamydia infections is recommended. Drugs in addition to those previously discussed for chlamydia with gonorrhea infections include ceftriaxone (250 mg) intramuscularly in a single dose or cefixime (400 mg) in a single oral dose or other single-dose injectable cephalosporins. All sexual partners should be treated simultaneously, and intercourse should be avoided or the man should use a condom until a cure is confirmed.

### Syphilis

Syphilis, caused by the spirochete *Treponema pallidum,* is divided into primary, secondary, and tertiary stages. The first sign of primary

## WOMEN WANT TO KNOW

### *Sexually Transmitted Diseases*

**What Are the Most Common Symptoms of Sexually Transmitted Diseases (STDs)?**

- Unexpected, nonbloody vaginal discharge (increased amount, unusual color, or odor) or vaginal bleeding
- Vulvar itching or swelling
- Pelvic pain, including painful intercourse, painful urination, and abdominal tenderness
- Skin eruptions or changes (rashes, ulcers, warts, blisters)
- Flu-like symptoms (fever, swollen or painful lymph glands, loss of appetite, nausea or vomiting)
- Presence of symptoms in a sexual partner, even if symptoms are absent in the woman

**What Are Common Methods of Diagnosis?**

- Culture (vaginal discharge, cervix, lesions) to identify organism; often combined with sensitivity to determine best medication therapy
- Blood test (serology) to determine if antibodies for specific diseases are present
- VDRL, RPR, or FTA-ABS test for syphilis, test for human immunodeficiency virus (HIV)
- Genetic tests from blood samples, such as visualization of chromosomes, analysis to identify abnormal sequences in genes or abnormal levels of genes associated with a specific disorder

**How Can STDs Be Prevented?**

- Limit number of sexual partners.
- Establish monogamous relationship with uninfected partner.
- Use mechanical and chemical barriers, such as a latex condom, with every act of intercourse.
- Remember that one episode of an STD offers no protection from future infection.
- Make sure partner is simultaneously treated to prevent reinfection.

**What Are the Most Important Things to Know About the Treatment?**

- The entire course of medication must be completed even if symptoms subside.
- Comply with follow-up care as the healthcare provider recommends.
- Sexual intercourse should be avoided until free of active infection.
- Partner should be examined, treated, and a follow-up evaluation performed before sexual intercourse is resumed.
- Side effects of medications, such as skin rashes, difficulty breathing, or headaches, should be reported.
- Not all STDs can be cured (herpes, HIV/AIDS, human papillomavirus), and treatment is aimed at slowing the disease and preventing complications.

**Are There Measures That Provide Comfort and Prevent Secondary Infections?**

- Keep the vulva clean but avoid strong soaps, creams, and ointments unless prescribed by healthcare provider.
- Keep the vulva dry. A hair dryer turned on low may help.
- Wear absorbent cotton underwear and avoid pantyhose and tight pants.
- Take analgesics (e.g., ibuprofen or acetaminophen) as directed by healthcare provider.
- Cool or tepid sitz baths may provide relief from itching.
- Wipe vulva from front to back after urination or defecation and then carefully wash hands.

*AIDS,* Acquired immunodeficiency syndrome; *FTA-ABS,* fluorescent treponemal antibody absorption; *RPR,* rapid plasma reagin; *VDRL,* Venereal Disease Research Laboratory

syphilis is a painless chancre that develops on the genitalia, anus, or lips or in the oral cavity. At this time, diagnosis is made by identifying the spirochete on dark-field microscopy in material scraped from the base of the chancre. A serologic test is generally negative in the primary stage. If untreated, the chancre heals in approximately 6 weeks. The disease is highly infectious during the primary stage.

Although the chancre disappears, the spirochete lives and is carried by the blood to all parts of the body. Approximately 2 months after the initial infection, infected people exhibit symptoms of secondary syphilis, including enlargement of the spleen and liver, headache, anorexia, and a generalized maculopapular skin rash. Skin eruptions, called *condylomata lata,* develop on the vulva during this time. Condylomata lata resemble warts; they contain numerous spirochetes and are highly contagious. Serologic tests are generally positive at this time.

If untreated, the disease enters a latent phase that can last for several years. Tertiary syphilis, which follows the latent phase, can involve the heart, blood vessels, and central nervous system. General paralysis and psychosis may result.

In addition to identification of the spirochete in material scraped from a chancre, diagnosis is also made by serology. The usual screening test is the Venereal Disease Research Laboratory (VDRL) serum test, which is based on the detection of antibodies produced in response to the infection. The rapid plasma reagin (RPR) and fluorescent treponemal antibody absorption (FTA-ABS) tests are more specific and are commonly performed to confirm a positive VDRL.

The best treatment for all stages of syphilis is with parenteral penicillin G. Ceftriaxone and doxycycline are second options for people who cannot take penicillin. Tetracycline can be given to women who are not pregnant. A woman who is allergic to penicillin can be admitted to the hospital for desensitization to penicillin and followed by administration of the drug.

### Herpes Genitalis

Herpes genitalis is an STD caused by the herpes simplex virus (HSV). Two types of HSV have been identified: type 1 and type 2. HSV 2 usually causes genital lesions, and HSV 1 usually causes oral-pharyngeal infection. However, either organism can infect the less-frequent location. Transmission occurs through direct contact with an infected person; the infected partner often is not yet aware of the infection. Diagnostic tests to detect either HSV antigen are most accurate before HSV lesions begin healing. Some diagnostics distinguish between HSV 1 and HSV 2, whereas others are less specific.

Within 2 to 12 days after the primary infection, vesicles (blisters) appear in a characteristic cluster on the vulva, perineum, or perianal area. The lesions of the primary infection cause severe vulvar pain and tenderness as well as dyspareunia. Lesions can also occur on the cervix or in the vagina. With primary infection, the woman may also experience flu-like symptoms, including fever, general malaise, and enlarged lymph nodes. The vesicles rupture within 1 to 7 days and form ulcers that take an average of 7 to 10 days to heal.

When symptoms abate, the virus remains dormant in the nerve ganglia and periodically reactivates, particularly in times of stress, fever, and menses. Recurrent episodes are seldom as extensive or painful as the initial episode, but they are just as contagious. Diagnosis is often based on clinical signs and symptoms and confirmed by viral culture of fluid from the vesicle. No cure is available, but the antiviral drugs acyclovir, famciclovir, and valacyclovir help reduce or suppress symptoms, shedding, and recurrent episodes. Women should be advised to abstain from sexual contact while lesions are present. For an initial infection, they should continue to abstain until they become culture-negative, because prolonged viral shedding can occur in such cases.

### Human Papillomavirus (HPV)

Condylomata acuminata, also known as *venereal* or *genital warts,* are caused by human papillomavirus, or HPV. The dry, wart-like growths may be small, discrete, and asymptomatic, or they may cluster and resemble cauliflower. Common sites include the vagina, labia, cervix, and perineal area.

Condylomata acuminata are of particular concern because of the association of HPV with cervical cancer. Colposcopy is usually done to evaluate abnormal cervical tissue and detect HPV. Women with HPV are advised to have Pap tests more frequently to detect cervical dysplasia (abnormal tissue development).

The goal of treatment is to remove the warts, which easily transmit the virus back and forth between sexual partners. Topical treatments applied to the warts by the woman include podofilox solution or gel, imiquimod cream, and sinecatechins ointment. Treatments by the healthcare provider may include application of podophyllin gel, trichloroacetic acid (TCA), or bichloracetic acid (BCA) to warts. More extensive warts or those that do not respond to topical therapy may require removal by cryotherapy (tissue destruction by extreme cold), electrodesiccation, electrocautery, or laser. Interferon, an antineoplastic drug, is sometimes used to treat condylomata acuminata in women older than 18 years who have not responded to conventional therapy.

The woman must understand that none of these treatments eradicates the virus and that she may have recurrences. Furthermore, all sexual partners must be treated. Sexual contact should be avoided until all lesions are healed, and condom use is recommended to reduce transmission.

Two vaccines are now available, a bivalent vaccine (Cervarix) against types 16 and 18, which cause 70% of cervical cancers, and a quadrivalent vaccine (Gardasil) against types 6, 11, 16, and 18 to also protect against 90% of genital warts caused by HPV. The vaccine is not as effective if a female has been exposed to one of the four types, and testing is not available to know of previous exposure. The CDC currently recommends immunizing males and females aged 9 to 26 years using a total of three doses (CDC, 2015a). Current cost to the private sector is $130 per injection. Health insurance or governmental health programs may cover the cost. Current costs for both pediatric and adult vaccines can be found at http://www.cdc.gov/vaccines/programs/vfc. VFC refers to the Vaccines for Children site, but adult vaccines are also listed. Costs in the list do not reflect the cost of administration in a medical office or clinic.

### Acquired Immunodeficiency Syndrome

Acquired immunodeficiency syndrome (AIDS), caused by HIV, remains the most devastating STD in the world today, although new treatments have improved the outlook considerably. HIV has been isolated from blood, semen, vaginal secretions, urine, saliva, tears, cerebrospinal fluid, amniotic fluid, and breast milk. The primary modes of transmission are intimate contact with infected bodily secretions, exposure to infected blood and blood products, and perinatal transmission from mother to infant.

HIV testing is routine for all pregnant women so treatment can be started if needed, possibly avoiding transmission to the fetus. A woman's risk for infection through a heterosexual relationship has surpassed the risk that her HIV infection stems from injectable drug use. Diagnosis of another STD is an indication for HIV testing, as is repeated infections such as herpesvirus or candidiasis. The healthcare provider should address concerns if a pregnant woman refuses testing or if she refuses retesting with subsequent pregnancies because the first test was negative. Consent for HIV testing should be incorporated into the plan of care (verbally or written). Patients also have the right to decline or "opt-out" of routine HIV testing. Assent is inferred unless the patient verbally declines testing (CDC, 2015c; ACOG, 2015).

No medications have been shown to cure HIV and AIDS. Research continues to investigate the benefits and safety of drug regimens that interrupt production of the virus. See Chapters 26 and 30 for a discussion of HIV and AIDS management in pregnant women and neonates. Updated guidelines for HIV and AIDS treatment in the pediatric, adult, and perinatal groups can be found at the AIDS Info website, a service of the National Institutes of Health: http://www.aidsinfo.nih.gov/guidelines.

### Nursing Considerations

In their role as teachers and counselors, nurses can play a major part in preventing the spread of STDs and in treating specific infections. For best patient care, nurses must:

- Teach the signs and symptoms that require medical attention.
- Explain diagnostic or screening tests and follow-up testing that may be needed.
- Teach treatment, follow-up care, and preventive measures for specific infection(s).

## Pelvic Inflammatory Disease (PID)

Pelvic inflammatory disease (PID), infection of the upper genital tract that can cause chronic pelvic pain, is a serious health problem in the United States. Acute PID occurs in 750,000 women each year, and 10% to 15% of these sexually active women have additional complications such as infertility and ectopic pregnancy. Approximately 15% to 25% of these women are likely to have chronic pelvic pain (CDC, 2015e; Sharp, 2008). Some are asymptomatic.

### Etiology and Pathophysiology

The primary sources of infection are *C. trachomatis* and *N. gonorrhoeae*. These sexually transmitted organisms invade the endocervical canal and cause cervicitis. Bacteria ascend and infect the endometrium, fallopian tubes, and pelvic cavity. The chronic inflammatory response results in extensive tubal scarring and peritubal adhesions that interfere with conception and transport of the fertilized ovum through the obstructed fallopian tubes. Cytomegalovirus (CMV) and a number of common vaginal organisms, such as *G. vaginalis*, also may be found in women with PID. Because the narrow fallopian tubes are often infected, a woman's risks for ectopic pregnancy or infertility increase.

### Manifestations

Some women with PID are asymptomatic or have subtle, mild symptoms. Others experience pelvic pain, fever, purulent vaginal discharge, nausea, anorexia, and irregular vaginal bleeding. Findings during physical examination may include abdominal or adnexal tenderness (accessory organs to the uterus such as fallopian tubes and ovaries) and pain of the uterus and cervix when moved during bimanual examination (cervical motion tenderness). Laboratory evaluation may reveal marked leukocytosis and an increased sedimentation rate. Urinalysis is needed to rule out urinary tract infection. Cultures for *N. gonorrhoeae, C. trachomatis,* or other suspected infectious organisms help diagnose and best treat PID. HIV testing is often done.

### Therapeutic Management

Women with serious infection, as manifested by fever, abdominal pain, and leukocytosis, may be admitted to a hospital. They are treated initially with IV combinations of antibiotics such as cefoxitin, cefotetan plus doxycycline, or clindamycin plus gentamicin. IV antibiotic treatment can be changed to oral treatment 24 hours after improvement, and the total duration of antibiotic therapy should be 14 days. Surgery may be needed for women who have a pelvic abscess or other persistent problems. Outpatient treatment is appropriate for many women who are able to comply with the recommended regimen (CDC, 2015c).

### Nursing Considerations

Nurses can play an important role in preventing PID by teaching women how to prevent STDs. Primary prevention involves avoiding exposure to these diseases or preventing infection during exposure. Measures include limiting the number of sexual partners and avoiding intercourse with those who have had multiple partners. Barrier methods (such as latex condoms) used consistently and correctly during all sexual activity reduce some STDs.

Secondary prevention for PID involves preventing a lower genital tract infection from ascending to the upper genital tract. Nurses should advise women to seek medical attention promptly after having unprotected sex with someone suspected of having an STD and when unusual vaginal discharge or genital lesions are apparent. Additional measures include taking medication as prescribed and returning for follow-up evaluation. Periodic medical evaluations may be recommended for a woman who is asymptomatic yet engages in sexual activity that increases risk.

## Toxic Shock Syndrome

Although toxic shock syndrome (TSS) is rare, it is a potentially fatal condition caused by toxin-producing strains of *Staphylococcus aureus*. The toxin alters capillary permeability, which allows intravascular fluid to leak from the blood vessels, leading to hypovolemia, hypotension, and shock. The toxin also causes direct tissue damage to organs and precipitates serious defects in coagulation. *S. aureus* is infrequently carried in the vagina, and only approximately 2% of women have the strain that can produce the toxin that causes TSS.

If toxin-producing strains of *S. aureus* inhabit the vagina, certain factors increase the risk that the toxin will gain entry into the bloodstream. Use of tampons or barrier contraceptives for a prolonged time can trap and hold bacteria that can multiply. Individuals having had nasal surgery or previous *S. aureus* wound infections also have a greater risk.

Signs and symptoms of TSS include a sudden spiking fever (38.9° C [102° F]) and flu-like symptoms (headache, sore throat, vomiting, diarrhea), hypotension, a generalized rash resembling sunburn, and skin peeling from the palms of the hands and the soles of the feet 1 to 2 weeks after the onset of the illness.

Vaginal and site-specific cultures are needed to determine the best therapy. General treatment consists of fluid replacement, administration of vasopressor drugs, and antimicrobial therapy. Corticosteroids can be used to treat skin changes. The case mortality rate has decreased with therapy but remains at 3% (CDC, 2012; Eschenbach, 2008).

### Nursing Considerations

Nurses are often responsible for providing information that may help prevent TSS and should instruct all women to do the following:

- For tampon use:
  - Wash the hands thoroughly to remove bacteria before inserting tampons.
  - Change tampons at least every 4 hours to prevent excessive bacterial growth on the tampon.
  - Do not use superabsorbent tampons at any time because they may be left in the vagina for a prolonged period, allowing bacteria to proliferate.

- Use pads rather than tampons during hours of sleep, which usually exceed the 4-hour segments of tampon use.
- For diaphragm use:
  - Wash the hands thoroughly before inserting the diaphragm.
  - Do not use a diaphragm during menstrual periods.
  - Remove the diaphragm within the time recommended by the healthcare provider.
  - For the woman with a history of TSS, reinforce warnings about recurrent episodes and that she should not use tampons.

## KEY CONCEPTS

- *Health maintenance* refers to examinations and screening procedures that allow early detection of specific conditions, such as breast or cervical cancer, and allow for prompt treatment that increases the chance of long-term survival.
- A major role of nurses is to explain screening procedures and to encourage women to have them on a regular basis. The most common screening procedures include breast self-examination, clinical breast examination, mammography, and often ultrasound examinations for breast cancer; vulvar self-examination to detect precancerous conditions or infections; pelvic examination to detect abnormalities of the uterus or ovaries; Pap test for cervical cancer; and screening for fecal occult blood.
- Disorders of the breast may be benign, such as fibrocystic changes that occur in relation to the menstrual cycle, or malignant. The discovery of any breast disorder creates anxiety in women, and nurses must be prepared to explain diagnostic procedures.
- Breast cancer develops in one in eight women in the United States. Besides sex, the greatest risk factors are advancing age and previous history of breast cancer. Additional factors include family history of breast cancer; specific genetic abnormalities; and previous uterine, ovarian, or colon cancer.
- Management of breast cancer includes surgical removal of the tumor plus varying amounts of surrounding tissue and lymph nodes. Adjuvant therapy includes radiation, chemotherapy, and drugs such as hormonal therapy or immunotherapy that block factors that promote growth of cancer cells.
- Breast reconstruction is an integral part of the surgical options related to breast cancer. Reconstruction methods include tissue expansion procedures, in which fluid-filled prostheses are placed, and tissue flap procedures, in which the woman's own tissue is used to create a graft for a new breast. Some women receive a combination of tissue expansion and tissue flap procedures for best reconstruction.
- Nursing care for women with cancer of the breast focuses on providing emotional support and accurate information.
- Cardiovascular disease is the leading cause of death in both women and men in the United States. Almost twice as many American women die of heart disease and stroke as from all forms of cancer, including breast cancer. Preventive measures that can be modified include control of weight, glucose, and hypertension, smoking cessation, becoming more active, and for many women, daily low-dose aspirin.
- Menstrual cycle disorders include amenorrhea, abnormal uterine bleeding, cyclic pelvic pain, and premenstrual syndrome (PMS). Some of the disorders, such as PMS, respond to lifestyle alterations such as changes in diet, exercise habits, and stress management.
- Elective termination of pregnancy can be performed by medical or surgical methods. Elective termination of pregnancy is associated with social and ethical conflicts.
- The *climacteric,* the time that precedes the final menstrual period that denotes menopause, is a combination of endocrine, somatic, and psychic changes that occur at the end of the reproductive cycle. A state of estrogen deficit accelerates during the climacteric and can result in bone loss (osteoporosis).
- Hormone replacement therapy may be prescribed to manage the symptoms of estrogen deficit, such as hot flashes and atrophic vaginitis, and to decrease osteoporosis. However, adverse effects of estrogen-progesterone therapy have been found to include a greater risk for cardiovascular disease and breast and uterine cancers. For women who decline or should not take hormone replacement, including estrogen-only medications, alternative measures are needed to control the symptoms of menopause.
- Relaxation of pelvic support structures, often occurring because of childbirth trauma, becomes troublesome as the woman ages and her falling estrogen levels cause genital atrophy.
- Benign disorders of the reproductive tract include cervical polyps, uterine leiomyomas (fibroids), and ovarian cysts. Malignant disorders include cancer of the cervix, uterus, and ovaries.
- Although some infections of the reproductive tract are related to a change in the pH or the flora of the vagina, such as candidiasis, many are transmitted by sexual contact.
- Pelvic inflammatory disease (PID) is often a complication of STDs, particularly chlamydial infection or gonorrhea. It can result in infertility or ectopic pregnancy because the fallopian tubes become scarred by inflammation during the infection.
- Toxic shock syndrome (TSS) is a life-threatening condition resulting from infection with toxin-producing strains of *S. aureus.* The infection is related to the use of high-absorbency tampons, cervical caps, and diaphragms that trap and hold bacteria in nutrient-rich menstrual blood for an extended time.

## REFERENCES AND READINGS


American Cancer Society. (2009). *Breast reconstruction after mastectomy*. Retrieved from http://www.cancer.org.

American Cancer Society. (2010). *Cervical cancer: Prevention and early detection*. Retrieved from http://www.cancer.org.

American Cancer Society. (2014a). *Ovarian cancer*. Retrieved from http://www.cancer.org.

American Cancer Society. (2014b). *Breast cancer: Early detection*. Retrieved from http://www.cancer.org.

American Cancer Society. (2014c). *Detailed guide: Breast cancer in men*. Retrieved from http://www.cancer.org.

American Cancer Society. (2014d). *Detailed guide: Cervical cancer*. Retrieved from http://www.cancer.org.

American Cancer Society. (2014e). *Endometrial (uterine) cancer*. Retrieved from http://www.cancer.org.

American Cancer Society. (2014f). *Non-cancerous breast conditions*. Retrieved from http://www.cancer.org.

American Cancer Society. (2014g). *Vulvar cancer*. Retrieved from http://www.cancer.org.

American College of Obstetricians and Gynecologists. (2009). *Misoprostol for postabortion care, Committee Opinion No. 427.* Washington, DC: Author.

American College of Obstetricians and Gynecologists. (2010). *Premenstrual syndrome (ACOG Practice Bulletin No. 15).* Washington, DC: Author.

American College of Obstetricians and Gynecologists. (Reaffirmed 2013). *Prevention of deep vein thrombosis and pulmonary embolism (ACOG Practice Bulletin No. 84).* Washington, DC: Author.

American College of Obstetricians and Gynecologists. (Reaffirmed 2014a). *Management of endometriosis (ACOG Practice Bulletin No. 114).* Washington, DC: Author.

American College of Obstetricians and Gynecologists. (Reaffirmed 2014b). *Osteoporosis. (ACOG Practice Bulletin No. 129).* Washington, DC: Author.

American College of Obstetricians and Gynecologists. (2014c). *Management of menopausal symptoms (ACOG Practice Bulletin No. 141).* Washington, DC: Author.

American College of Obstetricians and Gynecologists. (2014d). *Colonoscopy and colorectal cancer screening strategies. (ACOG Committee Opinion No. 609).* Washington, DC: Author.

American College of Obstetricians and Gynecologists. (Reaffirmed 2015). *Human immunodeficiency virus (ACOG Committee Opinion No. 389).* Washington, DC: Author.

American Heart Association. (2011). *What your cholesterol levels mean.* Retrieved from http://www.heart.org.

Amir, B., & Bent, A. (2008). Nonsurgical management of urinary incontinence and overactive bladder. In R.S. Gibbs, B.Y. Karlan, & A.F. Haney (Eds.), *Danforth's obstetrics and gynecology* (10th ed., pp. 890–899). Philadelphia: Lippincott Williams & Wilkins.

Archer, D.F. (2014). Commentary on 'menopausal hormone treatment in postmenopausal women: risks and benefits'. *Southern Medical Journal, 107*(11), 696–697 2p. doi:10.14423/SMJ.0000000000000191.

Carne, K. (2015). Osteoporosis and fractures: diagnosis and management. *Practice Nurse, 45*(5), 42–46 5p.

Cass, H., & Karlan, B.Y. (2008). Ovarian and tubal cancers. In R.S. Gibbs, B.Y. Karlan, & A.F. Haney (Eds.). *Danforth's obstetrics and gynecology* (10th ed., pp. 1022–1060). Philadelphia: Lippincott Williams & Wilkins.

Cedars, M.I., & Evans, M. (2008). Menopause. In R.S. Gibbs, B.Y. Karlan, & A.F. Haney (Eds.), *Danforth's obstetrics and gynecology* (10th ed., pp. 725–741). Philadelphia: Lippincott Williams & Wilkins.

Centers for Disease Control and Prevention. (2012). *Toxic shock syndrome.* Retrieved from http://www.cdc.gov.

Centers for Disease Control and Prevention. (2015a). *Cervical cancer screening in women ages 30 and older.* Retrieved from http://www.cdc.gov.

Centers for Disease Control and Prevention. (2015b). *High blood pressure.* Retrieved from http://www.cdc.gov.

Centers for Disease Control and Prevention. (2015c). Sexually transmitted diseases treatment guidelines 2010. *MMWR: Morbidity and Mortality Weekly Report, 64*(3), 1–140.

Centers for Disease Control and Prevention. (2015d). *Women and heart disease: CDC fact sheet.* Retrieved from http://www.cdc.gov.

Centers for Disease Control and Prevention. (2015e). *HPV Vaccine questions and answers.* Retrieved from http://www.cdc.gov.

Centers for Disease Control and Prevention. (2015f). *Overweight and obesity.* Retrieved from http://www.cdc.gov.

Centers for Disease Control and Prevention (2015g). *Pelvic inflammatory disease: CDC fact sheet.* Retrieved from http://www.cdc.gov.

Chichester, M., & Ciranni, P. (2011). Approaching menopause (But not there yet!). *Nursing for Women's Health, 15*(4), 320–324.

Cohen, D.P. (2008). Amenorrhea. In R.S. Gibbs, B.Y. Karlan, & A.F. Haney (Eds.), *Danforth's obstetrics and gynecology* (10th ed., pp. 648–663). Philadelphia: Lippincott Williams & Wilkins.

Compston, J. (2015). Obesity and fractures in postmenopausal women. *Current Opinion In Rheumatology, 27*(4), 414–419 6p. doi:10.1097/BOR.0000000000000182.

Cromer, B. (2011). Menstrual problems. In R.M. Kliegman, B.F. Stanton, & J.W. St. Geme III (Eds.), *Nelson textbook of pediatrics* (19th ed., pp. 685–692). Philadelphia: Saunders.

Crowder, B. (2009). Assessment of the cardiovascular system. In J.M. Black, & J.H. Hawks (Eds.), *Medical-surgical nursing: Clinical management for positive outcomes* (8th ed., pp. 1354–1384). St. Louis: Saunders.

Davis, A.J. (2008). Pediatric & adolescent gynecology. In R.S. Gibbs, B.Y. Karlan, & A.F. Haney (Eds.). *Danforth's obstetrics and gynecology* (10th ed., pp. 555–566). Philadelphia: Lippincott Williams & Wilkins.

DeLancy, J.O.L. (2008). Epidemiology, pathophysiology, and evaluation of pelvic support. In R.S. Gibbs, B.Y. Karlan, & A.F. Haney (Eds.), *Danforth's obstetrics and gynecology* (10th ed., pp. 818–838). Philadelphia: Lippincott Williams & Wilkins.

DeMartinis, J.E. (2009). Management of clients with hypertensive disorders. In J.M. Black, & J.H. Hawks (Eds.), *Medical-surgical nursing: Clinical management for positive outcomes* (8th ed., pp. 1290–1306). St. Louis: Saunders.

DeVon, H.A., Saban, K.L., & Garrett, D.K. (2011). Recognizing and responding to symptoms of acute coronary syndromes and stroke in women. *Journal of Obstetric, Gynecologic, and Neonatal Nursing, 40*(3), 372–382.

Eschenbach, D.A. (2008). Pelvic and sexually transmitted infections. In R.S. Gibbs, B.Y. Karlan, & A.F. Haney (Eds.),. *Danforth's obstetrics and gynecology* (10th ed., pp. 604–624). Philadelphia: Lippincott Williams & Wilkins.

Gemignani, M.L. (2008). Disorders of the breast. In R.S. Gibbs, B.Y. Karlan, & A.F. Haney (Eds.), *Danforth's obstetrics and gynecology* (10th ed., pp. 932–957). Philadelphia: Lippincott Williams & Wilkins.

Gish, B.A. (2011-2012). Interstitial cystitis/bladder pain syndrome. *Nursing for Women's Health, 15*(6), 496–507.

Giuntoli, R.L., & Bristow, R.E. (2008). Cervical cancer. In R.S. Gibbs, B.Y. Karlan, & A.F. Haney (Eds.), *Danforth's obstetrics and gynecology* (10th ed., pp. 971–988). Philadelphia: Lippincott Williams & Wilkins.

Goldstein, S.R. (2008). Abnormal uterine bleeding. In R.S. Gibbs, B.Y. Karlan, & A.F. Haney (Eds.), *Danforth's obstetrics and gynecology* (10th ed., pp. 664–675). Philadelphia: Lippincott Williams & Wilkins.

Haney, A.F. (2008). Leiomyomata. In R.S. Gibbs, B.Y. Karlan, & A.F. Haney (Eds.), *Danforth's obstetrics and gynecology* (10th ed., pp. 916–931). Philadelphia: Lippincott Williams & Wilkins.

Holmquist, S., & Gilliam, M. (2008). Induced abortion. In R.S. Gibbs, B.Y. Karlan, & A.F. Haney (Eds.), *Danforth's obstetrics and gynecology* (10th ed., pp. 586–603). Philadelphia: Lippincott Williams & Wilkins.

Jessup, M., & Antman, E. (2014). Reducing the risk of heart attack and stroke: the American heart association/American college of cardiology prevention guidelines. *Circulation, 130*(6), e48–e50 1p. doi:10.1161/CIRCULATIONAHA.114.010574.

Keresztes, P.A., & Weisel, M. (2009). Management of clients with functional cardiac disorders. In J.M. Black, & J.H. Hawks (Eds.), *Medical-surgical nursing: Clinical management and positive outcomes* (8th ed., pp. 1410–1449). St. Louis: Saunders.

McCormish, E. (2011-2012). Cervical cancer: Who's at risk? *Nursing for Women's Health, 15*(6), 476–483.

McSweeney, J.C., Pettey, C.M., & Souder, E. (2011). Disparities in women's cardiovascular health. *Journal of Obstetric, Gynecologic, and Neonatal Nursing, 40*(3), 362–371.

Mutch, D.G. (2008). Uterine cancer. In R.S. Gibbs, B.Y. Karlan, & A.F. Haney (Eds.), *Danforth's obstetrics and gynecology* (10th ed., pp. 1002–1021). Philadelphia: Lippincott Williams & Wilkins.

Nager, C.W., & Kane, A.R. (2008). Operative management of urinary incontinence. In R.S. Gibbs, B.Y. Karlan, & A.F. Haney (Eds.), *Danforth's obstetrics and gynecology* (10th ed., pp. 877–889). Philadelphia: Lippincott Williams & Wilkins.

National Center for Health Statistics. (2013). *Health United States 2013, with special feature on death and dying.* Hyattsville, MD: Author.

National Institutes of Health: Institute on Aging. (2012). *Hormones and menopause: Tips from the National Institute on Aging (NIH publication 09–7482).* Retrieved from http://www.nih.gov.

National Institutes of Health: Institute on Aging. (2010). *Age page: Menopause.* Retrieved from http://www.nih.gov.

National Institutes of Health: National Cancer Institute. (2002). *Bethesda System 2001: A revised system for reporting Pap test results aims to improve cervical cancer screening.* Retrieved from http://www.cancer.org.

National Institutes of Health: National Institute of Arthritis and Musculoskeletal and Skin Diseases. (2011). *Osteoporosis overview.* Retrieved from http://www.niams.nih.gov.

National Institutes of Health: National Institute of Diabetes and Digestive and Kidney Diseases. (2013). *Urinary incontinence in women (NIH Publication No. 08–4132, update 2013).* Bethesda, MD: National Kidney and Urologic Diseases Clearinghouse.

Norton, P.A. (2008). Female urinary incontinence: Epidemiology and evaluation. In R.S. Gibbs, B.Y. Karlan, & A.F. Haney (Eds.), *Danforth's obstetrics and gynecology* (10th ed., pp. 870–876). Philadelphia: Lippincott Williams & Wilkins.

Nygaard, I.E. (2008). Nonsurgical treatment of pelvic organ prolapse. In R.S. Gibbs, B.Y. Karlan, & A.F. Haney (Eds.), *Danforth's obstetrics and gynecology* (10th ed., pp. 866–869). Philadelphia: Lippincott Williams & Wilkins.

Pagana, K.D., & Pagana, T.J. (2011). *Mosby's diagnostic and laboratory test reference* (10th ed.). St. Louis: Mosby.

Pazol, K., Creanga, A., Burley, K., et al. (2013). Abortion surveillance—United States, 2010. Retrieved from *MMWR: Morbidity and Mortality Weekly Report, 62*(SS08), 1–44, Retrieved from http://www.cdc.gov.

Psaroudakis, D., Hirsch, M., & Davis, C. (2014). Review of the management of ovarian endometriosis: paradigm shift towards conservative approaches. *Current Opinion In Obstetrics & Gynecology, 26*(4), 266–274 9p. doi:10.1097/GCO.0000000000000078.

Raymond, J.L., & Couch, S.C. (2012). Medical nutrition therapy for cardiovascular disease. In K.L. Mahan, & S. Escott-Stump (Eds.), *Krause's food & nutrition therapy* (13th ed., pp. 742–781). St. Louis: Saunders.

Reid, R.L. (2008). Premenstrual syndrome. In R.S. Gibbs, B.Y. Karlan, & A.F. Haney (Eds.), *Danforth's obstetrics and gynecology* (10th ed., pp. 672–681). Philadelphia: Lippincott Williams & Wilkins.

Schenken, R.S. (2008). Endometriosis. In R.S. Gibbs, B.Y. Karlan, & A.F. Haney (Eds.), *Danforth's obstetrics and gynecology* (10th ed., pp. 716–724). Philadelphia: Lippincott Williams & Wilkins.

Sharp, H.T. (2008). Chronic pelvic pain. In R.S. Gibbs, B.Y. Karlan, & A.F. Haney (Eds.), *Danforth's obstetrics and gynecology* (10th ed., pp. 759–767). Philadelphia: Lippincott Williams & Wilkins.

Strohbehn, K., & Richter, H.E. (2008). Operative management of pelvic organ prolapse. In R.S. Gibbs, B.Y. Karlan, & A.F. Haney (Eds.), *Danforth's obstetrics and gynecology* (10th ed., pp. 839–869). Philadelphia: Lippincott Williams & Wilkins.

Wilton, J.M. (2011). Denosumab. *Nursing for Women's Health, 15*(3), 249–252.

# 33 Physical Assessment of Children

http://evolve.elsevier.com/McKinney/mat-ch/

## LEARNING OBJECTIVES

*After studying this chapter, you should be able to:*

- Apply the principles of anatomy and physiology to the systematic physical assessment of a child.
- Describe the major components of a pediatric health history.
- Identify the principal techniques for performing a physical examination.
- Use a systematic and developmentally appropriate approach for examining a child.
- Describe the general sequence of the physical examination of an infant, a young child, a school-age child, and an adolescent.
- Describe normal physical examination findings.
- List common terms used to describe the findings on physical examination.
- Record physical examination findings in a systematic way.

Nurses perform physical assessments of infants and children in various settings—the clinic, hospital, school, and home. The physical examination may be part of a well-child assessment, the admission examination when a child enters the hospital, or an initial assessment for home healthcare. The physical examination provides objective and subjective information about the child. The ability to perform a physical examination is fundamental to the nursing care of the child. Findings from a thorough physical examination help to determine a child's health status, which is the basis of all nursing interventions.

## GENERAL APPROACHES TO PHYSICAL ASSESSMENT

As when providing any nursing care for infants and children, the nurse applies the knowledge of growth and development when preparing the child and parents for performance of the physical examination. Involving parents as much as possible in the examination and allowing the child to handle safe, clean instruments, such as the stethoscope, reduce anxiety and increase the likelihood of examining a cooperative child.

The physical examination is often the first direct contact between the nurse and child. Establishing a trusting relationship between the child and examiner is important. Throughout the examination the nurse needs to be sensitive to the cultural needs of and differences among children. Providing a quiet, private environment for the history and physical examination is important. The classic systematic approach to a physical examination is to begin at the head and proceed through the entire body to the toes. However, when examining a child, the examiner tailors the physical assessment to the child's age and developmental level.

### Infants From Birth to 6 Months

Infants aged birth to 6 months are responsive to human faces, are increasingly interested in their environment, and do not mind being undressed (see Chapter 6). Therefore, their examination should be relatively easy. If the infant is nursing or asleep in the parent's arms, auscultate the heart, lungs, and abdomen without waking the baby. Even if the infant is awake, effective examination can still be accomplished with the infant lying or sitting in the parent's arms or on the lap. As body parts are examined, incorporate evaluation of the primitive reflexes—palmar grasp, plantar grasp, placing, stepping, and tonic neck reflexes. Leave all uncomfortable procedures, such as abduction of the hips, speculum examination of the tympanic membranes, and elicitation of the Moro reflex, until last. Before beginning the examination, undress the infant, leaving the diaper on a male child. Refocus an unhappy infant by calmly talking in a soft voice, distracting with a rattle, or offering a pacifier.

### Infants From 6 to 12 Months

For an older infant, follow the same procedures used for the infant from birth to 6 months, but keep in mind that infants 6 months and older feel stranger anxiety and so are more difficult to examine. Distracting a child of this age with a toy or object may be useful. It is easier to do as much of the examination as possible with the child held on the parent's lap. Leave ear, oral, and other uncomfortable procedures until last.

### Toddlers

Toddlers are the most challenging to examine because they are least likely to cooperate (see Chapter 7). To form a supportive relationship with the parent and toddler, the examiner begins by sitting or standing

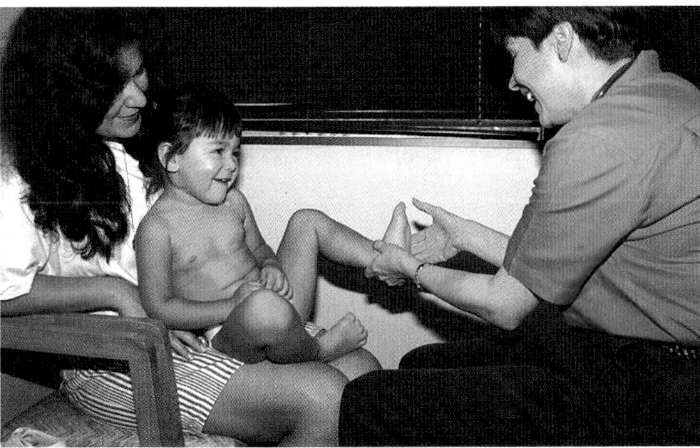

FIG 33.1 During the assessment, the nurse allows the child to remain on her mother's lap, enlisting the child's trust and increasing the likelihood of a successful physical examination. (Courtesy Parkland Health and Hospital System, Community Oriented Primary Care Clinics, Dallas, TX.)

**! NURSING QUALITY ALERT**

***Adapting the Physical Examination to the Child***

The classic systematic approach to the physical examination is to begin at the head and proceed to the toes. For children, painful or frightening procedures should be left until last. Involving parents by asking them to hold or stand by the child can decrease children's anxiety and assist them in relaxing.

next to the parent (Fig. 33.1). To facilitate relaxation, the examiner can provide a few toys and books and encourage the child to explore. Allowing the child to handle objects used during the examination can decrease fears. Communicating with the child, using age-appropriate words to describe what is about to be done, can also help decrease fear.

Portions of the examination can be done before the child is totally undressed. The order of the examination is flexible, proceeding from least to most invasive procedures. Resistance and crying are common with toddlers. The nurse assures the parent that the child's response to the examination is normal. The parent is the best resource for gaining the child's cooperation during the examination. Parents' use of familiar approaches to soothing and comforting a child can do much to facilitate examination.

### Preschoolers

Preschool children are usually more cooperative than toddlers but still like to have their parents nearby (see Chapter 7). Preschool children are happy to show nurses that they can undress themselves. They can also be expected to cooperate. The nurse can proceed with the examination from the head to the toe but should still save the more invasive procedures, such as the speculum ear examination and the oral examination, until last. The examiner can reinforce the child's interest by allowing the child to participate in the examination and by praising the child for cooperating.

### School-Age Children

To establish trust with the school-age child, the examiner asks the child questions the child can answer. Children in elementary school will talk about school, favorite friends, and activities (see Chapter 8). Older school-age children might need encouragement to talk about their school performance and activities. The examiner encourages the parent to support and reinforce the child's participation in the examination.

The examination proceeds from head to toe. Children of this age prefer a simple drape over their underpants or a colorful examination gown, and the examiner should be sensitive to the child's modesty. The examination is a wonderful opportunity to teach the child about the body and personal care. The nurse answers questions openly and in simple terms.

### Adolescents

Adolescents are most comfortable with a straightforward, noncondescending approach (see Chapter 9). Decisions about who should be present during the examination should be openly discussed with the adolescent. In most cases adolescents should be examined without the parent present. However, the parent should be given the opportunity to talk to the nurse about any concerns. The order of the examination is the same as for the school-age child.

It is best to incorporate the genital examination into the middle of the examination. If possible, proceed from the abdominal examination to the genital examination, to allow ample time for questions and discussions about this part of the examination. The physical examination provides the opportunity to assure the pubertal child about normal developmental stages and to answer concerns children this age frequently have about what is happening to their bodies. The adolescent is expected to undress and wear a gown. The adolescent is draped appropriately during the examination.

## TECHNIQUES FOR PHYSICAL EXAMINATION

When performing the physical assessment, the nurse uses the four basic techniques of inspection, palpation, percussion, and auscultation, generally in that order. During the abdominal examination, the sequence is altered; inspection is performed first, and then auscultation, percussion, and palpation. The sequence of the abdominal examination is changed so as not to alter bowel sounds before determining their presence and characteristics. Percussion is performed to determine the size of abdominal organs before palpation.

### Inspection

Most information is gathered during the physical examination by systematic and deliberate visual observations. The nurse first surveys an entire area of the body and then focuses on specifics, such as color, shape, size, and movement. Inspection can be both direct and indirect. Direct inspection relies on the examiner's senses of sight and hearing. Indirect inspection is accomplished with the use of special equipment, such as an otoscope, to examine a specific body area.

### Palpation

During palpation, the nurse uses the sense of touch to make judgments about pulsations and vibrations and to locate structures and masses. Palpation allows the nurse to determine characteristics such as size, texture, warmth, mobility, and tenderness of various areas of the body.

Different parts of the hands are used to detect different characteristics. The finger pads are used to palpate the breast, while fingertips are used to palpate the lymph nodes and pulses. The back of the hand is used to assess temperature. The palm of the hand is used to detect vibrations.

The type of palpation used is governed by the structure to be examined and the need to avoid any unnecessary discomfort to the child. Light palpation is accomplished by gently applying fingertip pressure to depress the skin surface approximately ½ to ¾ inch and then moving the fingertips in a circular motion.

Deep palpation identifies abdominal structures such as the liver, spleen, and kidneys and detects abdominal masses. Deep palpation follows light palpation. The surface is depressed approximately 1½ to

**! NURSING QUALITY ALERT**

***Using the Hands for Palpation***

- Finger pads are used to palpate the breast.
- Fingertips are used to palpate lymph nodes, and pulses.
- The back of the hand is used to assess temperature.
- The palm of the hand is used to identify vibrations.

2 inches to identify underlying masses and abdominal structures. Bimanual palpation is performed with both hands. The examiner superimposes one hand over the other to increase pressure or places one hand near the other to capture and trap a mass or structure between them, such as a kidney or the spleen.

### Percussion

To percuss, the nurse uses quick, sharp tapping of the fingers or hands to produce sounds. Percussion is performed to locate the position, size, and density of underlying structures. The three basic methods are as follows:

- *Mediate,* or *indirect, percussion,* in which the finger of one hand is placed against the body surface and the finger of the other hand acts as the hammer
- *Immediate percussion,* performed by striking the finger of one hand directly against the body
- *Fist percussion,* in which the ulnar aspect of the fist is used to deliver a firm blow directly to the area

The method used depends on the area to be percussed. The nurse uses quick, light blows to create vibrations that penetrate approximately 2 inches below the surface. Sounds identified by percussion are classified as *flat, dull, resonant, hyperresonant,* or *tympanic* (Box 33.1).

### Auscultation

Auscultation entails eliciting and listening to body sounds created in the lungs, heart, blood vessels, and abdominal viscera. The most common way to auscultate is to use a stethoscope. Most auscultated sounds result from air or fluid movement within the body. The diaphragm of the stethoscope is most effective in assessing high-pitched sounds, such as heart and breath sounds. The bell of the stethoscope is most effective in hearing low-pitched sounds, such as blood pressure and vascular sounds. Auscultation requires a quiet environment. The nurse places the stethoscope on the skin in the appropriate area. Sounds heard are described according to pitch, intensity, duration, and quality.

### Smell

While examining the child, the nurse uses the sense of smell to detect general body odors, common in children who are neglected or dirty. Odor may also indicate infection. Odors from the mouth, urine, or feces can be important. In particular, some diseases are characterized by odors coming from the mouth (Ball et al., 2015).

## SEQUENCE OF PHYSICAL EXAMINATION

### General Appearance

During the first contact with the child and parent, the examiner forms an initial impression by making a general survey. The nurse determines the child's age, sex, and race, and identifies clues concerning the child's behavior and health status. Because each child is a unique human, individual differences in behavior and health status related to growth and development will be evident. During the general survey, the examiner continually notes the parent-child interaction and the way the parent responds to the child's needs and behavior. Physical and emotional neglect, as well as inadequate parental supervision for the child's age, can be subtle or overt. These observations, together with other indicators of the child's health status, can provide clues to distress or abuse (Box 33.2).

### History Taking

Taking an accurate history is the single most important component of the physical examination. Practitioners obtain three different types of health histories: the complete, or initial, history; the well, interim history; and the episodic, or problem-oriented, history.

In the *complete* or *initial history* (Box 33.3), data are gathered about the child from the time of conception to the child's current status. The *well, interim history* includes data gathered about the child from the last well visit to the current visit. When doing a well, interim history, the examiner assumes that a database is in place. In a *problem-oriented* or *episodic* history (Box 33.4), information is gathered about a current problem. Information about the specific problem is then added to the existing database.

**? CRITICAL THINKING EXERCISE 33.1**

Ann Maloney, a 17-year-old single mother, brings her 6-month-old daughter, Kerrie, to the clinic. This is Kerrie's first visit. Ms. Maloney made several earlier appointments for Kerrie but was always unable to keep them. She states, "I am very busy trying to work and care for Kerrie. I had to miss work because Kerrie has lots of colds. I hate to take time off when she is well. My supervisor at work said that it is important for her to have her immunizations and a physical examination. I guess I messed up."

1. What assumptions could the nurse make about Ms. Maloney?
2. How should the nurse respond to Ms. Maloney's comment?
3. How can the nurse best act as an advocate for both Kerrie and her mother?

**BOX 33.1 Sounds Identified During Percussion**

*Flat:* High-pitched, soft-intensity sound elicited by percussing over solid masses, such as bone or muscle

*Dull:* Medium-pitched, medium-intensity sound elicited when percussing over high-density structures such as the liver

*Resonance:* Low-pitched, loud-intensity sound elicited over a hollow organ such as the lungs

*Hyperresonance:* Very low, very loud, with a booming quality heard over the lungs in young children

*Tympany:* High-pitched, loud-intensity sound heard over air-filled body parts such as the bowel or stomach

**BOX 33.2 Potential Indicators of Child Abuse**

*Dress:* Inappropriate for the weather; ragged or excessively dirty

*Grooming and personal hygiene:* Dirty teeth; broken and dirty fingernails; matted and dirty hair

*Posture and movements:* Crouching in a corner; slow, concentrated movements

*Body image distortion:* Being thin but describing self as fat

*Speech and communication:* Answering questions in words of one syllable; looking to others to respond first; seeking approval for answers

*Facial characteristics and expressions:* Fearful, anxious, tearful, sad, or angry expressions

*Psychological state:* Labile, demanding, bizarre, overly dramatic, or condescending

**BOX 33.3 The Complete History**

The complete or initial history includes the following:

1. *Statistical information:* Name, age, address, telephone number, birth date, names of parents or guardians, and source of support.
2. *Patient profile:* Times the child eats and sleeps, educational level, developmental level, race, ethnicity, nationality, religion, economic status, and health status perception. If an interpreter is used to gather the health history, the person's name is included in the record, usually in this section of the history. Also included is a statement about the reliability of an informant, such as an older sibling who answers questions concerning a younger sibling or an aunt or uncle who answers questions regarding a child.
3. *Health history:* Birth history, growth and development, common childhood illnesses, immunizations, previous hospitalizations, accidents or injuries, and allergies or allergic reactions and exact symptoms the allergy produced. The person taking the history should ask about medications taken daily or for an acute episode of an illness and should list all medications being taken, including dose and frequency. The parent should name both prescription and over-the-counter medications as well as herbal remedies and supplements. The examiner also asks whether the child has ever had a blood transfusion or has received any blood products. For any hospitalizations, serious illnesses, and injuries, the nurse should obtain the following information:
   a. Reason for admission
   b. Place of admission
   c. Length of stay
   d. Surgical procedures
   e. Other treatments
   f. Outcomes
   g. Follow-up
4. *Family history:* Information concerning the health status of the child's mother, father, siblings, and specific blood relatives such as aunts, uncles, and grandparents. If any are deceased, the history includes the age and cause of death. The purpose is to determine constitutional and hereditary factors that are likely to affect the child's health.
5. *Lifestyle and life patterns:* The child's interaction with the social, psychological, physical, and cultural environment. Growth and development; use of street drugs, alcohol, and tobacco; roles and relationships; and family life information are all important.
6. *Review of systems:* A systematic review of the major anatomic and physiologic parts. A head-to-toe review focusing on the health function and maintenance of each body part should occur in this order:
   a. General appearance
   b. Head
   c. Hair
   d. Face
   e. Eyes
   f. Ears
   g. Nose and sinuses
   h. Mouth
   i. Throat
   j. Neck
   k. Lungs
   l. Heart
   m. Breasts
   n. Abdomen
   o. Kidneys and bladder
   p. Bowels, rectum, and anus
   q. Genitals
   r. Extremities

**BOX 33.4 Problem-Oriented History**

*Chief complaint:* Use the child's own words.
*Body location:* Place the problem somewhere on the body.
*Quality:* Define what the problem is like for the child.
*Quantity:* Describe the intensity of the problem for the child.
*Chronology:* Determine when the problem began, the periodicity and frequency, and the course of symptoms.
*Setting:* Identify where the problem occurs.
*Aggravating and alleviating factors:* Find out what makes the problem better or worse.
*Associated manifestations:* Document other related information.
*Treatment:* Document what has been used to treat the problem. Be sure to ask about complementary therapies as well as traditional approaches.

## Recording Data

The information gathered during the history is documented concisely to provide all necessary information from pregnancy to the child's current status. Milestones in growth and development, immunizations, and family status are always included in the child's history.

## Vital Signs

Vital signs are taken for every child during every visit in ambulatory care settings and are monitored throughout the day in a hospitalized child. Assessment of vital signs (temperature, pulse, respirations, and blood pressure) is an important way to measure and monitor vital body functions. Measuring vital signs provides the basis for decisions concerning the child's overall health and illness. In children, changes in vital signs are important signs of changes in health status. Table 33.1 describes normal vital signs by age, and Chapter 37 details the procedure for taking vital signs in children.

### Temperature

The method for measuring children's temperature varies from one setting to another. Some parents are comfortable taking a rectal or axillary temperature with a digital thermometer (American Academy of Pediatrics [AAP], 2016). Healthcare providers might use a tympanic membrane or temporal artery sensor or an electronic, digital thermometer. Currently, parents are encouraged to take axillary rather than rectal temperatures. Reasons for the recommendation are the invasive nature of rectal temperature measurements, the risk of injury, and their questionable accuracy with febrile children because feces retain body heat for hours after a fever has diminished. Axillary temperatures, when taken correctly, provide accurate information concerning changes in the child's health status.

Temporal artery thermometers frequently are used in the healthcare setting (Battra & Goyal, 2013; Hurwitz, Brown, & Altmiller, 2015) because they can accurately measure body temperature in infants and children older than three months and are less invasive and more time efficient than rectal or axillary temperatures. They function using infrared technology and are considered to be very accurate (Hurwitz et al., 2015). Tympanic temperature measurements can be used as well. When recording a tympanic temperature, the nurse notes the side on which the temperature was elicited. Variation can occur from one ear to the other in the same child.

## TABLE 33.1 Normal Vital Signs by Age

| | TEMPERATURE* | | | | |
|---|---|---|---|---|---|
| **Age** | **Degrees Fahrenheit** | **Degrees Celsius** | **Pulse Rate[∞] (Beats/min)** | **Respiratory Rate[∞] (Breaths/min)** | **Blood Pressure Range (mm Hg)[+α]** |
| Newborn | 97.7-99.1 (axillary) | 36.5-37.3 (axillary) | 100-150 | 35-55 | Systolic: 65-95[†]<br>Diastolic: 30-60[†] |
| 2 yr | 97.5 – 98.6 (axillary) | 36.4-37 (axillary) | 70-110 | 20-30 | *Girls*<br>Systolic: 85-91<br>Diastolic:43-47<br>*Boys*<br>Systolic: 84-92<br>Diastolic: 39-44 |
| 4 yr | 97.5-98.6 (axillary) | 36.4-37 (axillary) | 65-110 | 20-25 | *Girls*<br>Systolic: 88-94<br>Diastolic: 50-54<br>*Boys*<br>Systolic: 88-97<br>Diastolic: 47-52 |
| 10 yr | 97.5-98.6 (oral) | 36.4-37 (oral) | 60-95 | 14-22 | *Girls*<br>Systolic: 98-105<br>Diastolic: 59-62<br>*Boys*<br>Systolic: 97-106<br>Diastolic: 58-63 |
| 16 yr | 97.5-98.6 (oral) | 36.4-37 (oral) | 55-85[‡] | 12-18 | *Girls*<br>Systolic: 108-114<br>Diastolic: 64-68<br>*Boys*<br>Systolic: 111-120<br>Diastolic: 63-67 |

*The normal range of the child's temperature depends on the method used. Temperatures exhibit circadian rhythms at all ages.
[+]Blood pressures represent values for the 50th percentile for age and height percentiles.
[∞]Data from: Hartman, M., & Cheifetz, M. (2016). Pediatric emergencies and resuscitation. In R. Kliegman, B. Stanton, J. St. Geme, et al. (Eds.), *Nelson textbook of pediatrics* (20th ed., Chapter 490). St. Louis, MO: Elsevier.
[α]BP data from: National Heart Lung and Blood Institute. (2004). *The fourth report on the diagnosis, evaluation and treatment of high blood pressure in children and adolescents.* Retrieved from http://www.nhlbi.gov.
[†]Taken by Doppler measurement.
[‡]After age 12 yr, a boy's pulse is 5 beats/min slower than a girl's.

An oral thermometer can be used with older children, usually starting at 5 or 6 years of age. For oral temperature measurements, an electronic thermometer has the benefits of being unbreakable and registering quickly. (See Chapter 37 for a discussion of various methods of assessing temperature.)

### Pulse

Apical pulse rates are measured in children younger than 2 years and in any child who has an irregular heart rate or known congenital heart disease. Radial pulse rates can be taken in children older than 2 years. To compensate for normal irregularities, the nurse counts the pulse for 1 full minute. Chapter 37 details the procedure for measuring the pulse rate.

Arterial pulses are palpated to determine pulse rate and rhythm and to evaluate blood flow, arterial wall elasticity, and vessel patency. To determine the position of the heart in the anterior precordium, the nurse palpates the apical impulse in infants and children younger than 6 years. In the acute care setting, an apical impulse is always palpated in every child, and the location of the apical impulse is noted. Simultaneously, the examiner palpates and compares femoral, radial, and carotid pulses in children of any age. The nurse can also compare a carotid pulse with a femoral or radial pulse for equality of pulses. In infants, the nurse notes the pulsating anterior fontanel. The pulse can increase significantly above normal in infants and children with anxiety, fever, exercise, inflammatory illnesses, shock, or heart disease. The resting heart rate changes with increasing age.

The rhythm of the heartbeat is assessed for equal spacing between consecutive beats. Irregular cardiac rhythms are not uncommon in children and are often related to changes in rhythm that occur in response to respiratory inspiration and expiration.

### Respirations

The nurse observes the rate, depth, and ease of respiration in the child. Respirations vary with age. The respiratory rate, like the heart rate, is significantly influenced by emotion and exercise. In infants, the rate can be determined by observing abdominal excursion. In toddlers and older children, the nurse observes thoracic excursion. Because the movements are irregular, the rate should be assessed for 1 minute in infants and young children. Respirations are best counted when the child is not paying attention to the examiner. Respirations should be counted while the examiner continues to keep fingers on a pulse or the stethoscope on the chest, as though checking the pulses. This effort will ensure that the child is unaware that the examiner is counting respirations.

The depth and rhythm of respirations are determined subjectively and compared with norms for a particular age-group. The ease or difficulty of respirations is a somewhat subjective observation. Respirations should be quiet and appear effortless. Stridor, a crowing noise heard on inspiration and heard louder over the neck, is worrisome in a child and may be a sign of croup or a late sign in epiglottitis (Roosevelt, 2016) (see Chapter 45). Inspiratory stridor indicates a partial obstruction of the airway. Continuous inspiratory and expiratory stridor can be related to delayed development of the cartilage in the tracheal rings or to a relatively small larynx.

### Blood Pressure

Although the United States Preventive Services Task Force (USPSTF) found no evidence that routine measurement of blood pressure in asymptomatic children who have no predisposing physical condition is beneficial (Moyer & USPSTF, 2013), the AAP (2012, 2013) continues to recommend routine blood pressure measurement for all children beginning at age 3 years according to current recommendations from the National High Blood Pressure Education Program Working Group (2004). Blood pressure measurements are taken for all children at every ambulatory visit; in an acute-care setting, blood pressure is measured at least daily, and often more frequently, depending on the child's condition. The appropriate-size cuff must be used in order to obtain an accurate blood pressure. Blood pressure measurements in healthy ambulatory children are compared with standard norms (see Table 33.1 for the effects of age on vital signs). An auscultated blood pressure measurement that is equal to or exceeds the 90th percentile for the child's sex, height, and age must be confirmed before the child is described as being hypertensive. An average of at least three abnormal blood pressure measurements taken on separate occasions requires further evaluation. If an adolescent's blood pressure is greater than 120/80 mm Hg, the adolescent is considered to be prehypertensive even if this value is below the 90th percentile (American Academy of Pediatrics [AAP], National High Blood Pressure Education Program Working Group on High Blood Pressure in Children and Adolescents, 2004).

The size of the cuff is important. Cuffs that are too small will cause falsely elevated values; those that are too large will cause inaccurate low values (see Chapter 37 for determining appropriate cuff size). To alleviate potential anxiety about the measurement procedure that might result in inaccurate measurement, the nurse can use distraction, such as allowing the child to first take a blood pressure on a doll, a stuffed animal, or the parent.

### Pain Assessment

For children in acute and ambulatory care settings, the initial and ongoing assessment of pain is essential (The Joint Commission, 2014) (see Chapter 39). The American Pain Society introduced the phrase "pain as the 5th vital sign" to emphasize the importance of assessing pain along with the standard four vital signs (American Pain Society, n.d.). Use of a pain assessment tool that is developmentally appropriate for the pediatric patient is recommended (Zeltzer, Krane, & Palermo, 2016). See Table 39.2 for a list of pain assessment tools.

## Anthropometric Measurement

Anthropometrics entails measuring the human body and assessing nutritional status, as well as growth and development. Weight, height, and head circumference are always measured in children and are compared with averages for age-group and gender. The amount of body fat should be measured on the basis of the body mass index (BMI), which is calculated according to a simple formula:

$$\text{BMI} = \frac{\text{Weight (kg)}}{\text{Height (m)}^2} \text{ or BMI} = \frac{\text{Weight (lb)} \times 703}{\text{Height (in)}^2}$$

Midarm muscle circumference, skinfold thickness, and weight provide information about three body tissues (subcutaneous tissue, muscle, and fat) altered by nutrition. Because children's body fat varies with age and gender, anthropometric measurements are most valuable when plotted on a growth curve and evaluated serially so that trends can be monitored.

Measuring height, weight and BMI are routine procedures that provide valuable information about a child's health. Children grow and develop rapidly, and this growth and development must be constantly evaluated. A child's serial physical measurements reflect the rate of growth. A failure in growth, an acceleration in growth, or any change in growth pattern can be the first clue to serious health problems. When a child's weight or height stops following the child's own growth curve, this is the most significant indicator of a change in health status. Measurements must be correct and accurate and are taken at every visit from birth to adulthood.

### Use of Growth Charts

Documentation of measurements provides an accurate record of a child's overall pattern of growth. The Centers for Disease Control and Prevention (CDC) provides growth charts (http://www.cdc.gov/growthcharts/clinical_charts.htm), a series of percentile curves for selected measurements, which are used to assess body size and monitor growth in infants, children, and adolescents in the United States (CDC, 2010).

The CDC recommends that healthcare providers use the World Health Organization (WHO) growth standards to monitor growth for infants and children aged 0 to 2 years and the CDC growth charts for children age 2 years and older. The data collected for the WHO growth charts represent infants and children who were breastfed during their first year of life, and this is considered to be the optimal standard of measurement for comparison (CDC, 2010).

Separate sets of growth charts are available for girls and boys. WHO growth charts for ages birth to age 2 years, plot length, weight, and head circumference measurements for age. They also plot the weight to length relationship, which can be used as an indicator of overweight or obesity in children. The CDC charts for ages 2 through 20 years, plot measurements of stature (height), weight, and BMI for age. BMI is used primarily to screen for children who are overweight, although it can also be used to describe children who are underweight (CDC, 2015). Special growth charts for premature, very-low-birth-weight infants (<1500 g) and children with special needs are available, but may be based on old or inconsistent data (CDC, 2013); normal growth charts can be used, with the infant's age corrected for gestational age (AAP, 2015).

Plotting on a growth chart proceeds as follows: The child's exact age (or gestational age) is located on the chart's horizontal axis. The corresponding measurement is noted on the chart's vertical axis. The chart is marked where the two lines intersect. The percentile lines on these charts indicate the number of children whose measurements are expected to fall above and below the child's measurement.

Weight and height measurements above the 97th percentile or below the 3rd percentile on a standard growth chart indicate a growth disturbance that needs further investigation. Brain growth can be assessed by serial head circumference measurements (see Chapter 52). BMIs from the 85th to below the 95th percentile indicate a risk for being overweight; BMIs at or above the 95th percentile in children older than 2 years indicate overweight (CDC, 2010).

### Height

The methods used to measure a child's stature vary with age. Infant and toddler length is best measured with the child lying down on a flat measuring board. This method is used until the child is able to stand independently. The child's head is held securely to the headboard, and the movable footboard is stretched to touch the child's heel. If a measuring board is not available for the infant and young child, it is possible to position the child's body on a flat surface, mark the point where the heel touches the surface, and then mark the point where the top of the head is lying on the surface, taking care to ensure that the child's legs and body are straight on the surface. The examiner then removes the child and measures the distance between the two points with a measuring tape. Measuring the length of the child in this manner is not as accurate as using a measuring board.

**! NURSING QUALITY ALERT**

***Importance of Anthropometric Measurements***

Anthropometric measurements reflect any change in the growth pattern and may be the first clue to a serious problem. Measurements must be taken at every healthcare visit from birth to adulthood. If a child's weight or height stops following the child's own growth curve, it is a significant indicator of a change in health status.

When a child is able to cooperate and stand without support, around age 2 years, the examiner stands the child in stocking feet next to a standard measuring tape that begins at the child's heel and is not displaced by room molding. A flat, hard surface is used to reach from the top of the child's head to the tape so that the examiner does not guess or add height because of the hair. Commercial measurement methods also are available and might provide a more accurate measurement. If this is the first standing measurement, there may be a slight discrepancy from the lying measurement.

Once the measurement is taken, it must be plotted on a standardized growth chart appropriate for length or height measurement. Height and weight are evaluated by determining whether the child is following a predictable percentile curve on a growth chart. Height and weight are related to hereditary factors and will vary from child to child.

### Weight

The method and equipment for weighing vary with the child's age. All scales must be balanced or zeroed first before weight is measured. Infants are placed in a lying position on a regular baby scale with all their clothing removed. Older children who are able to stand or walk without support may be weighed on the adult standing scale. On the older child, remove all clothing except underwear. Like height, weight is plotted on a standardized growth chart.

### Head Circumference

Head circumference is measured in all children from birth to age 36 months and is plotted on a standard growth chart on all visits. In the child older than 3 years with any questionable head size (macrocephaly or microcephaly), the head circumference should be measured at every visit. To measure the head circumference, a nonstretching measuring tape is wrapped above the supraorbital ridges and over the most prominent part of the occiput (Fig. 33.2).

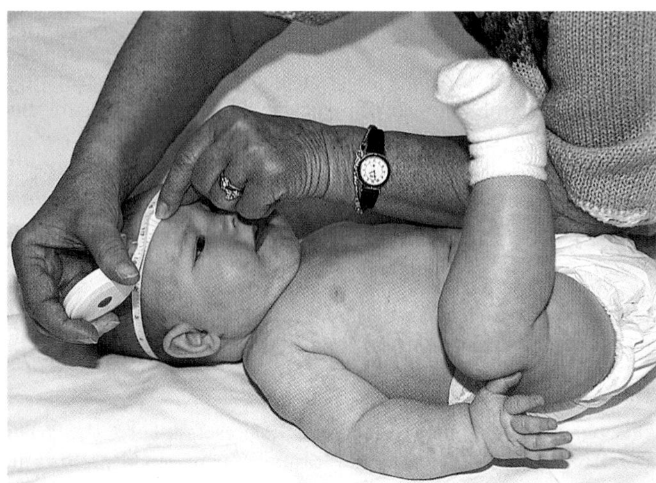

**FIG 33.2** Measuring head circumference. The head circumference is measured from birth through age 36 months. The nurse uses a nonstretching tape and measures in a "hat band" position, just above the eyebrows and around the occipital prominence in the back. Chest circumference is also routinely measured in the newborn; it is usually smaller than the newborn's head circumference. (Courtesy The University of Texas at Arlington College of Nursing, Arlington, TX.)

During the first year of life, the head circumference normally increases by 1.2 cm (0.5 inch) each month. Head circumference can reflect an abnormal rate of development, give some indication of nutritional status, and possibly indicate tumor growth or an abnormal accumulation of cerebrospinal fluid (CSF) known as hydrocephalus. Any marked increase in head circumference measurements during infancy requires referral for evaluation.

### Chest Circumference

Chest circumference is routinely measured only in the newborn infant. The newborn's head circumference is larger than the chest circumference. Chest circumference is almost equal to head circumference after age 1 year. To measure chest circumference, the measuring tape is wrapped around the chest at the nipple line. The measurement is taken between inspiration and expiration.

### Midarm Circumference

Midarm circumference reflects muscle mass and fat. To measure midarm circumference, the midpoint on the arm between the acromial process and the olecranon process is determined. Then, with the arm hanging loosely at the side, it is measured at the midpoint using a tape measure. The measurement is recorded in centimeters. With a decrease in fat or muscle atrophy, the midarm circumference decreases. It will increase with weight gain.

### Triceps Skinfold

Triceps skinfold thickness indicates total body fat because at least half of body fat is directly below the skin. Metal calipers are used to obtain this measurement. On the nondominant arm, the midpoint of the arm is determined with the same method that is used for measuring midarm circumference. With the arm hanging loosely at the side, a fold of skin at the midpoint on the posterior aspect of the arm is grasped. To avoid error, the child is asked to flex the arm muscle after the examiner grasps the skin. If contraction is felt, muscle as well as fat has been grasped. The examiner applies the caliper and takes a reading after waiting 3 seconds. Fat stores decrease with long-term undernutrition and malnutrition.

**BOX 33.5 Skin Color Terminology**

*Vitiligo:* Areas of depigmentation
*Nevi:* Areas of increased pigmentation
*Jaundice:* A yellow discoloration of the skin, best seen in the sclera of the eyes
*Cyanosis:* A blue discoloration of the skin, best seen in all races in the mucous membranes of the mouth, particularly under the tongue
*Carotenemia:* An orange color of the skin, best seen on the soles of the feet and palms of the hands
*Pallor:* Loss of skin color
*Erythema:* Diffusely red
*Mottling:* Discolored areas of the skin

## Skin, Hair, and Nails

### Skin

Skin assessment includes inspection and palpation. The entire skin surface is examined for color, texture, turgor, and presence of lesions. This examination may be combined with assessment of other areas of the body.

**Inspection.** The nurse observes the color and pigmentation of the skin. Skin color reflects the amount of melanin and can range from pink to black (Box 33.5). In dark-skinned infants and children, erythema appears dusky red or violet, cyanosis appears black, and jaundice appears diffusely darker. In dark-skinned infants and children, it is best to determine the normal skin color and then compare any color change with the normal color. Increased pigmentation and thickening of the skin on the posterior neck, the armpits, and behind the knees and elbows (acanthosis nigricans) can be an indication of type 2 diabetes mellitus in children (Dickey & Chu, 2016). Skin color changes can be related to sun exposure or tattooing.

**! NURSING QUALITY ALERT**

**Skin Inspection in Dark-Skinned Children**

- *Erythema:* Dusky red or violet
- *Cyanosis:* Black or dusky
- *Jaundice:* Diffusely darker than the child's normal color

**Palpation.** The examiner palpates the skin to assess moisture, temperature, texture, turgor, edema, and lesions, as follows:

*Moisture* is assessed by lightly stroking the skin surface and body creases. The external skin on exposed areas is normally drier than unexposed areas of the skin.

*Temperature* is assessed by using the back of the hand because it is more sensitive to skin changes. The two sides of the child's body are compared.

Normal *texture* of the skin is described as being smooth and soft. Scars or excessive scar tissue should be noted.

*Turgor* is assessed by grasping the skin between the thumb and index finger and quickly releasing it (see Fig. 40.1). The skin normally returns to place without excessive skin markings. Skin that "tents" when released indicates dehydration. The abdomen and upper arm are the best places to test for tissue turgor on a child.

*Edema* is the accumulation of excessive salt and water in the interstitial spaces. It is identified by pressing the thumb into an area of the body that may appear swollen and noting whether the indentation persists after the release of pressure. The extremities and buttocks are classic areas to palpate for edema in the child. Periorbital edema is observed on the eyelids.

*Lesions* are identified, noting configuration, distribution, color, and size. Skin lesions are identified as primary lesions, arising from normal skin (e.g., freckle), or secondary lesions, resulting from an alteration of a primary lesion (e.g., scab). Configuration of a skin lesion is the arrangement or position of several lesions in relation to one another or to the arrangement of a single lesion. Distribution is the body location and the symmetry or asymmetry of lesions.

### Hair

Hair normally covers the entire body except for the palms, soles, and parts of the genitalia. Hair is examined for texture, changes in color, unusual distribution, and cleanliness.

Scalp hair has a wide range of normal textures, including straight, curly, and kinky. The hair is usually shiny, silky, and strong. The examiner should keep in mind the child's age and development. Fine, downy hair is normal for a newborn infant, whereas in an older child it would lead the examiner to consider nutritional and endocrine abnormalities. Brittle hair, identified when the hairs break off easily when bent between the fingers, suggests endocrine or nutritional abnormalities.

The color of the hair is genetically determined and can be anything from pale blond to black. Changes in color can be caused by depigmentation, hereditary factors, or chemicals applied to the hair. Hair texture varies widely with race.

The distribution of the hair over the head is identified. In most children, the hair begins in a whorl and then is distributed over the head. Some children have more than one whorl. Scalp hair does not grow beyond the nape of the neck or down to the eyebrows. *Hirsutism* is defined as excessive hair growth; *alopecia* is unusual hair loss.

The hair is separated and examined for cleanliness, signs of trauma, lesions, and scaling. The scalp should be clean and free of any infestations. Most cases of head lice *(Pediculosis capitis)* are first detected when one or more children are seen scratching the head. Closer observation reveals nits adhering to the hairs. Depending on their distance from the scalp, these are the whitish to sand-colored empty shells of eggs that have hatched (see Chapter 49 for further discussion of the integumentary system).

### Nails

Nails are inspected and palpated for shape and contour. The nail surface is normally flat or slightly convex. The edges of the nails should be smooth, rounded, and clean. Clubbing of fingernails can be identified by looking at the index finger to see if the nail bulges upward. If the angle between the nail base and the fingertip is greater than 160 degrees, clubbing is present. On palpation, the base of the fingernail should be firm. On touching the index fingernails back to back, a diamond of light below the knuckle and above where the fingernails touch will be present. In early clubbing, the diamond shape is decreased or not apparent (see Chapter 45).

Press and release on the nail edge to assess capillary refill; the nail will blanch, and then color will normally return to the nail within 1 to 2 seconds. A capillary refill time of more than 2 seconds may be caused circulatory compromise, fluid imbalances, and an impediment to peripheral circulation (Ball et al., 2015).

## Lymph Nodes

Lymph nodes are inspected and palpated. Lymph tissue is found all over the body and must be evaluated as the examiner assesses body systems. The examiner should always assess for enlarged lymph nodes

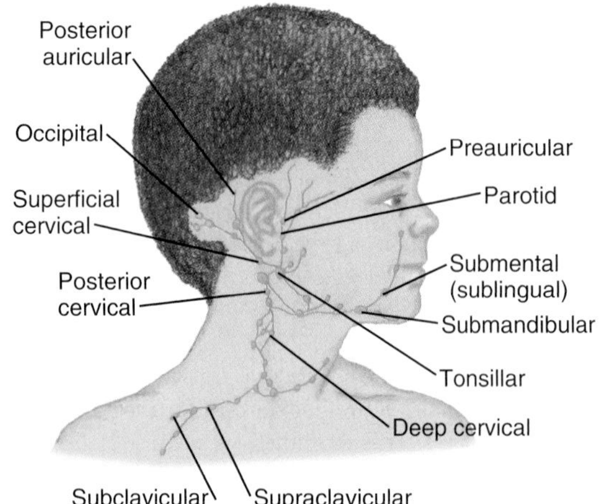


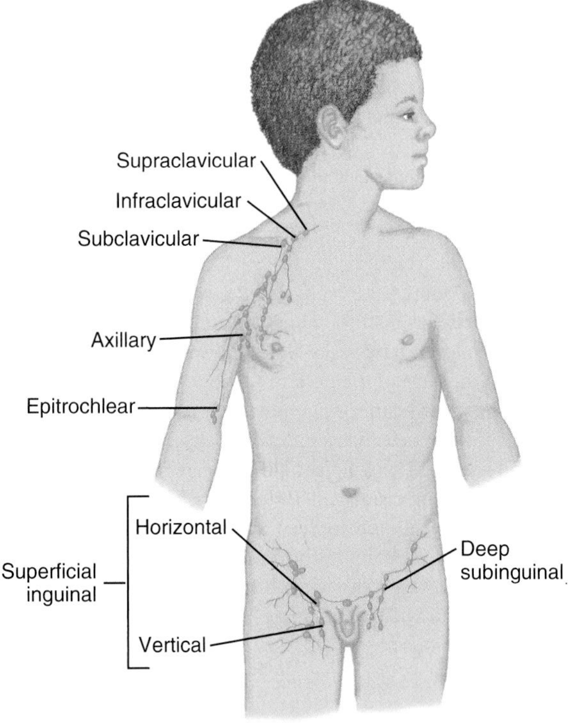


**FIG 33.3** Location of superficial lymph nodes.

in the head and neck, the supraclavicular area, the axillary region, the arms, and the inguinal region (Fig. 33.3). At the time these areas are examined, the lymph nodes are assessed as well. When an enlarged lymph node or a mass is found during examination, its characteristics should be described (Box 33.6).

To palpate for most lymph nodes, the examiner uses the distal portion of the fingers and gently but firmly moves the fingers in a circular motion to determine the node's characteristics and mobility.

Lymph nodes that are enlarged, warm, firm, and fluctuant indicate infection. Lymph nodes that are small, firm, and shotty (freely palpable and very small) are often palpable in healthy infants and children. Lymph nodes in children are, in general, not concerning until they are larger than 1 to 1.5 cm in size (Tower & Camitta, 2016). An enlarged supraclavicular lymph node on the left in young children is called the *sentinel node* because it may suggest a Wilms tumor or other neoplastic disease.

**BOX 33.6 Characteristics of Enlarged Lymph Nodes and Masses**

*Location:* Identify the anatomic location of the enlarged lymph nodes or mass. Use imaginary body lines or body axes to assist in locating findings.

*Size:* Describe in three dimensions: length, width, and thickness. Describe the shape: round or irregular.

*Surface characteristics:* Describe the surface as smooth, nodular, or irregular on palpation.

*Consistency:* Describe the nodes or masses as hard, soft, firm, resilient, spongy, or cystic on palpation.

*Symmetry:* Evaluate paired anatomic structures for symmetry.

*Fixed or mobile:* If a fixed mass is found, note whether it is fixed to underlying or overlying tissue. If a mobile mass is found, describe it in centimeters and describe its direction.

*Tenderness and pain:* Describe whether the tenderness or pain is present on direct palpation or occurs without stimulation. Identify referred pain and rebound tenderness.

*Erythema:* Describe the extent of any color change.

*Heat:* Palpate with the back of the hand to identify any abnormal warmth.

*Pulsatile nature:* Describe pulsations, if present, particularly when they are in an area where pulsations are not expected. All pulsating masses are auscultated for bruits.

*Increased vascularity:* Describe the prominence of overlying veins or the presence of cyanosis of the area.

*Transillumination:* If the mass is in an anatomic structure that can be transilluminated, record the results of the procedure.

**BOX 33.7 Head Shape Terminology**

*Normocephalic:* Normal-size head
*Microcephalic:* Head small for body size and age
*Macrocephalic:* Abnormally large head
*Bossing:* Frontal enlargement

## Head, Neck, and Face

### Head

The head is inspected and palpated. To examine the head, the examiner must see and feel. The head is evaluated from the front, the back, and the sides. The head is examined for symmetry, paralysis, weakness, and movement (Box 33.7).

Symmetry is assessed by looking at and feeling the entire head. If any lumps or bumps are seen or felt, the examiner notes their exact location, size, and density. The suture lines in infants should be palpated. Sutures are felt as prominent ridges in the neonate but usually flatten by 6 months of age.

Paralysis and weakness of the head are directly related to the condition of the neck muscles. That is, paralysis and weakness of the head occur with paralysis or weakness of the neck muscles.

Head movement is evaluated by observing the child's spontaneous head movement. Head control is observed with the infant in a supine position and while the examiner grasps the infants hands and pulls the infant into a sitting position. An infant younger than 4 months may show some head lag, but the infant in an upright position should be able to maintain the head upright for several seconds. Head lag after age 6 months suggests poor muscle development. However, increased neck extensor and axial tone in the young infant make head control appear better than it actually is and is suggestive of neuromuscular problems such as cerebral palsy (Johnston, 2016). The head should be

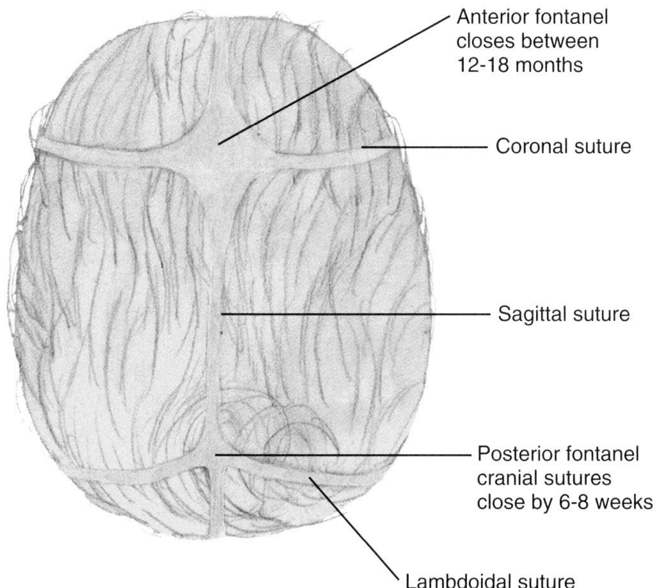


**FIG 33.4** Fontanels are inspected and palpated for size, tenseness, and pulsation.

put through a full range of motion by asking the older child to look up, down, and sideways. After age 4 months, inability to move the head or to hold the head in an upright position may be related to paralysis or weakness of the neck muscles.

The fontanels are inspected and palpated for size, tenseness, and pulsation (Fig. 33.4). The posterior fontanel is closed by age 2 to 3 months. The anterior fontanel should be soft and flat when the child is sitting. Measure the width and length of an open anterior fontanel. The anterior fontanel should be less than 5 cm in length and width after age 12 months and should be completely closed at approximately 12 to 24 months of age with the average age of closure at 18 months (Lehman & Schor, 2016). A sunken fontanel is associated with dehydration, and a bulging fontanel is associated with increased intracranial pressure. A bulging fontanel is normally seen when an infant cries, coughs, or vomits. Inability to palpate the anterior fontanel may be an indicator of premature closure known as craniosynostosis (see Chapter 52).

### Neck

The neck is inspected and palpated for symmetry, size, and shape, which are directly related to use or disuse of the neck muscles. The infant's neck is relatively short and lengthens as the child grows. The neck is viewed from the front, back, and both sides. Webbing of the neck, the presence of an extra fold of skin posteriorly, is associated with some chromosomal abnormalities such as trisomy 21, or Down syndrome.

The neck is mobile and supple. While palpating the child's neck, the examiner palpates the thyroid gland by identifying the isthmus of the thyroid across the trachea. To identify an enlarged thyroid in a child, the examiner gently displaces the thyroid gland laterally and palpates thyroid tissue with the opposite thumb and fingers. The lobe may be more palpable when the child swallows.

### Face

The child's face is inspected and palpated for dysmorphic features. Spacing and symmetry of facial features are noted. The face is observed for any changes in color or the presence of edema, such as cellulitis. The eyes are examined for size, position, and configuration. *Hypertelorism* is a condition in which the eyes are unusually widely spaced; in *hypotelorism*, the eyes are unusually close together. The child's nostrils should be oval in shape and equal in size, with no evidence of a hypoplastic philtrum (shallow crease or absence of a crease below the nose). The lips should be equal on either side of the midline. The child's ears are inspected for alignment. Low-set ears are identified when the auricle of the ear does not cross or touch the eye-occiput line. The position of the auricle should be almost vertical, with no more than a 10-degree lateral posterior angle (Fig. 33.5).

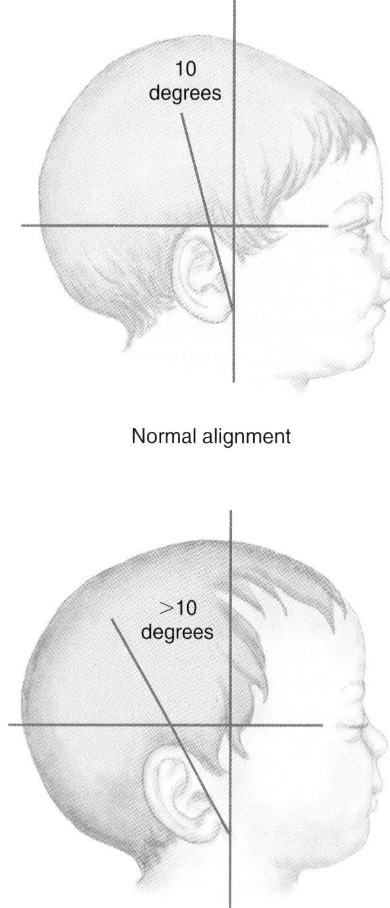


**FIG 33.5** The child's ears are inspected for alignment. Low-set ears could indicate an intellectual disability or renal anomalies.

The functions of cranial nerve V (trigeminal nerve) and cranial nerve VII (facial nerve) are evaluated during assessment of the face. Cranial nerve V is evaluated by observing chewing or sucking, which demonstrates the strength of the temporomandibular joint, and by touching the child's forehead and cheeks with a piece of cotton. The child should move the head or bat the object away. Cranial nerve VII is evaluated by asking a child to frown, smile, or make a face while the examiner observes for symmetry of movement. Having the child puff out the cheeks or whistle also allows the examiner to evaluate cranial nerve VII (Jarvis, 2012).

## Nose, Mouth, and Throat

### Nose

The examiner should wear gloves when doing the nasal examination, noting any drainage coming from the nose and describing the amount, color, and consistency.

The external nose is inspected and palpated. Patency can be determined by occluding one nostril and having the child sniff, and then repeating on the other side. The external nose is observed for symmetry, deformity, inflammation, or skin lesions. The "allergic salute," frequent wiping of the nose because of drainage, produces a transverse crease on the child's nose and is suggestive that the child has allergies. The entire external nose is palpated for septal deviation or other deformities. The sense of smell is mediated by cranial nerve I. This function can be evaluated by having the child close the eyes, occlude one nostril, and identify familiar odors, such as cinnamon, peppermint, orange, and cherry.

The nasal cavity can be examined by inserting the short, wide-tipped speculum on the otoscope into the nasal vestibule, with precautions taken to not put pressure on the nasal septum. The nasal mucosa is inspected for color and moisture. The nasal mucosa is normally smooth and moist, with a bright pink color. In children with allergies, the mucosa is pale and appears boggy. With infectious diseases (viral or bacterial), the mucosa is erythematous and swollen; the nasal drainage may be yellow or green. The nasal septum is examined for intactness and for any deviation.

The *frontal* and *maxillary sinuses* are inspected and palpated (Fig. 33.6). The areas over the sinuses are examined for color and swelling. Puffiness and redness over the sinuses and dark circles under the eyes may indicate an inflammatory process in children. The frontal sinuses are palpated by pressing over the sinuses below the eyebrow. The maxillary sinuses are palpated by pressing upward with the thumbs under the maxillary bones.

### Mouth and Throat

Assessment of the mouth in a young child should be performed at the end of the physical examination because it can cause anxiety. The examination should proceed from the anterior structures to the internal structures of the mouth.

The *philtrum,* the little notch between the nose and upper lip, should be intact. In children with dysmorphic features, the philtrum is absent or shallow.

The examiner should wear gloves when doing the oral examination. A tongue blade and a penlight assist with visualization of the oral cavity. When the child opens his or her mouth, the examiner evaluates mouth odors. The mouth and internal structures are examined by inspection, palpation, and smell.

Lips are inspected for symmetry, color, moisture, cracking, and the presence of any lesions. The alveolar frenulum, which attaches the lips to the gums, should be intact. The lips are palpated to identify any masses.

The *buccal mucosa* is examined by holding the cheeks open with a tongue blade and observing for color, nodules, and lesions. Significant mouth odors should be noted. For many children, this part of the examination can be unpleasant. To facilitate the child's cooperation, the examiner may want to demonstrate on a doll or on the parent or allow the child to place the tongue blade in the parent's mouth. The buccal mucosa should be pink, smooth, and moist. Dark-skinned children may have patchy areas of hyperpigmentation. The opening of the *parotid gland* is found as a small dimple on the buccal mucosa opposite the upper second molar. The entire surface of the buccal mucosa is palpated for changes in consistency or masses.

Teeth are inspected for number, cavities, tooth formation, and occlusion. The number and characteristics of the teeth will change with growth and development (Fig. 33.7). The eruption of deciduous teeth begins around the sixth month of extrauterine life; all 20 deciduous

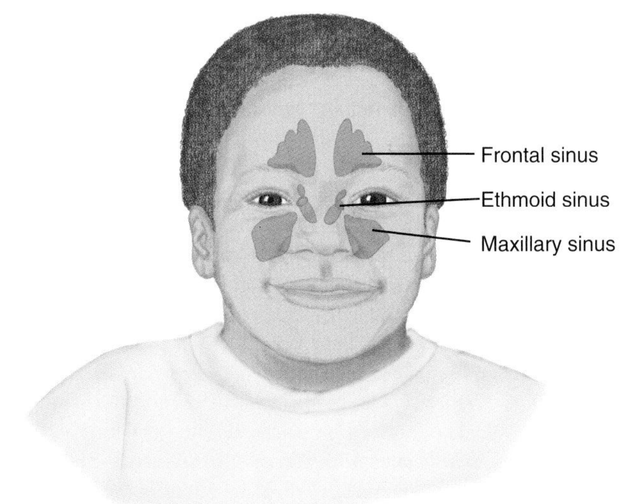


**FIG 33.6** The frontal, ethmoid, and maxillary sinuses.

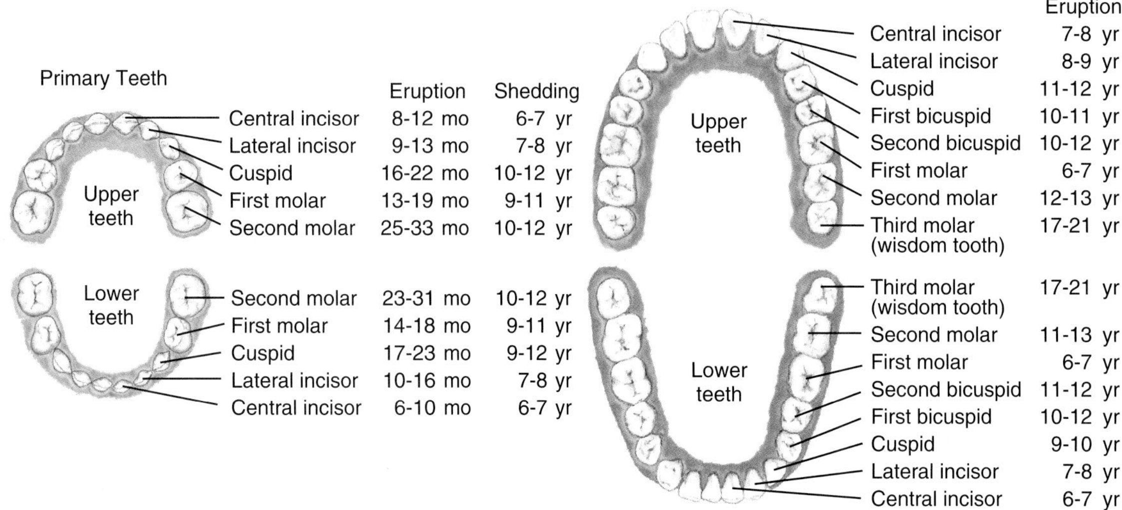


**FIG 33.7** Sequence of eruption of primary and secondary teeth. (Data from American Dental Association. Retrieved from http://www.ada.org.)

teeth are present by age 30 months. After having the child bite down, the examiner gently parts the lips and notes the position of the teeth. The upper teeth slightly override the lower teeth. The color and shape of each tooth should be noted. The crown is white, with some variation from person to person. Permanent teeth are larger and have a darker color than deciduous teeth. Brown or black discoloration of the teeth is usually caused by dental caries. Long-term use of certain medications (i.e., tetracycline, iron) can stain teeth. Excessive fluoride ingestion can cause a mottled appearance to the enamel of the permanent teeth. The shape of a tooth is determined by age, development, and the amount of wear.

## ! NURSING QUALITY ALERT

### *Normal Findings in Children*

- Small, firm, nontender, and shotty (freely palpable and very small) lymph nodes might be palpated.
- Tonsils of varying sizes; often larger in young children.
- Pupils of equal size, round, and reactive to light and accommodation (PERRLA).
- Pulses in upper and lower extremities; bilaterally symmetrical.

The gums *(gingivae)* are inspected and palpated for color and swelling. The gum surface has a pink, stippled appearance and feels firm. Some dark-skinned children have a dark-pigmented line along the gingival margin.

The floor of the mouth can be inspected by asking the child to lift the tongue to the roof of the mouth. The examiner observes the frenulum, the sublingual ridge, and Wharton's ducts, which lie on either side of the frenulum. The color of the floor of the mouth is pink.

The tongue is inspected and palpated. The dorsum of the tongue should appear dull red, moist, and glistening, with a white coat. The anterior portion of the tongue should have a slightly roughened appearance with papillae and small fissures. The tongue is palpated for indurations or ulcerations. While palpating the mouth of a young child, the examiner can prevent being bitten by holding the child's cheeks.

Cranial nerve XII *(hypoglossal nerve)* is examined by asking the child to stick out the tongue as though licking a lollipop and observe for any deviation of the tongue to one side. The examiner can determine the strength of the tongue by placing a finger to the side of the child's cheek and asking the child to press the tongue against the examiner's finger. The tongue should feel equally strong on the two sides.

To evaluate the hard palate, soft palate, and uvula, the examiner asks the child to tilt the head back. The examiner inspects the hard palate for shape and color. The hard palate is whitish and convex, with transverse rugae. The examiner palpates the hard palate for the height of the arch and for intactness. The examiner can allow the infant to suck on a gloved finger while palpating the hard palate to determine the strength of the sucking reflex. The soft palate is continuous with the hard palate and is concave and pinker. The uvula varies in length and thickness and is located in midline as a continuation of the soft palate. Cranial nerves IX *(glossopharyngeal nerve)* and X *(vagus nerve)* are evaluated at this time. The child is asked to say "ah"; normally, the soft palate and the uvula rise symmetrically and phonation of "ah" is understood.

A tongue blade is used to depress the tongue and observe the oropharynx. This action can be unpleasant for the child. To minimize discomfort, the examiner slides the tongue blade along the side of the tongue until it reaches the soft palate and then compresses the tongue to elicit the gag reflex (cranial nerve X) and observe the back of the throat. The tonsillar pillars are inspected with particular notation of size and color of tonsils. The tonsils are pink.

The size of tonsils varies; large tonsils are common in young children. Tonsils may have crypts where food particles collect. With inflammatory processes, the crypts can contain exudate. A child whose parents comment on the child's snoring or being awakened by snoring may have grossly enlarged tonsils. The posterior wall of the pharynx should be smooth and shiny, and pink in color; irregular spots of lymphatic tissue and small blood vessels may be observed (Ball et al., 2015).

## Eyes

The eyes are inspected, palpated, and evaluated for visual acuity and extraocular muscle function. A family history of eye disorders should be obtained at every well visit beginning with the newborn visit (AAP Committee on Practice and Ambulatory Medicine et al., 2016).

### External Eye

The external eye is evaluated for position and placement (Fig. 33.8). The examiner notes whether the eyes are set wide apart or close together. Epicanthal folds are seen in Asian children and in some non-Asian children as well. The slant of the eyes is determined by drawing an imaginary line across the inner canthi (see Fig. 33.8).

The eyebrows are inspected for symmetry and hair growth and eyelashes for even distribution. The *lacrimal apparatus* is assessed by asking the child to look down. The outer part of the upper lid is palpated along the bony orbit for any discomfort, swelling, or redness. The *punctum* (tear duct) on the inner canthus is palpated for obstruction in the infant.

The eye globe is palpated for firmness and can be gently pushed into the orbit without causing discomfort. Palpation of the eye can cause anxiety in small children and should not be done unless there is a serious concern about the size of the eye.

*Eyelids* are inspected for color, swelling, discharge, and lesions. The position of the eyelids on the globe should be noted. With the eyelids open, the upper lid normally falls below the superior limbus but does not cover any of the pupil. The lower lids normally fall just at the inferior limbus. The limbus is the point where the sclera of the eye meets the color portion of the iris. When closed, the eyelids approximate each other completely, without tremor, **fasciculations**, or tics.

The *conjunctiva* has two portions to evaluate. The palpebral portion of the conjunctiva lines the lids. The palpebral conjunctiva is examined by pulling down as the child looks up. It is normally clear, with a pink color, and several small blood vessels may be visible. The upper lid can be inspected by everting the upper eyelid over a cotton-tipped applicator. Eversion of the upper eyelid is not normally done because eye manipulation may cause apprehension in a child. The bulbar portion of the conjunctiva is transparent and lies over the sclera, allowing the white of the sclera to be clearly visible.

The following anterior structures of the eye are inspected: sclerae, cornea and lens, anterior chamber, and irises. The sclerae are white. The sclerae of dark-skinned children can have gray-blue or "muddy" color variations. Some dark-skinned children have small brown macules around the limbus (where the iris meets the sclera). These variations are normal. The corneas are clear, transparent, and very sensitive. Shining a light obliquely across the cornea highlights any abnormal irregularities on the corneal surface. The examiner illuminates the anterior chamber by shining a light across the eye from the temporal side to illuminate the entire iris without producing a shadow. The irises are round and contain muscle fibers that contract or expand in response to light. The pigmentation of the irises is unique for each individual. The two irises are similar in color but may exhibit some variation.

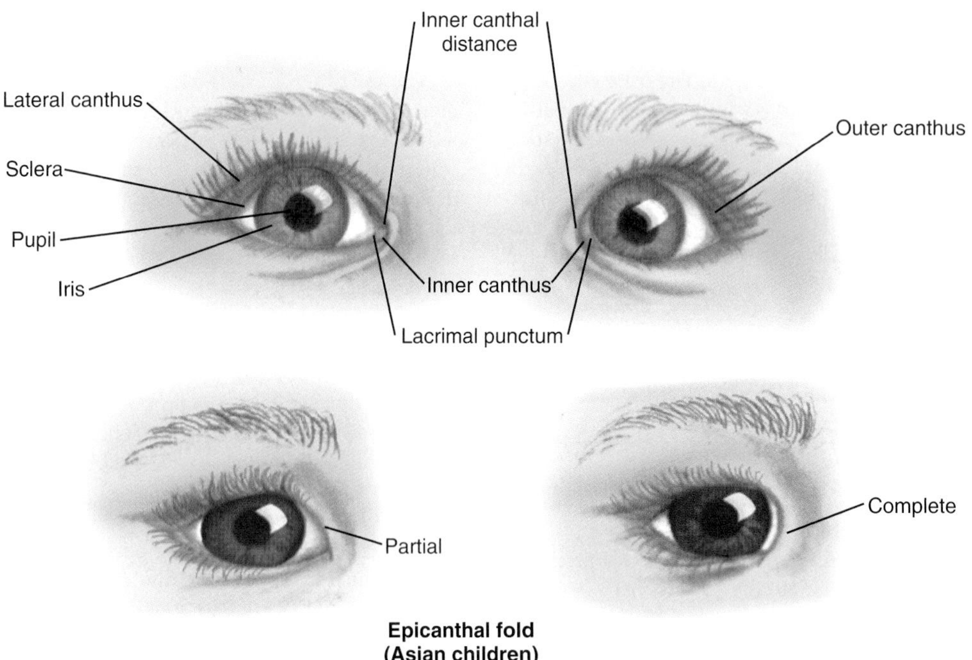


**FIG 33.8** External structures of the eye.

Pupils appear round, regular, and of equal size in the two eyes. The *pupillary light reflex* is tested by darkening the room and asking the child to gaze into the distance. A light is brought from the side (temporally), and the examiner notes the change in the size of the pupil. Shining a light directly into a pupil causes the pupil to constrict (direct light reflex). The procedure is repeated while the opposite eye is observed. The opposite eye constricts (consensual light reflex) in response to the light shone in the first eye. Pupils should constrict at equal speeds and to the same degree.

Pupil size should be the same in both eyes. In some children, pupils of unequal size are normal, but in general, unequal pupils call for a consideration of central nervous system injury. Asking the child to focus on a distant object can test accommodation. The pupils normally dilate. An object such as a puppet or a finger brought into the line of vision approximately 10 cm from the nose should cause pupillary constriction and convergence of the axes of the eyes (Ball et al., 2015).

### Ophthalmoscopic Examination

The ophthalmoscopic examination requires a cooperative child, practice, and patience. Lights in the room should be dim. Most children enjoy playing with the light of the "flashlight," and having them watch the light as the examiner moves it around the room facilitates cooperation. Minimally, all practitioners view the red reflex, but the procedure requires demonstration and practice. When the ophthalmoscope is placed in front of the pupil and the light hits the lens, a red color is reflected from the retina to the examiner. The retina, choroid, optic disc, macula, fovea centralis, and retinal vessels are also visible with the ophthalmoscope.

### Binocular Vision and Strabismus

Extraocular muscle function is evaluated to test binocular vision and the presence of strabismus. Strabismus, or "crossed eyes," is the abnormal or incomplete development of binocular visual alignment. Three tests are performed: the corneal light reflex (Hirschberg) test, field-of-vision test, and cover/uncover (alternate cover) test.

***Corneal light reflex test.*** The corneal light reflex is assessed by shining a light directly onto the irises from a distance of approximately 40.5 cm (16 inches). The reflection of the light should appear in exactly the same spot on both eyes. If the light falls off center in one eye, the eyes are malaligned. Children with *epicanthal folds*—vertical folds that partially or completely cover the inner canthi (see Fig. 33.7)—can give a false impression of malalignment (pseudostrabismus).

***Field-of-vision test.*** The six cardinal fields of vision are tested by holding the child's chin so that the head does not move and asking the child to follow a puppet or a familiar object held approximately 12 inches away from the face as the object is moved to each of the six cardinal positions. As the object is moved to the margins of each cardinal position, the examiner holds it momentarily in that position before proceeding back to the center. The eyes will track in a parallel fashion to each position. As the eyes are in the margins of each position, the examiner can note *end-stage nystagmus,* a gentle oscillation of the eye, which is considered normal. Children younger than 2 to 3 years may not be able to cooperate with this test.

***Tests for eye muscle function.*** Testing for extraocular muscle function in children younger than 5 years is critical to identifying any muscle imbalance so that it can be corrected at an early age to preserve vision. Extraocular muscle function evaluates three cranial nerves: cranial nerve VI, the *abducent* nerve, which innervates the lateral rectus muscle (responsible for abducting the eye); cranial nerve IV, the *trochlear* nerve, which innervates the superior oblique muscle (responsible for downward and inward movement of the eye); and cranial nerve III, the *oculomotor* nerve, which innervates the superior, inferior, and medial rectus and the inferior oblique muscles (Ball et al., 2015).

The cover/uncover test is used to detect deficits in binocular vision by interrupting fusion of the eyes as they gaze at a fixed object. One eye is covered with an opaque card while the child stares straight ahead, at which time the examiner observes the uncovered eye. A steady, fixed gaze is maintained by the uncovered eye. Next the covered eye is uncovered and observed for any movement; it should continue to stare straight ahead (Fig. 33.9). The procedure is repeated with the opposite

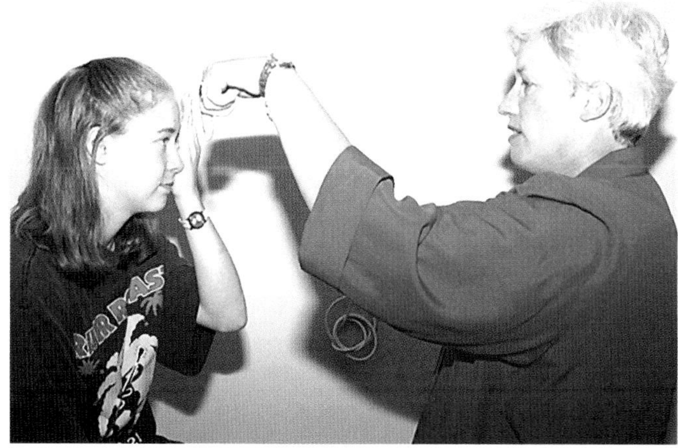

FIG 33.9 The cover/uncover test detects small degrees of eye-alignment deviation. With one eye covered, the child gazes straight ahead with the uncovered eye. The cover is then removed, and the eye should continue to stare straight ahead. Movement in either eye suggests muscle weakness. Extraocular muscle function is controlled by cranial nerves III, IV, and VI.

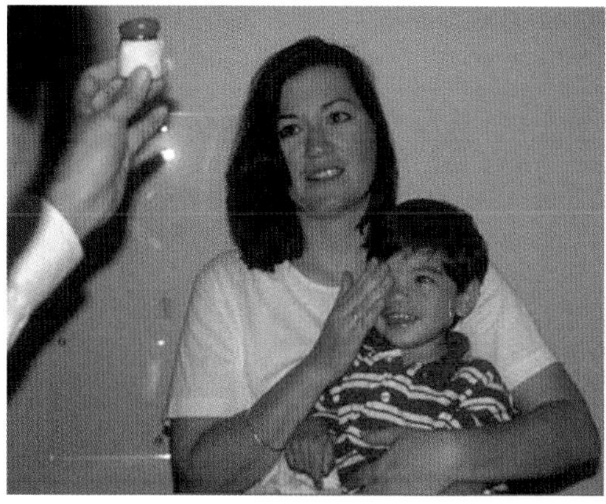

FIG 33.10 Visual fields (cranial nerve II) are tested in each eye separately. One eye is covered as the child stares straight ahead. An object is slowly moved from the side of the head into the field of vision. The child says "now" upon first seeing the object. (From Liu, Grant T., Volpe, Nicholas J., Galetta, Steven L., (2010). *Neuro-Ophthalmology: Diagnosis and Management* (2nd ed., pp. 7–36). London-Wall: Saunders.)

eye. Any movement in either eye in the process of covering or uncovering may indicate muscle weakness.

### Peripheral Vision

Visual fields are evaluated in older children to identify peripheral vision. The examiner's face is positioned directly in front and on the level of the child, approximately 2 feet away. The child's visual fields should roughly mirror those of the examiner. The examiner covers one eye and has the child mimic by covering the opposite eye. A puppet or some other test object is slowly brought from the periphery into the child's field of vision. The object should come from a position slightly behind the child's head, and the child is asked to say "now" when the object is in view (Fig. 33.10). Testing for visual acuity and visual fields evaluates cranial nerve II, the optic nerve, which mediates vision.

### Visual Acuity

Visual acuity can be difficult to evaluate in a young child. Acuity develops over time, and evaluation requires the child's cooperation. The infant from birth to age 1 or 2 months gazes at black-and-white contrasting figures and faces. At age 4 weeks or older, an infant fixates on a brightly colored object and follows it.

Visual acuity testing for all children beginning at age 3 years (if child is able to cooperate) is recommended (AAP Committee on Practice and Ambulatory Medicine et al., 2016). Items needed for evaluating a child's visual acuity are an eye cover and vision charts (Box 33.8). The chart chosen is determined by the child's age and development.

Visual acuity tests that have evidence to support reliability and validity for preschool children include the Lea chart, and the HOTV matching test (Donahue et al., 2016). The U.S. Preventive Services Task Force (2011b) recommends screening for all children for visual impairment at least once between the ages of 3 and 5 years, to detect the presence of amblyopia or its risk factors.

Preschool children can be tested using the HOTV chart at 10 feet (see Box 33.8). A card printed with *H, O, T,* and *V* is given to the child to hold. One eye is covered, and the child is instructed to match the letters on the held card with the chart at 10 feet using the uncovered eye. The child holds the card, or it is placed on a table directly in front of the child. Screening is begun at the 20/50 line for children younger than 4 years, the 20/40 line for children 4 to 5 years, and the 20/30 line for older children (Donahue et al., 2016). The child passes the screening if the child correctly identifies four of the five symbols.

Older children's visual acuity can be tested by use of the Snellen chart, placed on a wall 20 feet away from the child. The chart should have no glare and should be well illuminated. No other materials

#### BOX 33.8 Types of Eye Charts

*Snellen chart:* A standardized chart with graduated letters for testing far vision of children at 20 feet. Used with children older than 6 years.

*Lea chart:* A chart with four different symbols. Used for preschool-age children. Designed for use at 10 feet.

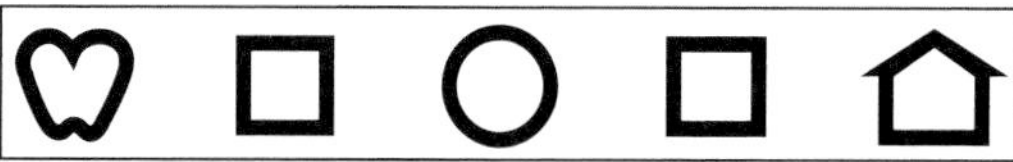

*HOTV chart:* A standardized chart with the letters *H, O, T,* and *V* in graduated sizes. Designed for use at 10 feet with children aged 3 to 6 years.

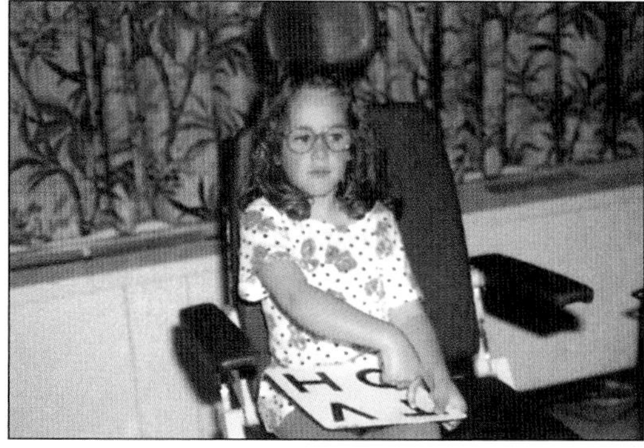

The letters *H, O, T,* and *V* are presented at a distance, and the child points to the corresponding letter on the card resting on her lap.*

*Ishihara chart:* A series of polychromatic cards with a pattern of dots printed against a background of many-colored dots. Designed to test for color vision between ages 4 and 6 years.

*From Goldbloom, R.B. (2011). *Pediatric clinical skills* (4th ed.). Philadelphia: Saunders.

should be around or near the chart. Both eyes are tested together first, and then each eye is tested separately. If the child has corrective lenses, the procedure should be repeated with the corrective lenses on. Unless the child is known to have very poor vision, testing is begun at the line on the chart for 40 feet. To determine at what level the child cannot see, the examiner finds the distance at which the child misses half plus one of the symbols on a line of the chart. The visual acuity is then designated as the smallest line at which the child is able to identify more than half the symbols on the line. For corrective lenses, the examiner notes the last date the child was examined for a prescription. Findings are recorded by noting the distance of the line correctly read for both eyes (i.e., right eye 20/20, left eye 20/20). This annotation means that the child has correctly interpreted the letters on the chart for 20 feet at a distance of 20 feet, which matches what the average child can see at that distance. If the child correctly identifies the letters on the line labeled *40 feet,* that child can see at 20 feet what the average child can see at 40 feet (20/40). Visual acuity changes with age and varies according to the test used. Normal ranges are as follows:

- *Birth:* fixates on objects (8 to 12 inches), 20/100 to 20/150
- *4 months:* 20/50 to 20/80
- *1 year:* 20/40 to 20/70
- *4 years:* 20/40 to 20/50
- *5 years:* 20/20 to 20/30

### Color Vision

Color vision deficit, less correctly termed *color blindness,* is an inherited recessive X-linked trait that, in varying degrees, can affect the child's ability to discern traffic lights, brake lights, and color-coordinated clothing. Color discrimination occurs through integration of information from the cone pigments in the retinal layers of the eye. The genes for some colors are located on the X chromosome, and because boys have only one X chromosome, they are more likely to have color vision deficit. Color vision deficit can affect learning if the learning is color related. The condition is very rare in females but affects 8% to 10% of males.

Color vision is evaluated by Ishihara charts—a series of polychromatic cards. These cards have a pattern of colored pictures embedded in the charts. Children between ages 4 and 8 years are tested once and are asked to touch or identify the embedded patterns. A child with this deficit cannot see the patterns against the field of color.

## Ears

Assessment of the ears includes inspection and palpation of the external ear, examination of the internal ear with the otoscope, and testing for hearing acuity.

### External Ear

The external ear is inspected and palpated. Ear placement and position are evaluated during assessment of the face (see Fig. 33.5), but the external ear is also examined for any malformations or unusual markings (Fig. 33.11). Any discharge coming from the auditory meatus is noted, and its amount and characteristics are described. Soft, yellow-brown cerumen (ear wax) is normally seen in the external auditory meatus.

The bony prominence of the mastoid process behind the ear is palpated for tenderness. The auricles are gently pulled to determine whether this action causes discomfort.

### Otoscopic Examination

The *tympanic membrane* is examined with the otoscope (Fig. 33.12). Many children are apprehensive about this examination. If necessary, a small child is positioned on the parent's lap, and the parent secures the child's arms. The examiner uses the largest speculum that will fit comfortably into the ear canal. In a child younger than 3 years, the ear canal is straightened by pulling the pinna of the ear down and back. If a child is 3 years or older, the pinna is pulled up and back. As much of the canal as possible should be visible before the speculum is inserted into the auditory meatus.

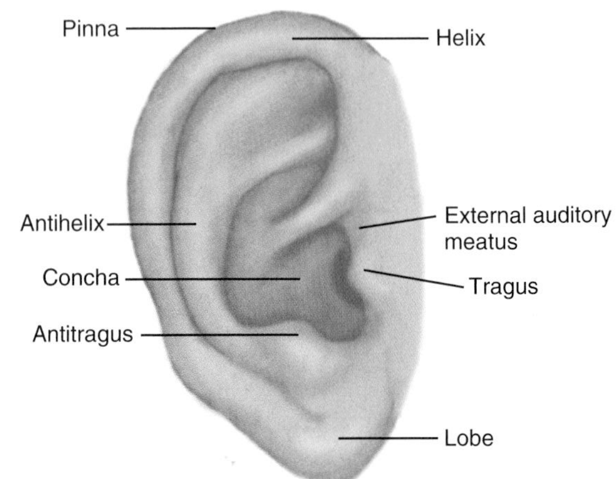


**FIG 33.11** Landmarks of the external ear.

The canal is inspected for any lesions and for cerumen. The tympanic membrane is inspected for landmarks, color, and mobility. A puff of air is injected into the canal with an insufflation bulb, and the tympanic membrane is observed for movement. Normally, the tympanic membrane moves inward with a slight puff and outward with a slight release.

### Hearing Acuity

***Infant assessment.*** Newborn infants born in a hospital are tested for response of the acoustic nerve at the time of birth and before discharge. In an older infant, hearing is assessed by asking the parent to speak to the infant from behind and observing the infant's response to the parent's voice. The examiner can stand behind the infant and ring a bell or make a sound the infant is familiar with and observe the infant turning to locate the sound. A very young infant, younger than 4 months, may demonstrate a startle reflex to loud sounds.

***Preschool and school-age assessment by audiometry.*** In preschool and school-age children, the audiometer gives a precise (quantitative) assessment of the ability to hear. The child is placed in a soundproof room and is asked to identify tones of different frequencies played at a specific decibel level (usually 20 db) (American Academy of Audiology [AAA], 2011).With the audiometer, two tests are used to evaluate hearing: the sweep test and the pure tone hearing test. The *sweep test* is used to screen for hearing losses. The *pure tone test* is used to determine the exact extent of the hearing loss. If a child misses a tone, the test should be repeated, but no more than four times (AAA, 2011). Tympanometry, which measures middle ear pressure, can confirm hearing loss, especially that due to middle ear effusion (see Chapter 55).

***Preschool, school-age, and adolescent assessment: the whisper test.*** The examiner stands approximately 0.6 m (2 feet) behind the child (to prevent lip reading); then exhales and whispers a series of three numbers and letters (i.e., 4-K-2). If the child correctly repeats the letter/number series, hearing is considered normal. Adaptations for preschool children may be necessary; the examiner whispers a command such as "Please put the toy on the floor" and then observes to see if the child follows the command, indicating normal hearing.

***Conduction tests (tuning fork hearing tests).*** Tuning fork tests are qualitative tests that determine the ability to hear by air conduction

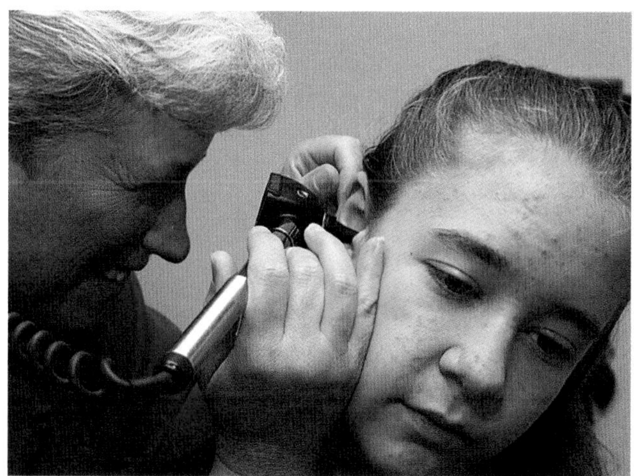

To straighten the ear canal of a child older than 3 years, the nurse pulls the child's pinna up and back.

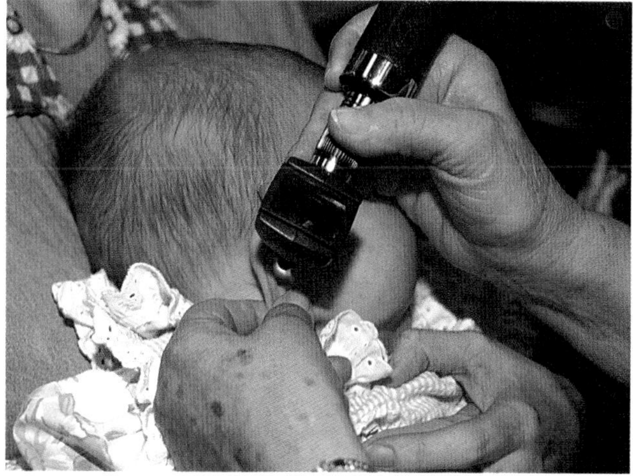

For children younger than 3 years, the pinna is pulled down and back.

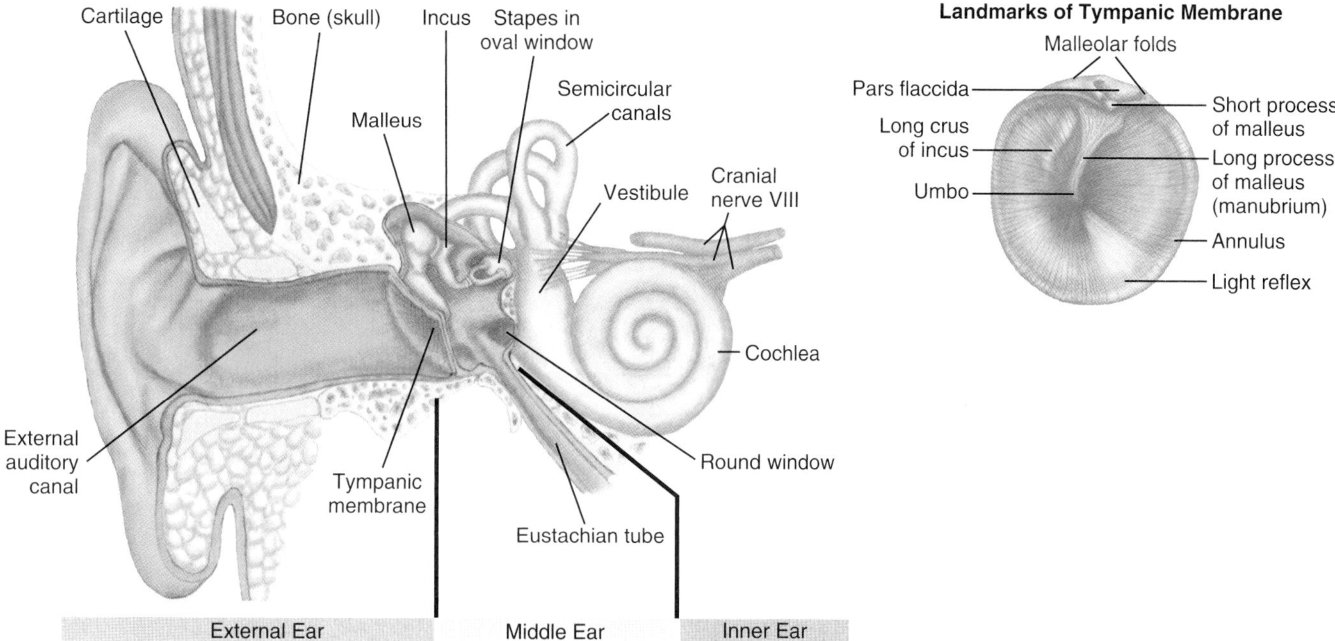


**FIG 33.12** Inspection of the tympanic membrane with the otoscope. The auditory canal is inspected before the otoscope is inserted to see the child's tympanic membrane.

and by bone conduction. In the normal child, air conduction of sound is greater than bone conduction. The *Rinne hearing test* is used to determine whether air conduction is greater than bone conduction. The *Weber hearing test* determines the child's ability to hear by bone conduction. Testing the child's hearing evaluates cranial nerve VIII *(acoustic nerve)*.

## Thorax and Lungs

Assessment of the thorax and lungs consists of inspection, palpation, percussion, and auscultation, although not necessarily in that order, to optimize the accuracy of findings. For example, in a sleeping infant, the nurse is wise to seize the opportunity to inspect and auscultate breath sounds. To assist with localizing findings on the thorax, anatomic landmarks such as the ribs and intercostal spaces are identified, and imaginary lines are drawn on the surface (Fig. 33.13, p. 734).

Location of lung tissue depends on the child's age and development. In an infant, lung tissue on the anterior chest can be located from the apex, above the clavicle, to the level of the fifth rib in the midclavicular line. By age 6 years, lung tissue is assessed from the apex to the level of the sixth rib in the midclavicular line. Laterally, lung tissue is assessed from the axilla to the level of the eighth rib. Posteriorly, lungs are assessed from the level of the first thoracic vertebra to the tenth thoracic vertebra.

### Inspection

The child's shirt or clothing covering the chest is removed. In adolescent females, the breasts should be kept covered and exposed only when necessary. Inspection of the chest includes observing the child for any cough, stridor, grunting, hoarseness, snoring, wheezing, and type and amount of any sputum, if present. Respiratory rate and pattern are observed. In young children and infants, breathing is more diaphragmatic or abdominal (see Table 33.1 for the effect of age on vital signs). The chest wall should expand symmetrically during respiration. Respirations should be easy, regular, and without apparent distress. Rapid respirations, retractions, nasal flaring, and head bobbing may indicate respiratory difficulty.

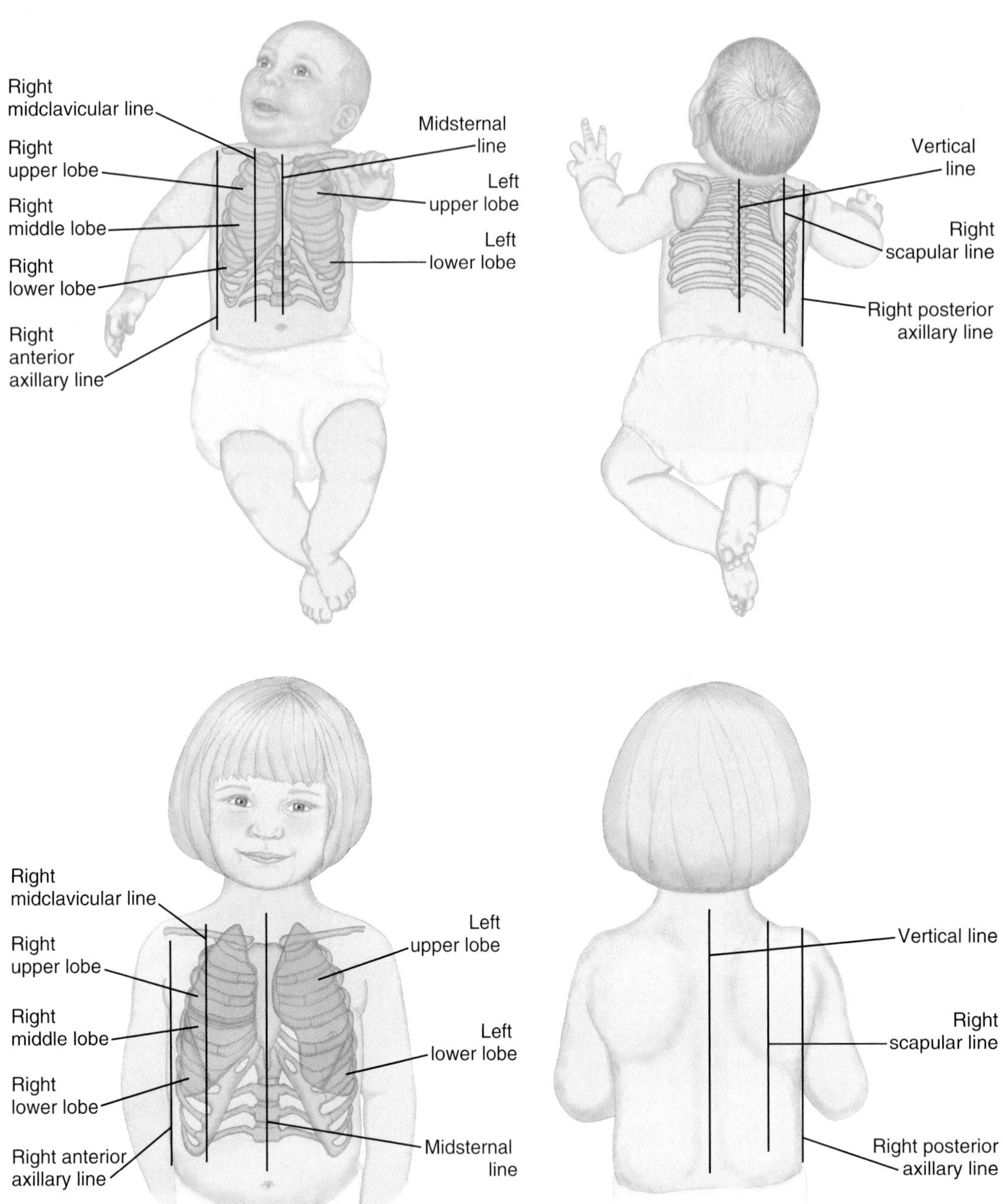


**FIG 33.13** Anatomic landmarks of the thorax in infants and children.

Thoracic configuration is evaluated by determining the shape and symmetry of the chest from the front, sides, and back (Fig. 33.14, p. 735). In infants and young children the thorax is more rounded. Some children have "Harrison groove," a horizontal line in the rib cage extending from the sternum to the midaxillary line. Two common alterations in structure in the anterior chest are *pectus carinatum* (pigeon chest) and *pectus excavatum* (funnel chest). *Scoliosis,* a lateral S-shaped curvature of the thoracic and lumbar vertebrae, is a common alteration of the posterior chest that may cause impaired pulmonary function.

## Palpation

Palpation of the chest begins with the posterior chest. To alleviate fear in a young child, the examiner should stand in a position that allows the child to see the examiner at all times. The posterior chest is palpated for areas of tenderness, tactile **fremitus**, and chest excursion.

To palpate for tenderness, the examiner touches the entire thorax with the palmar aspects of the fingers. This process elicits any points of discomfort or pain. The examiner notes any masses or edema (Fig. 33.15, p. 735). The presence or absence of tactile fremitus, vibration felt on the chest wall when the child is crying or speaking, indicate airway alterations, and thus, must be assessed.

Percussion of the chest is performed by advanced practitioners to determine changes in sound produced by the density of the underlying tissues. Hyperresonance is normal in the infant and young child because of the thin chest wall.

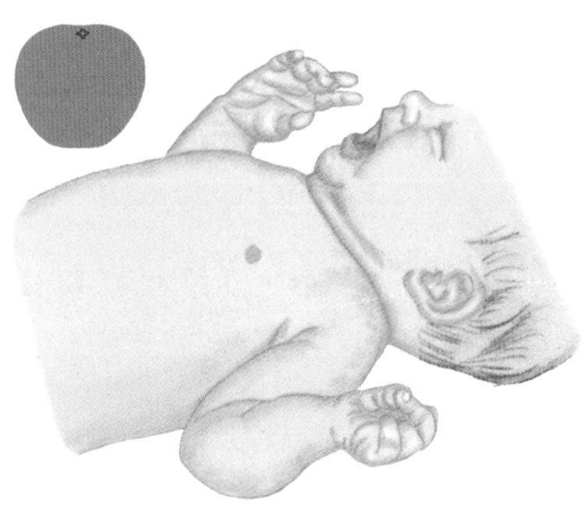

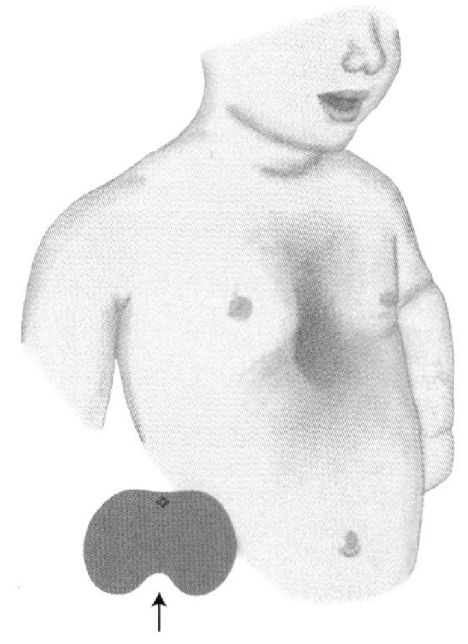

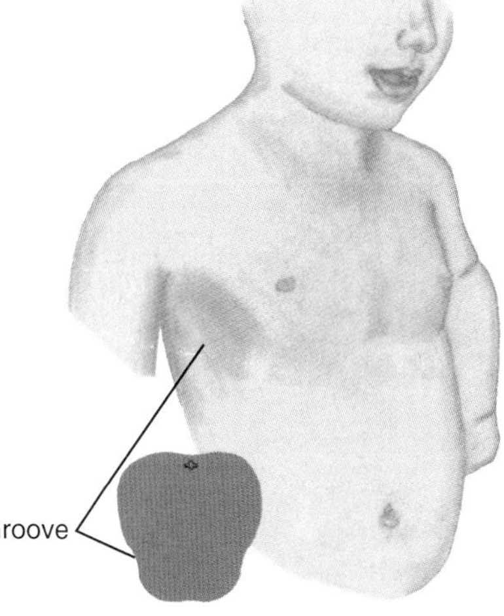


**Normal infant:** The chest of the normal infant is approximately round or barrel-shaped in cross section. A barrel chest in a child older than 6 years suggests a chronic pulmonary disease, such as asthma or cystic fibrosis.

**Funnel chest (pectus excavatum):** A funnel chest has a depression in the lower portion of the sternum. Compression of the heart and great vessels may cause murmurs.

**Pigeon chest (pectus carinatum):** In pigeon chest, the sternum is displaced anteriorly, increasing the anteroposterior diameter. Grooves in the chest wall accentuate the deformity.

FIG 33.14 Common alterations in chest configuration.

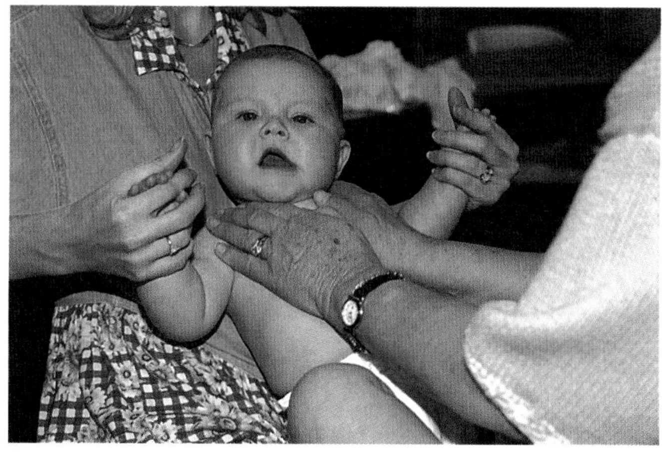

FIG 33.15 To identify areas of fremitus, tenderness, symmetry, and depth and equality of expansion, the nurse palpates the child's posterior and anterior chest. When palpating any area, warm hands increase the child's comfort. (Courtesy The University of Texas at Arlington College of Nursing, Arlington, TX.)

### Auscultation

Auscultating the chest with a stethoscope determines the characteristics of breath sounds. Breath sounds heard with the stethoscope are made by the flow of air through the respiratory tree and are characterized by intensity, pitch, quality, and duration.

It is best to listen to breath sounds with the child sitting upright if possible. Infants and toddlers can be held in the parent's lap; have the parent assist with removal of clothing and positioning of the child. The examiner's position is on the side of the child, allowing the child to observe the examiner's movements. Before touching the chest, the examiner allows the young child to hold or play with the stethoscope and warms the stethoscope before placing it on the child's chest. The head of the stethoscope is cleaned with alcohol between patients.

An anxious or frightened child might cry during this part of the examination. Distracting the child or having the young child focus on another activity can facilitate listening. For the inconsolable child, the examiner listens to breath sounds between cries. If the young child is sleeping or comfortable in the parent's arms, the examiner listens to the chest first, before proceeding to the rest of the examination.

For listening to the posterior thorax, the child is positioned with the head bent forward and hands folded in front. Having the child raise the arms overhead while sitting erect allows the examiner to listen laterally. To auscultate the anterior chest, have the child sit erect with the shoulders back (Fig. 33.16, p. 736).

The examiner begins on the posterior thorax and has the child open the mouth and breathe in and out while the examiner listens with the diaphragm of the stethoscope. Having the young child blow bubbles, pretend to blow out birthday candles, or blow a tissue increases breath sounds. Compressing the hand holding the stethoscope on the chest wall while placing the other hand on the opposite side of the chest accentuates expiration, making it easier to hear end-expiratory sounds (e.g., wheezes). Having the child inhale deeply and then blow the breath out forcibly assists with identification of adventitious breath sounds. Lung auscultation follows a zigzag pattern, comparing sounds from right to left. The usual sequence for listening to breath sounds is posterior chest, right and left lateral chest, and anterior chest (Fig. 33.17, p. 736); however, adjustments can be made to encourage the child's cooperation.

### Adventitious Breath Sounds

In addition to normal breath sounds, *adventitious sounds* may be audible with the stethoscope. Table 33.2 describes the origin and characteristics of adventitious sounds. Adventitious sounds are additional sounds heard in an abnormal clinical state. They are described by their quality. The examiner notes whether they are continuous or discontinuous and where they occur in the respiratory phase. The effects of coughing are also noted. When adventitious sounds are heard, they are described as to location, timing, and intensity.

## Heart

The techniques for assessing the heart are inspection, palpation, and auscultation. The sequence of this examination depends on the age, growth, and development of the child being examined. For an infant or

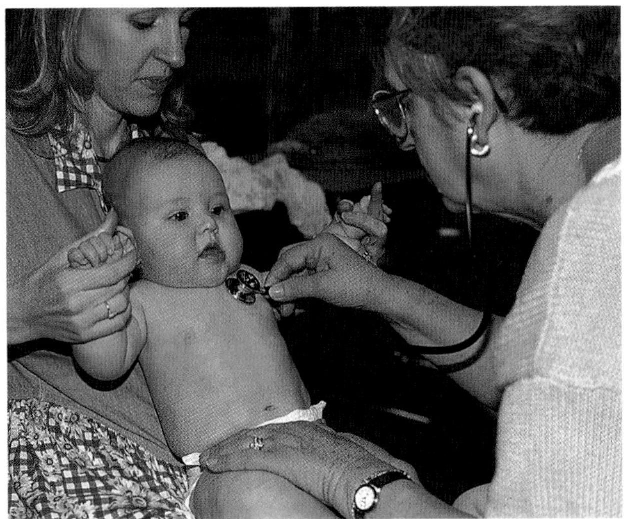

Infants and toddlers can be held sitting upright in the parent's lap while the nurse listens to breath sounds.

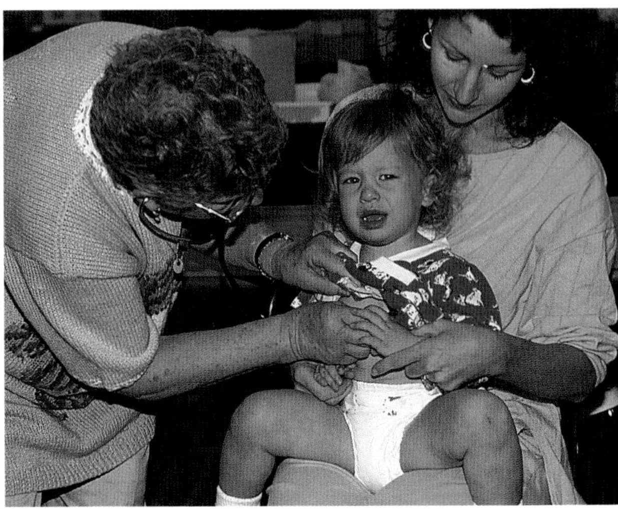

If the child is upset, the examiner may have to listen to breath sounds between cries. Keeping this child in the comfort of her mother's arms lessens distress.

**FIG 33.16** Auscultation is most easily done when the child is quiet, so this part of the examination is best performed first if the child is quiet or asleep. To allay fears, the child can play with the stethoscope first and can be distracted with a toy while the nurse is listening. Warming the stethoscope bell increases comfort. (Courtesy The University of Texas at Arlington College of Nursing, Arlington, TX.)

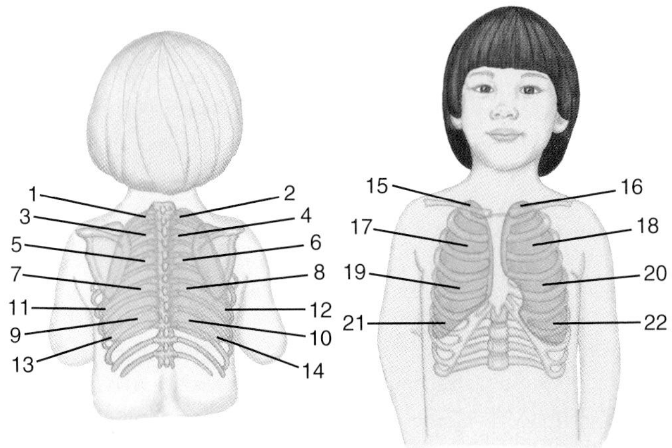


**FIG 33.17** Sequence for listening to breath sounds.

young child, the examiner might want to listen to the child's heart while the parent is holding the child, before doing other parts of the examination. Infants and children have varying degrees of dependence on parents and may be fearful of the examination. Percussion of the heart indicates primarily the size and shape of the heart and is not routinely done. The heart is assessed with the child three different positions: supine, left lateral recumbent, and sitting while leaning forward slightly.

## Inspection

The anterior chest is systematically inspected, with special attention paid to the following five areas: second right intercostal space (aortic area), second left intercostal space (pulmonic area), left sternal border (right ventricular area), fifth left intercostal space in the midclavicular line (apex), and just below the xiphoid process (epigastric area). The location of these areas will differ with a child's age (Fig. 33.18, p. 738). During infancy, the heart is more horizontal in the thorax, and the apex is one or two intercostal spaces above the fifth intercostal space and lateral to the midclavicular line. The examiner locates the second intercostal space by identifying the sternal angle. The second rib is attached to the sternum just below or at the sternal angle. The second intercostal space is below the second rib. Other ribs and intercostal spaces are identified by their relationship to the second rib.

The precordium (anterior chest overlying the heart and great vessels) is inspected for *bulges, lifts, heaves,* and *apical impulse.* The apical impulse is seen as a pulsation of the anterior chest wall every time the heart beats. The location of the apical impulse will change gradually as the child matures, and by age 7 years, it can be seen at the fifth intercostal space in the midclavicular line.

## Palpation

The examiner palpates the precordium with the fingertips for the presence of any pulsations at each individual area (see Fig. 33.18). The examiner locates the apical pulse, sometimes identified as the *point of maximal impulse (PMI),* or the point where the light tapping of the heart is felt the best. The location of the PMI varies with age. In a child younger than 7 years, the PMI is located in the fourth intercostal space, lateral to the midclavicular line. The PMI in a child older than 7 years is located in the fifth intercostal space in the midclavicular line. Using the palmar aspect of the hand to feel for *thrills* (palpable vibrations of the heart), the examiner then palpates each area of the precordium.

## Auscultation

The heart is auscultated by listening both with the bell and with the diaphragm of the stethoscope as the child is lying supine, in a left lateral recumbent position, and sitting up. To auscultate heart sounds, the examiner uses a systematic approach. Sounds heard with the stethoscope are predominantly produced with the closing of the heart valves. The four traditional areas for listening to heart sounds are the aortic valve area in the second right intercostal space, the pulmonic valve area in the second left intercostal space, the tricuspid valve area in the left lower sternal border, and the mitral valve area in the fifth intercostal space at the left midclavicular line (see Fig. 33.18). The position for listening to these areas depends on the age of the child. It is best to listen to heart sounds by inching the stethoscope across the

**TABLE 33.2 Origin and Characteristics of Adventitious Breath Sounds**

| Sound | Description | Mechanism | Clinical Example |
|---|---|---|---|
| **Discontinuous Sounds** | | | |
| Crackles (rales, crepitations); heard when fluid is in airways | Discontinuous, high-pitched, short, crackling, popping sounds heard during inspiration and not cleared by coughing. You can simulate this sound by rolling a strand of hair between your fingers near your ear or by moistening your thumb and index finger and separating them near your ear. Described as discrete (short), discontinuous. | Inhaled air collides with previously deflated airways; airways suddenly pop open, creating crackling sound as gas pressures between the two compartments equalize. | *Late inspiratory* crackles occur with restrictive disease: pneumonia, congestive heart failure, and interstitial fibrosis. *Early inspiratory* crackles occur with obstructive disease: chronic bronchitis and asthma. |
| Pleural friction rub | A very superficial sound that is coarse and low-pitched; it has a grating quality, as if two pieces of leather were being rubbed together. A pleural friction rub can sound just like crackles that are closer to the ear. It sounds louder if you push the stethoscope harder into the chest wall. | Caused when pleurae become inflamed and lose their normal lubricating fluid. Their opposing roughened pleural surfaces rub together during respiration. This sound is heard best in the anterolateral wall, where lung mobility is greatest. | Pleuritis; accompanied by pain with breathing (Rub disappears after a few days if pleural fluid accumulates and separates pleurae.) |
| **Continuous Sounds** | | | |
| High-pitched wheeze heard with narrowing of the air passages from fluid, swelling, spasm, and tumors | High-pitched, musical squeaking sounds that predominate in expiration but may occur in both expiration and inspiration. Coughing frequently will change the character of the sound. | Air squeezed or compressed through passageways narrowed almost to closure by collapsing, swelling, secretions, or tumors. The passageway walls oscillate in apposition between the closed and barely open positions. The resulting sound is similar to that produced by a vibrating reed. | Obstructive lung disease such as asthma. |
| Low-pitched wheeze (sonorous rhonchi) | Low-pitched, musical snoring, moaning sounds. They are heard throughout the cycle, although they are more prominent on expiration and may clear somewhat with coughing. | Airflow obstruction as described by the vibrating reed mechanism. The pitch of the wheeze does not correlate with the size of the passageway that generates it. | Bronchitis |

NOTE: Although nothing in clinical practice seems to differ more than the nomenclature of adventitious sounds, most authorities concur on two categories: 1. Discontinuous, discrete crackling sounds and 2. Coarse or wheezing sounds.

precordium in a Z-shaped pattern, from the base of the heart across and down, or from the apex upward. All areas are auscultated with both the bell and the diaphragm of the stethoscope.

Sounds produced by the closing of the valves can be heard all over the precordium, so it is necessary to concentrate on one heart sound at a time. The heart sounds are divided into two components, the first heart sound ($S_1$) and the second heart sound ($S_2$), and are auscultated using the diaphragm of the stethoscope. $S_1$ is heard best at the apex of the heart in the tricuspid and mitral area, and $S_2$ is heard best at the base in the aortic and pulmonic area (see Fig. 33.18). $S_1$, phonetically described as *lub,* is produced by the closing of the mitral and tricuspid valves. $S_2$, phonetically described as *dub,* is produced by the closing of the aortic and pulmonic valves.

The physiologic splitting of $S_2$, an audible pause between the closing of the aortic and pulmonic valves, frequently heard in children of all ages, is considered normal. Splitting of $S_2$ can be heard best at the pulmonic area because ejection times on the right side of the heart are slightly longer than on the left side. Splitting of $S_2$ is greatest at the peak of inspiration and decreases or goes away during expiration.

The routine for assessing heart sounds follows this sequence:

1. Identify the rate and rhythm.
2. Identify $S_1$ and $S_2$.
3. Assess $S_1$ and $S_2$ separately to determine where they are best heard.
4. Listen for extra heart sounds.
5. Identify murmurs.

***Normal rate and rhythm.*** The normal rate of a child's heart is different at various ages (see Table 33.1). Children's heart rates often increase with inspiration and slow down during expiration. To decrease the irregular rhythm associated with respirations, the examiner has the child hold the breath as the examiner continues to listen to the heart.

***Extra heart sounds, including murmurs.*** Extra sounds (sounds heard over and above the normal heart sounds) are described as opening snaps, ejection clicks, midsystolic to late systolic clicks, and murmurs. Snaps and clicks are short, high-pitched sounds heard with valve disorders and do not vary with respirations. *Murmurs* are blowing, swooshing sounds that occur because of turbulence of the blood flow into, through, or out of the heart and are best heard with the bell of the stethoscope. Innocent or functional heart murmurs are frequently heard in children. Innocent murmurs occur during systole, are heard best along the left sternal border, do not radiate, and change with position change. To describe and classify extra heart sounds, the nurse needs advanced training and practice.

## Peripheral Vascular System

Arterial pulses are examined for decrease or absence of pulses. Pulses are palpated, with the examiner noting the rate, rhythm, elasticity of the vessel wall, and equal force of bilateral pulses. The pulse force should be symmetrical and should be the same for upper and lower extremities. Comparison of opposite pulses is necessary in children. The examiner compares one femoral pulse with the opposite radial

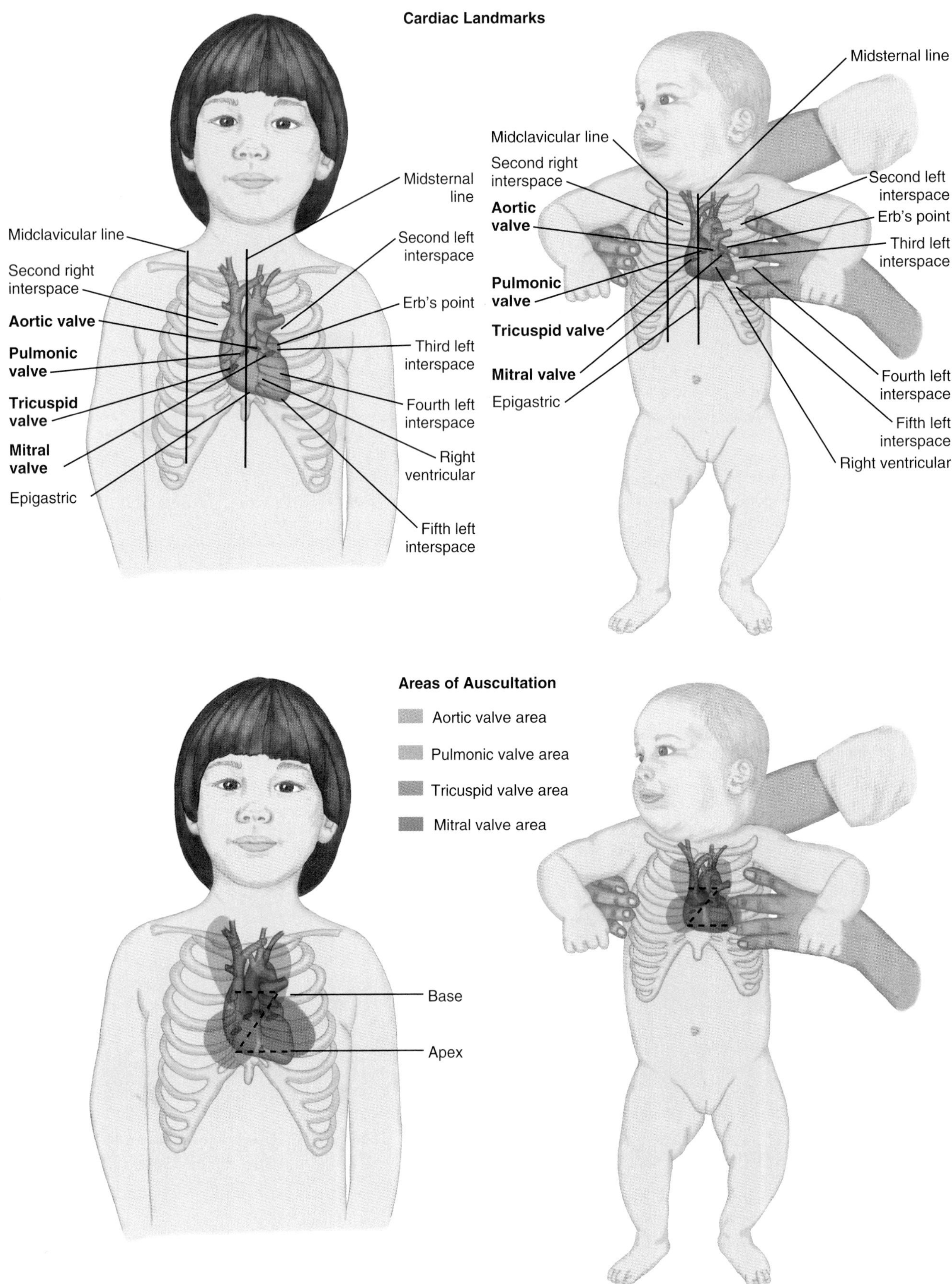


**FIG 33.18** Location of the heart within the thorax in the infant and the older child, showing landmarks and areas of auscultation.

pulse for equality and compares one lower extremity pulse with an upper extremity pulse for equality. A femoral pulse that is diminished (or absent), in comparison to the radial pulse, can be the sole indication of coarctation of the aorta in infants and children (see Chapter 46).

## Breast

The examiner inspects and palpates breast tissue. Developmental differences occur in response to circulating hormones and affect the appearance of breast tissue. In infants of both sexes, the breasts may appear engorged because of maternal estrogen crossing the placenta. *Thelarche,* or breast development, marks the beginning of puberty in preadolescent girls and can occur as early as age 7 years.

The examiner inspects the nipples for position and appearance. In infants, the nipple is flat and symmetrical with darker areolar pigmentation. In preadolescent and adolescent girls, the Tanner sexual maturity rating is used to evaluate developmental levels (see Table 9.1). The nipples should be symmetrical on the chest and should point in the same direction. Nipples can appear to be inverted or everted. An inverted nipple is significant if the inversion has occurred recently. The breast skin should be smooth and free of any dimpling. Some asymmetry is common during growth.

All adolescent girls should be taught how to do breast self-examination once they have reached menarche. Teaching self-examination to the adolescent and reinforcing its importance at every visit are important roles for the nurse. Many adolescents do not conduct breast self-examinations because of lack of knowledge or fear of finding something wrong. Once the adolescent is familiar with how her breasts look and feel, the natural and normal changes that occur in the breast as a result of hormonal fluctuations can be easily identified. The adolescent girl is taught to do breast self-examination 3 to 4 days after menses because the breasts usually are least tender and sensitive at that time.

The examiner uses the same technique to palpate the breast tissue and the axilla of the adolescent boy. In the male, the examiner expects to feel a thin layer of fatty tissue overlying the muscle. During puberty, some boys experience *gynecomastia,* an enlargement of breast tissue, felt as a smooth, firm, movable disk. It frequently affects only one breast and can be temporary.

## Abdomen

The child's comfort should be considered during the abdominal examination. Abdominal relaxation is enhanced if the child's bladder is empty, the examiner's hands are warm, and the child is positioned supine on the examining table with a pillow under the head and the knees flexed. For an infant or young child, most of the abdominal examination can be done while the child is lying in the parent's lap. For an older child, the genitalia and breasts are draped. The child and parent should be asked about urinary and bowel patterns.

The abdomen is divided into four quadrants that correlate with underlying anatomic structures (Fig. 33.19). Because bowel sounds are disturbed by percussion and palpation, the sequence of techniques differs in abdominal assessment. The abdomen is first inspected, then auscultated, then percussed, and last palpated.

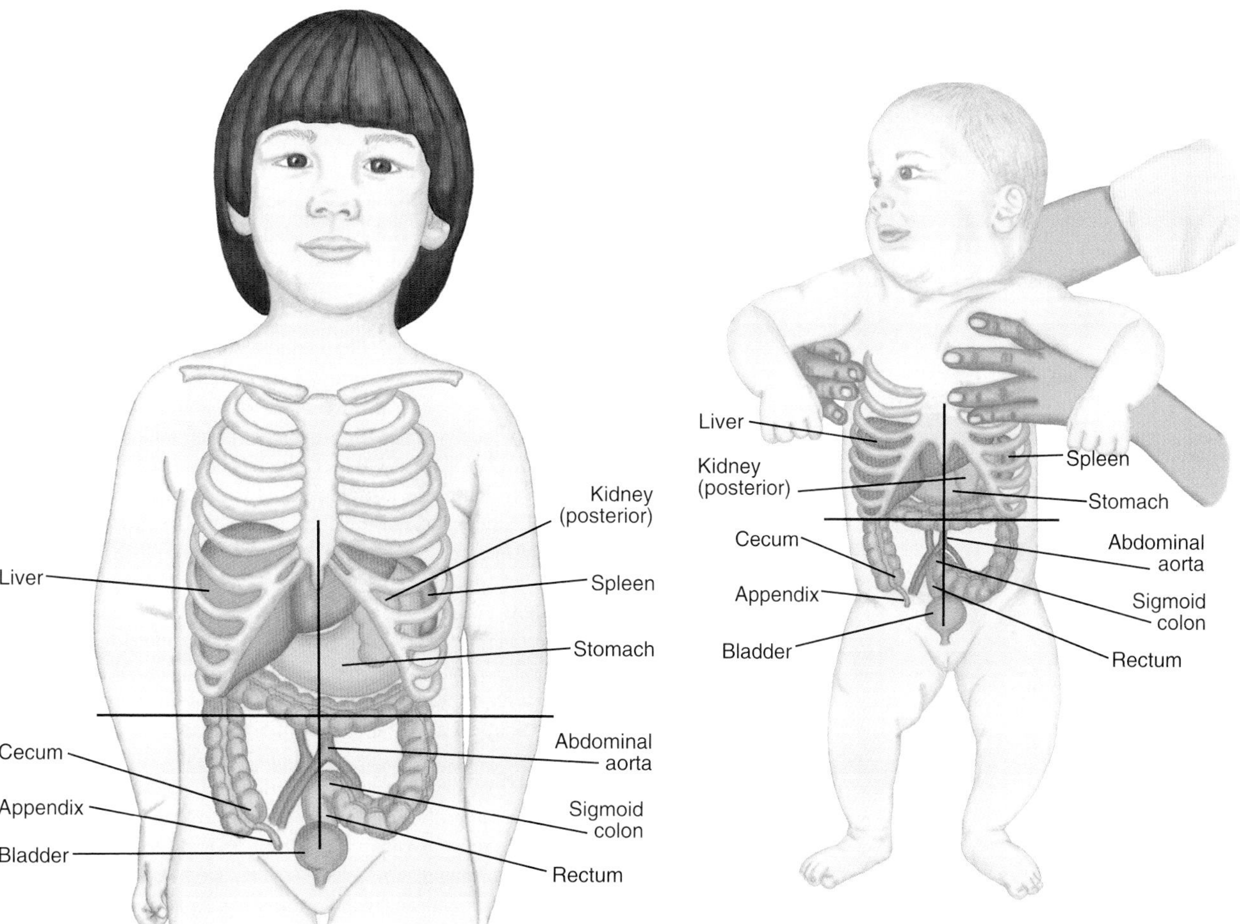


**FIG 33.19** Abdominal quadrants and structures.

### Inspection

Abdominal inspection assesses contour, symmetry, characteristics of the umbilicus and skin, pulsations or movement, and hair distribution. *Contour* is the profile of the abdomen from the rib margin to the pubic bone and is best determined by looking tangentially across the abdomen. The contour is described as flat, scaphoid, rounded, or protuberant (Fig. 33.20). The abdominal contour provides an overall indicator of nutritional state. The abdomen should be bilaterally symmetrical. The examiner looks for distention, bulging, a visible mass, and asymmetrical shape. A protuberant abdomen is typical for the toddler.

The umbilicus is normally midline and inverted. There should be no signs of discoloration, inflammation, or hernia. Throughout the neonatal period, the umbilical cord is inspected for signs of infection and bleeding.

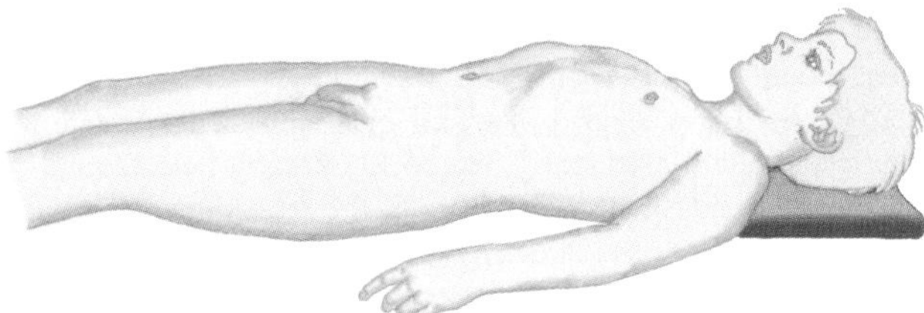

Flat: Thin child

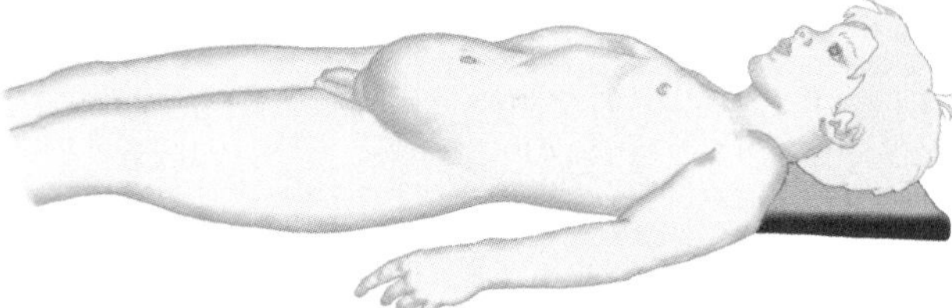

Rounded: Normal appearance of abdomen in a young child

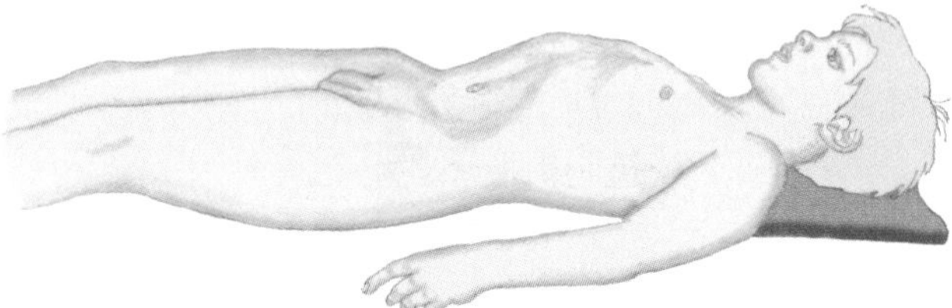

Scaphoid: Emaciated or malnourished child

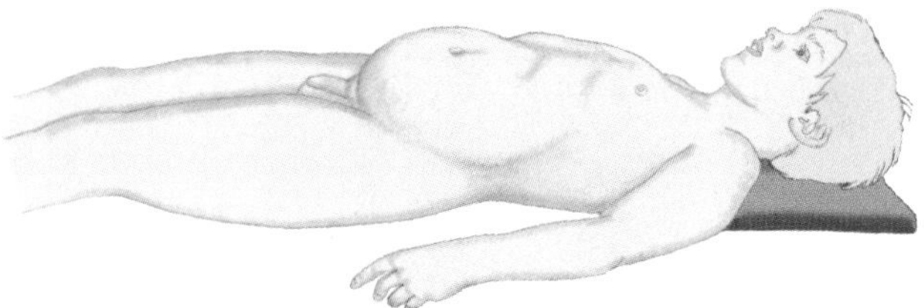

Protuberant: Recent distention with flatus; or extremely obese child (If adolescent female, may indicate pregnancy.)

**FIG 33.20** Abdominal contours. The contour of the abdomen provides an indication of the child's overall nutritional state.

The skin of the abdomen is inspected for color and the presence of scars, lesions, and striae. A fine venous network may be seen in infants and small children.

The abdomen is inspected for pulsations and movement. In thin children, the examiner may see the pulsations from the aorta beneath the skin in the epigastric area. Most children have abdominal movement with respirations. Peristalsis of the abdomen should not be visible.

### Auscultation

Auscultation of the abdomen follows inspection. The diaphragm of the stethoscope is held lightly against the skin to note the character and frequency of bowel sounds. Bowel sounds are high-pitched, gurgling sounds heard in all four quadrants. They are irregular and occur from 5 to 34 times per minute. The examiner begins in the lower right quadrant and listens in all four quadrants. To determine that there are no bowel sounds, the examiner must listen for up to 5 minutes in an area where no bowel sounds are heard.

The bell of the stethoscope is used to listen for bruits over the aortic, renal, iliac, and femoral arteries. The examiner also listens in the epigastric region and around the umbilicus for a venous hum—a soft, low-pitched, continuous sound.

### Percussion

Advanced practitioners perform abdominal percussion. The technique reveals tympany, liver span, and splenic dullness.

### Palpation

Abdominal palpation can identify any mass or tenderness and determine the size, consistency, and location of certain organs. The examiner should have warm hands before palpating the abdomen. Palpation of the infant or young child can be done with the child in the lap of the parent and examiner, who sit facing each other. The child lies with the head and thorax across the parent's legs and the child's abdomen and legs extending across the examiner's legs. The child's knees are flexed to prepare the child for palpation of the abdomen.

Fear and anxiety may cause the child to resist when the examiner touches the abdomen. Distracting the young child with a toy or by talking is helpful. Beginning with light palpation shows the child that palpation will not hurt.

The examiner asks an older child who is anxious or ticklish to assist with this part of the examination. The child places a hand on the abdomen, and the examiner places a hand, with fingers touching the abdomen, on top of the child's hand and asks the child to push as the examiner pushes. This technique allows the child some control as the examination begins, and it reduces the sensation of tickling. To assist with relaxation of the abdominal muscles, the examiner can ask the child to take deep breaths.

The examiner begins with light palpation of all four quadrants using light, even pressure and pressing the palmar surface of the fingers no more than 1 cm into the abdomen. The hand is lifted while moving from area to area. Sudden jabs should be avoided. As the examiner circles around the abdomen, the abdomen should feel soft and smooth. Light palpation is useful in identifying areas of tenderness and muscular resistance. Guarding, resistance, or tenderness should alert the examiner to move cautiously with deeper palpation.

Tenseness can be either voluntary or involuntary. In a child, tenseness and rigidity can be caused by fear and anxiety. Distracting the child or waiting for the child to breathe helps determine whether the tenseness is voluntary or involuntary. The examiner gently indents the fingers into the abdominal wall during inspiration. With even pressure, the abdomen should feel soft. Rigidity, a constant, board-like hardness, of the abdomen is usually associated with an acute inflammation of the peritoneum.

Using the same techniques, the examiner performs deep palpation of the abdomen. The examiner pushes down approximately 5 to 8 cm into the abdominal wall, beginning in the right lower quadrant. The entire abdomen is examined to identify palpable organs and masses.

To palpate the liver's edge, the examiner begins at the level of the umbilicus in the midclavicular line, using the side of the hand to indent the abdomen approximately 5 to 8 cm. With deep penetration of the abdominal wall, the hand is gently inverted toward the costal margin. Then the examiner progresses upward with the same maneuver until palpating the border of the liver. The edge of the liver is felt as soft and smooth. The firm border moves downward when the child takes a deep breath. In infants and young children, the examiner begins at the costal margin and, using the palmar aspects of the fingers, indents the abdominal wall approximately 5 to 8 cm. The examiner should move down from the costal margin until the hand falls off the edge of the liver border. In infants and toddlers, the liver edge is palpable 1 to 3 cm below the costal margin.

While palpating the abdomen, the examiner checks skin turgor and palpates the femoral pulses and inguinal lymph nodes. Advanced practitioners palpate the spleen and kidneys to determine the presence and size of masses and enlargement.

When areas of tenderness are elicited during palpation, a special procedure for identifying rebound tenderness is used. A site away from the identified tenderness is chosen. The examiner places a hand perpendicular to the abdomen, pushes down slowly and deeply into the abdomen, and then lifts the hand quickly. With peritoneal inflammation, the sudden release of the pressure will cause severe pain and muscle rigidity.

The child is turned over, and the buttocks are inspected. The buttocks in children are full, with symmetrical folds. No evidence of scars or ecchymosis should appear on the buttocks. The sacrococcygeal area is examined for dimples and tufts of hair.

## Male Genitalia

The approach to examining the male genitals depends on the child's growth and development. For an infant, toddler, or young child, the nurse tells the child what will occur and then the parent or guardian concurs that the nurse should proceed to examine the child's genitalia.

Objective signs of pubertal changes and the adolescent's perception of these changes affect their understanding of the physical signs experienced at this age. Adolescent boys are normally apprehensive about the genital examination. Concerns arise from modesty, fear of pain, negative judgment, or a previous uncomfortable experience. A matter-of-fact approach and direct communication will facilitate this part of the physical examination. The genital examination is performed during or immediately after the abdominal examination. In the adolescent, the physical examination should not conclude with the genital examination, so as to allow further opportunities for communication. A good practice is to conclude the physical examination with the musculoskeletal and neurologic examination after the genital examination has been completed.

Gloves should be worn during every genital examination. The examiner begins by inspecting the penis. The size of the penis is directly related to age and to growth and development. In infants and young boys, the penis is approximately 2 to 3 cm. Genital hair distribution is noted. The adolescent shows a wide variation in normal development of the genitals. Tanner stages are used for determining the level of development in the adolescent (see Chapter 9).

The skin on the penis normally appears wrinkled, hairless, and without lesions. In the adolescent, a dorsal vein may be prominent. Any indurations on the penile shaft should be noted. In the circumcised male, the glans looks smooth and without lesions. In an uncircumcised infant, the glans may not be visible. By the time the male is age 5 to 6 years, the foreskin may be easily retractable behind the corona of the glans. The adolescent is asked to retract the foreskin himself.

The meatus is evaluated by compressing the glans between the thumb and forefinger anteroposteriorly. The adolescent may be requested to compress the glans so that the examiner can see the meatus. The meatus in the male has a slit-like or tear-shaped configuration and is located on the ventral surface, just millimeters from the tip of the glans. The meatus opening is pink, smooth, and without discharge.

The scrotum is inspected for size and configuration, which changes with growth and development. In the infant or young boy, the proximal portion of the scrotum is wider and the distal portion narrower. In the adolescent boy, the proximal portion is narrower and the distal portion wider. Asymmetry of the scrotum is normal, with the left half slightly lower than the right. The scrotum is movable and, to maintain optimal temperature of the testes, moves closer to or away from the body in response to environmental temperature.

The contents of the scrotum are palpated. The *cremasteric* reflex in young boys may cause the testes to withdraw into the inguinal canal, making palpation more difficult. If the boy is old enough, have him sit in a cross-legged or "tailor" position, which will help prevent the cremasteric reflex by stretching the muscle, thereby preventing its contraction. In infants and young boys, before beginning the abdominal examination, the examiner warms the hands, blocks the inguinal canal with one hand, and palpates for the scrotal contents (Fig. 33.21). The examiner uses the thumb and first two fingers to palpate each testis and epididymis. The testes should be smooth, rubbery, and free of nodules. The size of the testes changes with growth and development. Tanner growth and development stages are used for appropriate interpretation. Because of the high incidence of testicular tumors in young men, adolescents should be taught to do testicular self-examination.

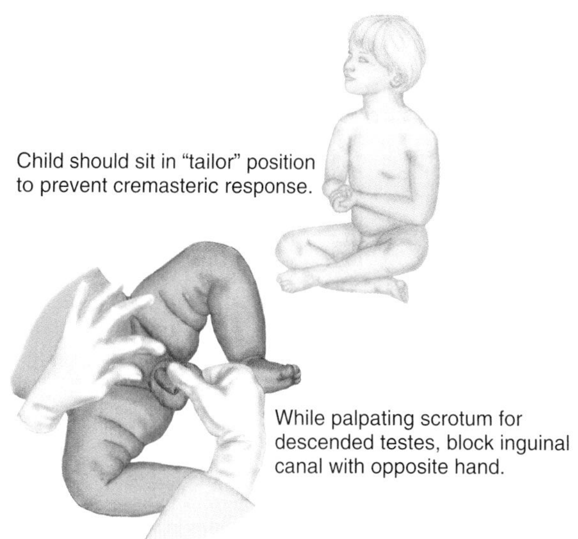

Child should sit in "tailor" position
to prevent cremasteric response.
While palpating scrotum for
descended testes, block inguinal
canal with opposite hand.


**FIG 33.21** When a boy's scrotum is examined, the cremasteric reflex may cause the testes to withdraw into the inguinal canal. To prevent this reflex, the examiner can have the boy sit in a tailor position. The examiner uses one hand to block the inguinal canal and the other to palpate.

## Female Genitalia

In general, the anogenital examination of prepubescent girls is limited to visual inspection and gentle palpation of the external area. The appearance of the external genitalia in females varies from child to child and with growth and development. A relaxed, caring attitude on the part of the examiner will reassure both the child and parent.

To safeguard privacy, reinforce modesty, and decrease anxiety, the child is draped appropriately. The examiner communicates to the child what will be done, and the parent or guardian concurs that it is appropriate to examine the genitalia. With the child in different positions, the genitals differ in tone, relaxation, and appearance. Generally, the genitalia in a young girl are examined with the child supine; the legs are gently drawn up onto the abdomen to expose the genitalia.

The examiner dons gloves and begins by inspecting the *mons pubis* and *labia majora.* The skin should be smooth and clean. The examiner notes the distribution of pubic hair. Tanner stages are used to determine appropriate growth and development (see Chapter 9).

In the newborn infant, the labia majora and minora may be edematous, with the *labia minora* often more prominent. In the infant, the *hymen* may protrude and appear thick and vascular. The clitoris may appear relatively large. The hymen is centrally located and is approximately 0.5 cm in diameter. The examiner determines whether the hymen has an opening.

In the young girl or adolescent, the labia majora may be gaping or closed, shriveled or full, dry or moist, depending on the age and development of the child. The labia majora are usually symmetrical (Fig. 33.22).

The examiner uses the fingers to gently spread the labia majora and then inspects and palpates the labia minora, the *clitoris,* the urethral orifice, and the *vaginal introitus.* The labia minora should appear symmetrical, dark pink, and moist. On palpation, the tissue should be soft and homogeneous with no tenderness.

With the labia majora spread, the examiner inspects the clitoris for size and length. The clitoris varies with growth and development. Moving toward the anus, the examiner locates the urethral meatus, which may be close to or inside the vaginal introitus. The urethral meatus is usually in the midline and appears as a dimple posterior to the clitoris.

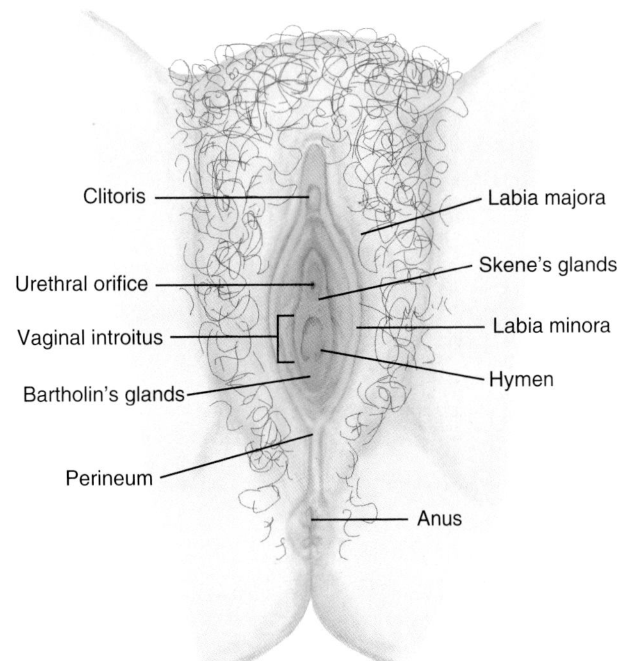


**FIG 33.22** Postpubertal female genitalia.

The vaginal introitus may be a thin, vertical slit or a large orifice with irregular edges, depending on the characteristics of the hymen. The hymen may or may not be stretched across the vaginal opening. By menarche, the opening should be at least 1 cm wide. The tissue is usually moist. The amount and characteristics of any vaginal discharge depend on the circulating hormones in the child. A normal vaginal discharge is odorless and may be cloudy or clear, thick or thin, and there may be a slippery sensation around the time of ovulation.

Normally, *Skene's glands,* located just inferior to the urethral meatus, are not seen or felt and have no discharge. Any discharge from Skene's glands indicates an infection. The examiner inspects and palpates *Bartholin's glands,* located in the posterolateral portion of the labia majora. Bartholin's glands should not be swollen or tender.

A speculum examination of the internal reproductive organs is not indicated for girls. The adolescent girl has special needs during the genital examination, which is performed by advanced practitioners.

## Musculoskeletal System

The musculoskeletal system is composed of the bones, joints, cartilage, ligaments, and muscles. Joint motions are defined as flexion, extension, abduction, adduction, internal rotation, external rotation, and circumduction. The musculoskeletal examination focuses principally on the upper and lower extremities and the spinal column. Musculoskeletal evaluation begins with observing the child during play or history taking. Observation of the child climbing, jumping, hopping, rising from a sitting position, and manipulating toys and other objects provides evidence of joint function, range of motion, bone stability, and muscle strength. The examiner assesses both fine and gross motor development in relation to usual developmental milestones.

General inspection begins with visual scanning of the body with the use of a *cephalocaudal* (head-to-toe) organization. The child can be dressed in shorts or underwear during the examination. The examiner compares the two sides of the body for symmetry, contour, size, and involuntary movement. The examiner then inspects the two sides for areas of swelling or edema and for ecchymoses or other discolorations. The structural relationship of the feet with the legs and the hips to the pelvis, upper extremities, shoulder girdle, and upper trunk are evaluated.

Common deformities of the extremities are *varus* and *valgus* deformities. With the reference point of the midline of the body, a varus deformity is a medial adduction, or turning inward. A valgus deformity is a medial abduction, or turning outward (see Chapter 50).

Injuries to the extremities caused by overexertion and strenuous movements are common in children. Sprains are the most common injury, followed by fractures, dislocations, and lacerations. Overuse injuries, common in school-age children and adolescents, are caused by repetitive microtrauma that exceeds the body's rate of repair. Overuse injuries occur most frequently in sports emphasizing repetitive motion such as swimming, running, gymnastics, and skating. Children's participation in sports should be evaluated for the specifics of conditioning and training.

Deformities of the spine include *scoliosis, kyphosis,* and *lordosis,* which are discussed in Chapter 50.

Palpation of the skull, extremities, and ribs for tenderness, swelling, deformity, and crepitus is performed on any child if injuries are suspected or if there are circumstances that point to possible abuse.

### Infants

During infancy, symmetrical flexion of the arms and legs is noted. Limbs should be freely movable, with symmetry of the axillary, gluteal, femoral, and popliteal creases. The examiner inspects the hands, noting the shape, number, and position of the fingers and palmar creases. The clavicle should feel smooth, regular, and without crepitus. By age 2 months, the infant can lift the head while prone.

The examiner observes range of motion as the infant spontaneously moves the extremities. The infant with normal muscle strength wedges securely between the examiner's hands when lifted under the axilla. The examiner checks the hips for congenital dislocation by comparing leg lengths. The baby's feet are placed flat on the table, and the knees flexed up. The examiner looks for the top of the knees to be the same height (Allis test). Posterior gluteal folds should be equal on both sides. The *Ortolani* and *Barlow maneuvers* are performed by a trained examiner on every visit until the infant is 1 year old (see Fig. 21.11).

### Toddlers, Preschoolers, and School-Age Children

The examiner may want to start with the child's hands and arms by checking for range of motion and the presence of pain while the child is sitting. Children are willing to show their hands, so this is an excellent way to make contact with the child.

The child should stand so that the examiner can observe the posture from behind. The shoulders should be level and the scapulae symmetrical. Lordosis is common in young children. Anteriorly, the examiner begins with the feet and observes for adduction and pronation of the foot. Pronation is common between ages 12 and 30 months because of the young child's broad-based stance. Adduction, or toeing in, is demonstrated when the child walks on the lateral side of the foot. Adduction tends to correct itself by age 3 years as long as the foot is flexible. *Genu varum* (bowleg) is present when a space of more than 2.5 cm is measured between the knees as the medial malleoli are held together. Genu varum is normal after the child has begun to walk and may persist until the child is 3 years old. With *genu valgum*, more than 2.5 cm remains between the medial malleoli when the knees are held together. Genu valgum is present between ages 2 and 3½ years (see Chapter 50).

The child is instructed to stand on one leg and then the other while the examiner watches from behind. The iliac crest should stay level when the weight is shifted.

### Adolescents

For adolescents, the examiner follows the sequence described for school-age children but with special attention to the spine. Adolescents frequently have kyphosis (see Fig. 50.5) caused by poor posture. Although the U.S. Preventive Services Task Force (2011a) recommends against routine screening for scoliosis in asymptomatic adolescents, the AAP, along with the Scoliosis Research Society, the American Academy of Orthopedic Surgeons, and the Pediatric Orthopedic Society of North America, has issued a position statement affirming evidence demonstrating that nonsurgical curve progression preventive interventions (e.g., bracing, exercises) can be successful (Hresko, Talwalker, & Schwend, 2015). Hresko et al. (2015) recommend screening by the primary provider twice for girls aged 10 to 12 years and once for boys aged 13 to 14 years. Therefore, the nurse needs to know the correct screening procedure. While standing, the child is told to bend forward, allowing the shoulders to droop with the arms hanging freely. The nurse looks for unilateral elevation of the lower thoracic ribs and flank (Box 33.9).

### Range of Motion

The examiner notes the child's ability to perform active range-of-motion movements when the child is sitting, standing, and moving about the examination room. The quality of movement for each joint and equality of movement for contralateral joints should be noted. There should be no pain, limitation of movement, spastic movement, joint instability, deformity, or crepitation during movement. Passive range-of-motion movements are performed on joints in which limitations are noted. Passive range-of-motion movement is accomplished by the examiner, who anchors the joint with one hand while using the other hand to slowly move the joint to its limit. Active and passive ranges of motion should be the same.

### Muscle Strength and Mass

The examiner assesses the strength of each muscle group. The child is asked to flex the muscle and then resist as opposing force is applied against flexion. Muscle tone should be firm on palpation. When appropriate, the evaluation of muscle strength is integrated with examination of the associated joint for range of motion. The motor segment of cranial nerve V *(trigeminal nerve)* is evaluated by the application of opposing force to the temporalis muscle while the child clenches the teeth. Cranial nerve XI *(accessory nerve)* is tested by assessing the strength of the sternocleidomastoid and trapezius muscles, during rotation of the head from side to side and from chin to shoulder.

When atrophy or hypertrophy is suspected, the examiner measures muscle mass. Muscles are best measured at their greatest circumference. With the joint used as a landmark, the distance from the joint to a point on the extremity is measured and compared with the opposite muscle. One measurement is not as significant as a series of measurements to determine changes in size of muscles.

### Joints

The examiner palpates each joint for temperature, tenderness, swelling, crepitation, and masses. In children, fatigue, stiffness, or weakness, along with heat and redness, are frequently associated with disorders of the joints. Children usually will not move a joint if it is painful.

### Gait

Assessment of the child's gait and the ability to ambulate is an essential part of both the musculoskeletal and the neurologic assessments. The developmental acquisition of the ability to walk follows a prescribed sequence in infants and toddlers (Table 33.3) (see Chapters 6 and 7).

Gait is assessed in two phases—stance and swing. The stance phase begins when the heel strikes the floor; then the weight is transferred to the ball of the foot, and the toes push off the floor. The swing phase occurs when the foot is off the floor and consists of acceleration, swing through, and deceleration.

## Neurologic System

The purpose of the neurologic examination in the child and adolescent is to identify any nervous system malfunction and to ascertain the extent of nervous system development and functioning. In cases of neurologic deficit, the examiner needs to determine the degree, type, and location of nervous system lesions. In the child, the examiner determines the degree to which the nervous system is functioning so that the healthy portion of the nervous system can be used for habilitation or rehabilitation. For the child younger than 5 years, neurologic functioning is best evaluated with a reliable and valid developmental screening test (see Chapter 5). For the child older than 5 years, the sequence of the neurologic examination is adapted to the child's ability to understand and cooperate.

Brain dysfunction in infants and young children can be manifested by apnea, loss of consciousness, and seizures. Very young children may have milder nonspecific clinical signs, such as irritability, recurrent vomiting, fever, and loss of appetite.

Testing cerebral function, cranial nerves, and cerebellar function gives a picture of nervous system functioning above the spinal cord.

### BOX 33.9 Screening Procedure for Scoliosis

Screening for scoliosis in children aged 9 through 15 ensures early detection and treatment. At greatest risk are girls aged 10 years old through adolescence.

The child should be unclothed or wearing only underpants so that the chest, back, and hips can be clearly seen. Have the child stand with his or her weight distributed equally on the feet, with legs straight and arms hanging loosely at the sides. Observe for the following signs of scoliosis:

- Nonpainful lateral curvature of the spine.
- Visible curve with one turn (C curve) or two compensating curves (S curve).
- Rotation of vertebrae, seen by looking at the rib position, as well as the spinal column itself.
- Unequal shoulder heights.
- Asymmetry of the scapulae
- Unequal waist angles, hip level appears higher on one side
- Unequal elbow to flank spaces
- Unequal rib heights when the child stands in Adam's position (see photograph).

The physical examination should also include the following:

- Observation for equal leg lengths
- Examination of the skin for hairy patches, nevi, café au lait spots, lipomas, and dimples
- Neurologic examination
- Cardiac examination for Marfan syndrome
- Congenital scoliosis is visible in the infant lying prone; the condition is sometimes more prominent if the infant is suspended prone.

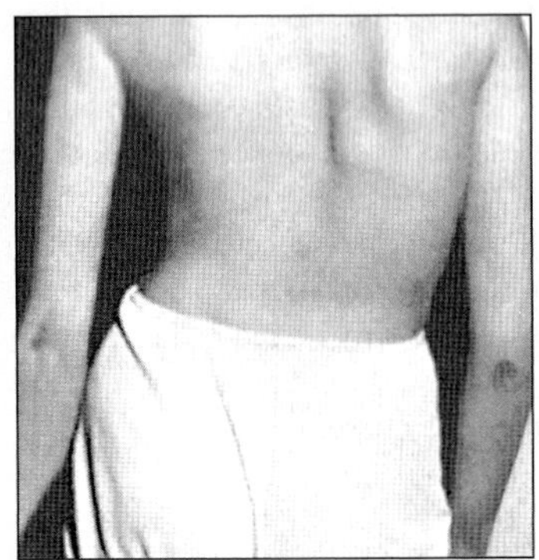

Lateral curvature of thoracic and lumbar segments of the spine, usually with some rotation of involved vertebral bodies. Functional scoliosis is flexible; it is apparent with standing and disappears with forward bending. It can be compensatory for other abnormalities such as leg-length discrepancy.

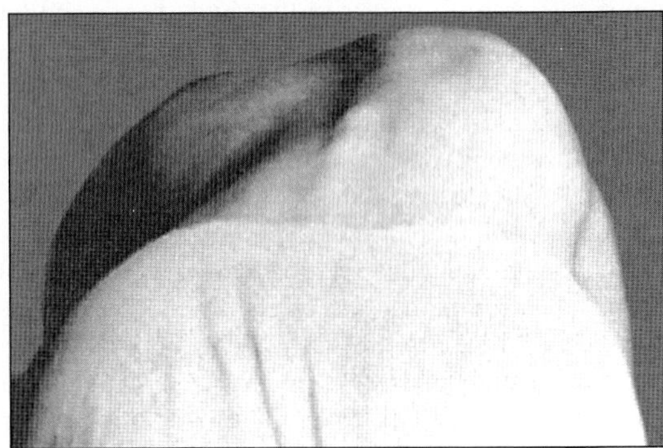

Adams' position demonstrates the rib hump of structural scoliosis. Structural scoliosis is fixed; the curvature is evident both when the individual stands and also bends forward. Note the rib hump on the right side with forward flexion. When the child is standing, unequal shoulder elevation, unequal scapulae, obvious curvature, unequal elbow level and unequal hip level are seen.

Data from Burns, C. (2008). Musculoskeletal disorders. In C. Burns, A. Dunn, M. Brady, et al. (Eds.), *Pediatric primary care* (4th ed.). Philadelphia: Saunders; Mustovich, R.J., & Spiegel, D. (2016). The spine. In R. Kliegman, B. Stanton, J. St. Geme, et al. (Eds.), *Nelson textbook of pediatrics* (20th ed., Chapter 679). St. Louis, MO: Elsevier. Photographs from Delp, M.H., & Manning R.T. (1981). *Major's physical diagnosis: An introduction to the clinical process* (9th ed., pp. 450). Philadelphia: Saunders.

The child's age and development determine the sequence of the neurologic examination. Infants and younger children are not able to cooperate with neurologic testing. A review of developmental milestones attained helps establish the rate and consistency of development in the infant and younger child. The 3- or 4-year-old child cooperates with testing when it is approached as a game.

### Cerebral Function

The evaluation of cognitive function focuses on appearance, behavior, orientation, speech patterns, memory, logic, and affect. The examiner needs to obtain information from the primary caregiver about changes in the child's behavior, personality, appearance, and age-appropriate school performance. Evaluation of cognitive function in the older child and adolescent is based on observation of level of consciousness, awareness, thought processes, and communication.

The degree of response to sensory stimuli provides information about the older child's or adolescent's level of consciousness. The child is described as alert, lethargic, **obtunded**, stuporous, or comatose.

The older child and the adolescent have the ability to understand, think, feel emotions, and appreciate sensory information about self and surroundings. Awareness is evaluated by observing the older child's or adolescent's level of orientation in relation to person, place, and time. The normally functioning child is oriented to person, place, and time.

Thought processes include abstract thinking, problem solving (simple calculations and concentration), insight, memory (recent and remote), and judgment. The child's school performance may or may not be an accurate indicator of thought processes. Factors that may influence thought processes are attention span, communication, perceptual problems, and emotional withdrawal and depression.

Language ability is evaluated through speech patterns and comprehension. The child is questioned about reading and writing ability. Is the child's speech intelligible? Does the child answer questions appropriately for age and developmental level? Typically, older children and adolescents are able to speak fluently, name objects correctly, and write their name and address (Box 33.10).

### Cranial Nerves

Assessment of the cranial nerves (Table 33.4) should be incorporated into the examination of the system each nerve affects. Games, such as making faces and performing tests on a parent or the examiner, will enhance cooperation.

**TABLE 33.3 Gross Motor Development in the Infant: Progression to Walking**

| Activity | Age |
|---|---|
| Raises head and holds position | 2 wk-2 mo |
| Moves all extremities, kicking arms and legs when prone | 2 mo |
| Draws up knees and raises abdomen off table; rocks back and forth while up on hands and knees; rolls over | 3-6 mo |
| Sits alone, using hands for support (tripod fashion) | By 7 mo |
| Lurches forward and pulls legs to chest in "inchworm" fashion, may move backward in same fashion; creeps and rolls | By 9 mo |
| Crawls in one-sided manner (moves arm and leg on same side of body, then other side) | 6-9 mo |
| Crawls in regular fashion, alternating arm and opposite leg | 6-9 mo |
| Begins to pull up | By 11 mo |
| Cruises: attempts to walk with support or holding onto something stable | By 12 mo |
| Momentarily lets go and maintains balance for a few seconds | Once comfortable standing and holding on |
| Takes first steps (a broad stance with arms flexed for balance) | Once standing balance accomplished |
| Sits from a standing posture | By 12 mo |
| Walks alone | By 15 mo |

**BOX 33.10 Specific Cerebral Function Tests**

*Sound recognition:* Can the child identify familiar sounds with the eyes closed?

*Auditory and verbal comprehension:* Does the child answer questions and carry out instructions appropriate for age?

*Recognition of body parts and sidedness:* Does the child recognize the parts of the body? Does the child know right from left?

*Performance of skilled motor acts:* Can the child drink from a cup, button clothes, use a common tool?

*Visual object recognition:* Can the child identify a familiar toy or object (e.g., ball)?

*Visual and verbal comprehension:* Can the child read appropriately and explain the meaning?

*Motor speech:* Does the child imitate different sounds and phrases?

*Automatic speech:* Can the child repeat a series of learned words (e.g., nursery rhymes, days of the week)?

*Volitional speech:* Does the child answer questions relevantly?

*Writing:* Can the child write his or her name or the name of an object?

**TABLE 33.4 Assessing Cranial Nerves***

| Cranial Nerve | Procedure |
|---|---|
| I (olfactory nerve) | The child is asked to identify familiar odors with the eyes closed. Each side of the nose is tested separately. |
| II (optic nerve) | Visual acuity is tested using the Snellen chart, or the Lea or HOTV chart for young children. Each eye is tested separately and then both eyes together. If corrective lenses are worn, the eyes are tested both with and without correction. |
| III, IV, VI (oculomotor, trochlear, abducent nerves) | The child is asked to follow a toy or the examiner's finger as the object moves in all directions of gaze (six cardinal fields of gaze). |
| V (trigeminal nerve) | The child is asked to identify a wisp of cotton on the face. Corneal reflex is tested by observing for blinking when the examiner approaches the face closely. The masseter and temporal muscles' strength can be evaluated by having the child bite down on a tongue blade as the examiner tries to remove it. |
| VII (facial nerve) | The child is asked to imitate the examiner's frown, wrinkled forehead, smile, and raised eyebrow. The child tries to keep the eyes closed while the examiner attempts to open them, to test the strength of the eyelid muscles. The sensory portion of the facial nerve can be evaluated by having the child identify the taste of sugar and salt placed on the anterior part of the tongue on each side. |
| VIII (acoustic nerve) | Cochlear nerve tests assess hearing. Audiometric testing is a quantitative evaluation of hearing. The Weber (lateralization) and Rinne (air and bone conduction) tests are qualitative evaluations of hearing. |
| IX, X (glossopharyngeal nerve, vagus nerve) | The glossopharyngeal and vagus nerves are tested together. With a tongue depressor, the gag reflex is tested by touching the posterior pharyngeal wall. The palatal reflex is tested by stroking each side of the mucous membrane of the uvula. The side touched should rise. Normal function of the vagus nerve is revealed by the child's ability to swallow and to speak clearly. |
| XI (accessory nerve) | The examiner palpates and notes the strength of the trapezius and sternocleidomastoid muscles against resistance, or the child shrugs the shoulders against resistance. |
| XII (hypoglossal nerve) | The child is asked to stick out the tongue, and the examiner notes any lateral deviation when it is protruded. The strength of the tongue is assessed by having the child push the tongue against the examiner's finger pressed against the cheek. |

*Cranial nerves are tested during assessment of the system in which they occur.

### Cerebellar Function

Proprioception, balance, and coordination are tested by having the child perform specific movements. The cerebellum controls balance and coordination. Proprioception evaluates laterality and orientation in space. The techniques used vary with the child's age and development. The child should attempt the technique and show continued improvement with maturation (Box 33.11).

### Motor System

Muscle size, muscle tone, involuntary movements, and muscle strength are assessed during the musculoskeletal examination.

While the child is at rest, the muscles are inspected and palpated for size, consistency, and possible atrophy. The examiner notes symmetry of posture and of muscle contours and outlines.

Muscle tone is evaluated by palpating the muscles at rest and noting resistance to passive movement. The examiner inspects the muscles for involuntary movements. Muscle strength is tested first without resistance and then against resistance. Corresponding muscles on the two sides are compared. The examiner then tests the major joints for flexion, extension, and other movements.

### Sensory System

Sensory testing depends on the child's perception and interpretation of the stimuli and on the child's age and development. Sensory tests should first be done in an educational practice session before being done in a testing situation. Sensory testing compares the two sides of the body, corresponding extremities, and the sensitivity of the distal and proximal parts of each extremity for each form of sensation. Sensory testing is performed to determine whether sensory changes involve one entire side of the body, are *dermatomal* (along nerve pathways in the skin) in distribution, or are confined to the peripheral nerves (Box 33.12). In an older child, primary forms of sensation such as superficial tactile, superficial pain, sensitivity to temperature, sensitivity to vibration, deep pressure pain, and motion and position can be tested. Cortical and discriminatory forms of sensation require interpretation by the cerebral cortex. They are evaluated by two-point discrimination, point localization, texture discrimination, *stereognostic* (touch recognition of objects) function, *graphesthesia* (identification of figures traced on the skin), and extinction phenomenon.

### Reflex Status

Most brain growth occurs in the first year of life. Primitive reflexes in the neonate are inhibited when more advanced cortical functions and voluntary control take over as the child matures and grows. Commonly elicited reflexes are illustrated in Table 33.5.

Motor maturation proceeds in a cephalocaudal direction. The ability to elicit a reflex requires an intact afferent nerve fiber, functional synapses in the spinal cord, intact motor nerve fibers, functional neuromuscular junctions, and competent muscle fibers. The examiner compares the responses on the right and left sides, which should be equal. Diminished or hyperreflexic responses are reported for further evaluation.

### Neurologic "Soft" Signs

Neurologic "soft" signs are findings that indicate the child's inability to perform certain activities related to the child's age. They can provide subtle clues to an underlying central nervous system deficit or neurologic maturation delay.

Children with neurologic "soft" signs need evaluation and monitoring because some children with medical, mental, or emotional problems also demonstrate such signs (Box 33.13).

## CONCLUSION AND DOCUMENTATION

When the physical examination has been completed, the examiner should ask the parents and child, if age appropriate, whether they have any questions concerning the examination. Findings are documented in a complete and concise manner. Deviations from normal and risk factors should be identified and documented. Depending on the setting, referrals may be made.

### BOX 33.11 Cerebellar Function: Tests of Balance and Coordination

Balance and coordination are tested by having the child perform the following movements:

- *Finger-to-nose test.* Child performs first with one hand, then with the other; first with the eyes open, then with the eyes closed. Ask child first to touch her finger to her nose and then to your finger as you change the position of your finger. Repeat this action with increasing rapidity. The tests are performed with each hand.

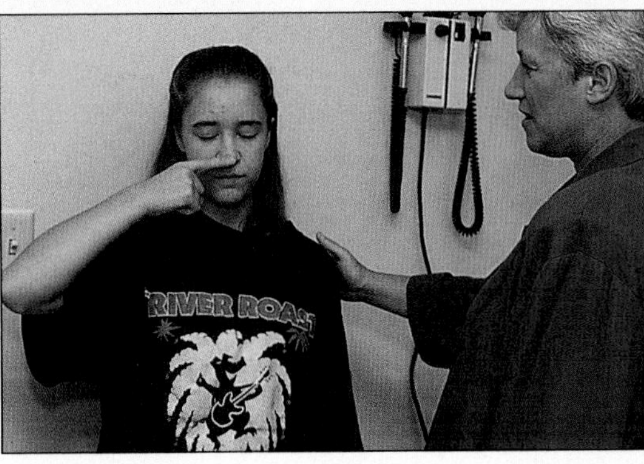


- *Rapid alternating movements.* Ask the child to rapidly pat her knee with the palms and backs of her hands by pronating and supinating the hands *(demonstrate first).* Ask the child to touch her thumb to each of her fingers in rapid succession *(demonstrate first).*

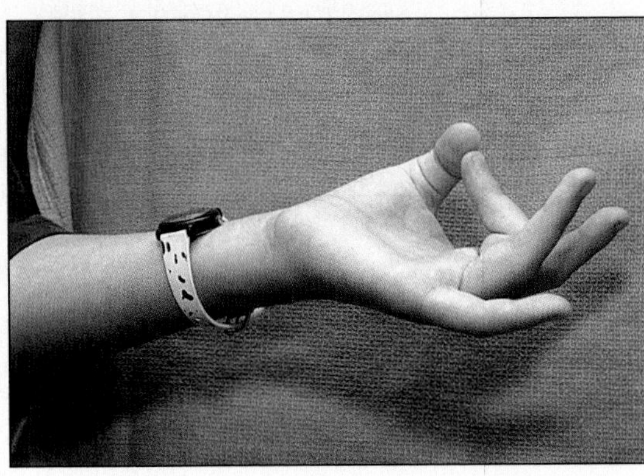

## BOX 33.11 Cerebellar Function: Tests of Balance and Coordination—cont'd

- Ask the child to stand erect, first with the eyes open and then with the eyes closed. Stand near the child to prevent injury if the child begins to fall.

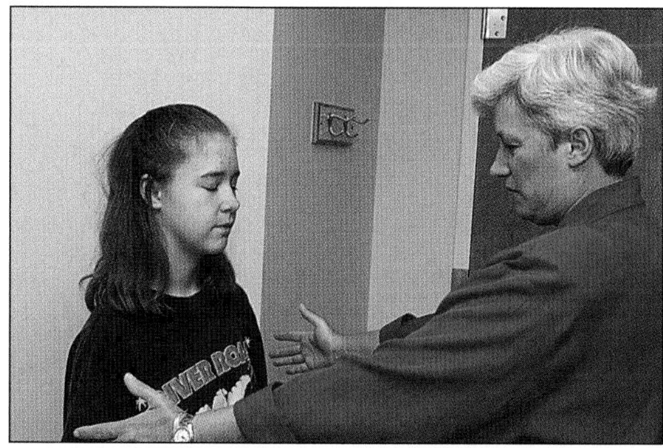

- Ask the child to walk in tandem fashion, placing her heel immediately in front of her opposite foot's toe and alternating while walking a straight line.

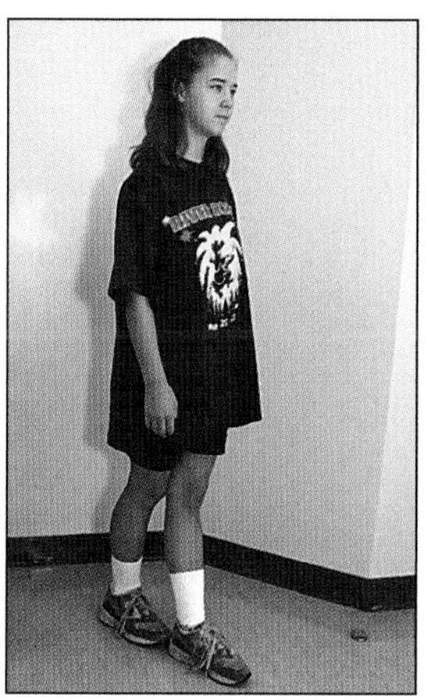

- Ask the sitting child to run each heel down the opposite shin. With the child lying down, ask the child to point to your hand with each big toe.

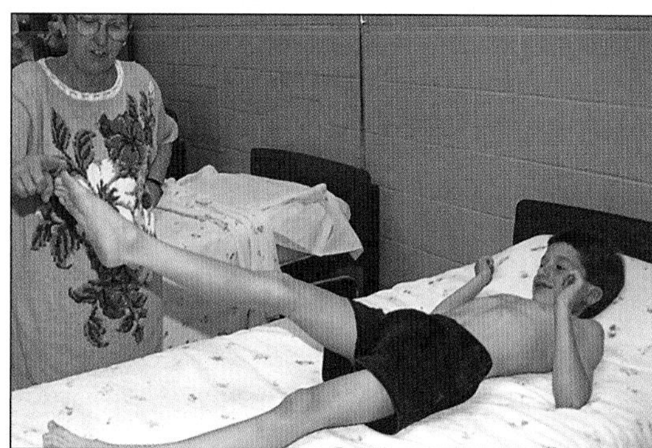

## BOX 33.12 Tests for Evaluating Sensory Function

### Primary Forms of Sensation

Check in sequence the hands, forearms, upper arms, trunk, thighs, lower legs, and feet for the following:

*Superficial tactile sensation:* Touch the child with a wisp of cotton.

*Superficial pain:* Touch the child with a pin or other sharp object. Be careful not to injure or frighten the child.

*Sensitivity to temperature:* Touch the various parts of the child's body with test tubes containing warm and cold water. This test is infrequently done with children because of the difficulty of keeping water warm or cold enough for the child to distinguish the difference.

*Sensitivity to vibration:* Hold a vibrating tuning fork to the bony prominences, noting the child's ability to perceive the vibration and tell you when the vibration stops.

*Deep pressure pain:* Press the tip of your fingernail against the child's fingernail. The child will feel discomfort. You may also squeeze the Achilles tendon, calf, and forearm muscles, noting sensitivity.

*Motion and position:* Hold the sides of the toes, thumbs, and fingers by grasping them between your index finger and thumb. Move the fingers and toes passively and ask the child to tell you the final position of the digit.

### Cortical and Discriminatory Forms of Sensation

These forms of sensation are complex somatic sensory impressions that require interpretation by the cerebral cortex.

The following sensations can be evaluated, depending on the age and development of the child being tested:

*Two-point discrimination:* Can the child differentiate between one and two points? With the child's eyes closed, various parts of the body are touched simultaneously with two sharp objects. Then alternate touching the child with one point or two points is done. Different areas of the body vary in the distance by which the child can differentiate one from two points. This test is more appropriate for older children.

*Point localization:* With the eyes closed, can the child locate the spot where she or he was touched?

*Texture discrimination:* Can the child recognize with the hands the difference in the feel of materials such as cotton, wool, and silk?

*Stereognostic function:* Can the child identify familiar objects placed in each hand? Place several objects in a paper bag, and have the child identify them with each hand and show you the object.

*Graphesthesia:* Can the child identify letters or numbers traced on the palm or back of the hand with a blunt point? Numbers are easier than letters for a young child to recognize.

*Extinction phenomenon:* With the eyes closed, can the child identify touch on both sides? Touch opposite sides of the body in identical areas simultaneously. This test is used for older children only.

**TABLE 33.5 Evaluating Common Reflexes**

| Reflex | Evaluation |
|---|---|
| Deep tendon reflexes | Evaluation elicited by tapping briskly on a tendon or a bony prominence, evoking a sudden stretching of certain muscles and their resulting contraction. For an adequate response, the limb should be relaxed and the muscle partially stretched. The reflex is stimulated by directing a sharp blow of the reflex hammer onto the muscle's insertion tendon. |
| Biceps reflex 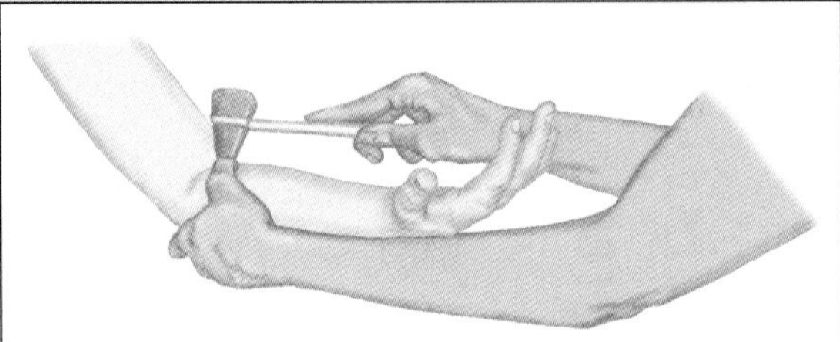 | The child's arm should be flexed up to 45 degrees at the elbow. The biceps tendon in the antecubital fossa is palpated. The thumb is then placed on the biceps tendon, and a blow is struck on the thumb. The response is a visible or palpable flexion of the forearm. |
| Triceps reflex 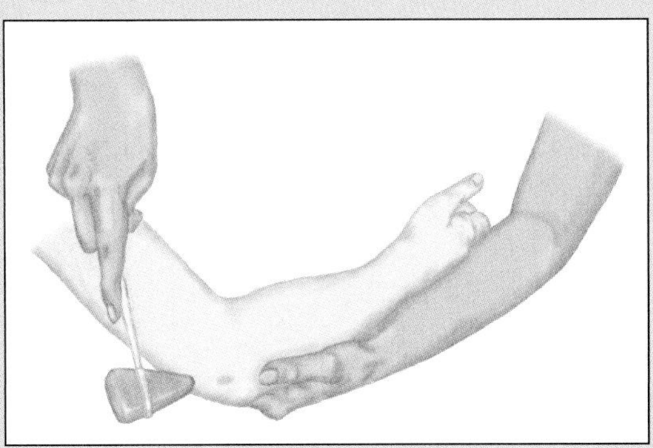 | The arm is suspended by holding the upper arm and instructing the child to just let the arm "go limp." Alternatively, the forearm can be supported on the examiner's arm. The triceps tendon is struck directly just above the elbow. The response is extension of the forearm. |
| Brachioradialis reflex 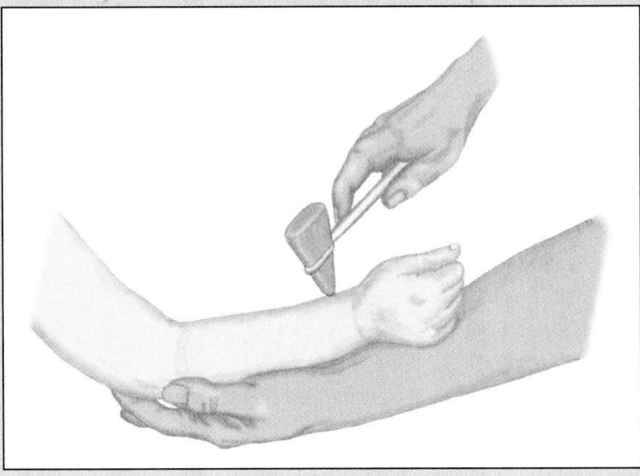 | The child's arm is supported on the examiner's arm, and the elbow is flexed up to 45 degrees. The brachioradial tendon is struck with the reflex hammer 2.5-5 cm (1-2 in) above the radial styloid process. The response is pronation and flexion of the elbow. |

**TABLE 33.5 Evaluating Common Reflexes—cont'd**

| Reflex | Evaluation |
|---|---|
| Patellar reflex 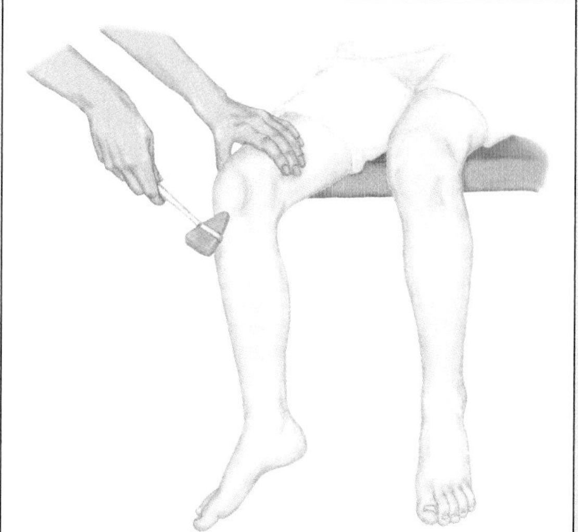 | The lower leg is allowed to dangle freely by flexing the child's knee up to 90 degrees. The examiner supports the upper leg with the hand and strikes the patellar tendon just below the patella. The response is extension of the lower leg. |
| Achilles reflex 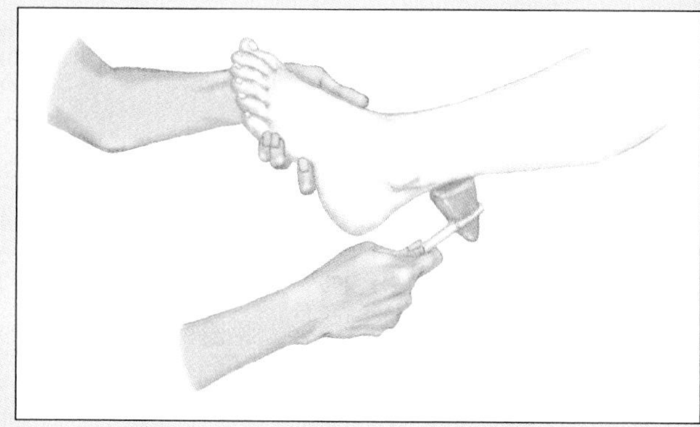 | The hip is externally rotated, and the foot is held in dorsiflexion. The Achilles tendon is struck directly. The response is plantar flexion of the foot. An alternative way to elicit this reflex is to have the child kneel on a chair with the toes pointing toward the floor; the examiner then strikes the Achilles tendon directly. |
| Clonus reflex | A *clonus*—a continued, rapid flexion and extension of the foot and hand—can be elicited in children. Clonus is elicited by suddenly and briskly dorsiflexing the foot or hand and applying sustained and moderate pressure. No rhythmic oscillating movements should be palpated. |
| Superficial reflexes | Tested by stroking the skin with an object that is moderately sharp but not sharp enough to break the skin. The receptors are in the skin rather than the muscles. |

Continued

**TABLE 33.5 Evaluating Common Reflexes—cont'd**

| Reflex | Evaluation |
|---|---|
| Upper and lower abdominal reflexes and cremasteric reflex 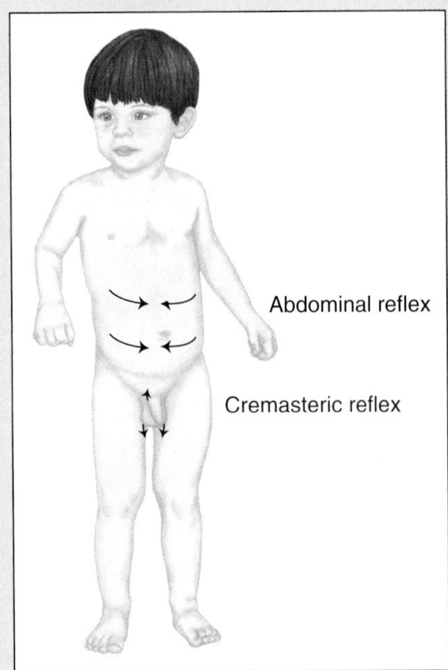  | *Upper and lower abdominal reflexes:* While the child is in a supine position and with the abdomen exposed and knees slightly bent, the skin of the abdomen is stroked. Stroking is directed from the side of the abdomen toward the midline at both the upper and lower abdominal levels. The response is ipsilateral contraction of the abdominal muscle, with an observable movement of the umbilicus toward the side being stroked.<br>*Cremasteric reflex:* In the male, light stroking of the inner aspect of the thigh causes the ipsilateral testicle to elevate. This reflex may cause withdrawal of the testicles into the inguinal canal when the abdomen is touched with very cold hands. |
| Plantar (Babinski) reflex 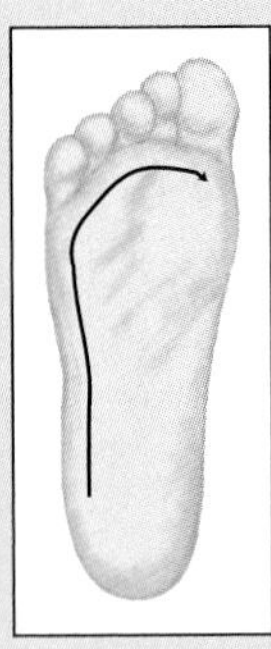 | The lateral aspect of the sole of the foot, from the heel to the ball of the foot, is stroked in a movement curving medially across the ball. A fingernail or the wooden end of an applicator stick is used. The response in an infant is dorsiflexion, fanning of the toes, and hyperextension of the great toe. Once a child is walking, the response is plantar flexion of the toes. Some children withdraw from this stimulus by flexing the hip and the knee. |
| Gluteal reflex | When the buttocks are separated, the skin tenses at the gluteal area. |

**BOX 33.13 Examples of Neurologic "Soft" Signs**

- Short attention span
- Poor motor coordination
- Clumsiness
- Frequent falling
- Hyperkinesis, voluntary or involuntary
- Uneven perceptual development
- Incomplete laterality, with no side clearly dominant
- Language disturbances: articulation disorders, dyslexia
- Motor outflow (movements involving more muscles than intended)
- Mirroring movements of the extremities (e.g., both hands in motion when only one is performing a function)

## KEY CONCEPTS

- Systematic physical examination is tailored to the child's developmental level, includes all body systems, and generally proceeds from head to toe.
- Developmentally appropriate assessment of children requires flexibility and creativity on the part of the examiner.
- Collection of accurate subjective and objective data is foundational to identifying nursing needs of children.
- Vital signs should be assessed during each visit in ambulatory care settings and monitored on a regular basis in the hospitalized child.

## KEY CONCEPTS—cont'd

- Assessment of vital signs is an important way to measure and monitor vital body functions.
- Examination findings are recorded completely and concisely. Deviations from normal and risk factors are identified, documented, and, when appropriate, reported for further evaluation.
- Serial recordings of growth, development, anthropometrics, and nutritional status provide important clues to a child's health status.
- The skin is inspected and palpated to determine color, moisture, temperature, turgor, edema, and lesions.
- A child's general appearance is observed for signs of abuse, both physical and psychological.
- Lymph nodes are palpated as part of the examination of different anatomic areas of the body.
- The head is inspected for symmetry, movement, control, and shape.
- The fontanels are inspected and palpated for size, tenseness, and pulsation.
- The eyelids, eyebrows, palpebral fissures, nasolabial folds, mouth, and nose are inspected for spacing and symmetry.
- The nasal mucosa is inspected for color and moisture.
- Assessment of a young child's mouth is performed at the end of the examination, as it can cause anxiety.
- Selection of an eye chart to assess visual acuity is based on the child's age and developmental level; it must be reliable and valid.
- Assessment of the thorax and lungs entails inspection, palpation, percussion, and auscultation.
- The heart is auscultated using both the bell and diaphragm of the stethoscope, with the child in the supine, left lateral recumbent, and sitting upright positions.
- An empty bladder, a warm room, and a supine position with a pillow under the head and knees flexed will enhance abdominal relaxation.
- Examination of the genitalia evokes concern in some children. A matter-of-fact approach and clear communication of what will occur will help create a positive experience.
- The musculoskeletal examination is directed predominantly toward the upper and lower extremities and the spinal column.
- The neurologic examination is done to identify any nervous system malfunction and to evaluate current nervous system development.
- When the physical examination has been completed, the examiner should ask the child and parents whether they have any questions concerning the examination.

## REFERENCES AND READINGS


American Academy of Audiology. (2011). *Childhood hearing screening guidelines.* Retrieved from http://www.audiology.org.

American Academy of Pediatrics. (2012). *Health issues: High blood pressure in children.* Retrieved from http://www.healthychildren.org.

American Academy of Pediatrics. (2013). *U.S. Preventive Services Task Force updates recommendation on blood pressure screening for children.* Retrieved from http://www.aap.org.

American Academy of Pediatrics. (2015). *Corrected age for preemies.* Retrieved from http://www.aap.org.

American Academy of Pediatrics. (2016). *Best ways to take a temperature.* Retrieved from http://www.healthychildren.com.

American Academy of Pediatrics Committee on Practice and Ambulatory Medicine, Section on Ophthalmology, American Association of Certified Orthoptists, American Association for Pediatric Ophthalmology and Strabismus, & American Academy of Ophthalmology. (2016). Visual system assessment in infants, children, and young adults by pediatricians. *Pediatrics, 137*(1), 28–30.

American Academy of Pediatrics, & National High Blood Pressure Education Program Working Group on High Blood Pressure in Children and Adolescents. (2004). The fourth report on the diagnosis, evaluation, and treatment of high blood pressure in children and adolescents. *Pediatrics, 114*(2), 555–576.

American Pain Society. (n.d.). *Pain: Current understanding of assessment, management, and treatments.* Retrieved from http://www.ampainsoc.org/education/enduring-materials.

Ball, J., Dains, J., Flynn, J., et al. (2015). (Eds.). *Seidel's guide to physical examination* (8th ed.). St. Louis: Elsevier Mosby.

Battra, P., & Goyal, S. (2013). Comparison of rectal, axillary, tympanic, and temporal artery thermometry in the pediatric emergency room. *Pediatric Emergency Care, 29*, 63–66.

Centers for Disease Control and Prevention. (2010). *WHO growth standards are recommended for use in the U.S. for infants and children 0 to 2 years of age.* Retrieved from http://www.cdc.gov.

Centers for Disease control and Prevention. (2013). *Frequently asked questions about the 2000 CDC growth charts.* Retrieved from http://www.cdc.gov.

Centers for Disease Control and Prevention. (2015). *About child and teen BMI.* Retrieved from http://www.cdc.gov.

Dickey, B., & Chu, Y. (2016). Acanthus nigricans. In R. Kliegman, B. Stanton, J. St. Geme, et al. (Eds.), *Nelson textbook of pediatrics* (20th ed., Chapter 657). St. Louis, MO: Elsevier.

Donahue, S. Baker, P., Committee on Practice and Ambulatory Medicine, American Association of Certified Orthoptists, American Association for Pediatric Ophthalmology and Strabismus, & American Academy of Ophthalmology. (2016). Procedures for the evaluation of the visual system by pediatricians. *Pediatrics, 137*(1), 1–9.

Hresko, M., Talwalker, V., & Schwend, R. (2015). *Position statement – screening for the early detection of idiopathic scoliosis in adolescents.* Retrieved from http://www.srs.org

Hurwitz, B., Brown, J., & Altmiller, G. (2015). Improving pediatric temperature measurement in the ED. *AJN, 115*(9), 48–55.

Jarvis, C. (2012). *Physical examination and health assessment* (6th ed.). St. Louis: Saunders.

Johnston, M. (2016). Cerebral palsy. In R. Kliegman, B. Stanton, J. St. Geme, et al. (Eds.), *Nelson textbook of pediatrics* (20th ed., Chapter 598). St. Louis, MO: Elsevier.

Lehman, R., & Schor, N. (2016). Neurological evaluation. In R. Kliegman, B. Stanton, J. St. Geme, et al. (Eds.), *Nelson textbook of pediatrics* (20th ed., Chapter 590). St. Louis, MO: Elsevier.

Moyer, V., U.S. Preventive Services Task Force. (2013). Screening for primary hypertension in children and adolescents: U.S. Preventive Services Task Force recommendation statement. *Pediatrics, 132*(5), 907–914.

Roosevelt, G. (2016). Acute inflammatory upper airway obstruction (Croup, laryngitis, epiglottitis, and bacterial tracheitis). In R. Kliegman, B. Stanton, J. St. Geme, et al. (Eds.), *Nelson textbook of pediatrics* (20th ed., Chapter 385). St. Louis, MO: Elsevier.

The Joint Commission. (2014). Clarification of the pain management standard. *Joint Commission Perspectives, 34*(11), 11.

Tower, R., & Camitta, B. (2016). Lymphadenopathy. In R. Kliegman, B. Stanton, J. St. Geme, et al. (Eds.), *Nelson textbook of pediatrics* (20th ed., Chapter 490). St. Louis, MO: Elsevier.

U.S. Preventive Services Task Force. (2011a). *First annual report to congress on high priority evidence gaps for clinical preventive services.* Retrieved from http://www.uspreventiveservicestaskforce.org.

U.S. Preventive Services Task Force. (2011b). *Visual impairment in children ages 1-5: Screening.* Retrieved from http://www.uspreventiveservicestaskforce.org.

Zeltzer, L., Krane, E., & Palermo, T. (2016). Pediatric pain management. In R. Kliegman, B. Stanton, J. St. Geme, et al. (Eds.), *Nelson textbook of pediatrics* (20th ed., Chapter 62). St. Louis, MO: Elsevier.

34

# Emergency Care of the Child

http://evolve.elsevier.com/McKinney/mat-ch/

## LEARNING OBJECTIVES

*After studying this chapter, you should be able to:*

- Describe general principles that encourage cooperation and help make examination and treatment of children in emergency settings more comfortable for a child and family.
- List significant developmental issues when caring for infants, toddlers, preschool and school-age children, and adolescents in emergency care settings.
- Compare the child's airway anatomy with that of an adult and explain the significance of these differences in managing the pediatric airway.
- Assess the early signs of shock in infants and children, thereby recognizing that changes in heart rate and skin signs are more accurate signs of early shock than decreased blood pressure.
- Define *triage* and list the most important factors to assess when obtaining an overall ("across the room") impression of an infant's or child's condition.
- Describe the general guidelines for cardiopulmonary resuscitation in infants and children and discuss what additional precautions and procedures are required for infants and children with traumatic injuries.
- List indications that suggest a child brought into the emergency care setting has been neglected or abused, and discuss the nurse's responsibility for reporting possible neglect or abuse.
- Identify several possible roles for nurses in preventing traumatic injuries, poison ingestion, and environmental injuries.

## CLINICAL REFERENCE

### GENERAL GUIDELINES FOR EMERGENCY NURSING CARE

Many factors affect the psychological impact of an emergency on both the child and family. In addition to the expected fears children have at various developmental stages (e.g., separation, pain, altered body image); an overriding concern expressed by both children and parents in emergency care settings is fear of the unknown. The suddenness with which the child and family come in contact with emergency personnel, the necessity for rapid assessment and intervention, and the relative seriousness of the child's condition can intensify a fearful response and overwhelm normal coping mechanisms. In addition, children and families are unfamiliar with the setting, staff of the healthcare facility, equipment, and procedures. Emergency nurses can use some simple interventions to make examination and treatment of children in the emergency setting more comfortable for a child and family and to decrease the adverse psychological effects of the experience.

*Communicate an attitude of calm confidence.* This attitude can be difficult to maintain when the situation is critical, but families in crisis look to nurses for reassurance and expect competent, professional behavior. Speak quietly and calmly to the child and parents and remain firmly in charge. Remember to talk to the family often throughout the visit; silence is a form of communication that is easily misinterpreted. Create a communication plan with the parent or family that specifies when they should be called if they are away from the department and that lists numbers where they can be reached. Acknowledge and address the child's and family's fears. Emergency settings require healthcare providers to rapidly treat patients while trying to establish a relationship with the patient and their family with little knowledge of the patient's medical history (Schinasi, Kolaitis, & Nadel, 2015). This situation can lead to ineffective communication. Poor communication is the cause of 70% of medical errors; therefore, effective and timely communication is essential for safe patient care, especially in high-risk areas such as emergency settings (Eppich, 2015).

*Establish a trusting relationship with the child and family.* Make eye contact with the child and family when you speak to them. Call the child by name to personalize care. Treat the child and family kindly and gently. To establish a trusting relationship, check back with the family often and provide periodic updates if the child and family are separated. When parents are confident that they are being kept informed, they are less likely to make demands for additional attention and information. When speaking to the child and family, use simple, nonmedical terms and remember that children (and sometimes adults) can have inaccurate ideas of how their bodies function and the location of body parts. Providing comfort measures to the family members also builds a trusting relationship. It is important to protect their privacy, direct them to a public telephone or cafeteria, and provide space where they can talk quietly.

*Encourage caregivers to stay with the child.* Family-centered care recognizes the partnership between healthcare workers and family in ensuring the well-being of the child. Nursing care is driven by the needs of the family and child rather than controlled by healthcare providers. According to comfort levels and ability, include the parents as partners in their child's treatment. Unless the child does not want a parent in the room (e.g., some adolescents), a parent can help calm the child, and many examinations and procedures can be performed with the child on a parent's lap. Although having the family remain with the child can be calming and supportive, respect the family's right to leave if the child's condition or the painful nature of a procedure provokes more anxiety than the family member is able to handle. Recent research demonstrates that families prefer to remain with their child. The presence of family members during procedures and resuscitations is becoming increasingly promoted as an integral part of family-centered care (Young, 2014).

For parents who do not know exactly how to be of assistance in these situations, it can help to explain how a parent might help, such as "I think he might stay calmer if you hold his hand and tell him a story while I clean this burn" or "Try counting to 10 with her while I start this intravenous line."

Whenever possible, designate one staff member as the child's caretaker and liaison to the parents. In the unfamiliar emergency setting, the child and family find that having one contact person is less confusing. Consistency is helpful in a crisis because the child and family may feel overwhelmed in the busy and sometimes confusing emergency department environment.

*Tell the truth.* To establish a trusting relationship, be as honest as possible. If a procedure will be painful, tell the child (usually shortly beforehand). Only then can the child believe healthcare providers when they say that a procedure will *not* be painful. When a painful procedure is completed, tell the child you are finished and there will be no more pain. Keeping a child informed of what will occur by describing sensations (e.g., "This will feel cold and wet as I clean your arm.") is more helpful than describing the actual procedure.

*Provide incentives and rewards.* Provide positive feedback when either the child or the parents are being helpful. Children from 3 to 12 years of age especially appreciate verbal praise and concrete rewards for good behavior, such as stickers, fancy bandages, or inexpensive toys. Adults also appreciate being thanked for their patience and for their assistance in their child's care. All these techniques help create as positive an experience as possible.

*Assess the child's unspoken thoughts and feelings.* Try to determine what the child is thinking or feeling but not verbalizing. Encourage the child to express thoughts and feelings; sometimes the child might be misinterpreting a situation or need to express emotions.

However, in some cases, the child's and family's coping mechanisms break down, causing inappropriate behavior. If violence or abusive behavior is an issue, you might need to obtain assistance from law enforcement or hospital security officers. For an emotional crisis that does not involve abusive or aggressive behavior, the following simple rules apply:

- Encourage the person in crisis to move to a quiet place. Observers and stimuli from other sources tend to aggravate a crisis.
- Encourage the child or parent to talk about feelings, as well as the "facts" of the situation. Use reflective statements.
- Avoid defensiveness, explanation, or justification of your own or others' behavior.
- Speak in simple sentences. Use sentences of no more than five words, with words no longer than five letters (e.g., "Let's sit down over here," "Let me help," "Please let go of that").
- Set limits. Avoid "yes" or "no" responses. Rather than saying, "Will you take this medicine?" (the small child will probably say "NO!"), ask "Would you rather take the pink or the yellow medicine first?"

When interacting with families in distress, a good general rule is to try to listen rather than talk. Simply being present for children and families and empathizing with them are useful interventions. Help families identify specific problems and their effective coping mechanisms and assist them to explore reasonable solutions.

However, when coping mechanisms break down entirely, some direction is necessary. Consulting social services, spiritual counselors (e.g., chaplain), or crisis intervention professionals can be helpful. Early intervention and support for appropriate coping mechanisms are far easier and less time consuming than intervening after a child's or parent's emotional decompensation.

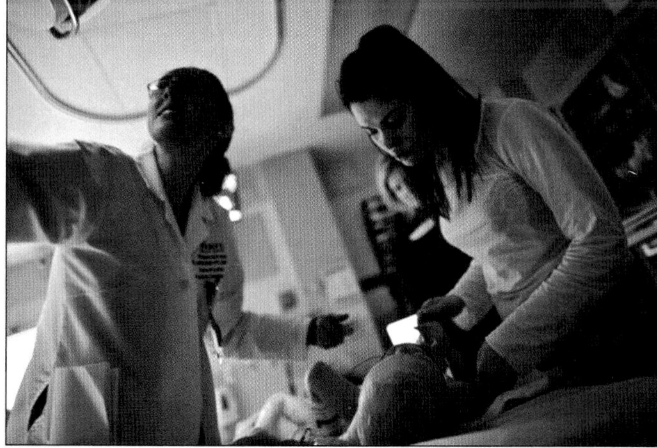

Encouraging parents to remain with their child in the emergency setting can bolster the family's coping. (Courtesy Children's Medical Center, Dallas, TX.)

## Pediatric Emergency Equipment

Airways
- Oropharyngeal airway: sizes 4-10 cm
- Nasopharyngeal: sizes 12-36 Fr
- Laryngeal mask airway: sizes are weight based
  - Size 1: <5 kg
  - Size 2: 5-10 kg
  - Size 2.5: 20-30 kg
  - Size 3: 30-50 kg
  - Size 4: 50-70 kg
  - Size 5: 70-100 kg

Endotracheal tubes: internal diameter (ID) in mm

$$\text{Size} = \frac{16 + \text{age in years}}{4}$$

- Depth = ETT size × 3
- For cuffed ETT, use 0.5 cm smaller.

Laryngoscope with blades
- Straight (Miller): sizes #0-3
- Curved (Macintosh): sizes #2-3

Magill forceps

Oxygen equipment: infant, pediatric, and adult masks and cannulas

Bag-mask ventilation device: infant, pediatric, and adult sizes

Chest tubes: sizes 8-30 Fr

Flexible suction catheters: sizes 5-14 Fr (tracheal)

Yankauer suction tip (oropharyngeal)

Pediatric peripheral IV equipment and solutions (cannulas: 18-24 gauge)

Intraosseous device: 15-18 gauge

Nasogastric tubes: sizes 5-18 Fr

Urinary catheters: sizes 5-12 Fr

Length-based resuscitation tape (Broselow)

Defibrillator with adult and pediatric pads/paddles

Electrocardiogram (ECG) monitors with pediatric-sized electrodes and sensors

Pulse oximeter

Capnometer to measure exhaled carbon dioxide ($CO_2$)

Heating source
- Fluid warmer
- Infrared lamp
- Overhead warmer

Data from Kleinman, M.E., Chameides, L., Schexnayder, S.M., et al. (2010). Part 14: Pediatric advanced life support: 2010 American Heart Association guidelines for cardiopulmonary resuscitation and emergency cardiovascular care. *Circulation, 122*(3), S876–S908; Susil, G. (2009). Emergency management. In J. Custer, & R. Rau (Eds.), *The Harriet Lane handbook* (18th ed., pp. 3–17). Philadelphia: Mosby.

## Pediatric Emergency Medications

| Medication | Use |
|---|---|
| Adenosine | Supraventricular tachycardia<br>Pearl: must be given via rapid flush technique at access point closest to the heart due to ultra-short half-life |
| Amiodarone | Pulseless arrest, supraventricular and ventricular tachycardia |
| Atropine sulfate | Symptomatic bradycardia and toxins/overdose (i.e., organophosphates) |
| Calcium chloride 10% | Hypocalcemia, hypermagnesemia, hyperkalemia, and calcium channel blocker overdose |
| Dextrose (25%, 50%) | Hypoglycemia, a common complication of dehydration, sepsis, and resuscitation |
| Inotropic agents | Hypotension or hypoperfusion, severe congestive heart failure, or cardiovascular shock |
| Epinephrine (1:1000 [endotracheal], 1:10,000 [intravenous/intraosseous]) | Bradycardia or pulseless arrest, hypotensive shock, anaphylaxis, toxins/overdose (i.e., beta blockers, calcium channel blockers) |
| Lidocaine | Pulseless ventricular tachycardia, ventricular fibrillation, or wide complex tachycardia (with pulses) |
| Magnesium sulfate | Torsades de pointes dysrhythmia, hypomagnesemia, or severe asthma |
| Naloxone hydrochloride | Reverses effects of opiate narcotics |
| Sodium bicarbonate | Severe metabolic acidosis, hyperkalemia, and sodium channel blocker overdose<br>Pearl: must use 0.5 meq/mL concentration if under 1 year old due to risk of IVH. If unavailable, can dilute standard concentration with equal volume saline |

Data from de Caen, A.R., Berg, M.D., Chameides, L., et al. (2015). Part 12: Pediatric Advanced Life Support 2015 American Heart Association Guidelines Update for Cardiopulmonary Resuscitation and Emergency Cardiovascular Care. *Circulation, 132*(2), S526–S542. doi:10.1161/CIR.0000000000000266.

Very few experiences are as frightening to a family as a child's sudden illness or injury. Therefore, caring for children and families in the emergency setting presents special challenges to the healthcare team. Nurses play an important role in emergency settings because they are most often responsible for the initial contact, triage, and continuing care throughout an emergency visit. The goals of emergency nursing care include addressing the child's physical problems, supporting the child's and family's coping mechanisms, and creating an atmosphere in which the family is valued and kept as intact as possible.

## GROWTH AND DEVELOPMENT ISSUES IN EMERGENCY CARE

Emergency nursing care of children needs to address both the physiologic and psychological differences in children in terms of age and development. Paying close attention to developmental issues assists in obtaining a more accurate assessment and can affect the course of care (see Chapters 6 through 9 for approaches to children of different ages). The nurse treats each child as an individual and avoids becoming judgmental when a child regresses to a "safer" developmental level. Although children of the same age-group are similar, differences in past experiences, cultures, and maturity levels result in a range of behaviors. One toddler might be much more mature than another, and one adolescent might lean more toward school-age behaviors than another (Box 34.1).

### The Infant

An infant experiences the world through the senses; hunger, satiation, cold, warmth, quiet, and noise affect the infant's comfort or discomfort. An infant has not learned patience and has little tolerance for physical or emotional discomfort, including pain (see Chapter 39 for management of pain in infants and children). Crying can be stressful for caregivers; pacifiers are an adequate self-comforting measure when analgesia is not indicated. Stress can cause increased metabolic demands in the infant, so offer rest periods during procedures to maintain normothermia.

### BOX 34.1 Working With Children in Emergencies: Developmental Guidelines

**Infants**

- Allow the use of a pacifier.
- Use a quiet, soothing voice.
- Touch, rock, or cuddle the infant. Holding the infant securely or swaddling a young infant can also be comforting.
- Keep the infant warm; if the infant must be left undressed, use warming lights to ensure a comfortable temperature.
- As much as possible, allay parents' fears so they will not be communicated to the infant.
- Remember that infants feel pain (see Chapter 39 for pain interventions).

**Toddlers**

- Give treatments and perform procedures with the toddler sitting up on the stretcher or examining table or on the parent's lap.
- Perform the most distressing or intrusive parts of the examination last.
- Reassure family members as much as possible; the child will benefit from their confidence.
- Allow the child to have familiar objects (transitional objects) such as a blanket, doll, or toy to help feel safe.
- Keep frightening objects out of the child's line of vision. Also try to keep machines that make loud noises away.
- Praise (e.g., "You are being so brave") and distraction (e.g., bubbles, puzzles) will decrease anxiety and increase cooperation.

**Preschoolers**

- Explain a procedure or treatment a few seconds rather than minutes beforehand, because allowing the young child time to think about it may result in frightening fantasies or exaggerations.
- Talk to preschool children throughout procedures, describing the sensations they are feeling or will feel and telling them how they can help.
- Distract the child with noises or bright objects. For some preschool children, counting with them can help calm them during procedures.
- Avoid criticizing the preschool child for crying, struggling, or fighting during a procedure.
- Reassuring a child that he or she did try his or her best to cooperate will help to build a positive self-image.
- Encourage the preschool child to talk about how the illness or injury occurred. If the child is inappropriately taking responsibility for the illness or injury, try to reassure that he or she is not to blame for the situation.
- Remember that preschool children can appear to understand more than they actually do. Healthcare providers often overestimate comprehension in a child of this age, so be sure to explain things in words the child understands.
- Use positive terms, such as "make better" and "help," and avoid more frightening terms, such as "shot" and "cut."
- Use adhesive bandages over small wounds and injection sites. Preschool children might imagine their blood leaking out through puncture wounds.

**School-Age Children**

- Offer simple choices whenever possible to help the child feel more in control. The school-age child is capable of deciding in which arm to have an injection or in which hand to hold a nebulizer. Talk directly to the child, explaining procedures in simple terms. When explaining treatments or care options to the parent, include the child.
- Ask the child about his or her level of understanding and allow time for questions.
- Address the child's fears or concerns directly rather than treating them as foolish or inconsequential.
- Give rewards, such as a sticker or an inexpensive toy, after a procedure, regardless of the child's behavior. Think of this gesture as a reward for undergoing the procedure, not as a judgment of "good" or "bad" behavior.

**Adolescents**

- Preserve the adolescent's modesty; offer adolescents a choice regarding whether they want their parents present when obtaining history and during the examination.
- Consider the legal issues regarding the right to privacy for pregnant adolescents and adolescents with sexually transmitted diseases.
- Provide an opportunity for questions.
- Listen to the adolescent's concerns nonjudgmentally and without belittling.
- Developing a teasing relationship with an adolescent is often a temptation, but this has potential for harm; the adolescent is easily embarrassed.
- Explain procedures or treatments carefully and allow choices. Adolescents are capable of complex abstract thinking and can make intelligent and reasoned decisions about their own care.

Although infants are able to discriminate their parents from others, older infants (9 to 18 months of age, or earlier in some infants) can exhibit signs of both separation and stranger anxiety. The nurse should allow the parent to hold the infant as much as possible for examination and treatment. This arrangement may not be possible in a critical situation, but nurses need to remember to reunite parent and child whenever feasible.

### The Toddler

Toddlers are just beginning to explore the world and seem to have limitless energy and curiosity. They are also beginning to have a clearer image of themselves as autonomous and distinct beings. For this reason, they do not respond well to restrictions and tend to push any limits imposed. This tendency can be a problem in the emergency setting because some nursing care might involve securing and restraining the toddler, making them feel vulnerable. The nurse should be sure to remove any restriction or restraint as soon as safety permits. Toddlers have little understanding of time, so procedures should be introduced just before they are initiated.

### The Preschooler

The preschool child is talking and beginning to be more independent. However, this outward appearance of organization is somewhat misleading because the preschool period is also the stage of fear and fantasy. Because of their imaginative nature, preschoolers need little time lag between the explanation of a procedure and its completion. Additionally, avoid using terms such as "stick" or "cut" to prevent literal misinterpretations of meanings. Preschoolers are strong believers in cause-and-effect relations and tend to blame themselves for illnesses and injuries.

The preschool child may be more willing than the toddler to be separated from parents, but the nurse should keep this separation as brief as possible. The nurse can include the parents in treatments and provide them with instructions on calming the child if they seem unsure. The nurse should not ask a parent to restrain the child because this role may be confusing to the child and difficult for the parent.

### The School-Age Child

School-age children are interested in learning and gradually acquire reasoning skills, including some abstract thinking. They are able to understand the cause of illness and injury and are much less likely to fantasize and exaggerate. School-age children have extensive vocabularies, and they can understand simple explanations of procedures. They are also able to make decisions about their own care. By this time, they have developed personal techniques to help them through painful times. The nurse helps them use coping techniques that work for them. Because risk-taking behaviors begin at this age, caregivers must stress the importance of injury prevention behaviors.

### The Adolescent

Although adolescents are at varying stages of puberty, they begin to resemble adults in appearance. They are also beginning to explore the adult world and develop their own unique identities. However, the nurse needs to remember that even though adolescents appear physically mature, they might not be emotionally mature, and they continue to require support. Coping with extraordinary changes in their physical appearance, they are often concerned with whether they are "normal" and whether others have similar thoughts and feelings.

Although this is an age of risk taking, which can make them prone to serious injury, adolescents can be quite fearful of death. Although they are aware of the possibility of their own death, they avoid thinking about its reality. Adolescents consider themselves invincible, and many experience overwhelming emotions when a friend dies unexpectedly.

Adolescence is an age of extremes; teenagers might either exaggerate or underplay the seriousness of a condition. Sometimes assessing the full extent of an adolescent's illness or injury is difficult. Expert care of the adolescent requires sensitivity to both verbal and nonverbal cues. Adolescents' privacy should be respected; nurses should approach them as one would an adult, giving them full attention and respect for their thoughts and feelings.

Adolescents are increasingly using emergency department settings for non-urgent care, and many of these adolescents demonstrate high-risk behavior. In addition, the prevalence of depression is high among adolescents. Therefore, it is crucial that nurses screen for high risk behavior and mental health concerns. Behavioral and mental health issues can be assessed using technology-based emergency-room screening tools, which may provide more privacy (Goyal, 2015).

## THE FAMILY OF A CHILD IN EMERGENCY CARE

Stress on the family results directly and indirectly from the child's illness or injury. The way a child perceives an illness or injury often is related to the parents' attitude, so caring for the child requires assessment of and intervention with the family.

The most common emotions experienced by parents of children cared for in emergencies are fear and anxiety. Past experiences may lessen or increase these emotions. Parents are afraid of the following possibilities:

- Their child might die. This fear is the greatest source of anxiety and can be present even when death is highly unlikely, such as in the case of minor illnesses or injuries. This anxiety is often the underlying cause of parents' anger toward healthcare providers.
- Their child might experience pain. As a rule, parents try very hard to protect children from pain. Even when pain is necessary, it is difficult for parents to understand and accept.
- The child's body may be permanently altered. Parents often fear that their children will have permanent scars or body changes.

Parental guilt is another frequently seen emotion. Parents can feel guilty for the following reasons:

- They feel responsible for their child's illness or injury.
- They are submitting their child to a painful experience.
- They do not have enough knowledge to make educated decisions about their child's care.

In addition, parents may have had negative experiences with healthcare providers in the past or have other concerns about siblings, financial arrangements, and work schedules.

The particular causes of stress for families in emergencies are unique to the circumstances and to the family involved. The nurse needs to define the family (e.g., single parent, two parents, grandparent, other caregiver), identify the decision makers (e.g., family members, religious leaders), and communicate accordingly. All the stressors combined might stretch parents' coping mechanisms to the limit and result in anger, withdrawal, or tearfulness. Stress also can manifest in hyperactivity—making numerous phone calls, repeating questions, and involving a large number of people.

Including family members in their child's care can reduce feelings of helplessness and promote positive coping mechanisms. Nurses should facilitate family presence during procedures and encourage them to support their child. Although it is not appropriate to solicit family members to help hold or restrain a child for a procedure, they can offer emotional support. Early assessment and appropriate support before problems occur are advantageous for both healthcare workers and the family.

## EMERGENCY ASSESSMENT OF INFANTS AND CHILDREN

In the emergency setting, assessment of the ill or injured child must be rapid and accurate to identify abnormal findings quickly. In children, initial evidence of life-threatening conditions can be subtle, with few signs of impending respiratory or cardiopulmonary arrest. Making as many initial observations as possible without touching the child is extremely important so that assessments can reflect the child's baseline, or resting condition. For an apparently stable infant or young child, most of the examination required for general triage can be performed with the child on the parent's lap. The nurse also observes the relationship between the parents and child during the examination process.

The triage nurse usually performs the initial observation in the emergency setting and decides the level of care needed for the child. Triaging is an important skill that improves with experience. The nurse bases much of the initial assessment on an overall sense of how the child looks—sick or well (an "across the room" assessment). Because children do not try to cover up how they feel or how they look, the nurse immediately receives a fairly accurate impression of illness or wellness.

Three essential factors combine to form a first impression: respiratory rate and effort, skin color, and response to the environment. Abnormalities are compared with the parent's or caregiver's perception ("Is this his normal color?"). If results of this assessment appear to be normal, the nurse completes a more thorough and in-depth evaluation. If the general impression is that the child is seriously ill, the nurse must intervene immediately and combine any additional evaluation with interventions.

### Primary Assessment

Primary assessment, which is part of the initial triage assessment, consists of assessing the ABCDEs—*a*irway, *b*reathing, *c*irculation, level of consciousness (*d*isability), and *e*xposure. Because the two most common pathways to death in children are respiratory failure and shock, interventions include providing respiratory and circulatory support. When head, neck, or back trauma is suspected, cervical spine protection should be initiated by maintaining the spine in a neutral position. Cervical and spinal cord injury can be difficult to detect without radiologic intervention in children who cannot effectively verbalize their pain or symptoms.

#### Airway Assessment

Although determining the cause of respiratory distress or failure in an ill child ultimately will be important, recognizing symptoms and signs of respiratory distress is more important. In the emergency setting, initial treatment is the same regardless of the cause. Remember that apparent respiratory distress can originate from causes such as rib fractures and metabolic acidosis.

Because of some differences in airway anatomy and physiology, children are at a greater risk of airway problems than adults (Table 34.1). When assessing children's airways, the nurse pays particular attention to breath sounds (often audible to the naked ear) as well as snoring, stridor, wheezing, and grunting. Snoring is caused by obstruction in the upper airway (often the tongue relaxing against the posterior pharynx) and can be heard in a child with decreased mental status. Stridor is a high-pitched sound heard on inspiration (laryngeal obstruction) or on both inspiration and expiration (midtracheal obstruction). Wheezing, a high-pitched, musical sound heard primarily on expiration, signals obstruction of the lower airway. Crackles or rales are fine, popping noises heard on inspiration; they usually indicate fluid in the lungs, as in pneumonia.

**! NURSING QUALITY ALERT**

***Initial Observations for Triage***

*Respiratory rate and effort:* Is the child's breathing rapid or shallow, or is the child using accessory muscles? What is the child's position of comfort? When children are having difficulty breathing, they use accessory muscles to help. Substernal, intercostal, or subclavicular retractions are all signs of serious breathing difficulties. Nasal flaring, head bobbing, grunting, stridor, upright position, and prolonged expirations signal increased work of breathing. A slow respiratory rate is of great concern; a child who seems to be breathing at a rate normal for an adult is almost certainly hypoventilating. This respiratory rate can signal imminent respiratory arrest. Observe for abnormal breath sounds, and assess oxygen saturation by pulse oximeter.

*Skin color:* Is the child's skin pale, mottled, or cyanotic? Abnormal skin color could result from the two greatest threats to a child's life: respiratory distress or failure and inadequate tissue perfusion (shock).

*Response to the environment:* Is the child alert, interactive, crying, sleepy, or limp? Is the child smiling and able to play? Does the child make eye contact and interact appropriately? Although response to the environment is more difficult to evaluate in the preverbal child, responsiveness is an important component of the assessment. A well child should look around, fixate on objects, and appear to recognize caretakers. An anxious-appearing child may be in respiratory distress; a flaccid, disinterested child may be in respiratory failure or frank shock.

#### Breathing Assessment

Level of consciousness, rate and depth of breathing, breath sounds, and the child's respiratory effort are indicative of relative oxygenation. Anxiety or decreased responsiveness suggests hypoxia. A rapid respiratory rate with shallow breathing indicates respiratory distress. Very slow breathing in an ill child is an ominous sign, indicating respiratory failure. A slowly breathing child might no longer have the energy for adequate ventilation. Increased work of breathing with quiet breath sounds may indicate an absence of air entry into lung fields. Abdominal breathing is normal in the infant or young child, so the nurse observes the rise and fall of the abdomen instead of the chest.

The use of accessory muscles for breathing invariably indicates respiratory distress. The child's chest wall is relatively weak and unstable, so retractions occur with increased work of breathing. Assessment of breathing includes observing the child for intercostal, substernal, suprasternal, supraclavicular, and infraclavicular retractions. As a child becomes exhausted, retractions may diminish, usually indicating respiratory failure. Nasal flaring with inspiration is another form of accessory muscle use. Grunting, a sound made by the expiration of air against partially closed vocal cords, is a sign of hypoxemia and represents the body's effort to improve oxygenation by generating positive end-expiratory pressure.

The nurse observes the child's preferred body posture. A child in respiratory distress is upright with the jaw thrust forward, leaning forward on outstretched arms—the tripod position. This position, often referred to as "tripoding," helps maximize airway opening and the use of accessory muscles of respiration.

Once the work of breathing has been carefully observed, listening to the chest provides some useful information. Children have small chests, and breath sounds can be transmitted throughout the chest. Therefore, the nurse auscultates a child's chest at both sides of the body at the midaxillary line and over the trachea to confirm equality of breath sounds and distinguish upper from lower airway noises.

Normal respiratory rates for children vary by age and are faster than for adults (see Table 33.1). However, a respiratory rate greater than 60

TABLE 34.1 **Primary Assessment in Pediatric Emergencies**

| Assessment | Pediatric Differences | Nursing Implications |
|---|---|---|
| **A: Airway** | | |
| Patency, positioning for air entry, audible sounds, airway obstruction (blood, mucus, edema) | The child's airway is narrower than an adult's and more easily obstructed by foreign bodies, small amounts of mucus, and tissue edema. Infants are preferential nasal breathers for the first several months of life; therefore, nasal secretions can cause respiratory compromise. Children are more susceptible to infectious respiratory diseases that contribute to risk of airway obstruction. Edema and mucus in a narrow airway cause incrementally more obstruction than in a wider one.<br>The tongue is relatively large in relation to the oral cavity and can more easily fall into the airway in the unconscious child.<br>Cartilage of the child's larynx is relatively soft, and the larynx is higher and more anterior, increasing the risk of obstruction and aspiration. Compared to an adult, the trachea is thinner and more flexible.<br>The submandibular area is softer and can be more easily compressed to occlude the airway.<br>Deciduous teeth are poorly anchored and easily dislodged.<br>Altered mental status is an early sign of hypoxia. | Allow the child to maintain a position of comfort or manually position the airway (jaw thrust or head-tilt/chin-lift); encourage the child to avoid flexing or hyperextending the neck; use spinal immobilization and airway adjuncts as required. |
| **B: Breathing** | | |
| Decreased level of consciousness, increased or decreased work of breathing, nasal flaring, use of accessory muscles of respiration (retractions), rate, pattern, quality, oxygen saturation | The chest wall is thin, softer, and more compliant. Rib alignment is more horizontal. The younger child is more susceptible to respiratory distress and failure. Retractions commonly occur with respiratory distress and can compromise the ability to increase tidal volume.<br>The diaphragm is the predominant muscle of respiration. Pressure above or below the diaphragm can impede respiratory effort.<br>Infants and children have a higher metabolic rate and increased oxygen demand. Hypoxia occurs more rapidly. | Provide supplemental oxygen; initiate assisted ventilation with bag-valve-mask ventilation device, and prepare for intubation as indicated; provide gastric decompression with orogastric or nasogastric tube; provide comfort measures; encourage family presence to decrease anxiety. |
| **C: Circulation** | | |
| Skin color, temperature, and capillary refill (<2 sec); rate and strength of peripheral and central pulses | The child's circulating blood volume per body weight is much larger than an adult's, even though actual blood volume is much smaller. Therefore, small volume losses have more severe circulatory consequences.<br>A higher percentage of fluid is located in the extracellular compartment, causing more rapid fluid shifts.<br>A higher metabolic rate and oxygen demand require an increased heart rate; tachycardia is the first compensatory mechanism for decreased oxygenation—not hypotension. | Control bleeding through application of direct pressure; obtain vascular access; initiate volume replacement; perform chest compressions; defibrillate or provide synchronized cardioversion; initiate drug therapy. |
| **D: Disability** | | |
| Level of consciousness or activity level; response to the environment (especially parents); pupillary response | A larger head-to-body ratio and weak neck muscles contribute to more serious head injury from shaking or impact.<br>The anterior fontanel remains open until approximately age 18 mo. An open fontanel allows for expanded cranial volume, so signs of increased intracranial pressure, which indicate underlying traumatic brain injury, may be delayed.<br>A thinner skull predisposes the child to more severe injury.<br>Nerve myelinization is incomplete during infancy; unmyelinated tissue is more vulnerable to shearing injury. | Treat the underlying cause (e.g., signs of increased intracranial pressure; fluid or blood volume deficit; hypoglycemia; hypothermia; hypoxia); compare assessment with parent's perception (a deeply sleeping child may be difficult to arouse, which is "normal" to parents). |
| **E: Exposure** | | |
| To identify underlying injuries or additional signs of illness | Bulging fontanel, periorbital edema, unusual rashes, and edema or exudate in the pharynx can indicate a variety of severe childhood communicable diseases.<br>Bruising, unusual burns, vaginal tearing, rectal bleeding, and discharge suggest child abuse.<br>Swelling, deformities can indicate underlying trauma to vital organs. | Remove all clothing, including diapers; save any clothing needed for evidence; maintain an appropriately warm environment. |

Data from Emergency Nurses Association. (2012). *Emergency nursing pediatric course provider manual* (4th ed.). Des Plains, IL: Author.

breaths per minute is abnormal for any age. Another important adjunct for respiratory assessment is the pulse oximetry reading (see Chapter 37). Measuring exhaled carbon dioxide ($CO_2$) using capnography (even in non-intubated patients) may provide a more sensitive detection of hypoventilation, impaired gas exchange and perfusion, metabolic acidosis, and carbon monoxide poisoning ("Is Capnography Used," 2011; "Monitoring $ETCO_2$," 2011).

### Cardiovascular Assessment

Cardiovascular assessment includes observing the child's skin color and temperature, checking capillary refill, and assessing central and peripheral pulse rate and quality. A child can compensate more effectively for fluid loss than an adult through increased heart rate and peripheral vasoconstriction. Tachycardia and decreased peripheral perfusion are early signs of cardiovascular compromise in a child and require immediate intervention to prevent decompensation. Hypotension is a late finding in a child with shock. Hypotension manifests only after significant fluid loss because of the compensatory mechanisms that result in vasoconstriction (de Caen et al., 2015a). Hypotension in children suggests that compensatory mechanisms are no longer adequate to maintain cardiac output.

### Disability: Neurologic Assessment

The infant's or child's level of consciousness is an essential component of the primary assessment. An altered level of consciousness (irritability or agitation, lethargy, or inability to recognize parents or caregivers) can be the first sign of respiratory compromise or worsening condition.

A rapid neurologic assessment consists of two components: (1) pupillary reactivity and size; and (2) a brief mental status assessment (*AVPU: a*lert, responds to *v*oice, responds to *p*ain, *u*nresponsive). More thorough and sophisticated means of assessment are used later if needed (see Chapter 52). Serial assessment is imperative. Progressive loss of consciousness can be the result of hypoxemia, hypercapnia, hypoglycemia, increased intracranial pressure, or another life-threatening condition.

### Exposure

Primary assessment ends with exposure, or removing the child's clothing to identify additional injuries or indicators of illness. The nurse needs to preserve the child's clothing appropriately if it will be needed for evidence in any potential civil or criminal proceeding. Infants and children have a larger body surface-area-to-weight ratio, making them at higher risk for hypothermia. Maintaining body temperature by shivering increases metabolic needs, requiring more oxygen and glucose, and the child has limited reserves. The risk of hypoxia and hypoglycemia is higher in neonates from the utilization of brown fat for nonshivering thermogenesis and from an increased metabolic demand secondary to an infectious or physiologic process. Methods to help the child maintain a normothermic state or help with warming include overhead warmers and heat lamps, warmed intravenous (IV) fluids and humidified oxygen, removal of wet clothes, and providing warmed blankets.

## Secondary Assessment

After the primary assessment is complete and interventions (if necessary) have stabilized the child, the nurse begins the secondary assessment. Components of the secondary assessment include vital signs, assessing for pain, history and head-to-toe assessment, and inspection (Table 34.2).

### Vital Signs

Vital signs are useful in the triage assessment of the child, but because age variations make their significance more difficult to interpret, they are not as reliable an indicator as for adults. This variation is especially marked with regards to temperature. For example, an infant has an immature thermoregulatory system and may not have a fever or may even be hypothermic in the presence of infection, so the nurse needs to be alert to supporting signs. The nurse remembers that an alteration in one part of the vital signs may result in abnormal values in other parts. For example, an abnormally high heart rate and respiratory rate may result from hyperthermia, crying, pain, hypoxemia, or hypovolemia (see Chapter 37 for methods of obtaining a temperature).

When taking a child's vital signs, the nurse observes the respiratory rate first and then obtains the pulse; the nurse obtains the temperature and blood pressure last because these procedures can be more upsetting for children and can alter the other vital signs. The nurse should be certain to use the correct size blood pressure cuff and take both the respiratory and heart rates for 1 full minute because subtle differences are important in the child. Normal pediatric respiratory and heart rates are faster than adult rates, whereas the blood pressure is lower on average (see Table 33.1 and http://www.nhlbi.nih.gov/files/docs/guidelines/child_tbl.pdf). An accurate weight should be obtained at

**TABLE 34.2 Secondary Assessment in Pediatric Emergencies**

| Assessment | Nursing Implications |
|---|---|
| **F: Full Set of Vital Signs; Family Presence** | |
| Evaluate the child's vital signs, including temperature, for abnormal findings; obtain weight in kilograms. Family presence: assess the needs of the family for support and inclusion in care. Focused Adjuncts: continuous physiologic monitoring. | Continuously monitor the child's vital signs, including temperature; weigh child or obtain estimated weight if child's condition prohibits measured weight. Facilitate family presence and support in a culturally appropriate way. Evaluate need for monitoring and additional procedures in response to the patient's condition. |
| **G: Give Comfort Measures** | |
| Discomfort is usually related to the underlying problem; use pain assessment scales for children. | Frequently monitor pain level and response to pain-relief measures; include nonpharmacologic techniques for reducing pain. |
| **H: Head-to-Toe Assessment; Obtain History** | |
| Perform a complete head-to-toe assessment and obtain a history; during triage assessment, a focused assessment related to the chief complaint can be used. | Continuously monitor the child for changes in condition; assess for any unusual odors. |
| **I: Inspect Posterior Surfaces** | |
| Observe the back for obvious or hidden injuries; assess for communicable illness or susceptibility to illness (immunocompromised patients). | Reinspect the back as indicated. |

Data from Emergency Nurses Association. (2012). *Emergency nursing pediatric course provider manual* (4th ed.). Des Plains, IL: Author.

this time, and monitors, such as a cardiac or pulse oximeter, should be applied as indicated.

### History and Head-to-Toe Assessment

A brief history provides information about prior illness or injury that might affect the emergency care of the child. One format often used for pediatric patients is the mnemonic *SAMPLE:*

**S** signs and symptoms
**A** allergies
**M** medications taken (prescription, over the counter, and herbal or home remedies) and immunization history
**P** prior illness or injury
**L** last meal and eating habits
**E** events surrounding this injury or illness (e.g., length of illness, mechanism of injury)

This mnemonic gives sufficient information to determine whether the child's medical history will play an important role in assessing and treating the current illness or injury. In emergency departments that care for children, a list of immunizations and the appropriate ages from the CDC (2016a) should be posted in a convenient location (see http://www.cdc.gov/vaccines/schedules/index.html).

After obtaining an appropriate history, the nurse begins to perform a head-to-toe assessment, documenting any findings that might affect the child's condition. Assessment findings are compared with the history to aid in diagnosis and look for inconsistencies. The nurse inspects all body surfaces, looking for fractures, lacerations, contusions, and penetrating injuries. The nurse also observes the skin for petechiae, purpura, or rashes. The presence and pattern of any pain are described. The nurse pays particular attention to signs of pneumothorax or hemothorax (e.g., decreased breath sounds on the affected side, signs of hypoxemia, and signs of shock). The nurse then palpates the child's abdomen and auscultates for the presence of bowel sounds. Any sign of hematuria suggests genitourinary injury or infection. Blood found at the urinary meatus suggests disruptive injury of the lower urinary tract, and a urinary catheter should not be inserted.

### Diagnostic Tests

Once the child has arrived in the emergency setting and has undergone initial assessment and interventions, diagnostic tests are performed that assist in the evaluation process. Standard protocols for laboratory tests usually include a complete blood count (CBC) with differential count, serum electrolytes, glucose (checked at the bedside), and urinalysis. Additional studies may be necessary for the child who has multiple trauma and could include laboratory tests for coagulation profiles, blood urea nitrogen (BUN), creatinine, glucose, amylase, lipase, aspartate aminotransferase (AST), alanine aminotransferase ALT), and blood type and crossmatch.

Radiologic films might be obtained, depending on the presenting problem and assessment data. Placement of a gastric tube, urinary catheter, or other device may be required. Orogastric tubes should be placed in children with suspected head trauma because of the risk of misplacement and injury with a nasogastric tube in children with basilar skull and facial fractures. Gastric tubes are placed to reduce gastric inflation that can place pressure on the diaphragm and decrease ventilation effectiveness, as children are diaphragmatic breathers.

### Weight

Determining the child's weight is essential in emergency care because all medication dosages and fluid amounts are calculated according to the child's weight in kilograms. The nurse weighs the child on an appropriately calibrated scale, if possible, following agency procedures for measuring and recording weight (e.g., with or without clothing, diaper on vs. diaper off).

Another way to determine the child's weight and medication dosages is through the use of a length-based resuscitation tape such as the Broselow tape. Tapes with precalculated medication doses calculated at various lengths have been proven more accurate in the prediction of body weight than provider or parent estimate-based methods (de Caen et al., 2015b). A length-based resuscitation tape is placed on a gurney or stretcher next to the child, and the child's length is measured. The length is keyed to emergency medication dosages, usually listed on the tape. The tape also indicates fluid bolus volumes, defibrillation energy levels, and sizes of the pediatric airway, bag-valve-mask ventilation device, laryngoscope, endotracheal tube, gastric tube, urinary catheter, chest tube, and IV catheter. The validity of length-based resuscitation tapes is questioned with the growing trends in childhood obesity, and these tapes should be used with caution in overweight children.

### Parent-Child Relationship

Rapid triage assessment of the child also includes observation of the child in relation to the parents. If the relationship does not appear to be close, comfortable, and trusting, the nurse may want to explore this further.

## CARDIOPULMONARY RESUSCITATION OF THE CHILD

### Airway and Breathing

#### Initial Assessment and Intervention

While lethal arrhythmias related to heart disease are the most common causes of cardiopulmonary arrest in adults, factors leading to shock and respiratory failure are the most common causes of cardiopulmonary arrest in children. Early recognition of and intervention for respiratory distress and compensated shock can be lifesaving for the child. Assistance with ventilation and administration of fluids may prevent further deterioration in the child's condition. Once the child progresses to respiratory failure and shock, **cardiopulmonary resuscitation** (CPR) is necessary. Resuscitation of children requires attention to the differences between adults and children (see Table 34.1).

If a child is unresponsive and not breathing, basic life-support measures will be initiated. However, the child with spontaneous respiratory effort or a pulse will require more evaluation to determine the need for CPR. Cardiac arrests in infants and children are more commonly caused by asphyxiation; thus, the recommendations from the American Heart Association (AHA) differ regarding the resuscitation of children and adults. The pediatric recommendations updated in 2015 continue to include the sequence of "CAB" (circulation, airway, breathing), although this remains controversial. Chest-compression only CPR is not recommended in children, in recognition of the high frequency of cardiac arrest caused by initial respiratory arrest in children (Atkins, Berger, Duff, et al., 2015).

Because of the proportionately larger size of the child's head with a weaker supporting muscle structure, repositioning the head and placing a rolled-up towel under the child's shoulders can often facilitate improved air exchange. Additionally, the tongue of the young child is larger in relation to the oropharynx and is often the cause of airway obstruction. When administering assisted ventilations, the nurse should stop inflating the lungs when the chest just begins to rise and allow enough time for exhalation (longer than inhalation). Endotracheal intubation by a provider skilled in the technique is necessary if the child cannot be ventilated adequately with these measures or if

## EVIDENCE-BASED PRACTICE

The triage area in an emergency department is extremely busy, and nurses working in that area are subject to many distractions from patients, families, and the environment itself. The purpose of triage is to make a rapid and accurate assessment of patients and a decision about the level of care needed. Because data collected at the point of care in triage are used subsequently by professionals treating the child, it is essential that important information be accurately assessed and documented. One critical piece of information is whether or not a child is allergic to medication.

Recent research had demonstrated "significant gaps" in the assessment and communication of children's medication allergy in an emergent care setting. Researchers have documented that errors (both positive and negative) identified during triage can be carried throughout the treatment phase. Several communication issues that apply specifically to nurses have been identified:

- Many parents identify their child as being allergic without describing data that support a hypersensitivity reaction, or are not able to identify specific medications to which the child may be allergic. Listing the patient's reaction to an allergen can differentiate between allergies, adverse drug reactions, and normal medication side effects, such as nausea, that are interpreted as allergies. Pediatric drug allergy claims frequently overestimate the real incidence of hypersensitivity reactions resulting in unnecessary avoidance of medications (Arikoglu, Aslan, Batmaz, et al., 2015).
- If nurses are not precise with terminology when asking about medication allergy, or if nurses do not clarify specific allergic manifestations, they risk identifying an allergy incorrectly or not identifying an allergy that actually exists.
- Reviewing an allergy history at all phases of an encounter to validate initial reports can assist with identification of incorrect allergy information.

Sastic (2014) describes an online educational program that nurses and support staff take to improve documentation of patient medication allergies. Better allergy reporting can assist in optimizing medication therapy, decreasing the incidence of adverse drug reactions, and ultimately improve overall patient care (Sastic, 2014). Asking "Has your child ever had a problem or reaction to any medicine that was given?" rather than "Does your child have any allergies?" decreases the risk of error related to parents' incomplete understanding of what constitutes an allergy. It also provides an opportunity for the nurse to clarify the child's specific history of reactions to medications. When caring for an infant in the emergency setting, there is a greater risk of poor communication with the family as well as among the heathcare providers which can lead to adverse events.

Think about how you have obtained a child's allergy history on admission to the hospital. Could you have been more precise in identifying or clarifying information provided by the parents? What methods do you think are essential for conveying medication allergy information to other nurses and healthcare providers? What is the potential influence of cultural or language differences? How might electronic health information technologies streamline the process of gathering key information as well as improve the accuracy of documentation? How can the nurse ensure accurate assessment of the patient's allergy status in the emergency setting?

References: Arikoglu, T., Aslan, G., Batmaz, S.B., et al. (2015). Diagnostic evaluation and risk factors for drug allergies in children: from clinical history to skin and challenge tests. *International Journal of Clinical Pharmacology, 37*(4), 583–591. doi:10.1007/s11096-015-0100-9; Sastic, C. (2014). Appropriate Assessment of Patient Medication Allergies. *Hospital Pharmacy, 49*(4), 322–323.

prolonged ventilation is anticipated. Ventilations should be given at a rate of 12 to 20 per minute or approximately 1 breath every 3 to 5 seconds; each breath should be given over 1 second (Atkins et al., 2015).

A pressure gauge attached to the bag-valve-mask ventilation device helps deliver breaths at the correct pressure, especially for infants and young children. Choosing the appropriate-size mask and the correct volume bag is important. The mask should cover the child's mouth and nose but not place pressure on the eyes. A good fit ensures a seal around the face and under the chin. Gastric decompression by use of an orogastric or nasogastric tube is indicated during assisted ventilation, as distention of the abdomen can make ventilation more difficult.

### Obstructed Airway Management

Inability to inflate the lungs suggests airway obstruction, a life-threatening emergency. When ventilation is not possible, the infant or child will die in a very short time.

Management of airway obstruction depends on the cause and on the child's age. Definitive treatment depends on diagnosis. While adults more commonly choke while eating, children can choke while eating or playing. Foreign body aspiration, for example, is a problem frequently seen in young children, with a large number of aspirations attributed to coins, small toy parts, and certain foods, particularly candy, nuts, and grapes. Choking is a leading cause of pediatric deaths in children younger than 4 years of age, accounting for 73% of cases in children under 3 years of age (Schroeder & Holinger, 2016). When a child is unable to ventilate adequately and aspiration of a foreign body is suspected, the nurse initiates maneuvers to remove the obstruction.

Although controversy remains about how to clear a foreign body from the airway, for conscious children older than 1 year, the AHA recommends using the Heimlich maneuver. CPR should be initiated for all unresponsive infants and children with a foreign body aspiration. The rescuer tries to visualize the foreign body for removal before each ventilation sequence (Atkins et al., 2015). Removal of a foreign body from an infant involves placing the infant in a downward slant position and giving five back blows alternating with five chest compressions. Abdominal thrusts are not used in infants because of the risk of liver injury. Blind finger sweeps used in an attempt to remove a possible foreign object are not recommended because of the risk of forcing the object farther down the airway or causing injury to the supraglottic area. If an object is seen, it should be removed.

If obstruction continues after these maneuvers, subsequent actions include direct laryngoscopy and use of a Magill forceps to remove the foreign body. Tracheostomy is used as a last resort. When the lower airway is obstructed because of a disease process, such as asthma, medication to open the airway may be necessary.

## SAFETY ALERT

### *Airway Obstruction in Children*

When a child is in significant respiratory distress but is coughing or able to breathe adequately despite partial obstruction, she or he should be allowed to maintain *whatever position is comfortable* until specialized care is available. In the smaller child, this position may be in the parent's or caregiver's arms. The nurse remains with the child and encourages her or him to remain calm by reassuring in a soothing manner.

### Circulation

The nurse feels for the pulse in the child older than 1 year by palpating the carotid or femoral artery and looking for signs of circulation such as movement. For an infant younger than 1 year, the nurse uses the brachial artery because the infant's relatively short, thick neck makes palpation of the carotid artery difficult. The nurse begins chest compressions if no pulse is palpated after approximately 10 seconds, or if the infant's or child's heart rate is less than 60 beats per minute (bpm) and perfusion is poor. Compressions should be administered at a rate of at least 100 compressions per minute with enough pressure to depress at least one third of the chest and allowing complete recoil after each compression (deCaen et al., 2015b) (Table 34.3).

Automatic external defibrillators (AEDs) are becoming increasingly more available in community settings. They are effective for correcting serious rhythm disturbances in adults and are recommended for use in infants and children as well. AEDs with high specificity in recognizing pediatric shockable rhythms and a system to decrease or attenuate the delivery of energy (shock) are best for use in children younger than 8 years of age (Atkins et al., 2015). In a witnessed arrest, the AED should be used as soon as it is available. If the arrest is not witnessed, CPR should be performed for at least 5 cycles (2 minutes), with minimal interruptions in chest compressions before the AED is used (Atkins et al., 2015).

Rapid venous access for fluid resuscitation and medication administration is essential in the child with compromised circulation. Because peripheral venous access can be challenging in critically ill children, attempts should be limited, and intraosseous (IO) access should be established during CPR or treatment of severe shock (de Caen et al., 2015a). An IO line placed in the anteromedial tibia or distal femur serves as a rapidly accessible and safe form of vascular access in children. Immediate availability of a fluid access site is more important than the route of administration. Children should be given IV fluid (usually lactated Ringer's or normal saline solution), 20 mL/kg, as a rapid bolus for symptoms of shock. The nurse administers additional boluses as needed after reassessing cardiovascular status and warms the solution before any rapid infusion if time permits. If more than three boluses are required for hemodynamic stability, administration of blood products may be required.

Epinephrine is the drug of choice for the management of cardiac arrest, arrhythmias, and hemodynamic instability. It can be given through the endotracheal tube when necessary. Atropine diminishes vagally mediated bradycardia. Sodium bicarbonate is given on the basis of arterial blood gas results, and dextrose can be used on the basis of blood glucose results for children unresponsive to other resuscitative efforts.

Although cardiac rhythm disturbances in children are rare, rapid heart rates can occur, including sinus tachycardia, supraventricular tachycardia, and ventricular tachycardia. Cardiac output is a function of stroke volume and heart rate. Because children are unable to increase stroke volume, they can increase cardiac output only by increasing their heart rate. As heart rates increase, cardiac filling time decreases and cardiac output ultimately falls.

Sinus tachycardia usually requires observation and determination of the cause (e.g., fever, shock, toxic ingestion). Vagal maneuvers (e.g., applying ice water to the face), synchronized cardioversion at 0.5 to 1.0 joules/kg, or adenosine may be necessary to treat symptomatic supraventricular tachycardia (heart rate greater than 200 bpm) (de Caen et al., 2015b). Ventricular tachycardia in a child is usually the result of congenital abnormalities, toxic ingestion, or chronic cardiac disease and requires complex interventions.

Resuscitation of the child requires a team effort. Training and rehearsal as in mock codes are needed. National courses such as the AHA's Pediatric Advanced Life Support (PALS) program, Pediatric Fundamental Critical Care Support (PFCCS) and the Emergency

**TABLE 34.3 Healthcare Professional Basic Life Support Elements for Infants and Children**

| Element | Infant (<1 Yr) | Child (1 Yr-Onset of Puberty) | Adult (Adolescent) |
|---|---|---|---|
| Discovery | Unresponsive<br>No breathing or only gasping<br>No brachial pulse palpated in 10 sec | No carotid or femoral pulse palpated in 10 sec | No carotid pulse palpated in 10 sec |
| **Sequence for CPR = C-A-B Circulation-Airway-Breathing** | | | |
| **Circulation** | | | |
| Compressions | | At least 100 compressions/min "Push fast" "Push hard" | |
| Location | Compress just below nipple line | Use automatic external defibrillator (AED)<br>Compress in center of chest between nipples | |
| Technique | Two fingers, or two thumbs encircling hands around chest with two rescuers | Heel of one or two hands (stacked) | Heel of two hands (stacked) |
| Depth | Approximately 1.5 in (4 cm) | Approximately 2 in (5 cm) | At least 2 in (5 cm) |
| Ratio | 30:2 one rescuer; 15:2 two rescuers | 30:2 one rescuer; 15:2 two rescuers | 30:2 one rescuer or two rescuers |
| Compressions/ Ventilations | | Allow chest to fully recoil after each compression<br>Limit interruptions in compressions to under 10 sec | |
| **Airway** | | Head-tilt/chin-lift (if trauma is present, use jaw thrust) | |
| **Breathing** | | 8-10 breaths/min; not correlated with chest compressions | |
| Advanced airway in place | | 1 breath every 6-8 sec<br>1 sec for each breath; look for chest to rise | |
| Defibrillation | Defibrillate as soon as possible; use manual defibrillator or AED with pediatric dose attenuator | Defibrillate soon as possible; use automatic external defibrillator (AED) | |
| Foreign body airway obstruction | Back blows, chest compressions | Heimlich maneuver (abdominal thrusts) | |

Data from Atkins, D., Berger, S., Duff, J., et al. (2015). Part 11: Pediatric basic life support: 2015 American Heart Association guidelines for cardiopulmonary resuscitation and emergency cardiovascular care. *Circulation, 132*, S519–S525.

Nursing Pediatric Course (ENPC) provided by the Emergency Nurses Association (ENA) are available.

## THE CHILD IN SHOCK

Shock is an acute, complex, unstable physiologic state of inadequate oxygen delivery to tissues. Decreased tissue perfusion (circulation of blood through the vascular bed of tissue) leads to a cascade of physiologic consequences and, if prolonged, irreversible tissue and organ damage (Turner & Cheifetz, 2016). The causes of shock can be classified into three major categories: hypovolemic, cardiogenic, and distributive, with some overlaps (Turner & Cheifetz, 2016). Regardless of the cause, the body will respond similarly to compensate for the alterations in the perfusion and transport of oxygen and metabolic substrates that have occurred.

### Etiology

#### Hypovolemic Shock

Hypovolemic shock is the most common cause of shock in children and is characterized by an overall decrease in circulating blood or fluid volume. Hemorrhage, burns, and dehydration are the most common causes of hypovolemic shock. Blood loss can be caused by trauma or surgery; fluid and plasma losses can occur with vomiting and diarrhea, burns, and diabetic ketoacidosis.

#### Distributive Shock

Distributive shock is the result of an abnormality in the distribution of blood flow or inability of the body to maintain vascular tone through vasoconstriction.

Septic shock is the most common form of distributive shock and occurs when microbial toxins (from bacteria, viruses, fungi, or rickettsiae) are present in the blood. These toxins cause a cascade of metabolic, hemodynamic, and clinical changes, resulting in impaired organ perfusion and hypotension. Despite major advances in vaccines in the past two decades, septic shock continues to be a frequent reason for admission to pediatric intensive care units. Organisms responsible for septic shock vary with age and immunocompetence, but include group B beta-hemolytic streptococci, enteric gram-negative rods (*Escherichia coli, Klebsiella,* Enterobacteriaceae), *Listeria monocytogenes,* and *Staphylococcus aureus* in neonates and *Streptococcus pneumoniae, S. aureus, Neisseria meningitides,* and group A *Streptococcus* in infants and children (Turner & Cheifetz, 2016). At greatest risk for developing septic shock are infants and children with debilitating illnesses, prolonged hospitalizations in the intensive care unit with many invasive lines, and those who are immunosuppressed. Anaphylaxis, central nervous system or spinal injury, and drug intoxication are other forms of distributive shock.

#### Cardiogenic Shock

Cardiogenic shock occurs when myocardial function is impaired and cardiac output is not sufficient to meet the body's metabolic demands. It is characterized by low cardiac output, cyanosis, respiratory distress, differentiated extremity blood pressures, poor tissue perfusion, and poor response to fluid resuscitation (Turner & Cheifetz, 2016). The causes of cardiogenic shock include structural abnormalities related to congenital heart disease, infectious and noninfectious cardiomyopathies, intractable arrhythmias, trauma, ischemia, metabolic abnormalities, drug intoxication, and impaired cardiac function after intracardiac surgical repair.

## PATHOPHYSIOLOGY

### *Shock*

#### Hypovolemic Shock

Hypovolemic shock results from an abnormal decrease in circulating fluid volume. Water constitutes a much greater portion of an infant's or a child's body weight than it does an adult's, and because the bulk of fluid volume in young children is located in the extracellular tissue spaces, they are more susceptible to hypovolemic shock. Infants, with their large body surface area and increased metabolic rate, also experience increased insensible fluid loss, thus compounding hypovolemia. Because of their small body size, even relatively small blood losses can result in hypovolemia.

When intravascular volume is reduced, the body initially compensates by increasing the peripheral vascular resistance, stroke volume, and heart rate and redistributing the blood flow to the vital organs (brain, heart). If fluid resuscitation is not initiated within an appropriate time frame, altered sensorium and oliguria will be noted, and hypovolemic shock will eventually result in irreversible tissue and organ damage (Turner & Cheifetz, 2016).

#### Distributive Shock

Septic shock, the most common form of distributive shock, occurs when an invading organism infects a susceptible host, overwhelms the host's first and second lines of defense, and enters the bloodstream. The body's response to toxins or organisms in the blood, including endocrine, metabolic, and immunologic reactions, can result in inflammatory and coagulation abnormalities. Endotoxins released by the lysis of bacteria cause maldistributed blood flow, cardiac dysfunction, oxygen supply-and-demand imbalance, and metabolic alterations. The result can be organ ischemia, multiple organ dysfunction syndrome, and death (Turner & Cheifetz, 2016).

#### Cardiogenic Shock

Cardiogenic shock is characterized by low cardiac output and hypotension, which result in inadequate oxygen delivery to the tissues. Unlike hypovolemic shock, the compensatory mechanisms that occur in a child with cardiogenic shock can cause further myocardial dysfunction. These compensatory mechanisms redistribute blood away from the peripheral, splenic, and mesenteric circulation to help maintain the circulation to the vital organs: the heart and brain. Initially, compensatory mechanisms increase the heart rate, myocardial contractility, and vasoconstriction. Subsequent events result in sodium and fluid retention, producing a greater workload on the left ventricle (afterload). The increased workload causes increased oxygen demands on the myocardium in response to a depleted oxygen supply. This process leads to myocardial ischemia, which further depresses cardiac function, thereby establishing a vicious cycle.

An alteration in contractility, as seen in an injury to the myocardium or myocarditis, results in a decreased stroke volume and the inability of the ventricle to eject blood.

References: Kleinman, M.E., Chameides, L., Schexnayder, S.M., et al. (2010). Part 14: Pediatric advanced life support: 2010 American Heart Association guidelines for cardiopulmonary resuscitation and emergency cardiovascular care. *Circulation, 122*(3), S876–S908; Turner, D., & Cheifetz, I. (2016). Shock. In R. Kliegman, B. Stanton, J. St. Geme, et al. (Eds.). *Nelson textbook of pediatrics* (20th ed., pp. 516–528). Philadelphia: Elsevier.

**BOX 34.2 Manifestations of Shock in Children**

**Hypovolemic Shock**
- Dry mucous membranes
- Depressed fontanel
- Cold, clammy skin
- Oliguria
- Poor skin turgor
- Delayed capillary refill

**Distributive (Septic) Shock: Early**
- Vasodilation
- Extremities that are warm to the touch
- Tachycardia, tachypnea

**Septic Shock: Late**
- Rapid, thready pulse
- Cyanosis
- Cold, clammy skin
- Purpuric skin lesions
- Narrow pulse pressure
- Oliguria or anuria

**Cardiogenic Shock**
- Hepatomegaly
- Cardiomegaly
- Increased central venous pressure
- Periorbital edema
- Crackles
- Diaphoresis
- Oliguria
- Reduced capillary refill
- Differences in proximal and distal pulses

**TABLE 34.4 Assessing a Child's General Appearance: "Looks Good" Versus "Looks Bad"**

| | "Looks Good" | "Looks Bad" |
|---|---|---|
| Color | Pink mucous membranes<br>Consistent color over the trunk and extremities | Mottled color, "gray" or pale |
| Skin perfusion | Warm<br>Brisk capillary refill (<2 sec) | Cold (peripheral to proximal cooling)<br>Sluggish capillary refill (>2 sec) |
| Activity | Age-appropriate (may be frightened, unhappy, unwilling to be separated from parents)<br>Will engage in play | Fretful, then lethargic |
| Responsiveness | Age-appropriate | Irritable (early), then lethargic<br>Decreased response to painful stimulus is worrisome |
| Infant feeding | Eats well | Weak suck<br>Tires during feeding<br>May have respiratory distress during feedings |

Data from de Caen, A.R., Berg, M.D., Chameides, L., et al. (2015a). Part 12: Pediatric Advanced Life Support 2015 American Heart Association Guidelines Update for Cardiopulmonary Resuscitation and Emergency Cardiovascular Care. *Circulation, 132*(2), S526–S542. doi:10.1161/CIR.0000000000000266.

## Manifestations

Recognition of the clinical manifestations, with early intervention, is imperative for optimal treatment of shock (Box 34.2). In the early stages, the child is able to compensate with tachycardia, tachypnea, and vasoconstriction to maintain cardiac output. If the condition cannot be reversed, a decompensated state arises, with altered perfusion (delayed capillary refill, weak pulses, cool extremities, and hypotension) and profoundly altered mental status. Progression results in cardiovascular collapse and death. Table 34.4 presents the general appearance of a child in shock.

**SAFETY ALERT**

***Hypotension in Children With Shock***

Because children can compensate for a 25% blood loss with an increase in heart rate and peripheral vascular resistance, hypotension is a late sign of shock (ENA, 2012). The lower limits for systolic blood pressure (BP) in children are as follows (ENA, 2012):
- Infants younger than 1 month: >60 mm Hg
- Infants ages 1 to 24 months: >70 mm Hg
- Children older than 24 months: 70 mm Hg plus the number that is double the child's age in years (e.g., 10-year-old child: 70 + 20 = 90 mm Hg)
- Children older than 10 years: >90 mm Hg

## Diagnostic Evaluation

The diagnosis of shock in infants and children is established chiefly on the basis of clinical manifestations and medical history. A chest radiograph may help differentiate cardiogenic shock from hypovolemic or distributive shock. In cardiogenic shock, the heart is usually enlarged, and the chest x-ray may show signs of pulmonary edema. In hypovolemic or distributive shock, the chest radiograph is usually normal or shows signs of infiltrates (indicative of pneumonia), and the heart is smaller than normal (indicative of a decrease in circulating volume). An echocardiogram can identify underlying structural cardiac disease.

Laboratory studies used in a differential diagnosis include blood cultures and cultures of other sites that may be the source of infection (e.g., spinal fluid, urine, sputum, wound drainage), arterial and venous blood gas values, glucose levels, electrolytes, BUN, creatinine levels, CBC, and coagulation studies.

## Therapeutic Management

The therapeutic management of the child in shock includes basic life support (maintaining circulation, airway, and breathing) and treating signs and symptoms.

Monitoring with pulse oximetry and increasing ambient oxygen are indicated in most cases. If vascular access cannot be obtained, an IO line can be used until the child is resuscitated, at which time the temporary IO line can be replaced with an IV line.

### Hypovolemic Shock

Once the airway, breathing, and circulation are established, the next priority is adequate vascular access. An IV crystalloid infusion of normal saline or lactated Ringer's solution should be promptly initiated. If hypovolemic shock is caused by hemorrhage and symptoms persist after administration of crystalloid boluses, blood transfusions may be considered (Hartman & Cheifetz, 2016).

Colloids (albumin, blood products) are protein-containing fluids that are used in volume resuscitation after the initial treatment with crystalloids.

### Distributive Shock

The therapeutic management of distributive shock involves restoring hemodynamic status with fluid resuscitation and promptly treating the underlying cause. For septic shock, parenteral antibiotics are administered promptly. Inotropic medications and vasodilators are used to manage the cardiovascular instability. Vasoconstrictors can be used to increase vascular tone and counteract the effects of toxins. Steroids, medications to treat hypoglycemia and electrolyte imbalances, and the administration of blood products may be required to combat complications of distributive shock (Hartman & Cheifetz, 2016). Maintaining a secure, patent airway may be necessary if significant respiratory distress occurs. Surgery also might be indicated to eliminate the source of infection (e.g., an abscess) or stabilize a central nervous system and/or spinal injury.

### Cardiogenic Shock

Supplemental oxygen, vascular access, hemodynamic monitoring, and frequent assessments are imperative in shock management. The nurse uses assessment skills to recognize early signs of deterioration and response to therapeutic interventions. Invasive monitoring of central venous pressure, arterial blood pressure, and pulmonary artery pressure helps to identify hemodynamic changes and the subtle clinical signs and symptoms of decreased cardiac output (e.g., cyanosis, decreased skin temperature, and delayed capillary refill).

With an excess of intravascular fluid volume, diuretics may be prescribed.

The heart rate must be in the normal range or higher than normal to improve the cardiac output. Children, especially infants younger than 6 months, have a decreased ability to increase stroke volume, and thus, depend much more on an increased heart rate as a compensatory mechanism to improve cardiac output. Pharmacologic therapy is the mainstay of medical treatment for children with cardiogenic shock. Frequently, a combination of pharmacologic agents is necessary to stabilize the child. Dopamine, dobutamine, and milrinone are the initial drugs of choice for treating cardiogenic shock (Hartman & Cheifetz, 2016).

Extracorporeal life support (ECLS) is a means of providing short-term circulatory and respiratory support for infants and children with underlying cardiac disease and/or when other methods of treatment are not effective. ECLS has been used successfully in distributive and cardiogenic shock. Vital organ perfusion is maintained by ECLS to allow for prolonged delivery of oxygen to tissues (Hartman & Cheifetz, 2016).

## NURSING CARE

### The Child in Shock

#### Assessment

Nursing assessment of a child in shock should be thorough, with attention focused on the child's cardiopulmonary system and neurologic status. A changing level of consciousness is one of the first indicators of a worsening condition, and early identification and treatment of shock in infants and children are crucial to decreasing morbidity and mortality rates. Initial concerns are ensuring a patent airway and monitoring the child's respiratory effort to confirm adequate air exchange with good chest expansion. Central circulation is assessed by checking a brachial, carotid, or femoral pulse. Assessments of the level of consciousness are performed serially to detect early changes.

***Hypovolemic shock.*** A child in hypovolemic shock often has a history of trauma, vomiting, diarrhea, or anorexia. The parent might report a decrease in wet diapers or explain that the child has not voided recently. With trauma, the child can demonstrate obvious signs of injury or bleeding or covert symptoms suggestive of blunt trauma.

The child in hypovolemic shock requires frequent assessment of vital signs, including blood pressure (every 15 to 60 minutes). Skin color, turgor, and temperature should be closely monitored. The anterior fontanel (if present) should be assessed to determine whether it is depressed or full. A depressed fontanel may be a manifestation of dehydration, whereas a full or level fontanel usually suggests that fluid volume is adequate.

In addition, the nurse assesses and monitors the child's neurologic status closely. A decreased or deteriorating level of consciousness should be reported promptly. The nurse auscultates heart and lungs and palpates peripheral pulses. Capillary refill time, moistness of mucous membranes, and general muscle tone and strength should be assessed and urine output closely monitored. In very young children, the diapers are weighed to quantify urine output. If the child has diarrhea, a urine bag or indwelling (Foley) catheter should be placed to monitor urinary output. The abdomen should be palpated and auscultated for the presence of bowel sounds. Abdominal injury must be ruled out, especially if the abdominal girth appears to be increasing, with evidence of abdominal distention. Any abnormal bruising or obvious trauma must be recognized quickly, because blunt abdominal trauma is a major cause of shock in children.

***Distributive shock.*** Early signs of distributive shock include hyperthermia or hypothermia. The temperature should be closely monitored. In early shock (the hyperdynamic phase), the skin is typically warm and flushed. In late shock (the hypodynamic phase), skin is ashen and cold. An exception is in the case of spinal injury, in which the body cannot maintain a normal temperature. Shock of any etiology can cause microcirculatory dysfunction leading to abnormal function of coagulation factors and platelets. Therefore, the nurse observes the skin closely for signs of petechiae, oozing of blood from invasive lines, or purpuric lesions. The presence of petechiae that are spread diffusely over the body indicates severe sepsis. In children, hypotension is a late sign of all types of shock.

***Cardiogenic shock.*** A child with cardiogenic shock requires close monitoring of the heart and lungs for adventitious sounds. The liver should be palpated and its size measured. The child's respiratory effort must also be assessed. Retractions, grunting, and nasal flaring may be apparent. Periorbital and peripheral edema or other signs of cardiac failure may be present. Close monitoring of the peripheral pulses and capillary refill is extremely important.

#### Nursing Diagnosis and Planning

The following nursing diagnoses and expected outcomes may be appropriate after assessment of the child with shock:

- Ineffective Tissue Perfusion (cardiopulmonary, cerebral, peripheral) related to decreased fluid volume (in hypovolemic shock); abnormal distribution of blood flow, metabolic acidosis, or both (in distributive shock); or decreased cardiac contractility (in cardiogenic shock).

***Expected outcome.*** The child will maintain adequate tissue perfusion, as evidenced by strong peripheral pulses, appropriate skin turgor, normal capillary refill time, pink and warm mucous membranes and nail beds, vital signs within normal limits for age, and no evidence of dyspnea or altered mental status.

- Impaired Gas Exchange related to possible decreased pulmonary blood flow, increased interstitial fluid in alveoli, and inflammatory response of alveoli.

***Expected outcome.*** The child will have adequate gas exchange, as evidenced by oxygen saturation level between 95% and 100% and normal arterial blood gas measurements.

- Risk for Infection related to invasive venous and arterial lines, indwelling catheters, presence of endotracheal tube, possible incisional wounds, and compromised state.

***Expected outcome.*** The child will remain free from signs of infection, as evidenced by normal temperature, white blood cell (WBC) count within normal limits, no signs of redness or purulence from access sites, and negative blood cultures.

- Anxiety related to threat of a possible grave prognosis in a critically ill child.

***Expected outcome.*** The child (if verbal) and parents will verbalize symptoms of anxiety, seek information to ensure understanding of the condition, and demonstrate adequate coping skills.

### Interventions

Interventions for the child in shock are directed toward maintaining tissue perfusion by improving cardiac output, ensuring adequate oxygenation, preventing infection, and enhancing child and family coping.

***Maintaining tissue perfusion.*** The nurse's careful and frequent observation of the child's cardiovascular status is essential. Vital signs are checked and circulation assessed every 1 to 2 hours. After establishing adequate IV access, appropriate fluid replacement is administered. The nurse maintains strict intake and output records and reports urine output that is abnormal for age (see Chapter 40) or any major discrepancy between intake and output. The child is weighed daily on the same scale; any rapid weight gain is reported immediately to the provider.

Because infants have high glucose requirements and low glycogen stores, alterations in glucose metabolism are frequently seen in response to stress. The nurse monitors blood glucose levels every 2 to 4 hours.

Ordered medications are administered by IV pump to ensure appropriate delivery of medication. Because vasoactive drugs can cause tissue necrosis if infiltration occurs in peripheral tissues, these agents are best administered through a central line.

***Ensuring oxygenation.*** The nurse observes and records respiratory rate and effort, skin color, chest expansion, and aeration. If signs of respiratory distress are present, they are noted and promptly reported to the provider. Oxygen is administered as ordered, ensuring that the delivery mode is appropriate for the child's age. Monitoring of oxygen saturation, arterial blood gases, and hemoglobin levels is ongoing. Maintenance of a patent airway is essential; emergency endotracheal intubation and ventilation equipment are available. The nurse ensures normothermia and controls pain and anxiety to decrease oxygen demands. A gastric tube can be placed to decompress the stomach and allow full expansion of the thoracic cavity.

***Preventing infection.*** Because children in compromised states are prone to infection, the nurse must maintain strict aseptic technique when handling IV lines, invasive tubes, and incisional or puncture sites. The child's temperature is closely monitored, and any rectal temperature greater than 38° C (100.4° F) or less than 36° C (96.8° F) is reported. The nurse observes secretions and body fluids, incisions, and puncture sites for erythema, edema, or purulent drainage. Positive culture results and elevated WBCs are reported promptly to the provider. Ordered antipyretics are administered when indicated, and adequate caloric intake is provided. If the child is unable to tolerate oral or nasogastric feedings, the nurse discusses alternative methods of feeding with the provider.

***Enhancing coping.*** The nurse provides concise, accurate information to parents at frequent intervals. Further, the nurse determines the child's developmental level and level of comprehension and provides simple explanations of procedures to the child and parents before initiating them. Information is given in a calm, relaxed, and empathetic manner. All questions are answered honestly, allowing the child and parents to express their feelings, concerns, and anxieties. Parents are encouraged to participate in the child's care as appropriate (e.g., bathing, combing hair, feeding). This assistance provides them with some degree of control. The nurse must be nonjudgmental in response to parents' actions. Available resources (e.g., social worker, chaplain, and other family members) are used to help calm parents who are exhibiting uncontrolled feelings.

The nurse elicits the parents' perceptions of the events and provides reassurance or clarifies any misconceptions. The availability of support systems is determined and their use encouraged. The nurse helps the parents identify coping mechanisms that have been effective in the past and encourages parents to use these mechanisms during the current crisis.

### Evaluation

- Does the child demonstrate pink mucous membranes, brisk capillary refill, alertness, responsiveness, and normal vital signs for age?
- Is the oxygen saturation at least 95% on room air, and are blood gas values within normal limits?
- Does the child demonstrate a normal breathing rate, pattern, and work of breathing?
- Is the child afebrile with negative culture results?
- Can the parents and child express their feelings to staff and significant others?
- Is the family demonstrating decreased anxiety by using available resources and effective coping mechanisms?

## PEDIATRIC TRAUMA

Despite a marked decline in injury deaths among children since 1980, unintentional injuries are still the leading cause of morbidity and mortality among children in the United States (Albert & McCaig, 2014). The Centers for Disease Control and Prevention (CDC) has consistently found that motor vehicle injuries have the highest death rate in all children younger than 19 years of age (CDC, 2012a; Hagan & Duncan, 2016). For infants younger than 1 year of age, two thirds of deaths are caused by suffocation, and drowning is the leading cause of injury deaths in those 1 to 4 years of age. Burns, poisoning, and falls are other unintentional injuries that are leading causes of fatal as well as nonfatal injuries requiring emergency department treatment (CDC, 2012a). Over one-third of ED visits made by children under 18 were injury related in 2009–2010 (Albert & McCaig, 2014). The term *injury* is used in preference to *accident* when describing trauma because some trauma is not accidental and much of it is preventable. Serious and fatal motor vehicle injuries can be reduced by over half with the use of age- and size-appropriate car and booster seats (Sauber-Schatz, Thomas, & Cook, 2015).

Injury prevention and education have been credited with a decrease in unintentional deaths among children. Despite this improvement, much more needs to be done to prevent injuries. Successful prevention and educational steps include motor vehicle safety restraints, firearm education, bicycle helmet programs, safety caps and locked medications, and eliminating potential hazards, such as old refrigerators and unfenced pools. Up-to-date educational resources can be obtained through organizations and websites such as those offered by the national Safe Kids USA campaign, the CDC, and the U.S. Consumer Product Safety Commission. When child victims of trauma are discharged from the emergency department, the nurse provides injury prevention information to the families. Injury prevention is also discussed at every well-child visit through adolescence (see Chapters 6 through 9).

## Mechanism of Injury

Injuries can be categorized as *blunt, penetrating,* and *multiple trauma.* The most common areas of bodily injury (in order of frequency) are head, musculoskeletal system, abdomen, and thorax (ENA, 2012). Knowing the mechanism of injury and recognizing anatomic and physiologic differences in the pediatric population help identify common injury patterns and predict the child's needs and outcomes.

### Blunt Trauma

Blunt or penetrating force causes tissue trauma. Blunt trauma occurs more frequently than all other injuries combined (Roskind, Dayan, & Klein, 2016). Injuries sustained from blunt trauma are often less apparent but, nevertheless, can be extremely serious.

**Motor vehicle trauma.** A common cause of blunt trauma is acceleration–deceleration force, often from motor vehicle collisions or falls. Just before a motor vehicle collision, both the occupant and the vehicle are traveling at the same speed. When the vehicle meets an opposing force, the speed of both the occupant and the vehicle rapidly decelerate. When this change occurs, four collisions take place: (1) the moving vehicle collides with the opposing object; (2) the occupant's body collides with the interior portion of the vehicle; (3) the occupant's internal organs and tissues collide with rigid internal structures; and (4) loose objects in the vehicle become projectile forces. Factors that affect the severity of motor vehicle collision injuries are the individual's location in the vehicle, impact speed, stopping distance, vehicle type, and restraint use (ENA, 2012).

Unrestrained occupants in a motor vehicle collision have a higher incidence of injury than do restrained occupants because they are tossed around the interior of the vehicle or are ejected at the point of collision. This principle applies also to children riding unrestrained in the back of open pickup trucks; they become missiles ejected out of the vehicle into oncoming traffic or onto the road. Children who are held on an adult's lap during a motor vehicle collision can be instantly crushed between the rigid part of the automobile and the moving adult.

Child safety seats and safety belts, *when appropriately sized and correctly installed,* can prevent injury and save lives. From 1990 to 2003, there were 227 confirmed cases reported to the National Highway Traffic Safety Administration (NHTSA) where deployment of an airbag resulted in a fatal injury; 62% of these cases were children under the age of 12 years (Kindelberger, Chidester, & Ferguson, 2012). Since then, airbags have been redesigned and improved, and the NHTSA has launched a national safety campaign educating parents about placing every child under age 13 years in the rear seat of an automobile in an appropriate child restraint system (NHTSA, 2012).

In 2011, the American Academy of Pediatrics issued recommendations for best safety practices related to child restraint systems and passenger vehicle safety: (1) rear-facing car safety seats for most infants up to 2 years of age; (2) forward-facing car safety seats for most children through 4 years of age; (3) belt-positioning booster seats for most children through 8 years of age; (4) lap-and-shoulder seatbelts for all who have outgrown booster seats; and (5) all children younger than 13 years ride in the rear seats of vehicles (Durbin, 2011).

**Pedestrian injury.** Pedestrian injuries in children are also a significant problem, causing 60,000 emergency department visits per year, with the largest number of incidences occurring in children 5 to 14 years of age (Hagan & Duncan, 2016). Many of these injuries occur as the child darts out into the middle of the street between parked cars or stands unnoticed behind a vehicle backing out of a driveway. In general, pedestrian injuries occur in urban areas, at non-intersections, in normal weather conditions, and at night.

When a child is hit by a motor vehicle, a triad of injuries, referred to as Waddell's triad, occurs (Fig. 34.1). This one traumatic event results in three different types of injuries:

1. After being struck by the bumper and hood of the car, the child sustains abdominal or thoracic injuries.
2. The child is then propelled into the air, lands on the ground, and sustains femur or other leg injury, as well as surface trauma.
3. As the child is propelled like a missile to the ground, the large size and weight of the child's head result in skull fracture or closed head injury to the contralateral side of the head.

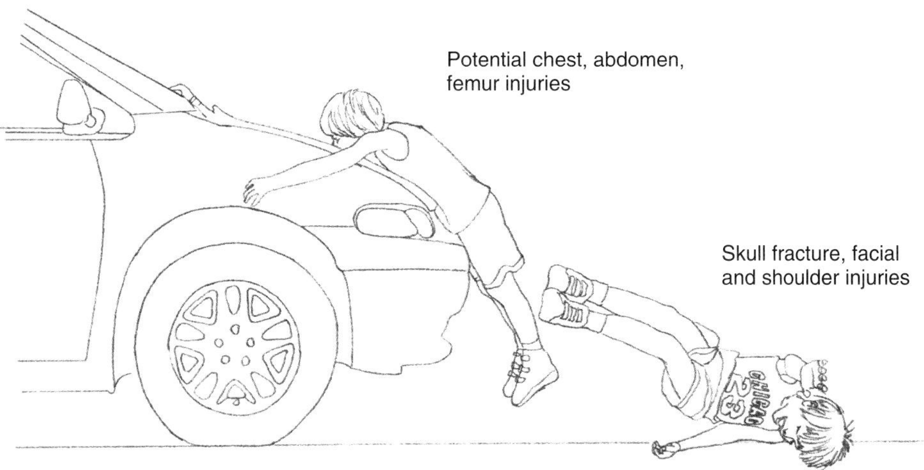


**FIG 34.1** Waddell's triad of injuries.

### Penetrating Trauma

Penetrating trauma includes stabbing, firearms, blasting, and impaling injuries. Damage to the body tissue can result from the penetrating object itself and secondarily from radiating energy forces along the pathway of the penetrating object. The severity of an injury depends on the location of impact and the type of object. For example, with gunshot wounds, what might seem like a fairly innocuous wound can actually be severe, depending on factors such as projectile, fragmentation, type of tissue struck, and striking velocity. The severity of injuries from a stab wound depend on the length of the instrument, applied velocity, and angle of entry. Penetrating injuries account for 22% of pediatric injuries and represent the fifth leading cause of death in children younger than 14 years of age. The incidence of gunshot wounds and nonfatal stabbing injuries is on the rise as a result of increased violence in younger children (ENA, 2012).

## Multiple Trauma

A child with multiple trauma incurs injuries to more than one body system. A positive outcome for a child who has sustained multiple trauma depends on rapid assessment and intervention, which begin at the scene of the accident and continue through the trauma center emergency department, the critical care and acute care units, and the rehabilitation phase. Ideally, a critically injured child should be rapidly transported to a trauma facility with the personnel, equipment, and commitment to provide specialized care to children.

At the trauma center, and even in the emergency department of the community hospital, the presence of qualified trauma team members to assess and treat the trauma patient is crucial. A trauma team consists of skilled surgeons, other physicians, nurses, social workers, and other healthcare professionals, each with a specific role and duties during trauma resuscitation. The team assembles after notification of a patient's pending arrival by prehospital personnel and readies the trauma room with appropriate personnel and equipment.

All children with multiple trauma require a rapid, complete, and thorough assessment to determine the extent of injuries. The assessment of a child with multiple trauma includes primary and secondary surveys, with concurrent suitable interventions.

### Primary Survey

The goal of the primary survey is to assess and manage life-threatening injuries. The primary assessment (see "Primary Assessment" section on p. 757) proceeds with the following additions.

***Airway assessment and management.*** Airway management is the priority. The airway is opened and maintained using the jaw-thrust maneuver to prevent movement of the cervical spine. The nurse inspects for loose teeth or other potential airway obstructions. Because the child's lower airway is narrow and easily obstructed by edema and mucus, oral suctioning may be required to keep the airway clear. All unresponsive and/or nonverbal trauma patients should have cervical spine protection until definitive diagnosis can be made (ENA, 2012). Cervical spine injury is uncommon, but the long-term results can be devastating. A pediatric cervical collar and immobilization board secure a child when spinal cord injury is a concern (Fig. 34.2). To determine a correct fit, the cervical collar is measured for maximal stability: The chin must rest securely in the chin holder, with the collar below the ears and the lower end not extending below the upper part of the sternum. Any movement can worsen spinal cord injury and compromise the airway. The cervical immobilization device and spinal immobilization device (long backboard) must remain in place until spinal injury has been ruled out. Because of children's proportionately large occiput (head), it may be necessary to place padding under the shoulders for neutral alignment of the cervical spine to prevent flexion and airway compromise.

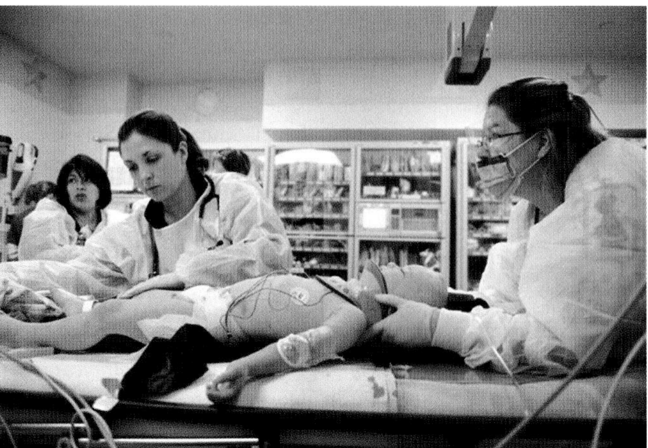

FIG 34.2 The child with multiple trauma injuries must remain on an immobilization board (long backboard) with a cervical immobilization device in place until the child has been evaluated for spinal injuries. (Courtesy Children's Medical Center, Dallas, TX.)

When an alert child is brought to the emergency setting in a car seat, the nurse places rolled towels on either side of the child's head and secures these with tape to maintain cervical immobilization without removing the child from the seat. The child can then remain in the car seat until radiographs have shown no injury to the cervical spine or until a change in status is noted.

***Breathing assessment and management.*** Pulse oximetry readings are an adjunct to evaluating ventilation and adequate oxygenation. Oxygen use in the child with multiple trauma is not contraindicated; therefore, the nurse starts supplemental oxygen at a rate of 10 to 15 L/min by mask. If the child is alert and does not tolerate the mask, using blow-by oxygen with the tubing only or using a plastic cup attached to the end of the tubing might be less threatening to the child.

If ventilation is inadequate or absent, the nurse begins to ventilate the child (see Table 34.1) using a bag-valve-mask ventilation device with a reservoir and high-flow oxygen. An oropharyngeal or nasopharyngeal airway maintains patency in a child with altered consciousness.

Endotracheal intubation may be needed for airway control and oxygenation in children with altered levels of consciousness, lack of spontaneous respirations, or severe head injuries. The nurse assists in evaluation of endotracheal tube placement after the procedure.

While observing the child for respiratory difficulty, the nurse checks the neck for obvious injuries. Jugular vein distention or tracheal deviation is difficult to assess in a child because they have shorter necks than adults. If visualized, both findings are late signs of a tension pneumothorax. Because respiratory difficulty can be caused by chest injury, the nurse observes the chest for contusions, penetrations, abrasions, and paradoxical movement. Chest tube insertion or interventions for cardiac tamponade can be indicated for a penetrating chest injury, or an occlusive dressing can be taped on three sides for an open pneumothorax.

Severe facial trauma, although rare in children younger than 5 years, can be life threatening, primarily because of the potential obstruction to ventilation. Both fractures and soft tissue injury can cause narrowing of the airway. Facial trauma in children is treated as is in adults. Nursing interventions include ensuring an adequate airway and breathing, observing for possible progressive obstruction, and keeping the injured areas clean to prevent infection.

*Circulation assessment and management.* Cardiovascular assessment of the child focuses on early recognition and treatment of hypovolemia. Blood loss in children is usually caused by internal abdominal or chest injury, severe injuries to the extremities, or surface head trauma. Early indicators of shock in children are tachycardia, increased capillary refill time (longer than 2 seconds), mottled skin, agitation or apprehension, pallor, and cool extremities. Decreased level of consciousness, dusky skin color, clammy extremities, bradycardia, and hypotension are late signs, indicating that cardiac arrest is imminent.

**! NURSING QUALITY ALERT**

***Artificial Airways***

*Oropharyngeal airway:* Used in the unconscious child only. Determine the length of the airway by measuring the distance from the corner of the mouth to the tip of the earlobe. Use a tongue blade to depress and displace the tongue while inserting the airway curve down (in the anatomic position) and over the tongue.

*Nasopharyngeal airway:* Select an airway with a diameter slightly less than the diameter of the child's nares, and determine the length of the airway by measuring the distance from the nares to the tragus of the ear. Make sure the bevel faces the septum regardless of which nare is used. Nasopharyngeal airways should be avoided in children with suspected or actual facial or head trauma.

Cardiac monitoring and frequent cardiovascular assessments are necessary during the acute stage. During this stage, any external hemorrhage is noted and controlled, and IV or other access to the circulatory system is obtained.

The nurse assesses extremities for fractures and decreased peripheral circulation and splints any suspected fracture, assessing peripheral circulation after applying a splint. Assessment includes motor (Can the child move the extremity? Does the child feel pain?), circulatory (Does the child have good color, a strong pulse, and good capillary refill?), and neural function (Is sensation to the area intact? Does the child have any numbness or tingling in the extremity?). If neurovascular or circulatory compromise is present, immediate intervention is necessary.

*Disability.* During the primary survey phase, a brief neurologic examination is performed to establish level of consciousness, pupil size and reactivity, and muscle movement. AVPU can assess mental status. Sudden changes, such as agitation or somnolence, indicate hypoxia or decreased cerebral perfusion.

### Secondary Survey

After exposing the child by removing all of his or her clothing and providing warming measures, the trauma staff assesses for pain, carefully inspects and documents all signs of injury by performing the head-to-toe assessment (including log rolling the child to inspect the back), and obtains a history of the injury.

*Obtaining a history of the injury.* Determining the degree and severity of injuries is both an art and a science. Diagnosis depends on knowing the mechanism of injury as well as the presenting signs and symptoms. Nurses can obtain a comprehensive history by asking specific questions (Box 34.3). Thorough assessment depends on a systematic trauma evaluation, which takes place along with lifesaving intervention.

*Trauma scoring.* On-site emergency medical personnel and nursing staff perform and document various kinds of scoring as part of the assessment process. A trauma score is used as an objective measure of the severity of the injury caused by a traumatic event and may be used to decide the facility most appropriate for treating the child. Most scoring systems are for the assessment of injury to adults and do not take into account the anatomic differences of children (Box 34.4).

**BOX 34.3 History of Injury Questions**

**For a Victim of a Motor Vehicle Collision**
- Was the child wearing a seatbelt or in a child's car seat?
- What was the type of seatbelt (lap, lap-and-shoulder, or car seat)?
- What was the speed of the motor vehicle?
- With what did the motor vehicle collide?
- At what location on the motor vehicle was the point of impact?
- Where was the victim seated in the motor vehicle?
- How much damage was done to the motor vehicle?

**For a Victim of a Fall**
- How far did the child fall?
- How did the child land (on what part of the body)?
- On what type of surface did the child land?
- Was the child's fall broken by any objects?

**For a Victim of a Penetrating Injury**
- How long and how wide was the blade of the knife?
- How far away was the gun when it was fired?
- What type of gun was used, and what was the caliber of the gun?

**BOX 34.4 Trauma Scoring Systems**

**Trauma Score (TS)**
- Adult scoring tool sometimes used with children
- Assesses respiratory rate and effort, blood pressure, and capillary refill
- Includes the Glasgow Coma Scale (GCS)

**Revised Trauma Score (RTS)**
- Composed of the GCS, blood pressure, and respiratory rate

**Pediatric Trauma Score (PTS)**
- Adapted for the pediatric patient
- Assesses size, airway, central nervous system response, systolic blood pressure, open wounds, and skeletal fractures

*Assessing for child abuse.* Child maltreatment can be a cause of injury (see Chapter 53 for an in-depth discussion of child abuse). Nurses working in emergency settings play an important role in both the assessment and reporting of child maltreatment. However, it is rare to have adequate time to assess parent-child interactions or observe at length the child's behavioral indicators, although these actions may provide important information. The following important indicators raise the suspicion of child maltreatment in the emergency setting:

- A history inconsistent with physical findings
- Activity reportedly leading to the trauma that seems inconsistent with the age and condition of the child
- Delay in seeking treatment for the trauma
- A history of other emergency department visits

The following physical findings should also raise the level of suspicion for child maltreatment:

- Fractures in various stages of healing noted on radiography
- Injuries rarely found in children (e.g., long bone or rib fractures) when the history is not appropriate for the injury
- Patterns of injury indicating that a specific object caused injury (e.g., belt marks, cigarette burns)

The nurse carefully assesses these indicators in the context of the injury and in relation to the effect on the child and family. Bruises are the most common injury experienced by abused children and are often the first indicator of abuse, but they must be carefully evaluated in the appropriate developmental context (Wood, Fakeye, Mondestin, et al., 2015). Children younger than 9 months old rarely have bruising, but toddlers who are beginning to crawl and walk may have bruising on bony prominences. Caution should be used when evaluating the stages of bruising, as increasing evidence suggests that it is very difficult to precisely determine the age of bruises (Dubowitz & Lane, 2016). Bleeding conditions, Mongolian spots, and brittle bone disease can mimic the signs of abuse and should also be considered. The nurse observes the family's reaction to the child and staff, keeping in mind that people behave differently depending on culture, ethnicity, experience, and psychological makeup. Above all, healthcare providers do not assume an investigative role—that is law enforcement's responsibility. However, nurses are required to report the suspicion of child maltreatment and must carefully document all observations in detail. When child maltreatment is suspected, the intervention of child protective services is essential to ensure the safety of the child (and that of other children in the home) and to prevent additional injury.

### Nursing Considerations

#### The Child and Family

The most critical aspect of nursing care of the child with traumatic injury is continuous assessment of the respiratory, circulatory, and neurologic status. The nurse observes injured children for the early signs of shock and intervenes immediately to prevent rapid and irreversible deterioration. Preparing for the many procedures and examinations required and observing the equipment used for monitoring should not interfere with close and continuous observation of the child's signs and symptoms.

Nursing care of the child also requires care of the family. When the family arrives at the hospital, one staff member should become the contact person and provide regular updates. The hospital staff supports family members when they visit their critically ill child. Information concerning their child's condition should be provided simply but completely, incorporating the family's educational and emotional status and readiness to learn. Family members are encouraged to touch and talk to their child if they so desire. Family presence during resuscitation and invasive procedures has been shown to facilitate healthy grieving and support the belief that everything possible was done in the event that their child dies as a result of injury or illness (ENA, 2012). Additionally, healthcare providers report there is no interruption in care delivery when someone (e.g., chaplain, social worker) is designated to stay with the family and provide updates. Remember that informed consent must be obtained from the families of children for all procedures unless the intervention is required to save the child's life.

#### The Child During Recovery

Regardless of the cause of the injury, most children with traumatic injury do well unless the injuries are extremely severe. Their cardiovascular systems are strong, and their bodies are growing, allowing them to compensate for even the most serious injuries. Even children with severe traumatic brain injuries (TBIs) have far more favorable chances of recovery than do adults. According to the CDC (2016b), 3,000 children and youth die from TBI; 29,000 are hospitalized, and 400,000 are treated in hospital emergency departments annually. Children and their families require nursing support to recover from both the physical and psychological effects of trauma; the need for rehabilitation must be considered from the moment the child arrives in the emergency setting.

## INGESTIONS AND POISONINGS

The term *poison exposure* is defined as the ingestion of or contact with a substance that can produce toxic effects. The combination of small weight and size, curiosity, lack of fear, and evolving mobility places all children at risk of injury or death from toxic exposure and ingestion. However, differences exist in types of incident by age-group. Younger children (1 through 5 years of age) are indiscriminately curious and can innocently ingest a toxic substance in a matter of seconds. As children grow, they gradually learn from parents to avoid dangerous substances, but accidental ingestions and exposures still can occur. In adolescence, the risk is higher for deliberate ingestion.

> **CRITICAL THINKING EXERCISE 34.1**
>
> You are working in a small emergency department when a father brings in his 6-year-old daughter who was struck by a car while riding a bicycle. She is in her father's arms, her eyes are closed, and she is pale with mottled lower extremities. Blood is on the father's clothes.
>
> 1. What are the key elements of your primary assessment? What are you looking for?
> 2. What questions would you ask the father to obtain the history?
> 3. What do you think is wrong with her? Is this an emergency? Why or why not?
> 4. What interventions would you do? Which would you do first? Why?
> 5. What responses to your interventions would be expected? Why?

### Incidence

Poisoning accounts for 3.9% of childhood deaths worldwide and is the number one cause of death in the United States (Hagan & Duncan, 2016; Kostic, 2016). More than half of all poison exposures occurred in children younger than 6 years. The mortality rate from poisonings is higher in the adolescent population as a result of adolescents using poisons to cause self-harm (Mowry, Spyker, Brooks, et al. 2014). More than 90% of all poison exposures occur in homes, with most resulting from oral ingestion. Ocular or dermal exposure, inhalation, parenteral exposure, and envenomation (e.g., an animal or insect bite) account for the remainder of poisoning incidents. Children are poisoned by plants; household and personal care products such as cosmetics, cleaning substances, and medicines; lead; and carbon monoxide. Adolescent poisoning tends to occur as a result of alcohol and prescription and nonprescription drug ingestion.

### Manifestations

Assessment and treatment of toxic exposure and ingestion go hand in hand. Although identification of the type and amount of the exposure is important, the child must initially be treated on the basis of physical signs and symptoms.

An accurate history of the ingestion is useful in planning for the child's care. History given by the child, parent, friend, or caretaker may not always be accurate or complete—areas of confusion are often present, especially in cases of unwitnessed ingestions. The information obtained in the history of the ingestion is combined with the child's presenting physical assessment to provide a complete picture of the event and plan treatment. Laboratory analysis in some cases may provide definitive diagnosis.

Most ingestions seen in emergency settings occur acutely, and the child is brought in immediately or when parents realize the event has occurred. An exception to this is lead poisoning. Although lead poisoning is relatively common, with an estimated 1 million children having elevated levels, it is rarely identified in the emergency setting. A child who has unusual neurologic signs or symptoms, neuropathy, or anemia that cannot be attributed to other causes may have lead poisoning. Elevated blood lead levels result primarily from exposure to lead-based paint or lead-contaminated dust and soil. Older miniblinds, improperly glazed pottery, folk remedies, toys, artificial turf, and cosmetics are also reported sources of lead poisoning (National Center for Environmental Health [NCEH], 2013). A careful history can assist in the diagnosis of lead poisoning, but testing serum lead levels provides the only accurate diagnosis. Recent studies have shown that low blood lead levels (BLL) can have adverse health effects on young children. Subsequently, the CDC now recommends that the health status of children ages 1 to 5 years with a BLL of equal or greater than 5 mcg/dL should be monitored and their environments investigated for lead exposure sources (CDC, 2012b). The child with a markedly elevated lead level usually is admitted to the hospital. Chelation therapy, if needed, is administered on an inpatient basis to remove lead from the blood and tissue. When a child is found to have elevated lead levels, other children in the home should be tested as well because of the environmental nature of the ingestion.

## Diagnostic Evaluation

In cases of known or suspected ingestion, laboratory tests can be performed to assess serum levels of the substance and the effects of the toxin on body systems. Regional poison control centers and clinical pharmacists should be included as members of the treatment team. Measurements of serum glucose level and toxicology analysis of urine, serum, and stomach contents are the most common laboratory tests ordered for possible toxic exposure or ingestion. Blood gases and chest radiographs are required if the child is hypoventilating, has other respiratory difficulties, or has been exposed to a hydrocarbon (e.g., gasoline) or bleach. Baseline liver enzymes and kidney function tests may be checked if the suspected substance is known to be toxic to these organs.

## Therapeutic Management

The first step in treatment of a toxic exposure or ingestion is to assess ABCDEs and stabilize the child. Oxygen can be given and breathing supported with a bag-valve-mask ventilation device, if necessary. If the child's level of consciousness is altered, endotracheal intubation may be necessary to protect the airway. When the child has ingested a sufficient amount of a substance to cause rapid deterioration in mental status, intubation equipment should be at the bedside even when the child is awake and alert. If the child is in shock or shows signs of compensated shock, IV fluid resuscitation is initiated. Cardiac rhythm disturbances can result from many ingested substances, so placement of a cardiac monitor and pulse oximeter is also indicated. Seizure precautions should be instituted in exposures to toxins with neurologic or metabolic side effects.

Care of the child who has been exposed to or ingested a toxic substance depends on the amount ingested and the toxicity of the substance (Table 34.5). After initial stabilization, removing the poison, preventing its absorption, and limiting complications are primary goals. Several methods frequently used to treat toxic exposures and ingestions include removal of dermal and ocular toxins, dilution of the toxin, administration of activated charcoal, and administration of an antidote. For most pediatric poison ingestion cases, gastric lavage is no longer recommended because of the risk of aspiration and further injury (Kostic, 2016).

### Removal of Dermal and Ocular Toxins

Removing the child from a toxic environment, including removing contaminated clothes, brushing chemical powders from skin and liberal washing, is mandatory with skin exposure. Copious irrigation of the eyes with water or normal saline is imperative with an ocular exposure. In cases of exposure to an alkaline substance, irrigation proceeds until the eyes return to a normal pH (see Chapter 55).

### Diluting the Ingested Toxin

Acid or alkali substances, when ingested, can cause burning of tissue along the gastrointestinal tract. Because these caustic substances continue to cause damage until neutralized, inducing emesis is contraindicated.

Administration of syrup of ipecac in the home setting is no longer recommended. Parents are advised to call the poison control center immediately if they suspect their child has ingested a poisonous substance.

### Activated Charcoal

Activated charcoal is a charcoal substance with a porous surface that binds to the toxin and passes it through the gastrointestinal system. It is most effective when administered within 60 minutes of ingestion. Activated charcoal can bind to the toxin at any point along the gastrointestinal tract; administration with sorbitol facilitates elimination of the bound substances and prevents constipation. Administering activated charcoal is a nursing challenge because the substance is unpalatable to young children in both taste and appearance. If airway protective reflexes are in doubt, charcoal must not be administered due to risk of aspiration. In the toddler, having the child sit on a parent's lap and administering charcoal by oral syringe may be successful. Mixing the activated charcoal with chocolate milk or other flavoring sometimes makes it easier to drink. Placing the charcoal in a covered opaque or decorated container prevents the child from seeing the substance while drinking. Activated charcoal administration can be repeated, especially in delayed release suspensions, to prevent reabsorption of the toxin from fluid secreted in the biliary tract. Reported use of activated charcoal has declined from 3.7% of pediatric cases in 1993 to just 0.8% in 2014 (Mowry et al., 2014).

### Antidotes

Specific antidotes can be used to inhibit the absorption of the toxin at the receptor site or to lower its concentration. Examples of commonly used antidotes are *N*-acetylcysteine (Mucomyst) for significant acetaminophen ingestion and naloxone (Narcan) for narcotics (see Table 34.5).

## NURSING CARE

### The Child Who Has Ingested a Toxic Substance

#### Assessment

Accurate and rapid assessment of the poisoned child can mean the difference between life and death. The nurse starts by assessing ABCDEs and taking frequent vital signs. Respiratory or circulatory support is initiated as needed. Because the ingestion of many different toxic substances results in shock, the blood pressure, tissue perfusion, and urine output are carefully monitored. The nurse observes and documents the child's mental status frequently to determine any changes in level of consciousness. Changes in pupil size or reactivity, as well as the occurrence of seizures, are assessed on a regular basis.

The nurse needs to take the responsibility for assessing the cause of poisoning. A poison exposure is extremely distressing to parents. If the ingestion was purposeful, psychological consultation and referral should be provided. In some cases, child abuse must be ruled out.

**Nursing Diagnosis and Planning**

The following diagnoses apply to the child and family:

- Risk for Injury related to insufficient parental knowledge about first aid for toxic ingestion and accidental poisonings.

**Expected outcome.** The parent will describe how to assess the child and access appropriate treatment if accidental poisoning occurs.

- Ineffective Breathing Pattern related to effects of toxic substances.

**Expected outcome.** The child will breathe in a way that maintains adequate oxygenation and ventilation, as evidenced by normal arterial blood gases and serum pH or pulse oximetry readings.

- Risk for Deficient Fluid Volume related to effects of ingested substances, treatment modalities, or decreased fluid intake.

**TABLE 34.5 Common Poisonous Substances**

| Substance | Pathophysiology | Clinical Manifestations | Treatment |
|---|---|---|---|
| **Acetaminophen (Tylenol, in Many Over-the-Counter Products)** | | | |
| Toxic dose: uncertain, do not exceed recommended levels<br>Seriousness of ingestion determined by amount ingested and length of time before intervention, and if toxicity is acute or cumulative<br>Other factors, such as decreased oral intake, have been linked with hepatotoxicity | Metabolic by-products deplete liver glutathione and cause damage to hepatic cells.<br>Children younger than 6 yr seem to be more resistant to development of hepatotoxicity than older children and adults. | *First stage* (first 24 hr): malaise, nausea, vomiting, sweating, pallor, weakness.<br>*Second stage* (24-48 hr): latent period with a rise in liver enzymes (aspartate and alanine aminotransferase) and bilirubin; right upper quadrant pain; prolonged prothrombin time.<br>*Third stage* (3-7 days): jaundice, liver necrosis, signs of hepatic failure.<br>*Fourth stage* (5-7 days): recovery or progression to death. | Administer antidote: *N*-acetylcysteine (Mucomyst) as ordered.<br>IV fluids.<br>Within 1-2 hr post-ingestion, administer activated charcoal.<br>Sodium-restricted, high-calorie, high-protein diet. |
| **Salicylates (Aspirin, in Many Over-the-Counter Products, Oil of Wintergreen)** | | | |
| Toxic dose: single dose exceeding 200-280 mg/kg<br>Peak gastric absorption occurs within 2 hr of ingestion | *First stage:* stimulation of respiratory center, leading to respiratory alkalosis.<br>*Second stage:* loss of potassium; increase in metabolic rate; accumulation of ketones leading to metabolic acidosis, hypokalemia, and dehydration.<br>Inhibition of prothrombin formation, decreased platelet levels and adhesiveness, capillary fragility (chronic poisoning). | Gastrointestinal effects: nausea, vomiting, thirst.<br>Central nervous system effects: hyperventilation, tinnitus, confusion, seizures, coma, respiratory failure, circulatory collapse.<br>Renal effect: oliguria.<br>Hematopoietic effects: bleeding tendencies.<br>Metabolic effects: sweating, dehydration, fever, hyponatremia, hypokalemia, dehydration, hypoglycemia. | Administer activated charcoal to decrease absorption.<br>IV fluids, sodium bicarbonate (enhances excretion), potassium replacement; volume expanders as needed to support circulation.<br>Vitamin K for bleeding tendencies (chronic poisoning).Glucose for hypoglycemia.<br>Hemodialysis in severe cases if child unresponsive to therapy. |
| **Corrosives (Toilet and Drain Cleaners, Bleach, Ammonia)** | | | |
| Extent of damage depends on causticity of substance and amount ingested | Severe chemical burns of mouth, throat, and esophagus. "Splash" burns of eyes and skin.<br>Alkaline substances can continue to cause damage after initial contact.<br>If damage is severe, long-term care is needed, including gastric button or tube, repeated esophageal dilations, and surgical repair of esophagus, sometimes with colon tissue transplant (done when child is older). | Whitish burns of mouth and pharynx, color darkens (red, swollen, oozing as ulcerations form and tissue erodes).<br>Edema, difficulty swallowing, drooling.<br>Respiratory distress, pain.<br>Residual difficulty swallowing; subsequent healing of burns can produce esophageal strictures.<br>Severe burns causing perforation can lead to vascular collapse and shock. | IV fluids while NPO.<br>Analgesics, steroids, antibiotics, nasogastric tube feedings. |
| **Hydrocarbons (Gasoline, Paint Thinner, Lighter Fluid, Turpentine, Furniture Polish)** | | | |
| | Chemical pneumonitis from aspiration of hydrocarbon.<br>Pneumonia and acute hemorrhagic necrotizing disease, usually in 24 hr. | Burning sensation in mouth and pharynx.<br>Characteristic petroleum breathe odor.<br>Nausea, vomiting, anorexia, central nervous system depression, fever.<br>Respiratory distress, wheezing. | Prevent vomiting.<br>Support ventilation; administer oxygen.<br>IV fluids. |

**TABLE 34.5 Common Poisonous Substances—cont'd**

| Substance | Pathophysiology | Clinical Manifestations | Treatment |
|---|---|---|---|
| **Lead (Paint Chips From Older Homes, Soil Contaminated With Lead, Lead Solder Used in Plumbing, Vinyl Miniblinds, Improperly Glazed Pottery, Toys)** | | | |
| Diet high in fat and low in iron and calcium increases lead absorption<br>Serum lead level: ≥5 mcg/dL, considered harmful; 5-15 /dL, more frequent screening and environmental investigation indicated; 15-20 mcg/dL, nutritional and educational interventions; 20 mcg/dL, possible removal and treatment | Gastrointestinal tract is major route of absorption.<br>Lead is deposited in blood, bone, and soft tissue.<br>Major toxic effects occur in bone marrow, nervous system, and kidney.<br>Amount of lead ingested, particle size, and repeated ingestion over time contribute to severity of lead poisoning. | Symptoms may be vague, with insidious onset.<br>Central nervous system effects: irritability, lethargy, hyperactivity, cognitive and perceptual motor difficulties, clumsiness, seizures, coma, and death (associated with blood level of 100 mg/dL).<br>Hematopoietic effect: anemia.<br>Gastrointestinal effects: anorexia, nausea, vomiting, constipation, lead line along gums.<br>Skeletal effects: increased density of long bones, lead line in long bones.<br>Renal effects: glycosuria, proteinuria, possible acute or chronic renal failure. Kidney damage is reversible early in the disease, but with continued lead exposure, permanent kidney damage can occur. | Level >25 mcg/dL: remove child from lead source, hospitalize if level is significantly higher.<br>Administer chelating agents: Succimer (Chemet) orally for lead level of 35-45 mcg/dL; EDTA for level >70 mcg/dL given IV over several hours for 5 days (causes lead to be deposited in bone and excreted by kidneys); bronchoalveolar lavage every 4 hr for six doses for level >70 mcg/dL. Monitor kidney function because EDTA is nephrotoxic; monitor calcium levels because EDTA enhances excretion of calcium.<br>Provide adequate hydration.<br>Calcium, phosphorus, and vitamins C and D.<br>Anticonvulsants.<br>Oral or intramuscular iron for anemia.<br>Follow-up lead levels to monitor progress (lead is excreted more slowly than it accumulates in the body). |
| **Battery Ingestions (Most Commonly 20-mm–Diameter Button Batteries)** | | | |
| Toxic Substance: alkaline corrosives in cylindrical batteries<br>Lithium batteries can cause tissue injury and necrosis within hours. | Battery can lodge in the esophagus, causing tissue necrosis and possible death. The majority of patients are under the age of 4 yr.<br>Batteries can also cause damage when inserted in the ear canal and nasal canal (Sharpe, Rochette, & Smith, 2012). | Injury occurs rapidly with asymptomatic or non-specific symptoms until injury progresses over several hours.<br>Button batteries have an external current, causing electrolysis of tissue fluids that produces hydroxide, leading to tissue damage. Leakage of alkaline electrolyte causes further damage such as esophageal perforation, stricture, and fistula (Sharpe, Rochette, & Smith, 2012). | Prompt identification and removal of the battery. Education about battery safety. Battery compartments should be securely shut and taped. |
| **Carbon Monoxide** | | | |
| Most often from improperly ventilated heaters; also from poorly ventilated vehicles.<br>Cause of the exposure should be determined and eliminated. | An odorless, colorless gas that binds to hemoglobin more effectively than does oxygen, thereby causing hypoxia. | Headache, visual disturbances.<br>Altered level of consciousness, cherry-red lips and cheeks, nausea, and vomiting. | 100% oxygen by nonrebreather mask.<br>Serum carboxyhemoglobin levels, hyperbaric chamber treatment may be necessary for patients with high carboxyhemoglobin levels.<br>Other interventions based on signs and symptoms.<br>Prevention: carbon monoxide detectors in every home. |

*EDTA*, Ethylenediaminetetraacetic acid; *IV*, intravenous; *NPO*, nothing by mouth

***Expected outcome.*** The child will maintain an hourly urine output appropriate for weight and age, with age-appropriate specific gravity.

- Compromised Family Coping related to sudden hospitalization and emergency aspects of illness.

***Expected outcomes.*** The family will appropriately discuss the child's condition and treatment, verbalize feelings and concerns, and remain with the child as much as possible.

- Risk for Poisoning related to insufficient parental knowledge about poisoning prevention.

***Expected outcome.*** The parent makes the necessary changes in the home environment to prevent future poisoning.

#### Interventions

Stabilization is the nurse's priority in caring for the child who has ingested a poisonous substance. Nursing care also includes reducing the child's and the family's fear and anxiety, providing preventive teaching concerning the storage of poisons and supervision of children, and removal of the poison from the child's skin and mucous membranes to reduce further injury.

**! NURSING QUALITY ALERT**

***Assessment of Poison Ingestion***

Obtain information about the following:

- Substance ingested, if known
- Amount ingested (how many pills are missing?)
- Approximate time of ingestion
- Change in the child's condition
- Treatment administered at home
- What other substances are available in the home?

Parents usually are overwhelmed by feelings of guilt, fear, and anger when their child has ingested a poisonous substance. Providing an opportunity for them to express their feelings in a nonjudgmental atmosphere helps parents cope with this experience. Some aspects of treatment, such as placement of a gastric tube or support of ventilation, are disturbing and frightening to parents. Support is offered by explaining treatment, including the parents in care (as appropriate), and informing them about their child's status.

Ideally, nurses intervene with parents (and other caregivers such as grandparents, older siblings, and childcare providers) before a poison exposure occurs. Knowledge of safety and "safe proofing" the child's environment is important. Discussion of safe storage of medications and other potentially toxic substances and age-appropriate supervision of children are essential aspects of poison prevention. The nurse advises the parents to post the poison control phone number clearly and to call the poison center before treating the child. This and other injury prevention information should be readily available in daycare, primary care, and emergency care settings and should be given to families proactively. Education through community programs to prevent poisoning and reduce drug abuse should be directed to the parents and caretakers of young children, as well as to adolescents. Simple ideas such as storing medication in the original containers and placing in locked cabinets; labeling all cleaning product containers and placing these out of the reach of children; and never calling medication "candy," should be promoted.

### Evaluation

- Do parents describe the appropriate actions to take in the event of a future poisoning?
- Are the child's oxygen saturation, blood gas measurements, and level of consciousness within normal limits?
- Is the child's hourly urine output appropriate for age and weight?
- Are family members remaining with the child and able to provide adequate support?
- Can parents and other caregivers describe poison prevention (e.g., keeping common poisonous household hazards out of the child's reach)? Do they have easy access to the poison control telephone number?

## ENVIRONMENTAL EMERGENCIES

Active children are exposed to a variety of environmental hazards. Injuries from animal and snake bites, submersion injuries, and sun- and heat-related illnesses account for the majority of **environmental injuries**. This section focuses on animal, human, snake, and spider bites; submersion injuries; and heat-related illnesses. Sunburn is discussed in Chapter 49.

### Animal, Human, Snake, and Spider Bites

#### Etiology

***Animal and human bites.*** Both animal and human bites involve soft tissue damage from crushing, lacerations, and puncture wounds. All animal bites have the potential for infection. Although human bites are relatively rare, they carry the greatest risk of infection if they break the skin, particularly if they are on the scalp, face, hands, wrists, or feet. Serious injury can result from any type of bite, but most bites are not life threatening.

***Snake and spider bites.*** Envenomation of children on land is usually from snakes, scorpions, and spiders. Envenomation can also result from marine animals such as jellyfish, sea urchins, and stingrays. Fatalities from envenomation are rare, with most occurring from snake bites.

#### Incidence

Animal bites in children are most often from dogs and have the highest incidence in boys 5 to 9 years of age (CDC, 2015). There are relatively few fatalities as a result of dog bites, and most injuries in children are in the head and neck region (CDC, 2015).

Bites from pet birds, rats, ferrets, pigs, hamsters, turtles, fish, alligators, snakes, horses, and many other animals have been seen in emergency settings, as have bites from a variety of wild animals, such as raccoons, skunks, and coyotes.

In the United States, there are two groups of poisonous snakes: Crotalids, or pit vipers, such as rattlesnakes, water moccasins, and copperheads; and Elapids, such as coral snakes. Children should be taught to avoid snakes, and healthcare providers should be familiar with snakes indigenous to their area. Bites from only two types of spiders in the United States can cause significant illness: the black widow spider and the brown recluse spider.

#### Manifestations

***Animal and human bites.*** Because of the risk of infection, human bites are more serious and can be differentiated from dog bites by the distance between the canine teeth; in human bites, the distance is generally greater than 3 cm. A human bite is horseshoe shaped and rarely breaks the skin. Localized tissue damage and multibacterial infections are serious manifestations of animal and human bites. Dog bites run an additional risk because of the crush injuries that ensue.

***Snake bites.*** To determine the cause of envenomation, medical staff in emergency settings should have some knowledge of the venomous snakes likely to be encountered in the surrounding geographic area.

Smaller children are usually bitten on the hand or foot, whereas older children are more commonly bitten on lower extremities.

Regardless of whether the snake can be positively identified, treatment should be based on physical assessment and symptoms. The following local signs and symptoms most commonly suggest envenomation from a snake:

- Bite marks that look like fang marks
- Burning at the site
- Ecchymosis and erythema
- Pain or numbness
- Progressing edema

The following systemic signs and symptoms suggest severe envenomation:

- Nausea, vomiting
- Sweating, chills
- Numbness, paresthesia of the tongue and perioral region
- Hypotension
- Coagulopathies

When a substantial amount of venom has been injected and treatment is delayed, envenomation can progress to coagulopathies, respiratory failure, renal failure, seizures, shock, and (rarely) death. Because of advancements in antivenin preparation and availability, significant injury can be prevented with early treatment. However, any child with a suspected or actual venomous snake bite should be monitored closely in the hospital for at least 24 hours even if antivenin has been administered (Schroeder & Norris, 2016).

*Spider bites.* Bites from neurotoxic spiders such as the black widow, are very painful. Possible systemic effects include hypertension, tachycardia, bradycardia, diaphoresis, increased salivation, and muscle spasms. A bite from a brown recluse spider can cause significant local tissue necrosis and, in rare cases, systemic toxicity with presenting signs of fever, chills, nausea, malaise, rash, and petechiae progressing to hemolysis, coagulopathy, and renal failure (Schroeder & Norris, 2016).

### Therapeutic Management

*Animal bites.* Emergency care for animal bites depends on the type of bite but usually includes thorough irrigation and debridement. The affected extremity should be kept in a dependent position to prevent changes in toxicity related to gravity or circulatory impairment. Tetanus prophylaxis is given if the child's immunization is not up to date or if documentation is unavailable. Antibiotics are prescribed when a high probability of infection exists. Smaller bite wounds are often left open rather than sutured because puncture wounds and wounds closed with sutures have more potential for infection. A specialist should be consulted if tendon, bone, or compartment injury is suspected. Treatment of the child for rabies may be necessary, especially in cases of wild-animal (e.g., raccoon, rat, and skunk) bites.

*Snake bites.* The following three factors influence the severity of bite from a venomous snake:

- The child's age, size, and general health
- Size of the snake (larger snakes produce more venom)
- Location of the injury (peripheral injuries account for 90% of the bites and are less severe)

When assessing the child with a snake bite, identification of the type of snake is helpful, but this is not always possible. In most cases, an expert in the treatment of snake bites should be consulted. Emergency treatments (e.g., use of a tourniquet, incision, and extraction of the venom; electric shock therapy; cryotherapy) are not recommended and can result in complications (Schroeder & Norris, 2016). First aid (after assessment and maintenance of the ABCs) includes washing with soap and water; immobilization of the extremity in a dependent position; removal of clothes, rings, and other constricting items; and rapid transport to an emergency facility.

In the hospital setting, emergency management continues assessment and maintenance of the ABCs, insertion of an IV line if envenomation is suspected, and laboratory studies, including CBC, coagulation studies, electrolytes, creatinine phosphokinase (CPK), and urinalysis, to assist in determination of need for antivenin therapy. Children with symptoms should be admitted to the hospital. In cases of moderate to severe envenomation, the negative side effects of antivenin must be weighed against the positive effects. Antivenin therapy is the mainstay of treatment for snake bites. Indications for administration include worsening injury, coagulation abnormalities, or systemic effects.

*Spider bites.* Supportive care is the focus for the management of spider bites. In severe cases, antivenin may be administered to reduce pain and reverse systemic effects from a black widow spider bite. The wound from a brown recluse spider bite requires daily cleansing and intermittent ice therapy for the first three days; antibiotics are given to prevent a secondary bacterial infection. Systemic disease is managed with medications and IV fluids because recluse spider antivenin is not available in the United States.

### Nursing Considerations

With severe bites, significant envenomation, or anaphylaxis, nursing interventions for bites and envenomation begin with attention to the ABCDEs and support of vital body functions. With envenomation, nursing care includes keeping the child as calm as possible to help prevent spread of the toxin or venom. Hospitals may not have sufficient antivenin for severe envenomations, so nurses should ensure that available protocols include the location of centers to contact for additional antivenin.

The injury site of all bites is carefully cleaned, and tetanus prophylaxis is administered if immunizations are not up to date. When the bite or envenomation is located on an extremity, the nurse immobilizes the extremity. Measuring the circumference of the affected extremity every 20 to 30 minutes will track the progression of the injury, as well as the results of the treatment.

If antivenin is to be administered, a thorough history of allergies is obtained because the most common antivenins are made from horse serum. Antivenin is most effective if given within 4 to 6 hours after injury, but it may be repeated if coagulopathies or bleeding is present. The nurse documents the type and location of the injury, the length of time since the injury, and the signs and symptoms resulting from the injury. All children who require antivenin should be monitored in an intensive care setting. To assess hypersensitivity, a small test dose of antivenin is given intradermally before the full dose.

Education concerning avoiding snake habitats, wearing protective clothing, and avoiding provocative behavior around snakes should be emphasized.

In most states, notification of the local animal control agency is required for animal bites. The rabies immunization status of the animal, if available, should be documented in nursing notes. Quarantine of the animal responsible for the attack may be necessary if the animal can be found. Nurses should advise parents to observe the child closely for changes in behavior and refer for counseling, if needed.

Discharge instructions should include observation for signs and symptoms of infection and wound care. The nurse provides injury prevention education to all families. This includes giving parents information about how to teach their children to avoid animal bites by avoiding strange animals and provocative behavior in dealing with enraged animals.

## Submersion Injuries (Near Drowning)

Known as the "silent event," submersion injury is the second leading cause of unintentional death in children 1 to 4 years old (CDC, 2014; Safe Kids Worldwide, 2016). *Drowning* is submersion that results in asphyxia and death within 24 hours. If the child survives longer than 24 hours after submersion, the event is referred to as *near drowning.*

One of the most important nursing responsibilities related to drowning is prevention of injury, including water safety education and training, support of legislative efforts to pass drowning prevention measures, and teaching CPR to families. Nurses must emphasize the importance of adequate adult supervision when children are in or around bodies of water.

### Etiology

Most drownings occur in residential swimming pools, although drownings can occur in any body of water, including hot tubs, spas, bathtubs, toilets, and even buckets. Open water sites, such as lakes, rivers, and oceans, are more likely to be the site of accidents among teenagers. Alcohol is often a factor in teenage drownings because it alters judgment and increases risk-taking behaviors.

### Incidence

Every day, approximately 2 children under the age of 14 years die from unintentional drowning (CDC, 2014). Nearly 40% of these children are in the toddler age-group. Boys are two to four times more likely than girls to die from drowning. Swimming pools, lakes, ponds, and bathtubs are common locations of drownings.

### Manifestations

The child's condition after near drowning varies with the extent of injury. Factors that may contribute to the child's eventual prognosis are: (1) age, (2) submersion time, (3) water temperature, (4) elapsed time before resuscitation efforts are instituted, and (5) neurologic status. A child with the poorest prognosis is one who was submerged longer than 10 minutes, received CPR for longer than 25 minutes, arrived at the emergency department in deep coma (Glasgow Coma Scale score of 5 or lower), and did not regain consciousness within the first 48 to 72 hours of hospitalization (Caglar & Quan, 2016).

The child who is conscious with adequate respirations might have mild hypothermia, show slight pulmonary changes on radiography, and demonstrate minor blood gas alterations. Children who are unconscious (stuporous or comatose) demonstrate consequences related to whether respirations are present or absent. If respirations are adequate, the child may have mild to moderate hypothermia and mild to moderate respiratory distress with abnormal chest radiography and arterial blood gas results. The child who required resuscitative efforts is in markedly poorer condition, with altered mental status, metabolic acidosis and other arterial blood gas abnormalities, electrolyte disturbances, possible seizures, or shock, and may develop disseminated intravascular coagulation. Death is the result of complete cardiopulmonary arrest or cerebral anoxic-ischemic injury. Most long-term sequelae of near drowning are neurologic in origin (Caglar & Quan, 2016).

## PATHOPHYSIOLOGY

### *Submersion Injury*

Hypoxia is the cause of organ system injury when drowning occurs. Drowning progresses in a predictable sequence of events. Drowning victims panic, struggle, and attempt to hold their breath. In doing so, they begin to swallow water, which is then vomited and aspirated. This process can cause laryngospasm, which leads to hypoxia, seizures, and death (called *dry drowning* because laryngospasm prevents large amounts of water from entering the respiratory system). If the child becomes unconscious before laryngospasm, hypoxia causes loss of airway reflexes and subsequent aspiration of large amounts of water (leading to *wet drowning*). As hypoxia and acidosis progress, cardiopulmonary arrest occurs. Swallowing large amounts of fresh water also causes electrolyte shifts into the intracellular spaces, resulting in hyponatremia and cerebral edema.

Submerged children lose body heat quickly in cold water because of their relatively large body surface area. Severe hypothermia offers some protection to the brain through the diving reflex, which is stimulated when the face is submerged in cold water. This neurologic reflex shunts blood away from the periphery, increasing blood flow to the brain and heart. The diving reflex is stronger in young children. Irreversible brain damage usually occurs after 4 to 6 minutes of submersion, but some children have had a complete recovery after lengthy submersion (10 to 40 minutes) in very cold water.

### Therapeutic Management

***Prehospital emergency management.*** Treatment begins at the scene of the submersion with rescue and removal from the water. The prehospital care that the child receives can significantly affect the chances for a normal recovery. Prompt initiation of CPR and activation of the emergency medical system are imperative. The goal of prehospital care is to maintain adequate oxygenation and circulation, minimize secondary organ damage, and take proper precautions to stabilize possible cervical spine injuries.

Every child with a submersion injury is considered hypoxic. When the brain is deprived of oxygen for even a short period, irreversible brain damage can occur. After the child's airway is open, the nurse suctions the child's oropharynx to remove mucus and fluid and delivers 100% oxygen by mask or by bag-valve-mask ventilation device in the child with inadequate respiratory rate or effort. Overinflation of the lungs must be avoided to prevent a pneumothorax. Pulse oximetry may not be available in prehospital management or may be inaccurate in the child with hypothermia. Assessment of breath sounds, chest symmetry and rise and fall, and central color are more reliable indicators of adequate respirations.

Elevating the head of the bed to 30 degrees may help lower intracranial pressure but should be done only if no spinal injury or shock is present. Intubation should be performed for unconscious and/or nonbreathing children.

A cardiac monitor is used for ongoing assessment of heart rate and rhythm. Ventricular fibrillation or asystole that is unresponsive to resuscitative efforts can occur in the severely hypothermic (28° C [92.4° F]) child. Resuscitative efforts continue while aggressive warming measures are instituted. Children have been successfully resuscitated up to 40 minutes after a cold-water immersion. Because the presence of a cardiac rhythm does not ensure perfusion of the tissues, the prehospital team assesses the child's cardiovascular status at regular intervals in addition to observing the rhythm on the cardiac monitor.

The wet clothes are removed, and the child is covered with warm blankets. Increasing the ambient temperature of the transport vehicle may be indicated. Rapid transport to the local emergency department or tertiary care center is critical for the severely hypothermic child.

Two IV lines should be started immediately in critically ill children with submersion injuries. Because of the electrolyte and fluid shifts into the intracellular space, children can become hypovolemic, and fluid resuscitation is required. Adequate circulation is necessary to maintain organ perfusion. The rescuer may obtain blood for laboratory analysis while inserting the IV lines. Standard blood studies for the submerged child include CBC, serum electrolytes, BUN, creatinine level, and serum amylase. If the child is in shock or has experienced significant trauma, typing and crossmatching of two to four units of blood should be included.

Both air and water can be swallowed during a submersion incident. Air may also be forced into the stomach with resuscitative efforts. Because gastric distention resulting from air and water in the stomach can prevent full expansion of the lungs, a gastric tube should be inserted to decompress the stomach, ensure full respiratory excursion, and prevent aspiration of stomach contents from vomiting.

***Hospital management.*** On reaching the emergency department, emergency care continues the prehospital goals of maintaining adequate oxygenation and circulation. Additional treatments are initiated on the basis of laboratory and radiologic findings. Arterial blood gases may indicate the need to correct acidosis with sodium bicarbonate administration. Continued hypothermia is addressed by providing warmed IV fluids and oxygen, overhead lights, and warmed blankets. Fluid and electrolyte corrections can be instituted.

The child is admitted to the hospital for observation, even if in stable condition after initial rescue and emergency treatment.

## NURSING CARE

### The Child With a Submersion Injury

Nursing care of the child with a submersion injury requires obtaining an accurate history, ensuring adequate oxygenation and tissue perfusion, and maintaining body temperature.

### Assessment

Assessment of the child with a submersion injury focuses on the respiratory system. Airway and breathing are the priorities. The nurse observes the child for rate and depth of respiration, work of breathing, and any change in mental status. Cardiovascular assessment includes assessment of capillary refill and heart rate. The child's temperature is taken as soon as possible to determine any hypothermia.

Obtaining an accurate history of the injury is important although often difficult. Whether the submersion incident occurred in salt or fresh water is irrelevant for early treatment, but subsequent intensive care may vary somewhat depending on the immersion fluid.

### Nursing Diagnosis and Planning

The following diagnoses are applicable to the child with a submersion injury:

- Impaired Gas Exchange (actual or potential) related to bronchospasm, aspiration of fluid, surfactant elimination, or pulmonary edema.

***Expected outcome.*** The child will demonstrate normal oxygen saturation, blood gas measurements, and clear breath sounds.

- Risk for Imbalanced Fluid Volume related to electrolyte imbalances that cause volume shifts from interstitial to intravascular space.

***Expected outcome.*** The child will maintain hourly urine output appropriate for weight and age and vital signs within normal limits; electrolytes will return to normal.

- Hypothermia related to prolonged exposure to cold water.

***Expected outcome.*** The child will maintain body temperature between 36.5° C and 37.4° C (97.7° F to 99.3° F).

- Compromised Family Coping related to the child's critical status.

***Expected outcome.*** The family will verbalize feelings (including feelings of guilt and anger) and concerns appropriately, exhibit an attitude of confidence in the care being provided, and provide support to the child.

### Interventions

After the initial assessment and emergency management have been completed, the nurse monitors for changes from the baseline, anticipates the development of complications, and implements therapeutic management.

***Providing respiratory support.*** Because hypoxia is the primary problem, with potential for damage to all major organ systems, attention to the pulmonary system is a priority. The nurse assesses the child's level of consciousness and listens for adventitious breath sounds, which can signal the development of complications such as pulmonary edema, atelectasis, or pneumonia. Persistent hypoxemia, dyspnea, tachycardia, and respiratory alkalosis can also signal these pulmonary complications. If the child is intubated, airway maintenance is a priority with frequent observations for signs of tube displacement or pneumothorax.

***Restoring appropriate circulatory status.*** Cardiovascular monitoring includes measuring vital signs, pulses, level of consciousness, skin temperature, color, and urine output. The well-perfused child is alert, with age-appropriate behavior, and has a capillary refill time of less than 2 seconds and urine output according to age (see Chapter 40). The nurse maintains IV lines and administers fluid volume replacement as ordered.

***Identifying and preventing neurologic consequences.*** The neurologic system is monitored frequently. Common parameters include level of consciousness, pupillary response, movement of extremities, reflexes, and vital signs. The nurse anticipates signs and symptoms of increased intracranial pressure up to 24 hours after the submersion event. Conventional measures to prevent increased intracranial pressure, such as positioning the head in the midline, elevating the head of the bed 20 to 30 degrees, preventing or managing elevated body temperature, and controlling pain and agitation, are instituted as ordered.

***Restoring fluid balance.*** As a result of ingestion of large amounts of water during the near-drowning event, the child is at risk for development of alterations in fluid and electrolyte balance. The nurse carefully monitors urine output, laboratory data, and physical signs and symptoms. Hyponatremia and water intoxication should be anticipated, particularly with a freshwater submersion. The nurse observes for changes in central nervous system functioning, especially seizures, as the serum sodium level drops.

***Controlling infection.*** The acutely ill child is at risk for local or systemic infection. Complications from organ damage, intubation and ventilation tubes, invasive monitoring lines, and urinary catheters are possible sources for infection. If infection is present, antibiotic therapy is started. The nurse must monitor the child's response to this therapy.

***Maintaining nutritional status.*** In the gastrointestinal system, hypoxia leads to decreased blood supply to the bowel. Stress ulcers and gastrointestinal (GI) bleeding are not uncommon. GI function in all areas must be monitored. This includes intake (nothing by mouth [NPO], oral or enteral feedings), internal systems (bowel sounds, residual feedings), and output (presence or absence of GI bleeding; amount, color, and consistency of stool).

The child's increased metabolic demands, along with disruption of GI functioning, can result in a nutritional deficit. Nutritional therapy is implemented as ordered in the form of enteral feedings or total parenteral nutrition. If enteral feedings are ordered, weight gain, residuals, amount and consistency of stools, and vomiting must be monitored to ascertain tolerance of the feedings. If total parenteral nutrition is ordered, the nurse checks the product label with the order, administers the solution as ordered, monitors laboratory values, and assesses for any side effects.

***Providing emotional care for the family.*** Because seriously ill children brought to the emergency department may not have a positive outcome, an important element of nursing care is psychological intervention and support for the child's family. The most important nursing interventions with the family of any critically ill or injured child initially include attention to the family's physical needs and provision of information and hope.

Families should be encouraged to participate in the decision regarding their presence in the treatment area, especially if the child is likely to die and the family may not have an opportunity to see the child alive again. If the parents choose to be brought into the resuscitation room, one person should be their liaison, bringing them into the room, answering questions, and escorting them out at appropriate times. The AHA guidelines for CPR and emergency care state that often families do not ask to be present during resuscitative efforts; nurses should be sensitive to this and offer the opportunity for family members to be present (deCaen et al., 2015a).

Be honest with the family. If the child is in full arrest, make a simple statement such as, "Your child (use the child's name if possible) is not breathing and has no heartbeat. We are supporting his breathing and helping his heart to beat right now." This statement is far better than "We're doing everything we can," which leaves much more room for doubt.

Parents react in many different ways, according to their cultures, religious beliefs, individual personalities, and past experiences. Denial can initially be protective and allows the family to accept information gradually. Family members are asked if they want other family members or clergy to be contacted. Religious rites, including baptism, may be extremely important to families. A list of clergy from a variety of religions should be readily available for use by the nursing staff in emergency care settings.

Providing hope for the family is always important. At times, the only hope may be that the child is not suffering, or did not suffer, and that the child is, or was, not alone. If the child survives the incident, the parents will have ample time to adjust to any adverse consequences, so insisting on their acceptance is not necessary at this point. Many miraculous recoveries have occurred after lengthy submersions, usually in very cold water. However, in the emergency setting, predicting the ultimate outcome for a child is impossible. The nurse needs to convey to the family a realistic, positive attitude, while acknowledging the strong possibility of long-term effects for the child.

### Evaluation

- Does the child demonstrate adequate oxygenation and independent breathing? Are lung sounds clear?
- Is the child's urine output appropriate for weight and age? Have electrolyte levels returned to normal?
- Is the child's body temperature between 36.5° C and 37.4° C (97.7° F to 99.3° F)?
- Do the parents verbalize their feelings and concerns appropriately, and do they provide appropriate support for the child?

**! NURSING QUALITY ALERT**

***Needs Expressed by Families of Critically Ill Children***

The highest ranked need identified for families in most research studies is the need for hope. Needs for privacy and comfort are also consistently identified as extremely important by the families of critically ill and injured children; these needs are usually ranked higher than the need for psychological support from nursing staff. Another commonly cited need is to have a contact person to provide updates and answer questions.

## HEAT-RELATED ILLNESSES

Heat-related illnesses include sunburn, heat cramps, heat rash, heat exhaustion, and heat stroke. The most serious types are heat exhaustion and heat stroke, both of which can ultimately result in death. Two important factors in evaluating the possibility of heat-related illnesses are environmental temperature and humidity. If the body is unable to maintain normal temperature through evaporation of sweat, as in the case of high humidity and exertion, thermoregulation systems can be overwhelmed, creating a cascade of potentially life-threatening events (Landry, 2016).

### Incidence

Children's anatomic and physiologic differences make them more susceptible to sun- and heat-related illnesses. In the US, there are on average 688 deaths a year due to heat-related illnesses (ENA, 2012). The majority of pediatric deaths are a result of small children being left alone in closed vehicles. Infants and young children are sensitive to the effects of high temperatures related to rapid fluid loss and impaired compensatory mechanisms. They rely on others to regulate their environments and provide adequate liquids. Prophylactic measures such as use of sunscreen and adequate fluid and electrolyte intake should be carried out. Both parents and children, early in life, should be taught to use these prophylactic measures. This section focuses on heat-related illnesses; sunburn is discussed in Chapter 49.

Children involved in physical activity sweat less, create more heat in proportion to their body size and weight, and take longer to adapt to warm environments than do adults (Landry, 2016). In addition, younger children have a greater body-surface-area-to-mass ratio, which causes their bodies to gain heat rapidly from the environment on a hot day. Obese children are vulnerable because of increased insulation. Active children may continue playing without feeling the need to drink adequate amounts of fluids, even in extremely hot environments.

### Manifestations and Therapeutic Management

Symptoms of heat-related illness are wide ranging and, if left unrecognized or untreated, can quickly progress to heat exhaustion and the life-threatening state of heat stroke. Management of heat-related illness is dictated by the severity of symptoms. The first priority in all cases is to move the child to a cool place and start cooling measures such as loosening and removing wet clothes and applying cool cloths. Rehydration is instituted, either by oral rehydration solution in cases of overexertion or by IV fluid and electrolyte administration if the child is unable to tolerate the oral route. In cases of heat stroke, this is not sufficient. The child's temperature-controlling mechanisms are not working, the child is unable to sweat, and brain damage and death could result if the body is not cooled rapidly. Concurrent assessment and prompt stabilization of cardiopulmonary circulation are critical (Table 34.6).

### Nursing Considerations

The nurse caring for a child with a heat-related emergency will initially assess and possibly intervene in stabilizing the ABCDEs, provide cooling measures aimed at progressively decreasing core body temperature without causing shivering or increased metabolic demands, give the child fluids with electrolytes as indicated, and provide emotional support for the child and family.

Depending on the severity of symptoms, the nurse will assess for respiratory compromise and intervene with the appropriate method of oxygen delivery. In the hospital setting, the child with heat exhaustion may benefit from cool oxygen blow-by or nasal cannula, whereas the child with heat stroke will require oxygen by nonrebreathing mask or even intubation in the case of insufficient respiratory effort. The nurse performs serial assessments of circulation and disability to determine the effectiveness of oral and/or IV fluid resuscitation.

As in other pediatric emergencies, the family should be involved early and to the extent they are comfortable. Family presence is encouraged, with the nurse or other member of the healthcare team available to provide clear explanations of procedures, answer questions, and give support.

Following stabilization of the child's condition, the nurse provides education to the family and child regarding prevention of heat-related illnesses. Even in cool temperatures, young children should *never* be left alone in a car or other type of vehicle. Even with the windows partially opened, the interior temperature can increase by 20 degrees (F) in the first 10 minutes, putting children at great risk for heat stroke and death. Parents, children, and members of the community need to gain an understanding about the dangers of sun and heat exposure and the importance of adequate fluid and electrolyte intake, wearing light-colored, loose-fitting clothing, and adjusting activity levels according to temperature and humidity of the environment.

**TABLE 34.6 Heat-Related Illness**

| Type | Pathophysiology | Clinical Manifestations | Treatment |
|---|---|---|---|
| Overexertion | Muscles generate heat during strenuous exercise; body fluids are being lost through sweating; rapid breathing; increased metabolic demands | Dizziness; flushed skin; diffuse muscle cramps | Move to cool environment; offer oral fluids; loosen clothing |
| Heat exhaustion | Increased loss of body fluids; increased blood flow to the skin with resulting decreased oxygen and blood flow to vital organs | Heavy sweating; nausea; vomiting; dizziness or fainting; exhaustion; headache; cramps; cool, moist, or flushed skin; core body temperature may be slightly elevated | Move to cool environment; apply cool, moist cloths to skin; remove clothing or change to dry clothing; elevate legs; offer oral rehydration fluids if no altered mental status or vomiting |
| Heat stroke | Thermoregulation is ineffective; sweating has stopped; vascular collapse and severe central nervous system abnormalities are noted because of hyperthermia and insufficient circulating volume | Hot, dry, red skin; change in level of consciousness or coma; rapid, weak pulse; rapid, shallow breathing; elevated core body temperature: 40.6° C (≥105° F) | Emergency transport to an emergency care setting; rapid cooling with moist, cool cloths and fans; administer oxygen by nonrebreather mask, or intubate for respiratory insufficiency; aggressive intravenous (IV) rehydration; intervene as needed to maintain vital functions |

**CRITICAL THINKING EXERCISE 34.2**

You are at a seventh-grade baseball game when you are asked by a parent to look at her previously healthy child who is reporting nausea, leg and arm cramps, and dizziness. His baseball uniform is wet, and the child is sweating profusely. It is 33.3° C (92° F) outside, and it had rained earlier in the day.

1. What do you think is wrong with the child? Why?
2. What are your interventions while on the baseball field?
3. If he starts vomiting, what interventions should be anticipated?

## DENTAL EMERGENCIES

### Incidence and Etiology

Injury to the teeth, particularly the anterior teeth, is common in children with 10% of children between 18 months and 18 years sustaining dental trauma (Tinaoff, 2016). Toddlers, because of their lack of coordination, receive dental injuries from falling from or onto furniture. School-age children are more likely to have their teeth injured on playgrounds and during sports activities. The first teeth begin to erupt at approximately 6 months of age. By approximately 2 years of age, a child has all 20 primary teeth. Permanent teeth come in at approximately 5 or 6 years of age. By adolescence, a child usually has the full complement of 32 permanent teeth, although the eruption of wisdom teeth may be delayed. Injury to primary and permanent teeth is considered equally serious. Teeth are embedded in the bones of the maxilla and mandible. Injuries to teeth are usually divided into the following categories:

*Concussion:* The tooth is not displaced, but pressure may cause pain.

*Subluxation:* The tooth is moveable within the socket but is displaced less than 2 mm. The socket is not damaged.

*Intrusion:* The tooth is pushed into its socket with injury to the underlying structures.

*Extrusion:* An upper tooth is dislodged downward from the socket, or a lower tooth is dislodged upward.

*Luxation:* The tooth is moved laterally with tearing of the periodontal ligament.

*Avulsion:* The tooth is no longer in the socket, and the socket itself may be damaged.

### Therapeutic Management

Dental emergencies require specialized care, which is often difficult to obtain immediately. Survival of the tooth depends on the periodontal ligament attachment, so concussion, subluxation, lateral luxation, and extrusion, in which the periodontal ligament is still attached, have a better prognosis than complete avulsion of a tooth. Intrusion of a tooth may damage underlying structures to a greater extent and diminish chances for tooth survival.

Time is of the essence in caring for dental injuries. With injury to a child's mouth, the nurse observes for missing teeth. If a missing tooth cannot be found in the oral cavity, possible aspiration should be considered in the presence of dyspnea. To determine whether other teeth are loose or malpositioned, the nurse gently palpates (using Standard Precautions) the teeth for movement and asks the child to check. A tooth that is loose in the socket should not be removed. If the position is not correct, repositioning may be necessary by a specialist.

In general, primary teeth are not replanted because damage to the developing tooth bud can occur. Complete avulsion of a permanent tooth requires care of the socket and the tooth itself. Survival of an avulsed tooth depends on prompt evaluation and replacement. Irreversible damage to the periodontal ligament because of dehydration of the open socket can occur after 60 minutes.

Emergency care by the dentist includes cleaning the tooth and socket, placing the tooth in the socket, and splinting the tooth. Tetanus immunization is given if needed, and an antibiotic may be prescribed.

### Nursing Considerations

Parents should be instructed to keep the tooth moist. The tooth can be immersed in saline, water, milk, or a commercial tooth-preserving liquid. The tooth should not be cleaned or scrubbed. These actions increase the chances of tooth survival. The child should see a dentist, if possible, or should go to an emergency facility for care without delay.

Parents should be given careful discharge instructions and appropriate referrals for continuing dental care. When appropriate, reassure the family that with proper care, a good cosmetic outcome is possible with injury to or loss of a child's primary as well as secondary teeth.

## KEY CONCEPTS

- Nursing care of ill and injured children may seem more complicated than care of adults because of their size, medication dosing, equipment, and age-related psychological differences.
- Familiarity with the issues related to the child's growth and development and careful organization of pediatric equipment can improve the care of children in emergency settings.
- Airway management is the most critical element in pediatric emergency care.
- Shock must be recognized early and must be taken into account when children begin to decompensate.
- Care of the family and the child's developmental stage should always be considered when providing nursing interventions in the emergency setting.
- Trauma assessment of the child includes the standard primary and secondary survey and intervention but must also include skin assessment, level of consciousness, and prevention of hypothermia.
- Injury prevention plays an important role in the nursing care of children. Motor vehicle injuries, ingestions, poisonings, and environmental injuries are largely preventable.

## REFERENCES AND READINGS


Albert, M., & McCaig, L. (2014). *Injury-related emergency department visits by children and adolescents: United States 2009-2010.* NCHS Data Brief No. 150, May 2014.

Arikoglu, T., Aslan, G., Batmaz, S.B., et al. (2015). Diagnostic evaluation and risk factors for drug allergies in children: from clinical history to skin and challenge tests. *International Journal of Clinical Pharmacology, 37*(4), 583–591. doi:10.1007/s11096-015-0100-9.

Atkins, D., Berger, S., Duff, J. et al. (2015). Part 11: Pediatric basic life support: 2015 American Heart Association guidelines for cardiopulmonary resuscitation and emergency cardiovascular care. *Circulation, 132,* S519–S525.

Caglar, D., & Quan, L. (2016). Drowning and submersion injury. In R. Kliegman, B. Stanton, J. St. Geme, et al. (Eds.), *Nelson textbook of pediatrics* (20th ed., pp. 561–568). Philadelphia: Elsevier.

Centers for Disease Control and Prevention. (2012a). *CDC childhood injury report.* Retrieved from http://www.cdc.gov/safechild/ChildInjuryData.html.

Centers for Disease Control and Prevention. (2012b). *Low level lead exposure harms children: A renewed call for primary prevention. Report of the advisory committee on childhood lead poisoning.* Retrieved from http://www.cdc.gov/nceh/lead/ACCLPP/Final_Document_030712.pdf.

Centers for Disease Control and Prevention. (2014). *Unintentional drowning: get the facts.* Retrieved from http://www.cdc.gov/HomeandRecreationalSafety/Water-Safety/waterinjuries-factsheet.html.

Centers for Disease Control and Prevention. (2015). *Preventing dog bites.* Retrieved from http://www.cdc.gov/features/dog-bite-prevention/index.html.

Centers for Disease Control and Prevention. (2016a). *Recommended immunization schedule for persons aged 0 through 18 years.* Retrieved from http://www.cdc.gov/vaccines/schedules/hcp/imz/child-adolescent.html.

Centers for Disease Control and Prevention. (2016b). *Traumatic brain injury in the united states: assessing outcomes in children.* Retrieved from http://www.cdc.gov/traumaticbraininjury/assessing_outcomes_in_children.html#3.

de Caen, A.R., Berg, M.D., Chameides, L., et al. (2015a). Part 12: Pediatric Advanced Life Support 2015 American Heart Association Guidelines Update for Cardiopulmonary Resuscitation and Emergency Cardiovascular Care. *Circulation, 132*(2), S526–S542. doi:10.1161/CIR.0000000000000266.

deCaen, A., Machonochie, I., Aickin, R., et al. (2015b). Part 6: Pediatric Basic Life Support and Pediatric Advanced Life Support: 2015 International Consensus on Cardiopulmonary Resuscitation and Emergency Cardiovascular Care Science with Treatment Recommendations. *Circulation, 132*(1), S177–S203.

Dubowitz, H., & Lane, W.G. (2016). Abused and neglected children. In R. Kliegman, B. Stanton, J. St. Geme, et al. (Eds.), *Nelson textbook of pediatrics* (20th ed., pp. 236–249). Philadelphia: Elsevier.

Durbin, D. (2011). Policy statement from the American academy of pediatrics, committee on injury, violence, and poison prevention: child passenger safety. *Pediatrics, 127*(4), 788–793.

Emergency Nurses Association. (2012). *Emergency nursing pediatric course provider manual* (4th ed.). Des Plains, IL: Author.

Eppich, W. (2015). "Speaking up" for patient safety in the pediatric emergency department. *Clinical Pediatric Emergency Medicine, 16*(2), 83–89.

Goyal, M.K. (2015). Communicating with the adolescent: consent and confidentiality issues. *Clinical Pediatric Emergency Medicine, 16*(2), 96–101.

Hagen, J.F., & Duncan, P.M. (2016). Maximizing children's health: screening, anticipatory guidance, and counseling. In R. Kliegman, B. Stanton, J. St. Geme, et al. (Eds.), *Nelson Textbook of Pediatrics* (20th ed., pp. 37–47). Philadelphia: Elsevier.

Hartman, M., & Cheifetz, I. (2016). Pediatric emergencies and resuscitation. In R. Kliegman, B. Stanton, J. St. Geme, et al. (Eds.), *Nelson textbook of pediatrics* (20th ed., pp. 489–506). Philadelphia: Elsevier.

Is capnography used by ED nurses? It may give life-saving information. (2011, December). *ED Nursing, 15*(3), 13–15.

Kindelberger, J., Chidester, A., & Ferguson, E. (2012). *Air bag crash investigations: National Highway Traffic Safety Administration.* Retrieved from http://www.nhtsa.gov/DOT/NHTSA/NRD/Articles/ESV/PDF/18/Files/18ESV-000299.pdf.

Kostic, M.A. (2016). Poisoning. In R. Kliegman, B. Stanton, J. St. Geme, et al. (Eds.), *Nelson textbook of pediatrics* (20th ed., pp. 447–467). Philadelphia: Elsevier.

Landry, G. (2016). Heat injuries. In R. Kliegman, B. Stanton, J. St. Geme, et al. (Eds.), *Nelson textbook of pediatrics* (20th ed., pp. 3354–3355). Philadelphia: Elsevier.

Monitoring ETCO2 may mean fewer treatments. (2011, December). *ED Nursing, 15*(3), 15.

Mowry, J., Spyker, D., Brooks, D., et al. (2014). 2014 Annual report of the American association of poison control centers' national poison data system: 32nd annual report. *Clinical Toxicology, 53*:10, 962–1147.

National Center for Environmental Health. (2013). *Lead.* Retrieved from http://www.cdc.gov/nceh/lead/default.htm.

National Highway Traffic Safety Administration. (2012). *Air bag safety.* Retrieved from http://www.safercar.gov/Air+Bags.

Roskind, C.G., Dayan, P.S., & Klein, B.L. (2016). Acute care of the victim of multiple trauma. In R. Kliegman, B. Stanton, J. St. Geme, et al. (Eds.), *Nelson textbook of pediatrics* (20th ed., pp. 545–553). Philadelphia: Elsevier.

Safe Kids Worldwide. (2016). *Drowning prevention fact sheet.* Retrieved from http://www.safekids.org/our-work/research/fact-sheets/drowning-prevention-fact-sheet.html.

Sastic, C. (2014). Appropriate Assessment of Patient Medication Allergies. *Hospital Pharmacy, 49*(4), 322–323.

Sauber-Schatz, E., Thomas, A., & Cook. L. (2015). Motor vehicle crashes, medical outcomes, and hospital charges among children 1-12 years – crash outcome data evaluation system, 11 states, 2005-2008. Retrieved from *MMWR: Morbidity and Mortality Weekly Report,*

*64*(SS08), 1–32, Retrieved from http://www.cdc.gov/mmwr/preview/mmwrhtml/ss6408a1.htm?s_cid=ss6408a1_w.

Schinasi, D.A., Kolaitis, I.N., & Nadel, F. (2015). Difficult conversions in the emergency department: spotlight on the disclosure of medical errors. *Clinical Pediatric Emergency Medicine*, *16*(2), 90–94.

Schroeder, B., & Norris, R. (2016). Envenomations. In R. Kliegman, B. Stanton, J. St. Geme, et al. (Eds.), *Nelson textbook of pediatrics* (20th ed., pp. 3452–3459). Philadelphia: Elsevier.

Schroeder, J.W., & Holinger, L.D. (2016). Foreign bodies in the airway. In R. Kliegman, B. Stanton, J. St. Geme, et al. (Eds.)., *Nelson textbook of pediatrics* (20th ed., pp. 2039–2041). Philadelphia: Elsevier.

Sharpe, S.J., Rochette, L.M., & Smith, G.A. (2012). Pediatric battery-related emergency department visits in the United States, 1990-2009. *Pediatric*, *129*(6), 1111–1117. doi:10.1542/peds.2011-0012.

Tinaoff, N. (2016). Dental Trauma. In R. Kliegman, B. Stanton, J. St. Geme, et al. (Eds.), *Nelson textbook of pediatrics* (20th ed., pp. 1776–1778). Philadelphia: Elsevier.

Turner, D., & Cheifetz, I. (2016). Shock. In R. Kliegman, B. Stanton, J. St. Geme, et al. (Eds.). *Nelson textbook of pediatrics* (20th ed., pp. 516–528). Philadelphia: Elsevier.

Wood, J.N., Fakeye, O., Mondestin, V., et al. (2015). Development of hospital-based guidelines for skeletal survey in young children with bruises. *Pediatrics*, *135*(2), e312–e320. doi:10.1542/peds.2014–2169.

Young, K.D. (2014). Observed study of family member presence for pediatric emergency department procedures. *Pediatric Emergency Care*, *30*(7), 449–452.

35

# The Ill Child in the Hospital and Other Care Settings

http://evolve.elsevier.com/McKinney/mat-ch/

## LEARNING OBJECTIVES

*After studying this chapter, you should be able to:*

- Discuss the nurse's role in various settings where care is given to ill children.
- List common stressors affecting hospitalized children.
- Describe the child's response to illness.
- Discuss the stages of separation anxiety.
- Describe the factors that affect children's responses to hospitalization and treatment.
- Discuss the psychological responses of families to the illness of a child in the family.

Because of current trends in healthcare management, the care of ill children continues to shift from the traditional acute-care hospital setting to community-based settings and the home. Hospitalized children are more acutely ill than in the past, and their stays are shorter. In addition, the hospitalized child is more likely to have a chronic or terminal disease or to have special needs that require specialized care. These changes do not mean that the need for pediatric nurses has diminished; their role is ever changing and expanding. Pediatric nurses will continue to care for children in hospitals, schools, clinics, and homes.

All children experience some form of illness at some time. The ways in which stressors and developmental needs are addressed are important factors in resolving the immediate crisis and in dealing with future illnesses. The nurse is often the first person the child sees when the child enters the healthcare system, and the nurse spends more time with an ill child than does any other healthcare provider. Therefore, the nurse has a unique opportunity to influence that child's physical and emotional health.

## SETTINGS OF CARE

### The Hospital

Entering the hospital is somewhat like visiting a foreign country. The language, culture, activities, and expectations may be unfamiliar to the child and the family. The nurse acts as a coordinator and provides a safe environment, both physically and emotionally. Being the coordinator includes activities as diverse as explaining the jargon (e.g., NPO, IV, "vitals"), explaining procedures that are often painful, and facilitating the parents' access to hospital resources, such as social services, case managers, child life specialists, spiritual counselors, and ethics specialists. Above all, the nurse must educate the child and family about the disease process, its treatment, hospital procedures, and discharge issues.

Hospitalizations can be categorized according to length of stay, planned or unplanned admission, surgical or medical intervention, and outpatient (day) or inpatient status. Although they overlap, these categories provide a framework for examining the child's experience.

Another variable is the type of facility. Children may be hospitalized in a pediatric hospital, on a pediatric unit within a general hospital, or in a general hospital that occasionally admits children. Pediatric units within a general hospital or hospitals that do not have a specific pediatric unit may not have as many child-oriented services as does a pediatric hospital. Special play areas and child-size equipment and fixtures are often not available in general hospitals. Also, staff members who do not care for children routinely may feel less comfortable in the relevant roles.

The nurse in this situation is aware of these challenges and can provide support for the child and the family. Examples include taking extra time when the child is admitted to explain routines and procedures and placing the child in a room close to the nurses' station. This support might include moving a cot into the room for the parent and ordering special foods for the child. Ultimately, providing support means being sensitive to the needs of the child and the family.

### Pediatric Observation Units or 24-Hour Observation

Many children with acute illnesses become ill quickly and recover quickly. The number of patients who stay one night or less has increased to 30% of all pediatric hospital stays (AAP, 2012). For this reason, they may need acute-care for a short time, as in cases of dehydration or acute asthma. At the end of 24 hours, the child is evaluated to determine whether further hospitalization is needed or discharge with home care instructions is appropriate. Some hospitals have designated special areas or units to care for patients. Benefits include reduced admissions in in-patient units and reduced crowding in emergency care units (AAP, 2012).

The nurse must prepare the child and family for discharge and assess the parents' ability to care for the child at home. Instructions should be written in the language the parent can read, and the parent should be encouraged to ask questions. The nurse informs the parent about when to notify the primary healthcare provider in the event that the child's condition worsens. An awareness of cultural and language differences enhances the nurse's ability to assess the child's and family's educational needs and to develop an individualized teaching plan. For example, is the parent smiling because of contentment, or is the parent embarrassed to ask a question? Are parents nodding because they understand or are they too embarrassed to say they cannot understand English or cannot read? Many children's hospital units have a policy of contacting caregivers 1 to 2 days after the child is discharged, especially if the child left the facility after a 24-hour stay. Arrangements are made with the parent for a convenient time to be contacted. This policy allows the nurse to check on the child's condition and reinforce discharge teaching.

### Emergency Hospitalization

An emergency admission can be distressing, as there is little time for the child and family to prepare. The admission can be the result of traumatic injury or acute illness. The family may arrive at the hospital with little money, clothing, or other resources. Siblings may also be present, competing with the sick child for the parent's attention. In addition to caring for the sick child, the staff may be called on to help meet the family's basic needs for food, clothing, and a place to stay. A social service referral is appropriate in such situations.

Because of the intense level of activity in emergency departments, care of the family is often overlooked. The family may fear that the child will die or be permanently disabled. Although nurses see many similar situations each day in which children do well, they must be sensitive to the family's fears, keep the family informed of the child's condition and care, and encourage a family member to stay with the child.

The time for preparing a child is usually limited in emergencies. Nurses must seize every opportunity to prepare children for the care they will receive. Holding and touching the child, talking softly, distracting the child, and involving the child in the procedure are methods of support used in emergencies. After the child is stable, the nurse returns and uses therapeutic communication to talk about the event. A child life specialist may also help the child express feelings. The use of dolls, puppets, and hospital equipment can aid children in communicating their feelings. (Chapter 34 provides more detailed information about caring for children and their families in an emergency setting.)

A 7-year-old boy was admitted to the general pediatrics unit after spending several hours in the emergency department because of acute asthma. Although his mother brought him to the hospital, she had his younger brother and sister with her and could not stay with him in the room. The boy remained quiet, but the nurse noticed that he watched every move she made. In such a case, the nurse might say, "Some kids say it's scary to come to the hospital and especially to be in the emergency room, with the bright lights and everyone rushing around. If you'd like, I can spend a little time with you and we can talk about being in the hospital."

### Outpatient and Day Facilities

Outpatient facilities have evolved in an effort to keep children out of the hospital unless absolutely necessary. The outpatient facility may be part of a hospital, or it may be free standing. The child arrives in the morning, undergoes a procedure, test, or surgery, and goes home by the evening. Common procedures performed during such admissions include tympanostomy tube placement, hernia repair, tonsillectomy, cystoscopy, and bronchoscopy.

This mode of care has three main advantages: (1) it minimizes separation of the child from the family, (2) it decreases the risk of infection, and (3) it reduces cost. A disadvantage is that outpatient facilities that are not connected to a hospital may not be equipped for overnight stays. If complications develop that require continued observation and treatment, the child may have to be transferred to a hospital.

Although the procedure may be short, teaching the child and the parent is as important as in the acute-care setting. When possible, a tour of the facility before the procedure can decrease fear of the unknown. Parents have indicated that although they like the idea of outpatient care, taking a child home afterward can be frightening.

Assessing the parent can assist the nurse in deciding whether the parent is capable of managing the child's care at home or whether home healthcare is needed. Written instructions specific to the child and procedure are helpful and reassuring. At the very least, a follow-up phone call to the home should be required. Parents must also be encouraged to call the facility if they have any concerns, and they should be given other resources to contact after the facility closes. Families who live far from the healthcare facility may want to spend the night at a nearby hotel or consider an overnight admission.

### Rehabilitative Care

After a serious illness or trauma, a child's ability to function sometimes changes. After the acute situation has resolved, the child may be admitted to a rehabilitation hospital. Staff members from nursing, medicine, physical therapy, occupational therapy, and other areas collaborate to develop a treatment plan by which the child, family, and health professionals work to help the child regain previous abilities. Children with neurologic injuries, such as head injuries, or children with serious burns may thrive in this environment, which usually resembles a home setting with facilities available for the child to relearn activities of daily living.

Nurses in rehabilitative settings must balance nurturing and firm discipline as they help children reclaim independence. Parents often need encouragement and support because they are torn between "doing for" their child and watching the child struggle to function independently. Overprotection is a common reaction, and parents can be assisted in understanding the child's developmental need to master the environment. The focus should be on what the child can do rather than on the child's limitations.

### The Medical-Surgical Unit

Children admitted to the hospital are usually acutely ill or have a chronic disease or disability that requires frequent, often long-term hospitalizations. (Care of the child with a chronic disease is discussed in Chapter 36.) The average length of hospital stay for the acutely ill child has shortened significantly, and the need for teaching has increased in proportion.

Preparation for a planned hospitalization is essential. Some hospitals provide an opportunity for the child to visit the hospital before admission, and many pediatric hospitals host preoperative tours or classes to introduce children to the strange sights and sounds they will experience during surgery. Literature is available from public libraries and hospital sources. Videos are sometimes available for family members to view together and then discuss. Parents should encourage the child to talk about the hospitalization and answer questions honestly.

Two concepts that are increasingly used in the hospital setting are family-centered care and shared decision making. In the 1960s Bolwby and Robertson described the negative consequences of hospitalization on the child and family. Subsequently, much research has focused on the effects of hospitalization on children. The goal of family-centered care is to become more knowledgeable and assume increased care of the child with the assistance of the nurse who must determine the level of involvement that the parent chooses to assume (Mikkelsen & Frederiksen, 2011).

### The Intensive Care Unit

When a child is admitted to the intensive care unit, both the child and the family can experience increased stress related to factors such as the seriousness of the admitting diagnosis, the rapid onset of the illness, and the high-technology, unfamiliar environment. In addition, the child often is experiencing pain, uncomfortable procedures, noise, and constant lighting. In many instances, the child cannot eat or talk. Meanwhile, the parents are experiencing a parent's worst fear—the possible loss of a child.

The child and family need intense emotional support. All the normal responses to hospitalization are magnified and need to be assessed. When possible, planned admissions to the intensive care unit (e.g., for cardiac surgery) should be preceded by visits to the unit or special classes that provide information about procedures and operations at a level the child can understand.

The parent should be encouraged to remain with the child and be kept informed of the child's condition (Fig. 35.1). Procedures, equipment, and treatments should be explained, in appropriate language, to both the child and the parent. If the parent leaves and the child's condition changes or a new tube or piece of equipment has been added, the nurse should prepare the parent for the change before the parent sees the child. Nurses need to encourage parents to provide care and to touch their child as much as possible. The nurse's active listening is essential.

Siblings of the seriously ill, hospitalized child can easily be overlooked. Siblings may need to talk, to be comforted, or to have the hospital experience explained to them. Parents can feel pulled between the ill child and the rest of the family. Family members often want to help but do not know what to do. Suggesting that a grandparent or other relative relieve a parent so that the parent has time with the ill child's sibling can help both the parent and the child. Supporting parents by discussing options can relieve stress and may lead to solutions. Inclusion of family members in the provision of care, such as bathing and feeding, is important to both the family members and the child.

Recent research determined that family conferences in the pediatric intensive care settings are vital in facilitating communication with patients and their families (Michelson et al., 2013). Family conferences involve sharing information about the patient, discussing the treatment plan, and identifying family values and perspectives. Difficult medical decisions can be made with ample time for questions and answers, especially when discussing difficult end of life care decisions (Michelson et al., 2013).

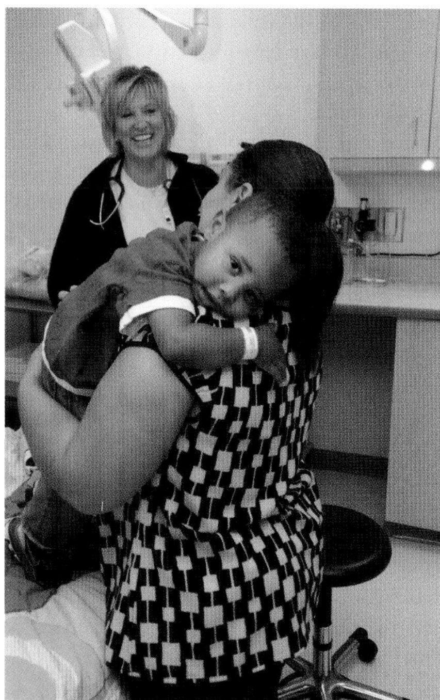

FIG 35.1 Parents are encouraged to stay with their child whenever possible. This mother is holding her child in the postanesthesia recovery room, a setting that in the past was off limits to parents. (Courtesy St. Louis Children's Hospital, St. Louis, MO.)

## School-Based Clinics

The traditional areas of school health nursing that are still prevalent in many school systems include the following:

- *Health screening:* Vision, hearing, and growth checks can provide information about problems that may affect a child's ability to learn. When problems are identified, referral and follow-up services are provided.
- *Emergency care:* School nurses are the first to provide care for children experiencing an unintentional injury, both on the playground and in the school building. Excellent assessment skills are necessary to determine the need for healthcare provider visits or emergency care.
- *Communicable disease management:* The nurse must assess children for illnesses that can be transmitted to other children, provide care and isolation until the parent can pick up the child from school, and give advice concerning the safe time for re-entry into the school setting.
- *Healthcare advice:* The school nurse can be a source of referral for families in need of services.
- *Provision of specialized care for children with chronic health needs:* School attendance by children with many healthcare needs, including catheterization, gastric tube feedings, and suctioning, requires variation in the school nurse role to provide or supervise these specialized services.

School-based clinics have been part of healthcare for more than 25 years, but with the recent changes in healthcare delivery, this setting is now a site for expanding primary care. The Patient Protection and Affordable Care Act of 2010 included provisions to expand school-based clinics across the United States (Parasuraman & Shi, 2014). School-based clinics play an important role in providing care for children in remote rural communities and in underserved inner-city areas and are key to improving student health by implementing policies and practices to reduce health-risk behaviors (Brener, Wechsler, & McManus, 2013). School nurses, nurse practitioners, physicians, social workers, and other healthcare providers typically staff these clinics. This area of practice will continue to grow, and many believe that school-based clinics are the perfect setting for providing primary care for selected groups of children and adolescents; they are well situated to influence the health and well-being of underserved or disadvantaged students and can have a profound impact on health outcomes later in life (Parasuraman & Shi, 2014).

Prevention remains the focus of school-based care as children learn healthy habits to prevent development of acute problems. Nurses identify children who need immunizations and provide immunizations when necessary. Screening that once required referral can often be handled on-site. Through school-based clinics, children can receive medical services in a timely manner and avoid expensive emergency visits. For example, a child with an earache at school can be seen on-site, treated, and sent home, if warranted. The child's adherence to treatment can be monitored and a follow-up visit scheduled to determine whether treatment has been effective.

Nurses in school-based clinics must be sensitive to parental concerns about certain topics in healthcare, especially areas related to sexuality (e.g., birth control, sexually transmitted diseases, abortion). Community involvement and support can dispel concerns and assist in setting guidelines for such clinics. School-based clinic nurses must also be team members who act in collaboration with other healthcare providers and have a strong background in preventive healthcare and the ability to think critically.

The school-based clinic provides a setting for parental education in preventive healthcare, growth and development, anticipatory guidance, parenting skills, and care of acutely and chronically ill children. The nurse respects the rights and wishes of the parents, but respecting parents' wishes can be a challenge when the value systems of the healthcare provider and the parent differ. The pediatric nurse is a child advocate but must exercise caution unless the child is being harmed. (Child abuse is discussed in Chapter 53.)

The school nurse is an integral part of the health education program addressing both health and educational goals for school children. A comprehensive health education program is an important part of the curriculum in most school systems, for children in kindergarten through high school (AAP Healthy Children, 2010). The goals for this program are to increase students' health knowledge, generate positive attitudes toward health maintenance, and encourage healthy behaviors. To achieve these goals, active participation by students and involvement of parents are essential. Topics addressed include nutrition, disease prevention, physical growth and development, reproduction, mental health, drug and alcohol abuse prevention, consumer health, and safety (crossing streets, riding bikes, first aid, the Heimlich maneuver) (AAP Healthy Children, 2010).

Evidence supports the concept of school-based mental health services to assist students' social-emotional health and to improve academic functioning. The benefit of this service is improved access to care, improved coordination of care, and interventions and prevention strategies to improve overall health (Ballard, Sander & Klimes-Dougan, 2014).

## Community Clinics

Community health clinics provide primary care for children and their families. In these settings, nurses, nurse practitioners, and physicians provide both case management of illness and health promotion. Community-based care is a very important way to address population health in a culturally sensitive manner. Community-based health promotion focuses on the health and education of the community where community members are empowered to promote community health and safety (Shannon, 2014). Support services and groups (e.g., social services, a dental clinic, daycare) can be made available in the same center, and referrals to medical specialists and other healthcare providers are also available.

Although many children seen at community health clinics are ill, nurses must use the opportunity to obtain a health history, determine if immunizations are up to date, and assess nutritional status, growth, and development. Needs for anticipatory guidance and education are evaluated as well. If the child is ill at the time of the visit, the nurse can set an appointment for the child to return for immunizations or other care that cannot be given when the child is ill (see http://www.cdc.gov/vaccines/recs/schedules/child-schedule.htm).

In some urban areas, nurses are involved in primary prevention and offer information and education about childhood immunization, the signs and symptoms of childhood illnesses, injury prevention, and parenting skills (Fig. 35.2). The Institute of Medicine (2010) recommends that nurses be exposed to these areas of care in their education to help them fully understand the impact on public health (Shannon, 2014).

## Home Care

Pediatric home care is the provision of skilled care within the child's home. Nurses in this setting are part of a multidisciplinary team that often comprises physicians, respiratory therapists, physical therapists, speech therapists, occupational therapists, and social workers. Children cared for at home include those receiving respiratory therapy, having dressing changes, receiving total parenteral nutrition, or needing skilled care because of a chronic illness or an injury.

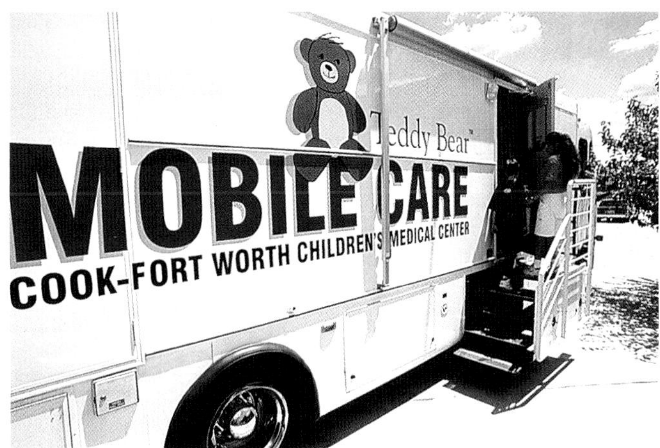


**FIG 35.2** Nurses today help take healthcare on the road to provide services to those who otherwise might not obtain them. This mobile van is stationed at a public school, where it offers health screenings and prevention services to children. (Courtesy Cook Children's Medical Center, Fort Worth, TX.)

Nurses who work in home care should have previous hospital experience in their practice area. The nurse must be able to make independent decisions and think critically and should have good clinical, documentation, communication, and teaching skills. To meet the needs of each child and family, the nurse must understand multiple cultures and socioeconomic backgrounds.

Although the separation of the child from the family is not a problem in home healthcare, the child may display many other effects of illness, such as fear of the unknown, loss of control, anger, guilt, and regression. In addition, care is taking place in the family's domain, and the nurse is a guest in the home. Family members may have to adjust to unfamiliar noises and equipment, such as special beds, ventilators, and intravenous (IV) pumps, in their home. They may feel that they have lost their privacy and cannot "be themselves" because someone outside the family is frequently present. Awareness of siblings' needs is also a nursing goal in this setting.

The nurse's role as a teacher is especially important because many tasks that the nurse might perform in the hospital are delegated to the family, with the nurse monitoring the care. In this case, the nurse acts as a case manager and coordinator of care.

With regards to coordinating the medical care of a child, a medical home is a model of care consisting of increased accessibility and family centeredness that results in favorable outcomes such as decreased emergency department use and hospitalization rates. The medical home provides continuity of care in a compassionate and culturally sensitive way that enhances the patients and families experience with the healthcare setting (Hadland & Long, 2014).

# STRESSORS ASSOCIATED WITH ILLNESS AND HOSPITALIZATION

Age, cognitive development, preparation, coping skills, and culture influence a child's reaction to illness. Previous experience with the healthcare system and the parent's reaction to the illness also affect the child.

Each child is unique, so predicting reactions to an illness is often difficult. In general, hospitalization can create a number of threats or fears for children, which fall into five main categories: (1) bodily injury and pain, (2) separation from parents, (3) fear of the unknown, (4) uncertainty about limits and expected behaviors, and (5) loss of control and autonomy (Visintainer & Wolfer, 1975). Educating parents about what to expect when their child is hospitalized and supporting their participation in their child's care decreases parental stress and enables them to better facilitate their child's adjustment.

**! NURSING QUALITY ALERT**

***Children's Responses to Illness***

- Fear of the unknown
- Separation anxiety
- Fear of pain or mutilation
- Loss of control
- Anger
- Guilt
- Regression

Nurses can help decrease stress for patients and their families by implementing interventions and supporting parents, whose stress can impair their ability to care for their child. One way to identify parental stress is to administer assessment tools such as the Parental Stressor Scale developed by Carter, Miles, Buford, et al. (1985). Higher parental stress levels were identified for unexpected hospitalizations, observing a painful procedure, and the altered behavior of their child (Agazio & Buckley, 2012). Interventions to decrease parental distress will result in improved ability to provide emotional support and care for their child (Agazio & Buckley, 2012).

Although preschoolers and young school-age children experience separation anxiety, it is most significant in infants and toddlers, especially those aged 6 to 30 months. In times of stress, anxiety related to separation increases.

Each age-group has its own fears related to pain and injury. The past decade has seen an expansion of knowledge about pain and its treatment, negating many erroneous beliefs about children and pain. Children quickly learn to associate healthcare activities and professionals with pain and injury. The fear is usually focused on injections ("shots"). (Chapter 39 discusses issues related to pain.)

Although specific fears are related to the child's age, hospitalization puts all children at high risk for fears related to their unfamiliarity with the people, surroundings, and events. The child has not developed trust in the healthcare provider, and thus, does not know what to expect. The child may have fear of real or imagined threats. Will the nurse know when I am hungry or hurting? Will the nurse hurt me?

Medical fears are prevalent and often increase with age. Children commonly fear needles, which can increase perceived pain (McMurtry, Noel, Chambers, et al., 2011). Nurses must provide appropriate interventions based on their assessment of the child's emotional understanding and cognitive status (McMurtry et al., 2011).

## The Infant and Toddler

### Separation Anxiety

Infants and toddlers, especially those between 6 and 30 months of age, often experience separation anxiety. Separation is this age-group's major stressor, and it is traumatic to both the child and the parent. The child passes through several stages in reaction to the separation: protest, despair, and detachment (Box 35.1).

In the initial phase, known as protest, the child demonstrates distress by crying and rejecting anyone other than the parents (Fig. 35.3). The child appears angry and upset. During the despair phase, the child feels hopeless and becomes quiet and withdrawn. Crying decreases and

**BOX 35.1 Stages of Separation**

- Protest: Child is agitated, resists caregivers, cries, and is inconsolable.
- Despair: Child feels hopeless and becomes quiet, withdrawn, and apathetic.
- Detachment: Child becomes interested in the environment, plays, and seems to form relationships with caregivers and other children. If parents reappear, the child might ignore them.

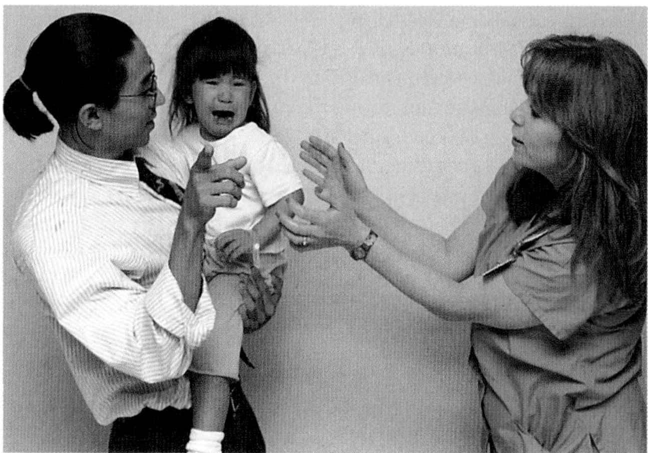

A toddler exhibits separation anxiety by reacting with protest to leaving her parent's arms.

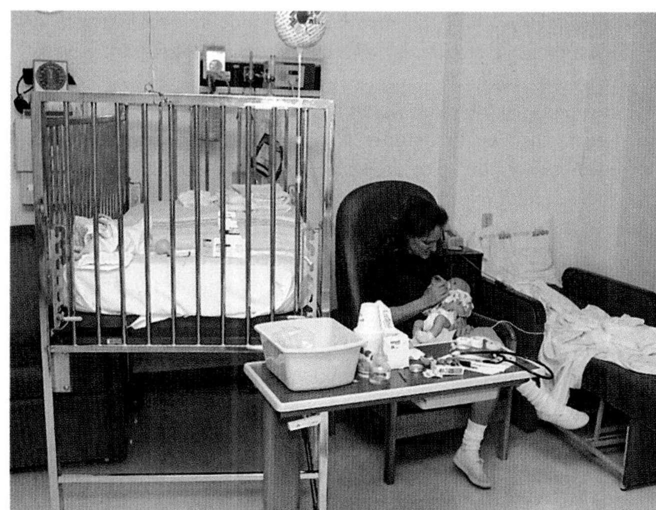

Rooming-in reduces the stress of hospitalization and provides opportunities for parent teaching.

**FIG 35.3** Separation is one of the stressors of hospitalization that affects both child and parent. (Courtesy T.C. Thompson Children's Hospital, Chattanooga, TN.)

the child becomes apathetic. If separation from the parent continues, the child enters the detachment phase. During this phase, the child again becomes interested in the environment and begins to play. Nurses may misinterpret this phase as a positive sign that the child has adjusted to the hospitalization. In reality, the child has "given up." If the parents return during this stage, the child may ignore them, and the parents may think that the child does not want to see them. However, this reaction is a coping mechanism to protect the child from further emotional pain related to the separation.

Nurses in acute-care settings see the first two stages of separation—protest and despair—much more frequently than the final stage, detachment, which is more common in long-term separations. Parents may misunderstand their child's behavior. They may even perceive the child's reaction as a behavior problem. Nurses need to reassure parents that this reaction is a normal response to separation and that most children will not have any permanent effects from the event. As understanding of separation anxiety has evolved, visiting times for hospitalized pediatric patients have changed from structured hours to more flexible rooming-in situations (see Fig. 35.3).

Most practitioners believe that if separation can be avoided, the child will be much more resilient during hospitalization. Infants and toddlers go through the stages of separation. For this age-group, the older the child, the more elaborate the child's protests. The child not only cries but also may cling to the parent, kick, and generally create a scene. Parents need to understand that this behavior is a sign of healthy parent-child attachment. The toddler may resist bedtime and eating and have temper tantrums more frequently than normal for this age. Regression may occur in toileting and eating. Nurses need to explain to parents that regression is normal and to encourage parents to reinforce appropriate behavior while allowing the regressive behavior to occur.

A parent might ask whether someone from the family needs to be with a hospitalized toddler all the time and may be especially concerned because the parents work and have other children. The nurse responds, "We encourage parents to stay with their children when they are in the hospital. However, if you have to leave, we will spend time with your child and check on your child frequently. You may call us at any time, day or night. When you return, perhaps you could bring a favorite toy or stuffed animal and something that reminds the child of you. A picture or a piece of clothing [transition object] will make your child feel more secure because it is familiar."

### Fear of Injury and Pain

Previous experiences, separation from parents, restraint, and preparation affect the reaction of infants and toddlers to pain and bodily injury. The young child views injury and pain concretely. Nurses who have worked with toddlers know that most toddlers react to any intrusive procedure, whether it is painful or not. (See Chapter 39 for a more extensive discussion of pain in infants and toddlers.)

### Loss of Control

According to Erikson (1963), the major task of the toddler is to develop autonomy. Control is a major issue with this age-group. The toddler experiences the environment through all the senses and loves to explore the environment. At the same time, toddlers need sameness (rituals, routines). Because of the changes in growth and development taking place in the toddler, familiar rituals and routines (e.g., those for eating, sleeping, playing) provide reassurance and stability.

Hospitalization, which has its own set of rituals and routines, can severely disrupt the toddler's life. The child may be confined to a crib, and the crib may have a cover over it. Because of safety issues, the child is not allowed to run in the halls. If the parents are unable to be with the child, the way the child is put to bed or bathed may be unfamiliar. Information obtained from parents about routines for feeding, going to bed, and playing can assist the nurse in maintaining usual and comforting routines. When children are unable to do things themselves, their sense of control and autonomy is weakened. They are frustrated and may have temper tantrums. Choices, even simple ones, can return some control to the child.

The child's sense of lack of control is often exhibited in behaviors related to feeding, toileting, playing, and bedtime. The nurse should remember that each of these activities may have associated rituals and routines and that the child may also show some regression in these areas.

## The Preschooler

### Separation Anxiety

Separation anxiety occurs among preschoolers, but it is generally less obvious and less serious than in the toddler. Although the preschooler may already be spending some time away from parents at a daycare center or preschool, illness adds a stressor that makes separation more difficult. Young children have a good recall of their medical experiences, so nurses must help to make their healthcare experiences positive by allowing children an outlet for their feelings and stress (Nabors et al., 2013).

The preschooler expresses the same protest as the toddler but tends to be less direct. The nurse may find a preschooler quietly crying because the parents have told the child to "act like a big boy (girl)." Children of this age may refuse to eat or take medications, and can be generally uncooperative. They may repeatedly ask when their parents will be coming for a visit; with access to a phone, the child might constantly call the parents. All these behaviors are signs that the child is having difficulty coping with the situation.

### Fear of Injury and Pain

The preschooler fears mutilation. The child who must have surgery affecting a limb or other body part feels greater fear. The preschooler generally does not understand body integrity. Children of this age report a predominant fear of pain and procedures that may cause pain such as injections (shots) and the drawing of blood (McMurtry et al, 2011). Procedures that could be painful should be performed in the treatment room so children see their hospital rooms as safe places. Because of their literal interpretation of words, they often imagine treatments to be much worse than they are. A child's imagination can become extremely active during illness. The preschooler may believe that the illness occurred because of some personal deed or thought or perhaps because the child touched something or someone. (The preschooler's specific reactions to pain are discussed further in Chapter 39.)

**! NURSING QUALITY ALERT**

***Maintaining a Safe Place***

A designated safe area can enhance the child's security. For example, intrusive procedures that can cause discomfort or anxiety might better be done in the treatment room rather than the child's room. The playroom should also be a place for playing, not treatments or administration of medications. Nurses should consider the child's age, developmental level, coping skills, and parent/child preference when deciding where to perform procedures that may be painful or distressing.

Adapted from Fanurick, D., Schmitz, M., Martin, G., et al. (2000). Hospital room or treatment room: Where should inpatient pediatric procedures be performed? *Children's Health Care, 29*, 103–111.

### Loss of Control

The preschooler has attained a good deal of independence in self-care and has been given more independence at home, preschool, or daycare. Some children expect to maintain their independence in the hospital. For example, the preschooler may like to wander about the unit and is not happy when restricted to the bed or room. Like the toddler, a preschooler likes familiar routines and rituals and can show some regression if not allowed to maintain some areas of control.

One 5-year-old boy refused to have his dressing changed by the nurse who had cared for him the previous day. She reported that he cried, pulled up the covers, and said that she was "mean." This behavior was unusual for him, and the nurse suspected that he had been told to do too many things and had not been given choices. In response, the nurse might say, "I know there have been many changes for you since you came to the hospital. Today, we are going to decide together what is going to happen. I see you have chosen a video to watch. Would you like me to change your dressing before you watch the video or after?" This approach gives the preschooler a choice and some control while maintaining boundaries.

### Guilt and Shame

Because their thinking is egocentric and magical, preschoolers may believe that their illness is somehow related to a thought or deed. This belief can lead to feelings of guilt, shame, and increased stress at a time when the child has to cope with several other stressors. Because the child typically does not share these feelings with adults, parents and caregivers must be aware of the possibility of guilt and shame in this age-group.

The nurse's role is to assess the child for this type of thinking and, through therapeutic communication, assist the child in identifying unfounded fears and beliefs. The child might be able to relate perceptions of what is happening. The use of puppets, dolls, and drawings can help children deal with their feelings. A tremendous decrease in anxiety can result when the nurse helps the child identify a perceived punishment and then reassures the child that nothing the child did could cause the illness.

## The School-Age Child

### Separation

The school-age child is accustomed to periods of separation from parents, but, as with the preschooler, the separation becomes more difficult as stressors are added. The younger school-age child may already have been feeling separation anxiety related to starting school.

Older children may be more concerned with missing school and the fear that their friends will forget them. However, the unfamiliar environment coupled with the regression seen in ill children increase the likelihood that some separation anxiety will take place.

### Fear of Injury and Pain

The school-age child is concerned with body disability and death. The child is more relaxed about having a physical examination or having the eyes or an ear examined but is uncomfortable with any type of genital examination. School-age children want to know the reasons for procedures and tests, and they ask relevant questions about their illness. Because they can understand cause and effect, they can relate actions to becoming ill. Their parents may tell them that if they do not get enough rest, wear warm clothes, or eat nutritious meals, they will get a cold. If they become ill, they associate their actions with the disease. (For further discussion of pain in the school-age child, see Chapter 39.)

### Loss of Control

School-age children are "movers and shakers." They control their self-care and typically are highly social. They like being involved, and most fill their days with activities. Illness can change all these patterns. If children of this age have physical limitations, they can feel helpless and dependent (Fig. 35.4). Anxiety in response to loss of control, environmental changes, and the hospitalization experience can alter the way school-age children appraise both the experience and the amount of resulting stress. School-age children can view the hospital experience as a threat. Children use coping strategies that include sleeping, talking with others, distraction (e.g., television, music, video games), and play. School-age children are better able to deal with the stressors of hospitalization because of their ability to reason and communicate their needs and feelings. They are better able to understand the explanations provided by the healthcare providers. They are often unsatisfied when they are lacking information about their care (Agazio & Buckley, 2012).

Friends are important to children of this age-group, and school-age children may think that their friends will forget them while they are ill. They are also accustomed to making choices about meals and activities. By capitalizing on their abilities and needs, the nurse can encourage children of this age to become involved in their own care. School-age children can select their own menus, assist with some treatments, keep their rooms neat, and visit with other children when it is appropriate for both. With these opportunities for independence, children retain a sense of control, enhance their self-esteem, and continue to work toward achieving a sense of industry.

## The Adolescent

### Separation

Adolescents often are unsure whether they want their parents with them when they are hospitalized. Some enjoy the freedom and the period of independence. Others, in response to the stress of illness, become more dependent and want their parents nearby. A third group cannot decide what they want, and this situation can be frustrating to parents. All of these responses are consistent with normal adolescent growth and development.

Because of the importance of the peer group, separation from friends is a source of anxiety to the adolescent. Ideally, the peer group will support the ill friend. Some adolescents are reluctant to visit friends in the hospital, either because of their own health fears or because the reality of illness in someone their age is difficult for them to handle. Hospitalized adolescents may be upset if their friends simply go on with their lives, excluding them. It is important to provide special activity areas and other opportunities for the adolescent to meet and interact with other hospitalized adolescents (see Fig. 35.4).

### Fear of Injury and Pain

To the adolescent, appearance is crucial. Therefore, an illness or injury that changes an adolescent's self-perception can have a major impact. Even children who have seemingly adjusted to a chronic disease in their earlier years may have difficulty during adolescence simply because they do not want to be different. The adolescent who has diabetes may not want to eat different foods or take time out from an activity for injections. Adolescents do not want attention drawn to them, so they may eat the wrong foods and skip their medication.

Adolescents can also give the impression that they are not afraid, even if they are terrified. Adolescents may think that being "cool" means being in control. They may question everything or appear overly confident. Because of their concern with their bodies, they are guarded when any areas connected with sexual development are examined.

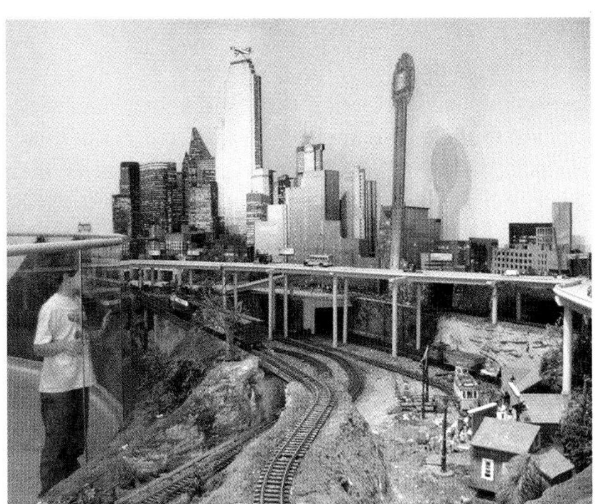

This model railroad "trainscape" in a pediatric hospital provides children and adults with a welcome respite from real-life stresses.

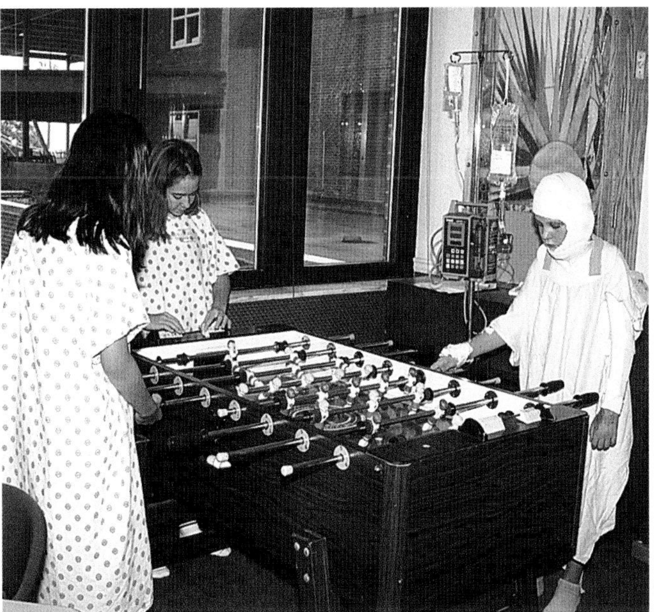

Hospitalized teens need to interact with their peers, as they do when they are well. A lounge area that is separate from the playroom used by younger children fulfills this need.

**FIG 35.4** Activities for the hospitalized child are important for growth and development, stress relief, socialization, and a sense of control. (Courtesy Frolin Marek, Marek Mountain RR, http://www.Frolin.com.)

Nurses need to be sensitive to adolescents' concerns and reassure them that they are normal, if in fact they are. Some adolescents also believe that they are invincible and that nothing can hurt them or cause death. They might take risks and be nonadherent to treatment because they do not see the consequences of their behavior. (Pain management is discussed in Chapter 39.)

### Loss of Control

Control is important to the adolescent. Thus, nurses must understand that many of the challenges they face caring for an ill adolescent stem from control issues. Giving the adolescent some control avoids endless power struggles. Behaviors exhibited in response to loss of control include anger, withdrawal, and general uncooperativeness. Adolescents desire autonomy, social acceptance, and increased self-esteem. Including adolescents in discussions regarding their plan of care helps them take control. Asking about the adolescent's perspective will lead to feelings of involvement and responsibility (Rich, Gonclaves, Guardiani, et al, 2014).

Control issues can cause a major conflict between adolescents and parents. Parents often feel like "ping-pong balls" as they are bounced back and forth by a child who wants help one minute and rejects it the next. Parents who do not understand growth and development can become frustrated and angry over such behavior.

Adolescents may also feel that they are losing control of their social lives as they sit on the sidelines of activities. Time to plan for the separation (e.g., scheduled surgery) allows a greater sense of control than an unplanned hospitalization (e.g., trauma).

### Fear of the Unknown

The sights and sounds of the hospital can be frightening and confusing to children. The child may have many questions, such as: Why are the nurses wearing masks? Why does that alarm keep ringing? Am I dying? Why are they putting tubes in me?

With disruptions in the child's routines and rituals, he or she might wonder what will happen next. Understanding these fears can assist the nurse in structuring care and teaching in a way that avoids unnecessary anxiety.

### Regression

Children may regress in toileting or cry for a bottle although they have been weaned for several months. They might want more attention at bedtime or have temper tantrums. The older child might react to separation by clinging or crying or have fears about shadows on the walls or noises in the halls.

Parents may be overly concerned about regression. They should be told that the child might continue some regressive behaviors at home for a period of time following hospital discharge. The child might need more emotional support while the parent slowly reintroduces the child's normal routines. If the child has regressed in toileting, the parent should wait until the child has returned to a daily routine and then begin the toilet training again. Behavior that is appropriate for the child's age should be reinforced.

The nurse might explain, "I know that you are concerned because your son has been soiling his pants since he has been in the hospital. This is an expected reaction to the stress of being ill and in the hospital. When he returns home and things return to normal for him, he will likely resume his previous schedule for using the toilet."

## FACTORS AFFECTING A CHILD'S RESPONSE TO ILLNESS AND HOSPITALIZATION

Each child responds to illness or hospitalization differently. The expression "perception is everything" certainly applies to the ill child. How children perceive an incident will affect their responses before, during, and after the illness or hospitalization. How a child reacts is often related to the parents' response to the illness and the child's age, level of cognitive development, preparation, previous experiences, and coping skills.

For children who have had a previous illness or hospitalization, how that event unfolded and the child's response to it will greatly affect the child's view of future experiences. Children with chronic diseases who undergo multiple hospitalizations have a different perception of illness than those who have an occasional cold (see Chapter 36). A visit to a pediatrician's office will show the wide range of responses that children exhibit. Some older children have more negative responses as they begin to associate certain people, colors, and surroundings with what was for them an unpleasant experience. The environment of the healthcare setting is an important aspect of how the child responds to the experience. It is often quite intimidating to a child to be in a healthcare facility, but a well-built facility that endeavors to make children less anxious and fearful and provides a space that engages children in a cognitively appropriate way will result in a positive experience for children and their families (Norton-Westwood, 2012). Private spaces with a lounge, rooms that have natural light, and windows with a view are therapeutic. Playrooms that encourage children to explore and engage in therapeutic play positively affect the child's experience. Access to school-like or classroom settings with unrestricted phone and computer use is much appreciated by older children (Norton-Westwood, 2012).

## Age and Cognitive Development

Children's developmental levels affect their reactions to illness. Developmental differences should be considered during the planning of nursing care. Preparing a toddler for hospitalization or a procedure differs from preparing a school-age child. The content, the time frame, the setting, and the method of preparation are all based on the child's growth and development. Pediatric nurses must have a clear understanding of the cognitive abilities of children in each age group (Box 35.2).

## Parental Response

Children have sharp observation skills and know when their parents are anxious and upset. This anxiety is transferred to the child, and the child's anxiety then increases. If the parents talk outside their child's room or within hearing range but in whispers, the child begins to imagine what the parents are saying. All children, but especially preschoolers, who have very active imaginations, can invent elaborate stories to explain what is happening.

The parent who does not answer the child's questions or who does not tell the truth for fear it will frighten the child only confuses the child and weakens the child's trust in the parent. The child wants to believe that someone is in control and that he or she can trust that person. Some parents cannot be honest with their children because of their own fears and insecurities. The nurse needs to assess for all of these issues.

## Preparing the Child and Family

*Stress* has been defined as a nonspecific response of the body to any demand made on it. Perceived stressors, the conditioning factors brought to the situation, and the coping mechanisms used to adapt all

## EVIDENCE-BASED PRACTICE

An integral part of the nursing process is evaluation. Following implementation of a patient's nursing care plan, the nurse carefully evaluates whether the expected outcomes for the patient have been met. This process then allows the nurse to revise the plan of care as indicated to optimize nursing care. Findings from qualitative research studies (Chappuis et al., 2011; Mattsson, Forsner, Castrén, et al., 2013) provide pediatric nurses with the unique opportunity to evaluate their behaviors and actions from the perspective of their patients—hospitalized children whose voices are not often directly and clearly heard.

Chappuis et al. (2011) conducted surveys and interviews of 136 children ages 6 to 12 years of age who were in the hospital for a minimum of 2 nights. Boys and girls were equally represented. The aim of the study was to explore the child's point of view regarding his or her hospitalization to better understand which areas in nursing care can be improved.

The analysis of the children's responses highlighted two main areas for improvement in nursing care. The first is understanding what mattered most to children during their hospitalization. The second is the need to assess the opinions of children separate from parents to meet their healthcare needs (Chappuis et al., 2011). Most children (90%) evaluated nurses in a positive manner. Children felt that the attitude of the nurse and their relationship with them took precedence over technical care. Emphasis was placed on the way children were welcomed to the unit. Areas for improvement include the sleep environment, pain management, and food. Another recurrent theme from the study was childrens' fears. Fears are common during hospitalization and nurses must assess for and mitigate fears by listening to and supporting children. This can decrease stress levels and speed recovery times (Chappuis et al., 2011).

Mattsson et al. (2013) sought to understand the meaning of nursing care though the concerns of the nurse caring for children in the pediatric intensive care unit (PICU). Results show that when treated in a holistic manner, children demonstrated feelings of value and hope. Nurses can better serve their patients by responding to all the needs of the child, acknowledging the child as a whole being, and avoiding medically oriented care that focuses on the illness.

These studies offer the following guidance for pediatric nursing practice:

- Welcome the child to the unit and remember to enter a child's room with a smile and establish eye contact.
- Ask children directly how they feel and what they need. This provides them with a voice and choices in the care they receive.
- Do not assume that because a child's parent or caregiver is present, the need for individualized, sensitive nursing care and presence is diminished.
- Acknowledge children with each interaction by using each child's name and engaging them in conversation about their concerns related to hospitalization and their life outside of the hospital.
- Provide age-appropriate diversion and friendly interaction.
- Provide basic needs in a gentle, organized manner.
- Step into a child's room frequently, even if only for a brief moment, to ensure the child's safety and well-being.
- Remember that older children continue to need physical comfort, reassurance, and conversation and that they appreciate the advocacy roles that nurses assume.
- Children and teens respect professionalism in their nurses and want to be respected as individuals.
- Make special efforts at the time of hospital admission to explain the role of the nurse to children inexperienced with hospitalization.
- Provide children with age-appropriate explanations of treatments, timely care, truthful responses, and privacy.

References: Chappuis, M., Vannay-Bouchiche, C., Flückiger, M., et al. (2011). Children's Experience Regarding the Quality of Their Hospital Stay: The Development of an Assessment Questionnaire for Children. *Journal of Nursing Care Quality, 26*(1), 78–87; Mattsson, J., Forsner, M., Castrén, M., et al. (2013). Caring for children in pediatric intensive care units: An observation study focusing on nurses' concerns. *Nursing Ethics,20*(5), 528–538.

## BOX 35.2 Developmental Approaches to the Hospitalized Child

### Neonate

- Anticipate needs and fulfill them in a timely manner.
- Provide opportunities for nonnutritive (comfort) sucking and oral stimulation with a pacifier.
- Provide swaddling, with the infant's hands drawn to the midline and close to the face. Use soft talking to soothe.
- If the infant is very ill, provide a quiet, soothing environment. Pay close attention to light and sound stimulation.
- When stimulation is appropriate, provide stimulation for each sense (e.g., mobiles, music, smell, soft stuffed animals). Use contrasting colors and textures.
- Watch for cues of overstimulation, such as eye avoidance, extension of arms, splaying of fingers, and "zoning-out" behavior.
- Before painful procedures, provide comforting touch and nonnutritive sucking. Follow painful procedures with tucking, holding, and cuddling.
- Model and share appropriate behaviors with family members regarding stimulation, touch, verbalization, and feeding.
- Provide consistent caregivers when parents are not available.
- Collaborate with parents on ways to provide care to the neonate.
- Involve the parents in the care of their neonate as much as possible.
- Encourage parents to room-in if possible.

### Infant

- For the younger infant, provide the same care given for a neonate.
- The older infant will begin to anticipate painful procedures and fight. Use sheets and blankets to provide swaddling if necessary. Allow nonnutritive sucking for comfort.
- Expect regression and inform parents to expect it and why.
- Limit the number of caregivers to whom the infant must adjust.
- Request that parents bring the infant's security object (e.g., blanket, stuffed animal).
- Encourage parents to be present during procedures.

### Toddler

- Expect regression and inform parents about behaviors.
- Follow home routines and rituals.
- Involve parents in the care of the toddler.
- Provide for rooming-in if possible.
- Allow opportunities for mobility when it can be done safely.
- Use all possible methods of pain control when the child must have a painful procedure.
- Anticipate temper tantrums when the child's frustration level is high.
- Maintain a safe environment for the toddler's physical acting out and temper tantrums.
- Encourage the child to be independent (e.g., feed self, use potty chair, put on socks).
- Provide support when the toddler needs to be dependent (e.g., hold after a procedure, comfort if parents leave).
- Approach with a positive attitude ("I am going to give you your medicine.").

### Preschooler

- Provide safe ways to act out aggression (e.g., with punching bags, painting, clay).
- Take time for communication. Answer questions with simple, concrete explanations. Explain all procedures honestly. Allow for choices whenever possible.
- Expect egocentric behavior.
- Provide for a safe and secure environment (e.g., with a night light, view of others, objects from home).
- Be consistent.
- Ask the parents how the child usually copes in new situations.
- Tell the child that he or she did not cause the illness.
- Involve parents in care and follow home routines.
- Place the child with other children of the same age if possible.
- Provide for play activities in the playroom and in the room.
- Accept regression if it occurs and explain it to parents.
- Encourage the child to be independent (e.g., feeding, dressing, toileting).

### School-Age Child

- Inform the child of limits, and enforce them (e.g., no water fights, no wheelchair races, no leaving the unit).
- Involve the child in planning and implementing care (e.g., allow child to choose from menu and assist with some procedures).
- Explain all procedures and allow the child time for questions and answers. Use medical and scientific terminology and diagrams, body outlines, or anatomically correct dolls to explain the procedure.
- Accept regression but encourage independence.
- Provide privacy.
- Encourage the child to assist in keeping the room and belongings in order.
- Assist the child in contacting friends. Encourage parents to contact the teacher and have school friends send mail.
- If the child's condition supports visits and calls from friends, encourage this contact.
- Provide for the child's educational needs by encouraging parents to bring in the child's homework and by scheduling study times. If the child will have a prolonged period of hospital or home care, arrange for a teacher to work with the child. Some hospitals have a hospital-based teacher.

### Adolescent

- Provide privacy for care and visiting.
- Encourage the adolescent to wear street clothes and perform normal grooming.
- Encourage questions about appearance and the effects of illness on the adolescent's future.
- Use scientific and medical terminology to prepare the adolescent for procedures.
- Use body outlines and diagrams and give the rationale for the procedure.
- When possible, provide for a special activity area that is limited to adolescent use. Introduce the child to other adolescents on the unit.
- Encourage peers to call and visit if the adolescent's condition can tolerate this action.
- Assist parents in communicating, supporting, and guiding adolescents by providing them with information about growth and development.
- Allow favorite foods to be brought in if the adolescent does not need a special diet.
- Approach the adolescent with caring, understanding, and acceptance.
- Provide for educational needs, as for a school-age child.

affect each person's adaptation to a stress-producing situation. Preparing for an event (in this case, hospitalization) can decrease stress in several ways. During preparation, the child's and parents' perceptions of the event can be explored. In addition, previous experiences that might affect the impending hospitalization and the use of previous coping strategies can be identified and discussed.

The depth and method of preparation needed varies between children and is based on an understanding of the child's individual needs. Variables that the nurse should consider are the child's age and developmental level, involvement of the family, timing, child's physiologic status and psychological status, setting, sociocultural factors, and the child's past experiences with illness and hospitalization.

Preparation sessions should be planned. Teaching is more effective if the nurse and family develop trust. Honesty and use of language appropriate for the child's age are imperative. When possible, all of the child's senses should be involved. The child should be allowed to see the intensive care area or surgery area before being admitted, to take the blood pressure of a stuffed animal, or to handle the mask that will be used in surgery. The nurse should avoid using medical terms that children and their parents might not understand. Literal interpretations of some words can be confusing and scary to some children, especially preschoolers (see Chapter 4). Some children assume that certain procedures involve pain. Explanation and the opportunity to handle equipment, when possible, can help children master the fear of hospitalization and treatment.

### Coping Skills of the Child and Family

Coping is the process of contending with difficulties in an effort to overcome or work through them. How the child copes with illness or hospitalization is related to age, perception of the event, previous hospitalizations and encounters with the healthcare profession, support from significant others, and the child's and parents' coping skills.

Depending on age, children use words, behaviors, and physical actions to help them through stressful situations. The child might also cope by ignoring or negating the event. Stress reactions depend on the child's age and developmental level (Kaulen, 2014). The younger child is more likely to use emotional expression, while the older child and adolescent are more likely to withdraw or practice more self-control behaviors. For example, although the younger child might scream and kick during a procedure, the older child might remain stoic and say that it did not hurt, even though it did. Some children try to appear brave and meet self-imposed or parental expectations.

Breathing (e.g., blowing bubbles, pinwheels, party blowers) or singing helps with relaxation and offers a focus for the child. Teaching coping mechanisms and practicing them before a procedure can help a child feel more in control and successful. Distraction (e.g., games, books, music) and imagery (e.g., tapes, scenarios) for older children are effective tools for coping. Parents, nurses, and child life specialists all can serve as facilitators of these techniques. Child life specialists play an important role in helping the patient and their family with all aspects of the hospitalization. They encourage parents to comfort their child and provide security. Child life specialists prepare a child for a procedure by incorporating the five senses into their explanations. They encourage the child to have some control by offering appropriate tasks and use play as a way of normalizing the experience (Kaulen, 2014).

### Psychological Benefits of Hospitalization

Some think that hospitalization causes only negative psychological effects. The stress of illness and hospitalization can actually enhance growth and development by promoting a child's use of coping skills and bolstering self-esteem. Children can increase their self-confidence as they overcome anxiety related to hospitalization and perhaps master some self-care skills. They feel positive about their recovery or increased ability to cope with any disability they have. In addition, hospitalization offers an opportunity for children to ask questions and obtain new information. Some even become interested in a career in healthcare while observing professionals caring for them. Hospitalization can also be an opportunity to teach parents about children's growth and development, improve parenting skills, and assess the child's well care and immunizations.

## PLAY FOR THE ILL CHILD

Play is an extremely important part of the hospitalization of a child. Play can help reveal how a child is coping with the stress of the hospitalization. Unstructured play is an outlet for the child to control events, ideas and relationships (Potasz, De Varela, De Carvalho, et al., 2013). Play allows time for children to process and express their feelings and fears. It gives the child control over his or her perception of the experience and provides an outlet for emotional release (Nabors et al., 2013). Siblings can also benefit from play. Nurses can evaluate how children and their siblings are coping with the hospitalization by observing their play and identifying any educational or further support needs (Nabors et al., 2013).

Play for the ill child is believed to decrease the potential negative effects of hospitalization by promoting expression of feelings and enabling control over stressful experiences (Bolig, Ferne, & Klein, 1986). Because play is familiar and comfortable for children, child life programs provide opportunities for play in a variety of healthcare settings, including inpatient units, intensive care units (ICUs), outpatient clinics, emergency departments, and presurgical waiting areas (AAP Child Life Council and Committee on Hospital Care, 2006). Preferred play activities vary according to the stage of development. For example, a young child engages in make-believe play, a school-age child joins others in a structured game, and an adolescent uses a computer to communicate electronically with peers outside the hospital (AAP Child Life Council and Committee on Hospital Care, 2006).

### Playrooms

Hospitals and clinics often provide playrooms where children can go to play with toys, participate in age-appropriate arts and crafts, and socialize with other children. Children should always see this area as a safe place where procedures and treatments do not take place. When their condition is stable, children can be taken to the playroom in their beds and wheelchairs (Fig. 35.5). A separate activity area should be provided, when possible, for adolescents to listen to music, play video games, use computers to access e-mail and Internet sites, and visit with their peers. If playrooms are not available, a supply of developmentally appropriate toys, games, and books should be maintained so nurses can give them to pediatric patients.

### Therapeutic Play

When a child is hospitalized, one component of the child's plan of care is the use of **therapeutic play**. Therapeutic play differs from normal play in its design and intent. Members of the healthcare team guide it, and activities are planned to meet the physical and psychological needs of the child. Interpretations of the child's play behavior and some types of play therapy require guidance by a trained play therapist. Therapeutic play can provide an emotional outlet, instruct, and improve physiologic abilities (AAP Child Life Council and Committee on Hospital Care, 2006). Supervised play with medical equipment helps reduce fear and separate reality from fantasy.

Child life specialists are available in many hospitals to share their expertise in child growth and development and the use of play. Child

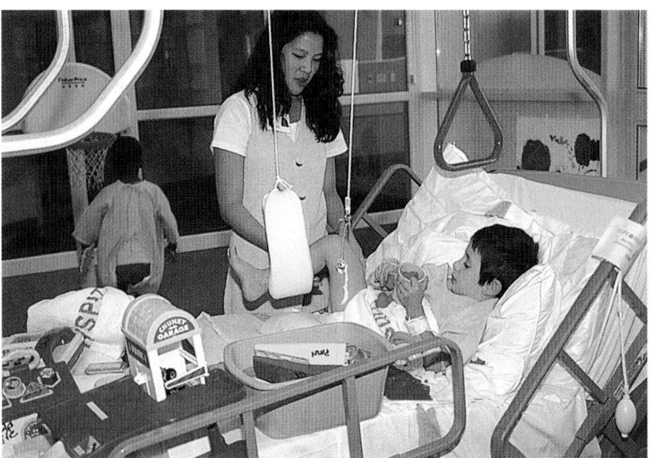

FIG 35.5 To provide diversion and allow interaction with other children, the play therapist wheels the child, while still in bed with traction in place, to the playroom. (Courtesy Parkland Health and Hospital System, Dallas, TX.)

life program goals include maintaining normal living patterns, minimizing psychological trauma, and promoting optimal development of the child.

### Emotional Outlet Play

Emotional outlet play is often called dramatic play. During this type of play, the child acts out or dramatizes real-life stressors. These might include emotional stressors, such as abuse or neglect, or a painful physical stressor, such as a bone marrow aspiration. A child who has been sexually abused might not be able to communicate the experience verbally but may be able to use an anatomically correct doll to show what happened. Terminally ill children have been reported to use play to tell their stories and to express thoughts and feelings, an important part of the emotional healing process for children and parents (Nabors et al., 2013).

Many commercially crafted toys are available for dramatic play. Anatomically correct dolls and puppets are available. Some dolls have removable parts that enable the child to see the various organs of the body.

Injection play is an appropriate intervention with the child who has to undergo frequent blood work, injections, IV therapy, or any other therapy involving syringes and needles. If a needle is used for this type of activity, safety is of the utmost importance, and the nurse should assess the child's growth and development level before using this type of directed play. An adult is always present if a needle is used. The child can give a doll an injection and thereby work through anger and anxiety. Wooden hammers and pegboards, foam (Nerf) balls, and boxing gloves are all avenues for release of stress or anger.

### Teaching Through Play

Play can also be used to educate. It can be used in preoperative teaching and teaching before a new, painful, or extensive procedure (Fig. 35.6). The nurse assesses the child's cognitive level before this type of teaching, and the play should be appropriate to the child's level.

Hospital equipment is often used in this type of play. The nurse might demonstrate taking a blood pressure on the child's stuffed animal before putting the cuff on the child. A breathing treatment might be "given" to the child's doll before the child is given the treatment. The nurse might use drawings and diagrams to explain procedures or surgery. Use of play for children experiencing invasive, painful procedures such as IV line insertion has been shown to be effective in teaching what to expect before the procedure and to improve coping skills (Nabors et al., 2013). Some hospitals have preoperative visits during which children come to meet the people who will be taking care of them and see the physical surroundings. They can see the scrub gowns and masks worn by the surgical staff and visit a typical room. Children and parents can ask questions and meet other children and parents who are going through a similar experience as they tour the area.

### Enhancing Cooperation Through Play

Children with illnesses that require unpleasant or painful therapies often are uncooperative. Developing a plan that will stimulate and engage such a child in the activity is a challenge. The nurse should include age-appropriate growth and development activities when planning care. The school-age child who loves competition and games is more likely to increase range of motion of an arm if points can be made each time a foam ball is thrown through a hoop.

Allowing the child to blow bubbles, a whistle, or a pinwheel or to simulate blowing out the nurse's penlight can enhance deep-breathing exercises. Range of motion can be accomplished by throwing foam balls, beanbags, and paper balls. The child who needs to increase intake can sometimes be motivated to drink more fluids if a graph shows the amount taken in and the child receives a reward when a selected goal is reached. Including the child in planning and identifying rewards and goals enhances motivation. Colorful stickers, baseball cards, small toys, and special pencils can be used as rewards.

### Unstructured Play

In addition to therapeutic play, the nurse encourages unstructured play in the hospital setting. Through unstructured play, children can control events, ideas, and relationships. Music therapy can give children choices to play instruments, such as drums and bells, or to join in while a music therapist leads songs and plays a guitar. Animal therapy is another popular type of play where the child can interact with animals and their trainers.

### Evaluation of Play

Therapeutic play should be reflected in the child's nursing care plan. During the evaluation step of the nursing process, the nurse looks at the outcome criteria to determine whether play has facilitated the achievement of goals. Is the child coughing and deep breathing every 2 hours? Is the child expressing feelings over the separation from parents? Is the child eating or sleeping? If the pediatric patient's goals have been achieved, the interventions have been effective.

## ADMITTING THE CHILD TO A HOSPITAL SETTING

### Taking the History

The admission procedure sets the tone for the hospitalization. It should not just consist of a series of questions but rather serve as a time of collaboration between the nurse and the family. The amount of time the family has spent in the emergency department, the seriousness of the illness, and other family needs (e.g., other children staying with grandparents or left with neighbors) will affect the interview process.

The nurse should acknowledge a parent's concerns. For example, the nurse might say to a parent, "I know you're concerned about your other children. Would you like to call your neighbor to check on them before I ask you some questions about your daughter and her illness?"

Most hospitals provide an admission interview form. Some of the information is essential for providing immediate care, and some can

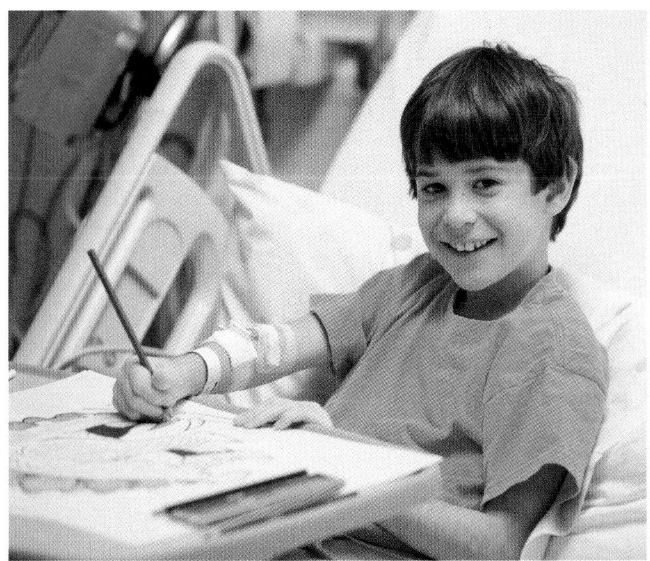

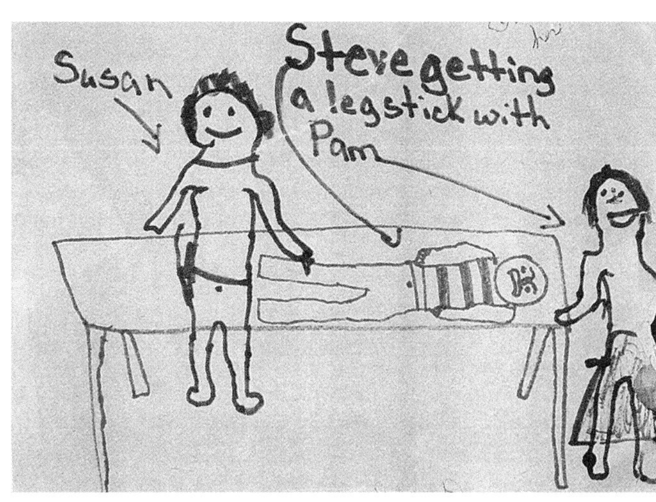


Art materials allow children to express their thoughts and feelings about illness and hospitalization. (©2016 Getty Images. Reprinted with permission.)

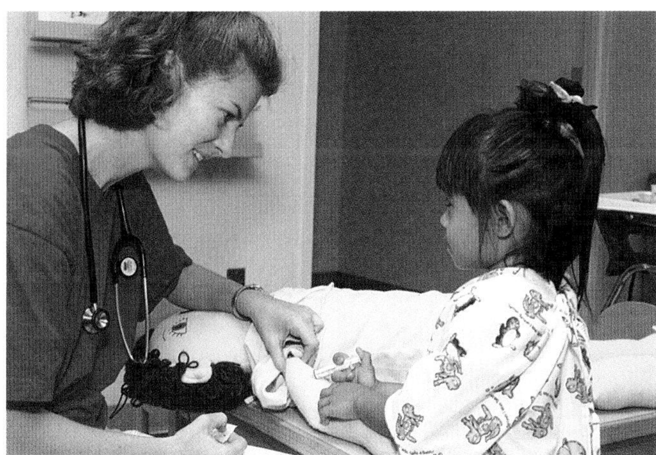

Giving a doll an injection can help a child work through anxiety and anger about injections she is receiving.

**FIG 35.6** Therapeutic play can be used to teach children about medical procedures or help them work through their feelings about what has happened to them in the healthcare setting. Child life specialists are often members of the team in children's hospitals to provide expert guidance for therapeutic play.

be collected later. By recognizing the family's needs, the nurse can structure each admission to fit the child and family. If the parent has entered the system through the emergency department, some of the questions may have been answered previously. Looking at the information already obtained by other departments can prevent repetition. However, critical data regarding allergies, medications taken at home, and recent illness history must be obtained again.

Although hospitals have policies and procedures for admission, the routine may need to be altered because of the child's condition. For example, an IV infusion should be started for a severely dehydrated child, and a child in pain should be medicated immediately. The primary needs of the child and family may be emotional. A parent who has just been told that her child may have a terminal disease might have difficulty remembering the dates of the child's immunizations. In this situation, the nurse should provide the parent with support and assistance in mobilizing coping mechanisms and support systems rather than focusing on data gathering.

After the child and family are made comfortable (Fig. 35.7), the nurse obtains a thorough physical, health, and psychosocial history.

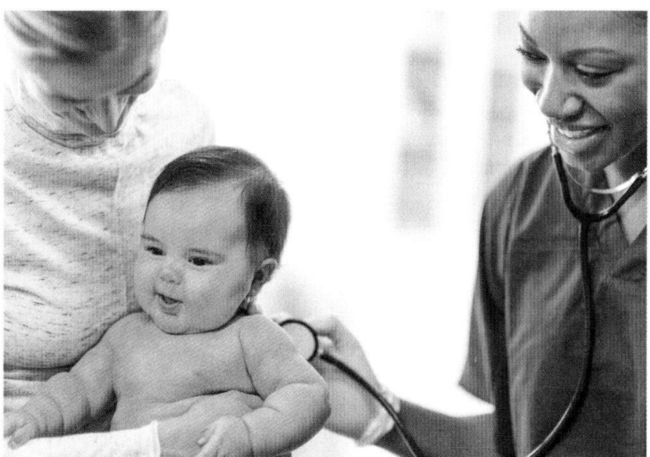

**FIG 35.7** To reduce the stress of unfamiliar surroundings and people, the nurse assesses the child who remains in the security of her mother's arms. (©2016 Getty Images. Reprinted with permission.)

This interview is followed by a detailed physical examination. For all types of admissions, the history is recorded on an admission data sheet that, depending on the facility, may be in electronic format. The format of the admission data sheet varies from hospital to hospital, but most admission forms ask for much of the same information, including past medical history, allergies, nutrition, sleep, elimination, and psychosocial factors.

## Physical Examination

### Initial Inspection

The initial inspection determines the need for any immediate or emergency care that must be provided before other information can be obtained.

### Baseline Data

The physical examination should be thorough, and special attention should be given to the body system or systems involved in the child's chief complaint. Many admission forms have an outline of the child's body on which the nurse should indicate any bruises, scratches, or other skin markings that provide specific objective data. (The process of interviewing, taking a history, and physical assessment is explained in Chapter 33.)

Data collected at admission are used to formulate nursing diagnoses and the child's plan of care and should be accessible to all healthcare providers. Placing the information in a location that is difficult to access diminishes its importance for care planning.

## NURSING CARE PLAN

### *The Child and Family in a Hospital Setting*

**Focused Assessment**

- Provide a comprehensive hospital admission assessment of the child and family.
  - Review the child's past medical history and records of previous hospital experiences.
  - Analyze physical examination data.
- Assess factors that affect the hospitalized child.
  - Nutrition: calorie intake compared to requirements for age and weight; height and weight percentiles; favorite foods; mealtime rituals; cultural or religious customs
  - Elimination: bowel and bladder control norms; terms child uses for elimination; signs of regression and whether regression is distressing to the child or family
  - Sleep: usual sleep patterns, bedtime, hygiene practices, and rituals (rocking, prayers, snacks, stories); compare to norms for age; changes in hours of sleep per day
  - Self-Care: typical level of function (e.g., eating, bathing, dressing, brushing teeth); note any alterations due to stress
  - Emotional/Social Status: signs of anxiety or fear of hospital setting (crying, tantrums, withdrawal, not communicating); participation in activities/play; maintaining contact with peers
- Assess factors that affect the family's adjustment to their child's illness and hospitalization.
  - Stress levels of parents
  - Stress levels of siblings and other family members
  - Quality of past hospital experiences
  - Concerns about severity of child's illness and prognosis
  - Need for sleep, food/fluid intake, healthcare, psychosocial/spiritual support, financial assistance, information and education

**Nursing Diagnosis**

Imbalanced Nutrition: Less Than Body Requirements related to unfamiliar foods, separation from caregiver, strange environment, or disease process.

**Planning**

***Expected Outcomes***

The child will eat the appropriate number of calories and variety of nutrients according to age and maintain prehospital weight.

**Interventions and *Rationales***

1. Identify the cause of the child's decreased intake.
   *Finding the cause of any decrease in appetite can facilitate problem solving.*
2. Encourage parents to bring foods from home and to be with the child during meals.
   *The parents' presence simulates the home environment and increases the likelihood that the child will eat.*
3. Allow the child to select food from the menu. Communicate to other staff the foods the child likes to eat.
   *This gives the child control and may prompt the child to eat.*
4. Offer frequent, nutritious snacks and encourage the parents to do the same.
   *Children need to eat foods with high nutritious value during meals and snacks.*
5. Offer small portions. Use colorful, small dishes, cups, and utensils.
   *Children may be overwhelmed by large portions and refuse to eat. Child-size tableware, which is decorated, is more appealing to children.*
6. Request a consultation with the dietitian.
   *Registered dietitians can assist in planning age-appropriate nutritious meals.*

**Evaluation**

Is the child's nutritional intake appropriate for age?
Did the child maintain baseline body weight during hospitalization?

**Nursing Diagnosis**

Delayed Growth and Development, regression in toilet training or self-care skills, related to separation and hospitalization.

**Planning**

***Expected Outcomes***

The child will maintain usual self-care activities of feeding, toileting, dressing, and bathing. Any regression reverses quickly after discharge.

**Interventions and *Rationales***

1. Follow home routines of elimination, when possible.
   *Cooperation will increase and anxiety will decrease if the child's normal routines are maintained.*
2. Support the child if regression in toileting skills occurs. Provide diapers and incontinence pads as needed.
   *Incontinence (day and/or night) may occur as a result of the stress of hospitalization and illness.*
3. Explain to parents that some temporary regression in self-care activities is expected for ill and hospitalized children.
   *Parents may be concerned about the child's regression, and this can increase their child's anxiety.*

*Continued*

## NURSING CARE PLAN—cont'd

### *The Child and Family in a Hospital Setting*

4. Encourage the child to participate in self-care activities according to developmental abilities. Provide assistance when factors related to illness impair performance.
   *Self-care increases the child's self-esteem and feeling of control. Fatigue, pain, and other symptoms may limit the child's ability to perform self-care independently.*
5. Provide the necessary equipment for self-care and place it within reach of the child.
   *Accessible equipment makes it easier for the child to engage in self-care activities and facilitates independence.*
6. Offer choices and allow the child to make decisions when appropriate.
   *Making choices increases the child's sense of control and may decrease anxiety.*

**Evaluation**

Is the child able to feed, toilet, dress, and bathe at the same level as before the illness?

Does the child readily participate in self-care activities?

**Nursing Diagnosis**

Disturbed Sleep Pattern related to unfamiliar environment, anxiety, or discomfort.

**Planning**

***Expected Outcome***

The child will sleep the appropriate number of hours for age.

**Interventions and *Rationales***

1. Plan for periods throughout the day for sleep and group nursing care activities together.
   *Planning to perform multiple tasks while in the child's room (i.e., measure vital signs, conduct shift assessment, and give medications) provides time for uninterrupted sleep.*
2. Post a sign on the door when the child is asleep to prevent staff and visitors from waking the child. Eliminate other distractions.
   *Minimizing staff and environmental distractions (blinds closed; TV, phone, and lights turned off; door closed, if safe) will facilitate uninterrupted sleep for the child and parents.*
3. Reassure the child and family that the nurses will closely monitor the child during periods of sleep, day and night. Provide a night light if indicated.
   *Feelings of security are increased if the child and family understand that the nurses are watching and available. Some children fear darkness and need a light on to be comfortable.*

**Evaluation**

Does the child take naps and sleep an appropriate amount of time according to age requirements?

**Nursing Diagnosis**

Anxiety related to fear of the unknown and separation from significant others and familiar surroundings.

**Planning**

***Expected Outcomes***

The child will display decreased indicators of distress (e.g., crying, withdrawal, irritability), verbalize feelings of anxiety, and play appropriately and maintain contact with peers.

**Interventions and *Rationales***

1. Orient the child and family to the hospital's layout and unit routines.
   *Familiarity with the environment and routines will decrease anxiety caused by fear of the unknown.*
2. Prepare the child for all procedures and events in an age-appropriate way. Educate parents in advance. Preparation for events decreases anxiety and fear.
   *Parents can better support their child if they are knowledgeable.*
3. Encourage parents to stay with the child when possible and to be involved in the child's care.
   *The presence of parents supports the parental role and decreases the child's separation anxiety.*
4. Hold, rock, and cuddle the infant or young child.
   *Physical contact increases feelings of security.*
5. If the parents cannot stay with the child, provide for a consistent caregiver.
   *Continuity of care provides the child the opportunity to develop a trusting relationship.*
6. Follow home routines and rituals when possible.
   *Familiar routines help the child predict events, resulting in decreased anxiety caused by the unfamiliar setting.*
7. Encourage parents to honestly tell their child when they must leave and when they will return. Obtain contact information from parents. Encourage parents to telephone their child and the nurses while away.
   *Trust is increased and anxiety and fear are decreased when parents are honest with their child. Open communication between the parents and nurses can decrease stress.*
8. Encourage parents to provide their child with transitional objects (e.g., blanket, teddy bear) and reminders of family (e.g., pictures, scarf, handkerchief).
   *Transitional objects and family reminders give the child a feeling of security and comfort, which can decrease anxiety particularly during times of separation.*
9. Plan play activities for the child throughout the day. Take children to the playroom; promote interaction with other children. Provide toys and other items (books, coloring books, crayons, video games) as well as time for play in the hospital room if the child cannot leave.
   *The playroom provides a safe place for the child to engage in activities that facilitate expression and distraction. Interaction with other children can support adaptation to the environment. All children need to be encouraged and given time for play.*
10. For the older child, arrange for peer contact through visits, phone calls/texts, e-mails, and cards/letters.
    *The older child may fear losing contact with peers. Maintaining contact supports positive self-esteem and security.*
11. Offer choices and allow the child to make some decisions.
    *Making choices increases the child's sense of control.*
12. Encourage children to wear their own clothes and to decorate their hospital room.
    *Giving children an opportunity for self-expression helps them feel more comfortable in the hospital environment.*
13. Provide opportunities for the older child to verbalize feelings about the illness and hospitalization; inform the child life specialist about the child's concerns and needs.
    *Fear and anxiety may decrease if the child has an opportunity to communicate feelings, have them validated, and participate in problem-solving techniques.*

## NURSING CARE PLAN—cont'd

### *The Child and Family in a Hospital Setting*

**Evaluation**

Is the child playing and communicating with other children and staff and showing decreased signs of distress?

Is the child able to express feelings of anxiety either verbally or through play?

**Nursing Diagnosis**

Interrupted Family Processes related to the child's hospitalization and illness.

**Planning**

***Expected Outcomes***

The parents and family members will participate in the child's care, maintain a baseline level of physical health, use appropriate support systems, identify ways to cope, and assist the child to move from a sick role to a well role.

**Interventions and *Rationales***

1. Orient the parents and family to the hospital and provide information related to their physical needs (e.g., fluids/food, sleep, bathing, medications).
   *The parents' and family's physical needs must be met so they can meet their emotional needs, and then meet the child's needs.*
2. Encourage family members (parents, siblings) to express their feelings and to ask questions about the child's illness.
   *Open communication decreases anxiety and clarifies misconceptions.*
3. Provide the family with information about the child's condition, treatment, and support systems. Begin to prepare them for the child's discharge.
   *Information gives parents a sense of control and decreases their anxiety.*
4. Identify with the family the ways in which they are coping; support their parenting skills.
   *Individuals are not always aware of their coping mechanisms, and the nurse should help the family evaluate the effectiveness of their coping skills.*
5. Refer the family to other professionals (e.g., social worker, clinical psychologist, clinical specialist, child life specialist, psychiatrist, clergy) when meeting their needs is not within the scope of nursing practice.
   *Early identification of family problems that require specialized intervention can decrease the possibility of escalation. Collaboration with other health professionals can facilitate a holistic approach to the care of child and family.*
6. Provide information to the parents about diagnosis, treatment, and prognosis. Attend to their needs for sleep and nutrition.
   *The child is affected by parents' anxiety. Helping the parents cope will help decrease their anxiety, which will in turn decrease the child's anxiety.*

**Evaluation**

Are the parents and family members able to participate in the child's care while meeting their own basic physical needs?

Do family members support each other and seek other resources when necessary?

Are family members able to describe and use positive coping skills?

Are the parents able to assist the child to move from a sick role to a well role?

## THE ILL CHILD'S FAMILY

Through family-centered care, the nursing care is provided to the child in the context of the family. The nurse's patient is the entire family. Further, the nurse acknowledges that the parents and family are the primary and continuing providers of care for the child. Occasionally, the parents are not able to stay with their hospitalized child due to outside obligations such as work, caring for other children, or lack of transportation. This separation can greatly increase the stress on the child, especially for young children. Older school-age children and adolescents are more accustomed to parental absence. Nurses often need to be more vigilant in ensuring the child is safe and coping with the absence of the parents as well as the hospitalization (Roberts, 2012).

### Parents

A child's illness can create a situational crisis for the family. If the illness leads to hospitalization, either planned or unplanned, the family's anxiety increases. Ill children become the parents' central focus; parents can become very vigilant and committed to protecting the child and ensuring optimal care. The parental role often changes when the child is admitted to the hospital. The parent who had been in control before the admission is now in an unfamiliar environment. Parents have identified significant stress regarding their ability to fulfill their parental role and care for their ill child. Parents may be confused as to what they can and cannot do. Can they bathe their child? Can they hold their child, or will they dislodge the tubes?

Parents play a vital role in helping their children cope with their hospitalization. Parents assist their child in various ways such as emotional support, distraction, and returning to the child's normal routine (Marsac, Donlon, Winston, et al., 2011). One of the most reported stressful aspects of hospitalization for parents was the relinquishing of the care of their child to health professionals. Other factors included the limited or absence of opportunity to participate in decision making regarding the care of their child and insufficient information regarding their child's medical status (LeGrow, Hodnett, Stremier, et al., 2014). The Institute of Medicine has made shared decision-making a research area priority to alleviate this cause of parental stress (Russell & Simon, 2014).

Nurses are responsible for ensuring that children and parents are prepared for hospital experiences, allowed to participate in care activities, and kept informed regarding the child's response to treatment. Use of medical interpreters can improve care for these children (Fig. 35.8).

Parents have varied responses to a child's illness. They may have guilty feelings related to the belief that if they had sought treatment earlier, the child would not be so ill, or they may initially deny that their child is ill. A period of denial can be followed by anger. This anger can be directed at the nurse, at another family member, or, sometimes, at a deity. When the immediate crisis is over, a period of depression can occur. Many times parents become exhausted, both physically and psychologically, from spending long hours at the hospital in addition to working and caring for their other children. Support can include encouraging parents to express their feelings, active listening, assistance with processing feelings, and referral for counseling and social work services. Helping parents to use reflective parenting to enhance the parent–child relationship by enabling the parents to understand their child's thoughts, feelings, and intentions is beneficial (Ordway, Webb, Sadler, et al., 2015).

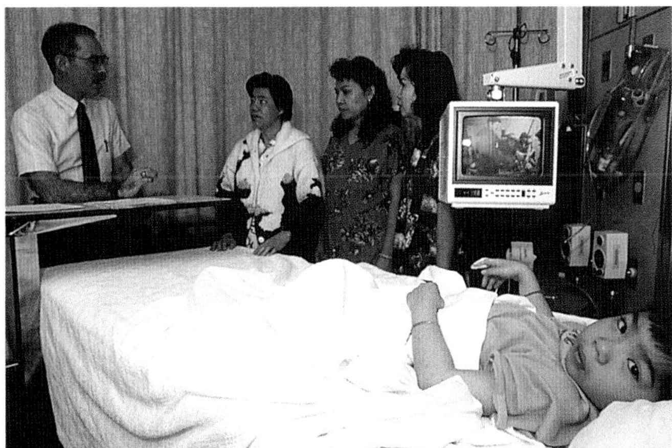

FIG 35.8 The family of a hospitalized child may not speak the prevailing language. Interpreters are available (on-site or on-call) at many hospitals to help parents and children communicate with healthcare team members. This arrangement provides a familiar link to the parents' and child's culture and language. (Courtesy Cook Children's Medical Center, Fort Worth, TX.)

The needs of fathers are sometimes forgotten. The father might come to the hospital only after he has spent a day at work and then, after a short visit, needs to go home to be with other children. He may not be there when the primary care physician makes rounds, and thus, receives most of his medical information from someone else. The father may think that he needs to be the strong one in the family and not show his fear and anxiety. In some families, the mother works outside the home while the father stays with the child. In either case, an awareness of each parent's role will assist the nurse in identifying the individual needs of the parents.

## PARENTS WANT TO KNOW

### *Information for Discharge*

After assessing the family's knowledge, the nurse provides the information families need and want to know to help the child's transition from hospital to home:

- Information about the illness or trauma and expected outcomes. Tell the parents when they should consult the primary care physician or nurse.
- Medications or treatments to be given at home and information about times, route, side effects, and any special care to be taken when giving the medication. Providing written information is valuable.
- Information about any special nutritional needs.
- Specific activities the child may or may not participate in.
- The date when the child may return to school.
- The date to bring the child back to the hospital, clinic, or office for follow-up care.
- Information about any referral agency needed for the child or family.
- The unit phone number and primary nurse's name.

The nurse explains, demonstrates, and then requests a return demonstration by the parents (and child, if age-appropriate) of any treatments or procedures that will be done at home. This teaching should be a continuing process and not left until the time of discharge because learning takes place at different rates.

Because of dual roles, long separations, increased stress, and numerous other factors, the parents' marriage can be strained. This situation is especially likely in marriages that are already at risk. Even when both partners are at the hospital, they may not have any time alone.

Many children have stepmothers and stepfathers or are cared for by grandparents. In such cases, all caregivers need recognition, support, and education. How the family copes with the child's illness depends on the use of coping strategies. A family that is already in crisis or one without support systems (e.g., family, friends, church) will have more difficulty adjusting to the change than a family that is organized and adjusted. A family that deals successfully with the crisis is strengthened by the experience. (For further discussion of the effects of illness on the family, see Chapter 3. For a discussion of the family with a child with a chronic illness, see Chapter 36.)

## CRITICAL THINKING EXERCISE 35.1

Tommy, 4 years old, was admitted to the hospital with pneumonia. Tommy has cystic fibrosis. His family has recently moved to the area, and this is his first admission to your hospital. Tommy loves to play with his dinosaur collection and spends much of his day playing and watching his favorite DVDs. His mother visits for short periods during the lunch hour, and his father visits in the evening. Tommy cries when his parents leave. You mention to a colleague that you think Tommy's parents should spend more time with him. She responds, "We don't know what their other responsibilities are."

1. What other responsibilities might the family have?
2. What are some of the nursing interventions that would support a family with a child in the hospital?

## Siblings

The illness or hospitalization of a brother or sister can be difficult for children. The ill child's siblings might experience jealousy, insecurity, resentment, confusion, and anxiety. Children often have difficulty understanding why their ill sibling is getting all the attention and why their parents have so little time for them. They may worry that if their sibling could get sick, so could they. Preschool children, who engage in magical thinking, might worry that they somehow caused the illness. All of these thoughts and feelings are compounded by children's difficulty expressing their feelings (Box 35.3). Siblings often feel guilty because they are "healthy." Worrying excessively about their ill sibling is common. Current research demonstrates that siblings can also be envious of the attention that the ill child is receiving, causing anger and feelings of loneliness as the parents' focus shifts to the ill child (Nabors et al., 2013). Although there are many documented negative behaviors demonstrated by siblings of ill children, there can also be some positive experiences, including having a closer relationship with the ill child and the family as a whole and becoming more empathetic and sensitive to the needs of other family members (Nabors et al., 2013). Nurses must take the time to address the needs of the sibling because lack of information leads to feelings of frustration and a lack of understanding of what the ill sibling is experiencing (Bugel, 2014).

The ability of siblings to cope with stress can vary with their age, developmental level, relationship with the ill child, and frequency of visits to see the ill child. In addition, parents significantly influence how siblings cope. Siblings are a part of the family unit, and their needs must be assessed so that appropriate interventions by nurses and other healthcare team members can be provided.

## BOX 35.3 Caring for the Siblings of an Ill or Hospitalized Child

**Factors That Add to the Stress of Siblings**

- Age younger than 10 years
- Emotional closeness to the hospitalized child
- Receiving only a limited explanation of the experience
- Fear of getting the illness themselves
- Being cared for outside their own home
- Perceiving that their parents are acting differently toward them
- Having a sibling who is progressively ill

**Nursing Care Guidelines for Meeting the Needs of Siblings**

- Encourage caregivers to have the ill child retell what happened. This experience may be uncomfortable for the adult, but it helps the sibling put the illness or accident in perspective.
- If the sibling has feelings of guilt, address the child's concerns directly. If the feelings of guilt continue, suggest a consultation with a counselor.
- Give parents educational materials, and show them how to use them with the sibling.
- Schedule a time for the sibling to visit. Prepare the sibling for the medical equipment and any changes in the ill child's appearance that may cause concern.
- If the sibling cannot visit, send photographs.
- Encourage the sibling to talk with the child on the telephone.

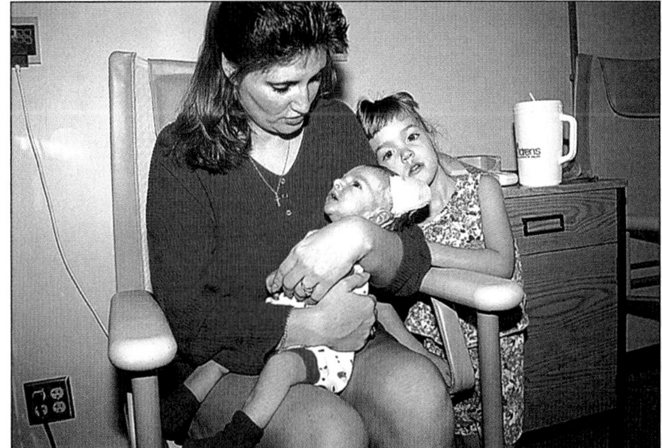

Siblings of ill children may experience jealousy, insecurity, resentment, confusion, and anxiety. The nurse can help them cope by assessing and implementing care to meet their needs. (Courtesy Children's Medical Center, Dallas, TX.)

Modified from Craft, M., Wyatt, N., & Sandell, B. (1985). Behavior and feeling changes in siblings of hospitalized children. *Clinical Pediatrics, 24,* 374–378.

## KEY CONCEPTS

- Pediatric nurses provide specialized care for children in different settings—hospital, school, community, and home.
- Common stressors that affect hospitalized children are separation anxiety, fear of pain or mutilation, fear of the unknown, and loss of control.
- Children may respond to illness with anger, guilt, and regression.
- The stages of separation anxiety are protest, despair, and detachment.
- With increased stress, children have more difficulty separating from their parents.
- A child's reactions to pain and fear of injury are related to developmental stage, previous experiences, separation from parents, restraint, and preparation.
- When ill children feel they have control, they are more likely to be cooperative.
- Children commonly return to an earlier stage of behavior (regression) when stressed by illness.
- Children's responses to illness and hospitalization are affected by their perception of events, age, developmental level, cognitive ability, preparation, previous experiences, coping skills, and parent and family responses.
- Nursing care of the ill child focuses on promoting self-care, minimizing separation anxiety, understanding growth and development, providing diversion by means of play, involving family, allowing control, and managing pain.
- Parents may feel guilt, denial, anger, and depression when their child is hospitalized.
- Therapeutic play allows for emotional expression and enhances development. It is used by nurses to educate children and prepare them for procedures.
- The nurse provides family-centered care to the entire family including the ill child, the parents, the siblings, and other family members.

## REFERENCES AND READINGS

Agazio, J., & Buckley, K., (2012). Revision of a Parental Stress Scale for Use On a Pediatric General Care Unit. *Pediatric Nursing, 38*(2), 82–87.

American Academy of Pediatrics. (2008). Policy statement: Role of the school nurse in providing school health services. *Pediatrics, 121*(5), 1052–1056.

American Academy of Pediatrics, Child Life Council and Committee on Hospital Care. (2006). Child life services. *Pediatrics, 118*(4), 1757–1763.

American Academy of Pediatrics, Committee on Hospital Care and Committee on Pediatric Emergency Medicine. (2012). Pediatric Observation Units. *Pediatrics, 130*, 172–179.

American Academy of Pediatrics, Healthy Children. (2010). *Ages and stages: Teaching health education in schools.* Retrieved from http://www.healthychildren.org/English/ages-stages/gradeschool/school/pages/Teaching-Health-Education-in-School.aspx.

Ballard, K., Sander, M., & Klimes-Dougan, B. (2014). School-Related and Social-Emotional Outcomes of Providing Mental Health Services in Schools. *Community Mental Health Journal, 50,*145–149.

Bolig, R., Ferne, D., & Klein, E. (1986). Unstructured play in hospital settings: An internal locus of control rationale. *Children's Health Care, 15*(2), 101–107.

Brener, N.D., Wechsler, H., & McManus, T. (2013). How School Healthy Is Your State? A State-by-State Comparison of School Health Practices Related to a Healthy School Environment and Health

Education. *Journal of School Health, 83*(10), 743–749.

Bugel, M.J. (2014). Eperiences of School-Aged Siblings of Children with a Traumatic Injury: Changes, Constants, and Needs. *Pediatric Nursing, 40*(4), 179–186.

Carter, M.C., Miles, M.S., Buford, T.H., et al. (1985). Parental environmental stress in pediatric intensive care units. *Dimensions of Critical Care Nursing, 4*(3), 180–188.

Chappuis, M., Vannay-Bouchiche, C., Flückiger, M., et al. (2011). Children's Experience Regarding the Quality of Their Hospital Stay: The Development of an Assessment Questionnaire for Children. *Journal of Nursing Care Quality, 26*(1), 78–87.

Craft-Rosenberg, M., & Krajicek, M.J. (2006). (Eds.). *Nursing excellence for children and families.* New York: Springer.

Erikson, E. (1963). *Childhood and society* (2nd ed.). New York: Norton.

Hadland, S., & Long, W. (2014). A Systemic Review of the Medical Home for Children Without Special Health Care Needs. *Maternal Child Health Journal, 18, 891–898.*

Institute of Medicine (2010). *"Front Matter:" The future of nursing: Leading change, advancing health.* Washington, DC: National Academies Press.

Kaulen, D., (2014). Child Life Experts Offer Tips For Calming Care of Children During Hospitalization. *Contemporary Pediatrics, 31*(6), 20.

LeGrow, K., Hodnett, E., Stremier, R., et al. (2014). Evaluating the feasibility of a parent briefing intervention in a pediatric acute care setting. *Journal for Specialist in Pediatric Nursing, 19,* 219–228.

Marsac, M., Donlon, K., Winston, F., et al. (2011). Child coping, parent coping assistance, and post-traumatic stress flowing paediatric physical injury. *Child: care, health and development 39*(2), 171–177.

Mattsson, J., Forsner, M., Castrén, M., et al. (2013). Caring for children in pediatric intensive care units: An observation study focusing on nurses' concerns. *Nursing Ethics,20*(5), 528–538.

McMurtry, C., Noel, M., Chambers, C., et al. (2011). Children's Fear During Procedural Pain: Preliminary Investigation of the Children's Fear Scale. *Health Psychology, 30*(6), 780–788.

Michelson, K., Clayman, M. L., Haber-Baker, N., et al. (2013). The Use of Family Conferences in the Pediatric Intensive Care Unit. *Journal of Palliative Medicine. 16*(12), 1595–1601.

Mikkelsen, G., & Frederiksen, K. (2011). Family-centered care of children in hospital- a concept analysis. *Journal of Advanced Nursing, 67,*(5) 1152–1162.

Nabors, L., Bartz, J., Kichler, J., et al. (2013). Play as a Mechanism of Working Through Medical Trauma for Children with Medical Illnesses and Their Siblings. *Issues in Comprehensive Pediatric Nursing, 36*(3), 212–224.

Norton-Westwood, D. (2012). The health-care environment through the eyes of a child-Does it soothe or provoke anxiety? *International Journal of Nursing Practice, 18,* 7–11.

Ordway, M.R., Webb, D., Sadler, L.S., et al. (2015). Parental Reflective Functioning: An approach to Enhancing Parent-Child Relationships in Pediatric Primary Care. *Journal of Pediatric Health Care, 29*(4), 325–334.

Parasuraman, S., & Shi, L. (2014). The Role of School-Based Health Centers in Increasing Universal and Targeted Delivery of Primary and Preventitive Care Among Adolescents. *Journal of School Health, 84*(8), 524–532.

Potasz, C., Varela, M., Carvalho, L., et al. (2013). Effect of play activities on hospitalized children's stress: a randomized clinical trial. *Scandinavian Journal of Occupational Therapy, 20,* 71–79.

Rich, C, Gonclaves, A., Guardiani M., et al. (2014). Teen Advisory Committee: Lessons Learned by Adolescents, Facilitators, And Hospital Staff. *Pediatric Nursing, 40*(6), 289–296.

Roberts, C. (2012). Nurses' Perceptions of Unaccompanied Hospitalized Children. *Pediatric Nursing, 38*(3), 133–137.

Russell, C., & Simon, T. (2014). Care of Children with Medical Complexity in the Hospital Setting. *Pediatric Annals, 43*(7), e157–e162.

Shannon, C. (2014). Community-Based Health and Schools of Nursing: Supporting Health Promotion and Research. *Public Health Nursing, 31*(1), 69–78.

Visintainer, M., & Wolfer, J. (1975). Psychological preparation for surgical pediatric patient: The effect on children's and parents' stress response and adjustment. *Pediatrics, 56*(2), 187–202.

36

# The Child With a Chronic Condition or Terminal Illness

http://evolve.elsevier.com/McKinney/mat-ch/

## LEARNING OBJECTIVES

*After studying this chapter, you should be able to:*

- Define chronic illness.
- Analyze the effects of a chronic illness on the child and family.
- Discuss the concerns and needs of the child and family dealing with a chronic illness.
- Compare the stages of death and dying.
- Apply the concepts of death and dying as they relate to the pediatric patient.
- Explain the concerns and needs of the child and family facing an impending death.
- Analyze the nurse's response to death and dying in the pediatric population.
- Use the nursing process to describe nursing care of the chronically ill and dying child.

Rapid advances in healthcare have changed the experience of chronic illness in childhood. Increasing numbers of children who previously would have died from their illnesses early in their lives are living longer, with an estimated 90% of children with chronic conditions reaching their twentieth birthday (Broger & Zeni, 2011). Improvements in early diagnostic testing and treatment have enhanced their quality of life, as well as longevity.

## CHRONIC ILLNESS DEFINED

A **chronic illness or condition** is long term, persisting more than 3 months. It does not spontaneously resolve, is usually without complete cure, frequently has residual characteristics that limit activities of daily living (ADLs), and requires adaptation or special assistance. Box 36.1 lists some of the common chronic conditions of childhood. The severity varies among chronic conditions. Many, such as epilepsy, diabetes, or sickle cell disease, although not physically apparent, have a tremendous impact on the child and family. A chronic condition that is terminal but lasts only a short time also has serious long-term effects on the surviving family. Although the first section of this chapter refers only to chronic conditions, this information also applies to terminal conditions. The U.S. Department of Health and Human Services, Health Resources and Services Administration, Maternal and Child Health Bureau (2008) developed the following definition regarding the special needs of chronically and terminally ill children for planning and advocacy purposes.

Children with special healthcare needs are those who have or are at increased risk for a chronic physical, developmental, behavioral, or emotional conditions and who also require health and related services of a type and amount beyond that required for children generally.

## THE FAMILY OF THE CHILD WITH SPECIAL HEALTHCARE NEEDS

### Family Dynamics and Impact on the Family

Children with special health needs are a growing population that requires many resources, both in the healthcare setting and in the home. It is estimated that 10.2 million children or approximately 14% of children in the US have special healthcare needs (Willits et al., 2013). Improvements in technology, reimbursement provisions (e.g., insurance, state and federal funding), and allocation of healthcare resources have all affected the family's role in caring for the child with a chronic illness. In 2010, the Health Care and Education Reconciliation Act provided access to health insurance and coverage to children with pre-existing conditions which will help alleviate some of the struggles families face with the increasing cost of healthcare insurance (DeRigne, 2012). Children with special needs can now be safely cared for in the home setting, with minimal periods of hospitalization. Recent research has focused on the improved delivery of care through the use of a medical home. In 1967 the AAP developed the concept of the medical home and in 2002 defined a medical home as primary care that is "accessible, continuous, comprehensive, family-centered, coordinated, compassionate, and culturally affective" (Drummond, Looman, & Phillips, 2012, p. 267). There are many benefits to having children with special healthcare needs cared for in a medical home, including improved communication between providers and between providers and families, increased access to care, and decreased parental stress. Based on these benefits, the Department of Health & Human Services has identified access to a medical home for children with special healthcare needs as a "national health objective " (Drummond et al., 2012). Although improved quality of life and longevity are positive developments, they do present certain difficulties. Despite healthcare advances, the child and family must live with a constant physical problem and uncertainty that require consistent, ongoing attention and adaptation. The course of a chronic illness and the impact on the lives of all those involved is referred to as the **illness trajectory**. For children, it is difficult to accurately predict the progression of many serious, long-term illnesses (Ullrich, Duncan, Joselow, et al., 2016).

Chronic illness is stressful and can create situational crises for families. A situational crisis is an unexpected crisis for which the family's usual problem-solving abilities are not adequate. However, studies show that some families reorganize and actually become stronger in response to a situational crisis. These families are considered resilient;

### BOX 36.1 Common Chronic Conditions of Childhood

- Attention-deficit/hyperactivity disorder (ADHD)
- Attention-deficit disorder (ADD)
- Asthma (reactive airway disease)
- Autism
- Bleeding disorders (e.g., hemophilia)
- Bronchopulmonary dysplasia
- Cancer
- Cardiac disorders
- Cerebral palsy
- Chronic renal failure
- Congenital heart disease and other heart conditions
- Cystic fibrosis
- Developmental delay
- Diabetes mellitus
- Down syndrome
- Hepatitis
- Human immunodeficiency virus (HIV) infection
- Acquired immunodeficiency syndrome (AIDS)
- Hydrocephalus
- Inborn errors of metabolism
- Juvenile arthritis
- Lupus erythematosus
- Intellectual impairment (formerly, mental retardation)
- Muscular dystrophy
- Neural tube defects
- Phenylketonuria
- Seizure disorders
- Sickle cell disease

that is, they are able to recover from adversities associated with chronic illness. They do this through **normalization**, making necessary changes in their lives and adjusting to the presence of the chronic illness. They actively work on responses that will help counteract the illness and the resulting abnormal behaviors to maintain social roles that are appropriate and valued.

Family resiliency implies present and future success at managing complex aspects of a crisis, such as having a child with a chronic condition. Resilient families are able to withstand or recover from traumatic stress such as the illness of a child (Rosenburg, Baker, Syrjala, et al., 2013). Resilient families exhibit many important traits, but a predominant trait is family cohesiveness. This cohesion is achieved through active efforts to keep the family intact by sharing the new responsibilities related to the chronic condition as well as the routine, enjoyable activities of family life. Although family life may be altered by the crisis, resilient families become skilled at successfully managing day-to-day tasks, even though roles within the family structure might need to be altered. Families accomplish these changes by developing protective factors to counteract the stress inherent in caring for a child with a chronic illness and by accessing resources to assist them. Processes that enhance family resilience include the following (Drummond, et al., 2012):

- Establishing and accessing both internal and external sources of physical, social, and financial support
- Reframing the situation to identify positive rather than negative aspects
- Successful coping that increases family self-efficacy, or the belief that the family can problem solve in new ways to meet the new challenges
- Maintaining high-quality and open communication patterns
- Being flexible
- Maintaining social integration
- Preserving family boundaries

Maintaining social integration involves balancing the needs of the family with the needs imposed by the child's condition, as well as reciprocal interactions with the community relative to the child's needs. Resilient families are careful in allocating resources, including money, time, and energy, as they balance various needs. This balance ensures that no child in the family, ill or well, is neglected or overindulged. Additionally, it ensures that the condition-related needs of the ill child are balanced with normal growth and development needs and that needs are met without overprotection. Parents might view the ill child with perceptions of vulnerability termed "vulnerable child syndrome," which can affect parenting and cause parents to doubt their ability to care for their child (Cousino & Hazen, 2013). In resilient families, the child's condition-related needs are incorporated into the family's daily life; they do not become the focus around which the activities of the entire family revolve. This integration helps achieve and maintain the family's new normality imposed by the illness. In such a family setting, baseball practices, school activities, ballet recitals, and other activities do not stop for either the ill child or the well siblings. Rather, care of the child, medical appointments, and treatments for the ill child are arranged around these activities to the degree possible. When conflicts do arise, parents (or other family members or friends) alternate responsibility for maintaining the activities of both the ill child and well siblings.

Equitable allocation of care giving and encouragement of parental involvement with each other and the well siblings help maintain appropriate family boundaries. When either of the two parents becomes primarily involved in meeting the needs of the ill child, the parental relationship suffers. To keep these boundaries intact, resilient families pay specific attention to maintaining a positive parental relationship. They also work to avoid showing favoritism toward the ill child.

Single-parent families may encounter additional difficulties that heighten the risks that the chronic condition will negatively affect resilience and impede normalization. Social support may not be inherent in the family structure, so these families are at increased risk for social isolation. Healthcare providers can refer single parents to support groups, put them in contact with other parents who have a child with a similar chronic condition, or organize group-sharing experiences between parents knowledgeable in the care of the child with a particular chronic condition and parents of newly diagnosed children.

Boundary problems of a different sort can arise when the need for outside care and assistance increases, as with the presence of home health or hospice personnel. Whether they are in the home around the clock or for various shifts throughout the week, external family boundaries can be negatively affected. However, difficulties can be minimized if family members adopt an assertive role in managing the child's care and, along with the healthcare personnel, work to maintain professional relationships and boundaries with caregivers.

Resilient families consistently work to ensure appropriate communication, which can be more difficult because of new, condition-related language (medical or otherwise); an increased need for problem-solving–based communication; and, most important, the need to express emotions. Accepting the validity of all emotions and learning suitable means of expressing them may be difficult. However, many families report that the experience of living with a chronic illness brings about positive life changes, such as increased empathy, increased family unity, and new meanings to life.

Even when positive meaning is attached to a child's chronic condition, much flexibility is required of family members regarding family roles and expectations. This flexibility is also required of the healthcare team, both for the benefit of the family and as a means of achieving a positive, collaborative relationship between the team and the family. The team becomes an integral part of family life. The quality of this relationship may affect how the entire family adapts to and copes with the child's condition.

For resilient families, coping is an active process that entails learning about their child's illness and available resources. These families do not sit idly by, letting others meet their child's needs. They are also the strongest advocates for their child. Subsequently, they have a tremendous need for any information concerning their child's condition. The nurse has an important role in helping families educate themselves and learn to meet their child's special healthcare needs.

At times of extreme stress, such as periods of unexpected physical setbacks, exacerbations, worsening or relapse of the condition, as well as at the time of death, families may slip into less effective patterns of behavior and coping that can affect family functioning. The association between increased parental stress and adverse sequelae for both the caregiver and the child is well documented (Cousino & Hazen, 2013). Therefore, gentle reminders, support, and encouragement may be all the assistance that a resilient family needs to help members resume the behaviors that foster resiliency despite the many ongoing stressors and uncertainties of a chronic condition.

## Coping and the Grieving Process

The most important aspect of a chronic illness is that it affects the entire family, not just the ill child. This scope of concern necessitates consistent family-centered nursing care (see Chapter 3). All family members respond to the child's chronic condition. However, responses of individual family members vary according to their age and developmental level, their relationship and involvement with the ill child, and any previous experiences they have had with a healthcare problem. Fathers are becoming more and more involved in the care of their children, and a father's ability to cope is integral in family-centered care. Studies show that fathers' inability to cope was often related to fear, anxiety, uncertainty, and lack of communication (Broger & Zeni, 2011). Nurses need to include fathers in all aspects of care and encourage paternal involvement and assess their coping mechanisms (Broger & Zeni, 2011).

Chronic and terminal conditions involve the loss of health and result in grief. Grief is a normal psychophysiologic process that occurs in response to a specific loss. A normal and frequent response to such conditions includes the five stages of grief as defined by Elisabeth Kübler-Ross (1969). Her work identified the stages in relation to the anticipated death of an adult. However, they can apply to children as well as adults and to the grief associated with a chronic condition as well as a terminal illness. The ill child, siblings, parents, and other family members may experience these stages.

The stages include denial, anger, bargaining, sadness or depression, and acceptance. During the first stage, *denial,* individuals react with disbelief and shock. Feelings of "no, not me" and "no, not my loved one" occur whether the person is explicitly told of the diagnosis or, in the case of some children, they figure it out on their own. *Anger* usually follows denial. This may include feelings of rage and resentment directed at themselves or at others. At this point, the questions of "why me?" and "why my loved one?" may also occur. Anger may recur at any time during the process of the illness. *Bargaining* then happens, whereby the individual attempts to postpone the inevitable. Although most bargaining is with a spiritual deity, bargaining with oneself or others may also take place.

*Depression* is the next stage. Such sadness can be for either past losses or those impending. Past losses can include physical losses, such as a change in appearance (e.g., hair loss), lifestyle changes, or changes in physical ability. Impending losses include the imminent loss of loved ones and preparing loved ones for the absence created by death. The last stage is *acceptance,* whereby the individual is no longer depressed or angry. Although acceptance is not necessarily a happy stage, it is generally a time of comfort and peace.

Individuals need different periods of time to work through and resolve the feelings of one stage before proceeding to the next. The stages are not always experienced sequentially. Some fluctuation can occur across stages before acceptance and comfort are reached. Acceptance of a chronic illness can take place even in the presence of noticeable denial. Such denial might appear to be maintained throughout the course of the illness. Because children have less predictable and more variable protective mechanisms, they may use denial more frequently than adults. An individual who has a positive, optimistic outlook and who focuses on concerns and tasks of the day rather than on fears about the condition may appear to be adjusting well; however, he or she may be using denial as a protective coping mechanism. As adjustment to the condition progresses, many parents experience chronic sorrow related to the unending nature of the child's condition and the ongoing feelings of loss. There is a deep sense of sadness that is common in bereavement; from this sadness comes solace (Klass, 2013). Chronic sorrow is a normal process that may never resolve. However, adaptation to the presence of the illness occurs. The family establishes a "new normal," and the family's life continues. However, chronic sorrow is not the same as prolonged or chronic grief. Chronic grief refers to mourning that is of excessive duration and interferes with the individual's ability to return to normal living, after the death of a significant person. Poor grief outcomes can be identified by stress-related symptoms such as anxiety, poor sleeping, insecurity, fatigue, and depression (Bugge, Haugstvedt, Røkholt, et al., 2012). An adolescent's grief over the death of a sibling can go unrecognized and become complicated as the adolescent has trouble acknowledging the death of their sibling. These adolescents are at increased risk for suicide (Balk, 2011).

The first step in supporting families and helping them deal with chronic sorrow is to listen and then recognize and acknowledge their emotions. The family can be assisted to recognize the normality of such feelings and emotions themselves. Family members should be gently encouraged to acknowledge and express feelings of chronic sorrow, to the degree with which they are comfortable. However, at the same time, they should be encouraged and assisted to verbalize and demonstrate realistic hopes and dreams. It is important to stress the nonlinear nature of grieving so parents understand that they may revisit the different stages of grief many times in subsequent years (Stroebe, Schut, & Finkenauer, 2013). Studies suggest that the average length of parental bereavement of a loss of a child is 18 years. In some cases the parents struggle with their relationship following the death of a child while others support each other and cope well as a couple (Stroebe et al., 2013). Nurses have a role in consoling family members by using soothing words, physical touch, and being present in an open and honest manner that will instill trust (Klass, 2013). Support groups offer much beyond the information related to the child's condition. The nurse should introduce the family to such services and, as necessary, assist them to use these services fully. Other bereaved parents can offer the parents support and are better able to understand what the parents are feeling, since others who have not experienced the death of a child cannot truly understand what they are experiencing (Klass, 2013). Conversely, a family's decision not to use support services should be respected.

Supportive services may be particularly important when observation and assessment of family behaviors indicate problems that may necessitate referral to a mental health professional. In caring for children with chronic or terminal illnesses and their families, one issue that is frequently overlooked is that death may occur unexpectedly or earlier than anticipated. This is an important but difficult issue to address with families. It should be done in the early stage of the condition to prepare them if the death does happen in an unexpected manner. The nurse should support children and their families through all stages of the grief process. Supporting the family requires understanding the family's current knowledge base, coping skills, and personal beliefs, as well as recognizing and attending to the grief-related problems that arise.

## THE CHILD WITH SPECIAL HEALTHCARE NEEDS

### Coping and Growth and Development Concerns

Children with chronic disorders have many different concerns and needs related to their conditions, not the least of which is successful navigation of the stages of growth and development. Children's responses to illness are influenced by their age at the onset of the disorder, as well as growth and development considerations throughout the course of the illness. Nursing care is planned accordingly.

Chronic and terminal conditions often span a number of years and developmental stages. Regardless of the stage, concerns related to self-esteem, self-reliance, and autonomy are prevalent among children with chronic conditions. Many will experience altered body awareness and body image as a result of physical changes related to the illness or treatment. These changes frequently have a negative impact on children's self-esteem. Control and autonomy can be decreased by hospitalizations and treatment regimens that offer few decision-making opportunities for the child. Socialization activities and adjustment may be limited as a result of hospitalization and the side effects of the illness or treatment. Side effects, including altered appearance, decreased physical ability, or increased susceptibility to infection, can interfere with age-appropriate socialization. There can be times when a medical condition (e.g., infection risk, bleeding risk) does not keep the child from participating, but the child declines to do so because of fears regarding his or her appearance or physical abilities.

Such factors can profoundly affect a child's acquisition of age-appropriate growth and developmental skills, especially during adolescence. An important goal is to minimize the effects of illness and hospitalization and to maximize the child's developmental potential. This is true regardless of the age or developmental stage, and the nurse should understand issues concerning self-esteem and autonomy in relation to each stage of growth and development (Box 36.2).

Despite the understanding and interventions of family and staff, a variety of consequences may frequently occur among children with a chronic condition or illness. Most are minimal, short lived, and expected as a part of the course of a chronic condition. For example, stranger anxiety may be heightened or may reappear months after previous resolution among infants and toddlers.

Temporary regression may be seen with children of all ages, including adolescents. However, it is more prevalent among older infants through the young school-age years. Toddlers use regression frequently as they attempt to cope with the stress of a serious illness. Despite the normalcy of regression, it may be unsettling to the child and family because it involves the loss of recently acquired skills or the reappearance of behaviors seen when the child was younger. Common regressive behaviors include reverting back to a bottle, pacifier, or thumb-sucking; a change in toileting skills; an increased incidence of bed-wetting; and an increased use of "baby talk" or communication techniques more appropriate for younger children.

Another possible difficulty is a fluctuation in the child's age-appropriate communication patterns between family and members of the healthcare team. Lack of communication or altered communication patterns with healthcare providers can occur in the clinic or hospital setting, with regular patterns of communication resuming at home. Among older preschoolers, a lack of communication can be a form of withdrawal or an expression of stubbornness and a refusal to cooperate. This problem is also being seen in school-age children and adolescents, usually related to issues involving independence and self-esteem.

Some children with special healthcare needs will benefit from a care plan developed with the assistance of the family. For instance children with Autism Spectrum Disorder can demonstrate difficult behavior while in the healthcare setting, especially during hospitalization (Chun & Berrios-Candelaria, 2012). These types of challenging behaviors are often a way of communicating their frustration with the experience. Nurses can assist parents in teaching children acceptable coping behaviors which can improve healthcare visits. Some methods are showing pictures to communicate, introducing change slowly, providing an outlet for stress and frustration, decreasing wait times and developing individualized health plans to assist healthcare teams (Johnson & Rodriguez, 2013).

### Coping and Parental Responses to Developmental Issues

Regardless of the developmental stage or the number of years that a chronic illness has existed, the basic guidelines for child rearing still apply to all children in the family. Boundaries, discipline, and consistency are equally important to both the ill child and the well siblings. A good example is the mother of a 3-year-old with cancer who would frequently remind both the ill child and her older sibling that cancer is no excuse for bad manners! However, for some parents, this is difficult, and they adapt a more permissive style of parenting with lower expectations for children with chronic illnesses (Rempel, Ravindran, Rogers, et al., 2012).

Experiencing a chronic illness is confusing, especially for children whose cognitive abilities are not sufficiently developed to allow understanding that could help them cope with the stress. When changes in a child's world begin to affect the family, the only constant he or she knows, it is often reflected in the child's behavior. Negative behavior can result from the stress of the illness and changes in the family and environment. Previously existing negative behaviors may worsen, making treatment and a positive, cooperative relationship with healthcare team members difficult. Future behavior and long-term development may be affected as well. At the time their child is diagnosed, parents should be reminded about the importance of maintaining previous rules and expectations. Chronically ill children are more likely to experience behavioral and psychological issues. Nevertheless, most children with chronic health problems will experience the same level of behavioral and psychological issues as other children in the same age-group (Chamberlain & Wise, 2016).

**! NURSING QUALITY ALERT**

***Goals for Chronic Care***

**Goals for the Child**

- Achieve and maintain normalization
- Obtain the highest level of health and function possible—physically, emotionally, and psychosocially

**Goals for the Family**

- Remain intact
- Achieve and maintain normalization
- Maximize function throughout the course of the illness

## THE CHILD WITH A CHRONIC ILLNESS

The goals for any child with a chronic illness are to achieve and maintain the highest level of health and function possible—cognitively, emotionally, physically, and psychosocially. The aim is similar for the

**BOX 36.2 The Illness Experience: the Child and Adolescent**

**Infant**

*Developmental task:* Achievement of awareness of being separate from significant other

*Impact of illness:* Potential distortion of differentiation of self from parents or significant others

*Cognitive age/stage:* Sensorimotor (birth to 2 years).

*Major fears:* Separation, strangers

*Interventions:* Provide consistent caregivers. Minimize separation from parents and significant others. Decrease parental anxiety, which is projected to infant. Maintain crib and nursery as "safe place" where no invasive procedures are performed.

**Toddler**

*Developmental task:* Initiation of autonomy.

*Impact of illness:* Interference with or loss of developing sense of control, independence

*Cognitive age/stage:* Preoperational (2 to 7 years): egocentric, magical, little concept of body integrity

*Major fears:* Separation, loss of control

*Concept of illness:* Phenomenism (2 to 7 years)—perceives external, unrelated, concrete phenomena as cause of illness (e.g., "being sick because you don't feel well"). Contagion—perceives cause of illness as proximity between two events that occurs by "magic" (e.g., "getting a cold because you are near someone who has a cold").

*Interventions:* Minimize separation from parents or significant others. Keep security objects at hand. Provide simple, brief explanations. Explain and maintain consistent limits. Encourage participation in daily care. Provide opportunities for play.

**Preschooler**

*Developmental task:* Creation of a sense of initiative

*Impact of illness:* Interference with or loss of accomplishments, such as walking, talking, controlling basic body functions

*Cognitive age/stage:* Preoperational thought—egocentric, magical, tendency to use and repeat words child does not understand, providing own explanations and definitions; literal translation of words; inability to abstract.

*Major fears:* Body injury and mutilation, loss of control, the unknown, the dark, being left alone

*Concept of illness:* Phenomenism, contagion

*Interventions:* Provide simple, concrete explanations. Advance preparation is important; days for major events, hours for minor events. Verbal explanations are usually insufficient, so use pictures, models, actual equipment, and medical play.

**School-Age Child**

Developmental task: Sense of industry

Impact of illness: Potential feelings of inadequacy or inferiority if autonomy and independence are compromised

Cognitive age/stage: Concrete operational thought (7 to 10 years)

Major fears: Loss of control, body injury and mutilation, failure to live up to expectations of important others, death

Concept of illness: Contamination—perceives cause as a person, an object, or an action external to the child that is "bad" or "harmful" to the body (e.g., "getting a cold because you didn't wear a hat"). Internalization—perceives illness as having an external cause but being located inside the body (e.g., "getting a cold by breathing in air and bacteria").

Interventions: Provide choices whenever possible to increase the child's sense of control. Emphasize contact with peer group. Use diagrams, pictures, and models for explanations because thinking is concrete. Emphasize the "normal" things the child can do because the child does not want to be seen as different. Reassure children that they have done nothing wrong; hospitalization, for example, is not punishment.

**Adolescent**

*Developmental task:* Achieving a sense of identity

*Impact of illness:* Potential alteration in or relinquishment of newly acquired roles and responsibilities

*Cognitive age/stage:* Formal operational thought (11+ years): beginning of ability to think abstractly; presence of some magical thinking (e.g., feeling guilty for illness) and egocentrism

*Major fears:* Loss of control, altered body image, separation from peer group

*Concept of illness:* Physiologic—perceives cause as malfunctioning or nonfunctioning organ or process; can explain illness in sequence of events. Psychophysiologic—realizes that psychological actions and attitudes affect health and illness

*Interventions:* Allow adolescent to be an integral part of decision making regarding care. Give information sensitively because adolescents react both to the content of information and to the manner in which it is delivered. Allow as many choices and as much control as possible. Be honest about treatment and its consequences. Stress the importance of cooperation and adherence. Additionally, emphasize decision making in which the adolescent can participate, as well as the areas in life over which control can be maintained. Assist in maintaining contact with peer group.

Data from Bibace, R., & Walsh, M.E. (1980). Development of children's concepts of illness. *Pediatrics, 66*(6), 912–918; Gibbons, M.B. (1993). Psychosocial aspects of serious illness in childhood and adolescence. In A. Armstrong-Dailey, & S. Goltzer (Eds.), *Hospice care for children.* New York: Oxford University Press.

family system, including parents or guardians, siblings, and extended family members. Goals for the entire family are to remain intact, achieve and maintain normalization, and maximize function throughout the illness. Attaining this goal necessitates a family-centered approach to nursing care.

The nursing process for the child with a chronic illness is ongoing for the duration of the illness. It may be more complex because the goals are both physical and psychosocial. The psychosocial environment is significant in that it greatly influences the manner in which the child relates to others and copes with stress. In addition, the entire family is involved, as well as the ill child. Care is provided over a span of years and must often incorporate rapid changes in the child's growth and development. The nurse is prepared for a changing assessment, both physical and psychosocial, related to the duration of care and fluctuations in the illness.

The planning and implementation of nursing care are based on several factors. The child's physical condition is the first consideration. Generalization across broad categories of illnesses, such as cancer, respiratory conditions, or cardiac problems, is not possible. Each illness has specific implications, including subsequent disabilities that affect the child's growth and development across the span of the illness. Additionally, the needs, coping mechanisms, and available resources of child and family are influencing factors. Nursing care includes assisting the child and family to accept, understand, and incorporate the illness appropriately into each stage of growth and development, regardless of the child's age at diagnosis.

## Ongoing Care

Evaluations, as well as subsequent modifications in the planning and implementation of nursing care, often take place on a daily basis because of the child's frequent physical changes. Unexpected setbacks, such as an exacerbation, a relapse, a critical infection, an undesirable response to medication, a lack of physical progress, or the need to undergo a medical or surgical procedure unexpectedly or sooner than anticipated, can be standard parts of the chronic illness. Goals may have to be repeatedly altered. All changes can be stressful and difficult for the child and family to handle, even though they have been coping with an illness for a long period of time. Continuous support and reassurance are necessary throughout the course of the illness.

### Education

With an illness that continues for several years, numerous changes occur because of the child's physical condition or increasing age. Education involves the child and family, addressing both physical and psychosocial needs. It is imperative that the family has an accurate knowledge base to provide care to the child at home.

One important consideration in relation to education and support for the ill child and siblings is involvement of a child life specialist (Fig. 36.1). The child life specialist uses methods that are educational, supportive, and therapeutic. These include medical play and art, and therapeutic play and art. All are similar in that they present the ill child with opportunities for learning, for increased expression of feelings, and for developing additional coping methods. The nurse can also use some of these techniques in daily care or when a child life specialist cannot be present.

### Communication

Communication with the ill child may be more difficult than the physical care (see Chapter 4). Communication is the most important factor in establishing a good relationship with the child and family. *Appropriate communication involves both honesty and compassion. It is always based on the child's age and development.* Following these principles can help decrease the child's fears and misunderstandings and increase the child's confidence in nurses and other members of the healthcare team. Increased cooperation with the therapeutic regimen is an additional benefit. If fears and misunderstandings are not alleviated at the beginning and caregivers do not gain the child's trust, establishing trust at a later date can be more difficult. This is particularly true when the nursing care involves unpleasant or painful medications and treatments.

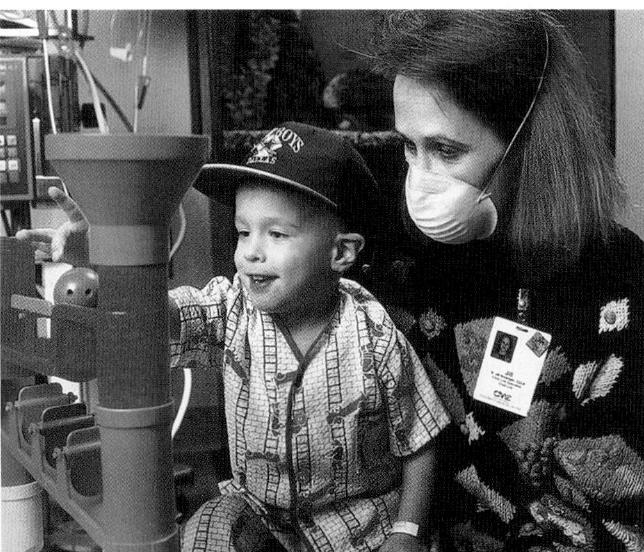

FIG 36.1 The nurse or a child life specialist can use therapeutic play, medical play, and therapeutic art to enhance self-expression, education, and growth and development. (Courtesy Norm Tindell for Cook Children's Medical Center, Fort Worth, TX.)

To prevent misinterpretations and misunderstandings, the nurse can ask children to explain what they know and understand. The nurse should also strive to understand what the child is really asking. Clarifying questions can help the nurse avoid providing more information than the child wants or can handle emotionally. Providing too much information can be overwhelming and frightening to the child and might inhibit future questions and interaction with the nurses.

Honesty and trust must be maintained at all times when caring for the child. These principles should be encouraged among the family and other members of the healthcare team. Complete honesty causes problems for some family and staff members, especially when they face the difficult questions that often arise when caring for a chronically or terminally ill child. The most difficult and feared questions are usually centered on whether the child is going to die and why he or she became sick and is dying. These questions are followed closely by those concerning the deaths of other children whom the child has known or with whom the child has developed a close relationship.

Children are often reluctant to ask questions of adults and to ask questions when they fear the answers. Often, the child already knows the answer, so the question is really a test concerning honesty and a point of reference in the child's relationship with the adult (parent or healthcare provider). As with adults, children need honesty to establish trust. They may not understand the use of dishonesty as a means of protecting them against emotional pain or unpleasantness. Once children have experienced dishonesty from an adult, they can feel that they cannot and will not trust any of the adults around them, parents or healthcare providers. Dishonesty can have damaging effects, particularly when trying to reassure a child and gain cooperation. If a chronic condition becomes terminal, the child's trust can be paramount to achieving comfort and peace.

For children with a chronic condition, honesty can increase their emotional pain to some degree and, conversely, help comfort them at the same time. Honest answers to a child's difficult questions are not always handled well by family members. The nurse strives to help family members understand the importance of maintaining the child's trust, to explore their feelings about providing honest answers to the child's questions, and to establish communication guidelines. The family might give instructions about communication that brings about conflict for the nurse, both professionally and personally. The family might ask that the nurse answer deceitfully concerning the serious nature of the illness or the fact that the child is expected to die. In many situations, a compromise is reached in that the nurse will not initiate conversations that could lead to questions about whether the child is expected to die. However, if the child initiates the conversation and asks questions directly, the nurse will reply honestly, in terms approved by the family. This approach may not work with some families. In such instances, other members of the healthcare team (physicians, child life therapists, social workers, pastoral care providers) can become involved to make communication decisions that best suit the needs of all involved.

### Caring for Parents

Healthcare professionals can support parents in the following ways (Broger & Zeni, 2011):

- Increase parents' confidence
- Acknowledge each parent as a person
- Acknowledge the parents as the child's healthcare provider and the experts on the child
- Ease the parents' daily worries by providing information and easy access to the healthcare provider when questions and problems arise
- Acknowledge the child as valuable and unique
- Help the parents see the child's potential and abilities
- Help the parents understand the child's normal growth and development needs
- Encourage the parents and healthcare team to reach mutually set goals

### Grief Education and Support

Nursing care should include education about the child's condition and treatment, as well as education concerning any grief issues. The nurse helps all family members, including the child, to understand and express their grief in the manner most comfortable for them. Taking time to provide care and support in this area is as important as physical care. Many adults have not experienced illness or death before the child's diagnosis and are not accustomed to the idea of grief, much less grief as a normal, healthy process. In addition, some family members may have had a previous experience with dying, death, and grief that they perceived as negative and distressing. Both situations can increase the support needs among the family.

The nurse educates the family about the importance of the grief process and provides opportunities for grieving. Nursing care can include conversations and time "being present" with family. Being present for all family members as the need arises entails the important aspect of listening and sitting in silence. Many times family members do not need or want conversation; they just want to be with someone who knows their child and is familiar with what they might be experiencing. This may be true even for siblings. Children who just want to be with an adult may require only that the person sit with them while they play. The expression of emotions is recognized to be more beneficial for most individuals than holding the emotions inside. However, for some, emotional expressions are not a normal or comfortable part of their lives before their child's illness. The nurse accepts each family member's choice to express or not express emotions while letting them know that a caring individual is available at any time should the need for talking and sharing arise.

### Cultural and Religious Beliefs

Culture and religion influence the meaning of illness and death, as well as customs observed by the family. Assessing the perceptions of the child and family regarding chronic illness, hospitalization, and disability in light of the family's culture facilitates culturally sensitive nursing care. When faced with an unfamiliar culture or religion, the nurse becomes familiar with beliefs and practices honored and used by the family. The nurse and the entire healthcare team should communicate acceptance of the family's beliefs. Team members must not assume that a family belongs to a particular religion or denomination based solely on their cultural background. In addition, they should not assume that a family adheres to all beliefs and practices of its religion or denomination. If in doubt, the nurse should ask questions of the family, stressing the need for information to provide the most comprehensive and appropriate care possible. Language barriers can lead to poor communication and adverse health outcomes. Nurses must ensure that health disparities do not exist due to language barriers by identifying patients and families with limited English proficiency (Bonilla & Edwards, 2011).

### Referrals

To the degree possible, the nurse should endeavor to make sure that the physical, emotional, psychosocial, and cognitive needs of the child and family are met. Additionally, nursing care includes assisting family members to provide for the child's physical and psychosocial needs. The nurse works as a member of an extensive healthcare team and determines when referrals need to be made to professionals with expertise needed by the child and family. For example, the child with a chronic illness and the family may need services from clergy members, psychologists, and social workers. Hospital chaplains generally have access to information on various religious beliefs, as well as to clergy members from different religious groups. Psychologists can provide ongoing counseling to the child and family on an individual or group basis. Social workers are able to provide information concerning available resources for the family related to finances, insurance, government assistance, housing, transportation, and medical care and supplies.

### Schooling

The face of public education and the child with special healthcare needs has changed dramatically. The Education for All Handicapped Children Act (PL 94-142), now codified as Individuals with Disabilities Education Act (IDEA), and subsequent amendments (most notably the Individuals with Disabilities Education Act, 1997) ensure a free, public education for each child with a disability or other chronic condition. The act also mandates that special education and support services be provided in the least restrictive environment for children ages 3 years and older. Consequently, children with a wide variety of physical needs are able to receive appropriate educational services and attend public school. These needs range from relatively simple needs (e.g., medication administration, respiratory treatments) to more extensive needs (e.g., gastrostomy tube feedings, management of tracheostomy tubes, ventilators). Facilitating the start or return to school for the child with special needs requires preparation and assistance from a healthcare team that includes the child, family, hospital or clinic nurse, school nurse, teacher, counselor, and director of special education for the school district.

A specific, structured plan of care is developed before the child's return to school. This plan is accomplished by the school system through a legally mandated process referred to as an *individualized educational program* (IEP) or *admission, review, and dismissal* (ARD) meeting. This plan is developed with input from members of the healthcare team, who are encouraged to attend the actual meeting, if possible. It addresses cognitive and physical needs in relation to the child's school attendance and includes learning goals that might require some modifications as a result of the child's special needs and chronic condition, as well as the specific tasks for achieving such goals. The plan also addresses any special healthcare that needs to be provided while the child is in school, such as medications, feedings, or breathing treatments. Planning conferences are held before the child is scheduled to start school for the first time after his or her condition has been diagnosed. After the initial plan, an IEP or ARD meeting must take place at least once a year and when changes in the child's condition occur that will necessitate changes in the schooling plan. Most schools offer children the opportunity to attend school full or part time as their conditions allow and to receive homebound instruction when necessary. Regardless of the type of school services the child is receiving, the hospital or clinic nurse may need to provide ongoing education and support to the school nurse and other school personnel.

Special considerations are given in the school setting for a child who is immunosuppressed, whether related to a disease or to treatment. Preventing the infection that can occur with immunosuppression is a challenge in the school setting, regardless of the age of the child. Reasons include the crowded conditions in school classrooms and the often inadequate infection control practices of children (e.g., good hand hygiene). The school nurse should alert teachers to be particularly vigilant and notify the nurse if any children with infectious diseases are present in the classroom. Families of all school children are asked to notify the school if their children contract a serious communicable illness such as strep throat and to keep their children out of school until their disease is no longer contagious. The school nurse may also visit classrooms and present health-teaching modules on general infection-prevention practices. The school nurse must obtain information about the specific signs to look for when monitoring the condition of the chronically ill child and how to contact the child's healthcare team directly and quickly if concerns arise.

Ongoing psychosocial support can also be necessary for the child and family in relation to school. Some parents experience mixed emotions regarding their child's return to school. They are likely to be pleased and excited that the child is well enough to attend school. At the same time, they can be concerned about the child's well-being during school hours, particularly whether the child's special healthcare needs will be met appropriately. For children with a terminal condition, parents can also experience a degree of sorrow about being apart during what limited time they have with their child. The child's siblings can experience similar feelings. The nurse can best provide support by maintaining ongoing communication with the family and recognizing that problems and concerns with school vary over time. Referral to a spiritual counselor, social worker, or mental health professional may also be helpful for the psychosocial support of the child and family.

For hospitalized children, the nurse must also consider the child's educational needs. School is an integral part of a child's life from a very early age. It is often the child's first concept of structure in their world (Eaton, 2012). What is the effect of missing school on a child with a chronic illness? Studies show that the effect is great, citing it as the top stress-related concern (Eaton, 2012). Therefore, in 2008, the Joint Commission required hospitals to arrange for a child to receive academic education. One way hospitals can assist children who are missing school is to use distance learning resources and complete homework and other activities online. Many hospitals employ teachers as liaisons between the hospital and the school system. The benefit of these services are many, especially the message to chronically or terminally ill children that they have purpose and will continue to live a normal life with education as a central feature, thereby maintaining structure and support (Eaton, 2012). Nurses who care for children with a life-threatening illness can support the school community by addressing their educational needs. If a student dies, the school community needs time to grieve, and it is important to understand that students express their grief in different ways and will need to be supported (Heller, Coleman, Best, et al., 2014).

### The Nurse as Liaison

The nurse is a liaison for the family in many different situations. However, the most important liaison work is to link the family with other members of the healthcare team, particularly the physician. In this capacity, the nurse can help guarantee that family members receive accurate information and have an appropriate understanding of their child's condition, as well as resulting psychosocial and physical needs. These efforts can facilitate the family's healthcare planning, working relationship with the healthcare team, communication with care providers, and compliance with the treatment plan.

### Caring for Siblings

The concerns and needs of siblings in relation to their brother or sister's chronic illness vary according to age and developmental stage. Thus, fluctuations are common when the child's chronic condition exists for several years. Siblings may have many of the same anxieties and fears as their parents.

Siblings often have feelings of guilt regarding their perceived role in the ill child's condition. Many children have had thoughts of what life would be like without having to share material possessions and parental love with their sibling(s). When a sibling then becomes ill, the guilt and associated emotions can be overwhelming. The well siblings should be reassured about the normalcy of such feelings and that the illness is not the result of anything that they said, thought, or did.

Nursing care of siblings involves education regarding the ill child's condition, treatment, physical changes, disabilities, and expected disease progression. The siblings should ideally be kept up to date regarding changes in the ill child's condition, both positive and negative. The same principles of honest communication apply both to siblings and to the child with the illness. However, what information is ultimately shared with siblings is at the parents' discretion. The hospital setting's rules, equipment, and personnel must also be explained to siblings in terms appropriate for their developmental level. If possible and suitable, siblings may be allowed to participate in the physical care of the ill child.

Siblings sometimes regress in developmental stage and activities. Parents frequently do not expect such behavioral changes from a well sibling. They might need to be reminded that in the presence of a stressful event, regression is a normal coping mechanism for all children, both ill and well.

The nurse can help siblings understand that illness creates stress that can result in difficult or painful emotions such as anger and jealousy. Children need to know that these emotions are a normal part of life, although they are often perceived as negative and harmful. Siblings must be allowed to have and express these feelings (Fig. 36.2). Healthcare professionals and the family must provide care and support to meet the psychosocial and emotional needs of the siblings to prevent added stress for the family that could negatively affect the ill child.

The nurse and family should include siblings as much as possible in the life and activities of the ill child, whether the child is hospitalized or receives outpatient care. The family will require education and input from the healthcare team regarding the pros and cons of sibling involvement. Spiritual or cultural beliefs may affect this type of decision. Many families choose to minimize siblings' time and involvement in the healthcare setting as a means of keeping the siblings' lives as normal and uninterrupted as possible. Other families try to maintain the existing degree of closeness between the siblings and the ill child and choose to have the siblings closely involved in the ill child's care at the hospital, including siblings being present during the day and for overnight visits, if permitted. Studies have found that time spent in the hospital with the sibling can be enjoyable and provides a way for the sibling to be involved and become closer to their family (Bugel, 2014). The family's decisions related to sibling involvement should be supported by the healthcare team.

The nurse ensures that siblings receive appropriate education to decrease misunderstandings and fears related to the ill child's condition and treatments as well as the emotions and behaviors of their parents and other adults. Medical play, therapeutic play, and therapeutic art are excellent means of educating and providing support

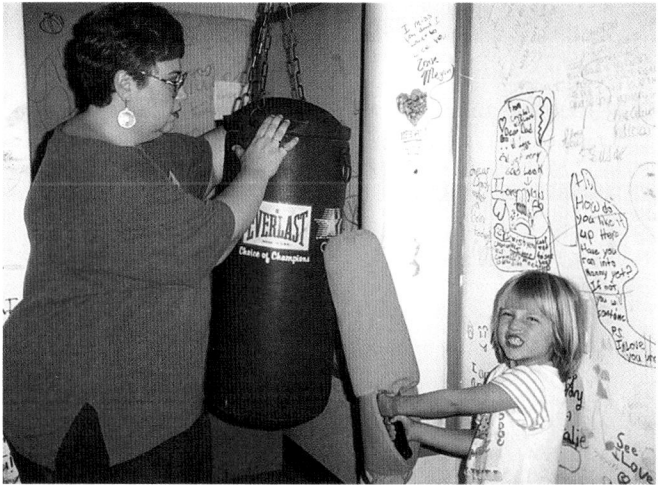

FIG 36.2 Chronic illness is stressful for the siblings of an ill child. Siblings' emotional needs may be overlooked. Siblings should be given the opportunity to express negative feelings such as anger and jealousy through therapeutic art and play, as well as through physical outlets such as striking a punching bag, as this little girl is doing. (Courtesy Gwen T. Martin, RN, Fort Worth, TX.)

to the siblings. These interventions can also help siblings understand their intense and confusing emotional responses, as well as how to express them in a healthy, appropriate manner. Nurses striving to teach, support, and include siblings in the care of the ill child should collaborate with the child life specialist.

Extensive sibling involvement can also bring additional risks. Siblings might be exposed to the ill child's severe physical and emotional experiences, which can have emotional consequences. Close attention from the healthcare team and family members can help determine whether siblings have needs for interventions by nurses, physicians, child life specialists, clergy, social workers, or professional counselors.

The relationship between the ill child and siblings can be altered because of normal feelings of resentment, jealousy, and competition as the siblings see the ill child receiving additional attention. They may resent being left in the care of other family members as the parents are consumed with the care of the ill child. Siblings may experience guilt and shame about such feelings. Siblings often are left out of the communications, leading to a lack of information that increases their anxiety. One study cited the lack of greeting by nurses and other medical staff as leading to feelings of insignificance and loneliness (Bugel, 2014). It is important for the nursing staff, child life specialist, social worker, and chaplain to give individual attention to the siblings separately from the ill child. Siblings can also be referred to support groups. These interventions provide siblings the opportunity to gain understanding and accept the normality of their feelings by verbalizing emotions, interacting with caring, nonjudgmental adults, and talking with peers who share similar experiences. In assessing family needs, it is important to assess the needs of the sibling and the parent's wishes for the amount of involvement of the siblings (Bugel, 2014).

Because the ill child often receives extra attention, including gifts, from family and friends, the siblings may associate illness with extra attention and gifts and subsequently experience real or imagined illnesses as a bid for similar attention. The nurse should encourage family and friends to give attention and gifts to the siblings as well as to the ill child. It is also helpful to acknowledge siblings' accomplishments and special times, such as birthdays. Encouraging the parent to spend some time every day with each sibling is essential for the family to maintain positive relationships.

**! NURSING QUALITY ALERT**

***Nursing Care for Children With Chronic Conditions and Their Families***

- Care for a child with a chronic condition means attending to the needs of the family system. Both parents and siblings may need additional support.
- The age and developmental level of the chronically ill child affect both the child's understanding and the family's needs. Goals may need to be frequently revised to meet the child's changing developmental needs.
- The nurse should listen carefully to the child's perception of the condition. A child's illness experience does not always match an adult's view of the physical limitations and emotional stress.

**CRITICAL THINKING EXERCISE 36.1**

How can the nurse apply the principles of family-centered nursing to the family with a chronically ill child?

Maintaining close contact with each sibling's school personnel and keeping them up to date regarding the current circumstances of the ill child are important. This communication can help personnel understand and support the siblings if behavioral issues are noted in school or if increased absences occur due to circumstances with the ill child. Siblings might also turn more frequently to their teacher and other school personnel for support. School personnel working with the siblings need similar educational support as those working with the ill child. The hospital or clinic nurse and child life therapist can make school visits and provide education to personnel, as well as to the siblings' peers and classmates. The family and members of the healthcare team determine the extent of information given to the children.

## THE TERMINALLY ILL OR DYING CHILD

### Coping and the Child's Concept of Death

An understanding of death and dying in relation to childhood is necessary when caring for the child approaching death. The established and accepted guidelines concerning children's concepts of death are based on the stages of growth and development. As Wass (1985) explains, these concepts correlate with age and cognition (Table 36.1). In addition, a child's response to death is affected by culture, environment, social setting, spirituality, and personal experiences with death (Bluebond-Langner, 1978).

#### Infants and Toddlers

Infants and toddlers view death in relation to the loss of a caregiver and the subsequent emptiness in their lives. They are also affected by the loss of comfort measures, as when they experience pain or cold. Consequently, time with primary caregivers is quite important. As they approach death, they often sense the severity of their condition through their parents' nonverbal communication. Children of this age can react to the dying process based on the sadness, anger, and anxiety conveyed by their parents. Reactions will be expressed through crying, attachment to the primary caregiver, and separation anxiety.

#### Preschoolers

Preschoolers view death as a separation or departure and believe it to be only temporary. Death is also seen as reversible. Magical thinking

## NURSING CARE PLAN

### The Child With a Chronic Condition in the Community Setting

#### Focused Assessment

- Provide a comprehensive and collaborative assessment of the chronically ill child.
  - Involve child, family, school personnel, and multidisciplinary healthcare team members.
  - Assess the child's development level and cognitive, physical, and psychosocial abilities.
  - Use assessment as a baseline for developing a hospitalization plan or school individualized education program (IEP).
  - Determine expectations and the level of assistance the child will require.
- Assess the child's perception of physical changes related to the chronic illness and treatments.
  - Address impact on self-esteem, self-reliance, and autonomy.
  - Determine if altered body awareness or image negatively affects self-esteem.
  - Assess over time the perception changes that occur at different developmental stages and school (grade) levels.
- Assess the child and the entire family system for:
  - Communication and behavior patterns and emotional concerns
  - Existing coping and adaptive mechanisms; when child is at home, school, or hospital
  - Inappropriate coping behaviors, considering interventions to support change to beneficial and healthy coping mechanisms.
- Explore family's response to the child's illness.
  - Verify the family's recognition that the illness affects the entire family system.
  - Determine each family member's understandings about the disease process and treatment regimen, correcting misinformation or misinterpretations.
- Assess coping over the course of the chronic disease.
  - Consider the physiologic progression of the disease.
  - Note that as the child's condition changes, the impact on the family will change, and different coping mechanisms will be needed.
- Evaluate and document the family's community support system.
  - Address the influence on family's beliefs, responses, and coping methods.

#### Nursing Diagnosis

Risk for Delayed Development related to the effects of chronic illness or disability.

#### Planning

***Expected Outcomes***

The child will:

1. Experience minimal disturbance of normal growth and development (physical, cognitive, emotional, and psychological), as evidenced by minimal delays and documented by an age-appropriate and reliable developmental screening tool.
2. Experience minimal disturbance of normal growth and development, as evidenced by ability to interact in an age-appropriate manner cognitively, emotionally, physically, and socially to the degree allowed by the existing disability.
3. Experience minimal disturbance of normal growth and development, as evidenced by the ability to perform usual, age-appropriate activities of daily living (ADLs) as allowed by the existing disability.

#### Interventions and *Rationales*

1. Educate the child and family about the physical conditions, expected physical changes or disabilities, and prescribed treatment. Education should be in a manner appropriate for the child's cognitive abilities.
   *This education encourages a sense of control and acceptance of the physical changes as well as increased cooperation with treatment. Some children with chronic conditions have cognitive abilities beyond their chronologic age and are able to discuss medical matters knowledgeably.*
2. Involve the child, family, school personnel, and interdisciplinary healthcare team in setting reasonable goals for improving and maximizing abilities in relation to the existing disability.
   *Goal setting assists children and families to increase their abilities and self-esteem through successful accomplishment of tasks. It may also increase a sense of situational control.*
3. Assist the child in developing a sense of pride in existing physical abilities and to set goals expanding the range of activities.
   *Focusing on regaining skills and participating in preferred activities can provide incentive for achieving new goals (e.g., obtain a driver's license).*
4. Collaborate with the child and school personnel to modify school routines to better fit the child's educational and social schedule and needs.
   *Involving the child in setting meaningful goals will support achievement.*
5. Offer child as many choices and opportunities to make age-appropriate treatment decisions as possible.
   *Offering choices and opportunities to the child promotes autonomy and situational control that are often lost as a result of limitations imposed by the condition or treatment and may improve self-esteem.*
6. Encourage the child to engage in age-appropriate ADLs and self-care. Provide and teach the child to use assistive devices, at home and school.
   *Self-care encourages independence and gives the child an opportunity to practice and improve abilities.*
7. During hospital stays, provide child's own clothes and items from home for grooming, eating, and recreation. Encourage completion of schoolwork and peer visits (e.g., invite peers to special events).
   *Use of personal items, maintaining school involvement, and engaging with peers promote normalization, minimize disturbances in usual routines, and maximize the child's sense of control. School nurses or child life therapists can educate and support peers if fears exist.*

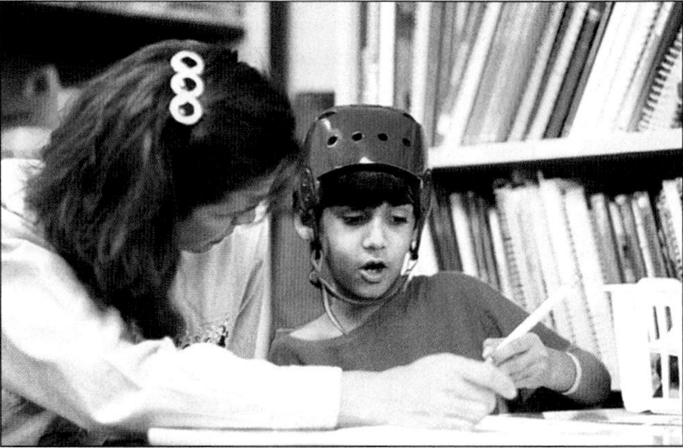

Because more children with chronic conditions are living longer, more attend public school. However, these children are likely to be frequently hospitalized, so hospitals often provide an area where teachers can help them with their studies. (Courtesy Cook Children's Medical Center, Fort Worth, TX.)

8. Provide social activities both in and out of the hospital and encourage peer interactions to the degree allowed by the child's physical condition or treatments. Advise family to schedule clinic visits and treatments to avoid conflicts with social events.

## NURSING CARE PLAN—cont'd

### The Child With a Chronic Condition in the Community Setting

*Ongoing social activities (e.g., sports, school clubs or activities, church, social groups) and peer connections encourage maintenance and acquisition of developmental skills as well as contribute to the child's positive self-esteem and autonomy.*

9. Encourage the child to join general or disease-specific peer support groups and attend special camp programs for children with chronic illness. Respect the decision if the child decides to not participate.
*Support, acceptance, understanding, and learning can be derived from regular interactions with peers who have similar chronic conditions. Support groups may be most beneficial after initial diagnosis, when fears and concerns are high. Considering the individual needs for each child is essential.*

**Evaluation**

Does the child exhibit minimal developmental delays?

Does the child exhibit age-appropriate cognitive, emotional, physical, and social interactions?

Does the child perform age-appropriate ADLs as allowed by the existing disability?

**Nursing Diagnosis**

Interrupted Family Processes related to intermittent situational crisis of chronic illness.

**Planning**

***Expected Outcomes***

The child and family will:

1. Experience normal family functioning, as evidenced by maintaining usual family routines, meeting developmental needs of all family members, and maintaining usual expectations for the ill child.
2. Experience appropriate psychosocial adjustment, as evidenced by expressing feelings, identifying ways to cope effectively, and using appropriate support systems.

**Interventions and *Rationales***

1. Provide information to the family that facilitates a positive, realistic view of their child in relation to the chronic condition. Discuss appropriate behavioral expectations for the chronically ill child.
*Education decreases fears and misconceptions, encourages appropriate interactions between family members and with the healthcare team, and prompts adherence to treatment.*
2. Assist the family to identify and express fears and emotions pertaining to the child's illness. Convey acceptance of feelings and explain that expression is a healthy part of coping.
*Verbalization of feelings, with positive feedback, can help decrease stress and facilitate resolution of negative emotions.*
3. Act as a role model for appropriate, accepting, positive attitudes and behaviors concerning the child.
*A positive role model can facilitate acceptance and adjustment by the family of a chronically ill child.*
4. Discuss with the family approaches to maintaining usual routines for the chronically ill child and the entire family.
*By including some adaptations, families can maintain usual routines and meet the needs of all family members.*
5. Refer the family and child to resources (e.g., social worker, clergy, counselor) for additional psychosocial interventions, as indicated.
*Psychosocial assistance beyond the nurse's scope of practice, or as requested by the family, may be needed for certain families and children.*

**Evaluation**

Is the family able to maintain its usual routine and meet the needs of all family members?

Does the family treat the ill child as normally as possible to avoid overdependence?

Do family members express their feelings? Has the family identified and used appropriate coping mechanisms, and are they using appropriate support systems?

**TABLE 36.1 The Child's Concept of Death**

| Age | Cognitive Stage | Concept |
|---|---|---|
| Infancy and toddlerhood (0-2 yr) | Sensorimotor | Death as loss of the caregiver |
| Early childhood (2-7 yr) | Preoperational | Death as a reversible and temporary separation |
| Middle childhood (school-age; 7-12 yr) | Concrete operations | Death as sad and irreversible but not necessarily inevitable |
| Adolescence (12+ yr) | Formal operations | Death as inevitable and irreversible but often a distant event |

and egocentricity at this age often lead to guilt and shame because children can believe that their thoughts or actions caused the death. The child's first exposure to death frequently involves a dead animal, such as an insect, bird, or pet.

Preschoolers facing impending death frequently view their condition as punishment for behaviors or thoughts. They respond with guilt, anger, sadness, and fear. Their self-imposed guilt can lead them to believe that others, including parents, see them as "bad" and are angry with them. Feelings are kept inside, and children this age may withdraw from everyone, including those they love and on whom they depend. Their anger at those they care about and the intensity of that anger frightens them. Great patience and understanding are required of their parents and nurses, particularly when emotions are labile and subject to frequent, sudden changes. Indeed, all children feel greater security when adults maintain discipline and suitable, customary limits; this is especially true for dying children who are experiencing multiple changes and discrepancies in their daily lives.

### School-Age Children

By the school-age years, death begins to be understood as a sad and irreversible event, yet its inevitability is not yet understood. Children at age 10 years begin to understand that they too can die. Some associated feelings of guilt often persist for school-age children. They may continue to believe that thoughts or actions can cause death or that death serves as a punishment for wrongdoing.

The school-age child has increased cognition and other resources necessary to cope with the dying process. However, these same abilities can lead to additional questions and fears. School-age children might wonder why they are ill and must die so young. Fear about the process of dying and what follows can also arise. Even in children who have a foundation of spiritual beliefs, this fear may persist because they do not have a concrete knowledge of what it is like after a person dies. The school-age child may fear being without the love and support of parents and other close family members. Moreover, school-age children may feel vulnerable and doubt their ability to cope with the knowledge of their impending death, as well as the experience itself.

#### Adolescents

Most adolescents have a fully developed understanding of death as inevitable and irreversible. However, many adolescents view death as a distant event and may consider themselves invulnerable to death, related to their increasingly independent frame of reference. Although adolescents may understand death and dying, they do not necessarily have an emotional acceptance of their impending death. Adolescents who are attempting to separate from their parents often test and break rules as they strive for independence. This process can cause guilt for the dying child, especially when contemplating the spiritual aspects of life and death.

As the result of their illness, adolescents can become isolated from their peers. The terminal illness or disability of a peer forces healthy adolescents to abruptly and unwillingly face and question their own mortality. Discomfort can prompt the healthy adolescent to decrease or stop contacting and visiting even a close friend who is seriously ill. Adolescents who are dying may become isolated from caring adults, family, and healthcare providers because they feel adults do not understand them. Consequently, many feel lonely and fear that they will die without the love and support they need and desire. Realizing that they are facing death when their lives are just beginning, adolescents can respond with anger and sadness, particularly when considering what they will never be able to experience as an adult. These feelings can contribute to the onset of depression.

## Coping and Responses to Death and Dying

The process of dying, as well as the actual death of a child, is a unique and complex situation. The responses of all persons involved—the child, family, and healthcare providers—are affected by multiple factors, including personal and spiritual beliefs, previous experiences with illness and death, the quality of the relationship with the dying child, and experiences with this child during the current illness and dying process. Another very important factor is the individual's progression through the stages of grief. At any given time, the child, parents, and siblings may all be experiencing a different stage of grief and expressing that grief in different ways.

### The Child's Response

A child who is dying wants to feel safe and does not want to be alone or in pain. These concerns are frequently more intense for school-age children and adolescents. The child's responses to death and dying will be multiple and varied, not always fully correlating with the child's chronologic age and expected stage of development and cognition. The traumatizing experiences associated with a chronic condition and treatments tend to make children more mature and "wise beyond their years." As dying children work through the five stages of grief, they may reach a point where they consider their illness and treatment to be worse than dying and then experience relief and acceptance of death. The responses and actions of the dying child are also affected by the behaviors and feelings of those around them, particularly family, friends, and healthcare providers.

The child's response to dying and the resulting actions are often more precocious than would be expected, particularly among preschool children. Family or hospital staff members may consider precocious actions to be inappropriate and some statements of a spiritual nature to be unbelievable. They possibly attribute these responses to physical changes, such as a low hemoglobin level, altered neurologic status, or medications such as analgesics or sedatives.

Spiritual beliefs can influence the child and be reflected in conversations and actions. Children might speak of seeing or even interacting with angels or the Higher Being recognized by their specific faith. They might also speak of going to heaven to be with the angels or other spiritual beings. In addition, children might speak of going to play or be with another child or relative who has already died. This type of conversation can take place anywhere from several weeks to days or hours before death, with children actually giving specifics as to when they will see or be with deceased individuals. Such behaviors are commonly referred to as *nearing death awareness.*

Dying children often experience a heightened sense of understanding and awareness, particularly as death nears. Many know specifically when they will die. As seen with adults, death often occurs after children have successfully achieved closure of some type. Closure can be a special event in their life or that of a loved one, such as a graduation, holiday, or birthday. Frequently, closure also involves resolution of unfinished business, such as interacting with a loved one who has been absent or apologizing for things they have said or done.

One concept of pediatric death that families may have difficulty understanding and accepting is "allowing" their child to die. As noted by Kübler-Ross (1983), children are afraid not of death but of abandonment. Children who are enveloped by hope, joy, and love may sustain their grasp on life. For most children, allowing them to die means giving the child permission to die. Accordingly, some children, particularly those who are younger, need verbal "permission" to die, reassurance that it is safe to do so, and a description of what to expect as they die and in the time afterward. Children might also need to know that the family, friends, and loved ones who are left behind will grieve and yet will be all right and will take care of each other. Equally important to children of all ages is the knowledge that loved ones will remember them always.

### The Parents' Response

When a child is initially diagnosed with any condition that is life threatening, every parent faces and begins to cope with the *possibility* of their child's death. When they are informed that nothing more can be done medically to treat their child's illness, parents face the *reality* of their child's death. They begin to experience **anticipatory grief**, the processes of mourning, coping, interacting, planning, and psychosocial reorganizing that occurs as part of the response to the impending death of a loved one.

The stages of grief associated with the child's illness must now be experienced in relation to the child's death. Acceptance does not always occur. Some parents may find it difficult or unacceptable to discontinue treatment. They might choose to continue treatment of a curative rather than a palliative nature. However, such a choice does not always indicate denial. It might simply represent a belief system based on spiritual or personal convictions. Legally, emotionally, and psychosocially, the family's decision must be upheld and supported by members of the healthcare team. However, such treatment could prolong and worsen the child's dying experience by causing pain or other uncomfortable symptoms. The healthcare team should strive as diligently as possible to remain the child's advocate, looking carefully at whether treatment is *doing for* the child as opposed to *doing to* the child.

At such times, the team's experience with other children in similar situations can be useful in gently guiding the parents toward **palliative** care services. In 2013, the AAP issued guidelines on pediatric palliative care to improve quality of life and decrease the stress on patients and their families when dealing with life-threatening or life-shortening care (AAP, 2013). It is estimated that 8,600 children are eligible for palliative care each day (Crozier & Hancock, 2012). All patients with chronic and life threatening illnesses should be referred to palliative care early in the course of illness to improve the care of the patient and family (Crozier & Hancock, 2012). Palliative care can be provided throughout the disease process and can occur while a child with a life-threatening illness is still receiving treatment focused on sustaining life. The interdisciplinary palliative care team provides comprehensive physical, psychological, social, and spiritual care to the entire family including the child, with consideration of cultural, religious, and family values (Ullrich et al., 2011). Research shows that parents retrospectively would have preferred earlier involvement in palliative care (Wolfe, 2012). Better experiences with palliative care have been reported when conversations about prognosis and the goals of care occur early (Crozier & Hancock, 2012). The palliative care team should include physicians, nurses, social workers, case managers, spiritual care providers, ethical care providers, bereavement specialists, and child life specialists (AAP, 2013).

Treatments are aimed at (AAP, 2013):

- Relieving suffering, including physical, psychological, social, and spiritual
- Improving the child's quality of life
- Facilitating informed decision making including end-of-life decisions
- Assisting with coordination of care

Parents will exhibit the need to talk about their child and the experience of their child's illness and death. They talk to assimilate the experience, but more important, they talk to remember their child.

When a chronic condition has extended over time, the parents' initial reaction to their child's death is often relief that the child is no longer suffering, physically or emotionally, and that the uncertainty of the illness has ended. Many times, this relief and feeling of peace may begin when death is known to be inevitable and imminent. Such relief can evoke feelings of guilt. Support and explanations regarding the normalcy of these feelings might be necessary for parents. Relief at the death is followed by numbness, intense sadness, and a sense of profound loss and emptiness. Since losing a child negatively affects all aspects of a parent's life, parents adopt coping strategies such as adopting a new role, having another child, or helping other families with similar experiences (Stroebe et al., 2013). The grief of the child's grandparents can be greater than that of the parents, because they grieve the loss of their grandchild and also grieve for *their own child,* the parent, who has experienced the death of a child.

### The Siblings' Response

The responses of siblings to death and dying, as well as their progression through the stages of grief, vary according to age and developmental level. Although children usually experience all five stages of grief, this may not necessarily occur in the given sequence. Frequently, children move between the stages in a seemingly random fashion, often experiencing one stage several times. This process is an appropriate coping mechanism for some children. Issues that were dealt with successfully earlier in the course of the illness, such as concerns about causing the illness or death of the brother or sister may resurface. Siblings can experience emotions similar to those experienced by their parents; however, they might not yet have the cognitive and developmental abilities to understand and work through the grieving process. The result is unresolved grief that can contribute to emotional problems in adult life.

Because children work through the grieving process differently than adults, siblings often need guidance and support from parents and others to resolve issues and complete the grieving process. Grief support centers are available to provide assistance to children who have experienced the death of a loved one, including a sibling. Healthcare providers and professional counselors can also intervene as indicated. Siblings should be prepared for the death of a sibling to facilitate bereavement and encourage adjustment to the loss of their sibling (O'Quinn & Giambra, 2014).

The most important aspect of providing support to a grieving sibling is acknowledging that the loss experience of the sibling is *just as significant* as the loss experience of the parents. Such validation of the sibling's grief can support their successful navigation of the grieving process.

## Caring for the Dying Child

Despite medical advances and current technology, many chronic disorders ultimately end in death. Providing nursing care to the child with a terminal illness who is nearing death, as well as to family members, requires a heightened level of understanding, compassion, and support. A family's coping abilities are often tested beyond measure. Nursing care includes assisting the child and family to withstand the intense pressures and emotional demands of the situation (Fig. 36.3).

### Nursing Professionalism and Boundaries

Caring for dying children involves certain stressors for all involved, including the nurse. An important aspect of self-care is for nurses to recognize and acknowledge the impact of these stressors. Caring for the child who is approaching death can be rewarding, but it can also severely test the nurse's coping skills. Compassion is necessary, but also essential are awareness and maintenance of professional boundaries. These boundaries are necessary for the nurses to provide clinically sound, compassionate care while maintaining their own emotional, physical, and spiritual health.

To maintain professionalism and boundaries, nurses must understand and accept their own feelings and beliefs about death. The psychological, spiritual, and ethical needs of the healthcare professional

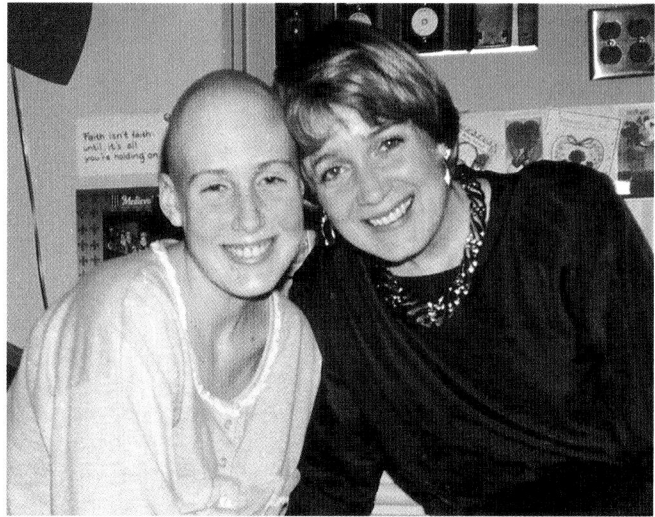

FIG 36.3 The family of the child with a terminal condition needs compassion and support from the nurse. Nursing care includes physical care and support of the family's care giving efforts and assistance with the grieving process. (Courtesy Gwen T. Martin, RN, Fort Worth, TX.)

should be addressed by the palliative care team (AAP, 2013). Hospital resources for nurses seeking support and assistance include the pastoral care team, social workers, and nursing support groups. Attending patient care conferences or ethics committee meetings can help the nurse better understand and participate in patient care decisions. The nurse also learns more about the education and services the family is receiving and how these are supporting their decision-making process. In some situations, nurses choose to obtain personal counseling services privately or through a hospital employee support program.

### Communication

Nursing staff and family members must be aware of, understand, and accept the dying child's communication needs and patterns. The dying child should consistently be reassured that the illness and approaching death are not the result of any action or omission committed by the child. Parents and nurses must make certain that dying children know they will never be left alone; a family member or healthcare professional must always be with these children.

Children who are dying need to experience complete love and acceptance; they must receive assurances that their feelings and thoughts are not wrong. Children, parents, and siblings may need assistance to understand their intense emotions, especially anger and guilt. Parents, other adult family members, and siblings need opportunities away from the dying child to express their feelings. This can help to minimize or prevent the dying child from feeling responsible for the emotions of others, particularly the parents. The goal is to have the child and family together in an environment that is as soothing, comfortable, and stress-free as possible.

Most dying children will follow the family's rules and patterns for communication. As death approaches, communication between child and family can decline in both extent and effectiveness. The nurse should consider communication strategies the family has used effectively during previously stressful times (e.g., at diagnosis, with relapses), and encourage the family to use those same approaches again. The nurse carefully evaluates each child and family on an individual basis and assists them to experience effective, comfortable communication.

The most common issue that arises when a family is facing the impending death of their child is whether to inform the child of the grave prognosis. Although the needs of the parents, siblings, other family members, and healthcare providers are considered, the needs of the dying child must take precedence. One suggested approach is to allow the child to maintain open communication with trusted individuals who are comfortable talking with the child about death. This supports the child's need for someone to acknowledge that the child is dying and be willing to talk with the child at the child's request. Simultaneously, it allows mutual pretense and decreased communication with those who prefer to not talk about the child's death. This flexible approach has been found to be effective and is prevalent.

Nurses can be caught between children who wish to talk about their death and parents who forbid any such conversation. As the caregiver and primary advocate, the nurse should first meet the child's needs. Any skirting of the issues or dishonesty with the child could damage the nurse-patient relationship, possibly denying the child a much-needed source of comfort and support. It is critically important that the nurse maintain the trust of the dying child to provide the child with optimal nursing care, including administering medications to manage pain and other symptoms. Nurses should inform parents that they will not initiate any discussion of the child's death but need and intend to respond openly and honestly if the child asks questions or wants to talk. This practice allows nurses both to respect the wishes of the parents and provide support to the child when needed.

Words are not always necessary to provide assistance and care to the dying child. Presence—simply sitting with the child—or a light touch, such as holding a hand, may be exactly what the child needs. The silence itself might be a therapeutic intervention, or it might help open the door for desired verbal communication.

### Family Dynamics, Beliefs, and Practices

To fully support parents during the time surrounding the death of their child, nursing care must impart consistent respect and acceptance, regardless of any differences between the spiritual or cultural beliefs and practices of the family and those of the nurse (Box 36.3).

The nurse will encounter different beliefs and practices surrounding death and the grieving process. Such practices include wearing prayer cloths, the laying on of hands, use of holy water or oil, viewing religious pictures, icons, or other objects, extemporaneous prayer gatherings, or the preparation and serving of certain foods. Some practices may be of concern to the nurse and the healthcare team related to safety and the child's emotional state. Each practice by each family must be evaluated individually, addressing the potential emotional or spiritual benefits to the child and family and potential safety issues.

Many parents have difficulty moving from active treatment that is aimed at curing the disease to palliative care with an emphasis on comfort and quality of life for the dying child. Some parents' final attempts to find a cure for their child's illness include the use of unproven medications or treatments, some of which are available in other countries. Although these treatments may not be approved by the U.S. Food and Drug Administration (FDA), many will not cause physical harm to the child. Indeed, they may be emotionally beneficial to both parent and child, providing affirmation that everything possible was tried to cure the child's terminal disease. These efforts may instill hope, which is vitally important to the child and family. If any of these unapproved medications or treatments is potentially harmful to the child, the healthcare team might choose not to allow their use. The decision and the rationale are explained compassionately yet firmly to the family, noting the decision was made in the best interest of the child.

Family beliefs and practices, as well as strong emotions, influence their decision making regarding do-not-resuscitate (DNR) orders. A DNR order means that cardiopulmonary resuscitation (CPR) or other interventions designed to initiate heartbeat and respirations after a cardiopulmonary arrest are not performed. Families who acknowledge their child's impending death may still have great difficulty and uncertainty about the decision to not resuscitate their child. They might change their decision several times regarding the DNR order. The healthcare team members need to educate family members regarding the possible choices and encourage them to discuss their feelings and explore their wishes for their child. A DNR order does not mean withholding treatment *while the child is alive.* Rather, it involves not initiating treatment *after the child has died.* Parents are reminded that if a DNR order is chosen, they can revoke the order at any time. Most important, the healthcare providers assure the family that their child will be cared for and comfort will be maintained regardless of the presence or absence of a DNR order.

Parents can make treatment decisions that do not seem to be in the best interest of the child. For example, parents might not allow their child to receive pain medication because they want the child to be more alert. They might request continued treatment that is traumatic and is not likely to provide long-term survival for the child. These situations can cause emotional, spiritual, and professional distress for the nurse, particularly when there is conflict with the nurse's beliefs. To provide the appropriate care, the nurse must use coping strategies or seek assistance in resolving these distressing feelings. If resolution is not

## BOX 36.3 Resources on Death and Dying for Families and Health Professionals

**Internet Resources**

Children's Hospice International (U.S.): http://www.chionline.org
Information regarding children's hospice, palliative, and end-of-life care.

Compassionate Friends (U.S.): http://www.compassionatefriends.org/home.aspx
Brochures for parents and siblings in both English and Spanish. Discussion support groups and chat rooms are available for siblings.

Baby Steps (Canada): http://www.babysteps.com
Extensive book list, sharing rooms, and grieving rooms.

**Book Selections for Children**

Alley, R.W. (1998). *Sad isn't bad.* St. Meinrad, IN: Abbey Press.

Barber, B. (2012). *My life about me: A kid's forever book.* Washington, DC: Magination Press. (memory book for school-age children)

Buscaglia, L. (2002). *The fall of Freddie the leaf: 20th anniversary edition.* Thorofare, NJ: Slack Inc. (all ages)

Fitzgerald, H. (2000). *A guide for teenagers and their friends.* New York: Simon & Schuster. (teens)

Hale, N., & Sternberg, K. (2004). *Oh Brother: Growing up with a special needs sibling.* Washington, DC: Magination Press. (older school-age children)

Mills, J., & Pillo, C. (2003). *Gentle willow: A story for children about dying.* Washington, DC: Magination Press. (young children)

Peterkin, A., & Middendorf, F. (1992). *What about me? When brothers and sisters get sick.* Washington, DC: Magination Press.

Raschka, C. (2007). *The purple balloon.* New York: Schwartz & Wade.

Simon, J. (2001). *This book is for all kids, but especially my sister Libby. Libby died.* Kansas City, MO: Andrews McMeel. (preschool)

**Book Selections for Adults—Parents and Nurses**

Bluebond-Langner, M. (2000). *In the shadow of illness.* Princeton, NJ: Princeton University Press.

Coloroso, B. (2000). *Parenting through crisis: Helping kids in times of loss, grief, and change.* New York: Harper Collins.

Grollman, E.A. (1990). *Talking about death.* Boston: Beacon Press.

Hilden, J.M., Tobin, D.R., & Lindsey, K. (2002). *Shelter from the storm: Caring for a child with a life-threatening condition.* Cambridge, MA: Perseus Press Group.

Ilse, S., & Leininger, L. (1985). *Grieving grandparents.* Maple Plain, MN: Wintergreen Press.

Power, P.W., & Dell Orto, A.E. (2003). *The resilient family: Living with your child's illness or disability.* Notre Dame, IN: Sorin Books.

Rothman, J. C. (1997). *The bereaved parent's survival guide.* New York: Continuum.

Schive, K., & Klein, S.D. (2001). (Eds.). *You will dream new dreams: Inspiring personal stories by parents of children with disabilities.* New York: Kensington.

Seibeti, D., Drolet, J.C., & Fetro, J.V. (2003). *Helping children live with death and loss.* Carbondale, IL: Southern Illinois University Press.

Sourkes, B.M. (1996). *Armfuls of time: The psychological experience of the child with a life-threatening illness.* Philadelphia: University of Pittsburgh Press.

**Book Selections for Nurses**

D'Avanzo, C. (2007). *Mosby's pocket guide to cultural health assessment* (4th ed.). St. Louis: Mosby.

Field, M.J., & Behrman, R. (Eds.), (2003). *When children die: Improving palliative and end-of-life care for children and their families.* Washington, DC: National Academies Press.

Giger, J.N., & Davidhizar, R.E. (2007). *Transcultural nursing: Assessment and intervention* (5th ed.). St. Louis: Elsevier.

possible, the nurse should be given the option of not participating in the child's care.

### Pain Control

The interventions that are seen as most important by the child with a terminal illness and the family involve pain management. The nurse educates the child and family regarding pain control methods and then provides consistent reassurance that all appropriate interventions will be done to provide for the child's continued comfort. Families and older children might express concerns about inadequate pain relief as well as fears about addiction when opioids are prescribed. The nurse reassures the child and family members that treating the child's pain symptoms is the top priority and that addiction is unlikely to occur when medications are given to the child for pain caused by the illness.

The child and family must be informed that the pain associated with terminal conditions can escalate acutely and often, leading to a corresponding decrease in pain relief from opioids and other medications. For this reason, it is necessary at times to increase the medication dosages or change the medication regimen to control escalating pain. The nurse ensures that the child and family understand that the child's pain will be assessed frequently and the pain control methods will be evaluated regularly to make needed changes to keep the child comfortable (For further information and discussion of pain control for children, see Chapter 39). Education regarding appropriate pain management, including myths and realities, should begin when pain medications are first used during the course of the child's illness. This previous education allows the nurse to simply reinforce information already learned during the terminal phase of the child's illness.

### Hospice Care

For many terminally ill children and their families, being outside the hospital environment, either in a home hospice program or at a hospice facility, is the preferred choice for meeting their complex needs during the dying process. Palliative care teams refer patients in the last six months of life for hospice services (Crozier & Hancock, 2012). **Hospice care** is a specialized, comprehensive system of care that provides support and assistance to patients and their families during the last phase of a terminal illness. The use of hospice care for children is increasing. The first pediatric hospice was established in Virginia in 1978 (Crozier & Hancock, 2012), and there are now over 3,000 hospices that provide care to children (O'Quinn & Giambra, 2014). Specialized nursing and physician care is the cornerstone; however, other care providers and services are available. Hospice team members include social workers, chaplains, home health aides, physical and occupational therapists, child life specialists, bereavement counselors, and volunteers. Families can receive pharmacy prescriptions, healthcare supplies, and medical equipment that are delivered to their home.

A child's home or a hospice care facility can provide a more comfortable and relaxed environment than the acute-care hospital unit. At home, children have family, pets, friends, and the comfort of their own bedrooms and possessions nearby. Hospice care is provided in a freestanding facility or in a separate unit of an acute-care hospital. Many families prefer end-of-life care outside of the acute-care setting when offered a choice (Gupta, Harrop, Lapwood, et al., 2013). Families choose a hospice care facility for the following reasons:

- The child's physical care requirements and the emotional burdens are too great for family caregivers to manage.

- The child's physical symptoms require aggressive management, or the child has pain requiring intensive and complex medication control.
- The home is not conducive to adaptations needed for the child's care (e.g., hospital bed, oxygen equipment, a private room).

Brief periods of inpatient hospice care also can be used to meet a family's needs for respite, providing an environment for the dying child that is less threatening and more home-like than an acute-care hospital setting. It is essential that family members take care of their physical and emotional needs so they are able to care for and support their children.

Hospice care should always be offered to families along with the information necessary for making an educated choice. Some families choose home-based hospice care but later admit the child to a hospital during the final hours or days of life. This choice, which always remains available to families, is often related to concerns about pain control, the adequacy of physical care for the child, and the emotional aspect of a death occurring in the home. Parents can be particularly anxious regarding how they or the siblings will cope with living in their home once their child's death has occurred there. This concern can lead parents to choose hospitalization, even if their child prefers to die at home. Healthcare team members need to discuss these concerns with the family early in the child's dying process to allow them time to explore their fears and emotions, ideally leading to a choice that is acceptable and comfortable for the child, siblings, and parents. Parents report that deaths occurring in hospice care are less chaotic, with home-like comfort, and enhanced dignity (Chavoshi, Miller, & Siden, 2013). If a family elects to hospitalize the child when death is imminent, healthcare providers must accept and support the decision.

### The Dying Process and the Time of Death

The care needs of the dying child are much like those of the chronically or seriously ill child. Much of the care is directed by the physical, emotional, and spiritual needs of the child and family. The goal of nursing care is to provide a comfortable, peaceful time for the child and family with minimal disruptions. Whether the death is occurring at home, in the hospital, or at a hospice care facility, the child's room should be secluded, comfortable, and quiet.

The family and child might express interest in creating lasting memories of the child that can be enjoyed by the family in the years to come. Child life specialists can assist families and children in legacy building activities such as journals, scrapbooks, photo albums, videos, and letters. Not only will the child and family enjoy spending time together creating the legacy, but the family may find solace in these memories after the child's death (Boles, 2014).

***Privacy for the child and family.*** Privacy without interruptions is important for the dying child and the family so that their physical, emotional, and spiritual needs can be met. The child's endurance will be greatly diminished, with increased needs for daytime napping and extended nighttime sleep, when possible. The child may experience sleep deprivation, frequent wakefulness, or nightmares. Privacy and careful control of the number and frequency of visitors will preserve the child's strength and promote rest and sleep. The child must be reassured that family members and care providers are close by and always accessible and available.

Disruptions by staff and possibly even by friends or extended family should be minimized to the extent desired by the child and family. Often, members of the immediate family will request private time with the dying child. Occasionally, this request causes others to become distraught or to insist on spending time with the child. The nurse, as an advocate for the child and family, takes responsibility for enforcing the request for privacy. Nurses also strive to facilitate communication between family members and with friends to convey the family's wishes and explain the need for privacy.

***Changes in family routines.*** The availability of loved ones becomes more important to the child with a terminal illness, who will experience more frequent periods of prolonged sleep. Regardless of the duration—moments, minutes, or hours—intervals spent with the child can become treasured memories. As much as possible, the nurse should facilitate maximizing the time for the parents, siblings, and dying child to be together. Special care must be taken to explain to siblings the reasons for rearranging life around the ill child's wakeful hours.

***Family concerns about oral intake.*** Lack of interest in eating and drinking is a normal part of the dying process, yet diminishing nutritional intake can be very difficult for family members to handle. They may hold misconceptions that the child will "starve to death" and that hunger or thirst will add to the child's discomfort. Fluid intake can actually cause discomfort for the child by increasing lung secretions that necessitate suctioning. The nurse must prepare the family by telling them that days before death children often lose the ability to swallow and oral intake ceases. If kidney function declines during the dying process, the child will retain fluids and feel uncomfortable; thus, fluid intake will need to be restricted.

***Fluids and oral care.*** There are important nursing implications regarding fluid intake and oral care for the dying child. If the child has a dry mouth or feels thirsty, small amounts of ice chips or fluids, given at the request of the child, can alleviate these symptoms.

Physical and emotional comfort can be enhanced by allowing the child who is terminally ill to drink favorite fluids, despite the risk of aspiration that exists if the ability to swallow is compromised. Promoting the child's independence and choices can give a sense of control that the child often loses during the dying process. If a lack of strength or coordination makes drinking from a glass or straw difficult, fluids can be provided using a "sippy" cup, spoon, medicine dropper, or syringe (oral or catheter-tip). Care must be taken not to deliver too much fluid at one time to avoid choking.

The nurse, with the help from the family, provides appropriate oral care to the dying child to promote comfort and prevent complications. Sponge swabs can be used to clean the lips and mouth and to provide moisture using artificial saliva preparations. Solutions that reduce pain and inflammation can also be applied with sponge swabs. Lip balms or medicated products can be applied to dry, chapped lips. Products that contain alcohol or fragrances should not be used in the mouth or on the lips; they can have a drying effect and cause irritation and pain to inflamed or cracked areas. Appropriate and frequent oral care will minimize mouth odor and improve the child's appearance. Providing oral care can give the family a feeling of usefulness and an opportunity for regular contact with the child. The nurse encourages the family members to decide the types and amount of physical care they wish to provide to their child.

***Responsiveness and communication.*** A child's level of awareness or wakefulness shortly before the time of death can be an overwhelming concern for family members. The child may be unresponsive in the days or hours before death or intermittently responsive until the actual moment of death. The nurse explains the possible variations to family members. Many children have been noted to experience a period of time (either a few hours or an entire day) immediately before they die when they are stronger, more alert, and show increased interest in their family members. This occurrence can cause family members to have unrealistic expectations for recovery; therefore, nurses must prepare and educate families about this possible event.

Although a dying child may appear unresponsive, hearing is the last sense to stop functioning before death. The nurse encourages the family members to talk to the child and maintain physical contact such as touching or holding the child's hand, until death occurs, and even after as desired by the family. Some family members may find this difficult because of personal fears or beliefs. Family members have different comfort levels in relation to the dying process, different needs for personal space, or different emotional expressions. The nurse assesses the needs of the family during the final moments of their child's death and offers assistance as indicated to facilitate contact and communication with the child.

## ! NURSING QUALITY ALERT

### *Nursing Care for the Dying Child and the Child's Family*

- The nurse should be available to assist both the dying child and the child's family but must not impose personal beliefs and expectations on either the child or the family members.
- The siblings of a dying child need time and attention. They, too, will experience grief and will need to resolve their feelings.
- Most family members need to talk about the experience of illness and death. Open communication helps support family resiliency and helps family members remember the child after death.
- Care for the dying child includes providing adequate pain control, oral care, privacy, and information. The family needs to be aware of the signs of imminent death and what to expect in the immediate postmortem period.
- After death occurs, family members should have as much time as they desire with the deceased child.

***Indicators of imminent death.*** Family members may find security and comfort in the knowledge of the physical indicators that usually signal that the time of death is imminent. The heart rate increases, with a concomitant decrease in the strength and quality of peripheral pulses. Blood pressure also decreases. Pulses and blood pressure may become difficult or impossible to palpate, a state that can last for hours. Cardiac changes generally occur before respiratory changes. Family members more readily notice respiratory changes, which are visible and audible. The force of the respiratory effort may decline. Increased work of breathing, along with apnea, may be noted. Respirations can fluctuate between the two states–rapid, increasingly shallow breaths, followed by cessation or Cheyne–Stokes respiration leading to respiratory arrest. Cheyne–Stokes respiration is a cyclic period of slowing respirations with apnea, followed by an increased respiratory rate to a peak, and then slowing and becoming apneic again. These respirations are often referred to as *agonal;* a description that can inaccurately imply that they are painful; thus, the term should not be used when family members are present.

As death nears, respirations can become more audible and can be accompanied by an expiratory sigh. This sigh often resembles moaning and can alarm family members because they interpret the sound to indicate pain. If the child is otherwise without verbal or physical indications of pain, the family should be reassured that the child's pain level is well controlled. The nurse educates the family as to the cause of the sounds and notes their correlation with each breath. All these variations in respiratory patterns will result in either hypoxia or hypercapnia. If hypoxic agitation occurs, it is treated with oxygen and morphine, intravenous (IV) or sublingual. Both measures provide physical comfort for the child and emotional comfort for the family. A rising carbon dioxide level can actually increase comfort because of sedative and analgesic effects. Continuing respiratory and cardiac changes can lead to cool extremities and cyanosis. These effects most often begin in the lower extremities and progress upward to the face. The nurse must prepare the family for the changes they are going to see.

Noisy breathing caused by the rattling secretions in the upper airway can be very distressing to family members. This rattling—often called the *death rattle*—occurs when the child has lost the strength and ability to clear airway secretions. The nurse educates the family about the causes of noisy breathing and that they may see secretions coming from the mouth. Even with education, hearing these sounds can be extremely difficult for the family to handle. Pharyngeal suctioning can help remove secretions but may need to be done very frequently. Medications such as atropine or diphenhydramine can be given to decrease the amount of secretions. The nurse can position the child in the side-lying position to facilitate the drainage of secretions. A cloth should be placed under the mouth to collect the secretions. The child is rarely aware of these respiratory changes; the focus of nursing care is symptom management and providing support to the family. When respirations stop, there may be a brief period of seconds or minutes until the heart stops beating. A final gasping noise can occur after respiratory and cardiac function have ceased. Reassure the family that this sound is normal and not painful.

***The family after death.*** After death has occurred, family members should have the opportunity to spend time with their child, even before the body is cleaned. It may be preferred to clean and prepare the body first because of the drainage, bleeding, and spontaneous elimination of body wastes that often occur at the time of death. Some families ask to make hand and foot prints or cut a lock of hair as a remembrance of the child. The nurse explains to the family what will be involved in the care of the body. Family members including siblings can be invited to assist in bathing the child's body. This final act of physical care can serve as a special means of closure. Some family members do not wish to assist with the bathing, and parents might not allow siblings to participate. The nurse respects whatever decisions are made by the family. On rare occasion, the family's time with the deceased child or ability to participate in after-death care is limited because of required procedures such as autopsy. Families should be provided information before the child's death if an autopsy will be required and how this will affect their time and involvement with their child after death occurs.

As family members prepare to hold the deceased child, the nurse discusses the physical changes that occur very quickly after death; cooling of the body, cyanosis or paleness, and stiffening. The nurse attempts to prevent further drainage of body fluids. The nurse prepares the family emotionally and provides towels and blankets to facilitate the family's comfort.

The nurse provides privacy for the family, but remains close by and returns as needed or requested. The nurse always offers the services of pastoral care or other appropriate hospital staff members. If a funeral home has not been chosen by the family, clergy and social services personnel can provide assistance.

The nurse informs the family that the child can go to the funeral home either in a hospital gown or in personal clothes. The family, including the siblings, can choose the clothes and a personal item such as a blanket or toy that will go with the child to the funeral home. The clothes and item will be returned to the family after the child is dressed for burial. Some hospitals and hospices hold periodic memorials for children who have died. Support for the family after the death of a child must be continued after leaving the hospital with bereavement follow-up (ENA, 2012).

### The Nurse's Response to the Dying Child

The AAP in collaboration with the American College of Physicians and the Emergency Nurses Association released a policy statement to guide

## NURSING CARE PLAN

### The Terminally Ill or Dying Child

**Focused Assessment**

- Provide a comprehensive assessment of the terminally ill child and family (parents and siblings).
  - Address family relationships and involvement with the child.
  - Assess the child's development level and cognitive, physical, and psychosocial abilities.
  - Determine the child and family's previous experiences with illness and death.
  - Examine recent experiences of the child and family related to the current illness.
- Explore the child and each family member's individual progression through the stages of grief in relation to the child's impending death.
- Assess the child and family for symptoms of anxiety and other negative psychosocial effects.
  - Examine child for indications that anxiety is exacerbating pain or triggering other physical symptoms (e.g., dyspnea).
  - Reassess level of anxiety or other concerns during times of increased stress (e.g., time of diagnosis, disease exacerbations, relapses).
- Assess the child's and family's coping strategies and adaptive mechanisms.

**Nursing Diagnosis**

Grieving related to the impending death of a child.

**Planning**

***Expected Outcomes***

The child and family will:

1. Experience appropriate progression through the five stages of grief, as evidenced by verbalization of an understanding of the five stages of grief, expression of emotions in an appropriate manner, and expression of feelings by each family member.
2. Exhibit behaviors indicating acceptance of the child's impending death, and the family will provide care and support—emotional, physical, and psychosocial—in the manner desired by the child.

**Interventions and *Rationales***

1. Explain the five stages of grief and the necessary grieving process, including resolution to acceptance.
   *Explanations of the normal grieving process should facilitate grief progression and guide behaviors in each stage.*
2. Identify the stage of grief being experienced and provide each family member the opportunity to verbalize feelings and receive positive feedback.
   *Verbalization of feelings and receiving positive feedback guide behaviors and facilitate progression through the grief stages.*
3. Explain to the family the stages of grief progression characteristic for children (the dying child and any siblings). Encourage patience with the extended period of grief for children.
   *Understanding the ways in which children's coping mechanisms differ from those of adults facilitates acceptance and understanding by parents.*
4. Offer the child and all family members the opportunity to verbalize and convey all emotions, in an appropriate manner. Exhibit a nonjudgmental attitude toward and acceptance of verbalizations and behaviors.
   *Venting of emotions helps decrease stress and facilitates the resolution of anger. An attitude of acceptance conveys care and support and encourages appropriate, needed expression of all emotions.*
5. Encourage open, honest communication with the child (to the degree requested). Demonstrate appropriate communication techniques.
   *Appropriate communication with the child will provide comfort and support as well as facilitate expression of needs and problem resolution.*
6. Offer family members the opportunity to participate in the child's physical care, as desired by both parties. Demonstrate providing gentle, supportive care.
   *Family members may fear the provision of physical care to a dying child. Observing the nurse can lessen fears and enhance care giving.*

**Evaluation**

Do the child (if cognitively able) and family verbalize an understanding of the five stages of grief and express emotions in an appropriate manner and in a communication style most comfortable for each individual?

Do the child and family exhibit behaviors that indicate acceptance of the impending death?

Does the family provide physical, emotional, and psychosocial care and support in the manner and environment desired by the child?

**Nursing Diagnosis**

Anxiety related to the threat of impending death.

**Planning**

***Expected Outcomes***

The child and family will:

1. Achieve anxiety control, as evidenced by open verbalization of all feelings and emotions and questions concerning the diagnosis and prognosis.
2. Verbalize physical, emotional, and spiritual comfort.

**Interventions and *Rationales***

1. Educate the child and family about the terminal phase of illness (e.g., what to expect in physical, emotional, and spiritual areas). Explain how needs will be met.
   *Misconceptions can lead to increased fear and family expressions of anxiety, which can cause increased distress for the dying child.*
2. Assure the child and family that the child will be kept safe and comfortable (with minimal pain), and will not be left alone. Provide frequent reassurance.
   *Fears about the child's comfort (pain level) and security are the most common. Frequent reassurances are often necessary as the disease and symptoms worsen.*
3. Provide as much privacy as possible for the family and the child dying in the hospital setting. Encourage parents and siblings to stay with the child if desired. Regulate visitations by those outside the immediate family, as necessary.
   *Immediate family members may need extended time for processing grief and to reach closure. Increased visitations can interfere with the time and privacy needed by the family when death is imminent. The nurse needs to manage the number of visitors because this often is too difficult for the family.*
4. Provide opportunities for family members to care for the child or to decline providing all or some aspects of care. As indicated, teach family members how to provide care in a suitable manner.
   *Children are usually most comfortable when cared for by family members. However, at times, the child and family may be more comfortable if the nurse provides certain aspects of care.*
5. Offer the family and child alternatives for care, such as hospice care in the home or an in-patient facility, if indicated.
   *Hospice care programs can be individualized to meet the needs of a dying child and the family.*

**Evaluation**

Do the child and family openly and appropriately verbalize all feelings, emotions, and questions concerning the diagnosis and prognosis?

Do the child and family exhibit physical, emotional, and spiritual comfort?

providers when dealing with a death of a child in the emergency setting. The principles focus on providing patient-centered, family-centered and team-oriented care. The statement emphasizes personal and compassionate support of the family (AAP, 2014).

Not all healthcare providers cope well with the reality of death. This limitation can hold serious implications for the nurse who chooses to work in an area where deaths occur frequently, such as the emergency department, oncology floors, and critical care units. Caring for dying children and their families can be stressful and emotionally demanding. Nurses working with terminally ill children need increased emotional and psychosocial strength, as well as clinical expertise.

The nurse's response to the dying process and death of a pediatric patient correlates to a certain degree with the stages of grief. The nurse who has become more accustomed to the reality and frequency of death may not experience each stage. Length of treatment and personal affinity can cause a nurse to become more involved with a certain child, and this can lead to a more intense response or a delay in the resolution of grief. Some nurses have difficulty maintaining appropriate boundaries between personal involvement and professional care. The nurse who is compassionate yet can maintain professionalism is better able to provide care on a continuing basis to children with terminal illnesses and their families.

Every nurse who cares for dying children will experience loss and grief and needs support. Nurses can provide mutual support through organized support programs as well as simple acts of respect, concern, and care among colleagues. When a nurse begins working with dying children for the first time, having a more experienced nurse mentor can be helpful. For nurses to provide high quality care to children with chronic or terminal illnesses and their families, nurses must also take care of their own physical and emotional health.

## KEY CONCEPTS

- Children with chronic conditions are living longer, often with conditions once considered fatal. Despite improvements in the quality and length of life, chronic illness remains a situational crisis for families.
- Chronic illness affects the entire family, not just the child.
- With a chronically ill child, all family members must work together to meet the physical and emotional needs of the child, provide care for the rest of the family, and manage financial burdens.
- The stages of grief are applicable to children, with special considerations. A child's concepts of death and dying are based on the developmental level as well as age, cognition, and life experiences. Both ill children and their well siblings fluctuate in their understanding of and responses to death and dying.
- The dying child, like the dying adult, desires the comfort, safety, and presence of loved ones.
- Parents must move from *fear* to *acknowledgment* of the child's impending death.
- For parents caring for a dying child, pain is the greatest concern.
- The grief of a sibling can be more difficult for the nurse to address, related to the developmental level, cognitive abilities, and changing needs, than the grief of parents.
- Each family member (adults and children) must process grief by understanding that the person who has died is gone and experience the resulting emotions. Family members must then reinvest in life and move forward.
- Caring for a terminally ill or dying child can be a stressful and demanding experience for the nurse. It is imperative that nurses attend to their own physical, emotional, and spiritual health so they can provide physical and psychosocial care to the child and family during this difficult time.

## REFERENCES AND READINGS


Academy of Pediatrics, Section on Hospice and Palliate Medicine and Committee on Hospital Care. (2013). Policy Statement: Pediatric Palliative Care and Hospice Care: Commitments, Guidelines, and Recommendations. *Pediatrics, 132*(5) 966–972.

American Academy of Pediatrics, Committee on Emergency Medicine. (2014). Policy Statement: Death of a Child in the Emergency Department. *Pediatrics, 134*(1) 198–201. doi:10.1542/peds.2014–1245

Balk, D. (2011). Adolescent Development and Bereavement: An Introduction. *The Prevention Researcher, 18*(3), 3–9.

Bluebond-Langner, M. (1978). *The private worlds of dying children*. Princeton, NJ: Princeton University Press.

Boles, J. (2014). Creating a Legacy For and With Hospitalized Children. *Pediatric Nursing, 40*(1), 43–44.

Bonilla, Z.E., & Edwards, P.D. (2011). Difficulties Encountered by Health Care Providers Serving Latino Families and Their Children With Craniofacial Conditions. *Hispanic Health Care International* 9(2), 61–71.

Broger, B., & Zeni, M.B. (2011). Father's Coping Mechanisms Related to Parenting a Chronically Ill Child: Implications for Advanced Practice Nurses. *Journal of Pediatric Health Care, 25*(2) 96–104.

Bugge, K.E., Haugstvedt, K.T, Røkholt, E.G, et al. (2012). Adolescent bereavement: embodied responses, coping and perceptions of a body awareness programme. *Journal of Clinical Nursing, 21,* 2160–2169.

Bugel, M.J. (2014). Experiences of School-Age Siblings Of Children with a Traumatic Injury: Changes, Constants, and Needs. *Pediatric Nursing, 40*(4) 179–186.

Chamberlain, L.J., & Wise, P.H. (2016). Chronic illness in childhood. In R. Kliegman, B. Stanton, J. St. Geme, et al. (Eds.), *Nelson textbook of pediatrics* (20th ed., pp. 252–256). Philadelphia: Elsevier.

Chavoshi, N., Miller, T., & Siden, H. (2013). Resource Utilization among Individuals Dying of Pediatric Life-Threatening Diseases. *Journal of Palliative Medicine, 16*(10), 1210–1214.

Chun, T. H., & Berrios-Candelaria, R. (2012). Caring for Children with Autism in Emergency Situations: What Can We Learn from... Broadway? *Contemporary Pediatrics, 29*(9), 56–64.

Cousino, M.K., & Hazen, R.A. (2013). Parenting Stress Among Caregivers of Children With Chronic Illness: A Systemic Review. *Journal of Pediatric Psychology 38*(8) 809–828.

Crozier, F., & Hancock, L.E. (2012). Pediatric Palliative Care: Beyond the End of Life. *Pediatric Nursing, 38*(4), 198–203, 227.

DeRigne, L. (2012). The Employment and Financial Effects on Families Raising Children With Special Health Care Needs: An Examination of the Evidence. *Journal of Pediatric Health Care 26*(4), 283–290.

Drummond, A., Looman, W.S., & Phillips, A. (2012). Coping Among Parents of Children With Special Health Care Needs With and Without a Health Care Home. *Journal of Pediatric Health Care, 26*(4), 266–275.

Eaton, S. (2012). Addressing the Effects of Missing School For Children with Medical Needs. *Pediatric Nursing, 38*(5), 271–277.

Emergency Nurses Association. (2012). *Emergency nursing pediatric course provider manual* (4th ed.). Des Plains, IL: Author.

Gupta, N., Harrop, E., Lapwood, S., et al. (2013). Journey from Pediatric Intensive Care to Palliative Care. *Journal of Palliative Medicine, 16*(4), 397–401.

Heller, K.W., Coleman, M.B., Best, S.J., et al. (2014). Supporting Children With Life Threatening Conditions in the Schools. *Journal of Hospice & Palliative Nursing, 16*(6), 355–361.

Johnson, N.L., & Rodriguez, D. (2013). Children with Autism Spectrum Disorder At a Pediatric Hospital: A Systemic Review of Literature. *Pediatric Nursing, 39*(3), 131–142.

Klass, D. (2013). Sorrow and Solace: Neglected areas in Bereavement Research. *Death Studies, 37*, 597–616.

Kübler-Ross, E. (1969). *On death and dying*. New York: Macmillan.

Kübler-Ross, E. (1983). *On children and death*. New York: Macmillan.

O'Quinn, L., & Giambra, B. (2014). Evidence of Improved Quality of Life With Pediatric Palliative Care. *Pediatric Nursing, 40*(6), 284–288, 296.

Rempel, G.R., Ravindran, V., Rogers, L.G., et al. (2012). Parenting under Pressure: a grounded theory of parenting young children with life threatening congenital heart disease. *Journal of Advanced Nursing, 69*(3), 619–630.

Rosenberg, A.R., Baker, K.S., Syrjala, K.L., et al. (2013). Promoting Resilience among Parents and Caregivers of Children with Cancer. *Journal of Palliative Medicine, 16*(6) 645–652.

Stroebe, M., Schut, H., & Finkenauer, C. (2013). Parents coping with the death of their child: From individual to interpersonal to interactive perspectives. *Family Science, 4*(1), 28–36.

Ullrich, C., Duncan, J., Joselow, M., et al. (2016). Pediatric palliative care. In R. Kliegman, B. Stanton, J. St. Geme, et al. (Eds.), *Nelson textbook of pediatrics* (20th ed., pp. 256–267). Philadelphia: Elsevier.

U.S. Department of Health and Human Services, Health Resources and Services Administration, Maternal and Child Health Bureau. (2008). *The national survey of children with special health care needs chartbook 2005–2006*. Rockville, MD: Author.

Wass, H. (1985). Concepts of death: A developmental perspective. *Issues in Comprehensive Pediatric Nursing, 8*(1–6), 3–25.

Willits, K.A., Platonova, E.A., Nies, M.A., et al. (2013). Medical Home and Pediatric Primary Care Utilization Among Children With Special Health Care Needs. *Journal of Pediatric Health Care 27*(3), 202–208.

Wolfe, J. (2012). Parents of Children with Serious Illness Are More Resilient than Credited. *Journal of Palliative Medicine, 15*(3), 258–259.

# 37

# Principles and Procedures for Nursing Care of Children

http://evolve.elsevier.com/McKinney/mat-ch/

## LEARNING OBJECTIVES

*After studying this chapter, you should be able to:*

- Describe how to prepare children and families for selected procedures frequently seen in an acute-care setting and a home-care setting.
- Compare anatomic and physiologic differences in children and adults as they apply to selected procedures.
- Identify psychosocial considerations unique to children undergoing selected procedures.
- Describe techniques useful for eliciting cooperation from the child undergoing selected procedures.
- Describe step-by-step nursing actions and the rationales for performing selected procedures.

Children need prior preparation and accurate information about any procedure that will be performed. This information is essential to promote a sense of security, decrease fear, elicit cooperation, and improve coping skills. Parents also need preparation because their anxiety about a procedure can be transferred to the child. Teaching before performing procedures increases the knowledge base of the child and family.

After assessing the child and family, the nurse plans how to conduct the procedure in the most effective manner. The nurse can implement strategies to help the child and parents through all phases of a procedure: the anticipation and preparation phase, the actual procedure, and the recovery period after completion.

## PREPARING CHILDREN FOR PROCEDURES

Preparing children and families for procedures, especially those that are painful, threatening, or invasive, starts with a thorough, individualized assessment. This process should include an assessment of the child's developmental stage, personality, existing level of knowledge, present level of understanding, past experiences, coping skills, and family situation. The nurse can then match explanations and teaching to the specific needs of the child and family. Determining the most effective communication approaches for the child and family is also important and should be based on the child's age and developmental level as well as the family's cultural preferences (see Chapter 4 for more information about communication).

### Explaining Procedures

Before preparing the child and family for a procedure, it is important for the nurse to review all the elements and hospital policies, if applicable. This is especially important if the procedure is new or performed infrequently. The nurse requests any needed medication for the child, gathers all supplies, and obtains assistance as necessary. Equipment is obtained and tested to ensure that it functions properly before beginning any procedure.

Explaining procedures includes demonstrating the equipment and describing anything the child will feel, see, hear, and smell. The nurse uses a developmentally appropriate approach and words the child will understand. Relating the experience to an object, or situation familiar or of interest to the child is an effective communication strategy.

Appropriately timing the explanation is critical. Many children respond better to procedures if the explanation is given either just before the procedure or step by step as the procedure unfolds. Some older children and adolescents like to be prepared well in advance in case they have questions and need more information. Advance preparation allows the child to express feelings about the procedure verbally or through role playing. Parents know their child best, so the nurse asks parents about the best timing and approach to use. Time should be allowed for the child to become familiar with the equipment and for the child and family to ask questions (Box 37.1).

**SAFETY ALERT**

***Standard Precautions***

Always use appropriate hand hygiene before a procedure and when the procedure is finished. Follow Standard Precautions.

Also important for a child's successful coping with an invasive or painful procedure is the presence of someone the child trusts. Time spent establishing a trusting relationship with a child is time well spent. Trust in healthcare providers enhances the child's unique coping strategies.

Before procedures, ensure the child's privacy by closing the door to the room and drawing a curtain around the bed. Taking the child to a treatment room is optimal if appropriate to the procedure and comfortable for the child and parent. The treatment room contains suitable equipment for invasive procedures and is a private area away from the safe haven of a child's room or the playroom (Fig. 37.1). The child life specialist is a good resource and can help prepare children for a

## BOX 37.1 Tips for Preparing and Supporting Children Undergoing Procedures

**Before the Procedure**

- Offer the child ways to cope with pain or discomfort. For example, some children can use coping strategies such as guided imagery. Others may listen to music, increasing the volume as the discomfort level increases. Give the child permission to cry or yell if necessary.
- Use developmentally appropriate words when discussing the procedure and expectations.
- Give the child as much choice as possible over what will happen. For example, when possible, the child could be allowed to choose an injection site or a site for intravenous catheter placement.
- Be sure the consent form has been signed, if applicable.
- Always use appropriate hand hygiene before beginning any procedure and follow Standard Precautions.

**During the Procedure**

- Talk to the child during the procedure if the child desires. However, if the child is using a coping strategy, such as guided imagery, talking will be a distraction and will decrease the child's ability to cope with what is happening.
- Keep the child informed of the procedure's progress.
- Tell the child when the procedure is nearly completed and the "worst is over."

**After the Procedure**

- Praise the child for attempts at cooperation, even if the child did not do anything you asked. Trying counts! Specifically praise the child for accomplishing an expected task.
- Provide an opportunity for the child to vent feelings about the procedure. Remember that expressing feelings of anger is appropriate. Tell the child that you understand if she or he does not want to talk with you right now and that you will return later.
- If the parents were not present during the procedure, reunite the child with the parents and allow them to provide comfort and support.
- Reward the child by using age-appropriate methods such as giving stickers.
- Document the preparation process and procedure performance, who performed the procedure, the child's tolerance of the procedure, and its outcomes.

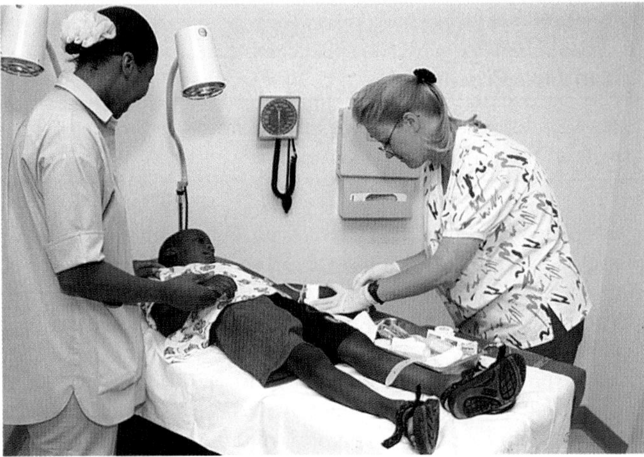

**FIG 37.1** Because a child should feel that the hospital room is a safe place, a treatment room is used for invasive or painful procedures. The parent is present not to restrain the child, but to provide emotional support.

procedure using anatomically correct dolls. Visitors should be asked to leave, and parents might also choose to leave, although parental participation is supported and encouraged.

Telling children and parents in advance what they can and should do during the procedure provides a sense of control and decreases potential feelings of powerlessness. For example, a child who is having an intravenous (IV) catheter placed or a blood specimen drawn is told that to "help," he or she must hold an extremity still and not move. Parents are asked to "help" the child by reminding him or her not to move. Even though the procedure will not be under the child's control, the child can control his or her breathing or use distraction through guided imagery (Shockey et al., 2013). Distraction can reduce children's pain during a procedure, which not only reduces the stress on children and their parents but also makes the procedure easier to perform (Ha & Kim, 2013). The minimization of pain and stress during procedures can have lasting effects on children, creating a positive association with the healthcare setting and future procedures (Nilsson, Enskär, Hallqvist, et al., 2013).

You might say to the child, "We have talked about why you need to have blood taken from your arm, but you need to know how important it is for you to hold your arm very still while we are doing this. I will tell you everything that is going to happen so you can be prepared and know when to help. Do you think you can help us, or do we need to ask someone to help you remember not to move your arm?"

The nurse offers choices to children when feasible. For example, a child is allowed to choose the type of colorful bandage that will cover an injection site or whether to have a procedure done before or after the next television show. Children are never threatened with punishment if they fail to cooperate. Nurses need to have realistic expectations that are based on the child's developmental level and capacity for cooperation.

Parents are encouraged to be involved as much as they want according to what is possible during procedures. For example, a child might be much more cooperative in taking oral medications if the mother administers them. By explaining what the parents will be seeing and what they can do, the nurse helps them feel comfortable staying with and supporting their child. However, the nurse should recognize that parents might be uncomfortable remaining with their child during a painful or invasive procedure. The nurse gives parents the permission to leave and assures them that they will be called if they are needed or as soon as the procedure is completed.

### Consent for Procedures

All surgical and invasive procedures, particularly those that involve risk to the child, require **informed consent**. Examples include lumbar puncture, chest tube insertion, and bone marrow aspiration. By law and ethics, the child (if appropriate) and the parents must be informed of the benefits and risks of the proposed procedure or treatment. Informed consent must be obtained from the parent or legal guardian before the procedure is performed.

Other procedures, such as IV line insertions, specimen collection, and medication and oxygen administration, are covered under the general consent to treat that is signed at admission. It is now also customary to obtain assent from children 7 years old and older. Assent means that the child has been fully informed about the procedure and concurs with those giving the informed consent. Laws on informed consent vary from state to state, so nurses should become familiar with the laws and policies of their institution. (See Chapter 1 for information related to consent and other legal issues.)

The person performing the procedure should obtain the consent. Nurses must check that the consent form is signed and witnessed, and they should answer questions relating to the procedure. Occasionally an emergency or life-threatening situation arises in which contacting the parents or legal guardian for consent is not possible. In such cases, administrative consent can be obtained to allow physicians to perform the indicated procedures. (See Chapter 1 for legal issues related to emergency consent provisions.)

## ! NURSING QUALITY ALERT

### *Preparation for Procedures*

- A treatment room is the preferred location for performing painful procedures. It is a private area away from the safe haven of a child's hospital room and contains the necessary equipment for a variety of procedures (see Fig. 37.1).
- Ensure that a person the child trusts is present for support.
- Use terminology appropriate for the child's developmental level. Avoid using words or phrases that the child might misinterpret (e.g., dye, put to sleep, stick).
- Offer the child choices, if appropriate.
- Tell the child and parents how they can help with the procedure.
- Do not threaten punishment for lack of cooperation.
- Encourage parental participation in the procedure, but do not force an unwilling parent to stay.

## HOLDING AND TRANSPORTING INFANTS AND CHILDREN

Infants can be held in several positions (Fig. 37.2). Before discharge from the hospital, the nurse teaches new parents how to hold the infant, and nurses working on pediatric units should hold infants in similar ways. Nurses hold infants securely, anticipating sudden movement. Because infants younger than 4 months old do not have well-established head control, supporting the head and neck is essential. Infants up to 2 to 3 months of age are cradled by holding them in a horizontal position, supporting the back, and grasping the thigh (see Fig. 37.2, *A*). When using the football hold, the infant is tucked between the nurse's body and elbow, with the arm carrying the infant's body and the hand supporting the head (see Fig. 37.2, *B*). When carrying the infant upright, the infant is erect against the nurse's chest (see Fig. 37.2, *C*). The infant's buttocks rest on the forearm, and the other arm supports the infant's head and shoulders. Even for infants with well-developed neck muscles and head control, this extra support prevents them from falling backward should they make a sudden move. Parents who use backpacks or front-facing baby carriers are advised to be sure that the infant's head is supported at all times when in the device.

Hospitalized infants and children sometimes must be transported to other areas within a hospital unit or even outside the unit. A change

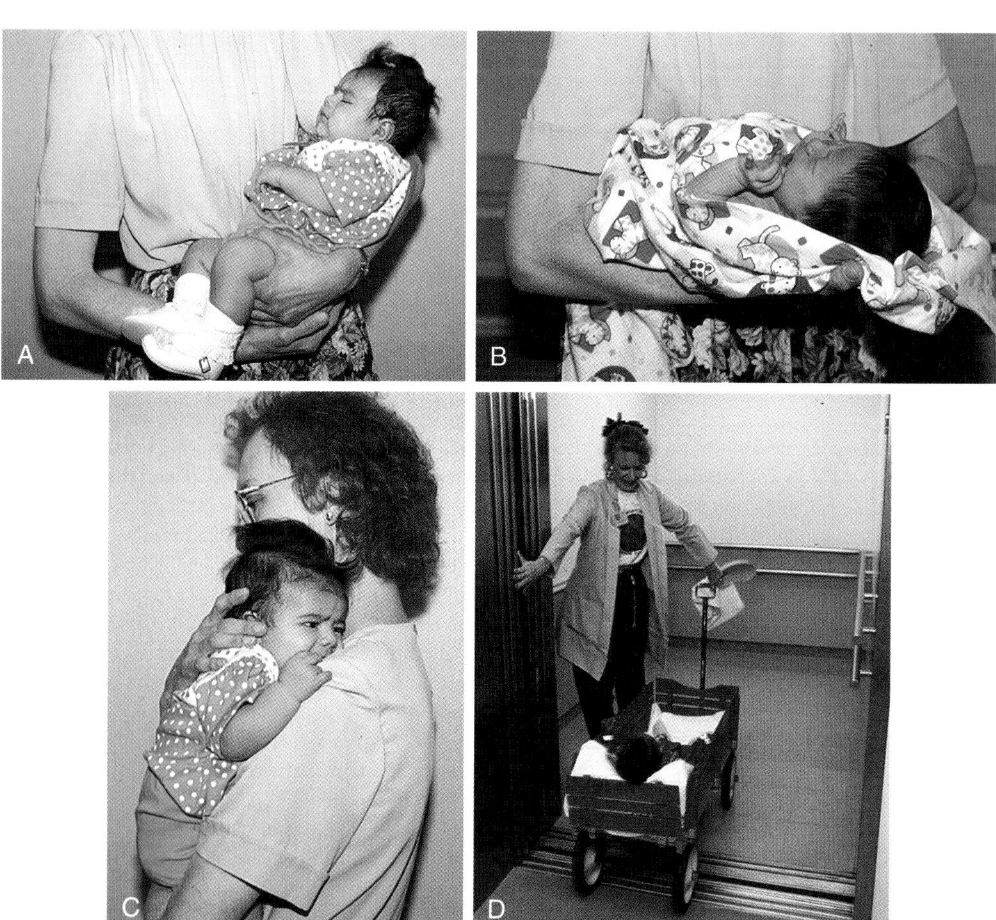


**FIG 37.2** Methods of transporting infants and children. The nurse carries the infant securely, anticipating sudden movement. **A,** Cradle carry. **B,** Football hold. **C,** Over-the-shoulder carry, which can be used until the infant is 6 to 7 months old. **D,** Transport can be fun for young children, especially when it is on wheels. (**A, B,** and **C,** Courtesy Parkland Health and Hospital System District Community Oriented Primary Care Clinic, Dallas, TX; **D,** Courtesy Cook Children's Medical Center, Fort Worth, TX.)

in location might be a response to changes in the child's condition or might be done to increase parental involvement in the child's care (e.g., rooming-in). Children might be transported to different areas on the same unit (e.g., treatment room, playroom) or other hospital departments for specialized care (e.g., rehabilitation) or for diagnostic testing.

The method of transportation will depend on the child's age, developmental level, and physical condition; the destination; safety factors; and whether equipment such as oxygen, an IV pump, or a cardiac monitor is needed to accompany the child. Any special accommodations should be arranged before the time of the planned transport.

Infants and toddlers can also be transported in a bassinet or crib. The rails should always be up in the highest position; for older infants and toddlers the protective top should be in place. Strollers and wagons can be used to transfer older infants and toddlers to other areas on the unit (see Fig. 37.2, *D*). Safety belts should be used, and the sides of the wagon should be in the raised position. An infant or a toddler is *never* left unattended in a wagon. With all transport methods, equipment is securely attached to a rolling cart or stand and then pushed or pulled along with the transporting vehicle. Equipment is *not* placed inside the transporting vehicle that infants or young children occupy.

Older children and adolescents are transported in wheelchairs or on stretchers with the side rails raised. In some cases, as for a child in traction, transporting the child in the bed is preferable. Safety belts *must* be used and side rails must be in the raised and locked position. Children of all ages are supervised when in a transport vehicle.

## SAFETY ISSUES IN THE HOSPITAL SETTING

Safety is of paramount concern for all children; infants and toddlers are at the greatest risk for injury. When an infant or toddler is in a crib, nurses and parents need to be especially vigilant about keeping crib side rails locked in the raised position to prevent the child from falling out of the crib. A hand is *always* placed on the back or abdomen of an infant or young child when the crib rails are down or when the small child is on an elevated surface such as a scale or treatment table. The nurse follows this practice consistently and teaches it to parents as well. As with adult patients, when children and adolescents are in hospital beds, they are maintained in the lowest position with the rails up on each side. Small objects, such as alcohol swabs and IV line caps, must be kept out of cribs and off of bedside tables, the floor, or any area within the young child's reach. Older infants and toddlers may put these small items in their mouths, causing a significant risk for choking.

When performing a procedure on a child, techniques such as distraction by a parent or child life specialist, can facilitate the child to stay calm and still (ENA, 2012; Shockey et al., 2013). Occasionally, to prevent trauma during a procedure, holding a child is necessary to restrict movement. If holding is required, it is important to enlist the cooperation of the child (if an appropriate age) and parent (Brenner, 2013). Some parents may be willing to hold their child on their lap for a procedure, or provide distraction while a second nurse holds the child. Parents should not be required to hold their child during a procedure, because this has been found to cause significant distress to the family (Brenner, 2013).

Restraints should be used only as a last resort for the protection of the child and others. Some infants and young children may require protection from pulling out a tube, removing a dressing, or disrupting a suture line by using a restraint. Covering the hands with mitts or using elbow restraints, which keep the elbows from bending so the child's hands cannot reach a vulnerable site, may be necessary. If a restraint is needed for the child's protection, most facilities require a physician's order stating why the restraint is needed and how long it will be in place. The restraint chosen should be the least restrictive device that will prevent injury.

Before applying any form of restraint, the nurse informs the parents and child, if appropriate, of the reason for the restraint, where it will be applied, what movement it will prevent, how long it will be in place, and how often a nurse will check on the child. The call button is made readily available so the child or parent can easily reach the nurse. Brenner (2013) described parents' experience with restraining a child, reporting that parents prefer good communication, precise directions on how they can assist, and seeing their children as individuals and not a task to be completed. The child's developmental needs (e.g., thumb-sucking) are assessed, and provisions are made to meet these needs when possible (e.g., restrain a toddler's arm so the thumb can still be placed in the mouth). Regardless of the type of restraint used, the nurse must remove the restraint and assess the patient on a regular and frequent basis (e.g., every 1 to 2 hours).

### SAFETY ALERT

#### *Using Restraints*

- Use the least restrictive restraint.
- Choose the proper device for the child's condition.
- Ensure proper fit of the device.
- Tie knots, if used, that can be easily untied for quick access.
- Secure ties to bed frames (not mattresses or side rails), to the frames of wheelchairs, or to another stable device.
- Check the extremity distal to the restraint for circulation, sensation, and motion every 15 minutes for the first hour and subsequently as agency policy dictates.
- Remove restraints every 1 to 2 hours for range-of-motion movement and repositioning and to offer the child food or the opportunity to use the bathroom.
- Document findings from neurovascular checks; restraint removal, repositioning and range of motion; and skin condition assessment.

Many hospitalized children are physically active and may be at risk for injury from falls. How hospitals define, classify, and measure fall injury rates for children varies considerably (Schaffer et al., 2012). Factors that can contribute to children's falls within the hospital setting include altered mental status (e.g., sedation, conditions that cause dizziness or confusion), age (younger than 3 years), need for mobility assistance, and inattentiveness by parents because of unfamiliarity with surroundings or anxiety (Schaffer et al., 2012). It is recommended that all children undergo a complete fall risk screen when admitted to the hospital. The Joint Commission recommends a proactive approach to the assessment and prevention of falls (Schaffer et al., 2012).

Recent research demonstrated that many falls in the hospital setting are preventable, which reinforces the need for vigilance in fall-prevention strategies (Jamerson et al., 2014). Nurses must ensure that children, parents, and other healthcare team members keep bedside and crib rails up. Infants or small toddlers can be placed in a crib with a plastic hood or higher extensions to the crib sides. Older children and adolescents at risk for falls are informed not to attempt to get out of bed without assistance and how to use the call system when they need help. Other preventive actions include keeping the floors free of objects and fluids, providing adequate lighting, using assistive equipment properly, wearing nonslip footwear, and frequent patient monitoring. For active children, prevention strategies might include using a sitter to stay with the child, behavior modification techniques such as a time-out, and diversional activities appropriate to the child's developmental level and condition (Jamerson et al., 2014).

## INFECTION CONTROL

### Hand Hygiene

Hand hygiene is the mainstay of infection control in healthcare settings and in the home. In 2009, the World Health Organization (2011) published guidelines regarding hand hygiene in healthcare settings as did the Centers for Disease Control and Prevention (CDC) in 2002. Based on studies demonstrating that organisms are present both in hospitalized patients and on environmental surfaces and that alcohol-based hand rubs are most effective for eliminating organisms, the CDC (2002) issued recommendations for hand hygiene. These recommendations have been updated in the clinical guidelines for preventing transmission of infection in the hospital (CDC, 2002) as follows:

1. If hands are contaminated with blood or body fluids or are visibly soiled, clean hands with soap and water.
2. If hands are clean, use an alcohol-based hand rub before and after touching potentially contaminated surfaces near the patient, before and after patient contact, before putting on gloves for a procedure, and after removing gloves.
3. Put alcohol-based hand rub on the hands, rub over all surfaces of hands and fingers, and allow to thoroughly dry (total time, approximately 20 seconds).

Procedures described subsequently in this chapter assume that the nurse will use appropriate hand hygiene both before and after each procedure.

### Standard Precautions

Standard Precautions that are used in institutions and the workplace for infection prevention apply to the following:

- Blood
- All body fluids, secretions, and excretions except sweat, regardless of whether they contain visible blood
- Nonintact skin
- Mucous membranes

This system includes two tiers of precautions. Standard Precautions, precautions in the first tier, apply to the care of all hospitalized patients, regardless of diagnosis or presumed infectious state. Second-tier precautions apply to the care of specific patients and are referred to as *Transmission-Based Precautions.* These precautions are used for patients known or suspected to be infected by pathogens that are transmitted through air or droplets or through contact with dry skin or contaminated surfaces.

### Implementing Precautions

When Transmission-Based Precautions are in effect, the items with which the infected child comes in contact are also contaminated. These items include the bed, linens, IV pump, sink, and toys. Therefore, the nurse who is going into the room to reset an IV pump, pick up soiled linens, and so forth must use whatever protective equipment is mandated by the type of precaution (e.g., gown, mask, gloves, goggles, face shield) (CDC, 2002).

Children placed on Transmission-Based Precautions often need extra attention to avert boredom. They need more diversional activities, such as games or movies, and more psychosocial support. Young children, for example, might think that they are being punished. Visitors might hesitate to enter the child's room and need additional support or reassurance from the nurse. Often, the amount of time spent on direct care of patients regarding contact precautions is considerably less than that provided to patients who are not on transmission-based precautions (Myers, 2014).

### Family Teaching

Family education is crucial for effective infection control and prevention. The nurse emphasizes to parents, visitors, and other healthcare providers that infection control precautions are important and must be closely followed. Parents often state that they are there to visit only their own child and do not understand the need to wear special clothing or equipment. The nurse needs to emphasize that the organisms that cause some diseases, such as respiratory syncytial virus, can live on inanimate objects such as clothing or crib rails for many hours. Thus, the disease can spread throughout the hospital or to the home if infection control or prevention measures are not followed. Family members are encouraged to visit the child frequently because visits will decrease the child's sense of isolation. Family members are taught that meticulous hand hygiene, both in the hospital setting and at home, is the best way to prevent infection.

## BATHING INFANTS AND CHILDREN

The nurse can use bath time to facilitate parent interaction with their infant. During the bath, the nurse demonstrates for the parents how to hold the infant securely and how to bathe the infant so that bath time is a positive experience for parents and children.

Strict observance of safety principles when bathing an infant or child can prevent falls, burns, or water aspiration. When bathing an infant or a child in the hospital setting, the nurse takes the opportunity to note any problems, such as altered skin integrity, surgical incisions, loss of sensation, abnormal skin color, bruising, paralysis, or any other condition that might warrant special consideration. Newborn infants can be immersed in water after the umbilical stump and circumcision sites (if applicable) have healed. The temperature of the bath water should not exceed 37.7° C (100° F) — warm, but not hot to the touch. If a bath thermometer is available, it should be used to check the temperature of the water. Otherwise, a temperature that is comfortable when tested on the inside of your wrist or elbow is appropriate.

Before bathing any child, assess the family's preferences and home practices. Factors to consider include the time of day usually set aside for the bath, bathing rituals, special equipment, any product allergies, and the type of bath preferred. This time is also used to determine the amount of assistance needed by the child and the family and to address any learning needs related to hygiene. Because bathing is one of the areas over which parents might be allowed to retain control when a child is hospitalized, it is important to allow them to make as many decisions as possible. Decision making also allows parents to maintain a part of the home routine with their hospitalized child.

An infant who cannot sit unaided can be given either a sponge bath or a bath in an infant tub. The infant's body and head are supported at all times during the bath (Fig. 37.3). Older infants and toddlers can be bathed in either an infant tub or a regular bathtub. Infants and small children are *never* left unattended in the bath. Older children can take showers if facilities are available. The nurse should use judgment in deciding how much supervision an older child needs while bathing. Privacy for the school-age child and adolescent is extremely important.

### Special Considerations

Bed baths are frequently used for hospitalized infants and children. When bathing a newborn or young infant, soap is not necessary. In fact, soap can be too drying to the skin if used frequently. If soap is necessary or desired by the parent, a gentle, non-alkaline soap should be used.

To prevent chilling when giving a sponge bath, be sure to keep the child covered with a cotton blanket. The entire body except for the

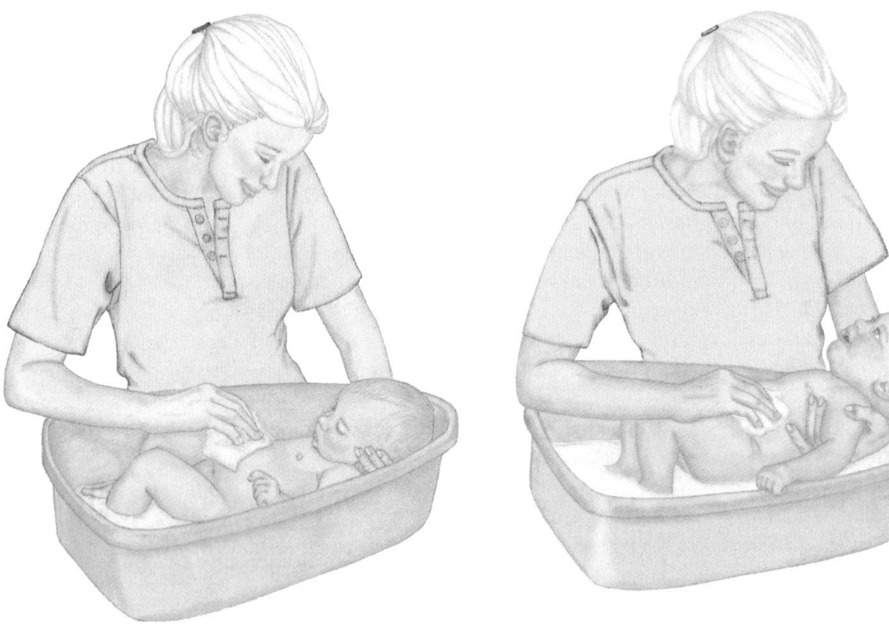


**FIG 37.3** Using hand to support infant's neck and head. When giving an infant a tub bath, the nurse supports the infant's body at all times.

body part being washed or rinsed is covered. The bath begins with the face, and the diaper area is cleaned last. If eye discharge is present, the nurse uses a clean, wet gauze for each eye, and cleans from the inner canthus outward. The outer ears can be cleaned with a wet face cloth.

If bathing an infant, line a plastic infant tub with a towel to provide comfort, as well as traction to prevent slipping. To prevent accidental drowning in case the infant slides down into the tub, fill the tub with no more than 2 to 3 inches of water.

When finished with the bath, the infant is wrapped in a dry towel or cotton blanket. Using the football hold and holding the infant over the tub, the nurse shampoos the infant's scalp and hair (including the area over the fontanel) with baby shampoo. Talcum powder, baby powder, and cornstarch are *not* used in the diaper area. When these substances get moist, they provide a medium for organism growth. Talcum powder and cornstarch, if accidentally inhaled, can result in respiratory complications.

Older children can choose to take a bath or shower, if their condition allows. The nurse ensures that the child has adequate towels, soap, and toiletries. Either the parent, nurse, or other staff member should remain nearby to provide assistance upon request. Instruct the child to pull the emergency light if assistance is needed.

Should an older child or adolescent require a bed bath, adjust the room temperature to a comfortable setting, and draw the curtain around the bed. As with any bed bath, the nurse begins with the face and proceeds in a head-to-toe progression. Obtain fresh water when it is time to rinse the child. Drape the child adequately for privacy and warmth. To prevent chilling, dry each body section as it is rinsed. The bath can be followed with application of lotion or deodorant if desired. The nurse performs the same assessment as with any child and provides assistance as necessary.

Some bathing restrictions might apply to children with surgical incisions, skin traction, IV catheters, casts, urinary catheters, artificial airways, or feeding tubes. Some children are restricted or unable to tolerate certain position changes because of their underlying conditions or treatments. It is imperative to assess for these special needs before beginning the bath.

### Documentation

Documentation includes the type of bath, child or parent participation, procedure tolerance, and any abnormal findings noted, such as bruising, rashes, or excoriation. Any lotions or other skin preparations used also should be recorded.

### Parent Teaching

General principles of hygiene and safety might need to be reinforced with some parents. Instruction in the use of special bathing equipment, such as infant bathtubs, safety bars, or tub grips, should be included as part of discharge teaching and preparation. To prevent injury or accidental drowning, appropriate supervision of the child should be maintained at all times. Parents are taught to *never* leave an infant or a young child alone in the bath; the risk of drowning, even in small amounts of water, is high. Infant bath seats that adhere to the floor of a regular bathtub by suction cups, are unsafe and should not be used because infants can slip out the sides and the seats can tip over.

## ORAL HYGIENE

To remove excess food and bacteria, the nurse wipes an infant's gums gently with a wet cloth after each feeding. After teeth erupt, brush a child's teeth with a smear or a grain-of-rice–sized amount of fluoride toothpaste and a pea-sized amount for children 3 years of age and older to clean the mouth and teeth after each feeding and before bed (AAP, 2014a). Until the parent is certain that the child can perform oral care correctly and independently, young children are supervised and assisted if needed. Even then, reminders to brush might be necessary.

Children frequently need reminders to brush their teeth. Toothbrushing should be done at least twice daily with a child's soft toothbrush. Children can ingest excessive amounts of fluoride if they are allowed to use large amounts of toothpaste or if they eat the toothpaste (CDC, 2011). Using the recommended amount of toothpaste and encouraging the child not to swallow the toothpaste will prevent fluorosis (brown spots on the teeth caused by too much fluoride).

Flossing is useful for cleaning between teeth and maintaining healthy gums. The child should begin to floss when all the primary teeth are in or when the child's molars begin to touch.

Immunosuppressed children, in particular, need excellent oral hygiene. Soft toothbrushes, sponge-covered Toothettes, or moistened gauze sponges can be used for dental care in the child who is at risk for gingival bleeding (see Chapter 48).

Since dental caries are the most common chronic disease in children, a caries risk assessment is an important part of an admission assessment (AAP, 2014a). Discharge teaching in the area of oral hygiene is important and yet often forgotten. Many parents do not realize that an infant's gums and teeth need to be cleaned. The American Academy of Pediatrics (AAP) recommends a dental visit by 1 year of age (AAP, 2014a). Thereafter they should be seen on a regular basis (every 6 months) for services that include checkups, professional cleaning, and fluoride application.

The risk of dental caries increases if formula, milk, or other liquids remain in a child's mouth overnight. Allowing an infant to fall asleep with a bottle containing one of these liquids can cause a condition known as bottle-mouth syndrome, which results in severely decayed primary teeth. Parents are instructed not to put a child to bed with a bottle of formula, juice, or sweetened liquid. If the child will not fall asleep without a bottle, advise the parent to use water only.

Good nutrition influences dental health. Avoiding sugary and carbonated drinks is important. Encourage parents to offer only water between meals (AAP, 2014a). Teaching about oral hygiene often provides an opportunity to educate the child and family about proper nutrition and general health maintenance.

## FEEDING

Mealtimes can be difficult for the hospitalized child. Changes in routine, diet, and surroundings, as well as dietary restrictions and illness, affect the child's ability and desire to eat. Refusing to eat might also be the way a child attempts to have some control.

The nurse assesses the child's preferences and dislikes on admission and before ordering meals. Mealtime rituals and routines, as well as cultural food variations are noted. Serving favorite and preferred foods and offering nutritious snacks can ensure appropriate caloric and nutrient intake.

The type and form of food chosen should be appropriate to the child's age and developmental level. (See Chapters 6 through 9 for a discussion of food types appropriate for each age-group.) When planning meals, the nurse must consider whether the child has any special needs or required restrictions.

Feeding a hospitalized infant seldom differs from feeding an infant at home. Types of foods, feeding schedules, and routines should mimic home schedules and routines when possible. If the infant's bottle or nipple brand is not available in the hospital, ask the parents to bring what the infant uses at home. Encourage parents to be present at mealtimes and feed their children if indicated. Feeding reinforces the special bond that develops between child and parent.

Nurses facilitate breastfeeding for infants by providing a private, quiet, and relaxed location so mother and infant feel comfortable and not rushed. If the mother is pumping breast milk for use when she is absent, the nurse meticulously follows hospital policy for labeling, storing, and administering pumped breast milk to the infant.

Unless medically contraindicated, infants should be held during feedings. Because of the risk of aspiration, bottles should *never* be propped; a pillow or rolled blanket must not be positioned next to an infant's mouth. Frequent burping during and after feedings can reduce the chance of regurgitation. To burp the infant, the nurse can use the upright hold and gently pat or rub the infant's back, or seat the infant on the nurse's knees with a hand supporting the infant's chin. After feeding, the infant can be positioned on the right side to facilitate the flow of the feeding toward the lower end of the stomach and allow any swallowed air to rise into the esophagus. However, if the nurse is placing an infant in the crib for sleep, the infant must be positioned supine, lying on his or her back. The supine position for sleeping infants has been shown to decrease the risk of sudden infant death syndrome. In 2011, the AAP expanded the "Back to Sleep" recommendations to include other risk factors for SIDS such as smoke exposure, avoidance of sleep positioners, and overheating. Nurses in the hospital setting should educate parents about the recommendations (Meadows-Oliver & Hendrie, 2013).

Toddlers and preschoolers often use food as a source of control. They might exhibit "food jags," during which they will eat only one or two items for a period of several days. They enjoy finger foods but are learning to use spoons or forks fairly competently. Colorful plates and cups can encourage a reluctant child to eat. Parents are encouraged to bring the child's own cups or utensils from home to simulate usual mealtime routines as closely as possible.

For young children, the nurse cuts foods into pieces appropriate in size and texture to decrease the risk of aspiration. Foods to avoid include hot dogs, popcorn, peanuts, and grapes, because if aspirated, these can occlude the airway. Young children *must* be supervised when eating. They are also secured at a table, in a highchair, or in bed using an overbed table during meals. "Roaming" while eating increases the risk of food aspiration and should be avoided. Children are prompted to feed themselves independently as much as possible. Mealtime is limited to 15 to 20 minutes and discontinued if the child is playing with and not eating the food.

Older children and adolescents seldom have difficulty expressing their dietary preferences. However, difficulty may arise when children this age are placed on a restricted or special diet. For example, the diabetic child often has difficulty staying on a restricted diet in the face of peer pressure. The nurse needs to provide support and clear limits to ensure cooperation. Referral to a dietitian may be necessary to help the child make appropriate food choices.

### Special Considerations

Keeping accurate intake and output (I&O) measurements is necessary for many hospitalized children. The nurse measures and records all intake; oral, **enteral**, and parenteral. All output, including output from urine and stool; drainage from tubes, stomas, or fistulas; and emesis, is also measured and recorded. When measuring urinary output for a child in diapers, weigh each wet diaper and subtract the weight of a dry diaper of the same size. One gram of weight equals approximately 1 mL of urine output.

### Documentation

Documenting the child's nutritional intake assists in determining the child's overall health. The nurse records food intake and preferences, as well as observations about the child's appetite and eating patterns. Older children and adolescents are assessed for any abnormal eating patterns, because eating disorders are more prevalent in these age-groups.

### Parent Teaching

Educating parents regarding feeding, special diets, and the nutritional needs of children is extremely important. The nurse should carefully instruct parents about how to manage any food or fluid restrictions, or special diets. A child with type 1 diabetes mellitus (see Chapter 51) or celiac disease (see Chapter 43) is at risk for injury if the prescribed diet is not closely followed.

## VITAL SIGNS

An underlying principle for obtaining vital signs in a child is to obtain the vital signs when the child is quiet, if at all possible. Sometimes this involves measuring the pulse and respirations when the child is asleep. If this timing is not possible, note any activity that affects accurate measurement (e.g., crying, playing). It is important for the nurse to monitor vital signs and compare them to the child's own baseline vital signs. The timing of vital signs is based on the policy of the hospital and the child's condition (Van Kuiken & Huth, 2013).

### Measuring Temperature

Temperature is an objective indicator of illness, and measuring temperature is an integral part of assessing children. Oral, rectal, axillary, temporal artery (infrared), and tympanic temperature readings are often obtained using different types of electronic, digital thermometers. Beginning in 2001 and reaffirmed in 2007, the American Academy of Pediatrics recommends that thermometers containing mercury not be used for children in hospital or home settings because of toxicity risks (AAP, 2007). Whatever temperature measurement method is chosen, the child's temperature should be measured at the same site and with the same device to maintain consistency and allow reliable comparison and tracking of temperatures over time. (See Table 33.1 in Chapter 33 for normal temperatures in children.)

Digital thermometers, which most often run on batteries, measure the temperature quickly (usually in less than 30 seconds). To prevent cross contamination, a child may have a single thermometer kept in the hospital room. If an electronic thermometer is used for multiple patients, a new disposable probe cover is used for each new patient. There is considerable variation in the types of thermometers used to measure the temperature of a hospitalized child. Factors to consider when selecting the route to use for obtaining a temperature reading include the child's age and ability to cooperate with the procedure, acuity of the illness, environmental factors (room conditions, food/fluid consumption), and equipment availability. Measuring body temperature can be time consuming for the nurse and stressful for the child. Therefore, it is imperative that nurses are trained in the use of the chosen device (El-Radhi, 2014). For all devices used to measure temperature by any route, the accuracy of the temperature reading is dependent on correct use of the equipment; the probe must be in the correct position and held steadily in place for the required period of time. For infants and children who are unable to properly hold an oral thermometer in their mouth, axillary, temporal artery, or tympanic thermometers are used (Fig. 37.4). Rectal temperatures are more accurate in measuring core body temperature, particularly in infants, and are the preferred site of measuring core body temperatures (El-Radhi, 2014). However, inserting a thermometer into a child's rectum is an invasive procedure and may be contraindicated for children at risk for anal or rectal injury, infection, or bleeding (El-Radhi, 2014). For this reason, many hospital units have policies that specify when a pediatric patient should have a rectal temperature measurement.

The advantage to temporal artery and tympanic temperature measurements is that they are obtained quickly, usually within a few seconds, and cause minimal discomfort to the child. Research has shown inconsistencies with tympanic temperature measurement (El-Radhi, 2014). The accuracy of temporal artery temperatures is still being evaluated; studies have indicated mixed results when comparing temporal artery measurements to other temperature measurements via rectal and other routes (Hamilton, Marcos, & Secic, 2013). Temporal artery measurement can be used for infants older than three months who show no signs of fever (Hurwitz, Brown, & Altmiller, 2015).

Axillary temperatures are appropriate for infants and children younger than 4 to 6 years or any child who cannot safely have or hold an oral thermometer in the mouth. Axillary temperatures are approximately 0.6° C (1° F) lower than the body's core temperature. For an accurate reading, the thermometer is held in the child's axilla for up to 5 minutes, which may be difficult for a child (El-Radhi, 2014). To help the child remain still, consider holding him or her on your lap and reading a story.

Temperatures are measured orally in most children ages 6 years and older, including adolescents. Keeping a thermometer in the correct location in the mouth can be a challenge for any child. The child is instructed to keep the mouth closed, with lips in a "kiss" position, and not to bite the thermometer. Intake of foods and liquids should be avoided for 30 minutes before the oral temperature measurement. Inaccurate oral temperatures may occur because of oral intake, oxygen

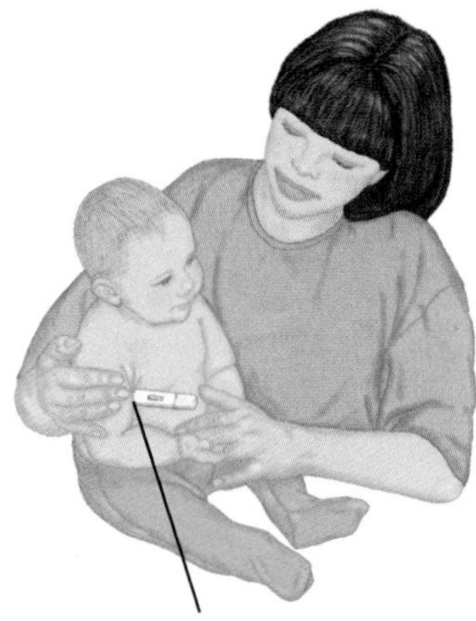

Axillary temperature
Place thermometer in the axilla and press child's arm close to body until reading is obtained.


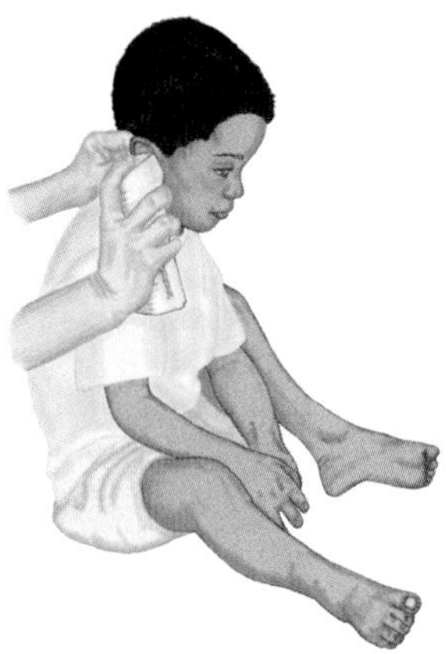

Tympanic temperature
Aim the thermometer tip toward tympanic membrane for accuracy.


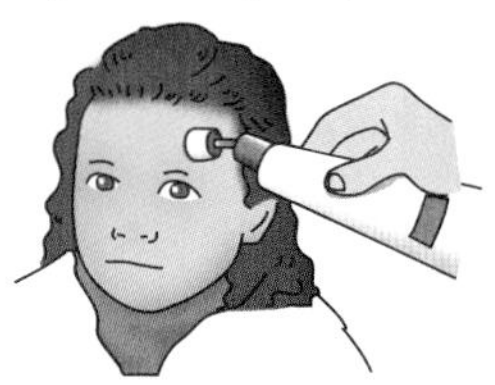

Temporal artery temperature
Place the thermometer probe flat on center of forehead and lightly slide horizontally across forehead to hairline.


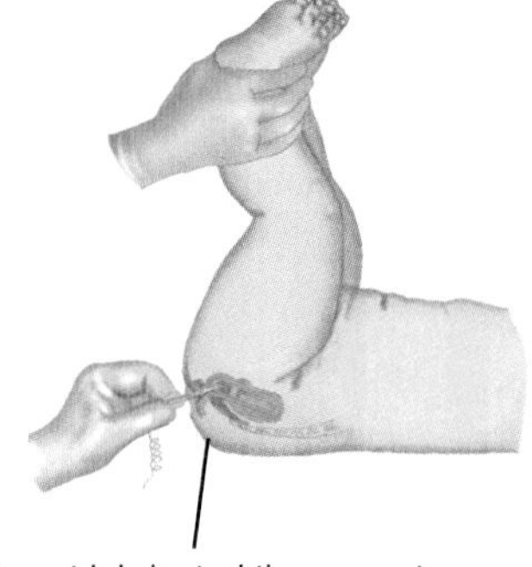

Rectal temperature
Insert lubricated thermometer no more than 1.25 cm in an infant and 2.5 cm in an older child.


**FIG 37.4** Four methods of temperature measurement.

administration, nebulized treatments, or crying. Oral temperature measurement should not be used in any child who has had oral or tonsillar surgery or in whom epiglottitis is suspected (see Chapter 45).

**! NURSING QUALITY ALERT**

***Measuring Temperature***

- If an elevated or low oral, axillary, temporal artery, or tympanic temperature reading is obtained, consider measuring the temperature via another route (including the rectal route), if possible.
- Report a temperature measurement of less than 36° C (96.8° F) or more than 38° C (100.4° F). Such reporting is critical for an infant younger than 3 months of age.

## Measuring Pulse

Apical pulse rate measurements (Fig. 37.5) are recommended for infants and children younger than 2 years of age and in any child who has an irregular heart rate or known congenital heart disease. It is best to auscultate the apical pulse when the child is quiet, counting for 1 full minute. The apical heart rate must be determined before administering certain medications, such as digoxin.

Radial pulse measurements are appropriate for children over 2 years of age (see Table 33.1 for normal pulse measurements).

## Evaluating Respirations

Infants often have irregular respiratory rates that change with stimulation, crying, and feeding. First, observe the pattern of inspiration and expiration to determine any irregular rhythm. Next, with an infant or young child who is quiet and at rest, measure the respiratory rate by auscultating for 1 full minute. For older children, either observe chest movement or auscultate respirations to obtain the rate (see Table 33.1 for normal respiratory rate measurements).

## Measuring Blood Pressure

The blood pressure (BP) of a well child is generally assessed just once per year during routine physical examination. For the hospitalized child, BP readings are obtained on admission and then at least every 24 hours. If abnormalities are detected or the child's condition is unstable, BP checks are done more frequently. When interpreting BP results, a child's age, gender, and height must be considered (see Table 33.1 for normal values). When obtaining a blood pressure the child's arm should be at the level of the child's heart, an appropriate size cuff should be selected and movement kept at a minimum. Children should be sitting with their legs uncrossed, though it is acceptable to have infants and young children lying down (Makic, Martin, Burns, et al., 2013).

Choosing the appropriate cuff size is required if accurate BP readings are to be obtained. A cuff that is too small may cause a BP reading to be falsely high, and a cuff that is too large may result in a falsely low reading. Recommendations for how to choose an appropriate cuff size vary, but the following is a suggested procedure (Makic et al., 2013):

- Find the midpoint of the right upper arm between the shoulder (acromion) and the elbow (olecranon).
- Holding the bladder of the cuff lengthwise, the bladder width should cover approximately 40% of the upper arm circumference at this point.
- When you wrap the cuff around the arm to take the BP, the bladder should encircle 80% to 100% of the arm without overlap. Nurses should note the markings on the cuff to determine the correct size.
- Palpate the brachial artery; place the stethoscope bell on the brachial artery below the cuff (medial aspect of the antecubital fossa).
- Measure the BP with the arm at heart level after the child has been at rest for 3 to 5 minutes.

For children, BP can be measured in the upper arm, lower arm, thigh, calf, or ankle (Fig. 37.6). If using a different site than the arm for BP measurement, the bladder should cover 40% of the circumference of the site used. Commercially designated BP cuffs are standardized widths, so select the closest standard width to the 40% circumference measurement. Table 37.1 illustrates average bladder widths of commercial BP cuffs.

To ensure consistency, take measurements in the same limb, in the same place, and with the child in the same position. BP measurements can differ depending on the site used, so the site must be documented (see http://www.nhlbi.nih.gov/guidelines/hypertension/child_tbl.pdf for normal results). For children, the systolic BP is determined by the onset of the first Korotkoff "tapping" sound, and the diastolic reading is the number at which the Korotkoff sound disappears. Mercury sphygmomanometers have been replaced by aneroid sphygmomanometers and automated oscillometric blood pressure monitors. Studies

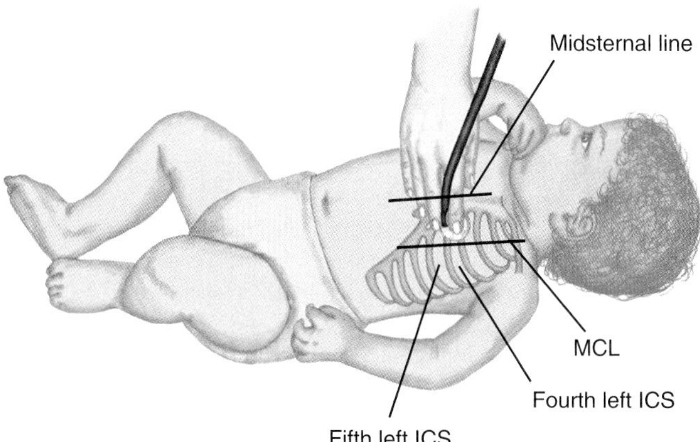
Apical pulse is lateral to the left midclavicular line (MCL) and fourth intercostal space (ICS) in children younger than 7 years and to the left MCL and fifth ICS in children older than 7 years.
Midsternal line
MCL
Fourth left ICS
Fifth left ICS

**FIG 37.5** Locating the apical pulse. Apical pulse is lateral to the left midclavicular line (MCL) and fourth intercostal space (ICS) in children younger than 7 years and to the left MCL and fifth ICS in children older than 7 years.

**TABLE 37.1 Recommended Dimensions for Blood Pressure Cuff Bladders**

| Age | Range Width (cm) | Length (cm) | Maximum Arm Circumference (cm)* |
|---|---|---|---|
| Newborn | 4 | 8 | 10 |
| Infant | 6 | 12 | 15 |
| Child | 9 | 18 | 22 |
| Small adult | 10 | 24 | 26 |
| Adult | 13 | 30 | 34 |
| Large adult | 16 | 38 | 44 |
| Thigh | 20 | 42 | 52 |

*Calculated so that the largest arm would still allow the bladder to encircle arm by at least 80%.

From National High Blood Pressure Education Program Working Group on High Blood Pressure in Children and Adolescents. (2004). The fourth report on the diagnosis, evaluation, and treatment of high blood pressure in children and adolescents. *Pediatrics, 114*(2), 557.

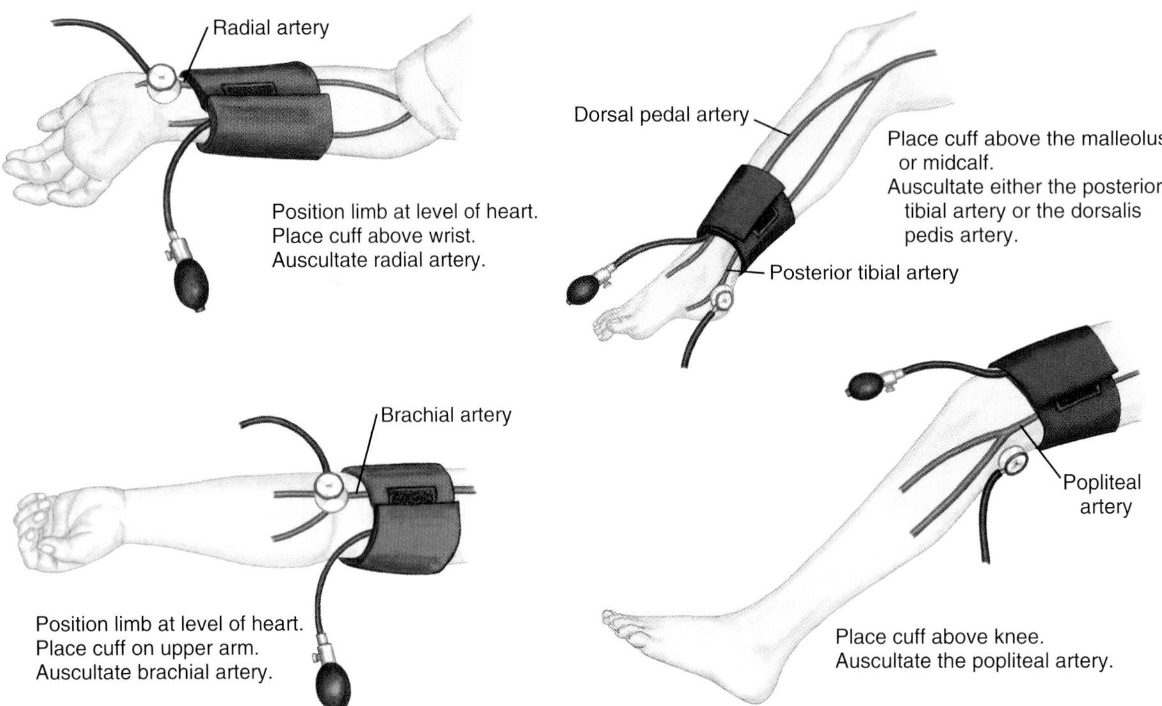
Radial artery
Position limb at level of heart.
Place cuff above wrist.
Auscultate radial artery.
Dorsal pedal artery
Place cuff above the malleolus or midcalf.
Auscultate either the posterior tibial artery or the dorsalis pedis artery.
Posterior tibial artery
Brachial artery
Position limb at level of heart.
Place cuff on upper arm.
Auscultate brachial artery.
Popliteal artery
Place cuff above knee.
Auscultate the popliteal artery.

**FIG 37.6** Blood pressures can be measured in the upper arm, lower arm, thigh, calf, or ankle. An appropriate-size cuff must be used to obtain accurate results.

show that there is variability in the blood pressure readings, and the results of either device should be confirmed with multiple measurements (Eliasdottir, Steinthorsdottir, Indridason, et al., 2013).

The AAP recommends BP measurements for early identification of hypertension. Approximately 1% to 5% of children and adolescents have hypertension and the prevalence is rising. These children and adolescents have a higher incidence of other cardiovascular risk factors putting them at risk for future cardiovascular disease (Thompson, Dana, Bougatsos, et al., 2013).

## Documenting Vital Sign Measurement

The nurse documents all vital signs in the child's paper or electronic medical record; the measurement result, the method used to measure each vital sign, the site where each measurement was obtained, and any action taken is included. It is essential that the nurse reports, as well as documents, any abnormal findings, or findings that are significantly different from the individual child's baseline.

## Preparing the Child and Family

The child and family are informed about the purpose of obtaining vital sign measurements. Children should be allowed to examine or handle the equipment while the nurse explains how it is used. Many children have toy medical instruments at home and may be familiar with the concept of taking vital signs.

Tell young children that the blood pressure cuff feels like a "hug" or a "squeeze" on their arm or leg.

## Parent Teaching

Some parents need to learn how to take the child's temperature at home. The nurse demonstrates how to take the child's temperature and then observes the parent performing the procedure. It is important to ensure that the parent is comfortable with the procedure and is able to read the thermometer accurately.

Some parents need to be taught how to correctly determine their child's heart rate and respiratory rate, as well as the acceptable range for their child. Special instructions relating to when parents should notify the physician may need to be provided for children who are taking certain medications, such as digoxin.

If the child's condition requires home BP monitoring, parents are taught to perform the procedure. The nurse provides information about the size of the BP cuff needed and ensures that the parents can read the dial accurately. Methods to involve the child in the procedure are discussed. For example, parents might make a smaller BP cuff for the child's favorite doll or stuffed animal.

### ! NURSING QUALITY ALERT

***Measuring Vital Signs***

- Temperatures should not be measured rectally in the immunosuppressed child or in any child who has had rectal surgery, diarrhea, or a bleeding disorder.
- Count respirations and measure the apical heart rate before taking other vital signs. Both signs are best measured on a sleeping or quiet child.
- Measure the apical heart rate for 1 full minute.
- Observe the child's respiratory rate and effort for 1 full minute while the child is quiet. Abdominal movement with breathing is normally observed in infants and young children, whereas thoracic movement can be noted in older children and adolescents.
- Evaluate the quality of respirations, symmetry of chest movement with each breath, and any noisy respirations (e.g., crackles, wheezes, friction rubs). Observe the child for any signs of respiratory distress, such as nasal flaring, grunting, stridor, retractions, increased work of breathing, cyanosis, or apneic periods.
- Always use a manual cuff and auscultation to verify electronically measured BPs that indicate hypertension or hypotension.

### Special Considerations: Cardiorespiratory Monitors

Some children need cardiorespiratory monitoring so that heart rate, respiratory rate, blood pressure, and temperature can be continuously measured. Children who are acutely ill or who are undergoing procedures might be placed on a monitor to help healthcare providers detect subtle changes in the child's condition.

The procedure and indications for attaching a child to a cardiorespiratory monitor are no different from those for an adult. Monitors sound an alarm to warn of changes in the child's cardiorespiratory status. In accordance with the child's age, alarm parameters for each measurement are often preset based on hospital policies and physician orders. It is important that the nurse verify settings and test that the monitor is functioning correctly. False alarms can occur. Whenever a monitor alarm sounds, the nurse must first look at the child and perform an assessment and then intervene if indicated. A flat line on the electrocardiogram (ECG) does not always signal a cardiac arrest, as it can be caused by a loose monitor lead. Check the manufacturer's recommendations for attaching leads and monitoring selected vital signs.

## FEVER-REDUCING MEASURES

The body's internal thermostat, the hypothalamus, attempts to keep the body's temperature between 36° C and 38° C (96.8° F and 100.4° F). This regulation is done through a complex series of interactions that result in heat gain or loss. The body's mechanisms for conserving or producing heat are vasoconstriction and shivering. Heat is lost through radiation, conduction, convection, and evaporation.

### Description of Fever

*Fever* is defined as a body temperature greater than 38° C (100.4° F) rectally or 37.5° C (99.5° F) orally that results from an insult or disease during which the body's set point temperature rises to a higher-than-normal level. After the cause of the fever is removed, the body resets its set point at the normal level.

The body's attempt to defend itself against illness is manifested by fever, which is triggered by endogenous pyrogens produced during the inflammatory response. Because research studies have not conclusively demonstrated whether fever is beneficial or detrimental, practitioners vary in their approach to managing fevers caused by infections. Mild degrees of fever may or may not require intervention, depending on the underlying cause and the child's response. Most fevers are brief and benign and resolve when the underlying infection resolves. Children with chronic cardiac or respiratory disease, those with neurologic disease, and those prone to febrile seizures should be treated for fever. Children with fevers of 40° C (104° F) or higher also should be treated.

Fever is uncomfortable and can make children irritable. For every 1° C of temperature elevation, the body's metabolic rate increases 10% to 13%, resulting in increased insensible fluid loss, increased oxygen consumption, and increased stress on the cardiovascular system (McDougall & Harrison, 2014). Regardless of the fever's cause, the child's comfort is the primary reason for treating a fever in a normally healthy child.

### Medications and Environmental Management

Treatment can consist of environmental measures, antipyretics, or a combination of interventions. Dressing the child appropriately (neither overdressed nor underdressed), providing adequate fluids, monitoring for signs of dehydration, and administering an appropriate antipyretic all are approaches to fever management. Studies have shown that the use of tepid sponging to reduce a fever can actually cause shivering and increased temperature as well as increased discomfort for the child (McDougall & Harrison, 2014).

Fevers in children are treated effectively with antipyretics such as acetaminophen or ibuprofen. Aspirin is not used to treat fever in children because of its association with Reye syndrome and viral illnesses (influenza and varicella). It is important to provide parents with written instructions regarding the correct dosing and dosing interval for antipyretics to avoid inaccurate dosing (Chang, Chen, Chang, et al., 2011).

Children with elevated temperatures often have a loss of appetite. Dehydration can occur from decreased oral intake and increased insensible water loss through the lungs and skin. To provide adequate hydration, offer the child oral fluids frequently, especially during times when their temperature drops (McDougall & Harrison, 2014). For those who refuse to ingest oral fluids or are unable to take in an adequate volume, evaluate the need for IV fluids.

To maintain body temperature and reduce heat loss, some infants are placed in radiant warmers or incubators (Isolettes). These microprocessor-based, servo-controlled temperature systems set the correct heating level by constantly monitoring the infant's temperature using a skin probe and the air temperature. Infants who are being cared for in these heating units must be carefully monitored, because accidental dislodgment of the skin probe can occur, resulting in excessive heating. Insensible water loss also is greatly increased for infants in these units, which must be considered when calculating fluid replacement.

**DRUG GUIDE**

***Acetaminophen (Tylenol, Tempra, Panadol)***

**Classification:** Non-narcotic analgesic and antipyretic.
**Action:** Unknown; may act on hypothalamic heat-regulating center.
**Indications:** Mild fever and pain relief.
**Dosage and Route:** Dosage is age and/or weight related; administered four or five times daily. Oral, rectal. Comes in a variety of oral preparations: oral suspension (160 mg/5 mL), chewable tablets (80 mg/tab), chewable tablets for older children (160 mg/tab), adult strength (325 mg/tab). Rectal suppositories in 80, 120, 325, and 650 mg.
**Absorption:** From the gastrointestinal tract; peak action in 1 to 3 hours.
**Excretion:** Duration approximately 4 to 5 hours.
**Contraindications:** Any previous sensitivity to the medication.
**Precautions:** Long-term use can cause liver damage. Other over-the-counter cold preparations can contain acetaminophen; if given concurrently they can increase the amount of acetaminophen above safe levels.
**Adverse Reactions:** Blood dyscrasias, hypoglycemia, rashes or urticaria, liver damage with prolonged use.
**Nursing Considerations:** Advise parents to be extremely careful not to confuse the liquid preparations; check the label carefully before giving the medication. Never refer to this or any other medication as "candy." Acetaminophen overdose must be treated immediately to prevent hepatic toxicity. Parents need to be aware that acetaminophen can affect home glucose readings. Parents should not continue to give their children this medication for fever that lasts longer than 2 days without checking with the child's primary care provider.

## SPECIMEN COLLECTION

Specimens are collected from children for the same reasons they are collected from adults, but children often need a more careful explanation of the procedures and reasons for specimen collection. All explanations should be given in age-appropriate language, and children should be prepared for any sensations that they might experience.

Regardless of the type of specimen to be obtained, Standard Precautions are used. The use of personal protective equipment (PPE) including gloves, gowns, masks, goggles or face shields, along with hand hygiene is required when there is the potential for the nurse to come in contact with blood and other body fluids that can contain infectious materials. The PPE used will vary according to the risk of contact with body fluids. For example, if a "splash" could possibly occur when collecting a specimen, a face shield and mask are worn in addition to gloves and a gown. The nurse should follow healthcare facility policies and procedures, based on Standard Precautions, when handling body fluids.

## Urine Specimens

### Voided Specimens

Infants and young toddlers are not yet toilet trained, and thus, unable to void on request, making urine specimen collection a challenge. A commonly used, noninvasive collection device is the urine collection bag. It consists of a plastic bag with an opening lined with adhesive so that it can be attached to the perineum. It is available in two sizes, infant and pediatric. Collection bags for a 24-hour urine specimen have a tube that extends from the end of the bag, allowing each void to be removed and placed in a designated, large container.

When using a urine collection bag to obtain a nonsterile specimen, the nurse first cleans the perineal area and then applies the bag (Procedure: Urine Specimen Collection from the Incontinent Child). If obtaining a specimen for urine culture, sterile gloves and cleansing solution plus a sterile urine collection bag should be used. Correct techniques when collecting, handling and transporting a urine specimen are essential to avoid contamination which may result in unnecessary and costly treatment (Dolan & Cornish, 2013). The AAP (2011) recommends the use of suprapubic aspiration (inserting a needle through the skin and directly into the bladder) to obtain a "sterile" urine specimen for culture from an incontinent child who is febrile with no other source for the fever.

Older children and adolescents often cooperate in the collection of urine specimens. Most can use a bedpan, urinal, or specimen cup with minimal assistance. Younger children and preschoolers who are toilet trained still have difficulty voiding on request. Parents can be helpful in obtaining urine specimens from their children. The nurse should use familiar terms, such as "pee pee," "tinkle," or "potty," when telling the preschool or young school-age child what is needed and have available a potty chair or a collection "hat" set in the toilet.

If the specimen must be collected using special techniques (e.g., a clean midstream urine sample), the nurse first carefully explains to the child and parent what preparation is needed and verifies understanding. A parent or nurse may need to assist the child during the collection. A young child may be able to sit on the toilet with the nurse or parent cleansing the perineal area and holding the specimen cup while the child voids. For a boy who wishes to stand while voiding, the cup can be held in the stream as he voids. If the specimen is to be carried to another area, place the cup in a plastic biohazard bag for transport.

### Urinary Catheterization

Reasons that a child needs a urinary catheter inserted include obtaining a sterile urine specimen for testing, accurately measuring urine output, and drainage of urine from the bladder (Procedure: Urinary Catheterization). Urinary catheterization can cause anxiety and discomfort in infants and children. Nurses need to take steps to ease the child's fears and discomfort through preparation of the child and family before the procedure, support during the procedure, selection of an appropriate-size catheter, and use of correct technique.

Children, based on their developmental level, and their parents need a complete explanation regarding the steps of procedure and what they need to do. This information includes instruction on how the child can relax pelvic muscles by blowing out, pressing the buttocks against the bed, or squeezing the abdomen as if having a bowel movement. Parents can provide distraction and comfort during the procedure by reading, singing, or holding the child's hand. A second nurse may be needed to gently hold the infant or child's legs to maintain them in the correct position.

## PROCEDURE

### *Urine Specimen Collection From the Incontinent Child*

**Purpose**

To obtain a voided urine specimen for testing.

1. Before beginning the procedure, provide adequate privacy. Some children are more relaxed if a parent is present. If both blood and urine specimens need to be obtained from the incontinent child, position the collection bag before drawing the blood. Infants and toddlers often void during a painful procedure.
2. Obtain the following equipment: nonsterile gloves, urine collection bag, sterile specimen cup, mild soap, warm water, washcloth, diaper and towel, and label and requisition form.
3. Perform hand hygiene. Put on gloves and clean the perineal area. Cleaning the perineum will remove any lotions or ointments and help the bag adhere. (If obtaining a specimen for urine culture, wear sterile gloves, use a sterile cleansing solution, and apply a sterile bag.)
   - For girls: Clean from front to back and from the urinary meatus to the labia majora (in to out).
   - For boys: Clean from the tip of the penis in a circular motion. Do not retract the foreskin of an infant or young child.
4. After the perineum has been cleansed, dry it thoroughly. The skin must be completely dry for the bag to adhere properly.
5. Remove the backing from the adhesive surface of the bottom half of the collection device.
6. Place the child in a frog-leg position to eliminate skin folds that may interfere with bag adherence. Apply the bottom half of the bag first and then remove the backing and apply the top half.

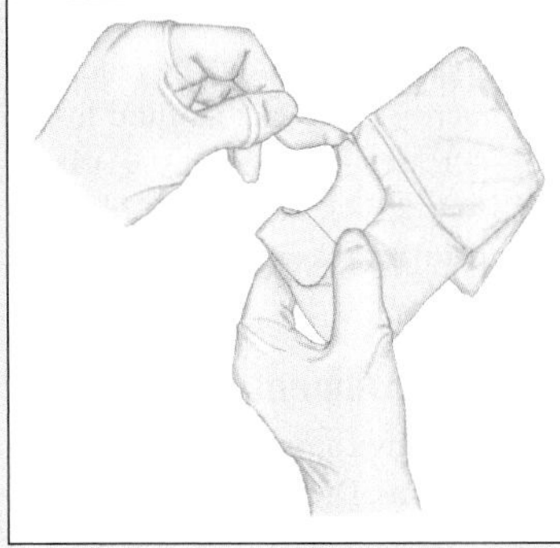

   - For girls: Hold the perineum taut and apply the adhesive portion of the bag, working outward. To keep feces from contaminating the specimen,

## PROCEDURE—cont'd

### *Urine Specimen Collection From the Incontinent Child*

the narrow "bridge" on the adhesive patch must be placed on the tiny area of skin between the anus and the genitalia.

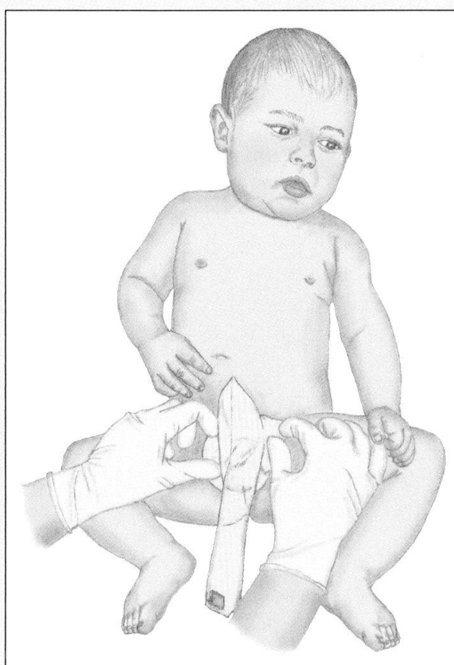

- For boys: Place the penis and scrotum (if small enough) inside the bag.

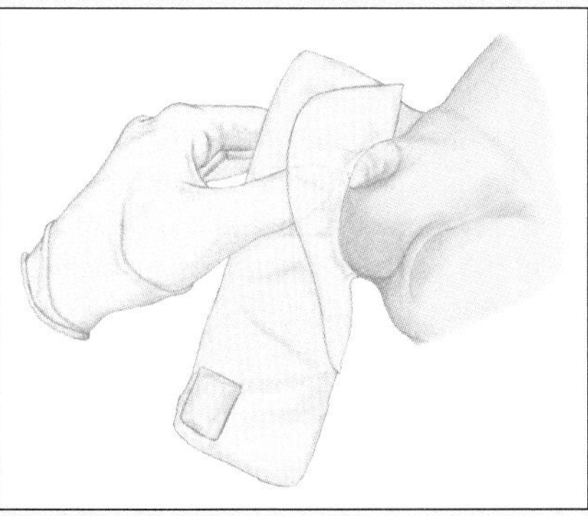

7. After the bag is attached, reapply a diaper. Cut a slit in the diaper and pull the end of the empty bag through the slit so that the bag protrudes from the diaper. This step reduces the chance of leaking and allows for observation of urine.
8. Check the bag every 30 minutes. Applying slight pressure over the suprapubic area or stroking along the older infant's spine will often induce voiding. As soon as urine is noticed in the bag, don gloves and gently remove the bag from the perineum.
9. Transfer the urine into a sterile specimen cup. Most bags have a small tab that can be removed to allow the urine to be poured. If the bag does not have a tab, clean the outside of the bag with an alcohol swab and withdraw the urine with a needle and syringe for placement in the appropriate container. Remove gloves and perform hand hygiene.

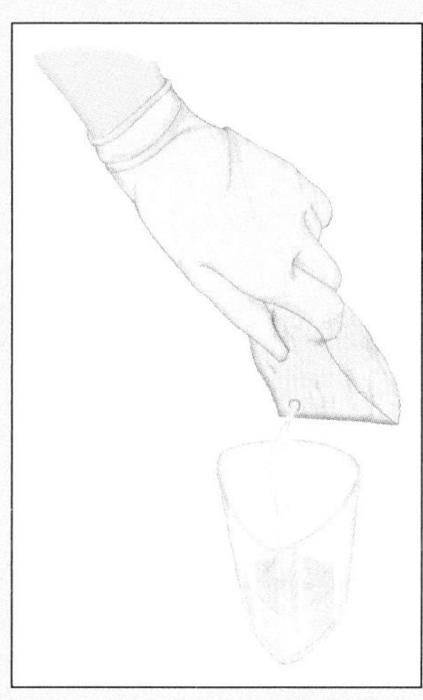

10. Label the urine specimen cup with the child's name, date, and time of collection. Place in a biohazard bag and deliver it promptly, together with a requisition form, to the laboratory. Urine for culture that cannot be tested within 30 minutes should be refrigerated.
11. Record the collection of the specimen in the child's chart. Include the date and time of collection and the amount, color, and appearance of the urine.

#### Home Adaptations

If a urine specimen is to be obtained at home, give instructions to the parent and provide the appropriate equipment. Parents can keep the urine collected at home in the refrigerator until they are asked to bring it to the laboratory. The specimen should be kept chilled during transport (i.e., placed in a cooler or plastic bag packed with ice).

## PROCEDURE

### *Urinary Catheterization*

#### Purpose

To monitor urine output accurately or obtain a sterile urine sample.

1. Prepare the child for the procedure by using age-appropriate methods. Explain what the child will feel and what the child can do to "help." Demonstrating the procedure on a teaching doll may be helpful. Teach the child to take slow, deep breaths during the procedure, and have the child practice breathing before the procedure. Encouraging the child to sing also helps relax the appropriate muscles. The child might feel a need to urinate during the catheter insertion. Reassure the child that the feeling is normal. The assistance of another adult is often necessary with younger children.
2. Make sure the area has good lighting, and gather all necessary equipment. If equipment is not contained in the catheterization kit, obtain the appropriate-size catheter, sterile gloves (extra pairs in case of contamination), sterile cleansing solution with applicators, drapes, specimen cup, sterile topical

*Continued*

## PROCEDURE—cont'd

### *Urinary Catheterization*

lubricant, label, and requisition form. If the child is to have an indwelling catheter placed, use of a closed system with the catheter already attached to the drainage tube and bag is preferred. Begin by performing hand hygiene.

3. The procedure is the same as for catheterizing an adult, with the following additions:
   - When preparing to insert an indwelling catheter, the nurse considers if the balloon integrity should be tested by injecting fluid from a prefilled syringe into the balloon port and then removing this fluid by aspirating with the syringe. This step is controversial because the balloon can stretch, forming ridges that can result in injury to the urethra during catheter insertion. It is recommended that the nurse follow the manufacturer's recommendations as well as hospital policy.
   - Take extra care to be gentle when cleansing the meatus or glans penis.
   - Choose the appropriate-size catheter. Apply the lubricant according to manufacturer's directions.
   - In girls, direct the catheter slightly upward and insert it gently through the meatus 1 to 2 inches (2.5 to 5 cm) or until urine appears. In boys, hold the penis at a 90-degree angle from the boy's body and gently insert the catheter 2 to 4 inches (5 to 10 cm) (longer in older boys) or until urine appears. Never force the catheter. The older child can assist in relaxing the external sphincter by bearing down.
4. Once urine is observed, advance the catheter approximately another ½ inch and hold until the urine stops flowing. If obtaining a specimen, be sure urine is collected in a sterile specimen cup. For an indwelling catheter, advance to the bifurcation of drainage and balloon inflation ports before inflation of the balloon (if applicable). This will be approximately 2 inches (5 cm) for girls, 3 to 4 inches (7.5 to 10 cm) for boys, newborn to preschool, and 5 inches (12.5 cm) for older boys. These distances reduce the risk of inflating the balloon in the urethra. Inflate the balloon slowly using the amount of fluid in the prefilled syringe that is recommended by the manufacturer. After inflating the balloon, remove gloves and perform hand hygiene.
5. Comfort the child if needed, offer praise for cooperation, and a reward, such as a sticker.
6. Label the specimen cup, place in a biohazard bag, and deliver promptly, together with the requisition form, to the laboratory. Refrigerate the specimen if transport to the laboratory is not immediate.
7. Document the date and time the procedure was performed, as well as the size of catheter used and the amount, color, and appearance of the urine. Note how the infant or child tolerated the procedure.

#### Home Adaptations

Catheterizing at home is usually a clean rather than sterile procedure used for children who have spina bifida, neurogenic bladder, or incomplete bladder emptying. Some families choose to use a new, packaged catheter each time; however, this can be extremely expensive when a child has to be catheterized several times per day. The alternative is to thoroughly rinse, clean, and dry the catheters and keep them in a clean, covered container or a plastic bag. The parent needs to follow physician protocols for cleaning the perineum; mild soap and water are often used. The infant or young child can be catheterized on a changing table, with the urine allowed to empty into a diaper or small container; the older child can be catheterized on the toilet.

## BOX 37.2 Guidelines for Urinary Catheter Selection by Age

- Infants up to 1 year old: 5 to 8 Fr
- Children 1 to 5 years old: 8 Fr
- School-age children: 8 to 12 Fr
- Adolescents: 10 to 14 Fr

Pediatric catheterization kits often contain a completely closed drainage system (with the catheter already attached to the drainage tube and bag). It is important that the nurse choose a urinary catheter that is the proper size for the child based on age. It should be small enough to be easily inserted into the meatus but large enough to prevent leakage of urine around the catheter (Box 37.2).

The catheter tip must be sufficiently lubricated to facilitate passage through the urethra and lessen discomfort. Some facilities recommend topical and intraurethral application of an anesthetic lubricant, such as 2% lidocaine hydrochloride gel, to diminish pain during catheterization.

Catheter associated urinary tract infections (CAUTI) have been identified as a hospital-acquired condition; therefore, reimbursement is no longer issued. In 2015, healthcare settings that continue to have CAUTI will be penalized (Strouse, 2015). Therefore, it is imperative that nurses provide meticulous hygiene to prevent urinary tract infections through appropriate insertion, removal, and maintenance techniques (Strouse, 2015).

Some children, particularly those who undergo multiple urinary tract catheterizations, are at high risk for developing latex sensitivity. At-risk children and others with known or suspected latex allergy should be identified early so that only latex-free catheters are used.

## Stool Specimens

Stool specimens are obtained to test for the presence of fat, blood, viruses, bacteria, parasites, or reducing substances in the stool. If a stool specimen from an incontinent child is needed, it often can be scraped from a diaper and placed in an appropriate container. If the stool is watery, a specimen can be collected by placing a piece of gauze in the diaper to absorb some of the stool or by applying a urine specimen collection bag over the anus.

A bedpan or a specimen collector "hat" set in the toilet can be used to obtain a specimen from an older child. Because older children can be embarrassed about providing a stool sample, the nurse should use a calm, matter-of-fact manner when explaining why the specimen is needed and the procedure for handling the specimen.

## Blood Specimens

Nurses use a variety of techniques to collect blood samples from children. Because blood collection is an invasive procedure, it should be performed in a treatment room if available.

Regardless of the sampling procedure used, most children find blood collection distressing. Some are concerned about the pain involved, and others fear the perceived loss of body fluid. Since most hospitalized children will have a venipuncture, it is important for the nurse to minimize the pain associated with it by involving the child life specialist, using distraction, administering analgesics or applying external cold devices such as Buzzy (MMJ Labs, Atlanta, GA) (Inal & Kelleci, 2012; Jeffs et al., 2011). The use of a topical anesthetic cream, such as eutectic mixture of local anesthetics (EMLA), can reduce the child's discomfort. To be effective, anesthetic creams generally must remain on the site for a minimum of 60 minutes before the needle is inserted (Baxter et al., 2013). Several studies show that distraction is also an effective technique when performing a venipuncture (Yoo, Kim, Hur, et al., 2011; Jeffs et al., 2011).

Children who need long-term venous access for nutrition or medications will often have a central venous catheter or port in place; the nurse can obtain blood for laboratory studies from this type of catheter or port.

Venipuncture in children for blood specimen collection is often performed using a butterfly catheter (Procedure: Venipuncture). The most commonly used sites are the veins of the hand and the antecubital area. The nurse always follows Standard Precautions when performing or assisting others with blood specimen collection.

### Jugular and Femoral Venipuncture

Jugular and femoral venipuncture are performed by a physician, with the nurse assisting and monitoring the child. If obtaining blood from one of the large superficial external jugular veins, assistance from a second nurse is necessary. The child's head is hyperextended to the side opposite the site, over the edge of a table or a small pillow (Fig. 37.7). After the venipuncture, pressure must be applied to the site for 3 to 5 minutes or longer until bleeding stops. Care is taken to not overextend the head, because this can cause airway problems.

For a femoral venipuncture, the child is placed supine in the frog-leg position to expose the groin area (see Fig. 37.7). The nurse stands above the infant's head, holding the infant's arms with the elbows and the infant's legs with the hands. To protect the venipuncture site if the infant urinates, a cloth diaper is placed over the perineal area and tucked under the buttocks, with one groin site exposed. Once the procedure is finished, the nurse applies pressure to the site for 5 minutes using a sterile gauze pad.

### Capillary Blood Sampling

When a small blood sample is needed, a commercial lancing device (Microlet lancet) designed to puncture at the proper depth can be used for a child's finger (Procedure: Capillary Blood Sampling) or an infant's heel (see Chapter 21, Procedure: Obtaining Blood Samples from the Newborn by Heel Puncture). The child's hand or the infant's heel is warmed first to increase blood flow. For finger punctures, the third (ring) finger of the nondominant hand should be used. The puncture is done just to the side of the finger pad rather than at the tip. Fewer nerve endings are in this location, and the area is highly vascular. When using the lateral aspect of an infant's heel, the puncture site chosen must avoid major nerves, blood vessels, and bone. The heel

## PROCEDURE

### *Venipuncture*

**Purpose**

To obtain a blood sample for laboratory testing with minimal trauma to the child.

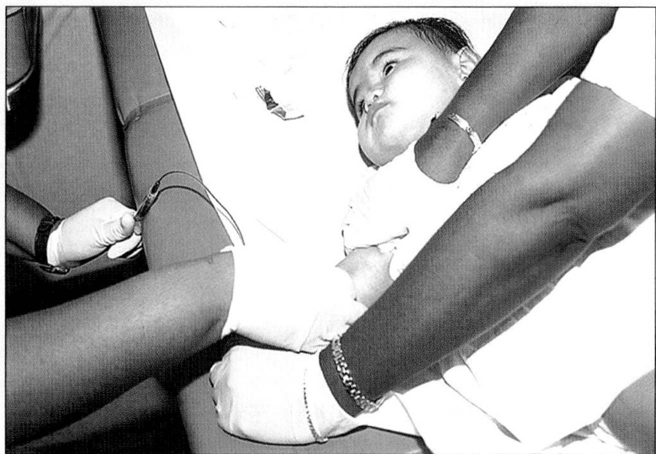

(Courtesy Parkland Health and Hospital System Community Oriented Primary Care Clinic, Dallas, TX.)

1. As with any procedure, prepare the child using age-appropriate language. Be sure to include what the child will see and feel. Ask the parents whether it is better to prepare their young child in advance or to describe what you are doing as you are performing the procedure. Assistance to hold the child is often necessary during the procedure. Parents are given the choice to stay with their child during the procedure or leave the room. If eutectic mixture of local anesthetics (EMLA) is to be used, it must be applied at least 60 minutes in advance of the procedure; follow the timing directions for other topical anesthetics if used.
2. Take the child to the treatment room. Have the following equipment available: 23- or 25-gauge butterfly catheter (or needle), gloves, antiseptic swabs, syringe or Vacutainer, sterile gauze, labels, appropriate collection tubes, requisition form, and tourniquet. (NOTE: Most tourniquets are composed of rubber tubing that is ½ - to 1-inch wide—rubber bands should not be used for infants because they can abrade the skin.)
3. Hold the child by having a nurse place one gloved hand under the child's arm (usually at the shoulder) and the other gloved hand on the child's hand. The second nurse is then able to draw the blood with less likelihood of missing the vein. The vein of the antecubital area or hand is commonly used for venipuncture in children.
4. Perform hand hygiene, put on gloves, and apply a tourniquet that is tight enough to restrict venous blood flow toward the heart and distend the veins, but not so tight as to cause pain or restrict arterial blood flow. To facilitate easy removal, the tourniquet should be looped when applied. To prevent hemoconcentration, a tourniquet should be left in place no longer than 2 minutes.
5. Lightly pat or rub the sample site to help the veins become more visible.
6. With a circular motion, clean the site with an antiseptic swab and allow to dry.
7. Insert the needle of the butterfly catheter into the vein, bevel side up.
8. When blood begins to flow into the catheter, wait until the blood reaches the end of the catheter, attach the syringe, and slowly draw the appropriate amount of blood into the syringe. The tourniquet can be released when blood begins to flow into the syringe.
9. After obtaining the required amount of blood, withdraw the needle and apply pressure to the puncture site using a sterile gauze pad until the bleeding has stopped. Fill the appropriate specimen tubes or containers. Be sure to dispose of needles in the sharps container and contaminated gauze in the biohazard receptacle. Remove gloves and perform hand hygiene.
10. Comfort the child and offer praise for cooperation. Encourage the parent to provide comfort. Adhesive bandages are important because they help prevent bleeding from the puncture site. Specially colored or cartoon character bandages are available commercially and are appropriate for children's "boo-boos." The nurse can also give the child a reward, such as a sticker.
11. Label the specimen with the child's name, place in a biohazard bag, and send to the laboratory with the requisition form for the test(s) to be performed.
12. Document the date and time of collection, the amount of blood collected, the site used for puncture, and the reason blood was drawn (e.g., diagnostic test). Note the child's reaction to the procedure and the number of attempts made before a specimen was obtained.

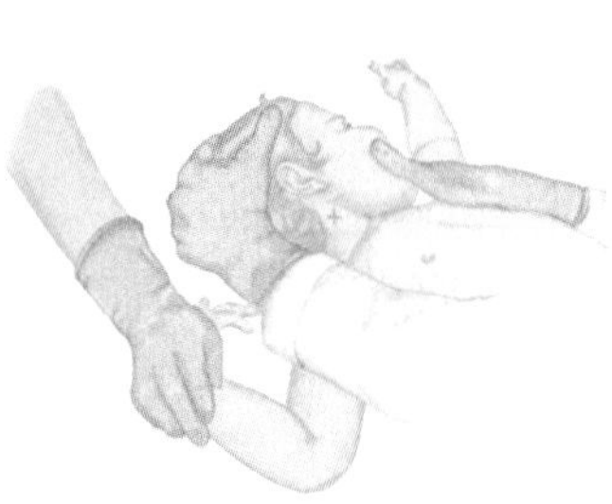

Infant positioned for jugular venipuncture

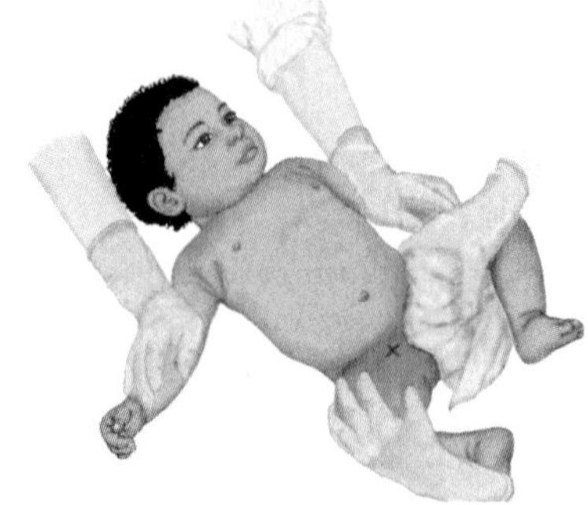

Infant positioned for femoral venipuncture

**FIG 37.7** Two additional sites for obtaining blood specimens from infants and young children are the large superficial external jugular veins and the femoral veins.

is not used once the infant is walking because calluses make it more difficult to puncture.

## Sputum Specimens

Sputum specimens are most frequently obtained to identify or rule out a respiratory infection. When obtaining any specimen, Standard Precautions are followed. If splashing is anticipated, wear a mask and goggles or face shield in addition to gloves.

Obtaining sputum in the older child is relatively easy because older children and adolescents can cough deeply and produce a sputum sample, which can then be placed in the appropriate container. Specimens are easily obtained from children with artificial airways by attaching a mucus or suction trap to a suction catheter and suctioning the airway to obtain the specimen. A cough can be elicited by placing a suction catheter into the back of the throat in an infant or a young child.

Because younger children and infants can seldom produce a deep cough on demand and often swallow those secretions, obtaining sputum samples often requires a nasal washing, or lavage (Procedure: Nasal Washing). Nasal washing is particularly used to obtain a sample for identifying respiratory syncytial virus (RSV), influenza, and pertussis.

## Throat and Nasopharyngeal Specimens

Throat cultures can identify the causative agent of sore throats or tonsillitis in children. Nasopharyngeal cultures are mainly used to identify pertussis (Procedure: Throat or Nasopharyngeal Culture).

## PROCEDURE

### *Capillary Blood Sampling*

**Purpose**

To obtain a small sample of capillary blood.

1. Prepare the child appropriately for the procedure by using developmentally appropriate explanations ("finger poke"). You can warm the site before proceeding or have the older child wash the hands in warm water.

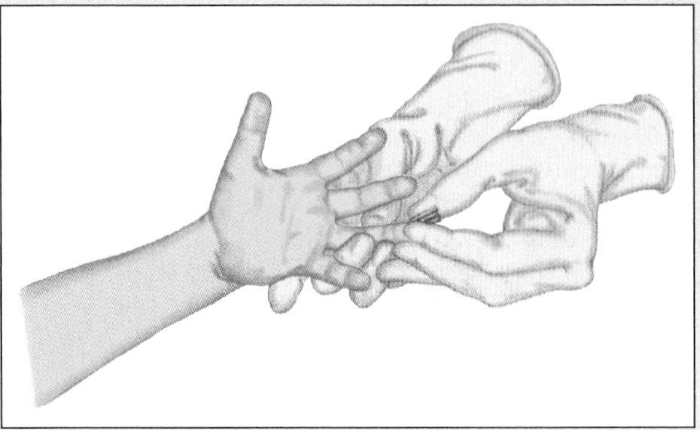

2. Bring the child to the treatment room, where the following equipment should be available: disposable lancing device, antiseptic swabs, sterile gauze, clean gloves, warm washcloth, Band-Aid, specimen containers/tubes, biohazard bag, and label and requisition form.
3. After performing hand hygiene and putting on gloves, cleanse the site, dry with sterile gauze or allow time to dry, and locate the puncture site. Use the child's third (ring) finger of the nondominant hand and puncture halfway between the center of the ball of the finger and its side. Do not use fingers that are bruised, edematous, or abraded, and avoid old puncture sites.
4. Puncture the child's finger with a lancing device that penetrates to a controlled depth and will not pierce the bone (approximately 2 mm). If possible, place the used lancing device in a sharps container before proceeding with the procedure.
5. To collect the blood sample, follow agency policy regarding whether to wipe away the first drop of blood with sterile gauze, how to collect the sample, the appropriate containers/tubes to use, amount of blood to be collected, and proper handling of the containers/tubes. To ensure adequate blood flow, it may be necessary to gently massage the finger from its base to the tip. Excessive squeezing of the finger must be avoided.
6. Once collection is complete, apply pressure with sterile gauze until the bleeding stops.
7. Provide for the child's comfort. Apply a decorative Band-Aid on the finger, if the child desires. Offer the child praise for cooperation and a reward such as a sticker.
8. Discard the lancing device in the sharps container and contaminated gauze and gloves in the biohazard receptacle. Perform hand hygiene.
9. Label the specimen with the child's name, birth date, medical record number, and the time and date of collection. Place in a biohazard bag and send to the laboratory with the requisition form for the test(s) to be performed.
10. Document the date and time, amount of blood collected, site used for the puncture, if more than one puncture was done, reason for the blood draw, and the child's reaction to the procedure. (For capillary blood sampling by heel puncture, see Chapter 21, Procedure: Obtaining Blood Samples from the Newborn by Heel Puncture.)

## PROCEDURE

### *Nasal Washing*

**Purpose**

To obtain a nasopharyngeal secretion sample from an infant or a young child.

1. Prepare the child for the procedure by using developmentally appropriate language and describing any expected sensations (the procedure will make the child sneeze).
2. Gather the following equipment: sterile syringe; sterile saline; gloves; mask; goggles or face shield; gown; small, sterile bulb syringe; sterile specimen container or pertussis kit; and labels and requisition form.
3. Ask for assistance to hold the child, or mummy wrap an infant to restrain the arms and legs.
4. Fill the syringe (without needle) with 1 to 3 mL of sterile saline.
5. Perform hand hygiene and don gloves, gown, mask, and goggles or face shield. Place the child in a supine position; gently place the tip of the syringe into one nostril.
6. Instill the saline into the nostril and immediately aspirate secretions with a small, sterile bulb syringe.
7. Place the saline and secretions into a sterile container. Remove gloves and perform hand hygiene.
8. Comfort the child and offer praise and a reward, such as a sticker, for cooperation.
9. Label the specimen with the infant or child's name, birth date, medical record number, and the time and date of collection. Place in a biohazard bag and send to the laboratory with the requisition form for the test(s) to be performed.
10. Document the amount of saline instilled and the method of collection used. Note the date, time, amount, color, and consistency of secretions.

## PROCEDURE

### *Throat or Nasopharyngeal Culture*

**Purpose**

To obtain a specimen for culture.

1. Explain the procedure to the child in appropriate language. For a throat culture, explain that the child will look up toward the ceiling, open the mouth very wide, and might feel like coughing or gagging. Emphasize that the procedure is not painful. For a nasopharyngeal swab, tell the child to look up and explain that you will be inserting the swab into the nose. The child will feel like sneezing. Do not do these procedures immediately after the child has taken medication, eaten, or had something to drink. Assistance may be needed to hold a younger child. Encourage the parent to support and comfort the child during and after the procedure.
2. Gather the following equipment: tongue depressor, throat or nasopharyngeal swab (cotton-tipped swab with a flexible wire extension), collection containers and labels (if not included with the swab), gloves, mask, goggles or face shield, and sterile saline.
3. An older child can sit in a chair or sit upright in bed for the culture. A younger child should be placed supine on a bed or examining table.
4. **Throat Culture**
   - Put on gloves, mask, and goggles or face shield, and have the child open the mouth and say "ahhh." Eliciting a cry from an infant will give optimal access to the pharyngeal area. Insert a tongue depressor into the mouth with the nondominant hand so that it covers the anterior half of the tongue, and depress the tongue to allow observation of the pharyngeal area. Swab the area quickly, avoiding the tongue, buccal mucosa, and palate. If the child opens the mouth wide enough for adequate visibility, a tongue depressor may not be needed. Only one swab should be used for each culture.
5. **Nasopharyngeal Culture**
   - Ask the child to look up. Bend the wire so that when the swab is inserted, the tip will go beyond the back of the nares and into the pharyngeal area. Dip the swab tip into saline and gently insert it into one nostril, down to the posterior nasopharynx. Leave it in place for several seconds and then remove.
6. After the specimen is obtained, place the swabs in the appropriate culture medium. Remove gloves and perform hand hygiene.
7. Comfort the child as needed and offer praise for cooperation and a reward, such as a sticker. If possible, offer the child cool fluids to drink after the procedure.
8. Label the specimen with the infant/child's name, birth date, medical record number, and the time and date of collection. Place in a biohazard bag and send to the laboratory with the requisition form for the test(s) to be performed.
9. Document the date and time, the appearance of the specimen, and the child's response to the procedure.

## SAFETY ALERT

### *Throat Cultures*

- Before obtaining a specimen for throat culture, assess for the presence of high fever of sudden onset, drooling, muffled voice, and erythema or exudate (signs of epiglottitis).
- Never attempt to obtain a throat specimen for culture in a child for whom a diagnosis of epiglottitis is suspected because the procedure could precipitate sudden airway obstruction.

## Cerebrospinal Fluid Specimens

Physicians and qualified advanced practice nurses perform lumbar punctures to examine the cerebrospinal fluid (CSF) for bacteria or abnormal cells, measure pressure within the cerebrospinal cavities, or inject certain medications (e.g., for pain control, to prevent or eradicate specific diseases, or as contrast agents for scans). A hollow spinal needle, inserted into the subarachnoid space between the third and fourth lumbar vertebrae, provides fluid exit and collection. An attached stopcock and manometer are used to measure spinal fluid pressure.

To minimize pain and trauma to the child, a topical anesthetic cream or spray should be used at the site of needle insertion. It is important that the topical agent be left in place the correct amount of time so the skin is numbed (see Chapter 38). Young children may require sedation because it is critical that the child not move during this procedure.

Because a lumbar puncture is frequently performed when a child is acutely ill, as with meningitis or leukemia, the child and family may experience a high level of stress. The physician or nurse practitioner explains the procedure and obtains an informed consent from the parents or guardians. The nurse provides support and additional information to the child and family as well as assists by positioning, holding/

restraining, and monitoring the child (see Chapter 52). Parents are most concerned with being able to keep their child calm before and during the procedure, thereby decreasing their child's distress both immediately and in the long term (Harper et al., 2013).

### Bone Marrow Aspiration

Bone marrow aspiration is performed to obtain specimens of marrow for diagnostic testing, for evaluation of response to treatment, or for transplantation (see Chapter 48). The most common site of bone marrow aspiration in the child is the posterior iliac crest. Other sites include the anterior iliac crest and the tibia.

To tolerate this procedure, children receive drugs selected from a wide range of sedative, analgesic, and/or topical anesthetic agents based on their age, developmental level, severity of illness, and hospital protocols. The World Health Organization (WHO) describes bone marrow aspiration as a moderate to painful procedure; therefore, adequate pain medication is necessary to avoid negative consequences for the child (Kato et al., 2014). Because the reasons for a bone marrow aspiration include ruling out serious diseases such as leukemia or assessing the progress of cancer treatment, the nurse needs to provide thorough preparation to the child and family and a great deal of support during and after the procedure.

## GASTROINTESTINAL TUBES AND ENTERAL FEEDINGS

Because of prematurity, illness, or injury, some infants and children are unable to tolerate adequate quantities of oral nutrition, and an alternative method of feeding may be indicated. Enteral feedings are an option for infants and children with a variety of conditions, including congenital anomalies, gastrointestinal disorders, swallowing impairments, neurologic diseases, and postoperative status. Feedings are given through an orogastric (OG), nasogastric (NG), transpyloric (nasointestinal), gastrostomy (G), or gastrojejunostomy tube (GJ) or a skin-level button (MIC-KEY) (see Chapter 43).

### Tube Route and Placement

Placement of a gastrostomy tube or gastrostomy button is a surgical procedure performed by a physician. A nurse usually inserts the OG, NG, or nasointestinal tube (Procedure: Feeding Tube Insertions). NG tubes are commonly used short-term because with nasal placement it is easier to secure the tube and keep it in place. However, nasal placement can potentially interfere with respiratory function. Children with head or nasal anomalies or injuries and infants who are still preferential nose breathers (usually those 4 months old or younger) may require an OG tube. A nasointestinal tube is more difficult to insert because it must pass through the stomach's pyloric sphincter to enter the small intestine.

Controversy exists regarding measurement of the length of the NG tube to be inserted. The two most common methods of measurement are (1) from the nose tip to the earlobe and then to the end of the xiphoid process and (2) from the nose tip to the earlobe and then to a point midway between the xiphoid process and umbilicus. Many consider the second method to be more accurate (Hannah & John, 2013). Based on a child's age and height, mathematical predictors have been developed for nurses to use for determining the correct NG tube length (Hannah & John, 2013).

### Tube Selection

Many types and sizes of tubes are commercially available. Factors influencing the selection of a feeding tube include the child's age and size, the viscosity of the formula to be administered, the reason for the enteral feeding, and whether an infusion device will be used. A feeding tube of size 5 Fr to 8 Fr is used in infants, and the size increases proportionately for older children, with 10 Fr to 12 Fr used in adolescents (Hannah & John, 2013). Selecting the smallest-diameter tube possible for the infusion and a tube of soft material will decrease the child's discomfort and help avoid leaking around the insertion site (Hannah & John, 2013).

### Safety Issues Related to Tube Placement

After a tube is initially inserted and *before* an enteral infusion is started or medication given, verification that the tube is located in the stomach or small intestine is essential. Radiographic confirmation is the most reliable method to assess tube location and is recommended following initial tube insertion and if there is doubt that a tube is in the correct position (Clifford, Heimall, Brittingham, et al., 2015; Hannah & John, 2013; Makic, Rauen, Watson, et al., 2014).

## PROCEDURE

### *Feeding Tube Insertions*

**Purpose**

To provide enteral nutrition.

1. Using developmentally appropriate language, explain the procedure to the child and parents and assess their needs and concerns (e.g., previous experience with tube insertion, ability to assist with the procedure, need for holding). Therapeutic play can be used to allay the fears of the child and parents related to the procedure.
2. Gather the following equipment before starting the procedure: feeding tube of appropriate size and type, ¼- or ½-inch hypoallergenic tape, 30-mL syringe, sterile water for oral use, stethoscope, water-soluble lubricating jelly (for nasal insertion only), pH reagent strips, gloves, gown, mask, and goggles or face shield, feeding pump and setup (enteral feeding bag), and the enteral fluid to be administered.
3. Position the child on the back or right side with the head of the bed elevated in the high-Fowler's position, if tolerated. To facilitate cooperation and decrease fear, a small child can be held in a parent's arms, with the child's head on the parent's shoulder. An older child may sit up in the bed. Have another staff member or parent hold the child, if necessary.

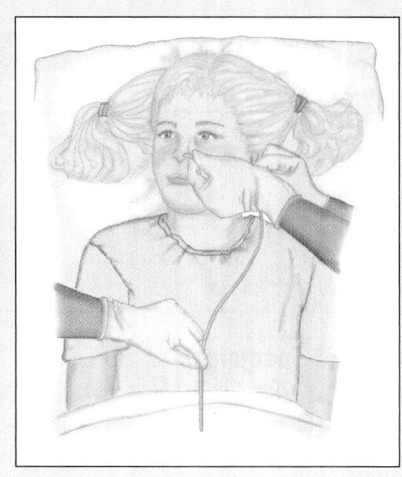

## PROCEDURE—cont'd

### *Feeding Tube Insertions*

4. Measure the length of the catheter to be inserted. Mark the total insertion distance with an indelible, waterproof marker or tape:
   - To place a nasogastric tube in a child or an orogastric tube in an infant, measure the distance from the tip of the nose to the earlobe and to a point midway between the end of the xiphoid process and the umbilicus.
5. Put on gloves and other personal protective equipment (PPE). To facilitate passage through the nasopharynx, lubricate the tube with water or water-soluble lubricant. In neonates and for orogastric placement, use water only.
6. Insert the tube gently but firmly through the mouth or nose and down the throat. If you encounter obstruction or if the tube curls in the mouth, remove the tube and repeat this step. If the child gasps, coughs, gags, or turns cyanotic, withdraw the tube and wait for the response to subside before proceeding.
7. Direct the tube toward the back of the throat. Continue to advance the tube gently to the predetermined mark. While advancing the tube, ask the cooperative child to swallow repeatedly when the tube reaches the pharynx, or give small sips of water through a straw if not contraindicated. Swallowing will ease insertion into the esophagus. Giving an infant a pacifier will encourage swallowing. Advance the tube 5 to 10 cm with each swallow. Temporarily secure the tube with tape to stabilize it while checking the tube position.
8. Attach the syringe to the end of the tube and insufflate 1 to 5 mL (more for an older child or adolescent) of air. Then, after withdrawing the air, aspirate the gastric contents for observation and pH testing. Monitor the child for signs of respiratory distress, choking, or soundless coughing that may indicate placement in the trachea.
9. Check the pH of the aspirate to confirm gastric or intestinal placement. Administration of antacid and gastric acid inhibitors will alter the pH of the aspirate, thus affecting the reliability of the pH test. Obtain radiographic confirmation of correct placement according to hospital policy and physician orders.
10. If a nasointestinal tube with a guide wire has been used, remove the guide wire by holding the tube at the child's nostril or the corner of the mouth and slowly removing it. To allow gravity to assist in the advancement of the tube into the duodenum, keep the child on the right side. An abdominal x-ray will be ordered by the physician to confirm tube placement in the duodenum.
11. Once tube placement is confirmed, tape the tube securely in place and label the tube with the date and time of insertion. Refer to your facility's policy and procedure manual for recommended frequency of tube changes. With indelible marker or tape, mark the tube just below the insertion site. This will assist with future assessments of tube placement. Remove gloves and perform hand hygiene.
12. Comfort the child and offer praise for cooperation after initial tube placement and following radiographic confirmation of position. Encourage the parent to provide comfort during and after the procedure. The nurse can also give the child a reward, such as a sticker.
13. Document the size and type of tube used, route, and placement, air insufflation results, pH testing results, observations of gastric aspirate, assessment of respiratory status, measurement of visible tube length, date and time of insertion, child and family teaching, and the child's tolerance of the procedure.

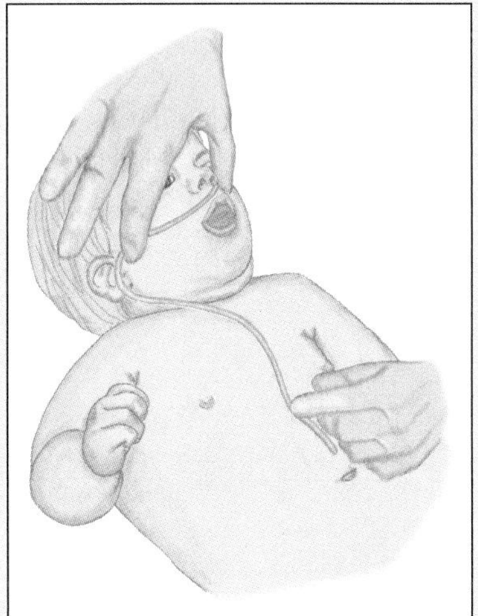

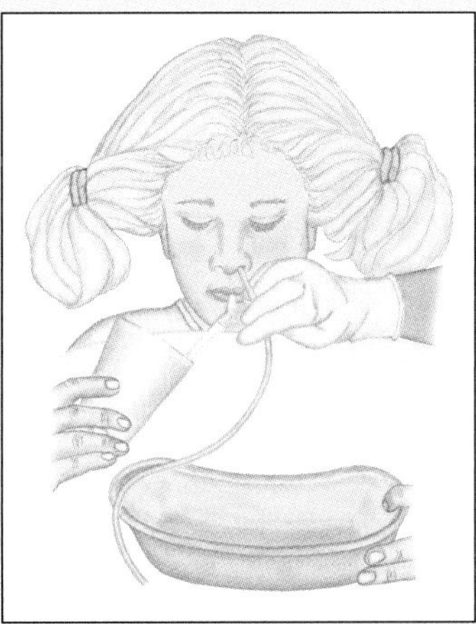

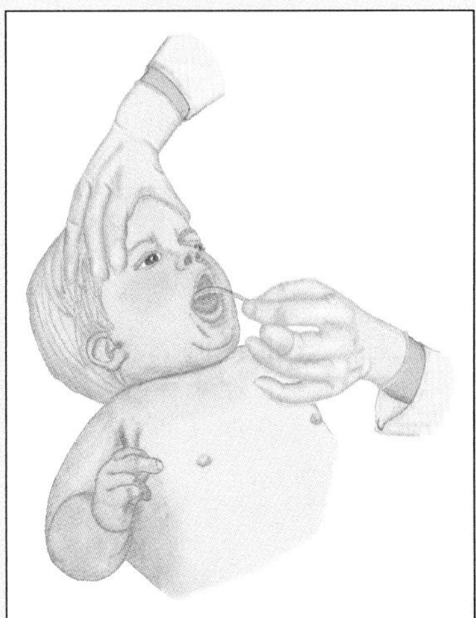

**Home Adaptations**

If the child is to receive enteral nutrition at home, teach the parent how to insert and check placement of the tube. Tube placement should be confirmed before each feeding or medication administration. Describe comfort measures that may be helpful. Be sure to have the parents give a return demonstration of tube placement including use of pH strips before taking the child home. Explain to parents how to contact a healthcare provider with questions about the tube placement.

Tube location should also be checked anytime a feeding is interrupted, before each bolus feeding or medication administration, and every 4 to 8 hours during continuous feedings (Clifford et al., 2015; Hannah & John, 2013). The American Association of Critical Care Nurses recommends that nurses use a variety of bedside methods to verify tube location (Clifford et al., 2015). These methods include assessing the patient for signs of respiratory distress (indicating the tube is in the respiratory tract); checking for a change in length of the external portion of the tube (movement from the marked position); observing the volume, appearance, and color of the aspirate from the tube; and testing the pH of the aspirate. Generally, gastric fluid is grass-green or clear (colorless), with a pH of 5 or less; however, occasionally the pH is higher. Auscultation as a verification method is not recommended (Lyman, Yaworski, Duesing, et al., 2016).

Respiratory secretions also can appear clear, but the pH is typically greater than 6. Small-intestine fluid is often bile stained (yellow or greenish-brown) with a pH of 6 or more. Keep in mind that both formula and certain medications can alter the pH of enteral secretions (Clifford et al., 2015). Although used in many settings, studies have shown that auscultating over the epigastric area for air insufflated through the tube is not reliable in distinguishing between tube placement in the respiratory tract and in the stomach (Clifford et al., 2015; Hannah & John, 2013).

NG tube placement is more of a risk in children who have a decreased level of consciousness; are uncooperative or restless; have recently been intubated or extubated; or demonstrate decreased swallowing, cough, or gag reflexes. Measuring, marking, and documenting the external length of the tube immediately after insertion will assist in determining whether the tube has lost its original position. However, nurses cannot assume that a feeding tube remains in the proper position just because the external position has not changed. Tubes can become dislodged with suctioning, retching, or vomiting (Clifford et al., 2015; Hannah & John, 2013).

### Contraindications to Tube Placement

It is crucial that the nurse determine if the child has any preexisting contraindications to tube placement such as previous surgeries, trauma, or congenital anomalies (e.g., choanal atresia, tracheoesophageal fistula, esophageal strictures) that could interfere with passage of the tube. If any of these findings is present, a physician may elect to use fluoroscopy to guide the insertion. If a tube that was placed during or through a surgical repair becomes dislodged, the nurse does not attempt reinsertion and notifies the surgeon immediately.

### Enteral Feedings

Following tube placement and verification, the nurse administers the enteral feeding either as a bolus (intermittent) or as a continuous feeding (Procedure: Administering Enteral Feedings [via the Orogastric, Nasogastric, or Nasointestinal Route]). Key steps start with preparing the child and family, and then aspirating stomach contents to check the residual volume from the last feeding. During the feeding, the nurse or parent/caregiver should hold the infant or young child, when possible, to associate the feeding with pleasant sensations and facilitate bonding. A pacifier is given to infants to promote non-nutritive sucking. The nurse encourages older children to sit at a table during meals to promote normal development and socialization.

### Gastrostomy Tubes and Buttons

The procedure for gastrostomy feedings is similar to that for OG, NG, and nasointestinal feedings. Because the gastrostomy tube or button is surgically placed percutaneously into the stomach, verifying the location of the tube is a simpler process. Most gastrostomy tubes and buttons are sutured to the skin and have an internal inflated balloon; however, dislodgement can occur. The nurse should check external tube length and observe for indications of change from the correct position. The nurse must also assess the aspirate for volume, appearance, and color.

Special considerations for children with gastrostomy tubes or buttons include skin care around the insertion site. The nurse assesses the site for abnormal findings such as leakage of formula, skin redness, drainage, bleeding, and skin breakdown. The stoma is cleaned with ½ hydrogen peroxide and ½ normal saline for the first 1 to 2 weeks, after which the site is cleansed with soap and water at least once daily and when soiled (Hannah & John, 2013).

Capped gastrostomy tubes extend several inches from the insertion site. The nurse checks to ensure that the external tube has no tension. If necessary, the tube is coiled and taped near the exit site. Gastrostomy buttons are placed close to the skin surface. They have a one-way valve that eliminates the need for clamping and provides a secure connection for extension tubing between the button and the feeding pump. Once the feeding is complete, the tube is flushed and the extension tube is removed and the button is capped. Gastrostomy buttons are easy for parents to use and allow children to participate in many activities.

It is important to watch for signs that the tube or button needs to be replaced and to report these to the physician. The signs include leaking, tube occlusion, malfunction of the antireflux valve, or abnormal tube position. Many children are discharged home with gastrostomy tubes or buttons (see Chapter 43). Parents must be educated so they can provide all required care, including checking for the correct position and monitoring the insertion site, recognizing symptoms that should be reported, and knowing what to do if dislodgement occurs. Information booklets are available to assist families. Parent teaching is a major part of nursing care for a child with a feeding tube.

#### ! NURSING QUALITY ALERT

***Enteral Feedings***

- Begin the feeding only after tube placement in the stomach has been properly verified.
- Discontinue feedings and notify the physician if signs of respiratory distress, cyanosis, abdominal distention, or vomiting occurs.
- Provide a pacifier to infants so that they can associate sucking with feeding. Encourage older children to sit at a table during meals to promote the normal socialization associated with eating.
- To avoid accidental overfeeding should the infusion pump malfunction, use only an amount of formula appropriate for a 4-hour feeding. Discard any formula that has been opened for more than 4 hours.
- Follow the facility's policies and procedures or physician's orders regarding discarding of residual volumes and the prescribed frequency for changing feeding equipment.

## ENEMAS

Enemas are given when stool needs to be removed from the bowel because of severe constipation or in preparation for a diagnostic procedure or surgery. The differences between giving an enema to a child

## PROCEDURE

### *Administering Enteral Feedings (via the Orogastric, Nasogastric, or Nasointestinal Route)*

**Purpose**

To provide adequate nutrition to a child who cannot tolerate oral feedings.

1. Using developmentally appropriate language, explain the procedure to the child and parent. Assess their needs and concerns related to the procedure, including previous experience with enteral feedings and the ability of the child to cooperate with the procedure. Use therapeutic play to prepare the child and family for the procedure.
2. The following equipment is needed: stethoscope, irrigation syringe, room-temperature formula, sterile water, pacifier for neonates and infants, electronic feeding pump (for continuous tube feedings), pH testing strips, and gloves.

**Intermittent Feedings (Bolus)**

3. Technique:
   a. Position the child on the back or right side with the head of bed elevated and remove the syringe or cap from the tube. Perform hand hygiene and put on gloves.
   b. Check for proper tube placement using multiple bedside methods in accordance with hospital policy. Be sure the mark indicating insertion length is in its original place relative to the exit site. Aspirate residual volume from the previous feeding; note quantity and characteristics, and document. Follow hospital policy or physician's orders regarding whether the next feeding should be given based on the quantity of residual and if residual fluid should be discarded or reinfused.
   c. Remove the plunger from the syringe and attach the syringe to the tube.
   d. Pour room temperature formula into the syringe and allow it to flow slowly into the tube (usually over a period of 15 to 30 minutes) via gravity. Raising or lowering the level of the syringe increases or decreases the flow of formula. Encourage the infant to suck on a pacifier during the feeding. Discontinue the feeding if signs of respiratory distress, cyanosis, abdominal distention, or vomiting occur, and notify the physician.
   e. After the prescribed volume has been infused, flush the tube with sterile water and clear the tube by injecting 1 to 5 mL of air.
   f. Discard the used syringe and close or clamp the tube unless otherwise indicated. Remove gloves and perform hand hygiene.
   g. Place the child lying on the right side with the head of the bed elevated for 30 to 60 minutes after the feeding. Monitor the child closely for nausea, emesis, or respiratory difficulties during this time.

**Continuous Feedings**

4. Technique:
   a. Position the child on the back or right side with the head of bed elevated. Perform hand hygiene and put on gloves. Check for proper tube placement using multiple bedside methods in accordance with hospital policy. The pH is a less reliable indicator of placement when a child is on continuous feedings. Be sure the mark indicating insertion length is in its original place relative to the exit site. Aspirate the residual volume and note quantity and characteristics; it may appear like curdled milk if the tube is in the stomach or appear bile stained if the tube is in the intestine. It is likely that a small quantity of residual will be present. Follow hospital policy or physician's orders regarding whether the next feeding should be given based on the quantity of residual and if the residual fluid should be discarded or reinfused.
   b. Fill the feeding bag, volume-control set, or syringe with the prescribed formula. Attach to infusion pump if applicable. Prime the infusion tubing with formula.
   c. Connect infusion tubing to the feeding tube and begin the infusion at the prescribed rate. Remove gloves and perform hand hygiene.
   d. Check tube placement and residual volumes every 4 to 8 hours. Flush with sterile water according to hospital policy or physician orders.
   e. To reduce the incidence of reflux and aspiration, keep the child positioned on the right side with the head of bed elevated. Encourage the infant to suck on a pacifier periodically while receiving the feeding. Monitor the child periodically for nausea, emesis, or respiratory difficulty.
5. Praise the child for cooperation during the feeding process.
6. Document the amount, color, and consistency of any residual fluids and note whether it was reinfused (returned) or discarded. Document the type and amount of formula given, the amount of sterile water given, the position the child was in after or during the feeding, and the child's tolerance of the procedure.

**Home Adaptations**

Assess the parent's ability to perform enteral feedings. Parents should be encouraged to make this as normal a procedure as possible (e.g., by holding the infant during feedings). Ask the parent to demonstrate the procedure before discharge. Complications are common, reported as high as 83%; proper education of the patient and parents is essential in preventing complications (Schweitzer et al., 2014). Assistance with home care can be provided by a home health agency. Advise the parent to follow manufacturer's recommendations about refrigerating and discarding opened, unused formula.

## ? CRITICAL THINKING EXERCISE 37.1

The assessment of feeding tube placement has historically been a nursing responsibility, although the only totally accurate assessment measure is radiographic confirmation.

1. What is the nurse's legal and ethical responsibility regarding feeding tube placement confirmation?
2. How does the nurse make the "best judgment" about what action to take if placement is questionable?

and giving an enema to an adult are the type and amount of fluid administered and the distance that the enema tip is inserted into the rectum.

## Enema Administration

Rectal damage and perforation can occur with improper insertion of the enema tip. The tip is lubricated and then gently inserted 2.5 cm (1 inch) to 10 cm (4 inch), depending on the age and size of the child (Table 37.2). Commercially prepared, single-use enemas come with prelubricated tips of appropriate lengths.

**TABLE 37.2 Recommended Volume and Depth for Enema Tip Insertion, by Age**

| | Volume (mL) | Depth of Insertion |
|---|---|---|
| Infants | 120-240 | 1 in (2.5 cm) |
| 2-4 yr | 240-360 | 2 in (5 cm) |
| 4-10 yr | 360-480 | 3 in (7.5 cm) |
| 11 yr + | 480-720 | 4 in (10 cm) |

### Solutions and Volumes

The amount of the enema solution will vary with the age and size of the child. Unless the physician's orders specify a different amount, the recommended volume of enema solution based on the child's age is listed in Table 37.2. Only isotonic solutions should be used with children to avoid electrolyte abnormalities (Freedman, Thull-Freedman, Rumantir, et al., 2014). Plain tap water, a hypotonic solution, should never be used because it can cause rapid fluid shifts and fluid overload.

After completing enema administration, a diaper is placed on the infant. Toddlers can use the bedpan, "potty" chair, or toilet. Older children and adolescents can use the bedpan, bedside commode, or bathroom toilet. The nurse documents the date and time the enema was given, the type and amount of solution, the amount and characteristics of the "returned" stool, other findings (e.g., presence of blood, mucus, foreign bodies, worms in the stool), and how the child tolerated the procedure.

## OSTOMIES

Urinary and fecal diversion is needed when normal methods of elimination are temporarily or permanently interrupted. Some conditions requiring the creation of a fecal stoma (ileostomy or colostomy) include imperforate anus, Hirschsprung disease, necrotizing enterocolitis, some cases of intestinal atresia, intussusception, Crohn's disease, and ulcerative colitis (see Chapter 43). The anatomic location of the stoma will dictate the consistency of the stool. The higher the stoma is located in the intestinal tract, the more liquid the stool.

Urinary diversion is usually the result of obstructive uropathy, congenital anomaly, or neurogenic bladder (see Chapter 44). The ureters can be brought out through the abdominal wall (ureterostomy) or connected to a segment of small bowel (ileal conduit).

Nursing care of the child with an ostomy focuses on teaching the child and family to perform the procedures involved in the care of the ostomy. The nurse uses developmentally appropriate terminology to explain the procedures to the child and parents. A teaching model, such as a doll with a stoma, can facilitate education.

Ostomy care includes the selection and effective use of the right type and size of appliance. Maintaining the integrity of the skin around the stoma is of great importance. The parents and the child need encouragement and support as they become active participants in the treatment regimen. The nurse should make referrals to an enterostomal therapist or other support services, as indicated. The nurse must assess the needs and assist the child in adjusting to having a stoma; communication with the nurse, family, and school community is necessary as the child enters or returns to school (Bennett, 2011).

## OXYGEN THERAPY

Hypoxemia, resulting from apnea or inadequate ventilation, occurs rapidly in children because of their high metabolic rate and increased

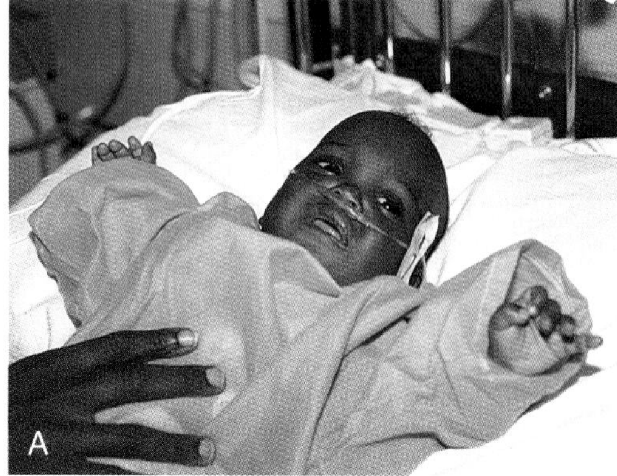


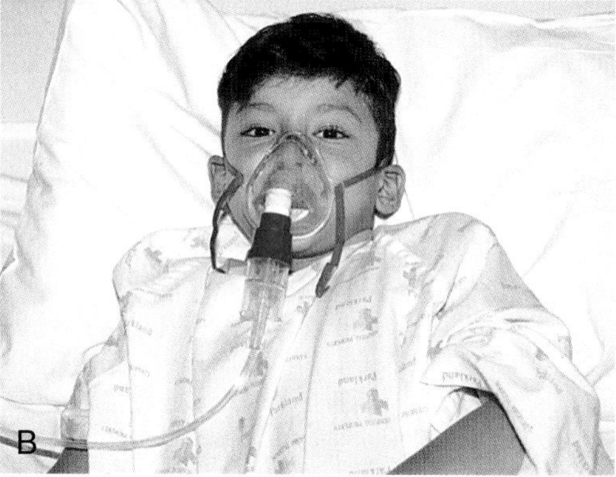


**FIG 37.8** When administering oxygen to children, special consideration is given to the size and type of equipment selected and the needs of the child and family for education and support. **A,** Nasal cannula. **B,** Simple facemask. (Courtesy Parkland Health and Hospital System, Dallas, TX.)

oxygen consumption. Cardiopulmonary arrest often follows progressive respiratory dysfunction in a child; thus, it is vital that nurses recognize the early, subtle signs and symptoms of respiratory distress.

For infants and children who are unable to maintain a normal arterial oxygen pressure ($Pa_{O_2}$), supplemental oxygen may be needed. A physician's order is generally required for the administration of oxygen. Some facilities have policies that permit nurses to start oxygen therapy in certain emergency situations.

### Oxygen Administration

Oxygen is commonly administered to children by nasal cannula, facemask (simple, nonrebreather, "blow-by" tube, partial rebreather, Venturi, or aerosol), an oxygen hood, or an oxygen tent (Fig. 37.8). Oxygen can also be given to a child with an artificial airway such as an endotracheal tube or tracheostomy using a specialty device (e.g., a tracheostomy collar) or a ventilator (see Chapter 45). The method of delivery depends on the concentration of oxygen needed and the child's ability to cooperate with the chosen method. The nurse must always check the physician's orders for the percentage of oxygen to be delivered and the method of delivery to be used, if specified.

In some facilities, a respiratory care therapist is responsible for the setup, maintenance, and management of oxygen equipment. However, the nurse needs to have a working knowledge of the oxygen administration systems used.

Oxygen administration equipment comes in a variety of sizes designed to provide a correct fit for children in different age groups. When delivering oxygen by mask, the correct size of mask that ensures a tight fit is selected. Masks are available in preemie, newborn, infant, child, small adult, and adult sizes. To determine the proper size for a child, the nurse determines that the mask extends from the bridge of the nose to the cleft of the chin. Nasal cannulas are also available in a variety of pediatric and adult sizes.

Different types of devices are used to meet the child's individual needs. Blow-by oxygen often is used to provide maximal oxygenation for neonates and infants. Older infants, toddlers, and preschoolers tend to tolerate oxygen via a nasal cannula, blow-by oxygen, or facemask. Some school-age children and adolescents prefer a nonrebreather mask to achieve maximal oxygenation.

A child experiencing difficulty breathing may be reluctant to have a mask or cannula placed on the face. The nurse must first explain to the child and parents, in developmentally appropriate language, what will happen, why the mask is needed, and how it will feel. The nurse encourages the child and parents to handle the equipment and to assist the nurse with placement. If needed, supports are provided to keep the oxygen delivery system in place, such as putting elbow restraints on an infant or taping nasal cannula tubing to the side of the child's face.

A nasal cannula is a low-flow delivery system indicated for infants and children who need modest amounts of supplemental oxygen (up to 40%, or a flow rate of 1–6 L/min). The loop of the cannula can be enlarged and then slipped easily over the child's ears. Prongs are placed in the nares and the loop tightened slightly. Flow rates should not exceed 6 L/min; higher flow rates can irritate the nasopharynx and cause gastric distention and regurgitation.

The simple facemask and the Venturi mask are indicated for infants and children who need modest amounts of supplemental oxygen (35% to 60%, or a flow rate of 6 to 10 L/min). The Venturi mask can be adjusted to deliver specific concentrations of oxygen (e.g., 24%, 28%, 35%, 50%, or 60%). The nurse attaches the mask to the humidified oxygen source and adjusts the flow rate to the prescribed level. The mask is placed on the child's face and then the nose clip and head strap are adjusted. A minimum flow rate of 4 to 6 L/min must be maintained to prevent rebreathing of exhaled carbon dioxide.

A partial or full nonrebreather mask is a facemask with an attached reservoir that allows a portion of exhaled gas to remain in the bag and mix with oxygen. Partial nonrebreather masks supply oxygen concentrations of 50% to 60% at a rate of 10 to 12 L/min. A full nonrebreather system can deliver close to 100% oxygen at a flow rate of 10 to 15 L/min if a tight seal can be maintained.

In the rare circumstance that a child needs a high-humidity environment with oxygen, a cool mist tent may be indicated. The nurse must ensure that the sides of the tent are completely tucked in to prevent escape of oxygen. To keep the child as dry as possible, cotton clothing is used, and clothing and bed linens are changed when needed.

With the use of any oxygen administration system, safety is of great concern. Signs stating "oxygen in use/no smoking" are posted outside the child's door and over the bed. Although healthcare facilities are nonsmoking facilities, parents and visitors are reminded that smoking is not allowed in the room. Toys that have the potential for producing a spark, including those that are battery powered, should not be permitted near the oxygen.

### Documentation

Documentation in the nurse's notes includes the date and time oxygen was started; the type of oxygen administration system used; the percentage of oxygen delivered and the flow rate; the child's vital signs, skin color, respiratory effort, and lung sounds; the child's response to the procedure; and any teaching done with the child or family.

### Parent Teaching

Infants and children often receive home oxygen therapy. The nurse and other healthcare providers such as respiratory care therapists educate the parents and caregivers about the operation of equipment to be used at home, equipment cleaning, safety factors, cardiopulmonary resuscitation, and available support services.

## ASSESSING OXYGENATION

Pulse oximetry is a sensitive, reliable, noninvasive means of measuring arterial oxygen saturation ($SaO_2$) in the blood. Oxygen saturation is the percentage of hemoglobin that is carrying the full complement of oxygen molecules (completely saturated = 100%). The pulse oximeter measures the absorption of light waves as they pass through highly perfused areas of the body. It provides the nurse with valuable information regarding a child's oxygenation status and can serve as an early warning sign of hypoxemia (Fig. 37.9; Procedure: Pulse Oximetry).

A pulse oximeter can be used to measure oxygen saturation at intervals or on a continuous basis. The relationship between oxygen saturation and actual oxygenation (as measured by $PaO_2$) is not 1:1. In general, a small decrease in oxygen saturation can represent a much larger decrease in $PaO_2$. Nurses must immediately report significant decreases in oxygen saturation and intervene according to the physician's orders and hospital policies (see Chapter 45).

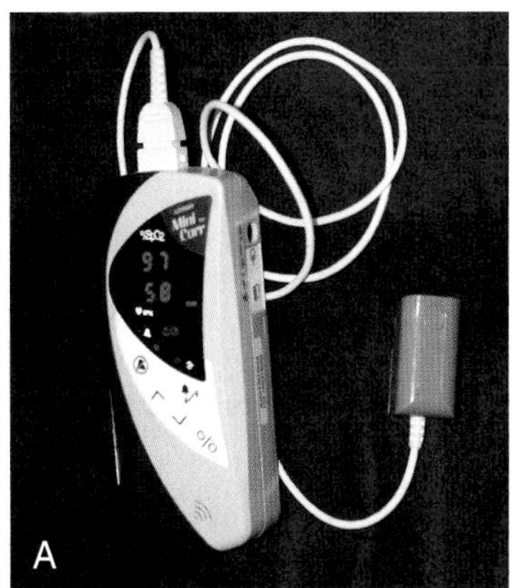


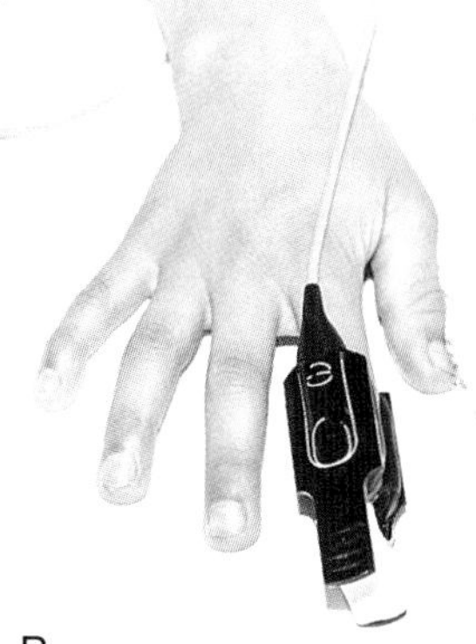


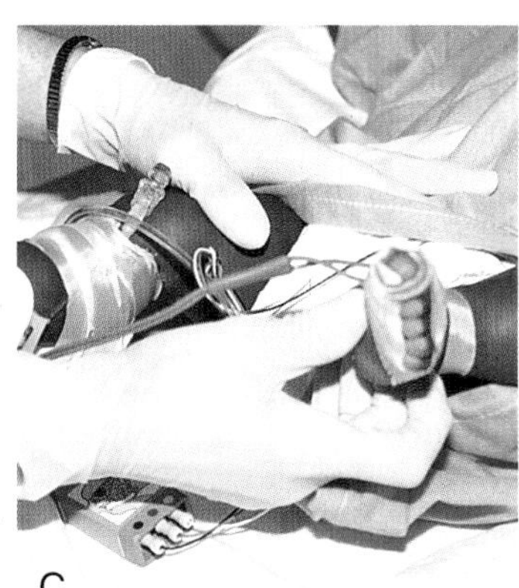


**FIG 37.9** The pulse oximeter is a reliable, noninvasive method that allows periodic or continuous measurement of blood oxygen saturation **(A)**. The sensor is applied to a child's finger **(B)** or an infant's toe **(C)**. (**A,** Courtesy Randall W. Nelson, N. Richland Hills, TX; **B** and **C,** Courtesy Parkland Health and Hospital System, Dallas, TX.)

## PROCEDURE

### Pulse Oximetry

**Purpose**

To assess the child's oxygen saturation.

1. Explain to the child and parents the indication for the procedure.
2. Bring the oximeter and sensor (finger probe, adhesive probe, or ear clip) to the child's room and allow the child to gently handle the equipment. The sensor will differ depending on whether the oximetry is intermittent or continuous.
3. Set the parameters for the alarm on a continuous measuring oximeter.
4. Place the probe on the finger, toe, or earlobe. Avoid placing the probe on an extremity with an arterial line, blood pressure cuff, or intravenous (IV) line in place. Fingernail polish or artificial nails will need to be removed before placing the sensor. Do not wrap the sensor so tightly as to prevent venous flow and cause inaccurate readings.
5. Observe and document the pulse rate and oxygen saturation. The pulse rate on the oximeter should coincide with an apical pulse or pulse rate on a cardiac monitor. If no pulse is detected, reposition the sensor.
6. To check the skin condition, remove the sensor from the site at least every 2 hours. If using a portable oximeter, be sure to clean the sensor with the manufacturer's recommended cleaning solution.
7. Document the child's response to the procedure and the pulse oximetry reading obtained, the percentage and flow rate of oxygen (if being administered), and the activity level of the child. Report any abnormal findings to the physician based on the individual child's condition. In general, a pulse oximeter reading of less than 95% is considered abnormal.
8. Inform the child and family that an alarm will sound if the child's oxygen saturation falls below the set parameters. The alarm may also sound if the child is particularly active or the sensor becomes dislodged.
9. Praise the child for cooperation with the procedure.

Pulse oximeter measurements reflect the child's oxygen saturation as well as perfusion status. Potential sources of error in measurements include an abnormal hemoglobin value (e.g., in hyperbilirubinemia or carbon monoxide poisoning), decreased peripheral perfusion (e.g., in hypotension or hypothermia), ambient light interference, motion artifact, and skin breakdown from the adhesive used to secure the sensor. To eliminate the effects of ambient light, an opaque shield can be placed over the sensor site. Sites, which include the finger, toe, pinna, ear lobe, and the sole of the foot in young infants, should be rotated to prevent skin breakdown (Fouzas, Priftis, & Anthracopoulos, 2011).

Under certain circumstances, arterial or capillary blood gases and pH may need to be measured to establish correlation of oxygenation with pulse oximetry readings and to monitor the child's acid-base balance. Both arterial and capillary blood sampling are invasive procedures; obtaining a capillary blood specimen is an easier procedure and less painful.

A sample of arterial blood can be obtained from an indwelling arterial catheter or an arterial puncture. The preferred site in children is the radial artery, although alternative sites (e.g., brachial artery) can be used. Based on the child's age and size, an appropriate needle length and gauge should be selected for use.

Specially trained respiratory care therapists, nurses, or other personnel must draw arterial blood samples. Nurses are often responsible for supporting and holding or restraining the child as well as assisting with the procedure. Once the specimen has been obtained, the nurse must hold pressure on the arterial puncture site for at least 5 minutes. The arterial blood gas specimen must be placed on ice immediately and then transported to the laboratory.

## ! NURSING QUALITY ALERT

### Assisting With Arterial Blood Gas Sampling

- Position the child's wrist with the palm up but not hyperextended. Stabilize the extremity, allowing neither twisting of the wrist nor jerking of the shoulder.
- Do not hold the child's arm too tightly because a tight grip occludes arterial blood flow.
- The skin is punctured at an angle of 15 to 45 degrees. When the needle is withdrawn, it is withdrawn slowly to decrease the incidence of arterial spasm.
- After the needle is withdrawn, apply direct pressure to the site using a sterile 2 × 2-inch sterile gauze for at least 5 minutes.
- Place the sample on ice until the laboratory analysis is performed.
- Record the puncture site and the child's activity level at the time of the sampling.

## TRACHEOSTOMY CARE

A tracheostomy is a surgically created opening (stoma) in the trachea. It is performed in children to bypass an upper airway obstruction, facilitate pulmonary secretion removal, or optimize mechanical ventilation. A tracheostomy can be either temporary or permanent.

Pediatric tracheostomy tubes vary in size and type. The tube most commonly used is made of Silastic (plastic), which is soft and flexible. It consists of two pieces: the outer cannula, which stays in the trachea to keep the stoma open, and an obturator, which guides the tube into place during tube changes. Some tubes have an inner cannula that can be removed for cleaning. Tracheostomy tubes with inner cannulas are often used for older children and for those who have increased mucus production.

Shiley or Bivona single-lumen tracheostomy tubes are often used for children. Tube size is categorized by the internal diameter (ID) of the tube measured in millimeters (mm). Pediatric sizes range from 2.5 mm for newborns to 5.5 mm for children. Adult-size tubes, with a 6- to 8-mm ID, are often used for adolescents.

### Suctioning

When a child has a tracheostomy, suctioning is often required to remove secretions and keep the airway patent. Suctioning should not be done on a routine basis; the frequency of suctioning is determined by the needs of the individual child (McClean, 2012). The nurse should frequently assess the child's breath sounds, respiratory rate, and character of respirations as well as the quantity and quality of secretions (sputum) to determine if a child needs suctioning.

Use of appropriate techniques and equipment for suctioning can prevent complications such as hypoxia, tissue damage, and infection (Procedure: Suctioning a Tracheostomy Tube). The suctioning of infants and children requires the use of smaller suction catheters and lower suction pressures than for adults. Catheter sizes range from 5 Fr to 14 Fr, with smaller sizes used for smaller tubes. To avoid total airway occlusion, catheter size should be approximately half the inner diameter of the tracheostomy tube. Recommended pressures for tracheostomy suctioning vary by age:

- Neonates and infants: 60 to 80 mm Hg
- Children: 80 to 100 mm Hg
- Adolescents: 80 to 120 mm Hg

The suction catheter should not be inserted beyond the end of the tracheostomy tube. Standard Precautions are used; PPE includes mask, goggles or face shield, and sterile gloves on both hands. The sterile suction catheter must be held in a sterile-gloved hand that remains

## PROCEDURE

### *Suctioning a Tracheostomy Tube*

**Purpose**

To maintain patency of the tracheostomy tube.

1. After using developmentally appropriate language to explain the procedure, its purpose, and other pertinent information to the child and parent, gather the following equipment: a sterile suction catheter of appropriate size, sterile gloves, mask, goggles or face shield, sterile normal saline, and sterile cup. Have equipment available to administer oxygen and a bag-valve-mask device, if applicable. Perform hand hygiene.
2. Auscultate the child's breath sounds. Assess respiratory rate and effort, and the presence of secretions.
3. Administer oxygen to the child, if indicated, using a tracheostomy collar. Adjust the suction vacuum pressure to the prescribed level and put on a mask and goggles or face shield. Pour normal saline into the sterile cup. Put on sterile gloves.
4. Remove the tracheostomy collar with the nondominant hand. Hold the catheter in the other hand covered in a sterile glove. Lubricate the catheter with normal saline, then insert the catheter the length of the tracheostomy tube (pre-measure another tracheostomy tube of the same size) with the suction off.
5. Withdraw the catheter using a twisting or twirling motion and apply intermittent suction. Limit insertion and suctioning time to 5 seconds to prevent hypoxia.
6. Reapply the tracheostomy collar and reoxygenate, as indicated. Allow time for the child to rest and take a few breaths. If needed, give oxygen using a bag-valve-mask device by "bagging" the child. If the child is on a ventilator, "bagging" is imperative.
7. Auscultate the child's breath sounds and assess respiratory rate and effort to determine effectiveness of suctioning and if secretions are still present. A pulse oximeter can be used to assess oxygenation status, if indicated. Repeat the procedure again to clear the airway, rinsing the suction catheter with sterile normal saline before the second insertion.
8. The oral cavity often requires suctioning as well. Oral cavity suctioning is performed at the end of the procedure, *after* suctioning of the tracheostomy is completed. The catheter is inserted into the mouth, and then suction is applied while the catheter is withdrawn.

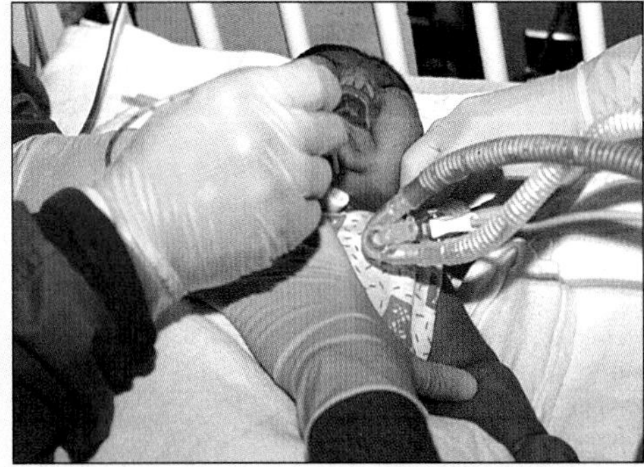

(Courtesy Parkland Health and Hospital System, Dallas, TX.)

9. Discard the suction catheter, sterile gloves, other equipment, and personal protective equipment (PPE) in an appropriate receptacle. Perform hand hygiene.
10. Comfort the child and offer praise for cooperation. Encourage the parent to provide comfort to the infant or child.
11. Document in the child's medical record, the date and time the procedure was performed, the amount and characteristics of the secretions obtained, the character of the breath sounds before and after suctioning, the child's response to the procedure, and any teaching done with the child and parents, as well as their level of understanding and their response to the teaching.

**Home Adaptations**

Tracheostomy suctioning at home is a clean rather than sterile procedure, although a new, sterile suction catheter is used each time. The family will need a powered suction apparatus, suction catheters of appropriate size, normal saline, and gloves. The procedure for suctioning is as previously discussed, including presuctioning and postsuctioning assessments.

sterile throughout the procedure. Instillation of saline into the tracheostomy to thin secretions has been linked to decreased oxygen saturation and should not be done on a routine basis (Cooper & Haut, 2013). Providing a humidified environment keeps secretions thin and easier to remove with suctioning.

### Stoma Care

Tracheostomy site care (Procedure: Care of a Tracheostomy) includes assessing the stoma area for signs of infection and skin breakdown, changing tracheostomy ties or velcro straps, cleaning the tracheostomy site and inner cannula, changing the tracheostomy tube, and suctioning. The areas around the tube and the inner cannula are cleaned, the ties changed, and a new, precut drain sponge applied as often as necessary to keep the site clean and dry. To prevent the tube from being accidentally dislodged while the ties are being changed, an assistant should be present to hold the child and keep the tube in place. The tracheostomy tube is usually changed weekly, often by the physician or respiratory care therapist. Because tracheostomy care is often tiring, the child is allowed to rest after the procedure.

An extra tracheostomy tube that is the same size or slightly smaller than the child's current tube is kept at the bedside (or taped to the head of the bed) for easy access if an emergency reinsertion is required. Because of the risk of aspiration and possible obstruction of the trachea, the child with a tracheostomy should not play with small toys or toys with small parts and should not use plastic bibs or bedding. In addition, powders and aerosol products should not be used near children with tracheostomies because of the risk of inhalation injury from breathing the particles.

## SURGICAL PROCEDURES

Although each child is unique and each surgical procedure is different, there is a general body of knowledge relevant to all children undergoing surgery. Surgery can be a traumatic event for children of all ages and their families. Stressors associated with surgery include separation from family members, care by strangers, unfamiliar surroundings, fear of the unknown, disruption in routine, lack of privacy, preoperative testing and medications, pain, and fear of mutilation, disfigurement, or disability. The nurse must identify the individual needs that the child and the family have for nursing care associated with the disorder and surgical treatment of the disorder.

Surgery can be scheduled weeks or months in advance or be performed on an emergency basis. Often, surgery for a child takes place

## PROCEDURE

### *Care of a Tracheostomy*

**Purpose**

To maintain a patent airway and prevent infection.

1. Using developmentally appropriate language, explain the procedure, its purpose, and other pertinent information to the child and parents. Some hospital facilities use videos (DVDs) and stoma dolls to demonstrate the procedure.
2. Obtain a tracheostomy care kit with the following: cotton-tipped applicators, pipe cleaners or a brush for cleaning the inner cannula, tracheostomy ties, sterile precut drain sponge, sterile gauze, gloves (sterile and nonsterile), towel or blanket roll, hydrogen peroxide, sterile normal saline, mask, and goggles or face shield.
3. To hyperextend the head and neck to expose the site, position the child with a towel or blanket under the shoulders.
4. Use appropriate hand hygiene and open the tray, creating a sterile field.
5. Pour equal parts of normal saline and hydrogen peroxide in one small tray and normal saline in the other small tray. Use the large tray for holding cotton-tipped applicators, clean tracheostomy ties, and sterile gauze.
6. Don nonsterile gloves, mask, and goggles or face shield, and remove the dressing around the tracheostomy, if present. Discard the dressing and gloves according to hospital policy. Assess the stoma for redness, drainage or discharge, and skin breakdown. Perform hand hygiene.
7. Don sterile gloves and using cotton-tipped applicators moistened in half-strength hydrogen peroxide solution, clean the child's neck under the tracheostomy tube flanges and tracheostomy ties, and dry with sterile gauze. If the child has a tracheostomy without an inner cannula, skip steps 8 and 9.
8. Unlock the inner cannula (if using a three-piece tracheostomy system) by rotating it counterclockwise. Remove the inner cannula and, using pipe cleaners or a brush, quickly clean it in half-strength hydrogen peroxide solution. (Alternatively, it may be replaced with a new inner cannula.) Rinse the cannula thoroughly in sterile normal saline and inspect it for cleanliness. Repeat the cleaning procedure if necessary.
9. To remove excess moisture, tap the cleaned inner cannula on the edge of the sterile container. Do not dry the outside of the inner cannula because moisture will act as a lubricant during reinsertion. Reinsert the inner cannula into the tracheostomy tube and lock it in place by rotating it clockwise.
10. It is recommended for two people to change ties. While the assistant (wearing sterile gloves, mask, and goggles or face shield) gently holds the tracheostomy tube in place, remove the existing ties from the flanges by untying or cutting with clean safety scissors. Clean and dry the skin under the ties or straps, and inspect the skin for breakdown caused by the ties.
11. Loop the new tracheostomy ties through the flange on one side of the tracheostomy. Bring the ties around the back of the child's neck and tie them securely to the opposite flange, on the side of the neck. Ties must be tight enough to keep the tracheostomy tube in the correct position; only one finger should be able to be inserted between the ties and neck. Use a double square knot to prevent accidental untying and dislodging of the tracheostomy.

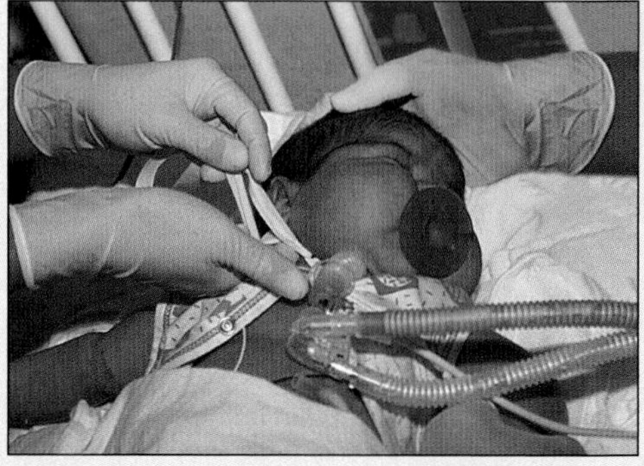

(Courtesy Parkland Health and Hospital System, Dallas, TX.)

12. If an assistant is not available, the soiled tracheostomy ties are removed *after* the new ties are securely tied and are maintaining the tracheostomy tube in the correct position.
13. Discard used supplies and personal protective equipment (PPE) in appropriate receptacles. Perform hand hygiene.
14. Comfort the child and offer praise for cooperation. Encourage the parent to provide comfort and support. The nurse can also give the child a reward, such as a sticker.
15. Document in the child's medical record the date, time, and type of procedure; the condition of the stoma and skin; any abnormal findings or complications and the nursing action taken; and the child's tolerance of the procedure. Document child and family teaching as well as their understanding of and involvement in the tracheostomy care.

**Home Adaptations**

Assess the parents' ability to perform the procedure. It may be necessary to engage the assistance of a home health agency. Begin to teach tracheostomy care early in the child's hospitalization, and teach more than one family member. Provide clear, written instructions. It is imperative to observe all caregivers during return demonstrations of the procedure before discharge from the hospital. All those caring for the child must have cardiopulmonary resuscitation (CPR) training.

The family may need a great deal of support and encouragement to feel comfortable with suctioning and tracheostomy care. The child can take baths, but care should be taken to prevent water from entering the trachea. Showers are not recommended. To avoid tracheal spasm, the tracheostomy can be covered loosely during cold or windy days.

in the operating room of an acute-care facility, with at least one overnight stay in the hospital. However, surgery performed on an outpatient basis is increasing. Ambulatory, or same-day, surgery adheres to the same standards of care as inpatient surgery but has the added benefits of the child spending less time away from home and family, lower infection rates, and reduced costs.

## Preparation for Surgery

Family-centered preparation involves educating and preparing all children and their families before the surgical procedure. Overall goals are to increase knowledge and decrease anxiety for the child and the parents (Copanitsanou & Valkeapää, 2013). A multidisciplinary approach is used that involves parents and other family members, nurses, child life specialists, physicians, anesthesiologists, and other specialists. In determining how to best prepare the child and family, the nurse considers the type of procedure to be performed, the setting (inpatient or outpatient), intensity of the child's illness or injury, the child's age and developmental level, and family coping skills (see Chapter 35).

Preparing the child and parents for surgery establishes a foundation of trust between the nurse, the child, and the family. Education sessions generally start 1 week before a scheduled surgery, although younger children may need preparation closer to the day of surgery.

There are a variety of ways to educate children and their families, including not only physical tours but also virtual tours, which are often the preferred method for younger children (Tourigny, Clendinneng, Chartrand, et al., 2011). Often, a tour of the perioperative area is included. Children are allowed to see and touch some of the equipment that will be used. Therapeutic play is an essential tool and can be facilitated by nurses, child life therapists, and parents (see Chapter 35). Adequate time must be provided so that questions posed by the child and family can be answered and they feel ready to undergo the procedure.

With the increase in same-day surgery, parents are often the primary educators for their child's surgical experience. Parents need to explain to the child as clearly as possible why she or he is going to the hospital or surgery center and what will happen during the stay. Nurses educate the parents first and then offer them additional support and assistance. Books and videos written for children that explain hospitalization and surgery can be used by parents to prepare their child. The child's primary care provider is often a good source of information as well as an advocate for the child during the process (AAP, 2014b).

On the day of surgery, the nurse reviews key points with the child and family. The nurse verifies that the parents or guardians have been fully informed and have signed the surgical consent form. According to the child's age and hospital policy, the nurse ensures that the child has assented to the procedure as well. Involving nurses and child life therapists who participated in the child's preparation will promote continuity of care and trust. If a waiting period is required before the scheduled surgery time, it is important to keep the child busy (distracted) in order to reduce anxiety. Age-appropriate toys and activities should be provided in the holding area or in the child's room.

Children often require physical preparation before surgical procedures. Routine preoperative activities include laboratory testing (complete blood cell count, chemistry profile with electrolyte levels, urinalysis, and chest x-ray); withholding food and/or drink for a specified number of hours before surgery; and administering preoperative medications ordered by the physician. Nurses are also responsible for checking the child's identification, confirming that the consent form is completed and signed, obtaining laboratory results, and gathering other documentation. Most hospitals and surgical centers have preoperative checklists that assist the nurse in documenting the child's preparation for surgery.

Because infants and children are at greater risk for dehydration, the period during which they can have nothing by mouth (NPO) may be shorter than for adolescents and adults (see Chapter 40) (Crenshaw, 2011). This period varies according to the protocols of the facility and the anesthesiologist (Box 37.3). It is critical that the nurse frequently monitors the hydration status of the infant or child who is NPO and waiting to go to surgery.

### BOX 37.3 Guidelines for Preoperative Fasting

1. Fast from solid food and full liquids from the night before as directed. Some physicians allow a light breakfast early in the morning if surgery will be late in the afternoon (at least 6 hours after ingestion).
2. Stop breastfeeding at least 2 hours before the hospital arrival time. Unless otherwise instructed, stop formula feeding from the night before surgery.
3. Clear liquids, such as water, broth, ice pops, gelatin, and clear juices, can be taken up to 2 hours before the time of arrival at the hospital.

## Preoperative Medication and Anesthesia Induction

Since many children experience distress at the induction of anesthesia (Scully, 2012), two interventions are used to manage their anxiety just before surgery: preoperative sedative medication and parental presence during anesthesia induction. When providing family-centered care, the decision regarding which intervention to use should be jointly made by the parents and the anesthesiologist (AAP, 2014b). Other concerns about giving a child sedative medications include uncomfortable side effects (dizziness, nausea), the child's fear of injection pain, fall risk, and possible airway obstruction. After the preanesthetic medication has been administered, the child must be constantly monitored by the nurse and parents, with the side rails raised on the bed or stretcher. The most commonly used medication in children is midazolam (Mountain, Smithson, Cramolini, et al., 2011).

When a parent is with the child during the start of anesthesia, it is important that he or she remains calm. Parents must have preparation in advance regarding what they will see happen to their child as anesthesia begins to take effect (e.g., sudden muscle relaxation, intubation) and what their role is in supporting their child (AAP, 2014b). Once the child is "asleep," the parent is escorted from the operating room to the surgical waiting area. Parents should be informed of the anticipated length of the surgery and receive periodic status reports throughout the course of the procedure.

## Postanesthesia Care

After surgery, the child is taken to the postanesthesia care unit (PACU) or recovery room. As the child gradually regains consciousness, the nurse performs frequent assessments of his or her neurologic, cardiorespiratory, and circulatory systems. Once the child is "awake," the parents should be present to comfort and calm the child. The child may also want a favorite toy or object. Providing warm blankets and a rocking chair as comfort measures can assist both the child and the parent. Pain medication should be given as indicated, since most children experience significant postoperative pain (Chorney, Tan, Martin, et al., 2012; Twycross, Finley, & Latimer, 2013) (see Chapter 39). Depending on the procedure performed, the child may be discharged to the home from the PACU or admitted to an inpatient unit.

## Postoperative Care

Most inpatient units have a specific protocol for postoperative care that is followed after a child has been transferred from the recovery room. At regular intervals, the child's vital signs are monitored, the surgical site is checked for drainage, fluid and electrolyte status is evaluated, and the pain level is assessed. The use of patient-controlled analgesia (PCA) and the routine administration of analgesics can provide acceptable pain control, which is important in the child's recovery (Chieng, Chan, Liam, et al., 2013). It is imperative for the nurse to assess and document the child's pain level within a designated time period following medication administration to evaluate effectiveness. (See Chapter 39 for a more detailed discussion of pain management in children.)

Atelectasis, a common complication of surgery, can result from the effects of anesthesia combined with other factors such as inadequate lung expansion due to pain. Frequent lung auscultation is done to identify adventitious breath sounds or areas of diminished or absent breath sounds. A pulse oximeter can be used to check oxygen saturation. Children are prompted to perform deep breathing and coughing. The use of an incentive spirometer and games where the child blows cotton, a pinwheel, or bubbles can facilitate air exchange and lung expansion. Sitting the child up on the side of the bed or in a chair as well as early ambulation can also prevent atelectasis.

To facilitate their recuperation, children are discharged from the hospital as soon as safely possible after surgery. It is essential to thoroughly educate the child and family regarding how to monitor the child's condition and provide appropriate care at home. The parents must receive clear information on what signs and symptoms, if present, indicate a possible complication and require that the physician or another healthcare team member be contacted. The nurse should review with the parents written schedules and instructions for medications, incision care, bathing, diet, and activity, allowing time for questions. Regarding procedures such as dressing changes, the nurse should instruct and demonstrate first and then allow the parents to perform a return demonstration before leaving the hospital.

When a child undergoes outpatient surgery, the parents manage the postoperative recovery of their child at home, including pain management. Studies have shown that parents and children can have misconceptions about pain medications, resulting in inadequate pain management (Joestlein, 2015; Vincent et al., 2012). Children may refuse to swallow a pill or liquid suspension, and parents can be reluctant to administer pain medications because of concern over side effects, especially when administering narcotics. More complete education on pain medications is needed before discharge, provided at a time when the child and parents are able to focus and comprehend (Joestlein, 2015).

With decreased lengths of stay, discharge planning has to begin at the time of admission. The nurse identifies the child and family's specific needs and determines the resources that are required to support home care for the child. Some children need specialized services after discharge. Home healthcare agencies can provide supplies and equipment, additional family education, and nursing care in the home. The overall goal of discharge planning is a smooth transition from hospital to home for the child and family.

## KEY CONCEPTS

- Whenever possible, procedures are performed in the treatment room, not in the child's room.
- Certain procedures require informed consent. Children aged 7 years and older may need to assent to some procedures. Nurses must be familiar with state laws and the policies of their institution.
- Use of developmentally appropriate language when preparing children for procedures is essential.
- Children need to be praised for attempts at cooperation during a procedure and for accomplishing an expected task.
- Documentation of a procedure includes recording the preparation, key elements of the procedure, the person who performed the procedure, and the way the child tolerated it.
- Standard Precautions are followed when collecting all specimens. Transmission-Based Precautions are used with patients known or suspected to have an infection that can be spread to others.
- Restraints are used only as a last resort to protect the child and others.
- Safety is of paramount concern for all children. Nurses must strictly observe safety principles when caring for children in a hospital setting.

## REFERENCES AND READINGS


American Academy of Pediatrics. (2007). *Technical report: reaffirmed. Mercury in the environment: implications for pediatricians—2001*. Retrieved from http://aappolicy.aappublications.org/cgi/content/full/pediatrics;120/3/683#SEC5.

American Academy of Pediatrics. (2011). *Clinical practice guidelines: clinical practice guidelines for the diagnosis and management of the initial UTI in febrile infants and children 2-24 months*. Retrieved from http://pediatrics.aappublications.org/content/128/3/595.

American Academy of Pediatrics, Section on Anesthesiology and Pain Medicine. (2014b). *Policy statement: the pediatrician's role in the evaluation and preparation of pediatric patients undergoing anesthesia*. Retrieved from http://pediatrics.aappublications.org/content/134/3/634.

American Academy of Pediatrics, Section on Oral Health. (2014a) *Policy statement: maintaining and improving the oral health of young children*. Retrieved from http://pediatrics.aappublications.org/content/134/6/1224.

Baxter, A.L., Ewing, P.H., Young, G.B., et al. (2013). EMLA application exceeding two hours improves pediatric emergency department venipuncture success. *Advanced Emergency Nursing Journal, 35*(1) 67–75.

Bennett, Y. (2011). Supporting children with a stoma in the school setting. *British Journal of School Nursing, 6*(3), 127–130.

Brenner, M. (2013). A need to protect: parents' experiences of the practice of restricting a child for a clinical procedure in hospital. *Issues in Comprehensive Pediatric Nursing, 36*(1-2), 5–16.

Centers for Disease Control and Prevention. (2002). Guideline for hand hygiene in health care settings. *MMWR: Morbidity and Mortality Weekly Report, 51*(RR16), 1–44.

Centers for Disease Control and Prevention. (2011). *Dental fluorosis*. Retrieved from http://www.cdc.gov/fluoridation/safety/dental_fluorosis.htm#6.

Chang, M.C., Chen, Y.C., Chang, S.C., et al. (2011). Knowledge of using acetaminophen syrup and comprehension of written instruction among caregivers with febrile children. *Journal of Clinical Nursing, 21*, 42–51.

Chieng, Y.T., Chan, W.C., Liam, J.L., et al. (2013). Exploring influencing factors of postoperative pain in school-age children undergoing elective surgery. *Journal for Specialists in Pediatric Nursing, 18*, 243–252.

Chorney, J., Tan, E.T., Martin, S.R., et al. (2012). Children's behavior in the postanesthesia care unit: the development of the child behavior coding system-PACU (CBCS-P). *Journal of Pediatric Psychology, 37*(3), 338–347.

Clifford, P., Heimall, L., Brittingham, L, et al. (2015). Following the evidence: enteral tube placement and verification in neonates and young children. *The Journal of Perinatal & Neonatal Nursing, 29*(2), 149–161.

Cooper, V.B., & Haut, C. (2013). Preventing ventilator-associated pneumonia in children: an evidence-based protocol. *Critical Care Nurse, 33*(3) 21–29.

Copanitsanou, P., & Valkeapää, K. (2013). Effects of education of paediatric patients undergoing elective surgical procedures on their anxiety- a systematic review. *Journal of Clinical Nursing, 23*, 940–954.

Crenshaw, J.T. (2011). Preoperative fasting: will the evidence ever be put into practice. *American Journal of Nursing, 111*(10), 38-43.

Dolan, V.J., & Cornish, N.E. (2013). Urine specimen collection: how a multidisciplinary team improved patient outcomes using best practice. *Urologic Nursing, 33*(5) 249–256.

Emergency Nurses Association. (2012). *Emergency nursing pediatric course provider manual* (4th ed.). Des Plains, IL: Author.

El-Radhi, A. (2014). Determining fever in children: the search for an ideal thermometer. *British Journal of Nursing, 23*(2), 91–94.

Eliasdottir, S.B., Steinthorsdottir, S.D., Indridason, O.S., et al. (2013). Comparison of aneroid and oscillometric blood pressure measurements in children. *The Journal of Clinical Hypertension, 15*(11), 776–783.

Fouzas, S., Priftis, K., & Anthracopoulos, M.B. (2011). *Pulse oximetry in pediatric practice.* Retrieved from http://pediatrics.aappublications.org/content/128/4/740.

Freedman, S.B., Thull-Freedman, J., Rumantir, M., et al. (2014). Pediatric constipation in the emergency department: evaluation, treatment, and outcomes. *Journal of Pediatric Gastroenterology & Nutrition, 59*(3), 327–333.

Ha, Y.O., & Kim, H.S. (2013). The effects of audiovisual distraction on children's pain during laceration repair. *International Journal of Nursing Practice, 19*(3), 20–27.

Hamilton, P.A., Marcos, L.S., & Secic, M. (2013). Performance of infrared ear and forehead thermometers: a comparative study in 205 febrile and afebrile children. *Journal of Clinical Nursing, 22*, 2509–2518.

Hannah, E., & John, R.M. (2013). Everything the nurse practitioner should know about pediatric feeding tubes. *Journal of the American Association of Nurse Practitioners, 25*, 567–577.

Harper, F., Peterson, A.M., Uphold, H., et al. (2013). Longitudinal study of parent caregiving self-efficacy and parent stress reactions with pediatric cancer treatment procedures. *Psych-Oncology, 22*, 1658–1664.

Hurwitz, B., Brown, J., & Altmiller, G. (2015). Improving pediatric temperature measurement in the ED. *American Journal of Nursing, 115* (9), 48–55.

Inal, S., & Kelleci, M. (2012). Relief of pain during blood specimen collection in pediatric patients. *Maternal-Child Nursing,37*(5) 339–345.

Jamerson, P.A., Graft, E., Messmer, P.R., et al. (2014). Inpatient falls in freestanding children's hospitals. *Pediatric Nursing, 40*(3), 127–135.

Jeffs, D., Wright, C., Scott, A., et al. (2011). Soft on sticks: an evidence-based practice approach to reduce children's needlestick pain. *Journal Nursing Care Quality, 26*(3) 208–215.

Joestlein, L. (2015). Pain, pain, go away! evidence-based review of developmentally appropriate pain assessment for children in a postoperative setting. *Orthopaedic Nursing, 34*(5), 252–259.

Kato, Y., Maeda, M., Aoki, Y., et al. (2014). Pain management during bone marrow aspiration and biopsy in pediatric cancer patients. *Pediatrics International, 56*, 354–359.

Lyman, B., Yaworski, J. A., Duesing, L., et al. (2016). Verifying NG feeding tube placement in pediatric patients. *American Nurse Today, 11*(1) 1–3.

Makic, M.F., Martin, S.A., Burns, S., et al. (2013). Putting evidence into nursing practice: four traditional practices not supported by the evidence. *Critical Care Nurse, 33*(2), 28–44.

Makic, M.F., Rauen, C., Watson, R., et al. (2014). Examining the evidence to guide practice: challenging practice habits. *Critical Care Nurse, 34*(2), 28–30, 32–46.

McClean, E.B. (2012). Tracheal suctioning in children with chronic tracheostomies: a pilot study applying suction both while inserting and removing the catheter. *Journal of Pediatric Nursing, 27*, 50–54.

McDougall, P., & Harrison, M. (2014). Fever and feverish illness in children under five years. *Nursing Standard, 28*(30) 49–59.

Meadows-Oliver, M., & Hendrie, J. (2013). Expanded back to sleep guidelines. *Pediatric Nursing, 39*(1) 40–49.

Mountain, B.W., Smithson, L., Cramolini, M., et al. (2011). Dexmedetomidine as a pediatric anesthetic premedication to reduce anxiety and to deter emergence delirium. *AANA Journal, 79*(3), 219–224.

Myers, F.E. (2014). Contact precautions reconsidered. *Nursing Management,45*(12) 33-35.

Nilsson, S, Enskär, K., Hallqvist, C., et al. (2013). Active and passive distraction in children undergoing wound dressings. *Journal of Pediatric Nursing, 28*, 158–166.

Schaffer, P.L., Daraiseh, N.M., Daum, L., et al. (2012). Pediatric inpatient falls and injuries: a descriptive analysis of risk factors. *Journal for Specialists in Pediatric Nursing, 17*, 10–18.

Schweitzer, M., Aucoin, J., Docherty, S.L., et al. (2014). Evaluation of a discharge education protocol for pediatric patients with gastrostomy tubes. *Journal of Pediatric Health Care, 28*(5), 420–428. doi: 10.1016/jpedhc.2014.01.002

Scully, S. (2012). Parental presence during pediatric anesthesia induction. *AORN Journal, 96*(1), 26–33.

Shockey, D.P., Menzies, V., Glick, D.F., et al. (2013). Preprocedural distress in children with cancer: an intervention using biofeedback and relaxation. *Journal of Pediatric Oncology Nursing, 30*(3), 129–138.

Strouse, A. (2015). Appraising the literature on bathing practices and catheter-associated urinary tract infection prevention. *Urologic Nursing, 35*(1) 11–17.

Thompson, M., Dana, T., Bougatsos, C., et al. (2013). *Screening for hypertension in children and adolescents to prevent cardiovascular disease.* Retrieved from http://pediatrics.aappublications.org/content/131/3/490.full.html.

Tourigny, J., Clendinneng, D., Chartrand, J., et al. (2011). Evaluation of a virtual tour for children undergoing same-day surgery and their parents. *Pediatric Nursing, 37*(4), 177–182.

Twycross, A., Finley, G.A., & Latimer, M. (2013). Pediatric nurses' postoperative pain management practices: an observational study. *Journal for Specialists in Pediatric Nursing, 18*, 189–201

Van Kuiken, D., & Huth, M.M. (2013). What is "normal" evaluating vital signs. *Pediatric Nursing, 39*(5) 216–224.

Vincent, C., Chiappetta, M., Beach, A., et al. (2012). Parents' management of children's pain at home after surgery. *Journal for Specialists in Pediatric Nursing, 17*, 108–120.

World Health Organization. (2011). *Clean care is safer care: clean hands protect against infection.* Retrieved from http://www.who.int/gpsc/clean_hands_protection/en/index.html.

Yoo, H., Kim, S., Hur, H., et al. (2011). The effects of an animation distraction intervention on pain response of preschool children during venipuncture. *Applied Nursing Research, 24*, 94–100.

38

# Medication Administration and Safety for Infants and Children

http://evolve.elsevier.com/McKinney/mat-ch/

## LEARNING OBJECTIVES

*After studying this chapter, you should be able to:*

- Describe different methods of administering medications to children.
- List the advantages and disadvantages of each route of administering medication to children.
- Describe the physiologic differences between children and adults that affect medicating a child.
- Describe the psychosocial interventions for teaching and successful medication administration for each age group.
- Describe quality and safety issues associated with medication administration in children.

Medicating infants and children is one of the nurse's most important responsibilities. The nurse plays a key role in administering medications, supporting the child and family during the experience, and teaching the child and parents about pharmacologic aspects of the child's care. Although physicians or nurse practitioners prescribe medications, the nurse or caregiver is responsible for their administration. The nurse has a legal responsibility to administer medications safely and accurately. Safe administration of medications to children requires an understanding of the dosages used for children and the expected actions, possible side effects, and signs of adverse reactions or toxicity. Nurses should use reliable sources of information (e.g., pharmacists, drug handbooks, hospital formularies, electronic drug databases) when administering medications and should ask the prescribing practitioner questions about orders that are unclear, inaccurate, or potentially incorrect before administering the medication.

Giving medications to children requires special skills. To gain the child's cooperation and to administer the medication in the least traumatic manner, the nurse needs to understand the physical characteristics and psychological needs of children at each developmental level. The nurse should use developmentally appropriate strategies to manage children's fears, prevent injury, and enhance coping. Involving the parent in distracting the child is not only preferred by the child and family but also cost effective for the healthcare setting (McCarthy et al., 2014).

It is vitally important to provide parents with information about medications used in their child's treatment and to encourage parents to support their child during experiences related to medications. Involving parents in the task of eliciting their child's cooperation not only makes the job easier but also gives the family a sense of self-management and control. If the parents will need to administer medications to their child at home, the nurse ensures that the parents receive complete instructions and correctly demonstrate medication administration techniques before the child is discharged.

Adherence to taking the full course of a medication to treat an acute illness or following a medication regimen for chronic illness management continues to be a challenge for children, adolescents, and their families (Ingerski, Perrazo, Goebel, et al., 2011; McGrady & Hommel, 2013). Barriers to effective adherence to medications include cost, medication taste, inability to read or comprehend directions, misunderstanding about the correct dose or number of times to take the medication, and lack of understanding about the illness and need for the medication (McGrady & Hommel, 2013).

Factors that improve medication adherence include allowing adequate time for the healthcare provider to educate the parent and child, continuity of care, availability of the health provider to answer questions about the medication, a medication schedule that fits the family's lifestyle, low cost, oral route, palatable taste for oral drugs, and low potential for side effects. Any medication regimen should consider the child's developmental needs. Further, a variety of administration, educational, and behavioral strategies need to be used; these include simple dosing schedules that correlate with daily routine, explanation of treatment goals, negotiation of treatment regimens, teaching ways to minimize side effects, supervised practice of skills by child and family, providing cues for monitoring adherence, promoting adherence through positive reinforcement, and encouraging self-management for older children and adolescents. The nurse must ask the family about the reasons for poor adherence to help the family overcome barriers, especially since long-term self-management practices are learned in childhood and adolescence (Ingerski et al., 2011).

## PHARMACOKINETICS IN CHILDREN

An understanding of pharmacokinetics and pharmacodynamics guides appropriate interventions in children. Pharmacokinetics refers to the actions of a drug (e.g., movement, biotransformation) within the human body over time, and pharmacodynamics is the behavior of a drug as it interacts with the biochemical and physiologic milieu of the body. The pharmacokinetic actions of absorption, distribution, metabolism, and excretion are influenced by the physiologic environment in which the drug moves, and this environment differs between adults and children (Fig. 38.1). The physiologic differences in body systems are most striking in the neonate.

It is important to note that many approved pharmaceuticals in the US have not been tested in children, resulting in inadequate guidelines

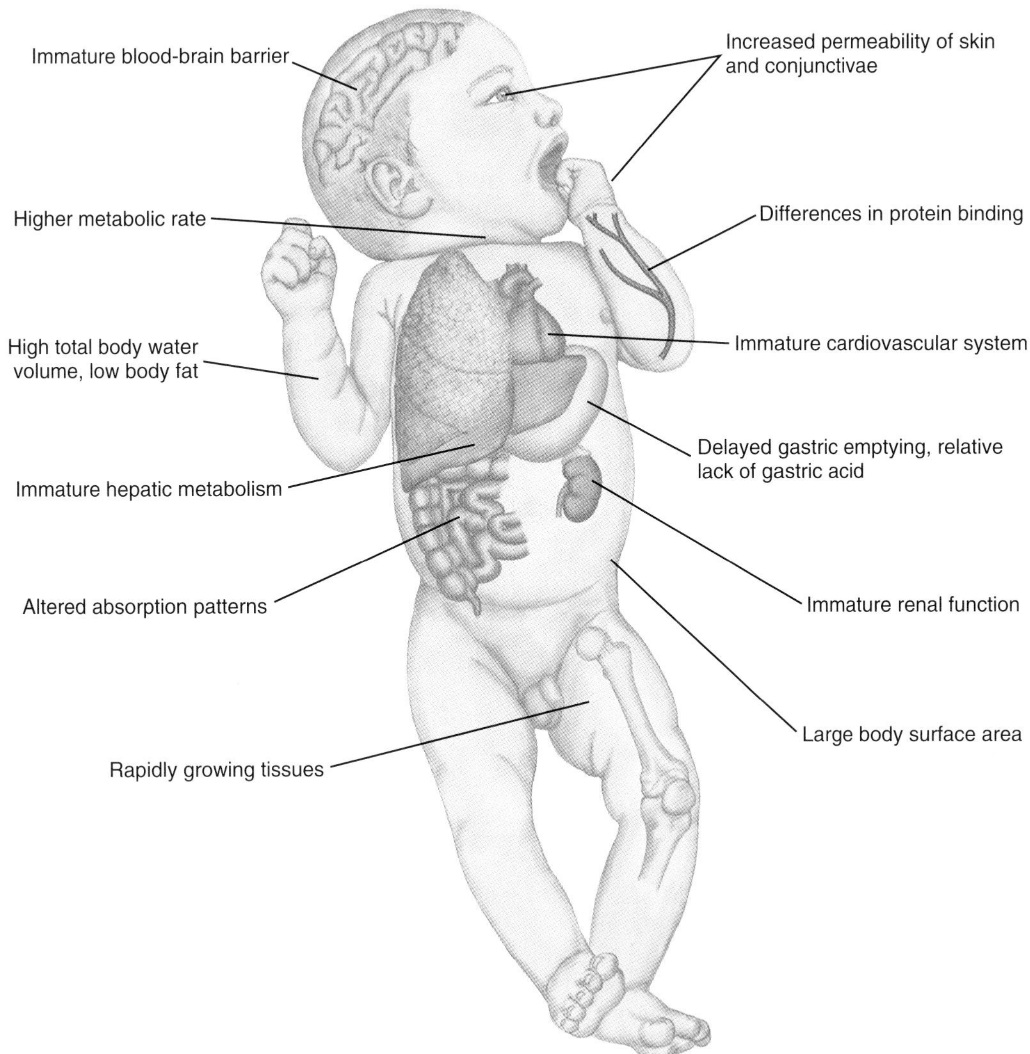


**FIG 38.1** Physiologic differences between children and adults affect drug absorption, metabolism, distribution, and excretion. These differences are most significant for infants.

for use in children. Since children do not metabolize drugs in the same manner as adults, this difference causes an increased risk of adverse drug reactions (Turner, 2013). To remedy this the *Best Pharmaceuticals for Children Act* and the *Pediatric Research Equality Act* were passed with the goal of increasing the number of pediatric clinical trials resulting in more safe and appropriate medication guidelines for children (Ivanovska, Rademaker, Dijk, et al., 2014). In 2007, the World Health Organization launched the "*Make Medicines Child Size*" project to address the need for drugs formulated for children (WHO, 2012).

Pharmacogenomic testing is an area of research that is helping providers understand how the child will metabolize certain medications. This testing is currently being used to treat patients who have cancer and human immunodeficiency virus (Turner, 2013).

## Absorption

### Oral Route

When a medication is given orally, several factors influence its absorption along the gastrointestinal (GI) tract. Because most medication absorption occurs in the small intestine, the drug must reach that location in a form suitable for maximum absorption. Four factors influence this process.

- Gastric acidity
- Gastric emptying time
- GI motility, or transit time through the GI tract
- Function of the pancreatic enzymes

***Gastric acidity.*** The gastric secretions of infants are less acidic than those of older children or adults. Secretions slowly increase in acidity during the first 2 years of life. Children, particularly infants and toddlers, tend to eat more frequently than adults, and thus, often have food and digestive enzymes present in their stomachs. Formula or milk can increase the alkalinity of gastric secretions, decreasing the absorption of medications that require a more acidic environment, and enhancing the absorption of medications that require a more alkaline milieu. These factors can greatly affect serum drug levels.

***Gastric emptying.*** Gastric emptying is intermittent and unpredictable in infants; it does tend to be slower than in older children. This slower pace can prolong the time it takes a medication to reach the intestinal absorption site.

***Gastrointestinal motility.*** Depending on whether an infant or young child has eaten recently, peristaltic activity in the intestine can be faster or slower than in an older child or adult. Infants up to 8 months of age tend to have prolonged motility. Certain adverse health conditions, such as diarrhea, can alter intestinal motility by increasing peristalsis. The longer the transit time in the intestine, the more medication is absorbed. Conversely, a shortened transit time decreases medication absorption.

***Enzyme activity.*** Pancreatic enzyme activity is variable in infants for the first 3 months of life as the GI system matures. Medications that require specific enzymes for dissolution and absorption might not be converted to a suitable form for intestinal action.

### Other Routes

Adequate absorption of medication administered intravenously (IV) depends on adequate peripheral perfusion. Medications given IV are immediately available for absorption into the child's bloodstream. Compared to that of an adult, a child's peripheral circulation is less reliable and more responsive to environmental changes. As a result, vasoconstriction or vasodilation can occur, altering the absorption of parenteral medications. Also, the cardiovascular system is less able to accommodate large or rapid changes in volume, and fluid overload can result from poorly controlled IV infusions. A child has a smaller muscle mass than an adult; an infant's body weight is approximately 25% muscle, compared to an adult whose body weight is approximately 40% muscle. Thus, infants have fewer sites available for intramuscular (IM) injections. Further, blood flow to muscle tissue can be erratic in young children, which can increase or decrease the absorption of IM medications.

Infants and young children have a thinner outer skin layer (stratum corneum) and a larger body surface area (BSA) to weight ratio. Infants have more skin surface area relative to weight than adults; thus, the absorption of topical medications is much greater than adults. Skin pH varies with age and can affect the absorption of topical medications as well. Children also are more prone to skin irritation, resulting in more frequent contact dermatitis and other allergic reactions. Irritated or open skin can enhance the absorption of topical medications.

## Distribution

Distribution refers to the general and specific concentration of the medication in body fluids and tissues. Medications are distributed to body tissues through blood and body fluids.

### Differences in Body Fluids

Fluid differences between children younger than 2 years and older children must be considered when the nurse determines medication dosages. The body fluid content ranges from 75% of body weight in infants to 60% of body weight in children 2 years and older (see Chapter 40). Because of their greater fluid volume per weight, children need a higher dose per kilogram of a water-soluble medication to achieve the desired distribution effects.

A higher percentage of the young child's body fluid is located in the extracellular fluid compartment. During certain illnesses, this extracellular fluid can be lost rapidly, causing fluid depletion. It is important to adjust medication dosages accordingly in an ill infant or young child to avoid overdosing or underdosing.

### Differences in Fat Percentages

Percentages of fat also change as the child grows. Fat makes up approximately 16% of an infant's weight, although total body fat varies from child to child. The percentage of fat per body weight is increased in a 1-year-old as compared to an infant, but then decreases in a preschool child. The percentage of body fat affects the distribution of fat-soluble medications in children. Because body fat must be saturated with a fat-soluble medication before the drug becomes detectable in the blood, dosages often must be varied to achieve desired effects.

### Differences in Proteins

Medications bind to plasma proteins, mainly albumin, for distribution. Only free, unbound medication can be absorbed by the body. Because preterm and newborn infants have lower levels of plasma proteins than do older children, more unbound drug circulates; the amount of medication needed to maintain a therapeutic drug level is thereby altered and can increase the infant's vulnerability to adverse drug effects.

### Blood–Brain Barrier

The **blood–brain barrier** does not fully mature until a child is approximately 2 years old. This immaturity causes the barrier to be less selective, allowing the distribution of medications into the central nervous system. As a result, encephalopathy can occur with some medications.

The relative immaturity of the nervous system also can lead to paradoxical effects from certain medications. For example, medications that normally cause sedation in adults may have the opposite effect in some children, causing hyperactivity.

## Metabolism

Most medications are metabolized in the liver. Metabolic enzyme systems are less mature in newborn and premature infants, so they may not properly metabolize all the medication in a given dose. Older infants, toddlers, and preschoolers metabolize certain drugs (e.g., pain medications) more rapidly than adults. For this reason, larger dosages or more frequent administration of certain drugs might be needed for young children to achieve desired therapeutic outcomes.

## Excretion

Most medications are excreted through the renal system. A newborn's renal system is immature, with a lower glomerular filtration rate and less efficient renal tubular function. Adult levels of renal function are not reached until between 1 and 2 years of age. In addition, infants and young children are less able to concentrate urine as compared to older children or adults (see Chapter 44).

Because of renal immaturity, adequate quantities of a given medication are not filtered out of circulating blood to be excreted in the urine (the primary method of medication excretion). As a result, a medication can circulate longer and reach toxic levels in the blood. Fluid volume loss (dehydration) can also decrease a child's ability to excrete medications and can adversely affect serum drug levels.

## Concentration

To safely administer medications to children, nurses need to know the concentration of certain medications in the bloodstream. Maintaining serum levels within a safe, therapeutic range maximizes the desired effect of a medication while reducing the risk of toxicity. With certain medications, the physician will order measurements of peak and trough serum levels to monitor medication concentrations. The peak concentration is not necessarily the highest concentration, but the concentration of the medication after it has been distributed. A medication reaches its peak concentration at a specified time after administration.

The medication trough is the level at which the serum concentration is lowest. Trough levels usually are obtained just before the next medication dose is scheduled to be administered. Knowing the peak and trough range for a specific medication will assist the nurse to accurately assess the child's response and potential toxic effects.

## PSYCHOLOGICAL AND DEVELOPMENTAL FACTORS

Growth and developmental principles and differences among age-groups must always be considered when medicating a child. Eliciting support from the parents often will help ease the child's concerns and fears.

Always approach children according to their developmental level, providing appropriate explanations about medication procedures. To decrease feelings of powerlessness, give the child as many choices as possible. For example, ask if a preschooler wants to hold the cup or have the nurse or a parent hold it while drinking the medicine.

Restraints are seldom necessary for administration of medications. It is appropriate to ask a staff member to assist the child to hold still during an injection because the child's movements could jeopardize safe administration of the medication (see Chapter 37). Parents can help to distract and comfort their child.

Honesty, praise, and reward are important elements of the medication administration process. The nurse should give honest explanations and tell the child if a medication has an unpleasant taste, when a procedure will be painful or uncomfortable, approximately how long the pain will last, and what the child can do to help during medication administration (e.g., not move, hold the cup). Terminology that is familiar and understandable (e.g., "pinching" or "stinging") should be used.

Praising the child after the medication administration for attempts at cooperation is important and helps gain trust and cooperation for future procedures. Even if the child had difficulty during the process, comment on at least one positive behavior (e.g., "I see that you did your best to take your medicine.").

Rewards following a procedure often serve to encourage the child and reinforce appropriate behavior. The reward should be safe and appropriate for the child's age. Stickers are usually a good choice for younger children. For an older child, providing time for a favorite activity, such as watching a video, may serve as a suitable reward.

### Infants

Administering medications to young infants can be relatively easy because of their small size. However, the use of appropriate administration techniques is essential to prevent aspiration of liquid or oral medications or adverse effects from injections (see Chapter 6). Giving medications safely to a squirming, older infant can pose a great challenge, requiring the nurse to obtain help from other staff members to hold the child. Parents need to be informed about all medications their infant is receiving, especially since children less than one year of age are at greatest risk for medication errors (Smith et al., 2014). Cuddling and comforting the infant before and after the procedure are also important interventions.

### Toddlers and Preschoolers

Older toddlers (2 to 3 years of age) are prone to magical thinking and might view the administration of medication (especially if the procedure is invasive) as punishment for "bad" thoughts (see Chapter 7). The nurse prepares toddlers with age-appropriate explanations, using play if possible. Allowing older toddlers to examine the equipment before the procedure may enhance cooperation. Toddlers can prefer to sit on the parent's lap when receiving medications. Helpful approaches for toddlers include praise and cuddling after procedures as well as giving rewards, such as stickers.

**PARENTS WANT TO KNOW**

***Medication Administration and Parent Roles***

Parents want to know how they can help their children during a procedure for administering medication. They may become concerned if the child refuses to take a medication that is intended to help the child recover from an illness. Nurses should do the following to empower parents:

- Obtain information from parents before administering a medication to their child:
  - Child's medication allergies and sensitivities
  - The child's ability to take medications (e.g., can the child swallow pills?)
  - Methods parents use to administer the medication (e.g., mixing it with a small amount of flavored syrup or jelly)
- Give parents a thorough explanation about all medications before administration. Include why the child needs the medication, anticipated therapeutic effects, possible side effects, how the medication will be administered (route, etc.), and expected location (e.g., injection site).
- Encourage parents to ask questions and express any concerns they may have, such as concern that a medication might not be effective or that it might be making their child ill. Parents know their children and often are aware of subtle changes before healthcare team members see them.
- According to the child's developmental level, explain to the child why a certain medication is needed. Be firm that the child must take the medication but offer allowable choices whenever possible, such as what juice the child can drink after an oral medication or which leg can be used for an injection.
- If preferred by the child, allow parents to administer certain medications (e.g., oral, otic, ophthalmic). Check five of the "six rights" of medication administration (right patient, right drug, right dose, right time, and right route) *before* you allow a parent to administer a medication.
- Show parents the most acceptable position for their child when administering a particular medication. Assist the child to maintain this position as needed.
- To increase cooperation, recommend the use of positive reinforcements, such as rewards or stickers, after the child has taken a medication.
- Complete the sixth right of medication administration—the right documentation—by documenting all required information in the child's medical record.

Preschoolers (3 to 5 years of age) continue to use magical thinking. They fear the unknown, and they fear painful procedures (see Chapter 7). This age-group benefits greatly from therapeutic play and participation. The nurse should offer the child as much control over the procedure and as many choices as possible (e.g., "Do you want to take your medication with juice or milk?"). The preschoolers may be able to hold still for an invasive procedure, although it is best to have a staff member ready to assist. Adhesive bandages after an invasive procedure, such as an injection, are important to children in this age-group because many believe a Band-Aid will "make it better;" an example of magical thinking.

### School-Age Children

School-age children fear loss of control, pain, and injury. At this age, a child can understand more complex explanations (see Chapter 8) as to why they need to take medication to recover from illness. Offering the child as much choice as possible is of great importance. School-age children often cooperate fully, even with invasive procedures, but often need a source of distraction (e.g., squeezing a person's hand, listening to music, talking about a subject of interest) and support (see Chapters 37 and 39). School-age children still appreciate receiving praise and rewards.

## Adolescents

Adolescents fear separation from peers and loss of control (see Chapter 9). Persons in this age-group understand adult explanations and can assist in making decisions about their nursing care. However, often adolescents exhibit a hyper-response to procedures that can seem inconsistent with their age. It is important to praise their cooperation, offer distractions, and help them find outlets for their frustrations (e.g., drawing, writing). Adolescents have increasing abilities to care for themselves due to their developing social, emotional, physical, and mental maturity (Altay & Çavusoglu, 2013).

# CALCULATING DOSAGES

Since the 1999 IOM report *To Err is Human,* there has been a much greater focus on patient safety (AAP, 2011). The Joint Commission (2015) published *National Patient Safety Goals* which include improving the safety of using medications in an effort to decrease medication errors. The AAP (2011) recognizes that medication errors cause great harm in children and have released several policy statements in an effort to reduce errors by focusing on an environment that embraces learning, understands human fallibility, and reports errors. An AAP policy statement noted that the most common causes of oral medication errors were due to volumetric dosing errors and the use of incorrect dosing delivery devices (AAP, 2015).

The nurse must always verify the accuracy of the ordered dose of medication before administration. First, the recommended dosage for the medication in mg/kg/day is checked and a calculation performed based on the child's weight to ensure that the right dose has been ordered. Second, the recommendation for the number of divided doses (e.g., every 4 hours, three times a day, every 12 hours) is confirmed. Last, the nurse ensures that route of administration is correct.

Dosages can also be calculated based on body surface area (BSA) (milligrams per square meter [$mg/m^2$]). Fig. 38.2 shows how to use a nomogram to obtain the BSA for a child. To calculate a medication dose on the basis of BSA, use the following formula:

$$\text{Appropriate dose} = \frac{\text{BSA of child } (m^2)}{1.7 \times \text{Adult dose}}$$

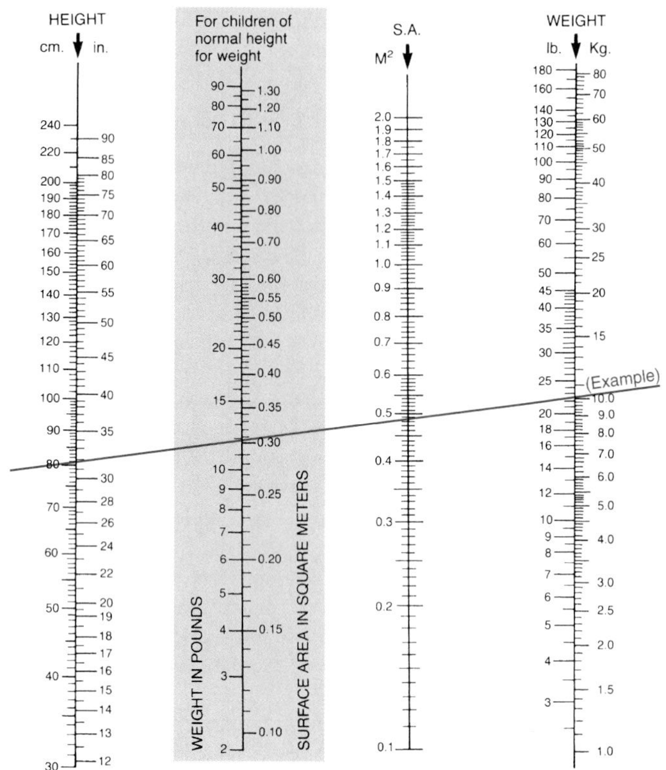


**FIG 38.2** Nomogram for calculating body surface area (BSA), which is used for determining medication dosages for infants and children. (From Custer, J., & Rau, R. (2009). (Eds.). *The Harriet Lane handbook: A manual for pediatric house officers* [18th ed., pp. 1032]. Philadelphia: Elsevier.)

# MEDICATION ADMINISTRATION PROCEDURES

To avoid errors in medication administration, follow these general procedures:

- Adhere to the "six rights" of medication administration: right patient/child, right drug, right dose, right time, right route, and right documentation.
- Check the orders to be sure that all information is correctly transcribed. Note any allergies.
- Always double-check medication calculations before administration. Be sure the child's weight is accurately recorded.
- Double-check dose calculations provided by the pharmacy in a unit dose form. Consult with the physician or pharmacist if there is any question about a dose.
- Ask another nurse to perform a second check for the following medications and any others as required by agency policy (Institute for Safe Medication Practices [ISMP], 2015a):
  - Insulin (subcutaneous and IV)
  - Oral hypoglycemic agents
  - Dextrose hypertonic IV solutions (20% or greater)
  - Narcotics/opioids (transdermal, IV, and oral)
  - Medications administered via epidural/intrathecal route
  - Chemotherapeutic agents (oral and parenteral)
  - Digoxin or other inotropic medications
  - Anticoagulants
  - Anesthetic and moderate sedation agents (inhaled and IV)
  - Potassium chloride, hypertonic sodium chloride, and magnesium sulfate for injection

## Medication Reconciliation

When admitting children to a hospital unit, the nurse obtains a list of all prescription and over-the-counter medications as well as any herbal preparations a child is taking at home. To ensure patient safety, the nurse compares the medications the child has been receiving at home to the list of medications prescribed for the child's hospital stay, identifying and communicating any discrepancies. This process is referred to as 'medication reconciliation' and is of paramount importance to preventing medication errors, according to the Joint Commission (AAP, 2011). The Joint Commission's national patient safety goals include an entire section on medication reconciliation, listing detailed performance elements designed to ensure that accurate medication information is maintained and communicated among healthcare team members, patients, and their families (2015).

The nurse must also assess the parents' knowledge of all the medications (and herbal remedies) the child is taking. This information includes the name of the medication, the dose, number of times a day the child is taking the medication, knowledge of side effects, the child's allergies, any adverse reactions the child might have experienced, and the time the medication was last administered. To facilitate medication reconciliation, parents are encouraged to bring all of their child's medications to the hospital or clinic visit. At discharge, medication reconciliation includes providing clear, detailed, written instructions to parents about all medications to be given at home as well as communicating precise medication information to the next healthcare provider.

Children are at greater risk than adults for medication errors and adverse drug events causing harm because of pharmacokinetics, dosages by weight or body mass, and narrow therapeutic-to-lethal ranges for many medications (Institute for Safe Medication Practice, 2015b). The Joint Commission (2015) has indicated that a significant percentage of pediatric adverse drug events are preventable. Recommendations to reduce the risk of pediatric medication errors include the following:

- Establish and implement standardized medication procedures and processes for drug administration.
- Limit the number of concentrations and dose strengths of high alert medications.
- Use oral syringes to administer oral medications.
- Enable dose/dose range software programs to provide alerts for potentially incorrect dosages.
- Educate healthcare providers (nurses) about the use of IV infusion pumps; recognize that medication errors can still occur.
- Use consistent physiologic monitoring (e.g., pulse oximetry) with age- and size-appropriate equipment for children under sedation.
- Use bar-coding technology that is adapted to pediatric processes and systems.
- On admission, weigh children in kilograms (kg) and use weight in kg for prescriptions, dose calculations, medical records, and staff communication.
- Use pediatric-specific medication formulations and concentrations.
- Comprehensive pediatric specialty training for all healthcare team members.

Major reasons for the increased use of computer systems such as patient electronic medical records (EMRs) and computerized physician order entry (CPOE) include reducing medication errors, improving communication, and improving medication adherence (Johnson & Lehmann, 2013; Wurster, Groner, & Hoffman, 2012). EMRs that include electronic medication administration records (EMARs) can improve the communication of patient medication lists and other information, such as allergies, between different healthcare providers working in the same facility or in other settings. Although electronic systems have shown great potential to significantly reduce the incidence of medication errors, they have limitations and cannot eliminate all errors (Johnson & Lehmann, 2013). These systems do not replace the responsibility of physicians and nurses for clear and complete medication orders, accurate dose calculations, and correct administration of medications to children.

## Administering Oral Medications

The oral route is the most widely used method of administering medications. It is also one of the least reliable methods of administration because absorption is affected by the presence or absence of food in the stomach, gastric emptying time, GI motility, and stomach acidity. The oral route is also less predictable because of potential medication loss to spillage, leaking, or spitting out.

Oral medications are available in liquid (elixir or suspension), tablet or capsule, chewable tablet, and sprinkle (powder) forms. If the child cannot swallow tablets or capsules, the nurse finds out whether the medication is available in a liquid form or as a chewable tablet. If not, the nurse determines if the tablet can be crushed or if the contents of a capsule can be emptied. It is not recommended to crush **time-release medications** (e.g., extended-release [XR], controlled-release [CR], sustained-release [SR]), as well as enteric-coated tablets.

Before administering oral medications, the nurse assesses the child's gag reflex and ability to swallow. The specific form of oral medication used should be tailored to the child's developmental level and ability to successfully take a particular form. An assessment of the way the child takes medications at home will help determine the best form to use.

### CRITICAL THINKING EXERCISE 38.1

The father of a 3-year-old boy calls the ambulatory care clinic with questions for the triage nurse. His son is refusing to take his medication because it tastes "yucky," and the father asks the physician to change the medication to something that tastes better. When asked, the father explains that the medication is penicillin liquid and that the child is taking it for the treatment of "strep throat." The father says the child is feeling much better now.

1. What information should the nurse give this father about the child's medication regimen?
2. What actions would the nurse advise the father to take that will encourage his son to take his medication?

### Preparation

When preparing to administer an elixir or a suspension, the nurse first ensures that the correct dose is drawn for administration. Physicians' orders often specify the dosage in milligrams (mg), *not* milliliters (mL), for liquid medications. It is important to calculate the mL dose properly based on the concentration (mg/mL) for the available liquid medication.

The AAP recommends using milliliter only systems with oral dosing syringes to avoid dosing errors (Yin et al., 2014). For volumes of 5 mL or less, an oral syringe designed for oral medication administration only should be used. Larger volumes are poured into calibrated plastic medicine cups, which generally hold up to 30 mL (1 oz).

The nurse can mix a sprinkle, powder, or crushed tablet with a small amount (e.g., 1 to 3 teaspoons) of a nonessential food such as applesauce or pudding or with a liquid. Mixing medications with necessary foods including formula is avoided because this can alter the food's taste; thus, the child may refuse further intake of that food. The medication's compatibility with food must be determined before mixing and administering.

### CRITICAL THINKING EXERCISE 38.2

You need to administer oral ibuprofen, 150 mg, to your 5-year-old patient. Ibuprofen is available in a liquid form with 100 mg in 5 mL.

1. How many milliliters (mL) will you administer?
2. When the child is discharged, how many teaspoons will you instruct the parent to administer for each 150 mg dose?

### Administration

The method for administering oral medications differs according to the child's age and developmental level. Infants usually receive elixir or suspension forms that are administered using an empty nipple or oral syringe. First, the infant is placed in an upright or semi-upright position, similar to the position used for feeding. The nurse opens the infant's mouth by applying gentle pressure to the chin or cheeks. If using a nipple, it is placed in the infant's mouth and the medication added to the empty nipple when the baby begins to suck. If using an oral syringe, it is gently placed in the infant's mouth along the side of the cheek, and the nurse pushes the medication in slowly as the infant sucks (Fig. 38.3). It may be necessary to hold an infant or young child in order to safely administer an oral medication. As seen in Fig. 38.3, the child's head is cradled between the nurse's nondominant arm and body; the nurse holds the child's hand with his or her nondominant hand and then administers the oral medication using the dominant hand.

Toddlers and preschoolers can easily take liquid medications from an oral syringe or a medicine cup. Allowing children to take their own medication, giving rewards as incentives, and providing choices that fit into the medication regimen enhance autonomy and cooperation.

Preschoolers and young school-age children can usually manage chewable tablets without difficulty. Many older, school-age children can swallow tablets or capsules; however, the nurse must assess a child's ability to swallow pills on an individual basis. If a child cannot swallow pills, the availability of other forms of oral medications, such as liquid suspensions or elixirs and powders, should be investigated.

Oral medications are given with the child in an upright or slightly recumbent position to facilitate swallowing and prevent aspiration. After administration of the medication, the child is given a food or fluid item such as formula, juice, or an ice pop, if not contraindicated.

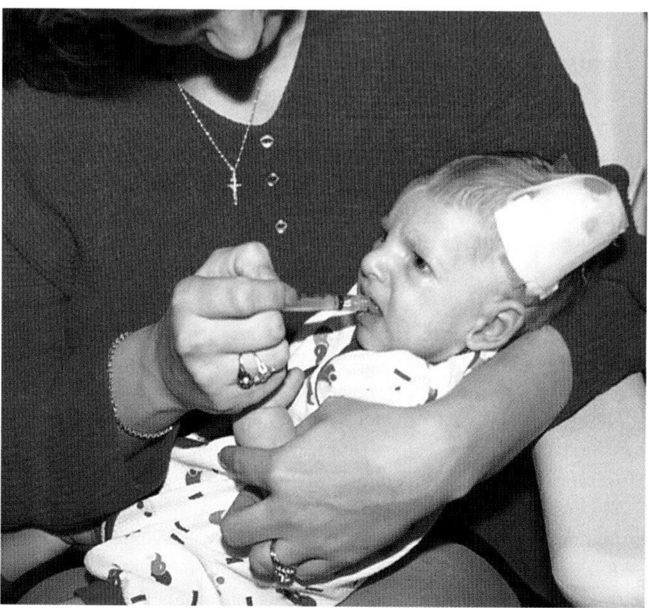

**FIG 38.3** Administering an oral medication to an infant using an oral syringe. (Courtesy Parkland Health and Hospital System, Dallas, TX.)

Children are allowed to select what they would like to eat or drink after taking oral medications, whenever possible.

If a child vomits or spits up after administration of an oral medication, the nurse notifies the physician. Another dose may be needed, depending on how long it has been since administration, the type of medication, and the amount of emesis.

### Alternative Routes for Oral Medications

Oral medications can be administered directly into the GI tract through a feeding tube. If the medication is to be administered through a feeding tube, verify tube placement before administration (see Chapter 37) and, depending on the type of tube, determine whether the tube is the proper route for the ordered medication. Before and after the medication is administered, the tube is flushed with water to ensure that the medication has reached the GI tract and to prevent blockage of the tube.

## Administering Injections

Injected medications are rapidly absorbed by diffusing into either plasma or the lymphatic system. Although injections result in faster and more reliable absorption than the oral route, injections are stressful and threatening to children and are not preferred. Injections are used most often for one-time doses of antibiotics (e.g., ceftriaxone for the initial treatment of severe infection), immunizations, insulin administration for diabetics, purified protein derivative (PPD) tuberculosis skin test, and allergy skin testing.

Appropriately preparing the child for an injection can reduce emotional and anticipatory concerns. Depending on the child's developmental level, explain the reason for the injection, any sensations the child might experience, and the length of time they are anticipated to last. Facilitate the child's understanding that an injection is not punishment but is needed to help the child get well or stay healthy. Practice distraction techniques such as deep breathing and singing with the child in advance.

Offer parents the option to stay with their child during the procedure or leave if they feel unable to cope with the stress. Many parents prefer to remain and help distract, comfort, and reassure their child who is receiving an injection.

To reduce the risk of injury, it is sometimes necessary to limit the child's movement before and during the administration of an injected medication. This restraint can be accomplished by swaddling the child and/or obtaining the assistance of other healthcare professionals. Some parents request to help hold their child while receiving an injection (Fig. 38.4). Parents who feel confident in their ability to hold their child

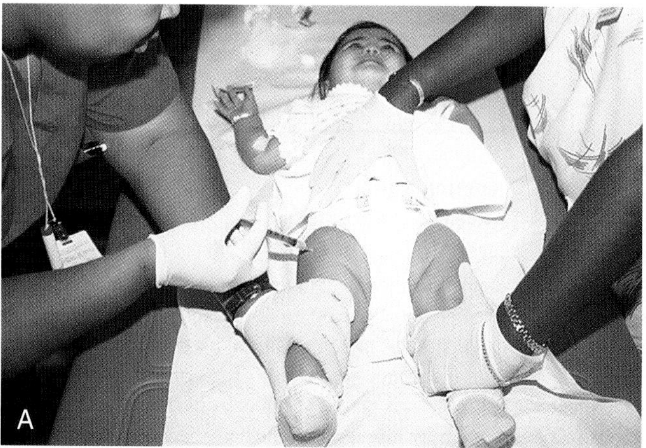



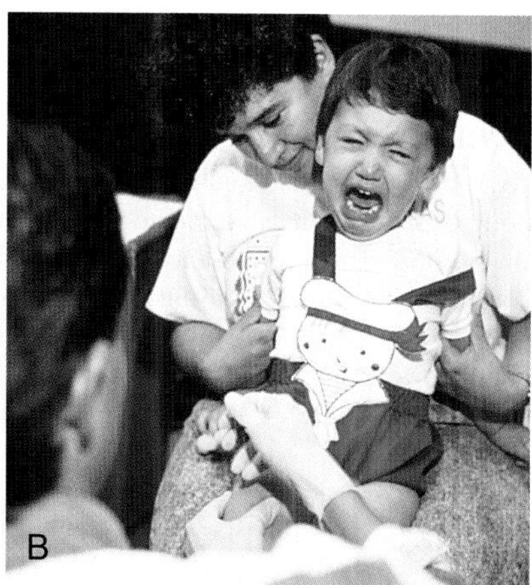



**FIG 38.4** Two methods of holding a child for an intramuscular (IM) injection at the vastus lateralis site. (**A,** Courtesy Parkland Health and Hospital System Community-Oriented Primary Care Clinic, Dallas, TX; **B,** Courtesy Cook Children's Medical Center, Fort Worth, TX.)

and prevent injury can be given this option. However, parents should not be required to restrain their child during a procedure.

Many children have great fears related to injections and perceive them to be very painful. Even with the best preparation and use of distraction techniques, it is hard for some children to cope with the pain of an injection, even if it lasts for only seconds. Use of oral sucrose for infants, vapocoolants, and topical anesthetic agents such as eutectic mixture of local anesthetics (EMLA) cream for all children has been shown to be effective in reducing or even eliminating injection pain (see Chapter 39) (Rishovd, 2014).

The child who must receive multiple injections might benefit significantly from therapeutic play during which the child uses a syringe to give "shots" to a doll. Therapeutic play is an effective approach to prepare a child for an injection (see Chapters 35 and 37). It can also help the child gain a sense of mastery over the experience of receiving injections, thus decreasing anxiety.

Documentation following an injection should include the amount of medication injected, the site used, and how the child tolerated the procedure. Federal vaccine regulations require nurses to record the vaccine manufacturer and lot number for each immunization given, as well as record and report any vaccine/immunization reactions. Premedicating a child with acetaminophen is not recommended because of the potential to decrease the immune response (Rishovd, 2014).

### Intramuscular Injections

Determine the injection site in advance, before initiating the injection procedure. The site should be soft and well vascularized with healthy, intact skin. The child's age, size, and muscle mass, along with the volume and properties of the medication to be injected, will influence the choice of the intramuscular (IM) injection site. It is essential to accurately locate and inject at an appropriate IM site to avoid injecting an IM medication into subcutaneous tissue or puncturing a blood vessel, nerve, or bone. The preferred IM injection sites in children are shown in Table 38.1. The preferred site for infants and toddlers is the vastus lateralis, while the deltoid is preferred for children 3 to 18 years of age (Rishovd, 2014; Jackson et al., 2013). Of note, the dorsogluteal site is not recommended due to potential injury to the sciatic nerve, and the rectus femoris is not recommended for use in children (Rishovd, 2014)

Selection of the appropriate needle size and length will depend on the child's size, the amount of body fat (distance between skin surface and muscle), the injection site to be used, and the child's muscle mass at the IM site. It is important to always use the smallest size needle and the shortest length that will safely and comfortably administer the medication. In general, the needle size used for children will be 22 to 25 gauge, with the length between ½ and 1½ inches. Use of a larger gauge needle may be indicated for viscous medication.

Safe volumes for IM injections range from 0.5 mL for infants and young children to 3 mL for adolescents; however, each child's size and muscle mass must be individually assessed. After performing hand hygiene, don gloves and clean the skin at the injection site with an antiseptic swab or pad and allow it to dry. Insert the needle at a 90-degree angle with a quick darting motion. Several agencies, including the AAP strongly, discourage the practice of aspirating before IM injections (Rishovd, 2014). Give the injection slowly, at a rate of 1 mL/10 seconds. Remove the needle and apply gentle pressure at the site with a dry gauze pad; do not massage. If the child will receive several IM injections over time, it is important to rotate sites to prevent tissue irritation and possible muscle atrophy and wasting.

### Subcutaneous Injections

A subcutaneous injection is given into the connective tissue that lies just below the dermal layer of the skin. This type of administration is used for medications that provide a sustained effect (e.g., heparin, insulin) or for certain immunizations. A subcutaneous injection should be given only into healthy tissue that is free from infection, bruising, and scarring. If circulation is impaired because of conditions such as shock or vascular disease, a subcutaneous injection should not be used because absorption will be altered.

Preferred subcutaneous injection sites for children include the outer posterior aspects of the upper arms and the anterior aspects of the thighs (Fig. 38.5). The abdomen, excluding a 2-inch radius around the umbilicus, is another site that is often used for children who require frequent subcutaneous injections (e.g., type 1 diabetics). Systematically rotating sites can facilitate consistent drug absorption. The site of each subcutaneous injection must be recorded for proper site rotation.

Subcutaneous injections are typically given with a 25- to 27-gauge needle that is ⅜- to ⅝-inch long. The subcutaneous injection volume is usually 0.5 mL; the maximum volume is 1 mL.

After performing hand hygiene, don gloves and clean the site in a circular pattern using an antiseptic swab, and allow the skin to dry. Gently pinch the tissue to raise the subcutaneous tissue from the muscle. The angle of needle insertion is usually 45 degrees; some nurses use a 90-degree angle with a ½-inch needle. Insert the needle with the bevel up using a dart-like motion. Release the tissue and inject the medication. After removing the needle, gentle pressure can be applied to the site using a dry gauze pad; do not massage.

### Intradermal Injections

Intradermal injections enter the dermis layer of skin, which is just below the epidermis, and usually on the inner aspect of the forearm or on the upper back. They are most often used for allergy testing or tuberculosis (TB) screening (PPD). The needle used is 25 or 27 gauge and ⅜- to ⅝-inch in length. The maximum volume injected is 0.1 mL. After performing hand hygiene, don gloves and clean the site in a circular pattern using an antiseptic swab, and allow the skin to dry. Turn the bevel of the needle up, and insert gently at a 5- to 15-degree angle, barely penetrating the skin (Fig. 38.6). Inject the medication slowly to form a bleb or wheal.

#### SAFETY ALERT

***Guidelines for Maximum Safe Volumes for Intramuscular Injections****

| | SITE | | |
|---|---|---|---|
| **Age** | **Deltoid** | **Ventrogluteal** | **Vastus Lateralis** |
| Premature | — | — | 0.5 mL |
| Neonate | — | — | 0.5-1 mL |
| Infant (1-12 mo) | — | — | 1 mL |
| Toddler (13-36 mo) | 0.5 mL | 1 mL | 1-1.5 mL |
| Young child (3-6 yr) | 0.5-1 mL | 1.5 mL | 1.5-2 mL |
| Older child (6-14 yr) | 0.5-1 mL | 1.5-2 mL | 1.5-2 mL |
| Adolescent (15 yr-adult) | 1 mL | 2-3 mL | 2-3 mL |

*Evaluate the individual child's muscle mass before injection.

#### CRITICAL THINKING EXERCISE 38.3

You need to immunize an infant with the hepatitis B vaccine. The dose ordered for the infant is 2.5 mcg. The vaccine you have available has 5 mcg/mL. How many milliliters (mL) will you administer to the infant via an intramuscular (IM) injection?

### TABLE 38.1 Preferred Intramuscular Injection Sites in Children

| Site | Key Points |
|---|---|
| Vastus lateralis 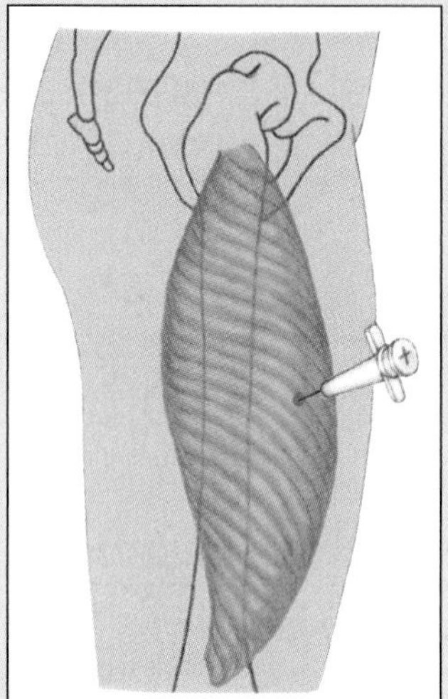 | Location is the anterior lateral thigh.<br>Well-developed muscle at birth.<br>Often used for infants and children younger than 2 yr, but acceptable site for all ages.<br>Can tolerate larger fluid volumes.<br>Not located near large nerves or blood vessels.<br>Easy to access.<br>Locate greater trochanter and knee joint; divide space into thirds; give the injection in the outer aspect of the middle third of the leg. |
| Ventrogluteal 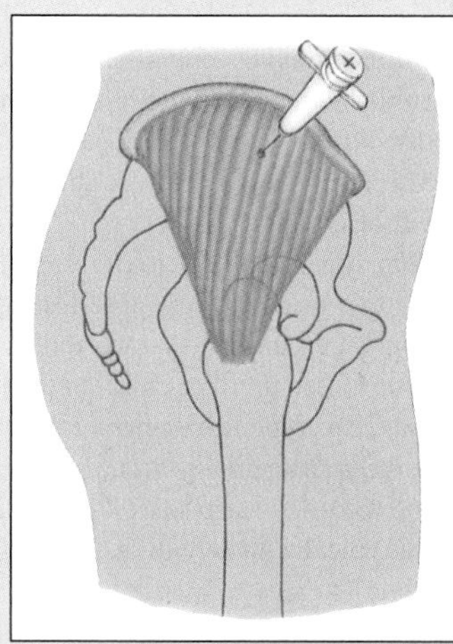 | Location is the gluteus medius muscle of the hip.<br>Can be used for infants, children, and adolescents.<br>Can generally hold larger fluid volumes.<br>Free of major nerves and vascular structures.<br>Some reports of less pain than vastus lateralis site.<br>Locate by placing heel of hand on greater trochanter with fingers pointed up and thumb pointed toward the groin. Place index finger over anterior superior iliac spine and middle finger along posterior iliac crest to form a V between the two fingers; give the injection in the center of the V. |
| Deltoid 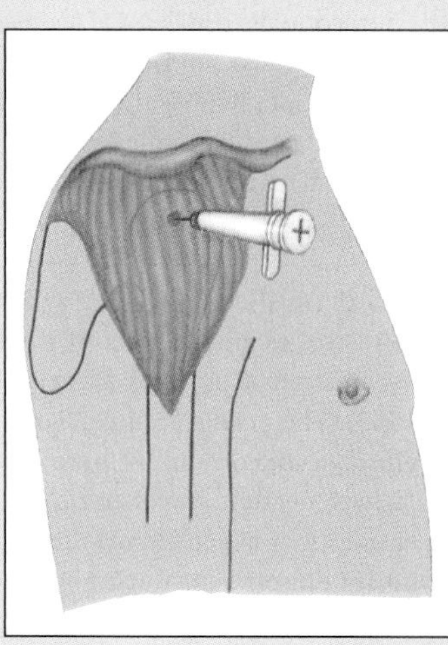 | Location is the deltoid muscle of the upper arm.<br>Recommended for use in children older than 2 yr.<br>Muscle mass is small; only use for 0.5-1 mL of fluid.<br>Close to radial and axillary nerves.<br>Easy to access with minimal clothing removal needed.<br>Less pain and local side effects from vaccines than vastus lateralis site.<br>Faster absorption than ventrogluteal site.<br>Locate acromion process at the top of the upper arm; inject in the middle of muscle section that is two fingerbreadths below acromion process but above the axilla. |

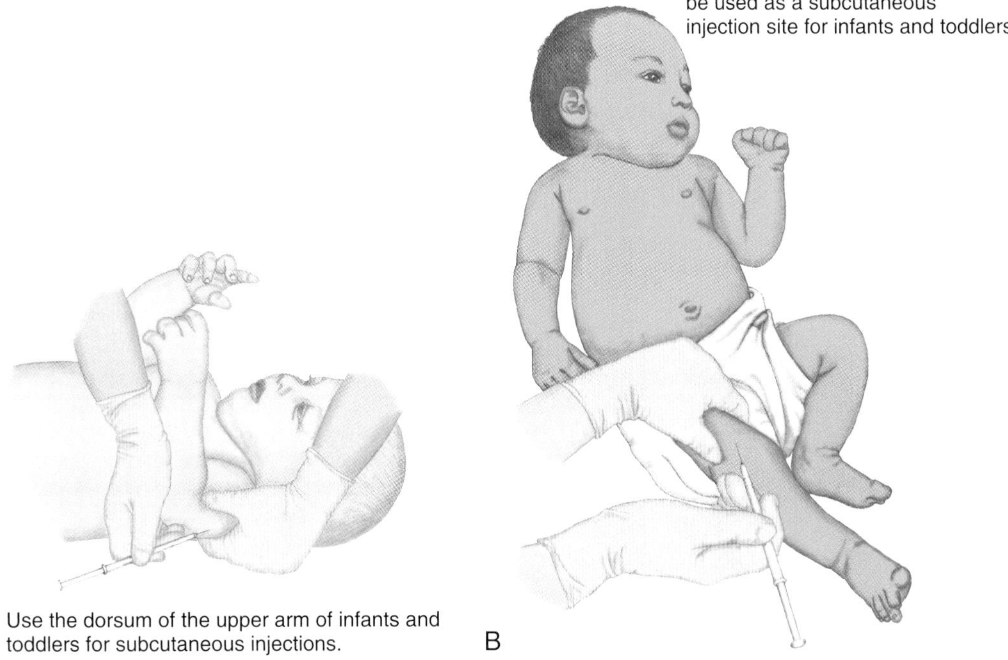

The anterior of the thigh can also be used as a subcutaneous injection site for infants and toddlers.
A Use the dorsum of the upper arm of infants and toddlers for subcutaneous injections.
B


FIG 38.5 Two of the preferred subcutaneous injection sites for infants and toddlers.

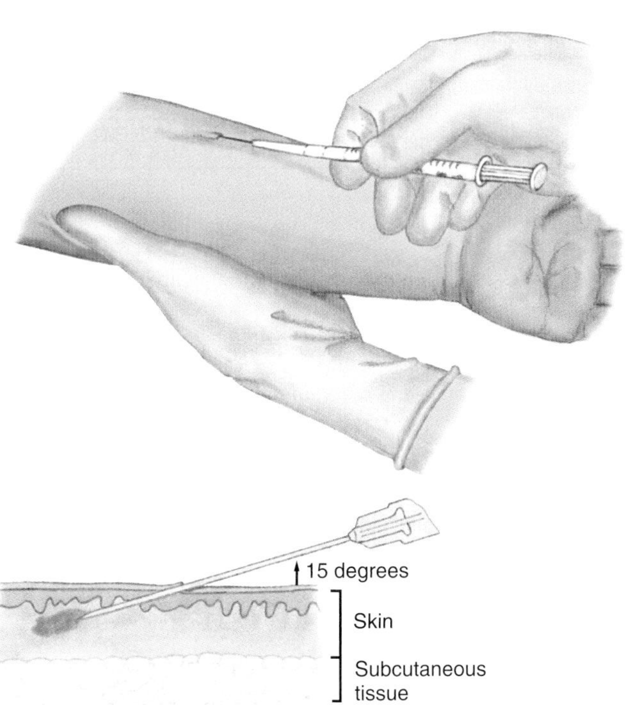


FIG 38.6 Intradermal injection site and technique.

## Rectal Administration

Medications given rectally can have a localized effect on the GI tract such as prompting defecation. They also can have a systemic effect such as decreasing fever, although absorption of medication administered by the rectal route is not as reliable as the oral route. Per rectum medication administration is usually reserved for times when a child cannot eat or drink or is unable to tolerate oral intake because of nausea and vomiting. Rectal administration carries a risk of injury to the anal and rectal tissues. This route should not be used if the rectum is full of stool. Also, rectal medication is contraindicated in children with rectal disease or those who have had rectal surgery.

Rectal administration is stressful for children because they fear intrusive procedures. Carefully prepare the child and explain the reason the medication is being given via this route, the steps of the procedure, and what the child can do to help.

Position the child on the left side with the right leg slightly flexed, exposing the anal area sufficiently for visibility. Adequate draping is essential for preschool and older children. Distraction and deep-breathing exercises can help the child relax the external sphincter.

Perform hand hygiene and don gloves. Place water-soluble lubricant on the suppository. Advise the child to take a deep breath or bear down, if possible, to relax the sphincter. Then, depending on the size of the child's anus, use either the index finger or little finger to gently insert the suppository through the anus and past the internal sphincter (approximately 1.5 to 2.5 cm). After insertion, hold the infant or young child's buttocks together for at least 5 minutes. Instruct older children and adolescents not to expel the suppository for 5 to 10 minutes.

## Vaginal Administration

The vaginal route is used primarily for school-age or adolescent girls who require topical treatment with an antiinfective agent for a vaginal infection. It is essential to explain the procedure, why it is indicated, and how the child can help.

Ask the child to void and then assist her into a supine position with the soles of her feet together and her knees resting on the bed (frog-leg position). Remember to use drapes and provide for privacy. After hand hygiene and donning gloves, gently spread the labia so that the vaginal orifice is visible. Lubricate the tablet, suppository, or applicator with a water-soluble lubricant. Have the patient take a deep breath and then gently insert the vaginal medication approximately 7.5 to 10 cm along the posterior wall of the vagina.

After the procedure is completed, the child may need to remain in a supine position for at least 10 minutes. Older school-age children and adolescents can be taught to instill their own vaginal medications.

## PROCEDURE

### *Administering an Ophthalmic Preparation*

**Purpose**

To treat an eye infection, dilate pupils for diagnostic testing, or keep eyes moist.

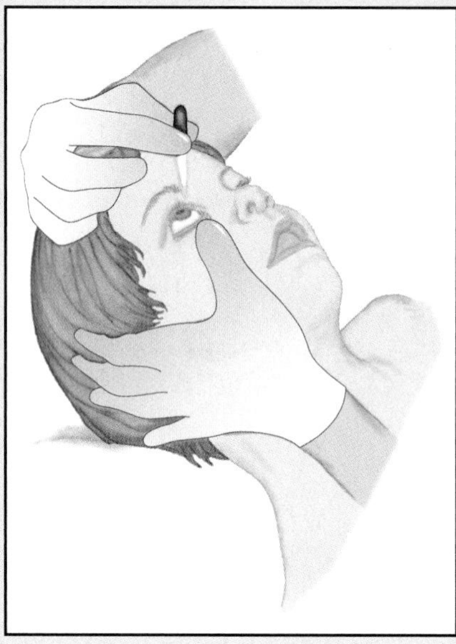

1. Explain the purpose for the medication or lubricating drops. Explain any expected sensations to the child in developmentally appropriate terms (e.g., "It will feel like there is something in your eye for just a minute"). Explain that the child might have blurred vision for a short time afterward. Tell the child how to help with the procedure ("Be sure to not rub your eyes"). Assistance in holding a young child might be necessary.
2. Gather needed equipment: eye drops or ointment, gloves, gauze pads, sterile saline solution for irrigation, and tissues. Use appropriate hand hygiene and don gloves.
3. Assist the child into the supine position with the neck slightly hyperextended (e.g., by placing a rolled towel or small blanket under the shoulder blades).
4. If the drops are to be instilled into the eye of an infant or young child, obtain assistance in holding the child's arms and head or use a mummy wrap if necessary.
5. If crusts or exudates are observed, use a sterile gauze pad that has been moistened with sterile saline and gently remove the crusts and drainage. Perform hand hygiene and don a new pair of gloves.
6. Instruct an older child to look upward and gently pull the lower lid down and away from the eye.
7. Place the drops into the space between the eye and lower lid, the conjunctival sac, taking care not to contaminate the end of the dropper.
8. Place a ribbon of ointment on the inside edge of the lower eyelid moving from the inner to the outer canthus, taking care to not contaminate the end of the ointment tube. If both drops and ointment are ordered, the drops should be administered first.
9. Have the child look down as the lower lid is released. Encourage the child to close both eyes gently and keep them closed for several seconds. Carefully blot any excess medication. Remove gloves and perform hand hygiene.
10. Praise the child for cooperation and assistance. Document all pertinent information, including how the child tolerated the procedure and responded to the medication, in the child's medical record.

## Ophthalmic Administration

For children, most ophthalmic medications come in the form of drops or ointment. If these preparations are refrigerated, allow them to warm to room temperature before instillation. After hand hygiene and putting on gloves, gently remove any exudates by wiping the child's eye with a sterile gauze pad (move from inner to outer canthus) using a different pad for each eye. Shake all suspensions well before instillation. Eye drops are instilled into the conjunctival sac. Eye ointment is applied along the inside edge of the lower eyelid from the inner to the outer canthus (Procedure: Administering an Ophthalmic Preparation).

## Otic Administration

When instilling medications into the ear (otic), the child is positioned supine with the head turned to allow access to the appropriate side (Procedure: Administering Otic Drops). If drainage is present, which can occur if the tympanic membrane is ruptured, gloves must be worn, following hand hygiene, to instill eardrops. First, gently clean any exudates from the outer ear with a sterile gauze pad. Never attempt to clean the ear canal by placing any item such as a cotton-tipped applicator (Q-tip) inside the ear. To avoid pain, otic solutions should be allowed to warm to room temperature before administration.

## Nasal Administration

Generally, nose drops and sprays are used for localized treatment of the nasal passages. However, the mucous membranes inside the nose allow for fairly rapid systemic absorption of medications. A wide range of medications can be given to children intranasally, including antidiuretic hormone (deamino-D-arginine-vasopressin [DDAVP]), fentanyl, ketamine, midazolam (Versed), and lorazepam.

Before administering nose drops to an infant, the nurse removes any excess mucus by gently suctioning the nares with a bulb syringe. To make eating more comfortable for a congested infant, saline nose drops are given, followed by gentle suction, 20 to 30 minutes before feedings.

Nose drops can cause an uncomfortable sensation when administered, which can be stressful for young children. Provide a thorough explanation of what the child will feel, how the medication will make it easier to breathe through the nose, and what the child needs to do to help. Assistance with holding may be necessary for young children.

Place the child supine with the head in the midline position and the neck slightly hyperextended. After hand hygiene and putting on gloves, instill the number of drops ordered into each naris. Keep the child's head in this same position for 1 minute. Instruct the child not to blow the medication out the nose. Praise all efforts at cooperation.

## Topical Administration

Topical medications (creams, lotions, ointments, patches, and pastes) can produce local as well as systemic effects when absorbed through the skin. Adhesive, transdermal patches release medication on a continuous basis over a prescribed time period (hours or even days). They are changed at scheduled intervals; thus, the child is cautioned to keep the patch in place. The patch is applied to clean, dry skin free of bruises,

## PROCEDURE

### *Administering Otic Drops*

**Purpose**

To treat inflammation or infection of the ear canal, relieve pain, or prevent otitis externa.

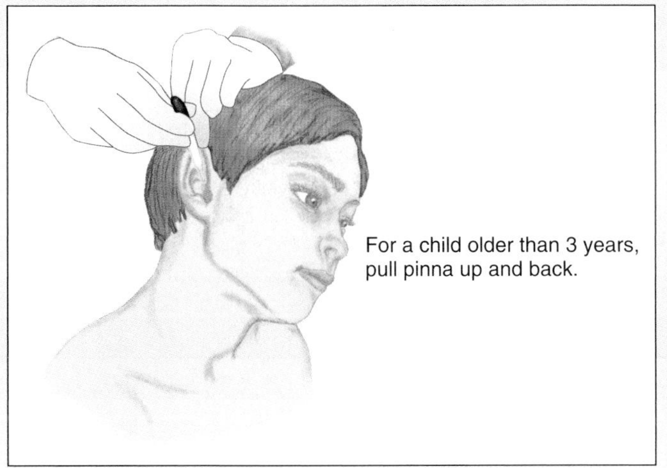

For a child older than 3 years, pull pinna up and back.

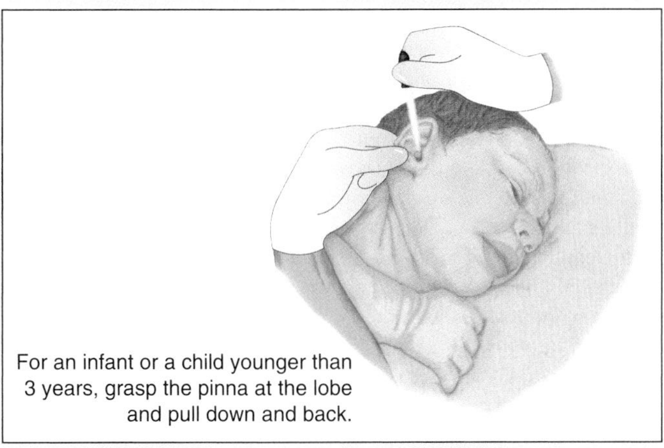

For an infant or a child younger than 3 years, grasp the pinna at the lobe and pull down and back.

1. Explain any expected sensations to the child in developmentally appropriate terms (e.g., "It may sound like there is a butterfly flying inside your ear"). Describe how the child can help. Assistance in holding a young child might be necessary.
2. Gather the following equipment: otic drops, gloves, sterile gauze pad, sterile cotton-tipped applicator, and cotton pieces. Use appropriate hand hygiene and don gloves. Ensure that the otic drops are at room temperature.
3. If drainage is noted in the ear, remove it from the external ear *only* with a sterile gauze pad or cotton-tipped applicator. Perform hand hygiene and don a new pair of gloves.
4. Position the child lying down with the affected ear up or sitting with the head turned so the affected ear is up.
5. Brace the administering hand against the child's head above the ear.
6. If the child is 3 years old or younger, pull the pinna of the ear down and toward the back of the head, holding near the lobe. If the child is older than 3 years, pull the pinna up and toward the back.
7. Insert the required number of drops, taking care not to contaminate the end of the drops container. Then gently massage or apply slight pressure to the tragus (anterior portion) with the index finger.
8. Place cotton loosely into the outermost portion of the canal, if ordered. Instruct the child not to remove the cotton or place anything inside the ear.
9. Keep the child on the unaffected side for 5 to 10 minutes after administration. (If medication is to be administered in both ears, repeat the procedure in the other ear.)
10. Remove gloves and perform hand hygiene.
11. Praise the child for cooperation and assistance. Document all pertinent information, including how the child tolerated the procedure and responded to the medication, in the child's medical record.

abrasions, and irritation. The nurse must wear gloves during the application of a transdermal patch.

A variety of prescription and over-the-counter creams, lotions, and ointments are used to treat skin irritation, dryness, or infection. Once the procedure has been explained to the child, perform hand hygiene, don gloves, cleanse the skin to remove any exudates, scales, or other residue, and allow it to dry. Don a new pair of gloves and apply the ointment or cream per orders or instructions. Encourage the child to avoid touching the treated areas.

## Inhalation Therapy

Respiratory medications, used frequently in children, are delivered by a nebulizer or a metered-dose inhaler, a hand-held device that delivers "puffs" of medication for inhalation (see Chapter 45). Although many inhaled medications have an unpleasant taste or smell, this route is a relatively nonthreatening form of medication delivery. Monitoring for desired therapeutic effects as well as systemic side effects is essential.

Nebulized medications are diluted in normal saline solution and administered with a hand-held, small-volume nebulizer. The nebulizer aerosolizes the medication for the child to inhale. Medication can be delivered through a facemask or through a plastic mouthpiece held between the lips or close to the face (Fig. 38.7). Encourage the child to breathe deeply and slowly during the treatment.

Nebulized medication can be delivered along with supplemental oxygen to a hospitalized child with an acute episode of respiratory distress. Nebulized medications can also be delivered to an unconscious or intubated child by inserting the aerosol administration device in-line between the child and a bag-valve-mask device or ventilator.

Metered-dose inhalers offer a portable means of delivering inhaled medications. Many people, particularly children, have difficulty using a metered-dose inhaler correctly. The effectiveness of these medications is increased with the use of a spacer device. A spacer is a cylindrical piece of hard or expandable plastic that attaches to the inhaler on one side and a mouthpiece or facemask on the other side. The child depresses the inhaler, and the medication enters the spacer, allowing the child time to deeply inhale the medication that is now mixed with air (Procedure: Using a Metered-Dose Inhaler).

Initial and ongoing education of the parent and child is important to ensure the effectiveness of inhalation therapy. The techniques for using home nebulizers and metered-dose inhalers and spacers must be demonstrated by the healthcare provider and then a return demonstration given by the child and parents. Parents must also be taught how

## PROCEDURE

### *Using a Metered-Dose Inhaler (MDI)*

**Purpose**

To deliver medication directly to the respiratory system.

1. Verify the physician's order for the medication(s) to be administered and the number of puffs prescribed.
2. If one of the medications is an inhaled steroid, administer it last.
3. Explain the procedure to the child and parents. It is often helpful to demonstrate the use of the inhaler and to explain specifically what the child is expected to do.
4. Perform hand hygiene. Shake the inhaler well and remove the cap.
5. Hold the inhaler upright and attach it to the spacer. Tell the child not to inhale too quickly or the spacer will whistle.
6. Ask the child to tilt the head back slightly, take a deep breath, and then exhale ("big breath out") slowly. Place the spacer mouthpiece in the child's mouth or the spacer mask over the face. The child might be more comfortable holding the spacer and helping you.
7. Tell the child that you will now depress the inhaler and release the medication into the spacer. Then direct the child to inhale ("big breath in") slowly, over 3 to 5 seconds, and deeply.
8. Encourage the child to hold his or her breath for approximately 10 seconds or until you finish counting slowly to 5.
9. Remove the inhaler and ask the child to exhale slowly through the nose.
10. Wait at least 1 to 2 minutes and then repeat the complete procedure if another puff is ordered. Praise the child for cooperating and helping.
11. Encourage the child to rinse his or her mouth with water. Rinse the inhaler adapter and spacer with cool water and allow it to dry. Perform hand hygiene.
12. Praise the child for cooperation and assistance. Document all pertinent information, including how the child tolerated the procedure and responded to the medication, in the child's medical record.

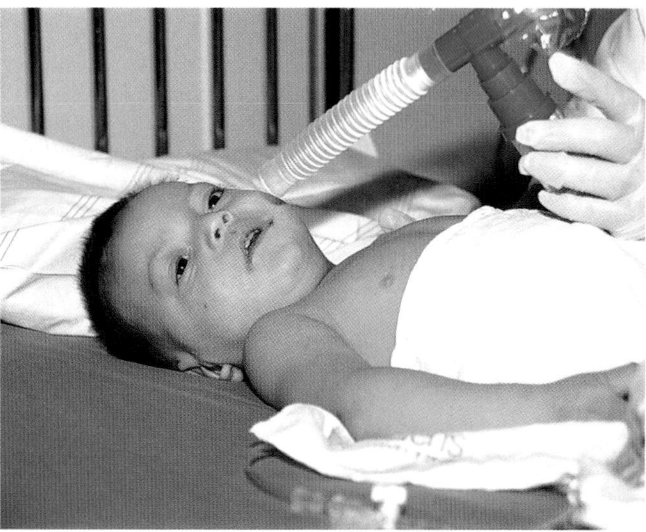

**FIG 38.7** Administration of nebulized medication to an infant. (Courtesy Children's Medical Center, Dallas, TX.)

to clean and maintain a home nebulizer. Correct use of the metered-dose inhalers and spacers must be reviewed at each physician's office or clinic appointment.

## INTRAVENOUS THERAPY

Intravenous (IV) therapy is widely used for children. Fluids and electrolytes, total parenteral nutrition (TPN), blood products, and medications can be delivered by the IV route. When used to administer medications, IV therapy produces consistent therapeutic blood levels. Some medications can only be given via the IV route. IV medications have a nearly immediate onset of action. The risks of IV therapy include fluid overload, adverse drug reactions, septicemia, and inflammation or infection at the IV catheter insertion site.

### Intravenous Catheter Insertion

Typically, over-the-needle IV catheters, 22 to 26 gauge, are used for children's peripheral IV lines. Vein size and the kind of fluid to be infused guide catheter selection. Generally, the smallest catheter through which fluids and medications can be safely infused should be used.

Venous access sites in children are shown in Fig. 38.8. The rate and type of fluid to be infused, the projected length of time the IV line will be needed, and the availability of veins often determine site selection in children. The nurse also considers the child's developmental level. For example, placement of an IV line into a toddler's foot is often a poor choice because it inhibits walking, a newly learned skill. Inserting IV lines into a child's dominant hand is avoided so as not to interfere with activities of daily living. The hand, forearm, and antecubital sites are frequently used in infants and children. Scalp veins can be used for infant IV lines; they can be adequately secured to allow the infant to move without dislodging the IV catheter. Scalp veins have no valves and can be infused in either direction.

Before an IV catheter is inserted, the nurse explains the procedure to the child and parent, including all available information about why the catheter is being placed, what the child will see and feel during each step of the procedure, where it will be inserted, how long it will be in place, what function(s) it will perform, and if additional equipment (e.g., an infusion pump) will be used. The parents are reassured that once the IV catheter is inserted and secured in place, they will be able to hold their child. It is explained to the child how participating in play activities and self-care is still possible.

The nurse assesses the child's level of fear and anxiety and has the child practice coping strategies in advance. Pharmacologic interventions are essential to reduce or eliminate pain from IV catheter insertion. Topical anesthetic agents such as EMLA or other devices such as the J-Tip, which delivers buffered lidocaine to the skin, must be used. Nonpharmacologic interventions including guided imagery (e.g., putting on an imaginary "magic glove" that keeps the hand from hurting) and distraction (e.g., music, videos, books) should be used as well (see Chapter 39).

The nurse must determine whether the child will be able to hold the arm (or foot) still during the procedure. Holding still is of major importance to prevent injury and to successfully insert the IV catheter. In most cases with young children, the nurse will need another health-care provider to hold the child and the extremity during the insertion procedure until the IV catheter is completely secured.

This procedure should be performed in the treatment room of the hospital unit. The nurse should have all the needed equipment ready in advance: IV catheter of appropriate size, ordered IV solution, primed

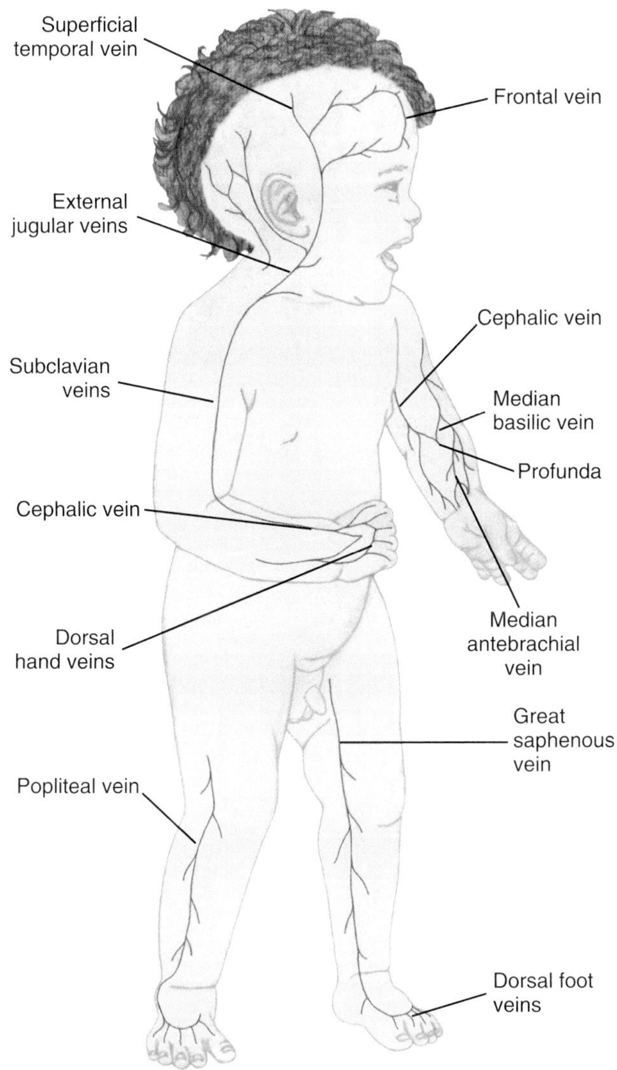


**FIG 38.8** Venous access sites in children.

## ! NURSING QUALITY ALERT

### *Using EMLA Anesthetic Cream*

- Choose a site for the procedure where there is intact, healthy skin. Clean the site with soap and water, then dry. Perform hand hygiene and don gloves.
- Place a mound of EMLA cream (2.5 g; half of a 5-g tube) on the selected skin site and cover it with an occlusive, transparent dressing. Do not rub it into the skin.
- Leave the EMLA in place for a minimum of 1 hour and no longer than 4 hours.
- Perform hand hygiene, don gloves, take off the dressing, and remove all of the EMLA cream from the site.
- Begin the venipuncture procedure. The anesthetic (numbing) effect will last for 1 to 2 hours.
- If the child is receiving IV therapy in an ambulatory care setting, provide the parent with a prescription for EMLA and directions for use. The parent should apply the cream at least 1 hour before the child's appointment.
- Use EMLA with caution in infants younger than 12 months. Do not apply to mucous membranes. Prevent accidental ingestion by older infants and young children. Do not administer EMLA to any child with methemoglobinemia.

infusion set, primed extension tubing, 3 to 5 mL of normal saline for injection in a syringe, strips of tape, sterile transparent occlusive dressing, a padded arm board, a clear plastic "IV house" shield, a tourniquet, antiseptic swabs (2% chlorhexidine gluconate [ChloraPrep] often is used), and gloves.

Parents often want to remain with the child during an IV insertion, if they feel able to cope with the stress of the situation. Parents should not be expected to restrain the child during the procedure. Explain the procedure to the child and parents at each step. The nurse applies the tourniquet and selects the IV site, beginning with the most distal veins of the nondominant hand or forearm. Veins can be identified using transillumination, near infrared light, or ultrasound to enhance success (Peterson, Phillips, Truemper, et al., 2012). The nurse then cleanses the skin at the chosen site and proceeds with the IV catheter insertion (see Chapter 37, Procedure: Venipuncture, for more detailed information). Catheter placement is confirmed by a blood return; a normal saline solution flush verifies that there is no infiltration. After the catheter is placed, it is secured in place with tape and a sterile, transparent, occlusive dressing. The clear dressing allows for adequate visibility and ongoing monitoring of the insertion site. Alternative types of securement devices (such as the STATLOCK stabilization device) can be used to avoid accidental dislodgement (Hetzler, Wilson, Hill, et al., 2011). The catheter extension tubing is taped to the extremity, maintaining access to the plastic clamp.

A well-padded arm board is commonly attached to the child's extremity to prevent injury and keep the IV catheter intact (Fig. 38.9). This practice is particularly important for active children. The extremity is placed in the anatomically correct position on the arm board and secured firmly but not so tight as to impair circulation or damage nerves. Placement also should allow some restricted use of the extremity. For example, an arm board for an IV near the wrist would be positioned to prevent the child from bending the wrist but allow use of the fingers and thumb. A clear plastic shield (such as an IV House UltraDome) placed on top of the IV insertion site adds further protection for the IV catheter while allowing the nurse to visualize the site.

The nurse documents in the child's medical record the location of the IV catheter; the antiseptic used to prep the site; the number of IV insertion attempts; if blood return occurred; use and amount of normal saline flush; the condition of the skin at the site; the type, length, and gauge of the IV catheter; the date and time it was inserted; and how the child tolerated the procedure.

## Intravenous Catheter Monitoring

The nurse should assess and document a child's IV catheter site at least every hour (Tofani et al., 2012), looking specifically for signs and symptoms of infiltration, phlebitis, and/or infection. By gently touching the site on top of the dressing, the nurse can detect warmth or coolness as well as any hardness of the vein. Observations are made for any redness, blanching, swelling, and/or exudates. If there is pain at the site, the nurse assesses the quality of the pain (sharp or dull) as well as the degree of pain using a pain scale. In accordance with hospital policy, the nurse documents in the child's medical record the IV site assessment findings. One way to assess for infiltration is by observing for symmetry in the size and shape of limbs or scalp as well as gently touching the site to determine whether it is soft or taut or whether the scalp site is boggy. If signs and symptoms of complications (e.g., edema, erythema, pain, blanching, coolness, purulent drainage, or red streaking of the skin above the vein) are noted, the IV infusion is discontinued and the physician is notified.

Because of the fragility of children's veins, the difficulty of finding new sites, and the stress of insertion, children's IV sites are to be changed only when clinically indicated (O'Grady et al., 2011). IV fluid

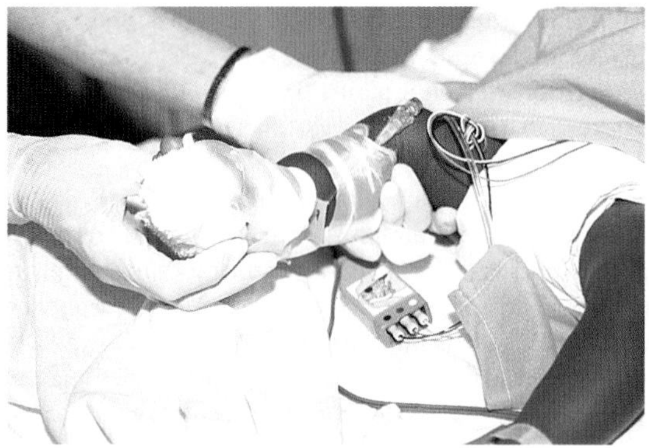
A foot vein is an acceptable IV site for an infant who is not walking or crawling.

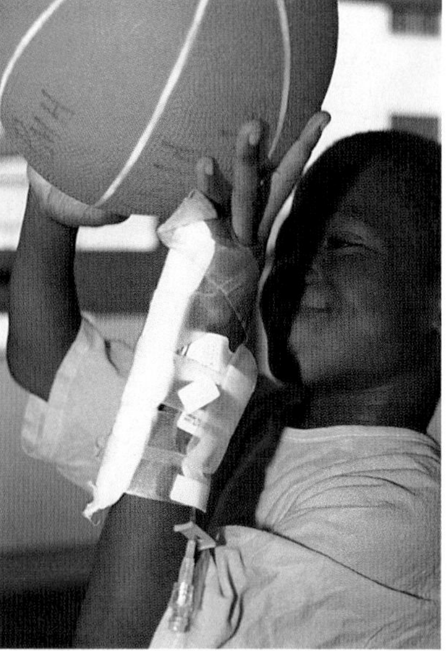
A padded arm board gently limits movement of the hand, and a plastic shield allows visibility yet keeps the IV site intact.

**FIG 38.9** Intravenous (IV) sites in children are secured and well protected to allow for activities and prevent dislodging the IV catheter. (Courtesy Parkland Health and Hospital System, Dallas, TX.)

bags, in general, are changed every 24 hours. It is now recommended to change IV tubing no more frequently than every 96 hours but at least every 7 days (O'Grady et al., 2011) to minimize the risk of intravascular infection. However, hospital policies do vary. IV bags and tubing should be changed more frequently (e.g., every 24 hours) when TPN, lipids, or blood products are administered (O'Grady et al., 2011).

## Intravenous Infusion Monitoring

To accurately control the infusion rate for IV fluid or medication administration, infusion pumps that deliver a preset volume at a set rate are used for infants and children (Fig. 38.10). Infusion pumps are programmed with IV fluid limits to prevent accidental fluid overload. Many hospitals have policies that require a child's IV pump be set to infuse no more than a 2-hour fluid volume.

## Infusion Rates and Methods

Physicians order hourly IV fluid infusion rates based on a child's daily maintenance fluid requirements, and additional fluid needs to replace deficits, if applicable. Box 38.1 illustrates how the nurse can use the formula to determine maintenance fluid requirements and corresponding IV rates based on a child's weight. The nurse verifies the IV rate with the physician's order and documents on the child's medical record the type of IV solution, the location of the site, the ordered rate (which should be the same as the rate set on the infusion pump), and the actual quantity of IV fluid that the child has received. *Even if the child is receiving IV fluids through an infusion pump, the nurse verifies the amount of fluid administered to the child at least hourly.* Pumps can malfunction, risking fluid overload if not meticulously monitored.

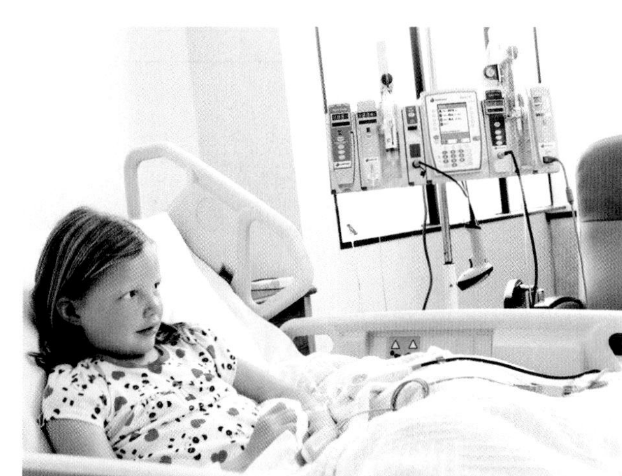
**FIG 38.10** Alaris® System intravenous (IV) infusion pump. (Courtesy CareFusion, San Diego, CA.)

## Administering Intravenous Medications

IV medications can be administered as a continuous infusion or intermittently. Bolus and intermittent infusion are the methods used for intermittent administration of IV medications. The appropriate method must be chosen to meet the needs of the child and to accommodate any restrictions posed by the medication and the volume of fluid.

When administering IV medications to children, the nurse must consider the compatibility of the medication with IV solutions, the type of IV tubing to be used, the recommended concentration for IV administration, the volume of the diluted medication, the suggested administration rate, and the amount of flush needed. Hospital policies and procedures may establish the type of administration to be used and the amount of flush needed. Reference information about the administration of specific IV medications can be obtained from pharmacists or the hospital formulary.

### Intravenous Bolus Administration

Medications delivered by IV bolus (push) are given over a defined period of time (a few minutes) directly into the IV catheter through the port closest to the child's insertion site. The volume of medication infused is small, usually 5 mL or less, and the effects can be seen immediately. It is imperative that the nurse verify the administration rate for an ordered medication to ensure that it can be safely given IV push. The use of needleless systems is recommended to access IV tubing (O'Grady et al., 2011).

## BOX 38.1 Daily Maintenance Fluid Requirements and Rates

### *Formula for Calculating Daily Fluid Requirements**

| Child's Weight | Maintenance Fluids |
|---|---|
| 10 kg or less | 100 mL/kg/day |
| Over 10-20 kg | 1000 mL/day + 50 mL/kg/day for each added kg over 10-20 kg |
| Over 20 kg | 1500 mL/day + 20 mL/kg/day for each additional kg over 20 kg |
| **Example 1:** | |
| Child's weight = 7.2 kg | Maintenance fluids |
| First 10 kg of body weight | 7.2 × 100 mL/kg/day = 720 mL/day |
| Hourly rate | 720 mL/day (24 hr) ÷ 24 = 30 mL/hr |
| **Example 2:** | |
| Child's weight = 15 kg | Maintenance fluids |
| First 10 kg of body weight | 10 × 100 mL/kg/day = 1000 mL/day |
| Added 5 kg of body weight | 5 × 50 mL/kg/day = 250 mL/day |
| Total | 1250 mL/day |
| Hourly rate | 1250 mL/day (24 hr) ÷ 24 = 52 mL/hr |
| **Example 3:** | |
| Child's weight = 23 kg | Maintenance fluids |
| First 10 kg of body weight | 10 × 100 mL/kg/day = 1000 mL/day |
| Added 10 kg of body weight | 10 × 50 mL/kg/day = 500 mL/day |
| Added 3 kg of body weight | 3 × 20 mL/kg/day = 60 mL/day |
| Total | 1560 mL/day |
| Hourly rate | 1560 mL/day (24 hr) ÷ 24 = 65 mL/hr |

*Holliday-Segar method Source: Custer, J., & Rau, R. (2009). (Eds.). *The Harriet Lane handbook: A manual for pediatric house officers* (18th ed.). Philadelphia: Mosby.

Before administering the medication, the nurse checks the IV site for any signs of infiltration or phlebitis and determines that the IV line is intact and patent. The nurse performs hand hygiene and dons clean gloves. The access port is then scrubbed thoroughly with an antiseptic swab, allowed to dry, and the sterile tip of the syringe containing the medication is connected to the port—actions designed to prevent catheter-associated intravascular (bloodstream) infections (O'Grady et al., 2011). The nurse occludes the IV line by pinching it just above the injection port while pushing the medication and then releases the tubing to allow IV fluids to infuse when not pushing the medication (Perry & Potter, 2011). If the medication is not compatible with the infusing IV fluid or is going into an intermittent infusion port, the nurse flushes the tubing with approximately 2 to 3 mL of normal saline solution before and after administering the medication. The access port is scrubbed with an appropriate antiseptic (and allow to dry) *each* time the port is about to be entered.

The nurse must administer the IV medication *exactly* at the prescribed rate over the *required* time period per the physician's orders. The child is closely assessed during and immediately after administration for intended as well as potential adverse effects of the medication. Reassessment of the child is performed at frequent intervals.

### Intravenous Intermittent Infusion Administration

Programmable infusion pumps are frequently used to facilitate safe intermittent infusion of IV medications for children via the "piggyback" method. These pumps have dual programming capabilities that allow a secondary line attached to an IV bag containing medication, diluted to the correct concentration, to run concurrently or sequentially with a primary infusion of IV fluids. It is essential that the nurse verify that the medication is compatible with the IV solution being used. Another type of IV pump often used with children is the syringe pump. The nurse places a syringe containing medication that has been mixed and properly diluted by the pharmacist, along with primed, low-volume tubing, into the pump. After connecting the tubing to the child's IV line, the nurse programs the pump to deliver the volume of medication in the syringe over a specified time period.

Many hospitals use "smart" pumps (see Fig. 38.10) with preprogrammed drug libraries that assist in the prevention of medication errors by alerting the nurse if a medication dose or IV administration rate exceeds parameters recommended by the hospital pharmacy. Thus, a "smart" pump that contains an individual child's profile (weight, list of ordered medications) would not "allow" the nurse to set the pump to administer an incorrect medication, the wrong dose, or an inappropriate rate. Although an IV pump is an excellent safety tool, the nurse must still adhere to the six rights of medication administration. For IV medications, the nurse verifies that the "right" dose includes that the medication is correctly diluted and is running at the recommended rate of infusion.

When performing intermittent infusion of IV medications, the nurse will often flush the IV tubing with fluid using the smart pump to complete the delivery of all the medication to the child. When the medication infusion is done, many pumps are set to sound an alarm so that the nurse can return to complete the flush. The volume needed for the flush varies according to the type of IV tubing used. All volumes, including the IV medication, added fluids for dilution, and flush or flushes used, need to be counted and documented as fluid intake. The total volume infused should be within safe limits for the child.

Before administering any IV medication, determine that the IV line is functioning properly and that the IV catheter site is free of complications. If the child does not have a running IV line but is receiving intermittent medication infusions, the nurse flushes the IV catheter with normal saline to ensure patency, before attaching the secondary infusion set. Hospital policies regarding labeling and flagging the syringe or IV bag containing the medication must be followed. In addition to documenting the medication given in the child's medical record, all volumes of the different IV fluids infused are recorded as well.

## CRITICAL THINKING EXERCISE 38.4

The physician has ordered ampicillin 1.4 grams (g) intravenous (IV) every 4 hours for your patient.

1. The ampicillin for injection is available in a vial that has 2 g in 5 mL. How many mL will you need to withdraw from the vial for the 1.4-g dose?
2. You add the ampicillin you withdrew from the vial to a 50 mL IV bag of normal saline. The physician's order specifies to infuse this IV bag with ampicillin over 30 minutes. At what rate (in mL/hr) will you set the IV pump?

## Venous Access Devices

### Intermittent Infusion Ports

Intermittent infusion ports allow drugs to be administered IV without the need for a running IV line. The intermittent infusion port is an IV catheter that is placed, flushed with normal saline (White, Crawley, Rennie, et al., 2011) to maintain patency, and then locked with an adapter. The port is accessed when needed for fluid or medication infusion. When the port is accessed, meticulous procedures are used, including hand hygiene and thorough cleansing of the port's hub with antiseptic solution to prevent catheter-associated bloodstream infections. IV site monitoring and site care are the same as for any IV catheter.

The frequency of flushing with saline is determined by hospital policy. Routine flushing with normal saline to maintain patency is generally performed every 8 to 12 hours. The device is also flushed with normal saline before and after medication administration and may be flushed at the end of the procedure with a heparinized saline solution if ordered or in accordance with hospital policy.

### Central Venous Access Devices

Central venous access devices are catheters placed directly into major blood vessels. They are most often used to administer medications, blood products, IV fluids, and parenteral nutrition to children over a prolonged period of time. These devices can be tunneled or nontunneled central catheters and implanted infusion ports. All central venous access devices need routine care (dressing changes, flushing) according to hospital protocols. Although the insertion site is assessed several times per day, dressing changes are done on a scheduled basis; frequency varies. When a transparent dressing is used, some institutions recommended cleaning the site and changing the dressing every 7 days. In most cases, each lumen of a central venous line is flushed with heparinized saline at least every 24 hours and after medication administration or a blood draw.

Because these devices enter the central venous system, all procedures are done using strict aseptic technique. Central-line–associated bloodstream infections are a common type of nosocomial infection (Saffer, 2012). The CDC issued *Guidelines for the Prevention of Intravascular Catheter-Related Infections* to decrease the incidence of infections (O'Grady et al., 2011). Use by healthcare providers of groups or "bundles" of aseptic practices for central venous line insertion as well as dressing changes and port access have been shown to significantly decrease the incidence of infection. These practices include proper hand hygiene, 10-minute scrubs of access ports before use, and prompt removal of unneeded lines.

Tunneled central lines (such as Broviac or Hickman catheters) are surgically placed lines that are held in place by a Dacron cuff located in a subcutaneous tunnel. They are most commonly placed in an external jugular vein but may also be placed in the cephalic, axillary, subclavian, femoral, saphenous, or internal jugular veins. The tip of the tunneled catheter is threaded until it rests at the junction of the superior vena cava and right atrium. Short-term or nontunneled central catheters are most frequently placed in the subclavian or femoral veins. These lines involve the placement of a large-gauge catheter that is then sutured in place.

An implanted venous access device (such as a Port-A-Cath) consists of a catheter that is connected to a port or reservoir. As with the tunneled catheter, the catheter tip rests at the junction of the superior vena cava and right atrium. The port is under the skin and is accessed with a noncoring needle placed through the skin into the port. The needle is then covered with a biocclusive dressing, and an extension set is attached to the end. When the port is no longer needed for infusions or obtaining blood specimens, it is flushed with a heparin solution, and the needle is withdrawn. The child with an implanted port can participate in typical childhood activities except those with a potential for high-impact contact with the chest (e.g., tackle football).

A peripherally inserted central catheter (PICC) line is often used for a child who needs IV access for a period longer than a peripheral IV catheter can be maintained (Klee, 2011). A PICC is a long catheter made of polyurethane or silicone that is threaded through an introducer placed in a peripheral vein of the upper arm (basilic, cephalic, or brachial vein). It is usually inserted by a specially trained nurse. The catheter is threaded so that the tip is located in the superior vena cava; the introducer is then removed. The catheter at the insertion site is covered with a Biopatch and then a transparent dressing. Placement is verified by x-ray examination. Several times per day, the insertion site and dressing are assessed for redness, moisture, drainage, or swelling, and catheter integrity is verified. Generally, the dressing is changed at 24 hours postinsertion and then every 7 days if it remains dry and intact. These catheters can be usually left in place for several weeks to months and frequently are used for home antibiotic therapy. The major complications of this type of line are phlebitis, infection, thrombosis, and catheter occlusion.

## ADMINISTRATION OF BLOOD PRODUCTS

Before administering blood products to a child, it is essential to prepare the child and family for the procedure. A child may be disturbed or frightened by seeing blood products in IV bags and tubing. The nurse explains to the child at a developmentally appropriate level, and to the parents, the reason the child needs to receive blood products; how long it will take; what the child will feel, see, and hear; and the type of blood products to be given. Information about the child's blood transfusion history including reactions is obtained from the family.

The nurse confirms the child's ABO blood type and Rh factor. Meticulous procedures must then be followed to ensure that the child receives a donor blood product that is ABO and Rh compatible and has been crossmatched specifically for the intended recipient. In most healthcare settings, it is required that two nurses (or a nurse and physician) identify the child and verify ABO/Rh type, donor number, and blood expiration date and time. The child needs a patent IV line; catheters as small as 22 to 24 gauge can be used, although the infusion rate may be slower for packed red blood cells (Makic, Martin, Burns, et al., 2013). Blood administration tubing is used that includes a filter to remove particulates from the blood and a "Y" connection that allows normal saline to be available for infusion. An IV pump is often used to facilitate precise regulation of the infusion rate and prevent too-rapid transfusion.

Children must be monitored closely during blood product administration for potential complications that include hemolytic (transfusion) reactions, allergic reactions, febrile reactions, circulatory overload, hypothermia, and electrolyte disturbances. Guidelines for nursing care include the following:

- Obtain baseline vital signs, including blood pressure, before administering blood products. Take vital signs every 15 minutes for the first 1 to 2 hours and then hourly until the infusion is complete.
- The rate of infusion of packed red blood cells is approximately 5 mL/kg/hr over no more than 4 hours.
- Monitor the child closely for signs and symptoms of an adverse reaction: fever or chills, headache, nausea, pain at the IV site, or difficulty breathing. The child should not be left alone while receiving blood products.
- If a reaction is suspected, stop the transfusion immediately and notify the physician. Infuse normal saline solution through new tubing to keep the IV line patent. Continue to monitor vital signs. Check urine output hourly and send samples of the child's blood and urine to the laboratory per physician orders.

## CHILD AND FAMILY EDUCATION

It is a key nursing responsibility to educate and prepare children and families for medication administration at home before discharge from the hospital, clinic, or physician's office. Studies have determined that parents make unintentional but frequent errors in the dose of oral medications given to their children (Yin et al., 2014). Further, it has been shown that parents with lower health literacy (level of health information and understanding) make more dosing errors (Yin et al., 2014).

Teaching the family about medications begins with a thorough assessment of all medications the child is currently taking, including over-the-counter medications and herbal preparations. Any history of allergies to medications should be noted to prevent potential drug interactions. The nurse must provide thorough verbal and written information and instructions to the family regarding the medications to be given, the dosage, when to administer, therapeutic effects, and potential side effects and adverse reactions. The child and family members are encouraged to ask questions to guide additional instruction.

The nurse must emphasize that all medications should be taken exactly as ordered. Information to be highlighted includes finishing the full course of a prescribed antibiotic, not changing dosages without consulting the physician, and returning for follow-up appointments.

The nurse problem-solves with the family to develop acceptable schedules for medication administration, to determine the best methods of administering oral medications (e.g., liquid or crushing and mixing with food), and to identify foods or fluids that might be mixed with the medication or given immediately after the medication is taken. The family is then provided a written schedule for medication administration.

The nurse also needs to demonstrate how to measure the correct dosage of a liquid medication using an oral syringe and then have the parents perform a return demonstration. Since pharmacies dispense different measuring devices with prescriptions, it is important to know which device a parent will be using to administer the medication (Wallace, Keenum, DeVoe, et al., 2012). If teaching a child or adolescent and parents to do subcutaneous injections (as for insulin), supervised practice of the injection procedure and ongoing education is essential.

It is essential to reinforce general safety information, such as keeping medications in a locked cabinet that is out of the reach of children and keeping all medications in their original pharmacy containers. The nurse evaluates interventions by asking questions of family members to determine their level of understanding regarding all aspects of the medication and the administration process. Careful observations of return demonstrations by the child and family help the nurse to judge teaching effectiveness. All teaching provided and validation of understanding should be specifically documented in the child's medical record.

The nursing student is responsible for understanding the importance of safety when administering medications to children. The wide range of doses based on weight must be accurately calculated, especially with IV medications, where most errors occur (Gill et al., 2012; Pauly-O'Neill & Prion, 2013). To assist students in learning to administer medications in the pediatric population, clinical opportunities along with simulation can provide opportunities. Simulation can enhance the clinical experience by providing students with psychomotor skills, improving clinical reasoning, and building confidence in a more structured environment. New technology, especially smart pumps, can help prevent many but not all errors. Students who are able to visualize the calculation problem are better able to make sense of it, decreasing the risk of miscalculation (Pauly-O'Neill & Prion, 2013). Research has shown that mixed methods of education such as lecture, clinical experiences, and simulation can increase a student's proficiency and self-confidence, especially when administering medications (Pauly-O'Neill & Prion, 2013).

### PARENTS WANT TO KNOW

#### *Medication Administration at Home*

Address the needs of parents to determine the best way to administer medication to their child at home before the child leaves the hospital or ambulatory care setting. This plan can help prevent medication errors and ensure that the child and family will follow the physician's orders for the home treatment plan. Provide the parents (and child according to the developmental level) the following information:

- Name of the medication (trade and generic)
- Why it has been prescribed for the child
- What the desired "therapeutic" effects are
- How to take the medication (how much, how often, how long to take it, techniques for administering the medication)
- Acceptable measuring device for home administration of oral medications (oral syringe; or small, calibrated medicine cup)
- How to use oral syringes to measure and give the right amount of medication
- Expected or potential side effects and what to do if they occur
- When the parents should notify a nurse or physician if the child had an adverse reaction
- Any dietary or activity restrictions

If the child will need to take medication during the school day, the physician must provide a written order that the parents give to the school nurse along with a parental permission form authorizing administration of the medication at school. The school nurse should also receive complete written information and instructions that include a description of the medication, the intended purpose of the treatment, potential side effects and adverse reactions, and when the medication should be given. Parents are required to provide the medication in the original pharmacy container. The school nurse also needs a complete list of all the medications the child is taking at home as well as at school.

## KEY CONCEPTS

- Standardized dosage ranges for many medications have not been established for children.
- Children respond differently to medication than adults.
- The nurse must incorporate principles of growth and development when administering medications to children.
- The margin of safety for medication administration is narrow for children.
- Based on developmental level, different types of devices and techniques are used to administer oral medications to children.
- Injections are stressful to children and used for a limited number of medications and immunizations.
- Site selection for IV insertion is influenced by the rate and type of fluid to be infused and the accessibility of veins.
- Although an infusion pump is used to control the rate and quantity of IV fluids administered to children, the nurse must assess the actual fluid administered hourly.
- Infants and children must be closely monitored when receiving IV medications because of the immediate onset of action.

*Continued*

## KEY CONCEPTS—cont'd

- Using "bundles" of aseptic practices, including hand hygiene and scrubbing the port's hub before accessing an IV line, can prevent catheter-associated bloodstream infections.
- A child undergoes a comprehensive, baseline assessment before blood product administration.
- Education of the child and parents is important to ensure that medications are administered accurately and in accordance with the physician's orders and the treatment plan

## REFERENCES AND READINGS


Altay, N., & Çavusoglu, H. (2013). Using Orem's self-care model for asthmatic adolescents. *Journal for Specialists in Pediatric Nursing 18*,233–242. doi: 10.1111/jspn.12032.

American Academy of Pediatrics. (2011). *Policy statement: Principles of Pediatric Patient Safety: Reducing Harm Due to Medical Care* Retrieved from http://aappolicy.aappublications.org/content/127/6/1199.full.html.

American Academy of Pediatrics. (2015). Policy statement: metric units and the preferred dosing of orally administered liquid medications. *Pediatrics, 135*(4) 784–787. doi:10.1542/peds.2015-0072.

Gill, F., Corkish, V., Robertson, J., et al. (2012). An exploration of pediatric nurses' compliance with a medication checking and administration protocol. *Journal for Specialists in Pediatric Nursing 17*, 136–146.

Hetzler, R., Wilson, M., Hill, E.K., et al. (2011). Securing pediatric IV catheters-application of evidence-based practice model. *Journal of Pediatric Nursing, 26*, 143–148. doi:10.1016/j.pedn.2010.12.008.

Ingerski, L., Perrazo, L., Goebel, J., et al. (2011). Family strategies for achieving medication adherence in pediatric kidney transplantation. *Nursing Research, 60*(3), 190–196.

Institute for Safe Medication Practices. (2015a). *ISMP's medication safety alert.* Retrieved from http://ismp.org/newsletter/acutecare/showarticle.aspx?id=112.

Institute for Safe Medication Practices. (2015b). *ISMP's list of high-alert medications.* Retrieved from http://ismp.org/Tools/highalertmedications.pdf.

Ivanovska, V., Rademaker, C.M., van Dijk L., et al. (2014). Pediatric Drug Formulations: A Review of Challenges and Progress. *Pediatrics, 134*(2) 361-372. doi: 10.1542/peds.2013-3225.

Jackson, L.A., Peterson, D., Nelson, J.C., et al. (2013). Vaccination site and risk of local reactions in children 1 through 6 years of age. *Pediatrics, 131*(2), 283–289. doi:10.1542/peds.2012-2617.

Johnson, K.B., & Lehmann, C.U. (2013). Technical report: electronic prescribing in pediatrics: toward safer and more effective medication management. *Pediatrics, 131*(4) 1350–1356. doi: 10.1542/peds.2013-0193.

Klee, S.J. (2011). The ideal use of the power injectable peripherally inserted central catheter in the pediatric population. *Journal of the Association of Vascular Access, 16*(2), 86–93. doi: 10.2309/java.16-2-5.

Makic, M.B., Martin, S.A., Burns, S., et al. (2013). Putting evidence into nursing practice: four traditional practices not supported by the evidence. *Critical Care Nurse, 33*(2) 28–44. doi: http://dx.doi.org/10.4037/ccn2013787.

McCarthy, A.M., Kleiber, C., Hanrahan, K., et al. (2014). Matching doses of distraction with child risk for distress during a medical procedure. *Nursing Research, 63*(6), 397–407.

McGrady, M.E., & Hommel, K.A. (2013). Medication adherence and health care utilization in pediatric chronic illness: a systematic review. *Pediatrics, 132*, 730–740. doi:10.1542/peds.2013-1451.

O'Grady, N., Alexander, M., Dellinger, E.P, et al. (2011). *Centers for disease control and prevention: guidelines for the prevention of intravascular catheter-related infections.* Retrieved from http://www.cdc.gov/hicpac/pdf/guidelines/bsi-guidelines-2011.pdf.

Pauly-O'Neill, S., & Prion, S. (2013). Using integrated simulation in a nursing program to improve medication administration skills in the pediatric population. *Nursing Education Perspectives, 34*(3), 148–153.

Perry, A., & Potter, P. (2011). *Mosby's pocket guide to nursing skills and procedures* (7th ed.). St. Louis: Mosby.

Peterson, K.A., Phillips, A.L., Truemper, E., et al. (2012). Does the use of an assistive device by nurses impact peripheral intravenous catheter insertion success in children? *Journal of Pediatric Nursing, 27*, 134–143. doi: 10.1016/j.peds.2010.10.009.

Rishovd, A. (2014). Pediatric intramuscular injections: guidelines for best practice. *Maternal Child Nursing, 39*(2), 107–112. doi:10.1097/NMC.0000000000000009.

Saffer, M. (2012). Preventing central line infections in outpatients. *Pediatric Nursing, 38*(6), 336.

Smith, M.D., Spiller, H.A., Casavant, M.J., et al. (2014). Out-of-hospital medication errors among young children in the United States, 2002-2012. *Pediatrics, 134*(6), 867–876. doi:10.1542/peds.2014-0309.

The Joint Commission. (2015). *National patient safety goals effective January 1, 2015: Hospital accreditation program.* Retrieved from http://www.jointcommission.org/assets/1/6/2015_NPSG_HAP.pdf.

Tofani, B.F., Rineair, S.A., Gosdin, C.H., et al. (2012). Quality improvement project to reduce infiltration and extravasation events in a pediatric hospital. *Journal of Pediatric Nursing, 27*, 682–689. doi: 10.1016/jpedn.2012.01.005.

Turner, R.M. (2013). From the lab to the prescription pad: genetics, CYP450 analysis, and medication response. *Journal of Child and Adolescent Psychiatric Nursing, 26* 119-123. doi:10.1111/jcap.12028.

Wallace, L.S., Keenum, A.J., DeVoe, J.E., et al. (2012). Women's understanding of different dosing instructions for a liquid pediatric medication. *Journal of Pediatric Health Care, 26*(6) 443–450. doi:10.1016/j.pedhc.2011.06.006.

White, M.L., Crawley, J., Rennie, E.A., et al. (2011). Examining the effectiveness of 2 solutions used to flush capped pediatric peripheral intravenous catheters. *Journal of Infusion Nursing, 34*(4), 260–270.

World Health Organization. (2012). Paediatric Medicines. *WHO Drug Information, 26*(1), 15–21.

Wurster, L.A., Groner, J., & Hoffman, J. (2012). Electronic documentation of trauma resuscitations at a level 1 pediatric trauma center. *Journal of Trauma Nursing, 19*(2), 76–79. doi: 10.1097/JTN.0b013e31825629ab.

Yin, H.S., Dreyer, B.P., Ugboaja, D.C., et al. (2014). Unit of measurement used and parent medication dosing errors. *Pediatrics, 134*(2) 354–361. doi: 10.1542/peds.2014-0395

# 39

# Pain Management for Children

http://evolve.elsevier.com/McKinney/mat-ch/

## LEARNING OBJECTIVES

*After studying this chapter, you should be able to:*

- Define *pain.*
- Discuss the gate control theory of pain.
- Discuss the myths and realities of pain and pain management.
- Discriminate between acute and chronic pain.
- Explain pain assessment in children according to developmental stages.
- Describe common pain assessment tools.
- Discuss non-pharmacologic and pharmacologic interventions that are used for pediatric pain management.
- Use the nursing process to describe nursing care of the child in pain.

Assessing and treating pain in children is a vital part of the nursing care of children, although at times it can be difficult. Many sources, including the Joint Commission, American Pain Society [APS], and the Agency for Healthcare Research and Quality [AHRQ], consider pain as the fifth vital sign (Freitas, Castro, Castro, et al., 2014; Vael & Whitted, 2014). Infants and children are often unable to communicate the presence, location, type, or intensity of pain. Parents may be hesitant to allow suitable pain management because of fears related to side effects from the use of opioids, including inaccurate fears regarding addiction. Additionally, nurses and other healthcare providers continue to have misconceptions about opioid pharmacokinetics and unwarranted concern about the adverse effects of opioid use in infants and children (Stanley & Pollard, 2013; Van Hulle, Wilkie, & Wang, 2011).

Comprehensive research and gains in knowledge over the past 10 to 15 years have greatly improved the assessment and treatment of pain in children. Yet, despite the increasing knowledge regarding safe and effective pain management in children, as well as widespread anecdotal experience, children remain at risk for unrecognized and undertreated pain. It is well documented that the youngest children have the greatest probability of receiving insufficient pain medications, that pain medication administration varies with age, and that pain medication is underused for many children (APS, 2011a; Stanley & Pollard, 2013).

Individual nurses vary in their ability to assess pain. Some of these differences have been linked to the lack of or inaccurate clinical knowledge regarding pain, inappropriate stereotyping of patients who require treatment for pain, and lack of nursing experience (Habich & Letizia, 2015). Additionally, consistent, appropriate use of pediatric pain assessment tools is not always seen among pediatric nurses, and many nurses feel that they are not knowledgeable enough about pain assessment tools to use them accurately (Stanley & Pollard, 2013).

Recent increases in quality pediatric pain research have led to more precise pain assessment and improved prescribing and administering of analgesics. Age-appropriate adjuvants are being used more frequently. However, the most current resources and strategies for pain management are not always implemented, emphasizing the continuing need for educating all healthcare providers. Nurses, having frequent interaction with physicians and other healthcare providers, can facilitate a significant improvement in pain management for infants and children. They can also play a vital role in educating other healthcare providers, as well as parents and children, with regard to appropriate pediatric pain management (Stanley & Pollard, 2013). Computer-based education programs and the implementation of a pain assessment protocol can improve pediatric pain management (Habich & Letizia, 2015).

## DEFINITIONS AND THEORIES OF PAIN

There are many definitions of pain. The International Association for the Study of Pain (IASP) (1979, p. 249) defines pain as "an unpleasant sensory and emotional experience associated with actual or potential tissue damage, or described in terms of such damage." In a commonly accepted definition, pain is whatever the person experiencing the pain says it is, existing whenever the person says it does (Pasero & McCaffery, 2011). Pain involves hormonal, neurochemical and electrophysical changes that can affect how a child heals. The management of acute pain is important in preventing harmful effects on the child and the development of chronic pain (Twycross, Finley, & Latimer, 2013). The pain threshold varies between individuals. Both definitions underscore the fact that pain is complex, multidimensional, subjective, and personal. The pediatric pain experience involves the interaction of behavioral, developmental, physiologic, psychological, and situational factors (APS, 2011a).

### Gate Control Theory

Pain or nociceptive impulses travel between the initial site of injury and the brain, and certain mechanisms affect pain intensity (Swift, 2015). According to the gate control theory proposed by Melzack and Wall in 1965, a gating mechanism at the level of the dorsal horn in the spinal cord can facilitate or dampen the transmission of pain signals. Stimulation of the larger afferent nerves, which carry benign sensations, can blunt the transmission of pain signals. The gating mechanisms are influenced by the relative activity in the sensory fibers. Input from the large fibers closes the gate, whereas input from the small fibers opens it (Moayedi & Davis, 2013). For example, rubbing an injured part activates large-fiber activity, which decreases the ability of small-fiber activity to open the gate, thus decreasing the pain. The theory further postulates that cognitive processes, such as attention, emotion, and memory, influence the gating mechanism and have an impact on the transmission of pain. The gate control theory has led to further research on understanding and treating pain (Moayedi & Davis, 2013).

### Acute and Chronic Pain

Nursing assessment and interventions will vary based on the nature of the pain. Children can have acute or chronic pain. Acute pain usually has a sudden onset, is from an identifiable trauma, and continues for a limited time. Resolution generally occurs with healing of the trauma. Frequently, the acute pain experienced by children in healthcare settings is a result of invasive procedures (e.g., injections) or complications (e.g., tissue injury from IV infiltration). Pain from such procedures particularly affects children with cancer and other chronic illnesses that require frequent medical care. Acute pain is also experienced with acute disease states, after surgery, and after trauma (such as falls or nonaccidental injury from child abuse). Events that cause acute pain may persist, leading to the development of chronic pain.

Chronic pain continues for an unpredictable period beyond the expected recovery period, is unlikely to resolve quickly, and can adversely affect the child's daily activities of living. Causes and types of chronic pain vary widely. Children with conditions such as juvenile arthritis, sickle cell disease, and cancer have chronic, repeated exacerbations of acute pain (American Society for Pain Management Nursing, 2012). Neuropathic pain is one of the most complex types of chronic pain to treat (Hyde, Price, & Nicholl, 2012). Chronic pain in childhood is much more prevalent than previously realized. A survey of the general pediatric population indicates that approximately 15% to 25% of children are living with chronic pain (Sieberg, Williams, & Simons, 2011).

Accurate assessment and successful treatment of chronic pain is very difficult. It remains a significant, unsolved challenge in pediatric pain management, leading to concerns regarding the long-term functional consequences of chronic childhood pain. The American Pain Society (APS) (2011b) has issued a position statement with the intent of increasing awareness and improving treatment of chronic pain in children. It advocates for increased education of all health professionals and more research on pediatric pain management.

Children with chronic pain are at increased risk for anxiety disorders that can affect their everyday lives, contribute to school avoidance, and often cause poor family functioning (Jacobson et al., 2013; Mano et al., 2012; Palermo, Valrie, & Karlson, 2014). Improvements in pain management have enabled children with pain related to chronic conditions to achieve a higher quality of life. They are able to enjoy a greater degree of normalcy by spending less time in the hospital and actively participating in school, play, and other activities of childhood (see Chapter 36). Nurses who work in the school, home healthcare, and hospice settings have added resources (e.g., knowledge, medication, equipment) that facilitate pain control, resulting in more comfortable, satisfying lives for these children and their families.

### Research on Pain in Children

Over the past three decades, there has been a proliferation of pediatric pain-related research that has led to clinical practice guidelines and additional standards of care for both acute and chronic pain (see publications from the World Health Organization [WHO] at http://www.who.int/publications/en, the American Pain Society [APS] at http://ampainsoc.org/education/guidelines/overview, the American Academy of Pediatrics [AAP] at http://www.aap.org/en-us/professional-resources/Pages/Professional-Resources.aspx, the American Society for Pain Management Nursing at http://www.aspmn.org/Pages/positionpapers.aspx, and the International Association for the Study of Pain (IASP) at http://www.iasp-pain.org/PublicationsNews).

The WHO's (2010) three-step analgesic ladder was developed in 1986 to improve treatment for cancer pain. The ladder suggests nonopioid analgesics for mild pain, weak opioids for mild to moderate pain, and opioid analgesics for severe pain, along with accessory medications to prevent breakthrough pain (Freitas et al., 2014). These guidelines are the basis for pain management of children and adults, particularly related to multidrug therapy. Beginning in 1999, the APS has developed and published clinical guidelines related to the care of pediatric (and adult) patients with acute and chronic pain associated with sickle cell disease, cancer, juvenile chronic arthritis, and fibromyalgia syndrome (APS, 2011c). The AAP and APS issued a joint position statement in 2001 with recommendations for the assessment and management of acute pain in infants, children, and adolescents (APS, 2011b). Since 2001, The Joint Commission accreditation standards have continued to address both pain assessment and management by requiring healthcare agencies to provide pain management education and guarantee all hospitalized patients the right to developmentally appropriate, comprehensive pain assessment and management, from admission until discharge (The Joint Commission, 2011).

Recent research demonstrates that up to 81% of hospitalized children experience moderate to severe pain yet nurses administer only 23% to 43% of analgesics that are ordered (Stanley & Pollard, 2013). Postoperatively, 77% of children experience moderate to severe pain at home (Van Hulle et al., 2012). To define the under-treatment of pain, Wilson and Pendleton coined the term *oligoanalgesia* (Gorodzinsky, Davies, & Drendel, 2014). Children who experience pain are at risk for increased pain sensitivity later in life (Van Hulle et al., 2011).

Advances in research, knowledge, and clinical expertise have led to significant increases in academic literature, research studies, and practice guidelines and standards regarding pediatric pain management. However, improvements are still needed in the following areas: research on nurse-physician collaboration for pediatric pain management and barriers to suitable pain management; education of healthcare providers about appropriate, effective pain management; increased information about pain management in neonates and infants; and testing for the safety and efficacy, specifically in children, of new analgesics as they are introduced.

## OBSTACLES TO PAIN MANAGEMENT IN CHILDREN

Obstacles to appropriate pain management in children include belief in myths; knowledge deficits, especially with regards to pharmacologic properties of pain management medications often used in children; inaccuracy of pain assessment and pain assessment measures; insufficient awareness of pain management interventions; lack of confidence regarding the efficacy of pain management; lack of communication with children and their parents; and personal attitudes and beliefs about pain (APS, 2011a; Jongudomkarn, Forgeron, Siripul, et al., 2012; McNamara, Harmon, & Saunders, 2012; Mosiman & Pile, 2013; Stanley & Pollard, 2013; Twycross & Collins, 2013; Twycross & Finley, 2014).

The two beliefs of parents and nurses that are most likely to interfere with the provision of adequate pain relief in infants and children are fear of respiratory depression and fear of addiction. In addition, many nurses believe that children over-report their pain (Stanley & Pollard, 2013; Twycross & Finley, 2013). Table 39.1 lists and refutes other prevalent myths about pain and pain management in children.

One strategy used by pediatric institutions to provide a comprehensive pain management program is a pain management team. The team can be composed of nurses certified in pain management,

**TABLE 39.1 Pain and Pain Management in Children: Myths and Realities**

| Myth | Reality |
|---|---|
| Neonates do not feel pain because of incomplete myelinization in peripheral nerves and the central nervous system (CNS). | Myelinization is not necessary for pain perception. Central and peripheral structures required for nociception are present and functional early in gestation. Therefore, infants have the neurologic capacity for pain perception at the time of birth, even those born prematurely (Mosiman & Pile, 2013; Stanley & Pollard, 2013; Tobias, 2014a; Wong, Lau, Palozzi, et al., 2012). |
| Children have no memory of pain. | Feeding and sleeping differences have been reported in studies of infants who experienced pain, suggests that the procedure had consequences extending beyond the event (Cong et al., 2013; Reavey et al., 2014; Van Hulle et al., 2011). |
| There is a correct or standard amount of pain associated with a specific injury or procedure. | The amount of pain a child experiences varies and cannot be predicted because of individual cognitive, developmental, and emotional factors affecting the child (Pasero & McCaffery, 2011; Twycross & Collins, 2013). |
| Children can easily become addicted to narcotic analgesics. | There is no identified characteristic of childhood physiology or development that indicates any increased risk of physiologic or psychological dependence. The actual risk of addiction is very low (Czarnecki et al., 2011a; Van Hulle et al., 2012). |
| Narcotic administration can easily cause respiratory depression. | No data support the belief that children are at higher risk for respiratory depression than adults. Respiratory depression is rare (Stanley & Pollard, 2013). |

**BOX 39.1 Pain Management Resources on the Internet**

- American Academy of Pain Medicine: http://www.painmed.org
- American Pain Foundation: http://www.painfoundation.org
- American Pain Society: http://www.ampainsoc.org
- American Society for Pain Management Nursing: http://www.aspmn.org
- Center for Pediatric Pain Research: http://pediatric-pain.ca
- International Association for the Study of Pain: http://www.iasp-pain.org
- Special Interest Group on Pain in Childhood: International Association for the Study of Pain: http://childpain.org
- NIH (National Institutes of Health) Pain Consortium: http://painconsortium.nih.gov

advanced practice nurses (APNs), physicians, pharmacists, and other healthcare practitioners. The team educates patients, families, nurses, physicians, and other healthcare providers. Parents often feel that communication with the nurses about the pain management plan for their child is lacking or inconsistent (Twycross et al., 2013). Further, the team offers pain management recommendations based on the most current knowledge. Availability and personalization of education can provide motivation for changes in beliefs and attitudes among healthcare providers as well as patients and families (Van Hulle et al., 2012; Voepel-Lewis, 2011). Pain management team members can also train resource nurses from each hospital unit to provide advice and support to their colleagues on best practices in pain management for children.

Nurses who recognize the importance of implementing appropriate pain management strategies need ongoing access to the most current information. The Internet can be a powerful tool for accessing instant, up-to-date information. Nurses and families are cautioned to ensure that they obtain information from trustworthy websites. Box 39.1 lists some suggested Internet resources. Given the rapidity with which Internet information changes, it is essential to verify the appropriateness of the website and accuracy of the information presented.

## ASSESSMENT OF PAIN IN CHILDREN

Pain in children is multidimensional and subjective (APS, 2011a). It is affected by the type and duration of pain, developmental level, emotional status, previous pain experiences, culture and ethnicity, personality type, gender, genetic variations, and parental response to the child's pain. These factors should all be taken into consideration when assessing an infant or a child in pain. Consequently, assessing pain in infants and children is more challenging than in adults. The nurse's role is to assess for pain, provide non-pharmacologic and pharmacologic interventions along with the healthcare team and evaluate the effectiveness of those interventions (Stanley & Pollard, 2013). Infants and young children may not have the language or cognitive abilities to communicate their pain. Their crying and verbal responses occur for many other reasons including hunger, sleepiness, and anxiety. Accordingly, the nurse must use a combination of behavioral and physiologic signs together with an appropriate pain assessment tool to determine the pain level in infants and some children (Van Hulle et al., 2011) (Box 39.2).

Vital signs data such as heart rate, blood pressure, respiratory rate, and oxygen saturation have been reported to provide information about acute pain (Stanley & Pollard, 2013). However, these physiologic signs are also affected by other factors such as illness, fever, and medications, and there is little evidence to support using changes in vital signs to assess pain (Herr, Coyne, McCaffery, et al., 2011).

Behavioral and some physiologic signs can play an important role in the assessment of pain in children who are giving a verbal report of pain that differs from their nonverbal behaviors. An example is a child who gives a verbal report of little or no pain out of concern that someone will become angry or that pain medication might involve an injection. Visually, the nurse might see the child grimacing, perhaps with tears, lying rigidly in bed and not moving. Such nonverbal behaviors would lead the nurse to speak and interact gently with the child about the actual level of pain to ensure appropriate pain management. Children who suffer from chronic pain may not demonstrate behavioral changes that are noticeable to the nurse, and they may be unable to accurately describe their pain level. It is important to assess the impact of pain on a child's daily life including sleeping, eating, attending school, social and physical activities (e.g., play or sports), and interactions with family and peers (APS, 2011b). Changes in these areas, such as being unwilling or unable to play with peers and impaired school functioning, may be subtle signs that a child is experiencing pain (Palermo et al., 2014).

Although older children may be able to verbalize their discomfort, they are often afraid of treatment that includes a painful procedure such as an injection (Melby, 2011). They may have also been told to

## BOX 39.2 Indicators of Pain According to Developmental Levels

**Neonate and Infant**

- Usually demonstrate changes in facial expression, including frowns, grimaces, wrinkled brow, expression of surprise, and facial flinching
- May demonstrate increases in blood pressure and heart rate, and decrease in oxygen saturation
- High-pitched, tense, harsh crying
- Tend to demonstrate a generalized or total body response to pain that becomes more purposeful as the infant matures
- May thrash extremities and exhibit tremors
- Older infants may localize the pain, rubbing the painful area, or pull away and guard the involved part

**Toddler**

- Likely to demonstrate loud crying
- Able to verbalize words that indicate discomfort such as "ouch," "hurt," "boo-boo"
- May attempt to delay procedures perceived as painful
- May demonstrate generalized restlessness
- May guard the site
- May touch painful areas
- May run from the nurse

**Preschooler**

- May think the pain is punishment for something he or she said or did
- Likely to cry and struggle
- Able to describe the location and intensity of pain (e.g., "ear hurts bad")
- May demonstrate regression to earlier behaviors, such as loss of bladder and bowel control
- May demonstrate withdrawal
- May deny pain to avoid taking oral medicine or a possible injection
- May have been told to "be brave" and deny pain, even if pain is present

**School-Age Child**

- Able to describe pain and quantify pain intensity
- Fears bodily injury
- Has an awareness of death
- May demonstrate stiff body posture
- May demonstrate withdrawal
- May procrastinate or bargain to delay procedure

**Adolescent**

- Perceives pain at a physical, emotional, and cognitive level
- Understands cause and effect
- Able to describe pain and quantify pain intensity
- May have increased muscle tension
- May demonstrate withdrawal and decreased motor activity
- May use words such as "sore," "ache," or "pounding" to describe pain

"be brave" and not verbalize or demonstrate the pain they are experiencing. Increasingly, children as young as 5 or 6 years may be fearful of taking pain medication because of the emphasis on "saying no" to drugs. Such an emphasis is meant to focus on illegal substances or inappropriate use of prescription medications. Nevertheless, some children translate this message to mean they should not use any drugs, even appropriate and necessary pain medications. Nurses need to provide developmentally appropriate education to children and their parents to overcome barriers to pain assessment and management. It is important to discuss individual strategies and goals for pain management with children and their families (Avansino, Peters, Stockfish, et al., 2013; Czarnecki et al., 2011a; Twycross & Finley, 2013).

Pain assessment and treatment are influenced by the cultural beliefs and practices of children and their families. Working to understand the impact of cultural differences on pain management is a crucial aspect of pediatric nursing care (Czarnecki et al., 2011a; Sadhasivam et al., 2012; Sng et al., 2013). Transcultural nursing literature can assist nurses to understand the diversity in nonverbal expressions of pain (facial expressions and other body language), words used for pain, descriptions of pain, and rating of pain noted among different cultures. Evidence supporting the validity of pain assessment scales for children from different cultures needs to be examined as a basis for nursing practice.

## Assessment According to Developmental Level

### Neonates and Infants

The fact that neonates and young infants have immature central nervous systems that lack myelinization of pain fibers led clinicians in the past to believe that they are incapable of perceiving pain. However, in recent years, substantial research has demonstrated that neonates and infants do feel pain (Cong, McGrath, Cusson, et al., 2013) and that infants whose pain is not addressed can experience long-term, negative consequences (APS, 2011a; Czarnecki et al., 2011a; Kesavan, 2015; Tobias, 2014a).

Assessing acute pain in neonates and infants is difficult and is primarily based on behavioral and certain physiologic indicators. Rapid changes in an infant's behavioral state and sleep/activity patterns signal the likelihood of pain. Behaviors that often serve as indicators of infant pain include crying, fist clenching, grimacing, wrinkling of the forehead, fussiness, and restlessness (Cong et al., 2013). Facial expression is considered the most consistent cue available when judging pain in infants and children (Cong et al., 2013). Facial expression, in combination with short latency to onset of cry and a long duration of the first cry cycle, typifies infants' reactions to painful procedures. Cries associated with pain are higher pitched, tense, and harsh, differing from those associated with hunger, discomfort, and stress. Therefore, parents and nurses may be able to differentiate between the usual cries of infants and the cries of pain.

Motor movements associated with pain in the neonate and infant progress from a generalized body response to more purposeful movements. For example, infants aged 9 to 12 months can use their hands to push the nurse away if they perceive a painful action is about to begin. The responses of neonates to painful stimuli are sometimes described as total body responses (Fig. 39.1). The infant's extremities may thrash about, and some infants exhibit tremors. Older infants may rub the painful area, pull away, or guard the involved body part.

Neonates who are experiencing prolonged or persistent pain may not exhibit the usual behavioral signs of pain seen in neonates who are experiencing acute pain and, instead, exhibit signs and symptoms of energy conservation (Herr et al., 2011).

Physiologic changes may be more difficult to assess and serve as just one part of a complete pain assessment. A nurse should suspect that an infant experiences pain before physiologic changes are observed. Increases in blood pressure, heart rate, and respiratory rate and

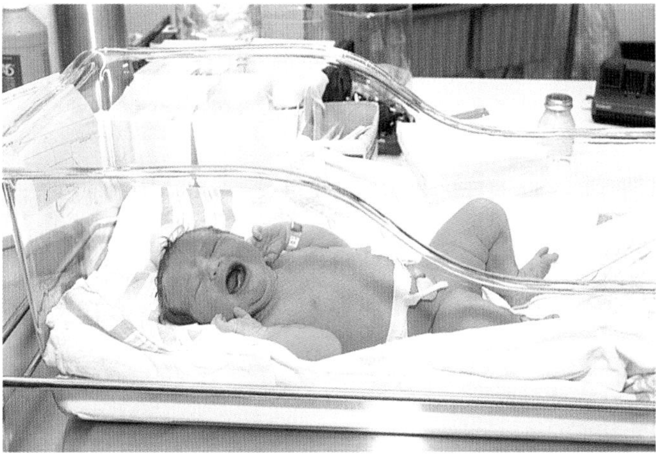

**FIG 39.1** Infant total body response to pain with arms thrashing, tremors, and vigorous crying.

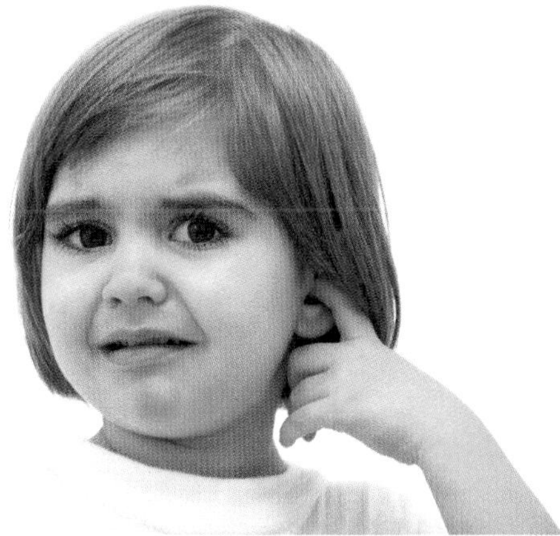

**FIG 39.2** Toddlers and preschoolers may express pain by guarding or touching the painful area. The toddler touching her ear is a characteristic expression of ear pain from otitis media. (©2016 Getty Images. Reprinted with permission.)

decreases in arterial oxygen saturation have been associated with pain in neonates, although these changes can be linked to other alterations such as agitation. Crying can also affect the infant's physiologic responses. Distinguishing between pain and agitation is sometimes difficult. If an infant is simply agitated yet is treated for pain, the cause of the agitation may remain untreated.

The behavioral and physiologic indicators discussed are components in several different pain assessment tools used for the preverbal or nonverbal child. The reliability and validity of these assessment tools have been studied extensively. To provide high-quality care, it is important that nurses use pain assessment tools rather than rely on personal, subjective appraisals of infant behavioral and physiologic indicators.

### Toddlers

Preverbal toddlers are often unable to describe their pain which puts them at risk for untreated pain (Vael & Whitted, 2014). The toddler in pain tends to cry longer than the infant. As verbal abilities become more advanced, the toddler can vocalize displeasure when a painful experience occurs. The toddler may ask for parents, use words that indicate discomfort ("ouch," "hurt"), and even verbalize negative emotions about the nurse. The toddler may also try to delay the nurse's implementation of a procedure judged as painful. The older toddler can often localize the pain and point to the body part that hurts.

## CRITICAL THINKING EXERCISE 39.1

You are about to care for Tanika, a full-term neonate (weight = 3500 g) who underwent surgery 24 hours ago for a fundoplication and placement of a gastrostomy tube. The nurse reports that Tanika has slept for short periods throughout the shift, sucks vigorously on her pacifier, and occasionally cries. The nurse notes that she has not medicated Tanika for pain because she does have periods when she sleeps for 15 to 30 minutes. Her blood pressure is 98/74, pulse rate 170, and respiration rate 50.

1. What would be your first nursing action?
2. What principles related to pediatric pain management would apply to this infant?

Generalized restlessness, guarding the site, and touching the painful area are signs of pain in the toddler (Fig. 39.2). The toddler may associate discomfort with a particular procedure, such as a dressing change, and might run from the nurse when approached. The toddler's facial expressions can indicate anger and fear. The child might avoid eye contact or look sad. In response to discomfort and pain, the toddler can also demonstrate regression to earlier, more comfortable behaviors such as lying on a parent's lap in a fetal position.

### Preschoolers

Preschoolers are egocentric. Relating only to the present, they have difficulty associating discomfort with any positive outcome, and this can intensify their pain experience. For example, the preschooler will not understand that debriding a painful burn will ultimately have a positive effect. Children in this age group are able to describe the location and intensity of pain, for example "a little" or "a lot" (Obrecht, Van Hulle, & Ryan, 2014).

Preschoolers tend to think pain will magically go away and that experiencing pain is punishment for some previous thought or deed. They also fear body mutilation, particularly of the genitals. Preschoolers may deny pain from a surgical incision, for example, in order to avoid an invasive procedure such as a pain medication injection. They may also cry and struggle in an attempt to escape from the procedure. Preschoolers can regress to earlier, more comfortable behaviors, such as thumb sucking, in response to pain, or they can withdraw and not participate in play activities.

### School-Age Children

School-age children can describe pain accurately and relate it to a specific body part, as well as quantify pain intensity (Palermo et al., 2014). They are beginning to understand the need for painful procedures. They fear body harm and have an awareness of death. Therefore, they may appear to overreact to illness or injury. As in other age-groups, the school-age child remembers previous pain experiences, which will affect the current response. The child's culture, gender, and cognitive abilities will also affect the pain experience.

Nonverbal and behavioral cues are very important in assessing a school-age child's pain. The child may exhibit a stiff body posture, withdraw, or be found quietly sobbing (Fig. 39.3). The school-age child who resists a treatment, cries loudly, or otherwise acts in an aggressive manner might later deny the behavior. School-age children might also attempt to procrastinate or bargain to delay a painful procedure. As with younger children, the school-age child may demonstrate regressive behaviors when experiencing pain. They also can have difficulty functioning in school (Palermo et al., 2014),

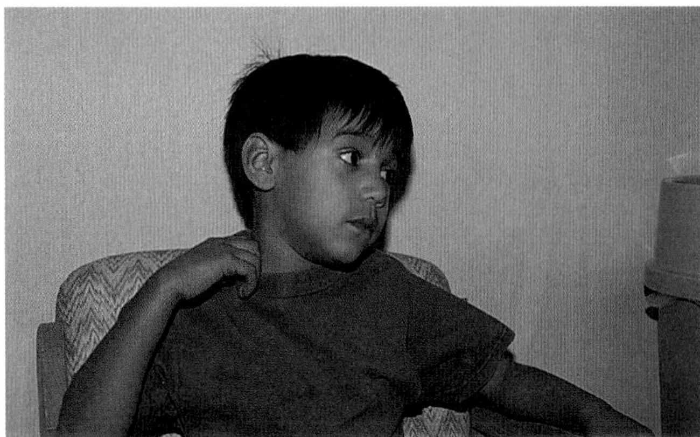

**FIG 39.3** School-age children may become very quiet and withdrawn when ill or in pain. The child with asthma is not attentive or active; his mother knew that something was wrong because of his withdrawn behavior. (Courtesy Parkland Health and Hospital System Community-Oriented Primary Care Clinic, Dallas, TX.)

### Adolescents

Adolescents can think abstractly and understand cause and effect. They can describe and quantify pain intensity and their feelings about pain. They can also discuss the strategies to help manage their pain. They are able to perceive and understand pain at a physical, emotional, and cognitive level. However, having these abilities does not mean the adolescent will use them. Adolescents are often confused by control issues and are uncertain of their roles as they move from childhood to adulthood. Regression can also occur at this age in relation to pain. Adolescents often are conflicted between striving for autonomy and having their parents involved in their care (Palermo et al., 2014).

Because adolescents are egocentric, they tend to think that others focus on their behaviors; therefore, adolescents may suppress the manifestations of pain. In addition, they might not report pain because they believe that the nurse knows when they hurt; subsequently, they expect to receive pain medication when they *need* it and not just when they ask for it. Adolescents tend to exhibit fewer outward signs of pain as compared to younger children. Possible signs include increased muscle tension, withdrawal, and decreased motor activity. Hospitalized adolescents use words such as "sore," "like an ache," "pounding," and "miserable" to describe pain.

**! NURSING QUALITY ALERT**

***Assessing Pain in Children***

- The use of a pain assessment tool is imperative in the assessment of pain in children and the evaluation of pain management interventions. The tool used is documented in the patient's medical record.
- If the child is unable to express or quantify pain, use parents as one of the first resources to assist in assessing the child's pain and response to interventions.
- Behavioral changes, such as guarding, body positioning, crying, grimacing, and other altered facial expressions, and changes in activity level may or may not be seen in a child experiencing pain.
- Physiologic changes are only one source of information when assessing pain in the neonate or infant. Other states, such as fear and anxiety, can also cause physiologic changes. Physiologic changes tend to occur during an acute pain experience and then return to normal; they may not be valid indicators of sustained or chronic pain.

### Assessment Tools

Consistent, appropriate use of a pain assessment tool is essential to pediatric pain management. A number of valid and reliable pain assessment tools are available to help the nurse make a more accurate pain assessment. Both self-report and behavioral instruments are available. Self-report of pain is ideal and considered the gold standard for assessing pain (Vael & Whitted, 2014). Examples of these tools are detailed in Table 39.2. Children benefit when pain assessment tools are used because they are given a simple and effective way to communicate the pain they are experiencing. Assessment tools provide more objective data, reducing the chance that discreet signs of pain will be overlooked. Unfortunately, they are not always used consistently and correctly in clinical settings. Using a tool in a way other than the developer intended can invalidate the pain assessment. Pain management is enhanced in acute care settings by limiting the number of pain assessment tools and providing routine education on the implementation of each tool (Mosiman & Pile, 2013).

An assessment tool should be used that corresponds to the child's developmental abilities. The crucial factors concerning selection of a pain assessment tool are that it is appropriate for the child's developmental level and can facilitate the development of an effective pain management plan based on the information gathered from the assessment. Varieties of tools are available for infants and the preverbal or nonverbal child, such as those who are neurologically unresponsive, developmentally delayed, or unable to speak because of medical treatment (e.g., intubation) (Herr et al., 2011). Tools for infants and preverbal children usually are based on behavioral cues (e.g., facial expression, motor responses, intensity of cry). One such tool, the Face, Legs, Activity, Cry, Consolability (FLACC) scale, has been examined numerous times for reliability and validity. It has been shown to be an appropriate, effective tool for the preverbal or nonverbal child (Herr et al., 2011) and is used with increasing frequency.

Cognitively impaired children are at increased risk for untreated pain, and nurses should use an appropriate tool such as the revised Faces, Legs, Activity, Cry, and Consolability (rFLACC) scale, which includes parent input of indications of pain in addition to appearance and behaviors of the child (Chen-Lim et al., 2012; Crosta, Ward, Walker, et al., 2014; Ely et al., 2012; Tobias, 2014a).

Children verbalize words for pain by approximately 18 months of age, and cognitive development is sufficient for reporting the extent of pain by 3 to 4 years of age. Self-report tools are effective in children older than 3 years. Pictures can be helpful in describing the location of pain (Mesko, Eliades, Libertin, et al., 2011). The Oucher pain scale, the Poker Chip Tool, and the FACES Pain Rating Scale are examples of tools for preschoolers and school-age children. The Oucher pain scale (Fig. 39.4), which has seven versions including five different ethnic groups, as well as different sexes for some of the scales, may facilitate a more culturally sensitive assessment (Joestlein, 2015; Nash, 2012). The Wong-Baker FACES Pain Rating Scale has been translated into 10 different languages. Matching the tool to the child's ethnicity and primary language can provide better information about pain experienced by children from diverse populations and promote better pain control (Wong-Baker FACES Foundation, 1983). Baker and Wong (1987) also developed the QUEST pneumonic to describe important pieces of pain assessment: question the child, use pain rating tools, evaluate their behavior, sensitize their parents, and take action.

School-age children can understand concepts of order and number and can use numeric rating scales, word-graphic rating scales, and visual analog scales (Tobias, 2014a). Table 39.2 describes pain assessment tools and lists the age or developmental level of children

**TABLE 39.2 Pain Assessment Tools**

| Tool | Description | Age |
|---|---|---|
| Adolescent and Pediatric Pain Tool (APPT) (see Fig. 39.6) | Three-part tool composed of a body outline, an intensity scale, and a pain descriptor word list (Savedra, Tesler, Holzemer, et al., 1992). | 8-17 yr |
| CRIES pain scale | Five behavioral categories: *C*rying, *R*equires $O_2$ for $SaO_2$ <95%, *I*ncreased vital signs, *E*xpression, *S*leepless; 0-2 for each category, with a total score from 0-10. A higher score indicates greater pain or distress (Krechel & Bildner, 1995). | Neonates; 0-6 mo |
| COMFORT Behavior Scale | Six categories are scored: Alertness, Calmness/Agitation, Respiratory response (if on ventilator) or Crying (if breathing spontaneously), Physical Movement, Muscle Tone, Facial Tension; 1-5 points for each category, with a total score from 6-30. A higher score indicates greater pain or distress (Van Dijk, Peters, & Van Deventer, 2005). | Infants and children in critical care settings |
| FLACC | Five behavioral categories: *F*ace, *L*egs, *A*ctivity, *C*ry, *C*onsolability. Each scored from 0-2 points, resulting in a total score from 0-10. A higher score indicates higher pain or distress (Merkel, Voepel-Lewis, & Malviya, 2002). | Infants and preverbal or nonverbal children |
| FACES Pain Rating Scale(see Fig. 39.5) | Six cartoon faces with neutral to gradually increasing painful expressions, corresponding to an analog scale with words ranging from a happy face (0; No Hurt) to a crying face (5 or 10; Hurts Worst). Accommodates a 0-5 or 0-10 system (Hockenberry & Wilson, 2009). | 3 yr and older |
| Numeric Rating Scale (NRS) | Patient is asked to give a number that reflects the pain level: 0 = no pain; 1-3 = mild; 4-6 = moderate; 7-10 = severe (Pasero & McCaffery, 2011). | Child 9 yr and older |
| Oucher pain scale (see Fig. 39.4) | A poster with a 0-100 scale for older children and a six-picture photographic scale for young children who cannot count to 100; 0 is no pain and 100 is the greatest pain. Five versions available: Caucasians/Whites, Asians (boy or girl), First Nations (boy or girl), Hispanics, and African-Americans/Blacks (Beyer, Villarruel & Denyes, 2009). | 3-12 yr |
| Poker Chip Tool | Four poker chips are used, with each chip representing a piece of hurt. One poker chip represents a little hurt, and four chips represent the most hurt the child could have (Hester et al., 1998). | 4-12 yr |
| Visual Analog Scale (VAS) | Usually a 10-cm line, with one end representing "no pain" and the opposite end "the worst pain" (Cline, Herman, & Shaw, 1992). | 7-18 yr |

appropriate for its use (Figs. 39.5 and 39.6). The same tool should be used each time a child is assessed to obtain consistent data and to avoid confusing the child. Whenever possible, the child should be taught how to use the rating tool before pain is experienced. This can be a part of preprocedure or preoperative education for the child and family.

In assessing pain and obtaining the pain history, the nurse should first ask the child and family which words the child uses to indicate pain. A child may use words such as "owie" or "ouchie" when describing pain or hurt. A child's word(s) must be used consistently by the nurse in any future discussions with the child regarding pain. In interviewing the parents and family, the nurse should address the presence and involvement of different family members, cultural and/or spiritual beliefs, and practices regarding pain and pain relief. Box 39.3 describes how to obtain a pain experience history from both the child and parents. Information to be gathered includes the child's past experiences with pain, how the child reacts to pain, the person the child tells about pain, how the parents know when their child is in pain, and what works best to take the child's pain away. Nurses must ensure that pain is assessed regularly. Documentation includes the tool used to assess pain. Pain should be reassessed in a timely manner in children, since undetected pain is often untreated (Joestlein, 2015; Shomaker, Dutton, & Mark, 2015). Computerized documentation that alerts the nurse when to reassess pain is helpful in increasing compliance (Reavey et al., 2014). Parental discharge education about the pain tool and discharge medications is vital to continued pain management in the home setting (Stapelkamp, Carter, Gordon, et al., 2011).

## NON-PHARMACOLOGIC AND PHARMACOLOGIC PAIN INTERVENTIONS

Pain management for children needs to be "multimodal," using an effective combination of a quiet, calm environment and both non-pharmacologic and pharmacologic approaches (APS, 2011a; The Joint Commission, 2014). The nurse's assessment helps determine the suitable intervention. If pharmacologic interventions are determined to be the first and best option, non-pharmacologic interventions can always be presented as an adjuvant for the chosen analgesic. Doing so may offer the child a sense of accomplishment and control that can replace the sense of helplessness that often accompanies the presence of pain, illness, and hospitalization.

### Non-Pharmacologic Interventions

The nurse caring for a child in pain can provide non-pharmacologic interventions in addition to pharmacologic interventions. Use of non-pharmacologic interventions in preparing the child for procedures and treatments can help minimize or relieve pain by reducing anxiety and fear of the unknown (see Chapter 35). Non-pharmacologic interventions must be suitable for the child's stage of development, personality, and his or her circumstances.

Parents play a very important role in assessing and providing pain management for their children. They are a resource for determining what methods of pain relief were effective in the past. They can help the nurse assess their child's current pain status and the need for intervention. Repositioning, holding, touching, massage, warm or cold compresses, breathing techniques, distraction, guided imagery, and muscle relaxation are all techniques that can be used by the person the child usually trusts the most—a parent. Many techniques require preliminary instruction by the nurse or other qualified individuals but then are easily learned and put into practice by parents. This practice also gives parents "hands-on" involvement and a sense of control when their child is hospitalized. Swaddling, breastfeeding and infant kangaroo care (holding with skin-to-skin contact) are examples of effective pain reduction interventions that can easily be provided by the mother (Harrington et al., 2012).

Distraction can be one of the more effective adjuvants for pain management (Fig. 39.7). It is also one of the simplest to accomplish. Distraction works by refocusing the child's attention from the pain to something else. For example, a child brought to the emergency department after an accident is invariably frightened. Even if the injury is minor, the fear and pain are real to the child. By using distraction, the nurse can decrease the child's anxiety, and the pain subsequently decreases. Some children experiencing pain will engage in activities on their own in an effort to ignore or "forget" their pain. It is important not to discount the pain experienced if a child is able to use distraction effectively to control it.

The form of distraction used should be appropriate for the child's developmental level. Techniques include blowing bubbles; looking through a kaleidoscope; listening to music or stories; reading; playing number, video, or board games; watching a video; and even doing multiplication tables or spelling words. Another distraction method used during a procedure or treatment involves allowing the child to help by handing, opening, or holding objects. This should be done only when it is safe and there is no danger of contaminating the materials or the treatment site.

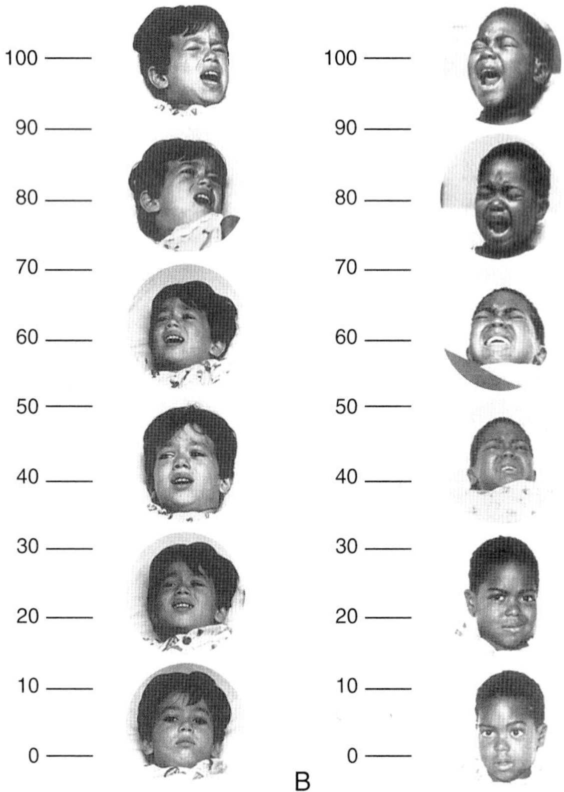


**FIG 39.4 A,** The Hispanic version of the Oucher pain scale. **B,** The African-American version. (**A,** Developed and copyrighted by Antonia M. Villarruel, RN, PhD, and Mary J. Denyes, RN, PhD, 1991. **B,** Developed and copyrighted by Mary J. Denyes, PhD, RN, FAAN [Wayne State University], and Antonia Villarruel, PhD, RN, FAAN [University of Pennsylvania] at the Children's Hospital of Michigan in 1990. Cornelia P. Porter, PhD, RN, and Charlotta Marshall, MSN, RN, contributed to the development of this scale.)

## PATIENT-CENTERED TEACHING

### *Pain Management for Children at Home*

- Parents are given a pain assessment tool with instructions regarding its accurate use. They should verbalize understanding about the tool and give a return demonstration using the tool with their child.
- The dose, route, and schedule for all pain medications are explained to the parents verbally and in writing. *All instructions should be in the appropriate language for the family, using clear, straightforward terminology that is at an educational level suitable for the parents.*
- Non-pharmacologic interventions that are appropriate and comforting for the child's pain (e.g., massage, warm or cold compresses, repositioning) are explained and demonstrated. Written instructions are provided as necessary.
- Parents are instructed to notify the primary healthcare provider if interventions for pain management are ineffective or if the child shows behavior or physiologic changes not consistent with the expected outcomes for the child.
- Parents are given a phone number where they can contact a nurse or other healthcare provider if they have any questions about their child's condition once the child is in the home setting.

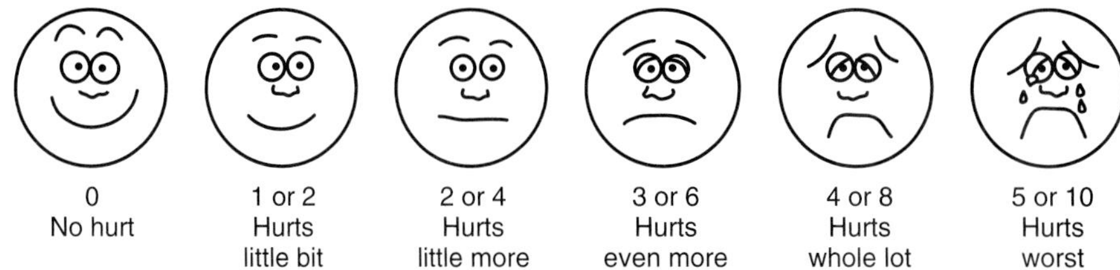


**FIG 39.5** FACES Pain Rating Scale. Explain to the child that each face is for a person who feels happy because he or she has no pain (hurt) or sad because he or she has some or a lot of pain. Ask the child to choose the face that best describes his or her own pain. (Wong-Baker FACES Pain Rating Scale reference manual describing development and research of the scale is available from City of Hope Pain/Palliative Care Resource Center, 1500 East Duarte Road, Duarte, CA 91010; 626-359-8111, ext. 3829; fax: 626-301-8941; http://www1.us.elsevierhealth.com/FACES.)

CODE ______________

DATE ______________

**Adolescent and Pediatric Pain Tool (APPT)**

**INSTRUCTIONS:**

**1. Color in the areas on these drawings to show where you have pain. Make the marks as big or small as the place where the pain is.**

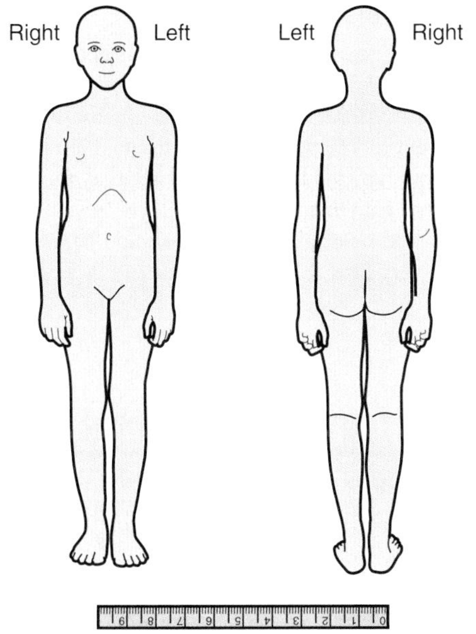

Right Left Left Right

**2. Place a straight, up and down mark on this line to show how much pain you have.**

No pain | Little pain | Medium pain | Large pain | Worst possible pain

**3. Point to or circle as many of these words that describe your pain.**

1
annoying
bad
horrible
miserable
terrible
uncomfortable

2
aching
hurting
like an ache
like a hurt
sore

3
beating
hitting
pounding
punching
throbbing

4
biting
cutting
like a pin
like a sharp knife
pin like
sharp
stabbing

5
blistering
burning
hot

6
cramping
crushing
like a pinch
pinching
pressure

7
itching
like a scratch
like a sting
scratching
stinging

8
shocking
shooting
splitting

9
numb
stiff
swollen
tight

10
awful
deadly
dying
killing

11
crying
frightening
screaming
terrifying

12
dizzy
sickening
suffocating

13
never goes away
uncontrollable

14
always
comes and goes
comes on all of a sudden
constant
continuous
forever

15
off and on
once in a while
sneaks up
sometimes
steady

If you like, you may add other words:

______________

______________

______________

For office use only.

BSA: ______

IS: ______

| | | | |
|---|---|---|---|
| #S (2-9) | ____ | /37= ____ | % |
| #A (10-12) | ____ | /11= ____ | % |
| #E (1,13) | ____ | /8= ____ | % |
| #T (14,15) | ____ | /11= ____ | % |
| Total | ____ | /67= ____ | % |

**FIG 39.6** Adolescent and Pediatric Pain Tool (APPT). Use with 8- to 17-year-olds. (From Savedra, M.C., Tesler, M.D., Holzemer, W.L., et al. [1992]. *Adolescent and pediatric pin tool: user's manual.* San Francisco: University of California, San Francisco, School of Nursing. ©1989, 1992.)

## BOX 39.3 Pain Experience History

**Child Form***

- What word(s) do you use to describe your pain?
- Tell me what pain is.
- What does a child with pain look like?
- How do you feel when you have pain?
- Have you ever had pain just like this before? Tell me about a time when you had pain.
- Is the pain you have now different than pain you have had before?
- Do you tell others when you hurt? Who do you tell?
- What helps the most to take your hurt away?
- What do you do for yourself when you are hurting?
- What do you want other people to do for you when you hurt?
- What don't you want other people to do for you when you hurt?
- Did anyone tell you that you might have pain? If yes, who told you and how did they tell you?
- Is there anything else at all you want to tell me about pain? (If yes, have child describe.)

**Parent Form**

- What word or words does your child use to describe pain?
- Describe the pain experiences your child has had in the past.
- Does your child tell you or others when in pain?
- How do you know when your child is in pain?
- How does your child usually react to pain?
- What do you do when your child is in pain?
- What does your child do when he or she is in pain?
- What works best to take away your child's pain?
- Is there anything special that you would like me to know about your child and pain? (If yes, describe.)

*Substitute the word *pain* or *hurt* with the word the child uses (e.g., "owie" or "ouchie").

Modified from Cheng, S., Foster, R.L., Hester, N.O., et al. (2003). A qualitative inquiry of Taiwanese children's pain experiences. *Journal of Nursing Research (Taiwan Nurses Association), 11*(4), 241–250; Hester, N.O., & Barcus, C.S. (1986). Assessment and management of pain in children. *Pediatrics: Nursing Update, 1*(14), 2–8.

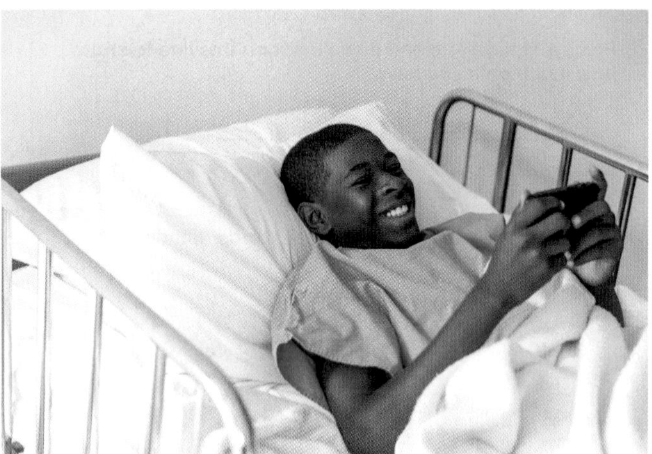

FIG 39.7 The boy plays a video game, which serves as a distraction to refocus attention and reduce pain. (©2016 Getty Images. Reprinted with permission.)

If a child has a favorite doll or stuffed animal, it can be used to create a story or a game. Children love to talk about their pets, and the nurse can ask the child to tell a favorite story about the pet. Engaging a child in conversation that is meaningful to the child not only aids in pain control but also facilitates development of a therapeutic nurse–patient relationship. Although each child is different, cues or verbal instruction from the child and the parent can indicate whether the nurse should hold the child's hand, touch the child's head, or provide some other interventions that are appropriate and comforting to the child. A child life specialist is a great resource in providing effective coping techniques tailored to the child, such as the use of play and self-expression activities (Madhok, Scribner-O'Pray, & Teele, 2011).

Once both the child and nurse can communicate personally, the nurse might say, "I see you have a baseball shirt." If the child expresses an interest in the game, the nurse can continue, "What is your favorite team?" The nurse should be comfortable with the topic because the child will sense a lack of genuine interest. If it is appropriate on the basis of the child's developmental level and degree of egocentricity, the nurse might interject a personal note such as "I enjoy going to baseball games with my family." This conversation could go on for 10 to 15 minutes, certainly long enough for minor procedures such as suturing a laceration, to be completed. The child will not be focusing as much on the procedure as on baseball. The topic must be of interest to the child to distract the child's attention away from pain.

Considerable research has studied the use of oral sucrose with or without nonnutritive sucking (NNS) on pacifiers as a non-pharmacologic adjuvant for neonatal and infant pain management. Several studies provide evidence that giving oral sucrose alone and with NNS before and during a procedure are safe and effective interventions that reduce procedural pain in infants (Mosiman & Pile, 2013).

Table 39.3 lists additional non-pharmacologic approaches to pain management for infants and children., Regardless of the technique used, it is important for the nurse to remember to evaluate its effectiveness and change the intervention if the chosen technique does not provide sufficient pain relief.

## Pharmacologic Interventions

Reluctance to administer analgesics to infants and children stems from the fears of many nurses and physicians that analgesics will cause respiratory depression and/or lead to addiction. Some healthcare providers incorrectly believe that a child does not experience enough pain to justify analgesic administration. If a procedure, surgery, or trauma causes pain in an adult, it will cause pain in a child, and analgesic medications are necessary. However, it is important to ensure that the correct medication and dose are ordered and administered. In some cases, the analgesic is underdosed, and the child still experiences untreated, unwarranted pain. Increased pain management experience and research have taught that a combination of medications (multidrug therapy) is often far more effective than a single analgesic. However, no one analgesic or combination of analgesics will provide optional pain management for all patients or in all circumstances. The chosen analgesic therapy must have a prompt onset of action, a predictable duration of action, manageable side effects, and an appropriate reversal agent.

### Administration of Analgesics

Analgesics can be administered by various routes—oral, rectal, intranasal, topical, transdermal, intravenous (IV), intramuscular (IM), subcutaneous, and epidural (see Chapter 38 for a discussion of the common routes). The least invasive route that provides optimum analgesia should always be chosen. As soon as the child can tolerate oral nutrition, pain medication should be given by the oral route whenever possible. Rectal medication should be avoided because this route can be very disturbing to children and is generally disliked. The IM route is used infrequently because many children are very afraid of injections ("shots").

**! NURSING QUALITY ALERT**

***Disadvantages of Intramuscular (IM) Analgesics***

- Most children have a significant fear of pain associated with IM injections.
- Fluctuations in tissue absorption lead to peaks and troughs in analgesia.
- Children may not have enough suitable sites for IM injections.
- Some medications can cause injury to tissues and nerves.
- IM analgesics have a shorter duration of action than oral analgesics.
- IM analgesics are contraindicated in children with low platelet counts and bleeding disorders such as hemophilia.

***Patient-controlled analgesia.*** One of the most effective ways of administering opioids is by use of a patient-controlled analgesia (PCA) pump. The pump administers an IV bolus of pain medication either with or without a continuous infusion of the same medication. The patient controls the infusion of the bolus. An underlying safety principle associated with PCA is that a sedated or sleeping patient will not be able to activate a bolus dose (Wuhrman & Broglio, 2015), thereby decreasing the risk of overdose.

When the child needs pain medication, a small dose of the opioid medication is received after a button connected to the pump is pushed (Fig. 39.8). After each dose, there is "lock-out" time during which the pump will not release the medication even if the button is pushed. The pump also has a maximum amount of medication that can be given over a designated period—usually 1 hour. If the maximum amount of medication for the designated time period has been reached, the pump will not release medication even if the button is pushed.

After checking to ensure that all doses are within appropriate range for the child, two registered nurses (RNs) must check the bag or syringe of medication before hanging it. After a PCA pump is programmed, it must then be double-checked by a second RN. Box 39.4 gives an example of orders for a PCA infusion. The opioid bag or syringe is

TABLE 39.3 **Non-Pharmacologic Pain Relief Techniques**

| Technique | Description | Nursing Considerations |
|---|---|---|
| Distraction | Related to the gate control theory, use of distraction techniques "closes the gate" by focusing the child on the distraction rather than on the pain experience. Active methods are more effective than passive (Moayedi & Davis, 2013; Olmstead, Scott, Mayan, et al., 2014).<br>Wide range of techniques (e.g., playing with toys, video games, blowing bubbles, watching videos, listening to music, singing, reading). | Relatively easy to use and often employed by nurses and other healthcare providers to help children cope with pain. Distraction must be developmentally appropriate for the child. |
| Regulated (controlled) breathing | Provides a focal point for distraction and produces relaxation. A simple mode for biofeedback. | Teach the child how to achieve a slow, rhythmic breathing pattern; teach parents the technique and how to help their child. |
| Guided imagery | The child is encouraged to remember or imagine the sounds, sights, and smells of an enjoyable item or experience such as playing in the water or a birthday celebration (Wohlheiter & Dahlquist, 2013). The facilitator talks in a soft, calm voice while "guiding" the child's imagination. Can be coupled with relaxation techniques such as rhythmic breathing. | Facilitated by trained healthcare providers (e.g., nurse, child-life therapist). Studies have shown reductions in children's pain from a variety of causes. |
| Biofeedback | Involves measurement of physiologic indicators (e.g., blood pressure, heart rate, skin temperature, sweating, and muscle tension) using specialized equipment. Alerts patients instantly to early signs of tension so they can commence relaxation techniques; the child learns to control physiologic responses based on the biofeedback. Has proven effective for treatment of headaches and other types of pain (Knox et al., 2011). | Requires trained personnel to administer and teach tension recognition and relaxation techniques. |
| Progressive muscle relaxation | Progressive, systematic, purposeful relaxation of one muscle group at a time through contraction and then relaxation of muscles; usually proceeds from head to toe; increases pain threshold. Often used effectively for migraine and tension headaches (Dolbier & Rush, 2012). | Teach the older child and adolescent the technique; encourage frequent practice. |
| Hypnosis | Focused, narrowed attention and an altered state of consciousness that facilitates relaxation. Used in association with painful procedures and treatments, postoperatively, or for chronic pain. | Hypnotists receive special training; children can be taught self-hypnosis. |
| Acupuncture | Based on traditional Chinese concepts of energy balance; insertion of very thin needles through the skin to stimulate anatomic points (meridians). Limited research in children (Gorodzinsky, Bernacki, Davies, et al., 2012). | Treatment is done by a trained acupuncturist; children may have concerns about the use of needles. |
| Topical heating and cooling | Application of cold or heat to a painful area provides pain relief and comfort; the mechanism of action is uncertain (Mosiman & Pile, 2013; Wong et al., 2012). | Used by nurses, physical therapists, sports trainers, and other clinicians. |
| Massage | Purposeful manipulation of the body, providing tactile and kinesthetic stimulation. Evidence regarding benefits is varied; strongest effect is anxiety reduction (Cong et al., 2013; Gorodzinsky et al., 2012). | Performed by massage therapists; nurses may provide basic massage. |
| TENS (transcutaneous electrical nerve stimulation) | Small amounts of electrical energy are delivered to the skin via electrodes. By interfering with the transmission of pain signals, TENS completely or partially blocks the sensation of pain rapidly in the stimulated area (Johnson, 2014). | Usually administered by physical therapists. Used frequently for children and adults. |
| Techniques for neonates and infants | Several noninvasive techniques used during and/or after a painful procedure or experience include breastfeeding; oral sucrose; nonnutritive sucking on a pacifier; skin-to-skin contact (kangaroo care) with the infant positioned directly on the mother's chest; holding and rocking by a parent or caregiver; and tucking or swaddling where the infant is wrapped with the extremities close to the trunk (Harrington et al., 2012). | Nurses may use a variety of techniques separately or in combination to distract the infant and reduce the severity of the pain experience. Parents can be taught to use techniques. |

locked into the PCA pump, and the pump itself is locked to the IV pole. The specialized PCA tubing does not have IV access ports.

The child is monitored frequently to ensure that pain control is effective and that the equipment is functioning correctly. The nurse should also carefully assess the child for signs of overmedication (especially depressed respiratory rate or inability to awaken) and the side effects that can accompany opioid administration. Vital signs should be assessed every 2 to 4 hours. Some institutions require hourly documentation of respiratory rate.

Additionally, many institutional policies require that children receiving PCA therapy be placed on continuous pulse oximetry, cardiac and respiratory monitoring, or both. Oxygen, a bag-valve-mask device, and IV naloxone (Narcan) should be readily available. Naloxone will reverse opioid-related analgesia and respiratory depression; it must be administered slowly until the first sign that respiratory depression is reversed. Because it has a short half-life, administration may need to be repeated every 30 to 60 minutes. Many institutions mandate that naloxone must be given in the presence of a physician because too-rapid infusion can result in cardiac arrest.

Frequent pain assessment is essential, usually every 1 to 4 hours and with any bolus dose, to assess the effectiveness of PCA therapy in general and of the bolus. Charting will include hourly documentation as to the number of bolus doses received and the number of bolus attempts made by the child. Total milligram dosages of the medication

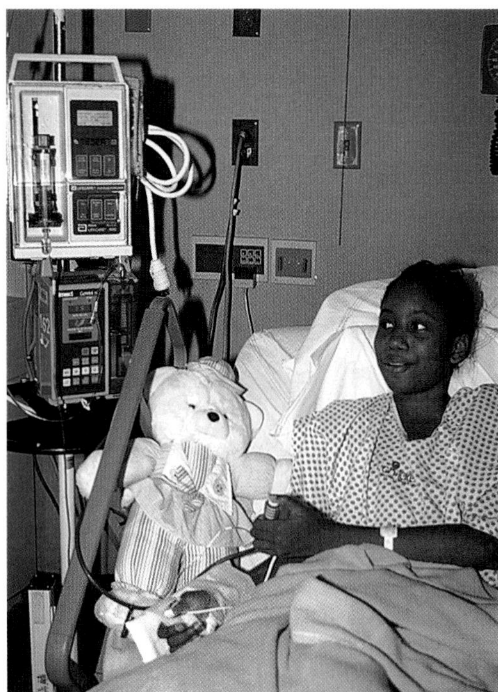

FIG 39.8 Patient-controlled analgesia (PCA) allows the child greater control over her own pain management. (Courtesy Children's Medical Center, Dallas, TX.)

**BOX 39.4 Aspects of Patient-Controlled Analgesia (PCA) Orders**

Medication/concentration: ____________________
Mode: PCA only ________ PCA and basal infusion ________
Continuous infusion only ________________
Dosages:
PCA bolus ____________ mg (recommended starting dose is 0.02 mg/kg/dose for morphine)
Basal rate or continuous infusion ____________ (recommended starting dose is 0.02 mg/kg/hr for morphine)
Lock-out: __________ minutes (usual is 6-10 minutes as needed)
1-hour limit: __________ mg PCA and basal rate combined (usual is 0.075 mg/kg for morphine)

received will be noted every 1 to 4 hours and documented on the medication administration record.

Most hospitals permit the use of PCA by children 5 to 7 years of age or older, when developmentally appropriate (Tobias, 2014b). For younger children or those not able to operate a PCA pump independently to control their own analgesia, family or healthcare providers can administer PCA by proxy (for the child). Because of adverse events that have occurred with PCA by proxy, The Joint Commission recommended that hospitals implement strict protocols for patient selection and institute a warning system that alerts unauthorized staff and families not to administer bolus doses for the patient. The American Society for Pain Management Nursing has issued recommendations for the use of authorized agent-controlled analgesia (AACA) by carefully selected nurses or family members (nurse-controlled analgesia or caregiver-controlled analgesia) (Czarnecki et al., 2011b). These include (1) developing stringent guidelines for selecting and educating nurses or appropriate family caregivers; (2) providing oral and written instructions that address how to assess when the child needs to receive a bolus and when the child should not receive a bolus; (3) selecting a single nurse or caregiver who will be with the patient consistently and can assess for medication effects and potential adverse consequences; and (4) documenting teaching and supervision of the person giving the AACA (Wuhrman & Broglio, 2015).

***Topical anesthetic agents.*** Several noninjection-based, topical anesthetic agents are available for use before painful procedures. These agents have been found to effectively reduce in children the pain associated with invasive procedures such as injections, venipunctures, lumbar punctures, and bone marrow aspirations (Czarnecki, Turner, Collins, et al., 2011c). Further, many pediatric institutions mandate that numbing agents be used for all IV catheter insertions, unless it is on an emergency basis.

Lidocaine–prilocaine 5% cream (eutectic mixture of local anesthetics [EMLA]) was the first agent that demonstrated efficacy for numbing the skin for invasive procedures. Additional topical agents used for children include 4% amethocaine gel (Ametop), liposomal lidocaine 4% or 5% cream (LMX4 or LMX5), and the Synera patch with 70 mg of lidocaine and 70 mg of tetracaine (Czarnecki et al., 2011c; Mosiman & Pile, 2013).

A cream or patch is applied to intact skin with no open wounds, burns, abrasions, cuts, or inflammation. The technique for application and amount of time the agent must be in contact with the skin varies according to the agent used (see Chapter 38). Generally, an anesthetic cream is placed on the skin at the procedure site ideally for 60 minutes to 120 minutes and provides a numbing effect for 1 to 2 hours after removal. Parents can apply an agent at home before a scheduled procedure, such as an immunization injection, to prevent pain. Parents are instructed to wear gloves when applying anesthetic creams. Young children must be supervised so they do not remove the dressing, rub the cream in their eyes or ears, or eat the cream, which may look like cake frosting.

The main side effect seen with any of the topical anesthetic creams is skin redness or blanching, with normal skin color returning in a few hours. The child should be monitored for burning, swelling, itching, or a rash at the application site; if seen, this would necessitate immediate removal of the cream from the skin.

A vapocoolant spray is used to provide immediate numbing of the skin for urgent procedures (Mosiman & Pile, 2013). Cold spray is sprayed either directly on the skin at the site or on a sterile cotton ball, which is then applied to the site for 15 seconds. The onset of action is immediate, and the numbing effect lasts approximately 15 seconds.

Needleless systems are also used to painlessly deliver anesthetic medication below the surface of the skin. Lidocaine hydrochloride 2% with 1:100,000 epinephrine topical solution (Numby Stuff) comes in an electrode patch and uses iontophoresis, a mild electric current, to push lidocaine and epinephrine into the skin to a depth of 10 mm. A newer approach is the J-Tip jet device, which delivers 1% buffered lidocaine into the skin at a depth of 5 to 8 mm via a carbon dioxide gas-driven plunger. Some studies have shown use of the J-Tip to reduce pain for children during IV catheter insertions, although its efficacy over other topical anesthetics is still being investigated (Czarnecki et al., 2011c). These methods can only be used in healthcare settings.

Optimal care for children undergoing painful, invasive procedures requires the combined use of several different interventions. Although topical anesthetic agents significantly reduce or even remove pain, children can still experience fear and anxiety, which in turn causes distress for the entire family. Use of topical agents along with distraction or other non-pharmacologic methods, and parental presence, work together to alleviate pain and stress for the child and family (Czarnecki et al., 2011c).

### Acetaminophen and Antiinflammatory Drugs

Acetaminophen (brand name Tylenol) is the most commonly used analgesic for mild to moderate pain as well as the drug of choice for treating children's fevers in the United States (Anderson, Rolfe, & Brennan-Hunter, 2013). It has a minimal antiinflammatory effect. The short-term use of acetaminophen is safe, even in neonates. It does not have the gastric irritation and gastrointestinal (GI) bleeding side effects of other analgesics. Usually related to overdosage, acetaminophen can cause hepatic damage. It is of critical importance to monitor the total amount of acetaminophen a child is receiving, because it is often combined with other prescription and over-the-counter medications to treat pain, fever, and other symptoms associated with upper respiratory infections and influenza.

Nonsteroidal antiinflammatory drugs (NSAIDs) reduce pain, fever, and inflammation by inhibiting the production of prostaglandins. Ibuprofen, naproxen/naproxen sodium (Aleve, Naprosyn, Anaprox), and ketorolac (Toradol) are the NSAIDs that are frequently used to treat mild to moderate pain in children. NSAIDs often are the preferred drugs to treat bone and inflammatory pain associated with bone injuries, arthritis-like conditions, and certain types of cancer (see Chapter 50). NSAIDS should not be given to infants under 6 months of age.

Although aspirin (acetylsalicylic acid) is an effective antiinflammatory drug, it is not recommended for use in children to treat pain or fever because of an association with Reye syndrome (see Chapter 52).

### Opioids

Opioids are natural or synthetic opium derivative analgesics that bind to central nervous system (CNS) opioid receptors and control pain by depressing pain impulse transmission. Opioids are the cornerstone drugs in the management of moderate to severe acute and chronic pain, including postoperative pain, posttraumatic pain, the pain of sickle cell vaso-occlusive crisis, and cancer pain. Opioids commonly used for children include fentanyl, hydrocodone, hydromorphone, methadone, morphine, and oxycodone. In pain management, *opioid* is the correct term for this class of medications. The antiquated term "narcotic" is often associated with illegal drug use and trafficking; referring to analgesics as narcotics may deter patients and families from appropriate use of these analgesics.

Opioids can be administered by most routes. However, the oral route should be used when appropriate if the child is able to take and tolerate oral opioids. Sustained-release forms of morphine and oxycodone, which last 12 to 24 hours, are available. These are supplemented with a short-acting form of these analgesics for "break-through" pain, resulting in longer pain-free periods for children with moderate to severe, long-term pain (e.g., cancer pain). Short-acting liquid opioids

#### DRUG GUIDE

#### *Acetaminophen*

**Classification:** Analgesic, antipyretic.
**Action:** Unknown, thought to produce analgesia by blocking generation of pain impulses.
**Indications:** Mild pain or fever.
**Dosages and Routes:** By mouth or rectal suppository dosage 10-15 mg/kg/dose every 4-6 hours (every 6-8 hours for neonates). Maximum dose of 90 mg/kg/24 hours; not to exceed 4000 mg/day.
**Absorption:** Rapid and almost complete absorption from gastrointestinal (GI) tract; less complete absorption from rectal suppository; peak effects in 1-1.5 hours.
**Excretion:** 90%-100% of drug excreted as metabolites in urine; excreted in breast milk; effects last 4-6 hours.
**Contraindications:** Hypersensitivity to acetaminophen or phenacetin; administration to patients with anemia or hepatic disease; cautious use in arthritic or rheumatoid conditions affecting children younger than 12 years; thrombocytopenia.
**Adverse Reaction:** Negligible with recommended dosage; rash.
**Nursing Considerations:** Can be crushed. Chewable tablets should be thoroughly chewed and wet before swallowing. With high doses or long-term therapy, periodic tests of hepatic, renal, and hematopoietic function are advised. Caution the parents about giving other medications that also contain acetaminophen. No more than six doses in 24 hours should be given to children unless prescribed by a physician.

#### DRUG GUIDE

#### *Ibuprofen*

**Classification:** Nonsteroidal antiinflammatory drug (NSAID), analgesic.
**Action:** Blocks prostaglandin synthesis.
**Indications:** Relief of mild to moderate pain for children >6 months of age. Chronic, symptomatic rheumatoid arthritis and osteoarthritis.
**Dosages and Route:** By mouth dosage 5-10 mg/kg/dose every 6-8 hours. Not to exceed 40 mg/kg/24 hours. Juvenile arthritis dosage 30-50 mg/kg/24 hours. Medication comes in liquid form for young children.
**Absorption:** 80% absorbed from gastrointestinal (GI) tract; peak action in 1-2 hours.
**Excretion:** Excreted primarily in urine; some biliary excretion.
**Contraindications:** Contraindicated in children less than 6 months of age. Contraindicated in children in whom urticaria, severe rhinitis, bronchospasm, angioedema, nasal polyps are precipitated by other NSAIDs; active peptic ulcer; bleeding abnormalities.
**Precautions:** Hypertension, history of GI ulceration, impaired hepatic or renal function, chronic renal failure.
**Adverse Reactions:** Heartburn, nausea, vomiting, epigastric or abdominal discomfort or pain, GI ulceration.
**Nursing Considerations:** Give with meals or milk to decrease GI intolerance. If the child is unable to swallow a tablet, administer the medication in liquid form. Ibuprofen that is not enteric-coated can be crushed and mixed with a small amount of food or liquid before swallowing.

#### DRUG GUIDE

#### *Ketorolac*

**Classification:** Nonsteroidal antiinflammatory drug (NSAID), analgesic.
**Action:** Blocks prostaglandin synthesis.
**Indications:** Short-term management of moderate acute pain.
**Dosages and Route:** Children older than 6 months, IV dosage 0.5-1 mg/kg one time, up to 30 mg followed by 0.5 mg/kg/dose every 6 hours, up to a maximum of 60 mg/24 hours.
**Absorption:** Peak action in 15 minutes.
**Excretion:** Excreted in the urine; effects last 4-6 hours.
**Contraindications:** Contraindicated in patients in whom urticaria, severe rhinitis, bronchospasm, angioedema, nasal polyps are precipitated by other NSAIDs; active peptic ulcer; bleeding abnormalities, severe renal impairment.
**Precautions:** Cautious use with history of ulcers, impaired hepatic or renal function.
**Adverse Reactions:** Drowsiness, dizziness, nausea, gastrointestinal (GI) pain, hemorrhage.
**Nursing Considerations:** Do not administer longer than 5 days. Monitor renal and liver function studies, signs and symptoms of GI upset or bleeding.

can be used for children who cannot swallow tablets. When the oral route is contraindicated, IV or subcutaneous opioids (morphine, fentanyl, hydromorphone, methadone) can be given by bolus or continuous infusion. The IM route should only be used when absolutely necessary because of the great fear and pain of injections seen in many children (Mudd, 2011).

The starting dose for opioids is determined according to the child's body weight, physiologic development, and medical situation. The goal is to control pain as rapidly as possible, so the starting dose should be optimal (APS, 2011a). Weight-based starting doses have empirically been shown to be safe; however, they are not maximum doses. Opioids do not have a ceiling effect; further doses should be titrated based on the child's response. The dose should be titrated upward if pain is not significantly reduced or relieved, or titrated downward if a child experiences intolerable side effects.

The nurse should remember that opioids can produce sedation and respiratory depression in addition to analgesia. Other adverse effects can include constipation, pruritus, nausea, vomiting, cough suppression, and urinary retention. Although children experiencing adverse effects must be closely monitored, most can tolerate these medications if their dosages are adjusted. Pruritus, nausea, sedation, and urinary retention tend to be time limited and resolve spontaneously within 1 to 3 days. Until that time, antiemetics and antipruritics can be provided. Constipation does not resolve spontaneously. The nurse must remain vigilant and advocate for the use of laxatives and bowel stimulants to prevent constipation.

Hydrocodone is the most commonly given oral opioid for moderate pain. It is only available in combination with acetaminophen or ibuprofen, in tablet and liquid forms. As with all opioids, the nurse should carefully check dosing parameters for both the hydrocodone and the acetaminophen or ibuprofen that is prescribed. Oxycodone is also used to control moderate pain and comes as single agent or in combination with acetaminophen. It is also available as a sustained-release tablet.

## DRUG GUIDE

### *Hydrocodone*

**Classification:** Opioid analgesic.

**Action:** Binds to opiate receptors in the central nervous system (CNS) to diminish pain.

**Indications:** Mild pain to moderate pain; acute pain

**Dosage and Routes:** By mouth dosage, 0.1-0.2 mg/kg every 3-4 hours. Maximum dosage dependent on acetaminophen or ibuprofen content of product.

**Absorption:** Onset 10-20 minutes; duration 4-6 hours.

**Excretion:** Excreted in the urine; half-life, 3.5-4.5 hours.

**Contraindications:** Hypersensitivity to codeine, hydromorphone, or other morphine derivatives, addiction.

**Precautions:** Addictive personality, increased intracranial pressure, respiratory depression, hepatic disease, renal disease. Cautious use in head injuries, increased intracranial pressure, asthma, and other respiratory conditions.

**Adverse Reactions:** Nausea, vomiting, constipation, pruritus, dizziness, lightheadedness, confusion, hallucinations, mood changes, sedation, respiratory depression, dependence.

**Nursing Considerations:** Nausea is a common side effect; report if this is accompanied by vomiting. Because dizziness and lightheadedness can occur, supervision of ambulation and other safety precautions may be necessary. Assess respiratory status carefully; assess for CNS changes and implement appropriate safety measures.

## DRUG GUIDE

### *Oxycodone*

**Classification:** Opioid analgesic.

**Action:** Inhibits ascending pain pathways in the central nervous system (CNS), increases pain threshold, alters pain perception.

**Indications:** Moderate to severe pain. Acute or chronic pain.

**Dosage and Routes:** By mouth starting dosage, 0.1-0.2 mg/kg/dose every 4-6 hours; maximum starting dose, 10 mg.

**Absorption:** Onset 10-20 minutes; duration 4-6 hours.

**Excretion:** Excreted in the urine; half-life, 3.5-4.5 hours.

**Contraindications:** Hypersensitivity to oxycodone, codeine, or other morphine derivatives; hepatic or renal dysfunction, addiction.

**Precautions:** Addictive personality, increased intracranial pressure, respiratory depression, hepatic disease, renal disease. Cautious use in patients with head injuries, increased intracranial pressure, asthma, and other respiratory conditions.

**Adverse Reactions:** Nausea, vomiting, constipation, pruritus, dizziness, lightheadedness, confusion, hallucinations, mood changes, sedation, respiratory depression, dependence.

**Nursing Considerations:** Nausea is a common side effect; report if this is accompanied by vomiting. Because dizziness and lightheadedness can occur, supervision of ambulation and other safety precautions may be necessary. Assess respiratory status carefully; assess for CNS changes and implement appropriate safety measures. Titrate dosage up or down to maximize pain relief and minimize adverse effects.

Codeine, which is classified as a weak opioid, is no longer recommended for use in children because of the potential overdose that can occur in patients who have the ultrarapid-metabolizer phenotype (Anderson, 2013; Berde et al., 2012; Racoosin, Roberson, Pacanowski, et al., 2013; Tobias, 2014b).

Morphine is the preferred opioid for children. It reaches its peak effect 10 to 20 minutes after IV administration and 1 hour after oral administration. It can produce sedation along with the analgesia. If sedation occurs, maximum respiratory depression will happen 7 minutes after IV administration. Naloxone (Narcan) should be available to reverse sedation or respiratory depression, if necessary. Hydromorphone (Dilaudid) is very similar to morphine but is approximately six times more potent. It may be used as a first-line opioid for moderate to severe pain or as an alternative for patients who experience intolerable adverse effects from morphine.

Fentanyl and its analogs (sufentanil, alfentanil) have a shorter duration of action than morphine and are 50 to 100 times more potent. Because much less histamine is released in response to these agents, they cause less pruritus. The short duration of effect makes IV use of these drugs appropriate when a brief, severely painful procedure is to be performed (e.g., bone marrow aspiration, inserting a chest tube, changing a burn dressing) and when children are critically ill. Fentanyl should be administered in a closely monitored setting. The fentanyl patch (Duragesic) is indicated for chronic pain; experience with its use in children is limited. Although administered to children as young as 2 years old, it is usually prescribed for adolescents. Transdermal fentanyl, 25 mcg/hr system, is approximately equal to 15 mg of IV morphine in 24 hours or 90 mg of oral morphine in 24 hours. Intranasal fentanyl has been shown to be as effective as IV fentanyl or morphine in providing pain control, making it an appropriate option for acute or procedural pain control in children (Mudd, 2011).

Methadone is metabolized very slowly, and thus, has a prolonged duration of action. It is absorbed well after oral administration and can be given via the IV route as well. Because of its long duration,

## DRUG GUIDE
### *Morphine*

**Classification:** Opioid analgesic.
**Action:** Binds with central nervous system (CNS) opiate receptors; alters physical and emotional response to pain.
**Indications:** Moderate to severe pain. Acute and chronic pain.
**Dosages and Routes:** By mouth or per rectum intermittent dosage, 0.2-0.5 mg/kg/dose every 4-6 hours; extended-release dosage, 0.3-0.6 mg/kg/dose every 8-12 hours.
Intravenous (IV) or subcutaneous intermittent dosage, 0.05-0.1 mg/kg/dose every 2-4 hours; maximum dose, 15 mg/dose. Continuous IV infusion dosage, 0.01-0.05 mg/kg/hr.
**Absorption:** Variable absorption from the gastrointestinal (GI) tract; peak action 60 minutes orally, 10-20 minutes IV.
**Excretion:** Excreted primarily in the urine; 7%-10% excreted in bile. Effects last up to 7 hours.
**Contraindications:** Hypersensitivity to opioids, increased intracranial pressure, seizure disorders, chronic pulmonary disease, respiratory depression.
**Precautions:** Cautious use with cardiac arrhythmias, reduced blood volume, addictive personality.
**Adverse Reactions:** Primarily CNS symptoms: dizziness, lightheadedness, drowsiness, sedation, lethargy, euphoria, agitation, restlessness, respiratory depression. GI symptoms; nausea, vomiting, constipation. Genitourinary (GU) symptoms: urinary retention. Pruritus.
**Nursing Considerations:** Nausea is a common side effect; report if this is accompanied by vomiting. Because dizziness and lightheadedness can occur, supervision of ambulation and other safety precautions may be necessary. Assess respiratory status carefully and frequently; assess for CNS changes and implement appropriate safety measures. Monitor intake and output related to urinary retention and constipation. Begin with the lowest dosage and titrate dosage up or down to maximize pain relief and minimize adverse effects.

it must be carefully titrated according to the patient's pain level; thus, diligent pain assessment is required. It is equal in potency to morphine.

Meperidine (Demerol) should be used only for short-term pain control (e.g., postoperatively) in children who have shown an allergy or intolerance to other opioids. The duration of analgesia is shorter than with morphine. Meperidine has been associated with convulsions and dysphoria after as few as two doses. It also has been known to cause hallucinations and agitation (Tobias, 2014b). Meperidine is infrequently prescribed for children.

Opioid prescriptions for children and adolescents have increased recently, which may be the result of better pain management in this population. With this change comes an increased risk of potential adverse events and misuse of the medication. Nurses must remain vigilant in assessing for signs of misuse and educate parents about recognizing important adverse effects (Voepel-Lewis, Zikmund-Fisher, Smith, et al., 2015).

### Procedural Sedation

Procedural sedation is a medically controlled state of depressed consciousness that allows the patient to respond appropriately to verbal and tactile stimulation and to maintain oxygenation and airway control independently. The child retains protective airway reflexes (e.g., cough and gag reflexes). There is a continuum of sedation levels: minimum, moderate (referred to as conscious sedation), and deep.

Procedural sedation is generally achieved through IV administration of a sedative-hypnotic (midazolam, propofol), an analgesic

## DRUG GUIDE
### *Hydromorphone*

**Classification:** Opioid analgesic.
**Action:** Inhibits ascending pain pathways in the central nervous system (CNS), increases pain threshold, alters pain perception.
**Indications:** Moderate to severe pain, acute and chronic pain.
**Dosages and Routes:** By mouth or subcutaneous dosage, 0.03-0.08 mg/kg/dose every 4 hours, with maximum starting dose of 7.5 mg. Intravenous (IV) intermittent dosage, 0.015 mg/kg/dose every 3-6 hours. IV continuous infusion dosage, 3-5 mcg/kg/hr.
**Absorption:** Onset 15-20 minutes; peak 0.5-1 hours; duration 4-5 hours.
**Excretion:** Excreted in the urine, half-life 3.5-4.5 hours.
**Contraindications:** Hypersensitivity, addiction.
**Precautions:** Addictive personality, increased intracranial pressure, respiratory depression, hepatic disease, renal disease. Cautious use in head injuries, increased intracranial pressure, asthma, and other respiratory conditions. Impaired renal or hepatic function.
**Adverse Reactions:** Nausea, vomiting, constipation, pruritus, dizziness, lightheadedness, confusion, hallucinations, mood changes, sedation, respiratory depression, dependence, increased urine output, urinary retention, seizures, palpitations, bradycardia, tachycardia, hypotension, other changes in blood pressure.
**Nursing Considerations:** Nausea is a common side effect; report if this is accompanied by vomiting. Because dizziness and lightheadedness may occur, supervision of ambulation and other safety precautions may be necessary. Assess respiratory status carefully; assess for CNS changes and implement appropriate safety measures. Titrate dosage up or down to maximize pain relief and minimize adverse effects.

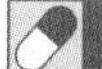

## DRUG GUIDE
### *Fentanyl*

**Classification:** Opioid analgesic.
**Action:** Opioid agonist with actions similar to morphine and meperidine, but action is faster and less prolonged.
**Indications:** Moderate to severe pain, particularly for brief procedures and when children are critically ill or high risk. Transdermal fentanyl is for moderate to severe chronic pain only; experience with children is limited.
**Dosages and Routes:** Intramuscular (IM), intravenous (IV), intranasal (IN) intermittent dosage, 1-2 mcg/kg/dose every 30-60 minutes. IV continuous infusion dosage, 0.05-3 mcg/kg/hr. Transdermal patch dosage, 25 mcg/hr system; used only in opioid-tolerant children older than 2 years.
**Absorption:** Absorbed rapidly after IV administration; 6-8 hours transdermally.
**Excretion:** Excreted in the urine. Lasts 30-60 minutes IV; 72 hours transdermally.
**Contraindication:** Hypersensitivity, addiction, patients who have received monoamine oxidase inhibitors within 14 days.
**Precautions:** Addictive personality. Use cautiously in children with head injuries, increased intracranial pressure, respiratory problems, hepatic and renal dysfunction.
**Adverse Reactions:** Nausea, vomiting, constipation, pruritus, dizziness, lightheadedness, confusion, hallucinations, mood changes, sedation, respiratory depression, dependence, increased urine output, urinary retention, seizures, palpitations, bradycardia, tachycardia, hypotension, other changes in blood pressure.
**Nursing Considerations:** Watch carefully for signs and symptoms of respiratory distress and depression. Have oxygen, resuscitative equipment, and naloxone available. Administer slow IV push to prevent chest wall rigidity.

## DRUG GUIDE

### *Methadone*

**Classification:** Opioid analgesic.
**Action:** Depresses pain impulse transmission at the spinal cord level through interaction with opioid receptors, thus producing central nervous system (CNS) depression.
**Indications:** Severe acute and chronic pain, opioid withdrawal.
**Dosages and Routes:** By mouth, subcutaneous, intramuscular (IM) and intravenous (IV) dosage, 0.05-0.1 mg/kg/dose every 4-6 or 12 hours. Maximum single dose, 10 mg.
**Absorption:** Variable absorption from the gastrointestinal (GI) tract; peak action, 60 minutes orally, 20 minutes IV.
**Excretion:** Excreted in the urine, crosses the placenta, excreted in breast milk. Half-life is 15-30 hours.
**Contraindications:** Hypersensitivity to this drug, chlorobutanol injection, addiction.
**Precautions:** Cautious use with addictive personalities, increased intracranial pressure, respiratory depression, hepatic or renal disease.
**Adverse Reactions:** Sedation, dizziness, confusion, euphoria, seizures, respiratory depression, hypotension, bradycardia, palpitations, nausea, vomiting, constipation, urinary retention.
**Nursing Considerations:** Carefully and frequently assess level of sedation and respiratory status. Assess cough reflex. Monitor intake and output checking for urinary retention and constipation. Titrate dosage up or down to maximize pain relief and minimize adverse effects.

(opioid), a dissociative (ketamine) medication, or a combination of these medications (Johnson, Miller, & Hagemann, 2012). However, multiple routes can be used: IV, intranasal, rectal, IM, oral, and sublingual. Frequently used for sedation as well as induction of general anesthesia, midazolam (Versed) is a short-acting sedative-hypnotic that can be given by multiple routes. Midazolam is often used for procedural sedation because it has minimal side effects, is short-acting, and can be used without IV access. It has no analgesic properties; therefore, for painful procedures, it should be given in combination with an opioid.

Children receiving procedural sedation require the care of clinicians with advanced skills in airway management, such as trained physicians, anesthesiologists, or nurse anesthetists. The level of sedation is not dose dependent. Children given recommended doses may remain alert and only experience reduced anxiety, or they may become moderately to deeply sedated. The nurse's role in administering and monitoring patients receiving sedation agents varies with agency policies and state regulations. It is important that nurses participate in the frequent assessment and documentation of the child's vital signs, oxygen saturation, capnography (concentration of exhaled carbon dioxide), and level of consciousness both during and after procedural sedation (Jest & Tonge, 2011).

## NURSING QUALITY ALERT

### *Pain Management for Children*

- The preferred route of administering analgesics to children is oral or intravenous (IV).
- As soon as the child can tolerate oral intake, pain medication should be changed from the IV to the oral route.
- After starting with the recommended initial dose for opioids, the dose is adjusted (titrated) to achieve best pain management with the fewest side effects.
- Opioids do not have a dose limit. The maximum dose is the dose that causes unacceptable side effects.
- Infants and children receiving epidural opioids should be monitored by a cardiac and apnea monitor and pulse oximetry.
- A cardiac and apnea monitor and a pulse oximeter may be required to monitor certain infants and children receiving IV opioids (e.g., neonates, children who are opioid naïve, children with a history of apnea or other respiratory difficulties). The risk of respiratory depression is greatest during the first 24 hours of administration.
- If respiratory depression occurs with opioid use, naloxone hydrochloride should be administered for reversal, if oxygen and stimulation of the child are ineffective.

### Epidural Analgesia

Pain medication (usually an opioid, a local anesthetic, or both) can be administered through an epidural catheter inserted into the epidural space of the spinal canal and secured to the child's back with an occlusive dressing. Because the medication is administered directly to the nerves that transmit pain, smaller doses are required for pain control, with fewer side effects than are usually associated with systemic (IV) opioid administration. Epidural analgesia is used for children following abdominal, anal, and genitourinary surgeries and procedures; open-heart and thoracic surgeries; and orthopedic surgeries of the lower limbs.

Nursing care of the child with an epidural catheter is similar to that for a child receiving PCA therapy. The child is attached to a continuous cardiac monitor and pulse oximeter. It is essential that the nurse assess the child for adequate pain relief, the presence of adverse effects (particularly decreased respirations), and for complications related to the epidural catheter placement (Schreiber, 2015). Possible side effects include constipation, nausea, vomiting, urinary retention, motor block, and sensory block. The child's dermatome level (the level of sensory blockade) and motor responses are checked at least every 4 hours. It is important to avoid any action that could pull or place tension on the catheter. The epidural catheter insertion site must be inspected frequently. Displacement (slippage), bleeding, leakage of cerebrospinal fluid, or a hematoma must be reported to the child's physician or anesthesiologist immediately.

## KEY CONCEPTS

- Pain is whatever the experiencing person says it is, existing whenever the person says it does.
- According to the gate control theory of pain, there is a gating mechanism in the spinal cord that facilitates or inhibits pain transmission. Stimulation of larger afferent nerves can dull pain.
- Two prevalent myths that children receiving pain medication are at a high risk for respiratory depression and that they are at an increased risk for addiction are not supported by evidence yet interfere with adequate pain management for infants and children.
- Pain assessment in infants and children takes a multidimensional approach. The child and parent are both interviewed, and behavioral and physiologic changes are evaluated.
- A developmentally appropriate pain assessment tool is used to assess, implement, and document effective pain management for an infant, child, or adolescent.
- Both pharmacologic and non-pharmacologic measures should be used together in the treatment of pain in children.

## REFERENCES AND READINGS


American Pain Society. (2011a). *The assessment and management of acute pain in infants, children, and adolescents: a position statement from the American academy of pediatrics committee on psychosocial aspects of child and family health and American pain society task force on pain in infants, children and adolescents.* Retrieved from http://www.ampainsoc.org/library/bulletin/sep01/article1.htm.

American Pain Society. (2011b). *Pediatric chronic pain: A position statement from the American pain society.* Retrieved from http://www.ampainsoc.org/library/bulletin/jan01/posi1.htm.

American Pain Society. (2011c). *Publications: clinical practice guidelines.* Retrieved from http://www.ampainsoc.org/pub/cp_guidelines.htm.

American Society for Pain Management Nursing. (2012). *Assessment and management of children with chronic pain.* Retrieved from: http://www.aspmn.org.

Anderson, B. (2013). Is it farewell to codeine? *Archives of Diseases in Childhood*, 1–3. doi: 10.1136/archdischild-2013-304974.

Anderson, C., Rolfe, P., & Brennan-Hunter, A. (2013). Administration of over-the-counter medication to children at home- a survey of parents from community health centers. *Journal of Community Health Nursing, 30*, 143–154. doi:10.1080/07370016.2013.806716.

Avansino, J.R., Peters, L.M., Stockfish, S.L., et al. (2013). A paradigm shift to balance safety and quality in pediatric pain management. *Pediatrics, 131*(3), e921–e927. doi:10.1542/peds.2012-1378.

Baker, C.M., & Wong, D.L. (1987). Q.U.E.S.T.: A process of pain assessment in children. *Orthopaedic Nursing, 6*(1), 11–20.

Berde, C.B., Walco, G.A., Krane, E.J., et al. (2012). Pediatric analgesic clinical trial designs, measures, and extrapolation: report of an FDA scientific workshop. *Pediatrics, 129*(2), 354–364. doi:10.1542/peds.2010-3591.

Beyer, J., Villarruel, A., & Denyes, M. (2009). *The Oucher: user's manual and technical report.* Retrieved from http://www.oucher.org/downloads/2009_Users_Manual.pdf.

Chen-Lim, M.L., Zarnowsky, C., Green, R., et al. (2012). Optimizing the assessment of pain in children who are cognitively impaired through the quality improvement process. *Journal of Pediatric Nursing, 27*, 750–759. doi:10.1016/j.pedn.2012.03.023.

Cline, M.E., Herman, J., & Shaw, E. (1992). Standardization of the visual analogue scale. *Nursing Research, 41*(6), 378–379.

Cong, X., McGrath, J. M., Cusson, R., et al. (2013). Pain assessment and measurement in neonates. *Advances in Neonatal Care, 13*(6), 379–395. doi:10.1097/ANC.0b013e3182a41452.

Crosta, Q.R., Ward, T.M., Walker, A.J., et al. (2014). A review of pain measures for hospitalized children with cognitive impairment. *Journal for Specialists in Pediatric Nursing, 19*, 109–118. doi:10.1111/jspn.12069.

Czarnecki, M.L., Simon, K., Thompson, J.J., et al. (2011a). Barriers to pediatric pain management: a nursing perspective. *Pain Management Nursing, 12*(3), 154–162. doi:10.1016/j.pmn.2010.07.001.

Czarnecki, M.L., Salamon, K.S., Mano, K.E., et al. (2011b). A preliminary report of patient/nurse-controlled analgesia (PNCA) in infants and preschoolers. *Clinical Journal of Pain, 27*(2), 102–107.

Czarnecki, M.L., Turner, H.N., Collins, P.M., et al. (2011c). Procedural pain management: a position statement with clinical practice recommendations. *Pain Management Nursing, 12*(2), 95–111. doi:10.1016/j.pmn.2011.02.003.

Dolbier, C.L., & Rush, T.E. (2012). Efficacy of abbreviated progressive muscle relaxation in a high-stress college sample. *International Journal of Stress Management, 19*(1), 48–68. doi:10.1037/a0027326.

Ely, E., Chen-Lim, M.L., Zarnowsky, C., et al. (2012). Finding the evidence to change practice for assessing pain in children who are cognitively impaired. *Journal of Pediatric Nursing, 27*, 402–410. doi:10.1016/j.pedn.2011.05.009.

Freitas, G.R., Castro, C.G., Castro, S.M., et al. (2014). Degree of knowledge of health care professionals about pain management and use of opioids in pediatric. *Pain Medicine, 15*, 807–819.

Gorodzinsky, A.Y., Bernacki, J.M., Davies, W.H., et al. (2012). Community parents' use of non-pharmacological techniques for childhood pain management. *Children's Health Care, 41*, 1–15. doi:10.1080/02739615.2012.643286.

Gorodzinsky, A.Y., Davies, W.H., & Drendel, A.L. (2014). Parents' treatment of their children's pain at home: pharmacological and nonpharmacological approaches. *Journal of Pediatric Health Care, 28*(2), 136–146. doi:10.1016/jpedhc.2012.12.007.

Habich, M., & Letizia, M. (2015). Pediatric pain assessment. in the emergency department: a nursing evidence-based practice protocol. *Pediatric Nursing, 41*(4), 198–202.

Harrington, J.W., Logan, S., Harwell, C., et al. (2012). Effective analgesia using physical interventions for infant immunizations. *Pediatrics, 129*(5), 815–822. doi:10.1542/peds.2011-1607.

Herr, K., Coyne, P., McCaffery, M., et al. (2011). Pain assessment in the patient unable to self-report: Position statement with clinical practice recommendations. *Pain Management Nursing, 12*(4), 230–250. doi:10.1016/j.pmn.2011.10.002.

Hester, N.O., Foster, R.L., Jordan-Marsh, M., et al. (1998). Putting pain measurement into clinical practice. In G.A. Finley, & P.J. McGrath (Eds.), *Measurement of pain in infants and children* (Vol. 10). Seattle: International Association for the Study of Pain Press.

Hockenberry, M., & Wilson, D. (2009). *Wong's essentials of pediatric nursing* (8th ed.). St. Louis: Mosby.

Hyde, C., Price, J., & Nicholl, H. (2012). Neuropathic pain management in children. *International Journal of Palliative Nursing, 18*(10), 476–482.

International Association for the Study of Pain (Subcommittee on Taxonomy). (1979). Pain terms: a list with definitions and notes on usage. *Pain, 6*(3), 249–252.

Jacobson, C.J., Farrell, J.E., Kashikar-Zuck, S., et al. (2013). Disclosure and self-report of emotional, social, and physical health in children and adolescents with chronic pain: a qualitative study of PROMIS pediatric measures. *Journal of Pediatric Psychology, 38*(1), 82–93. doi:10.1093/jpepsy/jss099.

Jest, A.D., & Tonge, A. (2011), Using a learning needs assessment to identify knowledge deficits regarding procedural sedation for pediatric patients. *AORN Journal, 94*(6), 567–574. doi:10.1016/j.aorn.2011.05.020

Joestlein, L. (2015). Pain, pain, go away! evidence-based review of developmentally appropriate pain assessment for children in a postoperative setting. *Orthopaedic Nursing, 34*(5), 252–259. doi:10.1097/NOR.0000000000000175.

Johnson, M. (2014). Transcutaneous electrical nerve stimulation: review of effectiveness. *Nursing Standard, 28*(40), 44–53.

Johnson, P., Miller, J., & Hagemann, T.M. (2012). Sedation and analgesia in critically ill children. *AACN Advanced Critical Care, 23*(4), 415–434. doi: 10.1097/NCI.0b013e31826b4dea.

Jongudomkarn, D., Forgeron, P.A., Siripul, P., et al. (2012) My child you must have patience and kreng jai: Thai parents and child pain. *Journal of Nursing Scholarship, 44*(4), 323–331. doi:10.1111/j.1547-5069.2012.01467.

Kesavan, K. (2015). Neurodevelopmental implications of neonatal pain and morphine exposure. *Pediatric Annals, 44*(11), e260–e264. doi:10.3928/00904481-20151112-08.

Knox, M., Lentini, J., Cummings, T.S., et al. (2011). Game-based biofeedback for paediatric anxiety and depression. *Mental Health in Family Medicine, 8*, 195–203.

Krechel, S.W., & Bildner, J. (1995). CRIES: A new neonatal postoperative pain measurement score. Initial testing of validity and reliability. *Paediatric Anaesthesia, 5*(1), 53–61.

Madhok, M., Scribner-O'Pray, M., & Teele, M. (2011). No needless pain: managing pediatric pain in minor injuries. *Contemporary Pediatrics, 28*(6), 24–31.

Mano, K.E., Evans, J.R., Tran, S.T., et al. (2012). The psychometric properties of the screen for child anxiety related emotional disorders in pediatric chronic pain. *Journal of Pediatric Psychology, 37*(9), 999–1011. doi:10.1093/jpepsy/jss069.

McNamara, M.C., Harmon, D., & Saunders, J. (2012). Effect of education on knowledge, skills and attitudes around pain. *British Journal of Nursing, 21*(16), 958–964.

Melby, V. (2011). Acute pain relief in children: use of rating scales and analgesia. *Emergency Nurse, 19*(6), 32–36.

Melzack, R., & Wall, P. (1965). Pain mechanisms: A new theory. *Science, 150*(699), 971–979.

Merkel, S., Voepel-Lewis, T., & Malviya, S. (2002). Pain assessment in infants and young children: The FLACC scale: a behavioral tool to measure pain in young children. *American Journal of Nursing, 102*(10), 55–58.

Mesko, P.J., Eliades, A.B., Libertin, C.C., et al. (2011). Use of picture communication aids to assess pain location in pediatric postoperative patients. *Journal of Perianesthesia Nursing, 26*(6), 395–404. doi:10.1016/j.jopan.2011.09.006.

Moayedi, M., & Davis, K.D. (2013). Theories of pain: from specificity to gate control. *Journal of Neurophysiology, 109*, 5–12. doi:10.1152/jn.00457.2012.

Mosiman, W., & Pile, D. (2013). Emerging therapies in pediatric pain management. *Journal of Infusion Nursing, 36*(2), 98–106. doi:10.1097/NAN.0b013e31828a8a5.

Mudd, S. (2011). Intranasal fentanyl for pain management in children: a systematic review of the literature. *Journal of Pediatric Health Care, 25*(5), 316–322. doi: 10.1016/jedhc.2010.04.011.

Nash, L. (2012). How to assess pain in children and young people. *Emergency Nurse, 20*(2), 19–22.

Obrecht, J.A., Van Hulle V.C., & Ryan, C.S. (2014).Implementation of evidence-based practice for a pediatric assessment instrument. *Clinical Nurse Specialist*, 97–104. doi:10.1097/NUR.0000000000000032.

Olmstead, D.L., Scott, S.D., Mayan, M., et al. (2014). Influences shaping nurses' use of distraction for children's procedural pain. *Journal for Specialists in Pediatric Nursing, 19*, 162–171. doi:10.1111/jspn.12067.

Pasero, C., & McCaffery, M. (2011). *Pain assessment and pharmacologic management.* St. Louis: Mosby.

Palermo, T.M., Valrie, C.R., & Karlson, C.W. (2014). Family and parent influences on pediatric chronic pain. *American Psychologist, 69*(2), 142–152. doi:10.1037/a0035216.

Racoosin, J.A., Roberson, D.W, Pacanowski, M.A., et al. (2013). New evidence about an old drug-risk with codeine after adenotonsillectomy. *New England Journal of Medicine, 368*(23), 2155–2157.

Reavey, D.A., Haney, B.M., Atchison, L., et al. (2014). Improving pain assessment in the NICU. *Advances in Neonatal Care, 14*(3), 144–153.

Sadhasivam, S., Chidambaran, V., Ngamprasertwong, P., et al. (2012). Race and unequal burden of perioperative pain and opioid related adverse effects in children. *Pediatrics, 129*(5), 832–838. doi:10.1542/peds.2011-2607.

Savedra, M.C., Tesler, M.D., & Holzemer, W.L. (1992). *Adolescent and pediatric pain tool: User's manual.* San Francisco: University of California, San Francisco, School of Nursing.

Schreiber, M.L. (2015). Nursing care considerations: the epidural catheter. *MedSurg Nursing, 24*(4), 273–276.

Sieberg, C.B., Williams, S., & Simons, L.E. (2011). Do parent protective responses mediate the relation between parent distress and child functional disability among children with chronic pain? *Journal of Pediatric Psychology, 36*(9), 1043–1051.

Shomaker, K., Dutton, S., & Mark, M. (2015). Pain prevalence and treatment patterns in a US children's hospital. *Hospital Pediatrics, 5*(7), 363–370. doi:10.1542/hpeds.2014-0195.

Sng, Q.W., Taylor, B., Liam, J.L., et al. (2013). Postoperative pain management experiences among school-aged children: a qualitative study. *Journal of Clinical Nursing, 22*, 958–968. doi:10.1111/jocn.12052.

Stanley, M., & Pollard, D. (2013). Relationship between knowledge, attitudes, and self-efficacy of nurses in the management of pediatric pain. *Pediatric Nursing, 39*(4) 165–171.

Stapelkamp, C., Carter, B., Gordon, J., et al. (2011). Assessment of acute pain in children: development of evidence-based guideline. *International Journal of Evidence-Based Healthcare, 9*, 39–50. doi:10.1111/j.1744-1609.201000199.

Swift, A. (2015). Pain management 1: how the body detects pain stimuli. *Nursing Times, 111*(39) 20–23.

The Joint Commission. (2011). *Facts about pain management.* Retrieved from http://www.jointcommission.org/assets/1/18/Pain_Management.pdf.

The Joint Commission. (2014). Clarification of the pain management standard. *Joint Commission Perspectives, 34*(11), 11.

Tobias, J.D. (2014a). Acute management in infants and children-part 1: pain pathways, pain assessment, and outpatient pain management. *Pediatric Annals, 43*(7), e163–e168. doi:10.3928/00904481-20140619-10.

Tobias, J.D. (2014b). Acute management in infants and children-part 2: intravenous opioids, intravenous nonsteroidal anti-inflammatory drugs, and managing adverse effects. *Pediatric Annals, 43*(7), e169–e175. doi:10.3928/00904481-20140619-11.

Twycross, A., & Collins, S. (2013). Nurses' views about the barriers and facilitators to effective management of pediatric pain. *Pain Management Nursing, 14*(4), e164–e172. doi:10.1016/jpmn.2011.10.007.

Twycross, A., & Finley, G.A. (2013). Children's and parents' perceptions of postoperative pain management: a mixed methods study. *Journal of Clinical Nursing, 22*, 3095–3108.

Twycross, A., & Finley, G.A. (2014). Nurses' aims when managing pediatric postoperative pain: Is what they say the same as what they do? *Journal for Specialists in Pediatric Nursing, 19*, 17–27. doi:10.111/jspn.12029.

Twycross, A., Finley, G.A., & Latimer, M. (2013). Pediatric nurses' postoperative pain management practices: an observational study. *Journal for Specialists in Pediatric Nursing, 18*, 189–201. doi:10.111/jspn.12026.

Vael, A., & Whitted, K. (2014). An educational intervention to improve pain assessment in preverbal children. *Pediatric Nursing, 40*(6), 302–306

Van Dijk, M., Peters, J., & Van Deventer, P. (2005). The COMFORT behavior scale: a tool for assessing pain and sedation in infants. *American Journal of Nursing, 105*(1), 33–36.

Van Hulle V.C., Chiappetta, M., Beach, A., et al. (2012). Parents' management of children's pain at home after surgery. *Journal for Specialists in Pediatric Nursing, 17*, 108–120. doi: 10.1111/j.1744-6155.2012.00326.

Van Hulle, V.C., Wilkie, D.J., & Wang, E. (2011). Pediatric nurses' beliefs and pain management practices: an intervention pilot. *Western Journal of Nursing Research, 33*(6), 825–845. doi:10.1177/0193945910391681.

Voepel-Lewis, T. (2011). Bridging the gap between pain assessment and treatment: time for a new theoretical approach? *Western Journal of Nursing Research, 33*(6), 846–851. doi:10.1177/0193945911403940.

Voepel-Lewis, T., Zikmund-Fisher, B., Smith, E.L., et al. (2015). Opioid-related adverse drug events: do parents recognize the signals? *Clinical Journal of Pain, 31*(3), 198–205. doi:10.1097/AJP.0000000000000111.

Wohlheiter, K.A., & Dalquist, L.M. (2013). Interactive versus passive distraction for acute pain management in young children: the role of selective attention and development. *Journal of Pediatric Psychology, 38*(2), 202–212. doi:10.1093/jpepsy/jss108.

Wong, C., Lau, E., Palozzi, L., et al. (2012). Pain management in children: part 1- pain assessment tools and a brief review of nonpharmacological and pharmacological treatment options. *Canadian Pharmacists Journal, 145*(5), 222–225.

Wong-Baker FACES Foundation. (1983). *Translations of the Wong-Baker FACES pain rating scale.* Retrieved from http://www.wongbakerfaces.org/wp-content/uploads/2010/12/FACES_translation1.pdf.

World Health Organization. (2010). *WHO's pain ladder.* Retrieved from http://who.int/cancer/palliative/painladder/en.

Wuhrman, E., & Broglio, K. (2015). Patient-controlled analgesia helps manage pain. *Nursing 2015 Critical Care, 10*(4), 38–42. doi:10.1097/01.CCN.0000466767.85553.95.

40

# The Child With a Fluid and Electrolyte Alteration

http://evolve.elsevier.com/McKinney/mat-ch/

## LEARNING OBJECTIVES

*After studying this chapter, you should be able to:*

- Identify the regulatory mechanisms that maintain fluid and electrolyte balance in the body.
- Compare those differences in body fluid and electrolyte composition and regulation between infants or children and adults that make infants and children more vulnerable to imbalances.
- Describe dehydration and acid–base imbalance.
- Differentiate among the various types of acid–base disturbances.
- Describe the processes and nursing care of a child with diarrhea or vomiting.
- Integrate assessment findings with nursing implementation to determine the success of therapy.
- Describe nursing interventions to prevent fluid and electrolyte imbalances.

## CLINICAL REFERENCE

### REVIEW OF FLUID AND ELECTROLYTE IMBALANCES IN CHILDREN

Characteristics unique to infants and young children make them more vulnerable than adults to fluid and electrolyte imbalances. Under normal conditions, the amount of fluid ingested during a day should equal the amount of fluid lost through sensible water loss (e.g., urine output) and insensible water loss (through the respiratory tract and skin). Insensible water loss per unit of body weight is significantly higher in infants and children. The faster respiratory rates of infants and young children also result in higher evaporative water losses. Any condition that prevents normal oral fluid intake (e.g., vomiting) or results in fluid losses (e.g., diarrhea, hyperventilation, burns, hemorrhage) is especially significant because it depletes the body's store of water and electrolytes much more rapidly in infants and young children than in adults.

Body water is located in two major compartments: within the cell, in the intracellular compartment; and outside the cell, in the extracellular compartment. These two compartments are separated by the cell membrane, across which body fluid is continually exchanged. Extracellular fluid (ECF) is located in several places: in interstitial spaces (surrounding the cells [e.g., lymph fluid]), intravascularly (within the blood vessels or plasma), and transcellularly (e.g., cerebrospinal fluid, pericardial fluid, pleural fluid, synovial fluid, sweat, digestive secretions). A child is more likely to lose ECF than intracellular fluid (ICF). ECF is lost first when fluid loss occurs (e.g., through illness, trauma, fever). The intracellular compartment is more difficult to dehydrate.

In the neonate, approximately 40% of body water is located in the extracellular compartment compared with 20% in the adolescent and adult. In the infant, half of the ECF is exchanged, while an adult exchanges one sixth of the ECF in the same amount of time. Because approximately 50% of this ECF is exchanged daily in an infant, dehydration can occur very suddenly and rapidly if fluid intake is inadequate or fluid losses are excessive. Because of the infant's higher metabolic rate, the rate of water turnover is rapid. Depletion of ECF, often caused by gastroenteritis, is one of the most common problems among infants and young children. In adults and older children, because a greater proportion of fluid is located in the intracellular compartment, severe fluid depletion does not occur as rapidly. Maturity in body space distribution is usually reached around age 3 years.

Body fluids have 2 primary components: water and solutes. *Water* is the primary constituent, with the infant's weight being approximately 75% water to the adult's 55% to 60%. In general, the volume of total body water to total body weight decreases with increasing age. An inverse relationship exists between total body water and total body fat. Compared with adults, neonates, particularly premature infants, have a lower proportion of fat.

The *solutes* include both electrolytes and nonelectrolytes. Most of the body's solutes are electrolytes, primarily sodium ($Na^+$), potassium ($K^+$), chloride ($Cl^-$), calcium ($Ca^{2+}$), and magnesium ($Mg^{2+}$). The primary electrolyte of the ECF is sodium; potassium and magnesium are the primary electrolytes in the ICF. The extracellular compartment contains more sodium and chloride during infancy, which increases the vulnerability of infants to electrolyte imbalances. Changes in the concentration of these electrolytes may result in cellular dysfunction and illness. Problems of fluid and electrolyte balance involve both water and electrolytes; thus, treatment includes the replacement of both, calculated according to serum electrolyte laboratory values.

### ALTERATIONS IN ACID–BASE BALANCE IN CHILDREN

Alterations in the acid–base balance can affect cellular metabolism and enzymatic processes. The body's ability to regulate this status is

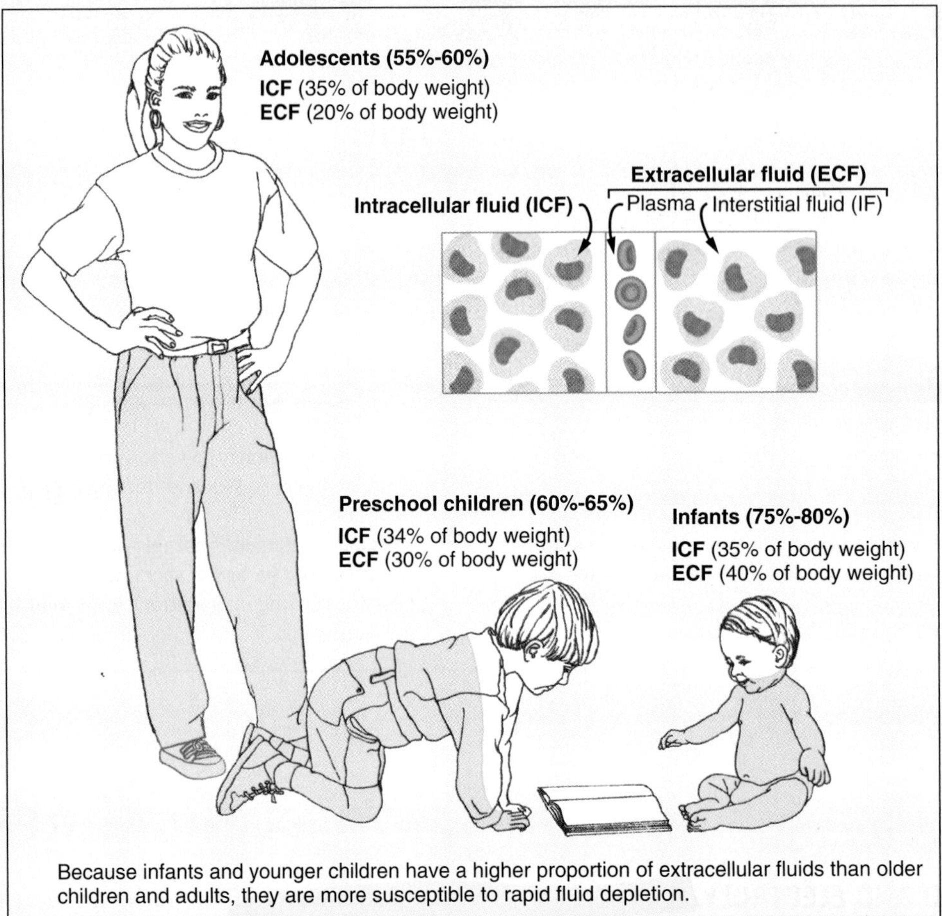


Because infants and younger children have a higher proportion of extracellular fluids than older children and adults, they are more susceptible to rapid fluid depletion.

## Pediatric Differences Related to Fluid and Electrolyte Balance

**Infants**

- Because of the higher percentage of water in the extracellular fluid (ECF), infants can lose fluids equal to their ECF within 2 to 3 days.
- Infants are less able to concentrate urine because of immature renal function.
- Infants have a higher rate of peristalsis than do older children.
- Infants have an immature lower esophageal sphincter, making them more prone to gastroesophageal reflux, which can lead to dehydration and electrolyte disturbances.
- Infants have a harder time compensating for acidosis because of their decreased ability to acidify urine.

**Infants and Children**

- Infants and young children have a higher metabolic turnover of water relative to adults because of a higher metabolic rate. (If losses are not replaced rapidly, imbalance occurs.)
- Infants and young children are unable to verbalize or communicate thirst.
- In comparison with adults, infants and children have a proportionately greater body surface area in relation to body mass, resulting in a greater potential for fluid loss through the skin and gastrointestinal tract.
- Infants and children have a higher proportionate water content (premature infants, 90%; term infants, 75% to 80%; preschool children, 60% to 65%; and adolescents and adults, approximately 55% to 60%), with a larger proportion of fluid in the extracellular space.
- The immune system of infants and children is not as robust as an adult's immune system, rendering young children more susceptible to infectious diseases, fever, gastroenteritis, and respiratory infections, all of which can result in fluid and electrolyte disturbances and fluid-volume deficit.
- Infants and children are at higher risk because of increased exposure to infections in a daycare or nursery setting.

crucial. Numerous pathologic conditions can cause an acid–base imbalance in children. The pH, or measure of acidity or alkalinity of body fluids, is regulated within a narrow range (normal blood pH is 7.35 to 7.45). Maintenance of serum pH within normal limits is crucial to maintaining cellular function, enzyme activity, and neuromuscular membrane potentials. Chemical buffers, the respiratory system, and the kidneys work together to keep the blood pH within normal range. Acid is constantly produced as a byproduct of metabolism. The body attempts to maintain blood pH within normal limits by reducing the buildup of acid. Extracellular and intracellular buffer systems minimize the effect of alterations in blood pH by neutralizing excess acids and bases that accumulate in body fluids. Two of the most significant buffers are bicarbonate and proteins. Bicarbonate, the most important buffer for plasma and interstitial fluids, is responsible for most ECF buffering and can exert its effects relatively quickly (within minutes).

When alterations in pH become too much for the buffer systems to handle, compensatory mechanisms in the respiratory and renal systems are activated. The respiratory system works rapidly to compensate for acid–base disturbances. If the blood pH drops below normal (causing **acidosis**), the respiratory rate and depth will increase, removing carbon dioxide and raising blood pH. Conversely, in the presence of **alkalosis**, the respiratory rate and depth decrease, thus lowering blood pH.

Kidneys regulate bicarbonate and remove hydrogen ions from the blood. If the blood is too alkaline, the kidneys conserve hydrogen ions, thus lowering blood pH. In the presence of acidosis, the kidneys excrete hydrogen ions and conserve bicarbonate, raising blood pH. Renal compensatory processes work more slowly than respiratory mechanisms—usually within 1 to 2 days. If compensatory mechanisms are ineffective, acid–base imbalances occur. When a dysfunction results in decreased hydrogen ion concentration in the blood, the arterial pH increases (causing alkalosis). When a dysfunction results in an increase in hydrogen ions, the arterial pH decreases (causing acidosis). It is important to remember the following when an acid-base imbalance occurs:

- Normal values from which to interpret blood gases: $Paco_2$, 35 to 45 mm Hg; pH, 7.35 to 7.45; bicarbonate, 22 to 26 mEq/L.
- When metabolic compensation occurs, assume origin in respiratory alteration.
- When respiratory compensation and release of tissue buffers occur, assume metabolic origin.

## ! NURSING QUALITY ALERT

### *Treatment Goals in Acid–Base Imbalance*

The treatment of metabolic acid–base disturbance is oriented toward correcting the underlying problem. The treatment of respiratory imbalance is directed toward reestablishing alveolar ventilation.

## Overview of Fluid and Electrolyte Disorders

| Disorder | Precipitating Events | Clinical Manifestations |
|---|---|---|
| Hyponatremia (sodium <135 mEq/L) | Fever<br>Increased water intake without electrolytes<br>Decreased sodium intake<br>Diabetic ketoacidosis<br>Burns and wounds<br>SIADH<br>Malnutrition<br>Cystic fibrosis<br>Renal disease<br>Vomiting, diarrhea, nasogastric suction | Neurologic:<br>• Usually do not show signs until sodium reaches 125 mEq/L<br>• Behavioral changes: irritability, lethargy, headache, dizziness, apprehension<br>Cardiovascular:<br>• Increased heart rate<br>• Decreased blood pressure<br>• Cold, clammy skin<br>Muscle cramps (especially abdominal)<br>Nausea |
| Hypernatremia (sodium >150 mEq/L) | Water loss or deprivation<br>High sodium intake<br>Diabetes insipidus<br>Diarrhea<br>Fever<br>Hyperglycemia<br>Renal disease | Intense thirst<br>Oliguria<br>Agitation, restlessness<br>Flushed skin<br>Peripheral and pulmonary edema<br>Dry, sticky mucous membranes<br>Nausea and vomiting<br>Serum sodium 150 mEq/L: disorientation, seizures, hyperirritability when at rest |
| Hypokalemia (potassium <3.5 mEq/L) | Stress<br>Starvation<br>Malabsorption<br>Excessive loss of GI fluids through vomiting, diarrhea, sweat, nasogastric tube<br>Administration of diuretics (especially furosemide, ethacrynic acid, thiazide diuretics)<br>IV fluids without added potassium<br>Administration of corticosteroids<br>Diabetic ketoacidosis | Muscle weakness, paralysis<br>Leg cramps<br>Decreased bowel sounds, nausea<br>Weak and irregular pulse, tachycardia or bradycardia, cardiac dysrhythmias<br>Hypotension<br>Ileus<br>Irritability, fatigue<br>Decreasing blood pressure |
| Hyperkalemia (potassium >5 mEq/L) | Increased intake of potassium (e.g., salt substitutes)<br>Decreased urine excretion<br>Kidney failure<br>Metabolic acidosis<br>Hyperglycemia<br>Potassium-sparing diuretics<br>Dehydration (severe)<br>Too rapid IV administration of potassium<br>Burns | Irritability, anxiety, increased restlessness<br>Twitching, hyperreflexia<br>Weakness, flaccid paralysis<br>Nausea, diarrhea, abdominal cramps<br>Bradycardia, irregular pulse<br>Decreased blood pressure<br>Cardiac arrest (concern if potassium >8.5 mEq/L)<br>Apnea, respiratory arrest |

*Continued*

## Overview of Fluid and Electrolyte Disorders—cont'd

| Disorder | Precipitating Events | Clinical Manifestations |
|---|---|---|
| Hypocalcemia (calcium <8.5 mg/dL, ionized calcium <4.5 mg/dL) | Inadequate intake of calcium<br>Vitamin D deficiency<br>Renal insufficiency<br>Calcium losses (e.g., infection, burns)<br>Alkalosis<br>Administration of diuretics<br>Hypoparathyroidism | Numbness and tingling of fingers, toes, nose, ears, circumoral area<br>Hyperactive reflexes, seizures<br>Muscle cramps, tetany<br>Laryngospasm<br>Lethargy and poor feeding in the neonate<br>Positive Trousseau's and Chvostek's signs<br>Hypotension<br>Cardiac arrest |
| Hypercalcemia (calcium >11.0 mg/dL, ionized calcium >5.5 mg/dL) | Milk-alkali syndrome (chronic ingestion of calcium carbonate antacids or milk)<br>Excessive IV or oral calcium administration<br>Acidosis<br>Prolonged immobilization<br>Hypoproteinemia<br>Renal disease<br>Hyperparathyroidism<br>Hyperthyroidism | Lethargy, weakness, anorexia<br>Thirst<br>Itching<br>Behavioral changes: confusion, personality change, stupor<br>Nausea, vomiting, constipation<br>Bradycardia, cardiac arrest |

*GI*, gastrointestinal; *IV*, intravenous; *SIADH*, syndrome of inappropriate secretion of antidiuretic hormone

## Assessment of Fluid Disturbances

| Parameter | Fluid Volume Deficit | Fluid Volume Excess |
|---|---|---|
| Weight | Loss: Percentage suggests degree of dehydration | Gain: Related to retention of interstitial and vascular fluid volume |
| Heart rate/pulse | Rapid, weak, thready | Rapid, bounding |
| Respirations | Normal | Moist breath sounds, dyspnea |
| Blood pressure | Normal to decreased (late sign of impending shock) | Increased |
| Skin and mucous membranes | Pale, cool, poor turgor, prolonged capillary refill (>2 sec), dry mucous membranes | Edema |
| Salivation or tearing | Decreased to absent | Normal |
| Sensorium changes | Thirst, irritability, lethargy; stupor or coma if associated metabolic acidosis | Fatigue |

Data from Porth, C. (2011). *Essentials of pathophysiology* (3rd ed.). Philadelphia: Wolters Kluwer.

## Common Laboratory and Diagnostic Tests for Fluid and Electrolyte Imbalance*

| Test | Description | Indications | Normal Findings |
|---|---|---|---|
| Urine osmolality | 24-hr urine collection or random test | Altered fluid status | 300-900 mOsm/kg |
| Urine sodium | 24-hr urine collection or random urine specimen | Altered fluid status, hyponatremia | 50-130 mEq/L |
| Urine specific gravity | Random urine specimen | Altered fluid status | 1.002-1.030 |
| Urea nitrogen | Random blood specimen | Altered fluid status, renal function | 5-18 mg/dL |
| Serum osmolality | Random blood specimen | Altered fluid status<br>Measures solute concentration of blood | 275-295 mOsm/kg |

*None of these studies have any specific nursing considerations, although the nurse may be required to collect and transport the specimen; there is no advance preparation for collection

## Selected Laboratory Values for Acid–Base Disturbances

| Test | Metabolic Acidosis | Metabolic Alkalosis | Respiratory Acidosis | Respiratory Alkalosis |
|---|---|---|---|---|
| ABG: pH | <7.35 | >7.45 | <7.35 | >7.45 |
| $Paco_2$ (mm Hg) | <40 | >45 | >45 | <35 |
| $Pao_2$ (mm Hg) | WNL or slightly decreased | Decreased | Decreased | Decreased |
| $HCO_3^-$ (mEq/L) | <22 | >26 | WNL or slightly increased | Decreased |
| $K^+$ (mEq/L) | >4.0 | Decreased | WNL | Slightly decreased |
| $Na^+$ (mEq/L) | Varies according to condition | Decreased | WNL | Slightly decreased |
| $Cl^-$ (mEq/L) | Usually increased | Decreased | WNL | Slightly decreased |

*ABG*, arterial blood gas; *$HCO_3^-$*, bicarbonate; *$K^+$*, potassium; *$Paco_2$*, partial pressure of carbon dioxide in arterial blood; *$Pao_2$*, partial pressure of oxygen in arterial blood; *WNL*, within normal limits.

## Acid–Base Disturbances: Principal Causes, Clinical Manifestations, and Treatment

| Condition | Principal Causes | Compensatory Mechanisms | Clinical Manifestations | Principal Treatment Methods |
|---|---|---|---|---|
| Metabolic acidosis | Ketoacidosis (DKA, alcohol-induced ketoacidosis)<br>Increasing metabolic rate from fever, RDS, seizures<br>Interference with normal metabolism: ketosis, tissue hypoxia<br>Loss of bicarbonate from diarrhea, ileostomy, or fistula drainage<br>Acute and chronic renal failure<br>ECF expansion and decreasing $HCO_3^-$ concentration | Hyperventilation causes decreased $PaCO_2$ | Increasing heart rate, dysrhythmias (fibrillation)<br>Hyperventilation<br>Kussmaul respirations<br>Cold, clammy skin (mild to moderate acidosis)<br>Warm, dry skin (severe acidosis)<br>Level of consciousness changes from weakness, fatigue, and confusion to stupor and coma | Identify and treat the underlying disorder<br>Provide $NaHCO_3^-$, $K^+$ replacement, and mechanical ventilation as indicated |
| Metabolic alkalosis | Volume depletion related to various conditions (vomiting, pyloric stenosis, gastric drainage, and diuretics)<br>Increased alkali intake<br>Medical conditions (cystic fibrosis) | Hypoventilation causes increased $PaCO_2$ | Dysrhythmias (atrioventricular with prolonged QT interval)<br>Increasing heart rate<br>Decreased respiratory rate and depth<br>Change in level of consciousness from apathy and confusion to stupor<br>Muscular weakness | Treatment depends on underlying cause; mild to moderate alkalosis usually does not require treatment<br>Use of fluids with NaCl and KCl, along with isotonic saline solution, an $H_2$-receptor antagonist (e.g., cimetidine) to decrease gastric hydrochloric acid, acidifying agents, and potassium-sparing diuretics (e.g., spironolactone [Aldactone], mannitol) |
| Respiratory acidosis | Pulmonary disease (BPD, RDS, asthma, cystic fibrosis, croup)<br>Airway obstruction<br>Chest conditions (flail chest, pneumothorax)<br>Acute and chronic respiratory failure<br>Neuromuscular abnormalities (Guillain–Barré syndrome, toxins, drugs, paralysis)<br>CNS depression from sedative overdose, trauma, anesthesia | Release of $HCO_3^-$ and increased renal reabsorption of $HCO_3^-$ and acid excretion | Increasing heart rate<br>Dysrhythmias with hypotension<br>Increasing rate and depth of respirations, forceful use of accessory muscles with retraction and cyanosis<br>Increasing intracranial pressure | Correction of ventilation problem: use of oxygen, intubation, mechanical ventilation, $NaHCO_3^-$ |
| Respiratory alkalosis | Hyperventilation from CNS stimulation such as emotions, fear, hysteria, pain, salicylate poisoning<br>Decreased lung compliance and hypoxemia from conditions such as pulmonary edema, HF, pneumonia, asthma, pulmonary emboli<br>Pregnancy<br>Compensation from metabolic acidosis<br>Sepsis | Decreased renal reabsorption of $HCO_3^-$ | Dizziness, paresthesias, lightheadedness, diaphoresis<br>Dysrhythmias (changes in ST-T wave) | Mild to moderate respiratory alkalosis usually does not require specific treatment<br>For hyperventilation-induced conditions, provide oxygen, rebreathing oxygen masks, breathing into a paper bag, psychological reassurance<br>Institute mechanical ventilation if condition is severe<br>Give sedatives or tranquilizers for anxiety-induced condition, acetazolamide to prevent motion sickness |

*BPD*, bronchopulmonary dysplasia; *HF*, heart failure; *CNS*, central nervous system; *DKA*, diabetic ketoacidosis; *ECF*, extracellular fluid; *$HCO_3^-$*, bicarbonate: *$K^+$*, potassium; *KCl*, potassium chloride; *NaCl*, sodium chloride; *Na $HCO_3^-$*, sodium bicarbonate; *$PaCO_2$*, partial pressure of carbon dioxide in arterial blood; *RDS*, respiratory distress syndrome.

A Normal: B
pH 7.35 - 7.45
$CO_2$ 45 - 35
$CO_3$ 22 - 26

Normal:
sodium (Na+) 135-145
K+ 3.5-5.0
Ca 9.0-10.5

## DEHYDRATION

Dehydration, or fluid loss in excess of fluid intake, results most frequently from severe gastroenteritis, and is one of the most common causes of hospitalization in infants and children. Decreased fluid intake or increased fluid loss can cause dehydration. Dehydration produces both fluid and electrolyte deficiencies. Dehydration is classified as isonatremic, hyponatremic, or hypernatremic (Table 40.1), according to the status of the serum sodium concentration. In isonatremic dehydration, the most common type of dehydration in children, water and electrolytes are lost in approximately the same proportion as they exist in the body, and serum sodium levels remain within the normal range of 138 to 145 mEq/L. In hyponatremic dehydration, the electrolyte loss is greater than the water loss, resulting in a serum sodium concentration less than 135 mEq/L. In hypernatremic dehydration, the water loss is greater than the electrolyte loss, and the serum sodium concentration is more than 150 mEq/L.

### Etiology and Incidence

Dehydration has many causes. Common alterations that can lead to dehydration reflect disturbances in the following systems:

- *Gastrointestinal tract:* Vomiting, diarrhea, pyloric stenosis, malabsorption
- *Endocrine system:* Fever, diabetes mellitus, cystic fibrosis

**TABLE 40.1 Types of Dehydration: Etiology, Clinical Manifestations, and Laboratory Values**

| Isonatremic Dehydration | Hyponatremic Dehydration | Hypernatremic Dehydration |
|---|---|---|
| **Etiology** | | |
| Vomiting, diarrhea, insensible fluid loss from respiratory and integumentary systems<br>Decreased oral intake with increased activity | ***Renal Losses***<br>Diuretics, hyperglycemia, nephritis, adrenal insufficiency<br>***Extrarenal Losses***<br>Vomiting, diarrhea, third spacing, burns, tube drainage<br>***Other***<br>HF, SIADH, nephrosis; administration of large amounts of electrolyte-free solutions (plain water) during illness or postoperatively | ***Renal Losses***<br>Osmotic diuretics, diabetes insipidus, diabetes mellitus<br>***Extrarenal Losses***<br>Vomiting, diarrhea<br>***Other***<br>Fever, increased sodium in formula, diet, or tube feeding; administration of hypertonic sodium IV fluids; burns; ineffective breastfeeding |
| **Clinical Manifestations** | | |
| Mild thirst | Increased thirst | Greatly increased thirst |
| Skin turgor poor | Skin turgor very poor | Skin turgor fair |
| Dry skin | Skin usually clammy | Skin texture thickened or "doughy" |
| Decreased urine output | Decreased urine output | Decreased urine output |
| Dry mucous membranes | Mucous membranes dry to slightly moist | Mucous membranes parched |
| Skin temperature cold | Skin temperature cold | Skin temperature cold or hot |
| Body temperature afebrile or febrile | Body temperature afebrile or febrile | Body temperature afebrile or febrile |
| Lethargy | Very lethargic, possible seizures | Lethargic, hyperirritable with stimulation |
| **Laboratory Values** | | |
| Serum sodium: 138-145 mEq/L | ***Renal Losses***<br>Serum sodium <135 mEq/L<br>Plasma osmolality decreased | ***Renal Losses***<br>Serum sodium >150 mEq/L |
| Urine Sodium usually within normal limits<br>Specific gravity slightly elevated<br>Osmolality usually within normal limits<br>Volume usually within normal limits or slightly decreased | Urine sodium increased<br>Urine specific gravity decreased<br>Urine osmolality decreased<br>Urine volume increased<br>***Extrarenal Losses***<br>Serum sodium <135 mEq/L<br>Urine sodium decreased<br>Urine specific gravity increased<br>Urine osmolality increased<br>Urine volume decreased<br>***Other***<br>Serum sodium <135 mEq/L<br>Urine sodium decreased<br>Urine specific gravity increased<br>Urine osmolality increased<br>Urine volume decreased | Urine sodium increased<br>Urine specific gravity decreased<br>Urine osmolality decreased<br>Urine volume increased<br>***Extrarenal Losses***<br>Serum sodium >150 mEq/L<br>Urine sodium decreased<br>Urine specific gravity increased<br>Urine osmolality increased<br>Urine volume decreased<br>***Other***<br>Serum sodium >150 mEq/L<br>Urine sodium decreased<br>Urine specific gravity increased<br>Urine osmolality increased<br>Urine volume decreased |

Data from Greenbaum, L. (2016). Deficit therapy. In R. Kliegman, B. Stanton, J. St. Geme, et al. (Eds.), *Nelson textbook of pediatrics* (20th ed., Chapter 55). St. Louis, MO: Elsevier.
*HF,* Heart failure; *IV,* intravenous; *SIADH,* syndrome of inappropriate secretion of antidiuretic hormone.

- *Skin:* Burns
- *Lungs:* Tachypnea
- *Kidneys:* Renal failure
- *Heart:* Heart failure

Children of any age can be affected, but neonates and infants, as discussed previously, are especially vulnerable to the effects of dehydration. Gastroenteritis with resulting dehydration results in 9% of the total deaths worldwide in children and is the second leading cause of death globally (Bhutta, 2016).

## Manifestations

Classifications of the severity of dehydration vary according to the published source. In general, for infants and young children with isonatremic dehydration, the fluid deficit is described as mild, moderate, or severe, depending on the percentage of body weight lost (Greenbaum, 2016):

- *Mild dehydration:* Less than 5% loss of body weight
- *Moderate dehydration:* 5% to 10% loss of body weight
- *Severe dehydration:* Greater than 10% loss of body weight

One milliliter of body fluid is approximately equal to 1 g of body weight, so a weight loss or gain of 1 kg (2.2 lb) in 24 hours represents a 1-L fluid loss or gain.

Older children have a lower total body water content and ECF volume than do infants and younger children. Therefore, an equivalent percentage of body weight lost from dehydration represents a more severe fluid depletion in the older child. Isonatremic dehydration in the older child is classified as *mild* if less than 3% of body weight is lost, *moderate* if 3% to 6% of body weight is lost, and *severe* if more than 6% of body weight is lost (Greenbaum, 2016).

The signs and symptoms associated with degree of isonatremic dehydration are listed in Table 40.2. As with impending shock, the most essential manifestations are changes in heart rate; general appearance, behavior, or sensorium; urine output; skin and mucous membrane qualities; and, in infants, sunken or depressed fontanels. In infants and children with moderate to severe dehydration, decreased to absence of tears are a sign of dehydration, but lack of tears is not an accurate sign in very young infants, who may not produce tears until approximately 2 to 3 months of age.

### SAFETY ALERT

**Signs of Impending Shock in the Dehydrated Child**

Because of the child's ability to compensate and maintain an adequate cardiac output, changes in heart rate, sensorium, and skin color are earlier indicators of impending shock than is blood pressure.

## Diagnostic Evaluation

Key factors to consider in determining the type and severity of dehydration in children include the following:

- A history of acute or chronic fluid loss
- Clinical manifestations
- Child's weight
- Serum electrolyte values for moderate to severe dehydration

Although weight is used as the primary sign of the extent of dehydration, research suggests that it can be inaccurate, because often the provider cannot obtain a precise weight prior to the dehydration episode (Freedman, Vandermeer, Milne, et al., 2015; Tam, Wong, Plint, et al., 2014). Abnormal serum electrolyte values, which include decreased bicarbonate, decreased potassium, and decreased glucose, are not unusual in the dehydrated child, although in isonatremic dehydration, the sodium level remains within normal limits (Felver, 2013). Serum pH levels provide information about acid–base balance in an infant or a child suspected of being acidotic or alkalotic. An elevated urine specific gravity (>1.020) suggests dehydration.

### PATHOPHYSIOLOGY

**Dehydration**

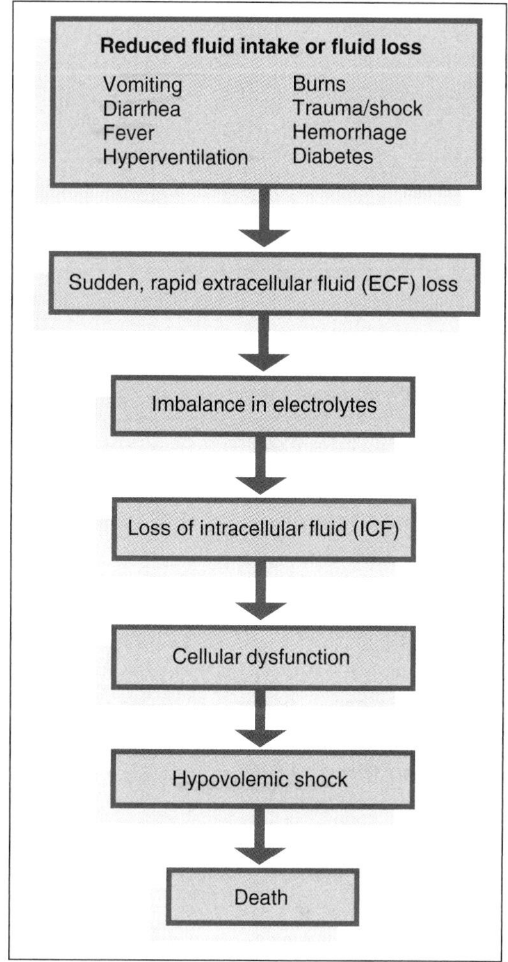


In the early phases of dehydration, fluids, with some electrolytes, are lost from the extracellular fluid (ECF). If the fluid loss continues, loss of intracellular fluid (ICF) can occur. Dehydration can lead to hypovolemic shock (see Chapter 34).

## Therapeutic Management

Management is directed toward correcting the fluid and electrolyte imbalance and then treating the causative factors.

### Minimal Dehydration

Treatment of minimal dehydration consists of continuing breastfeeding or age-appropriate diet, along with fluid replacement for each episode of fluid loss (stool, emesis) (Table 40.3). Regardless of the child's age, fluids are replaced with an oral rehydration solution (ORS) (CDC, 2014b), such as the World Health Organization's solution, Rehydralyte, Gastrolyte, Pedialyte, or Infalyte. ORSs have changed from the days of homemade recipes (mixtures of water, salt, sugar, and

**TABLE 40.2 Assessment of the Severity of Dehydration**

| Clinical Signs | Minimal or No Dehydration | Mild to Moderate Dehydration | Severe Dehydration |
|---|---|---|---|
| Weight loss | <3% | <5%-10% | >10% |
| Vital signs | | | |
| Pulse | Normal | Normal to increased, weak | Tachycardic, bradycardic in most severe cases; thready |
| Respiratory rate | Normal | Normal to fast | Rapid and deep |
| Blood pressure | Normal | Normal | Markedly decreased as a sign of hypovolemic shock |
| General appearance | Well, alert; drinks normally, might refuse liquids | Fatigued, restless, irritable; thirsty and eager to drink | Apathetic, lethargic, unconscious; drinks poorly or unable to drink |
| Mucous membranes | Normally moist | Dry | Parched |
| Anterior fontanel | Normal | Sunken | Markedly depressed |
| Eyes | Normal, tears present | Slightly sunken, tears decreased | Markedly sunken, tears absent |
| Capillary refill | <2 sec; extremities feel warm | Prolonged; extremities cool | Prolonged, minimal; extremities cold; mottled or cyanotic |
| Skin turgor (see Fig. 40.1) | Normal | Prolonged recoil | Tenting |
| Urine output | Mildly decreased | Decreased, concentrated urine | Minimal |

Modified from Centers for Disease Control and Prevention. (2003). Managing acute gastroenteritis among children: Oral rehydration, maintenance, and nutritional therapy. *MMWR: Morbidity and Mortality Weekly Report, 52,* Table 1, p. 5. Retrieved from http://www.cdc.gov; Greenbaum, L. (2016). Deficit therapy. In R. Kliegman, B. Stanton, J. St. Geme, et al. (Eds.), *Nelson textbook of pediatrics* (20th ed., Chapter 57). St. Louis, MO: Elsevier.

**TABLE 40.3 Oral Replacement and Rehydration Therapy in Children With Vomiting or Diarrhea**

| Minimally Dehydrated | Mild to Moderate Dehydration | Severe Dehydration |
|---|---|---|
| **Oral Rehydration Therapy (ORT)** | | |
| Not necessary unless not taking other fluids well | 50-100 mL/kg of oral rehydration solution (ORS) plus replace continuing losses rapidly over a 3- to 4-hr period | Intravenous (IV) therapy: bolus (or multiple boluses) of 20 mL/kg of normal saline or lactated Ringer's solution; begin ORT for the remaining deficit (100 mL/kg over 2-4 hr) when child is stable and alert and can take oral fluids; alternatively, infuse 5% dextrose in half-strength normal saline solution, initially in a bolus of 20 mL/kg over 2 hr, then at a rate that replaces the remaining fluid deficit over the next 24 hr; keep IV line in place until child is drinking well |
| **Continuing Losses** | | |
| 60-120 mL ORS for child weighing <10 kg, 120-240 mL for child weighing >10 kg to replace fluid loss from each episode of diarrhea or vomiting, **or** lost volume is measured and replaced (1 mL/g fluid loss) | 60-120 mL ORS for child weighing <10 kg, 120-240 mL for child weighing >10 kg to replace fluid loss from each episode of diarrhea or vomiting, **or** lost volume is accurately measured and replaced (1 mL/g fluid loss) | 60-120 mL ORS for child weighing <10 kg, 120-240 mL for child weighing >10 kg to replace fluid loss from each episode of diarrhea or vomiting, **or** lost volume is accurately measured and replaced (1 mL/g fluid loss); if unable to drink, administer replacement through nasogastric tube **or** infuse 5% dextrose and quarter or half-strength normal saline solution; potassium 20 mEq/L may be needed after urination established |
| **Feeding** | | |
| Continue age-appropriate diet | Continue breastfeeding; resume age-appropriate diet as soon as dehydration is corrected | Continue breastfeeding if able to take oral fluids; resume age-appropriate diet as soon as dehydration is corrected and able to take oral foods |
| **Reevaluate Hydration and Estimate Continuing Fluid Losses** | | |
| As necessary | Every 1-2 hr | Continuous evaluation; must evaluate after each bolus of IV solution |

Modified from Centers for Disease Control and Prevention. (2003). Managing acute gastroenteritis among children: oral rehydration, maintenance, and nutritional therapy. *MMWR: Morbidity and Mortality Weekly Report, 52,* 1–16. Retrieved from http://www.cdc.gov; Greenbaum, L. (2016). Deficit therapy. In R. Kliegman, B. Stanton, J. St. Geme, et al. (Eds.), *Nelson textbook of pediatrics* (20th ed., Chapter 57). St. Louis, MO: Elsevier.

cereals) to today's commercially available, lower-osmolality fluids. Because of their osmotic effect, the high carbohydrate content in fluids such as apple juice or colas may further aggravate diarrhea and cause additional fluid loss.

Electrolyte or sports drinks (e.g., Gatorade) have long been accepted oral rehydration formulations for older children. However, recent studies suggest that sports drinks are not the best solutions for rehydration and may in fact worsen diarrhea because of their high percentage of sugar and carbohydrates. These supplements greatly increase the osmotic load in the intestines and further aggravate diarrhea (CDC, 2014b).

### Mild to Moderate Dehydration

Treatment of fluid and electrolyte imbalances in children with mild to moderate dehydration should include rapid oral rehydration therapy (ORT) with an ORS in addition to replacing fluid losses due to episodes of vomiting or diarrhea. Suggested rehydration for children with mild to moderate dehydration is 50 to 100 mL/kg (based on the degree of dehydration) of ORS over 3 to 4 hours, with evaluation of the child's hydration status at least every 1 to 2 hours (CDC, 2003 as cited in Bhutta, 2016). Breastfeeding infants should continue to breastfeed during oral rehydration; an age-appropriate diet should be offered to all other children once the hydration status has improved (CDC, 2014a). The resumption of solid food promotes more rapid resolution of diarrhea (Bhutta, 2016). An alternative to oral rehydration is rehydration through nasogastric tube using an oral rehydration solution, which is as effective as oral rehydration in infants or children who are vomiting (Bhutta, 2016; CDC, 2014b). Evidence also suggests that a dose of oral ondansetron (Zofran) given to the vomiting child improves outcomes of oral rehydration therapy (Danewa et al., 2016).

### Severe Dehydration

If the child is severely dehydrated or unable to take fluids by mouth and continuing fluid replacement is needed, parenteral fluid and electrolyte therapy is initiated. Initial therapy is aimed at treating or preventing shock. Either lactated Ringer's solution or 0.9% sodium chloride solution is the fluid of choice for parenteral rehydration and restoration of circulation. Sodium chloride (0.9%) solution may be ordered initially in boluses (20 mL/kg; 10 mL/kg in frail or ill infants) until the child's hydration status has improved (as assessed by improved level of consciousness). Both the CDC (2014b) and the World Health Organization (WHO) (2016) recommend providing oral rehydration simultaneously with parenteral rehydration as long as the child is alert enough to drink. If not, oral rehydration should begin as soon as the child becomes alert (WHO, 2016). If the child cannot tolerate oral fluids, the remainder of the fluid replacement (maintenance requirement plus deficit less fluid amount already given) is provided intravenously over the next 24 hours (Greenbaum, 2016). If necessary, potassium is added to the intravenous (IV) solution once urine output is adequate, and additional fluid losses (by diarrhea or vomiting) are replaced as well. Box 40.1 lists daily fluid requirements by body weight and age-appropriate urine output.

The type of dehydration determines the rate of administration of replacement fluids. For the child with hyponatremic or hypernatremic dehydration, lost fluids may be replaced more slowly, with the amount of replacement fluid tied to the change in serum sodium levels (Greenbaum, 2016). For hypernatremic dehydration, the goal is to decrease serum sodium concentration by no more than 12 mEq/L in each 24 hours (Greenbaum, 2016). Fluid can be replaced over several days. Potassium losses must also be replaced; this process should proceed slowly to avoid hyperkalemia. Potassium replacement should begin only after urine output is adequate (see Box 40.1) and should be administered with extreme caution. If the child is anuric, potassium is retained, causing elevated potassium levels.

**BOX 40.1 Maintenance Fluid Requirements and Minimum Urine Output**

**Daily Fluid Requirements by Body Weight**

| | |
|---|---|
| ≤10 kg | 100 mL/kg |
| 10-20 kg | 1000 mL + 50 mL/kg for each additional kilogram between 10 and 20 kg |
| >20 kg | 1500 mL + 20 mL/kg for each additional kilogram over 20 kg |

**Minimum Urine Output by Age-Group**

| | |
|---|---|
| Infants and toddlers | >2-3 mL/kg/hr |
| Preschoolers and young school-age children | >1-2 mL/kg/hr |
| School-age children and adolescents | 0.5-1 mL/kg/hr |

**SAFETY ALERT**

***Guidelines When Administering Potassium***

- Do not administer potassium chloride if urine output is not age appropriate. See Box 40.1 for adequate urine output.
- *Never* give potassium by intravenous (IV) push.
- Give no more than 40 mEq/L, at a rate no faster than 1 mEq/kg/hr.
- Always check the dose and dosage calculations of potassium chloride. (Incorrect placement of a decimal point can result in a dose lethal to a child.)
- To avoid the risk of inadequate mixing, add potassium chloride to IV fluids with the plastic IV bag in the upright (noninfusion) position rather than in the down (infusion) position. (Inadequate mixing could result in the child's receiving an excessive amount of potassium chloride in the first few minutes.)
- Because of irritation of the vessel walls and potential phlebitis, IV solutions containing more than 30 mEq/L of potassium chloride should not be given through a peripheral IV line.

## NURSING CARE

### The Child With Dehydration

#### Assessment

Because dehydration can develop very quickly in infants and young children, the nurse must be alert for early signs of dehydration in children with conditions in which fluid losses are likely to occur, such as diarrhea, vomiting, burns, diabetes, trauma, and fever. The condition of infants and young children can change rapidly when fluid and electrolyte imbalances occur. It is particularly important to assess the following:

- *Intake and output:* Measure all fluid intake and losses accurately (including vomitus, urine, stools, nasogastric drainage, and wound drainage). The practitioner must also consider insensible water loss.
- *Urine output and specific gravity:* Output of less than 2 to 3 mL/kg/hr in infants and toddlers, 1 to 2 mL/kg/hr in preschoolers and young school-age children, and 0.5 to 1 mL/kg/hr in school-age children or adolescents or a specific gravity greater than 1.020 may indicate dehydration. However, glucose, large amounts of protein, and radiographic dyes elevate the specific gravity and can interfere with its accuracy.

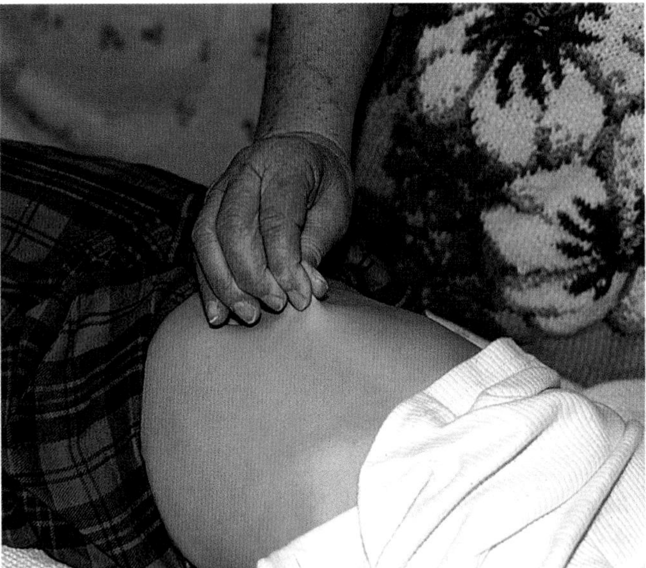

FIG 40.1 Testing skin turgor. Turgor refers to the elasticity of the skin, which is affected by the extent of hydration. The nurse tests turgor by gently grasping the skin. When the skin is released, it should instantly spring back into place; if it does not, tissue turgor is considered poor. (Courtesy University of Texas at Arlington School of Nursing.)

- *Weight:* Weight is a crucial indicator of fluid status. Accurate measurements of the weight of the unclothed child, using the same scale at the same time of day, are essential. Changes in weight related to changes in IV lines or dressings should be identified by recording 'with IV.' Weight gain during illness can indicate fluid retention or pulmonary or generalized edema. The weight should be rechecked, and the child should be assessed for pulmonary crackles and periorbital edema.
- *Stools, vomitus:* Frequency, type, amounts, and consistency should be assessed and recorded.
- *Sweating:* Estimate from dampness of clothing and linen.
- *Serum electrolytes:* See p. 890.
- *Skin:* Assess color, temperature, turgor (Fig. 40.1), moisture, and capillary refill.
- *Mucous membranes and presence of tears:* Dry or sticky mucous membranes and the absence of tears indicate dehydration. Absence of tears is not significant in an infant younger than 2 to 3 months because infants of this age often do not manufacture tears.
- *Anterior fontanel:* A sunken or depressed fontanel in infants indicates dehydration. Cranial suture lines may also become prominent with dehydration.
- *Vital signs:* Fever increases the metabolic rate and fluid requirements. With dehydration, the pulse is rapid, weak, and thready. An increase in the respiratory rate compensates for metabolic acidosis, which often accompanies dehydration. Blood pressure may be decreased in moderate and severe dehydration, but it is a late sign of hypovolemia.
- *Behavior:* Irritability, lethargy, confusion, or seizures may be present. The child may have a high pitched, weak cry.

### Nursing Diagnosis and Planning

- Deficient Fluid Volume related to gastric or intestinal infection or inflammation, hemorrhage, burns, or failure of fluid regulatory mechanisms.

*Expected outcome.* The infant or child will display adequate fluid volume, as evidenced by age-appropriate urine output, age-appropriate urine specific gravity, elastic skin turgor, and moist mucous membranes; serum pH and electrolyte levels within normal limits, and weight gain.

- Deficient Knowledge related to incomplete understanding of preventive measures for fluid loss.

*Expected outcomes.* The parent or caregiver will describe how to appropriately administer fluids to prevent dehydration. The parent or caregiver will describe concerning signs and symptoms and seek medical assistance when needed.

### Interventions

Teach parents how to prevent dehydration (see Patient-Centered Teaching: Dehydration). Parents should be taught to give infants and young children extra fluids during hot weather, to avoid overdressing their children, and to encourage frequent rest periods during high-energy playtimes. During minor illness, providing additional fluids to a child with fever can prevent the development of more serious problems. Teach parents how to identify the early signs and symptoms of dehydration, and instruct them to seek professional help if these signs and symptoms should occur.

## PATIENT-CENTERED TEACHING

### *Dehydration*

**Signs and Symptoms of Dehydration**

Watch for the following signs and symptoms of dehydration:

- Fewer wet diapers (especially no wet diaper for more than 6 to 8 hours)
- No tears when your child is crying if older than 2 to 3 months
- Inside of mouth dry or sticky
- Irritability; high-pitched cry
- Difficulty in awakening
- Increased respiratory rate or difficulty breathing
- Sunken soft spot, sunken eyes with dark circles
- Abnormal skin color, temperature, or dryness

Because a young child's condition may worsen faster than an older child's, seek professional assistance early if your child is younger than 6 months old.

Teach parents how to replace fluids when the child is mildly dehydrated. Oral rehydration formulations, such as Rehydralyte, Infalyte, Gastrolyte, or Pedialyte, contain the appropriate concentration of electrolytes and should be used. Parents need to understand that giving plain water alone or in large amounts can be extremely dangerous and why it is dangerous. The infant or child needs to continue to eat, as tolerated.

When caring for the hospitalized child with fluid and electrolyte imbalance, the nurse assumes the responsibility of continuously monitoring the child's condition and administering oral and IV fluids safely (see Chapter 38 for a discussion of IV therapy). When caring for children with conditions such as fever, burns, diarrhea, vomiting, or trauma, the nurse must continuously assess for signs of dehydration.

### Evaluation

- Is the child alert?
- Is urine output appropriate for age with a specific gravity within normal limits?
- Is the skin elastic and soft?
- Are the mucous membranes moist?
- Are serum pH and electrolyte levels within normal limits?

## DIARRHEA

Diarrhea, one of the most common disorders in childhood, is defined as an increase in the frequency, fluidity, and volume of stools. Worldwide, especially in developing countries, diarrhea is a significant cause of childhood mortality (Bhutta, 2016)). Deaths occur in children younger than 5 years old from complications related to diarrhea, most specifically dehydration. Diarrhea accompanies many childhood disorders and is acute or chronic, inflammatory or noninflammatory. Diarrhea caused by infection is usually called *gastroenteritis.* Viral gastroenteritis is the major cause of diarrhea in children older than 1 year of age. In the United States, the most common cause of gastroenteritis is norovirus infection (CDC, 2013). Rotavirus infection, formerly the most frequent cause of infectious diarrhea, has diminished due to the effects of widespread immunization with the rotavirus vaccine (CDC, 2013).

If not treated, acute diarrhea in infants and children can lead to dehydration, electrolyte imbalance, and hypovolemic shock. Acute diarrhea can be life threatening in infants and small children if gastrointestinal fluid losses are not adequately replaced.

### EVIDENCE-BASED PRACTICE

In the emergency department setting, finding a rapid, but accurate, way of assessing the severity of dehydration in young children (younger than 5 years old) might direct the initiation of appropriate treatment. Clinicians have found that, although weight is the "gold standard" for determining dehydration and response to treatment, often exact weights are not possible to obtain. Two recent studies have attempted to assess the reliability, validity and usefulness of an abbreviated dehydration scale – the Clinical Dehydration Scale (CDS). The four dehydration descriptors used in the CDS include general appearance (normal to drowsy), eyes (normal to sunken), mucous membranes (moist to dry) and tears (present to absent); each category is scored from 0 to 2, relating to no, moderate, or severe dehydration. Each characteristic of dehydration is given a precise definition so that well-trained nurses can reliably and quickly assign a score. Kinlin & Freedman (2012) tested inter-rater reliability of the scale by having a nurse and physician simultaneously assess and score the level of dehydration on 226 children who were receiving intravenous rehydration. They found that the scale correlated significantly with improvement in weight over the course of treatment and also with sodium bicarbonate levels; however, the scale was not so accurate for predicting the degree of dehydration to make treatment decisions. They did find moderate agreement between the nurses and physicians using the scale.

Tam et al. (2014) investigated correlations between the CDS and laboratory tests that might predict the level of dehydration. Their study was a case-comparison study where 73 children in a dehydration group were compared with 143 children without dehydration. A research nurse collected the physiologic data. Similar to the Kinlin and Freedman study, these researchers found a relationship between the CDS and sodium bicarbonate levels. They concluded that the scale was useful in assisting with determining degree of dehydration. Sometimes it takes several research studies to definitively determine whether a measurement scale is reliable and valid.

Think about the ways in which nurses can participate in clinical research. What types of clinical problems might you identify that would be of interest to a nurse researcher? Think about how sources of error could be controlled in clinical research studies.

References: Kinlin, L., & Freedman, S. (2012). Evaluation of a clinical dehydration scale in children requiring intravenous rehydration. *Pediatrics, 129*(5), e1211–e1219; Tam, R., Wong, H., Plint, A., et al. (2014). Comparison of clinical and biochemical markers of dehydration with the clinical dehydration scale in children: A case comparison trial. *BMC Pediatrics, 14,*149–158.

### CRITICAL THINKING EXERCISE 40.1

You have admitted a 9-month-old child who has been diagnosed with moderate dehydration to the emergency department. The physician has ordered oral rehydration therapy (ORT) for this child based on a weight of 9.5 kg at 50 mL/kg over 4 hours. In addition, the physician has ordered replacement fluid of 120 mL for each episode of diarrhea or vomiting. Over the first 4 hours of observation, the child had two episodes of diarrhea. How many milliliters would the child be expected to receive over the 4-hour period?

### Etiology and Incidence

There are many causes of both acute and chronic diarrhea (Table 40.4). Diarrhea with ensuing dehydration is a leading killer of children worldwide and is a major cause of morbidity, as well as a primary sign of many other conditions. Diarrhea can be either a short-term or a long-term condition. Infectious gastroenteritis can spread extensively and rapidly in schools and other highly populated settings (Lepkowaska, 2014).

### PATHOPHYSIOLOGY

#### Diarrhea

- Increased motility and rapid emptying of the intestines result in impaired absorption of nutrients and water and in electrolyte imbalance. Water, sodium, potassium, and bicarbonate are drawn from the extracellular space into the stool, resulting in dehydration, electrolyte depletion, and metabolic acidosis.
- Diarrhea occurs when there is excess fluid in the small intestine. This condition can result from a number of processes:
  - Bacterial toxins stimulating active transport of electrolytes into the small intestine: Cells in the mucosal lining of the intestines are irritated and secrete increased amounts of water and electrolytes.
  - Organisms invading and destroying intestinal mucosal cells, decreasing intestinal surface area, and impairing the intestine's capacity to absorb fluids and electrolytes.
  - Inflammation, which decreases the intestine's ability to absorb fluid, electrolytes, and nutrients. This condition occurs in malabsorption syndromes.
  - Increased intestinal motility, resulting in impaired intestinal absorption.

### Manifestations

Diarrhea can manifest either quickly or insidiously. Its manifestations include the following:

- *Integumentary:* Dry, hot skin; changes in skin texture and turgor; dry mucous membranes
- *Small intestine:* Cramps, nausea, vomiting; large-volume stools, light in color, loose to watery in texture; stools that tend to be soupy, greasy, or foul-smelling
- *Large intestine:* The urge to defecate with insignificant stool present; mushy, jelly like, or even bloody fecal matter; stool that is usually dark in color; stool that is rarely foul-smelling
- *Other:* Increased heart and respiratory rates, decreased tearing, fever

### Diagnostic Evaluation

Most infectious causes of diarrhea are self-limiting, making comprehensive testing of minor cases of diarrhea impractical. Because of the different possible causes, the diagnostic workup is frequently geared

**TABLE 40.4 Causes and Manifestations of Diarrhea in Infants and Children**

| Causes of Diarrhea | Manifestations |
|---|---|
| Intestinal infection | Watery stools containing mucus and possibly blood |
| Bacterial (*Campylobacter jejuni,* Salmonella,* Shigella,* Escherichia coli)* | Pain, cramps, nausea, vomiting, fever (>38.7° C [101.6° F] with bacterial infection); risk of dehydration, electrolyte imbalance, and shock |
| Viral (norovirus,* most common cause in U.S. children; rotavirus*; enteric adenovirus) | |
| Parasitic (*Giardia lamblia,* Cryptosporidium,** high incidence of both in daycare centers) | |
| Fungal overgrowth | |
| Food intolerance (lactose intolerance, overfeeding, introduction of new foods) | Diarrhea, increased mucus in stools, flatus, pain after ingestion of lactose or offending food |
| Malabsorption (cystic fibrosis, disaccharide deficiencies, celiac disease) | Diarrhea, cramps, distention, steatorrhea occurring after meals<br>Anorexia, weight loss, fatigue |
| Medications (antibiotics, chemotherapy) | Diarrhea after administration of medications, which usually stops when medications are discontinued |
| Colon disease (ulcerative colitis, Crohn disease, enterocolitis) | Inflammation and ulceration of intestinal walls, increased motility<br>May have 10-20 stools per day<br>Abdominal pain, fever, chills, anorexia, weight loss |
| Irritable bowel syndrome | Diarrhea alternating with constipation or normal bowel function<br>Pain, distention, nausea may be present |
| Intestinal obstruction (including intussusception) | Partial obstruction may result in diarrhea caused by increased intestinal motility<br>Pain, nausea, and sometimes bloody stool; may note mucus in stools |
| Emotional stress (anxiety, fatigue) | Increased motility |
| Infectious disease (otitis media, upper respiratory infection, urinary tract infection) | Diarrhea frequently accompanies other infections |

*Most common causative organisms.

toward ruling out infectious agents and anatomic and physiologic causes such as allergies, food intolerance, and bowel problems. Tests to be performed after an initial history has assessed for food intolerance, stress, or school- or work-related problems include the following:

- *Stool:* Cultures (for bacteria, ova, parasites), pH, red blood cells, leukocytes, glucose (Clinitest), blood (guaiac test or Hemoccult), various immunoassays for viral causes such as rotavirus or norovirus
- *Blood tests:* Especially blood cell counts, electrolytes, blood urea nitrogen, glucose, and blood cultures (if an infectious agent is suspected)
- *X-ray films:* Check for possible bowel abnormalities

## Therapeutic Management

The treatment of diarrhea is aimed at maintaining and restoring fluid and electrolyte balance and returning the bowel to normal function. Preventing the spread of infection to others is an important component of care, with meticulous hand hygiene (washing with soap and water) being critical. Parents must be informed of specific fluid intake requirements and signs of dehydration, which signal a worsening of the child's condition. Treatment of diarrhea and prevention of dehydration include replacing fluids, continuing feedings, and close monitoring and observation. Infants should continue to be given breast milk or regular-strength formula.

The continued feeding of a normal diet can prevent dehydration, reduce stool frequency and volume, and hasten recovery. It does not prolong diarrhea, and there is evidence that it can decrease the duration of diarrhea (CDC, 2014a). If adding milk to the diet increases diarrhea, transient lactose intolerance is possible, although it is not as common as was once thought. Common foods that are especially well tolerated during diarrhea are bland but nutritional foods, including complex carbohydrates (e.g., rice, wheat, potatoes, cereals), yogurt containing live cultures, cooked vegetables, and lean meats. This recommendation is a change from the formerly recommended BRAT diet, which consisted of bananas, rice, applesauce, and toast. The BRAT diet can be tolerated but is low in energy, density, fat, and protein.

Preventing dehydration is a primary issue in the management of the infant or child with diarrhea. ORS is given to replace each loose stool. In addition to continuing an age-appropriate diet, children weighing less than 10 kg should have losses replaced with 60 to 120 mL of ORS for each episode of diarrhea. Children weighing more than 10 kg should receive 120 to 240 mL of ORS (CDC, 2014a). For infants with mild to moderate diarrhea who have not become dehydrated, fluid loss replacement is started at home.

If an infant or a child has become mildly to moderately dehydrated and requires a visit to a clinic or an emergency room, ORT is recommended as described previously and in Table 40.3. At the end of each hour of rehydration, hydration and replacement losses should be assessed. Initial rehydration may require limiting the intake to smaller volumes (sips) to reduce any incidence of associated vomiting (e.g., 5 mL every 2 to 5 minutes) with a gradual increase in volume as tolerated. Nasogastric administration of ORS may be necessary to provide slow, steady, continuous administration to rapidly hydrate the child and avoid hospitalization.

Feeding of solids or formula is started as soon as the child is rehydrated. Children should be encouraged to eat frequently—every 3 to 4 hours. Parents should be instructed that, although stool output may increase, feeding will not prolong diarrhea and the child will be absorbing necessary nutrients and calories. For a child with severe dehydration and continuing losses, ORT is not recommended. Such children are usually admitted to a hospital for observation and IV therapy.

If bacteria, parasites, or fungi cause the diarrhea, other types of medication along with antibiotics may be ordered. The use of antidiarrheal medication is not recommended in children because of the binding nature of these products and the potential for toxicity (Bhutta, 2016). Antidiarrheal medications have not been found to shorten the course of the diarrhea, and in cases where the diarrhea is caused by pathogens, they may increase fluid and electrolyte loss by interfering with the body's attempt to rid itself of the organism and allowing the pathogen to remain in the body longer.

## Prognosis

Most children with diarrhea and subsequent dehydration have a relatively quick recovery, provided that the cause of the diarrhea is determined and therapy is started as soon as possible. Oral rotavirus vaccine is recommended by the CDC for prevention of diarrhea caused by rotavirus. There are two approved rotavirus vaccines: RV1 and RV5. Each is effective for preventing rotavirus, although their dosage scheduling differs. RV5 rotavirus vaccine is given to infants at ages 2, 4, and 6 months, whereas the RV1 vaccine is given at 2 and 4 months only (Advisory Committee on Immunization Practices [ACIP], 2016).

## NURSING CARE

### The Child With Diarrhea

#### Assessment

When a child is admitted to a hospital setting, the child's condition and hydration status should be the first area of assessment. The primary concern about dehydration is the potential for shock. The child and family should be questioned about possible food allergies, intolerance to foods, foods eaten over the past 24 hours, and outbreaks of diarrhea in the nuclear or extended family or daycare setting. If diarrhea is present, stools should be assessed for amount, color, consistency, and time (ACCT) and odor. When assessing and monitoring for ACCT, note the quantity and quality of the stool, its color (e.g., green, brown, clear, blood tinged), consistency (watery, loose), the presence of mucus, and the length of time since the stool's consistency has changed.

Other continuing assessments include documenting intake and output; assessing the current weight and comparing it with the last known weight; assessing for thirst, along with skin turgor and texture and mucous membranes; and observing the child's level of activity. The nurse also monitors electrolyte values, if ordered. If diarrhea is severe, it may be necessary to apply a urine bag to measure urine output and to obtain urine to measure specific gravity. Skin integrity must be monitored, especially if a urine bag is to be used. Observe the skin in the perineal area for color, texture, lesions, or drainage with each diaper change. Assess family members' knowledge of the transmission of infection by questions or testing. Observe family members as they use Contact Precautions, especially hand hygiene. Ask the family if any other members have cramping or diarrhea.

#### Nursing Diagnosis and Planning

The following nursing diagnoses and expected outcomes may be appropriate in the treatment of diarrhea in a child:

- Deficient Fluid Volume related to increased stool output.

  *Expected outcome.* The child will maintain fluid balance within normal limits, as evidenced by age-appropriate urine output, capillary refill time less than 2 seconds, elastic skin turgor, moist mucous membranes, and weight gain.
- Impaired Skin Integrity related to exposure to stool.

  *Expected outcome.* The child will have no sign of skin breakdown, as evidenced by intact perineal and perianal skin, or will exhibit signs of healing on affected or excoriated areas.
- Risk for Infection (in others) related to lack of knowledge about transmission prevention.

  *Expected outcome.* Family members will show no signs of infection and demonstrate correct precaution and hand hygiene technique (contact precautions).
- Imbalanced Nutrition: Less than Body Requirements related to decreased intake and inability of body to absorb fluids.

  *Expected outcome.* The child will tolerate the diet, as evidenced by weight gain and no recurrence of diarrhea.

#### Interventions

The child with diarrhea should be weighed unclothed on admission and daily on the same scale and at the same time each day to precisely determine changes in weight. To accurately determine fluid losses with each episode of diarrhea in untrained infants and children, weigh the diaper after each voiding and liquid stool and compare to the weight of the same type of diaper dry (each gram of excess diaper weight is equal to 1 mL of fluid output). Measuring amounts of liquid stool may be required for the older child. Accurate accounting of losses is necessary to maximize the effectiveness of the ORT and to prevent deficits and imbalances in electrolytes. Document the child's intake, as well as output.

Signs of dry mucous membranes, decreased tearing, and sunken fontanel (if appropriate) or eyes are often the first of indicators of dehydration and should be immediately reported. Vital signs should be measured every 4 hours, or as needed. Stool cultures and other tests to are used to determine the cause of diarrhea and specific management approaches.

Infants and young children can develop skin excoriation resulting from continual contact with loose stools. Nursing intervention includes providing meticulous skin care. Gently wash the area with warm water and mild soap after each loose stool and pat dry. Apply an ointment to protect the child's skin and, if ordered, a medicated cream to heal the skin. Some children benefit from exposing damaged skin to the air for small periods of time to promote healing. Turning every 2 hours keeps pressure off the skin and facilitates circulation to the affected area.

Nursing interventions, along with the prescribed therapy, work together to achieve the expected outcomes of managing any dehydration, decreasing the number of stools, and returning the bowel to normal function. ORT may be initiated in a hospital setting after or concurrent with IV rehydration. Administer the ORS as ordered, increasing the volume as tolerated. If the child refuses or is unable to tolerate the ORS, nasogastric therapy may be considered.

Most cases of diarrhea in children can be managed at home. Parent teaching needs to be clear, concise, and specific (see Patient-Centered Teaching: Caring for a Child with Diarrhea). Education about appropriate oral replacement fluids should include avoidance of sugary drinks, apple juice, sports beverages, and colas. Fluids should be offered in small amounts to prevent gastric distention and at room temperature to prevent increased stimulation of peristalsis.

Additional education should be provided regarding prevention of illness in the nuclear and extended family or daycare setting. In most instances, preventing infection transmission includes handwashing with soap and water. Handwashing is considered to be more effective against organisms that commonly cause diarrhea in children than antibacterial hand sanitizer (CDC, 2011). Instruction in careful handwashing technique before and after caring for the sick child will prevent spread of infection or reinfection. Proper disposal of and cleaning of contaminated articles and surfaces decreases the spread of infection.

## PATIENT-CENTERED TEACHING

### *Caring for a Child With Diarrhea*

**Diet**

Diet depends on the age of the child and the severity of the diarrhea.

**Mild Diarrhea (Mushy Stools) in Children of Any Age**

Continue with an age-appropriate diet. Continue breastfeeding, formula, or milk. Encourage increased intake of fluids. Avoid fruit juices, because they can worsen diarrhea. Provide a variety of nutritious foods, including foods containing complex carbohydrates, such as rice, potatoes, bread, and cereals. Avoid fatty or spicy foods.

**Moderate Diarrhea (Watery or Frequent Stools) in Children Younger Than 1 Year**

Continue breastfeeding or formula and age-appropriate diet. Provide additional fluids such as Infalyte, Pedialyte, Rehydralyte, or other similar commercially prepared oral rehydration solutions if urine output begins to decrease. If the diarrhea is severe and the child is uncomfortable with cow's-milk–based formulas, soy formula (e.g., Isomil, ProSobee) may be considered. Feed infants older than 6 months with such bland foods as applesauce, strained carrots, rice cereal, and yogurt with live cultures. Watch closely for signs of dehydration and report these immediately to your healthcare provider.

**Moderate Diarrhea (Watery or Frequent Stools) in Children Older Than 1 Year**

Continue age-appropriate diet with foods that are nutritional, bland, and high in starch. Suggested foods include breads, crackers, rice, mashed potatoes, noodles, yogurt with live cultures, cooked vegetables, and lean meats. Avoid beans, spices, and fatty foods. Avoid sports drinks, colas, and apple juice. Give additional fluids in the form of Infalyte, Pedialyte, or Rehydralyte. Watch closely for signs of dehydration and report these immediately to your healthcare provider.

**Preventing the Spread of Infection**

Infectious diarrhea is highly contagious. Some of the infectious agents can live on toys, water fountains, and other inanimate objects for several days. Thorough handwashing after diaper changing or using the toilet is crucial to prevent others in the household from getting diarrhea. All family members should be taught the importance of thorough and frequent handwashing. Diapers should be changed on a surface designated for that purpose, *not* on the kitchen counter where food is prepared. Changing areas should be cleaned with disinfectant after each diaper change.

**Skin Care**

To prevent breakdown of the sensitive skin in the diaper area, diarrhea stools should be completely washed off with mild soap and water after each bowel movement. (Washing the child under running water in the bathtub makes the job easier. The tub should be cleaned with disinfectant before anyone else uses it.) The skin should be patted dry and a layer of A & D ointment or other protective or "barrier" ointment applied.

Changing diapers immediately after bowel movements is important to prevent skin breakdown. The use of commercial baby wipes should be avoided because they may further irritate and cause additional breakdown of the skin. To prevent overflow of diarrhea from the diaper, diapers should be applied snugly.

**When to Call the Physician**

Call the physician immediately if any of the following occurs:

- The child does not urinate for longer than 6 hours.
- Crying produces no tears, or the mouth becomes dry.
- The infant's fontanel appears sunken.
- The child's behavior or mental status changes.
- Blood or pus appears in the diarrhea, or the diarrhea becomes severe and lasts longer than 24 hours.
- Severe abdominal cramps occur.
- The child has a fever (>39° C [102° F]).

**Oral Rehydration Therapy**

Giving plain water alone or in large amounts can be extremely dangerous because it does not contain needed electrolytes. Instead, commercially available oral rehydration solutions should be given.

Data from Centers for Disease Control and Prevention. (2011). Updated norovirus outbreak management and disease prevention guidelines. *MMWR: Morbidity and Mortality Weekly Report, 60*(RR03), 1–15; National Digestive Diseases Information Clearinghouse. (2011, January). *Diarrhea*. NIH Publication 11-2749. Retrieved from http://digestive.niddk.nih.gov.

### Evaluation

- Are weight, urine output, and specific gravity within normal limits for age?
- Is the capillary refill time less than 2 seconds?
- Is skin turgor elastic, and are mucous membranes moist?
- Have signs of excoriation, redness, blisters, pruritus, and infection been reduced or eliminated?
- Are family members free of infection?
- Do family members correctly practice Contact Precaution and appropriate hand hygiene technique on a consistent basis?
- Can the child retain food and fluids?
- Are normal bowel elimination patterns present?
- Has the child maintained or shown an increase in weight?

## VOMITING

Vomiting is the forcible ejection of stomach contents through the mouth. It involves a complex reflex associated with sweating, salivation, and often tachycardia (all symptoms of autonomic nervous stimulation). Terms that are used to differentiate vomiting episodes include *spitting up* [or *chalasia*], which is a normal process during infancy), *regurgitation* (associated with gastroesophageal reflux or overfeeding), and, if severe, *projectile vomiting* (usually indicative of obstruction, tumor, pyloric stenosis, or increasing intracranial pressure). Isolated incidents of vomiting are usually of little concern. However, the consequences of persistent or prolonged vomiting can be serious.

### CRITICAL THINKING EXERCISE 40.2

Mrs. Peters calls the clinic regarding 8-month-old David. She states that David has had diarrhea for 2 days and that she does not know what to do. She also states that her neighbor said she should stop breastfeeding and give David clear liquids. Mrs. Peters tells you that she is afraid she may have done something to cause David to get sick.

1. What questions should you ask Mrs. Peters about her infant?
2. What teaching can you do to help Mrs. Peters?

### Etiology

Vomiting, which occurs frequently in children, is usually a sign of some other underlying problem or disease. Vomiting has many possible causes, including infections, obstructions, motion sickness, metabolic alterations, and psychological alterations. If vomiting occurs in association with diarrhea, it may be related to gastroenteritis. Vomiting can also result from allergic reactions or occur as a side effect of medications (e.g., chemotherapy), as a toxic effect of medications or ingested substances, and from certain eating disorders.

### Manifestations

Sour milk curds without green or brown color and undigested food from the stomach are manifestations of vomiting. Green emesis usually indicates the presence of bile and possible intestinal obstruction below the ampulla of Vater. A fecal odor indicates lower intestinal obstruction or peritonitis. Emesis may be blood tinged, or the color may be bright red or look like coffee grounds. Bright red blood indicates that the blood has not been in contact with gastric juices.

The force of vomiting varies. Regurgitation, a backward flow of undigested food, can be caused by overfeeding. Forceful vomiting can indicate an obstruction. Projectile vomiting can indicate obstruction (see Chapter 43), tumor, or increased intracranial pressure. Continuous vomiting in a young child, in the absence of diarrhea, can contribute to metabolic alkalosis.

### Diagnostic Evaluation

Vomiting in children is usually of brief duration and not severe. However, if vomiting continues and the child starts to look deficient in fluid or electrolytes, the following tests may be indicated:

- Complete blood cell counts and electrolyte studies, blood urea nitrogen, glucose levels, and urine tests
- Radiographic studies (if an obstructive or neurologic process is suspected)
- Blood cultures (if an infectious disease is suspected)
- Arterial blood gas determinations

### Therapeutic Management

The primary focus of managing vomiting is detecting and treating the cause, with the secondary intent of preventing complications. ORT, as indicated for the treatment of diarrhea (see Table 40.3), is also appropriate for the vomiting child. Most episodes of vomiting can be managed at home, with small, frequent amounts of ORS to prevent dehydration (Bhutta, 2016), then resuming a regular diet as tolerated. Adequate fluid intake and replacement of continuing losses from emesis are necessary. In the hospital setting, the practitioner and parents must estimate the volume of emesis and replace it. Reevaluation and continuing loss replacement should be done every 1 to 2 hours for a mild to moderately dehydrated child. As the vomiting decreases in frequency, the amount and interval between feedings can increase. However, if the vomiting is severe or prolonged in neonates and young infants, IV therapy may be initiated.

Most children will respond well to treatment, but some will need antiemetics. Administration of ondansetron (Zofran) can facilitate the success of oral rehydration and decrease vomiting episodes, need for IV fluid resuscitation, and time spent in the emergency room (Danewa et al., 2016). To freshen the mouth and rid it of the hydrochloric acid, the parent should rinse the child's mouth and brush the child's teeth after each episode of vomiting.

## PATHOPHYSIOLOGY

### *Vomiting*

Vomiting is under the control of the emetic center, located in the reticular core of the medulla (in the brainstem). The emetic center receives stimuli from one of three sources:

- The vagal and sympathetic afferent nerves, as in stimulation from irritation, distention, obstruction, or inflammation
- Chemically, from drugs (e.g., ipecac, opioids), cerebral hypoxia, inner ear disturbances, or increased intracranial pressure
- From the higher cortical centers, with stimuli such as sights, odors, and fright or fear

The mechanism of vomiting occurs in the presence of several complex reflexes:

- Autonomic nervous system discharge, which causes salivation, sweating, pallor, and an increased heart rate
- Contraction of the stomach antrum and duodenum
- Relaxation of the remainder of the stomach, esophagus, and sphincters
- Closure of the glottis and soft palate
- Contraction of the diaphragm and abdominal muscles, which increases intraabdominal pressure and compresses abdominal contents, thus propelling them into the esophagus and out the mouth

## NURSING CARE

### The Vomiting Child

#### Assessment

Major concerns with vomiting are dehydration and fluid and electrolyte imbalance; therefore, it is essential that hydration status be carefully assessed, including accurate assessment of intake and output, weight, fontanels in infants, general behavior, dryness of mucous membranes, skin turgor, eyes, and urine output. Ask the parent to describe the type and force of vomiting (e.g., "spitting up" as opposed to regurgitation, forceful vomiting, or projectile vomiting) and the character (using the acronym ACCT: amount, color, consistency, time) of the vomitus. Because vomiting is often associated with gastric distention, the relationship, if any, with infant feeding should be assessed (e.g., poor feeding techniques, failure to bubble or burp, regurgitation with burp or "wet burp," improper positioning). Inquire about any other signs or symptoms the child may have.

## ! NURSING QUALITY ALERT

### *Caring for the Child Who Is Vomiting*

Nursing care of the child who is vomiting is directed toward the following:

- Observing and reporting vomiting
- Assessing for associated problems, such as dehydration
- Implementing measures to reduce the vomiting
- Recording accurate intake and output
- Evaluating the effectiveness of therapy
- Preventing aspiration

#### Nursing Diagnosis and Planning

The following nursing diagnoses and expected outcomes may be appropriate in the treatment of the vomiting child:

- Deficient Fluid Volume related to increased loss of gastrointestinal contents.

  **Expected outcome.** The child will maintain fluid balance within normal limits, as evidenced by age-appropriate fluid intake, and will have age-appropriate urine output, a capillary refill time of less than 2 seconds, elastic skin turgor, and moist mucous membranes.

- Imbalanced Nutrition: Less Than Body Requirements related to vomiting.

  **Expected outcome.** The child will maintain electrolyte and acid–base balance within normal limits, as evidenced by adequate amount of calories absorbed, steady weight gain or lack of weight loss, and decreased vomiting episodes.

### Interventions

The vomiting child should be placed in an upright or side-lying position to prevent aspiration. Nursing interventions are frequently determined by the cause of the vomiting, and thus, may be very specific. For example, if the vomiting is found to be caused by incorrect feeding techniques, the nurse's role is to educate the family regarding appropriate feeding techniques (e.g., adequate bubbling and burping and positioning after the feeding) and preparation of formulas. Once the cause of vomiting has been determined, nursing interventions are directed toward ensuring a continued reduction in the vomiting and preventing dehydration. Advise the parent to offer an ORS (see Table 40.3) in small, frequent feedings to avoid gastric distention and to continue age-appropriate diet as tolerated. The parent can gradually increase the amount of fluids and foods as vomiting episodes decrease. Another important consideration is education for the child and family about avoiding certain foods (e.g., fatty, acidified, or seasoned foods) and minimizing stimuli such as stress, anxiety, or unfavorable-smelling foods. Avoidance of food or activities that might upset the stomach, either directly or by association, may be helpful in decreasing nausea and vomiting. If the child repeatedly vomits or vomits large volumes, or if the child begins to exhibit signs of dehydration, the parent should notify the physician.

### Evaluation

- Is the child taking in age-appropriate amounts of fluid without vomiting?
- Is the child's urine output age appropriate?
- Is the child's skin turgor elastic, with a capillary refill time of 2 seconds or less?
- Does the child have moist mucous membranes?
- Is the child tolerating an age-appropriate diet?

## KEY CONCEPTS

- Infants and children are at a much greater risk than adults for fluid and electrolyte disturbances.
- The three mechanisms by which acid–base balance is maintained are chemical buffering, respiratory control of carbon dioxide, and renal regulation of bicarbonate and secretion of hydrogen ions.
- The two major forms of acid–base disturbance are acidosis and alkalosis, either of which may be respiratory or metabolic.
- The treatment of metabolic disturbances is directed toward correcting the underlying problem. Interventions for respiratory alterations are implemented toward reestablishing alveolar ventilation.
- Dehydration may be classified as isonatremic (the most common form), hyponatremic, or hypernatremic.
- Assessment of intake and output, vital signs, and level of activity (or sensorium) is crucial in appropriately managing the child with a fluid or electrolyte disturbance.
- Diarrhea can lead to loss of bicarbonate (and subsequently to acidosis).
- Oral rehydration therapy is indicated for the child with diarrhea, dehydration of any degree, and vomiting.

## REFERENCES AND READINGS


Advisory Committee on Immunization Practices. (2016). *Recommended immunization schedules for persons aged 0 through 18 years.* Retrieved from http://www.cdc.gov.

Bhutta, Z. (2016). Acute gastroenteritis in children. In R. Kliegman, B. Stanton, J. St. Geme, et al. (Eds.), *Nelson textbook of pediatrics* (20th ed., Chapter 340). St. Louis, MO: Elsevier.

Centers for Disease Control and Prevention. (2003). Managing acute gastroenteritis among children: Oral rehydration, maintenance, and nutritional therapy [Electronic version]. *MMWR: Morbidity and Mortality Weekly Report, 52,* 1–16.

Centers for Disease Control and Prevention. (2011). Updated norovirus outbreak management and disease prevention guidelines. *MMWR: Morbidity and Mortality Weekly Report, 60*(RR03), 1–15.

Centers for Disease control and Prevention. (2013). *Norovirus is now the leading cause of severe gastroenteritis in U.S. children.* Retrieved from http://www.cdc.gov.

Centers for Disease Control and Prevention. (2014a). *Guidelines for management of acute diarrhea after a disaster.* Retrieved from http://www.cdc.gov.

Centers for Disease Control and Prevention. (2014b). *Rehydration therapy.* Retrieved from http://www.cdc.gov.

Danewa, A., Shah, D., Batra, P. et al. (2016). Oral ondansetron in management of dehydrating diarrhea with vomiting in children aged 3 months to 5 years: A randomized controlled trial. *Journal of Pediatrics, 169,* 105-109.

Felver, L. (2013). Homeostasis and imbalances. In L. Copstead & J. Banasik (Eds.), *Pathophysiology* (5th ed., Chapter 24). St. Louis, MO: Elsevier Saunders.

Freedman, S., Vandermeer, B., Milne, A., et al. (2015). Diagnosing clinically significant dehydration in children with acute gastroenteritis using non-invasive methods: a meta-analysis. *Journal of Pediatrics, 166,* 908–916.

Greenbaum, L. (2016). Deficit therapy. In R. Kliegman, B. Stanton, J. St. Geme, et al. (Eds.), *Nelson textbook of pediatrics* (20th ed., Chapter 57). St. Louis, MO: Elsevier.

Kinlin, L., & Freedman, S. (2012). Evaluation of a clinical dehydration scale in children requiring intravenous rehydration. *Pediatrics, 129*(5), e1211–e1219.

Lepkowaska, D. (2014). "Winter vomiting bug": limiting norovirus outbreaks in schools. *British Journal of School Nursing, 9*(9), 448–449.

Porth, C. (2011). *Essentials of pathophysiology* (3rd ed.). Philadelphia: Wolters Kluwer.

Tam, R., Wong, H., Plint, A., et al. (2014). Comparison of clinical and biochemical markers of dehydration with the clinical dehydration scale in children: a case comparison trial. *BMC Pediatrics, 14,* 149–158.

World Health Organization. (2016). *Paediatric emergency triage, assessment and treatment.* Retrieved from http://www.who.int.

# The Child With an Infectious Disease

http://evolve.elsevier.com/McKinney/mat-ch/

## LEARNING OBJECTIVES

*After studying this chapter, you should be able to:*

- Analyze the infectious process.
- Compare between infectious diseases the mode of transmission, incubation time, and infectious period.
- Analyze the pathophysiology, clinical manifestations, complications, and nursing management of childhood infectious diseases.
- Analyze the pathophysiology, clinical manifestations, complications, and nursing management of sexually transmitted diseases.
- Use the nursing process to describe the nursing care of a child with an infectious disease.

## CLINICAL REFERENCE

## REVIEW OF DISEASE TRANSMISSION

Microorganisms are present throughout the environment. Most are harmless residents and a normal part of human flora. However, an organism that invades body tissue, causing tissue damage and disease, is a **pathogen**. For pathogens to invade a **host**, they must breach the normal host defenses by either attaching to or penetrating the host. The power of these pathogens, known as their **virulence**, depends on their ability to overcome the host defense mechanisms. Thus, a highly virulent organism can cause disease with relative ease.

Microorganisms that cause infectious diseases are of five classifications: bacteria, viruses and rickettsiae, fungi, protozoa, and helminths.

*Exogenous pathogens* are transmitted from outside the body to the host by various mechanisms. Exogenous organisms are present in contaminated air, food, water, and body fluids and on objects contaminated by these substances. *Endogenous pathogens* are found within the human body. Microorganisms (normal flora) are present on the skin and in the nose, mouth, gastrointestinal tract, and urogenital tract. For example, *Staphylococcus epidermidis* inhabits the skin, and *Escherichia coli* are found in the intestines. These microorganisms are beneficial and play an important role in the body's defenses. They help prevent virulent pathogens from colonizing by maintaining an acidic environment to discourage pathogen attachment, taking up epithelial space to prevent the growth of pathogens, and stimulating the immune system. However, situations may arise in which these normally benign organisms become virulent and harmful to the host.

### Chain of Infection

For a pathogen to maintain its infectious state, it must be transmitted to another host. Certain factors and conditions must be present for a disease (**infection**) to begin. These components and their relations are often referred to as a chain of infection. The major variables in the chain of infection include the agent (organism), reservoir (environment in which the agent resides and multiplies), portal of exit (route by which the agent leaves the host), transmission mode, portal of entry (route by which the agent enters the new host), and host susceptibility (internal and external environmental factors that increase or decrease the likelihood the host will develop disease). Changes in any one variable result in a change in the presence, intensity, and frequency of the entire infectious disease process.

### Transmission of Pathogens

Infection transmission occurs through several modes, or routes. For example, pathogens from the respiratory tract are shed through sneezing, coughing, and talking. If the pathogens survive in the air, they can infect others who inhale them (airborne route). Because this mode of transmission is relatively uncontrollable, infections can easily be spread in crowded conditions.

Pathogens can also be shed in fecal matter. When personal hygiene is poor and hand hygiene is not routinely practiced, pathogens have ample opportunities to enter through the mouth (fecal-oral transmission). Unclean hands can also contaminate food, which is then ingested.

Sexual activity involving direct mucosal contact is the most common means of transmission of sexually transmitted diseases (STDs) (direct contact transmission). If the mother's birth canal is infected, newborn infants can be infected by direct contact during birth. Saliva is another avenue of transmission, as is direct contact with infected skin. Pathogens can also be present in breast milk and can infect a nursing infant.

A tick, mosquito, mite, or animal can inject pathogens into the skin and blood of the host. Organisms carried in this way are considered to be **vector** borne. For example, a certain species of mosquito carries the malaria parasite; likewise, certain bats carry the rabies microorganism.

Contamination by blood of an infected host can occur through transfusions, blood products, and the use of contaminated needles (direct inoculation). A pregnant woman can transmit such pathogens through the placenta. Other modes of transmission include the transfer of spores found in soil (e.g., tetanus).

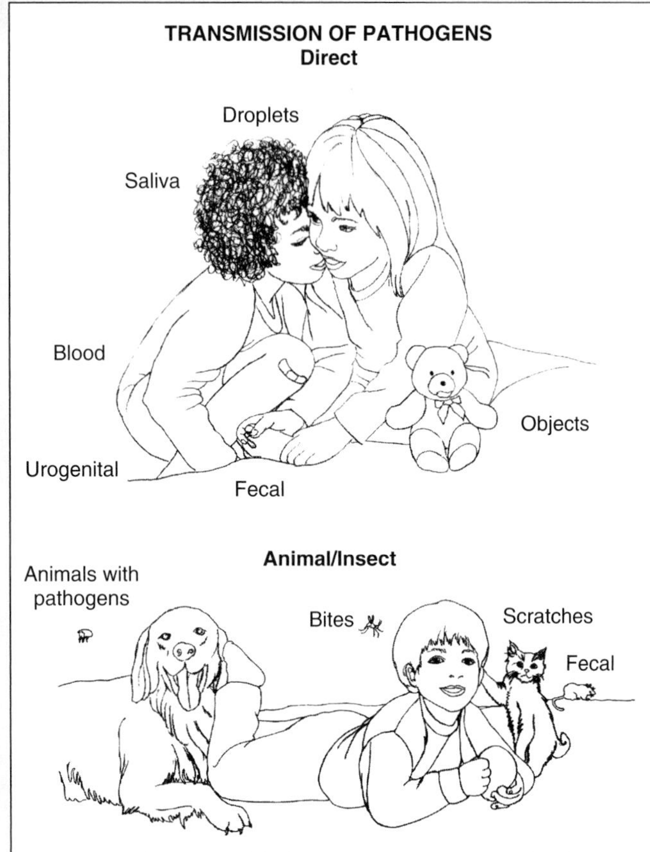


Infectious diseases are a major reason healthcare is sought for infants and children. Although most infections are not life threatening, fatal complications can develop, especially in infants or children with an immature or compromised immune system. Moreover, a child's illness directly affects the family and caregivers. Absence from work for the parent of a sick child can jeopardize job security, and the accompanying missed income can be devastating for both single- and two-income families.

Nurses play a major role in preventing pediatric infectious diseases and decreasing the incidence of disability and death in both community and hospital settings. Regardless of their clinical setting, nurses must be able to confidently recognize the sometimes subtle signs and symptoms of infectious diseases in children and initiate appropriate treatment, ensure appropriate precautions are implemented to prevent the spread of infectious diseases and provide evidence based nursing care. Nurses must also provide education about accessing appropriate community resources and limiting exposure of other children and community members.

In addition, because of the growing number of uninsured and underserved children in the United States, nurses may be the first and sometimes only healthcare professionals to evaluate and treat children in community-based settings. School nurses are frequently required to notify parents and caregivers when their children have been exposed to infectious diseases. Regardless of the particular type of infection, underlying principles of nursing care are similar.

### Epidemiologic Investigations

Epidemiology is the study of the distribution of health and illness within a population and the factors that determine the population's health status. Nurses may not realize that they are contributing to this process when they gather patient history information as part of the nursing assessment process. The data nurses collect help the entire healthcare team identify, treat, and prevent disease processes as well as promote health. Moreover, the specific steps of the epidemiologic process mirror the steps in the nursing process and include defining the condition; determining the condition's natural history; identifying critical control points; and designing, implementing, and evaluating control strategies.

## INFECTION AND HOST DEFENSES

The first stage of infection begins with colonization of the host by the pathogen. Microorganisms invade either by adhering to tissues or by invading cells. Initially, replication of the pathogen does not cause tissue damage, and colonization can occur without development of a clinical infection. As the host "recognizes" the invasion, the defense system—the immune response—is activated. The two components of the immune response are the innate, nonspecific immune response and the adaptive, specific immune response: cell mediated and humoral (see Chapter 42).

The first lines of defense in the innate immune system are the skin and intact mucous membranes. The skin serves as a barrier, preventing colonization of most pathogens. The acid secreted in sweat and by sebaceous glands inhibits pathogen invasion. Smooth muscle contraction and ciliary actions, such as those seen in bladder and bowel emptying and coughing and sneezing, remove pathogens mechanically. Physical and chemical barriers are provided through mucus production by goblet cells in mucous membranes. Nevertheless, the innate system may be unable to prevent the invasion. *Phagocytosis,* the process by which phagocytes digest and thereby destroy foreign microorganisms, can be overwhelmed. Large numbers of pathogens or their toxins can inhibit phagocytosis. Under such conditions, the adaptive immune system is activated. This system "recognizes" and responds to pathogens by destroying them. The adaptive immune system "imprints" on these pathogens so that if the body encounters them again, the response will be rapid and specific.

## IMMUNITY

Immunity is the body's resistance to the effects of harmful agents. It occurs as an antigen-antibody reaction that takes place whenever a foreign agent or its toxins enter the bloodstream. Immunity can be either active or passive. Active immunity occurs as a result of immune system stimulation from exposure to antigens, either naturally or through vaccine administration. Passive immunity is a form of infection protection acquired through the administration of serum containing antibodies.

Some childhood diseases have been significantly reduced and some nearly eliminated through the administration of vaccines producing active or passive immunity. A variety of preparations of disease-specific vaccines and preparations can artificially accomplish active or passive immunity (see Chapter 5).

## VIRAL EXANTHEMS

Viruses are small parasitic organisms with unique characteristics that are quite different from other organisms. They contain only genetic material, made up of one type of nucleic acid—either deoxyribonucleic acid (DNA) or ribonucleic acid (RNA). This lack of reproductive machinery prevents them from reproducing on their own. Instead, a host cell is needed to allow the virus to replicate.

The replication process begins with the virus first attaching itself to a host cell. After the initial attachment, a virus must invade the interior of the cell. Replication of the virus's DNA or RNA begins after the envelope and capsule (capsid) are shed and the genetic material of the virus is released into the cell; the host cell then assists in the replication and translation of the virus's genetic material. New capsules are then formed and released into the host's cell. The infected host cell can respond to the viral invasion by cell death (lysis) and destruction, or the infected cell can remain alive and continue to function while new viral particles are slowly released. This slow release occurs in an asymptomatic person who is a carrier of the virus. Some viruses are selective about the cells to which they attach. For example, the human immunodeficiency virus (HIV) prefers to attach to the T cell (see Chapter 42).

A virus can also invade a host and remain dormant until a trigger stimulates it to begin replicating. The triggering factors for many viruses are not fully understood. However, some triggers have been identified. An example is the effect of stress in herpes simplex (a viral disease), resulting in the formation of cold sores.

### Nursing Considerations for the Child With a Viral Exanthem Infection

An exanthem is an eruption or rash on the skin. Several childhood infectious diseases are characterized by rashes with distinctive characteristics. Nurses need to be aware that rashes have more than one characteristic and should obtain a detailed history of the characteristics of the rash, including its onset, initial location, and progression, as well as any associated physical signs or symptoms. Specific characteristics of the rash should be documented, including color, elevation, pattern or shape, size (in centimeters), location and distribution on the body, and any drainage. Vital signs, including temperature, should be taken and recorded. Also record the child's general state of health, recent exposures to illnesses, any prescribed or over-the-counter medications, and treatments taken and their results. Perform a general physical assessment to look for associated signs of inflammation, which may include abnormal enlargement or tenderness of the spleen, liver, or lymph nodes.

Children with typical uncomplicated viral exanthems are usually cared for at home. Hospitalization is indicated when complications occur or the exanthema is known to be associated with severe disease. Nurses who care for hospitalized children with an infectious disease should not also care for high-risk (immunosuppressed) children to prevent any possible cross transmission by the nurse.

Whether the child is cared for in the hospital or at home, any specific isolation measures will be determined by the child's specific infectious disease process.

### Rubeola (Measles)

| | |
|---|---|
| Causative agent | RNA virus |
| Incubation period | 8 to 12 days from exposure to onset of symptoms |
| Infectious period | Ranges from 3 to 5 days before the appearance of the rash to 4 to 6 days after appearance of the rash |
| Transmission | Transmitted between individuals by direct contact with infectious droplets or less frequently by airborne spread |
| Immunity | Natural disease or live attenuated vaccine |
| Season | Winter and spring |

#### Manifestations

The measles virus enters the body and slowly spreads. Respiratory symptoms appear after an average of 10 days. Typically, children have a prodrome period with fever that rises gradually and the "three Cs" (coryza [profuse runny nose], cough, and conjunctivitis) that lasts between 2 and 4 days. Children are most contagious during this time (Cherry, 2014) and are usually quite ill. Koplik spots appear approximately 1 to 4 days before the appearance of the rash (Fig. 41.1 on p. 906). Koplik spots are small, blue-white spots with a red base that cluster near the molars on the buccal mucosa. These spots increase in number before disappearing at approximately 3 days, after which they slough off. As prodromal symptoms reach a peak, the exanthem appears and is characterized by a deep-red, macular rash that usually begins on the face and neck and spreads down the trunk and extremities to the feet. The rash blanches easily with pressure and will gradually turn a brownish color. The duration of the rash is approximately 6 to 7 days.

A partially immune child, such as an infant younger than 9 months who has passively acquired maternal antibodies or a child given immune gamma globulin, may contract modified measles. The prodromal period is shorter and the symptoms are minimal, with few to no Koplik spots. The rash progression follows the pattern of regular measles.

#### Complications

Although considered a relatively rare disease in the US since vaccine became available, measles is still a concern due to its worldwide prevalence. Most cases occur when someone who is unvaccinated brings the disease home to the US after time abroad or someone who comes to the US after contracting the disease in another country; therefore, it is considered "imported" (Lindberg, Lanzi, & Lindberg, 2015). According to the CDC, there were 667 cases of measles in the US in 2014, a significant increase from the 187 cases in 2013. Fortunately, the number of cases in the US decreased in 2015 to 189 reported cases (Centers for Disease Control and Prevention [CDC], 2015a). Because of respiratory involvement, secondary infections such as otitis media, bronchopneumonia, and laryngotracheobronchitis (croup) can occur, especially in infants and younger children, as well as cardiac manifestations such as myocarditis and pericarditis. Rarely, central nervous system (CNS) complications such as encephalitis develop during the prodromal period and can lead to long-term sequelae such as brain death. The most common cause of death from measles is pneumonia (Lindberg et al., 2015). Measles can cause premature birth and miscarriage in pregnant women, but, unlike Rubella, it does not cause birth defects (Lindberg et al., 2015).

#### Therapeutic Management

The treatment of measles is symptomatic, whether the child is hospitalized or remains at home. If hospitalized, the child will require airborne isolation precautions. During the febrile period, the child should be restricted to quiet activities and bed rest. Fluids are encouraged, and humidification and antitussives are used to relieve the cough (Cherry, 2014).

Low levels of vitamin A are associated with measles and with an increase in disease severity. Vitamin A deficiency is common in

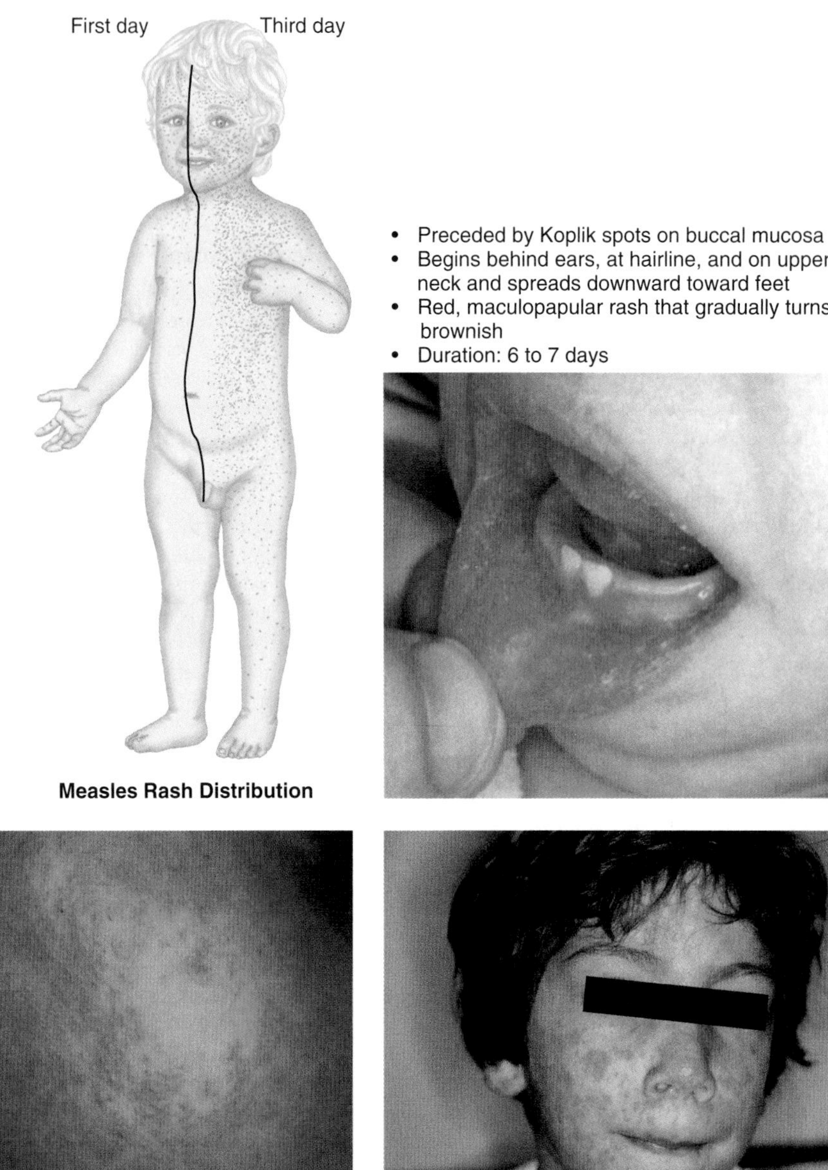

First day
Third day
Measles Rash Distribution
• Preceded by Koplik spots on buccal mucosa
• Begins behind ears, at hairline, and on upper neck and spreads downward toward feet
• Red, maculopapular rash that gradually turns brownish
• Duration: 6 to 7 days
Measles Rash, Dark Skin
Measles Rash, Light Skin


**FIG 41.1** Rubeola (measles) lesions and rash distribution. (Reprinted from Feigin, R., & Cherry, J. [Eds.], [2009]. *Feigin and Cherry's textbook of pediatric infectious diseases* [6th ed.]. Philadelphia: Saunders; from Paller, S.A. [2012]. *Hurwitz clinical pediatric dermatology: a textbook of skin disorders of childhood and adolescence* [4th ed.]. Philadelphia: Saunders.)

developing countries. Recent studies demonstrate that many children in the US also have vitamin A deficiency, prompting the World Health Organization (WHO) and the American Academy of Pediatrics (AAP) to recommend vitamin A supplementation for all measles patients, regardless of the country of residence (Mason, 2016).

Children can be protected against measles and other vaccine-preventable diseases by receiving all their immunizations during routine well-child checkups. Two doses of measles, mumps, and rubella (MMR) vaccine are required for full protection. The first MMR is recommended routinely at 1 year of age. The second dose of MMR is recommended at 4 to 6 years but can be administered during any visit if at least 4 weeks has elapsed since the first dose and both doses are administered beginning at or after 1 year of age. Children who have not previously received their second MMR dose should complete the schedule on or before 6 years of age (AAP, 2015a).

In 2005, the U.S. Food and Drug Administration (FDA) licensed a combination measles-mumps-rubella-varicella vaccine. Studies reveal that there is a very slight increased risk of fever and febrile seizures 7 to 10 days after vaccination in children age 12 to 24 months compared to the separate MMR and varicella vaccines. Therefore, history of

## NURSING CARE PLAN

### *The Child With an Infection in the Community Setting*

**Focused Assessment**

Obtain a complete history, focusing on the following:

- Child's usual state of health
- Any signs or symptoms of developing disease (prodrome)
- Vital signs, especially body temperature
- Description of any skin lesions or rashes, including color, pattern, or shape; size, location, and distribution on the body; presence of any drainage or erythema; and any changes since initial eruption
- Any other family members, classmates, or playmates (friends) showing signs or symptoms
- Any other associated signs or symptoms (arthralgia, malaise, pain, vomiting, headaches)
- History of exposure to illness or environmental vectors
- Medications or treatments tried and their effects

**Nursing Diagnosis**

Risk of Infection (cross-contamination of self or others) related to insufficient knowledge of how to avoid the spread of infectious disease.

**Planning**

***Expected Outcomes***

1. The child's contacts will remain free from symptoms of infection.
2. The child will demonstrate absence of infection, as evidenced by vital signs within normal parameters, resolving lesions with no evidence of complications, and age-appropriate behavior.
3. The family and child (if age-appropriate) will:
   - State symptoms of infectious disease and symptoms of secondary bacterial infections and appropriate disease-containment procedures.
   - Verbalize understanding of written health promotion information, including contact information for local community agencies and resources.

**Interventions and *Rationales***

1. Teach the family and child (if old enough) the symptoms of secondary bacterial infections and complications of infectious diseases that should be promptly reported to their primary medical caregiver (e.g., redness, warmth, swelling, tenderness or pain, new onset of drainage or change in drainage from wound, increase in body temperature, malaise, abdominal pain, vomiting or diarrhea, enlarged glands, changes in skin lesions including sores or wounds that do not heal). Provide the phone number or numbers to call if complications occur.
   *Promptly recognizing and reporting signs and symptoms of secondary bacterial infections can decrease complications.*
2. Teach the family and/or child about the underlying concepts of infection transmission (e.g., airborne, fecal-oral, direct contact), including how and to whom the infection should be reported.
   *Understanding promotes cooperation with infectious disease containment issues, policies, and procedures (e.g., child with chickenpox may not return to daycare or school until the sixth day after onset of rash or sooner if all lesions have dried and crusted).*
3. Emphasize the importance of and encourage the child and family to complete the full course of any prescribed medication unless experiencing adverse side effects.
   *Not taking a complete course of antibiotics may result in incomplete resolution of disease and contributes to antibiotic resistance.*
4. Model and teach the child and family infection-prevention behaviors, such as frequent and meticulous hand hygiene, disposal of used dressings to prevent spread of infectious disease to others, proper disposal of tissues, and covering the mouth when coughing or sneezing. (Follow Standard Precautions guidelines during any contact with blood, mucous membranes, nonintact skin, or any body substance except sweat; use goggles, gloves, and gowns when appropriate; help the family access these if needed.)
   *Demonstration and active participation are more effective teaching strategies than verbal instruction alone (parents will retain information better if they "use" the instruction). Nurses must assume all people are carrying blood-borne pathogens such as HIV or hepatitis B or C virus (HBV, HCV). Standard Precautions apply to everyone. Alcohol-based gels may provide as effective hand hygiene as washing with soap and water in most instances.*
5. Review the child's plan of care, including provision of rest, proper nutrition, fever control, recognition of the development of secondary infection, and when the child can resume normal activities. Provide written information about any instructions for treatment, medication administration, and any scheduled follow-up visits with the child's primary healthcare provider.
   *Providing written information assists with adherence to the plan after discharge.*
6. Provide health promotion information and education (e.g., routine immunization schedule) for the family and child.
   *Refer the family and child to local community agencies (health departments, clinics) as appropriate. Maintenance of an ongoing relationship with a primary care provider provides continuity of care and methods for access to care for the well and sick child as needed.*

**Evaluation**

Have any of the child's contacts contracted the disease?

Is the child free from infection, afebrile, and exhibiting age-appropriate behavior?

Have the parents and/or child verbalized an understanding of the infectious process and disease-containment procedures?

Are the family and/or child cooperative with written contact information and accessing follow-up and preventive healthcare and appropriate community resources?

Can the child and family members describe and demonstrate proper hand hygiene?

**Nursing Diagnosis**

Ineffective Health Maintenance related to insufficient knowledge about how to obtain needed information about infectious disease and its management.

**Planning**

***Expected Outcomes***

The child and family will:

1. Follow an agreed-upon infection-control plan.
2. Meet goals for health maintenance.

**Interventions and *Rationales***

1. Teach the family or child skin and wound assessment and ways to monitor for signs and symptoms of infection, complications, and healing.
   *Early assessment and intervention help prevent serious problems from developing (e.g., sexually transmitted diseases [STDs] in the adolescent girl can result in sterility). Providing information and encouragement promotes understanding and adherence to the treatment plan, thus preventing secondary infection or adverse consequences from infection.*
2. Teach adolescents health-promoting and health-seeking behaviors to reduce the risk of contracting an STD; education includes a description of the direct contact transmission mode and recognition of complications.
   *Providing information and establishing a nonjudgmental environment encourage future health-seeking behaviors. Long-term complications (e.g., sterility, chronic abdominal pain from untreated STDs) can be avoided with early detection, treatment, and appropriate follow-up care.*

*Continued*

## NURSING CARE PLAN—cont'd

### *The Child With an Infection in the Community Setting*

3. Screen for STDs as appropriate (e.g., a prepubescent girl with signs and symptoms of an STD). For prevention, teach children that it is not all right for someone to look at or touch their private parts.
   *Signs and symptoms of problems with the genital area (itching, rash, vaginal or penile discharge) should always be explored by the nurse with a complete history of symptoms to rule out sexual abuse, especially in prepubescent children. Sexual abuse of a child is a reportable offense and must be ruled out.*
4. Provide health promotion information and education (e.g., Papanicolaou [Pap] tests for sexually active adolescents). Refer the family or child to local community agencies (e.g., health departments, clinics) as appropriate.
   *Maintenance of an ongoing relationship with a primary care provider provides continuity of care and methods for access to care for health promotion and disease prevention.*

**Evaluation**

Do the child and family follow the agreed-on infection control plan?
Are they able to meet goals for health maintenance?

**Nursing Diagnosis**

Risk for Ineffective Thermoregulation related to infection.

**Planning**

***Expected Outcome***

The child will be afebrile and exhibit age-appropriate behavior.

**Interventions and *Rationales***

1. Teach the family and/or child normal temperature parameters (e.g., What is a fever?) and temperature-monitoring techniques (see age-appropriate guidelines in Chapter 37).
   *Consistently monitoring and promptly recognizing and reporting fever higher than normal parameters allow for early intervention and can decrease the potential for disability or death.*
2. Teach the family the signs and symptoms of hyperthermia and the complications that should be promptly reported to their primary medical caregiver (e.g., visual disturbances, headache, nausea, vomiting, muscle flaccidity, absence of sweating, delirium, coma). Provide the phone number(s) to call if complications occur.
   *Understanding promotes cooperation and adherence to the child's treatment and care plan.*
3. Teach the family about specific comfort measures (cool environment, light clothing) and medication administration (antipyretics) for fever. Teach parents the appropriate use of antipyretics (see Chapter 37). Use acetaminophen or ibuprofen as directed for fever control. Avoid aspirin products because of the possibility of developing Reye's syndrome (see Chapter 52). Check all over-the-counter medicines to be sure they do not contain aspirin or salicylate. Provide written information that explains the various preparations available (suspension, chewable tablets, suppositories) and the appropriate dose and administration intervals for their child. For example: The dosage of acetaminophen for a 2- to 3-year-old child is 160 mg. Any one of the following can be given every 4 to 6 hours as needed for fever or discomfort:
   Suspension liquid (80 mg in ½ tsp) = 1 tsp
   Children's chewable (80 mg each) = 2 tablets
   Suppository (80 mg each) = 2 suppositories
   *Appropriate teaching promotes cooperation and adherence to the child's treatment and care plan and can also prevent innocent administration of readily available, potentially lethal over-the-counter medication to a child with a viral illness. Providing information and creating awareness of self-care steps the family or adolescent can take to maintain or regain health promotes positive health-seeking behaviors. Because of the many different formulations of both of these over-the-counter medications, parents are frequently confused and inadvertently give the wrong dose, sometimes resulting in overdosing or underdosing and inadequate fever control.*
4. Teach the importance of and specific techniques for maintaining adequate hydration (monitoring the child's intake and output, frequently offering cool liquids, ice pops).
   *Maintaining adequate hydration will help maintain a normal body temperature. An elevated temperature is associated with increased metabolism and fluid use.*
5. Provide written health promotion information and education about fever control and when to access the healthcare system.
   *Maintenance of an ongoing relationship with primary care provider provides continuity of care and methods for access to care for well- and sick-child care as needed.*

**Evaluation**

Has the child maintained a body temperature within normal parameters?
Is the child's behavior within normal parameters for age?

**Nursing Diagnosis**

Fatigue related to discomfort associated with the infectious disease.

**Planning**

***Expected Outcomes***

The child will experience an increase in comfort level and energy, as evidenced by verbalization of decreased discomfort, a relaxed body posture, ability to rest appropriately, decreased crying and irritability, and an interest in age-appropriate activities.

**Interventions and *Rationales***

1. Teach and provide written information for comfort measures (cool environment; lightweight, cool clothing); treatments (monitoring the child's temperature); or medication administration (antipruritics, antipyretics).
   *Appropriate teaching promotes cooperation and adherence to the child's treatment and care plan. Maintaining adequate hydration will help maintain a normal body temperature. An elevated temperature is associated with increased metabolism and fluid use.*
2. Encourage energy conservation during the healing process of an infectious disease; children usually pace their own activity levels when ill. Provide age- and energy-appropriate activities depending on the child's level of wellness.
   *Energy conservation promotes the healing process and provides comfort to children with discomfort, pain, or fever. Using nonpharmacologic techniques, such as distraction, provides pain relief.*
3. Teach the child's family personal hygiene principles to promote the healing process and maintain health after the infectious disease process. Keep the child's skin clean, and change linens and clothing frequently. Wash clothes and linen in mild detergent, and double rinse.
   *Clean clothing helps prevent the spread of secondary infections. Double rinsing reduces the potential irritants in the clothing, thereby minimizing irritation in children with pruritus related to skin manifestations.*

**Evaluation**

Has the child experienced relief from discomfort by demonstrating a relaxed body posture, an interest in age-appropriate play, and verbalization of an increased comfort level?

**Nursing Diagnosis**

Social Isolation related to the confinement for the duration of the communicable disease.

## NURSING CARE PLAN—cont'd

### *The Child With an Infection in the Community Setting*

**Planning**

***Expected Outcomes***

1. The child and family will describe the reasons for isolation and incorporate the resulting restrictions into their home management.
2. The child will participate in age-appropriate activities within the restrictions imposed.
3. The family will contact community agencies for assistance if appropriate.

**Interventions and *Rationales***

1. Encourage the family and child to maintain contact with friends and family by telephone, mail, email, or text while the child is isolated.
   *Maintaining contact with family and friends helps the family adjust to activity limitations, reduces boredom, and provides emotional support.*
2. Provide written information to family about age- and energy-appropriate activities.
   *Providing age-appropriate activities prevents boredom and promotes normal growth and development.*
3. Provide information about community resources for respite and/or sick child care.
   *Providing resources for the family assists in caregiver relief and could result in the family's primary wage earner (especially in single-parent families) returning to work with less loss of income and decrease in the financial burden on the family.*

**Evaluation**

Can the child and family describe the reasons for the isolation, and have they incorporated the appropriate restrictions?

Is the child engaging in age-appropriate activities?

Is the family able to maintain contact with family and friends?

Have support systems been mobilized, both within the family and in the community?

## PATIENT-CENTERED TEACHING

### *How to Care for the Child With a Viral Exanthem*

- For elevated temperature, the child's activity should be restricted to age-appropriate, quiet activities and bed rest. As the fever decreases, the activity level can be gradually increased to a normal level.
- Generally, fever can be controlled with acetaminophen or ibuprofen (no aspirin products because of the risk of developing Reye's syndrome), sponge baths, decreased clothing, decreased environmental temperature, and increased fluid intake. Bed linens may need to be changed frequently during periods of high fever. Over-the-counter antipyretic acetaminophen comes in several different formulations. Read the label carefully and ask your primary healthcare provider if you have any questions regarding medication administration. Seizure precautions should be taken if your child has had a seizure previously.
- The amount of skin irritation and discomfort will vary. Lukewarm baths with colloid preparations (Aveeno), oatmeal, or baking soda (½ cup in tub of water) may help relieve itching. Soothing lotions (Lubriderm, Curel, Aveeno) may also provide comfort. Avoid the use of topical corticosteroids unless ordered by your primary healthcare provider. Use superfatted soaps for sensitive skin (Dove, Basis, Neutrogena, Aveeno). Fingernails should be short. If the child continues to scratch, cotton mittens or socks can be applied to the child's hands. Skin integrity must be maintained to prevent any secondary infections. If secondary infections occur, antibiotic therapy may be necessary.
- Administer antihistamines or antipruritics as prescribed.
- Dress your child in lightweight clothing that is not irritating. Avoid wool and scratchy materials.
- Coughing can be managed with cool humidification of the room and antitussives for children over 4 years of age.
- For arthralgia, antiinflammatory medications may be used. Involvement of weight-bearing joints may warrant bed rest.
- Some viral exanthems cause photophobia. In such cases, keeping the room dimly lit or providing sunglasses for the child may be helpful. If the child has conjunctivitis, secretions or crusts should be removed with tepid water and a clean cloth to prevent contamination.
- Fluid intake is important for successfully managing febrile stages of the disease. Encourage your child to drink cool liquids frequently. If the child's mucous membranes are involved, soft, bland foods may be beneficial.
- As your child progresses through the stages of illness, diversional activities will be necessary during the period of isolation. Choose activities that your child likes and can participate in without becoming unduly tired.
- Call your physician if your child develops any severe symptoms, such as high fever, dry mouth, decreased urine output, persistent cough, seizures, or nonresponsiveness.

seizures in a patient or close family member is a contraindication for the MMRV (AAP, 2015a).

### Rubella (German Measles, 3-Day Measles)

| | |
|---|---|
| Causative agent | RNA virus |
| Incubation period | 14 to 21 days |
| Infectious period | Ranges from 7 days before onset of symptoms to 14 days after appearance of the rash |
| Transmission | Airborne particles or direct contact with infectious droplets, transplacental transmission; small number of infants with congenital rubella continue to shed the virus for months after birth |
| Immunity | Natural disease or live attenuated vaccine |
| Season | Late winter and early spring |

### Manifestations

Rubella is usually a mild disease in children and adults. The virus enters the host, producing a rash after approximately 14 to 21 days. Young children are often asymptomatic until the appearance of the rash. Older children may report profuse nasal drainage, diarrhea, malaise, sore throat, headache, low-grade fever, polyarthritis, eye pain, aches, chills, anorexia, and nausea. Children of all ages usually have impressive posterior cervical, posterior auricular, and occipital lymphadenopathy.

The rash manifests as a pinkish rose maculopapular exanthem that begins on the face, scalp, and neck and is often pruritic (Fig. 41.2). It spreads downward to include the entire body within 1 to 3 days. As the rash spreads to the trunk, the rash on the face begins to fade. Petechiae (spots), which are red or purple color and pinpoint in size, may occur on the soft palate. Their appearance is sometimes referred to as Forchheimer's sign.

### Complications

The availability of rubella vaccine has effectively eliminated rubella in the United States (CDC, 2014b). Rubella has relatively few complications. The most common are arthritis and arthralgia, which occur more often in adult women than in children or adolescents. Mild thrombocytopenia may also occur but is usually self-limiting and of short duration. A rare complication is encephalitis, which is usually less severe than measles-related encephalitis.

The importance of recognizing and respecting this viral illness is not the morbidity of the disease itself but rather the consequences that can occur to a fetus during maternal infection. The most devastating form of rubella is congenital rubella syndrome (CRS) that occurs after maternal infection, usually during the first 12 weeks of pregnancy. One of the most common manifestations of CRS is intrauterine growth retardation. These infants typically weigh less than 2500 g and continue to have failure to thrive in infancy. Mortality is highest during the first year. Common causes of death include pneumonia, heart defects, encephalitis, and immune deficiency (Cherry & Adachi, 2014).

### Therapeutic Management

Treatment is generally supportive and symptomatic, with the disease being self-limiting with resolution within 5 days. Recommendation for exclusion of affected children from school or child care is 7 days after the rash begins. Infants with CRS are presumed contagious until age 1 year or nasopharyngeal and urine cultures for the rubella virus are repeatedly negative. Primary prevention of rubella can be accomplished through administration of the rubella vaccine in combination with measles and mumps vaccine (MMR), as previously discussed. There is a global initiative to eliminate rubella thereby eliminating CRS by vaccination, since only half of infants born globally are vaccinated (Grant, Reef, Dabbagh, et al., 2015).

**SAFETY ALERT**

***Congenital Rubella Syndrome***

The rubella virus can cross the placenta and infect the fetus, causing fetal death or abnormalities.

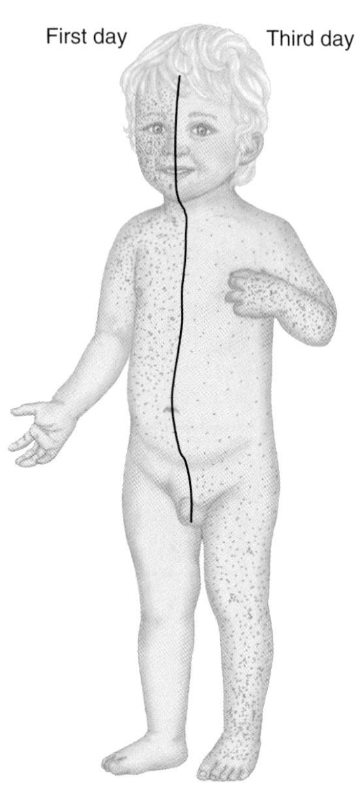


**German Measles Rash Distribution**

- Begins on face, neck, and scalp and spreads downward to entire body; fades on face as it spreads to trunk
- Pinkish, maculopapular rash
- Reddish, pinpoint petechiae may occur on soft palate (Forschheimer's sign)

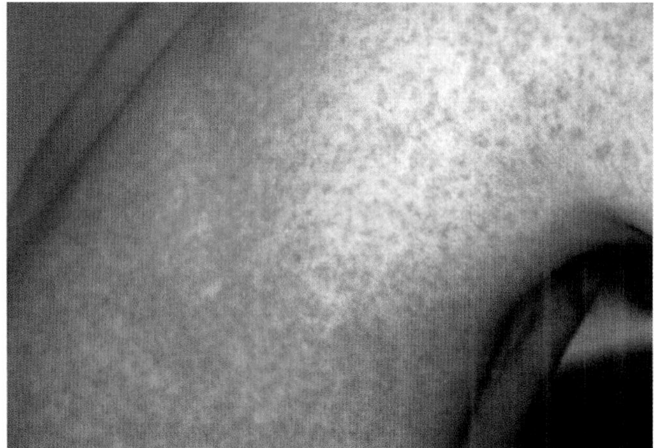

**FIG 41.2** Rubella (German measles) lesions and rash distribution. (From Paller, S.A. [2012]. *Hurwitz clinical pediatric dermatology: a textbook of skin disorders of childhood and adolescence* [4th ed.]. Philadelphia: Saunders.)

## Erythema Infectiosum (Fifth Disease, Parvovirus B19)

| | |
|---|---|
| Causative agent | Parvovirus B19 |
| Incubation period | 4 to 17 days but can be up to 28 days |
| Infectious period | Shedding of virus occurs between days 5 and 12 of the infection; usually from the prodromal period until the rash appears |
| Transmission | Airborne particles, respiratory droplets, blood, blood products, transplacental transmission |
| Immunity | Natural disease is thought to provide antibodies for immunity |
| Season | Late winter and early spring |

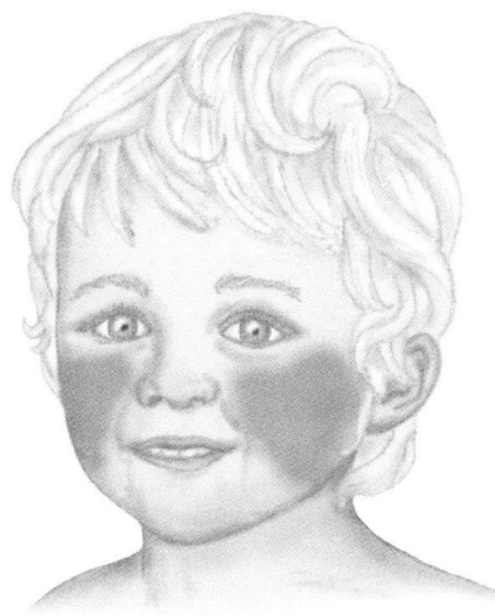


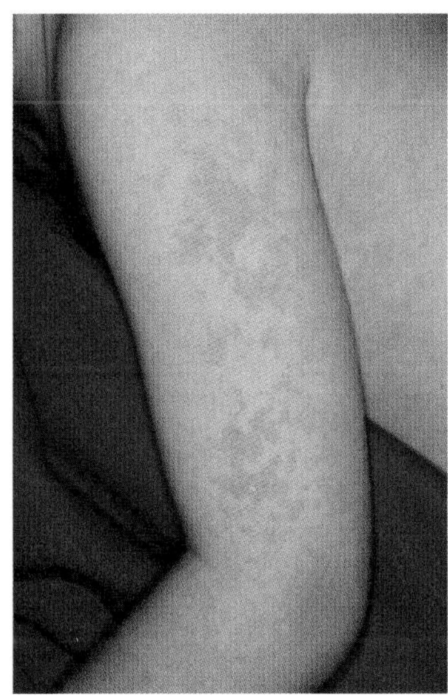

• Presents with fiery-red, edematous rash on cheeks—"slapped cheek" appearance
• Followed in 1-4 days by erythematous, maculo-papular, lacy rash on trunk and extremities


**FIG 41.3** Erythema infectiosum lesions and rash distribution. (From Paller, S.A. [2012]. *Hurwitz clinical pediatric dermatology: a textbook of skin disorders of childhood and adolescence* [4th ed.]. Philadelphia: Saunders.)

This disease is most common in children ages 5 to 15 years but can also occur in adults (O'Grady, 2014).

Fifth disease is a relatively mild systemic disease. Typically, the child appears well but has an intense, fiery red, edematous rash on the cheeks, which gives a "slapped cheek" appearance (Fig. 41.3), or a history of a rash that "comes and goes." Before the appearance of the rash, many children are asymptomatic or have nonspecific symptoms such as headache, runny nose, malaise, and mild fever. Approximately 1 to 4 days after the facial rash appears, an erythematous, maculopapular rash appears on the trunk and extremities. The rash fades with a central clearing area, resulting in a lacy appearance. The rash lasts 2 to 39 days and can reappear when aggravated by environmental factors such as heat, exercise, warm baths, rubbing of the skin, and stress.

### Complications

Because the disease is mild, complications are not usually reported, especially in children. Patients with sickle cell disease or beta-thalassemia are at risk for anemia and aplastic crisis. Patients with a poor immune system are also at risk for anemia. Because pregnant women are at risk for intrauterine infection, the nurse should obtain a careful history, with an emphasis on identifying any pregnant family members, teachers, or friends to prevent intrauterine infection and fetal death. Many school districts notify pregnant staff if they have been exposed to a child with fifth disease and recommend that they contact their healthcare provider. Parvovirus B19 occurs in approximately 1.5% of pregnancies (O'Grady, 2014). If a pregnant woman tests positive for Parvovirus B19, she should be closely monitored with serial ultrasounds by her obstetric provider (AAP, 2015b).

### Therapeutic Management

The disease is generally benign and self-limiting. Treatment is symptomatic and supportive.

## Roseola Infantum (Exanthem Subitum, 3-day fever)

| | |
|---|---|
| Causative agent | Human herpesvirus 6 (HHV-6) |
| Incubation period | 5 to 15 days |
| Infectious period | Unknown but thought to extend from the febrile stage to the time the rash first appears |
| Transmission | Most likely by contact with secretions (saliva, cerebrospinal fluid [CSF]) of asymptomatic close contacts |
| Season | Throughout the year without a distinctive seasonal pattern |

### Manifestations

HHV-6 appears to be the major causative agent, although other viruses have been implicated as well. Most clinical cases of roseola occur in children 6 to 18 months old. The child has a sudden high fever (103° F to 106° F [39.4° C to 41.1° C]), malaise, and irritability but may remain active and alert. An intermittent or constant fever may persist for 3 to 5 days. The child may also have a mild cough, runny nose, abdominal pain, headache, vomiting, and diarrhea. After 3 to 5 days, the fever subsides, and within several hours to 2 days, a rash appears. The rash consists of rose-pink maculopapules or macules that blanch with pressure (Fig. 41.4). The rash occurs predominantly on the neck and trunk and may be surrounded by a whitish ring. It normally persists for 24 to 48 hours before fading.

### Complications

Complications associated with roseola are uncommon. Febrile seizures (see Chapter 52) can occur.

### Therapeutic Management

Treatment is symptomatic. Family members should be taught about fever control and management.

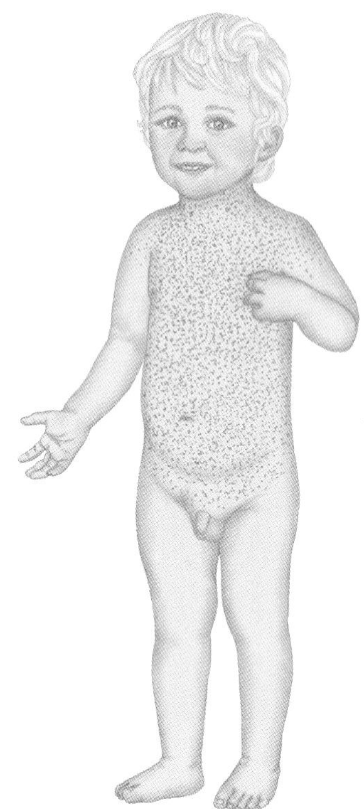

Rash appears several hours to 2 days after fever subsides
Erythematous maculopapular or macular rash may be surrounded by whitish ring
Blanches with pressure
Predominantly on neck and trunk
Usually persists for 24-48 hours


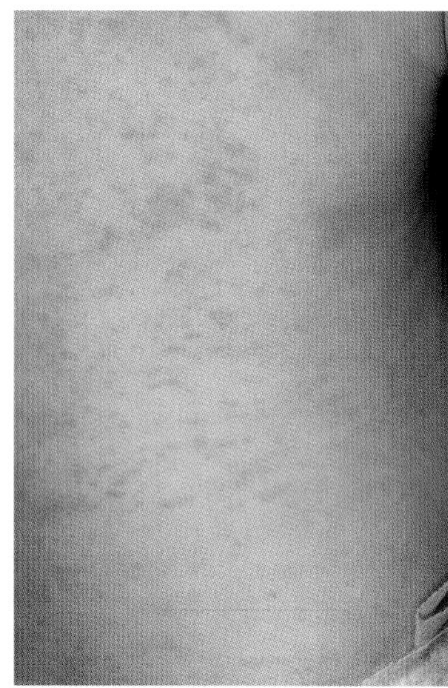

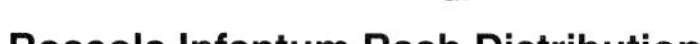


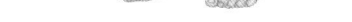

**FIG 41.4** Roseola infantum lesions and rash distribution. (From Paller, S.A. [2012]. *Hurwitz clinical pediatric dermatology: a textbook of skin disorders of childhood and adolescence* [4th ed.]. Philadelphia: Saunders.)

Antipyretic medications, lightweight clothing, cooler environmental temperatures, and increased fluid intake all assist with fever control. Temperature monitoring, medication administration (prescription and over-the-counter medications), and other comfort measures should be discussed. The nurse verifies that the child's family has access to a thermometer and knows how to use it. In addition, parents should be given information regarding the absolute avoidance of any form of aspirin (including over-the-counter medications containing salicylates) because of the potential risk of developing Reye's syndrome (see Chapter 52). Anticipatory guidance should include alerting the parent to the possibility of febrile seizures and teaching about seizure precautions (especially if the child has a history of previous febrile seizures).

Parents' understanding of the care necessary for their child is important, particularly regarding measures to control and prevent the spread of infection. Teach the parents how to recognize the signs and symptoms of complications so they can seek medical treatment when warranted. Providing parents with written instructions that they can refer to at home can be helpful.

## Enterovirus (Nonpolio) Infections (Coxsackieviruses, Group A and Group B), Echoviruses, and Enteroviruses

| | |
|---|---|
| Causative agents | RNA viruses including 23 group A coxsackieviruses (types A1 to A24, except type A23), six group B coxsackieviruses (types B1 to B6), 31 echoviruses (types 1 to 33, except types 10 and 28), and four enteroviruses (types 68 to 71) |
| Incubation period | Usually 3 to 6 days |
| Infectious period | Unknown, but fecal viral excretion and transmission can continue for 7 to11 weeks after the onset of infection |
| Transmission | Spread by fecal-oral and possibly by oral-oral (respiratory) routes. Contact precautions are implemented for infants and young children. |
| Season | In temperate climates infections are most common in the summer and fall, but no seasonal pattern is evident in the tropics |

### Manifestations

Common presentations in both infants and children include nonspecific febrile illnesses with a wide variety of respiratory, gastrointestinal, cardiac, neurologic, skin, oral, and eye signs and symptoms.

A frequently seen pattern of illness in young children is hand-foot-and-mouth disease, caused by coxsackievirus A16 or other enteroviruses. Inflammation and lesions in the mouth (Fig. 41.5), on the palms of the hands, and on the soles of the feet are the hallmarks of this syndrome, along with mild fever; some children experience small lesions on the buttocks. Lesions become vesicular over the course of several days and usually resolve by 1 week (Abzug, 2016). If lesions are particularly widespread in the oropharynx, the child may refuse to eat or drink; the potential for dehydration is present in very young children.

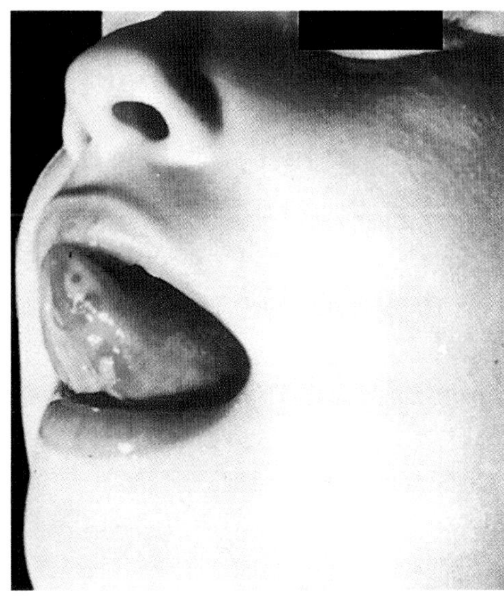

**FIG 41.5** Coxsackievirus mouth lesions. (Reprinted from Feigin, R., & Cherry, J. [Eds.], [2009]. *Feigin and Cherry's textbook of pediatric infectious diseases* [6th ed.]. Philadelphia: Saunders.)

### Complications

Although each of these groups of symptoms can be associated with different enteroviruses, complications can occur from specific strains. Young infants with a history of prematurity are at higher risks for complications and death. Serious complications such as myocarditis, hepatitis, and encephalitis are often the cause (Abzug, 2016).

### Therapeutic Management

Currently, no specific therapy is available for enteroviral infections, but clinical trials are evaluating the effectiveness of pleconaril, an antiviral drug, and immunoglobulin for neonates with severe disease (Azbug, 2016). Parents and caregivers should be given educational information regarding the importance of hand hygiene and personal hygiene, especially after diaper changes and trips to the bathroom.

Management of hand-foot-and-mouth disease is symptomatic. The parent can provide comfort and pain relief with acetaminophen and frequent administration of cool liquids. Milk-based ice cream is especially palatable. Extensive oropharyngeal lesions that prevent adequate oral intake can be treated with a salt and water mouth rinse or a topical solution of equal parts lidocaine gel, diphenhydramine liquid, and a liquid antacid (mixed by prescription) either applied directly to lesions or used as a mouthwash.

### Nursing Considerations

The nurse needs to obtain a detailed history of the onset of symptoms with a focused assessment on the particular body systems involved. Children with an enterovirus infection can be challenging because of the wide variety and degree of signs and symptoms. Supportive care is similar to that of any child with a viral exanthem. Parents and caregivers should be given educational information about disease transmission, school or daycare attendance policies, and any available community resources (sick-child care).

## Varicella-Zoster Infections (Chickenpox, Shingles)

| | |
|---|---|
| Causative agent | Varicella-zoster virus<br>Double-stranded DNA virus |
| Incubation period | 10 to 21 days |
| Infectious period | 1 to 2 days before the onset of rash until all lesions are dried (crusted over), usually 5 to 7 days |
| Transmission | Direct contact, droplet, airborne particles |
| Immunity | Natural disease of varicella; same virus causes zoster, and child may contract zoster at a later time; varicella vaccine |
| Season | Late winter through early spring |

Primary infection with the varicella-zoster virus causes chickenpox. Before 1995, when the vaccine became available, chickenpox was one of the most common childhood diseases in children 5 to 9 years old and was responsible for 100 to 125 deaths each year in the US (AAP, 2015c). Zoster (shingles), which is the reactivation of the latent varicella-zoster virus, occurs most frequently in the elderly population but can occur in children as well, especially adolescents and young adults. Generally, varicella and zoster in children are not life threatening.

### Manifestations

*Varicella.* During the 24 to 48 hours before the appearance of lesions, symptoms may include a slightly elevated body temperature, malaise, headache, and anorexia. A rash generally first appears on the trunk and scalp (Fig. 41.6), followed by the appearance of lesions, which quickly become teardrop vesicles with an erythematous base. The vesicles then become pustular, after which they begin to dry and develop a crust. The lesions appear in crops over the course of usually 3 to 4 days and can be seen to be in different stages of development. The number of lesions varies from child to child but usually average approximately 300. Children in the household with secondary cases generally have rashes that are more extensive than that of the child with the primary case. The lesions can appear on the mucous membranes in the mouth, genital area, and rectum. Second attacks are rare and are more common in immunocompromised children. Breakthrough attacks in immunized children are also rare, and the disease presentation is mild, with few lesions (LaRussa & Marin, 2016).

*Herpes zoster (shingles).* During the primary infection with varicella, the varicella-zoster virus enters the sensory nerve ending and the dorsal root ganglion and establishes a latent infection. Activation of the infection causes herpes zoster (shingles). Zoster manifests with tenderness along the involved nerve and surrounding skin for approximately 2 weeks before the appearance of the lesions. If pain is present, its intensity can range from an unpleasant, abnormal sensitivity to touch to burning, tingling, itching, sharp knife-like prickling, or even deep pain. Unilateral crops of lesions appear along a single dermatome of one or more sensory nerves. These lesions progress through the same stages as varicella. There may be enlargement and tenderness of the lymph nodes in the same region.

Risk factors for shingles are a history of chickenpox, age over 50 years, weakened immune system, stress or trauma, and being treated for cancer. Zoster is thought to be an infection of elderly people, but there are cases when children can get zoster.

### Complications

The most common complication of varicella-zoster virus infection is secondary bacterial infection of the skin lesions. Staphylococci and group A beta-hemolytic streptococci are the usual causative agents. CNS complications have been associated with mild to severe varicella infections. Encephalitis with ataxia, tremor, and nystagmus can occur

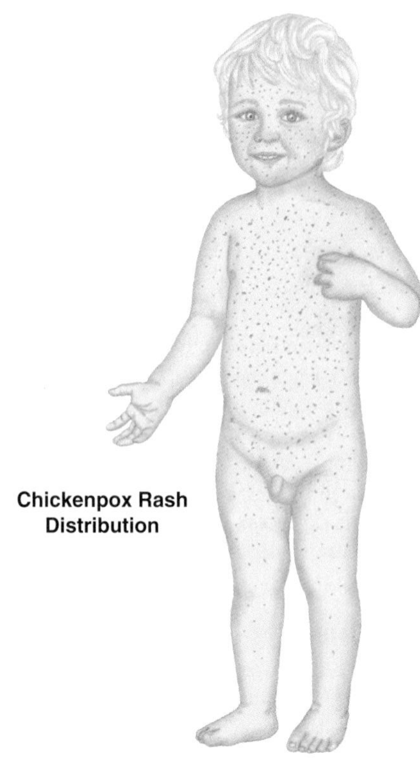

Chickenpox Rash
Distribution
• Macular rash 24-48 hours after slight fever, malaise, anorexia
• Lesions appear in "crops," first on trunk and scalp, then moving sparsely to extremities; may appear in mucous membranes (mouth, genital area, rectum)
• Generally three successive eruptions over 3-4 days
• Lesions begin as a macular rash, develop into a red papular rash, then move quickly into tear-drop vesicles with erythematous base; vesicle becomes pustular and begins drying, and a crust develops
• Rash varies from child to child


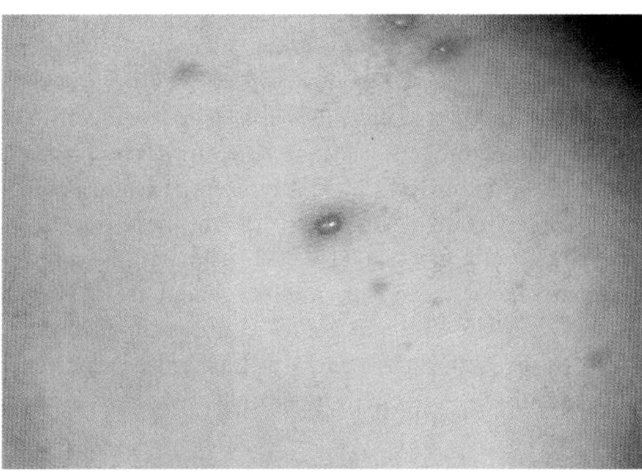


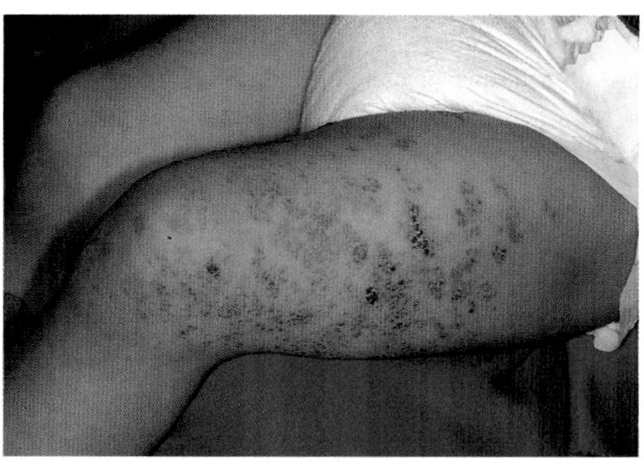


**FIG 41.6** Chickenpox and shingles lesions and rash distribution. (From Paller, S.A. [2012]. *Hurwitz clinical pediatric dermatology: a textbook of skin disorders of childhood and adolescence* [4th ed.]. Philadelphia: Saunders.)

in the first week. The prognosis is generally positive unless CNS involvement is severe—usually manifested by convulsions and coma. Children with these complications may have future CNS difficulties, including seizures, intellectual disability, or behavior disorders.

Varicella pneumonia, a common complication in adults, rarely occurs in children. Reye's syndrome has been known to occur after varicella infection (see Chapter 52), particularly if aspirin is given. Corneal involvement can occur if lesions involve the eye.

Complications of herpes zoster are rare but involve the same difficulties with secondary infections that occur with varicella.

Parents should be given educational information regarding the absolute avoidance of any form of aspirin (including over-the-counter medications containing salicylates) because of the potential risk of developing Reye's syndrome.

### Therapeutic Management

Treatment is symptomatic and supportive for the healthy child. Frequent bathing in an oatmeal bath and use of antihistamines can relieve itching and prevent secondary bacterial infections. Acetaminophen to control fever is the best option because aspirin must be avoided. Although oral acyclovir is not routinely recommended for healthy children with varicella, it can be considered for use in severe cases, people with chronic illnesses, those receiving long-term aspirin therapy, or children on short-term corticosteroid treatment. For immunocompromised children, acyclovir is given intravenously because the oral route is less reliable for these children (Gershon, 2014). The decision to use these medications, along with the duration and route, is individually determined by the primary healthcare provider. Response to antiviral drugs is good, provided that the treatment is started early in the illness, because antiviral drugs have a limited "window of opportunity."

In the hospital setting, children with varicella or zoster infections should be placed in a private room with strict isolation (Airborne and Contact Transmission Precautions). The nurse assigned should not simultaneously care for immunocompromised patients to decrease the risk of varicella transmission.

The CDC recommends that varicella vaccine can be given to healthy, nonimmune children (1 year of age or older) immediately after exposure and before 3 to 5 days; in some cases this will reduce the severity of the disease.

Primary prevention of varicella includes screening and administering the vaccine at routine well-child visits (see Chapter 6). Varicella vaccine is recommended at any visit on or after the first birthday for healthy susceptible children without a reliable history of actual disease or immunization and without contraindications to receiving the vaccine. A booster dose is given between 4 and 6 years of age. In 2005, a combination vaccine with MMR was licensed.

### Nursing Considerations

Care of children in a community with varicella can be challenging, because the condition is very contagious. A single case can quickly spread to others who are not immune, so prevention is essential. The nurse needs to educate parents of children with varicella about skin care to prevent secondary bacterial infections and emphasize the importance of absolute avoidance of any form of aspirin (including over-the-counter medications containing aspirin).

In the hospital setting, all contaminated materials must be bagged and labeled before reprocessing. Hands should be washed after contact with the child and before contact with another patient. Hospitalized children who have been exposed to varicella should be kept in strict isolation for 8 to 21 days after the onset of rash in the infected individual. At birth, neonates with mothers who have active varicella infections should be placed in strict isolation. In addition, Airborne Precautions and Contact Precautions should be in effect for children with herpes zoster infections.

**SAFETY ALERT**

***Varicella and the Immunocompromised Child***

Immunocompromised children who contract varicella may have large hemorrhagic lesions. Primary varicella pneumonia is a frequent complication. Some children develop an acute form of varicella with disseminated intravascular coagulation (DIC) that is fatal, often before antiviral therapy can be started.

## OTHER VIRAL INFECTIONS

### Mumps

| | |
|---|---|
| Causative agent | Paramyxovirus, single-stranded RNA |
| Incubation period | Usually 16 to 18 days but can be 12 to 25 days |
| Infectious period | From 7 days before swelling (parotitis) to 9 days after onset |
| Transmission | Airborne droplets, salivary secretions, possibly urine |
| Immunity | Natural disease or live attenuated vaccine |
| Season | Late winter and spring |

#### Manifestations

Prodromal manifestations include fever, myalgia, headache, and malaise. The classic clinical sign of parotid glandular swelling (parotitis) often follows these, although a substantial number of individuals have no such swelling. When parotid swelling occurs, it can be accompanied by fever.

#### Complications

Mumps generally affects the salivary glands but can involve multiple organs. The most common complication is aseptic meningitis, with the virus identified in the CSF. Signs of CNS involvement include nuchal rigidity, lethargy, and vomiting. Children with these manifestations usually completely recover. A less common CNS complication is meningoencephalomyelitis manifested by fever, headache, nausea, vomiting, nuchal rigidity, and changes in sensorium. These complications are treated symptomatically and generally have an uneventful recovery period.

The potential complication of most concern to parents is orchitis (inflammation of a testis). Orchitis is a complication frequently seen in adolescent boys and almost never before puberty; however, sterility is uncommon. Rarely, mumps can cause ovarian or breast inflammation in postpubertal girls. Although infrequent, mumps can cause sensorineural hearing impairment. Increased fetal mortality is noted in the first trimester (Cherry & Quinn, 2014).

#### Therapeutic Management

Uncomplicated mumps may require only symptomatic care and encouragement of adequate hydration. Avoidance of acidic foods such as orange juice is helpful. Droplet Precautions are indicated until 9 days after the onset of the parotid swelling. Parents should be given educational information regarding the absolute avoidance of any form of aspirin (including over-the-counter medications containing salicylates) because of the potential risk of developing Reye's syndrome.

Orchitis requires bed rest, intermittent application of ice packs, pain management, emotional support, and diversional activities. CNS complications require neurologic evaluations and vital sign measurement as indicated by the child's condition when the complications require hospitalization.

#### Nursing Considerations

The nurse should obtain a history of the onset of symptoms, examine the child's ears and throat, and perform a neurologic assessment. The child's vital signs (including temperature), usual state of health, and characteristics of the lymph nodes in the neck should be documented. In boys, an examination of the testes should be included in the initial assessment.

Typically, children with mumps are not hospitalized unless they have complications. Therefore, meticulous hand hygiene technique should be taught to the child, the family, and close contacts to prevent transmission. Hospitalized children are placed in isolation according to the facility's policies (usually Droplet Precautions).

Primary prevention of mumps can be accomplished through administration of the mumps vaccine in combination with measles and rubella vaccine (MMR vaccine), as previously discussed.

### Cytomegalovirus (CMV)

| | |
|---|---|
| Causative agent | Human cytomegalovirus (CMV), double-stranded DNA virus |
| Incubation period | Unknown, except for 3 to 12 weeks after blood transfusions and 4 weeks to 4 months after organ (tissue) transplantation |

| | |
|---|---|
| Transmission | Saliva, urine, blood, semen, cervical secretions, breast milk, organ transplants |
| Immunity | None, although CMV immune globulin, used only in seronegative transplant patients, has had moderate effectiveness |
| Season | Can occur during any season |

CMV is a common cause of congenital infection in infants and is a leading cause of hearing loss and intellectual disability in the United States. A child can become infected with the virus during the prenatal, perinatal, or postnatal period. Only infections in utero cause permanent infection. Approximately one third of women with primary CMV infections transmit CMV to the fetus. The prevalence in the United States is 1 in 150 live births, approximately 40,000 newborns causing permanent disability in 8,000 and death in 400 (Alex, 2014; Harrison, 2015). Only 5% to 15% of infants with congenital CMV infection have symptoms evident at birth; some infants who appear asymptomatic at birth later manifest signs of CMV. Asymptomatic infants have a better prognosis, but 10% to 15% may still develop hearing loss (Harrison, 2014). Among children, CMV is the leading nongenetic cause of deafness. Signs and symptoms in the infant include jaundice, lethargy, seizures, enlarged spleen and liver, petechial rash, respiratory distress, microcephaly, and intracerebral calcifications. The child can continue to shed the virus for up to 5 years.

During the postnatal period, the infant can acquire CMV from a maternal or nonmaternal source. The virus can be transmitted through the breast milk of an infected mother. Blood transfusions, which can be numerous in the premature infant, can also be a source of CMV infection. Children who are not infected congenitally or perinatally often acquire the virus during their toddler or preschool years. Because of sexual activity, the teen years are another period of potential acquisition. Affected adolescents are generally asymptomatic but can have a mononucleosis-like syndrome with fever, hepatosplenomegaly, and mild hepatitis.

### Therapeutic Management

The treatments for CMV are directed at early detection of disabilities and appropriate interventions to maximize developmental potential. Hearing aids, cochlear implants, and speech therapy are used to treat hearing loss. Assessments to detect learning disabilities and early intervention with physical, speech, and cognitive therapy play an important role. Recent studies have shown that children who receive treatment with antiviral drugs such as ganciclovir develop fewer developmental delays. Treatment with CMV immune globulin as well as antivirals is being studied to treat pregnant women with CMV. Using CMV-negative donors for neonatal transfusions can reduce the risk of exposure associated with bloodborne viral transmission. Several vaccines are currently being investigated, and the Institute of Medicine cited CMV as one of the highest priorities for vaccine development (Harrison, 2015). Presently, education regarding congenital CMV and the promotion of good hygiene practices are the best sources of prevention. Nurses must use proper precautions to avoid transmission of the disease, although there is no evidence that healthcare workers are at an increased risk of infection.

### Nursing Considerations

The nurse should obtain a history of the child's symptoms and possible exposures. Children with congenitally acquired CMV can develop a wide range of manifestations, so nursing care will vary according to the child's specific needs. In cases involving developmental delay, intellectual disability, neurologic deficit, or hearing loss, the nurse can help coordinate the healthcare team's efforts to meet the child's needs. Parents will need support and education in caring for a child with developmental deficits. The nurse will play a key role in identifying the need for referral and any resources available in the community, including parental support groups.

## Epstein-Barr Virus (Infectious Mononucleosis)

| | |
|---|---|
| Causative agent | Epstein-Barr virus (EBV, a herpes-like virus); double-stranded DNA |
| Incubation period: | 4 to 7 weeks |
| Infectious period | Unknown; the virus is commonly shed before clinical onset of disease until 6 months, then intermittently for life; asymptomatic carriers are common |
| Transmission | Saliva, intimate contact, blood |
| Immunity | Natural disease |
| Season | Can occur during any season |

Epithelial cells and the B lymphocytes are the primary sites of infection in infectious mononucleosis. EBV is well recognized as the causative agent in 90% of cases of infectious mononucleosis (Marshall & Foxworth, 2012). It also is associated with other diseases, especially outside North America. EBV has been identified as a cofactor in Hodgkin disease; in Burkitt lymphoma, often seen in Africa; and in cases of nasopharyngeal carcinoma, seen in China and Southeast Asia. EBV alone cannot cause the lymphomas or the carcinoma, but it acts in association with other factors.

### Manifestations

Infectious mononucleosis typically occurs in otherwise healthy individuals, most commonly in older children and young adults, with the highest prevalence in 15- to 19-year-olds. Clinical signs include fever, exudative pharyngitis, lymphadenopathy (cervical, axillary and inguinal), and hepatosplenomegaly. The severity of the clinical signs can range from asymptomatic and mild to severe and fatal. Some children develop a maculopapular rash, especially after treatment with an aminopenicillin antibiotic such as ampicillin or amoxicillin. Children may report malaise, headache, fatigue, nausea, and abdominal pain. The acute illness usually lasts 2 to 4 weeks and is followed by a gradual recovery. EBV can remain dormant after the infection and recur during times of suppressed immunity. The prognosis is generally excellent if no complications occur.

### Complications

Common complications, which are rare, include exanthems and hepatitis. More serious complications involve the pulmonary, neurologic, and hematopoietic systems. The risk of splenic rupture associated with EBV infection occurs most frequently during the first to third weeks of the illness. Patients with a palpable spleen are at a higher risk for rupture. Swelling of the pharynx and tonsils can be severe enough to compromise respiration. The outcome of these complications depends on the severity of the infection and the course of the complications.

### Therapeutic Management

The illness is generally self-limiting; therefore, treatment is supportive. Antivirals have little effect on the illness. Complications are addressed with appropriate medical treatment. Use of steroids to treat acute tonsillar swelling and other symptoms of infectious mononucleosis is effective in managing inflammation (Marshall & Foxworth, 2012). Strenuous physical activity and contact sports should be avoided during the acute illness and for at least one month or as long as the spleen is enlarged to minimize the risk of splenic rupture.

### Nursing Considerations

The history should include presenting signs and symptoms. Physical examination of the pharynx should be performed, with documentation of any redness or swelling. Note any rashes, including a description of their distribution and appearance. The spleen and liver should be evaluated for enlargement. The child's body temperature should be recorded and nutrition and hydration status evaluated.

Because EBV infection is self-limiting, nursing care is mainly supportive. Most children are cared for at home. Hospitalization with standard precautions for hydration therapy may be necessary if the child is unable to swallow. Care in both settings involves bed rest, hydration, and relief of discomfort.

Education and reinforcement regarding the importance of avoiding contact sports, including roughhousing at home with family and friends, should be given to older children or adolescents to help them understand the risks involved (see Patient-Centered Teaching: How to Care for the Child with Infectious Mononucleosis).

### PATIENT-CENTERED TEACHING

#### *How to Care for the Child With Infectious Mononucleosis*

- Prolonged rest is indicated during the acute stage of the illness.
- Acetaminophen may be useful in controlling discomfort caused by fever and enlarged tonsils.
- Activity restrictions include no contact sports of any type, including roughhousing at home with siblings or friends, to protect the child's enlarged spleen from rupture. With improvement in clinical signs, the child should be allowed to gradually resume normal activities as tolerated.
- The parents and child need to be prepared for a slow and gradual recovery. Fatigue may continue, necessitating a gradual return to school activities.
- Hydration should be monitored and encouraged.
- In children with a sore throat, soothing liquids, bland foods, and milkshakes may be better tolerated than a regular diet.
- Anxiety related to missed schoolwork should be anticipated. Homebound school programs should be arranged if the child will be absent from school for a prolonged period.
- The parents should have an understanding of the disease and the usual course of recovery. They may need support in exploring options for caring for their child during a lengthy recovery period, including referrals for alternative child-care arrangements, to decrease lost income and maintain job security.

## Rabies

| | |
|---|---|
| Causative agent | Rhabdovirus (RNA virus) |
| Incubation period | 5 days to more than 1 year; incubation can extend to 6 years, but the average is 1 to 3 months |
| Infectious period | 10 days (if the animal is still healthy, rabies is unlikely); however, bats can harbor the virus for a longer period |
| Transmission | Bites with contaminated saliva, scratches from claws of infected animals, airborne transmission in laboratory settings and in bat-infested caves, transplantation of corneas from undiagnosed donors |
| Immunity | Human diploid cell vaccine (HDCV), purified chick embryo cell vaccine (PCECV), and rabies vaccine absorbed (RVA) |
| Season | Can occur during any season |

Rabies is caused by a virus that can infect any warm-blooded animal. In the United States, the reservoir consists of skunks, bats, raccoons, foxes, squirrels, and woodchucks. Over the past few decades, most cases of rabies have been caused by bats. Dogs and cats can also be reservoirs, but the use of animal vaccines makes them a less common source of infection.

### Manifestations

The rhabdovirus results in a slowly developing infection. The virus travels up the axons of the motor or sensory neurons to the brain. For this reason, bites that occur on the feet or lower extremities are associated with longer incubation periods than are bites on the face. Incubation periods are shortened in children.

When left untreated, the virus will cause vague signs and symptoms. The child may report not feeling well. The child may have a sore throat, headache, fever, discomfort at the site of the bite, hyperactivity, anxiety, muscle spasms, or convulsions. The decreased ability to swallow results in drooling or aspiration, which explains the use of the term *hydrophobia* in connection with rabies. Once the disease has established itself, it is almost always fatal. Once symptoms appear, the disease generally lasts 2 weeks before progressing to death.

### Therapeutic Management

The focus of rabies management is preventive and includes educating adults and children to avoid touching and petting strange animals, especially those in unusual settings exhibiting strange behaviors. When an animal bites a child, a determination must be made regarding whether to treat that child. Factors to be considered include the geographic area, type of animal, circumstances of the bite, and the animal's vaccination record. If the animal is available, it can be observed for 10 days or killed for microscopic examination of the brain.

The bite wound should be cleaned with copious amounts of soap and water and vigorous rubbing for 10 to 15 minutes. Human rabies immune globulin (HRIG) is given. One half of the dose is infiltrated locally around the wound, and the other half is administered intramuscularly. Rabies vaccination should be administered as early as possible after exposure, preferably within 24 hours. Additional doses of the vaccine are given into the deltoid muscle on days 3, 7, and 14 after the first vaccine. Immunocompromised children should receive a fifth dose on day 28 (Michos & Zaoutis, 2011). Rabies vaccine is the only vaccine that can be given after exposure and result in successful immunity.

### Nursing Considerations

A complete history of the event should be obtained, including the type of animal involved, identification of the animal as wild or domestic, immunization record of the animal, and the present location of the animal (if known). This information will determine the course of action. The wound should be examined and a description noted in the child's record.

For the child who will undergo a complete series of vaccinations, the nurse can use a variety of distraction techniques (e.g., counting, singing). Allowing the child to administer injections to a doll may help relieve some anxiety associated with multiple injections. For the older child, an explanation of the injection process and reasons for treatment may be adequate.

Primary prevention of rabies includes anticipatory guidance focusing on teaching children to avoid petting or touching unknown animals. Responsible pet care, including vaccination, and stray animal control will assist in decreasing the risk of exposure. A good resource for children and families is http://www.cdc.gov/rabiesandkids.

For the child who develops rabies, nursing actions are supportive, including support of the child and family through the dying process (see Chapter 36). The child is placed in strict isolation, and Contact Precautions are instituted. The family will need support in preparing for the child's inevitable death and in coping with feelings of guilt.

## BACTERIAL INFECTIONS

Bacteria are abundant in the environment, yet relatively few cause diseases in humans. Bacteria are organisms that contain both DNA and RNA. They lack a nuclear membrane but have a complex cell wall. The properties of the cell wall determine the bacterium's classification as either gram positive or gram negative. Gram-positive bacteria have a thicker wall that helps resist bile activity, drying, and other environmental factors. Gram-positive bacteria can cause chronic inflammation of dermal tissue, fever, and shock. Gram-negative bacteria have a thinner cell wall.

Outside the cell wall, many bacteria have flagella, which help propel them through their environment. Some have pili—rigid projections that assist in attachment to the host cell or other bacteria. Capsules help hide the bacteria's presence from the host and make phagocytosis by the host cell more difficult.

Bacteria excrete toxins. Exotoxins are highly poisonous substances that cause cell damage by cell lysis, inhibition of protein synthesis, or interference with the passage of nerve impulses. Endotoxins, which are a portion of the gram-negative cell, cause fever, shock, and DIC.

### Pertussis (Whooping Cough)

| | |
|---|---|
| Causative agent | *Bordetella pertussis* (a gram-negative bacillus) |
| Incubation period | 6 to 20 days |
| Infectious period | Catarrhal stage (1 to 2 weeks) until the fourth week |
| Transmission | Direct contact or respiratory droplets from coughing |
| Immunity | Bacteria or vaccine, both of which provide varying degrees and duration of immunity against pertussis |
| Season | Can occur during any season, but usually in the summer and fall |

#### Manifestations

The three stages of pertussis are catarrhal, paroxysmal, and convalescent, lasting a total of 6 to 12 weeks (Box 41.1). The classic stages are not commonly seen in infants younger than 3 months (Long, 2016). Diagnosis is through positive nasopharyngeal culture.

#### Complications

The most frequently seen complication of pertussis is pneumonia. Other respiratory complications occur to varying degrees, ranging from atelectasis to interstitial or subcutaneous emphysema to pneumothorax. Hypoxemia can lead to CNS involvement. Malnutrition and dehydration can result from extensive vomiting and can be quite dangerous, especially for infants. Other complications include otitis media, ulcers of the frenulum of the tongue, epistaxis, hernia, and rectal prolapse. Infants younger than 6 months of age are at greatest risk for complications and are more likely to acquire pertussis because they do not receive maternal immunity and may be incompletely immunized.

**BOX 41.1 Stages of Pertussis Manifestations**

**Catarrhal**
- Duration: 1 to 2 weeks
- Symptoms: Symptoms of upper respiratory tract infection (rhinorrhea, lacrimation, mild cough, low-grade fever).

**Paroxysmal**
- Duration: 2 to 6 weeks
- Symptoms: Increased severity of cough. Repetitive series of coughs during a single expiration, followed by massive inspiration with a whoop (older children may not manifest this). Cyanosis, protrusion of tongue, salivation, distention of neck veins. Coughing spells may be triggered by yawning, sneezing, eating, or drinking. Coughing may induce vomiting.

**Convalescent**
- Duration: 1 to 2 weeks
- Symptoms: Episodes of coughing, whooping, and vomiting that decrease in frequency and severity. Cough may persist for several months.

#### Therapeutic Management

Primary prevention of pertussis can be accomplished through administration of five doses of the pertussis vaccine in combination with tetanus and diphtheria (DTaP). Because of waning immunity in the adolescent population, the AAP in 2006 recommended a booster, called Tdap, for children age 11 to 12 who completed a primary series of DTaP. It seems that immunity begins to wane approximately 2 to 5 years after the administration of the vaccine (Bass, 2015).

Erythromycin, azithromycin, or clarithromycin (depending on age), if given during the catarrhal stage, will eliminate the organism from the nasopharynx within 5 days, thereby reducing communicability. Infants and young children who are exposed to pertussis should continue their routine schedule of immunization. Erythromycin, azithromycin, or clarithromycin is also given to all close contacts, which include most children older than 13 years, because the immunity conferred by the childhood immunization declines by early adolescence.

Hospitalization and supportive care for the infant may be necessary, especially those 6 months and younger since they are at an increased risk of mortality, to monitor airway patency. Older children can usually be cared for at home. Respiratory status is monitored using a cardiopulmonary monitor and pulse oximeter. Droplet Precautions are observed.

#### Nursing Considerations

The nurse obtains a complete immunization history and any recent known exposures to illnesses. Pertussis often goes unrecognized in adolescents and adults, increasing the risk of exposure in the community. For this reason, it is vital for families and caregivers of young infants to be immunized against pertussis. Of note, recent studies show that siblings are now the most common mode of transmission (Skoff et al., 2015). Documentation also includes the parent's description of any respiratory events before admission and indicators such as coughing, secretions, cyanotic episodes, and the child's activity level. Assessment of the child's respiratory, fluid, nutrition, output, and neurologic status should be done.

The child's respiratory status needs monitoring with a cardiopulmonary monitor and pulse oximeter. If the child is hospitalized, the limits of the monitor should be checked frequently. Explain any monitoring devices to the child (if age appropriate) and parents to help alleviate anxiety. Suction and oxygen equipment should be readily available. Supplemental oxygen therapy could be ordered if the child's oxygen saturation falls below an acceptable range (especially during any coughing episodes). If the child needs oxygen therapy, instruct the parent about any oxygen equipment and the timing and possible length of treatment. Some children will need additional oxygen only during the paroxysmal spells.

Because the child's coughing paroxysms can be triggered by noises or frightening experiences, a quiet environment and a calm, reassuring approach should be used when caring for the child and supporting the parents. Paroxysmal episodes should be monitored for any drop in oxygen saturation levels. Parents and children will need additional support and reassurance that assistance is near and ready if needed during the child's coughing spells because these episodes can be extremely frightening.

The infant's nutritional status should be closely monitored. Small, frequent feedings may benefit infants if the feeding process becomes exhausting. If the child's intake becomes insufficient, nutritional support (gavage or parenteral) may be needed to prevent dehydration or weight loss. If the child has vomiting episodes when coughing, frequent oral care will be necessary.

Nursing care activities should be clustered, if possible, to allow the child and parent to rest. Diversional activities should be age appropriate. Parents may need emotional support to deal with feelings of guilt, especially if they chose not to immunize their child.

## Scarlet Fever

| | |
|---|---|
| Causative agent | Group A beta-hemolytic streptococci |
| Incubation period | 1 to 7 days (average of 3 days) |
| Infectious period | Acute stage until 24 hours after antimicrobial therapy has begun |
| Transmission | Airborne (inhalation or ingestion), direct contact |
| Immunity | None |
| Season | Late fall, winter, and spring |

### Manifestations

Abrupt fever, vomiting, headache, abdominal pain, pharyngitis, and chills characterize the onset of scarlet fever. The fever reaches a peak by the second day and returns to normal within 5 to 6 days. Within 24 hours, a fine red papular rash appears in the axillae, groin, and neck, which feels like sandpaper to the touch. The rash then spreads peripherally to cover the entire body (Fig. 41.7). The rash will blanch on pressure except in areas of deep creases (Pastia's sign). *Desquamation,* peeling of the skin, may begin on the face at the end of the first week, and flaking proceeds down the trunk. This process may continue for up to 6 weeks. The tongue is initially coated with a white, furry covering with red projecting papillae (so-called white strawberry tongue). By the fourth day the papillae slough off, leaving a red, swollen tongue (so-called strawberry tongue). The tonsils are edematous and may be covered with a gray-white exudate, which can spread to the pharynx. Petechial hemorrhages cover the soft palate.

### Complications

Complications generally result from extension of the streptococcal infection. They include sinusitis, otitis media, mastoiditis, peritonsillar abscess, bronchopneumonia, meningitis, osteomyelitis, rheumatic fever, and glomerulonephritis.

### Therapeutic Management

Rapid streptococcal screening in an office setting, usually with laboratory confirmation (generally by a throat culture) if the rapid screen is negative, is recommended for children with sore throats because of the similarity of symptoms between viral and group A beta-hemolytic streptococcal sore throats. The preferred treatment for any streptococcal infection is penicillin. Children allergic to penicillin can be given erythromycin a cephalosporin. Supportive care for symptoms is indicated. Children with streptococcal infections (throat, skin) may return to school or daycare 24 hours after beginning antibiotics, when they are no longer considered contagious. Droplet Precautions should also be observed until the child has been on antibiotics for 24 hours. Complications for an untreated Group A beta-hemolytic streptococci infection include acute rheumatic fever and acute poststreptococcal glomerulonephritis (Shulman, 2016).

### Nursing Considerations

The nurse should obtain and document a complete history of symptoms. The nurse also assesses the child's throat, tongue, rash, nutritional and fluid intake, vital signs, and level of general wellness. Any history of sensitivity to penicillin should be thoroughly explored and prominently noted on the child's records.

Generally, children with scarlet fever are cared for at home. Comfort measures include encouraging fluids (especially cool, nonacidic liquids) and administering antipyretics for fever control.

Analgesics may be given for discomfort, and antipruritic comfort measures may be necessary. Parents should understand the typical course of disease and any treatment measures, including the importance of completing the full course of any antibiotics prescribed (to prevent growth of resistant bacteria). Bed rest and quiet activities may be beneficial during the acute stage (see Patient-Centered Teaching: How to Care for the Child with Scarlet Fever).

**PATIENT-CENTERED TEACHING**

***How to Care for the Child With Scarlet Fever***

- The entire course of antibiotic therapy (usually 10 to 14 days) must be taken to destroy all the bacteria and decrease the risk of complications. If a partial course of antibiotics is given (antibiotic stopped by parent when child is feeling better), the bacteria can become resistant and fail to be eradicated with subsequent attempts.
- Cool drinks and liquid refreshments (ice pops, milkshakes) may be soothing and help maintain hydration.
- Acetaminophen, ibuprofen, throat lozenges, antiseptic throat spray (e.g., Chloraseptic), and cool mist may be used to relieve discomfort.
- Encouraging quiet activities will help prevent fatigue.
- In providing oral care, acidic preparations should be avoided. Saline rinses can provide comfort and promote hygiene.
- A soft, bland diet should be offered.
- Call your primary healthcare provider if your child develops drooling or great difficulty swallowing or acts very sick. After 48 hours of antibiotic therapy, your child should not have a fever.
- Your child is no longer contagious after 24 hours of antibiotic therapy. The rash is not contagious.

Some children with severe symptoms and complications need hospitalization and supportive care. In such cases, vital signs, especially body temperature, should be monitored.

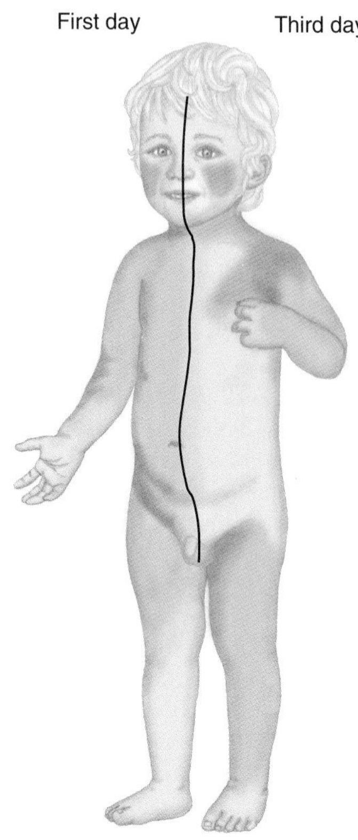


Scarlet Fever Rash Distribution

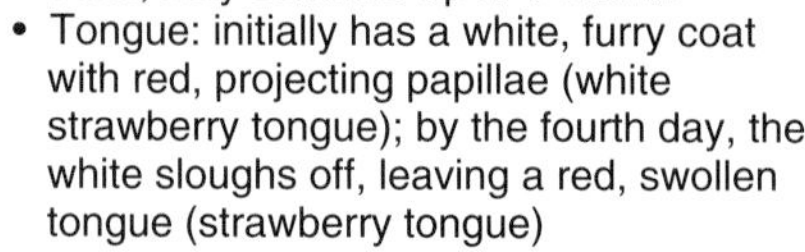

- Red, fine, papular rash appears within 24 hours of fever and other symptoms; in dark skin, rash is often seen as punctate papular elevations
- Begins in axillae, groin, and neck and spreads to cover entire body
- Desquamation begins on face at end of first week, and flaking proceeds down trunk; may continue up to 6 weeks
- Tongue: initially has a white, furry coat with red, projecting papillae (white strawberry tongue); by the fourth day, the white sloughs off, leaving a red, swollen tongue (strawberry tongue)

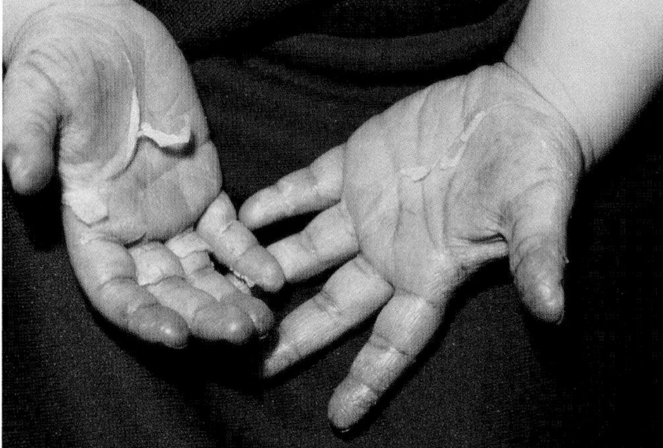

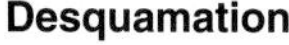

Desquamation

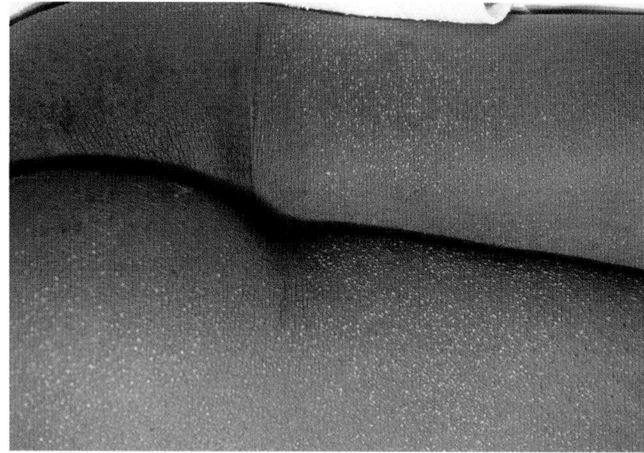

Rash, Light Skin

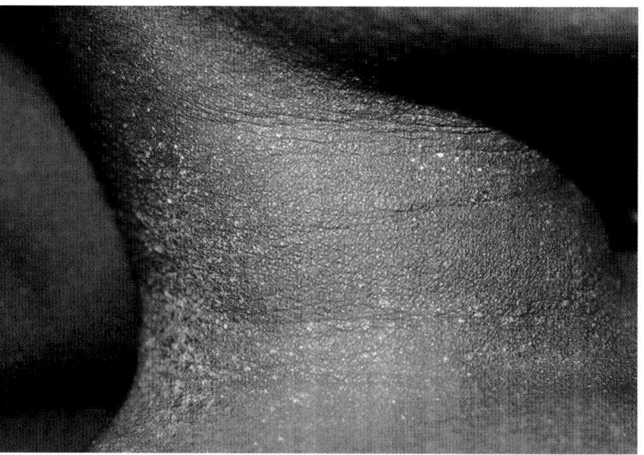

Rash, Dark Skin

**FIG 41.7** Scarlet fever rash distribution and appearance. Note the characteristic skin peeling. (From Paller, S.A. [2012]. *Hurwitz clinical pediatric dermatology: a textbook of skin disorders of childhood and adolescence* [4th ed.]. Philadelphia: Saunders.)

## Methicillin-Resistant *Staphylococcus aureus* (MRSA)

| | |
|---|---|
| Causative agent | *Staphylococcus aureus* (gram-positive cocci) |
| Transmission | Contact |
| Immunity | None |
| Season | No seasonal pattern |

Methicillin-resistant *S. aureus* (MRSA) was first identified in the 1960s and became increasingly prevalent in hospital settings. MRSA is categorized as either hospital-acquired or community-acquired. The first case of community-acquired MRSA (CA-MRSA) was documented in 1998, and its incidence has tripled over the past decade. The community strains are believed to have mutated from community-based methicillin-susceptible *S. aureus*. CA-MRSA has surpassed hospital-acquired MRSA (HA-MRSA) as the source of the most skin and soft-tissue infections. The criteria necessary for diagnosing CA-MRSA include being diagnosed in an outpatient setting or within 48 hours of hospital admission, no present use of medical devices, and no history of previous MRSA infection.

### Manifestations

HA-MRSA is often the cause of medical-device–related infections, pneumonia (including ventilator-associated pneumonia), and catheter-related bloodstream infections. The most common CA-MRSA infections are skin and soft tissue infections (furuncles, carbuncles, and abscesses) and, less commonly, urinary tract infections (UTIs), pneumonia, and bacteremia. Some of the more serious and potentially fatal complications include osteomyelitis, endocarditis, and necrotizing fasciitis.

Risk factors for MRSA include a history of a chronic illness, immunocompromised status, participating in close-contact team sports, and attendance at a daycare center.

### Therapeutic Management

A clinical practice guideline for the treatment of adults and children with MRSA contains evidence-based treatment recommendations (Liu, Bayer, Cosgrove, et al., 2011). HA-MRSA is difficult to treat, as it is resistant to beta-lactam and cephalosporin antibiotics; therefore, treatment, after incision and drainage of a cutaneous lesion or abscess, includes IV vancomycin or linezolid, among others (Liu et al., 2011). For more severe infections or bacteremia, IV vancomycin is used; follow-up blood cultures monitor the resolution of the bacteremia. Infectious endocarditis (see Chapter 46) is a risk (Liu et al., 2011).

For most skin and soft tissue infections acquired in the community, incision and drainage with culture and sensitivity is the option of choice, and antibiotic administration is not considered necessary unless there is severe disease present, the infection progresses rapidly, or the wound does not respond to incision and drainage alone (Liu et al., 2011). If necessary, CA-MRSA can be treated with a 5- to 10-day course of oral vancomycin, clindamycin, sulfamethoxazole-trimethoprim, or linezolid. Patients who are colonized, along with their family members, are instructed to disinfect their bodies using daily chlorhexidine gluconate baths and nasal mupirocin twice a day for 5 days (Kaplan, Hulten, & Mason, 2014).

### Nursing Considerations

Education on proper hand hygiene is of utmost importance in reducing the spread of MRSA. Athletes should avoid sharing of personal equipment and towels. Coaches must ensure that all equipment is properly cleaned. Useful information from the CDC for families and coaches can be found at http://www.cdc.gov/mrsa/community/index.html. Protocols to ensure the early identification of cases are vital to prevent the spread of MRSA in the hospital setting.

## *Clostridium difficile*

| | |
|---|---|
| Causative agent | *Clostridium difficile* (gram-positive anaerobic bacterium) |
| Transmission | Contact (fecal-oral) |
| Incubation period | Unknown |
| Immunity | None |
| Season | No seasonal pattern |

*C. difficile* is an increasingly common cause of diarrheal disease in infants and children. In the past, it was only associated with the healthcare setting and antibiotic use, but in recent years it has been more commonly seen in previously healthy infants and children. In 2011, the CDC found that *C. difficile* caused half a million infections in the US, resulting in 29,000 deaths; children accounted for 17,000 infections (CDC, 2015b). *C. difficile* is the most common cause of antimicrobial-associated diarrhea. Children ages 1 through 4 are most often affected.

### Manifestations

Although some patients can be asymptomatic, many have watery diarrhea, abdominal cramps, fever, and possible systemic toxicity. *C. difficile* is associated with antibiotic administration in young children, and its growth results from reduction of the normal bowel flora. Symptoms usually begin while the child is receiving a course of antibiotics, but can occur after the course is complete. Complications are more common with immunocompromised patients or those with inflammatory bowel disease and include intestinal perforation and toxic megacolon, both of which can be fatal.

### Therapeutic Management

Diagnosis of *C. difficile* is through identification of the specific toxin in the stool. Infants younger than 12 months of age are commonly colonized with *C. difficile* in their gastrointestinal tract and are usually asymptomatic. Therefore, infants that age are not usually tested for *C. difficile*. The initial treatment is cessation of the antibiotic course (if applicable), which is effective in approximately a quarter of the cases. Almost all antibiotics have the potential to cause *C. difficile*-associated diarrhea (CDAD), but clindamycin, third-generation cephalosporins, and penicillin are more often associated with CDAD. The antibiotics used for treatment of CDAD include 7 to 10 days of oral metronidazole for mild to moderate disease and vancomycin for more severe disease. Resistance to either of these agents is rare. Reinfection can occur within 4 weeks of treatment (Mezoff & Cohen, 2014). A new initiative by the CDC hopes to reduce outpatient prescribing of antibiotics by 20% in the next 5 years with the goal of reducing *CDAD*.

### Nursing Considerations

Patients are placed on Contact Precautions Plus (requires hand hygiene with handwashing as well as alcohol-based hand sanitizer) in the hospital setting. Proper hand hygiene is crucial. Because the *C. difficile* spores are not killed by alcohol-based hand sanitizer, it is recommended that healthcare workers use soap and water for hand hygiene after contact with a patient who has CDAD. Parents of young patients are cautioned about proper cleaning techniques (use of bleach-based products).

## Serious Bacterial Illness in Infants

| | |
|---|---|
| Causative agent | Multiple organisms include streptococci, *E. coli, S. aureus* |
| Incubation period | Unknown |
| Transmission | Placental, perinatal, postnatal from mother or environment |

Serious bacterial illness in infants usually is diagnosed in the newborn and referred to as neonatal sepsis, although sepsis can occur in older infants (>3 months of age) as well. Neonatal sepsis occurs when bacteria or their poisonous products, known as *endotoxins,* gain access to the bloodstream, causing systemic signs and symptoms. Evaluation of the newborn for the presence of bacterial sepsis is a common occurrence in the newborn nursery and presents challenges for the healthcare team in both the evaluation and treatment procedures. The challenges are the result, in part, of the varied and frequently nonspecific subtle signs and symptoms of the infant with neonatal sepsis. Neonatal sepsis is discussed in detail in Chapter 30.

Infants beyond the newborn period can also experience serious bacterial illness, which, if unidentified, can cause serious complications. The primary sign of serious bacterial illness is fever. Infants younger than 3 months of age who have a temperature equal to or higher than 100.4° F (38° C) should be seen by a provider for evaluation.

The approach used to evaluate an infant for sepsis is generally called a *sepsis (or septic) workup*. The exact approach varies with each infant, but all are based on assessment of clinical signs, careful history, and appropriate laboratory findings. Diagnostic tests, including cultures (blood, urine, nasopharyngeal, CSF [if indicated]) and additional blood tests (complete blood count [CBC] with white blood cell [WBC] count and complete differential count, C-reactive protein [CRP]) are obtained; a lumbar puncture is performed in the symptomatic neonate and can be done in asymptomatic infants if the infant's condition warrants. A recent report from the Agency for Healthcare Research and Quality (AHRQ) (2012) recommends that febrile infants be categorized as low or high risk for serious illness using these criteria, and that management differs depending on the category. Infants who appear well, have no observable infection site, and who have laboratory tests that do not indicate severe infection could be treated on an outpatient basis with a long-acting antibiotic, such as ceftriaxone. Follow-up within 24 hours is essential. High risk infants usually require hospitalization for IV antibiotics and observation. Management and nursing considerations for febrile infants are similar to that for newborns with neonatal sepsis.

### Rare Viral and Bacterial Infections

Table 41.1 presents several rarely seen viral and bacterial infections. Many of these have been nearly eliminated as a result of vigorous vaccination and immunization programs.

## FUNGAL INFECTIONS

Fungi are free-living organisms that can be found throughout the environment. Some species of fungi are part of the normal human flora, especially those in the mouth, intestine, vagina, and skin. A fungus is transmitted through inhalation or penetration of tissue as a result of trauma. Fungi grow quite slowly, so clinical symptoms may appear only after a prolonged period. They are aerobic, can grow in a wide range of temperatures, and are resistant to most antibiotics. Pathogenic fungi include two types of organisms: molds and yeasts.

Infections caused by fungi are classified into four groups:

1. Opportunistic: caused by a defect in host immunity
2. Systemic: involving deep tissues and organs
3. Subcutaneous: limited to deep subcutaneous tissue
4. Superficial: limited to skin, hair, and nails

Common fungal infections include tinea capitis, tinea pedis, and candidal infections (see Chapter 49).

## RICKETTSIAL INFECTIONS

Rickettsiae are small, parasitic bacteria that are transmitted to human beings by blood-sucking arthropods. A vertebrate is not necessary for the survival of the bacteria, and the host arthropod (usually a tick) appears not to be affected adversely by the rickettsiae. Replication of the rickettsiae in the new host cell causes cell death, which can lead to

**TABLE 41.1 Rare Viral and Bacterial Infections**

| Disease | Transmission | Manifestations | Complications | Therapeutic Management and Nursing Considerations |
|---|---|---|---|---|
| Smallpox<br>Variola virus | Transmitted through droplets via direct and prolonged face-to-face contact with an infected person; less commonly, smallpox transmitted through contact with contaminated objects<br>Most contagious when lesions rupture | Prodrome of fever, malaise, headache, muscle pain, prostration, and often nausea, vomiting, and backache<br>Fever of 101°F (38.3°C) but can be higher<br>Lesions appear as red spots in the mouth and on the tongue, develop into sores and break<br>After a few days a generalized vesicular rash appears (Fig. 41.8)<br>Lesions progress into pustules, then form scabs; complete scabbing of pustules by end of second week | Can be fatal | Supportive care<br>Infection control and prevention<br>Isolate exposed individuals as soon as fever appears<br>Place patient in negative air pressure room with airborne and contact precautions<br>Wear N95 respiratory protection<br>Only vaccinated healthcare workers can care for patients<br>Vaccinate all exposed contacts |
| Poliomyelitis<br>Poliovirus | Fecal-oral, oral-oral (respiratory) | Fever, malaise, anorexia, nausea, headache, sore throat, and generalized abdominal pain, which begin as mild symptoms, then grow more intense<br>Flaccid paralysis, especially of lower extremities | Cervical involvement, called bulbar polio, affects the respiratory and vasomotor centers, resulting in potential damage to respiratory centers and inability to breathe | No specific treatment<br>Respiratory paralysis is treated with mechanical ventilation<br>Physical therapy helps maintain muscle integrity and prevent contractures<br>Prevention through routine immunization<br>Risk for postpolio syndrome |
| Diphtheria<br>*Corynebacterium diphtheriae* (a gram-positive, nonmotile bacillus) | Contact with carrier or disease, droplets | Nasal manifestations initially resemble the common cold, then gradually begin to include discharge of foul-smelling mucopurulent material<br>Low-grade fever is common<br>Hallmark sign: thin, gray membrane on the tonsils and pharynx, causing "bull neck," or neck edema<br>Respiratory compromise due to a narrowing of the upper airway | Upper airway obstruction<br>Myocarditis<br>Peripheral neuropathies | Intravenous (IV) diphtheria antitoxin and antibiotics (e.g., erythromycin or penicillin G) within 3 days of the onset of symptoms<br>Prevention through routine immunization and boosters at regularly recommended intervals |

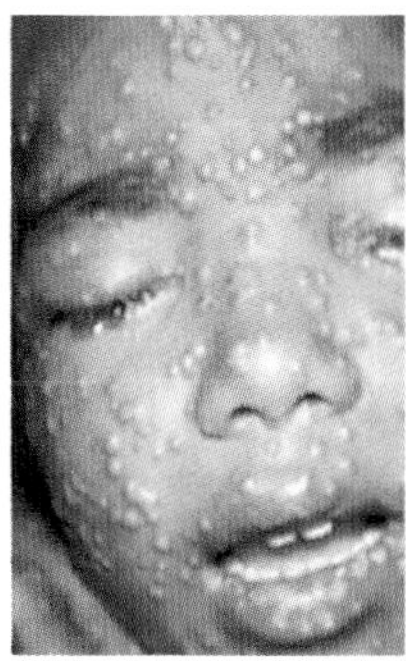
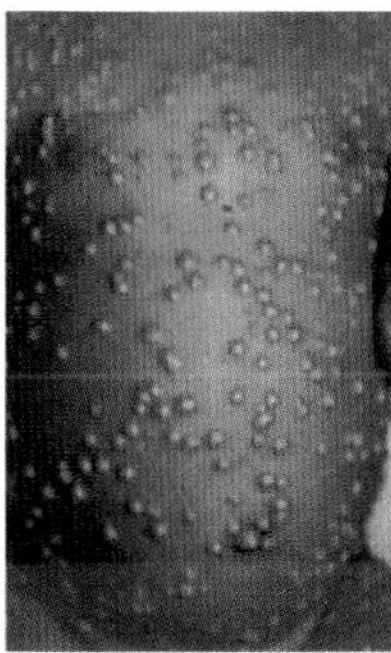
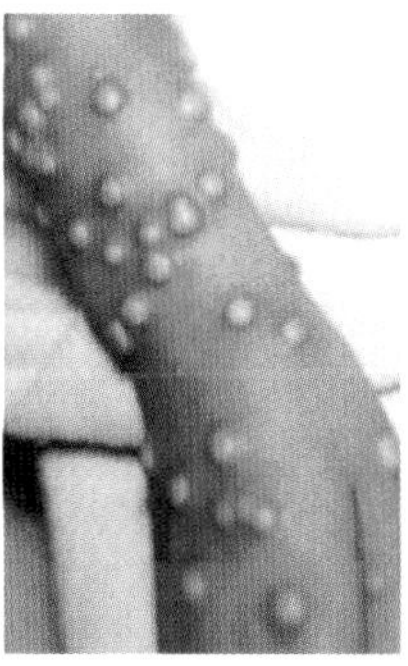

**FIG 41.8** Lesions of variola are at the same stage of development on all body parts. (Reprinted from Centers for Disease Control and Prevention. [2002]. *Evaluating patients for smallpox.* Atlanta: Author.)

vasculitis with thrombosis, increased permeability, tissue edema, hemorrhage, circulatory failure, and meningoencephalitis. Rickettsial diseases cannot be transmitted from person to person.

## Rocky Mountain Spotted Fever

| | |
|---|---|
| Causative agent | *Rickettsia rickettsii* |
| Reservoir | Wild rodents, dogs |
| Vector | Tick (wood, dog, Lone Star) |
| Incubation period | 2 to 14 days (average of 7 days) |
| Transmission | Bite of infected tick |
| Season | April through September |

### Manifestations

The onset of Rocky Mountain spotted fever (RMSF) is marked by nonspecific signs and symptoms such as headache, fever, anorexia, and restlessness. Generally, on the third day a characteristic maculopapular or petechial rash appears. This rash begins on the extremities (usually the wrists, palms, ankles, and soles) and spreads to the rest of the body. As the rash progresses, hemorrhagic and necrotic lesions can appear. Approximately 60% of cases have a history of a tick bite or exposure to tick-infested habitats. Many cases are caused by ticks that are carried by the family dog. Children under the age of 15 account for two thirds of all cases, with a peak age of 5 to 9 years. The prognosis is excellent when treated within the first 5 days of symptoms. This rate is increased in cases in which diagnosis is delayed beyond 1 week (Lantos & McKinney, 2014).

### Therapeutic Management

With early detection and treatment in children (within 5 days of the beginning of the illness), the likelihood of positive resolution increases. Doxycycline is the recommended treatment with a fluoroquinolone as an alternative. Treatment usually lasts 7 to 10 days. Doxycycline is used with caution in children younger than 8 years because of staining of the teeth (Lantos & McKinney, 2014). However, if vascular damage has already occurred, the drugs may not alter the course of the disease. There is no vaccine available at this time to prevent RMSF, and avoiding ticks is the most effective way to prevent RMSF (Lantos & McKinney, 2014).

### Nursing Considerations

The assessment of children with symptoms indicating RMSF should include obtaining a complete history of skin eruptions, medications taken, exposure to infectious diseases, and recent hiking or other activities in wooded areas. Any rashes or skin lesions should then be examined, with documentation of distribution and morphology. The child's vital signs, especially body temperature, should also be assessed and noted.

**BOX 41.2 Preventive Measures to Avoid Insect and Tick Bites**

- Children should wear tightly woven clothing consisting of long pants, long-sleeved shirts, long socks, and a hat when in wooded and grassy areas. Pants should be tucked into socks. Clothing should also be light-colored so ticks are easily visible.
- Paths should be followed and dense areas avoided if possible. Avoid known tick-infested areas.
- Insect repellents that contain diethyltoluamide (DEET) and permethrin should be used; apply before any possible exposure and every 1 to 2 hours sparingly according to manufacturer's directions. Care should be taken to avoid contact of repellent with the child's eyes or mouth. The repellent should not be applied to the hands to avoid contact with the eyes and mouth. Wash hands and skin after the child goes indoors.
- Repellents should be used with caution in infants because of the risk of encephalopathy.
- Insect repellent should not be applied to wounds or irritated skin.
- The body (especially exposed hairy regions) should be inspected periodically for ticks, which may resemble small moles or blood blisters. Early removal can prevent transmission of disease from an infected tick.
- Ticks should be removed with tweezers. The tick should be removed as close to the skin as possible using steady upward pressure. Ensure that all mouthparts are removed from the skin.
- Care should be taken to avoid handling the tick with bare hands or crushing the tick's body.
- Ticks may be preserved in alcohol for later identification.
- Pets should be kept free of ticks by dipping and spraying during tick season.
- Yards should be kept free of brush and undergrowth.

Hospitalized children will require supportive care for their symptoms. Straws should be used, and the mouth should be flushed if tetracycline is administered because it can stain the teeth. Parents should be cautioned to give the full course of any antibiotic to decrease the risk of complications and ensure that the disease is eradicated. Education regarding the control measures for prevention of tick-borne infections is vital (Box 41.2).

# *BORRELIA* INFECTIONS

*Borrelia* is a genus of spiral bacteria that are transmitted to human beings by arthropods. The diseases caused by *Borrelia* are relapsing fever and Lyme disease.

## Relapsing Fever

Relapsing fever is spread from person to person by lice or ticks. The bacteria are introduced into a bite wound when the bite is rubbed. This infection is spread when people fail to wash thoroughly and do not change clothes. The incubation period is 4 to 18 days.

Tick-borne relapsing fever *(Borrelia hermsii, B. turicatae)* results from tick exposures in rodent-infested cabins in western mountainous areas of the United States, including state and national parks. *B. turicatae* infections occur less frequently, with the majority of cases in Texas.

### Manifestations

The abrupt onset of high fever (up to 106.7° F [41.5° C]), shaking chills, sweats, headache, muscle and joint pains, and progressive weakness characterize relapsing fever. The symptoms resolve within a week, reoccur 1 to 2 weeks later, and continue to reoccur at intervals until treated. As the fever episode begins to resolve, two classic phases occur quickly: the chill phase, which includes an extremely high fever and possible confusion, and the flush phase, in which the fever decreases rapidly, causing the child to sweat profusely (CDC, 2012). Often the duration of symptoms decrease and the length of time between episodes increases with each subsequent episode (Krause, 2014)

### Therapeutic Management

Several antibiotics provide effective treatment. These include penicillin, doxycycline, tetracycline, erythromycin, and chloramphenicol for children older than 8 years and erythromycin for younger children.

### Nursing Considerations

Assessment should include a complete history of rash onset and characteristics, medications taken, and living environment, including available bathing and washing facilities. Fever, headache, and arthralgia should be treated with antipyretics and analgesics. Antibiotics should be given as ordered. Education includes personal hygiene, the use of pediculicides or insect repellent, and eradication methods.

## Lyme Disease

| | |
|---|---|
| Causative agent | *Borrelia burgdorferi* (spirochete) |
| Vector | Tick (Fig. 41.9) |
| Incubation period | 1 to 31 days |
| Transmission | Bite of infected tick (person-to-person transmission not possible) |
| Season | April to October |

Of the tick-borne diseases seen in the United States, Lyme disease is seen most frequently. The main cause of transmission in the northern or eastern United States is the deer tick, while the western black-legged tick transmits the disease to those on the Pacific coast. Lyme disease is a multisystem illness that affects the skin and the musculoskeletal, cardiovascular, and nervous systems.

### Manifestations

The manifestations of Lyme disease can be divided into three stages (early localized, early disseminated, and late disseminated). In the first stage (early localized), the skin lesions are most prominent; in the second stage (early disseminated), cardiac and neurologic findings are prominent; and in the third stage (late disseminated), arthritis is the main manifestation (Sood & Krause, 2014).

In the early localized stage of Lyme disease, local reactions to an infected tick bite occur, along with vague, flu-like symptoms (headache, chills, fatigue, and vague muscle aches and pains). An erythematous macule or papule forms at the site of the tick bite within 1 to 31 days (Fig. 41.10). This rash can enlarge to 16 to 68 cm in diameter, with a clearing in the center (erythema migrans, or "bull's eye" rash). It may itch, prickle, or burn. The rash generally lasts for 3 to 4 weeks, during which time it gradually fades.

In the early disseminated stage (generally 1 to 4 months after the bite), neurologic symptoms may be the first to occur. CNS symptoms can include severe headaches with myelitis, nausea, vomiting, facial nerve paralysis (Bell's palsy), forgetfulness or decreased concentration, and cerebral ataxia. General lymphadenopathy and joint and muscle pain may also be present. Lyme arthritis generally affects the large joints, with the knee being the most often involved. Children infrequently manifest carditis. The signs and symptoms generally resolve over a few days, but many individuals have recurrences. Skin lesions may recur but are smaller and more diffuse than the initial ones.

Symptoms of late disseminated Lyme disease (occurring months to years after the initial infected tick bite) occur intermittently and include chronic arthritis, profound fatigue, and chronic neurologic manifestations. The debilitating effects frequently affect a child's ability to participate in normal activities (e.g., sports) because of extreme fatigue or cardiac complications.

### Therapeutic Management

Primary prevention of Lyme disease includes anticipatory guidance and information about routine preventive measures to avoid insect bites. Early identification and treatment with antibiotics results in a rapid resolution of symptoms, especially in the early stages of the infection. A course of doxycycline, amoxicillin, or cefuroxime is commonly used for oral treatment. The length of treatment is usually 14 to 21 days, although a shorter 10-day course may be as effective. If the patient has neurologic or cardiac symptoms, IV ceftriaxone for 2 to 3 weeks is recommended (Sood & Krause, 2014). In addition, disease identified in early stages and treated with antibiotics does not progress to the more debilitating stages. The characteristic rash of Lyme disease linked to other symptoms leads to a diagnosis, except in cases where the child has atypical manifestations of the disease (e.g., one septic joint, usually the knee).

### Nursing Considerations

Assessment should include a complete history of rash onset and characteristics; medications taken; recent exposures to infectious diseases;

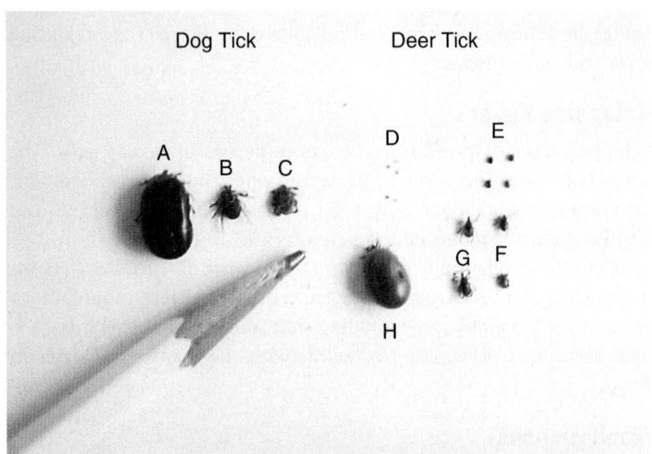


**FIG 41.9** Dog (wood) ticks and deer (black-legged) ticks compared with a pencil. Dog ticks: **A,** engorged female; **B,** female; **C,** male. Deer ticks: **D,** larvae; **E,** nymphs; **F,** males; **G,** females; **H,** engorged female. (Courtesy Lyme Disease Foundation, http://www.lyme.org.)

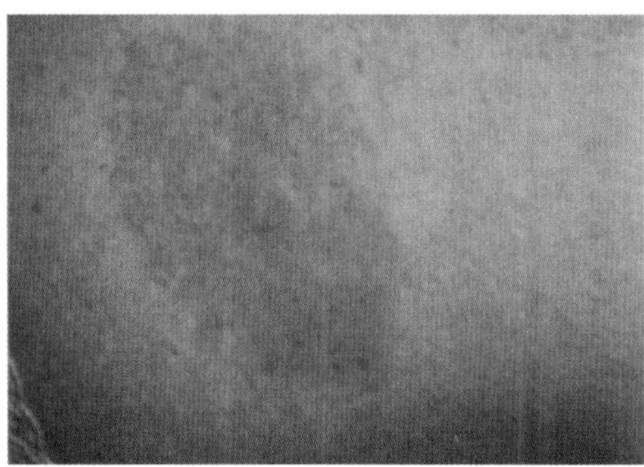

**FIG 41.10** Characteristic lesion of Lyme disease. (Reprinted from Larson, W.G., Adams, R.M., & Maibach, H.I. [1991]. *Color text of contact dermatitis.* Philadelphia: Saunders.)

**TABLE 41.2 Common Helminths**

| Class and Typical Agent | Transmission | Manifestations | Diagnosis | Treatment |
|---|---|---|---|---|
| Roundworm (*Ascaris lumbricoides*) | Ingestion of eggs from contaminated soil or food, transfer to mouth from fingers, toys, or other vectors | Abdominal pain or distention, abdominal obstruction, vomiting with bile staining, pneumonitis | Fecal smear | Mebendazole, albendazole, ivermectin |
| Pinworm (*Enterobius vermicularis*) | Ingestion or inhalation of eggs, transfer from hands to mouth | Nocturnal anal itching, sleeplessness | Cellophane tape test and microscopic examination | Pyrantel pamoate, mebendazole, albendazole |
| Tapeworm (*Taenia saginata*) | Ingestion from handling or eating infected beef or pork | Asymptomatic, segments of worms seen in stool, abdominal pain, nausea, anorexia, weight loss, insomnia | Fecal smear or microscopic examination | Praziquantel, niclosamide |
| Hookworm (*Necator americanus*) | Skin penetration from direct contact with contaminated soil | Dermatitis, blood loss leading to iron deficiency and anemia, pneumonitis, malnutrition | Fecal smear or microscopic examination | Mebendazole, albendazole pyrantel pamoate |

and recent hiking, working (forestry, farming, outdoor construction or maintenance), or vacationing (camping [e.g., Boy Scouts or Girl Scouts], hunting) in a known endemic area or heavily wooded area. Because ticks must be attached for longer than 36 hours to transmit the disease, parents must be vigilant in inspecting the skin after exposure to wooded area. Proper use of insect repellents such as diethyltoluamide (DEET) should also be stressed. Fever, headache, and arthralgia should be treated with antipyretics and analgesics. Parents should have a complete understanding of the course of treatment, including the importance of administering medications and antibiotics as prescribed. The importance of completing the entire course of antibiotic treatment should be stressed. Generally, affected children will be treated at home. Parental and caregiver education is important to prevent further exposures and to facilitate early recognition of disease symptoms.

## HELMINTHS

Helminths are worms that live as parasites. The three groups with the greatest impact on humans are tapeworms, flukes, and roundworms (Table 41.2). Children are more commonly infected than adults, primarily as a result of frequent hand-to-mouth activity and the likelihood of fecal contamination. Transmission occurs by oral-fecal ingestion, ingestion of contaminated tissue from another host, skin penetration, or the bite of a blood-sucking insect.

### Therapeutic Management

Treatment consists of the administration of oral medications effective against a specific helminth. Treatment is provided to the entire family. Anticipatory guidance to prevent reinfestation and education about the prevention of the spread of disease (basic enteric isolation procedures) for the family and primary caregivers, along with personal hygiene and sanitary practices, are also necessary (see Patient-Centered Teaching: How to Prevent Parasitic Infections).

### Nursing Considerations

A thorough history, including the child's general wellness, personal hygiene practices, and the availability of running water and bathing and laundry facilities, along with nutritional intake, should be obtained.

Most parasites are identified in fecal smears obtained from stool specimens. If the family or caregiver is to bring a stool specimen in for laboratory testing, the nurse should provide specific, clear instructions and provide a container if needed. Sample size and number, as well as proper storage, should be clearly explained. Stool specimens that have not been contaminated with urine are ideal. Obtaining urine-free specimens may be difficult, especially in infants or very young children. Plastic wrap can be placed over the toilet bowl or a potty chair, or specimens can be collected from a diaper using a clean tongue blade and placing in a container. The container should be marked with the child's name and the date and time of collection. It should then be refrigerated until it is delivered to the laboratory.

Education for the parents and primary caregivers should focus on medication administration, primary prevention of future reinfestations, and resource identification with referral to available community and social services for any basic living needs (running water, bathing facilities). The rationale for evaluating and treating the entire family for infection and the usual mode of transmission must be discussed to prevent future reinfestation or cross contamination of family members. Anticipatory guidance regarding primary prevention and teaching about prevention (personal hygiene and health habits) should be covered with the child's family. The nurse should help the family identify any resources (access to care, social services) necessary and initiate referral if appropriate.

**PATIENT-CENTERED TEACHING**

***How to Prevent Parasitic Infections***

- Handwashing (including under the fingernails) with soap and water should be done before eating or handling of food and after using the toilet.
- Placing hands in the mouth and nail biting should be discouraged.
- Toilets or other appropriate bathroom facilities should be used for elimination.
- Toilets or bathroom facilities should be cleaned with agents containing bleach.
- Scratching the anal area with bare hands should be discouraged.
- Dogs and cats should be kept at a distance from play areas and sandboxes, and the latter need to be covered when not in use.
- Shoes should be worn when outside.
- All fruits and vegetables should be washed before being eaten.
- Diapers should be changed frequently and disposed of properly (out of children's reach).
- Swimming facilities that allow diapered children should be avoided.
- Only bottled water should be used during camping outings.

## SEXUALLY TRANSMITTED DISEASES

The rates of infection of many STDs, or infections transmitted through sexual activity, are highest among adolescents. Those adolescents at highest risk are male homosexuals, sexually active heterosexuals, younger sexually active adolescents, and IV drug users. The CDC estimates that one in four women between the ages of 14 and 19 years has an STD (Sales et al., 2012). Not only do young adolescents have biologic factors that increase their risk of STDs, they often lack knowledge of methods for preventing STDs as they begin their sexual decision making (Sales et al., 2012). Moreover, the use of drugs and alcohol in this population increases the risk for unsafe and unprotected sex. Adolescents' developmental stage and sense of invulnerability lead to risky behavior and risk taking (see Patient-Centered Teaching: Sexually Transmitted Diseases). Recent research shows that good parent-adolescent communication about sexual behaviors and STD risk factors is protective in reducing adolescent's risk of contracting STDs (Sales et al., 2012).

### PATIENT-CENTERED TEACHING

#### *Sexually Transmitted Diseases*

- Sexually transmitted diseases (STDs) are infections that can be transmitted through body fluids (semen, vaginal fluids, blood) and contact with infected mucous membranes (mouth, vagina, anus).
- Not all STDs have symptoms. Many people with chlamydia (an STD) do not have any symptoms. Transmission of an STD that you do not know you have to someone else is possible.
- STDs can be painful, unpleasant, and dangerous to those who have them. Some can even cause sterility, neurologic (brain) damage, cancer, or death.
- STDs can infect anyone, regardless of race, religion, sexual preference, social status, or gender.
- Because many STDs can be transmitted through sexual intercourse, through oral sex, and skin-to-skin contact, even the most careful individuals can be susceptible to infections.
- Some STDs, such as gonorrhea, chlamydia, and syphilis, can be cured fairly easily by completing a course of medication. Others, such as herpes, genital warts, and human immunodeficiency virus (HIV), cannot be cured, although some treatments are available to reduce their symptoms.
- Abstinence is the only 100% effective way to prevent both pregnancy and STD transmission.
- Abstinence means never engaging in any form of sexual contact with a partner.
- Deciding if and when to have sex is an important issue to think about.
- No one should ever be pressured to have sex.
- If you choose to have sex, a male or female condom can reduce (not eliminate) your chances of acquiring or passing on an STD.
- Some symptoms that might mean you have an STD are unusual discharge, swelling, pain, sores, or a rash in your genital area; unusual nonmenstrual bleeding; pain when you urinate or have a bowel movement; or a sore throat for several weeks.
- If you are sexually active and note any of these symptoms, see your primary healthcare provider as soon as possible. Detecting and treating an STD early will decrease the chances of permanent damage.

Neonates are at risk for transplacental transmission of STDs from an infected mother or from direct contamination during the birthing process. Sexual abuse should be suspected in children who acquire STDs after the neonatal period (see Chapter 53).

### Chlamydial Infection

| | |
|---|---|
| Causative agents | *Chlamydia trachomatis, Chlamydophila psittaci, Chlamydophila pneumoniae* |
| Incubation period | 7 to 21 days |
| Transmission | During birth if mother is infected; through sexual activity |

Chlamydial infections are the most prevalent STDs in the United States. *Chlamydia* affects up to 20% of sexually active adolescents and young adults (Hammerschlag, 2016). There were 2941 cases per 100,000 in women aged 15 to 19 years in 2014 in the US. This age group was surpassed only by women aged 20 to 24 (CDC, 2015c). Therefore, the U.S. Preventative Services Task Force (USPSTF) recommends screening all sexually active females younger than age 25 years (LeFevre, 2014). Infants are infected during the birthing process. Half of all infants born vaginally to infected mothers will develop the disease. Chlamydial infection can cause morbidity in the infant and is responsible for neonatal eye infections and interstitial pneumonia.

#### Manifestations

Many people with a chlamydial infection have few or no symptoms, but chlamydia can cause urethritis and pelvic inflammatory disease (Beharry, Shafii, & Burstein, 2013). As a result, the disease may go undiagnosed until complications develop.

Neonatal conjunctivitis develops anywhere from a few days to several weeks after birth and manifests with a watery discharge that becomes purulent. Eyelids are edematous, and the conjunctiva may become inflamed. Mucoid rhinorrhea may be associated with the infection. Many infants with conjunctivitis will develop infection of the nasopharynx, which can progress to pneumonia. These infants may have a history of a cough and congestion. Long-term abnormalities of pulmonary function may result in chronic respiratory problems.

Urethritis with dysuria, urinary frequency, or mucopurulent discharge may indicate chlamydial infection. Any identification of this organism in young children indicates possible sexual abuse.

#### Therapeutic Management

In infants with conjunctivitis or pneumonia, a 14-day course of oral erythromycin is recommended; for incomplete eradication, a subsequent course of erythromycin may be necessary. For uncomplicated genital tract infection, a single dose of azithromycin is effective for children and adolescents, and a 7-day course of doxycycline may also be used for older children (older than 8 years) and teenagers (AAP, 2015d; Hammerschlag, 2016). Follow-up for a repeat culture is indicated if symptoms persist, because reinfection is common.

It is important that the nurse counsel the patient about the need to treat all sexual partners contacted in the last 60 days or greater if it is a current sexual partner and to abstain from sexual intercourse for 7 days and until all symptoms have resolved (Hammerschlag, 2016). The USPSTF recommends offering behavioral counseling to all adolescents diagnosed with an STD to address safe sex practices to help reduce the risk for reinfection and contraction of other STDs (LeFevre, 2014).

### Gonorrhea

| | |
|---|---|
| Causative agent | *Neisseria gonorrhoeae* (gram-negative diplococcus) |
| Incubation period | 2 to 7 days |
| Transmission | Intimate contact (perinatally, through sexual abuse, by sexual intercourse) |

Gonorrhea can be transmitted three different ways:

*Perinatally:* Transmission can occur during birth of a neonate whose mother is infected or with premature rupture of the membranes. The neonate can acquire the disease through aspiration of vaginal secretions, which leads to sepsis; through direct contact through the conjunctiva; or through direct contact through attachment of a fetal scalp electrode.

*Sexual abuse:* Any child with a positive culture and without a previous history of voluntary sexual behavior should be considered a potential sexual abuse victim until proven otherwise. Transmission through sexual play with children has been documented but is rare. Almost all children diagnosed with gonorrhea at age 1 year or older have experienced sexual abuse.

*Voluntary sexual activity:* This route of transmission remains the primary route of infection among adolescents. However, sexual abuse should not be excluded as a possibility.

The United States Preventive Services Task Force (USPSTF) recommends screening sexually active females aged 24 years or younger (LeFevre, 2014). Gonorrhea is the second most common STD after chlamydia, and rates have been on the rise in the US (Woods, 2014).

### Manifestations

Ophthalmia neonatorum is the most common type of gonorrheal infection in the infant, manifesting 2 to 5 days after birth. A thick, purulent discharge from the eyes may be present and, if not treated promptly, will progress to corneal ulceration, rupture, and blindness. Ophthalmia neonatorum has been controlled through prophylactic treatment with an ophthalmic antibiotic given immediately after birth. In older children, ophthalmic infection can be the result of self-inoculation from the genital site.

Girls with gonorrheal infection may have a purulent vulvovaginitis, whereas boys often have urethritis. A history of purulent discharge with burning during urination is often elicited. Adolescent girls may exhibit cervicitis, urethritis, perihepatitis, and salpingitis. One serious complication of gonorrhea is pelvic inflammatory disease (PID), which is an infection of the female upper genital tract. PID can lead to ectopic pregnancy, infertility, and chronic pelvic pain (Beharry et al., 2013).

### Therapeutic Management

Because hepatitis B, HIV, syphilis, and *Chlamydia* infection are also often present in individuals with gonorrhea, testing should take place for those diseases. Both penicillin and fluoroquinolones are no longer used as a treatment because of an increased incidence of resistance in the United States. Currently, ceftriaxone is recommended for children and adolescents with cefotaxime as an alternative in infants (Woods, 2014). Patients should also be treated with azithromycin or doxycycline for presumed *Chlamydia* infection. Adolescents coinfected with syphilis are treated appropriately as well. Sexual partners should be treated.

## Herpes Simplex Virus

| | |
|---|---|
| Causative agent | Herpes simplex virus, type 2 (see Chapter 49) |
| Incubation period | 2 to 14 days |
| Transmission | Direct sexual contact with an infected person |

Herpes simplex virus (HSV), type 2, is the predominant cause of genital herpes. Genital herpes is one of the most frequently seen STDs in the United States. It is especially problematic because an infected mother can transmit it to her newborn during vaginal delivery, causing multisystem disease. The highest risk for transmission is during the first infection with active lesions (Chua, Arnolds, & Niklas, 2015). Women with active HSV infection as labor and delivery approach may be advised to have a cesarean delivery. Congenital infections can cause preterm labor, spontaneous abortion, or stillbirth (Chua et al., 2015).

### Manifestations

At the initial infection, lesions occur in the genital area, usually on the vulva, perineum, or perianal area. However, lesions may also occur in the vagina and on the cervix, areas where they cannot be seen. Pain and tenderness in the affected area may coincide with lesion eruption. Vesicles erupt, rupture, and then ulcerate over the course of 1 to 7 days. The virus is shed for 2 to 3 weeks. Occasionally, flu-like symptoms (fever, malaise, dysuria, enlarged lymph nodes) can accompany vesicular eruption. After the acute phase has passed, the virus can remain dormant in the nerve ganglia, where it can reappear later in response to stressful triggers.

### Therapeutic Management

Viral culture from vesicular fluid can confirm the diagnosis. There is no cure for HSV 2, but administration of acyclovir (Zovirax) can diminish symptoms and reduce shedding time. Infected neonates are treated with parenteral acyclovir; those with ocular involvement receive a topical ophthalmic drug as well. Adolescents are treated for 10 days with oral acyclovir, valacyclovir, or famciclovir. Infected individuals should refrain from all sexual contact until the lesions have healed completely. Because the shedding time in an initial infection is prolonged, abstinence is recommended for several weeks. Current research shows that patients diagnosed with HSV are at significant risk for acquiring HIV. Recurrent infections can be controlled by the use of daily oral acyclovir, valacyclovir, or famciclovir (Stanberry, 2016).

### CRITICAL THINKING EXERCISE 41.1

Adolescents with a sexually transmitted disease (STD) may seek out school- or community-based healthcare. Their symptoms can be vague, with generalized feelings of malaise or fever; or specific, with reports of painful urination or vaginal or penile discharge. Often they hope that the nurse will ask about sexual activity because they feel they cannot trust other adults. What challenges does the nurse face when caring for these adolescents?

## Human Papillomavirus

| | |
|---|---|
| Causative agent | Human papillomavirus (HPV); there are in excess of 120 types, 40 infect the genital tract |
| Incubation period | 3 weeks to many months |
| Transmission | Direct sexual contact, perinatal contact during delivery |

HPV is responsible for the common wart and for genital warts (condylomata acuminata). Anogenital warts can be contracted primarily through direct sexual contact, and having multiple sex partners increases the risk. Children with anogenital warts should be investigated for sexual abuse. A person can get common warts through autoinoculation from other body sites. A break in skin integrity is necessary for infection to occur. Genital HPV infection has become endemic in the United States. The CDC estimates that most sexually active women will develop HPV, with adolescence through young adulthood being the period of greatest risk (CDC, 2016).

### Manifestations

Anogenital warts begin as small papules that grow into soft, clustered lesions. They are found in moist areas, such as the labia minora, vagina, cervix, anus, rectum, and glans penis. Common warts are frequently found on fingers, palms of the hands, and soles of the feet. Most common warts in children resolve within several years. Adolescents usually clear low-risk types in 4 to 5 months and high-risk types in 8 to 10 months, but warts may persist for longer.

HPV types such as HPV-6 and HPV-11 are associated with genital warts and do not cause cancer. Of the more than 120 types, approximately 35 have been associated with neoplastic lesions. HPV-16 and HPV-18 cause approximately 70% of cervical cancers (Moscicki, 2016).

### Therapeutic Management

In many instances, genital warts resolve spontaneously in 1 to 2 years (Nash, Harrison, Alexander, 2014). Treatment, which is often difficult, can include topical gels or creams such as imiquimod, cryotherapy, electrocautery, laser treatment, and various types of surgical removal. For sexually active individuals, transmission can be decreased by the use of condoms. Screening for cervical cancer with a Papanicolaou (Pap) test can detect cervical cancer in an early form and prevent progression to cervical cancer. The CDC recommends that women have yearly Pap tests starting at age 21 and every 23 years thereafter until the age of 29 (Nash et al., 2014).

There are three licensed vaccines against HPV in the United States. In 2006, the quadrivalent HPV-6/11/16/18 vaccine (Gardasil, Merck) was approved by the FDA for females and males aged 9 to 26 years. In 2009, a bivalent vaccine (Cervarix, GlaxoSmithKline) against HPV-16 and HPV-18 was approved for females age 9 to 25 years. Most recently an expanded 9-valent HPV vaccine was licensed in 2014 (Gardasil 9, Merck). The CDC's Advisory Committee on Immunization Practice recommends that females age 11 to 12 be immunized with one of the three HPV vaccines; males should receive either the HPV 9 or HPV 4 vaccine (AAP, 2015e). All vaccinations are given in a three-dose series. Unfortunately, the completion rates of the HPV vaccine fall well short of the *Healthy People 2020* goal of 80% coverage; therefore, current research is focusing on ways to increase rates (McRee, Gilkey, & Dempsey, 2014).

## Bacterial Vaginosis

| | |
|---|---|
| Causative agent | Specific cause is not clearly identified; however, the normal vaginal flora is replaced by an overgrowth of organisms such as *Gardnerella vaginalis, Mycoplasma hominis,* or anaerobic bacteria; a corresponding decrease in the concentration of lactobacilli occurs |
| Incubation period | Unknown |
| Transmission | Presumed to be transmitted through sexual contact because it is uncommon in females who are not sexually active |

Bacterial vaginosis can occur alone or concurrently with infections that result in vaginal discharge, such as trichomoniasis; it is a common diagnosis in adolescent girls who are sexually active.

### Manifestations

Bacterial vaginosis is characterized by a profuse, white, malodorous (having a fishy smell) vaginal discharge that sticks to the vaginal walls. Bacterial vaginosis may be asymptomatic and is not usually associated with abdominal pain, skin rashes, itching, or painful urination. Because other STDs can occur simultaneously, sexually active adolescents with bacterial vaginosis should be tested for coexisting STDs. Bacterial vaginosis is a risk factor for PID.

Bacterial vaginosis in a prepubertal girl is commonly caused by poor hygiene, a vaginal foreign body, or other infections.

Bacterial vaginosis responds well to oral metronidazole or to vaginal gels and creams (5- and 7-day administration schedules). Use of clindamycin cream, which is oil based, can alter the effectiveness of latex condoms for at least 5 days after the last application (AAP, 2015f). Male partners do not need to be treated, but patients should be aware of the risk of recurrence.

## Syphilis

| | |
|---|---|
| Causative agent | *Treponema pallidum* |
| Incubation period | Acquired primary infection: 10 to 90 days (average, 21 days) |
| Transmission | Intimate contact, transplacentally, or sexually |

Congenital syphilis can be transmitted transplacentally by an infected mother at any time during pregnancy or birth. Acquired syphilis is contracted through sexual contact. In children, syphilis diagnosed after the neonatal period can almost always be linked to sexual abuse.

### Manifestations

If untreated during pregnancy, congenital syphilis can cause stillbirth or neonatal death. Infants with congenital syphilis can be asymptomatic or exhibit signs and symptoms within the first 3 months of life. The classic signs are rhinitis, a maculopapular rash, and hepatosplenomegaly. Diagnostic radiographs may show osteochondritis, periosteitis, or metaphyseal changes, especially in the long bones of the femur and humerus. Late manifestations are a result of the scarring from the systemic disease process. The bones, teeth, eyes, and eighth cranial nerve are involved. The teeth are notched (Hutchinson's teeth), and hearing loss can occur suddenly at approximately 8 to 10 years of age. Acquired syphilis is divided into three stages and has the same clinical course in children as in adults. The primary stage is characterized by one or more painless ulcers that heal spontaneously. One to 2 months later, in the secondary stage, a generalized rash appears on the palms and soles. The final stage is latent syphilis, in which there are no clinical manifestations (AAP, 2015g).

### Therapeutic Management

Syphilis responds well to a single dose of benzathine penicillin G intramuscularly (the preferred treatment for children and adults). Aqueous crystalline penicillin G or procaine penicillin is effective with congenital syphilis. Acquired syphilis can be treated with benzathine penicillin G. Tetracycline and doxycycline for 14 days are options for the child older than 8 years but should not be used in younger children because of the greater risks of permanent tooth staining. In addition, the effectiveness of drugs other than penicillin and tetracycline remains unproven.

Education regarding potential long-term effects of partially or untreated syphilis must be discussed. Resources should be available and care should be accessible to ensure completion of treatment and eradication of disease. All women should be screened for syphilis in early pregnancy (AAP, 2015g).

## Trichomoniasis

| | |
|---|---|
| Causative agent | *Trichomonas vaginalis* (flagellated protozoan) |
| Incubation period | 5 to 28 days (average of 1 week) |
| Transmission | Perinatal contact during delivery, sexual activity |

### Manifestations

Infections with *Trichomonas* are frequently asymptomatic. Most males with the infection are asymptomatic. When symptoms occur, they may include dysuria, vaginal itching and burning (in females), and a frothy, yellowish green, foul-smelling discharge. Infected mothers can transmit the disease to their newborn infants during birth. Children with a positive culture for *Trichomonas* should be investigated for possible sexual abuse.

### Therapeutic Management

A single dose of metronidazole (Flagyl, Protostat) or tinidazole is the treatment of choice for adolescents; they have an approximate cure rate of 90% to 95%. For prepubertal girls, metronidazole is given in two or three divided doses. Sexual partners should also be treated, and patients are counseled to avoid sexual contact until they and their partners are asymptomatic.

Education regarding the potential presence of other STDs should be thoroughly discussed, especially with the adolescent patient, in a respectful and confidential manner.

### Nursing Considerations

Prevention, early identification, and treatment are the goals of nursing care associated with any STD. The nurse plays a key role in educating young people about STDs. Often, the school nurse is the healthcare professional whom adolescents feel they can trust; therefore, school nurses may be the care providers in the best position to educate this population. Establishing rapport with the teenager by using a nonjudgmental approach and reassurance of confidentiality is key. The nurse must be aware of symptoms and assist in identifying those adolescents who are at risk for STDs. Encouraging abstinence in those who are not sexually active and condom use in sexually active adolescents is a way to prevent STDs. The nurse may be the one to assume responsibility

## EVIDENCE-BASED PRACTICE

Human papillomavirus (HPV) is one of the most frequently seen sexually transmitted diseases (STDs) in the United States, with one quarter of 14 to 19 year-olds acquiring HPV. Although some cases of HPV are asymptomatic, many can cause genital warts or lead to several different types of cancer later in life. With the licensing of three HPV vaccinations, pediatric primary care providers are able to prevent not only genital warts and the painful procedures used to treat them, but also certain types of cancer, such as cervical, vaginal, anal, and penile cancers, as well as those of the head and neck.

The U.S. Food and Drug Administration (FDA) approved the first quadrivalent vaccination in June 2006 and a second, bivalent vaccine in October 2009 and a third 9-valent HPV vaccine in 2014. Recent data from the Centers for Disease Control and Prevention (CDC) show that only 33% of adolescent females and 7% of adolescent males completed the vaccination series (McRee, Gilkey, & Dempsey, 2014). These statistics demonstrate that adolescents and their parents are frequently not following the recommendation of the CDC's Advisory Committee on Immunization Practices (ACIP) for routine vaccination of females, and now males, age 11 to 12 with catch-up vaccination for those 13 through 26 years. Studies are being conducted to assess the effectiveness of a two-dose series of the 9-valent HPV vaccine in hopes of improving completion rates (Suryadevara, Paton, & Domachowske, 2015).

There are many arguments both for and against HPV vaccination of children; providers are in a position to assist parents in making an informed decision by educating them on HPV and the HPV vaccination.

Many parents report that they receive information regarding the HPV vaccination through TV, print news, and the Internet. Often these sources provide erroneous information, especially concerning adverse side effects, which can lead to declining HPV vaccination rates. The concern regarding the safety of the vaccine is very important in parents' decision whether or not to vaccinate their child.

Another parentally perceived barrier to receiving the HPV vaccination is the cost ($360 for the three-dose series) and whether it will be covered by the parents' health insurance carrier. The cost is covered by Medicaid and those eligible for the Vaccines for Children program.

However, there are persuasive arguments for vaccinating children against HPV. First and foremost is the protection against HPV-related cancers. All vaccinations are 100% effective against the HPV types included in the vaccine. With high immunization rates, there will be a significant decrease in morbidity and mortality. Approximately 26,000 new cancers diagnoses are attributed to HPV each year in the United States (CDC, 2014a). Recent economic studies show that there is a significant savings related to healthcare costs. Despite parental concerns that the vaccine will promote sexual activity in adolescents, data show that a significant number of high school students already report having sexual intercourse, despite various approaches to sex education.

Pediatric primary care providers bear the responsibility for educating parents and adolescents by providing accurate, up-to-date information. Several studies have indicated that the most important reason parents cite when deciding whether to vaccinate their adolescents is a healthcare provider's recommendation and unfortunately, only half of all adolescents receive such recommendations (McRee et al., 2014).

Cassidy, Braxter, Charron-Prochownik et al. (2014) designed a quality improvement initiative to evaluate if evidence based education can increase HPV vaccine rates. The study used a convenience sample of 24 parents of preteen females for the intervention group and 29 parents of preteen females for the control group. The researchers developed an educational brochure, an electronic reminder system along with a 1:1 intervention script with parents and providers to discuss barriers to vaccination. The study used a retrospective and a prospective review to compare vaccine initiation and completion rates between the two groups. The results demonstrated the intervention group was much more likely to initiate and complete the vaccination series (Cassidy et al., 2014).

As a healthcare provider, you will need to decide when is the appropriate time to vaccinate patients and to have productive conversations about their sexuality and the importance of safe sex. Providers may be concerned about lengthy discussions that take precious time from already short well care visits.

When providing evidence-based information to parents and their children, think about what you would recommend:

If a parent asks you about the HPV vaccination, what information would you provide?

Would you recommend the vaccination to children and adolescents age 9 through 26?

References: Cassidy, B., Braxter, B., Charron-Prochownik, D., et al. (2014). A quality improvement initiative to increase HPV vaccine rates using an educational and reminder strategy with parents of preteen girls. *Journal of Pediatric Health Care, 28*(2), 155–164. doi:10.1016/jpedhc.2013.01.002; Centers for Disease Control and Prevention. (2014a). *Human Papillomavirus.* Retrieved from http://www.cdc.gov/mmwr/preview/mmwrhtml/mm6304a1.htm?s_cid=mm6304a1_e; McRee, A.L., Gilkey, M.B., & Dempsey, A.F. (2014). HPV vaccine hesitancy: findings from a statewide survey of health care providers. *Journal of Pediatric Health Care, 28*(6), 541–549. doi:10.1016/jpedhc.2014.05.003; Suryadevara, M., Paton, L., & Domachowske, J.B. (2015). Adolescent immunization: 2015 and beyond. *Pediatric Annals, 44*(4), e82–e88. doi:10.3928/00904481-20150410-09.

for helping the adolescent obtain proper medical treatment and gain an understanding of the importance of completing the entire course of medication, as well as treatment of partners.

An issue that has become increasingly concerning is the number of young adolescents who practice oral sex. Research on this subject suggests that approximately 7% of young adolescents have been either active or passive participants in oral sex, and many of these teens do not understand or believe that they are at risk for STDs from this behavior. Health providers need to assess adolescents for oral sex participation and provide appropriate information about the risks involved in the same way information is provided about vaginal sex.

## KEY CONCEPTS

- Infectious diseases can be transmitted by direct contact with another infected person, by contact with animal or insect carriers, by ingestion of contaminated food or water containing the pathogens, and by contact with a contaminated object.
- Vaccines can be live or attenuated, killed or inactivated toxoids, human immune globulin, or animal serums or antitoxins.
- Assessment of the child with an infectious disease includes a thorough history (recent exposure, other family members or friends exhibiting signs or symptoms, environmental causes) and documentation of the type, configuration, and distribution of any lesions; the child's temperature; and any associated signs and symptoms.
- Children with infectious diseases usually can and should be cared for at home.
- STDs can be transmitted to neonates from exposure to organisms during delivery, but children who acquire an STD after the neonatal period should always be evaluated for possible sexual abuse.
- Abstinence is the only 100% effective way to prevent both pregnancy and STD transmission. Sexually active individuals should use barrier protection to prevent STDs.

## REFERENCES AND READINGS


Abzug, M.J. (2016). Nonpolio enteroviruses. In R. Kliegman, B. Stanton, J. St. Geme, et al. (Eds.), *Nelson textbook of pediatrics* (20th ed., pp. 1561–1568). Philadelphia: Elsevier.

Agency for Healthcare Research and Quality. (2012, March). *The diagnosis and management of febrile infants (0-3 months)*. Retrieved from http://www.ahrq.gov.

Alex, M.R. (2014). Congenital cytomegalovirus: implications for maternal-child nursing. *The Journal of Maternal Child Nursing, 39*(2), 122–129. doi: 10.1097/NMC.0000000000000008.

American Academy of Pediatrics. (2015a). Measles. In D.W. Kimberlin, M.T. Brady, M.A. Jackson, et al. (Eds.), *Red book 2015 report of the committee on infectious diseases* (30th ed., pp. 228–230). Elk Grove Village, IL: AAP; 2015.

American Academy of Pediatrics. (2015b). Parvovirus B19. In D.W. Kimberlin, M.T. Brady, M.A. Jackson, et al. (Eds.), *Red book 2015 report of the committee on infectious diseases* (30th ed., pp. 593–596). Elk Grove Village, IL: AAP; 2015.

American Academy of Pediatrics. (2015c). Varicella-Zoster virus infections. In D.W. Kimberlin, M.T. Brady, M.A. Jackson, et al. (Eds.), *Red book 2015 report of the committee on infectious diseases* (30th ed., pp. 846–860). Elk Grove Village, IL: AAP; 2015.

American Academy of Pediatrics. (2015d). Chlamydia trachomatis. In D.W. Kimberlin, M.T. Brady, M.A. Jackson, et al. (Eds.), *Red book 2015 report of the committee on infectious diseases* (30th ed., pp. 288–294). Elk Grove Village, IL: AAP; 2015.

American Academy of Pediatrics. (2015e). Human Papillomaviruses. In D.W. Kimberlin, M.T. Brady, M.A. Jackson, et al. (Eds.), *Red book 2015 report of the committee on infectious diseases* (30th ed., pp. 576–583). Elk Grove Village, IL: AAP; 2015.

American Academy of Pediatrics. (2015f). *Bacterial vaginosis*. In D.W. Kimberlin, M.T. Brady, M.A. Jackson, et al. (Eds.), *Red book 2015 report of the committee on infectious diseases* (30th ed., pp. 256–258). Elk Grove Village, IL: AAP; 2015.

American Academy of Pediatrics. (2015g). Syphilis. In D.W. Kimberlin, M.T. Brady, M.A. Jackson, et al. (Eds.), *Red book 2015 report of the committee on infectious diseases* (30th ed., pp. 755–768). Elk Grove Village, IL: AAP; 2015.

Bass, P.F. (2015). Pertussis makes a nasty comeback [Electronic version]. *Contemporary Pediatrics, 32*(03), 9.

Beharry, M.S., Shafii, T., & Burstein, G.R. (2013). Diagnosis and treatment of chlamydia, gonorrhea, and trichomonas in adolescents. *Pediatric Annals, 42*(2), 26–33. doi: 10.3928/00904481-20130128-09.

Cassidy, B., Braxter, B., Charron-Prochownik, D., et al. (2014). A quality improvement initiative to increase HPV vaccine rates using an educational and reminder strategy with parents of preteen girls. *Journal of Pediatric Health Care, 28*(2), 155–164. doi: 10.1016/jpedhc.2013.01.002.

Centers for Disease Control and Prevention. (2012). *Tick-borne relapsing fever: information for clinicians*. Retrieved from http://www.cdc.gov.

Centers for Disease Control and Prevention. (2014a). *Human Papillomavirus*. Retrieved from http://www.cdc.gov/mmwr/preview/mmwrhtml/mm6304a1.htm?s_cid=mm6304a1_e.

Centers for Disease Control and Prevention. (2014b). *Rubella*. Retrieved from http://www.cdc.gov/vaccines/pubs/surv-manual/chpt14-rubella.html.

Centers for Disease Control and Prevention. (2015a). *Measles Cases and Outbreaks*. Retrieved from http://www.cdc.gov/measles/about/overview.html.

Centers for Disease Control and Prevention. (2015b). *Tracking Clostridium difficile Infection*. Retrieved from: http://www.cdc.gov/hai/organisms/cdiff/tracking-Cdif.html.

Centers for Disease Control and Prevention. (2015c).*Chlamydia Statistics*. Retrieved from http://www.cdc.gov/std/chlamydia/stats.htm.

Centers for Disease Control and Prevention. (2016). *Human Papillomavirus*. Retrieved from http://www.cdc.gov/std/hpv/stdfact-hpv.htm.

Cherry, J. (2014). Measles Virus. In J. Cherry, G. Harrison, S. Kaplan, et al. (Eds.), *Feigin and Cherry's textbook of pediatric infectious diseases* (7th ed., pp. 2373–2395). Philadelphia: Elsevier Saunders.

Cherry, J., & Adachi, K. (2014). Rubella Virus. In J. Cherry, G. Harrison, S. Kaplan, et al. (Eds.), *Feigin and Cherry's textbook of pediatric infectious diseases* (7th ed., pp. 2195–2225). Philadelphia: Elsevier Saunders.

Cherry, J., & Quinn, K.K. (2014). Mumps Virus. In J. Cherry, G. Harrison, S. Kaplan, et al. (Eds.), *Feigin and Cherry's textbook of pediatric infectious diseases* (7th ed., pp. 2395–2407). Philadelphia: Elsevier Saunders.

Chua, C., Arnolds, M., & Niklas, V. (2015). Molecular diagnostics and newborns at risk for genital herpes simplex virus. *Pediatric Annals, 44*(5), e97–e102. doi: 10.3928/00904481-20150512-08.

Gershon, A.A. (2014). Varicella-Zoster Virus. In J. Cherry, G. Harrison, S. Kaplan, et al. (Eds.), *Feigin and Cherry's textbook of pediatric infectious diseases* (7th ed., pp. 2021–2033). Philadelphia: Elsevier Saunders.

Grant, G., Reef, S.E., Dabbagh, A., et al. (2015). Global progress toward rubella and congenital rubella syndrome control and elimination- 2000-2014. *MMWR, 64*(37), 1052–1055.

Hammerschlag, M.R. (2016). *Chlamydia trachomatis.* In R. Kliegman, B. Stanton, J. St. Geme, et al. (Eds.), *Nelson textbook of pediatrics* (20th ed., pp. 1493–1497). Philadelphia: Elsevier.

Harrison, G.J. (2014). Cytomegalovirus. In J. Cherry, G. Harrison, S. Kaplan, et al. (Eds.), *Feigin and Cherry's textbook of pediatric infectious diseases* (7th ed., pp. 1968–1991). Philadelphia: Elsevier Saunders.

Harrison, G.J. (2015). Current controversies in diagnosis, management, and prevention of congenital cytomegalovirus: updates for the pediatric practitioner. *Pediatric Annals, 44*(5), e115–e125. doi: 10.3928/00904481-20150512-11.

Kaplan, S.L., Hulten, K.G., & Mason, E.O. (2014). *Staphylococcus aureus* infections. In J. Cherry, G. Harrison, S. Kaplan, et al. (Eds.), *Feigin and Cherry's textbook of pediatric infectious diseases* (7th ed., pp. 1113–1130). Philadelphia: Elsevier Saunders.

Krause, P.J. (2014). Relapsing Fever. In J. Cherry, G. Harrison, S. Kaplan, et al. (Eds.), *Feigin and Cherry's textbook of pediatric infectious diseases* (7th ed., pp. 1739–1742). Philadelphia: Elsevier Saunders.

Lantos, P.M., & McKinney, R. (2014). Rickettsial and ehrlichial diseases. In J. Cherry, G. Harrison, S. Kaplan, et al. (Eds.), *Feigin and Cherry's textbook of pediatric infectious diseases* (7th ed., pp. 2647–2654). Philadelphia: Elsevier Saunders.

LaRussa, P.S., & Marin, M. (2016). Varicella-Zoster virus. In R. Kliegman, B. Stanton, J. St. Geme, et al. (Eds.), *Nelson textbook of pediatrics* (20th ed., pp. 1579–1586). Philadelphia: Elsevier.

LeFevre, M.L. (2014). Screening for chlamydia and gonorrhea: U.S. preventative services task force recommendation statement. *Annals of Internal Medicine, 161*(12), 902–910. doi: 10.7326/M14-1981.

Lindberg, C., Lanzi, M., & Lindberg, K. (2015). Measles: still a significant health threat. *The American Journal of Maternal Child Nursing* (5), 298–305. doi: 10.1097/NMC.0000000000000162.

Liu, C., Bayer, A., Cosgrove, S.E., et al. (2011). Clinical practice guidelines by the infectious disease society of America for the treatment of methicillin-resistant *Staphylococcus aureus* infections in adults and children: executive summary. *Clinical Infectious Diseases, 52*(3), 285–292.

Long, S.S. (2016). Pertussis (*Bordetella pertussis* and *Bordetella parapertussis*). In R. Kliegman, B. Stanton, J. St. Geme, et al. (Eds.), *Nelson textbook of pediatrics* (20th ed., pp. 1377–1382). Philadelphia: Elsevier.

Marshall, B.C., & Foxworth, M.F. (2012). Epstein-Barr virus-associated infectious mononucleosis [Electronic version]. *Contemporary Pediatrics, 52–62.*

Mason, W.H. (2016). *Measles.* In R. Kliegman, B. Stanton, J. St. Geme, et al. (Eds.), *Nelson textbook of pediatrics* (20th ed., pp. 1542–1552). Philadelphia: Elsevier.

McRee, A.L., Gilkey, M.B., & Dempsey, A.F. (2014). HPV vaccine hesitancy: findings from a statewide survey of health care providers. *Journal of Pediatric Health Care, 28*(6), 541–549. doi: 10.1016/jpedhc.2014.05.003.

Mezoff, E.A., & Cohen, M.B. (2014). *Clostridium difficile* infection. In J. Cherry, G. Harrison, S. Kaplan, et al. (Eds.), *Feigin and Cherry's textbook of pediatric infectious diseases* (7th ed., pp. 1434–1439). Philadelphia: Elsevier Saunders.

Michos, A., & Zaoutis, T. (2011). Bats and rabies: what rabies prophylaxis in needed and when? [Electronic version] *Contemporary Pediatrics,* 46–55.

Moscicki, A.B. (2016). *Human Papillomaviruses.* In R. Kliegman, B. Stanton, J. St. Geme, et al. (Eds.), *Nelson textbook of pediatrics* (20th ed., pp. 1618–1622). Philadelphia: Elsevier.

Nash, C.B., Harrison, G.J., & Alexander, K.A. (2014). *Human Papillomaviruses.* In J. Cherry, G. Harrison, S. Kaplan, et al. (Eds.), *Feigin and Cherry's textbook of pediatric infectious diseases* (7th ed., pp. 1871–1887). Philadelphia: Elsevier Saunders.

O'Grady, J.S. (2014). Fifth and sixth diseases: more than a fever and a rash. *The Journal of Family Practice, 63*(10), 1–5.

Sales, J.M., Brown, J.L., DiClemente, R.J., et al. (2012) Age differences in STDs, sexual behaviors, and correlates of risky sex among sexually experienced adolescent African-American females. *Journal of Pediatric Psychology, 37*(1), 33–42.

Shulman, S. (2016). Group A Streptococcus. In R. Kliegman, B. Stanton, J. St. Geme, et al. (Eds.), *Nelson textbook of pediatrics* (20th ed., pp. 1327–1332). Philadelphia: Elsevier.

Skoff, T.H., Kenyon, C., Corcoros, N., et al. (2015). Sources of infant pertussis infection in the United States. *Pediatrics, 136*(4), 635–641. doi: 10.1542/peds.2015-1120

Sood, S.K., & Krause, P.J. (2014). Borrelia. In J. Cherry, G. Harrison, S. Kaplan, et al. (Eds.), *Feigin and Cherry's textbook of pediatric infectious diseases* (7th ed., pp. 1729–1739). Philadelphia: Elsevier Saunders.

Stanberry, L.R. (2016). *Herpes simplex virus.* In R. Kliegman, B. Stanton, J. St. Geme, et al. (Eds.), *Nelson textbook of pediatrics* (20th ed., pp. 1572–1579). Philadelphia: Elsevier.

Suryadevara, M., Paton, L., & Domachowske, J.B. (2015). Adolescent immunization: 2015 and beyond. *Pediatric Annals, 44*(4), e82–e88. doi: 10.3928/00904481-20150410-09.

Woods, C.R. (2014). *Gonococcal Infections.* In J. Cherry, G. Harrison, S. Kaplan, et al. (Eds.), *Feigin and Cherry's textbook of pediatric infectious diseases* (7th ed., pp. 1271–1301). Philadelphia: Elsevier Saunders.

# 42

# The Child With an Immunologic Alteration

http://evolve.elsevier.com/McKinney/mat-ch/

## LEARNING OBJECTIVES

*After studying this chapter, you should be able to:*

- Describe how the immune system attempts to maintain homeostasis of the internal and external environment and what happens when it overfunctions or underfunctions.
- Explain how neonates acquire active and passive immunity.
- Delineate how to prevent the spread of organisms in children with an immune deficiency.
- Describe how to prevent, test for, care for, and support children with human immunodeficiency virus and their families throughout the entire spectrum of illness.
- Outline critical information needed by families with children receiving long-term corticosteroid therapy.
- Describe nursing interventions to help prevent the sudden death of a child having an anaphylactic reaction.

# CLINICAL REFERENCE

## REVIEW OF THE IMMUNE SYSTEM

The body's network of first-line, or external, defenses—intact skin and mucous membranes and the processes such as sneezing, coughing, and tearing—helps keep it free of disease. When a foreign substance penetrates first-line defenses, the immune (lymphoreticular) system, or internal defense system, provides secondary and tertiary protection through nonspecific and specific responses. The immune system is able to distinguish the body's own cells, or self, from foreign substances, or nonself; activate a response to detect and destroy foreign substances; suppress a response against the self; and memorize and store information.

Foreign substances, or antigens, possess unique configurations on their cell surfaces that mark them as foreign. The immune system first responds to the invader through nonspecific immune functions. If the antigen survives the action of the nonspecific response, the immune system initiates specific immune functions. It begins producing proteins called *antibodies*, also known as *immunoglobulins*. Each antibody is specific for a particular antigen, contains sites that are complementary, and can combine, or bind, with the antigen. This combination of antigen and antibody is called the *antigen-antibody complex* or *immune complex*. The immune complex prevents the antigen from binding to receptors on vulnerable cells.

The major organs and tissues of the immune system include the bone marrow, thymus, spleen, lymph nodes, and lymphoid tissue. Both the circulatory system and the lymphatic system connect these organs and tissues to one another. Specific types of cells are also important to the immune system.

### Nonspecific Immune Functions

The body's innate immune system consists of nonspecific immune functions that are protective barriers activated in the presence of an antigen but not specific to that antigen. These nonspecific immune functions include chemical barriers such as bactericides, fungicides, and enzymes in body secretions; interferon, a protein produced in response to viruses; and inflammation, involving increased capillary permeability, vasodilation, phagocytosis (cell eating), and elimination of cell products.

During an inflammatory response, vasodilation of small capillaries at the site of invasion increases circulation to the site. The resulting alteration in microvascular pressure facilitates movement of plasma cells into tissue, where they accumulate. Neutrophils are the first phagocytes that arrive at the site. Complement is a series of serum proteins involved in enzyme action and antigen death. Antigens activate the complement system, and this system acts as an inflammation stimulator to attract neutrophils to the site. Complement also promotes the increase in circulation and vascular permeability involved with the inflammatory response (Porth, 2014).

Phagocytosis can occur alone or as part of the inflammatory response. Phagocytes ingest the antigen and either survive or die. In dying, the phagocytes release additional chemicals that draw more phagocytes to the area.

Increased capillary permeability and vasodilation result in redness and edema. The products of phagocyte antigen death include toxins that give rise to fever, pain, and purulence. As the antigens are destroyed, the toxins are cleared from the lymph nodes, which often become enlarged. If the immune response is effective, the inflammation subsides.

### Specific Immune Functions

If the antigen survives within the phagocyte, two types of specific immune functions can recognize and destroy it: humoral and cell mediated. These responses are closely related.

Lymphocytes, which are a sub-classification of leukocytes (white blood cells) function in both types of immune response. Lymphocytes

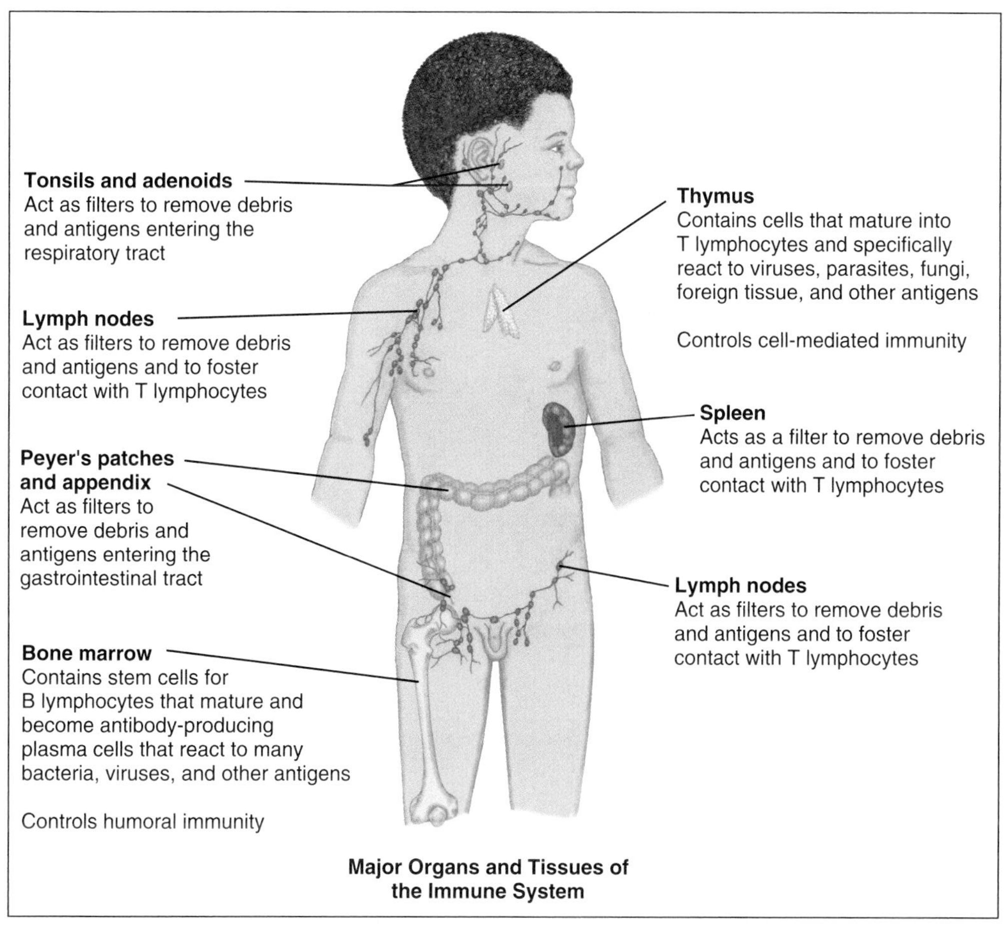
Tonsils and adenoids
Act as filters to remove debris and antigens entering the respiratory tract
Lymph nodes
Act as filters to remove debris and antigens and to foster contact with T lymphocytes
Peyer's patches and appendix
Act as filters to remove debris and antigens entering the gastrointestinal tract
Bone marrow
Contains stem cells for B lymphocytes that mature and become antibody-producing plasma cells that react to many bacteria, viruses, and other antigens
Controls humoral immunity
Thymus
Contains cells that mature into T lymphocytes and specifically react to viruses, parasites, fungi, foreign tissue, and other antigens
Controls cell-mediated immunity
Spleen
Acts as a filter to remove debris and antigens and to foster contact with T lymphocytes
Lymph nodes
Act as filters to remove debris and antigens and to foster contact with T lymphocytes
**Major Organs and Tissues of the Immune System**

circulate in the blood and the lymphatic system. They make up 53% to 57% of white blood cells during the first year of life, when specific immunity develops rapidly, but only 25% to 30% after 12 months of age. Two classes of lymphocytes are involved in the immune response: B lymphocytes (B cells) and T lymphocytes (T cells).

B cells, which promote the humoral response, originate in the bone marrow or liver but mature in the lymphoid tissue, becoming plasma cells. When exposed to antigens, some of the plasma cells produce antibodies, whereas others become memory cells. Antibodies are classified as immunoglobulins G, M, A, D, and E, often abbreviated IgG, IgM, IgA, IgD, and IgE. Immunoglobulins bind to antigens and facilitate their destruction.

T cells, which are responsible for the cell-mediated response, originate in the bone marrow and mature in the thymus, where they react specifically to viruses, fungi, parasites, foreign tissue, and other antigens. The three major types of T cells are effector (helper T cells [CD4+] and cytotoxic T cells [CD8+]), regulatory T cells, and memory T cells (Rote & McCance, 2014).

Natural killer cells, or large granular lymphocytes that resemble T lymphocytes, can recognize and directly destroy infected or malignant cells. They are not antigen-specific cells (Buckley, 2016; Rote & McCance, 2014).

### The Humoral Response

The humoral response involves chiefly B cells, although the cooperation of helper T cells is almost always necessary. Macrophages ingest antigens and introduce them into the circulation. In response, the B cells and helper T cells interact. The helper T cells secrete substances that cause B cells to multiply and differentiate into plasma cells, which produce vast quantities of antibodies specific to the antigen. These antibodies combine with the antigens to form immune complexes. The antibodies promote phagocytosis and destroy the antigens. Destruction and elimination of antigen eventually result in a decrease in the chemical factors that enhance the humoral response, "turning off" the response when it is no longer needed (Porth, 2014).

### The Cell-Mediated Response

A cell-mediated response is initiated by macrophages presenting antigens to T lymphocytes. Once activated, helper T cells secrete substances that facilitate macrophages to destroy antigens as well as stimulate the production and circulation of additional macrophages. One set of T cells, called *cytotoxic T cells,* tracks down and kills viruses, tumor cells, and other pathogens directly. Regulatory T cells, interacting with other immune components, draw the immune response to a close (Porth, 2014).

## Development of Immunity

By 8 weeks of gestation, B cell differentiation begins. The normal fetus can produce IgM by 20 to 24 weeks of gestation. The neonate's immune protection comes from prenatal transfer of maternal antibodies (IgG) and breast milk transfer of IgA. Gradually, the normal newborn infant's own humoral and cell-mediated responses to infections begin; immunity is acquired both actively and passively.

### Active Acquired Immunity

When the body reacts to an antigen through either a humoral or a cell-mediated response, it is developing **active immunity**. Active immunity is long lived and measured in months, years, or even a lifetime; it follows exposure to environmental antigens or vaccines. Immediately after exposure, there is a latency period when antibody levels are low. When the body recognizes the antigen as foreign, it makes antibodies. The first antibodies produced are predominantly IgM and subsequently, IgG. After a second exposure to the antigen, antibodies appear at a faster rate, and the latency period is shortened or nonexistent. The antibody levels remain high and persist for much longer periods. The predominant antibody in a secondary response is IgG.

Infants receive specific live or attenuated vaccines on a recommended schedule to induce immunity against the antigens in the vaccine (see the recommended schedule on the CDC website http://www.cdc.gov/vaccines/schedules/downloads/child/0-18yrs-child-combined-schedule.pdf).

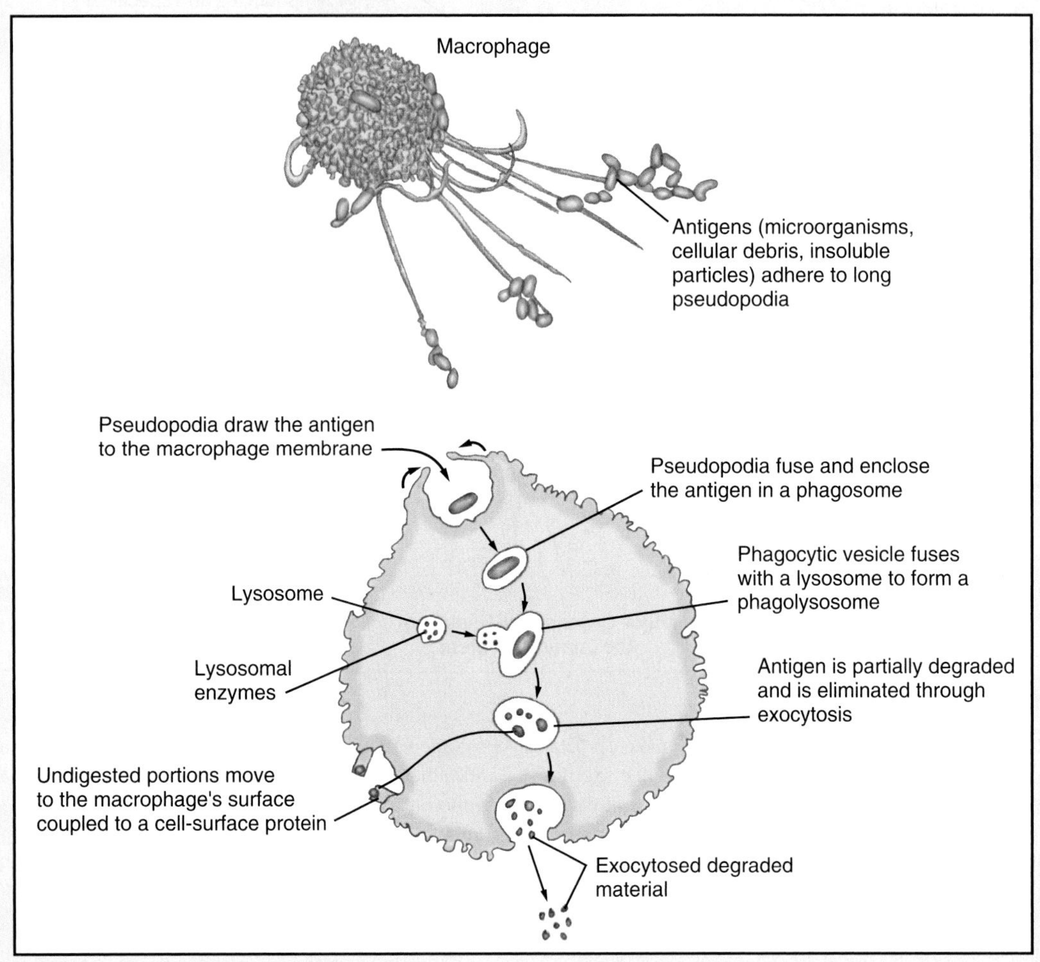


## Cells Involved in the Immune Response

| Cell Type | Nonspecific Immune Response (Innate Immunity) |
|---|---|
| **Granulocytes** | |
| Neutrophils | First leukocytes to respond to tissue damage |
| | Ingest and destroy antigens, especially bacteria, by phagocytosis |
| | Increase in number during acute inflammation, bacterial infection, and necrosis |
| | Immature neutrophils are called bands. Increased bands (shift to the left) indicate infection. |
| Eosinophils | Help control the inflammatory response |
| | Neutralize histamine |
| | Increase in number during hypersensitivity reactions and kill parasites directly. |
| Basophils | Secrete histamine, heparin, and serotonin in inflammation and immediate hypersensitivity reactions |
| | Basophils located in tissue rather than in blood are called mast cells, which activate the inflammatory allergic response. |
| **Agranulocytes** | |
| Monocytes/macrophages | Monocytes, immature macrophages, are large phagocytic agranulocytes. |
| | Monocytes ingest and introduce antigens into the circulation for recognition by B and T lymphocytes. |
| | Macrophages engulf bacteria and cellular debris to finish the cleanup process started by the neutrophils. |
| Natural killer (NK) | Recognize and directly kill viruses, tumor cells, and other abnormal cells. |

## Cells Involved in the Immune Response—cont'd

| *Cell Type* | *Specific Immune Response (Adaptive Immunity)* |
|---|---|
| B lymphocytes | Found primarily in lymphoid tissue.<br>Noncirculating, short-lived cells responsible for humoral immunity<br>Contain receptor sites that recognize specific foreign substances<br>Differentiate into plasma cells capable of secreting antibodies against bacteria. First responder to viral infection. Some become memory cells for long-term recognition of specific antigens. |
| T lymphocytes | Mature in the thymus then migrate to lymphoid tissue.<br>Responsible for cellular immunity.<br>Interact with specific antigens on cell surfaces and directly attack invading microorganisms<br>Respond to viruses, fungi, parasites, and foreign tissue.<br>Regulatory functions mobilize or deactivate other cells in the immune system |
| Helper ($CD4^+$) T cells | Recognize antigens that have been processed and presented to them<br>Secrete cytokines that stimulate B cells to manufacture antibodies<br>Facilitate function of most other cells in the immune system |
| Regulatory T cells | Inhibit the immune response<br>Help keep the immune system cells in check |
| Cytotoxic ($CD8^+$) T cells | Kill target cells directly<br>Particularly effective with viruses and malignant cells |

Data from Banasik, J. (2013). Inflammation and immunity. In L. Copstead, & J. Banasik (Eds.), *Pathophysiology* (5th ed., pp. 157–192). St. Louis: Saunders; Porth, C. (2014). *Essentials of pathophysiology* (3rd ed.). Philadelphia: Wolters Kluwer.

## Pediatric Differences in the Immune System

### The Organs of the Immune System Mature During Infancy and Childhood

- Lymphoid tissue increases in mass during infancy and early childhood. It reaches adult size by 6 weeks of age, grows larger during the prepubertal years, and involutes at puberty.
- The thymus reaches its peak mass before puberty and then involutes.
- The spleen reaches its full size during adulthood.
- The number of Peyer patches increases until the adult mean is exceeded during adolescence.

### Immaturity of the Immunologic System Places the Infant and Young Child at Greater Risk for Infection

- The infant has a limited capacity to mount an antibody response. The ability to respond to infections develops gradually as the infant acquires immunity actively and passively.
- Because of the immaturity of the inflammatory response in neonates, the more common signs and symptoms of infection (e.g., fever) are less pronounced, making diagnosis more difficult.
- The neonate's diminished nonspecific immune response allows a more rapid spread of infection, potentially leading to sepsis.
- The term newborn infant receives an adult level of IgG as a result of transplacental transfer from the mother. This level begins to disappear during the first 6 to 8 months, causing a physiologic drop in IgG.
- Premature infants are more susceptible to neonatal infections because of lower levels of transplacental transfer of IgG from the mother and a more severe physiologic drop in IgG.
- IgM, IgE, and IgD are normally in low concentration at birth. IgM, IgE, IgA, and IgD do not cross the placenta. The immunoglobulins approach adult levels at different ages*:
  - *IgM:* 1 year
  - *IgA:* 6 to 7 years
  - *IgG:* 7 to 8 years
  - *IgE:* 6 to 7 years
- Absolute lymphocyte counts reach a peak during the first year. Helper T cells reach adult levels by 6 years of age.
- Passive placental transfer of IgG can affect the infant's response to active immunization (i.e., pertussis or diphtheria).
- Immature or inexperienced immune cells affect the reliability of delayed hypersensitivity skin reactions. For this reason, allergy skin tests are not routinely used with infants.

### Disorders of the Immune System Manifest Differently in Children Than in Adults

- Primary immunodeficiencies typically manifest during the first 6 months of life.
- HIV infection, the major secondary immunodeficiency in children, typically (1) infects an infant through the mother, not sexually; (2) is diagnosed by measuring a feature of the virus, not antibodies as in adults; and (3) has a shorter latency period in infants, with several different AIDS-defining illnesses.

*Buckley, R. (2016). The T-, B-, and NK-cell systems. In R. Kliegman, B. Stanton, J. St Geme, et al. (Eds.), *Nelson textbook of pediatrics* (20th ed., pp. 1006-1032). Philadelphia: Elsevier.

### Passive Acquired Immunity

Passive immunity results from antibody transfer from one person to another. Transfer of antibodies from a woman to her fetus is an example of passive immunity. The fetus receives maternal IgG antibodies across the placenta, providing protection against many infections. Most maternal antibodies dissipate in the infant by 6 to 9 months of age, but some persist for up to 18 months. The duration depends on the level of a particular antibody in the maternal plasma. Protection against measles, for example, may last through the second year of life, whereas protection against certain bacterial infections may last only 1 to 2 months. The reason neonates are so susceptible to infections by bacteria such as *Escherichia coli* is that the respective antibodies do not cross the placenta.

Other sources of passive acquired immunity include administration of immune globulin to produce temporary protection after an exposure and certain other disease-specific antibodies (e.g., rabies).

## COMMON LABORATORY AND DIAGNOSTIC TESTS OF IMMUNE FUNCTION

### Immunodeficiencies

A variety of laboratory tests evaluate immune system function. Laboratory evaluation determines intactness of its major functions: B cell immunity, T cell immunity, and phagocytosis. Many values vary significantly with age, especially during infancy. Among these are the differential in the complete blood cell count, the amount of various immunoglobulins, the lymphocyte surface antigen count (e.g., $CD4^+$ count), and the total lymphocyte count.

### Allergy

Measurement of eosinophilia and IgE levels, along with a radioallergosorbent test (RAST) and skin testing, is helpful in diagnosing allergic reactions.

**Immunoglobulin Function and Pediatric Implications**

| Immunoglobulin Type* | Percent (%) of Total Ig* | Function and Pediatric Significance | Location |
|---|---|---|---|
| IgG | 80-85 | Comprises approximately 80% of circulating immunoglobulin<br>Contains most antibodies against bacteria, viruses, and fungi in blood and body spaces<br>Crosses the placenta<br>Provides maternal antibody protection to infants<br>Responsible for Rh reactions<br>Longer and stronger response than that of the other immunoglobulins | Appears in all internal body fluids<br>Present in majority of B cells |
| IgM | 5-10 | Earliest immunoglobulin produced in response to bacterial and viral infections<br>Responsible for transfusion reactions in the ABO blood typing system<br>Does not cross placenta, so values are low in neonates<br>Produced early in life<br>Level increases after 9 mo of age<br>Presence in cord or infant blood suggests infection in utero or in newborn period | Appears mostly in the circulation<br>Attached to B cells<br>Released into plasma during immune response |
| IgA | 10-15 | Prevents infection across mucous membranes (local immunity)<br>Especially important in antiviral protection<br>Passes to neonate in breast milk | Appears in body secretions (nasal and respiratory secretions, saliva, tears, breast milk) |
| IgE | 0.004 | Leads to release of histamines, producing an allergic response<br>Elevation suggests allergy in children<br>Plays a role in defense against parasites | Found on the surface membranes of basophils and mast cells<br>Produced by plasma cells in mucous membranes and tonsils and in lymphoid tissue |
| IgD | 0.2 | Poorly understood<br>Thought to influence B-cell differentiation | Appears in small amounts in serum<br>Attached to B cells |

*Normal immunoglobulin values differ for age.

Data from Tosi, M. (2014). Immunologic and phagocytic responses to infection. In R. Fegin, J. Cherry, G. Demmler, et al. (Eds.), *Textbook of pediatric infectious diseases* (7th ed., pp. 40–41). Philadelphia: Saunders.

### Common Laboratory and Diagnostic Tests of Immune Function

| Test | Function | Nursing Considerations |
|---|---|---|
| Serum immunoglobulins (IgG, IgM, IgA, IgE) | Tests humoral immunity function<br>Measures levels of immunoglobulins by separating them through immunoelectrophoresis | Immunization and toxoids received in the past 6 mo and blood transfusions, tetanus antitoxin, and gamma globulin received can affect results and should be noted on the laboratory requisition |
| Lymphocyte surface antigen | Determines the types and subtypes of lymphocytes present in blood<br>Names of lymphocyte surface antigens based on "clusters of differentiation" (CDs))<br>CD antigens on a lymphocyte allow identification<br>Two most frequently found surface antigens and the cell types they identify: $CD4^+$, helper T cells; $CD8^+$, cytotoxic T cells | CBC required to determine the number of a particular type of cell |
| Serum antibody titer to commonly received antigens in vaccines (e.g., tetanus, diphtheria) | Used to evaluate humoral immune function | Tests antibody level to specific antigens |
| Skin tests to *Candida*, tuberculosis | Used to evaluate cell-mediated immune function | Administered intradermally<br>Size of induration is measured at daily intervals for 3 days |
| Differential WBC count | Part of the CBC<br>Describes the relative amounts of the five types of WBCs (leukocytes) in the blood: neutrophils, eosinophils, basophils, monocytes, and lymphocytes<br>Differential WBC count expressed as number per cubic millimeter ($mm^3$) and as a percent of the total number of WBCs | Helps identify infection, immune status, and allergy |
| Allergy skin tests | On administration of minute amounts of antigen into the skin, tests either immediate or delayed-type hypersensitivity | Because anaphylactic reactions can occur even in the presence of minimal allergen exposures, emergency equipment and medications should be immediately available |
| RAST | Measures the quantity and increase of antigen-specific IgE present in the serum<br>Determines exact quantities of antibodies to pollens, foods, and other allergens | More expensive than traditional allergy skin testing but provides precise information without risk of hypersensitivity reaction |

Data from Pagana, K., & Pagana, T. (2014). *Mosby's manual of diagnostic and laboratory tests* (5th ed.). St. Louis: Mosby.

### Laboratory and Clinical Screening Tests for Allergy

| Test | Findings Suggestive of Allergy |
|---|---|
| CBC, differential | Excess eosinophils (>5% of WBCs) |
| Total eosinophil count | >450 μL eosinophils |
| Nasal smear | Excess eosinophils (>4% in young children, >10% in adolescents) |
| Serum IgE | Elevated for age |
| RAST, antigen-specific IgE | Increase in antigen-specific IgE in the serum |
| Skin testing | Urticarial wheal appears on skin within 20-30 min after administration of selected potential allergens<br>Reaction can be immediate or delayed and can even include anaphylaxis |

*CBC,* Complete blood cell count; *RAST,* radioallergosorbent test; *WBC,* white blood cell.

Immunologic alterations typically are chronic, lasting from months to years and interfering with a child's life. Physical signs range from simple, such as impaired skin integrity, to complex, such as overwhelming infection. Intervals of wellness, relapses, and sometimes a decline in health should be expected. Repeated office visits and hospitalizations, disruptions in family routines, altered social interactions, and emotional and financial strain often are coupled with anxiety about the future.

Initially, the nurse helps the family adjust to a new, often devastating diagnosis. Care during the acute phase of the illness may be critical in nature, as underlying organisms are diagnosed and treated and fevers and pain are controlled. Once the acute crisis has resolved, the nurse prepares the family for discharge by teaching home management and identifying community resources and referrals for continuing support. The nurse also teaches the family how to prevent the spread of microorganisms through infection control practices at home and describes parameters for when to call the health provider. The nurse discusses ways to maintain the child's skin integrity, the body's first line of protection against microorganisms, and recommends a diet that supports immune cell growth. The nurse must keep abreast of current information because the field of immunology continues to evolve. Nurses also play a vital role in advocating for children with conditions such as human immunodeficiency virus (HIV) infection.

Despite all efforts, rehospitalization is often inevitable. The family is an integral part of the multidisciplinary team, keeping the physicians, nurses, and social workers informed of changes in the child's condition, administering medications, providing respiratory care, and often making difficult decisions about continued treatment and comfort.

## HUMAN IMMUNODEFICIENCY VIRUS INFECTION

HIV infection is an acquired cell-mediated immunodeficiency disorder that causes a wide spectrum of manifestations in children, ranging from no signs or symptoms to mild and moderate to severe signs and symptoms. Because of improved medical approaches to this condition, HIV infection is viewed as a chronic condition with ongoing challenges. Acquired immunodeficiency syndrome (AIDS) is the most advanced manifestation of this infection.

### Etiology

HIV, present in an infected individual's blood or body fluids, can enter an uninfected adult's or adolescent's body in several ways, including sharing of needles or syringes, engaging in unprotected sexual activity with an infected person where body fluids are shared, or receiving an infected blood product. Infected women can transmit the virus to a fetus across the placenta during pregnancy, to the infant at delivery, and to the young child through breastfeeding. The incidence of perinatal transmission has decreased markedly since 1994, when it became practice to administer zidovudine (ZDV) to infected mothers prenatally and intrapartally and to the newborn infant (Centers for Disease Control and Prevention [CDC], 2016). Increases in prenatal counseling and testing and a combination antiretroviral regimen during pregnancy, combined with specific obstetric interventions designed to prevent transmission during labor, have reduced the transmission risk to less than 2% (CDC, 2016). Children are still at risk of acquiring HIV infection through sexual abuse.

> **CRITICAL THINKING EXERCISE 42.1**
>
> The standard of care now includes HIV testing of all women, along with other tests done prenatally to identify possible communicable disease. HIV testing is done on an "opt out" basis, meaning that the test will be done unless the pregnant woman chooses not to be tested. What might be the primary goal of this type of testing? What are the major issues that should be considered if a woman decides to decline testing when it is offered?

### Incidence

The incidence of HIV infection in infants and children in the United States is approximately 200 children annually; of these cases, 91% are the result of perinatal transmission (CDC, 2016). In the United States, approximately 10,000 children younger than 19 years of age are living with HIV/AIDS (CDC, 2014), posing challenges for children, families, and health professionals alike.

Heterosexual intimacy and infection through intravenous (IV) drug use are the most common transmission modes of HIV for women and adolescent girls. In the United States, African-American children younger than age 13 years are disproportionately affected, followed by Hispanic children (CDC, 2014).

**PATHOPHYSIOLOGY**

***HIV Infection***

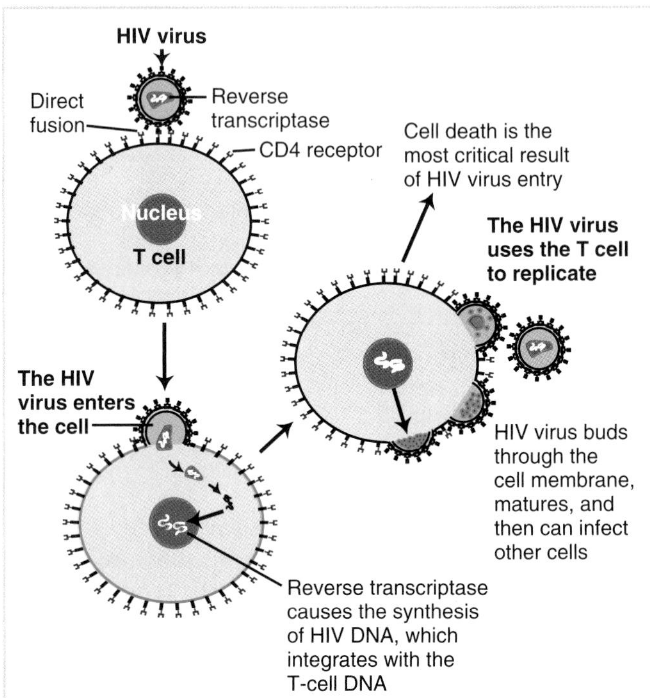


HIV is a retrovirus that contains RNA and the enzyme reverse transcriptase, which plays a key role in viral replication. HIV gains entry into a $CD4^+$ cell by direct fusion of the viral envelope to $CD4^+$ receptors on the cell surface. This fusion allows the viral RNA and other enzymes to enter the $CD4^+$ cell. Within the $CD4^+$ cell, reverse transcriptase conducts the synthesis of HIV DNA. This HIV DNA then integrates into the DNA of the $CD4^+$ cell. The virus then uses the $CD4^+$ cell to make more copies of itself. The new viruses assemble at the host cell surface. As the viruses bud through the cell membrane, they mature, are released, and can infect other $CD4^+$ cells. The most critical result of HIV entry into the $CD4^+$ cell is cell incapacitation and death.* Because $CD4^+$ cells primarily enhance cell-mediated immunity, severely infected infants and children will exhibit symptoms of viral or fungal infection. In addition, $CD4^+$ helper cells interact with the humoral immune response. Immunoglobulins become nonfunctional, making the child extremely vulnerable to bacterial infections.

*Kumar et al. as cited in Porth, C. (2014). *Essentials of pathophysiology* (3rd ed.). Philadelphia: Wolters Kluwer.

### Manifestations

Box 42.1 lists findings associated with general immunodeficiency. Children with HIV manifest most or all of these signs. HIV infection in children and adults differs in several ways (Working Group on Antiretroviral Therapy and Medical Management of HIV-Infected Children, 2014; Yogev & Chadwick, 2016):

- The progression of HIV infection to AIDS is faster in infants and children younger than 5 years of age. One factor contributing to the rapid progression in children is a higher viral load.
- Signs in children may include physical and developmental failure to thrive.

**BOX 42.1 Clinical Findings Associated With Immunodeficiency**

**Frequently Present, Highly Indicative Signs**
- Repeated or persistent respiratory tract infection
- Repeated or persistent otitis media or sinusitis
- Severe bacterial infections
- Opportunistic infections, such as *Pneumocystis jiroveci* (PCP) or cryptosporidiosis
- Poor response to appropriate therapy

**Frequently Present, Somewhat Suggestive Signs**
- Skin lesions
- Failure to thrive or grow
- Chronic diarrhea
- Thrush
- Hepatosplenomegaly
- Anemia, thrombocytopenia, neutropenia
- Small or absent lymph nodes, tonsils, and adenoids

- Children have early opportunistic infections (e.g., chronic oral candidiasis), a greater number of bacterial infections from childhood illnesses, and lymphoid interstitial pneumonitis (LIP), a condition in which the child can be asymptomatic or have parotid gland enlargement, hypoxia, and digital clubbing.
- *Pneumocystis jiroveci* (formerly *carinii*) pneumonia (PCP) in children with perinatally acquired HIV infection can occur early in infancy and is the most commonly reported opportunistic infection in children (Seeborg, Paul, & Shearer, 2014).

The CDC classifies the clinical manifestations of HIV infection as not symptomatic, mildly and moderately symptomatic in children younger than 13 years (Panel on Antiretroviral Therapy and Medical Management of HIV-Infected Children, 2015). Mild signs of the illness can be nonspecific and include lymphadenopathy, hepatomegaly, splenomegaly, dermatitis, parotitis, and recurrent or persistent upper respiratory infection, sinusitis, or otitis media. In moderate disease, some signs are considered to be important if they persist or recur, particularly anemia, neutropenia, or thrombocytopenia; diarrhea; fever for longer than 1 month; herpes simplex; and oral candidiasis in children older than 6 months. Other signs of moderate infection include bacterial meningitis, pneumonia, or sepsis (one episode); cardiomyopathy; complicated chickenpox; herpes zoster; hepatitis; nephropathy; LIP; and toxoplasmosis onset before age 1 month (Panel on Antiretroviral Therapy and Medical Management of HIV-Infected Children, 2015). In addition to LIP, the most common indicators of AIDS in children younger than 13 years are serious confirmed bacterial infections (multiple or recurrent), PCP and other opportunistic infections, encephalopathy, lymphomas, Kaposi sarcoma, and severe nutritional deficits with fall-off on growth percentiles (wasting syndrome) without evidence of another cause (Panel on Antiretroviral Therapy and Medical Management of HIV-Infected Children, 2015).

## Diagnostic Evaluation

Because most HIV infections in infants and children occur as a result of perinatal transmission, HIV-positive pregnant women must be identified, educated, and treated. Early identification and treatment of women reduce the HIV transmission rate, enabling early diagnosis and treatment of infected infants. Recommendations for preventing HIV transmission to neonates now include universal testing of all pregnant women (unless they "opt out") and HIV counseling. Women who are found to be at risk for HIV are tested a second time at 36 weeks' gestation. If a woman does not receive HIV counseling and treatment during pregnancy, providing these as soon as possible after delivery facilitates optimal management of the newborn (Panel on Treatment of HIV-Infected Pregnant Women and Prevention of Perinatal Transmission, 2015).

### Diagnosing HIV-Exposed Infants

Diagnosing HIV through traditional HIV antibody measurement by enzyme-linked immunosorbent assay (ELISA) or Western blot assay is not accurate in infants younger than 18 months because of the presence of maternal antibodies. Instead, virologic assay tests are used. These include HIV deoxyribonucleic acid polymerase chain reaction (DNA PCR) or HIV ribonucleic acid (RNA) assay.

For infants who have been exposed to HIV, virologic testing is performed when the infant is 14 to 21 days old, at 1 to 2 months, and again at 4 to 6 months; healthcare providers should consider performing virologic studies immediately after birth for infants known to be at risk for exposure (Panel on Antiretroviral Therapy and Medical Management of HIV-Infected Children, 2015).

Two positive virologic assays obtained on two separate occasions establish a positive diagnosis. Two negative virologic assays from separate specimens taken at 1 month of age and older and again at 4 months of age and older in nonbreastfed infants can establish negative HIV status; some specialists will follow up with an antibody test between 12 and 18 months of age to confirm (Panel on Antiretroviral Therapy and Medical Management of HIV-Infected Children, 2015). Two negative HIV antibody tests from separate specimens can rule out HIV infection in a child older than 6 months. HIV antibody measurement can be used if the child is older than 18 months. For all these tests, infants must not show any clinical signs of HIV infection (Panel on Antiretroviral Therapy and Medical Management of HIV-Infected Children, 2015).

### Ongoing Diagnostic Monitoring

$CD4^+$ lymphocyte counts and HIV RNA assays assess an infected young child's immune status, response to therapy, risk for disease progression, and need for PCP prophylaxis after 1 year of age. Low $CD4^+$ counts or a decreased percentage indicate reduced immune function. $CD4^+$ counts are measured at diagnosis and every 3 to 4 months thereafter, except in adolescents who have stable immune function; counts in stable and medication-adherent adolescents can be done less frequently. Monitoring may occur more often for infants younger than 12 months old, when a deterioration in physical condition is suspected, and when making decisions to treat or change treatment (Panel on Antiretroviral Therapy and Medical Management of HIV-Infected Children, 2015). Although the $CD4^+$ lymphocyte counts vary by age in children younger than 5 years old, the $CD4^+$ cell percentage does not; thus, the percentage is considered to be a more accurate assessment for childhood disease progression in children of this age-group (Panel on Antiretroviral Therapy and Medical Management of HIV-Infected Children, 2015).

The amount of virus in peripheral blood is called the *viral burden*. The HIV viral burden is measured by plasma HIV RNA copy number and is determined by use of a quantitative HIV RNA assay. The HIV RNA copy numbers work in tandem with the $CD4^+$ percentage to provide independent information about prognosis and guide treatment decisions. HIV RNA copy number is assessed immediately after positive virologic diagnosis of HIV and every 3 to 4 months subsequently, or more often, depending on the child's clinical and treatment status (Panel on Antiretroviral Therapy and Medical Management of HIV-Infected Children, 2015). Infants who are infected perinatally initially have a high viral burden; this burden decreases gradually over several years. A high viral burden (>100,000 copies/mL) in infants younger than 12 months of age may be related to more rapid disease progression (Panel on Antiretroviral Therapy and Medical Management of HIV-Infected Children, 2015).

## Therapeutic Management

The goals of management are directed toward rapidly decreasing the viral load to below detectable levels with the lowest risk of drug toxicity, preserving immune function, facilitating normal growth and development, and preventing medication resistance (Panel on Antiretroviral Therapy and Medical Management of HIV-Infected Children, 2015). Viral suppression that is ineffective can result in medication resistance; a dosage schedule that is the least complex to manage while providing maximum benefit with fewest toxic effects results in improved adherence to a medication regimen.

If a mother's HIV status is unknown when she begins labor, she should be tested for the HIV antibody, and her infant should be treated as if HIV exposure was confirmed. If maternal antibody test results are negative, treatment for the infant can be discontinued (Panel on Treatment of HIV-Infected Pregnant Women and Prevention of Perinatal Transmission, 2015).

### HIV-Exposed Infants

In addition to giving IV ZDV to the mother during labor, all infants of known HIV-positive mothers should receive oral ZDV therapy within 6 to 12 hours after birth. This should continue for 6 weeks or until the infant is positively diagnosed with HIV, at which time the regimen is changed to a combination of medications (Panel on Antiretroviral Therapy and Medical Management of HIV-Infected Children, 2015; Panel on Treatment of HIV-Infected Pregnant Women and Prevention of Perinatal Transmission, 2015).

In general, to decrease the risk of transmission to an infant during labor, HIV-positive women who have a high viral load (HIV RNA copies exceeding 1000 copies/mL) near delivery should be considered for cesarean section at 38 weeks (Panel on Treatment of HIV-Infected Pregnant Women and Prevention of Perinatal Transmission, 2015). Discussion about treatment options and recommendations should not be threatening. The mother makes the final decision about the use of antiretroviral medications. Women who decide not to accept treatment with ZDV or other drugs should not face punitive action or denial of care (Panel on Treatment of HIV-Infected Pregnant Women and Prevention of Perinatal Transmission, 2015).

Because HIV-exposed infants, whether infected or uninfected, are more prone to acquiring opportunistic infections from an HIV-infected mother, prophylaxis of opportunistic infections is an important focus (Siberry et al., 2013). HIV-exposed infants are at particular risk from PCP, certain strains of tuberculosis, bacterial and viral infections, and fungal infections, such as *Candida*. The CDC (Siberry et al., 2013) strongly recommends testing HIV-exposed infants for tuberculosis (TB) at 3 months of age, or if exposed to contagious TB. If positive, anti-TB medications are initiated. The CDC also recommends that varicella-zoster immune globulin be given to unimmunized infants within 96 hours of exposure to varicella or zoster infection.

Perhaps the most serious infection acquired by HIV-exposed infants is PCP. The CDC (Siberry et al., 2013) strongly recommends that all HIV-exposed infants receive PCP prophylaxis with trimethoprim-sulfamethoxazole beginning at 4 to 6 weeks of age until the infant reaches 1 year. HIV-exposed infants for whom HIV infection has been ruled out may have PCP prophylaxis discontinued once HIV-negative status has been confirmed. After 1 year of age, infected children receive PCP prophylaxis according to $CD4^+$ percentage or count, and prophylaxis can be discontinued with close monitoring if the child has been determined to have an acceptable percentage or count for 3 consecutive months (Siberry et al., 2013).

### HIV-Infected Infants and Children

The Panel on Antiretroviral Therapy and Medical Management of HIV-Infected Children, available from http://www.aidsinfo.nih.gov, updates treatment recommendations regularly.

***Treatment considerations.*** Treatment is directed toward suppressing viral load with medications or combinations of medications that are in an acceptable and palatable form for children, have the greatest effect while minimizing toxicity, have an administration routine that maximizes the child's and family's quality of life, and reduce the risk for medication resistance. Other goals of management for infants and children infected with HIV include facilitating optimal growth and development, providing ongoing support for the child and family, and referring the child for clinical trials as they become available (Panel on Antiretroviral Therapy and Medical Management of HIV-Infected Children, 2015). Infants and children who are HIV infected should be cared for by a multidisciplinary team of providers (physicians, nurses, social workers, pharmacists, dentists, nutritionists, psychologists, and outreach workers) led by specialists in pediatric HIV management (Panel on Antiretroviral Therapy and Medical Management of HIV-Infected Children, 2015).

More potent and improved antiretroviral medications have benefited HIV-infected children who have immunologic or clinical symptoms of HIV infection. These benefits include enhanced survival, improvements in growth and development, and reduced opportunistic infections and other complications related to HIV infection. Highly active antiretroviral therapy (HAART) has dramatically affected HIV-infected children's health, although its rigorous treatment schedules are challenging for children and families to maintain. There are also associated short- and long-term toxicities that can affect children (Panel on Antiretroviral Therapy and Medical Management of HIV-Infected Children, 2015).

Considerations of drug resistance and adherence are of primary importance. Before a medication routine is initiated, all infants and children with HIV should be tested for antiretroviral drug resistance. The rationale for this is that infants can acquire a drug-resistant strain of HIV from their HIV-infected mother or can develop drug resistance while receiving prophylaxis in anticipation of a diagnosis (Panel on Antiretroviral Therapy and Medical Management of HIV-Infected Children, 2015). Drug resistance testing should also be done when consideration is being given to changing a medication regimen. Resistance testing can help the specialist to choose the most appropriate antiretroviral drugs for an individual child (Panel on Antiretroviral Therapy and Medical Management of HIV-Infected Children, 2015).

One of the most important factors to consider when deciding on a treatment approach is the child's and the caregiver's ability to adhere to the prescribed regimen, because failure to follow the regimen can result in the development of drug resistance and subsequent treatment failure. Adherence issues need to be addressed before a decision to start therapy is made, and adherence needs to be assessed and discussed at each visit (Panel on Antiretroviral Therapy and Medical Management of HIV-Infected Children, 2015). The Panel on Antiretroviral Therapy and Medical Management of HIV-Infected Children (2015) describes multimethod strategies for improving adherence, which include choosing a medication regimen that fits as much as possible into the child's and family's lifestyle, using adherence aids (e.g., pillboxes, alarm watches, stickers), and providing ongoing teaching, support, and encouragement. A multidisciplinary team including physicians, nurses, pharmacists, and sometimes peers is the most helpful to families. Strategies focus on both the child and the caregiver and must address any social issue that is affecting the family's adherence to the prescribed regimen.

The Panel strongly recommends that the provider verify adherence by at least one means other than viral load monitoring at each visit. Verification strategies include having the parent or child make available a medication log (self-report), doing pill counts or checking the refill history with a pharmacist, or using a modified form of directly observed treatment (m-DOT) (Panel on Antiretroviral Therapy and Medical Management of HIV-Infected Children, 2015). Adherence during adolescence can be even more challenging, so re-evaluation of regimens may be necessary at that time.

***Treatment initiation.*** Currently, approximately 27 antiretroviral agents have been approved for treating children with HIV infection (Panel on Antiretroviral Therapy and Medical Management of HIV-Infected Children, 2015). Drug classes include nucleoside analog reverse transcriptase inhibitors (NRTIs, NtRTIs), nonnucleoside reverse transcriptase inhibitors (NNRTIs), protease inhibitors (PIs), entry and fusion inhibitors, pharmacokinetic enhancers, and integrase inhibitors. The preferred drug combination for initial treatment of infants and children with HIV infection includes the following (Panel on Antiretroviral Therapy and Medical Management of HIV-Infected Children, 2015):

- *For neonates 42 weeks gestation and 14 days to younger than 3 years of age:* two NRTIs plus lopinavir/ritonavir. *For children 3 years of age or older:* two NRTIs plus lopinavir/ritonavir or two NRTIs plus efavirenz (not for adolescent girls).
- *For children 6 years of age or older:* two NRTIs plus efavirenz (not for adolescent girls) or two NRTIs plus lopinavir/ritonavir, or two NRTIs plus atazanavir and low-dose ritonavir.
- Two NRTIs plus an NNRTI (nevirapine, but only if not used for primary prophylaxis) can be used at any age as an alternative.

Doses for infants and children are individualized according to age and growth considerations. Doses for adolescents are determined by multiple factors, including the adolescent's size, weight, age in relation to adult dosing, risk of pregnancy, use of contraceptives, and Tanner stage (see Chapter 9).

For perinatally infected infants, ZDV is discontinued as soon as HIV status has been confirmed, and combination therapy is started. In the past, treatment of asymptomatic HIV-infected infants with normal immunologic status was controversial; current recommendations call for aggressive treatment for all infants younger than 1 year of age irrespective of clinical or virologic status (Panel on Antiretroviral Therapy and Medical Management of HIV-Infected Children, 2015). Because the disease progresses more rapidly in children than in adults and the laboratory studies are less precise in predicting disease progression for children, they are treated aggressively. Table 42.1 presents current recommendations for initiating antiretroviral therapy in infants and children infected with HIV. Treatment is based on a combination of symptoms, $CD4^+$ percentage, and viral load as determined by HIV RNA copy number.

### Additional Issues Related to the Child With HIV Infection

***Multigenerational problems.*** One of the unique aspects of perinatal HIV infection is the multigenerational nature of the disease, in which both the mother and child may be infected. The transition to motherhood is challenging under normal circumstances and may be exacerbated when the mother has HIV.

When considering the special needs of the mother-infant dyad, the nurse should be aware of the mother's concerns both during pregnancy and after delivery to provide optimal nursing care.

Another important but difficult area to be addressed is planning for the future. Planning can include exploring the efficacy of standby guardianship, kinship care, or foster and adoptive placement. In addition, for children with advanced HIV disease, families have to make difficult decisions about an infected child's continuing care. Should aggressive treatment continue, or should the goal of treatment be to make the child comfortable? These decisions are best made in consultation with a multidisciplinary team that can identify areas of concern

**TABLE 42.1 Recommendations for Routine Immunization of Human Immunodeficiency Virus-Infected Children in the United States**

| Age Group | Criteria for Initiation | Treatment Recommendations |
|---|---|---|
| <12 mo | Regardless of clinical symptoms, immune status, or viral load | Treat |
| 1 yr to <5 yr | AIDS or significant HIV symptoms* | Treat |
| | Meet age-related $CD4^+$ threshold for initiating treatment, irrespective of symptoms or plasma HIV RNA level† | Treat |
| | Asymptomatic or mild symptoms‡ and $CD4^+$ ≥25% and plasma HIV RNA ≥100,000 copies/mL | Treat |
| | Asymptomatic or mild symptoms‡ and $CD4^+$ ≥25% and plasma HIV RNA <100,000 copies/mL | Consider§ |
| ≥5 yr | AIDS or significant HIV symptoms* | Treat |
| | $CD4^+$ count ≤500 cells/mm$^3$ | Treat |
| | Asymptomatic or mild symptoms‡ and $CD4^+$ count >500 cells/mm$^3$ and plasma HIV RNA ≥100,000 copies/mL | Treat |
| | Asymptomatic or mild symptoms‡ and $CD4^+$ count >500 cells/mm$^3$ and plasma HIV RNA <100,000 copies/mL | Consider§ |

Conditions for initiating treatment for children who have been deferred include the following:

- Increasing HIV RNA levels (e.g., HIV RNA levels approaching 100,000 copies/mL);
- Rapidly declining CD4 count or percentage to values approaching the age-related threshold for consideration of therapy;
- Development of clinical symptoms; and
- The ability of caregiver and child to adhere to the prescribed regimen.

*CDC Clinical Category C and most B conditions (except for single episode of serious bacterial infection), irrespective of $CD4^+$ percentage or count or plasma HIV RNA level.

†Age-related $CD4^+$ percentage for treatment initiation in children 1 to <5 years, <25%; $CD4^+$ count for children ≥5 years, <500 cells/mm$^3$.

‡CDC Clinical Category A or N or the following Category B condition: single episode of serious bacterial infection.

§Clinical and laboratory data should be reevaluated every 3 to 4 months.

From Panel on Antiretroviral Therapy and Medical Management of HIV-Infected Children. (2015, MARCH 5). *Guidelines for the use of antiretroviral agents in pediatric HIV infection.* Retrieved from http://www.aidsinfo.nih.gov.

and develop strategic approaches that incorporate family culture, beliefs, available physical and emotional resources, and knowledge.

***Disclosure.*** Initial reactions to an HIV diagnosis can include confusion, anger, denial, and despair. Informing a child about a shared HIV status may be intimidating in light of the parent's and child's physical, emotional, and social experiences. Unlike disclosure about other chronic illnesses children and adolescents may experience, disclosure of HIV status brings fear of social stigma (Andrinopoulos et al., 2011). Now that children with HIV are surviving into adolescence, the issue of disclosure becomes a vital part of their healthcare management, particularly considering the prevalence of adolescents who engage in sexual activities. The American Academy of Pediatrics (AAP) Committee on Pediatric AIDS has issued a policy statement regarding disclosure of illness status to HIV-infected children and adolescents (AAP, 1999/2005). Based on research that suggests a more positive emotional status in both children and parents who have disclosed, the AAP recommends that disclosure be considered in light of the child's cognitive and psychosocial development and clinical status, as well as the multitude of factors affecting the parent's decision to disclose. Although healthcare professionals respect the wishes of parents regarding disclosure, it is important to create a continuing supportive environment in which disclosure issues can be discussed and adequate preparation for eventual disclosure can occur (AAP, 1999/2005). The AAP recommendations for disclosure strongly emphasize encouraging disclosure to school-age children and state the ethical responsibility of pediatricians to fully disclose HIV status to affected adolescents (AAP, 1999/2005). Parents and other guardians of an HIV-infected child should be counseled by a knowledgeable healthcare professional about disclosure to the child. Repetition of such counseling may be necessary throughout the course of the child's illness.

## NURSING CARE PLAN

### *The Child With HIV Infection in the Community*

#### Focused Assessment

- Regardless of setting (home, school, daycare), assess development and well care, particularly immunization status (Table 42.2).
- Assess adherence to the anti-HIV medication regimen.
- Obtain a history of recent exposure to any communicable disease and whether the child is adhering to medication prophylaxis against opportunistic infections.
- At each well or ill visit, ask the caregivers about any fever, nausea, vomiting, diarrhea, ear pulling, or changes in appetite, sleep pattern, or behavior that might suggest a secondary infection.
- Assess the family's understanding about the HIV-related spectrum of illness, including immunologic status and treatment options.
- Inquire how the family is coping financially and emotionally, and whether referral may be needed for additional support.
- At hospital admission, focus the assessment on the following:
    - *Hydration status:* Intake, output, skin turgor
    - *Respiratory status:* Signs of respiratory distress, adventitious or diminished breath sounds, oxygen saturation
    - *Mucous membranes:* White patches on tongue or inside cheeks, blisters on the lips, or lesions on the tonsils or soft palate
    - *Skin:* Lesions (especially in diaper area; blotchy, red, flat areas, blistering, dryness, rashes or vesicles)
    - Pain by self-report using an developmentally-appropriate pain scale

#### Nursing Diagnosis

Deficient Knowledge about the natural history of pediatric HIV infection, potential complications associated with HIV infection, and current treatment modalities related to emotional reaction to the diagnosis.

#### Planning

***Expected Outcome***

The family will demonstrate knowledge acquisition, as evidenced by explaining what has been taught about HIV infection and playing an active role in determining the plan of care for the child.

#### Interventions and *Rationales*

1. Determine the family's knowledge about HIV infection, treatment modalities, and home care (see Patient-Centered Teaching: How to Care for the Child with an HIV Infection).
   *Teaching needs to begin at the family's level of understanding. It is important to note that because the majority of HIV-infected children are infected perinatally, the nurse may also be educating parents about their own disease process.*
2. Teach the family about HIV infection, its signs and symptoms, progression, and treatment.
   *Knowledge and understanding of HIV may increase cooperation and adherence to the often-complicated treatment regimens that are necessary to achieve viral suppression and will also serve to reduce anxiety.*
3. Identify the family's areas of concern (e.g., a new diagnosis, fear of transmission by casual contact within the family).
   *Addressing family concerns decreases misinterpretation. First, educate about the lack of transmission by household contact and correct any myths or misperceptions that may exist.*
4. Use teaching strategies that will maximize the potential for success (e.g., medication sheet that details medication name, dosage, how often to give, why the child is on the medication, and hints for administering unpalatable tasting medication).
   *Written information may assist the family to ensure that the correct medication regimen is being followed.*
5. Educate the family about the signs or problems that necessitate calling the healthcare provider for management advice.
   *Early identification of potential problems may prevent serious complications from developing.*

#### Evaluation

Can the family describe the natural history of HIV, systems affected by HIV, current treatment modalities, and care for the child at home?

Can the family administer the correct doses of medications at the appropriate times?

Does the family readily participate in developing and carrying out a plan of care for the child?

Does the family contact healthcare providers when the child is ill and in need of services?

#### Nursing Diagnosis

Anxiety (primary caregiver) related to fear of disclosure.

#### Planning

***Expected Outcomes***

The family will:

1. Share the diagnosis with those family members, healthcare professionals, and school staff who need to know.

## NURSING CARE PLAN—cont'd

### The Child With HIV Infection in the Community

2. Move through the stages of disclosure and feel comfortable sharing their feelings about the diagnosis with appropriate people.
3. Answer the child's questions honestly and share the diagnosis when the time is right.

**Interventions and *Rationales***

1. Listen quietly when the family talks about the diagnosis of HIV. Note their stage of disclosure (secrecy, exploratory, readiness, or full disclosure).
   *Sharing the diagnosis occurs on a continuum, with secrecy at one end and full disclosure at the other. Families initially may want to keep their feelings about the diagnosis private. However, a time may come when they wish to talk; the nurse should develop rapport and gain trust.*
2. Maintain confidentiality concerning the HIV diagnosis. Ask the primary caregiver what individuals know about the diagnosis and what specific information they have. Encourage the family to share the diagnosis with healthcare professionals.
   *Healthcare professionals who plan and coordinate care need to know the diagnosis to facilitate an optimal treatment plan.*
3. Help family members decide who needs to know the child's diagnosis and offer them education and support in the process of disclosure. Encourage peer support groups when the family is ready.
   *Do not assume that all family or friends accompanying the child to the clinic or hospital know the child's or parent's diagnosis. Although many people would like to know the diagnosis, only a few need to know. Ask families to consider the following when choosing whom to tell: the child's age, clinical condition, and healthcare requirements; the likelihood that bloody injuries will occur; and the use of Standard Precautions.*
4. Encourage the family to be honest with the child and to explain the reason for physician visits and procedures.
   *When to tell the child the diagnosis is a personal choice, but families need to understand that children will worry more if no one talks with them or if they sense dishonesty; ethical considerations make it important that adolescents be aware of their diagnosis.**
5. Encourage the family to listen to the questions the child is asking and to answer the questions briefly, using words the child can understand. Look for readiness cues indicating that the child wants to know more.
   *It is important for families to understand what their children are asking and to answer their questions, keeping responses short and simple.*
6. Encourage the family to speak with a healthcare professional when the child asks questions that are difficult to answer. Suggest that the parent seek counseling to help find the appropriate language for answering the child.
   *Role playing is a useful technique that allows families to practice potential responses to difficult questions. The nurse can offer to accompany them if they decide to share the diagnosis.*
7. Promote normal routines at home.
   *Children with HIV infection can go to school, church, and parties; play sports, and games; and develop or maintain friendships.*

**Evaluation**

Is the family able to share the diagnosis with all appropriate healthcare professionals and at least one significant person?

Does the family appear to be moving through the stages of disclosure and seeking out support from peers?

Is the family able to seek social and health services for which they qualify on the basis of their HIV/AIDS status?

Can family members answer the child's questions in a developmentally appropriate way?

**Nursing Diagnosis**

Ineffective Therapeutic Regimen Management: Nonadherence related to lack of support systems or denial of the illness.

**Planning**

***Expected Outcomes***

1. The mother who is infected with HIV will keep her own healthcare appointments and those of her child.
2. The family will work toward accepting the diagnosis.
3. The family will view themselves as valued members of the healthcare team.
4. The child/family will adhere to the medication regimen.

**Interventions and *Rationales***

1. Use language that shows respect. Offer information in a language that can be understood by the child and family. Use a translator as needed.
   *Families affected by HIV do not want their children called innocent victims or AIDS babies, nor do they want to be judged as promiscuous or substance abusers. Labels can create barriers, which can result in nonadherence with healthcare recommendations.*
2. Encourage the HIV-infected mother to keep her own healthcare appointments.
   *HIV-infected women often neglect their own healthcare needs as they attend to those of their children.*
3. Accept the parents' use of denial during periods of emotional respite. Refer for counseling to assist with the grieving process.
   *The diagnosis of HIV brings a series of losses, including the loss of the future and all that the future holds for a child. Denial is a coping mechanism.*
4. Maintain realistic hope when possible.
   *With new prophylaxis agents for HIV-positive pregnant women and their infants, HIV infection develops in fewer than 2% of all perinatally HIV exposed babies, and antiretroviral treatments have been successful in preserving immune function in infected infants.*
5. Refer the family to social services for assistance with finances, transportation, food, housing, clothing, medical care, and respite care as needed.
   *Many families simply lack the basic resources for adherence to a treatment regimen. Problems that affect the caregiver's ability to manage the therapeutic plan include inadequate or inconsistent housing or transportation and personal HIV disease. In some instances, substance use or abuse or mental illness can affect adherence. Guilt about passing HIV on to a child can interfere with providing the structure and discipline necessary for establishing a successful regular medication regimen.*
6. Teach the family how to give antiretroviral agents at home, keep a log, and adjust the schedule to accommodate school schedules, if necessary.
   *Give suggestions about helpful devices, such as daily or weekly pill boxes that can be prefilled, alarm watches, and pictorial medication reminders.†*
   *The antiretroviral regimen may include a combination of medications in addition to other medications a child may be taking. A daily log or other medication reminder device helps families keep track.*
7. Monitor medication adherence every visit.
   *A multifaceted approach works best in adherence issues. Palatability of the medication, ability to meld the medication schedule with existing routines, denial, guilt, and embarrassment about the diagnosis are all barriers to appropriate cooperation with the medication regimen.*

*Continued*

## NURSING CARE PLAN—cont'd

### *The Child With HIV Infection in the Community*

8. Suggest ways to make medications more palatable to children:
   - Encourage early pill taking.
   - Mix medication with chocolate syrup or follow with chocolate candy.
   - Give ice or ice pop before giving the medication.
   - Use an oral syringe to place the medication back in the mouth away from taste buds.
   - Avoid mixing medications in food or drink, fighting with the child, and skipping medication doses.

   *Making the medication and medication routine palatable to children and families enhances adherence.*
9. Liquid formulations of HIV medications may be foul tasting or have a gritty texture.

   *Unlike short-course medications, these medications must become part of the family's everyday routine for years.*

**Evaluation**

Is the mother able to take care of herself?

Has the patient or caregiver been able to move from denial to anger to acceptance of the diagnosis?

Are the primary caregivers active, participatory, and valued members of the healthcare team?

Do the child and family adhere to the medication regimen?

*Butler, A., Williams, P., Howland, L., et al.; Pediatric AIDS Clinical Trials Group 219C Study Team. (2009). Impact of disclosure of HIV infection on health-related quality of life among children and adolescents with HIV infection. Pediatrics, 123, 935-943.

†Panel on Antiretroviral Therapy and Medical Management of HIV-Infected Children. (2011, August 11). *Guidelines for the use of antiretroviral agents in pediatric HIV infection.* Retrieved from http://www.aidsinfo.nih.gov.

**TABLE 42.2 Recommendations for Routine Immunization of Human Immunodeficiency Virus-Infected Children in the United States**

| Vaccines | HIV Infection | Comments |
|---|---|---|
| Hepatitis B | Yes | Post-vaccination testing 1 to 2 mo after last dose; revaccinate (three doses) if anti-HBs level is <10 mIU/mL |
| Hepatitis A | Yes | Beginning at 12 months; two doses should be separated by at least 6 mo |
| DTaP | Yes | Tdap should be given to adolescents as a booster dose at 11 to 12 yr (5 yr after the primary series) |
| IPV | Yes | |
| MMR | Yes | Can be given to children who are not severely immune depressed ($CD4^+$ <15% or <200 cells/μL); administer close to the first birthday and 1 mo later |
| Hib | Yes | |
| Rotavirus | Consider risk/benefit | No safety or efficacy data available |
| Pneumococcal | Yes | Pneumococcal polysaccharide vaccine (PPSV) should be given to children 2 yr or older, ≥2 months after last PCV dose; older children and adolescents may receive one dose of PPSV if not previously immunized and one booster dose of PPSV if they had the PPSV series previously |
| Influenza | Yes | Use trivalent inactivated vaccine (TIV) only; immunize eligible close contacts |
| Varicella | Consider risk/benefit | Can be given to children with $CD4^+$ percentages ≥15% or count ≥200 cells/μL; give first dose near the first birthday and second one 3 mo later; do not give to immunosuppressed children ($CD4^+$ percentage <15% or count <200 cells/μL) |
| Meningococcal (MCV) | Yes | Two-dose series (3 months apart) of MCV4 for children 9 mo to 23 mo if at risk for meningitis; additional booster after 3 years and every 5 years thereafter if child remains at risk. For at-risk children 2 years and older, give 2 doses 2 months apart followed by boosters after 3 years and every 5 years if child remains at risk. At-risk children older than 7 years who have had the primary series should have a booster every 5 years while at risk. All children who have not received the vaccine should receive it at age 11 to 12 yr with a booster at age 16 yr |
| Human papillomavirus vaccine (HPV) | Yes | HIV-infected females older than age 9 yr, three-dose schedule; HPV4 series for males at 11 to 12 yr |

NOTE: Always check the most current immunization schedule.

*DTaP,* Diphtheria-tetanus-acellular pertussis; *Hib, Haemophilus influenzae* type B; *IPV,* inactivated poliovirus vaccine; *MMR,* measles, mumps, and rubella; *PCV,* pneumococcal conjugate vaccine; *Tdap,* tetanus-diphtheria-pertussis.

Data from Siberry, G.K., Abzug, M.J., Nachman, S., et al. The panel on opportunistic infections in HIV-exposed and HIV-infected children. (2013). Guidelines for the prevention and treatment of opportunistic infections in HIV-exposed and HIV-infected children. *The Pediatric Infectious Disease Journal, 32*(02); Advisory Committee on Immunization Practices Vaccines for Children Program. (2011, June). *Vaccines to prevent meningococcal disease* (Resolution No. 6/11-1; pp. 1-3). Retrieved from http://www.cdc.gov; Centers for Disease Control and Prevention. (2012). *Recommended immunization schedule for persons aged 7 through 18 years–United States 2012.* Retrieved from http://www.cdc.gov.

## PATIENT-CENTERED TEACHING

### *How to Care for the Child With an HIV Infection*

Review the following information and health practices at the time of initial testing and subsequent visits.

**Transmission**

HIV can be spread by the following:

- Unprotected sexual activity
- Sharing of needles
- An infected mother to her baby
- Breastfeeding
- Open wounds (if there is blood-to-blood contact)

HIV cannot be spread by the following:

- Sharing knives, forks, spoons, or cups
- Using the same toilet seats, bathtubs, or showers
- Coughing or sneezing
- Hugging, holding, or touching people

**Prevention**

The best way to prevent the spread of HIV is to do the following:

- Abstain from sex and from sharing needles, or
- Use latex condoms with nonoxynol 9, and
- Avoid reusing needles or wash needles in a 1 : 10 bleach solution

The best way to prevent pregnancies is to do the following:

- Abstain from sex, or
- Use a latex condom
- Use contraception

If infected with HIV, follow these precautions:

- Do not breastfeed
- Do not donate blood, sperm, or organs

**Testing**

- The most common HIV tests used for older children and adults are the enzyme-linked immunosorbent assay (ELISA) and the Western blot assay, which measure levels of antibodies to the virus.
- The most common HIV tests used for infants and children younger than 18 months are the HIV DNA polymerase chain reaction (PCR) and HIV RNA quantitative assays, which detect the presence of the virus itself.
- $CD4^+$ counts or percentage indicate how well the immune system is working.

**Illness (AIDS)**

Children with HIV infection might initially be asymptomatic. Mild and moderate symptoms include the following:

- Persistent upper respiratory and ear infections
- Thrush
- Skin conditions
- Vomiting and diarrhea
- Enlarged liver, spleen, lymph nodes, and parotid glands
- Growth and development problems
- Lymphoid interstitial pneumonitis (LIP): a rare lung disease

Some severe symptoms of the illness include the following:

- Opportunistic infections such as *Pneumocystis jiroveci* pneumonia (PCP) and cytomegalovirus (CMV)
- Recurrent bacterial infections such as sepsis, meningitis, and pneumonia
- Severe developmental delay or neurologic symptoms
- Wasting syndrome/failure to thrive

**Medications**

- Resistance testing
- Adherence to schedule (keep a written record of missed doses)
- Proper administration
- Safe and proper storage
- Side effects

**Home Care**

Offer a high-calorie, high-protein diet if growth is a problem:

- Mix formula as directed.
- Do not add extra water or cereal to formula.
- Give supplemental vitamins and minerals as ordered.

Practice basic infection control measures and follow Standard Precautions, including the following practices:

- Avoid touching blood.
- Do not share toothbrushes, pierced earrings, razors, or nail clippers.
- Use a barrier when caring for a cut or a bloody nose.
- Cover open sores.
- Leave scabs alone.
- Wipe up blood spills with a paper towel, wash the area with soap and water, rinse with bleach and water, and air dry.
- Wrap disposable materials soiled with blood in newspaper, tie off in a plastic bag, and throw away in a plastic-lined trash can.
- Wash hands with soap and water if you touch blood.
- Rinse blood-soiled clothing with hydrogen peroxide or cold water and then wash as usual.
- Allow blood to air dry on dry-clean-only clothing.

Keep your child's immunizations up to date. Your child should also receive the following:

- Pneumococcal vaccine at 2 years of age, if not given during infancy
- Flu shot each fall
- Immune globulin after measles exposure
- Varicella-zoster immune globulin after chickenpox exposure
- Tetanus immune globulin for tetanus-prone wounds

Call the physician if any of the following symptoms occur:

- Fever higher than 38.3° C (101° F)
- Vomiting and diarrhea
- Decreased appetite, difficulty swallowing, drooling
- Rashes, bumps, lumps, or sores on the skin
- Coughing or chest congestion
- Ear pain, pulling on the ears, or drainage from the ears
- Wounds that will not heal
- Exposure to measles or chickenpox

Give prophylaxis against PCP and antiretroviral drugs as ordered.

***HIV and school settings.*** As the population of children living with HIV/AIDS gets older, there are more HIV-infected children and adolescents in school systems. Parents of these children strive to maintain normal in-school and out-of-school routines as much as possible. Children who have HIV are protected by the federal Individuals with Disabilities Education Act and may not be discriminated against in the school. The National Association of State Boards of Education (NASBE) in 2001 produced an excellent guide to education policy and HIV infection that asserts that HIV is not a significant risk to others in the school setting when school personnel follow appropriate guidelines, and affirms the right of children and adults with HIV to fully participate in both the education and extracurricular programs at school.

## NURSING CARE PLAN

### *The Adolescent With HIV Infection*

**Focused Assessment**

- Assess the adolescent's knowledge of the disease and disease process.
- For the adolescent who was infected perinatally, assess growth and development.
- Inquire about the adolescent's risk-taking behaviors, especially those that could potentially transmit the virus to others.
- Pay particular attention to the adolescent's adherence to any antiretroviral therapy; use confirmatory methods for assuring adherence in addition to self-report.
- Assess the adolescent's understanding of the importance of regular medical follow-up.
- Obtain information about any specific concerns.

**Nursing Diagnosis**

Deficient Knowledge about the effect of HIV on adolescents, current treatment options available, and preventing transmission of virus to others.

**Planning**

***Expected Outcomes***

1. The adolescent and family will explain in their own words what has been taught about HIV infection, including potential treatment regimens, goals of preserving or restoring immune function, and issues related to adolescent risk taking and adolescent sexuality.
2. The adolescent and family will adhere to a mutually agreed-upon treatment regimen.

**Interventions and *Rationales***

1. Document the adolescent's and family's knowledge of HIV infection and associated concerns and emphasize the necessity for regular well care, developmental monitoring, nutritional support, medication adherence, and immunizations.
   *Teaching should be geared toward the adolescent's cognitive and emotional readiness to learn about HIV, its treatment, and prevention of complications.*
2. Identify the adolescent's specific concerns and address them first.
   *Acknowledging the adolescent's concerns can help allay fears and anxiety and help begin to develop a trusting relationship.*
3. Educate the adolescent about potential symptoms and problems to report to the healthcare provider.
   *Early identification of problems may prevent development of serious complications.*
4. Establish readiness to adhere to medication regimen. Include the adolescent in decision making about a treatment routine that will maximize adherence (e.g., compatibility with daily routine, minimum number of required pills and capsules, fewest side effects).
   *Adherence to medication regimens is critical to prevent development of viral resistance. Doses for adolescents are determined using either the Tanner stage of puberty (see Chapter 9), weight, or adult dose. Because of normal developmental issues of adolescence, the adolescent may deliberately not take medication or forget to do so because of lifestyle issues.*
5. Discuss high-risk behaviors that could result in transmission of HIV to others (e.g., sexual activity, intravenous [IV] drug use) and methods of prevention of transmission.
   *Frank discussions can empower the adolescent to assume responsibility for reducing the risk for transmission to others by encouraging safer behaviors in sexual practices and drug use.*
6. Offer participation in peer support groups.
   *The adolescent might benefit from sharing thoughts and feelings about living with HIV, difficulties in taking medications, and other issues, with others.*
7. Encourage school attendance and promote normal routines at home.
   *Promoting normalcy whenever possible assists in meeting developmental needs, as well as preventing social isolation.*
8. Refer the adolescent and family to an appropriate transition team that will manage transition into adult HIV care.
   *HIV infection has become a chronic condition, and many HIV-infected adolescents will need a period of time to transition from pediatric to adult care. Transition issues are similar to those of any adolescent with a chronic condition who must be on a lifelong medication regimen.*

**Evaluation**

Can the adolescent and family explain what HIV is and its treatment goals?

Can the adolescent describe appropriate measures to reduce disease transmission to others?

Does the adolescent state adherence with the prescribed therapeutic regimen?

This document is in current use. Most states have written policies based on this document, and these state-specific policies can be accessed through the NASBE. Privacy provisions are clearly stated and maintain that no one is required to disclose HIV status, nor will HIV antibody testing be required for any reason (NASBE, 2001). Strict confidentiality and health record keeping and storage procedures will be followed for all in the school setting according to the law, and a person's HIV status will not appear in educational records without consent. Schools will operate according to the standards promulgated by the U.S. Occupational Safety and Health Administration for the prevention of bloodborne infections. Because most HIV medications are now given once or twice daily under most circumstances, it is no longer necessary for school nurses to be involved in the administration of a child's medications.

## CORTICOSTEROID THERAPY

Corticosteroids, given as part of a treatment regimen, act as natural products of the adrenal glands, reducing local and systemic inflammatory symptoms.

### Incidence

Topical steroids are applied to the skin or mucous membranes to reduce edema and redness and to counteract itching. They may be used to treat ophthalmic reactions and skin conditions such as eczema. Hydrocortisone cream is one example of a topical steroid. Systemic steroids reduce the inflammatory symptoms of generalized allergic reactions (e.g., asthma, hives, severe contact dermatitis). Systemic steroids are also given increasingly to treat malignant or autoimmune disorders. An example of a systemic steroid is prednisolone (see Drug Guide). Long-term oral corticosteroid therapy is associated with adverse effects, and children should be screened for them periodically (Liu, Covar, Spahn, et al., 2016).

Inhaled corticosteroids produce a very strong local action and can control symptoms in children with asthma and allergic rhinitis. An example of an aerosol steroid is beclomethasone (see Chapter 45). Studies have varied as to whether long-term use of inhaled corticosteroids results in growth delay, with the general consensus being that there may be an initial period of growth delay but little effect on eventual height (National Heart, Lung, and Blood Institute & National

Asthma Education and Prevention Program, 2007; Fuhlbrigge & Kelly, 2014). Inhaled corticosteroids have a possible long-term effect on bone density, although the effect is not as great as with the long-term use of oral steroids (Fuhlbrigge & Kelly, 2014).

## Pathophysiology

Corticosteroids have many different effects but are usually prescribed for their antiinflammatory or immunosuppressive properties. As antiinflammatories, they inhibit chemical mediators and the occurrence of edema, capillary dilation, phagocytic activity, and the migration of leukocytes associated with the inflammatory response. As immunosuppressives, they decrease monocyte and macrophage differentiation and block lymphokine production, leading to T cell inhibition.

### DRUG GUIDE

#### *Prednisolone (Pediapred, Prelone)*

**Classification:** Corticosteroid

**Action:** Decreases inflammation; suppresses the immune response; affects bone marrow and the metabolism of proteins, carbohydrates, and fats.

**Indications:** Given for severe allergic and inflammatory conditions (e.g., asthma, eczema, juvenile arthritis), immunosuppression, and some autoimmune disorders.

**Dosage and Route:** Pediatric, oral: 0.5 to 2 mg/kg daily in divided doses; comes in syrup (15 mg/5 mL) or tablets (1 mg, 5 mg, 25 mg).

**Absorption:** Rapid absorption from the gastrointestinal tract.

**Excretion:** Half eliminated in 2 to 4 hours; metabolized in the liver and excreted in the urine.

**Contraindications:** Do not give if the child has a systemic fungal infection or is sensitive to any of the ingredients.

**Precautions:** Children taking prednisolone are more prone to infection. Avoid exposure to measles or chickenpox while on prednisolone; immunize the child with live-virus vaccines (measles, mumps, rubella; varicella) before beginning corticosteroid treatment. Avoid giving with nonsteroidal antiinflammatory drugs or aspirin because they increase the risk of gastrointestinal bleeding.

**Adverse Reactions:** Gastrointestinal distress, cushingoid state (moon face, buffalo hump), delayed wound healing, skin eruptions, carbohydrate intolerance, fluid retention, growth delay in children. Acute adrenal insufficiency can occur when the child is under stress or if the medication is withdrawn abruptly. Do not discontinue this medication without tapering the dose.

**Nursing Considerations:** Teach the parent to have the child take the medication with food or milk. Store the medication in a cool, dry location. Teach the parent to notify the physician if the child exhibits any of the following: fever, other signs of infection, fatigue, muscle weakness, sudden weight gain, severe gastric irritation, slow wound healing, or growth delay, or if the child is experiencing increased stress.

The side effects of steroids vary widely with the child and the medication. Generally, the higher the dose and the longer the medication is taken, the more serious are the side effects. More knowledge about reactions and a broader selection of steroids and alternatives have significantly reduced untoward reactions in recent years.

## Manifestations

Clinical manifestations of excess topically administered steroids include skin atrophy, delayed wound healing, telangiectasis, or dilation of the cheek blood vessels, striae, and excess absorption leading to any of the clinical manifestations of systemic use.

Some clinical manifestations of excess steroid administered systemically include the following:

- Edema, particularly in the face
- Gastrointestinal irritation, even bleeding
- Bruising and delayed wound healing
- Susceptibility to infections
- Growth limitations
- Hypertension
- Loss of muscle mass
- Increased appetite and weight gain
- Amenorrhea
- Pancreatitis
- Joint pain and osteoporosis (may lead to bone fractures)
- Cataracts

## Diagnostic Evaluation

The diagnosis of corticosteroid excess is suspected when clinical manifestations appear, and it is confirmed by administering a bolus of adrenocorticotropic hormone (ACTH) to the child. ACTH challenges the adrenal gland to respond to pituitary stimulation. If serum cortisol levels do not rise after administration of ACTH, adrenal suppression (cortisone excess) is present.

## Therapeutic Management

Every effort is made to prevent corticosteroid excess by observing the following:

- Short-term, high-dose therapy (for 1 week or less) is preferred over long-term therapy if there is a strong indication for the use of steroids.
- If long-term use is necessary, alternate-day administration may be prescribed.
- At the time of an acute infection or surgery, supplementary steroids are indicated for children who have received them over a long period.
- Because of immunosuppression, killed-virus vaccines are substituted for live-virus vaccines for children receiving high-dose or long-term steroids.

Children and adolescents who are receiving long-term oral or inhaled corticosteroids steroids must be meticulous about taking recommended calcium and vitamin D. In addition, the height growth rate should be assessed on a regular basis.

## NURSING CARE

### The Child Receiving Corticosteroids

#### Assessment

Assessment of a child receiving long-term steroid therapy includes measuring the height, weight, and blood pressure at each visit. In addition, the nurse observes the child for facial puffiness, abdominal pain, increased appetite, blurred vision, and increased thirst or urination. Families may report recent illnesses, bruising, or delayed wound healing.

#### Nursing Diagnosis and Planning

The nursing diagnoses and expected outcomes that may be appropriate after assessment of a child receiving corticosteroid therapy are as follows:

- Ineffective Therapeutic Regimen Management: Nonadherence related to associated complications.

*Expected outcome.* The child will take all medications as directed.

- Disturbed Body Image related to changes caused by treatment.

*Expected outcome.* The child will share feelings about any changes in appearance.

- Risk for Infection related to immunosuppression.

*Expected outcome.* The child will be afebrile and free of signs of secondary infections.

- Risk for Injury (adrenal insufficiency, delayed wound healing) related to insufficient knowledge.

*Expected outcome.* The child will not experience injury as a result of too-rapid withdrawal of medication or delayed wound healing. The parent can explain the reason for not withdrawing the medication abruptly.

- Risk for Delayed Growth and Development related to growth suppression and muscle wasting.

*Expected outcome.* The child will continue to grow according to his or her own height and weight curve.

#### Interventions

The nurse should provide the family with written instructions that specifically state what to do if a dose is missed and when to decrease dosages. In general, if a dose is missed, the child should take it as soon as it is remembered; if it is almost time for the next dose, the child should skip the dose altogether. The nurse should emphasize that corticosteroid therapy should not be discontinued abruptly. The child should take the medication with foods or milk to minimize the risk of gastrointestinal bleeding. Because the child's appetite may increase, encourage eating low-calorie snacks throughout the day. The nurse should remind the family that salt intake can increase fluid retention. Liquid forms of systemic corticosteroids can seem unpalatable to children. In this instance, the child may prefer a crushed tablet that has been put into a very small amount of a sweet food, or the liquid can be mixed with a sweet drink. Be sure to tell parents to mix the medication in 1 teaspoon or less of food or only a small amount of liquid to ensure that the child receives all the medication.

Changes in appearance are temporary and reversible. The nurse can compare changes in appearance and weight gain at each visit and encourage expression of the child's feelings. Weight and height monitoring of the child receiving long-term corticosteroid therapy is important; fluid retention can mask muscle wasting and growth suppression.

Corticosteroids can also mask infections. The family should be instructed to call the physician in the event of temperature elevation, cough, runny nose, ear tenderness, decreased appetite, nausea, vomiting, diarrhea, or behavioral change, or even if the child just "does not seem right." The child's skin should be checked routinely for bruising and signs of wound infection, and lesions that do not resolve as expected should be reported. The family should not treat the child with over-the-counter products without consulting the physician. The child receiving long-term therapy should avoid others who are sick; parents should promptly report any exposure to a communicable disease, such as measles or chickenpox, to the healthcare provider.

Because of possible impact on growth and bone density, the child should have a diet high in calcium-rich foods. Most young children receive vitamin D supplements, which enhance the absorption of calcium; children who are taking corticosteroids may need to be evaluated for increased requirements for calcium and vitamin D.

Potential environmental hazards and accident prevention strategies based on the child's developmental age should be emphasized. If the child gets a cut, the parent should hold gentle pressure to the site for 3 to 5 minutes to stop the bleeding and prevent hematoma formation. The child should wear a medical-alert bracelet stating the key clinical manifestations of corticosteroid excess or adrenal insufficiency.

**SAFETY ALERT**

***The Child Taking Oral Corticosteroids***

Long-term corticosteroid therapy causes adrenal insufficiency because exogenous (outside the body) use reduces the need for endogenous (within the body) production. Abrupt cessation of corticosteroid use without allowing for a gradual increase in adrenal production can cause insufficiency.

- Taper the dose to allow for a gradual return of adrenal function.
- Carefully monitor the child during the tapering process for the following: fatigue, muscle weakness, joint pain, dizziness, anorexia, nausea.
- Supplemental glucocorticoids might be necessary during times of increased stress to prevent adrenal insufficiency.

#### Evaluation

- Is the child taking corticosteroids as directed?
- Is the child able to express feelings about any changes in appearance?
- Does the child remain afebrile and free of any signs of secondary infection?
- Are any wounds healing at a normal rate?
- Is the child displaying any signs of adrenal insufficiency, and can the parent explain why the medication should not be withdrawn abruptly?
- Is the child growing at a rate appropriate for age as measured on a standard growth chart?
- Is the child obtaining an appropriate amount of calcium and taking recommended vitamin D supplements?

## IMMUNE COMPLEX AND AUTOIMMUNE DISORDERS

### Immune Complex Disorders

Immune complexes are clusters of interlocking antigens and antibodies. Under normal conditions, immune complexes are removed from the blood. In some circumstances; however, immune complexes continue to circulate. Eventually, they become trapped in the tissues of the kidneys, lungs, skin, joints, or blood vessels. There they set off reactions that lead to tissue inflammation and damage.

Deposition of immune complexes is considered to be a precipitator for several different conditions in childhood. Both Kawasaki disease (see Chapter 46) and acute poststreptococcal glomerulonephritis (see Chapter 44) are thought to be caused by immune complex deposition in tissues.

### Autoimmune Disorders

Sometimes the immune system's ability to differentiate self from nonself breaks down, and the body begins to make antibodies against its own cells, tissues (particularly connective tissue), and organs. Such antibodies are known as autoantibodies. Autoantibodies are common in conditions such as rheumatic fever (see Chapter 46), juvenile arthritis (see Chapter 50), and systemic lupus erythematosus.

It is still unclear what initiates an autoimmune response. Several theories have been proposed:

- Activation of immature B cells that do not develop antigen-specific receptors
- Alteration of normal cells by infection or another process, causing them to become antigenic
- Similarity between the structures of some infectious organisms and self-antigens, causing a cross-reaction
- Genetic predisposition to defective immune regulation

The response is exacerbated by a malfunction of helper T and regulatory T cells when there are too many helper cells and not enough suppressor cells to turn off the immune response. Some autoimmune disorders also manifest with increased tissue deposits of immune complexes.

## SYSTEMIC LUPUS ERYTHEMATOSUS

Systemic lupus erythematosus (SLE) is a chronic, multisystem autoimmune disease characterized by inflammation of the connective tissue. SLE varies in severity and is marked by remissions and exacerbations.

### Etiology

Although the etiology of SLE is not known, genetic, environmental, hormonal, and immune response factors are likely to be responsible. Environmental factors include exposure to the sun, ultraviolet light, stress, fatigue, viruses, bacteria, certain medications, and some food additives.

### Incidence

The overall prevalence of SLE is 1 to 6 per 100,000 (Sadun, Ardoin, & Schanberg, 2016). The condition is relatively rare in young children and has an average age of onset between 11 and 12 years. In young children, the female-to-male ratio is 2 to 5 : 1; after puberty, this ratio increases to 9 : 1. More Blacks, Hispanic, Native American, and Asian children are affected than white children (Sadun et al., 2016).

### Manifestations

Malaise, arthralgia, and recurrent fever of unknown etiology are among the frequent early manifestations of SLE. These manifestations can be easily confused with signs of other childhood illnesses. Neurologic manifestations such as headaches, mood disorders, cognitive disorders, and seizure disorders are often seen in children with SLE (Sadun et al., 2016). In general, the signs and symptoms depend on what organs the immune complexes affect and can include the following (Sadun et al., 2016):

- Malar butterfly rash: A fixed, red, flat, or raised rash over the cheeks and the bridge of the nose (Fig. 42.1)
- Discoid rash: Red, round, raised patches that spread
- Photosensitivity: Skin rash from sun exposure
- Oral and nasal ulcers: Usually painless lesions
- Arthritis: Painful, swollen joints with edema
- Pleuritis, pericarditis, or peritonitis
- Renal disorder: protein, casts, or red blood cells in urine
- Neurologic disorders: Headaches, personality changes, seizures, or psychosis
- Hematologic disorders: Anemia, leukopenia, lymphopenia, or thrombocytopenia
- Immunologic disorders
- Positive antinuclear antibody (ANA) assay

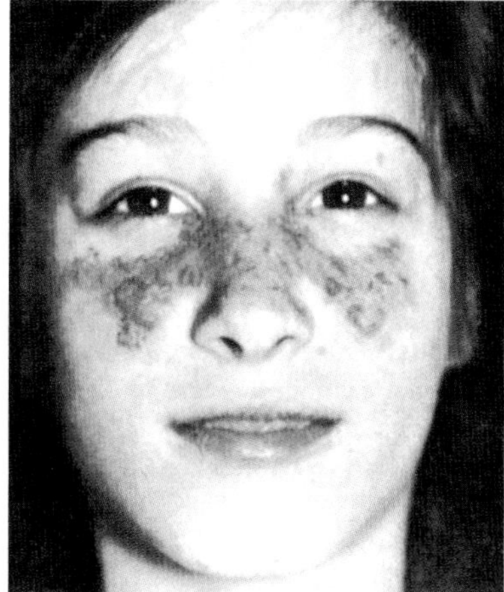

FIG 42.1 The butterfly rash of systemic lupus erythematosus. (From Behrman, R.E., Kliegman, R.M., & Jenson, H.B. [2004]. [Eds.]. *Nelson textbook of pediatrics* [16th ed., pp. 810]. Philadelphia: Saunders.)

**PATHOPHYSIOLOGY**

***Systemic Lupus Erythematosus***

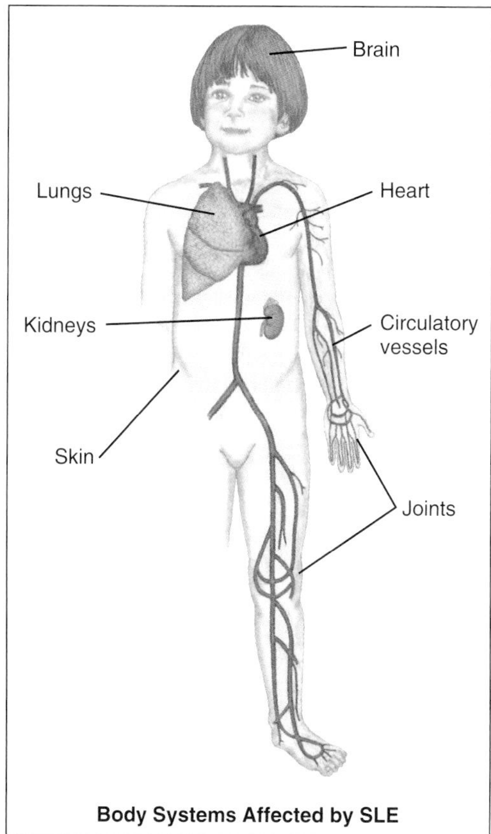


**Body Systems Affected by SLE**

Many abnormalities in the immune system are associated with systemic lupus erythematosus (SLE). Autoantibodies, referred to as antinuclear antibodies (ANAs), act against DNA and other cell nucleus components. Abnormal immune complex formation and nonspecific activation of B lymphocytes cause an increase in immune globulins, a process that triggers autoantibodies. This response is exacerbated by a reduction in the number of suppressor T cells. These autoantibodies produce inflammation and damage tissues and organs, including the skin, joints, heart, lungs, kidneys, brain, and circulatory vessels.

A child with SLE can have weight loss, growth impairment, headache, and memory problems. Occasionally, children will have Raynaud phenomenon, in which the digits of the hands and feet suddenly change color (mottled to white to blue) in response to cold. The most serious complications of SLE include renal disease and neurologic problems.

### Diagnostic Evaluation

Conforming with the American Rheumatism Association 1982 criteria for diagnosis, the presence of four or more of the clinical manifestations just listed, regardless of whether they occur simultaneously, is suggestive of SLE. In addition, a number of tests can be used to diagnose and monitor the progress of SLE. A positive ANA test, the presence of anti-DNA antibody, and the presence of antiphospholipid antibodies is highly suggestive of SLE. Blood urea nitrogen levels, gamma globulin levels, and the erythrocyte sedimentation rate can be elevated. Complement levels (C3 and C4) can be decreased. Pathologic changes compatible with SLE can be confirmed by electrocardiography, computed tomography, and magnetic resonance imaging and by skin and renal tissue biopsy specimens demonstrating immune complexes.

### Therapeutic Management

The treatment of SLE is tailored to the organ system or systems affected and is aimed at preventing exacerbations and complications. The goal of treatment is to use the least amount of pharmacologic intervention needed. Helping the child and family develop long-term coping strategies is important.

Systemic corticosteroids are most often given to control the inflammatory response. When steroid treatment is not effective or renal progression is rapid, cyclophosphamide (Cytoxan) might be considered. Nonsteroidal antiinflammatory drugs, excluding ibuprofen, are sometimes used to treat arthritis, serositis, and febrile attacks. Because these drugs can cause liver damage, they are used with caution and careful monitoring. Children with renal and neurologic disorders generally receive anticonvulsant and antihypertensive therapy, whereas those with skin lesions and joint problems take antimalarial drugs such as hydroxychloroquine (Plaquenil). Killed-virus vaccines rather than live-virus vaccines are used in affected children. A low-salt diet may reduce fluid retention and prevent elevated blood urea nitrogen levels; a low-protein diet helps preserve renal function.

The long-term prognosis for children with SLE is positive; the 5-year survival rate is close to 95% (Sadun et al., 2016). Close monitoring is essential for positive outcomes. Adverse outcomes include delayed growth and onset of puberty, decreased bone mass, atherosclerosis, and decreased quality of life (Sadun et al., 2016).

## NURSING CARE

### The Child With Systemic Lupus Erythematosus

#### Assessment

During a period of disease exacerbation, a child with SLE can become acutely ill. The nurse monitors the child's vital signs, mobility, activity level, and pain and completes a neurologic examination that assesses for decreased sensation, weakness in the extremities, and changes in behavior. Of equal importance is evaluation of the effect of living with a chronic illness on a young child's self-image and interaction with peers.

#### Nursing Diagnosis and Planning

The nursing diagnoses that apply to the child with SLE are as follows:

- Disturbed Body Image related to changes secondary to the disease process and treatments.

*Expected outcome.* The child will share feelings about altered appearance or function.

- Powerlessness related to memory and emotional alterations.

*Expected outcome.* The child and family will seek assistance in managing memory or emotional problems.

- Activity Intolerance related to the effects of the disease process.

*Expected outcome.* The child will participate in activities to the extent possible.

- Chronic Pain related to arthritis and numbness of the hands and feet.

*Expected outcome.* The child will be free of pain, demonstrating an acceptable level on an age-appropriate pain assessment tool and the ability to gain appropriate rest and participate in age-appropriate activities.

- Ineffective Therapeutic Regimen Management: Nonadherence related to associated complications and developmental level.

*Expected outcome.* The child will take all medications as directed and describe the medication plan and any medication side effects.

#### Interventions

The nurse needs to help the child and family understand the importance of drug therapy and activity restriction during acute exacerbations. Avoiding triggers that cause exacerbations is essential (e.g., avoiding exposure to sun or avoidable sources of infection). Wearing an appropriate sunscreen is a necessity (sun protection factor 30, waterproof, para-aminobenzoic acid free, ultraviolet A and ultraviolet B protective). Raynaud phenomenon can be prevented by dressing warmly in cold weather, paying particular attention to hat, gloves, and warm socks. An adolescent will have difficulty achieving a balance between the need to take risks and be accepted by peers and the realities of a chronic illness (see Chapter 36). The teenager with a chronic illness needs to participate as fully as possible in activities at home, at school, and in the community. Documenting episodes of fatigue along with associated activities allows young people to gain some control. They can then use this information to make sensible decisions about participation in extracurricular activities. The adolescent should be encouraged to plan an appropriate and convenient medication self-administration schedule and should be able to describe the side effects of the prescribed medications.

Anger about the diagnosis and alienation from peers are common. Wearing makeup can mask rashes and improve appearance. Keeping a diary also helps the young person vent anger. An affected peer who is in remission can offer support, as can national SLE organizations. The Internet is also a source of support and information.

#### Evaluation

- Does the child share feelings about her (or his) appearance or function?
- Do the child and family seek assistance as needed for related memory or emotional problems?
- Does the child participate in sports and extracurricular activities without becoming overly fatigued?
- Is the child free of pain as documented on an age-appropriate pain assessment tool?
- Is the child taking all medications as directed, and can the child describe the medication plan and side effects of the medications?

## ALLERGIC REACTIONS

Allergy is the immune response to an antigen called an *allergen* that causes a hypersensitivity reaction in various body systems. This hypersensitivity reaction, which occurs with a second exposure to an antigen, can be immediate or delayed. The classification of allergic reactions often reflects the pathophysiologic features of each type (Table 42.3). In most children with allergies, there is a genetic link. Common allergic conditions include allergic rhinitis, hives, eczema, asthma, colic, and migraines (Table 42.4).

Allergic rhinitis is an immediate hypersensitivity reaction to allergens trapped by the hairs and mucus that line the inside of the nose (see Chapter 45). Anaphylaxis is a life-threatening allergic response. Allergic reactions are related to the antibody IgE.

## ANAPHYLAXIS

Anaphylaxis, a severe, immediate hypersensitivity reaction to an excessive release of chemical mediators, affects the entire body.

**TABLE 42.3 Classification of Allergic Reactions**

| Type | Pathophysiology | Examples |
|---|---|---|
| I. Immediate (anaphylactic) hypersensitivity | IgE attaches to mast cells and basophils, causing rupture and release of all contents (i.e., histamines). | Allergic rhinitis, acute anaphylaxis, hives, eczema, asthma |
| II. Cytotoxic hypersensitivity | An allergen (e.g., red blood cell) stimulates IgE or IgM to react and mobilize complement to destroy the allergen. | Transfusion reaction after receiving incompatible blood |
| III. Arthus hypersensitivity (immune complex) | Immune complex is formed and can destroy tissues. | Serum sickness, glomerulonephritis |
| IV. Delayed cell-mediated hypersensitivity | An allergen reacts with T lymphocytes, and these lead other cells to produce damage. | Contact dermatitis (e.g., poison ivy) |

### Etiology

Food allergy is a major cause of anaphylaxis in children (Gupta, Dyer, Jain, et al., 2013). Other causes include penicillin or other antibiotics, insect stings, immunizations, allergy immunotherapy (desensitization), chemotherapeutic agents, blood products, and diagnostic contrast media. Peanuts (including peanut butter) and tree nuts (e.g., cashews, almonds, walnuts, pecans, pistachios) are particularly potent substances, causing anaphylaxis in increasing numbers of children. Other frequently seen food allergies include milk, eggs, wheat, shellfish, and other fish. Anaphylactic reactions to products containing latex have increased in incidence, especially among children with spina bifida (see Chapter 52) and with abnormalities of the urinary tract.

### Incidence

Approximately 8% of children in the United States have severe allergic reactions to foods (Gupta et al., 2013). In many cases, previous exposure to the allergen is undocumented, so the child has anaphylaxis presumably on first documented exposure. In the child who is allergic to foods, the allergen usually is small particles of food protein (Gupta et al., 2013). For children with allergies to peanuts or other nuts, an anaphylactic reaction can occur with exposure to nut oils, surfaces contaminated with nuts, shell fragments, or cooking and serving utensils used previously for nut products.

The incidence of anaphylaxis in the United States from all causes is considered to be 50 per 100,000 (Sampson, Wang, & Sicherer, 2016). Food-induced anaphylactic reactions cause 150 deaths per year in the United States (Broome, Lutz, & Cook, 2015).

### Manifestations

The onset of anaphylaxis is sudden, usually occurring within seconds to minutes after exposure to an allergen. The median time for

**TABLE 42.4 Common Allergic Conditions in Children**

| Allergens | Manifestations | Diagnosis |
|---|---|---|
| **Inhalants** | | |
| Pollen, dust, mold, dander | Sneezing; red, itchy nose, eyes, pharynx, and palate; edematous nasal passages; tongue clicking; runny or congested nose; mouth breathing; chronic cough; dark circles under eyes; nose wrinkling; pale, boggy nasal mucous membranes | Allergic rhinitis |
| **Applicants** | | |
| Heat, cold, wool, cosmetics, solutions for hair permanents, sunscreens, plants, grasses | Well-defined red, raised skin or mucosal lesions | Hives<br>Contact dermatitis |
| **Foods** | | |
| Milk, wheat, eggs, strawberries, tomatoes, oranges, chocolate, nuts, shellfish | Intestinal cramping, nausea, vomiting, diarrhea<br>Bronchospasm<br>Red patches on cheeks, face, wrists, neck, hands, extremities; swelling; itching; weeping; scales and crust<br>Well-defined red, raised skin or mucosal lesions<br>Vascular headaches | Colic<br>Asthma<br>Eczema<br>Hives<br>Migraines<br>Possible anaphylaxis |
| **Medicines** | | |
| Penicillin, cephalexin, immunizations, allergy immunotherapy, chemotherapy | Redness, swelling, pain<br>Weakness, restlessness, edema, laryngospasm, cardiovascular collapse | Local inflammation<br>Anaphylaxis |
| **Insects** | | |
| Stings of bees, wasps, hornets | Redness, swelling, pain<br>Weakness, restlessness, edema, laryngospasm, cardiovascular collapse | Local inflammation<br>Anaphylaxis |

## PATHOPHYSIOLOGY

### *Anaphylaxis*

Anaphylaxis occurs when an allergen binds with IgE on mast cells and basophils, causing degranulation and release of histamines and other chemical mediators. Histamine action precipitates respiratory signs of bronchoconstriction, with bronchospasm and edema (especially laryngeal edema) from increased vascular permeability. Other systems most affected during an anaphylactic response include gastrointestinal (itchiness and tingling along the gastrointestinal tract, vomiting, diarrhea, pain) and integumentary (urticaria). Anaphylaxis can lead to circulatory collapse and death if not promptly managed. An allergen that has previously provoked a response, or one that has not, can cause anaphylaxis.

symptoms to begin is 5 minutes to 2 hours after ingestion of a food allergen (Keet, 2011). Initial symptoms of impending anaphylaxis include the following:

- Sneezing
- Tightness or tingling of the mouth or face, with subsequent swelling of the lips and tongue
- Severe flushing, urticaria, and itching of the skin, especially on the head and upper trunk
- Rapid development of erythema
- A sense of impending doom

These symptoms might be followed by gastrointestinal and respiratory symptoms, which include nausea, vomiting, diarrhea, and cramping, as well as rhinorrhea, stridor, wheezing, and hoarseness.

The most serious features of anaphylaxis are laryngospasm, edema, cyanosis, hypotensive shock, vascular collapse, and cardiac arrest. Several hours after the initial phase of anaphylaxis resolves, a second, or biphasic, reaction can occur. This second reaction can be as severe as the initial reaction, affects similar body systems, and can occur hours up to several days after the initial episode.

## Diagnostic Evaluation

Anaphylaxis occurs suddenly, allowing no time for diagnosis. The etiology is determined later by obtaining a history of the exposure. Serum studies may reveal an elevated IgE for the agent of exposure. In some cases, the allergen can be confirmed by skin tests or RAST. For children with food allergy, a combination of skin-prick testing, allergen-specific serum IgE levels, and oral food challenge are best to confirm a diagnosis (Gupta et al., 2013).

## Therapeutic Management

Treatment of anaphylaxis must begin immediately because it can be only a matter of minutes before shock occurs. In the community setting, immediately activate the emergency response system. Injectable epinephrine is the first drug of choice in the acute treatment of anaphylaxis. In addition to epinephrine, oral diphenhydramine, a histamine inhibitor (e.g., ranitidine, cimetidine), and/or corticosteroids may be indicated.

Epinephrine (0.01 mg/kg/dose of 1 : 1000 concentration) is administered to children with suspected anaphylaxis. Children with known severe allergic reactions should have an EpiPen or other preloaded, automatic delivery system available at all times. The EpiPen (0.3 mg) is appropriate for children who weigh more than 25 kg, and the EpiPen Jr. (0.15 mg) can be administered to children who weigh 10 to 25 kg (Sampson et al., 2016).

In a hospital or emergency setting, managing anaphylactic shock includes the following:

- Ensure an adequate airway, possibly by endotracheal intubation (see Chapter 34).
- Administer epinephrine. If reaction is caused by an insect sting, place a tourniquet proximal to the site of the sting and administer epinephrine in the uninvolved extremity and in the area of reaction, with repeat dosing within 5 to 10 minutes.
- Administer oxygen if available.
- Administer corticosteroids and antihistamines as ordered.
- Keep the child warm and lying flat or with feet slightly elevated.
- Start an IV line.

Children who have had life-threatening insect sting anaphylaxis and demonstrate venom-specific IgE antibodies on skin studies or RAST are candidates for venom immunotherapy. All children experiencing episodes of anaphylaxis in the community should be transported by ambulance to an emergency facility (see Chapter 34) and kept for observation at least 4 to 6 hours after the episode is resolved to ensure prompt intervention should a biphasic reaction occur.

## NURSING CARE

### The Child With Anaphylaxis

#### Assessment

The child should be observed closely for airway obstruction and vascular collapse during the acute phase of anaphylaxis. Assessment includes noting airway patency, respiratory rate and effort, heart rate, peripheral pulses, capillary refill time, oxygen saturation, urine output, and level of consciousness. After emergency efforts, the nurse can try to determine the cause of the attack by correlating when the symptoms first occurred with foods ingested, medications administered, and the possibility of an insect sting.

#### Nursing Diagnosis and Planning

The nursing diagnoses that apply to the child with anaphylaxis and to the family are as follows:

- Ineffective Breathing Pattern and Decreased Cardiac Output related to an excessive hypersensitive reaction to an allergen.

*Expected outcome.* The child will maintain a patent airway and adequate cardiac output (short term).

- Deficient Knowledge about allergens and prevention through risk reduction related to inexperience.

*Expected outcome.* The child and family will describe the child's allergic reaction and initiate a management plan for avoiding allergens and treating reactions (long term).

#### Interventions

Initially, the nurse maintains an adequate airway by administering oxygen and assisting with aerosol treatments and intubation as necessary. A laryngoscope, an intubation tray, and a tracheostomy kit should be available, and the code cart should be nearby. In the case of an insect sting or injected medication, a tourniquet applied to the affected extremity just proximal to the site might help confine the allergen. It is important to have IV access with a large-bore needle in at least one site, preferably two, for medication administration. The nurse administers IV fluids, epinephrine, corticosteroids, and antihistamines as ordered and informs the physician of the child's improvement or deterioration. Extra fluids (crystalloids or colloids) and plasma expanders should be administered if the child shows signs of vascular collapse (see Chapter 34). Because epinephrine causes vasoconstriction and an increase in cardiac output, a child receiving the drug might have heart palpitations and tachycardia. This is frightening and aggravated by the emergency nature of the situation. The nurse should offer gentle reassurance to the child and provide the family with frequent reports about the child's condition.

After an initial anaphylactic episode, the nurse should assure the child and family that they were not at fault for the anaphylactic reaction and discuss how to prevent recurrences. Any child who has experienced anaphylaxis should have and learn to use injectable epinephrine. The EpiPen Jr. for children (weighing less than 25 kg) delivers 0.15 mg of epinephrine through a spring-loaded injector, and the EpiPen (for children weighing more than 25 kg) provides 0.3 mg of epinephrine. The dosage chosen by the provider is based on the child's weight. Teach the parent or child to hold the injector against the skin of the upper outer region of the child's thigh for 10 seconds after administering the injection to deliver the medication completely. The EpiPen can be injected through clothing. A medical alert bracelet alerts others to the child's allergy.

Caring for the child at school presents an additional challenge (Patient-Centered Teaching: Communicating with the School about Peanut Allergies). The school nurse must be aware of and communicate information to others, as appropriate, about any child who has had anaphylaxis. Policies regarding storage of and access to the EpiPen in the school setting differ in each school district. Some school districts train nonmedical personnel to administer the epinephrine if the child goes on a field trip; other school districts require a parent of a child who cannot self-administer epinephrine to accompany the child on a field trip. It is necessary for the school nurse to notify teachers and school nutrition personnel if a child or children in the school have allergies to peanuts or other foods. In some instances, the child may be so highly allergic that lunch must be eaten in the school health office, away from even the odor of peanut butter. Most commercial fast-food establishments post signs if pastries or other foods contain peanuts or other allergenic substances.

### Evaluation

- Is the child awake and alert with adequate oxygenation and a patent airway?
- Are the child's vital signs within normal limits for age?
- Is the family taking appropriate steps to reduce the risks of another anaphylactic reaction (Patient-Centered Teaching: How to Prevent Insect Stings)?
- Do the child, family, and other appropriate adults demonstrate the proper use of the insect sting kit?

#### PATIENT-CENTERED TEACHING

##### *Communicating With the School About Peanut Allergies*

If your child has had a severe reaction to peanuts or other nuts, it is important for you to talk to your healthcare provider about whether the child should have medication available at home and school.

Epinephrine, the medication that relieves a severe allergic reaction, is available in an easy-to-use automatic injector, which older children can self-administer and teachers or other school personnel can be taught to administer.

Important things to remember when using automatically injected epinephrine are as follows:

1. If using an EpiPen, the injection can be given through the child's clothing.
2. After starting the injection, you must continue to hold the EpiPen against the child for at least 10 seconds for all the medication to be delivered.

Your child should have an allergy action plan readily available at school. You can obtain a sample action plan from http://www.foodallergy.org.

Talk to the school nurse about the severity of your child's reaction and work with the nurse to create a way your child can avoid contact with peanuts while not singling the child out for special attention.

Many school districts have policies that prohibit sharing of food or eating food on school buses. Other practices available at certain schools include peanut-free classrooms and a peanut-free area in the school cafeteria. Your school nurse can help you decide what modifications are appropriate for your child.

#### PATIENT-CENTERED TEACHING

##### *How to Prevent Insect Stings*

- Select clothes with white or khaki colors, not dark or brightly decorative ones.
- Wear fitted clothes with long sleeves, pants, and shoes.
- Use unscented soaps, lotions, and deodorants.
- Apply insect skin protection.
- Avoid orchards, flowers, blooming trees, and shrubs.
- Stay away from picnic areas.
- Stay out of the garden.
- Keep car windows closed while driving.
- Place screens on all windows.
- Cover all garbage cans.
- Move away slowly from approaching insects.

## KEY CONCEPTS

- The immune system maintains homeostasis of the internal and external environment through nonspecific functions (inflammation, phagocytosis) and specific functions (humoral and cell-mediated immunity). Any derangement results in an immunologic imbalance whereby the immune system either underfunctions or overfunctions.
- When the immune system underfunctions, the susceptibility to infections increases (immunodeficiency). When the immune system overfunctions, it produces antibodies against cells of the body in autoimmune disease or against external sensitizing agents, forming the basis for allergies.
- Children with acquired or congenital immunodeficiency are vulnerable to bacterial and viral infections. The best way to prevent the spread of organisms is to practice appropriate hand hygiene routinely and to follow basic infection control practices based on three principles: (1) prevent contact with organisms, (2) create barriers if contact is unavoidable, and (3) kill organisms if contact is made.
- HIV infection is the best-known acquired immunodeficiency disease. It causes a wide spectrum of illness in children, ranging from no symptoms to mild and moderate symptoms to severe symptoms.

*Continued*

## KEY CONCEPTS—cont'd

- Standard treatments for HIV infection include a modified immunization program, antiretroviral therapy, PCP prophylaxis, and aggressive use of antibiotics.
- For children with HIV, nurses have the challenging tasks of respiratory management, promoting normal growth and development, preventing infections, and providing comfort. In addition, nurses must support families in dealing with a stigmatizing illness that is chronic in nature.
- Children who acquired HIV when they were born are now reaching teen years. Nurses must discuss issues of infection transmission and medication adherence with these teens.
- Corticosteroids have immunosuppressive and antiinflammatory properties. Tapering the dose during both long-term and short-term therapy regimens allows for the gradual return of adrenal function.
- Emergency treatment takes priority in an anaphylactic reaction because it is only a matter of minutes before the child will go into shock. In a community setting, epinephrine is administered to children with a known prior anaphylactic episode, and the emergency service system is activated. Initially, the goal is to maintain an adequate airway, sometimes necessitating endotracheal intubation. This action is followed by the administration of epinephrine.

## REFERENCES AND READINGS


American Academy of Pediatrics Committee on Pediatric AIDS. (1999, reaffirmed 2005). Disclosure of illness status to children and adolescents with HIV. *Infection Pediatrics, 103*, 164–165.

Andrinopoulos, K., Clum, G., Murphy, D., et al. The Adolescent Medicine Trials Network for HIV/AIDS, I. (2011). Health related quality of life and psychosocial correlates among HIV-infected adolescent and young adult women in the US. *AIDS Education & Prevention, 23*(4), 367–381.

Banasik, J. (2013). Inflammation and immunity. In L. Copstead, & J. Banasik (Eds.), *Pathophysiology* (5th ed., pp. 157–192). St. Louis: Mosby.

Broome, S. B., Lutz, B. J., & Cook, C. (2015). Becoming the Parent of a Child with Life-Threatening Food Allergies. *Journal of Pediatric Nursing, 30*, 532–542. doi.10.1016/j.pedn.2014.10.012.

Buckley, R. (2016). The T-, B-, and NK-cell systems. In R. Kliegman, B. Stanton, J. St Geme, et al. (Eds.), *Nelson textbook of pediatrics* (20th ed., pp. 1006–1032). Philadelphia: Elsevier.

Centers for Disease Control and Prevention. (2014). *Diagnosis of HIV infection in the United States and dependent areas.* Retrieved from *HIV Surveillance Report*, Retrieved from http://www.cdc.gov.

Centers for Disease Control and Prevention. (2016). *One test two lives.* Retrieved from http://www.cdc.gov.

Fuhlbrigge, A.L., & Kelly, H.W. (2014). Inhaled corticosteroids in children: effects on bone mineral density and growth. *The Lancet Respiratory Medicine, 2*(6), 487–496.

Gupta, R.S., Dyer, A.A., Jain, N., et al. (2013). Childhood food allergies: current diagnosis, treatment, and management strategies. *Mayo Clinic Proceedings, 88*(5), 512.

Keet, C. (2011). Recognition and management of food-induced anaphylaxis. *Pediatric Clinics of North America, 58*(2), 377–388. doi.10.1016/j.pcl.2011.02.006.

Liu, A.H., Covar, R.A., Spahn, J.D., et al. (2016). Childhood asthma. In R. Kliegman, B. Stanton, J. St Geme, et al. (Eds.), *Nelson textbook of pediatrics* (20th ed., pp. 1095–1115). Philadelphia: Elsevier.

National Association of State Boards of Education. (2001). *Someone at school has AIDS: A complete guide to education policies concerning HIV infection.* Retrieved from http://www.nasbe.org.

National Heart, Lung, and Blood Institute & National Asthma Education and Prevention Program. (2007). *Expert panel report 3: Guidelines for the diagnosis and management of asthma.* Retrieved from http://www.nhlbi.nih.gov.

Panel on Antiretroviral Therapy and Medical Management of HIV-Infected Children. (2015, March 5). *Guidelines for the use of antiretroviral agents in pediatric HIV infection.* Retrieved from http://www.aidsinfo.nih.gov.

Panel on Treatment of HIV-Infected Pregnant Women and Prevention of Perinatal Transmission. (2015, August 6). *Recommendations for use of antiretroviral drugs in pregnant HIV-1 infected women for maternal health and intervention to reduce prenatal HIV transmission in the United States.* Retrieved from http://www.aidsinfo.nih.gov.

Porth, C. (2014). *Essentials of pathophysiology* (4th ed.). Philadelphia: Wolters Kluwer.

Rote, N. & McCance K.L. (2014). Adaptive immunity. In K. McCance, S. Huether, & V. Brashers (Eds.), *Pathophysiology the biologic basis for disease in adults and children* (7th ed., pp. 224–261). St. Louis, MO: Elsevier Mosby.

Sadun, R.E., Ardoin, S.P., & Schanberg, L.E. (2016). Systemic lupus erythematosus. In R. Kliegman, B. Stanton, J. St Geme, et al. (Eds.), *Nelson textbook of pediatrics* (20th ed., pp. 999–1006). Philadelphia: Elsevier.

Sampson, H., Wang, J., & Sicherer, A.H. (2016). Anaphylaxis. In R. Kliegman, B. Stanton, J. St. Geme, et al. (Eds.), *Nelson textbook of pediatrics* (20th ed., pp. 1131–1136). Philadelphia: Elsevier.

Seeborg, F.O., Paul, M.E., & Shearer, W.T. (2014). Human immunodeficiency virus and acquired immunodeficiency syndrome. In J. Cherry, G. Harrison, S. Kaplan, et al. (Eds.), *Feigin and Cherry's textbook of pediatric infectious diseases* (7th ed., pp. 2591–2619). Philadelphia: Elsevier.

Siberry, G. K., Abzug, M. J., Nachman, S., et al. The panel on opportunistic infections in HIV-exposed and HIV-infected children. (2013). Guidelines for the prevention and treatment of opportunistic infections in HIV-exposed and HIV-infected children: *The Pediatric Infectious Disease Journal, 32*(02).

Working Group on Antiretroviral Therapy and Medical Management of HIV-Infected Children. (2014, May). *Guidelines for the use of antiretroviral agents in pediatric HIV infection.* Retrieved from http://www.aidsinfo.nih.gov.

Yogev, R., & Chadwick, E. (2016). Acquired immunodeficiency syndrome (human immunodeficiency virus). In R. Kliegman, B. Stanton, J. St. Geme, et al. (Eds.), *Nelson textbook of pediatrics* (20th ed., pp. 1645–1665). Philadelphia: Elsevier.

43

# The Child With a Gastrointestinal Alteration

http://evolve.elsevier.com/McKinney/mat-ch/

## LEARNING OBJECTIVES

*After studying this chapter, you should be able to:*

- Describe the development of the gastrointestinal system and its relation to selected congenital defects.
- Describe the anatomy and physiology of the gastrointestinal system in an infant and a child.
- Describe the common diagnostic and screening tests used to detect alterations in gastrointestinal function.
- Discuss and demonstrate an understanding of the structural and functional alterations in the gastrointestinal system.
- Discuss and demonstrate an understanding of the pathophysiology, etiology, clinical manifestations, diagnostic evaluation, and therapeutic management of malabsorption and infectious problems affecting the gastrointestinal system.
- State expected nursing diagnoses for gastrointestinal alterations.
- Use the nursing process to develop nursing care plans and teaching guidelines for the child with gastrointestinal alterations.
- Develop home care guidelines for a child with gastrointestinal alterations.
- Implement child and family teaching.
- Develop nursing implications for common medications used with a child having gastrointestinal alterations.
- Demonstrate critical thinking skills to manage a given patient care situation.

## CLINICAL REFERENCE

## REVIEW OF THE GASTROINTESTINAL SYSTEM

### Upper Gastrointestinal System

The upper gastrointestinal (GI) system includes the mouth, esophagus, and stomach. Its primary functions are to take in food and fluids, begin the digestive process, and propel food into the intestines, where nutrients are absorbed. The mouth or buccal cavity is the entrance to the GI tract. Here food is broken up and mixed with saliva. This process starts the digestion of carbohydrates. The submandibular, parotid, and sublingual glands secrete saliva in response to the smell, taste, or thought of food. The tongue contains taste buds that distinguish salt, sweet, sour, and bitter sensations. The tongue is essential for swallowing.

At birth, the esophagus measures approximately 10 cm in length; it lengthens to 18 to 25 cm by adulthood. The upper third of the esophagus consists of striated voluntary muscle; the lower two thirds consist of smooth muscle. The upper esophageal sphincter (UES) prevents the reflux of esophageal contents into the pharynx and lungs and prevents esophageal distention during respiration; the lower esophageal sphincter (LES, or cardiac sphincter) prevents the reflux of gastric contents into the lower esophagus.

Swallowing is under both voluntary and involuntary control. As food is chewed, it forms a small bolus, or mass; the tongue propels the bolus toward the oropharynx. The presence of this mass in the oropharynx stimulates the medulla, causing the soft palate to rise. The nasal passages close, the pharyngeal muscles contract, the larynx closes, and respiration is inhibited. Together, these processes propel the food into the esophagus. Through **peristalsis**, the bolus moves on to the LES, the muscle relaxes, and the bolus enters the stomach.

The stomach lies in the epigastric, umbilical, left hypochondrial region of the abdomen. It is a muscular pouch, shaped somewhat like a gourd, where the bolus is received. As the LES and the **pylorus** contract, the stomach muscles churn the contents. The contents mix with the digestive juices to form chyme. The chyme moves on to the pylorus and into the duodenum.

A mucous-bicarbonate barrier in the stomach provides a thick layer of mucus and a buffer zone to neutralize acid. Stomach acids diffuse slowly through this layer toward the gastric wall. They are neutralized by bicarbonate ions from the surface epithelial cells. Thus, a neutral pH is maintained at the gastric epithelial surface.

### Lower Gastrointestinal System

The lower GI system includes the duodenum, liver, gallbladder, pancreas, jejunum, ileum, cecum, appendix, ascending colon, transverse colon, descending colon, sigmoid colon, rectum, and anus. The primary functions of the lower GI tract are to digest and absorb nutrients, detoxify and excrete unwanted waste, and aid in fluid and electrolyte balance.

The duodenum, the first part of the small intestine, extends from the pylorus to jejunum. Partially digested chyme from the stomach enters the duodenum, where pancreatic enzymes and bile are excreted to further break down fats, carbohydrates, and proteins. The pancreas is an oblong gland lying behind the stomach that secretes enzymes to digest food and secretes glucagon and insulin to control motility and absorption.

The liver, the largest organ in the body, is located under the right diaphragm. The liver lies predominantly in the right upper quadrant, with the left lobe extending into the left upper quadrant. It is divided into two lobes separated by the falciform ligament. Within each lobe are numerous lobules that form the functional units of the liver.

The liver is unique in that it is supplied with blood from two sources: (1) the hepatic artery, which supplies oxygenated blood; and (2) the hepatic portal vein, which supplies deoxygenated blood with absorbed nutrients from the GI tract. The liver has numerous functions, including phagocytosis, bile production, detoxification, glycogen storage and breakdown, and vitamin storage. The production of bile is essential for the absorption of fat and the excretion of the end products of blood cell breakdown. The primary function of the gallbladder, a sac-like structure attached to the underside of the right lobe of the liver, is to store bile for secretion into the duodenum when stimulated by the presence of fat in its lumen.

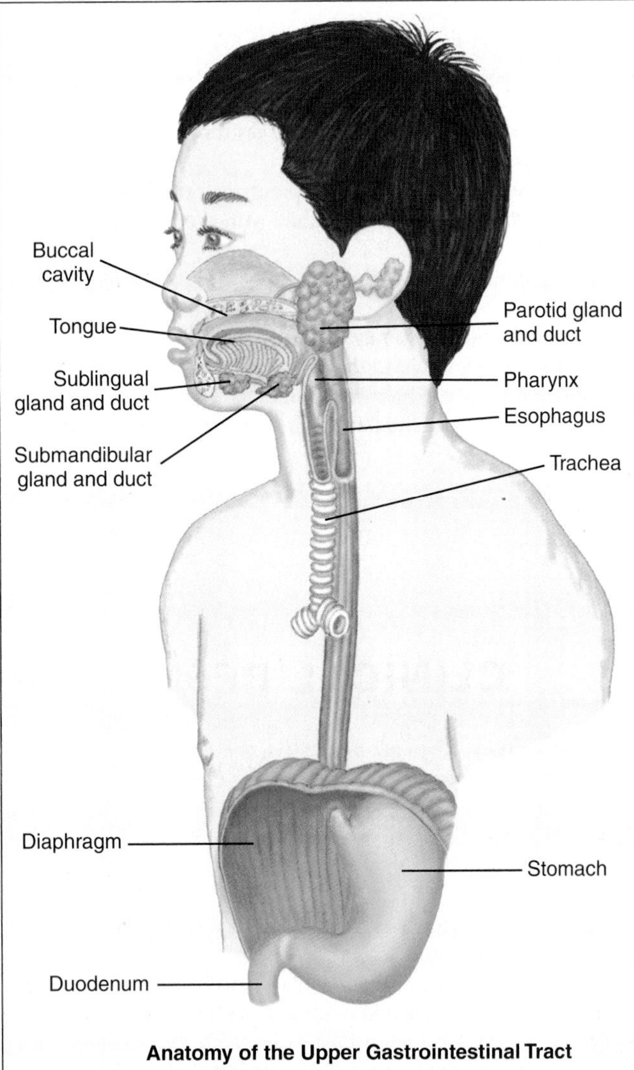


**Anatomy of the Upper Gastrointestinal Tract**

The jejunum and ileum form the remainder of the small intestine. Absorption of all nutrients and vitamins occurs here through the villi and microvilli by the processes of diffusion and active transport. Absorption of vitamin $B_{12}$ occurs only in the terminal ileum.

The large intestine starts with the cecum. This blind pouch, 2 to 3 inches long, begins at the ileocecal valve, which prevents reverse peristalsis into the small intestine. Attached to it is the appendix, a worm-like tube approximately 3 inches long. The open end of the cecum attaches to the remainder of the colon, which is divided into four sections: the ascending, transverse, descending, and sigmoid colon. One major function of the large intestine is water reabsorption, which occurs mostly in the cecum and ascending colon. Intestinal bacteria ferment the remaining carbohydrates and aid in the synthesis of vitamins B and K. Final breakdown of bile occurs here. Mucus secretion and peristalsis of wastes are also important functions.

The rectum is the last 7 to 8 inches of the intestine, and the anal canal refers to the last 1 to 2 inches. Stool is stored in the rectum until distention of the rectal walls initiates the defecation reflex—the final stage of the GI processes.

## Prenatal Development

The primitive gut is formed from the endoderm during the first 4 weeks of embryonic development. The primitive gut then gives rise to the following three sections of the GI tract, each having an individual blood supply and rate of development:

- Foregut: From the pharynx to the duodenum, including the liver, pancreas, and biliary tract
- Midgut: From the duodenum to the transverse colon
- Hindgut: Descending colon, rectum, and anal canal

Problems in the development of each of these three sections give rise to specific malformations and disease states. Anatomically, development is complete at birth, but physiologically, the neonate's GI tract is immature.

Fetal swallowing, intestinal motility, and defecation are detectable in the second trimester of gestation, but the most rapid and extensive development of the GI system occurs in the third trimester. The newborn must be able to adapt from total parenteral nutrition to total enteral nutrition because the placenta no longer performs nutrient exchange and waste removal.

### Common Laboratory and Diagnostic Tests for GI Disorders

| Test | Description | Normal Findings | Indications | Preparation and Nursing Considerations |
|---|---|---|---|---|
| **Stool** | | | | |
| Culture and sensitivity | Organisms from a small sample of stool are grown in culture media. | Normal GI flora | To identify infectious organisms and determine their antibiotic sensitivity | No patient preparation is necessary. The sample is delivered to the laboratory immediately; it must be kept free from contamination. |

## Common Laboratory and Diagnostic Tests for GI Disorders—cont'd

| Test | Description | Normal Findings | Indications | Preparation and Nursing Considerations |
|---|---|---|---|---|
| Reducing substances (Clinitest) | Stool is diluted with water and then tested for undigested carbohydrates with Clinitest tablets. | Negative | Used to diagnose malabsorption syndromes | No preparation is necessary.<br>The test is done by the nurse, who checks for a color change in the solution. |
| Occult blood (guaiac, Hematest) | Stool is smeared on filter paper and prepared with solution. | Negative | Used in inflammatory conditions and bowel necrosis | No preparation is necessary.<br>The test is done by the nurse; a blue color is positive. |
| Ova and parasites (O&P) | Stool is examined microscopically for presence of parasites or their eggs. | Negative | To identify enteric parasites in child with diarrhea or abdominal pain | No patient preparation is necessary.<br>Sample must be free from water or urine contamination.<br>The sample is delivered to the laboratory either fresh or in preservatives.<br>Barium, antacids, mineral oil, and antibiotics may interfere with results.1-3 samples are collected. |
| **Urine** | | | | |
| Urobilinogen | Dipstick or laboratory analysis is performed to determine bile byproducts in urine. | Negative | Levels determined in hepatic dysfunction and obstruction | No preparation is necessary. The test is done by the nurse. |
| **Blood** | | | | |
| Liver function tests | Serum levels are measured to give an indication of liver function. | AST: child <9 yr, 15-55 U/L; child >9 yr, 5-45 U/L<br>ALT: 5-45 U/L<br>Total bilirubin: 0.2-1.0 mg/dL<br>Ammonia: 29-70 mcg/dL in children; 90-150 mcg/dL in newborns | Tests performed when liver problems are suspected | No preparation is necessary.<br>Venipuncture is performed. |
| **Endoscopy** | | | | |
| Fiberoptic upper GI endoscopy | Study allows direct viewing of the lining of the esophagus, stomach, and proximal duodenum.<br>It also provides a means to obtain material for biopsies and cultures. | Normal mucosa | Used to rule out various upper GI tract disorders | Preparation includes teaching, keeping the child on NPO status for at least 6 hr before the examination, providing conscious sedation, and monitoring the child's respiratory function during sedation. |
| Colonoscopy | The colon is viewed directly by a fiberoptic scope and camera inserted rectally. | Normal mucosa and patent bowel | Performed to detect mucosal changes and abnormalities in the lumen of the colon | Preparation includes teaching, keeping the child on NPO status, bowel cleansing, and providing conscious sedation. |
| Biopsy (gastric, jejunal, rectal, liver) | A small piece of tissue is removed for analysis. | No abnormal tissue | Determines the amount of mucosal inflammation and the absence of ganglion cells | Preparation includes teaching, bowel cleansing, and providing sedation or anesthesia if the procedure is done percutaneously (liver). |

*Continued*

## Common Laboratory and Diagnostic Tests for GI Disorders—cont'd

| Test | Description | Normal Findings | Indications | Preparation and Nursing Considerations |
|---|---|---|---|---|
| **Radiologic Examinations** | | | | |
| Abdominal flat plate | Anterior and posterior radiographs are obtained. | | Radiographs demonstrate stool and gas patterns, inflammation, and patency of the GI tract.<br>It is commonly performed in cases of abdominal pain, imperforate anus, intussusception, and appendicitis. | Usually no preparation is necessary other than teaching. |
| Barium swallow examination | Radiopaque contrast medium or air (or both) is swallowed. | Normal swallowing, no anatomic defects | Identifies esophageal abnormalities, swallowing difficulties, and sphincter function | Preparation includes teaching and keeping the child on NPO status for 2-4 hr before the examination.<br>Adequate fluids are essential after the examination to prevent barium impaction. |
| Upper GI examination | Radiopaque contrast material is swallowed or inserted by NG tube. | Normal gastric emptying and no other abnormalities | Study outlines the stomach and pyloric canal and can be used to determine gastric emptying time. | Preparation includes teaching and keeping the child on NPO status for 4 hr before the examination.<br>Adequate fluids are essential after the examination to prevent barium impaction. |
| Barium enema, air-contrast barium enema examination | Radiopaque contrast material or air (or both) is placed in the large intestine via the rectum. | Patent bowel and no abnormalities | Study is used to identify abnormalities on the surface of the bowel lumen and to determine bowel patency.<br>It also provides hydrostatic reduction of intussusception. | Preparation includes teaching, keeping the child on NPO status, and bowel cleansing.<br>Adequate fluids are essential after the examination to prevent barium impaction. |
| CT scan | Oral radiopaque contrast material often used.<br>May also use IV or rectal contrast. | Normal anatomy without evidence of inflammation | Used to identify inflammatory conditions and appendicitis. | No patient preparation other than teaching.<br>Sedation can be used if child unable to remain still.<br>Can be completed in less than 15 min. |
| **Other** | | | | |
| Ultrasound | Study uses sound waves noninvasively to image anatomy and inflammation. | No abnormalities | Performed to identify anatomic abnormalities and inflammatory conditions | Preparation includes teaching.<br>For pelvic ultrasound, a full bladder is needed to improve imaging of pelvic organs. |
| Breath hydrogen test | Carbohydrate solution is given by mouth and exhaled.<br>Breath samples are collected over 3 hr. | Less than 20 ppm above baseline | Used to diagnose maldigestion or malabsorption syndromes<br>Inadequately digested carbohydrate produces hydrogen when acted on by GI flora. | Nursing preparation entails teaching about the procedure.<br>The child prepares by fasting for 4½ hr.<br>The study is noninvasive. A facemask can be worn to collect expired air. |

ALT, Alanine transaminase; AST, Aspartate transaminase; CT, Computed tomography; GI, gastrointestinal; IV, intravenous; NG, nasogastric; NPO, nothing by mouth.

## Major Digestive Enzymes

| Location | Enzyme | Function |
|---|---|---|
| Mouth | Amylase | Converts complex carbohydrate to simple carbohydrate |
| Stomach | Pepsin | Converts proteins to proteases |
| Small intestine | Enterokinase | Activates trypsin |
| | Peptidases | Convert peptides to amino acids |
| | Sucrase, maltase, lactase | Convert disaccharides to monosaccharides |
| Pancreas | Trypsin | Converts peptides to amino acids |
| | Lipase | Converts fat to fatty acids and glycerol |
| | Amylase | Converts carbohydrates to disaccharides |
| Liver, gallbladder | Bile | Emulsifies fat, allowing the lipase to function |
| | | Increases fat and fat-soluble vitamin absorption |

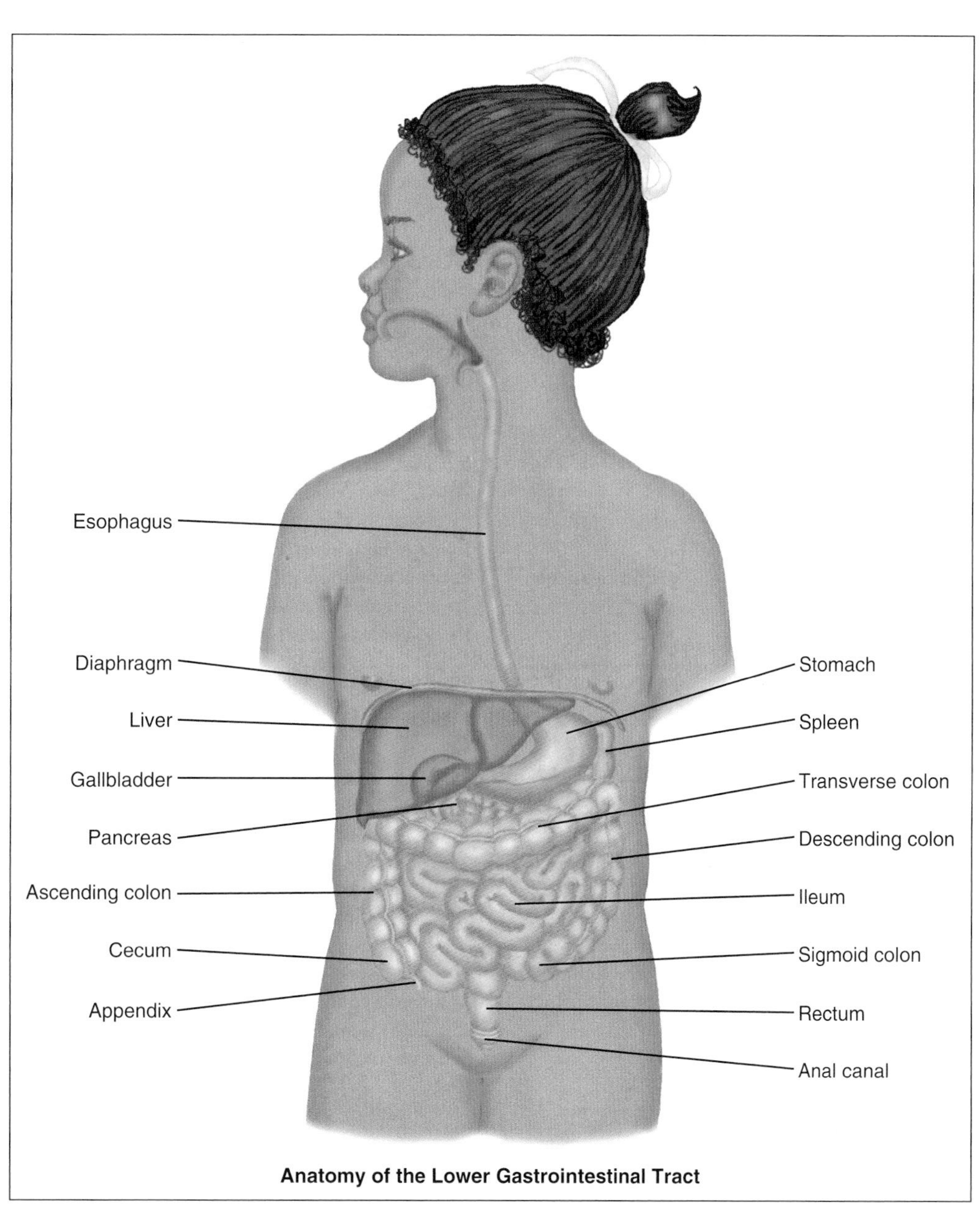


**Anatomy of the Lower Gastrointestinal Tract**

## Age-Related Differences in the Pediatric Gastrointestinal System

- Infants have minimal saliva.
- Swallowing is not under voluntary control until 6 weeks.
- Infants and children have less stomach capacity:

| Age | Stomach Capacity (mL) |
|---|---|
| Newborn | 10-20 |
| 1 wk | 30-90 |
| 2-3 wk | 75-100 |
| 1 mo | 90-150 |
| 3 mo | 150-200 |
| 1 yr | 210-360 |
| 2 yr | 500 |
| 10 yr | 750-900 |
| 16 yr | 1500 |
| Adult | 2000-3000 |

- The stomach lies transversely and is horizontal in the infant's abdomen; the abdomen is round in infants and toddlers.
- Peristaltic waves can reverse in infants, causing regurgitation and vomiting. In infants, peristalsis is faster and food remains in the stomach for a shorter period.
- Hydrochloric acid concentration is low until school age.
- Fever increases the rate of propulsion.
- The immature neonatal liver is not yet efficient in its detoxifying ability, resulting in less vitamin and mineral breakdown than in older children.
- The large intestine is relatively short, with less epithelial lining to absorb water from a fecal mass. As a result, stools have a soft consistency and peristalsis is more rapid.

Children with GI alterations and their families have many special requirements. Some GI problems begin at birth, with life-threatening consequences. Some require the parents to accept their child's altered appearance. Other problems develop after birth and provide long-term challenges in management and treatment. Sudden, unexpected surgery may be necessary. GI alterations cause anxiety and affect nutrition, elimination, respiratory status, skin integrity, body image, family processes, growth and development, and educational needs.

Upper and lower GI conditions can be categorized as follows:

- Developmental problems, such as cleft lip and palate, hernias, esophageal atresia, tracheoesophageal fistula, imperforate anus, and abdominal wall defects
- Problems affecting motility, such as gastroesophageal reflux, constipation, encopresis, and irritable bowel syndrome
- Inflammatory or infectious conditions, including ulcers, gastroenteritis, appendicitis, inflammatory bowel disease, and necrotizing enterocolitis
- Obstructive disorders, such as pyloric stenosis, intussusception, and Hirschsprung disease
- Malabsorption conditions, such as lactose intolerance and celiac disease
- Hepatic disorders, such as hepatitis, biliary atresia, and cirrhosis

Disorders that involve the liver and biliary tract can be the result of congenital malformations or acquired infection. Because the liver is important to metabolism, alterations in its function can affect many body systems, including the cardiovascular, integumentary, renal, neurologic, hematologic, and immunologic systems. These disorders can also have significant effects on growth and development. Nursing care may involve nutritional support, infection control, developmental stimulation, family support, and intensive physiologic care during a period of crisis.

## DISORDERS OF PRENATAL DEVELOPMENT

### Cleft Lip and Palate

Cleft lip, cleft palate, and cleft lip and palate are separate anomalies that are closely related in etiology, pathophysiology, and nursing care. These distinct problems are all abnormal openings in the lip or palate. The defects can occur unilaterally (on either side) or bilaterally and are the most common congenital craniofacial deformity.

#### Incidence

The incidence ranges from 1 in 750 white births for cleft lip and palate and 1 in 2,500 white births for cleft palate alone (Tinanoff, 2016). Cleft lip is seen predominantly in male infants, while cleft palate predominantly affects female infants. The prevalence of cleft lip and/or palate is higher in Asians and Native Americans and lower in Blacks. The etiology of cleft lip and palate malformations is thought to be multifactorial, including both genetic and environmental factors (Tinanoff, 2016). Although there appears to be a genetic pattern or familial risk involved, environmental factors such as maternal smoking have been found to be associated with an increased risk of oral cleft defects (Cleft Palate Foundation, 2014). Approximately 10% to 15% of infants who are affected with cleft lip and palate have other associated defects (Cleft Palate Foundation, 2014).

#### Manifestations and Diagnostic Evaluation

Cleft lip has the following manifestations: a notched vermilion border, variably sized clefts that involve the alveolar ridge, and dental anomalies (usually deformed, supernumerary, or absent teeth). Cleft palate includes nasal distortion, midline or bilateral cleft with variable extension from the uvula and soft and hard palates, and exposed nasal cavities.

The diagnosis of cleft lip and cleft palate is based on observation at birth and complete examination in the neonatal period. Diagnosis can also be made in utero with ultrasound. Cleft lip is readily diagnosed through inspection of the lip. The first sign of cleft palate may be milk or formula coming out of the nose. A gloved finger placed in the mouth to feel the defect of the palate or visual examination with a flashlight confirms the diagnosis.

#### Therapeutic Management

Management is based on the severity of the defect. A number of professionals are involved in this process, including surgeons; nurses; geneticists; psychologists or psychiatrists; ear, nose, and throat specialists; audiologists; and occupational and speech therapists. Orthodontists

## PATHOPHYSIOLOGY

### *Cleft Lip and Palate*

Cleft lip and cleft palate occur from embryonic developmental failures related to multiple genetic and environmental factors. These developmental failures result in an abnormal opening in the lip, palate, and, sometimes, nasal cavity. Cleft lip results when the medial nasal and maxillary processes fail to join at 6 to 8 weeks of gestation. Cleft palate results from failure of the primary palatal shelves, or processes, to fuse at 7 to 12 weeks of gestation.

Each of these abnormalities appears as a distinct malformation, but they can also appear together. Achieving suction during feedings may be impossible, and fluids can enter the nose, putting the child at risk for aspiration, feeding difficulties, and respiratory distress.

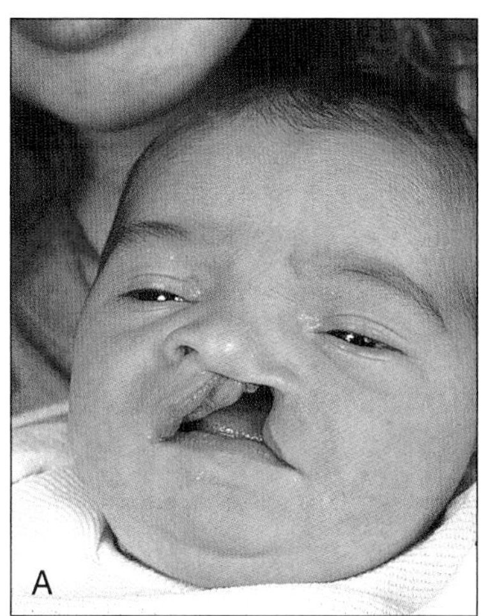


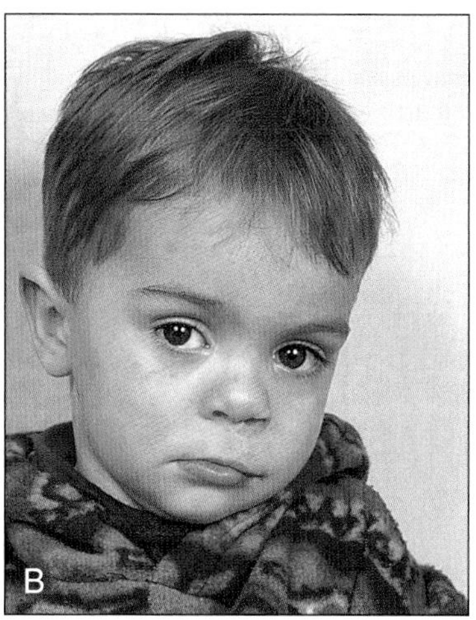


Child born with a cleft lip and palate, before **(A)** and after **(B)** repair. Repair of facial clefts usually requires multiple surgeries at different stages in the child's growth. Early repair of a cleft lip facilitates parent–infant bonding and improves feeding. Children generally experience good outcomes with today's surgical, orthodontic, and speech therapy techniques. (Courtesy Children's Medical Center, Dallas, TX.)

and plastic surgeons become involved in the long-term management of associated problems. Pediatricians provide ongoing child healthcare.

The first intervention involves the modification of feeding techniques as needed to allow adequate growth. Use of special feeding techniques, obturators, and unique nipples and feeders can usually accomplish this goal and allow early discharge home with parents (Fig. 43.1). These modified techniques can decrease the energy required for the infant to take in adequate nutrition. Before surgical repair, removable orthopedic devices such as a Latham device may be used to expand and realign parts of the palate or decrease the size of a wide lip cleft. It is important that families get adequate education regarding proper feeding techniques and support from healthcare professionals with expertise in feeding starting at the time of diagnosis until good feeding techniques are established (Lindberg & Berglund, 2013).

Cleft lip repair is usually performed by age 3 to 6 months. Early repair can improve bonding and makes feeding much easier. The surgical technique involves the use of a staggered suture line to minimize scarring. Some cosmetic modifications may be needed again at age 4 to 5 years.

Cleft palate repair is individualized and based on the degree of deformity and size of the child. Closure is completed between ages 6 and 24 months. Most teams recommend repair by 1 year of age. Earlier closure facilitates speech development.

After surgery, the priority is to keep the suture line clean and intact, avoiding tension on the sutures. Gentle aspiration of the nasopharynx reduces the chance of atelectasis (Tinanoff, 2016).

Concurrent treatment of altered dentition, recurring otitis media, speech dysfunction, emotional issues, and cosmetic concerns completes the ongoing therapy. Children with cleft palate are at high risk for developing chronic otitis media, which can cause long-term hearing loss.

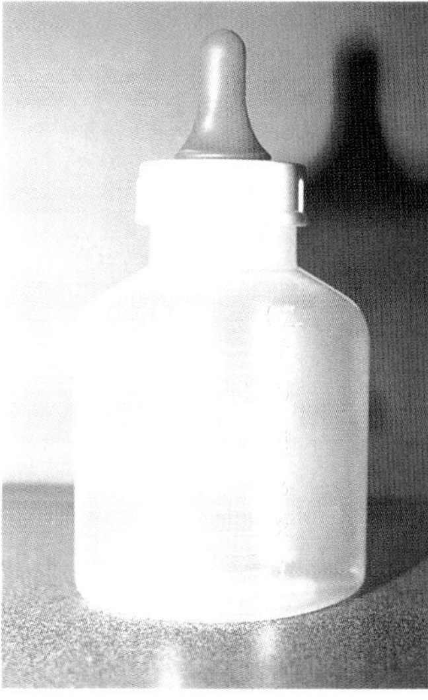

**FIG 43.1** Before and after repair of a cleft lip or palate, special feeding techniques are essential for adequate nutrition. A feeder with compressible plastic sides allows gentle squeezing of the sides of the bottle to help eject the breast milk or formula. A slightly longer nipple allows the milk to be swallowed with less chance of milk entering the nasopharynx and without stimulating the gag reflex.

## Esophageal Atresia With Tracheoesophageal Fistula

Esophageal atresia (EA) and tracheoesophageal fistula (TEF) are congenital malformations in which the esophagus terminates before it reaches the stomach and/or a fistula is present that forms an unnatural

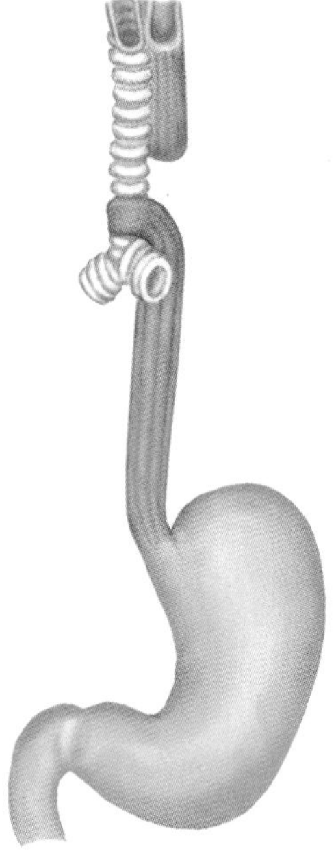

Esophageal Atresia with Distal TEF
Incidence: 85%-88%
Clinical Manifestations: Feeding causes regurgitation and coughing. Constant flow of saliva. Gastric distention.
Diagnostic Findings: Contrast reveals blind pouch. Air on abdominal x ray.
Surgical Treatment: One-stage surgical repair to ligate fistula and anastomose esophagus.


**FIG 43.2** Most common type of esophageal atresia (EA) and tracheoesophageal fistula (TEF).

connection between the esophagus and the trachea. Fig. 43.2 portrays the most common type of EA which is when the esophagus ends in a blind pouch and there is a distal TEF (Khan & Orenstein, 2016a).

### Etiology and Incidence

The cause of TEF and EA is unknown. EA occurs in 1.7/10,000 live births, with more than 90% having an associated TEF (Khan & Orenstein, 2016a). Nearly half of infants born with EA have other associated anomalies of the cardiac, GI, and central nervous systems. Prematurity and low birth weight are frequent concomitant problems that significantly affect long-term prognosis.

### Manifestations

- Failure to pass suction catheter, nasogastric (NG) tube at birth
- Excessive oral secretions, coughing, choking and respiratory distress
- Vomiting
- Abdominal distention
- Airless, scaphoid abdomen (atresia without fistula)

### Diagnostic Evaluation

A history of maternal polyhydramnios is a significant prenatal clue. If TEF is suspected prenatally, diagnosis can be made at the ideal time—in the delivery room. Atresia should be suspected if an NG tube cannot be passed 10 to 11 cm beyond the gum line. This suspicion is confirmed with an abdominal radiograph that will identify a proximal esophagus dilated with air (atresia) or abdominal distention (fistula). The radiologist can identify the specific type of defect after instilling less than 1 mL of a water-soluble contrast medium into the NG tube and documenting its movement into the tracheal tree and the proximal pouch. The medium is then withdrawn from the pouch to minimize the risk of aspiration. Laryngotracheobronchoscopy and endoscopy are also used to identify and assess fistulas and identify common secondary airway anomalies (Hseu, Recko, Jennings, et al., 2015). The infant should have diagnostic testing for commonly associated cardiac and other congenital anomalies that often are seen with this type of anomaly (Kahn & Orenstein, 2016a).

## PATIENT-CENTERED TEACHING

### *Home Care of the Child With Cleft Lip or Palate*

Your infant may require a special feeding method to maximize growth while waiting for surgery. It is helpful to practice the feeding method to be used after surgery until the incision heals. The feeding method you use will be based on what works for your child and what your physician recommends. In general, the following apply:

- Breastfeeding may be possible if your child has a small cleft lip or palate.
- A soft plastic, compressible bottle will prevent your child from having to suck vigorously because the breast milk or formula can be squeezed into the mouth, if needed.
- A longer nipple often allows the milk to be swallowed without entering the nose. It must not be so long that it causes gagging. Enlarging the nipple hole or "cross-cutting" a nipple can also be effective.
- A syringe with a rubber tip can also be used, especially after surgery.
- Feed your child slowly and provide short periods of rest for swallowing; children usually develop a feeding pattern of sucking, swallowing, and resting that helps them become more efficient eaters.
- Try to keep your child in an upright position during feedings to allow gravity to assist in the feeding and decrease the chance of choking.
- Burp your child frequently because excess air is often swallowed.

Before surgical repair, devices might be placed in your child's mouth to help line up the cleft in the palate for better surgical repair or to decrease the size of the lip cleft. Some of these devices require special care and cleaning. Consult your cleft team and nurses for specific instructions about your child's device.

After surgery, elbow restraints ("no-no's") can be used so that your baby cannot touch the stitches. The following are recommendations:

- Do not apply the restraints too tightly. They should be loose but still prevent elbow bending.
- Remove "no-no's" every 2 hours for 10 to 15 minutes and play games with your child that encourage movement of the elbows. Look for any skin irritation every time you remove an elbow restraint.
- Remove only one elbow restraint at a time.

Position your child for sleep on the back so the stitches are not rubbed on the linens. An infant seat can be used.

Do not brush your child's teeth for 1 to 2 weeks after surgery. Feeding a small amount of water after meals will help keep the teeth clean. Clean your child's lip as recommended by your physician. If ordered, you can use a cotton swab and a gentle rolling motion down the suture line and then apply antibiotic ointment using the same technique.

Make use of the many support professionals in following your child for speech, hearing, dental, or orthodontic problems.

Contact the American Cleft Palate-Craniofacial Association and the Cleft Palate Foundation at http://www.cleftline.org for further information.

### Therapeutic Management

Keeping the infant supine with the head of the bed elevated decreases the chance of gastric secretions entering the lungs. An NG tube must be in place and aspirated every 5 to 10 minutes to keep the proximal pouch clear of secretions and to avoid aspiration. Intravenous (IV) fluids and antibiotics to prevent pneumonia are essential (Khan & Orenstein, 2016a). Normal newborn care is appropriate, with special attention to keeping the infant warm and oxygenated.

Surgical repair is the mainstay of treatment. Initial repair includes ligation of the fistula and end-to-side anastomosis of the atresia to decrease the severity of stricture formation. If the gap between the two parts of the esophagus is too large, primary anastomosis may not be possible. Recent advances use traction suture ends to stimulate rapid growth of the esophageal ends over a 7- to 10-day period, allowing

## NURSING CARE PLAN

### *The Child With a Cleft Lip or Palate*

**Focused Assessment**

- During examination of the newborn with cleft lip and/or cleft palate, assess and document:
  - Degree of involvement
  - Infant's ability to suck, swallow, and breathe without distress
  - Infant's ability to handle normal secretions
- Assess and document:
  - Parent's initial reactions to the infant's appearance
  - Parent's interactions with the infant (i.e., touching, holding, examining)

**Nursing Diagnoses**

Imbalanced Nutrition: Less Than Body Requirements related to inability to suck and to the surgical repair.

Deficient Knowledge about feeding techniques and surgery related to unfamiliarity with the information.

**Planning**

***Expected Outcomes***

The child will:

1. Drink the desired amount of fluid within 30 minutes.
2. Be content during and after feeding.
3. Gain weight and height according to the normal growth curve.

The parents will:

4. Express satisfaction with progress of feedings.
5. Understand expected preoperative and postoperative feeding techniques.

**Interventions and *Rationales***

1. Describe the degree of cleft lip and/or palate and impairment of sucking.
   *Infants with cleft lip alone or simple cleft dental arch may be successful with breastfeeding or bottle feeding without modifications.*
2. Keep care and teaching simple and as closely related to normal infant feeding as possible.
   *Nutrition, parent-infant relationship, and adherence may be improved if normal techniques can be used.*
3. Provide alternative assistive feeding devices as needed and ordered.
   *Some infants may be able to breastfeed successfully. Techniques and equipment vary among institutions. Use what is available and effective for each child. Encourage breastfeeding first because breastfeeding confers added immune protection.*
4. Burp the infant frequently, and hold the infant in a more upright position.
   *Burping minimizes air swallowing and gastrointestinal (GI) flatus and minimizes risk of aspiration.*
5. Document the feeding program in written form for parents to use at home, and provide the plan to other health professionals.
   *Documentation provides consistency at home and at other times when the family is in contact with numerous medical professionals treating the child.*
6. Provide emotional support and positive reinforcement to parents as they learn to feed their child.
   *Self-care and bonding are improved when parents can assume total care.*
7. Keep an accurate record of the child's growth by using a growth chart.
   *A chart identifies growth changes early, when intervention can be most effective.*
8. Explain preoperative and postoperative procedures: oral feedings withheld for 6 hours, placement of intravenous (IV) lines, use of elbow restraints, appearance of repair in the immediate postoperative period.
   *Explanation decreases parental anxiety and encourages involvement.*
9. Postoperatively:
   a. Keep straws, pacifiers, spoons, or fingers away from the child's mouth for 7 to 10 days. Do not take temperatures orally.
      *Avoiding contact with the incision site reduces stress on surgical repair and prevents accidental tearing of very fine sutures.*
   b. Advance the child's diet as ordered and tolerated from clear liquids to a normal soft diet.
      *A normal diet minimizes nutritional deficits and stress on the child. No foods that can tear surfaces are offered.*
   c. After repair of a cleft lip, resume preoperative feeding techniques.
      *Little evidence shows that sucking causes excess suture stress.*
10. After repair of a cleft palate, provide short nipples that do not rest on palatal sutures; give baby food or baby food mixed with water.
    *Prevents direct contact with surgical site.*

**Evaluation**

Is the infant following the appropriate growth curve?

Is the infant happy and content during and after feedings?

Do the parents express satisfaction with the feeding technique used and the time required to complete a feeding?

Can the parents explain and demonstrate expected preoperative and postoperative care?

**Nursing Diagnosis**

Interrupted Family Processes related to the emotional reaction to an infant with a visible defect.

**Planning**

***Expected Outcomes***

The parents will:

1. Demonstrate positive behaviors toward the infant.
2. Access appropriate support.

**Interventions and *Rationales***

1. Encourage parents to discuss their fears, concerns, and negative emotions.
   *Grief, anxiety, confusion, guilt, denial, and anger are not uncommon and should be expressed.*
2. Encourage touching and holding.
   *Contact encourages bonding and prevents a delayed attachment.*
3. Make appropriate referral to a cleft lip and palate team of nurses, physicians, and other specialists as soon as possible.
   *A healthcare team can provide accurate information and begin to outline a plan of action.*
4. Express acceptance of the baby by modeling feeding and close physical contact.
   *These interventions assist parents with the adaptation process.*
5. Refer parents to community resources and parent groups.
   *Sharing with others in similar situations facilitates acceptance and adaptation.*
6. Encourage parents to share concerns about long-term care and emotional and financial stress.
   *Long-term concerns require extensive follow-up and can strain many families' resources. Identifying concerns early can increase problem-solving options.*

**Evaluation**

Can the parents identify their infant's positive characteristics?

Do the parents hold, cuddle, and make eye contact with the infant?

Have the parents sought personal, community, or organizational support?

*Continued*

## NURSING CARE PLAN—cont'd

### *The Child With a Cleft Lip or Palate*

**Nursing Diagnoses**

Impaired Skin Integrity related to the surgical repair.

Risk for Infection related to the surgical repair and aspiration.

**Planning**

***Expected Outcomes***

1. The repair site will heal without complications.
2. The infant will show no signs of infection as evidenced by a clean and intact suture line, absence of fever, and clear breath sounds.

**Interventions and *Rationales***

1. Clean the lip repair site according to physician protocol. Many physicians recommend cleaning with sterile water using a cotton swab or saline after feeding and as ordered. Use a rolling motion vertically down the suture line. Have parents demonstrate this cleaning technique.
   *The procedure decreases the medium for bacterial growth, decreases crusting, and minimizes scarring.*
2. Apply antibiotic ointment as ordered.
   *Antibiotic ointment prevents infection, crusting, and scarring.*
3. Use elbow restraints (no-no's) to keep the child from touching the repair site. Continue for 6 to 8 days. Remove every 2 hours for 10 to 15 minutes. Remove restraint from only one elbow at a time, with a parent or nurse in constant attendance.
   *Elbow restraints prevent accidental rupture or tear of sutures. Periodically removing restraints promotes contact with the child, decreases anxiety, and allows the nurse to assess skin integrity and circulation.*
4. Do not brush the child's teeth for 1 to 2 weeks.
   *Avoiding brushing prevents accidental tear of palatal sutures.*
5. Keep the child in a supine position or in an infant seat.
   *Careful positioning prevents contact of suture lines with bed linens.*
6. Observe for redness, swelling, excessive bleeding, drainage, respiratory distress, or fever.
   *Signs of infection must be identified early because additional inflammation can increase scarring.*
7. To clean the palate repair site, rinse the child's mouth with water after feedings.
   *Rinsing after feeding removes food and residual sugars from suture lines, reducing the risk of infection.*
8. Encourage the parents to hold and cuddle the child as the child desires.
   *Crying puts additional stress on the suture line.*
9. Maintain lip protective devices if ordered.
   *Protective devices prevent separation of lip suture lines.*

**Evaluation**

Is the suture site clean, dry, and without redness, heat, or drainage?

Is the suture site intact and healing without crusting or excessive scarring?

Is the infant afebrile and demonstrating clear breath sounds?

**Nursing Diagnosis**

Acute Pain related to the surgical incision and elbow restraints.

**Planning**

***Expected Outcome***

The child will be free from pain as evidenced by ability to sleep, eat, and respond in a positive way.

**Interventions and *Rationales***

1. Describe and document pain with appropriate tools (see Chapter 39).
   *Infants and young children do not react to pain in typical adult ways, so alternative observations are needed to validate assessment findings. Parents are the best resource to validate the nurse's assessment of their infant.*
2. Provide comfort measures, especially holding, rocking, and parental voices.
   *Comforting increases parental involvement, relieves discomfort, and reduces stress on sutures caused by crying.*
3. Provide analgesics and sedatives on a regular basis as ordered. Pain should decrease significantly after 24 to 48 hours.
   *Administering medication on a regular basis can prevent peaks of pain that cannot be managed appropriately.*
4. Report pain not managed by usual means.
   *Pain may indicate hematoma formation or other complications of the repair.*

**Evaluation**

Does the child participate in age-appropriate activities?

Is the child responding well to pain medication?

Does the child appear relaxed and content at rest?

Does the parent describe a child who is not in pain?

**Nursing Diagnosis**

Ineffective Health Maintenance related to the need for long-term care.

**Planning**

***Expected Outcomes***

1. The parents will seek continued follow-up care to evaluate and manage long-term complications.
2. The child will demonstrate normal speech and hearing.

**Interventions and *Rationales***

1. Make appropriate and early referrals for any problems with speech impairment or language-based learning disabilities.
   *Speech and language learning impairments are common complications of cleft lip and palate. Early intervention minimizes harm.*
2. Monitor for recurrent or chronic otitis media.
   *Schedule frequent hearing tests. Because of craniofacial deformities, otitis media can occur frequently and must be treated to prevent language and learning problems.*
3. Encourage early speech attempts. Arrange speech therapy as needed.
   *Cleft palate can make speech difficult to understand, and the child may feel self-conscious about speech errors. Practice improves development.*
4. Encourage good dental care.
   *With abnormalities of teeth and the alveolar ridge, malocclusion and dental caries are a major concern.*

**Evaluation**

Do the parents continue to seek follow-up care (ear, nose, and throat [ENT] specialist; speech therapy; dental)?

Does the child demonstrate age-appropriate speech?

Does the child have normal hearing?

Does the child have normal dentition?

**Nursing Diagnosis**

Anxiety (parental) related to special care needs and surgery.

## NURSING CARE PLAN—cont'd

### *The Child With a Cleft Lip or Palate*

**Planning**

***Expected Outcomes***

The parents will:

1. Express concerns and fears.
2. Express control over special care needs.

**Interventions and *Rationales***

1. Use a calm, reassuring, accepting approach with the infant and family.
   *Being calm and accepting encourages communication and reinforces to parents that their child is worthwhile.*
2. Explain all procedures and their rationale, including sensations likely experienced by their child.
   *Uncertainty and loss of control contribute to increased levels of anxiety.*
3. Listen actively to parents and their concerns. Encourage verbalization of feelings, perceptions, and fears.
   *Talking and sharing may decrease anxiety.*
4. Encourage parents to stay with their child in the immediate preoperative and postoperative periods.
   *Staying with the child encourages parent participation and control over as much as possible.*

**Evaluation**

Do the parents express concerns and fears?
Do the parents seek information to decrease anxiety?
Do the parents demonstrate ability to care for their child?

primary anastomosis. If a staged repair is necessary, a gastrostomy tube (G-tube) and cervical esophagostomy are placed. Later, anastomosis, colon interposition, and dilation can be expected. Esophageal motility dysfunction, gastroesophageal reflux, strictures, bronchitis, and pneumonia can occur as the child grows, requiring evaluation and treatment.

## PATHOPHYSIOLOGY

### *Esophageal Atresia and Tracheoesophageal Fistula*

Tracheoesophageal fistula is the result of an embryonal failure to differentiate the foregut into the trachea and esophagus and the incomplete fusion of them into distinct organs. The failure occurs between the fourth and fifth week of pregnancy and can be manifested in several ways (see Fig. 43.2 for most common type).

The presence of a fistula between the esophagus and trachea allows oral intake to enter the lungs or large amounts of air to enter the stomach. Coughing, choking, and severe abdominal distention can occur. Eventually, aspiration pneumonia and severe respiratory distress will develop in the untreated child, and death can result without surgical intervention. Esophageal atresia occurring alone causes respiratory distress attributable to the aspiration of saliva and any oral fluids given before diagnosis.

## PATIENT-CENTERED TEACHING

### *Home Care of the Child With a Gastrostomy Tube*

Your child's gastrostomy tube will require special care depending on the type of tube that is used. Your nurse and physician will help you learn the following skills:

- For a new gastrostomy, clean the site daily with soap and water. If crusty drainage appears, use half-strength hydrogen peroxide to clean. Apply antimicrobial ointment if indicated. Gently rotate or turn the tube in each direction every day (Hannah & John, 2013).
- After 1 to 2 weeks, tub baths can be used to clean the site. Clean with warm water and gentle soap and dry carefully. Stomahesive Protective Powder can be used to decrease moisture.
- Keep the tube open during the initial postoperative period.
- While the site is healing, make sure the tube is stabilized. The proper stabilization technique varies with the type of gastrostomy tube.
- When the tube is well healed, it can be secured as directed for specific tube type (tape or OpSite dressing may be used).
- Use skin barriers around the stoma to prevent skin breakdown.
- Assess the site every day and report any drainage, leakage of formula, redness, or pain to your physician.
- Ask your enterostomal therapist for help in making the best choices for your child.

Remember to use a pacifier or very small amounts of fluid in a bottle every day to allow your baby to practice sucking and swallowing.

## NURSING CARE

### The Infant With Tracheoesophageal Fistula

#### Assessment

The infant with TEF is at constant risk for aspiration. Assessment for respiratory distress in the immediate period after birth is essential. The nurse must examine the infant for excessive oral secretions, choking, and cyanosis. Difficulty swallowing, regurgitation, vomiting, and unexplained cyanosis after an initial feeding in the infant who is not diagnosed at birth are important assessment findings that must be reported to the physician immediately. Abdominal distention should be measured and the infant continually assessed for distress (vital signs, respiratory effort, nasal flaring, retractions, cyanosis). A newborn assessment should be completed, with special attention to identifying any concomitant congenital defects.

Family assessment for anxiety, fears, concerns, and knowledge level will provide important information for planning nursing care and teaching.

#### Nursing Diagnosis and Planning

The nursing diagnoses and expected outcomes appropriate after assessment of the infant with TEF include the following:

- Risk for Aspiration related to TEF.

**Expected outcome.** The infant will not aspirate, as evidenced by control of oral secretions without coughing, cyanosis, or adventitious breath sounds.

- Imbalanced Nutrition: Less Than Body Requirements related to possible feeding difficulties.

**Expected outcome.** The infant will gain weight and follow growth chart at appropriate level.

- Risk for Impaired Skin Integrity related to G-tube and esophagostomy.

**Expected outcome.** The infant will maintain skin integrity, as evidenced by intact skin around the G-tube and esophagostomy.

- Risk for Infection related to surgical repair.

*Expected outcome.* The surgical site, G-tube site, and esophagostomy in the infant will remain free from infection, as evidenced by clean, intact skin without drainage, exudate, or redness.

- Acute Pain related to surgical repair.

*Expected outcome.* The infant will be free from pain, as evidenced by resumption of normal activities, ease of comforting, and relaxed facial features.

- Anxiety (parental) related to neonatal surgical emergency.

*Expected outcome.* The parents will express feelings and concerns.

- Deficient Knowledge related to home care needs and follow-up care.

*Expected outcome.* The parents will demonstrate procedures for safe G-tube feedings and site care.

**SAFETY ALERT**

***Assessing and Managing the Child With Esophageal Atresia and Tracheoesophageal Fistula***

Any child who exhibits the "three Cs" of coughing, choking with feedings, and cyanosis should be suspected of having a tracheoesophageal fistula (TEF). Esophageal atresia (EA) and TEF represent a critical neonatal surgical emergency. While the baby is awaiting transfer to a neonatal unit and surgery, management of the condition centers on preventing aspiration.

### Interventions

Nursing interventions are different in the pre- and postoperative periods. In the immediate period after birth, placing the newborn in a radiant warmer and administering humidified oxygen are essential to relieve respiratory distress. The child is prepared for surgery, remains on nothing by mouth (NPO) status, and is hydrated with IV fluids. Maintaining thermoregulation and fluid balance is essential, so monitoring temperature and other vital signs, using radiant warmers, and keeping accurate intake and output records are important.

*Minimizing aspiration risk.* The risk of aspiration must be minimized. A chalasia board that helps keep the child at a 30-degree angle while supine can be useful to decrease reflux. Placing a suction catheter in the proximal pouch and mouth will keep secretions to a minimum. Constant assessment of respiratory status and antibiotic administration to prevent pneumonia are essential. Even after surgical repair, these children are prone to gastroesophageal reflux.

*Postoperative care.* In the immediate postoperative period, monitoring respiratory status, supporting fluid balance and nutrition, maintaining thermoregulation, providing pain relief, monitoring for infection, and promoting bonding with parents take priority. The child will probably have a chest tube in place; patency must be maintained, suction monitored, and output documented. Respiratory rate and effort and the presence of abnormal breath sounds should be documented. Thermoregulation can significantly affect respiratory status in the newborn, so monitoring and maintaining temperature with a radiant warmer may be necessary.

IV fluids, antibiotics, and parenteral nutrition may be ordered. The nurse must maintain patency of the IV line; monitor intake and output; and assess for signs of fluid and electrolyte alterations, including sunken fontanel and increased urine specific gravity measurements. Daily weights and measurement of head circumference can aid in assessing growth. Pain medications must be administered as needed on the basis of objective pain assessment measures.

If a cervical esophagostomy has been performed as the first stage of a surgical repair, it is kept covered with gauze to absorb saliva and provide skin care. Frequent cleaning and assessing for redness, breakdown, or exudate are essential because the skin in this wet area can easily become macerated and infected. Referral to an enterostomal therapist can be helpful in teaching parents esophagostomy care.

*Gastrostomy tube use.* In the immediate postoperative period, the G-tube is left open to drainage to allow gastric contents and air to escape; this setup promotes comfort and decreases the risk of pressure at the anastomosis. A pacifier satisfies sucking needs, provides early training in swallowing, makes later feeding easier, and provides comfort through distraction. Pacifiers should not be offered until the child can manage oral secretions.

Numerous types of G-tubes are available for placement, either percutaneously (percutaneous endoscopic gastronomy [PEG] tube) or during surgery. Among these are traditional G-tubes, which are anchored in place by an air- or saline-inflated balloon, as well as more innovative tubes that use various means for anchoring. The skin-level gastrostomy button (MIC-KEY) enables the secure connection of extension tubing to the gastrostomy site and is easy for parents to use (Fig. 43.3). Tube selection is usually made by the physician, but long-term successful care and use of the tube are nursing and parental responsibilities.

*Home care.* Parents should be taught the techniques of G-tube feeding and care (see Patient-Centered Teaching: Home Care of the Child with a Gastrostomy Tube). Skin care at the site may include using half-strength hydrogen peroxide to remove crusty drainage, rotating the tube, and using a skin barrier product, as well as other ostomy skin care products. Redness, exudate, pus, heat, or leakage of formula should be reported.

Parent education and support are critical components. Home care between stages of repair requires extra support from community healthcare providers and demonstration of parental proficiency in skin care, suctioning, gastrostomy feedings, and cardiopulmonary resuscitation. Such support should include discussing feelings and anxieties, providing information about home care, practicing special techniques, providing stimulation to the infant, and using appropriate resources such as enterostomal therapists and dietitians.

### Evaluation

- Can the child coordinate sucking and swallowing?
- Is the child tolerating oral feedings without choking, coughing, or becoming cyanotic?
- Is the child growing according to the growth chart?
- Is the surgical site clean, dry, intact, and free of redness, drainage, or exudate?

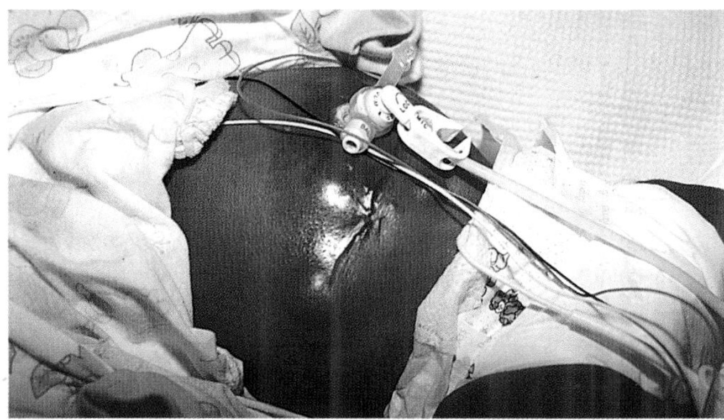

**FIG 43.3** The skin-level gastrostomy button is good for children who require long-term gastrostomy feeding. It is relatively flat, reduces skin breakdown, increases comfort, and is fully immersible in water. (Courtesy Parkland Health and Hospital System, Dallas, TX.)

- Is the skin intact and without breakdown around the G-tube and esophagostomy?
- Is the child resting contently without pain medication?
- Can the parents explain the need for the surgical procedure?
- Do parents demonstrate appropriate care of the G-tube?
- Have parents assumed all care responsibilities?

## Upper Gastrointestinal Hernias

A hernia is an abnormal protrusion of part of an organ or tissue through the structures that normally contain it. Hernias can be either congenital or acquired. Some hernias can be reduced; others become incarcerated, and the protruding organ segment cannot be returned by manipulation to the anatomically correct location. A medical emergency occurs when a hernia becomes strangulated and blood supply is cut off. This condition can occur suddenly and requires immediate treatment. The most common hernias of the upper GI tract are discussed in Table 43.1.

## Other Developmental Disorders

Table 43.2 discusses other developmental disorders of the upper and lower GI tracts.

## PATIENT-CENTERED TEACHING

### *Care of the Child With Infectious Gastroenteritis*

If your child has infectious gastroenteritis, you must do the following:

- Wash your hands frequently and thoroughly and insist that your child do so as well. Always wash your hands after changing diapers.
- Allow your child to use a separate bathroom if available.
- Continue to follow these measures for several weeks because bacterial diarrhea is sometimes communicable for several weeks after symptoms disappear.
- Administer oral fluids with appropriate rehydration solutions (e.g., Pedialyte, Rehydralyte) in small, frequent amounts (every 30 minutes). If your child is vomiting, administer 1 teaspoon of fluid every 5 to 10 minutes. Give one half cup for each watery stool.
- Do not give your child fruit juices, cola, sports drinks, tea, or sugary drinks.
- Continue to feed your child, but avoid high-fat or high-sugar foods. Breast milk and formula can be continued.
- Do not give over-the-counter medications without notifying your physician.

Call your physician if the following pertain:

- Your child is younger than 6 months.
- Your child has a fever.
- Diarrhea worsens.
- Diarrhea has blood in it.
- Vomiting increases or your child cannot keep down any fluid.
- Your child reports severe abdominal pain.
- Your child shows signs of dehydration, such as no tears, sunken eyes, or decreased urination.

## TABLE 43.1 Upper GI Hernias

| Description | Clinical Manifestations | Therapeutic Management | Nursing Management |
|---|---|---|---|
| **Hiatal Hernia** | | | |
| Protrusion of a portion of the stomach through the esophageal hiatus of the diaphragm | Vomiting<br>Abdominal pain<br>Coughing, wheezing, short periods of apnea<br>Failure to thrive | Medical management similar to that for the child with reflux<br>Surgical repair of defect if medical treatment fails | Monitor intake and output. Document vomiting. Observe for respiratory distress. Provide routine postoperative care for GI surgery.<br>Teach parents about surgery and medical treatment of reflux. |
| **Congenital Diaphragmatic Hernia (CDH)** | | | |
| Opening in the diaphragm through which abdominal contents herniate into the thoracic cavity during prenatal development; usually involving abnormal development at 6 to 10 weeks gestation (Sfakianaki, 2012).<br>Results in some degree of pulmonary hypoplasia and pulmonary hypertension, determined by the timing and size of the herniation.<br>Mortality rate: 50%-80%; 40% if extracorporeal membrane oxygenation (ECMO) used.<br>Degree of pulmonary hypoplasia determines outcome.<br>Incidence: 1 in 2000-5000 live births (Maheshwari & Carlo, 2016). | Clinical findings depend on severity of defect.<br>• Abdominal organs in chest (by fetal ultrasonography)<br>• Diminished or absent breath sounds on affected side<br>• Bowel sounds that are heard over the chest<br>• Cardiac sounds heard on the right side of the chest<br>• Respiratory distress developing soon after birth—dyspnea, cyanosis, nasal flaring, tachypnea, retractions<br>• Scaphoid abdomen | If diagnosed prenatally, mother moved to tertiary care center before delivery<br>In utero surgery possible<br>Neonatal emergency NG intubation with suction<br>High-frequency ventilation required<br>Acidosis managed with bicarbonate and ventilation<br>ECMO<br>Liquid ventilation<br>Manage pulmonary hypertension; inhaled nitric oxide may be used.<br>Surgical reduction of hernia after physiologically stable; often delayed until 6-18 hr after birth.<br>Respiratory support and ECMO until lungs are functioning after surgery | Identify clinical findings and report immediately.<br>Place child in semi-Fowler position on affected side with head of bed elevated.<br>Maintain patency of NG tube.<br>Monitor IV fluids.<br>Maintain mechanical ventilation, ECMO, chest tubes.<br>Assess oxygenation.<br>Do not use facemask or bag-valve-mask for ventilatory support because air can enter stomach and further impair respiratory function.<br>Provide minimal stimulation.<br>Provide routine postoperative care.<br>Monitor for signs of infection, respiratory distress, and feeding difficulties; report to physician.<br>Support family mourning loss of perfect child.<br>Provide clear, truthful information to parents.<br>Encourage parents to see and touch the infant.<br>Use prescribed feeding techniques.<br>Provide referral to support groups.<br>Provide discharge teaching. |

*GI*, Gastrointestinal; *IV*, intravenous; *NG*, nasogastric.

**TABLE 43.2 Developmental GI Defects**

| *Imperforate Anus* | *Gastroschisis* | *Omphalocele* | *Umbilical Hernia* |
|---|---|---|---|
| **Pathophysiology, Etiology, and Clinical Manifestations** | | | |
| Incomplete development or absence of the anus in its normal position in the perineum.<br>Defect can be high (above the levator ani muscle) or low (below the levator ani muscle).<br>Symptoms include failure to pass meconium stool, absence of anorectal canal, presence of an anal membrane, external fistula to the perineum.<br>Condition is diagnosed during the newborn examination with radiography, ultrasound, or CT scan used to determine the level of the lesion and associated anomalies. | Embryonal weakness in abdominal wall causes herniation of intestines on one side of umbilical cord during early development, most commonly on right side.<br>Viscera are outside the abdominal cavity and are not covered with the sac. | Large herniation of intestines into umbilical cord.<br>Viscera are outside the abdominal cavity but inside translucent sac, covered with peritoneum and amniotic membrane. | Imperfect closure of umbilical ring allows intestines to push outward at umbilicus during straining and crying.<br>Viscera are inside the abdominal cavity and under the skin.<br>The hernia is usually 1–3 cm and easily reduced. |
| **Incidence** | | | |
| 1 in 4000-5000 live births<br>More common in male infants | 4.9/10,000 live births<br>Incidence is increasing (Jones et al., 2016) | 1.5-3 in 10,000 live births (Spatz & Schmidt, 2012) | Most common in low birth weight and black infants |
| **Associated Anomalies** | | | |
| Genitourinary, sacral, or additional GI anomalies | Prematurity<br>Malrotation of intestines<br>Decreased abdominal capacity<br>Higher incidence of Meckel diverticulum<br>Atresia, stenosis, and other anomalies rare | Malrotation of intestines<br>Decreased abdominal capacity<br>Atresia and stenosis common<br>Higher incidence of Meckel diverticulum<br>Cardiac, genitourinary, or chromosomal anomalies in ⅓ to ½ of cases<br>Associated with Beckwith-Wiedemann syndrome (hypoglycemia, macrosomia, macroglossia) | Commonly occurs in children with Down syndrome, hypothyroidism, Hurler syndrome. |
| **Morbidity and Mortality** | | | |
| Prognosis depends on the level of the lesion.<br>Complete continence may be impossible. | Mortality rate 10%-15%.Death due to massive bowel loss and intestinal necrosis (Ledbetter, 2012) | Mortality rate 20%-30%.<br>Sepsis and intestinal obstruction common | Minimal |
| **Therapeutic Management** | | | |
| Anal stenosis is treated with repeated dilations.<br>All other defects require surgical intervention.<br>High defects may require a colostomy and bowel pull-through procedure. | IV and NG tubes are placed immediately.<br>TPN is provided.<br>Synthetic material (Silastic) is used to cover the intestines.<br>If defect is large, it is closed surgically after all contents have been returned to the abdominal cavity, which takes days or weeks.<br>Even if the defect is small, immediate surgical repair may be done in several stages.<br>If the condition is diagnosed prenatally, a C-section is recommended.<br>Necrotic bowel requires surgical removal. | IV and NG tubes are placed.<br>TPN is provided. Silastic is used to cover the sac if ruptured or if the defect is large. Surgical correction is similar to gastroschisis.<br>C-section delivery if diagnosed prenatally. | Most umbilical hernias disappear spontaneously by age 1 yr.<br>No surgical repair is necessary unless the hernia causes symptoms, persists past age 5 yr, becomes strangulated, or enlarges. |

**TABLE 43.2 Developmental GI Defects—cont'd**

| *Imperforate Anus* | *Gastroschisis* | *Omphalocele* | *Umbilical Hernia* |
|---|---|---|---|
| **Nursing Care** | | | |
| Report any skin dimples or the presence of stool in the urine or vagina.<br>Determine anal patency if meconium is not passed in the first 24 hr after birth.<br>Assess for other GI or genitourinary anomalies.<br>Facilitate bonding.<br>Provide appropriate postoperative care, including care of the colostomy. | Thermoregulation is critical because significant heat loss can occur through the exposed intestines. Use warmers and monitor the child's temperature.<br>Use sterile technique in dealing with the defect; immediately cover it with warm, moist, sterile gauze and wrap with plastic to keep moist.<br>Minimize movement of the infant and handling of the intestines.<br>Assess for circulatory compromise, obstruction, sepsis.<br>Monitor temperature, pulses, capillary refill time, skin color, changes in respiratory patterns, heart rate.<br>Observe for respiratory distress from high intraabdominal pressure as the intestines return to the peritoneal cavity.<br>Fluid volume management is a crucial nursing responsibility.<br>Monitor intake and output and daily weights, assess fontanels, monitor electrolytes, and maintain IV line.<br>Postoperatively, monitor and manage ileus, which commonly lasts for 2-4 wk.<br>Maintain NG tube for decompression, monitor bowel sounds and stools, measure abdominal girth.<br>Maintain TPN to sustain growth.<br>Recent research demonstrates improved success with earlier initiation of enteral feedings, especially when human milk is used (Kohler, Perkins, & Bass, 2013).<br>Offer pacifier to meet sucking needs.<br>Provide emotional support for parents as they deal with the loss of the "perfect child."<br>Encourage parents to provide care so they can talk to, touch, and hold the infant, when appropriate. | Same as for gastroschisis. | Binding is not effective in reducing or minimizing the bulge.<br>Monitor for changes in size of hernia.<br>Assess for changing bowel sounds and presence of an irreducible mass, which suggests strangulation. |
| **Teaching and Home Care** | | | |
| Teach parents colostomy care.<br>Demonstrate anal dilation (use only prescribed dilator, insert no more than 1-2 cm, and use a water-soluble lubricant).<br>Refer parents for counseling and support (March of Dimes Birth Defects Foundation, http://www.marchofdimes.org).<br>Provide guidance for toilet training. | Encourage parents to hold, cuddle, and bond with infant as soon as possible.<br>Provide developmental stimulation during long-term hospitalization.<br>Assist parents in dealing with feelings of guilt and disappointment.<br>Use pictures to help parents understand the defect.<br>Contact national support groups and community resources (e.g., March of Dimes).<br>Teach parents signs of bowel obstruction: vomiting, pain, irritability, anorexia, firm abdomen.<br>Provide follow-up from nutritional support personnel as needed. | Same as for gastroschisis. | Teach parents signs of strangulation: vomiting, pain, irreducible mass at umbilicus.<br>Contact physician immediately if strangulation is suspected. |

*CT*, Computed tomography; *GI*, gastrointestinal; *IV*, intravenous; *NG*, nasogastric; *TPN*, total parental nutrition.

## MOTILITY DISORDERS

### Gastroesophageal Reflux Disease

Gastroesophageal reflux (GER) is regurgitation of gastric contents back into the esophagus. GER is a normal physiologic phenomenon; all adults and infants periodically experience reflux, especially after meals. GER disease (GERD) is a more severe and chronic form that causes symptoms such as irritability, frequent back arching, esophagitis and failure to thrive. Reflux can be divided into two types: physiologic GER and pathologic GERD (Box 43.1).

#### Etiology

Many factors contribute to the development of GERD. Neurologic impairments such as cerebral palsy, Down syndrome, and head injury can affect the transmission of neural signals to the lower esophageal sphincter (LES). Delayed gastric emptying of a liquid meal because of distention can contribute. Partial or incomplete swallowing dysfunction or drugs such as theophylline or caffeine can also trigger LES relaxations. Increased intraabdominal pressure incurred while straining, crying, coughing, or slumping tends to promote increased episodes of GER. These postural effects are most likely primary contributing factors in infants. Obesity and hiatal hernias also promote GERD. Finally, during the first 6 months of life, the LES pressure undergoes maturational development. Because infants have a short abdominal LES, they have GER more often. As the infant grows, the LES matures and the reflux improves. The prognosis is likely related to the severity of symptoms. Reflux from maturational causes will likely resolve by 1 to 2 years of age.

#### Incidence

Approximately 67% of healthy infants aged 4 to 5 months have signs of GER. The peak incidence of GER occurs at approximately 4 months of age and decreases thereafter, so that less than 5% of children experience symptoms by the time they reach 1 year old (Neu, Corwin, Lareau, et al., 2012). The incidence of neonatal GER is higher in infants with medical comorbidities and in those who are born prematurely (Halbert, 2011).

#### Manifestations and Diagnostic Evaluation

Vomiting or spitting up after a meal, hiccupping, and recurrent otitis media related to pooled secretions in the nasopharynx during sleep are the hallmarks of GERD. In addition, the infant with pathologic GERD can experience weight loss, failure to thrive, irritability, discomfort, and abdominal pain. Severe GERD can result in hematemesis or melena and anemia. Frequently, respiratory illness or asthma is associated with GERD, and the child may experience coughing, choking, asthma, wheezing, pneumonia, apnea, or bradycardia.

A variety of chronic and acute illnesses have been associated with GERD. GERD should be confirmed only after other major conditions have been ruled out. In infants, signs and symptoms obtained through a comprehensive feeding and nutritional history can establish the diagnosis (Kahn & Orenstein, 2016b). Diagnostic tests in older children or those infants and children not amenable to treatment are classified as diagnostic tests to measure reflux events (pH monitoring, barium fluoroscopy, scintigraphy) or the consequences of the reflux events (esophagogastroscopy) (van der Pol, Smits, Vanmans, et al., 2013).

> **BOX 43.1 Types of Gastroesophageal Reflux**
>
> **Physiologic (Gastroesophageal Reflux [GER])**
> - Painless emesis after meals
> - Parents might be unconcerned or think it is normal
> - Rarely occurs during sleep
> - No failure to thrive
> - 40% asymptomatic by 3 months
> - 70% asymptomatic by 18 months
> - Pharmacologic and medical management very effective
>
> **Pathologic (Gastroesophageal Reflux Disease [GERD])**
> - Failure to thrive
> - Aspiration pneumonia and/or asthma
> - Apnea, coughing, and choking
> - Frequent emesis, abdominal pain, and crying
> - May require surgery and pharmacologic treatment

#### Therapeutic Management

Therapy for GERD is based on the severity of symptoms and includes dietary alterations, positional changes, medications, and surgery. Early treatment may prevent or lessen complications such as failure to thrive, esophagitis, and strictures. Many infants suspected of functional GER are treated conservatively with pharmacologic support. The American Academy of Pediatrics supports the North American Society for Pediatric Gastroenterology, Hepatology, and Nutrition (NASPGHAN) positioning guidelines for managing the child with gastroesophageal reflux.

***Diet.*** Small, frequent feedings with frequent burping are often tried as the first line of treatment. These smaller feedings can help to minimize the frequency of reflux but may be impractical for the caregiver. Severe restrictions in feeding can adversely affect the child's weight gain. NASPGHAN guidelines support the trial of hydrolyzed or amino acid formula in formula-fed babies with recurrent regurgitation and vomiting. Breastfed infants may benefit from a trial of withdrawal of cow's milk protein and eggs from the maternal diet. Feedings thickened with rice cereal (1 tbsp/oz) may decrease the frequency of daily regurgitation and emesis (Halbert, 2011; Neu et al., 2012). Thickened feedings also tend to decrease crying and increase weight gain in infants (Kahn & Orenstein, 2016b). Concentrated, high-calorie formulas and NG-tube feedings provide nutritional supplementation for the child with failure to thrive. Caffeinated, carbonated, acidic, spicy, and fatty foods all lower LES pressure and should be eliminated.

***Positioning.*** Much attention has been given to the best positioning for GER. Although prone positioning more effectively reduces reflux, current recommendations from the American Academy of Pediatrics and NASPGHAN are that infants younger than 12 months should be placed supine to sleep to reduce the risk of sudden infant death syndrome (SIDS), even if an infant is diagnosed with GERD. The only exception to this recommendation would be if the risk of death from aspiration or other complications of GERD greatly outweighed the increased risk from the prone positioning (Kahn & Orenstein, 2016b). However, when infants are awake, the use of the prone position with monitoring or the upright carried position can decrease reflux (Halbert, 2011). Elevating the head of the bed improves the condition of older children with GERD.

***Medications.*** Although the U.S. Food and Drug Administration (FDA) has not approved many medications used in the treatment of GERD for children, their use in children is common, and many are now available over-the-counter. Medications are often added to the treatment protocol. These medications include antacids for symptom relief, proton pump inhibitors (e.g., omeprazole and lansoprazole), $H_2$-receptor antagonists (e.g., cimetidine, ranitidine) to decrease acid secretion, and prokinetic agents (e.g., erythromycin, metoclopramide) to accelerate gastric emptying and improve esophageal and intestinal peristalsis. Antidopaminergic agents (e.g., metoclopramide) facilitate gastric emptying.

*Treatment of acute bleeding.* Bleeding is a complication of long-standing GERD and esophagitis. Stomach lavage (washing) with an NG tube is commonly performed to evacuate blood and blood clots during an episode of upper GI bleeding. The use of iced saline lavage to stop bleeding is no longer advocated. Radiologic procedures or surgery to coagulate bleeding vessels may be needed.

## PATHOPHYSIOLOGY

### *Gastroesophageal Reflux*

The lower esophageal sphincter (LES), a zone of tonically contracted smooth muscle surrounding the distal esophagus, is innervated by vagal nerves and receives signals from multiple organs. A defect in this neural control can lead to dysfunction of the LES, with periods of transitory spontaneous relaxation. These periods of relaxation allow gastric contents to reflux back into the esophagus.

In addition, the esophagus traverses both the abdominal and thoracic cavities, with the LES positioned strategically between the two. Most of the LES is abdominal. The greater the length of intraabdominal esophagus, the more competent this valve becomes. Any condition that shortens the abdominal segment of the LES will increase the likelihood of reflux.

*Surgery.* Children who continue to have severe complications from GERD may be candidates for fundoplication surgery. A 270 degree partial wrap (Toupet Fundoplication) or the more common complete 360 degree wrap (Nissen Fundoplication) to the stomach fundus is made around the distal esophagus (Halbert, 2011). This procedure tightens the LES and prevents gastric reflux. Gas bloat syndrome may develop because of the child's inability to burp, and a G-tube may be temporarily needed for gastric decompression. Continuance of the pharmacologic treatment regimen may be needed after surgery.

## NURSING CARE

### The Infant With Gastroesophageal Reflux Disease

#### Assessment

The nurse initially obtains a thorough history related to feedings (amount, frequency, formula changes, positioning); the frequency, pattern, and characteristics of vomiting/emesis (i.e., projectile, painful, bloody); and respiratory illness/symptoms including pneumonia, asthma, apnea, wheezing, choking, coughing, or cyanosis. Unusual postural habits (head cocking, arching, arm thrashing) that can indicate discomfort due to esophagitis are assessed. The infant is observed during feedings to assess feeding behaviors, comfort (pain) level, dysphagia, and regurgitation. The chest is auscultated for adventitious breath sounds, and the infant is assessed for signs of respiratory distress, including retractions. The infant's length, weight, and head circumference are plotted on standard growth charts based on age. The nurse monitors the parent–child interactions and feeding styles. Parents are encouraged to discuss their feelings and concerns about caring for their infant with GERD.

#### Nursing Diagnosis and Planning

The following nursing diagnoses and expected outcomes may be appropriate after assessing the infant with GERD:

- Risk for Aspiration related to GERD.

*Expected outcome.* The infant will maintain a patent airway without signs of respiratory distress.

- Deficient Fluid Volume related to decreased intake and frequent vomiting.

*Expected outcomes.* The infant will swallow and retain each feeding with regurgitation of less than 10 mL. The infant will not become fluid-volume deficient.

- Imbalanced Nutrition: Less Than Body Requirements related to dysphagia and reflux.

*Expected outcome.* The infant will gain weight and grow according to standardized growth charts.

- Deficient Knowledge related to disease process, total care, and medications.

*Expected outcomes.* The parents will explain GERD and demonstrate appropriate techniques for feeding, medication administration, and cardiopulmonary resuscitation (CPR). The parents will state correct purpose, dosage, schedule, and side effects for prescribed medications.

- Anxiety (parents) related to long-term care of the infant with GERD.

*Expected outcomes.* The parents will exhibit effective coping mechanisms. Adequate support systems are in place.

#### Interventions

It is critically important that the infant be carefully monitored for any signs of respiratory distress or periods of apnea using a cardiac and/or apnea monitor plus frequent observation and vital signs checks by the nurse. Proper positioning (upright or prone, if awake) and minimal handling after feedings can decrease reflux and aspiration risk. Pacifier use reduces crying and encourages swallowing.

*Minimizing reflux.* Multiple measures that should be used to minimize reflux include small feedings (1 to 3 oz) every 2 to 3 hours, use of breast milk or predigested formulas that are thickened with rice cereal (1 to 3 tsp/oz), frequent burping, and medications. Bottle nipples are cross-cut to enlarge the opening for thickened formula. The infant with frequent reflux and vomiting must be thoroughly assessed for signs of fluid-volume deficit (dehydration): sunken fontanel, no tears when crying, dry mucous membranes (mouth), poor skin turgor, and low urine output (fewer wet diapers). Weight should be checked daily to assess stability and gains. Weight, length, and head circumference are periodically measured and plotted on charts to monitor nutritional status and growth.

*Family education and support.* Family education and support are vital. The nurse begins educating the parents so they learn what GERD is and how this chronic disease is managed. It is explained that different formulas, feeding routines, and medications will be tried to determine what works best for their infant. The possibility of surgical treatment is discussed. Parents are taught the purpose, dosage, schedule, and side effects for each medication prescribed. The nurse shows parents how to monitor and care for their infant and then encourages them to practice assessment, positioning, formula preparation, feeding techniques, and medication administration with supervision until they demonstrate proficiency. Training for parents in infant CPR is mandatory. Parents of infants with GERD may feel overwhelmed by the complex healthcare needs of their infant and anxiety regarding their ability to care for their child on a long-term basis. The nurse encourages open communication so that parents will share their concerns and fears. Referrals to community agencies and services can significantly increase parental competency. Support from other parents of children with GERD can improve coping.

#### Evaluation

- Is the infant's airway patent, without choking, coughing, cyanosis, or retractions?
- Can the infant swallow without incurring respiratory distress?

- Can the infant retain feedings with regurgitation of less than 10 mL?
- Is the infant adequately hydrated?
- Is the child growing according to growth charts?
- Is the child receiving medications as prescribed at the correct times and in the correct dosage?
- Can the parents explain GERD and the reasons for positioning and dietary modifications?
- Are parents using correct feeding techniques?
- Have the parents demonstrated the ability to provide total care for their infant?
- Have the parents expressed concerns and feelings related to caring for their infant?
- Do parents have adequate support systems and demonstrate effective coping strategies?

## Constipation and Encopresis

Constipation is defined as a delay or difficulty in defecation that has been present for 2 or more weeks. A major concern with constipation is the development of encopresis or fecal incontinence. Encopresis is repeated, involuntary defecation in a child older than 4 years who has a normal colon and rectal anatomy. With encopresis, children often report that soiling occurs without warning. Parents find the situation frustrating, and soiling often becomes a major issue between the parent and child. Often encopresis causes children to feel ashamed or embarrassed, and they may avoid situations in which embarrassment might be heightened, such as spending the night with a friend or even going to school. If the condition persists over a long period, it usually affects the child's self-esteem and may impair social relations. Parents can experience a range of emotions, including guilt, shame, disgust, or anger, and they may project these feelings onto the child.

### PATHOPHYSIOLOGY

#### *Constipation and Encopresis*

When stool passes into the rectum, distention of the walls stimulates mass peristaltic movements in the bowel. This process is called the defecation reflex. If defecation is not desired, the external sphincter contracts and voluntary retention of stool occurs. As the stool remains in the rectum, the rectum relaxes and the defecation reflex wanes. Water reabsorption from the colon continues, resulting in hard, dry stool that is difficult to pass. The eventual passage of that stool can cause pain or anal fissures. If retention of stool continues, more fissures develop or become worse, so that eventually even soft stool produces pain. A cycle of pain develops in which the stool is retained to avoid pain but the retention leads to even more difficult defecation. Over time, the rectum becomes enlarged. An enlarged rectum can result in failure to control the external sphincter, which in turn results in encopresis.

### Etiology and Incidence

Constipation can have many causes, such as changes in diet, dehydration, lack of exercise, emotional stress, certain drugs, pain from anal fissures, or excessive milk intake. If the child has no neurologic or anatomic disorders, encopresis is usually the result of recurrent fecal impaction and an enlarged rectum caused by chronic constipation. Factors predisposing to encopresis include inadequate or inconsistent toilet training or some type of psychological stress, such as starting school or the birth of a sibling.

Constipation can affect any child at any time. At least 3% of all visits to the pediatrician and at least 25% of pediatric gastroenterologist visits are related to constipation (Ambartsumyan & Rodriguez, 2014; Petersen, 2014). Encopresis affects an estimated 1.5% of young children, with six times more boys than girls affected (AAP, 2015a). Encopresis can be classified as primary (never been continent of stool) or secondary (incontinent after a period of continence). The incidence of encopresis is higher in lower socioeconomic classes and among children with learning disabilities.

### Manifestations

***Constipation.*** The principal symptoms of constipation are the absence of stool, abdominal pain and cramping without distention, and palpable, movable fecal masses with large amounts of stool in an enlarged rectum. The child may also experience diarrheal overflow, normal or decreased bowel sounds, malaise, anorexia, headache, nausea, vomiting, and anal fissures.

***Encopresis.*** Children with encopresis have evidence of soiled clothing and fecal odor without apparent awareness. Anal irritation leads to scratching or rubbing of the anal area. Social withdrawal and avoidance of extended contact with others (e.g., overnight stays, camp) are common. Urinary incontinence and urinary tract infections may also be present.

### Diagnostic Evaluation

Abdominal radiographs may demonstrate an enlarged rectum with large amounts of stool and gas. The definitive diagnostic procedure is a rectal examination. This is rarely performed because of its emotional impact on the child and the possibility of pain from anal fissures. A thorough history is usually sufficient for the diagnosis. In children presenting to the emergency department with abdominal pain, constipation is the most common diagnosis (Caperell, Pitetti, & Cross, 2013).

### Therapeutic Management

The best form of treatment is preventing the development of a chronic problem through appropriate diet, exercise, and regular toileting habits. Education about "normal" bowel function can prevent a psychogenic component from compounding the problem. Normal frequency is 1.2 stools per day for a child 4 years and older (Petersen, 2014). The focus of management is to remove the impaction, retrain the rectum so the child is aware when it is full, and help the child overcome the pain-retention cycle.

Treatment usually involves the following phases (Fiorino & Liacouras, 2016a; Petersen, 2014):

1. Disimpaction (critical prior to maintenance treatment for success of management)
   a. Enemas until impaction is cleared; use Fleet, 1 oz/5 kg; if the child is larger than 20 kg, use an adult size.
   b. Stool softener or laxative (osmotic and stimulant) including mineral oil, lactulose, magnesium hydroxide, GlycoLax, senna, and bisacodyl.
2. Education/demystification
   a. Extensive discussion with child and family about causes of constipation (diagrams are helpful) and discussion about feelings, social consequences, and embarrassment. The child and family need to be assessed for readiness to change.
3. Maintenance
   a. Mineral oil (1 to 3 mL/kg/day) twice a day for children older than 1 year with a low risk of vomiting or aspiration.
   b. Lactulose (10 g/15 mL), 1 or 3 mL/kg twice daily, or polyethylene glycol 3350 (1 to 2 g/kg/day).
   c. Dietary changes, including limiting milk intake, increasing water and fiber intake, and increasing residue.
4. Changing the retention habit

a. Sitting on the commode for 5 to 10 minutes approximately 20 to 30 minutes after meals.
b. Keeping a behavioral chart with positive rewards (daily stars may be helpful).
c. Avoiding negative reinforcement.
d. Using biofeedback, a potentially useful tool to reteach the feeling of rectal fullness.
e. Increasing physical exercise, relaxation activities, and the use of stress reduction approaches to decrease anxiety.

The goal is for the child to pass two or three soft stools per day without pain within the first month following treatment. Medications are withdrawn slowly over a 3- to 6-month period after the fear of pain is gone or significantly diminished.

For infant constipation, rectal stimulation is discouraged. For example, rectal thermometers and glycerin suppositories should not be used. Barley cereal can be substituted for rice cereal. Ingestions of fructose (prune juice) or lactulose can help. High-fiber fruits and vegetables will also decrease constipation.

## NURSING CARE

### The Child With Constipation or Encopresis

#### Assessment

Obtain a thorough history of the soiling events, including frequency, intensity, and duration. Because parent–child relationships are often strained, interview the parents and child separately to reduce the child's embarrassment. The nurse can explain to parents that a medical history and examination will be performed to rule out organic causes of the chronic constipation, such as Hirschsprung disease.

#### Nursing Diagnosis and Planning

The following nursing diagnoses and expected outcomes may be appropriate after assessing for constipation or encopresis in the child:

- Constipation or Bowel Incontinence related to inconsistent patterns of elimination, anxiety, or pain during elimination.

*Expected outcome.* The child will have normal bowel function, as evidenced by the passage of soft stools without pain or incontinence, maintenance of a well-balanced diet high in fiber and sufficient fluid intake, and decreased reliance on laxatives.

- Compromised or Disabled Family Coping related to persistent stress, guilt, and embarrassment about the child's elimination difficulty.

*Expected outcome.* The family will function effectively as a unit, openly discuss problems, and develop a plan to achieve control over incontinence.

- Social Isolation related to embarrassment, peer teasing, and odor from bowel incontinence.

*Expected outcome.* The child will verbalize positive, realistic feelings about self and verbalize appropriate ways to achieve control over bowel incontinence.

- Impaired Skin Integrity related to poor hygiene in anal area, bowel incontinence, and lack of knowledge.

*Expected outcome.* The child will maintain skin integrity, as evidenced by clean, intact skin.

#### Interventions

Because constipation and encopresis represent a continuum of the same problem, a variety of approaches can be tried as needed to treat the problem. Simple constipation may resolve with only dietary changes or changing a habit of retention. Severe encopresis may require that multiple interventions be continued for 3 to 6 months.

*Overcoming withholding.* Before bowel retraining can begin, the child's bowel must be evacuated of all hard stool and impactions. This goal is best accomplished with the use of an appropriate size Fleet or isotonic enema every 12 hours until the impaction is cleared, usually within 48 hours. As indicated, parents are taught to administer enemas at home. During this time, the child should be monitored for hypernatremia or hyperphosphatemia, which could result from the repeated use of Fleet enemas (see Chapter 37 for a discussion of enema administration).

After bowel cleansing has been achieved, the child older than 1 year may be started on mineral oil or another maintenance laxative. Lactulose may be used in infants at least 6 months old but younger than 12 months. Mineral oil is best tolerated when it is given chilled or mixed with cold drinks. The oil can be mixed with ice cream or chocolate milk, blended with ice cubes and fruit juice, or chilled to help disguise the taste. Mineral oil should not be given if the child is vomiting, as aspiration could lead to hydrocarbon pneumonia. The child may leak oil from the rectum when dosages are high, thus parents and children need to be aware that leakage does not constitute encopresis. At the end of this intervention, the child should pass soft stools without pain or incontinence. Parents should be advised to adjust the laxative doses based on the characteristics of stool.

*Dietary changes.* Dietary modifications are used as a part of the treatment. Increasing water and fiber intake by offering granola bars, dried fruits, whole-grain cereals, and fresh vegetables with low-fat dip can increase the bulk in stool and make it easier to pass. Decreasing sugar and milk intake also helps keep stools soft. It may be advised to supplement with fat-soluble vitamins when mineral oil is being used because the oil potentially interferes with vitamin absorption in the small intestine. Dietary guidelines are available at http://health.gov/dietaryguidelines/2015/guidelines/.

*Changing the retention habit.* To help reestablish a normal bowel habit, the child should sit on the toilet for 5 to 10 minutes after breakfast and dinner. This routine will allow the normal gastrocolic reflex to assist with defecation and will eliminate the need to be involved with retraining during school hours. Star charts and small prizes, such as stickers, may be helpful in rewarding success. These interventions are continued for at least 3 to 6 months, during which the rectum will resume its normal size and the child will relearn to attend to the defecation reflex. If fecal impaction occurs at any time, enemas are again administered and the dosage of mineral oil is adjusted.

*Emotional support.* The child and parents are encouraged to express their feelings of success and failure with the ongoing program. To minimize the damage to the child's self-esteem, the nurse encourages self-care as much as possible. To decrease embarrassment, school-age children should have a complete change of pants and underwear at school if leakage occurs. Age-appropriate support groups may be available in a center with a large patient population or encopresis clinic.

Although teaching is a major intervention, encouraging the child and parents to share feelings of embarrassment and other concerns is equally important. The child is provided developmentally appropriate anatomic information to assist with understanding the cause of the problem. Drawings and books may be effective ways to begin providing information and prompting the child to share feelings. Relieving the child of shame and embarrassment may improve cooperation with the plan of care.

*Home care.* Because this condition is managed at home, extensive education of the parents is required. The parents need to understand the correct way to administer enemas (see Chapter 37), adjust the child's diet, give medications, and initiate bowel retraining. They also need support in implementing and documenting the child's successes and setbacks. The child and parents need encouragement to continue the program, even when the successes seem few. This problem develops over time and takes time, patience, and perseverance to resolve.

### Evaluation

- Is the child passing soft stools without pain?
- Does the food diary indicate a well-balanced, high-fiber diet?
- Is the child experiencing any incontinence?
- Are enemas, laxatives, or mineral oil still needed?
- Is the child experiencing success with bowel control as a result of implementation of a family designed plan?
- Does the child more readily participate in age-appropriate activities and express increasing control over bowel incontinence?
- Is the skin in the anal area clean and intact?

## Recurrent Abdominal Pain/Irritable Bowel Syndrome

Recurrent abdominal pain is not unusual in children older than age 6 years, and in many cases the cause is unknown or unexplained (functional pain). Some children experience symptoms that resemble the characteristic symptoms of irritable bowel syndrome (IBS) seen in some adolescents and adults (Sreedharan & Liacouras, 2016).

### Etiology and Incidence

The exact etiology of IBS is not understood, but factors such as stress, emotional events, and infection are believed to be triggers. The condition tends to occur in families with a history of other bowel disturbances or infantile colic. The condition tends to resolve by late adolescence but is sometimes present in adults as IBS. IBS is the most common diagnosis in children with recurrent abdominal pain. The incidence of IBS is approximately 5% (Chogle, Mintjens, & Saps, 2014). Patients have altered bowel habits and can fluctuate between periods of diarrhea and constipation. Some present as either diarrhea predominant, constipation predominant, or mixed type (Chogle et al., 2014).

### Manifestations and Diagnostic Evaluation

Manifestations of IBS include diffuse abdominal pain unrelated to meals or activity; alternating constipation and diarrhea, with undigested food and mucus present in the stool; and normal growth.

The diagnosis is made based on the elimination of major GI pathologic conditions, including Crohn's disease, giardiasis, lactose intolerance, and genitourinary abnormalities. Abdominal ultrasound, stool for ova and parasites (O&P) and cultures, abdominal radiography, and a complete gynecologic assessment (if age-appropriate) are often ordered.

***Therapeutic management and nursing considerations.*** No definitive treatment is available for this poorly understood functional bowel problem. Management is aimed at identifying and reducing triggers and reducing bowel spasms, which decreases symptoms. The primary nursing intervention should be reassurance that it is a self-limiting, intermittent problem.

**PATHOPHYSIOLOGY**

***Irritable Bowel Syndrome***

The precipitating factors in irritable bowel syndrome are unknown but result in two distinct problems. The first is disorganized contractility, which causes spasmodic peristaltic rushes and lulls. This disorganization causes alternating diarrhea and constipation, with intermittent abdominal pain. The second component is excess mucus production in the lumen of the bowel. This produces maldigestion and the passage of incompletely digested food and nutrients.

Unless lactose intolerance is suspected, no dietary modifications are required other than the maintenance of a healthy, well-balanced, moderate-fiber, lower-fat diet. The child is instructed to eat slowly, to avoid caffeine products, and not to drink carbonated beverages. For children with diagnosed lactose intolerance, supplemental lactase can be provided (Almadhoun, 2012).

Medications are sometimes used to treat the symptoms of IBS. Antispasmodic medications such as dicyclomine and hyoscyamine improve IBS symptoms, including abdominal pain, in some children (Chogle et al., 2014). Peppermint oil may reduce abdominal pain by relaxing intestinal smooth muscle by blocking calcium channels (Chogle et al., 2014). Antidepressants are used in severe cases. Alternative and complementary therapies, such as cognitive-behavioral therapy, guided imagery, relaxation, biofeedback, and hypnotherapy can be helpful (Chogle et al., 2014; Sreedharan & Liacouras, 2016).

Family and psychosocial assessments may reveal a family that is worried about a serious life-threatening disease and is quite focused on the child's bowel habits. The family may not be reassured by the normal findings on a physical and developmental examination.

The primary nursing interventions are teaching and reassurance. Health promotion activities such as exercise, balanced nutrition, and school activities can have a positive influence on the disease. Because of the associated psychosocial component, referral to mental health and family counseling services can be beneficial for some children, particularly if other measures have not been effective. The child and family are encouraged to express feelings and concerns that will assist in evaluating the interventions.

# INFLAMMATORY AND INFECTIOUS DISORDERS

## Ulcers

A peptic ulcer is an area of sharply circumscribed loss of the mucosa, submucosa, or muscular tissue that occurs in regions of the digestive tract exposed to acid and pepsin. Peptic ulcers can be primary or secondary, gastric or duodenal. Primary, or idiopathic, ulcers occur in the absence of underlying systemic disease, tend to be chronic, and are usually located in the duodenum. Secondary ulcers tend to be acute in onset, occur in conjunction with serious illnesses or the use of nonsteroidal anti-inflammatory drugs (NSAIDs) and are found more often in the stomach.

**PATHOPHYSIOLOGY**

***Ulcers***

A thick mucous–bicarbonate barrier, a layer of mucus that provides a buffer zone for acid neutralization, lines the stomach and duodenum. Stomach acids diffuse slowly through this layer toward the gastric wall but are encountered and neutralized by slowly diffusing bicarbonate ions liberated from surface epithelial cells. The establishment of a neutral pH at the gastric epithelial surface provides protection from the combined effects of acid and pepsin. Ulcers result when any imbalance in the process occurs and erosions develop on the surface of the gastric or duodenal mucosa.

### Etiology

Known factors that can alter the mucous-bicarbonate barrier in the stomach and duodenum of children include the following:

- Excessive acid secretion caused by Zollinger–Ellison syndrome or gastrinoma and hyperparathyroidism.

- Bile salts break down the adherent mucous structure of the gastric duodenal lining and expose the mucosa to acid.
- Prostaglandins augment both the mucous gel lining and bicarbonate secretion. Deficiencies in mucosal prostaglandins can impair the mucous-bicarbonate barrier.
- Duodenal ulcers show a familial tendency. Genetic factors together with environmental factors can predispose children to ulcer formation. An association between ulcer activity and type O blood has also been noted.
- *Helicobacter pylori (H. pylori)* is a gram-negative spiral bacterium that has been identified in the gastric antrum of children with duodenal ulcers. It acts by weakening the gastric mucosal barrier and allowing acid and peptic digestion of the susceptible mucosa.
- Physiologic stress accounts for most secondary ulcers encountered during infancy and early childhood. They tend to be acute and occur in seriously ill children.
- Medications such as aspirin, NSAIDs, and indomethacin, as well as tobacco and alcohol, are known to affect the gastroduodenal mucosa adversely.
- Diet does not seem to influence the development of ulcer disease in children. Although certain foods may cause indigestion, no convincing data show that dietary factors cause, perpetuate, or reactivate ulcers, especially duodenal. However, colas, teas, and chocolate do increase acid secretions and may be contributing factors.
- The importance of psychological factors is questionable. They likely influence exacerbations or complications but not initial ulcer activity.

### Incidence

The true incidence of primary peptic ulcer disease in children is unknown because ulcers often spontaneously heal before a diagnosis is made. Only five to seven children are diagnosed with a gastric or duodenal ulcer per 2500 hospital admissions each year (Blanchard & Czinn, 2016). *H. pylori* infection has been found in approximately 80% of children with duodenal ulcers (Blanchard & Czinn, 2016). Secondary ulcers in children occur as a result of NSAID use or the physiologic stress associated with a critical illness such as severe burns, sepsis, shock, or an intracranial lesion (Blanchard & Czinn, 2016).

### Manifestations and Diagnostic Evaluation

Manifestations of ulcer disease in children include burning, cramping pain when the stomach is empty, awakening during the night or early morning with abdominal discomfort, and vomiting in children younger than 6 years. Hematemesis and melena are common in infants and young children.

Fiberoptic upper endoscopy is the diagnostic tool of choice for all children, including neonates. Endoscopy provides direct visual observation of the lining of the esophagus, stomach, and proximal duodenum and also is a means for obtaining biopsy or culture material. Ultrasound can be performed to rule out gallstones, tumors, or mechanical obstruction. The fecal occult blood test is performed to check for GI bleeding.

### Therapeutic Management

Medical management is the most common treatment for ulcer disease in children. Factors considered in ulcer treatment include drug safety, symptom relief, child and parent adherence to the prescribed regimen, and the prevention of complications or ulcer recurrence. A bland diet with milk and small, frequent feedings was long thought to be the mainstay of ulcer therapy. However, the protein and calcium in milk actually stimulate more acid secretions than they buffer. A regular diet low in caffeine is now generally prescribed because caffeine is a potent stimulant of acid secretion and exacerbates GERD. A diet high in fiber and polyunsaturated oils may also play a role in ulcer prevention.

Medications are now considered the first line of treatment. They include antibiotics, proton pump inhibitors, $H_2$-receptor antagonists, and mucosa protective agents. Four- to six-week treatment using the combination of a proton pump inhibitor, an appropriate antibiotic, and bismuth salts is considered to be optimal therapy for eradicating *H. pylori* (Blanchard & Czinn, 2016). Vaccines to prevent *H. pylori* infections are currently under development.

Surgery is indicated for the management of ulcer complications such as hemorrhage, perforation, and obstruction. Possible surgical procedures include vagotomy, pyloroplasty, ligation of a bleeding vessel, and closure of a perforation.

If the child is actively bleeding, an NG tube is inserted to remove blood, decompress the stomach, and estimate blood loss. IV fluids, oxygen, blood replacement, and vasoactive drugs such as vasopressin (Pitressin) may be given. Balloon tamponade with a Sengstaken–Blakemore tube is sometimes indicated. Blood or clots are removed with room-temperature gastric lavage. The use of iced saline lavage to stop GI bleeding is no longer advocated because it increases bleeding and clotting times and prolongs the prothrombin time. It also imposes a risk of hypothermia on an already compromised child.

### Nursing Considerations

Nursing assessment of the child with peptic ulcer disease begins with a thorough history, including a family history of ulcer disease, past episodes of abdominal pain, or recent stressful events in the home, school, or community. A complete assessment of pain includes a description of the nature of the pain and its location; its relationship to meals, defecation, or voiding; episodes of nocturnal pain; and medications used to effectively relieve the pain. The child is examined for the presence of epigastric tenderness, nausea, vomiting, abdominal distention, hematemesis, melena, or recent changes in appetite or eating habits.

All stools and emesis fluid should be checked for the presence of blood. Bowel sounds are auscultated for 5 minutes. If vomiting is present, the child is assessed for signs of dehydration. If bleeding is observed, the child is monitored for changes in vital signs, and the physician is notified immediately. Finally, the nurse assesses family members for their understanding of the disease, the presence of a viable support system, and their ability to participate in their child's care.

***Providing information.*** The major focus of nursing interventions is teaching. The nurse reviews with the family the pathophysiology of the disease, medication administration, and diet and assesses the child for complications.

Preparing the child for diagnostic tests is an important nursing intervention. Because fiberoptic endoscopy is often performed, the child must be prepared for conscious sedation. Keeping the child on NPO status for at least 6 hours, maintaining an IV line, and monitoring vital signs and respiratory function during the procedure are nursing responsibilities. Upper GI examinations and ultrasonography may also be performed.

***Home care.*** Ulcers are managed almost exclusively in the home environment, so teaching, follow-up, and home health referral are essential. The correct use of medications and dietary modifications are parental responsibilities that may require educational materials, emotional support, help with time organization, and encouragement to continue even when symptoms are relieved. The nurse emphasizes to the parent that the medications must be given for the full prescribed course and should not be stopped when symptoms improve.

The child should not be given aspirin or any other NSAID because they can cause bleeding. Parents are instructed not to use any over-the-counter or other drugs without contacting the physician first. Dietary modifications, such as avoiding foods with caffeine, carbonated beverages, and acidic foods, may relieve symptoms. Parents are taught to call the physician if the child exhibits "coffee-ground" vomitus, tarry stools, increased pain, diarrhea, vomiting, or unexplained weight loss.

### Infectious Gastroenteritis

Infectious gastroenteritis is caused by a group of viruses, bacteria, and parasites capable of causing serious communicable diarrhea, massive fluid and electrolyte loss, sepsis, and death (for further discussion of fluid and electrolyte alterations, see Chapter 40).

#### Etiology

Ingestion of contaminated food or water and person-to-person contamination are the most frequent causes of infectious gastroenteritis in the United States. High-risk groups include children in daycare centers, preschools, and long-term care facilities and those who are immunocompromised. *Giardia* is the most common pathogen seen in children in daycare settings. Rotavirus is the most common viral cause of gastroenteritis in all children and accounts for 29% of all deaths due to diarrhea among children younger than age 5 years (Bhutta, 2016). Vaccination against rotavirus has been recommended for infants in the United States since February of 2006 and has been effective in reducing hospitalization and mortality rates for gastroenteritis (Bhutta, 2016). In many cases, the pathogen causing gastroenteritis is not identified (Table 43.3).

#### Incidence

Gastroenteritis is one of the most common outpatient infectious diseases in children. The World Health Organization and the United Nations Children's Fund (UNICEF) estimate that nearly 1.7 billion episodes of diarrhea occur in children younger than 5 years of age annually in developing countries (Bhutta, 2016). Although the number of deaths from diarrheal illnesses is declining, it is estimated that 0.71 million childhood deaths still occur worldwide each year (Bhutta, 2016).

#### Manifestations

Gastroenteritis likely manifests with diarrhea of varying amount and consistency, vomiting, and abdominal pain. In addition, the child may experience **tenesmus** and fever. Dehydration is a severe consequence of gastroenteritis and occurs mainly in children younger than 2 years of age. A history of travel to other regions of the world can provide clues to the causative organism.

#### Diagnostic Evaluation

A definitive diagnosis can be made when a stool culture yields a pathogen, but these cultures are expensive and result in many false-negative findings. Ova and parasites are more reliably found. Usually, only children who appear to be in a toxic condition or have bloody stools, abdominal pain, or tenesmus undergo a diagnostic workup. A travel and exposure history is important in diagnosing the cause of gastroenteritis (Bhutta, 2016). The presence of white blood cells (WBCs) and blood in the stool can support the presumptive diagnosis on the basis of clinical findings. Blood cultures may also be needed in the acutely ill infant and young child. An unprepared sigmoidoscopy can be useful in determining the amount of mucosal involvement, obtaining more reliable samples for culture, and diagnosing the disease.

**PARENTS WANT TO KNOW**

***Care of the Child With an Ulcer***

Parents and older children need to understand the pathophysiology, causes, diagnosis, and therapeutic management of ulcers. When educating the parent and older child, follow these guidelines:

- Emphasize the relationship of the ulcer to acute illness.
- Help the older child identify sources of excess stress that can be modified.
- Teach stress-reduction activities such as relaxation and exercise and refer parents to support groups.

Directions for administering medications include the following:

- Do not administer antacids within 1 hour of other antiulcer medications.
- Do not stop medications when symptoms improve; continue for the full prescribed course.
- Do not use aspirin or other nonsteroidal antiinflammatory drugs because they can cause bleeding.
- Do not use over-the-counter medications without your physician's knowledge.
- Do not add other drugs because ulcer medications can alter your child's metabolism and absorption.

Help parents make changes in diet as prescribed by teaching the following:

- If your child has a poor appetite, provide a well-balanced diet with many choices.
- Seek assistance from dietary services as needed.
- Provide meals and snacks every 2 to 3 hours.
- Make sure your child avoids coffee, chocolate, and caffeine and any other foods that might cause discomfort.

Instruct parents to call their physician if their child experiences any of the following problems:

- "Coffee-ground" vomitus
- Weight loss
- Tarry stools
- Increased pain
- Diarrhea
- Vomiting

**PATHOPHYSIOLOGY**

***Infectious Gastroenteritis***

As the pathogen adheres to the mucosa of the intestine, it is no longer affected by peristaltic waves and is not removed from the site. Epithelial invasion occurs, causing an inflammatory response and epithelial cell death. This response leads to ulcerations, pseudomembranes, bleeding, and possibly sepsis. As the pathogens multiply, some produce toxins. Enterotoxins (e.g., cholera, *Shigella*) cause fluid and electrolyte shifts that result in increased secretion into the intestine and a simultaneous decrease in absorption caused by edema. The absorptive capacity of the colon is exceeded, and massive diarrhea and dehydration result. Cytotoxins (e.g., *Salmonella*) produce local edema, malabsorption, and dehydration. Some pathogens are also capable of producing neurotoxins (e.g., *Shigella*) that act outside the gastrointestinal (GI) tract.

#### Therapeutic Management

The priority therapy is to replace water and correct acid-base or fluid and electrolyte disturbances with IV fluids or oral (PO) electrolyte replacement liquids. The rate of replacement may be as high as 50 to

**TABLE 43.3 Characteristics of Infectious Gastroenteritis**

| Characteristics | Clinical Manifestations | Diagnostic Findings | Treatment |
|---|---|---|---|
| ***Shigella* (Enteroinvasive With Cytotoxin)** | | | |
| Incubation period 1-2 days<br>Most common in summer<br>Fecal–oral spread<br>Remains communicable for 1-3 weeks | Symptoms last 4-10 days<br>Diarrhea begins as watery, progresses to bloody, with mucus<br>Severe abdominal pain<br>High fever<br>Neurologic symptoms (headache, nuchal rigidity, convulsions)<br>Risk for sepsis, hemolytic uremic syndrome, rectal prolapse, and DIC | Blood, mucus, WBCs in stool<br>Positive stool culture in some cases | Supportive care<br>First-line treatment:<br>TMP-SMX, 8-10 mg/kg/day for 3-5 days *OR* ampicillin, 50-100 mg/kg/day for 3-5 days<br>Ceftriaxone, fluoroquinolones, or azithromycin for resistant strains<br>Contact Precautions<br>Identify source if possible |
| ***Salmonella* (Enteroinvasive)** | | | |
| Incubation 1-3 days<br>Most common in summer and fall<br>Usually foodborne<br>Infectious for duration of illness and variable period afterward | Symptoms last 4-7 days<br>Rapid onset<br>Secretory diarrhea<br>Abdominal pain, nausea, and vomiting common | Blood and PMNs in stool<br>Positive stool culture | Supportive care<br>Antibiotics given in certain cases (third generation cephalosporins, ampicillin)<br>Contact Precautions<br>Identify source if possible |
| ***Escherichia Coli* (Enteroinvasive With Enterotoxin)** | | | |
| Incubation period 1-3 days<br>Most common in summer<br>Foodborne most common | Symptoms for 3-7 days or longer<br>Green, watery, secretory diarrhea<br>Can cause hemorrhagic colitis<br>Fever | Blood and PMNs in stool | Supportive care<br>Contact Precautions<br>TMP-SMX and quinolones for severe cases<br>Monitor renal function, hemoglobin, and platelets |
| **Campylobacter** | | | |
| Incubation 2-5 days<br>Most common in infants and adolescents | Symptoms for 2-10 days<br>Consumption of contaminated foods or water<br>Severe abdominal pain<br>Foul-smelling, watery diarrhea<br>Fever | Blood and PMNs in stool | Supportive care<br>Possible treatment with azithromycin or quinolones<br>Contact Precautions |
| ***Giardia lamblia*** | | | |
| Incubation period 1-2 wk<br>Most common cause of parasitic diarrhea<br>Spread in contaminated food and water | Symptoms for days to weeks<br>Afebrile<br>Abdominal distention, cramps, and flatulence<br>Variable diarrhea | Ova and parasites found in stool<br>Parasites found on duodenal biopsy | Metronidazole (Flagyl) for 7 days<br>Contact Precautions<br>Treat all unknown water sources with chlorine/iodine before drinking |
| **Rotavirus** | | | |
| Incubation 1-3 days<br>Common in winter months<br>Fecally contaminated food | Symptoms usually last 3-7 days<br>Vomiting, diarrhea, low-grade fever<br>History of preceding or concurrent respiratory illness | Virus in stool detected by enzyme immunoassay | No pharmacologic treatment<br>Supportive care; maintain hydration and electrolyte balance<br>Contact Precautions<br>Rotavirus vaccine at 2, 4, and 6 mo of age; series needs to be complete by 32 weeks of age |
| ***Clostridium difficile* (See Chapter 41)** | | | |
| Antibiotic associated<br>Most common nosocomial diarrhea | Fever for 24-48 hr<br>Diarrhea develops after antibiotic treatment | Blood and PMNs in stool | Possibly treated with vancomycin for more severe cases or metronidazole (Flagyl) for 7-10 days<br>Contact Precautions Plus<br>Discontinuation of antibiotic that caused diarrhea |
| **Norwalk** | | | |
| Incubation 1-2 days<br>Common in winter in schools and other group settings<br>Fecal-oral route of transmission | Symptoms last 1-2 days<br>Nausea, vomiting, diarrhea<br>Headache, low-grade fever, muscle aches, chills | Virus in stool | No pharmacologic treatment<br>Contact Precautions |

*DIC,* Disseminated intravascular coagulation; *PMN,* polymorphonuclear leukocyte; *TMP-SMX,* trimethoprim-sulfamethoxazole; *WBC,* white blood cell.

100 mL/kg over a 4- to 6-hour period (1 to 2.5 times maintenance requirements). Because diarrheal fluid is high in sodium, potassium, and bicarbonate, oral rehydration solutions should be used to match losses (see Chapter 40). Hospitalization for treatment is not uncommon, especially for the infant or small child, to allow for continued assessment and management of symptoms or sepsis. Antimicrobial therapy is useful in cases of infection with *Shigella* and *Giardia* and in some cases of infection with *Clostridium difficile* and *Escherichia coli (E. coli)*, but not for rotavirus infection. The FDA licensed a rotavirus vaccine for use in infants in 2006. The Advisory Committee on Immunization Practices (ACIP) recommends that all infants be immunized with three doses of the vaccine at 2, 4, and 6 months of age.

## NURSING CARE

### The Child With Infectious Gastroenteritis

#### Assessment

Obtain an adequate history of the event, including the length of symptoms, frequency and consistency of stools, and the presence of blood or mucus in stools. Noting the amount, color, consistency, and time (ACCT) of each stool or episode of vomiting is a consistent way to document findings. The concurrent appearance of symptoms in other members of the family can be helpful in the diagnosis. Any travel to other countries or wilderness areas should be recorded. Evaluating formula and food preparation at home and in daycare facilities, as well as examining sanitation and hygiene in these places, can provide valuable information.

The child may appear moderately to severely dehydrated, with hyperactive bowel sounds and severe diarrhea, which is often bloody. Blood in the stool usually appears after the maximal fluid loss has occurred and can be useful in determining the stage of illness. The presence of abdominal pain, vomiting, tenesmus, and fever should be assessed. Headache, nuchal rigidity, irritability, and seizures are important symptoms of the neurotoxic effects of *Shigella*.

Assessment of hydration status is critical. Low urine output, high urine specific gravity, poor skin turgor, dry mucous membranes, crying without producing tears, a sunken or depressed fontanel in infants, and skin tenting can occur quickly with the large amount of fluid lost through diarrhea. Loss of bicarbonate from severe diarrhea and dehydration makes metabolic acidosis a major concern. The compensatory mechanisms of increased respiratory rate and effort are important to document.

#### Nursing Diagnosis and Planning

The following nursing diagnoses and expected outcomes may be appropriate for the infant or child with gastroenteritis:

- Deficient Fluid Volume related to severe diarrhea.

**Expected outcome.** The child will be adequately hydrated without electrolyte disturbance, as evidenced by moist mucous membranes; good skin turgor; urine output appropriate for age; return to normal weight; and normal serum sodium, potassium, and bicarbonate levels. The child will have soft, formed stools without diarrhea, blood, or mucus.

- Risk for Infection related to exposure of family members and others to infectious agents.

**Expected outcome.** The child will not transmit pathogens to others.

- Acute Pain related to hyperactive motility.

**Expected outcome.** The child will be free from abdominal pain, as evidenced by a return to normal activity and no reports of pain.

- Deficient Knowledge related to inadequate information about the disease and its control.

**Expected outcome.** The parents will describe how to prevent transmitting the condition to others and will use Standard Precautions and Contact Precautions when handling the child's excretions.

- Imbalanced Nutrition: Less Than Body Requirements related to malabsorption.

**Expected outcome.** The child will resume a normal diet and will regain weight lost during the acute phase within 1 week after symptoms abate.

- Risk for Impaired Skin Integrity related to skin contact with feces and the necessity for frequent cleansing.

**Expected outcome.** The child will maintain skin integrity, as evidenced by clean, dry, intact skin without redness, drainage, or breakdown.

#### Interventions

**Maintaining fluid balance.** Critical nursing interventions are related to the fluid volume deficit. Oral or parenteral rehydration with correction of acid-base imbalances is essential to establish homeostasis. Accurate intake and output and weight measurements are important. Monitoring skin turgor, urine output, and serum electrolyte levels provides evaluation criteria in this area (see Chapter 40 for a further discussion of fluid and electrolyte alterations).

**Decreasing risk.** Providing safety, assessing neurologic symptoms, and monitoring for seizures are also priorities for the child with *Shigella* infection. Preventing the spread of infection remains a critical nursing intervention. Thorough hand hygiene is a must. Contact Precautions must be strictly enforced for all staff and family members to minimize the risk of spreading the infection. These precautions must be maintained at home for up to 2 weeks; the time period may be less if antibiotics are given. Pain and fever may be treated with acetaminophen. Symptomatic treatment with antidiarrheal medications is not recommended because they tend to increase the length of symptoms. Parents and children need to be taught these interventions and given information about the disease process during this period. Depending on the organism causing the gastroenteritis, follow-up by the public health department may be necessary. Organisms such as *Salmonella* and *E. coli* can be found in food and present a significant public health concern. A dietary recall for possibly contaminated foods can be important in establishing the cause and minimizing the risk of spread to the public.

**Home care.** The most important intervention that can be implemented at home is proper rehydration to prevent the need for hospitalization and IV therapy (see Chapter 40 for a discussion of oral rehydration fluids and care for the child with dehydration).

Dietary changes for vomiting and diarrhea may not be necessary if the child does not demonstrate dehydration. Breast milk can be offered as needed, and formula should be given full strength. Oral rehydration therapy (ORT) can be used in addition to the usual diet to replace GI losses and prevent dehydration (see Chapter 40). Vomiting does not prevent oral rehydration because the child can be successfully rehydrated with 5 to 10 mL of rehydrating solution every 2 to 5 minutes. When diet is continued, foods with fats and high sugar concentrations should be avoided. Complex carbohydrates, starches, lean meats, and vegetables should be encouraged. *Lactobacillus*, which can be found in yogurt or as a supplement, assists in reducing diarrhea by restoring normal bowel flora.

Children who demonstrate mild or moderate dehydration may require ORT at a rate of 50 to 100 mL/kg rapidly over a 3- to 4-hour period in addition to replacing fluid losses from vomiting or diarrhea (Bhutta, 2016). Regular diet can be resumed as just described once the fluid deficit has been corrected. Once a dehydrated child has been rehydrated, resuming an age-appropriate diet enhances recovery. Severe dehydration sometimes requires parenteral therapy and hospitalization.

Preventing the spread of infection is also essential for home care (see Patient-Centered Teaching: Care of the Child with Infectious Gastroenteritis). Good hand hygiene; the disinfection of contaminated linens, clothes, and diapers; and the use of surface disinfectant sprays are important preventive measures.

### Evaluation

- Has the child returned to preinfection weight within 1 week after symptoms subside?
- Does the child have good skin turgor, moist mucous membranes, and a urine specific gravity of less than 1.030?
- Does the child have a serum sodium level of 135 to 145 mEq/L and a serum potassium level of 3.5 to 5 mEq/L?
- Is the child passing soft, formed stools without diarrhea, blood, or mucus?
- Are other family members free from infectious diarrhea, and is the family following the appropriate precautions to prevent transmission?
- Is the child reporting abdominal pain?
- Does the child guard the abdomen during palpation?
- Are parents and staff at the daycare facility practicing infection control procedures, if appropriate?
- Can the child tolerate an age-appropriate regular diet?
- Is the child's skin intact and free from areas of irritation and breakdown?

## Appendicitis

Appendicitis is the inflammation and infection of the vermiform appendix, a small lymphoid, tubular, blind sac at the end of the cecum. It is the most common cause of emergency surgery in children and adolescents.

### Etiology and Incidence

Common causes of obstruction and subsequent appendicitis include lymphoid swelling related to viral infection, impacted fecal material, foreign bodies, and parasites. In most cases no definitive cause can be identified at the time of surgery.

Appendicitis occurs with equal frequency in both sexes, with most cases occurring during adolescence and early adulthood. The incidence is 19-28 cases per 10,000 children younger than 14 years annually (Aiken & Oldham, 2016). Appendicitis is uncommon in children younger than 4 years, but in young children it is associated with a high frequency of perforation by the time of the first visit, most likely related to the difficulty in establishing the diagnosis.

### Manifestations and Diagnostic Evaluation

The cardinal symptom of appendicitis is periumbilical abdominal pain, progressing in intensity and localizing to the lower right quadrant at McBurney point (Fig. 43.4). The pain starts insidiously and worsens over time (Murphy & Berman, 2014). Associated signs and symptoms include nausea and vomiting, anorexia, diarrhea or constipation, and fever and chills. A careful physical exam may elicit a positive Rovsing sign (palpation of the left quadrant causes pain in the right quadrant), psoas sign (pain with extension of the right thigh), and obturator sign (pain with flexion and internal rotation of the hip) (Hansen & Dolgin, 2016). If the appendix perforates, the child will initially

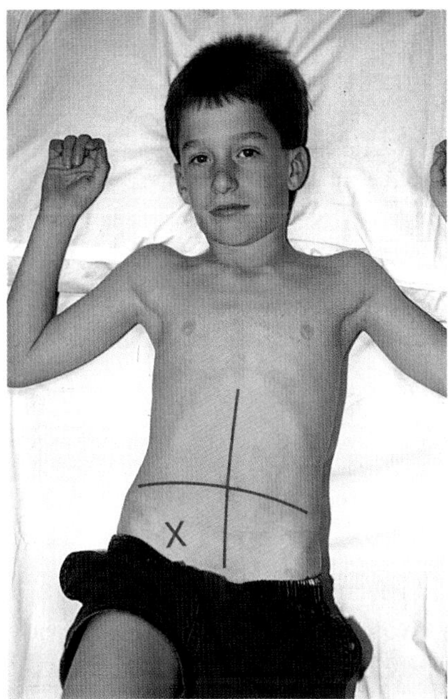


FIG 43.4 McBurney point is midway between the right anterior superior iliac crest and the umbilicus. It is usually the location of greatest pain in the child with appendicitis. (Courtesy University of Texas at Arlington College of Nursing, Arlington, TX.)

experience relief of pain. Other signs and symptoms will worsen, so that the child will appear acutely ill with high fever and signs of dehydration.

The diagnosis is usually made based on classic abdominal findings of pain localizing at the McBurney point, guarding, rebound tenderness, nausea, vomiting, and fever. A WBC count of 15,000 to 20,000/mm$^3$ supports the clinical findings. A quick, safe, and accurate diagnosis can usually be made with ultrasound as the first choice of imaging or with CT for complicated cases to limit radiation exposure (Bachur, Callahan, Monteaux, et al., 2015). Images show an enlarged, incompressible appendix that can be fluid filled and locally inflamed, which can be used to predict the severity of the disease (Murphy & Berman, 2014).

**PATHOPHYSIOLOGY**

***Appendicitis***

Obstruction of the appendix allows normal mucus secretions to accumulate in the appendix, producing distention. Distention eventually causes occlusion of the capillaries and engorgement of the appendix walls. Microabscesses form and can progress to abscesses and fistulas. Perforation occurs as a result of tissue breakdown and swelling. Bowel contents then contaminate the mesenteric bed and peritoneum, leading to peritonitis and sepsis.

### Therapeutic Management

The definitive treatment for appendicitis and suspected appendicitis is appendectomy. Preoperatively, the child is managed with fluid therapy, immobilization, pain control interventions, NPO status, antibiotics, and antipyretics, if indicated. The procedure is usually done laparoscopically or if necessary through an open abdominal approach, particularly if perforation is suspected (Hansen & Dolgin, 2016).

## NURSING CARE

### The Child With Appendicitis

#### Assessment

The nursing assessment will reveal a history of pain, fever, vomiting, and diarrhea or constipation. The physical examination discloses abdominal tenderness and guarding. The child may assume a supine position with the right leg flexed to decrease tension on the abdominal wall. The nurse must be keenly aware of the symptoms of perforation, including a sudden relief from pain followed by an increase in pain, rigid abdomen, and early shock symptoms. Behavioral changes and refusal to eat are important indicators in infants and toddlers.

Assess anxiety in the child and family members, who are most likely facing unexpected surgery. Because of the pain, the child may be uncooperative with abdominal assessment. The parents may have financial concerns related to the unplanned surgery.

#### Nursing Diagnosis and Planning

The following nursing diagnoses and expected outcomes may be appropriate after assessing the child with appendicitis:

- Acute Pain related to abdominal inflammation and surgical incision.

***Expected outcome.*** The child will be free from pain, as evidenced by resumption of normal activity and movement with no reports of pain.

- Risk for Infection related to rupture and surgery.

***Expected outcome.*** The child will have a clean, dry surgical incision that is free from redness, heat, or exudate, and the child will be afebrile with a WBC count of 5000 to 15,000/mm$^3$.

- Deficient Fluid Volume related to vomiting or diarrhea.

***Expected outcome.*** The child will be well hydrated, as evidenced by moist mucous membranes, good skin turgor, and hourly urine output appropriate for age (see Chapter 40).

- Anxiety related to unplanned surgery.

***Expected outcome.*** The parent or child will express feelings about surgery and will verbalize the need for emergency hospitalization.

**! NURSING QUALITY ALERT**

***Assessing Appendicitis in the Young Child***

Because symptoms of appendicitis can be vague and develop slowly over approximately a 12-hour period, the condition can be quite difficult to assess in young children. The complaint that "my tummy hurts" often is the only initial symptom. Appendicitis should be suspected if pain, anorexia, or nausea and vomiting, and fever occur simultaneously. If pain occurs before vomiting, appendicitis should be suspected. However, if vomiting precedes abdominal pain, gastroenteritis is more likely. The young child will usually refuse to play, preferring instead to lie down. Often, the child will lie in a knee-chest position to be comfortable. One way of helping the child describe the area of pain focus is to ask the child to stand on tiptoes and then drop to flat feet. The pain location elicited from this maneuver usually will be in the right lower quadrant.

#### Interventions

***Uncomplicated appendicitis.*** On admission, vital signs should be taken to monitor for sepsis or shock. The nurse institutes comfort measures, including topical cold application, pain medications, and positions of comfort. Enemas or laxatives should not be administered. No heat should be applied to the abdomen because it increases the chance of perforation as a result of vasodilation. IV fluid therapy is started to prepare the child for surgery and correct any existing fluid, electrolyte, or acid–base disturbances related to vomiting and diarrhea.

If the procedure is performed by laparoscopy, the nurse can expect the child to be discharged within 24 hours. Open surgery is often followed by a few days of recovery in the hospital. After either operation, the child will be on NPO status until bowel function has returned.

***Ruptured appendix.*** The child with a ruptured appendix needs specialized care. If perforation is suspected, prepare the child for NG tube insertion. The NG tube provides decompression before surgery and allows gastric content drainage postoperatively. The child will need IV antibiotics, which may be started preoperatively. For the child with a perforation, IV antibiotics are continued, and hospitalization can last 5 days, or longer if complications occur. After the NG tube is removed, the diet should be advanced gradually so that the child can tolerate a normal diet without vomiting or diarrhea.

Depending on the extent of the peritonitis, the child might have postoperative incisional drains. These drains are sometimes attached to suction, and aseptic technique and maintenance of patency are essential. The nurse carefully documents the drainage amount each shift. The wound is often left open and treated with sterile wet-to-dry or wet-to-moist (saline-soaked gauze) dressings and wound irrigation with antibacterial solutions.

Round-the-clock opioid analgesics provide relief from incisional pain and from pain caused by dressing changes (see Chapters 38 and 39). Continued reassessment of abdominal pain is essential for evaluating the presence of a wound infection, abscess, or fistula.

Monitor vital signs, including temperature, every 2 to 4 hours. Intermittent NG suction will likely be continued postoperatively until bowel sounds return. Positioning the child to facilitate drainage and minimize the spread of infection into the upper abdomen should be done by elevating the head of the bed or having the child lie on the operative side.

***Home care.*** After surgery and discharge, parents must be prepared to assume responsibility for the child's care. The surgical incision and any drain sites must be assessed for redness, drainage, dehiscence, or suture infections. Report any problems to the physician. Parents should advance the child's diet slowly, beginning with liquids and soft foods and progressing to the child's normal diet if tolerated without nausea or vomiting. Teach parents to watch for vomiting, abdominal pain, or distention as possible signs of bowel obstruction or peritoneal infection.

#### Evaluation

- Does the child report pain?
- Does the child demonstrate guarding on abdominal palpation?
- Has the child returned to a normal activity level?
- Is the surgical incision clean, dry, and free from redness, heat, purulent drainage, or dehiscence?
- Is the child afebrile, with a WBC count of 5000 to 15,000/mm$^3$?
- Is the child tolerating an age-appropriate regular diet without vomiting, diarrhea, or increased abdominal pain?
- Are the child and parents able to express relief from anxiety?

### Inflammatory Bowel Disease

Inflammatory bowel disease (IBD) is a chronic inflammatory condition of the small or large intestine. It includes two distinct conditions: ulcerative colitis and Crohn disease. Ulcerative colitis affects only the colon and involves both the mucosal and submucosal layers of the intestine. Crohn disease can occur anywhere in the GI tract, from the mouth to the anus, and is transmural, involving all layers of the intestine.

### Etiology

The exact cause of IBD is not known. Several triggers have been identified, including viral and other infectious agents, food allergies, vasculitis, increased intestinal permeability, immunologic dysfunction, and genetic factors. Increasing evidence demonstrates a connection between IBD and the effects of stress on the immune response.

### Incidence, Manifestations, and Diagnostic Evaluation

The incidence, manifestations, and diagnostic evaluation of both ulcerative colitis and Crohn disease are summarized in Table 43.4.

**TABLE 43.4 Crohn Disease and Ulcerative Colitis**

| Crohn Disease | Ulcerative Colitis |
|---|---|
| **Pathophysiology** | |
| Affects entire gastrointestinal (GI) tract, most common in the terminal ileum | Involves only colon, starting at the rectum and moving upward |
| Transmural involvement | Mucosa and submucosa only |
| Cobblestone appearance of mucosa | Mucosa lacking in most cases |
| Fistulas common | Fistulas rare |
| Remissions and exacerbations | Remissions uncommon |
| **Diagnostic Evaluation: Colonoscopy, Rectoscopy, Barium Enema, Biopsy** | |
| "Skip" lesions with deep fissures and granulomas | Inflammation and superficial ulceration; "cutoff" demarcation between areas of inflamed and normal colon |
| Biopsy–nonspecific chronic inflammation | |
| **Incidence** | |
| 5/100,000 in United States and increasing | 15/100,000 in United States |
| Equal gender distribution | Equal gender distribution. |
| Not seen in infants; peaks in teens, early 20s | Peaks between ages 15 and 25 yr |
| Clusters in families | Clusters in families |
| Associated with higher standard of living | Affects Whites more than others |
| **Clinical Manifestations** | |
| Abdominal pain | Abdominal pain unusual |
| Diarrhea, nonbloody | Diarrhea, occasionally with hemorrhage and anemia |
| Fever | |
| Palpable abdominal mass | No masses |
| Anorexia and severe weight loss | Moderate weight loss |
| Significant growth impairment | Mild growth impairment |
| Perianal and anal lesions | Perianal and anal lesions rare |
| Fistulas and obstructions | Fistulas and obstructions rare |
| Extraintestinal symptoms (arthralgia, arthritis) | Risk of toxic megacolon |
| **Morbidity** | |
| Regions of affected bowel increase | Remissions and exacerbations |
| Over time 50%-70% will eventually require surgery for obstruction or fistula | 10% chance of cancer after 10 yr |
| Surgery does not cure disease | Removal of colon can cure the disease |

### Therapeutic Management

Management for IBD is multidimensional and includes medication, dietary and nutritional support, and symptomatic treatment. Pharmacologic treatment includes antiinflammatory, antibacterial, antibiotic, and immunosuppressive drugs. The principal medications used to treat IBD include the following:

- 5-Aminosalicylic acid (5-ASA) medications such as sulfasalazine or mesalazine
- Corticosteroids such as prednisone
- Immune-modulating agents such as azathioprine, 6-mercaptopurine (6-MP), methotrexate, and cyclosporin A
- Tumor necrosis factor-alpha (TNF-α) antibody (infliximab)
- Antibiotics such as metronidazole (Flagyl) and ciprofloxacin (quinolones)

5-ASA and 6-MP are first-line immunosuppressants that allow selected children with Crohn disease to avoid steroids and their associated side effects. Infliximab (Remicade) has been approved for treatment of ulcerative colitis and Crohn disease in children. It binds to TNF-α to decrease inflammation and increase intestinal healing. Infliximab has been shown to be effective in moderate to severe acute disease and in children who do not gain results from corticosteroids (Judge, Giordano, & English, 2014). Nurses should monitor the patient closely when administering tumor necrosis factor, although it generally is well tolerated and safe with mild reactions that respond rapidly to intervention (Aschenbrenner, 2012).

Nutritional intervention is part of a holistic approach for children with Crohn disease and is a useful component with no side effects. Total parenteral nutrition (TPN) may be needed during acute flare-ups. Exclusive enteral nutrition with an elemental formula via NG tube or gastrostomy promotes healing of the mucosa and can control the disease as effectively as prednisone in some children with Crohn disease (Grossman & Baldassano, 2016a).

Crohn disease is best managed before permanent structural changes have developed. Malnutrition is a common problem and can involve protein, fat, carbohydrate, and vitamin deficiencies, leading to growth failure. Nutritional support and teaching are essential. Surgery is not curative, but partial bowel resections may be necessary to treat abscesses, fistulas, or chronic recurrent obstruction.

For ulcerative colitis, avoidance of milk products and ingestion of a hypoallergenic, low-fiber, low-fat, low-residue, high-protein, elemental diet can be useful. Surgical intervention for ulcerative colitis includes partial or total colectomy with creation of a colostomy or ileostomy. Optimally, a total colectomy is combined with an endorectal pull-through where the distal ileum is pulled down and sutured to the distal rectum, allowing the child to maintain continence (Grossman & Baldassano, 2016b).

## NURSING CARE

### The Child With Inflammatory Bowel Disease

#### Assessment

Recurrent or chronic diarrhea is the primary finding in the nursing history of a child with IBD. The major assessment findings are related to this diarrhea and the associated malabsorption that occurs. Weight loss, dehydration, anorexia, growth failure, vitamin deficiencies, and anemia are common. The severity of the GI symptoms and the amount and length of steroid use will have a significant influence on a child's growth rate. With ulcerative colitis, remissions and exacerbations of symptoms are common. Frank bleeding is also possible.

Intermittent cramping discomfort exacerbated by eating is common in Crohn disease. The child with Crohn disease may have oral lesions and perianal skin breakdown. Inflammatory changes also can occur outside of the GI system with arthralgia and arthritis, especially of the lower extremities, causing discomfort and mobility problems.

Depression, anxiety, fears about social interactions, and low self-esteem occur and are most likely related to the need to have quick access to restrooms at all times and to be close to home if an accident occurs. The chronic nature of this condition and its unknown prognosis can lead to family stress and tax the family's financial resources and support systems. Assessment should include questions about family and peer support, resources, and knowledge of the disease.

### Nursing Diagnosis and Planning

The following nursing diagnoses and expected outcomes may be appropriate for the child with inflammatory bowel disease and the child's family:

- Imbalanced Nutrition: Less Than Body Requirements related to chronic malabsorption.

  ***Expected outcome.*** The child will have acceptable bowel patterns, as evidenced by passing no more than four stools per day and being free from nocturnal diarrhea. The child will receive adequate nutrition, as evidenced by normal hemoglobin values and normal growth that follows the growth curve.
- Acute Pain related to cramping.

  ***Expected outcome.*** The child will be free from abdominal pain, as evidenced by resumption of normal activity and no reports of pain.
- Chronic Low Self-Esteem related to chronic diarrhea and colostomy.

  ***Expected outcome.*** The child will have a positive self-concept, as evidenced by leading an active lifestyle without depression.
- Delayed Growth and Development related to malnutrition, chronic illness, and steroid use.

  ***Expected outcome.*** The child will meet normal developmental milestones, as evidenced by progress on standard developmental screenings.
- Disturbed Body Image related to weight loss, water retention from steroid therapy, and colostomy or ileostomy.

  ***Expected outcome.*** The child will state reasons for changes in body appearance and will share concerns about changes with family and support personnel.
- Anxiety related to chronic diarrhea and risk for surgery.

  ***Expected outcome.*** The child will express concerns about the future and will contact support services as needed.
- Deficient Knowledge related to management of chronic disease.

  ***Expected outcome.*** The child will explain day-to-day management of disease and will demonstrate ability for self-care that is age-appropriate.

### Interventions

Nursing interventions focus on maintaining pharmacologic interventions, developing long-term nutritional management, educating, and providing emotional support.

***Medications.*** Teaching appropriate administration of medications is an important nursing role. Enemas are used before critical diagnostic tests and may serve as a method of medication administration. Any child who will be taking steroids (see Chapter 42) needs to understand the importance of regular administration as well as the risks associated with immunosuppression. Steroids should be given with food or antacids to prevent GI distress. The steroids, although beneficial in suppressing symptoms, may actually exacerbate the growth delays associated with inflammatory bowel disease.

***Nutritional management.*** Nutritional support varies with the disease and the child's tolerance of changes. In general, maintaining a low-fiber, low-residue, lowfat, milk-free, elemental diet provides some relief, although strict restrictions do not alleviate symptoms. A balanced, nutritious diet is recommended, as are vitamin, iron, and folate supplements.

During acute flare-ups or surgery, administration of TPN and lipids may be needed to restore a seriously malnourished child. These interventions do not change the course of the inflammation in the bowel but provide essential nutritional support. Elemental diets, which can be absorbed without significant digestion, may be used during acute episodes of Crohn disease to allow the bowel to rest. NG or G-tube feedings during the night may be necessary to prevent further growth impairment (see Chapter 37).

Continued assessments of nutritional status, growth patterns, and development are important elements of nursing care for children with this chronic problem. Assessing the number of stools, nutritional status, weight, developmental milestones, and pain will help evaluate the child's response to treatment.

***Family education and support.*** Because Crohn disease is a long-term health problem that requires numerous medical, pharmacologic, and surgical interventions, family support and financial resources can be strained to the limit. Appropriate community resources can provide education and assistance. The Crohn's and Colitis Foundation of America (CCFA) supplies educational materials and family information on local resources (including financial) and support groups. Long-term nursing care can be improved by providing consistent caregivers and encouraging the child to form relationships. Self-care and management should be major goals in working with children with IBD, as with other chronic diseases. A team approach that includes medical, nutritional, educational, rehabilitative, and psychological support is essential for success.

Another important resource for children with IBD is camp programs such as Camp Oasis sponsored by the CCFA (http://www.ccfa.org/get-involved/camp-oasis). With a dozen camps held each summer across the United States, children with IBD join together to learn more about their disease, create friendships with people who understand them, and gain self-confidence (CCFA, 2016).

***Home care.*** Home care is a mainstay of treatment as parents and child assume the responsibility for care. Teaching parents to administer steroids, including providing information on their inherent side effects and the importance of not discontinuing their use abruptly, should be a high priority. Also, techniques of enema administration and skin care for perianal lesions must be taught. Nutrition diaries can provide useful information. TPN may be administered at home, and parents need complete instructions and referral to a home nursing care agency to obtain equipment, supplies, and support.

In addition, helping children and parents know when to seek medical care is important. Sudden exacerbations of symptoms, weight loss, blood loss, and severe abdominal pain should be reported promptly to healthcare professionals. Stress management and the avoidance of triggers can help minimize the symptoms of the disease and its impact on the child.

The diagnosis of a chronic disease in adolescence can cause psychological distress during this critical time, when an adolescent seeks to gain an identity and begins to think in a more abstract manner; depression and isolation from peers can result (Ahmed, Sonnenburg, Foli, et al., 2016).

### Evaluation

- Is the child free from nocturnal diarrhea?
- Is the child passing fewer than four stools per day?
- Is the child gaining weight appropriately and following the growth chart?
- Is the child's hemoglobin value between 11 g/dL and 16 g/dL?

## PATHOPHYSIOLOGY

### *Inflammatory Bowel Disease*

A triggering factor, whether viral, allergic, or immunologic, causes the bowel to "respond" as if to an injury and results in capillary vasoconstriction and histamine release within the bowel. The histamine has two effects on the bowel. The first is vasodilation, which results in swelling that can cause malabsorption by distorting the surface area of the villi. Swelling then produces cell death and ulceration, which can progress to the development of fissures, strictures, fistulas, adhesions, and bowel obstruction. The second effect of histamine release is increased capillary permeability, which results in increased fluid in the intestine and subsequent diarrhea. Crohn disease affects all layers of the bowel; ulcerative colitis affects the mucosa and submucosa only.

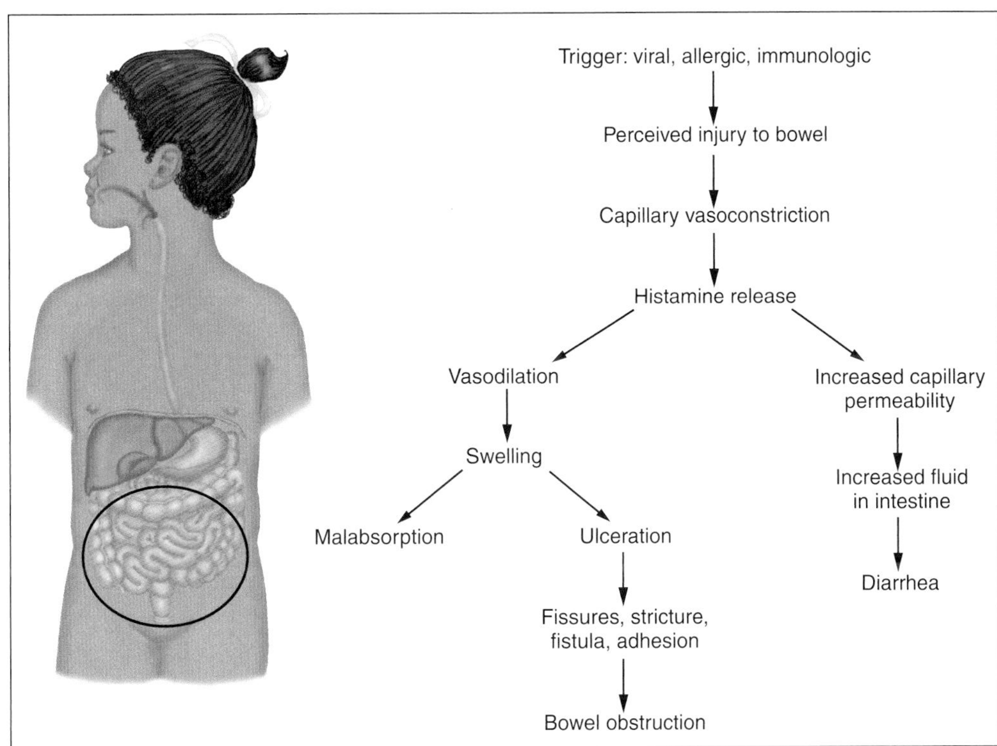


- Does the child report abdominal pain?
- Does the child participate in age-appropriate activities without evidence of depression?
- Is the child's development normal for age?
- Is the child able to share body image concerns with appropriate family members?
- Has the child or family sought external support through appropriate referral groups?
- Do the child and parent demonstrate appropriate skills for day-to-day management and make appropriate future plans for long-term management of disease?
- Do the child and family seek help when exacerbations occur?
- Does the child manage self-care appropriately for age?

## OBSTRUCTIVE DISORDERS

### Hypertrophic Pyloric Stenosis

Pyloric stenosis results when the circular area of muscle surrounding the pylorus hypertrophies and obstructs gastric emptying. This condition is one of the most common surgical disorders of early infancy.

#### Etiology and Incidence

The exact cause of pyloric stenosis remains unknown, but muscular hypertrophy is not present at birth. Pyloric stenosis may be associated with other GI anomalies such as malrotation, short bowel syndrome, esophageal and duodenal atresia, anorectal anomalies, hiatal hernia, and GER. Heredity and family predisposition seem to increase the risk of pyloric stenosis.

The incidence of pyloric stenosis is approximately 1 to 3 in every 1000 live births (Hunter & Liacouras, 2016). Children and offspring of an affected parent are at highest risk. Male infants are affected 4 to 6 times more often than female infants, and term infants are affected more often than premature infants. The incidence is also higher in white infants than in black or Asian infants.

#### Manifestations

Progressive projectile, nonbilious vomiting, usually starting after 3 weeks of age in a previously healthy infant, is the major manifestation of pyloric stenosis. The vomitus may become blood tinged if esophageal irritation occurs. A movable, palpable, firm, olive-shaped mass is felt in the right upper quadrant. This mass is most easily palpated when the stomach is empty and the infant is relaxed. Deep gastric peristaltic waves from left upper quadrant to right upper quadrant may be visible immediately before vomiting. The infant will be irritable and hungry a short time after being fed. If the condition progresses, the infant may become dehydrated and experience metabolic alkalosis. Hyperbilirubinemia is common and resolves after surgery (Hunter & Liacouras, 2016).

## PATHOPHYSIOLOGY

### *Hypertrophic Pyloric Stenosis*

Pyloric spasms cause milk curds to be propelled against a narrowed pyloric channel, with subsequent irritation of its sensitive mucosal lining. Edema of the pyloric mucosa results. This edema further reduces the size of the pyloric canal and creates resistance to the flow of milk. To promote gastric emptying and compensate for this resistance, the pylorus contracts with more force and gradually enlarges. This enlarged pyloric muscle slowly begins to constrict the pyloric channel, and when the mucosal edema subsides, the resistance to flow still remains. A vicious cycle develops and progresses to a high-level obstruction of the pyloric canal.

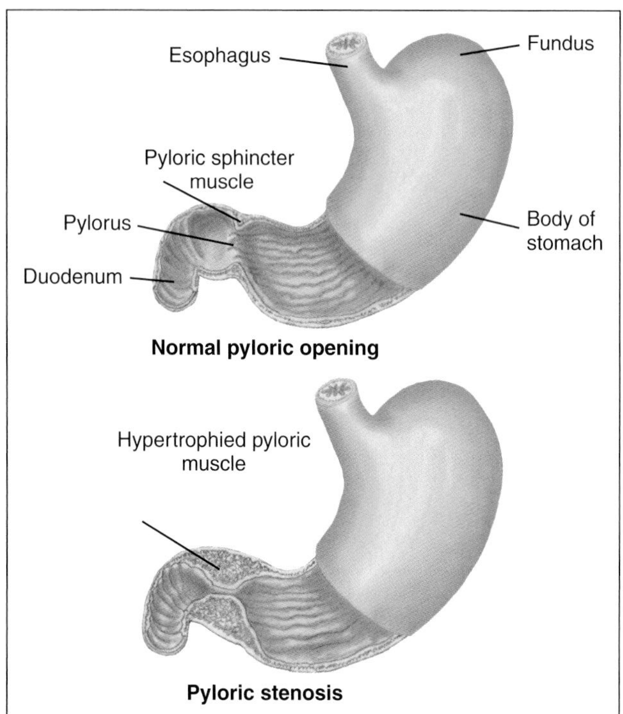


### Diagnostic Evaluation

The diagnosis is made based on a history of vomiting, visible peristaltic waves, and a palpable pyloric mass. When the mass cannot be palpated, ultrasonography will confirm the diagnosis (Markowitz, 2014). A flat plate of the abdomen will show a narrow pylorus with a dilated stomach and the absence of gas distal to the pylorus. A barium swallow examination will disclose the long, narrow pyloric canal and detect delayed gastric emptying. Laboratory findings may indicate metabolic alkalosis as a result of vomiting, including decreased serum potassium and sodium levels, increased pH and bicarbonate, and a decreased chloride level. Indirect bilirubin may be elevated.

### Therapeutic Management

Because pyloric stenosis is usually diagnosed early, few infants are seen in advanced stages of dehydration, malnutrition, and alkalosis. If present, these conditions must be corrected before surgery to prevent postoperative apnea (Hunter & Liacouras, 2016). An infant who is slightly dehydrated with a total serum or plasma carbon dioxide ($CO_2$) level of 25 mEq/L or less, or an infant who is moderately dehydrated with a $CO_2$ of 26 to 35 mEq/L is managed with replacement IV fluids and electrolytes and an NG tube for stomach decompression. Once the stomach is empty, most infants will stop vomiting. Surgery is usually delayed 24 to 48 hours until fluid and electrolyte deficits and acid–base imbalances are corrected. Severely dehydrated and malnourished infants with $CO_2$ levels above 35 mEq/L may need a 3- to 5-day course of IV fluids, electrolyte replacement, and infusions of plasma or packed red blood cells (RBCs) before surgical repair.

A pyloromyotomy, an incision of the pyloric muscle to release the obstruction, is the definitive treatment. Pyloromyotomy is not considered an emergency procedure but is usually performed without delay in well-hydrated infants. The surgery is performed laparoscopically with equal success (Hunter & Liacouras, 2016).

## ! NURSING QUALITY ALERT

### *Gathering Information From a Parent About Infant Vomiting*

Eliciting a description of the amount and characteristics of vomiting can be difficult because descriptive terms are nonspecific, and estimation of emesis amounts is very inconsistent. Useful questions include the following:

- Could you wipe the vomitus off the child with a diaper or cloth?
- Did it require a change of clothes for the infant or caregiver?
- If it was on a bed or sheet, how big a circle did it make?
- If it was on the floor, how big a circle did it make?
- Did it happen after every feeding?
- Did it look like what was just eaten, or was it curdled?
- What color was it?
- Did it appear to be under force and projected away from the child?

Encouraging the parents to keep a written record of answers to these questions can provide essential assessment information.

## NURSING CARE

### The Child With Hypertrophic Pyloric Stenosis

#### Assessment

Hypertrophic pyloric stenosis is suspected in infants with a history of **projectile vomiting**, especially after meals. A thorough nursing history includes the infant's feeding schedule with the type, amount, and frequency of fluid taken. Determine and document the relation of feedings to vomiting. Vomiting is assessed for frequency, amount, color, and consistency, as well as projection.

Assess for signs of dehydration, such as the absence of tears, a weak cry, a depressed fontanel, poor skin turgor, and dry mucous membranes. Signs of potassium, sodium, and chloride depletion should be noted. The abdomen is checked for distention, tenderness, bowel sounds, the presence of a pyloric mass, and gastric peristaltic waves. Family members are evaluated for their understanding of the disorder, a viable support system, and the ability to participate in their child's care.

#### Nursing Diagnosis and Planning

The following nursing diagnoses and expected outcomes are appropriate after assessment of the child with hypertrophic pyloric stenosis:

- Deficient Fluid Volume related to vomiting.

***Expected outcome.*** The infant will have a balanced intake and output, be free of signs of dehydration, and have a urine output greater than 2 to 3 mL/kg/hr.

- Imbalanced Nutrition: Less Than Body Requirements related to persistent vomiting.

***Expected outcome.*** The infant will tolerate regular feedings and will continue to show growth according to a growth chart.

- Impaired Skin Integrity and Risk for Infection related to surgical incisions.

*Expected outcome.* The infant will have clean, dry, intact incisions without redness or exudate.

- Deficient Knowledge related to insufficient information about the need for surgery or about pyloric stenosis.

*Expected outcome.* The parents will describe pyloric stenosis and the expected preoperative and postoperative care. Parents will assume total care of the infant before discharge.

- Acute Pain related to surgery.

*Expected outcome.* The child will not exhibit guarding to palpation and will be calm and content in parent's arms. The parent will be confident that the infant is pain free.

- Anxiety (parental) related to need for hospitalization and surgery.

*Expected outcome.* The parent will express feelings about the surgery and will list the reasons the infant needs to be hospitalized.

### Interventions

*Preoperative care.* Preoperatively, the infant is on NPO status and is stabilized with IV fluids and electrolytes. Measuring the vital signs, weighing the infant daily, and monitoring laboratory values and intake and output are essential nursing interventions. Intake and output should include all IV and PO fluids, blood products, emesis, urine output, stools, and NG drainage. The dehydrated infant is kept warm and quiet. The nurse should provide oral care because membranes are more susceptible to breakdown in their dehydrated state.

The head of the bed is elevated to reduce the risk of aspiration and blankets or towel rolls are used to maintain desired position. The NG tube should be patent and properly positioned. The nurse records the amount, color, and type of drainage. Frequent assessment for respiratory distress is performed.

The nurse explains procedures and plans to parents. Parents are encouraged to participate by holding and caring for their infant.

*Postoperative care.* Postoperatively, the care can vary according to the individual preferences of the surgeon. Most surgeons remove the NG tube immediately and order feedings within the first 4 to 6 hours after surgery if bowel sounds are present. Because gastric peristalsis is normally depressed for 12 to 18 hours after the pyloromyotomy, other surgeons delay feedings for 24 hours and leave the NG tube in place.

Feeding is started with small amounts of an oral electrolyte solution, such as Pedialyte, and the amount is slowly increased. Formula is offered in half-strength concentrations and advanced to full strength within 48 hours after surgery. If the child is receiving breast milk, dilution is not necessary. Feedings are not advanced until the child can tolerate the previous amount without vomiting. IV fluids are continued until the infant is taking and retaining sufficient amounts of formula or breast milk. Many infants have some vomiting during the early postoperative period, but it is usually temporary and without complications.

Postoperative nursing care follows the same guidelines as preoperative care, with accurate monitoring of all vital signs, laboratory values, respiratory status, and hydration. In addition, the nurse assesses the small surgical or laparoscopic incisions for redness, swelling, or drainage. Parents participate as much as possible in their infant's care; however, they may need educational and emotional support from the nurse in the unfamiliar environment of the hospital.

*Home care.* Because symptoms normally abate in the immediate postoperative period, parents may find taking care of their infant much easier than before surgery. However, they should be instructed to report any excessive vomiting, abdominal tenderness, fever, or incisional redness or drainage. If the child is discharged before the diet has been advanced to full strength, written instructions for advancing the diet are essential.

### Evaluation

- Does the child have a flat fontanel, good skin turgor, moist mucous membranes, a urine specific gravity of less than 1.030, and a sodium level within normal limits?
- Is the child tolerating oral feedings without vomiting?
- Has the child's weight returned to pre-illness level within 1 week?
- Is the surgical site clean, dry, intact, and without drainage or redness?
- Can the parents explain the need for surgery and routine preoperative and postoperative care?
- Is the child calm, content, and free from pain?
- Have the parents assumed all care responsibilities at home without assistance?

### CRITICAL THINKING EXERCISE 43.1

Andrew, age 5 weeks, is seen in the outpatient clinic of a large hospital. This is his first visit to the clinic since birth. Andrew's mother states that Andrew is her first child and that she has been concerned that Andrew "spits up" so much. She states she called the clinic approximately 2 weeks ago, but the nurse told her that all babies spit up and that she could talk with someone when she came in for Andrew's 1-month checkup. She missed the appointment because she could not get a ride to the clinic. She further states that the "spitting up" has increased, and for the past 2 days she has not been sure whether Andrew was keeping any of his feedings in his stomach. He has also been very fussy. After several unsuccessful attempts to speak to someone at the clinic by phone, she decided to bring Andrew in to be seen.

1. What will be your priority nursing action?
2. Identify two issues that you should address with Andrew's mother related to seeking care when healthcare information is needed.

## Intussusception

Intussusception is the invagination of a section of the intestine into the distal bowel, causing bowel obstruction. In children, this condition most often occurs as a section of terminal ileum telescopes into the ascending colon through the ileocecal valve. It is the most common cause of intestinal obstruction in children between the ages of 5 months and 3 years (Kennedy & Liacouras, 2016). Although relatively rare, it is a pediatric emergency with classic assessment findings.

### Etiology and Incidence

In young children, the cause of intussusception is unknown. Contributing factors include a preexisting upper respiratory tract infection or other viral infection. A pathologic condition within the colon, such as a mass or an anatomic defect, is the most likely cause in children older than 6 years.

Intussusception generally affects infants and young children, with 80% of cases occurring before age 2 years and rarely before age 3 months. This incidence is 1 to 4/1000 births, and it is more commonly seen in boys than girls (ratio is 3:1). Children with cystic fibrosis are at increased risk for intussusception (Kennedy & Liacouras, 2016).

### Manifestations and Diagnostic Evaluation

Intussusception occurs in children who are well nourished and without a history of GI problems. Paroxysms of pain occur, subside, and recur during the first several hours and then progress to a more constant severe pain. The child may vomit. The following are classic signs of intussusception:

- Abdominal pain
- Passage of bloody mucus ("currant jelly") stool and diarrhea, which may not occur until the postoperative period
- A sausage-shaped abdominal mass

Symptoms of shock and sepsis are present if obstruction has been present for longer than 12 to 24 hours. The child may be listless or lethargic. Older children can have pain without other symptoms.

Abdominal radiographs may show abnormal gas patterns related to the bowel obstruction or a soft tissue mass. Ultrasonography is useful in identifying the location of the intussusception and the amount of edema in the area. A definitive diagnosis can be made and treatment provided simultaneously with a barium enema or air enema examination.

### Therapeutic Management

The goal of treatment is to restore the bowel to its normal position and function as quickly as possible, preferably within the first 24 hours of the appearance of symptoms. In children who do not show symptoms of shock or sepsis, hydrostatic reduction is performed with an isotonic saline, or air enema under fluoroscopic or ultrasonic guidance, with an 80% to 95% success rate (Kennedy & Liacouras, 2016). If reduction fails or findings indicate damage to the bowel, immediate surgery is performed. If the intussusception is detected and reduced within 24 hours, morbidity is minimal. Laparoscopy is now being used if the enema fails to reduce the intussusception except where bowel necrosis is present. There is a 10% recurrence rate after hydrostatic reduction and a 2% to 5% recurrence rate after reduction surgery (Kennedy & Liacouras, 2016). Corticosteroids may play a role in preventing reoccurrence of intussusception (Kennedy & Liacouras, 2016).

## NURSING CARE

### The Child With Intussusception

#### Assessment

The nursing history typically reveals a previously healthy infant who suddenly began crying and flexing the legs in severe pain. This problem may resolve, only to recur a short time later and become more constant. The nurse should assess any child for a bowel obstruction with signs of vomiting, nausea, abdominal distention, and hypoactive or hyperactive bowel sounds. A palpable abdominal mass and passage of "currant jelly" stools will help confirm the diagnosis. The child's hydration status is assessed on admission. Fever, an increased heart rate, changes in level of consciousness or blood pressure, and respiratory distress should be reported immediately as they can indicate sepsis or peritonitis.

#### Nursing Diagnosis and Planning

The following nursing diagnoses and expected outcomes may be appropriate for the child with intussusception and the child's family:

- Risk for Ineffective GI Tissue Perfusion related to bowel compression.

***Expected outcome.*** The child will have a patent bowel, as evidenced by the passage of soft, formed, Hematest-negative stools.

- Acute Pain related to bowel obstruction and surgery.

## PATHOPHYSIOLOGY

### *Intussusception*

As the bowel telescopes inside itself, obstruction develops. In addition, the mesenteric vessels become trapped between the walls of the two layers, and ischemia occurs. This pressure on the bowel leads to bleeding and "currant jelly" stools. Mesenteric ischemia also causes edema and possible strangulation or infarction of the bowel, which can progress to perforation, peritonitis, sepsis, shock, and death.

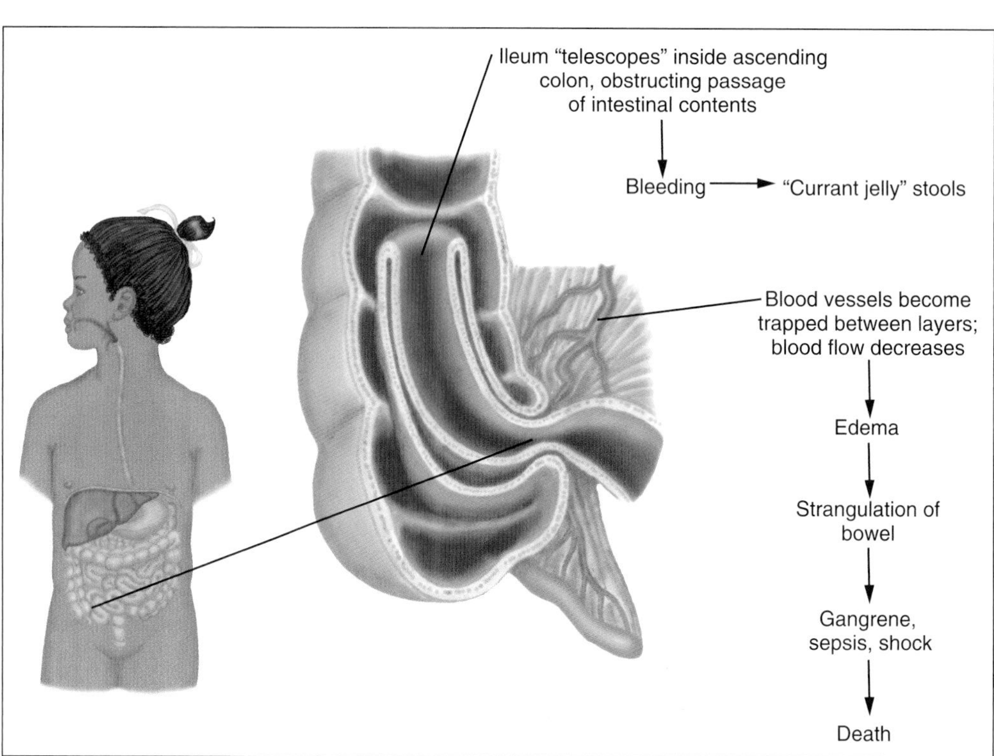

*Expected outcome.* The child will be free from abdominal pain, as evidenced by age-appropriate play and activity, and no guarding during palpation.

- Deficient Fluid Volume related to vomiting and diarrhea.

*Expected outcome.* The child will be able to tolerate age-appropriate food and fluids without vomiting or recurrence of symptoms and will be free from fluid and electrolyte disturbances, as evidenced by return to normal weight, moist mucous membranes, good skin turgor, and normal serum sodium level and hematocrit.

- Deficient Knowledge related to possibility of surgery and the need for immediate intervention.

*Expected outcome.* The parents will verbalize an understanding of the need for immediate intervention and will explain the mechanisms of intussusception and hydrostatic reduction.

- Anxiety (parental) related to the child's hospitalization or possible surgery.

*Expected outcome.* The parents will express concerns and fears and will seek appropriate support as needed.

- Disturbed Sleep Pattern related to colicky abdominal pain.

*Expected outcome.* The child will return to normal sleep patterns.

#### Interventions

*Initial care.* Once the diagnosis is made, immediate plans are made to admit the child to the hospital for hydrostatic reduction. Prompt assessment for dehydration, shock, and sepsis is essential, including documenting mental status, capillary perfusion, and urine output. The child is given IV fluids, and an NG tube is inserted if distention is present. During reduction, pain medications or sedation may be needed to decrease spasm. After reduction, clear liquids are started and the diet is advanced gradually as tolerated.

*Post reduction care.* The nurse observes for the passage of stool and notes the characteristics of the stool. The child is assessed for symptoms of bowel obstruction indicating a recurrence of intussusception. Resumption of a normal diet and activities and the passage of stool without blood indicate a successful outcome. If hydrostatic reduction is unsuccessful, the child must be prepared for abdominal surgery or laparoscopy. Because intussusception can resolve spontaneously in some cases, the nurse continues to monitor the child for return of normal bowel function, eliminating the need for surgery.

Postoperatively, the child is kept on NPO status until bowel function returns. Intermittent NG suction, IV therapy, pain medications, maintenance of respiratory function, frequent assessment, and meeting developmental needs remain nursing responsibilities.

*Family education and support.* During this difficult time for parents, relieving their anxiety by providing appropriate information is an essential nursing action. This includes describing the pathophysiology of intussusception, the process for hydrostatic reduction, and the expected recovery care for their child, including IV fluids, intermittent NG suction, and frequent vital sign checks and assessments. In addition, emotional support can be provided to the parents by encouraging participation in their child's care, listening to their concerns, and encouraging expression of their feelings during this stressful time.

To help parents visualize telescoping of the bowel with intussusception, the nurse can use a hospital glove, pressing one finger (representing the terminal ileum) into the inflated glove (the distal colon) and causing it to go inside itself. The same approach can show how hydrostatic reduction works. The nurse presses on the glove (the distal portion) with one hand, showing how the telescoped portion is pushed back into its normal position.

#### Evaluation

- In the preoperative period, does the child have moist mucous membranes, good skin turgor, and a urine specific gravity less than 1.030?
- Is the child passing soft, formed, Hematest-negative stools?
- Does the infant guard the abdomen during palpation?
- Is the child demonstrating age-appropriate activity levels, sleep patterns, and play?
- Is the child tolerating age-appropriate food and fluids without vomiting or recurrence of symptoms?
- Can the parents explain the rationale for hydrostatic reduction?
- Are all the parents' questions answered to their satisfaction?
- Are the parents able to resume care of their infant without stress or anxiety?

## Volvulus

Volvulus is a condition caused by a malrotation or twisting of the bowel that results in a bowel obstruction. It is the result of a defect in fetal development; the midgut, which normally rotates 270 degrees around the superior mesenteric artery, fails to rotate and fixes itself to the abdominal wall.

Affected infants usually manifest pain, bilious vomiting, and other signs of bowel obstruction. Surgery is essential to prevent bowel ischemia. The nursing care is similar to that for the child with intussusception who requires surgical treatment.

## Hirschsprung Disease

Also known as congenital aganglionosis or megacolon, Hirschsprung disease is the result of an absence of ganglion cells in the rectum and, to varying degrees, upward in the colon. Hirschsprung disease is the major cause of lower bowel obstruction in newborns (Fiorino & Liacouras, 2016b).

### Etiology and Incidence

The disease is a result of embryonic failure of migration of the hindgut ganglion cells to the most caudal portion of the GI tract, the rectum. The initiating factor in this failure is unknown.

Hirschsprung disease occurs in 1 in 5000 live births, with a 4:1 male-to-female ratio with short-segment disease and 2:1 male-to-female ratio with total colonic involvement (Fiorino & Liacouras, 2016b). It has a strong hereditary component and a higher incidence in children with Down syndrome.

### Manifestations and Diagnostic Evaluation

Delayed passage or absence of meconium stool in the neonatal period is the cardinal sign of Hirschsprung disease. Any child who does not pass meconium within the first 24 hours and who is prone to constipation or stool infrequency in the first month after birth is suspected of having Hirschsprung disease. The neonate, infant, or older child may exhibit signs of bowel obstruction, abdominal pain and distention, vomiting, and failure to thrive. Chronic constipation beginning in the first month of life results in pellet-like or ribbon-like stools that are foul smelling.

A rectal examination reveals a tight internal sphincter and the absence of stool, followed by an often explosive release of gas and feces related to the sudden but transient increase in rectal size. The definitive diagnosis is made by suction rectal biopsy. During biopsy, a small core or punch sample that contains all layers of the bowel mucosa is removed. Absence of ganglionic cells in the sample confirms the diagnosis of Hirschsprung disease. Some children require a full-thickness biopsy performed under anesthesia by a surgeon. The diagnosis of older children can be confirmed with a contrast barium enema that demonstrates retained contrast (Fiorino & Liacouras, 2016b). Anal rectal manometry (ARM) is helpful in the diagnosis of ultrashort-segment Hirschsprung disease, also known as anal achalasia. This is a test in which a catheter with a balloon is inserted into the rectum to test the nerves and sphincter pressure of the anus. Children with Hirschsprung disease will have a nonrelaxing internal anal sphincter.

### Therapeutic Management

Hirschsprung disease can involve the entire colon (total colonic Hirschsprung), a very short segment of the colon, or any amount in between. Treatment involves removing the aganglionic portion of the intestine in a one- or two-step surgical intervention. A one-step laparoscopic or transanal pull-through procedure is being used successfully with increasing frequency (Fiorino & Liacouras, 2016b). For neonates, a two-step surgical procedure is often used. First, to relieve the obstruction, a temporary colostomy is performed with the most distal section of normal bowel. Once the infant weighs 8 to 10 kg (18 to 22 lb), the final step, a pull-through procedure, is performed. All aganglionic portions of the bowel are excised, the normal bowel is reattached to the anal canal, and the colostomy is closed. Normal bowel function usually returns shortly after surgery. For children diagnosed after infancy, the type of surgical procedure and the time period between the steps of the pull-through procedure vary. Medical interventions such as botulinum toxin (Botox) injections to the internal anal sphincter (IAS) muscle are used to decrease the resting IAS pressures. Rectal irrigations to remove air and stool are sometimes needed to relieve symptoms associated with enterocolitis before surgery. Most patients are able to achieve bowel continence (Fiorino & Liacouras, 2016b).

## NURSING CARE

### The Child With Hirschsprung Disease

#### Assessment

The child with Hirschsprung disease will have constipation that has been present since the neonatal period and frequent passage of foul-smelling, ribbon-like or pellet-like stools. Nutritional status should be assessed because malnutrition can develop as a result of extreme distention or enterocolitis. Thin extremities, abdominal distention, and a history of poor feeding should be noted.

If the child is acutely ill on presentation, enterocolitis must be suspected and reported immediately, as this is a life-threatening complication. The nurse documents the assessment of bowel sounds and abdominal distention, the frequency of vomiting and diarrhea, and changes in abdominal circumference. Temperature readings must be obtained by a route other than rectal.

## PATHOPHYSIOLOGY

### *Hirschsprung Disease*

Ganglia provide parasympathetic innervation of the colon. In Hirschsprung disease, ganglia are absent from a variable length of colon extending proximally from the anus. Adequate peristalsis cannot occur in the affected colon, leading to a tonic contraction of the lumen that causes functional bowel obstruction, chronic constipation, and the passage of ribbon-like stools. Hirschsprung disease can cause complete bowel obstruction. Because of the constriction of the lumen, huge amounts of feces and gas collect proximal to the aganglionic portion, resulting in a gross enlargement of this segment (megacolon). The enlarged segment of colon is actually normal in its function.

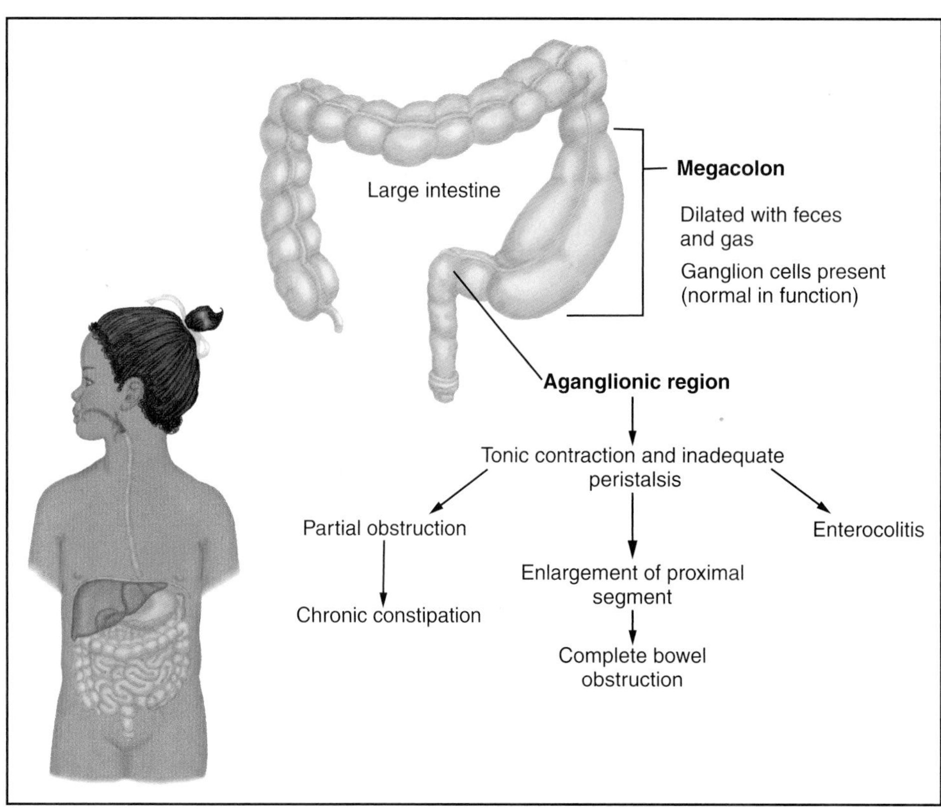

Family concerns and coping methods are assessed. This disease can drain family and financial resources during the diagnosis and surgical treatment. Mild disease can remain undiagnosed until the child is older, at which time the disease appears as chronic constipation. Assessing the older child's feelings about chronic constipation and its treatment is important.

### Nursing Diagnoses and Planning

The following nursing diagnoses and expected outcomes may be appropriate for the child with Hirschsprung disease:

- Constipation related to aganglionic bowel and inadequate peristalsis.

***Expected outcome.*** The child will pass soft, formed stools without retention.

- Risk for Deficient Fluid Volume or Excess Fluid Volume related to surgical preparation.

***Expected outcome.*** The child will be free from fluid and electrolyte disturbances related to presurgical bowel cleansing.

- Impaired Skin Integrity related to colostomy and surgical repair.

***Expected outcome.*** The surgical and colostomy sites will be clean and free from exudate, redness, or drainage. The colostomy site will be intact without bleeding or skin irritation.

- Risk for Infection related to surgical repair.

***Expected outcome.*** The child will be afebrile without signs of infection at the site.

- Imbalanced Nutrition: Less Than Body Requirements related to GI surgery.

***Expected outcome.*** The child will have normal bowel sounds, will pass stool, and will tolerate a regular diet.

- Acute Pain related to surgical incisions.

***Expected outcome.*** The child will be free from pain and will be able to participate in usual activities of daily living.

- Deficient Knowledge related to incomplete information about the need for surgery, irrigation, or care of the ostomy.

***Expected outcome.*** The parents will state the necessity for rectal irrigations or surgical intervention. The parents and child will assume responsibility for care of the ostomy and rectal irrigations, if indicated.

- Disturbed Body Image related to colostomy and irrigations.

***Expected outcome.*** The child and family will express feelings about irrigations, ostomy care, and the impact the condition has had on the child's body image.

- Anxiety (parental and child) related to the loss of the perfect child or need for surgery.

***Expected outcome.*** The parents will express fears and concerns and seek support as needed.

### Interventions

***Preparing the child for surgery.*** The nurse closely monitors and records the child's bowel elimination pattern. Isotonic saline enemas are administered preoperatively until the return is clear (see Chapter 37). An alternative bowel cleansing regimen is to administer a polyethylene-glycol–electrolyte lavage solution (GoLYTELY) orally or through the NG tube. This regimen is used only in children older than 5 years and is given at a dosage of 25 to 40 mL/kg/hr. Sodium phosphate (Fleets Phosphosoda) is another alternative requiring ingestion of only approximately 200 mL at one time for children older than 5 years. After bowel cleansing, the child is on NPO status until surgery. IV fluids are provided as needed and strict intake and output records are maintained.

***Preventing infection and maintaining skin integrity.*** Neomycin 1.0% solution given by rectum or stoma is administered preoperatively to sterilize the bowel for surgery. IV antibiotics also contribute to bowel sterilization as well as prevention of surgical incision site infection. The nurse monitors vital signs regularly and measures the child's abdominal circumference each time. The tympanic, temporal, oral, or axillary method for taking the temperature is used to avoid trauma to the rectal mucosa. The surgical site is checked for redness, swelling, and purulent drainage.

If the child has a colostomy, the stoma site is inspected for bleeding and impaired skin integrity. After the pull-through procedure, the nurse observes the anal site carefully for redness, discharge, and the presence of stool. To prevent skin breakdown, meticulous care of the skin of the abdomen and perineum is provided. Dressing changes are performed to keep incisions clean and dry. Ostomy sites are cared for by using appropriate-size, hypoallergenic ostomy supplies and appliances. The nurse encourages the parents and child to begin ostomy care as soon as possible.

***Maintaining nutritional and hydration status.*** Postoperatively, the child is on NPO status until bowel sounds return or flatus is passed. The NG tube is set to intermittent suction until peristalsis returns. The nurse monitors the child for signs of dehydration and acid–base disturbances. To prevent dehydration, the child remains on IV fluids until tolerating oral fluids well. Oral intake is then advanced from clear liquids to a regular diet as ordered.

***Reducing pain.*** Pain medications are administered as ordered along with other complementary interventions to provide effective pain management. Most school-age children can use patient-controlled analgesia (PCA) for effective pain control (see Chapter 39). The nurse encourages the use of nonpharmacologic pain control measures such as repositioning, back rubs, music, holding, rocking, massage, and quiet talking. If pain control is not achieved as anticipated, the child must be assessed for complications such as a bowel obstruction or infection.

***Providing education and relieving anxiety.*** Before the scheduled surgery, the parents may need to manage rectal irrigations at home. The parents must learn the procedure and observe for distention and signs of obstruction. Parents are prompted to express any concerns regarding the need for irrigations or their ability to perform them. The nurse teaches the parents and child about the surgery and recovery process. If the child is to have a colostomy, the child and parents are given the opportunity to see and manipulate the equipment before surgery.

Postoperatively, preschoolers and young school-age children are encouraged to draw pictures, use dolls, and engage in play to express concerns about body appearance, irrigations, and the colostomy. The nurse provides time for the child and family to share their fears, concerns, and questions; active listening is a critical nursing intervention. Colostomy care is taught in the immediate postoperative period, so the parents can participate in the child's care with assistance by the nurse. For the older child, self-care of the colostomy is initiated as soon as possible. Referral to an enterostomal therapist is recommended. The nurse also can refer the family to support groups for children with ostomies and other community resources.

### Evaluation

- Does the child pass soft, formed stools without retention after completion of the surgical correction?
- Has the child tolerated the bowel-cleansing regimen without signs of fluid and electrolyte imbalance, as evidenced by moist mucous membranes, good skin turgor, and an hourly urine output appropriate for age?
- Is the child afebrile, and are surgical sites free from redness, purulent drainage, excess heat, and dehiscence?

- Is the colostomy or anal pull-through area free from bleeding and skin breakdown?
- Are bowel sounds active and present in all four quadrants, and is the child tolerating an age-appropriate diet without vomiting or diarrhea?
- Does the child appear to be free of pain, as evidenced by the ability to sleep comfortably and participate in appropriate play activities when awake?
- Can the parents and child demonstrate all procedures needed for appropriate home care?
- Is the child able to express feelings about body changes related to treatments or procedures?
- Are the parents calm and able to resume all care of their child without anxiety?

## MALABSORPTION DISORDERS

### Lactose Intolerance

The inability to tolerate lactose, the sugar found in dairy products, is the result of an absence or deficiency of lactase, an enzyme found in the secretions of the small intestines that is required for the digestion of lactose. The four types of lactose intolerance are primary, secondary, congenital, and developmental. Congenital lactose intolerance, which is rare, appears at birth and involves a complete absence of lactase. Developmental lactose intolerance is a deficiency of lactase that appears in early to late childhood.

#### Etiology and Incidence

Most cases of lactose intolerance result from inadequate levels of lactase. The exact reason for this deficiency is unknown. The condition is likely to be more severe during and after other illnesses affecting the GI mucosa, such as viral gastroenteritis or food poisoning.

The condition appears to have an ethnic association, with an increased incidence in Asians, American Indians, Arabs, Jews, blacks, and southern Europeans (National Institute of Diabetes and Digestive and Kidney Diseases, 2014).

#### Manifestations and Diagnostic Evaluation

Manifestations of lactose intolerance include diarrhea that is frothy but not fatty, abdominal distention, cramping abdominal pain, and excessive flatus. The symptoms are not usually seen until lactase activity begins to decrease after age 3 years or during other GI illnesses. If the child has congenital lactose intolerance, symptoms will be seen immediately and can be severe.

A history of improvement after implementation of a lactose-free diet provides a presumptive diagnosis. A finding of 1+ or higher on the Clinitest stool test (0 to 4+ range) indicates intestinal malabsorption of sugar. Lactose tolerance testing (breath hydrogen test) involves giving the patient an oral lactose load and then measuring blood glucose levels and the amount of hydrogen in breath samples. Lower-than-expected blood sugar levels and high hydrogen content in breath samples point to poor lactose absorption in the small intestines.

#### Therapeutic Management

The treatment for lactose intolerance is removal of lactose from the diet. In most cases, total elimination is unnecessary. Removing milk as the beverage of choice often provides sufficient relief from symptoms. Additional dietary changes are sometimes necessary to provide adequate sources of calcium and, in the infant, protein and calories. Formulas that do not contain lactose (Isomil, Nursoy, Nutramigen, ProSobee, and other soy-based formulas) can be given to the infant suspected of having lactose intolerance. Breastfeeding mothers are urged to eliminate lactose products from their diet.

These dietary changes can be supplemented with the use of commercial lactase preparations (Lactaid, Dairy Ease, Lac-Dose) that can be taken with lactose-containing food to provide adequate lactase levels and variable relief from symptoms.

**PATHOPHYSIOLOGY**

***Lactose Intolerance***

An absence or a deficiency of lactase leads to the inability to digest lactose and the subsequent accumulation of lactose in the lumen of the small intestines. As a result, water is drawn into the colon, resulting in watery osmotic diarrhea containing undigested lactose. In addition, gastrointestinal (GI) bacteria break down lactose and release hydrogen, which causes excess gas production, bloating, and abdominal pain.

## NURSING CARE

### The Child With Lactose Intolerance

#### Assessment

Assessment will reveal a healthy-looking child with episodic abdominal pain and occasional diarrhea in the absence of nutritional deficiencies or other health problems. The child and family may or may not be able to correlate symptoms with food intake. With a congenital absence of lactase, the condition is likely to be more severe and diarrhea is a major concern. The neonate or infant may be extremely dehydrated, with severe diarrhea and weight loss.

**PARENTS WANT TO KNOW**

***Care of the Child With Lactose Intolerance***

- Your child must avoid all high-lactose foods (e.g., milk, ice cream). If you are unsure about whether a food contains lactose, examine labels for the presence of milk or milk products.
- You can use soy-based, lactose-free formulas as needed for your infant (e.g., Isomil, Nursoy, Nutramigen, ProSobee). If you are breastfeeding, limit your own intake of dairy products.
- Soy-based beverages (e.g., Silk) are available in most grocery stores.
- Your older child can obtain calcium through other foods besides milk. These foods include egg yolks, green leafy vegetables, dried beans, cauliflower, and molasses. Calcium supplements are also available.
- Once your child's symptoms have disappeared, you can gradually add yogurt, hard cheeses, and small amounts of milk to assess tolerance.
- If you are having difficulty determining what foods are lactose free or need help finding recipes that use lactose-free foods, ask for a dietary consultation.

#### Nursing Diagnosis and Planning

The following nursing diagnoses and expected outcomes may be appropriate for the infant or child with lactose intolerance:

- Acute Pain related to bloating and flatus.

*Expected outcomes.* The child will be free from abdominal pain, as evidenced by developmentally appropriate play and activity. The child will have normal bowel sounds with a soft abdomen that is not painful during palpation.

- Diarrhea related to maldigestion.

*Expected outcome.* The child will have soft, formed stools.

- Deficient Knowledge related to incomplete understanding about needed dietary changes.

*Expected outcome.* The child will take in a minimum of 800 mg of calcium per day, as reported in the dietary history. The child and family will state foods to be avoided or provided in small amounts. The child will receive adequate calcium sources in diet and appropriate lactase products.

### Interventions

The principal nursing intervention is teaching. Symptoms are often relieved after a lactose-free diet is followed for a short period. Foods containing small amounts of lactose can then be added gradually to assess the child's reaction. If small amounts of milk are tolerated, food or lactase preparations are given simultaneously with milk. These simple changes can offer instant relief.

After diagnosis and initial management, this condition is often perceived to be only a minor nuisance. However, emotional support for the family may be needed. Referring the family to self-help and information groups and encouraging family members to share successes and concerns are important nursing interventions.

### Evaluation

- Is the child happy, content, and free of excess gas and bloating?
- Can the parent state what foods are essential to avoid?
- Are the child's stools normal and formed?
- Does the food diary indicate an intake of at least 800 mg of calcium daily for a child age 1 to 10 years?
- Does the parent express satisfaction with control of the child's condition?

## Celiac Disease

Celiac disease (CD), also known as gluten enteropathy or tropical sprue, results from the inability to digest gluten. *Gluten* is a general term that refers to the storage proteins found in wheat, barley, and rye. This lifelong deficiency requires dietary modification to prevent chronic maldigestion and malabsorption.

### Etiology and Incidence

The etiology of CD is not fully understood, but it is considered to be an autoimmune disease that occurs in genetically susceptible patients (Hill, 2011). Some patients with CD carry either the *HLA-DQ2* or *HLA-DQ8* gene. However, many people who carry one of these genes do not develop CD despite recurrent gluten exposure. This observation suggests that the etiology of CD is multifactorial, including both environmental and genetic factors (Branski, Troncone, & Fasano, 2016). Delaying the introduction of gluten into the infant's diet and breastfeeding before and during that introduction can delay the appearance of symptoms in at-risk individuals but will not prevent celiac disease (Branski et al., 2016).

The incidence of CD varies in different regions. In the United States, the incidence is approximately 1% of the population (Branski et al., 2016; Allen, 2015). The incidence is much higher in Europe. Siblings and children of affected individuals are at highest risk for the disease (Allen, 2015).

### Manifestations

The major manifestations in the child with CD include diarrhea and growth failure. The child's growth usually is below the 25th percentile on growth charts.

Additional symptoms include abdominal distention, vomiting, anemia, irritability, anorexia, muscle wasting, edema, and folate deficiency. Symptoms are not seen until 3 to 6 months after the introduction of grains to the diet, usually at age 9 to 12 months. The child in celiac crisis exhibits profuse, watery diarrhea and vomiting, with eventual electrolyte imbalance and vascular compromise (Hill, 2011).

### Diagnostic Evaluation

Tests for the immunoglobulin A (IgA) antitissue transglutaminase (tTG) antibody or IgA antiendomysial antibody have replaced antigliadin antibody testing in children with CD. If children have a demonstrated IgA deficiency, the IgG anti-tTG test is used (Allen, 2015). Jejunal biopsy will unequivocally identify ulcerations in the GI tract. Monitoring the reaction to a gluten-free diet supports the diagnosis. Symptoms are often relieved in 1 week by removal of gluten from the diet.

Further diagnostic testing includes the breath hydrogen test to determine the amount of carbohydrate malabsorption occurring. This test is not specific for CD. D-Xylose testing indicates the amount of mucosal damage, allowing the remaining absorptive surface to be estimated.

### Therapeutic Management

Dietary management is the mainstay of treatment. All wheat, rye, barley, and oats should be eliminated from the diet and replaced with corn and rice. To correct deficiencies, vitamin supplements, especially with fat-soluble vitamins and folate, are sometimes needed in the early period of treatment.

Dietary restrictions are lifelong, although small amounts of grains might be tolerated after the ulcerations have healed. Adolescents have difficulty maintaining a gluten-free diet without having an unbalanced diet high in protein and fat. An adolescent on a strict gluten-free diet still has a risk for dietary imbalance; supplements and support from dietary services are essential for maintenance. Referral to a nutritionist who has experience with celiac disease is very important in helping children and their families as is support groups.

Occasionally, the nurse is the first to see a child in celiac crisis. Celiac crisis causes profuse, watery diarrhea and vomiting, which can quickly lead to severe dehydration and metabolic acidosis. The cause of the crisis, usually an infection or a hidden source of gluten, must be identified. The child is given IV fluids to correct fluid, electrolyte, and acid–base imbalances, albumin to treat shock, and corticosteroids to decrease severe mucosal inflammation.

## NURSING CARE

### The Child With Celiac Disease

#### Assessment

Assessment of the infant with celiac disease (CD) usually reveals an irritable, malnourished infant who exhibits failure to thrive by 9 to 12 months. Any child with diarrhea, especially one with foul-smelling, fatty stools and significant growth delays, should be suspected of having CD. A noticeable decline in the child's rate of growth as charted on the growth curve, associated with the addition of grains to the diet, is essential supportive evidence.

Abdominal assessment reveals distention and ascites with an increasing girth. Observations by the nurse often identify other signs of malnutrition, such as thin, edematous extremities, pallor, and muscle wasting. Anemia is a common finding.

The child with severe diarrhea, foul-smelling stools, vomiting, poor perfusion, edema, or changes in vital signs (shock or metabolic acidosis) should be referred for emergency care of celiac crisis.

## PATHOPHYSIOLOGY

### *Celiac Disease*

Gluten—the protein found in rye, oats, barley, and wheat—breaks down into gliadin and other by-products. Celiac disease results from an inability to digest gliadin. This condition results in the accumulation of glutamine in the intestine, which has a toxic effect on the mucosal cells. The villi atrophy, markedly decreasing the absorptive surface of the intestine. Malabsorption of fats, carbohydrates, and vitamins develops. Celiac crisis is the result of sudden accumulation of glutamine and the subsequent destruction of the mucosal cells, causing severe diarrhea and dehydration.

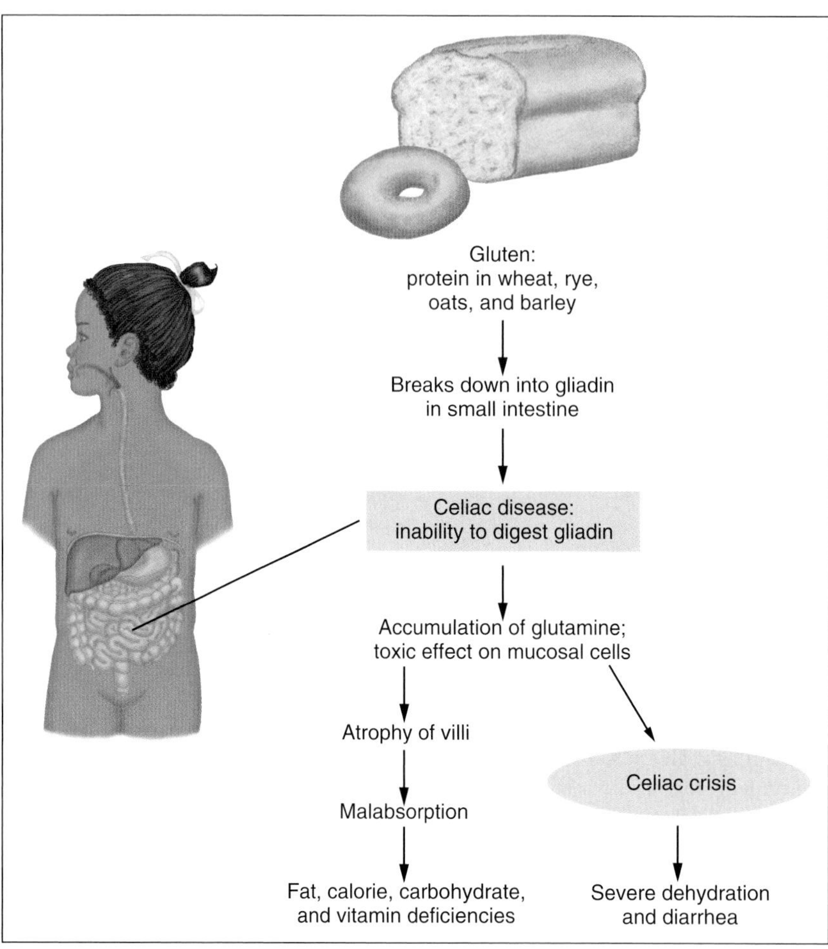


### Nursing Diagnosis and Planning

The following nursing diagnoses and expected outcomes may be appropriate for the infant or child with CD:

- Imbalanced Nutrition: Less Than Body Requirements related to malabsorption.

*Expected outcome.* The child will have soft, formed stools without diarrhea.

- Acute Pain or Chronic Pain related to abdominal distention.

*Expected outcome.* The child will be free from abdominal pain, as evidenced by age-appropriate play and activity level.

- Delayed Growth and Development related to malnutrition.

*Expected outcome.* The child will return to and follow a normal growth pattern according to a growth chart.

- Deficient Knowledge related to dietary changes.

*Expected outcome.* The family will offer appropriate foods to the infant or child, as evidenced by a food diary. The child and family will state the need for lifelong dietary changes and seek emotional and educational support as needed.

- Deficient Fluid Volume related to celiac crisis.

*Expected outcome.* The child will be adequately hydrated, as evidenced by moist mucous membranes and good skin turgor.

### Interventions

The most significant nursing intervention is teaching parents and the child to modify the child's diet. Pain will likely be quickly relieved by eliminating gluten from the diet. Involvement of nutritionists in teaching and follow-up care is important. Careful and consistent monitoring will be necessary to ensure that the infant or child resumes normal growth and development. When the child has normal stools without diarrhea and resumes a normal growth pattern, teaching will have been effective.

Because CD is a lifelong condition, support groups, camp programs, and other community resources can assist the child and family to manage the disease and sustain essential dietary modifications. The American Celiac Society is an excellent source of information and support. The nurse should refer the family to this group and other support organizations. The child and parents are encouraged to share their fears and concerns about the chronic nature of the disease and its impact on the family as a unit as well as each family member's life.

## PATIENT-CENTERED TEACHING

### *Care of the Child With Celiac Disease*

- You must eliminate all wheat, rye, barley, oats, and hydrolyzed vegetable protein from your child's diet. This includes most pasta, baked products, and many breakfast cereals.
- Gluten-free substitutes are available at specialized stores.
- You can substitute corn, rice, or millet as grains. These grains can be obtained as flour for baking.
- Your child should take vitamin supplements, especially folate and fat-soluble vitamins, because these vitamins will be hard to provide in your child's diet.
- You will need to read all labels on foods and medications carefully to avoid any unknown additives.
- When your child is old enough to understand, you will need to help your child make appropriate food choices. This challenge can be difficult for an older child or adolescent, because popular foods often contain ingredients that will make your child's condition worse. Encourage your child to talk with a nutritionist to plan a diet that is appropriate and not too different from the diet of peers.
- Support groups are available to provide information and resources.

### Evaluation

- Does the child have soft, formed stools without diarrhea or signs of dehydration?
- Is the child participating in age-appropriate activities?
- Has the child resumed a normal growth pattern according to a growth chart?
- Is the family able to verbalize an understanding of the child's dietary and emotional needs?
- Does a food diary indicate an intake of approximately 100 kcal/kg for the infant and for the child up to age 3 years?
- Do the parents use available support and education groups?
- Do the parents express satisfaction with the way they are coping with dietary changes?
- Does the child have good skin turgor, moist mucous membranes, and a urine output appropriate for age (see Chapter 40)?

## Short Bowel Syndrome

Short bowel syndrome (SBS) occurs as a result of congenital malformations of the GI tract or surgical resection that decreases the length of the small intestines (bowel). A loss of greater than 50% of the small bowel can result in symptoms of generalized malabsorption or deficiencies of certain nutrients related to the region of bowel that has been removed (Vanderhoof & Branski, 2016).

### Etiology and Incidence

SBS in newborns is caused by congenital short bowel syndrome, multiple GI tract atresias, and gastroschisis (Vanderhoof & Branski, 2016). Removing portions of the small bowel to treat conditions such as necrotizing enterocolitis (NEC), meconium ileus (associated with cystic fibrosis), intussusception, volvulus, long-segment Hirschsprung disease, Crohn disease, and trauma also cause SBS (Vanderhoof & Branski, 2016). The most common cause of SBS in preterm infants is NEC (National Institute of Diabetes and Digestive and Kidney Diseases, 2015) (see Chapter 29).

Determining the number of children and adults with SBS is difficult; most estimates are based on patients who require long-term TPN. Limited studies estimate three individuals with SBS per million population (Cagir & Sawyer, 2012; National Institute of Diabetes and Digestive and Kidney Diseases, 2015).

### Pathophysiology

The small bowel is 200 to 250 cm long at birth and grows to 300 to 800 cm long by adulthood (Vanderhoff & Branski, 2016). A small bowel that is too short has less mucosal surface area than normal, leading to inadequate absorption of fluids, electrolytes, and nutrients. Further, malabsorption of specific nutrients can occur, depending on the region of the bowel that has been removed. For example, resection of the proximal jejunum decreases the absorption of carbohydrates, proteins, iron, and water-soluble vitamins. Removal of the ileum can have a profound effect on fluid and electrolytes due to malabsorption of water and sodium (Vanderhoff & Branski, 2016).

### Manifestations

The most common symptom of SBS in infants and children is watery diarrhea (National Institute of Diabetes and Digestive and Kidney Diseases, 2015). Additional SBS manifestations are similar to those seen with other malabsorption disorders such as steatorrhea, bloating, excessive gas, foul-smelling stool, poor appetite, vomiting, weight loss or inability to gain weight, and fatigue. SBS complications include protein-caloric malnutrition, dehydration, electrolyte imbalances, gallstones, kidney stones, and high levels of bacteria in the intestines. Vitamin and mineral deficiencies can arise as evidenced by specific symptoms. For example, losses of vitamin D, magnesium, and calcium cause paresthesias and tetany; vitamin K depletion prolongs bleeding time, causing increased bruising.

### Therapeutic Management

During surgery, every effort is made to preserve as much small bowel length as possible. After surgery, the child's fluid and electrolyte balance must be restored and stabilized. The mainstay of treatment for infants and children is nutritional support. Total parenteral nutrition (TPN) is initiated as the primary source for all nutrients. It is infused daily over 10 to 12 hours or longer, often while the child is sleeping, using a central venous catheter (see Chapter 38). TPN is formulated to meet the child's nutritional needs as well as promote weight gain and growth.

Providing enteral nutrition as soon as possible following surgery is of key importance, as it allows for intestinal adaptation that increases the capacity of the small bowel to absorb nutrients. Continuous, small-volume enteral feedings are introduced as weaning from TPN begins. The child is given enriched formulas that provide for nutritional needs and contain components that stimulate growth of the bowel mucosal (Vanderhoof & Branski, 2016).

### Nursing Considerations

The child's nutritional therapy via IV and enteral routes must be carefully administered and monitored. TPN is generally infused through a central venous access device. Strict aseptic technique must be used when performing insertion site dressing changes and when administering TPN to prevent central-line–associated bloodstream infections (see Chapter 38).

Enteral feedings are generally infused through an NG tube, G-tube, or gastrostomy button (see Chapter 37 and Procedure: Administering Enteral Feedings). Verification of proper tube placement is essential before each feeding. For the child with SBS, enteral nutrition is advanced slowly while corresponding adjustments are made to the composition of the TPN. It is of critical importance to carefully assess and document the child's ability to tolerate enteral feedings noting any signs of dehydration, electrolyte imbalances, and nutritional deficits.

Infants and children with SBS need oral stimulation. The nurse provides opportunities for nonnutritive sucking and gives water and small amounts of solid foods to the infant or child orally. These interventions will promote learning to suck and swallow as well as help these children avoid oral hypersensitivity and food aversions.

Although some children need only a limited course of specialized enteral nutrition, others require prolonged TPN. If the child requires extended hospitalization, the nurse provides care that addresses the child's developmental and emotional needs as well as the psychosocial needs of the family. When long-term TPN and enteral feedings are required, the nurse develops and implements a teaching plan that will effectively prepare the family to provide the appropriate nutritional therapy in the home.

## HEPATIC DISORDERS

### Viral Hepatitis

Hepatitis is an acute or chronic inflammation of the liver caused by several different viruses, toxins, drugs, and disease states. Although each type of hepatitis is unique, assessment findings and treatment have many similarities.

#### Etiology

The most common causes of viral hepatitis are the hepatitis A, B, C, D, and E viruses (Table 43.5), with hepatitis A being the most prevalent in children (Jensen & Balistreri, 2016). Children can also have hepatitis caused by rubella, cytomegalovirus (CMV), herpes simplex virus, and Epstein-Barr virus.

In children, hepatitis A virus (HAV) is highly contagious and spreads readily in households and daycare centers. Infection with hepatitis B virus (HBV) can be transmitted perinatally. The incidence of HBV infection transmitted by blood transfusions has decreased in recent years as a result of improved blood product screening procedures. Contaminated body fluids splashed into the mouth or eyes can produce HBV infection. HBV can survive in the dried state for 1 week or longer; thus, percutaneous contact with contaminated objects can transmit infection.

**TABLE 43.5 Differentiation of Viral Hepatitis**

| Type/Etiology | Transmission | Incubation | Clinical Manifestations | Recovery Prognosis |
|---|---|---|---|---|
| Hepatitis A virus (HAV) | Person to person; fecal-oral route<br>Ingestion of contaminated food or water | 15-50 days (average, 28 days)<br>Most contagious 1-2 wk before and 1 wk after symptoms | Jaundice, fever, fatigue, anorexia, nausea, vomiting, abdominal pain, dark urine, clay-colored stools, joint pain<br>70% of children under 6 yr are asymptomatic with no jaundice | Self-limited disease, rarely fatal<br>No chronic carriers<br>Recovery provides lifelong immunity |
| Hepatitis B virus (HBV) | Percutaneous or mucosal contact with infectious blood or body fluids (e.g., semen, saliva) via injection (drug abuse), sexual intercourse, needle sticks, blood transfusions, and birth | 45-160 days (average, 90 days) | Same symptoms as HAV<br>Severity from mild illness to severe, acute or chronic illness<br>Most children <5 yr are asymptomatic; 30%-50% of children ≥5 yr have initial symptoms | Generally a full recovery.<br>Infected infants (90%) and children <5 yr (30%) will develop chronic carrier state<br>30%-90% of children <10 yr develop chronic hepatitis and are predisposed to cirrhosis and hepatocellular cancer |
| Hepatitis C virus (HCV) | Primarily by large or repeated percutaneous exposure to infectious blood via injection (drug abuse), blood transfusions, needle sticks, and birth | 14 days to 6 mo (average, 6-7 wk) | Same symptoms as HAV<br>Most persons with chronic HCV infection are asymptomatic.<br>Treatment for children 3-17 yr is combination therapy with peginterferon and ribavirin.<br>Newer treatments with direct-acting antiviral agents in adults have been very successful; however, they have not been adequately studied in children (AAP, 2015b; Jensen & Balistreri, 2016). | 75%-85% progress to chronic infection; 60%-70% develop chronic liver disease<br>Chronic HCV is the leading indication for liver transplantation in the United States. |
| Hepatitis D virus (HDV) | Percutaneous or mucosal contact with infectious blood or body fluids | 45-160 days (average, 90 days); coincides with HBV infection | Over half of infected children have chronic hepatitis.<br>Occurs only as coinfection with HBV, increasing the severity of disease.<br>BV vaccination reduces risk<br>Uncommon in the United States | More likely to develop fulminating hepatitis than other strains |
| Hepatitis E virus (HEV) | Fecal–oral<br>Ingestion of contaminated water | 15-60 days (average, 40 days) | Same symptoms as HAV<br>Outbreaks in countries with poor sanitation and contaminated water supply<br>Rare in the United States | High incidence of mortality in pregnant women<br>Children usually asymptomatic |

Data from Centers for Disease Control and Prevention. (2015). *Viral hepatitis*. Retrieved from http://www.cdc.gov/hepatitis.

### Incidence

The incidence of acute hepatitis B infection in the United States is 0.9/100,000 and has declined by approximately 81% since 1990 in all age-groups, with the greatest reduction of cases seen in children younger than 15 years of age (CDC, 2015). This decrease is the direct result of universal immunization of children against HBV, which began in 1991 (CDC, 2015). However, perinatal exposure to hepatitis-B–positive mothers is still a significant cause of infection in young children. The incidence of acute hepatitis A has decreased 92%, to approximately 0.4/100,000, since routine vaccination of children in the United States began in 1996 (AAP, 2015b; Dorell, Yankey, Byrd, et al., 2012). Because the virus is excreted for 1 to 2 weeks before the appearance of clinical signs and for 2 to 3 weeks afterward, outbreaks are common wherever good hand hygiene is not practiced.

### Manifestations

In infants and preschool-age children, HAV infection usually causes no symptoms or mild, nonspecific symptoms such as anorexia, malaise, and easy fatigability. In adults, the disease causes the more severe symptoms of nausea, jaundice, and malaise. Because most children with HAV infection have minimal to no symptoms, the disease is often not diagnosed until an outbreak of hepatitis occurs. Thus, spread of HAV infection can occur before the initial case is identified.

HBV infection has a wide range of clinical manifestations, from asymptomatic infection to acute fulminant hepatitis, which can be fatal. Symptomatic acute hepatitis occurs in two stages; the anicteric (without jaundice) phase and the icteric (jaundiced) phase.

During the anicteric phase, manifestations include anorexia, nausea, vomiting, right upper quadrant or epigastric pain, fever, malaise, fatigue, depression, and irritability. The anicteric phase lasts approximately 5 to 7 days. During the icteric phase, manifestations include jaundice, urticaria, dark urine, and light-colored stools. The child begins to feel better as jaundice becomes more apparent. Acute fulminating hepatitis is marked by bleeding abnormalities, encephalopathy, ascites, and acute hepatic failure. Fulminant hepatitis is caused primarily by HBV and hepatitis C virus (HCV).

The symptoms and clinical changes should return to normal within 3 months of onset. If not, a chronic state should be suspected. Infection with HBV, hepatitis D virus (HDV), and HCV can result in chronic hepatitis and cirrhosis. Chronic HBV infection can also cause hepatic carcinoma.

### Diagnostic Evaluation

A history of exposure to jaundiced individuals, confirmed outbreaks in daycare centers, or percutaneous exposure to blood or body fluids should raise the suspicion of hepatitis. Although no liver function test is specific for hepatitis, aspartate transaminase (AST), alanine transaminase (ALT), bilirubin levels, alkaline phosphatase, and sedimentation rate can indicate liver damage caused by hepatitis. Serum bilirubin levels peak 5 to 10 days after jaundice appears. A history of exposure and the course of the disease are essential in making the appropriate diagnosis.

Blood tests to diagnose hepatitis include identification of the viral antigens (e.g., hepatitis B surface antigen [HBsAg], hepatitis B early antigen [HBeAg], hepatitis B core antigen [HBcAg]), antibodies (e.g., anti-HAV, anti-HBcAg, anti-HCV), and genetic material (e.g., HCV RNA) associated with the disease. In hepatitis A, immunoglobulin M (IgM) anti-HAV antibodies are present at the onset of illness and are diagnostic (Jonas & Stoll, 2014). They usually disappear within 6 months, but can persist for 12 months. Children with hepatitis B are diagnosed by the presence of antigen (HBsAg) and IgM antibodies to HBcAg (Jensen & Balistreri, 2016). HCV serologic assays (e.g., polymerase chain reaction) are used to diagnose hepatitis C (Jensen & Balistreri, 2016).

Liver biopsy can be used to evaluate the chronic active forms of the disease and to determine the extent of liver damage in advanced or fulminant cases. Liver fibrosis increases with the duration of HCV infection.

## PATHOPHYSIOLOGY

### *Viral Hepatitis*

Hepatitis viruses cause necrosis of the parenchymal cells of the liver. The inflammatory response causes swelling and blockage of the drainage system in the liver, resulting in biliary stasis and further destruction of hepatic cells. Because the liver cannot excrete bile into the intestine, bile is present in the blood (causing hyperbilirubinemia), urine (as urobilinogen), and skin (causing hepatocellular jaundice).

Hepatitis infection can cause asymptomatic or mild illness, with complete regeneration of liver cells occurring within 2 to 3 months. More severe forms of hepatitis include fulminant hepatitis, in which hepatic necrosis and death can occur within 1 to 2 weeks and subacute or chronic hepatitis, which can result in permanent scarring of the liver and impaired liver function. Chronically infected individuals are carriers of the disease and are at increased risk for developing chronic liver disease (e.g., cirrhosis, chronic persistent hepatitis) or liver carcinoma later in life.

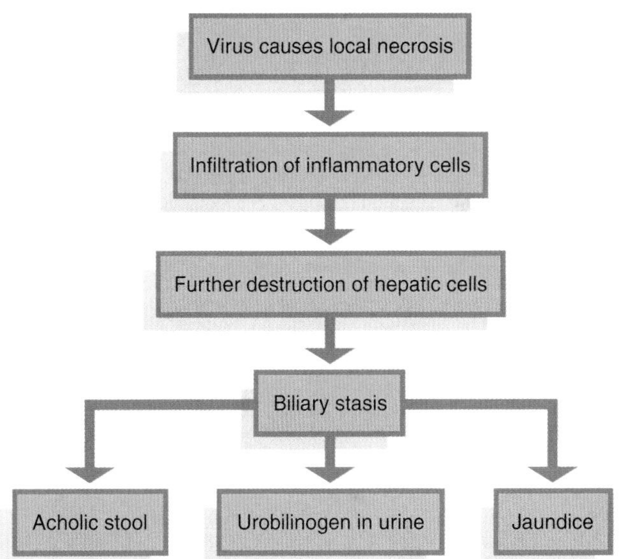


### Therapeutic Management

Acute viral hepatitis has no specific treatment. In uncomplicated viral hepatitis, treatment is mainly supportive because the disease is self-limiting. Treatment is aimed at maintaining comfort and adequate nutritional balance. A lowfat, balanced diet can be helpful if the child has nausea and anorexia. Hospitalization is rarely needed. All nonessential medications should be discontinued, and chemotherapy, corticosteroids, and alcohol should all be avoided during infection.

If needed, intensive care for fulminant hepatitis provides hemostasis, nutritional and fluid support, neurologic assessment, and management until the liver has time to recover.

***Hepatitis A.*** Control of further spread is essential. Because HAV can survive on contaminated objects for weeks, good hand hygiene and

**TABLE 43.6 Hepatitis Prophylaxis**

| Virus | Prevention of Spread | Immunization | Postexposure Prophylaxis |
|---|---|---|---|
| HAV | Hand hygiene; PPE; gloves<br>Identify infected food handlers | Given as two injections at age 1 yr and at least 6 mo later<br>Recommended for all children at age 1 yr and specific populations in high-risk areas | Within 2 wk, give hepatitis A immune globulin (HAIG), 0.02 mL/kg IM |
| HBV | Standard Precautions<br>PPE; gloves, mask, eye/face shield<br>Safe injections | Three injections at birth, age 1-2 mo, and age 6-18 mo<br>Recommended for all infants, children, and adolescents | For neonates of infected mothers, give hepatitis B immune globulin (HBIG) within 12 hr of birth followed by immunizations<br>HBIG, 0.06 mL/kg, within 24 hr of any percutaneous exposure |
| HCV | Standard Precautions<br>PPE; gloves, mask, eye/face shield<br>Safe injections | None | None |

Data from American Academy of Pediatrics. (2015b). Hepatitis. In D.W. Kimberlin, M.T. Brady, M.A. Jackson, et al. (Eds.), *Red book 2015 report of the committee on infectious diseases* (30th ed., pp. 391-432). Elk Grove Village, IL: AAP; 2015. Centers for Disease Control and Prevention. (2015). *The ABC's of Hepatitis.* Retrieved from http://www.cdc.gov/hepatitis/Resources/Professionals/PDFs/ABCTable.pdf. Jensen, M.K., & Balistreri, W.F. (2016). Viral Hepatitis. In R. Kliegman, B. Stanton, J. St. Geme, et al. (Eds.), *Nelson textbook of pediatrics* (20th ed., pp. 1942–1953). Philadelphia: Elsevier.

thorough disinfection of diaper-changing surfaces are imperative. Children and adults who have had direct contact with a person infected with HAV should receive immunoglobulin (Ig) as soon as possible after exposure. Immunization is currently recommended for all children beginning at age 1 year, as well other high-risk groups. Cases of hepatitis should be promptly reported to local public health officials. Daycare center employees suspected of infection and household contacts of infected persons should be tested for IgM anti-HAV antibodies (AAP, 2015).

***Hepatitis B.*** Children with acute or chronic HBV infection should be cared for with scrupulous Standard Precautions. The most effective means of preventing HBV infection is immunization. Immunization against HBV is recommended to start at birth; all children should receive this vaccine as early in childhood as possible. Other persons who should receive HBV immunization include IV drug users, healthcare and residential facility workers, household contacts and sexual partners of HBV carriers, inmates of correctional facilities, and international travelers. Hepatitis B immune globulin (HBIG) is effective in preventing HBV infection if given within 2 weeks after exposure. Hepatitis D can be prevented by preventing HBV (Table 43.6).

## NURSING CARE

### The Child With Viral Hepatitis

#### Assessment

The nursing history can be used to identify the source of infection. In children, flu-like symptoms of fever, malaise, anorexia, fatigue, and nausea might be the only indications of viral hepatitis. Abdominal assessment might disclose right upper quadrant tenderness and hepatomegaly. Stools will be pale and clay colored, and urine might be dark and frothy. Jaundice, if present, is best assessed in sclera, nail beds, and mucous membranes, and usually follows a cephalocaudal progression. In HBV infection, arthralgias are sometimes the presenting symptom.

Fulminant hepatitis will likely manifest as acute hepatic failure with associated encephalopathy, bleeding, fluid retention, ascites, and an icteric (jaundiced) appearance.

#### Nursing Diagnosis and Planning

The following nursing diagnoses and expected outcomes may be appropriate after assessing the child with viral hepatitis and the child's family:

- Imbalanced Nutrition: Less Than Body Requirements related to anorexia.

***Expected outcome.*** The child will be able to tolerate an age-appropriate diet without weight loss, vomiting, or abdominal pain and will return to a normal activity level.

- Risk for Infection related to exposure of family members to infectious agents.

***Expected outcome.*** The family will practice good hand hygiene and other necessary isolation procedures and will remain free from infection.

- Risk for Injury related to fulminant hepatitis.

***Expected outcome.*** The child will return to pre-illness weight and activity level.

- Deficient Knowledge related to incomplete information about home care and long-term prognosis.

***Expected outcome.*** The parents will verbalize a basic understanding of hepatitis and the importance of treatment and prevention.

#### Interventions

Unless fulminant hepatitis develops, children are usually treated at home, so parental education is crucial. Parents should be taught the importance of a nutritious, low-fat diet as tolerated by the child, adequate rest, and general supportive care. The child with hepatitis is often anorexic. Several small meals and snacks throughout the day are better tolerated than regular portions at mealtimes.

Fatigue and malaise can last for several weeks. Plenty of rest and sleep are important for recovery. Because HAV is no longer infectious within 1 week after the onset of jaundice, the child may return to school at that time if feeling well enough.

***Child and parent teaching.*** Teach the parents the danger signals that could indicate a worsening of the child's condition: changes in neurologic status, bleeding, and fluid retention. Jaundice sometimes worsens before it resolves, and parents should be prepared for this possibility. Also, teach parents not to give their child any over-the-counter medications such as acetaminophen because impaired liver function can prevent adequate metabolism and excretion of the medication. Caution adolescents not to drink alcohol during the illness or recovery period.

Preventing the spread of infection is an essential intervention for HAV. Prevention should include the use of Contact Precautions for at least 1 week after the onset of jaundice and meticulous hand hygiene. Hand hygiene is the most important preventive measure. Family members are taught how to institute appropriate precautions and to clean exposed household surfaces with a bleach solution. Diapers should not be changed on or near surfaces used for preparing or serving food. The nurse explains to family members the ways in which HAV (fecal-oral route) and HBV (parenteral route) are spread to others. Recommendations for hepatitis A and hepatitis B vaccination are discussed, and immunizations are provided to family members as indicated.

If the child has HBV infection, especially neonatal HBV, the parents are informed about the possibility of developing a chronic carrier state, cirrhosis, or hepatocellular cancer later in life. If a child or adolescent with HBV infection has a history of illicit IV drug use, the nurse has the responsibility of teaching about the risk of transmission of hepatitis and other infections via contaminated needles. Referral to a substance abuse program is advisable.

***Home care.*** Children with hepatitis are almost always managed at home. Nursing interventions include teaching parents hand hygiene skills, the use of gloves, and disinfection of contaminated surfaces and articles. Parents must learn to monitor their child for complications associated with hepatitis; provide a well-balanced, low-fat diet; and watch other family members for signs and symptoms of infection. As indicated, all family members and especially any siblings and children should be immunized against hepatitis A and B.

### Evaluation

- Has the child maintained a weight within 5% of the pre-illness weight?
- Is the child free of vomiting?
- Is the child participating in age-appropriate activities and play?
- Do family members practice good hand hygiene and adhere to procedures?
- Has the spread of hepatitis to other family members been avoided?
- Have all family members been immunized as appropriate?
- Can the parents describe the symptoms of hepatitis to watch for in other family members?

## Biliary Atresia

Biliary atresia refers to the obstruction or absence of the extrahepatic bile ducts. At birth, the liver itself is normal without inflammation, but the structural problem leads to significant cellular damage and eventual liver failure and death.

### Etiology and Incidence

The cause of biliary atresia is unknown. Because the problem originates during the prenatal period, viruses, toxins, and chemicals cannot be ruled out. The condition is unlikely to recur within the same family.

Extrahepatic biliary atresia occurs in 1 in 10,000 to 15,000 births, with a slightly higher incidence in female than male infants (Hassan & Balistreri, 2016). It is the most common cause of end-stage liver disease and the number one indication for liver transplantation in children (Wang, 2015).

### Manifestations

The child with biliary atresia appears healthy at birth. Manifestations that develop shortly afterward include jaundice, acholic stools (light in color because of the absence of bile pigment), bile-stained urine, and hepatomegaly.

### Diagnostic Evaluation

Investigation of liver function (bilirubin, aminotransferases [ALT, AST]) and clotting studies (prothrombin time [PT], partial thromboplastin time [PTT]) is important in establishing the diagnosis. Any newborn with conjugated hyperbilirubinemia should be thoroughly evaluated. To rule out inborn errors of metabolism (e.g., galactosemia and alpha$_1$-antitrypsin deficiency), which can have similar initial findings, metabolic screening is performed. Hepatitis B and other viral titers are also measured to rule out neonatal hepatitis. Urine and stool samples should be examined and urobilinogen levels checked to determine the degree of obstruction.

Percutaneous liver biopsy can provide a definitive diagnosis if bile plugs, edema, and fibrosis are found in the presence of normal hepatic lobular structure (Hassan & Balistreri, 2016). Cholangiography can be used to ascertain the extent of atresia.

### Therapeutic Management

During and after exploratory laparotomy, the size of the lesion can be identified, and drainage can be attempted. If no correctable lesion is found, a hepatic portoenterostomy (Kasai procedure) will be performed to allow bile to drain from the liver. This procedure allows bile to flow directly into the intestine through an anastomosis of the jejunum to the porta hepatis, the point at which the hepatic ducts join to form the common bile duct. The Kasai procedure does provide some long-term benefits, but hepatic dysfunction will persist. The main goal of the procedure is to allow growth and development of the child until liver transplantation can be performed. Approximately 80% of children with biliary atresia will need a liver transplant by 10 years of age (Wang, 2015).

Medical management involves treating the child's malnutrition and providing symptom relief. Medium-chain triglyceride (MCT) oil can be added to formula to increase calories, or TPN can be administered to provide essential nutrition. Vitamin malabsorption must be addressed to prevent night blindness (vitamin A), neuromuscular degeneration (vitamin E), rickets (vitamin D), and hypoprothrombinemia (vitamin K). Portal hypertension with its concomitant problems of ascites and variceal bleeding must be assessed and treated. Controlling bleeding, restricting salt intake, and using diuretics are essential in managing portal hypertension.

### Nursing Considerations

During the early phase of disease, in the first months of life, the infant with biliary atresia will appear jaundiced, with mild hepatosplenomegaly and increased abdominal girth. As the disease progresses, the child may appear thin, with failure to thrive, marked jaundice, and evidence of rickets caused by chronic vitamin D deficiency. Pruritus becomes a major problem; the child may develop skin infections or xanthomas (lipid deposits in the skin) as a result of retention of cholesterol in the skin.

After the Kasai procedure, the child should be assessed for evidence of portal hypertension, which can include the development of ascites and GI bleeding. Even after repair, acholic stools and bile-stained urine are not uncommon.

Psychosocial and family assessment must be a high priority. Biliary atresia is a life-threatening, chronic illness that requires surgical intervention, involvement of numerous healthcare providers, repeated hospitalizations, and eventually an extended wait for a liver transplant. The nurse gathers information about family structure and stability, financial resources, available support systems, and the feelings of the child and family about the management and progression of the disease.

Nursing interventions are directed toward six major areas: nutritional support, skin care, developmental stimulation, continued assessment, education, and emotional support.

***Nutritional support.*** Providing adequate calories, aiding in vitamin supply and absorption, and preventing hepatic encephalopathy are important goals. Calorie counts, daily weights, and abdominal girths are important assessment parameters that provide the data necessary to improve nutritional support. Concentrating calories by administering a glucose polymer (Polycose) and providing MCT supplements, which do not require the bile salts for digestion, can significantly improve the child's nutritional status. NG tube feeding or TPN might be necessary at times. Supplements of vitamins A, D, E, and K, as well as calcium, phosphate, and zinc, are essential for adequate nutrition. Limiting protein intake can prevent the development of hepatic encephalopathy. Plotting weight, length, and head circumference on growth charts monthly provides data to evaluate treatment effectiveness.

***Skin care.*** Bile acid binders such as cholestyramine aid in the excretion of bile salts and decrease pruritus and the development of xanthomas (Hassan & Balistreri, 2016). Colloidal oatmeal baths (e.g., Aveeno) can relieve severe itching. Preventing skin breakdown from severe scratching is essential. Wearing gloves during sleep and applying soothing lotions and creams for dry skin helps to prevent infection.

***Developmental stimulation.*** Teaching parents activities to provide developmental stimulation and accessing resources available through physical and occupational therapy are essential nursing responsibilities. As the child awaits a liver transplant, efforts should be made to facilitate achievement of developmental milestones related to gross and fine motor skills and social and emotional abilities. Routine screening tests document developmental growth and can be used to evaluate interventions.

***Continued assessment.*** Continuous monitoring for the development of portal hypertension is vital. The parents must be taught to watch for GI bleeding, severe edema, and ascites. If any of these conditions are noted, the physician must be notified immediately, as the child might need sodium intake restrictions, diuretics, IV albumin, or hospitalization.

***Family education and support.*** The family has many educational needs. The nurse helps family members understand the disease process, manage nutritional changes, provide skin care, assess for signs of complications, and enhance the child's development. Parents are given information about available resources. Organizations such as the Children's Liver Disease Foundation provide programs, educational materials, and referral to support groups for children with liver disease and their families.

The nurse plays a critical role by listening to parental concerns, providing information and support, and encouraging parents to participate in their child's daily care. Further, the nurse helps the parents focus on and prepare for their child's future liver transplant and related long-term care and treatment. Because transplantation usually occurs within the first 2 years of life, age-appropriate explanations for the toddler are also indicated.

The child and family should be prepared for the possible death of the child. Biliary atresia is a life-threatening condition, and some children succumb to the disease before liver transplantation can be performed. Further, management of the disease requires numerous hospitalizations, many diagnostic tests, and an extensive daily care

## PATHOPHYSIOLOGY

### *Biliary Atresia*

Obstruction of the extrahepatic bile ducts causes obstruction of the normal flow of bile out of the liver and into the gallbladder and small intestines. As a result, bile plugs form, causing bile to back up in the liver. This process causes inflammation, edema, and hepatic degeneration. Eventually, the liver becomes fibrotic, and cirrhosis and portal hypertension develop, leading to liver failure. The gradual degeneration of the liver causes jaundice, icterus, and hepatomegaly. Because bile is not present in the intestines, fat and fat-soluble vitamins cannot be absorbed. This condition leads to malnutrition, deficiencies in fat-soluble vitamins, and growth failure.

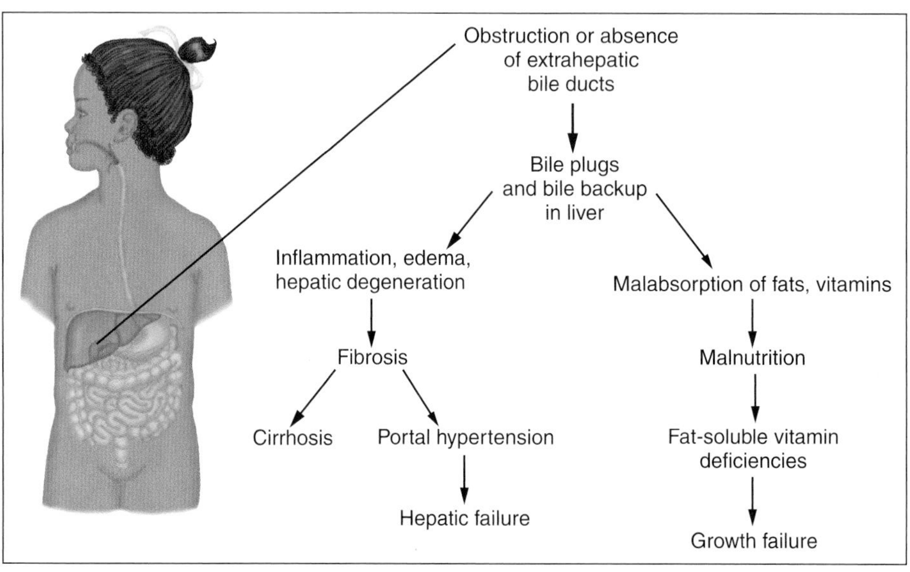

regimen. This situation places immense stress on families. Critical nursing interventions include arranging for and providing educational and emotional support to the child, and to the parents so that they can effectively care for their child.

*Home care.* The parents must be able to assume all home care responsibilities. They need to monitor nutritional intake, mix special formulas, manage NG feedings, provide skin care, give medications, and track their child's growth and development. Their ability to assess for GI bleeding, ascites, edema, and skin infections is critical so that treatment can begin promptly.

## Cirrhosis

Cirrhosis is a chronic, degenerative condition of the liver that results in the development of bands of fibrous tissue, firm nodules, and connections between the central and portal areas of the liver. This scarring causes irreversible damage to the liver.

### PATHOPHYSIOLOGY

#### *Cirrhosis*

Stasis of bile causes inflammation and hepatomegaly. If this condition continues, destruction of the liver begins. As the liver attempts to heal itself, fibrotic regeneration and nodules develop, impairing liver function. This scarring can cause altered hepatic blood flow and decreased liver cell function. Changes in hepatic blood flow can cause scarring and collapse of the hepatic vasculature, increased vascular resistance, and eventual portal hypertension. As the liver cells decrease in function, more cells die, and the liver cannot produce necessary proteins or bile, causing malabsorption and malnutrition. As liver cells continue to die, the cycle is repeated.

### Etiology

Cirrhosis in children usually results from chronic liver disease such as HBV infection, chronic hepatitis, or biliary atresia. Sickle cell disease, inborn errors of metabolism such as alpha$_1$-antitrypsin deficiency and disturbances in copper metabolism, cystic fibrosis, and Wilson disease are other possible causes of pediatric liver cirrhosis.

### Incidence

Cirrhosis is uncommon in children, but as the life spans of children with chronic disease continue to lengthen, the incidence of liver cirrhosis will rise.

### Manifestations

The symptoms are often nonspecific, vague, and slow to develop. They result from either liver cell failure or portal hypertension. Liver cell failure results in jaundice, intense pruritus, steatorrhea, abdominal distention, edema, anemia, bleeding tendencies, anorexia, frequent infections, and poor growth. Portal hypertension manifests as splenomegaly, esophageal varices, and GI bleeding. Both liver cell failure and portal hypertension contribute to the development of ascites.

### Diagnostic Evaluation

Because the most likely cause of cirrhosis in children is chronic biliary obstruction, evaluation is based on the history of preexisting conditions. A presumptive diagnosis of cirrhosis can be made based on the presence of clinical manifestations of chronic liver disease and a history of hepatitis or biliary atresia. The results of liver function tests such as bilirubin, aminotransferases, ammonia, albumin, cholesterol, and prothrombin time, can support the diagnosis. A liver biopsy that identifies fibrous scarring and changes of hepatic vasculature is indicative of cirrhosis.

### Therapeutic Management

No effective treatment is available to halt the progression of cirrhosis. Infections should be treated and obstructions repaired. Supportive care that includes rest, nutritional support, fluid management, and relief of symptoms, is provided. Management of life-threatening complications including bleeding varices, ascites, and hepatic encephalopathy, takes priority. Definitive therapy is a liver transplant. Liver function is carefully monitored to determine when the child will need liver transplantation. The risk of liver cancer is increased with cirrhosis (Pinto, Schneider, & da Silveira, 2015).

### Nursing Considerations

General appraisal will likely reveal a child with a history of failure to thrive and chronic biliary obstruction or HBV infection. The child may have varying degrees of distress and discomfort. Many children will have vague symptoms or be asymptomatic. The earliest findings of cirrhosis are likely to be anorexia, nausea, indigestion, fatigue, and right upper quadrant (RUQ) pain or fullness. Monitoring height and weight with a growth chart, gathering information on a typical day's food intake, and assessing sleep habits and activity levels can provide essential supportive evidence.

Abdominal palpation will likely reveal splenomegaly and RUQ tenderness or hepatomegaly. Distended superficial veins, edema, and tight, shiny skin are often seen. Jaundice and pruritus can be present, especially if the cirrhosis is the result of biliary obstruction. A complete skin assessment, including nail beds and sclera, can identify jaundice at its earliest stages. The skin should be examined for breakdown or infection caused by intense scratching. The amount and location of edema is also noted. Skin assessment may also reveal bruises related to thrombocytopenia and pale color related to anemia. A stool specimen can be used to identify the degree of bile obstruction and malabsorption.

The most critical assessment should be centered on detecting signs of the three major complications of cirrhosis: ascites, varices, and encephalopathy. The child with significantly increased abdominal girth, edema, bloody emesis, or changes in level of consciousness should be referred for emergency medical care related to these life-threatening complications.

The goal of nursing care is to sustain the child in optimal condition until liver transplantation can be achieved. The care can be divided into four areas: nutritional support, skin care, prevention of complications, and developmental and parental support.

*Nutritional support.* Providing optimal nutrition that allows the child to grow and develop is a major nursing intervention. The diet should be high carbohydrate, high calorie, normal protein, and low fat. Children with cirrhosis need up to 80% more calories than healthy children to achieve normal growth (Pinto et al., 2015). These changes put minimal stress on the liver while meeting the child's growth requirements. Protein intake should be limited if encephalopathy develops. Restricted sodium intake can help prevent edema. Multivitamin supplements containing vitamins A, D, E, and K are essential. Vitamin K injections can be administered, if indicated. Because of anorexia, creative food options, NG tube feedings, and TPN may be needed. Monitoring the child's weight on a daily and a weekly basis as well as recording intake and output provides critical information about edema and growth. Support from dietary personnel is valuable when working with these children and their families.

*Skin care.* Pruritus can be intense for the child with cirrhosis. Continued assessment for open lesions, scratch marks, bleeding, and ease of bruising is vital. Colloidal oatmeal baths and topical antipruritic lotions such as calamine can provide temporary relief.

Medications to treat pruritus are not usually given due to impaired liver function. Keeping the nails trimmed short or wearing cotton gloves during sleep can minimize injury to the skin from scratching.

***Prevention of complications.*** It is critical that the nurse prevent exposure of the child to infections as well as continuously monitor and immediately report fever or other signs of infection.

If the child is noted to be edematous, the nurse gives diuretics and albumin as ordered and maintains a low-sodium diet. The child who develops ascites will likely be hospitalized for treatment; key nursing interventions include tracking intake, output, and weight, maintaining fluid balance, and monitoring abdominal girth and distention.

Stool guaiac tests and careful observation will aid the nurse in identifying bleeding as soon as possible. To prevent bleeding, injections are avoided, the child is protected from injury, and vitamin K is given as ordered. For the hospitalized child, nursing care involves transfusing blood or blood products safely, maintaining fluid balance, monitoring pulse and blood pressure, administering oxygen therapy, and assisting with endoscopic sclerotherapy or the placement of a Sengstaken-Blakemore tube for compression of bleeding esophageal varices.

Encephalopathy occurs as a result of excess ammonia in the blood due to incomplete breakdown of protein by the liver. The nurse must frequently assess the child for changes in behavior and level of consciousness to detect encephalopathy. Per orders, limiting protein in the diet, giving lactulose to decrease the GI bacteria that produce ammonia, and administering antibiotics are important nursing responsibilities. Also, careful consideration must be given before any drugs are administered to the child with cirrhosis. Impaired liver function adversely affects the metabolism of many drugs; sedatives, opioids, acetaminophen (Tylenol), and alcohol are strictly avoided.

***Developmental and parental support.*** Children with cirrhosis are chronically ill and require much time and effort to maintain optimal health. Providing developmental stimulation on a daily basis is essential, and parents need education and support services to achieve this goal. In addition, parents need to be educated about the disease, its prognosis, the feasibility of a liver transplant, and the risk of complications. As the parents cope with the potential loss of their child, community resources and national support groups, such as the Children's Liver Disease Foundation, are helpful.

***Home care.*** The focus of nursing related to home care is education. Because the child will be cared for at home unless a serious complication arises or the child is hospitalized for a liver transplant, parents need complete information and instructions. Developing plans for meals and snacks that meet the child's special, daily nutritional needs can be difficult, and dietary personnel can provide invaluable assistance to parents. Nurses must teach parents how to prevent infection by sheltering their child from sources of infection and following hand hygiene and other disinfection protocols. The most critical nursing intervention is to educate parents so they can identify signs of complications such as GI bleeding, encephalopathy, and severe edema and know when they must immediately contact the physician. When the child with cirrhosis remains generally healthy, the family can facilitate progression of the child's developmental skills and prepare for liver transplantation.

## KEY CONCEPTS

- The GI system is formed in the first 4 weeks of embryonic development; this is when congenital defects occur.
- The anatomy of the GI tract is complete at birth but physiologically immature.
- Evaluating distress in small children must include a thorough history, physical assessment, pain assessment, and parents' perception of the child's pain.
- Fluid balance can rapidly shift in the child with vomiting, diarrhea, or anorexia; the nurse must thoroughly assess for changes frequently.
- Gastroesophageal alterations place the child at risk for respiratory distress. Assessment of respiratory function and maintenance of airway patency are critical interventions.
- Medications are essential in managing many GI diseases; the nurse must be knowledgeable of dosages, indications, side effects, and teaching needs.
- The emotional needs of the parents whose children have congenital anomalies should be addressed.
- Postoperative nursing care of children following GI surgery is focused on fluid balance, pain control, nutrition, parental involvement, and the child's developmental level.
- Parental anxiety can have a significant effect on the child with GI alterations and must be addressed.
- Correct use of Standard Precautions is essential to preventing the spread of GI infections.
- Some GI malabsorption disorders can be managed by dietary changes.
- Educating parents to care for their children with GI alterations at home is a priority nursing action.
- Referral to community resources is a vital aspect of nursing care for children with GI alterations.

## REFERENCES AND READINGS


Ahmed, A.H., Sonnenburg, K., Foli, K.J., et al. (2016). Managing ulcerative colitis in the adolescent: highlighting the developmental and self-management needs. *Holistic Nursing Practice, 30*(1), 39–46. doi:10.1097/HNP.0000000000000123.

Aiken, J.J., & Oldham, K.T. (2016). Acute appendicitis. In R. Kliegman, B. Stanton, J. St. Geme, et al. (Eds.), *Nelson textbook of pediatrics* (20th ed., pp. 1887–1894). Philadelphia: Elsevier.

Allen, P.J. (2015). Gluten-related disorders: celiac disease, gluten allergy, non-celiac gluten sensitivity. *Pediatric Nursing, 41*(3), 146–150.

Almadhoun, O. (2012). Managing chronic abdominal pain in children: understanding physical and behavioral components of functional abdominal pain [Electronic version]. *Contemporary Pediatrics, 29(3),* 18–23.

Ambartsumyan, L., & Rodriguez, L. (2014). Gastrointestinal motility disorders in children. *Gastroenterology & Hepatology, 10*(1), 16–26.

American Academy of Pediatrics (2015a). *Soiling (Encopresis).* Retrieved from https://www.healthychildren.org/English/health-issues/conditions/emotional-problems/Pages/Soiling-Encopresis.aspx.

American Academy of Pediatrics. (2015b). Hepatitis. In D.W. Kimberlin, M.T. Brady, M.A. Jackson, et al. (Eds.), *Red book 2015 report of the committee on infectious diseases* (30th ed., pp. 391–432). Elk Grove Village, IL: AAP; 2015.

Aschenbrenner, D.S. (2012). New pediatric indication for infliximab. *American Journal for Nursing, 112*(1), 25.

Bachur, R.G., Callahan, M.J., Monteaux, M.C., et al. (2015). Integration of ultrasound findings and a clinical score in the diagnostic evaluation of pediatric appendicitis. *The Journal of Pediatrics, 166*(5), 1134–1139. doi:10.1016/jpeds.2015.01.034.

Bhutta, Z. (2016). Acute gastroenteritis in children. In R. Kliegman, B. Stanton, J. St. Geme, et al. (Eds.), *Nelson textbook of pediatrics* (20th ed., pp. 1854–1875). Philadelphia: Elsevier.

Blanchard, S., & Czinn, S. (2016). Peptic ulcer disease in children. In R. Kliegman, B. Stanton, J. St. Geme, et al. (Eds.). *Nelson textbook of pediatrics* (20th ed., pp. 1816–1819). Philadelphia: Elsevier.

Branski, D., Troncone, R., & Fasano, A. (2016). Celiac disease (gluten-sensitive enteropathy). In R. Kliegman, B. Stanton, J. St. Geme, et al. (Eds.), *Nelson textbook of pediatrics* (20th ed., pp. 1835–1838). Philadelphia: Elsevier.

Cagir, B., & Sawyer, M. (2012). *Short-bowel syndrome.* Retrieved from http://emedicine.medscape.com/article/193391-overview#a0199.

Caperell, K., Pitetti, R., & Cross, K.P. (2013). Race and acute abdominal pain in a pediatric emergency department. *Pediatrics, 131*(6), 1098–1106. doi:10.1542/peds.2012-3672.

Centers for Disease Control and Prevention. (2015). *The ABC's of hepatitis.* Retrieved from: http://www.cdc.gov/hepatitis/Resources/Professionals/PDFs/ABCTable.pdf.

Chogle, A., Mintjens, S., & Saps, M. (2014). Pediatric IBS: an overview on pathophysiology, diagnosis and treatment. *Pediatric Annals, 43*(3), e76–e82. doi:10.3928/00904481-20140325-08.

Cleft Palate Foundation. (2014). *Prenatal diagnosis of cleft lip and cleft palate.* Retrieved from http://www.cleftline.org/wp-content/uploads/2012/03/PRE-01.pdf.

Crohn's and Colitis Foundation of America. (2016). *CCFA camp oasis.* Retrieved from http://www.ccfa.org/get-involved/camp-oasis.

Dorell, C.G., Yankey, D., Byrd, K.K., et al. (2012). Hepatitis A vaccination coverage among adolescents in the United States. *Pediatrics, 129*(2), 213–221. doi:10.1542/peds.2011-2197.

Fiorino, K.N., & Liacouras, C.A. (2016a). Encoporesis and functional constipation. In R. Kliegman, B. Stanton, J. St. Geme, et al. (Eds.). *Nelson textbook of pediatrics* (20th ed., pp. 1807–1809). Philadelphia: Elsevier.

Fiorino, K.N., & Liacouras, C.A. (2016b). Congenital aganglionic megacolon (Hirschsprung disease). In R. Kliegman, B. Stanton, J. St. Geme, et al. (Eds.), *Nelson textbook of pediatrics* (20th ed., pp. 1809–1811). Philadelphia: Elsevier.

Grossman, A., & Baldassano, R. (2016a). Crohn's disease (regional enteritis, regional ileitis, granulomatous colitis). In R. Kliegman, B. Stanton, J. St. Geme, et al. (Eds.), *Nelson textbook of pediatrics* (20th ed., pp. 1826-1831). Philadelphia: Elsevier.

Grossman, A., & Baldassano, R. (2016b). Chronic ulcerative colitis. In R. Kliegman, B. Stanton, J. St. Geme, et al. (Eds.), *Nelson textbook of pediatrics* (20th ed., pp. 1822–1826). Philadelphia: Elsevier.

Halbert, K.L. (2011). Nissen vs. Toupet fundoplication in the treatment of gastroesophageal reflux disease. *Pediatric Nursing, 37*(4), 171–174.

Hannah, E., & John, R.M. (2013). Everything the nurse practitioner should know about pediatric feeding tubes. *Journal of the American Association of Nurse Practitioners, 25,* 567–577. doi:10.1002/2327-6924.12075.

Hansen, L.W., & Dolgin, S.E. (2016). Trends in the diagnosis and management of pediatric appendicitis. *Pediatrics in Review, 37*(2), 52–57.

Hassan, H.H., & Balistreri, W.F. (2016). Neonatal cholestasis. In R. Kliegman, B. Stanton, J. St. Geme, et al. (Eds.), *Nelson textbook of pediatrics* (20th ed., pp. 1928–1936). Philadelphia: Elsevier.

Hill, I. (2011). Searching for celiac disease: whom to test and how to test. *Contemporary Pediatrics,* 20–26.

Hseu, A., Recko, T., Jennings, R., et al. (2015). Upper airway anomalies in congenital tracheoesophageal fistula and esophageal atresia patients. *Annals of Otology, Rhinology & Laryngology, 124*(10), 808–813. doi:10.1177/0003489415586844.

Hunter, A.K., & Liacouras, C.A. (2016). Pyloric stenosis and other congenital anomalies of the stomach. In R. Kliegman, B. Stanton, J. St. Geme, et al. (Eds.), *Nelson textbook of pediatrics* (20th ed., pp. 1797–1799). Philadelphia: Elsevier.

Jensen, M.K., & Balistreri, W.F. (2016). Viral hepatitis. In R. Kliegman, B. Stanton, J. St. Geme, et al. (Eds.), *Nelson textbook of pediatrics* (20th ed., pp. 1942–1953). Philadelphia: Elsevier.

Jonas, M., & Stoll, J. (2014). Hepatitis B and D viruses. In J. Cherry, G. Harrison, S. Kaplan, et al. (Eds.), *Feigin and Cherry's textbook of pediatric infectious diseases* (7th ed., pp. 1911–1933). Philadelphia: Elsevier Saunders.

Jones, A.M., Isenburg, J., Salemi, J.L., et al. (2016). Increasing prevalence of gastroschisis-14 states, 1995-2012. *Morbidity and Mortality Weekly Report, 65*(2), 23–26.

Judge, J., Giordano, B.P., & English, J. (2014). Crohn's disease masquerading as an acute abdomen. *Journal of Pediatric Health Care, 28*(5), 444–450. doi: 10.1016/jpedhc.2014.03.003.

Kahn, S., & Orenstein, S. (2016a). Esophageal atresia and tracheoesophageal fistula. In R. Kliegman, B. Stanton, J. St. Geme, et al. (Eds.), *Nelson textbook of pediatrics* (20th ed., pp. 1783–1784). Philadelphia: Elsevier.

Kahn, S., & Orenstein, S. (2016b). Gastroesophageal reflux disease. In R. Kliegman, B. Stanton, J. St. Geme, et al. (Eds.), *Nelson textbook of pediatrics* (20th ed., pp. 1787–1791). Philadelphia: Elsevier.

Kennedy, M., & Liacouras, C. (2016). Intussusception. In R. Kliegman, B. Stanton, J. St. Geme, et al. (Eds.), *Nelson textbook of pediatrics* (20th ed., pp. 1812–1814). Philadelphia: Elsevier.

Kohler, J.A., Perkins, A.M., & Bass, W.T. (2013). Human milk versus formula after gastroschisis repair: effects on time to full feeding and time to discharge. *Journal of Perinatology, 33,* 627–630. doi:10.1038/jp.2013.27.

Ledbetter, D.J. (2012). Congenital abdominal wall defects and reconstruction in pediatric surgery: gastroschisis and omphalocele. *Surgical Clinics of North America, 92,*713–727. doi:10.1016/jsuc.2012.03.010.

Lindberg, N., & Berglund, A.-L. (2013). Mothers' experiences of feeding babies born with cleft lip and palate. *Scandinavian Journal of Caring Sciences, 28,* 66–73. doi:10.1111/scs.12048.

Maheshwari, A., & Carlo, W.A. (2016). Diaphragmatic hernia. In R. Kliegman, B. Stanton, J. St. Geme, et al. (Eds.), *Nelson textbook of pediatrics* (20th ed., pp. 862–864). Philadelphia: Elsevier.

Markowitz, R.I. (2014). Olive without a cause: the story of infantile hypertrophic pyloric stenosis. *Pediatric Radiology, 44,* 202-211. doi: 10.1007/s00247-031-2834-7.

Murphy, E.K., & Berman, L. (2014). Clinical evaluation of acute appendicitis. *Clinical Pediatric Emergency Medicine, 15*(3), 223–230.

National Institute of Diabetes and Digestive and Kidney Diseases. (2014). *Lactose intolerance.* Retrieved from http://www.niddk.nih.gov/health-information/health-topics/digestive-diseases/lactose-intolerance/Pages/facts.aspx.

National Institute of Diabetes and Digestive and Kidney Diseases. (2015). *Short bowel syndrome.* Retrieved from http://www.niddk.nih.gov/health-information/health-topics/digestive-diseases/short-bowel-syndrome/Pages/facts.aspx.

Neu, M., Corwin E., Lareau, S.C., et al. (2012). A review of nonsurgical treatment for the symptoms of irritability in infants with GERD. *Journal for Specialists in Pediatric Nursing, 17,* 177–192. doi:10.1111/j.1744-6155.2011.00310.x.

Petersen, B. (2014). Diagnosis and management of functional constipation: a common pediatric problem. *The Nurse Practitioner,* 1–6. doi:10.1097/01.NPR.0000451909.40427.b0.

Pinto, R, Schneider, A.C., & da Silveira, T.R. (2015). Cirrhosis in children and adolescents: an overview. *World Journal of Hepatology, 7*(3), 392–405. doi:10.4254/wjh.v7.i3.392

Sfakianaki, A.K. (2012). Congenital diaphragmatic hernia [Electronic version]. *Contemporary OB/GYN,* 26–32.

Sreedharan, R., & Liacouras, C.A. (2016). Functional abdominal pain (nonorganic chronic abdominal pain). In R. Kliegman, B. Stanton, J. St. Geme, et al. (Eds.), *Nelson textbook of pediatrics* (20th ed., pp. 1884–1887). Philadelphia: Elsevier.

Spatz, D.L., & Schmidt, K.J. (2012). Breastfeeding success in infants with giant omphalocele. *Advances in Neonatal Care, 12*(6), 329–335. doi: 10.1097/ANC0b013e31826150c5.

Tinanoff, N. (2016). Cleft lip and palate. In R. Kliegman, B. Stanton, J. St. Geme, et al. (Eds.), *Nelson textbook of pediatrics* (20th ed., pp. 1771–1772). Philadelphia: Elsevier.

U.S. Department of Health and Human Services and U.S. Department of Agriculture. (2015). *2015–2020 Dietary guidelines for Americans.*

8th Ed. Retrieved from http://health.gov/dietaryguidelines/2015/guidelines/.

Vanderhoof, J., & Branski, D. (2016). Short bowel syndrome. In R. Kliegman, B. Stanton, J. St. Geme, et al. (Eds.), *Nelson textbook of pediatrics* (20th ed., pp. 1843–1844). Philadelphia: Elsevier.

van der Pol, R.J., Smits, M.J., Vanmans, L., et al. (2013). Diagnostic accuracy of texts in pediatric gastroesophageal reflux disease. *The Journal of Pediatrics, 162*(5), 983–987. doi:10.1016/jpeds.2012.10.041

Wang, K.S. (2015). Newborn screening for biliary atresia. *Pediatrics, 136*(6), e1663–1669. doi:10.1542/peds.2015-3570.

44

# The Child With a Genitourinary Alteration

http://evolve.elsevier.com/McKinney/mat-ch/

## LEARNING OBJECTIVES

*After studying this chapter, you should be able to:*

- Describe the anatomy and physiology of the infant's and child's genitourinary system.
- Describe the most common diagnostic and screening tests used to assess alterations in genitourinary function.
- Discuss frequently seen alterations in the genitourinary system.
- Use the nursing process to assess, plan, and provide nursing care to children with common genitourinary alterations.
- Develop home care guidelines for the child with a genitourinary alteration.

## CLINICAL REFERENCE

## REVIEW OF THE GENITOURINARY SYSTEM

The urinary system consists of the kidneys and ureters (upper urinary tract) and the bladder and urethra (lower urinary tract). A child's genitourinary system differs in structure and function from that of an adult in several ways.

### Pediatric Differences in the Genitourinary System

In a healthy infant, the kidneys operate at a functional level appropriate for body size; however, function is reduced when the infant is under stress.

By 6 to 12 months of age, kidney function is nearly like that of the adult.

In premature infants, the reabsorption of glucose, sodium, bicarbonate, and phosphate is reduced.

The young infant's kidneys cannot concentrate urine as efficiently as those of older children and adults because the loops of Henle are not yet long enough to reach the inner medulla, where concentration and reabsorption occur.* After the first few weeks of life, the ability of the kidneys to acidify the urine reaches adult levels. However, with acidosis, there is only a small increase in acid secretion, and susceptibility to acidemia rises.

The neonate's bladder, which is in the lower abdominal cavity, gradually sinks into the pelvic cavity during early childhood.

Young children have shorter urethras, which can predispose them to urinary tract infections (UTIs).

Children usually achieve complete bladder control by approximately 4 to 5 years of age.

Unlike adults, most children with acute renal failure regain normal function.

*Banasik, J. (2013). Renal function. In L. Copstead, & J. Banasik (Eds.), *Pathophysiology* (5th ed., pp. 568). St. Louis, MO: Elsevier Saunders.

### Structure

The bean-shaped kidneys are located on each side of the spinal column. In an adolescent or adult, the kidney is approximately the size of a fist; the infant's kidney is small but proportionally larger. The upper portion of the left kidney lies near the 12th rib, with the right kidney slightly lower. The *hilum,* the indentation in the kidney, is the area where the blood vessels, lymphatics, nerves, and *ureter* enter the kidney.

A thin, fibrous capsule encases the kidney. The outer region of the kidney is the cortex, and the inner region is the medulla; both can be observed with the kidney dissected longitudinally. The cortex contains the glomeruli and tubules, whereas the medulla contains the renal pyramids and portions of the tubules. The renal pelvis, located in the area of the hilum, is an extension of the upper end of the ureter.

The ureters extend downward from the kidney and enter the bladder wall. As the bladder fills with urine, it compresses the distal ureters, preventing urine reflux. The bladder is a muscular vessel with a rich blood supply. The bladder capacity for an infant or a child is approximately 10 mL/kg of body weight. The urethra leads from the bladder and contains an internal and an external sphincter, which control urination. Boys have a longer urethra than do girls.

The *nephron* is the kidney's functional unit. It consists of the Bowman's capsule, glomerulus, proximal tubule, loop of Henle, distal tubule, and collecting duct. Each kidney contains approximately 1 million nephrons.

Blood enters the kidney through the renal arteries, which branch off the abdominal aorta. The renal artery divides and subdivides, eventually culminating in the afferent arterioles, which feed into the glomerular capillaries. The glomerular capillaries empty into the efferent arterioles.

Peritubular capillaries surround the proximal tubule, the loop of Henle, and the distal tubules. The capillaries drain into the venous system. Blood returns to the heart through the renal vein, which enters the inferior vena cava.

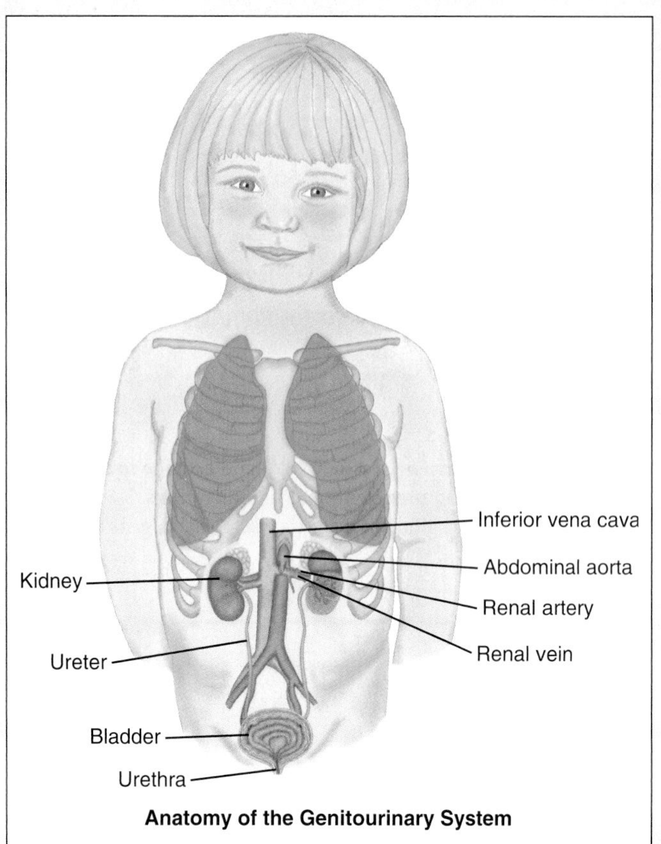

**Anatomy of the Genitourinary System**

## Function

The kidneys maintain fluid and chemical balance through glomerular filtration, tubular reabsorption, and secretion. The kidneys also have important hormonal functions:

- Production of *renin,* which helps with the regulation of blood pressure. Release of renin is stimulated primarily by decreased pressure in the afferent arterioles of the glomerulus.
- Production of *erythropoietin,* which stimulates red blood cell (RBC) production by the bone marrow.
- Metabolism of vitamin D to its active form, which is important in calcium metabolism.

Adequate renal function is important to the function of other body systems. When assessing a child for a possible genitourinary dysfunction, the nurse should consider such nonspecific assessment data as altered growth, skeletal anomalies, hypertension, skin lesions, and immune dysfunctions.

Genitourinary alterations in children encompass a wide range of conditions, from a single acute urinary tract infection (UTI) to end-stage renal disease (ESRD). The effects of illness on the child and family depend on the nature of the illness and on its severity and prognosis. Nursing care also varies. A child in an acute phase of nephrotic syndrome is sometimes hospitalized. Less severe genitourinary disorders may be treated at home. Therefore, the nurse can teach administration of an intravenous (IV) antibiotic or monitor adherence to a treatment plan.

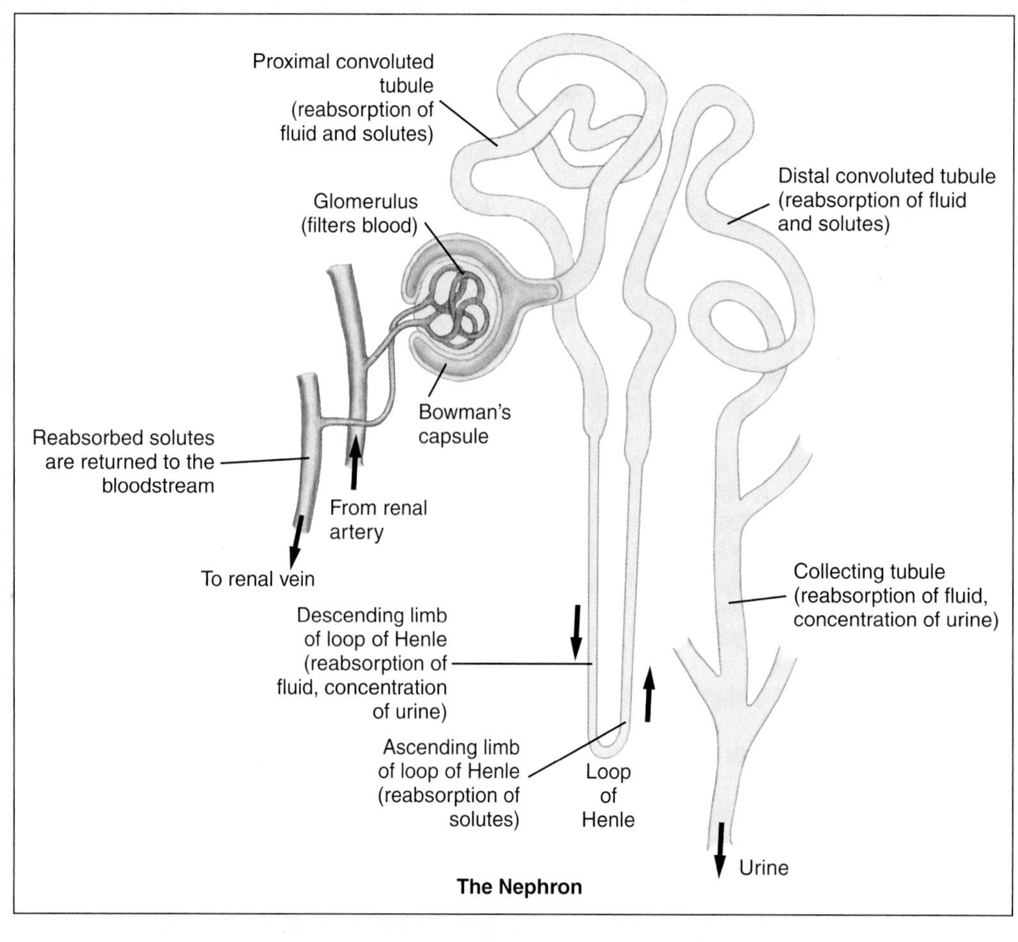

**The Nephron**

## Common Laboratory and Diagnostic Tests for Genitourinary Disorders

| Test | Description | Normal Findings | Indications | Nursing Considerations |
|---|---|---|---|---|
| **Urinalysis** | | | | |
| Specific gravity | Measurement of concentration of urine | 1.002-1.030 | Provides information regarding hydration and renal concentration ability | Specific gravity is higher if protein or glucose is present |
| pH | Determines acidity and alkalinity | 4.5-8.0 | Increases in urinary infections | Affected by diet |
| Protein | Detection of protein in urine | Negative or trace | May be first indication of renal disease | Early morning specimens preferable because they are more concentrated |
| Glucose | Detection of glucose in urine | Negative | Screens or confirms diabetes and monitors effectiveness of diabetes control; may be present in child with weight loss, dehydration, infection, renal disease | Nonspecific, needs further evaluation |
| Ketones | Formed in liver and completely metabolized; alteration in carbohydrate metabolism leads to excessive ketone production | Negative | Mainly associated with diabetes; may be present with fever, anorexia, diarrhea, fasting, starvation, prolonged vomiting | Children are more prone to developing ketonuria |
| Leukocyte esterase | Enzyme released during WBC breakdown | Negative | May be present when WBCs are in urine | Indicates possible UTI |
| Nitrites | Produced by select bacteria | Negative | May be present when bacteria are in urine | In infant and child, bacteria may not be present in bladder long enough to produce sufficient nitrites to yield positive results |
| WBCs | Microscopic finding of WBCs in urine | 0-2/high-power field | Seen with infection | Urine culture indicated |
| RBCs | Microscopic finding of RBCs in urine | 0-2/high-power field | Trauma, stones, infection, glomerulonephritis | Normal in menstruating females |
| Bacteria | Microscopic presence of bacteria in urine | None | UTI | Urine culture indicated |
| Casts | WBC casts and RBC casts originate in kidney tubules | None | Pyelonephritis, glomerulonephritis, renal infarction, collagen disease, interstitial inflammation of kidney | Helps in diagnosis |
| **Urine Culture and Sensitivity** | | | | |
| | Presence of bacteria or other pathogens | Negative or ≤100,000 colonies/mL of urine from clean-catch or sterile bag specimen | Isolation and identification of pathogens in urinary tract; identification of antibiotic sensitivity | Diagnoses UTI<br>See Chapter 37 for specimen collection guidelines |
| **Serum Studies** | | | | |
| BUN | End product of protein metabolism | Newborn: 3-12 mg/dL<br>Infant/Child: 5-18 mg/dL<br>Adult: 10-20 mg/dL | Gross indicator of renal function | Increases in renal insufficiency |
| Serum creatinine | By-product of muscle metabolism; production is constant as long as muscle mass remains constant | Newborn: 0.3-1.0 mg/dL<br>Infant: 0.2-0.4 mg/dL<br>Child: 0.3-0.7 mg/dL<br>Adolescent: 0.5-1.0 mg/dL<br>Adult female: 0.5-1.1 mg/dL<br>Adult male: 0.6-1.2 mg/dL | Increases in renal insufficiency | Should be assessed before giving nephrotoxic agents |
| Serum osmolality | Measurement of concentration of blood, determined by solute in blood | 275-295 mOsm/kg | Indication of fluid and electrolyte balance | Helpful in evaluating hydration status, liver disease, antidiuretic hormone function |

*Continued*

**Common Laboratory and Diagnostic Tests for Genitourinary Disorders—cont'd**

| Test | Description | Normal Findings | Indications | Nursing Considerations |
|---|---|---|---|---|
| **Radiography** | | | | |
| Kidney, ureter, bladder (KUB), flat plate film | Abdominal radiograph | Normal abdominal structures | Diagnoses renal stones; done before renal studies | No discomfort |
| **Cystoscopy** | | | | |
| | Bladder and urethra examined with cystoscope—a tubular, lighted, telescopic lens | Normal appearance | Examination of bladder and lower tract; visualization of tumor and stones; removal of small stones; biopsy of bladder or tumors; fulguration of bladder tumors and posterior urethral valves | Usually performed with child under general anesthesia; little pain involved; encourage fluids; assess ability to void after procedure |
| **Imaging Studies** | | | | |
| CT scan | Computerized calculations revealing a pattern of shades | Normal appearance | Renal tumors | Sedation may be required; child lies on back and should be still; oral contrast material may be administered; child is usually on NPO status because of sedation or oral contrast material |
| Voiding cystourethrogram (VCUG) | Contrast dye instilled in bladder; child or infant voids after bladder is full; serial films taken | Negative for reflux and dilation of posterior urethra, complete bladder emptying | Detects reflux of urine into ureters and its severity; detects bladder emptying problems; detects urethral problems | Can be done in nuclear medicine department to decrease radiation exposure; procedure is invasive; provide support and diversionary activities for child |
| Dimercaptosuccinic acid (DMSA) renal scan | Injection of radioactive agent technetium-99m ($^{99m}$Tc)-DMSA to allow visualization of kidney structures and function; serial films taken | Prompt uptake and excretion of radioactive agent | Evaluates blood flow and renal function; assesses renal scarring; identifies pyelonephritis | Minimal radiation exposure; child must remain still for procedure |
| Renal ultrasonography | Noninvasive; high-frequency sound waves directed at kidneys, ureters, and bladder | Normal size, shape, position, function of kidneys | Assesses position, size, and contour of kidneys, ureters, bladder; detects obstruction and stones; localizes for renal biopsy | Child lies on abdomen; if for transplanted kidney, child lies on back |
| **Urodynamic Studies** | | | | |
| | Invasive test involving urethral and rectal catheters and perineal surface electrodes; measures urine flow, bladder capacity, sensation, sphincter function, bladder pressures; measures voluntary and involuntary contractions | Normal bladder function | Voiding dysfunction, abnormal urinary tract | Inform child and family of procedure; provide support for child throughout procedure; provide diversionary activities |

*BUN,* blood, urea, nitrogen; *CT,* computed tomography; *NPO,* nothing by mouth; *RBC,* red blood cell; *UTI,* urinary tract infection; *WBC,* white blood cell.

## ENURESIS

Children with difficulties in urinary control are defined as having *enuresis.* Nocturnal enuresis occurs at nighttime during sleep, whereas diurnal enuresis occurs during the day, or in waking hours. *Primary enuresis* is defined as a child never having experienced a period of dryness, whereas *secondary enuresis* occurs when a 6- to 12-month period of dryness has preceded the onset of wetting.

### Etiology

Although there is no single cause for enuresis, several risk factors have been implicated. Physical factors include decreased bladder capacity, underlying urinary tract abnormalities, neurologic alterations, obstructive sleep apnea, constipation, urinary tract infection (UTI), pinworm infestation, diabetes mellitus, and voiding dysfunction. Emotional factors related to increased stress can contribute to secondary enuresis. These factors include family disruption, inappropriate pressure during toilet training, inadequate attention to voiding cues, and decreased self-esteem. Sexual abuse must be considered in a child with secondary enuresis.

### Incidence

Primary nocturnal enuresis is common, affecting approximately 15% of children at 6 years of age and decreasing spontaneously thereafter (Bayne & Skoog, 2014). It occurs more frequently in boys and in children with a family history of bed-wetting. Most children eventually outgrow bed-wetting without therapeutic intervention. Some children have diurnal (daytime) enuresis without nocturnal enuresis. Waiting until the last minute to void and not being able to access a bathroom quickly can be a factor in diurnal enuresis, but the main cause is an overactive bladder, a condition in which the child experiences bladder spasms or increased urgency (Elder, 2016). Primary enuresis often resolves spontaneously.

## PATHOPHYSIOLOGY

### *Enuresis*

Control of urination is related to the maturity of the central nervous system. By 5 years of age, most children are aware of bladder fullness and are able to voluntarily control voiding. Children usually achieve daytime urinary control first, with nighttime dryness occurring later. Girls seem to master this earlier than boys. Children who have primary nocturnal enuresis may have delayed maturation of this portion of the central nervous system.

A child with secondary nocturnal enuresis or with problems of daytime control and complaints of dysuria, urgency, or frequency should be evaluated for other conditions. Bladder infections can give rise to such symptoms. Excessive calcium loss in the urine can irritate the bladder and cause painful urination, urgency, frequency, or wetting. Secondary enuresis accompanied by excessive thirst and weight loss may indicate the onset of diabetes mellitus. Children whose bladders are very sensitive to urine volume may have uninhibited bladder contractions. Moderate to large amounts of urine in the bladder give rise to strong contractions of the bladder muscle. An anatomic abnormality in these cases is rare.

### Manifestations

#### Nocturnal Enuresis

Children with a continuing history of bed-wetting are not able to sense bladder fullness and do not awaken to void. Because physical maturation varies, nocturnal enuresis is not a matter for excessive concern unless the child is older than 6 years or has markedly decreased self-esteem.

#### Diurnal Enuresis

Children with urgency, frequency, and inappropriate wetting during the day may be seen rushing to the bathroom or tightly crossing their legs. Often these children cannot sit still and exhibit a constant odor of urine.

### Diagnostic Evaluation

The diagnosis of enuresis is based on the history and clinical symptoms. Urinalysis and urine culture can rule out possible UTI. Measurements of urine specific gravity and urine glucose are assessed for underlying diabetes. In addition, the child's urine should be checked for excessive calcium, and a pinworm evaluation should be done to exclude infestation.

If the child has daytime enuresis, voiding dysfunction with urge incontinence is explored. Bladder ultrasonography and measures of urine flow and bladder capacity may be indicated. Children with UTIs should have a workup for underlying structural abnormalities. Because enuresis can occur with constipation or encopresis, diagnosis includes a history of possible bowel dysfunction (Elder, 2016). Assessing the child's psychological state also is important because social or emotional situations can contribute to enuresis, and enuresis can alter a child's self-esteem (Elder, 2016).

### Therapeutic Management

Treatment of primary nocturnal enuresis often begins with general interventions, such as explaining theories underlying the problem in terms the child can understand. The child is reassured that, with assistance, the problem can resolve. Common sense approaches of limiting fluids after supper and voiding just before bedtime are encouraged. Diet modifications include avoiding extraneous sugar and caffeine intake after 4 PM, because these substances can act as bladder stimulants as well as diuretics (Elder, 2016). Also, the child can be trained to use imagery; thinking about what a full bladder feels like and picturing waking up and going to the bathroom. This imagery is done as the child lies in bed before drifting off to sleep. The child should keep a record of the number of dry and wet nights to measure progress.

Reward systems assume that bed-wetting is a voluntary behavior and have had varying results for the child with primary nocturnal enuresis. The child can be given a roll of favorite stickers to mark the dry nights on the calendar. The family decides on a special reward or outing when the child has achieved a certain number of consecutive dry nights.

Behavioral conditioning with the use of alarms has been successful in older children with nocturnal enuresis. A pad placed on the bed or device worn on the child's pajamas contains a moisture-sensitive alarm. As the child starts to void, the alarm goes off and the child awakens. The alarm system must be used consistently, often for three to six months, depending on the severity and response (March, Heering, & Pravikoff, 2016). Adherence is a major factor to successful resolution.

Desmopressin acetate (deamino-D-arginine vasopressin [DDAVP]) has also been helpful because of its antidiuretic effect. Desmopressin acetate is given as a tablet and is taken at bedtime. Pharmacologic treatment is not recommended for children under 6 years of age. Results improve when alarms and pharmacologic approaches are used concurrently (Elder, 2016; March et al., 2016).

Voiding frequently to keep a low volume of urine in the bladder can benefit children who are affected by uninhibited bladder contractions during the day. The use of an anticholinergic such as oxybutynin chloride, which relaxes the smooth muscle of the bladder, can be helpful for children with diurnal enuresis related to underlying bladder instability or small bladder capacity. Biofeedback also helps some children with diurnal enuresis, particularly those with dysfunctional voiding.

## NURSING CARE

### The Child With Enuresis

#### Assessment

The nurse should obtain a full set of vital signs and assess the child and parent for their understanding of enuresis, including the interventions they have already tried. The nurse asks the child and parent to describe voiding and bowel elimination patterns, establishing whether the enuresis is primary or secondary. The nurse should also ask whether the child participates in social activities with peers, such as sleepovers, and whether the child is concerned about the problem of wetting. Therapy is much more successful for the older child than for the younger child, who might not be bothered by bed-wetting. The nurse should assist the child in obtaining a urine specimen. The physical examination includes assessment for signs of sexual abuse or visible genital abnormalities. It also is important to observe the lower spine for the presence of a dimple or hair tuft that might suggest spina bifida occulta (see Chapter 52).

#### Nursing Diagnosis and Planning

The nursing diagnoses and expected outcomes that apply to the child with enuresis and the child's family are as follows:

- Situational Low Self-Esteem related to bed-wetting or urinary incontinence.

*Expected outcome.* The child will demonstrate positive self-esteem, as evidenced by a realistic description of the problem and positive self-statements.

- Impaired Social Interaction related to bed-wetting or urinary incontinence.

*Expected outcome.* The child will participate in age-appropriate activities such as sleepovers and overnight camp.

- Compromised Family Coping related to negative social stigma and increased laundry load.

*Expected outcome.* The family will identify strengths and will describe positive problem-solving strategies.

- Risk for Impaired Skin Integrity related to prolonged contact with urine.

*Expected outcome.* The child will have no rashes or redness in the perineal area.

#### Interventions

Enuresis can be a frustrating problem for both the child and family. The nurse can help by providing them with correct information about causes and therapeutic approaches. It is important that the family choose the treatment that will best meet its needs. Follow-up to determine the effectiveness of treatment is essential because becoming dry can be a long process, and the nurse is instrumental in providing support to the child and family over the entire course of therapy.

#### Evaluation

- Is the child able to describe ways to manage the condition?
- Is the child verbalizing a decrease in stress related to the enuresis, and does the child make positive self-statements?
- Is the child showing an increased interest in peer activities?
- Is the family able to identify its strengths and demonstrate appropriate problem solving?
- Is the child having increased dry nights?
- Does the child's skin remain intact, and is it free from redness and rashes?

### CRITICAL THINKING EXERCISE 44.1

Mr. Sampson brings his son Thomas in for his 5-year-old well-child visit. As the nurse is obtaining a history, Mr. Sampson expresses concern that Thomas wets the bed at night. He has been fully toilet trained for 1 year and does not have daytime urine accidents. Thomas refuses to wear a diaper at night because he "doesn't want to be a baby." As a result, he consistently sleeps in wet sheets and clothing.

1. What additional data would be helpful to obtain from Mr. Sampson?
2. What suggestions for an initial approach to the problem should the nurse give Mr. Sampson?

## URINARY TRACT INFECTIONS

Urinary tract infections (UTIs), which are characterized by the presence of bacteria in the urine along with systemic signs of infection, are commonly seen in children. In fact, UTIs result in significant morbidity in infants and children. These infections can have long-term complications that include renal scarring with decreased renal function, high blood pressure, and, rarely, end-stage renal disease (ESRD).

### Etiology

UTIs, except in newborn infants, are caused by bacteria ascending from outside the urethra into the bladder and from there into the upper urinary tract. Bacteria in the blood, which seeds in the kidney, can cause UTIs in newborn infants.

Fecal bacteria cause most UTIs, with *Escherichia coli* being the most prominent, especially in girls (Elder, 2016). Other bacteria known to cause UTIs are group B streptococci, *Klebsiella pneumoniae, Proteus* species, *Enterobacter* species, enterococci, and *Staphylococcus* species. Viruses and fungi, specifically *Candida* species, can rarely cause infections.

The following conditions predispose the infant or child to UTI:

- Urinary tract obstructions, which can be congenital or acquired. These include strictures, ureteropelvic narrowing, or other urinary tract anomalies. *Hydronephrosis* is dilation of the renal pelvis, usually caused by ureteropelvic junction obstruction. *Phimosis,* which is a narrowing of the prepuce opening, prevents the foreskin from being retracted.
- Voiding dysfunction resulting in urinary stasis. Conditions contributing to incomplete bladder emptying include neurogenic bladder and bladder instability. Constipation that causes pressure on the bladder can inhibit complete bladder emptying.
- Anatomic differences. Young girls have a short urethra, which expedites bacterial transit.
- Individual susceptibility to infection. Some infants and children have UTIs without any structural abnormality and may be more prone to bacterial adherence to epithelial cells in the urinary tract.
- Reflux. A primary contributing factor to upper UTI, or pyelonephritis, is vesicoureteral reflux (VUR).
- UTIs in toddler-age girls are more frequent during toilet training, most likely the result of urinary retention or incomplete bladder emptying (Elder, 2016). It is generally accepted that bacterial colonization of the prepuce of uncircumcised infants can increase the risk of UTI in infant boys younger than 1 year.
- Sexually active adolescent girls are at risk for UTIs.

### Incidence

The overall prevalence of UTIs in the United States is 1% to 3% in girls and 1% in boys. In girls, the first UTI generally occurs before 5 years of age, with an increase in the number of cases seen during infancy and toilet training. For boys, most UTIs occur during the first year of life, with a higher incidence in uncircumcised infants (Elder, 2016; Fisher & Steele, 2015).

## PATHOPHYSIOLOGY

### *Urinary Tract Infections*

Fecal bacteria colonize the perineal area or under the prepuce of uncircumcised infant boys. Bacteria adhere to epithelial cells in the urinary tract and then ascend through the urethra into the bladder, causing a bladder infection, or *cystitis*. In most circumstances, the bladder is emptied on a regular basis, which decreases the opportunity for bacterial growth. In children with incomplete bladder emptying, bacteria grow in the residual urine.

Bacteria ascending from the bladder into the ureters and up into the renal parenchyma cause pyelonephritis. Pyelonephritis is more frequently seen in children with vesicoureteral reflux (VUR) but can occur in its absence. Infants and young children (<24 months) are presumed to have pyelonephritis if they present with a febrile UTI. (Elder, 2016).

Scarring, as an inflammatory consequence of pyelonephritis, is more frequently seen in infants younger than 1 year and is a significant cause of hypertension during childhood. Scarring causes decreased arterial perfusion to the kidney, mimicking volume depletion. This triggers the renin-angiotensin mechanism to increase aldosterone release and cause sodium and fluid retention. The subsequent increase in circulating blood volume results in hypertension.

## Manifestations

Clinical manifestations of UTI vary widely (Box 44.1); factors include the child's age, sex, underlying anatomic or neurologic abnormalities, and frequency of recurrence. Signs in the young child and infant are more vague and nonspecific and can include disordered feeding, failure to thrive, odorous urine, and irritability (Fisher & Steele, 2015). Fever (100.4° F [38° C]) without a known focus for infection in infants and young children 2 to 24 months of age indicates the need for additional studies (American Academy of Pediatrics [AAP] Committee on Urinary Tract Infection, Steering Committee on Quality Improvement and Management, 2011). Suprapubic tenderness can be an accompanying sign in an infant. Signs and symptoms in a verbal child include abdominal pain, frequency, urgency, and dysuria (Fisher & Steele, 2015).

An abdominal mass in an infant can suggest hydronephrosis (Elder, 2016). Other signs and symptoms of hydronephrosis are similar to those for an infant with a UTI (see Box 44.1).

### BOX 44.1 Manifestations of Urinary Tract Infection in Infants and Children

**Infants**
- Nonspecific
- Fever or hypothermia in neonate
- Irritability
- Dysuria as evidenced by crying when voiding
- Change in urine odor or color
- Poor weight gain
- Feeding difficulties

**Children**
- Abdominal or suprapubic pain
- Voiding frequency
- Voiding urgency
- Dysuria
- New or increased incidence of enuresis
- Fever

**Children With Pyelonephritis**

Same symptoms as for children with uncomplicated urinary tract infection (UTI) plus:
- High fever, chills
- Back pain
- Costovertebral angle tenderness
- Nausea and vomiting
- Appears very ill

## PATHOPHYSIOLOGY

### *Hydronephrosis*

Obstruction at the ureteropelvic junction or other parts of the ureter causes dilation of the kidney. As the renal dilation increases, the risk of renal parenchymal damage and decreased renal function increases as well. In some instances, the obstruction is only partial, causing an initial dilation but no progressive renal function loss. Hydronephrosis can be associated with vesicoureteral reflux (VUR).

Ultrasonography has facilitated prenatal diagnosis of hydronephrosis.* Since urinary tract obstruction is often silent, these infants need a complete evaluation, including imaging studies, following birth.*

*Elder, J. (2016). Obstruction of the urinary tract. In R. Kliegman, B. Stanton, J. St. Geme, et al. (Eds.), *Nelson textbook of pediatrics* (20th ed., pp. 2567–2568). St. Louis, MO: Elsevier.

## Diagnostic Evaluation

Bacteria in the urine establish a diagnosis of UTI. Symptoms of UTI in the absence of bacteriuria can be caused by perineal inflammation, vaginitis, pinworms, or chemical irritation from bubble baths.

Urine dipstick that shows nitrites and/or leukocyte esterase can indicate a need for additional testing. If urinalysis is performed, hematuria and presence of white blood cells (WBCs) in addition to the nitrites and leukocyte esterase suggest a UTI. Urinalysis should be performed on a first morning urine specimen to be most accurate.

Urine culture is the single determining diagnostic study for a UTI. Any bacterial growth of a single-strain bacterium exceeding 100,000 colony-forming units/mL in a clean-catch urine specimen establishes a diagnosis of UTI. Obtaining a sterile urine sample is difficult in children, especially for those who are not yet toilet trained. A child who can void on demand can provide a midstream, clean-catch urine specimen. In infants and children who are not toilet trained, a sterile pediatric urine collection bag attached to the perineum can collect a urine specimen (see Chapter 37). Collecting urine by this method is less invasive but is clearly not as accurate for obtaining a culture as by other methods, and the urine specimen must be plated as quickly as possible. If the urine cannot be plated within 10 minutes of collection, it should be refrigerated.

When accurate determination of bacteria is the goal, more intrusive methods of bladder catheterization (see Chapter 37) or suprapubic aspiration are the collection methods of choice. If suprapubic aspiration is necessary, the area above the pubis is cleaned with an antiseptic solution, a needle attached to a syringe is inserted by the physician at a 90-degree angle into the bladder, and urine is aspirated. If catheterization or suprapubic aspiration is used to obtain a urine culture,

## PATHOPHYSIOLOGY

### *Vesicoureteral Reflux*

A valve-like mechanism at the junction of the ureter and bladder prevents urine reflux into the ureters. As urine fills the bladder or as the bladder contracts during voiding, pressure in the bladder occludes the opening to the ureter. When a defect occurs at the vesicoureteral junction, vesicoureteral reflux (VUR) results. The defect at the vesicoureteral junction is considered a congenital abnormality, although transitory VUR associated with a lower urinary tract infection (UTI) is also possible. VUR has a genetic component and is often seen in families.*

In VUR, two mechanisms contribute to UTI. Bacteria in the urine can be carried up to the kidney, causing pyelonephritis and renal damage with scarring. Also, when urine reflux into the lower ureter occurs, urine can return to the bladder, leaving residual urine that becomes a medium for bacterial growth.

The severity of VUR determines the potential risk for pyelonephritis and kidney damage. The International Classification of Reflux grades reflux on a scale of I through V. Grade I describes reflux into the ureter only with no dilation. Grade V, the most severe, includes gross dilation and reflux involving the kidney.

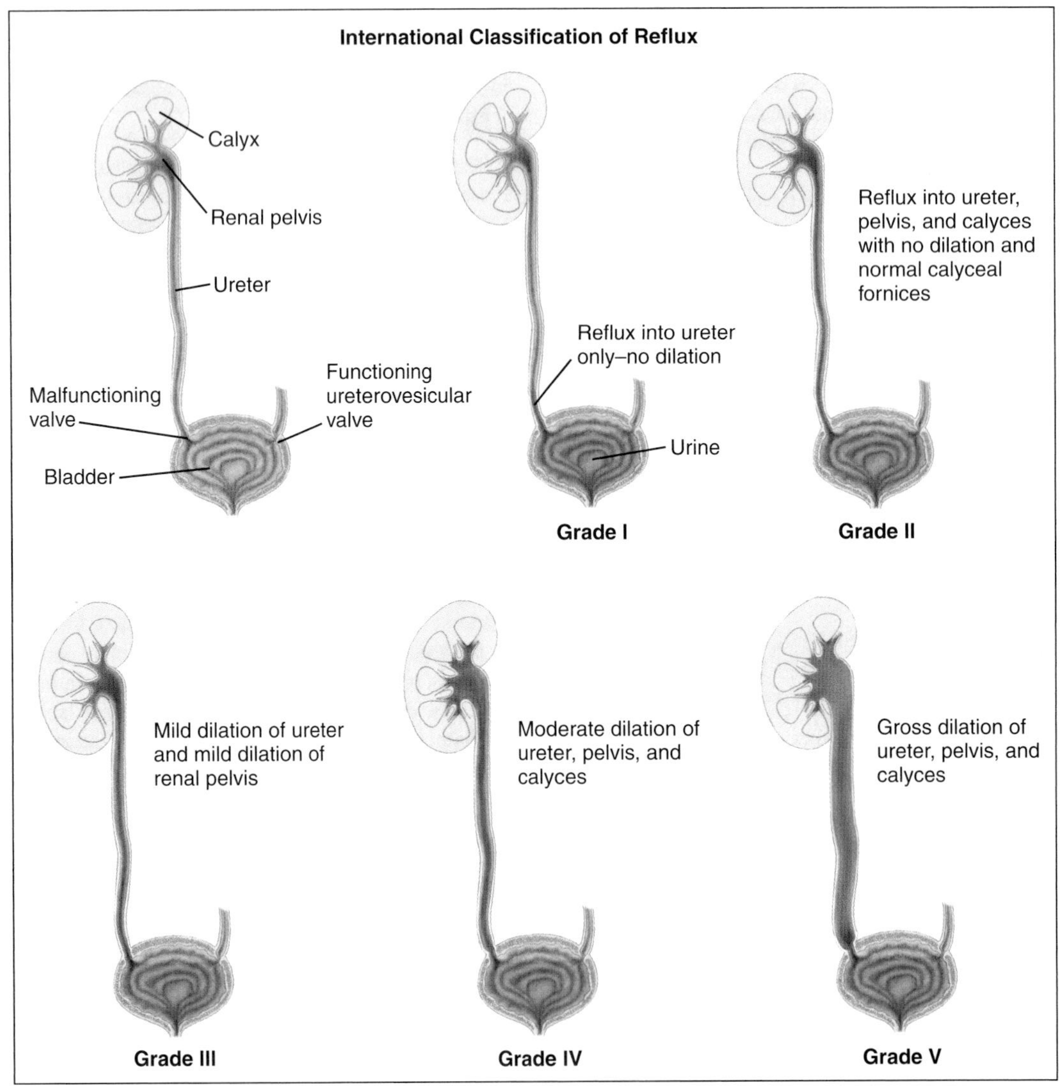


*Elder, J. (2016). Vesicoureteral reflux. In R. Kliegman, B. Stanton, J. St. Geme, et al. (Eds.), *Nelson textbook of pediatrics* (20th ed., pp. 2562–2566). St. Louis, MO: Elsevier.

positive nitrites and 50,000 colony-forming units/mL indicate infection (American Academy of Pediatrics [AAP] Committee on Urinary Tract Infection, Steering Committee on Quality Improvement and Management, 2011).

More intensive evaluation for underlying structural abnormalities is necessary for certain infants and young children with UTIs. Evaluative studies might include ultrasonography to detect kidney dilation resulting from obstruction, and a voiding cystourethrography (VCUG) or radionuclide cystography to detect VUR. It is important to diagnose UTIs quickly, as an ascending UTI can result in renal scarring.

### Therapeutic Management

A 3- to 5-day course of oral antibiotics is the treatment of choice for an uncomplicated UTI without systemic symptoms (Elder, 2016). The antibiotic chosen should be one to which the specific bacterium (identified by culture) is sensitive, should be easily administered, and should have minimal adverse effects. Oral trimethoprim-sulfamethoxazole, nitrofurantoin, and cephalosporins are frequently used.

Children with pyelonephritis often require initial treatment with parenteral antibiotics followed by oral antibiotic treatment. The older child who does not need hospitalization can receive daily intramuscular ceftriaxone for 1 to 2 days, followed by 10 to 14 days of oral antibiotics. Infants and children admitted to the hospital for treatment usually receive IV cephalosporin or an aminoglycoside (e.g., gentamicin) (Elder, 2016; Fisher & Steele, 2015). Some children are treated with a cephalosporin alone. Oral antibiotics follow this initial treatment with parenteral antibiotics for a total course of 7 to 14 days. Recent evidence (Shaikh et al., 2016) suggests that certain infants and children are at risk for antibiotic resistance to amoxicillin, sulfa, and first generation cephalosporins. The primary risk factor for antibiotic resistance is being an uncircumcised boy. The recommendation is to treat any young child with a febrile UTI with a second or third generation cephalosporin or other broad spectrum antibiotic (Shaikh et al., 2016).

When anatomic abnormalities are detected or UTIs recur, prophylactic antibiotic therapy might be initiated, although recent studies suggest that the risk of antibiotic resistance can be higher than the therapeutic value of prophylaxis (Brandstrom & Hansson, 2015). In addition, some studies have suggested that antibiotic prophylaxis contributes to, rather than prevents, subsequent UTI, even in children with low grade VUR because the organisms become resistant during treatment (Cara-Fuentes, Gupta, & Garin, 2015). Prophylactic antibiotics are sometimes given to children after their initial course of treatment while waiting for imaging studies to confirm an underlying structural abnormality. Children who have bowel and bladder dysfunction and those younger than one year of age might be candidates for antibiotic prophylaxis for UTI (Elder, 2016).

Because the majority of children with grades I through III VUR have a spontaneous resolution of the reflux, most physicians choose nonsurgical management of this condition (Elder, 2016). First-line surgical treatment for children with persistent grade I through III VUR is the endoscopic injection of bulking material into the submucosa of the affected ureter. The material, Deflux injectable gel, builds a protective wall inside the ureter to prevent the backflow of urine. Open surgical repair involving reimplantation of the ureter into the bladder is indicated for children who continue to have reflux and breakthrough UTIs despite antibiotic therapy, severe grade IV or V reflux, or two to three failed Deflux treatments (Elder, 2016).

## NURSING CARE

### The Child With a Urinary Tract Infection

#### Assessment

The nurse obtains a history from the child and family inquiring about age-specific signs and symptoms of UTI. Determining bowel elimination patterns is important as well, because constipation can increase the risk for UTI in certain children.

Physical assessment includes temperature, blood pressure, abdominal examination for masses, examination for costovertebral angle tenderness, and examination for genital abnormalities. It is important to obtain a urinalysis and urine culture before initiating antibiotics.

#### Nursing Diagnosis and Planning

The nursing diagnoses and expected outcomes that apply to the child with a UTI and the child's family are as follows:

- Risk for Injury to the kidney related to complications from the infectious process.

  **Expected outcome.** The child will be free of recurrent UTIs, as evidenced by the absence of voiding frequency and urgency, dysuria, and fever and the presence of a negative urine culture.
- Deficient Fluid Volume related to decreased intake and increased fluid loss from fever.

  **Expected outcome.** The child will maintain adequate intake of fluids and electrolytes for age, as evidenced by an output normal for age (see Chapter 40).
- Deficient Knowledge related to incomplete understanding of the disease process, diagnostic tests, antibiotic administration, and preventive measures for UTI.

  **Expected outcome.** The parent or child will explain the disease process, diagnostic tests, and preventive measures for UTIs. The family will follow through with appropriate follow-up care, including antibiotic administration and imaging studies, if recommended.

#### Interventions

Infants admitted to the hospital with fever of unknown source often are evaluated to rule out a focal infection or septicemia, as well as UTI, which is one of the most frequent causes of fever in infants. The evaluation includes blood studies and cultures, lumbar puncture, and urinary catheterization or suprapubic aspiration for urine culture. The parent already is anxious about the infant, so it is imperative that the nurse inform the parent about why procedures are being done. An IV line is established at the time of the workup because parenteral antibiotics are given while waiting for laboratory results and for several days thereafter if the child has a UTI.

The nurse encourages the parents to express concerns, and provides reassurance about the infant's condition. Every effort should be made to maintain the infant's routine; the mother continues to breastfeed, ensuring that the IV site is protected as she holds the infant. If the breastfeeding mother is unable to remain with the infant, she will need to pump her breasts. Allowing parents to participate in the infant's care provides them a measure of control in an uncertain situation. The infant with a documented UTI will require renal ultrasonography at the earliest convenient time.

Nursing care of the child who is not hospitalized includes ensuring administration of antibiotics, promoting comfort, maintaining good hydration, preparing the child and parent for diagnostic procedures, and monitoring for responses to treatment and possible complications.

Because repeated UTIs can contribute to renal damage, the nurse emphasizes the importance of adhering to the treatment regimen and obtaining follow-up studies, if ordered. The child and family are educated about the prevention of UTIs (see Patient-Centered Teaching: How to Manage and Prevent Urinary Tract Infections).

For the hospitalized child, optimal hydration is essential, especially if the child has been febrile, nauseated, vomiting, or feeding poorly. The nurse encourages oral fluid intake, if possible. IV hydration may be required, especially for young infants. The child must be observed for signs of dehydration: poor skin turgor, dry mucous membranes, a sunken fontanel, decreased output, and decreased peripheral perfusion. Daily weights, intake and output measurements, and urine specific gravity are indicators of the child's hydration status.

For children with VUR, the nurse explains the treatment plan, including medical or surgical management, to the parent and child in a simple, age-appropriate manner. If surgical treatment is required, the parents and child are given information regarding the procedure and preoperative and postoperative care. They need to understand that inpatient hospitalization is required. Medications are given for pain and bladder spasms, which frequently occur after surgery. Children

## PATIENT-CENTERED TEACHING

### *How to Manage and Prevent Urinary Tract Infections*

If your child has been diagnosed with a urinary tract infection, it is most important for you to do the following:

- Give your child the prescribed medication for the full number of days your physician or nurse practitioner recommends. Some children need to continue on a lower dose of the antibiotic after the initial treatment is finished.
- Take a follow-up urine culture to the laboratory if your physician or nurse practitioner has requested one. Use a sterile container to collect the urine. If the laboratory has not given you a sterile plastic container, you can use a glass container and a cover that have been sterilized. Make sure the urine stays refrigerated or in a cooler while you take it to the laboratory.
- Keep the appointment for follow-up studies of your child's urinary system, if ordered by the physician or nurse practitioner. These studies can help diagnose a structural problem with your child's urinary system or monitor the kidneys for any problems.
- Call your physician or nurse practitioner if your child has a fever or symptoms that make you think the infection has returned.

Preventing a urinary tract infection from recurring is important because repeated infections can cause kidney damage. Some suggestions that can help prevent a urinary tract infection are as follows:

- Wipe babies and teach young girls to wipe from front to back after going to the bathroom. This takes any germs away from the opening that leads into the urinary system. Be sure to keep the foreskin on uncircumcised baby boys as clean as possible without forcible retraction.
- Encourage your toilet-trained child to avoid "holding" urine and to urinate at least four times per day, emptying the bladder completely.
- Give your child lots of fluids throughout the day to help flush out the bladder.
- Avoid dressing your child in tight clothing or diapers. Use cotton underwear rather than synthetic fabric.
- Avoid bubble baths, which can irritate your child's urinary system.
- Emphasize proper hygiene if your daughter is sexually active and encourage her to urinate immediately after having sexual intercourse.
- Daily consumption of cranberry juice in a dose of 2 to 5 mL/kg/day might have protective action against UTI*

*Durham, S., Stamm, P., & Eiland, L. (2015). Cranberry products for the prophylaxis of urinary tract infections in pediatric patients. *Annals of Pharmacotherapy, 49*(2), 1349–1356.

who have had a ureteral implant for correction of VUR are normally discharged within two days. Discharge teaching is important, with emphasis on returning for any imaging studies postoperatively if warranted (Elder, 2016). Although controversial, antibiotic prophylaxis for UTI might be ordered for at-risk children, usually infants younger than one year of age or children with bladder and bowel dysfunction (Elder, 2016); if antibiotics are ordered, the nurse advises the parent to be meticulously adherent.

## ! NURSING QUALITY ALERT

### *Evaluation Follow-up for an Infant or Young Child With a Febrile Urinary Tract Infection*

Radiologic studies might be indicated for infants and children who are likely to have renal damage associated with structural abnormalities. Studies can diagnose underlying abnormalities and assess the extent of potential renal scarring. The following are recently recommended follow-up studies and evaluations*:

- For infants and children 2 to 24 months of age, ultrasonography is recommended after the first febrile UTI. Ultrasonography can assess renal scarring and extent of hydronephrosis, but is not accurate for VUR.
- Voiding cystourethrogram (VCUG) if the ultrasound is abnormal.
- VCUG after a second febrile UTI.
- Renal ultrasound and/or VCUG for siblings of children diagnosed with VUR

*Data from AAP Subcommittee on UTI, Steering Committee on Quality Improvement and Management. (2011). Urinary tract infection: clinical practice guideline for the diagnosis and management of the initial UTI in febrile infants and children 2 to 24 months. *Pediatrics, 128,* 595–610; Elder, J. (2016). Urologic disorders in infants and children. In R. Kliegman, B. Stanton, J. St. Geme, et al. (Eds.), *Nelson textbook of pediatrics* (20th ed., Part XXIV). St. Louis, MO: Elsevier; Nelson, C., Johnson, E., Logvinenko, T., et al. (2014). Ultrasound as a screening test for genitourinary anomalies in children with UTI. *Pediatrics, 133*(3), 394–403; Penny, S. (2016). The pediatric urinary tract and medical imaging. *Radiologic Technology, 87*(4), 425–444.

### Evaluation

- Is the child free of frequency, urgency, and dysuria?
- Is the urine culture negative?
- Is the child taking fluids in amounts expected for age?
- Is the child's urine output adequate (see Chapter 40)?
- Has the child continued on the prescribed antibiotic therapy regimen?
- Has the child received follow-up diagnostic testing?
- Can the parent or child describe symptoms of recurrence and measures to take if infection occurs?

## CRYPTORCHIDISM

Cryptorchidism (undescended or hidden testes) occurs when one or both testes fail to descend through the inguinal canal into the scrotal sac.

### Incidence

Congenital cryptorchidism is a common urologic problem, with approximately 1% to 5% of normal, healthy boys having at least one undescended testis discovered at birth (Kolon et al., 2014). Premature male infants have a significantly higher incidence (Fantasia, Aidlen, Lathrop, et al., 2015). Cryptorchidism is also seen more frequently in low-birth-weight or smaller-than-average-length newborns (Kolon et al., 2014). Most infants have spontaneous descent of their testes during the first 6 months of life. An increased incidence of acquired (ascending) undescended testes (testes descended at birth no longer remain in the scrotal sac) is being seen in boys ages 4 to 10 years (Elder, 2016; Kolon et al., 2014). Cryptorchidism has a multifactorial inheritance pattern, with genetic predisposition interacting with several potential environmental influences, such as maternal smoking and in utero exposure to pesticides (Fantasia et al., 2015; Kolon et al., 2014).

### Manifestations

Testes that are not palpable or not easily guided into the scrotum and a previously descended testis that ascends into an extrascrotal position

## PATHOPHYSIOLOGY

### Cryptorchidism

In normal fetal development, the testes begin their descent from the abdomen between 32 and 36 weeks of gestation. The exact reason for failure of the testes to descend is not known. Sperm production is decreased in the undescended testis, and there is increased risk for development of a malignancy when the child reaches adulthood. Inguinal hernias are commonly associated with cryptorchidism, as is testicular torsion.

are manifestations of cryptorchidism. Children with undescended testes are at increased risk for testicular malignancy and infertility.

### Diagnostic Evaluation

One or both testes may be undescended. If the testis is not palpable, it can be found at any point along the process vaginalis, in the abdomen, or might have followed an aberrant course and come to lie in the inguinal area, base of the penis, or perineum. When complete absence of the testes is discovered, the child needs immediate referral for diagnostic evaluation for a disorder of sexual development (DSD), most commonly congenital adrenal hyperplasia (CAH) (see Chapter 51). In this circumstance, the physician will order a karyotype, hormonal studies, and electrolytes (Kolon et al., 2014). Elevated follicle-stimulating hormone and luteinizing hormone levels accompanied by absent testosterone indicate testicular absence. True absence of both testes is rare.

### Therapeutic Management

Initially, the infant with cryptorchidism is managed by observation because spontaneous descent of the testes during the first 6 months of life is common. Recommendations from the American Urological Society (Kolon et al., 2014) include assessing for testicular presence at each well visit during childhood because a testis originally palpated in the scrotum can ascend (acquired cryptorchidism). If the condition persists beyond 6 months of corrected gestational age, an orchidopexy is performed to bring the testis down into the scrotal sac and suture it in place. Surgical correction before 12 months of age can reduce the risk for adverse consequences (altered fertility and malignancy) (Schneuer et al., 2016). This surgery is typically done on an outpatient basis using a laparoscopic approach; palpating for the testis position while the child is anesthetized and before beginning the surgical procedure assists in determining the type of surgery necessary (Kolon et al., 2014; Schneuer et al., 2016). Surgery can be done in one or two stages, depending on the ability to secure the testis in the correct anatomic position (Fantasia et al., 2015). If the position of the testis is high in the abdomen, an orchiectomy (removal) may be considered. The most common complications are bleeding and infection. A testicular implant can preserve the scrotal appearance and reduce psychological consequences (Elder, 2016). It is important for the adolescent male to perform testicular self-examinations throughout his life to screen for malignancy.

## NURSING CARE

### The Child With Cryptorchidism

#### Assessment

Absence of the testis in the scrotal sac can be discovered through routine physical examination of the newborn. The nurse also must assess the parents' knowledge of undescended testes and the importance of treatment.

## ! NURSING QUALITY ALERT

### Assessing for Cryptorchidism

Testes can retract into the inguinal canal if the infant is upset or cold. The cremasteric reflex, testicular retraction in response to tactile stimulation to the front inner thigh, can lead to a false diagnosis of cryptorchidism.

- Examine the infant in a warm environment. Be sure the infant is calm before the examination.
- Warm your hands before touching the infant.
- Milk each testis downward from the groin and document its distal point.
- Examine the older child in both a sitting and a frog-leg position (see Chapter 33).
- Most testes descend by the time the infant is 6 months old.

#### Nursing Diagnosis and Planning

The nursing diagnoses and expected outcomes that apply to the child with cryptorchidism and the child's family are as follows:

- Deficient Knowledge (parental) related to cause and management of cryptorchidism.

*Expected outcome.* The parents will be able to explain cryptorchidism, its management, and possible sequelae.

- Risk for Ineffective Health Maintenance related to possible decreased fertility and increased risk of testicular malignancy.

*Expected outcome.* The parents will help the child learn to perform regular testicular self-examination during adolescence, and the individual will seek referral for fertility testing as warranted.

#### Interventions

Nursing care should be directed at educating parents and providing them with information and resources. If the child has bilateral undescended testes or absence of testes, referrals to a counselor, psychologist, or specialist may be appropriate. The nurse provides routine postoperative care after orchidopexy, monitoring the child's voiding patterns, pain level, and swelling, and observing for signs of bleeding or infection.

#### Evaluation

- Are the parents able to explain cryptorchidism and its management?
- Do the parents state their responsibilities to guide their child when he is an adolescent to perform regular testicular self-examination and to seek fertility testing if appropriate?

## HYPOSPADIAS AND EPISPADIAS

Hypospadias is a congenital anomaly in which the actual opening of the urethral meatus is below the normal placement on the glans of the penis (Fig. 44.1). The degree of misplacement of the urethral opening can vary. The urethra may open only slightly ventral to the glans or as far back as the penoscrotal junction. *Chordee,* or downward curvature of the penile shaft, is usually seen in more severe forms of hypospadias. Associated anomalies include undescended testes and inguinal hernias. Dorsal placement of the urethral opening, or epispadias, also can occur but is less common.

### Etiology and Incidence

Hypospadias is one of the most common congenital anomalies, occurring in 1 of every 250 male children (Elder, 2016). Risk is increased if either the father or a sibling has the anomaly. Other contributing factors include maternal age older than 35 years, intrauterine exposure to environmental chemicals, and possible genetic mutation (Elder,

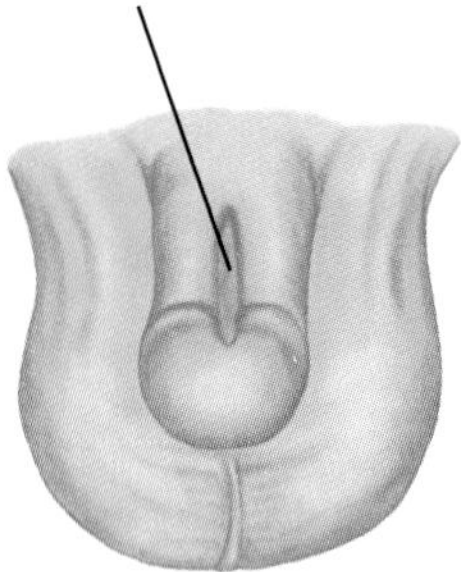


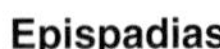

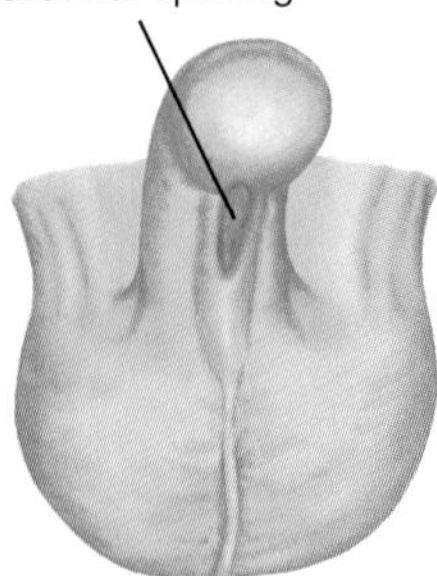


**FIG 44.1** Epispadias and hypospadias are congenital anomalies in which the urethral opening is above or below its normal location on the glans of the penis. Stenosis of the opening can occur, leading to possible urinary tract infections (UTIs) or hydronephrosis. Hypospadias might interfere with fertility if left uncorrected.

2016). Testes are undescended in 10% of affected children, and risk for inguinal hernias is increased. Epispadias is extremely rare and is often associated with bladder exstrophy.

## PATHOPHYSIOLOGY

### *Hypospadias*

Hypospadias occurs from incomplete development of the urethra in utero. The exact cause of the defect is not known, but it is thought to be influenced by genetic, environmental, and hormonal factors.*

The displacement of the urethral meatus does not usually interfere with urinary continence. However, stenosis of the opening gives rise to partial obstruction of outflowing urine. Further, ventral placement of the urethral opening might interfere with fertility in the mature man if left uncorrected.

*Elder, J. (2016). Urologic disorders in infants and children. In R. Kliegman, B. Stanton, J. St. Geme, et al. (Eds.), *Nelson textbook of pediatrics* (20th ed., Part XXIV). St. Louis, MO: Elsevier.

## Manifestations and Diagnostic Evaluation

Ventral placement of the urethral opening, altered urinary stream, and chordee are physical manifestations of hypospadias. A defect on the topside of the penis is indicative of epispadias, and the appearance of lower urinary tract structures outside the abdominal wall is seen with bladder exstrophy. Diagnosis is based on physical examination.

## Therapeutic Management

Correction of hypospadias is accomplished by surgical intervention, which is usually done in one stage and on an outpatient basis. The surgeon releases the chordee, lengthens the urethra, positions the meatus at the penile tip, and reconstructs the penis. The surgical procedure should be done before the age of toilet training because the location of the meatus may make it difficult for the child to urinate standing up. Surgery is ideally done when the child is between 6 and 12 months of age (Elder, 2016). Infants with hypospadias should not be circumcised because the foreskin can be used in the surgical reconstruction. After surgery, the child might have some type of temporary urinary diversion to allow for healing of the meatus. Indwelling urinary catheters or urethral stents are commonly used. In addition, the child's activity must be restricted for several days. These treatments are tolerated better by the younger child. The goal of surgery is to make urinary and sexual function as normal as possible and to improve the cosmetic appearance of the penis.

Surgical correction of epispadias can include bladder neck reconstruction and lengthening of the penis and urethra. If bladder exstrophy is present, surgical correction is more complex and may be performed in multiple stages; ongoing management of the urinary drainage system is required.

## NURSING CARE

### The Child With Hypospadias

#### Assessment

Hypospadias is usually discovered during the newborn examination. In the infant with hypospadias, the abdomen is palpated for a distended bladder or enlarged kidneys. The urinary stream should be observed, if possible. For the older infant with hypospadias, the parents are asked about UTIs, quality of urinary stream (whether it is steady or intermittent), dribbling, or family history of genitourinary problems. The nurse assesses the parents' understanding of hypospadias and the surgical procedure and follow-up care necessary for correction.

#### Nursing Diagnosis and Planning

The nursing diagnoses and expected outcomes that apply to the child with hypospadias and the child's family are as follows:

- Deficient Knowledge (parental) related to diagnosis of hypospadias, surgical procedure, and postoperative care.

**Expected outcome.** The parents will describe hypospadias and the reason for surgical correction. The parents will actively participate in the postoperative care.

- Risk for Infection related to indwelling catheter.

**Expected outcome.** The child will remain free of UTI, as evidenced by normal urinalysis and culture and absence of fever.

- Acute Pain related to surgery.

**Expected outcome.** The child will exhibit infrequent episodes of crying and demonstrate normal sleep patterns.

- Impaired Physical Mobility related to surgical procedure on the penis.

**Expected outcome.** The child will tolerate activity restriction, as evidenced by participating in developmentally appropriate bedside play.

#### Interventions

The nurse should provide parents with detailed preoperative teaching and encourage them to participate in the postoperative care of their child. To decrease edema, the child has a pressure dressing that is removed by the physician after approximately 4 days. Some infants have a stent that drains directly into the diaper, whereas others require a closed drainage bag system. The parents should be able to demonstrate proper care of the catheter or stent before discharge.

The nurse advises the parents to encourage the child to drink frequently. High fluid intake is necessary to maintain hydration and a free flow of urine. The parents are taught to monitor the child's temperature and observe urine for cloudiness or foul smell. Any signs of a UTI should be reported immediately. Postoperative prophylactic antibiotics may be prescribed.

The parents should provide the child with a variety of quiet diversional activities, being careful not to traumatize the site. The child is given medication as ordered for pain. The parents can provide environmental stimulation and a feeling of mobility by transporting the child in a carriage, wagon, or cart. Parents are encouraged to bring favorite toys or music to help the child feel less anxious.

### Evaluation

- Can the parents explain the surgical procedure and postoperative care of their child?
- Are the parents participating in the care of their child?
- Is the child afebrile, and are the child's urinalysis and culture within normal limits?
- Is the child happy, comfortable, and able to sleep?
- Is the child participating in age-appropriate play within restrictions?

## MISCELLANEOUS DISORDERS AND ANOMALIES OF THE GENITOURINARY TRACT

Other disorders and anomalies associated with the genitourinary tract are described in Table 44.1. Most require surgical correction. For both psychological and mechanical reasons, these defects are usually corrected at a young age; some may require more than one surgery.

## ACUTE POSTSTREPTOCOCCAL GLOMERULONEPHRITIS

The term *glomerulonephritis* refers to a group of kidney disorders characterized by inflammatory injury in the glomerulus. Infection or a systemic disease process, such as lupus erythematosus (see Chapter 42) or Schönlein-Henoch purpura (an autoimmune vasculitis), can cause glomerular inflammation. Acute glomerulonephritis refers to disorders that occur suddenly, are self-limiting, and resolve completely. Acute poststreptococcal glomerulonephritis, the most common type, is characterized by sudden onset of hematuria, proteinuria, hypertension, edema, and renal insufficiency (Pan & Avner, 2016).

### Etiology and Incidence

Acute poststreptococcal glomerulonephritis occurs as an immune reaction to a group A beta-hemolytic streptococcal infection of the throat or skin and streptococcal infection needs to be substantiated for a diagnosis. This disorder occurs most frequently in young children of preschool or early school age. Clinical symptoms usually develop 1 to 2 weeks after a streptococcal pharyngitis or 3 to 6 weeks after a streptococcal skin infection (pyoderma) (Pan & Avner, 2016). The incidence has decreased in the United States; however, the incidence in developing countries is high due to limited access to healthcare (Kausman & Powell, 2015).

### Manifestations

Hematuria, which is a cardinal sign of poststreptococcal glomerulonephritis, ranges in severity from microscopic to gross, as evidenced by

**TABLE 44.1 Miscellaneous Disorders and Anomalies of the Genitourinary Tract**

| Disorder or Anomaly | Therapeutic Management |
|---|---|
| **Hydrocele:** Painless swelling of the scrotum caused by a collection of fluid. | In the majority of infants, hydroceles resolve by 12 mo of age. A large, tense hydrocele or one that persists beyond 12-18 mo should be surgically repaired.* |
| **Phimosis:** Inability to retract the prepuce (foreskin) at an age when it should be retractable (usually 3 yr). | Accumulation of sebaceous gland secretions. Mild cases can be corrected through cleaning and gentle manual retraction. More severe cases require surgical enlargement of the phimotic ring or circumcision. |
| **Testicular torsion:** Rotation of the testicle that interrupts its blood supply, causing irreparable testicular damage if not corrected quickly. Manifests by sudden onset of severe, progressive scrotal pain, erythema, and edema. More common in adolescents and infants. | This is a surgical emergency. Surgery straightens and fixates the affected testicle and the other testicle to prevent torsion. If the affected testicle is necrotic, it is removed. |
| **Bladder exstrophy:** The extrusion of the urinary bladder to the outside of the body through a developmental defect in the lower abdominal wall. Associated with epispadias and other anomalies. | The exposed bladder tissue is covered with nonadhering plastic wrap until surgery. Surgical management is done in one or several stages and includes closing the abdominal defect and reconstructing the bladder and genitalia to allow the child to achieve urinary continence. It is important to address attachment issues with parents, who might be overwhelmed by their infant's appearance. Preventing UTI is essential. |
| **Disorders of sex development**† *46, XX DSD:* Normal internal female structures with virilized external genitalia. The most common cause is congenital adrenal hyperplasia (CAH) (see Chapter 51). *46, XY DSD:* Internal structures are testes; external genitalia are female, ambiguous, or demonstrate incomplete virilization. *Ovotesticular DSD:* Both ovarian and testicular tissues are present, with ambiguous external genitalia; most are genetically female. | Most infants are identified at birth because of ambiguous external genitalia or by signs of CAH. Because gender identity is influenced more by a combination of genetic, neurologic, family, and social factors, rather than external appearance, gender assignment is a complex process. It begins with karyotyping for sex chromosomes, and is followed by imaging studies to identify gonadal and reproductive structures, and a variety of hormonal studies. Decisions about surgical and other treatment approaches are based on potential fertility, external appearance, and the complexity of the proposed surgical reconstruction; parents and a variety of specialists (e.g., endocrinologist, surgeon, urologist, psychiatrist) are consulted. In some instances, surgery is postponed until the child is old enough to participate in the decision. Surgery can reconstruct external genitalia to match the gender assignment. Psychological support for the family should be provided on a regular basis throughout the child's life starting at birth. |

*Elder, J. (2016). Urologic disorders in infants and children. In R. Kliegman, B. Stanton, J. St. Geme, et al. (Eds.), *Nelson textbook of pediatrics* (20th ed., Part XXIV). St. Louis, MO: Elsevier.

†Data from Houk, C., Hughes, I., Ahmed, S., et al. (2006). Summary of consensus statement on intersex disorders and their management. *Pediatrics, 118*(2), 753–757; Donahoue, P. (2016). Disorders of sex development. In R. Kliegman, B. Stanton, J. St. Geme, et al. (Eds.), *Nelson textbook of pediatrics* (20th ed., Chapter 588). St. Louis, MO: Elsevier.

*UTI,* Urinary tract infection.

smoky or tea-colored urine. Edema, which is worse in the morning, affects primarily the eyelids and ankles. This condition can be accompanied by decreased urinary output. Hypertension can be severe. The child may be febrile. Many children experience fatigue. Pulmonary edema is a life-threatening complication.

## Diagnostic Evaluation

History, presenting symptoms, and laboratory results can establish the diagnosis of acute poststreptococcal glomerulonephritis. A urinalysis reveals macroscopic or microscopic hematuria with RBC casts, which indicates glomerular injury. Proteinuria is also present but not severe. Blood chemistry values are usually within the normal range. However, if renal insufficiency is severe, BUN and creatinine levels are elevated. Electrolyte disturbances, such as high serum potassium and low serum bicarbonate levels, can result from inadequate glomerular filtration.

The complete blood cell count usually demonstrates normal WBCs and mild anemia. The lower hemoglobin and hematocrit values reflect the dilutional effect of extra fluid in the blood as a result of decreased glomerular filtration.

Immunologic studies are important in diagnosing acute poststreptococcal glomerulonephritis. Serum complement (C3) may be low because of the fixation of complement in immune complexes. The values of an antistreptolysin (ASO) titer, which indicates the presence of antibodies to streptococcal bacteria, or Streptozyme test can be elevated. The ASO titer might not be elevated in a streptococcal skin infection, so a preferred test for children with antecedent skin infection is the antideoxyribonuclease B level (Pan & Avner, 2016). Culture of the throat or skin lesion (if present) may be helpful for isolating the bacterium; however, this is useful only if the infection is recent and the child has not received antibiotics. A renal biopsy may be indicated for those children whose signs and symptoms are not characteristic of acute poststreptococcal glomerulonephritis or for those children whose symptoms do not improve as expected.

## Therapeutic Management

There is no specific therapy for acute poststreptococcal glomerulonephritis. Supportive care and medical management are directed to the associated signs and symptoms and guided by the degree of renal dysfunction. A 10-day course of antibiotic therapy may be required. Children with acute renal failure should be hospitalized to allow for fluid and electrolyte management until their renal function has stabilized.

Antihypertensive therapy usually is necessary. Attaining appropriate blood pressure can best be accomplished by limiting sodium and water intake and by administering diuretics (Kausman & Powell, 2015); some children might require antihypertensives. The prognosis for children with acute poststreptococcal glomerulonephritis is excellent. The acute clinical episode is usually self-limiting, with diuresis signaling the beginning of resolution. Most children have a complete recovery; laboratory values usually return to baseline in 6 to 12 weeks, although microscopic hematuria can take up to two years to resolve (Pan & Avner, 2016).

## PATHOPHYSIOLOGY

### *Acute Poststreptococcal Glomerulonephritis*

Acute glomerulonephritis after a streptococcal infection is thought to occur as a result of an immunologic response. The body responds to the *Streptococcus* bacteria by forming antibodies, which combine with the bacterial antigens to form immune complexes. As these antigen-antibody complexes travel through the circulation, they become trapped in the glomerulus and activate an inflammatory response in the glomerular basement membrane. Products of the inflammatory response damage the glomerular capillaries and reduce the size of the capillary lumen. This process can cause a decrease in the glomerular filtration rate, leading to renal insufficiency. Sodium and fluid are retained, and the child exhibits edema and oliguria. In addition, injury to the capillary walls interferes with their permeability so that larger molecules and structures such as red blood cells (RBCs), casts, and proteins can pass through into the urine.

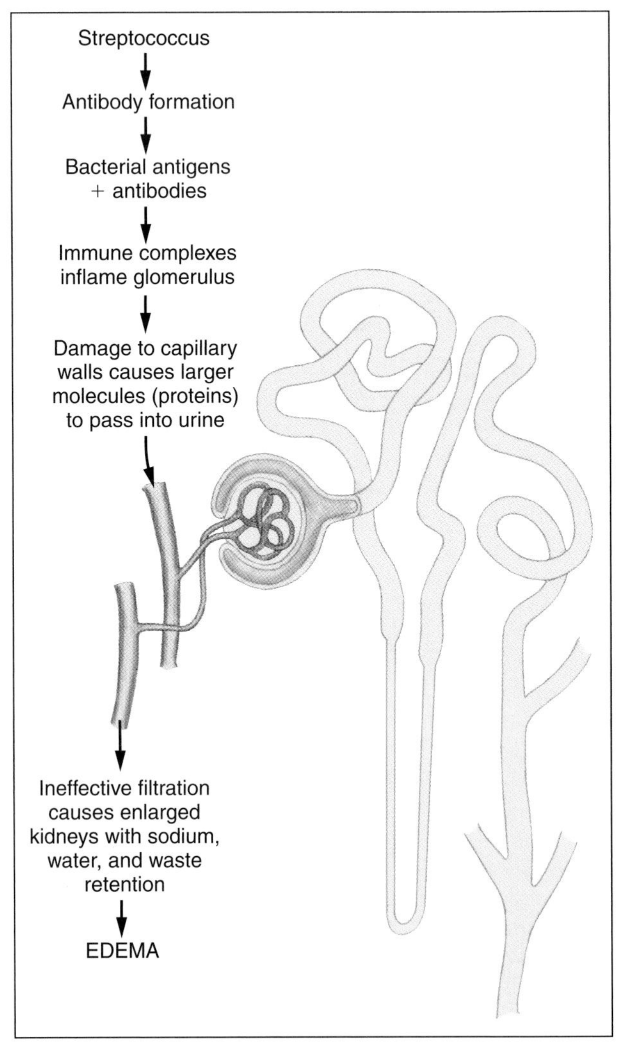


## NURSING CARE

### The Child With Acute Poststreptococcal Glomerulonephritis

#### Assessment

The nurse assesses the child for the presence of periorbital or lower extremity edema. Obtaining vital signs and monitoring daily weight are important for determining the degree of fluid retention and hypertension. An appropriate-size blood pressure cuff must be used to obtain accurate blood pressure measurements (see Chapter 37). The child's levels of fatigue and anxiety are monitored as well.

The child is evaluated for the presence of any respiratory difficulty, such as cough, increased respiratory rate, or increased work of breathing. Breath sounds are auscultated for crackles. Laboratory values, especially urinalysis and serum electrolytes, are monitored.

The nurse determines what the child and family understand about the illness and the reasons for hospitalization. The parents may be anxious about permanent damage to the child's kidneys as a result of this condition.

### Nursing Diagnosis and Planning

The nursing diagnoses and expected outcomes that apply to the child with acute poststreptococcal glomerulonephritis and the child's family are as follows:

- Risk for Imbalanced Fluid Volume related to retention of sodium and fluid and dietary fluid restriction.

*Expected outcome.* The child will maintain a normal fluid balance, as evidenced by urine output appropriate for age-group (see Chapter 40), moist mucous membranes, adequate skin turgor, normal blood pressure, no increase in weight, and no symptoms of respiratory distress.

- Risk for Activity Intolerance related to fatigue.

*Expected outcome.* The child will be rested, as evidenced by the ability to tolerate daily care and play activities.

- Risk for Impaired Skin Integrity related to edema and decreased activity.

*Expected outcome.* The child will exhibit no signs of skin breakdown, as evidenced by skin that is intact, normal color for race, and nontender to touch.

- Imbalanced Nutrition: Less Than Body Requirements related to diet restrictions.

*Expected outcome.* The child will have adequate nutrition, as evidenced by maintenance of weight at the pre-illness level.

- Anxiety related to insufficient knowledge about disease process or hospitalization.

*Expected outcome.* The child and parents will demonstrate decreased anxiety, as evidenced by cooperation with daily care and interest in developmentally appropriate play. Parents or caregiver will describe the disease process and its usual resolution.

### Interventions

*Preventing the consequences of fluid excess.* Frequent, accurate assessment of intake and output is essential for evaluating fluid volume status. Children with severe renal impairment might require measurement of intake and output every 1 to 2 hours. Fluid intake includes oral intake and IV fluids. If urine output is less than 1 mL/kg/hr, this must be reported to the physician (see Chapter 40), because oliguria suggests impending renal failure or inadequate fluid intake.

Comparing the child's weight each day is important for determining fluctuation in fluid balance. The nurse must obtain accurate daily weights, using the same scale at approximately the same time every day for maximum consistency. Infants and young children should be weighed without diapers, and older children should wear only a gown.

Because hypertension from fluid overload and glomerular damage is a severe consequence of this condition, the nurse measures blood pressure with an appropriate-size cuff every 4 to 8 hours and documents the results. Increased values are reported immediately to the physician. More frequent readings might be required if the child has significant hypertension or is receiving antihypertensive medication.

Breath sounds are auscultated every 4 to 8 hours, noting adventitious sounds and signs of increased work of breathing. Rapid respirations, retractions, nasal flaring, and crackles are signs of developing pulmonary edema, which can result from fluid overload.

Limits on fluid intake may be ordered. Such limitations can be difficult to enforce, as some children will "sneak" drinks or obtain beverages from people who are unaware of the restrictions. The nurse should inform parents, visitors, and hospital staff of the need to limit fluids. The child's favorite fluids are listed on the nursing care plan. The child is encouraged to consume fluids gradually, rather than drink large amounts all at once. The nurse provides the child with only the amount of fluids allowed for a given time period. Sodium intake can increase fluid retention. The nurse ensures that a low-sodium diet is followed if ordered and informs parents and visitors of any dietary restrictions.

*Providing adequate rest.* If fatigue is present, it is essential that the child is given ample opportunities to rest. Children with glomerulonephritis may tire easily when first hospitalized. Most children continue to participate in activities according to their level of fatigue. If needed, the nurse can limit play time to short periods and then extend the limits as the child's condition improves. The nurse should arrange daily care so that the child has some uninterrupted time for sleep and naps. Parents are asked to bring a favorite sleep toy or blanket for the child and to allow for nap time and bedtime to coincide with the child's home schedule as much as possible. Following home rituals can promote rest and sleep as well.

*Maintaining skin integrity.* Frequent position changes decrease pressure on bony prominences and help decrease edema in dependent areas. The nurse prompts the child to change position at least every 2 hours during the day. If the child has edema of the lower extremities, the extremities are elevated when the child is sitting or lying in bed. As the child's condition improves, engaging in activities that increase circulation and promote reabsorption of fluid from edematous areas is encouraged.

To prevent skin breakdown, the nurse maintains good hygiene by giving baths and cleaning the skin well after bowel movements and diaper changes. Using a small amount of lotion to massage the skin helps prevent dryness and promotes active circulation.

*Maintaining nutritional status.* Low-sodium foods taste different, and children may refuse to eat them. Offering a variety of low-sodium foods or treats may encourage the child to eat. The nurse consults with the dietary department about palatable low-sodium foods and drinks. Parents are allowed to bring favorite foods from home if they comply with the child's dietary restrictions.

A small fluctuation in weight can indicate fluid losses or gains as well as weight loss from decreased food intake. After obtaining the child's pre-illness weight, the nurse weighs the child daily to monitor for any fluid shifts or underlying weight loss. In addition, the nurse monitors the child for signs of dehydration (dry mucous membranes, listlessness, poor skin turgor, tachycardia) that would coincide with fluid restriction, diuretic administration, and diuresis.

*Relieving anxiety.* Allowing the parents and the child to voice their concerns provides support and a basis for evaluating their understanding of the disease process and prognosis. The nurse reassures the family that most children recover from this condition with no residual effects. Parents are encouraged to participate in the child's care, helping to make the child comfortable and providing suitable play activities and emotional support.

Information enables the child and parents to understand the course of the condition and to anticipate procedures and events. Knowing what to expect helps decrease anxiety. It is especially important to provide information and prepare the family for the child's care at home. If the child has been hypertensive or is to be discharged on antihypertensive medications, the nurse instructs parents on how to measure the child's blood pressure and emphasizes that blood pressure should be taken before medication administration. A blood pressure cuff of appropriate size and a stethoscope or an automated blood pressure device is obtained before discharge so the parents can learn how to use it. The nurse explains the parameters for when to withhold medication or when to call the physician regarding blood pressure readings.

### Evaluation

- Does the child demonstrate adequate urine output for weight and normal blood pressure for age?
- Are the child's mucous membranes moist, and does the child appear to be well hydrated?
- Is the child's respiratory status stable?
- Has the child's weight changed from the pre-illness weight?
- Is the child able to tolerate usual activities for age?
- Is the child's skin intact, appropriate color, and nontender to touch?
- Is the child relaxed enough to cooperate with care activities and maintain interest in play?
- Do parents participate appropriately in the child's care, providing comfort to the child?
- Can the parents describe the disease process and care required?

## NEPHROTIC SYNDROME

Nephrotic syndrome refers to a kidney disorder characterized by proteinuria, hypoalbuminemia, and edema. Nephrotic syndrome can be classified as primary or secondary. *Primary nephrotic syndrome,* or minimal change nephrotic syndrome (MCNS), results from a disorder within the glomerulus of the kidney and is the most common type seen in children. A child also can acquire nephrotic syndrome as the result of a systemic disease such as hepatitis, systemic lupus erythematosus, heavy metal poisoning, or cancer.

### Etiology

The cause of primary nephrotic syndrome is not fully understood, but it can arise from one of four types of renal lesions. Success in controlling the disease by the use of immunosuppressive drugs suggests the possibility of an immunologic component. In most children, minimal alterations of the glomerulus are seen on histologic examination. Accordingly, the most common disorder in children is idiopathic MCNS (Pais & Avner, 2016). Nephrosis can develop as a result of focal segmental glomerulosclerosis, membranoproliferative glomerulonephritis, or mesangial proliferation.

### Incidence

Primary nephrotic syndrome occurs most frequently during early childhood. The incidence is slightly higher in boys. The prognosis for children with MCNS is very good. Manifestations of the disease usually decrease with age, so relapses are rare in adolescence. Focal segmental glomerulosclerosis carries a poorer prognosis; the disease is progressive and often results in ESRD (Pais & Avner, 2016).

### Manifestations

Manifestations of primary nephrotic syndrome include edema, anorexia, fatigue, abdominal pain, respiratory infection, and increased weight. Unlike the child with glomerulonephritis, the child with nephrotic syndrome usually has normal blood pressure.

Edema is usually first noted in the periorbital spaces and dependent areas of the body; its onset is often insidious. Children awaken with facial edema and, as the day progresses, become edematous in the abdomen, genital area, and lower extremities. The pitting edema is most noticeable over the bony prominences of the lower extremities. Abdominal pain can occur from the presence of extra fluid in the peritoneal area. Edema of the bowel can cause diarrhea and decreased absorption of nutrients. Many children are misdiagnosed with allergies because of periorbital edema and respiratory symptoms.

### ! NURSING QUALITY ALERT

***Differences Between Children With Glomerulonephritis and Children With Nephrotic Syndrome***

The signs and symptoms of glomerulonephritis and nephrotic syndrome in children can be confusing. It is important for nurses to be able to discriminate between the two.

| Poststreptococcal Glomerulonephritis | Nephrotic Syndrome |
|---|---|
| **Manifestations** | |
| • Hematuria: cola-colored urine<br>• Proteinuria<br>• Edema: abrupt onset, mild periorbital or lower extremity<br>• Hypertensive<br>• Usually young school-age child | • Severe proteinuria: frothy urine<br>• Edema: insidious onset, massive edema from shift of fluid into interstitial spaces, worsens during the day<br>• Normotensive<br>• Hypovolemia<br>• Pallor, fatigue<br>• Toddler or preschool-age child |
| **Laboratory Findings** | |
| • RBCs, casts, small amount of protein in urine (0 to 3+)<br>• Normal serum albumin, cholesterol, and triglyceride levels; decreased or normal hemoglobin and hematocrit values<br>• Altered electrolytes, elevated blood urea nitrogen or creatinine levels<br>• Elevated ASO titer or Streptozyme, decreased complement | • Protein in urine (3+ to 4+), possible microscopic hematuria<br>• Hypoalbuminemia (less than 2.5 g/dL), elevated cholesterol and triglyceride, hemoglobin, hematocrit, and platelet levels<br>• Normal serum electrolytes, complement levels, ASO titer |
| **Management** | |
| • Supportive<br>• Antihypertensives and diuretics; antibiotic treatment for active streptococcal infection<br>• Low-salt diet<br>• Possible fluid restrictions | • Prednisone to initiate remission (less than 1+ protein in urine for 3 to 7 consecutive days)<br>• Diuretics, possible albumin administration<br>• Prevent infection and skin breakdown<br>• No-added-salt diet |

*ASO,* Antistreptolysin; *RBC,* red blood cell.

## Diagnostic Evaluation

Nephrotic syndrome is diagnosed based on clinical presentation, age of the child, and laboratory results. Urinalysis demonstrates protein (3+ to 4+), and the urine appears dark and frothy. Microscopic hematuria may be present. Serum cholesterol, triglycerides, hematocrit, and hemoglobin values are elevated. Serum albumin is markedly decreased (less than 2.5 g/dL). The child has normal electrolyte levels and a negative ASO titer or Streptozyme test. Serologic tests for hepatitis, human immunodeficiency virus, syphilis, and antinuclear antibody titers are performed to rule out underlying systemic disease.

In the event of an atypical presentation (a child older than 10 years or having gross hematuria or hypertension), a kidney biopsy might be performed if a lesion other than MCNS is suspected. A biopsy is also indicated for the child who does not respond as expected to pharmacologic treatment.

## Therapeutic Management

It is not unusual for the child with primary nephrotic syndrome to be hospitalized briefly during the initial onset of the disease to provide palliative treatment for the edema, perform necessary diagnostic testing, and initiate therapy. Parents are educated about the disease process and necessary home care. Before treatment begins, the child is tested for exposure to tuberculosis and varicella because treatment suppresses the immune system.

### Remission Induction

Therapy for remission includes prednisone 2 mg/kg/day at a maximum daily amount of 60 mg divided into two or three doses (Pais & Avner, 2016). This regimen is continued until the child is in remission—defined as less than 1+ urine protein for 3 to 7 consecutive days. Steroids usually are continued at the same daily dose for 4 to 6 weeks. After the initial treatment, the child's dose is decreased and changed to an alternate-day schedule and then slowly tapered. There has been some controversy over the length of time the child should remain on steroids because of their adverse effects. Some studies have suggested that treatment for an initial episode should be longer than two months. However, more recent data (Hoyer, 2015) and a Cochrane Review (Hodson, Willis & Craig, 2015) have demonstrated that there is no significant risk for relapse between children taking steroids for 2 to 3 months and those prescribed a longer treatment.

In the event of a relapse, steroid therapy is less prolonged. Once remission is achieved, dosing decreases to alternate days and is tapered more quickly to minimize prednisone side effects (see Chapter 42). There is some evidence to support changing from an alternate day to daily dose at the onset of a viral infection to minimize relapse (Hodson, Willis & Craig, 2015).

Some children respond to steroids quickly and achieve remission in 5 to 7 days, whereas others may not respond for 4 weeks. If proteinuria continues beyond 8 weeks of daily steroid therapy, the child is said to be steroid resistant; a kidney biopsy is performed to determine the exact nature of the disease.

Children who initially respond to steroid therapy but have relapses while on a tapering schedule or shortly after stopping steroids are said to be *steroid* dependent (Fig. 44.2). These children may benefit from a course of an alkylating agent such as cyclophosphamide; cyclosporine or rituximab (a monoclonal antibody) might be used instead (Kausman & Powell, 2015; Pais & Avner, 2016). The risks and benefits of this therapy must be carefully considered, and the parents should be informed of all possible side effects. A kidney biopsy is usually performed before therapy is started. The use of cyclosporine in children who remain steroid dependent despite a course of an alkylating agent, has proven to be effective in maintaining remission.

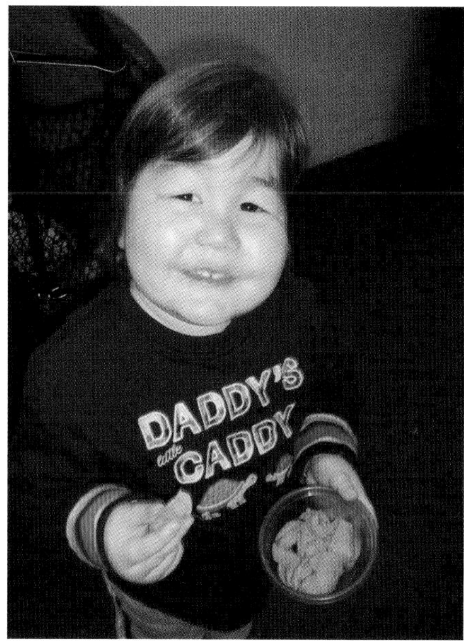


FIG 44.2 This child has nephrotic syndrome. He previously received steroid therapy and is now receiving CellCept immunosuppressant therapy to control the process. During the acute phase of the nephrotic syndrome, the child can have massive edema because blood proteins are lost to the urine. Skin pallor is also common. (Photo courtesy Cook Children's Pediatric Nephrology, Dialysis, and Transplant Services, Fort Worth, TX.)

### Additional Therapy

A no-added-salt diet is indicated. The parents should not use salt when cooking; the child should not be permitted to use the salt shaker, and the parents should avoid serving high-sodium foods such as pickles, salted chips, and cured meats. If edema is severe or if the child is hypertensive, sodium intake might be further restricted and the child might be placed on fluid restriction.

Diuretics might be administered until urinary protein loss is controlled. If the edema is marked and causes the child to have decreased mobility, poor oral intake, or decreased urine output, salt-poor albumin can be given intravenously. Albumin helps restore normal plasma osmotic pressure and promotes the movement of interstitial fluid back into the intravascular compartments. Furosemide is given intravenously after the albumin infusion to enhance diuresis and decrease the chance of fluid overload.

Severe edema in the lower extremities can give rise to cellulitis because of fluid stasis and poor circulation. Peritonitis, a severe complication, can develop from stasis of ascitic fluid, which functions as a culture medium for organisms such as *Streptococcus pneumoniae.*

Live-virus vaccines are contraindicated in children receiving steroid therapy. In addition to routine killed-virus vaccines, the child should receive pneumococcal immunization to prevent pneumococcal infection in the event of a relapse. The child with nephrotic syndrome should receive an influenza vaccine each year because an exacerbation of the disease can occur after an infection. Live virus vaccines can be administered when the steroid dose reaches 1 mg/kg/day but should be avoided if the child is taking agents other than corticosteroids (Pais & Avner, 2016).

## PATHOPHYSIOLOGY

### *Nephrotic Syndrome*

Primary nephrotic syndrome occurs from an insult to the glomerular basement membrane. Damage to the membrane causes increased permeability and loss of substances that would normally prevent negatively charged proteins from crossing the membrane. Negatively charged proteins, particularly albumin, are cleared at an increased rate, resulting in loss of plasma proteins and in proteinuria. Proteinuria is essential for the diagnosis of nephrotic syndrome.

Blood albumin values are low (hypoalbuminemia) because of the loss of albumin through the defective glomerulus and the liver's inability to synthesize proteins to balance the loss. Decreased levels of albumin reduce the plasma oncotic pressure so that the intravascular fluid moves into the interstitial spaces. This shifting of fluid reduces the intravascular volume, causing hypovolemia and subsequent decreased renal blood flow. In an effort to increase blood volume, the kidney stimulates renin production. Renin causes increased excretion of aldosterone, resulting in renal tubular reabsorption of sodium, which in turn causes water retention. The net effect of this phenomenon is edema.

In addition, the serum values of cholesterol and triglycerides are elevated. This change is thought to result from increased stimulation of lipoprotein production because of the decrease in oncotic pressure. Loss of immunoglobulins into the urine is common in nephrotic syndrome. Most notably, levels of immunoglobulin G are decreased, which makes these children more susceptible to infection. Before the use of antibiotics, infection was a frequent cause of death in these children.

Children with nephrotic syndrome are in a hypercoagulable state, predisposing them to venous thrombosis. This tendency occurs as a result of several factors, including decreased intravascular volume (hypovolemia), which causes increased concentrations of red blood cells (RBCs) and platelets and slowing of circulation. Urinary loss of proteins that inhibit coagulation also contributes to the risk of thrombus formation.

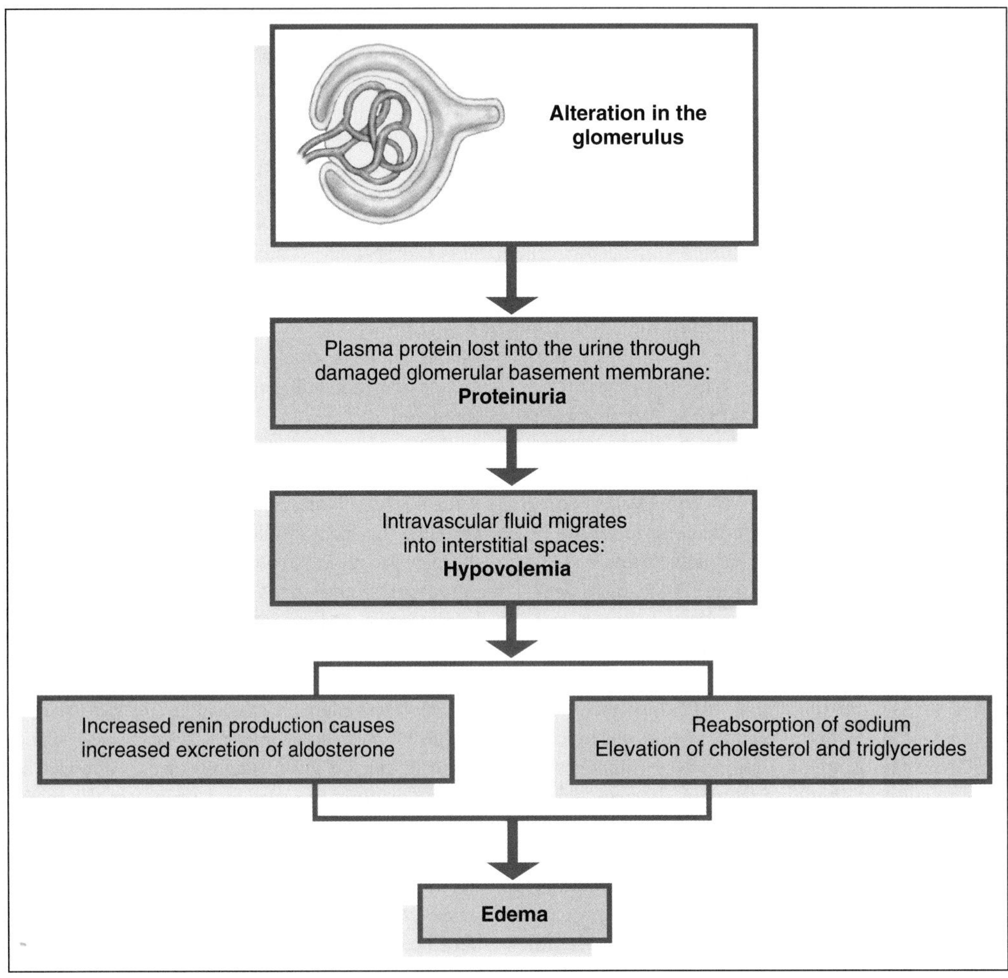


## ACUTE KIDNEY INJURY

*Acute kidney injury* (AKI), formerly acute renal failure (ARF) is defined as the sudden, severe loss of kidney function (Sreedharan & Avner, 2016). In AKI, the kidneys can no longer filter waste products, regulate fluid volume, or maintain chemical balance. Most children with AKI regain renal function, depending on the underlying cause.

### Etiology and Incidence

The three types of AKI are prerenal, intrinsic renal and postrenal. Causes of prerenal failure are dehydration, perinatal asphyxia, hypotension, septic shock, hemorrhagic shock, and renal artery obstruction. Nephrotoxins (e.g., aminoglycosides, contrast dye), lupus erythematosus, hemolytic uremic syndrome (HUS), glomerulonephritis, and pyelonephritis all can cause intrinsic renal failure. Postrenal failure is

## NURSING CARE PLAN

### *The Child With Nephrotic Syndrome*

**Focused Assessment**

- Monitor child for early signs of infection every 4 to 8 hours.
  - Vital signs (temperature)
  - Laboratory data (white blood cell [WBC] count)
- Assess fluid balance every 4 to 8 hours.
  - Monitor vital signs for indicators of hypovolemia (increased pulse rate, low blood pressure [BP]) or fluid overload (elevated BP)
  - Check laboratory data (hemoglobin, hematocrit)
  - Accurate daily weights.
  - Strict measurement and documentation of fluid intake and urine output
  - Auscultate breath sounds and observe for respiratory distress
- Assess the amount of edema present and condition of skin every 4 to 8 hours.
  - Check periorbital areas, abdomen, genitalia, and lower extremities
- Daily check laboratory data for amount of protein in the urine
  - Indicates severity of disease if increased or effectiveness of treatment if decreased
- Obtain a nursing history
  - Immunizations received
  - Recent exposure to communicable diseases
- Assess understanding of the child and family regarding the disease process and treatment
  - Determine need for referrals to appropriate support services
  - Evaluate educational needs

**Nursing Diagnosis**

Risk for Impaired Skin Integrity related to edema and decreased circulation

**Planning**

***Expected Outcome***

The child will remain free from skin breakdown, as evidenced by the absence of redness, tenderness to touch, and ulceration.

**Interventions and *Rationales***

1. Ensure that the child changes position every 2 hours.
   *Frequent position change decreases pressure on body parts and helps relieve edema in dependent areas.*
2. Maintain good hygiene by giving baths and changing linen daily. Use non-alcohol-based lotion for dry skin.
   *Body secretions and debris on linens can irritate the skin. Gentle massage when bathing and applying lotion helps increase circulation.*
3. Support or elevate edematous body parts while the child is in bed or sitting in a chair.
   *Edema is gravity dependent. Elevation helps move fluid away from dependent body parts.*
4. Promote physical activity as the child is able to tolerate by providing developmentally appropriate play activities.
   *Increased activity helps promote circulation.*

**Evaluation**

Is the child's skin intact without redness or tenderness?

**Nursing Diagnosis**

Risk for Infection related to urinary loss of gamma globulins and immunosuppressive therapy.

**Planning**

***Expected Outcome***

The child will be free of signs of an infection, as evidenced by normal WBC count, normal body temperature, and absence of abdominal pain and cough.

**Interventions and *Rationales***

1. Screen visitors for signs of infection, such as upper respiratory symptoms, sore throats, or exposure to communicable diseases.
   *Communicable diseases pose a serious threat because the child receiving immunosuppressive therapy is not able to respond appropriately to infection.*
2. Administer antibiotics as ordered.
   *Antibiotics are usually given for peritonitis prophylaxis during the edematous phase.*
3. Use thorough hand hygiene techniques and instruct family members to do the same.
   *Hand hygiene helps decrease transmission of organisms.*
4. Monitor child for fever, cough, sore throat, and complaints of abdominal pain, and check laboratory values (complete blood count [CBC], differential) every 8 hours.
   *Frequent monitoring ensures early detection of infectious processes. Abdominal pain can be an indication of peritonitis.*

**Evaluation**

Does the child maintain normal body temperature and exhibit normal laboratory values?

Is the child free from cough, pain, or other signs of infection?

**Nursing Diagnosis**

Risk for Deficient Fluid Volume (intravascular) related to proteinuria, edema, and effects of diuretics.

**Planning**

***Expected Outcome***

The child will maintain adequate fluid volume, as evidenced by normal blood pressure measurement, urine output appropriate for age, and normal hematocrit and hemoglobin values.

**Interventions and *Rationales***

1. Monitor vital signs, including blood pressure and pulse, every 4 to 8 hours. Report variance from baseline.
   *Low blood pressure and increased heart rate are signs of hypovolemia. Blood pressure may be elevated because of renin release.*
2. Monitor intake and output every 4 to 8 hours. Report if child has output of less than 1 to 2 mL/kg/hr of urine (see Chapter 40).
   *Accurate intake and output measurement is essential for evaluating fluid status.*
3. Monitor laboratory values, particularly hemoglobin and hematocrit.
   *Increasing values of hemoglobin and hematocrit may indicate hemoconcentration or low intravascular volume.*
4. Observe for signs of dehydration such as dry appearance of mucous membranes, poor skin turgor, increased capillary refill time, and decreased level of activity. (Capillary refill may be altered because of edema; assess in nonedematous area.) Report abnormal findings to the physician.
   *The pathophysiologic mechanisms of nephrotic syndrome may predispose the child to decreased intravascular volume. This condition is compounded by the use of diuretics.*

**Evaluation**

Are the child's vital signs and hematocrit and hemoglobin within normal limits?

Is the urine output normal for age-group (see Chapter 40)?

Does the child have moist mucous membranes and appropriate skin turgor?

*Continued*

## NURSING CARE PLAN—cont'd

### *The Child With Nephrotic Syndrome*

**Nursing Diagnosis**

Excess Fluid Volume related to decreased excretion of sodium and fluid retention.

**Planning**

***Expected Outcome***

The child will not exhibit signs of fluid overload, as evidenced by stable daily weights and normal respiratory pattern.

**Interventions and *Rationales***

1. Monitor intake and output every 4 to 8 hours.
   *Accurate intake and output are essential for evaluating fluid balance.*
2. Obtain accurate daily weights. Weigh child on the same scale, at same time each day in a gown only.
   *Daily weights are necessary to detect changes in fluid volume status. Clothing or presence of wet diaper can alter weight. Readings of weight can vary from scale to scale and time of day.*
3. Adhere to no-added-salt diet and fluid restriction if ordered.*
   *Excessive sodium intake can increase amount of water retention. If the child is hyponatremic, fluid restriction may be indicated.**
4. Measure and record abdominal girth each day. Ensure accuracy by measuring in the same area each time.
   *Edema commonly occurs in the abdomen. Ascites may increase during course of the disease.*
5. Monitor blood pressure at least once every 8 hours.
   *Increased total-body fluid volume and concurrent steroid therapy can result in increased blood pressure.*
6. Administer diuretics as ordered. Ensure adequate potassium intake.
   *Diuretics may aid in the elimination of excessive fluid. Diuretics can increase excretion of potassium.*
7. Monitor respiratory status every 4 to 8 hours. Auscultate breath sounds checking for crackles. Observe for signs of increased work of breathing (retractions, nasal flaring, increased respiratory rate) and cough.
   *Fluid overload can result in pulmonary edema.*

**Evaluation**

Does the child maintain a stable weight?

Is the child free from respiratory distress?

**Nursing Diagnoses**

Anxiety (parental) related to hospitalization of child and caring for a child with a chronic disease.

Deficient Knowledge about home management related to incomplete understanding.

**Planning**

***Expected Outcomes***

1. The parents will demonstrate decreased anxiety, as evidenced by participating in the care of their child and explaining the normal course of the disease process.
2. The parents will be able to explain principles of home management.
3. The child will gain understanding of disease management per developmental level.

**Interventions and *Rationales***

1. Allow parents to verbalize frustration and fears; encourage them to ask questions. Provide the parent and child with information about nephrotic syndrome and its treatment.
   *Verbalization of fears is often therapeutic. Information helps decrease anxiety by reducing fear of the unknown.*
2. Incorporate the parents into the child's daily care including urine protein testing with Albustix reagent strips, taking blood pressures, and assessing edema. Involve the child in care activities that are developmentally appropriate.
   *Nephrotic syndrome can be a chronic condition and it is usually managed at home. It is important for the parents to feel comfortable providing care for their child.*
3. Arrange for a dietary consultation.
   *Steroid therapy stimulates appetite. Children should be informed about low calorie snacks and portion size. Encourage the parents to cook without salt and remove the salt shaker from the child's access.*
4. Teach parents how to maintain a daily calendar of urine protein readings, obtain daily weights, administer approved medications only, and perform hand hygiene and other actions to prevent infection. Encourage parents to report any exposure to communicable disease.
   *Education allows the family to manage the child's care. The child's urine protein results are monitored for signs of relapse. Parent must check with the nephrologist before giving any over-the-counter medications; some can aggravate hypertension. Children receiving steroids are immunosuppressed and may require prophylactic treatment if exposed to communicable diseases.*

**Evaluation**

Can the parents describe their child's condition and required treatment?

Do the parents actively participate in the child's care?

Do the parents accurately demonstrate procedures they will be required to do at home?

Does the child participate in care activities?

*Pais, P., & Avner, E. (2016). Idiopathic nephrotic syndrome. In R. Kliegman, B. Stanton, J. St. Geme, et al. (Eds.), *Nelson textbook of pediatrics* (20th ed., pp. 2524-2526). St. Louis, MO: Elsevier.

associated with structural abnormalities such as ureteropelvic junction obstruction, ureterovesical obstruction, posterior urethral valves, neurogenic bladder, and outlet obstruction by stones, tumor, or edema (Sreedharan & Avner, 2016).

The incidence of AKI is difficult to determine in infants and children because of differences in diagnostic criteria. AKI is estimated to occur in 8% of critically ill neonates and 2% to 3% of critically ill children (Sreedharan & Avner, 2016). HUS is one of the most frequent causes of AKI in children (Sreedharan & Avner, 2016). This acute disorder is characterized by anemia, thrombocytopenia, and AKI. HUS is often associated with Escherichia coli *(E. coli)* infection that results from improperly cooked meat or contaminated dairy products.

## Manifestations

Manifestations of AKI include electrolyte abnormalities, fluid volume shifts, increased BUN and serum creatinine levels, acid–base imbalances, and nonspecific symptoms such as poor feeding, decreased appetite, vomiting, lethargy, seizures, and pallor. In children with HUS, gastrointestinal illness is characterized by abdominal pain, fever, vomiting, and bloody diarrhea.

## Diagnostic Evaluation

Determining the underlying cause of AKI is very important. If the cause can be reversed, renal function usually returns to normal.

## PATHOPHYSIOLOGY

### *Acute Kidney Injury*

Acute kidney injury (AKI) is categorized as prerenal, intrinsic, or postrenal. *Prerenal AKI* is the result of conditions that decrease perfusion of the kidney. The kidney must have adequate blood flow to effectively function. The decreased blood flow and subsequent ischemia cause cellular swelling and injury and possible cell death. *Intrinsic AKI* is the result of actual damage to kidney tissue from certain diseases, many with inflammatory, hypoxic, or ischemic components. *Postrenal AKI* is the result of obstruction of urine outflow. The obstruction increases pressure within the kidney, which decreases renal function.

Impaired perfusion markedly decreases the glomerular filtration rate (GFR), triggering oliguria (markedly decreased urine output), **azotemia** (elevated blood levels of urea, creatinine, and uric acid), and associated electrolyte imbalances. Tissue injury further magnifies the damage and the decreased perfusion.

As the underlying problem is treated, recovery of the renal endothelial and tubular cells begins, and renal function gradually improves. Because the GFR returns to normal faster than the tubular transport mechanisms, diuresis occurs first with the child voiding large amounts of dilute urine. This puts the child at increased risk for dehydration related to the fluid loss. In most cases, renal function progressively returns to normal.

## PATHOPHYSIOLOGY

### *Hemolytic Uremic Syndrome*

Most affected children have an associated prodrome of gastrointestinal symptoms, including bloody diarrhea, which suggests that an infectious gastrointestinal agent may be the cause of hemolytic uremic syndrome (HUS). Two important characteristics of the O157:H7 strain of *E. coli* contribute to the development of HUS. First, because this bacterium attaches itself to the intestinal mucosa, its clearance through normal intestinal peristalsis is decreased, allowing the bacteria to grow and multiply. Second, the bacteria produce a toxin that damages the endothelial cells of capillary walls, and the subsequent inflammatory response results in occlusion of capillaries. This process is especially significant in the renal glomeruli. The occlusion of glomerular vessels decreases filtration which results in acute renal failure. However, it is important to understand that the vascular process seen in HUS can affect any organ. Anemia results from fragmentation of red blood cells (RBCs), which are damaged as they try to pass through the occluded vessels and are removed from circulation by the spleen. Thrombocytopenia occurs because the platelets get trapped within the small vessels.

### History

The history often gives an indication of the underlying cause of the AKI. Vomiting, diarrhea, and fever may indicate dehydration and prerenal AKI. It is necessary to ascertain any recent history of bloody diarrhea that might suggest HUS.

### Fluid Volume Status

Prerenal AKI is usually associated with dehydration, whereas children with intrinsic AKI from glomerulonephritis often are fluid overloaded and have edema, crackles, and hypertension. Urine output can be normal, increased, or oliguric (less than 1 mL/kg/hr) (see Chapter 40).

### Laboratory Data

Serum creatinine and BUN levels are increased. BUN, an end product of protein catabolism, may reflect the child's nutritional status. Metabolic acidosis can occur, as indicated by low serum bicarbonate. Serum potassium may be increased. Serum sodium may be increased or decreased, depending on fluid volume status. The child with HUS exhibits hemolytic anemia, thrombocytopenia, hematuria, proteinuria, and in some cases, a stool culture that is positive for *E. coli.*

To aid in diagnosis, providers may use the pRIFLE list of diagnostic criteria. pRIFLE describes the categories of AKI based on estimated changes in glomerular filtration rate (eGFR) from baseline: Risk, 25% decrease in eGFR within seven days; Injury, 50% decrease in eGFR; and Failure, 75% decrease in eGFR (Thomas et al., 2015). Some specialists use comparable percentages of estimated creatinine clearance (Sreedharan & Avner, 2016).

### Physical Examination

The child might be hypertensive. Edema resulting from decreased urine output and fluid overload can be present. The child might be in respiratory distress because of fluid overload.

### Imaging Studies

Renal ultrasonography may help with the diagnosis of obstruction and postrenal AKI. A renal scan can be helpful in determining the cause of all AKI types. It can assess blood flow, kidney function, and obstruction.

## Therapeutic Management

Many children in AKI are managed without dialysis. Therapeutic management focuses on correcting imbalances.

### Fluid Imbalances

Maintaining a normal fluid volume status is critical for the child with AKI. If the child is dehydrated, precise fluid replacement is performed. Fluid restriction is necessary for a child who has decreased or absent urine output and is adequately hydrated or fluid overloaded. Fluid intake is calculated to replace insensible fluid loss and urinary output. Maintaining fluid restrictions can be difficult for some children. Giving small amounts of fluids as often as possible is helpful. Older children can participate in decisions about the type and frequency of fluids.

### Electrolyte Imbalances

***Potassium.*** Most children with ARF have a high serum potassium level, requiring intervention when the level reaches 6 mEq/L. Potassium is restricted from the diet and IV fluids. Interventions to remove potassium include gastric suction; administration of an exchange resin, such as Kayexalate; and administration of sodium bicarbonate, glucose, and insulin.

***Sodium.*** The serum sodium level may be elevated or decreased. A decreased sodium level is more common because of fluid overload, in which case fluid restrictions help improve the sodium level. Any replacement sodium is adjusted to maintain a normal serum sodium level.

***Acid–base imbalances.*** Children with AKI are unable to excrete hydrogen ions and ammonia through the kidney, so metabolic acidosis (low serum bicarbonate) develops. Additional sodium bicarbonate can be administered orally or intravenously.

### Nutrition

Nutritional support of children with AKI is critical. Foods should be low in sodium, potassium, and phosphorus; protein for growth is essential (National Institute of Diabetes and Digestive and Kidney Diseases [NIDDK], 2014).

The underlying principle of nutritional therapy for these children is to provide maximum calories. If the child is critically ill, parenteral hyperalimentation with essential amino acids can be administered (Sreedharan & Avner, 2016).

**! NURSING QUALITY ALERT**

***Indications for Dialysis in Acute Kidney Injury***

- Severe fluid overload
- Pulmonary edema or congestive heart failure caused by fluid overload
- Severe hypertension
- Metabolic acidosis not responsive to medications
- Hyperkalemia not responsive to medications
- Blood urea nitrogen level greater than 120 mg/dL

### Dialysis

Dialysis is a process of removing waste products and excess body fluid and regulating electrolytes and minerals. The two principal types of dialysis are hemodialysis and peritoneal dialysis.

### Nursing Considerations

Most children with AKI are cared for in special-care units. Principles of nursing care include (1) monitoring and maintaining fluid, electrolyte, and acid–base balances, (2) preventing infection, (3) providing adequate nutrition, (4) reducing parent and child anxiety, and (5) teaching about the disease process, treatment, and dialysis (Box 44.2).

## CHRONIC KIDNEY DISEASE (CKD) AND END-STAGE RENAL DISEASE

CKD is an irreversible loss of kidney function that usually occurs over months to years. It can be managed conservatively with medications and diet restrictions. CKD progresses to end-stage renal disease (ESRD), which is the permanent, irreversible loss of kidney function such that conservative treatment alone can no longer sustain the child's health and life. ESRD usually is diagnosed when the glomerular filtration rate (GFR) decreases to 10%.

### Etiology

The causes of CKD in children differ from those in adults. The most common causes, especially in younger children, are congenital anomalies such as obstruction, VUR, and renal dysplasia. CKD can develop in children from diseases such as glomerulonephritis, pyelonephritis, and HUS. In general, secondary causes of ESRD, such as diabetes and high blood pressure, are not seen in children.

### Incidence

The incidence of CKD with ESRD among children younger than 19 years is approximately 18 in 1 million (Sreedharan & Avner, 2016). The incidence is higher in adolescents, in boys, and in Whites.

### Pathophysiology

Regardless of the initial cause of kidney damage, CKD progresses to ESRD. The exact mechanisms are unclear. Factors that contribute to the development of ESRD include continuing immunologic injury, hyperfiltration (the overwork of the remaining nephrons), high dietary phosphorus intake, persistent proteinuria, and hypertension.

### Manifestations

Manifestations of CKD and ESRD include electrolyte abnormalities, fluid volume shifts (dehydration or fluid overload), acid–base imbalances, renal osteodystrophy (rickets), anemia, poor growth, hypertension, fatigue, decreased appetite, poor feeding, nausea and vomiting, and neurologic symptoms from accumulation of wastes in the blood.

### Diagnostic Evaluation

Chronic kidney disease may manifest nonspecifically. Physical examination sometimes reveals short stature and failure to thrive. The child might be hypertensive. Blood work reveals electrolyte abnormalities (varying according to the underlying disease process), calcium and phosphorus abnormalities (decreased calcium and bone calcium resorption, elevated serum phosphorus), and anemia. Rising serum creatinine and BUN levels suggest ESRD. Creatinine clearance testing measures the ability of the renal system to excrete metabolic products; it gives an approximation of the GFR. As renal function deteriorates, creatinine clearance decreases. Bone radiographs diagnose renal osteodystrophy. The child may have normal fluid volume, be dehydrated, or have fluid overload.

The history may or may not include known renal disease. Diagnostic tests can determine the etiology and prognosis. Such tests include a voiding cystourethrogram (VCUG), renal ultrasonography, renal scan, and renal biopsy.

### Therapeutic Management

#### CKD

The diet of a child with CKD is individualized and modified because of the decreased ability of the kidneys to regulate fluids, electrolytes, minerals, and waste products. Reductions in sodium and fluid intake are necessary to prevent fluid overload and hypertension. Phosphorus is restricted to manage bone disease (renal osteodystrophy). Serum potassium levels are closely monitored, and decreased intake may be required because of impaired excretion by the kidneys. Protein intake is carefully regulated to decrease the accumulation of waste products while providing the child with essential amino acids and other nutrients.

Diuretics may be indicated to control fluid overload, and antihypertensives are given for hypertension. Sodium bicarbonate tablets are taken to maintain acid–base balance. Synthetic, active vitamin D and phosphorus-binding medications are given to increase serum calcium, decrease phosphorus blood levels, control parathyroid gland activity, and treat renal osteodystrophy.

Children with CKD should receive all childhood immunizations and a yearly influenza vaccine, unless immunosuppressive treatment precludes live-virus vaccines. It is advantageous to administer live-virus vaccines as soon as possible within the normal childhood schedule so the child is fully immunized before undergoing kidney transplantation, which requires lifelong immunosuppressant therapy (Sreedharan & Avner, 2016).

Advances in the treatment of infants and children with chronic renal failure, such as recombinant erythropoietin and recombinant growth hormone, have improved the quality of life of these children (Sreedharan & Avner, 2016). Recombinant erythropoietin is used to treat anemia, thus improving the energy level and avoiding repeated blood transfusions. The use of recombinant growth hormone has significantly improved the growth of children with chronic renal failure (Sreedharan & Avner, 2016).

### End-Stage Renal Disease

The diagnosis of ESRD is made by monitoring serum creatinine levels, glomerular filtration rate (GFR), and the quality of the child's life. Dialysis or kidney transplantation is required once ESRD is diagnosed with only 5% to 10% of kidney function remaining.

### Kidney Transplantation

Transplantation is the therapeutic goal for most children with ESRD; it offers the best opportunity for a relatively normal life and continued growth and development. Unfortunately, transplantation is not a

## BOX 44.2 Dialysis

Dialysis removes waste products and excess body fluids and regulates electrolytes and minerals. It is sometimes necessary in acute renal failure. When chronic kidney disease progresses to end-stage renal disease (ESRD), dialysis or kidney transplantation is required. The two principal types of dialysis are hemodialysis and peritoneal dialysis.

### Hemodialysis

Hemodialysis cleanses the blood by circulating it through a special filter called an *artificial kidney*. Blood is pumped through the artificial kidney and returned to the body. Hemodialysis occurs through a surgically placed, vascular access, such as a double-lumen central line or an **arteriovenous fistula** or shunt. Children who receive long-term dialysis usually receive treatments three times per week for 3 to 4 hours each time.

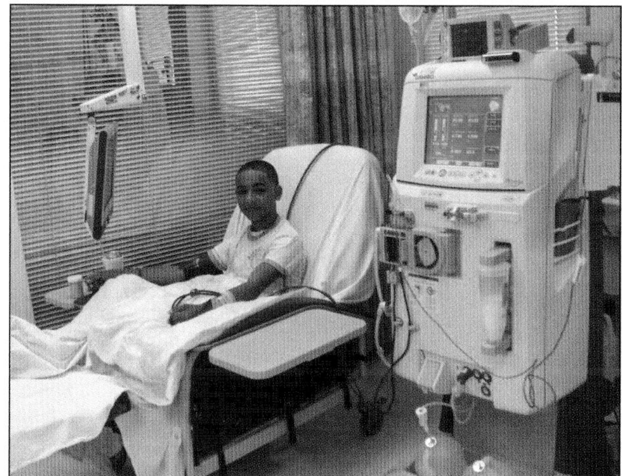

Teenager receiving hemodialysis. (Photo courtesy Cook Children's Pediatric Nephrology, Dialysis, and Transplant Services, Fort Worth, TX.)

The major complications of hemodialysis include access infection and access obstruction. In addition, school, social, and family lives are disrupted because of the treatment schedule. However, children treated with hemodialysis in a specialized pediatric unit can thrive. Hemodialysis is technically more difficult for infants and small children, and fluid and electrolyte shifts are more pronounced.

Hemodialysis is more efficient and requires less time than peritoneal dialysis. In addition, the family has less direct responsibility for the actual dialysis process because it is performed by personnel in a dialysis center.

### Peritoneal Dialysis

In peritoneal dialysis, fluid enters the peritoneal cavity through a catheter that is placed in the child's abdomen, at the bedside or in the operating room. The dialysis fluid remains in the cavity for a prescribed time (dwell time), during which waste products, chemicals, and fluid pass through the peritoneal membrane into the fluid. The fluid is then drained out of the body, and the process is repeated.

In children receiving long-term dialysis, the exchanges are often performed at home every night with an automated cycler while the child is asleep.

Peritoneal dialysis is technically easier than hemodialysis. Advantages over hemodialysis include more independence for the child and family and a more stable physiologic state because of more frequent dialysis. The disadvantages include the risk of infections (peritonitis, catheter exit site) and the stress often experienced by the family and child due to treatment demands.

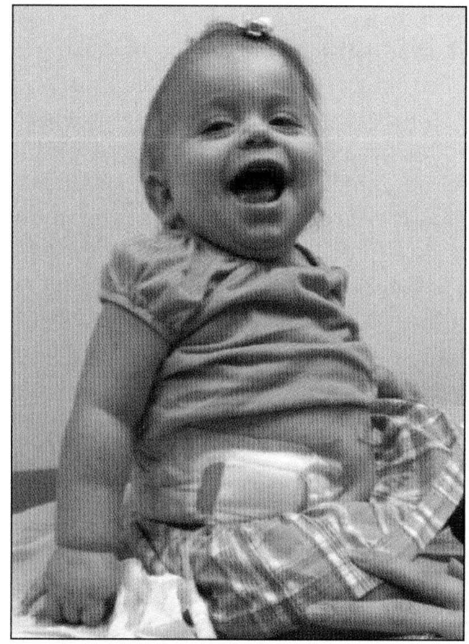

Peritoneal dialysis. Implanted line allows instillation of the dialyzing fluid into this child's peritoneal cavity. (Photo courtesy Cook Children's Pediatric Nephrology, Dialysis, and Transplant Services, Fort Worth, TX.)

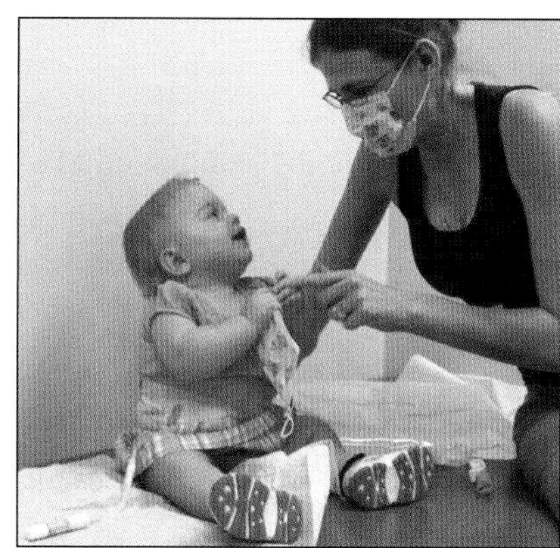

Infection of the peritoneal cavity is the chief hazard of peritoneal dialysis. When the lines are open to begin or end the dialyzing cycle, both adult and child wear masks. (Photo courtesy Cook Children's Pediatric Nephrology, Dialysis, and Transplant Services, Fort Worth, TX.)

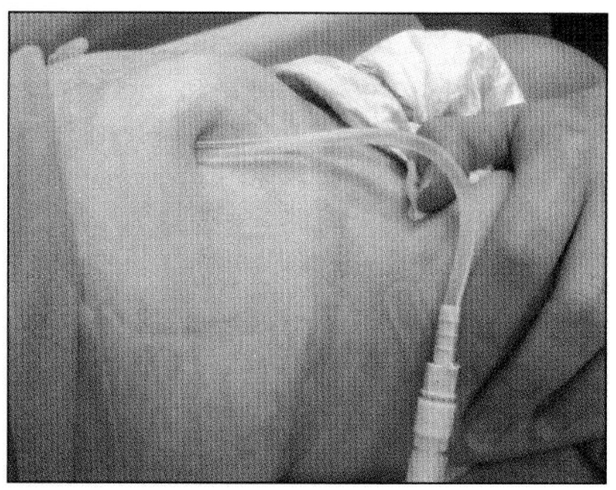

Peritoneal dialysis catheter exit site. (Photo courtesy Cook Children's Pediatric Nephrology, Dialysis, and Transplant Services, Fort Worth, TX.)

cure. Children with kidney transplants must continue to take immunosuppressive medications daily, have frequent blood tests, and attend regular clinic appointments.

Kidneys come from either living donors or cadaveric donors. A living donor is often someone in the child's family, such as a parent, older sibling, or grandparent, although persons without a biologic relationship can also donate a kidney. The donor must be in good health and have healthy kidneys. A cadaveric donor kidney is obtained from a person who has been declared brain dead and whose family has consented to the donation. The cadaveric donor kidney must have normal function. The blood and tissue types of the donor and recipient must be compatible. Transplants with kidneys from living, related donors are generally more successful in children than transplants using cadaveric donor kidneys.

Rejection of the transplanted kidney by the child's immune system is the most common complication. Immunosuppressive medications are taken to prevent rejection; these include cyclosporine (Gengraf or Neoral), prednisone, tacrolimus (Prograf), and mycophenolate (CellCept or Myfortic).

As with all medications, immunosuppressive medications have side effects. When the immune system is suppressed, the risk of infection is increased because of the body's decreased ability to fight infection. Children with renal transplants should be monitored for infection and might take antiinfective medications routinely.

High blood pressure is also a complication of transplantation. Underlying renal disease, the transplanted kidney, or immunosuppressive medication side effects can cause high blood pressure.

## NURSING CARE

### The Child With Chronic Kidney Disease and End-Stage Renal Disease

#### Assessment

The assessment of the child with CKD or ESRD is directed toward clinical manifestations of the renal failure and its possible complications. Blood is monitored for abnormalities and response to interventions. Monitoring hemoglobin and hematocrit assesses for potential anemia and assesses response to therapy in the child receiving recombinant erythropoietin. Serum calcium and phosphorus, alkaline phosphatase, and parathyroid hormone levels and bone radiographs are obtained to monitor for renal osteodystrophy.

The nurse assesses fluid volume status for fluid overload and dehydration by obtaining the child's weight, monitoring blood pressure and heart rate, and observing and documenting findings related to edema, skin turgor, mucous membranes, and fontanels.

Accurate weights and height measurements are obtained regularly and plotted on growth curves to assess the child's growth and development. Parents are asked to provide the child's dietary and caloric intake history. Information regarding attainment of developmental tasks, school performance, and peer relationships is important to include in the nurse's assessment.

#### Nursing Diagnosis and Planning

The nursing diagnoses and expected outcomes that apply to the child with CKD and ESRD and the child's family are as follows:

- Imbalanced Nutrition: Less Than Body Requirements related to decreased appetite and dietary restrictions.

  **Expected outcome.** The child will receive adequate nutrition for growth and health as measured by appropriate growth for age.
- Deficient Knowledge about disease process, treatment, or dietary restrictions related to anxiety or incomplete understanding of principles.

  **Expected outcome.** The child and parents will be able to explain the disease process, its treatment, and dietary restrictions.
- Risk for Imbalanced Fluid Volume related to fluid and electrolyte shifts secondary to renal dysfunction.

  **Expected outcome.** The child will exhibit no signs of fluid overload or deficit, as measured by weight, blood pressure, and absence of edema or signs of dehydration.
- Delayed Growth and Development related to restricted diet, chronic illness, and anemia.

  **Expected outcome.** The child will continue to grow and develop at acceptable rates according to standard measuring instruments.
- Interrupted Family Processes related to having a child with a chronic and potentially life-threatening disease.

  **Expected outcome.** The child and family will use successful coping strategies, as measured by their ability to care for the child, meet the needs of other family members, and access appropriate support.
- Risk for Impaired Skin Integrity related to edema and poor nutrition.

  **Expected outcome.** The child's skin will be intact and without redness, irritation, or breaks.

#### Interventions

The care of the child with CKD is complex and requires a multidisciplinary team. Maintaining adequate nutritional intake within the dietary restriction parameters is a challenge. The nurse individualizes the diet of the child with chronic renal failure and includes foods the child likes. Small, frequent meals are helpful. Diet supplements may be necessary to meet caloric needs. Administration of recombinant growth hormone may allow the child to have adequate growth.

Children with CKD and their families have multifaceted information requirements. The parents need information regarding diet, medications, potential adverse effects of the renal failure, and side effects from treatment. Most children with chronic renal failure will need dialysis. Children and their families will be most successful with dialysis if the method chosen fits their lifestyle (NIDDK, 2014). The goal is to optimize physical, social, and emotional development while addressing complex physical requirements. Additionally, children and parents need to be informed about other treatment options, including transplantation.

The nurse is diligent in providing the correct amount of fluid intake and ongoing assessment of fluid volume status. The child and family are educated about fluid restrictions and hydration assessment parameters such as weight, blood pressure, and appearance of edema.

The child is encouraged to participate in school and other age-appropriate activities. Parents might find it difficult to allow their child to be independent, needing assistance in this area.

Children with CKD and their families need support from a multidisciplinary team of healthcare providers. They need opportunities to ask questions, verbalize feelings, and express concerns. Involving children in their own care and decisions regarding treatment is beneficial. It is important to determine the coping strategies used successfully by the family in the past and then encourage family members to use those same strategies again. The nurse considers making referrals to social workers, child life specialists, play therapists, psychologists, or psychiatrists when the need for additional support is indicated.

#### Evaluation

Does the child maintain the age-appropriate growth percentile on a growth chart despite dietary restrictions?

- Can the parents and the child discuss the disease course and management?
- Is the child adapting to diet restrictions?

- Is the child free of edema?
- Has the integrity of the child's skin been maintained?
- Does the child have moist mucous membranes and adequate urine output (see Chapter 40)?
- Does the child continue to achieve age-appropriate developmental milestones?
- Is the family involved in the child's care?
- Has the family demonstrated appropriate coping strategies to meet the needs of all family members, and do they access appropriate support?

## KEY CONCEPTS

- The kidneys reach near-adult function at 6 to 12 months of age.
- Infants cannot concentrate urine as efficiently as older children and adults.
- With therapeutic intervention, nocturnal enuresis can be resolved for most children.
- The clinical manifestations of UTI vary in relation to the child's age, gender, underlying anatomic or neurologic abnormalities, and frequency of recurrence.
- UTI is the most common clinical manifestation of vesicoureteral reflux (VUR).
- To prevent UTI, nurses educate the parents and child about perineal hygiene, increased fluid intake, emptying the bladder, and wearing cotton underwear.
- Cryptorchidism will spontaneously resolve in most infants during the first year of life.
- Goals for hypospadias corrective surgery are normal urinary and sexual function and improved cosmetic appearance of the penis.
- Children with glomerulonephritis should be assessed for signs and symptoms of hypertension and fluid overload.
- Children with edema should have their position changed at least every 2 hours and their lower extremities elevated when they are sitting or lying in bed.
- Edema related to nephrotic syndrome is first noted in the periorbital spaces and dependent areas of the body. Prednisone usually induces remission in the child with nephrotic syndrome.
- Most children with acute kidney injury regain renal function.
- Children with CKD and End Stage Renal Disease (ESRD) and their families require multidisciplinary care.

## REFERENCES AND READINGS


AAP Subcommittee on UTI, Steering Committee on Quality Improvement and Management. (2011). Urinary tract infection: clinical practice guideline for the diagnosis and management of the initial UTI in febrile infants and children 2 to 24 months. *Pediatrics, 128,* 595–610.

Bayne, A., & Skoog, S. (2014). Nocturnal enuresis: an approach to assessment and treatment. *Pediatrics in Review, 35*(8), 327–335.

Brandstrom, P., & Hansson, S. (2015). Long-term, low-dose prophylaxis against urinary tract infection in young children. *Pediatric Nephrology, 30,* 425-432.

Cara-Fuentes, G., Gupta, N., & Garin, E. (2015). The RIVUR study: A review of its findings. *Pediatric Nephrology, 30,* 703-706.

Durham, S., Stamm, P., & Eiland, L. (2015). Cranberry products for the prophylaxis of urinary tract infections in pediatric patients. *Annals of Pharmacotherapy, 49*(2), 1349–1356.

Elder, J. (2016). Urologic disorders in infants and children. In R. Kliegman, B. Stanton, J. St. Geme, et al. (Eds.), *Nelson textbook of pediatrics* (20th ed., Part XXIV). St. Louis, MO: Elsevier.

Fantasia, J., Aidlen, J., Lathrop, W., et al. (2015). Undescended testicle: clinical and surgical review. *Urologic Nursing, 35*(3), 117–126.

Fisher, D., & Steele, R. (2015). *Pediatric urinary tract infection.* Retrieved from http://emedicine.medscape.com.

Hodson, H., Willis, N., & Craig, V. (2015). Corticosteroid therapy for nephrotic syndrome in children (Review). *The Cochrane Library, 3,* 1-30.

Hoyer, P. (2015). New lessons from randomized trials in steroid-sensitive nephrotic syndrome: clear evidence against long steroid therapy. *Kidney International, 87,* 17-19.

Kausman, J., & Powell, H. (2015). Paediatric nephrology: the last 50 years. *Journal of Paediatrics and Child Health, 51,* 94–97.

Kolon, T., et al. (2014). *Evaluation and treatment of cryptorchidism: American Urological Association guideline.* Retrieved from http://www.auanet.org.

March, P., Heering, H., & Pravikoff, D. (2016). *Enuresis nocturnal: behavioral intervention—alarms. evidence-based care sheet.* Glendale, CA: Cinahl Information Systems.

National Institute of Diabetes and Digestive and Kidney Diseases. (2014). *Overview of kidney disease in children.* Retrieved from http://www.niddk.nih.gov/Pages/default.aspx.

Nelson, C., Johnson, E., Logvinenko, T., et al. (2014). Ultrasound as a screening test for genitourinary anomalies in children with UTI. *Pediatrics, 133*(3), 394–403.

Pais, P., & Avner, E. (2016). Idiopathic nephrotic syndrome. In R. Kliegman, B. Stanton, J. St. Geme, et al. (Eds.), *Nelson textbook of pediatrics* (20th ed., Chapter 527). St. Louis, MO: Elsevier.

Pan, C., & Avner, E. (2016). Glomerulonephritis associated with infections. In R. Kliegman, B. Stanton, J. St. Geme, et al. (Eds.), *Nelson textbook of pediatrics* (20th ed., Chapter 511). St. Louis, MO: Elsevier.

Penny, S. (2016). The pediatric urinary tract and medical imaging. *Radiologic Technology, 87*(4), 425–444.

Schneuer, J., et al. (2016). Age at surgery and outcomes of an undescended testis. *Pediatrics, 137*(2), e20150164.

Shaikh, N., et al. (2016). Predictors of antibiotic resistance among pathogens causing urinary tract infection in children. *Journal of Pediatrics, 171,* 116-121.

Sreedharan, R., & Avner, E. (2016). Renal failure. In R. Kliegman, B. Stanton, J. St. Geme, et al. (Eds.), *Nelson textbook of pediatrics* (20th ed., Chapter 535). St. Louis, MO: Elsevier.

Thomas, M. et al. (2015). The definition of acute kidney injury and its use in practice. *Kidney International, 87,* 62–73.

45

# The Child With a Respiratory Alteration

http://evolve.elsevier.com/McKinney/mat-ch/

## LEARNING OBJECTIVES

*After studying this chapter, you should be able to:*

- Describe the differences in the anatomy and physiology of the respiratory system of infants and children that increase their risk for respiratory disease.
- Outline nursing care for a child with allergies to inhalants.
- Discuss the pathophysiology, clinical manifestations, and therapeutic management of common acute and chronic respiratory alterations.
- Identify the nursing care needs of infants and children with acute and chronic respiratory alterations.
- Develop guidelines for the home care of a child with an acute respiratory alteration.
- Identify common triggers of asthma symptoms.
- Apply measures that can be taken to prevent and treat asthma episodes.
- Identify teaching needs for children with asthma and their families.
- Describe the nursing care of the child with cystic fibrosis.
- Discuss measures to maintain adequate oxygenation and provide appropriate developmental stimulation for the child with bronchopulmonary dysplasia.
- Describe the correct method of administering and evaluating tuberculosis skin tests.
- Identify ways to prevent the transmission of tuberculosis and explain the importance of administering antituberculosis medications as prescribed.

## CLINICAL REFERENCE

### REVIEW OF THE RESPIRATORY SYSTEM

The respiratory system consists of the nose, pharynx, larynx, trachea, bronchi, and lungs. It is further divided into the *upper respiratory tract* (nose, pharynx, larynx) and the *lower respiratory tract* (trachea, bronchi, lungs).

#### The Upper Airway

Air enters the body through the *nares,* or nostrils, two nasal cavities lined with mucous membrane. In older infants and children, air can also enter through the mouth into the *pharynx,* or throat. The *nasopharynx* is located immediately behind the nasal cavity; the *oropharynx* is located behind the mouth. The *laryngeal pharynx* lies below the oropharynx and opens into the larynx toward the front and into the esophagus toward the back.

The *larynx* is located between the pharynx and the trachea. The vocal cords are at the upper end of the larynx. The proximity of the upper esophagus to the upper respiratory system can put an individual at risk for inhaling food or liquids, but the *epiglottis* covers the larynx during swallowing and helps keep food out of the lower respiratory tract.

*Cilia* are hair-like processes that move mucus and fluid. Damage to cilia interferes with the removal of mucus from the respiratory tract. Ciliated mucous membranes line the larynx and filter dust and other particles from the air. The particles are then carried to the pharynx to be removed by sneezing, blowing, or coughing. After being filtered, the air that enters the respiratory system is humidified and warmed before proceeding into the lungs.

The posterior oropharynx contains three types of tonsils: the oval *palatine tonsils,* located on either side of the pharynx; the *lingual tonsil,* located below the palatine tonsils at the base of the tongue; and the *pharyngeal tonsils,* or *adenoids,* located at the nasopharyngeal border. The tonsils are composed mainly of lymphoid tissue. They help filter the circulating lymph of bacteria and other foreign material that enter the body, especially through the mouth and nose.

#### The Lower Airway

The *trachea* conducts air between the larynx and the lungs. It divides into right and left main *bronchi* at its lower end, the *carina.* The right main bronchus is shorter and wider than the left. The main bronchi divide into the *lobar bronchi, segmental bronchi,* and *bronchioles* and terminate in *alveoli.* Mucus-secreting goblet cells line the bronchi and protect the lungs from dust and bacteria.

The *lungs* are two cone-shaped structures within the thoracic cavity. The right lung has three *lobes* (upper, middle, and lower); the left lung has two lobes (upper and lower). The *pleurae* are composed of two layers, the *parietal pleura* and the *visceral pleura.* The parietal pleura lines the entire thoracic cavity; the visceral pleura encases each lung. The pleurae help maintain lung stability. Negative pressure within the intrapleural space prevents the lungs from separating from the thorax. *Diffusion* of gases takes place in the lungs. Terminal bronchioles lack mucus-secreting goblet cells and cilia, and gas exchange does not take place here.

Distal to the terminal bronchioles are the alveoli, where most gas exchange occurs. The thinness of the alveolar walls aids in gas exchange.

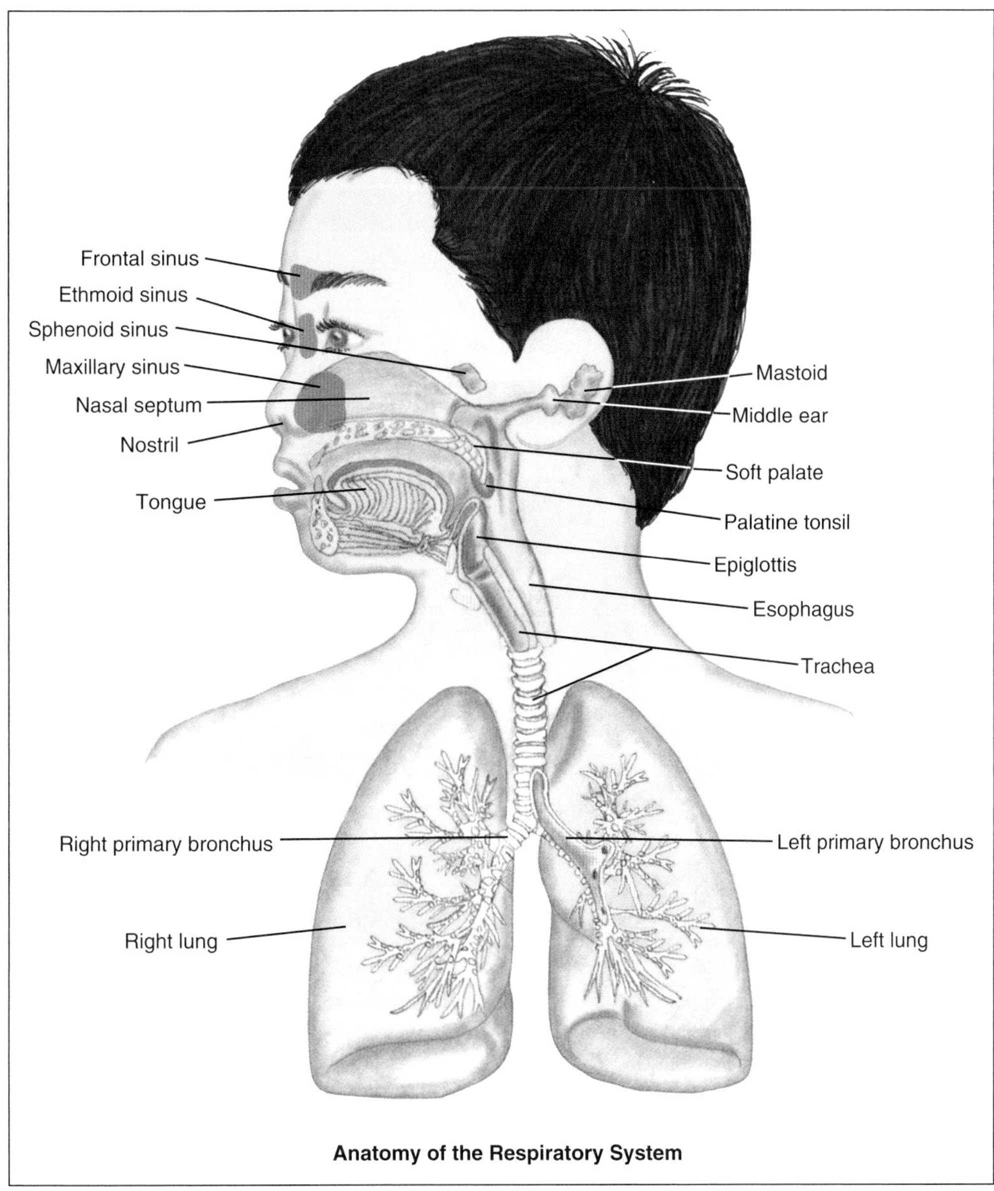


**Anatomy of the Respiratory System**

A nearly solid sheet of capillaries resides within the alveolar walls, localizing alveolar gases proximate to the capillary blood.

## Prenatal Respiratory Development

The respiratory system must mature before birth for the neonate to survive. The placenta performs oxygenation *in utero*, but to adapt to extrauterine life, the neonate must be able to inflate the lungs, establish continuous breathing, and transfer the gases needed to meet metabolic needs.

## Postnatal Respiratory Changes

Postnatal changes in the respiratory system occur as follows:

1. Compression of the thorax during vaginal delivery forces out some of the fetal lung fluid.
2. Respirations are stimulated by hypoxemia, hypercarbia, cold, tactile stimulation, and possibly by the decrease in the plasma concentration of prostaglandin $E_2$.
3. Inflation of the normal lung is complete within a few breaths, and most alveoli have expanded within the first hour of life.
4. Surfactant in the lung liquid lowers surface tension and facilitates lung expansion.
5. Pulmonary blood flow increases.
6. Closure of the foramen ovale and the ductus arteriosus (see Chapter 46) establishes the pulmonary and circulatory systems.

## Gas Exchange and Transport

Two-way diffusion takes place between the walls of the alveoli. *Diffusion* is the movement of molecules from an area of higher concentration to one of lower concentration. Blood entering the lung capillaries is relatively low in oxygen. Oxygen will diffuse from the alveoli, where its concentration is higher, into the blood. Similarly, carbon dioxide moves out of the blood and into the alveoli. Most oxygen that diffuses into the capillary blood in the lungs is bound to the hemoglobin of red blood cells. A small percentage is dissolved in

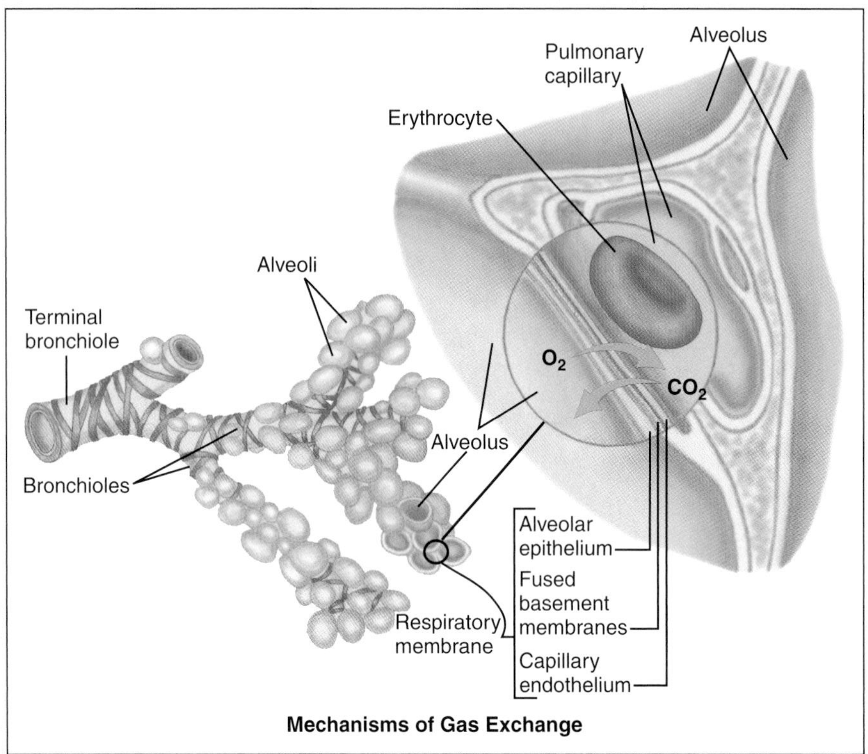

Mechanisms of Gas Exchange

## Pediatric Differences in the Respiratory System

- Surfactant is lacking in premature infants. Infants born before 34 weeks of gestation have a higher risk of respiratory distress syndrome (RDS).
- Smaller lower airways and undeveloped supporting cartilage predispose the child to an increased risk for obstruction by mucus, edema, and foreign bodies. The neonate's airway is 50% smaller than that of adults. A premature infant has a more compliant chest wall and weaker respiratory muscles than a term infant.
- Lung size is proportional to body height. Therefore, lung volumes and capacities do not vary from age to age.
- Infants are obligatory nose breathers; they have difficulty breathing through the mouth. If the infant has nasal congestion, breathing becomes more difficult.
- The diaphragm is the neonate's major respiratory muscle. Intercostal muscles are not well developed. **Retractions** are more common in the infant than in older children and adults.
- Brief periods of apnea (10 to 15 seconds) are common in the neonate. The respiratory pattern may be irregular.
- Children's normal respiratory rate is higher than that of adults.
- An increased metabolic rate increases oxygen needs.
- Alveoli develop from approximately 20 million to 200 million by age 3 years. Alveolar development gradually decreases after age 3 years; few develop after age 8 years.
- The lung surface increases until age 5 to 8 years. Actual lung growth continues into the adolescent years.
- Eustachian tubes are relatively horizontal, which increases the risk for bacteria entering the middle ear.
- Tracheal size approximately triples by adulthood.
- Tonsillar tissue is normally enlarged in early school-age children.
- Infants and children use abdominal muscles to inhale until approximately 5 to 6 years of age.
- The child's flexible larynx is more susceptible to spasm.

plasma. For oxygen to enter the cells, it must separate from hemoglobin. Carbon dioxide diffuses into the blood from the tissues and is transported to the lungs by the blood. Hemoglobin serves as a buffer that enables the blood to take up carbon dioxide without significantly altering the blood pH. The uptake and delivery of gases by the blood is a continuous process.

Ventilation occurs through *inspiration* and *expiration.* During inspiration, the diaphragm contracts and flattens, expanding the vertical dimension of the chest; the lung volume increases. During expiration, the diaphragm and chest wall relax, decreasing the thoracic volume. Intrathoracic pressure increases, and gas flows out of the lungs, taking with it the carbon dioxide that was delivered to the lungs by the blood. Ventilation of the lungs is intermittent. Inspired air is 21% oxygen; end-expired air is 16% oxygen and 35% carbon dioxide.

## Common Laboratory and Diagnostic Tests for Respiratory Disorders

| Test | Description | Normal Findings | Indications | Nursing Considerations |
|---|---|---|---|---|
| Chest radiography, posterior, anterior and lateral views | Shows airways, lungs, heart, great vessels | Normal appearance of internal structures of chest | To detect respiratory disease of lungs | Assist in holding child. |
| Computed tomography | Shows lesions in chest wall, pleural space, mediastinum, and lung parenchyma | Normal cross section of lung tissue | To image tumors or masses; to evaluate response to therapy aimed at defined lesions | Assist with sedation and immobilization of child. Withhold feedings 3-4 hr before the test because of frequent use of contrast medium. |
| Bronchoscopy | Provides viewing of tracheobronchial tree through a scope | Normal appearance of tracheobronchial tree or successful removal of foreign body or mucous plugs | To view a lesion and obtain biopsy material for culture; to remove foreign body or mucous plugs | Rigid bronchoscopy is usually performed with child under general anesthesia.<br>Fiberoptic flexible bronchoscopy can be performed while child is awake or sedated.<br>Observe child closely for signs of airway obstruction.<br>Mist may be given to decrease swelling and edema. |
| Laryngoscopy | Provides direct viewing of larynx with a scope | Normal appearance of larynx | To identify cause of stridor and local abnormalities | Mirror (indirect) laryngoscopy can be performed on children age 4 yr or older. In infants and younger children, direct laryngoscopy or transnasal laryngoscopy with flexible bronchoscope will give much better results.<br>General anesthesia is usually required; topical anesthesia and mild sedation can be provided for fiberoptic examination.<br>Fluids and foods are withheld until effects of local anesthetic have worn off and gag reflex has returned. |
| Cultures | Throat, blood, nasopharyngeal, sputum, induced sputum | No culture growth or normal flora only | To isolate and identify pathogens | See Chapter 37 for procedures. |
| RAST for IgE | Measures quantity of IgE antibodies in serum after exposure to specific antigens | If the child is not allergic to the antigen, IgE antibody is not detected.<br>A test result is positive in relation to a specific antigen if the value is above 400% of control | To identify specific allergens; systemic reactions to insect venom, drugs, and chemicals; to monitor response to desensitization procedures; also performed at the onset of asthma, hay fever, or dermatitis | Prepare child for peripheral blood sample to be drawn.<br>Determine whether child has undergone any radioisotope tests within past week because such tests can alter the results. |
| Pilocarpine iontophoresis (sweat test) | Measures sweat electrolyte concentration for diagnosis of CF<br>Sweating is stimulated on the child's forearm with a small electrical current and pilocarpine; a sweat sample is then collected on preweighed, dry, sterile gauze or filter paper and the amounts of sweat sodium and chloride are measured | Normal chloride: <40 mEq/L<br>Suggestive of CF: 40-60 mEq/L<br>Positive for CF: >60 mEq/L | To diagnose cystic fibrosis | No physical preparation is needed. Offer parents and child support as they face the implications of a positive diagnosis.<br>Inform child and parents that the test is painless and that it is usually performed twice to ensure accurate results.<br>Because an adequate amount of sweat is difficult to obtain from infants, the sweat test is usually unreliable in infants younger than 2 wk. |

*Continued*

**Common Laboratory and Diagnostic Tests for Respiratory Disorders—cont'd**

| Test | Description | Normal Findings | Indications | Nursing Considerations |
|---|---|---|---|---|
| Mantoux test | Skin test for TB<br>PPD: 5 TB units (0.1 mL) is injected intradermally into volar surface of forearm with short, 26- to 27-gauge needle, beveled side up.<br>A wheal 6-10 mm in diameter should appear during injection.<br>The site is checked in 48-72 hr by a healthcare professional.<br>Results are recorded in millimeters (not simply as positive or negative). The reading is based on induration (hardness), not redness. | Positive result: area of induration ≥15 mm (in children 4 yr of age and older); area of induration ≥10 mm in children younger than 4 yr or at high risk for exposure; area of induration ≥5 mm in highest risk group.<br>Negative result: Mantoux test cannot rule out the presence of TB, particularly in young infants. | To screen and test individuals suspected of having TB or of having been exposed to TB | Test is fairly difficult to administer.<br>After PPD is injected, withdrawal of needle should be delayed 2-3 s to minimize leakage of PPD at the puncture site.<br>In most children, skin testing will elicit positive reaction 3-6 wk after initial infection.<br>Steroids and immunosuppressants given within 4-6 wk can cause false-negative skin test results.<br>Positive tuberculin reactivity usually continues for person's lifetime, even with treatment. |

*CF,* Cystic fibrosis; *IgE,* immunoglobulin E; *PPD,* purified protein derivative; *RAST,* radioallergosorbent test; *TB,* tuberculosis.

## DIAGNOSTIC TESTS

In most instances, respiratory tract disorders are diagnosed from findings on physical examination and clinical manifestations. However, sometimes specific diagnostic tests are needed.

### Blood Gas Analysis

Arterial blood gas analysis plays an important role in the investigation of pulmonary function. Arterial blood gas values most frequently determined include the partial arterial oxygen pressure ($PaO_2$), the partial pressure of carbon dioxide in arterial blood ($PaCO_2$), the acid–base balance (pH), and bicarbonate ($HCO_3^-$). Arterial blood is more reliable than capillary or venous blood for these tests, especially in children with poor peripheral perfusion. Arterial blood gas values are used primarily to determine acid–base balance, not oxygen saturation (see Chapter 40).

### Pulmonary Function Tests

Two of the most useful measures of ventilatory function are the *vital capacity* and the *expiratory flow rate,* both measured by spirometry. Spirometry can be performed at an acceptable level by most preschool-aged children (Nierengarten, 2016). Accurate measurements are difficult to obtain in younger children because they are unable to follow commands. Infant pulmonary function testing is performed at many institutions with use of conscious sedation. Pulmonary function tests assess the degree of pulmonary disease, the response to therapy, and the presence of restrictive or obstructive disease. They are also done to test the child's response to bronchodilators should pulmonary function be affected.

The child must be given instruction and practice in blowing, pushing, and holding respirations. The child should become familiar with the mouthpiece and the nose clip to feel comfortable with their use.

### Pulse Oximetry

Pulse oximetry is a simple, noninvasive, intermittent or continuous method for measuring oxygen saturation for the purpose of determining the need for or response to oxygen therapy (see Chapter 37). The goal of treatment for most respiratory conditions is an oxygen saturation value greater than 95%. However, for children with chronic respiratory disease, a realistic goal may be slightly lower.

### Transcutaneous Monitoring

Transcutaneous monitoring continuously checks oxygen and carbon dioxide concentrations in the body through an electrode placed on the child's skin. Electrode sites must be changed every 3 to 4 hours to prevent burning the skin, and the machine must be recalibrated each time electrodes are changed. The readings may not be accurate if tissue perfusion is poor.

### End-Tidal Carbon Dioxide Monitoring

End-tidal carbon dioxide monitoring, often used in conjunction with pulse oximetry, noninvasively measures carbon dioxide in the exhaled breath. It is useful for verifying endotracheal tube position, evaluating asthma, and during procedural sedation. End-tidal carbon dioxide measurement can also be a primary indicator of worsening respiratory distress or impending respiratory failure because the results are thought to detect respiratory distress and hypercarbia earlier than does pulse oximetry (Walsh, Crotwell, & Restrepo, 2011).

## RESPIRATORY ILLNESS IN CHILDREN

Respiratory alterations are the most common causes of illness in the infant and child. Upper respiratory disorders affect the ears, nose, pharynx, and larynx; lower respiratory disorders include those that involve the trachea, bronchi, and lungs.

Infants and children younger than 3 years are at greater risk than older children and adults for developing respiratory infections because of their immature immune systems, smaller upper and lower airways, and underdeveloped supporting cartilage. Although most respiratory infections are self-limiting, respiratory distress can occur quickly in infants and young children, as mucus and edema obstruct their small airways.

Parents should be taught preventive measures, including adequate rest, optimal nutrition, and good hygiene, with an emphasis on hand hygiene. However, even with the most careful hygiene and preventive practices, most children will have some type of respiratory infection each year. School nurses often see children with respiratory problems in the school health office and may be the primary healthcare providers for these children.

Most children can be cared for at home by their parents and do not need hospitalization. Those children who are hospitalized are being discharged earlier in their recovery than in the past. The current healthcare environment necessitates that nurses teach parents appropriate home care techniques, including careful observation and recognition of signs that indicate the need to contact healthcare providers. Parents, especially first-time parents, often are frightened by the sudden onset of respiratory symptoms, which can indicate a severe problem. Teaching parents the signs and symptoms of serious illness will help them develop appropriate decision-making skills.

Children with chronic conditions have many special needs, and the child with a chronic respiratory disease is no different. Medications and treatments become a way of life for many of these children. Their activity level is often altered, and some may have a shortened life span.

Children with chronic respiratory conditions are now becoming adults with those same conditions. As advances in treatment modalities are made and children with these conditions are living longer, the transition to adult care becomes a necessity.

The nurse plays an important role in the care of the child with a chronic respiratory disease. Beyond giving acute care to the hospitalized child, the nurse must coordinate and facilitate the child's long-term care. Because of current advances in the treatment of chronic pediatric respiratory conditions, the treatment and care of children affected by these disorders are constantly changing and improving, requiring the nurse to stay current in these areas.

## ALLERGIC RHINITIS

Allergic rhinitis is an inflammatory disorder of the nasal mucosa that is usually seasonal, recurrent, and triggered by specific allergens (see Chapter 42). It is sometimes referred to as *intermittent allergic rhinitis* or *hay fever*. Some children have symptoms year round *(persistent allergic rhinitis)*.

### Etiology and Incidence

Agents that commonly cause allergic rhinitis include dust mites, feathers, animal dander, mold spores, and pollens of trees, grasses, and weeds. There is usually a family history, as seen in individuals with atopic dermatitis and asthma. Slightly over one third of children with allergic rhinitis also have asthma (Milgrom & Sicherer, 2016).

The onset of allergic rhinitis usually occurs during childhood but rarely before age 2 years. An estimated 20% to 40% of children have this type of allergic response, which is also associated with elevated levels of allergen-specific IgE (Milgrom & Sicherer, 2016).

**PATHOPHYSIOLOGY**

***Allergic Rhinitis***

Allergens (pollens, molds, spores, dust mites, animal dander) are deposited on the nasal mucosa, causing local inflammation and increased capillary permeability. Local immunoglobulin E (IgE) is produced, and sensitization of the respiratory tissues occurs. Mast cell mediators are released, producing vasodilation, mucosal edema, mucus secretions, stimulation of itch receptors, and a reduced threshold for sneezing.

### Manifestations

The classic symptoms of allergic rhinitis are clear rhinorrhea with itching of the nose, eyes, ears, and palate, and paroxysmal sneezing not associated with an upper respiratory infection. Additional signs and symptoms include the "allergic salute"—an upward rubbing of the nose with the palm of the hand, which can leave a crease below the bridge (Fig. 45.1); allergic shiners—dark circles under the eyes from congestion and edema; dry lips from mouth breathing; pale, boggy nasal mucous membranes; and nasal obstruction. Children with allergic rhinitis have symptoms as long as they are exposed to the allergen.

It is important to distinguish allergic rhinitis from viral *nasopharyngitis* (the common cold), which is usually caused by a rhinovirus and is spread by droplets or contact with contaminated items. Children with nasopharyngitis usually have the associated symptoms of sore throat, fever, cough, and fatigue. The condition is self-limiting and usually resolves within 2 weeks. The quality of the nasal discharge in children with nasopharyngitis often changes from clear to cloudy or yellow. Management is supportive. Because young infants are obligatory nose breathers, the infant's blocked nasal passages should be cleared by the instillation of normal saline solution drops followed by gentle bulb suction.

### Diagnostic Evaluation

A thorough personal and family history usually elicits a description that suggests an allergic rather than infectious pattern. The nasal smear

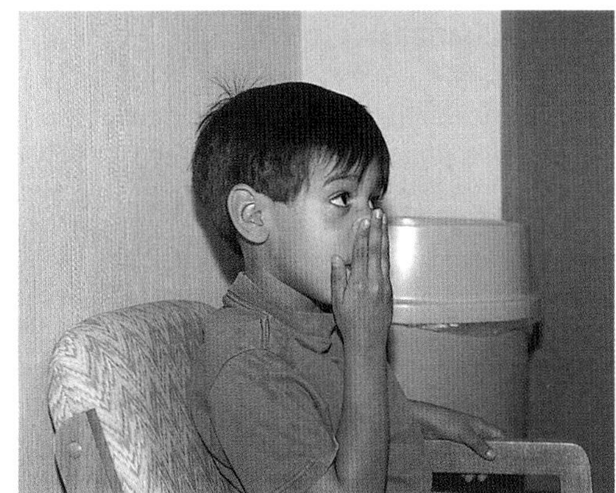

FIG 45.1 Children with allergic rhinitis often have dark circles under their eyes, called *allergic shiners,* and may be seen rubbing their noses upward with the palm—the "allergic salute." (Courtesy Parkland Health and Hospital System Community Oriented Primary Care Clinic, Dallas, TX.)

may demonstrate eosinophils. Allergy skin testing is done if signs and symptoms continue after treatment with medication. The radioallergosorbent test (RAST) is used only when skin testing is difficult because of generalized dermatitis, the young age of the child, or the child being too ill for skin testing. A complete blood cell count might reveal elevated eosinophils, a finding associated with allergic manifestations.

## Therapeutic Management

The treatment of choice is to eliminate the allergen from the child's environment. When this goal is impossible, as in the case of pollen in the air, medication can control symptoms.

Antihistamines and/or intranasal corticosteroids can be effective in treating allergic rhinitis (Lierl, 2014). Antihistamines are most effective when given before or very early in an allergic episode. Because they can cause drowsiness, they should be given at night. Some of the newer antihistamines (e.g., loratadine, cetirizine, fexofenadine) are long acting, have fewer side effects, and require only one or two doses daily. They are prescribed according to the child's age. Decongestants can be effective in relieving nasal congestion but are not recommended in young children. Decongestants have side-effect profiles that include insomnia, behavior problems, and even cardiac events (Milgrom & Sicherer, 2016).

Short-term topical intranasal corticosteroids (e.g., fluticasone, mometasone, and budesonide) are highly effective and can be used as first-line therapy for children with allergic rhinitis (Greener, 2015). Several days of treatment are required before the child feels the effects of topical corticosteroids.

Leukotriene inhibitors (e.g., montelukast [Singulair]) can be used to treat allergic rhinitis, although the results are sometimes suboptimal. These medications have a good safety profile and seem to work well for children with both allergic rhinitis and asthma (Greener, 2015; Milgrom & Sicherer, 2016).

Finally, immunotherapy (allergy shots) may be considered for children whose condition is not responsive to either environmental modification or medication. Immunotherapy involves injecting the child with progressively larger doses of the allergen in an effort to reduce the magnitude of the body's allergic response. Injections are given once or twice a week until a maintenance dose is reached; monthly maintenance injections can continue for several years. As a newer alternative, immunotherapy is accomplished through sub-lingual administration of the allergen; after the initial dose is administered, additional daily doses are administered at home (Lierl, 2014).

### PATIENT-CENTERED TEACHING

#### *How to Implement Environmental Modifications*

To reduce your child's exposure to allergens, take the following measures:

**Pollen and Dust**

- Wash your child's sheets and blankets weekly in hot water.
- Avoid using wool and down blankets.
- Encase pillows and mattresses in dust-proof covers.
- Replace carpet with wood, tile, slate, or vinyl.
- Replace drapes and blinds with curtains and shades.
- Replace upholstered furniture with wood or plastic.
- Keep closet doors shut.
- Cover hot air vents with filters.
- Install air cleaners.
- Use multilayer vacuum bags.
- Clean with a towel treated to attract dust.
- Run an air conditioner.
- Keep household humidity at 40% to 50%.

**Mold**

- Clean with a mold inhibitor.
- Dry everyone's shoes thoroughly.
- Use a moisture remover in closets.
- Encourage your child to stay out of the basement.
- Replace foam rubber mattresses with inner spring mattresses.
- Run an air conditioner.
- Keep the humidity below 35%.
- Run a dehumidifier.
- Ventilate the house.
- Store firewood outside.
- Limit the number of indoor plants.

**Dander**

- Keep pets outside if possible.
- Ventilate the house.
- Install air cleaners.
- Encase mattresses and pillows in dust-proof covers.

For further information, contact Allergy & Asthma Network/Mothers of Asthmatics Inc. website: http://www.allergyasthmanetwork.org, a family site that provides information on asthma products, kits and books.

## Nursing Considerations

Nursing care focuses on early identification of the clinical signs and symptoms of allergic rhinitis and the therapeutic management of the condition. The nurse assesses and records the applicable history and helps the family identify allergens to which the child is sensitive. Once the allergens are known, the nurse counsels parents regarding medication administration, environmental control, and immunotherapy, as appropriate (see Patient-Centered Teaching: How to Implement Environmental Modifications). Allergies, including allergic rhinitis, can negatively affect the quality of life and school performance. Children with allergic rhinitis, especially if also affected by other allergic disease, are at risk for developing both anxiety and depression (Nanda et al., 2016); nurses should be alert to signs of these conditions in young children.

Side effects of medications used to treat allergic rhinitis can further impair functioning. Drowsiness, the most common side effect of antihistamines, can usually be alleviated if the child takes the medication at night. Some children have dry mucous membranes or excitability. Warm water or saline solution irrigations of the nasal passages can be used to moisten mucous membranes, soften crusted secretions, and wash out irritants. Saline solution can be mixed by adding ¼ teaspoon of salt to a cup of warm water. Saline solution nose drops are also available without prescription.

When specific allergens have been identified, they should be eliminated or controlled. During the pollen season, the child should stay indoors as much as possible, and the windows should be kept closed if the house is air conditioned. After being outdoors, the child should shower and wash his or her hair to remove pollens from the body. Animals that have been outside are also be a possible source of contamination.

Receiving immunotherapy by injection can be a traumatic experience for a child. It is often difficult for children to understand how an injection will help them. Allergy injections must be given in a physician's office because of the risk of an anaphylactic reaction to the allergy serum. Monitor the child closely (vital sign changes, difficulty breathing) for 20 to 30 minutes after the injection in case anaphylaxis develops. Keep emergency epinephrine ready.

## SINUSITIS

Sinusitis, although not itself a serious disorder, can lead to life-threatening complications. Inflammation and infection of the sinuses can be acute or chronic.

### Etiology and Incidence

Acute sinusitis often follows an upper respiratory tract viral infection. Children with chronic sinusitis often have allergic rhinitis or otitis media with effusion (OME) as well. Hypertrophied adenoids, immune deficiencies, and foreign body obstruction of the nose also predispose one to sinusitis. Children with cystic fibrosis have a high incidence of sinusitis because of highly viscous mucus secretions and nasal polyps. The most common causative organisms are *Streptococcus pneumoniae, Haemophilus influenzae, Moraxella catarrhalis,* and *Staphylococcus aureus* (Pappas & Hendley, 2016).

Sinus infections can occur in infancy as well as in childhood and are seen frequently in preschool and school age children as a result of group exposure to upper respiratory infection (Pappas & Hendley, 2016).

### Manifestations

Sinusitis is characterized by signs and symptoms of a cold that do not improve after 10 days, low-grade fever, nasal congestion with purulent nasal discharge, halitosis, cough (which usually increases when the child is lying down), headache, and tenderness and a feeling of fullness over the affected sinuses. Young children may become irritable. Occasionally, children have facial edema or complications such as orbital cellulitis or central nervous system symptoms. Children with chronic sinusitis have many of the same symptoms except that the cough is chronic and the headache is recurrent. The child's sense of taste or smell may be impaired, and the child may be fatigued.

**PATHOPHYSIOLOGY**

***Sinusitis***

Acute sinusitis occurs when the sinus cavity is invaded by bacteria, causing mucosal inflammation and edema that block narrow sinus channels. The volume of secretions increases, and the affected sinuses fill with purulent material. Inflammation and infection interfere with the protective cleansing action of the cilia covering the sinus mucous membranes. Impaired mucociliary transport leads to stagnation of secretions within the sinuses; the stagnant secretions provide a medium for bacterial growth.

Chronic sinusitis is usually a complication of acute sinusitis. Prolonged or repeated infections result in irreversible changes in the mucosal lining of the sinus. Nasal polyps, a deviated septum, and enlarged adenoids inhibit sinus drainage, which can lead to infections. The frontal and sphenoid sinuses are most often involved in children.

Infection from sinusitis can spread to the middle ear, causing otitis media. Serious complications occur when infection spreads either directly through the bone or along the venous channels of the skull into adjacent structures, such as the orbit or the central nervous system.

### Diagnostic Evaluation

Imaging studies are not recommended for diagnosing sinusitis (Pappas & Hendley, 2016; Wald et al., 2013) because evidence suggests that the diagnosis can be made using criteria that distinguish it from an upper respiratory infection. The American Academy of Pediatrics (AAP) has defined the diagnostic criteria for acute sinusitis as follows: *Persistent* – symptoms for more than ten days without improvement; *Worsening* – symptoms that become worse after initial improvement, or symptoms along with a late-appearing fever; or *Severe* – purulent discharge along with fever for three consecutive days (Wald et al., 2013). MRI or CT scans may be appropriate for children who experience central nervous system complications (Pappas & Hendley, 2016).

### Therapeutic Management

Most cases of acute sinusitis are self-resolving and do not require antibiotics (Wald et al., 2013). The AAP allows for a watch and wait period of three days for persistent sinusitis before prescribing antibiotics, if the parent is willing. When a prescription is required, amoxicillin or amoxicillin–potassium clavulanate (Augmentin) is used most frequently. In addition to antibiotics, treatment includes analgesics, hydration, and the application of moist heat. Antihistamines may be used to treat allergy symptoms associated with chronic sinusitis, but they tend to impair sinus drainage by thickening secretions. Saline nasal irrigation might relieve symptoms, but the evidence for this effect is equivocal (Pappas & Hendley, 2016). Steroid nasal sprays may be used to reduce inflammation, but their efficacy has not been demonstrated consistently for children (Wald et al., 2013). Surgical correction via balloon sinuplasty may be considered for children with chronic sinusitis who have not responded to antibiotic therapy (Armstrong & Christian, 2014). If orbital cellulitis develops, the child should be hospitalized immediately and parenteral antibiotic therapy begun (Pappas & Hendley, 2011).

### Nursing Considerations

The nurse assesses the location of pain or fullness. Pain can occur in the forehead or over the cheek bones or upper teeth, or it may radiate to the top of the head. Inspect and palpate the face for edema, document any fever, and inspect the nose and throat for purulent discharge. The nasal mucous membranes are inspected for erythema and edema.

Nursing care focuses on teaching the parents antibiotic administration, comfort measures, how to monitor for response to treatment, and how to identify complications. Emphasize the importance of the child's taking the antibiotics as prescribed. Sinus drainage is facilitated by increasing the child's intake of clear fluids and by using a bedside humidifier.

Warm, moist compresses applied two or three times daily help decrease swelling and pain. Acetaminophen is given for fever and discomfort. Breathing warm mist in a hot shower or through hot, moist towels can help liquefy and mobilize nasal mucus, as can saline solution nose drops. The nurse teaches the parent to administer nose drops after the nasal passages have been gently cleaned. The amount, color, and consistency of nasal drainage should be noted and evaluated to determine whether the child is responding to treatment.

Carefully evaluate the child's response to treatment and the development of complications. Advise parents to contact the physician promptly if symptoms become worse, if the child has any periorbital redness or edema, or if the child does not seem to be feeling better after 3 to 4 days.

## OTITIS MEDIA

Otitis media is one of the most common illnesses of infancy and childhood. The term *otitis media* refers to *effusion* (fluid) and infection or blockage of the middle ear. *Acute otitis media* (AOM) is effusion and inflammation in the middle ear that occurs suddenly and is associated with other signs of illness. *Otitis media with effusion* (OME) refers to the presence of fluid behind the tympanic membrane without signs of infection. Otitis media with effusion often follows an episode of AOM and usually resolves in 1 to 3 months.

## Etiology

The bacterial pathogens that usually cause AOM are *S. pneumoniae, H. influenzae,* and *M. catarrhalis,* although since the introduction of pneumococcal immunization *S. pneumoniae* as a cause has decreased (Kerschner & Preciado, 2016). Although viruses do not cause otitis media, they are thought to predispose the child to ear infection by altering host defenses and contributing to eustachian tube dysfunction. Allergies are also thought to precipitate otitis media.

Attendance at daycare centers predisposes children to otitis media because of the close contacts children have with others. Infants younger than 1 year who attend daycare have a significant risk for acquiring AOM. Other risk factors include age (highest in 6- to 20-month-olds), ethnicity (higher in Native Americans, Alaskan and Canadian Inuit, and indigenous people of Australia), exposure to household cigarette smoke, and poverty (Kerschner & Preciado, 2016).

Bottle feeding can contribute to ear infection because of the position of the infant during feeding. Reflux of formula into the eustachian tube from the nasopharynx occurs when the infant swallows while supine. Breastfeeding offers some protection from ear infection by providing maternal antibodies and by decreasing the incidence of allergy; also, the more upright position of the infant while nursing or bottle feeding may be protective against ear infection (Kerschner & Preciado, 2016).

## Incidence

The incidence of otitis media peaks between ages 6 months and 2 years. Most initial episodes occur at approximately 6 months of age, when maternal antibody levels decline. Early onset of AOM (during infancy) increases the risk for recurrent episodes; by the end of the first year of life, up to 85% of children have experienced at least one episode of AOM (Kerschner & Preciado, 2016). Boys have a slightly higher incidence of otitis media than girls. The incidence of otitis media is highest in winter and spring and lowest in the summer months.

## Manifestations

AOM is characterized by the following:

- Otalgia (earache); infants may pull their ears or roll their heads.
- A bulging, opaque tympanic membrane that usually looks red, with decreased mobility; diffuse light reflex; and obscured landmarks (Fig. 45.2).
- Drainage, usually yellowish green, purulent, and foul smelling (indicates perforation of the tympanic membrane).

These signs and symptoms might also be accompanied by irritability, sleep disturbances, persistent crying in infants, fever, vomiting, anorexia, or diarrhea (especially in infants).

OME differs from AOM in that there are no signs of acute infection. The tympanic membrane appears retracted and either dull gray or yellow, and an air-fluid level or air bubbles may be visible through the tympanic membrane. The mobility of the tympanic membrane is

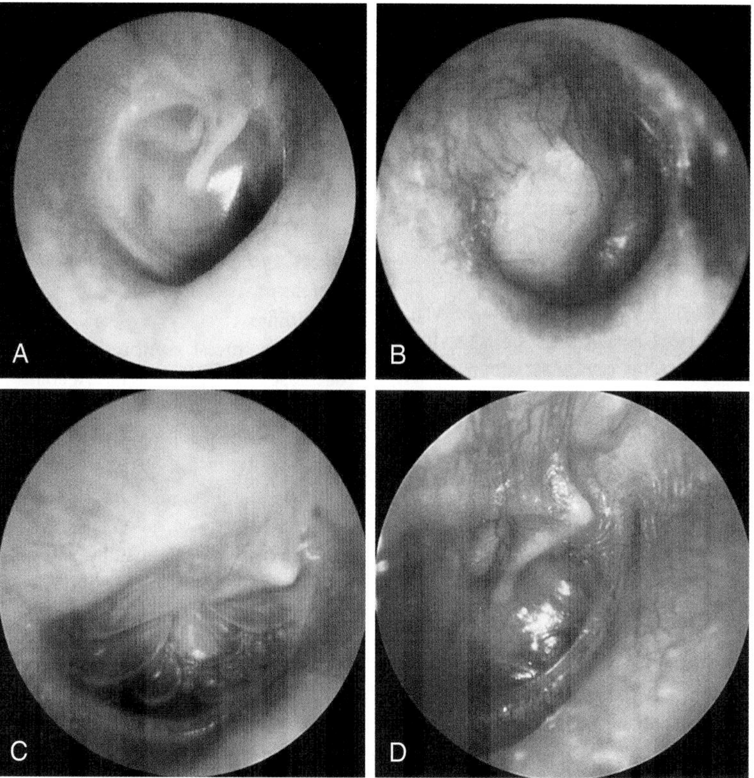


**FIG 45.2** Appearance of tympanic membrane in otitis media compared with normal tympanic membrane. **A,** Normal right tympanic membrane and middle ear. **B,** Acute otitis media: bulging right tympanic membrane. **C,** Otitis media with effusion: air-fluid level and bubbles visible through right retracted, translucent tympanic membrane. **D,** Otitis media with effusion: severely retracted, opaque right tympanic membrane. (From Bluestone, C.D., & Klein, J.O. [1995]. *Otitis media in infants and children* [2nd ed.]. Philadelphia: Saunders.)

## PATHOPHYSIOLOGY

### *Otitis Media*

The immature anatomy of the child's middle ear and eustachian tube predisposes infants and toddlers to otitis media. When the eustachian tube is obstructed, as frequently occurs with enlarged adenoids or mucosal edema from an upper respiratory tract infection, effective drainage and ventilation of the middle ear cannot occur. Air that is normally present in the middle ear is absorbed by the blood, causing a vacuum or negative pressure in the middle ear. Effusion accumulates within the middle ear space, creating a medium for bacterial growth. After an upper respiratory tract infection, pathogens travel from the nasopharynx to the eustachian tube. In the presence of effusion, negative pressure in the middle ear draws mucus through the eustachian tube whenever the child cries, yawns, or sucks forcefully on a nipple. Purulent fluid accumulates in the middle ear space, causing the pressure and pain of acute otitis media.

If the eustachian tube remains nonfunctional for a prolonged period, the fluid within the middle ear becomes thick and dark (glue ear). Mild temporary conductive hearing loss (see Chapter 55) often occurs in otitis media with effusion because of the decreased mobility of the ossicles and the tympanic membrane. Permanent conductive hearing loss can result from repeated episodes of otitis media, interfering with the development of language and cognitive skills. Chronic otitis media with effusion is the most common cause of hearing loss in children.

Older child
The eustachian tube normally ventilates the middle ear by opening and closing regularly. This equalizes pressure and permits middle-ear drainage. It also protects the middle ear from nasopharyngeal secretions and sound pressure.
Middle ear
Eustachian tube
Infant/toddler
Efficient drainage is inhibited by shorter and more horizontal eustachian tube.
Eustachian tube is more distensible in the infant.
Lack of cartilage support causes eustachian tube to collapse easily, restricting drainage.

Complications of otitis media include conductive hearing loss and sensorineural hearing loss. The infection of acute otitis media can spread to surrounding tissues, causing mastoiditis or intracranial complications such as meningitis or brain abscess. Inflammation and pressure from otitis media may result in *tympanosclerosis* (scarring of the tympanic membrane), perforation of the tympanic membrane, and *cholesteatoma* (a cyst formed from pus and debris in the middle ear).

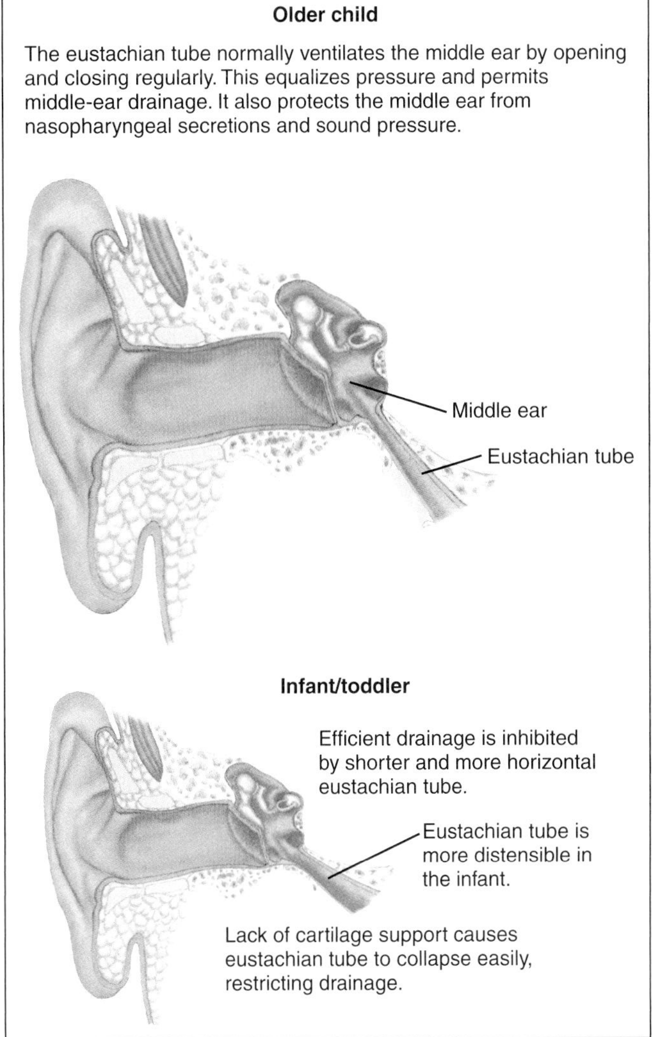


decreased, and landmarks are distorted. Associated signs and symptoms can be subtle and can include the following:

- Tinnitus, popping sounds
- Hearing loss (usually conductive) below 35 decibels; in the older child, hearing loss may manifest as behavior problems, poor school performance, disturbed sleep, irritability, and decreased responsiveness
- Mild balance disturbances that may result in delays in motor skills
- A flattened tracing and negative pressure on the tympanogram (a graphic representation of tympanic mobility and middle ear pressure)

AOM is considered to be persistent if the child experiences symptoms while being treated or within 1 month after treatment is complete. AOM is viewed as recurrent if the child experiences more than three episodes over a 6-month period or four episodes in a year (Lieberthal et al., 2013).

### Diagnostic Evaluation

Due to some confusion in the diagnosis and subsequent management of infants and children with AOM, the AAP updated its diagnosis and management guidelines (Lieberthal et al, 2013). Based on an extensive review of evidence, changes in diagnostic criteria have occurred. To diagnose a child with AOM, the provider must visualize the child's tympanic membrane. A moderate to severely bulging tympanic membrane establishes a diagnosis of AOM. In addition, AOM can be diagnosed in a child who has a tympanic membrane that is mildly bulging and/or has substantial erythema, and who is experiencing pain (Lieberthal et al., 2013). Children with acute otitis media also have decreased mobility of the tympanic membrane diagnosed by pneumatic otoscopy. In pneumatic otoscopy, a small puff of air is blown into the ear canal through the otoscope; the examiner can discern the appearance and mobility of the tympanic membrane. In addition to pneumatic otoscopy, tympanometry or tympanography can be used to confirm what was seen with the eye.

### Therapeutic Management

The emergence of resistant organisms has created much discussion around the use of antibiotics to treat AOM because spontaneous resolution of the infection occurs in a large majority of children. Research has demonstrated that the administration of antibiotics has little influence on the child's experience of pain (Venekamp, Sanders, Glaziou, et al., 2015), and updated guidelines for the management of AOM from the AAP (Lieberthal et al., 2013) place more emphasis on pain relief. Current recommendations include the following (Lieberthal et al., 2013):

- Accurate diagnosis of AOM before treatment decisions are made
- Optimal pain relief with an appropriate analgesic for children with AOM
- Symptomatic treatment and observation for 48 to 72 hours after diagnosis as an alternative to initiating antibiotic therapy for selected children
- Reassessment and treatment initiation for children with positive AOM after the 48- to 72-hour observation period
- Use of amoxicillin at a dose of 80 to 90 mg/kg/day for 5 to 10 days when treatment is indicated, or a cephalosporin for children allergic to penicillin
- Encouraging reduction of risk factors as a method for preventing AOM episodes
- The AAP guidelines (Lieberthal et al., 2013) specify criteria for management with antibiotics to include:

*Infants and Young Children (>6 months to <24 months):* Initiate antibiotics if the child has a positive diagnosis of AOM along with pain and fever (>39° C) for 48 hours, or bilateral AOM with mild symptoms. For children with unilateral AOM with mild symptoms, collaborative decision-making with the parent can include a "watch and wait" without antibiotics for 48 to 72 hours, ensuring sufficient follow-up of the child's condition.

*Older Children:* Initiate antibiotics for children with severe symptoms as previously described. Collaborative "watch and wait" may be used for 48 to 72 hours instead of antibiotics for older children with unilateral or bilateral AOM with mild symptoms.

For children with recurrent AOM, providers can offer surgical placement of tympanostomy tubes because of the connection between effusion and the occurrence of AOM (Lieberthal et al., 2013; Wallace et al., 2014).

For OME that persists for more than 3 months and is associated with hearing loss, *myringotomy* with insertion of *tympanostomy tubes* (pressure-equalizing tubes) may be performed (Kerschner & Preciado, 2016). During this operation, mucoid material is removed from the middle ear and a tympanostomy tube is inserted through the tympanic membrane. A tympanostomy tube is a small polyethylene tube that is inserted into the middle ear to equalize the pressure on both sides of the tympanic membrane and to keep the ear aerated. Negative pressure in the middle ear is relieved, allowing the middle ear mucosa to return to normal and growth of the eustachian tube to occur. The tube usually falls out spontaneously in 6 to 12 months. This period may provide enough time for the effusion process to resolve, but some children need repeated insertions of tympanostomy tubes because of persistent eustachian tube dysfunction. Tympanostomy tubes are inserted with the child under general anesthesia, usually in an outpatient surgery setting.

One little-known preventive intervention for children who experience episodes of AOM is the use of xylitol, a sugar-like substance that interferes with organism adherence to mucous membranes (Danhauer et al., 2015). Xylitol comes in several different types of preparations, which include chewing gum, syrup, nasal spray, and lozenges. The issue is that in order to be effective, it must be administered to the child between three and five times a day, a regimen that is difficult for parents. However, this treatment has shown promise in reducing episodes of otitis media (Danhauer et al., 2015).

## NURSING CARE

### The Child With Otitis Media

#### Assessment

Ask the parent whether the child has had a recent upper respiratory tract infection or previous ear infections. Assess the child for fever and pain. Because signs of ear infection can be subtle in infants, the nurse should assess not only for obvious signs of ear pain, such as head rolling and pulling at the ear, but also for nonspecific findings, such as irritability, diarrhea, and decreased appetite. Older children may complain of pain or a feeling of fullness in the affected ear. The nurse should examine the ear with a pneumatic otoscope, noting the color, mobility, and translucency of the tympanic membrane and the appearance of the external canal. The tympanic membrane should be inspected carefully for signs of perforation. The nurse can obtain a culture of any drainage and notes the color, consistency, and odor. Hearing and language development should be assessed.

#### Nursing Diagnosis and Planning

The nursing diagnoses and expected outcomes that may be appropriate for the family and infant or child with otitis media are as follows:

- Acute Pain related to inflammation and pressure in the middle ear.

**Expected outcome.** The child will be free of pain, as evidenced by sleeping through the night, not pulling at the ears, and decreased crying. The child's tympanic membranes will appear shiny and pearl-gray, with normal landmarks, a visible light reflex, and normal mobility on tympanography.

- Deficient Knowledge related to incomplete understanding of the disease process and treatment regimen.

**Expected outcome.** The parents will demonstrate (1) methods of feeding the infant that decrease the risk for otitis media, (2) how to keep the child's ears dry if tympanostomy tubes are in place, and (3) ways to follow the treatment regimen, including administering the entire course of antibiotics.

- Risk for Imbalanced Body Temperature related to inflammation.

**Expected outcome.** The child will display a normal body temperature.

- Risk for Deficient Fluid Volume related to elevated temperature and decreased intake.

**Expected outcome.** The child will have moist mucous membranes, good skin turgor, and appropriate intake and output for age.

#### Interventions

Teach the parents the importance of giving prescribed antibiotics on time and for the prescribed number of days. Because the child usually feels much better after a few days of medication, parents may believe that the antibiotics are no longer necessary and stop giving them. Increase adherence by giving written and oral instructions for administering medications. Providing a medication record form on which to record doses taken and a calibrated measuring device for liquid medications is also helpful.

The nurse also advises the parents to discard any unused antibiotic rather than save it and not to give the child an antibiotic without consulting the physician first.

Acetaminophen can be given to relieve discomfort. The child's fluid intake should be increased if fever is present. Advise the parents to notify the physician if the child's condition has not improved after 48 hours of observation without antibiotics, after 48 hours of antibiotic treatment without improvement in symptoms, or if there is drainage from the affected ear. If a follow-up visit is recommended, emphasize the importance of keeping the appointment.

The nurse can enhance medication adherence through specific teaching about administration of antibiotics. For example, the nurse might say, "After a few days, your child may seem to be well and show no signs of the ear infection. If you stop giving the antibiotic at that time, some of the germs that caused the otitis media might still be alive, and your child could have a relapse."

If the child is undergoing myringotomy with insertion of tympanostomy tubes, the nurse prepares the child and parents as for any outpatient surgical procedure. Explain the procedure in clear terms and answer questions simply and honestly.

Postoperatively, the child is monitored for ear drainage. A small amount of reddish drainage is normal for the first few days after surgery, but the parents should report any heavier bleeding or bleeding that occurs after 3 days. The parents should also be instructed to report any fever or increased pain. The child should avoid blowing the nose for 7 to 10 days.

Most physicians prefer that the child's ears be kept dry if tubes are in place, but some believe that a small amount of water in the ears is not harmful. However, bath and lake water are potential sources of bacterial contamination, and chlorinated swimming pool water can be irritating to tympanic membranes with tubes. The usual recommendation is to place ear plugs or cotton balls covered with petroleum jelly in the ears during baths and shampoos. Swimming is allowed only with ear plugs and the physician's approval. Diving and swimming deep under water are prohibited. The size and appearance of the tympanostomy tubes should be described to the parents, and they should be reassured that if the tubes fall out it is not an emergency but that the physician should be notified.

Otitis media is usually a chronic problem, with frequent recurrences of infection and effusion. The nurse teaches the parents the early signs of ear infection and the importance of seeking care if these signs should occur. Because hearing impairment from middle ear effusion can be very difficult for parents to detect, the child with chronic otitis media should undergo periodic hearing evaluations.

The nurse should teach parents methods to decrease the risk for recurrent otitis media, such as breastfeeding during infancy, discontinuing bottle feeding as soon as possible, feeding the infant in an upright position, and refraining from giving a bottle to the infant in bed. Parents should be told not to smoke in the child's presence because passive smoking increases the incidence of otitis media.

### Evaluation

- Is the child sleeping an appropriate amount of time for age with decreased episodes of crying or pulling at ears?
- Have otoscopic findings returned to normal?
- Did the parents complete the treatment regimen by giving the entire dose of the prescribed antibiotic, and are they able to demonstrate appropriate feeding methods?
- Were follow-up appointments kept to determine the resolution of the otitis media?
- Is the child afebrile?
- Does the child appear well hydrated with moist mucous membranes and good skin turgor?

## PHARYNGITIS AND TONSILLITIS

Pharyngitis, inflammation of the pharynx and surrounding lymphoid tissue, can be viral or bacterial in origin. Although pharyngitis is a self-limiting and relatively minor disorder, streptococcal infections can have serious complications—among them, rheumatic fever and acute glomerulonephritis.

*Tonsillitis* is the term commonly used to describe inflammation and infection of the two palatine tonsils. *Adenoiditis* refers to infection and inflammation of the pharyngeal tonsils, or adenoids, which are located above the palatine tonsils on the posterior wall of the nasopharynx. The purpose of these lymphoid tissues is to filter and protect the respiratory and digestive tracts from invasion by pathogens, but often the tonsils become a site for infection.

### Etiology

A variety of viruses play a role in pharyngitis, most notably adenoviruses, coronaviruses, enteroviruses (e.g., coxsackievirus), and respiratory syncytial virus. Group A beta-hemolytic streptococcal (GABHS) bacteria are an important and most frequently seen bacterial cause of pharyngitis (Tanz, 2016). Streptococcal pharyngitis is rare before age 3 years. Streptococcal infection is spread by close droplet transmission. Tonsillitis, like pharyngitis, can be bacterial or viral in origin.

The incidence of pharyngitis and tonsillitis peaks during middle childhood, when most children begin preschool and elementary school and have increased exposure to microorganisms. Group A beta-hemolytic streptococcal infection occurs most frequently in the winter and is spread more readily in crowded living situations. The incidence of tonsillitis decreases during middle childhood as the lymphoid tissue undergoes normal shrinkage.

### Manifestations

Signs and symptoms differ between viral and bacterial pharyngitis (Table 45.1). Not all children with pharyngitis complain of a sore throat, particularly if they are of preschool age. Instead, the child may complain of a stomachache or simply refuse to eat. The child with tonsillitis demonstrates the following:

- Sore throat, which can be persistent or recurrent
- Tonsils enlarged and bright red; may be covered with white exudate or cryptic plugs
- Difficulty swallowing
- Mouth breathing and an unpleasant mouth odor

**TABLE 45.1 Comparison of Viral and Bacterial Pharyngitis**

| Viral Pharyngitis | Bacterial Pharyngitis |
|---|---|
| Gradual onset | Abrupt onset (may be gradual in children <2 yr old) |
| Sore throat (reaches a peak on the second or third day) | Sore throat (usually severe) |
| Erythema and inflammation of the pharynx and tonsils (may be slight), vesicles or ulcers on tonsils | Erythema and inflammation of the pharynx and tonsils |
| Fever (usually low grade but may be high) | Fever (usually high, 39.4-40° C [103-104° F], but may be moderate), begins early in illness and usually lasts 1-4 days |
| Hoarseness, cough, rhinitis, conjunctivitis, malaise, anorexia (early) | Abdominal pain, vomiting, headache |
| Cervical lymph nodes may be enlarged and tender | Cervical lymph nodes may be enlarged and tender |
| Usually lasts 3-4 days | Usually lasts 3-5 days |

- Enlarged adenoids, which may cause a nasal quality of speech, mouth breathing, hearing difficulty, otitis media, snoring, or obstructive sleep apnea

Older children and adolescents can have a *peritonsillar abscess* associated with pharyngitis or tonsillitis. A peritonsillar abscess usually is unilateral, with the enlarged tonsil displacing the uvula to the opposite side. The child might refuse to talk or swallow because of severe pain that often radiates to the ear. There is a risk of airway obstruction and dehydration with this condition.

## PATHOPHYSIOLOGY

### Pharyngitis

Pharyngitis often accompanies the common cold. Tonsillitis is usually present with pharyngitis. Infection and inflammation of the tonsils cause them to enlarge. The palatine tonsils may meet in the midline ("kissing tonsils") and cause difficulty swallowing and breathing. If adenoids enlarge, they can obstruct the eustachian tubes, resulting in otitis media and hearing impairment. Hypertrophy of the adenoids can also block the passageway between the nose and the throat, causing mouth breathing or obstructive sleep apnea.

### Diagnostic Evaluation

The only reliable means of determining whether a case of pharyngitis is viral or bacterial in origin is with a throat culture; however, rapid antigen diagnostic testing (RAPDT) for streptococcal infection is considered to be highly specific (correctly diagnoses streptococcal infection), negating the necessity for a more expensive throat culture (Lean, Arnup, Danchin, et al, 2014). Rapid strep tests can give false-negative results; therefore, if the child's symptoms suggest a streptococcal infection or there is a family history of infection or exposure, throat swab for testing should be done using two swabs simultaneously to allow for a follow-up throat culture if needed. Because a small percentage of children carry group A beta-hemolytic streptococci in their throats, a positive throat culture is not proof of active infection.

### Therapeutic Management

During the acute phase of pharyngitis or tonsillitis, treatment is symptomatic, focusing on pain relief and rest. Acetaminophen or ibuprofen is used for pain; older children may find gargling with warm saline solution comforting. Cool, bland liquids are tolerated best because of the discomfort caused by swallowing solids or irritating liquids.

Antibiotics should be restricted to those children who test positive on rapid detection tests or cultures. The primary reason for treating streptococcal pharyngitis is to prevent acute rheumatic fever and its consequences (see Chapter 41). Streptococcal pharyngitis is most frequently treated orally with penicillin V given two to four times daily, depending on weight and age, for 10 days. Amoxicillin given daily for 10 days is considered to be as effective but more acceptable in taste for children (AAP Committee on Infectious Diseases, 2015). Cephalosporin, clindamycin, or erythromycin can be used for children who are allergic to penicillin; if using azithromycin, a 5-day course is effective as well (AAP Committee on Infectious Diseases, 2015). A single intramuscular dose of procaine penicillin and benzathine penicillin G might be considered in children for whom adherence is expected to be a problem. Children given penicillin therapy are noninfectious to others 24 hours after therapy is initiated.

Surgical removal of the tonsils, or tonsillectomy, is controversial. Although some physicians think that a tonsillectomy is warranted in cases of recurrent tonsillitis, the prevailing attitude is more conservative, and the procedure is generally reserved for cases of upper airway obstruction, peritonsillar abscess, obstructive sleep apnea, or other serious problems. Tonsillectomy is generally not performed in children younger than 3 years because of the tendency for remaining tonsillar tissues to hypertrophy. Contraindications to tonsillectomy include active infection and cleft palate (see Chapter 43). Surgical removal of the tonsils while they are infected can result in spread of the infecting organism and sepsis. In children with cleft palate, the tonsils help prevent air escape during speech. Adenoidectomy alone may be performed in cases of recurrent otitis media caused by eustachian tube obstruction or for persistent nasal or airway obstruction.

Many parents believe that a tonsillectomy will solve their child's problems of frequent sore throats, mouth breathing, and poor weight gain. There is no evidence that a tonsillectomy reduces the incidence of recurrent pharyngitis, but only for one to two years (Tanz, 2016). The nurse should be prepared to discuss the current treatment philosophy with parents and address their concerns. If tonsillectomy is chosen as the method of treatment, the procedure is often done in a day-surgery setting.

### Nursing Considerations

Assessment of the child with pharyngitis or tonsillitis includes inspecting the pharynx for erythema, exudate, or petechiae. The skin should be inspected for rash and color changes. Some children with streptococcal pharyngitis have a pink, sandpaper-like rash on the trunk (see Chapter 41) that peels after several days. The child is questioned about the onset and location of throat, ear, or abdominal pain. The parent of a preverbal child may report that the child refuses to eat or begins to cry during feedings. The nurse also assesses the child's temperature and respiratory status and asks the older child or parent about the onset of symptoms and any known contact with streptococcal infection in the school or family. Also ask whether the child has been taking any antibiotics at home, because antibiotics will interfere with the results of the throat culture.

Measures to relieve throat discomfort include administering acetaminophen, warm salt water gargles (¼ teaspoon of salt per 8-oz glass of water), and warm or cool compresses applied to the neck. The child should not be forced to eat. Offer cool, bland liquids to prevent dehydration. Soft foods such as gelatin, soup, mashed potatoes, puddings, Cream of Wheat, and flavored ice pops appeal to children the best. Bed rest is advisable while the child has a fever. The nurse should advise the parents to call the healthcare provider if the child has difficulty breathing or increased difficulty swallowing or if the fever has lasted more than 3 days. If a fever, sore throat, or headache develops in any family members, they should have a throat culture. Instruct the parents that leftover antibiotics from siblings or friends should never be used.

Moist mucous membranes and adequate urine output are signs of proper fluid balance. At the end of treatment, the child should be free of signs of infection and show no signs of complications of the disease.

## NURSING CARE

### The Child Undergoing a Tonsillectomy

#### Assessment: Preoperative Period

A complete history is taken, with special attention given to allergy symptoms, difficulty swallowing, or airway obstruction. The child is assessed for signs of active infection (fever, elevated white blood cell [WBC] count) and redness and presence of exudate in the throat. The child should be questioned about the presence of pain in the throat or ears. Because the tonsillar area is so vascular, any bleeding history must be recorded and communicated to the primary physician.

Laboratory results (prothrombin time, partial thromboplastin time, platelet count, hemoglobin, hematocrit, urinalysis) are reviewed, and the child should be checked for loose teeth to decrease the risk for aspiration during surgery. A complete current medication list should be reviewed as well.

### Nursing Diagnosis and Planning: Preoperative Period

The nursing diagnoses and expected outcomes that may be appropriate for the child undergoing a tonsillectomy and the child's family are as follows:

- Anxiety related to surgery.
  *Expected outcome.* The child and parents will exhibit a decreased level of anxiety, as evidenced by relaxed body posture and involvement in play activities.
- Deficient Knowledge related to surgery and procedures.
  *Expected outcome.* The child and parents will restate preoperative teaching.

### Interventions: Preoperative Period

The nurse reassures the child that talking will not be a problem after surgery. Providing the child a way to communicate will reduce postoperative anxiety. Emphasize to the child that it is important to drink liquids after surgery, although the child's throat will be sore (see also Chapter 40). It is important to maintain hydration postoperatively to promote healing. Teach the child's family about postoperative pain assessment and appropriate analgesia administration because many parents undermedicate their children. Undermedication can interfere with optimal postoperative recovery.

### Evaluation: Preoperative Period

- Does the child demonstrate relaxed body posture and the ability to engage in play while waiting for surgery?
- Can the parents describe what to expect during the postoperative period?

### Assessment: Postoperative Period

Immediately after surgery, the child should be assessed for bleeding and ability to swallow secretions. Postoperative hemorrhage is a dangerous complication that will need immediate attention. If bleeding occurs, the child is returned to surgery for recauterization. The rate and quality of respirations and breath sounds should be assessed. Vital signs, including blood pressure, should be monitored frequently until discharge. Suction equipment should be available, but do not suction unless there is airway obstruction. The child is assessed for bleeding (frequent swallowing; restlessness; a fast, thready pulse; or vomiting bright red blood). When visually assessing the site for clots or bleeding, use a flashlight for illumination and avoid using a tongue depressor if at all possible. If a tongue depressor is necessary, use a sterile tongue depressor and keep it as far forward in the mouth as possible.

**SAFETY ALERT**

***Caring for the Child Who Has Had a Tonsillectomy***

Assessing the child for postoperative bleeding is most important. Because the operative site is not as readily visible as other sites, the nurse needs to look for the following:

- Excessive swallowing
- Elevated pulse; decreasing blood pressure
- Signs of fresh bleeding in the back of the throat
- Vomiting bright-red blood
- Restlessness that does not seem to be associated with pain

### Nursing Diagnosis and Planning: Postoperative Period

The nursing diagnoses and expected outcomes that may be appropriate for the child who has undergone a tonsillectomy and the child's family are as follows:

- Risk for Injury (hemorrhage) related to surgery.
  *Expected outcome.* The child will experience minimal postoperative bleeding, as evidenced by vital signs within normal limits and absence of excessive swallowing, bright red vomitus, or restlessness.
- Ineffective Airway Clearance related to throat discomfort.
  *Expected outcome.* The child will maintain a clear airway without jeopardizing the operative site.
- Acute Pain related to surgical removal of tonsils.
  *Expected outcome.* The child will describe relief from pain and will be able to rest.
- Risk for Deficient Fluid Volume related to difficulty swallowing and nothing-by-mouth (NPO) status before surgery.
  *Expected outcome.* The child will have adequate fluid intake for age and minimal fluid loss.
- Deficient Knowledge related to home care.
  *Expected outcome.* The parents will describe how to care for their child at home.

### Interventions: Postoperative

The child should be placed in a prone or side-lying position to facilitate drainage. Although not all clinicians are in agreement, straws and forks may be withheld to prevent trauma to the surgical site. If bleeding occurs, the child is turned to the side and the physician notified.

Vomiting of old blood ("coffee grounds" emesis) is common. Antiemetics are given as ordered to decrease throat pain caused by retching. If vomiting occurs, keep the child on NPO status for 30 minutes and then resume clear liquids.

Nonaspirin analgesics (e.g., acetaminophen, ibuprofen) are given as ordered. Adequate analgesia increases fluid intake. It is common to prescribe the analgesic every 4 hours (or every three hours if alternating acetaminophen with ibuprofen) for the first 24 hours because throat discomfort is expected. An ice collar can be applied for comfort.

Provide clear, cool liquids when the child is fully awake. Avoid citrus drinks, carbonated drinks, and extremely hot or cold liquids because they may irritate the throat. Milk and milk products (puddings, ice cream) can coat the throat, causing a need to clear the throat, and thus, increasing the risk for bleeding. Adequate fluid intake promotes healing and maintains hydration. The nurse teaches the parents the principles of home management and ensures that the child is retaining fluids before discharging the child from the surgical unit. Be sure to tell the parent to monitor the child for postoperative bleeding both within the first 24 hours and again 7 to 10 days after surgery (see Patient-Centered Teaching: Caring for a Child after a Tonsillectomy).

### Evaluation: Postoperative

- Does the child have minimal bleeding, nausea, and vomiting, and are vital signs within normal limits?
- Is the child taking clear liquids and avoiding liquids that irritate the throat?
- Are the child's complaints of pain and irritability minimal?
- Can the parents describe home care measures?

## LARYNGOMALACIA (CONGENITAL LARYNGEAL STRIDOR)

Flaccidity of the epiglottis and supraglottic aperture and weakness of the airway walls contribute to laryngomalacia, the most common cause

## PATIENT-CENTERED TEACHING

### *Caring for a Child After a Tonsillectomy*

- Encourage your child to participate only in quiet activities for 1 week after surgery.
- Encourage abundant liquid intake. Avoid citrus juices, which irritate the throat, for 10 days.
- Avoid red liquids, which will give the appearance of blood if your child vomits.
- Add full liquids (cream soups, gelatin, puddings, and other soups) on the second day and soft foods (mashed potatoes, soft cereals, eggs) as your child tolerates them. Avoid rough or scratchy foods (bacon, chips, popcorn), citrus foods, or spicy foods for 3 weeks.
- Encourage your child to chew and swallow because this exercises pharyngeal muscles and promotes healing.
- Do not give your child any straws, forks, or sharp pointed toys that could be put in the mouth.
- Use acetaminophen for pain relief, or alternate acetaminophen with ibuprofen (Liu & Ulualp, 2015)
- Pain should not persist past the first week. Notify your physician if pain persists.
- Discourage your child from coughing, clearing the throat, or gargling.
- Bad mouth odor is normal and may be relieved by drinking more liquids.
- Earache and slight fever are common.
- Call your physician for any bleeding, persistent earache, or fever greater than 38.3° C (101° F).
- Bleeding caused by tissue sloughing during the healing process can occur 7 to 10 days after surgery. Such bleeding requires immediate medical attention.
- Keep your child away from crowds for 2 weeks to avoid catching a cold.
- Your child may return to school when directed by the physician, usually in approximately 10 days.
- Bring your child for a follow-up appointment in 1 to 2 weeks.

## CRITICAL THINKING EXERCISE 45.1

Discharge teaching following a tonsillectomy should include pain management. Inadequate pain relief at home is a major nursing concern.

1. What factors can contribute to inadequate pain relief?
2. What effects might inadequate pain relief have on the child?

of inspiratory stridor in the neonatal period (Schroeder & Holinger, 2016). Laryngomalacia may be caused by immature neuromuscular development in the airway.

### Manifestations

Noisy, crowing inspiratory respiratory sounds (**stridor**) are present, with or without retractions. The infant usually remains acyanotic despite the stridor. Stridor is usually present at birth but may begin as late as age 2 months. Symptoms increase when the infant is supine or when the infant is crying. There may be associated reflux or dysphagia. The diagnosis is based on a thorough history and on findings on direct laryngoscopy.

### Therapeutic Management

Symptoms usually resolve without treatment by age 18 to 24 months. In rare instances, endotracheal intubation or tracheostomy may be required.

### Nursing Considerations

The nurse observes the neonate for stridor, retractions, and dyspnea, noting any signs of acute respiratory distress. Because some infants have feeding problems, the infant should be observed for feeding difficulties and appropriate growth and development patterns. The infant's respiratory status is assessed, and findings are recorded every 2 hours and as needed. Obstruction may increase during crying or when the child has a respiratory infection. Stridor may increase when the child is supine with the neck flexed. Positioning with the neck hyperextended improves the child's breathing by reducing the obstruction, and thus, improves the stridor.

As part of discharge teaching, parents are taught the signs of respiratory distress so that they can monitor for changes that might indicate respiratory tract infection. If the bottle-fed infant has feeding difficulties, the parents can try using a smaller nipple. Smaller, more frequent feedings are sometimes better tolerated by infants with respiratory difficulties. Reassure the parents that the condition usually resolves by the time the child is 2 years old. The ability of parents to comfortably care for their child indicates the effectiveness of the discharge teaching.

## CROUP

Croup refers to a group of conditions characterized by inspiratory stridor, a harsh (brassy or croupy) cough, hoarseness, and varying degrees of respiratory distress (Table 45.2). The major types of croup are acute spasmodic croup, laryngotracheobronchitis, bacterial tracheitis, and epiglottitis. Although epiglottitis is a type of croup, it is discussed separately because it is a bacterial infection with unique symptoms and treatment.

### Etiology and Incidence

Parainfluenza viruses cause most cases of viral croup. The cause of acute spasmodic croup is unknown.

Laryngotracheobronchitis, the most common form of croup, usually affects infants and toddlers; it is one cause of airway obstruction in children ages 6 months to 6 years. The incidence of croup is higher in boys than in girls, and the disease occurs more often during the winter than in other seasons (Roosevelt, 2016).

Acute spasmodic croup occurs most often in children ages 1 to 3 years. Spasmodic croup occurs more often in anxious and excitable children. There seems to be hereditary predisposition to spasmodic croup (Roosevelt, 2016).

Bacterial tracheitis is less common than laryngotracheobronchitis and acute spasmodic croup. It progresses from an upper respiratory tract infection and may be confused with laryngotracheobronchitis because of similar manifestations. Treatment for laryngotracheobronchitis is not effective if the child has bacterial tracheitis.

The following discussion focuses on acute spasmodic croup and laryngotracheobronchitis, the most common types of croup leading to hospitalization.

### Manifestations

Croup often begins at night and may be preceded by several days of symptoms of upper respiratory tract infection. The child with laryngotracheobronchitis may have a gradual onset and a fever along with other signs and symptoms; occasionally the fever is as high as 40° C (104° F). Children with spasmodic croup do not have a fever. Other manifestations include the following:

- The sudden onset of a harsh, metallic barky cough; sore throat; inspiratory stridor; and hoarseness

**TABLE 45.2 Comparison of Types of Croup**

| | Acute Spasmodic Laryngitis (Spasmodic Croup) | Acute Laryngotracheobronchitis (Ltb) | Acute Epiglottitis | Acute Tracheitis |
|---|---|---|---|---|
| Age usually affected | 1-3 yr | 3 mo-3 yr | 3-7 yr | 1 mo-6 yr |
| Location of swelling and inflammation | Subglottic (below vocal cords) | Vocal cords, subglottic, and tissue below vocal cords, including bronchi | Supraglottic (above vocal cords) | Mucosa of upper trachea |
| Cause | Viral, emotional, or genetic predisposition | Usually viral but may be bacterial | Bacterial (usually Hib) | *Staphylococcus* (most common) |
| Assessment | Sudden onset, usually at night.<br>Child awakens with harsh cough, inspiratory stridor, dyspnea, and hoarseness | Gradual onset, usually at night.<br>Child awakens with harsh cough and inspiratory stridor | Sudden onset, which can rapidly progress to complete airway obstruction and death.<br>Sore throat, dyspnea, high fever | Progresses from upper respiratory infection (1-2 days).<br>High fever<br>Stridor<br>Croupy cough<br>Purulent secretions |
| Treatment | Increased fluids<br>May treat at home | Racemic epinephrine<br>IV fluids during respiratory distress<br>Hospitalization may be necessary | IV antibiotics<br>Artificial airway<br>IV fluids<br>Emergency hospitalization | Humidified oxygen<br>Antipyretics<br>IV antibiotics<br>May require intubation |

Hib, *Haemophilus influenzae* type B; IV, intravenous.

- The use of accessory muscles (substernal, intercostal, suprasternal retractions) to breathe
- Frightened appearance
- Agitation
- Cyanosis

### Diagnostic Evaluation

The diagnosis is made mainly from observation of clinical symptoms. Differentiation between viral croup and bacterial epiglottitis is very important because treatment differs. However, the use of the *H. influenzae* type B (Hib) vaccine has reduced the incidence of epiglottitis. A croup score is often used to describe the severity of respiratory distress. Arterial blood gas values or pulse oximetry readings may be monitored to detect decreased $PaO_2$ levels.

### Therapeutic Management

The goal of treatment is to maintain a patent airway. Children with acute spasmodic croup can usually be cared for at home. Treatment for acute spasmodic croup includes a calm approach and increased oral fluid intake if the child is not in respiratory distress. Taking the child out into the cool, humid night air may relieve mucosal swelling (Roosevelt, 2016).

Crying aggravates the airway obstruction. Children who develop stridor at rest, cyanosis, severe agitation, fatigue, moderate to severe retractions, or are unable to take oral fluids should be seen in the emergency department. For mild croup, oral dexamethasone in a single dose of 0.15 to 0.6 mg/kg or inhaled budesonide decreases airway inflammation and reduces the necessity for hospitalization for many children (Garbutt et al., 2013; Nierengarten, 2015).

Children with laryngotracheobronchitis, usually a more severe type of croup, are more often hospitalized than are those with acute spasmodic croup. Racemic epinephrine nebulized with oxygen can be given to decrease the laryngeal edema and bronchospasm. The child must be observed closely for changes in respiratory status and should not be treated with epinephrine on an outpatient basis because the effects of epinephrine are temporary. Croup symptoms can reoccur after approximately 2 hours, so children who receive epinephrine should be observed in the emergency department for at least 3 hours after treatment and should not be discharged if stridor or retractions are present. Antibiotics are not indicated unless a bacterial infection is present. Acetaminophen is given to reduce fever.

For children with more severe symptoms (progressively worsening stridor, cyanosis, decreased oxygen saturation, retractions), hospitalization is necessary. Humidified oxygen and intravenous (IV) fluids are given until respiratory distress subsides and the child can take adequate fluids by mouth. Sedatives are contraindicated because they depress respirations and could mask restlessness, an early sign of hypoxia.

If signs of moderate or severe hypoxia develop, the child is intubated immediately and is transferred to an intensive care unit. Usually, the tube remains in place for 3 to 5 days and is removed when the child can breathe around the tube and the inflammation subsides.

## NURSING CARE

### The Child With Croup

#### Assessment

A nursing history typically reveals a recent upper respiratory tract infection. Assess the child for inspiratory stridor, barking cough, hoarseness, and increased heart and respiratory rates. Record any signs of respiratory distress, such as the use of accessory muscles; substernal, intercostal, and suprasternal retractions; nasal flaring; restlessness and irritability; and pallor or cyanosis. Cyanosis, increased heart rate and respiratory rate, extreme restlessness, or evidence of fatigue or listlessness are signs of hypoxia and should be reported to the physician immediately (Nierengarten, 2015). The lungs should be auscultated for adventitious breath sounds or areas of decreased breath sounds. Temperature and hydration status should also be assessed.

#### Nursing Diagnosis and Planning

The diagnoses and expected outcomes that may be appropriate for the child with croup and the child's family are as follows:

- Ineffective Airway Clearance related to mucosal swelling and obstruction of the upper respiratory tract.

## PATHOPHYSIOLOGY

### Croup

Croup is a viral infection of the upper airway. Although the entire upper, or nonreactive, airway is involved to some extent in all forms of croup, each type is named according to the anatomic area most severely involved. For example, laryngotracheobronchitis affects the larynx, trachea, and bronchi. In acute spasmodic croup, the larynx is the area of most severe inflammation.

In all forms of croup, mucosal inflammation and edema cause narrowing of the airway. This narrowing is more dangerous in infants and young children than in adults because of their small airway diameter and flexible larynx, which is more susceptible to spasm.

Symptoms are usually worse at night and better in the day; they may recur for several nights. Croup usually lasts 3 to 4 days.

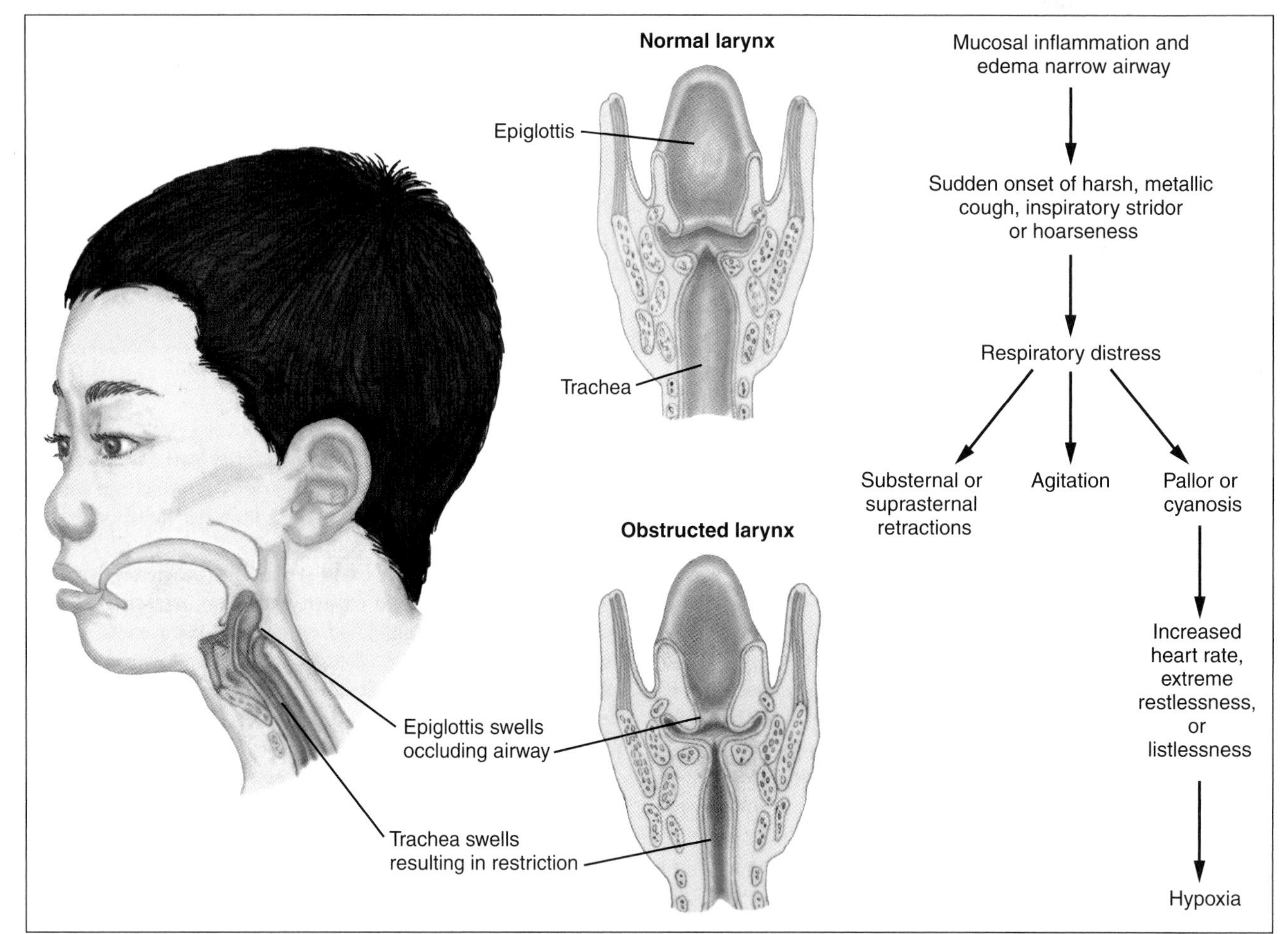


***Expected outcome.*** The child will breathe without difficulty and have a heart rate and respiratory rate within normal limits for age.

- Risk for Deficient Fluid Volume related to inadequate oral intake and tachypnea.

***Expected outcome.*** The child will have adequate fluid intake for age and weight.

- Fear related to dyspnea and hospitalization.

***Expected outcome.*** The child will appear less fearful, as evidenced by resting quietly, decreased crying, and cooperating with nursing care as appropriate for age. The parent will demonstrate decreased fear, as evidenced by their ability to assist the child to deal with stressors of hospitalization and illness.

- Deficient Knowledge related to the course of croup and home care.

***Expected outcome.*** The parents will have accurate knowledge of croup symptoms, state that they are comfortable in home management of croup, and seek assistance appropriately if symptoms become severe.

#### Interventions

***Facilitating airway clearance.*** The nurse monitors the child's breathing continuously for signs and symptoms of increased respiratory distress (increased respiratory rate, stridor at rest, nasal flaring, retractions, cyanosis, changes in level of consciousness or increased irritability, decreased or adventitious breath sounds, tachypnea). A child with respiratory distress should never be left alone, and the physician should be notified immediately. If epiglottitis is suspected, the physician should be contacted and the throat should not be inspected because such examination can result in laryngospasm and airway obstruction. The nurse should administer humidified oxygen at the ordered flow rate. Record vital signs and pulse oximetry readings frequently. There should be emergency intubation equipment (e.g., intubation tray, oxygen, suction, manual resuscitation bag-valve-mask) closely available should the child's condition change rapidly. Aerosolized racemic epinephrine is often administered to decrease laryngeal edema, and dexamethasone is given as an antiinflammatory agent. The child should be observed for recurrence of obstruction, which may occur within a few hours after administration of racemic epinephrine.

The child should be kept as quiet as possible because crying can aggravate laryngospasm and increase hypoxia. Encourage parents to stay nearby. Maintain a calm, quiet environment. Observe the child closely but disturb as little as possible. Support the child in an upright position with the head of the bed elevated to facilitate respiration.

***Maintaining fluid balance.*** Tachypnea causes insensible water loss, and difficulty swallowing leads to decreased intake. Therefore, the nurse monitors the child's hydration status with intake and output and urine specific gravity measurements. Check mucous membranes, skin turgor, and presence of tears. Weigh the child daily on the same scale and at the same time of day. Offer the child clear, room temperature liquids as tolerated when the child no longer exhibits signs of respiratory distress. Observe the child's ability to swallow because tachypnea and laryngospasm often cause dysphagia. IV fluids are administered in the acute phase of croup because oral fluids are contraindicated in the setting of severe respiratory distress that heightens the risk for aspiration. The child's temperature is taken every 4 hours, and acetaminophen is administered as ordered.

***Decreasing fear.*** Maintain a calm, restful environment for the child and organize nursing care so as to disturb the child as little as possible and allow for periods of uninterrupted rest. Encourage parents to touch and cuddle the child, because a parent's presence is important in reducing fear in infants and young children. Also, encourage parents' participation in care and explain ways that they can make their child more comfortable. Caring for a child in the hospital is exhausting for parents, and fatigue magnifies feelings of anxiety and helplessness. Therefore, provide parents with breaks as needed and assure them that their child will be cared for in their absence. Allow the child to keep a favorite toy or blanket and use developmentally appropriate communication techniques (e.g., play, puppets) when explaining treatments and procedures. Allow the child and parents to ask questions and to discuss fears and concerns, because croup symptoms can be frightening and parents sometimes feel guilty for not having brought the child in for treatment sooner.

***Providing teaching.*** The nurse determines the parents' level of understanding of croup and previous experiences in coping with the illness. Teach the parents that once a child has had an attack, croup may recur. Teach the parents that maintaining a stable environmental temperature and humidity and keeping the child well hydrated may help decrease the severity of attacks. Teach that croup is a viral infection and that avoiding large groups of people and practicing good health habits to prevent infection may decrease the risk for recurrence of croup. Teach parents the signs and symptoms of respiratory distress and symptoms that should prompt a call to the physician:

- Increased difficulty breathing or worsening of symptoms
- Retractions (tugging in of the skin between, above, or below the ribs with inspiration)
- Lips turn bluish or dusky
- Breathing cool or warm mist does not improve symptoms in 20 minutes
- Inability to drink much over the past 24 hours
- Drooling or difficulty swallowing
- Fever (greater than 39.4° C [103° F])
- Lethargy, listlessness, or severe agitation

The nurse emphasizes the importance of adequate hydration and nutrition. Parents are taught that acetaminophen or ibuprofen is effective in reducing fever and will help the child feel more comfortable. Cough syrups and cold medicines are avoided because they can dry and thicken secretions.

### Evaluation

- Are the child's respiratory rate and heart rate within normal limits for age, and is the oxygen saturation greater than 95%?
- Does the infant have moist mucous membranes, good skin turgor, and urine output appropriate for age? (See Chapter 40.)
- Does the child exhibit decreased signs of agitation or being upset (less crying), and is the parent able to comfort the child?
- Can the parents explain the appropriate treatment for croup and when medical help is needed?

## EPIGLOTTITIS (SUPRAGLOTTITIS)

Epiglottitis, the acute inflammation and swelling of the epiglottis and surrounding tissue, is a life-threatening, rapidly progressive condition that can cause complete airway obstruction within a few hours of onset.

### Etiology and Incidence

Epiglottitis is almost always caused by *H. influenzae.* Other organisms, such as *S. aureus, H. parainfluenzae, S. pneumoniae,* and group A beta-hemolytic streptococci, cause the infection less frequently. Viral epiglottitis is rare.

Epiglottitis occurs most often in children ages 3 to 7 years. The incidence is approximately equal in boys and girls. The incidence decreased markedly after the introduction of the Hib vaccine; however, vaccine failure and the emergence of epiglottitis caused by atypical organisms make it a relevant topic for discussion.

### Manifestations

Unlike croup, epiglottitis has an abrupt onset with rapid progression of symptoms. Often parents report that the child was put to bed well and awakened with a severe sore throat and difficulty swallowing. The child demonstrates a high fever (39° C to 40° C [102.2° F to 104° F]) and appears to be in a toxic condition and very ill. The accompanying sore throat can progress to acute respiratory distress in a few hours. The child appears anxious and frightened and may be irritable or lethargic. One of the classic signs of epiglottitis is that the child insists on sitting upright, often in a tripod position (leaning forward supported on the arms), with the chin thrust out and the mouth open. Respiratory symptoms include nasal flaring; suprasternal, substernal, and intercostal retractions; pale skin color to cyanosis (depending on the degree of airway obstruction); and tachycardia. The epiglottis appears edematous and cherry red.

**SAFETY ALERT**

***Cardinal Signs and Symptoms of Epiglottitis***

**D**rooling
**D**ysphagia (difficulty swallowing)
**D**ysphonia (difficulty talking)
**D**istressed inspiratory efforts

Do not examine or obtain material for culture from a child's throat if epiglottitis is suspected because any stimulation with a tongue depressor or culture swab could trigger complete airway obstruction.

Do not leave a child with epiglottitis unattended.

### Diagnostic Evaluation

The most reliable diagnostic sign of epiglottitis is an edematous, cherry-red epiglottis. However, examination and visual observation of

## PATHOPHYSIOLOGY

### *Epiglottitis*

Epiglottitis is a bacterial form of croup. The epiglottis and surrounding structures become inflamed as bacterial infection invades the soft tissue. The epiglottis becomes edematous and cherry red and may become so swollen that it completely covers the glottis and obstructs the airway. Secretions pool in the hypopharynx and larynx. As the disease rapidly progresses, swelling becomes so severe that the child is unable to swallow and begins to drool. The child's voice is muffled, and the throat is very sore. Inspiratory stridor, cough, and irritability are present. Complete airway obstruction can occur rapidly, resulting in hypoxia, acidosis, and death.

The onset of epiglottitis is usually sudden. The child may have had symptoms of a mild upper respiratory tract infection for a few days before symptoms began. Children with epiglottitis can progress from wellness to complete airway obstruction within 2 to 6 hours.

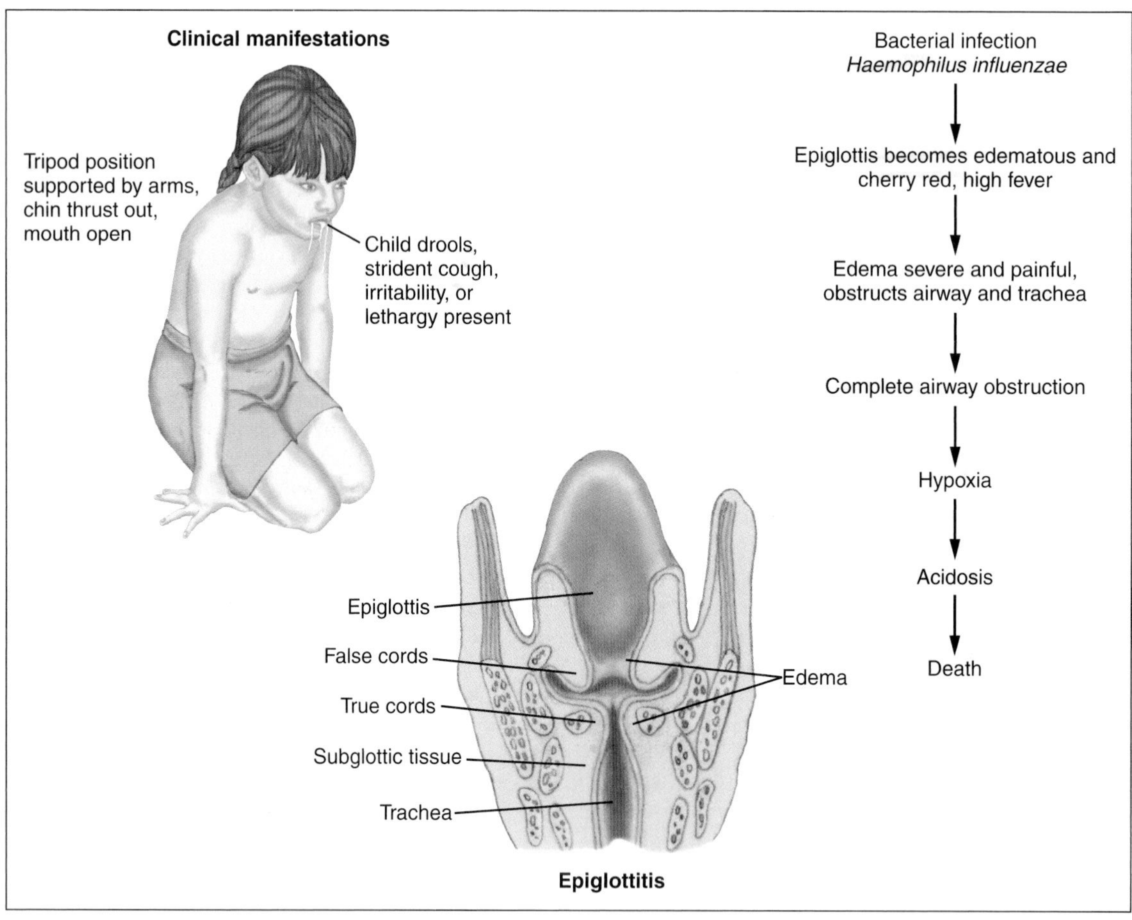


the epiglottis *are contraindicated* until emergency intubation equipment and qualified personnel are available to support the child in case of sudden airway obstruction. The child's WBC count is usually elevated (20,000 to 30,000/mm$^3$).

### Therapeutic Management

Treatment for epiglottitis should achieve a patent airway as quickly as possible. The child with epiglottitis has an edematous epiglottis that can completely obstruct the airway at any time. Radiographs are best obtained at the bedside, where the child can be constantly monitored and emergency equipment is readily available. The danger of airway obstruction is so great that usually all invasive procedures, such as venipuncture, are postponed until the child is intubated. Once the airway is secured, the child is transferred to the intensive care unit. Oxygenation status is closely monitored with arterial blood gas values or pulse oximetry, and humidified oxygen is administered. Mechanical ventilation is sometimes instituted.

Throat and blood specimens are obtained for culture after the child is intubated. Antipyretics are given for fever. Antibiotics, usually a cephalosporin, are administered IV until the child is extubated, then continued orally for a 10-day course (Roosevelt, 2016). Usually the child improves dramatically after 48 hours of antibiotic therapy and can be extubated at this time. Discharge occurs in approximately 3 to 7 days.

### Nursing Considerations

The nurse should continuously assess for signs of respiratory distress (stridor, nasal flaring, tachypnea, tachycardia, retractions, drooling, changes in level of consciousness, cyanosis). A sudden decrease in respiratory effort may be a sign of exhaustion and impending respiratory arrest. Arterial blood gas values and pulse oximetry findings are monitored. On pulse oximetry, the oxygen saturation should remain above 95%, with the $Pao_2$ between 80 and 100 mm Hg.

Maintenance of a patent airway is essential. The nurse should also keep the child as calm and quiet as possible. If temperature is taken, it should be by the axillary or tympanic route rather than the oral route. The child should be supported in a position of comfort, usually sitting straight up (orthopneic); never force the child to lie down. Children who are anxious and in respiratory distress are often less fearful sitting on their parents' laps. Parents should be encouraged to hug and comfort their child. The parents' anxiety level must be assessed and controlled because their anxiety is easily transferred to the child.

Humidified oxygen is delivered in high concentrations. Oxygen therapy is usually less upsetting if the parent holds the oxygen tubing in front of the child's face. All procedures are explained to the parent and child clearly, calmly, and according to the child's level of understanding.

Emergency intubation equipment (i.e., oxygen, laryngoscope, endotracheal tube, suction equipment) should be immediately available in case of complete airway obstruction. Worsening of the child's condition should be reported to the physician immediately.

Antipyretics are given rectally for fever. Because of the risk for aspiration, the child is kept on NPO status, and fluids are given intravenously. The nurse must closely monitor the ordered IV rate and the urine specific gravity and other indicators of hydration. IV antibiotics are administered as ordered.

If the child has an artificial airway, with either an endotracheal tube or a tracheostomy, the nurse must observe the child closely for respiratory distress and suction the airway as needed. The endotracheal tube must be securely taped to decrease movement of the tube and to minimize the chance of accidental extubation. Once intubated, the child needs to be restrained and sedated to prevent accidental extubation. It may be impossible to reintubate the child because of the severe swelling of the epiglottis. The endotracheal tube is usually kept in place for approximately 24 to 48 hours. After extubation, the child must be watched carefully and may be placed in a mist tent for 24 hours before being transferred to a pediatric unit. Normal respiratory rate and rhythm and normal color serve as evaluation criteria.

Because epiglottitis progresses rapidly and acute respiratory distress is frightening, the parents and child all have high anxiety levels. The nurse cares for the child calmly and efficiently and offers the family much-needed support during hospitalization. On discharge, the parents need to be taught how to administer the child's oral antibiotics. Reassure them that epiglottitis rarely recurs. The child should be free of respiratory difficulty, resting well, and without other distress. The nurse encourages parents of young children to have their children immunized against *H. influenzae* (see Chapter 5) to decrease the risk for contracting epiglottitis. Prophylaxis with rifampin is given to under-immunized contacts or family members younger than 4 years old and to any child contact who is immune depressed (Roosevelt, 2016).

## BRONCHITIS

Bronchitis is a disease that rarely exists by itself but occurs together with other conditions of the upper and lower respiratory tracts. It can be confused with asthma. A cough is the major sign; it usually resolves without therapy in approximately 2 weeks.

### Etiology and Incidence

Acute bronchitis is usually viral in origin. Rhinoviruses are the most common causative organisms. Other viruses thought to cause bronchitis include respiratory syncytial virus, influenza virus, parainfluenza virus, and adenovirus. Most bacterial infections occur secondary to a primary viral infection or some other airway problem. They can also occur as a result of foreign body aspiration. Air pollution has also been implicated in the disease.

The disorder is more frequent in young children and boys. It can occur anytime but is more common during the winter months than in other seasons.

### PATHOPHYSIOLOGY

#### *Bronchitis*

Inflammation of the trachea and major bronchi is present in bronchitis. Mucus production is increased, and the mucosa is congested. Because of nonspecific leukocytic migration, purulent secretions can occur even in the absence of a bacterial infection.

Acute bronchitis is a self-limiting disease. Chronic bronchitis in children may indicate an underlying chronic respiratory dysfunction.

### Manifestations and Diagnostic Evaluation

Bronchitis is characterized by the gradual onset of rhinitis and a cough that is initially nonproductive but may change to a loose cough with increased mucus production. Auscultation can reveal coarse and fine, moist crackles and high-pitched rhonchi (resembling the wheezing of asthma). Associated symptoms include malaise, low-grade fever, and increased mucus, which can be purulent.

Chest radiographs are usually normal. The diagnosis is based on the clinical findings.

### Therapeutic Management

Treatment is mainly symptomatic and includes rest, humidification, and increased fluid intake. Exposure to cigarette smoke should be avoided. Cough suppressants are not recommended unless the cough interferes with the child's ability to rest. Antihistamines should be avoided because of their drying effect on secretions. Antibiotics should be given only if a bacterial infection is confirmed by culture or if the clinical findings support the diagnosis.

### Nursing Considerations

The nurse should assess temperature, appearance of secretions, and respiratory effort every 2 to 4 hours. The child's intake should be monitored, and the nurse should observe for signs of sleep deprivation related to the persistent cough.

Advise the parents to encourage fluids by frequently offering small amounts of the child's favorite liquids and to humidify the child's room. The child should be assessed for signs of dehydration; this includes taking daily weights if the child is hospitalized. Acetaminophen is administered for an elevated temperature (usually above 38.3° C [101° F]). Quiet activities should be provided for diversion.

## BRONCHIOLITIS

Bronchiolitis, or inflammation of the bronchioles, is a significant cause of hospitalization in infants younger than 1 year. Respiratory syncytial virus (RSV) is the causative agent in more than half of cases (Coates, Camarda, & Goodman, 2016).

### Etiology and Incidence

Infants usually acquire the disease from an older child or adult, particularly a family member or daycare contact, who has a minor respiratory illness. RSV infection is easily communicable and is acquired mainly through contact with contaminated surfaces and hand-to-hand transmission. Nosocomial outbreaks in pediatric hospitals are common. RSV can live on skin or paper for up to 1 hour and on cribs and other nonporous surfaces for up to 6 hours. Although it is not airborne, it is highly communicable. It is usually transferred by inadequately washed hands. Meticulous hand hygiene decreases the spread of organisms.

## PATHOPHYSIOLOGY

### *Bronchiolitis*

In bronchiolitis, edema and the accumulation of mucus and cellular debris cause obstruction of the bronchioles. Infants' bronchioles are very small and can become obstructed quickly. Airway resistance is increased during the inspiratory and expiratory phases of respiration because of the small air passages. Hyperinflation of the lungs results from air trapping because the bronchioles constrict during expiration. Atelectasis can occur if obstruction becomes complete and trapped air is absorbed. Normal gas exchange is impaired, and the infant becomes hypoxic. Some infants have mild respiratory alkalosis; more frequently, metabolic acidosis is observed.

The child with bronchiolitis is most acutely ill during the first 48 to 72 hours after the onset of the disease. Improvement usually occurs in a few days. Symptoms may last for 10 to 14 days. Mortality rate is less than 1%. Some children who experience bronchiolitis as infants develop asthma later in childhood (Coates et al., 2016).

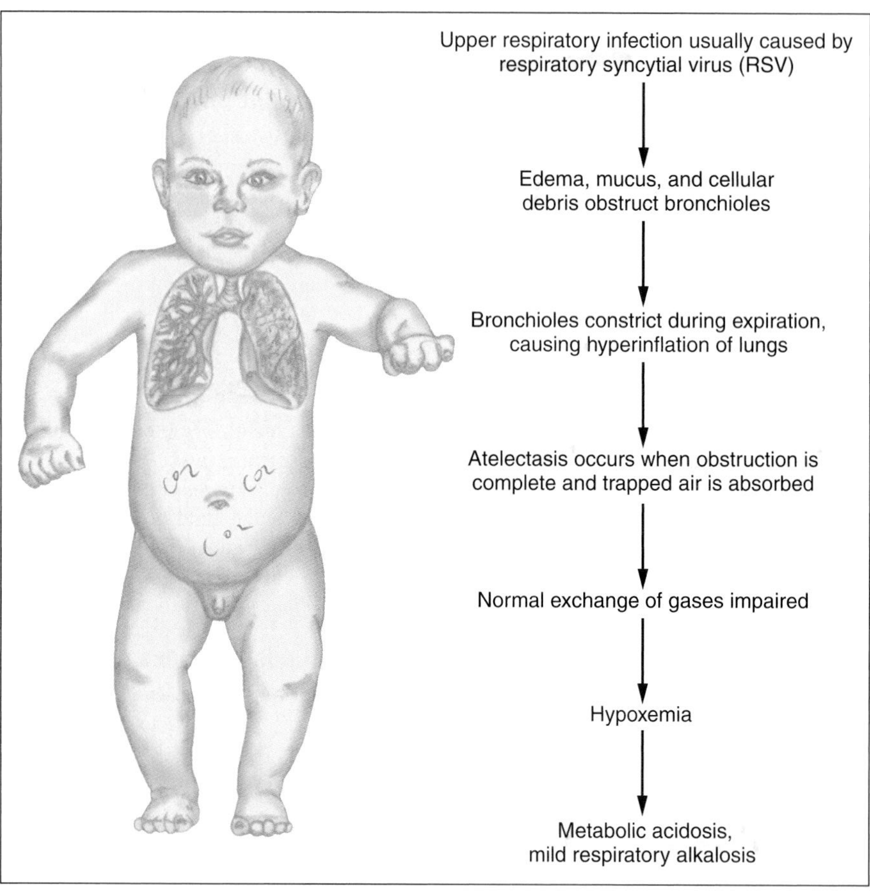


Reference: Coates, B., Camarda, L., & Goodman, D. (2016). Wheezing in infants: Bronchiolitis. In R. Kliegman, B. Stanton, J. St. Geme, et al. (Eds.), *Nelson textbook of pediatrics* (20th ed., Chapter 391.1). St. Louis, MO: Elsevier.

In addition to RSV, other causative organisms include *Mycoplasma*, parainfluenza virus, and some adenoviruses. RSV infection occurs in annual epidemics during the winter and early spring, mainly from November to March in northern climates. The incidence peaks at age 6 months. By age 2 years, nearly 100% of children will have had RSV. Immunity does not occur, but the incidence and severity decrease with age.

## Manifestations

A mild upper respiratory tract infection usually precedes the development of bronchiolitis. Serous nasal drainage, sneezing, low-grade fever, and anorexia are present for several days, followed by the onset of acute respiratory distress, manifested by the following signs and symptoms:

- Tachypnea—respiratory rates of 60 to 80 breaths/min
- Tachycardia—heart rate greater than 140 beats/min
- Wheezing, crackles, or rhonchi
- Intercostal and subcostal retractions with or without nasal flaring
- Cyanosis

Feeding may be difficult because of increased respirations, which interfere with sucking and swallowing. The body temperature varies from hypothermic to as high as 41° C (105.8° F).

## Diagnostic Evaluation

The clinical presentation and the age of the child suggest the diagnosis. Chest radiographs are not usually indicated, unless the child is suspected to have an atelectasis or pneumonia (Ralston et al., 2014a,b).

## Therapeutic Management

Infants with mild bronchiolitis can be treated at home with fluids, humidification, and rest. Infants with respiratory distress are hospitalized for supportive treatment. Cool, humidified oxygen is delivered if the oxygen saturation decreases to less than 90% on room air to relieve

## EVIDENCE-BASED PRACTICE

Bronchiolitis, or lower airway inflammation, in infants and young children is a major cause for hospitalization, primarily because of the risk for respiratory distress and airway obstruction (Coates, Camarda, & Goodman, 2016). Because bronchiolitis results from a viral infection, treatment is symptom-based and supportive, with interventions directed toward improving respiratory status and preventing dehydration. Improvement in respiratory status is the direct result of a combination of airway clearance and oxygen administration. Three nurse-led interdisciplinary and evidence-based quality improvement (QI) projects demonstrate how consistency in approach can standardize practice, improve patient outcomes and nurse satisfaction, and decrease overall costs for patients with bronchiolitis.

Believing that deep nasopharyngeal suction, a common practice for infants with bronchiolitis, is detrimental to small airways, Jarvis et al. (2014) developed a QI project with the goal of substituting nasal suction with saline and a bulb syringe for nasopharyngeal suction, except in cases where respiratory distress is evident or respiratory symptoms worsen after nasal suctioning. Based on extensive literature review, the team devised a standardized airway clearance procedure based on clear criteria for determining respiratory distress (e.g., retractions, labored breathing). They introduced the changes to nurses and determined that the protocol was being followed a large majority of the time. Decrease in nasopharyngeal suctioning over the study time period was significant at 11%.

Concerned about inconsistency in administering bronchodilators to children with bronchiolitis, Pinto et al. (2014) developed an algorithm to assist nurses in clinical decision-making regarding administration of an inhaled bronchodilator. Consistent with the evidence, a bronchodilator such as albuterol generally does not provide airway relief in children with bronchiolitis. These QI developers educated staff about consistency in assessing signs of respiratory distress to determine whether a bronchodilator is warranted and measured bronchodilator use before, during, and after the implementation of the protocol. As a result of the protocol, bronchodilator use decreased significantly.

Finally, Martin et al. (2015) looked at overuse of pulse oximetry and inconsistent protocols for weaning children from oxygen in preparation for discharge. Using an oxygen saturation goal of 91%, their algorithm called for using continuous pulse oximetry only for children in severe respiratory distress; for children with mild distress or stable moderate distress, the recommendation was to conduct spot checks either in conjunction with taking vital signs or routinely every four hours. To wean children from oxygen, the protocol called for standard decreases in oxygen to room air with rechecks of respiratory status for children with oxygen saturations greater than 91%; maintenance of current oxygen levels with rechecks for those with saturations of 91%; and increases in oxygen for children whose saturations were greater than 91%. Even though their study sample was small, both the use of continuous pulse oximetry and use of oxygen decreased by 50%.

These studies demonstrate how QI projects can expand knowledge and improve patient outcomes. Think about problems in your clinical area that might be amenable to a QI project. How would you initiate the process?

References: Coates, B., Camarda, L., & Goodman, D. (2016). Wheezing in infants: Bronchiolitis. In R. Kliegman, B. Stanton, J. St. Geme, et al. (Eds.), *Nelson textbook of pediatrics* (20th ed., Chapter 391.1). St. Louis, MO: Elsevier; Jarvis, K., et al. (2014). Change to a standardized airway clearance protocol for children with bronchiolitis leads to improved care. *Journal of Pediatric Nursing, 29,* 252–257; Martin, S., Martin, J., & Seigler, T. (2015). Evidence-based protocols to guide pulse oximetry and oxygen weaning in inpatient children with asthma and bronchiolitis. *Journal of Pediatric Nursing, 30,* 888–895; Pinto, J., Schairer, J., & Petrova, A. (2014). Comparative effectiveness of implementation of a nursing-driven protocol in reducing bronchodilator utilization in hospitalized children with bronchiolitis. *Journal of Evaluation in Clinical Practice, 20,* 267–272.

dyspnea, hypoxemia, and insensible water loss from tachypnea (Coates et al., 2016). Inhalation of hypertonic (3%) normal saline solution may improve respiratory status and decrease the hospital stay of infants with bronchiolitis (Pinto et al., 2014).

Parenteral administration of fluids may be necessary for acutely ill infants who are dehydrated from tachypnea or poor intake (Ralston et al., 2014a). The infant should be positioned with the head and chest at a 30- to 40-degree angle and the neck slightly extended to maintain an open airway and decrease pressure on the diaphragm.

Antibiotics are not given unless there is a secondary bacterial infection. Although some healthcare providers routinely prescribe bronchodilators, epinephrine, or corticosteroids, randomized clinical trials have failed to demonstrate clinical efficacy in the use of these medications (Ralston et al., 2014b).

RSV prevention is of the utmost importance to reduce hospitalizations for young, at-risk infants and children. Intramuscular palivizumab (Synagis) administered monthly throughout the RSV season has significantly reduced the hospitalization risk for some premature infants (less than 35 weeks of gestation) younger than 6 months and children younger than 24 months with chronic lung disease or congenital cardiac disease (Coates et al., 2016). Prophylaxis is done on an outpatient basis.

## NURSING CARE

### The Child With Bronchiolitis

#### Assessment

The nurse assesses the infant for signs and symptoms of respiratory distress (tachypnea, dyspnea, retractions, cyanosis, nasal flaring) every 1 to 2 hours during the acute phase and as needed if changes occur. Auscultate the lungs for breath sounds. Apnea monitoring and cardiorespiratory monitoring are indicated for the infant with acute disease. Make sure that the alarms on the cardiorespiratory monitor are appropriately set, and document any periods of apnea.

Assess the infant for signs of dehydration (dry mucous membranes, decreased urine output, sunken fontanel, weight loss) and monitor body temperature. The infant should be placed in a room near the nurses' station for easy observation. Assess the family's understanding of the disease and family members' level of anxiety. Observe the infant for signs of anxiety, restlessness, or irritability.

#### Nursing Diagnosis and Planning

The diagnoses and expected outcomes that may be appropriate for the infant with bronchiolitis and the infant's family are as follows:

- Impaired Gas Exchange related to airway edema and increased mucus.

**Expected outcome.** The infant will have adequate gas exchange, as evidenced by oxygen saturation above 95% on room air.

- Ineffective Airway Clearance related to increased secretions.

**Expected outcome.** The infant will exhibit clear breath sounds and normal respiratory rate, depth, and rhythm.

- Deficient Fluid Volume related to decreased intake and insensible loss.

**Expected outcome.** The infant will maintain adequate hydration, as evidenced by moist mucous membranes, a flat fontanel, urine output normal for age, and stable weight.

- Ineffective Thermoregulation related to illness.

**Expected outcome.** The infant will demonstrate a body temperature within normal limits.

- Anxiety related to hospitalization and the child's dyspnea.

***Expected outcome.*** The infant will demonstrate decreased anxiety, as evidenced by adequate sleep and stable vital signs. The parents will verbalize understanding of the infant's condition and be able to participate appropriately in the infant's care.

### Interventions

Many hospitals are now using clinical pathways for children with respiratory disease. Even when using a clinical pathway, the nurse needs to focus on appropriate nursing interventions.

***Facilitating gas exchange.*** The nurse documents the infant's vital signs and respiratory status every 1 to 2 hours or more often as needed. Particularly note the rate, quality, and depth of respirations along with any adventitious breath sounds and the presence of retractions. Close monitoring with a cardiorespiratory monitor or regular pulse oximetry measurement will ensure early identification of impending respiratory distress.

Oxygen administration is indicated for infants who are hypoxic or in respiratory distress. Administer humidified oxygen (at 35% to 40% concentration) in the manner most comfortable for the infant (by hood, mask, or nasal prongs) to decrease hypoxia and bronchial edema. Positioning the infant's head at a 30- to 40-degree upright angle with the neck slightly extended will maintain an open airway and ease respirations by decreasing pressure on the diaphragm. Scheduling periods of uninterrupted rest between care episodes decreases oxygen demand.

***Preventing transmission.*** Isolate the infant with RSV infection in a single room or place the infant in a room with other RSV-infected infants. Meticulous hand hygiene is imperative. Nurses caring for these infants should not care for other high-risk children. Maintaining Contact Precautions (i.e., wearing a gown and gloves) reduces nosocomial transmission of RSV.

Emphasize to parents and other visitors that touching the infant or surfaces within 3 feet of the infant can transmit the organism to the hands and clothes. It is essential to stress the importance for parents and visitors to use protective gloves and gown and practice meticulous hand hygiene before entering the infant's room and after removal of the gown and gloves to avoid transmitting the infection to others.

***Maintaining fluid balance.*** Most infants with bronchiolitis can take fluids orally; IV fluids are administered if respiratory distress is severe enough to risk aspiration. If the infant's nasal passages are blocked with mucus, instill saline solution nose drops (one or two drops in each nostril, followed by gentle suctioning with a bulb syringe) before feeding. Offer the infant frequent, varied clear liquids (juices, Pedialyte, Ricelyte). Older infants may enjoy frozen electrolyte pops. The infant's hydration status (skin turgor, fontanel, mucous membranes) and electrolyte values are monitored, and daily weights and intake and output are documented.

***Reducing fever.*** The nurse takes the infant's temperature every 2 to 4 hours and as needed. Control environmental temperature by maintaining the room temperature between 22° and 24° C (72° and 75° F) and dress the infant in light clothing. Oral fluid intake is encouraged, if respiratory rate is within normal limits, and liquid acetaminophen or ibuprofen is administered as ordered to reduce fever.

***Decreasing anxiety.*** Encourage the parent to stay with the infant when possible and to participate as much as possible in the infant's care. Hospital routines and all procedures and treatments should be explained to reduce fear of the unknown. Because adult anxiety can be transferred to the infant, maintain a calm environment and encourage parents to do the same. Parents need to be allowed to express concerns.

### Evaluation

- Does the infant demonstrate adequate oxygenation (oxygen saturation greater than 95%), clear breath sounds, and stable respiratory status?
- Does the infant have moist mucous membranes, good skin turgor, stable weight, a flat fontanel, and urine output of at least 2 to 3 mL/kg/hr? (For appropriate urine output in older children, see Chapter 40.)
- Is the infant's body temperature within normal limits?
- Does the infant demonstrate reduced crying or irritability and increased rest?
- Do the parents verbalize understanding of the disease, have a relaxed appearance, and demonstrate comforting behaviors toward the infant?

## PNEUMONIA

Pneumonia is an inflammation of the lung parenchyma that can occur as a primary or a secondary disease. Pneumonias are classified by anatomic distribution or by the agents that cause them. Environment, immune system status, and the child's age are factors in the pathogenesis of the disease.

The two most common types of infectious pneumonia are *viral* and *bacterial* (Table 45.3). Viruses are the most common causative agents in infants and children younger than 5 years old, particularly influenza and RSV (Kelly & Sandora, 2016). Community-acquired pneumonia is a significant problem worldwide, especially in developing countries. In the United States, the prevalence of pneumonia in children has decreased markedly with the institution of routine vaccination with pneumococcal conjugate and other vaccines (e.g. influenza, Hib, measles) during infancy (Kelly & Sandora, 2016). Children with chronic and acute conditions, such as acquired immunodeficiency syndrome, cystic fibrosis (CF), congenital defects, and foreign body aspiration, are at increased risk for development of pneumonia. Opportunistic infections (*Pneumocystis jiroveci* [formerly *carinii*] pneumonia) are associated with acquired immunodeficiency syndrome (see Chapter 42). Secondary pneumonia can result from aspiration of hydrocarbons contained in household products or lipids (e.g., mineral oil given to treat severe constipation).

## NURSING CARE

### The Child With Pneumonia

#### Assessment

Every 2 hours, or more frequently depending on the severity of respiratory distress, assess the child's breath sounds, respiratory rate and rhythm, color, vital signs, and degree of restlessness. Immediately report any signs of increased respiratory distress, including dyspnea, tachypnea, cyanosis, use of accessory muscles of breathing, diminished breath sounds, and crackles. Also note any fever, tachycardia, malaise, anorexia, discomfort, and changes in condition.

#### Nursing Diagnosis and Planning

The nursing diagnoses and expected outcomes that may be appropriate for the child with pneumonia and the child's family are as follows:

- Ineffective Airway Clearance related to bronchial obstruction.

***Expected outcome.*** The child will have clear airways, as evidenced by the absence of abnormal breath sounds and dyspnea.

- Ineffective Breathing Pattern related to increased mucus production and pain with inspiration.

***Expected outcome.*** The child will demonstrate effective breathing, as evidenced by respiratory rate and rhythm within normal limits for age and absence of retractions.

- Impaired Gas Exchange related to increased mucus and accumulation of exudate.

***Expected outcome.*** The child will maintain adequate gas exchange, as evidenced by decreased restlessness, appropriate

**TABLE 45.3 Comparison of Types of Pneumonia**

| Etiology and Incidence | Pathophysiology | Manifestations | Therapeutic Management |
|---|---|---|---|
| **Viral** | | | |
| Most often caused by influenza viruses, parainfluenza virus, and RSV. Viruses cause 80%-85% of all pneumonias.<br>Most common in children younger than 3 yr. | Cell destruction with sloughing of cellular debris into lumen of terminal airways and alveoli causes patchy infiltrate that affects multiple lobes. | Low to high fever, cough, crackles, wheezing (more common with RSV), headache, malaise, myalgia, abdominal pain.<br>Infiltrates seen on chest radiography.<br>WBC count <20,000/mm$^3$.<br>Usually lasts 5-7 days. | Supportive. No antibiotics are prescribed unless coexisting bacterial infection is suspected.<br>Severely ill infants and children may be hospitalized for oxygen and fluid therapy. |
| **Bacterial and Bacterial-Like** | | | |
| Caused primarily by *Streptococcus pneumoniae* in infants and children younger than 5 yr. *Mycoplasma pneumoniae and Chlamydophila pneumoniae* are more commonly seen in children older than 5 yr. Also caused by *Haemophilus influenzae* and group A streptococci.<br>*Chlamydia trachomatis* is seen mainly in infants. | Alveoli fill with fluid and cells in small segment or entire lung.<br>Bacteria enter bloodstream through pulmonary lymphatics.<br>Vital capacity and lung compliance decrease as consolidation increases. | Preceded by upper respiratory infection.<br>Abrupt onset of high fever, chills, cough, chest pain, decreased breath sounds, signs of respiratory distress (retractions, nasal flaring, tachypnea), restlessness, and apprehension.<br>Symptoms may be vague in infants; older children can have gastrointestinal symptoms, chest pain, and abnormal breath sounds.<br>Onset of the bacterial-like pneumonias can be more insidious.<br>Radiography reveals consolidation; WBC count is elevated. | Oral antibiotic therapy, usually with high dose amoxicillin, cefuroxime, or amoxicillin/clavulanate for mild episodes; erythromycin for penicillin-allergic children; azithromycin or fluoroquinolone for older children or adolescents.<br>IV cefotaxime or parenteral ceftriaxone for children needing hospitalization.<br>Hospitalization for severely ill infants and children who will need oxygen and fluid therapy. Chest tube drainage of fluid or purulence from pleural cavity may be necessary (particularly for children with staphylococcal pneumonia). |

*IV*, intravenous; *RSV*, respiratory syncytial virus; *WBC*, white blood cell

oxygen saturation, and improved mucous membrane and nail bed color.

- Deficient Fluid Volume related to fever, decreased intake, and tachypnea.

  **Expected outcome.** The child will maintain fluid balance, as evidenced by moist mucous membranes, good skin turgor, urine output appropriate for age, and maintenance of age-appropriate weight.

- Deficient Knowledge related to the disease process and home care.

  **Expected outcome.** The parents will explain the disease process and describe the child's care.

- Anxiety (parental) related to infant's dyspnea and hospitalization.

  **Expected outcome.** The parents will show a decrease in anxiety, as evidenced by decreased irritability and increased periods of rest. The parents will verbalize and demonstrate comfort and ease when caring for the child.

- Acute Pain related to coughing and difficulty breathing secondary to disease process.

  **Expected outcome.** The child will have decreased pain, as evidenced by less irritability, verbalization of increased comfort (if age appropriate), and a relaxed body posture.

### Interventions

The severity of the illness and the cause of the disease direct the nursing care of the child with pneumonia. Many children will be cared for at home, whereas others will be hospitalized on a general pediatric unit or special care area.

For the hospitalized child, elevating the head of the bed and changing the child's position every 2 hours assist respiratory effort and promote pulmonary drainage. Older children may assume a position of comfort but still must change their position every 2 hours. The use of infant seats should be avoided because pressure may be placed on the diaphragm, thus actually decreasing lung expansion.

The older child should be assisted with coughing and deep breathing and splinting as necessary to ease discomfort. Oxygen should be humidified and monitored. Pulse oximetry aids in monitoring oxygen saturation and the adequacy of air exchange. A cardiorespiratory monitor is used when available (Ensz & Crusse, 2016).

Oral or IV fluids are given as ordered. IV fluids may be indicated when oral intake increases the stress put on an already compromised body. The nurse monitors intake and output and observes for signs of dehydration (oliguria, poor skin turgor, dry mucous membranes, sunken fontanels, weight loss). Weight should be measured daily. The specific gravity of urine also is checked to monitor hydration status.

Because conserving energy aids oxygenation, nursing care is planned to provide for periods of rest. Quiet diversional activities, such as reading, puzzles, videos, and board games, are suggested. The nurse maintains a quiet and cool environment and limits visitors to allow the child maximum rest. Visits by anyone with an infection should be restricted.

Administer antipyretics, antibiotics, and analgesics as ordered. Normal breathing may cause discomfort. If an analgesic is not ordered, the physician should be notified of any discomfort the child has. Splinting of the affected side by lying on that side may decrease discomfort. Diversional activities and manipulation of the environment are often effective for pain relief.

The family and child (if of appropriate age) need to receive information about the disease and its treatment. The nurse explains all procedures and treatments and encourages the parents to stay with their child and participate in the child's care. The nurse conveys empathy for the family's feelings and concerns. The nurse also teaches the family about home management of the infant or child (see Patient-Centered Teaching: Home Management of the Child with Pneumonia).

### Evaluation

- Are the child's vital signs and respiratory status within normal limits?
- Is the child's oxygen saturation greater than 95%?

- Does the child appear hydrated, with moist mucous membranes, good skin turgor, and adequate urinary output for age?
- Can the parents describe home care techniques?
- Do the parents appear relaxed, and are they able to fully participate in the child's care?
- Can the child comfortably participate in quiet activities and rest quietly when appropriate?
- Is the child in pain?

## PATIENT-CENTERED TEACHING

### *Home Management of the Child With Pneumonia*

- Provide rest.
- Increase your child's fluid intake. Offer favorite fluids more frequently than usual, and be sure your child is urinating appropriate amounts. Warm liquids (lemonade, apple juice, Pedialyte, Ricelyte) help loosen secretions. Call your healthcare provider if the child's mucous membranes appear dry or if urination decreases.
- Administer acetaminophen for fever and discomfort.
- Administer antibiotics as ordered; give the correct dose and the entire prescribed amount.
- Avoid exposing your child to cigarette smoke.

## BOX 45.1 Common Items of Aspiration

- Nuts
- Pins
- Screws
- Coins
- Seeds
- Grapes
- Bones
- Earrings
- Small toys
- Chunks of food
- Parts of toys
- Hard candy
- Latex balloons
- Popcorn
- Hot dogs
- Carrots

## FOREIGN BODY ASPIRATION

Foreign body aspiration is seen most frequently in children ages 6 months to 5 years. Children who play, run, or laugh with objects in their mouths are at risk. Certain items have an increased incidence of aspiration by infants and children (Box 45.1).

### Etiology and Incidence

Children's curiosity, oral needs, and occasionally lack of supervision contribute to the occurrence of foreign body aspiration. Infants and children love to explore and investigate objects. Exploration often includes putting objects into their mouths. Children also have the uncanny ability to remove small parts from toys and to find other objects that parents thought were out of their reach (e.g., pins, screws, nuts, coins, earrings). Adults might give infants and small children foods they are not developmentally prepared to ingest (hard candy, popcorn, uncooked carrots, hot dogs, peanuts). Latex balloons account for a significant number of deaths from aspiration per year. Childhood aspiration can occur at any age, but it occurs most frequently in children younger than 4 years of age (Paul, Sanjeevaiah, & Routly, 2013).

### Pathophysiology

Most foreign bodies become lodged in the bronchi. The right main bronchus is a more common site than the left main bronchus because of its anatomic development. Objects lodged in the larynx cause edema and inflammation. Bronchial obstruction manifests as obstructive emphysema, pneumonia, or atelectasis. Failure to remove an obstructing foreign object is almost always fatal. Most can be removed mechanically without complications; a delay in treatment can lead to aspiration pneumonia and airway trauma.

### Manifestations

Immediate signs and symptoms include sudden, violent coughing; gagging; wheezing; vomiting; brief episodes of apnea; and possibly cyanosis.

After aspirating a foreign object, the child can remain asymptomatic for hours or weeks. If the object is not found and removed, signs and symptoms related to edema and increased irritation and obstruction may develop. Signs and symptoms of laryngeal and tracheal obstruction include choking, dysphagia, hoarseness, croupy cough, stridor, and possibly dyspnea with cyanosis. Coughing, wheezing, unilaterally decreased breath sounds, pneumonitis, and possibly respiratory arrest can indicate bronchial inflammation and obstruction.

### Diagnostic Evaluation

The diagnosis is based on an accurate history and the clinical manifestations. Fluoroscopy, magnetic resonance imaging (MRI), computed tomography (CT) scan, or chest radiography can be used to reveal the presence of a foreign object in the respiratory tract. Radiographs are not always helpful, because a nonmetallic object can be invisible. Rigid bronchoscopy confirms the diagnosis and might provide an avenue for removing the object.

### Therapeutic Management

Foreign bodies are removed from the respiratory tract by direct laryngoscopy or bronchoscopy. After the procedure, the child should remain hospitalized for observation for laryngeal edema and respiratory distress. Antibiotics are unnecessary unless respiratory signs and symptoms suggest an infection. Cool mist and administration of bronchodilators or corticosteroids 24 to 48 hours after the removal of the foreign body may be indicated.

### Nursing Considerations

The degree of obstruction should be assessed to determine the appropriate action to take. If the child is aphonic (not speaking) and not breathing, the nurse should follow the current guidelines for managing an obstructed airway (see Chapter 34). Children with a partially obstructed airway are observed for signs of increasing obstruction.

After the object has been removed, the child is observed for signs of obstruction caused by laryngeal edema and soft tissue swelling (restlessness, dyspnea). The child should be placed on a cardiorespiratory monitor.

Liquids are withheld until the child's gag reflex returns after anesthesia. Oral fluids should be started slowly and increased as the child tolerates the intake. Intake and output should be recorded. If the child refuses to drink because of a sore throat or is unable to take fluids orally, the physician should be notified so that IV fluids may be started. The parents' knowledge of respiratory distress is also evaluated before discharge.

Parental anxiety and guilt are common after an episode of aspiration. In addition to supporting the parents, the nurse assesses their knowledge of safety. Prevention is the key to reducing the incidence of aspiration. Safety is discussed at every well-child visit (see Chapters 6 through 9).

## PULMONARY NONINFECTIOUS IRRITATION

Although we think of foreign body aspiration as the most common type of pulmonary noninfectious irritation in children, other forms

**TABLE 45.4 Pulmonary Noninfectious Irritants**

| Acute Respiratory Distress Syndrome (ARDS) | Passive Smoking | Smoke Inhalation |
|---|---|---|
| **Clinical Manifestations** | | |
| Acute, subacute, and chronic phases<br>Pulmonary manifestations may be minimal during acute phase but will move toward respiratory distress (dyspnea, tachypnea, retractions, grunting, cyanosis).<br>Severe hypoxemia and, occasionally, hypercapnia may develop.<br>Note that there is a primary disease, and manifestations of that disease process will also be present. | Increased respiratory infections<br>An effect on respiratory function and growth in infants and small but significant reduction in airway function in older children<br>Possible negative effect on linear growth of children with CF | Singed nasal hair<br>Cough<br>Hoarseness<br>Hemoptysis<br>Soot in sputum<br>Cyanosis<br>Wheezing<br>Carbon monoxide effects:<br>Mild: Headaches, mild dyspnea, visual changes, confusion<br>Moderate: Irritability, diminished judgment, dim vision, nausea<br>Severe: Hallucinations, confusion, ataxia, collapse, coma<br>Can contribute to ARDS |
| **Therapeutic Management** | | |
| Need to be treated in ICU<br>Treat underlying cause<br>Oxygen/mechanical ventilation<br>Continuous positive pressure<br>Pulse oximetry<br>Maintain cardiac function<br>Stabilize hematocrit<br>Prevent infection | Awareness of problem and preventive teaching<br>Effective programs to prevent smoking in parents and minors | 100% oxygen by mask<br>Close monitoring of carboxyhemoglobin levels<br>Arterial blood gases<br>Intubation and tracheostomy equipment available<br>Aerosolized bronchodilators<br>Continuous positive pressure<br>Balance fluid therapy between need for large volume of fluid and need to limit fluid to decrease pulmonary edema<br>Prophylactic antimicrobial therapy is controversial |
| **Nursing Care** | | |
| Monitor respiratory status<br>Monitor blood gas analysis<br>Psychological support of child and parents<br>Monitor urine output, capillary filling, perfusion | Involvement in community projects to designate "no smoking" ordinances in public places<br>School-based prevention programs<br>Education of parents as part of anticipatory guidance of dangers of smoking, both active and passive<br>Role modeling no smoking | Respiratory assessment<br>Support of pulmonary therapy<br>Psychological support of child and family as a result of the fear of the trauma of the fire or insult that caused the injury<br>Children who have lost a family member will need long-term psychological support |
| **Prognosis** | | |
| High mortality rate, usually more than 50%<br>Those who survive have a good chance of full recovery | Increased numbers of studies have shown correlation between smoking and respiratory disease; more studies needed to show long-term effects | Most will return to near-normal pulmonary function<br>Few will have long-term problems associated with the injury |

*CF*, Cystic fibrosis; *ICU*, intensive care unit.

of irritation can cause respiratory difficulties. These include acute respiratory distress syndrome (ARDS), passive smoking, and smoke inhalation.

## Acute Respiratory Distress Syndrome

Although there is not uniform agreement as to what constitutes acute respiratory distress syndrome (ARDS), it is generally agreed that ARDS represents severe diffuse lung injury precipitated by a variety of illnesses. The mechanism of lung injury in children is similar to that of adults and usually occurs from 8 to 48 hours after the initial illness, which may be, but is not limited to, aspiration, trauma, drug ingestion, shock, and massive transfusions.

### Pathophysiology

The mechanism that initiates and perpetuates the lung injury is not understood. There is a breakdown in the alveolar-capillary barrier with fluid accumulation in the interstitium and alveoli. ARDS has acute and chronic stages. Initially there is capillary congestion and pulmonary edema. Fibrosis of the lungs develops in children who do not recover from the acute stage.

Table 45.4 discusses clinical manifestations, therapeutic management, nursing care, and prognosis.

## Passive Smoking

Increased attention has been paid to the role of passive smoking in the development of respiratory disease in children. Children with a history of exposure to cigarette smoke, both prenatally and postnatally, have more frequent upper and lower respiratory complications, more hospitalizations for those complications, and a greater tendency to develop wheezing than do nonexposed children.

### Pathophysiology

Smoke is an irritant that can cause increased airway reactivity and inflammation.

**TABLE 45.5 Apnea of Prematurity Compared With Infant Apnea**

| Etiology and Incidence | Pathophysiology | Therapeutic Management |
|---|---|---|
| **Apnea of Prematurity** | | |
| Most common type of apnea; occurs in neonates of 24-32 wk of gestational age, with onset usually within first 2 wk of life. It usually resolves by 37 wk.<br>Although neonate age may be similar to the age at greatest risk for SIDS, apnea of prematurity is not considered to predict risk for SIDS. | Varies among neonates but can be caused by upper airway obstruction, immaturity of central control mechanisms, compliant chest wall, or abnormal response during REM sleep.<br>Apnea often occurs during feeding because of immaturity of breathing, sucking, and swallowing coordination. | Gentle cutaneous stimulation is used to stimulate breathing in neonates with mild apnea (<10 episodes/day with little desaturation). For persistent apnea, use oxygen administration, cardiorespiratory monitor; consider CPAP for neonates with severe apnea.<br>Drug therapy may include caffeine, oral theophylline, or IV aminophylline to increase central respiratory drive and improve carbon dioxide sensitivity. |
| **Infant Apnea** | | |
| Most infant apnea has no known cause. Underlying conditions such as cardiac abnormalities, gastroesophageal reflux, seizures, hypoglycemia, respiratory infection, environmental exposures (e.g., cigarette smoke), or child abuse should be ruled out. | Three types:<br>• Central: Absence of respiratory effort and air movement.<br>• Obstructive: Apparent respiratory efforts without air movement or sound.<br>• Mixed: Absence of respiratory effort and nasal air movement followed by resumption of respiratory effort without air movement.<br>Short episodes of apnea are usually central apnea; apnea episodes that last 15 s or more are usually mixed. | Identify any underlying cause. If no underlying disorder is identified and the infant returns to normal behavior, no hospitalization or home apnea monitoring is needed. Offer CPR training and education to parent/caregiver. |

*CPAP,* continuous positive airway pressure; *IV,* intravenous; *REM,* rapid eye movements; *SIDS,* sudden infant death syndrome
Data from: Carlo, W. (2016). Apnea. In R. Kliegman, B. Stanton, J. St. Geme, et al. (Eds.), *Nelson textbook of pediatrics* (20th ed., Chapter 385). St. Louis, MO: Elsevier; Tieder, J, et al. (2016). Brief resolved unexplained events (formerly apparent life-threatening events) and evaluation of low risk infants. *Pediatrics, 137*(5), e1–e32.

See Table 45.4 for a discussion of clinical manifestations, therapeutic management, nursing care, and prognosis.

### Smoke Inhalation

As many as 50% of all fire-related deaths are caused by smoke injuries. The severity of lung injury is related to the nature of the material inhaled, the products of incomplete combustion that are generated, and the child's confinement in a closed space. Besides the noxious gases, fine particles of soot can also be inhaled; these particles might be contaminated with toxic gases and also can cause thermal burns.

#### Pathophysiology

Because the upper airway has a built-in cooling system, most thermal airway injury is limited to the areas above the larynx. Steam inhalation injury is an exception. Combustion of the materials involved causes a wide variety of noxious gases. These include but are not limited to oxides of sulfur and nitrogen, corrosive alkalis, and carbon monoxide. Exposure to and inhalation of these gases can cause mucosal edema, airway obstruction, atelectasis, necrosis of the pulmonary mucosa, and pulmonary edema (Antoon & Donovan, 2016). Smoke inhalation can lead to ARDS.

Carbon monoxide poisoning is a complication of smoke inhalation caused when carbon monoxide combines with hemoglobin to form carboxyhemoglobin, causing severe hypoxia.

See Table 45.4 for a discussion of clinical manifestations, therapeutic management, nursing care, and prognosis.

## APNEA

### Manifestations

Apnea is the cessation of breathing for a period of 20 seconds or longer, or for a shorter period but accompanied by bradycardia or cyanosis. True apnea differs from periodic breathing, which might be seen in premature infants. In periodic breathing, there is a shift from regular rhythmic breathing to brief episodes of apnea. This type of breathing pattern consists of three or more respiratory pauses of longer than 3 seconds, with less than 20 seconds of respiration between pauses. Rarely, periodic breathing is associated with changes in heart rate or color. Periodic breathing is common in premature infants and decreases as the infant's gestational age increases. The cause is unknown; periodic breathing may be a normal event.

Brief resolved unexplained events (BRUE) (previously referred to as apparent life-threatening events) are sudden episodes characterized by apnea (cessation or markedly decreased breathing lasting less than one minute), a color change, a change in muscle tone, and altered state of responsiveness in an infant who otherwise appears healthy and who returns to normal behavior and status after the event (Tieder et al., 2016, p. e3). The observer of the event relates the belief that the infant would have died if not for intervention. BRUEs most often occur in infants older than two months of age (but younger than 1 year old), who might have been born prematurely (but ≥ 32 weeks), and who have no apparent underlying health condition by history and physical examination (Tieder et al., 2016). Two categories of true apnea events are apnea of prematurity and infant apnea (Table 45.5).

### Diagnostic Evaluation

The AAP (Tieder et al., 2016) has issued guidelines for the identification and management of low-risk infants who have experienced a BRUE. Based on an extensive evidence review, the AAP recommends evaluation by a provider as soon as possible after the event, including health history (child and family), physical examination, and inquiry about any possible social issues. If the provider is confident that there are no underlying issues, the infant may not need hospitalization or home monitoring. A brief observation period (approximately one to four hours) with pulse oximetry in the emergency department might be warranted, depending on the child's condition (Tieder et al., 2016). The provider needs to follow-up within 24 hours of the event. Providing education and CPR training to the parents can make them more confident of their ability to manage any subsequent episode (Tieder et al., 2016).

Tests are not routinely ordered for older infants with apnea unless the provider determines the infant is at risk due to an underlying medical condition (Tieder et al., 2016). For young infants, if testing is warranted, tests are selected for the clinical indication. These could include cardiorespiratory and neurophysiologic studies, such as chest radiography, blood chemistry, electrocardiography, and electroencephalography.

## NURSING CARE

### The Infant With Apnea

#### Assessment

The hospitalized infant's heart rate and respirations are monitored continuously. The nurse should ascertain that the alarms on the cardiorespiratory monitor are set to avoid false alarms. Resuscitative equipment should be available.

If an apneic episode is observed, the nurse should record the time and duration of the episode, the skin color change, heart rate, and oxygen saturation. The nurse should also describe what the infant was doing before the episode and any actions the nurse took to stimulate breathing.

#### Nursing Diagnosis and Planning

The nursing diagnoses and expected outcomes that may be appropriate for the infant with apnea and the family are as follows:

- Ineffective Breathing Pattern related to apnea secondary to prematurity of respiratory control mechanisms (premature infant) and related to apnea of known or unknown etiology (term infant).

  ***Expected outcome.*** The infant will have regular breathing patterns, as evidenced by respiratory rate and rhythm within normal limits for age.
- Anxiety (parental) related to the possibility of the infant's death.

  ***Expected outcome.*** The parents will verbalize feelings concerning the infant's periods of apnea.
- Deficient Knowledge (parental) related to unfamiliarity with apnea monitoring equipment and cardiopulmonary resuscitation (CPR).

  ***Expected outcome.*** The parents will learn how to perform infant CPR and how to operate the apnea monitor.

#### Interventions

The nurse sets the heart rate parameters of the cardiorespiratory monitor according to the infant's age and the respiratory pause at greater than 15 seconds. Resuscitative equipment should be available, and the nurse should be proficient in using it.

The apneic infant can be stimulated by gently tapping the infant's foot or trunk or turning the infant over. The infant should not be shaken vigorously. If breathing does not resume, institute bag-and-mask ventilation.

Maintain a neutral thermal environment while the infant is hospitalized and avoid suctioning if possible. Several studies have shown that feeding affects ventilation. Therefore, infants should be monitored closely when being fed.

Home apnea monitoring remains controversial, and there are few clear guidelines related to which infants would benefit most from home monitoring. If home apnea monitoring is ordered, the family should be instructed in the use of the monitor and in CPR before the infant is discharged (Fig. 45.3). Stimulating action should be taken if the infant becomes bradycardic, even if the apnea monitor does not alarm. Emphasize to the parents that when the monitor alarm is triggered, they should immediately assess the infant rather than focus on the machine.

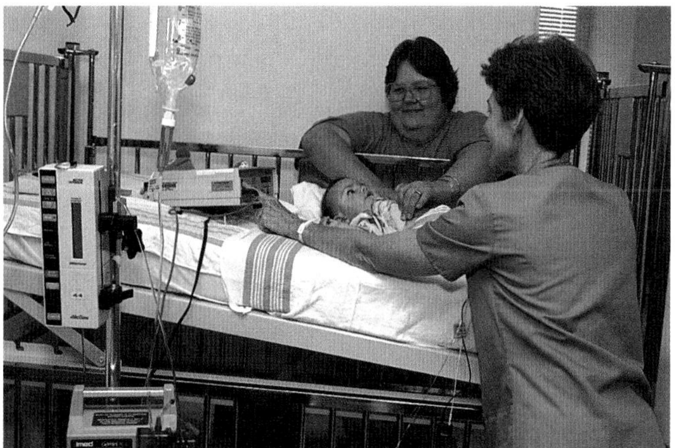

**FIG 45.3** Teaching the family about using an apnea monitor and how to respond to alarms is an important element in caring for the child with infant apnea. The nurse must assess the parents' ability to tolerate the stressors of living with a child who is prone to apnea and support them as they deal with these stressors.

Parents of infants who are monitored at home may have emotional needs that need to be met. Witnessing their infant during an apneic episode can be frightening and traumatic for parents. Referral for psychological support might be beneficial.

#### Evaluation

- Does the infant demonstrate normal respiratory rate and rhythm?
- Have the parents verbalized their fears associated with the infant's apnea?
- Have the parents demonstrated the ability to operate monitoring equipment and to perform CPR?

## SUDDEN INFANT DEATH SYNDROME

Sudden infant death syndrome (SIDS), which accounts for 44% of deaths in the general category of sudden unexpected infant death (SUID), is defined as the sudden and unexplained death of an infant younger than 1 year (Centers for Disease Control and Prevention [CDC], 2016b). The exact cause is unknown despite a thorough investigation that includes a complete autopsy, examination of the death scene, and review of the clinical history. It is sometimes referred to by the public as *crib death.* SIDS usually occurs during sleep.

### Etiology and Incidence

Despite a marked decline in the incidence of SIDS since the AAP issued preventive guidelines, it remains the fourth leading cause of infant death in the United States (CDC, 2015). SIDS occurs most frequently between the second and fourth months of life, with 95% of cases occurring before age 6 months. It is more common in boys, low-birth-weight infants, and infants from lower socioeconomic groups. It occurs more often during the winter months. American Indians and Alaskan Natives have the highest incidence, followed by Non-Hispanic Blacks (CDC, 2016b). Infant deaths from accidental suffocation or strangulation in bed are in a different cause of death category than SIDS (25% of infant deaths) (CDC, 2016b).

Although numerous theories have been proposed, the cause of SIDS is unknown. It is generally accepted that SIDS is the result of an interaction between nonmodifiable (intrinsic) factors, developmental maturity, and modifiable (extrinsic) risk factors (Goldstein et al., 2016). Intrinsic risk factors include genetic predisposition, male gender, and prematurity; extrinsic factors include prone sleeping position, bed sharing, use of soft bedclothes or mattresses, putting the infant to sleep on upholstered furniture or adult mattresses, and prenatal or postnatal exposure to cigarette smoke or alcohol (Goldstein et al., 2016). Trachtenberg et al. (2012) state that a significant number of infants who have died of SIDS manifested one risk factor, and a majority had at least one intrinsic and two extrinsic risks.

Numerous reports from countries outside the United States have found a significant association between a prone sleeping position and the incidence of SIDS. The AAP guidelines (2016) recommend that infants should be placed on their backs to sleep. Other sleep environment recommendations from the AAP (2016) include the following:

- Avoid bed-sharing; put the infant in a safe bassinet or crib in the parent's room for sleeping. The infant should be kept in the parents' room a minimum of six months and ideally up to one year of age.
- Use only a firm mattress fitted specifically to the crib frame; do not place any soft bedding (e.g., blankets, pillows, crib bumpers) in the crib or bassinet; sleep wear designed to keep the infant warm can be used.
- Provide a pacifier for sleep; wait a few weeks for breastfeeding to be established before introducing a pacifier.
- Do not put the infant to sleep in a car seat, infant carrier or swing; be sure infants who are being carried in a sling have their faces exposed and that no fabric is blocking the infant's mouth or nose.

## PATHOPHYSIOLOGY

### *Sudden Infant Death Syndrome (SIDS)*

There is no single cause of SIDS. Autopsy findings in infants who have died of SIDS vary. Nonspecific findings such as mild pulmonary edema and petechial hemorrhage are found fairly consistently. Other, less frequent, findings include physical and biochemical markers for asphyxia or hypoxemia and altered neurotransmitter action affecting respiratory and cardiac function and arousal.

Prevention is of the utmost importance. Nurses must be role models and teachers about infant sleep positioning and other risk factors associated with SIDS. Teaching begins at the earliest contact the nurse has with the infant and parents and as soon as possible after delivery.

Reference: Hunt, C., & Hauck, F. (2016). Sudden infant death syndrome. In R. Kliegman, B. Stanton, J. St. Geme, et al. (Eds.), *Nelson textbook of pediatrics* (20th ed., Chapter 375). St. Louis, MO: Elsevier.

Recent studies have suggested that the marked decrease in the prevalence of SIDS, while greatly correlated with the Back to Sleep Campaign and AAP recommendations, is also related to changes in other intrinsic and extrinsic factors (Goldstein et al., 2016). Improvements in prenatal care contributing to a decrease in premature births, decreased prevalence of smoking, more sophisticated medications that address respiratory immaturity, and increased breastfeeding all have influenced the decreasing incidence of SIDS (Goldstein et al., 2016).

### Manifestations

The principal manifestation of SIDS is silent death. The child may be found in any position and may be clutching bedding.

### Diagnostic Evaluation

Diagnosis is confirmed through autopsy. A medical history of the infant and family should be taken. The infant is examined for signs of illness or trauma. The death scene is also investigated.

## NURSING CARE

### The Family of the Infant Who Has Died of SIDS

#### Assessment

The nursing care involved in a SIDS case is family-centered, not patient-centered. When an infant is brought into the emergency department with suspected SIDS, the family is often confused. If resuscitation was begun at home, they may assume that it was effective and that their infant is alive. Assessment of the family's understanding of the situation is necessary to plan for teaching and support. The nurse should assess the family's emotional status and coping strategies.

The nurse interviews the family in a calm, slow, and nonthreatening manner. Questions should not imply negligence or any involvement in the death. Parents need to be given time to think before they answer questions. Because the parents will be overwhelmed, questions may need to be repeated for clarity.

#### Nursing Diagnosis and Planning

The nursing diagnoses and expected outcomes that may be appropriate for the family of the infant victim of SIDS are as follows:

- Interrupted Family Processes related to death of a child.

*Expected outcome.* The parents and family will verbalize feelings related to the death of the infant.

- Compromised Family Coping related to death of a child.

*Expected outcome.* The parents and family will identify strengths and accept support of other family members, friends, professionals, and support groups.

- Deficient Knowledge related to not understanding the cause of death.

*Expected outcome.* The parents will verbalize an understanding of the cause of their child's death.

#### Interventions

The nurse working with a family whose child has died of SIDS should provide calm and compassionate support. The parents are confused about the death and are trying to cope with many emotions. Most parents will experience a combination of guilt, anger, and emotional pain.

A quiet room with dim lighting and a rocking chair should be provided for the family, and someone should remain with them. Assist the family to call family, friends, or clergy. The nurse should accompany the physician when the parents are told their infant is dead. At this time the parents should also be told that the apparent cause of death is SIDS and that nothing could have been done to prevent the death. This information may help minimize feelings of guilt.

Parents should be given the opportunity to say good-bye to their child. Because the parents may not think to ask to see their infant, the nurse should provide this opportunity.

The nurse might say, "Would you like to have some time alone with your baby? We will bring him to you, and you can take as long as you would like to hold him."

The infant should be cleaned and wrapped in a blanket and brought to the parents. Parents who are not given the opportunity to hold their child and say good-bye often regret it later, but parents who do not want time alone with their baby should have their decision respected.

The nurse should accept the parents' decision in this matter. Each parent will cope in an individualized way.

The need for an autopsy should be explained. The autopsy will verify the cause of death and confirm for the parents that they did not cause the death.

Before the parents leave the hospital, arrangements for follow-up care should be made. Many hospitals have a team consisting of a social worker, chaplain, and nurse that is called when a suspected SIDS death occurs. Often, referral to a visiting nurse for follow-up can assist the family to cope. The purposes of the home visit include listening to family concerns, clarifying what the family members know about SIDS, providing education and support for the family to work through grieving, and allaying any feelings of guilt (Stastny, Keens, & Alkon, 2016).

The nurse may refer the family to a local SIDS program for information, support, and counseling (American SIDS Institute, 509 Augusta Dr., Marietta, GA 30067; website: http://www.sids.org). Nurses who are involved in home visiting can encourage the family to communicate their feelings. Siblings should not be overlooked; parents may be so overwhelmed with their own grief that they forget their other children. The nurse can suggest local grief counseling resources that target siblings specifically. Another reaction might be to overprotect their other children. The nurse should guide the family in identifying the members' various responses and in treating them at the appropriate developmental level. Children in the family who perhaps resented the new baby may have tremendous guilt feelings. The loss of a sibling can be especially traumatic to a toddler, who does not understand the changes that are taking place in the family. Routines and rituals that are important to the toddler may be disrupted.

### Evaluation

- Is the family able to verbalize feelings associated with the death of the child?
- Has the family joined a support group or identified a support system?
- Has the extended family mobilized to support the family?
- Is the family using effective coping skills to work toward an understanding of the child's death?

## ASTHMA

Asthma is a leading cause of acute and chronic illness in children and the most frequent admitting diagnosis in children's hospitals. Despite advances in medical treatment, the prevalence of asthma has plateaued (Akinbami, Simon, & Rossen, 2016).

### Etiology

It is unclear why some children's airways are more reactive than others. However, it is known that asthma is caused by an interaction between genetic and environmental factors, and the underlying physiologic alteration is inflammatory. The chronic inflammatory process can contribute to periodic obstruction of the airway (Liu, Covar, Spahn, et al., 2016).

An asthma episode can be triggered by a variety of stimuli, including cold air, smoke, allergens (e.g., pollen, dander, cockroach droppings, dust, mold), viral infection, stress, exercise, odors, and environmental pollutants (Liu et al., 2016). Foods are occasionally the trigger in infants but less commonly in older children.

The immature anatomy of infants and small children predisposes them to increased distress from asthma. Children's smaller, narrower airways and decreased elastic lung recoil make them more prone to airway obstruction. The child's flexible rib cage and underdeveloped chest muscles and diaphragm lead to exhaustion when respiratory effort increases. Although asthma is not actually outgrown, the severity of asthma attacks often decreases as the child gets older because of increased airway size, improved diaphragmatic support, and better clearing of mucus. Asthma is considered a lifelong condition and can become increasingly severe after a period of remission.

### Incidence

Approximately 8.3% of children in the United States have asthma. The incidence of asthma is highest in children 10 to 17 years of age and higher among non-Hispanic Blacks and children from poverty who live in urban areas, where they are exposed to a variety of adverse environmental and psychosocial triggers (Akinbami et al., 2016). Risk factors present in early childhood can result in ongoing asthma; these factors include parental history of asthma, presence of allergy or atopy, previous severe lower respiratory infection (e.g., pneumonia or bronchiolitis), and isolated wheezing (Liu et al., 2016). Asthma is more common in boys. Exposure to tobacco smoke can exacerbate inflammation in the respiratory passages.

### Manifestations

The manifestations of asthma vary. A child with an asthma episode may have only a dry cough. Wheezing is a classic sign of asthma, but other signs can be present, including shortness of breath, cough, or dyspnea on exertion. Other manifestations may have a sudden or insidious onset:

- Retractions, nasal flaring, or stridor
- Nonproductive cough (with or without wheezing) that later becomes productive
- Tachypnea, orthopnea
- Restlessness, apprehension, diaphoresis
- Abdominal pain resulting from the strain placed on the abdominal muscles during labored breathing
- A hunched-over sitting position with arms braced (tripod position)
- Fatigue and difficulty performing simple tasks such as eating, walking, or even talking, because of shortness of breath
- A feeling of chest tightness followed by a dry cough, wheezing, and dyspnea
- Worsening of symptoms after the child goes to bed at night because of increased narrowing of the airways at night and pooling of secretions

At the beginning of the asthma episode, wheezing might be heard only with a stethoscope. As the severity of the episode increases, wheezing may become audible to the unaided ear. Children in severe respiratory distress may not demonstrate wheezing because of decreased air movement; decreased wheezing in a child who is not improving clinically can signal an inability to move air. This is referred to as a *silent chest* and is an ominous sign during an asthma episode. With treatment, increased wheezing may actually signal that the child's condition is improving.

### Diagnostic Evaluation

For children older than 5 years, an objective measure of airflow by spirometry is necessary for diagnosis. Improvement of symptoms in response to nebulized bronchodilators is strongly suggestive of asthma as opposed to other pulmonary disease (Nierengarten, 2016). History of associated allergic manifestations or family history of asthma supports the diagnosis. Other conditions that cause a chronic cough in young children, such as gastroesophageal reflux disease (GERD) (see Chapter 43) and sinusitis, need to be ruled out. However, both of these

## PATHOPHYSIOLOGY

### Asthma

Asthma is a reversible obstructive airway disease characterized by the following:

- Increased airway responsiveness to a variety of stimuli
- Bronchospasm resulting from constriction of bronchial smooth muscle
- Inflammation and edema of the mucous membranes that line the small airways and the subsequent accumulation of thick secretions in the airways

#### Immediate Reaction (Early Phase Response)

Allergens or other trigger substances activate immunoglobulin E (IgE) receptors on sensitized airway mast cells, causing mast cell degranulation and release of chemical mediators (histamine, leukotrienes, prostaglandins). These mediators cause bronchoconstriction shortly after exposure to the trigger; the bronchoconstriction resolves within 1 to 2 hours.

#### Delayed Reaction (Late-Phase Response)

Chemical mediators attract immune system cells (eosinophils, neutrophils, basophils) to the respiratory tract. Infiltration by these cells and their release of additional inflammatory substances damage the epithelial and smooth muscle cells, causing airway edema, mucous plugging of small airways, and additional inflammation. Bronchoconstriction recurs and can persist for several hours. The airway hyperresponsiveness resulting from this inflammatory process can last several weeks or months.

Late asthmatic responses can occur without a previous early (immediate) response. When asthma is precipitated by nonallergenic stimuli (exercise, cold air), bronchospasm usually lasts less than 1 hour and is not followed by a late response.

During an asthma episode, the mucous membranes lining the bronchioles become edematous and secrete large amounts of thick mucus. As a result, the airways narrow, leading to increased airway resistance and respiratory distress. Because small airways are normally wider on inspiration than expiration, the child is able to inhale but has difficulty exhaling through the narrowed bronchioles. Wheezing can be heard as air is forced through the narrow passages during expiration. Air becomes trapped, causing hyperinflation of the alveoli.

Airway obstruction is more severe in some parts of the lungs than in others, and air flows more easily into areas with the least resistance. The blood that flows to the less-ventilated portions of the lungs is inadequately saturated with oxygen. Thus, a mismatch between ventilation and perfusion in poorly ventilated areas of the lung occurs, resulting in incompletely saturated blood entering the systemic circulation and decreased oxygen partial pressure ($Po_2$) (hypoxia).

As the child struggles to get enough air, the respiratory rate increases (tachypnea). Tachypnea lowers carbon dioxide levels in the blood **(hypocapnia)**. As the child tires from the increased work of breathing, hypoventilation occurs and carbon dioxide levels increase. Increased levels of carbon dioxide in the blood **(hypercapnia)** during an asthma episode are a sign of severe airway obstruction and impending respiratory failure.

conditions can coexist with asthma in children and need to be managed (Liu et al., 2016).

Chest radiographs are usually normal except in cases of severe asthma, in which hyperinflation of the airways can be seen. Pulmonary function tests reveal a decreased forced expiratory volume in 1 second, increased residual volume from air trapping, and decreased vital capacity (the maximum amount of air exhaled after a maximum inhalation). Other pulmonary function test results might be altered as well. The peak expiratory flow rate (PEFR) is used to monitor children with chronic asthma.

Rhinitis, sinusitis, and nasal polyps are often present in children with asthma. Eosinophilia is present in both the blood and the sputum. Skin tests are often performed to identify specific allergens. The RAST may be used to identify specific antigens. Arterial blood gas measurements may be ordered in children having a severe asthma episode because of initial respiratory alkalosis and subsequent metabolic acidosis. Pulse oximetry values provide information about oxygenation.

## Therapeutic Management

The National Heart, Lung, Blood Institute (NHLBI) and National Asthma Education and Prevention Program (NAEPP) periodically update guidelines for asthma management. The current recommendations, EPR-3, were published in 2007 with updates added in 2008. Management is based on four interacting components: (1) accurate assessment of severity and regular monitoring for control of symptoms; (2) creating and maintaining a partnership for care that includes the child, parent, health provider, and school nurse; (3) management or elimination of environmental triggers and coexisting conditions; and (4) pharmacologic therapy (NHLBI & NAEPP, 2007).

### Acute Asthma Episode

A child who is having an episode of wheezing along with other symptoms of asthma is usually seen at a physician's office or an emergency department. First, a bronchodilator, usually a short-acting beta$_2$-adrenergic agonist (SABA) such as albuterol, is administered by a powered nebulizer or metered-dose inhaler (MDI) as often as every 20 minutes for 1 hour or continuously. Oxygen is administered as well. Close monitoring of the child's respiratory status after each course of medication assesses resolution of the episode.

If the child improves (PEFR greater than 70% of baseline, sustained oxygen saturation greater than 92% on room air for 4 hours), the child can return home with a SABA prescription and instructions for assessing respiratory status or with instructions for administering the SABA more frequently along with routine asthma medications. A short course of an oral corticosteroid (liquid preparations are available for infants) and an inhaled corticosteroid, if not part of the child's usual therapy, are prescribed (Liu et al., 2016). If symptoms continue to worsen, administration of the bronchodilator every 20 minutes for an additional hour is warranted. Indicators for hospital admission include increasing respiratory distress (tachypnea, tachycardia, retractions, inspiratory and expiratory wheeze), PEFR less than 40%, agitation, and breathlessness at rest (Liu et al., 2016; NHLBI & NAEPP, 2007).

Once the child is hospitalized, humidified oxygen is administered at 30%, either by nasal prongs or by facemask, to keep the oxygen saturation at 95% or greater. An IV line delivers fluids and provides venous access for parenteral medications (e.g., methylprednisolone) as ordered, although most children, if not in severe respiratory distress, can manage oral steroids. Chest radiography, arterial blood gas determinations, or pulse oximetry may be performed to further evaluate the child's oxygenation status. The child receives a bronchodilator by nebulizer every 20 minutes to 1 hour initially, with the interval between doses increased as the child's condition improves. Some providers choose to deliver the nebulized bronchodilator continuously at a dose of 5 to 15 mg/hr (Liu et al., 2016). Ipratropium bromide (Atrovent), an anticholinergic agent, has been found to be an effective bronchodilator when administered along with albuterol in some children with severe exacerbations.

Increasingly severe asthma that is unresponsive to vigorous treatment measures is termed *status asthmaticus.* Status asthmaticus is a medical emergency that can cause respiratory failure and death. Hospitalization, usually in an intensive care unit, is indicated. The child is placed on a continuous cardiorespiratory monitor and continuous pulse oximeter. Blood gas and serum electrolyte values are monitored, as is fluid status. In addition to the previously discussed measures, the child may receive continuous nebulized albuterol and ipratropium bromide every 6 hours. If the child's condition does not respond to these medications, oral or IV steroids are then administered. Endotracheal intubation with mechanical ventilation may be necessary, along with other adjunctive approaches (Liu et al., 2016). Antibiotics may also be administered to treat concurrent infection (e.g., pneumonia).

### Long-Term Management

Long-term asthma treatment should minimize and control symptoms, prevent acute asthma episodes, avoid the side effects of therapy, and help the child maintain a normal lifestyle. The NHLBI and NAEPP (2007) recommend an in-depth and regular education process that facilitates self-management of asthma. Beginning with the first and second follow-up visits after diagnosis, the provider teaches about the etiology of asthma, the goals of management and control, environmental assessment, triggers, self-assessment of symptoms, and medications. These are reviewed at every follow-up visit thereafter (NHLBI & NAEPP, 2007). A resource for parents is the Asthma and Allergy Foundation of America, 1233 20th St. NW, Washington, DC 20036; website: http://www.aafa.org.

#### *Environmental control*

**Irritants and allergens.** Children with asthma and their parents can decrease the frequency and severity of asthma episodes by recognizing and controlling the triggers that precipitate symptoms. Common environmental irritants include cigarette smoke, smoke from wood-burning stoves and fireplaces, fumes, deodorants, overhumidified air, and perfume. Allergenic triggers, such as animal dander, cockroaches, dust mites, seasonal pollens, and molds, often cause problems (Liu et al., 2016).

The extent of environmental control needed depends on the severity of the asthma. If the asthma is mild, prohibiting smoking in the house and controlling dust with frequent house cleaning may be adequate. If the child continues to have problems after these interventions, additional steps should be taken to minimize environmental triggers.

Immunotherapy (allergy shots) can be helpful in decreasing asthma symptoms caused by specific allergens the child cannot avoid. Immunotherapy is used in conjunction with, not in place of, other asthma therapies.

**Exercise.** Exercise can be a trigger of asthma in asthmatic children. Exercise-induced bronchospasm is triggered by rapid breathing of large volumes of cool, dry air (e.g., with mouth breathing during exercise). The symptoms of exercise-induced asthma usually begin after 5 to 10 minutes of exercise and often last from 30 to 60 minutes.

Measures to prevent exercise-induced asthma include the following:

- Warming the air by breathing through the nose or covering the mouth and nose with a scarf when exercising in cold weather
- Using an inhaled beta$_2$-adrenergic agonist 30 minutes before exercise
- Practicing techniques to decrease hyperventilation (e.g., progressive muscle relaxation, diaphragmatic breathing)

Because athletics and active play are important parts of a child's life, children with asthma should not be restricted from physical activity. Exercise not only increases physical fitness but also enhances self-esteem and offers valuable opportunities for socialization. Swimming is frequently recommended as an ideal sport for children with asthma because the air is humidified, and exhaling underwater prolongs exhalation and increases end-expiratory pressure. Other sports that do not require sustained exertion, such as gymnastics, baseball, and weight lifting, are also well tolerated, and, if asthma is well controlled, the child can usually participate in any type of sport.

**Infection.** Viral respiratory infections are the most frequent triggers of pediatric asthma. It is advisable for children with frequent or severe asthma to avoid exposure to individuals with a viral respiratory infection. Children with asthma also benefit from influenza vaccine.

**Emotions.** Asthma is not caused by psychosocial problems. However, emotional upset can exacerbate asthma symptoms. Laughing, crying, or shouting can act as mechanical triggers of bronchoconstriction. Also, a child with asthma may become angry or frustrated and refuse to take medication or adhere to a treatment regimen. Moreover, anxiety during an episode may cause the child to hyperventilate, aggravating asthma symptoms.

***Monitoring symptoms.*** Asthma symptoms can be best treated if they are detected early. Children and their parents should be taught the subtle early symptoms of an asthma episode (itchy chest or chin, cough, irritability or tired feeling, increased breathing rate, dry mouth, unusually dark circles under the eyes).

A useful device for monitoring breathing capacity is the peak flow meter, which measures the flow of air in a forced exhalation in liters per minute. Peak flow monitoring can help identify the start of an asthma episode, often before the child is aware of symptoms. It can also help determine the need for treatment modification. Home monitoring of PEFR can be performed several times a day. The results are compared with the child's normal predicted level and with results obtained over the preceding several days, providing an objective assessment of respiratory status (Box 45.2). Children with moderate to severe persistent asthma should do daily PEFR monitoring. Ideally,

### BOX 45.2 Monitoring Breathing Capacity With a Peak Flow Meter

The peak flow meter is a device to help children monitor their asthma on a daily basis. Results gained from daily monitoring are related to an overall action plan (see Fig. 45.4) prescribed by the child's provider.

**Procedure**

1. Remove gum or food from the mouth and stand up.
2. Move the pointer on the meter to 0, its lowest point.
3. Hold the meter horizontally, being sure to keep your fingers away from vent holes and the marker.
4. Relax and take a few slow, deep breaths. Then, slowly take the deepest breath you possibly can with your mouth wide open.
5. While holding your breath, place the mouthpiece of the meter on your tongue, and close your lips tightly around the mouthpiece.
6. Blow out as hard and fast as possible. Give a short, sharp blast, like blowing a loud whistle, not a slow blow. (The meter records the fastest blow, not the longest.) Look at the number by the marker on the numbered scale. Write it down.
7. Repeat two more times. Wait at least 10 seconds between attempts. (Be sure to move the pointer to 0 after each try.)
8. Record the highest of the three readings in your daily asthma diary.
9. It is best to take peak flow readings every day, preferably in the morning and before and after you take a bronchodilator.

PEFR results should be compared with the child's "personal best" value. This value is the number on the meter reached most often over a 2-week period, when the child is feeling well.

Even with teaching, parents and children sometimes do not appropriately recognize or provide appropriate treatment for worsening asthma signs and symptoms. This observation underscores the need for thorough teaching guidelines for home asthma management, including the following (NHLBI & NAEPP, 2007):

- A written asthma action plan (Fig. 45.4) that includes details of home management and lists indications for seeking physician or emergency department care
- Daily use of a peak flowmeter (in children older than 5 years) to monitor pulmonary status and response to treatment
- Home initiation of inhaled beta$_2$-adrenergic agonists, and oral steroids when daily control medications are ineffective for resolving symptoms
- Prompt communication with the healthcare provider for deteriorating respiratory status or reduced response to medication

## SAFETY ALERT

### *Emergency Asthma Management*

The following symptoms indicate the need for emergency treatment of asthma:

- Worsening wheeze, cough, or shortness of breath
- *No* improvement after bronchodilator use
- A peak flow rate that decreases or does not change (even after use of an inhaled beta$_2$-adrenergic agonist) or that is less than 60% of the child's predicted baseline level or personal best
- Difficulty breathing (the child's chest and neck are pulled in with each breath, or the child hunches over or struggles to breathe)
- Trouble with walking or talking
- Discontinuation of play without the ability to resume activity
- Listlessness and weak cry in an infant; refusal to suck bottle or breast
- Gray or blue lips or fingernails (in which case the child needs emergency treatment *immediately!*)

***Medications.*** Initiating daily pharmacologic treatment is based on classification of severity and usually begins when the child exhibits symptoms of mild and persistent asthma. In general, for children, the decision to initiate long-term therapy is based on the following (NHLBI & NAEPP, 2007, pp. 72 and 73):

- Presence of symptoms or need for SABA more than 2 days/week but not as often as daily
- Wakes at night because of symptoms, from one time or fewer to four times per month (depending on age)
- Experiences minor limitations in usual activity
- Frequent exacerbations (more than two every 6 to 12 months, depending on age) that require short bursts of oral steroids or, in children younger than 5 years, more than four episodes of wheezing a year lasting longer than 24 hours and presence of asthma risk factors

Generally, asthma is treated with a combination of medications from two categories: bronchodilators and antiinflammatory agents. The first-line treatment recommended to all children for long-term control of persistent asthma, regardless of severity, is an inhaled corticosteroid in a dose that reflects the severity of the asthma (Liu et al., 2016). Other control medications are determined using a "stepwise" system, a flexible approach to asthma control in which approaches and pharmacologic intervention increase or decrease based on the severity of symptoms (NHLBI & NAEPP, 2007). The medication regimen depends on the classification of the child's asthma and can be changed at home according to symptoms and peak flowmeter readings (Box 45.3). It is important to differentiate rescue medications (those used for immediate relief of an exacerbation) and routine medications.

**Rescue medications.** Some medications used to relieve an asthma episode are described here:

- *SABAs:* albuterol (Ventolin, Proventil), levalbuterol (Xopenex), and terbutaline (Brethine, Brethaire) relax bronchial smooth muscle and inhibit the release of mediators from mast cells. They are delivered by MDIs (metered dose inhalers) or by nebulizer three or four times daily if the child is symptomatic or before exercise.
- *Anticholinergic:* Ipratropium bromide (Atrovent) is used in combination with beta$_2$-adrenergic agonists in older children (older than 12 years) with severe asthma.
- *Mast cell inhibitors:* Cromolyn sodium (Intal), an inhaled nonsteroidal antiinflammatory drug, prevents asthma symptoms by blocking the release of mast cell mediators. It can be given 30 minutes before exposure to triggers. Another antiinflammatory asthma medication, nedocromil sodium (Tilade), is available for use in children age 12 years or older.

## BOX 45.3 Classification of Asthma Severity

**Intermittent**

- Symptoms less than or equal to twice per week or only with exercise
- Asymptomatic with normal peak expiratory flow rate (PEFR) between episodes; PEFR 80% of predicted rate during exacerbation
- Brief episodes
- Infrequent use of bronchodilator (<2 days a week)
- Few missed school days
- Rare activity limitation
- Symptoms rarely disturb sleep (less often than twice monthly)

**Mild Persistent**

- Symptoms more often than twice per week but less than once per day
- Exacerbations may begin to affect activity
- Exacerbations that require a burst of oral corticosteroids experienced more frequently (≥2/year; more often in children younger than 4 years)
- Nighttime symptoms one to four times per month depending on age
- PEFR >80% predicted

**Moderate Persistent**

- Daily symptoms occur and bronchodilator used daily; exacerbations requiring a corticosteroid burst ≥2 times yearly
- More than 9 school days missed per year
- Some activity limitation
- Sleep disturbed by symptoms more than once per week
- PEFR 60% to 80% of predicted

**Severe Persistent**

- Throughout the day on a daily basis
- Use of bronchodilator several times per day
- Severely limited physical activity
- Frequent sleep disturbance
- Exacerbations requiring corticosteroid bursts occur frequently (≥2 a year)
- PEFR less than or equal to 60% of predicted

Modified from National Heart, Lung, and Blood Institute & National Asthma Education and Prevention Program. (2007). *Expert panel report 3: guidelines for the diagnosis and management of asthma.* Retrieved from http://www.nhlbi.nih.gov.

## Asthma Action Plan

For: ____________ Doctor: ____________ Date: ____________

Doctor's Phone Number ____________ Hospital/Emergency Department Phone Number ____________

**GREEN ZONE**

### Doing Well

- No cough, wheeze, chest tightness, or shortness of breath during the day or night
- Can do usual activities

**And, if a peak flow meter is used,**

**Peak flow:** more than ____________ (80 percent or more of my best peak flow)

My best peak flow is: ____________

**Take these long-term control medicines each day (include an anti-inflammatory).**

| Medicine | How much to take | When to take it |
|---|---|---|
| | | |
| | | |
| | | |
| | | |
| | | |
| Before exercise: ❒ ____________ | ❒ 2 or ❒ 4 puffs ____________ | 5 to 60 minutes before exercise |

**YELLOW ZONE**

### Asthma Is Getting Worse

- Cough, wheeze, chest tightness, or shortness of breath, or
- Waking at night due to asthma, or
- Can do some, but not all, usual activities

**-Or-**

**Peak flow:** ________ to ________ (50 to 79 percent of my best peak flow)

**First** **Add: quick-relief medicine—and keep taking your GREEN ZONE medicine.**

____________ (short-acting $beta_2$-agonist) ❒ 2 or ❒ 4 puffs, every 20 minutes for up to 1 hour ❒ Nebulizer, once

**Second** **If your symptoms (and peak flow, if used) return to GREEN ZONE after 1 hour of above treatment:**

❒ Continue monitoring to be sure you stay in the green zone.

**-Or-**

**If your symptoms (and peak flow, if used) do not return to GREEN ZONE after 1 hour of above treatment:**

❒ Take: ____________ (short-acting $beta_2$-agonist) ❒ 2 or ❒ 4 puffs or ❒ Nebulizer

❒ Add: ____________ (oral steroid) mg per day For ________ (3–10) days

❒ Call the doctor ❒ before/ ❒ within ________ hours after taking the oral steroid.

**RED ZONE**

### Medical Alert!

- Very short of breath, or
- Quick-relief medicines have not helped, or
- Cannot do usual activities, or
- Symptoms are same or get worse after 24 hours in Yellow Zone

**-Or-**

**Peak flow:** less than ____________ (50 percent of my best peak flow)

**Take this medicine:**

❒ ____________ (short-acting $beta_2$-agonist) ❒ 4 or ❒ 6 puffs or ❒ Nebulizer

❒ ____________ (oral steroid) mg

**Then call your doctor NOW.** Go to the hospital or call an ambulance if:

- You are still in the red zone after 15 minutes AND
- You have not reached your doctor.

**DANGER SIGNS**

- **Trouble walking and talking due to shortness of breath**
- **Lips or fingernails are blue**
- **Take ❒ 4 or ❒ 6 puffs of your quick-relief medicine AND**
- **Go to the hospital or call for an ambulance** ____________ (phone) **NOW!**

**FIG 45.4** Asthma action plan. (From National Heart, Lung, and Blood Institute. [2007, April]. *Asthma action plan,* NIH Publication No. 07-5251. Washington, DC: USDHHS.)

- *Systemic corticosteroids:* Prednisone and prednisolone decrease airway inflammation. They are preferably given in short-burst courses of 5 to 7 days.

**Routine medications.** Additional medications are recommended for long-term asthma control:

- *Inhaled corticosteroids:* Beclomethasone, budesonide, fluticasone, flunisolide, and triamcinolone acetonide deliver topical antiinflammatory action directly to the airway.
- *Long-acting beta$_2$-adrenergic agonists (LABAs):* Salmeterol (Serevent) and formoterol (Foradil).
- *Combination medications:* budesonide and formoterol (Symbicort, a combination inhaled corticosteroid and LABA), fluticasone and salmeterol (Advair, a combination inhaled corticosteroid and LABA)
- *Leukotriene blockers:* Montelukast diminishes the mediator action of leukotrienes. Montelukast is available in sprinkles and chewable tablets and can be given to children as young as 1 year old.
- *Anti-immunoglobulin E (anti-IgE) antibody:* Omalizumab (Xolair) for allergic-type moderate to persistent asthma is approved for use in children older than 12 years. It is administered subcutaneously every 2 to 4 weeks.

Children with intermittent asthma use a SABA as needed for symptom relief. Children and families need to be cautioned not to overuse these medications and to notify the healthcare provider if the medications are needed more than twice per week or more frequently than every 3 to 4 hours during a 12-hour period.

Children with mild to moderate persistent asthma should take daily antiinflammatory medications. Beclomethasone by MDI (children older than 5 years) or nebulized budesonide for younger children is preferred. It can take up to 3 weeks of daily dosing to realize a therapeutic effect. In addition, SABAs are used to relieve symptoms. For moderate persistent asthma in children older than 5 years, a LABA is added to keep the inhaled corticosteroid (ICS) dosage lower. A leukotriene modifier may be given as an alternative to the LABA (Liu et al., 2016; NHLBI & NAEPP, 2007).

PEFR monitoring helps the child with mild to moderate asthma monitor symptoms and pulmonary function. The family is given a written management plan.

Children with persistent severe asthma take daily ICSs and LABAs or leukotriene blockers. Oral corticosteroids are considered for management of exacerbations.

**Medication delivery.** Inhaled medications are delivered either by nebulizer (see Parents Want to Know: Tips on Using a Nebulizer) or by MDI (see Chapter 38). Both can be used for older and younger children. A spacer attached to an MDI may make it easier for younger children to use the MDI. It also provides a more even distribution of medication. If using a spacer, the child attaches the spacer to the outlet of the MDI, closes the lips around the spacer mouthpiece, activates the canister, and then inhales.

Dry-powder inhalers (DPIs) are now available as well. They are easier to use than MDIs because the medication only disperses when the child inhales. In addition to the single-dose DPI, a multidose inhaler (for budesonide) and a multidose disk-shaped inhaler (for fluticasone and salmeterol) are available.

## BRONCHOPULMONARY DYSPLASIA

Bronchopulmonary dysplasia (BPD) is a chronic obstructive pulmonary disease that occurs as a result of acute lung injury in some infants who have received supplemental oxygen and mechanical ventilation. BPD is now commonly referred to as *chronic lung disease of infancy.*

### Etiology

Lung immaturity and impediments to appropriate lung development seem to be a key factors in the development of BPD, but many other factors affect its development as well. Some major risk factors for BPD are premature birth, respiratory infection, oxygen supplementation, mechanical ventilation, and patent ductus arteriosus (see Chapter 46). Research suggests a possible genetic predisposition as well (Khetan, Hurley, & Spencer, 2016). Because lung development varies between

**PARENTS WANT TO KNOW**

***Tips on Using a Nebulizer***

- Wash your hands before setting up the nebulizer equipment. You should have available the nebulizer machine, clean tubing (attached to the nebulizer), and the reservoir for medication with dome cover attached to the t-shaped mouthpiece, or mask, if preferred.
- Unscrew the reservoir from the dome and place the ordered amount of liquid medication in the reservoir; most medications will have additional normal saline solution added.
- Reattach the dome cap tightly, attach to the tubing, and turn on the machine. You will see mist begin to come out of the mouthpiece.
- Ask the child to put the mouthpiece in the mouth with the lips forming a seal around the mouthpiece. The child should be sitting upright, if possible, or on your lap.
- Your child should breathe at a normal rate, but deeply. As the treatment progresses, condensation may build up on the sides of the reservoir. Gently tap the reservoir so the liquid drops to the bottom.
- Most nebulizer treatments take approximately 15 to 20 minutes.
- When the treatment is complete, be sure to clean the equipment carefully according to manufacturer recommendations and store it in a clean, dry place.

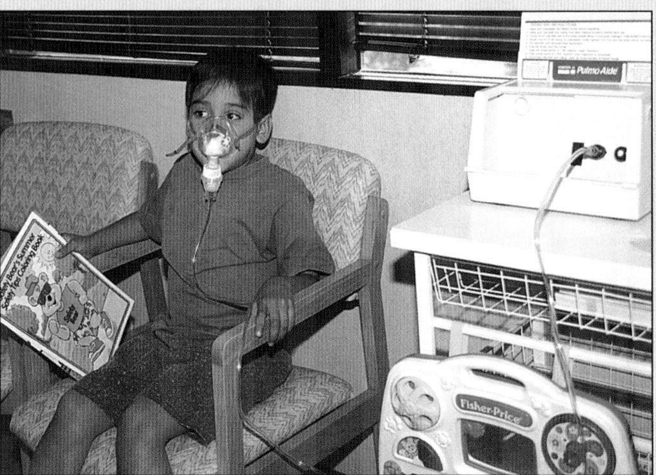

The powered nebulizer delivers a bronchodilator to the child who is having an acute asthma episode. This boy has a viral respiratory infection, which is a common trigger of acute asthma episodes in the pediatric population. (Courtesy Parkland Health and Hospital System Community Oriented Primary Care Clinic, Dallas, TX.)

## NURSING CARE PLAN

### *The Child Hospitalized With Asthma*

**Focused Assessment**

- Obtain a thorough history, including family history of asthma or allergy, past asthma or allergy episodes.
- Document treatments used and their effectiveness.
- Assess vital signs, oxygenation, level of consciousness, and respiratory status.
- Assess for signs of impending respiratory distress (retractions, nasal flaring, tachypnea, dyspnea, and fatigue).
- Auscultate breath sounds and document adventitious or diminished breath sounds.
- Assess fluid status (urine output, status of mucous membranes, presence of tears, skin turgor, and weight).
- Document the child's usual routines, previous hospitalizations, and the emotional states of the child and family.
- Determine any child or family teaching needs.

**Nursing Diagnoses**

Ineffective Airway Clearance related to bronchospasm and mucosal edema.
Impaired Gas Exchange related to air trapping in the bronchioles.

**Planning**

***Expected Outcomes***

1. The child will be able to clear the airway, as evidenced by a respiratory rate and rhythm appropriate for the child's age, the ability to expectorate mucus, and normal vital signs for age.
2. The child will have improved gas exchange, as evidenced by clear breath sounds, a pulse oximetry value of greater than 95% on room air, no use of accessory muscles, pink mucous membranes and nail beds, and a capillary refill time of less than 2 seconds.

**Interventions and *Rationales***

1. Monitor respiratory rate and effort, color, heart rate, and blood pressure every 15 to 30 minutes, with the interval lengthened as the child improves. Auscultate the chest for breath sounds. Monitor arterial blood gas values, pulse oximetry values, and pulmonary function test results. Notify the physician of any significant change (increased respiratory rate and effort, changes in wheezing, retractions, nasal flaring, severe cough, decreased alertness, cyanosis, increased dyspnea, apprehension).
   *Subtle changes in the child's condition may serve as an early warning of increased airway obstruction.*
2. Administer humidified oxygen at the ordered flow rate. If the child has chronic carbon dioxide retention, do not exceed 2 L/min.
   *Supplemental oxygen decreases hypoxia caused by airway edema, mucus, and bronchospasm. Administration of oxygen to a child with chronic carbon dioxide retention may lead to respiratory depression by decreasing the stimulus to breathe.*
3. Help the child assume an upright position or position of comfort. The older child may be most comfortable leaning forward on a pillow or an overbed table.
   *An upright position aids in expansion of the lungs and decreases pressure on the diaphragm.*
4. Administer medications as ordered and monitor for effectiveness. Assess whether medications are effectively relieving the child's symptoms. Monitor the child for side effects.
   *Short-acting bronchodilators provide relief fairly quickly. Oral or intravenous (IV) prednisolone begins to reduce airway inflammation.*
5. Keep the child on nothing-by-mouth (NPO) status during periods of severe respiratory distress, as ordered by the physician.
   *Oral intake is contraindicated for the child in severe respiratory distress because of the risk for aspiration.*
6. Obtain and maintain IV access.
   *IV access is necessary for administering medications and fluids.*
7. Ensure that respiratory treatments are given as ordered. Listen to and document the child's breath sounds before and after treatments. Encourage the child to cough and deep-breathe, especially after treatments. Suction as needed.
   *Breathing treatments help loosen or eliminate secretions and re-expand lung tissue. Mucous plugs can cause atelectasis and alveolar collapse.*
8. Ensure that emergency equipment is available (e.g., appropriate-size ventilation bag, endotracheal tubes, laryngoscope, emergency medication).
   *The child's condition can deteriorate rapidly. Immediate resuscitation may be necessary in the event of severe respiratory distress.*
9. Keep the child as calm as possible. Offer support during periods of respiratory distress.
   *Anxiety increases bronchospasms.*

**Evaluation**

Does the child have clear breath sounds with free movement of air?
Does the child expend minimal respiratory effort?
Does the child maintain a patent airway?
Is the respiratory rate within normal limits for age, and is the oxygen saturation greater than 95%?

**Nursing Diagnosis**

Fatigue related to hypoxia and increased work of breathing.

**Planning**

***Expected Outcome***

The child will exhibit decreased fatigue, as evidenced by less irritability and restlessness, uninterrupted sleep periods, and ability to perform usual activities.

**Interventions and *Rationales***

1. Observe the child for signs and symptoms of hypoxia, including restlessness, fatigue, irritability, increased heart rate, and increased respiratory rate.
   *Irritability and agitation may be early signs of hypoxia. Prompt treatment of hypoxia decreases fatigue.*
2. Organize nursing care to provide periods of uninterrupted rest and sleep.
   *Periods of quiet decrease stress and promote rest.*
3. Encourage the parents' presence, particularly if the child is young.
   *The parents' presence decreases fear and anxiety.*
4. Provide for the child's physical comfort. Encourage quiet, age-appropriate play activities as the child's condition improves.
   *Physical and emotional comfort confers a sense of well-being and promotes rest.*
5. Implement measures to relieve respiratory distress. Monitor the frequency of nebulized medications.
   *Restlessness, agitation, and inability to sleep are side effects of some asthma medications.*

***Evaluation***

Is the child able to play or perform usual activities without undue fatigue?

***Nursing Diagnosis***

Risk for Deficient Fluid Volume related to increased respiratory rate, diaphoresis, and decreased oral intake.

*Continued*

## NURSING CARE PLAN—cont'd

### *The Child Hospitalized With Asthma*

**Planning**

***Expected Outcomes***

1. The child will drink adequate fluid for age and weight.
2. The child will not become dehydrated.

**Interventions and *Rationales***

1. Monitor intake and output, status of mucous membranes, body weight, tearing, and urine specific gravity. Maintain urine specific gravity at 1.002 to 1.030. Monitor electrolyte levels. Observe the child's sputum for color, tenacity, and amount.
   *Rapid respiratory rate, diaphoresis, and increased pulmonary secretions can cause dehydration and increased viscosity of excretions.*
2. Maintain IV infusion at the ordered flow rate. Avoid excessive amounts of fluid.
   *Adequate hydration enhances liquefaction of secretions, and thinner secretions are more easily expectorated. Excessive fluids can lead to pulmonary edema.*
3. Encourage oral fluids when the respiratory distress has decreased, with the amount consumed being determined by the child's calculated needs. Offer favorite fluids. Provide liquids at the bedside.
   *Oral fluids are contraindicated during acute respiratory distress to minimize the risk for aspiration. Children are most likely to drink fluids if they are offered fluids they like.*
4. Offer liquids at room temperature. Avoid milk and milk products.
   *Cold liquids can aggravate bronchospasm. Milk sometimes causes increased coughing and mucus production.*
5. Provide a humidified atmosphere.
   *Humidification helps liquefy secretions and helps maintain hydration.*

**Evaluation**

Does the child ingest adequate fluid for age and weight?
Does the child maintain a urine specific gravity of 1.002 to 1.030?
Does the child maintain pre-illness weight?
Are moist mucous membranes and good skin turgor present?
Does the child have urinary output appropriate for age? (See Chapter 40.)

**Nursing Diagnosis**

Anxiety related to hospitalization and respiratory distress.

**Planning**

***Expected Outcomes***

1. The child will exhibit reduced anxiety, as evidenced by a relaxed body position and a decrease in negative behaviors.
   The parents will demonstrate reduced anxiety by verbalizing an accurate knowledge of asthma and participating in the child's care in a calm manner.

**Interventions and *Rationales***

1. Teach the child techniques to control panic and anxiety and to slow the breathing rate (e.g., visually imagining staying calm, breathing exercises, pursed-lip breathing, belly breathing).
   *Concentration on such activities during an asthma episode calms the child and decreases the fear of suffocation.*
2. Maintain a calm, quiet environment and a reassuring manner. Stay with the child. Provide care efficiently and calmly.
   *The ability to remain calm decreases the child's oxygen demand and work of breathing.*
3. Reassure the child that there is someone nearby to assist if breathing difficulties develop. To allay any fears about going to sleep, tell the child that someone will be watching at night. Make the call light available for older children.
   *Calm reassurance by the nurse can decrease the child's fear of suffocation and facilitate rest.*
4. Use play therapy.
   *Therapeutic play allows the child to work through fears in a nonthreatening manner.*
5. Encourage the parents to stay with the child. Praise the parents for rooming-in and supporting the child.
   *The presence of a familiar person can decrease fear and anxiety.*
6. Keep parents informed of treatments, routines, and the child's condition.
   *Reassuring the parents can help calm the child because parental anxiety is quickly transferred to the child. Frequent and accurate updating of the child's condition reassures parents and decreases fear of the unknown.*
7. Encourage expression of feelings by child and parents.
   *Expressing feelings can help relieve stress and guilt.*
8. Avoid the use of sedatives.
   *Sedatives can depress respirations.*
9. Explain all procedures in an age-appropriate manner.
   *Procedures and an unfamiliar hospital setting may produce anxiety. Explanations decrease fear of the unknown.*
10. Facilitate trust by being truthful and acknowledging the discomfort of procedures.
    *Honesty fosters trust.*

**Evaluation**

Does the child cooperate with and participate in treatment and appear relaxed?
Does the child obtain adequate rest and sleep?
Do the parents verbalize decreased anxiety about the hospitalization and the child's condition?

**Nursing Diagnosis**

Interrupted Family Processes related to the possibility of a chronic illness.

**Planning**

***Expected Outcomes***

The family will demonstrate the ability to cope with the child's illness and adhere to management in a way that promotes the child's normal growth and development.

**Interventions and *Rationales***

1. Provide opportunities for the family to express feelings. Recognize and accept negative feelings about the child and the illness.
   *This nonjudgmental approach helps the family work through fear, guilt, anxiety, and economic problems.*
2. Explore previous coping mechanisms used in times of stress.
   *Identification and review of previously successful coping skills can assist the family in dealing with the current crisis.*
3. Explain all procedures and treatments.
   *A thorough explanation decreases fear of the unknown and anxiety.*
4. Keep parents informed of the child's condition.
   *Knowledge gives parents a sense of control.*
5. Arrange for the family to meet with others affected by asthma. Identify available community resources.
   *Meeting others with asthma can assist with problem solving and provide support.*

## NURSING CARE PLAN—cont'd

### *The Child Hospitalized With Asthma*

**Evaluation**

Is the family able to provide necessary care?
Can the family describe how to access helpful resources?

**Nursing Diagnosis**

Deficient Knowledge about the disease process and home management related to inexperience with asthma.

**Planning**

***Expected Outcomes***

1. The family will identify asthma triggers.
2. The family will describe home management principles.

**Interventions and *Rationales***

1. Determine the child's and parents' understanding of asthma. Explain unfamiliar procedures and equipment at the child's level of understanding. Teach the family about the disease, its triggers, and prescribed medications and treatments.
   *Understanding increases adherence to treatment.*
2. Help the family identify precipitating factors (e.g., exercise, infections, allergens, weather changes).
   *An awareness of triggers may decrease future asthma episodes.*
3. Explain the role of emotions and stress in the development of asthma symptoms.
   *Stress and emotional upset can trigger bronchospasm.*
4. Teach the child and family about the importance of taking medications as prescribed. Assess ability to afford medications. Provide written information and instructions about medications (names, side effects, dosages, times of administration). Teach the family to recognize signs and symptoms that warrant notification of the physician. Reinforce the need to keep follow-up appointments.
   *Knowledge of medications increases adherence to the therapeutic regimen; adherence helps maintain serum drug levels within a therapeutic range.*
5. Assist in developing an exercise program for the child. Medication may be needed before exercise. Teach the importance of a healthy lifestyle (regular exercise, adequate fluids and nutrition, rest, prevention of infection).
   *Exercise promotes pulmonary and cardiovascular health and assists the child in leading a normal life.*
6. Refer the family to a support group.
   *Meeting with other children and families affected by asthma provides an avenue for expressing feelings and sharing information.*
7. Teach self-management of asthma. Teach the necessary skills for home care. Encourage the child to take charge of asthma. The child should know what triggers to avoid, early warning signs of an episode, the correct use of treatment aids (metered-dose inhaler [MDI], dry-powder inhaler [DPI], nebulizer, peak flow meter), and proper administration of medications and techniques for stress reduction and relaxation. Encourage the child and family to participate in programs designed to develop effective self-management and decision-making skills.
   *Knowledge of asthma decreases anxiety during acute episodes. The frequency and severity of episodes will be minimized if the child knows the appropriate actions for controlling symptoms. Learning about the condition can help decrease anxiety during episodes and increase the child's ability to take appropriate action to control symptoms. The frequency and severity of asthma episodes will be minimized if the child knows what triggers to avoid, the early warning signs of an episode, and the correct treatment of symptoms.*
8. Teach the importance of follow-up care and routine health maintenance, such as keeping immunizations up to date.
   *Preventing infection and practicing healthy living habits help decrease asthma triggers.*

**Evaluation**

Do the child and family verbalize an accurate knowledge of asthma and its treatment?
Do the child and family keep follow-up appointments?
Does the child resume normal daily activities?

infants, gestational age alone does not always predict the development of BPD.

## Incidence

BPD is a significant cause of morbidity and death among very low-birth-weight infants (less than 1000 g) and infants who have survived respiratory distress syndrome (RDS) (see Chapter 29). It is the most frequently seen chronic lung condition in infants. The true incidence of BPD is unknown because of differences in how the condition is categorized (Poindexter & Jobe, 2015). The extent of very premature births increases the incidence.

## Manifestations

Manifestations of BPD include tachycardia and tachypnea related to decreased oxygenation; an increased work of breathing, retractions, and prolonged exhalation with the increased use of abdominal and accessory muscles; pallor associated with chronic hypoxia; and cyanosis and activity intolerance (feeding, handling). Affected infants also exhibit weight loss or poor weight gain related to the increased metabolic workload, hypoxia, and poor feeding; restlessness and irritability related to hypoxia; wheezing (intermittent or chronic) associated with a hyperresponsive airway; and puckering or pursing of the mouth with flaring of the nares (early signs of impending respiratory distress).

## PATHOPHYSIOLOGY

### *Bronchopulmonary Dysplasia*

The pressure of mechanical ventilation damages the bronchial epithelium. Macrophages and polymorphonuclear inflammatory cells invade the airways, causing airway edema. Alveolar walls become thickened, and fibrotic changes occur in the airways and alveoli. The continued use of oxygen affects the growth and development of lung structures, significantly reducing the number of developing alveoli.

Cystic and atelectatic areas develop in the lungs, predisposing the infant to pulmonary hypertension. Loss of ciliated cells also can occur, which decreases the lungs' ability to remove mucus and leads to mucous plugs, atelectasis, and pneumonia.

## Diagnostic Evaluation

The diagnosis is based on clinical manifestations and radiographic abnormalities. BPD is categorized according to severity, which differs according to whether the infant was born earlier than 32 weeks' gestation or after 32 weeks (Khetan et al., 2016; Lestrud, 2016):

- Mild: requires supplemental oxygen for at least 28 days, but no longer requires it by 36 weeks of gestational age (<32 weeks' gestation); or oxygen for 56 days after birth (>32 weeks' gestation)

- Moderate: requires supplemental oxygen for at least 28 days, but less than 30% oxygen at 36 weeks' gestational age (<32 weeks); or less than 30% oxygen for 56 days after birth (>32 weeks).
- Severe: requires supplemental oxygen for at least 28 days, and greater than 30% oxygen at 36 weeks, and needs nasal CPAP, or mechanical ventilation (<32 weeks); or requires greater than 30% oxygen at 36 weeks, and needs nasal CPAP, or mechanical ventilation for 56 days after birth (>32 weeks).

Chest radiographs may show infiltrates.

## Therapeutic Management

Prevention of BPD is related to RDS prevention in very low-birth-weight infants. Precautions include provision of corticosteroids to the mother before birth, postnatal surfactant, and administration of vitamin A, as well as the use of nasal continuous positive airway pressure (CPAP) when the infant is intubated as well as after extubation (Carlo & Ambalavanan, 2016).

Treatment goals for the infant with BPD include maintaining adequate oxygenation to promote growth and development, preventing further lung disease, and promoting healing of the damaged lungs. Treatment consists of oxygen therapy, drug therapy, and nutritional support.

Positive-pressure ventilation should be discontinued as soon as possible. If mechanical ventilation is necessary to maintain life, the lowest possible inflation pressures should be used, together with expiratory times that allow the lung to empty completely. Weaning from the ventilator may be a slow process, requiring constant attention to subtle changes in the infant; however, earlier weaning strategies may lead to more positive outcomes (Carlo & Ambalavanan, 2016; Khetan et al., 2016).

### Oxygen Therapy

Oxygen can be administered through a hood, facemask, or nasal cannula. Oxygen saturation rates should be monitored closely and are usually maintained at a target of 92% (Khetan et al., 2016). Many infants are discharged from the hospital while still oxygen dependent.

### Medications

Diuretics and fluid restriction are initiated to treat pulmonary interstitial edema. Furosemide is the most common diuretic used, with some physicians attempting to change the medication to chlorothiazide and spironolactone once enteral feeding is tolerated. Because infants with BPD often have fluid overload and edema, fluid and electrolyte status should be monitored closely. Supplemental calcium, potassium, and chloride may be indicated for the infant receiving diuretics.

Inhaled bronchodilators, especially albuterol, sometimes in conjunction with ipratropium, can lessen airway resistance and decrease the possibility of lung damage. Theophylline or caffeine can be used to enhance lung compliance and improve respiratory status by relaxing the smooth muscles. Administration of dexamethasone is no longer recommended, but an ICS might be helpful to hasten extubation (Carlo & Ambalavanan, 2016).

Infants with BPD have frequent infections related to increased susceptibility and exposure to invasive treatments and procedures. After the initial stages of BPD, the risk for infection is probably the greatest risk to survival for these infants; hospital readmissions are frequent. RSV prophylaxis is recommended.

### Nutrition

The infant needs increased nutritional intake for lung growth and repair beyond that required for normal infant growth. Other factors, such as frequent respiratory exacerbations and feeding problems, also increase caloric needs. A calorie intake of approximately 150 kcal/kg/day to produce a weight gain of 20 to 30 g/day is an appropriate goal. High-calorie formulas (24 or 27 cal/oz) or fortified breast milk assist with meeting this requirement, especially in infants with fluid intake restrictions. The addition of medium-chain triglyceride oil or glucose polymers to the formula increases the calories per ounce. Some infants with BPD experience GERD (see Chapter 43), requiring therapy with an appropriate antacid medication (Lestrud, 2016).

## Prognosis

Most infants with BPD do improve. Death usually results from pulmonary complications. Most infants with BPD will require continuing therapy at home. Some will develop chronic airway hyperreactivity, which can progress to bronchial asthma. Many infants with BPD are rehospitalized during the first year of life because of acute respiratory tract infections. Some infants with BPD have growth retardation and developmental delay as well.

## Nursing Considerations

Because of their low birth weight and possible RDS, most neonates with BPD are initially cared for in a special-care nursery. Nursing intervention before discharge includes meticulous planning for home care, coordinating referrals, and teaching home management.

Home care of the infant with BPD decreases the risk for hospital-acquired infection and reduces healthcare costs. Care at home also improves social development by encouraging interaction between the child and family.

Preparation for discharge and home care requires a great deal of education and reassurance. Educating the family with a chronically ill or technology-dependent child must begin early with basic care—feeding, bathing, holding, and playing. This care progresses to medical, nursing, and respiratory procedures. The infant might continue to receive supplemental oxygen at home or may have a tracheostomy. Some infants are discharged while they are still ventilator dependent. Families must be taught the necessary precautions for safe use of oxygen in the home (see Patient-Centered Teaching: Safe Use of Oxygen at Home). Before hospital discharge, the nurse contacts emergency services, utility companies, and the telephone company to notify them that a technology-dependent child will be living in their area (Fig. 45.5). Required actions for contacting these services in case of emergency should be reviewed with the family.

Evaluating the family's response to the infant's illness and their coping strategies is critical for optimal home management of the infant with a chronic condition. The nurse should help the family identify physical and psychological strengths and weaknesses. Because the care of an infant with BPD can be extraordinarily expensive, the nurse should consider referring the family to social services for access to potential financial assistance.

# CYSTIC FIBROSIS

Cystic fibrosis (CF), the most common lethal genetic disease in Whites, is a chronic multisystem disorder affecting the exocrine glands. The mucus produced by the exocrine glands (particularly those of the bronchioles, small intestine, and pancreatic and bile ducts) is abnormally thick, causing obstruction of the small passageways of these organs. Although CF is incurable, the life expectancy of affected children has increased dramatically. The survival age is 40 years, making CF a disease not only of children but also of young adults (Cystic Fibrosis Foundation, 2016). The discovery of the mutated gene, *cystic fibrosis transmembrane conductance regulator* (CTFR), which encodes

**ELECTRIC COMPANY**
**REQUEST FOR SPECIAL CONSIDERATION**

Date: ______________________________

Name: ______________________________

Address: ____________________________

____________________________________

Phone: ______________________________

Account Number: ______________________

**Attention: Customer Service**

Our infant/child, ______________, is under the care of

Dr. ____________________ at ____________________ for ____________________

This condition(s) requires the use of a cardiorespiratory monitor and/or other life support equipment, specifically:

______________________________________________________________________

The necessary equipment selected for home care is equipped with a battery back-up system that will power the equipment in the event of a power failure for a **limited period of time.** If a power failure occurs, it is imperative to restore service to this home as soon as possible. Please place this home on a priority list for restoration of electric service. If you have advance warning of a temporary interruption in electric service, please notify the parents so alternative arrangements can be made. If you have questions regarding the specifications of the equipment provided, please contact our equipment provider, Pediatric Home Care Associates.

Thank you for your cooperation.

Sincerely yours,

OUR EQUIPMENT PROVIDER IS:

**FIG 45.5** Example of a letter that can be used to notify the local public service company that a technology-dependent child is living in the service area. (Courtesy Pediatric Home Care Associates, Garfield, NJ. From Barnhart, S.L., & Czervinske, M.P. [1995]. *Perinatal and pediatric respiratory* care [p. 662]. Philadelphia: Saunders.)

a defective chloride channel in epithelial cells, has improved clinicians' understanding of the pathophysiologic features of CF and has significantly aided diagnosis.

## Etiology

CF is transmitted as an autosomal recessive trait, which means that both parents must carry the gene for the child to be affected. If both parents carry the CF gene, each pregnancy has a 25% chance of producing an affected child. There are more than 1800 mutations of the CF gene, many of which determine the severity of disease symptoms. The most common mutation is the F508del mutation (Egan, Green, & Voynow, 2016). The test for carriers of CF can identify this and nearly 40 other frequently seen mutations (Cystic Fibrosis foundation, 2016).

## Incidence

The incidence of CF in white children is approximately 1 in 3500 live births (Egan et al., 2016). The prevalence in Blacks, Hispanics, and Asians is lower than that in the white population (Egan et al., 2016). Approximately 1 in 29 people in the United States are carriers (Cystic Fibrosis Foundation, 2016). Early diagnosis is possible, and more than three quarters of affected children are diagnosed before they reach age two years (Cystic Fibrosis Foundation, 2016).

## Manifestations

Signs and symptoms of CF, the extent of specific organ system involvement, and the age at which symptoms begin vary widely among affected children. Symptoms gradually worsen as the disease progresses, and the outcome is eventually fatal, as there is no cure.

### Respiratory System

Signs and symptoms of respiratory involvement include wheezing and a dry, nonproductive cough (earliest pulmonary manifestations), repeated bouts of bronchiolitis, pneumonia and bronchitis, and purulent and copious sputum accompanying chronic bacterial infections. The cough at this stage is wet and paroxysmal and may be followed by vomiting. As the disease progresses, symptoms include crackles, wheezes, diminished breath sounds, accessory muscle use, retractions, hypoxia, and cyanosis. Cough increases and, dyspnea and tachypnea occur. Emphysema and atelectasis may develop as the airways become increasingly obstructed with secretions; cor pulmonale and congestive heart failure resulting from fibrotic lung changes can be seen in later stages of the disease. Spontaneous pneumothorax or hemoptysis (blood-stained sputum) is seen in later stages as well. Nasal polyps, sinusitis, digital clubbing (Fig. 45.6), and a barrel chest (increased anteroposterior chest diameter) are also noted.

### Digestive System

Digestive system involvement is marked by steatorrhea (frothy, foul-smelling stools two to three times bulkier than normal) and flatus. Malnutrition and growth failure may be evident despite normal caloric intake; deficiencies in the fat-soluble vitamins A, D, E, and K are caused by an inability to absorb fats. Vitamin A deficiency can lead to

## PATIENT-CENTERED TEACHING

### *Safe Use of Oxygen at Home*

| Safety Guidelines | Rationale |
|---|---|
| Secure the oxygen tank in an upright position. | Oxygen tanks are highly explosive. If a horizontally positioned tank explodes, the rapid release of oxygen can catapult it through both animate (human bodies) and inanimate (walls) objects. |
| Keep oxygen tanks at least 5 feet from heat sources and electrical devices (e.g., space heaters, heating vents, fireplaces, radios, vaporizers). | |
| Ensure that no one smokes in the room or in the area of the oxygen tank. | Smoking increases the risk for fire, which could cause the tank to explode; escaped oxygen would feed the fire. |
| Avoid using alcohol-based substances or oil to relieve dryness around your child's mouth (e.g., petroleum jelly, vitamin A & D ointment, baby oil). | Both alcohol and oil are flammable and increase the risk of fire. |
| Keep a fire extinguisher readily available. | A fire extinguisher may be needed to put out a fire immediately. |
| Turn off both the volume regulator and the flow regulator when oxygen is not in use. | If the volume regulator is on when the oxygen is turned on, the child might receive a rapid, forceful flow of oxygen in the face that could be frightening and uncomfortable. Oxygen leakage, which might not be detected because oxygen is odorless, can cause a fire. |

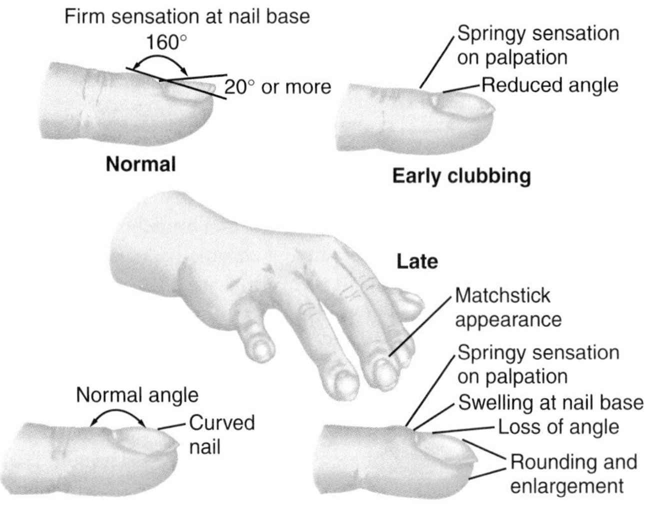

**FIG 45.6** Digital clubbing can be an indication of hypoxia, which often occurs in cystic fibrosis and other respiratory disorders.

xerophthalmia (abnormal thickening of eye tissue), and vitamin K deficiency can result in bleeding, especially in infants. Children with CF are usually thin and underweight, but with adequate treatment most attain normal height. A protuberant abdomen, barrel chest, wasted buttocks, and thin extremities are common.

Meconium ileus in the neonate is the earliest clinical manifestation of CF. Intestinal obstruction later in life, called *meconium ileus equivalent,* sometimes occurs and is the result of impacted feces at the ileocecal junction. Rectal prolapse and intussusception can also occur. Liver disease, as manifested by biliary cirrhosis, portal hypertension, and esophageal varices, resulting from obstruction of the bile ducts is commonly seen in the first decade of life, with a prevalence of 30% (Egan et al., 2016). Diabetes mellitus has evolved as a complication because of increased longevity.

### Exocrine Glands

Abnormally high concentrations of sodium and chloride in sweat are an early sign of CF (mothers often report that their infants taste salty when kissed). The risk of electrolyte imbalance during hot weather is high; infants are especially prone to developing hyponatremia and hypochloremia, as well as dehydration. Many children complain of a dry mouth and have an increased susceptibility to infection.

### Reproductive System

Involvement of the reproductive system is marked by an average 2-year delay in the development of secondary sex characteristics. Females with CF may have difficulty becoming pregnant because of the thick cervical mucus, which acts as a barrier to sperm. This impairment of fertility should not be relied on as a birth control method. Women with mild CF can carry a pregnancy to term with conscientious prenatal care. Sterility caused by lack of sperm is noted in approximately 95% of male patients with CF; otherwise, sexual function is normal (Egan et al., 2016).

## Diagnostic Evaluation

CF has been called the great imitator because failure to thrive and chronic respiratory infection are signs of many other childhood conditions. In some infants, CF is evident at birth because of symptoms of severe bowel obstruction (meconium ileus) caused by intestinal plugging by thick, tenacious secretions. Nearly all U.S. states now test for CF in routine newborn screening. The current test uses the immunoreactive trypsinogen assay; if elevated, this test is followed by deoxyribonucleic acid (DNA) testing for gene mutations (Nakano & Tluczek, 2014). Early diagnosis and treatment of CF make a difference in the quality and length of life for these children.

The diagnosis of CF requires a combination of clinical signs, close family history of CF, or positive newborn screening plus a positive sweat test result (obtained on two separate occasions), or DNA testing that identifies two CF mutations (Egan et al., 2016; Nakano & Tluczek, 2014). The sweat test, *pilocarpine iontophoresis,* measures the amount of sodium and chloride in sweat and is simple, painless, and reliable. A chloride level greater than 60 mEq/L is considered to be diagnostic for CF; a level of 40 to 60 mEq/L is suggestive of CF and requires a repeat test. A sample of at least 50 mg of sweat is required for accurate results. Because this amount is difficult to obtain from small infants, the sweat test is usually not reliable in infants younger than 2 weeks.

In addition to the sweat test, the following studies may also be performed: 72-hour fecal fat determination, liver function tests (alanine aminotransferase and aspartate aminotransferase), fasting blood glucose test, chest radiography, sputum culture (for identification of infective organisms), and pulmonary function tests.

DNA analysis of chorionic villi samples or amniotic fluid testing can establish a diagnosis prenatally. DNA analysis (by buccal smear or blood sample) can also determine whether siblings of the affected child are carriers.

## PATHOPHYSIOLOGY

### *Cystic Fibrosis*

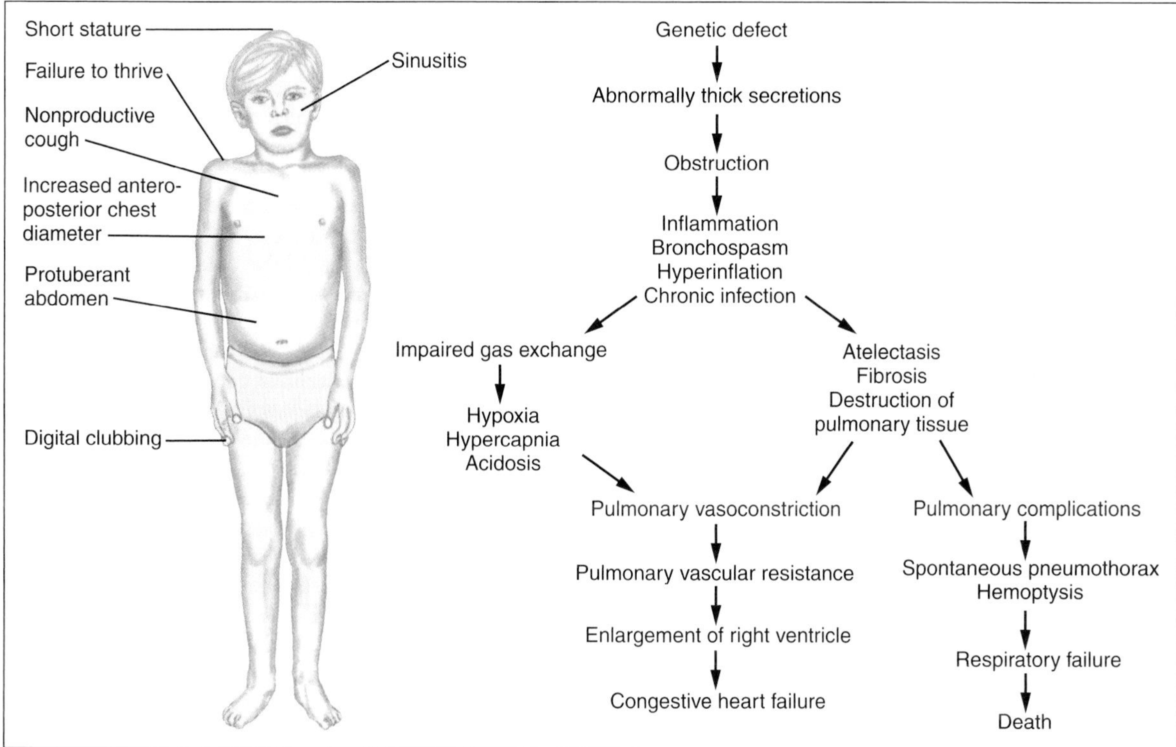


Cystic fibrosis (CF) affects the exocrine glands throughout the body and causes respiratory, digestive, integumentary, and reproductive dysfunction and damage.

#### Respiratory System

Abnormally thick, sticky secretions cause obstruction of both the small and large airways. Stasis of secretions from bronchial obstruction provides a medium for bacterial growth. Chronic infection causes the release of toxic chemicals that damage lung tissues and alter host defenses within the airways, thus exacerbating the infection and inflammation. Inflammation can also cause bronchospasm, worsening airway blockage. Because airways dilate on inspiration and constrict on exhalation, air is trapped in the peripheral airways narrowed by mucus secretions. Hyperinflation is one of the first findings on chest radiographs of a child with CF. Chronic infection leads to atelectasis and eventual fibrosis and destruction of pulmonary tissue.

As the disease progresses, the lungs of almost all children with CF eventually become colonized with *Pseudomonas aeruginosa*, an organism that most clinicians believe can never be completely eradicated from the respiratory tract but can be controlled with vigorous antibiotic therapy. Chronic respiratory tract infection and impaired oxygen and carbon dioxide exchange cause varying degrees of hypoxia, hypercapnia, and acidosis. Fibrotic lung changes occur as the disease worsens and hypoxia increases. Alveolar hypoxia leads to pulmonary vasoconstriction, increasing pulmonary vascular resistance. Increased pulmonary vascular resistance causes the right side of the heart to work harder to pump blood into the lungs. Enlargement of the right ventricle in response to increased pulmonary resistance (cor pulmonale) results. Heart failure may develop. Pulmonary complications include sinusitis, spontaneous pneumothorax, and hemoptysis. Death in individuals with CF is almost always the result of respiratory failure.

#### Digestive System

Blocked by thick mucus, the pancreatic ducts are unable to secrete trypsin, amylase, and lipase into the small intestine. Without these digestive enzymes, proteins, carbohydrates, and fats are poorly absorbed. Bowel obstruction from thickened intestinal mucus and pancreatic insufficiency may be present at birth (meconium ileus). The islets of Langerhans in the pancreas are normal in patients with CF, but they may decrease in number as the disease progresses and the pancreas undergoes fibrotic changes. Type 1 diabetes sometimes develops in older children with CF. Abnormalities of the gallbladder are common.

#### Integumentary System

The sweat glands of children with CF secrete normal amounts of sweat. However, the levels of sodium and chloride in the sweat are two to five times the normal range.

#### Reproductive System

Ninety-five percent of males with CF are sterile because of obstruction of the deferent ducts and seminal vesicles. Females have reduced fertility because of abnormally thick cervical mucus, which impedes sperm penetration of the cervical canal.

## Therapeutic Management

Therapy is individualized for each child and is aimed at preventing and treating pulmonary infections, maintaining optimal nutritional status, and promoting psychological adjustment. Children with CF are cared for at home most of the time. They are hospitalized during acute pulmonary infections, periodically for IV antibiotic treatment and vigorous chest physiotherapy (CPT), and for end-stage disease.

### Respiratory Problems

Because chronic respiratory infection is a major cause of lung damage in patients with CF, treatment goals are to relieve airway obstruction by mobilizing secretions, to decrease the number of bacteria by removing secretions, and to treat infections by administering antibiotics.

Airway clearance techniques (ACT) include segmental percussion and postural drainage. These, preceded with inhalation therapy, are performed several times a day to loosen secretions and move them from the peripheral airways into the central airways where they can be expectorated (Cystic Fibrosis Foundation, 2016). Controversy has existed over the effectiveness of chest physiotherapy for children with respiratory illness. Systematic reviews of randomized clinical trials suggest that, although generally ineffective for such conditions as asthma and bronchiolitis, chest physiotherapy has positive short-term effects on secretion mobilization in children with cystic fibrosis (Roque i Figuls, Gine-Garriga, Granados, et al., 2012). Newer airway management techniques such as forced exhalation and positive expiratory pressure (PEP) devices (PEP valve, Flutter device, Acapella device) have been successful in mobilizing mucus. Mucolytic agents (inhaled recombinant DNase or dornase alfa [Pulmozyme]), inhaled bronchodilators, and antiinflammatory agents (ibuprofen, steroids, macrolides) are often used with postural drainage to decrease the viscosity of secretions or clear the airways (Egan et al., 2016).

Exercise is an important part of pulmonary treatment. Regular aerobic exercise such as jogging, swimming, and/or weight training can improve or maintain lung function (Egan et al., 2016). Children with CF who exercise regularly have fewer pulmonary exacerbations and generally feel better than those who do not.

Antibiotics have played a major role in increasing the life expectancy of children with CF. Depending on the course of the child's condition, the symptoms and history, and the underlying organism involved, organism-sensitive oral antibiotics may be prescribed intermittently or continuously (Egan et al., 2016). Children with CF frequently need higher-than-usual doses of antibiotics because of their rapid metabolism of these drugs. Aerosolized antibiotics (tobramycin and aztreonam) are used to control organisms that are resistant to oral antibiotics, most specifically *Pseudomonas aeruginosa* (Cystic Fibrosis Foundation, 2016).

IV antibiotics are the usual treatment of choice during acute pulmonary exacerbations. IV antibiotics are usually administered during hospitalization, but home IV therapy is becoming more widely accepted, offering substantial savings and minimizing disruption of daily activities. Aerosolized antibiotics may be used as an adjunct to IV therapy (Egan et al., 2016).

Because they decrease inflammation in the lung, steroids are sometimes prescribed when pulmonary symptoms are unresponsive to antibiotics and increased CPT; however, adverse side effects, including growth retardation and altered glucose tolerance, are problematic with long-term steroid treatment. Long-term ibuprofen administration has demonstrated positive benefits in delaying disease progression. Azithromycin has been found to decrease the length of hospital stay (Egan et al., 2016).

Advances in medication approaches include newly developed therapies directed toward specific mutations. They act by correcting the defective action of proteins produced by the CF gene mutation (Nakano & Tluczek, 2014). Ivacaftor, which can be prescribed for children older than two years, is used to treat CF caused by ten different gene mutations and is only effective in children with these specific mutations. Lunacaftor/ivacaftor, taken by older children (>12-years-old) is specific for the more common F508del mutation (Cystic Fibrosis Foundation, 2016). Oxygen therapy is used with caution because many children with CF have chronic carbon dioxide retention and are at risk for oxygen-induced carbon dioxide narcosis.

### Digestive Problems

Early in the course of CF, the child may exhibit a huge appetite but not gain weight. Chronic pulmonary infections, increased work of breathing, and malabsorption place an increased calorie and protein demand on the child with CF. The child's calorie requirements are approximately 150% of the normal recommended daily allowance. Children with CF are managed with a high-calorie, high-protein diet, pancreatic enzyme replacement therapy, fat-soluble vitamin supplements, and, if nutritional problems are severe, nighttime gastrostomy feedings or total parenteral nutrition. Fats are not restricted unless steatorrhea cannot be controlled by increased pancreatic enzymes. Because CF causes malabsorption of fat soluble vitamins, supplementation with A, D, E, K is required (Egan et al., 2016)

Infants are sometimes given a predigested formula (Pregestimil, Nutramigen), which is more easily absorbed than regular formula. Formulas may also be concentrated to provide more calories. For the older child, caloric intake can be increased with food supplements or enteral tube feedings. The administration of growth hormone has shown significant improvement in both height velocity and weight gain in children with CF (Egan et al., 2016).

Enteric-coated microencapsulated pancreatic enzyme preparations (Creon, Pancreaze) are administered with every meal and snack. Enzyme dosage is adjusted according to stool formation: fewer enzymes with constipation; more enzymes with loose, fatty stools. Still, the enzyme dosage should be individualized for each child and kept as low as possible while still maintaining the child's nutritional status. Often, histamine-2 receptor blockers (ranitidine) or proton-pump inhibitors are prescribed to decrease the overly acidic intestines, because enzymes will only work in an alkaline environment. Extra salt is added to the diet in extremely hot weather or when the child exercises vigorously.

## NURSING CARE

### The Child With Cystic Fibrosis

#### Assessment

The child with CF should be assessed for signs and symptoms in each of the systems usually affected by the disease and for psychosocial adaptation to this chronic condition.

***Respiratory assessment.*** The child may have had frequent episodes of pneumonia or bronchitis. Auscultate the chest to detect any crackles, wheezes, areas of diminished breath sounds, or a prolonged expiratory phase of respiration. Note signs of long-standing respiratory difficulty, such as barrel chest or digital clubbing. The respiratory status is assessed by noting the rate, depth, and ease of respirations; the color of the nail beds and mucous membranes; and pulse oximetry. The characteristics of the child's cough and the color, amount, and quality of sputum should be documented, along with any fever. Exercise tolerance and the child's ability to sleep lying down at night should also be assessed.

***Digestive assessment.*** The nurse weighs and measures the child, plotting the results on a standardized growth chart. Signs of malabsorption (e.g., steatorrhea; loose, bulky stools; protuberant abdomen with thin extremities) should be noted. A diet history is useful in assessing the child's caloric intake. The use of vitamins and dietary supplements should be recorded. Determining the number and consistency of stools assesses the adequacy of intestinal enzyme replacement. Because ulcers and intestinal obstruction often accompany CF, complaints of abdominal pain, blood in the stools, and constipation should be noted. Use of antacids, $H_2$-receptor blockers, or antireflux medications should also be assessed.

***Reproductive assessment.*** Girls should be assessed for vaginal itching or drainage, which may indicate a vaginal infection. Contraception should be discussed with affected sexually active adolescents.

### Nursing Diagnosis and Planning

The nursing diagnoses and expected outcomes that often apply to children with CF are as follows:

- Ineffective Airway Clearance related to increased pulmonary secretions.

***Expected outcome.*** The child will be able to remove secretions from the airway.

- Impaired Gas Exchange related to air trapping within the alveoli secondary to obstruction of the airways by thick mucus.

***Expected outcome.*** The child will maintain an oxygen saturation level of greater than 95%.

- Risk for Infection related to tenacious secretions and altered body defenses.

***Expected outcome.*** The child will remain free of infection.

- Imbalanced Nutrition: Less Than Body Requirements related to poor intestinal absorption of nutrients.

***Expected outcome.*** The child's nutritional status will improve, and the child will exhibit normal growth; the child's stools will be of normal consistency, frequency, and color.

- Activity Intolerance related to pulmonary congestion and poor absorption of nutrients.

***Expected outcome.*** The child will rest comfortably and will engage in age-appropriate activities.

- Situational Low Self-Esteem related to physical changes from chronic illness.

***Expected outcome.*** The child will demonstrate a positive self-concept and feelings of independence, as demonstrated by participating in self-care and in age-appropriate activities.

- Ineffective Coping (individual) and Compromised Family Coping related to chronic illness.

***Expected outcome.*** The child and family will adhere to the treatment regimen, verbalize feelings about the impact of the illness on their lives, and use available support systems and community resources.

- Anticipatory Grieving related to a potentially fatal diagnosis.

***Expected outcome.*** The child and family will make realistic plans for the future and will be able to discuss feelings about the child's prognosis.

### Interventions

***Facilitating airway clearance and gas exchange.*** Perform CPT two or three times a day and as needed; perform treatments at least 1 hour before or 2 hours after meals to reduce gastrointestinal upset (description of the chest physiotherapy procedure can be found at http://www.cff.org). Administer bronchodilators and mucolytics before or during CPT; administer antibiotics afterward (Cystic Fibrosis Foundation, 2016). The child's respiratory status should be determined before and after CPT. Note the child's tolerance of the procedure. Teach "huffing" (forced expiration) to mobilize secretions. The child should take a deep breath and then exhale rapidly while whispering the word "huff." There are now many techniques from which to choose to facilitate airway clearance. These include PEP devices, autogenic drainage, active cycle of breathing, high-frequency vibratory vest, and even exercise (Cystic Fibrosis Foundation, 2016).

To facilitate gas exchange, administer humidified, low-flow (2 L/min or less) oxygen as ordered. The recommended amount of oxygen should not be exceeded because too much oxygen administered to children who are chronically hypoxic can depress respirations. If the child is dyspneic, elevate the head of the bed or support the child in an upright position. Be sure to stay with the child during coughing episodes.

***Preventing infection.*** Children with CF are prone to respiratory infection, especially airway colonization with *P. aeruginosa*, and oral or inhaled antibiotic therapy may be routine. IV antibiotics may be required during acute exacerbations. Pay meticulous attention to hygiene measures, especially hand hygiene, and teach the child and family to do the same. Monitor the child for signs of respiratory infection (fever, chills, increased respirations, dyspnea, cough, purulent secretions, increased WBC count). Advise the family to avoid exposing the child to others who are ill. Children with CF should receive all routine childhood immunizations at ages recommended by the AAP (see http://www.cdc.gov). An annual influenza vaccine also is appropriate, based on the recommendations by the Centers for Disease Control and Prevention.

***Providing optimal nutrition for growth.*** Provide a well-balanced diet that is high in calories, protein, and carbohydrates and includes the child's favorite foods. Oral or enteral high-calorie supplements can increase the child's calorie intake.

The child needs to take pancreatic enzymes (which come as enteric-coated capsules containing the enzyme beads) as ordered within 30 minutes of eating all meals and snacks. The child should not mix the enzymes with hot foods because enzymes are inactivated by heat. Older children can swallow the enteric-coated pancreatic enzyme capsules. For children who cannot swallow capsules, the capsules can be opened to display the beads, which are then mixed with a small amount of a nonprotein, non-acidic, food. Because prolonged contact with enzyme beads can cause excoriation of oral mucosa, wipe off any beads that remain on the child's lips. Advise the family to note the color, consistency, and frequency of the child's stools because enzyme replacement correlates with the child's bowel elimination pattern (e.g., an acceptable pattern is one or two stools daily in older children and more often in infancy). The enzyme dosage should be increased when high-fat foods are eaten. Administer multivitamins; water-miscible, fat-soluble vitamins; and iron supplements as ordered. Monitor the child's appetite and food intake. Extra salt and fluid are required when the weather is hot.

***Promoting increased exercise tolerance.*** For the child in acute exacerbation, provide rest periods between treatments and organize nursing care to ensure periods of uninterrupted rest. The child's activity level is increased as tolerated. Arrange age-appropriate activities geared to the child's energy level. When the child is feeling well, encourage active play and activities such as swimming and gymnastics.

***Meeting the child's and family's emotional needs.*** Encourage the child to express feelings about the chronic illness and its effect on feelings of self-worth. Identifying a support system is especially important for adolescents as they begin to take responsibility for their health (Kirk et al., 2012). Helping the child identify personal strengths and areas of accomplishment will increase the child's self-esteem. Teach parents the importance of fostering their child's independence. As the child grows, encourage discussion about areas of concern, such as dating, sexuality, and peer acceptance. Assist families with the child's transition from pediatric to adult healthcare providers.

Introducing the family to other families affected by CF can increase problem-solving strategies and facilitate support. Provide information about available community resources, such as the Cystic Fibrosis Foundation and the American Lung Association. The family also should be encouraged to communicate with personnel at the child's school to ensure coordination of care between home and school.

Although tremendous progress has been made in treating CF, it remains a chronic disease with no cure. Provide the family with honest information about the disease and its prognosis. Refer the family for counseling and listen if they wish to discuss feelings about the disease, the future, and possible death.

***Home care.*** Preparation for home care involves teaching family members how to carry out CPT, how to provide breathing treatments, and how to give medications at home. Written instructions should describe the specifics of all aspects of the child's care. Families may need assistance in obtaining home care equipment.

### Evaluation

- Does the child exhibit improved breath sounds, oxygen saturation greater than 95% on room air, and stable respiratory status?
- Are the child's body temperature and WBC count within normal limits? Has the sputum amount decreased?
- Is the child growing in height and weight along the normal growth curve?
- Are the child's stools of normal consistency, frequency, and color?
- Is the child able to engage in appropriate physical activity?
- Does the child appear to be developing age-appropriate cognitive, emotional, and social skills and an appropriate level of self-care?
- Does the child demonstrate an attitude of acceptance of self and of the illness?
- Does the family demonstrate appropriate coping strategies, adherence to the child's treatment plan, and the ability to access needed resources?
- Can the parents demonstrate CPT, inhalation therapy, and other treatments to be performed at home?
- Are the child and family able to appropriately express feelings of anger, sadness, and fear without guilt?

## TUBERCULOSIS

Tuberculosis (TB) is a reportable contagious disease with high morbidity and mortality rates throughout the world. World-wide, 9.6 million people are infected with TB, with the highest incidence in the poorer countries (World Health Organization [WHO], 2016). Approximately five percent of the cases in the United States are in children, primarily those younger than five years and older than ten (CDC, 2014).

### Etiology

*Mycobacterium tuberculosis,* an acid-fast bacillus, causes TB. Contamination occurs chiefly through inhalation of droplets from a person with active TB. Droplets produced by coughing and sneezing remain suspended in the air. When inhaled, they can reach the bronchioles and alveoli.

The risk of infection by the organism is thought to depend on several physiologic and socioeconomic factors. Most children are infected by a family member, babysitter, or other person with whom they have frequent contact (Box 45.4).

### Incidence

In the United States, there is a disparity in incidence between people born in the United States and those born in other countries, with foreign-born people having a two-thirds higher incidence (CDC, 2016a). For U.S.-born citizens, the incidence is highest in non-Hispanic Blacks and Whites; for foreign-born people living in the United States, the highest incidence is found in the Asian populations (CDC, 2016a). The incidence of tuberculosis in the United States has plateaued after many years of decline (Salinas et al., 2016). In the pediatric population, TB occurs most frequently in infants and adolescents and in children with immunosuppressive conditions. Of particular concern is the increase in multidrug-resistant TB. Because resistance is most often caused by poor adherence to drug therapy, directly observed treatment (DOT) is indicated for anyone being treated for tuberculosis disease (Hatzenbuehler & Starke, 2016).

### Manifestations

Children aged 3 to 15 years are usually asymptomatic, have normal chest radiographs, and can be identified only through a positive skin

**BOX 45.4 Risk Factors for the Development of Tuberculosis**

- Contact with adults with infectious tuberculosis (TB)
- Chronic illness, immunosuppression, human immunodeficiency virus (HIV) infection
- Malnutrition
- Age (infancy, adolescence)
- Nonwhite racial and ethnic groups; immigration from areas with a high incidence of TB
- Urban, low-income living conditions
- Incarcerated adolescents
- Children in close contact with any of the following groups of adults: HIV-infected persons, users of intravenous (IV) or other street drugs, poor or medically indigent city dwellers, residents of nursing homes, migrant farm workers

**PATHOPHYSIOLOGY**

***Tuberculosis***

The bacillus multiplies in lung tissue, alveoli, and regional lymph nodes. After an incubation period of 2 to 10 weeks, hypersensitivity develops; at that time, skin tests of the infected child will be positive. Most infected children are asymptomatic at the time of the initial positive skin test result.

The *disease* of tuberculosis (TB) is differentiated from TB *infection* by the presence of clinical manifestations. The risk for development of TB disease is highest in the first 2 years after infection, but many infected children never progress to clinical disease.

The immunologic response of most people is usually strong enough to keep the bacteria from multiplying and spreading. If the host response is adequate, the organism is walled off and the tubercle becomes a healed calcified mass. TB bacilli can remain dormant and cause active disease at a later time if the child's resistance is lowered. If the lesion does not heal and is not walled off, it may continue to enlarge and spread into nearby tissues or enter the blood and spread to other sites (middle ear, brain, kidney, bones, joints, skin).

TB disease destroys host tissue. When tubercle bacilli multiply, they can damage tissue so badly that the center of the infected area turns to liquid pus. When this liquid escapes through an airway, it is coughed up as sputum, leaving a tiny hole (cavitation) in the lung. The bacteria-laden sputum is infectious. Children rarely have active TB with cavitation, in which case they can be infectious to others. Because children with primary pulmonary TB have small lesions and minimal cough, they are not contagious (AAP Committee on Infectious Diseases, 2015). The duration of infectivity of treated adults and adolescents depends on the drug susceptibility of the infecting organism and cough frequency. Although infectivity usually lasts only a few weeks after treatment is begun, it can last longer if the person fails to take the prescribed medication or is infected with a resistant strain.

American Academy of Pediatrics Committee on Infectious Diseases. (2015). In D. Kimberlin (Ed.), *Red book 2015 report of the committee on infectious diseases* (30th ed., pp. 732–742). Elk Grove Village, IL: American Academy of Pediatrics.

test. Some children have malaise, fever, night sweats, a slight cough, weight loss, anorexia, lymphadenopathy, or more specific symptoms related to the site of extrapulmonary infection (e.g., kidneys, brain, bone).

## Diagnostic Evaluation

Skin testing is the initial method of screening and testing for TB. Skin testing is performed on children with known risk factors (see Box 45.4). In most children, the skin test will become positive 2 to 10 weeks after the initial infection; once positive, tuberculin reactivity usually continues throughout life, even with treatment.

Skin testing with 5 tuberculin units of purified protein derivative (PPD) (Mantoux test) is the preferred method of screening. The PPD is administered by intradermal injection on the forearm. The skin reaction is read by an experienced professional 48 to 72 hours after placement. A 15-mm induration in any child older than 4 years is considered a positive sign of TB, whether or not the child has known risks. Induration of more than 5 mm suggests TB in children younger than 4 years and in certain populations of children. A negative tuberculin skin test does not rule out TB, particularly in infants (Box 45.5). For at-risk children who have been immunized with Bacillus Calmette-Guérin (BCG) vaccine, which can cause a false-positive TB skin test, an interferon-gamma release assay (IGRA) is used; if positive, the child is considered to be infected (AAP, Committee on Infectious Diseases, 2015).

Children with positive skin-test results undergo follow-up examinations, which include periodic chest radiography and sputum cultures and smears for the presence of acid-fast bacilli. Because children often swallow sputum rather than expectorate it, gastric washings to obtain swallowed sputum are sometimes done. A thorough history should be obtained, and all contacts of the affected child should be tested for the disease.

### BOX 45.5 Definition of a Positive Mantoux Skin Test

**Area of Induration ≥5 mm Considered Positive in:**
- HIV-infected persons
- Recent contact of a person with tuberculosis (TB) disease
- Persons with fibrotic changes on chest radiograph consistent with prior TB
- Persons who are immunosuppressed for other reasons (e.g., taking the equivalent of >15 mg/day of prednisone for 1 month or longer, taking tumor necrosis factor-alpha antagonists)

**Area of Induration ≥10 mm Considered Positive in:**
- Recent immigrants (<5 years) from high-prevalence countries
- Injection drug users
- Residents and employees of high-risk congregate settings
- Mycobacteriology laboratory personnel
- Persons with clinical conditions that place them at high risk
- Children <4 years of age
- Infants, children, and adolescents exposed to adults in high-risk categories

**Induration ≥15 mm Considered Positive in:**
- Any person, including persons with no known risk factors for TB.

From Centers for Disease Control and Prevention. (2012). *Tuberculin skin testing*. Retrieved from http://www.cdc.gov.

## Therapeutic Management and Nursing Considerations

Understanding the differences between TB exposure, infection, and disease is important. *Exposure* is recent and significant contact with an individual diagnosed with contagious TB. The skin test is often negative at this point, and the child is asymptomatic. TB *infection* is defined by a positive skin test. The child continues to lack signs and symptoms of TB, and there might be no chest radiograph changes at this time. Prophylactic treatment is instituted to prevent the progression to disease. TB *disease* is defined by chest radiograph changes along with signs and symptoms of disease and a positive skin test.

### Tuberculosis Infection

After a chest radiograph is obtained, asymptomatic children with positive tuberculin tests and no previous history of TB receive daily isoniazid (INH) for 9 months. Children with drug-resistant TB need an individualized treatment regimen; the most commonly used alternative drug is a 4-month daily course of rifampin. Rifampin can alter the efficacy of oral contraceptives, so alternative methods of birth control must be used if an adolescent girl requires treatment with this medication (AAP Committee on Infectious Diseases, 2015).

Household contacts, especially those who are younger than 4 years or immunosuppressed, should undergo skin testing and chest radiography. Even if the skin test is negative, asymptomatic contacts should receive INH for at least 8 to 10 weeks after exposure, after which skin testing should be repeated. If the test is still negative and there is no clinical evidence of TB, the INH may be discontinued, so long as the contact is not immunosuppressed. Immunocompromised children may need to complete the full regimen of INH (AAP Committee on Infectious Diseases, 2015). Reporting cases of TB is required by law in all states in the United States. Nurses should assist in searching for the source case and others infected by the source case.

BCG vaccine is the only anti-TB vaccine available. Unfortunately, the vaccine varies in the immunity it provides and has resulted in serious reactions. In the United States, it is used mainly for children who test negative for tuberculosis but who are continuously exposed to (1) contacts who are not treated or undertreated for contagious pulmonary TB and the child cannot be removed or take antituberculosis medications; and (2) contacts who have INH and rifampin-resistant pulmonary TB (AAP Committee on Infectious Diseases, 2015).

### Tuberculosis Disease

The mainstays of treatment include a 6-month course of combination antituberculosis medications (INH, rifampin, ethambutol, and pyrazinamide for the first 2 months; INH and rifampin for the next 4 months), optimal nutrition, and preventing exposure to infection, which could further compromise the child's already-challenged immune system (AAP Committee on Infectious Diseases, 2015). Most children are treated at home. The nurse should emphasize to the family the importance of following the prescribed medication regimen meticulously and for the appropriate length of time because inappropriate medication dosing contributes to the growth of drug-resistant organisms. The AAP Committee on Infectious Diseases (2015) recommends DOT for all children taking medication for tuberculosis. In most cases, supervision of medication administration is done by a visiting nurse or public health nurse.

Children with TB are sometimes hospitalized, depending on the severity of the disease, the age of the child, the need for more extensive testing, and the child's family and social environment. Unless the child is acutely ill, bed rest is not required. Isolation usually is not required because children with TB are rarely contagious.

### Prevention and Screening

The focus of disease prevention includes prompt identification of cases and appropriate treatment. Because most children are infected by a family member, the best way to stop transmission of the disease is to identify those who are infected and to provide TB therapy.

Early detection of the disease is accomplished by screening. Children at high risk for TB should be tested annually with the Mantoux test. Annual skin testing of children in low-prevalence areas who have no risk factors is not indicated.

## KEY CONCEPTS

- Infants and children younger than 3 years are at increased risk for development of respiratory tract infections because of their immature immune system, smaller airways, and underdeveloped supporting cartilage.
- At birth, the neonate must inflate the lungs, establish continuous breathing, and transfer the gases needed to meet metabolic needs.
- The severity of allergic rhinitis can be decreased through the early identification and treatment of manifestations.
- The only reliable way to determine whether pharyngitis is viral or bacterial in origin is with a throat culture.
- Manifestations of bleeding after a tonsillectomy include frequent swallowing; restlessness; a fast, thready pulse; and the vomiting of bright-red blood.
- The mucosal edema associated with croup can sometimes be decreased by taking the child out into the cool, humid night air.
- Children with croup who have stridor at rest, cyanosis, severe agitation or fatigue, moderate to severe retractions, or are unable to take oral fluids should be seen in the emergency room.
- The four *D*s of epiglottitis are *d*rooling, *d*ysphagia, *d*ysphoria, and *d*istressed inspiratory efforts.
- Visual examination of the epiglottis is contraindicated if epiglottitis is suspected because the examination tools can provoke laryngospasm and airway obstruction.
- Because RSV infection is highly communicable, during RSV season hospitalized infected children should be placed on Contact Precautions. Good hand hygiene should be emphasized and gowns worn when there is a chance that clothing might be soiled.
- Oxygen needs can be decreased in the child in respiratory distress by scheduling nursing care to allow the child periods of rest.
- If a child is aphonic and not breathing, the guidelines for management of an obstructed airway should be followed.
- During an apneic episode, the time and duration of the episode, color change, bradycardia, oxygen saturation, what the infant was doing before the apneic period, and any actions that stimulated breathing should be recorded.
- Healthy infants should be placed on their backs for sleeping to reduce the risk of SIDS.
- When interviewing parents of an infant suspected of dying of SIDS, the nurse should avoid any implication of fault on the part of the parents.
- Asthma is the most common chronic disease of childhood. Asthma is characterized by bronchospasm, edema of the bronchiolar mucous membranes, and increased secretion of mucus in the airways.
- Asthmatic symptoms signaling spasm of the smooth muscle of the bronchi and bronchioles may be triggered by a variety of stimuli, including allergens, cold air, weather changes, infection, exercise, fatigue, and emotional distress.
- Status asthmaticus (continued severe respiratory distress despite medical treatment) places the child in imminent danger of respiratory arrest and requires immediate hospitalization.
- Nursing care of the child with a severe asthma episode includes administration of inhaled bronchodilators and IV or oral corticosteroids, as ordered; providing oxygen therapy; providing IV fluids; and assisting with intubation and mechanical ventilation.
- Nursing care of the child with chronic asthma includes administration of prescribed medications and treatments and education of the child and family about medications, how to avoid triggers of asthma symptoms, how to recognize early warning signs of an asthma episode, and measures that can be taken to prevent severe asthma episodes.
- BPD is a chronic lung disease characterized by thickening of the alveolar walls and bronchiolar epithelium. BPD occurs primarily in premature and low-birth-weight infants who have been mechanically ventilated for prolonged periods.
- Nursing care of the infant with BPD includes supportive interventions to maintain adequate oxygenation and the provision of appropriate stimulation to promote normal growth and development.
- CF is an inherited (autosomal recessive), multisystem disorder characterized by widespread dysfunction of the exocrine glands. Abnormal secretion of thick, tenacious mucus causes obstruction and dysfunction of the pancreas, lungs, salivary glands, sweat glands, and reproductive organs.
- Nursing care of the child with CF includes maintaining a patent airway by administering bronchodilators and performing or supervising respiratory treatments, administering antibiotics and pancreatic enzymes, and teaching the child and family about CF and its treatment.
- Nursing care of the child with TB includes administering and evaluating TB skin tests and administering anti-TB medications as ordered. The nurse also instructs the child and family about the importance of adequate rest, a nutritionally adequate diet, adherence to the medication regimen, and ways to prevent the transmission of TB infection.

## REFERENCES AND READINGS


Akinbami, L., Simon, A., & Rossen, M. (2016). Changing trends in asthma prevalence among children. *Pediatrics, 137*(1), 1 ac 7.

American Academy of Pediatrics Committee on Infectious Diseases. (2015). In D. Kimberlin (Ed.), *Red book 2015 report of the committee on infectious diseases* (30th ed., pp. 732–742). Elk Grove Village, IL: American Academy of Pediatrics.

American Academy of Pediatrics Task Force on Sudden Infant Death Syndrome. (2016). SIDS and other sleep-related infant deaths: Updated 2016 recommendations for safe infant sleeping environment. *Pediatrics, 132*(5), 1–12.

Antoon, A., & Donovan, M. (2016). Burn injuries. In R. Kliegman, B. Stanton, J. St. Geme, et al. (Eds.), *Nelson textbook of pediatrics* (20th ed., Chapter 75). St. Louis, MO: Elsevier.

Armstrong, M., & Christian, D. (2014). What's new in sinus surgery? *OR Nurse, 8*(3), 36–46.

Carlo, W. (2016). Apnea. In R. Kliegman, B. Stanton, J. St. Geme, et al. (Eds.), *Nelson textbook of pediatrics* (20th ed., Chapter 101.2). St. Louis, MO: Elsevier.

Carlo, W., & Ambalavanan, N. (2016). Respiratory tract disorders. In R. Kliegman, B. Stanton, J. St. Geme, et al. (Eds.), *Nelson textbook of pediatrics* (20th ed., Chapter 101). St. Louis, MO: Elsevier.

Centers for Disease Control and Prevention. (2014). *TB in children in the United States.* Retrieved from http://www.cdc.gov.

Centers for Disease Control and Prevention. (2015). *Health United States, 2015.* Retrieved from http://www.cdc.gov.

Centers for Disease Control and Prevention. (2016a). *Basic TB facts.* Retrieved from http://www.cdc.gov.

Centers for Disease Control and Prevention. (2016b). *Sudden unexpected infant death and sudden infant death syndrome: data and statistics.* Retrieved from http://www.cdc.gov.

Coates, B., Camarda, L., & Goodman, D. (2016). Wheezing in infants: Bronchiolitis. In R. Kliegman, B. Stanton, J. St. Geme, et al. (Eds.), *Nelson textbook of pediatrics* (20th ed., Chapter 391.1). St. Louis, MO: Elsevier.

Cystic Fibrosis Foundation. (2016). *What is cystic fibrosis?* Retrieved from http://www.cff.org.

Danhauer, J., et al. (2015). Will parents participate in and comply with programs and regimens using Xylitol for preventing acute otitis media in their children? *Language, Speech, and Hearing Services in Schools, 46*, 127–140.

Egan, M., Green, D., & Voynow, J. (2016). Cystic fibrosis. In R. Kliegman, B. Stanton, J. St. Geme, et al. (Eds.), *Nelson textbook of pediatrics* (20th ed., Chapter 403). St. Louis, MO: Elsevier.

Ensz, C., & Crusse, E. (2016). Do you know the common causes of increased work of breathing for infants, children, and adolescents? Just think bad coughs. *Nursing Made Incredibly Easy*, 43–51.

Garbutt, J.M., et al. (2013). The comparative effectiveness of prednisolone and dexamethasone for children with croup: a community-based randomized controlled trial. *Clinical Pediatrics, 52*(11), 1014–1021.

Goldstein, R., Trachtenberg, F., Sens, M, et al. (2016). Overall postneonatal mortality and rates of SIDS. *Pediatrics, 137*(1), 1-aa-10.

Greener, M. (2015). Looking at the impact and management of allergic rhinitis. *British Journal of School Nursing, 10*(3), 119–121.

Hatzenbuehler, L., & Starke, J. (2016). Tuberculosis (*Mycobacterium tuberculosis*). In R. Kliegman, B. Stanton, J. St. Geme, et al. (Eds.), *Nelson textbook of pediatrics* (20th ed., Chapter 215). St. Louis, MO: Elsevier.

Hunt, C., & Hauck, F. (2016). Sudden infant death syndrome. In R. Kliegman, B. Stanton, J. St. Geme, et al. (Eds.), *Nelson textbook of pediatrics* (20th ed., Chapter 375). St. Louis, MO: Elsevier.

Jarvis, K., et al. (2014). Change to a standardized airway clearance protocol for children with bronchiolitis leads to improved care. *Journal of Pediatric Nursing, 29*, 252–257.

Kelly, M., & Sandora, T. (2016). Community acquired pneumonia. In R. Kliegman, B. Stanton, J. St. Geme, et al. (Eds.), *Nelson textbook of pediatrics* (20th ed., Chapter 400). St. Louis, MO: Elsevier.

Kerschner, J., & Preciado, D. (2016). Otitis media. In R. Kliegman, B. Stanton, J. St. Geme, et al. (Eds.), *Nelson textbook of pediatrics* (20th ed., Chapter 640). St. Louis, MO: Elsevier.

Khetan, R., Hurley, M., Spencer, S., et al. (2016). Bronchopulmonary dysplasia: within and beyond the neonatal unit. *Advances in Neonatal Care, 16*(1), 17–25.

Kirk, S., Beatty, S., Callery, P., et al. (2012). The effectiveness of self-care support interventions for children and young people with long-term conditions: a systematic review. *Child: Care, Health, and Development, 39*(3), 305–324.

Lean, W., Arnup, S., Danchin, M., & Steer, A. (2014). Rapid diagnostic tests for group A streptococcal pharyngitis: A meta-analysis. *Pediatrics, 134*(4), 771-781.

Lestrud, S. (2016). Bronchopulmonary dysplasia. In R. Kliegman, B. Stanton, J. St. Geme, et al. (Eds.), *Nelson textbook of pediatrics* (20th ed., Chapter 416). St. Louis, MO: Elsevier.

Lieberthal, A., et al. (2013). Clinical practice guideline: The diagnosis and management of acute otitis media. *Pediatrics, 131*(3), e964–e999.

Lierl, M. (2014). New developments in the treatment of pediatric allergic rhinitis and conjunctivitis. *Pediatric Annals, 43*(8), e192–e200.

Liu, A., Covar, R., Spahn, J. & Sicherer, S. (2016). Childhood asthma. In R. Kliegman, B. Stanton, J. St. Geme, et al. (Eds.), *Nelson textbook of pediatrics* (20th ed., Chapter 144). St. Louis, MO: Elsevier.

Liu, C., & Ulualp, S. (2015). Outcomes of an alternating ibuprofen and acetaminophen regimen for pain relief after tonsillectomy in children. *Annals of Otology, Rhinology, and Laryngology, 124*(0), 777–781.

Martin, S., Martin, J., & Seigler, T. (2015). Evidence-based protocols to guide pulse oximetry and oxygen weaning in inpatient children with asthma and bronchiolitis. *Journal of Pediatric Nursing, 30*, 888–895.

Milgrom, H., & Sicherer, S. (2016). Allergic rhinitis. In R. Kliegman, B. Stanton, J. St. Geme, et al. (Eds.), *Nelson textbook of pediatrics* (20th ed., Chapter 143). St. Louis, MO: Elsevier.

Nakano, S., & Tluczek, A. (2014). Genomic breakthroughs in the diagnosis and treatment of cystic fibrosis. *AJN, 114*(6), 36–43.

Nanda, M., et al. (2016). Allergic diseases and internalizing behaviors in early childhood. *Pediatrics, 137*(1), 1–10.

National Heart, Lung, and Blood Institute & National Asthma Education and Prevention Program. (2007). *Expert panel report 3: guidelines for the diagnosis and management of asthma.* Retrieved from http://www.nhlbi.nih.gov.

Nierengarten, M.B. (2015). Diagnosis and management of croup in children. *Contemporary Pediatrics*, 31–33. Retrieved from http://contemporarypediatrics.modernmedicine.com.

Nierengarten, M.B. (2016). Spirometry establishes asthma control in children. *Contemporary Pediatrics, 33*(3), 20–24.

Pappas, D., & Hendley, O. (2011). Sinusitis. In R. Kliegman, B. Stanton, J. St. Geme, et al. (Eds.), *Nelson textbook of pediatrics* (19th ed., pp. 1436–1438). Philadelphia: Saunders.

Pappas, D., & Hendley, O. (2016). Sinusitis. In R. Kliegman, B. Stanton, J. St. Geme, et al. (Eds.), *Nelson textbook of pediatrics* (20th ed., Chapter 380). St. Louis, MO: Elsevier.

Paul, S., Sanjeevaiah, M., & Routly, C. (2013). Ingestion or aspiration of foreign bodies by children. *Emergency Nurse, 21*(7), 32–36.

Pinto, J., Schairer, J., & Petrova, A. (2014). Comparative effectiveness of implementation of a nursing-driven protocol in reducing bronchodilator utilization in hospitalized children with bronchiolitis. *Journal of Evaluation in Clinical Practice, 20*, 267–272.

Poindexter, B., & Jobe, A. (2015). The conundrum of bronchopulmonary dysplasia. *The Journal of Pediatrics, 167*(3), 517–518.

Ralston, S.L., et al. (2014a). Clinical practice guideline: the diagnosis, management, and prevention of bronchiolitis. *Pediatrics, 134*(5), e1474-e1500.

Ralston, S., Comick, A., Nichols, E., et al. (2014b). Effectiveness of quality improvement in hospitalization for bronchiolitis: a systematic review. *Pediatrics, 134*(3), 572–581.

Roosevelt, G. (2016). Acute inflammatory upper airway obstruction (croup, epiglottitis, laryngitis, and bacterial tracheitis). In R. Kliegman, B. Stanton, J. St. Geme, et al. (Eds.), *Nelson textbook of pediatrics* (20th ed., Chapter 385). St. Louis, MO: Elsevier.

Roque i Figuls, M., Gine-Garriga, M., Granados, R., et al. (2012). Chest physiotherapy for acute bronchiolitis in paediatric patients between 0 and 24 months old. *Cochrane Database of Systematic Reviews*, 1–33.

Salinas, J., et al. (2016). A leveling of tuberculosis incidence – United States 2013-2015. *MMWR, 65*, 273–278.

Sarnaik, A.P., Clark, J., & Sarnaik, A.A. (2016). Respiratory distress and failure. In R. Kliegman, B. Stanton, J. St. Geme, et al. (Eds.), *Nelson textbook of pediatrics* (20th ed., Chapter 71). St. Louis, MO: Elsevier.

Schroeder, J., & Holinger, L. (2016). Laryngotracheomalacia. In R. Kliegman, B. Stanton, J. St. Geme, et al. (Eds.), *Nelson textbook of pediatrics* (20th ed., Chapter 386.1). St. Louis, MO: Elsevier.

Stastny, P., Keens, T., & Alkon, A. (2016). Supporting SIDS families: the public health nurse SIDS home visit. *Public Health Nursing, 33*(3), 242–248.

Tanz, R. (2016). Acute pharyngitis. In R. Kliegman, B. Stanton, J. St. Geme, et al. (Eds.), *Nelson textbook of pediatrics* (20th ed., Chapter 381). St. Louis, MO: Elsevier.

Tieder, J., et al. (2016). Brief resolved unexplained events (formerly apparent life-threatening events) and evaluation of low risk infants. *Pediatrics, 137*(5), e1–e32.

Trachtenberg, F., Haas, E., & Kinney, H. (2012). Risk factor changes for sudden infant death syndrome after initiation of the back-to-sleep campaign. *Pediatrics, 129*(4), 630–638.

Venekamp, R., Sanders, S., Glaziou, P., et al. (2015). Antibiotics for acute otitis media in children. *Cochrane Database of Systematic Reviews,* (6), CD000219.

Wald, E., et al., (2013). Clinical practice guideline for the diagnosis and management of acute bacterial sinusitis in children aged 1 to 18 years. *Pediatrics, 132*(1), e262–e280.

Wallace, I.F., et al., (2014). Surgical treatments for otitis media with effusion: a systematic review. *Pediatrics, 133*(2), 296–311.

Walsh, B., Crotwell, D., & Restrepo, R. (2011). Capnography/capnometry during mechanical ventilation: 2011. *Respiratory Care, 56*(4), 503–509.

Williamson, I., et al. (2015). Effect of nasal balloon autoinflation in children with otitis media with effusion in primary care: an open randomized controlled trial. *CMAJ, 187*(13), 961–969.

World Health Organization. (2016). *Tuberculosis.* Retrieved from http://www.who.int.

46

# The Child With a Cardiovascular Alteration

http://evolve.elsevier.com/McKinney/mat-ch/

## LEARNING OBJECTIVES

*After studying this chapter, you should be able to:*

- Describe the anatomy and physiology of the normally functioning heart.
- Describe the major circulatory changes that occur in the fetus during the transition from intrauterine to extrauterine life.
- Discuss specific techniques used in a comprehensive cardiac assessment.
- Explain the various classifications of congenital heart disease, describe their underlying mechanisms, and list the associated congenital cardiac defects.
- Discuss the nursing process used for an infant or child with congestive heart failure.
- Discuss the major physiologic features and the therapeutic management of a child with a heart defect, including left-to-right shunting lesions, right-to-left shunting lesions, and obstructive or stenotic lesions.
- Discuss the importance of early recognition and treatment of infective endocarditis.
- Describe nursing care of a child with rheumatic fever, Kawasaki disease, or hypertension.
- Explain why high cholesterol is an important health issue for children and adolescents, and describe the assessment and nursing management of this problem in children in the community.
- Explain the effects of childhood obesity on future cardiovascular health.

## CLINICAL REFERENCE

## REVIEW OF THE HEART AND CIRCULATION

### Normal Cardiac Anatomy and Physiology

The heart is a muscular pump that is divided into four chambers. The two upper chambers are the atria, and the two lower chambers are the ventricles. The atria are referred to as the filling chambers and the ventricles as the pumping chambers. The heart has two atrioventricular (AV) valves, the tricuspid and mitral valves, and two semilunar valves, the pulmonary and aortic valves. In normal blood flow, desaturated venous blood returning from the body flows from the superior vena cava and inferior vena cava into the right atrium. It then moves through the tricuspid valve into the right ventricle and is pumped into the main pulmonary artery and branch pulmonary arteries to the pulmonary circulation. In the lungs, carbon dioxide is removed and oxygen is added to the blood. This richly oxygen-saturated blood returns from the pulmonary circulation to the left side of the heart through the pulmonary veins and into the left atrium. From the left atrium, it flows through the mitral valve into the left ventricle and is pumped into the aorta and systemic circulation.

Mechanical contraction of the heart muscle starts with electrical stimulation. This electrical stimulation is normally initiated by a group of cells called the *sinus node,* located at the superior vena cava and right atrial junction. The electrical impulse spreads through the atrium to the relay station, the AV node, and is then transmitted to the ventricles through the bundle of His, the bundle branch system, and finally the Purkinje fibers. The result is rhythmic atrial electrical stimulation and then contraction, followed by ventricular stimulation and contraction.

The electrocardiogram records this electrical activity. The P wave reflects atrial depolarization; the QRS complex reflects ventricular depolarization; the T wave reflects ventricular repolarization. Each cardiac cycle consists of this electrical activity, which produces depolarization and subsequent repolarization of the cardiac muscle—more simply, a heartbeat.

The venous (or right) side of the heart is normally a lower-pressure system than the higher arterial (or left) side of the heart. The range of

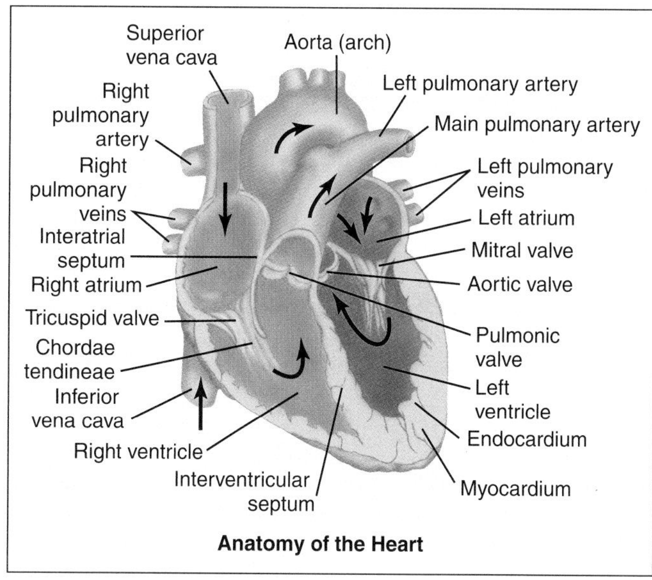


**Anatomy of the Heart**

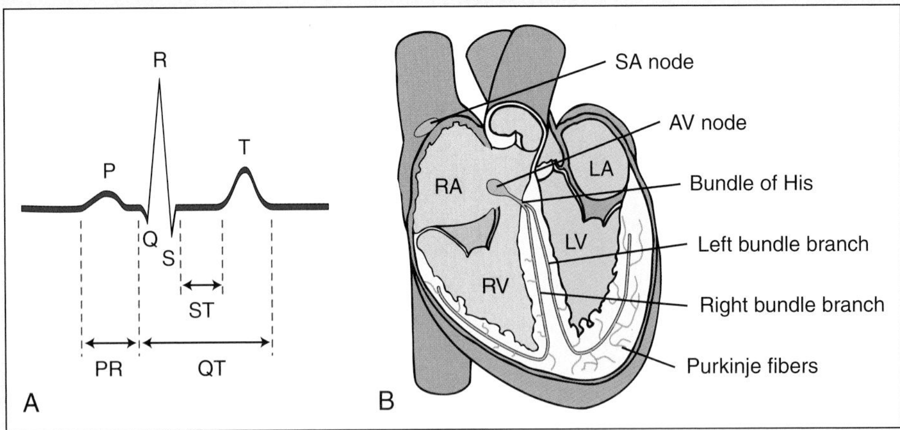


**A,** Normal heart cycle, represented as an electrocardiographic configuration. **B,** Cardiac electrical conduction system. (Modified from Park, M.K., & Guntheroth, W.G. [2006]. *How to read pediatric ECGs* [4th ed., pp. 11]. St. Louis: Mosby.)

normal pressure in the right ventricle is 18 to 30/0 to 5 mm Hg, while that of the pulmonary artery is 20 to 30/8 to 12 mm Hg. The range of normal pressure of the left ventricle is 90 to 140/5 mm Hg (age dependent), and that of the aorta is 100/60 mm Hg (age dependent). On an average, the left-side pressures are four to five times higher than those on the right side. In addition, the venous circulation normally has lower oxygen saturation, in the range of 65% to 80% compared to the arterial circulation, which is 95% to 100%. Congenital or acquired malformations or anomalies in any of the cardiac structures can affect blood flow, pressures, and oxygen saturations, thereby altering hemodynamic stability.

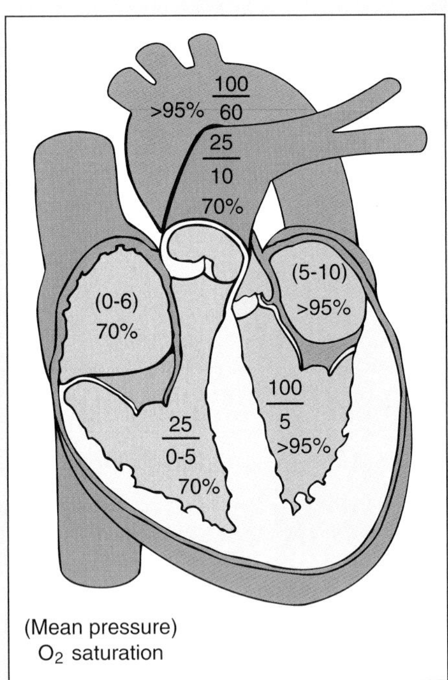


Normal pressures (mm Hg) and saturations (%). (Modified from Ko Chiang, L., & Ensor Dunn, A. [2000]. Cardiology. In G.K. Siberry, & R. Iannone [Eds.], *The Johns Hopkins Hospital Harriet Lane handbook* [15th ed., pp. 154]. St. Louis: Mosby.)

## Fetal Circulation

Fetal circulation differs from neonatal circulation in three aspects: the process of gas exchange, the pressures within the systemic and pulmonary circulations, and the presence of anatomic structures that assist in the delivery of oxygen-rich blood to vital organ systems. In the fetus, oxygenation (gas exchange) occurs at the placenta. Oxygen and nutrients are carried by the blood in the umbilical vein, which travels through the fetal liver to the inferior vena cava. A small amount of blood travels into the hepatic circulation to provide oxygen and nutrients to the hepatic tissue. Liver function is minimal in the fetus; therefore, very little blood supply is required. The remainder of the blood flows into the inferior vena cava through a fetal structure, the *ductus venosus.*

The inferior vena cava empties blood into the right atrium. The trajectory (direction) of the blood flow, as well as the pressure in the right atrium, propels most of this blood through a second fetal structure, the *foramen ovale,* into the left atrium. This richly oxygenated blood travels through the left ventricle into the aorta, feeding the coronary arteries and the brain—the two most oxygen-needy organ systems.

Blood returning from the upper body enters the right atrium through the superior vena cava. This blood is primarily directed through the tricuspid valve and the right ventricle into the pulmonary artery. Resistance in the pulmonary circulation is very high because the lungs are collapsed and filled with fluid. A very small amount of blood flows through the branch pulmonary arteries to provide oxygen and nutrients to the pulmonary tissue. Most of the blood flows through a third fetal structure, the *ductus arteriosus,* to the descending aorta. This blood is then distributed to the organ systems and tissues in the lower portion of the body and returns to the placenta for gas exchange through two umbilical arteries.

## Transitional and Neonatal Circulation

Major changes in the circulatory system occur at birth. With the neonate's first breath, gas exchange is transferred from the placenta to the lungs. The fetal shunts (ductus venosus, ductus arteriosus, foramen ovale) functionally close in response to pressure changes in the systemic and pulmonary circulations and to increased blood oxygen content. Pulmonary vascular resistance begins to decrease and pulmonary blood flow markedly increases. Closure of the ductus arteriosus, along with the increased pulmonary blood flow, enhances left ventricular filling. The increase in systemic arterial pressure as a result of clamping the umbilical cord at delivery and the placental separation from the fetus increases the workload of the left ventricle, and the neonatal heart now functions on its own. The neonatal circulation is now normal. In some neonates, it may take several days for the fetal shunts to close.

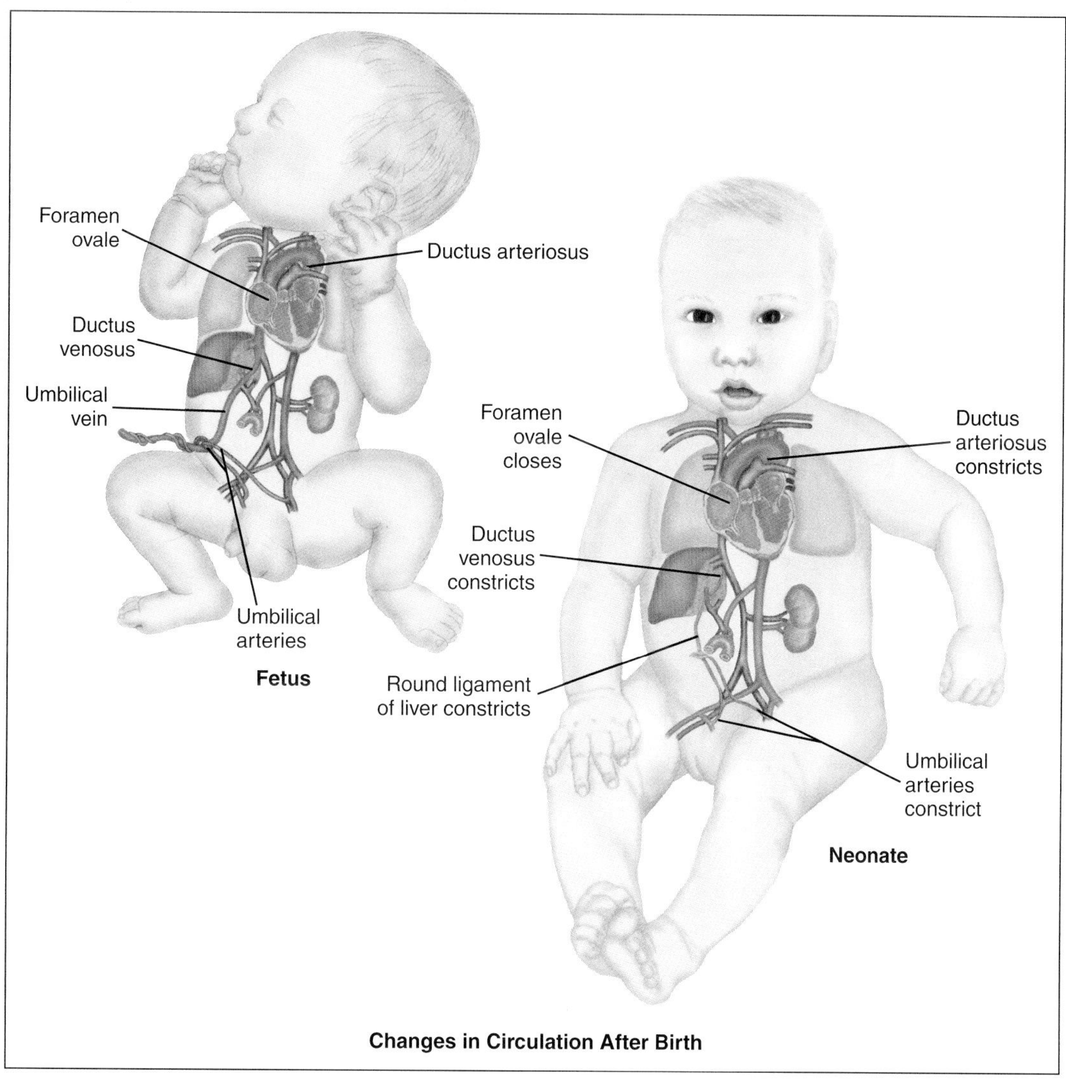


Changes in Circulation After Birth

## Differences in the Heart and Circulation of Neonates and Infants

- The heart and the great vessels develop during the first 3 to 8 weeks of gestation. The fetus is most vulnerable to cardiac malformations during this period.
- Heart sounds in the neonate are higher pitched and of greater intensity than in the adult, and the pulse rate is higher. Many variations in these parameters are both possible and normal.
- The chest wall of infants and young children is thin because of the relative lack of subcutaneous fat and muscle tissue. Innocuous murmurs can be auscultated in structurally normal hearts because of the wall thinness.
- The neonate and infant's myocardial muscle is less efficient. The myocardial cells are smaller and contain fewer contractile elements; therefore, neonatal and infant hearts have decreased myocardial contractility. This feature makes neonates and infants particularly dependent on adequate heart rate and rhythm to maintain their cardiac output because they cannot increase their stroke volume as effectively as the older child or adult (Cardiac output = Stroke volume × Heart rate).
- The neonatal heart is highly dependent on calcium, glucose, and volume for optimal cardiac function.
- In a very sick child, the cardiac output should be evaluated as either adequate or inadequate to meet metabolic demands. Shock can be present even when the cardiac output is normal or high.
- Blood pressure is not a reliable indicator of clinical decompensation.
- Hypotension can indicate decompensated shock.
- Increased pulmonary vascular resistance in the neonate increases pressure on the right side of the heart. This circumstance can delay detection of left-to-right shunts in the newborn period because increased right-sided pressure decreases the left-to-right shunting and the intensity of cardiac murmurs. Normally, pulmonary vascular resistance decreases to the adult range over the first 4 to 6 weeks of life. Obvious signs and symptoms of left-to-right shunting may not be present until that time.

## Common Diagnostic Tests for Cardiac Disorders

| Test | Description | Preparation and Nursing Considerations | Comments |
|---|---|---|---|
| Electrocardiogram (ECG) | Provides recording of heart's electrical activity from outside surface of body. Electrodes are placed over precordium and on the four extremities; electrodes are attached to lead wires. Lead wires are attached to an electrocardiograph that records and prints electrical activity. | Best done when the child is quiet and cooperative.<br>Skin should be free of lotions and oils. | Displays heart rate and rhythm.<br>Detects chamber enlargement and deviations in axis caused by congenital or acquired heart defects or disease. |
| Holter monitor | Continuously records heart rate and rhythm for 24 hr. Electrodes and leads are attached to the child, who wears a compact recorder. | Same as for ECG. | Child or parent records times of activities, symptoms, or other events in a diary to be returned with the monitor. Important that diary be accurately completed. |
| Chest radiography | Provides x-ray picture of heart and associated organs and structures in the chest cavity. | Remove electrodes and lead wires if attached.<br>Encourage the parent or family member to accompany the child to x-ray department. | Provides information about heart size; blood flow to lungs; sidedness of the stomach, liver, and heart. |
| Echocardiography (ECHO) | Uses high-frequency sound waves (ultrasound) to generate an image of the heart and associated structures.<br>The study assesses location and relationship of intracardiac and extracardiac structures, cardiac function; measures size of cardiac chambers, valve function, size of septal or other defects; estimates gradients across structures and blood flow direction. | Must be done when the child is quiet and cooperative.<br>If not cooperative, sedation may become necessary. | Methods of echocardiograms:<br>• M-mode<br>• Two-dimensional<br>• Doppler<br>Types of echocardiograms:<br>• Transthoracic<br>• Transesophageal<br>• Directly on cardiac muscle<br>• Fetal |
| Magnetic resonance imaging | A strong magnetic field surrounds the child; the field promotes rotation of nuclei (that normally spin) at predictable speed, allowing visualization of soft tissue, tumors, shunts, myocardial thickness, structure, and valve function. | Teaching about the procedure.<br>Nothing-by-mouth status for at least 4 hr before procedure if requiring sedation.<br>Assessment for allergy if contrast medium is to be used.<br>All metallic items must be removed. | The child must be able to lie still for up to 1 hr or will require sedation. |
| Ventilation-perfusion scan | IV injection of isotope, which reveals distribution of pulmonary blood flow and ventilation; assists in quantifying percentage and pattern of pulmonary blood flow. | Requires an IV line for radioisotope injection. | The child must be able to lie still for a short time for the scan. |
| Pulse oximetry | A bandage probe is attached to a digit or earlobe; measures oxygen saturation of blood noninvasively. | No specific preparation.<br>The extremity needs to be relatively motion free for accurate reading.<br>All nail polish must be removed. | If alarms (high or low), validate the child's heart rate corresponds to the monitor.<br>Know the expected saturation range for the child's cardiac defect. |

*IV*, Intravenous.

Cardiovascular alterations in children are either congenital or acquired. Congenital heart disease (CHD) denotes one or more structural abnormalities that develop before birth, although clinical symptoms may not be present in the newborn. Acquired heart disease, such as cardiomyopathies, Kawasaki disease, or rheumatic fever, develops after birth and is seen in both children with normal hearts and those with CHD. Over the past 3 decades, there have been major advances in the diagnosis and management of CHD. Because of these advances, approximately 85% to 90% of infants born with CHD can be expected to live into adulthood (Boyle, Kelly, Reynolds, et al., 2015). To appreciate each defect or combination of multiple defects and their effects on a child's life requires an understanding of normal cardiac anatomy and physiology, including the development of the heart, circulation (including fetal, transitional, and postnatal), normal structures, and function.

## CONGENITAL HEART DISEASE

Congenital cardiac defects are some of the most frequently seen congenital defects in infants and children, with an overall incidence of 8 in every 1000 live births (American Heart Association [AHA], 2015; Bernstein, 2016a). As interventional cardiology becomes more effective, more adults are living with congenital heart disease (CHD). The AHA estimates that 1 in 150 adults are now living with CHD (Boyle et al., 2015).

Newborn screening for critical congenital heart disease was recommended to be added in 2011 by the Secretary of the US Department of Health and Human Services. Following this addition, the AAP issued Strategies for Implementing Screening for Critical Congenital Heart Disease. A pulse oximeter reading of a newborn's oxygen saturation should be obtained no earlier than 24 hours after birth and before discharge (AAP, 2016a). Although the nongenetic etiology and risk factors for CHD are not completely known, maternal diabetes mellitus, maternal infection during pregnancy, maternal smoking, maternal obesity, and maternal exposure to some chemicals and pollutants have been implicated (AAP, 2016b). Children with certain genetic conditions or defects have an extremely high incidence of cardiac disorders, including those with chromosome aberrations. Among children with trisomy 21 (Down syndrome), the incidence of CHD is approximately 40 to 50% (CDC, 2016; Park, 2014). Other congenital conditions that increase the risk for CHD include Turner syndrome in girls (single X chromosome), Klinefelter variant in boys (additional X chromosomes), and children with Marfan syndrome or velocardiofacial syndrome (DiGeorge syndrome) (Park, 2014). A maternal history of CHD increases the risk of cardiac disorders to as high as 15% (Park, 2014).

### Classification of CHD

Congenital heart defects can be classified according to structural abnormalities, functional alterations, or both (Table 46.1). Historically, defects were simply classified according to whether they were cyanotic or acyanotic. Currently, these classifications are subdivided into groups defined by blood flow patterns, including increased pulmonary blood flow, normal to decreased pulmonary blood flow, obstructive lesions, and miscellaneous complex lesions.

Clinical signs of congenital cardiac defects can manifest any time during the newborn period, infancy, or early childhood. The degree of symptoms, indications for medical, surgical, or transcatheter interventions, and chronicity of the condition depend on the diagnosis.

#### Shunting: Saturation Considerations

Abnormal blood flow from one part of the circulatory system to another is called a shunt. A shunt occurs when (1) there is an abnormal opening or connection between the cardiac chambers or great arteries, (2) the pressure is higher on one side of the heart than the other (pressure gradient), and (3) the oxygen saturation is increased in blood that is normally desaturated or decreased in blood that is normally fully saturated. It is important to remember that the venous (right side) is usually a low-pressure, desaturated (average 70%) system and the arterial (left side) is usually a high-pressure, fully saturated (95% to 100%) system. The combination of pressure differences and the size of the abnormal opening determine the extent of shunting.

#### Blood Flow Considerations

Generally, the amount of blood flow to the lungs through the pulmonary artery is the same as the amount of blood flow to the systemic circulation through the aorta. This ratio of pulmonary to systemic blood flow is described as the *pulmonary-to-systemic ratio* (QP/QS ratio) and is usually 1 : 1. Patients with CHD can have normal, increased, or decreased QP/QS blood flow ratios. Understanding the principles of shunting and normal saturations in each of the heart's chambers helps clarify the blood flow direction in CHD.

## PHYSIOLOGIC CONSEQUENCES OF CHD IN CHILDREN

The two primary physiologic consequences of CHD in children are heart failure and cyanosis.

### Heart Failure

The definition of *heart failure* (HF) is the heart's inability to circulate blood sufficient to maintain the metabolic demands of the body. Despite the causes of HF, the heart initially responds to the need for increased cardiac output by increasing the heart rate. Over time, the heart may become enlarged (cardiomegaly), causing the muscle walls of the heart to grow weak and inefficient. This inefficiency decreases the blood volume in the body, causing the body's arteries to constrict and force the heart to work even harder. This poor function causes congestion in the body and/or lung tissues (pulmonary edema).

### Etiology

The etiology of HF in neonates, infants, and children differs from that in adults. In infants and children, HF is most often related to an underlying congenital cardiac defect that causes volume or pressure overload but other etiologies are possible, including acquired heart disease. Examples of acquired heart disease include cardiomyopathies, dysrhythmias, infections (e.g., endocarditis, myocarditis), and tumors. Damage to the heart also can occur as a result of inborn metabolic disorders and exposure to certain drugs or toxins (CDC, 2016; Park, 2014). The symptoms often can be treated with drugs. For an anatomic defect, correction of the cause either by surgery or transcatheter intervention is often needed.

Defects that lead to volume overload and cause HF symptoms in infants and children include left-to-right shunts (e.g., atrial septal defects [ASDs], ventricular septal defects [VSDs], common AV canal defect [CAVC], and patent ductus arteriosus [PDA]). These defects allow excess blood to pass from the left side of the heart to the right, causing the heart to work harder to pump this extra volume to the lungs.

Defects that lead to pressure overload and cause symptoms of HF mainly include left-side heart obstructive lesions (e.g., critical aortic stenosis, severe aortic coarctation, congenital mitral stenosis, and hypoplastic left heart syndrome). These defects require the heart to pump harder against an obstruction to get blood to the body. Over

**TABLE 46.1 Classification of Congenital Heart Disease**

| Defect | Underlying Mechanism | Examples |
|---|---|---|
| Left-to-right shunting lesions (lesions that increase pulmonary blood flow) | A defect in the atrial septum or persistence of a PDA causes saturated blood to shunt through this opening. This left-to-right shunting of blood results in a volume overload in the right side of the heart and in the pulmonary artery; cardiac workload (including ventricular strain, dilation, and hypertrophy) increases to manage the additional volume (pressure overload). This abnormal increase in highly saturated blood combined with the increased fluid volume in the lungs, results in altered gas exchange. One of the major consequences of left-to-right shunting lesions is HF. Other consequences include pulmonary vascular disease, pulmonary hypertension, Eisenmenger syndrome, and frequent upper and lower respiratory infections that can progress to respiratory failure. | ASD<br>VSD<br>PDA<br>AVSD (endocardial cushion defect) |
| Obstructive or stenotic lesions, or lesions that decrease cardiac outflow | *Stenosis*, the narrowing or constriction of an opening, can occur in a valve or vessel constricting or obstructing blood flow through the area. Pressure rises in the area behind the obstruction; blood flow distal to the obstruction may be decreased or absent. Stenotic lesions can occur in the right or left side of the heart; obstruction on the left side of the heart decreases the amount of available blood for systemic perfusion. Physiologic effects of stenotic lesions include increased cardiac workload and ventricular strain, with clinical consequences of HF, decreased cardiac output, and pump failure. | Pulmonary stenosis<br>Aortic stenosis<br>Coarctation of the aorta |
| Cyanotic lesions with decreased pulmonary blood flow | These lesions arise from an error in fetal development that results in *hypoplasia* (incomplete development), malalignment, or obstruction on the right side of the heart, decreasing the amount of blood flowing to the lungs. Pulmonary blood flow may require a PDA. The left side of the heart has abnormally low oxygen saturation. Physiologically, the child manifests hypoxemia, increased cardiac workload, and ventricular strain. The hypoxemia results in cyanosis, and even with oxygen administration, saturations do not approximate normal. Other clinical findings include upper respiratory infection, severely limited pulmonary blood flow, and marked exercise intolerance. | Tetralogy of Fallot<br>Tricuspid valve abnormalities<br>Pulmonary atresia with intact ventricular septum |
| Cyanotic lesions with increased pulmonary blood flow | When the fetal heart fails to develop into separate pulmonary and systemic circulations or when there is a reversal of circulation so that desaturated blood goes to the systemic circulation and saturated blood to the pulmonary circulation, cyanosis occurs. Sometimes classified as mixing lesions, these defects cause increased cardiac workload, ventricular strain, and decreased cardiac output. Lesions are usually discovered early in the neonatal period. The infant might appear ruddy or cyanotic, with increased respiratory effort, or, if systemic circulation is compromised, may be dusky or gray and in cardiogenic shock (see Chapter 34). To support life, these complex cardiac defects require intervention that allows for mixing of arterial and venous blood. | Truncus arteriosus<br>Hypoplastic left heart syndrome*<br>Transposition of the great arteries |

*Also classified as a lesion that decreases cardiac outflow.
*ASD*, Atrial septal defect; *AVSD*, atrioventricular septal defect; *HF*, heart failure; *PDA*, patent ductus arteriosus; *VSD*, ventricular septal defect.

time, this extra work will cause the heart muscle to enlarge (hypertrophy) and become inefficient.

Defects that are acquired and cause symptoms of HF include primary myocardial diseases that attack and weaken the heart muscle. **Dysrhythmias** disrupt the delicate balance of the electrical or conduction system of the heart, causing the heart rate to be slow, fast, or erratic. Over time, dysrhythmias lead to poor cardiac output. The incidence of HF in infants and children is difficult to estimate because of improvements in surgical options.

### Manifestations

The earliest clinical manifestations of HF are often subtle. Mild tachypnea (70 to 100 breaths/min) at rest and difficulty feeding are present in some infants. Parents may report that feedings take longer and the child requires frequent rest periods. This type of history describes a scenario in which fewer calories are consumed even though metabolic demands are increased. Therefore, feedings provide little satisfaction, and the infant may appear hungry and irritable soon after a feeding. Over time, the infant fails to gain weight and eventually develops a condition known as failure to thrive (FTT).

Children with HF can also exhibit respiratory-related symptoms. Some complain of dyspnea (particularly on exertion) and tachypnea. They are often described as having less energy than their peers. They may exhibit diaphoresis and complain of decreased appetite. These symptoms are caused by chronic abdominal pain, usually related to poor circulation and decreased perfusion to the abdominal organs. This condition can also prevent normal weight gain. Other clinical manifestations of HF include an abnormal cardiac rhythm known as a gallop, periorbital and facial edema, neck vein distention (in older children), hepatomegaly, splenomegaly, decreased peripheral perfusion, decreased urine output, mottling, cyanosis, and pallor.

### Diagnostic Evaluation

The diagnosis of HF is based on the clinical history, physical examination, chest radiographic appearance, electrocardiography (ECG), and echocardiography (ECHO). Chest x-rays can reveal cardiomegaly with increased pulmonary vascular markings. These markings reflect increased interstitial pulmonary fluid. Laboratory studies used to determine the presence of HF in children include determinations of arterial blood gas values, serum electrolyte levels, complete blood cell

## PATHOPHYSIOLOGY

### Heart Failure

When a child develops heart failure (HF), hemodynamic and neurohormonal changes occur in response to decreased cardiac output. Cardiac output is a function of stroke volume and heart rate. Stroke volume (SV) is defined as the amount of blood ejected from the heart with each heartbeat. It is expressed in liters per minute (L/min). Cardiac output equals heart rate multiplied by stroke volume. Other factors affecting cardiac output include preload, afterload, and contractility.

Neurohormonal changes include the stimulation of both the sympathetic nervous system and the renin-angiotensin system. Maintaining blood pressure, blood flow, and oxygen delivery to vital organs is the goal of this compensatory system. With decreased cardiac output, there is stimulation of the sympathetic nervous system. Initially, this stimulation leads to increases in the heart rate, contractility, and stroke volume; increased systemic vascular resistance (afterload); and selective peripheral vasoconstriction. Tachycardia, although beneficial to compensate for early HF, increases myocardial oxygen consumption, decreases the diastolic filling time and resting phase of the heart, and decreases coronary artery perfusion.*

Decreased cardiac output also causes decreased renal blood flow and a diminished glomerular filtration rate, leading to increased stimulation of the renin-angiotensin-aldosterone system. Sodium and water are reabsorbed, causing fluid retention and thereby increasing intravascular volume. Initially, this volume retention increases preload and cardiac output. Later, the myocardium becomes more edematous, and ventricular function decreases from volume and pressure overload.

The pulmonary system is also affected by this increased volume, and interstitial edema develops. In addition, myocardial oxygen consumption increases and may exceed the oxygen availability. Finally, myocardial muscle can undergo cellular and muscular mass changes, or hypertrophy. Without intervention, heart failure progresses until the compensatory mechanisms are no longer effective.

*Bernstein, D. (2016b). Heart failure. In R. Kliegman, B. Stanton, J. St. Geme, et al. (Eds.), *Nelson textbook of pediatrics* (20th ed., pp. 2282–2288). Philadelphia: Elsevier.

count, erythrocyte sedimentation rate (ESR), serum glucose and calcium levels, and urinalysis.

### Therapeutic Management

Management of a child with HF involves correcting the underlying problem as soon as possible. The medical management of HF is directed toward decreasing cardiac workload and improving cardiac output through the manipulation of the hemodynamics and neurohormonal responses. Supplemental oxygen can be helpful for increasing oxygen saturation, but it should be used with caution in children with left-to-right shunts. Because oxygen is a vasodilator, it can increase pulmonary blood flow. Pharmacologic agents used include positive inotropes (e.g., digoxin), diuretics, and angiotensin-converting enzyme (ACE) inhibitors (Bernstein, 2016b). Digoxin is now used less frequently in favor of ACE inhibitors because of the risk of toxicity (Bernstein, 2016b). In addition, optimizing nutritional intake to meet the metabolic demands and improve growth is of paramount importance. A persistence of symptoms and lack of weight gain are indications for surgical intervention.

Digoxin is a cardiac glycoside that increases cardiac output and improves cardiac effectiveness by several mechanisms. It has a positive inotropic effect that strengthens the force of myocardial contractions. It has a negative chronotropic effect that slows the heart rate and, at higher doses, slows conduction of cardiac impulses through the AV node, allowing the ventricles more time to fill with blood. It also improves blood flow to the kidneys and enhances diuresis.

Obtain a baseline ECG before initiating digoxin. Digoxin is administered intravenously or orally. The effectiveness of digoxin depends on achieving and maintaining a therapeutic serum drug level. A loading or digitalizing dose according to the child's age and weight is administered in divided doses over 12 to 18 hours, and maintenance doses are given daily, usually in two divided doses. The range between therapeutic and toxic digoxin levels is narrow, with a therapeutic range of 0.8 to 2.0 ng/mL (Park, 2014). To avoid a falsely elevated serum digoxin level, serum digoxin levels should be measured at a minimum of 6 hours from the previous dose. Measurement in the first 3 to 5 days after digitalizing can also yield elevated results; thus, ECG changes are a more accurate sign of an elevated serum digoxin level during this time (Bernstein, 2016b; Park, 2014). Levels are generally obtained when assessing for toxicity or medication adherence. If a child is receiving digoxin and is having dysrhythmias, the digoxin level should be measured. Hypokalemia and hypomagnesemia can increase the risk for digoxin toxicity. In children with altered renal function, the dose should be decreased.

Diuretics are administered to eliminate excess water and sodium through increased urine production, thereby reducing systemic and pulmonary congestion. Furosemide is a potent loop diuretic and is preferred for initial diuretic therapy. Another class of diuretics, the thiazides, acts at the distal renal tubules. These can be less potent than loop diuretics. These drugs cause the kidneys to waste potassium, placing the child at risk for hypokalemia. Potassium-sparing diuretics, such as spironolactone, are weak diuretics. This class of diuretics is often given with loop diuretics or thiazides to decrease the potential for hypokalemia. Potassium supplements can also be given in tandem with diuretics to replace these losses.

Vasodilators such as hydralazine, captopril or enalapril can be used to relax vascular smooth muscles and reduce afterload (Bernstein, 2016b; Park, 2014). Captopril and enalapril are called ACE inhibitors because they block the conversion of angiotensin I to angiotensin II and reduce vasoconstriction and sodium retention. In addition, ACE inhibitors decrease norepinephrine release from the sympathetic nervous system.

### Pulmonary Hypertension

Pulmonary hypertension (PAH) is elevated blood pressure in the blood vessels of the lungs. PAH is diagnosed when the mean pulmonary arterial pressure exceeds 20 mm Hg at rest (normal at rest, 15 mm Hg). PAH in children is most commonly idiopathic or familial, followed by CHD as the cause (Bernstein, 2016c). Initially, infants with a significant left-to-right shunting defect have reversible pulmonary vasoconstriction and increased pulmonary blood flow that causes elevated pulmonary artery pressure. PAH occurs over time when vascular changes eventually lead to vessel wall thickening, severe irreversible vasoconstriction, and vascular obstruction. This severe condition leads to a reversal of the cardiac shunting, becoming right-to-left (called *Eisenmenger syndrome*), with less blood pumped to the lungs, so that a previously acyanotic child becomes cyanotic as oxygen-poor blood gets pumped to the body (Bernstein, 2016d). It is critical to time any surgical intervention before the development of irreversible vascular changes. This information is assessed clinically and in the cardiac catheterization laboratory. Repair of lesions with large left-to-right shunts is generally recommended in the first 3 to 6 months of life.

Children with large left-to-right shunting lesions, particularly at the ventricular level, have high pulmonary artery pressures but low

## NURSING CARE PLAN

### *The Child With Heart Failure*

**Focused Assessment**

- Closely assess vital signs, cardiovascular status, and pulmonary status
- Observe the child for the worsening signs and symptoms of tachycardia, tachypnea, poor feeding, diaphoresis during feeding, and increased irritability or fatigue
- Obtain a history of the child's fluid and nutritional status, feeding patterns, and growth
- Strictly monitor intake and output
- Weigh daily and report any weight increases

**Nursing Diagnosis**

Decreased Cardiac Output related to heart failure (HF) or decreased myocardial function.

**Planning**

***Expected Outcome***

1. The child will have adequate cardiac output, as evidenced by pink or baseline cyanotic (in cyanotic heart disease) mucous membranes and nail beds, a capillary refill time of less than 2 seconds, warm extremities, easily palpable peripheral pulses, adequate urinary output, no edema, appropriate heart rate, and an activity level within the normal limits of the defect.

**Interventions and *Rationales***

1. Observe and document peripheral perfusion by palpating peripheral pulses, noting temperature, color changes, and capillary refill time.
   *Poor peripheral perfusion is usually evidenced by decreased or absent pulses in the extremities. Color and temperature changes (e.g., cyanosis, coolness, mottling) may be present in all extremities. Prolonged capillary refill time is an additional sign of poor perfusion.*
2. Assess whether heart rate is appropriate for level of activity.
   *Tachycardia occurs in an attempt to maintain adequate cardiac output.*
3. Monitor and document hourly urine output.
   *Altered renal perfusion caused by decreased cardiac output results in decreased urinary output.*
4. Maintain a neutral thermal environment; use a warmer bed or incubator for the neonate; treat fever promptly.
   *Episodes of hypothermia or hyperthermia increase oxygen demands and increase the cardiac workload.*
5. Time nursing interventions to allow the infant or child rest periods. Anticipate and respond quickly to stressful events, crying, or restlessness.
   *Rest periods reduce cardiac workload. Organizing nursing activities to promote rest results in decreased stress and fatigue for the child.*
6. Administer digoxin (Lanoxin) as prescribed. Ascertain that the dosage is within safe limits. Count the apical rate for 1 full minute. Check the dosage with a second nurse. Withhold the dose and notify the provider if the heart rate is less than 100 beats/min in infants; the heart rate at which the medication should be withheld varies in older children and adolescents. If the withholding pulse rate is not ordered, withhold the medication and call the provider if the pulse rate is progressively decreasing or markedly lower than previous rates. Observe for signs of toxicity, and monitor for hyperkalemia in the child taking potassium-sparing diuretics.
   *Digoxin is effective within a narrow therapeutic range (0.8-2 ng/mL),* although the pediatric range is not well defined. Safety in dosing is achieved by double checking the dose and counting the apical heart rate for a full minute. Digoxin toxicity can manifest with slow pulse, vomiting, and dysrhythmias.*

**Evaluation**

Are mucous membranes and nail beds pink or baseline cyanotic?
Is the capillary refill time less than 2 seconds?
Are peripheral pulses easily palpated, and is the child alert and active?
Is the heart rate in the expected range for activity?

**Nursing Diagnosis**

Excess Fluid Volume related to volume overload and HF.

**Planning**

***Expected Outcome***

1. The infant or child will remain free of evidence of fluid overload (e.g., infrequent urination, inappropriate water weight gain, inadequate balance between intake and output, edema [periorbital, hepatomegaly], respiratory distress, poor feeding).

**Interventions and *Rationales***

1. Administer diuretics as prescribed, ensuring correct dosage, route, and effectiveness.
   *Diuretics help the body eliminate excess fluid. Their effectiveness is evaluated from the urine output (either by measuring the amount of urine or by weighing diapers), weight, decreasing edema, decreasing respiratory distress, and improved feeding.*
2. Maintain accurate intake and output records. The fluid intake and output should be about the same.
   *If intake grossly exceeds output, the diuretics may need to be altered, the child may need fluid restriction, or both.*
3. Maintain fluid restriction, if ordered.
   *Fluid restriction will decrease pulmonary and liver edema.*
4. Using the same scales, weigh the child daily at approximately the same time. Notify the provider of excessive weight gain (infants, >50 g/day; children, >200 g/day).
   *Excess fluid volume is not always overtly visible. Weight changes may indicate fluid retention. Weighing the infant or child on the same scales at the same time each day ensures consistency.*
5. Provide skin care and change position frequently.
   *Edematous areas are extremely prone to skin breakdown because of stretching and opacity. Frequent position changes will prevent undesirable pooling of fluid in certain areas.*
6. Monitor for increased or decreased edema (in infants and young children, edema is usually periorbital) and hepatomegaly; generalized edema in the preoperative patient is extremely rare.
   *Changes in the amount of edema can indicate the effectiveness or ineffectiveness of therapies and interventions.*
7. Monitor serum electrolyte levels, especially potassium.
   *Diuretics may stimulate potassium loss.*

**Evaluation**

Is the child urinating frequently in comparison with age-related norms (see Chapter 40)?
Is the child edematous?
Has the child lost or gained weight?
Are intake and output balanced?

**Nursing Diagnosis**

Ineffective Breathing Pattern related to pulmonary congestion.

**Planning**

***Expected Outcomes***

The child will:

1. Demonstrate a respiratory rate within normal limits for age and a normal respiratory effort.
2. Have satisfactory rest periods.
3. Have color that remains pink or baseline cyanotic.

## NURSING CARE PLAN—cont'd

### *The Child With Heart Failure*

**Interventions and *Rationales***

1. Monitor respiratory rate and rhythm, the presence or absence of retractions or nasal flaring, the use of accessory muscles, and the presence or absence of crackles or rhonchi.
   *Infants and children with HF have changes in their breathing pattern because of increased fluid retention in the lungs, liver, and other areas of the body.*
2. Position the infant or child with the head of the bed elevated 30 to 45 degrees. Avoid clothing that constricts the chest.
   *An elevated position lowers the diaphragm and maximizes chest expansion.*
3. Administer oxygen as needed.
   *Supplemental oxygen administration improves oxygen saturation and delivery to tissues. Cautious use of oxygen is indicated in left-to-right shunting lesions because of the effect of oxygen on lowering pulmonary vascular resistance, which can increase pulmonary blood flow and increase the degree of pulmonary congestion and symptoms of HF.*
4. Plan nursing interventions to allow maximum rest for the child. Feed the child when the child is rested. Avoid performing multiple interventions at any one time.
   *Clustering nursing activities decreases the child's fatigue, promotes feeding effort, and conserves metabolic demands.*
5. Prevent exposure to individuals with respiratory illnesses. Prevent nosocomial exposures and infections.
   *Respiratory infections with associated CHD can have a severe adverse effect on respiratory stability. Children with CHD are at a higher risk for nosocomial infections.*

**Evaluation**

Is the child's respiratory rate within normal limits for age?
Are the child's mucous membranes and nail beds pink or at baseline cyanosis?
Is the child breathing easily?
Is the child able to obtain an appropriate amount of rest?

**Nursing Diagnosis**

Imbalanced Nutrition: Less Than Body Requirements related to increased energy expenditure and increased feeding effort.

**Planning**

***Expected Outcome***

The infant or child will demonstrate appropriate weight gain and no significant loss of weight over a short period.

**Interventions and *Rationales***

1. Weigh the infant or child daily or before and after each feeding for breastfed infants. Use the same scale.
   *Using the same scale ensures consistency.*
2. Breastfeed or feed smaller volumes of concentrated formula (24 to 27 cal/oz) every 3 hours.
   *Increased caloric content of formula increases caloric consumption and enhances weight gain. May require 120 to 150 kcal/kg/day for adequate weight gain. Additives are available that increase the caloric content of breast milk.*
3. Use a nipple that the infant can comfortably adjust for flow rate and energy to express milk. May need a soft, large-hole nipple.
   *Infants with HF tire easily. An appropriate nipple for the infant minimizes the level of energy required to express milk at a rate of flow the baby can swallow comfortably. A soft nipple with a large hole may facilitate easy sucking and decrease energy expenditure during feeding.*
4. Implement gavage feedings if the infant tires before the recommended amount of feeding is consumed, takes longer than 30 minutes to feed, displays increased fatigue during or after feeding, or demonstrates poor weight gain on adequate caloric intake.
   *Gavage feedings decrease energy expenditure and allow calories consumed to be used for growth. Can be used in conjunction with timed nipple periods to maintain feeding skills.*
5. Time the feedings to allow for adequate rest. Every 3 hours is a frequently used interval.
   *Frequent disturbances increase oxygen consumption. Too frequent feedings disturb rest, whereas less frequent feedings require increased intake, which tires the infant.*
6. Monitor for feeding intolerance.
   *May not tolerate concentrated formulas. Also, gastroesophageal reflux may be present.*

**Evaluation**

Has the infant or child maintained a steady weight gain?
Is the feeding pattern stable or changing?
Is the infant or child tolerating feedings without vomiting or other signs of intolerance?

**Nursing Diagnosis**

Deficient Knowledge related to anxiety and unfamiliarity with the disease process, treatment, interventions, and home care.

**Planning**

***Expected Outcomes***

1. Parents will describe the cardiac defect and current and future interventions.
2. Parents will demonstrate an ability to perform treatments, including medication administration.

**Interventions and *Rationales***

1. Determine the parents' readiness to learn, anxiety level, knowledge needed to care for their child, and specific concerns. A baseline assessment of prior knowledge should be considered before developing a teaching plan.
   *Addressing special concerns initially can facilitate parents' comfort level and receptiveness to new knowledge. Decreasing anxiety assists with information processing.*
2. Provide brief, factual explanations of the child's defect or any treatments and interventions. Do so frequently.
   *Parents are most likely to retain consistent, repetitive explanations.*
3. Allow the parents and child to verbalize feelings and concerns related to hospitalization and caring for the child at home.
   *Hospitalization is a frightening experience. By allowing verbalization of feelings and concerns related to the experience, nurses can assist in allaying fears and addressing concerns. Discussing care at home can also assist in allaying fears and addressing concerns.*
4. Teach the parents to administer all necessary cardiac medications and explain their associated actions and potential adverse effects. Provide demonstrations and obtain return demonstrations by parents. Explain the use of oral syringes for accurate measurement of drugs. Provide a daily medication chart (which can be color-coded for specific medications) for children receiving multiple medications. Provide parents with written information (see Patient-Centered Teaching: Giving Your Child Digoxin Elixir).
   *Family members should be taught how to administer all cardiac medications before discharge. This allows for teaching appropriate medication dosage, questions, answers, and evaluation of their home care techniques. Written information provides an adjunct to individual teaching and a reference for the caregiver at home. Written information can be referred to during less*

*Continued*

## NURSING CARE PLAN—cont'd

### *The Child With Heart Failure*

*stressful times, when it may be more likely to be retained or used as a reference.*

5. Determine parents' understanding of instructions through return demonstrations and repeated information. This includes signs and symptoms requiring medical or nursing assessment.
   *Return demonstrations and repeated information validate that learning has occurred and that the parents are competent to provide care.*

**Evaluation**

Have the parents verbalized adequate and correct knowledge of the diagnosis and interventions?

Have the parents demonstrated confidence and competence in caregiving activities, including medicine administration?

Are the parents able to describe conditions that necessitate a call for medical or nursing advice?

*Skidmore-Roth, L. (2011). *Mosby's nursing drug reference* (24th ed.). St. Louis: Mosby.

## EVIDENCE-BASED PRACTICE

In 2013, the American Heart Association issued a statement promoting physical activity for children with congenital heart disease. The benefits of physical activity positively affect the health of a child both physically and psychologically. The benefits that are well researched include improved cardiovascular health, decreased risk of diabetes, decreased incidence of overweight and obesity, decreased incidence of depression, and many more. As the care of children born with congenital heart disease improves, most of these children are surviving into adulthood with an estimated one million children living with congenital heart disease. In caring for children with congenital heart disease, one area that patients and their families feel is lacking is information regarding the type, level, and amount of physical activity that is appropriate for the child. This lack of knowledge often leads to inappropriate restrictions on physical activity implemented by the parents, thereby placing the child at risk for obesity, diabetes, and cardiovascular disease.

Reducing the proportion of children and adolescents who are obese and overweight is one of the Healthy People 2020 objectives. Presently, 17% (or 12.7 million) of children and adolescents aged 2 to 19 years are obese (CDC, 2014). The CDC now recommends 60 minutes of daily activity. This recommendation is often not met by children in the United States, and even more so with children diagnosed with a congenital heart disease.

Children born with congenital heart disease tend to have a more sedentary lifestyle. Healthcare providers need to incorporate physical activity guidelines tailored to each child during all patient interactions. The benefits of physical activity need to be reinforced, and the appropriate type, level, and amount of physical activity should be discussed with both the child and their caregivers. Physical activity is not only important for the physical benefits but also for the psychological wellbeing of the child.

The barriers to physical activity include self-imposed activity restrictions, poor coordination, lack of knowledge regarding appropriate physical activities, and poor self-esteem. Parents of children with congenital heart disease often overprotect children, causing them to avoid physical activity and to have poor leadership skills. This limitation discourages independence at a critical time in childhood, especially as the child enters adolescence—a time when independence increases as the adolescent discovers his or her identity. The adolescent strives for acceptance and does not want to feel different than peers because they were born with a congenital heart disease (Caplan & Allen, 2011). Another barrier is that adolescents report that providers often speak to their parents and not directly to them, making them feel less valued in the decision making of their own care.

Ray, Green, & Henry (2011) conducted a cross-sectional study to identify the association between physical activity participation and body mass index (BMI) in 84 children aged 10 to 14 who were born with congenital heart disease. Several studies have noted that the incidence of obesity in children with congenital heart disease is similar to that of the general population (Ray et al., 2011). The participants self-reported their physical activity using the Previous Day Physical Activity Recall. Results showed that children with congenital heart disease had lower levels of physical activity, and those with more severe defects had the lowest levels of physical activity than compared to healthy children (Ray et al., 2011).

Collaboration between the cardiology clinic and the primary care clinic can enhance the opportunities for education about specific physical activity guidelines that are appropriate for the patient. Uncertainty about the amount and type of physical activity that is appropriate for a child causes concern about their abilities and anxiety about the severity of their illness. Misinterpretation of recommendations is a common barrier that can be alleviated with education about the type, level, and amount of physical activity that is appropriate for the child at each healthcare visit.

Think about the implication of this research on clinical practice. How can you, as the nurse, help coordinate the care between the cardiology provider and the primary care provider? What education about physical activity would you provide to a child with congenital heart disease and his or her caregivers? Are there other resources you can provide that could help the child maintain a healthy lifestyle? How can you motivate the child to implement the plan of care for physical activity?

References: Centers for Disease Control and Prevention. (2014). *Childhood obesity facts.* Retrieved from http://www.cdc.gov/obesity/data/childhood.html; Caplan, R., & Allen, P.J. (2011). Physical activity recommendations for adolescents with repaired tetralogy of fallot: review of the literature and guidelines for practitioners. *Pediatric Nursing, 37*(4), 191–199; Office of Disease Prevention and Health Promotion. (2014). *Nutrition and weight status.* Retrieved from http://www.healthypeople.gov/2020/topics-objectives/topic/nutrition-and-weight-status/objectives#4928; Ray, T.D., Green, A., & Henry, K. (2011). Physical activity and obesity in children with congenital cardiac disease. *Cardiology in the Young, 21,* 603–607. doi:10.1017/S1047951111000540.

## PATIENT-CENTERED TEACHING

### *Giving Your Child Digoxin Elixir*

**Medication:** Digoxin (Lanoxin)

**Your child's dosage:** ________ mL twice a day. Your child will be taking this medicine twice a day for several months to years.

**What it does:** Digoxin (Lanoxin) helps the heart pump blood more effectively, thereby improving the circulation of the blood, and promoting the normal elimination of excess fluid.

**What you need to know:**

- Digoxin (Lanoxin) is usually given every morning and evening. You may adjust the times to fit your and your child's schedule.
- Give the digoxin 20 to 30 minutes before a feeding. Give it at the same time every day so that it becomes part of your routine.
- The amount of digoxin you give your child must be measured carefully with a syringe, not the dropper provided with the medicine.
- Put a few drops of digoxin in your child's mouth and let the child swallow it before giving more.
- If you forget to give your child a single dose of digoxin, give the dose when you remember it; then resume your original schedule.
- If your child vomits after taking the digoxin, do not repeat the dose. Resume the digoxin at the next dosage time.
- *If you miss or your child vomits two doses in a row, call the cardiology department.*
- Rarely, children have too much digoxin in their body and can have vomiting. If your child vomits, call your pediatrician or cardiologist. You will be instructed what to do about your child's dosage.
- Keep the digoxin in a place where children living or playing in your home will not be able to reach it.
- If someone accidentally takes the digoxin, call poison control or take the person and the digoxin bottle to the emergency room.
- Obtain refills at least 1 week before you are out of medicine. Ask for new prescriptions as needed.

Modified and used with permission from Children's Hospital Oakland, Department of Cardiology, Oakland, CA. Developed and revised by Lili Cook, RN, MS, and Sally Higgins, PhD, RN, FAAN.

## ! NURSING QUALITY ALERT

### *Feeding the Infant or Child With Heart Failure*

Feed the infant or child in a relaxed environment. Time the feedings before multiple other activities to preserve the infant's energy. The infant with heart failure (HF) tends to tire easily during feedings. Frequent, small feedings can be less tiring. Holding the infant in an upright position causes less stomach compression and improves respiratory effort during the feeding. If the child is unable to consume an appropriate amount during a 30-minute feeding period every 3 hours, nasogastric (NG) or nasoduodenal (ND) feedings should be considered. Assess for increased tachypnea, diaphoresis, or feeding intolerance (vomiting). Concentrating formula from the basic level of 20 kcal/oz to 30 kcal/oz or higher can increase caloric intake without increasing the infant's work.

pulmonary vascular resistance. Initially, HF develops. Management is directed toward treating the symptoms of HF, including treatment with digitalis, calcium channel blockers, diuretics, warfarin, and supplemental oxygen. Additionally, the family is advised to have the child avoid strenuous exercise and high altitudes. Vasodilators can be helpful if the child demonstrates adequate response when these medications are given during cardiac catheterization (Bernstein, 2016c; Park, 2014). Inhaled nitric oxide has been shown to be an effective pulmonary vasodilator and is used in the treatment of persistent PAH of the newborn.

## ? CRITICAL THINKING EXERCISE 46.1

Lin, a 2-month-old infant, is seen in the pediatrician's office. She has gained 1 lb since birth and has a heart murmur. She is admitted to the pediatric unit with a diagnosis of heart failure (HF). You will obtain a health history and perform an admission assessment.

1. What specific questions should you ask Lin's parents about her feeding patterns and behavior?
2. What physical assessment findings would you expect in an infant with HF?
3. List nursing interventions that would address Lin's nutritional and comfort needs.

PAH can also be caused by heritable (genetic mutations) or idiopathic etiologies. Idiopathic disease is diagnosed when no underlying disease can be found. Conditions leading to PAH include alveolar hypoxia, such as pulmonary parenchymal disease or airway obstruction that leads to vasoconstriction. Pulmonary venous hypertension is seen in left heart outflow obstructive lesions and connective tissue disorders.

Many studies and ongoing trials are investigating PAH-specific therapies for children. With early surgical intervention, children with reversible PAH can have a return of normal pulmonary pressures postoperatively. Early intervention is important because the increasing pulmonary vascular resistance caused by pulmonary vascular changes puts children at higher risk for surgical morbidity and mortality and for the development of irreversible PAH. Management of children with idiopathic or advanced PAH remains challenging, as current pharmacologic therapies (e.g., IV epoprostenol or oral bosentan) have somewhat improved survival but have not adequately addressed disease progression (Bernstein, 2016c).

### Cyanosis

Cyanotic cardiac lesions produce cyanosis when desaturated blood from the venous system enters the arterial system without passing through the lungs, commonly through an abnormal opening that enables shunting of desaturated blood. Cyanosis, a bluish discoloration of the skin, nail beds, and mucous membranes, appears when tissues are deprived of adequate amounts of oxygen. Cyanosis becomes visible when hemoglobin that is not bound to oxygen reaches a level of approximately 5 g/dL blood and the measured oxygen saturation drops below 85%. The degree of cyanosis varies; some children will appear pale and mildly cyanotic, whereas others will be quite dusky. In anemic infants or children, desaturation will be higher before cyanosis is apparent (the lower total hemoglobin level in anemia means that a higher percentage must be desaturated before cyanosis is visible). Conversely, with significant *polycythemia* (increased red blood cells with resulting elevated hemoglobin), children will appear cyanotic when less desaturated (with the higher hemoglobin level in polycythemia, a lower percentage must be desaturated before cyanosis is visible).

Cyanosis can occur when blood flow to the lungs is decreased (e.g., in severe pulmonary artery stenosis, pulmonary atresia, tetralogy of Fallot, or tricuspid atresia) or desaturated blood is pumped to the body (e.g., in total anomalous pulmonary venous return, truncus arteriosus, and hypoplastic left heart syndrome). Cyanosis intensifies with crying in children with these defects and is not alleviated by the administration of 100% oxygen.

The clinical consequences of cyanosis include polycythemia, anemia, clotting abnormalities, hypercyanotic episodes, central nervous system

(CNS) injury caused by abscess or embolic events, PAH, and endocarditis. Developmental delay can be related to CNS injury, severe hypoxic events, or chronic illness.

Polycythemia is a compensatory response of the body to chronic hypoxia. The body attempts to improve tissue oxygenation by increasing the oxygen-carrying capacity of the blood—in other words, by producing additional red blood cells. Accelerated red blood cell production increases the viscosity of the blood and crowds the vascular space so there is less room for plasma and clotting factors. Children who are polycythemic are at a greater risk for bruising and prolonged bleeding because of decreased specific clotting factors.

Increased blood viscosity makes the peripheral circulation sluggish and places the child at risk for CNS injury from a brain abscess or cerebrovascular accident. Depletion of iron stores can also result, and anemia can develop if iron is not available to participate in hemoglobin formation.

Dehydration can rapidly occur in cyanotic heart disease. Hyperthermia (fever or environmental), poor oral intake, vomiting, and diarrhea can cause acute dehydration. Dehydration can be life threatening for the child with a cyanotic heart disease because the fluid loss can contribute to the relative viscosity of the blood. The increased viscosity can close a shunt that is necessary for pulmonary blood flow (shunt thrombosis). Once the shunt closes, there is no pulmonary blood flow, resulting in metabolic acidosis and severe hypoxemia that can lead to cardiopulmonary arrest.

### Hypercyanotic Episode

A serious, clinically significant, and dramatic event seen in children with cyanotic heart disease is the hypercyanotic episode. These events are often called *tet spells* because they frequently occur in children with unrepaired tetralogy of Fallot. The exact cause is unknown, but it is thought that the child has an acute spasm of the right ventricular outflow tract as a result of agitation or another adverse event that dramatically decreases pulmonary blood flow, causing hypoxia and metabolic acidosis (Bernstein, 2016e). These episodes last a few minutes to a few hours and include rapid and deep respirations, irritability and crying, peripheral vasodilation, increased systemic venous return, increasing cyanosis that can be very severe, and a decrease in the systolic murmur, reflecting decreased pulmonary blood flow (Bernstein, 2016e). As the child becomes more cyanotic, tachypnea and hyperpnea increase, which in turn increase the degree of right-to-left shunting. The incidence of hypercyanotic spells is not directly related to the degree of baseline desaturation and cyanosis.

Hypercyanotic episodes are seen most frequently in the first 2 years of life and seem to occur mainly in the morning. Often, the episode is preceded by crying, feeding, or defecation. The infant becomes agitated and may eventually lose consciousness. Although usually self-limiting, the spells can progress to a vicious cycle that can be fatal if not recognized and treated. Frequent or prolonged episodes can lead to diminished cerebral oxygenation and ischemic brain injury.

Treatment of the episode includes calming the infant, placing the infant in the knee-chest position (to increase systemic vascular resistance and force blood to the pulmonary system), and administering oxygen (pulmonary vasodilation). Morphine sulfate is administered to suppress the respiratory center and decrease the degree of hyperpnea (which contributes to vasodilation) (Huether & McCance, 2017; Park, 2014). Potent medications that cause vasoconstriction (e.g., phenylephrine) may be needed to increase systemic vascular resistance, decrease the degree of right-to-left shunting, and force blood into the pulmonary system. Propranolol which slows the heart and may reduce spasms has also been used with some success (Park, 2014). Preventing or treating hypovolemia is also an important factor. Hypercyanotic episodes indicate the need to surgically repair or palliate the defect.

## NURSING CARE

### The Child With Cyanosis

#### Assessment

The nurse must know the source of pulmonary blood flow when caring for a child with cyanotic heart disease. Infants and children who are dependent on a shunt for pulmonary blood flow are at risk for shunt thrombosis (as detailed earlier). Infants with right-to-left shunts are at increased risk for an arterial air embolus from an IV line because a small embolus can cross directly from the venous circulation to the arterial circulation through the shunt.

Evaluation of the child with cyanotic heart disease includes an assessment of baseline cyanosis and general appearance. Assess the level of activity, including irritability. Visible cyanosis is most easily seen in natural light and is evaluated by observing the skin of the central mucous membranes of the mouth and conjunctiva and the nail beds. General skin color is also assessed. Cyanotic children may be smaller than their peers and may demonstrate clubbing, thickening, and flattening of the fingertips and toes as a result of polycythemia (see Fig. 45.6). Oxygen saturation levels should be obtained and compared with the child's baselines. To prevent infective endocarditis, some children with unrepaired cardiac defects and those who have had infective endocarditis previously require antibiotic prophylaxis for certain dental and surgical procedures until the defect is repaired and for several months afterward.

The child can become dyspneic during feeding, crying, and other activities that require exertion and might have difficulty keeping up with peers. Some children with cyanosis have frequent respiratory infections, miss more school days, and, as a result, lag behind their classmates academically despite being developmentally normal. If the child requires an IV line for hydration or another indication, it is imperative that the nurse assess IV line patency and inspect IV tubing for the presence of air in the line because even a small amount of air in the circulation increases the risk of systemic air emboli that can cause a stroke or heart attack. The use of an air filter is recommended.

#### Nursing Diagnosis and Planning

Nursing diagnoses and expected outcomes typical for the child with cyanosis and the child's family include the following:

- Deficient Knowledge related to inexperience with the management of a child with a life-threatening illness.

*Expected outcome.* The parents, and child if age appropriate, will explain the disease process, treatment, and interventions and will demonstrate the ability to perform home care treatments, including medication administration.

- Interrupted Family Processes related to impact of an acute, chronic, or life-threatening disease.

*Expected outcome.* The parents will express positive feelings for their child and for each other and will demonstrate the ability to meet the needs of the child, each other, and other family members.

- Delayed Growth and Development related to altered oxygenation or inadequate cardiac output to meet metabolic needs.

*Expected outcome.* The child will demonstrate adequate growth according to an optimal growth curve for age and condition and will perform motor, social, and expressive skills typical of age-group within the scope of the child's present capabilities. The parents will describe any developmental delay or deviation and make plans for intervention.

- Ineffective Tissue Perfusion related to hypercyanotic episodes.

*Expected outcome.* The child will remain free of decreased tissue perfusion, as evidenced by the absence of profound cyanosis and by the child's activity level, affect, respiratory status, and oxygenation all being normal. The parents will list signs and symptoms that signal the onset of hypercyanotic episodes.

- Risk for Infection related to the presence of infection-promoting conditions created by the underlying defect.

*Expected outcome.* The child will remain free of endocardial infection. The parents will understand and carry out any ordered antibiotic prophylaxis; and the parents will list when to seek medical attention for fevers.

- Deficient Knowledge related to unfamiliarity with the systemic complications from increased risk of clotting.

*Expected outcome.* The parents will describe the signs and symptoms to report immediately, including increasing cyanosis, vomiting, and fever (signs of clotting of the pulmonary shunt), and new-onset facial or extremity weakness, slurred speech, clumsiness, or breathing difficulty (signs of a CNS clot).

### Interventions

Cyanotic heart disease is usually diagnosed during the newborn period. The initial nursing interventions are directed toward stabilizing and preparing the child for medical or surgical intervention. Pulmonary blood flow in cyanotic heart disease may depend on the persistence of the ductus arteriosus. Prostaglandin $E_1$ ($PGE_1$), a vasodilator, is often administered to maintain ductal patency and restore pulmonary or systemic blood flow. Continuous infusion of the drug can improve arterial oxygen saturation and tissue perfusion, allowing the infant to be stabilized in anticipation of further diagnostic and treatment interventions. $PGE_1$ is rapidly metabolized through the pulmonary circulation and excreted through the renal system. It must be infused by continuous IV administration. The major side effect is apnea, and infants frequently require intubation. The nurse is responsible for monitoring $PGE_1$ infusion flow and evaluating peripheral perfusion and respiratory status.

Parental teaching and support at the time of diagnosis are a priority. Parents receive complicated information and are often asked to make important decisions that affect their child's current therapy and, perhaps, future interventions. Parents need simple, yet thorough, explanations to help them make informed choices. The nurse may need to repeat the information several times. Help parents identify sources of emotional support and encourage communication within the family.

Parents of children with cardiovascular disease respond with a variety of reactions. Knowing this, the nurse has a responsibility to educate parents about their child's disease and to stress the importance of the child interacting with the environment as normally as possible. For effective planning and provision of care, the child's condition must be placed in the context of the family's life.

In the child with cyanosis, careful monitoring of fluid status is necessary to prevent hemoconcentration. Intake and output are closely monitored, and daily weights are often recorded during hospitalization. Teach parents to recognize illnesses that place their child at risk for dehydration and to seek medical attention when their child has fluid losses.

Parents have concerns about worsening cyanosis and fear hypercyanotic episodes. Teach parents to recognize events that can trigger an episode and to respond calmly and place the infant in a knee-chest position. Review indications to seek medical care. Because most children with cyanosis limit their own physical activities, parents do not need to strictly limit the child's activities.

Prevention of infective endocarditis is necessary for select patients and is accomplished through antibiotic prophylaxis. Parents are given a copy of the AHA prevention guidelines. Compared with previous guidelines, fewer patients are candidates to receive prophylaxis.

Children with cyanosis are prone to frequent respiratory infections. Respiratory infections can increase cardiac workload and lead to increased cyanosis and desaturation. Careful hand hygiene is necessary to reduce the risk of infection. Teach parents to avoid crowded areas and contact between their child and other people with respiratory infections.

The nurse's role includes the astute and vigilant assessment, monitoring, and collaborative treatment of a child with known or potential cardiovascular alterations. Rapid changes in acuity and **decompensation** can occur in children with certain congenital and acquired heart diseases. Thus, the skills required of the pediatric nurse must be focused and refined to identify clinically significant changes that may impact this often complex population.

### Evaluation

- Can the parent, or child (if appropriate), describe the cardiac defect and its implications?
- Are the parents able to monitor their child's condition, provide home treatments, administer medications, and support the child's fluid and nutritional needs?
- Are family members appropriately expressing feelings and supporting each other and the child, and can the parents meet the needs of siblings and each other?
- Is the child showing a steady increase in physical growth and attaining age-appropriate developmental milestones?
- Is the child undergoing any change in the level of cyanosis, activity, respiratory status, or oxygenation?
- Can the parents describe signs, symptoms, and management of hypercyanotic episodes?
- Is the child afebrile and free of other signs and symptoms of infection, and can the parents explain the necessity for seeking medical attention for any fevers?
- Are the parents able to list complications related to possible pulmonary shunt or CNS clotting?

## ASSESSMENT OF THE CHILD WITH A CARDIOVASCULAR ALTERATION

Serious congenital cardiac lesions usually become symptomatic early in infancy. Remarkable technologic advances in the understanding of the function and requirements of the cardiovascular system have led to refinements in the tools and techniques for detecting, diagnosing, and treating congenital heart defects. Invasive procedures are now required less for initial diagnosis but rather to obtain more detailed hemodynamic information and for interventional procedures. Nevertheless, no tool or technique replaces obtaining a comprehensive history from both the child and the parents and performing a thorough physical examination (Table 46.2).

The cardiac assessment should take place in a quiet and nonthreatening environment with a parent present if possible. Parents know their child best, and they can offer a time line of events and subtle clinical information that may not be evident on examination. The nurse should establish an atmosphere of trust and cooperation—cardiac assessment is best and most easily performed on a cooperative infant or child.

The room should be warm and well lit. Natural light from windows will allow the nurse to accurately assess skin color. The assessment should begin with the least threatening steps—the history and inspection. During the parent interview, the child has the opportunity to observe the interaction between nurse and parent and has time to become comfortable with the nurse's presence. The child should be allowed to participate in the assessment and encouraged to touch and inspect each piece of equipment to be used during the examination.

**TABLE 46.2 Cardiac Assessment for the Child With CHD***

| Assessment Guidelines | Findings and Comments |
|---|---|
| **Health History** | |
| Inquire about a family history of CHD, sudden death, or fetal/infant death. | Some families have an increased incidence of CHD. |
| Ask about prenatal care, maternal illnesses, infections, medications taken during pregnancy, alcohol consumption. | CHD is linked to chronic maternal illness (diabetes, lupus), perinatal infections (rubella), and certain medications (lithium). |
| Discuss pregnancy, birth history, associated birth defects or genetic anomalies. | The incidence of CHD is higher in children with certain genetic anomalies or birth defects. Cyanosis, murmur, or other cardiac events present at birth can indicate cardiac disease. |
| Discuss feeding difficulties (including decreased intake or increased rest periods during feeding), tachypnea or increased work of breathing, frequency of respiratory infections, poor weight gain, fatigue, exercise intolerance, color changes with crying or Valsalva maneuvers, diaphoresis. | Poor weight gain and failure to thrive are often associated with cardiac disease. Cyanosis may be more prominent with crying or Valsalva maneuvers. |
| **Inspection** | |
| *Color:* Assess skin color in natural light if possible. Pay special attention to oral mucous membranes, nail beds, and conjunctiva, which can reflect central cyanosis. Assess hands, feet, and face. Assess body for differential or demarcated cyanosis or color differences. | Central cyanosis can reflect cardiac or pulmonary alterations. Differential cyanosis may indicate complex heart disease that is dependent on PDA blood flow for systemic or pulmonary blood flow. Pallor, mottling, or ruddiness can indicate cardiac disease.<br>Acrocyanosis (a painless disorder caused by constriction or narrowing of small blood vessels in the skin) is sometimes seen in the healthy newborn.<br>Clubbing of nail beds can indicate chronic hypoxia. Usually present after 6 mo of arterial desaturation (see Fig. 45.6). |
| *Activity level:* Assess child while sitting and lying down. | Lethargy, irritability, or restlessness can indicate poor cardiac function. |
| Observe level of activity and position of comfort. Observe for color changes with activity, feeding, or crying. Observe for exercise tolerance, including any respiratory distress or frequent rest. | Squatting can indicate cyanotic heart disease and attempts to improve hypoxia. |
| *Chest:* Assess precordial activity, chest movement (including symmetry), and chest shape (including convex or concave).<br>Assess for sternotomy or thoracotomy incisions. | PMI (apical pulse) is sometimes seen in thin children. It is found at fourth left ICS in young children and fifth ICS in children older than 7 yr. In neonates, PMI does not correspond with apical pulse. It is found at fourth ICS and can be more midline toward xiphoid because of right ventricular dominance in the fetal and neonatal heart.<br>An active precordium suggests cardiac disease.<br>A convex chest cavity shape suggests cardiac disease. |
| *Respiratory pattern:* Observe work of breathing at rest and with activity, including feeding.<br>Look for signs of respiratory alteration or distress. (Tachypnea, retractions, nasal flaring, crackles, grunting, and head bobbing are late signs of distress, indicating impending respiratory failure.) | Increased work of breathing and respiratory difficulty can indicate HF. |
| **Auscultation** | |
| *Heart sounds:* Auscultate with both bell (for low-pitched sounds) and diaphragm (for high-pitched sounds) of stethoscope. | Heart sounds should be synchronous with palpable central or peripheral pulse.<br>Rhythm normally is regular. A normal variation is sinus dysrhythmia when the rhythm can alter and rate can increase with inspiration and decrease with expiration. |
| Identify first and second heart sounds. | Ask the older child to briefly hold a breath to allow the nurse to hear more clearly.<br>$S_1$ is heard best at apex of heart (fourth or fifth ICS at left midclavicular line) and reflects closure of mitral and tricuspid valves. Correlates with palpable pulse.<br>$S_2$ is heard best at base (right and left of sternum at second ICS) and reflects closure of aortic and pulmonic valves. |
| Identify additional heart sounds ($S_3$, $S_4$). These can be assessed with the child lying supine or on the left side. | $S_3$ can be heard at the LLSB or apex and can be a normal finding or reflect CHF. $S_4$ can be heard at the LLSB or apex and reflects cardiac disease.<br>A gallop is an extra heart sound ($S_3$ or $S_4$), common in HF. |
| Identify presence of murmurs, clicks, precordial friction rubs. | Murmurs are caused by turbulent blood flow.<br>Murmurs are described according to location, timing within cardiac cycle, intensity, pitch, quality, and duration.<br>Clicks reflect abnormal valve motion.<br>Precordial friction rubs can reflect pericardial inflammation. |

**TABLE 46.2 Cardiac Assessment for the Child With CHD—cont'd**

| Assessment Guidelines | Findings and Comments |
|---|---|
| **Palpation** | |
| *Temperature:* | |
| Compare temperature of trunk with temperature of extremities. | Cooler extremities can indicate poor perfusion because of decreased cardiac output.<br>If room is cold, cool extremities can result from vasoconstriction to conserve heat. |
| *Pulses:* | |
| Compare central and distal pulses. | Peripheral pulses may be diminished if cardiac output is impaired. Causes include HF and dehydration. |
| Assess pulses in all four extremities. | Weak or absent pulses in the lower extremities may indicate coarctation of the aorta. |
| *Blood pressure:* | |
| Assess in all four extremities during initial assessment. | Discrepancies between upper and lower extremity blood pressure can indicate cardiac disease, including coarctation of the aorta. |
| *Capillary refill:* | |
| Assess capillary filling in extremities; use fingertips to compress skin. | Normal is less than 2-3 sec. |
| *Chest:* | |
| With fingertips, locate the PMI. | PMI located lower than normal can indicate cardiac enlargement. |
| Assess for presence of vibratory thrills, heaves or lifts, or friction rubs. | Thrills are vibratory in nature.<br>Heaves or lifts are palpable chest wall movement, separate from the PMI, and reflect hyperactive precordium.<br>Friction rubs, caused by the presence of fluid in the cardiac or pleural space, produce a grating sound. |
| *Abdomen:* | |
| Locate the liver border. It should be at or slightly below the right costal margin in infants and young children. In the neonate the liver can be 2-3 cm below the right costal margin and still be normal. | Normally, the border is firm and smooth.<br>With HF, liver may be boggy with a poorly defined edge and palpable more than 1-2 cm below the right costal margin. |
| **Percussion** | |
| Percussion of the chest provides little useful data in a cardiac assessment. | PMI is a better indicator of heart size. |

*A thorough cardiac workup will often include chest radiography, electrocardiogram (ECG), and echocardiogram.
*CHD,* Congenital heart disease; HF, heart failure; *ICS,* intercostal space; *LLSB,* left lower sternal border; *PMI,* point of maximal impulse.

**! NURSING QUALITY ALERT**

***Assessing Murmurs***

Develop a systematic approach to assessing heart sounds with every examination. Abnormal heart sounds will be easier to detect once you can recognize a normal heart sound. Consider other clinical findings, including fatigue associated with anemia and fever, which can intensify a murmur by altering cardiac output.

Organic murmurs reflect an abnormality in the heart structures. Innocent (functional) murmurs do not reflect heart abnormalities but are the sounds made as the blood flows through the structurally normal heart. They can be loud or soft and are often vibratory in quality. Innocent murmurs do not affect growth or well-being and are common in children.

Assessment progression includes inspection, auscultation, and palpation; each step requires more touching. The nurse must remember to warm the stethoscope used for auscultation, as well as the hands, before touching the child's skin. This warming is particularly important when assessing a resting infant, who could be startled by the cold touch of the hands and stethoscope.

## CARDIOVASCULAR DIAGNOSIS

Tests used to diagnose cardiac problems in children have been described previously. Cardiac catheterization is still considered the gold standard by which all other therapeutic modalities are measured, although this diagnostic is changing with the advent of cardiac MRI. Catheterization usually constitutes the final definitive diagnostic test for many patients.

### Cardiac Catheterization

Cardiac catheterization began as an invasive diagnostic procedure. It is now used as a diagnostic, interventional, and therapeutic procedure. During cardiac catheterization, catheters are advanced, generally through the femoral vein or artery, through the venous or arterial system and directly into the heart. Interventional catheterization is now being used to treat fetal cardiac lesions such as aortic stenosis (Bernstein, 2016f). Data obtained and interventions performed during the procedure include the following:

- Measurement of oxygen saturations in cardiac chambers and great arteries
- Measurement of pressures in cardiac chambers and great arteries and determination of gradients
- Evaluation of cardiac output
- Angiography to identify detailed images of structures and blood flow patterns
- Electrophysiologic studies to map the cardiac conduction system and identify the locus of dysrhythmia-producing cells; radiofrequency catheter ablation is used for destruction of these cells
- Corrective, palliative, or therapeutic interventional procedures that include angioplasty of the pulmonary artery and branches, pulmonary valvuloplasty, aortic valve balloon angioplasty, stent placement to maintain patency of vessels, balloon/blade septostomy for creation of an atrial septal defect (indicated for certain complex congenital heart defects), percutaneous pulmonary valve replacements, device closure of septal defects, and coil embolization of a patent ductus arteriosus or collateral vessels

### Complications

Complications can occur both during and after the procedure. Potential complications of which the nurse should be aware include dysrhythmias, hemorrhage, vascular damage, vasospasm of the catheterized vessel, thrombus or embolus formation, infection, reaction to the dye, and catheter perforation. Dysrhythmias can be hemodynamically compromising. Vasospasm of the vessel results in poor perfusion to the affected leg. Thrombus formation at the catheter insertion site can impair perfusion to the affected limb and shed emboli that can travel anywhere in the vascular system, depending on the cardiac anatomy, including the lung or brain. A thrombus in the venous system can be indicated by swelling or inflammation of the affected limb. A thrombus in the arterial system can be indicated by coolness or discoloration of the extremity and loss of pulses distal to the thrombus. Thrombus formation can occur in the systemic-to-pulmonary artery shunts that provide pulmonary blood flow. Reactions to the dye include rash, pruritus, vomiting or, very rarely, severe anaphylaxis. Perforation by the catheter of the heart or vessels during the procedure can result in cardiac tamponade and cardiac arrest. Additional minor reactions to the procedure include anesthesia- or sedation-related nausea and vomiting or pressure ulceration of pressure points related to prolonged immobility and decreased subcutaneous tissue.

### Nursing Care

Prior to cardiac catheterization, patients should have a 12- lead electrocardiogram, a chest x-ray, and coagulation studies (Park, 2014). Because impaired peripheral perfusion is a possible consequence of cardiac catheterization, it is important for the nurse to locate and mark distal pulses before the procedure. Marking the location of pulses will assist the nurse with rapid postprocedure assessment.

After the procedure, the child is positioned with the affected leg straight for 4 to 6 hours; infants can be held prone on a parent's lap. Older children remain in bed with the head of the bed raised at only a 20-degree incline. IV fluid administration continues until the infant or child is taking and retaining adequate amounts of oral fluids. Vital signs should be obtained frequently (every 5 to 15 minutes) for the first hour, with continuous initial monitoring of heart rate, blood pressure, respiratory rate, oxygen saturation, and temperature.

The insertion site dressing should be observed frequently, at least every 5 to 15 minutes, during the early postprocedure hours. Assess for bleeding not only on the dressing but also on sheets. Look under the child to check for pooled blood. Pull back bed linens and remove the infant's diaper (if applicable) to check the perineal area for bleeding under the skin. If bleeding occurs, place a gloved heel of the hand firmly on the insertion site. Apply pressure for at least 10 to 15 minutes and assess distal perfusion of the extremity. Immediately notify the interventional cardiologist. Assess blood loss and the child's hemodynamic status.

Peripheral perfusion is also monitored. The affected extremity frequently will be mottled in appearance and cooler to touch than the other extremities. Distal pulses should be palpable, although they may be weaker than in the contralateral extremity. Nonpalpable distal pulses should be checked using Doppler technology. Notify the cardiologist if distal pulses are absent on the affected extremity, the temperature or degree of mottling has changed, or the child complains of increasing pain. Heparin drip infusions are initiated under certain circumstances, often related to pulse loss or catheter route, or with placement of stents, coils, or closure devices.

Children who have undergone a diagnostic cardiac catheterization are often discharged the same day. Children undergoing some types of interventional procedures or electrophysiologic studies might remain hospitalized overnight. The following day, the pressure bandage is removed and is replaced with an adhesive bandage (Band-Aid). Discharge instructions vary according to the institution but may include the following:

- Inspecting the catheter insertion site to assess healing or the presence of local infection
- Bathing limited to a shower, sponge bath, or brief tub bath (no soaking) for the first 1 to 3 days after the procedure
- Avoiding strenuous exercise (climbing trees, swimming, contact sports) for up to 1 week after the procedure or 6 weeks after a device is placed
- Returning to school on the third day after the procedure
- Notifying the cardiologist if the child has a fever above 38.3° C (101° F); bleeding or drainage (pus) from the catheter insertion site; or pallor, coolness, or numbness of the affected extremity
- Resuming normal feeding patterns and medication therapy, if applicable
- Reviewing the need to continue antibiotic prophylaxis for dental or other specific medical procedures
- Following up with a cardiologist at a scheduled visit

### Congenital Cardiac Defects

Table 46.3 presents the most frequently seen cardiac lesions in infants and children.

## THE CHILD UNDERGOING CARDIAC SURGERY

Most cardiac lesions are amenable to palliative or corrective repair, and the child with significant CHD will undergo a surgical or interventional catheterization procedure at some point during infancy or childhood. The timing of surgery is dictated by the child's clinical condition, but the trend in recent years is to intervene at an early age. The ultimate goal of intervention is for physiologic and anatomic correction to normal or near-normal circulation. Complex lesions can require multiple, palliated stages with the goal of separating the saturated and desaturated blood, correcting cyanosis, and optimizing pulmonary and cardiac function.

Families anticipate surgery as a means of achieving a more normal lifestyle, but they also feel anxiety about the child's postoperative course and ultimate outcome. The nurse can help both the child and the parents cope with this stressful and traumatic event through support and education.

### Preoperative Preparation

Preoperative teaching and preparation expose the child and family to the hospital environment and expected perioperative and postoperative care. The family should receive verbal, written, and visual information that describes the course of events throughout the hospitalization. Interpreter services should be used when indicated. It is important to evaluate the family's understanding of the surgical procedure and its expected outcomes. A multidisciplinary team, including physicians, nurses, a child life specialist, and social services, provides a comprehensive approach in the assessment of and interventions for the child and family. Barriers to hospitalization (e.g., financial, social, transportation) and discharge can be identified and interventions begun before the actual hospitalization. In addition, identifying positive coping mechanisms and providing anticipatory guidance can help the child and parent be empowered in their understanding and participation in care while the child is hospitalized. In family-centered care, the healthcare team works with the family in caring for the child.

*Text continued on p. 1102*

**TABLE 46.3 Congenital Cardiac Defects**

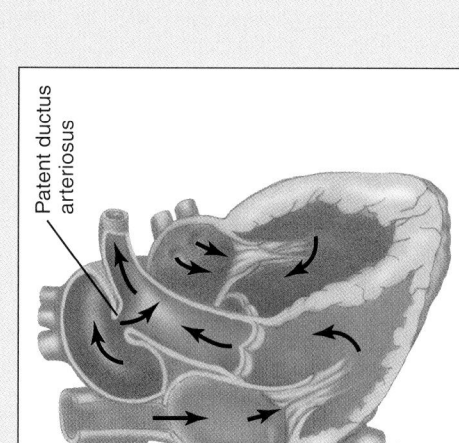

| Incidence and Pathophysiology | Altered Hemodynamics | Manifestations | Therapeutic Management |
|---|---|---|---|
| **Left-to-Right Shunting Lesions** | | | |
| ***Patent Ductus Arteriosus (PDA)*** | | | |
| 5%-10% of all congenital heart lesions*<br>Often present with other lesions<br>Caused by failure of the fetal ductus arteriosus to close completely after birth—normal closure within 24-72 hr after birth due to decreased prostaglandin (PG) levels and decrease in blood pressure (BP) in ductus lumen; eventual degeneration to the ductus ligamentum | Because of a drop in pulmonary vascular resistance and failure of the ductus arteriosus to close, increased systemic pressure moves saturated blood from the aorta into the pulmonary arteries (left-to-right shunt), the lungs, and the left side of the heart, causing both increased left-sided cardiac workload and increased pulmonary blood flow. | Signs of heart failure related to the size of the lesion and amount of left-to-right shunting;<br>Continuous murmur (machinery-like sound)<br>Widened pulse pressure (increased difference between systolic and diastolic readings)<br>Bounding pulses<br>Cardiac enlargement | *Medical Management*<br>Interventions to address HF<br>Administration of indomethacin (Indocin), a PG inhibitor, that constricts the ductus; used in premature infants but is not effective in term infants<br>Monitor respiratory status, renal function, and growth<br>*Interventional Cardiac Catheterization*<br>Standard of care is nonsurgical occlusion<br>A coil is placed to occlude the ductus. Tissue grows around the coil (endothelializes) forming permanent occlusion.<br>*Surgical Management*<br>Ligation of the ductus via left thoracotomy, usually within the first year of life |
| ***Atrial Septal Defect (ASD)*** | | | |
| 5%-10% of cardiac lesions; seen more often in girls<br>Abnormal opening between the atria; three types predominate: (1) ostium secundum (located in the middle of the septum) is most common; (2) ostium primum (located low in the septum), associated with endocardial tissue formation defect and cleft mitral valve; (3) sinus venosus (located high in the septum near superior vena cava) | 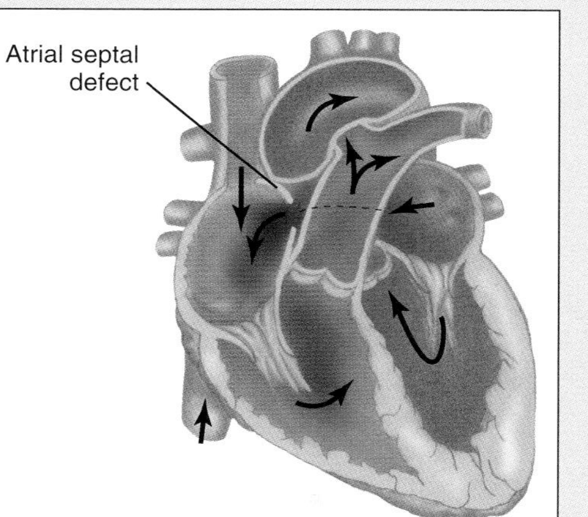<br>Decreased right ventricular compliance (ease of ventricular filling during diastole) compared to left ventricular compliance leads to left-to-right shunting across the abnormal septal opening; right atrium is enlarged and pulmonary blood flow increased | May be asymptomatic depending on size of lesion and the age of the child (symptoms usually do not to occur until age 3 to 4)<br>Fatigue, dyspnea on exertion, palpitations, atrial dysrhythmias<br>Recurrent respiratory infections related to increased pulmonary blood flow<br>Systolic murmur from increased blood flow across the pulmonary valve; diastolic murmur with large shunting<br>Mitral valve regurgitation is possible<br>HF may develop during young adulthood, if not repaired<br>Risk for stroke | *Medical Management*<br>Conservative, because spontaneous closure can occur (up to 80% close by 4 years)<br>Diuretics and digoxin for signs of HF<br>Antidysrhythmics for atrial dysrhythmias<br>*Interventional Cardiac Catheterization*<br>Occluder devices placed if criteria are met regarding size of lesion, significance of shunting, and availability of septal tissue to anchor the device; usually done between 2 and 5 yr of age<br>Daily low-dose aspirin for 6 months following procedure*<br>*Surgical Management*<br>Surgical placement of sutures or prosthetic patch through open heart procedure using cardiopulmonary bypass<br>Done only when occluder devise closure is not appropriate<br>Surgical complications include dysrhythmias and postpericardiotomy syndrome (inflammation with pericardial effusion) |

*Continued*

**TABLE 46.3 Congenital Cardiac Defects—cont'd**

| Incidence and Pathophysiology | Altered Hemodynamics | Manifestations | Therapeutic Management |
|---|---|---|---|
| ***Ventricular Septal Defect (VSD)*** | | | |
| 15%-20% of cardiac defects<br>Abnormal opening between the ventricles. Three types according to location: (1) conoventricular, (2) atrioventricular (AV) canal, and (3) muscular; Depending on size, complete absence of the septum results in a common ventricle.<br>Most common type of cardiac defect<br>Sometimes accompanied by other defects | 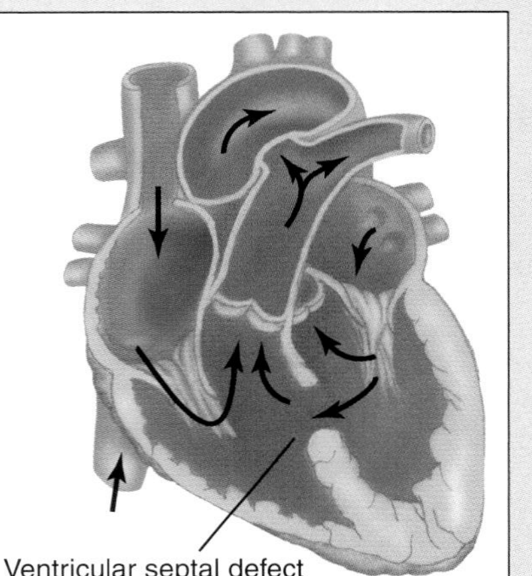<br>Ventricular septal defect<br>Decrease in pulmonary vascular resistance compared to systemic vascular resistance in the weeks after birth results in left-to-right shunting through the VSD. Increased pulmonary blood flow, pulmonary hypertension, and progressive pulmonary vascular disease can occur over time. | Signs and symptoms are related to the size of the defect; some children remain asymptomatic.<br>Loud, harsh systolic murmur<br>Varies in intensity and duration depending on degree of shunting and size of defect<br>Palpable thrill, diastolic murmur, and gallop rhythm sometimes present<br>HF can occur with moderate to large defects | *Medical Management*<br>Conservative—35% to 60% close spontaneously*<br>Diuretics, digoxin and medications for afterload reduction (e.g., angiotensin-converting enzyme [ACE] inhibitors)<br>Management of associated HF<br>*Interventional Cardiac Catheterization*<br>Occluder device can be inserted as a hybrid procedure, using a surgical approach to visualize and directly access the ventricle and catheterization to place the device.<br>*Surgical Management*<br>Suture or patch closure using open heart surgery with cardiopulmonary bypass<br>Consideration of pulmonary artery banding to reduce pulmonary blood flow for children with multiple defects and severe HF<br>Banding is no longer performed unless unable to repair the defect completely<br>Complications: residual VSDs, pulmonary hypertension, heart block that requires temporary or permanent pacemaker, abnormal rhythm (junctional ectopic tachycardia) that decreases cardiac output, postpericardiotomy syndrome |
| ***Atrioventricular Septal Defect (Endocardial Cushion Defect)*** | | | |
| 2% of cardiac defects<br>Often associated with genetic syndromes (e.g., Down syndrome)<br>Abnormal endocardial tissue development affecting the atrial and ventricular septum and mitral and tricuspid valves (AV valves).<br>Three types: (1) partial—ostium primum ASD and two separate AV valves but a mitral valve cleft; (2) intermediate or transitional—ASD, beginning connection between the two AV valves, no VSD; (3) complete—a single connected AV valve, ASD and VSD | 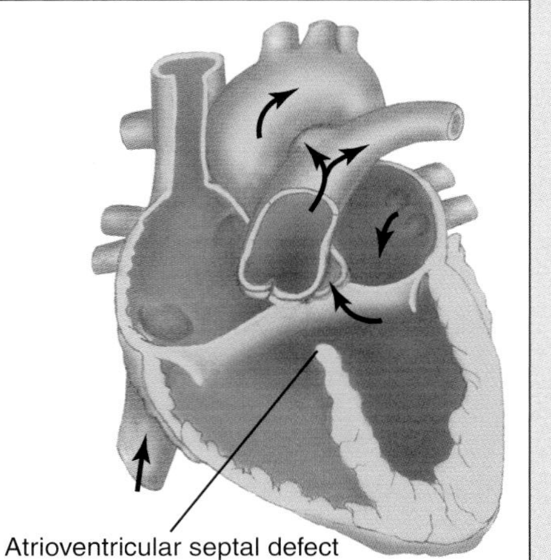<br>Atrioventricular septal defect<br>Partial defect—left-to-right shunting of blood with increased pulmonary blood flow related to differences in aortic and pulmonary pressure<br>Complete—markedly increased pulmonary blood flow with associated pulmonary hypertension and risk for pulmonary vascular disease; mixture of saturated and desaturated blood as pressures change and right-to-left shunting occurs | Varying degrees of HF related to the size and number of defects and pressure differences<br>Systolic pulmonary flow murmur that develops over a few weeks after birth<br>Intermittent cyanosis | *Medical Management*<br>Symptomatic treatment of HF with diuretics, digoxin, and ACE inhibitors<br>*Surgical Management*<br>*Partial*—if asymptomatic, ASD and mitral valve cleft are repaired in late infancy or early childhood<br>*Complete*—ASD and VSD are closed, construction of two separate AV valves from the common valve, possible mitral valve replacement; performed at 3-4 mo of age or later (but before pulmonary hypertension occurs) if child is asymptomatic<br>Children with small atria or ventricles may require palliative surgery (designed to relieve symptoms by directing venous blood return directly to the pulmonary artery)<br>Postoperative mortality is approximately 10% for complete repair; complications similar to VSD repair |

| Obstructive or Stenotic Lesions | | | |
|---|---|---|---|
| ***Pulmonary Stenosis***<br>8 - 10% of cardiac defects<br>Narrowing at entrance to the pulmonary artery at the valve, below the valve or above the valve<br>Valve can be normal (tricuspid), bicuspid, or dysplastic. | 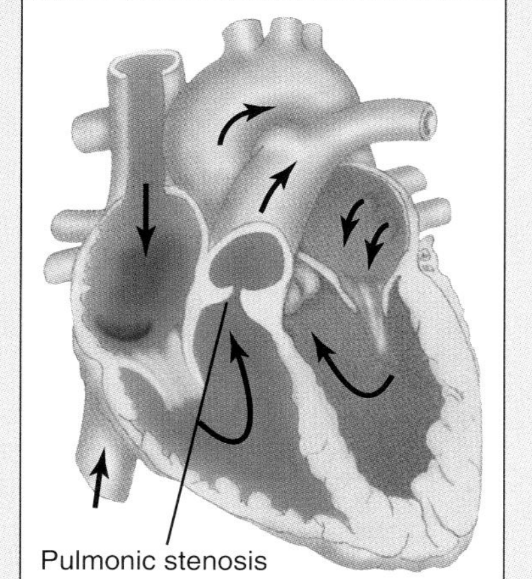<br><br>Obstruction causes resistance to blood flow at the right ventricular outflow track; increased pressure in the right ventricle leads to right ventricular hypertrophy.<br>Critically severe pulmonary artery obstruction elevates right ventricular pressure severely, causing blood to regurgitate into the right atrium; rising right atrial pressure forces the foramen ovale open, allowing blood to flow from the right to the left side of the heart. | Many asymptomatic; signs in symptomatic children include exercise intolerance, signs of right-sided HF<br>Systolic ejection murmur, possible palpable thrill<br>Cardiomegaly on radiograph<br>Cyanosis in severe cases | *Medical Management*<br>Cardiac observation and antibiotic prophylaxis for children who are asymptomatic<br>Additional intervention related to increasing pulmonary pressure gradient across the pulmonary valve<br>Interventional catheterization or surgical management for severe stenosis<br>Prostaglandin $E_1$ ($PGE_1$) infusion keeps the ductus arteriosus open so blood can return to lungs for oxygenation.<br>*Interventional Cardiac Catheterization*<br>Balloon valvuloplasty with dilation of the valve to decrease the pressure; pulmonary regurgitation is a possible complication; may have to be redone later<br>*Surgical Management*<br>Surgical **valvulotomy** for unsuccessful valvuloplasty or if stenosis is supravalvular<br>Placement of a shunt from aorta to pulmonary artery (systemic to pulmonary artery shunt) for critical pulmonary stenosis with small right ventricle or for children who must remain on $PGE_1$ after interventional cardiac catheterization |
| ***Aortic Stenosis***<br>10% of cardiac defects<br>Narrowing of the entrance to the aorta; may be supravalvular, subvalvular, or at the valve level (most common); thickened, rigid, with some fusion of the leaflets; the valve may be bicuspid | 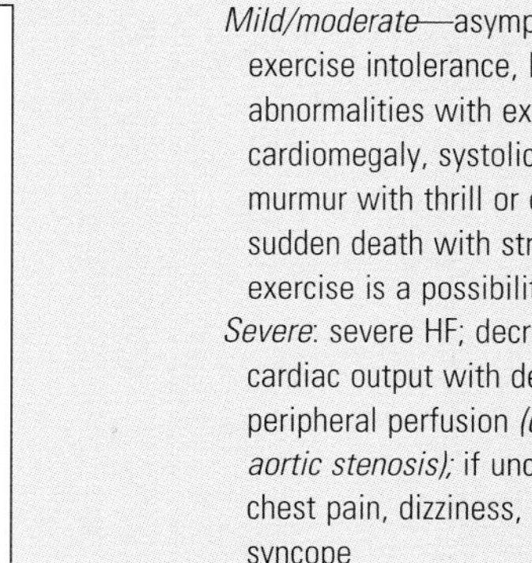<br><br>Blood has difficulty flowing through the aortic valve, causing increased pressure and hypertrophy in the left ventricle, decreased cardiac output, decreased blood supply to the coronary arteries | *Mild/moderate*—asymptomatic; exercise intolerance, ECG abnormalities with exercise, cardiomegaly, systolic ejection murmur with thrill or click; sudden death with strenuous exercise is a possibility<br>*Severe*: severe HF; decreased cardiac output with decreased peripheral perfusion *(critical aortic stenosis)*; if uncorrected, chest pain, dizziness, and syncope | *Medical Management*<br>Mild/moderate: regular follow-up, especially for athletes; restriction from competitive athletics depending on degree of stenosis and severity of signs and symptoms<br>*Interventional Cardiac Catheterization*<br>Aortic balloon valvuloplasty decreases stenosis and improves cardiac output; may be performed to delay surgical intervention; aortic insufficiency, thrombosis, infection or artery damage can occur<br>*Surgical Management*<br>Surgical valvulotomy<br>Aortic valve replacement for recurrent stenosis: (1) Mechanical valve replacement requires warfarin treatment; valve does not grow with the child; (2) use of child's pulmonary valve to replace the aortic valve; pulmonary valve homograft to replace the pulmonary valve; new aortic valve grows with the child; homograft will need later replacement |

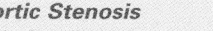

*Continued*

**TABLE 46.3 Congenital Cardiac Defects—cont'd**

| Incidence and Pathophysiology | Altered Hemodynamics | Manifestations | Therapeutic Management |
|---|---|---|---|
| ***Coarctation of the Aorta*** | | | |
| 8%-10% of cardiac defects<br>Aorta is constricted near the ductus arteriosus insertion site; associated with bicuspid aortic valve that can later become stenotic | 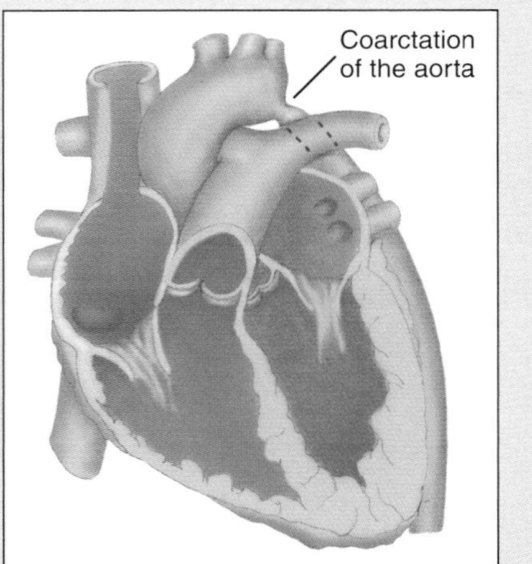<br>Narrowing of the aortic structure obstructs the left ventricular output, increasing afterload to left ventricle; blood supply is decreased in the abdominal organs and the lower periphery; left ventricular pressure increases; aortic pressure is high proximal to the constriction and low distal; pulmonary edema can occur<br>If coarctation is mild, collateral blood supply can develop to channel blood past the constriction | Left-sided HF with low cardiac output, poor lower extremity peripheral perfusion, metabolic acidosis, shock<br>If PDA present: right-to-left shunting with differential cyanosis (color and oxygenation differential between upper and lower extremities)<br>Asymptomatic children may show pulse and blood pressure differences between upper (systolic hypertension) and lower extremities; weakness, tingling, cramps in lower extremities<br>Systolic murmur accompanied by ejection click (with bicuspid aortic valve) or thrill | *Medical Management*<br>Diuretics and digoxin to improve cardiac output; $PGE_1$ infusion to open the ductus arteriosus and improve perfusion to the lower body<br>*Interventional Cardiac Catheterization*<br>Balloon dilation with placement of stent for recurrences; increased incidence of recurrence with balloon angioplasty used for the initial procedure*<br>*Surgical Management*<br>Performed shortly after diagnosis in most cases<br>Several surgical procedures available—end-to-end anastomosis, use of prosthetic patch, left subclavian artery patch (results in postoperative absence of left palpable pulse) |
| **Cyanotic Lesions With Decreased Pulmonary Blood Flow** | | | |
| ***Tetralogy of Fallot*** | | | |
| 5%-10% of congenital cardiac defects; most frequently seen cyanotic lesion<br>Constellation of lesions results from malalignment of the ventricular septum during fetal development: (1) ventricular septal defect, (2) right ventricular outflow tract obstruction (e.g., pulmonary stenosis), (3) overriding of the aorta (arises partially out of the right ventricle), (4) right ventricular hypertrophy | <br>Equal right- and left-sided ventricular pressures related to the pulmonary artery obstruction and size of the VSD; desaturated blood enters the systemic system by shunting right to left across the VSD, or into the overriding aorta | Onset and severity of signs and symptoms are related to the extent of the obstructed pulmonary blood flow, which causes the right-to-left shunting; if lesions are mild, shunting is decreased and saturations are mildly low (pink tet)<br>Signs become worse in the neonate as the ductus arteriosus closes<br>Cyanosis, extreme fatigue, hypercyanotic episodes, chronic hypoxemia<br>Harsh systolic murmur with a palpable thrill; boot-shaped heart on radiography (related to poor development of the pulmonary artery) | *Medical Management*<br>$PGE_1$ infusion to maintain patency of the ductus arteriosus and blood flow to the lungs; management of hypercyanotic episodes; treatment of iron deficiency anemia<br>*Surgical Management*<br>Primary repair of defects during infancy is the procedure of choice; surgery performed after 3- 4 mo of age and is timed according to the degree of cyanosis and other symptoms.<br>Surgery requires cardiopulmonary bypass.<br>For infants who are poor candidates for early primary repair, palliative shunt procedures increase pulmonary blood flow; modified Blalock–Taussig procedure (creation of a systemic-to-pulmonary-artery shunt using a Gore-Tex tube) is used.<br>Surgical complications: rhythm disturbances, residual VSD, low cardiac output, residual right ventricular outflow obstruction, pulmonary valve regurgitation, residual right-sided HF; mortality is low |

| | | | |
|---|---|---|---|
| ***Tricuspid Atresia***<br>1%-3% of cardiac defects<br>Nondevelopment of the tricuspid valve, patent foramen ovale or ASD, underdeveloped (hypoplastic) right ventricle, VSD of varying size, pulmonary artery located in normal position or transposed with the aorta, pulmonary stenosis of varying degrees | 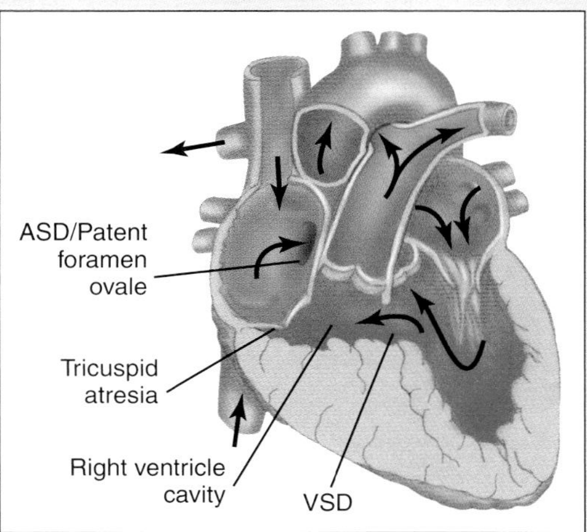<br>Desaturated blood enters the right atrium, shunts right to left through a patent foramen ovale into the left atrium; desaturated blood mixes with saturated blood in the left atrium, proceeds into the left ventricle and into the aorta; some blood shunts through the VSD to the right ventricle and into the pulmonary artery to the lungs; if the ductus arteriosus is open, some blood will flow from the aorta to the pulmonary artery; lesser pulmonary stenosis can contribute to pulmonary congestion | Profound cyanosis with decreased pulmonary blood flow<br>Single second heart sound because tricuspid valve does not close<br>Systolic murmur from the VSD; PDA murmur if ductus remains open | *Medical Management*<br>$PGE_1$ infusion to maintain patency of the ductus arteriosus<br>*Interventional Cardiac Catheterization*<br>Balloon atrial septostomy (creating an opening in the septum) if the foramen ovale begins to close; catheter is threaded through femoral vein, advanced into the right atrium, through the foramen ovale into the left atrium; balloon is inflated and pulled back into the right atrium through the foramen ovale, tearing the septum<br>Catheter blade septostomy to cut the septum tissue, if balloon septostomy is not effective<br>*Surgical Management*<br>Goal: to separate desaturated and saturated blood and to optimize ventricular function by decreasing the workload on the heart<br>Three-stage surgery: (1) Palliative systemic-to-pulmonary artery shunt (see Tetralogy of Fallot) (2) Creation of a connection between the superior vena cava and pulmonary arteries (bidirectional Glenn procedure); results in desaturated blood flow directly from the superior vena cava to the pulmonary artery and decreased volume in the left ventricle; performed at 4-6 mo of age; pulmonary hypertension may result (keep the child positioned with the head elevated postoperatively)<br>(3) Modified Fontan procedure during early childhood: connection created from the inferior vena cava to the pulmonary arteries<br>Surgical procedures result in a single ventricle and all desaturated blood going from the vena cavae directly into the pulmonary arteries.<br>Occasionally, a small connection (fenestration) between the venous and arterial circulation is kept to assist with adjustment to new flows and pressures; the fenestration is closed later. |

*Continued*

## TABLE 46.3 Congenital Cardiac Defects—cont'd

| Incidence and Pathophysiology | Altered Hemodynamics | Manifestations | Therapeutic Management |
|---|---|---|---|
| ***Pulmonary Atresia With Intact Ventricular Septum*** | | | |
| <1% of cardiac defects<br>Failure of the pulmonary valve to develop; hypoplastic development of the pulmonary artery and right ventricle; extremely high right ventricular pressures; possible associated underdeveloped tricuspid | 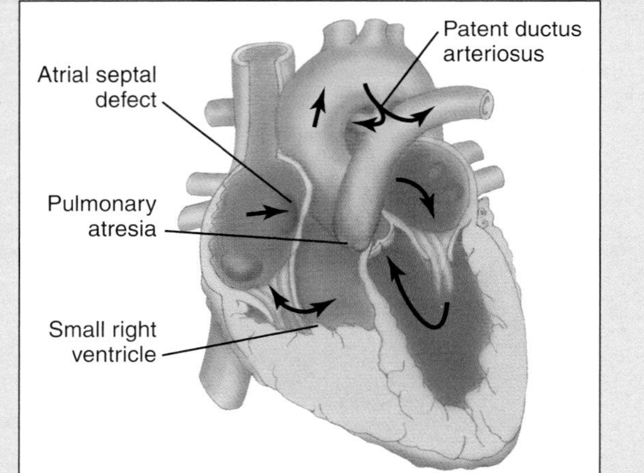<br>Desaturated blood flows through the tricuspid valve to the right ventricle but cannot enter the pulmonary artery because there is no pulmonary valve; blood backs up through the tricuspid valve back into the right atrium, shunts right to left through the foramen ovale to left atrium; mixed desaturated and saturated blood flow into the left ventricle and out the aorta; blood is oxygenated through a left-to-right shunt from the aorta through a patent ductus arteriosus to the pulmonary artery and lungs | Profound cyanosis; survival depends on a PDA<br>Single second heart sound<br>PDA murmur | *Medical Management*<br>Continuous $PGE_1$ infusion<br>*Interventional Cardiac Catheterization*<br>Laser wire and radiofrequency valvulotomy with balloon dilation of the valve in some children*<br>*Surgical Management*<br>Early management: pulmonary valvulotomy or systemic-to-pulmonary artery shunt (Blalock–Taussig procedure) in children with adequate right ventricle size[†]; as blood flow from the right ventricle to the pulmonary artery increases, the atrial right-to-left shunting decreases; later, the ASD and systemic-to-pulmonary shunt may be closed.<br>Bidirectional Glenn procedure or modified Fontan procedure if right ventricle remains small and cannot pump adequate blood to the pulmonary artery |

***Total Anomalous Pulmonary Venous Return***

<1% of cardiac defects

Defect of fetal development during first 8 wk of pregnancy; pulmonary veins do not connect with the left atrium but connect somewhere else, such as to the superior vena cava (most frequently seen)

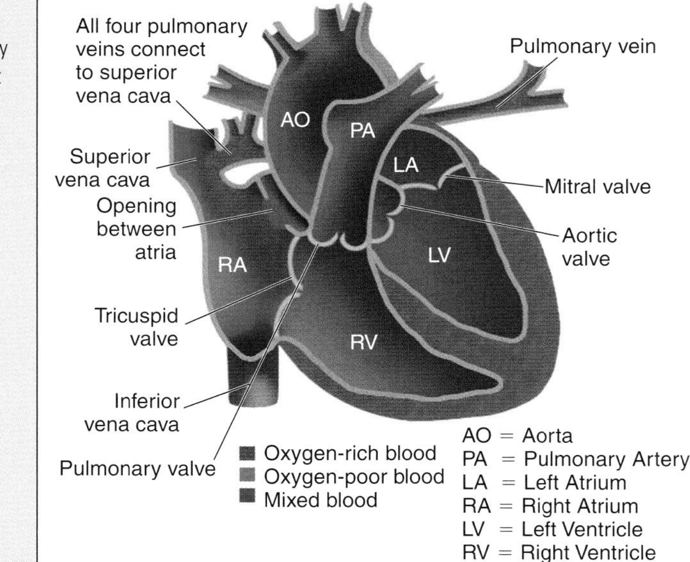


Oxygen-rich blood that would normally return to the left side of the heart mixes with desaturated blood in the right side of the heart; associated heart defects (ASD, VSD, PDA) allow for communication between the right and left sides of the heart, delivering mixed blood to the systemic circulation.

Cyanosis, severe respiratory distress, tachycardia, worsening pulmonary hypertension, progressive clinical deterioration with possible early death (first week to month after birth)

Murmur (systolic over the pulmonary area or tricuspid insufficiency murmur) may or may not be present

Decreasing peripheral pulses, increasing HF, enlargement of the liver, failure to thrive, frequent pulmonary infection in infants without pulmonary vein obstruction*

*Medical Management*

No treatment needed if asymptomatic

HF and pulmonary edema treated with digoxin, diuretics, oxygen, mechanical ventilation

Treatment of metabolic acidosis

Enlargement of the septal defect through balloon or blade septostomy can facilitate right-to-left shunting; $PGE_1$ infusion to maintain patency of the ductus arteriosus

*Surgical Management*

Surgery between birth and 6 mo of age, depending on extent of obstruction

Goal of surgery is to reroute blood from the abnormally placed pulmonary veins to the left atrium

Surgical procedure varies according to the site of the abnormal circulation; all involve cardiopulmonary bypass, hypothermia, and total circulatory arrest; the associated ASD is closed as well.

*Continued*

**TABLE 46.3 Congenital Cardiac Defects—cont'd**

| Incidence and Pathophysiology | Altered Hemodynamics | Manifestations | Therapeutic Management |
|---|---|---|---|
| **Cyanotic Lesions With Increased Pulmonary Blood Flow** | | | |
| ***Truncus Arteriosus*** | | | |
| 1% of cardiac defects<br>Failure of the common great vessel, the truncus arteriosus, to divide into the pulmonary artery and pulmonary valve and the aorta and aortic valve during fetal development; results in a single vessel and valve, which give rise to the pulmonary, systemic, and coronary circulations<br>Associated failure of septal development with VSD; the common vessel overrides the VSD and receives blood from both right and left ventricles | Desaturated blood enters the right atrium, and through the tricuspid valve to the right ventricle; saturated blood from the left atrium flows through the mitral valve into the left ventricle; saturated and desaturated blood mix in the ventricles at the level of the VSD and common ventricular outflow tract; mixed blood flows into the common vessel and is circulated to the systemic, pulmonary and coronary circulations<br>Ventricles are under pressure and volume overload; oxygen saturation depends on the volume of pulmonary blood flow and determines the signs of HF, decreased cardiac output, and coronary artery ischemia | Signs of HF and cyanosis in neonate—determined by the volume of pulmonary blood flow (the higher the flow, the greater the symptoms of HF); pulmonary vascular disease can develop in early infancy; pulmonary stenosis limits the blood flow and increases cyanosis<br>Harsh systolic murmur with thrill; diastolic murmur of truncal valve insufficiency may be heard; opening of the single truncal valve produces a click<br>Truncal valve insufficiency produces a bounding pulse and widened pulse pressure | *Medical Management*<br>ACE Inhibitors and diuretics for HF<br>Preventing polycythemia is important<br>Preventing frequent infections and assessing calcium and magnesium levels: this defect can be associated with DiGeorge syndrome, which causes immune system depression and hypocalcemia*<br>*Surgical Management*<br>Varies with truncus classification. In the more commonly seen type, the VSD is closed and blood flow from the left ventricle is directed into the truncal vessel; a connection (conduit) is made between the right ventricle and the pulmonary artery, creating a pulmonary circulation. The conduit may need revision as the child grows<br>Surgical mortality risk depends on the type of truncus and the extent of the required repair; mortality is higher with truncal valve stenosis or insufficiency. |

| | | | |
|---|---|---|---|
| ***Hypoplastic Left Heart Syndrome*** | | | |
| <1% of cardiac defects<br>Inadequate development of the left side of the heart results in one effective ventricle; associated with aortic valve atresia, hypoplasia of the left ventricle, hypoplasia of the ascending aorta and mitral valve stenosis or atresia*<br>Seen more often in males than females; associated with brain abnormalities; if untreated, most infants die within the first few months of life | <br>Saturated blood returns to the left atrium but is unable to flow to the remainder of the left side of the heart; blood is shunted from left-to-right through a patent foramen ovale or ASD to the right atrium, where it mixes with desaturated blood; mixed blood enters the pulmonary circulation—some goes to the lungs, some to the ductus arteriosus, which remains open, and to the systemic circulation | HF from increased pulmonary blood flow; tachypnea<br>Systemic hypoperfusion and shock as ductus arteriosus begins to close<br>Infant is grayish blue, has dyspnea and hypotension | *Medical Management*<br>Emergency management to correct acid-base and electrolyte imbalances; $PGE_1$ infusion to maintain ductus arteriosus patency until surgery<br>*Surgical Management*<br>Three options available: (1) no intervention with supportive care; (2) cardiac transplantation; (3) three-stage palliative repair that will result in a single right ventricle, with different portions of the pulmonary artery acting to facilitate both systemic and pulmonary circulation |
| ***Transposition of the Great Arteries*** | | | |
| 5%-7% of cardiac defects<br>Abnormal separation and rotation of the fetal common truncal vessel causes the aorta to arise from the right ventricle and the pulmonary artery to arise from the left ventricle<br>Associated VSD | <br>Desaturated blood returns to the right atrium, flows into the right ventricle and out the aorta to the systemic circulation; saturated blood returns to the left ventricle, out the pulmonary artery to the lungs<br>Survival depends on blood mixing through a patent foramen ovale/ASD and patent ductus arteriosus<br>Some infants have a VSD | Cyanosis at birth<br>Hypoxemia, despite oxygen administration<br>Progressive desaturation and acidosis; developing HF | *Medical Management*<br>Emergency $PGE_1$ infusion to maintain patency of the ductus arteriosus; oxygen administration<br>*Interventional Cardiac Catheterization*<br>Balloon atrial septostomy to enhance mixing of blood in some infants<br>*Surgical Management*<br>Arterial switch procedure, which places the aorta and pulmonary artery in their anatomically correct position and reimplants the coronary arteries in the new aorta<br>Long-term survival rates are positivePostoperative complications include low cardiac output, dysrhythmias related to decreased coronary artery perfusion and myocardial ischemia. |

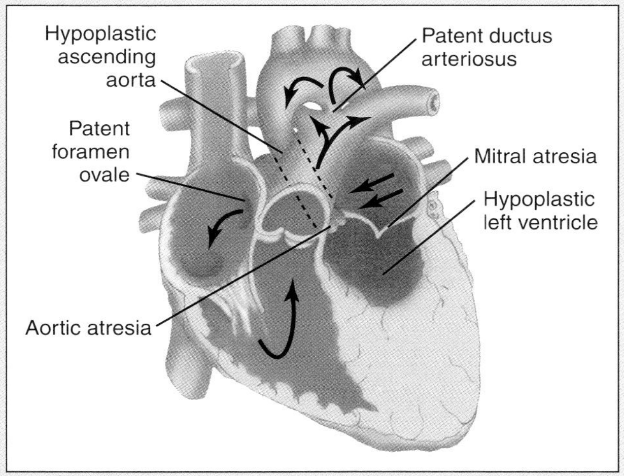

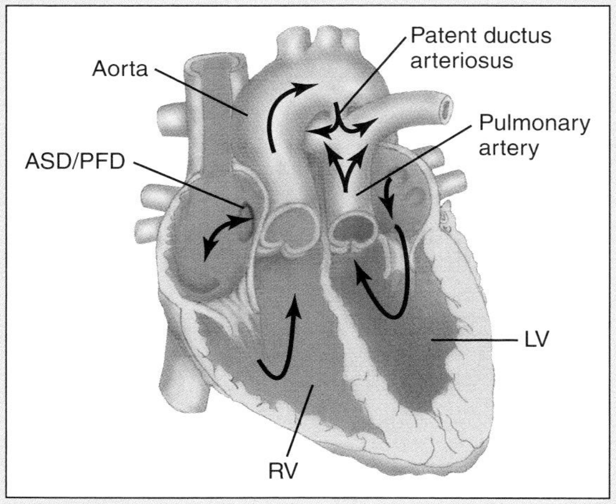

*Park, M. K. (2014). *Pediatric cardiology for practitioners* (6th ed.). Philadelphia: Elsevier.

†Bernstein, D. (2016). The cardiovascular system. In R. Kliegman, B. Stanton, J. St. Geme, et al. (Eds.), *Nelson textbook of pediatrics* (20th ed., pp. 2153–2303). Philadelphia: Elsevier.

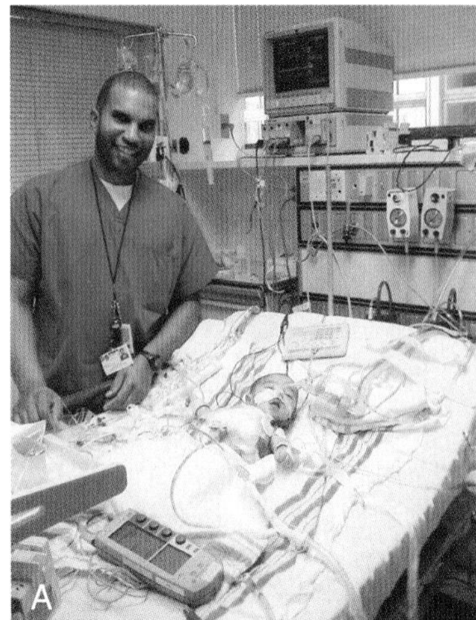


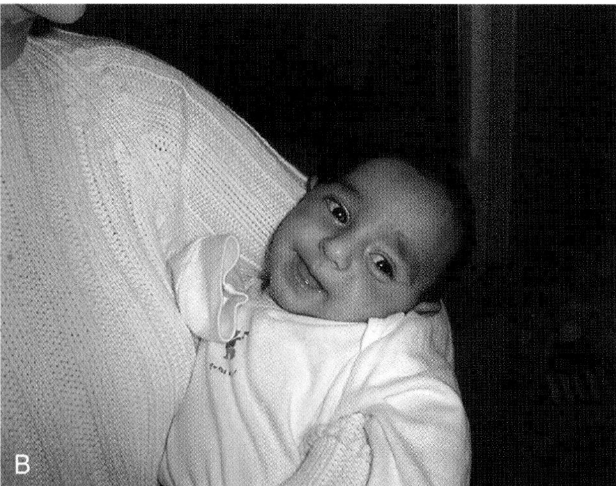


**FIG 46.1 A,** A preoperative visit to the intensive care unit and other units should be directed at an age-appropriate level for the child and the family before the child undergoes cardiac surgery. The experience prepares the family for the sights and sounds of the unit. **B,** Going home. (Courtesy Children's Hospital Oakland, Oakland, CA.)

The parents and child should tour the intensive care unit (Fig. 46.1) and other units where the child will reside during the hospitalization. This preparation allows them to become familiar with the physical environment and the noise and activity level. The visit should allow time for the family to meet members of the nursing staff and see equipment that will be used in the child's postoperative care. In addition, seeing other families and children who have undergone similar procedures as they progress and recover from the surgical process can be an encouraging experience.

Monitors, ventilators, and tubes should be described and shown to the family. Parents and children are reminded that invasive monitoring lines, chest tubes, and an endotracheal tube are inserted during surgery while the child is anesthetized, and they should be reassured that these tubes and lines will be removed as soon as the child's condition permits.

The sequence of events surrounding the day of surgery—when and where to arrive and where to wait during the procedure—should be reviewed. Parents should be assured that they will receive updates about their child's condition throughout the procedure and will be permitted to visit soon after the surgery is completed.

## Postoperative Management

Postoperative nursing management includes promoting hemodynamic and respiratory stability, preventing and identifying potential complications, providing comfort, ensuring pain assessment and interventions, and providing continuing educational and emotional support. Early postoperative care in the intensive care unit involves continuous monitoring of vital signs and cardiac output and frequent multisystem assessments. These assessments continue, with decreasing intensity, until discharge.

Cardiac surgical repair is either a closed heart or an open heart procedure. The underlying cardiac defect and anticipated surgical intervention are the determining factors in the type of procedure performed.

In a closed heart surgery, the heart continues to pump and maintain cardiac function during the repair. Some examples of closed heart procedures include repair of a PDA, coarctation of the aorta, and certain aorta-to-pulmonary artery shunts.

Potential complications include recurrent laryngeal nerve injury with associated vocal cord paralysis, pneumothorax, chylothorax, atelectasis, phrenic nerve injury and associated diaphragm paralysis, bleeding, infection, and, rarely, death.

Open heart surgery takes place with the child on a cardiopulmonary bypass machine. The machine takes over the roles of the lungs and heart—oxygenation and the delivery of blood to the body. Special cannulas are placed in the venous side of the heart, and venous blood is diverted into the bypass circuit. In the circuit, the blood is oxygenated and filtered and returned to the aorta, where it is pumped to the brain and systemic circulation. The principles of hemodilution, hypothermia, and anticoagulation are critical to use of cardiopulmonary bypass. In addition, myocardial preservation is critical. The heart is generally not pumping during cardiopulmonary bypass, and all systems are supported. Potential complications from cardiopulmonary bypass include bleeding, stroke, myocardial infarction, dysrhythmias, fluid and electrolyte imbalance, postpericardiotomy syndrome (an inflammatory process with the development of pericardial effusion), and death. Additional complications include those detailed for closed heart surgery (see previous paragraph). The majority of repairs are done with the child on cardiopulmonary bypass, including ASD, VSD, tetralogy of Fallot, and AV septal defect (AVSD).

### Monitoring Cardiac Output

The child's cardiac output is monitored through the assessment of vital signs and peripheral perfusion. Signs of low cardiac output include tachycardia, coolness and mottling of extremities, diminished peripheral pulses, delayed capillary refill time, hypotension, decreased urine output, metabolic acidosis, and changes in level of consciousness (difficult to assess in a sedated and intubated child). Intracardiac pressure monitoring is also used and assessed.

The components of cardiac output are heart rate, preload, contractility, and afterload. Problems with one or more of these components can develop during the early postoperative period. Changes in heart rate or rhythm affect cardiac function, and antidysrhythmic drugs or temporary cardiac pacing may be instituted to correct transient postoperative rhythm disturbances. Blood loss and leakage of fluid into the interstitial space can also influence preload. Transfusions of blood products, colloids, and crystalloids are frequently needed to maintain adequate circulating blood volume. Acid-base and electrolyte imbalances, as well as hypoxia, adversely affect contractility. Correction of these abnormalities may improve cardiac function, but most children will need some degree of continuous infusion of inotropic medications to support cardiac output. Changes in systemic and pulmonary vascular resistance influence afterload and the use of inodilators (medications with inotropic and vasodilator effects), such as milrinone, sometimes proves necessary.

### Supporting Respiratory Function

During cardiopulmonary bypass, the lungs are not ventilated and expanded, placing the child at risk for postoperative atelectasis. Fluid can accumulate in the pleural and interstitial spaces during and after cardiopulmonary bypass. For surgery, the child will be intubated and mechanically ventilated and often returns to the intensive care unit intubated.

Airway patency is maintained, in part, through prudent suctioning of the endotracheal tube. The nurse must pay strict attention to oxygen saturation readings (and know the anticipated saturations for the specific cardiac defect and surgical intervention), including during suctioning, to avoid episodes of transient hypoxia. Frequently, the child receives bolus or continuous infusions of analgesia (sedative medications) to help maintain comfort during this time.

Once extubated, the child is encouraged to deep breathe and cough. Incentive spirometry or therapy is often used to enhance lung expansion. Supplemental oxygen is administered initially and then tapered off as the child's condition permits. Pain medication is given before treatments and pulmonary exercises to allow the child to participate with minimal discomfort. The child can be encouraged to splint the chest during coughing by hugging a favorite stuffed animal.

Chest tubes are placed during surgery to evacuate drainage and air and assist with lung reexpansion. These tubes are inserted in either the mediastinal or pleural space, depending on the surgical approach, and are removed when lung reexpansion is confirmed and drainage has ceased.

Initial chest tube drainage is bloody and changes to serosanguineous and then serous over time. Drainage is heaviest during the first 12 to 24 hours postoperatively, and it is measured and the color evaluated hourly. Increased chest tube drainage can indicate surgical bleeding or clotting abnormalities and must be strictly monitored and rapidly resolved.

Chest tubes are uncomfortable while in place; they restrict movement and cause discomfort when the child's position is changed. Chest tube removal is a painful experience, and the child should be premedicated with an opiate analgesic before the procedure.

Pulmonary hypertension presents a complicated and potentially life-threatening problem postoperatively. Intensive monitoring of pulmonary status (while intubated and extubated), saturations, and pulmonary artery pressures is indicated. In addition, special precautions before suctioning or other noxious stimuli are indicated while caring for these children.

### Maintaining Fluid and Electrolyte Balance

Cardiac surgery and cardiopulmonary bypass affect fluid and electrolyte status. Blood loss and fluid shifts reduce circulating blood volume. Cardiopulmonary bypass stimulates secretion of aldosterone and antidiuretic hormone, resulting in water and sodium retention and potassium loss. Stress can increase calcium deposition in bone, placing the child at risk for hypocalcemia. In addition, administration of blood products can bind circulating calcium and lead to hypocalcemia.

Accurate recording of intake and output monitors fluid balance. Urine output is measured hourly, and weight is often measured daily. Fluid requirements are calculated based on the 24-hour intake and output and child's weight. The child with fluid-volume deficit can be treated with fluid boluses of crystalloid, colloid, or blood, whereas the child with fluid-volume excess is treated with fluid restriction and diuretic therapy.

Electrolyte imbalances adversely affect cardiac contractility. Serum electrolyte values are determined at regular intervals in the early postoperative period, and IV boluses of calcium or potassium are administered to correct abnormalities. Calcium chloride continuous infusions are often instituted in neonates who have undergone open heart surgery. These medications are delivered through a centrally placed venous line and given according to precise guidelines.

In addition, glucose is a critical factor in maintaining cardiac contractility, especially in the neonate and infant. Monitoring for and treating hypoglycemia are critical.

### Promoting Comfort

Postoperative pain management is an important nursing function in the care of the child undergoing cardiac surgery. The experience is frightening to both the child and parents. Parents worry that their child will be in constant, severe pain after the procedure.

Optimal pain management in the initial postoperative period may require the use of a continuous IV infusion of an opiate analgesic, such as morphine sulfate or fentanyl. This infusion is often accompanied by the administration of sedatives and antianxiety agents. In addition, nonsteroidal antiinflammatory agents can be used. This combination of drugs controls pain, relieves anxiety, and allows the child to rest. Scheduled pain medication, along with as-needed doses, often provides better pain control than as-needed pain medication alone.

Once invasive monitoring lines and tubes have been removed, pain control can usually be achieved through the use of oral analgesics. Acetaminophen with or without an opiate additive or nonsteroidal antiinflammatory agents are frequently the drugs of choice. The incision site sometimes determines the amount of pain medication the child will need to remain comfortable. A thoracotomy incision usually divides muscle and necessitates spreading of the ribs for exposure; children who have undergone this surgical approach frequently have more postoperative discomfort than those who have had a midsternotomy incision.

Pain should be assessed frequently throughout the hospitalization. Preverbal children are unable to express their discomfort, and older children may not be able to accurately describe their pain. Pain assessment tools should be used to accurately assess the child's pain. The nurse also must be alert to nonverbal pain behavior, which includes restlessness and irritability, difficulty resting and sleeping, guarding, rigidity, resistance to movement, an increase in heart rate and blood pressure, and lack of interest in eating and other activities. Consulting the parents can help the nurse validate the assessment. Parents know their child best and are familiar with their child's response to stressful situations.

### Promoting Healing and Recovery

A balance between rest and activity is necessary to promote healing. Children often feel fatigue during their postoperative recovery, and some benefit from a planned schedule of progressive activity. Parents should be encouraged to allow their child to gradually resume the preoperative activity level. Regularly scheduled administration of pain medication provides comfort during activity, allows the child to rest, and reduces fatigue and anxiety.

Nutritional intake is monitored, and the child is encouraged to resume normal eating patterns. Infants and children who were in significant HF preoperatively from large left-to-right shunting lesions sometimes demonstrate improved oral intake even before discharge home. Rarely, diet restrictions are implemented for the older child.

These restrictions may be related to long-term anticoagulation with warfarin (Coumadin) or salt restrictions. Discharge teaching is important to ensure that parents feel comfortable managing their child at home (see Patient-Centered Teaching: Care after Heart Surgery).

## ACQUIRED HEART DISEASE

Acquired heart disease encompasses all cardiac conditions that are not present at birth. Children with CHD can develop acquired cardiac problems, such as infective endocarditis and dysrhythmias. Children with structurally normal hearts can be affected by these conditions and by other cardiac conditions such as rheumatic heart disease, Kawasaki disease, hypertension, and cardiomyopathies. Some factors that play a role in triggering these problems include genetic tendencies, autoimmune responses, and infection.

### Infective Endocarditis

Infective endocarditis (IE) is an inflammation resulting from infection of the cardiac valves and endocardium by a bacterial or occasionally a fungal or viral agent. The infection can occur as the result of procedures such as dental work or invasive surgery to the respiratory tract; however, most cases are not attributable to an invasive procedure, and AHA-recommended IE-prevention guidelines now suggest that the risk is greater from poor oral hygiene (Bernstein, 2016g). Previously, a distinction was made between acute bacterial endocarditis, with a rapid fulminant course of days to weeks, and IE, with a slow, indolent course of several months' duration. The general term IE is now more accepted, with further classification based on the organism responsible for the infection.

#### Etiology

IE in children occurs most commonly in the presence of CHD. Those with prosthetic heart valves, complex cyanotic heart disease, surgically constructed systemic-to-pulmonary artery shunts, or a previous history of endocarditis are at greatest risk (Bernstein, 2016g). Acquired valvular disease with scarring (e.g., from rheumatic fever) also presents a risk for IE, but the incidence of this condition is decreasing, as the incidence of rheumatic fever has decreased (Bernstein, 2016g). The bacterial organisms most commonly responsible for IE are gram-positive organisms, including *Streptococcus viridans* and *Staphylococcus aureus,* (Bernstein, 2016g). Fungi are becoming more frequently implicated, most commonly after open heart surgery (Bernstein, 2016g; Park, 2014).

#### Incidence

The incidence of IE is variable depending on the population. Approximately 10,000 to 15,000 cases/yr occur in the United Sates (Slipczuk et al., 2013). However, IE is an important cause of hospitalization, with 0.5 to 1 in 1000 hospitalizations attributed to nonpostoperative IE (Park, 2014).

#### Manifestations

The clinical manifestations of IE are highly variable depending on the organism and the host immune response. Manifestations include fever; nonspecific complaints of anorexia, nausea, fatigue, and malaise; arthralgias; chest pain; HF; petechiae; neurologic impairment as a result of embolic events; and presence of, or change in, a heart murmur (Bernstein, 2016g). Because murmurs are present in many children with underlying CHD, it is important to detect a change in the quality of the murmur.

**PATIENT-CENTERED TEACHING**

***Care After Heart Surgery***

**Activity**
- Resume regular nap and sleep schedules and play activities (infants).
- Omit contact play for several weeks; allow quiet inside and outside play as tolerated. Avoid wrestling, jumping, tugging on arms. Also, avoid sandbox play or swimming until the incision is healed.
- Avoid activities where the child could fall (e.g., riding tricycles or bicycles, swinging, playing on monkey bars or jungle gyms, sliding) for 4 to 6 weeks after hospital discharge.
- Avoid ill contacts.
- Resume regular bedtime (children).
- Avoid large crowds of people for up to 4 to 6 weeks after discharge (including daycare and places of public worship), especially during winter months.

**Diet**
- Resume regular breastfeeding or fortified formula (as instructed) and baby foods (infant).
- Do not give any new foods until after the first checkup (infant).
- Encourage adequate liquid intake.
- Appetite should improve at home.

**Incision**
- Do not bathe the infant or child until instructed to do so.
- When instructed, bathe the infant or child with soap and water in the usual way. Pat the incision; do not rub it while it is healing.
- If the infant drools saliva or formula, cover incision with gauze to prevent excessive moisture.
- Do not use creams, lotions, or powders on incision until it is completely healed and without scabs.
- Report any redness, drainage, or signs of infection at the incision or suture sites.

**School**
- The child may return to school the second to third week after hospital discharge.
- The child may return to school for half days for the first few days.
- The child should not participate in physical education until 2 months after the operation.

**When to Call the Provider**
- Faster, harder breathing than normal when child is at rest.
- Temperature above 37.7° C (100° F).
- New, frequent coughing.
- Turning blue or bluer than normal.
- Any swelling, redness, or drainage of the incision.
- Frequent vomiting or diarrhea.
- Pain worse instead of better.
- Appetite worse than at time of discharge.

**Checkup**
- An appointment should be made for a 1- to 2-week follow-up at the time of discharge.
- No immunizations should be given for 4 to 6 weeks postoperatively.

## PATHOPHYSIOLOGY

### *Infective Endocarditis*

Children with congenital heart defects often have pressure gradients between the structures of the heart. A pressure gradient causes turbulence, which can erode underlying tissue and damage the endocardium or endothelium. A clot composed of fibrin and entrapped platelets sometimes forms at the site of the disruption. If bacteria are present (most commonly *Staphylococcus aureus* or *Streptococcus*), they can become entrapped in the clot and encircled by the fibrin and platelets. This structure is known as a vegetation. The vegetation increases in size as the microorganisms, fibrin, and platelets proliferate within a protective sheath of fibrin. The contained and protected bacteria can quickly destroy the surrounding tissue and valve structures. Because the vegetation is constantly exposed to pressure from blood flow, it can break off and migrate to other tissues. Particularly dangerous is a cerebral infarct.

### Diagnostic Evaluation

The diagnosis of bacterial endocarditis is established based on several blood cultures that yield the causative organism and on ECHO findings. Blood cultures should be obtained on 3 to 5 separate occasions (Bernstein, 2016g). In 90% of cases, the first two blood cultures will yield the causative agent if the patient has not received antibiotics (Bernstein, 2016g; Park, 2014). The visualization of a *vegetation* (an abnormal growth of infected tissue) on ECHO studies helps considerably in establishing the diagnosis, but a study that is negative for vegetations does not rule out IE. ECHO can help identify the subgroup of children who might require early surgical intervention to prevent further hemodynamic compromise or neurologic complications, such as those with large, mobile, left-sided vegetations. Other laboratory tests that help to confirm the diagnosis include complete blood count (CBC), ESR, ECG, and rheumatoid factor. The development of AV block suggests extension of disease into the myocardium, which can be helpful in identifying another subgroup of children who might benefit from early surgery. The Duke criteria lists major and minor criteria that help diagnose infective endocarditis (Bernstein, 2016g; Park, 2014).

### Therapeutic Management

Prevention is the most important therapeutic intervention for IE. Children at risk should establish and maintain an optimal oral hygiene routine to reduce the incidence of periodontal infections. Guidelines have changed the recommendations for antibiotic prophylaxis in at-risk infants and children. Recognizing that the risk for IE is higher from poor oral hygiene than from periodic invasive dental procedures and that adverse effects from antibiotics (e.g., allergy, resistance) are increasing, the guidelines recommend that antibiotic prophylaxis be given to the following patients only (Park, 2014):

- People who undergo prosthetic valve replacement or repair
- People who have unrepaired complex cyanotic heart disease or palliative shunts
- People who are within a 6-month postprocedure period for repair of a cardiac defect with a prosthetic device or material
- People who have residual defects near the site of a prosthetic repair
- People who have had IE previously
- People who have had a cardiac transplant with subsequent valve dysfunction

Additionally, prophylaxis is recommended only for dental procedures that involve "manipulation of gingival tissue or the periapical region of teeth or perforation of oral mucosa" (Park, 2014) and for invasive respiratory tract procedures such as tonsillectomy and adenoidectomy or biopsy. Prophylactic antibiotics are no longer recommended for gastrointestinal or genitourinary procedures unless an infection is present (Park, 2014). The standard general prophylactic agent is amoxicillin given orally 1 hour before the procedure. Clindamycin or azithromycin is the antibiotic of choice in children allergic to penicillin or amoxicillin (AAP 2015a; Bernstein, 2016g).

Treatment for IE caused by bacteria invariably includes parenteral administration of antibiotics for up to 6 weeks, depending on the pathogen and the clinical circumstances (Bernstein, 2016g). The prolonged course of antibiotics is necessary because total elimination of the bacteria is essential. Because the bacteria in vegetations are protected from host defense mechanisms by the deposition of platelets and fibrin, aggressive and prolonged treatment is necessary for bacterial eradication (Bernstein, 2016g).

Surgical interventions, such as excision of the vegetation or removal of an infected valve, may be indicated, particularly in the acute forms of endocarditis. Indications for surgery include severe, unresponsive HF, abscess, and evidence of valve involvement (Bernstein, 2016g).

## NURSING CARE

### The Child With IE

#### Assessment

Assessment of the child with IE requires close monitoring of temperature elevations and vital signs. Vital signs should be monitored every 2 to 4 hours, along with a thorough cardiovascular and neurologic assessment. If a heart murmur is present, any change in it should be reported to the provider.

#### Nursing Diagnosis and Planning

Nursing diagnoses and expected outcomes for the child with IE include the following:

- Ineffective Tissue Perfusion (peripheral and cerebral) related to hemodynamic instability as a result of impaired valvular or myocardial function and effects of a cerebral infarction.

**Expected outcome.** The child will have adequate peripheral tissue perfusion, as evidenced by pink mucous membranes and nail beds, a capillary refill time of less than 2 seconds, strong peripheral pulses, vital signs within normal limits, and adequate cerebral perfusion, as evidenced by mental status and a level of consciousness within normal limits and no evidence of focal neurologic deficits.

- Hyperthermia related to bacterial infection.

**Expected outcome.** The child will maintain a body temperature that is within normal limits.

- Acute Pain or Chronic Pain (headaches, arthralgias, myalgias) related to the body's immunologic response.

**Expected outcome.** The pain associated with headaches, arthralgias, and myalgias will be reduced or eliminated.

- Deficient Knowledge about home care of the child with IE related to unfamiliarity of the information.

**Expected outcome.** The parents will be able to administer medications and monitor the child's condition. They will explain the need for antibiotic prophylaxis and when it is indicated.

#### Interventions

The child will need vigilant monitoring of vital signs, peripheral perfusion, and hemodynamic stability. Any change in the vital signs, neurologic status, heart murmur, or tissue perfusion should be immediately reported to the provider. The child's activity level may be diminished, necessitating assistance with activities of daily living. Opportunities for quiet activities such as reading, watching videos, drawing, and doing puzzles, should be provided.

The child's temperature should be monitored every 2 to 4 hours and plotted on a graph. If the child is receiving an aminoglycoside antibiotic, serum peak and trough levels may be monitored. The nurse must administer the antibiotics at the appropriate time, with trough levels determined before and peak levels determined 1 hour after the dose is administered. Acetaminophen is administered as needed for fever, as ordered by the provider, once the initial blood samples have been drawn for culture. Acetaminophen can also be administered for persistent headaches, arthralgias, and myalgias. Reassure the child and parents that the aches and malaise will resolve.

Some children are discharged home receiving parenteral antibiotic therapy. It is imperative that the parents have access to adequate community resources. The nurse must confirm that they have undergone formal instruction in the use of the IV mode selected (e.g., saline lock, implanted venous access device, Hickman catheter, percutaneous line) and the proper administration of antibiotics. Provide reassurance and support to the family and child regarding the extensive and lengthy therapy that will be needed.

### Evaluation

- Have the child's vital signs improved?
- Does the child have a capillary refill of less than 2 seconds?
- Does the child have a negative neurologic examination?
- Is the child's body temperature within normal limits?
- Have symptoms of anorexia, malaise, arthralgia, and fever subsided?
- Can the parents demonstrate administration of medications and verbalize an understanding of the need and indications for antibiotic prophylaxis?
- Are the parents demonstrating the ability to manage their child's condition at home?

## DYSRHYTHMIAS

The identification of a dysrhythmia (a cardiac rhythm disturbance) in childhood is an important finding. The most important aspect is to recognize that a dysrhythmia is present and classify it quickly as life-threatening or non–life-threatening. Assessing the child hemodynamically is a critical factor in determining the interventions. Often, the nurse will note an abnormal rhythm during a child's or adolescent's well examination. After the assessment of an abnormal or irregular radial pulse measurement, the nurse should obtain an apical pulse, counting for a full minute.

### Etiology

Cardiac rhythm disturbances have numerous causes. Dysrhythmias can be associated with underlying CHD or occur in structurally normal hearts. Either abnormal impulse formation, abnormal conduction, or a combination of these two factors causes a dysrhythmia. Rhythm disturbances can be classified as tachydysrhythmic (rapid) or bradydysrhythmic (slow). Dysrhythmias lead to decreased cardiac output and can result in more serious and life-threatening arrhythmias (Van Hare, 2016).

Dysrhythmias are seen in the postoperative period after repair or palliation of a cardiac lesion. Postsurgical dysrhythmias result from injury to the conduction system, edema, ischemia, incision or suture placement, and acid–base or electrolyte imbalances.

Underlying acquired heart disease, such as myocarditis or cardiomyopathy, sometimes produces dysrhythmias. Abnormal electrical pathways in the heart can cause certain dysrhythmias. *Wolff–Parkinson–White syndrome* is the most common example. Abnormal electrical repolarization of the heart can cause disturbances such as prolonged QT syndrome, which can result in a life-threatening ventricular tachycardia. Such disturbances can have a genetic cause. Noncardiac causes of rhythm disturbances include fever, temperature instability, hypoxia, electrolyte and metabolic disturbances, increased intracranial pressure, hypovolemia, cardiac tamponade, and drug therapy or reactions.

### Incidence

Dysrhythmias in children are not uncommon, most are not life threatening, and most appear in children whose hearts are structurally normal. Supraventricular tachycardia is the most common primary symptomatic rhythm disturbance seen in infants and children. It occurs in 0.1% to 0.4% of otherwise healthy children (Paul, Blaikley, Peevers, et al., 2012).

### Manifestations

In tachydysrhythmias and bradydysrhythmias, cardiac output is diminished. The clinical presentation is of low cardiac output syndrome with poor end-organ perfusion. The earliest signs and symptoms may be subtle; later they can be quite dramatic. Clinical manifestations for the infant and toddler may include poor feeding, irritability, lethargy, pale or mottled color, poor peripheral perfusion (diminished pulses, mottling, cool extremities, delayed capillary refill time), decreased urine output, and HF.

In older children, palpitations, dizziness, syncope, and exercise intolerance may be demonstrated. Tolerance of rhythm disturbances is based on the type of rhythm, underlying cardiac condition, and duration of rhythm and the effect on cardiac output.

In absent rhythms, there is no cardiac output. This is a medical emergency. Cardiopulmonary resuscitation (CPR) and medical intervention must be initiated if the child is to survive.

### Diagnostic Evaluation

The primary tool for diagnosing pediatric dysrhythmias is the 12-lead ECG. Twenty-four-hour Holter monitoring and transtelephonic monitoring are useful for documenting intermittent episodes of cardiac rhythm disturbances.

### Therapeutic Management

Pediatric rhythm disturbances should be treated as emergencies if they compromise cardiac output or have the potential to degenerate into lethal (collapse) rhythms (e.g., ventricular fibrillation) (Van Hare, 2016). Management strategies include drug therapy, radiofrequency ablation, cardioversion, and pacemakers; the choice of treatment is guided by the origin of the dysrhythmia and the clinical consequences.

#### Fast Pulse Rate

***Supraventricular tachycardia.*** Supraventricular tachycardia (SVT) is a narrow QRS tachycardia. This narrow QRS configuration indicates that the impulse begins above the ventricles. Rates can be in the 220 to 300 beats/min (bpm) range. Children who are asymptomatic and hemodynamically stable can be treated conservatively. Vagal maneuvers can be used to terminate an episode of SVT by eliciting the diving reflex. Immersing the older child's face in ice water stimulates a vagal response that can stop the tachycardia; briefly placing an ice bag or bag of frozen vegetables over the infant's face accomplishes the same result. This maneuver should be done only while constantly monitoring the child and with emergency equipment available in case the child has a prolonged slow heart rate while converting to a normal rhythm.

If vagal maneuvers do not convert the child's heart to a normal rhythm, antidysrhythmics should be considered. Antidysrhythmic drug therapy can also suppress further episodes. Older children who

## PATHOPHYSIOLOGY

### Dysrhythmias

#### Tachydysrhythmias

Primary tachydysrhythmias can originate in either the atria or the ventricles. The most common atrial tachydysrhythmia is supraventricular tachycardia (SVT). SVT is triggered by an atrial ectopic focus (a group of irritable cells somewhere in the atrium) or a re-entry circuit (accessory pathway permitting abnormal conduction within the heart). Ventricular tachycardia is uncommon; it is seen in prolonged QT syndrome and in the preoperative or postoperative period in children with underlying structural heart disease. It also is seen with severe acidosis or in any scenario with severely reduced heart function, such as myocarditis, or from indwelling catheters such as PICC lines or broviacs.

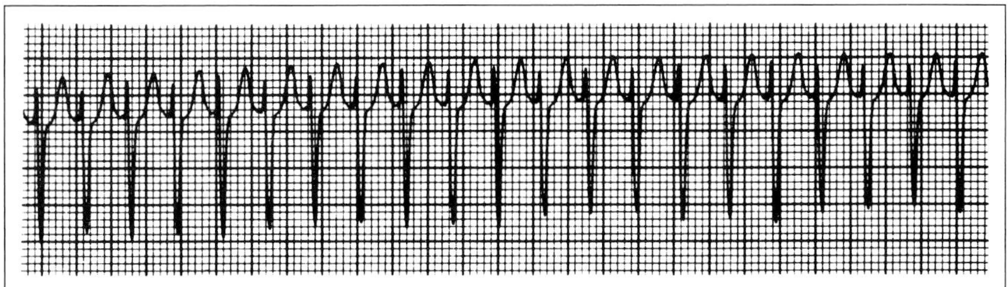

Supraventricular tachycardia. (Modified from Park, M.K., & Guntheroth, W G. [2006]. *How to read pediatric ECGs* [4th ed., pp. 224]. St. Louis: Mosby.)

#### Bradydysrhythmias

In children, primary cardiac bradydysrhythmias usually result from damage to the sinus node or the conduction pathway between the atria and the ventricles (AV block). Secondary bradydysrhythmias frequently result from surgery for congenital heart disease, especially surgery involving the atria. Children also can experience sinus bradydysrhythmia in which the pulse rate is markedly slower than expected for age. Bradycardia is a sign that a child is decompensating. As this condition can lead to cardiopulmonary arrest, early identification and treatment are imperative (ENA, 2012).

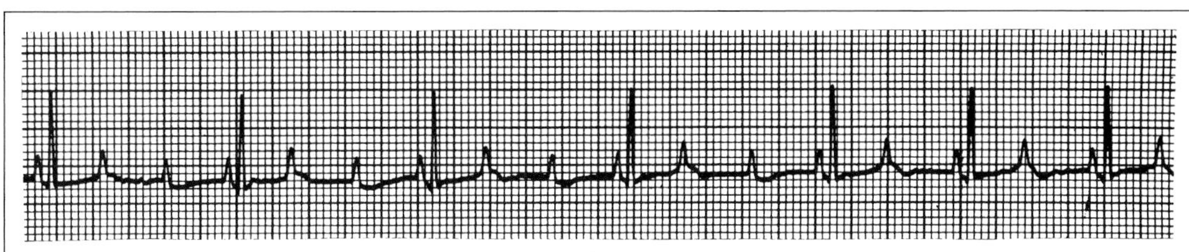

Heart block—two or three P waves for every QRS. Cardiac output is based on the rate of the QRS complexes—ventricular contraction. (Modified from Park, M.K., & Guntheroth, W.G. [2006]. *How to read pediatric ECGs* [4th ed., pp. 232]. St. Louis: Mosby.)

Data from Park, M. K. (2014). *Pediatric cardiology for practitioners* (6th ed.). Philadelphia: Elsevier.

continue to have episodes of SVT may benefit from radiofrequency ablation of the ectopic focus or accessory pathway.

Infants and children who are hemodynamically unstable require emergency intervention. If vascular access is present, the drug adenosine can be given. Adenosine is an effective antidysrhythmic because of its ability to slow conduction through the AV node and, in many cases, successfully terminate episodes of SVT rapidly and safely (Park, 2014; Van Hare, 2016). However, synchronized cardioversion remains the treatment of choice for the child with profound cardiovascular compromise.

*Ventricular tachycardia.* Ventricular tachycardia is a wide complex tachycardia, indicating that the impulse originates in the ventricle. The emergency management of ventricular tachycardia in unconscious children is synchronized cardioversion. Children with a wide complex tachycardia and absent pulse require CPR until defibrillation is available. Lidocaine, 1 mg/kg, can be administered before cardioversion, followed by a continuous infusion of the drug to prevent further episodes (Park, 2014). Once the tachycardia has been terminated, underlying causes should be explored.

### Slow Pulse Rate

*Bradydysrhythmias.* Primary cardiac bradydysrhythmias include the varying degrees of heart block and junctional or ventricular "escape" rhythms caused by sinus node dysfunction. These dysrhythmias are marked by dissociation between the P wave and the QRS complex, with the asynchrony between the atrial and ventricular contractions. Some are congenital, but they also are seen often in children who have undergone cardiac surgery, especially surgery of the atria. Temporary or permanent cardiac pacing may be necessary to maintain adequate cardiac output.

*Absent rhythms.* The classification of absent or collapse rhythms includes asystole, ventricular fibrillation, and pulseless electrical activity. In asystole, electrical cardiac activity is absent. Approximately 2,000 children die each year due to sudden cardiac arrest (ENA, 2012). Epinephrine is administered to stimulate cardiac activity. The heart is in electrical standstill, and there is no myocardial activity or cardiac output. The ECG rhythm strip is a "flat line." The emergency management of asystole is CPR and medical management. Epinephrine is administered to stimulate cardiac activity. The drug is given IV, intraosseously, or through an endotracheal tube.

Ventricular fibrillation, rare in children, is frequently the result of underlying cardiac disease. The emergency management of episodes of ventricular fibrillation is defibrillation and CPR. Drugs administered during resuscitation efforts include epinephrine, lidocaine, and other antidysrhythmic agents.

Pulseless electrical activity indicates a hemodynamically compromised state in which cardiac electrical activity is unable to generate effective myocardial contraction and cardiac output. The ECG rhythm strip shows what looks like a normal rhythm. When the nurse palpates for a pulse or listens for a heartbeat, there will be none. CPR must be initiated. The underlying cause is usually noncardiac (e.g., respiratory arrest), and it must be identified and corrected for the child to survive the episode.

## NURSING CARE

### The Child With a Dysrhythmia

#### Assessment

Children with dysrhythmias require a thorough cardiovascular assessment because they are at risk for developing cardiogenic shock. In a stable or compensated child with a dysrhythmia, it is important to obtain a comprehensive and accurate history of activity tolerance. Older children may have unexplained episodes of dizziness, palpitations, or syncope. Irregular pulse is sometimes noted. Nurses who have been trained to read pediatric ECG rhythm strips might observe signs of a particular dysrhythmia.

**SAFETY ALERT**

***Dysrhythmias***

If a child is having a dysrhythmia, assess responsiveness and remember CAB:

**CIRCULATION** assessment.

- Palpate and auscultate pulses for a maximum of 10 seconds.
- If no pulse, begin chest compressions.
- If slow pulse, assess the child's tolerance of slow pulse (including perfusion and pulses).

**AIRWAY** assessment.

**BREATHING** assessment.

- If no breathing, begin ventilation after first cycle of chest compressions.
- Obtain an ECG rhythm strip for assessment.
- Shock delivery if needed.

#### Nursing Diagnosis and Planning

Nursing diagnoses and expected outcomes for the child with a dysrhythmia include the following:

- Decreased Cardiac Output related to decreased ventricular filling or decreased rate of heart contractions.

*Expected outcome.* The child will have pink or baseline cyanotic mucous membranes and nail beds, brisk capillary refill, good-quality pulses, and a normal level of consciousness.

- Risk for Injury related to episodes of syncope.

*Expected outcome.* The child will remain free of injury during any episodes of syncope.

- Deficient Knowledge about Care of a Child with a Potentially Fatal Condition related to unfamiliarity with the information.

*Expected outcome.* The family will describe medication administration, will demonstrate an ability to identify signs and symptoms indicative of dysrhythmias, and will be able to perform CPR.

#### Interventions

Nursing interventions involve immediate care of the child who has the dysrhythmia and education of the child and family. The child and family will need information regarding monitoring for future signs and symptoms of dysrhythmias, administering medications as ordered, and appropriate emergency measures to initiate, including CPR, once the child has been discharged from the hospital.

Educating the child and family is imperative for those children with life-threatening dysrhythmias. Teach the child and family how to take a pulse or listen to the heart rate with a stethoscope. Teach the child and family to identify the signs and symptoms of dysrhythmia, including poor feeding, color changes, palpitations, syncope or dizziness, respiratory distress, and fatigue. These signs and symptoms should be reported to the parent or teacher as soon as possible, and medical attention should be sought. Children who take antidysrhythmics at home must adhere to the prescribed medication schedule closely and must be careful not to skip any doses. Medical alert bracelets should be worn by children who are in preschool or school. Parents and teachers also should be aware of signs and symptoms that indicate the early appearance of dysrhythmias. All caretakers should complete a formal course in CPR and know how to activate the emergency medical services system.

#### Evaluation

- Are the child's pulses of good quality and mucous membranes pink or baseline cyanosis, and does the child have a normal level of consciousness?
- Has the child remained free from injury related to falling as a result of syncope?
- Have the child, parents, and other caregivers demonstrated an understanding of medications, activity limitations, the possibility of a life-threatening episode, and how to activate the emergency medical services system?
- Have the child and parents demonstrated how to listen to the heart rate with a stethoscope or palpate a pulse?

## RHEUMATIC FEVER

**Rheumatic fever** (RF) is a diffuse inflammatory condition, most likely of autoimmune origin (see Chapter 42), of the connective tissue, primarily involving the heart, joints, subcutaneous tissues, brain, and blood vessels. The most serious complication is rheumatic heart disease, which can result in permanent damage to the cardiac valves, most commonly the mitral and aortic valves.

### Etiology

RF characteristically manifests 2 to 6 weeks after an untreated or partially treated group A beta-hemolytic streptococcal infection of the upper respiratory tract. The initial infection may or may not produce symptoms of pharyngitis. The major complication of RF is rheumatic heart disease.

### Incidence

RF has nearly disappeared from the United States and other developed countries. It occurs in 0.3 to 3% of children after GAS pharyngitis infection (Park, 2014). The incidence peaks between ages 5 and 15 years (Kogelschatz & King, 2012). However, it is endemic worldwide in countries with overcrowding, poor access to healthcare, poor sanitation, and persistent exposure to streptococcal infections; it is also present in indigenous populations within developed countries (e.g., Alaskan natives and native Americans in the United States).

## PATHOPHYSIOLOGY

### *Rheumatic Fever*

Infection by group A beta-hemolytic streptococci located in the pharyngeal area triggers an abnormal humoral and cell-mediated immunologic response in children who have rheumatic fever (RF). Immune complexes cross-react with normal tissue in the heart, brain, skin, and joints, causing inflammation in these sites. Although the disease is self-limiting, permanent damage to cardiac valve tissue can eventually occur. There may be a genetic predisposition to developing RF, although the evidence is unclear.

Reference Bernstein, D. (2016h). Rheumatic heart disease. In R. Kliegman, B. Stanton, J. St. Geme, et al. (Eds.), *Nelson textbook of pediatrics* (20th ed., pp. 2269–2271). Philadelphia: Elsevier.

## Manifestations

Major manifestations of RF include the following (Fig. 46.2):

- *Arthritis:* Tender, warm, erythematous joints, especially in the large joints, including the elbows, knees, ankles, and wrists; occurs in 75% of RF cases during the acute febrile period (first 1 to 2 weeks of illness). The typical presentation is a migratory polyarthritis, with inflammation moving rapidly from one joint to another and usually lasting less than 1 week for an individual joint before resolving.
- *Carditis:* Inflammation of the endocardium, including the valves, myocardium, and pericardium; can be subclinical and is usually diagnosed by the development of a cardiac murmur, cardiac enlargement or failure, or a pericardial friction rub. Mitral valve involvement is the most frequent manifestation of carditis.
- *Chorea:* Involuntary, purposeless, jerking movements of the legs, arms, and face, with speech impairment and emotional lability, caused by CNS involvement in RF. Also referred to as *Sydenham's chorea,* it is more common in girls and usually occurs in the absence of carditis or polyarthritis. Chorea has a longer latency period of up to 6 months after the initial streptococcal pharyngitis.
- *Erythema marginatum:* Red, painless skin lesions that start as flat or slightly raised macules, usually over the trunk. The erythema spreads at the margins of the lesion with central clearing.
- *Subcutaneous nodules:* Small, nontender lumps, attached to the tendon sheaths of joints and on bony prominences. They occur only rarely in RF and usually are associated with severe carditis.

Although arthritis is the most common manifestation, carditis is by far the most serious and the major cause of morbidity and mortality during both acute and chronic phases of the disease. Cardiac valvular disease is the major long-term consequence of RF (Bernstein, 2016h; Kogelschatz & King, 2012).

Minor criteria that assist in making a diagnosis of RF include a history of previous RF; arthralgias (joint pain) without arthritis; fever; elevated acute-phase reactants, including C-reactive protein and ESR; and first-degree AV block on ECG.

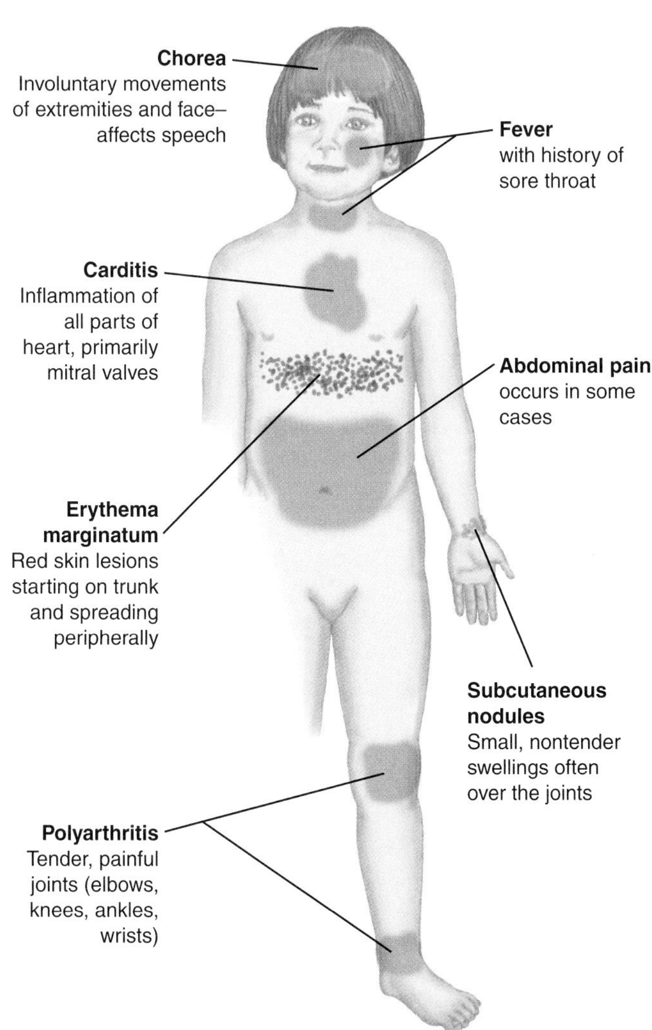


**FIG 46.2** Clinical manifestations of rheumatic fever.

## Diagnostic Evaluation

A diagnosis of RF is made using the Jones criteria in the presence of at least two major manifestations or one major and two minor manifestations, plus evidence of a recent streptococcal infection on the basis of at least one of the following diagnostic studies: positive throat culture; antistreptolysin O titer, streptozyme, or anti-DNase B assay; or by a history of scarlet fever (Box 46.1). In children with suspected carditis, a chest radiograph may show enlargement of the heart. An ECG may show rhythm abnormalities or the decreased voltages and ST-T abnormalities associated with myocarditis. An

### BOX 46.1 Diagnosis of Acute Rheumatic Fever by the Jones Criteria—1992 Update

**Major Manifestations**

- Carditis
- Polyarthritis
- Chorea
- Erythema marginatum
- Subcutaneous nodules

**Minor Manifestations**

- Fever
- Arthralgia
- Elevated erythrocyte sedimentation rate or positive C-reactive protein
- Prolonged P-R interval
- Plus supporting evidence of preceding streptococcal infection: history of recent scarlet fever, positive throat culture for group A streptococci, increased antistreptolysin O titer, or other streptococcal antibodies

From Park, M. K. (2014). *Pediatric cardiology for practitioners* (6th ed.). Philadelphia: Elsevier.

echocardiogram is essential in determining the extent of valvular, myocardial, and pericardial involvement, including the severity of mitral or aortic insufficiency, decreased ventricular function, or pericardial effusions.

### Therapeutic Management

The management of RF includes eradication of the streptococcal bacteria and treatment of other symptoms, such as joint inflammation, HF, and chorea. Once RF has been confirmed, the child receives a 10-day course of oral penicillin or a single dose of benzathine penicillin intramuscularly. Cephalosporins or erythromycin may be used in penicillin-allergic children (AAP, 2015b). Once the diagnosis is firmly established, antiinflammatory agents, including aspirin, or corticosteroids in the presence of significant carditis, are administered to speed resolution of the inflammatory process, although neither therapy has been proved to have an effect on the incidence or course of carditis. The duration of therapy is tailored according to the child's clinical course.

Children who have had RF are susceptible to recurrent attacks, risk further cardiac valve damage, and require secondary prophylaxis to prevent recurrence. The child without cardiac complications should receive antibiotic prophylaxis for 5 years or through age 21 years, whichever is longer. Those with rheumatic heart disease but no residual cardiac effects should continue prophylaxis for at least 10 years and until age 21 years (whichever is longer), and those with both rheumatic heart disease and residual cardiac issues continue prophylaxis for the longer of either 10 years or until 40 years of age (AAP, 2015b; Park, 2014). The AHA recommends prophylaxis for life for those who have contact with children who may have group A streptococcal infection, such as teachers, healthcare workers, and parents of school-age children. Penicillin is the drug of choice, either by monthly intramuscular injection (most reliable in terms of adherence) or an oral dose of 250 mg twice daily (AAP, 2015b).

## NURSING CARE

### The Child With RF

#### Assessment

Children with RF often are admitted to the hospital and maintained on bed rest during the acute phase. Initially, the nurse determines whether the child or any family members have had a sore throat or unexplained fever within the past 2 months. The child should be assessed for cardiac symptoms throughout the course of hospitalization. Temperature, pulse, respiration, and blood pressure are assessed, and the child is observed for signs of carditis, including tachycardia, heart murmur, friction rub, shortness of breath, or edema of the face, abdomen, or ankles. Examination of the joints may reveal very tender elbows, knees, ankles, and wrists, with subcutaneous nodules over extensor surfaces of the joints. RF can also cause red skin lesions on the trunk and rapid, purposeless, involuntary movements (chorea), either on observation or by history.

#### Nursing Diagnosis and Planning

Nursing diagnoses and expected outcomes for the child with RH include the following:

- Deficient Knowledge related to unfamiliarity with medications and activity restrictions.

  ***Expected outcome.*** The child will adhere to the medication regimen and activity restrictions.
- Ineffective Coping related to confinement.

  ***Expected outcome.*** The child will participate in quiet activities and will maintain social contact.
- Acute Pain related to polyarthritis.

  ***Expected outcome.*** The child will verbalize an increase in comfort and will indicate a decrease in pain using an age-appropriate pain tool.
- Risk for Injury related to subsequent streptococcal infection.

  ***Expected outcome.*** The child will inform parents at the first sign of a sore throat, and the family will adhere to antibiotic prophylaxis.

#### Interventions

The nurse administers antibiotics, analgesics, and antipyretics as ordered and reports to the provider any fever or pain. Children with RF require bed rest during the acute febrile stage of the illness and should not return to school while there is clear evidence of rheumatic activity. While the child's activities are restricted, the nurse and family should talk about limiting visitors and arranging for quiet yet enjoyable activities. Family members and friends may provide board and computer games, movies, puzzles, and crafts for the school-age child. Such activities will help minimize activity and cardiac demand. The child may benefit from a daily schedule that includes rest periods interspersed with these diverse activities and some limited exercise (e.g., passive range-of-motion exercises). An art or play therapist can work with the child who is extremely anxious because of confinement.

Nursing comfort measures include alternating application of heat and cold to affected joints, repositioning, massage, and providing distraction by use of guided imagery and relaxation. Seizure precautions are warranted if the child has chorea. At home, parents must practice safety measures. For example, the child who cannot control movements might need to sleep on a mattress on the floor and to be assisted going up and down stairs. The child might be embarrassed by uncontrolled movements, especially in front of peers, and will need reassurance that these symptoms are temporary.

Emphasize to parents the importance of adherence to antibiotic prophylaxis. The family might be allowed to offer an adolescent the choice of monthly injections versus daily oral administration. If the child chooses the oral route, instruct the family about the required dose, frequency of administration, duration, effects, side effects, and potential cardiac complications if the regimen is not followed precisely.

### ! NURSING QUALITY ALERT

#### *Streptococcal Prophylaxis for the Child With Rheumatic Fever*

Streptococcal prophylaxis is the most important aspect of therapeutic management in rheumatic fever (RF) because damaged valves can become further damaged with repeated infections. This prophylaxis can be lifelong if there is actual valve involvement. Intramuscular penicillin, administered monthly, is the drug of choice. Alternatives include oral penicillin taken twice daily or sulfadiazine taken orally once daily; sulfadiazine or erythromycin taken twice daily is appropriate for children who are sensitive to penicillin.

#### Evaluation

- Is the child taking antibiotics as ordered?
- Is the child following modified bed rest guidelines?
- Is the child playing board games, reading, and visiting with friends as tolerated?
- Has the child verbalized a decrease in pain and indicated decreased pain on an appropriate assessment tool?
- Does the child take antibiotic prophylaxis as ordered and notify the parent if experiencing a sore throat?

## KAWASAKI DISEASE

Kawasaki disease, also called *mucocutaneous lymph node syndrome,* is an acute, febrile, exanthematous illness of children involving generalized vasculitis of unknown etiology. Kawasaki disease is a major cause of acquired heart disease in children in the United States. Coronary artery aneurysms are seen in 20% to 25% of children with untreated Kawasaki disease (Son & Newburger, 2016).

### Etiology

The cause of Kawasaki disease remains unknown. However, recent evidence suggests that it is an immune-mediated vasculitis triggered by an acute infection or a bacterial toxin (see Chapter 42). Kawasaki disease may have a genetic component (Son & Newburger, 2016); it also has a seasonal component, being diagnosed most often in late winter and early spring.

### Incidence

Kawasaki disease is seen most frequently in children younger than 5 years of age and is diagnosed less frequently in children older than 8 years of age. Affected boys outnumber affected girls (1.5 to 1), and there is an increased incidence in children of Asian ancestry (Rowley, 2012).

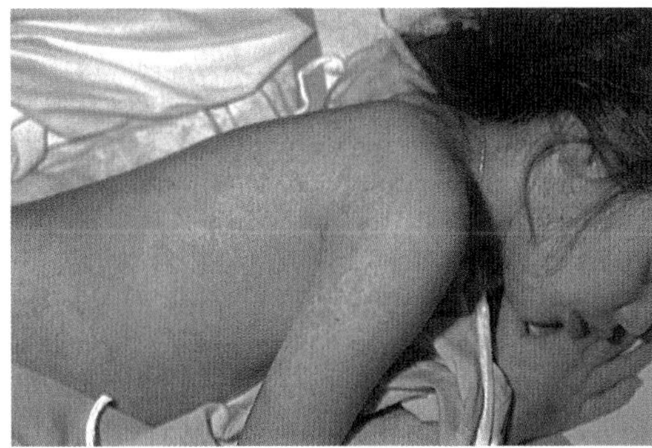

FIG 46.3 Erythematous rash of Kawasaki disease. (From Lookingbill, D.P., & Marks, J.G., Jr. [1992]. *Principles of dermatology* [2nd ed., pp. 223]. Philadelphia: Saunders.)

#### PATHOPHYSIOLOGY

***Kawasaki Disease***

An infectious or possibly toxic trigger initiates an immune system response that affects medium-size arteries, especially the coronary arteries. A generalized immune response becomes more specific, with increasing numbers of T lymphocytes and B lymphocytes infiltrating the smooth muscle cells of the vascular walls. The infiltration causes edema and inflammation, which progressively weaken the vascular walls, leading to aneurysms. As the disease progresses, fibrous connective tissue forms at the inflammatory sites, eventually thickening and scarring the vascular walls. These vascular changes, along with the increased platelets that occur as part of the disease process, can cause thrombus formation, myocardial infarction, and death in some children.

### Manifestations

Kawasaki disease manifests in three phases. The acute stage lasts approximately 10 days and is characterized by a high fever that persists longer than 5 days. The fever is unresponsive to antibiotic treatment. Clinical signs include bilateral, nonpurulent conjunctivitis; changes in the mucous membranes (i.e., erythema, fissures, and cracking of the lips; strawberry tongue); changes in the peripheral extremities, such as swelling of the hands and feet and erythema of the palms and soles; a generalized erythematous rash (Fig. 46.3); and enlarged cervical lymph nodes. Tachycardia and extreme irritability are also common.

The second or subacute phase lasts from approximately day 11 to day 25. The fever disappears, and most symptoms resolve. The phase is characterized by continued irritability, anorexia, desquamation of the fingers and toes, arthritis and arthralgia, and cardiovascular manifestations, including HF, dysrhythmias, and the typical coronary aneurysms (Park, 2014).

Coronary aneurysm formation begins early in the second phase with 20% of patients affected (Park, 2014). A baseline echocardiogram at diagnosis with repeat studies at 2 weeks, 6 to 8 weeks, and 6 to 12 months (optional) will help identify those with coronary artery involvement (Son & Newburger, 2016). Severe thrombocytosis occurs during this period and marks the period of highest risk for coronary artery thrombosis in the areas of aneurysm, resulting in myocardial infarction.

The final or convalescent stage begins when most symptoms have disappeared and lasts until the ESR returns to normal. Deep transverse grooves, called *Beau's lines,* may appear on the child's nails.

### Diagnostic Evaluation

Fever of 5 days duration in conjunction with at least four of the five following primary clinical findings for the acute phase establishes the diagnosis of Kawasaki disease (Son & Newburger, 2016):

- Bilateral nonpurulent conjunctivitis
- Oral mucosal alterations (e.g., strawberry tongue; pharyngeal erythema; dry, fissured lips)
- Redness of the hands and feet followed by desquamation
- Rash on the trunk
- Cervical lymphadenopathy with large nodes
- No other known disease process to explain the signs and symptoms

Laboratory data are nonspecific. The white blood cell count is elevated during the acute phase, as are the ESR and C-reactive protein level. There is sterile pyuria. The ECG in the acute phase may demonstrate first-degree heart block. Platelet levels dramatically rise during the subacute phase. Aneurysms are detected with ECHO.

### Therapeutic Management

Therapeutic management is directed toward preventing or reducing the coronary artery damage from Kawasaki disease. High-dose intravenous immune globulin (IVIG) in combination with aspirin has been shown to lower the prevalence of coronary artery abnormalities when given within 10 days of fever onset. At diagnosis, IVIG is given in a dosage of 2 g/kg over a 10- to 12-hour infusion (American Academy of Pediatrics [AAP] Committee on Infectious Diseases, 2015c). High-dose aspirin therapy is begun at the same time. Initially, the dosage is in the antiinflammatory range of 80 to 100 mg/kg/day in four evenly divided doses until fever resolves. The dosage is then reduced to an antiplatelet aggregation dose of 3 to 5 mg/kg/day once daily and continued through weeks 6 to 8 of the illness (AAP Committee on Infectious Diseases, 2015c). If coronary artery abnormalities are identified, this dosage is continued indefinitely (Park, 2014). Corticosteroids may be considered if the child is unresponsive to standard therapy; however, clear data regarding its administration is lacking (Son & Newburger, 2016).

## NURSING CARE

### The Child With Kawasaki Disease

#### Assessment

During the acute phase, the nurse must monitor the child's cardiac status closely, looking for clinical signs and symptoms of HF. Changes in pulse, respiration, blood pressure, and color, along with shortness of breath, chest pain, and decreased activity, suggest cardiac complications. It is important to examine the child's eyes, mouth, and skin for signs of infection and the joints for redness, swelling, and tenderness.

The nurse should determine the parents' anxiety level. Parents are often frightened by how sick the child is and the threat of a possibly devastating outcome. Families appreciate talking about their fears; learning about the cause of the illness, the treatment plan, and the prognosis; and participating in the child's care.

#### Nursing Diagnosis and Planning

Nursing diagnoses and expected outcomes for the child with Kawasaki disease and the child's family include the following:

- Risk for Deficient Fluid Volume related to fever.

  ***Expected outcome.*** The child will maintain fluid and electrolyte balance, as evidenced by normal laboratory values and intake and output appropriate for age.
- Acute Pain related to fever, skin manifestations, and joint inflammation.

  ***Expected outcome.*** The child will rest comfortably, as evidenced by periods of uninterrupted sleep, and will express decreased pain on an age-appropriate pain assessment tool.
- Fear related to changes in the child's behavior and uncertainty about the long-term prognosis.

  ***Expected outcome.*** The parents and child will discuss their fears related to having a serious disease with a long recuperative period.

#### Interventions

The nurse should administer aspirin with milk or food and infuse IVIG as ordered. During the infusion, it is important to monitor the child's vital signs and any adverse reactions to IVIG, including facial flushing, tightness in the chest, chills, dizziness, nausea, vomiting, diaphoresis, and hypotension. Blood pressure is checked every 15 minutes for the first hour and every 30 minutes thereafter until the infusion is complete. A precipitous fall in blood pressure can occur 30 to 60 minutes after the infusion has begun; this is often related to the rate of infusion. The provider will usually lower the prescribed rate of infusion if such a reaction occurs and order diphenhydramine (Benadryl) and acetaminophen to control side effects. Epinephrine is given for anaphylactic reactions. IVIG can interfere with achieving immunity from live-virus vaccines, so some immunizations (e.g., measles, mumps, rubella, varicella) should be delayed for 11 months after IVIG therapy (AAP Committee on Infectious Diseases, 2015c).

Nursing care focuses on comfort measures and adequate hydration. The nurse and parents must encourage fluid intake by offering ice pops or ice to numb affected mucous membranes, giving liquids that are high in calories and low in acid through a straw (avoiding citrus drinks and sodas), and offering favorite foods that are soft and bland. The nurse or family can apply salve to soothe cracked, dry lips.

Sponge baths with tepid water often decrease fever and relieve discomfort from skin manifestations. The child should be handled gently and only when necessary. If itching is severe, the provider should be notified.

Toddlers and preschool children fear hospitalization and body changes, often exhibiting regressive behavior and sleeping poorly. In addition, children with Kawasaki disease also manifest increased irritability during the acute phase. If possible, keep the environment calm by talking in gentle tones, playing soft music, and avoiding bright overhead lights. It may help to line the bed with soft blankets from home. Assure the family that the fever, pain, and irritability will eventually resolve and praise their hard work in keeping the child comfortable. Because the child's extreme irritability is an area of concern for parents, the nurse should provide support so the parent can take periodic breaks. Discharge instructions should include provisions for a cardiac follow-up. Parents' fears can be decreased through an understanding of the disease and treatment.

#### Evaluation

- Is the child taking adequate amounts of fluid and maintaining electrolyte balance?
- Is the child's urine output appropriate for age (see Chapter 40)?
- Is the child experiencing periods of uninterrupted rest?
- Does the child demonstrate decreased pain on an age-appropriate assessment tool?
- Are the parents able to verbalize their fears and discuss the course of the illness and their commitment to follow-up care?

## HYPERTENSION

*Hypertension* is defined as an average systolic or average diastolic blood pressure that exceeds or is equal to the 95th percentile for age, height, and sex based on measurements obtained on at least three occasions. Children with systolic blood pressure or diastolic blood pressure between the 90th and 95th percentiles are considered to be prehypertensive; prehypertension in adolescents is defined as blood pressure greater than or equal to 120/80 mm Hg (Lande, 2016). Normal blood pressure is defined as a systolic or diastolic pressure that is less than the 90th percentile for age, height, and sex (see http://www.nhlbi.nih.gov/guidelines/hypertension/child_tbl.htm). Hypertension is categorized into two types: *primary* (idiopathic) and *secondary* (symptom of underlying disease). Primary hypertension predominates among older adolescents, whereas secondary causes are overwhelmingly more common in the younger age-groups.

### Etiology

Pediatric hypertension that is not the result of an underlying disease is referred to as essential hypertension, similar to that seen in adults. The incidence of pediatric hypertension has been increasing in the United States, related intimately to the increasing prevalence of obesity (Lande, 2016). Essential hypertension is more prevalent among adolescents, teenagers, and those with moderately elevated blood pressure. The early development of essential hypertension is linked to childhood obesity, children with diabetes mellitus, and a strong family history of hypertension. Affected adults and children can exhibit exaggerated blood pressure responses to physical and emotional stresses compared with normotensive individuals. Some individuals with essential hypertension are negatively affected by increased levels of dietary sodium (Lande, 2016).

Height and weight are additional determinations of blood pressure in children. Children with elevated blood pressure are usually taller and heavier than their age-matched peers. The causes of secondary hypertension in children include various renal and renovascular diseases, coarctation of the aorta, endocrine and metabolic disorders, neurologic disease, and drug-related causes.

Of children with significant blood pressure elevations, the vast majority has renal or renovascular disease as the underlying cause. Renal arterial disease is a common etiology in the sick neonate and is usually caused by renal artery thrombosis resulting from the use of umbilical artery catheters or from polycythemia. Renal parenchymal diseases, including glomerulonephritis, obstructive uropathy, and hemolytic uremic syndrome, are the most common causes of hypertension in children before adolescence.

Coarctation of the aorta is the primary cardiovascular cause of hypertension. Coarctation should be ruled out early in the course of the evaluation, because this treatable cause of hypertension can result in fixed vascular changes if not detected before adolescence. The heart itself is primarily an *end-organ* in which hypertension can have long-term detrimental effects, as opposed to having any important etiologic role in hypertension. Endocrine causes include pheochromocytoma and congenital adrenal hyperplasia. Diabetes mellitus is frequently complicated by renal involvement and associated hypertension. Increased intracranial pressure from a tumor, trauma, or meningitis will produce acute, severe hypertension and is a medical emergency. Common causes of elevated blood pressure include the use of corticosteroids, oral contraceptives, and sympathomimetic drugs (e.g., those found in over-the-counter cold preparations), and cocaine or amphetamine abuse.

## Incidence

Hypertension is increasingly seen in children, with an overall prevalence of approximately 3 to 5 per 100 children (Gralia, Yehle, Ahmed, et al., 2015). A growing concern is the rapid increase in overweight children and adolescents, of which 30% are diagnosed with hypertension (Gralia et al., 2015). The majority of these children have only mild elevations of blood pressure, and those with significant blood pressure elevations often have secondary hypertension. Because adult hypertension is more prevalent in the black and Asian populations, adolescents from these racial groups should be monitored carefully. Children in families who have members with hypertension tend to have higher-than-normal blood pressures. Because of the increasing prevalence of hypertension in young children, the AHA recommends blood pressure measurements for all children beginning at 3 years of age, and earlier in children with underlying cardiac or renal disease or certain other underlying medical conditions (Lande, 2016).

## PATHOPHYSIOLOGY

### *Hypertension*

Systolic pressure reflects the stroke volume of the heart, the rate of blood ejected, and the elasticity of the aorta. Diastolic pressure reflects the resting pressure of the arterial system; it is affected by the peripheral vascular resistance or the diameter of the arteries and the heart rate. An increase in the heart rate decreases the diastolic or ventricular filling time. Together, these measurements form the arterial blood pressure and provide information about arterial function.

Hypertension, or increased arterial blood pressure over time, can cause cardiac enlargement and subsequent cardiac failure, cerebrovascular disease, renal disease and failure, retinal disease, accelerated atherosclerosis, and coronary heart disease. These effects are seen predominantly with primary or essential hypertension.

## Manifestations

Children with primary hypertension rarely have clinical evidence of disease; the elevated blood pressure is usually detected on a routine physical examination. However, high elevations of blood pressure can lead to the following manifestations:

- Essential or primary hypertension—dizziness, headaches, epistaxis, and visual disturbances. Late signs of severe or acute hypertension include neurologic deficits, extremity weakness, and cerebrovascular accidents.
- Secondary hypertension—*renal:* weight loss or failure to gain weight, facial or periorbital edema, pale mucous membranes, and unilateral or bilateral abdominal mass; *cardiovascular:* absent or decreased femoral pulses, decreased blood pressure in the lower extremities compared with the upper extremities, cardiomegaly, murmur, and signs and symptoms of HF.

## Diagnostic Evaluation

Differentiating primary from secondary hypertension requires a comprehensive medical history and physical examination. Blood pressure measurements are done on all four extremities and repeated twice if elevated. Blood tests (complete blood cell count; blood urea nitrogen, creatinine, uric acid, and electrolyte levels), urinalysis, ECHO, ultrasonography of the kidneys, and arteriography can rule out causes of secondary hypertension. Urinary catecholamines can be considered to rule out pheochromocytoma.

The diagnosis of primary, or essential, hypertension is established primarily by excluding an underlying disease. A hypertensive preadolescent or adolescent with a family history of hypertension is more likely to have primary hypertension as opposed to secondary hypertension. For younger age-groups, secondary causes of hypertension are much more prevalent.

## Therapeutic Management

### Primary Hypertension

Treatment of primary, or essential, hypertension during childhood emphasizes risk factor modification. Lifestyle counseling focuses on non-pharmacologic therapy that includes weight reduction, physical conditioning, dietary modifications, and stress modification. If the non-pharmacologic treatments are maximized, the need for pharmacologic therapy in children with hypertension should be reduced.

***Weight reduction.*** A direct relationship exists between obesity and hypertension. This relationship is caused in part by increased sympathetic nervous system activity. Weight maintenance (children) or gradual weight reduction (adolescents) plays an important role in lowering blood pressure. Weight loss requires a program of diet, exercise, and lifestyle changes, and it is often very difficult to achieve significant results in asymptomatic young people. Even so, a modest 5- to 10-lb weight loss can have a positive effect on blood pressure reduction. Because of the long-term nature of primary hypertension, efforts should focus on education regarding a healthy lifestyle and the gradual incorporation of good dietary habits and activity into the child's everyday life. Success frequently depends on support from healthcare professionals, nutritionists, and family members.

***Physical conditioning.*** An exercise program should be initiated in conjunction with a dietary weight reduction plan. Exercise not only facilitates weight loss, it also lowers blood pressure independent of weight loss. Thirty to 60 minutes of aerobic exercise several times per week can result in a consistently lower resting blood pressure. Recently, studies have also suggested that any increase in total physical activity during the day, such as climbing a flight of stairs several times per day instead of using an elevator, can show measurable benefit over months and years. The most successful approach in children and adolescents is to focus on activities that they enjoy and that provide a social outlet, such as organized sports or bike riding. Exercise in which the whole family can participate, such as walking or hiking, is also more likely to be successful in terms of maintaining a consistent lifestyle change.

***Dietary modification.*** Avoidance of a high sodium intake is recommended in hypertensive and normotensive children and adolescents.

Evidence suggests an association between alcohol and hypertension, believed to be related to alterations in the renin-angiotensin system and neurotransmitters. Smoking produces an aldosterone-like hypertension in young people. Therefore, avoidance of alcohol and tobacco is recommended.

**Relaxation techniques.** Relaxation techniques have resulted in modest reductions in blood pressure in the adult population. Information on efficacy in children is not yet available.

**Pharmacologic treatment.** Pharmacologic treatment of primary hypertension may be indicated if there is coexisting secondary hypertension, or if lifestyle modifications are ineffective. Diuretics, beta-adrenergic receptor blockers, and vasodilators are the mainstay of pharmacologic treatment. Pharmacologic therapy usually is begun with a diuretic and/or a beta-adrenergic receptor blocker; a vasodilator is added if these are not effective (Lande, 2016; Park, 2014).

### Secondary Hypertension

Treatment of the underlying process is the focus of therapy in secondary hypertension. If the secondary disease is coarctation of the aorta or renal artery disease, surgery may be indicated. Therapy in patients with renal parenchymal or endocrine pathologic conditions focuses on the disease process. Effective treatment will often result in secondary control of blood pressure.

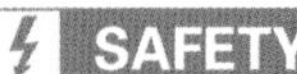

**SAFETY ALERT**

***Infusing Intravenous Antihypertensive Medications***

Intravenous antihypertensive medications must be infused very slowly, and an arterial line is often placed for continuous monitoring. Sudden hypotension can occur after initiation of antihypertensive drugs.

## NURSING CARE

### The Child With Hypertension

#### Assessment

**Blood pressure screening.** Blood pressure screening should be initiated when a child is 3 years old and should continue through adolescence. Blood pressure should be checked at least yearly and more often if the blood pressure reading is higher than recommended. The environment should be as quiet as possible, and the child's arm should be supported at the heart level. If an elevated blood pressure is found, measurement should be repeated two more times, allowing a 2- to 3-minute interval between blood pressure checks.

Cuff size is of critical importance. A too-small blood pressure cuff will result in an inappropriately high blood pressure reading. (See Chapter 37 for cuff measurement and selection.)

**Physical assessment.** Assessment of a child with hypertension includes inspection of the skin to detect evidence of underlying disease, including edema (renal disease) and the presence of café-au-lait spots (neurofibromatosis) or moon facies (Cushing syndrome, steroid administration). The pulses should be palpated for symmetry and strength. A child with coarctation of the aorta is likely to have bounding upper extremity pulses and diminished or absent femoral and pedal pulses. The heart and chest are auscultated to determine the heart rate and to detect any heart murmur, gallop, or aortic bruit. The abdomen is auscultated for renal bruits. A neurologic examination is urgently indicated in children with acute, severe hypertension to rule out increased intracranial pressure.

#### Nursing Diagnosis and Planning

Nursing diagnoses and expected outcomes for the child with hypertension include the following:

- Ineffective Tissue Perfusion (peripheral and cardiovascular) related to elevation in systolic or diastolic arterial blood pressure.

**Expected outcome.** The child will maintain normal tissue perfusion with blood pressure at a controlled level (below the 90th percentile for age).

- Ineffective Therapeutic Regimen Management related to excessive demands of dietary restrictions, physical conditioning, and a possible medication regimen.

**Expected outcome.** The child will describe and will engage in diet, physical conditioning, and medication therapy to lower blood pressure.

#### Interventions

Nursing interventions focus on education and family support and adherence to the treatment regimen. The nurse can consult a dietitian and collaboratively develop a teaching plan regarding a modified-sodium and weight-reduction diet if ordered. When the nurse counsels the family and child about dietary modifications, it is important to include the whole family in making dietary changes to increase motivation and adherence.

If a physical conditioning program is prescribed, physical activities the child enjoys are identified so that they can be incorporated into the plan. Family members and friends are encouraged to join the child in the exercise program. Praise the child for progress in weight loss and increased endurance. Encourage the child to express feelings about any possible problems related to home or school situations. Discuss methods for facilitating relaxation that may be helpful during periods of stress.

The child who is hospitalized with acute, severe hypertension often requires medications. Once the child has been stabilized after an acute hypertensive crisis, oral antihypertensive medications will likely be prescribed. During discharge planning, reinforce the importance of adherence to the medication regimen and of periodic follow-up evaluations.

#### Evaluation

- Does the child maintain blood pressure below the 90th percentile for age?
- Has the child achieved weight loss?
- Is the child adhering to a modified-sodium diet?
- Is the child engaging in regular physical exercise according to the prescribed regimen?
- Is the child adhering to the medication regimen?

## CARDIOMYOPATHIES

The cardiomyopathies are diseases of the heart muscle in which the cardiac pathologic condition is not the result of CHD, coronary artery disease, or other systemic disease. Cardiomyopathy is classified into three types on the basis of the size and function of the ventricles:

- *Dilated:* Decreased contractility and dilation of the ventricles without an increase in wall thickness (hypertrophy). There are congenital or genetic forms and acquired forms caused by infection or toxin exposure.
- *Hypertrophic:* Hypertrophy of the ventricles, generally with improved contractility but impaired ventricular filling because of increased "stiffness" of the ventricular walls. The interior chamber size of the ventricle may be decreased. Left ventricular outflow tract

obstruction can occur and cause sudden death. Hypertrophic cardiomyopathy is considered a genetic disorder.

- *Restrictive:* Impaired ventricular filling usually caused by infiltration of the muscle with abnormal material. The ventricular size and contractility are usually fairly normal. It can be congenital or acquired.

Hypertrophic cardiomyopathy (HCM), with a prevalence in adults of 1 in 500 is one of the major causes of sudden cardiac death in adolescents (Miller, Wang, & Ware, 2013). Approximately 50% of the cases of sudden death in athletes are related to HCM. Predicting sudden cardiac death from this cause is difficult because children with this disorder can have completely normal physical examination findings.

The assessment data that best predict whether a child or adolescent is at risk are a family history of early or sudden cardiac death or a family history of HCM; the condition has a genetic predisposition (Park, 2014). If the adolescent is symptomatic, the most frequently seen signs and symptoms include dyspnea or chest pain with exertion, palpitations, presyncope, and syncope. Infants and children may fatigue easily. The thickened left ventricle is poorly compliant (stiff) and has impaired filling, causing pulmonary venous congestion and associated exertional dyspnea and orthopnea. On auscultation, the heart sounds are normal, and there is often a systolic murmur at the left sternal border or apex. The murmur will characteristically vary in intensity depending on position or recent exertion.

The ECG can demonstrate left ventricular hypertrophy, deep Q waves, and ST-T abnormalities. Affected individuals should have a Holter monitor test to screen for asymptomatic ventricular dysrhythmias. The chest radiograph may show mild cardiomegaly. The diagnosis is usually established by echocardiogram, often with concentric or localized ventricular hypertrophy of the left and often the right ventricle.

All children with diagnosed HCM should be restricted from strenuous exertion and competitive sports. Beta blockade or calcium channel blockade (verapamil) is frequently used, especially in children with obstructive HCM, to decrease ventricular hypercontractility and outflow tract obstruction. Beta blockade is also used as prophylaxis against ventricular dysrhythmias. Prophylactic therapy may be started in asymptomatic children with HCM, especially in case of a family history of sudden death, though this remains controversial (Park, 2014).

Surgery is indicated in children who are symptomatic or have severe outflow tract obstruction despite medical management. The most common procedure is a septal myomectomy, which is the resection of a portion of the left ventricular septum to relieve obstruction. This procedure often results in an improvement in symptoms and carries low surgical mortality risk but does not decrease the mortality rate of the disease itself.

A newer intervention is insertion of a pacemaker, which, by depolarizing the ventricle, causes dyssynchronous ventricular contraction and decreased outflow tract obstruction. In addition, an implantable defibrillator pacemaker is available for children with life-threatening dysrhythmias. The surgical risk of pacemaker or defibrillator insertion is much lower than that of myomectomy, and these options are likely to be used increasingly as long-term outcome data become available.

## HIGH CHOLESTEROL LEVELS IN CHILDREN AND ADOLESCENTS

Preventive cardiology has become increasingly important during childhood and adolescence. Developing heart-healthy habits during these years reduces the risk of coronary artery disease and other cardiovascular problems during adulthood. Several major risk factors during childhood and adolescence appear routinely in the literature, including the following:

- Tobacco use
- High low-density lipoproteins (LDLs) and low high-density lipoproteins (HDLs)
- Hypertension (greater than the 90th percentile)
- Decreased physical activity
- Obesity
- Family history
- Type I or 2 diabetes mellitus

Recent statistics on overweight and obesity reveal that approximately 17% (12.7 million) of children and adolescents aged 2 to 19 years are obese (CDC, 2014).

### Assessment of Children at Risk

High cholesterol levels (dyslipidemia) can be the result of genetic or dietary factors or a combination thereof. Since 2011, the AAP has recommended that all children have a lipid profile checked once between the ages of 9 and 11 years and again between the ages of 17 and 21 years (Neal & John, 2016; Park, 2014). This recommendation is a change from the targeted approach, testing only those who were deemed high risk.

### Therapeutic Management

Children older than 2 years can follow a sensible, low-fat dietary program. Such a diet includes nonfat or low-fat dairy products; limiting red meat intake; and increasing the intake of fish, vegetables, whole grains, and legumes. Children should avoid excessive intake of fruit juices and other sweetened drinks, sugars, and saturated fats. Adequate intake of dietary fiber and avoidance of processed foods also contribute to lowering LDL levels (Neal & John, 2016). Young children with elevated or borderline LDL levels should have their saturated fat and dietary intake monitored more closely. These children should limit their intake of saturated fat to less than 7% of total daily calories and reduce cholesterol intake to less than 200 mg/day (Neal & John, 2016).

Other factors that contribute to a healthy lifestyle in children and adolescents include increased physical activity and avoidance of a sedentary lifestyle (e.g., excessive television watching) and monitoring for coronary heart disease risk factors.

Cholesterol-lowering medications are used for children who do not respond to dietary modifications after a period of 6 months (Neal & John, 2016). A variety of medications are used to treat high LDLs in children, and these include the statins, bile acid-binding resins (e.g., cholestyramine, colestipol), nicotinic acid, and cholesterol absorption inhibitors (Neal & John, 2016).

### Nursing Considerations

The most effective approach to decreasing risk factors during childhood and adolescence appears to be both population-based and individual-targeted, with continuing education about risk factors occurring in communities, schools, physicians' offices, and the media. Nurses play an important part in educating parents and children about healthy diets, the importance of regular exercise, and reducing other risk factors (see Chapter 8).

## KEY CONCEPTS

- With the neonate's first breath, gas exchange is transferred from the placenta to the lungs. The fetal shunts (ductus venosus, ductus arteriosus, foramen ovale) close, and resistance to flow in the pulmonary system decreases as systemic resistance increases. Pulmonary vascular resistance decreases, and a marked increase in pulmonary blood flow follows.
- Stenosis can occur in a valve or a vessel and can result in obstruction of blood flow through the area.
- In left-to-right shunts, blood is shunted to the right side of the heart because the pressure is lower on the right side and higher on the left. Oxygenated (saturated) and unoxygenated (desaturated) blood mix. Systemic saturations are normal.
- Poor weight gain with failure to thrive is a common sign of HF.
- Hypercyanotic episodes, or "tet spells," are characterized by increased respiratory rate, increased depth of respiration, and severe hypoxemia.
- Assessment of the family of a child with a congenital cardiac defect should begin at diagnosis and continue throughout the care of the child.
- Common nursing diagnoses associated with infants with congenital heart defects and their parents include Decreased Cardiac Output, Imbalanced Nutrition: Less than Body Requirements, Activity Intolerance, Deficient Knowledge, Anxiety, Interrupted Family Processes, Risk for Infection, and Risk for Ineffective Health Maintenance.
- Signs of HF include tachycardia, cardiomegaly, gallop rhythm, decreased peripheral perfusion, excessive diaphoresis, weight gain, ascites, liver and spleen enlargement, edema, neck vein distention, dyspnea, rales, tachypnea, intercostal muscular and sternal retractions, and wheezing.
- Measures to decrease the workload on the heart include limiting the time the child is allowed to breastfeed or bottle-feed, elevating the head of the bed, allowing for uninterrupted rest periods, allowing self-limiting activity, and providing oxygen (cautious use with left-to-right shunting lesions) during stressful periods.
- It is imperative to educate parents regarding medications, monitoring for signs and symptoms of HF, increasing cyanosis, dehydration, infection, dysrhythmias (when indicated), infective endocarditis prophylaxis, decreased nutritional intake, and decreasing ill contacts in the environment as the family is prepared for home discharge with infants or children with HF and CHD.
- Prophylaxis with penicillin is the most important aspect of therapeutic management for RF. Intramuscular injection is the route of choice. Oral medication is an alternative, if given precisely and faithfully.
- In Kawasaki disease, coronary aneurysms can occur approximately 11 days after the onset of fever.
- Nursing management of a child with Kawasaki disease includes administering IVIG and aspirin to reduce the formation of the aneurysms and fever.
- The initial management of children with primary hypertension includes diet modification, reduction of weight (when needed), physical conditioning, and relaxation techniques.
- An appropriate-size blood pressure cuff, two repeat blood pressure readings on all four extremities, and a careful medical history are important in assessment for a diagnosis of hypertension.
- The heart rate is usually faster in infants and children than in adults and decreases with age.
- Population-based education of children and parents is the most effective way to prevent the cardiac consequences of high cholesterol levels.

## REFERENCES AND READINGS


American Academy of Pediatrics Committee on Infectious Diseases. (2015a). Prevention of Bacterial Endocarditis. In L.K. Pickering, C.J. Baker, & D.W. Kimberlin (Eds.), *Red book 2009 report of the committee on infectious diseases* (30th ed., pp. 970–971). Elk Grove Village, IL: American Academy of Pediatrics.

American Academy of Pediatrics Committee on Infectious Diseases. (2015b). Group A Streptococcal Infections. In L.K. Pickering, C.J. Baker, & D.W. Kimberlin (Eds.), *Red book 2009 report of the committee on infectious diseases* (30th ed., pp. 732–744). Elk Grove Village, IL: American Academy of Pediatrics.

American Academy of Pediatrics Committee on Infectious Diseases. (2015c). Kawasaki disease. In L.K. Pickering, C.J. Baker, & D.W. Kimberlin (Eds.), *Red book 2009 report of the committee on infectious diseases* (30th ed., pp. 494-500). Elk Grove Village, IL: American Academy of Pediatrics.

American Academy of Pediatrics. (2016a). *Newborn Screening for Critical Congenital Heart Disease.* Retrieved from http://www.aap.org/en-us/advocacy-and-policy/state-advocacy/Documents/Newborn%20Screening%20for%20Critical%20Congenital%20Heart%20Disease.pdf.

American Academy of Pediatrics. (2016b). *Risk factors for CHD.* Retrieved from http://www.aap.org/en-us/advocacy-and-policy/aap-health-initiatives/chphc/Pages/Risk-Factors-For-CHD.aspx.

American Heart Association. (2015). *Understand your risk for congenital heart defects.* Retrieved from http://www.heart.org/HEARTORG/Conditions/CongenitalHeartDefects/UnderstandYourRiskforCongenitalHeartDefects/Understand-Your-Risk-for-Congenital-Heart-Defects_UCM_001219_Article.jsp#.VxKpxjArKM8.

Bernstein, D. (2016a). Congenital heart disease. In R. Kliegman, B. Stanton, J. St. Geme, et al. (Eds.), *Nelson textbook of pediatrics* (20th ed., pp. 2182–2187). Philadelphia: Elsevier.

Bernstein, D. (2016b). Heart failure. In R. Kliegman, B. Stanton, J. St. Geme, et al. (Eds.), *Nelson textbook of pediatrics* (20th ed., pp. 2282–2288). Philadelphia: Elsevier.

Bernstein, D. (2016c). Primary pulmonary hypertension. In R. Kliegman, B. Stanton, J. St. Geme, et al. (Eds.), *Nelson textbook of pediatrics* (20th ed., pp. 2239–2241). Philadelphia: Elsevier.

Bernstein, D. (2016d). Pulmonary vascular disease (Eisenmenger syndrome). In R. Kliegman, B. Stanton, J. St. Geme, et al. (Eds.), *Nelson textbook of pediatrics* (20th ed., pp. 2241–2243). Philadelphia: Elsevier.

Bernstein, D. (2016e). Cyanotic congenital heart lesions associated with decreased pulmonary blood flow. In R. Kliegman, B. Stanton, J. St. Geme, et al. (Eds.), *Nelson textbook of pediatrics* (20th ed., pp. 2211–2222). Philadelphia: Elsevier.

Bernstein, D. (2016f). Diagnostic and interventional catheterization. In R. Kliegman, B. Stanton, J. St. Geme, et al. (Eds.), *Nelson textbook of pediatrics* (20th ed., pp. 2180-2182). Philadelphia: Elsevier.

Bernstein, D. (2016g). Infective endocarditis. In R. Kliegman, B. Stanton, J. St. Geme, et al. (Eds.), *Nelson textbook of pediatrics* (20th ed., pp. 2263–2268). Philadelphia: Elsevier.

Bernstein, D. (2016h). Rheumatic heart disease. In R. Kliegman, B. Stanton, J. St. Geme, et al. (Eds.), *Nelson textbook of pediatrics* (20th ed., pp. 2269–2271). Philadelphia: Elsevier.

Boyle, L., Kelly, M.M., Reynolds, K., et al. (2015). The school age child with congenital heart disease. *Maternal Child Nursing, 40*(1), 16–23. doi:10.1097/NMC.0000000000000092.

Centers for Disease Control and Prevention. (2014). *Childhood obesity facts*. Retrieved from: http://www.cdc.gov/obesity/data/childhood.html.

Centers for Disease Control and Prevention. (2016). *Facts about Down syndrome*. Retrieved from http://www.cdc.gov/ncbddd/birthdefects/DownSyndrome.html.

Emergency Nurses Association. (2012). *Emergency nursing pediatric course provider manual* (4th ed.). Des Plains, IL: Author.

Gralia, N.M., Yehle, K.S., Ahmed, A., et al. (2015). Managing hypertension among obese children in primary care: updated evidence. *The Journal for Nurse Practitioners, 11*(3), 328–334. doi:10.1016/j.nurpra.2014.11.003.

Huether, S.E., & McCance, K.L. (2017). *Understanding pathophysiology*. St. Louis: Elsevier.

Kogelschatz, C.J., & King, M.A. (2012). Six-year-old girl with abnormal movements and emotional lability. *Contemporary Pediatrics, 29*(10), 4–50.

Lande, M.B. (2016). Systemic hypertension. In R. Kliegman, B. Stanton, J. St. Geme, et al. (Eds.), *Nelson textbook of pediatrics* (20th ed., pp. 2294–2303). Philadelphia: Elsevier.

Miller, E.M., Wang, Y., & Ware, S.M. (2013). Uptake of cardiac screening and genetic testing among hypertrophic and dilated cardiomyopathy families. *Journal of Genetic Counsel, 22*, 258–267. doi: 10.1007/s10897-012-9544-4.

Neal, W.A., & John, C.C. (2016). Disorders of lipoprotein metabolism and transport. In R. Kliegman, B. Stanton, J. St. Geme, et al. (Eds.), *Nelson textbook of pediatrics* (20th ed., pp. 691–705). Philadelphia: Elsevier.

Park, M. K. (2014). *Pediatric cardiology for practitioners* (6th ed.). Philadelphia: Elsevier.

Paul, S.P., Blaikley, S., Peevers, C., et al. (2012). Acute supraventricular tachycardia in children. *Emergency Nurse, 20*(6), 26–29.

Rowley, A.H. (2012). Kawasaki disease: genetics, pathology, and a need for earlier diagnosis and treatment. *Contemporary Pediatrics, 29*(12), 18–24.

Slipczuk, L., Codolosa, J.N., Davila, C.D., et al. (2013). Infective endocarditis epidemiology over five decades: a systematic review. *PLoS One, 8*(13), 1–17. doi:10.1371/journal.pone.0082665.

Son, M.B., & Newburger, J.W. (2016). Kawasaki disease. In R. Kliegman, B. Stanton, J. St. Geme, et al. (Eds.),. *Nelson textbook of pediatrics* (20th ed., pp. 1209–1214). Philadelphia: Elsevier.

Van Hare, G.F. (2016). Disturbances of rate and rhythm of the heart. In R. Kliegman, B. Stanton, J. St. Geme, et al. (Eds.), *Nelson textbook of pediatrics* (20th ed., pp. 2250–2261). Philadelphia: Elsevier.

Wilson, M., Taubert, K., Gewitz, M., et al. (2007). Prevention of infective endocarditis: Guidelines from the American Heart Association: A guideline from the American Heart Association Rheumatic Fever, Endocarditis and Kawasaki Disease Committee, Council on Cardiovascular Disease in the Young and the Council on Clinical Cardiology, Council on Cardiovascular Surgery and Anesthesia, and the Quality of Care and Outcomes Research Interdisciplinary Working Group. *Circulation, 116*, 1736–1754.

# 47

# The Child With a Hematologic Alteration

http://evolve.elsevier.com/McKinney/mat-ch/

## LEARNING OBJECTIVES

*After studying this chapter, you should be able to:*

- Describe the anatomy and physiology of the hematopoietic system.
- Discuss the pediatric differences related to blood and blood formation.
- Discuss the role of the nurse in the prevention of iron deficiency anemia.
- Describe common factors in the care of a child with anemia.
- Discuss the pathophysiology and therapeutic management of common hematologic alterations.
- List possible nursing diagnoses for children with hematologic alterations.
- Describe possible nursing care for children with hematologic alterations.

## CLINICAL REFERENCE

### REVIEW OF THE HEMATOLOGIC SYSTEM

Hematology is the study of the blood and blood-forming tissues. In fetal life, various tissues produce erythrocytes (red blood cells), but after birth, their production is controlled exclusively by the bone marrow, primarily in the long bones. With age, the more membranous bones of the vertebrae, sternum, and ribs assume red blood cell (RBC) production. Age, sex, and the altitude at which a person lives affect the number of RBCs.

Normally, RBCs are biconcave disks that are capable of changing shape as they flow through the microvasculature of the body. They have a fairly uniform size that is determined mainly by the amount of cellular content of substances, primarily hemoglobin. Their function is to transport oxygen to tissues. Essential to this ability to carry oxygen is an appropriate amount of hemoglobin, whose production depends on sufficient amounts of circulating iron. Iron is absorbed from dietary intake by the intestines and stored by the liver in both soluble and insoluble forms, to be used when necessary.

The stimulus for production of RBCs is a decrease in circulating oxygen, which in turn stimulates the kidneys to produce a hormone called *erythropoietin*. Erythropoietin stimulates the production of RBC precursors and causes them to mature rapidly. Disorders of the kidney can affect the individual's ability to produce this hormone, and thus, can affect RBC production by the bone marrow.

*Anemia* is a decrease in the number of RBCs, reduction in their hemoglobin content, or reduced volume of packed RBCs. Anemia results from one of two problems; either too rapid a loss of RBCs (by covert or overt bleeding or destruction) or too slow a production of RBCs. Anemias are categorized according to the size of the RBC (macrocytic, microcytic, normocytic) and the content of hemoglobin in the RBC (hypochromic, normochromic).

Polycythemia, which is an increase in the number of RBCs, is less frequently seen than anemia. *Polycythemia* can occur as a result of hypoxia, such as that experienced at high altitude or when oxygen is not sufficiently directed to the tissues, as in cyanotic heart disease.

White blood cells (WBCs) or leukocytes are formed in the bone marrow and in lymphatic tissue. They assist in the body's ability to distinguish "self" from "nonself." WBCs destroy foreign cells through the processes of phagocytosis and antibody production. Both phagocytes and antibodies destroy foreign cells and tissues perceived by the body as nonself (including, e.g., bacteria, fungi, viruses, parasites, and transplanted tissue) (see Chapter 42). WBC disorders result from an altered rate of production of WBCs (lymphocytosis or lymphopenia) or an alteration in cell function.

#### Pediatric Hematologic System

Three important types of cells are formed in the bone marrow: red blood cells (RBCs), white blood cells (WBCs), and platelets.

Red blood cells are produced initially in the marrow of all bones. After 5 years of age, RBC production in the shafts of the long bones (tibia, femur) is reduced, and production ceases in these locations entirely at the age of 20 years. After 20 years of age, **hematopoiesis** takes place primarily in the marrow of the ribs, sternum, vertebrae, pelvis, skull, clavicles, and scapulas.

The number of erythrocytes (RBCs) varies according to age. The fetus has a higher oxygen-carrying capacity than an infant because of their considerably higher number of RBCs, with proportionately elevated hemoglobin and hematocrit values.

The life span of RBCs in neonates is shorter than in older infants and children because of increased destruction during rapid growth.

By 2 months of age, **erythropoiesis** increases, leading to increased **reticulocytes** in the blood and a rise in hemoglobin.

## Types and Functions of White Blood Cells

- **Granulocytes:** Phagocytic cells produced in the bone marrow and found in the circulation. These cells include:
  - Neutrophils: Primary defense in bacterial infection; capable of phagocytizing and killing bacteria
  - Eosinophils: Influence the inflammatory process, fight parasites, and influence allergic hypersensitivity reactions
  - Basophils: Activate the inflammatory response; contain histamine; other roles are unclear
- **Agranulocytes:** Participate in inflammatory and immune reactions. These cells include:
  - Monocytes/macrophages: Phagocytize large cells, including necrotic tissue; therefore, important in fighting chronic infection
  - Lymphocytes: Found in bone marrow, spleen, thymus, lymph glands, tissues, and circulation
  - T cells: Made in the thymus and responsible for cell-mediated immunity
  - B cells: Responsible for humoral immunity (antibody production)
  - Natural killer cells: Lymphocyte-like cells that can kill certain types of tumor cells and viruses directly

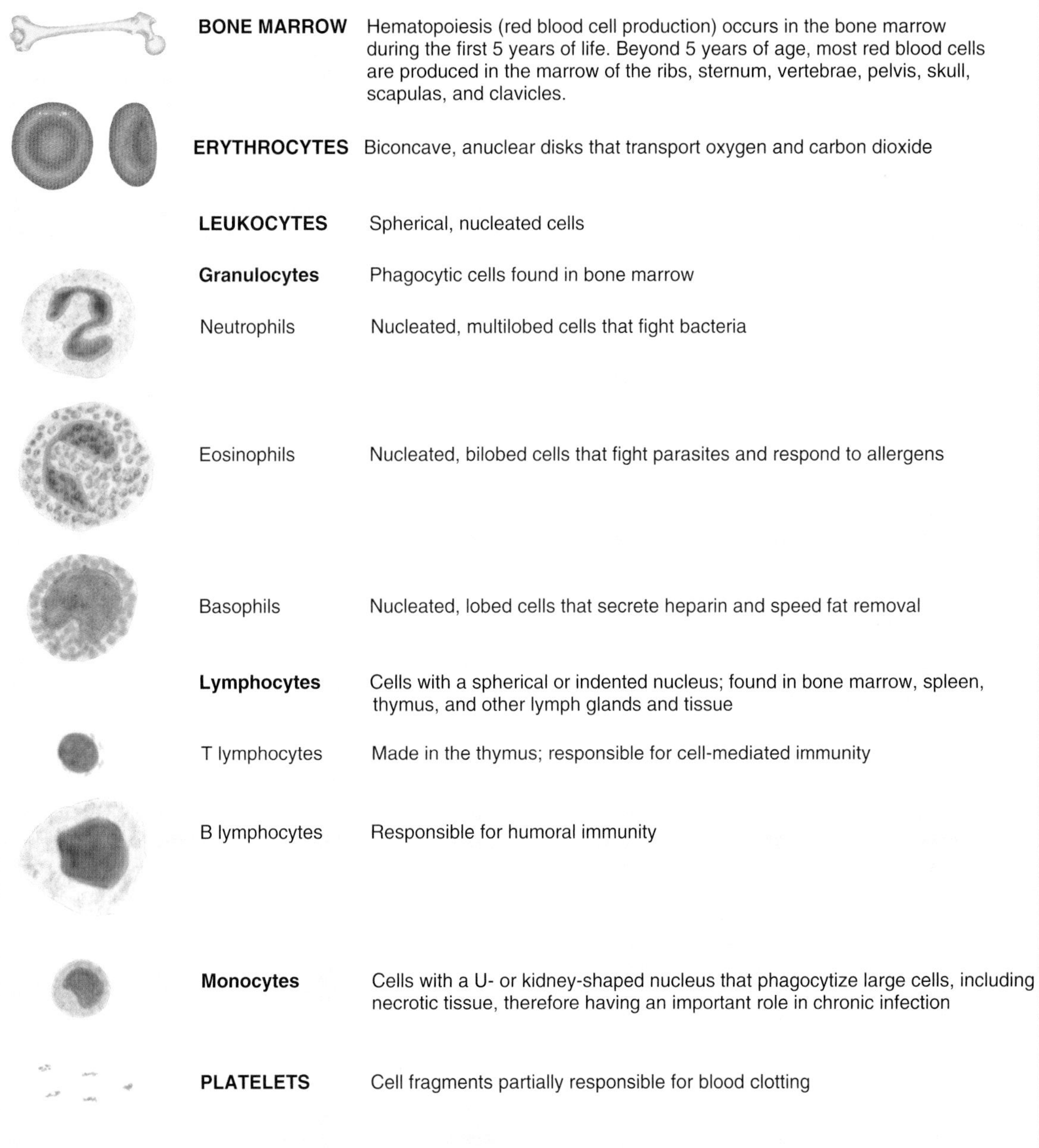

| | |
|---|---|
| **BONE MARROW** | Hematopoiesis (red blood cell production) occurs in the bone marrow during the first 5 years of life. Beyond 5 years of age, most red blood cells are produced in the marrow of the ribs, sternum, vertebrae, pelvis, skull, scapulas, and clavicles. |
| **ERYTHROCYTES** | Biconcave, anuclear disks that transport oxygen and carbon dioxide |
| **LEUKOCYTES** | Spherical, nucleated cells |
| **Granulocytes** | Phagocytic cells found in bone marrow |
| Neutrophils | Nucleated, multilobed cells that fight bacteria |
| Eosinophils | Nucleated, bilobed cells that fight parasites and respond to allergens |
| Basophils | Nucleated, lobed cells that secrete heparin and speed fat removal |
| **Lymphocytes** | Cells with a spherical or indented nucleus; found in bone marrow, spleen, thymus, and other lymph glands and tissue |
| T lymphocytes | Made in the thymus; responsible for cell-mediated immunity |
| B lymphocytes | Responsible for humoral immunity |
| **Monocytes** | Cells with a U- or kidney-shaped nucleus that phagocytize large cells, including necrotic tissue, therefore having an important role in chronic infection |
| **PLATELETS** | Cell fragments partially responsible for blood clotting |

**Review of the Hematologic System**

Platelets are the cells that promote hemostasis—the prevention of blood loss. They are formed in the bone marrow from megakaryocytes. Megakaryocytes later fragment into smaller cells known as *platelets,* either in the bone marrow or shortly after release into the systemic circulation. Platelets can circulate in the blood for approximately 10 days before they die; however, disease, fever, and infection can shorten a platelet's lifetime. Platelet disorders occur when the bone marrow cannot meet the production demands of the body.

When caring for infants and children with blood disorders, the nurse is challenged in the areas of preventive, acute, and chronic care. Depending on the disorder and the child's condition, care may be provided in the home, an outpatient setting, or the hospital. It is not unusual for a child to be seen in an outpatient setting (clinic, school), referred to a hospital for diagnosis and stabilization, and returned to the home for maintenance. Genetic counseling may be indicated for children or families with certain types of blood disorders.

Many medications for hematologic disorders can be given at home, including deferoxamine mesylate (Desferal), intravenous immune globulin (IVIG), intravenous (IV) antibiotics, coagulation factor products, and, in some instances, even blood transfusions. Parents are learning to manage infusion therapy in regard to initiating, monitoring, and discontinuing infusions when appropriate, with guidance from the collaborative efforts of the multidisciplinary healthcare team.

## IRON DEFICIENCY ANEMIA

Iron deficiency is the most common cause of anemia during infancy, childhood, and adolescence. Iron deficiency anemia (IDA) can be mild or marked.

### Etiology and Incidence

Several factors can contribute to IDA, including decreased iron intake, increased iron or blood loss, and periods of increased growth rate.

IDA related to inadequate dietary iron intake is rare before age 4 to 6 months because of the presence of maternal iron stores; it occurs most often in children age 9 to 24 months as iron stores are depleted. Premature infants can develop iron deficiency early in life because they are born with insufficient maternal iron stores (Sills, 2016). Delaying cord clamping by 1 to 3 minutes can decrease the risk for iron deficiency (Sills, 2016). Decreased iron intake is often related to the intake of large amounts of cow's milk instead of breast milk or fortified formula and iron-fortified foods (Powers & Buchanan, 2014). The incidence has dropped in recent years because of increased education about and availability of iron-fortified formula and cereals. Early transition from breast milk or infant formula to cow's milk can precipitate chronic diarrhea with occult intestinal bleeding in children younger than 2 years. This response results from exposure to a protein found in cow's milk (Powers & Buchanan, 2014). The rapid growth of infants and children younger than 2 years, if combined with decreased iron intake, further contributes to the increased incidence in this age-group.

Adolescents are also at risk for IDA because they too are undergoing increased growth and often have poor dietary habits. The situation is further complicated by the blood loss during menstruation in young women.

### Manifestations

The clinical manifestations of IDA vary with the degree of anemia but can include extreme pallor with porcelain-like skin, pale mucous membranes and conjunctiva, tachycardia, tachypnea, lethargy, fatigue, and irritability. Children with lead poisoning often have associated IDA. Consequences of undetected iron deficiency anemia are associated neurodevelopmental issues such as lower IQ and poor executive functioning (Powers, McCavit, & Buchanan, 2015).

### Diagnostic Evaluation

Any child with anemia should first have a complete history taken, with particular emphasis on assessment of nutritional intake. The results of a complete blood count (CBC) in individuals with IDA will show low hemoglobin levels (6 to 11 g/dL) and microcytic, hypochromic RBCs, reflected in a decreased mean cell volume (MCV) and decreased mean cell hemoglobin (MCH). The reticulocyte count is usually normal or slightly elevated. With these findings, serum ferritin levels and serum iron or iron-binding capacity should be assessed. The total iron-binding capacity (TIBC) is usually elevated as a result of decreased serum iron levels. Serum ferritin and serum iron are low. Hemoglobin electrophoresis can rule out causes other than IDA.

### Therapeutic Management

Therapy is directed toward increasing the dietary intake of iron and iron supplementation. The absorption of iron from dietary iron-rich foods is unreliable and does not rapidly provide the body with enough iron to correct an iron deficiency. Therefore, affected children are given a daily oral iron preparation of one of the available ferrous salts (ferrous sulfate, ferrous gluconate, or ferrous fumarate) based on the content of elemental iron (dose should be 3 to 6 mg/kg/day [2 to 4 mg/kg/day for premature infants] in three equally divided doses). Iron supplements should be given on an empty stomach 1 to 2 hours before or after meals with vitamin C-rich fluids for ideal absorption. Nurses should educate parents about common side effects of iron administration such as staining of the teeth, dark stools, and constipation (Powers & Buchanan, 2014).

Follow-up monitoring includes a CBC, reticulocyte count, and serum ferritin. The reticulocyte count should increase within days of the initiation of iron therapy. An increased hemoglobin level can be expected in 4 to 30 days. The response to iron therapy can often be positively predicted, so blood transfusions are rarely indicated to correct IDA. RBC transfusions are reserved for severe anemia and cardiovascular compromise. Oral iron therapy will be continued for 3 to 4 months after hemoglobin and hematocrit levels return to normal to replenish the child's iron stores. Thereafter, administration of a daily multivitamin with iron can be recommended.

## SICKLE CELL DISEASE

*Sickle cell disease* (SCD) is the generic term that refers to a group of genetic disorders characterized by the production of sickle hemoglobin (HbS), chronic hemolytic anemia, and ischemic tissue injury. The more common forms of SCD include homozygous sickle cell disease (HbSS) or sickle cell anemia, sickle hemoglobin C disease (HbSC), and the sickle beta-zero thalassemia syndromes. SCD is an inherited, lifelong disease that affects primarily individuals of African, Mediterranean, Indian, and

## PATHOPHYSIOLOGY

### *Iron Deficiency Anemia*

Iron is one of the components necessary for the synthesis of hemoglobin. Without an adequate amount of iron, the bone marrow continues to manufacture red blood cells (RBCs), but their content of hemoglobin is decreased, rendering these RBCs inefficient at carrying oxygen to the tissues. The constellation of clinical signs evident with iron deficiency anemia (IDA) results from compromised tissue oxygenation.

The full-term neonate is born with enough stored maternal iron to produce adequate amounts of hemoglobin for 4 to 6 months. The average life of an RBC is approximately 100 to 120 days. Thus, IDA is usually not seen in children before age 9 months.

As RBCs undergo **hemolysis**, intracellular iron is released into the circulation for use by the body. Adults are able to use this breakdown of RBCs as a primary source of iron. However, children grow very rapidly and expand their circulating blood volume at the same time. Because children must produce additional RBCs to accommodate for their physical growth, their need for iron to synthesize new hemoglobin for RBC production is increased. Therefore, children must increase their dietary consumption of iron. The American Academy of Pediatrics (AAP) recommends screening for anemia at 12 months of age or earlier if assessed at high risk for iron deficiency (Sills, 2016), but the US Preventative Services Task Force (USPSTF) in a 2015 statement concluded that there is insufficient evidence to assess the benefits versus the harm of routine screening for iron deficiency anemia in children aged 6 to 24 months (Siu, 2015).

Iron deficiency can also result from inadequate iron absorption. Various factors can contribute to a lack of absorption of iron by the gastrointestinal tract. When cow's milk is introduced into the diet before age 1 year in place of breast milk or formula, infants do not ingest sufficient iron because cow's milk is a poor dietary source of iron. Often, the potentially large amount of cow's milk replaces iron-fortified cereals and iron-rich baby food. Although iron from breast milk is well absorbed, it is not a complete source of iron, and dietary iron supplements must be introduced to augment its nutrients when the infant is 4 months old (Sills, 2016).

Iron deficiency can be the result of occult intestinal bleeding. Blood loss from an infant's intestine typically occurs very slowly and may have several causes. The immature intestine may be unable to tolerate the protein in cow's milk or milk-based infant formula. Irritation of the bowel results in hemorrhages of the microvasculature, resulting in blood loss in the stool. Although unusual, parasitic infections can also irritate the intestinal lining.

## PARENTS WANT TO KNOW

### *Home Care of the Child With Iron Deficiency Anemia*

**Dietary Changes**

- Provide iron-fortified formula or breast milk with iron-fortified food supplements if the child is younger than 12 months of age.
- If the child is older than 12 months of age, limit intake of cow's milk to 24 oz/day or less.
- Increase the child's intake of age-appropriate iron-rich foods, with selections based on the age of the child: liver, dried beans, Cream of Wheat, iron-fortified cereal, apricots and prunes (and other dried fruits), egg yolks, and dark-green leafy vegetables.

**Administration of Iron**

- Administer iron in one to three divided doses between meals.
- Give with vitamin-C–rich fluids such as orange juice.
- Administer iron through a straw or medicine dropper placed at the back of the mouth, away from the teeth. Brush or wipe off teeth because oral iron can stain the teeth.
- Recognize that iron supplementation causes black, tarry stools.
- Avoid administration of iron with milk or formula and cereal because iron binds with calcium, thus impeding absorption.

**Follow-Up Care**

- Keep appointments for follow-up evaluations.
- Expect blood work to be done at follow-up visits.

## ! NURSING QUALITY ALERT

### *Obtaining a Dietary Intake History*

Parents do not always respond readily or accurately to questions about their child's dietary intake. Ask the parents to begin the dietary history at the time the child awoke yesterday, describing the child's activities and exactly what the child ate. Correlating activities with diet enables the nurse to obtain a better history and become aware of feeding patterns for which counseling is indicated. Determine the number of bottles of milk or juice that the child is taking each day and the size of the bottles. Parents often underestimate the ounces of milk or juice that the child is taking in.

Children with iron deficiency anemia occasionally develop pica. Pica is an appetite for nonnutritive substances such as paper, cardboard, ice, or sometimes dirt. Ask about the intake of nonfood items, because parents may not openly share this information.

Middle Eastern descent. The morbidity and mortality rates for the severe forms of the disease have decreased as a result of newborn screening for the disease, routine prophylactic penicillin administration, and pneumococcal and *Haemophilus influenzae* vaccines.

## Etiology

SCD is a group of hemoglobinopathies in which normal hemoglobin A (HbA) is partially or totally replaced by abnormal hemoglobin, HbS. SCD is an inherited, autosomal recessive condition. Each affected individual carries two copies of the gene that directs the production of hemoglobin. The normal hemoglobin gene is *HbA*. If one parent has the HbS trait (one copy of the *HbA* and one copy of *HbS* gene, genotype *HbAS*) and the other parent does not (both copies *HbA*, genotype *HbAA*), each pregnancy has a 50% risk of the child inheriting the trait. If each parent carries the trait (both parents with genotype *HbAS*), there is a 25% chance that the child will be unaffected *(HbAA)*,

## NURSING CARE PLAN

### The Child With Iron Deficiency Anemia in the Community Setting

**Focused Assessment**

- Obtain history from parents addressing the following:
  - Decrease in child's activity level—more quiet than usual
  - Increased desire to be held
  - Infant given cow's milk before age 12 months
  - Increased milk consumption with exclusion of solid foods for infant and child
  - Child's heart "races" when at rest
- Conduct a physical examination and look for:
  - Pallor
  - Tired appearance
  - Mild to severe tachycardia
  - Heart murmur (due to severe anemia—is reversible)

**Nursing Diagnosis**

Imbalanced Nutrition: Less Than Body Requirements related to parents' lack of knowledge of age-appropriate nutritional needs.

**Planning**

***Expected Outcome***

The parents will have an understanding of the child's nutritional needs, as evidenced by verbal description of the child's dietary plan, including foods containing appropriate dietary iron.

**Interventions and *Rationales***

1. Obtain the child's past and current nutritional history. Instruct the caregiver to continue to give the infant iron-fortified formula or breastfeed and give supplementary iron-fortified foods until age 12 months. For a child older than 12 months, instruct parents to limit cow's milk intake to a maximum of 24 oz/day and increase consumption of iron-rich foods.
   *Cow's milk is poorly digested and is not rich in iron. The American Academy of Pediatrics (AAP) recommends continuing breast milk or iron-fortified formula until age 12 months. Decreasing milk intake will encourage the consumption of other iron-rich and iron-fortified foods (see Patient-Centered Teaching: Home Care of the Child with Iron Deficiency Anemia).*
2. Advise the parent to keep a dietary diary.
   *Keeping a record of food and fluid intake assists with a dietary evaluation and identifies areas for additional teaching.*
3. Explain to parents the need for iron in the manufacture of red blood cells (RBCs), how iron therapy affects laboratory test results, the potential outcome with no intervention, the lack of iron in cow's milk, and iron's effect on the body.
   *Explaining the rationale for therapy can often help improve adherence.*
4. Instruct the parents to administer oral iron supplements as ordered by the primary care provider. Allow parents to practice medication administration, and then evaluate their technique, providing additional instruction as indicated (see Patient-Centered Teaching: Home Care of the Child with Iron Deficiency Anemia).
   *Iron supplements immediately increase iron intake beyond that absorbed from formula or food. Practice and additional instruction will build the parents' skills and confidence in giving their child medication.*
5. Inform parents to give iron supplements with fruit juice and NOT with milk, formula, or cereal; when the child's stomach is empty.
   *An acid stomach environment facilitates absorption. Calcium in milk products binds with iron to decrease iron absorption.*
6. Instruct parents to administer vitamin C as ordered and encourage intake of foods rich in vitamin C.
   *Vitamin C increases the absorption of iron by the body.*
7. Instruct the parents to keep iron supplements (and all medications) out of reach of children and in a locked cabinet.
   *Iron poisoning is possible with overdose. This can be serious and possibly fatal.*
8. Instruct the parents to obtain follow-up laboratory tests when ordered, including reticulocyte count and hemoglobin and hematocrit levels.
   *The reticulocyte count should peak in 5 to 7 days. It is an objective test that can determine the degree of adherence to iron therapy. The hemoglobin level should increase in 4 to 30 days.*
9. Instruct the parents to monitor for and expect to see black, tarry stools. Verify that parents have observed this characteristic.
   *Iron therapy causes black, tarry stools. If absent, it may indicate lack of adherence to therapy.*
10. Refer to social services for enrollment in federal or state programs, if warranted.
    *Poor nutritional practices may be attributable to a lack of resources to obtain appropriate foods.*

**Evaluation**

Does the dietary diary reflect an increase in iron-rich and iron-fortified foods in the child's daily meal plan?
Does the child have normal iron, hemoglobin, and hematocrit levels?
Do the parents demonstrate adherence to the prescribed therapy and verbalize appropriate questions?
Has the child had a recurrence of iron deficiency anemia (IDA)?

## CRITICAL THINKING EXERCISE 47.1

Mrs. Anders has brought 18-month-old Jacob to the clinic because he is irritable, is running a low-grade fever and has a cough. In the process of assessing Jacob, you note that he seems lethargic and his skin is very pale. You obtain a 24-hour diet history and suspect the child does not have adequate iron intake. A complete blood count (CBC) and serum ferritin confirms a diagnosis of iron deficiency anemia (IDA).

1. What do you think Mrs. Anders is most concerned about?
2. What is the nurse's role when a child enters the healthcare system with an acute illness?
3. What opportunities are present when a child is brought to an ambulatory care setting because of an acute illness?

a 50% chance that the child will carry the trait *(HbAS)*, and a 25% chance that the child will have the disease (HbSS). Although not a disease in and of itself, the carrier state of SCD—sickle cell trait *(HbAS)*—can produce clinical symptoms (e.g., hematuria, bacteriuria) in times of extreme stress, during extremely vigorous exercise, and at high altitudes.

## Incidence

SCD affects approximately 1 in 500 Blacks (Shahine, Badr, Karam, et al., 2015). Sickle cell trait is found in 1 of 12 Blacks and is also prevalent in persons of African, Mediterranean, Indian, and Middle Eastern descent (MacMullen & Dulski, 2011). An estimated 90,000 people in the United States are affected by SCD, 90% of whom are of African descent (DeBaun, Frei-Jones, & Vichinsky, 2016a).

## PATHOPHYSIOLOGY

### *Sickle Cell Disease*

The normal red blood cell (RBC) is a smooth, biconcave disk that is capable of changing shape to enable it to flow easily through the microvasculature of the circulation. Under conditions of low oxygen concentration, acidosis, and dehydration, the RBCs in a child with sickle cell disease (SCD) assume a sickle shape similar to a half moon, which prevents them from flowing easily through the smallest blood vessels. Sickled RBCs are stiff and nonpliable. These sickled cells clump together, causing occlusions in the small vessels. With reoxygenation, most of the sickled RBCs resume their normal shape. After repeated sickling (deoxygenation) and unsickling (reoxygenation), the cells become irreversibly sickled, and their life span is reduced from approximately 100 to 120 days to 10 to 20 days (MacMullen & Dulski, 2011).

Sickled cells cause microvascular occlusion, leading to tissue ischemia, infarcts, and organ damage. The lungs, spleen, and brain are the organs most seriously affected by the complications of SCD. The normal spleen functions to filter bacteria in the blood. However, the spleen of a child with SCD does not function properly much beyond age 5 years because of this repeated microvascular occlusion and damage. The large vessels are also affected, leading to strokes and other vaso-occlusive events.

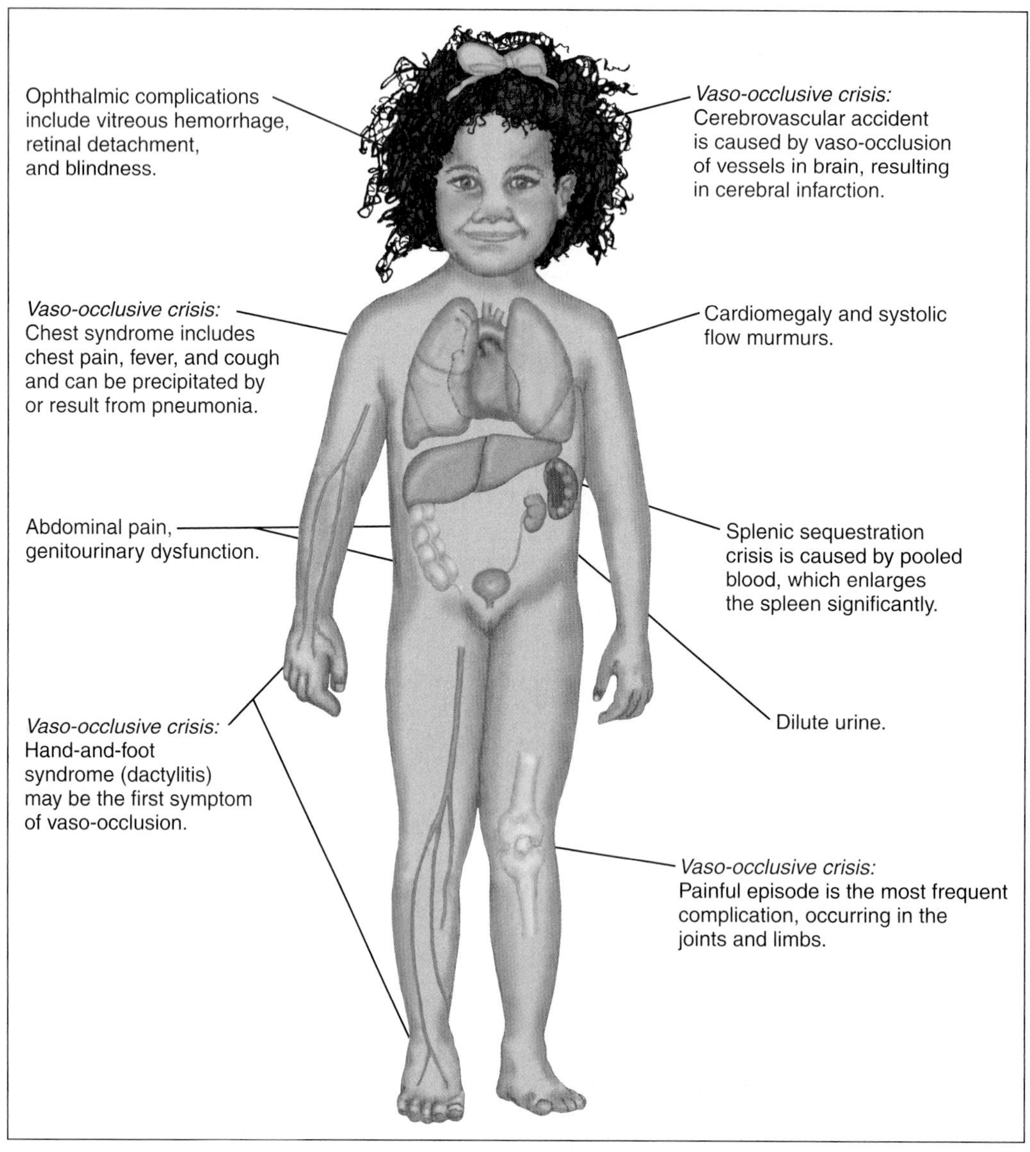
Ophthalmic complications include vitreous hemorrhage, retinal detachment, and blindness.
*Vaso-occlusive crisis:* Cerebrovascular accident is caused by vaso-occlusion of vessels in brain, resulting in cerebral infarction.
*Vaso-occlusive crisis:* Chest syndrome includes chest pain, fever, and cough and can be precipitated by or result from pneumonia.
Cardiomegaly and systolic flow murmurs.
Abdominal pain, genitourinary dysfunction.
Splenic sequestration crisis is caused by pooled blood, which enlarges the spleen significantly.
Dilute urine.
*Vaso-occlusive crisis:* Hand-and-foot syndrome (dactylitis) may be the first symptom of vaso-occlusion.
*Vaso-occlusive crisis:* Painful episode is the most frequent complication, occurring in the joints and limbs.

## Manifestations

All the clinical manifestations of SCD are a result of the obstructions caused by the sickled RBCs and the increased destruction of RBCs because of their shortened life span in SCD. Large amounts of fetal hemoglobin (HbF) present in the first few months of life obscure the presence of HbS, so symptoms of the disease usually do not appear until age 4 to 6 months, when the infant begins to manufacture hemoglobin S.

The disease affects most organ systems. Delayed growth and puberty are common. The child usually has small stature throughout adolescence but may attain normal growth in the early 20s.

The general manifestations of SCD are chronic hemolytic anemia, pallor, jaundice, fatigue, cholelithiasis, delayed growth and puberty, avascular necrosis of the hips and shoulders, renal dysfunction, and retinopathy. Sickling events can also progress to acute episodic exacerbations known as *sickle cell crisis.* Infection, dehydration, hypoxia, trauma, or general stress can precipitate a crisis episode. The crisis takes one of three forms: vaso-occlusive, acute sequestration, or aplastic.

A vaso-occlusive crisis occurs when blood flow to tissues is obstructed by sickled RBCs, leading to hypoxemia and ischemia. This ischemic event causes the child to experience pain in the affected body part.

An acute sequestration event occurs when blood flow from an organ, such as the liver, lungs, or spleen, is obstructed by sickled RBCs. These organs then become engorged with blood, leading to acute anemia and, when in the lungs, acute chest syndrome with potential respiratory failure. Acute chest syndrome is one of the most common causes of death and peaks in children age 2 to 4 years (Abbas, Kahale, Hosn, et al., 2013).

An aplastic event occurs when there is either increased destruction or decreased production of RBCs. Increased destruction can be related to fever or infection. Decreased production is frequently associated with a viral infection such as parvovirus B19 (also known as Fifth disease). Repeated vaso-occlusive crises and a virtually continual state of anemia produce long-term problems later in the life of the individual with SCD. Table 47.1 presents the clinical manifestations of SCD.

**TABLE 47.1 Clinical Manifestations and Therapeutic Management of Sickle Cell Disease Complications**

| Complication | Characteristics | Manifestations | Treatment |
|---|---|---|---|
| **Vaso-Occlusive Crisis** | | | |
| Painful episode | Most common type of crisis and reason for hospitalization<br>Typically produces bone or joint pain, but pain can occur anywhere<br>Pain may come and go<br>Frequency of pain is individualized<br>Pain is precipitated by infection, cold, stress, acidosis, local or generalized hypoxia | *Mild:* Joint or bone pain lasting a few hours<br>*Severe:* Joint or bone pain lasting days | Oral analgesics initially and, if ineffective, IV opioids (usually morphine), which are given by either intermittent or continuous infusion<br>Oral or IV NSAIDs<br>Oral and IV hydration<br>Aggressive incentive spirometry use (10 breaths every 2 hr when awake)<br>Consistent manner to assess subjective experience of pain is essential<br>Use of nonpharmacologic pain management strategies in addition to medications |
| Acute chest syndrome | Common cause of hospitalization<br>Sometimes confused with pneumonia<br>Can recur | Chest pain, fever, cough, abdominal pain | IV hydration (1-1½ times maintenance), antibiotics, oxygen, RBC transfusion, analgesics |
| Dactylitis (hand-and-foot syndrome) | Occurs in children aged 6 mo to 4 yr<br>Self-limiting complication | Swelling of hands or feet, pain, warmth in affected area | Oral analgesics, hydration (oral or IV), rest |
| Priapism (persistent erection of the penis) | Occurs if penile blood flow becomes obstructed | Persistent, painful erection | Analgesics; hydration<br>Avoid hot and cold packs<br>If prolonged, transfusion therapy |
| Cerebrovascular accident | Without treatment, mortality rate of 20%; 70% of patients have a recurrence | Hemiparesis or monoparesis, aphasia/dysphasia, seizures, alteration in level of consciousness, vomiting, vision changes, ataxia, headache | Long-term RBC transfusion therapy or erythrocytapheresis and possibly chelation therapy<br>Sometimes requires extensive rehabilitation |
| **Acute Sequestration Crisis** | | | |
| | Blood volume pooling in the spleen, causing splenic enlargement<br>Life-threatening condition of hypovolemic shock<br>Usually occurs in children aged 6 mo to 4 yr<br>One episode increases the risk of future occurrences | Decreased hemoglobin level, acutely ill-looking child, pallor, irritability, tachycardia, impressively enlarged spleen, hypovolemic shock | Emergency treatment to restore circulating blood volume with crystalloid and colloid (blood) infusion<br>Long-term transfusion therapy if recurrent<br>Eventual splenectomy in cases of persistent recurrence |
| **Aplastic Crisis** | | | |
| | Profound anemia caused by diminished erythropoiesis<br>Has been observed after parvovirus-like agent exposure | Pallor, lethargy, headache, fainting | RBC transfusions and treatment of symptoms |

*IV,* Intravenous; *NSAIDs,* nonsteroidal antiinflammatory drugs; *RBC,* red blood cell.

## Diagnostic Evaluation

In the past, many infants died from complications of SCD before being diagnosed with the disorder. However, newborn screening for SCD has significantly decreased the mortality rate. A laboratory diagnosis of SCD is established based on a CBC, isoelectric focusing, hemoglobin electrophoresis, and high-performance liquid chromatography. Children with SCD have elevated reticulocyte counts because of the shortened life span and destruction of sickled RBCs. Prenatal diagnosis is an option and is made by chorionic villus sampling at 8 to 10 weeks of gestation or amniocentesis at 15 weeks of gestation.

## Therapeutic Management

In SCD, the spleen often does not function properly because of obstruction of splenic blood flow or previous surgical removal for SCD-related complications (Ellison, 2012). Functional or actual asplenia places children and adults with SCD in an immunocompromised state at high risk for infection. Splenic dysfunction can begin at 6 months of age, and those with HbSS can have total dysfunction by age 5 years. Bacterial septicemia poses a severe health risk to children with SCD (DeBaun et al., 2016a; Ellison, 2012). The bacteria *Streptococcus pneumoniae* and *H. influenzae* are normally destroyed by the reticuloendothelial system of the spleen, but because the child with SCD does not have a properly functioning spleen, the child is considered to be more susceptible to infection with these bacteria.

The natural history of splenic dysfunction in children with HbSS places them at higher risk for fulminant septicemia and death during the first 3 years of life than children with HbSC. Prophylactic daily penicillin V therapy (given twice a day) is recommended for all children with suspected or actual diagnosis by age 2 months and is continued until at least age 5 years (DeBaun et al., 2016a; Ellison, 2012). Although views regarding the use of penicillin differ, some experts will continue penicillin prophylaxis throughout childhood in high-risk patients with asplenia.

Not all pneumococcal infections can be prevented by penicillin chemoprophylaxis because of the development of penicillin-resistant pneumococcal strains. The pneumococcal polyvalent vaccine (PCV13) is routinely recommended for children at ages 2, 4, 6, and 12 to 15 months of age. Routine vaccination against *H. influenzae* infections and routine immunization against hepatitis B are recommended as well. Moreover, children with SCD should receive the influenza vaccine annually and immunization against meningococcal disease after age 2 years because of their increased risk for related complications.

Stroke occurs in 8% of children with the HbSS form of SCD by the age of 10 years (Ellison, 2012). Stroke, caused by vaso-occlusion of blood vessels in the brain with sickled RBCs, leading to ischemia, can result in significant motor and neuropsychological deficits. The goal of treatment is early identification of those at increased risk and intervention to prevent the occurrence of a stroke. The risk for stroke can be predicted by the performance of a transcranial Doppler ultrasound. Those with abnormal results are often managed to reduce their risk for stroke by either monthly transfusions or erythrocytapheresis.

A child with SCD and a temperature of 101.3° F (38.5° C) or higher should receive prompt medical evaluation and treatment because of the overwhelming risk for infectious complications. Fever can be the first sign of bacteremia. Parenteral antibiotics, blood cultures, IV hydration, and general monitoring are the standard of care for children with SCD who have fever. Outpatient therapy with long-acting parenteral antibiotics may be provided in combination with rigorous evaluation and follow-up in those centers with the capabilities to do so. Children who are not eligible for outpatient therapy are those with the following signs and symptoms (considered at high risk for sequelae):

- Ill appearance
- Cardiovascular instability
- Age younger than 1 year
- Pulmonary infiltrate
- Prior splenectomy or history of pneumococcal sepsis
- Hemoglobin less than 5 g/dL
- Family's or child's lack of ability to adhere to outpatient therapy
- WBC count less than 500/$mm^3$ or more than 30,000/$mm^3$
- Dehydration

### PATIENT-CENTERED TEACHING

#### *Home Care of the Child With Sickle Cell Disease*

- Encourage fluid intake; increase fluid intake in hot weather or when there are other risks for dehydration.
- Expect frequent urination.
- Provide for adequate rest periods.
- Avoid cold, which can increase sickling, and extreme heat, which can cause dehydration.
- Avoid known sources of infection.
- Avoid prolonged exposure to the sun.
- Monitor the child's body temperature (know the proper use of a thermometer) and promptly notify the medical team in the event of a fever (avoid antipyretics until discussed with the medical team).
- Administer penicillin daily as ordered.
- Avoid use of aspirin; use acetaminophen or ibuprofen as an alternative.
- Be cautious when traveling with the child to avoid conditions or locations with decreased atmospheric oxygen.
- Call the primary caregiver if symptoms of infection are evident.
- Know the physician's telephone number.

Opioids and nonsteroidal antiinflammatory drugs (NSAIDs) (i.e., ibuprofen, ketorolac) are the mainstays of analgesic treatment, particularly in combination for painful crises. Morphine is the current opioid of choice. Meperidine (Demerol) is not recommended for long-term pain management because of its side-effect profile; codeine is avoided due to the association between genotype and codeine metabolism (DeBaun et al., 2016a). Opioids provide systemic relief, and the NSAIDs act locally to decrease inflammation at the site of vaso-occlusion and provide analgesia without the potential side effect of respiratory depression. Morphine has been very effective when administered intravenously, particularly when given using the patient-controlled analgesia method (see Chapter 39). Using techniques such as guided imagery in addition to medications can assist in reducing pain intensity and improving quality of life (Dobson & Byrne, 2014).

The treatment of SCD focuses on precise diagnosis, education about the disease, prevention of exacerbations, prompt identification of complications, and supportive care during crises (hydration, oxygenation, analgesia, RBC transfusion) (see Table 47.1). Education often is directed to parents only; therefore, nurses should assist children as they grow older to take responsibility for learning about their disease and how best to manage it (Jacob et al., 2013). Additional therapies currently under investigation include erythrocytapheresis (removal of sickled erythrocytes by an exchange transfusion technique), phenotyping RBCs for transfusion ("tissue typing" blood products that can potentially reduce alloimmunization), and hydroxyurea administration (increases the fetal hemoglobin [HbF] in RBC's, which interferes with the RBC sickling process and is considered to be protective against exacerbations and severity of symptoms) (Wang et al., 2013).

## NURSING CARE PLAN

### *The Child With Sickle Cell Disease*

**Focused Assessment**

- On initial diagnosis, obtain the history related to parents' concern that their child is in pain. Ask if the child:
  - Has joint swelling
  - Refuses to move an extremity
  - Cries out when a joint is moved or touched
  - Has a fever
  - Is irritable
- Ask parents of a child with sickle cell disease (SCD) for a more detailed history related to signs and symptoms of complications.
- Assess for possible causes of pain other than SCD.
- Assess the severity of the child's condition.
- When assessing pain in adolescents with SCD, consider the following:
  - They want to fit in with their peer group, but they are different because of SCD.
  - They may verbalize continued symptoms in an attempt to gain attention from healthcare providers, avoid peers, and delay a return to normal activities.
  - Obtain objective data specific to the type of painful episode.
- Teach parents (and child) to closely monitor the child's condition, assess for complications, and check the size of the child's spleen, reporting enlargement to the physician.

**Nursing Diagnosis**

Ineffective Peripheral Tissue Perfusion and Risk for Decreased Cardiac Tissue Perfusion related to red blood cell sickling.

**Planning**

***Expected Outcomes***

1. The child will demonstrate adequate tissue perfusion, as evidenced by palpable peripheral pulses; warm, dry skin; adequate urinary output for age; and oxygen saturation greater than 95%.
2. The child and family will describe the treatment regimen, including medications and their actions and possible side effects.

**Interventions and *Rationales***

1. Monitor the child's vital signs and respiratory status every 4 hours and as needed.
   *Vital signs and respiratory status are assessed frequently to detect changes in tissue perfusion and respiratory status. Signs of altered perfusion include increased respiratory rate, increased work of breathing, decreased oxygen saturation, poor color, mottled appearance, prolonged capillary refill time, decreased peripheral pulses, and altered level of consciousness. A change in the level of consciousness often indicates poor perfusion or oxygenation of the brain.*
2. Monitor oxygen saturation using pulse oximetry and administer oxygen to keep saturation greater than 95%.
   *Ensuring adequate oxygen can ease the child's work of breathing and facilitate tissue oxygenation. Oxygen does not reverse the sickling process but may prevent more sickling.*
3. Ensure adequate hydration by measuring intake and output and administering crystalloids and colloids (red blood cells [RBCs]) as ordered.
   *Measuring intake and output monitors renal function and level of hydration. Transfusions of crystalloids and (nonsickled) RBCs will increase the oxygen carrying capacity of the blood and decrease the relative number of sickled cells.*
4. Determine the child's and family's understanding of SCD and the treatment regimen and provide information or clarification as necessary.
   *Adequate understanding of SCD can increase adherence to preventive measures and prompt interventions during exacerbations and hospitalizations.*

**Evaluation**

Are the child's vital signs and oxygen saturation within normal limits?

Does the child demonstrate palpable peripheral pulses, capillary refill time less than 2 seconds, and warmth of extremities?

Can the child and family demonstrate their ability to administer medication and describe possible side effects?

Have the child and family requested additional information or clarification related to treatment?

**Nursing Diagnosis**

Acute Pain related to vaso-occlusion.

**Planning**

***Expected Outcome***

The child will have decreased pain, as evidenced by a lowered score on the selected pain assessment tool.

**Interventions and *Rationales***

1. Monitor and record pain level every 1 to 2 hours and more frequently if needed, using a pain assessment tool appropriate for the child's age.
   *Pain can be severe in vaso-occlusive crisis and is relieved for only short periods. An assessment tool that measures the subjective experience of pain is helpful in determining the child's level of discomfort (see Chapter 39 ).*
2. Administer analgesics as ordered.
   *Analgesics may be administered intermittently, by a patient-controlled analgesic (PCA) pump, and by continuous infusion through an intravenous (IV) line.*
3. Increase oral fluids, if able to tolerate, or administer fluids IV at a rate that is 1 to 1½ times the maintenance rate.
   *Increased fluid volume reduces the viscosity of the blood, thus alleviating sites of vascular occlusion and preventing further sickling caused by dehydration.*
4. Administer RBCs as ordered.
   *Maintaining an adequate hemoglobin level increases oxygen-carrying capacity to aid in further preventing sickling and microvascular ischemia.*
5. Incorporate the use of age-appropriate, non-pharmacologic pain relief measures.
   *Comfort measures often help distract the child from discomfort (see Chapter 39 ).*
6. Perform passive range-of-motion exercises and avoid exertion.
   *Passive range-of-motion exercises promote circulation without exacerbating fatigue.*

**Evaluation**

Does the child verbalize or demonstrate decreased pain?

Does review of the child's pain assessment tool rating show a decrease in discomfort?

**Nursing Diagnosis**

Risk for Infection related to chronic immunocompromised state.

**Planning**

***Expected Outcomes***

1. The child will remain free from infection, as evidenced by normal vital signs and activity for age.
2. The child and family will verbalize signs and symptoms of infection and when to notify the medical team.

**Interventions and *Rationales***

1. Monitor vital signs every 4 hours and more frequently as needed. Report any temperature elevations to the physician.

## NURSING CARE PLAN—cont'd

### *The Child With Sickle Cell Disease*

*Elevated temperature and increased respiratory rate may be signs of infection.*

2. Administer antipyretics and antibiotics as ordered.
   *Antibiotics may be given prophylactically because of the high risk for infection. Prompt intervention is critical in children with homozygous sickle cell disease (HbSS) and sickle beta-zero thalassemia during febrile illness.*
3. Administer penicillin daily as ordered. Administer preventive immunizations to decrease the risk for infection (pneumococcal, meningococcal, *Haemophilus influenzae* type b, influenza vaccines).
   *Children are at a high risk for pneumococcal infections and should receive long-term penicillin therapy. The pneumococcal, meningococcal, and H. influenzae type b vaccines can prevent sepsis, and the influenza vaccine can prevent complications from influenza.*
4. Teach the parents signs of infection to watch for and the proper way to obtain the child's temperature. Confirm that the parents have a thermometer. Instruct the parents when to notify the physician.
   *A comprehensive teaching plan is essential. Do not assume that the parent has a thermometer or knows how to accurately obtain a temperature reading.*

#### Evaluation

Is the child's body temperature within normal limits?

Can the child and family describe their plan to identify and respond to signs of infection?

#### Nursing Diagnosis

Ineffective Coping related to chronic illness.

#### Planning

##### *Expected Outcomes*

The child and family will:

1. Adhere to the treatment plan and follow-up visits.
2. Verbalize feelings about the impact of the illness on their lives.
3. Use available support systems and community resources.

#### Interventions and *Rationales*

1. Teach the family the necessity of and rationale for following the treatment as outlined by the healthcare team (see Patient-Centered Teaching: Home Care of the Child with Sickle Cell Disease).
   *Conscientious adherence to the treatment regimen decreases the frequency of hospitalizations and improves the child's health and longevity.*
2. Provide written instructions on all aspects of the child's care, complications to watch for, when to contact the healthcare team, and names and phone numbers of who to contact.
   *Education helps the family gain a sense of control and allows them to make informed decisions. Parents can refer to written instructions when less stressed and able to comprehend.*
3. Listen and encourage the child and family to verbalize their feelings and express their concerns regarding SCD. Answer questions honestly and openly. Make a referral to the social work team to provide additional supports, as needed.
   *Identifying concerns and clarifying misconceptions will help the family cope with the stress of chronic illness.*
4. Introduce the family to other families of children with SCD.
   *These families can offer support, suggestions, and strategies for dealing with problems.*
5. Encourage parents to contact healthcare team members when they have questions or concerns. Provide parents with the address and phone number of the local chapter of the Sickle Cell Foundation.
   *Knowing about available resources and how to access assistance decreases parents' feelings of frustration and helplessness.*

#### Evaluation

Are the child and family demonstrating adherence to the treatment plan?

Do the child and family demonstrate positive coping mechanisms?

Do the child and family use available resources?

Is the family able to discuss problems related to caring for a child with a chronic disease?

Does the child share fears and frustrations related to having SCD?

## EVIDENCE-BASED PRACTICE

Vaso-occlusive crisis (VOC) the hallmark of sickle cell disease (SCD) is often treated inadequately in the emergency department (ED). Starting in 2002, all patients with SCD reporting to Children's Hospital of Pittsburgh (CHP) ED were treated with VOC using a structured algorithm. Individual regimens were used and recorded for each patient. These plans were adjusted to patient response at subsequent VOC visits. Rates of hospitalization following an ED visit with readmission within 1 week after discharge with that of 4 comparable hospitals from the Pediatric Health Information (PHIS) database. Parents and patients completed surveys of satisfaction with pain management and with care. Between 2002 and 2008 there was a decline in the rate of admission of patients presenting to the ED Improvement in pain score during ED visit for pain management was 2.0 or more on Wong Baker scale of 0-5. Participants on average, rated quality of pain management as very good or higher. This study demonstrates that individual pain management plans in the ED are effective in delivering high quality management of VOC in the ED (Krishnamurti et al., 2014).

Reference: Krishnamurti, L., Smith-Packard, B., Gupta, A., Campbell, M., Gunawardena, S., & Saladino, R. (2014). Impact of individualized pain plan on the emergency management of children with sickle cell disease. *Pediatric Blood & Cancer*, *61*(10), 1747–1753 7p. doi:10.1002/pbc.25024

Research toward a cure continues; especially promising is gene therapy. Another promising area of research is hematopoietic stem cell transplantation, which has been a successful modality for a limited number of children. Logistic and ethical issues are involved in candidate selection for this potentially curative strategy.

Better management of SCD has increased the life expectancy in the United States to the mid 50s (Atoui et al., 2015). Therefore, nurses must educate patients about childbearing and the associated risks such as bleeding, infection, pre-term labor, and preeclampsia, in addition to worsening of their disease symptoms (Wilkie et al., 2013)

## THALASSEMIA

The thalassemias are a group of inherited disorders characterized by an abnormality in hemoglobin synthesis resulting in a reduction in or absence of one of the chains composing normal hemoglobin. These disorders are categorized by the site of the aberrant globin synthesis (e.g., alpha-thalassemia, beta-thalassemia). The homozygous form of beta-thalassemia, also known as *thalassemia major* or *Cooley anemia*, is the most common and severe form of thalassemia.

### Etiology and Incidence

Inheritance is through an autosomal recessive pattern. The child who inherits only one gene for beta-thalassemia may have only a mild anemia, hence the term *thalassemia minor*. The child who inherits two genes for beta-thalassemia will have severe anemia, hence the term *thalassemia major*. The worldwide prevalence of genetic carriers of beta-thalassemia is 3% (DeBaun et al., 2016b). The thalassemias are found primarily in people of Mediterranean descent, although they have been reported in Asian and African populations. In the United States, the incidence of thalassemia is approximately 1,000 cases/year (Carson & Martin, 2014).

### Manifestations

The clinical manifestations of beta-thalassemia include pallor, growth retardation, pubertal delay, severe anemia, characteristic facies (enlarged head, frontal and parietal bossing, severe maxillary hyperplasia, malocclusion), hepatosplenomegaly, and a bronze skin tone (Box 47.1).

**BOX 47.1 Characteristic Features of a Child With Beta-Thalassemia**

Features develop as a consequence of inadequate treatment:

- Frontal bossing (prominent and protruding forehead)
- Maxillary prominence
- Wide-set eyes with a flattened nose
- Hepatosplenomegaly
- Greenish yellow skin tone

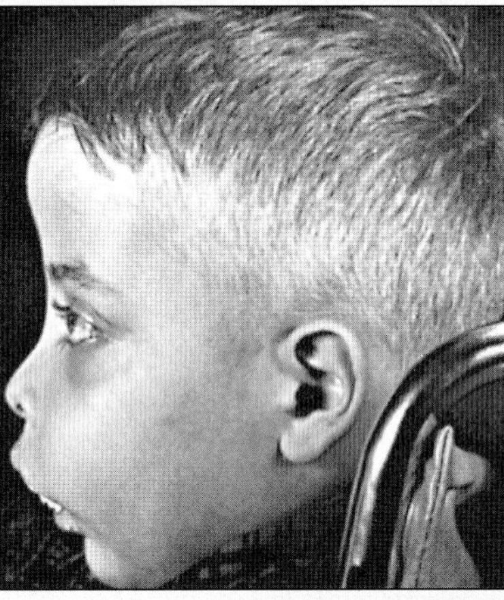

(Photo from Behrman, R.E., Kliegman, R.M., & Arvin, A.M. [1996]. [Eds.]. *Nelson textbook of pediatrics* [15th ed., pp. 1402]. Philadelphia: Saunders.)

### Diagnostic Evaluation

In addition to a CBC, laboratory testing should include quantification of reticulocyte count, serum iron level, total iron-binding capacity, hemoglobin electrophoresis, and HbA and HbF levels to confirm the diagnosis. The CBC will often reflect microcytic, hypochromic erythrocytes. A detailed family history sometimes reveals a history of anemia and delayed growth and maturation.

### Therapeutic Management

The management of beta-thalassemia centers on three techniques: (1) erythrocyte transfusions, (2) **chelation** therapy, and (3) splenectomy. To prevent the severe side effects and bony changes associated with the disease, the hemoglobin is maintained at approximately 11 g/dL, although this parameter is often individualized.

The major complication of long-term transfusion therapy is **hemosiderosis**. To prevent organ damage from excessive iron overload, these children must receive some form of chelation therapy.

The mainstay of chelation therapy is the drug deferoxamine (Desferal). It is most effective when given subcutaneously or intravenously. To avoid hospitalizing children who require deferoxamine therapy, the drug is often administered in the home by continuous subcutaneous infusion via a pump over an 8- to 12-hour period at night. This

**PATHOPHYSIOLOGY**

***Beta-Thalassemia***

Abnormal synthesis of the beta-polypeptide chain of hemoglobin impairs the erythrocytes' ability to carry oxygen. Thalassemia is classified by the degree of imbalance in the globin chain and can be minor, intermediate, or severe.

Typically, during the second 6 months of life, severe anemia develops. Erythrocytes are hemolyzed as they are produced. Because the body's natural response to a reduction in circulating hemoglobin is to produce more erythrocytes, the bone marrow begins massive production. Progressive disease constantly stimulates the bone marrow. The body perceives this as an inability to keep up with the need for erythrocytes. As a result, **extramedullary** (outside the bone marrow) sites of production of erythrocytes begin **erythropoiesis**. The result is a chronic state of production and destruction of erythrocytes that have an inadequate amount of normal hemoglobin.

Iron is necessary for the production of hemoglobin, and it is a by-product of the hemolysis of RBCs. Normally the intestines absorb small amounts of iron. However, in this disorder, the body increases the absorption of iron. When increased iron absorption is combined with the increased iron introduced into the circulation by the transfusions necessary to treat thalassemia, hemosiderosis occurs, usually during the second decade of life. Hemosiderosis is the deposition of excess amounts of iron in tissue.

The results of excessive erythropoiesis and hemolysis are considerable. The bones become thin and fragile from excessive erythropoiesis. Hepatosplenomegaly occurs as a result of extramedullary erythropoiesis and hemosiderosis. Growth is impaired and puberty delayed. Without proper management, multisystem organ dysfunction ensues.

approach can preserve some degree of normalcy in lifestyle for the family. Therapy is continued until the iron returns to an acceptable level. This goal can be accomplished within months of initiating chelation therapy. However, compliance with nightly subcutaneous infusions is often poor.

An oral chelation agent, deferasirox (Exjade), became available in the United States in 2005 for children older than 2 years. Compliance is improved with this once-a-day, orally administered medication (Eckes, 2011).

Splenectomy may be indicated in children who are not transfusion dependent to increase their hemoglobin level and avoid transfusions. Splenectomy is a therapy that should not be considered casually because susceptibility to infection with *S. pneumoniae, H. influenzae,* and *Neisseria meningitidis* increases after splenectomy in children, particularly in those younger than 2 years of age (Taher & Cappellini, 2014). Standard therapy for asplenic individuals includes immunizations, prophylactic penicillin, and a high index of suspicion and aggressive antibiotic therapy for febrile illnesses as described previously for children with SCD.

Bone marrow transplantation (BMT) is the only available cure for thalassemia at this time. BMT can cure over 85% of low-risk children with thalassemia which leads to an improved quality of life (Gooneratne et al., 2015).

## PATIENT-CENTERED TEACHING

### *Home Chelation Therapy*

**Subcutaneous Route by Infusion Pump**

- Know the technique for placing the subcutaneous needle, medication preparation, and infusion pump operation.
- Check needle security and placement.
- Check pump for proper infusion rate.
- Call the home care, clinic, or physician resource if the site becomes inflamed, red, or painful.
- Know indications for medication and side effects that require healthcare team notification; hearing loss or ringing in the ears, fever, diarrhea, visual disturbances, allergic reactions, and respiratory compromise.

**Intravenous Route: Totally Implantable or Tunneled Access Device**

- Know the technique for placing access needle or catheter connection, medication preparation, and infusion pump operation.
- Call the home care, clinic, or physician resource if the site becomes inflamed, red, or painful or the specific access device is obstructed.
- Have a list of home care resources for technique assistance, supplies, and problematic pump functioning.
- Know indications for medication and side effects that require healthcare team notification: hearing loss or ringing in the ears, fever, diarrhea, visual disturbances, allergic reactions, and respiratory compromise.

## NURSING CARE

### The Child With Beta-Thalassemia

#### Assessment

Subjective data can include the parents' observations that their child is not as active as other children of the same age. The child might sleep more than other children or want to be held often. The child appears pale, with laboratory values reflecting a microcytic, hypochromic anemia. Clinical symptoms are related to the degree of anemia, ranging from mild to severe.

An older child with the disease or a child who has not received adequate treatment will likely have characteristic facial deformities, including maxillary hyperplasia and malocclusion. These characteristics develop from extramedullary marrow expansion, a consequence of the marrow's effort to keep up with the demand for RBCs as a result of anemia. Hepatosplenomegaly is usually seen at this time in older children but not in infants.

#### Nursing Diagnosis and Planning

The nursing diagnoses and expected outcomes that may be appropriate after assessment of the child with thalassemia are as follows:

- Ineffective Peripheral Tissue Perfusion and Risk for Decreased Cardiac Tissue Perfusion related to anemia.

*Expected outcome.* The child demonstrates adequate tissue perfusion, as evidenced by palpable peripheral pulses; warm, dry skin; urinary output appropriate for age; and the absence of cardiorespiratory distress (oxygen saturation >95%).

- Disturbed Body Image related to altered appearance and the perception of having a chronic disease.

*Expected outcome.* The child and family will verbalize feelings related to changes in appearance and the limitations imposed by the disease process.

- Anxiety related to the diagnosis.

*Expected outcome.* The child and family will express feelings about the disorder, lifestyle disruptions as a result of treatment, and possible genetic transmission of the disease.

- Deficient Knowledge related to inadequate information about the disorder.

*Expected outcome.* The child and family will describe the disorder and its treatment regimen, including medications and their actions and possible side effects.

#### Interventions

Expect transfusions to begin immediately for an affected child while cardiovascular compromise from the anemia is being assessed. Preparing the child and family for diagnostic procedures will help alleviate fears. Once the diagnosis is made, education should begin. Parents need to understand the importance of proper and continuing follow-up. The family needs much support as they begin chelation therapy, which is very time consuming and interferes with family routines. The nurse must regularly monitor the family's adherence to therapy. If hematopoietic stem cell transplantation becomes an option, the parents will need referral to a specialty center and will need support from the entire healthcare team as they contemplate this course of treatment.

#### Evaluation

- Are the child's peripheral pulses palpable and oxygen saturation increased to 95%?
- Is the child's hemoglobin level improving?
- Is the child able to verbalize feelings associated with the treatment or the psychosocial implications of the disease?
- Is the child sharing feelings related to changes in appearance, limitations imposed by the disease, and having a chronic disease?
- Has the family sought genetic counseling?
- Does the family readily verbalize feelings about having a child with beta-thalassemia?
- Has the family demonstrated adherence to therapy?

## HEMOPHILIA

Hemophilia is a lifelong hereditary blood disorder with no cure. Hemophilia A is associated with the deficiency of coagulation factor

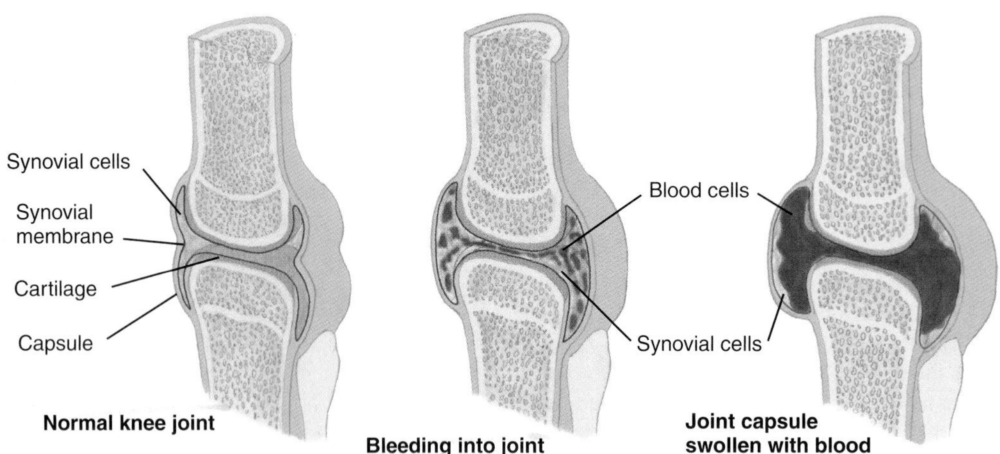


FIG 47.1 Hemarthrosis and joint destruction are characteristic of hemophilia.

VIII. Hemophilia B, a deficiency in factor IX, is associated with a constellation of symptoms similar to hemophilia A. A lack of factor XI, Hemophilia C, results in only mild bleeding tendencies (Bolton-Maggs, 2011). Hemophilia affects 1 in 5,000 males (Scott and Flood, 2016), and factor IX deficiency affects 1 in 25,000 to 30,000 males (Zaiden et al., 2011). Approximately 90% of these patients have hemophilia A (McCarthy & Mathew, 2011). Congenital deficiencies in these three factors account for approximately 90% to 95% of the bleeding disorders referred to as *hemophilia*.

## Etiology and Incidence

Hemophilia is an X-linked autosomal recessive disorder; carrier females pass on the defect to affected males. Women who never produce an affected male child can silently pass the gene on for generations, but typically there is a history of hemophilia in the family. Rarely, female offspring are born with the disorder, but only if they inherit an affected gene from the mother and are the offspring of a father with hemophilia.

## Manifestations

The disease severity is individual but tends to be familial. Bleeding occurs after surgery or serious trauma in all children with this disease. Bleeding occurs after tissue trauma in children with moderate and severe disease. Bleeding occurs spontaneously and for no apparent reason in children with severe disease. Affected children bruise easily, have episodes of epistaxis, and some have hematuria. They can also have bleeding with loss of deciduous teeth, even from minor lacerations, and from injections. Most commonly, bleeding develops in the muscles and joints (hemarthrosis), especially the knees, in those children with moderate and severe disease (Fig. 47.1). Recurrent bleeding commonly occurs in the same joint in severely affected children, causing swelling, pain, bleeding, and stiffness.

## Diagnostic Evaluation

Hemophilia is sometimes but not always diagnosed after circumcision, at which time prolonged bleeding may be observed. Because the most common sites of bleeding are in the muscles and joints, the diagnosis can be delayed until the toddler years, when the child becomes more active and the disease has an opportunity to manifest itself. By the preschool years, most affected children have had an episode of persistent bleeding from a minor traumatic laceration.

A diagnostic workup for the child with suspected hemophilia includes determining the prothrombin time (PT), partial thromboplastin time, bleeding time, fibrinogen level, platelet count, quantitative immunoelectrophoretic assay, and factor VIII and IX assays.

### PATHOPHYSIOLOGY

#### *Hemophilia*

More than 10 factors in the blood work in sequence to produce blood clotting. Factor VIII (antihemophilic factor) and factor IX (or plasma thromboplastin component), are the two missing or defective constituents in the blood that cause hemophilia A (classic hemophilia) and hemophilia B (Christmas disease). When these factors are missing or defective, blood does not clot as it should. The two disorders are inherited in the same way and have similar manifestations. Normal factor activity is described as a percentage. The percentage of factor activity is closely related to the level of factor in the blood (e.g., 100 units/dL factor equals 100% factor activity). Normal levels of factor VIII and IX are 50% to 150%. The severity of the disease is classified as follows:

*Severe:* Less than 1% factor activity
*Moderate:* 1% to 5% factor activity
*Mild:* 6% to 50% factor activity

## Therapeutic Management

The management of hemophilia is highly individual and depends on the severity of the illness. Therapy aims to prevent excessive bleeding and tissue damage by supplying the body with additional factor, substituting for factor (VIII or IX) that is missing or ineffective.

Previously, treatment involved transfusions of blood products or administration of freeze-dried preparations manufactured from blood products. One of the major risks associated with this type of factor replacement therapy was contracting hepatitis or human immunodeficiency virus infection. Because of this risk, manufacturers began to heat-treat the blood factor to reduce the risk for viral transmission. Monoclonal products were then developed that were found to be even safer than the heat-treated products. The most recent development in the treatment of hemophilia is the availability of recombinant antihemophilic factor, which is not derived from human plasma but is produced synthetically from the isolated gene. Recombinant factor eliminates the risk for virus transmission. Factor preparations must be reconstituted with sterile water before being given intravenously.

Prophylactic therapy is now being started in infants and young children with severe hemophilia to prevent joint problems. Some children with mild hemophilia A can use desmopressin acetate (1-deamino-8-D-arginine vasopressin [DDAVP]) intranasal spray, which has

## NURSING CARE PLAN

### *The Child With Hemophilia*

**Focused Assessment**

- Consider these parameters when assessing children for signs and symptoms of hemophilia:
  - For male newborns, observe the circumcision site and injection sites for prolonged bleeding.
  - For children learning to crawl and walk, explore parental concerns about bruising easily after minor falls.
  - Ask parents about previous cuts and abrasions to determine if child needed more than the usual pressure application or time for the bleeding to subside.
  - Inquire about a family history of bleeding disorders.

**Nursing Diagnosis**

Risk for Injury related to prolonged bleeding.

**Planning**

***Expected Outcome***

The child and family will recognize bleeding resulting from injury and promptly control it to prevent permanent tissue damage.

**Interventions and *Rationales***

1. Monitor the area of injury hourly for bleeding over a 24-hour period.
   *Bleeding may be prolonged and, especially in the case of head trauma, may not manifest immediately.*
2. Measure the circumference of an injured joint.
   *Joint measurement provides objective rather than subjective data for future comparisons.*
3. In the case of head trauma, assess the child's level of consciousness at least hourly and note any behavioral changes.
   *Decreased level of consciousness and unusual behaviors are early indicators of increased intracranial pressure resulting from hemorrhage.*
4. Apply gentle pressure for 10 to 15 minutes to small superficial wounds and assess the area for subcutaneous bleeding.
   *Small wounds may ooze blood into the subcutaneous tissue. Pressure facilitates clot formation.*
5. Administer factor replacement as ordered.
   *Factor must be reconstituted just before infusion. It may be given as a prophylactic measure even if no bleeding is apparent.*
6. When a child is hospitalized, monitor factor blood levels, as ordered.
   *With serious injuries, factor levels aid in prescribing dosages and establishing thresholds for the child.*
7. If a muscle or joint injury occurs, immobilize, elevate, and apply ice to the affected part, as ordered by the physician.
   *Initial immobilization will help prevent further injury until the bleeding resolves.*
8. Offer suggestions for establishing a safe home environment for the child (see Patient-Centered Teaching: Home Care of the Child with Hemophilia).
   *A safe home environment will help prevent injuries.*
9. Avoid rectal temperature measurement.
   *Rectal temperatures may cause bleeding from tissue trauma.*
10. Teach parents to provide for and expect behaviors consistent with normal growth and development per their child's age.
    *Parents may tend to overprotect or provide special treatment for their child. This unnecessarily limits the child's opportunities for normal psychosocial development and decreases self-esteem.*

**Evaluation**

Has the child had serious bleeding from injury?
Has the child adhered to the treatment regimen to control injuries?
Are there long-term complications from injury?

**Nursing Diagnosis**

Deficient Knowledge related to the need for information about disease diagnosis and treatment.

**Planning**

***Expected Outcomes***

The child and family will:

1. Explain the diagnosis.
2. Demonstrate adherence to the home care regimen.

**Interventions and *Rationales***

1. Determine the child's and family's readiness for learning. Create an environment conducive to learning.
   *The family may need time to adjust to the initial diagnosis before they are ready to be educated. Parents may need an educational setting away from the child so they can focus on learning.*
2. On initial diagnosis and with subsequent follow-up visits, spend time with the child and parents explaining the diagnosis, sequelae, and treatment. Offer written literature and other educational materials.
   *Education is ongoing and reinforcement is needed for stressed parents. Explaining the rationale for treatment and the disease's sequelae will help ensure adherence to therapy. Written or other forms of information (such as videos) can be reviewed later, improving parent comprehension.*
3. Offer encouragement and praise for prompt recognition and response to bleeding.
   *Praise will reinforce appropriate actions taken by the child and parents.*
4. Teach techniques for reconstitution and infusion of factor at home. The infusion technique will depend on type of venous access (peripheral infusion, central venous line, implantable infusion device [port]) (see Patient-Centered Teaching: Home Care of the Child with Hemophilia).
   *Parents (and child per developmental level) are taught techniques for accessing the venous line or port, infusing the factor, and heparinizing the line or port.*
5. Consider using a topical anesthetic, such as eutectic mixture of local anesthetics (EMLA), when accessing infusion ports or peripheral sites.
   *The use of topical anesthetics decreases pain, thus causing the child less trauma and anxiety.*

**Evaluation**

Are the child and family able to safely administer factor replacement at home?
Do the child and family promptly recognize and react to bleeding?

**Nursing Diagnosis**

Ineffective Coping related to chronic illness and guilt.

**Planning**

***Expected Outcomes***

The child and family will:

1. Adhere to the treatment plan, as evidenced by safety alterations being made in the home and community.
2. Use available support systems and community resources.

Family members will verbalize concerns about the impact of the illness on the family.

**Interventions and *Rationales***

1. Teach the family the need for safety precautions, correct response to injury, medication administration methods, and importance of following the treatment plan as outlined by healthcare providers (see Patient-Centered Teaching: Home Care of the Child with Hemophilia).
   *Conscientious adherence to the treatment regimen decreases the potential for long-term complications.*

*Continued*

## NURSING CARE PLAN—cont'd

### *The Child With Hemophilia*

2. Listen to and encourage the child and family to verbalize their feelings and express their concerns regarding hemophilia. Answer questions honestly and openly. Be alert for feelings of guilt expressed by the mother.
   *Identifying concerns and clarifying misconceptions help families cope with the stress of chronic illness. Mothers may experience guilt because of the genetic inheritance pattern of the disease.*
3. Introduce the family to other families of children with hemophilia.
   *Other families of children with hemophilia can offer support, suggestions, and strategies for coping.*
4. Provide referral to the state chapter of the Hemophilia Foundation.
   *Access to information and assistance can help the family deal with the potentially overwhelming financial and emotional burdens of caring for a child with hemophilia.*
5. Explore the child's feelings about restrictions in activities and participation in some sports due to having hemophilia. Assess the child's coping strategies and need for support.
   *Discussing feelings related to a chronic disease provides an opportunity for the child to explore options and improve coping strategies.*

**Evaluation**

Does the older child avoid contact sports and participate in other activities, such as swimming?

Has the family contacted the state chapter of the Hemophilia Foundation?

Is the child able to balance limitations with normal childhood activities?

## SAFETY ALERT

### *Acetylsalicylic Acid: Contraindication*

Acetylsalicylic acid (e.g., aspirin, aspirin-containing products) should not be given to children with factor disorders because it inhibits platelet function. Because some over-the-counter medications contain acetylsalicylic acid, it is important to read all labels carefully before giving medication to the child.

vasoconstrictor action, to stop bleeding. Children with hemophilia A or B can be given aminocaproic acid (Amicar) or tranexamic acid (Cyklokapron)—oral medications that stabilize oral clots and can also sometimes stop nosebleeds (Weiss, 2012).

In addition to factor prophylaxis, the child with hemophilia must try to avoid activities that induce bleeding. Special precautions can be taken to protect joints, thereby allowing the child to lead a more normal life. Prophylactic factor replacement therapy should also be given before surgery and some dental procedures. Bleeding is treated with rest, ice, elevation of the affected part, and compression (also referred to as *RICE: r*est, *i*ce, *c*ompression, *e*levation). More recent data suggest that low temperature impairs platelet function, so cold should be applied for no more than 15 to 20 minutes at a time (Kauffman, 2014).

## NURSING QUALITY ALERT

### *Interviewing a Child With Hemophilia*

Subjective data gathered from a child known to have hemophilia should include information about recent trauma and initial measures to stop bleeding. An important question is the length of time that pressure had to be applied before the bleeding subsided. Other questions to ask include whether the swelling increased after the surface bleeding stopped and whether swelling and stiffness occurred without apparent trauma.

## VON WILLEBRAND DISEASE

Von Willebrand disease (VWD) is the most commonly inherited bleeding disorder, with an estimated prevalence of 1.3% of the U.S. population; males and females are affected equally (Weiss, 2012).

### Etiology

VWD is an autosomal inherited disorder with both dominant and recessive variants (Weiss, 2012). VWD is classified into three categories, with 60% to 80% of those identified as Type 1, which results in mild to moderate bleeding (Flood & Scott, 2016). Most of the remaining population has Type 2, which results in moderate bleeding due to a defect in von Willebrand factor (Weiss, 2012).

### Pathophysiology

Children with VWD have either underproduction or dysfunction of von Willebrand protein. The von Willebrand protein occurs together with factor VIII in the circulation, making it a carrier protein for factor VIII. One of its most important functions is to bind and attract platelets to the site of endothelial tissue injury, thus facilitating the formation of a clot. Deficiency of von Willebrand protein can result in a corresponding functional deficiency of factor VIII.

### Manifestations

Clinical features and the need for treatment depend on the severity of the disorder. The clinical manifestations of VWD include a history of epistaxis, bleeding from the gums, prolonged bleeding from cuts, excessive bleeding after surgery or trauma, and menorrhagia (excessive menstrual bleeding) in females.

### Diagnostic Evaluation

A thorough history will ascertain whether the episode of bruising is proportional to the degree of trauma. A family history of bleeding disorders is important. Recently researchers have developed scoring systems for identifying those at risk for VWD. Positive history of epistaxis, skin bleeding, oral/dental bleeding, gastrointestinal bleeding, muscle/joint bleeding, central nervous system (CNS) bleeding, and significant bleeding after surgery are each evaluated and scored in these scoring systems. These scoring systems are not yet validated in children because they lack specificity and sensitivity.

Laboratory evaluations are obtained once it has been identified, based on bleeding history, that a child potentially has VWD. Possible laboratory tests include a bleeding time and a partial thromboplastin time, the results of which can be normal in children with VWD. Thus, children with a history of significant bleeding episodes must be further evaluated with more specific assays for von Willebrand factor. The most clinically useful and widely used laboratory tests for diagnosing this disorder are the enzyme-linked immunosorbent assay (ELISA) and the quantitative immunoelectrophoretic assay, which measure the quantity of von Willebrand factor antigen in the plasma (Weiss, 2012).

## PATIENT-CENTERED TEACHING

### *Home Care of the Child With Hemophilia*

- Apply gentle, prolonged pressure to superficial wounds until the bleeding has stopped.
- Call the physician in the event of blunt trauma, especially trauma involving the joints.
- Establish an age-appropriate, safe environment:
  - Pad table corners.
  - Pad crib rails.
  - Provide extra joint padding on clothes.
  - Remove items that can tip over or be pulled down on the child.
  - Do not leave a crawling or toddling child unattended.
  - Use a toothbrush with soft bristles and a Waterpik for dental care.
  - Instruct older children to avoid contact sports and to take precautions with other sports.
  - Pad the knees and elbows for physical education class.
  - Use protective helmets for any sport in which head injury could occur (e.g., bicycling, skating).
  - Use an electric razor for shaving.
- Call the physician if any head injury occurs.
- Reconstitute and administer factor through an intravenous (IV) line or the child's central venous access device.
- If a child has an implantable infusion device, caregivers should understand the following:
  - Site preparation
  - Sterile technique for insertion of access needle
  - Technique for verification of needle placement
  - Administration of factor by IV push
  - Saline solution and heparin flush
  - Removal and proper disposal of needle
- Keep current with the schedule of immunizations, dental hygiene, and routine well-child care.
- Allow your child to set personal safety limits when possible.
- Provide for normal growth and development opportunities (safe activities, time with other children, limit setting, independence).

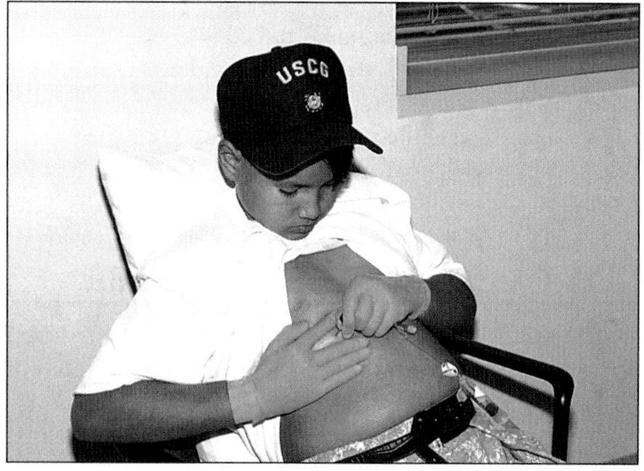

Control of deficient blood clotting in hemophilia requires injection of the missing clotting factors. This young man is injecting his factor into an implanted central venous access port. Sterile technique is essential. (Courtesy family of Jason Lee Davis.)

### Therapeutic Management

Therapy is aimed at controlling bleeding episodes and replacing the missing or dysfunctional factor in the blood. A concentrate of antihemolytic factors that have undergone purification to inactivate viruses or possibly fresh frozen plasma is administered before events that cause excessive bleeding such as surgery or after trauma with excessive bleeding (Weiss, 2012).

The treatment of choice is DDAVP, a synthetic derivative of the antidiuretic hormone vasopressin, which is administered intravenously, subcutaneously, or intranasally. The DDAVP products are given for type I and type IIA VWD only (Kauffman, 2014; Weiss, 2012). High-purity (not monoclonal or recombinant) factor VIII products that are specifically known to contain von Willebrand factor can be used to treat type IIB disease. (Only a minority of currently available factor VIII concentrates actually contain von Willebrand factor.) Adolescent females with menorrhagia can be treated with antifibrinolytics such as aminocaproic acid (Amicar) or tranexamic acid, which are available in both oral (Lysteda) and intravenous forms (Cyklokapron) (Weiss, 2012). Of note, one goal of *Health People 2020* is to increase the proportion of females who are diagnosed with VWD within a year of first bleeding episode (Khamees, Klima, & O'Brien, 2015).

## NURSING CARE

### The Child With Von Willebrand Disease

#### Assessment

A careful history detailing episodes of bruising and bleeding is essential. In addition, documenting a family history of bruising or bleeding can assist with identifying the condition (Weiss, 2012). Possible causes of any previous episodes of bleeding, if any can be identified, should also be discussed. The nurse asks how many times the child has had a nosebleed, how long the child bleeds from minor injuries, and whether there is a history of prolonged bleeding associated with surgery or trauma.

Physical examination usually reveals a healthy child except for evidence of bruising greater than expected for the degree of trauma. If the child is being seen after a major bleeding episode, signs of hemorrhage or a decreased hemoglobin level (or both) will be seen.

#### Nursing Diagnosis and Planning

The nursing diagnoses and expected outcomes that may be appropriate after assessment of the child with VWD include the following:

- Ineffective Protection related to abnormal clotting.

  ***Expected outcome.*** The child will remain free of life-threatening episodes of hemorrhage.
- Deficient Knowledge related to the disorder.

  ***Expected outcome.*** The child and family will explain the disorder, its management, and its chronic nature.

#### Interventions

Education of the family is aimed at producing an understanding of the precautions to take with the child and knowledge of when prophylactic therapy should be given before elective procedures. The child should wear a medical alert tag at all times. The degree of activity limitation will depend on the severity of the disorder. Possible limitations include avoidance of contact sports, especially football. Avoidance of prescription and over-the-counter medications that affect platelet function, such as aspirin and NSAIDs, is also recommended. The nurse should advise the parents to check the labels of all over-the-counter medications for presence of aspirin or ibuprofen. The family should be referred to the state chapter of the Hemophilia Foundation for support services.

### Evaluation

- Are episodes of bleeding minimal and controlled?
- Does the family communicate an understanding of the importance of avoiding medications that affect platelet function and avoiding activities that increase the risk for bleeding?
- Does the family seek appropriate resources for information about the condition and its management?

## IMMUNE THROMBOCYTOPENIC PURPURA

Immune thrombocytopenic purpura (ITP) is an acquired bleeding disorder characterized by thrombocytopenia (platelet count below 150,000/mm$^3$), a purpuric rash, normal bone marrow, and the absence of signs of other identifiable causes of thrombocytopenia. It is classified as acute or chronic, with chronic being defined as the persistence of thrombocytopenia for more than 6 months.

### Etiology and Incidence

ITP is one of the most common acquired bleeding disorders in children. The incidence of symptomatic disease is approximately 8/100,000 children/year (Buchanan, 2014). Acute ITP is more prevalent among children younger than 10 years, affects males and females equally, and is more prevalent during the late winter and spring. Chronic ITP affects adolescents more than younger children, with females being affected more frequently than males. The etiology of ITP is unknown, although in the majority of children, it follows a viral illness and is considered to be an autoimmune process.

### Pathophysiology

In general, ITP is caused by antibodies directed against platelet membrane antigens resulting in the destruction of platelets by macrophages in the liver and spleen (Buchanan, 2014).

### Manifestations

Clinical manifestations of ITP include the sudden onset of bruising and petechiae, with bleeding involving the mucous membranes and gums, in a child who is in otherwise good health (Fig. 47.2).

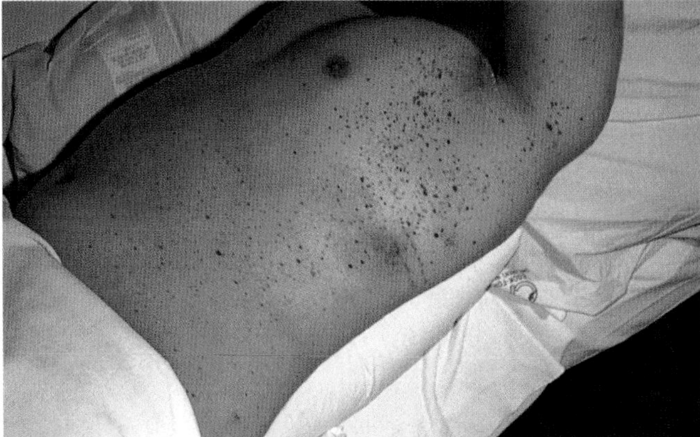

FIG 47.2 Multiple petechiae are characteristic of immune thrombocytopenic purpura. This disorder results in the destruction of circulating platelets and decreased bone marrow production of new platelets. (Courtesy Cook Children's Medical Center, Fort Worth, TX.)

### Diagnostic Evaluation

The initial diagnostic evaluation should include a thorough history and a CBC, including evaluation of a peripheral blood smear. A family history of ITP, information about any medications the child has taken that could cause thrombocytopenia, history of recent live virus vaccination, and any instances of illness, especially febrile illness, in the past month, are obtained. In an affected child, the initial CBC will reveal a low platelet count, often below 50,000/mm$^3$, but the remainder of the CBC will otherwise be normal. The physical examination findings will be normal, aside from the signs of bleeding.

If any data in the history or CBC are suggestive of a diagnosis other than ITP, the physician may obtain a bone marrow aspirate to rule out an oncologic disorder and to determine whether megakaryocytes, the precursors of platelets, are present. Routine bone marrow examination is not warranted in a child with findings consistent with acute ITP.

Physical examination of the affected child reveals bruising and petechiae, the severity of which depends on how low the platelet count is and the child's tolerance of the low platelet count. The spleen and liver are generally normal in size. The greatest risk for a low platelet count is intracranial hemorrhage, so a neurologic assessment is important.

### Therapeutic Management

The goal of treatment is to prevent rare, life-threatening bleeding events, such as intracranial bleeding. Additional goals include restoration of the platelet count to above 20,000/mm$^3$ in children with mucocutaneous bleeding and a reduction in the duration of thrombocytopenia. Treatment is based on the child's presenting condition.

Because most cases of ITP are self-limiting, with a normal platelet count returning within 6 months, no therapy is needed; however, platelet counts and bleeding status should be monitored frequently (Buchanan, 2014).

The mainstays of treatment are oral steroids and IVIG. Depending on whether the child is an inpatient or outpatient, IV or oral steroids may be administered over a 2- to 4-week period. Steroids block the autoimmune destruction of platelets. IVIG is administered once daily for 1 to 2 days. Often, the platelet count is dramatically increased after one dose of IVIG.

ITP is considered to be acute if recovery of a normal platelet count occurs within 6 months. The condition becomes chronic if recovery takes longer than 6 months. Children with chronic ITP may initially respond to steroids with an increased platelet count, but it will not reach normal levels. These children may go for long periods without excessive bleeding or a low platelet count; the count will then begin to decline again, at which time steroid therapy should be resumed.

When steroids and IVIG do not control the thrombocytopenia in a child with chronic ITP, a splenectomy may be indicated. Splenectomy will cure most children with chronic ITP because the spleen synthesizes the antiplatelet antibody that results in the destruction of circulating platelets. The risk associated with removal of the spleen is sepsis from those organisms that the spleen's reticuloendothelial system fights, so ITP is managed without splenectomy, if possible, until age 5 years. Platelet transfusions are given to children only when active, uncontrolled bleeding occurs.

## NURSING CARE

### The Child With Immune Thrombocytopenic Purpura

#### Assessment

Parents usually bring their child to the physician because they have noticed excessive bruising or a "red rash" in the child's mouth or on their body. Although this "rash" (actually petechiae) may look remarkable to a nurse, it often evolves so gradually that it escapes the immediate notice of a parent who sees the child every day. As a result, healthcare may not be sought until very significant bruising and petechiae, even hematomas, are present.

Affected children usually demonstrate normal activity levels for their age because they do not "feel bad." Assessment should include observation for signs of any further bruising or bleeding, including epistaxis, hematuria, or blood in the stools, as well as for signs of a decreasing level of consciousness, which could indicate intracranial hemorrhage.

### Nursing Diagnosis and Planning

The nursing diagnoses and expected outcomes that may be appropriate after assessment of the child with ITP are as follows:

- Ineffective Protection related to low platelet count.

*Expected outcome.* The child will exhibit no signs of active bleeding or intracranial hemorrhage, as evidenced by pulse and blood pressure within normal limits and an alert and responsive child.

- Risk for Infection related to chronic use of steroids or splenectomy.

*Expected outcome.* The family will identify signs of infection and notify the healthcare team, and the child will respond rapidly to treatment for infection.

- Deficient Knowledge related to insufficient information about the disorder and its therapeutic management.

*Expected outcome.* The child and family will describe ITP and the treatment plan.

### Interventions

The family is referred to a healthcare center to carry out medical treatments, and the family is educated about ITP and home care (see Patient-Centered Teaching: Home Care of the Child with Immune Thrombocytopenic Purpura).

An IV access line might be established for the purpose of administering IV steroids or IVIG. Establishing IV access in children with ITP can be quite challenging because merely puncturing the skin can result in a hematoma, which can be confused with "blowing" the vein. Careful evaluation of blood return and flushing of the IV catheter with normal saline solution will confirm proper placement of the catheter.

Restricting the activity of toddlers and young children can be a challenge. Extra-soft bristle toothbrushes or Toothettes should be used for mouth care on all children whose platelet count is below 20,000/mm$^3$. Until the platelet count returns to normal, activities such as bicycle riding, contact sports, and roller-skating should be curtailed.

Education includes teaching the family about the disease process of ITP, the side effects of steroids and IVIG if used, the need to restrict the child's activity, and the importance of proper follow-up evaluations. Steroids can mask the presence of an infection. Parents should be instructed regarding the signs and symptoms of infection and what actions they should take if fever and other signs of infection are seen.

#### SAFETY ALERT

**_Actions to Avoid in Children With Low Platelet Counts_**

- Avoid administering intramuscular injections, aspirin, aspirin-containing products, and nonsteroidal antiinflammatory medications (e.g., ibuprofen) to children with low platelet counts.
- Avoid measuring temperatures rectally, and perform invasive procedures with extreme caution.

The nurse ensures that parents and the child's primary care physician are informed if the child receives IVIG. The AAP recommends delaying the administration of routine measles immunization for up to 11 months after a child receives an immune globulin preparation because it can block the replication of live-virus vaccine immune response (AAP, 2015).

If a splenectomy is planned, both the pneumococcal and *H. influenzae* type B (Hib) vaccines are given if not previously administered. After the splenectomy, the child must take prophylactic penicillin daily. Any signs and symptoms of infection should be reported immediately to the physician so that proper therapy can be initiated before the infection becomes life threatening.

### Evaluation

- Are the child's vital signs within normal limits?
- Is the child responding in an age-appropriate manner?
- Have areas of ecchymosis and petechiae decreased?
- Does the family verbalize and implement a plan of care that decreases the risk of the child incurring an injury that is likely to cause hemorrhage?
- Does the family respond quickly to early signs of infection by notifying the primary healthcare provider?

#### PATIENT-CENTERED TEACHING

**_Home Care of the Child With Immune Thrombocytopenic Purpura*_**

- Eliminate participation in high-risk activities, such as contact sports, bicycle riding, roller-skating, and diving, if the child's platelet count is low.
- Avoid medications that can affect platelet function (ibuprofen, aspirin). Be sure to read over-the-counter medication labels to check for these medications, which can be included in combination products such as cold, flu, and upset stomach remedies.
- Use an extra-soft bristle toothbrush if the platelet count is less than 20,000/mm$^3$.
- Establish an age-appropriate, safe home environment.
- Pad table corners.
- Pad crib rails.
- Offer extra joint padding on clothes.

*For additional resources and information, contact the national organization for people with ITP (e.g., Platelet Disorder Support Association [PDSA] at http://www.pdsa.org).

## DISSEMINATED INTRAVASCULAR COAGULATION

Disseminated intravascular coagulation (DIC) is an acquired hemorrhagic syndrome characterized by uncontrolled formation and deposition of fibrin thrombi. The consumption of clotting factors results, leading to uncontrolled bleeding. In children, DIC does not have the high mortality rate seen in adults. The keys to recovery for children are identification and treatment of the underlying cause of the DIC.

### Etiology

DIC is triggered by any factor that causes endothelial damage, liberation of tissue thromboplastin, circulating endotoxins, or immune complexes. In children, the most common causes are trauma, hypoxia, necrotizing enterocolitis, shock, liver disease, overwhelming viral or bacterial infections, and acute promyelocytic leukemia.

## Manifestations

Manifestations of DIC involve an insidious onset that corresponds to changes in the platelet count and fibrinogen levels. Early indicators include excessive bruising and petechiae, oozing from puncture sites, oozing from sites of mild tissue trauma (e.g., site of insertion of a nasogastric tube), and mild gastrointestinal bleeding. As the disease progresses, manifestations of DIC include purpuric rash, worsening of bleeding, hemoptysis, hypoxemia, oliguria progressing to renal failure, progressive organ failure, and intracranial hemorrhage.

## Diagnostic Evaluation

The diagnosis of DIC is confirmed by laboratory testing (Box 47.2).

## Therapeutic Management

To control DIC, the clinician must identify and then treat the underlying cause of the condition. Treatment then becomes symptomatic and directed at replenishing consumed coagulation factors (Scott & Raffini, 2016). Depleted fibrinogen and other coagulation factors are replaced (e.g., fresh-frozen plasma) to normalize the prothrombin time (PT). RBCs and platelet transfusions can aid in replacing cells lost with hemorrhage. Exchange transfusions are used in neonates to minimize the excessive fluid volume required by replacing platelets, clotting factors, and RBCs. Vitamin K administration can also normalize the PT. The most frequent drug used to dissolve clots is heparin. However, heparin has a controversial role in the treatment of childhood DIC because it can increase the risk for bleeding.

### BOX 47.2 Confirmatory Laboratory Findings in Disseminated Intravascular Coagulation

- Decreased red blood cell (RBC) count
- Low platelet count noted on complete blood count (CBC)
- RBC fragments on the smear
- Prolonged prothrombin time (PT)
- Decreased fibrinogen level
- Elevated levels of fibrin degradation products (FDPs) and D-dimer

## Nursing Considerations

DIC typically develops in a child who is already hospitalized. The subjective and objective data assessed will depend entirely on the initial illness. The nurse must be cognizant of the child who is at risk for DIC. Evidence of bleeding at any site of integumentary interruption and at every orifice, must be assessed. The nurse also notes any changes in the pattern of vital signs. Adequate tissue perfusion should be confirmed because normal function of an organ is the end result of sufficient oxygenation of that organ. Children with full clinical manifestations of DIC are typically cared for in an intensive care setting owing to the multisystem sequelae and complex management of DIC.

Any areas of active bleeding should be located promptly and pressure applied, if possible. The nurse continues to monitor the child for overt and covert signs of bleeding. Care should be taken to avoid any unnecessary tissue trauma or injury. IV lines and indwelling tubes should be secured and protected to eliminate the additional trauma caused by reinsertion. Frequent monitoring of vital signs is necessary to identify changing patterns and ensure adequate cardiac output and end-organ perfusion. Laboratory results are also monitored carefully, with particular attention to the trending of values. Per physician orders, medications, blood products, and treatments are administered and the child's tolerance and outcomes are monitored closely. Because hypoxemia and acidosis can actually cause DIC, adequate ventilation must be ensured to prevent or reduce compromised respiratory function.

Because DIC can be life threatening, the nurse helps parents deal with their anxiety about their child's condition. It is essential that the nurse is available to answer questions and update the parents on the child's progress.

The morbidity and mortality rates in children with DIC depend on the underlying causative condition. With prompt recognition of both the underlying cause and the diagnosis of DIC and with proper management, these children can have favorable outcomes.

# APLASTIC ANEMIA

Aplastic anemia is a condition in which the bone marrow ceases production of the cells it normally manufactures. The result is peripheral **pancytopenia**, a condition in which all formed elements of the blood are simultaneously depressed.

### PATHOPHYSIOLOGY

#### *Disseminated Intravascular Coagulation*

Disseminated intravascular coagulation (DIC) is a consumptive disorder caused by abnormal activation of the clotting mechanism, which causes rapid depletion of platelets, prothrombin, and fibrinogen. It is a pathologic syndrome resulting from the formation of thrombin, subsequent activation and consumption of certain coagulant proteins, and the production of fibrin thrombi. DIC manifests with diffuse microvascular coagulation caused by depletion of clotting factors, resulting in impaired hemostasis.

The pathophysiology of DIC is complicated and often not easily understood because both excessive bleeding and excessive clotting are occurring at the same time. The syndrome of DIC leads to deposition of platelet and fibrin plugs in the vasculature and the simultaneous depletion of platelets and clotting factor proteins.

The process of blood coagulation follows either an intrinsic or an extrinsic pathway. Both pathways ultimately lead to the common pathway of prothrombin forming thrombin, which, in the presence of fibrinogen, forms fibrin. Alternately, fibrinolysis (clot destruction) requires the presence of thrombin. During this process, the enzyme *plasmin* lyses fibrin into fragments called *fibrin degradation products,* which interfere with the ability of platelets to adhere to one another. In DIC, initiation of the clotting process is stimulated by endothelial damage or some form of tissue injury. Platelets and clotting factors are subsequently depleted. As clotting is stimulated, the body perceives the need to produce substances to dissolve those clots, and there is an increase in the end result of clot lysis, fibrin degradation products. The overstimulation of both of these normal processes has four major effects on the body:

- Increased, uncontrolled bleeding resulting from the depletion of platelets and clotting factors and overstimulation of the fibrinolytic process
- Anemia caused by the excessive bleeding and the mechanical fragmentation of RBCs
- Organ damage resulting from the formation of emboli
- Tissue hypoxia leading to tissue necrosis

## Etiology and Incidence

Aplastic anemia can be congenital or acquired. Several rare, inheritable disorders are characterized by aplastic anemia. The most common of these is Fanconi anemia. Aplastic anemia can also be acquired, with a number of agents and conditions implicated as the probable cause. These most often include drugs or chemicals and, less often, radiation exposure, viruses (e.g., parvovirus B19), and immune diseases. Most cases (approximately 70%) of aplastic anemia in children are idiopathic—without an identifiable cause. Aplastic anemia results in a physiologic and anatomic failure of the bone marrow that prevents the development of granulocytes, erythrocytes, and megakaryocytes. In the United States and Europe, the annual incidence of aplastic anemia is only 2 cases per million (Hartung, Olson, & Bessler, 2013).

## Manifestations

The clinical manifestations of aplastic anemia include petechiae, ecchymosis, pallor, epistaxis, fatigue, tachycardia, anorexia, and infection.

## Diagnostic Evaluation

Although the diagnosis of aplastic anemia may be suspected from the child's history and the results of a CBC, bone marrow aspiration and biopsy must be performed for confirmation. Biopsy results should reveal the presence or absence of precursors of the mature cells found in a peripheral blood sample. In aplastic anemia, these precursors are notably absent from the marrow sample. This type of marrow is described as *hypocellular* and often contains a predominance of lymphocytes and yellowish fatty tissue.

## PATHOPHYSIOLOGY

### *Aplastic Anemia*

Aplastic anemia is characterized by cessation of hematopoiesis of granulocytes, erythrocytes, and megakaryocytes by the bone marrow. The disease is classified as mild, moderate, or severe, depending on the absolute counts of neutrophils, platelets, and reticulocytes. The diagnosis of severe aplastic anemia requires two of the following anomalies: granulocyte count less than 500/mm$^3$, platelet count less than 20,000/mm$^3$, and reticulocyte count below 1% (after correction for hematocrit).* In addition, the bone marrow biopsy specimen must contain less than 25% of the normal cellularity.

*Hord, J.D. (2016). The acquired pancytopenias. In R. Kliegman, B. Stanton, J. St. Geme, et al. (Eds.), *Nelson textbook of pediatrics* (20th ed., pp. 2370–2372). Philadelphia: Elsevier.

## Therapeutic Management

If the aplastic anemia is determined by history to be acquired, exposure to the causative agent is discontinued immediately. Treatment then is based on symptoms. Platelet and erythrocyte transfusions might be needed. Granulocyte transfusions are not used routinely because of their short life span in the circulation. When signs and symptoms of infection are suspected or present, antibiotics are administered after appropriate cultures are obtained.

Bone marrow or allogeneic hematopoietic stem cell transplantation remains the treatment of choice for children with severe aplastic anemia for whom a suitable donor has been identified (Hartung et al., 2013) (See Chapter 48 for a discussion of hematopoietic stem cell transplantation). An immunosuppressant medication regimen of cyclosporine and antithymocyte globulin (ATG) effectively treats acquired aplastic anemia in many children for whom a suitable bone marrow or stem cell donor is not available (Hord, 2016).

## NURSING CARE

### The Child With Aplastic Anemia

#### Assessment

The subjective assessment usually elicits parents' observations of bruising immediately after an event that would not normally result in a bruise. For example, an observant parent might have noted petechiae in the child's mouth while assisting the child in brushing the teeth. The parent might also have observed extreme fatigue, headaches, and dizziness upon rising. Information should be elicited about medications recently taken or recent exposures to environmental substances outside the child's usual realm in an effort to determine possible drug- or chemical-related causes for the pancytopenia.

Petechiae, bruising, pallor, lethargy, and tachycardia are the usual abnormal findings and are directly related to the degree of pancytopenia. A history of fever is also commonly present in the child with aplastic anemia. Otherwise, the results of the physical assessment are usually normal.

#### Nursing Diagnosis and Planning

The nursing diagnoses and expected outcomes appropriate for the child with aplastic anemia include the following:

- Risk for Infection related to inadequate secondary defenses or immunosuppression.

  ***Expected outcome.*** The child remains free from infection, as evidenced by being in the expected range for body temperature, neurologic assessment, cardiorespiratory assessment, gastrointestinal status, and genitourinary status.
- Ineffective Protection related to thrombocytopenia.

  ***Expected outcome.*** The child will remain free of bleeding episodes and will demonstrate appropriate precautions to prevent or decrease bleeding.
- Ineffective Peripheral Tissue Perfusion and Risk for Decreased Cardiac Tissue Perfusion related to anemia.

  ***Expected outcome.*** The child's tissues will be perfused, as evidenced by palpable peripheral pulses, capillary refill less than 2 seconds, urine output appropriate for age, and absent respiratory distress.
- Deficient Knowledge related to incomplete information about the disease process.

  ***Expected outcome.*** The child and family will describe the disease process and its potential complications.

#### Interventions

Nursing care initially focuses on providing supportive care and preventing any serious physiologic sequelae of pancytopenia. Because of the increased risk for bacterial and viral infection, affected children should be assigned to a private room, preferably a positive pressure room. All visitors as well as the child should be instructed in meticulous hand hygiene. Precautionary measures should be taken as for any individual with a low platelet count, including no injections; no rectal temperatures, examinations, or medications; use of an extra-soft bristle toothbrush or Toothette; abstinence from any contact sports or activity; and periodic assessment for increased bleeding.

Physician orders should be followed with regard to blood and platelet transfusions, acquisition of blood cultures, and antibiotic, antiviral, and antifungal medication administration. Usually, the platelet count will be maintained at a level greater than 20,000/mm$^3$ to prevent intracranial hemorrhage or active bleeding. The hemoglobin level is typically maintained above 7 g/dL. However, if a child is to receive a hematopoietic stem cell transplant, efforts are made to use blood transfusions only as necessary to avoid possible alloimmunization. If any symptoms of infection are present, blood should be drawn for culture. The decision to culture other body fluids or sites will be based on the child's clinical examination.

Antibiotics should be administered immediately to a febrile child with neutropenia because of the risk for rapid onset of overwhelming sepsis. Children who are hospitalized, febrile, and neutropenic should be assessed frequently for signs of septic shock. Assessment includes the quality of peripheral pulses compared with central pulses, extremity temperature, capillary refill time, level of consciousness, vital signs, condition of cannulation sites, and presence of skin breakdown.

Education of the family and child should include information about the disease process and the complications that must be reported promptly to the healthcare provider. Often, referral is made to a transplant center. If so, intense pretransplant education is indicated. The Aplastic Anemia and MDS International Foundation (http://www.aamds.org) is a good source of information for children, parents, and healthcare providers. Follow-up studies should include frequent CBC and physical examinations.

### Evaluation

- Is the child afebrile, and do cannulation or other skin sites remain free of redness or swelling?
- Are assessment data related to other body systems within normal ranges?
- Has the child had any major bleeding?
- Is the child able to participate in age-appropriate activities without injury?
- Does the child demonstrate palpable peripheral pulses, capillary refill less than 2 seconds, urine output appropriate for age (see Chapter 40), and oxygen saturation more than 95%?
- Has the family received instruction regarding the disease and home care and verbalized an understanding of the information?

## KEY CONCEPTS

- For RBCs to carry oxygen, there must be an adequate amount of hemoglobin, which depends on sufficient circulating iron.
- Anemia results from blood loss, decreased production of RBCs or hemoglobin, or increased destruction of RBCs.
- Caring for children with blood disorders requires an understanding of the anatomy and physiology of blood and blood-forming tissues, genetics, and chronic illness.
- The number of RBCs in the blood varies according to age, sex, and the altitude at which a person lives.
- Iron deficiency anemia can be prevented by providing children from birth to 12 months with iron-fortified formula, or breast milk with iron-fortified cereal and foods.
- Morphine is the drug of choice for children with a painful episode associated with SCD.
- Complications associated with sickle cell disease can be reduced through early screening, diagnosis, and treatment; routine and pneumococcal, meningococcal, and influenza immunizations; penicillin prophylaxis; and parent/child education.
- Children with decreased platelet counts and factor disorders should not receive aspirin or aspirin-containing products. To prevent hemorrhage, rectal temperatures must be avoided and invasive procedures done only when necessary, using extreme caution.
- Factor prophylaxis for infants and young children with hemophilia is warranted due to the risk for bleeding and joint damage.
- Bleeding associated with hemophilia is treated with rest, ice, compression, elevation, and factor replacement, as necessary.
- Family education about caring for a child with hemophilia at home should include management of bleeding episodes, environmental safety, administration of medications, health promotion, and normal growth and development.
- Educating the family of a child with ITP about activity restrictions and protection from injury is a major nursing challenge.
- Management of DIC is directed toward identifying and treating the underlying cause.
- Nursing care of the child with aplastic anemia focuses on the prevention of infection resulting from pancytopenia.

## REFERENCES AND READINGS


Abbas, H.A., Kahale, M., Hosn, M.A., et al. (2013). A review of acute chest syndrome in pediatric sickle cell disease. *Pediatric Annals, 42*(3), 115–120. doi:10.3928/00904481-20130222-11.

American Academy of Pediatrics. (2015) Active immunization. In D.W. Kimberlin, M.T. Brady, M.A. Jackson, et al. (Eds.), *Red book 2015 report of the committee on infectious diseases* (30th ed., pp. 13–56). Elk Grove Village, IL: AAP.

Atoui, M., Badr, L.K., Brand, T.D., et al. (2015). The daily experiences of adolescents in Lebanon with sickle cell disease. *Journal of Pediatric Health Care, 29*(5), 424–434. doi:10.1016/j.pedhc.2015.01.012.

Bolton-Maggs, P. (2011). *Hemophilia C*. Retrieved from http://emedicine.medscape.com/article/955690-overview.

Buchanan, G.R. (2014). Immune thrombocytopenia during childhood: new approaches to classification and management. *The Journal of Pediatrics, 165*(3), 437–439. doi:10.1016/j.jpeds.2014.05.030.

Carson, S. M., & Martin, M.B. (2014). Effective iron chelation practice for patients with ß- thalassemia major. *Clinical Journal of Oncology Nursing, 18*(1), 102–111. doi:10.1188/14.CJON.102-111.

DeBaun, M., Frei-Jones, M., & Vichinsky, E. (2016a). Sickle cell disease. In R. Kliegman, B. Stanton, J. St. Geme, et al. (Eds.), *Nelson textbook of pediatrics* (20th ed., pp. 2336-2345). Philadelphia: Elsevier.

DeBaun, M., Frei-Jones, M., & Vichinsky, E. (2016b). Thalassemia syndromes. In R. Kliegman, B. Stanton, J. St. Geme, et al. (Eds.), *Nelson textbook of pediatrics* (20th ed., pp. 2349–2353). Philadelphia: Elsevier.

Dobson, C.E., & Byrne, M.W. (2014). Using guided imagery to manage pain in young children with sickle cell disease. *American Journal of Nursing, 114*(4), 26–36.

Eckes, E.J. (2011). Chelation therapy for iron overload. *Journal of Infusion Nursing, 34*(6), 374–380. doi:10.1097/NAN.0b013e3182306356.

Ellison, A.M. (2012). Sickle cell disease: advise on handling emergencies. *Contemporary Pediatrics, 9*(9), 18–27.

Flood, V.H., & Scott, J.P. (2016). Von Willebrand disease. In R. Kliegman, B. Stanton, J. St. Geme, et al. (Eds.), *Nelson textbook of pediatrics* (20th ed., pp. 2390–2392). Philadelphia: Elsevier.

Gooneratne, L.V., Dissanayake, R., Jayawardena, A., et al. (2015). Allogeneic bone marrow transplant in a child with thalassaemia. *Ceylon Medical Journal, 60*, 74–75.

Hartung, H.D., Olson, T.S., & Bessler, M. (2013). Acquired anemia in children. *Pediatric Clinics of North America, 60*, 1311–1336. doi:10.1016/j.pcl.2013.08.011.

Hord, J.D. (2016). The acquired pancytopenias. In R. Kliegman, B. Stanton, J. St. Geme, et al. (Eds.), *Nelson textbook of pediatrics* (20th ed., pp. 2370–2372). Philadelphia: Elsevier.

Jacob, E., Pavlish, C., Duran, J., et al. (2013). Facilitating pediatric patient-provider communications using wireless technology in children and adolescents with sickle cell disease. *Journal of Pediatric Health Care, 27*(4), 284–292. doi:10.1016/j.pedhc.2012.02.004.

Kauffman, J. (2014). Management of surgical patients with bleeding disorders. *Infusion Nurses Society, 37*(2), 88–94. doi:10.1097/NAN.0000000000000023.

Khamees, D., Klima, J., & O'Brien, S.H. (2015). Population screening for Von Willebrand disease in adolescents with heavy menstrual bleeding. *Journal of Pediatrics, 166*(1) 195–197. doi:10.1016/jpeds.2014.09.026.

MacMullen, N.J., & Dulski, L.A. (2011). Perinatal implications of sickle cell disease. *Maternal-Child Nursing, 36*(4), 232–238. doi:10.1097/NMC.0b013e3182182215.

McCarthy, J., & Mathew, P. (2011). Treatment of hemophilia with inhibitors: an advance in options for pediatric patients. *Journal of Emergency Nursing, 37*(5), 474–476. doi:10.1016/j.jen.2010.03.004.

Powers, J.M., & Buchanan, G.R. (2014). Iron deficiency anemia: in toddlers to teens: how to manage when prevention fails [Electronic version]. *Contemporary Pediatrics, 31*(5).

Powers, J.M., McCavit, T.L., & Buchanan, G.R. (2015). Management of iron deficiency anemia: a survey of pediatric hematology/oncology specialists. *Pediatric Blood Cancer, 62*, 842–846. doi:10.1002/pbc.25433.

Scott, J.P., & Flood, V.H. (2016). Hereditary clotting factor deficiencies (bleeding disorders). In R. Kliegman, B. Stanton, J. St. Geme, et al. (Eds.), *Nelson textbook of pediatrics* (20th ed., pp. 2384–2389). Philadelphia: Elsevier.

Scott, J.P., & Raffini, L.J. (2016). Disseminated intravascular coagulation. In R. Kliegman, B. Stanton, J. St. Geme, et al. (Eds.), *Nelson textbook of pediatrics* (20th ed., pp. 2399–2400). Philadelphia: Elsevier.

Shahine, R., Badr, L.K., Karam, D., et al. (2015). Educational intervention to improve the health outcomes of children with sickle cell disease. *Journal of Pediatric Health Care, 29*(1), 54–60. doi:10.1016/j.pedhc.2014.06.007.

Sills, R. (2016). Iron-deficiency anemia. In R. Kliegman, B. Stanton, J. St. Geme, et al. (Eds.), *Nelson textbook of pediatrics* (20th ed., pp. 2323–2326). Philadelphia: Elsevier.

Siu, A.L. (2015). Screening of iron deficiency anemia in young children: USPSTF recommendation statement. *Pediatrics, 136*(4), 746–752. doi:10.1542/peds.2015-2567.

Taher, A.T., & Cappellini, M.D. (2014). Management of non-transfusion-dependent thalassemia: a practical guide. *Drugs, 74*, 1719–1729. doi:10.1007/s40265-014-0299-0.

Wang, W.C., Oyeku, S.O., Luo, Z., et al. (2013). Hydroxyurea is associated with lower costs of care of young children with sickle cell anemia. *Pediatrics, 132*(4), 677–683. doi:10.1542/peds.2013-0333.

Weiss, J.A. (2012). Just heavy menses or something more? raising awareness of Von Willebrand disease. *American Journal of Nursing, 112*(6), 38–44.

Wilkie, D.J., Gallo, A.M., Yao, Y., et al. (2013). Reproductive health choices for young adults with sickle cell disease or trait. *Nursing Research, 62*(5), 352–361. doi:10.1097/NNR.0b013e3182a0316b.

Zaiden, R., Besa, E., Crouch, G., et al. (2011). *Hemophilia B.* Retrieved from http://emedicine.medscape.com/article/779322-overview#a0156.

# 48

# The Child With Cancer

http://evolve.elsevier.com/McKinney/mat-ch/

## LEARNING OBJECTIVES

*After studying this chapter, you should be able to:*

- List common clinical manifestations of childhood cancer.
- Discuss the treatment modalities used in the treatment of children with cancer.
- List common late adverse effects of cancer treatment.
- Demonstrate an understanding of the nursing care associated with caring for a child with cancer.
- Discuss symptom management of the child with cancer.

## CLINICAL REFERENCE

### REVIEW OF CANCER

A *neoplasm* is any tumor that arises from new, abnormal cell growth. A tumor is either **benign** or **malignant**. The distinguishing feature of cancer is its ability to invade surrounding tissue and spread to distant sites. Cancer cells spread in one of two ways: (1) by *invasion,* in which cells grow in unrestricted, disorderly fashion at the site of origin; and (2) by *metastasis,* in which the cells grow in sites other than the site of the primary cancer. The cancerous cells grow progressively. The cells have lost the ability to perform their intended functions because changes in the cell's deoxyribonucleic acid (DNA) cause "wrong" information to be transmitted. As the cancerous cells continue to proliferate, they crowd out normal cells and compress vascular structures and vital organs, causing symptoms.

Tumor staging is based on the results of diagnostic studies and, in some cases, surgical examination. Staging describes the extent of disease locally, regionally, and systemically and guides the therapy for most solid tumors. Each tumor has its own specific system of staging, which assists in determining treatment and prognosis.

The cause of most childhood cancers is unknown. The three main categories that predispose children to cancer are genetic, environmental, and microbial (Barbel & Peterson, 2015). Certain alterations in normal DNA predispose a child to the development of cancer. A small percentage of cancers are associated with an inherited predisposition related to chromosomal abnormalities (Asselin, 2016). Known carcinogens, such as radiation, physical irritation, and chemical irritants, contribute to the development of cancer. Lifestyle choices also increase the risk of cancer. Studies have linked higher body mass index in childhood to solid tumors in adulthood (Chang & Davidson, 2015).

The cardinal signs of cancer in children differ from those seen in adults. Most adult cancers are carcinomas, and more screening tools are available to assist with their early detection. The difficulty in diagnosing cancer in children is that symptoms resemble those of common childhood illnesses. Children often are not brought for medical care until obvious signs and symptoms are present. Primary care providers are understandably reluctant to think about cancer as the cause of the child's illness.

#### Cardinal Signs and Symptoms of Cancer in Children

**Overt Signs**

- A mass
- **Purpura**
- Pallor
- Weight loss
- Whitish reflection in the eye
- Vomiting in early morning
- Recurrent or persistent fever

**Signs and Symptoms That Can Be Covert**

- Bone pain
- Headache
- Persistent **lymphadenopathy**
- Change in balance, gait, or personality
- Fatigue, malaise

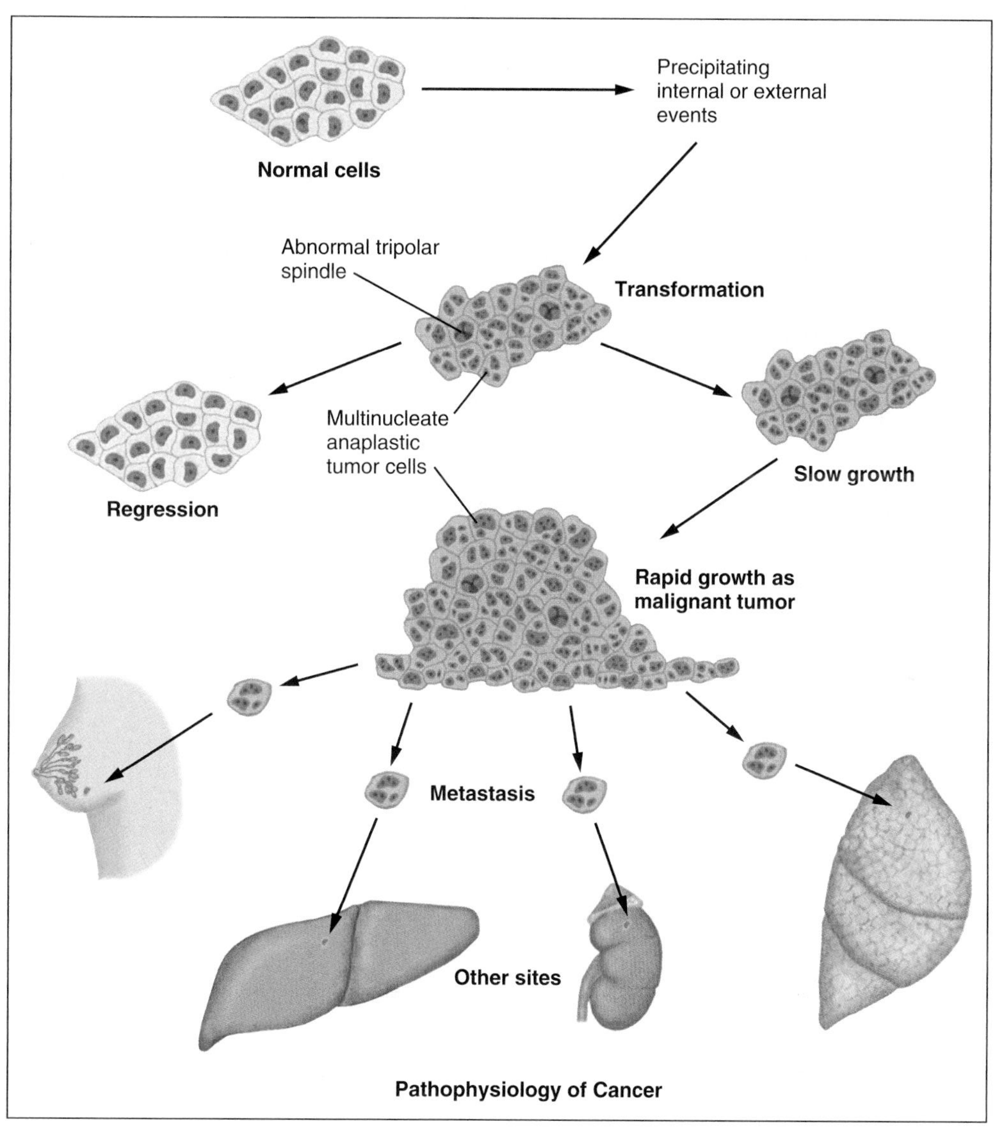


Pathophysiology of Cancer

## Diagnostic Tests and Procedures for Cancer

| Test | Description | Purpose | Nursing Considerations |
|---|---|---|---|
| Bone marrow aspiration | Bone marrow is aspirated from the anterior or posterior iliac crests (the tibia is sometimes used in infants). | Pathologic examination of the aspirated material shows the presence, absence, and ratio of cells that are specific to and diagnostic of certain diseases. Some conditions that can be diagnosed are leukemia, specific vitamin deficiencies, neoplastic diseases in which the marrow is invaded by tumor cells, and aplastic anemia. | 1. Describe the procedure to the child and parents. Check the signed consent. Allow parents to stay with the child if they wish.<br>2. Depending on the protocol of the facility, the child may receive a wide range of sedative or anesthetic agents. Some centers use local anesthesia with no systemic sedation; others use a combination of a sedative and an analgesic.<br>3. The child should be positioned prone with a small pillow under the hips to facilitate access to the posterior iliac crest, the usual site. Tell the child that the physician will clean the site and that it will feel cold. Just before the needle insertion, the child should be told that some discomfort will be felt when the needle is inserted and the marrow aspirated but that the discomfort will last only a few seconds; it will help for the child to sing, count, or take slow, deep breaths.<br>4. Apply a dressing to the area. If the child's platelet count is less than 50,000/mm$^3$, use a pressure dressing. Monitor vital signs until stable, and monitor the puncture site for bleeding and later for signs of infection. |
| Bone scintigraphy | A radiolabeled nucleotide is injected into the bloodstream. This tracer migrates to areas of the body in a predictable pattern. | Pattern of uptake in the axial skeleton is evaluated for variation from normal. Areas of increased uptake indicate increased cellular turnover related to growth, infection, trauma, or tumor activity. | Preparation similar to steps 1 and 2 for bone marrow aspiration.<br>The child will be asked to lie still for 45-60 min to complete testing. |
| Gallium scan | Similar to bone scintigraphy. | In Hodgkin disease, 60%-70% of patients will have uptake of this isotope in active areas at diagnosis. Used as a marker for disease during and after therapy. | Preparation similar to steps 1 and 2 for bone marrow aspiration.<br>The child will be asked to lie still for 45-60 min to complete testing. |
| Positron emission tomography (PET) scan | This study combines conventional nuclear medicine techniques with tomography and adds double-photon imaging, which displays metabolic activity. | PET scans reveal differences in metabolic processes. Glycolysis is accelerated in tumor cells compared with the tissues of origin. PET scans can be useful for diagnosis, staging, and follow-up monitoring. | Be sure the patient is not pregnant.<br>Younger children may need sedation. |
| Single-photon emission computed tomography (SPECT) | This study combines the techniques of conventional nuclear medicine imaging with that of computed tomography (CT) using gamma-emitting radioactive isotopes. | SPECT displays a normal organ in axial, parasagittal, and coronal sections. | Older children should be told about the scan and allowed to see the equipment. |

See Chapter 52 for information about other diagnostics tests (CT scan, lumbar puncture, magnetic resonance imaging [MRI]).

## THE CHILD WITH CANCER

Cancer in children is often difficult to diagnose, and healthcare providers must be aware of the clinical manifestations that should raise the suspicion of cancer. The signs and symptoms depend on the type of tumor, the location of the tumor within the body, the extent of the disease, and the child's age. Testing, diagnosis, and initiation of therapy may occur within a very short period. The diagnosis of cancer can be devastating to both the child and the family. The nurse becomes the informational lifeline for the child and the family as they go through the treatment process. Some resources that are beneficial to patients, families, and providers are the American Cancer Society (http://www.cancer.org), American Childhood Cancer Organization (http://www.acco.org), and National Cancer Institute (http://www.cancer.gov).

### Incidence

Cancer is uncommon in children; nevertheless, pediatric cancer is the second leading cause of death in childhood, after unintentional injuries, and is the leading cause of death from disease. Childhood cancer represents only approximately 1% of all new cancers diagnosed annually in both children and adults in the United States. The most common childhood cancers are leukemias, brain tumors, and lymphomas (Asselin, 2016) (Fig. 48.1). Treatment challenges include minimizing treatment-related side effects while maintaining the child's normal growth and development.

### Childhood Cancer and Its Treatment

Children with cancer are treated in a multidisciplinary setting. Pediatric oncology nurses play a prominent role in the care of children with cancer and their families. They support and educate the children and their families as they move through a stressful process. Pediatric oncology nurses are challenged to maintain a high level of technical competence and an ability to provide the psychological support required by the child and family. Working with children with cancer can be an emotional experience. According to one study, parents felt that a good nurse helped their child feel secure, used distraction techniques appropriately, and provided information that assisted in feeling more in control of the situation (Darcy, Knutsson, Huus, et al., 2014).

A great deal of research has been done over the past 30 years to improve the outcomes for children with cancer. Current survival rates are attributed to cooperative, systematic research through the Children's Oncology Group (COG) and the International Society for Pediatric Oncology. Each group meets twice a year to develop new research protocols and monitor the progress of current protocols; subgroups meet as needed throughout the year. Research protocols direct when drugs are to be given, how frequently, and in what dosages, and which diagnostic and follow-up studies are to be performed. Research has shown that children have better outcomes if they are treated by a scientifically derived protocol. To encourage the development of pediatric cancer treatments, legislative initiatives such as "Creating Hope Act" and the "Best Pharmaceuticals for Children Act" offer incentives for the pharmaceutical companies (Smith & Reaman, 2015).

Because of advances in treatment, the 5-year survival rate has increased to 83% (Barbel & Peterson, 2015). The marked improvement in childhood cancer survival rates has placed renewed emphasis on the importance of identifying the long-term sequelae of cancer treatment in children and initiating timely intervention (American Cancer Society, 2014).

Even with apparently successful treatment of cancer in children, the disease may recur. Recurrences can occur during therapy, shortly after therapy has been completed, or years later. A second tumor can be a new (or second) malignancy. Recurrence is the resurgence of the initial disease, whereas a second cancer is a likely result of the initial treatment. For example, some children with acute lymphocytic leukemia (ALL) develop acute myeloid leukemia (AML) after therapy is complete. Brain tumors develop in a small number of children with ALL who were treated with radiation to their central nervous system (CNS).

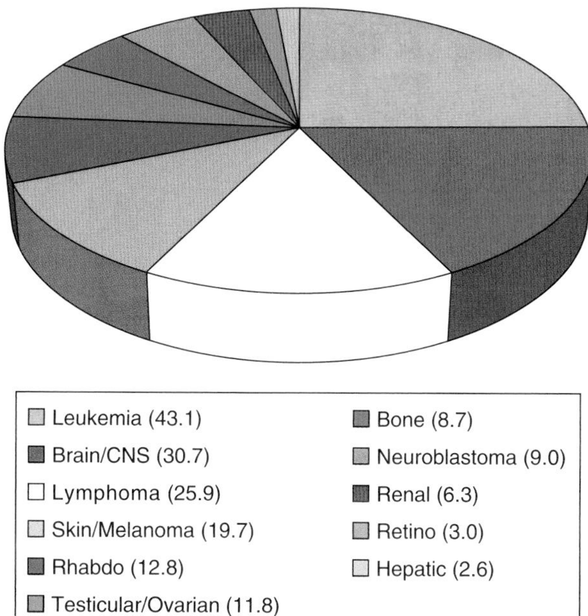


**FIG 48.1** Incidence of Cancers in Children. Rate per million children younger than age 20 years, 2005-2013. (Data from U.S. National Institute of Health, National Cancer Institute, Surveillance Epidemiology and End Results. [2016]. *SEER cancer statistics review 1975-2012.* Retrieved from http://seer.cancer.gov/csr/1975_2012/browse_csr.php?sectionSEL=28&pageSEL=sect_28_table.02.html.)

### Therapeutic Management

Chemotherapy, surgery, and radiation therapy are the primary treatment modalities for children with cancer. Hematopoietic stem cell transplantation (HSCT), steroid therapy, and biologic response modifiers are reserved for a specific subpopulation of children with cancer.

#### Chemotherapy

Chemotherapy is the use of drugs (antineoplastic agents) to kill cancer cells. Different drugs have different side effect profiles and modes of action. Combinations of drugs known individually to be active against the specific disease are used. Tumors can develop resistance to chemotherapy agents, so a variety of active drugs are frequently used. Chemotherapy is given orally, intravenously, intramuscularly, subcutaneously, or intrathecally (through the spinal column). Depending on the protocol, a child will receive chemotherapy either while hospitalized, as an outpatient, or at home.

The side effects of chemotherapeutic agents represent challenges to caregivers. Chemotherapy nonselectively kills rapidly dividing cells. In addition to cancerous cells, the cells most often affected include cells of the hematopoietic system, gastrointestinal (GI) tract, and integumentary system (Box 48.1).

The bone marrow is one of the rapidly proliferating tissues adversely affected by many chemotherapy agents. Bone marrow production may become suppressed, resulting in neutropenia, anemia, and thrombocytopenia. The *nadir*—the time of the greatest bone

## BOX 48.1 Common Side Effects of Chemotherapy and Radiation Therapy

Chemotherapeutic drugs and radiation therapy affect normal and abnormal cells, primarily cells that divide rapidly, such as cells of the gastrointestinal (GI) tract, hair follicles, and bone marrow. As a result, children undergoing these therapies frequently have the following:

### Chemotherapy Side Effects

- Bone marrow suppression
- Bruising
- Alopecia
- Malaise and fatigue
- Nausea
- Vomiting
- Anorexia
- Mucositis/Stomatitis

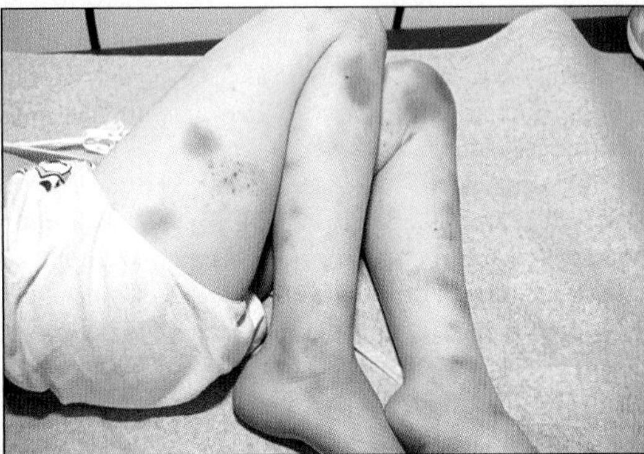

Suppression of the bone marrow because of chemotherapy or radiation therapy reduces the blood counts. Low platelet levels lead to spontaneous bruising, as shown. Nosebleeds and bleeding of the gums are other consequences. The nurse must make a special effort to observe for bruising in dark-skinned children because it will be more difficult to see.

### Radiation Side Effects

#### *Acute (During and Shortly After Irradiation)*

- Skin reactions
- Bruising
- Fatigue
- Bone marrow suppression
- Nausea
- Vomiting
- Anorexia
- Mucositis
- Brain edema
- Transient increase in neurologic symptoms

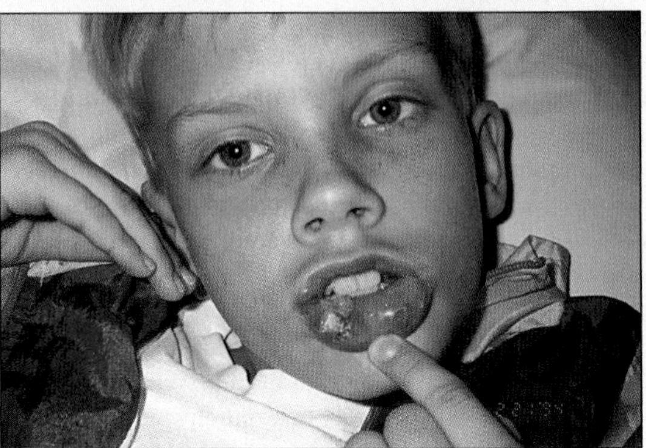

Mucositis (inflammation of the mucous membranes) and mouth ulcers are common side effects of chemotherapeutic drugs. Any mucous membrane can be affected.

#### *Subacute (1 to 6 Months After Irradiation)*

- Somnolence syndrome: pronounced drowsiness, nausea, and malaise (typically 4 to 8 weeks after completing radiation therapy)
- Fever
- Irritability
- Ataxia
- Anorexia
- Dysphasia

#### *Late Effects (More Than 6 Months After Irradiation)*

- Morphologic changes (e.g., cerebral atrophy, white matter degeneration, necrosis, calcification)
- Functional changes (e.g., encephalopathy, neuropsychological deterioration, focal neurologic deficits)
- Alopecia within the radiation field
- Mucositis of any mucous membrane and mouth ulcers

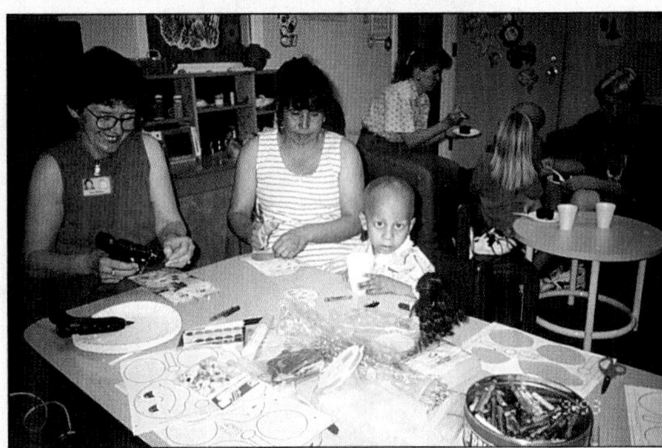

Hair loss is a distressing side effect of cancer treatment. School-age children and adolescents are most likely to feel this distress. Activities such as crafts or playgroups help children feel more normal and provide interaction with others in an accepting environment. (Courtesy Cook Children's Medical Center, Fort Worth, TX.)

marrow suppression when blood counts will be the lowest—generally occurs 7 to 14 days after chemotherapy administration, depending on the specific agent used. The greatest concern during the period of bone marrow suppression is infection.

Neutropenia places the child with cancer at risk for the development of opportunistic infections. Opportunistic infections are caused by nonpathogenic bacteria, viruses, and fungi that, because of compromised immunity, may invade and cause infection. Bacteria, generally present on the skin and within the intestinal tract, can invade the bloodstream through a break in the skin or mucous membranes, leading to a life-threatening infection. In the presence of markedly decreased white blood cells (WBCs), the usual inflammatory responses (erythema, edema, swelling) indicative of an infection is not present. Fever is frequently the only indication of infection. Healthcare providers and families must remain acutely aware of elevated body temperature and breaks in the skin during periods of neutropenia.

The GI tract is affected in a number of ways. Chemotherapy is a noxious stimulus that triggers nausea and vomiting. The treatment of nausea and vomiting was revolutionized in 1992 with the release of a class of nonsedating antiemetic drugs called *5-HT3 serotonin antagonists.* These drugs include ondansetron (Zofran), granisetron (Kytril), and dolasetron (Anzemet). 5-HT3 serotonin antagonists prevent serotonin from binding to vagus nerve receptors, consequently interrupting neurologic signals to the vomiting center of the brain. They have been more effective in combating chemotherapy-induced nausea and vomiting than earlier antiemetics.

Another nonsedating antiemetic drug has further improved the control of chemotherapy-induced nausea and vomiting. Aprepitant (Emend) belongs to a class of drugs known as substance P antagonists. Aprepitant works by binding to neurokinin 1 receptors in the central and peripheral nervous systems, thereby preventing activation of these receptors by substance P, which would trigger vomiting. Aprepitant is used in conjunction with 5-HT3 serotonin antagonists and has proven very effective at preventing chemotherapy-induced nausea and vomiting.

Anorexia is associated with nausea and a change in taste experienced by some people in response to certain chemotherapeutic agents. Anorexia can lead to malnourishment, resulting in weight loss and poor linear growth. Although antiemetics can be effective at preventing nausea and vomiting, they do not prevent alterations in taste that can occur with chemotherapy administration. This alteration in taste, often accompanied by an increased sensitivity to odors, contributes to anorexia.

Certain chemotherapeutic agents cause sloughing of the mucosal tissue of the GI tract, leading to the development of mucositis, both oral (stomatitis) and perianal, and esophagitis. These conditions can be painful and contribute to poor nutrition. Bacteria and yeasts, present as part of the normal digestive process in the mouth and intestinal tract, may cross the open skin or mucous membrane and be absorbed into the bloodstream. The presence of breaks in the integument can lead to bacterial infections of the blood, particularly alpha-hemolytic streptococcus.

Decreased activity, pain medication, and poor oral intake can contribute to the development of constipation. Certain chemotherapeutic agents (such as vincristine) also contribute to constipation. Passage of hard stool can cause abrasion of the delicate mucous membrane of the rectum. The stool is loaded with microorganisms as part of the digestive process. Again, the presence of breaks in the integument can lead to bacterial infections of the blood.

Hair loss (alopecia) has a tremendous psychological effect, especially on school-age children and adolescents. Some chemotherapeutic agents do not produce hair loss, but most do. Children should be reassured that their hair will grow back after the completion of therapy. Accommodations should be made to ease the child's transition to alopecia, including the use of wigs, hats, or scarves. Although young children may respond casually to hair loss, teenagers, particularly girls, often struggle with this dramatic change in their body image.

Changes to the appearance of the skin and nails are common while receiving chemotherapy. These changes include hyperpigmentation of the skin, especially of the hands. Striae, or stretch marks, are also common with treatment regimens that contain high-dose steroids. The nails may become brittle and appear either darkened or with whitish inclusions and/or scarring. These changes, with the exception of striae, typically resolve on completion of the chemotherapy regimen. In addition, many of the medications (such as methotrexate and trimethoprim-sulfamethoxazole) can lead to hypersensitivity to sunlight. The child should avoid excessive sun exposure by the use of long sleeves, hats, and sunscreen.

Treatment-related fatigue, which is thought to be related to loss of muscle mass and function, is distressing to patients and their family. Nurses should assist with educating patients and their families about ways to manage fatigue and reassure them that it lessens as the disease burden decreases (Hooke, Garwick, & Gross, 2011)

Nurses administering chemotherapeutic agents should have evidence of special chemotherapy training by the institution in which they work. The Association of Pediatric Hematology/Oncology Nurses (APHON) (2016) has developed a Pediatric Chemotherapy and Biotherapy Provider Program to help standardize nursing education regarding the administration of pediatric chemotherapy and biotherapy. The program includes a provider course and an instructor course. Nursing responsibilities and precautions related to chemotherapy administration are detailed in Box 48.2.

The more that is understood about the cycles of chemotherapy and the resulting signs and symptoms, the better the nurse can monitor, prevent, educate, and intervene.

### BOX 48.2 Nursing Responsibilities and Precautions for Chemotherapy

- Know Occupational Safety and Health Administration (OSHA) guidelines for administration of antineoplastic agents.
- Measure child's height and weight accurately.
- Confirm body surface area (BSA)—calculated in square meters and used to determine dosages.
- Always double-check the ordered dosage against protocol recommendations.
- Always double-check the medication against the original physician's order.
- A complete blood count (CBC) should be obtained within 48 hours preceding administration of chemotherapy.
- The white blood cell (WBC) and platelet counts need to be at a predetermined level before chemotherapy is given.
- Know the potential side effects of the drugs being administered and appropriate actions to ameliorate those effects.
- Before giving any drugs, ensure the patency of intravenous (IV) tubing by checking for blood return.
- If using an implantable infusion device, ensure that needle placement is secure and blood returns.
- Vesicants (agents that produce blisters) should be given through a new IV site.
- Have appropriate emergency drugs available.
- Know and follow your agency's policies for administration of high-alert medications.

### Surgery

Surgery is frequently part of cancer therapy for children. The surgery may be limited to a biopsy or involve the removal of a solid tumor mass. The purpose of a biopsy is to obtain a small piece of the tumor for microscopic examination. Examination of the tissue by a pathologist confirms the tumor type and influences therapy decisions. Surgery can also be used for debulking or resecting a solid tumor mass. In some diseases, the tumor cannot be resected at the beginning of therapy. After the child has received a few rounds of chemotherapy, the mass may decrease in size, and a less extensive surgical procedure can then be performed (see Chapter 37 for a discussion of preoperative care).

A central venous catheter (CVC) is frequently placed during an initial surgical procedure to facilitate chemotherapy administration. A CVC is a central line that provides easy access to the venous system; the proximal tip of the catheter ends in the large vein just above the heart, the superior vena cava. Three types of CVCs are available. In an external catheter, the distal portion exits the skin, and a tiny polyester cuff is "tunneled" under the exit site where the skin will adhere and hold the catheter in place. In an implanted venous access device (IVAD) or Port-A-Cath, the distal portion ends in a well or reservoir that is placed in the subcutaneous tissue of the anterior chest wall. A percutaneously (peripherally) inserted central catheter (PICC) is inserted into the brachial vein at or near the antecubital fossa using a technique that initially is similar to placement of a peripheral intravenous (IV) catheter. The PICC is then advanced up the veins of the arm until the tip ends in the superior vena cava. This placement procedure usually takes place in an interventional radiology unit.

Preparing the child and family for surgery includes providing information about what will occur before surgery (bowel preps, intake [nothing-by-mouth {NPO}] restrictions) and education regarding the postoperative expectations such as pain control, wound healing, signs and symptoms of bleeding. Because the risk of infection is higher for those receiving chemotherapy, the signs and symptoms of wound infection are important and may be subtle in an immunosuppressed child with a lower than usual WBC count. Such symptoms include warmth, redness, tenderness, and drainage. In addition, it is important for the nurse to check the most recent blood counts before surgery to ensure that the surgical timing is appropriate in relation to the last chemotherapy administration.

Clinical trials are underway to test a new tool that will assist neurosurgeons in identifying where brain tumors begin and end. This assessment will ensure that the entire tumor and all cancerous cells are removed with as little damage as possible to surrounding brain tissue (Zimlich, 2015).

### Radiation Therapy

Radiation can be administered to cure or eradicate disease or administered in low doses as a palliative therapy to prevent further growth of a tumor. To eradicate microscopic disease and promote bone marrow suppression, total body irradiation is given before some stem cell transplants. Radiation can be given in fractionated doses, in which the daily dose is split into smaller doses given more frequently to minimize side effects and increase tumor kill by decreasing the time for cell repair between doses.

Preparing the child and family for radiation involves education about the process in addition to the side effects. Some institutions provide an introductory tour (often called a *simulation*) of the radiation facility so the child can experience the room and surroundings before therapy begins. During the tour, children should be shown the window or monitor through which they will be observed while undergoing radiation alone in the room. Some children need to be sedated for radiation treatments; others can be coached to lie still with the help of child life specialists and parents. The child must lie still for what seems like long periods because the radiation oncologist must carefully control the depth and peripheral margins of the radiation site.

During the simulation, computed tomography (CT) scans and x-rays are performed to identify the site where the radiation therapy will be delivered. Some children receive skin markings with an indelible marker to help guide the radiation oncologists during each treatment. The markings are often covered with a transparent dressing. These markings (or tattoos) should be protected from inadvertent removal.

The side effects of radiation are dose and treatment site specific. As with chemotherapy, side effects result from radiation's effect on healthy, rapidly dividing cells. The side effects usually appear 7 to 10 days after the initiation of therapy. Most often, acute side effects dissipate a few days or weeks after the end of radiation therapy. Common side effects include fatigue, skin damage, hair loss, nausea and vomiting, and low blood counts. Children receiving cranial radiation are particularly affected by fatigue and an increased need for sleep during and shortly after completion of a course of radiation. Skin damage can include

#### EVIDENCE-BASED PRACTICE

For many years, nurses have assessed and provided interventions for fatigue, one of the most distressing symptoms in adult cancer victims. Fatigue and its effects on adolescents and children with cancer have only been recently studied. Hooke, Garwick, & Gross (2011) suggests that fatigue in children and adolescents with cancer is a significant symptom that interferes with the child or adolescent's quality of life.

Hooke et al. (2011) conducted a study to examine the relationship between physical performance and fatigue in children as they received chemotherapy. Hooke et al. (2011) used an exploratory study of 30 participants who were newly diagnosed with cancer and being treated with a minimum of three cycles of chemotherapy. Using the Childhood Fatigue Scale (CFS) for children and the Fatigue Scale for Adolescents (FS-A) for adolescents aged 13 to 18, the participants completed the instruments during their first and third cycles of chemotherapy. To assess physical performance, two measurements were used, the Timed Up and Down Stairs test and the 6-Minute Walk test. The fatigue scales were administered before the physical performance measurements.

Hooke et al. (2011) found that fatigue decreases early in treatment as the burden of disease and the side effects diminish. The study helps healthcare providers better understand the complex relationship between fatigue and physical performance and provides support for future studies to investigate the use of exercise interventions in treating fatigue and improving the quality of life for children and adolescents receiving chemotherapy.

Consider what the experience of fatigue would mean to a child or adolescent who continues to attend school. What types of modifications to the child or adolescent's schedule could facilitate learning while conserving energy? How might a school nurse work with the school administrators to advocate for the adolescent with cancer?

Reference: Hooke, M.C., Garwick, A.W., & Gross, C.R. (2011). Fatigue and physical performance in children and adolescents receiving chemotherapy. *Oncology Nursing Forum, 38*(6), 649–657. doi:10.1188/11.ONF.649-657.

changes in pigmentation (darkening), redness, peeling, and increased sensitivity. Extra care must be taken to avoid excessive skin exposure to heat, sunlight, friction (such as rubbing with a towel or washcloth), and creams or moisturizers. Only topical creams and moisturizers prescribed by the radiation oncologist should be applied to the radiated skin.

The decision regarding radiation dose, frequency, and location depends on the purpose of the radiation and the disease process being treated. In general, radiotherapy is used more cautiously during childhood because children's developing tissues and organs are more vulnerable to radiation's adverse effects (Bleyer, Ritchey, & Friehling, 2016).

Radiation therapy slows the growth of tumors and kills rapidly dividing cells nonselectively. Unfortunately, in a developing child, normal cell development may not be complete when radiation exposure occurs. Radiation therapy to developing brain tissue can alter the cognitive potential. In children younger than 3 years, the effect of radiation therapy can be cognitively devastating. Bone growth is altered if radiation therapy is delivered to areas of growth potential such as facial bones, the spine, and growth plates in long bones. The possible effects, appearing many years later, include skeletal malformations and failure to achieve anticipated growth.

Radiation exposure has been linked to the development of certain types of cancer, and radiation exposure to treat cancer can lead to the development of a second malignancy. Between 3% and 10% of children treated for cancer will have a second malignancy develop, usually 10 to 15 years after exposure (Chang & Davidson, 2015).

### Hematopoietic Stem Cell Transplantation

In recent years, the use of hematopoietic stem cell transplantation (HSCT) has become accepted therapy for the treatment of several hematologic and oncologic disorders. Transplantation allows extremely high doses of chemotherapy (with or without radiation) to be given without regard for bone marrow recovery because hematopoiesis will be restored through transplantation. Stem cells are harvested from bone marrow, peripheral blood, and umbilical cord blood. HSCT is often used interchangeably with bone marrow transplant (BMT) in the clinical setting even when referring to stem cells from cord or peripheral blood.

BMT uses bone marrow to reconstitute the immune function of the child after high-dose chemotherapy. Stem cell transplantation uses a unique immature cell present in the peripheral circulation to restore immune function in a similar manner. Stem cells are able to differentiate into any type of hematologic cell.

The healthy bone marrow cells or stem cells are infused into the bloodstream and migrate to the marrow space to replenish the child's immune function. The decision regarding the source of marrow or stem cells depends on the disease process being treated and the availability of an appropriate donor source.

Recent advances in the understanding of histocompatibility and advances in supportive care have improved outcomes in allogeneic (matched related or unrelated donor) transplants. The child's own harvested stem cells (an autologous transplant) using peripheral blood can be the source of stem cells in certain instances. Autologous transplant allows for aggressive chemotherapy that almost totally ablates the bone marrow. Peripheral blood stem cells (PBSCs) are then given back to "rescue" and restore hematopoietic function of the child's bone marrow.

Umbilical cord blood is another source of transplanted stem cells. Because of the ability to "bank" or store umbilical cord blood, this source is becoming more significant. Cord blood from infants is easily harvested and banked. The donor undergoes no risk during harvesting of the cord blood, and the graft is thought to be more immunologically "tolerant" than stem cells from older donors. A national or international search for a matched, unrelated donor can be done through the National Marrow Donor Program (NMDP).

In preparation for a transplant, the child begins a regimen of chemotherapy with or without radiation (called *conditioning*). The goal of conditioning is to eradicate any disease from the body with high-dose chemotherapy and radiation therapy. WBC, red blood cell (RBC), and platelet counts begin to drop as the chemotherapy and radiation exert their effects on the bone marrow. When the conditioning phase is over, the child receives the donor marrow or stem cells by IV infusion.

Once the marrow is infused, nursing care focuses on preventing profoundly immunosuppressed children from developing life-threatening infections and on minimizing treatment-related side effects. Parents and the child anxiously wait for the day when the complete blood cell counts begin to show signs of marrow engraftment. The production of WBCs, RBCs, and platelets from the transplantation of normal cells is evidence that the marrow has engrafted, or been accepted by the body. Typically, the child is hospitalized for at least one month (Bingen et al., 2012).

Common complications in the days and weeks after HSCT include mucositis, diarrhea, fevers, and nosebleeds. Children receive aggressive nutritional support because most will have substantial difficulty taking foods and fluids orally as a result of severe mucositis, GI discomfort, and diarrhea.

The major problem associated with allogeneic transplants is graft-versus-host disease (GVHD). GVHD is caused when the infused immunocompetent donor bone marrow recognizes the recipient's tissue as foreign and attacks the body, affecting numerous organ systems. Children can exhibit a wide variety of symptoms associated with GVHD, such as mild to severely elevated liver enzyme levels, mild to copious diarrhea, and maculopapular skin reactions ranging from rashes to full skin desquamation. Antirejection drugs such as prednisone, cyclosporine, and tacrolimus are given to prevent GVHD from occurring or lessen its severity.

Transplantation is currently standard therapy for children in first remission with Philadelphia-chromosome–positive ALL (a genetically specific type of ALL with a 90% relapse rate), AML, stage IV neuroblastoma, severe aplastic anemia, severe combined immunodeficiency syndrome, and certain other hematologic disorders (see Chapter 47). Transplantation is also used to treat children with certain solid tumors, Hodgkin disease, and non-Hodgkin lymphoma that are resistant to conventional chemotherapy and radiation, and to treat children who experience relapses. The long-term effects of HSCT include second malignancies and damage to the cardiovascular, respiratory, renal, endocrine, and nervous systems (Mallhi, Lum, Schultz, et al., 2015).

### Steroid Therapy

High-dose and/or long-term steroid therapy is a mainstay of treatment for children with leukemia, as an adjunct for control of nausea and vomiting, and for children with brain tumors complicated by increased intracranial pressure. High-dose steroids (dexamethasone and prednisone) cause a myriad of side effects that include increased appetite, fluid retention, weight gain, hypertension, insulin-dependent diabetes (usually reversible once steroid therapy is stopped), emotional lability (mood changes), sleep disturbances, changes in appearance (abdominal striae, cushingoid features), and immunosuppression.

It is important to educate the child and caregivers about these side effects, as they can be quite frightening (sleep disturbances such as vivid dreaming) and disruptive (mood shifts from angry to sad to happy in very short periods of time). In addition, the family should be prepared for changes in the child's diet such as cravings for high salt-containing foods that can contribute to increased fluid retention, weight gain, and hypertension. The family should be aware of the need to notify the healthcare team if the child has increased thirst and/or voiding at night, which suggest hyperglycemia. The physical changes associated with steroid use can create body image disturbances for children. These changes (cushingoid features) include puffy cheeks, abdominal weight gain, striae (stretch marks), increased acne, and a flushed, shiny appearance of the skin.

The child and caregivers should be reassured that these symptoms typically resolve over a period of weeks once the steroid therapy is stopped.

### Biologic Agents

More recent additions to cancer therapy are the biologic response modifiers. Biologic response modifiers are naturally occurring substances found in small quantities in the body that influence immune system functions (e.g., colony-stimulating factors [CSFs]).

Used to enhance cell recovery, different CSFs work on different types of blood cells to reduce the time and severity of bone marrow suppression. Granulocyte colony-stimulating factors (GCSFs) stimulate WBC recovery. GCSFs can reduce the length of time a child has neutropenia by stimulating production of neutrophils, a type of granulocyte. Other CSFs promote recovery of platelets or RBCs and subsequently reduce the need for blood products.

Over the past few years, a number of immune-modulating agents have been examined in the laboratory; some have translated into clinically beneficial treatment modalities. Certain "targeted" monoclonal antibodies are being used for very specific types of neoplasms and often are used in conjunction with other modalities, such as radiation and chemotherapy. They provide the advantage of effective treatment with less toxicity to normal tissue than other cancer modalities (Bleyer et al., 2016).

### Complementary and Alternative Medical (CAM) Therapies

Complementary therapies are proven therapies (based on research) or therapies that are not yet scientifically proven but are deemed not to be harmful as adjunctive treatment. Alternative therapies are those designed to replace conventional therapy in the treatment of individuals with cancer. The use of CAM therapies, although often harmless and potentially beneficial for the child and family, can negatively affect the efficacy of therapy. Therefore, it is important to determine if children are receiving CAM therapies. One approach is to build a supportive, open rapport with these children and their families. However, not all families will disclose their use of CAM therapies without direct, but supportive, questioning. Most pediatric oncology centers provide an informational notebook or handbook to the family at the time of diagnosis. One technique for eliciting discussion regarding the use of CAM therapies is to include a description of their use and to emphasize the importance of discussing this issue with the child's healthcare providers.

*Family-centered care* is the delivery of care with the intent of developing mutually beneficial partnerships between healthcare providers, families, and patients. The first family-centered approach regarding the use of CAM therapies includes the goal of preserving the dignity of patients and their families. The nurse can achieve this goal by validating the feelings of the child and family regarding their desire to achieve a cure for the child's cancer. The nurse first seeks to understand what CAM therapy the family has chosen and why the family has made the choice. The next family-centered care approach is information sharing. The nurse provides factual information and useful resources to families regarding CAM therapies and cancer. The ultimate decision regarding the use of CAM therapies rests with the family in consultation with the healthcare team. Nurses collaborate with the family in care planning that includes physician-approved CAM therapies.

### Follow-Up Care After Cancer Treatment

Care of the child with cancer continues long after the completion of the child's treatment. It is important that education is provided regarding the late effects of cancer treatment, which can affect growth and development, weight, cardiovascular, pulmonary, and hepatic systems, and dentition. A second malignancy, most commonly AML or solid tumors related to radiation therapy, develops in approximately 20% of children and is the most common cause of death in patients who survive greater than 15 years (Bass, 2014). Primary care providers who have supported children and their families through their journey must continue to monitor and screen children for the late effects of cancer treatment. To assist PCP's, the Children's Oncology Group (COG) developed guidelines for follow-up of pediatric cancer patients (http://www.survivorshipguidelines.org). This resource provides screening recommendations and follow-up care for the cancer survivor (Landier, Armenian, & Bhatia, 2015).

#### CRITICAL THINKING EXERCISE 48.1

When caring for children with cancer, nurses often encounter families who want to try (or are trying) a method of complementary or alternative medical (CAM) therapy to treat the child's cancer. It is not uncommon for families to try CAM therapies without disclosing this practice to the healthcare team for fear of alienating their providers. Families should be asked about the use of CAM therapies through direct questioning in a supportive, nonthreatening manner. Some CAM therapies can potentially decrease the efficacy of chemotherapy (such as folate supplementation in the child receiving methotrexate, an antifolate drug). Others include vitamin supplements that can be obtained inexpensively but perhaps were marketed to the family as a cure and are being provided at a very high cost. Unfortunately, even families in crisis are sometimes exploited. Think about the issues involved with the use of complementary and alternative therapies.

1. What is the difference between complementary and alternative medicine?
2. How might the nurse learn more about what particular CAM therapies can be incorporated into a child's plan of care?
3. As the nurse working with a parent of a young child with recurrent cancer that is resistant to conventional forms of therapy, how might you best assist the family to make decisions regarding the use of CAM therapies?

## LEUKEMIA

As the first disseminated cancer shown to be curable, the approaches to caring for children with childhood leukemia set the standard for principles of pediatric cancer diagnosis, prognosis, and treatment (Tubergen, Bleyer, Ritchey, et al., 2016). Leukemia is the most common form of cancer in children younger than 15 years of age with 2,500 to 3,000 new cases in the US each year (Alperstein, Boren, & McNeer, 2015). The cause of disease is an abnormal proliferation of immature WBCs (blasts), which compete with normal cells for space and nutrients. Bone marrow production of other cells is suppressed, so very low numbers of RBCs (anemia) and platelets (thrombocytopenia) may be seen at diagnosis. Considerable progress in treatment has been achieved through years of research. Leukemia was uniformly fatal in the 1960s. Today, children diagnosed with the most common form of leukemia, acute lymphocytic leukemia (ALL), can almost always achieve remission, with a 5-year disease-free survival rate of 80 to 85% (Alperstein et al., 2015; Cooper & Brown, 2015; Hunger & Mullighan, 2015).

### Etiology

The cause of childhood leukemia is unknown. Geographic distribution varies around the world, with leukemia being uncommon in developing countries but more common in industrialized countries. This variation might be related to underdiagnosis in developing countries, or could implicate exposure to agents in industrialized countries in the development of leukemia.

Genetic factors appear to play a significant role in the development of leukemia. When karyotyped, the leukemic cells in most children with the disease reveal chromosomal abnormalities. Some of these chromosomal abnormalities have become prognostic factors for the disease (Tubergen et al., 2016). Because of the genetic basis of this disease, identical twins have a significantly greater chance of sharing chromosomal abnormalities that later lead to disease. So, the risk of a second twin acquiring the disease after the first has been diagnosed in infancy is significantly higher than that of the general population (Tubergen et al., 2016). The fraternal twin of a child who has had ALL has a two to four times higher likelihood of developing the disease than other children. Children with Down syndrome have a 10 to 30 times greater risk of developing leukemia than the general population (Alperstein et al., 2015). Other less common preexisting chromosomal abnormalities, such as Fanconi anemia and neurofibromatosis, have been correlated with the development of leukemia.

Exposure to ionizing radiation and certain chemical toxins has been shown to increase the risk of leukemia development (Alperstein et al., 2015). Leukemia was well documented in both the child and adult survivors of the atomic bomb detonations in Japan during World War II. Chemical exposure to alkylating agents, a drug class used to treat cancer, has been shown to increase the risk of developing acute myeloid leukemia (AML).

Large epidemiologic studies are ongoing to examine links to pesticide exposure, electromagnetic fields, parental smoking, parental alcohol use, and parental exposures to occupational chemicals. Thus far, relationships between these exposures and leukemia have not been demonstrated.

### Incidence

Leukemias represent approximately 25% of all cancers in children in the United States, with the highest percentage of children diagnosed with leukemia having ALL (>75%) (Bhojwani, Yang, & Pui, 2015). ALL is more common in boys, and the peak incidence occurs between 2 and 5 years of age (Bhojwani et al., 2015; Hunger & Mullighan, 2015). With improvements in treatment, mortality in children younger than 15 years old has decreased markedly, and 80% survive beyond 5 years after diagnosis (Cooper & Brown, 2015). Fifteen to 20% of children relapse which is associated with a poorer prognosis (Hunger & Mullighan, 2015).

### Manifestations

Clinical manifestations of leukemia include fever, pallor, excessive bruising, bone or joint pain (usually leg or knee pain), lymphadenopathy, malaise, hepatosplenomegaly, abnormal WBC counts (either lower or higher than normal for age), and mild to profound anemia and thrombocytopenia. The severity of the clinical manifestations varies with the cell type of leukemia and the length of time before diagnosis.

### Diagnostic Evaluation

The diagnosis can be strongly suspected from a history of the clinical manifestations and an initial complete blood count (CBC). The confirmatory test for leukemia is microscopic examination of bone marrow obtained by bone marrow aspiration and biopsy. A bone marrow aspirate usually provides sufficient material to establish the diagnosis of ALL. A lumbar puncture is also performed to look for leukemic blast cells in the spinal fluid, which are indicative of CNS involvement.

Flow cytometry, the analysis of the bone marrow cells using a laser beam, is another test commonly performed on the initial bone marrow sample. Flow cytometry provides a rapid diagnosis by characterizing the type of leukemia within hours. In addition, a portion of the initial bone marrow sample is sent for cytogenetic analysis to determine the chromosomal changes that have occurred in the leukemic blast cells. These results typically take 2 to 3 weeks to receive, and thus, are not useful for making induction treatment decisions. However, this chromosomal information can be used to determine the intensity of the child's consolidation and maintenance therapy based on known prognostic indicators.

### Therapeutic Management

Combination chemotherapy is the preferred treatment for leukemia. The particular drugs used and their dose, route, and scheduling depend on the protocol that will be used for that specific type of leukemia. Children are placed into prognostic categories with specifically tailored therapies. This specificity helps to provide less toxic treatments when appropriate (Alperstein et al., 2015). Treatment of ALL is divided into phases: induction, consolidation, and maintenance. The aim of the first month of chemotherapy treatment, or induction, is to induce remission. Remission is the reduction of immature blast cells in the bone marrow to less than 5%. Approximately 98% of children with ALL achieve remission within 1 month (Tubergen et al., 2016).

**PARENTS WANT TO KNOW**

***Caring for the Child With Cancer***

- Reinforce teaching concerning diagnosis, treatment, and side effects of chemotherapy.
- Encourage parents to participate actively in the child's care.
- Provide written and verbal instructions concerning home care, and provide ample opportunity for parents to give return demonstrations of the following:
  - Central venous access dressing changes
  - Oral medication administration
  - Assessment of oral mucous membranes and rectal mucosa
  - Temperature measurement by axillary, oral, temporal, and tympanic routes
- Teach the signs and symptoms of infection and bleeding that require immediate treatment and how to access after-hours emergency treatment.
- Provide telephone numbers parents can call to obtain answers to questions concerning the diagnosis, treatment, and side effects of chemotherapy.
- Make appropriate referrals to social services, a chaplain or other religious figure, and a home health nursing agency.
- Encourage parents to use community resources.
- Stress the importance of preventing infection (Fig. 48.2) and bleeding and the need for follow-up visits.

Before induction, the child is treated for presenting signs, which include sepsis, anemia, hemorrhage, and metabolic abnormalities. Serum electrolyte levels are determined to ensure metabolic stability before chemotherapy is initiated. An elevated uric acid level, indicating rapid cell turnover, can be expected if the WBC count is very high. As WBCs break down in reaction to chemotherapy, they release uric acid. Uric acid has poor water solubility and can compromise kidney

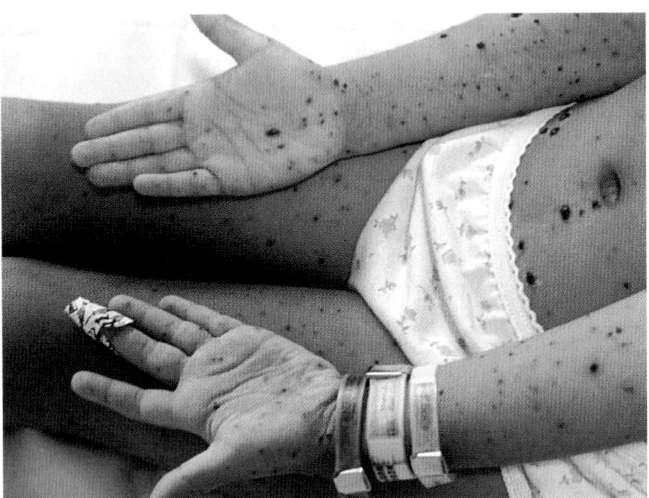

**FIG 48.2** Varicella (chickenpox) can be deadly in the immunocompromised child. Thrombocytopenia (low platelet count) associated with chemotherapy can cause the varicella lesions to be hemorrhagic, like those shown here. Secondary infections of the lesions are also common because of low white blood cell (WBC) counts. (Courtesy Cook Children's Medical Center, Hematology-Oncology Clinic, Fort Worth, TX.)

function (tumor lysis syndrome). When the WBC count is extremely high, allopurinol and IV fluids with sodium bicarbonate are given to decrease the serum uric acid level and alkalinize the urine before chemotherapy starts.

During induction, the hospitalized child receives the first doses of chemotherapy while the response to the drugs is assessed. Remission can be verified within the first 28 days after the initiation of chemotherapy by sequential bone marrow aspirates and lumbar punctures. If a significant number of blast cells are still present, a new and stronger drug regimen is given. The presence of more than 5% blasts in the marrow at day 28 is an ominous sign indicative of a poorer prognosis (Alperstein et al., 2015).

Once the child is medically stable, most chemotherapy treatment for ALL is given on an outpatient basis. Children are usually healthy and able to return to school and engage in most age-appropriate activities.

The consolidation phase of ALL therapy follows induction and remission. The goal of consolidation therapy is to maintain remission and prevent disease in extramedullary "sanctuary sites" such as the testes and CNS, where systemic therapy is not easily delivered. Intrathecal chemotherapy is given prophylactically to prevent relapse in the CNS. If the testes are involved, radiation therapy is administered.

*Text continued on p. 1155*

## PATHOPHYSIOLOGY

### *Leukemia*

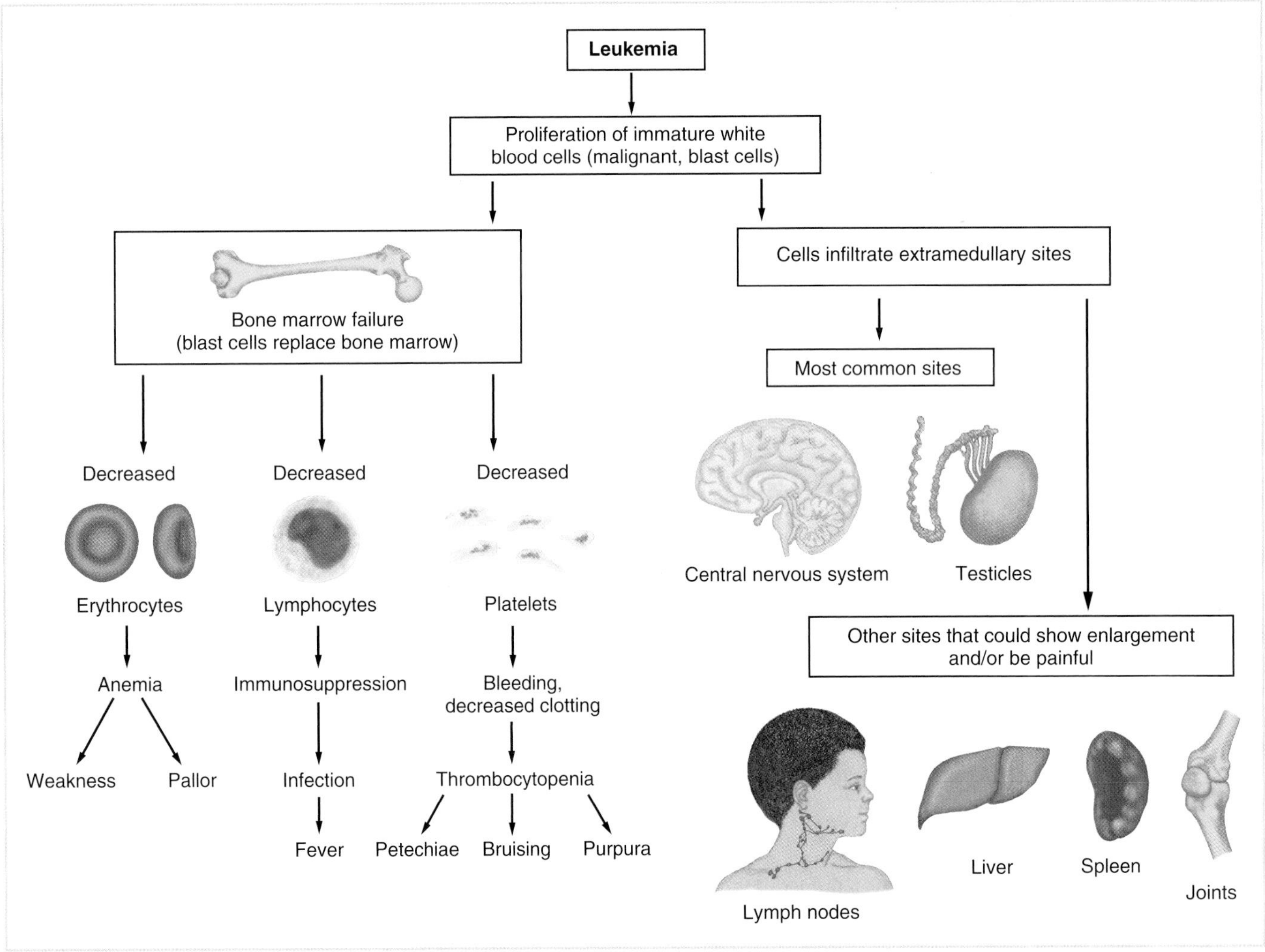

Leukemia

Proliferation of immature white blood cells (malignant, blast cells)

Bone marrow failure (blast cells replace bone marrow)

Decreased

Erythrocytes

Anemia

Weakness

Pallor

Decreased

Lymphocytes

Immunosuppression

Infection

Fever

Decreased

Platelets

Bleeding, decreased clotting

Thrombocytopenia

Petechiae

Bruising

Purpura

Cells infiltrate extramedullary sites

Most common sites

Central nervous system

Testicles

Other sites that could show enlargement and/or be painful

Lymph nodes

Liver

Spleen

Joints

## PATHOPHYSIOLOGY—cont'd

### *Leukemia*

Leukemia most likely arises from a fundamental alteration in the genetic makeup of a white blood cell (WBC). Cells produced from the altered WBC have a defect that prevents maturation. These cells tend to replicate quickly, forming immature cells, or blast cells, in the bone marrow. The blast cells do not respond properly to the body's feedback mechanism and continue to replicate in great numbers. Blast cells are then released into the peripheral circulation and appear in a complete blood count (CBC) test.

In leukemia, normal bone marrow is replaced by malignant blast cells. As the blast cells take over the bone marrow, eventually red blood cell (RBC) and platelet production is impaired, and the child becomes anemic and thrombocytopenic. The symptoms of the disease reflect bone marrow failure and organ infiltration.

In addition to being present in the blood and bone marrow, leukemia cells infiltrate **extramedullary** sites, most commonly the central nervous system (CNS) and the testicles. Although extramedullary leukemia is not common at first diagnosis, these are common sites of relapse.

Leukemias are classified by the type of WBC affected. Broadly, acute leukemias are classified as acute lymphocytic leukemia (ALL) and acute nonlymphocytic leukemia (ANLL). ALL is an abnormality of the lymphocytes. This type of leukemia is also referred to as acute lymphoblastic leukemia.

ANLL is a broad term for leukemias not originating from abnormal lymphocytes. Acute myeloid leukemia (AML) is an example of an ANLL. AML accounts for 25% of childhood leukemias and can be further classified as acute promyelocytic leukemia (APL), acute myelomonocytic leukemia (AMMoL), and acute monocytic leukemia (AMoL). ANLL tends to be less common in children, less responsive to therapy, more difficult to treat, and more likely to result in relapse than ALL.

Chronic leukemias are rare in children. The term *chronic* refers to the indolent nature of the disease. Whereas acute leukemias have a rapid onset to detectable disease, chronic leukemias have a slower onset of symptoms.

## NURSING CARE PLAN

### *The Child With Leukemia*

#### Focused Assessment

- Obtain history from parents of child's symptoms and the likely insidious onset of the disease.
- Possible symptoms include decreased activity level, persistent or recurrent fever of unknown cause, more bruises than usual, intermittent stomachaches, and leg pains with refusal to walk (parents might interpret as child trying to avoid school, having growing pains, or being lazy).
- Conduct physical examination and comprehensive assessment.
- Look for fever, fatigue, pallor, bruising on the extremities, **petechiae** in the mouth and sclera, hepatomegaly, very high white blood cell (WBC) count, and bleeding.
- Check mental and neurologic function due to risk of leukemic infiltration into the central nervous system (CNS).
- Provide ongoing psychosocial assessment of the child and family to determine needs for intervention and support.
- Parents may express guilty feelings that they delayed seeking treatment because they did not initially recognize their child's symptoms as signs of serious illness.
- Observe the child's and parents' reactions to the disease. Assess how each person copes with the illness and treatment. (Parents who are unable to cope often display a high level of anxiety that can be transferred to the child.)
- Include these critical factors in the child's assessment: age, developmental level, and experiences with the healthcare system or providers (child may exhibit increased anxiety if she or he had previous negative experiences).

#### Nursing Diagnosis

Risk for Infection related to the immunosuppressed state.

#### Planning

##### *Expected Outcomes*

1. The child will be free of signs of infection, as evidenced by an afebrile state, no redness of the integument, no redness or swelling at the site of insertion of a central venous catheter, and negative culture results.
2. The parents and the child will recognize and verbalize early signs of infection.

#### Interventions and *Rationales*

1. Monitor vital signs every 4 hours and as necessary if the child is hospitalized. Instruct parents to measure the child's temperature as needed at home (by the oral, axillary, temporal, or tympanic routes only).
   *In the presence of markedly decreased WBCs, and elevated temperature may be the only sign of infection. The risk of injury to the fragile mucous membranes is so great that only oral, tympanic, temporal, or axillary routes should be used to measure temperatures (NO rectal temperatures). Rectal abscesses can easily occur to friable rectal tissue. Report a single temperature of 38.5° C (101.3° F) or a temperature of 38.0° C (100.4° F) that continues for more than 1 hour.*
2. Monitor complete blood count (CBC) with differential as ordered. Report moderate to severe neutropenia.

| Absolute Neutrophil | Count (Anc) (Cells/mm$^3$) Risk |
|---|---|
| 1500-2000 | Not Significant |
| 1000-1500 | Minimal |
| 500-1000 | Moderate |
| <500 | Severe |

   *The risk of infection increases significantly with moderate and severe neutropenia. The absolute neutrophil count can be easily calculated using the results from the child's CBC and this formula: (a) add the percent of neutrophils and the percent of bands; (b) convert the summed percentage into decimal form (e.g., 55% = 0.55); then (c) multiply that figure by the WBC count (stated in thousands).*
3. Practice proper hand hygiene and teach this to the family.
   *Proper hand hygiene is the best way to prevent the spread of infection.*
4. Inspect the child's skin daily for breaks and redness.
   *Some neutropenic children will not produce erythema or purulent drainage. Because pus is made of WBCs, drainage cannot be used as a sign of infection. Skin provides a barrier against infection.*
5. Inspect the child's mouth daily for oral ulcers, and inspect the perineum for fissures. Teach older children to do self-examination. No suppositories should be given.
   *Mucous membranes are fragile and easily affected by chemotherapy and irradiation. Mouth ulcers and rectal fissures are common side effects of*

*Continued*

## NURSING CARE PLAN—cont'd

### The Child With Leukemia

*chemotherapy and radiation therapy and potential sites for bacteria entry because of the impaired mucosa.*

6. Encourage and monitor regular bowel habits.
   *Decreased activity, altered nutrition, and certain medications may predispose to constipation. The passage of hard stool may traumatize delicate rectal mucous membranes and create a potential site for entry of bacteria.*
7. Teach the parents and child meticulous oral hygiene at diagnosis. The child should use a soft-bristled toothbrush or Toothettes when performing oral hygiene four times each day. If the platelet count is low, a cotton-tipped applicator, finger cot, or washcloth wrapped around a finger is used instead of a toothbrush.
   *Prevention of dental caries and ulcerations on fragile oral mucosa will help prevent infections.*
8. At the first signs of mouth ulcers, begin a mouth care regimen four times daily, which includes use of an antifungal drug as ordered by the physician. Do not use alcohol-containing mouthwashes.
   *Fungal infections originating from the mouth or gastrointestinal (GI) tract can quickly become disseminated in immunosuppressed children. Over-the-counter mouthwashes may have high alcohol content and may be drying to oral mucosa, thus increasing the risk of breaking down the protective barrier of the skin.*
9. For the hospitalized neutropenic child, fresh flowers or plants are usually not permitted to decrease the risk of exposure to fungal spores. Do not use humidifiers.
   *Standing water and damp soil harbor Aspergillus and Pseudomonas organisms, to which these children are extremely susceptible.*
10. Use sterile techniques to change any dressings and intravenous (IV) lines.
    *A child with neutropenia is not able to fight infection normally; extra precautions must be taken.*
11. In general, the child should not receive live-virus or live bacterial vaccines such as the measles-mumps-rubella (MMR) and the varicella vaccines. Special circumstances are considered when risks of the disease outweigh risks of the vaccine. Siblings should receive inactivated polio vaccine and may also receive live (MMR) and varicella vaccines. Flu shots are recommended for the patient, family members, and close contacts.
    *Live MMR vaccine could produce infection in the severely immunocompromised child, but no virus shedding occurs to create a threat if given to the sibling. Exposure to a rash produced by the varicella vaccine does have the potential of causing varicella disease in an immunocompromised child. If rash should occur in a vaccinated sibling, the immunocompromised child should be separated from the sibling until the rash resolves.*
12. Keep any child with chickenpox or any child who has been exposed to the virus away from the child with cancer. Inform the teacher of the importance of notifying parents immediately if a case of chickenpox occurs in another child at school. Encourage vaccination of siblings who have not had varicella to create "herd" immunity.
    *Immunocompromised children are unable to fight varicella adequately; chickenpox is life-threatening to them (see* ***Fig. 48.2****). If a child who has not had chickenpox is exposed to someone with varicella, the child should receive varicella-zoster immune globulin within 96 hours of exposure.*
13. Obtain specimens for culture as ordered and monitor the results.
    *Physicians will order blood, urine, stool, and wound cultures as indicated when the neutropenic child has fever.*
14. Administer acetaminophen for fever.
    *Aspirin and ibuprofen given to a child who is thrombocytopenic can cause platelet dysfunction.*
15. Administer antibiotics as ordered after cultures have been obtained. Cultures should be obtained and antibiotics should begin as soon as possible. Once the culture results are available, anticipate that antibiotic therapy will be tailored to treat any identified organisms. Organisms are not always identified, necessitating the continuation of broad-spectrum antibiotics until the child is afebrile, has continued negative cultures, and demonstrates recovering neutrophil counts.
    *Cultures identify the specific organism so that the most effective antibiotic can be given. Appropriate antibiotic treatment should begin promptly.*

#### Evaluation

Is the child afebrile and free of redness or swelling at insertion sites or other integumentary sites?

Have the child and parents promptly recognized and responded to warning signs of infection?

#### Nursing Diagnosis

Risk for Injury related to thrombocytopenia.

#### Planning

##### *Expected Outcomes*

1. The child will have no excessive, uncontrolled bleeding.
2. The parents and child will understand risk for hemorrhage, as evidenced by making the home environment safe and by their ability to respond appropriately to bleeding.

#### Interventions and *Rationales*

1. Apply gentle, firm pressure to any puncture sites. Apply a pressure dressing to sites of bone marrow aspiration.
   *Additional pressure may be needed to stop bleeding if the platelet count is low.*
2. For the child who is severely thrombocytopenic (platelet count <20,000/mm$^3$), monitor closely for signs of bleeding including urine and stool checks for blood. Limit any activity that could result in injury and especially head injury; participation in contact sports is not allowed. Encourage the child to participate in quiet activities (e.g., reading books, watching videos, coloring). Provide a soft-bristled toothbrush or Toothettes for oral hygiene. Give stool softeners to prevent straining with constipation and do NOT use suppositories. Ensure the child avoids eating "sharp" foods such as chips that could cause injury to the oral mucosa.
   *A decreased platelet count increases the risk for bleeding and intracranial hemorrhage is a potential risk.*
3. Teach the child how to control nosebleeds and blow the nose gently.
   *One of the most common sites of bleeding is the nose. Blood loss can be reduced through avoidance of nosebleeds.*
4. Evaluate menstrual flow in adolescent girls.
   *Menstrual bleeding can be severe when girls have low platelet counts. Occasionally, hormone therapy is required to inhibit menses.*

#### Evaluation

Has the child had bleeding that could not be controlled?

Have the parents demonstrated what to do for a nosebleed?

Have the child and parents promptly recognized and responded to bleeding?

#### Nursing Diagnosis

Imbalanced Nutrition: Less Than Body Requirements related to nausea and vomiting, mucositis, or taste changes.

## NURSING CARE PLAN—cont'd

### *The Child With Leukemia*

**Planning**

***Expected Outcomes***

The child will:

1. Experience no more than 5% weight loss.
2. Eat palatable foods that provide nutrients for growth.

**Interventions and *Rationales***

1. Following physician orders, administer antiemetics prophylactically and as needed.
   *Antiemetics help decrease or prevent vomiting.*
2. When the child is nauseated, offer cool, clear liquids. Offer bland, soft foods at room temperature, served in small portions. Be creative with the liquids and foods offered to make them more interesting and inviting.
   *Cool liquids and foods are soothing and better tolerated than hot ones, and the risk of burning fragile mucosa is eliminated.*
3. Offer small, frequent meals of high protein and high calorie content. Fortify foods with nutritional supplements. Allow the family to bring favorite foods to the hospital.
   *Small, frequent meals are better tolerated than large ones. Protein promotes tissue healing. A large number of calories are needed for growth. Children are more likely to eat their favorite foods.*
4. Avoid offering favorite foods when the child is nauseated.
   *Foods eaten within hours of nausea will be associated with feeling "sick."*
5. Administer ordered mouth analgesics before oral intake.
   *If mouth sores are present, analgesics will increase comfort and enable interest in eating.*
6. Monitor daily weight. Keep strict intake and output records. Weigh the infant's diapers.
   *Strict measurement ensures adequate intake and provides an objective assessment to alert the nurse that further interventions may be needed.*
7. Involve the child in food selection.
   *Allow the child as much control as possible over the foods to eat; this may increase interest and participation in eating.*
8. Include a dietitian in the nutritional assessment and evaluation.
   *A dietitian provides specialized input into developing a nutrition plan and evaluating the child's nutritional status.*

**Evaluation**

Did the child have no more than 5% weight loss, as documented on a growth chart?

Does the child eat foods that provide appropriate nutrients for growth?

**Nursing Diagnosis**

Deficient Knowledge related to unfamiliarity with the disease process and treatment plan.

**Planning**

***Expected Outcomes***

The child and parents will:

1. Explain the diagnosis.
2. Demonstrate adherence to treatment.

**Interventions and *Rationales***

1. Determine the child's and parents' readiness for learning. Create an environment of learning.
   *After the initial diagnosis, family members may need time to adjust before they are ready for education.*
2. During each hospital and clinic visit, spend time with the family, explaining the diagnosis, its sequelae, and its treatment. Repeat key educational interventions for the child and family. Offer written information and videos of educational sessions.
   *The diagnosis of cancer in a child is overwhelming. The family receives a flood of information and needs time to process. Educational interventions are repeated over time as the family's stress decreases to reinforce learning and facilitate understanding.*
3. During education sessions with the family, demonstrate procedures required for the child's care, discuss ways to approach nausea, explain the management of fatigue and other side effects, and address ways to encourage the child's normal development. Explain rationale for treatment and anticipated sequelae.
   *Home care for the child is complex and the family needs comprehensive education. Understanding the rationale for treatment and expected outcomes encourages adherence to therapy.*
4. Determine the family's preferred method of learning (demonstration, reading, listening, observing). Keep explanations at the family's level of understanding.
   *Matching teaching techniques to preferred method of learning will facilitate the education process.*
5. Offer encouragement for parents' recognition of danger signs and parents' appropriate use of medical care, to reinforce these actions.
   *Parents want to know they are doing the right thing for their child.*

**Evaluation**

Have the parents and child demonstrated an understanding of the treatment protocols by adhering to therapy and seeking appropriate medical care for danger signs?

**Nursing Diagnosis**

Disturbed Body Image related to hair loss.

**Planning**

***Expected Outcome***

The child will adapt to alopecia, as evidenced by a return to socialization, and discuss concerns related to hair loss.

**Interventions and *Rationales***

1. Instruct the child and parents on the progression of hair loss and potential changes in color and texture when the hair regrows. (Cranial irradiation can result in patches of permanent hair loss.) Suggest obtaining a wig before hair is lost or bringing a clipping of hair with a recent photograph.
   *Knowing how hair loss occurs and that it is temporary for most children can be reassuring to the child and family. Matching a wig to original hair color, texture, and style is easier before hair is lost*
2. Encourage verbalization of feelings about hair loss. Enlist the help of a child life specialist to engage the child in play therapy.
   *Allowing the child to verbalize concerns about returning to a social environment or school is important. Play therapy is a safe way for the child to express feelings and fears.*
3. Discuss ways to minimize the reaction to alopecia by promoting creative solutions such as hats, wigs, or scarves.
   *Allowing children to create their own head coverings may reduce the negative impact of hair loss.*
4. Make visits to the child's classroom.
   *Preparation of classmates for the child's school reentry will lessen classmates' negative reactions, fears, anxiety, and lack of understanding. It will also increase the support they can give the ill child.*
5. Encourage a return to school as soon as possible.
   *The sooner the child returns to school, the less likely it is that the child will begin a pattern of absenteeism. If the child returns to school before major*

*Continued*

## NURSING CARE PLAN—cont'd

### *The Child With Leukemia*

*body changes take place, the changes may not be so noticeable to the other children, thus decreasing undesirable reactions.*

**Evaluation**

Is the child involved in prediagnosis social life?

Has the child discussed hair loss and feelings connected with body image?

Has the child experienced a successful reentry to school?

**Nursing Diagnosis**

Ineffective Coping (individual) or Compromised Family Coping related to chronic illness.

**Planning**

***Expected Outcomes***

1. The child will exhibit effective coping as evidenced by adherence to the treatment plan and identification of support systems (child life therapists, playroom activities, summer camps).
2. The parents will exhibit effective coping as evidenced by verbalization of their concerns about the impact of the child's illness on the family and use of support systems and community resources.

**Interventions and *Rationales***

1. Teach the family the necessity of adhering to the protocol. Teach the warning signs of problems and how to access after-hours emergency care.
   *Conscientious application of the treatment plan increases the chance of a positive outcome.*
2. Listen and encourage the child and family to verbalize their feelings and express their concerns. Answer questions honestly and openly.
   *Identification of concerns and clarification of misconceptions will help children and families cope with the stress of chronic illness.*
3. Introduce the family to other families of children with cancer.
   *Other families of children with cancer can offer suggestions and support.*
4. Consult social services, child life specialists, and a chaplain or other appropriate religious figure.
   *The financial and emotional burdens of caring for a child with cancer can be overwhelming.*
5. Offer a list of local support groups appropriate to the child's age and the family's individual needs.
   *Children and family members in similar situations can provide comfort and support to the child with cancer and the family.*

***Evaluation***

Is the family adhering to the treatment plan?

Do the family and child verbalize appropriate concerns and questions?

Has the family contacted a local support group?

**Nursing Diagnosis**

Acute Pain and Chronic Pain related to the disease process and procedures.

**Planning**

***Expected Outcome***

The child will experience decreased discomfort, as evidenced by periods of uninterrupted rest, verbalization of increased comfort, a reduced pain score on an age-appropriate pain assessment tool, and participation in play activities.

**Interventions and *Rationales***

1. Explain procedures to the child in an age-appropriate manner before performing them.
   *Honest explanations build rapport and reduce fear.*
2. Enlist a child life specialist's help before and during procedures.
   *Child life specialists are trained to use distraction techniques with children and represent a "safe" person for the child to be with during repeated painful procedures.*
3. Administer antianxiety drugs as ordered (see Chapter 39).
   *Anticipation of a painful procedure may worsen the pain, especially in the adolescent. Giving an antianxiety drug may help calm the child so the procedure is better tolerated.*
4. Monitor for signs and symptoms of pain such as inactivity for age, increased heart rate or blood pressure, grimacing, verbalization of discomfort, irritability, and crying. Use a developmentally appropriate assessment tool and nonverbal cues to evaluate pain.
   *Younger children will not be able to verbalize pain. Stoic children may not express discomfort. Nurses must watch for physiologic and behavioral signs of pain.*
5. Provide comfort measures as needed such as positioning, adjusting room temperature, and offering distractions appropriate for age.
   *Comfort measures can decrease the perception of pain and even decrease the amount of analgesic needed.*
6. Administer analgesics promptly as ordered. Use topical anesthetics for procedural pain. Ensure analgesia or nonpharmacologic strategies before painful procedures.
   *Analgesics reduce the pain of procedures and of the disease. Delays in analgesic administration can increase anxiety and thus increase pain. Nonpharmacologic interventions can decrease anxiety and pain.*
7. Explain the pain control regimen to the parents and child as age appropriate.
   *Parents know their child and can help the nurse assess pain promptly.*
8. Notify the physician if pain relief is not obtained with the ordered dose of analgesic.
   *Pain tolerance varies greatly among children. Dosage increases may be needed, especially in the child with chronic pain or the dying child.*

**Evaluation**

Does the child express decreased levels of discomfort, and have a reduced pain score on an appropriate pain assessment tool?

Is the child joining other children in play?

**Nursing Diagnosis**

Impaired Skin Integrity related to radiation therapy, chemotherapy, and immobility.

**Planning**

***Expected Outcomes***

1. The child's skin will remain free of breakdown.
2. The child and family will maintain the integrity of the child's skin.

**Interventions and *Rationales***

1. Assess and document the child's skin condition each shift. (Skin erythema is common with radiation therapy but should not progress to skin breakdown.)
   *Ongoing assessment and documentation will reveal early skin changes that require intervention to prevent skin breakdown.*
2. Use only approved lotions and creams on the skin.
   *Some commercial lotions can increase skin irritation and redness.*
3. Avoid excessive scrubbing of skin, hot water, and abrasive soaps.
   *Friction may increase skin breakdown. Hot water is uncomfortable to irritated tissue.*

## NURSING CARE PLAN—cont'd

### *The Child With Leukemia*

4. Offer loose clothing of soft materials.
   *Tight clothing or abrasive fabrics may further irritate the skin.*
5. Notify the physician if skin breakdown occurs.
   *Additional orders for therapeutic creams may be needed.*
6. If the child is immobile, gently turn and vary the position at least every 2 hours.
   *Immobility may increase pressure on skin and promote breakdown.*
7. Teach the parents how to regularly assess the condition of the child's skin. Provide oral and written instructions to the family on the skin care techniques listed above.
   *The family needs comprehensive education and detailed instructions in order to assess the child's skin and provide appropriate care.*

**Evaluation**

Has the child's skin remained intact?
Can parents describe skin assessment and care techniques?

**Nursing Diagnosis**

Impaired Oral (and Anal/Rectal) Mucous Membranes related to chemotherapy and radiation therapy.

**Planning**

***Expected Outcome***

The child will not exhibit side effects from treatment, as evidenced by intact oral and anal/rectal mucous membranes.

**Interventions and *Rationales***

1. Monitor the child's mouth and anus each shift for ulcers, erythema, or breakdown. Teach the parents and the child, if age appropriate, how to perform this assessment. Report ulcerations to the physician.
   *A breakdown in mucous membranes usually begins with erythema and progresses to ulcerations. Home care should include this assessment for the duration of therapy.*
2. Begin meticulous mouth care, avoiding alcohol-based mouthwashes, several times a day with a soft-bristled toothbrush or Toothettes.
   *Removing bacteria from the oral mucosa will decrease the risk of infection of irritated tissue.*
3. Offer bland, nonirritating foods and cool liquids.
   *Citrus products and spicy foods may be quite painful to an ulcerated mouth. Cool liquids are soothing. Ice pops and slushes are usually well tolerated.*
4. If ulcerations occur, administer medications, mouth rinses, and ointments per physician orders.
   *Immediate treatment is essential to prevent infection and other complications.*
5. Do not take a rectal temperature in a child undergoing chemotherapy or radiation therapy. Do not take oral temperatures if mouth ulcers are present. Teach parents how to take accurate axillary, temporal, or tympanic temperatures.
   *The introduction of a thermometer into the rectum or mouth of a child with fragile mucous membranes, no matter how carefully done, can tear tissue.*
6. If the anal/rectal mucosa becomes irritated, begin sitz baths several times a day and after bowel movements.
   *Lukewarm sitz baths keep the perineum clean and soothe irritated tissue.*
7. In diaper-wearing children, use only diaper wipes that do not contain alcohol or perfumes. If the perineum is very irritated, use only warm water wipes on the area.
   *Alcohol and perfumes will further irritate the skin and can cause great discomfort. Very few commercial diaper wipes are safe for these children.*

**Evaluation**

Has the child exhibited signs of oral mucosal or anal/rectal ulceration?

Generally, after the initial induction and consolidation phases of chemotherapy are complete, a maintenance phase begins. Maintenance chemotherapy usually consists of lower doses of chemotherapy given orally and possibly intravenously on a regular basis over a period of 2 to 3 years to "maintain" remission and prevent recurrence of the leukemia. Total treatment time for ALL is approximately 2½ years for girls and 3½ years for boys.

## BRAIN TUMORS

Brain tumors are the most common solid tumor and the second most common childhood malignancy after leukemia. Brain tumors are a diverse group of tumors described by their tissue of origin, location within the brain, and rate of growth. Unlike other neoplasms, primary brain tumors are confined to the brain and spine and rarely metastasize to bone marrow or other organs. The mortality rate is higher than any other pediatric malignancy (Cataudella & Zelcer, 2012).

### Etiology

The cause of brain tumors remains unknown. Heredity and environment both are associated with their development. Several inherited syndromes are associated with the development of brain tumors in children, such as neurofibromatosis and tuberous sclerosis. Additional risk factors include immune system suppression and cranial irradiation. Although exposure to electromagnetic fields has been suggested to increase a child's risk of a brain tumor, no confirming evidence supports this theory (Barbel & Peterson, 2015).

### Incidence

Approximately 4350 children younger than age 20 years of age are diagnosed with primary brain tumors annually (Chintagumpala & Gajjar, 2015). Approximately 50% of pediatric CNS tumors develop in the posterior fossa—the lower part of the brain that contains both the cerebellum and the brainstem (Ater & Kuttesch, 2016).

### Manifestations

Manifestations of brain tumors vary with tumor location and the child's age and development. Symptoms produced by tumors in the posterior fossa include ataxia (unsteady gait), poor coordination of the upper extremities, visual changes (nystagmus, diplopia, strabismus) (see Chapter 52), and occasionally head tilt. Posterior fossa tumors are associated with increased intracranial pressure (ICP) caused by the tumor mass itself or, more commonly, by the tumor obstructing the normal flow of cerebrospinal fluid (CSF). Increased ICP often causes headaches, vomiting, and lethargy. These symptoms are usually most intense on arising in the morning.

Symptoms of increased ICP caused by a brain tumor are frequently subacute and nonspecific (see Chapter 52). In infants, these include irritability, lethargy, poor feeding, increased head circumference, and bulging fontanels. Many younger children demonstrate loss of developmental milestones. Symptoms in school-age children include declining academic performance, fatigue, personality changes, and vague, intermittent headache. Cranial nerve deficits and hemiparesis are usually associated with brainstem involvement.

Supratentorial tumors characteristically cause headaches, seizures, or focal neurologic deficits. Especially with slow-growing tumors, symptoms can be subtle and initially attributed to more common childhood illnesses.

Neurocognitive deficits may not be evident until years after treatment and can affect the child's quality of life. Radiation to the brain is a risk factor for increased neurocognitive deficits; therefore, many children are treated with chemotherapy alone (Nelson, Compton, Patel, et al., 2013).

## Diagnostic Evaluation

Once a tumor is suspected, evaluation is considered to be an emergency. Relevant imaging techniques include magnetic resonance imaging (MRI), CT, and positron emission tomography (PET). MRI is currently the imaging modality most commonly used to evaluate brain tumors. During MRI, the child must lie motionless inside a dark tunnel for approximately 1 hour. This requirement is especially difficult for young children. In general, children younger than 6 years need sedation. A spinal MRI is performed to look for metastatic disease in the spine. A CSF sample obtained from lumbar puncture is examined for the presence of tumor cells. In some cases, the tumor produces tumor markers such as alpha-fetoprotein that can be identified in the CSF or blood.

Usually the diagnosis is suspected from the child's signs and symptoms and the location of the tumor (Fig. 48.3). Pathologic examination confirms the tissue type and tumor diagnosis. On the rare occasion when the tumor is not surgically accessible, the diagnosis must be made on the basis of location and radiologic evaluation alone.

## Therapeutic Management

Initial intervention for a child with a brain tumor is surgery. The goal is to remove as much of the tumor as possible while minimally disturbing the surrounding brain tissue so that the child's neurologic functioning is preserved to the highest degree possible. Complete removal of the

## PATHOPHYSIOLOGY

### *Brain Tumors*

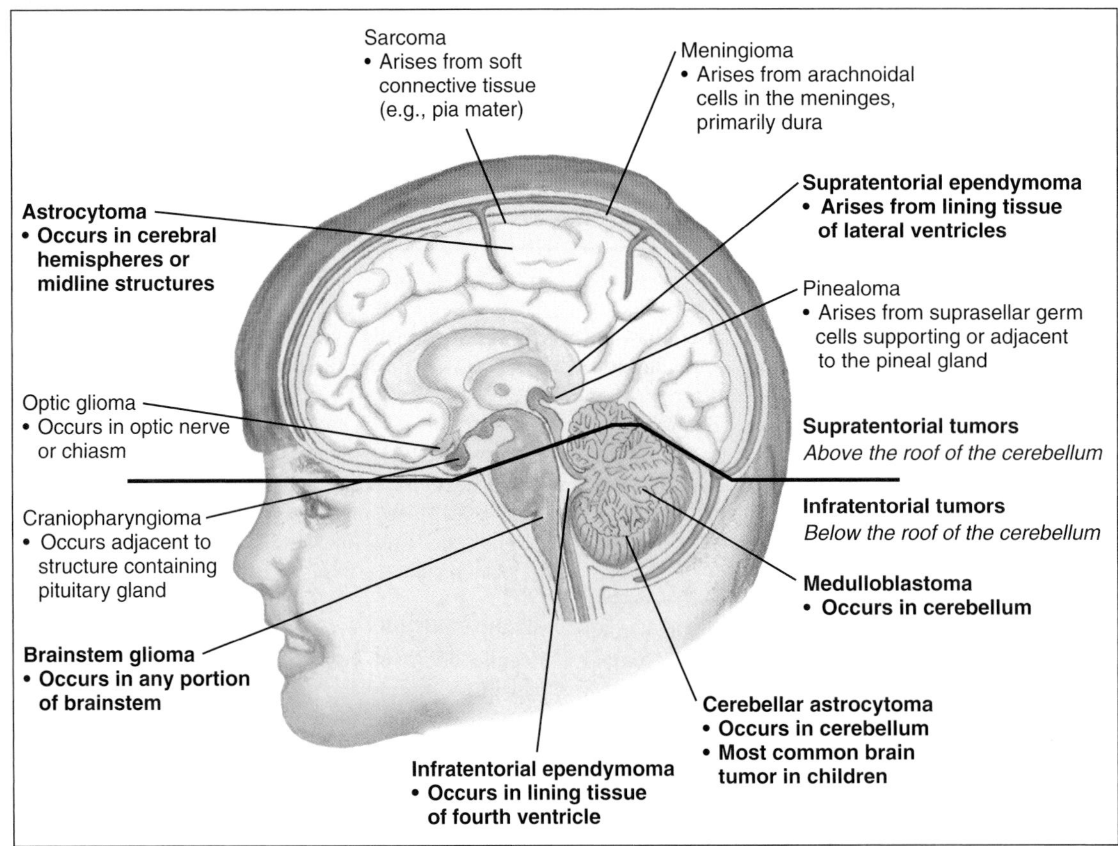
Sarcoma
• Arises from soft connective tissue (e.g., pia mater)
Meningioma
• Arises from arachnoidal cells in the meninges, primarily dura
Astrocytoma
• Occurs in cerebral hemispheres or midline structures
Supratentorial ependymoma
• Arises from lining tissue of lateral ventricles
Pinealoma
• Arises from suprasellar germ cells supporting or adjacent to the pineal gland
Optic glioma
• Occurs in optic nerve or chiasm
Supratentorial tumors
Above the roof of the cerebellum
Infratentorial tumors
Below the roof of the cerebellum
Craniopharyngioma
• Occurs adjacent to structure containing pituitary gland
Medulloblastoma
• Occurs in cerebellum
Brainstem glioma
• Occurs in any portion of brainstem
Cerebellar astrocytoma
• Occurs in cerebellum
• Most common brain tumor in children
Infratentorial ependymoma
• Occurs in lining tissue of fourth ventricle

Brain tumors are classified according to cell histology and rate of tumor proliferation. The most commonly seen brain tumors are pilocytic astrocytomas and medulloblastomas (Ater & Kuttesch, 2016).*

The histology of brain tumors ranges from benign to highly malignant. The effect these tumors have on the brain and the clinical symptoms they produce often have more to do with the tumor size and location than with the aggressiveness of the tumor. Most astrocytomas are low grade or slow growing; however, if they persist after treatment, they can produce significant neurologic deficits.

*Ater, J., & Kuttesch, J.F. (2016). Brain tumors in childhood. In R. Kliegman, B. Stanton, J. St. Geme, et al. (Eds.), *Nelson textbook of pediatrics* (20th ed., pp. 2453–2460). Philadelphia: Elsevier.

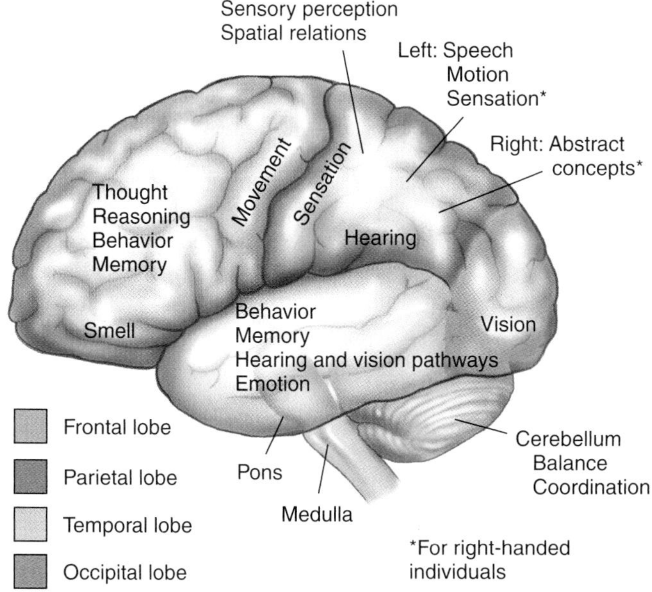


FIG 48.3 Lobes of the brain.

tumor is associated with the best prognosis. In the case of a brainstem tumor or an optic pathway glioma, the risk of postoperative neurologic dysfunction outweighs the benefits of resection, so surgery is not performed.

Depending on the location of the tumor and the extent of surgical resection, a ventriculoperitoneal (VP) shunt may be inserted to relieve hydrocephalus, an excessive accumulation of CSF in the ventricles of the brain and the symptoms associated with it (see Chapter 52). Children with tumors located above the roof of the cerebellum (supratentorial) are at risk for seizures from the tumor itself or from scar tissue formation after surgery. These children are prescribed anticonvulsants with monitoring of therapeutic levels.

The therapeutic regimen is based on the type of tumor, its location, the amount of residual tumor that remains after surgery, and the child's age. Some tumors, such as low-grade astrocytomas, require surgery alone if the tumor can be completely resected. However, for malignant tumors, treatment is often multimodal involving complete surgical removal of the tumor and then radiation therapy and chemotherapy as indicated (Ater & Kuttesch, 2016). Radiation therapy in children younger than 5 years of age can have toxic effects on the developing brain. Use of chemotherapy has emerged in recent years as an alternative or adjunct to radiation treatment (Nelson et al., 2013). Imaging is performed at intervals to help determine the response to therapy. Prognostic percentages vary with the type of tumor, whether all or only part of the tumor was resected, metastatic spread, child's age, child's physical status, and individual responses to treatment.

Although greater than 70% of children with brain tumors will be long-term survivors, more than half will experience chronic neurologic problems as a result of the tumor and its treatment with surgery, radiation, and chemotherapy (Ater & Kuttesch, 2016). Problems include seizure disorders, focal motor and sensory abnormalities, learning disabilities, developmental delays, and neuroendocrine dysfunction causing growth failure and delays in the onset of puberty (Ater & Kuttesch, 2016). These children need ongoing medical management to control seizures and correct endocrine deficits. Further, they will benefit from rehabilitation services and therapies as well as individualized education programs and neuropsychological testing. The results of such testing can be used to develop an appropriate Individual Education Plan (IEP) for the child (Nelson et al., 2013).

## ! NURSING QUALITY ALERT

### *Signs of Brain Tumor in Children*

The hallmark symptoms of children with brain tumors are headache and morning vomiting related to the child getting out of bed. The shift in intracranial pressure (ICP) with the change in position from lying flat (higher ICP) to standing up (lower ICP) causes the vomiting.

## NURSING CARE

### The Child With a Brain Tumor

#### Assessment

A thorough neurologic examination is paramount for any child diagnosed with a brain tumor. Knowing the location of the tumor heightens the nurse's understanding of neurologic deficits the child may have (see Fig. 48.3). A psychosocial and developmental history is important to obtain, including information regarding the child's neurologic symptoms, achievement of developmental milestones in younger children, and school performance in older children. Children who have insidious loss of vision may have learned to compensate well; excellent nursing skills will be needed to identify vision loss. The nurse addresses impaired balance and coordination, brainstem dysfunction, and any loss of vision when evaluating the child's safety. The nurse should be especially vigilant when assessing for signs and symptoms of increased ICP in children who have just been diagnosed with a brain tumor, who are in the immediate postoperative period following tumor resection, and who have a VP shunt that can malfunction. Many children with brain tumors have seizures at some time during their illness, so seizure precautions should be considered even in the child with no previous history of seizures (see Chapter 52). It is essential to assess the child's nutritional status and watch for weight loss throughout treatment.

#### Nursing Diagnosis and Planning

The following nursing diagnoses and expected outcomes may be appropriate for the child with a brain tumor and the child's family:

- Acute Pain and Chronic Pain related to increased ICP.

  **Expected outcome.** The child will verbalize a decrease in the severity of headaches.
- Risk for Infection related to surgery or immunosuppression after chemotherapy.

  **Expected outcome.** The child will remain free from signs of infection, as evidenced by body temperature within normal limits. The child and family will demonstrate infection prevention measures.
- Anxiety (child and parent) related to the surgery and diagnosis.

  **Expected outcome.** The child and parents will exhibit decreased anxiety about the outcomes of surgery and therapy, as evidenced by verbalization of decreased stress and an increased ability to problem solve.
- Deficient Knowledge about the disease process related to unfamiliarity with the information.

  **Expected outcome.** The child and parents will describe the disease process and its management.
- Disturbed Body Image related to a shaved head, hair loss, and/or neurologic deficits.

  **Expected outcome.** The child will demonstrate appropriate coping techniques for hair loss and changes in coordination or other abilities, as evidenced by maintaining social relationships and verbal statements indicating adaptation to the changed appearance.

### Interventions

Nursing care focuses on controlling acute symptoms, preparation for surgery, and postoperative management. The family will also need education and support to cope with the significant anxiety caused by fear of the potential impact of surgery on the child's neurologic system, treatment failure, and the child's death. Preoperative teaching at the child's developmental level prepares the child and family for the potential outcomes of surgery. The child should be educated about anesthesia and should be prepared to be in the intensive care unit following surgery. (See Chapter 37 for a discussion of preoperative care.)

The child's head will be shaved before surgery. Although every effort is made to shave only as much hair as necessary, hair loss may still be traumatic for the child. The nurse should be aware of this and assist the child in verbalizing fears. Some children enjoy wearing a favorite cap or hat and make it a special event to buy a hat. The child must be prepared to wake up with a large dressing covering the head after surgery.

In addition to postoperative concerns of pain, hemorrhage, and infection, the nurse must also monitor the child for signs and symptoms of increased ICP. Increased ICP (see Chapter 52) is a risk in the postoperative period related to cerebral edema, hydrocephalus, or hemorrhage. The nurse performs and records vital sign measurements, mental status exams, and neurologic function checks frequently after surgery. If indicators of increased ICP are noted, the nurse immediately notifies the physician and prepares the child for an evaluation, including an MRI or a CT scan. The child should not be placed in the Trendelenburg position since this can increase ICP and the risk of bleeding.

Many children return from the operating room with external ventricular shunts in place that temporarily remove CSF and reduce ICP. These external drains must be maintained at appropriate levels and CSF measured accurately. Normal CSF is colorless; bloody or discolored drainage can be a sign of contamination or bleeding and must be reported to the physician immediately. Many children require placement of a permanent VP shunt because of secondary hydrocephalus.

After the child's condition has been stabilized, the child is assessed for functional deficits resulting from surgery or damage to normal brain tissue by the tumor. These deficits can be somewhat predictable if the involved area of the brain and the function of that area are known (Box 48.3). If radiation therapy is delivered, families should be made aware of potential side effects and understand that acute side effects will resolve over time. Chemotherapy is delivered on an inpatient or outpatient basis; the nurse prepares the child and family for the side effects and how they are managed.

### BOX 48.3 Potential Functional Deficits Related to a Brain Tumor

After surgery, the child should be assessed for functional deficits in the following areas:

- Gait: Look for ataxia, including head control and truncal stability
- Bilateral extremity strength and purposeful movement
- Speech
- Ability to swallow
- Vision and hearing
- Presurgical developmental task mastery
- Receptive and expressive language

If the deficits are significant, the child may need rehabilitative therapy to regain function.

If neurologic deficits are significant and persist, rehabilitative therapy may be necessary to help the child regain function. Adequate academic support such as an individual education plan should always be considered for these children when they return to school.

### Evaluation

- Are both verbal and nonverbal indications of a positive comfort level present?
- Does the child's rating on a pain assessment tool indicate decreased pain?
- Has the child remained afebrile, and do the child and family demonstrate infection prevention measures?
- Have the child and family expressed decreased levels of stress and the ability to rely on coping strategies?
- Is the family able to discuss the treatment plan and concerns related to the disease and treatment plan?
- Is the child relating with peers in the same manner as before the diagnosis and hospitalization, and is the child expressing adaptation to the changed appearance?

## MALIGNANT LYMPHOMAS

Malignant lymphomas are neoplasms of lymphoid cells, a component of the immune system. Lymphomas represent 25% of childhood cancers in adolescents. Lymphomas are the third most common childhood malignancy (Hochberg, Giulino-Roth, Cairo, 2016). Lymphomas are divided into two main types; non-Hodgkin lymphoma (NHL) and Hodgkin lymphoma.

The average occurrence of NHL in children 19 years and younger in the United States is approximately 750 to 800 new cases/year (Hochberg et al., 2016). NHL originates from a proliferation of either B or T lymphocytes. The three subtypes of pediatric NHL are: (1) small, noncleaved cell (Burkitt, Burkitt-like) lymphomas; (2) large-cell lymphomas; and (3) lymphoblastic lymphomas.

Hodgkin lymphoma in 15- to 19-year-olds comprises approximately 15% of all cancers seen in this age-group, accounts for 5% of all cancers seen in children 14 years and younger, and is rarely seen in children under age 10 years (Hochberg et al., 2016). It represents approximately 40% of lymphomas. The presence of giant multinucleated cells (Reed-Sternberg cells) is the hallmark of Hodgkin disease.

The incidence of NHL increases gradually throughout life, unlike Hodgkin disease, which has a bimodal incidence curve (Hochberg et al., 2016). Because the incidence of Hodgkin disease peaks in children 15 years old and older, it accounts for a greater proportion of the lymphomas seen in older children. NHL in children younger than 5 years is uncommon.

### Non-Hodgkin Lymphoma

NHL differs greatly from Hodgkin disease in its clinical behavior, pathology, mode of metastasis, and responsiveness to therapy. This disease has a rapid onset with widespread involvement at diagnosis.

#### Etiology

Viral, immunologic, and genetic factors are believed to contribute to the development of NHL, although the exact cause is unknown (Barbel & Peterson, 2015; Hochberg et al., 2016). Children with congenital immunodeficiency syndromes or acquired immunodeficiency syndrome (AIDS), as well as those who have undergone organ transplantation and have chronically suppressed immune systems, are at higher risk for developing NHL and other lymphoproliferative disorders (Barbel & Peterson, 2015).

### Manifestations

Symptoms of abdominal disease include abdominal cramping, constipation, pain, anorexia, weight loss, ascites, and obstruction, with vomiting as a late sign. Painless, enlarged lymph nodes are found in the cervical or axillary region and less commonly in the inguinal area. If mediastinal disease is present, cough, respiratory distress, symptoms of bronchitis, and possibly significant tracheal deviation are seen. Bone marrow disease leads to a general decline in health and bone marrow suppression.

### Diagnostic Evaluation

In addition to a physical examination looking for enlarged lymph nodes and hepatosplenomegaly, extensive laboratory work is necessary. Especially with Burkitt lymphoma, the uric acid level is often high, indicating a rapid turnover of cells.

A chest radiograph is obtained to look for mediastinal disease and tracheal deviation. The extent of disease is further evaluated with a CT scan of the neck, chest, abdomen, and pelvis; PET scans; and flow cytometry to identify the cell origin. Bone marrow aspirations and biopsies are performed to assess involvement of disease in the marrow. A lumbar puncture is performed to assess the CSF for disease. Pathologic findings are confirmed with a lymph node biopsy.

### Therapeutic Management

Children with NHL, especially Burkitt lymphoma, often present in metabolic disarray because of the rapidity with which the disease progresses. These children are prone to tumor lysis syndrome from the large tumor burden, with rapid tumor cell turnover and cell death. With the lysis of the tumor cells, potassium, phosphorus, and nucleic acids are released into circulation causing metabolic alterations including hyperkalemia, hyperphosphatemia, hyperuremia and hypocalcemia, all of which must be stabilized before the initiation of chemotherapy (Allen, Kelly, & Bollard, 2015; Henry & Sung, 2015).

In children susceptible to tumor lysis syndrome, intensive hydration with an IV fluid containing bicarbonate alkalinizes the urine to help prevent the formation of uric acid crystals, which damage the kidney. There should be no potassium in the IV fluid. Oral allopurinol is started to decrease the uric acid level. Parenteral urate oxidase (rasburicase) is indicated if further degradation of uric acid is necessary (Henry & Sung, 2015). With the initiation of chemotherapy, serum electrolyte levels (electrolytes, calcium, magnesium, phosphorous, uric acid, and creatinine) may be checked several times a day to keep close surveillance on the child's metabolic state because these tumors respond rapidly to treatment. The urine sometimes turns milky white as the tumor cells are filtered through the kidneys. Children who cannot be hemodynamically monitored on the general unit are sometimes moved to the intensive care unit until metabolically stabile.

#### ! NURSING QUALITY ALERT

***Tumor Lysis Syndrome***

In tumor lysis syndrome, the intracellular contents are dumped into the extracellular fluid as the tumor cells are lysed, or killed. These intracellular contents have different electrolyte concentrations (higher potassium and phosphorus) than the extracellular blood. The high concentrations of electrolytes overload the kidneys and, if the condition is not monitored and treated carefully, cause acute renal failure. Common electrolyte abnormalities in tumor lysis syndrome include hyperkalemia, hyperphosphatemia, and hypocalcemia. Tumor lysis syndrome is most common in children with leukemias who have very high WBC counts and in children with non-Hodgkin lymphomas, especially when extensive disease is present.

The primary treatment modality for all histologic classifications and stages of NHL involves multiagent chemotherapy with intrathecal chemotherapy. Surgery is used to obtain a diagnostic biopsy. In general, these lymphomas present as generalized disease, making them less amenable to treatment with radiation therapy; irradiation is reserved for emergent situations resulting from CNS disease or airway compromise. Chemotherapy is given over a 6- to 24-month period, depending on the type of lymphoma. Typically, a CVC is placed to assist in delivering chemotherapy drugs. Frequent follow-up visits are made after the completion of treatment because the risk of recurrent disease is greatest immediately after therapy is stopped.

Survival rates of children with localized lymphoma approach 100%. Among children whose disease is advanced, the survival rate is between 60% and 95% (Hochberg et al., 2016).

## NURSING CARE

### The Child With Non-Hodgkin Lymphoma

#### Assessment

The parents of children with NHL will report an acute onset of symptoms that vary with the type of organ involved. Most parents will state that their child has become irritable and "just not himself." Children with metastatic disease often appear very ill. The nurse assesses lymph nodes and closely checks the respiratory system in a child with mediastinal disease, especially if the trachea is deviated. Signs of tumor lysis syndrome are considered and include subtle changes in behavior (restlessness and irritability) and changes in the sensorium. These are ominous signs indicative of electrolyte imbalances such as hyperuricemia, hyperkalemia, hyperphosphatemia, and hypocalcemia.

#### Nursing Diagnosis and Planning

The following nursing diagnoses and expected outcomes may apply to the child with NHL and the child's family:

- Ineffective Breathing Pattern related to mediastinal disease.

**Expected outcome.** The child's respiratory status will remain stable, as evidenced by normal breath sounds for age and stable respiratory rate and rhythm.

- Risk for Injury related to electrolyte imbalances secondary to tumor lysis syndrome.

**Expected outcome.** The child will maintain a normal fluid and electrolyte balance, as evidenced by a stable metabolic state and urine output appropriate for age.

- Risk for Infection related to the state of immunosuppression.

**Expected outcome.** The child will exhibit no signs and symptoms of infection, as evidenced by normal body temperature.

- Deficient Knowledge related to unfamiliarity with the disease process.

**Expected outcome.** The child and parents will describe the disease process and its management.

#### Interventions

Initial nursing care focuses on following the physician's orders for maintaining a stable metabolic state before and during the induction phase of chemotherapy. All children undergoing induction chemotherapy should have intake and output and serum chemistry values strictly monitored. Occasionally, children with Burkitt lymphoma will need a urinary catheter inserted for measurement of output. If a fever develops, urine and blood should be cultured to rule out an infection. The nutritional status of these children following chemotherapy induction must be carefully evaluated, and many will require enteral feedings. If necessary, total parenteral nutrition is given.

Parents will need support because the chemotherapy often makes the child seem more ill initially. The nurse answers the family's questions directly and honestly. Once the child starts to recover from the initial chemotherapy, the nurse can provide more extensive education to the family about the disease and its treatment.

Consultations with child life specialists, chaplains or other religious figures, and social workers can enhance the psychosocial care of these families. Realistic expectations of therapy and of the child's response to therapy can help parents deal more effectively with their fears and anxiety (see Nursing Care Plan: The Child with Leukemia, for other related nursing care).

#### Evaluation

- Has the child's respiratory status remained stable, with normal rate and rhythm and clear breath sounds?
- Is the child's urine output appropriate for age, and are electrolytes within normal range?
- Are the child's vital signs within normal limits?
- Are the parents asking questions about the disease process and the care of their child?

### Hodgkin Disease

Hodgkin disease has a more indolent course than NHL. It frequently presents as localized disease. Systemic symptoms include unexplained fevers, weight loss, and night sweats. These systemic signs are used in diagnostic staging.

#### Etiology

The cause of Hodgkin disease is unknown. However, the possibility of an infectious agent is being investigated. Herpesvirus 6, cytomegalovirus, and Epstein-Barr virus (EBV) are associated with Hodgkin disease, but the exact relationship remains unknown (Hochberg et al., 2016). As with other cancers, no single environmental agent can be said to precipitate the disease process.

**SAFETY ALERT**

***Prevention of Urinary Tract Infection in the Immunocompromised Child***

Urinary catheters are used very infrequently in immunocompromised children because of the risk of introducing organisms into the urinary tract system.

#### Manifestations

Painless, firm, movable adenopathy in the cervical and supraclavicular regions is the most common presentation. Mediastinal involvement, with or without airway obstruction, occurs in two thirds of children. From 20% to 30% of children have constitutional symptoms that include fever, drenching night sweats, and weight loss. Other manifestations include fatigue and signs of airway obstruction such as dyspnea and cough.

#### Diagnostic Evaluation

Biopsy of an involved lymph node and histologic classification of the tissue confirm the diagnosis. Often a chest radiograph is done prior to lymph node biopsy to identify a mediastinal mass. Laboratory tests include a CBC, renal and liver function tests, erythrocyte sedimentation rate (ESR), and serum copper and ferritin levels. Elevation of ESR or serum copper or ferritin level is useful for follow-up evaluation if it correlates with disease activity at diagnosis. A gallium scan is performed to investigate the extent of disease. When a tumor demonstrates gallium uptake at diagnosis, a gallium scan can serve as a staging study as well as disease response marker. PET scanning can be more sensitive and specific than CT or gallium scanning. Chest radiography and CT of the chest, abdomen, and pelvis are performed to determine the extent of disease. Bilateral bone marrow aspirations and biopsies are done only if constitutional symptoms are present (Hochberg et al., 2016).

**PATHOPHYSIOLOGY**

***Hodgkin Disease***

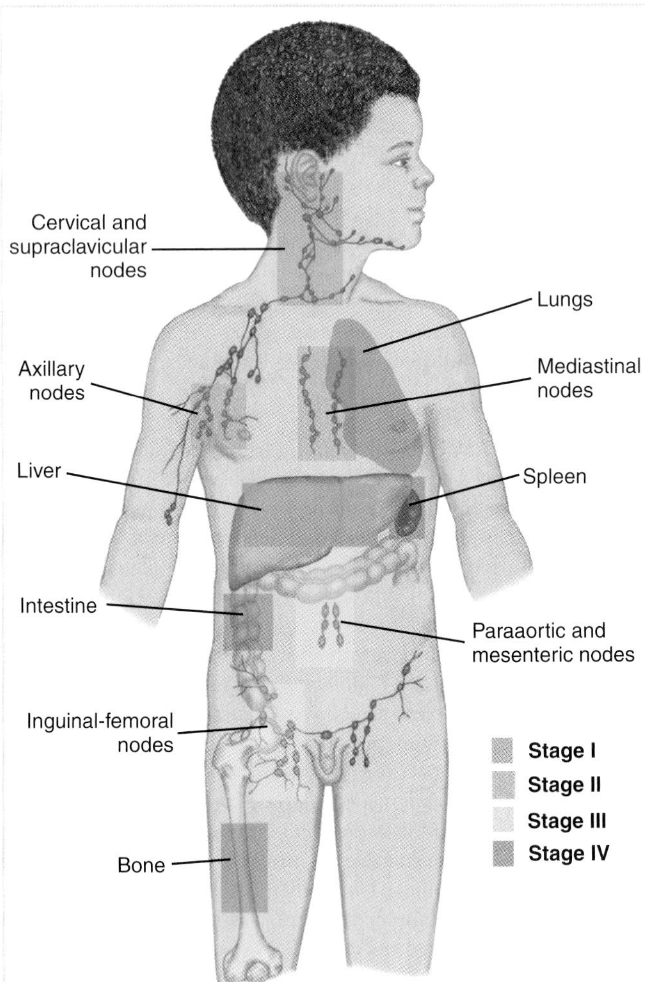


Hodgkin disease originates in a single lymph node or a group of lymph nodes in the same anatomic region. Hodgkin disease is characterized by giant multinucleated cells called *Reed-Sternberg cells* that are thought to represent activated B and T lymphocytes. Hodgkin disease spreads predictably from lymph nodes to nonnodal sites such as the spleen, liver, bone, bone marrow, lungs, and mediastinum.

#### Therapeutic Management

Therapy depends on the child's age at diagnosis, disease stage, and histologic type. If the mediastinal disease is expansive, it can compromise respiration. Radiation therapy can be used to shrink the tissue before any procedure requiring general anesthesia is performed. Recent studies conclude that radiation is not necessary in some lower-risk patients (Allen et al., 2015).

Most children are treated with chemotherapy alone or chemotherapy and low-dose, involved-field radiation therapy. High-dose, extended-field radiation therapy alone can be used if the disease is detected in a single site or in older adolescents who are full-grown. Long-term survival rates in excess of 95% can be expected in children with stage I or II disease and positive prognostic factors. For more advanced stages of disease, the long-term survival rate approximates 95% (Hochberg et al., 2016).

### Nursing Considerations

The onset of Hodgkin disease is insidious. Frequently, when asked about activity level, children report not noticing any change until it was brought to their attention. Typically, the child noticed lumps around the neck while bathing. Initial assessment of these children includes a thorough lymph node examination.

At least two thirds of children have some degree of mediastinal involvement. As with NHL, management of the airway is a concern if the child has any mediastinal disease. The nurse should assess the respiratory system for any changes in status with the child both sitting and lying down. If the airway is compromised, radiation therapy will be given locally to provide immediate relief.

Initially, the nurse should prepare the child for diagnostic procedures and a surgical biopsy. A CVC might be inserted at the time of diagnosis. Induction chemotherapy is begun as soon as the child is stable and staging of disease has been completed. In older children, a peripheral IV line can be placed at the time of each chemotherapy treatment to avoid a CVC placement.

Education includes an explanation of the therapeutic protocol. Questions asked by the child and family are answered honestly. Although improvements in care continue, 25% of children fail to respond or relapse (Allen et al., 2015). Realistic expectations of the response to therapy often help the child and family members cope more effectively. Hodgkin disease in first remission is treated in the outpatient setting at most centers. The nursing care is similar to that for a child with NHL.

## NEUROBLASTOMA

Neuroblastoma is the most commonly diagnosed malignancy in infants and is only found in infants and children (Zage & Ater, 2016). This embryonal cancer of the sympathetic nervous system presents in a range from very aggressive tumors that are unresponsive to treatment to tumors that spontaneously regress (generally in children younger than age 12 months).

### Etiology

The cause of neuroblastoma is unknown. Evidence for a familial form of neuroblastoma has been reported; children in families with one or more affected members may be at increased risk for the development of neuroblastoma. It is also associated with certain congenital syndromes and possibly with maternal and paternal occupational exposure to chemicals, farming items, and electronics, although no single environmental source is known to cause neuroblastoma (Zage & Ater, 2016).

### Incidence

Neuroblastoma represents approximately 8% to 10% of all childhood cancers, with an annual incidence of 600 new cases in the United States (Zage & Ater, 2016). It is slightly more common in boys and in white children. The median age of presentation is 22 months, with 90% of cases diagnosed by 5 years of age (Zage & Ater, 2016).

### Pathophysiology

Neuroblastoma arises from neural crest cells, which normally develop into the sympathetic nervous system and the adrenal medulla. Cells proliferate and begin to form a solid mass or tumor. These cells are immature and nonfunctional. Typically, the tumor infringes and infiltrates into adjacent normal tissue and organs. Metastatic disease may be present in the lymph nodes, bone marrow, bone, liver, and skin, and rarely, in the lung or brain (Zage & Ater, 2016). Greater understanding of the cellular genetic makeup of this tumor has provided insight into prognostic indicators that help with treatment planning.

### Manifestations

The manifestations of neuroblastoma depend on the extent of disease and the location of the tumor. In most cases, a primary abdominal mass and a protuberant, firm abdomen are present. Other manifestations include impaired range of motion and mobility, with pain and limping. Chest tumors can produce a cough and decreased chest expansion, with respiratory compromise. Compression of the superior vena cava results in facial and periorbital edema. Spinal cord compression can cause an inability to walk and impaired bowel and bladder function. Tumor infiltration can cause dark circles under the eyes, giving an appearance of "raccoon eyes." Bruising, drooping eyelids, or small pupils may be evident, along with opsomyoclonus, or "dancing" eye movements and myoclonic jerks. These children act restless and uncomfortable.

### Diagnostic Evaluation

The diagnostic workup includes chest radiography; CT or MRI of the chest, abdomen, and pelvis; and skeletal scintigraphy to determine the extent of disease. Bone marrow aspiration and biopsy, usually of both posterior iliac crests, are performed to evaluate marrow involvement.

Definitive diagnosis is made when tissue is obtained by biopsy. Tumor samples are sent to special reference laboratories to determine the genetic makeup of the tumor. The genetic information can sometimes reveal the aggressiveness of the tumor and help determine the prognosis and treatment plan.

### Therapeutic Management

The treatment of neuroblastoma depends on the presence and extent of metastasis. The International Neuroblastoma Staging System (INSS) is used to compare patients. Staging is graded I through IV, with stage I representing localized disease and stage IV denoting distant spread. Staging criteria include the extent and location of metastases, lymph node involvement, and whether the tumor is unilateral or crosses the midline. Early stage disease (stage I or II) without metastasis can require only surgical excision of the tumor and follow-up evaluations. Some children with later-stage (stage IV) disease undergo surgery to obtain tissue samples or to debulk a tumor for pain control.

Age at diagnosis is an important prognostic indicator. Children diagnosed before age 1 year have a better prognosis than children diagnosed at a later age. Approximately half of the infants diagnosed with neuroblastoma when younger than 1 year have a genetically less aggressive tumor type and are watched carefully or treated with low-dose chemotherapy.

Treatment plans for children with advanced disease (stage III or IV) can include radiation therapy to tumor sites and systemic chemotherapy for several months. Another attempt might be made to resect the tumor after combination chemotherapy has been administered to reduce the tumor size. Autologous stem cell transplantation (ASCT) after high-dose chemotherapy has been shown to improve survival rates over chemotherapy alone (Zage & Ater, 2016). Administration of the biologic modifier 13-*cis*-retinoic acid orally after ASCT is used to eradicate any residual disease by decreasing proliferation and inducing differentiation in neuroblastoma cell lines, which further increases survival rates (Zage & Ater, 2016).

Children with stage I or II disease who are without poor prognostic factors have a long-term survival rate of greater than 90%. Intermediate-risk children's long-term survival rate is approximately 70% to 80%. The long-term survival of high-risk children is approximately 25% to 35% (Zage & Ater, 2016).

## NURSING CARE

### The Child With Neuroblastoma

#### Assessment

Children with neuroblastoma typically appear pale, quite irritable, and uncomfortable. Parents might state that their child has wanted to be held more often than usual. Activity level and appetite are usually decreased. Because of large abdominal tumors, many have protuberant abdomens in which hard masses crossing the midline can be palpated. Range of motion and mobility are often impaired, so much so that the child cannot bear weight. If the tumor is compressing a nerve, neurologic changes may be noted. If the tumor is causing compression within the abdomen, vascular drainage can be compromised, with constipation or GI obstruction (Irwin & Park, 2015). Periorbital infiltration can cause characteristic ecchymosis or "raccoon eyes" (Zage & Ater, 2016).

#### Nursing Diagnosis and Planning

The following nursing diagnoses and expected outcomes may be appropriate for the child with a neuroblastoma and the child's family:

- Acute Pain related to tumor pressure.

  ***Expected outcome.*** The infant will exhibit pain relief, as evidenced by decreased crying and a relaxed body position.

- Anxiety (parents) related to a diagnosis of cancer, surgery, and the treatment plan.

  ***Expected outcome.*** The parents will express decreased anxiety about the outcomes of therapy.

- Deficient Knowledge related to unfamiliarity with the disease process and its management.

  ***Expected outcome.*** The parents will describe the disease process and its implications.

#### Interventions

Nursing care initially focuses on support of family members as they react and adjust to the diagnosis of cancer. The nurse facilitates the educational process to allay fears of the unknown. The child's initial care includes pain management, both preoperatively and postoperatively. The child with an abdominal tumor will return from surgery with a nasogastric (NG) tube in place. The nurse assesses the wound carefully for bleeding and signs of infection (see Chapter 37). In the case of tumors that are responsive to treatment, the child's condition and disposition will improve quickly.

Bowel habits can be altered because of pain, immobility, medication, surgery, and changes in nutritional patterns. Compression by large abdominal tumors can cause gastrointestinal obstruction. The nurse should obtain a history of bowel habits and notify the physician if bowel habits are dramatically altered.

Management of the airway is of concern if the child has any mediastinal disease. It is of critical importance that the nurse monitors the child's respiratory effort, color, and pulses and places the child in a position that facilitates effective respirations.

#### Evaluation

- Has the child exhibited decreased crying and irritability?
- Does the child rest quietly and comfortably in the parent's arms and have uninterrupted periods of rest?
- Are the parents verbalizing their fears and expressing decreased anxiety?
- Are the parents asking questions related to the child's disease and treatment and seeking the support of family and friends?

## OSTEOSARCOMA

Osteosarcoma (also called *osteogenic sarcoma*) is the most common primary bone malignancy in children. The symptoms of this disease in its earliest stage are almost always attributed to extremity injury or normal growing pains. Typically, unresolved pain attributed to trauma (often a sports-related injury) brings the tumor to the attention of medical personnel.

### Etiology

The cause of osteosarcoma is unknown, although associations have been made between radiation therapy for other diseases and osteosarcoma. Familial tendencies have been seen, suggesting that genetic factors are involved (Arndt, 2016a).

### Incidence

In the United States, osteosarcoma occurs at a rate of approximately 5.6 new cases/1 million children under 15 years of age per year (Arndt, 2016a). Osteosarcoma is rare in young children, peaks in the teenage years, and is more common in males than in females. Osteosarcoma occurs at an earlier age in girls than in boys, which corresponds to the earlier maturation of girls (Arndt, 2016a). If metastases are present, the lungs are the primary organ involved.

### Pathophysiology

Osteosarcoma originates from bone-producing cells that invade the medullary canal of the bone and form a solid tumor. The incidence is higher in the most rapidly growing bones in adolescents—that is, the distal femur, proximal tibia, and proximal humerus. Since the highest risk period for osteosarcoma is the adolescent growth spurt, there is a possible association between rapid bone growth and malignant transformation (Arndt, 2016a).

### Manifestations

Manifestations of osteosarcoma include progressive, insidious, or intermittent pain at the tumor site; a palpable mass; limping, if a weight-bearing limb is affected; progressive, limited range of motion; and eventually, pathologic fractures at the tumor site.

### Diagnostic Evaluation

Initially, radiographs of the primary site and chest are taken, followed by CT or MRI and skeletal scintigraphy. The CT scan includes the chest to search for pulmonary metastases, which helps stage the disease. A biopsy of the tumor must be performed with great care so that no local contamination of tissue by tumor occurs. Laboratory tests include a CBC, chemistry levels, and serum alkaline phosphatase and lactate dehydrogenase (LDH) determinations (HaDuong, Martin, Skapek, et al., 2015).

### Therapeutic Management

The goals of therapy are to remove the tumor and prevent the spread of disease. Osteogenic sarcoma is treated with a combination of surgery and chemotherapy. After biopsy of the tumor by an orthopedic oncology surgeon, chemotherapy is administered for approximately 3 months before surgical resection of the tumor. To address the presence of microscopic disease, chemotherapy then resumes after recovery from the surgical resection and continues for an additional 9 months (American Cancer Society, 2012). Continuing chemotherapy is aimed at preventing the spread of disease by killing any microscopic tumor cells present anywhere in the body. After resection, the tumor is sent to pathology for determination of the percentage of tumor necrosis (how well the tumor responded to chemotherapy). The optimal response is 100% tumor necrosis. Radiation therapy is used only for palliative pain control in advanced-stage disease, because osteosarcoma is generally unresponsive to irradiation.

Amputation was once the standard surgical intervention for osteosarcoma and is still necessary in some cases. Favorable tumor location allows specially trained orthopedic surgeons to perform a complex limb salvage operation. The affected tissue is removed with the certainty of clean margins, and limb function is preserved. The diseased bone is removed, and either bone grafts or surgically placed orthopedic devices are implanted.

The extent of disease at diagnosis, elevated LDH and alkaline phosphatase levels, and tumor necrosis found on surgical resection are the three most significant prognostic indicators. The cure rate is 75% for children with local disease and 25% for children with metastatic disease at diagnosis (HaDuong et al., 2015).

## NURSING CARE

### The Child With Osteosarcoma

#### Assessment

Subjective data to be gathered include a history of any injury to the affected limb and a history of discomfort. By the time children with osteosarcomas come to medical attention, they are often in considerable pain from the tumor. Warmth, erythema, and tenderness at the site of tumor are not uncommon. If the swelling is great, the skin can appear shiny and taut, with dilated blood vessels. Lung involvement is usually asymptomatic. As soon as a bone mass is identified, the child must become non–weight-bearing on the affected limb (preferably using crutches). The bone surrounding the tumor is weakened by the tumor and is susceptible to a pathologic fracture, which can cause spread of the cancer, necessitating amputation of the affected limb.

To prepare the child for the possible outcomes of surgery, an assessment of physical activity and sports involvement is essential, as is a psychosocial history. As for any child with cancer, body image changes, especially if the affected limb must be amputated, are of paramount importance. Preoperatively, the nurse should assess the child's values and fears and begin the process of preparing the child for postoperative lifestyle modifications.

#### Nursing Diagnosis and Planning

The following nursing diagnoses and expected outcomes may be appropriate for the child with an osteosarcoma and the child's family:

- Acute Pain related to disease process and procedures.

  **Expected outcome.** The child will have decreased pain, as evidenced by verbalization of adequate pain control and decreased pain rating on an age-appropriate pain assessment tool.
- Fear and Anxiety related to the potential loss or impairment of a limb and a diagnosis of cancer.

  **Expected outcome.** The child and parents will express decreased fears and anxiety related to the surgery and diagnosis.
- Risk for Infection related to chemotherapy or surgery.

  **Expected outcome.** The child will remain free from signs and symptoms of infection, as evidenced by normal body temperature and no redness or purulent drainage from the surgical site.
- Disturbed Body Image related to loss or impairment of a limb.

  **Expected outcome.** The child will have a positive body image, as evidenced by a return to appropriate social situations and statements that indicate adaptation to the altered appearance and function.
- Impaired Physical Mobility related to loss or impairment of limb function.

  **Expected outcome.** The child will regain maximal mobility, as evidenced by ability to perform activities of daily living.
- Deficient Knowledge related to unfamiliarity with the disease process and anxiety.

  **Expected outcome.** The child and parents will describe the disease process and potential postoperative adaptations.

#### Interventions

Initial care is focused on making the child comfortable. Preoperative teaching is extensive and procedure specific. If limb salvage is the procedure of choice, the surgeon and nurse will spend considerable time with the family explaining the planned procedure. The nurse reinforces preoperative and postoperative teaching.

In addition to the usual postoperative care, pain, infection, and potential hemorrhage are nursing concerns. The potential for postoperative pneumonia is increased in the child with pulmonary metastases.

If amputation occurs, phantom limb pain is a temporary condition that a child may experience. This sensation of burning, aching, or cramping in the missing limb is most distressing to the child. The child needs to be reassured that the condition is normal. Numerous pharmacologic agents are available to address postoperative neurogenic pain.

The child who undergoes amputation will be fitted with a permanent prosthesis once the surgical site has thoroughly healed. A temporary prosthesis is sometimes used to begin molding the stump for the permanent prosthesis. The temporary prosthesis enables the child to maintain use and strength of surrounding muscles in preparation for the permanent device. A prosthesis can positively affect the issue of body image disturbance and enable the child to become independent in activities of daily living. The nurse prepares the child for extensive work with physical therapists to achieve mobility with the prosthesis. Teenagers especially can be discouraged if they expect the prosthesis to allow them full mobility; some children will continue to have a limp or other awkward movements with the prosthesis.

It is imperative that the nurse help the child verbalize feelings about changes in body image and function. The child is encouraged to participate in age-appropriate decision making concerning care. Promoting interaction with other children of the same age that have the same disease (support groups) can facilitate adaptation. It is of key importance that the nurse provides opportunities for the family to participate in the child's care as well as provide support and encouragement.

Follow-up outpatient visits should include a careful assessment of psychosocial adjustment. Questions should include the topics of social interactions, school attendance and performance, and behavioral changes.

#### Evaluation

- Does the child have discomfort related to the surgical procedures?
- Does the child's pain rating on the pain assessment tool show decreased pain?
- Are the family and child discussing fears related to the disease and treatment?
- Is the child afebrile, and is the surgical site free of redness and purulence?
- Is the child relating with peers?
- Has the child made positive statements indicating beginning adaptation to the physical impairment?

- Is the child readily participating in physical therapy and returning to performing activities of daily living?
- Are the child and family asking questions related to the disease process?
- Do the family and child accurately describe the treatment regimen?

## EWING SARCOMA

Ewing sarcoma is the second most common bone tumor seen in children. The diagnosis is often challenging to make because this disease mimics infection and is difficult to differentiate from other malignancies. Ewing sarcoma can also manifest as a soft tissue mass. This tumor is also referred to as a peripheral primitive neuroectodermal tumor (PPNET).

### Etiology

Ewing sarcoma is proposed to be caused by random factors, as it is not associated with other preexisting congenital chromosomal abnormalities. However, the cause remains unknown.

### Incidence

The incidence of Ewing sarcoma in the United States is 2.1/1 million white children/year (Arndt, 2016a). The disease is very uncommon in African-Americans. Ewing sarcoma is rare in children younger than 5 years and yet is more common than osteosarcoma in children under age 10 years. Both Ewing sarcoma and osteosarcoma are more likely to occur in the second decade of life (Arndt, 2016a).

### Pathophysiology

The diagnosis of Ewing sarcoma is made after all other solid tumors have been excluded. Ewing sarcoma has no defining characteristics. As with osteosarcoma, this tumor invades the bone and is found most often in the flat bones of the axial skeleton such as the vertebrae, ribs, scapula, and pelvic bones. Gross metastasis is uncommon at diagnosis but does occur, most often to the lungs, bones, or bone marrow. As with osteosarcoma, microscopic disease is thought to be present early in the disease process.

### Manifestations

Manifestations of Ewing sarcoma include pain, soft tissue swelling around the affected bone, and fever. If metastatic disease occurs, anorexia, fever, malaise, fatigue, and weight loss are seen. If a vertebral tumor is present, neurologic symptoms will be seen. If a rib tumor is present, respiratory symptoms can be present.

### Diagnostic Evaluation

The diagnostic workup is the same as for osteosarcoma and a biopsy is necessary to differentiate Ewing sarcoma from other neoplastic processes.

### Therapeutic Management

A multidisciplinary approach with chemotherapy, surgery, and radiation is the basis of management. Treatment begins with chemotherapy to decrease the tumor bulk, followed by surgical resection of the primary tumor. Local control of the primary tumor site can be achieved with surgery or radiation therapy because this tumor is sensitive to radiation. Consideration is given to the expendability of the bone involved when surgery is a treatment option versus the potential late effects of radiation. Ribs and the proximal fibula are considered expendable and can be removed to excise a tumor without affecting function. Cure rates exceed 75% to 80% in children with small extremity tumors and no metastases (Arndt, 2016a). With gross metastasis, the cure rate decreases dramatically.

### Nursing Considerations

Nursing care is similar to that for children with osteosarcomas, with the addition of care for the child receiving radiation therapy.

## RHABDOMYOSARCOMA

Rhabdomyosarcoma is a malignancy of muscle or striated tissue that most often occurs periorbitally, in the head and neck in younger children, or in the trunk and extremities in older children. Long-term survival rates vary with the child's age, the histologic subtype, and the location of the tumor.

### Etiology

Although the exact cause is unknown, rhabdomyosarcoma is associated with familial cancer syndromes.

### Incidence

Rhabdomyosarcoma is the most common soft tissue malignancy in children and accounts for approximately 3.5% of all pediatric cancers (Arndt, 2016b). The annual incidence in the United States is estimated at 4.5 cases/1 million white children, with males affected greater than females (HaDuong et al., 2015). Two age-groups are predominant: children younger than 10 years and adolescents (American Cancer Society, 2011).

### Pathophysiology

There are two main histologic subtypes of rhabdomyosarcoma that occur in children. Approximately 60% of tumors are of the embryonal type and have an intermediate prognosis. Approximately 25% to 40% of cases are of the alveolar type, which is found most often in the trunk and extremities and has the poorest prognosis. Lesions in the extremities (alveolar type) are most often found in the adolescent age-group (Arndt, 2016b).

The prognosis depends on several factors other than histologic type. If the tumor is in a location where manifestations appear early, rather than deeply buried in a body cavity, the prognosis is better because the tumor is usually found before it has metastasized. Abnormalities in the DNA content of the tumor cells have prognostic significance. Staging of the tumor is based on whether the tumor was resected completely, was resected with residual microscopic disease, was incompletely resected, or had metastasized to distant sites. Local failure is more common if the tumor cannot be completely resected.

### Manifestations

The manifestations of rhabdomyosarcoma depend on the tumor location. Soft to hard, nontender, relatively immobile masses can be mistaken for a traumatic hematoma. If the lesion is periorbital, visual changes are present; the child might have ptosis, exophthalmos, or proptosis (bulging). The cranial nerve can be involved. If the lesion affects an extremity, range of motion will be limited. In the case of pelvic tumors, the function of organs around the tumor is disrupted.

### Diagnostic Evaluation

CT, skeletal scintigraphy, and bone marrow aspiration and biopsy are performed to determine the extent of disease. The diagnosis is made after biopsy or attempted surgical resection of the tumor. A decision about treatment is made depending on the location of the tumor, histologic subtype, and the presence of distant metastases. Laboratory studies include a CBC, urinalysis, and renal and liver function tests.

## Therapeutic Management

Rhabdomyosarcoma is treated with chemotherapy, surgery, and radiation therapy. Chemotherapy is used to decrease the tumor bulk and reduce the extent and morbidity of surgery. After surgical removal of the tumor, additional chemotherapy is provided. As with Ewing sarcoma, microscopic rhabdomyosarcoma is often present at the time of diagnosis. Discontinuation of chemotherapy after removal of the tumor generally results in recurrent disease. Tumor cells not removed by surgery are referred to as *residual disease.* Radiation therapy is used for children who have residual disease or whose tumor was not resectable. Only approximately 50% of children with metastatic disease at the time of diagnosis achieve initial remission, and of these, less than 50% are cured (Arndt, 2016b).

Follow-up care involves periodic CT or MRI studies to assess tumor response to therapy and monitor any development of disease progression. Most relapses occur within 2 years of diagnosis and during therapy, although late relapse (more than 5 years from therapy) is occasionally reported.

## Nursing Considerations

Parents might relate that their first indication that something was wrong was a decreased activity level in a young child unable to verbalize pain. If the tumor is more superficially located, the parents might have discovered a lump or swelling.

The physical examination findings will depend on the location of the tumor, but typically a soft to hard, nontender mass will be palpated. The surrounding lymph nodes should be palpated for enlargement, which suggests tumor involvement. The CBC is usually normal unless the tumor has extended into bone marrow, causing a decrease in hemoglobin and platelet values.

Nursing care initially focuses on support of family members as they react and adjust to the diagnosis of cancer. Second, the nurse facilitates the educational process to allay fears of the unknown.

Postoperative care of the biopsy or surgical site involves careful observation for signs of infection, hemorrhage, and edema. If surgery involves excision of an abdominal or pelvic tumor, the child will return from the operating room with an NG tube and possibly drains in place.

# WILMS TUMOR

Wilms tumor is the most common renal tumor in children. Much research has been done on this disease, and the subsequent changes in therapy have resulted in improved outcomes. Prognosis is related to the stage of disease at diagnosis, histopathologic features of the tumor, and child's age.

## Etiology

Most Wilms tumors occur in children with no unusual physical features and no family history of the disease. These are considered "sporadic" cases. In approximately 1% to 2% of children with this disease, there is a genetic predisposition and familial occurrence. Certain genes for Wilms tumor have been identified (Daw et al., 2016). Wilms tumor can occur in one or both kidneys; bilateral disease is more common in familial cases than in sporadic cases. Although the cause of Wilms tumor is unknown, it is associated with a variety of childhood syndromes and congenital anomalies including aniridia (absence of the irises), hemihypertrophy, cryptorchidism, and hypospadias (see Chapter 44).

## Incidence

Approximately 8 new cases/1 million children under age 15 years are diagnosed annually, representing 6% of childhood cancers (Daw et al., 2016). Most children are diagnosed between the ages of 2 to 5 years; however, Wilms tumor is seen in neonates, adolescents, and adults. Bilateral Wilms tumors are seen in 7% of pediatric cases (Daw et al., 2016).

## Pathophysiology

Wilms tumor arises from the renal parenchyma of the kidney. Categories of Wilms tumor are based on favorable and unfavorable histologic findings; children with favorable histologic findings (the majority of children with Wilms tumor) have a better prognosis (Daw et al., 2016). At the initial diagnosis, the disease is usually local, but metastasis to other organs occasionally occurs. The lungs are the most common site of metastasis. As with other tumors, a staging system directs treatment.

## Manifestations

The most common clinical presentation of Wilms tumor is an asymptomatic, mobile, abdominal mass discovered by the parent or other caregiver while bathing the child or by a primary care provider during a routine physical examination. Additional manifestations include microscopic or gross hematuria, hypertension, abdominal pain, fatigue, anemia, and fever.

## Diagnostic Evaluation

The diagnosis is suspected from data in the child's history. Abdominal ultrasonography is the initial study done to detect a solid intrarenal mass. Abdominal CT or MRI, chest radiography, and chest CT are performed to further evaluate extent of disease. Laboratory tests include a CBC, electrolyte levels, liver and kidney function tests, and urinalysis. A definitive diagnosis is made at the time of surgery on the basis of pathologic findings. Palpation or any pressure on the tumor before surgery must be avoided to prevent possible rupture and spillage of tumor cells into the peritoneum.

## Therapeutic Management

Treatment for Wilms tumor consists of surgery and chemotherapy alone or in combination with radiation therapy. In most cases, the tumor can be completely removed by surgical resection at the time of diagnosis. During surgery, the surgeon is careful to prevent rupture of the tumor and spillage, which might necessitate more aggressive treatment (Daw et al., 2016). In a few cases, complete surgical resection is considered too great a risk at the time of diagnosis and only a biopsy is performed to determine pathology. The goal of the initial chemotherapy treatments in these children is to reduce the tumor size before definitive surgery, although the COG now recommends surgery before chemotherapy treatments (Daw et al., 2016). All children receive chemotherapy after the tumor is surgically removed. Radiation therapy is added to the treatment of larger, more extensive tumors or those with an unfavorable histologic classification. Survival rates for children with Wilms tumors are higher than rates for children with many other forms of cancer. The overall survival of children with Wilms tumor is 90%; survival is higher among those with a more favorable prognosis (Daw et al., 2016).

**! NURSING QUALITY ALERT**

***Assessing the Child With a Wilms Tumor***

The tumor mass should not be palpated during the assessment because of the risk of rupturing the protective capsule. Excessive manipulation can cause seeding of the tumor and spread of cancerous cells.

## NURSING CARE

### The Child With Wilms Tumor

#### Assessment

Parents often report that when bathing or dressing their child they noticed the child's stomach seemed swollen. Some parents state that the diapers no longer fit easily around the child's abdomen. More often than not, the child's activity level and appetite have not changed. Except for a palpable abdominal mass that usually does not cross the midline, the child's physical examination is normal.

#### Nursing Diagnosis and Planning

The following nursing diagnoses and expected outcomes apply to the child with Wilms tumor and the child's family:

- Anxiety related to surgery with nephrectomy.

*Expected outcome.* The child and parents will express decreased anxiety about the outcome of surgery.

- Risk for Infection related to surgical interventions.

*Expected outcome.* The child will exhibit no signs and symptoms of infection, as evidenced by normal body temperature, intact incision site without redness and swelling, and absence of purulent drainage.

- Deficient Knowledge related to unfamiliarity with the disease process and treatment plan.

*Expected outcome.* The child and parents will describe the disease process and treatment plan.

- Risk for Deficient Fluid Volume related to having only one kidney postoperatively.

*Expected outcome.* The child will demonstrate fluid balance, as evidenced by moist mucous membranes, normal electrolyte and urine values, and hourly urine output appropriate for age.

#### Interventions

Because the child usually feels well, nursing care initially focuses on preoperative teaching for the parents and child. The nurse places a sign on the child's bed warning against palpating the abdomen. A nephrectomy is a serious surgical procedure, and family members will have anxiety about the child losing a kidney. Nurses must offer support and reassurance.

Postoperatively, the nurse monitors the child for GI activity, bowel sounds, stool production, abdominal distention, signs and symptoms of infection, hemorrhage, and changes in blood pressure. Careful assessment of urine output by the remaining kidney is essential. Intake and output are precisely measured and totaled at least every 4 hours. These children will probably return from surgery with an NG tube in place.

Once the tumor has been staged, the child is assigned to the appropriate therapeutic protocol. Teaching should center on the sequencing of tests and drugs on that protocol. The nurse provides support to the child and family and assesses their coping skills throughout the course of outpatient chemotherapy.

#### Evaluation

- Are the parents and child using coping skills and mobilizing support systems?
- Has the child remained afebrile?
- Is the incision site dry and intact and free from redness, swelling, and purulent drainage?
- Is blood pressure within normal limits for age?
- Does the child have moist mucous membranes, are electrolytes and urinalysis within normal limits, and is hourly urine output appropriate for age?
- Is the family asking questions and sharing concerns and fears?

## RETINOBLASTOMA

Retinoblastoma is a rare, malignant tumor of the embryonic neural retina. This tumor of the eye is found only in children. Observant parents may bring this disease to the attention of the physician when they look at a photograph and see a white reflection (leukocoria) in one of the child's eyes instead of the normal red color when the camera flash is reflected off the retina.

### Etiology

Retinoblastoma results from a series of genetic mutations. The majority of these genetic mutations are sporadic, occurring within a single retinal cell that then multiplies to form the tumor. Hereditary, or familial retinoblastoma occurs in individuals who have a germline mutation present. The mutation places the child at high risk of developing retinoblastoma, as well as other associated malignancies. A second mutation occurs in one or more of the retinal cells, which then multiply to form a tumor. Advances in genetic studies of this disease have led to genetic research on other forms of childhood cancer.

### Incidence

Retinoblastoma represents 4% of all pediatric cancers. Thirty percent of retinoblastomas are of the hereditary form, and 70% are nonhereditary (Barbel & Peterson, 2015). The majority of children (66% to 75%) have unilateral involvement. Over 90% of cases are seen in children less than 5 years of age; the median age at diagnosis is approximately 2 years (Tarek & Herzog, 2016).

### Pathophysiology

The human retina does not reach maturation until approximately age 3 years. During this early process of differentiation, cells are at risk for abnormal division and neoplasia. The tumor develops on the retina, growing inward toward the vitreous humor or out toward the subretinal space. Retinoblastoma can develop at a single site or as multiple independent tumors that originate within the globe of the eye. The process of cells breaking off from the main mass and forming additional independent tumors is called *seeding*. If diagnosis is delayed, these tumors can extend down the optic nerve and spread to CNS sites outside the eye (Tarek & Herzog, 2016).

### Manifestations

The most common findings of retinoblastoma are leukocoria and strabismus resulting from vision loss. In general, young children will not report vision loss limited to one eye. Manifestations also include pain, redness, and inflammation of the eye.

### Diagnostic Evaluation

Leukocoria or strabismus discovered by the parent or on a routine physical examination results in a referral to an ophthalmologist. A funduscopic examination with the child under general anesthesia is the best means of diagnosing and monitoring retinoblastoma. Ultrasound imaging confirms that the retinoblastoma tumors are present and determines their thickness and height. CT or MRI of the eyes, orbits, and brain is performed to evaluate the tumors within the eyes and search for extraocular spread (Tarek & Herzog, 2016).

### Therapeutic Management

As with other cancers, a staging system has been developed to standardize descriptions of the extent of disease confined to the eye and those tumors that have spread outside the eye and to other parts of the body. This system directs treatment and indicates prognosis.

The goals of treatment for retinoblastoma are to save the child's life and preserve the eye with useful vision. Treatment decisions are based on the size of the tumor and whether it is confined to the eye or has spread to other parts of the body. Enucleation, removal of the eye, is becoming less frequent with the successful use of focal therapies (cryotherapy or laser photocoagulation) alone for small lesions or in combination with multiagent chemotherapy for larger tumors (Tarek & Herzog, 2016). External-beam radiation therapy can be considered if chemotherapy plus focal therapy fails. Radiation can lead to orbital deformities and increased risk of secondary malignancies in children with familial retinoblastoma.

Enucleation is performed if there is no chance the child will have useful vision in the affected eye, if the tumor is unresponsive to nonsurgical treatment, or if the tumor recurs (Tarek & Herzog, 2016). When enucleation is performed, the child does not require any further therapy and is monitored closely for tumor recurrence with serial examinations.

Because intraocular penetration of systemic chemotherapy agents is poor and the tumors can develop multidrug resistance, alternative treatment options are under investigation. The prognosis for children with retinoblastoma (confined in the orbit) is excellent, with a 5-year survival rate of 95% (Tarek & Herzog, 2016). Retinoblastoma that extends to extraocular sites is associated with a poor prognosis. Routine eye exams for children under age 7 years can result in early detection of a tumor before it spreads and successful treatment (Tarek & Herzog, 2016).

## NURSING CARE

### The Child With Retinoblastoma

#### Assessment

Except for leukocoria (a whitish reflex in the pupillary area), the findings on physical examination are often normal. The nurse assesses for strabismus, isotropic, exotropia, or decreased vision (see Chapter 55). The child may have compensated for loss of vision in one eye; therefore, the nurse must be very astute when assessing vision in these children.

#### Nursing Diagnosis and Planning

The following nursing diagnoses and expected outcomes apply to the child with retinoblastoma and the child's family:

- Anxiety (child and family) related to cancer, enucleation, and fear of blindness.

  ***Expected outcome.*** The child and family will express decreased anxiety about outcomes of therapy.
- Risk for Injury related to visual changes caused by the tumor or enucleation.

  ***Expected outcome.*** The child will develop compensatory mechanisms for vision, as evidenced by the ability to safely perform activities of daily living.
- Deficient Knowledge related to unfamiliarity with the disease process and treatment.

  ***Expected outcome.*** The child and parents will describe the disease process and the treatment plan and will demonstrate the use of any prosthetic device, if required.

#### Interventions

Nursing care initially focuses on support of family members as they react and adjust to the diagnosis of cancer. Second, the nurse facilitates the educational process so families are informed of what to expect, decreasing fear and anxiety.

Postoperative care of the enucleated orbit entails careful observations for signs of infection, hemorrhage, and edema. The child will wear a patch over the socket for approximately 1 week postoperatively. To preserve the shape of the orbit for prosthesis, which will be fitted 5 to 6 weeks after surgery, a conformer is placed in the orbit. Nursing interventions include teaching the parents (and child if old enough) how to remove, clean, and reinsert first the conformer and then the prosthesis.

The nurse can reassure parents that children can generally accommodate to vision in only one eye. Protective eyewear must be worn when the child is participating in sports or other potentially hazardous activities, to protect the remaining eye.

Whatever the extent of involvement by tumor or the treatment modality used, careful follow-up with retinal examinations performed with the child under anesthesia and by CT, are indicated. Genetic counseling is recommended. If the retinoblastoma is found to be inherited, siblings should be examined periodically.

Children with familial retinoblastoma have a high incidence of developing second malignancies (primarily osteosarcoma) later in life because of the genetic origin of the disease. Although no specific screening is recommended, signs and symptoms should be carefully evaluated with a high index of suspicion.

#### Evaluation

- Are the child and family verbalizing fears and demonstrating a decrease in anxiety?
- Is the child able to compensate for loss of vision and safely continue daily activities?
- Is the child able to relate to peers and family?
- Are the child and family able to describe the disease and the treatment plan and demonstrate proper care of any prosthetic device?

## RARE TUMORS OF CHILDHOOD

Several tumors not mentioned in this chapter occur infrequently in the pediatric population. These include soft tissue sarcomas other than rhabdomyosarcoma, primary tumors of the liver (e.g., hepatoblastoma and hepatocellular carcinoma), and gonadal (ovarian and testicular cancer) and extragonadal germ cell tumors. Carcinomas and primary cancer of the lungs are a few of the cancers seen in adults that are exceptionally rare in children.

One cancer that has been steadily increasing (approximately 2%/year) in the adolescent population is melanoma (Hawryluk & Liang, 2014). This increased incidence may be due to an increase in sun exposure and a decrease in ozone protection (Gupta & Cohen, 2012). Providers must remain vigilant in detecting signs and symptoms of melanoma and educate patients and their families on safe sun practices.

Many of the key principles of nursing care—pain management, nutrition, comfort, infection control, and emotional support—remain constant for all pediatric cancer diagnoses.

## KEY CONCEPTS

- The signs and symptoms of childhood cancer vary according to the child's age, the type of tumor, and the extent of the disease.
- Childhood cancer is difficult to diagnose because most early symptoms can be attributed to common childhood illnesses.
- The decision to use allogeneic bone marrow, autologous peripheral blood stem cells, or umbilical cord blood stem cells is based on the disease process being treated and the availability of hematopoietic cells.
- Nursing care of children with BMTs focuses on preventing infection until the marrow engrafts and WBCs are produced. All organ systems must be monitored for GVHD and toxicities from pretransplant chemotherapy and radiation.
- Biologic response modifiers are naturally occurring substances found in the body that influence the immune system.
- Chemotherapy is nonselective in its cytotoxic effect.
- Fatigue is a common side effect of radiation therapy; children may need longer or more frequent rest periods.
- Children receiving chemotherapy or radiation are at risk for breakdown of mouth and anal mucous membranes. Meticulous mouth and anal care should be provided. No rectal temperatures and limited use of oral thermometers are indicated.
- After surgical removal of a brain tumor, the child is at risk for increased ICP related to edema, hydrocephalus, or hemorrhage. The nurse should frequently check vital signs, mental status, and neurologic status.
- The abdomen of a child with Wilms tumor should not be palpated, as this can lead to rupture of the protective capsule and seeding of the tumor.

## REFERENCES AND READINGS


Allen, C.E., Kelly, K.M., & Bollard, C.M. (2015). Pediatric lymphomas and histiocytic disorders of childhood. *Pediatric Clinics of North America, 62,* 139–165. doi:10.1016/j.pcl.2014.09.010.

Alperstein, W., Boren, M., & McNeer, J.L. (2015). Pediatric acute lymphoblastic leukemia: from diagnosis to prognosis. *Pediatric Annals, 44*(7), e168–e174. doi:10.3928/00904481-20150710-10.

American Cancer Society. (2011). *Retrieved from Rhabdomyosarcoma,* Retrieved from http://www.cancer.org/acs/groups/cid/documents/webcontent/003136-pdf.pdf.

American Cancer Society. (2012). *Retrieved from Chemotherapy for osteosarcoma,* Retrieved from http://www.cancer.org/Cancer/Osteosarcoma/DetailedGuide/osteosarcoma-treating-chemotherapy.

American Cancer Society. (2014). *Children diagnosed with cancer: Late effects of cancer treatment.* Retrieved from http://www.cancer.org/Treatment/ChildrenandCancer/WhenYourChildHasCancer/children-diagnosed-with-cancer-late-effects-of-cancer-treatment.

Arndt, C. (2016a). Malignant tumors of bone. In R. Kliegman, B. Stanton, J. St. Geme, et al. (Eds.), *Nelson textbook of pediatrics* (20th ed., pp. 2471–2474). Philadelphia: Elsevier.

Arndt, C. (2016b). Soft tissue sarcoma. In R. Kliegman, B. Stanton, J. St. Geme, et al. (Eds.), *Nelson textbook of pediatrics* (20th ed., pp. 2468–2470). Philadelphia: Elsevier.

Asselin, B. (2016). Epidemiology of childhood and adolescent cancer. In R. Kliegman, B. Stanton, J. St. Geme, et al. (Eds.), *Nelson textbook of pediatrics* (20th ed., pp. 2416–2418). Philadelphia: Elsevier.

Association of Pediatric Hematology/Oncology Nurses. (2016). *Pediatric chemotherapy and biotherapy provider program.* Retrieved from: http://www.apon.org/education/ped.cfm.

Ater, J., & Kuttesch, J.F. (2016). Brain tumors in childhood. In R. Kliegman, B. Stanton, J. St. Geme, et al. (Eds.), *Nelson textbook of pediatrics* (20th ed., pp. 2453–2460). Philadelphia: Elsevier.

Bass, P.F. (2014). Living past cancer: Late effects and long-term care [Electronic version]. *Contemporary Pediatrics, 31*(9), 4.

Barbel, P., & Peterson, K. (2015). Recognizing subtle signs and symptoms of pediatric cancer. *Nursing 2015,* 31–37. doi: 10.1097/01.nurse.0000461852.18315.b5.

Bhojwani, D., Yang, J.J., & Pui, C. (2015). Biology of childhood acute lymphoblastic leukemia. *Pediatric Clinics of North America, 62,* 47–60. doi:10.1016/j.pcl.2014.09.004.

Bleyer, A., Ritchey, A.K., & Friehling, E. (2016). Principles of treatment. In R. Kliegman, B. Stanton, J. St. Geme, et al. (Eds.), *Nelson textbook of pediatrics* (20th ed., pp. 2426–2436). Philadelphia: Elsevier.

Bingen, K., Kent, M., Rodday, A.M., et al. (2012). Children's coping with hematopoietic stem cell transplant stressors: results from the journeys to recover study. *Children's Health Care, 41,* 145–161. doi:10.1080/02739615.2012.656551.

Cataudella, D.A., & Zelcer, S. (2012). Psychological experiences of children with brain tumors at end of life: parental perspectives. *Journal of Palliative Medicine, 15*(11), 1191–1197. doi:10.1089/jpm.2011.0479.

Chang, V.Y., & Davidson, T.B. (2015), Childhood exposures and risk of malignancy in adulthood. *Pediatric Annals, 44* (11), e270–e273. doi:10.3928/00904481-20151112-10.

Chintagumpala, M., & Gajjar, A. (2015). Brain tumors. *Pediatric Clinics of North America, 62,* 167–178. doi:10.1016/j.pcl.2014.09.011.

Cooper, S.L., & Brown, P.A. (2015). Treatment of pediatric acute lymphoblastic leukemia. *Pediatric Clinics of North America, 62,* 61–73. doi:10.1016/j.pcl.2014.09.006.

Darcy, L., Knutsson, S., Huus, K., et al. (2014). The everyday life of the young child shortly after receiving a cancer diagnosis, from both children's and parent's perspectives. *Cancer Nursing, 37*(6), 445–456. doi: 10.1097/NCC.0000000000000114.

Daw, N.C., Huff, V., & Anderson, P.M. (2016). Wilms tumor. In R. Kliegman, B. Stanton, J. St. Geme, et al. (Eds.), *Nelson textbook of pediatrics* (20th ed., pp. 2464–2467). Philadelphia: Elsevier.

Gupta, A., & Cohen, B.A. (2012). Ultraviolet radiation exposure and melanoma: providing safer skin practices for children. *Contemporary Pediatrics, 29*(5), 10–14.

HaDuong, J.H., Martin, A.A., Skapek, S.X., et al. (2015). Sarcomas. *Pediatric Clinics of North America, 62,* 179–200. doi:10.1016/j.pcl.2014.09.012.

Hawryluk, E.B., & Liang, M.G. (2014). Pediatric melanoma, moles, and sun safety. *Pediatric Clinics of North America, 61,* 279–291. doi:10.1016/j.pcl.2013.11.004.

Henry, M., & Sung, L. (2015). Supportive care in pediatric oncology: oncologic emergencies and management of fever and neutropenia. *Pediatric Clinics of North America, 62,* 27–46. doi:10.1016/j.pcl.2014.09.016.

Hochberg, J., Giulino-Roth, L., & Cairo, M. (2016). Lymphoma. In R. Kliegman, B. Stanton, J. St. Geme, et al. (Eds.), *Nelson textbook of pediatrics* (20th ed., pp. 2445–2453). Philadelphia: Elsevier.

Hooke, M.C., Garwick, A.W., & Gross, C.R. (2011). Fatigue and physical performance in children and adolescents receiving chemotherapy. *Oncology Nursing Forum, 38*(6), 649–657. doi:10.1188/11.ONF.649–657.

Hunger, S.P., & Mullighan, C.G. (2015). Acute lymphoblastic leukemia in children. *The New England Journal of Medicine, 373*(16), 1541–1552. doi:10.1056/NEJMra1400972.

Irwin, M.S., & Park, J.R. (2015). Neuroblastoma. *Pediatric Clinics of North America, 62,* 225–256. doi:10.1016/j.pcl.2014.10.015.

Landier, W., Armenian, S., & Bhatia, S. (2015). Late effects of childhood cancer and its treatment. *Pediatric Clinics of North America, 62,* 275–300. doi:10.1016/j.pcl.2014.09.017.

Mallhi, K., Lum, L. G., Schultz, K.R., et al. (2015). Hematopoietic cell transplantation and cellular therapeutics in the treatment of childhood malignancies. *Pediatric Clinics of North America, 62,* 257–273. doi:10.1016/j.pcl.2014.10.001.

Nelson, M.B., Compton, P., Patel, S.K., et al. (2013). Central nervous system injury and neurobehavioral function in children with brain tumors. *Cancer Nursing, 26*(2), e31–e47. doi:10.1097/NCC.0b013e31825d1eb0.

Smith, M.A., & Reaman, G.H. (2015). Remaining challenges in childhood cancer and newer targeted therapeutics. *Pediatric Clinics of North America, 62,* 301–312. doi:10.1016/j.pcl.2014.09.018.

Tarek, N., & Herzog, C. (2016). Retinoblastoma. In R. Kliegman, B. Stanton, J. St. Geme, et al. (Eds.), *Nelson textbook of pediatrics* (20th ed., pp. 2476–2477). Philadelphia: Elsevier.

Tubergen, D., Bleyer, A., Ritchey, K., et al. (2016). The leukemias. In R. Kliegman, B. Stanton, J. St. Geme, et al. (Eds.), *Nelson textbook of pediatrics* (20th ed., pp. 2437–2445). Philadelphia: Elsevier.

Zage, P., & Ater, J. (2016). Neuroblastoma. In R. Kliegman, B. Stanton, J. St. Geme, et al. (Eds.) *m Nelson textbook of pediatrics* (20th ed., pp. 2461–2464). Philadelphia: Elsevier.

Zimlich, R. (2015). Clinical trial tests tool that sees cancer cells [Electronic version]. *Contemporary Pediatrics, 32*(6).

49

# The Child With an Alteration in Tissue Integrity

http://evolve.elsevier.com/McKinney/mat-ch/

## LEARNING OBJECTIVES

*After studying this chapter, you should be able to:*

- Describe the anatomy and physiology of normal skin.
- Contrast characteristics of the neonate's, child's, and adult's skin.
- Identify the manifestations of common skin disorders seen in infants and children.
- Discuss the management of skin disorders seen frequently in children, such as bacterial, fungal, and viral infections; infestations; inflammatory disorders; acne vulgaris; and insect bites and stings.
- Discuss common causes of burns in children and the prevention of burn injuries.
- Analyze the implications of burn injuries in children.
- Discuss the classifications of depth, extent, and severity of a burn injury.
- Describe the therapeutic management and nursing care of children with minor burns.
- Apply the nursing process to the care of infants and children with skin disorders.

# CLINICAL REFERENCE

## REVIEW OF THE INTEGUMENTARY SYSTEM

Knowledge of integumentary structure and function is necessary to understand the changes that occur with disease. There are a number of important differences between the skin of infants and young children and that of adults.

The skin has five major functions: (1) to protect the deeper tissues from injury, drying, and invasion by foreign matter; (2) to regulate temperature; (3) to aid in water excretion; (4) to aid in vitamin D production; and (5) to initiate the sensations of touch, pain, heat, and cold.

The skin is composed of two principal layers: the outer epidermis and the inner supportive dermis. Beneath these layers is the subcutaneous layer, which is composed largely of adipose tissue.

The epidermis is nonvascular stratified epithelium that is divided into two major layers. The outermost layer, the stratum corneum, is a tough, horny collection of dead keratinized cells that have migrated up from the underlying layers. Keratin, a fibrous protein, is also the principal component of nails and hair. Skin cells are constantly being shed and replaced with new cells from the layers below.

The stratum basale, or basal cell layer, anchors the epidermis to the dermis. It contains dividing, undifferentiated cells that migrate upward toward the stratum corneum, differentiating into keratinocytes on their way. Epidermal replacement is relatively rapid; the epidermis is completely replaced approximately every 4 weeks. The stratum basale also contains melanocytes—the source of melanin, the pigment that gives skin its color.

The dermis, composed of tough connective tissue, contains lymphatics and nerves. The highly vascular dermis nourishes the epidermis.

Appendages from the epidermis—sebaceous glands, sweat glands, and hair follicles—are embedded in the dermis. The sebaceous glands arise from the hair follicles and produce sebum, which lubricates the epidermis and is slightly bacteriostatic. Sebaceous glands are particularly abundant on the face and scalp. Hormones influence their activity, with testosterone increasing secretion and estrogen suppressing it.

There are two types of sweat glands. The eccrine sweat glands open directly onto the skin surface and produce sweat, which evaporates to reduce body temperature. Eccrine sweat glands are widely distributed over the body and are functionally mature by 2 months of age. The apocrine sweat glands produce a thick, milky secretion and open onto hair follicles. They are located mainly in the axillary and genital areas and become active during puberty.

Each hair is composed of a shaft and a root, which lie in a deep cavity of dermal cells called the hair follicle. There are several types of hair. Lanugo is the fine first hair that covers the body during fetal life and generally disappears before or shortly after birth. It is replaced by fine, nonpigmented vellus hair. Terminal hair covers all the ordinarily hairy parts of the body; it is coarse, long, and pigmented.

The subcutaneous layer, composed of fat cells, underlies the dermis. Adipose tissue helps cushion and insulate underlying structures.

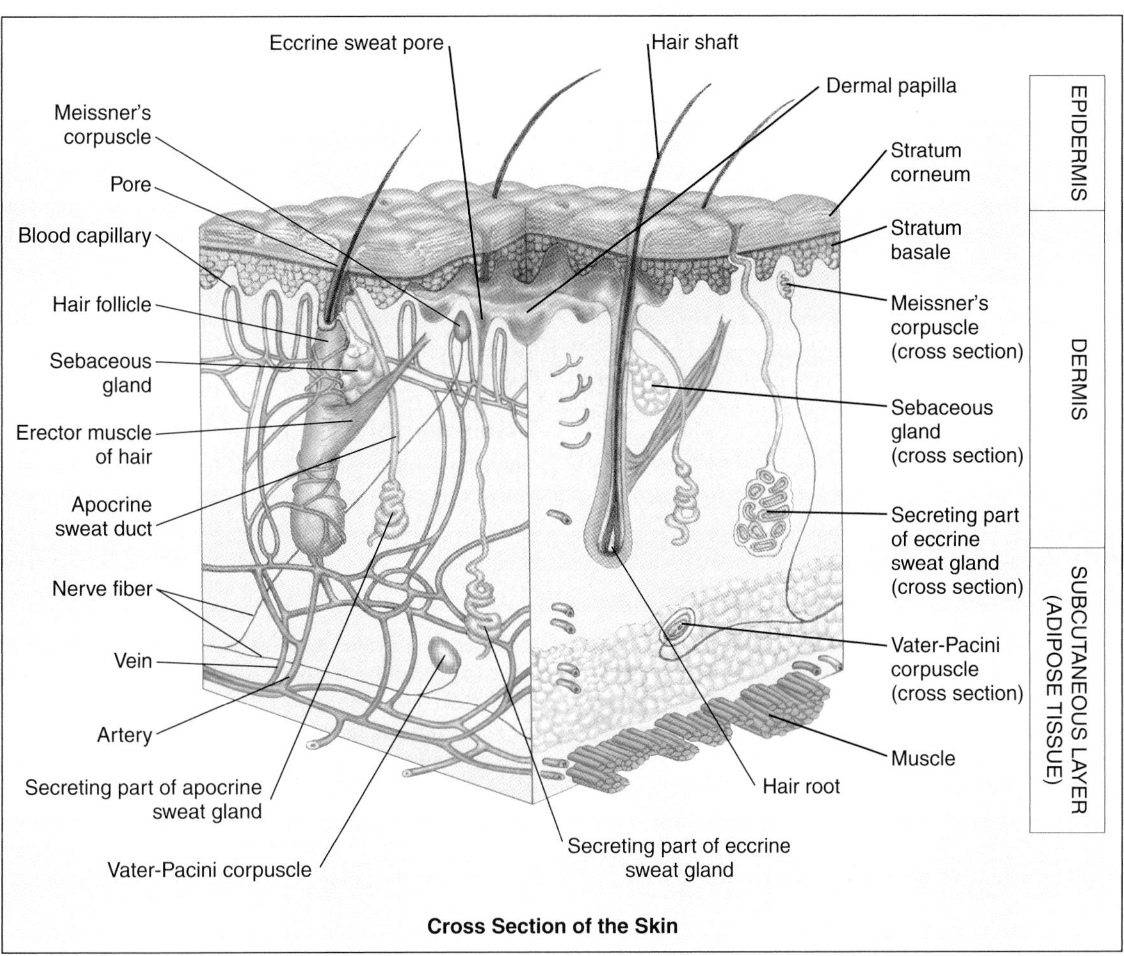


**Cross Section of the Skin**

## Pediatric Differences in the Skin

- The newborn's epidermis is thinner than that of adults, increasing its permeability to topical agents and water loss through the skin.
- The ratio of skin surface area to body volume is greater in infants and small children than in adults, contributing to the risk of greater absorption through the skin. Topical medications should not be used without a physician's order.
- Premature infants have a proportionately greater body surface area than older infants and children, which increases evaporative fluid losses. Premature infants also have fewer cell attachments, which increases the tendency to blister.
- Eccrine glands do not reach mature function until age 2 or 3 years, making infants and young toddlers less able to regulate body temperature.
- Infants have fewer melanocytes than adults, which increases photosensitivity.
- IgA, secreted by the epithelial cells of the mucous membranes, does not reach adult levels until age 2 to 5 years. Consequently, the infant is less resistant to organisms such as those occurring on the hands or other objects the infant might mouth.
- Hormonal changes during adolescence increase sebum production, which contributes to acne vulgaris.

Information from Puttgen, K. & Cohen, B. (2013). Neonatal dermatology. In B. Cohen (Ed.). *Pediatric Dermatology* (4th ed.). St. Louis, MO: Elsevier Saunders.

The skin is a sensitive indicator of a child's general health. Skin disorders are among the most common health problems in children. They may cause pain, pruritus, or changes in local sensation. Because the skin is visible and its disorders are often disfiguring, skin disorders can cause emotional and psychological stress for the child and family. Whether it is the discomfort and stress produced by an infant's eczema or the emotional upset caused by an adolescent's acne, these disorders can influence the child's psychological and social development.

Nurses caring for children are in a unique position to assess the condition of children's skin and to help children and families cope with skin disorders. Nurses can play an important role by teaching parents and children strategies to maintain healthy skin and prevent future skin problems.

## VARIATIONS IN THE SKIN OF NEWBORN INFANTS

Parents typically inspect every inch of their newborn infant's skin and continue to attend closely to variations in the skin of older infants. Regardless of whether the parent mentions it, the nurse may be sure the family is aware of spots, bumps, or rashes on the baby. Families frequently worry needlessly about skin lesions on infants, and the nurse can ease anxieties by pointing out and explaining the meaning and natural history of common skin variations.

## COMMON BIRTHMARKS

Most birthmarks are composed of cells of one or more of the skin's normal elements. Any of the skin's components can produce a birthmark, including melanocytes, blood vessels, epidermal cells, connective tissue, and hair follicles. The great majority of birthmarks are benign, although some signal congenital syndromes, some are associated with an increased risk for malignancy, and others interfere with function or are disfiguring.

### Etiology

Port-wine stains are the result of capillary malformation. Hemangiomas result from the proliferation of dilated capillaries and endothelial cells of the capillary linings. Salmon patches (nevus simplex) are caused by distended dermal capillaries that are believed to result from persistent fetal circulation. Mongolian spots are not vascular but the result of collections of pigment deep in the dermis. They occur as a result of arrested migration of melanocytes from the neural crest to the skin during embryonic development. Café-au-lait spots, light-brown pigmented areas, can appear anywhere on an infant's body. Six or more of these lesions, if larger than 5 mm in diameter, suggest an underlying disorder, such as neurofibromatosis, Noonan syndrome, or McCune-Albright syndrome.

### Incidence

Vascular birthmarks are extremely common, with most references estimating an incidence of occurrence in more than 1 in 10 neonates. Port-wine stains occur in 3 in 1000 live births (Vascular Birthmarks Foundation, 2015), and approximately 5% of all newborn infants have hemangiomas (Martin, 2016b). The most common vascular lesion is the salmon patch, which some references estimate to occur in as many as 40% of neonates. The incidence of Mongolian spots is proportional to the depth of the baby's pigmentation. As many as 80% of black, Asian, and American Indian infants are born with Mongolian spots. Fewer than 10% of white infants have Mongolian spots (Martin, 2016a).

### Manifestations

The port-wine stain is present at birth. At first it is only faintly colored and flat, but it becomes darker as the child grows. In some cases, underlying bone and tissue enlarge as well. The port-wine stain is permanent, and by middle age, the mark can be dark purple and rough or nodular. Hemangiomas, conversely, are not usually visible at birth but appear during the first few weeks of life and then grow during the first year. Generally, they begin to disappear spontaneously after 1 year of age and are gone by age 5 or 6 years of age. The salmon patch is a flat, pink, irregular-shaped spot on the nape of the neck, the forehead, between the eyes, on the eyelids, or around the nasolabial folds. Commonly called "stork bites" or "angel kisses," these lesions are benign and usually fade during the first year of life. Salmon patches typically appear darker when the child is crying. Mongolian spots are present at birth and appear as flat, gray-green or blue lesions similar to bruises. They are most commonly distributed on the lumbosacral regions or buttocks, although they can appear on any part of the body. Mongolian spots generally fade completely by the time the child is 4 to 5 years old.

### Diagnostic Evaluation

The appearance of most birthmarks is sufficient to make a diagnosis, although biopsy and histologic evaluation are definitive. Rarely, a hemangioma is a sign of a more serious, underlying disorder. Worrisome hemangiomas include those with large, segmented facial distributions, those with a beard distribution, and those that involve the gluteal cleft. Magnetic resonance imaging and Doppler ultrasound is typically performed to rule out underlying anomalies (Sethuraman, Yenamandra, & Gupta, 2014).

### Therapeutic Management

Other than education, treatment for salmon patches and Mongolian spots is not indicated. Treatment for port-wine stains is not indicated in the neonatal period, but their identification should prompt evaluation for associated congenital syndromes, such as Sturge–Weber, Beckwith–Wiedemann, and Klippel–Trénaunay syndromes. Conservative management of port-wine stains in older children includes instructions for concealing the lesions with makeup and psychotherapy if needed. Pulsed dye laser therapy is the treatment of choice for darker port wine stains (Martin, 2016b).

The treatment for hemangiomas includes simple observation as the lesion involutes (resolves) on its own, pharmacotherapy, surgical excision, radiation, and laser therapy. Active intervention is reserved for hemangiomas that interfere with function, such as those that obstruct the nose, mouth, or eyes, or lesions that tend to ulcerate and bleed frequently. Pharmacologic approaches include injection of steroids into the lesion, oral steroids, and topical imiquimod. The argon laser tends to relieve the symptoms of ulcerated hemangiomas in a matter of days, and involution typically follows. A rapidly growing, deep hemangioma may be a sign of Kasabach–Merritt syndrome, a coagulation disorder that results in thrombocytopenia, severe anemia, and the collecting of platelets within the hemangioma. This condition can be life threatening (Martin, 2016b).

### Nursing Considerations

Assess the child's entire body for the distribution, size, and shape of lesions. Assess hemangiomas for symptoms such as ulceration or bleeding and for the potential to obstruct function. Assess the extent of the parents' knowledge regarding the infant's birthmarks.

Parents are frequently anxious about newborn infants' skin lesions, and it is not unusual to discover that parents already have acquired misinformation from friends and family members about the meaning and prognosis of birthmarks. Common anxiety-provoking beliefs include the ideas that prominent lesions are malignant or that the mother caused the lesions by careless behaviors during her pregnancy.

The parents should receive a simple, scientific explanation for the skin lesions and instructions regarding the usual skin care for neonates (see Parents Want to Know: Care of Newborn and Infant Skin). Parents should be made aware of the expected course of their child's lesion, and their expectations should be explored. Nurses can reassure parents when the lesions are benign and educate them thoroughly about what to expect when treatment is indicated.

## SKIN INFLAMMATION

Inflammatory conditions that affect the child's skin can be acute or chronic. A primary nursing goal when caring for a child with an inflammatory skin condition is to prevent secondary infection.

## PARENTS WANT TO KNOW

### *Care of Newborn and Infant Skin*

Encourage parents to protect the infant's skin by teaching the following:

- Infants may be bathed and shampooed daily after the umbilical cord has fallen off. Use mild soap and warm water.
- Avoid overbathing, which dries the skin. Do not allow the infant to bathe longer than 10 minutes. Avoid bubble bath products; they dry and irritate the skin.
- Lotions, creams, and powders are not needed after the bath.
- Change diapers frequently and clean the diaper area with water at each change.
- Remove diapers for short periods during the day while the baby lies on a washable pad, to expose diaper area to air.
- Avoid hot environments and overbundling the baby. Infants do not sweat effectively, and heat results in rashes and problems with temperature regulation.
- Avoid direct exposure to the sun during the first 2 weeks of life and avoid sun exposure for more than 10 to 15 minutes daily thereafter during early infancy. Babies should wear hats or bonnets and shirts in the sun. Do not use sunscreen on infants younger than 6 months; keep them out of prolonged direct sunlight.

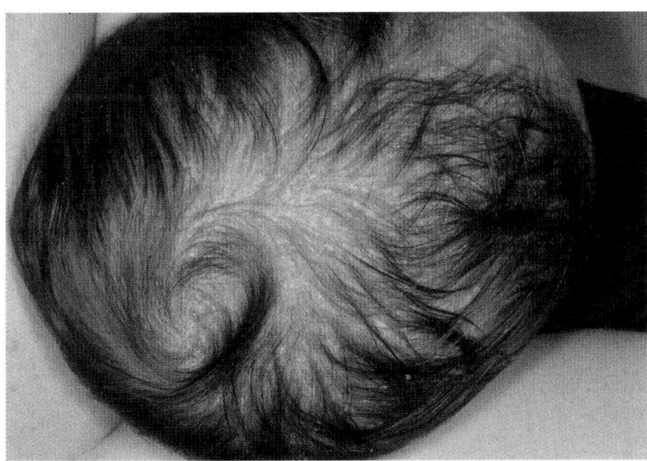

**FIG 49.1** "Cradle cap," the most frequent form of seborrheic dermatitis in infants. The condition often begins in the first 2 to 3 weeks of life and usually disappears by age 12 months. (From Paller, S.A. [2012]. *Hurwitz clinical pediatric dermatology: a textbook of skin disorders of childhood and adolescence* [4th ed.]. Philadelphia: Saunders.)

## Seborrheic Dermatitis

Seborrheic dermatitis is a chronic inflammatory skin condition seen frequently in infants. It is referred to as "cradle cap" when located on the scalp. It often begins in the first 2 to 3 weeks of life and usually disappears by age 12 months. Seborrhea in older children might appear on the face, behind the ears, around the umbilicus, or in any other area with a large number of sebaceous glands. Although the precise cause is unknown, seborrhea appears to be related to sebaceous gland dysfunction and overgrowth of the fungi *Candida* and *Malassezia ovalis* (Victoire, Magin, Coughlan, et al., 2014).

Seborrheic dermatitis is characterized by nonpruritic, oily, yellow scales that block sweat and sebaceous glands, causing retained secretions and inflammation in affected areas (Fig. 49.1). Confluent erythema is commonly present in the diaper and intertriginous areas and around the umbilicus (Fig. 49.2). Often, there is overgrowth of normal skin bacteria and yeast, which increases inflammation and leads to secondary infection.

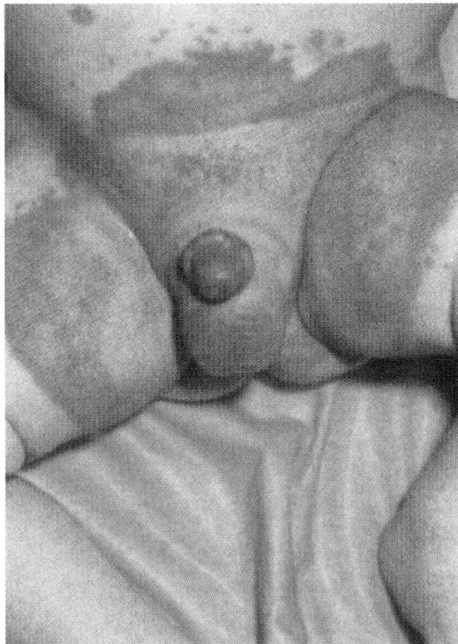

**FIG 49.2** Seborrheic diaper dermatitis. (From Moschella, S.L., & Hurley, H.J. [1992]. *Dermatology* [3rd ed., pp. 239]. Philadelphia: Saunders.)

The nurse inspects the infant's scalp or other affected areas for lesions and inflammation and questions parents about the frequency and technique of washing the infant's scalp. Instruct the parents to remove the scales daily by shampooing with a mild baby shampoo or an over-the-counter antiseborrheic shampoo containing sulfur and salicylic acid (Fostex Medicated Cleansing, P&S liquid, Sebulex), selenium, or tar (Neutrogena T/Gel, Polytar). Ketoconazole 2% shampoo has been reported to be safe in infants less than 12 months of age (Victoire et al., 2014). Massaging the scalp with warm mineral oil before shampooing helps loosen scales. Using a fine-tooth comb or a clean, soft-bristle toothbrush during the shampoo also helps loosen scales. Eyelid dermatitis (blepharitis) is treated with warm tap water compresses and cleansing with "no tears" baby shampoo. Care must be taken to keep topical medications out of the infant's eyes.

Teach the parents the importance of good hygiene when caring for the infant's scalp and skin to prevent recurrence. Reassure them that the fontanel is not fragile and will not be damaged by gentle pressure and washing. Advise the parents to contact the physician if the sites become infected. Skin lesions that do not clear with frequent washing can be treated with hydrocortisone cream applied twice a day.

Seborrheic dermatitis of the diaper area is often secondarily infected with *Candida albicans* and requires appropriate treatment. Lotions and creams tend to aggravate the condition and should not be used.

## Contact Dermatitis

Contact dermatitis is a skin inflammation that results from direct skin-to-irritant contact.

### Etiology

Contact dermatitis can be caused by hundreds of substances. Among the most common causes of contact dermatitis are rubber products, clothing dyes, nickel (in jewelry, bra strap hooks, jeans fasteners), and plant oils. Scented or strongly alkaline soaps, skin lotions, cosmetics, and wool clothing also are irritating to many children.

Diaper dermatitis (diaper rash) is a contact dermatitis from irritants such as moisture, friction, and chemical substances. Urine ammonia, formed from the breakdown of urea by fecal bacteria, is extremely irritating to sensitive infant skin. Ammonia alone does not cause skin breakdown. Only skin damaged by infrequent diaper changes and constant urine and feces contact is prone to damage from ammonia in urine. Inadequate fluid intake, heat, and detergents in diapers aggravate the condition.

## PATHOPHYSIOLOGY

### *Contact Dermatitis*

Contact dermatitis is an inflammatory reaction of the skin either caused by direct exposure to an irritant *(irritant contact dermatitis)* or a delayed hypersensitivity response to an allergen *(allergic contact dermatitis).*

Irritant contact dermatitis can occur in any person who has repeated or prolonged contact with a primary irritant. Examples of primary irritants include citrus juices, detergents, bubble bath formulations, and urine. Diaper dermatitis is an example of irritant dermatitis that results from prolonged exposure to urine. Teething infants can have dermatitis on the face and neck folds from drooling.

Allergic contact dermatitis, a delayed hypersensitivity reaction, occurs in susceptible individuals who are sensitized to a substance by a previous exposure to the contact allergen. *Rhus dermatitis* (caused by poison ivy, oak, and sumac), the most common type of allergic contact dermatitis in children, is caused by oleoresins contained in all parts of the plant. Lesions appear several hours to several days after contact.

### Incidence

Irritant contact dermatitis is more common in children than is allergic contact dermatitis. Although most infants develop some form of contact dermatitis, it occurs less often in infants who are breastfed (reasons unknown). Many children have at least one episode of diaper dermatitis, usually occurring between ages 3 and 18 months, although it is most common between ages 8 and 10 months (American Academy of Pediatrics [AAP] Patient Education Online, 2015).

### Manifestations

Manifestations of irritant contact dermatitis include dry, inflamed, and pruritic skin. The distribution of lesions correlates with the skin surface in contact with the offending agent (e.g., watchband, clothing). Diaper dermatitis begins with erythema in the perianal region and can progress to macules and papules, which form erosions and crusts (Fig. 49.3). Manifestations of allergic contact dermatitis include blistering; weeping lesions over an area of inflamed skin; intense pruritus; and crusted, scaly lesions that heal in 10 to 14 days without treatment. Rhus dermatitis (e.g., poison ivy, oak, sumac) can cause severe systemic reactions.

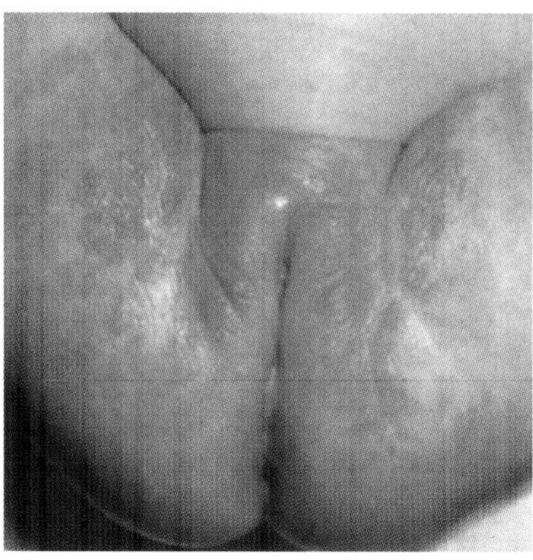

**FIG 49.3** Contact diaper dermatitis. (From Moschella, S.L., & Hurley, H.J. [1992]. *Dermatology* [3rd ed., pp. 239]. Philadelphia: Saunders.)

### Diagnostic Evaluation

The characteristic appearance of the lesions and a history of exposure to an irritating substance establish the diagnosis. Skin testing might be performed in children with persistent or recurrent dermatitis.

### Therapeutic Management

Discontinuing exposure to the offending agent treats contact dermatitis. The skin should be washed thoroughly if any irritant remains on the skin. Cool compresses of tap water or Burow's solution or steroid cream (e.g., triamcinolone 0.1% or fluocinolone 0.025%) may be applied several times a day after application of compresses. Severe contact dermatitis might require treatment with oral steroids, which should be tapered gradually. Desensitization therapy is usually not effective in managing contact dermatitis.

## NURSING CARE

### The Child With Contact Dermatitis

#### Assessment

Investigate new or continuing exposure to any potentially irritating substances. Assessment of skin lesions includes noting their distribution and configuration and looking for evidence of pruritus.

For a child with diaper dermatitis, carefully inspect the diaper area, noting the type and extent of lesions. It is important to assess the infant's hygiene and the parents' knowledge of care related to the infant's skin integrity. Question parents about the type of diapers used, laundering practices, and frequency and method of cleaning the diaper area. Any recent changes in the infant's care, such as new foods, soaps, detergents, or lotions, should be investigated.

#### Nursing Diagnosis and Planning

The nursing diagnoses and expected outcomes that may be appropriate for the child with contact dermatitis and the child's family are as follows:

- Acute Pain related to skin inflammation.

  **Expected outcome.** The child will have reduced skin irritation, as evidenced by decreased excoriation and increased healing. The child will exhibit decreased irritability, absence of scratching, and uninterrupted periods of sleep.

- Risk for Infection related to scratching of pruritic lesions.

  **Expected outcome.** The child will have no signs of secondary bacterial infection, as evidenced by clear, intact skin.

- Deficient Knowledge of management and prevention of future skin inflammation related to incomplete understanding of therapeutic principles.

  **Expected outcome.** The child and family will identify and avoid irritating substances and will carry out prescribed treatments correctly.

#### Interventions

Nursing care of the child with contact dermatitis is directed toward relieving itching, preventing infection, and identifying and removing offending substances. Cool compresses and tepid oatmeal (Aveeno) baths provide some relief from itching. Prescribed topical steroid creams should be applied in a thin layer. Antihistamines, such as diphenhydramine (Benadryl) or hydroxyzine (Atarax), also help the child rest. Because overheating increases itching, advise the parents to occupy the child with quiet activities and to keep the room temperature at a comfortable level.

Reassure the parents and child that the lesions are not contagious and cannot be spread to others or to other parts of the body by scratching. However, if oils from rhus plants remain on the skin, nails or on clothing, they may contact other parts of the child's body and cause new lesions at the point of contact. Keep the skin clean and help the child avoid scratching to prevent secondary infection. Instruct the parents to contact the health provider if the child has a fever or if the lesions produce purulent drainage.

Contact dermatitis is prevented by avoiding offending substances. Children should be taught to recognize plants of the rhus group. If the child is exposed to these plants, rinse the skin with cool water immediately (within 15 minutes) and wash clothing in hot, soapy water. Oleoresins in the plants can be spread not only by direct contact with the plant but also in the smoke of burning leaves or by touching pets that have contacted the plants.

Avoiding known irritants, such as cosmetics, jewelry, and canvas athletic shoes, can prevent other types of contact dermatitis. Nickel-sensitive children can usually tolerate 14-karat gold or sterling silver jewelry. Pierced earrings should have hypoallergenic or surgical stainless steel posts.

Diaper dermatitis is much easier to prevent than to treat. Successful treatment and prevention of diaper rash, regardless of the cause, depend on cleaning the diaper area thoroughly and keeping the skin dry. Prompt, gentle cleaning with water and mild soap (Dove, Neutrogena Baby Soap) after each voiding or defecation rids the skin of ammonia and other irritants and decreases the chance of skin breakdown and infection. Careful attention should be given to skin folds and creases. The parent should pat the skin dry with a soft cloth towel after washing. Air drying the skin and frequently exposing the skin to air and light promote healing of diaper rash. During bouts of diaper rash, the diaper may be left off during nap times.

A bland, protective ointment (A & D, Balmex, Desitin, zinc oxide) can be applied to clean, dry, intact skin to help prevent diaper rash. Ointments should not be applied to inflamed areas because they retain moisture. Occlusion increases the risk of systemic absorption of steroid; thus, steroid creams are rarely used for diaper dermatitis because the diaper functions as an occlusive dressing. Frequent diaper changes decrease irritation from urine and feces. Encourage the parent to check the newborn infant's diaper every hour and the older infant's diaper every 2 hours. Using disposable diapers does not eliminate the need for frequent diaper changes. Although the "wicking" action of disposable diapers pulls moisture away from the skin toward the liner, ammonia and other byproducts are left behind on the infant's skin, causing irritation. Rubber or plastic pants increase skin breakdown by holding in moisture and should be used infrequently.

If cloth diapers are laundered at home, the parent should wash them in hot water, using a mild soap and double rinsing. Soaking diapers before washing in a quaternary ammonium compound (Diaparene) decreases the ammonia in them.

Advise the parent to contact the health provider if the rash becomes solid and bright red, if it becomes raw or bleeds, if blisters or boils develop, if the rash does not improve in 3 days with treatment, or if the infant has a fever.

### Evaluation

- Is the child's skin intact, with healed lesions and no evidence of pain or pruritus?
- Is the child's skin free from signs of secondary infection?
- Does the parent demonstrate understanding of proper skin and diaper area care?

## Atopic Dermatitis

Atopic dermatitis, or eczema, is a common chronic inflammatory disease of the skin characterized by severe pruritus. Atopic dermatitis can have distressing psychosocial effects on the child and family.

### Etiology

The cause of atopic dermatitis (eczema) is unknown, but the disease is thought to be genetically determined and related to a malfunction in the body's immune system. Contributing factors include an inherited tendency for dry, sensitive skin; allergy; and emotional stress. Most children with atopic dermatitis have a family history of asthma, hay fever, or atopic dermatitis. Children with atopic dermatitis may present with asthma or allergic rhinitis. Although the role of allergy in the etiology of atopic dermatitis is controversial, immunoglobulin E (IgE)–mediated food allergy has been shown to be an exacerbating factor in some children (Leung & Sicherer, 2016).

### Incidence

The prevalence of atopic diseases, including asthma, allergic rhinitis, and atopic dermatitis, has increased substantially in the past 30 years. Atopic dermatitis usually begins in infancy and is most common between 3 and 6 months of age. Of the children affected, approximately 60% develop eruptions in the first 12 months, and 90% do so by the age of 5 years. Atopic dermatitis can persist through adolescence and adulthood. Atopic dermatitis affects all races. Symptoms tend to be worse during winter months (Eichenfield et al., 2014).

### Manifestations

During infancy, erythematous areas of oozing and crusting appear first on the cheeks and then on the forehead, scalp, and extensor surfaces of the arms and legs (Fig. 49.4). Papulovesicular rash and scaly, red plaques become excoriated and lichenified. The affected scalp area resembles seborrheic dermatitis, but unlike seborrheic dermatitis, atopic dermatitis is intensely pruritic. Infants begin manifesting symptoms at approximately age 1 to 4 months.

#### PATHOPHYSIOLOGY

#### *Atopic Dermatitis*

Atopic dermatitis is an allergic skin condition. In children who are genetically susceptible, there is excessive production of T-cells, which are attracted to the skin. The T-cells release cytokines and other chemicals that facilitate increases in mast cells and eosinophils. As the mast cells increase, they release substances that trigger an inflammatory response in the skin. This inflammatory response causes erythema, edema, and intense pruritus. Scratching increases itching, leading to an itch-scratch-itch cycle. Continual scratching and rubbing excoriate and damage the skin. Oozing, weeping, crusting, and cracking lesions develop. The skin of children with atopic dermatitis carries a higher-than-normal colonization of *Staphylococcus aureus*, and secondary infection is common. Impetigo and viral infections (herpes, molluscum contagiosum) occur frequently in these children.

Children who have atopic dermatitis after infancy have a rash pattern that differs from the rash seen during infancy. The flexor surfaces of the wrists, ankles, knees, and elbows are affected, as are the neck creases, the eyelids, and the dorsal surfaces of the hands and feet. There may be acute weeping areas, with or without secondary infection. Chronic lichenification results from persistent scratching.

Children and adolescents with atopic dermatitis readily experience intense itching, especially in response to sweating or contact with irritating fabrics, such as wool. Emotional upset increases sweating and precipitates itching and scratching. Dry skin is a hallmark of this condition.

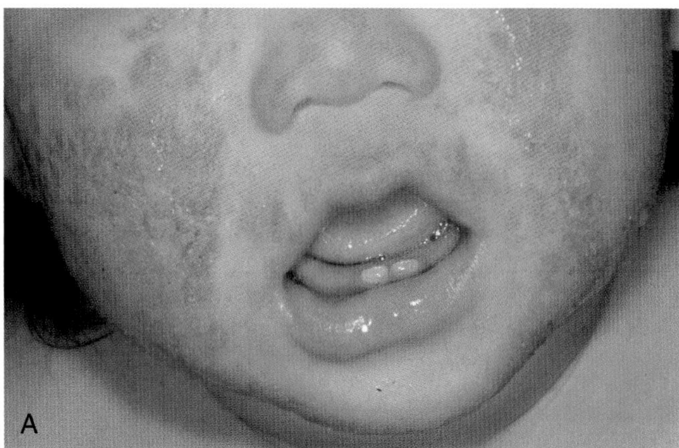


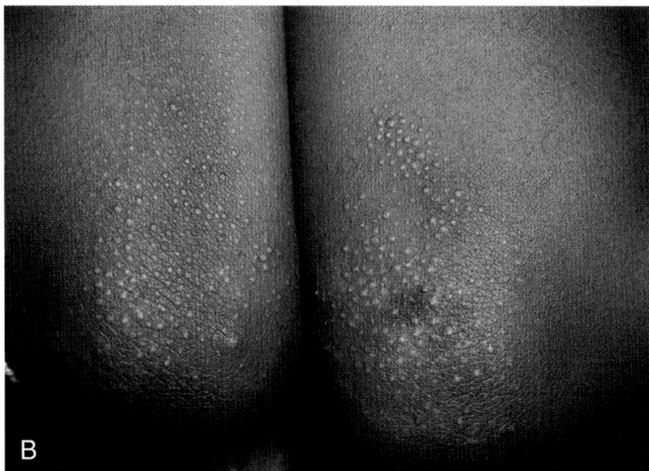


**FIG 49.4** Atopic dermatitis, an allergic skin condition, usually begins in infancy and clears by age 2 to 3 years. However, it can continue into childhood. **A,** Lesions on cheeks often spread to the forehead, scalp, and extensor surfaces of arms and legs. **B,** Flexor surfaces of wrists, ankles, knees, and elbows can be affected in the childhood form of the disease. (From Paller, S.A. [2012]. *Hurwitz clinical pediatric dermatology: a textbook of skin disorders of childhood and adolescence* [4th ed.]. Philadelphia: Saunders.)

### Diagnostic Evaluation

The diagnosis is based on the clinical features of intense pruritus, the appearance of the lesions, the pattern of remissions and exacerbations, and a family history of allergy. IgE levels and eosinophils are often elevated. Skin testing for food allergies—usually milk, eggs, wheat, soy, peanuts, and fish—can help identify potential food triggers.

### Therapeutic Management

The main goals of treatment are to control itching and scratching, moisturize the skin, prevent secondary infection, and remove irritants and allergens. Control of pruritus includes avoiding environmental triggers, such as overheating, soaps, wool clothing, and other skin irritants. Oral antihistamines, such as hydroxyzine (Atarax), diphenhydramine (Benadryl), and loratadine (Claritin), can be used to help break the "itch-scratch-itch" cycle. Nonsedating antihistamines, such as loratadine, may be preferred for school-age children. Itching is typically more severe at night; thus, antihistamines should be given before bedtime. Secondary infection is treated with antibiotic therapy.

Proper skin hydration is essential. Either a "dry" or "wet" approach can be used. The dry approach depends on avoiding bathing and the liberal use of emollients on dry skin. The wet approach is currently more popular. It permits bathing for limited periods of time, and the use of wet compresses and occlusive creams and ointments are the mainstays of treatment. In humid climates, bathing should be infrequent, and only lukewarm water and mild, nonperfumed soap (e.g., Purpose, white Dove, Basis) should be used. Emollients such as Eucerin cream or petroleum jelly applied to damp skin immediately after bathing help the skin retain moisture. Applying the moisturizer while the skin is still damp hydrates the skin. The child who lives in a dry climate should bathe frequently (several times a day) using a hydrophilic agent such as Cetaphil instead of soap and should moisturize with a moisturizing ointment or cream immediately after bathing. The child should avoid lotions that contain alcohol because these can contribute to skin dryness. Regardless of the approach used, moisturizing the skin is maintenance therapy for atopic dermatitis and should become a daily routine for the child.

Antiinflammatory corticosteroid creams and ointments are prescribed for inflamed or lichenified areas. These creams are more effective when applied to damp skin. The lowest potency that controls signs should be used, and topical steroids are usually reserved for treatment of episodic flares.

Topical calcineurin inhibitors (TCIs), such as tacrolimus and pimecrolimus, have antiinflammatory action and can be used in place of topical corticosteroids in children older than 2 years of age who do not respond well to other treatment approaches (Leung & Sicherer, 2016). Patients should avoid exposure to sunlight, tanning beds, sun lamps, and any other sources of ultraviolet light while taking these medications. They can be applied to 100% of the body surface if needed and can be used intermittently for longer periods of time than topical steroids. Topical immunomodulators do not cause skin atrophy. Although they can penetrate the skin enough to suppress local inflammation, they are only minimally absorbed into the circulation. An FDA black box warning cautions against using the medications off label in children younger than 2 years, because there are no long-term data on its safety in this age group (American Academy of Dermatology, 2015).

Identifying and eliminating allergens can be helpful. Allergy-proofing the home might be recommended (see Chapter 42). Because allergy to certain foods is an exacerbating factor in some children, such foods should be eliminated from the diets of sensitive infants. Breastfeeding for the first year is recommended for infants at risk for allergy. Solid foods should not be introduced until the infant is at least 6 months old.

## NURSING CARE

### The Child With Atopic Dermatitis

#### Assessment

Obtain a thorough history that includes information about allergies in the family. Question parents about any environmental or dietary factors that seem to worsen the child's condition. Determine what treatments have been tried and their effectiveness. Examine skin lesions for type, distribution, and evidence of any secondary infection. Assess the child's comfort level and the family's feelings and coping methods.

#### Nursing Diagnosis and Planning

The nursing diagnoses and expected outcomes that may be appropriate for the child with atopic dermatitis and the child's family are as follows:

- Impaired Skin Integrity related to environmental and immunologic factors.

  ***Expected outcome.*** The child's skin will exhibit decreased evidence of dryness, irritation, and excoriation.
- Acute Pain related to dry skin, secondary infection, and external irritations.

## DRUG GUIDE

### Topical Corticosteroids

**Classification:** Topical antiinflammatory.

**Action:** Reduce inflammation by causing vasoconstriction and inhibiting the movement of inflammatory cells from the bloodstream into local tissue.

**Indications:** Inflammatory skin diseases, such as atopic dermatitis.

**Dosage and Route:** Topical route; number of applications depends on the child's condition and the potency of the medication. Topical steroids are commonly divided into seven classes, with those of lowest potency assigned to the lowest (seventh) class.

***Class I:*** Optimized betamethasone dipropionate 0.05% (Diprolene cream or ointment)

***Class II:*** Triamcinolone acetonide ointment 0.5% (Kenalog); mometasone furoate ointment 0.1% (Elocon)

***Class III:*** Triamcinolone acetonide ointment 0.1% (Aristocort A); triamcinolone acetonide cream (Aristocort-HP); fluticasone propionate ointment 0.005% (Cutivate)

***Class IV:*** Hydrocortisone valerate ointment 0.2% (Westcort); mometasone furoate cream 0.1% (Elocon); desoximetasone cream 0.05% (Topicort-LP)

***Class V:*** Fluticasone propionate cream 0.05% (Cutivate); hydrocortisone valerate cream 0.2% (Westcort); triamcinolone acetonide cream 0.025% (Aristocort)

***Class VI:*** Desonide cream 0.05% (DesOwen); alclometasone dipropionate cream 0.05% (Aclovate)

***Class VII:*** Hydrocortisone cream 0.5%, 1% (Cortizone, Hytone, generic)

**Absorption:** Better absorbed through the skin immediately after bathing.

**Contraindications:** Never apply to diaper rashes or chickenpox lesions. Superpotent topical steroids (class I) are rarely used for children. Only low-potency agents should be used on the face.

**Precautions:** Unless directed by the physician, do not bandage, wrap, or otherwise cover areas being treated with topical steroids. In general, the more potent the medication, the shorter the treatment time will be.

**Adverse Reactions:** Systemic side effects can occur with short-term use of high-potency topical steroids or with long-term use of lower-potency topicals. Systemic effects include suppression of the hypothalamic-pituitary-adrenal axis, resulting in growth suppression; suppression of immune response; osteoporosis; moon face; and obesity. Locally, thinning of the skin, striae, telangiectasia, atrophy, and purpura can occur.

**Nursing Considerations:** Advise the parent to apply to the child's skin within 5 minutes of bathing, to meticulously follow the physician's directions for use, and to immediately report any side effects.

*Expected outcome.* The child will have minimal pain and pruritus, as evidenced by decreased irritability, absence of scratching, and uninterrupted periods of sleep.

- Risk for Infection related to skin excoriation.

*Expected outcome.* The child will have no signs of secondary bacterial infection, as evidenced by a normal body temperature and absence of purulent drainage.

- Deficient Knowledge about controlling itching, preventing secondary infection, and identifying aggravating factors related to anxiety or incomplete understanding of information.

*Expected outcome.* The child and family will identify and eliminate allergens and aggravating factors. The family will carry out prescribed treatments correctly. Family members will express any anxiety related to the child's condition.

- Interrupted Family Processes related to the child's pruritus and involved treatment.

*Expected outcome.* The child and family will discuss their feelings and concerns.

- Disturbed Body Image related to perception of appearance.

*Expected outcome.* The child will engage in activities with other children. The child will verbalize positive ideas about self.

#### Interventions

Care of the child with atopic dermatitis is demanding, and the entire family routine may revolve around the affected child. Parents need support and reassurance as they care for an uncomfortable, often irritable child.

Keeping the child's skin hydrated will help relieve itching. Instruct parents to apply a moisturizing cream, such as Eucerin, several times a day and immediately after the child is bathed. Reassure parents that moisturizing creams contain no harmful drugs and should be applied whenever the child's skin looks dry. Soaks and cool, wet compresses are soothing and can be applied to remove crusts, reduce inflammation, and dry weeping areas. Provide parents with explicit instructions on the use of soaks and topical medications. Strips of old cotton sheets moistened in lukewarm or cool tap water work well for wet dressings. Wet compresses should not be used for more than 3 days.

Rough clothing can aggravate eczema, particularly wool or other fabrics that cause sweating. Soft cotton or cotton-polyester blends are tolerated best. Undergarments with irritating seams can be turned inside out so that the soft seam is against the skin. Heat and sweating increase pruritus, so instruct parents to be careful not to "bundle up" the child in heavy blankets or clothing. Because detergents and fabric softeners can also aggravate atopic dermatitis, clothes should be washed in mild detergent and rinsed twice.

Advise the parents to keep the child's fingernails clean and short. Cotton gloves or mittens might be needed to prevent excoriation from scratching but should be used with caution, preferably only at night, because overuse could interfere with fine motor development. Lightweight, long-sleeved tops and one-piece outfits discourage scratching.

The child's skin must be kept clean to minimize secondary infection. Avoid using soap. Bath oil or emulsifying ointment can be used as a soap substitute but must be used with caution because these cause both the child and the tub to become slippery. Tepid bath water helps prevent the child from becoming overheated and itchy. Instruct parents to contact the physician at the earliest signs of skin infection (weeping skin, pustules) and to administer topical and oral antibiotics as prescribed.

Children with atopic dermatitis who swim should apply moisturizer before swimming and immediately on exiting the pool. Prolonged immersion in water (more than 20 minutes) can have a drying effect. A humidifier in the child's room during winter months can decrease skin dryness. The child should avoid the drying effects of sun exposure.

Children and families of children with atopic dermatitis exhibit frustration when the condition does not resolve quickly. The parent or child might be concerned about the child's appearance, as well as the child's discomfort.

Help parents take control of the child's condition by empowering them with knowledge about therapeutic management. Allowing parents to verbalize frustrations and helping them learn management techniques that do not disrupt family routine are important interventions.

Although studies do not consistently support emotional upset as a direct cause of atopic dermatitis flares, it is helpful to teach an older child stress reduction techniques to help cope with the frustration and discomfort of the condition. A resource for families of a child with atopic dermatitis is the National Eczema Association for Science and Education.

### Evaluation

- Is the child's skin intact and smooth?
- Have itching and pain been reduced?
- Is the child's skin free from redness or purulence that would indicate secondary infection?
- Do parents carry out prescribed treatments correctly?
- Are parents able to demonstrate appropriate coping techniques?
- Can the child demonstrate stress relief measures to decrease itching?

## SKIN INFECTIONS

Skin infections are common in childhood. Bacteria are normally present on healthy skin. The skin's susceptibility to bacterial infection depends on several factors, including the intactness of the skin, the virulence of the organisms, and the child's immune status. Children are susceptible to fungal and viral infections as well. Unlike bacterial infections, which generally respond fairly quickly to treatment, fungal and viral infections can be persistent and challenging to treat.

Although bacterial skin infections are caused by a variety of microbes, *Staphylococcus* is a major pathogen, accounting for most of the skin infections of childhood. The skin infections predominantly caused by *Staphylococcus aureus* range from minor, superficial lesions to severe generalized lesions with systemic effects. These skin infections include folliculitis, furuncles (boils), cellulitis, bullous impetigo, nonbullous impetigo, and staphylococcal scalded skin syndrome. Impetigo, a superficial, usually minor staphylococcal infection, is the most common bacterial skin infection of childhood. Folliculitis is inflammation of hair follicles. Furuncles, or boils, develop when the infection of an existing folliculitis progresses deeper. Cellulitis is an infection of the subcutaneous tissues.

### Impetigo

Impetigo often occurs as a secondary infection from another skin lesion, such as an insect bite. Close contact contributes to the spread of impetigo, which is highly contagious. Children in daycare facilities, schools, or camps and adolescent athletes are at increased risk. The incubation period for impetigo is 7 to 10 days, and it can spread to other parts of the child's skin or to others who touch the child, use the same towel, or drink from the same glass. Spread of the infection is fostered by poor hygiene, crowded living conditions, and a hot, humid environment. Lesions resolve in 12 to 14 days with treatment.

#### Etiology

Impetigo can be caused by *S. aureus,* group A beta-hemolytic streptococci, or a combination of these bacteria. *S. aureus* is the primary pathogen in most cases. Nonbullous impetigo, sometimes referred to as crusted impetigo, was formerly thought to be a result of streptococcal infection. More than 90% of impetigo cases are caused by *S. aureus,* which is the primary cause of both bullous and nonbullous impetigo (AAP, 2015b). Bullous impetigo is at the minor end of a spectrum of blistering disorders caused by the exfoliative toxins produced by some strains of *Staphylococcus.* Staphylococcal scalded skin syndrome is at the more severe end of that spectrum.

**PATHOPHYSIOLOGY**

***Impetigo***

Impetigo begins in an area of broken skin, such as an insect bite, scabies, or atopic dermatitis. The break in the skin allows for organism entry. The inflammatory process results in the formation of a pustular lesion. Honey-colored fluid from this lesion becomes crusted. In some children, nasal discharge containing the organism erodes healthy skin above the upper lip, allowing for organism entry.

#### Incidence

Impetigo occurs most often during hot, humid summer months. Toddlers and preschoolers are most commonly affected, often when recovering from an upper respiratory tract infection.

#### Manifestations

The primary lesions of impetigo occur in two forms. Bullous impetigo characteristically manifests as small vesicles that can progress to bullae. The lesions are initially filled with serous fluid and later become pustular. The bullae rapidly rupture, leaving a shiny, lacquered-appearing lesion surrounded by a scaly rim. Crusted impetigo appears initially as a vesicle or pustule that ruptures to become erosion with an overlay of honey-colored crust. The erosions bleed easily when crusts are removed (Fig. 49.5). Lesions are mildly pruritic. Scarring is uncommon but can occur if the child picks or scratches the lesions. Postinflammatory hyperpigmentation is a frequent sequela in dark-skinned children. The lesions are often located around the mouth and nose but can appear on any part of the body.

#### Diagnostic Evaluation

The characteristic appearance of the lesions usually confirms the diagnosis. Failure to respond to treatment suggests community-acquired methicillin-resistant *S. aureus* (CA-MRSA) (see Chapter 41), an increasing problem in children (Velez, VanGraafeiland, & Sloand,

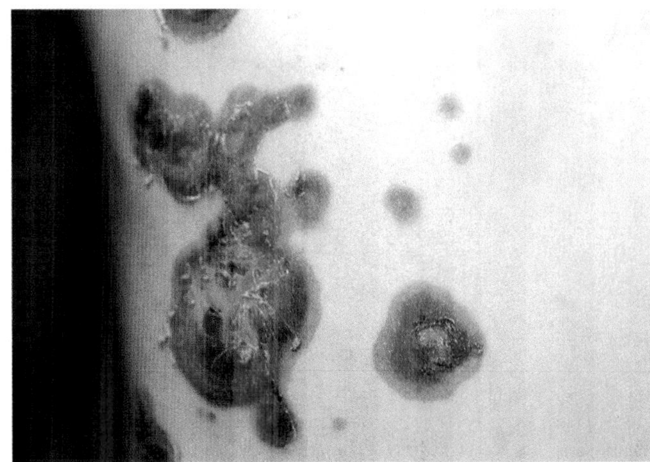

**FIG 49.5** Impetigo lesions are usually located around the mouth and nose but may be located on the extremities. (From Paller, S.A. [2012]. *Hurwitz clinical pediatric dermatology: a textbook of skin disorders of childhood and adolescence* [4th ed.]. Philadelphia: Saunders.)

2015). If a culture is ordered, the specimen should be obtained from beneath the crust or from the fluid inside the lesions.

### Therapeutic Management

Impetigo is treated with topical and oral antibiotics. The lesions should be gently washed three times a day with a warm, soapy washcloth and the crusts soaked and carefully removed. A topical ointment, such as mupirocin (Bactroban) or bacitracin (Baciguent), is then applied to the lesions. Topical therapy lasts 7 to 10 days. Severe cases of impetigo or cases of impetigo around the mouth are treated with oral antibiotics that are effective against both staphylococcal and streptococcal organisms. Impetigo that is extensive is treated with intravenous (IV) antibiotics. Antibiotic treatment of streptococcal impetigo does not prevent glomerulonephritis, but it does hasten healing of the lesions.

Good handwashing and careful hygiene are imperative to prevent spread of the infection and should be emphasized to the child and parents. The child should not attend school or daycare for 24 hours after beginning treatment (AAP, 2015c). The school should be notified of the diagnosis.

## NURSING CARE

### The Child With Impetigo

#### Assessment

Assess the child's skin for the size, distribution, and spread of impetigo lesions. If the child is taking systemic antibiotics, monitor for signs of adverse effects, such as rashes or diarrhea. Observe for periorbital edema or blood in the urine, which suggests the development of acute glomerulonephritis if the impetigo is caused by group A, beta-hemolytic streptococci.

#### Nursing Diagnosis and Planning

The nursing diagnoses and expected outcomes that may be appropriate for the child with impetigo and the child's family are as follows:

- Impaired Skin Integrity related to destruction of skin layers secondary to bacterial infection.

*Expected outcome.* The child will maintain skin integrity, as evidenced by confinement of the infection to the primary site. The area will heal without scarring or further infection.

- Deficient Knowledge related to unfamiliarity with measures to prevent spread of infection, care of impetigo lesions, and antibiotic administration.

*Expected outcome.* The child and family will adhere to measures to prevent the spread of infection. The parent will demonstrate care of the lesions and administration of medications.

#### Interventions

Teach parents to soak the crusts and then wash them off with a warm, soapy washcloth three times a day. Advise them to gently remove the crusts after soaking, taking care not to spread the infection to other parts of the body with the contaminated washcloth. Antibiotic ointment should then be applied to the lesions and the affected areas left open to air. A small amount of bleeding after crust removal is common.

The child should sleep alone and should be bathed daily, alone, with antibacterial soap. The caregiver should wear gloves when caring for the child. Emphasize the importance of administering the full course of topical or systemic antibiotics as prescribed.

#### Evaluation

- Are the lesions healing, and have they remained confined to the primary site?
- Do the child and family members practice handwashing and other techniques to prevent the spread of infection?

> **SAFETY ALERT**
>
> ***Caring for a Child With Impetigo***
>
> - The child can spread impetigo lesions merely by touching another part of the skin after scratching the infected area.
> - Keep the child's fingernails short and wash the child's hands frequently with antibacterial soap.
> - Emphasize good handwashing and careful hygiene for the child's entire household.
> - Discourage family members from sharing towels, combs, or eating utensils with the infected child.

- Do the parents appropriately explain the necessity for administering the full course of treatment?

## Cellulitis

Cellulitis is bacterial infection of the subcutaneous tissue and the dermis. It is usually associated with a break in the skin, although cellulitis of the head and neck can follow an upper respiratory tract infection, sinusitis, otitis media, or tooth abscess. Cellulitis occurs most commonly in the lower extremities and in the buccal (inside the cheek) and periorbital (around the eye) regions. Complications of cellulitis include septic arthritis, meningitis, and brain abscess. Periorbital cellulitis can lead to blindness.

### Etiology and Incidence

Since the introduction of the *Haemophilus influenzae* type B vaccine, group A streptococci and *S. aureus* have become the most common causes of cellulitis. Cellulitis is most frequent in children age 2 years and younger.

### Pathophysiology

Bacteria overwhelm the defensive cells that normally contain inflammation to local areas. The result is more extensive invasion of the causative organism as the infection moves from superficial tissue to deeper subcutaneous tissue.

### Manifestations

The affected area is red, hot, tender, and indurated. If *H. influenzae* is the suspected organism, the affected area might have a purplish tinge. Edema and purple discoloration of the eyelids and decreased eye movement are present in periorbital cellulitis. Lymphangitis may be seen, with red "streaking" of the surrounding area and enlarged regional lymph nodes (lymphadenitis). The child usually exhibits fever, malaise, and headache.

### Diagnostic Evaluation

Usually a complete blood cell count, blood cultures, and culture of the affected area are done. If no drainage is present, the affected area can be aspirated. Orbital cellulitis can be diagnosed by computed tomography of the orbit.

### Therapeutic Management

After an initial intramuscular or IV dose of an antibiotic, such as ceftriaxone, the child with cellulitis of an extremity is usually treated at home with a 10-day course of oral antibiotics (cephalosporin, cloxacillin, or dicloxacillin) and warm compresses. If the cellulitis involves a joint or the face, or if the child shows other signs of acute febrile illness, hospitalization and IV antibiotics are required. Incision and drainage of the affected area may be necessary. Community acquired MRSA (CA-MRSA) is an increasing problem in children and adolescents, particularly athletes. Several published reports have documented

CA-MRSA cases among military and sports communities (Velez et al., 2015). Lesions, especially abscesses, should be cultured for the presence of methicillin-resistant staphylococcal organisms because treatment of CA-MRSA is tailored to sensitivity results. Effective antibiotics for CA-MRSA infection in children include sulfamethoxazole-trimethoprim, clindamycin, vancomycin, and linezolid (see Chapter 41).

## NURSING CARE

### The Child With Cellulitis

#### Assessment

Record the history and question the parent regarding recent ear infections, dental caries, or trauma to the skin surrounding the affected area. Other pertinent data include when the inflammation started and how rapidly it has progressed. Examine the skin, noting any temperature increase, swelling, redness, and drainage. Assess for fever, pain, guarding, and irritability.

#### Nursing Diagnosis and Planning

The nursing diagnoses and expected outcomes that may be appropriate for the child with cellulitis and the child's family are as follows:

- Impaired Skin Integrity related to bacterial invasion
  ***Expected outcome.*** The child will exhibit signs of healing, such as decreases in redness, swelling, and fever.
- Acute Pain related to soft tissue swelling and inflammation.
  ***Expected outcome.*** The child will be able to sleep and will demonstrate decreased irritability.
- Deficient Knowledge related to unfamiliarity with the illness and treatment.
  ***Expected outcome.*** The family will describe measures to prevent the spread of infection, will describe how to administer antibiotics as prescribed, and will demonstrate the ability to carry out treatment measures.

#### Interventions

The child should rest in bed with the affected extremity elevated and immobilized. Warm, moist soaks applied every 4 hours increase circulation to the infected area, relieve pain, and promote healing. Acetaminophen can be given to control fever and pain. Frequent hand hygiene is essential to prevent the spread of infection. If the child is hospitalized, IV antibiotics should be administered accurately and on time to maintain a therapeutic blood level. If the child is being treated at home, the parents must understand the importance of administering the entire course of antibiotics as ordered. The child should be carefully monitored for signs of sepsis (increased fever, chills, confusion) and spread of infection.

#### Evaluation

- Does the child's skin exhibit signs of healing?
- Is the child free from signs of infection and pain?
- Does the parent administer prescribed medications and carry out appropriate home care?

## Candidiasis

Thrush (oral candidiasis) (Fig. 49.6) is a superficial fungal infection of the oral mucous membranes that is common in infants. Thrush occurs as a result of overgrowth of *C. albicans.* In addition to oral lesions, the child may exhibit lesions in the diaper area, which are caused by *C. albicans* passing through the intestine. Moisture and heat in the diaper area create an environment favorable to the development of *Candida* dermatitis. Persistent candidiasis suggests that the child might be immunocompromised.

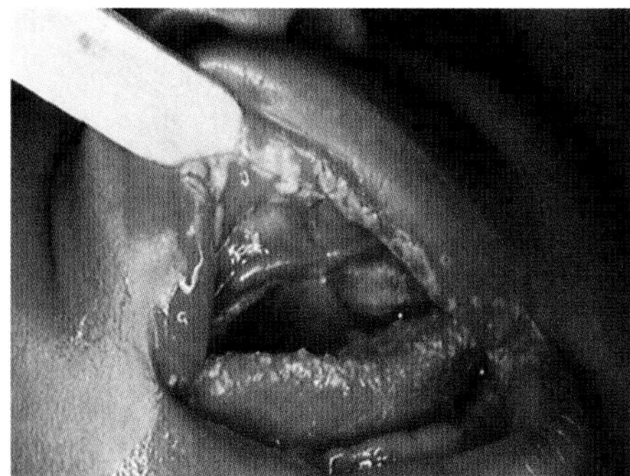

**FIG 49.6** White, curd-like plaques of thrush (oral candidiasis, oral moniliasis), a common fungal infection in infants. (From Paller, S.A. [2012]. *Hurwitz clinical pediatric dermatology: a textbook of skin disorders of childhood and adolescence* [4th ed.]. Philadelphia: Saunders.)

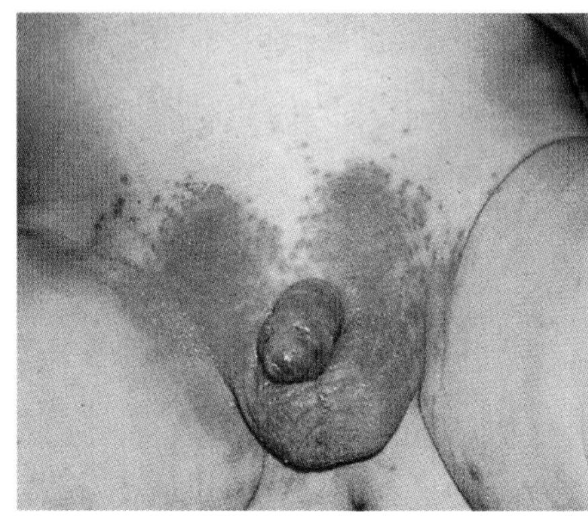

**FIG 49.7** Diaper candidiasis. (From Feigin, R.D., & Cherry, J.D. [2009]. [Eds.]. *Feigin and Cherry's textbook of pediatric infectious diseases* [6th ed., pp. 774]. Philadelphia: Saunders.)

### Etiology

A neonate can acquire candidiasis during delivery while passing through an infected vagina. An older infant can have a fungal overgrowth as a result of immunosuppression, during antibiotic therapy, from exposure to the mother's infected breasts, or from unclean bottles and pacifiers.

### Incidence

Candidiasis occurs most often in infants. Predisposing factors in all age-groups include antibiotic therapy, diabetes, and altered immune status.

### Manifestations

White, curd-like plaques are noted on the tongue, gums, and buccal mucosa in children with thrush. They can be distinguished from milk curds by the difficulty encountered in removing them and the bleeding of an erythematous base when plaques are removed. A child with severe infection may have difficulty eating. The lesions of *Candida* diaper dermatitis are usually bright red and coalesced, with some satellite lesions spreading out to the child's abdomen and thighs (Fig. 49.7).

### Diagnostic Evaluation

The diagnosis of thrush and candidal diaper dermatitis is made from the clinical appearance of the lesions.

### Therapeutic Management

Nystatin oral suspension (100,000 units/mL), swabbed onto the mucous membranes of the mouth, is effective in treating thrush. Because *Candida* is present in the gastrointestinal tract, oral nystatin is often prescribed to decrease the likelihood of recurrence. Oral fluconazole is an alternative therapy. Candidal diaper dermatitis is treated with a topical antifungal agent such as nystatin or clotrimazole (Lotrimin).

## NURSING CARE

### The Child With Candidiasis

#### Assessment

Nursing assessment includes obtaining a history of maternal and infant *Candida* infections. Question the mother regarding vaginal itching or discharge or any nipple tenderness or redness. Also discuss methods used to clean bottles and pacifiers. Examine the infant's mouth and diaper area and assess nutrition and hydration status.

#### Nursing Diagnosis and Planning

The nursing diagnoses and expected outcomes that may be appropriate for the child with candidiasis and the child's family are as follows:

- Impaired Skin Integrity related to the effects of fungal infection.

  ***Expected outcome.*** The infant will exhibit signs of healing lesions, as evidenced by pink, intact mucous membranes or resolution of diaper rash.
- Acute Pain related to oral lesions or skin irritation.

  ***Expected outcome.*** The infant will have reduced discomfort, as evidenced by ability to take feedings without difficulty, decreased fussiness, and improved ability to sleep.
- Deficient Knowledge related to incomplete understanding of the cause of the infection and administration of medication.

  ***Expected outcome.*** The family will demonstrate methods to prevent spread of infection and will administer the entire course of medication as prescribed.
- Imbalanced Nutrition: Less Than Body Requirements related to mouth irritation and altered taste.

  ***Expected outcome.*** The infant will accept feedings and will consume appropriate amounts of nutrients.

#### Interventions

Teach the parent to swab 1 mL of oral nystatin suspension onto the infant's gums, tongue, and buccal mucosa every 6 hours until 3 to 4 days after symptoms have disappeared. Because cotton-tipped applicators tend to absorb the medication, a more effective method of administration is to rub the suspension onto the mucous membranes with a gloved finger. To increase the amount of time the medication is in contact with the mucous membranes, nystatin should be applied after feedings. Alternatively, oral fluconazole administered once a day may be used for treatment of thrush in infants.

Pacifiers, nipples, and bottles should be thoroughly cleaned to decrease the chance of reinfection. Teach the parents the technique and importance of good hand hygiene. If the infant is breastfed, the mother's breasts should also be treated with nystatin.

Suggest small, frequent feedings for the infant or child with thrush who is uncomfortable. Cool liquids are soothing to the older child.

For the infant with candidal diaper dermatitis, suggest that the parent apply nystatin or clotrimazole cream. Leaving the diaper area exposed to air reduces the moisture that facilitates fungal growth.

Advise the parent to contact the healthcare provider if the infant refuses to eat or fever develops or if the candidiasis does not clear with treatment.

#### Evaluation

- Have the lesions disappeared, leaving intact skin and oral mucous membranes?
- Does the child appear to be comfortable, sleeping well, and less irritable?
- Can the parents demonstrate proper medication administration?
- Is the child increasing the amount of oral intake?

## Tinea Infection

Tinea is a superficial skin infection caused by a group of fungi known as dermatophytes. Tinea infections are designated by the word *tinea* followed by the Latin word for the affected part of the body. Fig. 49.8 illustrates various types of tinea infections.

### Etiology

Two types of dermatophytes, *Trichophyton* spp. and *Microsporum* spp., cause the majority of tinea infections. *Trichophyton* affects all keratinized tissue, including skin, nails, and hair. *Microsporum* invades the hair.

## PATHOPHYSIOLOGY

### *Tinea Infection*

Tinea infection occurs when the fungus causing tinea invades the hair, the stratum corneum of the skin, or the nails.

In *tinea capitis,* the fungus invades the hair shafts, causing the hairs to become brittle and to break off at the level of the scalp, leaving an area of stubby, black-dotted alopecia. An immune reaction to the fungus may develop in the form of a *kerion,* a boggy, red, tender scalp mass that may contain *Staphylococcus aureus* and is often accompanied by fever and lymphadenopathy. Children with allergies seem to be more susceptible to tinea capitis.

*Tinea corporis* (ringworm) is a fungal infection of the face, trunk, or extremities. It can be transmitted by humans or by dogs and cats. Most lesions of tinea corporis clear without treatment in several months, but some may become chronic.

*Tinea cruris* (jock itch) is characterized by an intense inflammatory reaction with severe pruritus.

*Tinea pedis* (athlete's foot) can become chronic, particularly in adolescents who wear unventilated athletic shoes. Tinea lesions can become secondarily infected with bacteria or *Candida.*

Tinea infections are transmitted from person to person, by animal contact, or by contact with contaminated fomites (e.g., combs, hats, headrests, pillows). Tinea cruris (fungal infection affecting the groin and scrotal area) is not highly contagious. Poor hygiene, friction from tight clothing, and obesity are predisposing factors. Tinea pedis (athlete's foot) is a fungal infection of toes and feet. It is contagious but rarely develops on healthy, dry skin.

### Incidence

Tinea capitis usually occurs in children ages 1 to 10 years, whereas tinea pedis and tinea cruris are most common in adolescent boys. Because a moist environment supports the growth of fungal infections, most tinea infections appear when the weather is hot and humid.

### Manifestations

Common manifestations of tinea capitis include erythema and scaling of the scalp and one or more round patches of alopecia that slowly increase in size. Small papules at the base of hair follicles become crusting pustules and red scales. In some cases, thick, broken hairs close to the scalp surface result in patches of black-dotted alopecia. Enlarged lymph nodes may surround a kerion.

Tinea corporis, commonly seen on the trunk, face, and extremities, is characterized by ring-like plaques with clear centers and scaly,

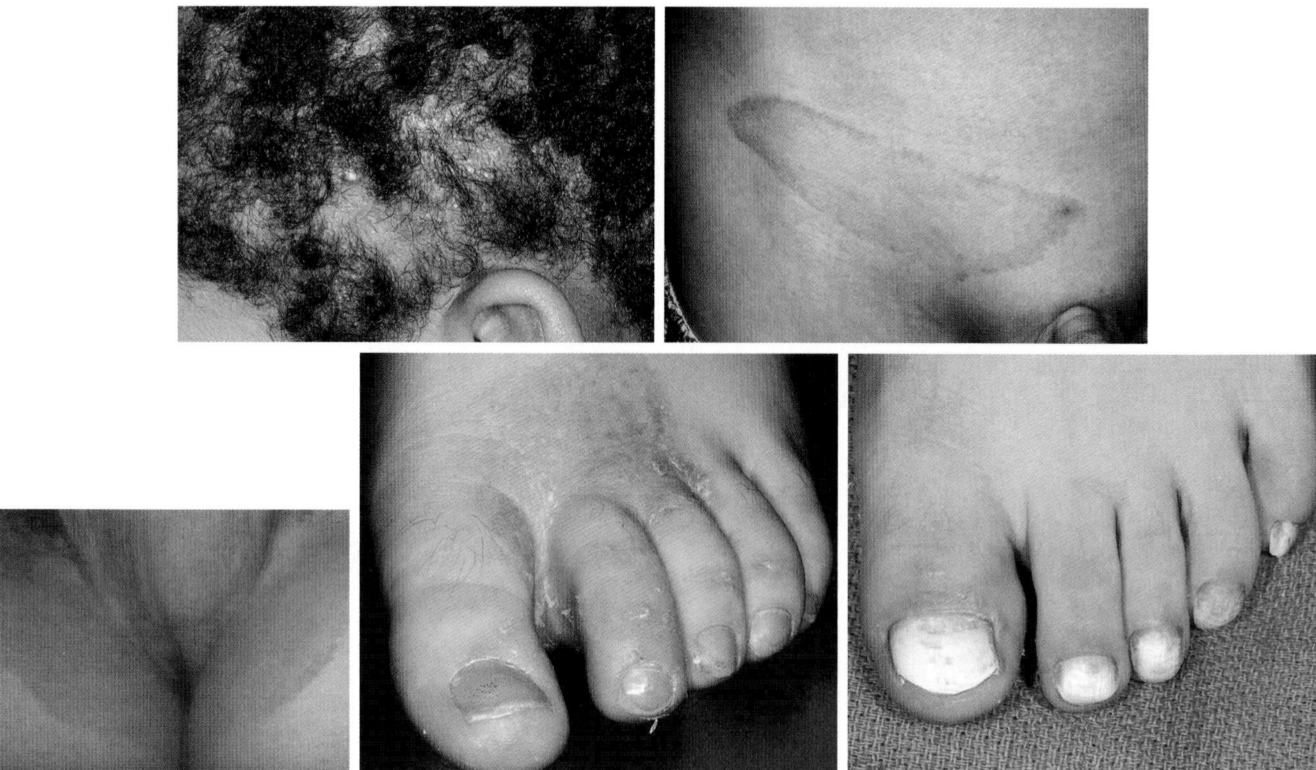

**FIG 49.8** Tinea (ringworm) is an infection caused by dermatophytes, a group of fungi. Tinea is classified according to the part of the body affected. Five common types of tinea are shown here: Tinea capitis (scalp); Tinea corporis (trunk, face, extremities); Tinea cruris (groin, buttocks, scrotum); Tinea pedis (feet); Tinea unguium (nails, nail beds). (Tinea cruris from Hurwitz, S. [1993]. *Clinical pediatric dermatology: a textbook of skin disorders of childhood and adolescence* [2nd ed., pp. 380]. Philadelphia: Saunders; remaining figures from Paller, S.A. [2012]. *Hurwitz clinical pediatric dermatology: a textbook of skin disorders of childhood and adolescence* [4th ed.]. Philadelphia: Saunders.)

red margins. Lesions are usually ½ to 1 inch in diameter and mildly pruritic.

Manifestations of tinea cruris include pink papules and scales on the inner thighs, groin, scrotum, and buttocks (but not the penis). Pruritus is also present.

Tinea pedis, commonly referred to as "athlete's foot," produces fine vesiculopustular or scaly lesions on the soles of the feet, between the toes, and under the nails. The webs between the fourth and fifth toes are most commonly involved. Peeling, fissures, and maceration appear in severe cases, and pruritus and burning are typically present.

### Diagnostic Evaluation

Most tinea infections can be diagnosed from the clinical appearance of the lesions. Fungal cultures or microscopic examination of skin scrapings prepared with potassium hydroxide confirms the diagnosis. *Microsporum* lesions fluoresce as a bright blue-green under a Wood light. However, the most common organism causing tinea today, *Trichophyton tonsurans*, does not fluoresce.

### Therapeutic Management

***Tinea capitis.*** For treatment to be effective, medication must penetrate the hair follicles. Topical therapy alone is not effective for tinea capitis. Oral griseofulvin administered daily for at least 6 weeks is the treatment of choice; it is the only drug approved by the FDA for treating tinea capitis. Because griseofulvin is insoluble in water, its absorption is increased if taken with a high-fat meal or with milk. Other antifungals, such as ketoconazole (Nizoral), terbinafine (Lamisil), or fluconazole (Diflucan), can be prescribed for older children who cannot tolerate griseofulvin or who fail to respond to it (AAP, 2015d). Ketoconazole and other azole antifungals are used with caution in children because of the risk of hepatotoxicity during long-term therapy. Selenium sulfide shampoo should be used twice per week for 2 weeks to eliminate spores and to decrease transmission.

***Tinea corporis.*** Local treatment is usually effective for tinea corporis. Antifungal preparations, such as clotrimazole (Lotrimin) or miconazole (Monistat), can be used twice a day for approximately 4 weeks (AAP, 2015d). Application of cream should extend 1 inch beyond the lesion borders to prevent spread. Infected pets should be treated as well, and the child should avoid close contact with infected pets.

***Tinea cruris.*** Management for tinea cruris is similar to that for tinea corporis. Topical antifungal preparations should be applied twice a day to the lesions and at least 1 inch beyond the borders. Care should be taken to apply the medication to all creases, and the adolescent should be advised to wear loose clothing.

***Tinea pedis.*** A prescribed topical antifungal agent, such as clotrimazole (Lotrimin), miconazole (Monistat), or oxiconazole (Oxistat), is applied twice a day until the lesions have been cleared for 1 week. If the lesions do not respond to topical therapy, oral griseofulvin may be given for 1 month or longer, to promote healing. Newer systemic antifungals, such as itraconazole (Sporanox), have demonstrated improved success over a shorter time than griseofulvin. If the affected area is inflamed and oozing, soaking the feet in Burow's solution can promote healing.

## NURSING CARE

### The Child With a Tinea Infection

#### Assessment

Obtain a history that includes a description of the skin lesions and possible contacts. Animals with which the child has played should be carefully inspected for ringworm. The child's siblings and playmates should also be examined.

#### Nursing Diagnosis and Planning

The nursing diagnoses and expected outcomes that may be appropriate for the child with a tinea infection and the child's family are as follows:

- Impaired Skin Integrity related to inflammation and excoriation.
  *Expected outcome.* The child will exhibit intact skin over impaired areas. The skin lesions will exhibit progressive healing.
- Impaired Comfort related to pruritic lesions.
  *Expected outcome.* The child will remain calm and will exhibit no evidence of discomfort or pruritus; scratching will decrease.
- Deficient Knowledge of the cause, treatment, and spread of the infection related to lack of information.
  *Expected outcome.* The child and family will verbalize accurate information about the child's skin condition. The child and family will demonstrate behaviors that prevent spread of the fungus. Treatments will be performed correctly.
- Disturbed Body Image related to alopecia or unattractive lesions.
  *Expected outcome.* The child will return to or continue with social involvement.

#### Interventions

Adequate teaching is essential for successful treatment of tinea infection (see Patient-Centered Teaching: Home Care for a Child or Adolescent with a Tinea Infection). In addition to teaching therapeutic management techniques specific for the child's particular type of tinea, emphasize to the parent that any prescribed oral medication regimen must be followed meticulously. Tinea infections are sometimes difficult to eradicate; discontinuing medication too soon risks recurrence. Treatment commonly continues for as long as 6 to 8 weeks and continues for months for difficult infections of fingernails or toenails. It is important to advise the parent and the older child that the child taking griseofulvin must avoid sun exposure because this drug makes the skin more susceptible to a photosensitivity reaction. If the child is taking itraconazole or longer courses of griseofulvin, the parent must ensure that the child undergoes any recommended liver function studies.

Fungus thrives in a warm, moist environment, so it is important to keep infected areas as dry as possible. Teaching proper hygiene is essential for preventing and treating fungal infections. Teach children to avoid sharing personal items, such as combs, hats, and hair ornaments. Children with tinea infections should sleep alone and should not share towels and washcloths with others. Feet should be washed daily and kept dry. Advise children to allow their nonventilated athletic shoes to dry thoroughly between wearings. Heavy cotton socks absorb sweat and keep the feet dry. If tinea pedis is present, the child should change socks at least twice a day and go barefoot or wear sandals as much as possible. Talcum powder or antifungal powder applied twice a day might help keep feet dry. If the child showers at school or at a gym, shower shoes should be worn.

Tinea cruris heals much faster if the groin area is kept dry. Loose-fitting cotton underwear should be worn, and athletic supporters and underwear should be washed frequently. The rash should be washed each day with plain water and carefully dried. Soap should be avoided. Scratching delays healing, so instruct the child to avoid scratching the area. Reassure the young man and his parents that tinea cruris is not related to sexually transmitted diseases.

Instruct parents to call the physician if the infection has not improved in 4 weeks or if it continues to spread after 1 week of treatment. Reassure parents that fungal infection is not an indication of poor hygiene or neglect. Avoid expressions of distaste or surprise when caring for children with severe alopecia or inflammation. Encourage parents to return the school-age child to school as soon as possible. Children with severe inflammatory tinea capitis may wish to wear a cap or scarf for a time until healing has progressed.

#### Evaluation

- Does the child have clean, intact skin?
- Is the child comfortable and without pruritus?
- Do the child and parents perform treatments correctly and verbalize ways to prevent the spread of infection?
- Does the child participate in usual social activities?

## PATIENT-CENTERED TEACHING

### *Home Care for a Child or Adolescent With a Tinea Infection*

When providing information to the parent or older child with tinea, emphasize the following:

- Keep the infected areas as dry as possible.
- Do not share personal items, such as towels, washcloths, combs, hats, or hair ornaments.
- Athlete's foot: Wash the feet daily, and keep them dry. Nonventilated athletic shoes should dry thoroughly between wearing. Wear heavy cotton socks and change socks at least twice a day. Talcum powder or antifungal powder applied twice a day might help keep feet dry.
- Jock itch: Keep the groin area dry. Wear loose-fitting cotton underwear. Wash athletic supporters and underwear frequently. Wash the rash each day with plain water and dry carefully. Do not use soap on the affected area. Avoid scratching.
- Take oral medication as directed, even if the condition has improved. Discontinuing medication too soon can allow the infection to reappear.
- Call your physician if the infection has not improved in 4 weeks or if it continues to spread after 1 week of treatment.

### Herpes Simplex Virus Infection

Herpes simplex virus types 1 and 2 (HSV 1, HSV 2) are responsible for a common, contagious, and often recurrent infection of the skin and mucous membranes. This infection can be asymptomatic or symptomatic and extremely painful. A wide spectrum of disease is caused by HSV: the common fever blister or cold sore (herpes labialis); corneal lesions; genital lesions (rare in children); and central nervous system infection.

#### Etiology

HSV is transmitted by infected body fluids and secretions coming in contact with breaks in the skin or mucous membranes. Delivery through an infected birth canal can cause infection in neonates. HSV can be transmitted by nurses who fail to practice careful hand hygiene.

Children with burns, eczema, or diaper rash or those who are immunosuppressed are particularly susceptible to HSV infection.

### Incidence

HSV is widespread. Infections in children are usually caused by HSV 1. Herpes labialis, commonly referred to as a "fever blister," is one of the most common manifestations of HSV 1. The primary infection with HSV 1 usually occurs before 20 years of age. HSV 1 is a highly infectious virus that is transmitted by oral to oral contact (Looker et al., 2015). Infection with HSV 2, which affects primarily the anal-genital area, is rare before age 14 years. Child sexual abuse should be considered in any child with a genital herpes infection.

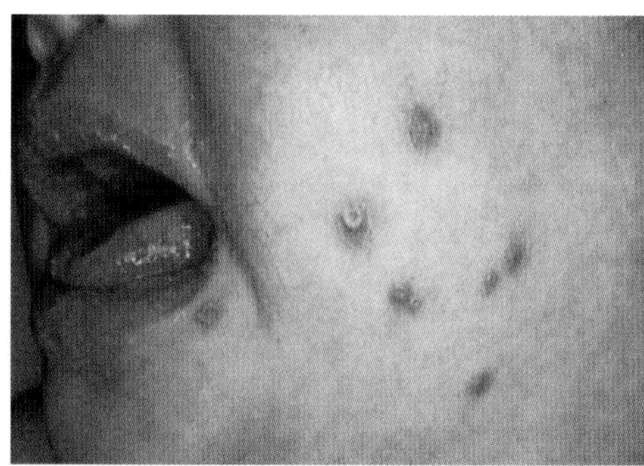

**FIG 49.9** Herpes simplex infection in an infant. (From Feigin, R.D., & Cherry, J.D. [2009]. [Eds.]. *Feigin and Cherry's textbook of pediatric infectious diseases* [6th ed., pp. 760]. Philadelphia: Saunders.)

## PATHOPHYSIOLOGY

### *Herpes Simplex Type 1 Infection*

The human herpes viruses include herpes simplex virus (HSV) types 1 and 2; cytomegalovirus; Epstein-Barr virus, which causes infectious mononucleosis; and varicella-zoster virus. HSV 1 causes the "oral" type of herpes and usually affects areas above the waist, producing cold sores, fever blisters, and corneal lesions. HSV 2 affects areas below the waist (anal-genital area). However, either type can affect any region of the body. After an initial HSV 1 infection, the virus remains dormant but alive within nerve cells that innervate the portion of the skin originally infected. Fever, stress, trauma, sun exposure, menstruation, or immunosuppression can reactivate the virus. When reactivated, the virus migrates to the skin area innervated by the ganglia that harbor it, near the site of the initial infection. The recurrent infection can be symptomatic or asymptomatic, but it is just as contagious as the initial infection. Recurrent infections tend to be less severe than the initial infection.

The immune status of the host determines the severity of HSV infection. HSV 1 infection in the neonate or immunocompromised child can be fatal. HSV 1 is a common cause of viral encephalitis in children.

*Herpetic whitlow,* a painful HSV 1 infection of the fingers, can be transmitted to a nurse during oral or tracheal care of a child with herpes infection. Thumb-sucking children with oral HSV 1 infection can also develop this condition. Healthcare personnel with herpetic whitlow should not have patient contact until the infection has healed because the infection is highly contagious.

### Manifestations

**Herpes labialis ("cold sore," "fever blister").** Prodromal symptoms of herpes labialis are burning, itching, or tingling; these symptoms occur up to several days before lesions appear. Symptoms appear 2 days to 2 weeks after exposure. Lesions appear in clusters of fluid-filled vesicles that ulcerate, dry, and crust within 7 to 14 days (Fig. 49.9). Usually one or two lesions are present on the lips, tongue, gingiva, or buccal mucosa. Pruritus and pain are present. Approximately 85% of active HSV 1 infections are asymptomatic.

**Herpetic gingivostomatitis.** Herpes gingivostomatitis is a severe oral infection that affects children younger than 5 years of age. Vesicles and ulcerations; an edematous throat; and enlarged, painful cervical lymph nodes are seen. Associated signs and symptoms include chills, fever, malaise, bad breath, and drooling.

**Herpetic ocular infection.** Herpetic ocular infection (keratitis) is typically the result of rubbing the eyes with contaminated fingers. Herpetic keratitis causes irritation and inflammation of the conjunctiva or cornea with associated tearing and photophobia. Vesicles appear on the eyelid and mucous membranes of the eye. Children with HSV keratitis are at risk for recurrent episodes and vision loss (Farooq & Shukla, 2012).

**Herpetic whitlow.** Symptoms of herpetic whitlow appear 3 to 7 days after exposure and include vesicles, swelling, pruritus, and severe pain of the affected fingers. Discomfort may continue for weeks after the vesicles have healed.

### Diagnostic Evaluation

Clinical manifestations and the child's history suggest the diagnosis. A Tzanck smear can confirm a herpes infection, but a positive smear cannot differentiate between varicella-zoster virus and HSV 1, and a negative smear does not rule out HSV infection. Immunofluorescence assay to detect HSV 1 antigen and polymerase chain reaction to detect HSV 1 deoxyribonucleic acid can be performed on blood samples, but tissue culture is still considered the primary standard for diagnosis. Brain imaging can be used to assist in the diagnosis of HSV encephalitis, and magnetic resonance imaging (MRI) is the preferred imaging study (Sanders & Garcia, 2014).

### Therapeutic Management

Treatment is symptomatic. The child with oral HSV 1 infection is usually cared for at home if able to take adequate fluids. If the child becomes dehydrated, IV fluids are needed.

Topical or oral acyclovir (Zovirax), if given early enough in the course of the infection, can reduce the time to recovery. Although there is no cure for HSV 1 infection, IV acyclovir (Zovirax) is used in immunocompromised children, neonates, and children with encephalitis to decrease the severity of the infection (Stanberry, 2016). Treatment of ocular HSV 1 infection is determined in consultation with an ophthalmology specialist.

Antibiotic ointment may be used to treat secondary bacterial infection of lesions. Corticosteroids are contraindicated because they can worsen HSV 1 infection. Oral or rectal acetaminophen, with or without codeine, is often prescribed, and topical anesthetics can be dabbed onto lesions to help relieve pain. A prescribed anesthetic mouth rinse of equal parts of diphenhydramine (Benadryl) elixir, bismuth subsalicylate (Kaopectate), and 2% viscous lidocaine can decrease pain and help the child eat. Topical anesthetics, such as viscous lidocaine, must be used with caution. Overuse of topical anesthetics in small children can depress the gag reflex and increase the risk of aspiration.

## NURSING CARE

### The Child With a Herpes Simplex Infection

#### Assessment

Obtain a history, and ask the parent or child about previous HSV infections or contact with an infected person. Examine the skin carefully for lesions. Inspect the eyes for corneal ulcerations and edema and assess the child's vision for pain, blurring, and photophobia. Referral to an ophthalmologist is necessary for suspected ocular HSV infection. For the child with herpes gingivostomatitis, pay particular attention to assessing hydration status.

#### Nursing Diagnoses and Planning

The nursing diagnoses and expected outcomes that may be appropriate for the child with a herpes simplex infection and the child's family are as follows:

- Impaired Skin Integrity related to inadequate secondary defenses.

**Expected outcome.** The child will demonstrate healing of lesions. The child will have no other signs of infection.

- Acute Pain related to inflammation and infection.

**Expected outcome.** The child will have minimal pain, as evidenced by adequate fluid intake, decreased verbalization of pain, and decreased restlessness and irritability.

- Risk for Infection related to changes in skin integrity.

**Expected outcome.** The child will have no signs of secondary bacterial infection, as evidenced by healing lesions and normal body temperature.

- Risk for Deficient Fluid Volume related to painful oral lesions.

**Expected outcome.** The child will maintain urine output appropriate for age and will exhibit moist mucous membranes and good skin turgor.

#### Interventions

Children with oral HSV infection can be extremely uncomfortable. Swallowing can cause severe pain, and dehydration is a real danger. Advise parents to contact the physician if the child has signs of dehydration. Fluid intake is very important, and the child must be encouraged to drink. Most children will accept ice pops, noncitrus juices, milk, and noncarbonated or "flattened" soft drinks. Frequent small feedings of bland, soft foods can be offered. Reassure parents that a few days without solid food will not harm the child as long as fluid intake is adequate.

To prevent secondary infection, the child's mouth should be rinsed often with normal saline solution, especially after eating. Hospitalized children infected with HSV should be placed on Contact Precautions. The child is considered contagious until the scabs from visible lesions have fallen off. Because scabs do not form on mucous membranes, these lesions are considered contagious until they are completely healed. All persons who have contact with the child should follow Contact Precautions meticulously and be particularly careful when touching the child near the lesions, when administering oral care or suctioning, and when handling bed linens or objects that might be contaminated with saliva or secretions from the lesions. Careful hand hygiene is essential.

Parents should take similar precautions when caring for the child at home to prevent spread of infection. Advise the parents to wash bottles, nipples, toys, eating utensils, and towels in hot, soapy water or in a dishwasher, if available. Family members should not share any of these items with the infected child.

Because the infection can be spread to other parts of the body, the child should not put his or her fingers near the mouth or infected area. Elbow restraints may be necessary for children too young to understand this. The child with HSV 1 infection is usually miserable and needs generous cuddling and comforting.

#### Evaluation

- Are lesions healed, with no sign of the infection spreading?
- Does the child demonstrate increased comfort?
- Does the skin remain free of signs of secondary infection (redness, swelling, drainage)?
- Is the child properly hydrated, with adequate fluid intake and hourly urine output? (See Chapter 40.)
- Can the parent or caregiver describe infection control measures?

## SKIN INFESTATIONS

Children can become infested with a variety of parasitic insects that feed on human blood and cause intense itching with subsequent alterations in skin integrity. Such parasites include lice and the mites that cause scabies. Infestations are extremely contagious and require a holistic management approach.

### Lice Infestation

Lice are small, blood-sucking insects approximately 2 to 4 mm in length. *Pediculosis* refers to infestation of lice on the scalp or body. Although pediculosis is not a serious health problem, it can cause embarrassment and often elicits an emotional reaction among parents and school personnel who mistakenly associate it with poor hygiene. Head lice are not responsible for the spread of any disease, although body lice are known to serve as vectors of several pathogenic bacteria (Centers for Disease Control and Prevention [CDC], 2013).

#### Etiology

Lice live only on humans and are transmitted by direct contact with infected persons and contact with infested objects (e.g., brushes, hats). Lice cannot jump like fleas, and clean hair is no deterrent to head lice.

#### Incidence

The precise prevalence of head lice is difficult to determine because it is not a reportable condition. However, it is estimated that millions of children worldwide are infested each year (CDC, 2013). Girls are affected twice as often as boys. All socioeconomic groups are affected. The peak incidence is in preschool and young school-age children. Pubic lice are usually seen in adolescents or young adults and are generally transmitted by sexual contact.

#### Manifestations

***Pediculosis capitis (head lice).*** Nits are visible and are attached firmly to the hair shafts near the scalp. They are tiny, silvery or grayish-white specks resembling dandruff, but they are more difficult to remove. They are commonly found behind the ears and at the nape of the neck. In active infestation, nits are found approximately ¼ to ½ inch away from the scalp surface (Fig. 49.10); nits found greater than ¼ inch from the scalp are considered to be nonviable (CDC, 2013). Adult lice are difficult to see because of their small size and the fact that they crawl very fast to avoid light. Scattered lesions on the scalp, behind the ears, or on the back of the neck cause intense pruritus. These lesions are often associated with posterior cervical lymph adenopathy. Secondary scalp infection can develop from scratching.

***Pediculosis corporis (body lice).*** Papular, rose-colored dermatitis, causing intense pruritus, appears on the skin in areas under tight clothing. Nits attach firmly to seams of the child's clothing or bedding.

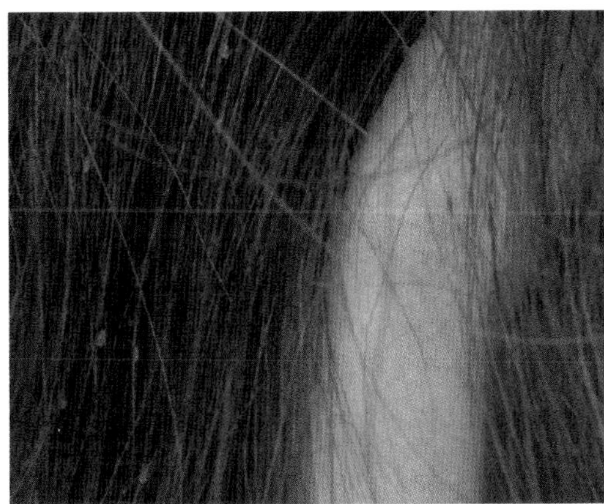

**FIG 49.10** Head lice (pediculosis capitis). Note the nits attached to the hair shafts. (From Callen, J., Greer, K.E., Hood, A.F., et al. [1993]. *Color atlas of dermatology* [pp. 373]. Philadelphia: Saunders.)

## PATHOPHYSIOLOGY

### Pediculosis

Pediculosis can involve the scalp (pediculosis capitis), the body (pediculosis corporis), or the pubic area and eyelashes (pediculosis pubis). A specific type of louse, each of which has a similar life cycle, causes each of these infestations. All lice pierce the skin and suck blood. Severe itching caused by bites can predispose the child to secondary infection.

Head and pubic lice spend their life cycles on the skin of the human host; body lice live in clothing, coming to the skin only to feed. The female head louse lays eggs (nits) at the base of the hair shaft. The egg is covered with a gelatinous material that hardens to semiopaque, tiny, pearly whitish masses; these egg cases stick tightly to the hair shaft (see Fig. 49.10). Eggs incubate for approximately 1 week, and lice reach sexual maturity in about 2 weeks.

Pediculosis pubis is spread through sexual contact. Half of all patients with pediculosis pubis have another sexually transmitted disease, usually gonorrhea.

Lice can spread as long as the lice and nits remain alive on the infested person or belongings. Lice can live only 48 hours off the human host. Nits shed into the environment are capable of hatching for 10 days.

*Pediculosis pubis (pubic lice, crab lice).* Pediculosis pubis is lice that can be found in pubic hair and facial hair, in axillae, and on the body surface. The presence of pubic lice in the eyebrows or eyelashes of a prepubescent child suggests sexual abuse. Pubic lice also cause intense pruritus. Maculae ceruleae (blue spots) may be seen on the thighs and trunk in cases of heavy infestation. Dark-brown spots on underwear and sheets are insect waste materials.

### Diagnostic Evaluation

The diagnosis of head lice is made by identification of nits or lice on the scalp. The examiner parts the hair with two tongue depressors and moves from side to side and front to back, paying particular attention to the crown, behind the ears, and the nape of the neck. The exposed scalp should be carefully examined under bright light or in a sunny area. A magnifying glass can assist in identification. Combing the hair with a fine-tooth nit comb can quickly aid in diagnosis (Devore, Schutze, & The Council on School Health and Committee on Infections Diseases, 2015). Unlike dandruff, nits are not easily removed from hair shafts. Pubic lice are diagnosed from a history of symptoms and visual inspection.

### Therapeutic Management

Management of the child with pediculosis focuses primarily on killing active lice and nits and preventing spread or recurrence by managing the environment.

*Killing active lice and nits.* Approaches to treating pediculosis are changing as a result of the development of pediculicide-resistant strains of lice and because prescription lindane (Kwell) persists as a poison in the environment and can be neurotoxic if absorbed through the skin. Lindane is an organochloride, and the AAP no longer recommends it as a pediculicide. Although the lindane shampoo 1% is approved by the FDA for the treatment of head lice, it is not currently recommended as a primary choice of treatment. Lindane can be toxic to the brain and other parts of the nervous system; its use should be restricted to patients who do not respond to other medications that pose less risk. Lindane should not be used in treatment of premature infants, persons infected with HIV, those with a seizure disorder, women who are pregnant/ breast–feeding, those who have very irritated skin or sores where the Lindale will be applied, or a person of any age who weighs less than 110 lb (CDC, 2015c).

An over-the-counter pediculicide, permethrin 1% (Nix, Elimite, Acticin), kills head lice and pubic lice and eggs with one application and has residual activity (i.e., it stays in the hair after treatment) for 10 days. Nix crème rinse is applied to the hair after washing with a conditioner-free shampoo. It is applied as a lotion to pubic hair. Crème rinse or lotion should be rinsed out after 10 minutes. The hair should not be shampooed for 24 hours after the treatment. Even though the kill rate is high and there is residual action, treat the hair again after 7 to 9 days (AAP, 2015a). Over-the-counter products containing pyrethrins (RID, Triple X, Tisit, R&C, Pronto) are safe and effective, but lice are becoming resistant to these products. Because they lack residual activity, treatment with these products must be repeated on days 7 to 9 after the initial treatment. Ovicides should not be used routinely in children younger than 2 years (AAP, 2015a); using a fine-tooth nit comb on wet, conditioned hair at least four times over a 2-week period is an evidence-based recommendation (Devore et al., 2015).

Pubic lice are treated similarly to head lice, with the exception of areas around the eyes, which can be treated with two to four applications a day of petroleum jelly (AAP, 2015a). Treatment and testing for other sexually transmitted diseases are required for sexual contacts of a person with pubic lice. For body lice, clothing and bedding should be washed in hot water and dried for 20 minutes at a hot dryer setting. Meticulous hygiene and regular laundering can eliminate body lice (AAP, 2015a).

The pesticide Malathion (Ovide) is approved for the treatment of lice in children older than 6 years, but it requires prolonged contact (8 to 10 hours) to be effective. It is also flammable, and families should be cautioned not to use hair dryers or allow the child near fires or heaters while hair is being treated. The AAP recommendations for the treatment of head lice are revised every 3 years, and the interested reader is referred to that source for current guidelines (http://www.aap.org).

*Addressing the environment.* Environmental objects, clothing, and bedding should be treated or washed. It is important to examine family members and others who might be in close contact with the infested child; only those with an observed infestation should be treated (Devore et al., 2015). The parent needs to notify the school if a child has an active case. Meticulous vacuuming of carpets in classrooms with affected children will help prevent transmission.

## NURSING CARE

### The Child With Pediculosis

#### Assessment

Examine children for lice in an unobtrusive and private manner. In a school setting, classmates should be brought to the school nurse's office and admitted one at a time, rather than being seen together in a general check in a classroom setting. Use disposable tongue depressors or ice-pop sticks to part the hair, and discard these implements between children. Check all family members for the presence of nits or lice.

Assess adolescents with pubic lice for signs of other sexually transmitted diseases and ask about sexual contacts, because they will need treatment as well.

#### Nursing Diagnosis and Planning

The nursing diagnoses and expected outcomes that may be appropriate for the child with pediculosis and the child's family are as follows:

- Acute Pain related to inflammatory response and pruritus.
  **Expected outcome.** The child will rest comfortably and will refrain from scratching.
- Risk for Infection related to scratching of scalp.
  **Expected outcome.** The child will have no signs of secondary bacterial infection, as evidenced by intact skin and normal-size cervical lymph nodes.
- Deficient Knowledge about the treatment of lice infestation and the prevention of recurrence related to anxiety or incomplete information.
  **Expected outcome.** The child or family will carry out the prescribed treatment. The parent will demonstrate measures taken to prevent reinfestation.
- Risk for Situational Low Self-Esteem related to social stigma associated with lice.
  **Expected outcome.** The child or family will verbalize self-acceptance and will engage in usual social activities.

#### Interventions

Advise parents to carefully follow directions that come with over-the-counter pediculicides or to follow the physician's instructions for using prescription products. Caution parents against applying the medication more frequently than recommended.

Reassure parents that lice infestation does not reflect poor hygiene or low socioeconomic status. Advise them that it is necessary to notify the school nurse if the child is infested.

If the parent believes it is necessary to remove nits, teach the parent to remove them by back-combing with a fine-tooth comb. One hour before combing, nits can be loosened with a mixture of half vinegar and half water or a commercial product, such as Clear or Step 2. It is easier to comb the child's hair for nit removal when the hair is damp rather than wet or dry. Lice and nits can be removed from eyelashes by applying petrolatum to the eyelashes twice a day for 8 days. Many schools have a "no nit" policy, which requires that a child be free of all nits before reentry, although such policies are strongly discouraged because of the missed school time and the low risk of transmitting the infestation to others (Devore et al., 2015).

Advise parents to wash clothing (especially hats and jackets), bedding, and linens in hot water, and dry them in a hot dryer setting. Dress-up clothes, hair ornaments, bicycle helmets, batting helmets, headphones, and similar objects should be also treated. Items that cannot be washed should be dry cleaned or sealed in plastic bags for 2 to 3 weeks.

Antilice sprays used for furniture and other environmental objects should never be used on a child. Thorough home cleaning is necessary to remove any remaining lice or nits. The parent should vacuum floors, play areas, and furniture to remove any hairs that might carry live nits. Combs and brushes should be boiled or soaked in antilice shampoo or hot water (greater than 60° C [140° F]) for at least 10 minutes. Routinely teach children not to share hats, combs, or hair ornaments with other children. At school, individually assigned lockers or separate hooks for coats can help inhibit the spread of lice.

The child should be rechecked for infestation in 7 to 9 days. Advise parents to call the physician if itching interferes with the child's sleep, if the condition does not clear up after 1 week, or if scalp lesions look infected. The National Pediculosis Association provides information about this condition. The CDC is a resource that provides reliable, up-to-date information on the recommendations for combating head lice at http://www.cdc.gov/lice/head/treatment.html#supplement.

#### Evaluation

- Is the child free of infestation, pain, and pruritus?
- Is the skin intact, and does the child exhibit normal-size cervical lymph nodes?
- Do parents carry out the prescribed treatments?
- Can parents describe measures to prevent the spread of lice to others?
- Do the parents and child realistically describe the cause of pediculosis and continue to engage in usual social activities?

### CRITICAL THINKING EXERCISE 49.1

The pediatric clinic receives a phone call from an obviously upset mother about her 4-year-old daughter, who is in preschool. This is the third time in 1 month that the parent has been called at work to take her child out of school because the child was found to have lice. The mother states that she has properly treated her daughter and other family members, and she insists that the child is catching the condition from someone at school. The school maintains that no other child has this problem.

1. What should be the nurse's approach to this mother?
2. What kind of information will the nurse need to obtain to help this mother with her problem?

## Mite Infestation (Scabies)

Scabies is a contagious condition that has been recognized for many centuries. It results from infestation with *Sarcoptes scabiei*, the "itch mite."

### Etiology

Scabies is transmitted by close personal contact with infected persons. Those who share a bed or live in crowded conditions are likely to transmit scabies to each other. The scabies mite cannot survive for more than 3 days away from human skin. For that reason, transmission of scabies by bedding or clothing is infrequent.

### Incidence

Scabies is widespread throughout the United States and prevalent in many schools. All socioeconomic groups are affected.

### Pathophysiology

The female mite burrows into the epidermis, lays her eggs, and dies in the burrow after 4 to 5 weeks. The eggs hatch in 3 to 5 days, and

## EVIDENCE-BASED PRACTICE

Pediculosis is a worldwide problem, and its treatment is challenging for families. The cost associated with treating a family for lice infestation can be high, sometimes more than $20.00 per treatment. In addition, resistance to pediculicides is increasing, potentially reducing the effectiveness of existing treatments. Treatment is effective only when 100% of adult lice are killed and eggs are prevented from hatching.

Nurses from the University of Texas Austin published a clinical practice guideline (Level V evidence) that addresses the diagnosis and treatment of pediculosis in children. Their recommendations for diagnosis and treatment of pediculosis are described. This guideline provides good evidence that persistent infestation usually results from incomplete following of directions for using pediculicides, pediculicide resistance, or reinfestation. They recommend strongly against "No nit" policies in schools, because evidence shows that, even though removal of nits after treatment may not be complete, living lice would be found only rarely. "No nit" policies in schools have contributed to interruptions in student education and achievement.

If you were doing a clinical placement in a school setting, where the school nurse was maintaining a "No nit" policy, what information might you want to give the nurse? How would you support your recommendation, and where might you refer the nurse for updated information? What kind of teaching might you do with families of children who have a problem with repeated infestations?

Reference: University of Texas School of Nursing Family Nurse Practitioner Program. (2013). *Guidelines for the diagnosis and treatment of pediculosis capitis (head lice) in children and adults – 2013.* Retrieved from http://www.guidelines.gov.

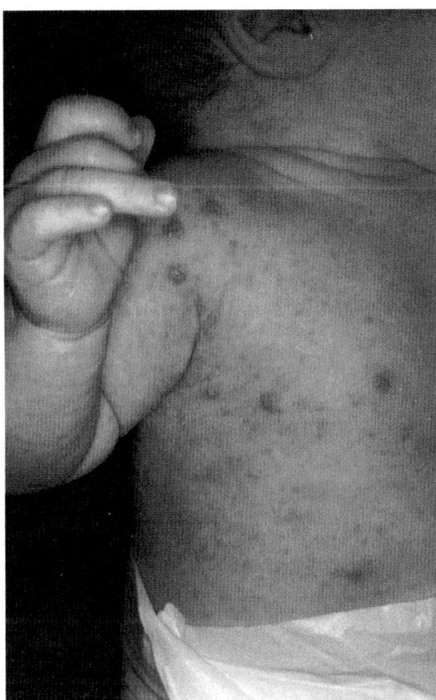

**FIG 49.11** Scabies lesions on an infant. (From Callen, J.P., Greer, K.E., Paller, A.S., et al. [2000]. *Color atlas of dermatology* [3rd ed., pp. 3283]. Philadelphia: Saunders.)

larvae migrate to the skin surface to mature and complete the life cycle. The mites, eggs, and their excrement cause intense pruritus. One of the major complications of scabies is impetigo resulting from scratching.

### Manifestations

Intense pruritus occurs, especially at night. Infants may be cranky, sleep fitfully, and rub their hands and feet together. Burrows (fine, grayish, thread-like lines) can be difficult to see because they are usually obscured by secondary changes of excoriation and inflammation. Papules, vesicles, and nodules are common (Fig. 49.11) and are located mainly on the wrists, in the finger webs, on the elbows, in the umbilicus, in the axillae, in the groin, and on the buttocks. In infants, the head, palms, and soles may be affected.

### Diagnostic Evaluation

The characteristic skin eruption and a history of intense pruritus, especially at night, are suggestive of scabies. The diagnosis is made by microscopic examination of scrapings of the lesions.

### Therapeutic Management

Scabies can be treated with topical application of permethrin 5% (Elimite); Ivermectin, Sulfur 5% to 10%, Crotamiton 10% lotion, and lindane cream 1% (Kwell) are used as alternatives if primary treatment with permethrin is not effective. Because of the risk of neurotoxicity, lindane should not be used in children younger than 2 years or in pregnant women and others weighing less than 110 lb (CDC, 2015b). The medication is applied to the body and head (depending on age), avoiding the eyes and mouth. The medication must remain on the child for 8 to 14 hours (depending on the medication prescribed) to be effective, so applying it at bedtime is recommended. It is washed off in the morning. Retreatment in 1 week is usually recommended. Pruritus lasts for several days to weeks after treatment and can be relieved with corticosteroid cream (e.g., hydrocortisone cream) and oral antihistamines.

Family members, even if asymptomatic, and daycare contacts (except for pregnant women) should also be treated. The child's bedding and clothing should be washed in hot water in a fashion similar to the environmental treatment for pediculosis.

### Nursing Considerations

Nursing care of the child and family with scabies is similar to that for pediculosis. Inspect the child's hands, elbows, umbilicus, groin, and buttocks for burrows. However, burrows are sometimes difficult to see, and persistent itching may be the only symptom. Evaluate an adolescent with scabies for sexually transmitted disease.

Instruct parents to use the scabicide according to the manufacturer's instructions. The lotion is applied all over the child's body, including the soles of the feet, the scalp, behind the ears, in intertriginous areas, and under the toenails and fingernails. The lotion should be kept on for the recommended time (4 to 8 hours for lindane; 8 to 14 hours for Elimite), followed by bathing. Infants should be clothed during treatment so they cannot lick their skin. To minimize absorption and the risk of toxic effects from lindane, the lotion should not be applied for at least 30 minutes after bathing and should be applied only to cool, dry skin. Advise the parent that persistent itching after treatment is expected for approximately 2 weeks and is not a sign of reinfestation or an indication for repeated application.

Scabies is usually cured with one treatment; however, a repeat application in 1 week is recommended. Clothing and bed linen should be dry cleaned or washed in hot water and dried at a hot dryer setting.

## ACNE VULGARIS

Acne is a disorder of the sebaceous hair follicles. Although acne is generally perceived as a minor disorder, it can cause significant anxiety

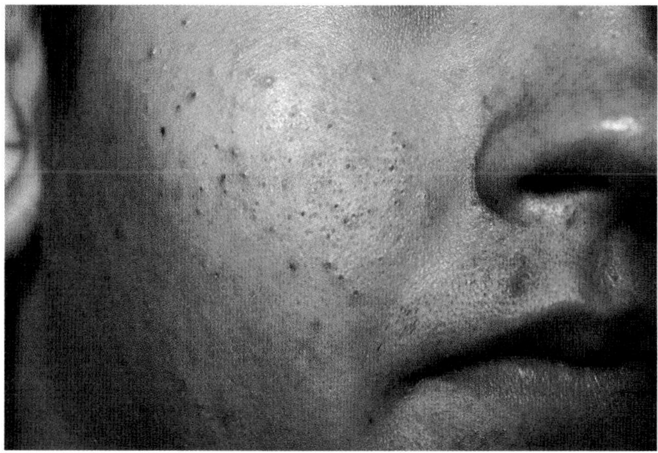

FIG 49.12 An adolescent with acne vulgaris. (From Paller, S.A. [2012]. *Hurwitz clinical pediatric dermatology: a textbook of skin disorders of childhood and adolescence* [4th ed.]. Philadelphia: Saunders.)

and emotional pain for affected adolescents. The disfiguring lesions of acne can lead to physical and emotional scarring.

## Etiology

Multiple factors play a role in the development of acne lesions, including abnormal sloughing of skin cells lining the sebaceous hair follicles, overgrowth of normal bacteria, and host factors, such as heredity, hormonal influences, and emotional stress. Neonatal acne is triggered by infection with fungi, such as *Pityrosporum* species. Foods do not appear to cause or increase the severity of acne. Acne is unrelated to the general cleanliness of the skin.

## Incidence

Acne affects approximately 85% of adolescents and up to 20% of neonates. Although acne can begin at any age, it usually develops during puberty and lasts into early adulthood. Acne is more common in boys than in girls. It tends to improve in summer and flare up in winter. Acne in newborn infants typically resolves spontaneously by 3 months of age.

## Manifestations and Diagnostic Evaluation

Acne consists of closed whiteheads, blackheads, papules, pustules, nodules, and cysts (Fig. 49.12). Not all adolescents have all types of acne, and treatment is based on the type of acne. The areas most often affected are the face, neck, back, shoulders, and upper chest. The diagnosis is based on examination of the lesions and the child's history.

## Therapeutic Management

The goal of treatment is to prevent scarring and to promote a positive self-image in the adolescent. Treatment must be individualized according to the severity of the condition, the types of lesion present, and the adolescent's gender. Improvement usually begins in 4 to 6 weeks, so the adolescent needs support to keep from feeling discouraged after treatment begins. Three to 5 months are needed for optimal results.

Topical therapy with a variety of agents is the primary treatment for acne. Commonly used agents include benzoyl peroxide, which reduces fatty acid production and is bactericidal for *Propionibacterium acnes,* and tretinoin (Retin-A), a vitamin-A derivative. Tretinoin reduces comedo formation and eliminates the lesions already present. Benzoyl peroxide comes in a gel, cream, lotion, or soap in various strengths. Lower-potency formulas are available over the counter. Tretinoin is available in cream, gel, or liquid form by prescription. Sunscreen should be used with tretinoin to reduce photosensitivity.

## PATHOPHYSIOLOGY

### *Acne Vulgaris*

Acne begins when sebaceous glands, stimulated by androgens at the onset of puberty, enlarge and secrete increased amounts of sebum. The sebaceous glands become plugged and dilated with sebum. When the enlarged gland is open to the skin surface, an open comedo, or blackhead, is formed. The characteristic black color is not a result of poor hygiene but is produced as fatty acids are oxidized on the skin. If the gland does not have an opening, a closed comedo, or whitehead, forms. Closed comedones are small, nonerythematous papules just beneath the skin surface. Because a closed comedo has only a microscopic opening on the skin surface, pressure from excess sebum and keratin causes the comedo walls to rupture. Fatty acids produced by bacterial action on sebum are released into the surrounding tissues, causing inflammation. If the rupture occurs close to the surface, a pustule is formed. Ruptures deep in the dermis result in cysts and abscesses, which can lead to significant scarring.

Bacteria, particularly *Propionibacterium acnes,* play a role in the development of acne lesions by increasing inflammation and disrupting the integrity of the follicle walls.

Depending on the severity of the acne, the provider might recommend a combination of agents. For example, when applied together to the skin, benzoyl peroxide and tretinoin have a potentially offsetting effect that can reduce the overall effectiveness of each individual agent. For this reason, the health provider may order that the two medications be applied on alternate days or that benzoyl peroxide be applied in the morning and tretinoin at bedtime. In most instances it will take approximately 8 weeks for topical preparations to be effective (Gailbraith, 2016).

Topical antibiotics, such as clindamycin and erythromycin, decrease the number of *P. acnes* organisms in hair follicles and are often used for inflammatory acne. Topical antibiotics are preferred over systemic antibiotics.

Oral antibiotics (tetracycline, minocycline, erythromycin, clindamycin) might be prescribed for adolescents with severe inflammatory acne or those who are unresponsive to topical treatment. These medications are used in conjunction with non-antibiotic topical treatment (Gailbraith, 2016). Exposure to sunlight should be avoided if tetracycline is used. Oral isotretinoin (Accutane) has dramatically improved the condition of adolescents with severe nodular/cystic acne. This drug suppresses sebum production and sebaceous gland activity. Because of the severity of side effects, isotretinoin is not indicated for all adolescents. Side effects include cataracts, cheilitis, dry skin, pruritus, conjunctivitis, nosebleeds, and depression. In some instances, depression associated with isotretinoin has possibly resulted in suicide (Gailbraith, 2016). Young women who anticipate becoming pregnant should not take isotretinoin because of its teratogenic effects. Sexually active female adolescents should use an effective form of contraception, or combination of contraceptive methods, from 1 month before treatment until 6 weeks after discontinuing treatment. A negative pregnancy test must be obtained before initiating therapy. Informed consent is recommended for treatment with isotretinoin.

Estrogen is prescribed for young women who are unresponsive to antibiotic therapy or who cannot take isotretinoin. Combination oral contraceptives (progestin and estrogen) are also indicated for treatment of some cases of acne. Although the dermatologist may mechanically express comedones, the adolescent should be cautioned not to pick or squeeze lesions. Although scars cannot be completely removed, techniques such as dermabrasion, plastic repair, and collagen implants can improve appearance.

## NURSING CARE

### The Adolescent With Acne Vulgaris

#### Assessment

Obtain a history that includes how long acne lesions have been present and the effect of menses, stress, and other aggravating factors on the severity and frequency of the lesions. Investigate acne treatments that have been tried and their effectiveness. Establish how often the adolescent washes the skin and hair and the type of cleansing agents used. Inquire about whether the adolescent uses cosmetics on a regular basis and what types of cosmetics are used. Try to assess the adolescent's understanding of the development and treatment of acne.

Examine the adolescent's face, chest, back, and neck for lesions. The depth of tissue involvement and the presence of pustules, papules, cysts, and scars should be noted. The adolescent's feelings about appearance and self-image and the effects acne may have had on social functioning should be explored.

#### Nursing Diagnosis and Planning

The nursing diagnoses and expected outcomes that may be appropriate for the adolescent with acne vulgaris are as follows:

- Impaired Skin Integrity related to increased sebaceous gland secretions, hormonal changes, and the action of bacteria on the contents of clogged follicles.

  ***Expected outcome.*** Affected areas will exhibit signs of healing.
- Risk for Infection related to inflammation of skin lesions.

  ***Expected outcome.*** The adolescent will have no signs of secondary bacterial infection, as evidenced by clear, intact skin.
- Disturbed Body Image related to appearance of skin lesions.

  ***Expected outcome.*** The adolescent will verbalize feelings and concerns and will participate in desired social activities.
- Deficient Knowledge about skin care and treatment regimen related to being too embarrassed to ask questions.

  ***Expected outcome.*** The adolescent will carry out the prescribed treatment regimen to control excessive sebaceous gland activity.

#### Interventions

Because acne is a long-term condition, the affected adolescent needs support and encouragement if the treatment regimen is to be effective. Improvement can take as long as 12 weeks, and exacerbations are common. Although there is no cure for acne, much can be done to control inflammation and reduce scarring.

Explain the cause of acne and the rationale for treatment at the outset, so the adolescent can help plan the treatment regimen. Providing written instructions and involving the adolescent in care can help improve adherence. The treatment must be individualized, but all treatment regimens include measures to reduce oil on the skin. Gently cleaning the face twice a day with mild antibacterial soap and shampooing the hair daily are important facets of care. Warn the adolescent to avoid vigorous scrubbing and picking or squeezing of lesions, which can rupture pilosebaceous ducts and cause secondary infection. Teach the adolescent how to apply topical medications and caution against overusing these products to speed results. Because oily cosmetics and creams add to the plugging of follicles, only water-based cosmetics should be used.

A healthy lifestyle, including adequate rest, exercise, and a balanced diet, promotes healing of lesions. Explore the adolescent's feelings about appearance and coping mechanisms. Reinforce positive self-image and self-esteem. Concerns and fears should be openly discussed and myths about acne dispelled. Provide parents with needed information about acne to clear up misconceptions and to prevent needless nagging of the adolescent.

#### Evaluation

- Do the acne lesions exhibit signs of healing without signs of infection?
- Is the adolescent able to express feelings and concerns about possible change in body image?
- Does the adolescent appear confident and assured as the process of healing is occurring?
- Does the adolescent carry out the treatment regimen to control acne and prevent scarring?

## MISCELLANEOUS SKIN DISORDERS

There are a large number of less common skin disorders of varied causes and manifestations. Several of these disorders, along with their manifestations, management, and special considerations, are listed in Table 49.1.

## INSECT BITES OR STINGS

Insects are found almost everywhere, and children often come in contact with them during play. The bites of most insects are not serious, usually causing only itching and mild pain; however, severe systemic reactions can occur in sensitized children. Systemic reactions to the venom of stinging insects, including wasps, honeybees, yellow jackets, hornets, and fire ants, is estimated to occur in nearly 1% of American children (Wang & Sicherer, 2016). Anaphylaxis from insect stings results in a number of deaths annually in the United States (Golden, Moffitt, & Nicklas, 2011). Children who are allergic to insect stings should wear a medical alert bracelet and be provided with an epinephrine autoinjector (EpiPen) and information on avoidance. Parents need to make certain that the autoinjector is actually with the child or a responsible adult when the child is outdoors. The expiration date on the autoinjector must be checked regularly, and families must know how to obtain replacements when the autoinjector is outdated. Patients with a clear history of anaphylaxis after *Hymenoptera* stings should be referred to an allergist for immunotherapy (Golden et al., 2011). (See Chapter 42 for additional information about anaphylaxis.)

Arachnids (scorpions, spiders, ticks, mites) are found in areas where children play. Most arachnids are not dangerous or aggressive. In the United States, only one type of scorpion and two types of spiders (black widow, brown recluse) cause life-threatening reactions.

Topical insect repellents are an important measure in preventing insect bites. The CDC recommends the use of products that contain active ingredients registered with the Environmental Protection Agency. Repellents containing high concentrations of diethyltoluamide (DEET) should not be used on small children because of the risk of toxic encephalopathy. Likewise, products containing oil of eucalyptus are not indicated for children younger than 3 years. The AAP Committee on Environmental Health recommends that repellents with DEET should not be used on infants less than 2 months old. Such repellents should not be applied near the face, and children should be cautioned not to put their fingers in their mouths when wearing diethyltoluamide (CDC, 2015c).

The bites and stings of common insects and arachnids are discussed in Table 49.2. The table includes information on manifestations, treatment, and prevention.

TABLE 49.1 **Skin Disorders**

| Disorder/Etiology | Manifestations | Management | Comments |
|---|---|---|---|
| **Stevens–Johnson Syndrome** | | | |
| Acute, sometimes recurrent autoimmune disease.<br>Can be triggered by infections or medications such as sulfonamides or anticonvulsants.<br>New lesions continue to erupt for 2-3 wk, followed by healing during the next 6 wk. | After a prodromal respiratory illness, bullae appear on the lips, mouth, eyes, and genitalia. Fever, chills, malaise, neutropenia, anemia, weakness. Purulent conjunctivitis is common. Skin lesions rupture and can lead to significant fluid loss. | Withdraw the triggering medication.<br>Treatment of skin lesions similar to that for extensive burns: aseptic technique, IV fluids, air/fluid bedding, nutritional support, pain management. Give antibiotics for secondary infections. Obtain ophthalmology consultation for eye lesions. | Reassure the child that the skin lesions will disappear. Inform parents about the possibility of recurrence and encourage them to avoid any implicated medications. |
| **Psoriasis** | | | |
| Chronic, inflammatory rash caused by rapid proliferation of keratinocytes. Hereditary predisposition; onset in first 2 decades of life.<br>Remissions and exacerbations; lasts throughout life.<br>Exacerbations associated with stress.<br>Arthritis is sometimes a complication. | Pruritus; erythematous, elevated plaques and silvery scales on the scalp, face, knees, elbows, and gluteal folds. Scales are attached at the center rather than edges and may bleed when removed. | Topical corticosteroids and tar preparations; keratolytic agents. Exposure to ultraviolet light and sunlight. Skin care to prevent secondary infection. Keratolytic agents enhance penetration of topical steroids. Sunlight can cause phototoxic reactions with tar preparations. To prevent tar folliculitis, tar should be applied down an extremity rather than up. | There is no cure for psoriasis. Cutaneous trauma and streptococcal infections (e.g., tonsillitis) are common aggravating factors. A resource for families of children with psoriasis is the National Psoriasis Foundation: http://www.psoriasis.org/home. |
| **Pityriasis Rosea** | | | |
| Acute, inflammatory, self-limited skin disorder. Etiology unknown; might be viral. | Sudden eruption of salmon-pink, irregular patches on trunk and proximal portions of extremities. Symmetric distribution of lesions, "Christmas tree" appearance on back. "Herald patch" precedes rash by 7-10 days. | No treatment required for asymptomatic children. Pruritus can be treated with antipruritic lotions, ultraviolet light, or sunlight. | Child generally feels well. Rash lasts 6-12 wk. |
| **Warts** | | | |
| Skin infection caused by human papillomavirus. Incubation period is 1-6 mo. Can persist from a few months to 5+ yr. | Painless, hyperkeratotic papule. Begins as a round, flesh-colored papule; later becomes brown or tan with a rough surface. Most common sites: dorsum of hands, fingers, feet, face, genitalia. | Various methods of treatment: daily application of lactic acid and salicylic acid (e.g., Compound W); freezing with liquid nitrogen; topical application of cantharidin for plantar or periungual warts. | Most warts disappear without treatment in 2-3 yr. With treatment, they usually resolve in 2-3 mo.<br>Picking at warts may cause them to spread to other areas of the body. Warts are not highly contagious to other people.<br>Immunocompromised children are more susceptible to warts. |
| **Molluscum Contagiosum** | | | |
| Viral infection of the skin and mucous membranes.<br>Transmitted by skin-to-skin and fomite-to-skin contact. May be transmitted by sexual contact. | Begin as pinpoint papules that increase in size to 2-3 mm or larger. Firm, solid, pink papules changing into soft, waxy, umbilicated papules.<br>Curd-like core of the lesion can be expressed.<br>Most common sites: face, trunk, extremities, oral mucous membranes, conjunctiva, genitalia. | Lesions are treated with cantharidin, cryotherapy, tretinoin, or imiquimod. Condition usually responds well to treatment. Spontaneous disappearance is common. | Lesions can spread to other parts of the body and can be transmitted to others.<br>Lesions disappear spontaneously over time. Children with eczema or impaired immunity are at risk for generalized spread of lesions (See Chapter 41 for additional discussion of genital warts [HPV]). |

*Continued*

TABLE 49.1 **Skin Disorders—cont'd**

| Disorder/Etiology | Manifestations | Management | Comments |
|---|---|---|---|
| **Frostbite** | | | |
| Freezing of tissue resulting from exposure to extreme cold. Exposed areas (fingers, toes, nose, cheeks, ears) are most often affected. Cold causes arteriolar vasoconstriction, resulting in tissue anoxia and destruction. | Early signs: blanching of skin; stinging sensation followed by numbness and white, mottled appearance. Area feels cold, hard; may be without sensation.<br>First-degree: redness and discomfort with return to normal in a few hours.<br>Second-degree: redness; blisters and bullae 24-48 hr after rewarming. Pain during rewarming.<br>Third-degree: cyanosis and mottling, followed by redness and swelling. Necrosis of epidermis, dermis, and subcutaneous tissue. Sensation is absent. Pain during rewarming.<br>Fourth-degree: complete necrosis with gangrene, possible loss of body part. | Immediately cover affected areas with warm hands and warm clothing. Massaging areas causes further damage and should be avoided.<br>Rapidly rewarm areas by immersion in a warm water bath (90° F-106° F [32.2° C-41.1° C]) until all frozen tissues are thawed and the skin appears flushed.<br>Pain during thawing can be severe and should be treated with analgesics and sedatives. Severely damaged areas are treated as burns. | Children in cold climates should be taught to prevent frostbite by wearing adequate warm, layered clothing; hat; gloves; and two pairs of socks (one cotton, one wool). Children should be taught to warm themselves when hands or feet begin to sting.<br>Young children should not be allowed to play outside in extremely cold temperatures. |
| **Foreign Bodies** | | | |
| Skin injury caused by penetration of splinters, gravel, cactus spines, bee stingers, glass, or other foreign objects. | Pain, erythema, possible secondary infection.<br>Foreign body may or may not be visible. | Area surrounding foreign body should be washed with soap and water before removal. Superficial splinters can be removed with a needle and tweezers disinfected with alcohol or flame. | Deeply embedded foreign bodies, fishhooks, and other difficult-to-remove objects may require medical attention.<br>Tetanus prophylaxis may be indicated. |

TABLE 49.2 **Skin Lesions Caused by Insects and Arachnids**

| Agent and Characteristics | Manifestations | Treatment and Prevention |
|---|---|---|
| **Insects** | | |
| ***Mosquitoes, Fleas, Flies, Gnats*** | | |
| Foreign protein in insect's saliva is injected as insect pierces skin to suck blood. | Itching, erythema, small wheal. Local reaction may occur that is difficult to distinguish from cellulitis. | Apply antipruritic lotions and cool compresses to relieve itching. Give antihistamines if needed for sleep.<br>Prevention: Wear insect repellent when contact is anticipated. Treat potential breeding places (standing water for mosquitoes; pets, furniture, yard for fleas). |
| ***Hymenoptera (Bees, Wasps, Hornets, Yellow Jackets, Fire Ants)*** | | |
| Venom is injected through a stinger. | Histamine and foreign proteins in venom cause local reaction of pain, swelling, redness, and itching. Systemic allergic reactions may be manifested by nausea, generalized edema, respiratory distress, and shock. | If visible, carefully remove stinger by scraping it out horizontally. Avoid squeezing stinger, because more venom will be released. Wash with soap and water. Paste made of powdered meat tenderizer and water is soothing. Apply ice and analgesics for discomfort, antihistamines for itching. For a systemic allergic reaction, give epinephrine and corticosteroids immediately; transport to emergency facility. Children allergic to *Hymenoptera* should wear medical identification.<br>Prevention: Treat known hives or nests. Avoid wearing colorful clothing and perfumes when outside. |

**TABLE 49.2 Skin Lesions Caused by Insects and Arachnids—cont'd**

| Agent and Characteristics | Manifestations | Treatment and Prevention |
|---|---|---|
| **Arachnids** | | |
| ***Brown Recluse ("Fiddle Back") Spider*** | | |
| Yellowish to reddish brown with a violin-shaped mark on its back.<br>Venom injected by fangs. Bites only when threatened. Lives in dark, protected areas (woodpiles, basements, closets, trash heaps). | Mild stinging at time of bite. Within 2-8 hr, area around bite becomes painful and erythema develops, followed by a blister. Venom is necrotoxic. Edema, redness, and purpura may involve entire limb.<br>Central portion of lesion develops an indurated wheal that progresses to deep, sloughing ulcer in 7-14 days. Ulcer often does not heal for several months. Usually results in a scar. | Immobilize and elevate affected extremity. Cool compresses, analgesics, tetanus prophylaxis.<br>Observe for secondary infection.<br>Skin graft may be necessary for large ulcers.<br>No antivenin available.<br>Prevention: Avoid areas inhabited by spiders. |
| ***Black Widow Spider*** | | |
| Shiny black with a red hourglass-shaped mark on abdomen.<br>Female's venom is very poisonous to humans. Males do not bite. Female builds irregular web in dark, sheltered spots and aggressively defends eggs. | Bite may be painless initially. Within 1 hr pain develops at site. Severe muscle pains and numbness spread from bite, and puncture site becomes red, swollen, and pruritic. Neurotoxic venom enters the bloodstream within 1 hr, causing dizziness, headache, nausea, vomiting, cramps, tremors, and rapid, shallow respirations.<br>Shock and renal failure may develop in young children. | Hospitalization for children. Antivenin if no allergy to horse serum. Supportive care, including IV calcium gluconate, morphine, muscle relaxants. Tetanus prophylaxis.<br>Prevention: Avoid areas infested by spiders (woodpiles, outhouses). Carefully check packaged fruits and produce before reaching into bags or boxes. |
| **Ticks** | | |
| Brown or gray; live in fields, pastures, woods.<br>Feed on blood of humans, dogs, livestock, or deer. Larvae feed on rodents. Tick buries head and mouth parts in the skin to suck blood. | Bites can cause local reactions or, rarely, systemic reactions (tick fever, tick paralysis). Ticks can transmit Lyme disease, babesiosis, Rocky Mountain spotted fever, Q fever, and tularemia. Also, depending on the type of tick, they can cause rare allergic reactions to certain foods (e.g., red meat). | Methods to remove ticks: Remove with tweezers as close to the skin as possible, taking care to remove head. If mouth parts remain, remove with sterile needle. Wash site with soap and water. There is some evidence that prompt removal of ticks decreases chance of disease transmission.<br>Prevention: Wear long sleeves and pants and use insect repellent when walking in tick-infested areas. Inspect clothing and hair for ticks after walking through fields or woods. (See Chapter 41 for additional discussion.) |
| **Scorpions** | | |
| Most scorpions are not dangerous. They rarely attack humans unless accidentally disturbed or stepped on. If disturbed, they inflict a painful sting. One type (found in Arizona), *Centruroides sculpturatus,* is extremely poisonous, and its sting can be fatal. Scorpions are found mainly in the southwestern United States. Scorpions hide by day in basements, garages, closets, crevices. Some varieties burrow and hide in gravel or children's sandboxes. | Sting is extremely painful.<br>Local reaction of swelling at puncture site. Some species cause systemic reactions: tachycardia, hypertension, dysrhythmias, irritability, seizures, pulmonary edema, coma.<br>Fatal reactions most often occur in children younger than 3 yr. | Ice packs and tourniquet applied proximal to the site slow the spread of venom. Wound should not be excised.<br>Topical steroids and antihistamines are used to relieve symptoms. For severe reactions, provide supportive care for pain, shock, seizures. Narcotic analgesics act synergistically with scorpion venom and are contraindicated. Antivenin is given for systemic reactions (available from the Antivenom Production Laboratory, Arizona State University).<br>Prevention: Wear shoes to prevent stepping on scorpions. Inspect shoes and clothing before dressing. Apply creosote to garages, basements. |
| **Chiggers (Harvest Mites)** | | |
| Live in tall grass and underbrush; burrow into hair follicles and skin pores to feed. | Tend to concentrate in warm areas where clothing is snug (underwear elastic). Cause erythematous papules and intense itching. | Antipruritic agents. Prevention of secondary infection.<br>Prevention: Insect repellent on clothing, ankles, legs. |

*HPV,* Human papillomavirus; *IV,* intravenous.

**BOX 49.1 Pediatric Differences in the Effects of Burn Injury**

- Very young children who have been severely burned have a higher mortality rate than older children and adults with comparable burns.
- Because a child's skin is thinner than that of an adult, lower burn temperatures and shorter exposure to heat or chemicals can cause a more severe burn.
- A larger body surface area compared with that of adult's places severely burned children at increased risk for fluid and heat loss. Children are also at increased risk for dehydration and metabolic acidosis from diarrhea, evaporative water loss, and increased fluid requirements.
- The higher proportion of body fluid to body mass in children increases the risk of cardiovascular problems because of their less effective cardiovascular response to changing intravascular volume.
- Burns involving more than 10% total body surface area (TBSA) require fluid resuscitation.
- Infants and children are at increased risk for protein and calorie deficiency because they have smaller muscle mass and lower body fat than adults. If they are not eating and their metabolism is increased, their protein and calorie needs will not be met.
- Hypertrophic scarring is more severe, and scar maturation is prolonged.
- An immature immune system means an increased risk of infection for infants and young children.
- A delay in growth may follow extensive burns.
- In children, Curling (gastroduodenal) ulcer occurs in the third or fourth week after a burn, which is later than in adults.

**TABLE 49.3 Age-Related Risks for Burn Injury**

| Injury Type | Risk Factors |
|---|---|
| **<5 Yr of Age** | |
| Flame | Playing with matches and cigarette lighters<br>Playing with fires in fireplaces, barbecue pits, trash fires |
| Scald | Kitchen injury from tipping scalding liquids<br>Bathtub scalds associated with lack of supervision or child abuse<br>Most pediatric burn patients are infants and toddlers younger than 3 yr burned by scalding liquids |
| **5-10 Yr of Age** | |
| Flame | Boys at increased risk<br>Often associated with fire play and risk-taking behaviors |
| Scald | Girls at increased risk<br>Likely to occur at home in kitchen or bathroom |
| **Adolescent** | |
| Flame | Injury associated with male peer-group activities involving gasoline or other flammable products<br>Gasoline sniffing possibly involved<br>Rarely occurs in female adolescents except in house fires or automobile accidents |
| Electrical | Occurs most often in male adolescents involved in dare-type behaviors, such as climbing utility poles or antennas<br>In rural areas, is associated with moving irrigation pipes that touch an electrical source |

## BURN INJURIES

Burn injury can involve a small, painful area that hurts until healing occurs, or it can involve most of a child's body, with resulting severe trauma or death. Infants and toddlers are at greatest risk for sustaining burns because they depend totally on others for safety.

Recovery from a major burn injury requires many months, and the child's appearance might be altered for life. Caring for a burned child entails a multidisciplinary approach with a focus on the child and the family. Nursing care involves treating the physical injury and its psychological effects on the child and family members. The challenges of burn nursing begin with acute burn care but continue through the rehabilitation phase until the child is restored to optimal function (Box 49.1).

### Etiology

Burn injuries in children can be unintentional or intentional. In children younger than 5 years, unintentional burns are likely to occur as a result of environmental situations that are not controlled by caretakers. The young child's curiosity and increasing mobility contribute to the risk (Table 49.3). A child can start a fire by playing with matches (Fig. 49.13) or flammable materials near open fires. A child might be the victim of a house fire while sleeping, or might be unintentionally scalded or electrocuted (Fig. 49.14) (See Chapters 5 through 9 for a discussion of safety). Recently, severe burns have resulted from contact with heat shields from gas fireplaces and outdoor fire pits. Both inattentive supervision and purposeful abuse can cause intentional burns (see Patient-Centered Teaching: Measures to Prevent and Initially Manage a Burn).

The extent of the injury determines whether burn-related problems are local or systemic. Other factors, such as the location of the burned area, whether the injury is electrical, whether there is a concurrent inhalation injury or trauma, and whether there is a preexisting medical condition, contribute to morbidity and mortality rates. Morbidity and mortality rates from burns are higher in children than in adults.

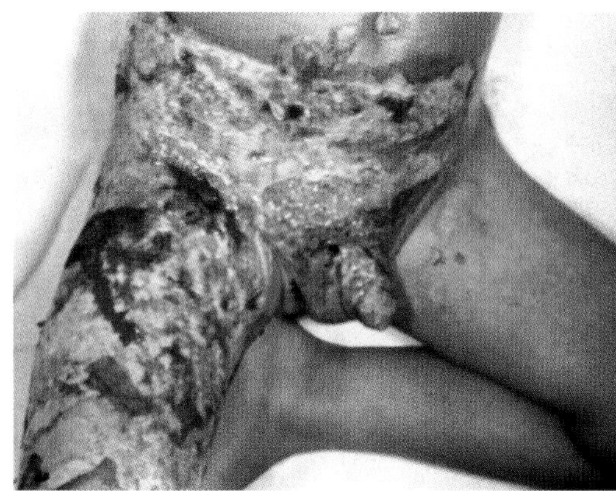

**FIG 49.13** These burns were sustained when the child's pajamas caught fire while he was playing with matches. (From Cosman, B. [1973]. *Management of the burned patient.* New York: MEDCOM.)

### Incidence

Fire and burn injuries are a leading cause of unintentional deaths in children ages 1 to 14 years in the United States (CDC, 2014). Scald burns are the most common burn injuries seen in pediatrics (Antoon

## PATIENT-CENTERED TEACHING

### *Measures to Prevent and Initially Manage a Burn*

**Prevention**

- Have periodic fire drills to teach your children how to evacuate the house in the event of a fire.
- Place child identification stickers, which can be obtained from most fire departments, on the outside of the bedroom door and in one window of each child's bedroom.
- Identify two or more exits from each room and a location to meet outside the house. Emphasize to your children that they should not return to the house under any circumstances, even if another family member or pet remains in the house.
- Be sure your child understands "stop, drop, and roll" as a measure to stop the burning process.
- Be sure to keep all matches and lighters out of reach. Check electrical cords regularly. Use outlet covers if children younger than 5 years of age are in the house.
- Check smoke and carbon monoxide detectors regularly and keep them clean. Replace the batteries regularly if they are battery operated.
- To reduce the number of scald burns, turn the hot water heater thermostat down to 120° F (48.8° C).
- Turn pot handles in and use back burners on the stove whenever possible.
- Do not sit a child on your lap while you are drinking a hot liquid.
- Keep your children away from outdoor grills and fire pits, and indoor wood-, gas-, or coal-burning stoves. Keep older infants from crawling near floor heating grates.

**Initial Emergency Burn Management**

- Apply cool compresses or submerge minor burns in cool water, not ice.
- To prevent scalding, remove clothing soaked with hot water as quickly as possible.
- Contact the physician for any child with a burn that has blistered.
- Cover a child who has a major burn with a clean sheet while waiting for emergency personnel.
- Do not try to remove clothing that is adhering to burned skin.

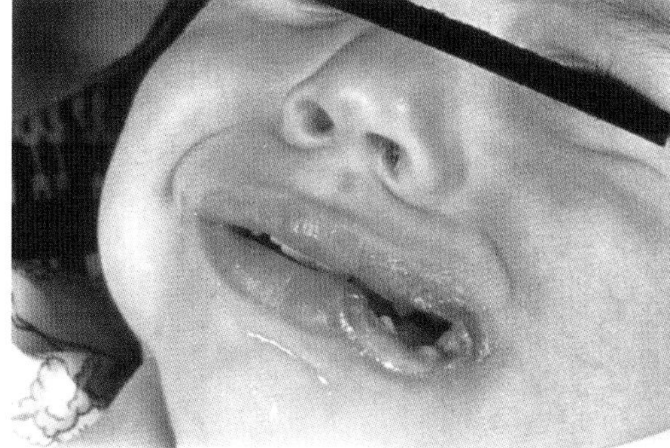

**FIG 49.14** These burns were sustained when the child sucked on an electrical socket. (From Cosman, B. [1973]. *Management of the burned patient.* New York: MEDCOM.)

& Donovan, 2016). Other burn injuries include those induced by flame, electrical, and chemical causes. Child abuse accounts for a significant portion of the scald and immersion burns in children (Gonzalez & Shanti, 2015). Most children with severe burns are treated in burn centers. The American Burn Association has outlined criteria for referral to a burn center (Box 49.2).

**BOX 49.2 Burn Center Referral Criteria**

The American Burn Association recommends that children with the following injuries be referred to a burn center after emergency assessment and stabilization:

- Second-degree burns greater than 10% body surface area
- Burns that involve major joints, face, hands, feet, genitalia, or perineum
- Third-degree burns
- Electrical burns, including lightning injury
- Chemical burns
- Inhalation injury with burns
- Preexisting medical disorders that might complicate recovery
- Coexisting trauma in which the burn injury poses the greatest risk to life or function
- Burned children in hospitals without qualified personnel to care for pediatric burn patients
- Children who will require specialized psychosocial or long-term rehabilitation

Modified from American Burn Association and American College of Surgeons Committee on Trauma. (2006). Guidelines for the operations of burn centers. *Resources for optimal care of the injured patient* (Chapter 14, pp. 79). Retrieved from http://www.ameriburn.org.

## Pathophysiology

In a burn injury, the injuring agent (flame, chemical, ultraviolet light, or electrical energy) denatures cellular proteins, destroying collagen linkages in connective tissue. As a result, osmotic and hydrostatic pressure gradients are disrupted, and intravascular fluid moves into interstitial spaces. Inflammatory chemicals are released from injured cells, increasing capillary permeability and adding to fluid shifts. Burn injuries are classified by depth and extent of tissue damage and by severity of injury. The combination of these factors determines referral and therapeutic management decisions.

### Depth of Burn Injury

Depth of burn injury describes local tissue damage and is determined by the duration of exposure and the temperature or destructive potential of the causative agent. Depth of injury is classified as superficial, superficial partial thickness, deep partial thickness, or full thickness (Table 49.4).

Superficial burns, usually sunburns, affect only the epidermis. No blisters form in a true superficial burn, and the surface of the injury is dry. The pain of sunburns is usually delayed for several hours after sun exposure. Partial-thickness thermal, chemical, or electrical injury to the skin interferes with the skin's ability to carry out its normal physiologic functions of protection from infection or injury, preservation of fluid balance, and temperature regulation. In addition, deep tissue injury damages sensory nerve endings and local circulatory patterns and adversely affects the skin's ability to regenerate or synthesize vitamin D.

## TABLE 49.4 Depth of Burn Injury

| | Superficial | Superficial Partial Thickness | Deep Partial Thickness | Full Thickness |
|---|---|---|---|---|
| Normal skin<br>Epidermis<br>Dermis<br>Subcutaneous<br>Muscle | Epidermis<br>Dermis<br>Subcutaneous<br>Muscle | Epidermis<br>Dermis<br>Subcutaneous<br>Muscle | Epidermis<br>Dermis<br>Subcutaneous<br>Muscle | Epidermis<br>Dermis<br>Subcutaneous<br>Muscle |
| Morphologic features | Destruction of epidermis; physiologic functions remain intact | Destruction of epidermis and some dermis | Destruction of epidermis and dermis | Destruction of epidermis, dermis, underlying tissue; may include fascia, muscle, tendon, bone |
| Blister formation | After 24 hr (e.g., from sunburn) | Within minutes; thin walled, fluid filled | May or may not appear as fluid-filled blisters; often they are flat, dehydrated, and like tissue paper; body fluids lost through burn tissue must be replaced | Rare; may appear as a tissue-paper–like layer that is flat and dehydrated |
| Appearance | Peels after 24-48 hr | Red to pale ivory, moist surface | Mottled, waxy white, dry surface | White, cherry red, or black |
| Healing time | 3-7 days | 7-21 days if no infection develops | 30 days to several months if no infection; if infected, this type of burn can convert to full-thickness burn | Will not heal; skin grafting required; very small areas may heal from edges after a period of weeks |
| Patient reaction | Moderate discomfort, pain; chills; nausea; vomiting | Can cause considerable pain | Severe pain on exposure to air or water because nerve endings are intact | No pain in area of full-thickness burn because nerve endings are destroyed; surrounding areas of lesser depth are painful |
| Scarring | None | Minimal; influenced by genetic predisposition | Greatest because the slow healing of these burns increases scar tissue; scar formation influenced by genetic predisposition | Autograft scarring is minimized by early excision and grafting; scar formation influenced by genetic predisposition |

### Extent of Burn Injury

The extent of injury refers to the percent of total body surface area (TBSA) burned. The standard "rule of nines" used in adults gives an inaccurate estimate for children because of the differences in body proportion between children and adults. Many burn facilities use the Lund and Browder chart, which is a body surface chart corrected for age (Fig. 49.15). Another method estimates burn percentage in smaller-area burns by calculating the complete palmar surface of the child's hand and assumes the area of the palmar surface equals 1% of the TBSA (Antoon & Donovan, 2016).

### Severity of Burn Injury

Severity of burn injury is determined by the degree to which the skin's physiologic functions are disrupted beyond the body's normal ability to respond with compensatory mechanisms. Burn injuries are classified as minor, moderate uncomplicated, and major. The severity of burn injury is related to a combination of factors. These include age,

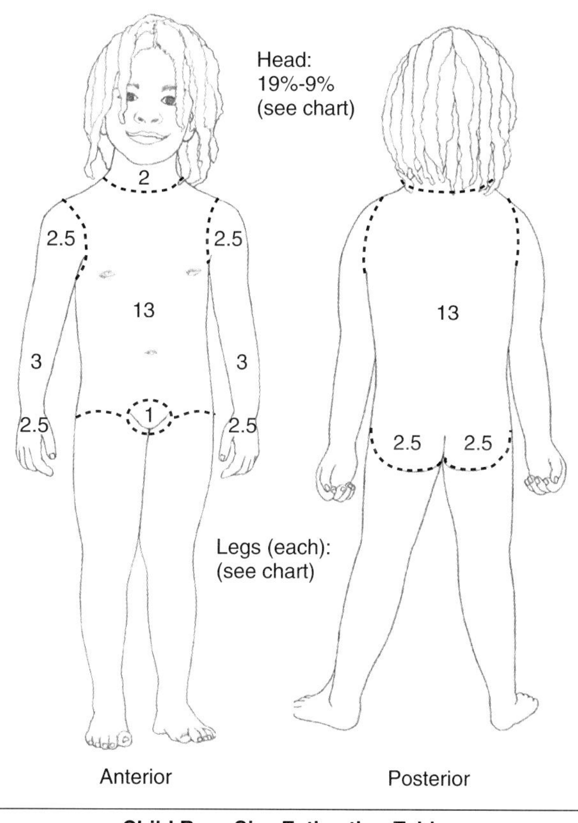


**Child Burn Size Estimation Table**
(percent total body surface area)

| | Age in Years | | | | | |
|---|---|---|---|---|---|---|
| | < 1yr | 1 | 5 | 10 | 15 | Adult |
| Head | 19 | 17 | 13 | 11 | 9 | 7 |
| Neck | 2 | 2 | 2 | 2 | 2 | 2 |
| Anterior Trunk | 13 | 13 | 13 | 13 | 13 | 13 |
| Posterior Trunk | 13 | 13 | 13 | 13 | 13 | 13 |
| Buttock | 2.5 | 2.5 | 2.5 | 2.5 | 2.5 | 2.5 |
| Genitalia | 1 | 1 | 1 | 1 | 1 | 1 |
| Upper arm | 2.5 | 2.5 | 2.5 | 2.5 | 2.5 | 2.5 |
| Lower arm | 3 | 3 | 3 | 3 | 3 | 3 |
| Hand | 2.5 | 2.5 | 2.5 | 2.5 | 2.5 | 2.5 |
| Thigh | 5.5 | 6.5 | 8 | 8.5 | 9 | 9.5 |
| Leg | 5 | 5 | 5.5 | 6 | 6.5 | 7 |
| Foot | 3.5 | 3.5 | 3.5 | 3.5 | 3.5 | 3.5 |

**FIG 49.15** Calculating total body surface area (TBSA) burned in children. The standard "rule of nines" and standard body surface charts must be adapted because of the difference in body proportions between adults and children. (From Deitch, E., & Rutan, R. [2001]. *The challenges of children: the first 48 hours.* Chicago: American Burn Association.)

medical history, extent and depth of burn, special care of the body area involved (e.g., face, hands), and the presence of associated trauma, such as fractures or head injury, sustained at the time of the burn. Burn severity relates to the child's eventual morbidity or mortality status.

## Manifestations

Table 49.5 lists the clinical manifestations associated with burns with respect to severity. Assessment of the distribution of scald burns is of particular importance in infants and toddlers because of the possibility of child maltreatment. The classic forced immersion burn occurs when a child's extremity or buttocks are held under hot water. These burns have a "stocking" or "glove" appearance with a relatively sharp line dividing the burned from unburned skin. There are usually no smaller, scattered burns ("splash marks") that indicate attempts to remove the extremity.

## Therapeutic Management

### Superficial Burn Injuries

The most common cause of a superficial (epidermal layer only) burn is sunburn. Although uncomfortable, sunburn rarely requires intensive burn treatment. Cool compresses and application of soothing topical lotions (especially those containing aloe) or mild topical corticosteroids provide symptomatic treatment. If the discomfort is disturbing the child's sleep, acetaminophen or ibuprofen can provide relief.

Preventing sunburn is especially important in children because frequent sunburn causes long-term damage to the skin. Children who are susceptible to sunburn are also susceptible to the later development of melanoma and nonmelanoma skin cancers (Skin Cancer Foundation, 2015). Children should avoid sun exposure, especially between the hours of 10 AM and 3 PM during the summer. During sun exposure, parents should apply to the child's skin an appropriate ultraviolet A and ultraviolet B protective sunscreen with a sun protection factor greater than 15. Hats and shirts are also desirable. Waterproof sunscreens are available for children who like to run in and out of the water, but frequent applications of sunscreen are still desirable. Recommend that parents check the date on the sunscreen to be sure it has not expired. Sunscreen is contraindicated for infants younger than 6 months. Parents should keep infants in the shade, away from reflecting sun rays.

### Superficial Partial-Thickness Burn Injuries

In general, children with a minor burn injury are treated as outpatients in a physician's office, clinic, or hospital physical therapy department unless the extent of injury warrants hospital admission. Therapy is aimed at promoting wound healing, preventing infection, and providing pain relief. Burn wound care requires aseptic technique. Because anaerobic and aerobic bacteria can grow at the interface between burned and healthy tissue, tetanus toxoid is given to children who have not received tetanus immunization during the 5 years preceding the burn injury.

***Wound cleaning.*** Burn wounds receive care at least daily until closure is achieved. After old dressings are removed, the burned skin is cleaned with sterile saline solution or mild soap and water. If the child is hospitalized, hydrotherapy (Fig. 49.16) can be used to remove old dressings and clean the wound and the child. During this cleaning process, the child can perform active range-of-motion exercises. Hydrotherapy can be done in a tank, tub, or shower. Some facilities use disposable plastic liners to prevent contamination between uses. Hydrotherapy should last no longer than 20 minutes to prevent electrolyte loss (through skin into water, as a result of osmosis). The

**TABLE 49.5 Classification of Severity of Burn Injury in Children**

| Type of Injury | Clinical Manifestations |
|---|---|
| **Minor** | |
| Partial-thickness burn of <10% of TBSA<br>Full-thickness burn of <2% of TBSA that does not involve special care areas (eyes, ears, face, hands, feet, perineum, joints)<br>Excludes electrical injury, inhalation injury, concurrent trauma, all poor-risk children (e.g., those of extremely young age or with concurrent disease) | Localized pain and blister formation in the area of injury; white or black full-thickness injury<br>No systemic effects<br>Little or no scarring, except in areas of full-thickness injury |
| **Moderate, Uncomplicated** | |
| Partial-thickness burns of 10%-20% of TBSA<br>Full-thickness burns of <10% of TBSA that do not involve special care areas<br>Excludes electrical injury, inhalation injury, concurrent trauma, all poor-risk children (e.g., those of extremely young age or with concurrent disease) | Open wound that is a potential source of infection and a site for loss of fluids and electrolytes<br>Pain that may interfere with routines of daily living<br>Wound healing rate influenced by nutritional status<br>Possible scarring in areas of partial- and full-thickness injuries |
| **Major** | |
| Partial-thickness burns of >20% of TBSA<br>All full-thickness burns of ≥10% of TBSA<br>All burns involving eyes, ears, face, hands, feet, perineum, or joints<br>All inhalation injury, electrical injury, concurrent trauma, all poor-risk patients | Life-threatening injuries with risk for severe complications and death<br>Volatile hospital course characterized by periods of relative physiologic stability followed, within hours, by life-threatening emergencies, such as shock<br>Repeated operative procedures for skin grafting that are accompanied by major blood loss requiring multiple transfusions<br>Potential risk for infection, either of the burn wound or related to pulmonary complications or systemic sepsis, until wound closure is achieved over 80% of the TBSA<br>Much higher mortality rate associated with burn injury accompanied by inhalation injury than with burn injury alone |

*TBSA*, Total body surface area.

room temperature is kept warm, and the child is covered and dried immediately after the procedure.

***Débridement.*** Débridement is the removal of dead material within a wound to promote healing. In a burn injury, there is necrosis of skin and subcutaneous tissue. The burned tissue is called **eschar**. Eschar releases chemical mediators that stimulate leukocytes to digest debris, but this process also damages capillaries and skin elements. Necrotic tissue within a wound prolongs inflammation and slows healing and epidermal coverage.

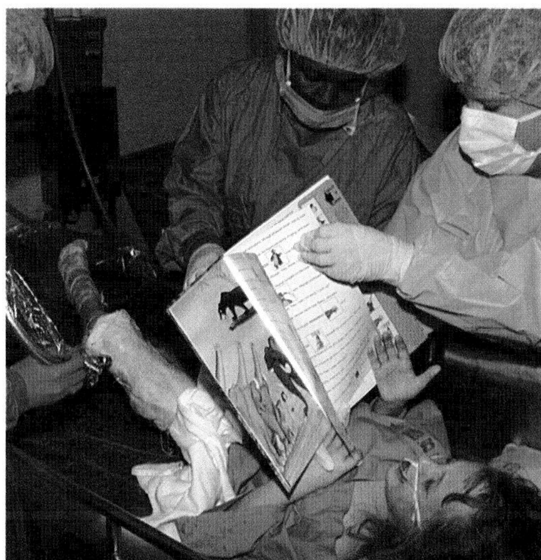

**FIG 49.16** Burn dressings can be changed in the hydrotherapy room. The room is kept warm because children who have been burned have poor body temperature control. The child life therapist reads a book to the child to distract her from the discomfort associated with the procedure. (Courtesy Parkland Health and Hospital System, Dallas, TX.)

The initial débridement might be performed in the office, emergency room, or hydrotherapy treatment room. The burned area is débrided of loose debris and necrotic tissue. Blisters, particularly on palmar skin, are usually left intact in superficial partial-thickness burns. Subsequent to rupture, they are débrided (Antoon & Donovan, 2016). Old creams and ointments must be removed as part of the débridement, and loose tissue is trimmed around the burned area.

***Application of antimicrobial agents and dressings.*** Topical antibacterial agents (Table 49.6) are placed on burn wounds to penetrate the eschar and to control bacterial growth in and around the burn wound. Silver sulfadiazine (Silvadene) is the most commonly used topical agent, but it is not typically used on the face or on electrical burns. Facial burns are covered with a light layer of antimicrobial ointment. Mafenide (Sulfamylon) is the topical agent of choice for burns to the ear or electrical burns because of its deep penetration into the eschar. Mafenide should not be applied to the face. Collagenase ointment, a topical enzyme, is an effective topical agent for débridement (Antoon & Donovan, 2016).

After application of the topical antibacterial agent, a dressing usually is applied. A variety of dressings, or membranes, some impregnated with silver, provide pain relief, reduce fluid and heat loss, and decrease bacterial colonization. For superficial or partial thickness burns, the dressings remain on the child for 7 to 10 days, but are checked frequently (Antoon & Donovan, 2016). Commonly used biologic dressings include human skin, pig skin, and fresh human amniotic membrane (from the placenta). Synthetic dressings include plastic films, hydrocolloids, hydrogels, and collagen-impregnated dressings. The major risk associated with these dressings is infection; thus, the wound must be clean and dry before dressing application.

For more severe burns, depending on the burn care protocol, dressings are changed one to three times a day. Because exposed nerve endings can cause significant pain, wound assessment and care should be done as quickly as possible. Narcotic or non-narcotic pain medications are administered 20 to 30 minutes before dressing changes to

**TABLE 49.6 Topical Antimicrobial Agents Commonly Used for Burns**

| Advantages | Side Effects and Disadvantages | Nursing Considerations |
|---|---|---|
| **Silver Nitrate Solution** | | |
| Effective against most gram-positive and some gram-negative organisms | Hyponatremia, hypokalemia, hypochloremia<br>Decreased penetration of eschar<br>Not effective against established infection<br>Requires large, bulky dressings that limit mobility | 0.5% solution in distilled water applied to wet dressing every 2 hr<br>Dressing changes twice daily<br>Can cause staining of linens and clothing and interferes with accurate wound assessment |
| **Mafenide Acetate Cream (Sulfamylon)** | | |
| Effective against a wide range of gram-positive and gram-negative organisms<br>Rapid penetration through eschar (improved effectiveness in established infections)<br>Permits open treatment of wound, thus increasing mobility | Painful on application<br>Causes hypersensitivity reaction in 5%-7% of patients<br>Associated with acid–base alteration (metabolic acidosis) | Applied to cleansed wound once or twice daily<br>Treated area usually left open; a light dressing may be used<br>Must be completely removed before reapplication<br>Check sensitivity to sulfonamides |
| **Silver Sulfadiazine Cream (Silvadene)** | | |
| Effective against a wide range of gram-positive and gram-negative organisms<br>Soothing on application<br>Moderate eschar penetration<br>Absorbed slowly, reducing the possibility of nephrotoxicity | Causes hypersensitivity reaction in 5%-7% of patients<br>Associated with initial decrease in leukocyte count (transient) | Applied to cleansed wound once or twice daily<br>Wound is left open or covered with light dressing<br>Check sensitivity to sulfonamides<br>Must remove all medication before reapplication |

ensure maximum pain control at the time of the procedure. The child life specialist can assist with teaching the child how to use nonpharmacologic pain relief techniques.

Besides pain control, measures to maintain the child's core body temperature, minimize shivering, and conserve energy also must be implemented as part of wound care activities. To the degree possible, the child's capacity for self-care should be optimized. Allowing the child to remove dressings provides a measure of control.

Aseptic technique is used during dressing changes. After dressings are applied to burn wounds, isolation is not necessary and the child does not need to be restricted to a room or to an area of the hospital.

## PATIENT-CENTERED TEACHING

### *Home Care for a Child With Burns*

Often it is the parents' responsibility to care for the burn wound at home, supported by daily visits to the office or clinic for débridement and wound assessment.

**Parents Will Need to Know the Following to Adequately Care for the Child:**

- Type of cleaning method used to remove old antimicrobial ointment
- Where to obtain the topical ointment and dressing supplies
- How often to visit the office or clinic (the nurse provides the telephone number and a list of scheduled appointments)

**Teach the Parents the Following:**

- Use principles of aseptic technique. Use sterile gloves and applicators and know where to obtain these supplies. Know how to put on the gloves; give a return demonstration.
- If required to change the dressing, give the child medication for pain (if needed) 20 to 30 minutes before starting the procedure. Enlist other family members to provide distraction or to help hold the child.
- Wash the area with mild soap and tepid water or sterile saline solution. The old dressing can be soaked in tepid water to loosen it and decrease the discomfort of its removal.
- Apply the prescribed ointment and a light gauze dressing. Cover the area with a tubular net bandage, if possible, rather than wrapping with flexible gauze.
- Recognize signs and symptoms of infection; provide adequate fluids, and be sure the child's nutritional needs are met.
- Encourage the child in activities appropriate for age and development.
- Keep follow-up appointments.

## NURSING CARE PLAN

### *The Child With a Minor Partial-Thickness Burn*

**Focused Assessment**

- Rapidly assess for burn severity, considering the following:
  - Minor burn: Pain, wound condition, and potential for outpatient management
  - Moderate burn: Pain, wound condition, and possible need for fluid resuscitation
  - Severe burn: Multisystem assessment and possible transfer to a burn center
- Assess vital signs, particularly temperature, and determine risk for rapid heat loss leading to hypothermia.
- Obtain neurologic signs: Child should be awake and alert.
- Regular pain assessment both before and after intervention.
- Assess extremity range of motion and child's ability to independently perform activities of daily living (ADLs).

**Nursing Diagnosis**

Risk for Infection related to thermal tissue injury.

**Planning**

***Expected Outcome***

The burn will heal without infection, as evidenced by normal temperature, lack of purulent drainage, normal granulating tissue, and restoration of the epithelial layer.

**Interventions and *Rationales***

1. Clean and débride the wound daily and apply antimicrobial ointments and dressings as ordered. Document and record healing and any signs of wound infection, particularly fever and any change in wound appearance (drainage, odor). Obtain specimens for culture if ordered.
   *Infection can be prevented by removing bacterial contamination, exudate, and previously applied medication. Early detection of infection will ensure proper treatment and prevention of complications.*
2. Maintain aseptic technique for wound care.
   *An open skin surface allows for organism entry.*
3. Make sure that the child's tetanus toxoid immunizations are current.
   *Anaerobic bacteria can cause infection at the interface between the burn wound and healthy tissue.*

**Evaluation**

Is the tissue pink and free from exudate?

Is the child free of fever and other signs of infection?

**Nursing Diagnosis**

Impaired Skin Integrity related to thermal tissue injury and scratching of a healing wound.

**Planning**

***Expected Outcome***

The skin will exhibit progressively normal granulation, and restoration of the epithelial layer.

**Interventions and *Rationales***

1. Administer antihistamines as ordered.
   *Itching persists for several months after burns heal as new nerve endings and dermal elements reestablish themselves. Antihistamines such as diphenhydramine hydrochloride (Benadryl) reduce itching.*
2. Apply soothing lotions, such as Nivea or Eucerin, to healing skin.
   *These lotions reduce dryness, which is a factor contributing to itching.*
3. Keep the child's hands clean at all times and the fingernails cut short. Encourage the child not to scratch or rub healing skin.
   *These actions reduce the risk of impairing skin integrity.*
4. Promote adequate fluid and nutritional intake. Offer, or encourage the parent to offer, high-calorie, high-protein meals and snacks. Provide foods that the

## NURSING CARE PLAN—cont'd

### *The Child With a Minor Partial-Thickness Burn*

child likes. Arrange the timing of meals so that they do not immediately precede or follow painful or distressing events.
*Healing occurs only in the presence of a positive nitrogen balance. The child's protein and calorie needs are elevated because of increased metabolism and catabolism.*

5. Perform active and passive range-of-motion exercises of the affected parts of the child's body; this can be done at the time of dressing change and between dressing changes.
*Using the burned area promotes edema reabsorption and prevents contracture deformity.*
6. Administer vitamins and minerals (vitamins A, B, and C and iron and zinc) as ordered, or encourage the parent to do so.
*Vitamin and mineral supplements facilitate wound healing and epithelialization.*
7. Instruct the child and parents to keep the healed burn wound out of the sun for at least 1 year.
*Burned skin is more sensitive to sunlight, which increases the risk of sunburn.*

**Evaluation**

Does the burn wound show signs of progressive healing?
Is the skin smooth and pink without excessive scar tissue?
Is the child's itching controlled in a way that reduces scratching?

**Nursing Diagnosis**

Acute Pain related to thermal injury and related procedures.

**Planning**

***Expected Outcomes***

1. The child will describe decreased pain on an age-appropriate pain assessment scale, except during procedures and physical therapy.
2. The child will exhibit age-appropriate behaviors, appropriate nutritional intake, and appropriate sleep patterns.

**Interventions and *Rationales***

1. Determine the child's pain level with an age-appropriate assessment tool.
*The child's developmental stage affects response to pain, and the child's response to various pain assessment tools is related to developmental level.*
2. Administer pain relief measures and medication on a scheduled basis rather than on demand. Premedicate the child at least 20 to 30 minutes before painful procedures and advise the parent to do the same before the physician visit.
*Regular administration of pain relief controls pain and prevents cyclic episodes of severe pain, which are more difficult to manage effectively.*
3. Minimize the time spent on wound manipulation and exposure.
*Exposure of the burned area to air or water causes pain because the nerve endings are exposed. Dressing changes should be done as quickly as possible to minimize pain.*
4. Use nonpharmacologic pain reduction measures.
*Distraction, relaxation techniques, therapeutic touch, and other measures may help alleviate pain.*
5. Perform passive and active range-of-motion exercises. Be careful that dressings are applied so as to preserve function of body parts.
*Exercise, although painful in the acute stage, reduces the likelihood of contracture formation and increases functional ability.*

***Evaluation***

Except during times of direct wound care and physical therapy, is the child pain free, as evidenced by decreased pain assessment score and normal sleep, play, and eating patterns?
Is the child able to cooperate with dressing changes and range-of-motion exercises?

***Nursing Diagnosis***

Risk for Deficient Fluid Volume related to fluid shifts into burned tissue.

**Planning**

***Expected Outcome***

The child will maintain normal fluid and electrolyte balance, as evidenced by intake and output measurements and serum electrolyte values within normal ranges, moist mucous membranes, and good skin turgor on unaffected area.

***Interventions and Rationales***

1. Administer fluids orally or intravenously as ordered.
*Fluids help maintain capillary circulation to the viable skin appendages and general circulation to the vital organs. Fluid replacement continues until wound coverage is achieved.*
2. Instruct the parents to monitor the child's intake and output frequently.
*Close monitoring is necessary to determine whether fluid resuscitation is adequate. Fluid intake sufficient to produce age-appropriate hourly urine output (see Chapter 40) ensures adequate tissue perfusion.*
3. Weigh the hospitalized child daily.
*Weight is an accurate measurement of hydration status. Increasing weight may indicate fluid overload.*
4. Monitor laboratory values for elevated electrolyte or hemoglobin levels.
*Early identification of abnormal laboratory values permits early treatment of fluid volume imbalances.*

**Evaluation**

Is the child's urine output adequate for age? (See Chapter 40.)
Are serum electrolyte values within normal ranges?
Does the child appear well hydrated with moist mucous membranes and appropriate skin turgor?
Does the child take fluids well?

**Nursing Diagnosis**

Disturbed Body Image related to altered appearance of the healing burn.

**Planning**

***Expected Outcomes***

1. The child will re-enter previous social settings and express a feeling of comfort in these areas.
2. The child will discuss feelings about others' reactions to the change in appearance.
3. The family will provide emotional support for the child.

**Interventions and *Rationales***

1. Encourage the child to verbalize feelings about appearance and about returning to school.
*Identifying the child's concerns and anxieties is the first step in developing effective coping strategies.*
2. Provide honest answers to the child's questions regarding appearance.
*Honesty builds trust and helps the child develop realistic expectations.*
3. Encourage the family's involvement in the child's care (see Patient-Centered Teaching: Home Care for a Child with Burns).
4. Encourage the child to provide age-appropriate self-care.
*Participating in self-care helps increase self-esteem.*
5. Identify support systems and coping mechanisms used in previous times of stress or crisis.

*Continued*

## NURSING CARE PLAN—cont'd

### The Child With a Minor Partial-Thickness Burn

*Strategies that were previously effective can be mobilized to aid the child and family through a stressful period.*

6. Engage the assistance of a child life specialist to work with the child to identify feelings.
   *Children can often best express feelings through play and art.*
7. Discuss ways in which the child can "cover up" any disfigurement through clothing and makeup.
   *Cosmetics can decrease or minimize the disfigurement.*
8. Visit the child's school before the child's return or remain in contact with the school nurse.
   *Prepare the child's classmates for the changes in the child's appearance and engage them in making the re-entry a positive experience through acceptance. If visiting is not possible, the school nurse can assist the child with the transition to school.*

**Evaluation**

Does the child express a desire to reengage social contacts?

Is the child able to express fears related to the reactions of others?

Does the family support the child emotionally and encourage her or him to express feelings?

## CONDITIONS ASSOCIATED WITH MAJOR BURN INJURIES

For a child with a major burn injury, initial assessment and care focus on the primary survey (see Chapter 34) and particularly establishing and maintaining the child's airway, breathing, and circulation. After an airway and IV access have been established, a catheter is inserted into the bladder to begin hourly urine output measurements, and a nasogastric tube is inserted into the stomach to prevent aspiration.

Burn shock is a hypovolemic condition that develops after a burn injury affecting more than 15% to 20% of TBSA in children. The mechanisms of burn shock are not well understood, but the sequence of major burn injury followed by massive capillary leakage of circulating fluid into the surrounding tissues is well recognized.

Within minutes of a major burn injury, all the capillaries in the circulatory system, not just those in the area of the burn, lose their capillary seal, resulting in leakage of intravascular body fluid into the interstitial spaces. Erythrocytes and leukocytes remain in the circulation and produce an elevated hematocrit and leukocyte count. The process of burn shock continues for approximately 24 to 48 hours, at which time the capillary seal is restored.

Treatment for burn shock is aimed at supporting the child through the period of hypovolemic shock until capillary integrity is restored. To maintain adequate circulating volume, IV fluids are administered at a rate greater than the rate of fluid loss. Fluid resuscitation depends primarily on crystalloid solutions, particularly during the first 24 hours after injury, although recent studies show that colloid resuscitation (plasma) has the potential to decrease the amount of fluids needed to maintain adequate urine output and prevent complications. Clinicians must continually aim for the ideal balance between over and under-fluid resuscitation in an attempt to obtain the best outcomes and avoid complications. Fluid resuscitation depends primarily on crystalloid solutions, particularly during the first 24 hours after injury, although evidence shows that colloid resuscitation (plasma) has the potential to decrease the amount of fluids needed to maintain adequate urine output and prevent complications, such as increased intraabdominal pressure (Bacomo & Chung, 2011). Various formulas are used to calculate the rate of fluid administration. The specific protocol for fluid resuscitation remains controversial. In the absence of clinical trials to identify best burn resuscitation practices, protocols are determined by the burn unit or healthcare facility. In general, the amount of fluid replacement in children is calculated according to body surface area. Typically, half the calculated fluid amount is given over the first 8 hours after the burn, and the remaining half is given over the next 16 hours.

Because urine output reflects end-organ tissue perfusion, IV fluids are administered at a rate sufficient to maintain the child's urine output at a value appropriate for age (see Chapter 40). Inadequate urine output during burn shock is usually the result of insufficient administration of resuscitative fluids. Renal failure is not an expected component of burn shock if an adequate volume of IV fluids is being administered for burn shock resuscitation. It should be recognized that burn shock fluid resuscitation formulas are guidelines; individual children may need more fluids during the first 24 hours after the burn.

Table 49.7 lists additional physiologic effects caused by moderate to major burns. Once a child with a moderate or major burn has been stabilized, he or she usually is transferred to a burn center for specialized care.

## CONDITIONS ASSOCIATED WITH ELECTRICAL INJURY

Electrical injury is a major injury that often results in instant death because the electrical current disrupts the electrical rhythm of the heart. The child who does not die instantly is at risk for four major complications during the acute phase:

- Cardiac arrest or dysrhythmia
- Tissue damage
- Myoglobinuria (globulin from muscle serum appearing in the urine)
- Metabolic acidosis

### Cardiac Arrest or Dysrhythmia

The immediate risk is cardiac arrest or dysrhythmia resulting from damage to the heart's electrical conduction system. If cardiac arrest occurs, standard cardiac life support measures are initiated (see Chapter 34).

### Tissue Damage

The electrical current follows the path of least resistance through the body. Entering through the skin, electricity causes heat damage to the skin layers, bone, nerves, tendons, and blood vessels. The heat of the electrical current coagulates blood vessels and leaves the affected area without a blood supply. Gangrene develops in necrotic tissue unless it is removed. Amputation is necessary in more than 90% of children sustaining electrical injuries. The location of the damage depends on the child's position and exposure. Electricity might enter one hand and exit from the other, for example, or travel through the body and exit from one or both legs. The greatest damage occurs at the entrance and exit sites.

**TABLE 49.7 Body System Alterations After Moderate to Severe Burns**

| System/Alteration | Cause | Management |
|---|---|---|
| **Respiratory** | | |
| Upper airway tissue injury with respiratory distress, possible obstruction | Edema from inhalation of superheated air | Establish adequate airway, provide moist mist with oxygen as needed |
| Lower airway tissue injury | Inhalation of smoke | Give oxygen as needed, place child in a head-elevated position, intubate with ventilatory support if necessary |
| Carbon monoxide inhalation, hypoxia | End products of combustion | Give 100% oxygen by mask; intubate and provide ventilatory support if necessary |
| Limited chest expansion | Circumferential burns | Escharotomy |
| **Cardiovascular** | | |
| Fluid volume deficit with decreased cardiac output; tachycardia | Fluid shifts from vascular to interstitial compartment; massive leaking of fluid through the burn wound | Provide fluid and electrolyte replacement with or without colloids; goal is to achieve urinary output appropriate for age and good capillary refill |
| Initial vasodilation, then vasoconstriction | Compensatory mechanism to preserve fluid volume and prevent shock | |
| Edema, compartment syndrome | Increased fluid in interstitial spaces | |
| Elevated hemoglobin, hematocrit levels | Hemoconcentration caused by fluid loss | |
| Increase followed by decrease in serum potassium levels | Release of destroyed tissue cells into extracellular space | |
| Decreased serum sodium levels | Trapped in edema fluids | |
| **Gastrointestinal** | | |
| Gastric dilation, paralytic ileus | Decreased perfusion to gastrointestinal tract as a result of hypovolemia | Restore fluid and electrolyte balance |
| Thirst | Hypovolemia | |
| **Renal** | | |
| Oliguria, elevated blood urea nitrogen and creatinine values | Reduced circulation to kidneys | Adequate fluid resuscitation |
| Risk for acute tubular necrosis | Obstruction of renal tubules | |
| **Metabolic** | | |
| Increased metabolic rate with elevated body temperature and massive evaporative heat loss | Insult of open wound | Provide caloric requirements two or three times basal requirements; provide high-protein diet or protein supplements; tube feed or use parenteral nutrition as necessary; provide vitamin C and vitamin A supplements |
| Catecholamine release | Burn stress; increased temperature and metabolic rate | |
| Hyperglycemia | Mobilization of glucagon and decreased insulin production | |
| **Hematologic** | | |
| Decreased hematocrit level follows initial hematocrit increase (from hemoconcentration) | Increased red blood cell (RBC) hemolysis, decreased RBC production, blood loss from wound care | Packed RBC transfusion for low hematocrit |
| Coagulation disorders | Decreased platelet count and serum clotting factors | |
| Increased immature neutrophils to digest products of injury | Depletion of mature neutrophils | |
| High risk for infection, wound sepsis, septic shock (disorientation, fever, diminished bowel sounds are first signs, temperature falls below normal as body's resistance to infection decreases) | Open wound; altered protective mechanisms; decreased circulation to the skin | Burn excision and débridement followed by application of topical antimicrobial agents; may need biologic or synthetic skin coverings, graft |
| **Pain** | | |
| | Tissue injury exposing nerve endings; edema; burn treatments | Meticulous pain management both around-the-clock and before treatments |

### Myoglobinuria

Myoglobinuria develops from release into the blood of products found in normal muscle; the release can be occasioned by electrical injury. Myoglobin is a large molecule that can mechanically obstruct the renal tubules and lead to acute tubular necrosis unless large amounts of IV fluid are administered to flush the myoglobin out of the kidneys. The administration of osmotic diuretics promotes increased urine volume. IV fluid is administered at a rate that maintains urine output at 2 mL/kg/hr until the myoglobinuria resolves.

### Metabolic Acidosis

Metabolic acidosis follows electrical injury because of the associated cellular destruction and hypovolemic shock. Ringer's lactate solution (the fluid used for fluid resuscitation) contains sufficient bicarbonate to manage the acidosis that accompanies burn shock but not enough to correct that associated with shock after electrical injury (i.e., pathophysiologic hypovolemic shock, not a "shock" from the electrical current).

### Other Complications

The four complications just described usually resolve within 24 hours after injury. Other complications that follow electrical injury include loss of short-term memory and altered emotional states. Children can usually remember events up to the time of injury, including the names of family members and their own address, telephone number, and personal information, but they are unable to recall more recent events. This loss of memory can be distressing to the child and frustrating to the family. For example, the child might be unable to remember visits by the family, and thus, feels abandoned by them. It is difficult for the child to follow instructions if they have difficulty retaining them; this condition can cause difficulty in planning care. Altered emotional states include an absence of affect and blank stares or the opposite type of emotional response—manic behavior, hyperactivity, swearing, physical violence, and feelings of paranoia. Emotional responses usually become normal after approximately 1 week but persist longer in some children. The electrical injury need not be to the head for these altered states to occur.

The long-term sequelae of electrical injury include neurologic deficits, amputations, and ocular cataracts. Ocular cataracts can occur in one or both eyes at varying times from 3 months to 18 months after injury. In the very young child, changes in visual acuity can go unnoticed; therefore, regular eye examinations should be scheduled every 3 months for the first year after injury.

## KEY CONCEPTS

- The functions of the skin include protection, thermoregulation, excretion, production of vitamin D, and sensation.
- The skin comprises two major layers—the outer epidermis and the inner supportive dermis. The dermis contains blood vessels, nerves, and sweat glands. Beneath these layers is subcutaneous tissue, which attaches the dermis to the underlying structures.
- Developmental differences cause the skin of infants and children to be more susceptible to external irritants and infection than adults' skin.
- Neonates frequently exhibit a variety of birthmarks. Many of these resolve spontaneously, but some are associated with other congenital syndromes.
- Diaper dermatitis is much easier to prevent than to treat. Successful treatment and prevention of diaper rash entail thorough cleansing of the diaper area and keeping the skin dry.
- Nursing care for the child with eczema includes frequent skin moisturizing and cautioning against the use of clothing, fabrics, or soaps that might irritate the skin. Identifying and eliminating allergens may be helpful.
- Impetigo, the most common skin infection of childhood, is highly contagious. Nursing care includes administration of topical or oral antibiotics and education regarding good hand hygiene to prevent spread of infection.
- Because the fungus that causes tinea thrives where it is moist and warm, infected areas should be kept as dry as possible. Proper hygiene should be taught and maintained to minimize the spread of infection.
- Herpes simplex virus is transmitted by infected body fluids coming in contact with breaks in the skin or mucous membranes. Careful handwashing and attention to hygiene decrease the risk of spreading infection.
- Preventing reinfestation is a primary goal in the treatment of pediculosis and scabies.
- Nursing care of the adolescent with acne includes teaching about regular, gentle cleansing of the skin, applying topical medications, and encouraging a healthy lifestyle with adequate rest, exercise, and a balanced diet. The nurse must be sensitive to the effect of acne on the adolescent's self-image.
- Insect bites and stings can cause severe systemic reactions in a sensitized child.
- Young children are at increased risk for burn injuries because they are curious, mobile, and totally dependent on their caretakers for safety.
- The extent of a burn injury (depth, severity) determines whether the child will have a local or a systemic reaction.
- The depth of a burn injury is classified as superficial, superficial partial thickness, deep partial thickness, or full thickness.
- Compared to adults, children who sustain burn injuries are at greater risk for fluid and heat loss, hypertrophic scarring, cardiovascular problems, infection, and protein and calorie deficiency.
- In calculating the TBSA burned, a body surface chart that is corrected for age should be used.
- A minor burn wound should be cleaned with mild soap and water, debrided of loose debris and tissue, and covered with an antimicrobial ointment and a sterile dressing.
- After stabilization, a child with a major burn is cared for in a burn treatment center because of multiple body system complications.

## REFERENCES AND READINGS


American Academy of Dermatology. (2015). *Atopic dermatitis: Topical calcineurin inhibitors recommendations.* Retrieved from https://www.aad.org.

American Academy of Pediatrics. (2015a). *Healthy children: Lice.* Retrieved from http://www.healthychildren.org.

American Academy of Pediatrics. (2015b). *Impetigo.* Retrieved from http://www.healthychildren.org.

American Academy of Pediatrics. (2015c). *Impetigo Care.* Retrieved from http://www.healthychildren.org.

American Academy of Pediatrics. (2015d). *Tinea Infections* Retrieved from http://www.healthychildren.org/.

American Academy of Pediatrics Patient Education Online. (2015). *Diaper rash.* Retrieved from http://www.healthychildren.org.

Antaya, R. (2014). *Capillary malformation.* Retrieved from http://www.emedicine.medscape.com.

Antoon, A., & Donovan, M. (2016). Burn injuries. In R. Kliegman, B. Stanton, J. St. Geme, et al. (Eds.), *Nelson textbook of pediatrics* (20th ed., Chapter 75). St. Louis, MO: Elsevier.

Bacomo, F.K., & Chung, K.K. (2011). A primer on burn resuscitation. *Journal of Emergencies, Trauma and Shock, 4*(1), 109–113. doi: 10.4103/0974-2700.76845.

Centers for Disease Control and Prevention. (2013). *Lice: body lice.* Retrieved from http://www.cdc.gov.

Centers for Disease Control and Prevention. (2014). *Ten leading causes of injury deaths by age group: highlighting unintentional injury deaths, United States – 2013.* Retrieved from http://www.cdc.gov.

Centers for Disease Control and Prevention. (2015a). *Parasites-lice-head lice.* Retrieved from http://www.cdc.gov.

Centers for Disease Control and Prevention. (2015b). *Parasites –scabies.* Retrieved from http://www.cdc.gov/parasites/.

Centers for Disease Control and Prevention. (2015c). *West Nile virus-updated information regarding mosquito repellents.* Retrieved from http://www.cdc.gov.

Devore, C.D., Schutze, G.E., & The Council on School Health and Committee on Infections Diseases. (2015). Head lice. *Pediatrics, 135*(5), e1355–e1365.

Eichenfield, L.F., Tom, W.L., Chamlin, S.L, et al. (2014). Guidelines of care for the management of atopic dermatitis: part 1 diagnosis and assessment of atopic dermatitis. *Journal of American Academy of Dermatology, 70*(2), 338–351. doi: 10.1016/j.jaad.2013.10.010.

Farooq, A.V., & Shukla, D. (2012). Herpes simplex epithelial and stromal keratitis: an epidemiologic update. *Survey of Ophthalmology, 57*(5), 448–462. doi: 10.1016/j.survophthal.2012.01.005.

Gailbraith, S. (2016). Acne. In R. Kliegman, B. Stanton, J. St. Geme, et al. (Eds.), *Nelson textbook of pediatrics* (20th ed., Chapter 669). St. Louis, MO: Elsevier.

Golden, D., Moffitt, J., & Nicklas, R. (2011). *Stinging insect hypersensitivity: a practice parameter update 2011.* Retrieved from http://www.aaaai.org.

Gonzalez, R., & Shanti, C.M. (2015). Overview of current pediatric burn care. *Seminars in Pediatric Surgery, 24,* 47–49.

Leung, D., & Sicherer, S. (2016). Atopic dermatitis (atopic eczema). In R. Kliegman, B. Stanton, J. St. Geme, et al. (Eds.), *Nelson textbook of pediatrics* (20th ed., Chapter 145). St. Louis, MO: Elsevier.

Looker, K.J., Magaret, A.S., May, M.T., et al. (2015). Global and regional estimates of prevalent and incident herpes simplex virus type 1 infections in 2012. *PLoS ONE, 10*(10), e0140765. doi: 10.1371/journal.pone.0140765.

Martin, K. (2016a). Diseases of the neonate. In R. Kliegman, B. Stanton, J. St. Geme, et al. (Eds.), *Nelson textbook of pediatrics* (20th ed., Chapter 647). St. Louis, MO: Elsevier.

Martin, K. (2016b). Vascular disorders. In R. Kliegman, B. Stanton, J. St. Geme, et al. (Eds.), *Nelson textbook of pediatrics* (20th ed., Chapter 650). St. Louis, MO: Elsevier.

Sanders, J.E., & Garcia, S.E. (2014). Pediatric herpes simplex virus infections: an evidence-based approach to treatment. *Pediatric Emergency Medicine Practice, 11*(1). Retrieved from http://www.slremeducation.org.

Sethuraman, G., Yenamandra, V., & Gupta, V. (2014). Management of infantile hemangiomas: current trends. *Journal of Cutaneous and Aesthetic Surgery, 7*(2), 75–85.

Skin Cancer Foundation. (2015). *Skin cancer.* Retrieved from http://www.skincancer.org.

Stanberry, L. (2016). Herpes simplex virus. In R. Kliegman, B. Stanton, J. St. Geme, et al. (Eds.), *Nelson textbook of pediatrics* (20th ed., Chapter 252). St. Louis, MO: Elsevier.

Vascular Birthmarks Foundation. (2015). *Port wine stain information.* Retrieved from http://www.birthmark.org.

Velez, R., VanGraafeiland, B., & Sloand, E. (2015). Using clinical guidelines and clinical acumen to manage community-acquired methicillin-resistant *Staphylococcus aureus* infection. *The Journal for Nurse Practitioners, 11*(1), 124–130.

Victoire A., Magin, P., Coughlan, J., et al. (2014). Interventions for infantile seborrhoeic dermatitis (including cradle cap). *Cochrane Database of Systematic Reviews,* 11, CD011380. doi: 10.1002/14651858.CD011380.

Wang, J., & Sicherer, S. (2016). Insect allergy. In R. Kliegman, B. Stanton, J. St. Geme, et al. (Eds.), *Nelson textbook of pediatrics* (20th ed., Chapter 146). St. Louis, MO: Elsevier.

White, S. (2011). The management of childhood atopic eczema. *Nurse Prescribing, 9*(10), 491–494.

50

# The Child With a Musculoskeletal Alteration

http://evolve.elsevier.com/McKinney/mat-ch/

## LEARNING OBJECTIVES

*After studying this chapter, you should be able to:*

- Describe the implications of the differences in the anatomy and physiology of the growing musculoskeletal systems of infants and young children in comparison to the mature musculoskeletal system.
- Describe the pathology, etiology, manifestations, diagnostic evaluation, and therapeutic management of musculoskeletal alterations frequently seen in infants, children, and adolescents.
- Identify characteristic assessments that indicate alterations in musculoskeletal function.
- State appropriate nursing diagnoses for children with an alteration in musculoskeletal function.
- Summarize the treatment modalities used to manage the child with a musculoskeletal alteration.
- Design, implement, and evaluate appropriate nursing interventions for the child with altered musculoskeletal function.

# CLINICAL REFERENCE

## REVIEW OF THE MUSCULOSKELETAL SYSTEM

The nursing care for a child with a musculoskeletal alteration requires an understanding of the structure and function of the musculoskeletal system, comprehension of growth and development, and an awareness of the differences in the musculoskeletal system of infants and children as compared to adults.

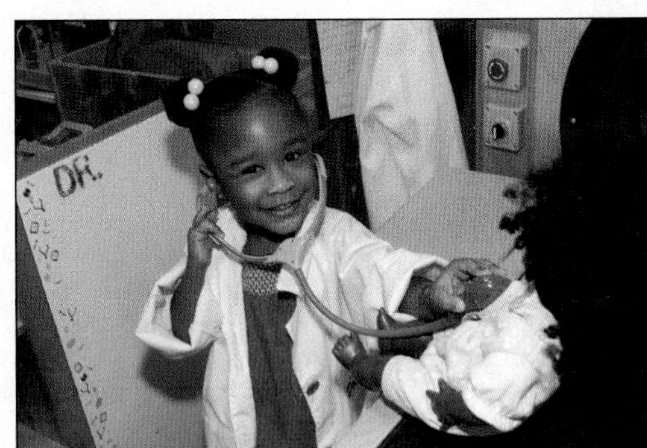

Child with hand differences.

### Skeletal System

The musculoskeletal system is composed of bones attached to joints, joints connected by ligaments, muscles supported by tendons, and cartilaginous tissues. The function of this system is to provide a skeletal framework to support the body, protect vital organs, and provide movement. It also supplies a storage space for the blood cell production and minerals responsible for regulating resorption and reformation of itself, as well as regulation of mineral and hormonal imbalances in the body (Huether & McCance, 2017).

Newborns are born with more bones than adults have, because cranial bones and other small bones, such as bones in the coccyx or sacrum, fuse during infancy and childhood, resulting in the adult complement of 206. The newborn's skeletal structure is mostly cartilaginous at birth, then evolves and ossifies through osteogenesis. There are two distinct types of **ossification**: intramembranous and endochondral ossification. Intramembranous ossification is the process in which osteoblasts form bone without the cartilaginous stage (Baldwin, Wells & Dormans, 2016a). Endochondral ossification occurs when the mesenchyme differentiates to cartilage, and cartilage then transforms into bone within primary and secondary ossification centers. Primary ossification occurs in the diaphysis (center of the bone), whereas secondary ossification occurs at the epiphysis (end of the bones). The physis, or growth plate, is formed between the primary and secondary ossification center and allows for longitudinal growth of long bones (Baldwin et al., 2016a). The growth plate absorbs shock and protects the joint surfaces from serious fractures. The metaphysis (above the growth plate) is composed mostly of cartilage and is the area that grows between the diaphysis and epiphysis to form solid bone in adulthood. Anatomic location is important for discussing sites of infection, neoplasm, fractures, and metabolic and endocrine disorders.

The periosteum is a vascular connective tissue that lines the outer surface of all bones. It has receptor nerve endings, and is the site of attachment for muscle, ligaments, and tendons (Scott et al., 2015). The periosteum contributes to bone development by appositional bone growth and has the capability to heal fractures and regenerate bone rapidly in children.

There are five classifications of bones: long bones, such as the femur; short bones, such as the carpals; irregular bones, such as the vertebrae; flat bones, such as the ribs; and sesamoid (sometimes

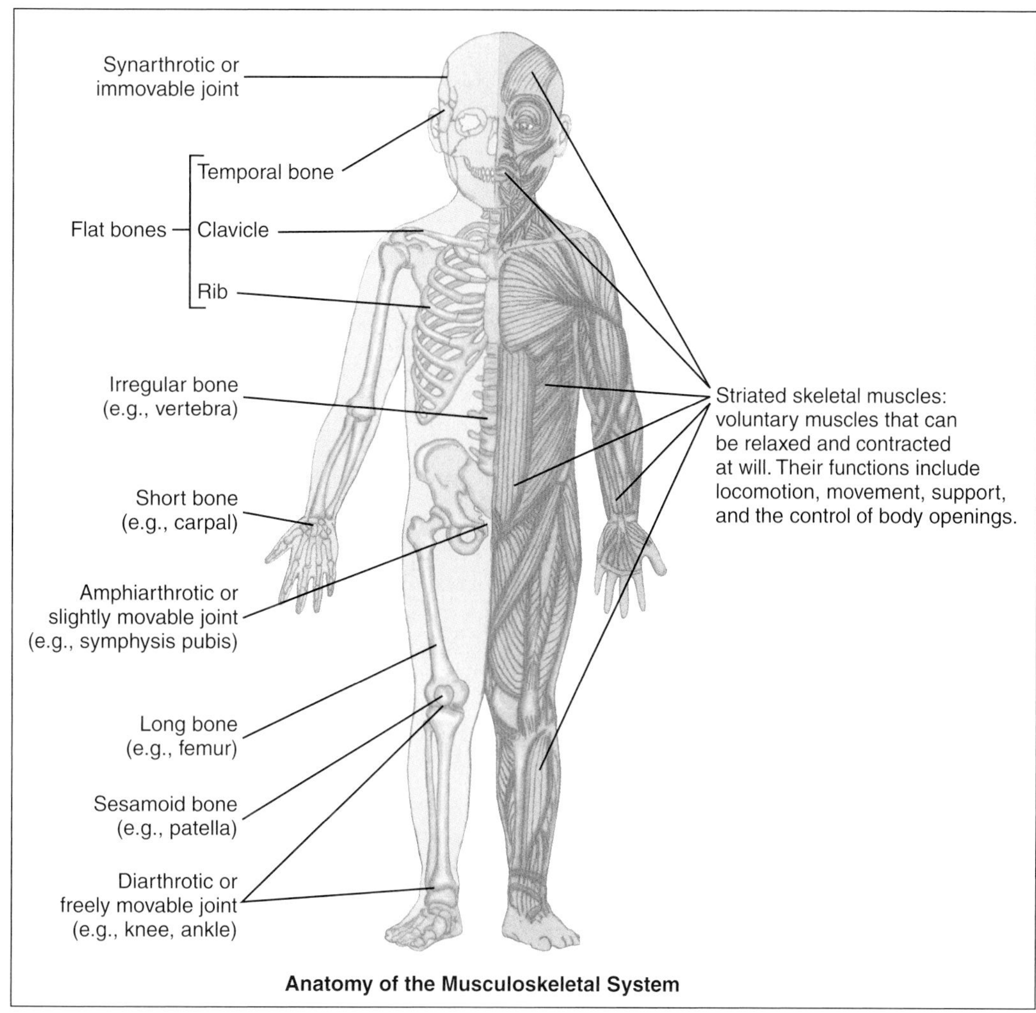


Anatomy of the Musculoskeletal System

classified as short) bones, such as the patella. There are also two major divisions to the skeletal system: the axial skeleton, which forms longitudinally and includes the vertebral column and the skull; and the appendicular system, which is attached to the axial skeleton and encompasses the pelvis, pectoral girdle, and upper and lower extremities (Huether & McCance, 2017).

## Articular System

Joints, which are composed of connective tissue and cartilage, connect two or more bones to one another and enable movement. Joints are classified by structure, function, and movement. In general, joints are freely movable (e.g., the hip) (Huether & McCance, 2017).

Alterations in joint movement and swelling require further evaluation. Defective joints are often seen in children with neuromuscular disorders such as spina bifida and arthrogryposis. Alterations in joint movement and swelling can also be indicative of trauma, infection, or arthritis.

## Muscular System

Muscles help stabilize joints and maintain contact between articular surfaces. Skeletal muscles are attached by tendons to bones. Ligaments bind one bone firmly to another, and the joints are further stabilized by the overlying tendons and muscles. The shape of the two ends of each muscle and of the joint determines the extent of movement or articulation. Skeletal muscles, which are composed of elongated fibers, function voluntarily and produce movement by contraction. Muscle disease in children presents as muscle weakness, spasticity, myoclonus, and myalgia (Baldwin, Wells, & Dormans, 2016b).

## Cartilage

Cartilage is dense connective tissue that develops at the epiphysis and is capable of withstanding considerable tension. During early fetal development, the skeletal structure is composed mostly of cartilage. In time it will largely convert to bone by ossification. Connective tissue is made up of collagen and proteoglycans (Matsiko, Levingstone, & O'Brien, 2013).

## Growth and Development

Knowledge of normal growth and development is essential when assessing, caring for, and evaluating the pediatric patient's musculoskeletal system. Infants experience the greatest growth rate. During childhood, growth slows and then increases rapidly again in adolescence with peak height velocity. Peak height velocity is the maximum growth that occurs during puberty. Growth in the length of the long bones continues at the epiphysis until adult height is reached (see Chapter 9).

Children should be weighed and measured for length or stature with each visit. The results of these measurements should consistently

## Pediatric Differences in the Musculoskeletal System

- In the fetus, bony tissue begins to develop as closely packed connective tissue. Connective tissue is replaced by cartilage, and cartilage is replaced by mineral salts, which give rise to solid bone. The infant's bones are only 65% ossified at 8 months of age and are neither as firm nor as brittle as those of the older child.
- The periosteum of the child's bone is much stronger than that of adults.
- New bony tissue is produced during periods of growth. The rate of growth varies at different ages. Skeletal growth is stimulated by pituitary growth hormone. Growth of the long bones occurs at the epiphyses, which are located at the ends of the bones and separated from the main portion of the bone by cartilage during the period of growth. Injury to the epiphyses can cause growth disturbances.
- Growing bones produce **callus** and heal quickly, making **internal fixation** of fractures unnecessary in most children. Fractures in children younger than 1 year are unusual due to the large amount of force necessary to break an infant's bone; abuse or underlying pathophysiology is often the cause of fractures in infants.
- The skull is not rigid during infancy, and the sutures of the cranium do not fuse completely until approximately 12 to 18 months of age. Increased intracranial pressure can separate the sutures, causing the infant's head to enlarge.
- Muscle tissue is almost completely developed at birth. Growth occurs because of an increase in size rather than number of the muscle fibers.
- Postural changes during infancy and childhood result from the development of neurologic control, bone and muscle growth, and the laying down of adipose tissue. Postural changes are a good indication of the level of development of the musculoskeletal and neurologic systems.
- Soft tissues are resilient in children, so dislocations and sprains are also less common than in adults.

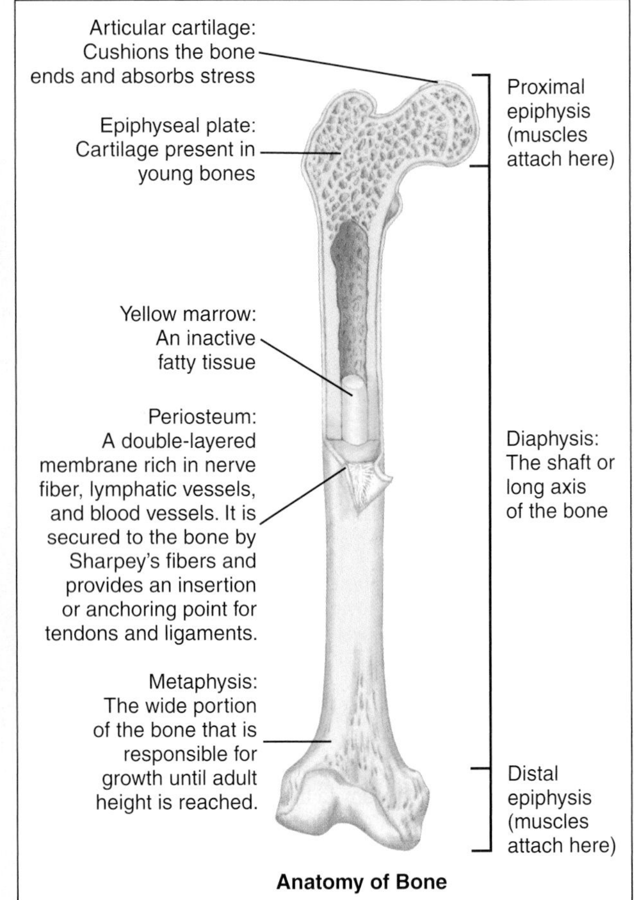

Anatomy of Bone

and correctly be plotted on appropriate growth and development graphs in order to be aware of any variations in height or weight (see Chapter 33).

A basic understanding of when children meet their major developmental milestones, especially for gross motor development, is crucial when assessing and treating the child with an alteration of the musculoskeletal system. Failure to meet these milestones in a timely manner can indicate hypotonia, cerebral palsy (hemiplegic), or a neuromuscular disorder. See Chapters 6 through 9 for developmental milestones in children of various developmental levels.

### Diagnostic and Laboratory Tests

Radiographs are the mainstay of an orthopedic evaluation. They provide important diagnostic evaluation after a clinical assessment when there is concern of a musculoskeletal abnormality. Studies have shown risks of cancer with radiation exposure in a growing child (Hendee & O'Connor, 2012). Several recommendations have been formulated to protect the child. Radiologists and technicians are to use the most diagnostically effective test with the least radiation exposure on children. In addition, care needs to be taken to shield the gonads, make sure the patient is placed in the correct anatomic position, use as low as possible dosing, take single radiographs instead of multiple views, and consult as needed with the provider ordering the x-rays (Dorfman et al., 2016). Noting the pediatric differences in plain films as compared to adults is important because the differences can lead to misinterpretation and over- or undertreatment. For example, children have open growth plates at the proximal and distal aspects of the long bones that can easily be confused with fractures. Furthermore, a periosteal reaction in the diaphysis after trauma or infection can be misinterpreted as normal (Schug et al., 2013).

Clinical laboratory tests are also useful in evaluating the patient with a suspected musculoskeletal alteration. Nurses must have a baseline comprehension of what the normal laboratory values are for each study to inform and educate the family about the results. Fasting is not required for these studies.

The hematology workup in orthopedics includes a complete blood count with a differential, C-reactive protein (CRP), and erythrocyte sedimentation rate (ESR) for musculoskeletal disorders (Baldwin et al., 2016b). CRP is a protein that appears in blood during an inflammatory process and is not seen in healthy people. The measurement is nonspecific, merely indicating the presence of inflammation. ESR is the rate at which erythrocytes settle out of unclotted blood, measured in millimeters per hour. Inflammation and necrotic problems cause an elevation in ESR levels.

Chemistry labs assist in the evaluation for metabolic conditions, such as rickets. These labs include studies of calcium, alkaline phosphatase (ALP), and phosphorus. ALP is an enzyme found mainly in bone, liver, placenta, and kidney. ALP levels are often elevated in bone disease, fractures, trauma, or liver disease and during periods of rapid growth. Tests might be ordered to differentiate between bone and liver problems.

Enzyme studies such as creatine phosphokinase (CPK) may be ordered. CPK is an enzyme found in heart and skeletal muscle; the CPK assay is a specific test for assessing cardiac and muscle damage.

## Common Diagnostic Procedures for Musculoskeletal Disorders in Children

| Purpose and Description | Nursing Implications |
|---|---|
| **Radiography (X-Ray)** | |
| *Purpose:* To detect abnormalities or to determine bone age.<br>*Description:* X-rays (gamma radiation) are passed through the body, reaching the film on the other side of the body and creating an image. Different densities of tissue absorb various amounts of radiation. The four densities of x-ray appear as follows:<br>Air: black<br>Fat: dark gray<br>Water: lighter gray<br>Bone: whitish | Noninvasive<br>Food and fluids are not usually restricted.<br>Clothing and jewelry that could interfere with the study are removed; a paper or cloth gown and shorts without metal are worn.<br>Young children may require assistance for proper positioning and immobilization.<br>Adequate preparation is essential to ensure cooperation. |
| **Ultrasound** | |
| *Purpose:* To demonstrate body tissue structure or for waveform analysis of Doppler studies<br>*Description:* The Doppler probe is held over the skin surface or in a body cavity, transmitting ultrasound waves to form two-dimensional images of muscles, tendons, cartilaginous tissues, bones, and internal organs. | Noninvasive<br>Food and fluid are not restricted except in small infants, who may be on nothing-by-mouth (NPO) status for 2-3 hr before the procedure so they can eat during the test.<br>Young children may require assistance for proper positioning and immobilization.<br>Adequate preparation is essential to ensure cooperation. |
| **Computed Tomography (CT)** | |
| *Purpose:* To visualize bony and soft tissue details<br>*Description:* Narrow-beam x-rays in a transverse plane are used to scan an area in successive layers. These images are then reconstructed by computer in the frontal plane and sagittal plane and can even be shown in three-dimensional cross section. *Disadvantages:* Greater radiation exposure; sedation may be required for infants and young children to keep still; significant costs | Noninvasive<br>Food and fluids are not restricted.<br>Although the procedure is painless, it may be frightening. Provide developmentally and culturally appropriate preparation and patient education. For example, "The machine looks and sounds like a large clothes dryer or washing machine."<br>Clothing and jewelry that may interfere with the study are removed; a paper or cloth gown and shorts without metal are worn.<br>The child must remain still during procedure, so young children need sedation and might be NPO for food and fluids for safety while sedated. Contrast medium is sometimes used. |
| **Magnetic Resonance Imaging (MRI)** | |
| *Purpose:* To clearly define organ structures; shows changes in soft tissue, such as edema, blood flow patterns, infarcts; demonstrates marrow, bone and soft tissue tumors, structure of muscles, ligaments, bones<br>*Description:* Performed by placing the patient on a moving table, which is pushed into a large cylinder that contains a huge magnet and radio waves that create an energy field that can be translated into a visual image. A variety of noises are heard during the procedure. In contrast to other diagnostic studies, it does not require radiation exposure.<br>*Disadvantages:* Cost | Noninvasive<br>Food and fluids are not restricted.<br>Patients are thoroughly screened to assure removal of any metal they might be wearing or have in their possession. The study is not done in children with metal implants, pacemakers, or prostheses. Provide developmentally and culturally appropriate preparation and patient education.<br>Procedure may take 1 hr or more. Adequate preparation, relaxation techniques, and parental presence decrease fear and feelings of claustrophobia. Use of a music headset or video can promote relaxation.<br>The child must remain still during procedure, so young children need sedation and may be NPO for food and fluids for safety while sedated. |
| **Radionuclide Scintigraphy (Bone Scan)** | |
| *Purpose:* To further investigate trauma with early stress fractures, tumors, and cysts to localize the lesion; infections, such as osteomyelitis and diskitis, **avascular necrosis** in Perthes; to screen for child abuse in some cases, and pain of unknown origin.*<br>*Description:* A radioactive material (technectium-99m) is administered intravenously, and then the body is scanned to evaluate for abnormal uptake after 3-4 hr.* | Encourage fluids 2-4 hr before the test to ensure the child is well hydrated and quickly eliminate radioactive material not absorbed by the bones. Child must void before the scan so that the pelvic bones can be seen.<br>Young children may need sedation. |
| **Arthrography** | |
| *Purpose:* To evaluate suspected joint damage, such as cartilage tears<br>*Description:* Dye is injected into the affected joint (usually the knee; sometimes the shoulder or other joint) to further evaluate the cartilaginous structure. | Check for allergies to iodine.<br>Provide developmentally and culturally appropriate preparation and patient education.<br>A local anesthetic is required. The child must remain still during the procedure, so young children may require assistance or sedation for proper positioning and immobilization. If sedated, the child may be NPO for food and fluids.<br>Joint should rest for approximately 12 hr; a compression dressing may be applied after procedure to reduce swelling. |

*Continued*

**Common Diagnostic Procedures for Musculoskeletal Disorders in Children—cont'd**

| Purpose and Description | Nursing Implications |
|---|---|
| **Joint Aspiration** | |
| Fluid is withdrawn for analysis, usually to detect infection, evaluate arthritis, or relieve pain. | Provide developmentally and culturally appropriate preparation and patient education.<br>A local anesthetic is required. The child must remain still during the procedure; so young children may require assistance or sedation for proper positioning and immobilization. If sedated, the child may be NPO for food and fluids. |
| **Arthroscopy** | |
| *Purpose:* To image the inside of a joint for diagnosis of injury or minor surgical repairs; arthrography is usually performed before arthroscopy.<br>*Description:* Fiberoptic endoscope is inserted to examine interior of joint. | Requires local or general anesthesia. The child must be on NPO status if general anesthesia is used; NPO status recommendations for local anesthesia vary with the practitioner.<br>Prepare the child for postoperative dressings, altered mobility, and pain.<br>Assess for infection. Prophylactic antibiotics may be ordered.<br>Use ice postoperatively to reduce swelling. |

*Texas Scottish Rite Children's Hosptial. (2014). Tachdjian's pediatric orthopaedics: from the Texas Scottish Rite Hospital for children: expert consult: online and print, 3- volume set (2 volumes in ... online only), 5th ed. Saunders.

Levels are elevated in trauma, myocardial infarction, and muscular dystrophy. Tests might be ordered to differentiate between cardiac (MB) and skeletal (MM) CPK.

Rheumatoid factor (RF) and a hematology workup are used to evaluate rheumatologic disorders (Baldwin et al., 2016b). RFs are antibodies that are associated with the destructive changes of rheumatoid arthritis. A positive RF with an elevated CRP and ESR is indicative of arthritis in children; however, RF is positive in less than 10% of these cases.

Musculoskeletal problems affect muscles, bones, joints, and tendons, all of which are necessary for movement, and thus, are critical to a child's development. Many musculoskeletal problems occur because of vigorous motor activities that are part of a child's daily life, but the rapid growth of the skeletal system also plays a significant role. Most musculoskeletal problems are short term, but a number of chronic musculoskeletal conditions require long-term treatment and nursing assistance.

The child with a musculoskeletal alteration presents a unique opportunity for nursing care. A general knowledge of the structure and function of the system is required to understand the rationale for the alteration. An awareness of normal versus abnormal growth and development patterns is necessary in order to recognize delays, variations, and medical conditions. An appreciation of the musculoskeletal differences exhibited in the pediatric patient in comparison to the adult is also essential. To implement nursing considerations, nurses should be familiar with the various diagnostic imaging procedures used in evaluating patients with musculoskeletal alterations. Knowledge of normal laboratory values commonly ordered for patients with musculoskeletal conditions is vital for providing prudent, good-quality, effective nursing care.

## CASTS, TRACTION, AND OTHER IMMOBILIZING DEVICES

Immobilizing a bone or joint helps achieve and maintain a more functional position or rests and protects an affected area during bone healing. Because many musculoskeletal problems require the application of an immobilizing device, the nurse should understand the general principles of care.

### Splints

Splints are used to stabilize and protect or rest an affected area, increase range of motion and function, and decrease pain (Texas Scottish Rite Children's Hosptial [TSRHC], 2014). Splints are fabricated of fiberglass, plaster of Paris, metal, or thermoplastic polymers. Splint materials are chosen for drapability, durability, softness, setup time, thickness, capacity for remolding, and color. Splinting is a safe, effective, and cost-saving alternative to casting for some conditions (Birrer, O'Connor, & Kane, 2016; von Keyserlingkl, Boutis, Willan, et al., 2016).

### Casts

A cast provides support and maintains anatomic position for bone healing or aids in correction of a deformity. Casts are also used to ensure adherence to treatment protocols or to protect a wound. The type and size of the cast are dictated by the child's age and size, type of fracture or injury, type of surgery, and amount of weight the extremity can bear.

Casts are made of synthetic materials, such as fiberglass, semirigid nonfiberglass (soft cast), or plaster of Paris (Birrer et al., 2016). Casting material comes in varied colors and patterns; casts can be wrapped and decorated to appeal to young children. The following equipment is needed for cast application:

- Tubular gauze/stockinette (optional)
- Waterproof lining (optional)
- Cotton under-cast padding material (e.g., Webril)
- Casting material, fiberglass and/or plaster of Paris (rolls and/or strips/splints)
- Water (clarify water temperature with professional applying cast)

- Moleskin
- Waterproof tape
- Scissors
- Cast remover (if needed to trim edges or split cast)

The cast is usually applied by the physician and another trained person, one to hold the extremity in correct alignment and one to apply the cast. It is very important not to move the affected area to be casted while applying the cast. A waterproof liner or stockinette is applied if desired. Waterproof linings for casts have been shown to be as effective as cotton lining for immobilization (Robert, Jiang, & Khoury, 2011). A thin layer of Webril is then applied over the initial lining. The material is rolled in a spiral fashion around the affected area, overlapping each layer by approximately 50%. Additional padding can be placed over bony prominences, making sure there are no wrinkles in any layer. Any wrinkles in the cast padding or cast material become "set" into the cast and can cause skin breakdown. Next, the casting material is dipped in water and applied over the cotton padding, making sure to leave a cotton edge at the top and bottom of the cast for patient comfort and to maintain skin integrity. A chemical reaction between casting material and water makes it feel warm and causes it to harden. The cast should not be covered while warm to prevent a burn.

Rough edges of casts must be trimmed to prevent injury. Petaling of cast edges with moleskin or latex-free tape decreases irritation and breakdown of adjacent skin and protects the edges of the cast from excessive wear.

Fiberglass casts dry quickly, usually set within 30 minutes of application. Fiberglass should be rolled onto the affected body part without stretching the fiberglass. Fiberglass is less forgiving in the presence of swelling; if the fiberglass is pulled "tight" or stretched during application, the neurovasculature can be compromised (TSRHC, 2014).

Fiberglass casts are lighter weight and more durable than plaster casts (TSRHC, 2014). Fiberglass casts are water-resistant, so the hard outer shell will not break down in water; however, the padding underneath the cast material is likely cotton and will absorb and hold water. Therefore, if a fiberglass cast becomes wet, inadequate airflow under the cast will prevent thorough drying of the padding and skin. Damp skin is more susceptible to skin breakdown and infection.

Plaster casts can be used when the physician wants to "mold" the cast to apply corrective forces to a body part, as in the treatment of a clubfoot or early onset scoliosis (TSRHC, 2014). Plaster casts will set within 10 to 15 minutes, but will not fully dry for 24 to 48 hours. Plaster is not water resistant and will break down if it gets wet.

## Traction

Effective immobilization can also be achieved with traction. Traction is a pull or force exerted on one part of the body. Traction can be applied to the skin or the bone. For treatment, traction can be applied to the spine, pelvis, or long bones of the upper and lower extremities. The angle formed by the placement of the pulley and the angle of the involved joint determines the direction of the pull or force. Once the direction of the pull or force has been determined, the traction is directed along the long axis of the bone.

An opposing pull or force (counter-traction) must be provided at the same time if the traction is to be effective. Counter-traction results in a two-way pull that maintains alignment of the affected extremity. The child's weight is usually sufficient to provide the counter-traction. If body weight is not sufficient, additional weights are used. Depending on the age of the child, restraining devices might be needed to maintain counter-traction. Some forms of traction, such as halo traction used for cervical spine injury, exert a force without the use of weights.

If traction is being applied while the child is in bed, the part of the bed that holds the traction apparatus is tilted or elevated, thereby assisting with counter-traction. For example, if the leg were being placed in traction, the foot of the bed would be elevated. Otherwise, the child would slide in the direction of the traction, disrupting the alignment of the extremity and reducing the effectiveness of treatment. In addition, the mattress should be firm, and a foot board or foot plate may be necessary to keep the extremity in the correct position.

Traction is either *continuous* or *intermittent*. Continuous traction exerts a constant pull and is used for fractures and dislocations. Intermittent traction provides a periodic pull or force and is used for contractures, low back pain, or muscle spasm. *The nurse should always assume that traction is continuous unless the physician states otherwise.* The removal of traction intended to be continuous could prove harmful to the child. If the force of the traction is altered, the muscles contract, and fracture alignment could be disrupted. The tissues around the fracture could also be injured, resulting in poor healing. The nursing care plan should always reflect the frequency and amount of time intermittent traction may be removed. When removing the traction apparatus, the nurse must maintain manual traction and pull on the body part.

The disadvantages of traction include prolonged immobility and the potential need for hospitalization. Currently, early casting and percutaneous pinning are replacing the use of traction for some musculoskeletal conditions (Nascimento et al., 2013).

### Skin Traction

Skin traction (Box 50.1) is noninvasive and well tolerated, and application does not require anesthesia (TSRHC, 2014). Skin traction is most

**BOX 50.1 Types of Skin Traction**

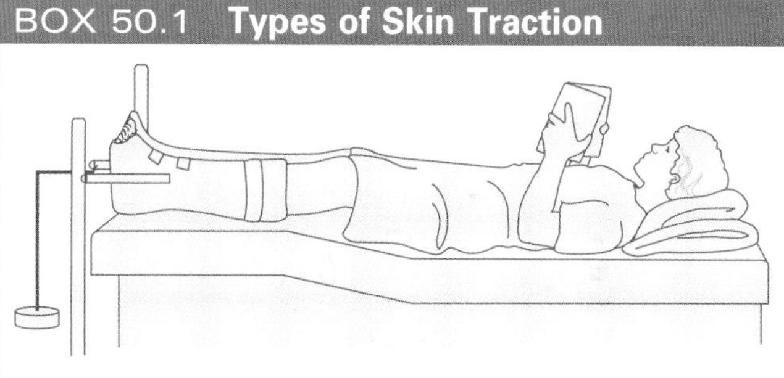

**Buck's Extension**

**Buck**

- *Purpose:* Used to treat some fractures, hip disorders, contractures, and muscle spasms.
- *Description:* Continuous or intermittent boot or circular wrap is applied to the skin. Traction is applied to boot or wrap. Rolled towels are placed on the external surface of the knee to prevent **external rotation** of the affected leg. Unless otherwise ordered, the mattress should be flexed at the knee (20 to 30 degrees).

**Bryant**

- *Purpose:* Used to treat very young children (younger than 2 years of age) with femur fractures or developmental dysplasia of the hip.
- *Description:* The child's affected lower extremity or extremities are wrapped. The child lies in bed (or crib) with hips flexed 90 degrees and the knees extended. Traction is applied overhead with just enough weight to elevate the buttock off the surface of the mattress.
- Is continuous for femur fractures, but can be intermittent for children with developmental dysplasia of the hip. Traction is used for 2 to 4 weeks to loosen muscles before a child goes to the operating room for closed or open **reduction** of the displaced hip.

effective for children who weigh less than 15 kg (33 lb) or are younger than 2 to 3 years. It can be applied to the pelvis, spine, or extremities (usually the long bones). Skin traction is preferred for conditions in which invasive procedures are contraindicated, such as hemarthrosis (collection of blood in the joint) as a result of hemophilia. Foam rubber straps, adhesive moleskin, elastic bandages, or cloth belts are applied to the skin and then attached to the weights and pulleys. If skin traction to the lower leg is needed, a foam rubber or fabric boot can be used; the fit should be secure.

Skin traction is not appropriate if the child has a skin infection, an open wound, or extensive tissue damage. Skin breakdown can develop as a result of skin traction. Applying tincture of benzoin to the intact skin before the traction is applied helps to protect against skin irritation.

If the traction has not been set up correctly, neurovascular impairment can result. Therefore, skin traction is not appropriate for patients with abnormal sensation in the lower extremities (TSRHC, 2014). Hyperextension of the knee and elastic bandages that have been wrapped too tightly are the most common causes of traction-related neurovascular impairment. A thorough assessment of the traction apparatus and the extremity should be conducted at least once each shift.

### Skeletal Traction

Skeletal traction (Box 50.2; Fig. 50.1) exerts greater force than skin traction and can be physiologically tolerated for longer periods. Skeletal traction helps maintain correct alignment of bony fragments and assists in proper healing. Traction is maintained by a metal device inserted into the bone. The fracture site determines the insertion site of the stainless steel wires, pins, or tongs. Common sites for skeletal traction include the skull, the proximal end of the ulna, the distal end of the femur, as well as the tibia and heel. General anesthesia is necessary for skeletal traction placement and removal.

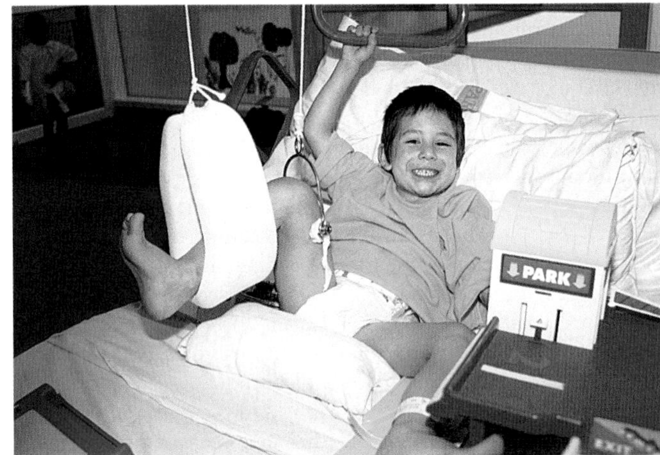


**FIG 50.1** Skeletal traction is used to reduce and immobilize fractures and allows greater pull than would be possible with skin traction. Because skeletal traction is invasive, osteomyelitis is a possible serious complication. (Courtesy Parkland Health and Hospital System, Dallas, TX.)

## BOX 50.2 Types of Skeletal Traction

**Halo**

- *Purpose:* To stabilize fractures or displaced vertebrae in cervical and thoracic areas. Also used to prepare the spine (muscles, vertebrae, and spinal cord) before spinal fusion, casting, or bracing in younger patients.
- *Description:* The halo is fitted with pins drilled directly into the skull. The halo is then attached by a rope to weights or a pulley above the head or to a special vest connected to the halo with rods. When the halo is attached to weights, the center of the curved metal bar over the halo must extend along the same planes as the spinal cord. Traction pull is always along the axis of the spine. The child must maintain straight body alignment.

**90/90 Femoral**

- *Purpose:* Most commonly used traction for complicated fractures of the femur; most effective in children older than 6 years. Within 2 to 3 weeks, callus formation is sufficient to allow application of a spica cast.
- *Description:* A pin or wire is inserted through the distal femur.

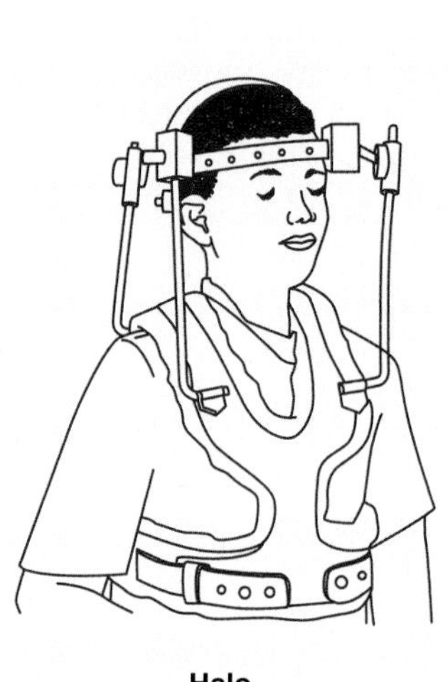

Halo

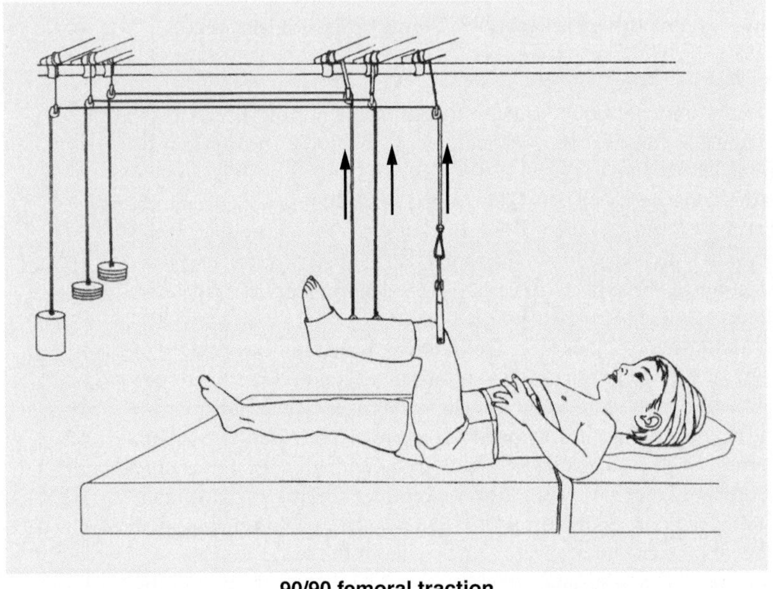

90/90 femoral traction

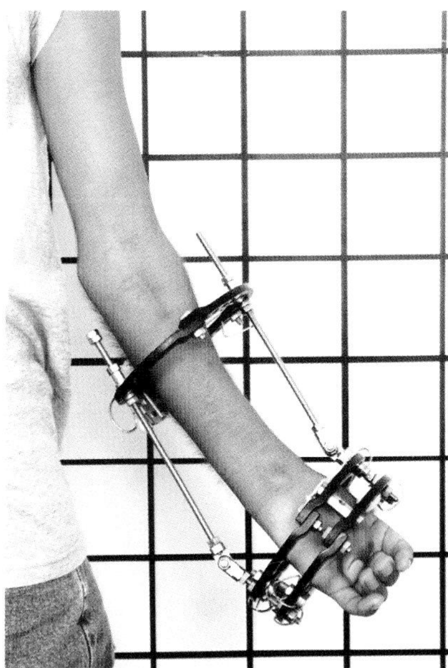

FIG 50.2 Ilizarov external fixator. (Courtesy Shriners Hospitals for Children, Houston, TX.)

The most serious complication associated with skeletal traction is *osteomyelitis,* an infection involving the bone. Organisms gain access to the bone systemically or through the opening created by the metal pins or wires used for traction. Clinical manifestations include localized pain, swelling, warmth, tenderness, unusual odor, fever, and irritability or lethargy in young children. To decrease the risk of infection, pin site care is required at least once per day. Pin care protocols involve inspecting each site for signs of infection (e.g., tenting or pulling around the pin, redness at the site, purulent drainage) and cleaning the skin around pin sites with one of various cleansing solutions (e.g., chlorhexidine gluconate, plain normal saline, soap and water), Upon practice review of pin-site–care protocols, there is no one method that is best for preventing infection at pin sites (Ferreira & Marais, 2012).

## External Fixation Devices

External fixation devices are used in the treatment of complex fractures, to lengthen bones, and to correct angular deformities that involve bone and soft tissue. These devices provide distraction, keeping the bone ends separated and in alignment so that healing can occur. External fixators also allow periodic changes in alignment and bone length. These devices, such as the Ilizarov external fixator (Fig. 50.2), consist of pins or wires inserted through skin, soft tissue, and bone that are secured on the outer limb surface to a rigid metal frame. General anesthesia is necessary for placement and removal of external fixation devices.

Because the pins or wires of the external fixator pass through the skin to anchor into the bone, meticulous assessment of entry sites for signs of inflammation, infection, or loose pins is necessary. Pin tract infection occurs in approximately 50% of cases (TSRHC, 2014). Pin site care similar to that for children in traction is recommended. To prevent injury to the other limb or to others, sharp protrusions from the fixator should be adequately covered.

## Nursing Considerations

Before the application of an immobilizing device, assess the child's and parents' knowledge about the procedure. Also assess the child's skin and note the presence of any bruises or abrasions that might be covered by the device.

### SAFETY ALERT

**The Child in a Cast or Traction**

Tissue ischemia and nerve damage are serious complications that can accompany immobilization in a cast or traction. Skin color and temperature, movement and sensation of the extremity, quality of pulses, and capillary refill time are related to neurovascular status and should be carefully assessed. Problems must be handled quickly to prevent permanent disabilities.

The five *P*s can be used as a guide for assessing neurovascular status:

***P***ain unrelieved by analgesia
***P***allor
***P***ulselessness or lack of capillary refill
***P***aresthesia
***P***aralysis or progressive loss of motion

Assessment that identifies any of these five *P*s of neurovascular compromise indicates possible tissue ischemia. Prompt referral to a physician and intervention is crucial if neurovascular impairment is to be prevented.

Reference: Johnston-Walker, E., & Hardcastle, J. (2011). Neurovascular assessment in the critically ill patient. *Nursing in critical care, 16*(4), 170–177.

## Neurovascular Status

After the device is applied, perform a neurovascular assessment (CSM—*c*irculation, *s*ensation, and *m*otion) at least every 2 hours during the first 48 hours. Assess the strength of the pulse distal to the site, and compare it with the pulse in the uninvolved extremity. A sluggish capillary refill time suggests neurovascular impairment.

Signs of circulatory impairment include coldness, pallor, blueness of the extremity, swelling, loss of motion, and numbness and tingling of the extremity. Touch the child's skin proximal and distal to the device to assess temperature; ask the child to move the fingers or toes. Paresthesia, or numbness, burning, and tingling, can be assessed by touching the fingers or toes and noting any decrease or loss of feeling. Paresthesia is of serious concern because paralysis can result if the problem is not corrected. Report a child's complaints of a pins-and-needles sensation or of the extremity "feeling asleep." Young children are not always able to describe a feeling or sensation, so avoid questions such as "Do you feel this?" Instead, ask a child to wiggle the fingers or toes to appropriately determine motor impairment.

## Special Considerations for the Child in Halo Traction

Children who must be in halo traction have additional neurovascular issues that must be addressed (Table 50.1).

***Assessing and managing compartment syndrome.*** Serious complications, such as nerve compression, circulatory impairment, and compartment syndrome, can result from swelling caused by trauma or an immobilizing device. The muscles and nerves of the upper and lower extremities are enclosed in compartments surrounded by tough, inelastic fascia (comparable to sausage casing). *Compartment syndrome* occurs when swelling causes pressure to rise within these closed fascial compartments, compromising vascular perfusion to the muscles and nerves (Johnston-Walker & Hardcastle, 2011). Compartment syndrome is a true surgical emergency that requires prompt diagnosis and intervention to prevent paralysis and tissue necrosis (Johnston-Walker & Hardcastle, 2011; TSRHC, 2014).

Signs of compartment syndrome include severe pain, often unrelieved by analgesics, and signs of neurovascular impairment (TSRHC,

**TABLE 50.1 Neurologic Assessment for Patients Requiring Halo Traction**

**Neurologic Assessments Are Usually Performed Three Times Per Day.**

- Obtain and document baseline assessment before first traction application.
- Assess patient in the morning approximately 30 min after the patient goes from bed to wheelchair or walker traction.
- Assess patient again after lunch.
- Assess patient for the third time in the evening after the patient goes from wheelchair or walker traction to bed.

**NOTE: All of these checks should be positive, except clonus and the Babinski sign should be negative (but Babinski can be positive up to age 2 yr).**

| | |
|---|---|
| Lateral gaze | Check eye movements. Ask patient to follow your finger with the eyes and move your finger side to side. |
| Tongue movement | (Cranial nerve XII: hypoglossal) Ask patient to stick out tongue and move tongue right, left, up and down. |
| Show teeth | (Cranial nerve VII: facial nerve) Ask patient to smile and show teeth. |
| Swallow | (Cranial nerve IX: glossopharyngeal) Patient should be able to swallow easily and effectively. Should not choke on solids, liquids, or saliva. Should not have difficulty swallowing. |
| Deltoid-shoulder strength | (Cranial nerve XI: spinal accessory nerve) Have patient abduct and adduct shoulders and move shoulders up against your hands to assess strength. |
| Grip strength | Have patient grasp your hands and squeeze both right and left hand at the same time. |
| Quadriceps | While patient is seated with legs dangling over the edge of bed or table, ask patient to extend each leg straight and resist your attempt to bend the leg. You can also check quadriceps strength by asking patient to raise the leg off the bed against your resistance. |
| Ankle flexion and extension | Ask patient to flex and extend ankle against your resistance. |
| Big toe | Ask patient to move a big toe down toward the floor and up toward the body—both independently of other toes. |
| Knee jerk | With leg bent at the knee, firmly tap knee with reflex hammer to elicit response from the lower leg. |
| Babinski | Using a blunt object (pen or end of a reflex hammer), run object along the sole of foot from the bottom of heel, up along the lateral edge, and over under the big toe. Toes will curl down for a negative Babinski and toes will fan out for a positive result. |
| Clonus | While holding foot in neutral position with your hand, gently but quickly dorsiflex the ankle. The "jumpy" or "bouncy" feeling you get from the sudden stretching of the Achilles tendon is clonus. |

2014). If extending the fingers or wiggling the toes produces pain, and/or the quality of the radial or pedal pulse is poor to absent, notify the physician. In addition, assess for pallor, paresthesia, and pulselessness as previously described. Paresis and paresthesias are late findings, typically a sign of permanent damage (TSRHC, 2014).

The diagnosis of compartment syndrome is made primarily on physical findings, but if physical findings provoke any question, diagnosis can be aided by measurement of the pressure within the affected compartment. The intracompartmental pressure at which compartment syndrome ensues is unknown, and the pressure can vary with the measurement technique (TSRHC, 2014). If compartment syndrome is suspected, the nurse should immediately elevate the extremity only to the level of the child's heart, loosen any restrictive bandages or dressings (if able), split the cast (if able), notify the physician immediately, and administer pain medication as ordered. The child will be kept on nothing-by-mouth (NPO) status for possible emergent surgical management.

### Immobility

Children in immobilizing devices are subject to the consequences of immobility. Immobility can affect several body systems. Appropriate assessment and intervention can prevent adverse effects (Table 50.2).

### Special Considerations for the Child in Traction

Children who are placed in traction are hospitalized from several days to weeks, depending on the underlying condition. It is imperative that the nurse check the amount of traction the patient is receiving against the physician's orders; all weights should be hanging free and not touching the floor or bed, and all ropes must be placed appropriately on the pulleys. Elevate the head or foot of the bed as indicated to maintain countertraction. It may be necessary to draw a line on the child's bed sheet and ask the parents to keep the child above that line. An older child can pull on an overhead trapeze to maintain proper position and alignment.

### Home Care

Most children are discharged home shortly after a cast application. The box entitled 'Parents Want to Know: Home Care for the Child in a Cast' presents the basic principles for caring for a child in a cast at home. Care for children discharged with an external fixator can involve frequent neurovascular assessments and possibly pin-site care. Parents must be able to describe how to care for the cast or fixator, when they should contact their physician, and how to contact any needed resources in the community (e.g., physical therapy, occupational therapy, school district personnel). The nurse can also help parents to select appropriate clothing and adaptive devices if needed. Encourage the parents to promote the child's self-care whenever possible.

## FRACTURES

Fractures in children are common and can vary in severity from benign to life threatening. A **fracture** is a break or disruption in a bone's continuity. Most fractures occur when excessive or traumatic force exceeds the strength of the bone.

### Etiology

Fractures in children are common because of their increased mobility and inadequate or immature motor and cognitive skills. Fractures can result from accidental trauma (e.g., falls, motor vehicle crashes, sports injuries), nonaccidental trauma (e.g., child abuse), or pathologic conditions that result in abnormally fragile bones (e.g., osteogenesis imperfecta, tumors, cysts).

Many biochemical and physiologic properties of pediatric bones differ from those of adults. Three essential differences contribute to the understanding of injury, fracture patterns, healing, and treatment (Baldwin, Wells, & Dormans, 2016c). First, children's bones are less brittle, with a higher collagen-to-bone ratio. This difference is

TABLE 50.2 **Consequences of Immobility**

| Assessment Criteria | Nursing Diagnosis | Intervention |
|---|---|---|
| **Integumentary** | | |
| Red or irritated skin, presence of ulceration or drainage | Impaired Skin Integrity | Reposition the child every 2 hr and as needed; encourage the child in traction to use a trapeze to facilitate movement.<br>Use an egg-crate–type or sheepskin mattress for comfort under the back and lower legs. If the child is not capable of any independent repositioning or has decreased sensation, use a pressure relief overlay or mattress. Pay particular attention to the heels to prevent skin breakdown.<br>Wash and thoroughly dry the areas twice a day; refrain from using lotion, powder, or talc, which can retain moisture.<br>Change the untrained child's diapers frequently to prevent skin breakdown. Examine and record the child's skin condition once per shift. |
| **Gastrointestinal** | | |
| Decrease in number or consistency of bowel movements because of decreased gastrointestinal motility | Risk for Constipation | Assess bowel sounds, abdominal distention, elimination pattern; be sure to know the child's normal pattern, usual stool consistency, and words used for defecation.<br>Provide a diet high in roughage and fiber and increase fluid intake with foods and fluids the child likes.<br>Position the child as upright as possible during defecation.<br>Administer laxatives and/or stool softeners if needed. |
| **Respiratory** | | |
| Decreased or altered respirations, shortness of breath, decreased breath sounds, adventitious breath sounds | Ineffective Breathing Pattern | Assess respiratory status at least once per shift.<br>Encourage coughing and deep breathing through the use of games, such as blowing bubbles or pinwheels; older children can use an incentive spirometer.<br>Reposition every 2 hr and as needed. |
| **Genitourinary** | | |
| Decreased urinary output from stasis or retention, concentrated or foul-smelling urine | Impaired Urinary Elimination | Maintain hydration levels.<br>Offer juices (cranberry, apple) and acid-ash foods (cereal, meats) that will acidify the urine.<br>Monitor the child's urinary output. |
| **Musculoskeletal** | | |
| Reduced strength and joint mobility, loss of muscle tone and potential for muscle atrophy, limited range of motion | Impaired Physical Mobility | Test muscle strength and joint mobility every shift and as needed.<br>Encourage active range-of-motion and stretching exercises of unaffected extremities.<br>Plan developmentally appropriate activities that require the use of unaffected extremities. Provide foods high in protein and calcium.<br>Use elastic stockings or thromboembolic disease hose to promote venous return and decrease circulatory stasis. |
| Developmental regression, irritability, anxiety, excessive dependence on others, passive behavior | Powerlessness | Recognize the child's need to regress in response to the immobility; help child regain previous developmental stages when ready.<br>Explain all routines and procedures to the child and parents and encourage them to participate in care.<br>Provide the opportunity for therapeutic play: modeling clay, paints, remote-control toys (which give the feeling of mobility and control), puppet play, storytelling, role playing.<br>Allow the child to use age-appropriate dishes and cups, clothing from home (might have to be adapted to fit over an immobilizing device), transitional object, night light.<br>Determine and follow the child's usual routine.<br>Encourage the school-age child and adolescent to keep up with schoolwork and stay in contact with peers.<br>Frequently provide a change in environment: move the bed to take advantage of a different view; move the bed into the playroom; keep side rails up for safety.<br>Allow and encourage the child's autonomy in decision making. |

## PARENTS WANT TO KNOW

### *Home Care for the Child in a Cast*

**Check the Edges of the Cast as Follows:**

- If they appear rough or are irritating the skin, "petal" the cast by overlapping moleskin or adhesive tape (1 to 2 inches in width; 3 to 4 inches in length with one rounded edge) around the cast edges.
- Waterproof tape should be used in the perineal area.

**To Assist with Drying the Cast, Do the Following:**

- Place the child on a firm mattress.
- Support the cast and adjacent joints with pillows.
- For a plaster cast, reposition every 2 to 4 hours to ensure thorough drying.
- Lift the cast with the palms of your hands.
- A fan directed toward the cast facilitates drying.
- Once dry, the cast should sound hollow and be cool to the touch.

**Swelling Generally Peaks within 24 to 48 Hours. To Prevent Problems, Do the Following:**

- Apply bagged ice to the casted area (be sure to keep melting ice from touching the cast or leaking underneath).
- Elevate the extremity at the level of the heart with pillows.
- Apply pressure to the nail bed of the child's casted extremity and count how long it takes for the color to return (it should take no longer than 2 seconds). Repeat every 2 hours for the first 24 to 48 hours.
- The casted extremity should be the same color and temperature as the other extremity.
- Check each finger or toe for sensation and movement several times each day for 2 days.

**Protect the Cast as Follows:**

- If the child is permitted to bathe or shower, be sure to cover the cast with plastic and waterproof tape to keep the cast dry.
- Do not put anything inside the cast. Keep small toys and sharp objects away from the cast. Supervise your child during mealtimes so the child does not get food underneath the cast.

**Contact the Physician If Any of the Following Occurs:**

- The cast feels warm or hot or has an unusual smell.
- Any drainage or blood suddenly appears on the cast.
- Your child reports pain, burning, numbness, or tingling.
- The extremity changes color or temperature, or any swelling persists.
- Any fever above 101.5° F (40° C) taken by mouth.
- Slipping of cast, inability to visualize toes or fingers.

**When Preparing to Remove the Cast, Do the Following:**

- Explain the cast removal to your child. The cast remover works by vibration that creates a warm, tickling feeling on the skin and sounds like a vacuum cleaner.
- Allow time for the child to adjust to the cast remover. Ask the technician or physician if your child can examine the cast remover and see how it works ahead of time.
- Once the cast is removed, the skin will be dry and flaky. Wash the area with warm water and soap. Discourage the child from scratching.
- The extremity will be stiff for a while and will look smaller because the muscles have not been used. It might need to be supported with a sling. Normal movement will correct the stiffness.

protective, making incomplete fractures more likely. Secondly, children have a stronger periosteum. This also makes complete fractures less likely or at least limits fracture displacement. The third essential pediatric bone difference is the epiphyseal plate or growth plate. The epiphyseal plate is the weakest part of the growing bone but often bears the brunt of children's bone injuries.

An understanding of growth and development is helpful when assessing trauma in specific age-groups. For example, fractures in infancy are generally rare because of the cartilaginous quality of the skeleton. Fractures in infants are usually the result of trauma during birth or nonaccidental trauma. Therefore, fractures that occur after the birthing process warrant further investigation to rule out the possibility of child abuse.

Clavicle fractures can occur at any age. Lack of movement or a pseudoparalysis of the upper extremity may be the only sign in an infant who has sustained a fractured clavicle during birth. It is important to assess the infant with clavicle fracture for brachial plexus palsy because the two are associated. An older child will report pain and show swelling on the clavicle at the site of the fracture. A common mechanism of clavicle injury in older children is blunt trauma from contact sports.

Another major cause of children's fractures is falls. The outstretched arm often receives the full force of the fall, even though this action is the result of the child's protective reflexes (Fig. 50.3). Although this force of impact can involve any part of the arm (wrist, elbow, shoulder), the supracondylar humeral fracture of the elbow is most commonly seen with this type of fall. Secondary complications of this injury include circulatory impairment, cellular necrosis, neurovascular damage, ischemic contracture (Volkmann contracture), and compartment syndrome.

Thorough and timely assessment of a fracture is important to prevent loss of function and disturbance to the bone growth of the pediatric patient regardless of age or type of skeletal injury. Understanding the etiology and location of the fracture is important to prevent complications.

## Incidence

Pediatric trauma is the leading cause of death and disability in children and one of the largest challenges to their health (Baldwin et al., 2016c; Sharma et al., 2011). The United States has the highest incidence of pediatric trauma among developing nations; musculoskeletal trauma makes up the largest portion of pediatric injuries, with 25% of children sustaining an injury annually and 8.5% to 25% of those injuries being fractures (Flynn, Skaggs, & Waters, 2015).

Fractures are common in children and adolescents because numerous gross motor activities place them at risk. Young children are acquiring new motor skills, whereas older children and adolescents are participating in risk-taking behaviors as part of their normal growth and development. It is estimated that 40% of boys and 25% of girls will sustain a fracture by 16 years of age (Flynn, Skaggs, & Waters, 2015). The distal forearm is the most common site to be fractured in children; the clavicle is second.

## Manifestations

The presentation of fractures varies with location, type, and cause of injury. General signs and symptoms include pain or tenderness at the site, immobility or decreased range of motion, deformity, and swelling. Other signs and symptoms include **crepitus**, ecchymosis, erythema, muscle spasm, and inability to bear weight.

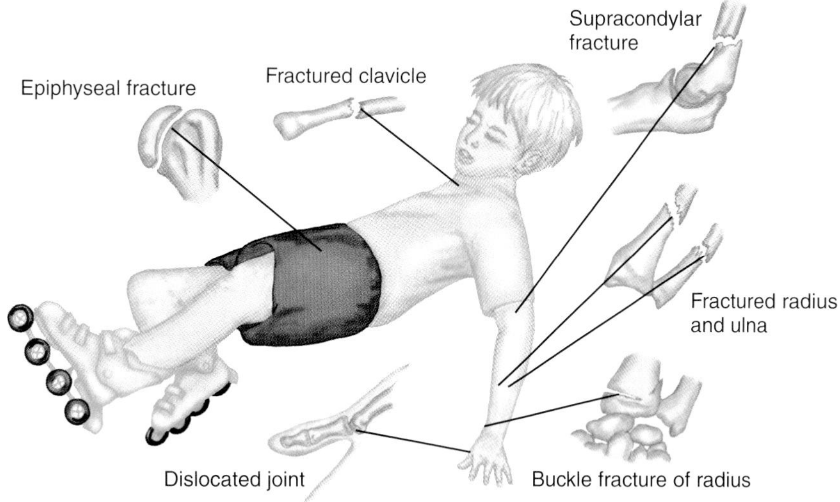


FIG 50.3 Upper extremity fractures in children often occur when the child attempts to break a fall with an outstretched arm.

The periosteum of children's bones is thicker and stronger than that of adults; therefore, fractures are less likely to be displaced. Local signs and symptoms of a fracture are not always present, which can make diagnosis of a fracture difficult. Radiography is the most effective tool for determining the type and location of a fracture. Fractures are not always visible on radiographs until healing begins. A radiograph of the unaffected extremity might be obtained for comparison purposes, especially when trying to determine whether a line on the radiograph represents a fracture or merely an epiphyseal line. Radiographs are also obtained after fracture reduction and during the healing process to assess progress.

## Therapeutic Management

The goal for managing fractures in children is to maintain function without affecting growth. The key to healing is the correct reduction and retention of the fracture. *Reduction* is the repositioning of the bone fragments into normal alignment. Retention entails the application of a device or mechanism that maintains alignment until healing occurs.

### Reduction Methods

Fractures are treated by either closed or open reduction. Closed reduction is accomplished by manual alignment of the fragments followed by immobilization. Simple or closed fractures are treated by closed reduction. Hospitalization is seldom necessary for closed reduction, and most of these fractures heal without complications.

Open reduction entails the surgical insertion of internal or external fixation devices such as rods, wires, or pins that help maintain alignment while healing occurs. When open reduction is used, hospitalization may be required to assess the child for postoperative complications. Complications after open reduction include delayed healing, nonunion, and infection. Close assessment by the healthcare team and strict adherence to sterile technique during dressing changes decrease the risk of postoperative problems and promote healing.

### Retention

Once the bone is aligned, the fracture site must be protected and the position of the fragments maintained. This stability is accomplished through the application of a splint, cast, external fixation device, or traction that effectively immobilizes the area while healing occurs.

## Nursing Considerations

### Initial Trauma Assessment

Nursing assessment of the child with a traumatic fracture should begin with a thorough primary survey (see Chapter 34). A complete history of the circumstances surrounding the fracture should be obtained to identify the mechanism of injury and rule out nonaccidental trauma.

Examine the fracture site for bruising, skin lacerations, and swelling. Most often, the child favors the extremity by cradling or guarding the limb. Many children report numbness and tingling distal to the fracture site. Movement and range of motion are often limited. The five Ps of neurovascular status should be assessed carefully and interventions initiated appropriately to prevent impairment.

### Assessing and Managing Complications

Fat embolism and resultant respiratory distress are commonly seen in adults with multiple or long-bone fractures but are rare in children (George, George, Dixit, et al., 2013). Fat embolism involves the escape of fat particles from the fracture site; they are carried through the circulatory system and lodge in the lung capillaries. Signs and symptoms of fat embolism are the same in a child as in adults. These include axillary petechiae, hypoxemia, and radiographic changes showing pulmonary infiltrates (George et al., 2013). These changes appear within several hours after the fracture. Rarely, fat emboli can lodge in the small capillaries in the brain or other vital organs. Hypoxemia and mental status changes are typically caused by other injuries or from overmedication with opioid analgesics rather than fat embolism. Minimal movement of fractured extremities can prevent or lessen the effects of fat embolism. Treatment is primarily supportive and includes volume resuscitation, respiratory support, and adequate oxygenation.

Another complication that can occur with an orthopedic injury is deep vein thrombosis. The incidence of deep vein thrombosis in children with lower extremity trauma is approximately 0.058% (Murphy, Naqvi, Miller, et al., 2015). Risk factors include prolonged central line placement, obesity, infection, and long-bone trauma (Murphy et al., 2015). Prevention includes elevation of the fractured extremity, early ambulation with support, and prompt initiation of postoperative physiotherapy. Pain management is an important adjunct for meeting this goal, as well as for promoting healing and shortening the hospital stay. Currently, there is no standard of care for deep vein thrombosis

## PATHOPHYSIOLOGY

### *Fractures and Physeal Growth Plate Injuries*

Fractures result in bone fragmentation and injury to the surrounding tissues. Torn blood vessels cause bleeding from the bone and tissues around the bone fragments. As blood clots at the site, fibrin strands provide a network for healing. **Osteoblasts** begin forming in immense numbers almost immediately after the injury. This increased osteoblastic activity results in the formation of new bone matrix between the bone fragments. Calcium salts are deposited in the new bone matrix, forming a *callus*. The callus provides stability and support of the fracture while healing occurs. Gradually, the callus is formed into new bone. Remodeling (the correction of an injury at the fracture site through the buildup of callus) occurs more rapidly in growing children.

Fractures are categorized as *simple* or *compound*. A *simple* (closed) fracture is one with the skin intact. A simple fracture still requires a thorough nursing assessment because of potential problems associated with this injury. Possible complications include internal hemorrhage, compartment syndrome, and neurovascular compromise.

When the skin, subcutaneous tissue, or muscle has been disrupted, the fracture is classified as *compound* (open). Infection is a risk with this type of fracture because organisms can enter the fracture site through the wound. Children with compound fractures are at risk for blood loss as a result of external hemorrhage.

Systemic risks associated with fractures, especially multiple fractures or femur fractures, are emboli and shock. Emboli can result from postinjury bleeding with clotting or from fat droplets released from the fractured bone marrow (fat embolism). The emboli enter the circulatory system and can travel to the lungs, heart, or brain. Hypovolemic shock is a possibility with both closed and open fractures.

A break or fracture between the shaft of the bone and epiphyseal plate is referred to as a *growth plate injury*. In a growing bone, the region of least resistance to stress is the area between the metaphysis and the cartilaginous epiphyseal plate. The amount of growth arrest associated with an epiphyseal injury is determined by the extent of the damage to the epiphyseal plate (Baldwin, 2016c). If the germinal cells remain with the epiphysis and appear uninjured, healing is rapid and growth is seldom affected. However, if the germinal layer is destroyed, growth disturbances will occur. The Salter-Harris classification system classifies epiphyseal growth plate injuries and their associated risk of growth disturbance.

**Pediatric fractures are seldom complete breaks. Rather, children's bones tend to bend or buckle because of increased flexibility. This flexibility is due to a thicker periosteum and increased amounts of immature bone.**

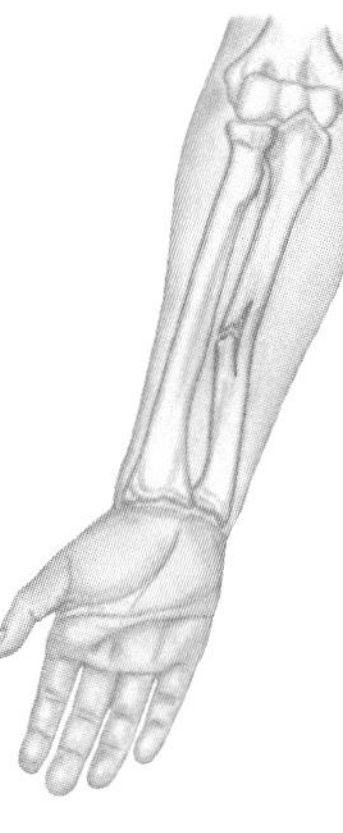

**Greenstick**

Break occurs through the periosteum on one side of the bone while only bowing or buckling on the other side. Seen most frequently in forearm.

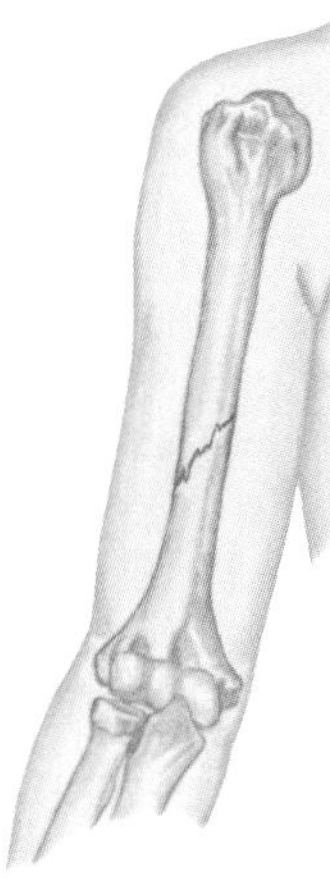

**Spiral**

Twisted or circular break that affects the length rather than the width. Seen frequently in child abuse.

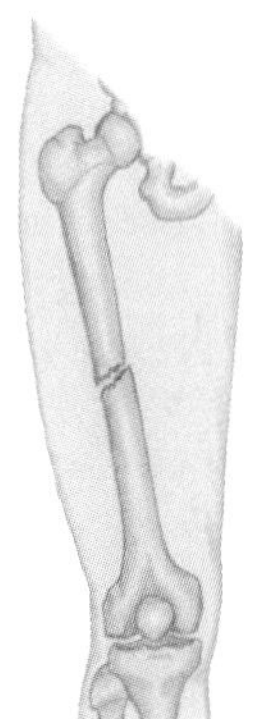

**Oblique**

Diagonal or slanting break that occurs between the horizontal and perpendicular planes of the bone.

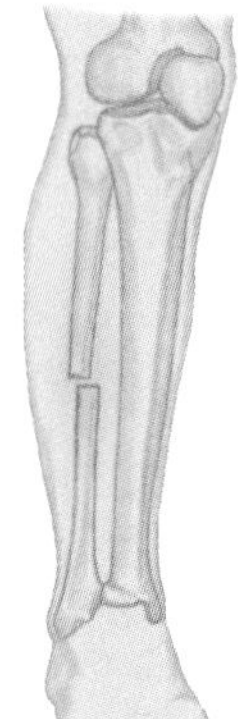

**Transverse**

Break or fracture line occurs at right angles to the long axis of the bone.

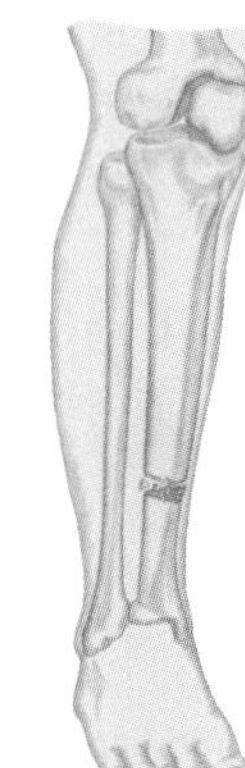

**Comminuted**

Bone is splintered into pieces. This is a rare occurrence in children.

## PATHOPHYSIOLOGY—cont'd

### *Fractures and Physeal Growth Plate Injuries*

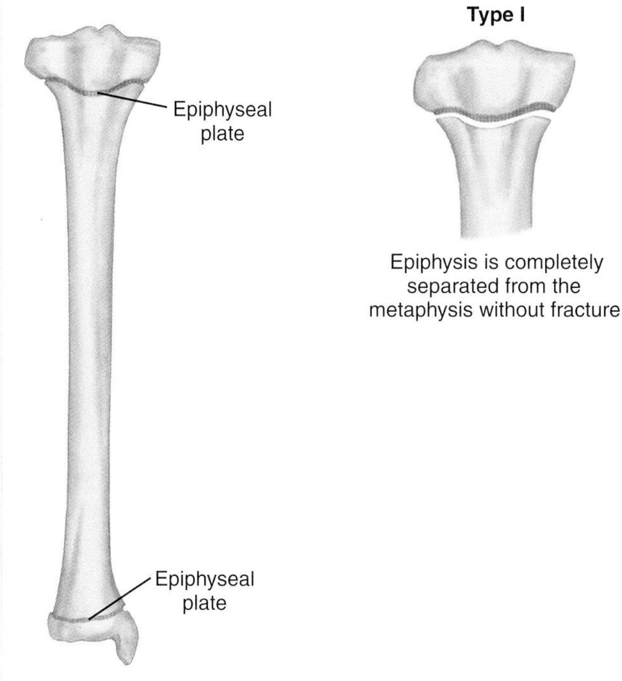


**Type I**

Epiphysis is completely separated from the metaphysis without fracture.

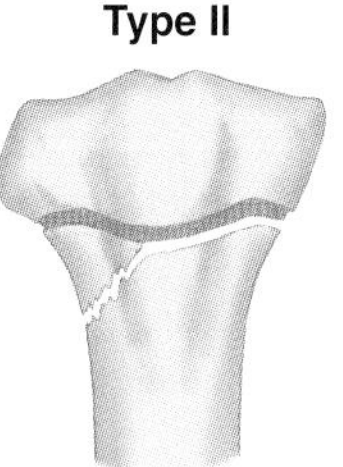

**Type II**

Transverse fracture extends through the separated epiphyseal plate producing triangular break.

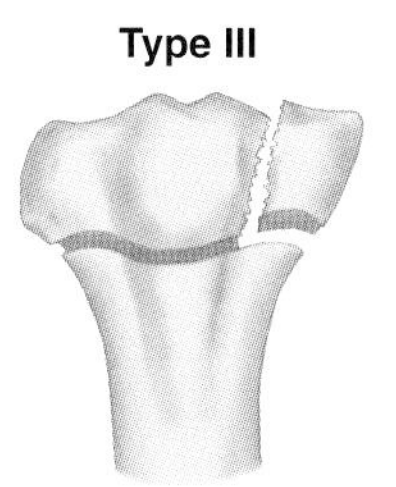

**Type III**

Fracture extends through part of the epiphyseal plate into the joint.

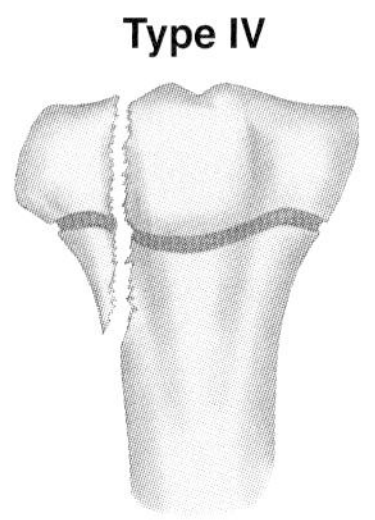

**Type IV**

Fracture extends through the epiphyseal plate and through the metaphysis.

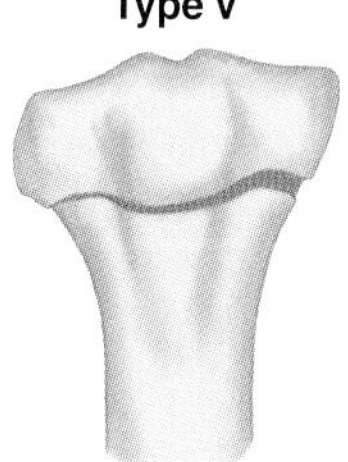

**Type V**

Epiphyseal plate is crushed, causing cell death in growth plate.

Reference: Baldwin, K.D., Wells, L., & Dormans, J.P. (2016c). Common fractures. In R. Kliegman, B. Stanton, J. St Geme, et al. (Eds.), *Nelson textbook of pediatrics* (20th ed., pp. 3314–3322). Philadelphia: Saunders.

**TABLE 50.3 Sport-Specific Injury Risk**

| Low | Low to Moderate | Moderate | Moderate to High | High | Very High |
|---|---|---|---|---|---|
| Swimming | Running | Ballet | Ice hockey | Cycling | Trampoline |
| Tennis | Inline skating | Baseball | Horseback riding | Diving | |
| | Strength training | Basketball | Skiing | American football | |
| | | Gymnastics | Snowboarding | Skateboarding | |
| | | Soccer | | Wrestling | |

Data from Staheli, L.T. (2008). (Ed.). *Fundamentals of pediatric orthopedics* (4th ed., pp. 90–92). Philadelphia: Wolters Kluwer/Lippincott Williams & Wilkins.

prophylaxis in the pediatric or adolescent trauma patient (Greenwald et al., 2012).

## SOFT-TISSUE INJURIES: SPRAINS, STRAINS, AND CONTUSIONS

Soft-tissue injuries are common among children and are usually related to play or athletic activities.

### Etiology

Sprains occur as a result of trauma to a joint in which ligaments are stretched or are partially or completely torn. *Strains,* also known as *pulls, tears,* or *ruptures,* result from an excessive stretch of muscle. *Contusions* occur when soft tissue, muscle, or subcutaneous tissue is damaged. Sprains and contusions frequently accompany each other. Dislocation occurs when a joint is disrupted in such a way that articulating surfaces are no longer in contact.

### Incidence

Sprains are not seen frequently in young children because of their poorly developed epiphyseal plates. A twisting or turning injury will more likely result in a fracture at the weak epiphyseal location than a sprain. Sprains and strains are more common in adolescents and are frequently the result of athletic injuries. Anterior cruciate ligament (ACL) tears are one of the most common types of knee injury, especially in adolescent athletes.

Rising participation in sports is associated with an increase in sports-related injuries in young children (Table 50.3). An estimated 2.6 million children receive medical treatment for a sports-related injury each year (CDC, 2013).

### Manifestations and Diagnostic Evaluation

Manifestations of soft-tissue injuries include pain, swelling, localized tenderness, limited range of motion, poor weight bearing, and a pop or snapping sound (sprain). The diagnosis is made based on the clinical picture. However, a radiographic examination might be ordered to rule out a fracture. Magnetic resonance imaging (MRI) or arthroscopy is sometimes necessary to diagnose knee-ligament tears.

### Therapeutic Management

The primary goal in managing a soft tissue injury is to control swelling and prevent further injury. External pressure (compression) is most beneficial before edema has accumulated (van den Bekerom et al., 2012). Swelling can inhibit healing by keeping the ligament ends separated and increasing fibrous scarring. The earlier the treatment is initiated, the less severe the swelling and immobility.

The injured area should be immediately wrapped with a compression bandage to support the joint and control swelling. Ice should be applied to the injured area to reduce swelling for no longer than 20 minutes at a time. The effects of the ice can last as long as 5 to 6 hours, and ice should be used repeatedly for several days. Nonsteroidal antiinflammatory drugs (NSAIDs) help to alleviate pain and reduce inflammation.

For more severe soft-tissue injuries, the child should avoid bearing weight for 3 days. Crutches are sometimes necessary to ensure that the affected limb does not bear weight. An *air cast* (a plastic, air-filled pressure cuff) can be used over the elastic wrap to support the joint and reduce swelling. The air cast or compression bandage should be worn for several weeks while the joint is healing. The child can begin stretching and isometric exercises to improve joint stability after the swelling and pain have diminished.

Immobilization of the injured joint and cold application are generally effective in the treatment of incomplete ligament tears. A complete rupture can require surgery to prevent excessive scar formation and long-term joint stability problems. Application of a cast or splint for 4 to 5 weeks may also be necessary, especially for knee injuries.

### Nursing Considerations

One of the major nursing functions when assessing a sprain is to determine the severity of the injury. Assess the child for neurovascular impairment and for diminished range of motion. The initial examination may reveal localized tenderness over the injured joint, as well as limited joint mobility.

Analgesics, such as ibuprofen or acetaminophen, are appropriate for pain management. Distraction and age-appropriate play activities can be effective in helping children cope with pain.

The nurse should keep the extremity elevated at the level of the heart. This position enhances venous return and aids in reducing the swelling. Pillows placed beneath the extremity provide support and comfort. Support and immobilization devices should be snug but not tight. Assess neurovascular status before and after application of any splint, compression wrap, or cast.

For the child who has undergone surgery for any type of knee ligament reconstruction, immediate postoperative use of a cold compression cuff and a continuous passive motion (CPM) machine—a machine that continuously moves the knee joint in flexion and extension—will likely be used. Nursing measures involve regular emptying and refilling of the cuff to maintain the cold temperature. The nurse must also check the settings on the CPM machine to ensure that they match the ordered degree of flexion and extension. Pain control is most important.

Stretching and strengthening exercises are helpful in maintaining joint and muscle integrity. These exercises are done passively at first. As healing progresses, teach the child active stretching and strengthening exercises. The effectiveness of parent and family teaching should be evaluated by return demonstration. Physical therapy referrals can be helpful as well.

The amount of time needed for healing is determined by the severity of the injury. Weight bearing is gradually increased as the pain subsides. More severe injuries can require partial weight-bearing exercises, with full weight bearing introduced once the swelling has resolved. Activities might be restricted as directed by the healthcare provider.

Review the principles of rest, support, and the application of ice with the parents and child. If wraps, splints, or air casts are used, teach the parents and child how to assess neurovascular status. If crutches are required, review the principles of crutch walking with both the parents and the child. Make sure all family members understand activity and sports restrictions. Discuss follow-up appointments and the importance of adhering to activity restrictions until the injury has healed and the child has been cleared for participation in sports.

**! NURSING QUALITY ALERT**

***The Child With a Soft Tissue Injury***

The first 6 to 12 hours after soft tissue injury are the most important in controlling swelling and reducing muscle damage. Treatment of soft-tissue injuries is summarized in the acronyms *RICE* and *ICES:*

| | |
|---|---|
| **R**est | **I**ce |
| **I**ce | **C**ompression |
| **C**ompression | **E**levation |
| **E**levation | **S**upport |

## OSTEOMYELITIS

Osteomyelitis is a bacterial infection of the bone that involves the cortex or marrow cavity. This serious problem can be difficult to diagnose and treat. Osteomyelitis has high morbidity and mortality rates. It is classified as *acute, subacute, chronic,* or *chronic recurrent multifocal* (TSRHC, 2014). This condition is considered chronic if the infection persists longer than 1 month or does not respond to the initial antibiotic protocol.

### Etiology

Bacteria infiltrate the bone through endogenous routes (e.g., skin or respiratory infections, abscessed teeth, acute otitis media) or exogenous routes (e.g., injury, surgical procedures). The infection is usually the result of vascular spread of the bacteria. Osteomyelitis also can occur as a result of direct entry (open fracture), injury to surrounding soft tissues (cellulitis), external fixation devices, and skeletal traction.

The most common causative organism for osteomyelitis and septic arthritis in all age-groups is *Staphylococcus aureus* (Kaplan, 2016). Cases of community-acquired methicillin-resistant *S. aureus* osteomyelitis have been reported (Sarkissian et al., 2015). *Streptococcus pyogenes, Haemophilus influenzae* (in unimmunized infants), *Kingella kingae, Escherichia coli,* and group B streptococci (in neonates) also can cause osteomyelitis. When the cause is trauma, the possible organisms include *Pseudomonas aeruginosa* and other organisms found in the soil. *Salmonella* is the most common causative organism for osteomyelitis in children with sickle cell anemia.

### Incidence

Osteomyelitis typically affects preschoolers and young school-age children, with a mean age of 6 years. Boys are affected more often than girls, possibly because of more risk-taking behavior leading to minor trauma (Kaplan, 2016).

## PATHOPHYSIOLOGY

### *Osteomyelitis*

Osteomyelitis occurs most frequently in the metaphyseal region of the long bones, especially the femur or tibia. Bacteria enter the metaphysis through small capillaries, and the inflammatory process begins. A preceding trauma can cause rupture of these capillaries, providing a medium for bacterial growth. Pus forms, and because it cannot move from the metaphyseal area into a joint, it spreads toward the medullary canal as well as the cortex of the bone. Pus accumulates under the periosteum and displaces it, causing it to separate and form an abscess.

The underlying blood supply is interrupted, which causes necrotic tissue to form *(sequestrum)*. New bone *(involucrum)* develops around the sequestrum, and the inflammatory process continues, causing further damage to surrounding bone tissue. Large sections of sequestrum may eventually become honeycombed with cavities or sinuses that contain infective material. These cavities are so effectively walled off that antibiotic therapy might not be successful. Thus, osteomyelitis can become chronic. Septic arthritis has the same basic pathophysiology, with the bacteria entering the joint.

### Manifestations

The manifestations of osteomyelitis in infants can be vague and nonspecific, such as fever, irritability, lethargy, and feeding difficulties. Some infants demonstrate signs of sepsis. In the older child, the major signs and symptoms include pain, warmth, erythema, and tenderness localized over the site of infection; favoring of the affected extremity; limited range of motion; and systemic manifestations such as fever and lethargy. Pain, usually localized, can radiate to adjacent areas of the body; radiating pain to an adjacent joint necessitates an assessment for possible septic arthritis (TSRHC, 2014).

### Diagnostic Evaluation

Imaging studies such as radiography, ultrasonography, radionuclide bone scans, MRI, and computed tomography (CT) scans diagnose and monitor the progress of osteomyelitis (TSRHC, 2014). Laboratory evidence of an infectious process (elevated ESR, elevated CRP level, and elevated white blood cell count) is usually found. Blood culture can positively identify the infecting organism. The physician can aspirate the affected area to obtain fluid for culture and sensitivity.

### Therapeutic Management

Intravenous (IV) antibiotics are usually started based on the probable organism and changed as needed according to culture results. This protocol makes obtaining the child's history a key component of case management. Controversy exists regarding the length of time required for antibiotic therapy, the need for IV versus oral antibiotics, and the role of bactericidal antibiotics and therapeutic blood levels. Nevertheless, therapy for osteomyelitis generally requires high-dose parenteral therapy, preferably through a peripherally inserted central catheter (PICC). The organism involved dictates the type of antibiotic and the length of treatment.

Assessment of the child's response to the antibiotics is an integral part of the treatment protocol. Peak and trough serum antibiotic levels are closely monitored. Children receiving aminoglycosides should be periodically assessed for side effects such as ototoxicity and nephrotoxicity. Renal and hepatic function should be monitored and blood cell counts measured frequently to determine bone marrow activity.

Physical activities depend on the child's clinical condition and pain control. Surgical intervention may be necessary if an abscess is present or if the infection does not respond to antibiotics. Invasive procedures include draining the abscess, débriding necrotic tissue, and performing a sequestrectomy (removal of the sequestrum). Osteomyelitis of the proximal femur generally requires some type of surgical decompression because septic arthritis of the hip can accompany this infection.

## NURSING CARE

### The Child With Osteomyelitis

#### Assessment

Because the organism is frequently transported through the bloodstream, a comprehensive history and physical, including dental history, is indicated. Although recalling every injury their child has experienced is difficult for parents, a thorough history of recent falls or traumas is helpful. The nurse should carefully examine the affected area and note any pain, tenderness, erythema, or swelling. Note if the pain or swelling involves the joint, as this can indicate septic arthritis. Usually, the child will protect the extremity, even tensing adjacent muscles and demonstrating reluctance to straighten or move it.

Document the child's neurovascular and pain status at least every 4 hours (more often if indicated). If the child is preverbal or not able to explain, the nurse should consult the parent. During the acute phase, the pain can be quite severe, and the nurse should assess the child's pain level and intervene before activities.

#### Nursing Diagnosis and Planning

The following nursing diagnoses and expected outcomes may be appropriate after assessment of the child with osteomyelitis:

- Acute Pain related to the infectious process.

**Expected outcome.** The child will experience a decrease in pain, as evidenced by a decreased pain score on an appropriate pain assessment tool and increased function.

- Impaired Physical Mobility related to the pain.

**Expected outcome.** The child will exhibit full range of motion and participate in self-care.

- Risk for Injury related to complications of antibiotic therapy.

**Expected outcome.** The parenteral insertion site will remain patent and free from signs of infection. The parents will properly store and administer the ordered antibiotics, care for the insertion site, and dispose of IV equipment.

- Deficient Knowledge about home management of long-term antibiotic therapy related to unfamiliarity with the procedures.

**Expected outcome.** The parents will demonstrate the correct administration of antibiotics, verbalize reportable adverse effects, and identify any other concerns or issues regarding home care.

#### Interventions

**Administering IV antibiotics.** A long-term IV site for antibiotic administration must be maintained. Therefore, the nurse must carefully and frequently monitor the site for signs of complications (see Chapter 38) and flush the line according to protocol.

The nurse should have a thorough knowledge of the antibiotic being given, which requires calculating the dosage based on body weight or surface area, reviewing side effects and adverse effects, and determining whether therapeutic blood levels are required. If the level of drug in the patient's blood exceeds the therapeutic range, the antibiotic should be withheld and the physician notified. Also notify the physician if the level is below the therapeutic level.

The child might receive multiple antibiotics. The nurse monitors compatibility and the total amount of fluids given. Allergies and any problems the child experienced during previous antibiotic administration should be evaluated. The nurse should periodically review current laboratory data to ensure adequate liver and kidney function. A complete blood cell count (CBC), CRP, and ESR should be measured on a regular basis to evaluate the child's response to treatment.

*Providing wound care.* Standard Precautions should be maintained at all times. Children with surgical wounds or drains need close monitoring. The color and consistency of the drainage and any unusual odor should be documented in the nurses' notes. A description of the wound should also be included.

*Maintaining nutritional status.* Meeting the child's nutritional needs is essential to facilitate growth and development and assist with the healing process. The child should receive a diet high in calories and protein. Frequent small meals and food that has been brought from home are helpful in stimulating the child's appetite.

*Teaching home management.* If the child is to receive IV antibiotic therapy at home, teach the parent how to set up the medication, how to maintain the IV line, and how to ensure that the infusion is being safely administered. Plan the teaching to fit the parent's schedule, and pay particular attention to signs of frustration or anxiety. Repetitive questions, poor eye contact, and nervous gestures are indicators that anxiety may be interfering with the parent's ability to retain information. Allow the parent to express feelings of concern and give positive feedback as the parent learns procedures. Before discharge, have the designated caregiver return demonstrate the administration of medications and catheter care. Make a home care referral to assist the family with the IV infusions.

Children who have had a favorable clinical response to IV antibiotics will occasionally be discharged with a course of oral antibiotics. Adherence to the medication regimen must be discussed with the parent. Emphasize the importance of follow-up care.

*Promoting optimal development.* Developmental issues should be addressed by the nurse. Discuss age-appropriate activities that will maintain current developmental levels. If the child is to remain at home for antibiotic therapy, advise and arrange for tutoring as soon as possible. School-age children need to continue with their schoolwork and maintain contact with their friends. Resources available to homebound children should be explored with the parent. If the child is exhibiting any residual fears or concerns related to hospitalization, therapeutic play activities might be needed.

### Evaluation

- Is the peripheral IV insertion site free from redness or swelling, and does the antibiotic infuse well?
- Can the parent describe and demonstrate proper antibiotic administration, care of the IV catheter, and disposal of associated equipment?
- Does the child indicate decreased pain on an appropriate pain assessment scale?
- Can the child exhibit full range of motion?
- Does the child participate in self-care?
- Does the parent provide developmentally appropriate activities for the child?
- Does the child exhibit any signs of developmental regression?
- Can the parent demonstrate all procedures needed for home care?

## SCOLIOSIS

Scoliosis is a lateral deviation, or curvature, of the spine that is greater than 10 degrees (Mistovich & Spiegel, 2016; Yang, Andras, Redding, et al., 2016). The extent of lateral curvature is determined using a Cobb angle measurement. In addition to lateral curvature, scoliosis involves actual rotation of the vertebral bodies in the spine; therefore, this deformity is considered to be three-dimensional (TSRHC, 2014). As a spinal curvature worsens, rotational structural deformities are seen in the vertebra and rib cage; severe rotational deformities can result in compromised respiratory function. Distortion of the intrathoracic and abdominal organs can also occur with severe deformity; however, this condition usually does not affect the function of these organs.

Classifications of scoliosis etiologies include congenital, syndromic, neuromuscular, and neural axis abnormalities; spinal tumors; thoracogenic (caused by a thoracotomy approach for surgical repair of an unrelated condition) (Table 50.4); and idiopathic. Idiopathic scoliosis can present at any point during a child's growth and is classified by the age at presentation: *infantile* (birth to 3 years of age), *juvenile* (3 to 10 years of age), and *adolescent* (10 years or older).

Early onset scoliosis (EOS), regardless of cause, occurs in infants and children up to 8 years of age. Children with EOS are at particular risk for *thoracic insufficiency syndrome,* which occurs when progressive rotation of the ribs or lack of thoracic growth (associated with congenital scoliosis) impairs growth of one or both lungs and

**TABLE 50.4 Classifications of Scoliosis**

| Classification | Curve |
|---|---|
| Congenital | Deformity occurs during fetal development<br>Present at birth<br>May have associated organ anomalies<br>Defect in vertebral formation and/or segmentation<br>Progression is unpredictable<br>Surgical management to halt progression |
| Syndromic<br>Idiopathic type (Marfan, neurofibromatosis, osteogenesis imperfecta)<br>Congenital type (VACTERL [VATER] syndrome, achondroplasia) | Idiopathic-like or congenital-like curve, depending on specific syndrome<br>Managed with observation and a variety of nonoperative and operative approaches |
| Neuromuscular | Long, sweeping curve, usually involves whole spine<br>Managed with observation, bracing, or fusion using laminar wires (not hooks and screws) |
| Neural axis abnormalities (syringomyelia [syrinx], tethered cord, diastematomyelia) | Idiopathic-like curve<br>Managed with a variety of nonoperative and operative approaches |
| Thoracogenic (related to a thoracotomy approach to repair an unrelated diagnosis) | Idiopathic-like curve<br>Managed with a variety of nonoperative and operative approaches |
| Postlaminectomy (typically for tumor removal or trauma) or postirradiation | Curve usually localized to immediate area or laminectomy, but may develop compensatory curve<br>Kyphotic deformity more common<br>Managed with a variety of nonoperative and operative approaches |

*VACTERL,* Vertebral, vascular, anal, cardiac, tracheoesophageal, renal, limb anomalies; *VATER,* vertebral defects, imperforate anus, tracheoesophageal fistula, radial and renal dysplasia.

interferes with respiration (TSRHC, 2014; Yang et al., 2016). Children with EOS must be examined frequently to assess for respiratory compromise. Both nonoperative and operative management are options for these children, with the goals being to halt the progression of the curve, facilitate thoracic growth, and improve pulmonary function.

## Adolescent Idiopathic Scoliosis

### Prevalence and Etiology

Adolescent idiopathic scoliosis (AIS) is the most common type of scoliosis. Radiographic evidence of curves of at least 10 degrees has established a prevalence of 2% to 3% in the general population (Weinstein & Dolan, 2015). The ratio of affected females to affected males increases with increasing curvature. Progressive curvature is more prevalent in females than males (TSRHC, 2014).

To date, there is no defined causative factor for idiopathic scoliosis. The most common proposed etiologies involve central neurologic dysfunction, connective tissue abnormalities, and genetic factors (TSRHC, 2014). Evidence indicates a strong genetic tendency toward idiopathic scoliosis in some families, as well as apparent autosomal dominant inheritance of adolescent idiopathic scoliosis and linkage between several chromosomes (Mistovich & Spiegel, 2016).

### Manifestations

The clinical manifestations of scoliosis include a visible curvature of the spine (Fig. 50.4). Other frequent manifestations include a rib hump that is visible when the child is bending forward, an asymmetrical rib cage, uneven shoulder or pelvic heights, prominence of the scapula, or hip, and leg-length discrepancy. A size difference in the space between the arms and the trunk is sometimes visible when the child is standing. Complaints of back pain are considered atypical and require a careful history and physical examination by the orthopedist. Impairment of respiratory function is also uncommon, as most patients are treated surgically before the curve progresses to a magnitude that would impair function.

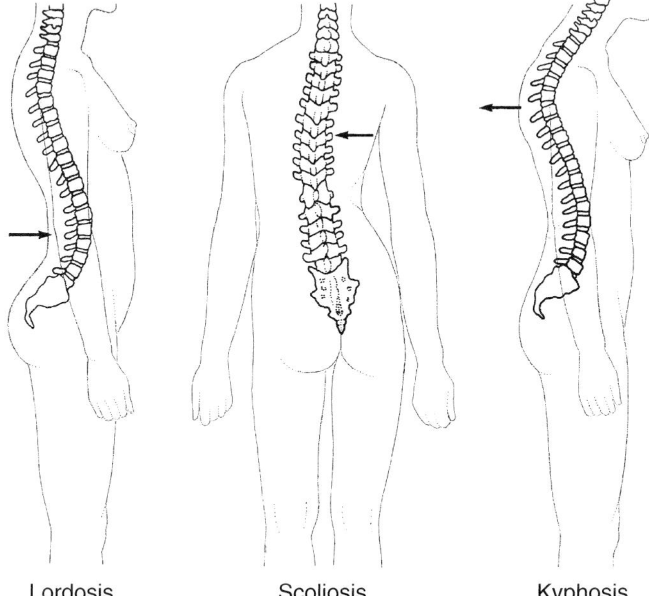


**FIG 50.4** Most spinal abnormalities in children are abnormal curvatures. In *scoliosis,* the spine curves laterally and the vertebrae rotate, pulling the ribs along. *Kyphosis* is a front-to-back rounding, usually of the thoracic spine; it is often accompanied by scoliosis. *Lordosis* is an exaggerated concave curvature of the spine, usually in the lumbar area.

### Diagnostic Evaluation

*School screening.* The American Academy of Orthopaedic Surgeons (AAOS), the Scoliosis Research Society (SRS), the Pediatric Orthopaedic Society of North America (POSNA), and the American Academy of Pediatrics (AAP) recognize the benefit of school screening for earlier detection of scoliosis (Scoliosis Research Society, 2015). They recommend that girls be screened twice, at 10 and 12 years of age (grades 5 and 7), and boys once, at age 13 or 14 (grades 8 or 9). Screening should always include the forward bending test, also known as an Adams forward bend test (see Chapter 33). A scoliometer, a small level-type device, can be used during the forward bend test to provide an angle of any vertebral rotation. Referral to an orthopedic surgeon is recommended for scoliometer readings of 7 or greater, indicating a 7-degree angle of trunk rotation. Because no single test is completely reliable for screening, a screening protocol should also assess for shoulder asymmetry, unequal scapular prominence, hip prominence or asymmetry, and the head not centered over the pelvis (see Fig. 50.4) (Mistovich & Spiegel, 2016; TSRHC, 2014). If asymmetry is detected, the parents should be informed, and orthopedic referral is recommended.

*Physical examination.* The orthopedist will view the entire back as well as the shoulders and iliac crests. To preserve the adolescent's modesty, a swimsuit or an examination gown is worn. The examination includes observing the shoulders and iliac crests for asymmetry, flank creases, rib hump, waist asymmetry, limb length discrepancy, and whether the head and/or trunk are centered over the middle of the pelvis. The patient is also assessed from the side to appreciate any decrease or increase in the natural curvature of the sagittal plane of the spine. A basic neurologic examination of strength and reflexes of the extremities will be performed. The patient's abdominal reflexes are assessed to rule out a neurologic cause of the scoliosis (idiopathic patients respond the same on both sides of the abdomen).

Spinal deformity progression is driven by growth; therefore, indicators of skeletal maturity are important factors in analyzing a patient with AIS. For girls, menarche is a crucial indicator; a premenarchal girl is still actively growing, whereas a postmenarchal girl is in the decelerated process of growth, and thus, has a lower chance of curvature progression. The sexual maturity of the patient is assessed using the Tanner system, which classifies breast and pubic hair development (see Chapter 9).

*Radiographs.* Plain radiographs will be obtained with a coronal and sagittal view, from the head down to the mid-thigh (Fig. 50.5). Possible findings include a single curvature or a main curvature with secondary or even tertiary curvatures surrounding it. These secondary curves can be structural or compensatory (meaning not a true manifestation of the disease but the body's response in trying to get the head level over the pelvis).

The orthopedist measures the degree of scoliosis seen on the radiographs using the Cobb angle technique. Cobb angle measurements are obtained for all curvatures shown on radiographs in both the coronal and sagittal views. Because scoliosis is a three-dimensional deformity, the amount of vertebral rotation as well as indicators of spinal balance are also assessed on the radiographs.

Radiographs are also examined for signs of skeletal maturity and growth status. An indicator called the Risser sign (grades 1 to 5) can assist with assessing the level of peak height velocity (PHV) (see Chapter 9), which can determine the probability of curve progression (Horne, Flannery, & Usman, 2014). After skeletal maturity, the rate of curve progression decreases significantly. Curvature size is also useful

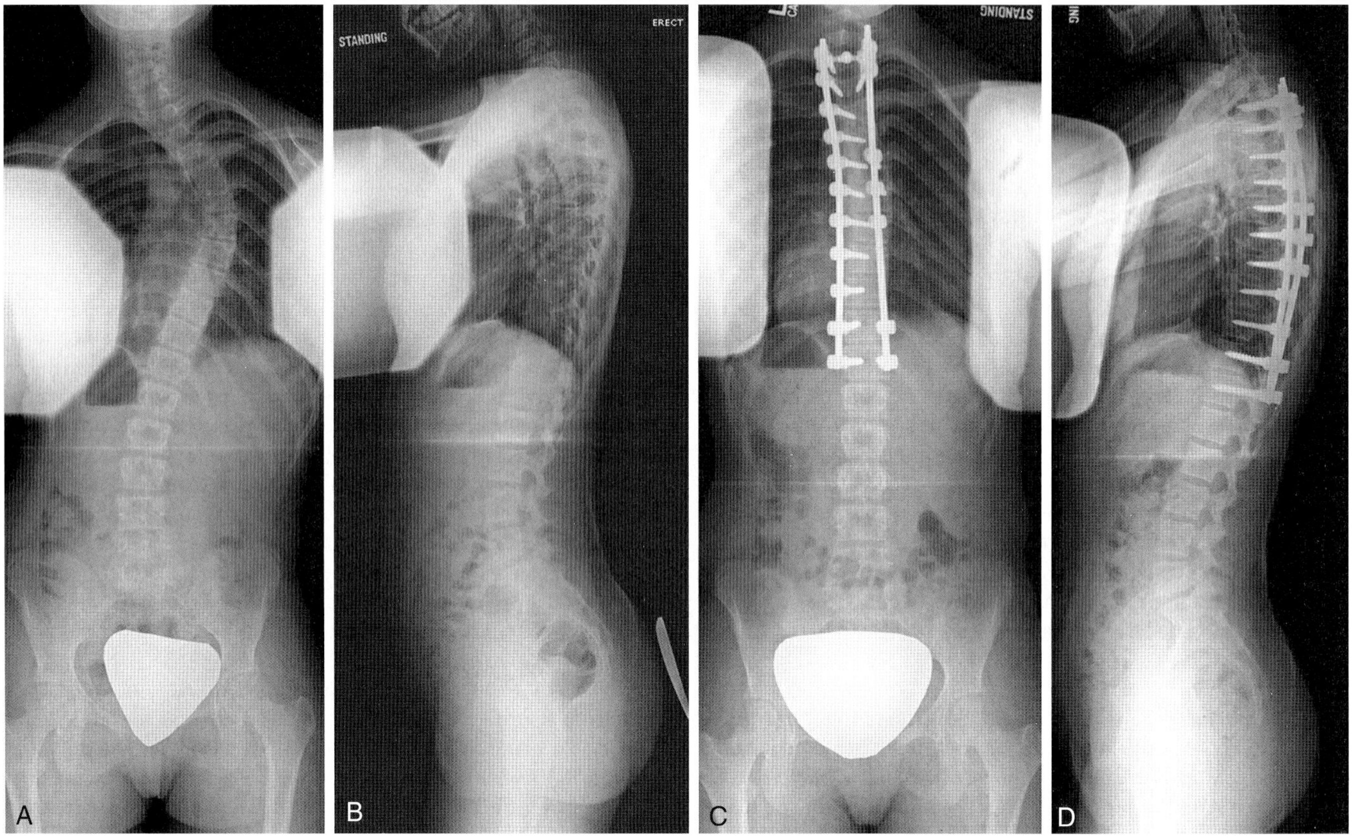

**FIG 50.5** Plain radiographs of scoliosis before **(A, B)** and after spinal fusion **(C, D)**. (Courtesy Texas Scottish Rite Hospital for Children, Dallas, TX.)

in predicting progression, as larger curves have a greater chance of progressing (Horne et al., 2014).

## Treatment

***Nonsurgical interventions.*** Curves less than 25 degrees require observation for progression, regardless of skeletal maturity (TSRHC, 2014). Patients closer to 25 degrees and who are skeletally immature will require more frequent radiographic observation than a patient with a smaller curvature who is skeletally mature. Progression is defined as a 7 to 10 degree increase in the Cobb angle.

Brace treatment is recommended for patients who present or progress in curve magnitude to 25 degrees or more and are still skeletally immature. The goal of treatment is to prevent further progression, which is accomplished by pads in the brace that push on the curve. Each brace is custom made for the individual patient curve(s) by an orthotist (Fig. 50.6). Patients with a lumbar curve typically wear a nighttime-only brace. Other curve patterns require that a brace be worn 22 to 23 hours a day. Patients are told to wear a form-fitting T-shirt underneath the brace to reduce skin breakdown and irritation. Wearing the brace is effective in preventing progression of the curve (Horne et al., 2014).

Radiographs are typically obtained every 4 months during rapid growth and then every 6 months as the patient reaches maturity. The patient is told not to wear the brace the night before the visit to see how the curve is responding. As the patient is growing, adjustments to the brace may be necessary, or a new brace may be required. For girls, brace wear is discontinued once she is 18 to 24 months postmenarchal, has a Risser grade suggesting she is near skeletal maturity, and has had

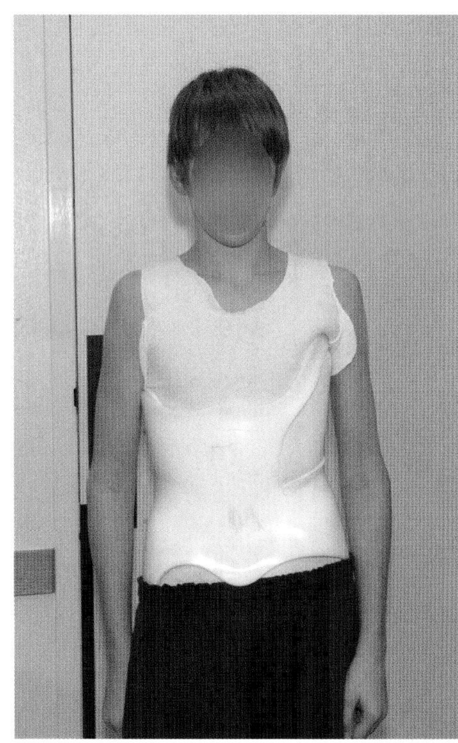

**FIG 50.6** Adolescent with scoliosis brace. (Courtesy Texas Scottish Rite Hospital for Children, Dallas, TX.)

no further increase in standing height. For boys, discontinuation is recommended after achieving a Risser grade of 5, which is typically in the later teenage years.

*Surgical intervention.* Surgery is considered for curvatures that reach 40 to 50 degrees. The primary goal is to reduce the size of the curve(s) and obtain a solid fusion of the treated part of the spine. A successful surgery might not completely correct the curvature but will provide the patient with a well-balanced spine that centers the patient's head, shoulders, and trunk over the pelvis (TSRHC, 2014).

Typically, the surgical approach is posterior down the length of the spine to be fused. An anterior approach is sometimes considered for a large, stiff curve; young age; or a curvature limited to the lumbar spine. In a posterior approach, implants (either hooks or screws) are placed on or in the vertebral body. These implants are then attached to two rods that are used to correct the deformity. To achieve a solid fusion of the corrected curvature, additional bone is needed to graft the fixed portion of the spine. Bone can be grafted from the patient (autograft). Common graft donor sites include parts of the vertebral body removed during surgery, the iliac crest, and ribs. Allograft in the form of frozen, bank-stored bone is becoming increasingly popular as it has proven safe, efficacious, and cost-effective (Fischer et al., 2013). Bone morphogenetic protein (BMP) is an additive that can be used to speed up and further solidify the fusion.

*Surgical complications.* Significant blood loss is common with spinal fusion surgery because of the vascular nature of the vertebrae and spinal canal. Several methods are used to reduce the need for donor blood transfusion intraoperatively; these include preoperative autologous blood donation (children donate their own blood before surgery), controlled hypotensive anesthesia, hemodilution, cell salvage of lost blood, and the use of antifibrinolytic agents (aprotinin or aminocaproic acid [Amicar]). Clinical indicators, not just hemoglobin values, inform the decision to transfuse (TSRHC, 2014).

A potential complication of surgical correction is insult or injury to the spinal cord. Intraoperative neuromonitoring (IONM) of motor and sensory function, with immediate corrective actions by the surgeon or the anesthetist should the changes be severe (Pastorelli et al., 2011), can reduce the chance of neurologic injury during surgery.

Other complications include lack of solid bone fusion (pseudoarthrosis), implant failure (rod breakage or pullout of a hook or screw), continued progression of the deformity, and infection (Cho & Egorova, 2015; Mistovich & Spiegel, 2016). Some infections require only a round of oral antibiotics, while others are extensive and require irrigation, débridement, and total implant removal.

*Postoperative management.* Postoperative pain is typically treated with analgesics and regional anesthesia (e.g., epidural) (Slinko, 2014). These methods of pain management are usually used up to postoperative day 2 or 3, at which time the patient is switched to an oral method of pain control. Patients are able to sit up in a chair on postoperative day 2 and typically go home by day 4 or 5.

*Follow-up care.* Patients return to the clinic within 1 to 6 weeks, depending on surgeon preference, and are usually followed for 2 or more years postoperatively or until reaching 18 years of age. Most patients return to school after 2 weeks. Patients are released to full activity by 6 months to 1 year postoperatively. Every patient is instructed to avoid tattoos and piercings. Although controversial, some surgeons will also require their patients to have prophylactic antibiotics before dental procedures to reduce the chance of infection (TSRHC, 2014).

## KYPHOSIS

*Kyphosis* is the natural curvature of the thoracic spine in the sagittal plane (see Fig. 50.4), although it also can occur in other areas of the spine. Normally, kyphosis ranges between 20 and 45 degrees by Cobb angle measurement. Hyperkyphosis is any angle greater than 45 degrees. Postural kyphosis is benign and can be corrected by proper posture techniques (actively contracting the erector spinae muscles and tightening the abdominal muscles) (TSRHC, 2014). Typically, this condition resolves if the patient follows a core-muscle–strengthening program.

### Scheuermann's Kyphosis

Scheuermann's disease is the most common cause of hyperkyphosis in adolescents (TSRHC, 2014). This condition involves a fixed angular kyphosis with a characteristic wedging of the anterior vertebra at the apex of the curve (middle). The incidence of Scheuermann's disease is reported as 0.4% to 10% of adolescents between 10 and 14 years of age. The etiology of this disease is unknown.

Patients can experience pain at the apex of the deformity and at the base of the neck. The kyphotic apex becomes apparent on an Adams forward bend. Most patients are given a core-strengthening program and need no further intervention, as the natural history of this disease is relatively benign. Follow-up includes clinical and radiographic observation on an annual basis.

For patients who have progressive kyphosis with the apex located in the thoracic area, bracing might be advised. However, correction gains made during bracing disappear when bracing is discontinued (TSRHC, 2014). Surgical treatment of Scheuermann's disease is reserved for patients with documented pain in a rigid curve of more than 70 degrees and a poor sagittal contour clinically (Mistovich & Spiegel, 2016). The goal of surgery is to provide a well-balanced spine in the sagittal plane. Typically, a posterior spinal fusion is performed in a manner similar to that for an AIS patient. Intraoperative neuromonitoring is key, as the hyperkyphosis presents a more stretched spinal cord than in scoliosis and can increase the risk for spinal cord injury. Potential complications, postoperative care, and follow-up are the same as those described for surgical treatment of AIS (Mistovich & Spiegel, 2016).

### Other Causes of Hyperkyphosis

Any of the etiologies that have been discussed as causing scoliosis can also cause hyperkyphosis. Typically, idiopathic-like syndromes, neuromuscular, and neural-axis abnormalities produce a more global hyperkyphosis, meaning that all of the thoracic spine and possibly some of the lumbar spine is involved (TSRHC, 2014). Kyphosis that is congenital, postlaminectomy, tubercular, or postirradiation is more localized or angular, such that two to five levels are involved. This condition can occur in any region of the spine. In global deformities, surgical intervention will depend on the curvature size and the amount of growth left in the spine. In angular deformities, surgical intervention is warranted if the curvature is compressing or stretching the spinal cord, causing neurologic symptoms.

## LIMB DIFFERENCES

Limb differences are common in children. Most alterations of arms and legs are mild variations of normal posture. Education and reassurance are the primary nursing interventions for patients with limb differences.

### Etiology and Incidence

Limb differences can be physiologic, congenital birth anomalies, or the result of trauma, infection, or radiation. These differences take many forms, including webbing (syndactyly), extra digits (fingers or toes; polydactyly), genu valgum ("knock-knees"), genu varum (bowlegs),

## NURSING CARE PLAN

### *The Adolescent Undergoing a Spinal Fusion*

**Focused Assessment**

***Preoperative Assessment***

- Assess anxiety related to surgery, hospitalization, and postsurgical issues (e.g., pain, appearance of the operative site, activity limitations, and altered appearance).

***Postoperative Assessment***

- Meticulously assess the neurologic status of the lower extremities.
- Assess pain, fluid balance, bleeding, and return of bowel function.
- Assess and document wound healing, ease of mobility, and nutritional status.
- Focus on respiratory assessment if the anterior/thoracic approach has been used and the adolescent has a chest tube.
- Determine discharge teaching needs and parent or adolescent understanding of follow-up care.

**Nursing Diagnosis**

Anxiety (preoperative) related to impending surgery.

**Planning**

***Expected Outcome***

The adolescent will have reduced anxiety, as evidenced by seeking information about the surgery and postoperative care and by identifying and using effective coping mechanisms to address it.

**Interventions and *Rationales***

1. Determine whether the adolescent is anxious about surgery.
   *The adolescent may not be anxious or may be hiding anxiety.*
2. Initiate a conversation with the adolescent about what anxiety feels like and how anxiety is a normal response to anticipated surgery.
   *The adolescent may need permission to discuss anxiety and may require assistance verbalizing feelings. Adolescents need to be assured that they are normal.*

For example,

"Many girls facing surgery are nervous about what it will be like to have this operation. Perhaps you would like to know more about what it will be like."

3. Assist the adolescent with identifying positive and effective means for resolving anxiety (e.g., talking with a friend, exercising, engaging in activities, practicing relaxation techniques).
   *By role modeling for the adolescent and discussing various possibilities for coping, the nurse allows the adolescent to find a comfortable means for expressing feelings.*
4. Identify and discourage negative behaviors associated with anxiety (e.g., verbal outbursts, physical aggression, withdrawal).
   *The adolescent needs to understand that expressing feelings can be done in acceptable and unacceptable ways.*

Try telling the adolescent,

"It's OK and normal to be anxious about surgery. This is hard for your parents, too. Let's talk about ways you might let your parents know how you are feeling."

5. Reassure the adolescent about specific fears ("Can my parents be with me?" "Will I get a shot?" "Will I have a huge scar?").
   *Reassurance and conversation may help resolve some fears.*
6. Determine the adolescent's need for specific information, particularly about postoperative care. Explain the reason for the various postoperative interventions:
   a. Neurovascular checks every 2 hours for the first 48 hours and every 4 hours thereafter
   b. Turning by log-rolling every 2 hours
   c. Deep breathing and use of incentive spirometer (chest tube if anterior approach is used)
   d. Wound dressing (if applicable)
   e. Brace application and skin care
   *Fears about the unknown may be reduced by increasing knowledge. Adolescents are more cooperative in the postoperative period if they know the reason for interventions.*
7. Have the adolescent (or parents and adolescent) demonstrate specific skills (e.g., coughing, recumbent log-rolling).
   *Allows the nurse to evaluate learning and allows the adolescent to gain confidence in being able to perform the maneuver; confidence in managing care decreases anxiety.*
8. Encourage the adolescent to ask questions and discuss concerns. Correct any inaccurate information.
   *Clarification of misperceptions decreases anxiety.*

**Evaluation**

Does the adolescent seek information about the surgery and its postoperative course?

Is the adolescent able to talk about anxiety or fears with parents, friends, or the nurse?

Can the adolescent use appropriate techniques to reduce anxiety?

**Nursing Diagnosis**

Acute Pain related to the operative procedure.

**Planning**

***Expected Outcomes***

The adolescent will indicate decreasing amounts of pain as measured on a pain scale, appear calm and relaxed, and participate in postoperative activities.

**Interventions and *Rationales***

1. Frequently monitor the adolescent's pain level by using an appropriate pain rating scale in the postoperative period. (Statements of pain, anxiety, an inability to cough, hyperalertness, reluctance or refusal to move, and sweating indicate pain.)
   *Adolescents may be unable or unwilling to verbalize their pain.*
2. Provide prescribed analgesics in a timely manner (children usually receive epidural analgesia or patient-controlled analgesia [PCA] initially after surgery).
   *The appropriate and timely use of analgesics provides optimal control of pain. Epidural analgesia provides more constant pain relief and prevents peaks and valleys of pain. Oral analgesics should be given on an around the-clock schedule to avoid peaks and valleys of pain control from prolonged onset and peak of action.*
3. Determine response to pain-relief measures and communicate with the physician about possible adjustments if needed. (See Chapter 39 for a thorough discussion of the nursing care of children and teenagers in pain.)
   *Adjustments may be necessary to achieve optimal pain relief.*

## NURSING CARE PLAN—cont'd

### *The Adolescent Undergoing a Spinal Fusion*

**Evaluation**

Can the adolescent use a pain scale to rate pain?
Does the adolescent appear calm and relaxed?
Is the adolescent able to participate in postoperative activities?

**Nursing Diagnosis**

Deficient Knowledge related to unfamiliarity with information about spinal fusion and postoperative management at home.

**Planning**

***Expected Outcome***

The family and adolescent will successfully manage treatment at home, as evidenced by demonstrating procedures, accessing appropriate community resources, and keeping follow-up appointments.

**Interventions and *Rationales***

1. Teach the family and adolescent the correct technique for wound care and the signs of wound infection (redness, swelling, drainage, fever); emphasize the role of a well-balanced diet in wound healing.
   *Proper wound care and good nutrition promote healing and decrease the chance of infection.*
2. Have the adolescent (or parents) demonstrate specific skills (e.g., brace application, skin care, daily exercises, performing activities without bending at the waist).
   *Allows the nurse to evaluate learning and encourages the adolescent to gain confidence in the ability to perform the appropriate skills.*
3. Discuss home care:
   a. Activity restrictions. (Initially, these adolescents will be restricted from participating in sports or gym or lifting more than 10 lb.)
   b. Be alert for signs such as skin breakdown, pain, numbness or tingling in the extremities, and other potential problems.
   *Home care instructions reduce the possibility of complications. Activity restrictions are usually maintained for 6 to 9 months depending on the type of surgery and the physician.*
4. Provide the name and telephone number of an easily accessible healthcare provider if questions arise at home. Inform the family about community resources available, including resources for tutoring. Referral to national scoliosis associations may be helpful. Schedule a follow-up appointment and emphasize the importance of keeping appointments.
   *Access to a healthcare provider and/or community resources decreases anxiety and improves adherence to treatment. Periodic evaluation is important to recovery.*

**Evaluation**

Can the family demonstrate the procedures necessary to care for the adolescent at home?
Can the adolescent and family demonstrate correct application of the brace (if required), proper wound and skin care, or prescribed exercise regimen?
Is the family aware of sources of help if needed?
Does the family keep follow-up appointments?

limb-length differences, and congenital absence of all or part of an extremity.

### Diagnostic Evaluation

Most congenital defects are readily apparent at birth. Mild defects and deformities that develop over time are usually identified by parents or school nurses and are evaluated by specialized clinicians. Radiographs may be necessary to evaluate limb defects fully and assist with developing a treatment plan.

### Therapeutic Management

The management of children with limb differences is related to the type of difference the child is manifesting (Table 50.5).

### Nursing Considerations

Nursing considerations for a child with a physiologic limb difference mainly include providing reassurance to the parent that the child's condition will self-correct and educating the parent about safety if the child has any gait disturbance. For children who require treatment, such as immobilization or surgical correction, teach the parent and the child, if appropriate, what to expect both before and after the procedure or surgery.

## DEVELOPMENTAL DYSPLASIA OF THE HIP

Developmental dysplasia of the hip (DDH) describes a variety of disorders that present in different forms at different ages. Dysplasia varies in severity from quite mild to severe dislocation. DDH can be present at birth (congenital), but in some children, it develops after birth—hence the term *developmental*.

### Etiology and Incidence

The exact cause of DDH is unknown, but genetic factors may play a role (Sankar, Horn, Wells, et al., 2016). Risk factors include being the first-born child, being female, breech position, and low levels of amniotic fluid *in utero* (Sankar et al., 2016). Estimates of the incidence of hip instability in the newborn range from 1 in 100 to 1 in 250, with an actual hip dislocation in approximately 1 to 1.5/1000 (Sankar et al., 2016). Higher incidences are reported when screening uses both clinical examination and ultrasonography. The incidence of DDH shows distinct geographic and racial variations. Children of African or Chinese descent have a low incidence of DDH, while other groups, including Native American children, have a high incidence. One or both hips can be involved.

### Manifestations

The symptoms of DDH vary according to age. In neonates, it is characterized by instability of the hip; the femoral head can be displaced partially (subluxated) or fully (dislocated) from the acetabulum by the examiner. The hip sometimes rests in a dislocated position and can be reduced on examination. This condition can be detected by performing the Ortolani and Barlow tests (see Chapter 21) or by observing significant changes in the morphology of the hip on sonograms.

**TABLE 50.5 Limb Differences**

| Description | Therapeutic Management |
|---|---|
| **Femoral Anteversion (Intoeing)** | |
| Forward position of the femoral neck in relation to the femoral shaft; results in internal rotation of the lower extremity; intoeing noticed when child begins to walk | No treatment necessary because the condition usually resolves with growth and skeletal maturity |
| **Tibial Torsion** | |
| Most common cause of intoeing or outtoeing; inward or outward rotation of the tibia; noticed when child begins to walk | Observation; spontaneously resolves in most cases |
| **Genu Varum (Bowlegs)** | |
| Legs are in bowed position (Fig. 50.7); more apparent when child stands or walks | Spontaneous resolution by 2 yr of age; reevaluation required if condition persists beyond age 2 yr or becomes progressively worse |
| **Genu Valgum (Knock Knees)** | |
| Valgus alignment (Fig. 50.8) can be normal until 8 yr of age | Correction with surgical *hemiepiphysiodesis* (slows the growth plate on the inside) if condition persists beyond 8 yr or if child has gait disturbance, difficulty running, or knee pain |
| **Tibia Vara (Blount Disease)** | |
| Growth retardation of the medial aspect of the tibial epiphysis; results in progressive or persistent bowing of the legs<br>• Infant form: Appears before 3 yr of age; more prominent in children of Afro-Caribbean or Scandinavian descent; child usually above 95th percentile for weight; lateral thrust of the knee resembles a limp<br>• Adolescent form: Appears after 10 yr of age | Infant form: If untreated, deformity progresses and growth retardation can occur; orthotic correction if condition is in an early stage; surgical **osteotomy** considered if condition persists beyond 3 yr<br>Adult form: Primarily surgical to restore physeal growth and prevent degenerative arthritis of the knee; osteotomy or lateral epiphysiodesis (slows growth on the outside of the growth plate) may be considered |
| **Leg Length Discrepancy** | |
| Inequality in the length of the two legs | No treatment if the discrepancy is 2-2.5 cm in a skeletally mature child; shoe lift is considered for toe walking; possible surgery for discrepancy larger than 2.5 cm includes epiphysiodesis on longer leg or femoral shortening with internal fixation; leg lengthening might be considered for discrepancy larger than 4 cm, but it has complications, so not done routinely |
| **Osteochondritis Dissecans of the Knee** | |
| Softened, loose, or separated cartilage and bone along the femoral articular surface; knee pain, parapatellar ache that worsens with sports or vigorous activity | Observation and activity restriction until symptoms resolve—lesions usually heal spontaneously over several months; immobilization or brace may be considered if symptoms persist; gradual resumption of activity; arthroscopy for persistent or unstable lesion |
| **Osgood-Schlatter Disease** | |
| Bilateral knee pain that occurs with running, jumping, or climbing stairs; associated with growth and more common in boys; pain and swelling at the tibial tubercle from inflammation at the tendon insertion site | Usually self-limiting—resolves with skeletal maturity; is not made worse with activity; NSAIDs for pain; knee immobilizer may be considered |

Infants beyond the newborn period exhibit asymmetry of the gluteal skinfolds when lying with the legs extended against the examining table (or when the infant is held upright with the legs dangling). The affected hip has a limited range of motion, and asymmetric **abduction** is present when the child is placed supine with the knees and hips flexed. The femur on the affected side appears to be shorter than that on the other side. The symptoms range from lax ligaments to contractures and stiffness in the affected hip joint or joints.

Any abnormalities in an older child's gait should be carefully evaluated as possible signs of the condition. Walking children may exhibit limping, toe-walking, or a waddling gait. Bilateral dysplasia is always more difficult to identify than unilateral dysplasia because there is not a normal hip to use for comparison.

### Diagnostic Evaluation

DDH can be difficult to diagnose in the neonate because the signs and symptoms are often quite subtle. A well-trained nurse or physician screens for DDH at birth and during each routine infant well-child visit by carefully performing the Barlow and Ortolani maneuvers.

An ultrasound of the hip is used to confirm DDH in infants (Sankar et al., 2016). Ultrasonography reveals the anatomy of the hip and the relationship of the femoral head and acetabulum. Current research indicates that ultrasonography is a more sensitive indicator of abnormalities of the infant hip than radiography. However, some authors argue that ultrasonography is too sensitive and results in overtreatment of hips that would otherwise develop normally.

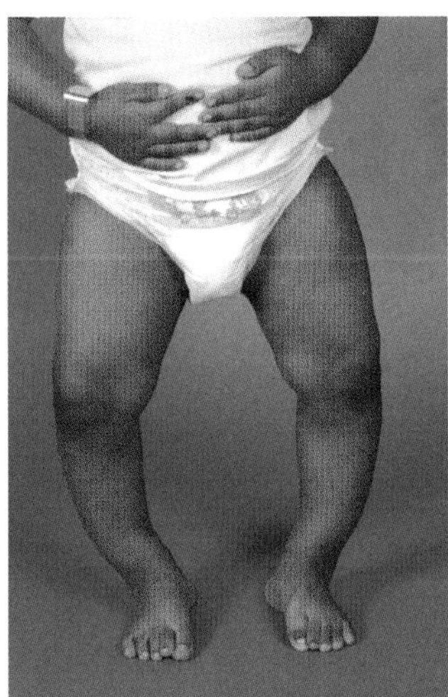

FIG 50.7 Genu varum (bowlegs). In the child with genu varum, or bowlegs, a persistent space is present between the knees when the ankles are together. Genu varum is a normal finding for 1 year after the child begins walking. (Courtesy Texas Scottish Rite Hospital for Children, Dallas, TX.)

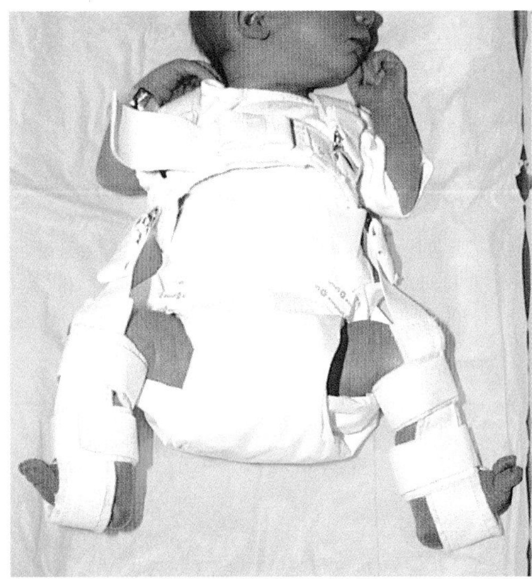

FIG 50.9 An infant in a Pavlik harness to treat developmental dysplasia of the hip.

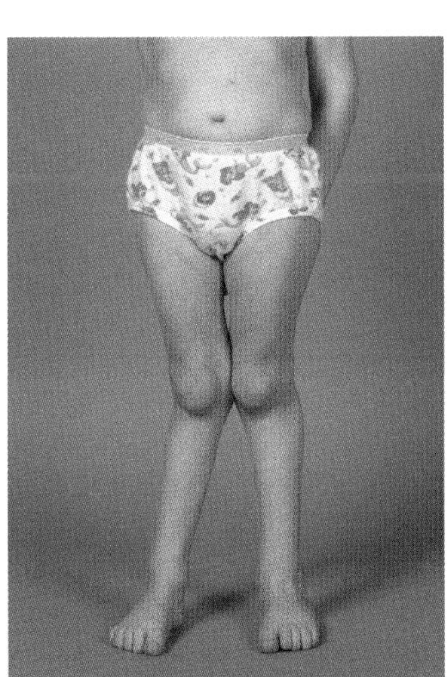

FIG 50.8 Genu valgum (knock knees). In the child with genu valgum, or knock knees, a space is present between the ankles when the knees are together. To remember the terminology, liken the r's and g's: genu va*r*um—knees apa*r*t; genu val*g*um—knees to*g*ether. (Courtesy Texas Scottish Rite Hospital for Children, Dallas, TX.)

Plain radiography of the pelvis usually reveals a frankly dislocated hip in individuals of any age, but because ossification is not complete in infancy, radiographs may only be diagnostic after 1 year of age. Some parents are concerned about radiation exposure in the course of treating their child's DDH. Reassure them that the increase in cancer risk from the cumulative radiographs taken to manage an average patient with DDH is less than 1%. CT and MRI are sometimes used in complex cases.

## Therapeutic Management

Early diagnosis and treatment of DDH are important for maximizing the likelihood of a successful outcome. Treatment depends on the age of the child at the time of diagnosis and on the severity of the dysplasia. The primary goal of treatment in DDH, regardless of age, is to facilitate normal development of the hip socket. This is accomplished through approaches that provide anatomic reduction of the hip and maintenance of the reduction. In newborns and infants younger than 6 months, a Pavlik harness is the treatment of choice for a hip that is dislocated and can be reduced by the examiner. The Pavlik harness maintains the hips in flexion, abduction, and external rotation. This device consists of chest and shoulder straps and foot stirrups (Fig. 50.9). Initially, the harness is worn continuously. This bracing method can be the only treatment necessary to allow the hip to mold and grow normally, promoting development of a functional hip socket and a well-formed femoral head. Hips that remain unstable become progressively deformed as the skeleton matures, resulting in functional disability.

Parents must be taught the proper use of the harness because improper positioning of the infant's hip can cause interruption of the blood supply to the head of the femur, resulting in *avascular necrosis* (tissue damage caused by an inadequate blood supply) or femoral palsy. Teach parents to observe for equal leg extension in and out of the harness. In addition, skin care; techniques for holding, feeding, and diapering; and the importance of vigilant follow-up must be emphasized.

Treatment is more complicated when the condition is diagnosed after the newborn period. Closed or open hip reduction surgery, preceded by home management with Bryant's traction (to release muscles and tendons), is usually necessary to manipulate the hip joint (TSRHC, 2014). Positioning and immobilization for 3 months in a spica cast follow the procedure. After reduction of a dislocated hip, the acetabulum begins to remodel in response to the pressure exerted by the femoral head. In some instances, this process is incomplete, and the acetabulum remains shallow.

Adolescent patients sometimes present with hip complaints, including groin pain (indicating pain coming from the hip joint) and lateral hip pain (usually indicating lateral abductor fatigue pain). For children with residual dysplasia and acetabular dysplasia diagnosed during adolescence, osteotomy (surgical cutting of the bone) and repositioning of the femur is recommended (Sankar et al., 2016). After certain surgeries, long-term immobilization in a spica cast is necessary until healing is achieved. Radiographs show the progress achieved with treatment. Follow-up monitoring is essential.

## PATHOPHYSIOLOGY

### *Developmental Dysplasia of the Hip*

In the normal infant hip, the head of the femur is well seated in the acetabulum (hip socket) and is stable. Developmental dysplasia of the hip occurs in varying degrees, ranging from instability of the hip joint to frank dislocation, defined as follows:

- *Instability of the hip* is the appropriate term when the head of the femur is located in the acetabulum but is subluxated (partially dislocated) or even dislocated with manual manipulation.
- *Dislocation of the hip* occurs when the head of the femur lies outside the acetabulum. It can occur as a late stage of developmental dysplasia of the hip or in children with certain neuromuscular disorders.
- **Subluxation** *of the hip* occurs when the head of the femur is positioned under the edge of the acetabulum. It is not well seated in the acetabulum, yet neither is it completely dislocated.

Interestingly, many unstable hips spontaneously resolve. If untreated, only approximately 20% will settle into a dislocated position.

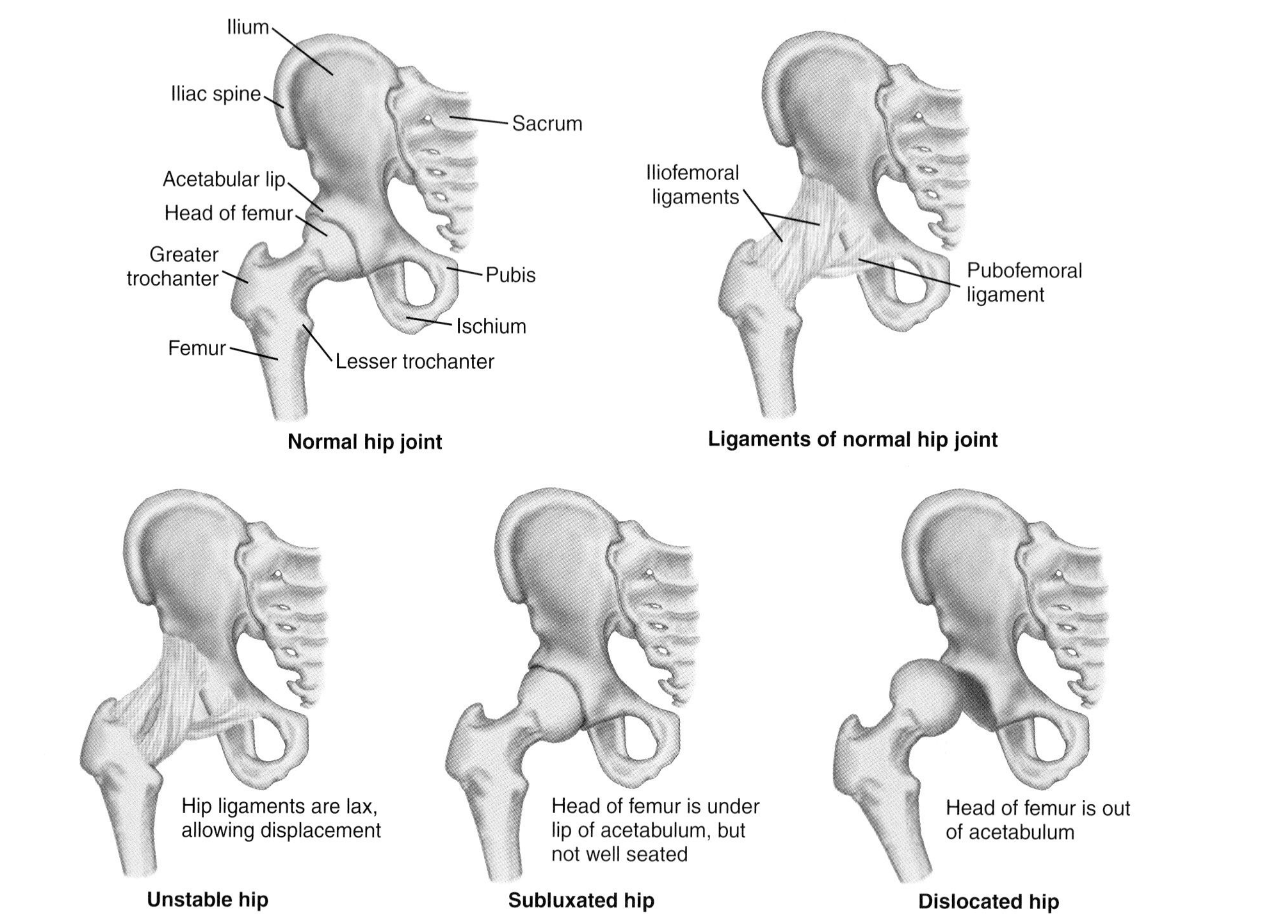


## NURSING CARE

### The Child With Developmental Dysplasia of the Hip

#### Assessment

All infants should be assessed for DDH during routine neonatal and well-child visits to ensure prompt diagnosis and treatment. Assessment procedures vary with the age of the child. Once the diagnosis is established, nursing assessment is directed to the parents' knowledge level, their anxiety and coping abilities, and ensuring that the treatment regimen is followed.

Because the needs of children with musculoskeletal disorders are often long term, parents usually have a good understanding of their child's progress. Questions such as "What concerns do you have about your child's progress today?" or "How are you doing at home?" acknowledge that the parents' feelings and ideas are valued and important. Information generated by such questions can become the focus for assessment and further intervention.

Monitor the skin integrity of an infant in a Pavlik harness or spica cast. When surgery becomes necessary, nursing priorities shift to assessing lower extremity circulation and pain.

#### Nursing Diagnosis and Planning

The nursing diagnoses and expected outcomes that may be appropriate for the child with DDH and the child's family include the following:

- Deficient Knowledge related to confusion regarding child's condition and ongoing treatment.

***Expected outcome.*** The parents will demonstrate understanding of DDH and the therapeutic use of a Pavlik harness (or spica cast). The parents will describe and demonstrate how to care for their child in a Pavlik harness (or spica cast). The parents can describe adverse effects, complications of treatment, and whom to contact with questions and concerns.

- Parental Anxiety related to guilt (for having a less-than-perfect child) and the need to provide complex care for an extended period.

*Expected outcome.* The parents will feel less anxious, as evidenced by being able to describe DDH and its treatment in lay terms to other family members, carry out treatment regimens, demonstrate increased self-confidence in the care of their child, treat the child as normally as possible, and interact with healthcare providers and others in a calm and friendly manner.

- Risk for Impaired Skin Integrity related to skin chafing by the Pavlik harness or spica cast.

*Expected outcome.* On follow-up visits, the cast will be reasonably clean and dry and the child's skin will be clear and intact, without abrasions or sores.

- Ineffective Tissue Perfusion (Lower Extremities) related to impaired circulation as a result of bracing, casting, or surgery.

*Expected outcome.* The circulation to the child's feet and toes will remain adequate as evidenced by a capillary refill time of less than 2 seconds and toes that are pink and warm.

- Risk for Injury related to improper positioning of a child in a Pavlik harness or spica cast.

*Expected outcome.* The child will be safe from falls and will be adequately restrained when traveling in an automobile.

### Interventions

*Teaching about the pavlik harness.* Demonstrate and teach the parents the proper care and application of the Pavlik harness, including how to position and fasten the chest halter (leave room for two fingers to rotate under this strap), fasten the shoulder straps (crossed in back) over each shoulder (leave room under the top of each shoulder strap for one finger), place the child's leg and foot into the stirrup and straps, and connect the straps to the chest halter. The requirements for harness use can change during therapy, so teaching, demonstration, and return demonstration are essential at every visit. Leg straps should be secure enough to keep the child's hips flexed without being tight. The harness should be worn 23 hr/day and should be removed only according to the physician's recommendation. Encourage the parents to hold and cuddle the infant as much as possible. An infant in a Pavlik harness can be fed in the usual positions.

Teach the parents to protect the child's skin and legs under the harness. A long T-shirt ("onesie") under the halter reduces harness rubbing. The diaper should go under the harness. Teach the parents to inspect the child's skin frequently for reddened or irritated areas and to reposition the child often.

*Teaching about spica cast care.* Caring for a child in a spica cast is similar to caring for a child in any other type of cast (as previously discussed), with some additional adaptations. Because the cast covers the entire lower half of the child's body with only a limited perineal opening, managing the child's elimination is a challenge. Excess urine can trickle under the cast, irritating and macerating the skin, resisting drying, and becoming malodorous. Advise the family to tuck a disposable diaper underneath the cast edges at the circular perineal opening; advise parents not to use sheet plastic under the cast, which can cause pooling of urine beneath the cast and subsequent skin breakdown. Place a sanitary napkin within the diaper that is tucked under the cast edges. Elevating the head of the bed helps urine and feces drain downward and away from the cast.

Monitor the child's neurovascular status frequently (Fig. 50.10), and teach the family the signs of neurovascular compromise. Fever, wound drainage, and discomfort are signs of infection and should be reported promptly. Teach the family ways to provide environmental and developmental stimulation (e.g., by moving the child to different areas during the day, placing appropriate toys within reach, and providing age-appropriate activities). Teach the family to ensure that the extremities within the cast are always supported with pillows, rolled-up towels, or "bean bag" chairs. Explain the importance of feeding the child a diet high in fluids, calories, calcium, protein, and fiber, and instruct parents to keep the child in an upright position for a minimum of 30 minutes after feeding. Explain ways to dress the child to accommodate climate, style, and other needs (e.g., by fitting socks over the toes of the cast, using Velcro closures on pants and shorts, or using clothing made of stretch fabrics). Give the parents the name and telephone number of an easily accessible healthcare provider in case questions arise at home.

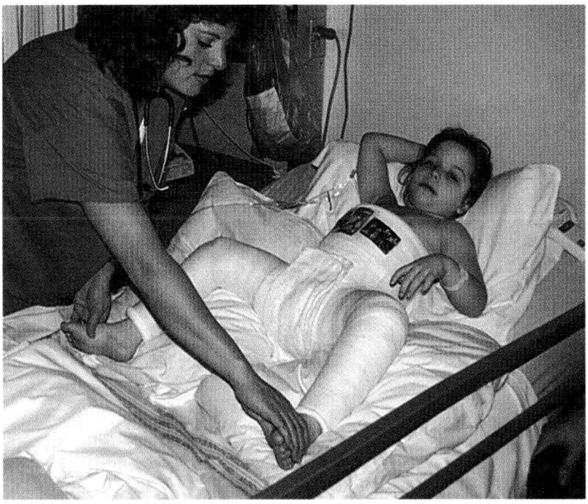

**FIG 50.10** Regular assessment of circulation, sensation, and movement in the lower extremities is essential when a child has a hip spica cast.

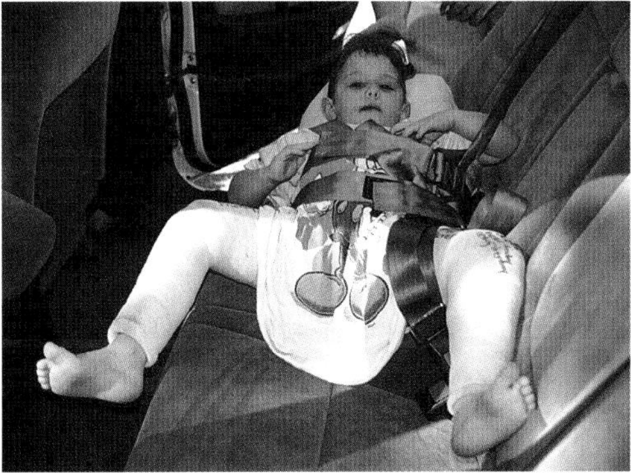

**FIG 50.11** Use a car seat that can accommodate the wide leg spread caused by the spica cast or a car vest restraint for older children.

*Alleviating anxiety.* Communicate information to parents in a clear, kind, and straightforward manner, because complex or ambiguous messages raise anxiety. Adjust teaching to accommodate parents' need for information and support. Reduce waiting time during follow-up visits and express interest in the child and parents. Preoperative teaching should include pictures of children in spica casts and showing a doll in a sample spica cast. Providing reliable, respectful, and empathetic care builds trust and reduces stress.

*Preventing injury.* Assume a proactive role, and advise parents of the potential for injury and the importance of taking safety precautions. Most infant-carrying devices are not suitable or safe for infants in spica casts. Assist parents in identifying strategies for transporting their infant in a safe and comfortable manner, including the use of a car seat that can accommodate the wide leg spread caused by the spica cast or a car vest restraint for older children (Fig. 50.11). During waking hours, teach parents to vary the child's position at least every 2 hours throughout the day. Remind parents that the child must never be left unattended; infants and young children often develop a surprising ability to move despite the restrictions imposed by a cast.

### Evaluation

- Do the parents demonstrate the use of the Pavlik harness or spica cast in a safe and therapeutic manner?
- Can the parents describe adverse effects or complications of treatment?
- Can the parents describe DDH and its treatment in lay terms to other family members, carry out the prescribed therapy to the greatest extent possible, and treat the child as a normal developing child?
- Do the parents and child appear calm and able to participate in care?
- Do the parents seek recommended healthcare and keep follow-up appointments?
- Is the child's skin clear and free of lesions or breakdown?
- Are the child's toes warm and pink, with capillary refill time less than 2 seconds, and can the child move the toes freely?
- Does the child remain injury free?
- Can the parents describe home care adaptations, and are these appropriate for the child's developmental level?

## LEGG–CALVÉ–PERTHES DISEASE

Legg–Calvé–Perthes disease is a condition in which an avascular event affects the epiphysis of the femur and prevents further growth of the ossific nucleus, resulting in increased bone density. As the bone is subsequently reabsorbed and replaced by new bone, the femoral head tends to flatten and enlarge. The child usually complains of a painful limp that is exacerbated by activities such as walking or running.

### Etiology and Incidence

The cause of Legg–Calvé–Perthes disease is unknown, but it is widely accepted to be a growth disorder. Children with Legg–Calvé–Perthes disease are usually shorter-than-average height, and many were low-birth-weight infants (less than 2.5 kg). Abnormalities in certain clotting mechanisms (tendency to develop or failure to lyse thrombi) might also contribute to this condition (Sankar et al., 2016; TSRHC, 2014). Studies have identified other factors related to the etiology of the disorder based on findings of abnormal growth and development, including trauma, infection, and transient synovitis but are unconfirmed (Sankar et al., 2016).

Legg–Calvé–Perthes disease occurs in approximately 1 in 1,200 children, with the incidence in boys 4 to 5 times that of girls (Sankar et al., 2016). Legg–Calvé–Perthes is most commonly seen in children between 4 and 8 years of age (Sankar et al., 2016). The earlier the condition is identified, the better the long-term prognosis (Sankar et al., 2016). Unilateral hip involvement is more common than bilateral involvement. This disease is rare in Blacks and Asians.

### PATHOPHYSIOLOGY

#### *Legg–Calvé–Perthes*

This disorder is classified by the extent of femoral head involvement and disease stage. The disorder usually progresses through five stages over a 1- to 2-year period. During *stage 1,* the epiphysis begins to show the results of ischemia. Synovitis produces stiffness and pain. Necrosis begins; radiographs show a reduction in size and increased density of the femoral head. Once necrosis occurs *(stage 2),* the bone weakens and dies, causing collapse of the femoral head. *Stage 3* is the fragmentation stage, in which avascular bone is reabsorbed. Healing occurs as new bone is formed. During the reossification stage, *stage 4,* the femoral head and neck begin to re-form. *Stage 5,* or the stage of reconstitution, results in final healing.

### Manifestations

The most common symptom of Legg–Calvé–Perthes disease is persistent pain of the hip that worsens with movement. Pain may be intermittent over a period of weeks or months and can be felt in other parts of the leg, such as groin, thigh, or knee. Patients may have a limp or limited range of motion.

The most serious complication of Legg–Calvé–Perthes disease is permanent deformity. If the femoral head protrudes outside the acetabulum and the healing process within the femoral head is incomplete, the femoral head will flatten over time and take on a misshapen appearance.

### Diagnostic Evaluation

In the majority of cases, plain radiographs of the femoral head will disclose the condition. A bone scan or MRI study can reveal necrosis and irregularity of the femoral head.

### Therapeutic Management

Treatment goals are to prevent deformity of the hip and delay the onset of arthritis and degenerative joint disease. The femoral head is contained and maintained in the acetabulum and protected from the stress of weight bearing during the healing process. However, some physicians do not believe that weight bearing is harmful as long as the femur remains in the acetabulum.

Initial treatment includes antiinflammatory medications (such as ibuprofen), range-of-motion exercises, and bed rest. If improvement is not seen within 7 to 10 days and the child is still unable to abduct the hip, alternative methods of treatment are considered. Traction, Petrie casts, or abduction braces may be recommended.

For children with severe necrosis, the femoral head is abducted and internally rotated in relation to the acetabulum through a type of containment device that uses the acetabulum to maintain the spherical shape of the femoral head. Containment prevents the acetabulum from rubbing against the weakened portion of the femoral head and creating a flat shape. Surgical procedures include an osteotomy, which places the femur more securely into the acetabulum, or an acetabular osteotomy, which rotates the acetabulum to cover the femoral head completely. Many physicians recommend surgical intervention because it reduces treatment time and eliminates problems with adherence to treatment.

## NURSING CARE

### The Child With Legg–Calvé–Perthes Disease

#### Assessment

Assessment of a child with Legg–Calvé–Perthes disease reveals loss of internal hip rotation and limited abduction. The nurse determines how long the child has been limping, as well as the pattern, timing, and severity of the pain. The pain may be referred to the thigh or knee. The child will describe the pain as increasing with activity and decreasing with rest. Physical examination of the extremity may reveal muscle wasting of the thigh and buttock—a reflection of disuse. Shortening of the extremity on the affected side indicates collapse of the femoral head.

#### Nursing Diagnosis and Planning

The following nursing diagnoses and expected outcomes may be appropriate after assessment of the child with Legg–Calvé–Perthes disease:

- Impaired Physical Mobility related to activity restrictions.

  **Expected outcome.** The child will maintain mobility and strength of all unaffected joints and tolerate activity restrictions.

- Anxiety related to deficient knowledge about the condition and home management.

***Expected outcome.*** The family will provide safe home care and provide age-appropriate activities for their child.

### Interventions

***Facilitating appropriate activity.*** Activity restrictions are one of the most problematic areas in the care of a child with Legg–Calvé–Perthes disease. The child may become frustrated and angry when unable to meet the physical and social demands of peers. Initially, the child may appear to adjust to the lifestyle restrictions, but the nurse must be alert to subtle indicators of rebellion and uncooperative behavior. Other children will adapt quickly. Do not construe a child's refusal to adhere to treatment regimens as maladaptive behavior. The demand to keep up with their peers is sometimes so great that children are simply unable to make appropriate choices regarding their health.

If a brace is prescribed, returning to school with a brace poses unique problems. The school nurse and the child's teacher should be involved in the discharge planning. The child should participate in as many school-related activities as possible. Acknowledging the child's mobility limitations and working with school officials to identify appropriate alternatives will ensure a successful school re-entry. Emphasizing hobbies and other creative activities provides ways for the child to excel and feel a sense of accomplishment.

***Teaching home management.*** Because the child will receive the majority of treatment as an outpatient, nursing care should focus on home care management. The family must clearly understand the need for care adherence and the role it will play in the healing process. Teach parents to perform neurovascular assessments. The nurse should also help parents identify skin and safety issues related to the child's mobility restrictions and the use of a brace. Physical and occupational therapists are important resources for the parents.

### Evaluation

- Does the child exhibit normal joint and muscular integrity, and does the child adhere to the treatment plan?
- Does the child participate in age-appropriate peer and school-related activities within activity limitations?
- Can the child appropriately express frustration or feelings about being different?
- Are the parents able to provide developmentally appropriate activities for their child?
- Can the parents describe and demonstrate brace care (if applicable) and neurovascular assessments?

## SLIPPED CAPITAL FEMORAL EPIPHYSIS

Slipped capital femoral epiphysis (SCFE) is a condition that occurs during a period of rapid growth in adolescence. Shearing stress causes the femoral capital epiphysis to displace from its normal position relative to the femoral neck.

### Etiology and Incidence

The cause of SCFE is unknown. Slippage appears to be related to increased stress on the proximal femur at a time when the epiphyseal plate is preparing for eventual closure. The weakness of the growth plate may be related to adolescent hormonal imbalance combined with mechanical stress on the hip during growth (Sankar et al., 2016). SCFE most frequently occurs in adolescent boys who are overweight; the majority of affected adolescents exceed the 90th percentile for weight (Sankar et al., 2016).

The incidence is approximately 2/100,000, although this rate varies according to race, sex, and geographic location (Sankar et al., 2016). SCFE occurs approximately two to three times more in young boys than young girls, and some families have an increased incidence. Although initially the condition is unilateral, over half become bilateral (Sankar et al., 2016).

### Pathophysiology

The epiphyseal plate begins to thin in response to hormonal influences during adolescence. Increased body weight and height place more stress on the epiphyses, causing a relative displacement (slip) of the femoral neck from the femoral head. The epiphyseal movement appears to be in a posterior and inferior direction. The usual deformity consists of an upward and anterior movement of the femoral neck on the capital epiphysis. The slip can occur gradually, acutely without previous symptoms, or acutely after an extended period of mild symptoms. SCFE requires immediate medical treatment.

### Manifestations and Diagnostic Evaluation

The classic symptoms of SCFE include a limp and pain. The pain usually is in the groin, thigh, or knee; it is intermittent and worsens with activity. Because knee pain can be the primary complaint, hip involvement may be overlooked. Often, the leg is externally rotated. The presenting symptoms along with characteristic growth signs suggest the diagnosis. Radiographs confirm the diagnosis. Radiographs are obtained with the legs in a frog-leg position.

### Therapeutic Management and Nursing Considerations

As soon as the diagnosis is made, the adolescent is admitted to the hospital and placed on bed rest to prevent exacerbation of the slip. Treatment is usually internal fixation; a pin or screw inserted across the growth plate secures the femoral head and prevents further slippage. More severe slips can require reconstruction of the femoral head, followed by pinning. Postoperatively, the adolescent uses crutches with partial weight-bearing for 4 to 6 weeks. Depending on the severity of the slip and extent of the osteotomy, some adolescents are required to be non–weight-bearing for 4 to 6 weeks, with transfers to a wheelchair only. The screw or pin can be removed after several years.

The nurse should assess for SCFE any time an adolescent reports knee or thigh pain. Interventions are similar to those for any child in traction or undergoing surgery. Postoperatively, the adolescent should be taught isometric exercises and crutch walking. Weight control may be an issue; the overweight adolescent needs to learn to develop good nutritional habits and avoid high-calorie foods. Referral to a dietitian may be helpful. Provide the adolescent and parent with written instructions before discharge.

### CRITICAL THINKING EXERCISE 50.1

Children often come to the ambulatory care setting reporting hip or knee pain and walking with a limp. Compare and contrast the three common hip disorders in children.

## CLUBFOOT

Clubfoot *(talipes equinovarus)* is characterized by rigid midfoot *C*avus, forefoot *A*dduction, heel *V*arus, and ankle *E*quinus (CAVE).

### Etiology and Incidence

Clubfoot represents a congenital dysplasia of all tissue (bone, muscle, ligaments, nerves, and blood vessels) below the knee. The incidence of clubfoot is 1 in 1000 live births. Both feet are affected in nearly 50% of

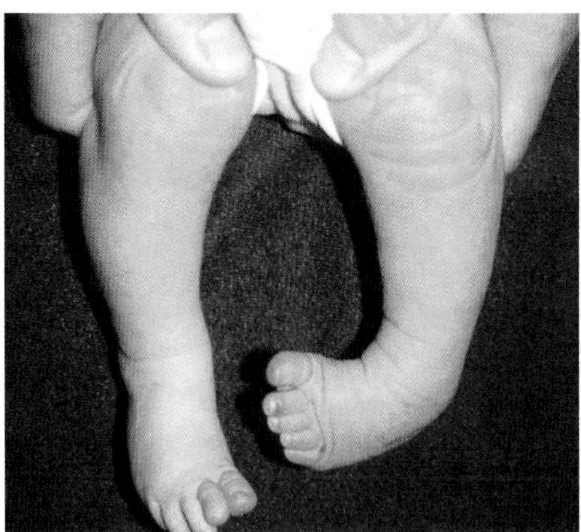

**FIG 50.12** An infant with left clubfoot. Note the positional difference between the two feet.

patients, and it is seen more commonly in males by more than a 2:1 ratio (Winell & Davidson, 2016). Although the means of transmission remains unknown, heredity and race, not environment (i.e., intrauterine packing), seem to play a factor in the occurrence of clubfoot. Clubfoot is seen least frequently in the Japanese population (0.87:1000) and most frequently in the Hawaiian population (6.8:1000). Many etiologic theories have been proposed, but none can fully explain this complex deformity. The cause is likely multifactorial (TSRHC, 2014).

## Manifestations and Diagnostic Evaluation

Clubfoot can be diagnosed prenatally by ultrasound. Radiographic imaging is rarely used or necessary for assessment of a clubfoot. The deformity is easily recognized on clinical examination (Fig. 50.12) (Winell & Davidson, 2016).

## Therapeutic Management

The goal of treatment for a child with a clubfoot is to reduce or eliminate all of the components of the deformity so the child has a functional, structural, mobile, pain-free foot (Aroojis, Pirani, Banskota, et al., 2014). Additionally, treatment goals include a satisfactory appearance, ability to wear normal shoes, and the avoidance of unnecessary or prolonged treatment.

Until the mid-1990s, the preferred treatment for clubfoot in the United States was predominately surgical. Because long-term complications and recurrence were found to occur after surgical correction, nonoperative treatment modalities are now used. The Ponseti casting method and the French physiotherapy method greatly decrease the need for extensive surgery in these patients (Winell & Davidson, 2016).

The French physiotherapy method, used by only experienced physical therapists in inpatient settings, involves daily sequential stretching, strengthening, and mobilization of the foot followed by taping and splinting to allow for gradual correction of the deformity (Winell & Davidson, 2016). Most of the correction is obtained by the physical therapist within the first 3 months of treatment, with full correction expected within 5 months. Committed, well-trained parents are an integral part of the technique, with parents being taught the technique early on and home therapy continuing until walking age. Splinting continues until 2 or 3 years of age in an effort to prevent recurrence of the deformity (TSRHC, 2014).

### Ponseti Casting Method

By far, the standard of care for clubfoot treatment is the Ponseti casting method (Ponseti, 1992) developed in the 1940s and essentially unchanged to this day. This method requires weekly, gentle stretching and manipulation of the misaligned bones followed by application of a well-molded, long-leg plaster cast (TSRHC, 2014). The cast maintains the correction obtained by the orthopedist and allows for further relaxation and softening of the tissues with atraumatic remodeling of the abnormal joint surfaces. Unlike other forms of nonoperative treatment, the Ponseti method corrects all the components of the deformity simultaneously, with the exception of the equinus, which is corrected last. Correction of the deformity is usually obtained within 6 to 8 weeks of casting, with a percutaneous tendoachillis lengthening (TAL) being frequently performed before the final cast application to correct the equinus contracture (Aroojis et al., 2014; Winell & Davidson, 2016). The TAL is generally performed in the clinic setting using a topical anesthetic cream (eutectic mixture of local anesthetic [EMLA]) or needleless injectable lidocaine (J-Tip) (TSRHC, 2014). A final cast is applied and maintained for 3 weeks. On completion of casting, the foot will appear overcorrected. Correction is maintained through the use of an abduction orthosis full-time for 3 months followed by 12-hour nightly use until at least 2 years of age in an effort to prevent recurrence of the deformity.

### Clubfoot Recurrence

Despite the differences between Ponseti casting and the French physiotherapy method, both have been shown by MRI to be effective in achieving and sustaining normal bone and joint alignment in the foot. Both have demonstrated satisfactory short-term outcomes with reduced need for extensive surgery; to date, neither has been shown to be superior to the other (Herring, Birch, Johnston, et al., 2015). Unfortunately, there are still clubfeet that ultimately require surgical intervention. Surgical correction can involve a limited posterior release, anterior tibialis tendon transfer, lateral column release, or complete posteromedial release (TSRHC, 2014).

## Nursing Considerations

Regardless of the method of treatment used, patients and their families will encounter many similar challenges that can be effectively managed with good nursing care. Nursing interventions include education and anticipatory guidance, reduction of infant discomfort and pain, and patient advocacy (Aroojis et al., 2014; Hockenberry & Wilson, 2014).

### Education and Anticipatory Guidance

Information about their child's clubfoot and treatment protocol can be helpful in reducing the anxiety and guilt experienced by many parents and facilitates treatment adherence, which leads to improved patient outcomes. When talking with families, use descriptive rather than scientific terms. Explain that the cause of clubfoot remains unknown and that children with idiopathic clubfoot are expected to develop normally and participate in normal activities. Prepare the families for expected disruptions in their child's care such as difficulties with dressing, sleep, and play often seen with the initiation of casting and bracing. Knowledge that their child will adapt, usually within 24 to 48 hours, is helpful to families. Families must receive thorough and ongoing education about proper neurovascular, skin, and pain assessment to help prevent potential problems. Positioning, bathing, and skin care must be addressed with clear verbal and written instructions. Inform families whom to contact with questions or concerns.

### Reduction of Discomfort and Pain

Both the Ponseti casting and French physiotherapy treatment methods obtain the best results when the infant is relaxed during manipulation of the foot. Infant feeding should be timed to coincide with the treatment session to aid in infant distraction and relaxation. This coordination may require alterations in feeding routines and necessitate breastfeeding mothers to pump or supplement with formula or a pacifier and 24% sucrose during casting sessions. Providing a calm, quiet, warm environment with dimmed lights, soft music, and parental involvement is comforting to infants and helps them relax, or even sleep during the session. If a TAL is required, premedication with a local anesthetic is indicated to decrease procedural discomfort (Aroojis et al., 2014).

If surgery is needed, the nurse oversees pain management in the immediate postoperative period. Elevate the child's feet postoperatively to reduce swelling and pain. Administer analgesics. Assess the neurovascular status of the toes at least every 2 hours in the immediate postoperative period.

### Patient Advocacy

Family involvement and commitment to the treatment is critical for a successful outcome. Nurses can advocate for their young patients and help improve family adherence through frequent reinforcement of treatment protocols and parental encouragement with ongoing education, phone calls to the home to address problems and concerns, frequent follow-up appointments, and facilitation of a parent support network.

## MUSCULAR DYSTROPHIES

Muscular dystrophies include more than 30 genetic diseases (National Institute of Neurological Disorders and Stroke [NINDS], 2015). These are progressively degenerative, inherited diseases that affect the muscle cells of specific muscle groups, causing weakness and atrophy.

### Etiology

Muscular dystrophies vary in their patterns of inheritance and age at onset, but most are identified in early childhood (Table 50.6).

### Incidence

Duchenne muscular dystrophy (DMD) is the most common muscular dystrophy, occurring in 1 in 3600 male children (Sarnet, 2016). This disease accounts for approximately 50% of all cases of muscular dystrophy.

### Pathophysiology

Despite differences in genetic transmission, age at onset, distribution of involvement, and clinical course, the changes in muscles are similar across all forms of muscular dystrophies (TSRHC, 2014). Early in this process, muscle fibers begin to leak the protein creatine kinase and take on excess calcium, causing further harm to muscle fibers. Over time, muscle fibers degenerate and are replaced by fat and connective tissue. As muscle fibers die, progressive weakness and wasting of symmetric groups of skeletal muscles result in increasing disability and deformity.

### Manifestations

In children with Duchenne muscular dystrophy, progressive, symmetric muscle wasting and weakness without loss of sensation first

**TABLE 50.6 Muscular Dystrophies of Childhood**

| Onset and Progression | Inheritance and Incidence | Clinical Manifestations |
|---|---|---|
| **Duchenne** | | |
| Onset: usually before 3 yr, manifests between 3-6 yr<br>Rapidly progressive; loss of walking by 9-12 yr; death in late teens from respiratory failure, heart failure, pneumonia | X-linked recessive<br>Most common hereditary neuromuscular disease; affects all races<br>Incidence: 1 in 3600 male infants | Progressive generalized weakness and muscle wasting affecting limb and trunk muscles first; calves often enlarged; waddling gait; lordosis; cardiomyopathy; Gower maneuver; cognitive disability common |
| **Becker** | | |
| Onset: usually 7-11 yr<br>Slowly progressive; maintain walking past early teens; life span into third decade | X-linked recessive Incidence: 1 in 20,000 male births | Almost identical to Duchenne but less severe; child is mobile at least until late teens; normal intelligence |
| **Congenital Myotonic** | | |
| Severe neonatal form<br>Onset: birth<br>Weakness at birth, may have paralysis of diaphragm<br>If child survives early weeks of life, steady improvement in motor function over the first decade, usually developing ability to walk; often survive to late adulthood | Autosomal dominant Incidence: 1 in 30,000 births | In the severe neonatal form, hypotonia and muscle weakness (especially of the face) at birth; difficulty swallowing, sucking, impaired breathing, absence of reflexes, skeletal deformities, such as club feet |
| **Steinert** | | |
| Onset: late adolescence to early adulthood | Autosomal dominant Incidence: 1 in 8000 births | May appear normal at birth; mild weakness in first few years, with progressive wasting of distal muscles; myotonia worsened by cold, fatigue, stress; cognitive disability in approximately half of cases |

Data from National Institute of Neurological Disorders and Stroke. (2015). *Muscular dystrophy: hope through research.* Retrieved from http://www.ninds.nih.gov/disorders/md/detail_md.htm; Texas Scottish Rite Hospital for Children. (2014). In Herring, J.A. (Ed.), *Tachdjian's pediatric orthopaedics* (5th ed.), Philadelphia: Saunders.

appear after walking is achieved (usually 3 to 7 years). The child must use the Gower maneuver to rise from the floor (child puts hands on knees and moves the hands up legs until standing erect) (TSRHC, 2014). The child has a waddling, wide-based gait. The calf muscles are characteristically weak but hypertrophied. The muscles of the pelvis and shoulders are also affected. Increasing disability and deformities include hip and knee contractures, foot deformities, scoliosis, and lordosis. Walking ability is lost by age 9 to 12 years. Associated signs and symptoms include moderate obesity, cognitive disability, cardiomyopathy, and shortened life span. Other forms of muscular dystrophy also affect the cardiopulmonary endocrine systems, the eyes, and other organs (NINDS, 2015). Cardiopulmonary complications are the most common cause of death.

### Diagnostic Evaluation

The gene loci for many muscular dystrophies have been identified, which makes the carrier status for women easier to determine. Children with a positive family history are especially at risk for muscular dystrophy and should be monitored for clinical symptoms. Serum creatine kinase (CK) levels are elevated in the early stages of the disease and then decrease as muscle bulk decreases. Electromyography and muscle biopsy may also assist with the diagnosis.

### Therapeutic Management

The therapeutic management of the child with a muscular dystrophy is aimed at maintaining ambulation and independence for as long as possible as muscle weakness progresses. Contractures further reduce mobility and independence. Surgery, bracing, and physical therapy contribute to keeping the child as mobile as possible. Later therapy is directed toward maximizing sitting capabilities, respiratory function, and self-care. The prevention of obesity to facilitate mobility and care is a priority. Prompt attention to infection, especially of the respiratory tract, is essential. Children with DMD are surviving longer due to current clinical management such as steroid use, ventilatory assistance, and scoliosis surgery (Romitti et al., 2015).

### Nursing Considerations

When muscular dystrophy is present in the family history, infants and young children should be monitored carefully for its occurrence. When a diagnosis is made, nursing interventions can become a major source of support for these children and their families. Nursing interventions for the child with muscular dystrophy include coordinating a variety of healthcare services. Anticipating the child's future needs requires a sensitive yet knowledgeable approach. The family's ability to cope with chronic illness and the poor prognosis of muscular dystrophy should be assessed. Over time, the child's mobility and self-care abilities should be monitored to ensure independence for as long as possible. Maintenance of activity and self-care functions is important to the child and the family, and independence must be fostered within the limits of safety. Activities such as swimming that promote range of motion and mobility for as long as possible are helpful. As the disease progresses and movement is increasingly restricted, the nurse can suggest activities that take less energy but keep the child involved with peers. The potential for weight gain and respiratory tract infection and the adequacy of support systems must be regularly assessed.

Children in the late stages of muscular dystrophy have difficulty moving. The nurse and family should assist with position changes every 2 hours to prevent injury to the skin and other tissues from prolonged pressure. Adequate fluid intake must be encouraged to prevent urine stasis. A bowel regimen, including stool softeners or laxatives, may be necessary.

The home environment, including bathing and toileting facilities, may need modification to allow wheelchair mobility. Creative approaches to clothing can simplify dressing while meeting the needs of a child trying to fit in with peers.

Specific suggestions about dietary modifications to control weight may be necessary. The nurse can educate families about how to make dietary changes without making food a source of controversy. To reduce the chance of life-threatening respiratory infections, the child should be protected from children with respiratory and contagious diseases. As disability progresses, pulmonary hygiene and respiratory exercises are needed to maintain respiratory function.

Regular monitoring by a multidisciplinary team helps meet the varying needs of the child and family as the child's condition changes. Therapy is individualized to address the child's specific needs. Genetic screening and counseling are recommended for parents and siblings of children with muscular dystrophy.

Parents should be taught how to perform basic nursing tasks and should be referred to agencies that can assist with home care and equipment, such as a motorized wheelchair. Extended family and support groups, such as the Muscular Dystrophy Association of America, can provide needed emotional support and specific assistance as parental energies are exhausted. In addition, the needs of the grieving family should be addressed.

## JUVENILE IDIOPATHIC ARTHRITIS

Juvenile idiopathic arthritis (JIA), formerly known as *juvenile rheumatoid arthritis,* is an autoimmune inflammatory disease with no known cause. The term *juvenile rheumatoid arthritis* is misleading because it implies a positive RF test. However, only approximately 5% of children with JIA test positive for RF. Arthritis in children appears in a number of different forms, each with a different treatment protocol and prognosis.

The term *arthritis* refers to swelling in a joint. There are many causes of joint swelling, including trauma and infection. To diagnose JIA, the child must be younger than 16 years of age and have swelling in at least one joint for at least 6 weeks with two or more signs of decreased range of motion, discomfort on movement, or increased warmth (Wu, Bryan, & Rabinovich, 2016).

JIA is one of the more common chronic diseases in children and the leading cause of childhood disability. With ongoing research and advances in treatment, the prognosis has improved over the past decade.

### Etiology

Despite extensive research, the cause of JIA remains unknown. The cause is most likely multifactorial, including genetic predisposition, abnormal immune response, and environmental triggering factors such as infection or trauma.

### Incidence

JIA affects approximately 100,000 children in the United States. The most common age of onset is between 2 and 4 years of age; for the most common subtype of JIA (pauciarticular), girls are three times more likely to experience the condition than boys (Wu et al, 2016).

### Manifestations

Persistent joint swelling in one or more joints that lasts 6 weeks or longer suggests JIA. The joints may be stiff, swollen, warm to the touch, erythematous, and have a limited range of motion. Stiffness is worse in the morning or after a prolonged period of rest. This feature is referred to as the "gel phenomenon," because the joints seem to gel into place. Identification of the subtype will guide management and prognosis.

**TABLE 50.7 Major Types of Juvenile Idiopathic Arthritis**

| Subtype of JIA | Gender | Age | Joints Affected | Other Manifestations |
|---|---|---|---|---|
| Oligoarticular, early onset | Females > males | 1-4 yr | Four or fewer joints affected; in ⅓ of patients involve single joint | ANA (+) in approximately 60% (increased risk of uveitis) |
| Enthesitis-related arthritis (late-onset oligoarticular) | Males > females | 9-12 yr | Often have four or fewer joints involved but can have a polyarticular course; possible sacroiliitis | May carry the *HLAB27* gene, enthesitis |
| RF (–) polyarticular | Females > males | 1-4 yr | Affects five or more joints, combination of small and large joints, often symmetrical involvement | RF (–) |
| RF (+) polyarticular | Females > males | 9-16 yr | Affects five or more joints, combination of small and large joints, often symmetrical involvement | RF (+), rheumatoid nodules, risk of bony erosions |
| Systemic-onset JIA | Females = males | | Usually polyarticular involvement | High daily or twice-daily spiking fevers, rash, risk of pericarditis, lymphadenopathy, hepatosplenomegaly |

*ANA,* Antinuclear antibody; *HLA-B27,* human leukocyte antigen B27; *JIA,* juvenile idiopathic arthritis; *RF,* rheumatoid factor.

**PATHOPHYSIOLOGY**

***Juvenile Idiopathic Arthritis***

The synovial joints are the primary structures involved in this process. Normally, joints are movable and contain synovium, a highly vascular tissue that produces a clear, viscous synovial fluid that nourishes and lubricates articular cartilage. In juvenile idiopathic arthritis (JIA), immune complexes in blood and synovial tissue initiate the inflammatory response, producing inflammatory cytokines. Phagocytosis and accumulation of immune complexes cause chronic inflammation and joint destruction.

As the synovium becomes inflamed, excessive fluid is produced. Unlike normal synovial fluid, this fluid is thin and watery. The synovium swells, and thickened villi and nodules protrude into the joint cavity. *Pannus* (inflamed granulating tissue) formation occurs over the articular cartilage. With further deterioration, the articular cartilage and contiguous bone become eroded and are destroyed.

Table 50.7 lists the associated signs and symptoms of the JIA subtypes (Wu et al., 2016). If untreated, *uveitis,* an associated inflammation of the eye structures in the uveal tract, can lead to vision loss.

## Diagnostic Evaluation

The early diagnosis of JIA depends on a comprehensive history and physical examination. The character, frequency, and severity of the systemic and articular manifestations are critical to the diagnosis and treatment. Laboratory markers such as the RF, antinuclear antibody (ANA), human leukocyte antigen B27 (HLA-B27), and anticyclic citrullinated peptide (anti-CCP) antibody are helpful in identifying the JIA subtype. CBC, ESR, and CRP can be useful in identifying the presence of inflammation. In addition, children with JIA need routine slit-lamp eye exams to screen for uveitis, which occurs more frequently in individuals who are positive for ANA.

## Therapeutic Management

This is no known cure for JIA. Therapeutic management is directed toward preserving joint function, controlling the inflammatory process, minimizing deformity, and reducing the impact of the disease on the child's development (Ringold et al., 2013). Management includes medication, physical and occupational therapy, family education, home care, and encouragement of age-appropriate activities as tolerated.

### Drug Therapy

Pharmacologic treatment is dependent on the severity of the disease and the number of joints involved. Although NSAIDs such as ibuprofen, naproxen sodium (Naprosyn), sulindac (Clinoril), and celecoxib (Celebrex) are the first line of treatment, other medications are often needed. If the child's condition does not improve after 4 to 6 weeks, methotrexate, a disease-modifying antirheumatic drug (DMARD) is added to the medication regimen. However, methotrexate is being used more often as a first line of treatment because it provides longer periods of disease control and clinical remission (Nierengarten, 2014). Additional medications, commonly referred to as biologics, are sometimes needed to completely control the child's arthritis. These drugs include etanercept (Enbrel), adalimumab (Humira), and infliximab (Remicade). Anakinra (Kineret) is a newer medication used in children with systemic-onset juvenile arthritis. Local corticosteroid injections are often used to reduce inflammation in selected joints.

### Physical and Occupational Therapy

In addition to drug therapy, physical and occupational therapy are also important interventions to preserve muscle integrity and joint mobility. Active disease processes can place the child with JIA at risk for impaired mobility, contractures, and altered growth and development. Rehabilitation is designed to prevent such problems. Depending on the disease process, a program of rest, proper positioning, exercises, and activity of daily living (ADL) modifications will be developed by occupational and physical therapists. To ensure effectiveness and cooperation, an individualized therapy program will take into consideration the child's limitations, abilities, home and school environment, and interests.

Exercise programs consist of gentle active and/or passive range of motion and strengthening. Active range of motion and rest are indicated during times of increased synovitis and pain. Gentle movement through available range will maintain joint mobility. Rest or frequent rest breaks will increase overall endurance and limit joint impact throughout the day. Inactivity can lead to the loss of joint motion and decreased muscle strength. Passive range of motion is not indicated in early stages of the disease or during times of active inflammation;

## DRUG GUIDE

### *Naproxen, Naproxen Sodium*

**Classification:** Nonsteroidal antiinflammatory drug (NSAID)
**Action:** Unknown; reduces inflammation and fever, possibly by inhibiting prostaglandin synthesis.
**Indication:** Juvenile idiopathic arthritis (JIA)
**Dosage and Route:** 10 mg/kg/day orally in two divided doses; medication comes in tablet or liquid suspension (125 mg/5 mL).
**Absorption:** Absorbed rapidly from the gastrointestinal tract with peak action in 1 to 4 hours.
**Excretion:** Effects last approximately 7 hours; eliminated primarily by the kidneys.
**Contraindications:** Contraindicated in any child who has had an allergic reaction to this drug or similar drugs or in children with a syndrome of asthma, rhinitis, and nasal polyps; naproxen should not be administered concurrently with naproxen sodium.
**Precautions:** Can prolong bleeding time, alter liver functions, and contribute to renal toxicity. Use cautiously if the child is also taking methotrexate, aspirin, anticoagulants, probenecid, or steroids.
**Adverse Reactions:** Primarily gastrointestinal irritation (gastrointestinal ulceration with bleeding from prolonged use); edema; headache, drowsiness, or dizziness; tinnitus; pruritus or skin rash; risk for renal failure.
**Nursing Considerations:** Assess for adverse reactions, particularly if the child is receiving long-term therapy. Advise the child to take the medication with food or milk to minimize gastrointestinal upset. Be aware that antiinflammatory medications can mask signs of infection. Teach the child and family signs of gastrointestinal bleeding.

instead, it is more advantageous to encourage play activities to increase the active range. A child may begin gradual strengthening once the synovitis is well controlled and a functional range of motion is obtained. Examples of low-impact strengthening activities are swimming and riding a bicycle.

In addition to exercise, modalities such as heat and splinting are helpful in reducing pain and maintaining the range of motion during painful episodes. Hot baths, whirlpools, moist hot packs, and paraffin baths are all examples of heat that can be used at home or in conjunction with therapy. Heat will also reduce joint stiffness and increase the elasticity of tissues surrounding the joints, making stretching more effective. Splinting is used to rest the joint, decrease pain, and align the joint in the proper position; it may also be helpful as a support when the child becomes more active.

The goal of rehabilitation is to maintain functional mobility and allow affected children to keep up with their peers. Children are naturally active, and children with JIA are no different. Activity that helps maintain normal muscle and joint integrity should be encouraged but might require modification.

### Surgical Treatment

Surgical intervention, although rare, is considered when the child or adolescent is having problems with joint contractures, micrognathia, or unequal growth of extremities.

## NURSING CARE

### The Child With JIA

#### Assessment

The nursing assessment focuses on the status of affected joints, the child's physical limitations, the level and intensity of pain, and the child's and family's response to the disease process. The nurse assesses the affected joints for warmth, tenderness, pain, and limited range of motion. Be alert for guarding of painful joints, refusal to bear weight, limping, and facial expressions of discomfort. The parent might describe the child as fussy and irritable in the morning. The young child may be reluctant to walk and want to be carried.

Assess joint stiffness, including the duration of the stiffness and the child's description of how difficult movement is after periods of inactivity. Assess the child for any indication of systemic involvement, such as a history of temperature elevations, especially in the late afternoon or evening. Determine whether a rash occurs with the fever. Also assess for anorexia, weight loss, and failure to grow.

#### Nursing Diagnosis and Planning

The following nursing diagnoses and expected outcomes may be appropriate to the child with juvenile arthritis and the child's family:

- Chronic Pain related to the inflammatory process.

**Expected outcome.** The child's pain will decrease, as evidenced by increased participation in usual activities and verbal report of decreased pain.

- Impaired Physical Mobility related to inflammation of the joint and associated muscle weakness.

**Expected outcome.** As a result of appropriate activity and an ongoing exercise program, the child's joints will remain mobile. The child will correctly use any appropriate adaptive equipment to accomplish ADLs and participate in a regular exercise program. The child will show no signs of the hazards of immobility.

- Delayed Growth and Development related to activity intolerance.

**Expected outcome.** The child will exhibit age-appropriate behaviors. The parents will support and maintain appropriate developmental activities for their child.

- Disturbed Body Image related to activity intolerance.

**Expected outcome.** The child will maintain relationships with peers and participate in age-appropriate activities when able.

- Deficient Knowledge about the care and treatment of JIA related to unfamiliarity with the condition.

**Expected outcome.** The parents will demonstrate safe home care and adherence to the treatment regimen and the prescribed exercise program.

#### Interventions

**Managing pain.** Teach parents to identify both verbal and nonverbal pain indicators. Nonverbal cues are more difficult to recognize but include restlessness, withdrawal, decreased attention span, increased crying, and decreased sleep. Maintaining a therapeutic blood level of pain medication is the most effective way to ensure maximal comfort. The nurse should teach parents the side effects of the prescribed medications and advise that most NSAIDs should be given with food or milk to prevent gastrointestinal irritation. Nonpharmacologic pain relief measures such as diversion, splinting, heat or cold application, imagery, and meditation are useful for some children.

**Promoting mobility.** Teach positioning of inflamed joints, appropriate application of heat or cold, and how to support and protect the affected joints. Encourage families to be consistent with exercise programs prescribed by the physical and/or occupational therapist. Emphasize that isometric exercises and passive range-of-motion exercises will prevent contractures and deformities. Help the family to identify when there is a flare in the child's condition, thus necessitating activity modification. If there are no restrictions per therapy, parents should promote the child's participation in age-appropriate activities.

The child may need more time than average to begin morning activities. Teach the parents to allow plenty of time for the child to awaken, take a warm shower or bath, and relieve morning joint stiffness. Keeping the child's room or bed warm is important. Administering the child's NSAID with a snack first thing in the morning and allowing the medication to take effect before the child arises may help reduce pain and stiffness.

***Managing potential infections.*** Some of the medications used to treat JIA cause immunosuppression, so teach the parents to recognize the signs of possible infection and whom to notify. Medications may need to be temporarily withheld if the child is actively infected. Live-virus vaccinations, including varicella, measles, mumps, and rubella (MMR), and flu-mist, must be held while the child is on any DMARD or biologic medication. Encourage yearly flu vaccination with the injectable form.

***Facilitating emotional and social development.*** Acknowledge the child's and family's anxiety and allow family members to express concerns. Encourage expressive therapeutic activities such as doll play, pounding boards, bean bags, clay, painting, and story composing. Therapeutic play provides a safe and effective mechanism for reducing the stress. The nurse should recognize that age, sex, and self-concept play a role in a child's adjustment to chronic illness. Use anticipatory guidance to help the child develop coping mechanisms that will foster the development of optimism and a sense of personal competence. Help the child identify strengths and areas of accomplishments to increase self-esteem. Identify creative hobbies or activities that will enhance the child's sense of self-worth.

Communicate with the school nurse about scheduling necessary rest periods for the child during the school day. The child might enjoy a short period of quiet activity in the school health office if allowed to bring a friend. School nurses can help with the child's transition to school by communicating with teachers about the child's needs.

***Family education.*** As part of the multidisciplinary approach, the nurse must take an active part in helping the child and parents learn how to cope with and adapt to the limitations of the disease. This support includes referring them at onset to sources of accurate information about the condition and its associated care. Information should be of a variety of types and appropriate for the child's developmental level. The Arthritis Foundation can provide information to parents and children. Parents also want to ensure that others in the community have an understanding of JIA. Increased understanding by others in the child's environment will increase his or her ability to maintain a normal, developmentally appropriate lifestyle.

Because most of the child's care takes place in the home, the success of the therapeutic plan will be determined by the parents. Planning begins as soon as possible in the course of the illness. The parents should be involved in as many nursing activities as possible to reduce their anxiety and increase their sense of control over difficult situations. Provide verbal and written instructions and use return demonstration to ensure parental understanding of procedures. Coordinate referrals and physical therapy with the child's and parents' routines and schedules.

Encourage the parents to provide a diet high in fiber, protein, and calcium and an adequate fluid intake. If the child has anorexia or pain while eating, consider smaller, more frequent high-calorie foods.

Emphasize regular visits to the ophthalmologist to evaluate the eyes for inflammation. Children with JIA should be referred to an ophthalmologist at diagnosis and for recommended periodic follow-ups (Wu et al., 2016).

### Evaluation

- Does the child experience pain control, as evidenced by report of decreased pain, increased sleep, decreased restlessness and irritability, and increased participation in age-appropriate activities?
- Is the child free from joint inflammation, and does the child demonstrate age-appropriate range of motion and muscle strength?
- During an exacerbation, is the child able to accept activity restrictions and participate in the exercise program?
- Is the child free from respiratory problems or other problems associated with immobility?
- Is the child able to perform age-appropriate self-care activities?
- Do the parents demonstrate the ability to facilitate the child's growth and development within the limitations posed by the child's disease?
- Does the child demonstrate age-appropriate behaviors, increased social interactions with friends, and appropriate adaptation to school?
- Are the parents able to articulate and demonstrate solutions to care for problems encountered in the home?

## SYNDROMES AND CONDITIONS WITH ASSOCIATED ORTHOPEDIC ANOMALIES

Several syndromes and other conditions are associated with various orthopedic anomalies (Table 50.8). Because people unfamiliar with osteogenesis imperfecta might assume that the child's fractures and old fractures are the result of child abuse, the nurse must be particularly careful with nursing assessments for all children with unexplained fractures.

**TABLE 50.8 Syndromes and Conditions With Associated Orthopedic Anomalies**

| Syndrome or Condition | Incidence | Orthopedic Anomalies |
|---|---|---|
| Achondroplasia | Most common form of dwarfism<br>1.3 in 100,000 to 1.5 in 10,000 live births | Angular deformity of lower extremities: genu varum and tibia vara more common than valgus<br>Cranial cervical stenosis<br>Mortality rate as high as 7.5%<br>Symptoms include hypotonia and sleep apnea<br>Elbow deformity: lack of full extension<br>Short stature<br>Spinal stenosis<br>• One third of patients with symptoms by 15 yr of age<br>• Symptoms include pain in lower back and legs exacerbated by activity<br>Thoracolumbar kyphosis: surgery indicated for persistent kyphosis |
| Arthrogryposis | 1 in 3000 live births | Congenital joint stiffness, typically all four extremities are involved; Varying degrees of muscle weakness; Normal to above normal intelligence; Goals of treatment: independent ambulation and function of upper extremities for activities of daily living |
| Down syndrome (see Chapter 54) | Genetic condition associated with intellectual disability<br>1 in 800 live births<br>40% have congenital heart defects | Hypermobility of the upper cervical spine<br>• Atlantoaxial (C1-C2), screen for instability before athletic or Special Olympics participation<br>• Occipital-atlanto, reported incidence varies widely<br>• Only indication for surgery is neurologic symptoms<br>Hypermobility and ligamentous laxity of hips<br>• 7.9% have some form of hip abnormality<br>• Recurrent, usually painless dislocations (see DDH*) occur in nearly 5%, typically between 2 and 10 yr of age<br>• Slipped capital femoral epiphysis<br>• Avascular necrosis<br>Patella femoral disorders<br>Clubfeet, may be resistant to nonoperative treatment<br>Flat feet |
| Marfan | Autosomal dominant<br>Prevalence 1 in 5000 live births<br>More may have subtle variations | Tall, lanky, abnormally long arms with reduced extension of the elbows<br>Generalized joint laxity<br>Protrusio acetabuli (increased depth of the acetabulum)<br>Arachnodactyly (long, slender, spider-like fingers)<br>Scoliosis, spondylolisthesis<br>Chest wall deformity, pectus deformities<br>Developmental dysplasia of the hips<br>Extreme myopia<br>Loud cardiac murmur, may have aortic dilation, an aortic aneurysm, and mitral valve prolapse |
| Neurofibromatosis | Hereditary<br>Type 1: 1 in 3,000 live births | Neurofibromatosis-1 associated with orthopedic conditions;<br>orthopedic conditions rare in children with neurofibromatosis-2<br>Spinal deformities, typically thoracic<br>Hemihypertrophy<br>Congenital pseudoarthrosis of the tibia |
| Osteogenesis imperfecta | Autosomal dominant or recessive, or spontaneous mutation<br>Incidence<br>Type 1: 1 in 30,000 live births<br>Type 2: 1 in 62,000 live births<br>Type 3: Very rare<br>Type 4: Unknown | Characterized by connective tissue defects and extreme bone fragility; 90% of those affected have a genetic defect in type I collagen formation<br>• Most common manifestation is frequent fractures with even the slightest injury; the earlier the fracture occurs, the more severe the disease<br>• Short stature<br>• Spinal and long-bone deformities, frequently require surgical intervention<br>• Osteoporosis<br>• Blue sclera<br>• Discolored teeth<br>• Conductive hearing loss<br>Infants with type 2 usually die during the perinatal period or early infancy<br>Older children need gentle handling and movement, injury prevention, nutritional management; enhance family and child coping with chronic condition IV bisphosphonate may increase bone density |

*DDH,* Developmental dysplasia of the hip; *IV,* intravenous.
*See the text section, "Developmental Dysplasia of the Hip."

## KEY CONCEPTS

- The neurovascular assessment of a child in traction or a cast includes assessment of skin color, capillary refill time, temperature, sensation, and movement of digits in casted hand or foot, if exposed. The quality of the pulse distal to the site should also be evaluated and compared with that of the uninvolved extremity.
- When evaluating neurovascular status, remember to assess for the five Ps of ischemia—pain, pallor, pulselessness, paresthesia, and paralysis.
- Consequences of immobility include alterations in the integumentary, gastrointestinal, respiratory, genitourinary, and musculoskeletal systems as well as children's growth and psychological development.
- Musculoskeletal problems are frequently caused by trauma. Nonaccidental trauma or child abuse may be involved. Therefore, nursing assessment should always begin with a primary emergency survey.
- Treatment of fractures involves repositioning the bone fragments (reduction) and applying a cast or traction to maintain alignment (retention) until healing occurs.
- Nursing care of the child with osteomyelitis includes assessment and documentation of the child's status, pain management, and administration of antibiotics without iatrogenic injury.
- Frequently seen musculoskeletal developmental disorders include scoliosis, limb differences, DDH, Legg–Calvé–Perthes disease, SCFE, and clubfoot. Splinting, traction, bracing, casting, or a combination thereof is often required. Similar approaches are used in the management of orthopedic anomalies related to various childhood syndromes.
- Nursing outcomes for a child with muscular dystrophy include maintaining physical activity, promoting respiratory function, managing weight, and reducing the impact of the disease on the child's development.
- Nursing outcomes for a child with JIA include keeping the child free from injury, controlling pain, enhancing physical mobility, and promoting age-appropriate developmental behaviors.

## REFERENCES AND READINGS


Aroojis, A., Pirani, S., Banskota, B., et al. (2014). Clubfoot etiology, pathoanatomy, basic ponseti technique, and Ponseti in older Patients. In *Global orthopedics* (pp. 357–368). New York: Springer.

Baldwin, K.D., Wells, L., & Dormans, J.P. (2016a). Growth and Development. In R. Kliegman, B. Stanton, J. St Geme, et al. (Eds.), *Nelson textbook of pediatrics* (20th ed., pp. 3241–3242). Philadelphia: Saunders.

Baldwin, K.D., Wells, L., & Dormans, J.P. (2016b). Evaluation of the child. In R. Kliegman, B. Stanton, J. St Geme, et al. (Eds.), *Nelson textbook of pediatrics* (20th ed., pp. 3242–3247). Philadelphia: Saunders.

Baldwin, K.D., Wells, L., & Dormans, J.P. (2016c). Common fractures. In R. Kliegman, B. Stanton, J. St Geme, et al. (Eds.), *Nelson textbook of pediatrics* (20th ed., pp. 3314–3322). Philadelphia: Saunders.

Birrer, R.B., O'Connor, F.G., & Kane, S.F. (2016). *Musculoskeletal and Sports Medicine For The Primary Care Practitioner, Fourth Edition* (Vol. 1). Boca Raton, FL: CRC Press.

Centers for Disease Control and Prevention. (2013). *A national action plan for child injury prevention: reducing sports and recreation-related injuries*. Retrieved from http://www.cdc.gov/safechild/NAP/overviews/sports.html.

Cho, S.K., & Egorova, N.N. (2015). The association between insurance status and complications, length of stay, and costs for pediatric idiopathic scoliosis. *Spine, 40*(4), 247–256.

Dorfman, A.L., Fazel, R., Einstein, A.J., et al. (2016). Use of medical imaging procedures with ionizing radiation in children: a population-based study. *Archives of Pediatrics & Adolescent Medicine, 165*(5), 458–464. doi:10.1001/archpediatrics.2010.270.

Ferreira, N., & Marais, L.C. (2012). Prevention and management of external fixator pin track sepsis. *Strategies in Trauma and Limb Reconstruction, 7*, 67–72.

Fischer, C.R., Cassilly, R., Cantor, W., et al. (2013). A systematic review of comparative studies on bone graft alternatives for common spine fusion procedures. *European Spine Journal, 22*(6), 1423–1435.

Flynn, J.M., Skaggs, D.L., & Waters, P.M. (2015). *Rockwood & Wilkins' fractures in children* (8th ed.). Philadelphia: Wolters Kluwer Health.

George, J., George, R., Dixit, R., et al. (2013). Fat embolism syndrome. *Lung India, 30*, 47–53.

Greenwald, L.J., Yost, M.T., Sonseller, P.D., et al. (2012). The role of clinically significant venous thromboembolism and thromboprophylaxis in pediatric patients with pelvic or femoral fractures. *Journal of Pediatric Orthopedics, 32*(4), 357–361.

Hendee, W.R., & O'Connor, M.K. (2012). *Radiation risks of medical imaging: separating fact from fantasy*. doi:10.1148/radiol.12112678.

Herring, J.A., Birch, J.G., Johnston, C.E., et al. (2015). A glimpse into Texas Scottish Rite Hospital's educational, clinical care, and research development. *Journal of Pediatric Orthopaedics B, 24*(2), 84–88.

Hockenberry, M.J., & Wilson, D. (2014). *Wong's nursing care of infants and children*. Elsevier Health Sciences.

Horne, J.P., Flannery, R., & Usman, S. (2014). Adolescent idiopathic scoliosis: diagnosis and management. *American Family Physician, 89*(3), 193–198.

Huether, S.E., & McCance, K.L. (2017). *Understanding pathophysiology*. St. Louis: Elsevier.

Johnston-Walker, E., & Hardcastle, J. (2011). Neurovascular assessment in the critically ill patient. *Nursing in critical care, 16*(4), 170–177.

Kaplan, S.L. (2016). Osteomyelitis. In R. Kliegman, B. Stanton, J. St Geme, et al. (Eds.), *Nelson textbook of pediatrics* (20th ed., pp. 3314–3322). Philadelphia: Saunders.

Matsiko, A., Levingstone, T., & O'Brien, F. (2013). Advanced strategies for articular cartilage defect repair. *Materials, 6*(2), 637–668. doi:10.3390.

Mistovich, R.J., & Spiegel, D.A. (2016). The spine. In R. Kliegman, B. Stanton, J. St Geme, et al. (Eds.), *Nelson textbook of pediatrics* (20th ed., pp. 3283–3297). Philadelphia: Saunders.

Murphy, R.F., Naqvi, M., Miller, P.E., et al. (2015). Pediatric orthopaedic lower extremity trauma and venous thromboembolism. *Journal of Children's Orthopaedics, 9*, 381–384.

Nascimento, F.P.D., Santili, C., Akkari, M., et al. (2013). Flexible intramedullary nails with traction versus plaster cast for treating femoral shaft fractures in children: comparative retrospective study. *Sao Paulo Medical Journal, 131*(1), 5–12. doi:10.1590/S1516-31802013000100002.

National Institute of Neurological Disorders and Stroke. (2015). *NINDS muscular dystrophy information page*. Retrieved from http://www.ninds.nih.gov/disorders/md/md.htm.

Nierengarten, M.B. (2014). Juvenile idiopathic arthritis: rethinking remission. *Contemporary Pediatrics*, 14–19.

Pastorelli, F., Di Silvestre, M., Plasmati, R., et al. (2011). The prevention of neural complications in the surgical treatment of scoliosis: the role of the neurophysiological intraoperative monitoring. *European Spine Journal, 20*(1), 105–114.

Ponseti, I. (1992). Current concepts review: treatment of congenital clubfoot. *Journal of Bone and Joint Surgery, 74-A*, 448–454.

Ringold, S., Weiss, P.F., Beukelman, T., et al. (2013). 2013 update of the 2011 American College of Rheumatology recommendations for the treatment of juvenile idiopathic arthritis: recommendations for the medical therapy of children with systemic juvenile idiopathic arthritis and tuberculosis screening among children receiving biologic medications. *Arthritis & Rheumatism, 65*(10), 2499–2512.

Schug, G.R., Blevins, K.E., Cox, B., et al. (2013). Infection, disease, and biosocial processes at the end of the Indus civilization. *PLoS One, 8*.

Robert, C., Jiang, J., & Khoury, J. (2011). A prospective study on the effectiveness of cotton versus waterproof cast padding in maintaining the reduction of pediatric distal forearm fracture. *Journal of Pediatric Orthopaedics, 31*(2), 144–149.

Romitti, P.A., Zhu, Y., Puzhankara, S., et al. (2015). Prevalence of Duchenne and Becker muscular dystrophies in the United States. *Pediatrics, 135*(3), 513–521. doi: 10.1542/peds.2014-2044.

Sankar, W., Horn, D., Wells, L., et al. (2016). The hip. In R. Kliegman, B. Stanton, J. St Geme, et al. (Eds.), *Nelson textbook of pediatrics* (20th ed., pp. 3274–3283). Philadelphia: Saunders.

Sarnet, H.B. (2016). Muscular dystrophies. In R. Kliegman, B. Stanton, J. St Geme, et al. (Eds.), *Nelson textbook of pediatrics* (20th ed., pp. 2975–2986). Philadelphia: Saunders.

Sarkissian, E.J., Gans, L., Gunderson, M.A., et al. (2015). Community-acquired methicillin-resistant *Staphylococcus aureus* musculoskeletal infections:... - Abstract - Europe PMC. *Journal of Pediatric Orthopedics.* doi:10.1097/BPO.0000000000000439.

Scoliosis Research Society. (2015). *SRS/AAOS position statement: screening for the early detection for idiopathic scoliosis in adolescents.* Retrieved from http://www.srs.org/about-srs/quality-and-safety/position-statements/screening-for-the-early-detection-for-idiopathic-scoliosis-in-adolescents.

Scott, J.R., van Gastel, N., Carmeliet, G., et al. (2015). Uncovering the periosteum for skeletal regeneration: the stem cell that lies beneath. *Bone, 70*, 10–18. doi:10.1016/j.bone.2014.08.007.

Sharma, M., Lahoti, B.K., Khandelwal, G., et al. (2011). Epidemiological trends of pediatric trauma: a single-center study of 791 patients. *Journal of Indian Association of Pediatric Surgeons, 16*, 88–92.

Slinko, S. (2014). Perioperative care of the orthopaedic surgery patient. In *Pediatric critical care medicine* (pp. 177–185). London: Springer.

Texas Scottish Rite Children's Hosptial. (2014). *Tachdjian's pediatric orthopaedics: from the Texas Scottish Rite Hospital for children: expert consult: online and print, 3- volume set (2 volumes in ... online only)*, 5th ed. Saunders.

van den Bekerom, M.P.J., Struijs, P.A., Blankevoort, L., et al. (2012). What is the evidence for rest, ice, compression, and elevation therapy in the treatment of ankle sprains in adults? *Journal of Athletic Training, 47*(4), 435-443. doi:attr-47-04-14.

von Keyserlingkl, C., Boutis, K., Willan, A.R., et al. (2016). Cost-effectiveness analysis of cast versus splint in children with acceptably angulated wrist fractures. *International Journal of Technology Assessment in Health Care, 22*(7) 101-107. doi:10.1017/S0266462311000067.

Weinstein, S.L., & Dolan, L.A. (2015). The evidence base for the prognosis and treatment of adolescent idiopathic scoliosis: the 2015 orthopaedic research and education foundation clinical research award. *The Journal of Bone Joint Surgery. American Volume, 97*(22), 1899–1903. doi:10.2106/jbjs.o.00330.

Winell, J.J., & Davidson, R.S. (2016). The foot and toes. In R. Kliegman, B. Stanton, J. St Geme, et al. (Eds.), *Nelson textbook of pediatrics* (20th ed., pp. 3247–3257). Philadelphia: Saunders.

Wu, E.Y., Bryan, A.R., & Rabinovich, C.E. (2016). Juvenile idiopathic arthritis. In R. Kliegman, B. Stanton, J. St Geme, et al. (Eds.), *Nelson textbook of pediatrics* (20th ed., pp. 1160–1171). Philadelphia: Saunders.

Yang, S., Andras, L.M., Redding, G.J., et al. (2016). Early-onset scoliosis: a review of history, current treatment, and future directions. *Pediatrics, 137*(1), 1–12. doi:10.1542/peds.2015-0709.

51

# The Child With an Endocrine or Metabolic Alteration

http://evolve.elsevier.com/McKinney/mat-ch/

## LEARNING OBJECTIVES

*After studying this chapter, you should be able to:*

- List the major hormones of the endocrine system.
- Describe negative feedback.
- Discuss nursing strategies to improve adherence with medication administration.
- Describe the signs and symptoms of hypothyroidism versus hyperthyroidism.
- Compare and contrast diabetes insipidus and syndrome of inappropriate antidiuretic hormone as they relate to fluid and electrolyte balance.
- Describe the psychosocial issues concerning children with precocious puberty.
- Identify the role of insulin in the metabolism of carbohydrates, fats, and proteins in both the fasting and postprandial states.
- Compare and contrast type 1 diabetes mellitus and type 2 diabetes mellitus.
- Identify management goals and nursing implications of insulin therapy, diet therapy, exercise, self-monitoring of blood glucose, and urine ketone monitoring in the care of the child with type 1 diabetes.
- Describe the signs, symptoms, causes, and treatment of hypoglycemia and hyperglycemia in the child with diabetes.
- Identify the pathophysiology of diabetic ketoacidosis, and describe the management and nursing care of the child in diabetic ketoacidosis.
- Identify management goals and nursing implications of medication, diet therapy, exercise, and self-monitoring of blood glucose in the care of the child with type 2 diabetes.

# CLINICAL REFERENCE

## REVIEW OF THE ENDOCRINE SYSTEM

The endocrine system is composed of various tissues that produce and secrete chemicals called hormones. The hormones stimulate and regulate the actions of other tissues—the target tissues.

The endocrine system and the autonomic nervous system function in tandem to regulate growth, metabolism, and reproduction. The hypothalamic-pituitary axis controls their activities. The autonomic nervous system reacts to a stimulus, transmitting its message to the hypothalamus. In turn, the hypothalamus manufactures and secretes the appropriate hormonal factors. These are transmitted to the anterior pituitary gland, which then stimulates or inhibits the release of the involved hormones.

### Pediatric Differences in the Endocrine System

The endocrine system is less developed at birth than any other body system.

Hormonal control of many body functions is lacking until 12 to 18 months of age. As a result, infants may manifest imbalances in the concentration of fluids, electrolytes, amino acids, glucose, and trace substances.

The principle of feedback control is involved in hormone production and secretion. In negative feedback, increasing levels of a specific hormone begin to inhibit the system responsible for releasing that hormone. As the hormonal secretion rises, the secretion and production of its stimulating hormone decrease. Conversely, when too little circulating hormone is present, the target gland is stimulated to secrete additional hormone.

The pituitary gland is composed of an anterior lobe and a posterior lobe. The anterior lobe secretes adrenocorticotropic hormone (ACTH), thyroid-stimulating hormone (TSH), follicle-stimulating hormone (FSH), luteinizing hormone (LH), growth hormone (GH), and prolactin. Four of these hormones (ACTH, TSH, LH, and FSH) in turn stimulate their target glands to secrete the appropriate specific hormones. The posterior pituitary lobe stores and releases antidiuretic hormone (ADH) and oxytocin, which are synthesized by the hypothalamus.

Congenital malformations, infections, and neoplastic or autoimmune processes can disrupt normal endocrine function of the hypothalamus, pituitary gland, or target gland.

Fetal endocrine systems develop and function *in utero*. Portions of the endocrine system are immature at birth but transition to more mature function after delivery.

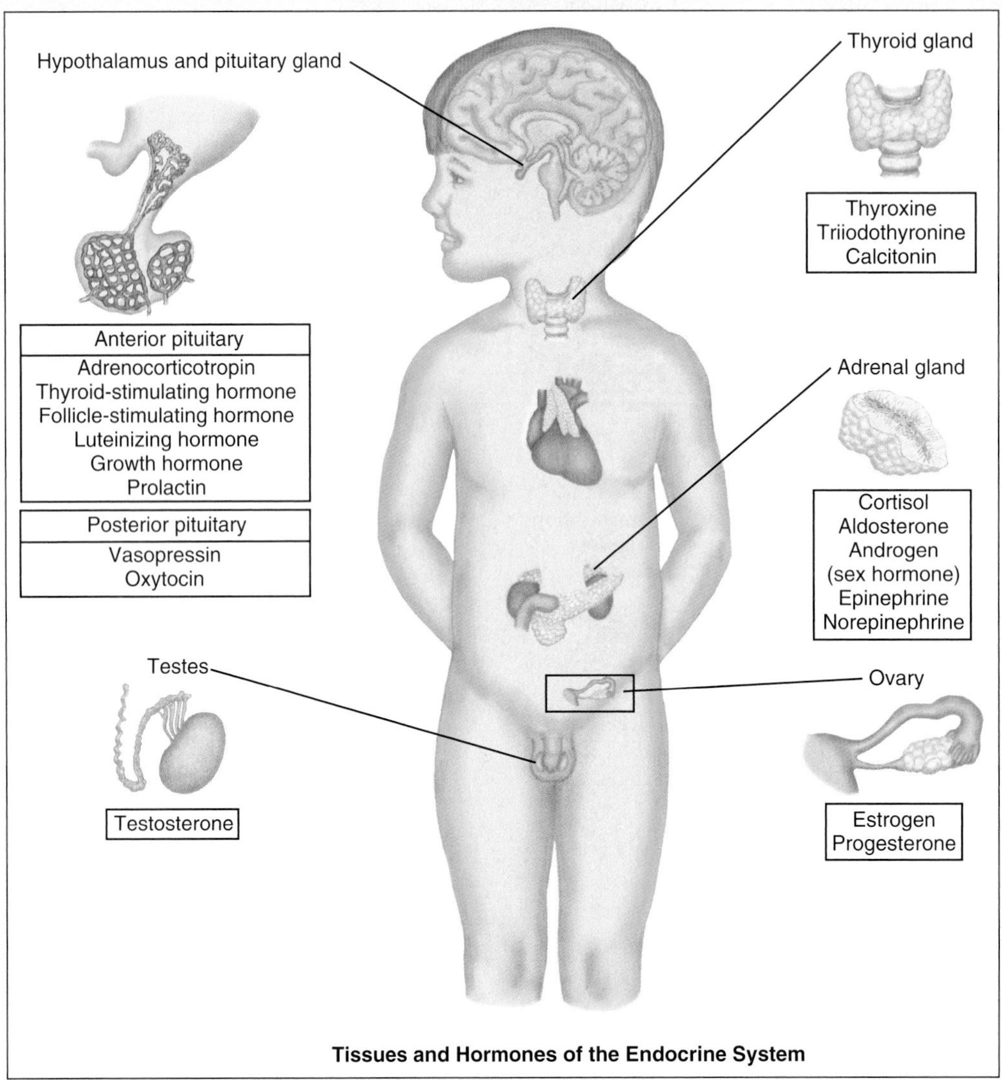

**Tissues and Hormones of the Endocrine System**

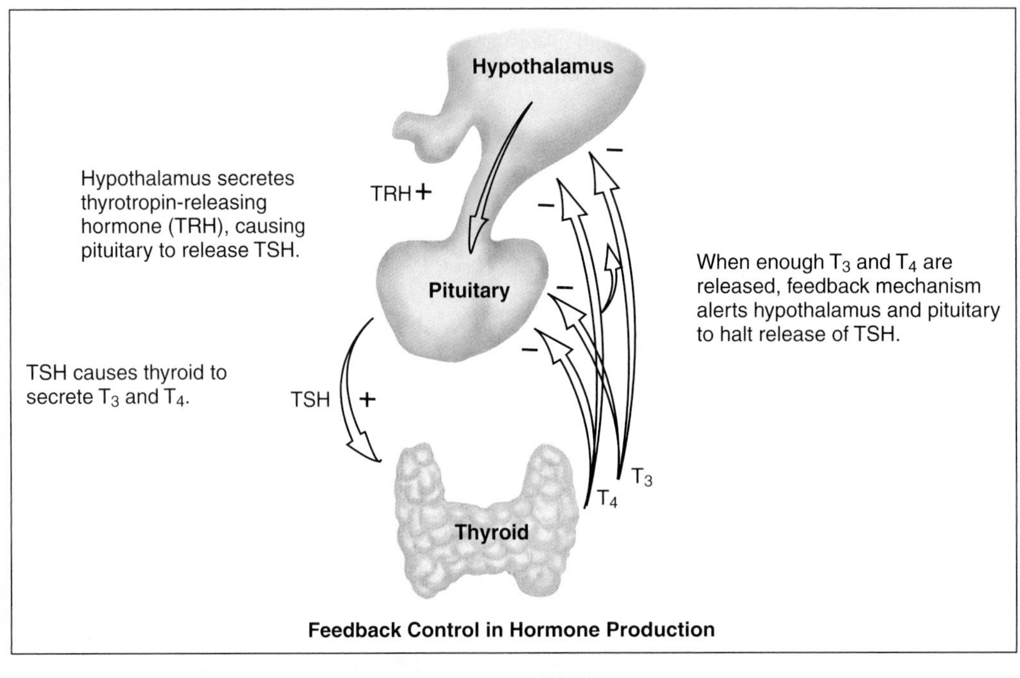

**Feedback Control in Hormone Production**

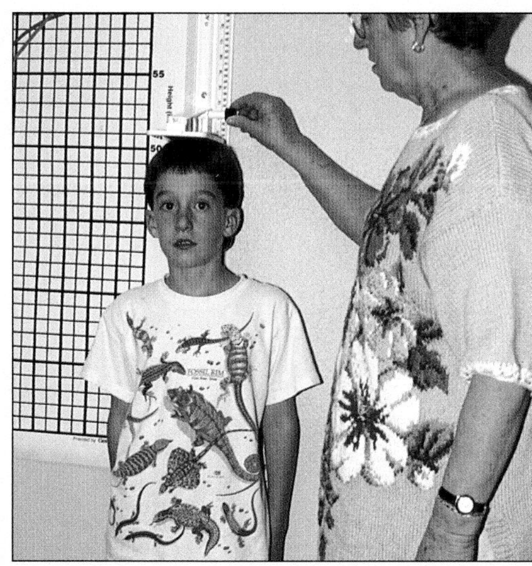

## DIAGNOSTIC TESTS AND PROCEDURES

Diagnosing endocrine dysfunction usually involves laboratory testing. Serum hormone levels are measured to determine if the amounts are adequate, deficient, or excessive. Laboratory screening is useful for diagnosing disease and monitoring children on hormone therapy.

Normal hormone levels are related to the child's age and stage of puberty. Because hormones are secreted at various times during the day or on a circadian rhythm, random blood samples can be difficult to interpret. Stimulation testing frequently demonstrates more accurate and definitive test results. With stimulation testing, a releasing factor or other agent is given to trigger the release or inhibition of a specific hormone. Serial blood sampling identifies the peak or trough level of the hormone, aiding in more accurate interpretation. A list of the common stimulation studies is provided in the accompanying table.

Other diagnostic tests include radiography and imaging techniques. Bone age radiographs can determine bone maturation, from which growth potential can be determined. Computed tomography (CT) scans and magnetic resonance imaging (MRI) are used to determine the presence of tumors or congenital malformations affecting the hypothalamus, pituitary, or target glands.

Accurate measurements of height and weight are essential when assessing the child for endocrine function. Evaluation of sexual development according to Tanner stages is also a part of the diagnostic workup (see Chapter 9). Developmental milestones and school performance should also be monitored because delays may be associated with endocrine disorders.

### Common Laboratory and Diagnostic Tests of Endocrine Function

| | Normal Findings | Indications | Preparation and Nursing Considerations |
|---|---|---|---|
| **GH Stimulation Test** | | | |
| An agent (e.g., insulin, arginine, clonidine) is given to stimulate release of GH. | One or more peak levels of GH >10 ng/mL | Evaluate GH production.<br>Identify GH deficiency. | Time specific; specimens must be drawn accurately.<br>NPO after midnight.<br>Notify provider if hypoglycemia or hypotension develops. |
| **ACTH (Cortrosyn) Stimulation Test** | | | |
| Cortrosyn (ACTH) is given to stimulate cortisol production. Tests ability of adrenal glands to function. | Cortisol should increase > 7 mcg/dL above baseline.<br>Cortisol < 18 mcg/dL suggests adrenal insufficiency. | Evaluate adrenal production of cortisol.<br>Identify infants with congenital adrenal hyperplasia. | Time specific; Cortisol level must be drawn before, 30 and 60 min after Cortrosyn administration. |
| **GnRH or GnRHa Stimulation Test** | | | |
| GnRH or GnRHa is administered to test the pituitary-ovarian axis for central precocious puberty (CPP). | LH should be <8 mIU/mL after GnRH or LH < 5 IU/L after GnRHa to not be consistent with CPP | Evaluate for central p recocious puberty. Clinical symptoms: Early thelarche (breast development), pubarche (pubic hair), bilateral testicular enlargement | Time specific; specimens must be drawn accurately at 1 and 3 hr after GnRH/ GnRHa administration. |
| **Water Deprivation Test** | | | |
| Child deprived of water and fluids for 7-8 hr | Decreased urine output, Increased urine specific gravity, Normal serum sodium and osmolality | Confirm diagnosis of central diabetes insipidus. | Strict monitoring of serum sodium and serum and urine osmolality.<br>Weigh child before, during, and after test.<br>Stop test if significant weight loss or change in vital signs or neurologic status develops. |

*Continued*

**Common Laboratory and Diagnostic Tests of Endocrine Function—cont'd**

| | Normal Findings | Indications | Preparation and Nursing Considerations |
|---|---|---|---|
| **hCG Test** | | | |
| Intramuscular hCG is administered serially to stimulate testicular production of testosterone. Allows test for conversion of testosterone to DHT. Tests function of undescended testes. | Low levels of testosterone and DHT in prelaboratory samples<br>Elevated levels of both testosterone and DHT—compare with known standards | Confirm testicular insufficiency.<br>Confirm 5-alpha-reductase deficiency.<br>Undescended testes may descend. | Time specific; draw samples before and after hCG.<br>Monitor for testicular descent and increase in phallic length. |

*ACTH,* Adrenocorticotropic hormone; *DHT,* dihydrotestosterone; *FSH,* follicle-stimulating hormone; *GH,* growth hormone; *GnRH,* gonadotropin-releasing hormone; *hCG,* human chorionic gonadotropin; *IV,* intravenous; *LH,* luteinizing hormone; *NPO,* nothing by mouth.

Pediatric endocrine disorders are generally managed in the outpatient setting. Most endocrine disorders are chronic conditions requiring long-term nursing management. The nurse assumes the roles of both educator and advocate for the child. Also important for the care of children with chronic medical problems is a careful psychosocial evaluation on a regular basis.

## PHENYLALANINE HYDROXYLASE DEFICIENCY (FORMALLY PHENYLKETONURIA)

Phenylalanine Hydroxylase Deficiency (PAH deficiency) is a genetic metabolic disorder that results in central nervous system (CNS) damage from toxic levels of phenylalanine (PHE) in the blood. PAH deficiency is characterized by a deficiency of phenylalanine hydroxylase, the enzyme needed to convert PHE to tyrosine.

### Etiology

PAH deficiency is an autosomal recessive disorder and is manifested only in the homozygote (individual who inherited two identical genes for a specific trait). With both parents carrying the recessive gene, each pregnancy has a 25% chance that the child will have PAH deficiency.

### Incidence

PAH deficiency occurs most commonly in whites, with an overall incidence of 1 in 10,000 live births. It is more prevalent in some European countries, including Turkey and Ireland (Vockley et al., 2014).

### Manifestations

The underlying metabolic alterations begin to have an immediate effect on the infant, although signs may not be apparent until the infant is approximately 3 months old. The first sign may be digestive problems with vomiting. These infants also can have a musty or mousy odor to the urine, infantile eczema, hypertonia, seizures, and hyperactive behavior. Older children can have hypopigmentation of the hair, skin, and irises; they are commonly blond with light blue eyes. Intellectual impairment is a long-term consequence of untreated PAH deficiency (Mitchell, 2013).

### Diagnostic Evaluation

Routine neonatal screening for PAH deficiency is mandatory in all 50 states of the United States. With early postpartum discharge, screening is often performed on infants younger than 2 days of age because of the concern that the infant will be lost to follow-up. Previously, when screening was performed before the third day of life there was a higher risk of a false-negative outcome. However, screening now uses tandem mass spectrometry that can quantify PHE concentrations as early as 24 hours after birth. A serum PHE level greater than 130 µmol/L indicates a positive result; however, this result alone is not diagnostic and indicates that the infant should be evaluated further (Vockley et al., 2014).

**PATHOPHYSIOLOGY**

***PAH Deficiency***

PAH deficiency refers to a group of biochemical diseases associated with enzymatic blocks in the conversion of the essential amino acid *phenylalanine* to *tyrosine.* Classic PKU consists of the absence of the enzyme *phenylalanine hydroxylase.* This deficiency results in the toxic accumulation of PHE in the bloodstream after the ingestion of protein containing PHE. Phenylalanine can adversely affect the myelinization process in central nervous system (CNS) development. Most of that process takes place during the first decade of life. Intellectual impairment occurs and progresses if treatment is not implemented.

### Therapeutic Management

Evaluation by a specialist should be instituted as soon as the diagnosis is confirmed because the best results are obtained with early management. Phenylalanine tolerance varies according to the infant and the severity of the enzyme deficiency. Treatment should be initiated if the infant's blood phenylalanine level exceeds 600 µmol/L (Rezvani & Ficicioglu, 2016). Infants and children with PAH deficiency are treated with a special diet that restricts PHE intake. The goal of therapy is to keep the serum PHE level between 120 and 360 µmol/L for patients of all ages. Phenylalanine intake should be limited but provide enough of this essential amino acid to meet the patient's growth requirements. Dietary management must be started early in neonatal life because the untreated infant will sustain CNS damage by several weeks of age. Historically, relaxation of PHE control and treatment was allowed because intellectual disability did not occur in patients that were well controlled throughout their childhood. However, it has been found that adverse neurocognitive and psychiatric outcomes do occur later in life in those with relaxed PHE control. Therefore, treatment and maintenance of appropriate PHE serum levels should continue throughout the lifespan. Cofactor tetrahydrobiopterin (sapropterin [Kuvan]), a medication that can lower blood PHE levels by increasing the metabolism of phenylalanine to tyrosine, is appropriate for some individuals with PAH deficiency (Rezvani & Ficicioglu, 2016). Large neutral amino acids and polyethyleneglycol-conjugated phenylalanine ammonia lyase are two other pharmacotherapies being studied to treat this disease (Vockley et al., 2014).

Another consideration is genetic counseling for women with PKU who become pregnant. Adolescent girls and women of childbearing age require counseling about fetal risks including mental deficiency, microcephaly, retarded growth, seizures, and an increased incidence of structural defects. The goal is to control phenylalanine levels before conception and maintain strict control during the pregnancy.

### Nursing Considerations

Although a family history of PKU would alert the caregiver to an infant at risk, most infants with PKU are not identified at birth. Neonatal symptoms are usually not present. A screening test, part of the newborn screen done in all states, is the first diagnostic procedure. Newborn screenings usually include testing for PKU and congenital hypothyroidism, as well as any other screening tests mandated by local and state public health departments, such as hemoglobinopathies (i.e., sickle cell disease or trait), galactosemia, and maple syrup urine disease. A positive screening result requires further diagnostic evaluation to verify the diagnosis.

A low-phenylalanine diet is initiated immediately; the infant with PKU is fed a low-phenylalanine formula and, as foods are introduced, the child must follow a protein-restricted diet. The child must avoid high-protein foods such as meats, fish, eggs, cheese, milk, and legumes. Because protein is also present in grains, low-protein breads, cereals, and pastas are used. Dietary staples are vegetables, fruits, and starches. To avoid the consequences of insufficient protein for growth, some children with PKU take a phenylalanine-free protein supplement. The growth pattern and neurobehavioral development of the affected child must be monitored closely.

Follow-up is provided for all infants if the initial screening result is abnormal. The nurse assists with referral to a genetic center that is capable of diagnosing and treating the infant.

Phenylalanine requirements change rapidly in the first months of life. Parents are encouraged to adhere to monitoring requirements for the infant diagnosed with PKU. Rigid regimens for diet control will not be successful unless the family accepts the changes required. The nurse helps the family deal with lifestyle changes by initiating referrals as needed (e.g., to social service agencies, registered dietitian, support groups). On-line support groups and chat rooms provide ideas for adapting recipes; specialized cookbooks are also available.

The nurse encourages the parents to express their feelings about the infant's diagnosis and the risk of PAH deficiency in future children. Family members need support to recognize the problems caused by the disease and identify strategies for dealing with the stress of having a child with a chronic illness. Physical measurements and neurologic and intellectual development should be documented through standardized testing. If control of the phenylalanine level is established early, normal infant growth and development should occur.

## INBORN ERRORS OF METABOLISM

In addition to PAH deficiency, there are other genetically transmitted metabolic diseases that rarely occur in newborns (Table 51.1). Nurses

**TABLE 51.1 Inborn Errors of Metabolism**

| Description | Management |
|---|---|
| **Galactosemia** | |
| A deficiency of galactose-1-phosphate uridyltransferase prevents the conversion of galactose to glucose in lactose digestion. Infants cannot properly digest milk or sugar. Although rare (1 in 40,000-60,000 live births), infants exhibit intrauterine growth retardation, hypotonia, liver damage, cataracts, and infections. The urine contains reducing substances. Vomiting and diarrhea occur after feedings. | The child is on a lifelong lactose-restricted diet and close monitoring for and treatment of infections. If untreated, the infant usually dies; infants who have been treated may have developmental or learning deficits. The condition is genetically transmitted through an autosomal recessive inheritance pattern; referral to a genetic counseling center is warranted. |
| **Maple Syrup Urine Disease** | |
| This is a very rare (1 in 250,000-300,000 live births) autosomal recessive inherited condition that affects metabolism of certain amino acids. Buildup of acids causes ketoacidosis, which appears 48-72 hr after birth. The infant is lethargic and can display poor feeding, vomiting, weight loss, seizures, and loss of reflexes. The urine smells like maple syrup. | Dialysis is needed to reduce accumulated acids. The child must be on a lifelong low-protein, limited amino acid diet. If untreated, the child can die quickly; children who have been treated can have neurologic deficits. Referral to a genetic counseling center is warranted. |
| **Tay-Sachs Disease** | |
| A genetic condition that affects primarily infants in the Ashkenazi Jewish population. It is caused by an abnormal buildup of gangliosides (normal constituents in nerve synapse membrane) in the neurons. After a 6-mo period of relatively normal development, the infant begins to demonstrate developmental delay and progressive neurologic deterioration. The infant usually exhibits macrocephaly, seizures, blindness, and deafness; death occurs during early childhood. | Management is symptomatic and supportive to the child and family. Referral to a genetic counseling center is essential. |

Data from Rezvani, I., & Rezvani, G.A. (2016). An approach to inborn errors of metabolism. In R. Kliegman, B. Stanton, J. St. Geme, et al. (Eds.), *Nelson textbook of pediatrics* (20th ed., pp. 634–6636). Philadelphia: Elsevier.

should create a climate in which parents can express their feelings about the lifelong care of their child, as well as concerns for future pregnancies. Families with affected infants are referred to genetic counseling centers. Many of these infants are identified through universal newborn screening or screening specific for at-risk infants. Additional nursing care is related to the particular disorder but is similar to that for the child with PAH deficiency.

## CONGENITAL ADRENAL HYPERPLASIA

Congenital adrenal hyperplasia (CAH) is a group of autosomal recessive disorders in which the adrenal gland is not able to manufacture adequate glucocorticoid (cortisol), and while working to make glucocorticoid, produces excess androgens (sex hormones). Mineralocorticoid (aldosterone) production can be either normal or low.

### Etiology

CAH is caused by a defect in the enzymatic pathway of adrenal steroid production. Diminished glucocorticoid production prompts increased ACTH production by the pituitary gland, further increasing adrenal androgen excess. Several enzymatic defects have been identified, the most common being 21-hydroxylase deficiency (21 OHD), accounting for more than 90% of cases. Infants with diminished mineralocorticoid production (specifically aldosterone) will waste salt through the kidneys, resulting in a "salt-wasting" crisis that manifests as poor feeding, vomiting, dehydration, failure to thrive, weight loss, hypotension, hyponatremia, and **hyperkalemia**. This condition accompanies the more life-threatening form of CAH, occurring in 75% of patients with 21 OHD CAH (Nimkarn, Lin-Su, & New, 2011).

### Incidence

The worldwide incidence of the classical type of 21 OHD CAH is between 1 in 15,000 to 1 in 20,000 live births (White, 2016). In contrast, the incidence of non-classical 21 OHD CAH is much higher, with 1 in 1,000 live births. Ashkenazi Jews and Hispanics are most afflicted by this disease (Nimkarn et al., 2011; White, 2016).

### Manifestations

CAH is marked by ambiguous genitalia of the newborn female infant, postnatal virilization in both sexes, and salt-wasting crisis (in the first few weeks of life) with low serum sodium, high serum potassium, hypovolemia, and eventual hypotensive crisis. Simple virilizing CAH is not associated with a salt-wasting crisis and manifests as a muscular body, advanced bone age, and premature pubic hair. Typically, this form is seen later in infancy or early childhood. Untreated or poorly treated CAH can result in an advanced bone age with ultimate adult short stature. A milder form of CAH (3-beta-hydroxysteroid dehydrogenase (3β-HSD) can cause symptoms during childhood or adolescence, with the child exhibiting hirsutism, menstrual irregularities, or delayed menses.

### Diagnostic Evaluation

The finding of ambiguous genitalia in the newborn infant should raise concern for the possibility of CAH. The diagnosis is confirmed by elevated levels of 17-hydroxyprogesterone, a glucocorticoid precursor. The corticoptropin stimulation test is the gold standard for diagnosis in non-classical or more ambiguous cases. CAH is a part of newborn screening in all 50 states. An appropriate evaluation includes obtaining serum electrolyte, carbon dioxide, and renin levels and performing a physical examination. Serum sodium levels in the infant suspected of CAH will be low, with elevated serum potassium. Serum renin levels will be elevated, indicating mineralocorticoid deficiency. A karyotype to determine genetic sex may be indicated, depending on the degree of genital ambiguity (Nimkarn et al., 2011).

### Therapeutic Management

An accurate diagnosis and prompt treatment of fluid and electrolyte abnormalities may avert a salt-wasting crisis. The child with CAH requires lifelong glucocorticoid therapy. Oral glucocorticoid (hydrocortisone acetate, cortisone acetate) dosage is prescribed on the basis of body size and is given two or three times per day in either a liquid suspension or tablet form. For children with salt-wasting CAH, mineralocorticoid replacement therapy is required using fludrocortisone acetate (Florinef), which is taken once or twice daily. Therapy effectiveness is evaluated with serum electrolyte, 17-hydroxyprogesterone level, and renin levels. Special sick-day instructions should be provided to the family. The glucocorticoid dosage is usually doubled or tripled when the child is ill, has a broken bone, or is undergoing a surgical procedure. Bone-age radiographs are performed yearly to assess skeletal maturity; poor adherence to the medication regimen or under-treatment can result in advanced bone aging and decreased final adult height.

### Nursing Considerations

All newborn girls should be assessed for ambiguous genitalia, fused labia, enlarged clitoris, or migration of the urethral opening. Infant boys and girls with unexplained dehydration and low serum sodium levels should be considered to have adrenal insufficiency and undergo careful assessment of fluid and electrolyte status.

**SAFETY ALERT**

***Congenital Adrenal Hyperplasia***

- Children with salt-wasting congenital adrenal hyperplasia (CAH) require glucocorticoid replacement to survive.
- In the event of significant stress, such as fever, broken bone, or surgery, children with CAH will require "stress dose" medical therapy.
- If the child with CAH begins to vomit, the glucocorticoid must be administered parenterally.
- Mineralocorticoid therapy is required in salt-wasting CAH.
- Supplemental sodium occasionally may also be required.

Infant girls with ambiguous genitalia might require reconstructive surgery. Depending on the degree of virilization, surgical correction is recommended in infancy or in early puberty. When appropriate, the nurse reassures the parents that the infant has appropriate internal structures and that external structures can be corrected surgically. Parents are encouraged to express their concerns. The nurse helps to facilitate parent-infant attachment.

Older children receiving glucocorticoid replacement therapy are assessed for linear growth and signs of early puberty. Serial height measurements can provide data about the adequacy of glucocorticoid supplementation. In children with salt-wasting CAH, serum renin levels should be closely monitored; effective treatment with mineralocorticoids will maintain these levels in or near the normal range (White, 2016). Nonadherence can cause early virilization, increased growth velocity, diminished final adult height, and menstrual irregularities in girls. Blood pressure monitoring is important for children receiving mineralocorticoid replacement therapy.

The nurse carefully instructs the parents about replacement hormone administration and the timing of medication. Parents are included in the development of a plan for sick-day dosages of medications. The infant with salt-wasting CAH may require salt supplements; the family needs instruction on preparation of these supplements.

Follow-up evaluations with the endocrinologist are scheduled for every 2 to 3 months in infancy and every 4 to 6 months in the older child. Parents of the child with CAH should be referred to a genetic counselor if they plan more pregnancies because future children are at risk for CAH. *Prenatal* treatment (dexamethasone taken by the mother) is available to prevent virilization of the female fetus (Nimkarn et al., 2011). If effective, this prenatal treatment eliminates the need for surgical correction of ambiguous genitalia in the affected female infant.

Adolescents are encouraged to assume increasing responsibility for medication administration. The nurse strongly emphasizes the importance of compliance. Surgical reconstruction of the genitalia and vaginal dilation may be required in the adolescent years. Careful explanations and preparation for these procedures will reassure affected adolescents and help them understand the expected outcomes following the procedures.

## CONGENITAL HYPOTHYROIDISM

Congenital hypothyroidism is a condition in which the thyroid gland does not produce sufficient thyroid hormone to meet the body's metabolic needs. The condition is present from birth and, if not treated, can lead to intellectual impairment.

### Etiology

Congenital hypothyroidism is caused by an absent (aplastic), underdeveloped, or ectopic thyroid gland. This group of congenital defects is referred to as *thyroid dysgenesis.* For unknown reasons, the fetal thyroid gland fails to develop properly or fails to migrate to the appropriate location. Other rare causes are hypothalamic or pituitary disorders in which TSH secretion is insufficient to stimulate the thyroid gland. Biochemical defects in thyroid hormone production also cause congenital hypothyroidism. Maternal intake of medications, such as propylthiouracil (PTU), during pregnancy to control maternal hyperthyroidism can cause transient hypothyroidism in the infant. Transfer of maternal antibodies to the fetus can also cause transient hypothyroidism (Leger et al., 2014).

### Incidence

The incidence of congenital hypothyroidism is 1 in 2,000 live births in countries with newborn screening availability (LaFranchi & Huang, 2016a). Untreated hypothyroidism causes intellectual impairment; to prevent this occurrence, all 50 states in the U.S. to carry this test on their newborn screening. Early detection and treatment favor increased intellectual function. Most occurrences are spontaneous, with a smaller percentage having a genetic (autosomal recessive) inheritance that results in defective thyroxine synthesis (Leger et al., 2014).

### Manifestations

The infant with congenital hypothyroidism often displays signs including skin mottling, a large anterior fontanel, a large tongue, hypotonia, slow reflexes, and a distended abdomen (Fig. 51.1). Other signs and symptoms include prolonged jaundice, lethargy, constipation, feeding problems, coldness to touch, umbilical hernia, hoarse cry, and excessive sleeping. The infant with congenital hypothyroidism may have none of these signs or symptoms; the newborn screening test is essential to recognize these infants (Leger et al., 2014).

### Diagnostic Evaluation

Congenital hypothyroidism is detected by elevated TSH (with or without T4 evaluation) on newborn screening that is collected after 24 hours of age, although the best time for testing is between 48 and 72 hours of age (Leger et al., 2014). Practitioners must be cautious with test interpretation because of the rise in TSH immediately after birth as part of the normal newborn transition. For a newborn with a low $T_4$ value, a TSH level will be obtained. A low $T_4$ level with TSH elevation is indicative of congenital hypothyroidism; further testing is often done to determine the cause (LaFranchi & Huang, 2016a). Thyroid scans can identify any functioning thyroid tissue. Treatment should never be delayed while waiting for scan results.

### Therapeutic Management

If capillary TSH on the newborn screen is greater than or equal to 40 mU/L, treatment should be initiated as soon as venous blood sampling can be obtained, without delay to wait for results. Treatment of children with congenital hypothyroidism consists of lifelong thyroid hormone replacement, usually in the form of levothyroxine. It is given as a single daily oral dose that varies with the weight and age of the child or adult (Leger et al., 2014). The dosage is titrated to maintain TSH and $T_4$ in a normal range.

## PATHOPHYSIOLOGY

### Congenital Hypothyroidism

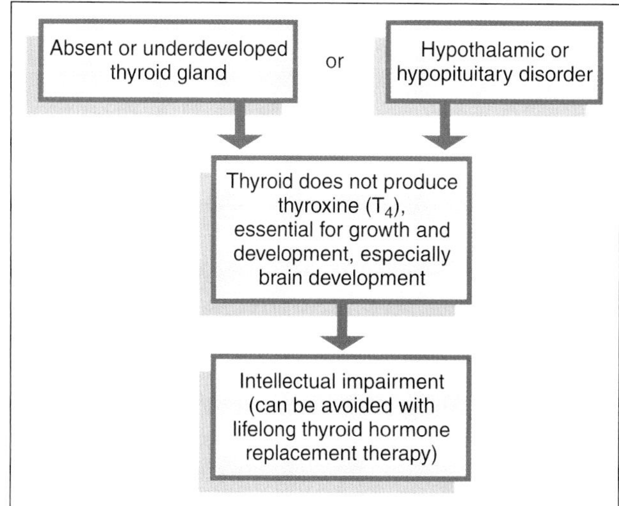


The thyroid gland is a butterfly shaped gland located in front of the neck. Thyroid-stimulating hormone (TSH), secreted by the pituitary, induces the thyroid to produce thyroxine ($T_4$) and triiodothyronine ($T_3$). The thyroid traps iodine and produces $T_4$, which is essential for normal growth and development, especially brain development, in the first 2 years of life. Immediately after delivery, TSH increases dramatically, likely related to the stress of the birth process. Within the first week of life, the TSH level gradually falls.

Underdevelopment of the thyroid gland or a hypothalamic or pituitary disorder causes inadequate production of $T_4$, which is essential for brain development. If not treated, this condition can cause intellectual impairment in the developing child. An infant with congenital hypothyroidism has elevated TSH and low $T_4$ levels.

## NURSING CARE

### The Infant With Congenital Hypothyroidism

#### Assessment

Nursing care of the infant with congenital hypothyroidism involves assessing growth and development and ensuring adherence to the

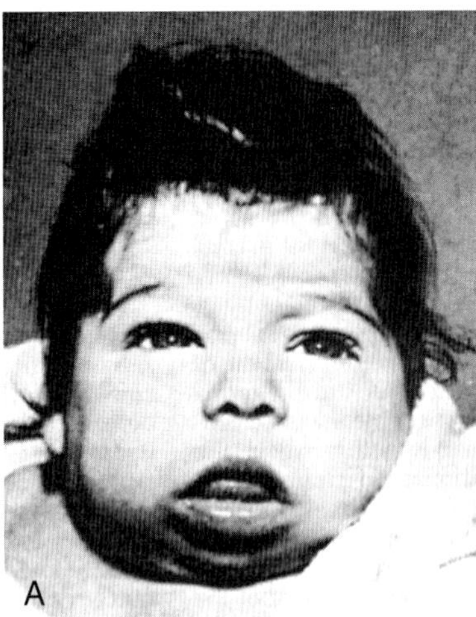


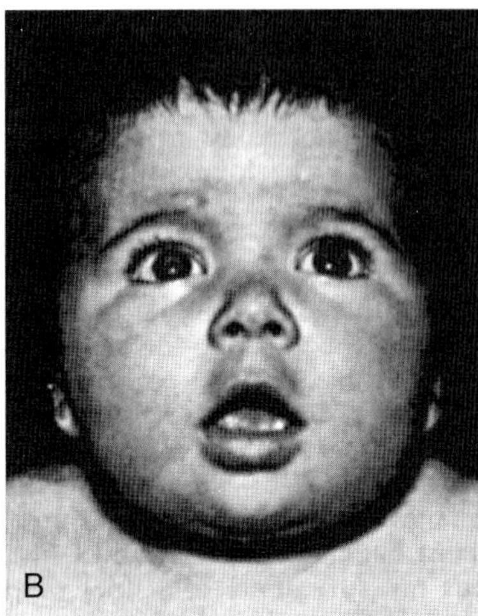


**FIG 51.1** **A,** This untreated 6-month-old infant with congenital hypothyroidism fed poorly and was constipated. She was lethargic and had no social smile or head control. Note her puffy face, large tongue, dull expression, and excessive hair growth (hirsutism) on the forehead. **B,** The same infant 4 months after treatment. Note the decreased facial puffiness, decreased forehead hirsutism, and alert appearance. (Data from LaFranchi, S.H., & Huang, S.A. (2016). Hypothyroidism. In R. Kliegman, B. Stanton, J. St. Geme, et al. [Eds.], *Nelson textbook of pediatrics* [20th ed., pp. 2665 51–2675]. Philadelphia: Elsevier.)

prescribed medication regimen. Nurses can play a major role in recognizing the infant with hypothyroidism. Intellectual impairment caused by untreated hypothyroidism cannot be reversed, but it can be prevented through early identification and proper treatment. Once a normal TSH concentration is achieved, infants with hypothyroidism typically are evaluated every 1 to 3 months for the first year of life, every 2 to 4 months to the age of three years, and then every 3 to 12 months thereafter. The nurse should obtain accurate measurements of height, weight, and head circumference at each visit. Frequent developmental assessments are also essential (Leger et al., 2014).

### Nursing Diagnosis and Planning

The following nursing diagnoses and expected outcomes may be appropriate for the infant with congenital hypothyroidism and the infant's parents:

- Deficient Knowledge related to unfamiliarity with the congenital disorder.

  ***Expected outcome.*** The parents will demonstrate the ability to monitor their infant for signs and symptoms of hypothyroidism and hyperthyroidism and give thyroid medication properly. The parents will verbalize an understanding of normal growth and developmental milestones and their child's lifelong needs for care and follow-up.

- Delayed Growth and Development related to disease process.

  ***Expected outcome.*** As a result of appropriate disease management, the infant will demonstrate growth and developmental milestones appropriate for age.

- Ineffective Thermoregulation related to decreased basal metabolic rate.

  ***Expected outcome.*** As a result of disease management, the infant will maintain a temperature within normal range.

### Interventions

The nurse instructs family members on the importance of medication adherence emphasizing that the medication is necessary for the child's growth, especially for the rapidly developing brain.

The family is taught how to administer levothyroxine orally as a single daily dose. It can be dissolved in a small amount of water and given by syringe or placed into the nipple of a baby bottle (see Chapter 38). When the infant is older, the medication can be given in a spoonful of baby food. Toddlers can usually chew tablets without difficulty. If the infant or child vomits within 1 hour of taking medication, the dose should be re-administered. Frequent missing of doses can lead to developmental delays and poor growth.

**! NURSING QUALITY ALERT**

***The Child With Congenital Hypothyroidism***

- Untreated hypothyroidism leads to intellectual impairment.
- Thyroxine ($T_4$) and thyroid-stimulating hormone (TSH) levels vary with age, but any infant with a low free $T_4$ OR an elevated TSH > 20 mU/L (even if normal free $T_4$) is considered to have primary hypothyroidism; treatment should be initiated immediately*

*LaFranchi, S.H., & Huang, S.A. (2016a). Hypothyroidism. In R. Kliegman, B. Stanton, J. St. Geme, et al. (Eds.), *Nelson textbook of pediatrics* (20th ed., pp. 2665–2675). Philadelphia: Elsevier.

The nurse also teaches the parents the signs and symptoms of both hypothyroidism and hyperthyroidism and when to notify the provider if symptoms occur. Hyperthyroidism can develop in infants receiving too much medication. Parents should be taught to determine their child's pulse rate and notify their healthcare provider if the rate is greater than the recommended parameter.

Because hypothyroidism is a lifelong condition, school-age children and teenagers should be made aware of the importance of taking their medication and of keeping regular follow-up appointments with the provider.

### Evaluation

- Have the parents demonstrated the ability to monitor the child's signs and symptoms, recognize growth and developmental problems, administer the medication, and discuss the child's lifelong needs for care and follow-up?
- Is the child developing appropriately for age according to growth charts and formalized developmental screening tests?

- Does the child have normal results on thyroid function tests?
- Is the child's body temperature within normal limits?

## ACQUIRED HYPOTHYROIDISM

Hypothyroidism is a condition in which the thyroid gland produces an inadequate amount of thyroid hormone to meet the body's metabolic needs.

### Etiology

Hashimoto thyroiditis is an autoimmune process and a common cause of acquired hypothyroidism, usually associated with a goiter. Other causes of acquired hypothyroidism include surgical thyroidectomy, radioactive iodine therapy for hyperthyroidism, radiation therapy for malignancies, and excessive iodine ingestion. Less frequently, decreased TSH secretion by the pituitary gland or decreased thyrotropin-releasing hormone (TRH) secretion by the hypothalamus causes hypothyroidism (Brown, 2012).

Autoimmune thyroiditis is the most common cause of acquired hypothyroidism in children and adolescents (LaFranchi & Huang, 2016b). It often occurs in families with a history of thyroid disease. Other family members may test positive for thyroid antibodies. Thyroiditis is more common in girls and most often occurs in chronic lymphocytic thyroiditis (Brown, 2012).

### Pathophysiology

Circulating autoantibodies known as TSH receptor blocking antibodies decrease thyroid gland production of triiodothyronine ($T_3$) and $T_4$. These antibodies bind at the TSH receptor sites on the thyroid gland, resulting in decreased thyroid hormone production. The cause of this antibody production is unknown (Brown, 2012).

In contrast to congenital hypothyroidism, adverse effects from hypothyroidism acquired after 2 to 3 years of age are often reversible. Goiter, an enlarged thyroid gland, occurs in response to increased TSH secretion, autoimmune attack of the thyroid gland, or goitrogens.

### Manifestations

Clinical manifestations of hypothyroidism include goiter (one lobe frequently larger than the other); dry, thick skin; coarse, dull hair; fatigue; cold intolerance; constipation; weight gain; decreased linear growth; edema of face, eyes, and hands; and irregular or delayed menses (Box 51.1).

**BOX 51.1 Indicators of Hypothyroidism or Hyperthyroidism**

| Hypothyroidism | Hyperthyroidism |
|---|---|
| Fatigue | Emotional lability, anxiety |
| Constipation | Diarrhea |
| Cold intolerance | Heat intolerance |
| Weight gain | Weight loss, increased appetite |
| Dry, thick skin | Smooth, velvety skin |
| Edema of face, eyes, hands (myxedema) | Prominent eyes |
| Decreased growth, delayed skeletal maturation and puberty | Accelerated linear growth |
| Decreased activity and energy | Hyperactivity |
| Muscle hypertrophy (pseudodystrophy) | Muscle weakness |
| Decreased heart rate | Increased heart rate |
| Increased need for sleep | High blood pressure |
| Ataxia | Tremor |

### Diagnostic Evaluation

Elevated TSH and low $T_4$ levels are diagnostic of hypothyroidism. Elevated TSH level is the most sensitive indicator of primary hypothyroidism.

Thyroiditis is diagnosed by the presence of circulating thyroid antibodies and is usually associated with a firm goiter. Initially TSH is elevated with normal $T_4$ levels, although $T_4$ decreases over time. With secondary or tertiary hypothyroidism, TSH is not elevated; therefore, thyroid-releasing hormone stimulation testing is usually required for diagnosis.

### Therapeutic Management

Management of the child with hypothyroidism involves thyroid hormone replacement, usually with levothyroxine. The dosage varies according to the child's age and weight and is given as a single daily dose. The dose is titrated to maintain $T_4$ in the upper half of the normal range and to maintain TSH in the normal range for age.

## NURSING CARE

### The Child With Acquired Hypothyroidism

#### Assessment

Care of the child with acquired hypothyroidism includes assessing response to treatment and adherence to the medication regimen. With treatment, the goiter should decrease in size. Signs and symptoms of hypothyroidism should also resolve with adequate thyroid hormone replacement. Monitoring height and weight, and conducting developmental screening at each clinic visit assesses the child's growth and development. The nurse should monitor school performance as well and maintain contact with the school nurse.

#### Nursing Diagnosis and Planning

The following nursing diagnoses and expected outcomes may be appropriate for a child with acquired hypothyroidism:

- Constipation related to decreased basal metabolic rate as a result of hypothyroidism.

*Expected outcome.* The child will maintain regular bowel movements of normal consistency as basal metabolic rate improves.

- Activity Intolerance related to fatigue.

*Expected outcome.* The child will maintain normal energy levels for age, as evidenced by the ability to exercise at the same level as peers.

- Disturbed Body Image related to weight gain/obesity.

*Expected outcome.* The child will verbalize feelings about body changes and will accept reassurances that changes will resolve with treatment.

- Ineffective Thermoregulation related to decreased basal metabolic rate secondary to hypothyroidism.

*Expected outcome.* As a result of appropriate disease management, the child will maintain normal body temperature.

#### Interventions

Parents and children who are school age or older should be instructed on the correct dose and timing of thyroid medication. Thyroid hormone levels are usually checked every 3 to 6 months. Laboratory values within the normal range indicate good response to therapy. The nurse educates the older child and parents on the signs and symptoms of hypothyroidism and hyperthyroidism and to notify the provider if symptoms occur. The child is reassured that signs such as constipation, fatigue, and weight gain will resolve as the medication becomes effective.

### Evaluation

- Has the child maintained regular bowel movements of normal consistency?
- Can the child tolerate exercise at the same level as peers?
- Does the child express feelings related to body changes and accept reassurances that problems will resolve?
- Has the child maintained normal body temperature?

## HYPERTHYROIDISM (GRAVES' DISEASE)

Graves' disease is an autoimmune condition in which excessive thyroid hormones are produced by an enlarged thyroid gland. It is the most common cause of hyperthyroidism in children.

### Incidence

The incidence of hyperthyroidism in children younger than 15 years is approximately 1 in 100,000 (Rivkees, 2014), with girls being more likely than boys to acquire the condition. Peak age for acquiring the condition is between 10 and 14 years. Graves' disease can have a familial tendency, and children with autoimmune disease are at risk for other autoimmune disorders. Neonatal Graves' disease is associated with maternal hyperthyroidism and is relatively uncommon, with an estimated incidence of 1 in 25,000 neonates (Srinivasan & Misra, 2015).

### Pathophysiology

Circulating autoantibodies known as *thyroid-stimulating immunoglobulins* (TSIs) stimulate the thyroid gland to make $T_3$ and $T_4$. These antibodies bind to the TSH receptor sites on the thyroid gland, resulting in excessive thyroid hormone production. The cause of this antibody production is unknown. In newborns, maternal TSI is transferred through the placenta to the fetus. TSIs bind to the TSH receptor, causing neonatal hyperthyroidism.

### Manifestations

Goiter, increased appetite, weight loss, nervousness, diarrhea, increased perspiration, heat intolerance, increased heart rate, muscle weakness, palpitations, tremors, exophthalmos, poor attention span, and behavior or school problems are common in Graves' disease (see Box 51.1). In the neonate, irritability, tachycardia, hypertension, voracious appetite with poor weight gain, flushing, prominent eyes, and thyroid enlargement are major signs. These signs are self-limiting, but cardiac failure and death can occur if the signs are unrecognized or poorly treated.

**! NURSING QUALITY ALERT**

***Autoimmune Thyroid Disorders***

- Treatment for Graves disease is either medical (antithyroid medications) or ablative (radioactive iodine or surgery).
- Adherence to medical therapy is problematic because of the requirement for twice-daily or three-times-daily dosing for protracted periods (2 to 3 years).
- Goiter can be present with either hypothyroidism or hyperthyroidism.
- Autoimmune thyroiditis resulting in either hypothyroidism or hyperthyroidism can be permanent or transient.

### Diagnostic Evaluation

Elevated serum $T_4$ and $T_3$ levels with suppressed TSH levels, associated with signs and symptoms of hyperthyroidism, suggest Graves' disease. Autoantibodies to thyroid tissue usually are positive. Thyroid uptake of radioactive iodine is increased (Srinivasan & Misra, 2015).

### Therapeutic Management

The three approaches to the management of Graves' disease are antithyroid drug therapy, radioactive iodine, or surgery. Antithyroid drug therapy with methimazole is the treatment of choice for childhood hyperthyroidism (Huang & LaFranchi, 2016b). Propylthiouracil (PTU) has an unacceptable risk for liver toxicity in children and its use is not recommended unless other therapies are not a suitable option or the child is allergic to methimazole. These drugs act by blocking thyroid hormone production by the thyroid gland. The medications usually are given three times per day, and they lower thyroid hormone levels in several weeks. Minor adverse effects include arthralgia, skin rash, pruritus, and gastric intolerance. Major adverse effects include neutropenia, hepatotoxicity, and hypothyroidism (Srinivasan & Misra, 2015).

A second approach to management is oral radioactive iodine treatment. Radioactive iodine ($^{131}I$) is given as an oral solution. It is typically used in children older than 10 years. With this therapy, the radioactive iodine is absorbed and concentrated by the thyroid gland, destroying the thyroid tissue in approximately 6 to 18 weeks. Hyperthyroid symptoms may intensify briefly after treatment. Hypothyroidism can result once the thyroid gland is irradiated, necessitating thyroid replacement therapy.

Subtotal or partial thyroidectomy, the surgical removal of thyroid gland tissue, is the third form of management. Inorganic iodine, given 7 to 10 days before surgery, decreases the gland's vascularity. Surgery carries the risk of bleeding, wound infection, vocal cord paralysis, and injury to the parathyroid glands, resulting in hypoparathyroidism including hypocalcemia. Calcium levels should be monitored after surgery (Srinivasan & Misra, 2015).

Recurrence of hyperthyroidism is uncommon but possible. Affected children also have a 60% to 80% chance for developing hypothyroidism, which can be treated with thyroid replacement therapy.

Follow-up evaluations correlate with response to therapy. As thyroid functions normalize, follow-up endocrine evaluations are recommended once or twice per year.

## NURSING CARE

### The Child With Hyperthyroidism

#### Assessment

The treatment goals consist of normalizing thyroid hormone levels, alleviating symptoms of hyperthyroidism, and decreasing the goiter. The nurse should assess for adherence to medical therapy and determine if the family understands that medical therapy might take several weeks to decrease thyroid hormone action. The child is closely monitored for adrenergic signs and symptoms. Propranolol, a beta-adrenergic blocker, may be prescribed to decrease adrenergic signs and symptoms (tachycardia, heat intolerance, tremor) until the antithyroid medication takes effect.

A child being treated with PTU has an increased risk of neutropenia and hepatotoxicity; regular blood counts and liver function studies are done to assess these risks. The nurse assesses the child for fever, joint pain, edema, rash, and excessive bruising. A child who acquires a fever or sore throat while receiving PTU should be evaluated by a healthcare provider and a complete blood count obtained to evaluate for agranulocytosis.

#### Nursing Diagnosis and Planning

The following nursing diagnoses and expected outcomes may be appropriate for a child with hyperthyroidism and the child's family:

- Ineffective Family Therapeutic Regimen Management related to nonadherence to the medication regimen.

***Expected outcome.*** The family will adhere to the medication regimen, as evidenced by normal thyroid hormone levels.

- Diarrhea related to increased basal metabolic rate secondary to hyperthyroidism.

***Expected outcome.*** The child will be euthyroid, as evidenced by normal results on thyroid function tests. The child will have normal bowel movements.

- Risk for Activity Intolerance related to loss of muscle mass from increased basal metabolic rate secondary to hyperthyroidism.

***Expected outcome.*** The child will be able to exercise at the same level as peers as basal metabolic rate returns to normal.

- Disturbed Sleep Pattern related to increased basal metabolic rate secondary to hyperthyroidism.

***Expected outcome.*** The child will sleep the appropriate amount of time for age as basal metabolic rate returns to normal.

- Ineffective Thermoregulation related to increased basal metabolic rate secondary to hyperthyroidism.

***Expected outcome.*** The child will regain normal body temperature as basal metabolic rate returns to normal.

### Interventions

The antithyroid drug PTU is usually given two or three times per day, whereas methimazole can be given once daily (Huang & LaFranchi, 2016b). A multiple-times-a-day medication regimen is difficult for some children and parents to follow. Use of pill dispensers and a watch with an alarm to remind the child to take the medication at specific times enhances compliance. The endocrinologist should evaluate the child and monitor thyroid function every 2 to 4 months while the child is undergoing treatment. Normal values for thyroid function tests and alleviation of symptoms indicate appropriate responses to therapy.

Once the child is euthyroid and asymptomatic, she or he should be evaluated once or twice a year. Medication dosages may be tapered after 2 to 3 years to evaluate for remission. Contact sports should be limited while the child is being treated to decrease the possibility of damage to the liver. Collaboration with the school nurse to facilitate medication administration is an important nursing function.

### Evaluation

- Does the child have normal results on thyroid function tests?
- Has the basal metabolic rate returned to normal?
- Does the child demonstrate normal bowel movements?
- Is the child able to exercise at an age-appropriate level?
- Does the child obtain an appropriate amount of sleep?
- Has the child maintained a normal body temperature?

## DIABETES INSIPIDUS

Diabetes insipidus (DI) is an inability to concentrate urine, accompanied by hypernatremia and dehydration. In central DI, the most common form, there is a deficiency of vasopressin, also known as antidiuretic hormone (ADH). In nephrogenic DI, the kidneys are insensitive to vasopressin (Breault & Majzoub, 2016a).

### Etiology

Both forms of DI can occur from inherited defects or acquired conditions (Breault & Majzoub, 2016a). Central DI frequently results from head trauma, tumors, or infection in the area of the hypothalamus. The most common type of tumor involving the hypothalamus that causes DI is craniopharyngioma. Cranial radiation for treatment of tumors can lead to ADH deficiency. Other causes include infections of the CNS such as meningitis or encephalitis, and congenital malformations such as septo-optic dysplasia or isolated pituitary malformation or ectopy. Several genetic mutations in the vasopressin gene causing DI have been identified. Central DI can also be caused by an idiopathic autoimmune process. Nephrogenic DI can be caused by genetic mutations or hypercalcemia, low protein diet, hypokalemia, the release of a ureteral obstruction or certain medications (Jain & Ravindranath, 2015).

**BOX 51.2 Indicators of Diabetes Insipidus or Syndrome of Inappropriate Antidiuretic Hormone (SIADH)**

| Diabetes Insipidus (High and Dry) | SIADH (Low and Wet) |
|---|---|
| Increased urination (polyuria) | Decreased urination |
| Nocturia | Hypertension |
| Increased thirst (polydipsia) | Weight gain |
| Dehydration | Fluid retention |
| Hypernatremia | Hyponatremia |
| Urine specific gravity <1.005 | Urine specific gravity >1.030 |
| Elevated serum osmolality (>300 mOsm/kg) | Decreased serum osmolality (<280 mOsm/kg) |
| Decreased urine osmolality | Increased urine osmolality |

### Incidence

DI is not common in the United States, occurring in 1 of every 25,000 individuals. Head trauma and cranial surgery account for the largest percentage of DI cases. Ten percent of cases are classified as idiopathic (Breault & Majzoub, 2016a).

### Manifestations

Increased urination (polyuria) and excessive thirst (polydipsia) are the classic manifestations of DI. Other signs and symptoms include nocturia and dehydration (Box 51.2).

### Diagnostic Evaluation

Diagnostic criteria include polyuria with associated hypernatremia (greater than 150 mEq/L) low urine specific gravity (less than 1.005), and serum osmolality greater than 300 mOsm/kg in the absence of hyperglycemia, hypokalemia, hypercalcemia, and chronic renal insufficiency. Urine should be checked for glucose to rule out hyperglycemia as a cause of increased urine output (Jain & Ravindranath, 2015).

A water deprivation test is sometimes necessary to confirm the diagnosis. In this 7- to 8-hour procedure, the child is deprived of all fluid intake. A normal response is decreased urine output with a high urine specific gravity and no change in serum sodium. The child with DI continues to produce large amounts of dilute urine (low urine specific gravity) during fluid restriction. The serum sodium level also increases. To ensure the child's safety, this test is done in a hospital setting with frequent monitoring of serum sodium, hematocrit, and osmolality. Urine osmolality and output are also measured. The child is weighed at the beginning, middle, and conclusion of the water deprivation test. Water deprivation should be stopped if the child loses more than 5% of baseline body weight, has intolerable thirst, becomes dehydrated, or demonstrates a significant change in vital signs or neurologic status (Jain & Ravindranath, 2015).

### Therapeutic Management

Treatment for central DI involves maintaining fluid balance and administering synthetic vasopressin (1-deamino-8-D-arginine-vasopressin [DDAVP]). The dose of DDAVP ranges from 5 to 20 mcg/day (intranasal) or 100 to 400 mcg/day (oral), divided into one or two doses per day. The oral form of DDAVP is also used for treatment of nocturnal enuresis in generally smaller doses. The half-life of DDAVP is 3.5 hours, the peak concentration is reached at 50 minutes, and the duration of action is 6 to 18 hours. Decreased urine output is seen 1 to 2 hours after administration. Excessive fluid intake should be avoided while on chronic DDAVP therapy due to the fixed urine osmolality of about 1000 mOsm/kg and risk of developing hyponatremia. Other treatments include thiazide diuretics, chlorpropamide, clofibrate, and carbamazepine; and hypo-osmolar with low sodium diets (Jain & Ravindranath, 2015).

Dosage is individualized on the basis of the child's age, size, urine output, and urine specific gravity. Doses are timed so that before the next dose, the child is allowed to have mildly increased urination to help prevent overtreatment and water retention. Parents are often taught to measure urine specific gravity at home to monitor the effectiveness of treatment.

**! NURSING QUALITY ALERT**

***Diabetes Insipidus***

- Hypernatremia (sodium > 150 mEq/L) and low urine specific gravity in the absence of hyperglycemia are diagnostic of diabetes insipidus.
- 1-Deamino-8-D-arginine-vasopressin (DDAVP) is the treatment of choice for central diabetes insipidus.
- Overtreatment with DDAVP will result in fluid retention and dilutional hyponatremia. If the hyponatremia is severe enough, seizures may occur.

The goals for the management of nephrogenic DI are to prevent severe dehydration and provide adequate calories for growth. With acquired disease, treatment is focused on eliminating the underlying cause; congenital nephrogenic DI is very difficult to treat (Breault & Majzoub, 2016a).

### Nursing Considerations

Nursing care involves assessing the understanding of the child and parents about DI. The nurse educates the family about the basic pathophysiology of water metabolism and the cause of DI. This education includes a description of signs and symptoms (increased thirst, polyuria, dehydration) and how they indicate the need for DDAVP, as well as signs and symptoms of excessive DDAVP administration (decreased urine output, headaches, water retention). The child must be closely monitored for these signs and symptoms of dehydration, and the parents must know the appropriate actions to take if dehydration occurs.

The family is taught how to correctly administer DDAVP and then provides a return demonstration of medication administration. If appropriate, the nurse instructs the family in the use of a refractometer to measure urine specific gravity. The child should wear a medical alert bracelet noting the diagnosis of DI. School personnel need to be aware of the diagnosis and must allow the child free access to water and toilet facilities.

## SYNDROME OF INAPPROPRIATE ANTIDIURETIC HORMONE

The syndrome of inappropriate antidiuretic hormone (SIADH) is the inability to excrete free water resulting from excessive production or release of ADH, or vasopressin.

### Etiology

Childhood SIADH is rare and usually related to an underlying cause. The most frequent cause is excessive use of vasopressin in the treatment of central DI (Breault & Majzoub, 2016b). Other causes include CNS infections (e.g., encephalitis and meningitis), head trauma, brain tumors, and generalized seizures (see Chapter 52). SIADH is usually transient and resolves when the underlying condition is corrected. However, brain surgery in the region of the hypothalamus or pituitary gland can cause the child to have transient SIADH but permanent DI. A triple response can occur after surgery: the child has DI, then experiences temporary SIADH, finally returning to permanent DI (Breault & Majzoub, 2016a).

### Manifestations

Manifestations that occur with SIADH include hyponatremia, decreased urine output, increased urine specific gravity, fluid retention with slightly elevated plasma volume, weight gain, and increased urine osmolality (see Box 51.2).

### Diagnostic Evaluation

SIADH should be suspected in children with CNS involvement, such as infections or head trauma, who have decreased urine output despite adequate intake. Laboratory diagnosis includes evidence of hyponatremia, hypochloremia, and low serum osmolality. Urine osmolality is usually greater than serum osmolality. Urine specific gravity is more than 1.030. Adrenal, thyroid, and renal function studies can rule out other causes of hyponatremia.

### Therapeutic Management

Initial treatment is correction of the underlying cause. The healthcare provider orders fluid restriction to correct hyponatremia. A child with severe hyponatremia may need an IV infusion of sodium chloride with slow correction of serum sodium (no faster than 0.5 meq/L/h) to avoid CNS damage such as central pontine myelinolysis. Drug therapy usually is not indicated for transient SIADH. Medications such as lithium and demeclocycline block the action of ADH at the renal collecting tubules and have been used in management; however, its use is discouraged in younger patients because of side effects (Ranadive & Rosenthal, 2011).

### Nursing Considerations

The nurse should assess the child with SIADH for signs and symptoms of fluid overload, including edema, weight gain, and urine specific gravity more than 1.030, and for dilutional hyponatremia by checking serum electrolyte levels frequently. The child with hyponatremia is at risk for injury related to seizures. The child's neurologic status is closely monitored every 2 to 4 hours by assessing and recording level of consciousness and observing for headache, irritability, or seizures (Box 51.3). The provider is alerted immediately if any changes in neurologic status occur. The nurse initiates seizure precautions if the serum sodium level drops below 125 mEq/L.

Additional interventions are directed toward maintaining fluid and electrolyte balance. The child's hydration status is carefully assessed.

**BOX 51.3 Signs of Hyponatremia**

| Mild (Early) | Moderate | Severe |
|---|---|---|
| Anorexia | Confusion | Seizures |
| Nausea | Lethargy | Coma |
| Headache | Irritability | |
| Vomiting | Altered level of consciousness | |

## PATHOPHYSIOLOGY

### *Diabetes Insipidus*

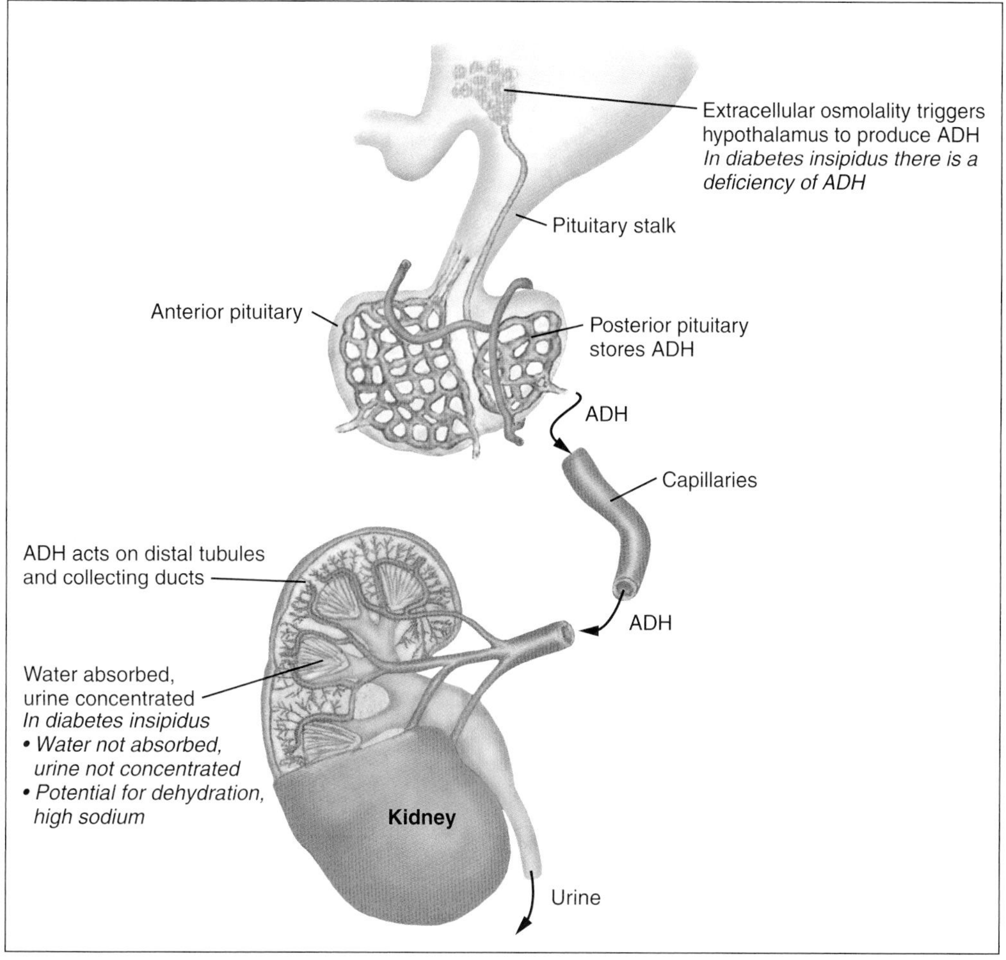


Antidiuretic hormone (ADH) is produced in the hypothalamus, transported through the pituitary stalk, and stored in the posterior pituitary. It is carried through the blood to the kidneys, where it acts on the distal tubules and collecting ducts to increase reabsorption of free water, thereby concentrating urine and decreasing urinary output.

ADH is under the control of osmoreceptors in the anterior hypothalamus. These osmoreceptors operate on a negative feedback system based on serum osmolality, particularly sodium concentration. When the serum osmolality is low, production of ADH decreases, causing increased urine output and normalizing osmolality; conversely, when serum osmolality is increased, ADH production increases, causing water retention and decreasing urine output. In diabetes insipidus, a deficiency of ADH makes the body unable to conserve water, which results in the excretion of large volumes of dilute urine. Loss of free water leads to an elevated serum sodium concentration. If the child has an intact thirst center, increasing oral intake might compensate for the large fluid loss. If the thirst drive is not intact or the child is unable to drink enough, the child can become dehydrated and develop a high serum sodium level.

A child with an intact thirst center is able to self-regulate fluid needs and intake. An infant who is too young or a child who had head trauma or surgery may not able to recognize thirst; the healthcare provider should prescribe a 24-hour fluid intake requirement to ensure adequate hydration.

## PATHOPHYSIOLOGY

### *Syndrome of Inappropriate Antidiuretic Hormone*

Excessive antidiuretic hormone (ADH) results in the kidney reabsorbing too much free water. This causes decreased output of concentrated urine, evidenced by a high urine specific gravity (greater than 1.030). The excess water also causes a slightly expanded intravascular fluid volume and a low serum sodium level. Once the sodium level falls below 120 mEq/L, the child can become symptomatic and have anorexia, nausea, weakness, weight gain, confusion, irritability, and seizures (Breault & Majzoub, 2016b).

Intake and output are accurately measured and recorded. The child is weighed at least daily to monitor fluid retention.

Fluid restrictions are strictly maintained. The child may have difficulty adhering to a decrease in fluid intake. The nurse explains to the child and parents the reasons for limiting fluids and that the restrictions are temporary. The nurse may give the child hard sugarless candies or apply wet washcloths to help keep mucous membranes moist.

Diet for the child with hyponatremia should include foods with high sodium content because extra sodium can help correct this

> **! NURSING QUALITY ALERT**
>
> ***Syndrome of Inappropriate Antidiuretic Hormone (SIADH)***
>
> - SIADH is characterized by low serum sodium (125 mEq/L or lower) and high urine specific gravity, as well as decreased serum osmolality and increased urine osmolality.
> - Seizures may develop with hyponatremia.
> - Treatment depends on strict fluid restriction to maintain serum sodium in a near-normal range. Frequent and precise measurements and recording of intake and output along with daily weights are critical to the evaluation and management of the child with SIADH.

problem. However, salty foods, such as chips, may make the child thirsty.

Evaluation of the child with SIADH should address a balanced intake and output, stable weight, and normal serum sodium levels. Urine specific gravity should be maintained between 1.010 and 1.020.

## PRECOCIOUS PUBERTY

Precocious puberty refers to the early onset of puberty, traditionally considered as the onset of puberty before 8 years of age in girls (7.5 years in Hispanics and Blacks) and before 9 years of age in boys (Chen & Eugster, 2015). Precocious puberty is defined as the premature appearance of secondary sexual characteristics, accelerated growth rate, and advanced bone maturation (Garibaldi & Chemaitilly, 2016). The major consequence of precocious puberty is rapid bone growth, which causes early growth plate fusion and ultimately short stature in adulthood compared with genetic height potential.

### Etiology

Central precocious puberty can be idiopathic or caused by CNS tumors (including benign hamartomas), head trauma, infection, septo-optic dysplasia, genetic mutations, or cranial radiation. Central precocious puberty is associated with several genetic syndromes: neurofibromatosis type I, tuberous sclerosis, and Sturge-Weber (Chen & Eugster, 2015). CNS abnormalities are seen with much greater frequency in boys than girls (Chen & Eugster, 2015). In girls, precocious puberty is idiopathic in 90% of cases (Garibaldi & Chemaitilly, 2016). Factors that contribute to precocious puberty in girls include obesity, ethnicity, genetic predisposition, psychosocial stress, and exposure to certain environmental chemicals that disrupt endocrine function (Fuqua, 2013).

The causes of the much less common precocious pseudopuberty (peripheral precocious puberty) include congenital adrenal hyperplasia; other abnormalities or tumors of the adrenal glands, ovaries, or testes; McCune-Albright syndrome; DAX1 genetic mutations; exogenous steroids; and untreated chronic hypothyroidism (Dhivyalashmi, Bhattacharyya, Reddy, et al., 2014).

### Incidence

Precocious puberty is ten times more likely to occur in girls than boys, affecting 0.2% of girls and less than 0.05% of boys (Chen & Eugster, 2015; Fuqua, 2013). Growing evidence indicates that the number of girls diagnosed with precocious puberty has increased over the years and that Black girls mature at an earlier age than do white girls (Fuqua, 2013).

### Manifestations

Manifestations of precocious puberty reflect gender differences:

| Girls | Boys |
|---|---|
| Breast development | Testicular enlargement |
| Enlargement of vagina, uterus, and ovaries | Penis enlargement |
| Pubic hair | Pubic hair |
| Axillary hair | Facial hair |
| Acne | Acne |
| Growth spurt | Deepening of voice |
| Adult body odor | Adult body odor |
| Onset of menstrual periods | Moodiness |
| Moodiness | |

### Diagnostic Evaluation

Diagnosis of precocious puberty begins with a thorough history, including onset of secondary sexual characteristics, and a physical examination. Bilateral testicular enlargement in males, and both bilateral breast development and pubic hair in females will be apparent. Blood tests are performed to evaluate for elevated levels of LH, FSH, testosterone, and estrogen. Unfortunately, because these hormones are released in small bursts during the day, random samples may not be adequate.

The gonadotropin-releasing hormone (GnRH) stimulation test is considered the gold standard for diagnosis; however, its lack of availability has led to the use of GnRH analogs (GnRHa) instead. GnRHa is administered intravenously or subcutaneously to stimulate the release of LH and FSH from the pituitary gland. Serial samples of LH and FSH are then obtained over a 2-hour period after IV administration. With subcutaneous administration, a single sample of LH and FSH is obtained using an ultrasensitive assay. Before the onset of puberty, the FSH peak is higher than the LH peak. With the onset of puberty, the LH peak is higher than the FSH peak. An LH/FSH ratio of greater than or equal to 2 or LH level is greater than or equal to 5 IU/L after GnRHa is consistent with central precocious puberty (Chen & Eugster, 2015).

Radiographic studies also support the diagnosis of precocious puberty. Radiographs of the wrist determine bone age and maturation and can assist in predicting final adult height. Skull radiographs screen for CNS lesions, although CT and MRI scans are more accurate in visualizing tumors. Abdominal ultrasound and pelvic ultrasound are beneficial in diagnosing adrenal and ovarian tumors or cysts. Pelvic ultrasound also provides evidence of pubertal changes in the uterus and ovaries. Finally, isolated pubic hair development and elevated androgen hormone levels suggest an adrenal origin for premature hair growth.

### Therapeutic Management

The primary goal of treatment of the child with precocious puberty is to preserve final adult height followed by stopping or reversing the development of secondary sexual characteristics. Observation is recommended initially since some patients can achieve normal adult height because they have a form of central precocious puberty that progresses slowly. Treatment in girls age 8 years and older is not indicated since they will not benefit (Chen & Eugster, 2015). Current therapy for central precocious puberty involves administration of a GnRH agonist, or blocker. GnRH blockers inhibit the binding of GnRH to the pituitary gland, causing decreased production of the pubertal hormones and slowing or reversing sexual development.

Several commercially available GnRH agonists can be administered by a monthly or 3-monthly intramuscular injection or by subcutaneous implantation every 1 to 2 years. Once therapy is initiated, GnRH secretion is suppressed within 2 to 4 weeks. The accelerated growth rate and bone maturation will slow, and some secondary sexual characteristics will regress within the first year of treatment. Nonadherence with medication therapy, such as missed or delayed administration of injections, can promote pubertal changes rather than suppress puberty. Oxandralone, growth hormone, and aromatase inhibitors have been studied as adjunctive therapies as well with need for further research (Chen & Eugster, 2015).

No evidence suggests that GnRH agonist therapy interferes with the child's reproductive function in the future. Once therapy is discontinued, pubertal progression resumes. For children with peripheral precocious puberty, treatment is aimed at correcting the underlying cause.

## NURSING CARE

### The Child With Precocious Puberty

#### Assessment

Nursing care of the child with precocious puberty addresses the physical and behavioral changes associated with puberty. A nurse working with these children may note that they feel more comfortable around older children than with peers their own age. They often experience teasing about their bodies and may limit social activities such as swimming. Boys often exhibit aggressive behavior. Children who go through early puberty appear older than their chronologic age and are often treated accordingly by adults. Because of their mature appearance, girls with precocious puberty are potentially at greater risk for sexual abuse and exploitation; however, current data do not consistently support this notion (Chen & Eugster, 2015).

If a child appears embarrassed or uncomfortable when being interviewed about sexual development, the nurse should explain to the child, "Everyone goes through body changes when growing up; it's just that these changes are happening to you sooner than most children. Can you tell me in your own words how you feel about your body?"

#### Nursing Diagnosis and Planning

The following nursing diagnoses and expected outcomes may be appropriate for the child with precocious puberty and the child's family:

- Deficient Knowledge about medication administration related to inadequate understanding of intramuscular or intranasal GnRH agonist.

*Expected outcome.* The parents will explain the need for the medication and will give an appropriate return demonstration of medication administration technique.

- Disturbed Body Image related to early sexual development.

*Expected outcome.* The child will describe the relationship between early sexual development and the underlying condition, express feelings about early sexual development, and verbalize acceptance of body appearance.

- Impaired Social Interaction related to appearing older than chronologic age.

*Expected outcome.* The child will adjust socially to body changes, as evidenced by exhibiting age-appropriate behaviors and social interactions.

#### Interventions

Many parents are not comfortable with their child's early development. The nurse explains the stages of puberty and each stage's associated behavioral changes. The nurse teaches parents that the child is experiencing normal changes at an earlier time than expected.

Explanations given to the child should be geared to the level of intellectual development. The nurse can direct the parent to books that explain sexual maturation in terms the child can understand. Psychological counseling might be necessary to help the family deal with the sensitive issues of sexuality.

The nurse also teaches the family about the prescribed medication regimen. In some instances, the parent is taught how to administer the injections. Injections might be stressful for the young child. The nurse demonstrates appropriate injection technique and teaches the child coping strategies to be used when the injection is given.

#### Evaluation

- Can the parents explain the need for the medication and demonstrate proper medication administration?
- Is the child able to relate the body changes to the underlying condition?
- Have the child and parents verbalized any concerns about the child's early sexual development?
- Is the child exhibiting age-appropriate social interactions?

## GROWTH HORMONE DEFICIENCY

Growth hormone (GH) deficiency results from inadequate production or secretion of GH, causing poor growth and short stature. Hypoglycemia is sometimes the manifestation of GH deficiency.

### Etiology

GH deficiency can be isolated or associated with an underlying cause. Such causes include hypopituitarism, congenital malformations of the pituitary gland, brain tumors (most commonly craniopharyngioma), and cranial irradiation. Other disorders associated with short stature that may respond to GH therapy include Turner syndrome, Prader-Willi syndrome, and chronic illnesses such as renal disease and inflammatory bowel disease.

### Incidence

Isolated growth hormone deficiency occurs in 1 in 4,000 to 1 in 10,000 live births, with 3% to 30% of cases being familial (Alatzoglou, Webb, Le Tissier, et al., 2014). No racial differences in incidence are apparent. Boys are much more likely to be diagnosed and treated for GH deficiency than girls; whether this difference is related to referral bias by parents and practitioners is unknown.

### Manifestations

Manifestations typical of GH deficiency include height below the fifth percentile for age and sex, diminished growth rate (2 or more standard deviations below the mean for age and sex), immature or cherubic facies, delayed puberty, hypoglycemia, diminished muscle mass with relatively increased body fat (adiposity), and micropenis (associated with hypopituitarism).

### Diagnostic Evaluation

Diagnosis of GH deficiency begins with careful measurements of growth over an extended period (usually 6 to 12 months). Height should be measured on a consistent scale, preferably with a calibrated stadiometer. Initial screening involves thyroid function tests, electrolytes, blood urea nitrogen (BUN), creatinine, complete blood count, insulin-like growth factor 1 (IGF-1) and IGF binding protein 3 (IGFBP-3), and a bone age radiograph. Normal thyroid function is essential for adequate growth; thyroid studies are essential when evaluating for

## PATHOPHYSIOLOGY

### *Precocious Puberty*

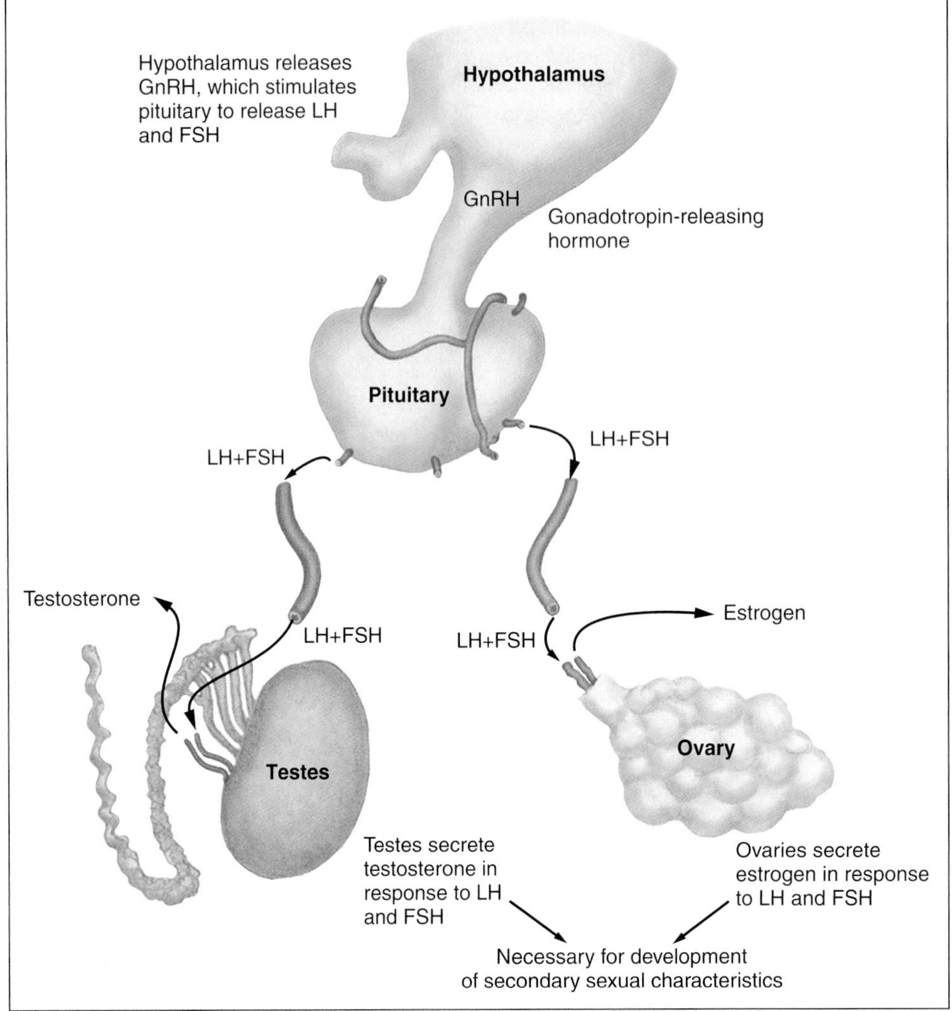
Hypothalamus releases GnRH, which stimulates pituitary to release LH and FSH
Hypothalamus
GnRH
Gonadotropin-releasing hormone
Pituitary
LH+FSH
LH+FSH
Testosterone
LH+FSH
LH+FSH
Estrogen
Testes
Ovary
Testes secrete testosterone in response to LH and FSH
Ovaries secrete estrogen in response to LH and FSH
Necessary for development of secondary sexual characteristics

Puberty occurs when the hypothalamus releases gonadotropin-releasing hormone (GnRH). This stimulates the pituitary gland to release luteinizing-hormone (LH) and follicle-stimulating hormone (FSH). In girls, FSH stimulates formation of ovarian follicles to produce estrogen. Estrogen is necessary for the development of secondary sexual characteristics such as breast development and maturation of the vagina and labia. LH is involved in the process of ovulation. In boys, FSH triggers the testes to support the development of sperm. LH stimulates the production of testosterone, which is necessary for the development of sexual characteristics and sperm production. Puberty development is classified according to Tanner stages 1 through 5 (see Chapter 9). The adrenal glands produce the hormone dehydroepiandrosterone (DHEA), which causes pubic and axillary hair growth. During puberty the growth rate increases, called a "growth spurt," in which a child grows an average of 4 to 6 inches/yr.

In precocious puberty the sex hormones that accelerate growth also cause the bone plates (epiphyseal plates) to close early. Usually the epiphyseal plates fuse at 14 years of age for girls and 17 years for boys; premature closure can lead to decreased linear growth with reduced adult height. With true precocious puberty, children have hormonal changes that mimic the onset of normal puberty. These hormonal changes may be central, arising from the hypothalamus, or peripheral, arising from the ovaries, testes, or adrenal glands.

## ! NURSING QUALITY ALERT

### *Precocious Puberty*

- Children with precocious puberty appear older than their chronologic age. Although they tend to be treated as older children, they should be treated according to their chronologic age.
- Other children often tease children with precocious puberty.
- Precocious puberty may occur in infancy or childhood.

short stature. Complete blood count and other specific blood screening for any systemic or chronic illness should be done. Electrolytes and renal function studies eliminate primary kidney dysfunction as a cause of poor growth. A karyotype (chromosomes) might be performed for girls to rule out Turner syndrome.

Because GH is normally secreted in pulses throughout the day and night, stimulation testing is necessary to confirm the diagnosis of GH deficiency. Agents used in provocative testing to stimulate GH production include insulin, arginine, clonidine, glucagon, and levodopa (L-dopa). Once the stimulating agent is given, serial GH levels are

## PATHOPHYSIOLOGY

### *Growth Hormone Deficiency*

Growth hormone (GH), thyroxine, cortisol, and sex hormones all influence growth. The hypothalamus secretes GH-releasing factor, which stimulates the pituitary gland to release GH. This hormone is secreted in pulses, with increased secretion during the night. In the presence of hypoglycemia, GH is secreted to counteract insulin and raise the blood glucose level. Many children with GH deficiency have hypoglycemia.

Most children with short stature have constitutional growth delay. Children with short stature or poor growth rates may also be deficient in other hormones. Normal thyroid function is essential for growth; therefore, hypothyroidism can cause short stature. Sex hormones are required for the growth spurt and sexual maturation that occur with puberty. Children lacking more than one hormone produced by the pituitary gland are referred to as having *hypopituitarism*. Rate of growth and final adult height depend on factors such as genetics (family heights), nutrition, and general health. Any child growing less than 5 cm/yr should be referred to an endocrinologist for further evaluation.

determined. Although diagnostic criteria vary, most clinicians accept a GH level less than 10 ng/mL as indicative of GH deficiency. Generally, two positive tests are required for diagnosis.

### Therapeutic Management

A child with GH deficiency requires replacement therapy. Synthetic GH comes in a powdered form that must be diluted for administration or a premixed liquid form. It is given as a subcutaneous injection daily, usually at bedtime; however, alternative forms are also available, requiring administration a few times or once weekly. Dosage ranges from 0.18 to 0.3 mg/kg/week, depending on the child's age, pubertal stage, and response to therapy (Parks & Felner, 2016). Once diluted, GH must be stored at 36° F to 46° F (2.2° C to 7.7° C). With treatment, the growth response is most evident in the first year, then gradually decreases; many children experience linear growth 200% of the pretreatment velocity during the first year. After several years of treatment, linear growth averages 150% from the baseline (Ergun-Longmire, & Wajnrajch, 2013). When treatment is started at a younger age, the child's height potential is increased. GH therapy continues until the child's growth plates close or the child reaches an acceptable or predicted final height.

## NURSING CARE

### The Child With Growth Hormone Deficiency

#### Assessment

Nursing care of the child with GH deficiency includes assessment of family attitudes and perceptions. Parental attitudes regarding the child's size can influence the child's self-esteem. Assessment of the child's attitude about height is essential. The nurse determines if height and growth concerns are voiced more by the parents or by the child. If parents place excessive emphasis on height, the child may be more self-conscious or demonstrate low self-esteem. Height issues can adversely affect a child's psychosocial adjustment, as demonstrated by poor school performance and lack of involvement in extracurricular activities. Short children often appear younger and are treated as such by adults. Affected children may be teased by their peers. The nurse might ask, "Have you ever been teased or been in any fights at school because of your height?" Once the child is receiving therapy, the nurse assesses adherence to the medication regimen, injection technique, and medication preparation and storage. These factors should be reviewed periodically and with each dosage change. As the child matures, self-injection techniques can be taught.

#### Nursing Diagnosis and Planning

The following nursing diagnoses and expected outcomes may be appropriate for the child with GH deficiency and the child's family:

- Delayed Growth and Development related to GH deficiency.
  **Expected outcome.** The child will receive and respond to treatment, as evidenced by increased linear growth rate.
- Disturbed Body Image related to short stature.
  **Expected outcome.** The child will demonstrate acceptance of body image, as evidenced by verbalization of acceptance of ultimate height.
- Situational Low Self-Esteem related to short stature.
  **Expected outcome.** The child will accept short stature, as evidenced by verbalizing appropriate feelings of self-esteem.
- Ineffective Family Therapeutic Regimen Management related to nonadherence to daily injection.
  **Expected outcome.** The child and parents will adhere to the injection schedule, as evidenced by appropriate record keeping and the child's steady growth.

## ! NURSING QUALITY ALERT

### *Criteria for Suspecting Growth Hormone Deficiency**

- Severe short stature: height < −3 standard deviations (SD) below mean
- Height < −1.5 below mid-parental height
- Height < −2 SD below mean + height velocity < −1 SD below mean over year OR decrease in height SD more than 0.5 SD over year
- If not short stature, height velocity < −2 SD below mean over year OR < −1.5 below mean over 2 years
- Neonatal hypoglycemia, microphallus, prolonged jaundice, or craniofacial midline abnormalities
- Consistently poor growth (less than 5 cm/yr)
- Signs of intracranial lesion
- Signs of multiple pituitary hormone deficiency

*Stanley, T. (2012). Diagnosis of growth hormone deficiency in childhood. *Current Opinion in Endocrinology, Diabetes, and Obesity, 19*(1), 47–52. doi:10.1097/MED.0b013e32834ec952.

#### Interventions

The nurse reassures the child and parents that adherence to the injections will improve growth rate. Reminders that the injections are temporary and are helping the child to grow are also helpful. Keeping a growth chart at home and noting the need for larger clothing sizes are physical signs the child can use to monitor growth. These indicators also can assist with adherence.

The nurse has an important role in educating children and families about the proper dilution and administration of the GH if needed. The nurse demonstrates the injection technique to the parents (and child if age-appropriate) and requests a return demonstration.

Effectiveness of therapy is evidenced by the child's growth rate. Children are evaluated approximately every 3 to 4 months by an endocrinologist; accurate measurements of height are essential. The use of a growth chart helps identify growth velocity. GH therapy is continued until the child reaches an acceptable adult height or radiographic evidence shows growth plate fusion.

### Evaluation

- Has the child exhibited increased linear growth rate?
- Does the child verbalize positive feelings regarding body image and self-esteem?
- Do the child and family adhere to the injection schedule?

### CRITICAL THINKING EXERCISE 51.1

Parents of young adolescent boys often are concerned about their child's current and eventual adult height. Boys who are significantly shorter than their peers during early adolescence can experience lowered self-esteem.

How should a nurse respond if parents ask whether giving growth hormone (GH) to their 13-year-old son with short stature will increase his eventual adult height?

## DIABETES MELLITUS

Type 1 and type 2 diabetes mellitus (DM) are chronic diseases requiring life-long management and care (see Chapter 36). Both types of DM involve abnormal carbohydrate metabolism and hyperglycemia. While the incidence of DM increases with age until mid-puberty, type 1 diabetes mellitus can occur at any age, including infancy.

The increasing prevalence of both types of diabetes mellitus worldwide is of concern. A study of 3300 adolescents ages 12 to 19 years revealed that the prevalence of prediabetes/diabetes (fasting blood glucose >99 mg/dL) increased significantly from 9% in 1999 to 23% in 2008 (May, Kuklina, & Yoon, 2012).

### Type 1 Diabetes Mellitus

Type 1 diabetes mellitus results when the pancreas is unable to produce and secrete an adequate amount of insulin. This form of diabetes, the most common childhood endocrine disorder, presents challenges in the areas of teaching, management, and adherence. Because of recent changes in the healthcare delivery system, meeting the needs associated with management of type 1 diabetes mellitus has become more complicated. Unless the newly diagnosed child is in diabetic ketoacidosis (DKA), hospitalization is not always necessary. The nurse must develop a plan of care that involves child and family education and support in either an inpatient or outpatient setting.

### Etiology

Type 1 diabetes mellitus is an inflammatory process in the insulin-secreting islet cells of the pancreas resulting from an autoimmune process that causes their eventual destruction. Although multiple genes are thought to play a role in the genetic predisposition to type 1 diabetes, an environmental trigger is thought to initiate the autoimmune destructive process. Possible triggers include viral and bacterial infections, dietary toxins, history of obesity, and certain chemicals (Knip & Simell, 2012). Current research is focused on identifying factors that increase susceptibility and exploring methods of interrupting or preventing the autoimmune response in susceptible individuals (first-degree relatives of a diabetic person). At this time, no prevention or cure is available; however, transplantation of islet cells and the pancreas is being explored. Children with type 1 diabetes mellitus are prone to developing other autoimmune conditions such as Graves disease, Hashimoto thyroiditis, and celiac disease (see Chapter 43).

### Incidence

More than 25 million children and adults in the United States have diabetes (American Diabetes Association [ADA], 2011). The CDC (2014) reported that in persons younger than 20 years old, 18,436 were newly diagnosed with Type 1 DM and 5,089 were diagnosed with Type 2 DM in 2014. Approximately 215,000 people younger than 20 years have diabetes, which is 0.26% of the population in this age group. Type 1 diabetes accounts for 90% of diabetes (Nierengarten, 2016) and is diagnosed in 0.17% of children and adolescents; the peak age of diagnosis is 12 years (Huether & McCance, 2017).

### Manifestations

Type 1 diabetes mellitus is manifested by the classic initial signs of hyperglycemia known as the three *P*s: *p*olyuria (or enuresis in a toilet-trained child), *p*olydipsia, and *p*olyphagia. The child's other symptoms include weight loss (despite increased food intake), fatigue, and blurred vision.

If the condition progresses without intervention, the child can exhibit signs and symptoms of DKA: nausea and vomiting, abdominal pain, acetone (fruity) odor to breath, dehydration, increasing lethargy, Kussmaul respirations, and coma.

Children who receive insulin for treatment of type 1 diabetes mellitus can have hypoglycemia. Table 51.2 lists the actions of insulin, and Table 51.3 compares hypoglycemia, hyperglycemia, and ketoacidosis.

### Diagnostic Evaluation

Diagnosis of type 1 diabetes mellitus is made on the basis of laboratory data: HbA1c greater than or equal to 6.5% OR a fasting blood glucose (FBG) exceeding 126 mg/dL OR a 2-hour oral glucose tolerance test greater than or equal to 200 mg/dL OR a random serum glucose of 200 mg/dL or more with classic hyperglycemia symptoms (Gregory, Moore, & Simmons, 2013). Ketonuria, although not diagnostic, is a frequent finding, as is glycosuria. Glucose tolerance testing is rarely used in diagnosing type 1 diabetes mellitus. The glycosylated hemoglobin ($HbA_{1c}$) value is elevated in response to prolonged elevations of blood glucose.

### Therapeutic Management

The American Diabetes Association (ADA) (2015) recommends that children newly diagnosed with diabetes mellitus be managed and educated by a multidisciplinary team of experts in pediatric diabetes. Children diagnosed with type 1 diabetes will be started on insulin therapy to reverse metabolic imbalances (Gregory et al., 2013). At the time of their initial type 1 diagnosis, one third of children present with DKA (Klingensmith et al., 2013) and require management in a pediatric intensive care unit.

**TABLE 51.2 Actions of Insulin**

| Anabolic Actions of Insulin | Catabolic Consequences of Insulin Deficit |
|---|---|
| Promotes glucose as a fuel source | Promotes fats and proteins as fuel sources |
| Promotes storage of glucose as glycogen | Allows glycogen stores to be broken down |
| Prevents breakdown of fat stores | Allows fat stores to be depleted |
| Increases protein synthesis | Allows protein breakdown into amino acids |

**TABLE 51.3 Comparison of Hypoglycemia, Hyperglycemia, and Ketoacidosis**

| Hypoglycemia | Hyperglycemia | Ketoacidosis |
|---|---|---|
| | **ONSET** | |
| *Rapid* | *Slow* | *Slow* |
| **Signs and Symptoms** | | |
| Adrenergic signs:<br>Trembling<br>Sweating<br>Tachycardia<br>Pallor<br>Clammy skin | Increased urination<br>Increased thirst<br>Fatigue<br>Weight loss (gradual, over several weeks)<br>Blurred vision | Hyperglycemia signs plus:<br>Abdominal pain<br>Chest pain<br>Kussmaul respirations<br>Nausea and vomiting<br>Acetone (fruity) breath odor<br>Signs and symptoms of dehydration:<br>Tachycardia<br>Tachypnea<br>Dry lips and mucous membranes<br>Sunken eyes<br>Sudden weight loss<br>Decreased urination |
| **Alterations in Sensorium** | | |
| Neuroglycopenic symptoms:<br>Personality change<br>Irritability<br>Drunken behavior<br>Slurred speech<br>Decreased level of consciousness to total loss of consciousness<br>Seizure activity | Emotional lability<br>Headache<br>Hunger | Increasing lethargy<br>Decreasing level of consciousness<br>Coma |
| **Laboratory Data** | | |
| Blood glucose <60 mg/dL | Blood glucose >160 mg/dL | Blood glucose >200 mg/dL<br>Urine ketones positive<br>Serum pH <7.30<br>Bicarbonate 15 mEq/L<br>Serum ketones positive |
| **Causes** | | |
| Too much insulin<br>Excessive activity without eating extra carbohydrates<br>Missed or delayed meal | Excessive intake of carbohydrates<br>Little or no exercise<br>Inadequate amount of insulin<br>Increased stress, either emotional or physical | Inadequate amount of insulin<br>Excessive stress |
| **Treatment** | | |
| 15 g of carbohydrate<br>*For loss of consciousness or seizure activity:*<br>Glucagon subcutaneous or intramuscular<br>Intravenous (IV) dextrose | Insulin<br>Exercise<br>Increased oral fluids | IV fluids<br>IV insulin<br>Electrolyte replacement<br>Generalized supportive care |

The goals of diabetes management for children with type 1 diabetes mellitus include the following:

- Facilitating appropriate growth (height, weight)
- Maintaining an age-appropriate lifestyle
- Achieving age-related near-normal $HbA_{1c}$ with minimal episodes of hypoglycemia
- Preventing acute complications (hypoglycemia, hyperglycemia, DKA)

## Insulin Therapy

The child with type 1 diabetes mellitus loses the ability to make insulin because of autoimmune destruction of the insulin-producing cells, the beta cells. Symptoms of hyperglycemia become evident when most of the beta cells are destroyed. After initiation of insulin therapy, the child may have a "honeymoon" phase characterized by hypoglycemia and a decreasing need for insulin. This phase usually lasts up until 7 months into therapy but the length is highly variable (Gregory et al., 2013). The nurse should prepare the child and family for the possibility of a honeymoon phase, both to avoid the misconception that the diabetes is "going away" and to provide instruction on recognition and treatment of hypoglycemia.

The goal of insulin therapy is to replace the insulin the child is no longer able to make in an acceptable physiologic pattern. Synthetic human insulin, made using recombinant deoxyribonucleic acid (DNA)

## PATHOPHYSIOLOGY

### *Type 1 Diabetes Mellitus*

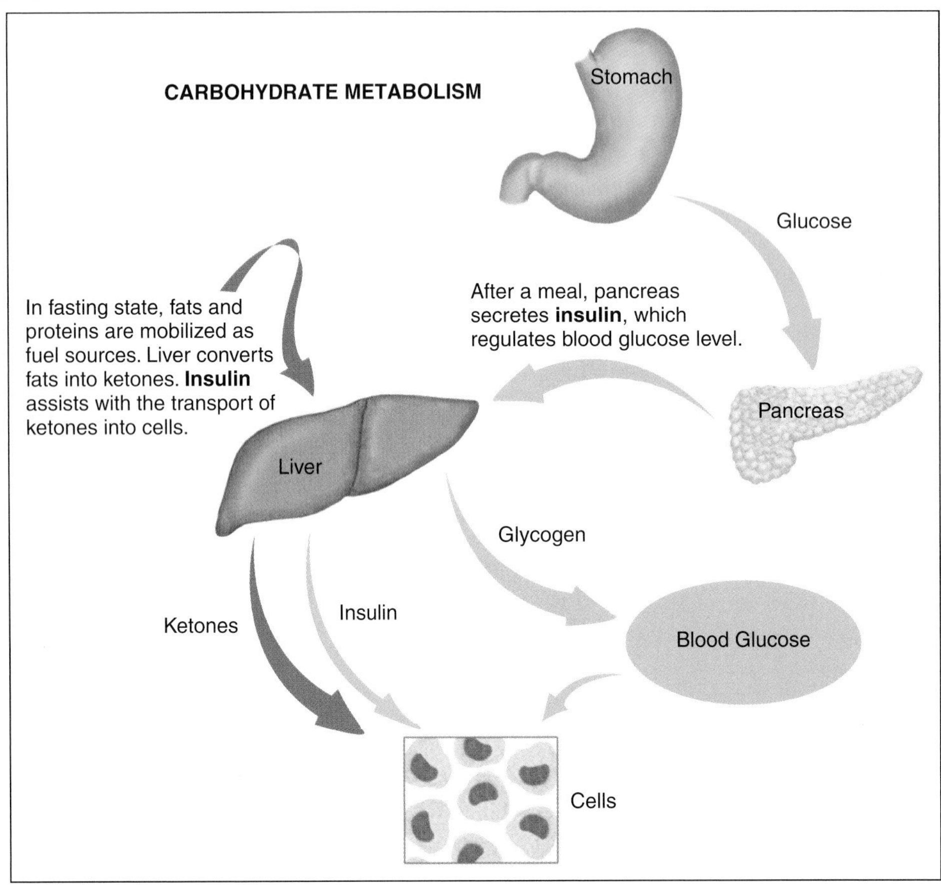
CARBOHYDRATE METABOLISM
Stomach
Glucose
After a meal, pancreas secretes **insulin**, which regulates blood glucose level.
In fasting state, fats and proteins are mobilized as fuel sources. Liver converts fats into ketones. **Insulin** assists with the transport of ketones into cells.
Pancreas
Liver
Glycogen
Ketones
Insulin
Blood Glucose
Cells

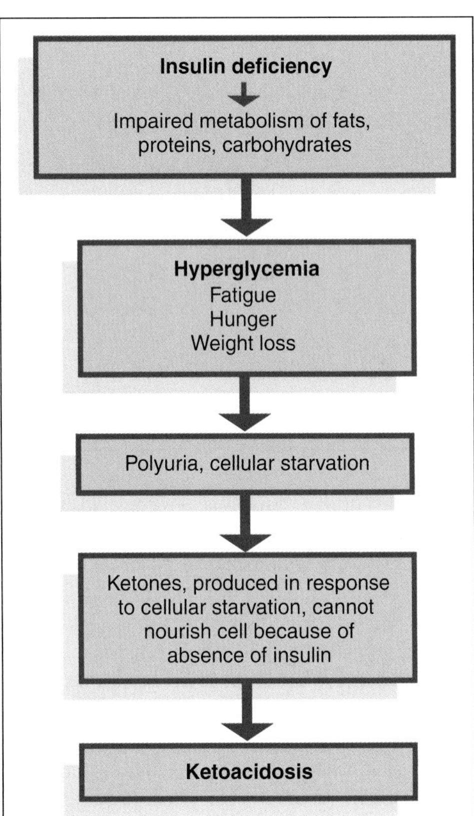
Insulin deficiency
Impaired metabolism of fats, proteins, carbohydrates
Hyperglycemia
Fatigue
Hunger
Weight loss
Polyuria, cellular starvation
Ketones, produced in response to cellular starvation, cannot nourish cell because of absence of insulin
Ketoacidosis

Glucose is the primary source of energy for body cells. Any extra glucose taken in by the body can be stored as glycogen in muscle or liver cells or in the form of fatty tissues. Glucose can be extracted from glycogen for periods of fasting (e.g., overnight). Once glycogen stores have been depleted, new glucose (gluconeogenesis) is made from amino acids released from muscle into the bloodstream. The energy for gluconeogenesis is supplied by the breakdown of stored fats.

Insulin, a hormone, is secreted by the beta cells of the pancreas. Its main function is to regulate the blood glucose level by controlling the rate of glucose uptake by cells. Little or no insulin is secreted by the beta cells when a person is in the fasting state; greater quantities are secreted after the person has eaten a meal. In the fasting state, with relatively small quantities of available insulin, the body mobilizes fats and proteins to be used as fuel sources. The liver then converts the fats into **ketoacids**, or ketones. With the assistance of insulin, ketones are transported into the cells and are used as an alternative source of fuel for cellular energy. This process ensures an energy source during long periods of fasting. Not all cells in the body are capable of using ketone bodies and require glucose as their primary fuel (see Table 51.2).

In the absence of insulin, the metabolism of fats, proteins, and carbohydrates is impaired. Glucose is unable to move into the intracellular space, resulting in hyperglycemia. As blood glucose levels exceed the renal threshold, glucose is "spilled" into the urine, causing osmotic diuresis and subsequent polyuria. Excessive thirst follows in response to fluid loss. Fatigue, hunger, and weight loss also accompany the onset of type 1 diabetes mellitus because cellular starvation continues in the absence of insulin.

Ketones (ketoacids), manufactured by the liver from adipose tissue, are produced in response to cellular starvation. In the absence of insulin, ketones are also unavailable to the cell for nourishment. Increasing blood levels of ketones (ketonemia) result in ketoacidosis.

**TABLE 51.4 Insulin Action by Type**

| Name | Type | Onset | Peak | Duration |
|---|---|---|---|---|
| Lispro/Aspart/Glulisine (Humalog/ Novolog/Apidra) | Rapid acting | 15 min | 30-90 min | 4-6 hr |
| Regular | Short acting | 30-60 min | 2-3 hr | 8-10 hr |
| NPH | Intermediate acting | 2-4 hr | 4-10 hr | 12-18 hr |
| Glargine/Detemir (Lantus/Levemir) | Long acting | 2-4 hr | No peak (Glargine)<br>3-9 hr (Detemir) | 20-24 hr (Glargine)<br>6-24 hr (Detemir) |

*NPH,* Neutral protamine Hagedorn.

technology, is free of animal impurities and is recommended for children. Oral hypoglycemic agents, although useful in the treatment of type 2 diabetes, are not effective in the treatment of type 1 diabetes.

The choice of insulin types and schedule of injections are determined based on the child's needs (Table 51.4). Daily self-monitoring of blood glucose aids in defining insulin requirements. The child in the honeymoon phase needs less insulin than the child who makes no endogenous insulin. The pubertal child requires larger insulin dosages.

***Schedule.*** Insulin requirements are commonly based on age, body weight, and pubertal status. In general, children who are newly diagnosed with type 1 diabetes typically need an initial total daily dose of approximately 0.5 to 1 unit/kg. Because dosages for infants and toddlers frequently are less than 1 unit, the insulin is diluted with an approved diluent to increase the volume to be administered and improve accuracy in dosing. Many children are managed through administration of insulin by three or more injections per day. Administration involves a combination of intermediate or long-acting insulin (basal) and rapid or short-acting insulin (bolus) injected multiple times per day before meals and snacks. More children are now receiving insulin through a continuous subcutaneous insulin infusion (CSII) pump. The insulin administration schedule is individually prescribed according to the child's age-related glycemic targets. The peak actions of these insulins are timed to correspond to the child's usual meal and snack times to minimize the possibility of hypoglycemia. To prevent hypoglycemia, a child must eat within 15 minutes of administration of rapid-acting insulin.

A recent option for the basal/bolus insulin regimen is using both rapid-acting analogs and long-acting insulin that has no peak action time. Glargine (Lantus), a long-acting peakless analog, has been approved for children ages 6 years and older and is given in the evening as the basal insulin and complemented during the day by a rapid-acting insulin (lispro or aspart) when the child eats carbohydrates (Gregory et al., 2013). This schedule provides improved glycemic control (Fig. 51.2) (ADA, 2015). Lantus insulin is not mixed in the same syringe with other types of insulin or solutions. Rapid-acting insulin analogs are also beneficial in the management of issues related to insulin resistance during puberty.

***Administration.*** Because insulin is a protein and would be digested if taken orally, it is given parenterally. Insulin is administered by subcutaneous injection using a specialized insulin syringe into the adipose tissue over large muscle masses. Preferred sites include the back of the upper arms, the top and outer portion of the thighs, the abdomen, and the hip (Fig. 51.3). To avoid injecting into the muscle or vascular space, a 45-degree angle of injection is used with a ½-inch needle or a 90-degree angle with a ⅜-inch needle. Rotation of injection sites helps prevent areas of adipose hypertrophy (fatty lumps), which interfere with insulin absorption. Various injection sites absorb insulin at slightly different rates. Absorption is also affected by body temperature and the level of muscle activity (exercise) under a given injection site.

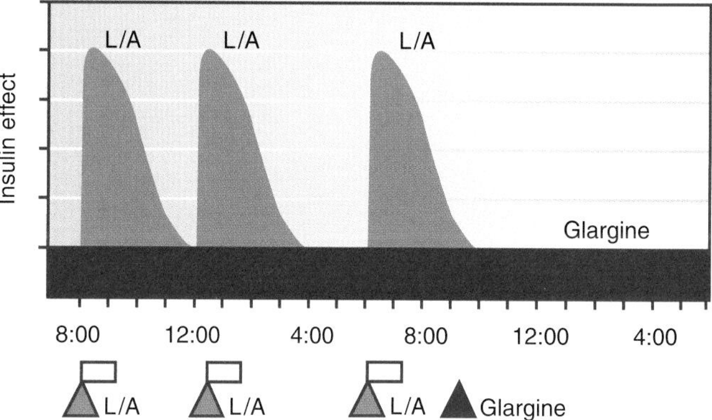


**FIG 51.2** Peak action of insulin injections is timed to correspond with the child's usual meal and snack times to minimize the chance of hypoglycemia. *L/A,* Lispro/Aspart (rapid-acting insulin). (Data fro: Svoren, B.M., & Jospe, N. [2016a]. Type 1 diabetes mellitus [immune mediated]. In R. Kliegman, B. Stanton, J. St. Geme, et al. [Eds.], *Nelson textbook of pediatrics* [20th ed., pp. 2763–2783]. Philadelphia: Elsevier.)

To help decrease variations in absorption, the child should use different locations within a major injection site for one day. For example, the child would inject insulin in one location on the back of the upper right arm for the morning injection, then rotate to another location on the back of the upper right arm for the afternoon injection, and a third location again on the upper right arm for the evening injection. The next day, another major site such as the top, outer portion of the right thigh may be used, depending on the site rotation schedule.

Insulin can be administered by an insulin syringe, air injector, or insulin pump. Disposable syringes are to be used only one time and then safely discarded (with the syringe/needle placed in a puncture-resistant, opaque container before placing in the trash). The air injector uses compressed air to deposit the insulin within the fatty tissue without the use of a needle. The child or family must learn to use the air injector device by correctly loading insulin, adjusting pressure settings to avoid intramuscular delivery, and cleaning.

The insulin pump is a battery-operated device that provides a continuous infusion of rapid-acting insulin (Gregory et al., 2013). Use of the pump in the pediatric population continues to increase. Evidence suggests that the insulin pump provides tighter control of blood sugar levels and more flexibility in lifestyle. The pump is a mechanical device, approximately the size of a pager, which is often worn on a belt or in a pocket. It delivers insulin to the body through an infusion set consisting of thin plastic tubing attached to a cannula or needle inserted into the subcutaneous tissue of the thigh, abdomen, or buttocks. A continuous basal rate of insulin infusion is maintained, and bolus dosages are infused as determined by blood glucose testing.

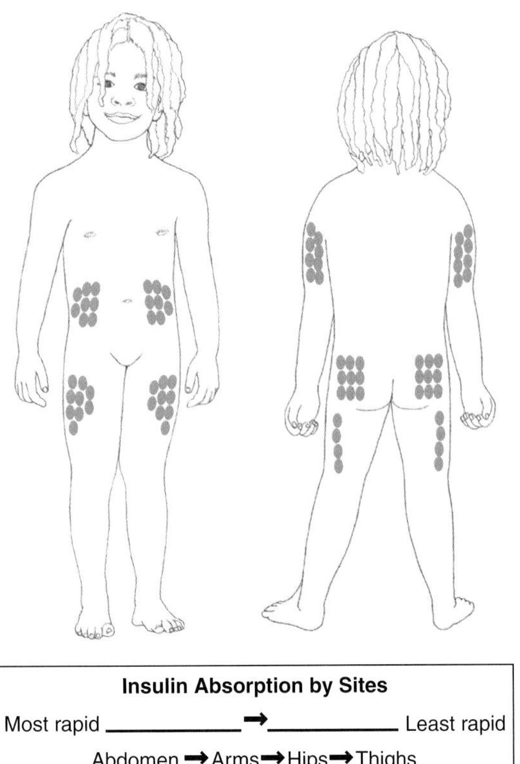

Insulin Absorption by Sites
Most rapid → Least rapid
Abdomen → Arms → Hips → Thighs


**FIG 51.3** Subcutaneous insulin injection sites most commonly used. Rate of absorption varies by site. (Chart modified from Albisser, A.M., & Sperlich, M. [1993]. Adjusting insulins. *Diabetes Educator, 18*[3], 211–227.)

The pump most closely mimics physiologic delivery of insulin (Gregory et al., 2013). A candidate for insulin pump therapy must be confident in diabetes management, willing to measure blood glucose meticulously (at least four glucose checks per day), be able to count carbohydrates and calculate appropriate insulin coverage, and have a supportive home environment. Parents and/or other caregivers are responsible for the insulin pump when used by infants and toddlers. Dietary recommendations are different for children or adolescents using an insulin pump and are based on carbohydrate counting.

### Nutrition Therapy

The goal of nutrition therapy is to promote normal growth, encourage healthy nutrition, prevent complications, and maintain near-normal blood glucose levels. Because the insulin dosage is balanced with food intake, the diet plan should stress a consistent intake, particularly of carbohydrate food products. The diet therapy chosen should be easy to understand and help the child and family learn to make healthy food choices. The individualized meal plan is based on the child's diet history and is tailored to food preferences, physical activity, cultural aspects, and schedules. As the child grows, the meal plan is tailored to meet changing dietary needs.

### Physical Activity

Exercise is an important aspect of diabetes management. Exercise enhances the action of insulin in lowering blood glucose levels. In addition, exercise promotes a greater sense of well-being, improves physical and cardiovascular fitness, and contributes to an improved lipid profile. The child with diabetes should be encouraged to participate in age-appropriate sports. Early enjoyment of a sport or activity can promote a lifelong active lifestyle. Because exercise lowers glucose levels, the child must be taught how to prevent hypoglycemia. The child should try to schedule activities to avoid exercising when an insulin dose is peaking. Proper hydration must be maintained while exercising.

**! NURSING QUALITY ALERT**

***Managing the Child With Type 1 Diabetes Mellitus***

**Insulin**

- Store insulin in a cool, dry place. Do not freeze or expose to excessive heat.
- Do not shake insulin. It is recommended to roll the vial back and forth to mix.
- Check the expiration date on the vial before using.
- Once opened, date the vial and discard as recommended.
- When mixing two different types of insulin in the same syringe, inject the appropriate amount of air into both vials, withdraw the short-acting (clear) insulin *first,* and then withdraw the intermediate-acting (cloudy) insulin.

**Nutrition**

- Meals and snacks are balanced with insulin action.
- Both the timing of the meal or snack and the amount of food are important in avoiding hyperglycemia or hypoglycemia.
- Adherence to a daily schedule that maintains a consistent food intake combined with consistent insulin injections aids in achieving metabolic control.

**Exercise**

- Avoid exercising during insulin peak-times.
- Add extra 15- to 30-g carbohydrate snacks for each 45 to 60 minutes of exercise.
- Blood glucose should be ≥100 to 120 mg/dL prior to exercise to decrease risk of hypoglycemia

**Blood Glucose Monitoring**

- Record blood glucose results in a diary.
- A 3- to 4-day alteration in glucose levels requires an adjustment of insulin doses.

The child and family are taught to add extra carbohydrate snacks that correlate to the duration of exercise. Coaches and teammates should be taught how to recognize and treat hypoglycemia. Delayed or nocturnal hypoglycemia can occur after strenuous activity. Additional carbohydrate intake might be required after exercise to maintain blood glucose levels. The child should always wear medical alert identification.

### Blood Glucose Monitoring

Self-monitoring of blood glucose (SMBG) provides an objective tool to assist with diabetes control. Monitoring is recommended before meals and before the bedtime snack. Monitoring is more frequent during prolonged exercise, during an illness, or if nighttime hypoglycemia is suspected.

Blood glucose goals must be tailored to the abilities of the caregivers and the age of the child. For example, goals for the infant or toddler are usually liberalized to help prevent severe hypoglycemia. The identified goals are a target range; not all glucose levels fall in this range, even in the child with excellent diabetes control. Preprandial (before meal) blood glucose goals are as follows (ADA, 2015):

- Non-diabetic: 70 to 110 mg/dL
- Children with type 1 diabetes mellitus: 90 to 130 mg/dL
- Infants and toddlers with type 1 diabetes mellitus: 100 to 180 mg/dL

Glucose test results should be recorded in a diary or record book. Patterns or trends in blood glucose levels outside the target range indicate a need to adjust the insulin dose. Three or 4 days of a consistent pattern of elevated glucose values (e.g., 200 mg/dL before the evening meal for 3 consecutive days) indicates a need to increase the dose of the appropriate insulin. The healthcare team may provide the family with guidelines for increasing insulin doses based on blood glucose patterns.

A majority of blood glucose meters can store multiple monitoring results so that blood glucose patterns can be evaluated. Blood glucose meters are accurate only if used according to manufacturer recommendations. Regardless of the brand selected, quality control procedures must be performed as recommended. Test supplies must be stored according to manufacturer specifications and discarded when outdated.

## Developmental Issues

***Infant and toddler.*** The infant or toddler with type 1 diabetes poses special challenges for diabetes management. The parents must adapt to the diagnosis and master the daily management needs of the child. Severe hypoglycemia occurs most often in this age group, so glucose target levels are liberalized.

Achieving consistency in dietary intake can be difficult. Inconsistent intake, particularly of carbohydrates, contributes to blood glucose variability. Food control issues can easily become a battleground between the child and the parent. A diet strategy that stresses carbohydrate consistency rather than specific food groups offers more flexibility.

Allowing the toddler to participate in making food choices (from perhaps two or three options) can provide the child a sense of control. The signs and symptoms of hypoglycemia are difficult to recognize in the infant; in a toddler, they can be mistaken for a temper tantrum. Establishing rituals and routines also helps the toddler feel more in control. Parents are encouraged to have a specific place to perform blood tests and to safely store supplies. Toddlers need to know when care activities will occur as well as participate according to their developmental level (Table 51.5).

***Preschooler.*** The preschool years are characterized by increasing motor maturity, a widening social circle, and magical thinking. The preschooler can understand simple explanations regarding diabetes. Such explanations help allay fears that the diabetes was caused by the child being "bad." Play therapy with dolls and diabetes equipment helps the preschooler express concerns regarding injections and finger sticks.

The preschooler has a more predictable appetite than the toddler and is frequently willing to try new foods. Nonetheless, supervision is necessary to ensure that meals and snacks are eaten, especially if the child is in a daycare setting with many distractions.

The preschooler may be able to identify the feelings associated with hypoglycemia. It is important to use the child's description as a code word for the onset of hypoglycemia symptoms. Preschoolers' preferences for high-energy activities put them at risk for hypoglycemia. The parents and other caregivers should be prepared with readily available carbohydrate foods, as well as emergency medications.

***School-age child.*** The school-age child and family face the challenge of incorporating diabetes care within a busy school day. To avoid

**TABLE 51.5 Examples of Diabetes Management Tasks Delegated to Child (With Supervision)**

| Developmental Characteristics | Management Task | Diet Task |
|---|---|---|
| **Toddler or Preschooler** | | |
| Likes rituals<br>Finicky eater<br>Not yet able to understand need for insulin | Chooses and cleans finger for puncture<br>Helps by holding still for injection<br>Identifies a word or phrase to describe a feeling of hypoglycemia | Helps by choosing foods |
| **School-Age Child** | | |
| Present oriented<br>Spends large amounts of time away from parents<br>Begins to develop self-concept | Performs finger puncture and blood glucose test<br>Chooses injection site according to rotation schedule<br>Pushes plunger on insulin syringe after the needle is inserted by parent or gives own injection<br>Performs ketone urine test | Recognizes need to eat on time to avoid hypoglycemia<br>Knows treatment for hypoglycemia |
| **Early Adolescent** | | |
| Looks to peer group for identity<br>Needs to conform to peer-group norms<br>Increased risk-taking behaviors | Records blood glucose values in diary<br>Draws up insulin with supervision<br>Performs insulin injection<br>Begins to manage insulin pump and carbohydrate counting | Knows meal plan<br>Can choose correct foods for snack<br>Adds extra snack for increased activity |
| **Middle or Late Adolescent** | | |
| Future oriented<br>Wants to take charge of life<br>Able to recognize consequences of behaviors and choices<br>Emotional separation from parents | Draws up and injects insulin<br>Looks for patterns in blood glucose values<br>Recognizes when to test for ketones in urine<br>Initiates treatment for ketones (fluids) | Can plan meals and snacks based on meal plan<br>Can choose appropriate foods at a party or when eating out |

singling out the child, the diabetes care should be as unobtrusive as possible while still maintaining a safe environment for the child. Children with type 1 diabetes mellitus fall under Section 504 of the Individuals with Disabilities Education Act and, as such, are entitled to services within the school setting (Nierengarten, 2016). The child should have a diabetes management plan that specifically describes the frequency of blood glucose testing, insulin doses, nutrition, and any other therapy or modifications associated with the diabetes (ADA, 2015). The family should communicate with school personnel about the child's diabetes. A school nurse or health aide should be identified to supervise before-lunch blood glucose monitoring, assist with insulin injections, and educate other school personnel in recognizing and treating hypoglycemia. Schools vary on the availability of nursing services. Parents may have to work with school personnel to identify appropriate staff to supervise their child's diabetes care.

Planning ahead for field trips, school parties, and athletic events allows the child with diabetes to participate safely in age-appropriate activities. For example, the child who has soccer practice three afternoons per week needs to plan how to prevent hypoglycemia during practice.

***Adolescent.*** The adolescent's developmental milestones are often in conflict with the recommendations for achieving diabetes control. The young adolescent is concerned with body image and peer-group acceptance and is moving away from the family for support and identity. Clothing, diet, lifestyle, and speech are areas in which the early adolescent strives to conform to peers.

The child in mid-adolescence might engage in risk-taking behaviors and more openly challenge parental authority. By late adolescence, the individual becomes more future oriented, with behaviors based more on abstract reasoning and less on peer-group demands.

## NURSING CARE PLAN

### *The Child With Type 1 Diabetes Mellitus in the Community Setting*

**Focused Assessment**

- Obtain history from family of signs and symptoms of hyperglycemia:
  - Polydipsia: requests water through the night
  - Polyuria: increased frequency of urination
  - Enuresis (if previously toilet trained)
  - Polyphagia
  - Weight loss
  - Fatigue
  - Nausea and vomiting
- Ask family about all medications the child is taking.
  - Certain drugs can cause hyperglycemia
- Perform a physical assessment and look for signs and symptoms of:
  - Dehydration
  - Acidosis
  - Infection
- Assess the child's and family's knowledge and ability to carry out the diabetes home management plan.
- Assess the child's and family's ability to cope with the diagnosis of a chronic illness.

**Nursing Diagnosis**

Deficient Knowledge related to unfamiliarity with home care needs of the child with type 1 diabetes mellitus.

**Planning**

***Expected Outcome***

The child and family will be able to successfully manage diabetes, as evidenced by demonstration of skills and verbalization of concepts necessary for home care (see Patient-Centered Teaching: Home Management of Type I Diabetes Mellitus box).

**Interventions and *Rationales***

1. Identify potential barriers to learning home care information and performing diabetes management skills. Specifically address language, literacy, manual dexterity, stressors, and fears.
   *Identifying and addressing these issues before education begins will optimize the family's learning. Additional resources may be needed such as translator services or counseling.*
2. Assess the family's knowledge of diabetes. Identify learning objectives with the child and family.
   *The education plan needs to be individualized. Specific objectives guide the learning process.*
3. Prepare the family to participate in diabetes education.
   *The child and family must learn home care strategies and skills.*
4. Present information that is suitable for the child's age and developmental level.
   *The child needs to understand diabetes and the management plan in order to engage in self-care at a developmentally appropriate level.*

**Evaluation**

Can the child and family successfully manage care, as evidenced by return demonstrations of knowledge and skills necessary to provide home care?

Are the child and family able to describe principles of diabetes management?

**Nursing Diagnosis**

Interrupted Family Processes related to the chronic healthcare needs of a child with type 1 diabetes mellitus.

**Planning**

***Expected Outcomes***

The child and family will cope with managing diabetes, as evidenced by recognizing stresses and constructing strategies for dealing with the stress of a chronic disease.

**Interventions and *Rationales***

1. Help the family identify diabetes management responsibilities appropriate to delegate to the child and those the parents must assume.
   *Delegation of responsibilities to the child occurs when the child is able to both perform the skill and understand the implications. Parental support and supervision are essential for all children.*
2. Help the child and family identify behaviors that the child recognizes as supporting adherence to the diabetes management plan.
   *Family communication and participation facilitates adherence (i.e., all family members follow the child's meal plan).*
3. Identify community support systems available for the child and family (i.e., summer diabetes camp, peer and parent support groups, community agencies, and financial resources).
   *Community resources offer a variety of services (see American Diabetes Association "In My Community" at http://www.diabetes.org/in-my-community/?loc=GlobalNavIMC for local resources). Peer support groups for the diabetic child and the family build motivation and self-esteem.*
4. Identify alternative care options that allow the primary caregiver to take a break from diabetes management responsibilities.

## NURSING CARE PLAN—cont'd

### *The Child With Type 1 Diabetes Mellitus in the Community Setting*

*Taking care of a child with diabetes is very stressful and demanding. Sharing responsibilities among family members and other caregivers helps decrease stress.*

**Evaluation**

Can the child and family verbalize a plan for sharing diabetes management responsibility?

**Nursing Diagnosis**

Imbalanced Nutrition: Less Than Body Requirements related to insulin deficit.

**Planning**

***Expected Outcomes***

1. The family and child will maximize nutritional status, as evidenced by demonstrating the ability to administer insulin, control diet and exercise, and perform blood glucose monitoring.
2. The child will be in nutritional balance, as evidenced by appropriate glucose levels and expected growth.

**Interventions and *Rationales***

1. Teach the child and family how food intake affects blood glucose level (i.e., carbohydrates raise blood glucose; fats and proteins have minimal effects).
   *Understanding the relationship of food to blood glucose levels provides the child and family the rationale for adhering to the diet plan.*
2. In conjunction with the child and family, develop an eating schedule for meals and snacks that also includes times for blood glucose testing, medications, and exercise.
   *The consistent timing of meals and snacks in relation to insulin injections and exercise is essential. Child and family involvement in schedule planning provides a sense of control and promotes adherence to the schedule.*
3. Ask the child to identify favorite foods and demonstrate how these can be incorporated into the meal plan.
   *Most foods can be incorporated into the meal plan, even if only in small amounts. Allowing some quantity of favorite foods encourages adherence.*
4. Observe whether the child's hunger is satisfied on the prescribed diet and adjust meal plan as needed.
   *The meal plan is tailored to the child's nutritional needs and activity level.*
5. Record height and weight measurements on the appropriate growth charts.
   *Monitoring the child's growth indicates whether the meal plan is meeting nutritional needs.*
6. Identify ideal blood glucose levels for the child. Ask the child and family to identify what changes could be made to diet, insulin, and/or exercise if the blood glucose level is out of the ideal range.
   *Diet, exercise, and insulin therapy are diabetic management tools that the child and family must learn how to use in order to attain ideal blood glucose levels.*

**Evaluation**

Do the child and family demonstrate appropriate insulin administration, diet therapy, and glucose monitoring?

Do the child and family adhere to the schedule for blood glucose testing, insulin injections, food intake, and exercise?

Do the child and family adhere to the meal plan?

Are the child's height and weight appropriate for age compared with growth chart percentiles?

**Nursing Diagnosis**

Risk for Injury related to hypoglycemia or hyperglycemia.

**Planning**

***Expected Outcomes***

1. The child will remain injury free as a result of appropriate recognition and management of hypoglycemia or hyperglycemia.
2. Family members will demonstrate knowledge of the signs, symptoms, and treatment of hypoglycemia and hyperglycemia and will initiate appropriate treatment.

**Interventions and *Rationales***

**For hypoglycemia (blood glucose level less than 60 mg/dL):**

1. Teach the child and family to recognize the signs and symptoms of hypoglycemia (see Table 51.3). Involve the daycare workers for young children and the school nurse, teachers, and other personnel in the care of a school-age child or adolescent.
   *Recognition of hypoglycemia signs and symptoms prompts the child, parent, or school personnel to perform a blood glucose check and rapidly initiate treatment for hypoglycemia, if indicated.*
2. Teach the child and family (as well as daycare and school personnel) to treat hypoglycemia immediately with oral intake of 15 g of easily digested (simple) carbohydrates. In 15 minutes, if symptoms are not relieved or blood glucose is 80 mg/dL or lower, repeat treatment. If the hypoglycemia occurs during the night, treat with 30 g of carbohydrate (½ simple and ½ complex) and with protein.
   *Early treatment reduces the possibility of a more severe reaction. There are 15 g of carbohydrates in 4 oz of 100% fruit juice.*
3. Teach the family as well as daycare and school personnel how to treat severe hypoglycemia for a child who is unconscious or having seizures. Place the child in the side-lying position. Rub glucose gel, frosting, or honey on the child's inner cheek and gums. If prescribed, glucagon can be injected subcutaneously or intramuscularly (onset of action is 10 to 15 minutes).
   *Urgent treatment is essential if a hypoglycemic child is unconscious or seizing. The child is positioned on the side to prevent aspiration. Glucose is rapidly absorbed through mouth epithelial tissues into the bloodstream. Glucagon is a pancreatic hormone that opposes the action of insulin and promotes conversion of liver glycogen to blood glucose.*
4. Help the child and family identify strategies to prevent and, if needed, treat hypoglycemia. Have the child wear medical alert identification at all times.
   *Many episodes of hypoglycemia can be averted by better planning of food intake and avoiding late or missed meals, excess insulin, or extra exercise. A diabetes box with hypoglycemia treatment instructions and supplies should be available at home and at daycare or school.*

**For hyperglycemia (blood glucose level higher than target range):**

1. Teach the child and family (as well as daycare and school personnel) to recognize the signs, symptoms, and causes of hyperglycemia (see Table 51.3).
   *Being aware of situations that may result in hyperglycemia can help distinguish the signs and symptoms of hyperglycemia versus hypoglycemia. The child's blood glucose level must be checked before starting treatment.*
2. Teach the child and family the correct procedure to test for ketones in the urine when the child is ill or the blood glucose level exceeds 250 mg/dL.
   *Ketones are formed in response to insulin deficit. Early recognition of ketonuria and treatment can prevent acute complications including diabetic ketoacidosis (DKA).*

*Continued*

## NURSING CARE PLAN—cont'd

### *The Child With Type 1 Diabetes Mellitus in the Community Setting*

3. Teach child and family how to treat hyperglycemia. Administer calorie-free oral fluids and additional short-acting insulin subcutaneously as ordered by the healthcare provider.
   *Fluids and insulin remove excess ketones. A child with nausea and vomiting cannot be treated with oral fluids; the physician must be notified due to the risk of dehydration.*
4. Instruct family on sick-day diabetes management. Explain to the family how and when a diabetes healthcare team member should be contacted (Box 51.4).
   *Stress due to infection or other causes can result in uncontrolled diabetes. Sick-day management is an effective prevention strategy.*
5. Evaluate the child's dosages and types of insulin prescribed and the administration schedule.
   *Persistent hyperglycemia may indicate the need to adjust the insulin regimen.*
   *The growing child will need periodic increases in baseline insulin dosages.*
6. Evaluate the family's diabetes home management knowledge, adherence to the recommended plan, home supervision of the child, and coping skills.
   *Frequent episodes of hyperglycemia (and DKA) may reflect a lack of understanding or nonadherence to the home management plan, inadequate child supervision, and ineffective coping strategies.*
7. Help the child and family identify strategies to prevent hyperglycemia. Provide additional interventions or refer to support services, as indicated.
   *Consistency in diet, exercise, and insulin injection times helps prevent hyperglycemia. The child and family may need additional services in order to successfully manage the child's chronic illness.*

**Evaluation**

Does the child remain injury free?

Are the child and family able to recognize and correctly and promptly treat hypoglycemia and hyperglycemia?

Is the child free of episodes of severe hypoglycemia or hyperglycemia?

## BOX 51.4 Sick-Day Management for the Child With Type 1 Diabetes Mellitus

1. Always give insulin injections, even if the child does not want to eat. If concerned that the child will become hypoglycemic with the usual dose, contact a diabetes healthcare team member for instructions. If ordered, use sliding scale, rapid- or short-acting insulin for hyperglycemia every 3 to 4 hours.
2. Test blood glucose level at least every 4 hours or more often if hypoglycemic or hyperglycemic.
3. Test for urine ketones with each voiding. Notify diabetes team member if moderate or large amounts of urine ketones are present. Additional regular insulin may be ordered.
4. Encourage intake of calorie-free liquids. Liquids aid in clearing ketones from the blood.
5. Follow the child's usual meal plan. If the child has a poor appetite, a sick-day diet replacing the usual grams of carbohydrate with simple carbohydrate foods is used.
6. Encourage rest. Exercising while ketones are present results in increased ketone formation.
7. Notify the diabetes healthcare team member of the following:
   - Nausea and vomiting
   - Fruity odor to the breath
   - Deep, rapid respirations
   - Decreasing level of consciousness
   - Moderate or high urine ketones
   - Persistent hyperglycemia

These normal milestones become dilemmas when diabetes control is affected. Missed injections, omitted blood tests, irregular meals, and dietary splurges are frequent complaints of parents of diabetic adolescents.

Parents and their adolescents must accept that diabetes management responsibility increasingly shifts to the adolescent. Parents are encouraged to work as partners with the adolescent to achieve diabetes control. It is essential to identify what is important to the adolescent and to use that information to motivate adherence. The adolescent is not motivated by predictions of complications in the distant future. Rather, motivation should focus on issues of current significance to the adolescent such as personal appearance, athletic ability, strength and muscle mass, endurance, or ideal weight.

### Delegating Diabetes Management Responsibilities

Children with diabetes are functionally able to perform diabetes management tasks far sooner than they can cognitively understand the implications of this action or consequences of omitting the action. Transfer of responsibility from the parents to the child should be on a step-by-step basis, according to the child's cognitive understanding and functional abilities. Diabetes management shifts from full parental responsibility to a partnership between parent and child and then to the acceptance of full responsibility by the young adult. Delegation of management responsibility to the child too soon can result in poor diabetes control and frequent DKA episodes. Ongoing parental support and supervision is essential (see Table 51.5).

## DIABETIC KETOACIDOSIS

DKA is the metabolic consequence of a severe insulin deficit leading to hyperglycemia and the presence of ketone bodies in the blood, followed by metabolic acidosis. For individuals with type 1 diabetes, DKA is seen more frequently in young children and adolescents than in adults (Klingensmith et al., 2013). DKA affects up to 40% of children diagnosed with new-onset type 1 diabetes mellitus (Svoren & Jospe, 2016a).

### Etiology

DKA results from an absolute or relative insulin deficit. In the younger diabetic child, the most common cause is insulin resistance, as in a stress response initiated by an infection. In the adolescent, the most common cause is one or more missed insulin injections.

### Manifestations

Table 51.3 lists the signs and symptoms of DKA, which include abdominal and chest pain, nausea and vomiting, fruity breath smell, decreased level of consciousness (LOC), Kussmaul respirations, and symptoms of dehydration.

## PATIENT-CENTERED TEACHING

### *Home Management of Type 1 Diabetes Mellitus*

The child and family are understandably overwhelmed with questions and fears about the diagnosis. Encourage all family members to participate in the educational process. Choose a comfortable location subject to few interruptions. Provide appropriate literature and materials for family members. DVDs, booklets, and pamphlets should be developmentally appropriate. Educational materials for the parents should also match the parents' literacy skills.

The following checklist of outcomes evaluates the family's understanding of the pertinent information:

- General information about type 1 diabetes mellitus
- How to administer and store insulin
- How to monitor blood glucose levels and use the equipment properly
- Signs and management of hypoglycemic episodes
- Signs and management of hyperglycemia
- Strategies for when the child is ill
- Nutrition and exercise principles
- Potential long-term complications
- Available resources for community services and emotional support

All family members should be given the opportunity to practice skills taught. Practicing procedures on themselves or each other helps allay fears and allows the child to supervise as a family member performs the procedure. Help develop problem-solving skills by using various scenarios that encourage decision making. Because education is an ongoing process, the family needs a contact person to whom they can turn for advice and support.

#### Outcomes

#### *General Information*

The child and family will be able to do the following:

1. Describe the action of insulin in the body.
2. Describe the characteristics of type 1 diabetes.
3. Identify three factors that can be used to control blood glucose levels.

#### *Medication Therapy*

The child and family will be able to do the following:

1. Name the types of insulin the child is using and identify the onset, peak, and duration of action for each.
2. State the storage recommendations for insulin.
3. State the recommended expiration date of the insulin.
4. Demonstrate accurate syringe or air injector preparation for a single type of insulin.
5. Demonstrate syringe preparation for two types of insulin.
6. Demonstrate subcutaneous insulin injection technique with syringe/needle or air injector.
7. Identify insulin injection sites and describe a pattern of rotation.
8. Identify a plan for safe syringe and needle disposal.
9. Identify recommended insulin dosages and injection times.
10. Describe the function and management associated with an insulin pump. Demonstrate setup and use of an insulin pump, if applicable.

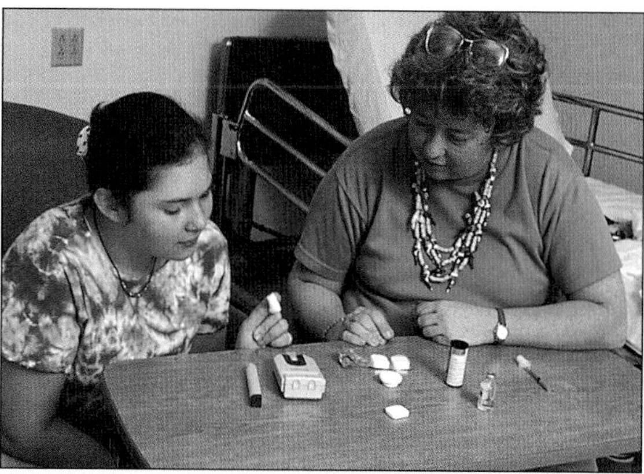

When other parts of the treatment regimen have become familiar, the injection technique can be taught. Initially, self-injecting insulin may be frightening for the school-age child, so the parent may insert the needle and have the child then push the plunger. The child can then progress to performing self-injection.

#### *Home Glucose Monitoring*

The child and family will be able to do the following:

1. Identify nondiabetic blood glucose levels and target goals for good glucose control.
2. Demonstrate the use, calibration, control testing, and cleaning of the blood glucose monitor.
3. Demonstrate finger-stick technique to obtain the blood sample.

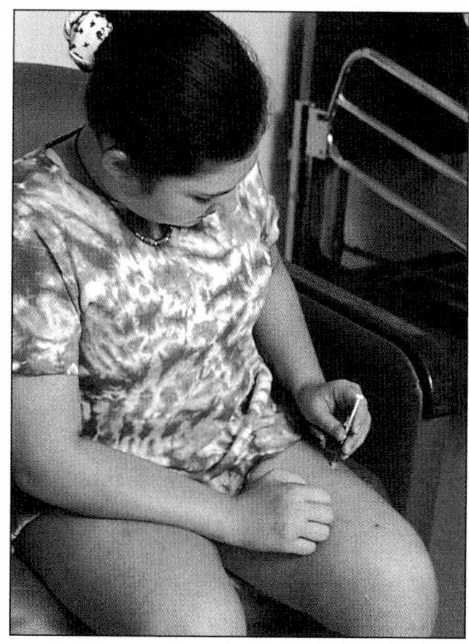

4. Identify a plan for recording blood glucose values.

The school-age child is usually able to perform daily self-monitoring of blood glucose with parental help. However, the child should not be expected to adjust the insulin dose based on the reading. By early adolescence, the child can be in charge of recording blood glucose values in the diary.

*Continued*

## PATIENT-CENTERED TEACHING—cont'd

### *Home Management of Type 1 Diabetes Mellitus*

***Hypoglycemia***

The child and family will be able to do the following:

1. Identify the signs and symptoms of a hypoglycemic reaction.
2. Describe appropriate treatment for both a mild and a severe hypoglycemic reaction.
3. Identify three potential causes of a hypoglycemic reaction.
4. Identify the importance of medical emergency identification.
5. Describe typical blood glucose trends during the honeymoon phase.

***Hyperglycemia***

The child and family will be able to do the following:

1. Identify the signs and symptoms of hyperglycemia.
2. Identify strategies to control hyperglycemia.
3. Describe the possible effects of stress or illness on diabetes control.
4. Demonstrate the procedure for ketone (urine, serum) testing.
5. State when to test for ketones.
6. State basic treatment if the child tests positive for ketones.
7. Describe the signs and symptoms requiring provider or other healthcare team contact.

***Nutrition/Exercise***

The child and family will be able to do the following:

1. State the effect of exercise on blood glucose levels.
2. State the benefits of an appropriate nutrition plan and describe precautions for exercise.
3. Identify the correlation of diet, exercise, and insulin with blood glucose control.
4. Generate a home schedule that identifies mealtimes and snack times, blood test times, and insulin injection times.

***Complications***

The child and family will be able to do the following:

1. Identify the role of glucose control in the prevention or delay of diabetes-related complications.
2. Identify appropriate healthcare follow-up for the child with diabetes.

***Psychological Adjustment and Family Involvement***

The child and family will be able to create a plan for the entire family to participate in diabetes care and management.

***Community Resources***

The child and family will be able to identify available community resources for ongoing diabetes services, education, and support.

### Diagnostic Evaluation

Diabetic ketoacidosis is confirmed by the following test results:

- Blood glucose ≥ 200 mg/dL
- Venous pH < 7.3
- Ketonuria
- Ketonemia
- Serum potassium: Elevated, normal, or low
- Serum phosphorus: Low
- White blood cell (WBC) count: Elevated as a result of stress demargination (higher with infection)
- Serum carbon dioxide: Low

### Therapeutic Management

The child in DKA usually is admitted to an intensive care unit. Management includes hourly glucose monitoring, hourly vital signs and neurologic checks, strict intake and output measurements, frequent assessment of fluid and electrolyte status, IV fluid replacement, potassium replacement if needed, and administration of continuous IV insulin (Wolfsdorf et al., 2014).

## LONG-TERM HEALTHCARE NEEDS FOR THE CHILD WITH TYPE 1 DIABETES MELLITUS

Serious complications are associated with long-term type 1 diabetes, including retinopathy, nephropathy, neuropathy, and cardiovascular disease. Studies have demonstrated that strict metabolic control of diabetes can decrease the severity of complications and/or delay onset (Sobotka, Danielson, Drum, et al., 2014). A team approach to diabetes management can best provide the tools to achieve metabolic control. The team includes the physician specialist, nurse educator, dietitian, and behavioral specialist. Regular checkups and frequent telephone communication between the diabetes team; the parents; and the child, if age-appropriate, are essential to address the needs of the growing child.

For children, glycemic control over time (3 months or longer), as assessed by $HbA_{1c}$, is critically important to reduce the cognitive sequelae of hypoglycemic episodes (ADA, 2015). Although the normal $HbA_{1c}$ for adults is considered to be approximately 7% or less, recommendations are less restrictive for children and adolescents. The ADA (2015) recommends a target $HbA_{1c}$ below 7.5% in all pediatric age groups and less than 7% only if reasonably achieved without excessive hypoglycemia.

Older children with type 1 diabetes should be screened to prevent long-term complications. The ADA recommends that children older than 10 years and those who are symptomatic be screened for microscopic albuminuria, autoimmune thyroid disease, retinopathy, hypertension, dyslipidemia, and celiac disease (Gregory et al., 2013). Early identification of and treatment for these conditions can minimize serious complications in adulthood.

Routine healthcare for the child with diabetes should also include yearly dental and ophthalmologic evaluations, as well as prophylactic interventions such as influenza vaccinations. Children and their families should be referred to other healthcare providers, counselors, other service providers, and community resources as specific needs are identified.

Diabetes research is aimed at preventing diabetes and finding a cure after diagnosis. Multiple immune intervention strategies are being identified and tested. In addition, pancreas and islet cell transplantation continues to be investigated as potential cures in the future.

## TYPE 2 DIABETES MELLITUS

Type 2 diabetes is an emerging problem in the pediatric population. The rise in the incidence of overweight and obese children is directly related to the increased number of children diagnosed with type 2

## NURSING CARE PLAN

### *The Child in Diabetic Ketoacidosis (DKA)*

**Focused Assessment**

- Assess for signs and symptoms related to:
  - Respiratory status
  - Level of consciousness
  - Hydration status
  - Electrolyte and acid-base balance
- Obtain the following history data from family:
  - Most recent blood glucose values
  - Urinary ketones test results and treatment
  - Time and amount of last insulin injection
  - Time and amount of last food eaten
  - Routine daily management plan (insulin dose/schedule, blood glucose checks, diet, and exercise)
  - Sick-day management plan
  - Family's understanding of diabetes management plan

**Nursing Diagnosis**

Deficient Fluid Volume related to abnormal fluid losses through diuresis and emesis.

**Planning**

***Expected Outcome***

The child will be safely rehydrated, as evidenced by normal weight, good skin turgor, appropriate urine output for age, and moist mucous membranes.

**Interventions and *Rationales***

1. Determine the child's hydration status, evaluating weight, skin turgor, mucous membranes, and urine output.
   *This identifies current hydration status. A comparison of the child's usual weight with the admission weight provides an estimation of percent body fluid loss.*
2. Encourage intake of calorie-free fluids if the child is not nauseated. Administer intravenous (IV) fluids as ordered (normal saline is given initially).
   *Rehydration is the initial step in resolving DKA. Fluid losses occur primarily from the osmotic diuresis with hyperglycemia. If acidosis has resulted in nausea and vomiting, IV fluids are required.*
3. Maintain strict intake and output monitoring.
   *Accurate intake and output records are essential in determining rehydration status.*
4. Observe for edema or pulmonary congestion.
   *These signs indicate overhydration.*
5. Weigh child on admission and every 8 to 12 hours.
   *Comparing admission weight to the child's usual weight indicates initial hydration status. Follow-up weights provide ongoing assessment.*

**Evaluation**

Is the child safely rehydrated, as evidenced by normal weight, urine output appropriate for age, good skin turgor, and moist mucous membranes?

**Nursing Diagnosis**

Risk for Injury from altered acid-base balance leading to ketone production and acidosis related to lack of insulin.

**Planning**

***Expected Outcome***

The child will have a resolution of ketosis and acidosis, as evidenced by laboratory results and clinical assessment.

**Interventions and *Rationales***

1. Test all urine samples for the presence of ketones. Monitor the child's breath for acetone. Observe for Kussmaul respirations.
   *Urinary ketones indicate possible acidosis. Serum ketone analysis, or beta-hydroxybutyric acid, is a direct measurement. When acetone, a ketoacid, is expelled, the child's breath has a fruity smell. High acid levels trigger rapid and deep breaths (Kussmaul respirations).*
2. Encourage calorie-free fluids if the child is able to drink. If ordered, begin IV fluids.
   *Fluids are essential in flushing ketones out of the blood.*
3. Initiate continuous IV infusion of regular insulin as ordered. Titrate to maintain blood glucose in safe range.
   *Insulin therapy starts after rehydration is underway. Blood glucose should drop no more than 80 to 100 mg/dL/hr to prevent rapid fluid shifts.*
4. Monitor blood glucose every hour during IV insulin infusion.
   *IV insulin acts quickly and can suddenly cause hypoglycemia.*
5. Provide glucose-containing IV fluids as ordered.
   *Insulin inhibits the production of ketones. When blood glucose reaches 230 to 300 mg/dL, glucose is added to the IV fluids to prevent hypoglycemia. Insulin infusion continues until serum ketones are cleared.*

**Evaluation**

Within 24 hours of admission, does the child display any evidence of ketosis (ketonuria, fruity breath, elevated blood glucose)?

**Nursing Diagnosis**

Risk for Injury related to electrolyte imbalance from emesis and acidosis.

**Planning**

***Expected Outcome***

The child will remain free from adverse consequences of electrolyte abnormalities, as evidenced by normal serum sodium and potassium values.

**Interventions and *Rationales***

1. Monitor potassium levels every 1 to 2 hours initially; look for signs and symptoms of hyperkalemia (bradycardia, muscle weakness, hyperreflexia, cardiac or respiratory arrest) and hypokalemia (muscle weakness, fatigue, hypotension). Monitor serum sodium levels at intervals.
   *During acidosis, potassium moves out of the cells to the intravascular space and then is excreted through diuresis. Initially, serum potassium levels may be acceptable; this does not reflect intracellular losses. With rehydration and correction of acidosis, potassium moves back into the cells, resulting in lower serum levels (see Chapter 40).*
2. Maintain child on a cardiac monitor to watch for abnormal electrocardiogram findings. Prepare for a rapid response if a medical emergency occurs.
   *Hypokalemia produces prolonged ST segments; notched, flat, or inverted T waves; and arrhythmias. Hyperkalemia produces flattened P waves or peaked T waves and ventricular fibrillation.*
3. Administer potassium as ordered, if child has urine output. If anuric, notify healthcare provider and *do not* give potassium.
   *Renal failure can result from severe dehydration. With anuria, potassium is retained, resulting in hyperkalemia.*

**Evaluation**

Does the child maintain a stable fluid and electrolyte balance, with serum sodium and potassium levels within normal limits?

**Nursing Diagnosis**

Risk for Injury related to cerebral edema from resolving DKA.

*Continued*

## NURSING CARE PLAN—cont'd

### *The Child in Diabetic Ketoacidosis (DKA)*

**Planning**

***Expected Outcome***

The child will remain free from adverse consequences of cerebral edema, as evidenced by appropriate level of consciousness, pupils equal and reactive to light, and absence of headache.

**Intervention and *Rationale***

1. Perform neurologic checks every 1 to 2 hours and observe for signs of cerebral edema (headache; decreased level of consciousness; nonreactive to light, unequal, or dilated pupils). Notify the provider immediately of any neurologic changes.
   *Cerebral edema is a complication of resolving DKA that can result in brain damage or death. Causes are unclear; may be related to overhydration, rapid fluid shifts, and electrolyte imbalances. Prompt recognition and treatment may prevent neurologic injury (see Chapter 52).*

**Evaluation**

Is the child alert, with equal and reactive pupils and without reports of headache?

diabetes (St. Onge, Miller, Motycka, et al., 2015). At the time of diagnosis in adolescents, only approximately 20% of the beta cells are still producing insulin. These children have a combination of insulin resistance and decreased insulin secretion (Elder et al., 2014).

## Etiology

The majority of children with type 2 diabetes are at risk for being overweight (body mass index [BMI] between 85th and 95th percentile) or are overweight (BMI greater than 95th percentile) at diagnosis and have glycosuria without ketonuria, absent or mild polydipsia and polyuria, and no or little recent weight loss. Type 2 diabetes is not caused by an autoimmune response. The pancreas still produces insulin, but in an amount insufficient to overcome persistent hyperglycemia. Genetics and familial factors, obesity, race and ethnicity, female sex, maternal gestational diabetes, and intrauterine growth retardation, along with a lack of physical activity in childhood and adolescence, seem to be crucial factors in the development of type 2 diabetes in children (ADA, 2015).

## Incidence

The incidence of Type 2 diabetes in pediatric patients continues to climb, with a substantial increase globally in the past 2 decades. The 2008 National Health and Nutrition Examination Survey discovered an increase in the prevalence of Type 2 diabetes among 12- to 19-year-olds from 9% (years 1999 to 2000) up to 23% (years 2007 to 2008). Type 2 diabetes onset is most prevalent between 15 to 19 years of age. In the United States, the SEARCH for Diabetes in Youth Study found that in 10- to 19-year-olds, the highest incidence of type 2 diabetes occurs in American Indians followed by Asian-Pacific Islanders and Black (St. Onge et al., 2015; Svoren & Jospe, 2016b).

## Manifestations

Children with type 2 diabetes are typically overweight and have acanthosis nigricans, a velvety darkening of the skin around the back and sides of the neck and other areas, including inguinal folds, axilla, umbilicus, knees, antecubital fossa, and backs of the hands. This condition is a marker for metabolic syndrome (as well as hypertension and dyslipidemia), also known as insulin resistance syndrome (Gregory et al., 2013). Other possible symptoms include fatigue, yeast infections, blurred vision, and frequent urination. Hypertension, elevated triglyceride and low-density lipoprotein levels, and polycystic ovary syndrome are common presenting signs.

## Diagnostic Evaluation

Diagnosis of type 2 diabetes depends on careful physical examination, elevated endogenous insulin levels, and no evidence of serum autoantibodies. A fasting blood glucose (FBG) over 126 mg/dL or a random serum glucose level of 200 mg/dL or more indicates diabetes, either type 1 or type 2. The fasting C-peptide level is usually elevated in type 2 diabetes (ADA, 2015).

## Therapeutic Management

The mainstays of treatment for children with type 2 diabetes are nutritional interventions for weight maintenance or weight loss (depending on age) and regular, moderate-intensity physical exercise (St. Onge et al., 2015).

Any child with severe hyperglycemia, ketonemia, and metabolic abnormalities, whether diagnosed with type 1 or type 2 diabetes, will need insulin therapy to reverse metabolic imbalances. Some children with type 2 diabetes require insulin; however, most are managed with oral agents that decrease insulin resistance or augment endogenous insulin production. Blood glucose monitoring and diet management are important aspects of therapy. If these children lose weight, some can be managed with diet and exercise alone.

The goals of type 2 diabetes management for children include the following:

- Achieving near-normal glycemic control (acceptable $HbA_{1c}$ according to age)
- Facilitating reasonable weight for height
- Achieving normal blood glucose levels
- Prevention of hyperlipidemia and hypertension
- Decreasing the frequency of microvascular and cardiovascular complications

### Medication Therapy

For the child with type 2 diabetes mellitus, oral hypoglycemic agents are used if the diabetes cannot be managed with diet and exercise. At present, metformin is the only type 2 diabetes medication approved by the U.S. Food and Drug Administration for use in children ages 10 years and older (St. Onge et al., 2015). It is commonly prescribed as the initial oral hypoglycemic medication if severe hyperglycemia is not present. Reduced serum triglyceride and cholesterol levels and weight stabilization or decrease are other effects of metformin use.

### Nutrition Therapy

Nutrition therapy goals for children and adolescents with type 2 diabetes are individualized, with emphasis on improved glycemic control and weight maintenance or loss through a reduced intake of calories. A dietary pattern that encourages consumption of fruits, vegetables, whole grains, legumes, and lowfat milk is recommended (ADA, 2015). Improved glycemic control can be achieved through carbohydrate counting. Reducing foods containing saturated and trans fatty acids, cholesterol, and sodium may lead to improvement in dyslipidemia and lower blood pressure (ADA, 2015). Participation of the entire family in a weight management program, which incorporates behavior modification strategies, is a key to success.

### Physical Activity

Increased physical activity by individuals with type 2 diabetes can improve glycemic control, decrease insulin resistance, and reduce cardiovascular disease risk factors (ADA, 2015). For children with type 2 diabetes, at least 60 minutes of moderate to vigorous physical activity daily and less than 2 hr/day of "screen time" sedentary activities (TV, computer, video games) are required for prevention and management of type 2 diabetes (St. Onge et al., 2015).

### Blood Glucose Monitoring

The frequency of blood glucose testing for a child with type 2 diabetes is based on blood glucose goals, as well as the child's and family's willingness and ability to perform the tests. Ideally, blood glucose levels should be checked two to three times daily and $HbA_{1c}$ levels monitored every 3 months (Gregory et al., 2013).

### Prevention

The ADA (2015) recommends routine monitoring of children for the presence or development of type 2 diabetes who are overweight and have two or more risk factors. These factors include a family history of type 2 diabetes, member of an at-risk race or ethnic group (Black, Latino/Hispanic, Native-American Indian, Asian-American, Pacific Islander), signs of insulin resistance or associated conditions (hypertension or dyslipidemia), and a mother who had gestational diabetes or diabetes starting at age 10 years or younger (with the onset of puberty). These children should be tested for HbA1c every 3 years (ADA, 2015).

Metabolic syndrome predicts the development of both type 2 diabetes mellitus and cardiovascular disease in adults. There has been great debate regarding the diagnostic criteria of metabolic syndrome, especially in pediatrics. Generally, an individual with at least three of the five risk factors/characteristics is considered to have metabolic syndrome: hypertension, dyslipidemia (hyperlipidemia, low HDL), insulin resistance (elevated fasting blood glucose), and central obesity with increased waist circumference. Due to difficulties with diagnosis, the underestimation of the prevalence of metabolic syndrome in children is of concern. Studies have found a prevalence ranging from 2% to 9% in the general population and an increased prevalence of 12% to 44% in obese children. Children and adolescents must be identified and early interventions provided to reduce their risk of developing chronic, debilitating diseases as adults (Lee, 2012).

## KEY CONCEPTS

- The six major hormones of the endocrine system secreted by the anterior pituitary gland are ACTH, TSH, FSH, LH, GH, and prolactin.
- The pituitary gland secretes stimulating hormones that cause target organs to produce specific hormones. Per the negative feedback system, when hormone levels are sufficient, secretion of stimulating hormones decreases.
- Pill dispensers and reminder watch alarms can improve adherence to daily medication regimens.
- Some signs and symptoms of hypothyroidism (fatigue, weight gain, constipation, cold intolerance) are opposite of those for hyperthyroidism (nervousness, weight loss, diarrhea, heat intolerance).
- DI is caused by deficient ADH leading to high output of unconcentrated urine and hypernatremia. SIADH occurs with excessive production of ADH and results in decreased output of concentrated urine and hyponatremia.
- Children with precocious puberty may experience psychosocial issues including self-consciousness about their bodies, being treated as older than their chronologic age, and aggressive behavior in boys.
- Without insulin, metabolism is impaired and glucose does not move into the intracellular space, resulting in hyperglycemia.
- Both type 1 diabetes mellitus and type 2 diabetes mellitus involve abnormal carbohydrate metabolism and hyperglycemia; however, causes, risk factors, treatment, and prevention differ significantly.
- The goals of diabetes management are to maintain glycemic control, reasonable weight for height, and an age-appropriate lifestyle as well as prevent acute and long-term complications.
- Hypoglycemia results from too much insulin, resulting in neuroglycopenic symptoms (personality changes, slurred speech, decreased LOC) and adrenergic signs (trembling, sweating, tachycardia, pallor, clammy skin); treat with ingestion of 15 g of easily digested carbohydrate.
- Hyperglycemia is caused by excessive carbohydrate intake and inadequate insulin, resulting in signs and symptoms of increased urine output, thirst, and hunger as well as fatigue, blurred vision, headache, and emotional lability; treat with insulin and increased fluid intake.
- DKA occurs as a result of severe hyperglycemia with ketones in the blood and metabolic acidosis. Management often requires intensive care to lower blood glucose, reverse acidosis, and correct fluid and electrolyte imbalances.

## REFERENCES AND READINGS


Alatzoglou, K.S., Webb, E.A., Le Tissier, P., et al. (2014). Isolated growth hormone deficiency (GHD) in childhood and adolescence: recent advances. *Endocrine Reviews, 35*(3), 376–432. doi:10.1210/er.2013-1067.

American Diabetes Association. (2011). *Diabetic statistics*. Retrieved from http://www.diabetes.org/diabetes-basics/statistics.

American Diabetes Association. (2015). Standards of medical care in diabetes—2015. *Diabetes Care, 38*(Suppl 1), S1–S93. Retrieved from http://care.diabetesjournals.org/content/suppl/2014/12/23/38.Supplement_1.DC1/January_Supplement_Combined_Final.6-99.pdf.

Breault, D.T., & Majzoub, J.A. (2016a). Diabetes insipidus. In R. Kliegman, B. Stanton, J. St. Geme, et al. (Eds.), *Nelson textbook of pediatrics* (20th ed., pp. 2644–2646). Philadelphia: Elsevier.

Breault, D.T., & Majzoub, J.A. (2016b). Other abnormalities of arginine vasopressin metabolism and action. In R. Kliegman, B. Stanton, J. St. Geme, et al. (Eds.), *Nelson textbook of pediatrics* (20th ed., pp. 2644–2646). Philadelphia: Elsevier.

Brown, R.S. (2012). Disorders of the thyroid gland in infancy, childhood, and adolescence. In L.J. DeGroot, P. Beck-Peccoz, G. Chrousos, et al. (Eds.), *Endotext* [Internet]. South Dartmouth, MA: MDText.com, Inc. Retrieved from http://www.ncbi-nlm-nih-gov.lp.hscl.ufl.edu/books/NBK279032/.

Centers for Disease Control and Prevention [CDC]. (2014). *National Diabetes Statistics Report: Estimates of Diabetes and its Burden in the United States, 2014*. Atlanta, GA: U.S. Department of Health and Human Services. Retrieved from http://www.cdc.gov/diabetes/pubs/statsreport14/national-diabetes-report-web.pdf.

Chen, M., & Eugster, E.A. (2015). Central precocious puberty: update on diagnosis and treatment. *Pediatric Drugs, 17*, 273–281. doi:10.1007/s40272-015-0130-8.

Dhivyalashmi, J., Bhattacharyya, S., Reddy, R, et al. (2014). Precocious pseudopuberty due to ovarian causes. *Indian Pediatrics, 51*(10), 831–833. Retrieved from http://www.indianpediatrics.net/oct2014/831.pdf.

Elder, D.A., Hornung, L.N., Herbers, P.M., et al. (2014). Rapid deterioration of insulin secretion in obese adolescents preceding the onset of type 2 diabetes. *Journal of Pediatrics, 166*(3), 672–678. doi:10.1016/j.jpeds.2014.11.029.

Ergun-Longmire, B., & Wajnrajch, M. (2013). Growth and growth disorders. *Endotext [Internet]*. Retrieved from http://www.ncbi-nlm-nih-gov.lp.hscl.ufl.edu/books/NBK279142/.

Fuqua, J.S. (2013). Treatment and outcomes of precocious puberty: an update. *The Journal of Clinical Endocrinology and Metabolism, 98*(6). 2198–2207. doi:10.1210/jc.2013-1024.

Garibaldi, L.R., & Chemaitilly, W. (2016). Central precocious puberty. In R. Kliegman, B. Stanton, J. St. Geme, et al. (Eds.), *Nelson textbook of pediatrics* (20th ed., pp. 2626-2658). Philadelphia: Elsevier.

Gregory, J.M., Moore, D.J., & Simmons, J.H. (2013). Type 1 diabetes mellitus. *Pediatrics in Review, 34*(5), 203–215. doi:10.1542/pir.34-5-203.

Huang, S.A., & LaFranchi, S.H. (2016). Hyperthyroidism. In R. Kliegman, B. Stanton, J. St. Geme, et al. (Eds.), *Nelson textbook of pediatrics* (20th ed., pp. 2680–2685). Philadelphia: Elsevier.

Huether, S.E., & McCance, K.L. (2017). *Understanding pathophysiology*. St. Louis: Elsevier.

Jain, V., Ravindranath, A. (2015). Diabetes insipidus in children. *Journal of Pediatric Endocrinology and Metabolism*, doi:10.1515/jpem-2014-0518.

Klingensmith, G.J., Tamborlane, W.V., Wood, J., et al. (2013). Diabetic ketoacidosis at diabetes onset: Still an all too common threat in youth. *The Journal of Pediatrics, 162*(2), 330–334. doi:10.1016/j.jpeds.2012.06.058.

Knip, M., & Simell, O. (2012). Environmental triggers of type 1 diabetes. *Cold Spring Harbor Perspectives in Medicine, 2*(7). doi:10.1101/cshperspect.a007690.

LaFranchi, S.H., & Huang, S.A. (2016a). Hypothyroidism. In R. Kliegman, B. Stanton, J. St. Geme, et al. (Eds.), *Nelson textbook of pediatrics* (20th ed., pp. 2665–2675). Philadelphia: Elsevier.

LaFranchi, S.H., & Huang, S.A. (2016b). Thyroiditis. In R. Kliegman, B. Stanton, J. St. Geme, et al. (Eds.), *Nelson textbook of pediatrics* (20th ed., pp. 2675–2677). Philadelphia: Elsevier.

Lee, L. (2012). Metabolic syndrome. *Pediatrics in Review, 33*(10). doi:10.1542/pir.33-10-459.

Leger, J., Olivieri, A., Donaldson, M., et al. (2014). European society for paediatric endocrinology consensus guidelines on screening, diagnosis, and management of congenital hypothyroidism. *The Journal of Clinical Endocrinology and Metabolism, 99*(2), 363–384. doi:10.1210/jc.2013-1891.

May, A., Kuklina, E., & Yoon, P. (2012). Prevalence of cardiovascular disease risk factors among US adolescents, 1999-2008. *Pediatrics, 129*(6), 1035–1041.

Mitchell, J.J. (2013). Phenylalanine hydroxylase deficiency. *Gene reviews*. Retrieved from http://www.ncbi.nlm.nih.gov/books/NBK1504/.

Nierengarten, M.B. (2016). Pitfalls in pediatric type 1 diabetes management. *Contemporary Pediatrics, 33*(4), 16–20.

Nimkarn, S., Lin-Su, K., & New, M.I. (2011). Steroid 21 hydroxylase deficiency congenital adrenal hyperplasia. *Pediatric Clinicals of North America, 58*(5), 1281–1300. doi:10.1016/j.pcl.2011.07.012.

Parks, J.S., & Felner, E.I. (2016). Hypopituitarism. In R. Kliegman, B. Stanton, J. St. Geme, & et al. (Eds.), *Nelson textbook of pediatrics* (20th ed., pp. 636–640). Philadelphia: Elsevier.

Ranadive, S.A., & Rosenthal, S.M. (2011). Pediatric disorders of water balance. *Pediatric Clinics of North America, 58*(5). 1271–1280. doi:10.1016/j.pcl.2011.07.013.

Rezvani, I., & Ficicoglu, C.H. (2016). Phenylalanine. In R. Kliegman, B. Stanton, J. St. Geme, et al. (Eds.), *Nelson textbook of pediatrics* (20th ed., pp. 636–640). Philadelphia: Elsevier.

Rivkees, S.A. (2014). Pediatric Graves' disease: management in the post-propylthiouracil Era. *International Journal of Pediatric Endocrinology, 1*, 1–10. doi:10.1186/1687-9856-2014-10.

Sobotka, S.A., Danielson, K.K., Drum, M.L., et al. (2014). Maternal body mass index (BMI) is independently associated with the control of diabetes mellitus in young patients. *Pediatric Nursing, 40*(4), 187–194.

Srinivasan, S., & Misra, M. (2015). Hyperthyroidism in children. *Pediatrics in Review, 36*(6), 239–248. Retrieved from https://www.ncbi.nlm.nih.gov/pubmed/?term=Srinivasan%2C+S.%2C+%26+Misra%2C+M.+(2015).+Hyperthyroidism+in+children.+Pediatrics+in+Review%2C+36(6).+239-248

St. Onge, E., Miller, S.A., Motycka, C., et al. (2015). A review of the treatment of type 2 diabetes in children. *Journal of Pediatric Pharmacology, 20*(1), 4–16. doi:10.5863/1551-6776-20.1.4.

Svoren, B.M., & Jospe, N. (2016a). Type 1 diabetes mellitus (immune mediated). In R. Kliegman, B. Stanton, J. St. Geme, et al. (Eds.), *Nelson textbook of pediatrics* (20th ed., pp. 2763–2783). Philadelphia: Elsevier.

Svoren, B.M., & Jospe, N. (2016b). Type 2 diabetes mellitus. In R. Kliegman, B. Stanton, J. St. Geme, et al. (Eds.), *Nelson textbook of pediatrics* (20th ed., pp. 2783–2785). Philadelphia: Elsevier.

Vockley, J., Anderson, H.C., Antshel, K.M., et al. (2014). Phenylalanine hydroxylase deficiency: diagnosis and management guideline. *Genetics in Medicine, 16*(2), 188–200. doi:10.1038/gim.2013.157.

White, P.C. (2016). Congenital adrenal hyperplasia due to 21-hydroxylase deficiency. In R. Kliegman, B. Stanton, J. St. Geme, et al. (Eds.), *Nelson textbook of pediatrics* (20th ed., pp. 2714–2723). Philadelphia: Elsevier.

Wolfsdorf, J.I., Allgrove, J. Craig, M.E., et al. (2014). ISPAD clinical practice consensus guidelines 2014 compendium: diabetic ketoacidosis and hyperglycemic hyperosmolar state. *Pediatric Diabetes, 15*(Suppl 20), 154–179. doi:10.1011/pedi.12165.

# 52

# The Child With a Neurologic Alteration

http://evolve.elsevier.com/McKinney/mat-ch/

## LEARNING OBJECTIVES

*After studying this chapter, you should be able to:*

- Describe the embryologic development of the nervous system.
- Describe the anatomy and physiology of the nervous system.
- Describe the normal compensatory mechanisms that keep intracranial pressure within a constant range.
- Identify the neurologic differences between the infant, child, and adult.
- Be able to perform a neurologic assessment of a child and record findings.
- Use the nursing process to assess, plan, and provide nursing care to children with common neurologic alterations.
- Discuss the nursing implications of medications frequently used in the management of neurologic disorders.
- Describe teaching strategies that can be used for the child with neurologic problems and the child's family.
- List the measures used to keep a child safe during a seizure.
- List the measures used to prevent or treat cerebral edema.
- Differentiate between abnormal flexion and extension posturing and discuss the significance of each.
- List the compensatory mechanisms that affect intracranial blood flow and extravascular fluid volume if hydrocephalus develops.

## CLINICAL REFERENCE

## REVIEW OF THE CENTRAL NERVOUS SYSTEM

### Embryologic Development

The nervous system is one of the first systems to form *in utero.* A neural tube remains hollow throughout development and eventually becomes the central nervous system. By the 4th week of gestation, the neural tube has closed at the anterior end to form the brain and at the posterior end to form the spinal cord.

During the second month of gestation, the brain becomes the prominent body structure. It grows rapidly and continues to grow until approximately the fifth year of life. Two periods of rapid brain cell growth appear to occur during gestation. Between the 15th and 20th weeks of gestation, the number of neurons increases significantly. At 30 weeks, the number of neurons increases again, continuing through 1 year of age. Appropriate prenatal care during periods of rapid neuronal increase can prevent developmental neurologic deficits.

### The Myelin Sheath

Myelin is the fatty substance that surrounds the nerves of both the central and the peripheral nervous systems. The myelin begins to form at approximately the 16th week of gestation. Myelin insulates the nerves and helps conduct electrical impulses. Coordination of fine and gross motor skills progresses with the deposition of the myelin sheath. Nerve fibers can conduct impulses in the absence of myelin; however, the impulses travel more slowly. Gross motor skills develop before fine motor skills as coordination and control advance throughout childhood. The myelin sheath can be destroyed by disease, drugs, and the aging process.

### The Neural System

The neural system develops multiple connections between the areas of the brain that control specific functions, including vision, hearing, movement, sensation, coordination, and speech. Each function is under the control of a specific area of the brain. The right half, or hemisphere, of the brain controls the left side of the body and is concerned with the social aspects of perception, intuition, and experience. The left hemisphere controls the right side of the body and is largely concerned with the acquisition and use of language and logical verbal reasoning.

The neonate's nervous system functions at a subcortical level. Spinal cord reflexes, such as sucking and cardiorespiratory functions, are present. Cortical functions, including memory and coordination, are only partially developed.

### The Axial Skeleton

The axial skeleton protects the underlying structures of the central nervous system (CNS). For convenience of study, the bones of the skull and the vertebral column are divided into regions that form the wall of the cranial cavity and the spinal column. The frontal, occipital, temporal, and parietal bones form the cranial vault. The floor of the cranial vault is composed of three compartments, or fossae—the anterior, middle, and posterior fossae. The anterior fossa houses the frontal lobes of the brain, the middle fossa contains the upper brainstem and the pituitary gland, and the posterior fossa contains the lower brainstem. Blood vessels and cranial nerves enter and leave the skull through the foramina.

At birth, the skull plates are not fused but are separated by nonossified spaces called *fontanels.* The posterior fontanel usually fuses by age 2 months and the anterior fontanel by 16 to 18 months. The fontanels allow the cranium to expand in response to rapid brain growth. Before fusion of the fontanels and sutures, an increase in intracranial pressure (ICP) will produce an increase in head circumference and can result in macrocephaly.

Because brain growth is rapid during infancy, the long-term sequelae of neurologic insults that occur to infants are difficult to

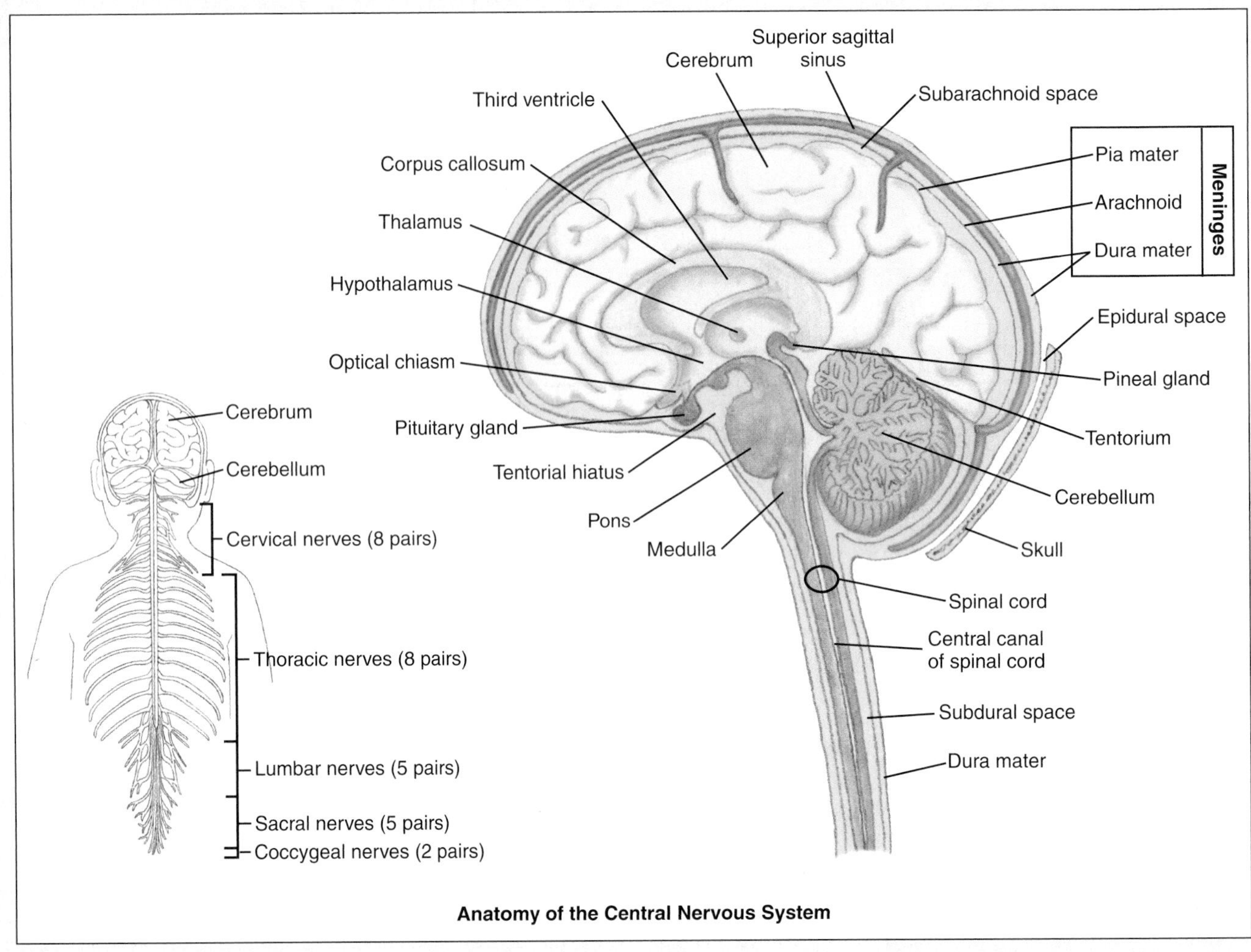


**Anatomy of the Central Nervous System**

## Pediatric Differences in the Central Nervous System

- The brain constitutes 12% of a newborn's body weight compared with only 2% of an adult's body weight.
- The brain of a term infant is two thirds the weight of an adult's brain. By the age of 1 year, it weighs 80% as much as an adult's brain, and by the age of 6 years, it weighs approximately 90% as much as an adult's brain.
- An infant has approximately 50 mL of cerebrospinal fluid (CSF) compared with 150 mL in an adult.
- The peripheral nerves are not completely myelinated by birth. As myelinization progresses, so do the child's coordination and fine muscle movements.
- The head circumference in a term infant is 34 to 35 cm. By the age of 6 months, the head circumference is 44 cm; by the age of 12 months, it is 47 cm.
- Papilledema rarely occurs in infancy because of the open fontanels and sutures, which can expand with increased intracranial pressure.
- The primitive reflexes of Moro, grasp, and rooting, present at birth, disappear at various times during the first 5 months. These primitive reflexes may reappear with neurologic disease.

predict. Brain growth can be assessed by head circumference measurements. These measurements are an important part of the routine physical examination of children and should be plotted on a growth chart. Insufficient or excessive head and brain growth indicate a potential neurologic problem. Premature closing of the fontanels or sutures can cause massive neurologic damage, and continued evaluation by the physician is needed.

### The Meninges

The meninges are the membranes that surround the brain and spinal column. The outer layer is the dura mater, a fibrous connective tissue structure containing many blood vessels. The dura mater consists of two layers having outer and inner meningeal components. Between the periosteum of the bone and the dura mater lies the epidural space. Sheets of dura also extend downward and inward to form partitions within the cranium. The falx cerebri separates the cerebral hemispheres, and the falx cerebelli separates the cerebellar hemispheres.

The tentorium is a tent-like structure that separates the cerebellum from the occipital lobe of the cerebrum. The large gap through which the brainstem passes is the tentorial hiatus.

The middle meningeal layer is the arachnoid, a delicate, avascular, web-like, serous membrane loosely covering the brain. Between the arachnoid and the dura lies the subdural space, which contains a small amount of fluid, just sufficient to prevent adhesion of the two membranes.

The innermost layer is the pia mater. It is a delicate, transparent membrane that adheres closely to the outer surface of the brain. The pia mater is a vascular membrane, consisting of arteries and veins.

Between the pia mater and the arachnoid is the subarachnoid space, which is filled with cerebrospinal fluid (CSF). The CSF acts as a cushion to reduce the force of trauma on the brain. Endothelial cells within the brain form a semipermeable **blood-brain barrier** that allows some substances to pass to the brain and prevents others from entering. The blood-brain barrier provides protection for the brain.

## The Brain

The three sections of the brain are the cerebrum, the cerebellum, and the brainstem. The cerebrum is the largest component, filling the upper portion of the skull. It is divided into two hemispheres, right and left, which are separated by a longitudinal fissure. The two hemispheres are joined by a band of commissural fibers called the *corpus callosum*. The cerebral hemispheres are further divided into lobes in relation to the cranial bones: frontal, parietal, temporal, and occipital. The cerebrum also includes part of the thalamus, the hypothalamus, the **basal ganglia**, and the olfactory and optic nerves.

The cerebellum is composed of white matter and gray matter. The gray matter is often referred to as the **cerebral cortex**. It is attached to the brainstem by paired bundles of fibers. The brainstem consists of the midbrain, the pons, the medulla, the thalamus, and the third ventricle.

## The Cranial Nerves

Twelve pairs of cranial nerves arise from the brain and brainstem, each with a specific function. Testing these nerves can indicate the location and degree of CNS injury (see Chapter 33).

## The Spinal Cord

The spinal cord is described as segmented into the cervical, thoracic, lumbar, and sacral regions. The spinal nerves are named for their corresponding vertebral segments.

The spinal cord transmits signals to and from the brain and responds to local sensory information through automatic motor responses called *reflexes*. The simplest type of spinal cord response is the reflex arc. Sensation is transmitted to the spinal cord from a sensory nerve fiber. It synapses with a motor neuron in the same cord segment, causing a muscle or tendon contraction in the corresponding motor nerve. Deep tendon reflexes are examples of the reflex arc.

Sensory innervation occurs as sensory nerves carrying body sensations enter the spinal cord on the dorsal surface. Most sensory fibers for pain and temperature ascend to the brain by lateral spinal tracts. Sensory fibers for touch and pressure ascend through anterior tracts. Almost all sensory fibers pass through the thalamus, where the perceptions of touch, pressure, and temperature are interpreted. Perceptions of texture, size, and weight are interpreted in the cortex.

Motor nerves are stimulated to respond after the brain receives a signal from a sensory nerve. The motor nerves cross over to the contralateral (opposite) side of the spinal cord from which they originate and then exit on the ventral surface of the spinal cord. The side of the body contralateral to the injured side of the brain will be the side affected by injury.

Functional differences exist between the upper and lower motor neurons. The outcome of a spinal cord injury is affected by the site of the injury. An injury between the brain and the dendrites (the nerve fibers that carry impulses toward the cell body) will render the brain incapable of signaling the muscle cells to cease responding reflexively, and the muscle will become contracted, or spastic. If the injury is to a section of the nerve between the muscle and axons (the nerve fibers that carry impulses away from the cell body), the muscles will become incapable of responding reflexively, causing them to become flaccid.

## Cerebrospinal Fluid

Cerebrospinal fluid (CSF) is a clear liquid produced in the choroid plexus of the ventricles at approximately 0.3 to 0.4 mL/min. The CSF aids in protecting the brain, spinal cord, and meninges by acting as a watery cushion surrounding them to absorb the shocks to which they are exposed. CSF also functions to maintain homeostasis as it drains unwanted substances away from the brain. It is reabsorbed through the arachnoid villi into the venous sinuses. The total volume of CSF is renewed approximately three times or more each day.

## Cerebral Blood Flow and Intracranial Regulation

The internal carotid arteries supply blood to all parts of the brain. Approximately 17% of cardiac output and 20% of body oxygen are transported to the brain. The brain requires approximately 10 times the oxygen used by the rest of the body.

Cerebral blood flow (CBF) is controlled by **cerebral perfusion pressure** (CPP), which is the difference between the mean arterial blood pressure (MBP) and the ICP.

**Autoregulation**, or self-regulation, is a unique physiologic capability. It allows cerebral arteries to change diameter in response to changes in the CPP. The cerebral vessels can maintain a steady blood flow to the brain during alterations in blood pressure and perfusion. However, autoregulation fails when the limits of cerebrovascular dilation are reached.

Autoregulation can be impaired as a result of trauma, ischemia, or increased intracranial pressure. It is influenced significantly by changes in partial pressure of oxygen in arterial blood ($Pao_2$) and partial pressure of carbon dioxide in arterial blood ($Paco_2$). An increase in $Paco_2$ (above 40 mm Hg) produces cerebral vasodilation and an increase in CBF. A decrease in $Paco_2$ (25 to 30 mm Hg) causes cerebral vasoconstriction, and thus, reduces blood flow to the brain. Alterations in $Pao_2$ between 80 and 100 mm Hg have little effect on CBF, although hypoxia dramatically increases CBF.

### CSF Analysis in Children: Normal Findings

| | NEONATE | | |
|---|---|---|---|
| Parameter | Preterm | Term | Child Older Than 6 mo |
| WBCs (per mm$^3$) | ≤25 | ≤19 (infants aged 6-28 days)<br>≤9 (infants aged 29-56 days) | ≤5 |
| Protein (mg/dL) | <150 | <170 | <45 |
| Glucose (mg/dL) | >30 | >60 | >40 |
| Pressure (mm Hg) | 50-80 | 50-80 | 100-280 |

## Cerebrospinal Fluid Analysis: Findings in Pathologic Conditions

| Condition | Appearance | Pressure | Cells | Protein | Glucose/Other |
|---|---|---|---|---|---|
| Traumatic tap | Bloody; supernatant fluid clear | Normal | Any red blood cells | 4 mg/dL rise per 5000 red cells | Not applicable |
| Acute bacterial meningitis | Cloudy to milky or yellow (xanthochromatic) | Usually elevated | Polymorphonuclear cells: ≥100/mm$^3$ | 100-500 mg/dL | Decreased compared with blood glucose |
| Viral meningitis | Clear | Normal or increased | Zero to a few hundred per mm$^3$, mostly leukocytes | 50-200 mg/dL | Normal |
| Encephalitis | Clear, colorless | Normal or slightly increased | Normal or increased | 50-200 mg/dL | <40 mg/dL |
| Subdural hematoma | Yellow to clear, colorless | Increased | Normal | Normal or increased | Normal |
| Diabetic coma | Clear, colorless | Decreased | Normal | Normal or slightly increased | May be 200-300 mg/dL |
| Guillain-Barré syndrome | Clear | Normal | <10 white blood cells per mm$^3$ | More than 2× normal | Normal |

## Common Diagnostic Tests and Procedures for Neurologic Disorders

| Test | Description | Purpose | Nursing Considerations |
|---|---|---|---|
| CT scan | Produces computer image of horizontal and vertical cross sections of brain at any axis. | To identify abnormal tissue and structures as in brain tumor, bleeding, or hydrocephalus. | Insert IV line if contrast medium is used. Notify the radiologist if the child is allergic to iodine. May need to sedate child. Consider number of previous CT scans and risk of radiation exposure; MRI sometimes preferred. |
| Angiography | After IV contrast dye is injected, a clear image of the vessels is obtained; view of all other tissues not infused with dye is eliminated. | To reveal vascular abnormalities. | NPO order is possible. Notify the radiologist if the child is allergic to iodine. Obtain signed permission form. Some restrictions on activity necessary after the test. |
| Echoencephalography | Echoes from ultrasonic waves are recorded as they reflect off various surfaces of the skull. | To identify abnormal structure, position, and function. | Painless procedure. No preparation. |
| EEG | Electrodes placed on the scalp conduct and amplify electrical activity; electrical potential of the brain is measured and recorded. | To identify abnormal electrical brain discharges, such as in seizures. | Child allowed regular diet and fluids but no caffeine or stimulants. Hair should be clean. May include sleep EEG; in this case, child should be sleep deprived the night before test. The procedure is painless. |
| Long-term video EEG | Continuous EEG with video of physical symptoms. Process can last 24 hr to several days. | To enable clinical events to be recorded and played back for in-depth review, as well as correlated with the presence of abnormal electrical activity. | Electrodes are secured with skin glue. Electrode sites should be evaluated and documented every shift. Child will have to stay in a small area during testing. Age-appropriate toys and activities are made available. |
| Lumbar puncture | CSF pressure is measured and a specimen obtained as a needle is inserted into the subarachnoid space between L3 and L4 or L4 and L5. | To determine pressure and analyze CSF. Can identify hemorrhage or infections. Procedure can be used to administer medications. | Obtain signed consent. Instruct the child to lie on the side with the knees up to chest. After the procedure, the child lies flat. If not fluid restricted, encourage fluids after the procedure. Use a topical anesthetic at needle insertion site to decrease pain, whenever possible. |
| MRI | Produces computer images of the brain by radiofrequency emissions from certain elements. | To demonstrate morphologic features of tissue and structures with high degree of detail. | The procedure is painless, but the child must not move; sedation may be necessary for children under the age of 8 yr. Inform child that loud clicking noises will be heard. The child's head will be restrained. |
| Nuclear brain scan (SPECT) | A radioactive substance is injected IV. Abnormal uptake indicates abnormal tissue or structure. | To identify focal brain lesions by allowing the visualization of blood flow through the brain. | The child must remain still during the test. An IV line is needed. The amount of the substance injected is measured and recorded. |

*CBC,* Complete blood count; *IV,* intravenous.

Reference: Lehman, R.K., & Schor, N.F. (2016). Neurologic evaluation. In R. Kliegman, B. Stanton, J. St. Geme, et al. (Eds.), *Nelson textbook of pediatrics* (20th ed., pp. 2791–2802). Philadelphia: Elsevier.

## Lumbar Puncture: Educating the Family

If the child is old enough to understand, explain the following:

- The child will need to lie on his or her side with body bent and knees and chin touching. Explain that you will help hold the child in that position by "hugging" the knees to the chin. If there is time, allow the child to practice the position. (An infant can be in a side-lying position or a sitting position with the infant facing you and your thumbs across the infant's scapulae; steady the infant's head against your body.) For an older child, consider demonstrating the procedure on a stuffed animal or doll.
- Tell the child that the physician will wash the child's back with a cool liquid. After that, the child might feel a "pinch" or "sting" as the needle is inserted. A topical anesthetic should be used whenever possible to decrease the pain caused by the needle. The child must remain still.
- Encourage the child to relax, sing, take deep breaths, or use guided imagery throughout the procedure to help decrease anxiety. The collection of CSF samples and pressure measurement usually takes several minutes. When the needle is withdrawn, the child will feel light pressure and the application of a small dressing.

Remember to do the following:

- Monitor the child's cardiorespiratory status throughout the procedure.
- Maintain the child's position with shoulders and hips aligned to prevent rotation of the spine.
- Help the parents comfort the child during and after the procedure.

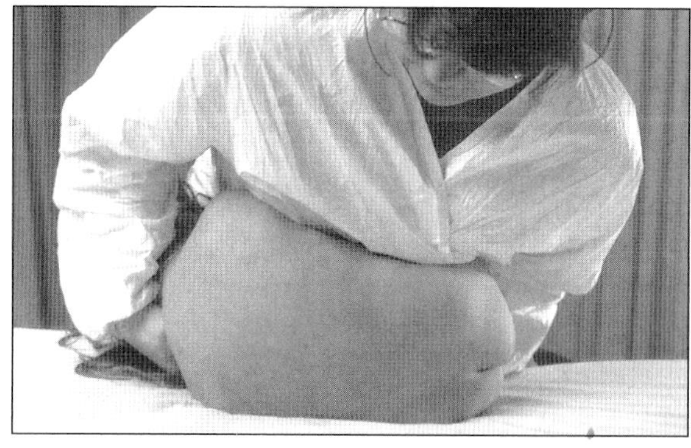

For the lumbar puncture: Place one hand farther down, under the child's neck. Your forearm moves behind the child's head to support the neck. Place the other arm farther under the child's upper thighs and curl the child's body by bringing the knees up to the head. Note that this nurse's weight is supported on the edge of the examination table, and the nurse leans slightly over the child, controlling the arms and legs. Because direct visibility of the child's respiratory status is limited in this position, a cardiorespiratory monitor must be used for the child. (Courtesy Cook Children's Medical Center, Fort Worth, TX. © Bob Lukeman, photographer.)

Care of the child with a neurologic problem requires knowledge of neuroanatomy, neurophysiology, and normal growth and development. The nurse plays an important role in the early recognition of pediatric neurologic problems, some of which have the potential for devastating long-term outcomes. The nurse assesses the child's condition by comparing the child's normal behavior with current behavior. The family is an invaluable source of information about the child's normal behavior and how current behavior deviates from that norm. The child and the family need support and understanding because the child's condition is a crisis in their lives. The family's ability to respond and influence the child's coping mechanisms directly influences the recovery and adaptation process.

Many conditions of the nervous system share common assessment data, diagnoses, and interventions. Principles of nursing care for the child with a nervous system disorder can be applied to a variety of situations.

## INCREASED INTRACRANIAL PRESSURE

Increased intracranial pressure (ICP) reflects the pressure exerted by the blood, brain, CSF, and any other space-occupying fluid or mass. Increased ICP results from a disturbance in autoregulation and is defined as pressure sustained at 20 mm Hg or higher for 5 minutes or longer.

### Etiology

Alterations in the brain can result from a space-occupying lesion, such as a brain tumor or hematoma. The brain can swell as a result of head trauma, infection, or a hypoxic episode. Overproduction of fluid, malabsorption of fluid, or a communication problem within the system can disrupt CSF dynamics. Aneurysms within the brain and acute liver failure can also lead to increased ICP.

### Manifestations

Signs and symptoms of increased ICP differ according to the child's developmental level (Box 52.1).

#### Level of Consciousness

Children with increased ICP often have an altered level of consciousness. The Glasgow Coma Scale (GCS) is a standardized scale that, in a modified form, is frequently used to assess level of consciousness in infants and children. It consists of a three-part assessment: eye opening, verbal response, and motor response (Table 52.1). Each level of response is assigned a numeric value. When the assessment of each response is complete, the scores are added, providing an objective measure of the child's level of consciousness and the severity of the injury (Ducharme-Crevier & Wainwright, 2015). The total scores

### BOX 52.1 Developmental Manifestations of Increased Intracranial Pressure

**Infant**

- Poor feeding or vomiting
- Irritability or restlessness
- Lethargy
- Bulging fontanel
- High-pitched cry
- Increased head circumference
- Separation of cranial sutures
- Distended scalp veins
- Eyes deviated downward ("setting-sun" sign)
- Increased or decreased response to pain

**Child**

- Headache
- Diplopia
- Mood swings
- Slurred speech
- Papilledema (after 48 hr)
- Altered level of consciousness
- Nausea and vomiting, especially in the morning

## NURSING CARE PLAN

### The Child With a Neurologic System Disorder

#### Focused Assessment

- Assess child's level of consciousness using the Glasgow Coma Scale (GCS) modified for children.
- Assess child's orientation, mood, and behavior.
  - Compare with normal developmental milestones for age.
  - Observe interactions with family and environment.
  - Note lethargy, drowsiness, hyperactivity, tremors, or jitteriness.
- Assess motor skills, balance, and coordination.
  - Observe child dressing, playing, throwing a ball, using a pencil, or touching finger to nose.
  - Observe child walking to assess gait (look for hemiplegia, scissors gait, wide-spaced gait).
  - Check muscle development, strength, and tone.
- Determine range of motion for all joints.
- Test deep tendon reflexes, comparing side to side.
- Assess for sensory function and symmetry of both sides of face, trunk, arms, and legs.
  - Test for vibration, superficial tactile sensation, superficial pain, and temperature.

#### Nursing Diagnosis

Risk for Ineffective Tissue Perfusion (cerebral) related to alteration of arterial or venous blood flow, cerebral infarction, hemorrhage, hematoma, increased intracranial pressure (ICP), cerebral edema, seizures, hypoventilation, or increased cerebral metabolism.

#### Planning

***Expected Outcomes***

The child will:

1. Have improved cerebral perfusion, as evidenced by absence of cranial nerve deficits, improved or normal level of consciousness, vital signs in baseline normal, and GCS score within normal limits.
2. Demonstrate appropriate behavior or thought patterns for age.

#### Interventions and *Rationales*

1. Determine the child's baseline age and developmental level.
   *Baseline age and developmental level will help the nurse gauge changes in neurologic status.*
2. Perform a baseline neurologic and level of consciousness (LOC) assessment and measure vital signs on admission.
   *Changes in neurologic signs can indicate deterioration or improvement in status. Changes are compared with baseline.*
3. Monitor factors that may further increase cerebral edema and ICP (hypoxia, fever, seizures, hypotension, hypercapnia).
   *Monitoring these factors allows for correction of conditions that increase ICP and keeps cerebral metabolic needs to a minimum.*
4. Maintain head of bed at a 30- to 45-degree angle.
   *Venous outflow drainage of the brain is facilitated by gravity.*
5. Avoid the prone or flat, supine position, neck flexion, or hip flexion.
   *These positions tend to increase ICP. Neck flexion can partially occlude the jugular vein and impairs drainage. Hip flexion can increase intraabdominal or intrathoracic pressure, thus increasing ICP.*
6. Organize nursing care around periods of low ICP. Decrease stimulation (noise, bright lights, touch, movement, pain) and avoid activities as much as possible that cause agitation and may increase ICP.
   *Nursing care such as suctioning, bathing, and repositioning, and other stimuli increase ICP; minimizing stimuli will decrease ICP.*
7. Monitor pupil size and reactivity to light every hour as needed or as ordered.
   *An increase in pupil size and no or sluggish constriction in response to light may indicate an increase in ICP.*
8. Monitor vital signs every 1 to 2 hours.
   *Acute changes in vital signs may indicate increased ICP.*
9. Measure head circumference daily or more often as needed, and record on age-appropriate growth chart.
   *If fontanels are open, cranial expansion takes place when the cerebrospinal fluid (CSF) is under pressure.*
10. Palpate the anterior fontanel every 8 hours if age-appropriate.
    *An increase in fontanel size and tenseness may indicate an increase in CSF accumulation.*
11. Palpate the cranial suture lines every 8 hours if age-appropriate.
    *The cranial sutures may separate with an increase in CSF volume or pressure.*
12. Observe the infant for irritability, lethargy, feeding intolerance, and decreasing GCS score.
    *These are signs of increasing ICP and deteriorating neurologic status.*
13. Place emergency equipment (oxygen, suction, bag-valve-mask) near the child's room or at the bedside.
    *Increased ICP can cause apnea and may lead to cardiopulmonary arrest.*

#### Evaluation

Does the child demonstrate an improved LOC?

Are vital signs within normal limits?

Does the child show intact cranial nerve function, an optimum level on the GCS, and behavior and thought patterns appropriate for age?

#### Nursing Diagnosis

Imbalanced Nutrition: Less Than Body Requirements related to restricted intake, neurologic impairment, swallowing or chewing difficulty, risk for aspiration, nausea, or vomiting.

#### Planning

***Expected Outcome***

The child will have adequate nutritional intake, as evidenced by maintaining stable or normal weight for age and height; exhibiting normal serum protein levels, moist mucous membranes, and adequate urine output; and being free of nausea and vomiting.

#### Interventions and *Rationales*

1. Determine the child's LOC before giving liquids.
   *A decreased LOC increases the risk of aspiration with swallowing.*
2. Weigh the child daily on the same scale, at the same time of day, and in the same clothes. Record on a growth chart.
   *Changes in weight indicate alterations in fluid balance and nutritional status. Being consistent with timing and type of clothing enhances accurate comparison. The nurse should weigh the child only if the procedure does not increase ICP.*
3. Monitor skin turgor, mucous membranes, eye orbits, urine output, urine specific gravity, and serum and urine electrolyte values.
   *These are indicators of fluid and electrolyte status.*
4. Consult a registered dietitian.
   *The dietitian will advise how best to meet metabolic demands and plan the most efficient way to provide the child with calories.*
5. Position the child or infant upright after feedings. If the child is old enough and the ICP is not elevated, the head should be slightly flexed and facing forward. Arms should be positioned forward with feet placed on a firm surface.

## NURSING CARE PLAN—cont'd

### The Child With a Neurologic System Disorder

*Proper positioning will decrease the risk of aspiration, enhance comfort, prevent contractures, and provide for safety while feeding/eating.*

6. Verify placement of any oral or nasogastric tube before tube feedings are initiated.
   *Incorrect placement of a nasogastric tube can result in placing feedings into the lungs (see Chapter 37).*
7. Provide a flexible feeding schedule with small feedings of favorite foods.
   *These techniques facilitate digestion, voluntary food intake by the child, and the ability to maintain adequate caloric intake.*
8. Minimize handling around feeding times.
   *Minimal handling during feeding decreases the likelihood of vomiting and aspiration.*
9. If swallowing is impaired, assist the child with chewing by holding the child's chin and jaw.
   *Swallowing may be facilitated by this method, because it keeps the child's head stabilized in an appropriate anatomic position.*
10. Obtain order to medicate for nausea and vomiting if necessary.
    *The child will be more likely to tolerate feedings when nausea is controlled.*

**Evaluation**

Does the child show normal growth for age, with no weight loss?
Does the child have age-appropriate caloric intake daily?
Does the child have proper hydration with moist mucous membranes and age-appropriate urine output for age?
Is the child free from nausea and vomiting?

**Nursing Diagnosis**

Risk for Impaired Skin Integrity related to neuromuscular impairment, decreased level of consciousness, inadequate physical activity, immobility, or improper fluid or nutritional intake.

**Planning**

***Expected Outcome***

The child's skin will remain intact and free from pressure breakdown.

**Interventions and *Rationales***

1. Use pressure-equalizing mattress or special flotation mattress to protect bony prominences. Reposition every 2 hours and as needed. Check for redness and pressure areas.
   *The child with a depressed LOC may not be active, and immobility can lead to skin breakdown.*
2. Observe skin condition every 2 hours with the repositioning of the child or infant.
   *Prolonged pressure on the skin will quickly lead to breakdown.*
3. Avoid putting temperature probes, cardiac monitor leads, or excessive tape over a ventriculoperitoneal shunt site.
   *Irritation from adhesives will contribute to skin breakdown and possible infection.*
4. Encourage parents to participate in passive range-of-motion exercises for the child, if appropriate.
   *Participating in the child's care enhances the parents' sense of control and the child's sense of well-being. Passive range-of-motion exercises provide emotional and physical support for the child and increase the child's activity.*
5. If braces or splints are used, assess the skin before and after the splints or assistive devices are put on and taken off.
   *Correct application of braces will minimize pressure points and reduce skin breakdown.*
6. Implement a daily skin care regimen. Teach parents or family to check skin frequently.
   *Bathing, moisturizing, and inspecting the skin will preserve skin integrity.*

**Evaluation**

Does the child have intact, clean, dry skin without pressure areas or ulcers?

**Nursing Diagnosis**

Anxiety (parental) related to change in the child's health status; the child's behavior changes, possible injury, seizures, neurologic impairment; threat to parental role identity, social isolation, or lack of privacy.

**Planning**

***Expected Outcome***

The parents will demonstrate management of anxiety, as evidenced by maintaining social and personal relationships, verbalizing relaxation, verbalizing feelings about the child's neurologic impairment, and demonstrating effective coping skills.

**Interventions and *Rationales***

1. Keep the parents informed of the child's progress, prognosis, and plan of care. Encourage parents to talk about concerns and ask questions. Allow parents to make decisions when possible.
   *Control over any event in the child's care helps the parents feel they are part of the caregiving team and lessens their anxiety.*
2. Encourage parents to participate actively in activities of daily living (e.g., oral hygiene, bathing, feeding), as the child's condition permits.
   *Touching the child and actively participating in the child's care lower parental anxiety.*
3. Orient the parents to hospital routine, and refer to clergy, social worker, and other team members.
   *A familiar environment is less threatening and will enable the family to more positively deal with the child's condition and prognosis.*
4. Encourage rooming-in when possible.
   *Rooming-in will involve the parents more in the child's care, facilitate collaboration with the healthcare team, and decrease the child's anxiety.*
5. Assist with anxiety-reduction techniques such as relaxation techniques, music, and guided imagery.
   *Such techniques facilitate coping and stress reduction.*

**Evaluation**

Are the parents able to discuss concerns and fears?
Do the parents plan with the team for the child's future and participate in decision making?
Are the parents able to state reduced feelings of anxiety?
Do the parents demonstrate coping and problem-solving skills?

**Nursing Diagnosis**

Deficient Knowledge related to unfamiliarity with infectious process, disease process, medication regimen, dietary or fluid needs, measures for prevention, or chronic illness of a child or infant.

**Planning**

***Expected Outcome***

The child and parents will verbalize and demonstrate an understanding of the child's disease process, as evidenced by stating age-appropriate, realistic

*Continued*

## NURSING CARE PLAN—cont'd

### *The Child With a Neurologic System Disorder*

factors about the child's condition; listing factors to decrease neurologic deficits and measures to prevent further occurrences of illness; and demonstrating medication administration and nutritional adaptations.

**Interventions and *Rationales***

1. Allow time for family education. If the child is to undergo surgery, provide preoperative teaching for the child and parents.
   *Teaching answers questions and reinforces information given to the parents by the physician. It includes the parents in the learning experience.*
2. Determine the parents' understanding of the child's condition, including the child's need for physical, speech, or occupational therapy.
   *Parents need to understand their child's intellectual and physical abilities and challenges in order to give informed consent or reinforce the need for rehabilitative therapies.*
3. Refer the parents to community and Internet-based support groups.
   *Support can be gained by seeing or hearing how others coped with similar situations.*
4. Supply the parents with telephone numbers to call for needed information once they are home.
   *Healthcare providers can help parents feel in touch and educate them at the same time by discussing the child's condition on the telephone.*
5. Teach the parents important signs and symptoms to monitor related to their child's condition, side effects of medications, and when to call the physician or nurse. Provide written instructions.
   *The parents need to state important signs and symptoms that indicate a change in the child's condition and be aware of when to seek medical attention. Anxiety reduces learning and attention span. A written copy of signs and symptoms and instructions provides an ongoing resource that can be referred to later.*
6. Review the signs and symptoms of wound infection.
   *Until the surgical incision is healed, the risk of infection is present.*
7. Instruct the parents to watch for signs and symptoms of urine retention or urinary tract infection.
   *Because of retention and reflux, the child may be at risk for urinary tract infections. Parents must seek treatment for the child if signs and symptoms of retention or infection are observed.*
8. Provide reliable and credible Internet resources for parents.
   *Credible Internet resources provide enhanced knowledge for parents and are available when parents are ready to learn more about their child's condition.*

**Evaluation**

Can the parents discuss the child's care appropriately?
Are the parents able to list situations in which the child should be seen by the physician or nurse?
Do the parents know how to contact community support?
Can the parents demonstrate an understanding of their child's disease and care requirements?

**TABLE 52.1 Glasgow Coma Scale Modified for Children**

| Child | Infant |
|---|---|
| **Eyes** | |
| 4 = Opens eyes spontaneously | 4 = Opens eyes spontaneously |
| 3 = Opens eyes to speech | 3 = Opens eyes to speech |
| 2 = Opens eyes to pain | 2 = Opens eyes to pain |
| 1 = No response | 1 = No response |
| ____ = *Score (Eyes)* | |
| **Motor** | |
| 6 = Obeys commands | 6 = Spontaneous movements |
| 5 = Localizes | 5 = Withdraws to touch |
| 4 = Withdraws | 4 = Withdraws to pain |
| 3 = Flexion | 3 = Flexion (decorticate) |
| 2 = Extension | 2 = Extension (decerebrate) |
| 1 = No response | 1 = No response |
| ____ = Score (Motor) | |
| **Verbal** | |
| 5 = Oriented | 5 = Coos and babbles |
| 4 = Confused | 4 = Irritable cry |
| 3 = Inappropriate words | 3 = Cries to pain |
| 2 = Incomprehensible words | 2 = Moans to pain |
| 1 = No response | 1 = No response |
| _____ = *Score (Verbal)* | |

Reprinted from James, H.E., Anas, N.G., & Perkin, R.M. (1985). *Brain insults in infants and children.* Orlando, FL: Grune & Stratton.

range from 15, indicating no change in level of consciousness, to 3, indicating a deep coma and poor prognosis. A score of 8 or less requires aggressive management and monitoring of ICP (Hartman & Cheifetz, 2016). This tool can help detect brain injury early to prevent permanent damage (Kochanek & Bell, 2016).

## NURSING QUALITY ALERT

### *Standard Terms for Level of Consciousness*

Level of consciousness should be described by the nurse using standard terminology:

- *Full consciousness:* Awake, alert, oriented, interacts with environment
- *Confused:* Lacks ability to think clearly and rapidly; usually oriented to person
- *Delirious:* Not oriented to person, place, or time; impairment of reality with auditory or visual hallucinations possible
- *Disoriented:* Lacks ability to recognize place or person
- *Lethargic:* Very drowsy and needs increased stimuli to be awakened
- *Obtunded:* Sleeps unless aroused; once aroused has limited interaction with the environment; answers questions with minimal response
- *Stupor:* Requires vigorous stimulation to arouse
- *Coma:* Vigorous stimulation produces no motor or verbal response

### Behavior

Changes in the child's normal behavior pattern may be an important early sign of increased ICP. Parents often are the first to notice a change in the child's behavior; therefore, a parent's comment that "he isn't acting like himself" should be taken seriously. Irritability, mild confusion, and agitation are symptoms that warrant further assessment. The child who no longer recognizes parents, cannot follow commands, or has minimal response to pain is deteriorating. Decreased responsiveness to painful stimuli is a significant sign of alteration in level of consciousness.

### Pupil Evaluation

As ICP rises, compression of the third cranial nerve occurs, resulting in pupil dilation with sluggish or absent constriction in response to light. A fixed, dilated pupil is an ominous sign in an unconscious child. This condition suggests **herniation** of the center section of the brain (also known as a transtentorial herniation). Other eye dysfunctions associated with increased ICP include ptosis and ovoid pupil. Older children might complain of blurry vision, diplopia, or decreased visual acuity.

### Motor Function

The child with increased ICP exhibits changes in motor function. Purposeful movement will decrease, and abnormal posturing may be observed. **Flexion**, or **decorticate posturing**, refers to flexion of the upper extremities (elbows, wrists) and extension of the lower extremities. Plantar flexion of the feet may also be observed. This type of posturing implies an injury to the cerebral hemispheres. **Extension**, or **decerebrate posturing**, involves extension of the upper extremities with internal rotation of the upper arm and wrist. The lower extremities will extend, with some internal rotation noted at the knees and feet. This type of posturing indicates damage to more areas of the brain, such as the diencephalon, midbrain, or pons. The progression from flexion to extension posturing usually indicates deteriorating neurologic function and warrants physician notification (Fig. 52.1). Flaccid paralysis indicates further deterioration in the child's condition.

### Vital Signs

Temperature elevation may occur in children with increased ICP. **Cushing's response**, which consists of an increased systolic blood pressure with widening pulse pressure, bradycardia, and a change in respiratory rate and pattern, is usually apparent just before or at the time of brainstem herniation. This response usually indicates an alteration in brainstem perfusion, with the body attempting to improve cerebral blood flow by increasing blood pressure. In children, Cushing's response is a late sign of increased ICP.

As ICP rises, the child's baseline respiratory pattern may change, exhibiting Cheyne-Stokes respiration, central neurogenic hyperventilation, or apneustic breathing. *Cheyne-Stokes respiration* refers to a pattern of breathing characterized by increasing rate and depth and then decreasing rate and depth with a pause of variable length. The cycle will be repeated again and again. *Central neurogenic hyperventilation* is identified by a rapid rate despite normal arterial blood gas values. This type of breathing pattern usually indicates midbrain or pontine involvement. *Apneustic breathing* occurs when the child demonstrates prolonged inspiration and expiration. As Cushing's response occurs, the child will develop apnea. Late signs of increased ICP include tachycardia that leads to bradycardia, apnea, systolic hypertension, widening pulse pressure, and flexion or extension posturing.

### Diagnostic Evaluation and Therapeutic Management

Diagnostic tests for increased ICP include computed tomography (CT), magnetic resonance imaging (MRI), lumbar puncture, serum and urine electrolytes, arterial blood gas determinations, a complete blood cell count, electroencephalography (EEG), and radiography. Normal blood gas levels are $Pao_2$ greater than 80 mm Hg and $Paco_2$ less than 45 mm Hg in a child with normal ICP.

The management of increased ICP is multimodal and is directed toward treating its underlying cause, reducing the volume of the CSF, preserving cerebral metabolic function, and avoiding situations that increase ICP. An intraventricular catheter may be used to measure ICP, drain CSF, and/or administer medications (Box 52.2).

The head of the child's bed should be elevated 30 degrees with midline positioning of the head, and normothermia should be maintained. The child may be given an osmotic diuretic (e.g., mannitol) or hypertonic saline, sedation and analgesia, and anticonvulsant medications (Kochanek & Bell, 2016). Blood glucose levels are closely monitored to maintain normal levels and prevent further increases in metabolic demands. Intravenous fluid boluses with normal saline are used for children with hypovolemia (Kochanek & Bell, 2016). Hyperventilation is used if there are signs of cerebral herniation (Kochanek & Bell, 2016). Corticosteroids are no longer used in the treatment of increased ICP due to traumatic brain injury (TBI) (Kochanek & Bell, 2016).



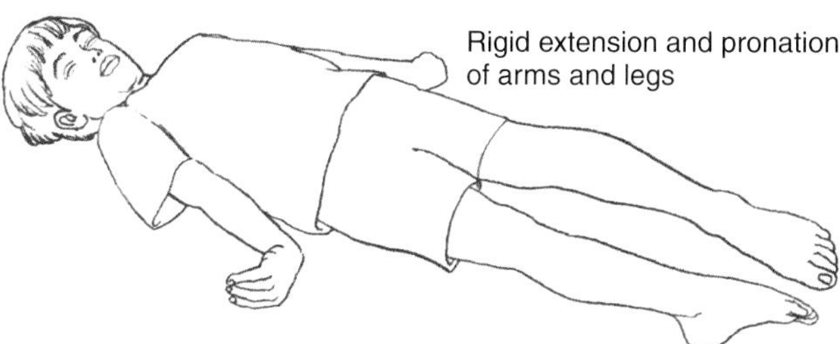


**FIG 52.1** Flexion and extension posturing.

## SPINA BIFIDA

Spina bifida is a congenital neural tube defect (NTD) characterized by incomplete closure of the vertebrae and neural tube during fetal

**BOX 52.2 Instruments for Monitoring Increased Intracranial Pressure**

| Subarachnoid Bolt | Intraventricular Catheter |
|---|---|
| The end of the bolt is placed in the subarachnoid space. The top of the bolt is attached to a transducer to conduct a waveform to the monitor. The neurosurgeon adjusts the transducer to produce a waveform on the monitor. | The catheter is placed in the lateral ventricle or subarachnoid space. The catheter provides a method for measuring pressure, as well as a conduit to drain off extra fluid into the drainage bag. The manometer and drainage bag are part of a sterile, closed system. |

## PATHOPHYSIOLOGY

### Increased Intracranial Pressure

The major pathophysiologic changes associated with increased intracranial pressure (ICP) result from alterations in the brain, cerebrospinal fluid (CSF) dynamics, and cerebral blood flow. To maintain cerebral pressure and volume within normal range, changes in one or more of the contents of the cranium must be compensated for by changes in the others; this is referred to as the **Monro-Kellie doctrine**.

Compensatory mechanisms include a reduction in CSF production, an increase in CSF absorption, and a reduction in cerebral mass as a result of fluid displacement. Once the limits of compensation are reached, any further increase in volume or pressure will cause a sudden increase in ICP and an associated decline in the child's clinical status. Ultimately, increased ICP will compromise cerebral perfusion and produce shifting of brain tissue, causing herniation. The consequences of herniation depend on its severity and location.

Herniation is classified into four types:

- *Transtentorial herniation* occurs when part of the brain herniates downward and around the tentorium cerebelli. This condition can be unilateral or bilateral, involving the anterior or posterior regions of the brain. If a large amount of tissue is involved, it can cause death because vital brain structures are compressed and become unable to perform their functions.
- *Temporal lobe herniation,* or uncal herniation, refers to a shifting of the temporal lobe laterally across the tentorial notch. This condition produces compression of the third cranial nerve and ipsilateral pupil dilation. If pressure continues to rise, flaccid paralysis, pupil dilation, pupil fixation, and death will result.
- *Tonsillar herniation* occurs when the cerebellar tonsils herniate through the foramen magnum. The child will develop nuchal rigidity, shoulder or arm numbness, and changes in heart and respiratory rates and patterns. Arnold–Chiari malformation, a condition sometimes associated with hydrocephalus, includes herniation of the cerebellar tonsils.

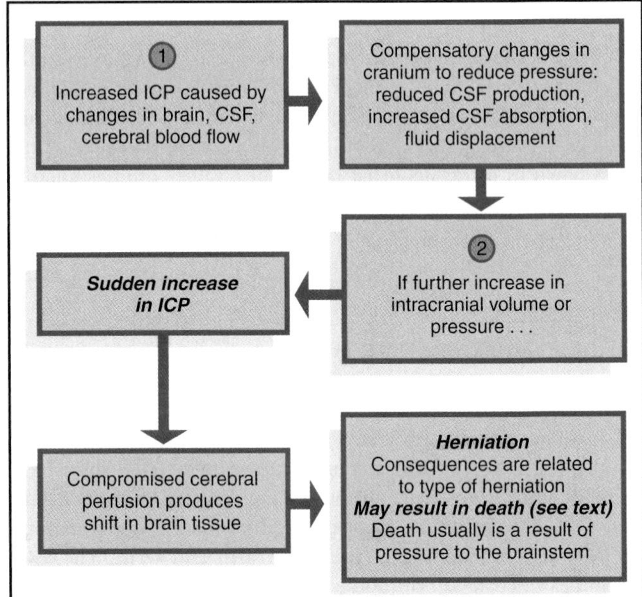


- *Brainstem herniation* through the foramen magnum results in death from compression of vital cardiorespiratory centers.

Infants are somewhat able to compensate for increasing ICP because their cranial sutures remain open. *Craniosynostosis* is premature closure of the cranial sutures. This abnormal skull development causes an abnormally shaped skull. In some cases, craniectomy is needed to manage the increased ICP.

## EVIDENCE-BASED PRACTICE

The Glasgow Coma Scale (GCS) (see Table 52.1) is one of the most widely used assessment tools for determining and monitoring changes in level of consciousness in patients who have sustained neurologic insult. First introduced in the mid-1970s, its original purpose of assessing the level of consciousness in an adult after a traumatic brain injury has been expanded in general use to include assessing diagnostic and prognostic criteria for individuals with traumatic brain injury. Because the *best verbal response* of the GCS was particularly difficult to assess in preverbal infants and children as well as in intubated children and adults, various modifications of the scale for use with these populations have been presented in the literature.

Research relating to reliability and validity of the original GCS has demonstrated varying results. GCS is useful for making decisions regarding neuroimaging, airway management, and return to play of injured athletes. However, studies recognize the limitations associated with verbal scoring, particularly in children younger than 5 years of age. The use of sedation can cause practitioners to underestimate scores. Furthermore, because evidence suggests that improper implementation can lead to inappropriate scoring, interrater reliability is also a limitation. Nurses in clinical practice should be certain the scale is used in a trustworthy manner and with high interrater reliability.

Several in-depth reviews of research on the GCS have suggested the following limitations that apply to clinical practice for nurses:

- Experienced personnel are more accurate and consistent in the application of the scale criteria than are inexperienced personnel.
- Several conditions (e.g., sedation, endotracheal intubation, fractures) interfere with accurate observation of parts of the scale, and thus, rely on individual clinician judgment for scoring.
- When assessing response to painful stimuli, nurses use a variety of methods to elicit the pain response, thus calling into question the consistency, accuracy, and reliability of the assessment.

What implications do these pieces of research have for clinical practice? The GCS is only one part of an overall neurologic assessment. Correlation of the patient's history, symptoms, and radiology study results are imperative components of a complete neurologic evaluation. Clinical agencies should consider first establishing a consistent and written procedure for assessing all components of the scale, then pairing inexperienced nurses with experienced nurses to ensure appropriate training and execution of the assessment procedure to increase interrater reliability.

References: Cicero, M.X., & Cross, K.P. (2013). Predictive value of initial Glasgow coma scale score in pediatric trauma patients. *Pediatric Emergency Care, 29*(1), 43–48; Kochanek, P.M., & Bell, M.J. (2016). Neurological emergencies and stabilization. In R. Kliegman, B. Stanton, J. St. Geme, et al. (Eds.), *Nelson textbook of pediatrics* (20th ed., pp. 507–514). Philadelphia: Elsevier; Woischneck, D., Firsching, R., Schmitz, B., et al. (2013). The prognostic reliability of the Glasgow coma score in traumatic brain injuries: evaluation of MRI data. *European Journal of Emergency Surgery, 39,* 79–86. doi:10.1007/s00068-012-0240-8.

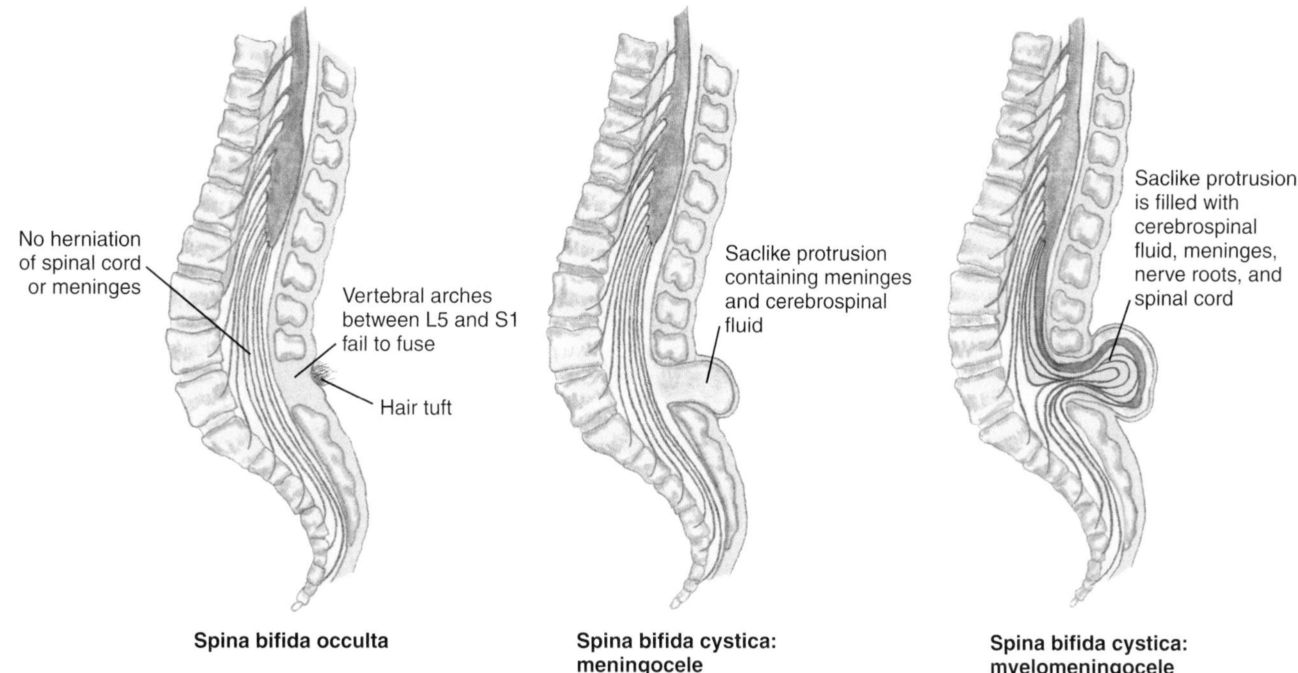
No herniation of spinal cord or meninges
Vertebral arches between L5 and S1 fail to fuse
Hair tuft
Spina bifida occulta
Saclike protrusion containing meninges and cerebrospinal fluid
Spina bifida cystica: meningocele
Saclike protrusion is filled with cerebrospinal fluid, meninges, nerve roots, and spinal cord
Spina bifida cystica: myelomeningocele

FIG 52.2 Three forms of spina bifida.

development. Spina bifida is classified as spina bifida occulta and spina bifida cystica (Fig. 52.2). Spina bifida occulta usually occurs between the L5 and S1 vertebrae, with failure of the vertebrae to completely fuse. Some children with spina bifida occulta have no sensory or motor defects. The only clinical manifestation may be a dimple, a small tuft of hair, a hemangioma, or a lipoma in the lower lumbar or sacral area, detected accidentally on routine radiographs. Spina bifida cystica is a more extensive defect with a range of sensory and motor impairments.

## Etiology and Incidence

The cause of spina bifida is unknown in most cases. Evidence suggests a possible genetic predisposition. Maternal folic acid deficiency has been strongly linked to neural tube defects. Daily consumption of 0.4 mg of folic acid by all women of childbearing age is recommended and 4 mg if the mother has had a previous child with a NTD. Evidence of a viral origin has prompted research, but other than folic acid, no cause or preventive measures have been identified.

## Manifestations

In addition to the appearance of the lesion, manifestations relate to the degree of deficit, which is determined by the level of the lesion (Fig. 52.3).

| | |
|---|---|
| T12: | Flaccid lower extremities, decreased sensation, and bowel and bladder incontinence |
| L1 to L3: | Hip flexion, flail feet |
| L2 to L4: | Hip adduction |
| L3 to S2: | Hip adduction, hip extension, knee flexion |
| S3 and below: | No motor impairment |
| Sacral roots: | Plantar flexion |

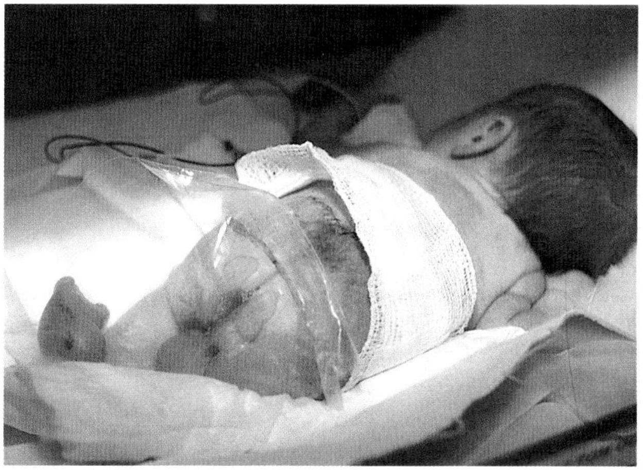

FIG 52.3 This infant has a repaired myelomeningocele. Note the left clubfoot. This deformity often accompanies the defect because normal intrauterine movement does not occur in the fetus with spina bifida, interfering with the development of the extremities. The legs are flaccid, and normal neonatal flexion is absent. The infant also dribbles stool and urine constantly. Hydrocephalus commonly accompanies these neural tube defects. (Courtesy Parkland Health and Hospital System, Dallas, TX.)

Children with spina bifida are at high risk for developing latex allergies because of frequent exposure to latex during catheterizations, shunt placements, and other operations. Latex allergy is estimated to occur in approximately 73% of children with spina bifida. Allergic reactions can range from mild signs and symptoms to anaphylactic shock. Children should be tested for latex allergy, and precautions should be taken from birth to decrease exposures. The nurse should check equipment and supplies for latex and select nonlatex alternatives for use. The Spina Bifida Association website (http://spinabifidaassociation.org/latex/) has good resources for parents about latex items

## PATHOPHYSIOLOGY

### *Spina Bifida*

Spina bifida occurs during the 4th week of gestation (days 24 to 28), when ventral induction of the neural tube fails to occur. The degree of impairment corresponds to the level of the defect on the spinal cord and the size of the defect. Ninety percent of spinal cord lesions are at or below the L2 vertebra. The lesion results in paralysis, partial paralysis, or varying sensory defects. Clubfeet, scoliosis, and contracture and dislocation of the hips often accompany the defect. Spina bifida cystica results in incomplete closure of the vertebrae and neural tube, evidenced by a sac-like protrusion in the lumbar or sacral area with varying degrees of nervous tissue involvement. Spina bifida cystica is further described as meningocele, myelomeningocele, lipomeningocele, and lipomyelomeningocele. Meningocele is a sac-like protrusion filled with spinal fluid and meninges. The most severe form is myelomeningocele, in which the sac is filled with spinal fluid, meninges, nerve roots, and spinal cord. Hydrocephalus and Arnold–Chiari malformation occurs in 80% of patients with myelomeningocele. The mortality rate is approximately 10% to 15%.

The incidence of myelomeningocele is 1 in 4000 live births. In the United States, this number is declining. Awareness of the importance of folic acid supplementation during pregnancy and prenatal diagnostic techniques have contributed to a reduction in children born with this defect. Nearly 80% of infants with myelomeningocele will require shunting to treat associated hydrocephalus.

Reference: Kinsman, S.L., & Johnston, M.V. (2016b). Myelomeningocele. In R. Kliegman, B. Stanton, J. St. Geme, et al. (Eds.), *Nelson textbook of pediatrics* (20th ed., pp. 2805–2806). Philadelphia: Elsevier.

found in the home, community, and hospital (Spina Bifida Association, 2015).

### Diagnostic Evaluation

Diagnostic tests include determining alpha-fetoprotein (AFP) levels in blood at 16 to 18 weeks of gestation. If the AFP screen is elevated, amniocentesis and fetal ultrasound are performed. After delivery, the infant may undergo a CT scan or myelography.

### Therapeutic Management

Prenatal microsurgical closure of the myelomeningocele, performed at approximately 19 to 25 weeks of gestation, shows promise for reducing the severity of Chiari type II malformations and incidence of hydrocephalus (Kinsman & Johnston, 2016a). Risks associated with prenatal surgery include premature birth, with its associated consequences, and possible fetal death. Maternal risks (e.g., abruptio placentae, preterm membrane rupture, preterm labor, wound infection, chorioamnionitis, uterine hemorrhage, loss of uterus, and damage to adjacent organs) are directly related to the hysterotomy.

Following birth, immediate surgical closure of the defect decreases the risk of infection, morbidity, and mortality. Other benefits are improved prognosis without further cord deterioration and earlier and easier physical handling and bonding between the newborn and the parents.

The child will need lifelong management of neurologic, orthopedic, and urinary problems and is best managed in a multispecialty outpatient setting. Urodynamic studies are performed early, and a bladder-emptying program is initiated, with close monitoring of the child's urinary tract infection status. In most instances, the child will require orthopedic bracing and possibly orthopedic surgery to maximize the child's mobility. Spina bifida clinics that coordinate care between the multiple providers to implement the plan of care for a patient in one visit have fewer complications and hospitalizations of patients and improved communication between providers and the patient and their family (Brustrom, Thibadeau, John, et al., 2012).

## HYDROCEPHALUS

Hydrocephalus develops as a result of an imbalance between the production and absorption of CSF. As excess CSF accumulates in the ventricular system, the ventricles become dilated and the brain is compressed against the skull. This results in enlargement of the skull if the sutures are open; it results in signs and symptoms of increased ICP if the sutures are fused.

### Etiology

Hydrocephalus may be congenital, acquired, or of unknown etiology. In infancy, hydrocephalus is most often congenital or related to prematurity. Congenital hydrocephalus results from developmental defects such as Arnold-Chiari malformations, congenital arachnoid cysts, congenital tumors, or aqueductal stenosis. In premature infants, neonatal meningitis or subarachnoid hemorrhage can result in hydrocephalus. Hydrocephalus is often associated with myelomeningocele. Intrauterine infection and perinatal hemorrhage cause hydrocephalus in some infants. In older children, hydrocephalus is usually acquired as a complication of meningitis, tumor, or hemorrhage.

### Incidence

The estimated prevalence of hydrocephalus is 1 to 2 in every 1,000 children in the United States (National Institute of Neurological Disorders and Stroke [NINDS], 2013a). Obstructive, or noncommunicating, hydrocephalus accounts for nearly all cases of hydrocephalus in children. Communicating hydrocephalus in a premature infant usually occurs because of a subarachnoid hemorrhage (Kinsman & Johnston, 2016a).

### Manifestations and Diagnostic Evaluation

Because of anatomic differences between infants and children, manifestations of hydrocephalus differ according to developmental stage (Table 52.2).

Diagnostic tests for hydrocephalus include serial measurements of head circumference, CT, MRI, ultrasonography, and lumbar puncture with pressure monitoring.

### Therapeutic Management

Therapy is aimed at preventing further CSF accumulation and reducing disability and death. The objective is to bypass the blockage and drain the fluid from the ventricles to an area where it can be reabsorbed into the circulation. A *ventriculoperitoneal shunt,* a tube leading from the ventricles out of the skull and passing under the skin to the peritoneal cavity, accomplishes this goal (Fig. 52.4). An alternative shunt, the *ventriculoatrial shunt,* which is used in older children, drains the fluid from the ventricles to the right atrium of the heart.

Shunt infection in the first 6 months occurs in 10% of infants, and shunt malformation in the first 2 years is also common; therefore, children should be monitored closely, especially for fever (Wenger, 2014). Shunt infection is decreasing with the use of antibiotic-coated ventroperitoneal shunts (Wenger, 2014). The shunt may need to be revised as the child grows. Long-term follow-up is essential.

A surgical procedure, endoscopic third ventriculostomy, facilitates the rerouting of CSF around the obstructed ventricular system

**TABLE 52.2 Early and Late Manifestations of Hydrocephalus**

| Early | Late |
|---|---|
| **Infant** | |
| Rapid head growth: increase in head circumference above the normal growth curve | Setting-sun sign: sclera visible above the iris |
| Full, bulging anterior fontanel | Frontal bone enlargement or bossing |
| Irritability | Vomiting, difficulty feeding and swallowing |
| Poor feeding | Increased blood pressure, decreased heart rate |
| Distended, prominent scalp veins | Altered respiratory pattern |
| Widely separated cranial sutures | Shrill, high-pitched cry |
| | Sluggish or unequal pupillary response to light |
| **Child** | |
| Strabismus | Seizures |
| Frontal headache that occurs in the morning and is relieved by emesis or by sitting upright | Increased blood pressure |
| Nausea and vomiting (can be projectile) | Decreased heart rate |
| Diplopia | Alteration in respiratory pattern |
| Restlessness | Blindness from herniation of the optic disc |
| Changes in ability to do schoolwork | Decerebrate, extension posturing and rigidity |
| Behavior or personality changes | |
| Ataxia | |
| Papilledema | |
| Irritability | |
| Sluggish and unequal pupillary response to light | |
| Confusion | |
| Lethargy | |

(Kinsman & Johnston, 2016a). This technique has become increasingly popular over the past 20 years. For this procedure, the surgeon creates a small burr hole in the skull through which an endoscope is passed. The third ventricle is visualized, and a small opening is created in its floor. This opening allows the CSF to bypass the fourth ventricle and return to circulation, where it is reabsorbed. The procedure is 50% to 80% successful in children older than 2 years. Other surgical techniques for treating hydrocephalus are preferred in some children, since a repeat of the procedure may be necessary (Kinsman & Johnston, 2016a).

## CEREBRAL PALSY

Cerebral palsy is a chronic, nonprogressive disorder of posture and movement. It is characterized by difficulty in controlling the muscles because of an abnormality in the extrapyramidal or pyramidal motor system (motor cortex, basal ganglia, cerebellum). Co-morbidities such as cognitive, hearing, speech, and visual impairments, as well as seizures, are common but vary widely from one affected child to another.

### Etiology and Incidence

The damage to the motor system can occur prenatally, perinatally, or postnatally (Box 52.3). Cerebral palsy (CP) is one of the most common chronic neurologic impairments in children, and more that 500,000 Americans are affected. The rate of cerebral palsy is 3.6/1000 live births (Johnston, 2016). Problems associated with prematurity and low birth weight are related to the occurrence of CP. Aggressive neonatal intensive care, administration of surfactant to mature infant lungs, and administering steroids to mothers before delivery has improved survival rates and also resulted in an increased prevalence of CP, with 59.5/1000 weighing less than 1000 g affected (CDC, 2015a). Infants with the lowest birth weights (less than 1000 g) may be at increased risk for CP because of intracerebral hemorrhage or periventricular leukomalacia (Johnston, 2016). However, in general, children diagnosed with CP are born at term after a normal labor and delivery (Johnston, 2016).

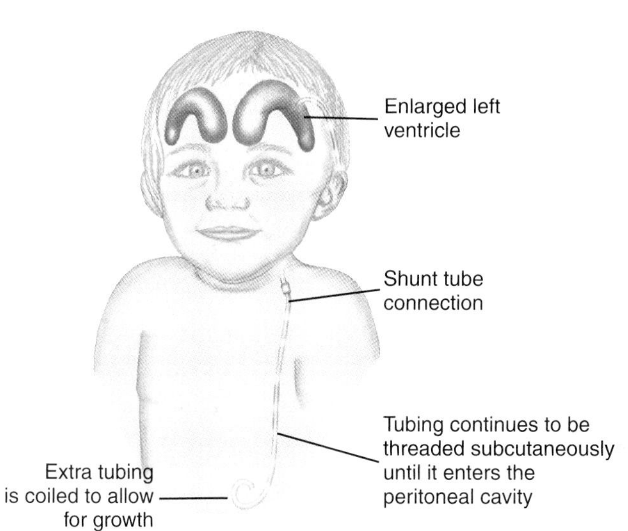


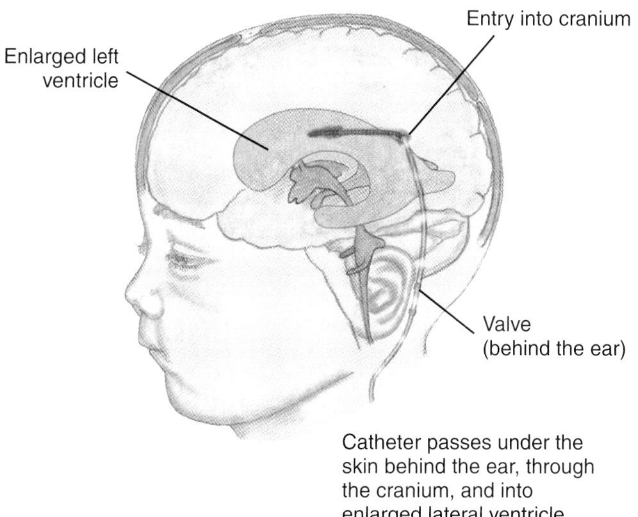


**FIG 52.4** A ventriculoperitoneal shunt may be implanted in the child with hydrocephalus to prevent excess accumulation of cerebrospinal fluid (CSF) in the ventricles. The tubing diverts the CSF from the ventricles into the peritoneal cavity, where it is reabsorbed. Nursing care includes monitoring for infection, obstruction, and pain, administering antibiotics and pain medications as ordered, and teaching the family how to change dressings and how to recognize shunt blockages or other problems.

## PATHOPHYSIOLOGY

### Hydrocephalus

Cerebrospinal fluid (CSF) is produced primarily by the choroid plexus, which lines the lateral ventricles. CSF circulates through the ventricular system and flows into the subarachnoid space around the brain and the spinal cord. It is then reabsorbed within the subarachnoid space.

Hydrocephalus results when either of the following conditions is present: (1) impaired absorption of CSF within the subarachnoid space *(communicating hydrocephalus)* or (2) obstruction of CSF flow within the ventricles that prevents CSF from circulating around the spinal cord and the subarachnoid space *(noncommunicating hydrocephalus)*. In rare cases, hydrocephalus is caused by overproduction of CSF because of a tumor of the choroid plexus.

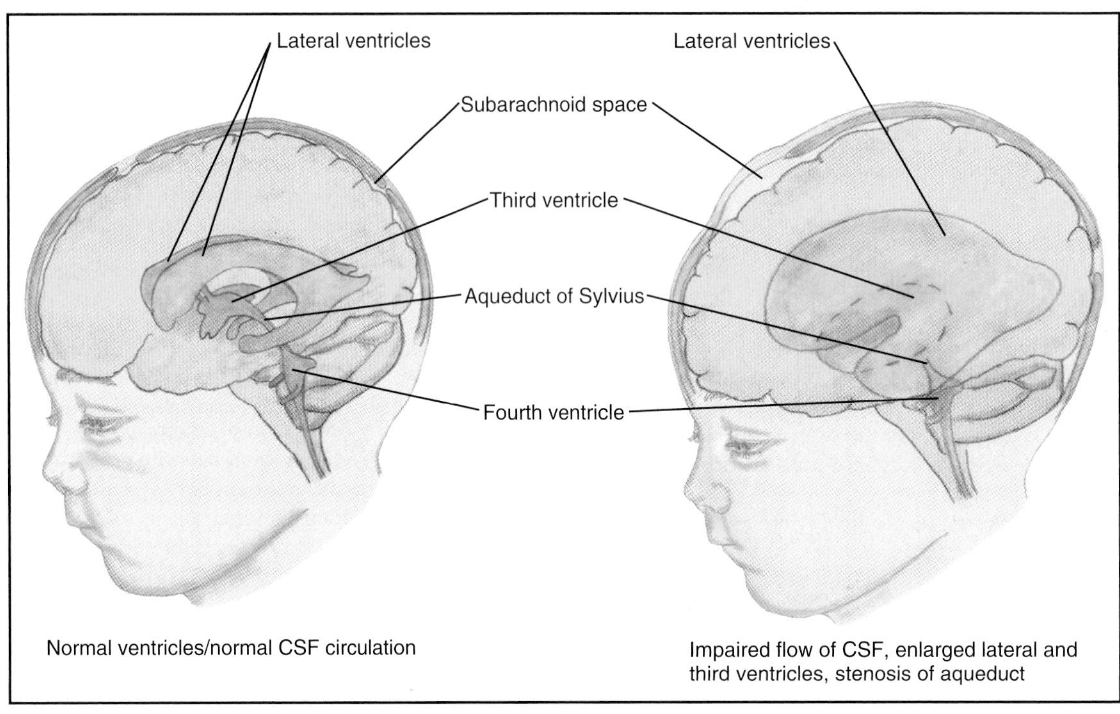


### BOX 52.3 Factors Associated With Cerebral Palsy

**Prenatal**
- Maternal diabetes
- Rh or ABO blood type incompatibility
- Rubella in the first trimester
- Genetic causes
- Intrauterine ischemic event
- Toxoplasmosis
- Cytomegalovirus
- Congenital brain abnormality
- Prenatal exposure to maternal infection
- Precipitous delivery
- Pregnancy-induced hypertension
- Birth trauma
- Anoxia
- Prolonged labor
- Perinatal metabolic condition (diabetes)
- Intracranial hemorrhage
- Other congenital anomalies

**Perinatal**
- Asphyxia
- Low birth weight
- Prematurity

**Postnatal**
- Infections
- Trauma
- Stroke
- Poisoning

### Manifestations

The manifestations of CP vary widely from one child to the other. A child with CP can have persistence of primitive reflexes, delayed gross motor development, abnormal muscle tone, and lack of progression through developmental milestones. Abnormal posturing with inability to maintain normal posture and balance may be present, as well as spasticity or uncontrollable movements in the extremities. Also seen are disturbances of gait (particularly ataxia and toe walking), seizures, attention-deficit disorder, sensory impairment, failure of automatic reactions (equilibrium), and speech and swallowing impairments.

### Diagnostic Evaluation and Therapeutic Management

A diagnostic evaluation includes EEG, CT scan or MRI, electrolyte levels, metabolic workup, a thorough history, and a complete neurologic examination. Additional genetic evaluation may be considered with patients who have congenital malformations. Assessment for developmental disorders is important since there is an increased incidence in children with CP (Johnston, 2016).

The goal of managing the child with CP is early recognition and intervention to maximize the child's abilities. Cerebral palsy often is not diagnosed before the child is 2 years old. Before age 2, the child may be diagnosed with *static encephalopathy,* a nonspecific term referring to permanent brain damage. Repetition of motor activities facilitates development of new brain pathways through alternative receptor sites and enhances appropriate motor function. The child might be intellectually intact, but this factor can be overlooked because of the child's physical limitations. Intrathecal baclofen, a skeletal muscle relaxant, administered via an infusion pump can be used to treat severe spasticity in children with CP. Benzodiazepines are also used to treat spasticity (Johnston, 2016) Botulinum toxin A injected into the muscle is an option for nonambulatory children to help with comfort and care (Edwards et al., 2015). Close monitoring of the child for infection and the pump for malfunction, as well as correct pump assembly and programming, are required.

A multidisciplinary healthcare team approach is necessary to meet the many needs of the child with CP. The team includes the child and family, pediatrician, neurologist, orthopedic surgeon, nurse, speech and hearing therapists, social worker, occupational therapist, physical therapist, educators, physiatrist, neurosurgeon, and orthotist.

## HEAD INJURY

Head injury refers to the pathologic result of any mechanical force to the scalp, skull, meninges, or brain.

### Types of Head Injuries

Types of head injury include the following:

- *Closed head injury:* Nonpenetrating injury to the head in which no break occurs in the integrity of the barrier between the outside environment and the intracranial cavity
- *Open head injury:* Penetrating injury to the head in which there is a break in the integrity of the barrier (skull, meninges) between the outside environment and the intracranial cavity; infection is a major concern
- *Coup injury:* Cerebral injury sustained directly below the site of impact

## PATHOPHYSIOLOGY

### *Cerebral Palsy*

A number of neuromuscular disabilities are associated with cerebral palsy. The alteration in voluntary muscular control is related to a cerebral insult. The area of the brain that is affected determines the type of neuromuscular disability.

The five classifications of cerebral palsy are dyskinetic, spastic, ataxic, rigid, and mixed:

- *Dyskinetic (athetoid) palsy* refers to a disorder in the basal ganglia. Slow, writhing, uncontrolled, involuntary movements involving all extremities characterize this type.
- *Spastic cerebral palsy* is the most common type. The affected area of the brain is the cortex. Spastic cerebral palsy is characterized by increased deep tendon reflexes, hypertonia, flexion, and sometimes contractures. The child's muscles are very tense, and any stimulus can cause a sudden jerking movement. The child has to make a conscious effort to relax. Scissors gait, hip flexion with adduction and internal rotation, or toe walking because of tight heel cords may be present.
- In *ataxic cerebral palsy,* the affected area of the brain is the cerebellum. This type of cerebral palsy is characterized by a loss of coordination, equilibrium, and kinesthetic sense. Overall, the child appears clumsy.
- *Rigid (tremor, atonic) cerebral palsy* is relatively rare in children. The child has rigidity of both flexor and extensor muscles. In a child with tremors, the tremors are apparent both at rest and during movement. The prognosis for a child with this type of cerebral palsy is poor because of associated deformities and lack of active movement.
- *Mixed* is more than one type of cerebral palsy. A common combination is spastic and dyskinetic.

Approximately half of children with cerebral palsy have other disabilities, including epilepsy, a cognitive disability, learning problems, poor attention span, hyperactivity, hearing or visual impairment, and emotional problems. Gastroesophageal reflux can occur (see Chapter 43). Intense movements that cause a high expenditure of calories along with feeding challenges can lead to a calorie deficit and poor nutritional status.

## NURSING CARE PLAN

### *The Child With Cerebral Palsy in the Community Setting*

**Focused Assessment**

- Monitor at risk infants for indications of cerebral palsy
  - Irritability, feeding difficulties, delayed development, poor motor development, abnormal posturing, persistent primitive reflexes, poor muscle tone, and ataxic gait
- Assess infants and children for delays in reaching developmental milestones (key indicator of cerebral palsy)
- For children with cerebral palsy, assess response to therapy
  - Monitor and document progress or lack of progress
- For school-age children with cerebral palsy, assess need for physical and learning adaptations in the school setting
  - Consider use of assistive devices (i.e., wheelchairs, walkers, communication boards, and computers)
  - Provide assessment on regular basis; the school nurse is member of educational team that develops the child's individual learning plan

**Nursing Diagnosis**

Impaired Physical Mobility related to spasticity and muscle weakness.

**Planning**

***Expected Outcomes***

1. The child will maximize ability for movement, as evidenced by freedom from contractures or injuries and no complications from immobility.
2. The parents will demonstrate how to do the child's exercises and notify the school nurse if any changes are made in the child's plan.

**Interventions and *Rationales***

1. Reinforce physical therapy exercises to strengthen and help coordination of muscles. These exercises may have to be performed in the school setting.
   *Early intervention and consistent therapy facilitate proper posture and circumvent the development of contractures.*
2. Encourage parents to be active in the child's daily physical and occupational therapies.
   *Active involvement in the child's care empowers the parents.*
3. Observe and record the child's response to physical therapy.
   *Changes in therapy may be made in a timely fashion for a higher degree of success.*

*Continued*

## NURSING CARE PLAN—cont'd

### *The Child With Cerebral Palsy in the Community Setting*

4. Determine the need for special equipment for reading, writing, eating, and mobility. Convey this information to the school evaluation team.
   *The use of special equipment improves the chance for successful self-care. Incorporating this into the child's education plan will maximize learning potential.*
5. Monitor the child for chronic pain resulting from surgical procedures and other interventions used to improve mobility and decrease spasticity.
   *Chronic pain can contribute to lack of well-being for the child and family.*

**Evaluation**

Have the child's joints remained mobile and free from contractures?
Does the child demonstrate improved mobility and self-care?
Can the parents demonstrate physical therapy techniques used for their child?
Have the parents notified the school about any changes in the child's plan of care?

**Nursing Diagnosis**

Delayed Growth and Development related to neuromuscular impairment.

**Planning**

***Expected Outcome***

The child will maximize potential for meeting growth and developmental milestones, as evidenced by participation in family, social, and school activities.

**Interventions and *Rationales***

1. Monitor the child's developmental level and cognitive abilities using specific and sensitive developmental screening tests, both on a routine basis and as needed.
   *The child with cerebral palsy should be given opportunities to learn and should be exposed to new experiences to maximize developmental progress.*
2. Encourage early intervention and refer for early intervention community programs. Promote participation in school programs including play and social activities involving peers.
   *Interventions by multidisciplinary providers will maximize the child's potential for learning. Involvement with peers is essential to achieving developmental milestones.*
3. Communicate and interact with the child at the child's functional level, not chronologic age.
   *A child with normal cognitive abilities can understand age-appropriate communication and speech, but a child with a decreased cognitive level may have different understanding than the chronologic age would indicate.*

**Evaluation**

Do the parents encourage social and developmental activities that maximize the child's potential?
Does the child attend public school and play with peers when possible?
Does the child participate in physical, speech, and occupational therapy at school?

**Nursing Diagnosis**

Risk for Injury related to spasticity, uncontrolled muscle movements, or seizures.

**Planning**

***Expected Outcomes***

1. The child will have a safe environment, as evidenced by freedom from injuries.
2. The parents will describe ways to adapt the child's environment to maximize safety.

**Interventions and *Rationales***

1. Teach the family principles for providing a safe environment (e.g., remove sharp objects and toys, pad sharp furniture edges).
   *A safe environment will reduce the risk of injury.*
2. Have the child wear a protective helmet and pads if falling occurs frequently.
   *A helmet protects against head injury.*
3. If the child is hospitalized, implement bedside seizure precautions. (Do not pad the rails with pillows.)
   *Keeping suction, oxygen, and airway equipment at the bedside and padding the side rails help prevent injury and allow for resuscitation of the child, if necessary. Pillows should not be used as pads because they may cause suffocation.*
4. Provide safe toys that are appropriate for age and developmental level.
   *No sharp, very small, or easily shattered toys should be allowed for the child who may fall because of erratic movements.*
5. Position the child upright during and after meals.
   *An upright position prevents aspiration from gastroesophageal reflux.*

**Evaluation**

Does the child remain free from injury?
Do the parents demonstrate safety measures for their child?
Have the parents adapted the child's environment to be safe and secure?

**Nursing Diagnosis**

Impaired Verbal Communication related to neuromuscular impairment and difficulty with articulation.

**Planning**

***Expected Outcome***

The child will maximize communication ability, as evidenced by appropriately expressing needs and developing methods for communicating with others.

**Interventions and *Rationales***

1. Use the child's usual mode of communicating, such as flash cards and talking boards, to facilitate communication.
   *Teaching aids help reinforce language and speech development and increase self-esteem.*
2. Refer the child to a speech therapist.
   *Early intervention maximizes speech capabilities.*
3. Encourage and reinforce speech therapy techniques, nonverbal methods of communication, and jaw control.
   *These techniques facilitate communication and decrease the child's frustration at not being understood.*
4. Encourage parents to convey in detail the child's communication techniques any time the child is in a new situation.
   *Sharing the child's communication techniques helps the child adjust to new situations.*

**Evaluation**

Does the child participate in groups using appropriate communication?
Does the child use various methods to communicate?
Do the parents allow time for the child to respond to questions and conversations?
Have the parents learned the same communication method that the child uses?

- *Contrecoup injury:* Cerebral injury sustained in the region or pole opposite the site of impact; caused by the rapid movements of the semisolid brain within the cranial vault
- *Missile injury:* Penetrating injury of the skull or brain, most often caused by a bullet
- *Impalement injury:* Penetrating injury caused by piercing of the scalp, skull, or brain by a sharp object

### Skull Fractures

Skull fractures include the following types:

- *Linear:* Straight-line fracture; dura not involved
- *Depressed:* Bone pressing downward, indented
- *Basilar:* Fracture of the base of the skull; symptoms are Battle sign, raccoon eyes, rhinorrhea, otorrhea, and hemotympanum (blood behind the eardrum)
- *Comminuted:* Fragmentation of the bone into many pieces or a multiple fracture line

### Contusion

Contusions are petechial hemorrhages along the superficial aspects of the brain. They can occur at the site of impact or in association with a lesion remote from the site of direct impact.

### Concussion

A concussion is transient and reversible neuronal dysfunction, with instantaneous loss of awareness and responsiveness.

### Intracranial Hemorrhage

Intracranial hemorrhages are defined as the following two types:

*Epidural:* Blood accumulates between the dura and the skull. Arterial damage is the usual type of injury; therefore, the hemorrhage develops rapidly (Fig. 52.5).

*Subdural:* Blood accumulates between the dura and the cerebrum. A subdural hemorrhage is usually caused by an injury to a vein and can be acute or chronic.

## Incidence

Multiple trauma is the leading cause of death in children beyond infancy. In the United States, nearly 500,000 children between infancy and 14 years of age are seen in emergency departments for assessment and treatment of traumatic brain injury (TBI); falls and motor vehicle crashes are the primary causes of TBI in this age-group (Atabaki, 2013; Geyer, Meller, Kulpan, et al., 2013; Mason, 2013). Other causes of head injuries include bicycle collisions, sports injuries, child abuse, and gunshot wounds.

## Manifestations

Head injuries are classified as minor, moderate, or severe as correlated with the GCS. Children with minor head injuries score 13 or higher on the GCS and can have a change in level of consciousness and also exhibit transient periods of confusion, irritability, vomiting, somnolence, and headache (Geyer et al., 2013). Moderate HI's score between 9 and 12, and a severe injury scores less than 8 (Geyer et al., 2013). Moderate to severe head injuries are marked by a decreased level of consciousness, changes in vital signs, signs of increased ICP, retinal hemorrhage, hemiparesis, and papilledema (Box 52.4). Seizures may occur within the first 7 days after a moderate to severe head injury (Geyer et al., 2013).

## Diagnostic Evaluation

A complete history of the event helps determine the mechanism of injury and whether the child lost consciousness. Spinal radiographs are obtained to ascertain any cervical spinal cord injury; these are followed by a complete neurologic examination. Any indication of increased ICP is quickly reported to the physician. CT scan and MRI are the most commonly used studies to evaluate head injury and rule out serious brain injuries such as intracranial hemorrhage and hematomas. When ordering a CT scan, providers must balance the risk of exposure to ionizing radiation and missing a clinically important head injury. Many guidelines agree that CT scans of the head are not routinely recommended and unnecessary CT scans in children should be avoided (Rivera, Roberson, Whelan, et al., 2015). Despite these recommendations, there has been a significant increase in the use of CT scans for

**BOX 52.4 Classification of Severity of Head Injuries Based on Glasgow Coma Scale (GCS)***

Minor (mild) head injury: GCS score = 13-15
Moderate head injury: GCS score = 9-12
Severe head injury: GCS score = 3-8

*Data from Atabaki, S.M. (2007). Pediatric head injury. *Pediatrics in Review,* 28(6), 215–224.

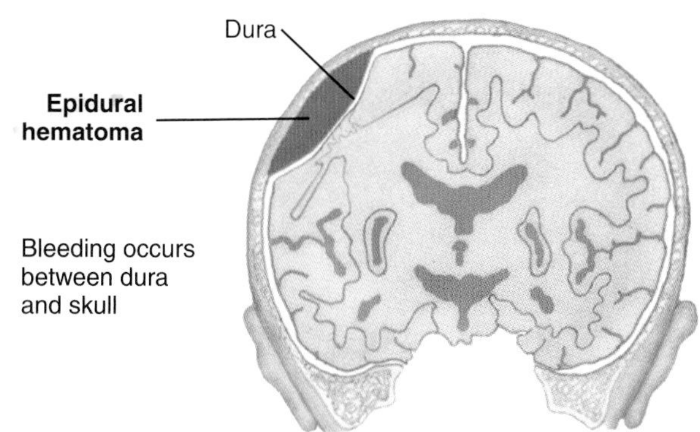


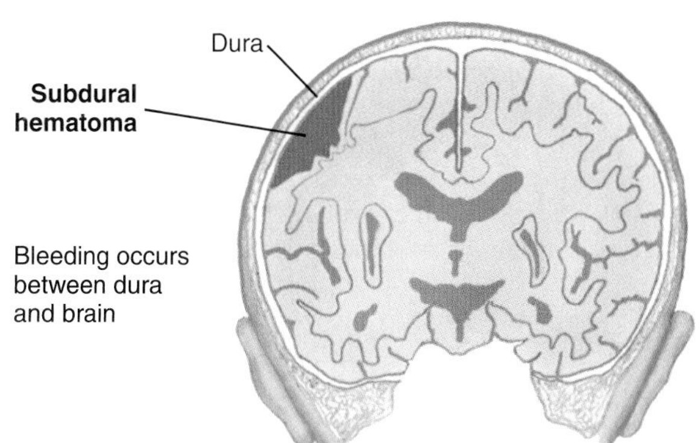


**FIG 52.5** Epidural and subdural hematomas are the two most common cranial hematomas, occurring in 6% to 7% of all children with head injuries. With *epidural hematoma,* a rapid decline in neurologic function can occur 4 to 8 hours after a brief period of lucidity. If untreated, the increased intracranial pressure (ICP) can cause death in a short time. A *subdural hematoma* is often caused when the head strikes an immovable object. A subdural hematoma (along with retinal hemorrhage) in an infant or child can occur as a result of child abuse involving aggressive shaking, blunt impact, or both (abusive head trauma).

children with a head injury in the past 2 decades (Atabaki, 2013). In response, recent studies have published prediction rules to identify children at risk for clinically significant head injury (Atabaki, 2013; Horeczko & Kuppermann, 2012).

### Therapeutic Management

Initial management of the child with a head injury includes assessment of airway, ventilatory function, neurologic status, and any other injuries present (see Chapter 34). Interventions to maintain vital functions, including adequate oxygenation and perfusion, are provided until all injuries are determined. The goal of treatment is to minimize long-term sequelae. Increased ICP or seizures can develop in a child with a head injury. In children with TBI, the presence of hypoventilation, hypoxemia, and hypotension is concerning and correlates with increased mortality (Geyer et al., 2013).

Because their brains are still developing, children and adolescents who suffer concussions are at risk for long-term complications that necessitate appropriate management (Gioia, 2012; Kerr, 2014; Master & Grady, 2012). Physical and cognitive exertion after a concussion may increase the metabolic demands causing strain on vulnerable cells in the brain. Most patients have an increase in symptom severity when returning to school in the first 2 weeks after a concussion. Therefore, a recommendation to stay home from school for 1 to 3 days or until the child can tolerate 30 minutes of cognitive activity without an increase in symptoms is beneficial (Grady, Master, & Gioia, 2012). Recovery occurs more quickly in those who rest immediately after the injury (Vidal, Goodman, Colin, et al., 2012).

Recommendations from the American Academy of Pediatrics (AAP, 2015a) state that all young athletes who have sustained a sport-related concussion must do the following:

- Be evaluated by a physician
- Be restricted from physical activity until they are asymptomatic at rest and with exertion
- Be allowed a minimum of 7 to 10 days and up to weeks and months to fully recover
- Be provided neuropsychological testing to obtain objective data
- Be informed there is no evidence that treatment with medications is safe or effective
- Be told to consider retirement from contact sports if multiple concussions have been sustained or if postconcussion symptoms have persisted for more than 3 months

Under no circumstances should a child or adolescent resume playing a sport the same day of the concussion; protocols have been developed to guide the gradual return of the young athlete to "return to play" after a concussion (Gioia, 2012; Kerr, 2014). All states have enacted legislation that requires school districts to have guidelines regarding concussion prevention and management. Many schools have implemented baseline cognitive function assessment tools to compare to post injury scores (McLaughlin, 2015).

To help coaches and athletes identify and manage concussions, the CDC developed the *Heads Up* concussion training course, which is free for coaches, officials, athletes, and parents (CDC, 2015b).

### Nursing Considerations

Initial and ongoing assessment of the child with a head injury includes evaluation of the *ABCDEs*; *a*irway, *b*reathing, *c*irculation, *d*isability (level of consciousness), and *e*xposure (see Chapter 34). The child's neck must be immobilized because there is a higher incidence of associated cervical spine injury with head trauma. The nurse obtains and records baseline vital signs, as well as other data as indicated by the child's clinical condition. A complete history and comprehensive neurologic examination should be performed. The child's level of consciousness (using the GCS), pupil size, and pupil reactivity to light are assessed frequently.

Cranial nerve function is tested to identify deficits resulting from the injury and monitor for increased ICP. The clinical signs and

## PATHOPHYSIOLOGY

### *Head Injury*

The cranium is a rigid structure that contains blood, brain tissue, and cerebrospinal fluid (CSF). The pressure exerted by these components on the cranium is between 2 and 10 mm Hg, depending on the age and activity level of the child. According to the Monro–Kellie doctrine, an increase in one of these components must be accompanied by a decrease in one of the other components to maintain intracranial pressure (ICP) within normal range. Cerebral function depends on adequate delivery of nutrients such as oxygen, glucose, and other substrates; an abnormal increase in ICP interferes with the balance and delivery of these nutrients.

Head injuries are either primary or secondary. *Primary head injuries* are those in which damage is sustained at the time of injury; *secondary head injuries* refer to the consequences of the primary injury, particularly increased ICP. The severity of the injury depends on the amount of stress to the cranium and brain. Head injuries include concussions, contusions, lacerations, fractures, and hematomas.

Motor vehicle collisions, falls, sports injuries, and child abuse cause most head injuries in children. *Acceleration–deceleration* is the term used to describe the mechanism of injury. The shearing force of the initial impact moves the brain forward in the brain, followed by a countering, backward movement of the brain in the skull. The shearing force produces bruising, tearing, and bleeding. Abusive head trauma (formerly referred to as shaken baby or infant syndrome) is a type of child abuse that can result in epidural hematomas and retinal hemorrhages (see Chapter 53).

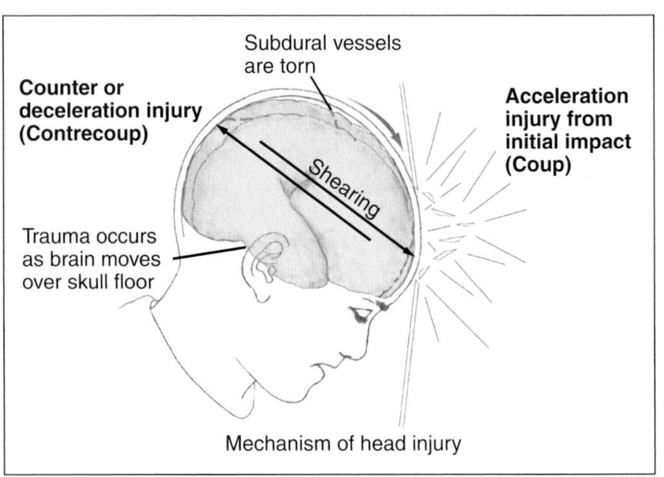

Mechanism of head injury

References: Fingarson, A., & Pierce, M.C. (2012). Identifying abusive head trauma: knowing what to look for can save babies from future harm [Electronic Version]. *Contemporary Pediatrics, 16–22;* Geyer, K., Meller, K., Kulpan, C., et al. (2013). Traumatic brain injury in children: acute care management. *Pediatric Nursing, 39*(6), 283–289.

## PARENTS WANT TO KNOW

### Guidelines for the Child With a Head Injury

After the injury, apply cold (cool pack wrapped in a towel or cool wet compresses) to the site for 20 minutes to prevent or reduce swelling. Clean any scrapes or cuts with soap and water. Encourage the child to rest and limit foods if vomiting. You will need to watch your child closely for the first 24 to 48 hours after the injury in case the child develops a problem and needs to be taken to the healthcare provider. Follow your health provider's directions as to whether the child should be awakened at night. Some providers suggest waking the child every few hours to be sure the child becomes alert and answers questions appropriately.

The following are signs of more serious injury, and you should call the physician or emergency transport immediately after the injury if the child:

- Has bleeding that does not stop after pressure has been applied for 10 minutes or is oozing from the nose or ears
- Needs sutures
- Is younger than 2 years
- Has trouble breathing
- Vomits or complains of a severe headache that does not go away
- Had a seizure after the head injury
- Was unconscious or confused
- Has a severe headache or vomiting
- Has slurred speech or blurred vision
- Has blood or watery fluid coming from the ear or nose
- Has unequal pupils or crossed eyes
- Has difficulty walking or crawling or weakness in the arms
- Becomes hard to wake up
- Becomes pale and remains that way for more than an hour
- Has other symptoms that concern you

**Postconcussion Syndrome**

Some children who have had a head injury can have an after-effect called *postconcussion syndrome*. If your child has this condition, he or she may be upset easily and become irritable if tired or stressed. Memory problems are common, as are learning difficulties, double vision, dizziness, headaches, fatigue, and light sensitivity. Younger patients are at greater risk. These symptoms can last many months.

**Second Impact Syndrome**

If your child is diagnosed with concussion, a second concussion that occurs before healing of the first can cause more harm to the brain and even lead to death. Be sure to talk with your health provider about whether and when the child can return to activities or sports.

Reference: McGuire, C.S., & McCambridge, T.M. (2011). Concussion in the young athlete: diagnosis, management, and prevention [Electronic Version]. *Contemporary Pediatrics,* 30–44.

symptoms of increased ICP, with or without actual measurement of the ICP, determine both the child's clinical status and medical and nursing interventions. Nasotracheal suctioning or placement of a nasogastric tube is contraindicated in a child with a basilar skull fracture; because of the nature of the injury, the suction catheter or tube could be introduced into the brain. CSF may leak from the nose or ears; packing or blowing of the nose is contraindicated.

Nursing care of the child with a head injury is similar to nursing care of any child with increased ICP. The nurse must closely monitor for signs and symptoms of increased ICP as well as avoid activities and stimuli that can elevate ICP. Positioning with the head of the bed elevated 30 to 45 degrees promotes venous drainage (see Nursing Care Plan: The Child with a Neurologic System Disorder).

Any child with a head injury needs to be assessed for fluid and electrolyte alterations. The child with a head injury can have a postinjury alteration in antidiuretic hormone (ADH). Possibly as a result of injury to the hypothalamus or posterior pituitary, the child can exhibit signs of excess ADH (syndrome of inappropriate antidiuretic hormone [SIADH]) or deficient ADH (diabetes insipidus) (see Chapter 51). The nurse carefully monitors intravenous and oral fluid intake, determines hourly fluid output, documents all data, and evaluates the child's fluid balance status. Laboratory data for serum electrolytes is frequently checked and abnormalities reported to the physician.

If the child develops SIADH, diuretics may be administered and fluids may be restricted to reduce the risk of increasing ICP from cerebral edema (Geyer et al., 2013). Fluid restriction is a nursing challenge because it involves the cooperation of parents and others involved in the child's care. Placing a sign at the child's bedside to alert others of the restriction is useful. The nurse selects fluids the child likes and distributes the allocated amounts over the course of the child's waking hours.

If the child is discharged from the emergency department, written instructions should be given to parents for home monitoring, signs and symptoms to be immediately reported to the physician, and follow-up care. Some children with severe head injuries require surgical intervention, intensive care, prolonged acute-care hospitalization, and multidisciplinary rehabilitative care in a specialized unit or facility.

## SPINAL CORD INJURY

Spinal cord injury can result from any trauma or injury to the spinal cord or its vascular supply or venous drainage.

### Etiology

Spinal cord injuries in children are usually caused by motor vehicle crashes, falls, diving accidents, sports injuries, tumor, congenital anomalies, gunshot or knife wounds, or attempted suicide. In the infant, a common cause of spinal cord injury is intentional, aggressive shaking by an older person.

### Incidence

Spinal cord injuries are less common in children than in adults, with 12,000 spinal cord injuries occurring each year in the Unites States (NINDS, 2013b). Most spinal cord injuries in children occur in the cervical spine, between the occiput and C3 (Rekate, 2016). Young children are more susceptible to upper spinal cord injury because of their larger head size in relation to body size. As the child grows older, the likely site of the spinal cord injury moves distally.

### Manifestations

Manifestations of spinal cord injury include loss of some or all movement or sensation below the level of injury, respiratory depression or apnea, hypotension and bradycardia, hypothermia, and neck pain. These signs vary with the level of injury as well as whether the spinal

## PATHOPHYSIOLOGY
### *Spinal Cord Injury*

Spinal cord injuries occur in children when vertebral bodies are fractured or subluxation of the vertebra occurs. Subluxation results in malalignment of contiguous vertebrae so that the spinal cord is compressed. The cord may be crushed, stretched beyond tolerance, or completely divided. All neurons carrying sensations from those parts of the body below the lesion are unable to pass their message on to the brain. A cord injury causes complete paralysis and complete loss of sensation below the level where the spinal cord was severely damaged or severed.

Flaccid paralysis of the affected limbs immediately follows a spinal cord injury. Paralysis is caused by spinal shock, which can last 4 to 6 weeks or longer. The flaccidity changes to spasticity when the spinal shock resolves. Hypotension, bradycardia, and peripheral vasodilation result from spinal shock and associated loss of vasomotor tone.

Reference: Pruitt, D.W., & McMahon, M.A. (2016). Spinal cord injury and autonomic crisis management. In R. Kliegman, B. Stanton, J. St. Geme, et al. (Eds.), *Nelson textbook of pediatrics* (20th ed., pp. 3400–3402). Philadelphia: Elsevier.

cord injury is complete or incomplete. If complete, the cord is completely severed and no spinal innervation is present below the injury. For example, with a complete injury at the C2 level (cervical vertebrae 2), the child is apneic and requires ventilatory support. With an incomplete spinal cord injury, the cord has some function remaining below the level of injury (NINDS, 2013b).

## Diagnostic Evaluation

After the nurse takes the history of the injury and performs a complete neurologic examination, the extent of the spinal cord injury is determined by radiography or MRI. The extent of the motor or sensory deficit may resolve somewhat as spinal shock resolves. Spinal cord injury without radiologic abnormalities (SCIWORA), which is more common in children, is a neurologic consequence of injury to the spinal cord related to anatomic differences in the structure of the spinal column and cord (Rekate, 2016).

## Therapeutic Management

Current treatment of spinal cord injury includes immobilization and steroid therapy. If used, steroids must be administered within 8 hours of the injury as a bolus of 30 mg/kg followed by a continuous infusion of 5.4 mg/kg/hr for 23 hours. Because of adverse effects associated with steroid administration, use of steroids is controversial. More research is needed to evaluate the effectiveness of steroid therapy for cervical spine injuries and to determine protocols for steroid administration times after spinal injury (Rekate, 2016). Until permanent surgical stabilization can be performed, other treatments such as halo traction (Fig. 52.6) and Gardner-Wells tongs might be used for temporary stabilization.

Autonomic dysreflexia (AD) is characterized by severe peripheral hypertension. AD can occur in children following spinal cord injuries at or above the T6 (thoracic vertebrae 6) level. Early signs include a sudden, significant rise in systolic and diastolic blood pressure, usually with bradycardia; flushing of the face, neck, and shoulders; goose bumps above T6; blurred vision; spots in the child's visual field; and nasal congestion. Recognition of these signs followed by emergency treatment to lower the blood pressure is essential to preventing cerebral and retinal hemorrhage, seizures, and myocardial infarction (Campagnolo, 2011; Pruitt & McMahon, 2016).

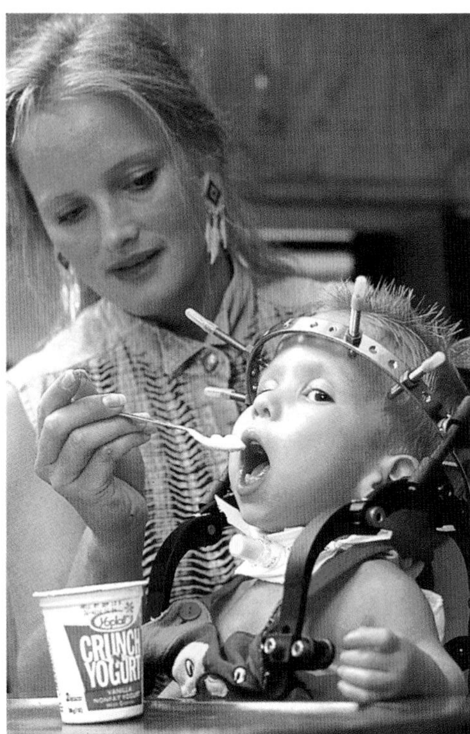


FIG 52.6 Children who have injuries or birth defects that involve the upper spine may be placed in halo traction to stabilize the spine and prevent added nerve damage. Spinal cord injury is a catastrophic event for the child and family; intense nursing support and education, as well as referral to support groups, will be needed. (Courtesy Cook Children's Medical Center, Fort Worth, TX.)

## NURSING CARE
### The Child With a Spinal Cord Injury
#### Assessment

The spine must be immobilized before any attempt is made to move the child. The airway is assessed immediately, and if intubation is necessary, it is done without hyperextending the neck (see Chapter 34). Circulation is then assessed; hypotension can result from either hypovolemia or neurologic shock. Bradycardia and hypothermia may occur. The nurse closely monitors the child's body temperature and oxygenation status.

The neurologic assessment by the nurse includes evaluating mobility, sensation, and reflexes. The nurse considers the suspected level of spinal cord injury and whether the injury is thought to be complete or incomplete. The neurologic assessment is ongoing and carefully documented so that changes can be promptly reported. The child is also assessed for other areas of trauma and the impact of the spinal cord injury on other systems including genitourinary, gastrointestinal, and integumentary.

#### Nursing Diagnosis and Planning

The following nursing diagnoses and expected outcomes may be appropriate after assessment of the child with spinal cord injury and the child's family:

- Ineffective Breathing Pattern related to weakness or paralysis of respiratory muscles after spinal cord injury.

**Expected outcome.** The child will not have respiratory distress, as evidenced by arterial blood gas (ABG) values within normal limits, stable vital signs, and adequate motor and sensory function.

- Risk for Impaired Skin Integrity related to immobility.

  *Expected outcome.* The child will maintain skin integrity, as evidenced by intact skin and absence of breakdown.
- Anxiety related to having a child with an acute condition.

  *Expected outcome.* The child and parents will have decreased anxiety, as evidenced by an ability to verbalize the impact the child's spinal cord injury will have on their lives.
- Interrupted Family Processes related to having a child with an acute and chronic injury.

  *Expected outcome.* The parents will show signs of adapting to their child's injury, as evidenced by participating in the child's care and seeking appropriate support within the community.
- Impaired Physical Mobility related to neuromuscular impairment.

  *Expected outcome.* The child will maximize his or her potential for improved mobility, as evidenced by involvement in physical therapy and occupational therapy.

### Interventions

The goals of nursing care are to minimize the potential for further injury, prevent the sequelae of immobility, and promote maximal spinal cord recovery. The spinal cord is first immobilized with the use of tongs or halo traction. The child remains in traction for several weeks (see Chapter 50). The nurse is responsible for maintaining proper alignment by monitoring the status of the traction every 1 to 2 hours. Towels and rolls can be useful to help position the child. The nurse should perform a motor and sensory assessment after each change of position (see Chapter 33).

If the child's condition becomes unstable, surgical stabilization may become necessary. Progressive neurologic deterioration is the major indicator for surgery.

The child who is immobilized and neurologically impaired is at risk for respiratory complications as a result of muscle weakness and immobility. Respiratory status and pulse oximetry readings are assessed and recorded every 1 to 2 hours. Supplemental oxygen may be indicated. Nebulizer, incentive spirometry, and intermittent positive-pressure breathing (IPPB) are administered as ordered. Some children need a tracheostomy for prolonged mechanical ventilation if the respiratory muscles are involved.

The nurse evaluates perfusion and neurologic integrity by continuously monitoring circulation, sensation, and motion. In addition, the nurse assesses hourly vital signs, color, core body temperature, skin, and intake and output. If alterations in perfusion occur; the child receives crystalloids by bolus infusion. Vasopressors can also be used and are often required for cervical spinal injuries.

Children with spinal cord injuries often have difficulty with body temperature control. Some are unable to maintain body heat because of dermal vasodilatation *(poikilothermia)* (Pruitt & McMahon, 2016). These children will need to be gradually warmed or cooled as indicated. If the child has an elevated temperature, samples of wound material and blood are obtained for culture. Sputum cultures might be ordered. Antipyretic and broad-spectrum antibiotic therapies are initiated after the specimens are sent to the laboratory.

Each time the child is repositioned (every 1 to 2 hours); the nurse thoroughly inspects the child's skin and administers skin care. Pressure on the bony prominences is minimized with the use of special mattresses and padding. Because of bladder muscle weakness or paralysis, an indwelling urinary catheter is often used to facilitate bladder emptying and permit accurate measurement of intake and output on an hourly basis. While the indwelling catheter is in place, care is taken to prevent infection. Intermittent catheterization may eventually be initiated.

The child may have a nasogastric tube in place with gravity drainage or low, intermittent suction. The nurse maintains tube patency and observes and records the characteristics and quantity of the drainage. Since these children are at risk for stress ulcers and gastrointestinal hemorrhage, the pH of the gastric fluid is tested and the child treated with antacids or histamine blockers as indicated. A bowel regimen is initiated and maintained to prevent impaction. Bowel training includes ingestion of a high-fiber diet (when the child is able to eat), the use of stool softeners, and increased water intake. Adequate nutrition is essential to the healing process. Caloric intake is monitored, and the child may receive nutrition by oral intake, tube feeding, or total parenteral nutrition. A good indicator of a favorable response to the nutrition is timely healing of wounds.

Spinal cord injury is a catastrophic event. The lives of the child and family have been suddenly and permanently altered. They will need intense assistance and support. These nursing care goals can be achieved through therapeutic play, promotion of independent functioning, referral to a multidisciplinary rehabilitation team, referral to support groups, psychological counseling, and thorough discharge planning. Following stabilization, most children are transferred to a rehabilitation unit for ongoing interdisciplinary care, therapy, and teaching in preparation for returning home.

### Evaluation

- Are body functions (respirations, elimination, muscle strength) maintained as normally as possible?
- Is the child's skin intact and free from breakdown?
- Do the child and parents verbalize feelings or emotions about the injury and the prognosis?
- Do the parents demonstrate the ability to provide physical and emotional support for the child?
- Has the child's neurologic function improved?

## SEIZURE DISORDERS

A seizure consists of brief paroxysmal behavior caused by excessive abnormal discharge of neurons. Epilepsy is marked by recurrent seizure activity that does not occur in association with an acute illness. Epilepsy is diagnosed after 2 or more unprovoked seizures (Doerrer & Kossoff, 2014). Seizures are classified into three major categories: focal, generalized, and unknown. Focal seizures occur in one part of the brain and may or may not alter consciousness. Generalized seizures occur over the entire brain and do alter consciousness (Mikati & Hani, 2016a). A seizure of the unknown type cannot be characterized as focal or generalized; epileptic and infantile spasms are examples (Berg & Scheffer, 2011).

### Etiology

Seizures are symptomatic of altered neuronal activity in the CNS. Seizures can occur for many reasons and are categorized according to etiology, genetics, structural/metabolic causes, or unknown (Berg & Scheffer, 2011). Genetic seizures occur as the direct result of a genetic defect (known or presumed). Structural/metabolic seizures are associated with specific conditions or diseases and including strokes, trauma, and infection. If the cause is not known, the seizure etiology is categorized as unknown, which accounts for one third of all epilepsies (Berg & Scheffer, 2011).

### Incidence

Approximately 120,000 children in the United States are evaluated for new-onset seizures each year (Chelse, Kelley, Hageman, et al, 2013). An estimated prevalence of 0.7% of children and adolescents aged

6 to 17 years have had a seizure (CDC, 2015). One third of those with first time seizure will be diagnosed with epilepsy. The prevalence of epilepsy in children in the United States is 1% (Hartman & Devore, 2016). The incidence of epilepsy increases to 70% with a second seizure (Sankaraneni & Lachwani, 2015). Most of the newly diagnosed cases of epilepsy in pediatrics occur in early childhood and adolescence. An estimated 2% to 5% of all children will have a febrile seizure, and the majority outgrow the tendency for this type of seizure by age 5 years (Patterson, Carapetian, Hageman, et al., 2013).

Because of the subtlety of neonatal seizures, the incidence is difficult to determine. Seizure manifestations are easily confused with normal infant behavior. More severe outcomes tend to be experienced by neonates who have seizures in the first few days of life as compared to those who develop seizures later in the neonatal period.

## Pathophysiology

During a seizure, excessive, self-limiting neuronal discharges occur. The result of these discharges is activation of associated motor or sensory organs. The extent of the seizure depends on the location and extent of the abnormal neuronal discharges. The brain consists of millions of nerve cells; electrical impulses are sent between many of these cells by neurotransmitters. When numerous nerve cells fire abnormally at the same time, a seizure can result.

## Manifestations

Many types of seizures occur. The International Classification of Seizures is used to divide seizures into the three major groups (Box 52.5).

*Febrile seizures* are generally seen in young children between the ages of 6 months and 3 years with a peak incidence of 18 months.

### BOX 52.5 International Classification of Seizures

**Generalized Seizures**

Onset at any age. Clinical features indicate involvement of both cerebral hemispheres. Consciousness is impaired.

***Tonic, Clonic, and Tonic-Clonic Seizures***

Formerly called *grand mal seizures,* tonic-clonic seizures cause an abrupt arrest of activity and impairment of consciousness. The *tonic phase* consists of a sustained, generalized stiffening of muscles, including the diaphragm, lasting a few seconds. The *clonic phase* is symmetric and rhythmic, consisting of alternating contraction and relaxation of major muscle groups. This phase usually ends spontaneously in less than 5 minutes. Respirations are irregular, and the child may have stridor. Sphincter incontinence (stool and/or urine) occurs in some. The tonic-clonic seizure is followed by a variable period of confusion, lethargy, and sleep (postictal phase).

***Atonic Seizures***

Atonic seizures cause an abrupt loss of postural tone, impairment of consciousness, confusion, lethargy, and sleep. A child might have multiple episodes of sudden and brief head drop or a drop attack, during which they fall to the ground, often face down, lose consciousness for a few seconds, and then get back up as if nothing happened.

***Myoclonic Seizures***

Myoclonic seizures are brief, random contractions of a muscle group, followed by loss of muscle tone and forward falling. They can occur on both sides of the body, singly or in clusters. Impairment of consciousness sometimes occurs during myoclonic seizures. Onset can be as early as age 2 months, but myoclonic seizures are more frequently seen in school-age children or adolescents than in very young children.

***Absence Seizures***

Formerly called *petit mal seizures,* absence seizures are very brief episodes of altered consciousness. Typically, no muscle activity occurs except for upward rolling of the eyes. The child has a blank facial expression. Absence seizures last only 5 to 20 seconds or less, but they can occur up to hundreds of times per day. Absence seizures account for 8% to 15% of childhood epilepsies. They are characterized by the immediate return to the activities the child was involved in just before the seizure. Children with atypical absence seizures might experience some myoclonic movements (eyelid fluttering) and muscle tone changes (head bobbing). The onset of absence seizures is usually between ages 4 and 10 years, with a peak incidence between 6 and 8 years. Eighty percent of children outgrow absence seizures by adolescence.

**Focal Seizures**

Onset is at any age. The clinical features suggest that only a limited functional area in one hemisphere of the brain is involved, with symptoms seen on only one side of the body. Focal seizures are described according to the features exhibited by the child during the seizure. Types of features are awareness/responsiveness (altered or intact), sensory/psychic (aura), motor, and autonomic. Impairment in consciousness or awareness and decreased responsiveness occur with some but not all focal seizures. An aura (the sensation of an upcoming seizure) is actually part of a focal seizure. Other sensory symptoms include a rising abdominal feeling, an unexplained sense of fear, déjà vu feeling, an odd taste in the mouth or odd smell, and visual/auditory hallucinations. Children under 7 years of age are less likely to report sensory symptoms; however, parents might observe them staring or looking around without purpose, being less responsive, and exhibiting automatisms.

Motor features, which are commonly seen, include involuntary, brief movements (tonic, clonic, or atonic) that are localized to one area, and turning eyes and head away from the side of the seizure. During a focal seizure, children can exhibit automatisms, repetitive, nonpurposeful movements of mouth and extremities such as lip smacking, chewing, teeth grinding, scratching, pulling at clothing or sheets, and shuffling. Salivation, dilation of pupils, and skin flushing occur as well. The average duration of a focal seizure is 1 to 2 minutes. A variable period of confusion, lethargy, and sleep follows the event.

A focal seizure can become a bilateral, convulsive seizure when the electrical impulses pass across the corpus callosum to the other hemisphere. In this case, the child may experience bilateral tonic and clonic movements, urinary and stool incontinence, and loss of consciousness.

**Unknown**

This classification is for seizures that cannot be characterized as generalized or focal. These include epileptic spasms (Lennox-Gastaut syndrome) seen in older children as well as infantile spasms (West syndrome) seen in infants aged 2 to 12 months. These infants will exhibit brief contractions of the neck, arms, trunk, and legs (myoclonic spasms) and eventually suffer developmental regression.

Data from Doerrer, S.C., & Kossoff, E.H. (2014). First seizure: dispel the myths [Electronic Version]. *Contemporary Pediatrics, 31*(2), 9; Park, J.T., Shahid, A.M., & Jammoul, A. (2015). Common pediatric epilepsy syndromes. *Pediatric Annals, 44*(2), e30–e35. doi:10.3928/00904481-20150203-09; Wolf, S.M., & McGoldrick, P.E. (2015). Seizure patterns in childhood. *Pediatric Annals, 44*(2), e24–29. doi:10.3928/00904481-20150203-08.

Febrile seizures occur more frequently in males and in those with a familial history. Children who have had a febrile seizure are at a slightly increased risk of epilepsy (Patterson et al., 2013). Febrile seizures are classified as simple or complex based on duration and symptoms. The height and rapidity of temperature elevation seem to be factors in precipitating febrile seizures. The temperature is usually elevated above 102°F (38.8°C). The seizure activity occurs during the temperature rise rather than after prolonged elevation, usually in the first 24 hours of the illness (Patterson et al., 2013). Most febrile seizures occur as a result of fever caused by otitis media, pharyngitis, or adenitis. The family of a child who has a febrile seizure should be given information about these seizures and instructed what to do if another seizure occurs. Rectal diazepam is often prescribed for use after complex febrile seizures, but the AAP does not recommend the use of antiepileptic drugs (Patterson et al., 2013).

*Neonatal seizures* are usually caused by an underlying pathologic process. The most frequent cause of neonatal seizures is perinatal asphyxia leading to hypoxic-ischemic encephalopathy. The second major contributing factor is intracranial hemorrhage. Other causes include metabolic disturbances, intrauterine and perinatal infectious disorders, cerebral infarcts, drug withdrawal, hyperthermia, hypoglycemia, sodium and potassium imbalances, congenital anomalies of the CNS, and inherited syndromes (Mikati & Hani, 2016b).

The mechanism of neonatal seizures is not clearly understood. Because of the overall anatomic and physiologic immaturity of the neonate's nervous system, including a lack of myelinization of fiber tracts, generalized tonic-clonic seizures are rare. Seizures in neonates may produce subtle signs such as sustained eye opening, tonic horizontal deviation of the eyes, blinking or eyelid fluttering, sucking, smacking, drooling, tongue thrusting, pedaling movements of the legs, swimming movements of the arms, and apnea. These manifestations are more common in preterm infants and infants with hypoxic-ischemic encephalopathy. Neonatal seizures occur in the first 28 days of life and can be focal, tonic, or myoclonic, with jerking movements of the extremities. The mortality rate is 9% to 15%, with poorer outcomes seen in premature neonates who have generalized tonic, myoclonic, and subtle seizures (Anand & Nair, 2014).

### Diagnostic Evaluation

The child's health history and family history are important parts of the initial workup. A thorough description of the child's behavior before, during, and after the seizure activity is important to delineate the type of seizure. Video recording and EEG monitoring help identify the seizure. Serum electrolyte determinations, complete blood count (CBC), blood glucose determination, lumbar puncture, and other laboratory tests are only needed if the child has additional concerning symptoms such as lethargy, vomiting, and dehydration, since these tests can help uncover metabolic causes. Both CT and MRI will indicate trauma, tumor, or congenital malformation; MRI provides a better detail of the brain structure and does not involve radiation (Doerrer & Kossoff, 2014). In neonates, several other laboratory tests may be included, such as *t*oxoplasmosis, *o*ther agents, *r*ubella, *c*ytomegalovirus, and *h*erpes simplex virus (TORCH) titers—to exclude congenital viral infections, as well as amino acid and organic acid studies to exclude inborn errors of metabolism.

### Therapeutic Management

The basic tenet of treatment for the child with seizures is to treat the whole child. Antiepileptic medications are commonly used to manage seizures. Treatment goals are to identify and correct the cause of the seizure, eliminate the seizure with a minimum of side effects and the least amount of medication, and normalize the lives of the child and the family (Table 52.3). The CDC provides patients and families with helpful resources which can be found at http://www.cdc.gov/epilepsy/basics/index.htm.

Vagus nerve stimulation (VNS) can significantly reduce the number and intensity of seizures in children age 12 years and older with focal seizures (Mikati & Hani, 2016c; Sharp, Samanta, & Willis, 2015). A generator is implanted in the chest wall, and a wire is clipped to the vagus nerve to deliver electrical impulses at regular intervals to the brain. Side effects include a tickling sensation in the throat, change in voice tone during stimulation, slight coughing during stimulation, and rarely, vocal cord paralysis and infection that requires removal of the device (Sharp et al., 2015). Positive effects include reduction in seizure frequency and severity, increased cognition and improved mood and behavior (Sharp et al., 2015). VNS therapy may decrease the need for pharmacologic intervention and emergency care.

A ketogenic diet is another treatment option for children with epilepsy. The diet is essentially carbohydrate-free, composed mostly of fat, and produces a state of ketosis that is thought to control seizures through the antiepileptic effects of ketone bodies on the brain (Sharp et al., 2015). This diet is very strict and considered mainly for children with epilepsy that is refractory to conventional treatment. It may be more readily accepted by children who have not developed taste preferences, those who are developmentally delayed, and those who are fed through gastrostomy tubes. Side effects include constipation, dehydration, vitamin deficiency, and kidney or gall stones (Epilepsy Foundation of America, 2012). Older children can use a modified Atkins diet, which is not as restrictive (Sharp et al., 2015).

Both the ketogenic diet, modified Atkins diet and VNS therapy are considered adjunctive therapies for epilepsy treatment. Antiepileptic medications will typically be continued for most children to achieve the best degree of seizure control.

The AAP recently made recommendations for the management of children in the school setting. It is important to have good communication between the patient and family, the primary care provider, and the school setting to ensure appropriate and individualized plans of care for children with epilepsy (Hartman & Devore, 2016).

Often the plan involves the administration of seizure rescue medications after a specific period of time to prevent the progression to status epilepticus. Examples of care plans can be found on the Epilepsy Foundation website (http://www.epilepsyfoundation.org). The school nurse should be familiar with the commonly prescribed rescue medications such as rectal diazepam, oral or intranasal midazolam, oral lorazepam, and clonazepam disintegrating tablets (Hartman & Devore, 2016). Privacy makes rectal administration less appealing. The care plan should also include when to seek further medical assistance and the adverse effects of the medications (Hartman & Devore, 2016).

## STATUS EPILEPTICUS

Status epilepticus is a medical emergency. It is marked by prolonged seizure activity, in the form of either a single seizure lasting 5 minutes or more or recurrent seizures lasting more than 5 minutes with no return to a normal level of consciousness between seizures (Mikati & Hani, 2016a). The most common form of status epilepticus is generalized status, which has the highest potential for complications and possible death.

### Etiology

The causes of status epilepticus are numerous. Acute CNS injury from head trauma, meningitis, or electrolyte imbalance frequently precipitates status epilepticus. The condition can also be caused by toxins,

**TABLE 52.3 Common Seizure Medications**

| Drug Name | Seizure Type | Side Effects | Nursing Implications |
|---|---|---|---|
| Carbamazepine (Tegretol) | Focal or generalized | Sedation, cognitive deficits, behavior outbursts, weight gain, leukopenia | Watch for change in behavior or decrease in school performance.<br>Child should not be given erythromycin, which causes an increase in drug level.<br>Monitor blood tests for therapeutic levels. |
| Rufinamide (Banzel) | Lennox-Gastaut (multiple seizure types) | Headache, tremor, dizziness, fatigue, sleepiness, double vision | Can be crushed and taken with food. |
| Felbamate (Felbatol) | Focal or generalized | Nausea and vomiting, weight loss, anorexia, agitation and aggression, aplastic anemia, liver failure | Shake oral suspension well. Associated with aplastic anemia and hepatic failure.<br>Monitor liver enzymes and CBC. |
| Ethosuximide (Zarontin) | Generalized; mostly childhood absence epilepsy | Nausea and vomiting, lethargy | Observe for excessive drowsiness; take with food. |
| Lamotrigine (Lamictal) | Generalized or focal; broad spectrum use | Rash (increased risk of severe rash in children with previous reaction to any drug or to another antiepileptic drug), dizziness, headache, double vision, nausea and vomiting, ataxia | Not affected by food absorption. Instruct parents to report any signs of rash immediately. |
| Gabapentin (Neurontin) | Generalized or focal | Drowsiness, dizziness, nystagmus, nausea and vomiting, ataxia | Dosage must be adjusted relative to renal function. |
| Levetiracetam (Keppra) | Focal, myoclonic, and generalized | Sleepiness, weakness, headache, infection | Monitor for side effects and frequency of seizures and renal dysfunction. |
| Phenobarbital | Generalized or focal | Sedation, cognitive deficits, behavior outbursts | Watch for excessive drowsiness, changes in school performance, and respiratory depression.<br>Monitor blood tests for therapeutic levels. |
| Phenytoin (Dilantin) | Focal, generalized, or status | Lethargy, nystagmus, ataxia, allergic reactions, hypertrophic gums, hirsutism, osteoporosis | Teach meticulous oral care to decrease gum hypertrophy.<br>IV form must be given in normal saline and filtered.<br>Monitor blood tests for therapeutic levels. |
| Topiramate (Topamax) | Focal or generalized tonic-clonic | Fatigue, nervousness, decreased attention, anorexia, renal stones, tremor, speech problems | Affects levels of other antiepileptic drugs.<br>Keep children well hydrated to decrease chances of renal stones. |
| Tiagabine (Gabitril) | Focal | Lethargy, sedation, double vision, ataxia | Monitor for generalized weakness. |
| Valproic acid (Depakene) | Generalized, focal, absence, myoclonic | Nausea and vomiting, tremor, weight gain, hair loss, menstrual cycle irregularities in women, thrombocytopenia, liver failure | Do not crush or cut pills/sprinkles. Can cause stomach ulcers.<br>Take with food.<br>Monitor blood tests for therapeutic levels. |
| Oxcarbazepine (Trileptal) | Focal | Fatigue, headache, dizziness, double vision, unsteadiness, nausea and vomiting, hyponatremia, rash | Interacts with other antiepileptic drugs; levels should be monitored. |

*CBC,* Complete blood count; *IV,* intravenous.

specific medications, chronic CNS injury, and sudden withdrawal from antiepileptic medications.

## Incidence

Status epilepticus occurs in 5% to 10% of children with epilepsy and occurs more often in children under the age of 5 years (Mikati & Hani, 2016a). The most common form in children younger than 3 years is febrile status epilepticus.

## Pathophysiology

Status epilepticus is caused by the random discharge of large numbers of neurons firing abnormally. The discharges cause abnormal repetitive motor activity. In the CNS, the metabolic rate increases, glucose stores are depleted, and oxygen consumption increases. If cerebral metabolic demands are not met, these changes cause neuronal injury. Prolonged seizures cause lactic acidosis, an altered blood-brain barrier, and increased ICP.

## Manifestations

See the International Classification of Seizures in Box 52.5.

## Diagnostic Evaluation

Diagnostic laboratory tests should include blood glucose, ABGs, electrolytes, anticonvulsant drug levels, a toxicology screen, and possibly lumbar puncture. Results may be similar to those of the child with increased ICP. An MRI might also be performed.

## Therapeutic Management

Generalized status epilepticus is a medical emergency. Treatment consists of maintaining optimal respiratory and hemodynamic function

## NURSING CARE PLAN

### *The Child With a Seizure Disorder in the Community Setting*

**Focused Assessment**

- Obtain a detailed prenatal, perinatal, and neonatal history to determine factors that may have caused the child's seizures.
  - Pathologic factors include hypoxia, cerebral trauma, high fever, lead poisoning, metabolic disorders, brain tumors, birth trauma, and central nervous system (CNS) infections.
  - Nonpathologic factors include overhydration, oversedation, drug abuse, alcohol intoxication, sleep deprivation, antihistamine drug use, and family history.
- Ask parents for detailed description of child's seizures. A video tape of the seizure activity.
  - Age at onset of child's seizure activity
  - Time of day when seizures occur
  - Precipitating event(s)
  - Child's behavior before, during, and after a seizure
  - How the child looks during the seizure
  - How the seizure progresses
  - How long the seizure lasts
- Perform comprehensive physical examination with emphasis on the nervous system.
  - Assess behavior, motor skills, and developmental level.
  - Assess emotional responses of the child and of the family to the child's seizure disorder.
- For the school-age child with a known seizure history, the school nurse maintains pertinent information in the child's record and communicates appropriate information to teachers, if needed.
- During a seizure, first provide for the child's safety. Observe the child closely and document findings; observations can assist with seizure management.

**Nursing Diagnosis**

Risk for Injury related to seizure activity.

**Planning**

***Expected Outcomes***

1. The child will remain free from injury through the use of appropriate injury prevention strategies.
2. The parents and older child will discuss seizure prevention and demonstrate appropriate safety interventions for seizures.

**Interventions and *Rationales***

1. If the child is hospitalized, institute seizure precautions that include padded side rails, bed in low position, and suction and airway at bedside. Instruct the parents that in case of a seizure at home, place the child on a soft surface or keep in bed. Remove sharp objects and keep furniture out of the way.
   *These actions make the environment safer for the child during the seizure.*
2. *Do not* put anything into the child's mouth during a seizure.
   *Forcing something into the child's mouth may injure the child's mouth, gums, or teeth or cause gagging and vomiting.*
3. During a seizure at home or at school, advise the parent or teacher to place the child on the side in a lateral position. Do not restrain the child. Loosen clothing around the child's neck.
   *Positioning the child on the side prevents aspiration because saliva or vomit will drain out the corner of the child's mouth. Restraints could cause injury to the child. The teacher or family may gently guide or protect the child's movements and may suction the child's mouth after the seizure is over if suction is available.*
4. Stay with the child who is having a seizure.
   *Staying with the child reduces the risk of injury and allows observation and documentation of the seizure.*
5. Record and instruct parents to record the time of seizures, precipitating factors, types of behavior including level of consciousness observed during and after the seizure, bladder or bowel incontinence, and frequency of seizures.
   *These observations help pinpoint the focus of the seizure and help the physician treat the seizure correctly.*
6. If a seizure lasts longer than 5 minutes, instruct parents to notify the physician immediately and administer rescue medications as ordered.
   *Medication may need to be administered to stop prolonged seizures. The main side effect of diazepam (Valium) and lorazepam (Ativan) is respiratory depression.*

**Evaluation**

Does the child remain injury free?
Do the child and family implement injury prevention strategies?
Do the parents monitor the seizure and record vital information?
Can the parents demonstrate safety interventions for seizures?
Can parents administer rescue medications as ordered?

**Nursing Diagnosis**

Deficient Knowledge related to the need for information about how to manage a child with a seizure disorder.

**Planning**

***Expected Outcomes***

The child and parents will:

1. Seek information about the child's management.
2. Describe how to meet the child's physical, emotional, and educational needs.

**Interventions and *Rationales***

1. Determine the educational needs of the child and parents.
   *Determining educational needs provides baseline information to develop a teaching plan.*
2. Provide an individual teaching plan for the child and parents for managing seizures.
   *An individualized teaching plan ensures that what is needed by the child and parents will be taught.*
3. Explore actual and potential problems that may arise and interfere with treatment.
   *Exploring possible problems facilitates adjustment and normalizes life; it also provides anticipatory guidance.*
4. Measure outcomes of education to ensure that learning has taken place and is facilitating acceptance of the child's condition.
   *Evaluation of teaching is an ongoing process to ensure continued learning.*
5. Refer to an epilepsy support group.
   *Social support is helpful for some families and may promote adjustment to lifestyle changes.*
6. Educate the child and parents about the medication regimen. Emphasize the importance of adhering to medical treatment and administering medications on time.
   *The goal of pharmacologic management is to raise the seizure threshold, thus preventing seizures from occurring.*
7. Identify the side effects of the medication and when medical attention should be sought.

*Continued*

## NURSING CARE PLAN—cont'd

### *The Child With a Seizure Disorder in the Community Setting*

*Knowledge of what is expected and normal will facilitate proper use of and adherence to the medication regimen.*

8. Identify the hazards of nonadherence to the medication regimen. Encourage the parents and child not to discontinue medications even if the child is seizure free.
   *Nonadherence will affect the serum levels of anticonvulsant drugs and may cause a seizure to occur.*
9. Emphasize to the child and parents the importance of regular medical evaluation and follow-up, including measurement of blood levels of the medication and evaluating for toxicity or side effects.
   *Regular medical follow-up facilitates maintenance of appropriate therapeutic blood levels of antiepileptics and identification of side effects of medication.*
10. Inform the parents about the need for a medical alert bracelet for the child.
    *Medical alert bracelets alert others to the child's condition in an emergency. If the child has a seizure in a public place, the bracelet will inform other people about appropriate actions to take on behalf of the child.*
11. Educate the parents about possible seizure triggers and avoidance of stressors. Many children are susceptible to having seizures when subjected to stress.
    *Lack of sleep, illness, and other stressors may increase the likelihood of seizures occurring.*
12. Encourage the family to find alternative activities besides contact sports for the child. The child should avoid swimming or climbing alone. Identify the child's strengths—not the child's limitations.
    *Appropriate activities reduce the risk of injury while promoting a positive self-image.*
13. Encourage verbalization of fears and concerns about having seizures.
    *Therapeutic communication may identify issues that need to be addressed.*
14. Teach the child and parent to educate other family members, friends, and teachers about seizures. Advise the family to provide necessary information to the school nurse.
    *Accurate information reduces the stigma associated with epilepsy and helps inform others of the seizure rescue plan.*

#### Evaluation

Does the child discuss having seizures, fears, and concerns about seizures, and life with the condition?

Does the child participate in the medical regimen by discussing medication side effects and dosage?

Does the child demonstrate a positive self-image?

Does the family administer antiepileptic medications safely and appropriately and know when to call the physician?

## PATIENT-CENTERED TEACHING

### *Guidelines for the Child or Adolescent Taking Seizure Medication*

- Oral care is very important for children taking phenytoin (Dilantin) because phenytoin can cause gum problems. Your child should brush with a soft brush and floss after every meal. Take your child to the dentist every 3 to 6 months for a checkup and teeth cleaning.
- Once your child has started taking the medication, blood levels should be monitored to determine that the medication has reached and maintained a therapeutic level and to monitor for a toxic level. In addition, other blood tests may be needed to ensure that the medication is not harming the liver or blood cells. Blood levels should be measured periodically as your physician recommends, if a seizure occurs, or if side effects are noticed.
- If your child is taking valproic acid, be alert for any signs of unusual bleeding or bruising. Valproic acid can affect the platelets (cells that help the blood clot) and cause the platelet counts to drop. Valproic acid can also increase the appetite. Offer healthy snacks and small meal portions.
- Be sure your child does not suddenly stop taking antiepileptic medications without discussing it with a physician or nurse. Suddenly stopping medications can cause the child to have a seizure or status epilepticus.
- Some states require a driver to be seizure free for a time ranging from a few months to a few years to obtain a driver's license. If your child is of driving age, discuss this matter with your healthcare provider.*
- Birth control pills can be less effective while taking antiepileptic medications. If sexually active, your adolescent should consult a nurse or physician for additional forms of birth control. Folic acid supplementation may be advised for teen females taking antiepileptic medications.
- Cognitive and behavior changes are sometimes seen with some of the antiepileptic medications. Attention span, memory, and interpersonal interactions can be impaired.
- Alcohol, marijuana, and street drugs lower the seizure threshold. These drugs should be avoided.
- Contact sports such as football and wrestling are not advised.
- Showers are preferred over baths for children who are concerned about privacy. Younger children with epilepsy should never be left alone in a tub of water. Swimming activities should be supervised by a strong swimmer who can rescue a child who has a seizure in the water.
- Depression is a diagnosis that often accompanies epilepsy and is associated with antiepileptic medications. Report any symptoms of depression to the physician.
- Maintaining a seizure diary that lists seizure frequency, associated triggers, and details of seizure activity is a good way for parents to collaborate with the healthcare team in determining the effectiveness of the treatment plan.
- Call 911 if your child has a seizure that does not resolve after 5 minutes.
- Your child should wear a medical alert bracelet to alert others of potential problems if they appear.†

*Krumholz, A. (2009). Driving issues in epilepsy: Past, present, and future. *Epilepsy Currents,* 9(2), 31–35. Retrieved from http://onlinelibrary.wiley.com/doi/10.111/j.1535-7511.2008.01283.x/full.

†Flower, D. (2009). Epilepsy part 3: Planning for emergencies. *British Journal of School Nursing,* 4(5), 164–168. Retrieved from www.internurse.com/cgi-bin/go.pl/library/contents.html?uid=2744;journal_uid=29.

**NURSING QUALITY ALERT**

***Observations and Nursing Care During a Seizure***

- As the seizure begins, look at your watch or a clock. You should be able to describe how long seizure activity lasts.
- Protect the child from injury by loosening clothing at the neck and turning the child gently onto the side, removing any obstacles in the child's environment. *Do not* restrain the child or insert any object into the child's mouth.
- Carefully observe in which body part the seizure begins, its progression, and how it ends.
- Be able to describe any preceding or accompanying sensory or motor manifestations.
- When the seizure is over, allow the child to rest if she or he desires. Record the child's behavior before, during, and after the seizure and the approximate duration of the seizure.
- In neonates, if the movement can be initiated by a stimulus, such as touch, it is probably a tremor. If the movement cannot be stopped or controlled with gentle restraint or passive flexion, it is probably a seizure.

and identifying and treating the causes of the seizure activity. Diazepam (Valium), lorazepam (Ativan), or midazolam (Versed) is given intravenously. If intravenous (IV) access cannot be obtained, medication can be given orally or rectally. Fosphenytoin (Cerebyx) or phenobarbital may be given IV as a second round of drugs if diazepam or lorazepam does not stop the seizures. The intramuscular route is not used because absorption of the medication is unpredictable.

## NURSING CARE

### The Child With Status Epilepticus

#### Assessment

On arrival at the hospital, the child will exhibit seizure activity and have unstable vital signs. Along with general seizure precautions, this child requires rapid assessment and vigorous supportive therapy. Supportive measures include assessing and maintaining a patent airway and administering oxygen. IV hydration and drug therapy are initiated to arrest the seizure activity.

#### Nursing Diagnosis and Planning

The following nursing diagnoses and expected outcomes may apply to the child with status epilepticus:

- Impaired Gas Exchange related to decreased respirations associated with seizures.

**Expected outcome.** The child will remain free from respiratory distress, as evidenced by pulse oxygen saturation remaining at or above 95%.

- Ineffective Breathing Pattern related to loss of muscle control associated with seizures.

**Expected outcome.** The child will maintain a normal breathing pattern, as evidenced by pulse oxygen saturation remaining at or above 95% and respiratory rate within normal range.

- Ineffective Airway Clearance related to possible aspiration during seizure.

**Expected outcome.** The child's airways will be clear, as evidenced by clear breath sounds.

- Risk for Ineffective Cerebral Tissue Perfusion related to lactic acidosis with prolonged seizure activity.

**Expected outcome.** The child will reestablish cerebral tissue perfusion, as evidenced by a return to normal levels of consciousness.

#### Interventions and Evaluation

The child will initially require establishment and maintenance of a patent airway. The nurse takes vital signs and performs neurologic checks frequently. Once the child is stable, nursing interventions and evaluation are similar to those described for the child with epilepsy.

**SAFETY ALERT**

***Drug Therapy for Generalized Status Epilepticus***

Generalized status epilepticus is a medical emergency. Intravenous (IV) diazepam (Valium), midazolam (Versed), or lorazepam (Ativan) is given. IV diazepam must be given directly into the vein (not the tubing, because it interacts with plastic) at a rate no greater than 1 to 2 mg/min. Diazepam should not be mixed with other drugs or solutions, and it can be diluted only with normal saline. Diazepam rectal gel can be administered in a community or hospital setting and is useful when the child does not have a readily accessible IV. Other pharmaceutical options for emergency treatment include buccal administration of midazolam and intranasal lorazepam. The use of newer antiepileptic drugs such as valproate and levetiracetam for the treatment of status epilepticus is an alternative. Resuscitation equipment should be at the bedside and the child's respirations closely monitored during IV antiepileptic drug administration.

Reference: Mikati, M.A., & Hani, A.J. (2016a). Status epilepticus. In R. Kliegman, B. Stanton, J. St. Geme, et al. (Eds.), *Nelson textbook of pediatrics* (20th ed., pp. 2854–2856). Philadelphia: Elsevier.

## MENINGITIS

Meningitis is the most common infectious process affecting the CNS. It can occur as a primary disease or as a result of complications of neurosurgery, trauma, systemic infection, or sinus or ear infections. A wide variety of bacteria and viruses can be responsible for the primary infection. Earlier diagnosis and prompt antibiotic therapy reduce mortality rates, which remain high, and the incidence of complications from bacterial meningitis (Richard & Lepe, 2013).

### Etiology

The primary organisms responsible for causing bacterial meningitis vary according to age. The organisms primarily responsible for neonatal meningitis are group B streptococci and *Escherichia coli.* Among children aged 2 months to 12 years, three pathogens seem to be the most prevalent; *Haemophilus influenzae* type B, *Neisseria meningitidis,* and *Streptococcus pneumoniae* cause 95% of the cases of purulent meningitis in this age-group. Tuberculous and *Borrelia burgdorferi* (Lyme disease) meningitis are becoming more common. These types of meningitis usually result from extension of a localized infection, such as otitis media, sinusitis, pharyngitis, or pneumonia, into the CSF.

Organisms also can be introduced directly after an injury in which the skin is broken and communication between skin, sinuses, and CSF occurs. Entry can occur in association with a lumbar puncture, skull fracture, or surgery.

Meningococcal meningitis caused by *N. meningitidis* usually occurs in older children and adolescents. Because it is transmitted primarily by droplet infection, the risk increases as the number of contacts increases. Viral meningitis is associated with the mumps virus, paramyxovirus, herpesvirus, and enterovirus. In rare cases, protozoa or fungi cause meningitis, usually in children with acquired immunodeficiency syndrome (AIDS).

## Incidence

Meningitis most commonly affects children between ages 1 month and 5 years, but it can occur at any age. Boys are affected more frequently than girls, and the incidence is higher among Black children than among white children. The incidence of *H. influenzae* type B meningitis has declined rapidly since the institution of routine immunization of infants.

## Manifestations

Signs and symptoms of meningitis vary according to the age of the child and the duration of the preceding illness. No single hallmark sign or symptom exists. In the neonate, infant, and young child, the symptoms of meningitis are frequently vague and nonspecific.

The clinical signs of meningitis in the neonate include poor feeding; poor sucking; vomiting; diarrhea; poor muscle tone; weak cry; hypothermia or hyperthermia; apnea; seizures; sepsis; disseminated intravascular coagulation (DIC); a full, tense, and bulging fontanel; and lethargy.

Clinical signs of meningitis in the infant and preschool-age child include fever, poor feeding, vomiting, irritability, seizures, a high-pitched cry, a bulging anterior fontanel, and lethargy. Early clinical signs of meningitis in children and adolescents include severe headache, photophobia, nuchal rigidity, fever, altered level of consciousness (lethargy, irritability), decreased appetite, vomiting, diarrhea, agitation, and drowsiness. Muscle or joint pain and purpura may be noted. Kernig sign (pain with extension of leg and knee) (Fig. 52.7) and Brudzinski sign (flexion of head causing flexion of hips and knees) are often exhibited. In the case of a meningococcal infection, a petechial or purpuric rash may be observed. Late signs include a decreased level of consciousness and seizures.

## Diagnostic Evaluation

The diagnosis is made by testing CSF obtained by lumbar puncture. Findings usually include increased CSF pressure, cloudy CSF (in the case of bacterial meningitis), high protein concentration, and low glucose level. Blood cultures are obtained; nose and throat cultures may be done, particularly if the CSF culture is negative.

## Therapeutic Management

Acute bacterial meningitis is a medical emergency requiring early recognition and prompt, aggressive management to avoid adverse outcomes. The child is placed in a private room on droplet transmission precautions, and these are maintained for at least 24 hours after antibiotics are initiated. Immediate initiation and uninterrupted IV administration of appropriate antibiotics are essential in cases of suspected

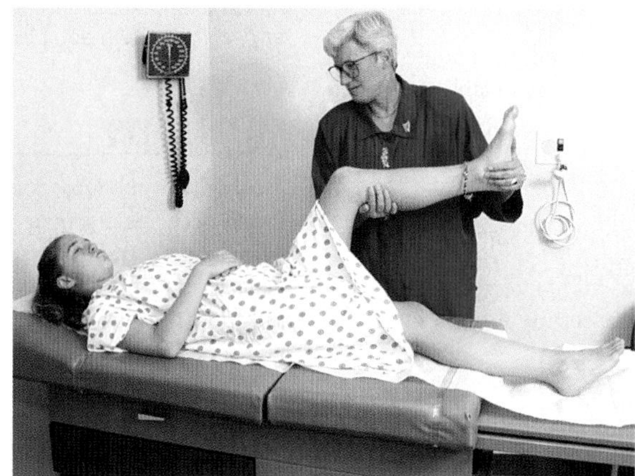

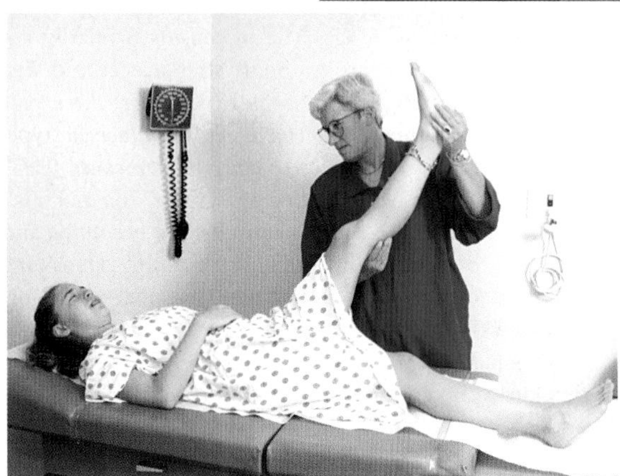

**Kernig Sign** The child can easily extend the leg when in the supine position. However, when the thigh is flexed toward the abdomen, pain prevents complete extension of the leg.

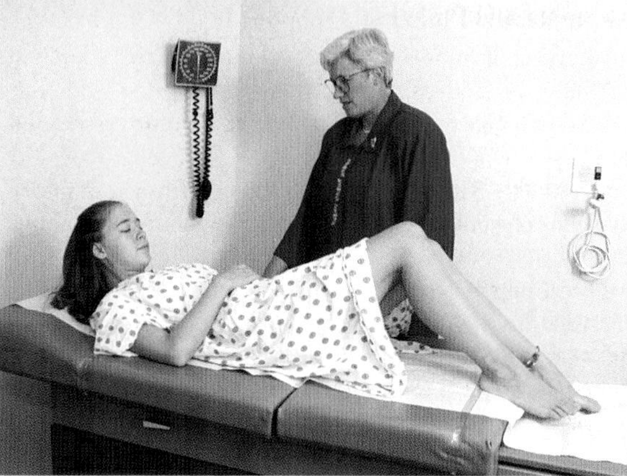

**Brudzinski Sign** In the supine position, the child bends her head toward her chest (in the younger child, the nurse can bend the child's head). This action usually produces involuntary hip and knee flexion in the child with meningitis.

**FIG 52.7** As part of the assessment for meningitis, the nurse can attempt to elicit the Kernig sign and Brudzinski sign. Both are early indicators of meningitis in children and adolescents. (Courtesy Parkland Health and Hospital System, Dallas, TX.)

bacterial meningitis; a delay could be fatal. Treatment is started before the causative organism is identified because cultures take up to 3 days to yield results. Selection of the broad-spectrum antibiotics initially used is based on the age of the child, the suspected pathogens most frequently encountered in the child's age-group, and the initial appearance of the CSF. If IV access is difficult to achieve, the first dose of antibiotics should be administered intramuscularly.

## PATHOPHYSIOLOGY

### *Meningitis*

Meningitis is an inflammation of the meninges of the brain that results from a pathogen entering the central nervous system (CNS) and causing a toxic response. As the process continues, increased intracranial pressure (ICP) develops along with subdural empyema. If the infection spreads to the ventricles, edema and tissue scarring around the ventricle cause obstruction of the cerebrospinal fluid (CSF) and subsequent hydrocephalus.

This process can happen quite rapidly; CSF is an excellent growth medium for bacteria because it contains nutrient substances such as protein and glucose. Leukocytes are unable to function as a defense mechanism in the fluid environment of the CSF. Leukocytes require a tissue surface to destroy bacteria, so there is little defense to stop the growth of bacteria, which multiply quickly.

As the infection spreads further into brain tissue, changes occur in the permeability of capillaries and blood vessels in the dura mater. These changes lead to increased passage of albumin and water into the subdural space, with a subsequent accumulation of protein and fluid that further increases the ICP.

Neurologic sequelae occur is approximately 10% to 30% of patients; the most common neurologic sequelae of meningitis are hearing loss, intellectual impairment, seizures, visual impairment, and behavioral problems (Richard & Lepe, 2013). Other complications include cranial nerve dysfunction, brain abscess, and syndrome of inappropriate antidiuretic hormone (SIADH). Meningococcemia, a fulminating manifestation of *Neisseria meningitides* infection that manifests with petechiae and purpura and signs of viral-type illness, can proceed in a matter of a few hours to adrenal insufficiency, bilateral adrenal hemorrhage (Waterhouse-Friderichsen syndrome), and septic shock.

Reference: Richard, G.C., & Lepe, M. (2013). Meningitis in children: diagnosis and treatment for the emergency clinician. *Clinical Pediatric Emergency Medicine, 14*(2), 146–156.

Treatment for neonatal bacterial meningitis consists of ampicillin and an aminoglycoside or a third-generation cephalosporin antibiotic. Monitoring of peak and trough antibiotic levels is essential to prevent ototoxicity and nephrotoxicity from aminoglycosides. For older children and adolescents, the treatment of choice is ampicillin, penicillin G, or a third-generation cephalosporin. When the culture and sensitivity test results are available, treatment regimens can be refined. Morbidity and mortality associated with bacterial meningitis is reduced by adjunctive treatment with dexamethasone, which can decrease intracranial pressure (Kim, 2014; Richard & Lepe, 2013). The treatment for viral meningitis is managed at home by providing symptomatic and supportive care, usually with complete recovery (Nigrovic, Fine, Monuteaux, et al., 2013).

Current recommendations are that children be vaccinated with meningococcal vaccine at the age of 11 to 12 years, or by the age of 18 years if previously unvaccinated. It is important that prospective college students receive meningococcal vaccine before college entry to prevent meningococcal meningitis and that children receive the *H. influenzae* type B (Hib) vaccine as part of their routine immunization schedule during infancy and early childhood (Centers for Disease Control and Prevention, 2015d).

## NURSING CARE

### The Child With Meningitis

#### Assessment

Baseline data are obtained from the history and physical examination and a complete neurologic assessment that evaluates headaches, photophobia, hearing loss, seizure activity, changes in level of consciousness, changes in pupil reactions and size, nuchal rigidity, and muscle flaccidity. Personality changes, irritability, changes in food and fluid intake, nausea, vomiting, and loss of appetite are also addressed. The nurse should review the history for past immunizations, recent illnesses including upper respiratory tract infection, otitis media, and skull fracture, and recent surgery or lumbar punctures.

#### Nursing Diagnosis and Planning

Nursing diagnoses that apply to the child with meningitis include those common to other neurologic disorders. (See Nursing Care Plan: The Child with a Neurologic System Disorder.) The following nursing diagnosis is specific to the child with meningitis and the child's family:

- Deficient Knowledge related to seriousness of meningitis, possible residual neurologic deficits, home management, and prophylaxis.
  **Expected outcome.** The parents' level of understanding of meningitis will increase, as evidenced by an ability to discuss the disease process and possible sequelae, treatment, home management, and possible implications for spread of the disease.

#### Interventions

The nurse discusses the disease process and prognosis with the parents after assessing their existing knowledge. The family is taught about the possible complications and sequelae of meningitis and the importance of follow-up care.

## ! NURSING QUALITY ALERT

### *Guidelines for the Child With Meningitis*

- The close contacts of the child with *Haemophilus influenzae* infection need prophylactic treatment with rifampin.
- In households with a person with *Haemophilus influenzae* infection where there is a household member younger than 48 months and unimmunized or incompletely immunized, rifampin is recommended for all household members.
- All close contacts of children with *Neisseria meningitidis,* regardless of age or immunization status, need prophylactic treatment, usually with oral rifampin or ciprofloxacin (AAP, 2015b).
- Rifampin colors the urine and sweat red-orange and will stain contact lenses.

Prophylaxis for the close contacts of the ill child with bacterial meningitis is necessary. Parents are asked to identify others exposed to meningitis and refer them for treatment. Close contacts must seek prompt medical attention because they might be incubating the infection.

The nurse educates the child, if age-appropriate, and parents about prescribed medications and treatments and provides written instructions. Parents must provide a return demonstration of all procedures they will perform at home, allowing the nurse to determine whether further education is needed. The nurse is aware that parents are often anxious about the child's illness and outcome so learning may be difficult. It is important to repeat information and allow time for practice in order to reinforce learning.

## CRITICAL THINKING EXERCISE 52.1

Pediatric nurses in the community often are in a position to answer questions about childhood illnesses. Recently, parents of high school children received a notice from the school nurse that a male student had been diagnosed with meningococcal meningitis. Close contacts of the student had been identified and treated appropriately. The nurse recommended that parents of children not in close contact with the student should be watchful but not overly concerned. Her letter advised parents to watch their children for 2 weeks and call the physician at any sign of illness.

1. Is this course of action prudent?
2. If so, why? If not, why not?

Complications of meningitis include hydrocephalus, vision and hearing loss, delayed growth and development, seizures, subdural effusions, and cranial nerve palsy. Vigilant assessment by the nurse and prompt notification of the physician can facilitate initiation of effective interventions if complications do occur. Early recognition and treatment of meningitis and its complications can substantially reduce morbidity and mortality rates.

### Evaluation

- Can the parents demonstrate the ability to administer the child's treatments and medications?
- Do the parents discuss the disease and treatments?
- Have the parents referred close contacts for treatment?

## GUILLAIN-BARRÉ SYNDROME

Guillain-Barré syndrome (GBS) is an autoimmune neurologic disorder of the peripheral nervous system characterized by rapidly progressing limb weakness and the loss of deep tendon reflexes. In rare cases, the motor and cranial nerves are also affected. Symptoms result from acute demyelinization of the nerves. In approximately half of the cases, the illness originates as an upper respiratory or gastrointestinal (GI) viral infection that is followed by signs of GBS in 2 to 4 weeks (Ryan, 2013). Associated viruses include rubella, enterovirus, Epstein-Barr virus, cytomegalovirus (CMV), mycoplasma, and varicella. *Campylobacter jejuni* is the most commonly identified pathogen linked to Guillain-Barré. The syndrome also occurs as a toxic response to seasonal influenza vaccines.

### Incidence

Guillain-Barré syndrome is rare and affects approximately 1 person in 100,000 each year worldwide (Morgan, 2015). It affects people of all ages, including infants, but the mean age of onset is 5 years (Morgan, 2015). It occurs moderately more often in males.

### Pathophysiology

The most prominent feature of Guillain-Barré syndrome is the infiltration of lymphocytes into peripheral nerves and subsequent inflammation. Initially, the myelin sheath becomes edematous; as further inflammation takes place, segmental demyelinization occurs. This process takes place along the membrane surrounding the Schwann cells. As the inflammatory process continues, myelin loss increases and results in axonal degeneration.

### Manifestations

- *Limb paresthesia and/or pain,* including numbness, tingling, and weakness of the lower extremities with an ascending loss of deep tendon reflexes leading to a flaccid paralysis.
- *Autonomic instability,* including blood pressure fluctuations, cardiac arrhythmias, postural hypotension, and urinary and bowel incontinence.
- *Cranial nerve dysfunction,* with facial nerve paralysis; dysphagia; and inadequate cough, gag, and swallow reflexes. In such cases, respiratory function will be impaired.
- *Respiratory failure* resulting from the progressive motor paralysis of the intercostal and phrenic nerves. Respiratory failure occurs in 15% to 25% of children with Guillain-Barré syndrome and is one of the major causes of mortality (Bilan, Barzegar, & Habibi, 2015).
- *Neuromuscular impairment* (bilateral ascending weakness or paralysis) usually progresses upward from the feet to the head. (As healing takes place, neuromuscular function returns gradually in reverse order—head to feet.)

### Diagnostic Evaluation

Bilateral ascending weakness or paralysis occurring 2 to 4 weeks after an upper respiratory infection or gastric illness is a diagnostic indicator. The paralysis can affect the respiratory muscles quickly, and any indications of respiratory distress should prompt elective intubation (Morgan, 2015). The CSF may demonstrate high protein levels. Nerve conduction studies, LP, and MRI can help confirm the diagnosis (Morgan, 2015).

### Therapeutic Management

Spontaneous recovery occurs with 2 to 3 weeks, and most patients regain full muscular strength (Sarnet, 2016). Children with rapidly progressing paralysis are treated with high-dose IV immune globulin (IVIG) for several days. A recent study showed that some children benefit from a second course of IVIG because of patient differences in pharmacokinetics (Morgan, 2015). For patients who fail to recover with IVIG, plasmapheresis is an alternative treatment (Morgan, 2015; Ryan, 2013). Medical management of the child with Guillain-Barré syndrome is supportive, with attention given to the neurologic, respiratory, and cardiovascular systems. Respiratory support is of critical importance because most deaths are attributed to respiratory failure.

## NURSING CARE

### The Child With Guillain-Barré Syndrome

#### Assessment

A complete history and physical examination are important to determine the presence of an antecedent viral illness and establish baseline clinical status. Special emphasis is given to evaluating the respiratory and neurologic systems. Respiratory status should be assessed hourly or more frequently in some cases because of the risk of respiratory compromise and the need for prompt action, including intubation and ventilator support, if the child's respiratory status deteriorates. Major assessment parameters include respiratory rate, chest excursion, energy expended to breathe, and breath sounds. Pulse oximetry assesses the effectiveness of gas exchange. Daily pulmonary function testing might be ordered. A thorough neurologic assessment is generally performed every 1 to 2 hours, although this may be done more frequently depending on the child's clinical condition. Neurologic parameters to address include cranial nerve function, motor capabilities, sensory perception, and deep tendon reflexes.

#### Nursing Diagnosis and Planning

The following nursing diagnoses and expected outcomes may apply to the child with Guillain-Barré syndrome and the child's family:

- Ineffective Breathing Pattern related to neuromuscular impairment.

*Expected outcome.* The child will remain free from respiratory distress, as evidenced by clear bilateral breath sounds, good chest expansion, and normal tidal volume.

- Decreased Cardiac Output related to autonomic instability.

*Expected outcome.* The child will maintain cardiac output, as evidenced by brisk capillary refill, normal urine output, good pulses in all extremities, and no arrhythmias.

- Risk for Impaired Skin Integrity related to immobility with paralysis.

*Expected outcome.* The child will maintain skin integrity, as evidenced by the absence of skin breakdown or pressure ulcers.

- Impaired Verbal Communication related to neuromuscular impairment.

*Expected outcome.* The child will maintain the ability to communicate, as evidenced by demonstration of new ways to communicate with available muscles, such as eye blinks or eye movements.

- Impaired Urinary Elimination related to paralysis.

*Expected outcome.* The child will have acceptable urinary elimination, as evidenced by an empty bladder, no urinary tract infection or distention of the abdomen, and urine output within normal limits for age (see Chapter 44).

- Anxiety related to increasing ascending paralysis.

*Expected outcome.* The child will display decreased anxiety, as evidenced by an ability to interact calmly with parents and healthcare providers and have decreased fretful periods and increased restful periods.

- Deficient Knowledge related to unfamiliarity with disease progression, treatment, and home care.

*Expected outcome.* The child and parents will have increased knowledge of the disease and treatment, as evidenced by an ability to make plans about discharge care and discuss the illness and possible complications.

- Interrupted Family Processes related to having a child with a prolonged illness.

*Expected outcome.* The parents will use coping strategies to adjust to their child's illness, as evidenced by discussing support systems and changes in the family.

### Interventions

The goals of nursing care for the child with Guillain-Barré syndrome are to achieve optimal neurologic function with an emphasis on maintaining independence in activities of daily living and to facilitate a recovery without complications.

Treatment is largely supportive, with a focus on assessing and monitoring the child's clinical status and preventing or minimizing complications. The nurse must be able to recognize any change in the child's condition and intervene in a timely and effective manner.

The nurse must anticipate possible deterioration in the child's respiratory status due to progressive muscle weakness leading to flaccidity. Resuscitation and ventilatory support might be urgently needed; appropriate emergency equipment and personnel should be available. Equipment, such as a bag-valve-mask device, oxygen, suction, endotracheal tubes with stylets, and a laryngoscope with a variety of blades, should be at the bedside. To prevent infection, chest physiotherapy should be done every 2 to 4 hours.

Interruption in the autonomic nervous system reflexes can cause circulatory changes, resulting in arrhythmias, hypotension, dizziness, and night sweats. Early detection of neurologic changes is made by serial assessments, and prompt action should be taken to correct problems and prevent complications.

The child with Guillain-Barré syndrome is at an increased risk for developing complications associated with immobility. Maintaining skin integrity is a priority. Turning, repositioning, passive range of motion, and monitoring pressure points are performed by the nurse at least every 2 hours. Use of special mattresses and managing incontinence will help prevent skin breakdown. To prevent contractures, daily physical and occupational therapy are included in the child's treatment plan. Range of motion, active exercises, correct alignment, and application of splints and braces are all part of the child's daily care.

The risk of pulmonary embolus as a result of deep vein thrombosis is always a threat. Frequent turning and repositioning, with special attention to positioning the child's legs to alleviate pressure on the dorsal aspect of the knees, are essential. Anticoagulant therapy may be initiated; if so, the nurse should monitor clotting times and watch for any signs of bleeding.

As cranial nerve function is altered and interference with gag and swallow occurs, nutrition becomes a vitally important issue. Adequate caloric intake is essential to prevent catabolism. Alternative methods of providing nutrition must be used. The physician might order nasogastric, nasojejunostomy, or gastrostomy feedings. The nurse monitors the type and amount of feeding, tube placement and patency, tolerance of feedings (residuals, abdominal distention, stools), and weight gain. Total parenteral nutrition is provided to the child during the acute phase of the illness or if alternative methods of nutritional support are not tolerated.

The progression of Guillain-Barré syndrome is unpredictable; the loss of function is frightening, and the recovery time varies from months to years. These factors can result in considerable anxiety for the child and family. The nurse provides educational and emotional support to the child and family, reassuring them that a full recovery from Guillain-Barré syndrome is possible. It is essential to keep them well informed and answer their questions. The nurse encourages the child and family members to verbalize feelings concerning the illness and hospitalization, and then supports and validates these feelings. Referrals to other healthcare providers, child life therapists, and counselors are often indicated.

Facilitating the child's development during the illness by normalizing the situation as much as possible is a key nursing intervention. As the child's clinical condition worsens and dependency on the parents and healthcare providers increases, the child is offered choices and encouraged to make decisions whenever possible. Communication is maintained with the child's teacher, classmates, and friends, and involvement in school work is continued.

The nurse supports the role of the parents as the primary caregivers by facilitating parental participation in the child's care. This helps the parents support their child. If the child's clinical condition requires transfer to a critical care unit, the nurse ensures that the child and family are prepared and takes other actions to lessen the family's anxiety. Compassionate and competent healthcare team members can optimize the child's recovery.

### Evaluation

- Does the child demonstrate normal respiratory function?
- Is the child able to communicate needs?
- Has the child's neurologic status returned to normal?
- Is the child's skin intact?
- Do the parents participate in and discuss the child's care?

## NEUROLOGIC CONDITIONS REQUIRING CRITICAL CARE

A number of neurologic conditions, including encephalitis, Reye syndrome, botulism, and tetanus, require critical nursing care. Children with these conditions are frequently admitted to hospital critical care units where the care is specialized (Table 52.4).

**TABLE 52.4 Neurologic Conditions Requiring Critical Care**

| Pathophysiology, Etiology, and Incidence | Manifestations | Therapeutic Management | Nursing Considerations |
|---|---|---|---|
| **Encephalitis** | | | |
| Inflammation caused by infection or toxin, resulting in cerebral edema and neurologic dysfunction.<br>Numerous agents are causative, including St. Louis encephalitis, CMV, and West Nile virus.<br>Peak incidence is in middle to late childhood, with a prevalence of 0.3-0.5/100,000 people in the United States*. | Headache, irritability, lethargy, altered level of consciousness, nuchal rigidity, seizures, fever, malaise, dizziness, nausea and vomiting, ataxia, sensory disturbances | Diagnosed by lumbar puncture and CSF culture; EEG alterations are not unusual.<br>Care includes hospitalization and monitoring for increased ICP.<br>Medication: cephalosporin or acyclovir (depending on causative agent), antiepileptics. | Care is similar to that for any child with increased ICP.<br>Care includes fever management with antipyretics; pharmacologic and nonpharmacologic headache relief measures; maintenance of fluid and electrolyte balance; support for anxious family members; assistance to the family with management of any long-term neurologic deficits; and facilitation of grieving for the family of a child with a poor prognosis. |
| **Reye Syndrome** | | | |
| Exposure to viral agent or toxin in at-risk children leads to liver cell damage with rising serum ammonia levels. The toxic serum ammonia levels result in cerebral dysfunction (encephalopathy, cerebral edema), fluid and electrolyte and acid–base imbalances, and coagulopathies.<br>The average age at onset is 6-7 yr.<br>Reye syndrome may be related to administration of aspirin to children with a viral disease. | Antecedent viral infection; malaise, nausea and vomiting, progressive neurologic deterioration.<br>Elevated serum ammonia levels, liver dysfunction on biopsy, hypoglycemia, altered coagulation times, increased ICP with respiratory dysfunction.<br>Reye syndrome is clinically staged from I (lethargy) to V (coma with flaccidity/extension posturing). | Care includes hospitalization for monitoring of neurologic status, increasing ICP, hydration and acid-base balance, and cardiorespiratory status. | Care is similar to that for any child with increasing ICP, with the potential addition of mechanical respiratory support.<br>Accurate, continuous monitoring of neurologic and cardiorespiratory status is essential because the child's condition can deteriorate suddenly.<br>Fluid replacement is achieved with IV hypertonic solutions if ICP is not increased.<br>Protect the child from coagulopathy-related injury. |
| **Botulism** | | | |
| Food poisoning caused by *Clostridium botulinum* toxin. The source is honey (in infants) or improperly sterilized canned foods.<br>Approximately 200 cases occur per year in the United States (Bork & Rega, 2012). | CNS symptoms 12-36 hr after ingestion include weakness, headache, double vision, vomiting, difficulty talking, respiratory paralysis, decreased deep tendon reflexes, impaired gag reflex. | Care is supportive and includes respiratory support and administering antitoxin.<br>Recovery after treatment takes an average of 1 mo. | Advise parents not to give infants honey or syrup in their milk or water.<br>Educate the public about proper food preparation techniques. |
| **Tetanus (Lockjaw)** | | | |
| Caused by endotoxin produced by the anaerobic, spore-forming, gram-positive bacillus *C. tetani.*<br>Entry sites include puncture wounds, burns, lacerations, and compound fractures.<br>Approximately 50 cases occur in the United States each year. The incubation period is 2 days to 2 wk (Arnon, 2016). | Painful muscular rigidity of masseter and neck muscles, facial spasms, dysphagia, laryngospasm, severe pain, respiratory arrest. | Care includes wound debridement, ventilatory and respiratory support. Medication: diazepam (Valium) or lorazepam (Ativan) for seizures; tetanus immune globulin. Penicillin G and metronidazole are the antibiotics used most frequently (Arnon, 2016). | Assess the child's ventilatory and neurologic status and provide respiratory support as needed. Provide fluids and electrolytes, seizure precautions, quiet environment. Educate the child and family about immunizations. |

*Tailor, Y.I., Suskauer, S.J., Sepeta, L.N., et al. (2013). Functional status of children with encephalitis in an inpatient rehabilitation setting: a case series. *Journal of Pediatric Rehabilitation Medicine, 6,* 163–173. doi:10.3233/PRM-130248.

*CNS,* Central nervous system; *CSF,* cerebrospinal fluid; *EEG,* electroencephalogram; *ICP,* intracranial pressure; *IV,* intravenous.

## HEADACHES

Headaches are a common disorder in children of all ages, and their prevalence has significantly increased in western countries and in Asia over the past 30 years. Up to 75% of children and adolescents complain of occasional headaches, with 20% of these children being affected by chronic tension and migraine headaches (Hershey, Kabbouche, & O'Brien, 2016; Kaczynski, Claar, & LeBel, 2013).

### Etiology

The three primary sources of recurrent headache are vascular, tension (stress), and increased ICP. Vascular headaches include migraines and headaches that occur as a result of arteriovenous malformations. Tension headaches frequently are the result of stress. Contributing factors to increased ICP are space-occupying lesions and hydrocephalus.

### Incidence

Migraine (vascular) headaches occur in approximately 8% of children and adolescents (Harding & Clark, 2014). Migraines in preadolescents are equally prevalent in males and females, but for adolescents, the incidence greatly increases for females. A family history of headaches is noted in a majority of these cases. Other frequent causes of headaches in children include tension-type headaches and nonmigrainous headaches.

### Manifestations

#### Migraine

Symptoms range from mild episodes, in which case the child can continue with daily activities, to episodes that force the child to go to a quiet, dark room for relief. In some cases, an aura occurs before the headache begins. The aura can include seeing flashing lights; smelling specific odors; blurry, double, or lost vision; and tingling in the arms or legs. Once the headache begins, the most common symptoms include throbbing pain, often on both sides of the head, nausea and vomiting, irritability, abdominal pain, photophobia, and phonophobia. The pain of a typical migraine lasts from 1 hour to more than 48 hours. Depression and anxiety frequently coexist with migraine headaches (Harding & Clark, 2014).

#### Tension-Type Headaches

The pain associated with tension-type headaches is usually more generalized than that of a migraine. The child may describe the pain as a band-like tightness or pressure, tight neck muscles, or soreness of the scalp. Nausea is rare, but fatigue and dizziness are common. These headaches can last for days or weeks but usually do not interfere with the child's regular activities.

### Diagnostic Evaluation

The International Headache Society published revised clinical criteria for classifying and diagnosing headaches in 2013 (third edition of the International Headache Classification [ICHD-3]). Clinical manifestations and diagnostic criteria are more precisely identified allowing for the development of targeted treatment plans (International Headache Society, 2013). In addition to addressing the signs and symptoms of headache as described in the ICHD-3, the child's blood pressure is evaluated and head size is measured, looking for evidence of chronically increased ICP. A detailed neurologic examination should be performed, with special attention given to auscultating for a bruit in the head (suggesting an arteriovenous malformation), assessing mental status, and examining both optic disks for papilledema. CT or MRI may be performed in children with chronic headaches or those with abnormalities found on the neurologic examination. A thorough assessment also includes asking questions about medication history, since daily use of analgesics can cause rebound headaches (Harding & Clark, 2014).

## NURSING CARE

### The Child With Headaches

#### Assessment

A detailed history of the child's headache and preheadache events is important to determine precipitating factors (e.g., poor diet, poor hydration, food sensitivities, altered sleep patterns, flashing lights). A social history of the child and family may identify triggering stressors (e.g., divorce; move to a new school; loss of a family member, friend, or pet). The child should receive a comprehensive physical examination with emphasis on the neurologic system.

#### Nursing Diagnosis and Planning

Nursing diagnoses that may apply to a child with a headache and the child's family include those common to other neurologic disorders, such as the following:

- Acute Pain or Chronic Pain related to underlying contributing factors.

*Expected outcome.* The child will have decreased pain related to headaches, as evidenced by an ability to identify triggering factors and demonstrate appropriate nonpharmacologic approaches.

- Deficient Knowledge related to unfamiliarity with the management of a child with headaches and the medication regimen.

*Expected outcome.* The child and parents will discuss the plan for managing the child's headaches including a description of the medication regimen.

- Risk for Injury related to headache symptoms (change in vision, dizziness).

*Expected outcome.* The child will have risk for injury reduced, as evidenced by parents verbalizing a safety plan for the child during a headache and when receiving medication for treatment of a headache.

#### Interventions

The nurse educates the child and family about factors that can trigger the onset of a headache (e.g., stress, food, menstruation, visual stimuli, fatigue, certain medications), and how to make lifestyle changes that will lower stress and avoid triggers. Keeping a diary of the child's headaches and preheadache events will help identify specific triggers; electronic diaries are increasingly common for children 8 years and older (Connelly & Bickel, 2011).

For mild or infrequent migraines and tension headaches, common analgesics, such as ibuprofen or acetaminophen are effective in alleviating half of moderate to severe headaches within 2 hours (Harding & Clark, 2014). For more severe migraine in adolescents older than 12 years of age, or those with persistent symptoms, the recommended treatment is nasal sumatriptan, almotriptan, or rizatriptan for children six years and older (Harding & Clark, 2014). If children have two or more severe migraine headaches per month, they may need daily prophylactic medication; Topiramate is the only FDA approved prophylactic medication and is approved for adolescents age 12 and older, although amitriptyline and propranolol are commonly used (Harding & Clark, 2014). Psychological evaluation followed by relaxation therapy, counseling, acupuncture, or biofeedback therapy helps some children (Harding & Clark, 2014).

The nursing care for a child with headaches is both acute and long term. Acute management includes placing the child in a dark, quiet environment and administering medication. Long-term management focuses on education about and elimination of trigger factors, stress relief measures, and medication administration. Teaching adolescents stress reduction and relaxation techniques can alleviate symptoms, thereby decreasing the social isolation that often accompanies headaches (Helvig & Minick, 2013).

### Evaluation

- Can the child and parents describe the management of headache and the medication regimen?
- Do the child and parents understand the need for following a safety plan to prevent injury during headache and when receiving treatment with medication?
- Are the child and parents learning to eliminate headache trigger factors?
- Can the child demonstrate and benefit from relaxation therapy and biofeedback?

## KEY CONCEPTS

- The CNS is composed of the brain and spinal cord. The bones of the skull do not become fused until 12 to 18 months of life. The brain and spinal cord are covered by a fibrous connective structure containing many blood vessels known as meninges.
- CSF surrounds the brain and spinal cord. The brain is composed of the cerebrum, cerebellum, and brainstem.
- The peripheral nervous system comprises 12 pairs of cranial nerves and 31 pairs of spinal nerves. The autonomic nervous system includes the sympathetic and parasympathetic systems.
- The physiologic process of autoregulation helps the body regulate blood flow. When autoregulation fails to change vascular diameter in response to changes in cerebral perfusion pressure, cerebrovascular dilation is impaired, and cerebral blood flow decreases.
- Hypercapnia or hypoxia leads to cerebral dilation and increased ICP. Hypocapnia leads to cerebral arterial constriction and decreased ICP.
- An infant's brain is two thirds the size of an adult's brain. The brain grows to 80% of adult size by age 1 year.
- Head circumference can change in the infant and young child, but the head of the adolescent and adult is unyielding. This change has implications for head circumference measurement for growth and development in the infant and young child.
- The spinal cord, cranial nerves, and peripheral nerves become longer during childhood; the spinal cord terminates at L3 in the newborn and L1 to L2 in the adult.
- Myelinization of nerves begins in the third month of gestation and is completed in adolescence, as demonstrated by progressive development and coordination.
- Neurologic changes may be more subtle in the infant or child than in the adult and can be indicated by irritability or poor feeding behaviors.
- The neurologic examination assesses level of consciousness, pupil size and reaction to light, cranial nerve function, motor and sensory functions, respiratory status and function, vital signs, and head circumference.
- Different seizure types are treated with specific antiepileptic medications to achieve optimal seizure control. These medications have many side effects. CBC, liver enzyme levels, and medication levels should be determined routinely.
- When antiepileptics are given via IV, the most common side effect is respiratory depression.
- Mannitol and furosemide (Lasix) are diuretics used to decrease ICP. Their effect is monitored through serum electrolyte levels and serum osmolality.
- Cerebral edema is decreased by maintaining adequate oxygenation and perfusion of the brain, administering diuretics, elevating the head of the bed 30 to 45 degrees, keeping the child in good alignment so that venous drainage is not impaired, and reducing agitation and noxious stimuli.
- Abnormal posturing (flexion or extension) is an ominous neurologic sign.
- Hydrocephalus can be communicating or noncommunicating. Enlarged ventricles and increased ICP can result. If the cranial sutures are not ossified, the head circumference will be abnormally large.
- Teaching for the child with a neurologic deficit and the child's family is begun after the child's and family's needs have been assessed. The family's grieving may be verbalized; emotions and fears should be expressed and validated. The nurse reinforces information that has been supplied by other members of the healthcare team.
- The nurse encourages parents in their caregiving efforts when appropriate, assists the family in setting realistic goals for the child, and identifies support systems and refers to community agencies.
- The nurse has family members demonstrate skills necessary for home care and encourages therapeutic play and peer contact. The nurse provides incentives for accomplishments and identifies the child's positive qualities and coping mechanisms.

## REFERENCES AND READINGS


American Academy of Pediatrics. (2015a). *Sports-related concussion: understanding the risks, signs & symptoms*. Retrieved from https://www.healthychildren.org/English/health-issues/injuries-emergencies/sports-injuries/Pages/Sports-Related-Concussion-Understanding-the-Risks-Signs-Symptoms.aspx.

American Academy of Pediatrics. (2015b). Meningococcal infections. In D.W. Kimberlin, M.T. Brady, M.A. Jackson, et al. (Eds.), *Red book 2015 report of the committee on infectious diseases* (30th ed., pp. 547–558). Elk Grove Village, IL: AAP; 2015.

Anand, V., & Nair, P.M. (2014). Neonatal seizures: predictors of adverse outcome. *Journal of Pediatric Neurosciences*, *9*, 97–99. doi:10.4103/1817-1745.139261.

Arnon, S.S. (2016). Tetanus (*Clostridium tetani*). In R. Kliegman, B. Stanton, J. St. Geme, et al. (Eds.), *Nelson textbook of pediatrics* (20th ed., pp. 1432–1434). Philadelphia: Elsevier.

Atabaki, S.M. (2013). Updates in the general approach to pediatric head trauma and concussion. *Pediatric Clinics of North America*, *60*, 1107–1122. doi:10.1016/j.pcl.2013.06.001.

Berg, A., & Scheffer, I. (2011). New concepts in classification of the epilepsies: entering the 21st century. *Epilepsia, 52*(6), 1058–1062. Retrieved from http://www.ilae.org/Visitors/Centre/ctf/documents/NewConcepts-Classification_2011_000.pdf.

Bilan, N., Barzegar, M., & Habibi, P. (2015). Predictive factors of respiratory failure in children with Guillain-Barré syndrome. *International Journal of Pediatrics, 3*(2-1), 33–37.

Bork, C.E., & Rega, P.P. (2012). An assessment of nurses' knowledge of botulism. *Public Health Nursing, 29*(2), 168–174. doi:10.111/j.1525-1446.2011.00988.x.

Brustrom, J., Thibadeau, J., John, L., et al. (2012). Care coordination in the spina bifida clinic setting: current practice and future directions. *Journal of Pediatric Health Care, 26*(1), 16–26. doi:10.1016/j.pedhc.2010.06.003.

Campagnolo, D. (2011). *Autonomic dysreflexia in spinal cord injury*. Retrieved from http://emedicine.medscape.com/article/322809-overview.

Centers for Disease Control and Prevention. (2014). *Epilepsy basics*. Retrieved from http://www.cdc.gov/epilepsy/basics/index.htm.

Centers for Disease Control and Prevention. (2015a). *Data and statistics for cerebral palsy*. Retrieved from http://www.cdc.gov/ncbddd/cp/data.html.

Centers for Disease Control and Prevention. (2015b). *Heads up to school sports*. Retrieved from http://www.cdc.gov/headsup/highschoolsports/index.html.

Centers for Disease Control and Prevention. (2015c). Seizures in children and adolescents aged 6- 17 years- United States, 2010-2014. *Morbidity and Mortality Weekly Report, 64*(43) 1209–1214.

Centers for Disease Control and Prevention. (2015d). *Meningococcal Vaccination*. Retrieved from: http://www.cdc.gov/vaccines/vpd-vac/mening/default.htm.

Chelse, A.B., Kelley, K., Hageman, J.R., et al. (2013). Initial evaluation and management of a first seizure in children. *Pediatric Annals, 42*(12), 244–248. doi:10.3928/00904481-20131122-08.

Cicero, M.X., & Cross, K.P. (2013). Predictive value of initial Glasgow coma scale score in pediatric trauma patients. *Pediatric Emergency Care, 29*(1), 43–48.

Connelly, M., & Bickel, J. (2011). An electronic daily diary process study of stress and health behavior triggers of primary headaches in children. *Journal of Pediatric Psychology, 36*(8), 852–862. doi:10.1093/jepsy/jsr017.

Doerrer, S.C., & Kossoff, E.H. (2014). First seizure: dispel the myths [Electronic Version]. *Contemporary Pediatrics, 31*(2), 9.

Ducharme-Crevier, L., & Wainwright, M. (2015). Acute management of children with traumatic brain injury. *Clinical Pediatric Emergency Medicine, 16*(1), 48–54.

Edwards, P., Sakzewski, L., Copeland, L., et al. (2015). Safety of botulinum toxin type a for children with nonambulatory cerebral palsy. *Pediatrics, 136*(5), 895–904. doi:10.1542/peds.2015-0749.

Epilepsy Foundation of America. (2012). *Ketogenic diet*. Retrieved from http://www.epilepsyfoundation.org/aboutepilepsy/treatment/ketogenicdiet/index.cfm.

Fingarson, A., & Pierce, M.C. (2012). Identifying abusive head trauma: knowing what to look for can save babies from future harm [Electronic Version]. *Contemporary Pediatrics, 16–22.*

Geyer, K., Meller, K., Kulpan, C., et al. (2013). Traumatic brain injury in children: acute care management. *Pediatric Nursing, 39*(6), 283–289.

Gioia, G.A. (2012). Pediatric assessment and management of concussions. *Pediatric Annals, 41*(5), 198-203. doi:10.3928/00904481-20120426-10.

Grady, M.F., Master, C.L., & Gioia, G.A. (2012). Concussion pathophysiology: rationale for physical and cognitive rest. *Pediatric Annals, 41*(9), 377–382. doi:10.3928/00904481-20120827-12.

Harding, A., & Clark, L. (2014). Pediatric migraine: common, yet treatable. *The Nurse Practitioner, 39*(11), 22–31. doi:10.1097/01.NPR.0000454980.88918.f0.

Hartman, A.L., Devore, C.D., & Section on Neurology & Council on School Health. (2016). Rescue medication for epilepsy in education settings. *Pediatrics, 137*(1), 1–5. doi:10.1542/peds.2015-3876.

Hartman, M.E., & Cheifetz, I.M. (2016). Pediatric emergencies and resuscitation. In R. Kliegman, B. Stanton, J. St. Geme, et al. (Eds.), *Nelson textbook of pediatrics* (20th ed., pp. 489–506). Philadelphia: Elsevier.

Helvig, A.W., & Minick, P. (2013). Adolescents and headaches: maintaining control. *Pediatric Nursing, 39*(1), 19–25.

Hershey, A.D., Kabbouche, M.A., & O'Brien, H.L. (2016). Headaches. In R. Kliegman, B. Stanton, J. St. Geme, et al. (Eds.), *Nelson textbook of pediatrics* (20th ed., pp. 2863–2873). Philadelphia: Elsevier.

Horeczko, T., & Kuppermann, N. (2012). To scan or not to scan: pediatric minor head trauma in your office, clinic, or emergency department [Electronic Version]. *Contemporary Pediatrics,* 40–47.

International Headache Society. (2013). *IHS classification: ICHD III*. Retrieved from http://www.ihs-headache.org/ichd-guidelines.

Johnston, M.V. (2016). Encephalopathies. In R. Kliegman, B. Stanton, J. St. Geme, et al. (Eds.). *Nelson textbook of pediatrics* (20th ed., pp. 2896–28910). Philadelphia: Elsevier.

Kaczynski, K.J., Claar, R.L., & LeBel, A.A. (2013). Relations between pain characteristics, child and parent variables, and school functioning in adolescents with chronic headache: a comparison of tension-type headache and Migraine. *Journal of Pediatric Psychology, 38*(4), 351–364. doi:10.1093/jepsy/jss120.

Kerr, H.A. (2014). Concussion risk factors and strategies for prevention. *Pediatric Annals, 43*(12), e309–e315. doi:10.3928/00904481-20141124-10.

Kinsman, S.L., & Johnston, M.V. (2016a). Hydrocephalus. In R. Kliegman, B. Stanton, J. St. Geme, et al. (Eds.), *Nelson textbook of pediatrics* (20th ed., pp. 2814–2817). Philadelphia: Elsevier.

Kinsman, S.L., & Johnston, M.V. (2016b). Myelomeningocele. In R. Kliegman, B. Stanton, J. St. Geme, et al. (Eds.), *Nelson textbook of pediatrics* (20th ed., pp. 2805–2806). Philadelphia: Elsevier.

Kim, K.S. (2014). Bacterial meningitis beyond the neonatal period. In J. Cherry, G. Harrison, S. Kaplan, et al. (Eds.), *Feigin and Cherry's textbook of pediatric infectious diseases* (7th ed., pp. 425–461). Philadelphia: Elsevier Saunders.

Kochanek, P.M., & Bell, M.J. (2016). Neurological emergencies and stabilization. In R. Kliegman, B. Stanton, J. St. Geme, et al. (Eds.), *Nelson textbook of pediatrics* (20th ed., pp. 507–514). Philadelphia: Elsevier.

Lehman, R.K., & Schor, N.F. (2016). Neurologic evaluation. In R. Kliegman, B. Stanton, J. St. Geme, et al. (Eds.), *Nelson textbook of pediatrics* (20th ed., pp. 2791–2802). Philadelphia: Elsevier.

Mason, C.N. (2013). Mild traumatic brain injury in children. *Pediatric Nursing, 39*(6), 267–282.

Master, C.L., & Grady, M.F. (2012). Office-based management of pediatric and adolescent concussion. *Pediatric Annals, 41*(9), 1–6. doi:10.3928/00904481-20120827-08.

McGuire, C.S., & McCambridge, T.M. (2011). Concussion in the young athlete: diagnosis, management, and prevention [Electronic Version]. *Contemporary Pediatrics,* 30–44.

McLaughlin, K. (2015). Pediatric concussions: can technology detect the impact? *Journal of Pediatric Nursing, 30,* 270–273. doi:10.1016/j.pedn.2014.10.008.

Mikati, M.A., & Hani, A.J. (2016a). Status epilepticus. In R. Kliegman, B. Stanton, J. St. Geme, et al. (Eds.), *Nelson textbook of pediatrics* (20th ed., pp. 2854–2856). Philadelphia: Elsevier.

Mikati, M.A., & Hani, A.J. (2016b). Neonatal seizures. In R. Kliegman, B. Stanton, J. St. Geme, et al. (Eds.). *Nelson textbook of pediatrics* (20th ed., pp. 2849–2854). Philadelphia: Elsevier.

Mikati, M.A., & Hani, A.J. (2016c). Treatment of seizures and epilepsy. In R. Kliegman, B. Stanton, J. St. Geme, et al. (Eds.), *Nelson textbook of pediatrics* (20th ed., pp. 2838–2849). Philadelphia: Elsevier.

Morgan, L. (2015). The child with acute weakness. *Clinical Pediatric Emergency Medicine, 16*(1), 19–28.

National Institute of Neurological Disorders and Stroke. (2013a). *Hydrocephalus fact sheet*. Retrieved from http://www.ninds.nih.gov/disorders/hydrocephalus/detail_hydrocephalus.htm.

National Institute of Neurological Disorders and Stroke. (2013b). *Spinal cord injury: hope through research*. Retrieved from http://www.ninds.nih.gov/disorders/sci/detail_sci.htm.

Nigrovic, L.E., Fine, A.M., Monuteaux, M.C., et al. (2013). Trends in the management of viral meningitis at United States Children's Hospitals. *Pediatrics, 131*(4), 670–676. doi:10.1542/peds.2012-3077.

Park, J.T., Shahid, A.M., & Jammoul, A. (2015). Common pediatric epilepsy syndromes. *Pediatric Annals, 44*(2), e30–e35. doi:10.3928/00904481-20150203-09.

Patterson, J.L., Carapetian, S.A., Hageman, J.R., et al. (2013). Febrile seizures. *Pediatric Annals, 42*(12), 249–254. doi:10.3928/00904481-20131122-09.

Pruitt, D.W., & McMahon, M.A. (2016). Spinal cord injury and autonomic crisis management. In R. Kliegman, B. Stanton, J. St. Geme, et al. (Eds.), *Nelson textbook of pediatrics* (20th ed., pp. 3400–3402). Philadelphia: Elsevier.

Rekate, H.L. (2016). Spinal cord injuries in children. In R. Kliegman, B. Stanton, J. St. Geme, et al. (Eds.), *Nelson textbook of pediatrics* (20th ed., pp. 2957). Philadelphia: Elsevier.

Richard, G.C., & Lepe, M. (2013). Meningitis in children: diagnosis and treatment for the emergency clinician. *Clinical Pediatric Emergency Medicine, 14*(2), 146–156.

Rivera, R.G., Roberson, S.P., Whelan, M., et al. (2015). Concussion evaluation and management in pediatrics. *Maternal Child Nursing, 40*(2), 76–86.

Ryan, M.M. (2013). Pediatric Guillian Barré syndrome. *Current Opinion in Pediatrics, 25*, 689–693. doi:10.1097/MOP.0b013e328365ad3f.

Sankaraneni, R., & Lachhwani, D. (2015). Antiepileptic drugs- a review. *Pediatric Annals, 44*(2), e36–e42. doi:10.3928/00904481-20150203-10.

Sarnet, H.B. (2016). Guillain-Barré syndrome. In R. Kliegman, B. Stanton, J. St. Geme, et al. (Eds.), *Nelson textbook of pediatrics* (20th ed., pp. 3010–3013). Philadelphia: Elsevier.

Sharp, G.B., Samanta, D., & Willis, E. (2015). Options for pharmacoresistant epilepsy in children: when medications don't work. *Pediatric Annals, 44*(2), e43–e48. doi:10.3928/00904481-20150203-11.

Spina Bifida Association. (2015). *Latex List.* Retrieved from http://spinabifidaassociation.org/latex/.

Vidal, P.G., Goodman, A.M., Colin, A., et al. (2012). Rehabilitation strategies for prolonged recovery in pediatric and adolescent concussion. *Pediatric Annals, 41*(9), 1–6. doi:10.3928/00904481-20120827-10.

Wenger, J.K. (2014). Spina bifida: top 10 things for physicians to know [Electronic version]. *Contemporary Pediatrics, 31*(12), 18–19.

Woischneck, D., Firsching, R., Schmitz, B., et al. (2013). The prognostic reliability of the Glasgow coma score in traumatic brain injuries: evaluation of MRI data. *European Journal of Emergency Surgery, 39*, 79–86. doi:10.1007/s00068-012-0240-8.

Wolf, S.M., & McGoldrick, P.E. (2015). Seizure patterns in childhood. *Pediatric Annals, 44*(2), e24–29. doi:10.3928/00904481-20150203-08.

53

# Psychosocial Problems in Children and Families

http://evolve.elsevier.com/McKinney/mat-ch/

## LEARNING OBJECTIVES

*After studying this chapter, you should be able to:*

- Identify risk factors for internalizing and externalizing (emotional and behavioral) disorders that emerge in childhood and during adolescence.
- Recognize symptoms, behaviors, and characteristics for internalizing and externalizing disorders.
- Identify individual and familial factors and behaviors that correlate with childhood depression, suicide, or suicide attempts.
- Delineate a nursing care plan for a child at risk for suicide and the child's family, as well as for the support of a family with a child who has committed suicide.
- Discuss the incidence, risk factors, symptoms, and nursing interventions for children with eating disorders and their families and describe their nursing care.
- Identify the primary symptoms and manifestations of children with attention-deficit/hyperactivity disorder and describe their nursing care.
- Identify signs and symptoms of substance abuse disorders and develop a nursing care plan.
- Describe the major types of abuse and neglect seen in children, their contributing factors, and nursing care for abused children and their families.

## CLINICAL REFERENCE

## OVERVIEW OF PSYCHOSOCIAL DISORDERS OF CHILDHOOD

Children with psychosocial disorders frequently manifest difficulty in functioning in social situations (school, play, family) and have problems communicating with other people. These problems affect and are affected by the child's psychologic or mental health. Mental health is a state of well-being in which a child has the ability to manage normal life stressors, engage in meaningful interactions, and achieve his/her full potential (World Health Organization, 2011). Mental health is more than just the absence of a specific disorder; it includes the ability to engage in activities of daily living, to manage emotions, to have meaningful interpersonal relationships, and to develop age-appropriate psychologic skills (American Nurses Association, 2014).

Psychosocial disorders or mental illness refer to disorders that affect a child's personal and social functioning or cause acute distress. Disorders that impinge on mental health are characterized by sustained disturbance, disruption, or alteration in cognition, **mood**, or behavior. These disturbances must be of sufficient intensity and duration to disrupt or impair the ability to engage in developmental life tasks and to impair social and emotional functioning.

In this sense, mental health and mental illness are not mutually exclusive states but rather exist on a continuum. Mental health disorders can result from biologic, neurologic, cultural, societal, or psychologic causes. Some of these disorders are genetic, while others are triggered by trauma or stressful events. A child without underlying mental illness may experience life events that trigger mental health disruptions, and these may require treatment. Likewise, a child who has a mental illness may exhibit areas of psychologic dysfunction, while at the same time may show areas of good or outstanding functioning in regard to school or activities of daily living.

Psychosocial disorders disrupt the normal functioning of the affected child and family. Children may lose interest in play and school activities, and relationships with family and friends are usually impaired. They may exhibit learning deficits related to behavior in school or inability to concentrate on learning. Some disorders manifest through somatic complaints, with no underlying physical cause. These symptoms include recurrent abdominal pain, headaches, or fatigue. Recurrent thoughts of death or suicide are sometimes reported and should always be taken seriously. Hospitalization may be required.

The emergence of a psychosocial condition has a powerful impact on parents, siblings, friends, teachers, and the child's school environment. Conversely, the reaction of parents, siblings, friends, and teachers has a powerful impact on the severity and course of the disorder. Effective assessment and timely intervention can change the course of the child's disorder and ultimately affect lifelong mental health. Nurses should always assess emotional and psychologic state when caring for a child, across all settings.

The first section of this chapter provides an overview of the psychosocial disorders that may emerge during childhood and adolescence. Issues pertaining to suicide are also addressed because these disorders present a risk for the emergence of suicidal impulses or thoughts. The second section of this chapter surveys substance abuse and eating disorders. Finally, nursing care related to the child and family in which child abuse or neglect is occurring is described.

### Psychosocial Disorders Typically Manifested in Childhood

- *Mood disorders*: Depression, dysthymia, adjustment disorder, bipolar disorder
- *Anxiety disorders*: Social anxiety disorder, separation anxiety disorder, posttraumatic stress disorder, phobias, obsessive–compulsive disorder
- *Attention-deficit/hyperactivity disorder*
- *Eating disorders*: Anorexia nervosa, bulimia nervosa

Data from American Psychiatric Association. (2013a). *Diagnostic and statistical manual of mental disorders* (5th ed.). Washington, DC: Author.

## Prevalence

The Centers for Disease Control (CDC) compiled estimates of children aged 3 to 17 years who have specific mental disorders (CDC, 2013). Their key findings include:

- Millions of American children live with a mental health issue.
- ADHD is the most prevalent current diagnosis.
- Incidence of a mental disorder increased with age, with the exception of the autism spectrum disorders.
- Boys were more likely to be diagnosed with ADHD, conduct disorders, autism spectrum disorders, anxiety, Tourette syndrome, and cigarette dependence.
- Adolescent boys (12 to 17 years) were more likely to die by suicide.
- Adolescent girls were more likely to be diagnosed with depression or an alcohol use disorder.

## Precipitating Factors

Psychosocial disorders can manifest as disturbances in feelings (e.g., depression, anxiety), body functions (e.g., constipation, encopresis, enuresis), somatic symptoms (e.g., headaches, stomachaches), behaviors (e.g., conduct disturbance, school avoidance, passive-aggressive behaviors), or performances (concentration problems, test-taking difficulties). Stress, and the child's response to stress, can be both an underlying and contributing factor to the experience of a psychosocial disorder.

The development of a psychosocial disorder generally results from complex interactions among inherited predisposition, age, developmental level, temperament, parental mental health, coping and adaptive abilities within the family, precipitating traumatic experiences, duration of stressors in the environment, stability and support within the family, and social supports outside the immediate family. Trauma and **posttraumatic stress disorder** (PTSD) correlate with the development of anxiety and **mood disorders** (Friedman, 2016).

## Diagnostic Evaluation

The nurse, as part of a multispecialty team, will gather information about the child's physical condition, developmental level, cognitive ability, and onset of specific symptoms. In addition to the overall assessment, a structured mental status examination of the child is usually indicated. Laboratory and diagnostic tests may also help provide some insight into differential diagnosis and determine whether pharmacologic and psychologic interventions are likely to be effective.

Accurate diagnosis is complicated by the fact that wide ranges of emotional, cognitive, and social ability are normal because the brain develops at a different pace for each child. This means that emotional and behavioral responses can be inconsistent and unpredictable. For this reason, the nurse should attend to the environment where the child will be interviewed. The nurse should plan time to establish a relationship as a caregiver and to establish a level of trust and comfort. Repeated assessments in a variety of situations and over time will provide the most accurate sense of what is "normal" for an individual child.

### Screening Questionnaires and Standardized Assessment Tools

Screening questionnaires and assessment tools are increasingly used as part of a developmental and psychosocial evaluation, and some have demonstrated reliability for children. Multidimensional tools assess from multiple perspectives, including attitude toward school, sensation seeking, locus of control, somatization, social stress, anxiety, depression, interpersonal relationships, self-esteem, and self-reliance.

One widely used method of assessing the emotional, psychologic and social development of a child is the Child Behavior Checklist (CBCL), which has versions for preschool children (Achenback & Rescoria, 2000) and children aged 6 to 18 years (Achenback & Rescoria, 2001). The checklist poses a number of statements about the child's behavior (e.g. Acts too young for his//her age), which are scored using a Likert scale (Achenback & Rescoria, 2000).

The Behavioral Assessment System for Children (BASC-3) screens behaviors and emotions and can include parent and teacher assessments (Reynolds & Kamphaus, 2015). The BASC-3 is a fully online version of the scale and can be convenient in many settings or for telehealth care (Reynolds & Kamphouse, 2015).

In addition to the use of standardized tools, a structured mental status examination conducted by a skilled child interviewer will provide important information for planning nursing care. The interview and assessment process involves gathering observations about behavior. The nurse's ability to interact with a child over an extended period of time can provide essential insight.

### Mental Status Examination of Children

- *Appearance:* Noting appropriateness of dress and grooming, ability to engage in greeting behaviors, eye contact, dress, gestures, posture, tics, other repetitive movements; physical presentation, such as age, stature, race, age-appropriate behaviors
- *Speech:* Fluency, tone, volume, vocabulary, age appropriateness, ability to articulate feelings
- *Mood or affect:* Predominant feelings, mood fluctuations, congruence between observed mood and verbalization of mood state
- *Manner of relating to the examiner:* Exploration of the child's understanding of the purpose of the interview, approach or avoidance behaviors, use of play materials available, verbalizations, ability to sit and talk and attend to the interview or to tasks
- *Intellectual skills:* Problem-solving abilities, conceptualization of causality, body image, memory, judgment, general fund of knowledge, insight (findings are compared with developmental norms)
- *Play:* Capacity for imaginative thinking and play, ability to interact during play
- *Sensory and motor development:* Fine and gross motor skills, symmetry and coordination of movement, hand and eye dominance, right-left discrimination
- *Perceptions and thought content:* Presence or absence of suicidal-homicidal ideation, intent, plan; delusions or illusions; hallucinations
- *Externalizing behaviors:* (aggression, impulsivity)

## EVIDENCE-BASED PRACTICE

Evidence-based practice refers to the use of high quality published research to inform clinical decision-making and practice. Translating research to practice requires first accessing multiple studies of varying levels of evidence, such as randomized controlled trials, systematic reviews, meta-analyses, identification of relevant qualitative studies, and expert opinion. Completing a thorough review of best practices and collaborating to reach consensus on a solution is just the first step in ensuring that clinical practice is based on best available information. Ensuring that best practices are adopted means that evidence must be reliably and readily available to those who will use it. Adapting the evidence to the unique setting of the practitioner is called "implementation science." For specific clinical problems, this process can result in change in practice. However, for public health issues affecting populations, not only does implementation science change practice, but it also can change policy.

A crucial issue health promotion for children is finding the best ways to apply emerging knowledge to practice settings. Governmental and private organizations gather scientists and clinicians, usually from a variety of disciplines, to discuss and debate the most effective ways to move knowledge forward to practice. One of the most challenging issues is the issue of "scale," or thinking about how policy makers can adapt research and implementation that works for relatively small populations to larger populations nationally and globally. Interventions that have shown benefit to small groups or communities of children may be difficult or impossible to translate to large groups, countries, or globally.

During 2016 the Forum on Investing in Young Children Globally (iYCG) through the National Academies of Sciences, Engineering and Medicine held several interdisciplinary workshops on the topic of early childhood programs. One workshop was titled *Moving from Evidence to Implementation of Early Childhood Development: Strategies for Implementation.* The overarching goal of the workshop was to discuss the bridge from research to practice to improve outcomes for children. Workshop topics included: generating global political priority for early childhood development; taking research to scale; and the role of research in policy making. Another was titled *Innovations in Investing in Young Children Globally,* which focused on best innovative practices for financing early childhood development programs.

Frequently, following these collaborative meetings, a group might publish a report that summarizes the discussions. The publication that evolved from the workshop on early childhood development is *Moving from Evidence to Implementation of Early Childhood Programs* (National Academies Press, 2016). The interdisciplinary report from the *Innovations in Investing in Young Children Globally,* is titled *Beyond Survival: The Case for Investing in Young Children Globally* (Huebner et al., 2016). It was published by 31 professionals across a variety of disciplines. This paper is a call to action about the strategic importance of investing global resources in young children, to gather relevant data, synthesize and debate that data, and find ways to bring the knowledge to practice.

This box identifies the process of implementation science, and discusses some issues that occur when best practices are disseminated. One issue is that of scaling. What examples can you identify that would affect scaling of early childhood development efforts from a rural setting to an urban setting? What about between countries with different cultures?

Now, go to https://nam.edu/beyond-survival-the-case-for-investing-in-young-children-globally. What argument or call to action do the authors make? In your opinion is this call to action justified? If not, why not?

References: Huebner, G., Boothby, N., Aber, J.L. et al. (2016). *Beyond survival: The case for investing in young children globally.* Washington, DC: National Academy of Medicine; National Academies of Sciences, Engineering, and Medicine (2016). *Moving from evidence to implementation of early childhood programs. Proceedings from a workshop-in brief.* Washington, D.C: The National Academies Press. Doi: 10.17226/23669.

The Institute of Medicine (2009) promoted a shift in the approach to childhood mental health issues from identification and treatment to an overall mental health promotion and illness prevention approach. Although this chapter is organized according to mental, emotional, and behavioral disorders, nurses should think about facilitating preventive measures and mental health promotion for all children beginning in infancy.

## INTERNALIZING DISORDERS

Nurses caring for children frequently encounter moods or behaviors that compromise a child's ability to function at appropriate developmental levels and successfully establish interpersonal relationships. Research consistently shows that most psychosocial disorders are caused by a combination of predisposing or inherent factors and environmental factors that trigger symptoms.

Psychosocial disorders often occur in children who have a familial or genetic predisposition toward the disease. This predisposition may become apparent if physical or emotional stressors create a vulnerability for manifestation of the disorder. In addition to genetic and familial traits, contributors to a psychosocial disorder include physical problems, such as head injuries, sleep disorders, birth defects, physical injuries, and chronic illness. Environmental stressors such as inconsistent or contradictory child-rearing practices, marital conflict, neglect, or traumatic events may also precipitate the development of a psychosocial disorder. Some cognitive, emotional, and behavioral manifestations are associated with genetic syndromes, such as fragile X syndrome. Other disorders, such as fetal alcohol syndrome (FAS), are associated with prenatal or infancy deficiencies or substance abuse by pregnant women (CDC, 2016; Williams &Smith, 2015). Still other disorders are related primarily to an inaccurate or inappropriate relationship between the child and significant others in the social environment.

Psychosocial disorders are classified into two broad categories: **internalizing disorders** and **externalizing disorders**. Children suffering with internalizing disorders will tend to keep their problems to themselves (internalize the problem). Externalizing disorders cause behaviors that are directed toward the environment. These are sometimes referred to as *disruptive behavior disorders*.

Internalizing disorders include depression, anxiety, obsessive–compulsive and related disorders, trauma and stress-related disorders, bulimia and anorexia (American Psychiatric Association [APA], 2013a). Characteristic symptoms include fear, sadness, depression, worry, somatic complaints, poor self-esteem, social withdrawal, and suicidal behaviors.

Organic causes should be ruled out before psychiatric diagnosis is assigned. These include hyperthyroidism, hyperglycemia, temporal lobe epilepsy, and extreme caffeine intake, as well as other disorders. However, the presence of mitral valve prolapse does not exclude the diagnosis of panic disorder (Kaplan et al., 2014), and both should be noted.

Externalizing disorders (disruptive behavior disorders include attention-deficit/hyperactivity disorder, oppositional defiant disorder, and conduct disorder (APA, 2013b). Symptoms of externalizing disorders include problems with attention, impulsivity, aggression (verbal or physical), theft, and fire-setting. It should be noted that these disorders have now been grouped together with the neurodevelopmental disorders (the autism spectrum disorders) in the DSM-5 (APA, 2013a). The externalizing disorders will be discussed later in this chapter; the autism spectrum disorders will be discussed in the succeeding chapter.

## Anxiety Disorders

Anxiety is a normal human emotion, the body's adaptive response to change or challenges. Anxiety can be expected during times of transition or times of achieving developmental milestones. Most people can identify anxiety as an uncomfortable feeling of worry, dread, fear, or apprehension that occurs in response to external or internal stimuli. Symptoms and displays of anxiety are expected and normal in children at specific times in development. For example, infants and children up to preschool age often show intense distress at times of separation from their parents or family members (see Chapter 35). In addition, it is common for young children to have short-lived fears related to darkness, storms, animals, and imaginary situations (see Chapters 7 and 8).

Anxiety is generally considered to occur in two subtypes: state and trait. *State* anxiety refers to transitory feelings of apprehension, tension, or worry. These feelings vary in intensity and often have an identifiable event contributing to them, and the anxiety fluctuates over time. *Trait* anxiety describes a condition of anxiety that is prevalent, stable over time, and less likely to be associated with a specific triggering event.

Predispositions to anxiety result from a confluence of genetic factors, petrochemical and hormonal imbalances, parental patterns of coping with stress, and societal influences (AACAP, 2015). The amygdala has a central role in the physical response to stress and fear, and some disorders may relate to amygdala activity (Aubry, Serrano, & Burghardt, 2016).

Nurses caring for children must differentiate normal or expected anxiety (rising from life stressors) from the chronic condition of anxiety. The identification, treatment, and management of an anxiety disorder will foster a child's enjoyment of life, including their social and educational success, and their adjustment to adult life.

Exposures to trauma and PTSD have been linked to the development of anxiety disorders (Friedman, 2016). Differentiation of normal anxiety from anxiety disorders is made when worry and distress become overwhelming or interfere with the child's ability to attend to tasks of daily functioning such as work, school, and home life. Symptoms such as muscle tension, increased respiratory rate, headaches, heightened startle reflex, tremors, and increased perspiration can be identified during the history and physical examination. Although school-age children typically express anxiety or fear of body harm or potentially real worries (e.g., thunder, lightning), adolescents may exhibit anxiety regarding social situations and acceptance (see Chapter 9).

### Social Anxiety Disorder

Social anxiety disorder (social phobia) is the most common of the anxiety disorders and usually shows its first symptoms in childhood or early adolescence. It is also a disorder that, untreated, has wide-reaching effects on the child's ability to make friends, successfully transition to school, play sports, be part of a peer group during adolescence, and make the transitions to dating and to college. Recent research suggests that social anxiety disorder results from a combination of genetic, biologic, cultural and developmental factors. Additionally, child temperament and parenting style can influence the child's negative perception of others' responses in social situations (Spence & Rapee, 2016). Social anxiety contributes to decreased social interaction. and some research indicates that anxiety disorders may create social isolation that precedes depression and predisposes to substance abuse (Spence & Rapee, 2016).

Symptoms of social anxiety can be generalized or focused on specific triggers. Generalized social anxiety is characterized by fearfulness or discomfort in many social situations. Nongeneralized social anxiety is characterized by severe anxiety about discrete situations or tasks, such as public speaking, test taking or socializing at parties, that people without social anxiety disorder can manage (Spence & Rapee, 2016).

Social anxiety can be misinterpreted as shyness. The child may seem aloof from groups of children or uninvolved in social situations. Children may avoid social or performance situations to such a degree that their daily routine is affected (e.g., by refusing to participate in physical education exercises or by failing to raise their hands to ask a question in class). Social phobia can result in social isolation for the child who has difficulty establishing and maintaining peer relationships.

Social anxiety disorder generally responds well to treatment, and several different treatment approaches have been shown to be effective. These could include cognitive-behavioral therapy, targeted training in social skills, as well as parent training (Spence & Rapee, 2016).

### Separation Anxiety

The essential hallmark of separation anxiety is disabling anxiety about being apart from one's parents or another significant person to whom the child is attached or anxiety about being away from home. It can develop spontaneously or under stress (e.g., in temporary relation to a move or a death in the family) and may last for several years, with symptoms developing and remitting in a cyclical pattern. Children with separation anxiety frequently fear that if they are apart from their parents, harm will come to the parent or themselves. Separation anxiety occurs in approximately 4% to 5% of children and young adults (Rosenberg & Chiriboga, 2016). Separation anxiety disorders in childhood are associated with increased risk for the subsequent development of panic disorders and depression (Rosenberg & Chiriboga, 2016).

School refusal is related to separation anxiety disorder (AACAP, 2013a) and may also be related to a social anxiety disorder. Persistent reluctance or refusal to go to school or elsewhere may be the primary reason families seek intervention for separation anxiety disorder. The child may complain of physical symptoms, cry, bargain, plead, or even exhibit panic symptoms as school time approaches. Symptoms resolve quickly if the child is allowed to stay home but will reappear the next morning. Sometimes the child may simply refuse to leave the home. Consideration of this diagnosis should rule out precipitating factors such as fear of bullying, fatigue, boredom, learning challenges, upsetting incidents that occur in the school setting, or upsets that are occurring in the home.

### Panic Disorder

The diagnosis of panic disorder is more frequently seen in adolescents than in children (Queen, 2010). Panic disorder (panic attack) is distinguished from other anxiety disorders by the rapid onset of physical, cognitive, and emotional symptoms. Once symptoms are triggered rapid, onset ensues, usually within a few minutes. The child's ability to cope may be quickly overwhelmed by the marked discomfort that includes physical symptoms such as cardiovascular (palpitations, chest pain) and respiratory (shortness of breath) distress, a choking sensation, dizziness, and psychologic symptoms characterized by a strong feeling of impending doom or fear of impending death (Rosenberg & Chiriboga, 2016).

### Posttraumatic Stress Disorder

PTSD is a disabling psychosocial disorder that follows a traumatic or overwhelming experience. Population studies estimate that exposure to at least one traumatic event is experienced by 14% to 43% of children and adolescents (National Center for PTSD, 2015). The development of PTSD correlates with the severity of trauma, proximity, repeated experience of trauma, and social supports. PTSD affects approximately 1% to 15% of children, with a higher incidence in girls (National Center for PTSD, 2015). A number of studies have linked the development of PTSD to sexual or physical abuse (National Institute of Mental Health [NIMH], 2016b), but PTSD also occurs as a sequel to other traumatic events, such as the experience of a natural disaster, life-threatening accidents, loss of a parent, or severe injury.

PTSD is characterized by four main clusters of symptoms: re-experiencing symptoms, arousal symptoms, avoidance symptoms, and cognition/mood symptoms, which are experienced for at least a month (NIMH, 2016b). Re-experiencing symptoms include nightmares, flashbacks (terrifying memories), and a feeling of depersonalization. Arousal symptoms include trouble sleeping, agitation, exaggerated startle response, or regressive behavior. Avoidance symptoms are characterized by avoidance of people, places, or triggers that remind the child of the perpetuating traumatic event. Cognitive or mood symptoms, such as decreased memory of the traumatic event details, feelings of guilt or responsibility, or signs of depression (NIMH, 2016b). Other symptoms of PTSD include intense fear, helplessness, or horror, along with physiologic symptoms. For example, the child may demonstrate determined avoidance of stimuli associated with the traumatic event but may have persistent nightmares or flashbacks. Children may reenact the event during play. Adolescents may exhibit antisocial or aggressive behaviors and may be at risk for using substances that they perceive will alleviate their feelings of distress (National Center for PTSD, 2015). PTSD interferes with the child's developing brain and ability to concentrate, can contribute to sleep problems, and can cause the child to be hypervigilant or agitated

### Obsessive–Compulsive Disorder

Affecting approximately 1% to 3% of children (Rosenberg & Chiriboga, 2016), obsessive–compulsive disorder (OCD) manifests as repetitive unwanted thoughts (obsessions) or ritualistic actions (compulsions), or both. Obsessions are recurrent intrusive thoughts, feelings, and ideas. Compulsions are behaviors or actions that are repetitive and recurrent. Compulsions are designed to relieve the anxiety that the child usually realizes is irrational. Because young children cannot adequately describe their uncomfortable thoughts or concerns, they manifest extreme distress, particularly when a ritual has been interrupted.

Children often go through transient stages of obsessive thinking or compulsive behavior, usually at times of anxiety or stress, and these transient symptoms do not warrant the diagnosis. Such thinking is usually manifests in the need to count or to check and recheck locks on doors.

OCD is considered when obsessions and compulsions are intractable, disturbing to the child, and interfere with activities and relationships. Several studies link OCD to depressive disorders, with the prefrontal cortex, the basal ganglia, and the limbic system as affected areas (Rosenberg & Chiriboga, 2016).

Pediatric autoimmune neuropsychiatric disorders associated with streptococcal infection (PANDAS) refer to the abrupt onset of OCD symptoms or tic disorder symptoms (see Chapter 54) following a group A beta-hemolytic streptococcal infection. Research suggests that the disease is not caused by the bacteria but rather by the antibodies that attack neural tissue in the basal ganglia of the brain (Rosenberg & Chiriboga, 2016). Research regarding the strength of the relationship between streptococcal infection and OCD has had varying results. Recent evidence suggests that PANDAS is actually a subtype of PANS (pediatric acute-onset neuropsychiatric syndrome), which is an abrupt onset of symptoms of OCD in children (Orefici, Cardona, Cox, & Cunningham, 2016).

## Mood Disorders

Mood disorders are characterized by lowering of mood or cycling between low mood and mania. Mood disorders are classified on the basis of severity of symptoms, the course of the illness, and the presence or absence of mania. The mood disorders include major depressive disorder, dysthymic disorder, bipolar disorder, and adjustment disorder.

### Major Depressive Disorder and Dysthymic (Persistent Depressive) Disorder

Major depressive disorder (MDD) and dysthymic disorder (DD) are diagnoses that have become increasingly prevalent in the adolescent age-group. Recent estimates for both disorders combined indicate a prevalence rate of 13% of 12- to 17-year-olds, with major depression seen more frequently in girls (Walter, Bogdanovic, Moseley, et al., 2016). The prevalence of depression in girls is nearly three times that of boys. In addition, the depression rates appear to increase with age; approximately 2% of children younger than 13 years of age are considered to be depressed (Walter et al., 2016).

The contributors to depression appear to be numerous, including genetic predisposition, familial situation, life events, physical or psychologic trauma, and head injuries. In young children, depression can be related to abuse, neglect, or other situational triggers. An episode of MDD increases the risk for subsequent episodes. Depression often manifests as a co-morbidity with substance abuse, so children who report depression should be assessed for substance abuse as well. The distinction between MDD and DD is based on the level of depression and the effect on the adolescent's functioning.

DD is considered to be a chronic lowered mood level that is persistent. Children or adolescents who exhibit a less severe but depressed or irritable mood for at least 1 year meet the criteria for DD. Children with DD are generally able to continue overall functioning, but energy and motivation may be low (Walter et al., 2016).

By contrast, MDD is a debilitating and severe depression that poses significant risk factors. Clinical signs and indicators include angry outbursts, irritability, loss of interest and enjoyment in usual activities, decreased energy, altered appetite, altered sleep patterns, decreased self-esteem, disengagement from family and friends, and thoughts of suicide. If the clinical presentation lasts at least 2 weeks (or longer), the child meets the criteria for MDD. Children and adolescents who are diagnosed with MDD should be carefully assessed for risk for self-harm, suicide, or aggression toward others.

### Adjustment Disorder

Adjustment disorders are maladaptive reactions to identifiable traumas or stressors. The *Diagnostic and Statistical Manual of Mental Disorders* (DSM-V) (APA, 2013) sets two conditions that are essential for consideration of the diagnosis: The response to the stress or trauma must be "abnormal" (that is, beyond the level of stress that most children would display), and in addition, the child must experience significant impairment in social and developmental functioning (APA, 2013). In the case of adjustment disorders, the stressors act as precipitating events.

Adjustment disorders are characterized by less severe mood disturbance, fewer overall symptoms, and a self-limiting course (generally 3 months or less). Manifestations of adjustment disorder include depression, anxiety, mixed depression and anxiety, and disturbance of conduct.

The incidence of adjustment disorders is difficult to estimate because other diagnoses are frequently co-morbid. Caretakers should be alert for signs of social isolation, withdrawal from socialization or affection, and suicidal thinking. Early identification, support, and intervention can be a powerful resource in minimizing the length and severity of mood disruption.

### Bipolar Disorder

The onset of bipolar disorder occurs most often in late adolescence or early adulthood but can be seen during early and middle childhood (Walter, Bogdanovic, & DeMaso, 2016). Bipolar disorder is characterized by chronic, fluctuating, and extreme mood disturbances. The disturbances are much more extreme than the child's usual fluctuations of mood. Depression and lowered mood alternate with episodes of elation, irritability, anger, and aggression. The child or adolescent experiencing a manic mood state may be overly elated, grandiose, easily distracted, irritable, and aggressive, and also may demonstrate increased risk-taking behavior, talk rapidly, and be unable to sleep (NIMH, 2016a). Impaired social relationships are common.

When these mood fluctuations have been present for 1 year and are not related to a physical or developmental condition, bipolar mood disorder may be diagnosed. However, normal mood swings that accompany some developmental stages, particularly early adolescence, may confound the ability to make an accurate diagnosis. A challenge also is that signs and symptoms of other psychiatric conditions, such as ADHD, can complicate assessment and diagnosis (Renk et al., 2014). In children, bipolar disorder most often manifests in rapidly changing, extreme mood swings (NIMH, n.d.). Other signs include irritability, anger, aggressive behavior, rapid speech, sleep disturbances, psychosomatic complaints, sadness, decreased energy, and suicidal ideation (NIMH, 2016a). Bipolar mood disorders affect approximately 0% to 3% of adolescents (NIMH, n.d.). Parents of children who have bipolar disorder are more likely to have bipolar disorder themselves (NIMH, 2016a).

## Etiology and Physiology of Internalizing Disorders

The contributing factors to internalizing disorders include biologic, environmental, and traumatic factors.

### Biologic Factors

Research supports the view that internalizing disorders have biologic components that affect brain structure and function; it is also possible that overwhelming events can interrupt brain development (Spence & Rupee, 2016). Biologic factors that contribute to mental disorders include genetic determinants, genetic predispositions (risk factors), traumatic brain injury, and disease states that affect brain function (AACAP, 2015). Other factors can influence behavior by affecting a child's physiologic processes. Stress perception, such as PTSD, and certain mood disorders, such as depression, are associated with increased cortisol levels over time, with emerging evidence that these increased cortisol levels contribute to alterations in structural brain development (Laurent et al., 2015).

### Environmental Factors

A family history of depression (particularly parental) is a significant risk factor for depression in children or adolescents, which increases their risk for suicide (Walter et al., 2016). Emotional and behavioral theories emphasize the importance of the interaction within the family system and quality of relationships with family members, especially parents (Dittman et al., 2011). Evidence suggests that children with a history of verbal, physical, or sexual abuse, frequent separation from or loss of loved ones, drug use, incarceration, lower socioeconomic status, homosexuality, chronic illness, behavioral disorders, and dysfunctional families are more likely than peers with healthy family patterns to have anxiety or depressive disorders (Walter et al., 2016).

### Traumatic Brain Injury

Growing evidence points to the secondary development of mood and behavioral disorders in children and adolescents who have sustained traumatic brain injury (TBI), including concussion. The impact of damage resulting from brain injury depends on a number of factors, including the extent, location, and treatment of the injury (Centers for Disease Control and Prevention [CDC], 2016a). One significant factor is the maturational stage of the brain at the time the damage occurs. Another physiologic factor is the length of time the brain tissue is impaired (as a result of swelling, hemorrhage, or tissue destruction). Finally, the specific area of the brain that is damaged determines the precise areas of deficit.

The severity of TBI can be mild, with only a brief change in mental status, or severe, causing long-term functional changes that can affect emotions, sensations, memory, or cognition. Damage can be cumulative over consecutive injuries (CDC, 2016a).

## Manifestations

Disruption in emotional state, including sadness, worry, fear, and somatic complaints, is often prominent in the clinical presentation of internalizing disorders, which include both anxiety disorders and mood (depressive) disorders. In addition, suicide risk is increased, particularly with mood disorders.

Anxiety disorders and mood disorders may present with mixed features (i.e., depression and anxiety are both present), which complicates establishing an accurate diagnosis. For example, the child who is anxious may be withdrawn, tearful, unwilling to engage in play, or prone to acting aggressively toward others. These same symptoms typically occur in children who are depressed. Moreover, it is often difficult to differentiate between normal mood changes that are the result of developmental maturation and adaptation and abnormal, persistent mood disturbances.

However, mood disturbance usually is more intense and persistent and interferes with social relations and daily functioning. Finally, the child or adolescent can have both anxiety and a mood disorder. Mood disorders are also varied and are classified according to the intensity or duration of depressive symptoms or the particular behaviors displayed by the child. For these reasons, careful assessment by a specialist in psychosocial disorders and the use of screening tools is essential.

## Therapeutic Management of Children With Internalizing Disorders

The management of depression and anxiety in the pediatric population is focused toward providing immediate symptom relief, stabilizing the family situation, and planning for supports that will help mitigate the intensity and frequency of recurrence. Interventions will vary based on the age, developmental level, and social support available to the child.

Recurrence of symptoms is common, with every recurrence increasing the likelihood of future events. For this reason, accurate identification, appropriate intervention, and long-term follow-up are essential to protect the child's physical, intellectual, and social development, because poor health behaviors and social isolation accompany the disorders.

## NURSING CARE

### The Child With an Internalizing Disorder

#### Assessment

In addition to the diagnostic methods described earlier in this chapter (see Diagnostic Evaluation), a thorough physical and developmental history should be obtained from the child and/or the family, with attention paid to previous episodes of the presenting problem. Children may initially be most comfortable having parents present, but once the child is comfortable with the nurse, a private interview should also be offered. Presenting emotional symptoms, physical symptoms (e.g., headaches, stomachaches), and precipitating events should be identified. Initial assessment should also include descriptions of the child's moods, patterns of daily activity, stressors, and coping style (Walter & DeMaso, 2016).

Gaining information regarding the risk for self-harm or suicide is important, particularly if the child shows symptoms of depression. Assessment of risk for self-harm and suicide includes questions about ideation (thoughts), impulses, or plans. Assessment of previous suicide attempts is essential because previous attempts increase the risk (Shapiro, Pinto, & Evans, 2016).

Family history provides a contextual framework for understanding the child's symptoms. Family history assessment should include identification of extended family members who may share living arrangements and questions about the family interaction patterns. Family (particularly parental) history of psychosocial disorder, mood or anxiety disorder, or substance abuse are all risk factors for a child's development of a psychosocial disturbance. Parents or caregivers should be asked to describe changes in the child's behaviors and when these changes began, as well as effects on the child's relationships with others. The use of appropriate screening tools can be a helpful adjunct for assessment. Other assessment areas include the presence of school difficulties, child temperament, child self-evaluation, and exposure to trauma (Walter & DeMaso, 2016). For a child who presents with symptoms of OCD or tic disorder, history of sore throats related to strep infection should be noted, along with whether OCD symptom onset was sudden or occurred after an illness (see PANDAS, this chapter).

### Nursing Diagnosis and Planning

The nursing diagnoses and expected outcomes that apply to children who are experiencing depression and anxiety include:

- Ineffective Coping related to loss of energy, sleep disturbance, biochemical imbalance, loss of control, or side effects of medication.

**Expected outcome.** The child will display adaptive ability, as evidenced by participation in and enjoyment of regular activities. The parent will describe any expected or unexpected side effects from the prescribed medication.

- Situational Low Self-Esteem related to cognitive distortions, inability to manage daily events, and a sense of hopelessness or guilt.

**Expected outcome.** The child will display increased self-esteem, as evidenced by verbalization of an increase in self-confidence and an increase in positive feelings about self.

- Risk for Self-Directed Violence related to suicidal ideation, guilt, or hopelessness.

**Expected outcome.** The child will demonstrate more positive moods and reduced anxiety levels and will talk to a responsible family member or professional about any thoughts of self-directed violence.

- Disturbed Sleep Pattern related to anxiety, depression, and inactivity.

**Expected outcome.** The child will exhibit appropriate sleep patterns, as evidenced by expressing feelings of being well rested, showing no signs of sleep deprivation (e.g., irritability, lethargy, restlessness), and showing no signs of excessive sleeping.

- Risk for Delayed Development related to poor concentration, fatigue, inability to participate in school

**Expected outcome.** The child will engage in appropriate play for developmental level, attend school, maintain educational progress, and continue positive relationships with peers.

### Interventions

Depending on the seriousness of the child's symptoms, functional impairment, and risk for harm, the child might be admitted to a mental health facility for initial stabilization and maintenance of safety. Once stabilized, the child can be transitioned to a community placement or to home to be managed by a primary care provider (DeMaso & Walter, 2016).

Treatment of internalizing disorders can include psychotherapy, pharmacologic therapy, family intervention, parenting support, and other methods, such as cognitive-behavioral therapy (CBT). Social skills training or group therapy may be most helpful for social anxiety. Children will often try to avoid anxiety by limiting social interactions, creating a cycle of avoidance and associated shame. Behavioral interventions for children with school phobias are directed toward keeping the child attending school, while offering interventions during school time to reduce anxiety symptoms, such as refusing to pick up the child from school, even if the child insists. This form of intervention is a type of desensitization therapy.

Controversy has surrounded the use of antidepressants. Most antidepressants have been studied in adult populations, and evidence is emerging that children may not metabolize these substances in the same manner as adults. A black box warning about the potential for increased risk for suicidal ideation and behavior in children, adolescents, and young adults appears on all dispensed prescription antidepressants. Schneeweiss, Patrick, Solomon, et al. (2010) conducted an extensive study of antidepressant use and suicide thoughts or acts in more than 20,000 children and adolescents and found that increased suicide risk does not differ between various classes of antidepressants. Therefore, the decision to prescribe a particular antidepressant should be based on its potential for therapeutic effects and not on its relative risk for suicide (Schneeweiss et al., 2010). The use of antidepressants to treat these disorders in children and adolescents is not prohibited; however, it is advised to keep a close watch on initiating any type of medication treatment in this population. With careful monitoring when drugs are introduced, use of selective serotonin reuptake inhibitors (SSRIs) for medication management is an appropriate and widely used treatment for depression and anxiety in children (Walter et al., 2016).

Children, parents, and clinicians may prefer to initiate psychotherapy before, and perhaps in lieu of, medications; however, the most effective treatment combines medication with psychotherapy or other supportive intervention (DeMaso & Walter, 2016). Individual therapy and family counseling are essential for children with suicidal ideation, persistent mood disturbances or disabling anxiety; in these cases, consideration of hospitalization is paramount to protect the child from harmful impulses (DeMaso & Walter, 2016). Increasingly, day treatment programs have become an alternative to hospitalization. Hospital and day treatment settings use cognitive-behavioral therapies (CBTs) to increase coping skills and social skills and to provide tools that can be used to manage stress. The underlying principle of CBT is that individuals, by consciously becoming aware of stressful thoughts and feelings associated with various events or situations, can learn to analyze behaviors related to these thoughts or feelings and begin to think and behave in more positive ways. CBTs have shown benefit for all of the internalizing disorders. They can be done individually or in groups. Other behavioral strategies for managing depression and anxiety include relaxation therapy, distraction strategies, self-talk, or cognitive strategies, parent training, and support from adults or friends who are safe and reassuring (Spence & Rapee, 2016).

### Evaluation

- Does the child exhibit an energy level that allows for interactions, play, and school?
- Does the child seem interested in people and events?
- Does the child communicate positive statements about self?
- Does the parent report that the child appears happier and more engaged?
- Does the child exhibit normal patterns of eating and sleeping?
- Can the parent describe the medication effects and side effects?

## SUICIDE

Suicide is a major public health problem, the second leading cause of death among adolescents between 15 and 24 years old and the third among children 5 to 14 years old. (National Center for Health Statistics, 2016). Among young people, the suicide incidence rises with age. Suicide by children younger than 10 years of age is uncommon. Suicide rates among adolescents in the United States have risen dramatically. Estimates of the prevalence of suicidal ideation (seriously considering) are 17.7%, and 14.6% of adolescents report having made a plan to commit suicide (CDC, 2016b).

Other differences are noted. For example, girls are twice as likely to consider committing suicide as boys (CDC, 2016b). Methods appear to vary by gender, with girls using poisons and boys using firearms most frequently, which is why boys are far more likely to die from a suicide attempt (CDC, 2015a).

Risk for suicide should be assessed by ascertaining previous suicide attempts, family history of suicide, history of depression, substance abuse, alcohol abuse, an overwhelming life stressor, access to methods, and history of arrest or incarceration (CDC, 2015b). The presence of risk factors does not mean that a suicide attempt is inevitable, but should raise the awareness of anyone who interacts with the child or adolescent.

### ! NURSING QUALITY ALERT

#### *Resources for People With Thoughts of Suicide*

Resources for anyone who is having thoughts of suicide are available through the National Suicide Prevention Lifeline (1-800-273-8255); through its website (http://www.suicidepreventionlifeline.org), or from the American Association of Suicidology at http://www.suicidology.org.

Of significant importance is that gay, lesbian, bisexual, and possibly transgender (LGBT) adolescents are twice as likely to experience suicide ideation and to attempt suicide than are their heterosexual peers (CDC, 2014). This trend appears to be linked to social stigma, feelings of isolation, increased bullying and level of vulnerability, and stress (CDC, 2014) Positive and accepting environments at school and at home assist LGBT youth to feel safe and prevent adverse emotional consequences (CDC, 2014). **Suicide potential** should always be assessed for a child with symptoms of a mood disorder, or multiple disorders (**co-morbidity**), or history of previous suicide attempts. Family history of psychosocial disorders (especially depression or a parent who has died by suicide) creates increased risk.

Underlying major depression, poor self-concept, and hopelessness appear to be the most significant factors contributing to suicide, regardless of age or sex. Long-standing family dysfunction is often present, with emotional detachment and isolation among family members. The suicide victim is typically a vulnerable individual who, under stress and unable to envision a solution, seeks and finds a way to die. In the case of children, risks are greatest when there is not adequate adult support to identify and intervene in the escalation of symptoms.

Most adolescent suicide attempts are impulsive: motivated by a desire to influence others, gain attention, communicate love or anger, or escape a difficult or painful situation. Suicide hotlines or drop-in centers can often serve to keep the young person safe until the impulse passes.

However, any verbalization or gesture of suicide should be taken very seriously and should never be ignored. Approximately 29% of children who die by suicide have told someone else about their thoughts in advance. Therefore, the young person should be encouraged to discuss the thought specifically to determine whether there is a plan and the lethality of the plan (Sheftall et al., 2016). Help should be obtained from qualified health professionals.

Suicide remains a rare phenomenon for young children, although a child who has lost a parent before the age of 13 years has increased risk for mood disorder and suicide. Until approximately the age of 6 years, most children do not have a realistic concept of death, although they may express thoughts about harming themselves. However, children as young as 3 years have tried to commit suicide and apparently understood what they were doing.

Knowledge regarding prevention of suicide is an essential role for the community health nurse and the school nurse, especially for nurses at the middle or high school level. It is imperative that school nurses educate school personnel about recognizing the subtle signs of an impending suicide attempt so intervention can occur. Considerations included in continuing education should be whom to contact if a teacher or other school worker suspects a child is considering suicide, who will interview and evaluate the child, and what personnel will notify the family. Often, schools have professional teams that perform the evaluation and make appropriate referrals. Suicide prevention and incidence reduction are two of the national goals described in *Healthy People 2020* (U.S. Department of Health and Human Services [USDHHS], 2010).

### Manifestations and Risk Factors

The risk for suicide should be considered if the following are present:

- Previous suicide attempts
- Past psychosocial hospitalization; overt signs of mental illness manifested as delusions or hallucinations
- A family member or friend who has committed suicide; exposure to violence in the home or social environment
- Death of a parent before the child reached 13 years of age
- Recent losses; these may include the death of a relative, a family divorce, a breakup, or any significant change or life event that disrupts the emotional status quo
- Preoccupation with death; statements about suicide or self-harm; suicidal clues, such as cryptic verbal messages, giving away personal items, and changes in expected patterns of behaviors (e.g., sudden calmness in a normally anxious teenager)
- History of risk-taking or self-abusive behaviors; use of alcohol or drugs to cope with emotions
- Overwhelming sense of guilt or shame; obsessional self-doubt
- Social isolation: the individual does not have social alternatives or the skills to find alternatives to suicide
- Handguns in the home, especially if accessible or loaded
- History of physical or sexual abuse
- Homosexuality, especially if the teen discovers same-sex orientation early in adolescence, experiences violence because of homosexual identity, or is rejected by family members as a result of sexual orientation

## Therapeutic Management

### Prevention

Recognition of risk factors for suicidal feelings by healthcare providers and at schools is one of the most significant prevention strategies. Children or adolescents who commit suicide have usually offered at least veiled information about their suicidal ideation or feelings of despair to classmates, teachers, or healthcare providers. Children or adolescents with suicidal ideation should undergo a thorough psychosocial evaluation by a mental health professional. The child may need pharmacotherapeutic agents such as antidepressants or antipsychotic medications. The use of medications in children at risk for suicide requires close monitoring, and medications should be distributed in small doses because they could be used in a suicide attempt or act (DeMaso, Wallter & Wharff, 2016). The decision to discharge a child for observation or to hospitalize is based on the nature of the ideation, the access to methods, and the ability of the family to provide a supportive and safe environment (DeMaso et al., 2016).

### When Prevention and Intervention Fail

A suicide attempt or death by suicide is a crisis event for all family members and friends. Counseling by a mental health specialist who is experienced in the area of suicide should be provided to all family members and the child's immediate friends. It is important that these services be offered quickly, preferably within the first 24 hours. In the event of a death by suicide, counselors should remain available for at least 1 year after the event. Grieving and emotional adjustments often take several months and may peak around the anniversary of the suicide event. The experience of losing someone by suicide creates an increased risk that others will act on similar impulses.

## NURSING CARE

## The Child or Adolescent at Risk for Suicide

### Assessment

The risk for suicide is best assessed by a systematic approach to behaviors, attitudes, and risk factors, as described previously. Several instruments have been developed to assess lethality and potentiality, lessening the likelihood of overlooking contributing factors. The instruments are similar and explore risk factors, stressors, lethality of method, coping mechanisms, and support systems. Subtle symptoms of depression or anxiety, such as decreased energy, persistent restlessness, or anger, should also be considered. It is important to explore thought content and organization, awareness and expression of feelings, perceived level and types of stress, perceived availability of support resources, previous suicidal behaviors, and medical status (Box 53.1).

### Nursing Diagnosis and Planning

The nursing diagnoses and expected outcomes that apply to the child or adolescent at risk for suicide and the family are as follows:

- Risk for Self-Directed Violence related to a desire to end emotional pain, to solicit the attention of others, or to avoid responsibility.

Expected outcome. The child or adolescent will indicate a decrease in the risk for self-directed violence, as evidenced by an ability to use effective communication techniques to express needs and feelings and to verbalize alternative solutions to problems.

- Situational Low Self-Esteem or Chronic Low Self-Esteem related to a perception of failure and hopelessness about the ability to change self or circumstances.

Expected outcome. The child or adolescent will demonstrate increased self-esteem, as evidenced by verbalization of ability to change self or circumstances.

**BOX 53.1 Questions to Assess Suicide Potential**

1. Have you ever thought of trying to hurt yourself? How might you do this?
2. Have you ever thought of killing yourself? How might you do this?
3. Have you known anyone who has committed suicide? When did this occur? What was it like for you?
4. Do you have access to firearms or knives?
5. Do you ever do things to deliberately place yourself in danger, such as driving when you are drunk or playing Russian roulette with a gun?
6. Have you ever told anyone about wanting to kill yourself?
7. Have you ever been hospitalized for suicidal behavior?
8. Can you describe how you feel right now?

- Anxiety related to current or anticipated events.

Expected outcome. The child or adolescent will have decreased anxiety, as evidenced by recognizing and expressing anxiety and use of effective coping mechanisms to decrease anxiety.

- Interrupted Family Processes related to relational disturbance or possible abuse or neglect.

Expected outcome. The child or adolescent and family will access and mobilize appropriate support systems in an effective manner.

- Ineffective Coping related to a sense of despair or limited availability of support.

Expected outcome. The child or adolescent and family will work with professionals to begin to identify and express feelings and strengths and to discuss appropriate actions when feelings become overwhelming.

### Interventions

Adolescents who are experiencing suicidal ideation and impulses are generally depressed, experiencing themselves as isolated and rejected. Caregivers should be empathic and nonjudgmental; voice and demeanor should be clear, direct, and supportive. At the same time, the ability to create a safe environment is the first priority if suicidal impulses are present. The nurse should ensure that potentially harmful objects are removed to prevent self-injury. It is important for the nurse to assess how closely a child needs to be monitored throughout the day, realizing that the potential for self-harm fluctuates. If the adolescent is not hospitalized, the nurse should ensure that the family has removed weapons from the home.

Results from the Treatment for Adolescents with Depression Study (March & Vitiello, 2009) have demonstrated that CBT alone or, even more effective, combined with medication therapy reduced the risk for suicide in adolescents with a history of a mood disorder. CBT can help individuals learn to consider alternative actions when thoughts of self-harm arise. The identification of trigger events and strategies to avoid or manage these events is important. Nursing interventions include exploration of coping strategies to be used when impulses arise. Planning alternative activities, avoiding isolation, and talking to the treatment team are all effective ways to manage thoughts of self-harm.

Families are also affected when a member harms or kills him- or herself. Individual as well as family meetings provide an opportunity to explore the issues raised and to learn to effectively provide emotional and social support to grieving family members. Grieving will occur even if the suicide attempt was unsuccessful. Individual and family therapy will also provide an opportunity to explore contributory factors that can be altered to reduce the suicide potential. Nurses, as members of the treatment team, work to help the parents regain their ability to assist their child and manage the home environment.

### Evaluation

- Is the child able to identify situations, events, or times when ideas or impulses are likely to occur? Does the child have a strategy for seeking help during these times?
- Does the child participate in activities that reduce feelings of despair and hopelessness?
- Does the child display evidence of positive self-esteem through positive self-statements or ability to describe how circumstances can be changed?
- Has the child or adolescent verbalized a decrease in anxiety?
- Is the family able to identify warning signs of suicidal risk?
- Do family members support one another, and can the family identify community resources to assist?
- Has the child or adolescent developed coping mechanisms and effective problem solving?
- Has the family developed a suicide prevention plan?

## EXTERNALIZING DISORDERS

Externalizing disorders involve symptoms that are behavioral in nature. The symptoms are observable, such as disruptive behavior, problems with attention, impulsivity, verbal or physical aggression, vandalism, and theft. (APA, 2013b). The externalizing disorders include attention-deficit/hyperactivity disorder, oppositional defiant disorder, and conduct disorder (APA, 2013b). These disorders have now been grouped together with the neurodevelopmental disorders (the autism spectrum disorders) in the DSM-5 (APA, 2013a).

All children misbehave at times; this is a normal feature of childhood development. Incidents of unacceptable or risky behavior are common, particularly among adolescents. Disorders affecting behavior are not incidents or stages of difficulty in behavior. Instead, externalizing disorders represent a chronic pattern of aggression, hostility, or disruption that is persistent, is unresponsive to parental controls, and has lasted for more than 6 months.

Children with externalizing disorders typically exhibit clusters of signs and symptoms that are primarily inattentive (attention-deficit disorder [ADD]), primarily impulsive/hyperactive (hyperactivity disorder [HD]), or a combination of both types of symptoms (attention-deficit/hyperactivity disorder [ADHD]).

Warning signs for externalizing disorders include (AACAP, 2011):

- Impulsive or overly aggressive behavior
- Harm, or threats of harm, directed at themselves or others
- Stealing, damaging or destroying property, or other violations of the rights of others
- Lying (sometimes compulsive lying)
- Poor school performance, avoiding school
- Early smoking, drinking, or drug use
- Early sexual activity
- Frequent tantrums and arguments
- Consistent hostility toward authority figures

Externalizing disorders include conduct disorders (aggressive and oppositional disorders), ADDs, and HDs. A mental health specialist with experience in the area should make the diagnosis of an externalizing disorder.

ADHD is the most common chronic externalizing disorder that emerges during childhood. ADHD is associated with significant problems in three areas: (1) attention and concentration, (2) impulse control, and (3) hyperactivity. Morbidity estimates of the prevalence of ADHD in children age 3 to 17 years old in the United States is 9.8%. The percentage of boys diagnosed at any time with ADHD is 13.4%, while that for girls is 6%. In epidemiologic studies, the male-to-female ratio is approximately 2:1 among referred children displaying ADHD symptoms (USDHHS, 2015).

Children with ADHD show symptoms related to attention and concentration, including trouble sustaining attention, trouble organizing tasks, appearing to not hear when spoken to, and losing items necessary to complete tasks, such as assignments, pencils, or books. Symptoms related to impulsivity include difficulty waiting, blurting out comments, interruptions, or intruding. Symptoms related to hyperactivity include fidgeting, excessive talking, excessive running, and an inability to engage in quiet activities (APA, 2013b). Symptoms generally emerge early in childhood, with the mean age at onset 3 or 4 years; however, medication treatment may not be started until the child is in a structured school setting. Parents, teachers, or pediatric caregivers may make referrals for ADHD, expressing concerns regarding frequent injuries, poor scholastic performance, and low performance motivation. In addition, reports may indicate associated symptoms, including depression or anxiety, aggressiveness toward peers, and antisocial or oppositional defiance toward authority figures.

A child affected with ADHD may have exceptional sensitivity to noises or disruptions in the environment. For example, ambient sounds such as an air conditioner switching on may disrupt attention to tasks. Rigid controls on physical activity or talking are likely to trigger symptoms. For this reason, the classroom setting is often the place where the disorder is identified. Teachers describe their frustration with having children call out answers (instead of raising their hand) or talking to other children. In situations where the structure is rigid or behavior is severely restricted, the child with ADHD becomes increasingly frustrated and symptoms increase.

### Etiology

ADHD occurs more commonly in first-degree biologic relatives of people with the disorder than in the general population, which suggests a genetic predisposition for the disorder. Other central nervous system (CNS) abnormalities, such as the presence of neurotoxins or epilepsy, and other neurologic disorders are thought to be predisposing factors, along with prenatal factors such as maternal substance use and complications related to labor or delivery (Urion, 2016). Chaotic or abusive environments may predispose to the appearance of ADHD.

### Manifestations

According to the DSM-V (APA, 2013a), a diagnosis of ADHD requires the exhibition of symptoms of inattention and impulsivity/hyperactivity.

- Inattention: Carelessness, inattention to details, difficulty attending to work or games, does not listen, poor follow-through with instructions or does not complete tasks, difficulty with organization skills, avoidance of tasks that require mental effort, misplaces equipment or supplies necessary to complete tasks, easily distracted, forgetfulness, poor planning.
- Impulsivity/hyperactivity: Fidgets with hands, feet, or hair; unable to remain in a seat for extended periods; runs and climbs excessively in inappropriate settings; difficulty in engaging in quiet activities; mostly "on the go"; talks excessively; blurts out questions or answers; cannot await a turn; interrupts conversations

Signs usually must be present for at least 6 months, have occurred before the age of 12 years, be present in two or more settings (e.g., home, school, recreation, church), not be associated with another mental or developmental disorder, and significantly impair at least one level of functioning (academic, social, occupational) (APA, 2013a).

Although the American Psychosocial Association calls this disorder ADHD, not all children with the disorder exhibit overt hyperactivity, although most demonstrate a degree of impulsivity. ADHD is frequently co-morbid with other disorders, such as motor disorders (tics), oppositional defiant disorder, mood disorders, and anxiety disorders. Therefore, children with ADHD should be screened for co-morbid depression, anxiety, and social impairment. Children with ADHD often have a diagnosed learning disability (Urion, 2016).

## Diagnostic Evaluation

Although high-resolution magnetic resonance imaging and blood and urine studies of metabolites of brain neurotransmitters have been performed in individuals with ADHD, none of these tests have provided consistent diagnostic information. The behaviors and symptoms of ADHD must be present in two of three areas—home, school, or social situations—to support the diagnosis. These reports are coupled with psychologic assessments conducted while the child is completing tasks requiring vigilance, attention, and concentration and those involving delayed gratification. Clinical interviews may be coupled with clinical trials of psychopharmacologic agents to determine the child's behavioral response. In addition, standardized questionnaires for parents and teachers allow in-depth information to be collected.

## Therapeutic Management

The goal of therapeutic management is to reduce the frequency and intensity of unsocialized behaviors. This requires achieving a balance between the child's temperament and environmental demands, expectancies, and supports. Therefore, treatment interventions must be targeted at enhancing the child's capabilities and self-esteem. Expectations that may be appropriate for a child without ADHD—"he should be able to sit still in school for 40 minutes," or "she should be able to handle 1 hour of homework"—may need to be modified for the child with ADHD. In every case, the nurse should work with the parents to modify the environment and to develop strategies that foster competencies in the child.

Most clinicians combine pharmacotherapy with behavior-oriented family therapy to achieve alterations in the child's internal functioning and external environment. Stimulant medications commonly used as part of the treatment plan include methylphenidate (Ritalin), dextroamphetamine (Dexedrine), and amphetamine/dextroamphetamine (Adderall). Newer timed-released formulas of methylphenidate (Concerta, Ritalin LA, and Metadate ER) and mixed amphetamine salts (Adderall XR) are advantageous for once-a-day dosing, thereby eliminating mid-day trips to the nurse's office. Medication treatment is most effective when it is used in conjunction with behavioral interventions. It is important to individually tailor the child's medication dosage to achieve maximum results with the fewest side effects. Initially, the dose should be the lowest appropriate for the child's age and weight, then increased over a period of weeks until symptoms are controlled (Urion, 2016).

The most common side effects associated with the use of the stimulant medications are weight loss, difficulty sleeping, decreased appetite and the emergence of motor disorders, particularly the tics Another concern is that children on ADHD medications can experience sudden cardiovascular events. For that reason medication monitoring by the child's provider should occur at least every three months.

## NURSING CARE

### The Child With ADHD

#### Assessment

The nurse documents the parent's description of the child's typical behavior while playing alone and with other children, during mealtimes, and while the parent is on the telephone or occupied with chores. The length of time it takes the child to bathe or dress and how often the child becomes distracted during these tasks are also explored. These behaviors are then compared with those exhibited when the child is engaged in highly stimulating activities and activities with frequent feedback, such as video and computer games. The child's behavior is also compared during novel versus routine activities.

The child's developmental and family history is explored in detail, with the nurse noting the age at which the child began to exhibit independent behaviors such as walking, getting out of bed alone, and exploring the environment. It is not uncommon for children with ADHD to explore the environment at an early age, with only limited need to return to the caregiver for support or approval. Family members who are diagnosed with ADHD or exhibit similar behaviors are noted. Observation within the home or school setting is likely to generate the most valid information because the clinic environment may be unfamiliar and, by the nature of the disorder, inhibit the child's natural tendency to explore, become distracted, or display limited motivation in task completion.

#### Nursing Diagnosis and Planning

The nursing diagnoses and expected outcomes that apply to the child with ADHD and the child's family are as follows:

- Impaired Social Interaction related to impulsivity, poor self-management skills, and aggressive behaviors.

**Expected outcomes.** The child will demonstrate an improvement in social interactions, as evidenced by improvement in impulse control and an ability to sustain attention on tasks. The child will relate in a more positive way with peers.

- Risk for Injury related to impulsivity, limited judgment skills, or excessive need for mobility and stimulation.

**Expected outcome.** The child will remain safe from injury, as evidenced by a decrease in injuries and implementation of a plan to prevent injuries.

- Compromised Family Coping or Disabled Family Coping related to the need for consistent and close supervision of the child, the child's hyperactivity, or social stigma of having a child with impulsive or aggressive behaviors.

**Expected outcome.** The family will mobilize coping strategies, as evidenced by an ability to discuss the child's needs and a plan to provide the needed support.

- Deficient Knowledge related to perceptions that the child is willfully defiant or disobedient in following directions or in testing limits.

**Expected outcome.** The family will increase knowledge related to their child's condition, as evidenced by a willingness to discuss the child's condition and display an understanding of the condition and its treatment.

#### Interventions

Living with a child who has ADHD can be challenging on a daily basis for parents and other family members. Because of their sometimes disruptive or oppositional behavior, children with ADHD often interact in provocative or intrusive manners. Social and family conflicts are common. Often, parents of children with ADHD have difficulties because their child's behavior offers fewer positive parenting experiences, decreases parenting self-confidence, and increases stress. These parenting outcomes can contribute to negative social, emotional, and educational outcomes in the child. One nursing goal is to teach the family about the disorder, and help them develop management strategies. Demonstrate ways to provide frequent positive reinforcement. Also important for parents and the child is instruction about medications and adaptations in the environment that are needed for the child to practice new skills.

The nurse may facilitate communication between the family and the school about ways to accommodate the child's shortened attention span and increased need for mobility and frequent breaks. Often CBT, provided by a specially trained professional, is helpful in identifying specific exercises that can reduce bothersome traits. Support groups for parents can help families cope with the child with ADHD and modify their interactions with and expectations of the child. Ordinarily, the positive effects of medication on the child's behavior are seen immediately; however, it may take several weeks to titrate the medication to the point that symptoms are controlled with the fewest side effects.

It is common for the family to observe a rapid change in the child's behavior and performance and to feel relief as manifestations subside. Continuing support is required, because this disorder is lifelong, and progress in self-control and behavioral patterns is usually slow. Parents and school nurses need to be actively involved in dispensing medication, even through adolescence, because children fluctuate in their willingness to adhere to therapy. Affected children also may have difficulty remembering to take the medication because of the attention deficits characteristic of the disorder.

Nutritional management is also an issue with children taking medication for the treatment of ADHD. Many of the medications suppress appetite, and the child may begin to refuse meals or snacks. Maintaining appropriate developmental weight gain is an issue of concern. The nurse advises the parent to encourage high-calorie breakfasts and more frequent but smaller meals. Some children prefer to eat a large snack after arrival home from school in the afternoon. Providing high-nutrient meals and snacks is preferred; referral to a nutritionist may be advisable.

Some parents and professionals prefer more conservative approaches, such as dietary changes, to pharmacologic treatment of ADHD. Although researchers continue to debate whether food additives and sugars have significant clinical influences on most children with ADHD, the general scientific consensus is that they do not. Medication is typically administered during the school day, but it has become increasingly recognized that attention, concentration, and alertness are needed for any learning task, such as learning to play baseball or learning to drive a car. The side effects and potency of the medications used to treat ADHD often make parents and physicians hesitant to administer medications other than during critical learning periods.

### Evaluation

- Does the child adhere to the cognitive and pharmacologic strategies designed to increase self-control, as evidenced by a decrease in impulsivity and an increase in attention to task?
- Does the child complete school assignments in less time than before, with less distractibility?
- Does the child demonstrate increased skill in peer relations, as evidenced by fewer conflicts and more frequent positive statements to and about peers?
- Does the family provide a safe and supportive environment within the home, as evidenced by adequate supervision and opportunities for meeting the child's mobility needs in a safe manner?
- Is the child maintaining developmentally appropriate weight gain?
- Does the family demonstrate acceptance of the child and the child's special needs?
- Does the family demonstrate an increased acceptance of the child's condition as a medical problem rather than a social or behavioral problem?
- Does the family adhere to the medication regimen?

## EATING DISORDERS: ANOREXIA, BULIMIA, AND OBESITY

Eating disorders include anorexia, bulimia, pica, and binge eating disorder. Anorexia, bulimia, and obesity are the most frequently seen eating disorders in children. Anorexia and bulimia have overlapping features and similar underlying mechanisms, but are separate disorders. Females are more likely to be affected by eating disorders. The prevalence of bulimia nervosa is approximately 3% to 5%; the prevalence of anorexia nervosa in girls is 0.5% to 1%. Eating disorders are less common in boys but comprise approximately 10% of their prevalence (Kreipe, 2016). Co-morbidities are common with all types of eating disorders, including depression and anxiety (Kreipe, 2016).

Anorexia is characterized by a deliberate refusal to maintain adequate body weight, a distorted body image, and amenorrhea (in females). Weight loss can be rapid, extreme, or dramatic. Bulimia is characterized by recurrent episodes of binge eating; a sense of lack of control over eating binges; self-induced vomiting or excessive use of laxatives, diuretics, or emetics to prevent weight gain; excessive exercise to prevent weight gain; and a persistent concern with body image, although body image is usually not distorted.

Children with eating disorders typically report shame and guilt about many life experiences, especially eating. Individuals with severe eating disorders, particularly anorexia, have a mortality rate up to 20% from complications of the disorder or suicide (National Association of Anorexia Nervosa Associated Disorders, 2016).

Treatment resistance is common because of the cognitive distortions that support the inaccurate body image. Secondary gains for the disorders include a heightened sense of self-esteem, attention from family and caregivers, cultural admiration given to thin people, envy, and control over others through eating patterns. Ritualistic behaviors are seen frequently, particularly around issues of food. For example, the child may eat only at a particular time of day, eat foods only in a certain order, of a single color, or insist on washing all foods before eating them. The rituals are often an attempt to control the portions, fat content, or nutrients ingested. The rituals also serve to enhance the individual's sense of control over food or dietary intake.

Children or adolescents with anorexia will go to extreme measures to prevent others from becoming aware of the weight loss or lack of food intake. For example, they may ingest large amounts of water or insert heavy objects in the vaginal cavity before weighing to give the impression of weight gain. The child or adolescent with either anorexia or bulimia may eat in front of people and then go to the bathroom to purge after the meal.

Obesity in children is a world-wide phenomenon; in the United States approximately 32% of children are overweight, 17% of them obese. The prevalence is higher in non-Hispanic black children, Hispanic children, and American Indian/Alaskan Natives (Gahagan, 2016). Obesity in children is identified through BMI percentile measures – overweight is between the $85^{th}$ and $94^{th}$ BMI percentile for age, obesity is equal to or greater than the $95^{th}$ percentile. The causes of obesity are multifactorial and include genetic, environmental (e.g., diet, family influences), and hormonal factors. The marked increase in childhood obesity also correlates with changes in food consumption, with many more foods having added sugar and fat (Gahagan, 2016).

Obesity, while the result of multiple influences, can be related to a binge eating disorder. Similar to bulimia, the child binges, eating enormous amounts of food; however, unlike bulimia, the child does not purge afterward (Kreipe, 2016). These children can gain significant amounts of weight. Children with a binge eating disorder often exhibit anxiety, depression, or OCD, any of which can contribute to the disordered eating (Gahagan, 2016). This type of disordered eating can be treated with medication (e.g., SSRIs) and CBT (Gahagan, 2016). See Chapter 8 for prevention and treatment of childhood obesity.

### Etiology

Disordered eating emerges from multiple risk factors including biologic, social, cultural, and psychological contributors. Children or adolescents with eating disorders often have a family history of internalizing disorders, such as major depression. The disorder is more common among sisters and mothers of those with the disorder than in the general population, suggesting some genetic predisposition.

Neurobiologic research has demonstrated that brain levels of serotonin and dopamine contribute to dysregulation of appetite, dysphoric mood, and difficulties with impulse control (Kaye, Wierenga, Bailer et al., 2013). Community-based studies indicate that gene abnormalities may create a predisposition toward eating disorders (Kreipe, 2016).

The development and severity of the risk for eating disorders appear to be related to the child's response to the biologic, psychological, and social demands of maturation. Other significant risk factors are earlier pubertal development and higher body fat, depressive tendencies, anxiety, rigidity, temperament (perfectionist personality) and cultural expectations to be thin (Kaye et al., 2013; Lock, LaVia and the AACAP Committee on Quality Issues, 2015).

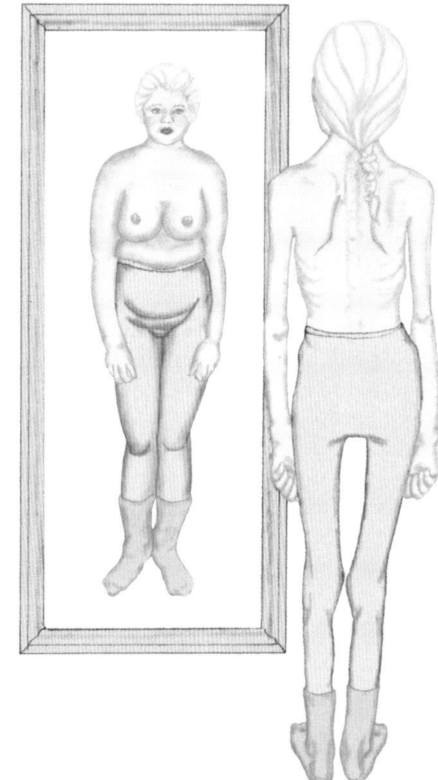


**FIG 53.1** In anorexia nervosa, the adolescent refuses to maintain adequate body weight, partly because of a distorted body image: She perceives herself as overweight when in fact she is below minimum weight.

### Manifestations

#### Anorexia

The hallmark of anorexia is the refusal to maintain a body weight that exceeds the minimal weight recommended for height (15% below expected weight). Intense preoccupation with and unrelenting fear of obesity and a disturbed body image (weight, size, or shape) that is obviously contrary to reality are also observed. Children who look in a mirror report seeing themselves as fat and are repulsed by the sight (Fig. 53.1).

Other clinical manifestations in females include amenorrhea; a misperception of internal and external stimuli, particularly food-related cues such as hunger; overwhelming feelings of ineffectiveness and inadequacy; lanugo, dry or flaky skin, and dull, brittle hair; and fatigue and muscle wasting (Kaye et al., 2013; Martin & Golden, 2014).

Boys with eating disorders demonstrate many behavior patterns similar to girls' behavior patterns, including weight loss through excessive dieting, compulsive activities, and purging, to get strong or to become more muscular (rather than to be thin, as reported by females) (National Eating Disorders Association [NEDA], n.d.).

#### Bulimia

The clinical manifestations associated with bulimia nervosa include recurrent episodes of rapid, compulsive, uncontrolled (binge) eating linked to purging; a sense of lack of control over eating behaviors during binges; and use of strategies to prevent weight gain (self-induced vomiting; use of laxatives, diuretics, or emetics; fasting; vigorous and excessive exercise). A minimum of two binge eating episodes per week for at least 3 months and persistent irrational concern with body shape and weight are also common factors. These children are also at increased risk for tooth erosion because of the effects of the acidic stomach contents on the teeth from induced vomiting. Some children with bulimia also use excessive exercise to control weight. Unlike children with anorexia, those with bulimia are mostly within normal weight percentiles.

#### Obesity

Obesity is caused by genetic, metabolic, behavioral, and environmental factors. The prevalence of obesity has risen at an alarming rate in the United States (Ogden, Carroll, et al., 2014). Obesity is not the same as overweight; obesity is defined purely by excess body fat and is linked to cardiovascular disease, diabetes, cancer, and adult obesity (CDC, 2015a).

### Diagnostic Evaluation

The medical history and physical assessment should be comprehensive, focusing on any medically based illness that mimics an eating disorder or exists concomitantly. Assessment of body image and identification of problems, substance abuse, and social support systems used by the child or adolescent are important components of the evaluation and treatment planning. A family history of eating disorders or other psychosocial illnesses should be noted. Family dynamics, including the level or quality of interaction, support, discipline, and individuation, should be explored in depth. Previous treatment attempts and successful coping strategies should be identified.

An electrocardiogram and chest radiograph are typically obtained if symptoms of bradycardia, hypotension, or hypothermia are noted. Complete liver and renal function tests, thyroid function tests, and serum electrolyte studies are usually included in the medical workup.

### Therapeutic Management

Children with severe eating disorders may need to be hospitalized to achieve physiologic stability. The priority for care is to stabilize body weight and protect from life-threatening complications (e.g., dysrhythmias, depression, or electrolyte imbalance).

One risk during this time is refeeding syndrome, which can be fatal if not recognized quickly and treated promptly. Refeeding syndrome is a fluid, electrolyte, mineral, and metabolic disturbance that results from introducing nutrition too rapidly to someone who has been starving (-Martin & Golden, 2014). This condition occurs most commonly in people who have lost weight rapidly. Starvation can drastically alter fluid, electrolyte, and metabolic balances and result in severe cardiovascular and neurologic complications with too rapid replacement of calories (Kreipe, 2016). A high index of suspicion for this syndrome is warranted, because electrolyte and fluid balances can strain the cardiac and respiratory systems. This syndrome can occur at the beginning of treatment when patients are reintroduced to a healthy diet.

Once stabilized, the child or adolescent is generally transferred to a day treatment program. Care focuses on restructuring cognitive perceptions, reducing opportunities to engage in ritualistic and self-injurious behaviors, and reestablishing physiologic homeostasis. The programs typically include interventions that enlist the adolescent's cooperation in a refeeding program. Nutritional consultation is provided to facilitate gradual weight gain. Intake and output, weight gain, vital signs, laboratory values, electrolyte status, and cardiac status are carefully monitored.

## NURSING CARE

### The Child or Adolescent With an Eating Disorder

#### Assessment

School nurses or nurses in community settings are in an optimal position for recognizing children with eating disorders. They become familiar with students they see on a regular basis and can assess changes in weight, emotional status, or behaviors. Once considered an adolescent problem, eating disorders are now observed in much younger children, so nurses in elementary schools need to be alert for early signs of the disorders. Awareness programs organized by school nurses offer opportunities for inquiries from children who might not normally speak about their eating problems or concerns about weight. Short and reliable screening tools are available to assist school nurses in identifying children who may be at risk for the disorder.

Children with eating disorders typically convey mistrust, ambivalence, and denial. It is generally better if the assessment is conducted in a structured and concrete manner (rather than as an open-ended exploration), with an emphasis placed on alliance building and periodic review.

Determining motivations for changing behaviors is crucial, and motives should be assessed for each specific behavior (i.e., weight gain, induced vomiting, altered self-perception of body). A mental status examination should also be included because the side effects of restrictive dieting can impair cognitive functioning and perpetuate emotional disturbances. Any history of self-injury should be noted. The nurse should assist the child or adolescent in gaining an understanding of impulse control problems and ritualistic and compulsive behaviors.

Before beginning a refeeding program, the nurse must assess baseline weight, electrolyte status, blood glucose, and vital signs. Assessment of intake and output is essential.

#### Nursing Diagnosis and Planning

The nursing diagnoses and expected outcomes that apply to the child or adolescent with an eating disorder follow:

- Imbalanced Nutrition: Less Than Body Requirements related to inadequate intake, malabsorption from extended periods of starvation, or distorted body image.

  **Expected outcome.** The child or adolescent will meet daily nutritional requirements, as evidenced by sufficient weight gain or maintenance of an adequate weight to sustain systemic homeostasis and physiologic health.
- Anxiety, Fear, or Powerlessness related to weight gain, sense of inadequacy, and lack of control over body and self.

  **Expected outcome.** The child or adolescent will display decreased anxiety, fear, and powerlessness, as evidenced by demonstration of the ability to seek help with anxiety management and demonstration of improved coping strategies, including open expression of feelings.
- Risk for Activity Intolerance or Disturbed Sleep Pattern related to fatigue, depression, and an excessive drive to exercise and expend energy.

  **Expected outcome.** The child or adolescent will have adequate rest, as evidenced by an ability to establish improved sleeping and activity patterns with a corresponding improvement in affect, energy, and sense of well-being.
- Deficient Fluid Volume related to excessive use of diuretics or laxatives or inadequate fiber and fluid intake.

  **Expected outcome.** The child or adolescent will maintain fluid and electrolyte balance, as evidenced by electrolyte levels within normal limits, normal skin turgor, and moist mucous membranes.

#### Interventions

The treatment of eating disorders initially focuses on disrupting the cycle of the eating disorder and addressing the secondary effects of self-induced vomiting, excessive use of diuretics and laxatives, and insufficient nutrients to sustain the function of body systems. Treatment may take place in an outpatient setting or an inpatient setting if the child's physical and emotional status requires more intensive treatment and monitoring (AACAP, 2015). Electrolyte levels and body chemistry values should be stabilized to prevent sustained damage to body systems, especially the cardiac, respiratory, and gastrointestinal systems. Adequate caloric intake is the next major goal of treatment and often requires strict monitoring to prevent sabotage of medical treatment. Fluids and foods are introduced gradually in order to reduce the risk for refeeding syndrome. Continuing intensive and highly individualized therapy helps the adolescent cope with complex issues. Family intervention usually is necessary. Finally, alteration of misperceptions about body image and a reorientation to issues of control and self-management are necessary. Follow-up therapy for the individual and family is indicated for a period of several months to 3 years. In general, the psychopharmacologic treatment of children with anorexia has not been effective, although the use of SSRIs has shown benefit for adolescents with bulimia (AACAP, 2015).

Support in exploring refeeding, sensations of fullness, bloating, and delayed gastric emptying and help in tolerating these feelings and body sensations are important. The nurse and child or adolescent jointly participate in monitoring affect, mood, and potential for suicide. They also agree to a contract specifying necessary interventions to ensure safety and to monitor daily food intake and feelings. These interventions may take the form of interacting with the staff at regular intervals or agreeing to approach the staff if suicidal ideation is present. The nurse will need to validate the adolescent's feelings of ambivalence, fear, and powerlessness. If hyperalimentation or nasogastric tube feedings are required to ensure adequate nutritional intake, the nurse should offer support regarding the discomfort and education about the importance of the interventions and should closely monitor feedings. As the child begins to show physical and cognitive gains, the nurse should provide educational information about the short-term and long-term effects of starvation.

The nurse is likely to participate in providing or supporting treatments, such as individual, group, and family therapy sessions. Especially in the early phase of treatment, the child or adolescent may be very resistant to efforts to increase nutritional intake, resorting to denial, trickery, or manipulation to prevent a weight increase or thwart adherence to dietary regimens. Observing the child or adolescent after meals may be necessary to prevent episodes of purging.

Families are informed and involved in treatment goals and apprised of progress toward these goals. Participation in family therapy is generally a required part of the treatment plan for eating disorders, because family patterns of communication and interaction can be contributory factors in success or relapse. The nurse supports the family in voicing concern for the child's health and well-being, while encouraging the view that the child needs an independent identity and sense of control.

### Evaluation

- Does the child or adolescent demonstrate an increase in food consumption adequate to sustain growth and developmental needs?
- Has the child or adolescent controlled impulses to overeat and purge?
- Can the child or adolescent demonstrate a positive alteration in self-perceptions and body image, as evidenced by verbalizing an increased sense of self-control and decreased anxiety about the present and the future?
- Does the child or adolescent demonstrate a decrease in ambivalence and mistrust about self and significant others?
- Does the child or adolescent show increased energy and display appropriate affect?
- Are electrolyte levels within normal limits, and are mucous membranes moist?

## SUBSTANCE ABUSE

Chemical agents that are typically abused by children and adolescents include alcohol, hallucinogens, sedatives, analgesics, anxiolytics, steroids, inhalants, and stimulants. The substance chosen depends on its availability and cost as well as social influences and parental behaviors or tolerance of drug use. Most professionals differentiate between substance abuse and substance addiction. However, the basic treatment concerns are similar. Substance abuse is generally considered to increase over time.

Great variation exists in the types of substances abused across sexes and ages (Table 53.1). Typically, boys consume alcohol more than girls do. Female junior high school students are increasing their use of tobacco, whereas tobacco use by their male counterparts has remained consistent.

The National Institute on Drug Abuse (NIDA) (2015) has tracked illicit drug use and attitudes toward drug, alcohol, and cigarettes among middle school and high school students nationwide since 1975. Each fall, the updated results of the *Monitoring the Future (MTF) Survey* are released. According to the 2015 survey, marijuana use has stabilized. However, there are continued increases in the rates of nonmedical use of prescription medications, particularly opioids (NIDA, 2015). The greatest concern in current trends of illicit drug use by teenagers is the increase in painkiller use. In its 2015 report, the NIDA reported the prevalence of illicit drug use among adolescents to be 8.1% of 8th graders, 16.5% of 10th graders, and 23.6% of 12th graders (NIDA, 2015). Use prevalence of over-the-counter (OTC) drugs, synthetic cannabanoids, alcohol, and heroin has decreased dramatically; however, an area of concern is the increase in e-cigarette use (NIDA, 2015).

**TABLE 53.1 Commonly Abused Drugs and Their Effects**

| Drug | Expected Behaviors and Effects | Special Considerations |
|---|---|---|
| Tobacco | Chronic cough, wheezing, increased phlegm production, atherosclerosis | Considered a gateway drug; initial use usually begins in elementary school |
| Alcohol | Amount-related effects include euphoria followed by depression or hostility, decreased inhibitions, impaired judgment, lack of coordination, and slurred speech | Considered a gateway drug; easily accessible |
| Marijuana | Relaxation, mild euphoria, loss of inhibition, decreased motivation, red eyes, dry mouth | Considered a gateway drug |
| Opiates | Euphoria, elation, pain relief, detachment and apathy, drowsiness, constricted pupils, constipation, slurred speech, impaired judgment | Long-term apathy about self, often leading to physical malnutrition and dehydration; criminal behaviors associated with obtaining drugs likely to occur; infections at injection sites common |
| Barbiturates | Similar to those associated with alcohol | Often used in conjunction with stimulants; may have a paradoxical effect of hyperactivity in children |
| Amphetamines | Euphoria, hyperactivity, agitation, irritability, insomnia, weight loss, tachycardia, hypertension | May have a paradoxical effect of depression in children |
| Cocaine | Euphoria, elation, agitation, hyperactivity, irritability, pressured speech, grandiosity, tachycardia, hypertension, diaphoresis, anorexia, weight loss, insomnia | Psychotic behavior possible if the dose is large; can be fatal if combined with other drugs |
| Hallucinogens (lysergic acid diethylamide [LSD], 3,4-met hylenedioxymethamphetamine ["ecstasy"]) | Distorted perceptions, heightened awareness, hallucinations, illusions, depersonalization, dilated pupils, hypertension, increased salivation | Psychotic behaviors, panic flashbacks long after drug use ceases, self-destructive behaviors |
| Phencyclidine hydrochloride (PCP) | Euphoria, distorted perceptions, agitation, violence, antisocial behaviors, hypertension, increased salivation, increased pain response | Panic, irrational behaviors, psychosis |

Heroin use increased in the United States, and the increase was seen across a wide range of demographic groups. Deaths from heroin overdose have also increased, particularly when combined with other substances such as alcohol and the opioid pain relievers, such as Fentnyl (Jones, Logan, Gladden, Bohm, 2015). Heroin use in the pediatric population has seen a decline in recent years, with heroin use among 8-12 graders declining, however the trend of increased heroin use is driven by the young adult population, 18-25 (Substance Abuse and Mental Health Services Administration, 2013).

Alcohol use remains a significant problem, with over 35% of 12th graders reporting its use (NIDA, 2015). The prevalence of marijuana use among 12th graders is approximately that of alcohol, at 34.9% (NIDA, 2015). Research consistently supports the hypothesis that drug use progresses from beer or wine to cigarettes or hard liquor and then marijuana, followed by other illicit drugs. These substances are sometimes referred to as gateway substances. Increasingly, research demonstrates that early use of these substances can do harm to the developing adolescent brain, particularly in the area of cognitive function. Substance abuse is also strongly associated with other high-risk behaviors in adolescence such as unintentional injuries and unprotected sex (Box 53.2).

Public awareness and emphasis on treatment and prevention seem to be working. Although these factors had very limited effect on teenagers in the 1990s, there is a promising increase in the belief that illicit drugs are harmful, and increased numbers of teenagers disapprove of their use. Reducing substance abuse is a national health goal identified in *Healthy People 2020* (USDHHS, 2010). An awareness of the possibility of substance abuse is the responsibility of the parent, teacher, and health professional. Knowing the clinical behavioral manifestations of substance abuse is essential, and much information is readily available to adults interested in prevention and early identification.

## Etiology

Drugs affect the brain by altering the biochemical pathways in the CNS. The brain regions most affected in substance abuse are located within the mesocorticolimbic system and include the hippocampus, ventral segmental area, nucleus accumbens, and medial prefrontal cortex. Biochemical alteration results in a complex interplay among dopamine, serotonin, norepinephrine, and γ-aminobutyric acid. Some drugs mimic natural neurotransmitters, thereby activating neurons. Other drugs, such as amphetamines and cocaine, cause the nerve cells to flood the synaptic space, greatly amplifying the normal effect. All drugs of abuse directly or indirectly target dopamine, the neurotransmitter present in areas of the brain that regulate emotion, cognition, movement, and pleasure. This overstimulation creates the euphoric, energized feeling sought by users (NIDA, 2014).

Substance abuse and substance dependence tend to cluster in families. For alcohol, as for most other drugs, evidence indicates that substance abuse often represents the child's or adolescent's attempt to cope with anxiety generated by impaired social skills, low self-esteem, poor interpersonal relationships, or lack of adaptive behaviors. Emotional and behavioral disorders, such as anxiety disorders, ADHD, depression, and conduct disorder, are associated with an increased risk for substance abuse.

### BOX 53.2 Phases of Substance Abuse

**Phase 1: Experimentation**
The drug is taken to see what it does or to appease peers.

**Phase 2: Early Drug Use**
A specific drug or various drugs are used with some regularity for their pleasurable effects or to reduce anxiety. Social use of drugs typically falls into this category.

**Phase 3: True Drug Addiction**
Drugs are used regularly, and physical dependence begins if characteristic of the drug. Social functioning revolves around a drug focus.

**Phase 4: Severe Drug Addiction**
The physical condition of the addicted child or adolescent deteriorates. All activities are related to obtaining or using the drug, with isolation from nondrug culture.

## Manifestations

The clinical manifestations of substance abuse are marked by increased antisocial behavior as the desire for social conformity and acceptance decreases and the need for the substance increases. Behaviors that may indicate substance abuse problems include irregular school attendance, low grades or poor school performance, aggressive or rebellious behavior, excessive dependence on peer influence, and deterioration of relationships with family members or former friends. Rapid or extreme changes in behavior or mood and loss of interest in hobbies, sports, or other favorite activities are often observed. Further possible factors include a lack of parental support and supervision and changes in eating or sleeping patterns that increase as manipulative behaviors increase, especially those related to the need to acquire desired substances.

### ! NURSING QUALITY ALERT
#### *Relapse Among Substance Abusers*

Substance abusers' rates of refusal to adhere to therapeutic recommendations, together with resulting relapses, are quite high. More than 60% of those completing a course of treatment continue to abuse substances throughout their lifetimes.

## Therapeutic Management

Treatment in a center specifically designed for substance abuse is recommended and includes individual, group, and family therapy. Participation in Alcoholics Anonymous or Narcotics Anonymous is advocated. These organizations also offer support groups geared toward helping family members, offering programs that promote alterations in the family system to decrease the likelihood of relapse.

Increased, and increasing, incidence of opioid overdose has created a public health issue that affects families, healthcare providers and first responders. States have legislated different pathways to managing the epidemic of heroin and opioid use. Approaches include state organized monitoring of prescription writing by providers, and databases by which providers can quickly access information about the opiates, doses and pharmacies where a patient has filled prescriptions.

In 2014 Attorney General Eric Holder called for all first responders to be equipped and trained in the use of naloxone (Narcan) as a tool to restore breathing while awaiting medical aid (U. S. Department of Justice, 2015). Since that time many states have trained police, firefighters and other likely responders in the use of this lifesaving intervention.

The relapse rate among youthful substance abusers is extremely high, and success in a short-term treatment program is not necessarily an indicator of long-term control. The incidence of relapse is generally reduced if the child and family maintain active, long-term involvement in support groups such as Alcoholics Anonymous, Alateen, Alatot, and

Narcotics Anonymous. Parenting groups may also be beneficial in providing counsel and support as parents navigate the numerous and often painful decisions they must make.

## NURSING CARE

### The Child or Adolescent With a Substance Abuse Problem

#### Assessment

Physical assessment should include evaluation of the respiratory rate, heart rate, blood pressure, activity level (hyperactive, hypoactive), mood, affect, judgment, speech, sensory responses, and memory. A thorough history of current and past drug use should be obtained. A family and social history, medical history, and legal history (e.g., past and current charges related to substance abuse) should be obtained as well. The possibility of pregnancy should also be considered, since drugs taken during pregnancy will also affect the neonate.

#### Nursing Diagnosis and Planning

The nursing diagnoses and expected outcomes that apply to the child or adolescent with a substance abuse problem follow:

- Disturbed Thought Processes related to the specific effects of the particular substance involved.

Expected outcome. The child or adolescent will exhibit behaviors indicative of the absence of substance abuse, as evidenced by the ability to maintain oriented to time, place, and person.

- Disturbed Sensory Perception related to the specific effects of the particular substance involved.

Expected outcome. The child or adolescent will remain free from sensory changes, as evidenced by the absence of falls or other injuries.

- Anxiety related to a decrease in sense of control over self or the environment.

Expected outcome. The child or adolescent will display decreased anxiety, as evidenced by verbalization of increased feelings of self-worth and the ability to change behavior.

- Ineffective Coping related to limited development of effective social interactions and problem-solving skills.

Expected outcome. The child or adolescent will increase ability to interact socially and to problem solve, as evidenced by an ability to identify current stressors leading to substance use or abuse.

- Impaired Social Interaction related to anxiety or limited social skills.

Expected outcome. The child or adolescent will begin to develop healthy social skills, as evidenced by an ability to identify alternative activities, people, and social situations that discourage substance abuse.

- Situational Low Self-Esteem or Chronic Low Self-Esteem related to limited social skills, ineffective coping skills, or a poor sense of self-management.

Expected outcome. The child or adolescent will increase self-esteem, as evidenced by replacing substance abuse with more appropriate social skills and developing meaningful relationships with nonabusing peers and family members.

#### Interventions

The nurse's responsibilities in caring for children or adolescents with substance abuse problems depend on the care setting, the severity of the abuse, and the treatment goals. Often, other students report a child's use or abuse of substances to the school nurse. In this instance, appropriate care and referral begin in the school setting and may include a thorough assessment and parent notification. The nurse can be a resource for parents and community members as to agencies within the community that can assist the child and family. Many school districts have a zero-tolerance policy for tobacco, drugs, and alcohol; in some instances, the school resource officer or local police will be called. Often a crisis team within the school that includes the school nurse as a participating member makes this decision. Most school districts actively incorporate alcohol and drug prevention programs in their curricula for students at various grade levels.

If the youth has been identified as a substance abuser and referred to a treatment facility, the nurse's primary responsibility will be to stabilize the physiologic status and support recommendations for treatment. Explaining the expectations and the types of services offered is important because most treatment programs increase child or adolescent and family responsibilities over time.

Initially, maintaining safety and an optimal level of physical comfort is necessary, especially if detoxification is required. Safety measures include close observation, removal of any potentially dangerous items, and monitoring vital signs. Being readily available to discuss thoughts, concerns, and perceptions is important to create an emotional sense of safety. Additional interventions include educating the child or adolescent and family members about necessary laboratory tests and providing information about the nature of substance abuse.

Another significant nursing intervention is to assist the child or adolescent and family in developing social support systems and refer them to appropriate resources that can offer additional support as they make long-term changes in their social and emotional patterns of relating. It is also essential to help the youth assume responsibility for the substance abuse problem rather than passing the blame on to others. Providing emotional support for the youth and family as they develop insight into their behaviors and the need for changes is important because these changes are often difficult to effect.

#### Evaluation

- Has the child or adolescent remained substance free and been oriented to time and place?
- Has the child or adolescent remained injury free as a result of sensory or perceptual changes?
- Is the child or adolescent able to identify stressors and use appropriate coping mechanisms?
- Has the child or adolescent assumed responsibility for changing behaviors related to the substance abuse?
- Is the child or adolescent participating in daily activities?
- Does the child or adolescent show improvement in peer and family relationships?
- Does the child or adolescent demonstrate an increased sense of self-confidence?

## CHILDHOOD PHYSICAL AND EMOTIONAL ABUSE AND CHILD NEGLECT

Child abuse includes emotional abuse, physical abuse, and sexual exploitation or molestation by caretakers or other individuals. Deliberate failure to provide for a child's physical, educational, or emotional needs is considered to be neglect. Although the federal definition of child abuse includes neglect, some states separately define neglect and each major type of abuse (USDHHS Administration for Children and Families, Administration on Children, Youth and Families, Children's Bureau, 2014).

### Etiology

Family dysfunction underlies most forms of child abuse or neglect. The family profile varies with the type of abuse, although it is not

**BOX 53.3 Characteristics of the Abusive Family**

- Isolation from community and social groups
- Intense competition for emotional resources within the family, such as affection, attention, and nurturing
- Low levels of differentiation among family members
- Low trust of outsiders and family members
- Unpredictable and unstable family environment
- Conflict resolution generally achieved through aggression or power struggle between family members
- Current focus and crisis-oriented actions for immediate gratification
- Communication often characterized by mixed or double messages, threats, or a focus on nonverbal communication rather than direct verbalization
- Family roles that are typically fixed and traditional, with rigid rules
- Frequent domination by a single family member who maintains control through manipulation, intimidation, deceit, and aggression

uncommon for multiple types of abuse to exist in a single family. Particular risk factors for child maltreatment include perpetrator alcohol or drug abuse, domestic abuse, and child disability (USDHHS Administration for Children and Families, Administration on Children, Youth and Families, Children's Bureau, 2014) (Box 53.3).

Socioeconomic factors also appear to influence the incidence and etiology of child abuse, with increased physical abuse observed during periods of economic hardship or external stress. The typical perpetrator is a direct relative of the child (78% were parents), with mothers being perpetrators more often than fathers (USDHHS Administration for Children and Families, Administration on Children, Youth and Families, Children's Bureau, 2014).

In sexual abuse, the perpetrator is more likely to be a family friend or neighbor (60%) than a parent (3%) (U.S. Department of Veteran's Affairs, 2015). Perpetrators are most often males who may have mental health issues; some were abused during childhood or adolescence (Center for Sex Offenders Management, 2015). The typical profile of an abused child is more difficult to determine.

A substantial percentage of children (27%) who have been maltreated are younger than 3 years, with girls and boys being victims at a similar rate (USDHHS, Administration for Children and Families, Administration on Children, Youth and Families, Children's Bureau, 2014). Some research indicates that the child who is maltreated often has mild physical abnormalities, is developmentally or physically delayed, or has behavior problems.

## Incidence

The reporting of child abuse to child protective services have increased. This increase is attributed to public awareness as well as increased awareness and willingness to report on the part of teachers and healthcare providers. In 2014, 62% of reports to child protective services nationwide were made by professionals, including medical, educational, and law enforcement (USDHHS Administration for Children and Families, Administration on Children, Youth and Families, Children's Bureau, 2014).

In 2014, approximately 700,000 children were identified as victims of substantiated physical, sexual, or emotional abuse or neglect. Of those identified, 75% suffered from neglect, 17% were physically abused, and 8.3% were sexually abused (USDHHS Administration for Children and Families, Administration on Children, Youth and Families, Children's Bureau, 2014). The national rate of victimization is 9.4 in 1000 children, with white, Hispanic, and black children having the highest incidence (USDHHS Administration for Children and Families, Administration on Children, Youth and Families, Children's Bureau, 2014).

Approximately 1500 children died from maltreatment in 2014. Seventy percent of the children killed were younger than 3 years (USDHHS, Administration for Children and Families, Administration on Children, Youth and Families, Children's Bureau, 2014).

## Manifestations

The indicators of specific types of child abuse can be both physical and behavioral. The health provider needs to be aware that there may be more than one type of abuse occurring simultaneously in a given child.

### Indicators of Physical Abuse

Physical signs that raise suspicion of physical abuse include the appearance of bruises, especially bruises in various stages of healing, bite marks, burns in unusual locations (e.g., back, palms of the hands) (Fig. 53.2), and signs and symptoms of skeletal injury (e.g., multiple bone fractures). The child may be unwilling, unable, or too frightened to explain the origin of the injuries. The child's behavior might demonstrate wariness or fear of adults and, if in school, the child may resist going home. In some cases, the child may report an inflicted injury. Interview with the child's parents may reveal an inconsistent story about how the child sustained the injuries. Parents may demonstrate inconsistent or overly harsh discipline when interacting with the child (USDHHS Child Welfare Information Gateway, 2013). Adolescents who are physically abused may cope by running away.

### Indicators of Neglect

Children experiencing neglect will most often show inadequate weight gain for age, poor growth pattern, and failure to thrive. Teachers may notice that the child comes to school inappropriately dressed for the weather (e.g., wearing shorts in winter, without shoes) or has signs of inadequate hygiene. The child may be lacking routine healthcare, such as immunizations or needed eyewear. Truancy may be a problem with neglected children. Children who are neglected may beg for money or steal food. The child may report being home alone for long periods of time unsupervised. Observation of parent–child interaction may reveal a parent who appears indifferent or unaware of the child's needs, or who demonstrates behaviors that indicate a possible emotional or substance abuse disorder (USDHHS Child Welfare Information Gateway, 2013).

### Indicators of Emotional Abuse

Signs of emotional abuse may include delays in both physical and emotional development. One hallmark of a child who is emotionally abused is that the child may behave in ways that are too adult in relation to the child's age (e.g., being protective of others), or too immature for age. Behavioral extremes (e.g., overly aggressive or overly compliant) are not unusual. The child may demonstrate repetitive habits, such as head-banging, rocking, biting, and sucking. The parent–child relationship appears to lack warmth or attachment, and parents may demonstrate an overly critical approach. Children who are emotionally abused are at high risk for suicide (USDHHS Child Welfare Information Gateway, 2013).

### Indicators of Sexual Abuse

The sexually abused child may exhibit difficulty walking or sitting and complain of pain on urination or in the genital area. Examination may reveal physical signs of bruising or laceration of perineal tissue (e.g., vaginal, anal) or the diagnosis of a sexually transmitted disease. Previously toilet-trained children may experience urinary accidents.

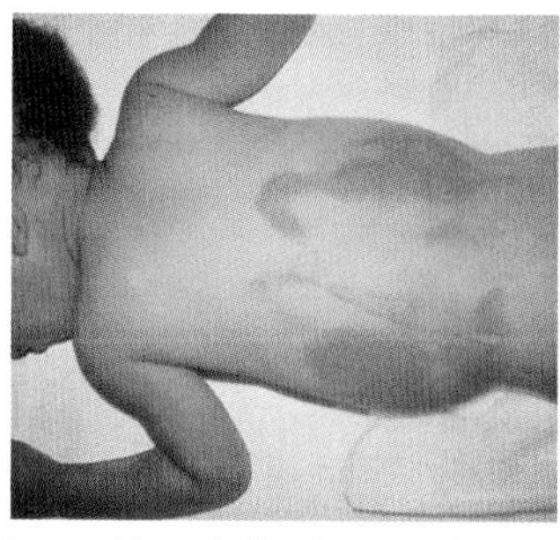
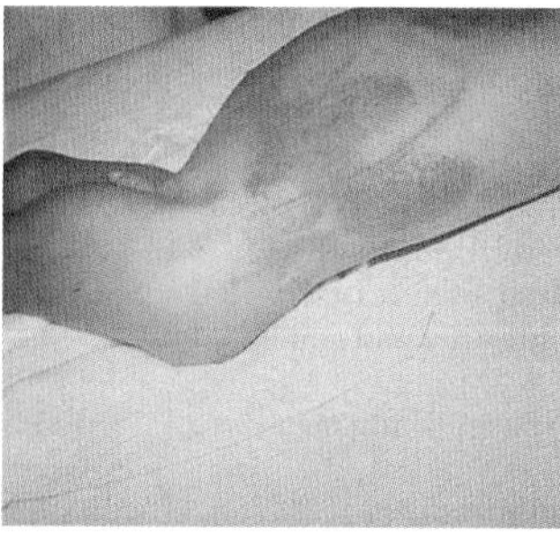

Nonaccidental distribution of bruises: All four surfaces of the torso are involved, but there are no bruises on arms and legs.

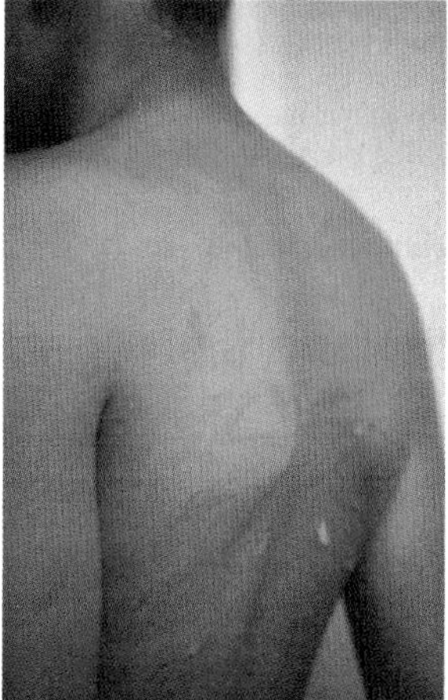
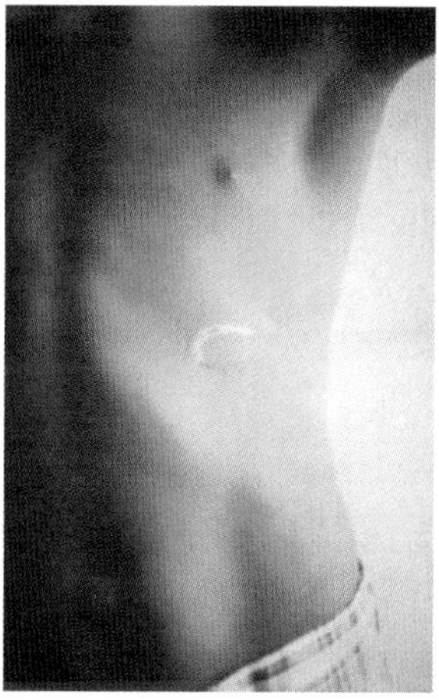

Pattern of injury: Linear scars of various ages indicate repeated abuse with a switch or a whip. The loop pattern on the boy's anterior torso is consistent with a looped electrical cord used as a whip.

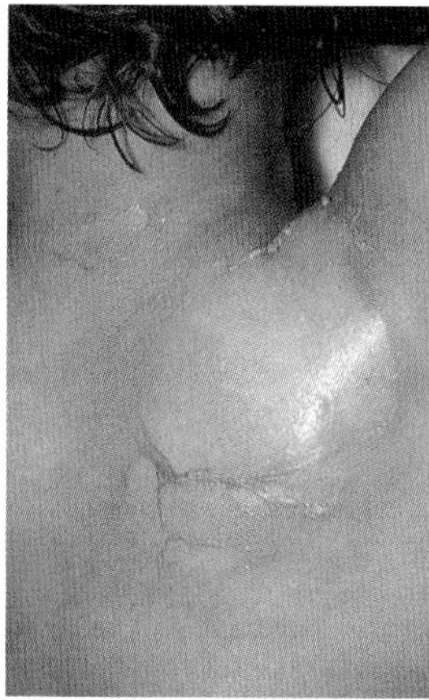

Scald burn of shoulder and neck: The typical distribution of a scald burn in a toddler. This type of injury occurs when a toddler pulls a cup of coffee or pan of water off a stove.

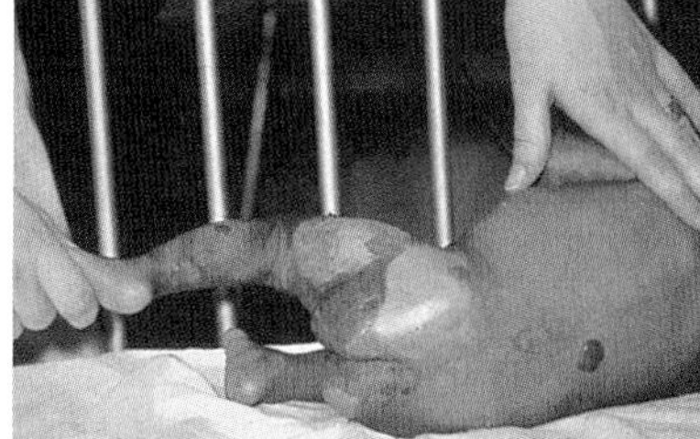

Nonaccidental immersion scald: Involvement of virtually the entire posterior surface of the legs indicates that the legs were held under scalding water; even an infant this young would flex the knees to avoid the hot water.

**FIG 53.2** Physical signs of child abuse. The nurse should be alert for the typical behavioral indicators of abuse. (Courtesy Barbara Tenney, MD. From Henry, M.C., & Stapleton, E.R. [1992]. *EMT: prehospital care* [pp. 675]. Philadelphia: Saunders.)

Nightmares or other sleep disturbances, decreased appetite, sudden refusal to participate in gym or other physical activities, and overt aggression are also behavioral indicators. The child may exhibit signs of emotional distress or self-destructive behaviors. Sexually abused children may use sexual language and innuendo that is not appropriate for age; sexually abused adolescents may be promiscuous. Behavioral indicators in the parents include being overly protective, isolating the child from other children, and exhibiting overly controlling behavior toward family members (USDHHS Child Welfare Information Gateway, 2013).

Children who are sexually abused may or may not report the abuse or may deny the abuse occurred, even with direct questioning. Sometimes memories of childhood abuse surface years later. The manner in which disclosure of sexual abuse occurs has important legal implications because in the absence of physical signs, reliance is on the child's report.

### Other Specific Abusive Situations

***Abusive head trauma.*** Abusive head trauma (AHT), formerly known as shaken infant or shaken baby syndrome, is a widely recognized form of physical child abuse that often is caused by vigorous shaking of the infant while the child is held by the extremities or shoulders. This type of physical abuse leads to whiplash-induced intracranial and retinal bleeding. There is usually no external sign of head trauma, which makes this syndrome difficult to detect. However, recent evidence suggests that if three of the major signs of head trauma are present in a child younger than three, it is more likely to be abusive head trauma (Crowley, Morris, Maguire, et al., 2015). Signs of concern include retinal hemorrhage, skull fracture, altered neurologic status, apnea, head or neck bruises, subdural hematoma, and seizures. The most common trigger for severe shaking is crying, especially if the child is colicky.

***Factitious disorder by proxy (munchausen syndrome by proxy, or medical child abuse).*** Factitious disorder (formerly Munchausen Syndrome) is a psychiatric disorder wherein people feign illness to gain attention. Factitious disorder by proxy occurs when a parent or caregiver falsifies illness in a child. This rare disorder may be the most difficult form of child abuse to diagnose. Most victims are children younger than school age.

### CRITICAL THINKING EXERCISE 53.1

Matthew, aged 2 years, is brought to the emergency department by his mother, Ms. Jackson, and her boyfriend. Ms. Jackson tells the nurse that Matthew has been crying and holding his arm since she picked him up at the babysitter's earlier in the evening. On further questioning, Ms. Jackson states "Matthew is all boy. You have to watch him every minute or he is into something. He is constantly climbing and falling."

On examination, the nurse notes several bruises on Matthew's right leg and right arm. He also has a small abrasion on his nose. Ms. Jackson is holding Matthew and seems concerned, as does her boyfriend. Matthew quiets when his mother holds him, and he drifts off to sleep. Ms. Jackson's boyfriend leaves the room and returns with a snack for both Matthew and Ms. Jackson. He offers to hold Matthew.

1. What are some of the possible reasons Matthew is crying and holding his arm? Support your assumptions with rationales.
2. If the nurse suspects child abuse, what added assessments should be performed?
3. What legal responsibility does the nurse have in cases of suspected child abuse?

The caretaker falsifies illness in the child through simulation or production of illness and then takes the child for medical care, claiming no knowledge of how the child became ill. The most common reasons these caretakers give for seeking medical treatment for the child include bleeding, seizures, CNS depression, apnea, diarrhea, vomiting, fever, and rash.

Some clinicians suggest that the syndrome be considered a form of medical abuse. Mortality rates are hard to estimate, but the long-term mortality rate in these cases is as high as 9% to 30% (Brannon, Abdulhamid, & Poirier, 2015). Under the supervision of other adults, the child exhibits no symptoms and may appear normal and healthy. The parent's behavior reflects a serious disturbance that requires specialized psychiatric treatment and removal of the child from the parent's care. A multidisciplinary team is the best approach to diagnosing this disorder (Dubowitz & Lane, 2016).

## NURSING CARE PLAN

### *The Abused Child*

#### Focused Assessment

- Examine the skin for any impaired integrity or bruising, especially of the scalp, bottoms of the hands and feet, front and back of the trunk, and genitalia.
- Obtain a baseline measurement of height and weight; document infant birth weight.
- Assess the child's anxiety level, ability to relate to the examiner, and emotional tone.
- Assess family supports: Patterns of interaction, belief systems, and social support systems.
- Unemotionally request information about bruises, injuries, and sexual abuse with particular attention to the child's need for privacy and dignity.
- Record the child's comments verbatim; these may be needed for legal proceedings later.
- Encourage the child to make self-care decisions and to discuss thoughts and feelings that might possibly have been repressed to survive the trauma (Fig. 53.3); facilitate a supportive environment for the child and family.
- Recognize that the child may have low self-esteem, feelings of inadequacy, fear, and a desire to protect the perpetrator.
- Use an appropriate assessment tool to identify behaviors typical of a sexually abused child.
- Report any suspected abuse to the appropriate authorities.

#### Nursing Diagnosis

Impaired Parenting related to immaturity, lack of knowledge, apathy on the part of parental caregivers, or limited or negative past parenting experience.

#### Planning

##### *Expected Outcome*

The family will exhibit appropriate parenting skills, as evidenced by describing the aspects of positive parenting models and responding to the child's needs in a timely and appropriate manner.

#### Interventions and *Rationales*

1. Elicit information about the parents' strengths and weaknesses, normal coping mechanisms, and the presence or absence of support systems. Special attention should be paid to:
   a. Expectations with regard to the child
   b. Comforting behaviors
   c. Response to the child
   d. General knowledge about the child
   *To provide optimal care for the child, involvement of the family is crucial. By understanding the needs of the family, the nurse can develop a plan of care, including referral to appropriate supportive agencies.*
2. Discuss with the parents the parenting they received as children.
   *Parenting is a learned skill.*
3. Observe the parents' interactions with the child.
   *Although parents may verbalize a positive relationship with their child, observation of actual interactions provides a more realistic view of the parent–child relationship.*
4. Provide an accepting environment.
   *Communication is encouraged by demonstrating acceptance.*
4. Provide information for parents regarding normal growth and development.
   *Parents who are abusers often have unrealistic expectations of their children, in part because of their lack of knowledge regarding growth and development.*
5. Include role modeling as a method of teaching parenting.
   *By observing the way the nurse touches and talks to the child in an affirming manner, the parents can observe firsthand the child's response to positive parenting-type skills.*
6. Devote part of the time spent with the child and family to focusing on the child's positive attributes. For example:
   *You might say "I appreciate how quietly you have played with your toys while I have been talking with mommy," or "Look at how nicely you are talking to your doll."*
7. Encourage the parents to participate in the child's care. Reinforce positive behaviors.
   *Strategies that encourage and reinforce positive parental participation in child care build self-esteem and confidence in parenting skills.*

#### Evaluation

Do the parents interact appropriately with the child through verbal, physical, and visual contact?
Have the parents described features of normal growth and development?
Do the parents make positive statements about the child?
Do the parents bring the child in for follow-up visits?

#### Nursing Diagnosis

Fear and/or Powerlessness related to the possible outcomes of disclosure, sense of shame, and possible loss of family.

#### Planning

##### *Expected Outcomes*

1. The child will verbalize the source of fear.
2. The child will express feelings related to shame and fear of loss of family.

#### Interventions and *Rationales*

1. Reassure the child in regard to personal safety.
   *Verbal reassurance can provide a sense of security.*
2. Identify specific strategies the child can use to maintain a sense of stability (i.e., stay with a trusted adult, refuse to answer intrusive questions, limit exposure to adults who are not trusted).
   *By providing some viable options, the nurse can help the child begin to gain a sense of control over the experience.*
3. Acknowledge the child's fear.
   *Acknowledgment helps the child identify feelings and opens up new areas of communication.*
4. Spend time with the child. Use both verbal and nonverbal forms of communication.
   *Actions of support provide comfort and encourage verbalization of feelings.*

## NURSING CARE PLAN—cont'd

### *The Abused Child*

5. Offer choices, when available, regarding activities of daily living, recreation time, and time with other children and adults.
   *Being offered choices gives the child a sense of control and diminishes feelings of powerlessness.*

**Evaluation**

Does the child participate in play activities?
Has the child verbalized specific fears related to abuse and disclosure?
Has the child verbalized fears related to being removed from the family?

**Nursing Diagnosis**

Deficient Knowledge about the child's realistic developmental abilities, how to access external support resources, or ways to manage internal and external stressors related to past inexperience with parenting.

**Planning**

***Expected Outcomes***

1. The family will increase knowledge related to growth and development, as evidenced by verbalization of an understanding of the child's developmental and emotional needs in a framework that is oriented to the child's welfare.
2. The family will identify support systems.

**Interventions and *Rationales***

1. Determine the parents' knowledge of child growth and development.
   *A baseline assessment must be done to develop a plan of care.*
2. Serve as a role model for positive parenting skills.
   *Learning can be enhanced through observing the application of parenting skills, which is more effective than listening to a lecture.*
3. Assist the family in identifying stressors and the support systems and resources that may help decrease the parents' stress level.
   *If the parents' level of stress is decreased, the risk for abuse is decreased.*
4. Refer the family to pertinent support groups, such as Parents Anonymous.
   *Lack of support and isolation are common among abusive families. A support group may decrease isolation.*
5. Involve the parents in the care of the child.
   *Participation in care will provide opportunities for positive reinforcement, teaching, and increased emotional attachment to the child.*
6. Provide education in the following areas: Growth and development, nutrition, care related to activities of daily living, routine well-child care, manifestations of illness, and need for care and loving.
   *Education in parenting skills may decrease unrealistic expectations, increase awareness of the needs of children, and increase the chances of positive parenting. Parents may not have had positive-parenting role models as children.*
7. Provide a consistent caregiver from among the nursing staff.
   *Consistency of care increases the child's feelings of trust and security and provides increased opportunities for the child to verbalize feelings.*

**Evaluation**

Can the parents describe normal child growth and development and developmental expectations?
Have the parents joined a support group?

**Nursing Diagnosis**

Risk for Injury related to a family with a history of physical abuse, physical neglect, emotional abuse, or sexual abuse.

**Planning**

***Expected Outcome***

Injury related to abuse will cease, as evidenced by the child remaining free from physical or psychological injury and neglect.

**Interventions and *Rationales***

1. Describe the child's physical and mental status.
   *All children should undergo a thorough physical assessment on presentation to the healthcare setting and should be assessed for bruises, burns, scars, and other signs of abuse. Children may enter the healthcare system for reasons other than injury.*
2. Observe the interactions between child and family.
   *Subtle signs of abuse may be detected in the way the child interacts with the abuser and other adults.*
3. Obtain a thorough history.
   *Frequent presentation of the child for injuries or signs of healed injuries may indicate a pattern of abuse.*
4. Use a nonthreatening, nonjudgmental manner when interacting with the child's parents.
   *By building a trusting relationship with the parents, the nurse can help the child. If the parents become suspicious or alienated, they may deny the child access to healthcare. They will become defensive and will not be open to teaching.*
5. Report all cases in which abuse is suspected.
   *All 50 states require healthcare professionals to report all cases of suspected abuse.*
6. Assist in removing children from an unsafe environment.
   *Suspected abuse should be evaluated immediately so that the child can be removed to an environment that is safe, thereby preventing further injury.*
7. Document the following: Results of the child's physical assessment, observations of interactions between the child and family and between the child and other adults and the child's reaction to hospitalization or the healthcare setting, direct comments made by the child and the family that pertain to the child or the child's injury, and child's developmental level.
   *Objective documentation is essential in all cases of suspected abuse.*
8. If the child is removed from the home, provide the child and family with support and opportunities to verbalize feelings. Play therapy may be used effectively with children.
   *Children who are removed from the custody of their parents will grieve their loss. Parents will need support in dealing with guilt and loss.*

**Evaluation**

Does the child remain free of inflicted injury?
Has the child been placed in a safe environment?
Has the child verbalized feelings regarding placement outside the home?
Has the family sought psychological counseling?

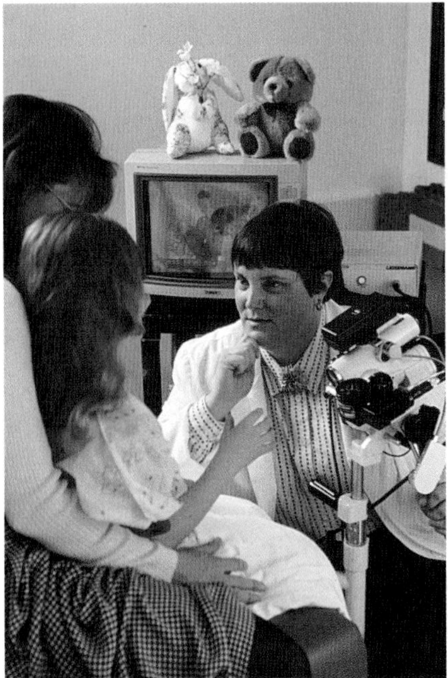

Note the communication techniques designed to reassure the child and give the child some power. The little girl is not immediately positioned for a genital examination. The physician first sits to talk with the child at her eye level and makes eye contact with her.

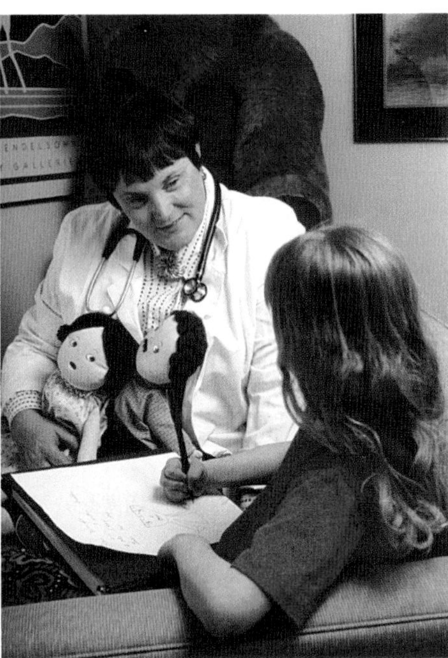

Drawings may help to identify the abused child and assist in therapy. Art can also help the child express what cannot be expressed in words.

**FIG 53.3** Disclosure of abuse may be slow because the child often has difficulty trusting any adult. Physical examination and interview of children who may be victims of sexual abuse require particular sensitivity because physical inspection of the child's genitalia to detect signs of injury or sexually transmitted disease may frighten the child, who associates handling of the genitalia with pain or shame. Anatomically correct dolls are often used in the assessment of abuse within a family. These dolls help children express what they cannot express in words; young children in particular have a limited vocabulary to use when describing the events that have occurred. (Courtesy Cook Children's Medical Center, Fort Worth, TX.)

## KEY CONCEPTS

- In children and adolescents, the behavioral manifestations of anxiety and depression can be similar. Children with both diagnoses may be withdrawn, tearful, unwilling to engage in play, and aggressive toward others.
- It is difficult to differentiate between normal mood changes resulting from developmental maturation and abnormal, persistent mood disturbances.
- Separation anxiety and school avoidance should be addressed if the problem becomes persistent or debilitating. Such anxiety is characterized by excessive fear, even panic, of being away from the parent or home.
- A suicide gesture or statement should never be ignored.
- Protecting a child or an adolescent from inflicting harm to self involves being emotionally and physically available, offering opportunities to discuss feelings and the suicidal event, and removing potentially harmful objects.
- Support for grieving families of suicidal or potentially suicidal children or an adolescent is best provided on both an individual and a group basis to allow exploration of personal issues and social support.
- ADHD is a behavioral disorder characterized by developmentally inappropriate degrees of inattention, overactivity, and impulsivity.
- Support groups are important in assisting families to cope with and modify expectations and interactions involving the child with ADHD.
- Educating the family about ADHD is a crucial component of caring for the child with this disorder.
- Anorexia nervosa is characterized by a deliberate refusal to maintain adequate body weight, a distorted body image, and amenorrhea (in female patients).
- One common factor among children with an eating disorder is a family system in which the individual is considered to be an extension of the parent or serves as a means of meeting the parents' needs, rather than being allowed to develop as an autonomous individual. The family is often disordered and chaotic, resulting in the child's sense of isolation.
- The focus of care for an adolescent with an eating disorder involves restructuring cognitive perceptions, reducing opportunities for engaging in ritualistic and self-injurious behaviors, and reestablishing physiologic homeostasis.
- During the early treatment phase of eating disorders, it may be necessary to observe the adolescent after meals to prevent episodes of purging.
- Common signs of substance abuse include low grades; irregular school attendance; aggressive or rebellious behavior; deteriorating relationships with family members or former friends; rapid or extreme changes in behaviors or mood; and loss of interest in hobbies, sports, or other activities.
- A child or an adolescent with a substance abuse problem, together with the family, should receive help in developing social support systems, with referral to appropriate resources that can offer additional support as they attempt to make long-term changes in their social and emotional patterns of relating.
- Physical child abuse tends to increase during times of economic hardship or external stress. Abusive families are often isolated, lack

## KEY CONCEPTS—cont'd

a support system, exhibit low levels of trust, resolve conflict through aggression, assume fixed and traditional roles within the family, and establish rigid rules.

- All suspected child abuse must be reported to the appropriate authorities.
- Abusive parents often have unrealistic expectations of their children, which may relate to lack of knowledge of normal growth and development.
- Modeling positive parenting skills is an effective intervention in the care of the child who has been abused.

## REFERENCES AND READINGS


Achenbach, T.M., & Rescoria, L.A. (2000). *Manual for the ASEBA preschool forms and profiles.* Burlington VT: University of Vermont, Department of Psychiatry.

Achenbach, T.M., & Rescoria, L.A. (2001). *Manual for the ASEBA school age forms and profiles.* Burlington VT: University of Vermont, Research Center for Children, Youth and Families.

American Academy of Child and Adolescent Psychiatry. (2011). *Facts for families: When to seek help for your child.* Retrieved from http://www.aacap.org.

American Academy of Child and Adolescent Psychiatry. (2013a). *School refusal.* Retrieved from http://www.aacap.org.

American Academy of Child and Adolescent Psychiatry. (2013b). *What causes pediatric bipolar Disorder?* Retrieved from http://www.aacap.org.

American Academy of Child and Adolescent Psychiatry. (2015). *Anxiety disorders resource center: What causes anxiety?* Retrieved from http://www.aacap.org.

American Nurses Association. (2014). *Psychiatric-Mental Health Nursing: Scope and Standards of Practice* (2nd ed.) nursesbooks.org.

American Psychiatric Association. (2013a). *Diagnostic and statistical manual of mental disorders*, 5th edition. Washington, DC.

American Psychiatric Association. (2013b). *Disruptive, impulse control and conduct disorders.* Diagnostic and statistical manual of mental disorders (5th ed.). Washington, DC: Author. doi:10.1176/appi.books.

Aubry, A., Serrano, P. & Burghardt, N. (2016). Molecular mechanisms of stress-induced increases in fear memory consolidation within the amygdala. *Frontiers in Behavioral Neuroscience.* doi:10.33389/fnbeh201600191.

Brannon, G., Abdulhamid, I., & Poirier, M. (2015). *Factitious disorder imposed on another.* Retrieved from http://www.emedicine.medscape.com.

Center for Sex Offenders Management. (2015). *What you need to know about sex offenders.* Retrieved from http://www.csom.org.

Centers for Disease Control and Prevention (2013). Mental health surveillance among children-United States, 2005-2011. *Morbidity and Mortality Weekly Report, 62* (02). Retrieved from http://www.cdc.gov.

Centers for Disease Control and Prevention. (2014). *LGBT youth.* Retrieved from http://www.cdc.gov.

Centers for Disease Control and Prevention (2015a). Childhood obesity facts. *Healthy Schools*, U.S. Department of Health and Human Services. Retrieved from http://www.cdc.gov.

Centers for Disease Control and Prevention. (2015b). *Suicide facts at a glance.* Retrieved from http://www.cdc.gov.

Centers for Disease Control and Prevention. (2016a). *Traumatic brain injury: Potential effects.* Retrieved from http://www.cdc.gov.

Centers for Disease Control and Prevention. (2016b). Youth Risk Behavior Surveillance United States 2015. *MMWR, 65*(6), 1-174.

Crowley, L., Morris, C. Maguire, S., et al. (2015). Validation of a predictive tool for abusive head trauma. *Pediatrics, 136*(2), 290–298.

DeMaso, D., & Walter, H. (2016). Psychological treatment of children and adolescents. In R. Kliegman, B. Stanton, J. St. Geme, et al. (Eds.), *Nelson textbook of pediatrics* (20th ed., Chapter 21). St. Louis, MO: Elsevier.

DeMaso, D., Wallter, H., & Wharff, E. (2016). Suicide and attempted suicide. In R. Kliegman, B. Stanton, J. St. Geme, et al. (Eds.), *Nelson textbook of pediatrics* (20th ed., Chapter 27). St. Louis, MO: Elsevier.

Dittman, C. et al. (2011). An epidemiological examination of parenting and family correlates of emotional problems in young children. *American Journal of Orthopsychiatry, 81*(3), 360-371.

Dubowitz, H., & Lane, W. (2016). Medical child abuse (factitious disorder, Munchhausen syndrome). In R. Kliegman, B. Stanton, J. St. Geme, et al. (Eds.), *Nelson textbook of pediatrics* (20th ed., Chapter 40.2). St. Louis, MO: Elsevier.

Friedman, M. (2016). *PTSD history and overview.* Retrieved from http://www.ptsd.va.gov.

Gahagan, S. (2016). Overweight and obesity. In R. Kliegman, B. Stanton, J. St. Geme, et al. (Eds.), *Nelson textbook of pediatrics* (20th ed., Chapter 37). St. Louis, MO: Elsevier.

Institute of Medicine. (2009). *Preventing mental, emotional, and behavioral disorders among young people: Progress and possibilities.* Retrieved from http://www.iom.edu/Reports/2009/Preventing-Mental-Emotional-and-Behavioral-Disorders-Among-Young-People-Progress-and-Possibilities: *Basic biology to clinical manifestations.* Retrieved from https://www.ncbi.nlm.nih.gov/books/NBK333433.

Kaplan, B., Saddock, V., & Ruiz, P. (2014). *Kaplan and Saddock's synopsis of psychiatry: Behavioral sciences/clinical psychiatry.* Baltimore, MD: Lippincott, Williams & Wilson.

Kreipe, R. (2016). Eating disorders. In R. Kliegman, B. Stanton, J. St. Geme, et al. (Eds.), *Nelson textbook of pediatrics* (20th ed., Chapter 28). St. Louis, MO: Elsevier.

Laurent, K., Gilliam, K., Wright, D., & Fisher, P. (2015). Child anxiety symptoms related to longitudinal cortisol trajectories and acute stress response: Evidence of developmental stress sensitization. *Journal of Abnormal Psychology, 124*, 68-79.

March, J., & Vitiello, B. (2009). Clinical messages from the treatment for adolescents with depression study (TADS). *American Journal of Psychiatry, 166*(10), 1118-1123.

National Center for Health Statistics. (2016). *Health, United States, 2015.* U.S. Department of Health and Human Services. DHHS publication no. 2016-1232.

National Center for PTSD. (2015). *PTSD in children and teens.* Retrieved from www.ptsd.va.gov.

National Institute of Mental Health. (n.d.). *Bipolar disorder among children: overall prevalence.* Retrieved from www.nimh.nih.gov.

National Institute of Mental Health. (2016a). *Bipolar disorder.* Retrieved from www.nimh.nih.gov.

National Institute of Mental Health. (2016b). *Eating disorders.* Retrieved from www.nimh.nih.gov.

Orifici, G., Cardona, F., Cox, C., & Cunningham, M. (2016). *Pediatric autoimmune neuropsychiatric disorders associated with streptococcal infections (PANDAS).* Retrieved from www.ncbi.nlm.nih.gov/books/NBK333433.

Queen, A. (2010). *Screening for adolescent panic disorder in pediatrics settings (Master's thesis).* Retrieved from http://scholarlyrepository.miami.edu/oa_theses/68.

Regier, D.A., Kuhl, E.A., & Kupfer, D.J. (2013). The DSM-5: Classification and criteria changes. *World Psychiatry, 12*: 92-98. Doi:10.1002/wps.20050.

Renk, K. et al. (2014). Bipolar disorder in children. *Psychiatry Journal, 2014*, 1-19.

Reynolds, C.R., Kmphaus, R.W. (2015). *Behavior Assessment System for Children.* (3rd ed.) Pearson Education Inc. http://www.pearsonclinical.com

Rosenberg, D., & Chiriboga, J. (2016). Anxiety disorders. In R. Kliegman, B. Stanton, J. St. Geme, et al. (Eds.), *Nelson textbook of pediatrics* (20th ed., Chapter 25). St. Louis, MO: Elsevier.

Schneeweiss, S., Patrick, A.R., Solomon, D.H., et al. (2010). Comparative safety of antidepressant agents for children and adolescents regarding suicidal acts. *Pediatrics, 125*, 876–888.

Shapiro, S., Pinto, M., Evans, D. (2016). Suicidality risk assessment in adolescents and young adults. *Advanced Emergency Nursing Journal, 38*(1), 4-9.

Sheftall, A., et al. (2016). Suicide in elementary school-aged children and early adolescents. *Pediatrics, 138*(4), e20160436.

Spence, S. & Rapee, R. (2016). The etiology of social anxiety disorder: An evidence-based model. *Behaviour Research and Therapy, 86*, 50-67.

Substance Abuse and Mental Health Services Administration. (2013). *Results from the 2012 National Survey on Drug Use and Health. Summary of National Findings.* Rockville, MD: Substance Abuse and Mental Health Services Administration.

Urion, D. (2016). Attention deficit/hyperactivity disorder. In R. Kliegman, B. Stanton, J. St. Geme, et al. (Eds.), *Nelson textbook of pediatrics* (20th ed., Chapter 33). St. Louis, MO: Elsevier.

U.S. Department of Health and Human Services. (2010). *Healthy people 2020: mental health and mental disorders.* Retrieved from http://www.healthypeople.gov.

U.S. Department of Health and Human Services. (2015). *Table C3a: Age-adjusted percentages (with standard errors) of ever having been told of having a learning disability or attention deficit hyperactivity disorder for children aged 3-17 years, by selected characteristics, 2015. National Health Interview Survey, 2015.* Retrieved from https://ftp.cdc.gov.

U.S. Department of Health and Human Services, Administration for Children and Families, Administration on Children Youth and Families, & Children's Bureau. (2014). *Child maltreatment* 2014. Retrieved from http://www.acf.hhs.gov.

U.S. Department of Health and Human Services Child Welfare Information Gateway. (2013). *What is child abuse and neglect? Recognizing the signs and symptoms.* Retrieved from http://www.childwelfare.gov

U.S. Department of Justice. (2015). *Attorney General Eric Holder delivers remarks at the 2014 Police Executve Research Forum.* Retrieved from http://www.justice.gov/iso/opa/ag/speeches/2014/ag-speech-140416.hml.

U.S. Department of Veterans' Affairs. (2015). *Child sexual abuse.* Retrieved from http://www.ptsd.va.gov.

Walter, H., & DeMaso, D. (2016). Assessment and interviewing. In R. Kliegman, B. Stanton, J. St. Geme, et al. (Eds.), *Nelson textbook of pediatrics* (20th ed., Chapter 20). St. Louis, MO: Elsevier.

Walter, H., Bogdanovic, N., Moseley, L., et al. (2016). Mood disorders. In R. Kliegman, B. Stanton, J. St. Geme, et al. (Eds.), *Nelson textbook of pediatrics* (20th ed., Chapter 26). St. Louis, MO: Elsevier.

Williams, J.F., & Smith, V.C. Committee on Substance Abuse.. (2015). Fetal Alcohol Spectrum Disorders. *Pediatrics.136*(5), American Academy of Pediatrics. Clinical Report doi: 10.1542/pes.2015-3133.

World Health Organization. (2011). *Mental health: a state of well-being. Geneva Switzerland.* Retrieved from http://www.who.int/features/factfiles/mental_health/en/index.html.

# 54

# The Child With an Intellectual Disability or Developmental Disability

http://evolve.elsevier.com/McKinney/mat-ch/

## LEARNING OBJECTIVES

*After studying this chapter, you should be able to:*

- Define the concepts of maturational and developmental disorders, including intellectual disability, developmental disorders, and autism spectrum disorders.
- Develop an understanding of the use of the terms *intellectual disability* versus *mental retardation.*
- Identify the various causes of intellectual and developmental disabilities.
- Identify educational and support resources for families with a child who has an intellectual disability or developmental delay.
- Develop appropriate nursing strategies for supporting the family and child with an intellectual disability or developmental delay.
- Develop nursing strategies for families caring for a child with Down syndrome.
- Identify behavioral characteristics and appropriate nursing actions when working with a child with fragile X syndrome.
- Identify characteristics and appropriate nursing interventions for an infant with fetal alcohol syndrome, and provide appropriate family assessment and intervention.
- Identify the basic diagnostic criteria for the autism spectrum disorders.
- Identify genetic aspects of intellectual and developmental disorders.
- Identify the major considerations in working with the family of a child with an intellectual or developmental disorder or disability.
- Develop home care interventions appropriate to the family's abilities and to the developmental needs of a child with an intellectual or developmental disorder or disability.

## CLINICAL REFERENCE

### GENETICS AND GENOMICS

The sequencing of the human genome opened a new window in our understanding of human traits, skills, and disabilities. Genetic breakthroughs will require nurses to be active participants in using genetic information in all aspects of providing patient care (American Association of Colleges of Nursing, 2008). Some nursing activities will include the assessment of genotypes, obtaining family history via a three-generation genogram, identification of signs of developmental or intellectual disorders, assisting patients and families to access appropriate resources, referral for care, and education of patients and families with the goal of maximizing individual development within a cultural context (Calzone, Jenkins, Prows, & Masny, 2011)). A number of resources are available for nurses to gain essential knowledge and skill in the area of genetics and genomics (see Chapter 10).

The human genome is the full set of DNA instructions that creates the characteristics of a human. However, the human genome has innumerable small variations called *genotypes.* Genotypes are small variations in specific parts of the genome's DNA sequences. These small changes account for the phenotype—the visible differences in eye color, skin color, height, and every other observable physical characteristic. The term genotype can be used to describe large groups of people who share common physical characteristics, or phenotypes. The phenotype is the visible representation of the genotype.

Changes *(mutations)* in a specific stretch of DNA occur through deletion, addition, or recopying. Some of these mutations do not result in any change in the individual's appearance or functioning. However, some small mutations create enormous negative effects in cell and individual development. These small mutations are the underlying cause of the intellectual (ID) and developmental disabilities (DD) that will be discussed in this chapter. Some of these genetic changes affect intellectual ability; some affect physical development or maturation.

## Common Diagnostic Tests for Intellectual and Developmental Disorders

| Test | Description | Normal Findings | Indications | Nursing Implications |
|---|---|---|---|---|
| Vision test | Assessment of vision, ocular pressure, and structural defects | Normal vision, normal structures | Children with Down syndrome; 40%-45% have refractive errors, cataracts, or other visual problems. | Explain pupil dilation. Provide protective eyewear after examinations. |
| Hearing test | Assessment of perception of sound frequency and volume | Normal hearing range | Children with Down syndrome; 70%-80% have hearing defects.<br>Children with autism and PDD often appear to have defective hearing despite normal hearing function, so hearing tests should be conducted. | Explain the test in simple terms.<br>The test may require that the child wear a headphone, which may be difficult to tolerate. |
| Thyroid studies | Blood serum tests to determine thyroid levels, serum thyroxine | Ages 1-3 yr: 6.8-13.5 μg/dL<br>Ages 3-10 yr: 5.5-12.8 μg/dL<br>Puberty to adulthood: 4.2-13.0 μg/dL | Children with Down syndrome; slowed growth rates are common. | These studies should not be performed within 7 days of a radionuclide scan. |
| Adaptive behavior scales* | Assessment of language, motor, social, and self-care skills | Age-expected skills within 1 SD from mean | Children with suspected developmental delays | Explain the test and how results will be interpreted. |
| IQ tests† | Assessment of intellectual abilities | Age-normal skills within 1½ SD from the mean | Children with suspected developmental delays | Explain the test and how results will be interpreted. |
| Bone roentgenography | Assessment of bone plates and joint spaces | Age-expected bone age | Children with Down syndrome; decreased growth rate is common. Children with Down syndrome have atlantoaxial instability. | The child must be motionless during the study; cervical spine radiographs should be done for all children with Down syndrome at a young age and before they participate in athletics. |
| Brain sonography | Ultrasonogram of cranium | Normal position of brain's midline structures and normal blood flow velocity, no hemorrhages | Microcephaly or macrocephaly, misshapen cranium, family history of hydrocephaly | The child must be supine.<br>Any jewelry or metal objects should be removed from the child's head.<br>The child may need sedation or restraint because this procedure takes 1 hr to complete.<br>Explain to the child that the test is not painful.<br>Keep the child warm during the procedure. |
| Genetic analysis | Cytogenic bonding, culture media analysis | Normal findings for gene product analysis | Suspected genetic or neoplastic disorders | Allow the child and family an opportunity to ask questions and express concerns about the possible results and implications of the testing. |
| Computed tomography | Special noninvasive radiographic technique that images brain tissue in very thin sections | No blood clots, tumors, or infections | Impaired development, such as microcephaly; family history of CNS malformations; possible tumors or subdural hematomas | The child may need to be sedated or restrained and must be supine. Scans require the use of contrast medium, requiring informed consent. |
| Magnetic resonance imaging | Noninvasive method used to create images corresponding to density of tissue | Normal anatomy and physiology of the brain and spinal column | Same as for computed tomography | The test requires informed consent.<br>Remove metal or magnetic objects from the child before the study.<br>Sedation of the child is usually required. |

**Common Diagnostic Tests for Intellectual and Developmental Disorders—cont'd**

| Test | Description | Normal Findings | Indications | Nursing Implications |
|---|---|---|---|---|
| Positron emission tomography | Noninvasive means of comparing cerebral brain flow and metabolic changes; used to localize seizure foci, visualize brain hemodynamics, and study brain pharmacology using radioisotopes | Normal metabolism of glucose in brain, normal blood flow and electrical activity | Seizures, hydrocephaly, evidence of cerebral dysfunction | The test requires informed consent. The child will need to be sedated. Liquids may be limited before the procedure. If not in diapers, the child will need to void before the procedure. Parents may be able to remain with the child during the procedure. |

*CNS*, Central nervous system; *IQ*, intelligence quotient; *PDD*, pervasive developmental disorders; *SD*, standard deviation.
*Adaptive behavior scales include the American Association on Mental Retardation (AAMR) test, the Minnesota Child Development Inventory Profile, the Denver Developmental Screening Test-II (DDST-II), the Wechsler Preschool and Primary Scale of Intelligence (WPPSI), the Wechsler Intelligence Scale for Children (WISC-III), and the Wechsler Adult Intelligence Scale—Revised (WAIS-R).
†IQ tests include the Bayley Scales (birth to 3 yr), the Stanford–Binet Scale (2 yr and older), the WPPSI (3-6 yr), the WISC-III (6-16 yr), and the WAIS-R (16 yr and older).

## INTELLECTUAL AND DEVELOPMENTAL DISORDERS

The prevalence of IDs and DDs continues to rise. Children living in poverty experience the highest rates of disability (102.6 cases/1000 population), but the largest increase in incidence is seen in households with incomes greater than 400% of the poverty level, an affluent population (Houtrow et al 2013). Children who have intellectual or developmental disorders experience genetic or external influences that may limit their potential abilities. However, these potential limits will be minimized or maximized by their interaction with the environment. Many intellectual or developmental disorders will respond to early and intensive intervention and close attention. However, children and families face lifelong challenges that require assistance from both healthcare and educational professionals to maximize the child's developmental potential. The family of a child with an intellectual or developmental impairment copes with frequent and exceptionally high demands, often including chronic medical and educational challenges that require lifelong management. Independence and self-management should be emphasized throughout childhood and adolescence so that, as the individual reaches adulthood, the possibility of independent living and gainful employment can be maximized.

### Developmental Disability and the Americans With Disabilities Act: the Impact of Public Policy

Historically, the intellectual, sensory and developmental disorders were considered to be distinct, although overlapping syndromes. In recent years, the term *developmental disability* has become an umbrella term to encompass children with intellectual disabilities, sensory deficits (hearing, vision, and speech), orthopedic problems, and conditions such as cerebral palsy and autism spectrum disorders. Uniting these disorders under the term *developmental disability* has important legal and policy implications because it unites a number of people who have similar psychosocial and developmental disorders and similar needs for services. From a health policy perspective, united groups are more powerful in gaining legislative and policy recognition. This effort was successful in the passage and enactment of the Developmental Disabilities Assistance and Bill of Rights Act of 2000 (PL 106-402) (2000). The purpose of this act is to attempt to ensure equal rights and accessibilities for all disabled individuals.

In this bill, the United States Congress defined a developmental disability as having the following components (Developmental Disabilities Assistance and Bill of Rights Act of 2000):

- The disability is severe and chronic and is attributable to mental or physical impairment or a combination of both.
- The impairment must be present before the individual turns 22 years old.
- The impairment is likely to continue, reflecting the need for lifelong individual services or support.
- There must be substantial functional limitations in three or more areas, such as self-care, receptive and expressive language, learning, mobility, self-direction, capacity for independent living, or economic self-sufficiency.

As a result of this bill and earlier legislative efforts such as the Individuals with Disabilities Education Act (IDEA) of 1997, every disabled child must have a written individualized education plan (IEP) that outlines specialized instruction and services the public school system will provide. The child's parents and school personnel design the plan following an educational assessment. School nurses often participate in IEP evaluations, providing expert advice about classroom adaptations or medical services needed for these children. When working with these children, teachers, families, and communities, the nurse may serve as a resource for identifying advocacy services.

Nursing goals when caring for children with an intellectual or developmental disorder or disability include accurate assessment of the specific cause and nature of the disorder or disability and the identification of possible co-morbidities and risk factors. Complete information enables the nurse to plan interventions that will maximize the child's development and adaptive functioning. Nursing care in this specialty area always includes assessment, referral, education and follow-up, and advocacy for the child and family members.

Intellectual and developmental disorders are frequently co-morbid (occurring together). These children are also at risk for psychosocial disorders. For example, a child who is diagnosed with Asperger syndrome is at risk for symptoms of depression. In the same manner, children who are diagnosed with autism frequently also show symptoms of intellectual disability.

The nurse is an integral part of the multidisciplinary team that manages the care of a child with a developmental disorder. The nurse is involved in early assessment of the child, support of the family, assistance with self-care training and behavioral training, referral to support services, and providing the necessary nursing care for other disabilities the child may have. School and community nurses need a broad range of knowledge to support children who have multiple intellectual and physical disabilities.

The first section of this chapter reviews **intellectual disability disorders** (ID), also known as **intellectual development disorders**. These were formerly referred to as disorders associated with mental retardation. The considerations in the care of a child with Down syndrome will illustrate nursing care for children with intellectual disabilities. The second section of the chapter gives an overview of developmental disorders that have clear genetic causes (fragile X syndrome, Rett syndrome). The third section looks at developmental disorders where the cause is related to environmental or prenatal toxins (fetal alcohol syndrome). The last section examines the autism spectrum disorders. The nursing care for a child with autism will demonstrate considerations in planning care that promotes maximal development for all children with developmental disorders and their capability to move through the expected stages of childhood development.

## Terminology

### Mental Age, Functional Age, Adaptive Functioning

Children with developmental disabilities can have impairments in motor skills or sensory ability that are minor and manageable or involve significant impairment in intellectual, functional, and adaptive development. *Mental age* and *functional age* are terms used to compare a child's current ability with children of the same chronologic age. These terms are generally more useful than references to the intelligence quotient (IQ), which can be misleading, especially for children with language disabilities. Mental age gives the caregiver information regarding level of intellectual understanding. For example, if an individual has a mental age of 5 years, the nurse's explanations should be simple and specific, regardless of chronologic age. However, if the individual has a mental age of 12 years, the nurse's explanations can be complex and use some abstractions. Functional age refers to the level of *adaptive function,* the level of coping that a child has developed that supports activities of daily living (ADLs), communication skills, and social skills (American Association on Intellectual and Developmental Disabilities [AAIDD], 2011). Maximizing the child's adaptive function by supporting identified strengths and supplementing weak areas will allow the child to develop realistically to full potential (AAIDD, 2011). It is possible for a child with a low mental age to function well beyond what would be expected. This is an example of a high level of adaptive functioning.

### Intellectual Impairment and Intellectual Disability

*Intellectual impairment* is a descriptive term that denotes a significant limitation in both intellectual and functional capacity. This term indicates that the impairment manifests in measured intelligence (i.e., IQ) and also in adaptive behavior. Intellectual impairment distinguishes intellectual or cognitive deficits from specific, limited sensory deficits (e.g., vision, hearing). It also differentiates emotional or psychological disability. Specific intellectual impairments are considered through assessment of language, cognition, academic ability, self-help skills, social behaviors, and motor performance.

The term is used to describe conditions that originate before the age of 18, with significant evidence of below-average intellectual functioning and adaptive functioning in areas such as communication, ability to work, home living, community use, health and safety, leisure, self-care, social skills, self-direction, functional academics, or work abilities (AAIDD, 2011). The level of intellectual disability may be mild, moderate, severe, or profound. Intellectual impairment can result from genetic mutations that cause malformations of the brain and central nervous system (CNS), or it may result from injury, infection, anoxia, poisoning, prenatal alcohol use, brain trauma, accidents, Down syndrome, or other inherited disorders. In some cases, the cause is unknown.

Children with intellectual disabilities require support and interventions to acquire self-care and adaptive skills; however, many children are educated, hold a job, and independently accomplish some self-care activities (Bitsko et al., 2016).

### Intellectual Development Disorder versus Mental Retardation

Intellectual disability has replaced the term *mental retardation* (MR) to describe people with below-average general intellectual functioning. Over time "mental retardation" has generally been removed as a clinical classification, and the term was formally removed from IDEA in 2010 (National Dissemination Center for Children with Disabilities, 2011). This decision is significant, and a number of rationales were cited for the change, including the scientific inaccuracy of the term *retardation* and the stigma associated with the term (AAIDD, 2011). As a result of this change in clinical classification, the American Association on Mental Retardation (AAMR) voted to change the name of its organization (and its publications) to the American Association of Intellectual and Developmental Disabilities (AAIDD, 2011).

### Autism Spectrum Disorders versus Pervasive Developmental Disorders

Pervasive developmental disorders (PDDs) vary widely in etiology and level or type of impairment. They are termed *spectrum disorders* because the impairment can range from mild to severe.

Some of the PDDs are clear genetic disorders, such as Rett syndrome, fragile X syndrome, and Down syndrome. These disorders are characterized by recognizable physical characteristics and usually by impairment in physical development and cognition, as well as by significant intellectual impairment.

The PDD classification also includes the autism spectrum disorders (ASDs), where genetic influence is likely but less definitive. The ASDs include attention-deficit disorder (ADD), attention-deficit/hyperactivity disorder (ADHD), Asperger syndrome, and autism. A third group within the PDD classification represents disorders that result from toxins or prenatal influences, such as fetal alcohol syndrome. Although these disorders have different features, they are linked as Autism Spectrum Disorders in the *Diagnostic and Statistical Manual of Mental Disorders* (DSM-V) (American Psychiatric Association [APA], 2013).

The PDDs discussed in this chapter include Rett syndrome, fragile X syndrome, fetal alcohol syndrome, failure to thrive, and the ASDs of Asperger syndrome and autism. ADD and ADHD are discussed in Chapter 53.

## Etiology of Intellectual Disabilities and Pervasive Developmental Disorders

These disorders can be the result of genetic mutations, prenatal environment, or congenital or early environmental factors such as maternal substance abuse or lack of stimulation in early childhood. They can also be the result of head injury, asphyxia, intracranial hemorrhage, infections, poisoning, or the presence or treatment of a brain tumor. Developmental disorders have more than 350 known causes, but a specific cause is unknown in nearly half of all diagnosed cases. New etiologies are being identified, and underlying mechanisms of known causes are becoming more clearly understood. Often the cause is a subtle but nonetheless significant biologic factor such as exposure to infection or viruses, chromosomal abnormalities, lead exposure,

**BOX 54.1 Causes of Intellectual Disability**

**Mild Disability – Environmental**

***Alterations Occurring During Pregnancy***

- Intrauterine infections: Congenital rubella, toxoplasmosis, herpes, HIV
- Exposure to environmental toxins: Fetal alcohol spectrum disorder, drug exposure
- Intrauterine growth restriction

**Neonatal Alterations**

- Prematurity/very low birthweight
- Perinatal insult or injury
- Other conditions present at birth: Hyperbilirubinemia, hypoglycemia, central nervous system (CNS) hemorrhage, ABO incompatibilities

**Severe Disability - Biologic**

***Genetic***

- Inborn errors of metabolism (e.g., Galactosemia, Tay–Sachs disease, phenylketonuria)
- Hereditary syndromes (e.g., Muscular dystrophy, tuberous sclerosis, neurofibromatosis)
- Chromosomal alterations (e.g., Down syndrome, fragile X syndrome [leading cause of intellectual impairment])

**Acquired Childhood Conditions or Diseases**

- Meningitis, encephalitis, pertussis, varicella or other complications from infection
- Lead or other poisoning
- Neurologic insult (e.g., trauma hydrocephalus, tumors)
- Conditions impairing cardiac or respiratory function (e.g., cardiorespiratory arrest, asphyxiation)

**Psychosocial Problems**

- Psychosocial deprivation
- Poverty and inadequate healthcare
- Parental neurosis, psychosis, character disorder
- Childhood psychosis, autism, other pervasive developmental disorders

**Unknown Causes**

Data from: American Psychiatric Association. (2000). *Diagnostic and statistical manual of mental disorders* (4th ed., Text revision). Washington, DC: Author; Shapiro, B., & Batshaw, M. (2016). Intellectual disability. In R. Kliegman, B. Stanton, J. St. Geme, et al. (Eds.), *Nelson textbook of pediatrics* (20th ed., Chapter 36). St. Louis MO: Elsevier.

**EVIDENCE-BASED PRACTICE**

Caring for children with a learning disability (LD) can be a challenge in the hospital environment. These children often have a wide range of intellectual functioning, as well as co-morbid physical, communication, sensory, or complex medical issues. Given the fast-paced nature of the inpatient environment, subtle changes in the child's condition might be overlooked, resulting in adverse complications associated with the medical diagnosis.

Wishing to begin to develop a model of care for children with LD in the hospital setting, Oulton, Sell, Kerry, and Gibson (2015) conducted an ethnographic qualitative research study with 27 healthcare personnel, including 10 nurses. Their goal was to describe how nurses can provide individualized care to children, incorporating the "little things" of importance that facilitate a safe and comfortable environment for children and families. Over a 12-month period of time, researchers used observation, structured and informal conversation, discussion with children and families, and evaluation of documentation to identify specific needs of hospitalized children with LD. Conversations lasted 30 to 70 minutes apiece and were audio-recorded, transcribed verbatim, and analyzed.

Oulton et al. (2015) identified six important themes that could provide a basis for optimal care. These included:

- Acquiring the knowledge and experience to care for children with special needs through formal and informal training
- Identifying the population with detailed individualized communication and documentation
- Focusing on the "little things" – non-medical comfort measures, such as maintaining routines, considering preferences, and appropriately communicating information specific to each child
- Creating a safe environment, including providing adequate supervision and incorporation of play according to the child's interests and abilities
- Using appropriate resources and non-medical adaptive equipment designed for the child's specific disability
- Developing a partnership with parents that focuses not just on obtaining information, but also on negotiating the conditions of the caregiving role while the child is hospitalized

If a parent were to tell you that her child was particularly sensitive to noises, think about how you could address this in an individualized care plan. What approaches would you suggest and how would you go about ensuring that this child's comfort needs are met.

Reference: Oulton, K., Sell, D., Kerry, S., & Gibson, F. (2015). Individualizing hospital care for children and young people with learning disabilities. *Journal of Pediatric Nursing, 30*(1), 78-86.

nutritional deficiencies, or exposure to numerous prenatal infections or trauma. Evidence suggests that early intervention programs that promote neurodevelopment can show benefit for later neurologic integrity and intellectual ability. Low socioeconomic status and related factors have also been consistently reported as influencing intellectual function (Box 54.1).

## Incidence of Intellectual and Developmental Disorders

The prevalence of childhood disorders has grown at a surprising rate, increasing by 15.6% between 2001 and 2011 and now affecting approximately 6 million U.S. children (Houtrow et al., 2013). Families with children or adolescents who are mildly or moderately impaired are likely to care for children at home. An increased incidence of intellectual disability is reported in the early school years; the incidence then declines in late adolescence as the children leave the formal education setting and are assimilated into the adult world. Most intellectually-impaired individuals are able to marry (often to individuals with normal intellectual functioning), maintain employment, and have satisfying relationships.

Psychiatric co-morbidity is common in people with both intellectual and developmental disorders, probably because underlying conditions that cause intellectual disabilities also affect areas of the brain that regulate emotional state. The most frequent accompanying diagnoses include disruptive behavioral disorders, depression, and atypical psychosis. Prevalence estimates for co-morbidity between psychosocial disorders and developmental disorders are as high as 60% to 70%, but the incidence is lower in children and adolescents compared to adults with developmental disorders (Sadock, Sadock, & Ruiz, 2015).

Developmental disorders increase the risk for child abuse (Centers for Disease Control and Prevention [CDC], 2016). Possible reasons for this strong relationship are the intense stress experienced by families of disabled children, parent isolation, and unrealistic expectations for

**BOX 54.2 Problems Related to Intellectual Disability**

**Mild**
- Self-esteem issues related to the presence or absence of physical features, largely determined by the cause of the intellectual disability
- Social isolation and loneliness
- Depression

**Severe**
- Self-injury
- Fecal smearing
- Tearing of personal clothes and objects
- Severe temper tantrums
- Disrobing

the child's performance because of a lack of knowledge about normal growth and development. Despite available funding and community support groups, families of children with developmental delays often feel isolated from supportive services and report that professionals have limited understanding of their children's needs. These factors further perpetuate the sense of helplessness and lack of control in these family systems, leading to a climate with a heightened potential for abusive behaviors.

## Manifestations

The cardinal sign of developmental disorders is delayed achievement of developmental milestones. Specific congenital malformations often result in specific clinical manifestations. Also, the severity of the impairment affects the types and frequency of problem behaviors (Box 54.2).

In addition to general clinical manifestations based on the degree of impairment, many syndromes are characterized by features that are helpful in determining the cause of the disability. Two genetic disorders in which intellectual disability is a central feature are Down syndrome and fragile X syndrome. An infant born with fetal alcohol syndrome (FAS) will show both intellectual and developmental disorders in addition to specific physical growth, facial, skeletal, and cardiac features.

Many disorders associated with intellectual disability can further limit a child's adaptive skills. Such disorders include cerebral palsy, visual deficits, seizure disorders, communication deficits, feeding problems, ASDs, failure to thrive, and ADHD. Speech and language development are often profoundly affected. Depending on the condition, seizure disorders frequently develop as the child matures.

Although children who are intellectually impaired can be generally physically healthy, the presence of associated disabilities may place these children at increased risk for illness (Fig. 54.1). For example, if a child who is intellectually impaired also has cerebral palsy, the risk for gastroesophageal reflux and aspiration pneumonia is high. Motor or swallowing problems may result in inadequate oral intake or insufficient weight gain.

## Diagnostic Evaluation

Diagnostic evaluations may be performed during pregnancy, during the neonatal period (based on risk factors), or after the child fails to achieve expected developmental milestones. Early identification is important so that early intervention treatment plans can be established. Tests may be general or specific for the neurologic or intellectual area in question. Several tests assess the child's current level of functioning and help the clinician anticipate persistent intellectual disabilities. These tests—which may involve pencil-and-paper tasks, motor tasks, sensory tasks, or some degree of intellectual processing—help determine both the severity and type of intellectual disability (Box 54.3). Learning disabilities are often identified using some of these same instruments, and many are available through the school system. Nurses also can learn to administer developmental screening tools. The American Academy of Pediatrics (AAP) recommends developmental surveillance at each well visit during infancy and early childhood and formal developmental screening for all children at ages 9 months, 18 months, and 30 months (American Academy of Pediatrics, 2016) (see Chapter 5). Often, the diagnosis of a developmental disorder is not made until the child begins school and has significant academic failure, prompting formal psychological and neurologic testing. However, routine assessment of development during pediatric visits is the best method of early detection.

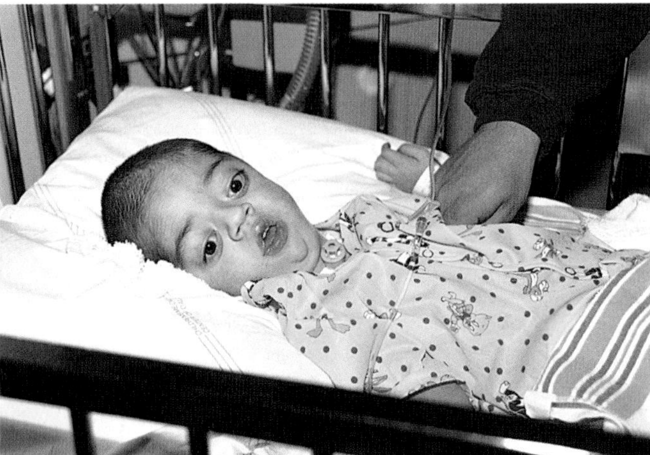

**FIG 54.1** Children with intellectual impairments may have other dysfunctions as well. The family of a child with an intellectual impairment often feels continual grief because the child does not meet their expectations. This child has additional dysfunctions that require respiratory and nutritional support. (Courtesy Children's Medical Center, Dallas, TX.)

## Management

Both general strategies and strategies designed to keep children safe provide the basis for managing children with intellectual or developmental disorders or disabilities.

### General Strategies

Therapeutic management depends largely on community and educational resources. However, obtaining services for these children requires multidisciplinary efforts and strong advocacy on the part of both parents and professionals. Reduction in the occurrence of developmental disorders is a national priority identified in *Healthy People 2020* (USDHHS, 2010). Adequate prenatal care is of primary importance. An additional priority related to children with disabilities is increasing the percentage of time these children spend in regular school programs (USDHHS, 2010).

For children with associated medical co-morbidities, medical strategies are directed toward preventing and treating infections, correcting structural deformities, and treating associated behaviors, such as aggressiveness. Corrective measures might include congenital heart surgery for malformations, inserting tympanostomy tubes, or placing splints on joints that are hypotonic and hyperextended. The treatment of behavioral difficulties and psychosocial disturbances may involve administration of medications.

**BOX 54.3 Expected Skills According to Adaptive Behavior and Required Supports**

**Mild Intellectual Disability – Minimal Support (IQ 50-~70)**

Slight delay in achieving developmental milestones but can communicate well and demonstrate some social skills

May require special education services with an emphasis on vocational and self-maintenance skills

Able to form and maintain adult relationships and can generally care for themselves

**Moderate Intellectual Disability – Limited to Moderate Support (IQ 36-49)**

Noticeable delay in motor and speech development by preschool age

Can communicate, although have less than adequate social skills

Usually can achieve cognitively at an elementary school level

Can live best as an adult in a supportive and supervised setting, such as a group home

Can perform unskilled work in a supervised setting, such as a sheltered workshop

**Severe Intellectual Disability – Daily Extensive Support (IQ 20To 35)**

Early and marked delay in all motor skills

Limited expressive speech and self-help skills

Constant supervision required, with group home living possible as an adult

**Profound Intellectual Disability – 24 Hour Support (IQ <20 to 25)**

May be able to walk

May have primitive speech

Often have physical limitations

Usually requires complete provision of activities of daily living

Modified from American Psychiatric Association. (2013). *Diagnostic and statistical manual of mental disorders* (5th ed.). Washington, DC: Author; Boat, T, & Wu, J. (Eds.) (2015). Clinical characteristics of intellectual disabilities. In *Mental disorders and disabilities among low income children* (Chapter 9). Washington, DC: National Academies Press.

### Safety Challenges

Children who are intellectually impaired are less capable of managing environmental challenges than are their peers who are unimpaired. Because of impaired executive and motor functioning, injuries are generally more common than in same-age children. However, among preschool-age children, injuries are less common in those with intellectual disability, perhaps due to parental oversight and less exposure to risk. Table 54.1 presents some safety issues to be taught in the home and in the community. Although the learning needs of children who are intellectually impaired are similar to those of children without disabilities, children with intellectual disabilities may need prolonged teaching, more demonstration during teaching, frequent verbal and visual reminders, and more practice. Resources for schools and teachers have been essential in helping children with intellectual or developmental disabilities integrate into classrooms (United States Department of Education, 2016).

**SAFETY ALERT**

***The Child With a Developmental Disorder***

Safety is a persistent concern of parents, teachers, and health professionals, because the child's maturation in anticipating danger, problem solving, and judgment is delayed and remains generally impaired across the life span. Children with motor disabilities are often unable to perform skills in ways that foster safety.

## DISORDERS RESULTING IN INTELLECTUAL OR DEVELOPMENTAL DISABILITY

Disorders that result in intellectual disability, developmental disability, or both can be classified and discussed according to any of a number of schemes. To facilitate understanding of their common features and specific differences, disorders are discussed in the following order:

- Disorder of intellectual impairment: Down syndrome
- Disorders of known genetic cause: Fragile X syndrome and Rett syndrome

**TABLE 54.1 Safety Concerns for Developmentally Delayed or Impaired Children**

| Site of Concern | Possible Injury | Education and Training Issues |
|---|---|---|
| **Home** | | |
| Kitchen | Burns<br>Poisoning | *Preschool age:* preventive education (i.e., instruct not to touch hot stove, not to ingest toxic substances)<br>*Elementary school age:* safe use of equipment, basic safety<br>*High school age:* cooking safety, emergency precautions |
| Bathroom | Falls<br>Burns<br>Cuts | *Elementary school age:* tub safety, precautions on wet floors<br>*High school age:* safe use of hair care equipment, shaving utensils, and similar objects |
| General | | Preschool and elementary school age: avoidance of electrical outlets, safe passage around objects |
| **Outdoors** | | |
| Yard or playground | Animal bites<br>Poisoning<br>Abduction | *Preschool age:* staying within boundaries, appropriate response to strange animals and people, safe use of equipment, avoidance of ingestion of berries<br>*Elementary school age:* stranger safety, bicycle safety, traffic safety, water safety |
| Vehicles | Cuts<br>Falls<br>Serious injury | *Preschool and elementary school age:* seatbelt use, keeping hands in car<br>*High school age:* traffic safety |

- Disorders related to environmental alterations: Fetal alcohol syndrome, nonorganic failure to thrive
- Disorders with little understood genetic influence: Autism spectrum disorders

## DOWN SYNDROME

Down syndrome (DS), also known as Trisomy 21, is caused by the presence of all or part of a third copy of chromosome 21. This disorder is the most common of the chromosomal disorders, and the most frequent cause of moderate to severe intellectual impairment (CDC, 2014). The assessment and nursing interventions for a child who is intellectually impaired are applicable to children with DS; however, additional issues need consideration.

Depending on the severity of the symptoms, most parents raise the child at home until early adulthood, after which group home placement is an option. Supported employment is encouraged, and parents are typically advised to initiate vocational training in elementary school. The partnership of parents and professionals is vital to managing the symptoms and providing the comprehensive services that are

### NURSING CARE PLAN

### *The Child With a Developmental Disorder or Disability in the Community Setting*

#### Focused Assessment: The Child

- Assess intellectual skills and level of adaptive functioning, especially social interaction, competence in independent activities of daily living (ADLs), and communication.
- Alternate between questions and demonstrations when conducting the assessment.
- Look directly at the child and speak in a direct and simple yet noncondescending manner in vocabulary appropriate for the child's developmental level, not the child's age.
- Ask the child for as much of the necessary information as possible, rather than relying solely on the parents to provide the information.

#### Focused Assessment: The Family

- Assess the family's level of functioning, particularly interaction patterns, available coping skills and the family's awareness of and involvement in addressing the child's needs.
- Observe and elicit information about signs of grief or anxiety related to the child's condition or changes in the child's developmental status.
- Explore the family's social and financial resources in a manner that is informative but respectful of privacy.
- Assess the family's requirements for short- and long-term assistance in the child's comprehensive management.
- Assess the family's ability to identify and maximize the child's strengths.
- Identify the need for interdisciplinary services, including genetic counseling, respite care, in-home services, parent training, and support groups.

#### Nursing Diagnosis

Risk for Injury related to level of self-care skills and inability to anticipate danger.

#### Planning

*Expected Outcome*

The parent and child will describe and avoid unsafe situations that lead to self-injury or unintentional injury.

#### Interventions and *Rationales*

1. Provide anticipatory guidance relative to the child's specific developmental abilities.
   *Parents may not be able to anticipate the child's intellectual or functional level accurately, particularly if they are inexperienced or have limited intellectual skills themselves.*
2. Keep safety rails up on hospital beds and on the bed at home if the child is predisposed to falling or roaming at night. Provide child-size furniture, and select age- and skill-related play equipment.
   *These strategies help prevent accidental falls.*
3. Give simple explanations about unsafe areas in the environment. Use the child's intellectual level as a key to what the child can understand or the degree of unsupervised freedom that can be allowed safely.
   *Young or intellectually delayed individuals can understand concrete explanations.*

#### Evaluation

Can the parent or child describe unsafe situations?
Has the child remained safe and free from injury?

#### Nursing Diagnosis

Deficient Knowledge (family members) related to unfamiliarity with the cause and likely outcomes of the child's intellectual disabilities, available support systems, or information about sexuality, vocational options, leisure skills, and so on.

#### Planning

*Expected Outcomes*

1. The family will describe and plan for the child's special needs.
2. The family will access and use personal and community resources to increase the child's ability to develop personal skills for appropriate social, leisure, and vocational abilities.

#### Interventions and *Rationales*

1. Provide information that is simple, concrete, and solution focused.
   *Stress may impair the family's adaptive coping skills.*
2. Explain any medical terms without assuming that the family knows the terminology. Give explanations to both the child and the parents. Use demonstrations and therapeutic play. If the child is hospitalized, communicate information about the child's intellectual and functional level to other team members.
   *The child may have a limited capacity to understand words but may be able to understand a demonstration.*
3. Select skills that enhance self-care and socially-appropriate behaviors. As the child reaches puberty, provide simple information about sexuality and physical changes. Support training in leisure skills.
   *Education that is practical and functional for the child's mental and chronologic age fosters self-esteem, compliance, and cooperation.*
4. Identify for the parents local and national resources for care, education, and training of intellectually-impaired children.
   *Additional services will be needed as the child grows or needs more specialized training. Families may have to find out-of-home placement if the child's disability is severe or destructive to the family.*

## NURSING CARE PLAN—cont'd

### *The Child With a Developmental Disorder or Disability in the Community Setting*

5. Provide parents with anticipatory guidance about developmental milestones and anticipated skills, including safety, sexuality, skills that can be expected, and behavioral changes throughout the developmental process.
   *Parents may have unrealistic expectations or expect too little from the child.*

**Evaluation**

Has the family made progress in describing and planning for the child's special needs?

Has the family used the resources available in the community to maximize the child's abilities?

**Nursing Diagnosis**

Impaired Social Interaction (child) related to an inability to initiate and maintain social relationships.

**Planning**

***Expected Outcomes***

1. The child will develop positive relationships with family and peers.
2. The child will have solitary leisure skills.

**Interventions and *Rationales***

1. Encourage the parents to support the child in participating in group activities that promote peer interactions (e.g., Special Olympics, special camps) (Fig. 54.2). The family will arrange social activities with other children (e.g., visiting the park with friends, inviting friends to the home to play).
   *To adapt to social expectations and demands, children who are intellectually impaired or developmentally disabled need to be exposed to children who are not impaired and to children with similar challenges.*
2. Encourage the parents to participate on a regular basis in interactive activities such as reading books and playing.
   *Families are likely to limit interactions because the child offers reduced reinforcements in social situations.*

**Evaluation**

Has the child demonstrated a sense of pleasure in social interactions with family members and with other individuals within the child's social sphere?

**Nursing Diagnosis**

Compromised Family Coping or Disabled Family Coping related to excessive emotional and financial strain on family members caused by caring for a child who is intellectually impaired, lack of acceptance by society, or an extended grieving process associated with diagnosis of a child with a chronic disability.

**Planning**

***Expected Outcomes***

1. The family will integrate the child in the family system in a manner that facilitates maximum growth and maturity.
2. The family members will express self-satisfaction in their family management.
3. The family will demonstrate social acceptance within the community.

**Interventions and *Rationales***

1. Provide anticipatory and continuing support for the grieving process. Parents should be told the diagnosis and be given needed information as quickly as possible. This information should be given when parents and supportive family members are available. The nurse may need to explain information in different ways (orally, in writing, with videos) to help parents grasp the meaning of the diagnosis.
   *Families typically experience a cycle of grieving that is repeated when milestones are not reached or when the child has an illness or a change in behavior.*
2. Assist in identifying appropriate resources for social interactions and social training (e.g., early intervention programs, special education programs, recreational programs for developmentally disabled children).
   *Individuals who are mildly or moderately impaired often feel loneliness and depression as a result of insufficient stimulation and social contact. Such programs can assist these children in reaching their maximum potential.*
3. Identify and refer the family to appropriate community resources for both emotional support and family and child education. The nurse may need to act as an advocate and referral center (regarding support groups, education consultants, home health agencies).
   *The grieving process and the need to accommodate the child's skill level are continuous; families often feel isolated and helpless in locating necessary resources.*
4. Assist family members to identify realistic short- and long-term goals for the child and themselves. Encourage the family to express feelings and concerns; provide hope when appropriate.
   *Stress, grieving, and limited knowledge may impair the family's ability to set reasonable goals without assistance.*
5. Educate the parents in monitoring the child for alterations in health status. Help the family recognize nonverbal signs of discomfort.
   *The child may be unable to verbalize pain typically associated with ear infections, colds, or major illnesses.*
6. Assist family members in exploring their choices for home care, a group home, or a residential facility.
   *Families may hesitate to discuss care options out of fear of being perceived as uncaring or unable to provide home care.*

**Evaluation**

Does the family integrate the child into the family system in a manner that facilitates growth and maturity to the greatest degree possible?

Does the family seek medical attention when needed and use several resources to meet the child's social, emotional, educational, and medical needs?

Is the family able to meet financial responsibilities?

Does the family participate in social activities outside the family?

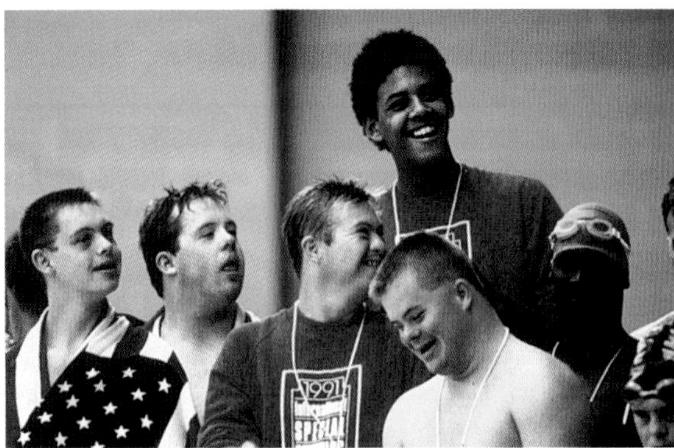

**FIG 54.2** Special Olympics International is the largest recreational program in the world for people with intellectual impairment. With more than 1 million athletes in 125 countries, Special Olympics offers opportunities for social interaction with peers and assists children who are intellectually disabled in reaching their maximum potential. (Courtesy Special Olympics, Inc.)

needed. In the past 10 years, advocacy groups have supported the integration and support for children and families with DS (National Down Syndrome Society [NDSS], 2012).

Services required throughout the life span include education and vocational training, transitional services, respite care, social services, financial supplements, psychotherapy, and preventive or corrective medical care (Box 54.4). This array of needed services may be overwhelming to the family, and the potential for frustration on the part of both the parents and the professional team is high. Communication and coordination of services are considered primary tasks for each team member (Fig. 54.3).

## Etiology

Several chromosomal alterations that result in DS have been identified. *Trisomy 21* accounts for approximately 95% of DS cases (NDSS, 2012). In trisomy 21, a gamete (e.g., an egg cell) is created that contains an additional copy (or part of a copy) of chromosome 21. This is termed *nondisjunction,* a failure of the chromosomes to separate normally during meiosis. This extra copy affects the physical and neurologic development of the baby. Most of the remaining 5% of DS cases result from either of the following, with mosaicism being the rarest:

- *Translocation,* in which an adult who appears normal carries a chromosome that is partially fused to another chromosome (generally chromosomes 21 and 14) (Lee, 2016). This type of transmission is not associated with maternal age or parental sex.
- *Mosaic DS (mosaicism),* a condition in which some of the cells in the body are normal but some have trisomy 21. Children who have mosaic DS may have fewer signs of the condition (Lee, 2016).

World Down Syndrome Day is observed annually on March 21. The date is chosen to reflect the origin of the syndrome, the result of three copies of the 21st chromosome, the unique genetic feature of people with DS (World Down Syndrome Day, 2016).

## Incidence

DS is the most common genetic cause of intellectual and developmental disability, occurring in 1 out of 691 births in the United States (NDSS, 2012). DS affects boys more often than girls and is highest in non-Hispanic white children (CDC, 2016b).

Maternal age has been consistently identified as one of the most significant risk factors associated with DS, although DS is not unusual in younger women. The risk of a 35-year-old woman bearing a child with DS is 1 in 353; by age 40 years, the risk increases to 1 in 85. The risk is higher also if parents already have one child with DS (March of Dimes, 2016). This statistic probably reflects the overall fertility of the age-group. Although maternal age is the greatest predictor of risk, some couples are at increased risk for producing multiple offspring with DS because of carrier genes.

### BOX 54.4 Medical Conditions Associated With Down Syndrome

**Conditions Frequently Identified During the Neonatal Period**

Cardiac conditions:
- Endocardial cushion defect
- Tetralogy of Fallot
- Atrial septal defects
- Patent ductus arteriosus
- Ventricular septal defects

Gastrointestinal conditions:
- Tracheoesophageal fistula
- Pyloric stenosis
- Imperforate anus
- Duodenal atresia
- Aganglionic megacolon (Hirschsprung disease)

Congenital cataracts
Hypothyroidism
Dysplastic hips
Leukemia-like conditions

**Conditions Frequently Identified During Childhood**

Endocrine disorders:
- Decreased growth
- Obesity resulting from overeating, insufficient exercise, or undetected hypothyroidism
- Thyroid dysfunction
- Infertility (male)
- Alopecia
- Thin hair

Sensitive skin and propensity for rashes
Ophthalmic problems, such as myopia, strabismus, nystagmus, cataracts, blepharitis, and keratoconus
Chronic serous otitis media
Hematologic abnormalities:
- Subtle immune deficiencies
- Acute nonlymphoblastic leukemia
- Acute lymphoblastic leukemia

Craniofacial defects:
- Malocclusions
- Delayed tooth eruption
- Periodontal disease and gingivitis
- Bruxism
- Sinusitis and rhinitis
- Sleep apnea as a result of cranial malformations

Musculoskeletal abnormalities:
- Hypotonia
- Joint laxity and dislocations
- Atlantoaxial subluxation or dislocation

Sensory deficits
Seizure disorders
Psychiatric disorders, particularly adjustment reaction disorders, anxiety disorders, depression, behavior disorders, dementia
Autism spectrum disorders (ASDs)

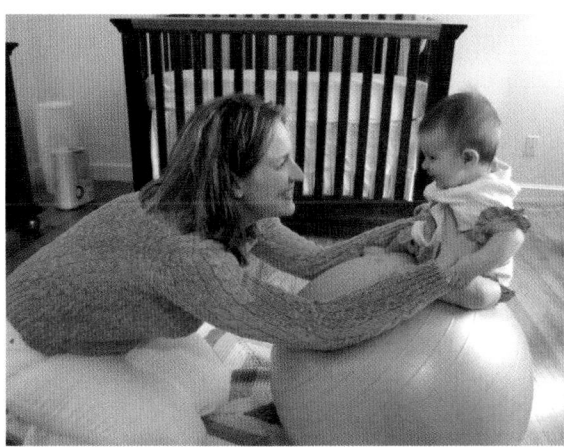

FIG 54.3 Children with delayed motor or cognitive function, whether temporary or pervasive, benefit from early and vigorous therapy to help them reach their maximum development.

Other than maternal age and genetic predispositions, no specific risk factors are known for DS, and no geographic or economic risks have been identified.

## PATHOPHYSIOLOGY

### *Down Syndrome*

Trisomy 21, or Down syndrome, occurs when three representatives of chromosome 21 are present instead of the usual two. Evidence suggests that a particular region of chromosome 21 is responsible for the facial features, heart defects, intellectual impairment, and dermatologic changes associated with Down syndrome. Many of the malformations in this disorder result from incomplete rather than abnormal embryogenesis. Examples include malformations of the atrioventricular canal, tracheoesophageal fistula, and imperforate anus. Alterations in neurotransmitters, particularly in the cholinergic system, are responsible for the premature aging and Alzheimer-type dementia that are common in individuals with Down syndrome.

A number of medical problems in the newborn period can seriously compromise health and survival. If the child survives these complications, a number of less serious difficulties are generally encountered in childhood.

### Manifestations

The phenotype for DS is often identified at birth by characteristic facial and head features, such as brachycephaly (disproportionate shortness of the head); flat profile; inner epicanthal folds; wide, flat, nasal bridge; narrow, high-arched palate; protruding tongue; and small, short ears that may be low set. In addition, children with DS may have other serious abnormalities that affect their development, including congenital cardiac defects, vision and hearing difficulties, and childhood leukemia.

In addition to facial and head features, certain body features also may be apparent in the child with DS. These include short stature; short, broad hands; singular transverse creases across the palm and the sole of the foot; wide gap between first and second toes; short, broad neck; increased likelihood of umbilical hernia; dry skin with a tendency to crack and fissure; hyperextensibility of joints with hypotonicity of muscles; and atlantoaxial instability (i.e., at the first and second cervical vertebrae).

Risks for associated medical conditions include malformations of the atrioventricular canal, tracheoesophageal fistula, and imperforate anus. Alterations in neurotransmitters, particularly in the cholinergic system, are responsible for premature aging and the concomitant increased risk for early development of Alzheimer disease.

Most children with DS have mild (IQ 50 to 70) to moderate (IQ 35 to 50) intellectual impairment. As they age, people with DS have declining intellectual abilities, reduced social and adaptive skills, and the onset of Alzheimer-type dementia. Prevalence is estimated at 25% of people with DS who are older than 35 years; by age 60, most people with DS show problems with thinking and memory (United states Department of Health and Human Services, n.d.).

### Diagnostic Evaluation

Prenatal testing includes amniocentesis or chorionic villus sampling. An abnormal triple maternal serum screen value (low α-fetoprotein, low unconjugated estriol, and increased human gonadotropin levels) may prompt additional testing. DS is usually evident at birth because of the characteristic phenotype facial features, although chromosomal analysis is conducted to confirm the diagnosis. Other diagnostic tests are conducted to identify associated medical conditions, such as nasopharyngeal abnormalities or cardiac defects.

To rule out associated disorders and to detect frequently encountered difficulties, clinicians recommend that the child be monitored frequently throughout the first 12 months of life, with an emphasis on gastrointestinal and cardiac symptoms. The diagnosis often requires a full cardiac workup initially and an electrocardiogram at the end of the first year. In the second to fourth years of life, the medical emphasis is on sleep and behavioral difficulties, along with annual thyroid screening and ophthalmologic assessment. Generally, the child is referred for dental assessments at 24 months; tooth development and alignment problems are common. Generally, children should be reevaluated medically and behaviorally on an annual basis.

### Therapeutic Management

Regular screening, early intervention, and active management of identified problems are essential, because there is no cure for the disorders caused by the syndrome. Surgery to correct cardiac abnormalities, gastrointestinal malformations, and craniofacial deviations has been used to prolong life, alleviate discomfort, and decrease the likelihood of further medical complications. Neck radiography should be performed before the child participates in any sports because children with DS are at risk for atlantoaxial instability.

## NURSING CARE

### The Child With DS

#### Assessment

Neonatal assessment is crucial in diagnosing DS on the basis of physiologic characteristics. A thorough physical examination should be conducted, including hearing and vision examinations. Children with DS are at increased risk for hearing deficits and refractive errors or cataracts. When DS is suspected or already confirmed on the basis of prenatal genetic testing, serum α-fetoprotein levels, or amniotic fluid samples, an assessment is conducted to determine the severity of the manifestations and the family's ability to cope with and accommodate the needs of the infant. Assessment for intellectual disability is also appropriate for the child with DS.

If a child with DS is hospitalized for surgical repair, infections, or injury, assess the child's typical coping patterns to support strategies already in place. Children with DS prefer routine and consistency, so an assessment of their daily routine is important; include times and habits related to mealtimes, bathing, and order of dressing. Assessing the child's understanding of language and ability to communicate is important for providing information that the child can understand. Knowing the child's words for specific body functions, such as voiding, defecating, and sleeping, will allow for greater comfort for the hospitalized child. It is important to assess the child's learning abilities before initiating any education or procedure-related play.

The child's motor skills are assessed to determine what procedures will be necessary to ensure the child's safety. Sensory deficits, such as vision or hearing difficulties, should be identified as part of routine regular follow-up. Some deficits can be detected by closely observing as the child reaches for objects, by listening to conversation, or by speaking the child's name. However, the child with DS may respond to sensory stimuli less noticeably than unimpaired children or may respond with a dulled affect, even if hearing or vision deficits are not present. Developmental delays in balance and coordination increase the risk for injuries from falls. Self-stimulating behaviors (e.g., picking at the arm) need to be identified because they are often used as coping strategies but may also be self-injurious.

Identification of areas of good functioning and adaptive behavior is important, because families need reassurance about developmental gains and emotional support for their efforts at care. A child with DS is most often a beloved member of the family, viewed by parents and siblings as a valuable addition. Nurses, who can offer important support for the normalization of the syndrome, can support these attachments. Assessment of the family and living environment is critical to ensure that both physical safety and stimulation of development are present. Affected children frequently do not seek out stimulation and may need encouragement through colors, sound, and motion. An assessment of social behaviors is also important and should include play, social judgment skills, and social interest in the environment. The child may demonstrate inappropriate behaviors similar to those associated with severe intellectual disability. Moreover, the child's natural curiosity may be diminished as a result of fear or frustration. Nursing care of the child with DS is similar to that for any child with an intellectual disability, with some specific additions.

### Nursing Diagnosis and Planning

The nursing diagnoses and expected outcomes that are appropriate for the child with DS and the child's family are as follows:

- Impaired Parenting related to the child's delayed development, physical appearance, and medical complications.

  ***Expected outcome.*** The family will demonstrate satisfying and supportive relationships that meet the physical and emotional needs of each family member.
- Self-Care Deficit (Bathing/Hygiene, Dressing/Grooming, Feeding, Toileting) related to intellectual immaturity.

  ***Expected outcome.*** The child will demonstrate the ability to independently meet needs related to bathing/ hygiene, dressing/grooming, feeding, and toileting.
- Delayed Growth and Development related to poor sucking abilities, mouth deformities, flaccid facial muscles, or other abnormalities.

  ***Expected outcomes.*** The child will maximize progress toward attaining developmental milestones and will demonstrate appropriate and measurable growth during childhood.

### Interventions

The stigma attached to DS can be pervasive and crippling, particularly for parents and caregivers. Nurses should be aware of their personal response to the diagnosis. It is not uncommon for parents to describe delivery room scenes in which medical and nursing staff "become quiet" at a time when the parents expect congratulations on the birth of their child. This reaction sends the message that the birth of the child is a tragedy. This experience creates anger at healthcare professional prejudice and is viewed by the parents as both cruel and inaccurate. Children with DS are frequently welcomed by their parents, siblings, and extended family. The goal of all nursing interventions is directed toward the goal of benefiting the child and the family in adaptation and assimilation.

When the diagnosis is made at birth, parents greatly benefit from support in accepting the diagnosis and quick identification of resources available to teach them the special care needs for their children. The nurse can encourage bonding and attachment by identifying the positive features and behaviors in the child; looking at the child's strengths from the beginning reduces the likelihood that parents will see the child negatively when milestones are not attained alongside others of the same chronologic age.

The nurse helps the parents explore options for fluid and calorie intake. Breastfeeding may not be possible if the child's muscle tone or sucking reflex is immature, although some children with DS can breastfeed adequately. As the child develops, special bottles or adaptive utensils may assist with feeding. Refer the parents for nutritional counseling as needed. Provide resources for behavioral training to encourage intake of new foods or the acquisition of new skills.

Children with DS benefit from regular schedules, and changes in the child's routine can cause frustration and decreased coping abilities. When the child is hospitalized, the nurse must try to keep the child's environment and routine as close to the home routine as possible; families can generally identify the important routines associated with waking, sleeping, eating, and conversation. An accurate and detailed description of these routines on the child's written care plan ensures consistency. Care plans are based on the child's unique personality, as well as the child's intellectual, developmental, and adaptive abilities. Chronologic age is generally not a good indicator, because the child's skills may be age appropriate in some areas but markedly delayed in others. Parents are encouraged to observe the child for signs of readiness to learn a new task (reaching for a cup, attempting to dress) and encourage self-care whenever possible. The child's level of coordination, muscle strength, and dexterity may not allow the child to zip, button, or self-feed in the usual way, so adaptive tools may be needed.

As the child grows, advise the parents to encourage participation in recreational activities that the child can manage. Be sure to advise them that the child will need to have neck radiography before participating in any active sports program.

### Evaluation

- Have the child and family demonstrated positive and mutually satisfying interactions?
- Are the parents able to identify the child's strengths and positive attributes?
- Do the parents state an interest and willingness to help the child learn new skills through demonstration, repetition, and much positive feedback?
- Does the child demonstrate continued development and a sense of competence in self-care skills?
- Does the child demonstrate steady progress toward attaining developmental milestones and appropriate measurable growth?

## FRAGILE X SYNDROME

Fragile X syndrome (FXS) is a common inherited cause of cognitive impairment and a known genetic cause of autism, although the syndrome can present with or without autism (Bacino & Lee, 2016). Males are generally more severely affected by the syndrome than females, who may be genetically protected from the most extreme manifestations of the disease by their double X chromosome. The majority of boys who inherit this disorder display significant cognitive and learning disabilities (Bacino & Lee, 2016). Females who are not affected by the syndrome can be carriers of the syndrome to their children.

## Etiology

The gene that causes FXS *(FXMR1)* is located on the X chromosome, and inheritance of the gene is through a sex-linked inheritance pattern (see Chapter 10). Because females carry two X chromosomes, the second X chromosome provides protection from full manifestation of the syndrome, which may be absent or present with only mild symptoms. A male child who inherits the X chromosome with a fragile site is not protected, because males carry one X and one Y chromosome. These children will usually exhibit the full effects of the syndrome.

A female child can inherit the gene from either parent. A girl who inherits the X chromosome that has a fragile site can be a carrier, passing on the abnormal X chromosome. Transmission of the syndrome occurs only through carrier mothers, because the fragile site is located on the X chromosome. This means that males who are not affected by the syndrome will not be genetic carriers, whereas females who are not affected may still be carriers of the fragile site.

## Incidence

FXS affects approximately 1 in 5000 male children (CDC, 2016d. Both males and females can carry the fragile X gene. The gene can be carried as either a partial or full mutation. In general, only males exhibit the full effects of this X-linked recessive disorder because their single X chromosome has the abnormal gene.

## PATHOPHYSIOLOGY

### *Fragile X Syndrome*

Fragile X syndrome is caused by an underlying single gene defect on the X chromosome. All affected individuals have this defect, which is located in the fragile X intellectual disability gene (*FXMR1*). The genetic defect involves excessive repetitions of the nucleotide cytosine-guanine-guanine (CGG) deoxyribonucleic acid (DNA) sequences.

## Manifestations

FXS, like the ASDs, can cause a number of different symptoms with varying levels of dysfunction. Overall, the areas of functioning that are affected span six categories:

- Intellectual functioning
- Physical characteristics
- Social and emotional relatedness
- Speech and language capability
- Sensory impairment
- Presence of co-morbid disorders commonly associated with the syndrome

### Physical Characteristics

Physical features associated with FXS include facial dysmorphism, often with large or prominent ears and a long, narrow face; a head circumference that may be disproportionate to the child's height and weight; lowered epicanthal folds; and prominent nasal alae (cartilaginous flap on the outer side of each nostril). In addition, the child may manifest enlarged testicles (postpubertal macro-orchidism), flat feet, lax ankles, hyperextensible fingers, soft and smooth skin, and mitral valve prolapse.

### Social and Emotional Relatedness

FXS is also a disorder of social connectedness; decreased activity is seen in the prefrontal regions of the brain that are related to social connections (Hahn, Brady, Fleming, & Warren, 2016). Characteristics include difficulty looking at people directly (gaze aversion) and difficulties with peer social relationships. This difficulty appears to be related to facial recognition—the ability to recognize a face that has been seen before (face encoding).

### Speech and Language Capability and Sensory Impairment

Language and sensory impairments likely contribute to the social and behavioral dysfunctions associated with FXS, which include disruptive behaviors such as temper tantrums; self-injury; extreme agitation; autism-like behaviors such as gaze avoidance, hand flapping, echolalia, and abnormal speech patterns; hyperkinetic behaviors, including restlessness, agitation, and attention deficits; hand biting; and sensory motor integration deficits such as poor coordination, motor planning deficits, and tactile defensiveness. The child may have strengths in visual memory but weaknesses in auditory processing abilities and abstract reasoning; improved performance with simultaneous, rather than sequential, processing; language delays; perseveration; tangential speech; and other communicative disorders. Girls manifest only mild intellectual deficits but with many variations. People with FXS experience worsening of symptoms across the life span, including high risk for progressive dementia.

### Co-Morbid Disorders

A variety of physical and emotional disorders can coexist with the signs and symptoms of fragile X. Anxiety and depression are not uncommon. Affected girls can experience primary ovarian insufficiency, postpubertal testicular enlargement is not unusual, and both girls and boys are at risk for seizures (March of Dimes, 2014).

## Diagnostic Evaluation

Deoxyribonucleic acid testing is the definitive method of diagnosing FXS. Identification of the *FMR1* gene mutation allows diagnosis in both carriers and those affected. Children with intellectual disability of unknown cause or learning disabilities, together with manifestations of FXS, should be considered for fragile X testing.

## Therapeutic Management

Treatment is provided through early intervention programs. Special education, vocational programs, and behavioral management classes are important to overall development. Speech and language evaluation and therapy are generally prescribed during the first year of life and are made available on a continuing basis. Sensorimotor integration therapy may be offered to enhance motor planning; joint stability; coordination; and integration of visual, auditory, and tactile information. Sensorimotor therapy is considered to be the intervention of choice for these children with learning disabilities.

There are no medications that can treat FXS itself, however medications are used to manage associated symptoms. These include medications that treat depression or anxiety, hyperactivity and seizures (Bacino & Lee, 2016).

## Nursing Considerations

The nursing care of children with FXS is similar to care for any child with an intellectual disability, with specific attention to the behavioral and intellectual difficulties presented by the individual child. The plan should include a multidisciplinary team approach to assessment. Anticipatory guidance should be provided, with a review of the support groups and services available. Special education services will be necessary to address the child's specific intellectual and academic difficulties, to foster continued skill development, and to reduce the stress created in the typical educational setting. Remediation services should include behavioral interventions specific to the child's needs, speech and language assistance, and possibly occupational and physical therapy to address visual-motor and motor skill deficits. Family members of children with FXS should receive genetic counseling and testing, because unaffected females may be carriers (National Fragile X Foundation, n.d.).

## RETT SYNDROME

Unlike FXS, which affects primarily males, Rett syndrome (RS) is almost exclusively linked to female sex, with an estimated 1:10,000 females affected (International Rett Syndrome Foundation [IRSF], 2016b). However, both disorders are related to the X chromosome. The syndrome is characterized by an initial period of normal development, with symptoms emerging between the ages of 6 and 18 months. Social and intellectual development stops, and seizures and physical disabilities emerge (IRSF, 2016a). The emergence of symptoms in a child who was developing normally is devastating for the families of children with these disorders.

RS is considered to be a developmental disorder as opposed to a degenerative disorder, because neurons are not destroyed (IRSF, 2016b). RS has been characterized as an ASD and is the only ASD for which the cause is known. Diagnosis is made by detecting mutations on the X chromosome, gene *MECP2,* combined with clinical evaluation for the characteristic clinical signs. These signs include stereotyped hand movements, gait disturbances, loss of fine motor control, and regression in speech; these signs occur in the absence of brain trauma and not during the first six months of life (IRSF, 2016a).

Nursing considerations for the child with RS are similar to those for the child with FXS or other child with an intellectual or developmental disability.

## FETAL ALCOHOL SPECTRUM DISORDER (FASD)

As with other spectrum disorders, the signs and symptoms related to prenatal alcohol exposure can range in effect from mild to severe. Fetal alcohol spectrum disorder is the most severe disorder experienced by the infant exposed to alcohol *in utero.* FASD refers to the classic defects of persistent symmetric growth retardation, malformations of the face and skull, skeletal and cardiac malformation, and CNS deficits, including intellectual and developmental disabilities.

### Etiology and Incidence

Maternal alcohol consumption is the cause of FASD. No safe level of alcohol consumption during pregnancy has been established. The incidence of FASD is believed to be grossly underestimated because of lack of awareness in diagnosis and underreporting of alcohol intake during pregnancy. The incidence of FASD varies by country and ethnic group, but it is estimated to be 0.2 to 1.5/1000 live births in the United States (CDC, 2016c).

### Manifestations

The infant with FASD exhibits prenatal and postnatal growth deficiency, microcephaly, joint anomalies, mild to moderate intellectual disability, tremulousness in the neonatal period, and irritability; the child with FASD exhibits hyperactivity. Infants may have characteristic facial features, including short palpebral fissures, a smooth philtrum (the vertical groove in the median portion of the upper lip), and a thin upper lip (Fig. 54.4). Other abnormalities associated with this syndrome include altered palmar crease patterns, short distal phalanges, cervical vertebral malformations, ear anomalies, cleft lip and palate, severe cardiac defects, renal anomalies, strawberry hemangiomas, and genital anomalies (Williams & Smith, 2015).

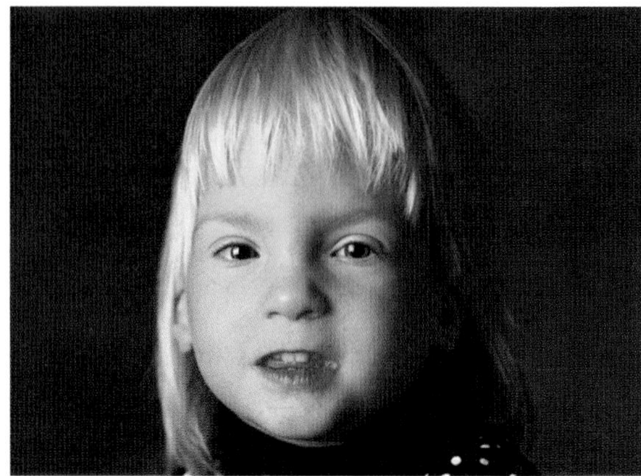

**FIG 54.4** Toddler with fetal alcohol syndrome spectrum disorder. Subtle indicators are a flat mid-face, indistinct philtrum, and low-set ears. (From Fortinash, K.M., & Holoday Worret, P.A. [2012]. *Psychiatric mental health nursing* [5th ed.]. St. Louis: Mosby.)

**PATHOPHYSIOLOGY**

***Fetal Alcohol Spectrum Disorder***

Alcohol and its metabolite (acetaldehyde) cross the placenta rapidly; therefore, the fetus has blood levels of alcohol equivalent to the maternal levels. Prenatal alcohol exposure is thought to affect protein synthesis, influencing the growth and development of the brain and other tissues. This effect can result in a decreased number of brain cells, diminished intelligence, and brain malformation.

Assessment should be performed for other related abnormalities, including cleft palate, foot deformities, hip dislocations and other conditions involving joint hyperextensibility, hernias, and hypertonia. These children may have seizures, so medications and educating the family about seizure disorders is warranted for some.

### Diagnostic Evaluation

Diagnostic features of FASD include the following criteria developed by the CDC (2014b). Alcohol exposure during pregnancy is established by self-report, reports by other reliable individuals, documented elevated blood alcohol level, alcohol treatment, or documentation of other known alcohol-related problems. However, confirmation of the use of alcohol is not totally necessary for a diagnosis of FASD (CDC, 2016c), because the diagnosis can be made if the child meets the criteria for diagnosis. An infant or child can be diagnosed with FAS if the following criteria are met (CDC, 2014b):

- *Three facial abnormalities:* Smooth philtrum, thin vermilion border, small palpebral fissures
- *Growth deficit:* 10th percentile or less for height, weight, or both
- *CNS abnormalities:* Head circumference at the 10th percentile or less; brain abnormalities identified by imaging studies; motor deficits or seizures from no other identified cause
- *Developmental milestones* below the expected range for the child's age, physical or psychosocial circumstances in at least three of the following: cognitive function, executive function, attention, motor function, and social skills. Associated problems, such as abnormal

sensitivities to taste and touch or inability to appropriately respond to facial expression or parenting techniques, compose the final criteria.

FASD is diagnosed through physical examination and perinatal history, and a referral is often made to a geneticist. Families require counseling to help them cope with the diagnosis and to help them understand the risks involved in future pregnancies if lifestyle changes are not made.

## NURSING CARE

### The Infant With FASD

#### Assessment

When FASD is suspected, an extensive diagnostic workup is required. Microcephaly, hypotonia, tremulousness, and irritability can raise the level of suspicion. Feeding difficulties may be encountered as well.

The family requires assistance in coping with the diagnosis and the inherent difficulties associated with caring for a child who may be difficult to soothe or has feeding problems. Special attention must be given to involving the parents in the care of the infant. As with other developmental disorders, there is evidence that early intervention will maximize the developmental potential of the nervous system.

#### Nursing Diagnosis and Planning

The nursing diagnoses and expected outcomes that apply to the infant with FASD and the family are as follows:

- Ineffective Infant Feeding Pattern related to congenital anomaly.

  ***Expected outcome.*** The infant will establish appropriate sleep-wake and feeding patterns, as evidenced by appropriate weight gain and growth.
- Delayed Growth and Development related to FASD.

  ***Expected outcome.*** The infant will develop to maximum potential, as evidenced by growth and development behaviors relative to age and potential.
- Deficient Knowledge (infant's anomalies and potential sequelae) related to lack of exposure to accurate information.

  ***Expected outcome.*** Parents will increase knowledge related to the child's disorder, as evidenced by recognition of FASD and acknowledgment of the potential for future problems.
- Interrupted Family Processes related to birth of a disabled child.

  ***Expected outcome.*** The family will use coping strategies to care for the child, as evidenced by an ability to mobilize their energies toward caring for the infant with FASD.

#### Interventions

Daily weight gain is monitored, and intake and output are measured and documented. Various feeding strategies (e.g., varying the positioning of the infant; trying smaller, more frequent feedings; using different nipples) should be attempted until the infant is successful with nipple feedings or breastfeeding. Because parents may become frustrated or feel inadequate in dealing with a difficult feeder, it is important to assist the parents with feeding in a supportive manner. Promoting early parent–infant attachment will support the child's well-being. Encourage the family to visit frequently and involve parents in caretaking activities.

The infant with FASD is likely to have severe permanent neurologic and developmental deficits. Discuss the infant's recognizable anomalies and the possible sequelae. Allow the parents to verbalize their concerns about their infant's future. Avoid encouraging unrealistic expectations; rather, acknowledge the infant's existing problems and suggest coping strategies.

The family is in a crisis situation, and the mother may feel guilt or be blamed by other family members for the infant's disability. Encourage family members to verbalize their feelings. Initiate referrals to appropriate community resources. The needs of the high-risk family are significant and require long-term follow-up.

#### Evaluation

- Are the infant's sleep patterns appropriate for age?
- Is the infant gaining weight at a rate that is appropriate for age?
- Is the child able to attain appropriate growth and development milestones?
- Are the parents discussing the cause and prevention of FASD?
- Is the family able to identify its own strengths and weaknesses, coping skills, and support systems?
- Have referrals to community resources been made and implemented?

## FAILURE TO THRIVE

The term *failure to thrive* is used to describe children whose weight or rate of weight gain is significantly below that of comparably-aged children. These children appear dramatically smaller than their peers. Failure to thrive can result from numerous organic or medical causes, including chromosomal abnormalities, defects in the heart or lung, CNS damage, or exposure to toxins. In the absence of organic causes, failure to thrive may be the result of a multifactorial interplay between child temperament, parental expectations, maternal emotional state, and sociodemographic factors (McLean & Price, 2016). Most clinicians agree that failure to thrive is not an actual diagnosis but rather a term that describes a cluster of concurrent symptoms. In practice, if a child is considered to be significantly smaller than peers or if a child fails to gain appropriate weight over time, the child is considered to be at risk for failure to thrive, and a more thorough evaluation is warranted (McLean & Price, 2016).

### Etiology

Failure to thrive can be organic, caused by an underlying physical problem, or nonorganic. The contributing factors to and interventions for physical growth delay have been described in detail in previous chapters. Failure to thrive can result in both intellectual and developmental delays.

### Incidence

It is difficult to estimate the number of children seen in general practice with symptoms of failure to thrive. Although failure to thrive occurs in children of all social classes, a disproportionate number of these children are from low-income families. Poverty affects nearly 20% of children, many of whom experience food insufficiency (Sirotnak, 2016).

### Manifestations and Risk Factors

Physical indicators of nonorganic failure to thrive include weight below the 5th percentile, a sudden or rapid deceleration in the growth curve, delay in reaching developmental milestones, and decreased muscle mass. Muscle hypotonia, abdominal distention, generalized weakness, and cachexia (general ill health and malnutrition) are additional signs.

Behavioral indicators of failure to thrive include avoidance of eye contact, avoidance of physical touch, intense watchfulness, and sleep disturbances. Lack of age-appropriate stranger anxiety, inappropriate lack of preference for one's own parents, and disturbed affect (e.g., apathy, extreme irritability, extreme compliance) may also be observed.

Repetitive self-stimulating behaviors, such as rocking, head banging, intense sucking, intense chewing on fingers or hands, and head rolling, are also seen.

### Diagnostic Evaluation

The differential diagnosis is generally made by a multidisciplinary team whose initial task is to search for an organic cause of the growth failure. If no cause is identified, the approach is to diagnose by response. Nutrition and nurturing are provided in a consistent manner, and if the infant gains the expected weight, nonorganic failure to thrive is considered to be the appropriate diagnosis.

### Therapeutic Management

Children with failure to thrive usually are managed in an outpatient setting. Treatment provides nutritional therapy to increase the child's caloric intake. The goal is for the child to grow at two to three times the average rate for age. Daily multivitamin supplements with minerals are often prescribed to ensure that specific nutritional deficiencies do not occur in the course of rapid growth. Caloric enrichment of food is essential, and formula may be concentrated in titrated amounts up to 24 cal/oz. Greater concentrations can lead to diarrhea and dehydration.

Family therapy may be indicated. Effective parenting classes can assist the parent to identify psychological and physical factors that have contributed to the child's condition.

### Nursing Considerations

In addition to assessing contributing factors that would suggest organic failure to thrive (e.g., age at onset, history of illness especially gastrointestinal illness, and dietary patterns), the nurse should complete a thorough psychosocial history that focuses on income, family (dis) organization, social isolation, stress factors, support systems, and family psychopathologic conditions such as maternal depression, family violence, or alcoholism. It is important to ask about the availability of food, especially around the time of arrival of a paycheck or other forms of income. Finally, the psychosocial history should include questions about facilities for storing and preparing food.

Assessment of parent–infant interactions should focus on the ways in which the child is held and fed, how eye contact is initiated and maintained, and the facial expressions of both the child and the caregiver during interactions. Observations of various kinds of interactions are also important and should include play, talk, and touch by both the child and caregiver and the other's reaction to these attempts to engage in interaction. The nurse should note the responses of the caregiver to the child's cues, such as when the child cries, reaches out, or looks toward the caregiver. A feeling of synchrony or harmony should be sensed in the interaction.

The focus for nursing intervention is to facilitate improvement in the child's physical and developmental status as well as enhancing positive parenting. If the child is hospitalized, providing a consistent caregiver from the nursing staff increases trust and provides the child with an adult who anticipates needs and is able to model child care to the parent. Role modeling and teaching appropriate adult-child interactions (including holding, touching, and feeding the child) will facilitate appropriate parent–child relationships and enhance parents' confidence in caring for their child and expression by the parents of realistic expectations based on the child's developmental needs.

## AUTISM SPECTRUM DISORDERS

Autism spectrum disorders (ASDs), as a significant part of the pervasive developmental disorders, range in severity from severe (autism disorder) to a milder form (Asperger syndrome). A child who has symptoms of either of these disorders but does not meet the criteria for either diagnosis is generally diagnosed with the classification PDD—not otherwise specified (American Psychiatric Association, 2013).

The CDC estimates that approximately 1 in 68 children in the U.S. are identified with an ASD (Christensen, Baio, Braun et al., 2016). All forms of ASD are characterized by atypical patterns of development and clusters of developmental problems and deficits. These features include difficulty developing and maintaining social relationships, disordered communication, and stereotyped interests and behaviors (APA, 2013). Symptoms are usually noticeable by 3 years of age and may be gradual or sudden in onset. Earlier screening as recommended by the American Academy of Pediatrics (2016) can identify symptoms at a much earlier age. Occasionally, the disorder is not identified until the child reaches school age, particularly in cases where gross motor skills show normal progression. ASDs are frequently linked to co-morbidity with intellectual, emotional, and behavioral disorders or other medical conditions (Sadock, Sadock, & Ruiz, 2015).

Indicators of ASDs include lack of social ability (e.g., poor eye contact), lack of verbalization (such as babbling), little interest in verbal interaction, inability to use toys, lack of smiling, excessive preoccupation with creating order, and lack of response to verbal interactions. Parents often express concern that their child does not appear to be attaching to them and does not seek comfort or cuddling. Social cues and gestures have little meaning to children with ASD.

### Asperger Syndrome

Historically, Asperger syndrome was classified as "high-functioning autism." New understandings of the disorder have led to the classification of Asperger syndrome as a distinct subcategory within the autism spectrum. Children with Asperger syndrome do not show the level of disability seen in autism, and these children typically show normal and often high levels of intellectual and language development. Symptoms are primarily social and emotional. Children with Asperger syndrome display an impaired ability to understand common social cues and an inability to behave according to social norms. They will often be fluent in language, but the content of conversations is fixated on the topic of interest to the child, with no regard for the reaction of the listener. They also frequently display rigidity regarding schedules, motor clumsiness, trouble handwriting, and organizational skill problems. Children with Asperger syndrome are often friendly and would like to establish peer relationships, but their inability to understand social cues creates difficulty in establishing and maintaining relationships (Autism Society of America, 2016).

### Autism

Autism is the most severe form of the ASDs. It is a complex disorder, with many potential causes, one of which may be genetic. To date, there is no evidence that autism can be cured, so treatment is generally lifelong and is characterized by varying degrees of success. Early diagnosis, with comprehensive and ongoing intervention targeted to presenting symptoms, appears to offer the best prognosis for educational and psychosocial outcomes (Table 54.2).

#### Etiology

Family child-rearing practices and parental personality characteristics were once believed to influence the development of autism. However, no controlled studies confirm this view, and the notion that autism has a psychogenic origin in family dysfunction has been largely discounted.

**TABLE 54.2 Differential Diagnosis of Autism, Intellectual Disability, and Schizophrenia**

| Autism | Intellectual Disability |
|---|---|
| Peaked skill profile | Flat skill profile |
| Lack of imitative skills | Imitation skills and gesturing |
| Nonsocial behaviors with little initiation | Social behavior, initiation of social contact |
| Abnormal communication and language | Limited language ability but sufficient for communication |
| Development of seizures possible during adolescence | Usually no seizures, Alzheimer-type dementia in adulthood |
| **Autism** | **Schizophrenia** |
| Onset before age 54 mo | Onset during pubescence or adolescence |
| No remissions | Remissions and relapses |
| Hallucinations and delusions rare | Hallucinations and delusions common |
| Absence of thought disorder | Thought disorder |
| No family history of schizophrenia | Family history of schizophrenia |
| Self-stimulating behaviors | Odd behavior but no self-stimulating behaviors |
| Medications of limited use | Medications often helpful in reducing symptoms |

Researchers theorize that the disorder can be caused by a wide range of prenatal, perinatal, and postnatal conditions, including maternal rubella, untreated phenylketonuria, tuberous sclerosis, anoxia during birth, encephalitis, seizures, and FXS (Sadock, Sadock, & Ruiz, 2015).

Other theories have proposed possible connections between autism and hazardous chemical exposures, including thimerosal in vaccines administered during infancy and childhood. Epidemiologic studies have examined the relationship between the occurrence of autism and administration of the measles, mumps, rubella (MMR) vaccine or vaccines preserved with thimerosal. Multiple epidemiologic studies have shown no correlation between the occurrence of autism and childhood vaccination. Recent research suggests that ASD and other developmental disorders may be related to maternal metabolic influences during pregnancy (Krakowiak, Walker, & Bremer, 2012), including obesity and diabetes mellitus. Other research has linked the prevalence of autism to low birth weight or prematurity (Pinto-Martin, Levy, Feldman, 2011). Research into the etiology of autism is ongoing.

There is a growing body of research directed toward identifying genetic mutations related to autism. The American Recovery and Reinvestment Act of 2009 allocated a significant amount of funding to address contributing factors to autism, including genetic and genomic factors (National Institute of Environmental Health Sciences [NIEHS], 2011).

Inherited genetic mutations have been thought to be contributory, particularly in families where multiple siblings have been affected by the disorder. However, in 2007 Sebat, Lakshmi, Malhotra et al. described tiny rare mutations that appear unpredictably across the genome; these mutations may be related to autism in families where only one child is affected. This discovery has led to the proposition that two subtypes of genetic disorders exist. The first spontaneous mutation is linked to families with single cases of autism (sporadic autism); the second subtype, inheritance, is linked to families with multiple members affected by the disorder (familial autism). Sebat et al. found spontaneous deletions and duplications that were 10 times more prevalent in children with the sporadic subtype than in healthy control subjects. The mutations were only twice as prevalent in children from families with multiple children affected by autism as compared to control subjects (Sebat et al., 2007). This evidence implies that autism may share common neurobiologic features with a variety of biologic and emotional disorders (Raviola, Trieu, DeMaso, et al., 2016).

### Incidence

Prevalence rates for autism have been difficult to establish. Most recent data looking at children with autism have established a prevalence of 11.3/1,000 children in the United States (Raviola et al., 2016). This number is a substantial increase over the previous several years. Autism is more common in boys than in girls and is highest in non-Hispanic white children, although this statistic might be related to the fact that black and Hispanic children do not have the same access to diagnosis as white children do (Christensen et al., 2016).

### Manifestations

Autism can be a severely incapacitating, lifelong developmental disability that is characterized by a qualitative impairment in the developmental areas of communication or language, social skills, and behavior, which includes abnormal responses to normal body sensations (AAP, 2012). Children may demonstrate evidence of cognitive capacity, but with absence or delay in language; abnormal ways of relating to people, objects, or events; and difficulty regulating emotions (CDC, 2016a).

The variety of forms that autism can take makes planning care difficult, because it must be individually targeted. A child may have a large vocabulary yet have no comprehension of the meaning of the words. Another child may be able to solve intricate mathematical problems but not be able to make change for a dollar. Children may be unresponsive to the sound of their own names but come running into the room at the sound of a truck. Generally, children with autism show a fixed, unchanging response to a particular stimulus. Self-stimulation is common and generally involves repetition of a particularly pleasing sensory stimulus, such as twirling a toy or rubbing the top of the head.

Apparently, interest is limited by nature, rather than by choice, to an extremely narrow range. The child with autism generally overreacts to any change within the environment. Often, autistic children do not have a typical sense of personal space and so may touch others on the face or stand face to face, with noses touching, even when encountering a total stranger.

Infants with ASD are generally thought to manifest subtle signs of social and language delays, which may be masked by normally developing motor skills (AAP, 2012). For this reason, the AAP (2016) recommends formal screening for ASD beginning at 9 months of age.

Impairment secondary to autism covers a wide range, with 75% of autistic children considered intellectually impaired. A few children with autism also have an extremely developed skill in a particular area, such as music or mathematics. These individuals are sometimes known as *autistic savants* because they have both a severe intellectual disability and an extraordinary intellectual skill or expertise. High-functioning autistic children were once considered to have Asperger syndrome, but these are now considered distinct disorders.

The child with ASD exhibits the following behaviors and characteristics; severity of symptoms also is considered (APA,2013).

*Social*

- Marked lack of awareness of the existence or feelings of others (e.g., child ignores emotions of others)

- Lack of or abnormal amount of comfort-seeking at times of distress (e.g., child does not show pain when hurt)
- Lack of or abnormal imitation of others' actions
- Lack of or abnormal social play (generally plays alone or involves others only as mere objects)
- Gross impairment in social peer relationships (appears not to want or need friends)

*Language*

- Lack of or impaired verbal communication and abnormalities in the production of speech (inappropriate volume, pitch, rate, rhythm, or intonation, such as a monotone voice or echolalia)
- Markedly abnormal nonverbal communication (e.g., the child uses no gestures or behavioral cues)
- Absence of imaginative play (no imitative or dramatic role playing)
- Impaired interactive speech and communication (the child does not allow for the normal give and take of conversation and tends to become preoccupied with a given subject or word out of context with the conversation)

*Restricted behavioral repertoire.* Presence of at least two of the following:

- Stereotyped body movements (e.g., spinning around, head banging, "flapping," rocking)
- Persistent preoccupation with characteristics of objects (smell, taste, texture) or an abnormal attachment to objects (e.g., piece of string, picture of a whale)
- Marked distress over a minor change in the environment (e.g., exhibiting tantrums when a light is turned on, refusing to look at a teacher who is wearing a new dress)
- Unreasonable insistence on routine (e.g., following a schedule exactly to the minute or second, refusal to attend an assembly during a scheduled mathematics class)
- Marked restriction in range of interests (e.g., may repeatedly align objects and cannot be diverted from doing so)

### Diagnostic Evaluation

A diagnosis of autism is usually established on the basis of specific behavioral manifestations, with evidence gained through parental consultation, patient history, and direct observation. Often, the family is interviewed initially, followed by observation of the child alone, with the parent, and interacting with the examiner or others in the environment. Interviews are coupled with observations and the clinician's rating scales. The onset of characteristic delays or of abnormal functioning must occur before age 3 years.

The AAP (2016) strongly recommends formal developmental screening for all children at well visits when the child is 9 months, 18 months, and 24 to 30 months old and autism-specific screening at 18 and 24 months. The use of screening tests that are sensitive and specific for developmental alterations should be used. Sensitive and specific screening tests include, but are not limited to, the Ages and Stages Questionnaires (ASQ) for children 4 to 60 months, Communication and Symbolic Behavior Scales—Developmental Profile (CSBS-DP) (ages 6 to 24 months), Pervasive Developmental Disorders Screening Test II (PDDST-II) (12 to 48 months), and the Modified Checklist for Autism in Toddlers (M-CHAT). These, along with parental concern about the child's development, and clinical observation, can assist with early diagnosis (CDC, 2016a).

A more complete diagnostic workup for a child with autism involves intelligence testing, although the ability to test intelligence levels is limited, because traditional tests such as the Wechsler Intelligence Scale for Children (WISC) rely heavily on language ability. Another test, the Raven's Progressive Matrices (RPM), is used to test "fluid intelligence" which is the ability to infer rules, set goals, and use high-level abstractions. Matrix tests do not rely on language, but rather on memory, attention, and executive functioning capacity.

### Therapeutic Management

Early identification of autism is essential. Treatment generally entails creating an environment that facilitates interaction and promotes replacement of stereotypical behaviors with more normal behaviors. Behavioral methods are typically used. Autistic people have a normal life span; consequently, they require significant financial resources for treatment and supervision.

Because of the severity of the social impairment and the ineffectiveness of normal environmental interventions, affected children are usually referred to special programs designed to offer stimulation, modify stereotypical behaviors, or establish routines for teaching as soon as the disorder has been identified. Programs usually focus on safety precautions for self-injurious behaviors such as head banging and the promotion of communication. Facilitative communication through the use of picture boards or keyboards is controversial but has been used in many educational settings to help autistic children interact with the environment.

### CRITICAL THINKING EXERCISE 54.1

You are a nurse working in a clinic and conducting a health assessment on a 9-month-old infant. As you provide the parent with information about the measles, mumps, and rubella (MMR) vaccine, which would be given to the infant at the 1-year well visit, the parent expresses concern that he has heard that the MMR vaccine causes autism.

1. What will be your response to this parent?
2. What kind of information can you give the parent to assist him in evaluating information he reads or hears about through the lay media?

## NURSING CARE

### The Child With Autism

#### Assessment

Because there are no classic physical features that highlight autism, the nurse must assess the child with possible autism as if no physical or intellectual disabilities are present. Such assessment is done before establishing a diagnosis. The primary characteristic of autism is lack of social interaction and awareness. For this reason, if the child is very young, the nurse who interacts only with the child's parents is unlikely to be aware of the child's degree of social disengagement. The assessment is performed in the same manner as with any normally developing child if the child has already been diagnosed as having autism and the purpose of assessment is to determine the severity of the disorder or if the assessment occurs before a procedure or hospitalization. However, the nurse will quickly become aware of the child's social detachment or lack of language as the assessment continues.

A systematic exploration of the child's skills and comparison with developmental norms are essential. For the staff nurse or school nurse, this process may include evaluating the child's ability to self-feed, dress, and toilet. The assessment should include the child's interactive patterns and verbalization skills. It is also important to note the child's motor skills, as they have major implications for safety and self-care. For the initial, generalized screening, using a reliable and valid developmental screening instrument may be helpful (see Chapter 5). A family history of autism or other mental disorders, family coping skills, and available social support systems should also be assessed.

### Nursing Diagnosis and Planning

The nursing diagnoses and expected outcomes that may be appropriate after assessment of the child with autism are as follows:

- Risk for Injury related to an inability to anticipate danger, a tendency for self-mutilation, and sensory perceptual deficits.

*Expected outcome.* The child's safety will be ensured, as evidenced by maintaining integrity of skin and avoiding self-injury or accidental injury.

- Impaired Social Interaction related to an inability to initiate and maintain social relationships and limited verbal skills.

*Expected outcomes.* The child will demonstrate improvement in communication skills and will begin to show appropriate interaction with others.

- Disturbed Thought Processes related to an inability to perceive self or others accurately and to intellectual and perceptual dysfunction.

*Expected outcomes.* The child will show progress in developing an interest in surroundings and the ability to acknowledge others in the environment; will demonstrate orientation to person, place, and time; and will perform ADLs appropriate to this orientation.

### Interventions

When working with autistic children in the hospital setting, the nurse should work closely with the family to determine the child's routines, habits, and preferences. The nurse should write down any specific cues that will help the child remain oriented to the environment and facilitate tolerance to change. For example, the nursing staff should be limited to as few individuals as possible. The child may need to perform toileting and self-care activities in a particular order. The child may need an environmental cue, such as stroking a favorite blanket, before being able to move from one activity to the next. The nurse can generally evaluate the child's tolerance of the situation by monitoring signs of anxiety or emotional comfort, as evidenced by such behaviors as attending or observing the nurse in the room or demonstrating a willingness to participate in self-care.

**! NURSING QUALITY ALERT**

***Maintaining Routine for the Child With Autism***

Children with autism often are unable to tolerate even the slightest change in routine and may become withdrawn, self-abusive, or violent if their routines are altered.

The nurse must work closely with the family to determine the specific ways in which the child communicates. The child may use sign language or pictures to specify needs if no verbal skills have developed. Children with autism are often reluctant to initiate or sustain direct eye contact, so the nurse may interpret this behavior as meaning that the child is not listening or is unaware of what is being said. In addition, the child may answer questions after several minutes' delay. The nurse should identify these behaviors, allow extra time, and be alert to differences in communication styles. Children with autism generally understand much more language than they are able to use expressively.

The child who demonstrates a tendency for head banging may need a helmet or side rolls. Meticulous observation may be necessary if the child is unable to remain in the bed at night. The nurse should help the parents understand and explain to their child any safety precautions that are unfamiliar to the child. The presence of a parent or older sibling is almost always necessary when an autistic child is hospitalized. Evaluating the child for safety is an ongoing nursing function. Reducing the adjustment demands for the child may be necessary if the nurse recognizes behaviors indicating stress or anxiety.

### Evaluation

- Has the child remained free of injury?
- Has the child developed a way to communicate needs?
- Does the child demonstrate an interest in surroundings?
- Does the child acknowledge the presence of others in the environment?
- Has the child developed the ability to perform ADLs?

## KEY CONCEPTS

- The causes of intellectual disabilities and developmental disorders can be genetic or environmental.
- Children with an intellectual disability may have limitations in both intellectual and adaptive functioning, which include social interactions, use of language for self-expression, and self-care abilities. If these limitations are severe, the child will need lifelong care by mature, caring adults.
- Children with intellectual impairment have many normal needs, including the need for positive attention and opportunities for self-discovery and growth. The active participation of the child and family is needed for the care and planning for the child's future.
- Primary nursing responsibilities when caring for a child with an intellectual disability and the child's family include facilitating initial grief, assistance with coping, and identifying resources to help meet the child's lifelong needs.
- Developmental disability is a legal term that encompasses intellectual disability as well as disability as a result of a developmental disorder.
- Early screening to identify children who may have a developmental disorder is imperative for facilitating maximum development, and the American Academy of Pediatrics recommends routine screening at certain intervals during infancy and early childhood.
- Conditions that cause intellectual or developmental disability include: (1) disorder of intellectual impairment—DS, (2) disorders of known genetic cause—FXS and RS, (3) disorders related to environmental alterations—FASD, failure to thrive, and (4) disorders with little understood genetic influence—ASDs.

## REFERENCES AND READINGS

American Academy of Pediatrics. (2012). *What are autism spectrum disorders and what are the symptoms?* Retrieved from http://www.aap.org.

American Academy of Pediatrics. (2016). *Recommendations for preventive pediatric health care.* Retrieved from http://www.aap.org.

American Association of Colleges of Nursing. (2008). *The essentials of baccalaureate education for professional nursing practice.* Washington, DC: Author.

American Association on Intellectual and Developmental Disabilities. (2011). *FAQ on intellectual disability*. Retrieved from http://www.aaidd.org.

American Psychiatric Association. (2013). *Diagnostic and statistical manual of mental disorders* (DSM-5). Washington, DC: Author.

Autism Society of America. (2016). *Asperger's syndrome*. Retrieved from http://www.autism-society.org..

Bacino, C., & Lee, B. (2016). Fragile X syndrome. In R. Kliegman, B. Stanton, J. St. Geme, et al. (Eds.), *Nelson textbook of pediatrics* (20th ed., Chapter 81.5). St. Louis MO: Elsevier.

Bitsko, R. et al. (2016). Health care, family, and community factors associated with mental, behavioral, and developmental disorders in early childhood – United States 2011-2012. *MMWR*, *65*(9), 221–226.

Calzone, K., Jenkins, J., Prows, C., & Masny, A. (2011). Establishing the outcome indicators for the essential nursing competencies and curricula guidelines for genetics and genomics. *Journal of Professional Nursing*, *27*(3), 179-191.

Centers for Disease Control and Prevention. (2014a). *Birth Defects: Data and statistics*. Retrieved from http://www.cdc.gov.

Centers for Disease Control and Prevention. (2014b). *Fetal alcohol spectrum disorders (FASD) diagnosis*. Retrieved from http://www.cdc.gov.

Centers for Disease Control and Prevention. (2016a). *Autism spectrum disorders*. Retrieved from http://www.cdc.gov.

Centers for Disease Control and Prevention. (2016b).*Down syndrome*. Retrieved from http://www.cdc.gov.

Centers for Disease Control and Prevention. (2016c). *Fetal alcohol spectrum disorders (FASD)*. Retrieved from http://www.cdc.gov.

Centers for Disease Control and Prevention. (2016d). *Fragile X syndrome data and statistics*. Retrieved from http://www.cdc.gov.

Christensen, D.L., Baio, J., Braun, K.V., et al. (2016). Prevalence and characteristics of autism spectrum disorder among children aged 8 years- Autism and developmental disabilities monitoring network, 11 sites, United States, 2012. *MMWR Surveillance Summaries 65*(3): 1-23. doi: 10.15585/mmwr.ss6503a1.

Developmental Disabilities Assistance and Bill of Rights Act of 2000 (PL 106-402). (2000). *Passed by U.S. Congress on October 30, 2000.*

Hahn, J., Brady, N., Fleming, K. & Warren, S. (2016). Joint engagement and early language development in young children with Fragile X Syndrome. *Journal of Speech, Language, and Hearing Research*, *59*, 1087-1098.

Houtrow, A.J., Larson, K., Olson, L.M., et al. (2013). Changing trends of childhood disability, 2001-2011. *Pediatrics*, *134*, 530–538.

International Rett Syndrome Foundation. (2016a). *About Rhett syndrome*. Retrieved from http://www.rettsyndrome.org.

International Rett Syndrome Foundation. (2016b). *What is Rett syndrome?* Retrieved from http://www.rettsyndrome.org.

Krakowiak, P., Walker, C., Bremer, A., et al. (2012). Maternal metabolic conditions and risk for autism and other neurodevelopmental disorders. *Pediatrics*, *129*(5), e1121–e1128.

Lee, B. (2016). Down syndrome and other abnormalities of chromosome number. In R. Kliegman, B. Stanton, J. St. Geme, et al. (Eds.), *Nelson textbook of pediatrics* (20th ed., Chapter 81.2). St. Louis MO: Elsevier.

McLean, H., & Price, D. (2016). Failure to thrive. In R. Kliegman, B. Stanton, J. St. Geme, et al. (Eds.), *Nelson textbook of pediatrics* (20th ed., Chapter 41). St. Louis MO: Elsevier.

March of Dimes. (2014). *Fragile X syndrome*. Retrieved from http://www.marchofdimes.org.

March of Dimes. (2016). *Down syndrome*. Retrieved from http://www.marchofdimes.org.

National Dissemination Center for Children With Disabilities. (2011). *Intellectual disabilities*. Retrieved from www.nichcy.org.

National Down Syndrome Society. (2012). *About the NDSS advocacy and policy center*. Retrieved from http://www.ndss.org.

National Institute of Environmental Health Sciences. (2011). *AARA investments in autism*. Retrieved from http://www.niehs.nih.gov/health/topics/conditions/autism/.

National Fragile X Foundation. (n.d.). *Testing for fragile X*. Retrieved from https://fragilex.org.

Pinto-Martin, J., Levy, S., & Feldman, J. (2011). Prevalence of autism spectrum disorders in adolescents born weighing less than 2000 grams. *Pediatrics*, *128*(5), 883–891.

Raviola, G., Trieu, M., DeMaso, D., et al. (2016). Autism spectrum disorder. In R. Kliegman, B. Stanton, J. St. Geme, et al. (Eds.), *Nelson textbook of pediatrics* (20th ed., Chapter 30). St. Louis MO: Elsevier.

Sadock, B., Sadock, V.A., & Ruiz, P. (2015). *Kaplan & Saddock's synopsis of psychiatry: Behavioral sciences/clinical psychiatry* (11th ed.). Philadelphia: Lippincott Williams & Wilkins.

Sebat, J., Lakshmi, B., & Malhotra, D. (2007). Strong association of de novo copy number mutations with autism. *Science*, *316*, 445–449.

Sirotnak, A. (2016). *Failure to thrive*. Retrieved from www.emedicine.medscape.com/article/915575.

United States Department of Education. (2016). *Ideas that work: Preparing children and youth with disabilities for success*. Retrieved from http://ccrs.osepideasthatwork.org.

United States Department of Health and Human Services. (n.d.). *Alzheimer's and Down Syndrome*. Retrieved from www.alzheimers.acl.gov.

U.S. Department of Health and Human Services. (2010). *Healthy people 2020*. Retrieved from http://www.healthypeople.gov.

Williams, J.F., & Smith, V.C. (2015). Fetal alcohol spectrum disorders. *Pediatrics*, *136*(5), e1395–e1406.

World Down Syndrome Day. (2016). *About WDSD*. Retrieved from http://www.worlddownsyndromeday.org.

# 55

# The Child With a Sensory Alteration

http://evolve.elsevier.com/McKinney/mat-ch/

## LEARNING OBJECTIVES

*After studying this chapter, you should be able to:*

- Describe the structure and function of the eye and ear.
- Describe the specific information required in a health history for a child with potential sensory alterations.
- Define the nurse's role in assessing for sensory alterations.
- Describe specific nursing care for children with health problems affecting the eye and ear.
- Describe how alterations in the sensory organs affect the child's ability to communicate.
- Identify potential growth and development interruptions that may occur with problems affecting the sensory organs.

## CLINICAL REFERENCE

## REVIEW OF THE EYE

### Structure and Function

The eye is attached to the skull by six accessory muscles. These muscles are used to move the eye to achieve vision. Ciliary muscles function to alter the shape of the eye to provide focus and accommodation at various distances. Cranial nerves II, III, IV, V, and VI all affect the eye (see Chapter 33 for cranial nerve assessment).

The orb, or eye, is made up of several parts. The cornea is the clear area located in the front of the eye, where light enters. The cornea and sclera (white outer covering) make up the eye's outer layer. The middle layer is composed of the choroid (vascular lining), the lens (a clear structure that changes shape to allow accommodation of light on the retina), and the iris (the colored muscular ring located behind the cornea that expands or contracts to control the amount of light entering the eye). The inner layer of the eye is known as the *retina.* This area contains the rods and cones. These receive light impulses and transmit them through the optic nerve (cranial nerve II) to the brain. The macula contains the greatest concentration of nerve endings. The cornea and lens focus light onto the macula. The optic disk is the area where the optic nerve enters the eye.

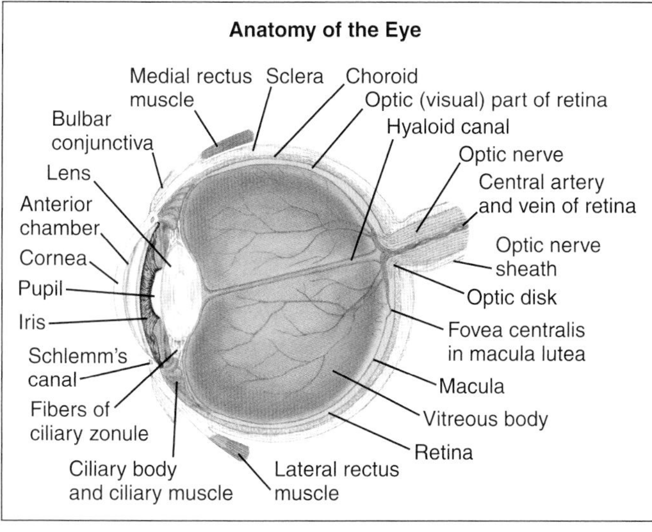


### Neonatal Development

The eyes begin to develop at approximately 22 days of gestation. The critical period for development is from days 22 to 50. Congenital abnormalities can be caused by either genetic or environmental factors or by a combination of the two. The eye is especially sensitive to teratogens, as in infections such as cytomegalovirus and rubella.

## REVIEW OF THE EAR

### Structure and Function

The ear is divided into three parts: the outer, middle, and inner ear. The outer ear includes the auricle and external ear canal. It is separated from the middle ear by the tympanic membrane (eardrum). The tympanic membrane vibrates to conduct sound waves to the middle ear. The middle ear contains the bones of hearing—the malleus (hammer), incus (anvil), and stapes (stirrup). These bones conduct sound waves from the tympanic membrane to the inner ear. The inner ear contains the nerve endings that conduct sound impulses to the brain. These nerve endings are located in a snail-shaped chamber (the cochlea) that is filled with fluid. The inner ear also controls balance. The eustachian tube connects the middle ear to the nasopharynx. It allows fluids to drain into the nasopharynx and assists in equalizing pressure between the outer ear and the middle ear.

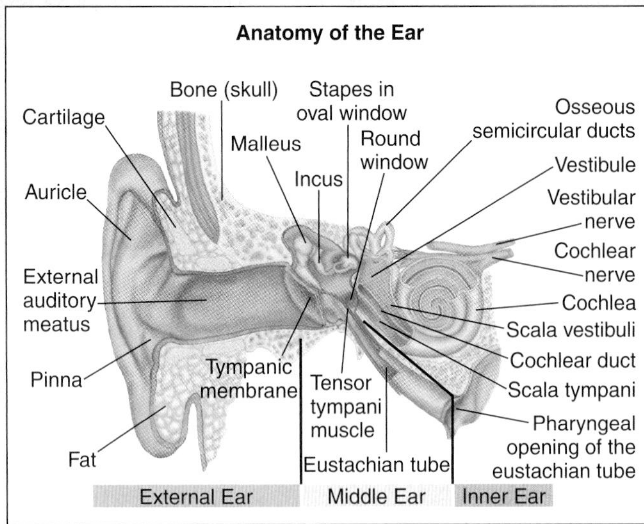


### Neonatal Development

The ear begins to develop during the 3rd week of gestation. The critical period for the development of the ear is between 4 and 6 weeks of gestation. Like the eye, the ear is highly sensitive to teratogens. It is innervated by the acoustic nerve (cranial nerve VIII). Congenital deafness is largely the result of genetic factors.

## SPEECH DEVELOPMENT

Because the fetus is capable of hearing during the second trimester of pregnancy and is able to hear voices and the mother's heartbeat, the infant is born with a sensitivity to variations in speech. Adequate hearing is essential for the development of speech. The infant begins to coo and vocalize quite early (birth to 4 months). Babbling begins at approximately 4 to 6 months. Babbling is followed by receptive language development (understanding words) and expressive language development (saying words; see Chapters 6 through 9 for specifics of speech development). Any hearing impairment can interfere with speech development, as can any alteration affecting the oral cavity.

### Pediatric Differences in Sensory Function

#### *Vision*

- Development of the eye is not complete at birth, but the newborn is able to fixate, follow an object to midline, and react to a change in intensity of light.
- By 3 months of age, the infant can follow moving objects; by 4 months of age, the infant can recognize familiar objects.
- Binocularity, the ability to fixate on one visual field with both eyes, is not present at birth but is established by 6 months of age. Frequent eye-crossing after 6 months of age is abnormal and indicates strabismus.
- Visual acuity changes with age:
  4 months 20/50 to 20/80
  1 year 20/40 to 20/70
  4 years 20/30 to 20/40
  5 years 20/20 to 20/30
- Lacrimal glands are not fully developed at birth. Tears are not often present with crying until after 1 to 3 months. Temporary obstruction of lacrimal ducts may cause overflow of tears.
- The size of the orbits doubles by the time the child is 1 year of age and doubles again by age 6 years. Eye growth is completed at 10 to 12 years of age.

#### Hearing

- Development of the ear begins during the 3rd week of gestation and is complete by the third month of embryonic life. Infection or other insult to the fetus during this time can cause irreparable damage to the ear. Ear development occurs at the same time as kidney development, so malformation in one system may indicate problems in the other.
- An infant as young as 3 days is able to distinguish between familiar and unfamiliar sounds and can recognize the mother's voice. The infant can distinguish between frequently heard words and other words (nonsense language) by 1 year.
- Basic auditory skills are in place by 3 years of age. Hearing can be evaluated by audiometry testing by this age.
- Infants and young children have shorter, more horizontal, and more flaccid eustachian tubes, predisposing them to otitis media.

#### Speech and Language

- Infants can imitate sounds heard by 3 to 5 months of age.
- Verbal dialogue similar to an adult's is noted by approximately 6 months of age.

Because a child learns so much through the senses, deficits in hearing and vision can have profound effects on development. Appropriate screening and early interventions are crucial. Early identification of vision and hearing deficits allows for early intervention—either correction or the provision of adaptive measures—to facilitate the child's "normal" growth and development. Because a child cannot report sensory deficits, nurses must carefully assess for vision or hearing alterations.

U.S. legislation PL 94-142 (Education for All Handicapped Children Act), passed in 1975 and subsequently updated as the Individuals with Disabilities Education Act (see Chapter 54), mandates special education services for children with severe sensory deficits. Identifying children at a young age who might be eligible for special educational services is important to maximize their education.

The health history of a child with a potential sensory deficit is essentially the same as for any child (see Chapter 33) but should include the following additional pieces of information:

- Thorough prenatal history
- Growth and developmental history
- History of any infections (including treatment, because many medications can cause sensory deficits)
- History of previous trauma to the eye or ear
- Changes noted in behavior (e.g., rubbing the eyes, turning up the volume on the television, decreased attention span)
- Changes in appearance (e.g., red, inflamed eyes; drainage from the eye or ear)
- Physical symptoms (e.g., reports of ear or eye pain, headache, nausea, and vomiting)

After carefully reviewing the health history, the nurse performs a thorough physical examination with age-appropriate measures of vision and hearing acuity (see Chapter 33).

## DISORDERS OF THE EYE

The nurse has an important role in the prevention and early detection of eye problems. All children should have sensitive and specific vision screening performed at well visits. The American Academy of Pediatrics (AAP), American Association of Certified Orthoptists, American Academy of Ophthalmology, American Association for Pediatric Ophthalmology and Strabismus, and Children's Eye Foundation (Donahue & Baker, 2016 a,b) recommend the following assessments:

- *At birth:* External and internal appearance for structural abnormalities, red reflex, fixation; family history of congenital eye disorders, as well as family history of amblyopia and strabismus
- *Age 3 to 6 months:* Fixation and ability to follow, alignment (cover/uncover test, corneal light reflex, photo screening)
- *Birth to 3 years:* All of the above with ocular history, instrument screening (photoscreening, autorefraction); may begin visual acuity testing at 10 feet if cooperative

The United States Preventive Services Task Force (USPSTF) (2011), along with the previously mentioned organizations (Donahue & Baker, 2016 a,b) recommend the following for older children:

*Age 3 years and older:* All of the above plus visual acuity using developmentally appropriate charts (HOTV matching test, LEA symbols) and ophthalmoscopy; stereopsis can be tested by using the random dot E test (see Chapter 33). Current recommendations for testing visual acuity and screening for amblyopia include the use of "crowding bars" on visual acuity charts. These are bars that surround each symbol and are sensitive for assessing amblyopia (Donahue & Baker, 2016a). Additionally, beginning the screening using the line the child would be expected to see according to age (critical line screening), rather than threshold screening (beginning with a large symbol and working down) provides more rapid screening and reduces attention distraction. For children who are uncooperative or who are otherwise unable to participate in traditional vision screening, photoscreening or autorefraction may be used. Neither of these procedures measures visual acuity, but both measure errors in refraction, and can determine when referral to a specialist is necessary. Photoscreening (photo refractive screening), a process of photographing images of eye light reflexes, can easily detect a variety of eye problems in young children. Photoscreening is particularly useful for detecting refractive errors, strabismus, and other conditions that contribute to amblyopia (Schwartz, Schuman, & Wei, 2014). Autorefraction is the process for estimating refractive error using ultrasound methods (Cotter et al., 2015). Photoscreening and autorefraction equipment are available in hand-held devices, which are easier to use in an outpatient setting, and smart phone applications are becoming more available (Schwartz et al., 2014). Refer children who do not pass structural or vision screening for complete ophthalmologic evaluation. Careful attention to behavior and appearance changes, as well as physical symptoms, assists in the early detection and treatment of eye disorders (Box 55.1). Children who have any symptoms should be referred for further evaluation.

### BOX 55.1 Signs and Symptoms of Potential Vision Problems

- Inability to fix both eyes on an object and follow the track of a moving object with both eyes
- Persistent discharge from one or both eyes, especially accompanied by redness of the sclera
- Excessive tearing, especially when accompanied by itchiness or pain
- Cloudiness or white areas in the pupil
- Deviation of the iris in an inward or outward direction (crossing)
- Head tilting or closing one eye to see
- Squinting
- Reports of headache or blurred or double vision
- The need to sit close to a television or blackboard to see
- Holding reading material close to the eyes
- Excessive fatigue with visual concentration

### ! NURSING QUALITY ALERT

**_Vision Screening_**

- Thoroughly explain the procedure to the child before beginning. If using a symbol chart (HOTV or LEA), show the child the symbols, and ask the child to identify or match them. If using a machine to test the child's vision, demonstrate in advance how it works.
- Take the child to a quiet, nondistracting area that has been marked for the appropriate distance from the chart (shorter distances for younger children).
- Have the child cover one eye. Use a colorful, opaque cover that completely blocks the child's vision. The parent can help hold the cover in place.

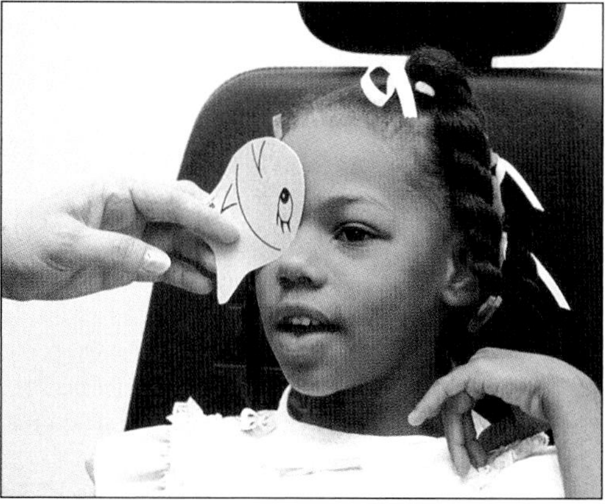

- Point to a symbol on the line a child of that age would be expected to see (critical line screening). Vary the direction (left to right, right to left) to reduce the likelihood that the child is memorizing the symbols.
- Give positive feedback. Perform the test as quickly as possible because small children lose interest quickly.
- Test both eyes. Refer for further evaluation if there is a discrepancy in two lines or if the child tests in the abnormal range on two successive screenings.

### Nursing Considerations for the Child With a Blocked Lacrimal Duct

A blocked lacrimal (tear) duct is characterized by excessive tearing (epiphora) and crusting on the eyelids on awakening. Parents may also note a small mass just below the inner aspect of the eye. Treatment usually consists of massaging the duct. If the duct remains blocked despite massaging or remains blocked after 1 year of age, the surgical opening of the duct is indicated.

The nurse should carefully assess the mucoid drainage. In a noninfected duct, the drainage is usually white or clear. However, if the duct has become infected, the drainage may be green or yellow. If the

**TABLE 55.1 Types of Refractive Disorders**

| Description | Clinical Manifestations | Treatment |
|---|---|---|
| **Myopia** | | |
| Nearsightedness | Difficulty seeing the blackboard or television clearly | Treated with biconcave lenses |
| Ability to see close objects more clearly than those at a distance | Decreased interest in activities requiring distance vision | New lenses may be required every 1-2 yr as the child grows |
| Caused by the image focusing in front of the retina | Squinting, head tilting, holding books close to eyes<br>Decreased attention span, poor school performance | |
| **Hyperopia** | | |
| Farsightedness | Most children are normally hyperopic until approximately 7 yr of age but are able to accommodate to see clearly | Most young children with hyperopia need no correction |
| Ability to see distant objects more clearly than those close up | | |
| Caused by the image focusing beyond the retina | Strabismus or amblyopia can develop from prolonged hyperopia | If correction is required, convex lenses are used |
| **Astigmatism** | | |
| Unequal curvature of the cornea or the lens causing light rays to bend in different directions | Mild astigmatism may be asymptomatic<br>Manifestations may be similar to myopia | Treated with special lenses to compensate for the unequal curvature of the cornea |
| May coexist with myopia or hyperopia | | |

drainage suggests an infected duct, treatment with antibiotic eyedrops or ointment is indicated.

The nurse teaches the parent about the proper technique for lacrimal massage. This process involves washing hands thoroughly and placing the index finger over the lacrimal duct (at the inner aspect of the eye by the bridge of the nose) and "milking," or gently massaging, the duct in an upward motion. Emphasize that massaging down the nasal bone has very little effect on the duct because the lacrimal system is intraosseous and unaffected by massage over bone. Other teaching includes monitoring for signs and symptoms of infection.

## Nursing Considerations for the Child With a Refractive Error

Refractive errors cause vision disturbances from alterations in the path of light rays through the eye. They usually result from an abnormally shaped orb; the orb may be flattened or elongated (Table 55.1). Refractive errors are often discovered when a child squints, frowns, or moves objects so they are more easily seen. Reports from the child or a teacher can also alert parents. *Legal blindness* is defined as a correction of 20/200 or worse in the better eye or a visual field of 20 degrees or less.

Nurses should assess children's vision at every well-child visit, particularly during the preschool years. Visual acuity can be reliably tested in a cooperative child as young as 3 years. When testing visual acuity, the nurse should remember that a vision discrepancy of two lines or more on the vision chart, even if one eye tests normal, is cause for referral. A child with this discrepancy could have *anisometropia*, a large refractive discrepancy between the eyes. If not corrected, this condition can lead to amblyopia.

School nurses routinely test children's vision and, in fact, annual vision screening is offered to children throughout the United States. The U.S. Preventive Services Task Force (2011) has recommended that vision screening begin early in the preschool years (at 3 years of age) to identify amblyopia and other associated vision alterations. Several states in the United States mandate that a child have an approved vision screening test (administered by a trained examiner) within the year before entering kindergarten. The HOTV matching test and LEA symbols are comparatively effective as screening measures for preschool age children (Donahue & Baker, 2016a). School nurses have used various methods of notifying families of children who do not pass a school vision screening (e.g., telephone call to parents, letter brought home by the child, letter mailed home). Ultimately, the parent is responsible for follow-through with a visit to a specialist. Nurses should be aware that some parents, for a variety of reasons, do not take the child for a follow-up comprehensive eye examination; for this reason, nurses in other settings must ask for details about the child's vision and previous vision testing.

Corrective lenses are used to improve the child's vision. Encourage the parent to look for impact-resistant eyeglasses with spring-loaded frames, which are less likely to bend or warp. Fitting glasses to an infant or young child can be challenging; the goal is to choose shatter-resistant lenses in a type of frame that can be closely fitted to prevent easy dislodging during activity. Infant frames often have elasticized straps to keep them properly positioned. Teach the parent and child, if appropriate, to always store the glasses in a case when not being used. Special directions for cleaning must be followed to avoid scratching the lenses.

Both gas-permeable and soft contact lenses provide an alternative for children old enough and responsible enough to care for contacts independently. The nurse should teach parents and children about appropriate care of corrective lenses and how to recognize and intervene with vision problems early.

Protective eyewear made of shatterproof polycarbonate should be worn by all who participate in sports that pose a risk for eye injury. A variety of prescription sports glasses are available for athletes; glasses chosen should adhere to the standards of the American Society of Testing and Materials. Cracked or old eyewear should be discarded and replaced. Protective eyewear should be selected according to the sport and the relative risk for injury (American Academy of Ophthalmology, 2016).

## Nursing Considerations for the Child With Color Deficiency

Colorblindness, or color deficiency, occurs in approximately 8% of the population and is nearly 20 times more prevalent in males (Albany-Ward & Sobande, 2015). Color deficiency is the genetic result of an alteration in the X-chromosome, which results in the brain's inability to discriminate various light wave lengths associated with colors (Albany-Ward & Sobande, 2015). It interferes with the ability to distinguish between colors within certain groups, such as red, blue, and green, and can contribute to learning difficulties.

Testing should be done if the clinician suspects a problem (i.e., a suspected optic nerve or retinal dysfunction) or the family has a history of color deficiency. Testing is routine in preschool boys. The most common detection test is the pseudoisochromatic (color confusion) test, in which color plates include patterns that are hidden to a person with a color deficit. Pseudoisochromatic plates are also available for children who cannot yet read. If a problem is detected, more sophisticated testing may be necessary to determine the exact type of color deficiency. Although color deficiency has no cure, certain types of tints used in contact lenses and glasses can help the child discriminate color differences.

Because color deficiency cannot be cured, nursing care focuses on adaptive and supportive measures. Encourage parents to have children tested if the family has a history of color deficiency or if the nurse suspects the child is having trouble distinguishing colors.

Parent and child education is important for the child with color deficiency. Teaching should focus on alternative ways to discriminate the deficient colors. For the older child who can dress without assistance, clothes can be labeled or organized so that items can be easily coordinated.

Safety is a major concern for the color-deficient child. For example, the child who cannot distinguish red and green must learn another way to distinguish traffic signals and other warning lights. Finally, anticipatory guidance is sometimes related to appropriate career choices. For example, color deficiency might prohibit an adult from becoming a pilot, police officer, or firefighter.

## Nursing Considerations for the Child With Amblyopia

Amblyopia, or "lazy eye," one of the most frequent causes of diminished vision in children, results from a variety of eye alterations seen in children whose visual acuity is impaired. The prevalence of amblyopia is between 2% and 4% in children (USPSTF, 2011). When both eyes are unable to focus simultaneously, the brain suppresses the image from the deviating eye to avoid double vision (diplopia). Amblyopia frequently accompanies strabismus, as well as other eye conditions such as congenital cataract and severe refractive error. If the underlying eye condition is untreated in a child younger than 4 years (the critical period for development of the visual cortex), permanent loss of vision from amblyopia can result; amblyopia can be treated in the older child but is more resistant to treatment at that time (Olitsky, Hug, Plummer, et al., 2016). Because the child loses binocular vision, depth perception might also be impaired. Early detection and treatment of strabismus or other underlying causes of amblyopia are essential to prevent loss of vision.

Two primary approaches, penalization (blurring) and occlusion, are used to correct amblyopia. Both approaches are designed to alter or obscure vision in the stronger eye to force the child to use the amblyopic eye. Atropine, which is a cycloplegic (paralyzes the ciliary muscles to dilate the eye), most often is used to blur the vision in the stronger eye. Wearing eyeglasses in which the lens over the stronger eye creates blurring has a similar effect.

Wearing lenses corrective for refraction error can improve amblyopia in some children (Stewart, Moseley, & Fielder, 2011) and is the first step in treating amblyopia (Olitsky et al, 2016). Patching combined with the use of corrective lenses has been demonstrated to have better outcomes than wearing corrective lenses alone for treating amblyopia caused by strabismus (Taylor & Elliott, 2011). Patching is used most often during the preschool years, when the visual cortex is developing. In this treatment, the normal eye is patched so that the child is forced to use the weaker eye. The schedule for patching is individualized. Because many children resist patching, the patching regimen recently has been reduced to only a few hours over a 24-hour period (Olitsky et al., 2016; Tailor et al., 2015). The patching regimen is prescribed by the ophthalmologist. Cooperation with the patching regimen is essential. Teaching should explain the reasons for patching or corrective lenses, the expected results of wearing the patch or lens, correct placement of the patch, the number of hours per day the patch or lens is to be worn, and the expected length of treatment (see Patient-Centered Teaching: Information about Eye Patching). The child should be taught that wearing the patch or lens is not negotiable. The nurse often must teach parents strategies for dealing with resistant behaviors.

### PATIENT-CENTERED TEACHING

#### *Information About Eye Patching*

- Your child will need to wear the eye patch for the exact time your physician has prescribed. Not adhering to the full wearing time could interfere with the treatment.
- Prescribed patching will not harm your child's stronger eye but will force the muscles of the weaker eye to be used.
- Apply the patch directly to your child's face, being sure to cover the whole eye. Do not leave any openings through which the child can peek.
- If your child wears eyeglasses as well, put the glasses on over the patch.
- It can be frustrating for the child to have to wear the patch. Try to be patient, understanding, and supportive. Patching must be nonnegotiable. Find decorative patches or put your own decoration on the patch. Praise your child frequently for cooperating with the treatment.

A newer, more acceptable, approach to managing amblyopia in children involves playing specially designed video games (Li et al, 2014; Tailor et al., 2015). Eyewear worn while playing the game alters the contrast (sharpness) in the better eye to balance with the amblyopic eye, thus creating binocular vision (Li et al., 2014). In preliminary studies, evidence suggests that visual acuity improves fairly rapidly (over a four-week time frame) and is maintained for at least three months thereafter. Randomized controlled studies are needed to demonstrate the long-term effect (Tailor et al., 2015)

## Nursing Considerations for the Child With Strabismus

Strabismus is a condition in which the eyes are not aligned because of a lack of coordination of the extraocular muscles. This condition occurs in approximately 4% of children younger than 6 years (Olitsky et al., 2016). Strabismus is most often caused by muscle imbalance or paralysis of the extraocular muscles but can also result from conditions such as a brain tumor, myasthenia gravis, or infection. Infants and children with strabismus often have a close relative with the condition. Other contributing factors include genetic abnormalities, neuromuscular disease, exposure to teratogens, and trauma; the prevalence is higher in children who were born prematurely or who were of low birth weight (American Academy of Ophthalmology [AAO], 2012). The type of deviation noted defines strabismus (Box 55.2). When assessing infants for strabismus, the nurse should remember that strabismus is normal in the young infant but not in those over approximately 3 months of age.

The corneal light reflex test, simultaneous red reflex test, cover-uncover test, and alternate-cover test (see Chapter 33) are used in the diagnosis of strabismus. The nurse should suspect strabismus when the child reports frequent headaches, squints, or tilts the head to see. The parent might suspect something is wrong when a flash photograph

## BOX 55.2 Types of Strabismus

- *Comitant strabismus:* Most common type of strabismus in children. Constant deviation in all fields of gaze; not associated with eye muscle paralysis. All extraocular muscles function but are not coordinated. Child has difficulty seeing at close range and often squints. Accommodative nonparalytic strabismus may develop between 2 and 4 years of age as a result of a large refractive error.
- *Paralytic strabismus:* Caused by a weakness or paralysis of one or more of the extraocular muscles. Usually involves dysfunction of one or more cranial nerves involved with ocular movement. The eye appears crossed when turned in the direction of the affected muscle. Can cause headache and poor coordination. Diplopia may cause child to close one eye or tilt the head.
- *Esotropia (convergent):* The eye turns inward; most common type of strabismus in infants. Can occur with hyperopia as the eyes compensate for the refractive error by overconvergence.

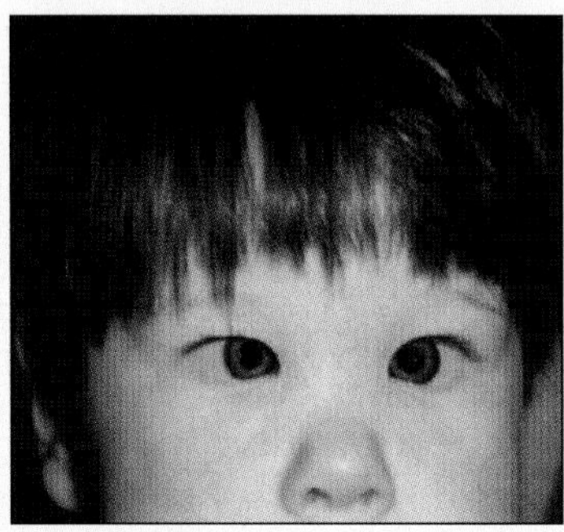

Child with early onset esotropia. The deviation may not be apparent until age 3 or 4 months.

- *Exotropia (divergent):* The eyes turn away from the midline; occurs most often when the child attempts to focus on a distant object. May be present at birth.

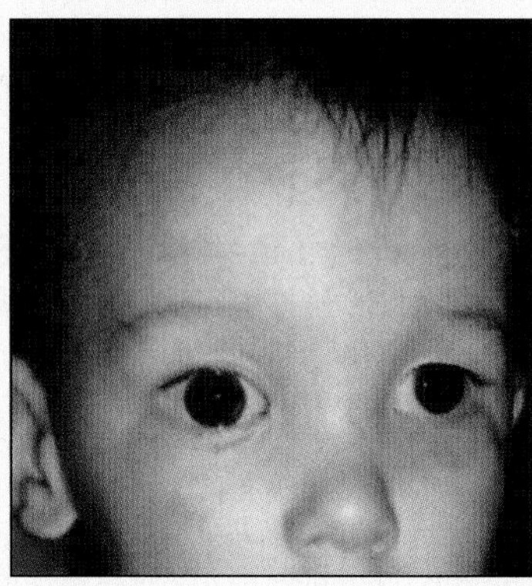

Child with left exotropia. Most exodeviations in childhood are intermittent.

- *Pseudostrabismus:* Not true strabismus. The eyes appear to deviate inward but are actually in alignment. Facial features, such as epicanthal folds and a broad, flat nasal bridge, can give the appearance of misalignment.
- *Phoria:* A tendency for the eye to deviate. More evident during times of stress, fatigue, or illness.
- *Tropia:* A continuous or intermittent misalignment of the eye.

Photographs from Albert, D.M., & Jacobiec, F.A. (1994). (Eds.). *Principles and practice of ophthalmology* (pp. 2731, 2733). Philadelphia, PA: Saunders.

of the child reveals unequal "red eye." Children who have family members with strabismus should be regularly assessed for development of the condition. Strabismus can contribute to amblyopia in the infant or young child.

Treatment of strabismus may include special corrective lenses, vision therapy, surgery, or pharmacologic therapy; the goal is to initiate treatment as early as possible to preserve vision and reduce the risk for amblyopia. If the deviation is caused by hyperopia, corrective lenses are indicated to correct vision. Eyeglasses with specially ground prism power might also be indicated. These glasses correct vision in the affected eye so that the brain receives the same image from both eyes.

Botulinum toxin (Botox) is one approach to treating strabismus. The toxin is injected into the eye muscle to produce temporary paralysis. This condition allows the muscles opposite the paralyzed muscle to straighten the eye. With successful treatment, the correction remains after the medication wears off (in approximately 2 months). The most common side effect is a drooping eyelid (ptosis), which usually resolves spontaneously.

Surgery might be indicated to realign the weakened muscles in a child with strabismus, most often when amblyopia is present. In this case, the surgery should be performed before the child is 2 years of age. The stronger eye can be patched before surgery to treat any existing amblyopia. Surgery might be required on the weakened eye only or on both eyes. More than one surgery is sometimes necessary. During the surgery, small incisions are made, and the weakened muscles are tightened or the stronger muscles are weakened and lengthened (AAO, 2013).

If the child is to have a surgical correction, the nurse should prepare the child and parents before surgery for what to expect after surgery and provide information about dressing changes, eye drops, corrective lenses, and any other required postoperative treatments. Interventions are similar to those for any child having eye surgery.

### Nursing Considerations for the Child With Glaucoma

Glaucoma is a condition in which the intraocular fluid pressure of the eye is increased. If left untreated, this increased pressure leads to atrophy of the optic disk and, ultimately, blindness. Glaucoma is a significant cause of blindness in children (Bhate &Wang, 2015).

Several types of glaucoma occur in children. **Congenital glaucoma**, often called infantile glaucoma, occurs during the first 3 years of life and is caused by a defect in the drainage network of the eye. Primary congenital glaucoma has a genetic origin, with an autosomal recessive inheritance pattern. **Secondary glaucoma**, which can be accompanied by other ocular anomalies, refers to disease that occurs after 3 years of age and results from an inherited disease (juvenile glaucoma) or is acquired from infection, trauma, or cataract removal (acquired glaucoma) (Olitsky et al., 2016).

Clinical signs of glaucoma include excessive tearing, light sensitivity, blepharospasm (muscle spasm causing involuntary closing of the eyelid), and enlargement of the globe and cornea. Parents often note excessive tearing or corneal haziness caused by edema and bring the child in for clinical evaluation. The child might also be brought to the practitioner for what appears to be conjunctivitis ("pink eye").

Physical examination includes an assessment of visual acuity, measurement of intraocular pressure (tonometry), assessment of corneal diameter and clarity, and an examination of the retina to assess for optic nerve cupping. Any infant with a visible iris diameter greater than 10.5 mm should be evaluated. If retinal edema is present, the light reflex is diffuse. Because young children may not be able to cooperate during an examination, they are often sedated. However, intraocular pressure should be measured only under light sedation because deeper sedation may alter readings (either high or low, depending on the agent used).

The preferred treatment for childhood glaucoma is surgery. Surgery should be performed as soon as possible after diagnosis to prevent loss (or further loss) of vision. The goal of surgery is to increase the outflow of the aqueous humor from the anterior chamber by correcting the structural abnormality causing the decreased outflow or to create a different route for the outflow (trabeculotomy) (Bhate & Wang, 2015). Medications such as cholinergic agents, beta-adrenergic blocking agents, or adrenergic agents may be indicated after surgery to maintain low intraocular pressure; however, these drugs can have systemic side effects, so the child must be watched carefully (Bhate & Wang, 2015).

The prognosis varies from child to child. With prompt treatment, most children attain appropriate vision, although repeated surgeries might be necessary. Decreased vision can result from damage to the optic nerve, opacity of the cornea or lens, or amblyopia resulting from refractive errors. Children with glaucoma must be followed closely over the long term to quickly identify any rise in intraocular pressure.

Nursing interventions are similar to those for any child having eye surgery. Postoperative nursing care includes monitoring for signs and symptoms of increased intraocular pressure (pain, nausea and vomiting, increased inflammation) and administering any ordered medications, such as miotic eyedrops (used to constrict the pupils) and antibiotic ointments or eyedrops. If the child's eyes are patched, the nurse pays special attention to the resulting sensory deficits. The nurse also considers safety to be an issue when eyes are patched.

Parental education is essential to maintain the appropriate intraocular pressure and prevent complications (including blindness). Education includes the use of any prescribed medications, patching, and any other measures designed to correct refractive errors. The importance of returning for follow-up care should be emphasized. The child and caregivers should also be taught signs and symptoms of increasing intraocular pressure. Any signs of increasing intraocular pressure or infection should be immediately reported to the ophthalmologist. Because certain types of glaucoma can be related to genetic abnormalities, referral for genetic counseling may be indicated.

### Nursing Considerations for the Child With a Cataract

A cataract is an opacity, or loss of transparency, of the lens. Causes include an inherited tendency (usually an autosomal dominant trait), infection (e.g., rubella), trauma, or a metabolic imbalance; the cause of the majority of congenital cataracts is unknown (Patel et al., 2014). Cloudiness of the lens may be noted during examination in the newborn nursery (indicated by a white instead of red reflex) or by the parents. Ophthalmoscopy may reveal a dark spot in the lens. Parents sometimes note that the infant exhibits visual inattentiveness and come in for an evaluation. Other clinical signs include nystagmus and strabismus. The cataract alters vision because it does not allow a sharp, clear image to be formed on the retina.

Treatment for cataracts in most instances is the surgical removal of the opaque lens as soon as possible and optimally within eight weeks of age (Patel et al., 2014). The resultant hyperopia is then dealt with by using a contact lens or, in older children, an intraocular lens implant. Any resulting amblyopia must also be addressed. Glasses may also be used to correct the resultant vision problem, although these can be difficult to manage in infants and small children (Olitsky et al., 2016; Patel et al., 2014).

Amblyopia can be a consequence of congenital cataract. In this case, the normal eye may be patched after surgery to develop the weakened eye.

Postoperative interventions are directed toward avoiding increased intraocular pressure. Measures include preventing coughing, straining, vomiting, and touching the surgical site. A patch and "hard shield" are usually in place after surgery to prevent injury to the surgical site. To prevent edema and pressure on the site, the nurse should elevate the head of the bed slightly and position the child so that the affected eye is not in a dependent position. Assess the child for signs and symptoms of infection (fever, drainage, redness). Medications, including antibiotics, mydriatics, and steroids, may be used after surgery.

Postoperative teaching includes how to insert, remove, and care for the child's contact lens. Parents need to be taught the signs and symptoms of infection and increasing intraocular pressure. To provide visual stimulation to the affected eye and prevent further loss of vision, the importance of adhering to any prescribed patching regimen should also be emphasized. Finally, the nurse teaches the importance of returning for follow-up visits to ensure that the lens fits correctly, the vision correction is appropriate, and no signs and symptoms of complications are present. As with glaucoma, the occurrence of some cataracts has a genetic component, so referral for genetic counseling may be indicated.

## EYE SURGERY

Several eye disorders, as mentioned previously, that are seen in infancy and childhood require surgical correction. Any surgical procedure is stressful for the child and family. Eye surgery is particularly stressful because the child's visual fields or acuity may be greatly reduced or absent for a period. If both eyes are affected, the child's ability to maneuver and perform activities of daily living independently is also affected.

The nurse should pay special attention to education. If the child is going home with patches, drops, or any other procedure that must be performed, the family needs to know how to perform this care and should also know the safety precautions involved.

## NURSING CARE PLAN

### *The Child Having Eye Surgery*

**Focused Assessment**

- Determine the child's and family's understanding of the planned surgical procedure and why surgery is necessary; include assessment of their knowledge of post-surgical and discharge care.
- Assess the child's and family's knowledge of strategies to maintain safety for a child who has a visual deficit.
- Assess potential discharge teaching needs.

**Nursing Diagnosis**

Disturbed Sensory Perception (visual impairment) related to eye patching or surgical procedure.

**Planning**

***Expected Outcomes***

1. The child and family will describe any anticipated temporary vision changes.
2. The child and family will demonstrate familiarity with the surroundings and associated sights and sounds.
3. The child will remain alert and oriented to time and place.

**Interventions and *Rationales***

1. Prepare the child and family before surgery for any changes expected in vision, including blurred vision or patched eyes.

*Continued*

## NURSING CARE PLAN—cont'd

### *The Child Having Eye Surgery*

*Preoperative preparation allows the child and family to know what to expect, thus lessening anxiety.*

2. Before surgery, orient the child and family to the surroundings, including the recovery room and hospital room. Describe any unfamiliar sounds the child may hear; have the child close his or her eyes and listen.
   *Preoperative orientation to surroundings allows the child a feeling of familiarity during the postoperative period.*
3. Provide reality orientation (time, day) for the child during the postoperative period, especially if vision is impaired or eyes are patched.
   *Providing a sense of time passage and orienting to day and night prevent the child from becoming disoriented and confused.*
4. Provide emotional support and allow expression of feelings of anger and frustration, possibly through play therapy and therapeutic communication.
   *Allowing the child and family to express their fears and frustrations provides an appropriate outlet and encourages the use of other senses.*

**Evaluation**

Can the child and family describe expected temporary postoperative vision changes?

Can the child describe the hospital and room environment and its associated sounds?

Does the child remain alert and oriented to time and place?

**Nursing Diagnosis**

Risk for Injury related to increased intraocular pressure resulting from bleeding, edema, hematoma, postoperative vomiting.

**Planning**

***Expected Outcome***

The child will remain free from injury (increased intraocular pressure, bleeding) through appropriate management of postoperative eye care, crying, nausea, and vomiting.

**Interventions and *Rationales***

1. Fully orient the child to surroundings and ensure that unsafe objects are removed from the environment.
   *Orienting the child to the environment and ensuring that the environment is safe prevents falls and other injuries when the child is out of bed.*
2. Ensure that the child wears eye patches or shields as ordered.
   *Eye patches and shields are often prescribed to prevent any further injury to the eye.*
3. Encourage the parents to remain with the child and to prevent the child from rubbing the eyes. Restraints are used as a last resort to prevent injury. Encourage the parent to keep side rails up at all times.
   *Rubbing the eyes can damage the surgical site. If restraints are needed, elbow restraints provide protection without total restriction.*
4. Monitor for signs and symptoms of increased intraocular pressure. Give ordered antiemetics if the child is nauseated. Administer intravenous fluids until the child is stable.
   *Increasing intraocular pressure can damage the eye and seriously impair vision. Vomiting can increase intraocular pressure.*
5. Approach the child in a calm and soothing manner. Assign personnel whom the child has met and trusts. Encourage the parent to soothe the child who is crying.
   *Avoidance of crying postoperatively reduces the risk of increasing intraocular pressure. Assigning the child to a familiar nurse reduces fear and anxiety that may lead to crying.*

**Evaluation**

Does the child remain free of physical injury?

Is the child's intraocular pressure within normal limits?

Is the child free from crying, nausea, and vomiting?

**Nursing Diagnosis**

Risk for Infection related to surgical incision.

**Planning**

***Expected Outcome***

The child will remain free from infection, as evidenced by normal temperature and absence of discharge and excessive tearing or edema.

**Interventions and *Rationales***

1. Monitor the child for signs and symptoms of infection, including redness, drainage, fever, and excessive tearing or edema.
   *These are physical signs that a postoperative infection is developing in the eye.*
2. Administer antibiotic therapy as ordered.
   *Antibiotics may be used as prophylaxis against infection.*

**Evaluation**

Is the child free from fever, redness, edema, and excessive eye drainage?

**Nursing Diagnosis**

Acute Pain related to surgical procedure.

**Planning**

***Expected Outcome***

The child will experience minimal discomfort during the postoperative period, as evidenced by an acceptable pain scale rating, normal vital signs, and participation in approved quiet activities.

**Interventions and *Rationales***

1. Monitor the child frequently (every 2 to 4 hours while awake) for pain using a verbal age-appropriate pain scale. Use a preverbal pain scale, in addition to self-reported pain, to assess pain level in infants and young children whose eyes are occluded. Monitor physiologic signs of pain in the young child (increased pulse, restlessness, inability to sleep, inability to play).
   *Pain can increase anxiety and restlessness that could lead to increased intraocular pressure. The young child who would ordinarily use a visual scale to rate pain is unable to do so if the eyes are patched.*
2. Administer pain medications as ordered.
   *Pain control decreases the child's need to rub or touch the eyes, which can cause trauma to the surgical site.*
3. Provide non-pharmacologic pain-relief measures, such as ice pack and moist heat, as indicated. Use distraction techniques frequently (music, stories).
   *Nonpharmacologic pain-relief measures can replace or augment pharmacologic measures. Verbal distraction techniques can decrease pain and take the child's mind off the bandages.*

**Evaluation**

Does the child express relief of pain with an age-appropriate pain scale?

Are the child's vital signs within normal limits, and can the child participate appropriately in approved quiet activities?

## EYE INFECTIONS

### Nursing Considerations for the Child With Conjunctivitis

Conjunctivitis ("pink eye") is an inflammation of the conjunctiva (the clear, membranous lining of the lid and sclera). Signs and symptoms of conjunctivitis may include itching, burning, light sensitivity (photophobia), "scratchy" eyelids, redness, edema, and discharge. It is caused usually by either allergy or infection. Accurate diagnosis before treatment is important because inappropriate treatment can lead to complications.

Conjunctivitis noted in the first few weeks of life is called ophthalmia neonatorum. In infants, conjunctivitis occurring in the first 24 hours of life is usually caused by chemical irritation from infection prophylaxis administered soon after birth. Either infection or a blocked lacrimal duct can cause conjunctivitis that occurs after the first 24 hours. Infants acquire infection during birth (from passing through the birth canal) or after birth. *Chlamydia* is responsible for most eye infections noted in infants (Dietrich, 2014). Medical treatment should be directed at the cause of the infection. Antibiotic or antiviral eyedrops or ointments are most often used to treat infectious conjunctivitis. However, if *Chlamydia* is the cause, systemic antibiotics (e.g., erythromycin) are also used to prevent pneumonia.

Conjunctivitis in older children has a variety of causes, including bacteria, viruses, allergy, infection, and trauma. Organisms most frequently implicated in bacterial conjunctivitis include *Haemophilus influenzae* and *Streptococcus pneumoniae* (Olitsky et al., 2016; Wong & Anninger, 2014), although with the introduction of *H. influenzae* type B (Hib) vaccine, *H. influenzae* has decreased as a major cause. As with the infant, treatment depends on the cause. The nurse obtains a detailed history to help determine the cause. Infection should be suspected if the child has recently been exposed to another person with conjunctivitis or has had an upper respiratory infection. Itching and tearing often identifies the cause as an allergic response. Although children with allergic conjunctivitis exhibit redness of the conjunctiva, they usually do not manifest the type of thick discharge seen in bacterial conjunctivitis (Utz & Kaufman, 2014).

Chlamydial conjunctivitis is rare in children older than 3 years. However, it may be suspected in a sexually active adolescent with persistent conjunctivitis. A diagnosis of chlamydial conjunctivitis in an older child who is not sexually active should signal the healthcare provider to assess the child for possible sexual abuse (Wong & Anninger, 2014).

Medical management depends on the cause of the conjunctivitis. If the cause is infection, antibiotic or antiviral eyedrops or ointment may be prescribed. If allergies are suspected, antihistamines, either oral or in the form of eyedrops, may be indicated. In severe cases of allergic conjunctivitis, steroid eyedrops and cromolyn sodium eyedrops might be helpful. The steroid eyedrops are tapered over an approximately 7-day period. Because steroids can worsen the severity of many infections, they are used with caution and only for a short time. Used over the long term, steroids can exacerbate glaucoma and contribute to cataract development.

Teach parents to keep the child's eye clean and administer any prescribed medications (see Chapter 38). The parent can gently remove crusted material from the eye with a cotton ball soaked in warm water. Teach the parent to wipe the eye from the inner to the outer aspect and wash the hands and use a new cotton ball for the other eye. Because bacterial or viral conjunctivitis is extremely contagious, the nurse should teach infection control measures. These include good handwashing and not sharing towels and washcloths. Bottles of eye medication should never be shared with another person. The tip of the dropper or ointment tube should not touch the child's eye or eyelid during administration. The child with purulent conjunctivitis should also be kept home from school or daycare until 24 hours after antibiotics are started (AAP Committee on Infectious Diseases, 2015).

Preventing injury from rubbing the eye is also important. Mittens can be used for infants. These can be fashioned from bootie-type socks or can be commercially made. Distraction and constant reminding are recommended for toddlers and older children. If the child wears contact lenses, advise discontinuing them until the infection has completely cleared. Securing new contact lenses eliminates the chance of reinfection from contaminated contact lenses and also lessens the risk of a corneal ulceration. Eye makeup should also be discarded and replaced because the chance of reinfecting eyes from contaminated makeup is high. Mascara should be replaced routinely at least every 3 months.

If the conjunctivitis is allergic in origin, cool compresses and dark glasses can also help lessen the irritation and photophobia. If cromolyn sodium eyedrops are prescribed, parents should be taught to begin using them *before* the allergy season because they need several weeks to reach full effectiveness. Ophthalmic nonsteroidal antiinflammatory preparations may also be helpful (Wong & Anninger, 2014).

### Nursing Considerations for the Child With Orbital Cellulitis

Orbital cellulitis is caused by an infection of the soft tissues of the orbit. It can occur as a result of trauma or, more commonly, an associated sinus infection (Olitsky et al., 2016). The usual infecting organisms are *Staphylococcus aureus* and *S. pneumoniae*. Clinical signs and symptoms include severe eyelid edema, erythema, and an anteriorly displaced eye. Decreased or absent vision, increased intraocular pressure, and pain can complicate the child's condition. The child is febrile and has an elevated white blood cell count. Orbital cellulitis is distinguished from periorbital (preseptal) cellulitis in that periorbital cellulitis is inflammation and infection of the superficial skin tissues that surround the eye (e.g., eyelids) and not the tissue of the eye itself (Wong & Anninger, 2014).

Computed tomography (CT) scanning of the eye and brain confirms the diagnosis, assesses complications, and assists with developing the treatment plan (Olitsky et al., 2016). After cultures have been taken, the child is treated with intravenous administration of an antibiotic designed to act on the major causative organisms (most frequently vancomycin or ceftriaxone); the treatment is individualized when the culture results are available. If the area is painful, analgesics may also be prescribed. Children with orbital cellulitis should be admitted to the hospital for observation and treatment because of the potential for rapid progression to systemic disease. Left untreated, the infection causing the orbital cellulitis can spread to the optic nerve and then directly to the brain, causing meningitis and blindness. Affected children need frequent vision assessments during treatment. Surgical intervention may be required.

Nursing care involves administering prescribed medications and assessing the child receiving intravenous therapy. The child also should be carefully monitored for signs and symptoms that the infection is spreading. This includes a thorough neurologic assessment. Finally, the nurse frequently assesses the child's pain status. Heat application four times a day and prescribed analgesics can relieve pain.

### Nursing Considerations for the Child With a Corneal Ulcer

Corneal ulcers are usually caused by ocular infection as a result of trauma. Signs and symptoms include pain, tearing, purulent discharge, and blurred vision. Besides trauma, risk factors for corneal ulceration include extended wearing of soft contact lenses, surgical procedures, and viral infection in the eye (usually herpesvirus type 1). Corneal ulcerations may be a sign of underlying systemic disease. If not properly and aggressively treated, corneal ulcerations can cause corneal scarring and blindness.

Treatment includes aggressive topical antibiotic therapy with a broad-spectrum antibiotic until cultures return. Treatment is started with potent fluoroquinolones: ciprofloxacin, ofloxacin, and norfloxacin. Topical antiviral preparations are used for ulcers caused by viral infection. Systemic acyclovir may be prescribed by the ophthalmologist to treat ocular herpesvirus infection. The nurse teaches the parent about the administration of any prescribed medications and the cause and prevention of future ulcerations. The parent needs to discourage the child from rubbing the eyes (which can worsen the injury). The child who wears contact lenses should avoid wearing them until the ulceration and infection are completely healed. Any lenses worn during the episode should be discarded.

## EYE TRAUMA

### Nursing Considerations for the Child With a Corneal Abrasion

Corneal abrasions usually result from a scraping or tearing of the cornea by foreign bodies, contact lenses, paper, or fingernails. The child may have light sensitivity, pain, excessive tearing, and decreased vision. The abrasion is diagnosed by instilling a fluorescein dye in the eye and examining the eye under a blue-filtered light (Wood lamp) to highlight the injury. If foreign bodies remain in the eye, they should be removed.

If the abrasion is small, treatment consists only of the instillation of an appropriate antibiotic ointment or drops four times a day for 1 to 2 days with a follow-up evaluation to check healing. Referral to an ophthalmologist should be considered with any eye injury, but particularly for a large abrasion or with the suspicion of a penetrating injury. Many authorities now recommend no patching unless the wound is large. When large abrasions are patched, the patch remains in place for 24 hours, and the eye is reexamined at the end of the 24-hour period. Failure to treat an abrasion can result in loss of visual acuity or permanent scarring and opacity of the cornea.

Parent education is important in caring for the child with a corneal abrasion. Because an abrasion increases the risk of infection, parents should be taught the importance of administering ophthalmic antibiotics as prescribed. The child should not rub the eye because rubbing can worsen an abrasion. If the eye is patched, advise the parents not to remove the patch for 24 hours, even to instill ointment. Keeping the patch in place prevents further damage to the eye from blinking. The nurse also reinforces injury prevention, especially wearing safety goggles during sports and other activities, such as woodworking.

### Nursing Considerations for the Child With Hemorrhage

Subconjunctival hemorrhages manifest as red areas beneath the conjunctiva. They are often the result of Valsalva maneuvers, such as coughing, vomiting, or straining. Subconjunctival hemorrhages resolve on their own within 2 to 3 weeks and require no treatment. Although they often appear worse than they actually are, they can be associated with other ocular or physical problems and should be evaluated.

Because these hemorrhages resolve spontaneously, care is aimed at reassurance. Parents should be told that the hemorrhage will appear to grow larger in the first few days because of the effects of gravity.

Hemorrhages can occur with nonaccidental eye injury as well. In a child suspected of having abusive head trauma (shaken baby syndrome), for example, retinal hemorrhaging of various types can occur. The child will manifest abnormal findings on funduscopic examination and may exhibit retinal detachment (Olitsky et al., 2016). The infant or child who receives a direct blow to the eye will usually demonstrate bruising around the eye. Hyphema and damage to the eye structures are a consequence of this type of trauma.

### Nursing Considerations for the Child With Hyphema

A hyphema is a hemorrhage resulting from a blow or penetrating injury to the eye. Symptoms include a recent history of injury, pain, light sensitivity, decreased vision, the presence of floaters, and excessive tearing. The child is usually sleepy. If the child has no known history of injury, the child should be assessed for a bleeding disorder, anticoagulant therapy, renal or hepatic disease, retinoblastoma, or child abuse. Children with sickle cell disease are prone to hyphema. An examination of the eye reveals blood in the anterior chamber (between the cornea and iris) of the eye. Traumatic hyphema usually fills less than one third of the anterior chamber.

Hyphema usually results from blunt trauma to the eye (Pons, 2011) but can result also from penetrating eye trauma (Olitsky et al., 2016). Any penetrating eye injury is an emergency, requiring rapid referral to an ophthalmologist and treatment to prevent blindness. At the scene of the injury, the eye should be immediately covered with a sterile dressing and an eye shield (manufactured rigid eye shield, Styrofoam or plastic cup). Keep the child's head as still as possible until emergency services arrive. Treatment for hyphema includes bed rest with the head elevated 30 to 40 degrees, sedation, and protective shielding of the eye. Treatment can be managed at home if the child is cooperative with bed rest; otherwise, hospitalization is indicated (Olitsky et al., 2016). There is a risk of a rebleed within five days after the trauma; children who experience a rebleed should be hospitalized (Grigorian, Patel, Lai et al., 2015).

Medications such as steroid eye drops, antifibrinolytic eyedrops (tranexamic acid is best for pediatric use), antiglaucoma medications, and cycloplegic eye drops (atropine) may also be used. The child should be closely monitored for side effects of medications, which will vary according to the prescribed therapy. Aspirin and nonsteroidal anti-inflammatory medications are contraindicated because of rebleed risk.

Careful assessment is required for the child with a hyphema. Assess the eye frequently for a secondary hemorrhage, or rebleed. This condition is characterized by an increase in the size of the hyphema, with bright-red "new" blood noted over the existing clot. Children who rebleed have a poorer long-term prognosis for vision because acute or chronic glaucoma can be a consequence. The child should also be monitored for signs and symptoms of increasing intraocular pressure (pain, nausea and vomiting, increased inflammation). The child is usually restricted to bed rest with bathroom privileges. Elevating the head of the bed 30 to 40 degrees helps settle the hyphema in the inferior anterior chamber angle. Television viewing may or may not be allowed, and reading and other close-up activities are usually forbidden. Therefore, boredom is a problem for most children. Offer diversional activities such as music and books on tape that do not involve reading or straining the eyes. If both eyes are covered, the nurse orients the child to the environment and provides for safety.

Discharge teaching includes use of prescribed home medications, shield regimen (the eye is usually shielded at night for 2 weeks after discharge), and prevention of further injury. The child can usually return to all normal activities several weeks after the injury. Eye protection is recommended for all children who participate in sports or other high-risk activities, but lifelong use of protective eyewear is recommended for the child who has had hyphema. The nurse should also emphasize the importance of follow-up because the child is at risk for complications such as glaucoma and cataracts.

Teaching to prevent eye injury is an important nursing intervention (see Parents Want to Know: How to Prevent Eye Injuries While Participating in Sports). Many school and recreational athletic organizations have policies regarding eye protection during sports activities. Teens who attend vocational schools must wear protective eye covering in shops where eye injury is a risk. Of more concern is the potential for eye injury occurring during unsupervised play.

**PARENTS WANT TO KNOW**

***How to Prevent Eye Injuries While Participating in Sports***

- The highest risk for eye injuries occurs when children participate in sports that do not require eye protection, such as basketball, baseball, lacrosse, racquet sports, martial arts, and boxing.
- The highest percentage of injuries is seen in basketball and baseball.
- Wear certified protective eyewear—such as goggles or eyewear made of hard polycarbonate lenses, helmets, and face shields—when possible.
- Wear sports goggles under helmets and with hockey masks.

Data from Turbert, D. (2016). *Eye health in sports and recreation.* Retrieved from http://www.aao.org.

### Nursing Considerations for the Child With a Chemical Splash Injury

Splash injury can occur any time infective, hot, or corrosive liquid splashes into a child's eye; burns of the eye constitute an ocular emergency. Burns can occur from any number of common household items, including bleach, ammonia, drain opener, and oven cleaner.

Initial care of the child with a splash injury to the eyes focuses on immediate irrigation with water or saline to prevent further injury. In a chemical splash, if the chemical is alkaline, irrigation may continue for several hours because the damaging action of alkaloids can be prolonged. Irrigation of a frightened child's eyes can be difficult and painful for the child. Pre-irrigation anesthetization of the eye can facilitate irrigation (Pons, 2011).

If the burn is mild, irrigate for at least 30 minutes using at least 2 L of irrigant; if the burn is severe, continue irrigating for 2 to 4 hours or with at least 10 L of irrigant (Olitsky et al., 2016). Periodically check the eye pH with litmus paper until the results are within normal range (7.3 to 7.7) (Olitsky et al., 2016). The cornea may appear cloudy after an alkali burn. Further treatment may include referral to an ophthalmologist for topical steroids, medications to dilate the pupils and decrease the risk of adhesions, antibiotic ointment, and patching. Oral antibiotics and analgesics may also be indicated. Nursing care focuses on prescribed medical treatments, comfort measures, and injury prevention (particularly if both of the child's eyes are patched).

Discharge teaching focuses on the prescribed medical treatments and the importance of adherence with long-term follow-up and injury prevention. Follow-up care includes monitoring visual acuity and for side effects such as increased intraocular pressure and cataracts.

## HEARING LOSS IN CHILDREN

### Etiology

Damage to, or impairment of, any part of the ear can cause hearing loss. Four types of hearing loss have been identified: conductive, sensorineural, mixed, and central. Each has a different treatment regimen and response to intervention (Box 55.3). Hearing loss can be congenital or acquired. In infants with sensorineural hearing loss, an autosomal recessive inheritance pattern is the cause in more than 80% of cases (Haddad & Keesecker, 2016). Infection, damage from ototoxic medications, head injury, and trauma from noise exposure are the major causes of acquired hearing loss in children (American Speech-Language-Hearing Association, 2015).

**BOX 55.3 Types and Etiology of Hearing Loss**

- *Conductive:* Outer or middle ear affected by damage, inflammation, or obstruction. Sound conduction is prevented from progressing from the outer ear to the inner ear. May be the result of excessive cerumen (wax), foreign bodies, perforated tympanic membrane, or otitis media (with or without effusion). Hearing loss is often temporary and reversible.
- *Sensorineural:* Result of damage or malformation of structures of the inner ear and/or auditory nerve. May be the result of heredity or environmental factors, such as infection (meningitis or intrauterine), exposure to loud noise, ototoxic medications, or prematurity. Meningitis is a significant cause of acquired sensorineural hearing loss in children. Hearing loss is usually permanent.
- *Mixed:* Combination of conductive and sensorineural loss. Conductive loss is often reversible, whereas sensorineural loss is not.
- *Central:* Result of damage to the conduction system between the auditory nervous system and cerebral cortex. Can be the result of trauma, neurovascular changes, or brain tumors. May cause difficulty in differentiation of sounds, auditory memory.

**SAFETY ALERT**

***Working With a Child Who Has a Visual Impairment***

- Orient the child to the hospital environment on admission. Orientation can be done by walking the child around the room and identifying objects such as the bed, bathroom, doorways, windows, and chairs.
- Never touch the child without first identifying yourself and explaining what you plan to do.
- When describing objects or the environment to a child who is blind or visually impaired, use familiar terms. For example, if the child is older and recently blinded, you may be able to use color when describing objects. If the child has been blind since birth, color has no meaning. Describing how many steps away something is or the placement of eating utensils on a tray are both useful tactics. Remember that parents are often the best resource for communication.
- Identify noises for the child because children who are visually impaired or blind often have difficulty establishing the source of a noise.
- Orient the child frequently to time and place. Confusion can be frightening.
- Keep all items in the room in the same location and order. Changing the order or spacing of objects may cause confusion or lead to injury.
- Provide detailed explanations and allow the child to progress through care in steps to learn the order.
- As with any child, allow as much control over the situation as possible.
- Supervise the child and counsel parents to supervise the child as needed.

### Incidence

The reported prevalence of mild or more severe hearing loss in children in the United States is 3.1%; the prevalence is higher in Hispanics and Black children and those of lower socioeconomic status (Haddad & Keesecker, 2016). Estimating the true prevalence of hearing loss in

**BOX 55.4 Risk Factors Indicating the Need for Hearing Screening**

- Parental/caregiver concern
- Family history of hearing loss
- In utero exposure to infection (e.g., TORCH infections)
- Craniofacial abnormalities
- Syndromes associated with hearing loss
- Neonatal intensive care unit for more than 5 days
- Post-natal infection
- Trauma
- Exposure to excessive noise
- Chemotherapy or other medication associated with hearing loss

Data from: Centers for Disease Control and Prevention. (n.d.). *Hearing loss in infants and children: Considerations for pediatric primary care providers.* Retrieved from http://www.cdc.gov.

infants and children is difficult because most newborn screening tools identify only those newborns with moderate to severe hearing loss. Although universal hearing screening has been successful in identifying infants with hearing loss, many identified infants do not access appropriate early intervention; therefore, children with mild or unilateral hearing loss may encounter difficulties with academic performance when they enter school (Krishnan & Von Hyfte, 2014).

Evidence suggests that many preschool and school age children experience hearing loss to the extent that their academic performance is affected when they begin school (American Speech-Language-Hearing Association [ASHA], 2015). As a result, the AAP (2016a) has taken the position through its Early Hearing Detection and Intervention (EHDI) program that pediatric providers must be proactive in assessing risk for hearing loss throughout childhood and refer as necessary. Box 55.4 lists criteria used to assess infants and children who may be at risk for hearing loss. The AAP recommends that all pediatric providers follow the CDC's 1, 3, and 6 guidelines: screening for hearing loss by 1 month of age, identification of hearing loss and referral to an audiologist by 3 months of age, and initiation of early intervention for documented hearing loss by 6 months of age (CDC, n.d.). The AAP (2016b) recommends newborn screening followed by annual hearing risk assessment up to age 4 years, formal screening from 5 to 7 years, then alternating screening with risk assessment through middle childhood.

## Diagnostic Evaluation

Evidence demonstrates that infants with hearing loss who have been identified and treated before 6 months of age have a better prognosis than those for whom treatment has been delayed. The use of risk criteria for screening infants for hearing loss helps identify only approximately 50% of infants affected (see Box 55.4). Many states have passed legislation making newborn hearing screening mandatory, and more than 95% of infants born in hospitals are screened before discharge (AAP, 2014).

Hearing screening for infants is challenging because of their inability to give accurate behavioral cues to indicate intact hearing. Historically, hearing assessment in the newborn or young infant often relied on eliciting a startle reflex with a loud noise. However, being certain that the response is actually caused by the sound itself is difficult. Two hearing screening tests can accurately identify infants with hearing deficits: the auditory brainstem response and the evoked otoacoustic emissions test (Box 55.5). Newer equipment has allowed these tests to be completed quickly and accurately in the hospital

**BOX 55.5 Hearing Tests Used for Infants**

**Auditory Brainstem Response**

- Electrodes, which record brain wave activity, are placed on the infant's head.
- Foam-padded earphones are placed over the ears.
- The earphones sound a click at a 35-dB volume.
- The resulting brain wave measurement is compared with the brain wave measurement from a normal infant.
- The test takes 10 to 60 minutes to administer, depending on the underlying testing objective.

**Evoked Otoacoustic Emissions**

- This test assesses the integrity of the inner ear structures by recording sounds (otoacoustic emissions) generated by the inner ear. It cannot assess the degree of hearing loss but can assess whether hearing is present.
- An ear probe, which contains a sound transmitter and microphone, is attached to a computer and placed in the ear.
- Click sounds evoke the emissions, which are displayed on the computer screen.
- Emissions are present in infants who can hear at 20 dB but not present in infants who hear only at 30 dB or higher.*
- The test takes approximately 5 minutes to administer.

*American Speech-Language-Hearing Association. (n.d.). *Hearing screening.* Retrieved from http://www.asha.org.

nursery. Both tests have a pass/refer option. If the infant does not pass after two tries (2 weeks apart), referral to an audiologist for more accurate testing is required. More sophisticated testing, such as visual reinforcement audiometry or conditioned-play audiometry, is performed by audiologists.

## PATHOPHYSIOLOGY

### *Hearing Loss*

Adequate hearing depends on intact auditory structures and quality of sound. Sound is described in terms that combine volume (expressed in decibels [dB]) and pitch, or frequencies (expressed in hertz [Hz]). Normal speech ranges in volume between 10 and 60 dB. Normal hearing ranges from −10 to +15 dB at a variety of frequencies. Most people can hear frequencies between 10 and 20,000 Hz. For screening purposes, inability to hear frequencies at 26 dB is cause for referral. Other hearing loss categories are:

*Moderate:* Failure to hear at 40 to 69 dB
*Severe:* Failure to hear at 70 to 89 dB
*Profound:* Failure to hear at more than 90 dB

A child with mild hearing loss may have difficulty hearing speech in a classroom setting. This deficit obviously poses academic problems for children who have not been identified as having a hearing loss and miss most of what a teacher says in a classroom.

Data from: Centers for Disease Control and Prevention. (2015). *Official MADDSP and MADD surveillance case definitions.* Retrieved from http://www.cdc.gov.

Hearing testing in the older child (age 3 years and older) is done by play audiometry (e.g., the child performs a play activity when the sound is heard) or conventional audiometry (Haddad & Keesecker, 2016). The child is presented tones of varying frequencies at a standard volume (usually 20 decibels [dB]). A quick screening test performed in a physician's office with a hand-held audiometer tests frequencies of 500, 1000, 2000, and 4000 hertz (Hz). If the child does not pass the screening, particularly at lower frequencies and lower volume, a tympanogram may indicate middle ear effusion (see Chapter 45). The problem with office audiometric screening is that it can miss hearing loss at higher frequencies, which is usually sensorineural. Therefore, when performing an audiometric screening of children, the nurse should perform the test in a quiet environment and determine ahead of time what signal the child will use to indicate hearing the tone. All infants and young children should be assessed regularly at well visits for any communication delay or academic difficulty that might be related to decreased hearing. Should problems arise, referral for complete audiologic examination is warranted (AAP, 2016b).

### Therapeutic Management

The goals of identification and management of infants and children with hearing loss are directed toward maximizing language development and preventing later problems with school performance and social interaction. Treatment of hearing loss depends on the type of loss. Conductive hearing loss is managed by medical or surgical correction of the underlying problem (otitis, cerumen). One device that has been successful with certain types of conductive and mixed hearing loss is a bone conduction hearing device (Finley, 2011). This device is attached to an ossified titanium screw implanted in the mastoid bone. Sound is conducted directly from the screw through bone to the inner ear, bypassing the outer and middle ear structures (Finley, 2011).

Sensorineural hearing loss, which is seldom reversible, requires a different approach. Hearing aids are often recommended for these infants (as young as two months of age) and children as soon as possible after diagnosis to help facilitate language development (Haddad & Keesecker, 2016). The type of aid chosen depends on the specific needs of the child. The aid should provide the best acoustics and be cosmetically appropriate. For example, an adolescent seldom chooses a body-type hearing aid if an ear-level aid (one inserted into the ear canal) suffices. The four types of hearing aids most commonly used for pediatric patients are behind-the-ear, ear-level (in the ear), eyeglass (aids attached to the temples of eyeglass frames), and body (a box with wires connected to an ear mold). Infants and young children often do better with ear-level hearing aids.

Cochlear implants offer an option for children with sensorineural hearing loss, even those with some residual hearing. The implant is a small electronic device surgically implanted into the cochlea. It delivers electrical stimulation to the inner ear, causing nerve impulses to travel to the brain, where they are interpreted as normal sound. Early cochlear implantation (before 2 years of age) allows for normal language development in a large majority of children (Geers, Nicholas, Tobey, et al., 2016; Haddad & Keersecker, 2016). For children with delayed language development, additional, or updated, implants assist with achieving normal language development (Geers et al., 2016). Ensuring appropriate immunization (PCV13) and an additional booster dose (PPSV23) of pneumococcal vaccine is essential for children receiving a cochlear implant due to the high risk of pneumococcal meningitis (Haddad & Keersecker, 2016).

### Nursing Considerations for the Child With Hearing Loss

Assess the child's hearing at each well-child visit and at other times when warranted (e.g., with chronic otitis media [see Chapter 45]). Note an infant's response to bells, rattles, clapping of hands, or horns held approximately 12 inches from the ear. Older children can be asked to repeat whispered words or phrases or listen for a ticking watch. Begin audiometry testing at 3 years of age or younger in a cooperative child.

Assess language-skill development. Infants who are deaf babble in the same way as hearing infants until approximately 5 to 6 months of age, at which time babbling is noted to cease. The nurse also questions parents about the child's attention span, disruptive behavior, and other behaviors, such as increasing the volume on the television. If the child appears to have hearing loss or is lagging behind in developmental milestones, refer for further evaluation by an audiologist and ear, nose, and throat specialist.

When caring for a child who is hearing impaired, the nurse should do the following:

- If the child has a hearing aid, encourage its use. Make sure it is in place before beginning to speak.
- Look directly into the child's face. To enhance lip reading, have the child's complete attention before beginning to speak.
- Speak clearly. Slow speech slightly. Do not speak loudly.
- Eliminate background noise.
- Use visual aids to assist communication. Such aids include pictures, hands, and written messages for older children.
- If the child uses American Sign Language to communicate, have a diagram of commonly used words readily available. Use an interpreter for more complex discussions.

An important nursing responsibility is to educate parents about preventable hearing loss. Mild sensorineural hearing loss can occur from exposure to loud noises, such as from firecrackers, firearms, loud infant squeak toys, outdoor yard equipment, boat and snowmobile motors, and rock music. People exposed to loud sounds over long periods need to wear protective ear coverings (e.g., ear plugs, mufflers). Advise teens to decrease exposure to loud rock music and to turn music volume down, especially when listening through earphones. Referral for genetic counseling is important if the child has congenital sensorineural hearing loss. Prevention also includes the appropriate prevention and treatment of prenatal infections and infections during infancy and early childhood. Children with hearing loss may need speech therapy; referral to a speech therapist or early intervention program should occur as soon as possible.

#### CRITICAL THINKING EXERCISE 55.1

At the recommendation of the Joint Committee on Infant Hearing, most U.S. states and many areas of Canada have implemented mandatory newborn infant hearing screening programs. As part of these programs, newborns are screened before hospital discharge. Consider the advantages and disadvantages of this issue. Why should nurses advocate that their states implement similar programs if they do not already exist?

## LANGUAGE DISORDERS

Until 10 to 12 months of age, a child is considered prelingual. The sounds the child makes have no direct meaning or connection to future language. They are, instead, practice of a learned skill. Before approximately 6 months of age, infants make few sounds other than crying. However, at approximately 4 to 6 months of age, they enter the babbling phase. These are the cooing, happy sounds that an infant makes when content. The first words appear at approximately 10 to 12 months of age. First sentences appear at approximately 18 months of age. By 2 years of age, most children have at least a 50-word spoken vocabulary.

Girls have more rapid language development until approximately 3 years of age, when the difference disappears. However, by adolescence, girls again show superior verbal skills. Although a correlation exists between developmental delay and verbal skills, the relationship between language development and intelligence is unclear. No scientific evidence seems to suggest that a child who talks early is brighter than one who does not. However, children who talk quite early do

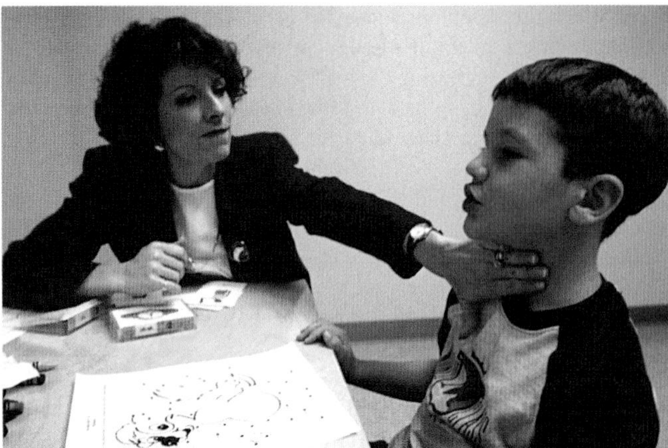

**FIG 55.1** Expressive speech disorders include disorders of voice, articulation, and fluency. A speech therapist works with the child to help the child speak more clearly and be better understood. Early intervention is important to correct speech disorders. Therefore, the nurse should assess speech patterns during each health screening. Referrals should be made for any problems noted. (Courtesy Cook Children's Medical Center, Fort Worth, TX.)

appear to be bright, whereas those who talk extremely late appear to have some developmental delay.

Language disorders in the child are usually of two types: receptive and expressive. A child with a receptive disorder has a decreased ability to comprehend language. A child with an expressive disorder cannot express thoughts through speech. Some children have a combination of both expressive and receptive language difficulty. Language disorders can result from genetic influences, infection, trauma, autism, hearing loss, and other etiologies (Simms, 2016).

Expressive disorders are most often of three types. The first is a disorder of the voice that involves an alteration in the pitch and intonation; such disorders can result from a medical condition, such as a cleft palate. The second is a defect of articulation, or the way in which words are pronounced. This type of speech defect is the most common and can be caused by a neuromuscular disease or structural abnormalities of the nose, throat, and mouth. Some articulation defects are idiopathic. Finally, fluency disorders interrupt the normal flow of speech. Included in this category are lisping and stuttering. If stuttering persists after 5 years of age, the child should receive appropriate referrals for speech evaluation (Fig. 55.1).

## PATIENT-CENTERED TEACHING

### *How to Encourage Language Development*

**Infancy to 2 Years**

- Talk to the child regularly using different types of voice inflection.
- Mimic the infant's sounds as vocalizations begin.
- Make frequent eye contact.
- Play social games—waving, hand-clapping games.
- Read, read, read.

**2 to 4 Years**

- Model clear speech with appropriate grammar; avoid talking baby talk.
- Clarify your child's comments.
- Expand the child's vocabulary by using descriptive words to build on simple ones the child is using.
- Talk about daily experiences as they are occurring—car rides, grocery store visits,
- Sing and teach your child simple songs.
- Encourage story-telling using pictures in books.

**4 to 6 Years**

- Attend to what your child is saying and insist the child attend to what you are saying.
- Give increasing number of simple directions.
- Encourage imaginary play.
- Answer questions with more complex vocabulary.
- Continue reading to the child frequently.

Remember language develops at different rates in different children. If you have any concerns, contact your health provider as soon as possible.

Data from: American Speech-Language-Hearing Association. (n.d.). *Activities to encourage speech and language development.* Retrieved from http://www.asha.org.

As with screens for hearing loss, the nurse should assess the child's communication patterns with each well-child visit. Any problems should be noted and referrals made to provide appropriate intervention as soon as possible. Encourage parents to take measures to encourage speech and prevent speech problems (see Chapters 6 to 9 for specific information about language development).

## KEY CONCEPTS

- Anything that alters a child's sensory perception can adversely affect growth and development.
- Sense organs develop quite early and are sensitive to teratogens. Any interference with development can result in later sensory alteration.
- Most screenings for sensory alterations are noninvasive and relatively painless.
- Vision screening begins at birth with examination of the newborn for structural abnormalities of the eye, red reflex and ability to fixate.
- Vision screening should be regularly assessed throughout childhood and adolescence using such screening methods as HOTV cards or LEA symbols. The child is also tested for color deficiency and stereopsis.
- Refraction errors are treated using corrective lenses.
- Strabismus, malalignment due to extraocular muscle imbalance, can lead to amblyopia if not treated early. Amblyopia results from the brain suppressing vision in one eye to reduce double vision and can lead to permanent loss of vision.
- Both congenital glaucoma and cataracts can have a genetic component, among other causes. Each of these conditions may require surgical intervention.
- The most frequently seen eye infections include conjunctivitis and orbital cellulitis. Orbital cellulitis is an emergent condition that requires aggressive intravenous (IV) antibiotic treatment to prevent the development of a more severe infection, such as meningitis.
- Traumatic injuries to the eye include corneal abrasion, hyphema, and chemical splash injury. Each must be treated promptly to prevent permanent consequences to vision.

- More than 95% of newborn infants in the United States are screened for hearing deficits shortly after birth; however, many children who pass the newborn hearing screen actually have mild to moderate hearing loss, which can affect both their language development and school achievement.
- Universal assessment for hearing risk should occur throughout infancy and childhood, with referral to an audiologist if risks are present.
- Objective hearing screening begins at approximately 4 years of age and is performed regularly during the school years.
- Special care should be taken when caring for the child with sensory alterations. Orientation to a new environment is essential for preventing stress and possible injury.
- Parent education and support are critical in assisting the child with sensory alterations to develop as normally as possible.
- Early intervention and special school supports for the child with sensory alterations allow for more normal growth and development.
- Health teaching should include injury prevention.

## REFERENCES AND READINGS


Albany-Ward, K., & Sobande, M. (2015). What do you really know about colour blindness? *British Journal of School Nursing, 10*(4), 197–199.

American Academy of Audiology. (2011). *Childhood hearing screening guidelines.* Retrieved from http://www.audiology.org.

American Academy of Ophthalmology. (2012). *Strabismus causes.* Retrieved from http://www.aao.org.

American Academy of Ophthalmology. (2013). *Strabismus surgery.* Retrieved from http://www.aao.org.

American Academy of Ophthalmology. (2016). *Know the score: Wearing eye protection helps athletes from getting benched due to ocular injury.* Retrieved from http://www.aao.org.

American Academy of Pediatrics. (2014). *Newborn hearing screening: Lost to documented follow-up: considerations for the medical home.* Retrieved from http://www.aap.org.

American Academy of Pediatrics. (2016a). *Early hearing detection and intervention.* Retrieved from http://www.aap.org.

American Academy of Pediatrics. (2016b). Recommendations for preventive pediatric health care. *Pediatrics, 137*(1), 25–27.

American Academy of Pediatrics Committee on Infectious Diseases (2015). *Red Book®: 2015 report of the Committee on Infectious Diseases* (30th ed., pp. 155-157.). Elk Grove Village, IL: American Academy of Pediatrics.

American Academy of Pediatrics Joint Committee on Infant Hearing (2007). Year 2007 position statement: Principles and guidelines for early hearing detection and intervention programs. *Pediatrics, 120*(4), 898–921.

American Speech-Language-Hearing Association. (n.d.). *Activities to encourage speech and language development.* Retrieved from http://www.asha.org.

American Speech-Language-Hearing Association. *Hearing screening.* (n.d.) Retrieved from http://www.asha.org.

American Speech-Language-Hearing Association. (2015). *Causes of hearing loss in children.* Retrieved from http://www.asha.org.

Bhate, D., & Wang, X. (2015). Surgery interventions for primary congenital glaucoma. *The Cochrane Library, (Issue 1)*, 1–48.

Centers for Disease Control and Prevention. (n.d.). *Hearing loss in infants and young children: Considerations for pediatric primary care providers.* Retrieved from http://www.cdc.gov.

Centers for Disease Control and Prevention. (2015). *MADDSP and MADDS surveillance case definition.* Retrieved from http://www.cdc.gov.

Chou, R., Dana, T., & Bougatsos, C. (2011). *Screening for visual impairment in children ages 1 to 5 years: Systematic review to update the 2004 U.S. Preventive Services Task Force recommendations.* Rockville, MD: Agency for Healthcare Research and Quality.

Cotter, S., Cyert, L., Miller, J., et al. (2015). Vision screening for children 36 to <72 months: recommended practice. *Optometry Vision Science, 92*(1), 6–16.

Dietrich, A. (2014). Common neonatal condition. *Pediatric Emergency Medical Reports.* Retrieved from http://www.ahcmedia.com.

Donahue, S., & Baker, C. (2016a). Procedures for the evaluation of the vision system by pediatricians. *Pediatrics, 137*(1), 1–9.

Donahue, S., & Baker, C. (2016b). Visual system assessments in infant, children and young adults by pediatricians. *Pediatrics, 137*(1), 28–30.

Donahue, S., & Ruben, J. (2011). U.S. preventive services task force vision screening recommendations. *Pediatrics, 127*, 569–570.

Finley, E. (2011). Bone-anchored hearing devices. *NASN School Nurse.* 338-339.

Geers, A., Nicholas, J., Tobey, E., et al. (2016). Persistent language delay versus late language emergence in children with cochlear implantation. *Journal of Speech, Language, and Hearing Research, 59*, 155–170.

Grigorian, P., Patel, A., Lai, K et al. (2015). *Hyphema.* Retrieved from http://www.aao.org.

Haddad, J., & Keesecker, S. (2016). Hearing loss. In R. Kliegman, B. Stanton, J. St. Geme, et al. (Eds.), *Nelson textbook of pediatrics* (20th ed., Chapter 637). St. Louis, MO: Elsevier.

Krishnan, L., & Von Hyfte, S. (2014). Effects of policy changes to universal newborn hearing screening follow-up in a university clinic. *American Journal of Audiology, 23*, 282–292.

Li, S., et al. (2014). A binocular iPad treatment for amblyopic children. *Eye, 28*, 1246–1253.

Olitsky, S., Hug, D., Plummer, L., et al. (2016). The eye. In R. Kliegman, B. Stanton, J. St. Geme, et al. (Eds.), *Nelson textbook of pediatrics* (20th ed., Chapters 621, 623, 627, 632, 634, 635). St. Louis, MO: Elsevier.

Patel, A., Stelzner, S., Epley, K., et al. (2014). *Cataracts in children, congenital and acquired.* Retrieved from http://www.aao.org.

Pons, J. (2011). Eye trauma. *Continuing Medical Education, 29*(2), 66–68.

Schwartz, R., Schuman, A., & Wei, L. (2014). Instrument-based vision screening: update. *Contemporary Pediatrics, 31*(2), 39-45.

Seltz, L., Smith, J., & Durairaj, V. (2011). Orbital cellulitis in children. *Pediatrics, 127*(3), e566–e572.

Simms, M. (2016). Language development and communication disorders. In R. Kliegman, B. Stanton, J. St. Geme, et al. (Eds.), *Nelson textbook of pediatrics* (20th ed., Chapter 35). St. Louis, MO: Elsevier.

Stewart, C., Moseley, M., & Fielder, A. (2011). Amblyopia therapy: An update. *Strabismus, 19*(3), 91-98.

Tailor, V., Bossi, M. Bunce, C., et al. (2015). Binocular vision versus standard occlusion or blurring treatment for unilateral amblyopia in children aged three to eight years. *Cochrane Database of Systematic Reviews,* (8) CD011347, 1–36.

Taylor, K., & Elliott, S. (2011). Interventions for strabismic amblyopia. *Cochrane Database of Systematic Reviews* (8) CD006461.

Turbert, D. (2016). *Eye health in sports and recreation.* Retrieved from http://www.aao.org.

U.S. Preventive Services Task Force. (2011). Screening for visual impairment in children ages 1 to 5: Recommendation statement. *Pediatrics, 127*, 340–346.

Utz, V., & Kaufman, A. (2014). Allergic eye disease. *Pediatric Clinics of North America, 61*(3), 607–620.

Wong, M., & Anninger, W. (2014). The pediatric red eye. *Pediatric Clinics of North America, 61*(3), 591–606.

# A APPENDIX

# NANDA-I Diagnoses and Definitions

**Activity intolerance:** Insufficient physiologic or psychologic energy to endure or complete the required or desired daily activities.

**Acute pain:** An unpleasant sensory and emotional experience associated with actual or potential tissue damage or described in terms of such damage (International Association for the Study of Pain); sudden or slow onset of any intensity from mild to severe with an anticipated or predictable end.

**Anxiety:** Vague, uneasy feeling of discomfort or dread accompanied by an autonomic response (the source is often nonspecific or unknown to the individual); a feeling of apprehension caused by anticipation of danger. It is an alerting sign that warns of impending danger and enables the individual to take measures to deal with the threat.

**Bowel incontinence:** Change in normal bowel habits characterized by involuntary passage of stool.

**Caregiver role strain:** Difficulty in performing family/significant other caregiver roles.

**Chronic pain:** Unpleasant sensory and emotional experience associated with actual or potential tissue damage or described in terms of such damage (International Association for the Study of Pain); sudden or slow onset of any intensity from mild to severe, constant or recurring without an anticipated or predictable end and a duration of more than 3 (>3) months.

**Compromised family coping:** A usually supportive primary person (family member, significant other, or close friend) who provides insufficient, ineffective, or compromised support, comfort, assistance, or encouragement that may be needed by the client to manage or master adaptive tasks related to his or her health challenge.

**Constipation:** Decrease in the normal frequency of defecation accompanied by difficult or incomplete passage of stool and/or passage of excessively hard, dry stool.

**Decreased cardiac output:** Inadequate blood pumped by the heart to meet the metabolic demands of the body.

**Deficient diversional activity:** Decreased stimulation from (or interest or engagement in) recreational or leisure activities.

**Deficient fluid volume:** Decreased intravascular, interstitial, and/or intracellular fluid. This refers to dehydration, water loss alone without change in sodium level.

**Deficient knowledge:** Absence or deficiency of cognitive information related to a specific topic.

**Diarrhea:** Passage of loose, unformed stools.

**Disabled family coping:** Behavior of the primary person (family member, significant other, or close friend) that disables his or her capacities and the client's capacities to effectively address the tasks essential to either person's adaptation to the health challenge.

**Disturbed body image:** Confusion in the mental picture of one's physical self.

**Disturbed sleep pattern:** Time-limited interruptions of sleep duration and quality because of external factors.

**Excess fluid volume:** Increased isotonic fluid retention.

**Fatigue:** An overwhelming, sustained sense of exhaustion and decreased capacity for physical and mental work at the usual level.

**Fear:** Response to perceived threat that is consciously recognized as a danger.

**Grieving:** A normal complex process that includes emotional, physical, spiritual, social, and intellectual responses and behaviors by which individuals, families, and communities incorporate an actual, anticipated, or perceived loss in their daily lives.

**Hopelessness:** Subjective state in which an individual sees limited or no alternatives or personal choices available and is unable to mobilize energy on his or her own behalf.

**Hyperthermia:** Core body temperature above the normal diurnal range because of failure of thermoregulation.

**Hypothermia:** Core body temperature below the normal diurnal range because of failure of thermoregulation.

**Imbalanced nutrition: less than body requirements:** Intake of nutrients is insufficient to meet the metabolic needs.

**Impaired comfort:** Perceived lack of ease, relief, and transcendence in physical, psychospiritual, environmental, cultural, and/or social dimensions.

**Impaired gas exchange:** Excess or deficit in oxygenation and/or carbon dioxide elimination at the alveolar–capillary membrane.

**Impaired home maintenance:** Inability to independently maintain a safe growth-promoting immediate environment.

**Impaired parenting:** Inability of the primary caretaker to create, maintain, or regain an environment that promotes optimum growth and development of the child.

**Impaired physical mobility:** Limitation in independent, purposeful physical movement of the body or of one or more extremities.

**Impaired skin integrity:** Altered epidermis and/or dermis.

**Impaired social interaction:** Insufficient or excessive quantity or ineffective quality of social exchange.

**Impaired urinary elimination:** Dysfunction in urine elimination.

**Impaired verbal communication:** Decreased, delayed, or absent ability to receive, process, transmit, and/or use a system of symbols.

**Ineffective airway clearance:** Inability to clear secretions or obstructions from the respiratory tract to maintain a clear airway.

**Ineffective breastfeeding:** Difficulty in providing milk to an infant or young child directly from the breasts, which may compromise the nutritional status of the infant or young child.

**Ineffective breathing pattern:** Inspiration and/or expiration that does not provide adequate ventilation.

**Ineffective childbearing process:** Pregnancy and childbirth process and care of the newborn that do not match the environmental context, norms, and expectations.

**Ineffective coping:** Inability to form a valid appraisal of the stressors, inadequate choices of practiced responses, and/or inability to use available resources.

**Ineffective family health management:** A pattern of regulating and integrating into family processes a program for the treatment of illness and its sequelae that is unsatisfactory for meeting specific health goals.

**Ineffective health maintenance:** Inability to identify, manage, and/or seek out help to maintain health.

**Ineffective infant feeding pattern:** Impaired ability of an infant to suck or coordinate the suck/swallow response, resulting in inadequate oral nutrition for metabolic needs.

**Ineffective peripheral tissue perfusion:** Decrease in blood circulation to the periphery that may compromise health.

**Ineffective protection:** Decrease in the ability to guard self from internal or external threats such as illness or injury.

**Ineffective sexuality pattern:** Expressions of concern regarding own sexuality.

**Ineffective thermoregulation:** Temperature fluctuation between hypothermia and hyperthermia.

**Interrupted breastfeeding:** Break in the continuity of providing milk to an infant or young child directly from the breasts, which may compromise breastfeeding success and/or nutritional status of the infant or young child.

**Interrupted family processes:** Change in family relationships and/or functioning.

**Parental role conflict:** Parental experience of role confusion and conflict in response to crisis.

**Powerlessness:** The lived experience of lack of control over a situation, including a perception that one's actions do not significantly affect an outcome.

**Readiness for enhanced childbearing process:** A pattern of preparing for and maintaining a healthy pregnancy, childbirth process, and care of the newborn for ensuring well-being, which can be strengthened.

**Readiness for enhanced family coping:** A pattern of management of adaptive tasks by the primary person (family member, significant other, or close friend) involved with the client's health change, which can be strengthened.

**Readiness for enhanced nutrition:** A pattern of nutrient intake, which can be strengthened.

**Readiness for enhanced parenting:** A pattern of providing an environment for children or other dependent person(s) to nurture growth and development, which can be strengthened.

**Risk for aspiration:** Vulnerable to the entry of gastrointestinal secretions, oropharyngeal secretions, solids, or fluids to the tracheobronchial passages, which may compromise health.

**Risk for bleeding:** Vulnerable to a decrease in blood volume, which may compromise health.

**Risk for constipation:** Vulnerable to a decrease in normal frequency of defecation accompanied by difficult or incomplete passage of stool, which may compromise health.

**Risk for deficient fluid volume:** Vulnerable to experiencing decreased intravascular, interstitial, and/or intracellular fluid volumes, which may compromise health.

**Risk for delayed development:** Vulnerable to a delay of 25% or more in one or more areas of social or self-regulatory behavior or in cognitive, language, gross, or fine motor skills, which may compromise health.

**Risk for disorganized infant behavior:** Vulnerable to alteration in integration and modulation of the physiologic and behavioral systems of functioning (i.e., autonomic, motor, state-organization, self-regulatory, and attentional–interactional systems), which may compromise health.

**Risk for imbalanced body temperature:** Vulnerable to failure to maintain body temperature within normal parameters, which may compromise health.

**Risk for impaired attachment:** Vulnerable to the disruption of the interactive process between parent/significant other and child that fosters the development of a protective and nurturing reciprocal relationship.

**Risk for impaired oral mucous membrane:** Vulnerable to injury to the lips, soft tissues, buccal cavity, and/or oropharynx, which may compromise health.

**Risk for impaired skin integrity:** Vulnerable to alteration in the epidermis and/or dermis, which may compromise health.

**Risk for ineffective cerebral tissue perfusion:** Vulnerable to a decrease in cerebral tissue circulation, which may compromise health.

**Risk for ineffective gastrointestinal perfusion:** Vulnerable to a decrease in gastrointestinal circulation, which may compromise health.

**Risk for ineffective peripheral tissue perfusion:** Vulnerable to a decrease in blood circulation to the periphery, which may compromise health.

**Risk for infection:** Vulnerable to invasion and multiplication of pathogenic organisms, which may compromise health.

**Risk for injury:** Vulnerable to physical damage because of environmental conditions that interact with the individual's adaptive and defensive resources, which may compromise health.

**Risk for poisoning:** Vulnerable to accidental exposure to or ingestion of drugs or dangerous products in sufficient doses, which may compromise health.

**Risk for situational low self-esteem:** Vulnerable to developing a negative perception of self-worth in response to a current situation, which may compromise health.

**Social isolation:** Aloneness experienced by the individual and perceived as imposed by others and as a negative or threatening state.

**Urinary retention:** Incomplete emptying of the bladder.

## REFERENCES AND READINGS

NANDA International, Inc. (2014) In T. H. Herdman, & S. Kamitsuru (Eds.), *Nursing Diagnoses: Definitions & Classifications 2015-2017* (10th ed.). 2014 NANDA International, Inc. John Wiley & Sons, Ltd. Companion website: www.wiley.com/go/nursingdiagnoses. In order to make safe and effective judgements using NANDA-I nursing diagnoses, it is essential that nurses refer to the definitions and defining characteristics of the diagnoses listed in this work.

# GLOSSARY

## A

**ABCDEs** Airway, breathing, circulation, disability, and exposure; critical components of the primary assessment that require interventions and evaluation in the stabilization of a critically ill or injured child.

**abduction** Movement of a limb away from the midline of the body.

**ablation** Destruction of diseased tissue.

**abortion** A spontaneous or elective termination of pregnancy before the 20th week of gestation, based on the date of the last menstrual period. Spontaneous abortion is frequently called *miscarriage*.

**abruptio placentae** Premature separation of a normally implanted placenta.

**abstinence syndrome** A group of symptoms that occurs when a person who is dependent on a specific drug withdraws or abstains from taking that drug.

**achalasia** Failure of smooth muscle fibers of the gastrointestinal tract to relax, resulting in a functional obstruction and difficulty in passage of food and chyme along the tract.

**acidosis** A condition resulting from the accumulation of acid (hydrogen ions) or the depletion of base (bicarbonate) in the blood or body tissues. The arterial blood pH measures acid–base balance.

**acme** Peak or period of greatest strength of a uterine contraction.

**acrocyanosis** Bluish discoloration of the hands and feet caused by reduced peripheral circulation.

**active immunity** Protection that forms in response to exposure to natural antigens or vaccines; protection can last months, years, or a lifetime.

**active listening** Listening empathically to gain a better understanding of both the actual and implied message.

**addiction** A neurobiologic disease state influenced by genetic, psychologic, and environmental factors characterized by impaired control over drug use, compulsive use, continued use despite harm, and cravings.

**adduction** Movement of a limb toward the midline of the body.

**adequate intake** Nutrient intake assumed to be adequate when a recommended daily allowance (RDA) cannot be determined.

**adjuvant** A pharmacologic or nonpharmacologic intervention with additive effects on pain management; designed to assist the primary pain management intervention.

**adjuvant therapy** Additional treatment that increases or enhances the action of the primary treatment.

**adnexa** Accessory organs of the uterus, such as the fallopian tubes and ovaries.

**adolescence** Period between the onset of puberty and the cessation of physical growth; the passage from childhood to adulthood.

**advocacy** Speaking or arguing in support of a policy or a person's rights.

**advocate** One who speaks on behalf of another.

**afterload** The amount of force against which the ventricles contract.

**afterpains** Cramping pain after childbirth, caused by alternating relaxation and contraction of uterine muscles.

**agonist** A substance that causes a physiologic effect.

**airway management** Correct positioning of the airway, appropriate interventions used to ensure patency of the airway, and adequate oxygenation and ventilation.

**alkalosis** Abnormal accumulation of base in or loss of acid from the body, with serum pH of more than 7.45.

**allele** Alternate form of a gene.

**allergy** A hypersensitivity reaction in various body systems, resulting from the immune system's response to exposure to an irritant (allergen).

**alopecia** Hair loss; a common side effect of chemotherapy.

**alpha-fetoprotein (AFP)** Plasma protein produced by the fetus.

**ambiguity (ambiguous)** Lack of clarity or certainty; having more than one meaning.

**ambivalence** Simultaneous conflicting emotions, attitudes, ideas, or wishes.

**amblyopia** Reduced visual acuity not correctable by refractive means and not attributable to structural or pathologic ocular anomalies.

**amenorrhea** Absence of menstruation. Primary amenorrhea is a delay of the first menstruation. Secondary amenorrhea is the cessation of menstruation after its initiation.

**amniocentesis** Transabdominal puncture of the amniotic sac to obtain a sample of amniotic fluid that contains fetal cells and biochemical substances for laboratory examination.

**amnioinfusion** Infusion of a sterile isotonic solution into the uterine cavity during labor to reduce umbilical cord compression; may be done to dilute meconium in amniotic fluid.

**amniotic fluid index (AFI)** Calculation of the amniotic fluid volume for adequacy at the gestational age.

**amniotomy** Artificial rupture of the amniotic sac (fetal membranes).

**analgesic** A systemic agent that relieves pain without loss of consciousness.

**anaphylactoid syndrome** A disorder in which amniotic fluid with its particulate matter enters the pregnant woman's circulation, lodging in her lungs. Also called *amniotic fluid embolism*.

**anastomosis** Surgical connection of separate tubular hollow organs to form a continuous channel, such as between two parts of the intestine or esophagus.

**anesthesia** Loss of sensation, especially pain sensation, with or without loss of consciousness.

**anesthesiologist** A physician who specializes in the administration of anesthesia.

**angioplasty** Procedure that dilates vessels.

**anorexia** Loss of appetite.

**anorexia nervosa** Refusal to eat because of a distorted body image and feeling of obesity.

**antagonist** Substance that blocks the action of another substance or of body secretions.

**antepartum** Refers to the period of pregnancy before the onset of labor.

**antibody** A protein that the immune system produces to bind to specific antigens and eliminate them from the body.

**anticipatory grief** The processes of mourning, coping, interacting, planning, and psychosocial reorganizing that occur as part of the response to the impending death of a loved one.

**anticipatory guidance** Providing the family with information on what to expect regarding a future event, a potential problem or issue, or a child's next developmental phase.

**antigen** A substance that possesses unique configurations, enabling the immune system to recognize it as foreign.

**antiphospholipid antibodies** Autoimmune antibodies that are directed against phospholipids in cell membranes. It is associated with recurrent spontaneous abortion, fetal loss, and severe preeclampsia.

**antipyretic** An agent that reduces or relieves fever.

**apical pulse rate** Heart rate determined by placing the stethoscope over the point of maximal intensity and counting for 1 minute.

**apneic spells** Cessation of breathing for more than 20 seconds or accompanied by cyanosis, pallor, bradycardia, or hypotonia.

**Arnold–Chiari malformation** Abnormalities of the fourth ventricle, lower cerebellum, and brainstem characterized by herniation of the cerebellum through the foramen magnum into the spinal canal; often associated with myelomeningocele.

**arteriovenous fistula** A connection between an artery and a vein, usually for the purpose of hemodialysis.

**asphyxia** Insufficient oxygen and excess carbon dioxide in the blood and tissues.

**asphyxiation** A state of suffocation that severely compromises oxygen delivery to the body.

**aspiration pneumonitis** A chemical injury to the lungs that may occur with regurgitation and aspiration of acidic gastric secretions.

**assisted reproductive techniques (ART)** Use of medical, surgical, laboratory, or micromanipulation techniques to handle the ovum and sperm to improve chances of conception.

**associative play** Group play without group goals.

**assumptions** Beliefs taken for granted without examination.

**astigmatism** Abnormal curvature of the cornea or lens.

**atelectasis** A collapsed or airless state of the lung that may involve all or part of the lung.

**atony** Absence or lack of usual muscle tone.

**atresia** Absence or abnormal closure of a normal body orifice or passage.

**atrophic vaginitis** Inflammation that occurs when the vagina becomes dry and fragile, usually as a result of estrogen deficit after menopause.
**attachment** Development of strong ties of affection as a result of interaction between an infant and a significant other (mother, father, sibling, or caretaker).
**attitude** Relationship of fetal body parts to one another, such as flexion or extension.
**augmentation of labor** Artificial stimulation of uterine contractions that have become ineffective.
**auscultate** To listen to body sounds (e.g., heart sounds, breath sounds) using a stethoscope.
**auscultation** Elicitation and evaluation of sounds produced by the body, frequently using a stethoscope to magnify body sounds.
**autism spectrum disorders** Pervasive developmental disorders characterized by impairment in communication skills, social interaction, and repetitive and stereotyped patterns of behavior; this term is generally replacing the term *pervasive developmental disorders.*
**autogenous graft** Tissue moved from one part of the body to another part of the same person's body.
**autoimmune disease** Disease that occurs when the immune system produces antibodies—called *autoantibodies*—against cells of the body.
**autonomy** Independent will and the capacity to be self-governing.
**autoregulation** The unique ability of the cerebral arteries to maintain a steady blood flow during changes in blood pressure and perfusion by adjusting their diameter in response to alterations in cerebral perfusion pressure.
**autosome** Any of the 22 pairs of chromosomes other than the sex chromosomes.
**avascular necrosis** Tissue damage caused by inadequate blood supply.
**axillary tail** Wedge of tissue extending from the breast into the axilla (also called the *tail of Spence*).
**azoospermia** Absence of sperm in semen.
**azotemia** The presence of urea and other nitrogenous bodies in the blood; an elevated blood urea nitrogen or creatinine level.

## B

**ballottement** Rebound of the fetus when the cervix is tapped during vaginal examination.
**baroreceptors** Cells that are sensitive to blood pressure changes.
**basal body temperature (BBT)** Body temperature at rest.
**basal ganglia** A major communication and sorting area for messages to and from the cerebral hemispheres composed of masses of gray matter; controls movement and participates in emotion and cognition.
**baseline data** Information that describes the status of the patient before treatment begins.
**baseline risk** The risk, usually in reference to birth defects or spontaneous abortion, of the general population of pregnant women who have no identified high-risk factors or invasive procedures.
**Battle sign** Bruising or hemorrhage over the mastoid, which may be indicative of a skull fracture.
**benign** Slow-growing cells, often almost normal in appearance, forming a tumor with distinct borders.
**bias** A prejudice that sways the mind.
**bicornuate (bicornate) uterus** Malformed uterus having two horns.
**bilirubin** Unusable component of hemolyzed (broken down) erythrocytes.
**bilirubin encephalopathy** Acute manifestation of bilirubin toxicity.
**bioethics** Rules or principles that govern right conduct, specifically those that relate to healthcare.
**biophysical profile (BPP)** Method for evaluating fetal status during the antepartum period based on five fetal variables: fetal heart rate variability, fetal breathing movements, gross body movements, muscle tone, and amniotic fluid volume (also known as *amniotic fluid index* or *AFI*).
**birth defect** Abnormality of structure, function, or body metabolism presenting at birth that results in physical or mental disability or is fatal (according to the March of Dimes).
**blast cells** Immature white blood cells, such as lymphoblasts, myeloblasts, or monoblasts.
**blood–brain barrier** Selective anatomic or physiologic capillary obstruction that prevents potentially harmful substances, such as certain medications, radioactive ions, and viruses, from entering the parenchyma of the brain.
**bloody show** Mixture of cervical mucus and blood from ruptured capillaries in the cervix. Bloody show often precedes labor and increases with cervical dilation.
**body image** Subjective image of one's physical appearance and capabilities derived from one's own observations and from the evaluation of significant others.
**bonding** Development of a strong emotional tie of a parent to a newborn; also called *claiming* or *binding in.*
**brainstem** Structure connected to the cerebral hemispheres by thick bunches of nerve fibers; all nerve fibers traverse through the brainstem from the hemispheres to the cerebellum and spinal cord.
**Braxton Hicks contractions** Irregular, usually mild uterine contractions that occur throughout pregnancy and become stronger in the last trimester. May be confused with true or false labor.
**bronchopulmonary dysplasia** Chronic pulmonary condition in which damage to the infant's lungs requires prolonged dependence on supplemental oxygen. Also called *chronic lung disease.*
**brown fat (or brown adipose tissue)** Highly vascular specialized fat found in the newborn that provides more heat than other fat when metabolized.
**bulimia** Eating disorder characterized by ingestion of large amounts of food, followed by purging behavior such as induced vomiting or laxative abuse.

## C

**café au lait spots** Light brown birthmarks.
**callus** Tissue that joins fractured bone ends or repairs damaged bone; begins as cartilaginous tissue and becomes hardened through osteoblastic activity.
**caput succedaneum** Area of edema over the presenting part of the fetus or newborn, resulting from pressure against the cervix. Usually called simply *caput.*
**carcinoma in situ** Malignant neoplasm in surface tissue that has not extended into deeper tissue.
**cardiomegaly** An enlarged heart.
**cardiopulmonary resuscitation** Protocol performed when an individual's respiratory and cardiovascular systems require support to maintain vital functions; airway management, ventilation, and chest compressions are provided to improve tissue perfusion until definitive care is available.
**caries** Decay of teeth.
**case management** A practice model that uses a systematic approach to identify specific patient needs and to manage patient care to ensure optimal outcomes.
**catabolism** A process that converts living cells into simpler compounds. Involved in the involution of the uterus after childbirth.
**cataract** A loss of transparency of the crystalline lens or its capsule.
**central venous access device** Venous access device in which the catheter is placed centrally rather than peripherally, usually in the superior vena cava or jugular vein; used for long-term intravenous therapy.
**cephalhematoma** Bleeding between the periosteum and skull from pressure during birth; does not cross suture lines.
**cephalocaudal** Progression from head to toe.
**cephalopelvic disproportion** Fetal head size that is too large to fit through the maternal pelvis at birth. Also called *fetopelvic disproportion.*
**cerclage** Encircling the cervix with sutures to prevent recurrent spontaneous abortion caused by early cervical dilation.
**cerebral cortex** Gray matter of the cerebrum where the higher functions of thinking occur.
**cerebral perfusion pressure** The difference between mean arterial blood pressure and intracranial pressure.
**cervical cap** A small cup-like device placed over the cervix to prevent the sperm from entering.
**cesarean birth** Surgical birth of the fetus through an incision in the abdominal wall and uterus.
**Chadwick's sign** Bluish purple discoloration of the cervix, vagina, and labia during pregnancy as a result of increased vascular congestion.
**chelation** Binding of a metallic ion with a structure so that the ion is inactivated.
**chemical dependence** Physical and psychologic dependence on substances such as alcohol, tobacco, or drugs, either legal or illicit.
**chemoreceptors** Cells that are sensitive to chemical changes in the blood, specifically changes in oxygen and carbon dioxide levels and in acid–base balance.

**chignon** Newborn scalp edema created by a vacuum extractor.

**choanal atresia** Abnormality of the nasal septum that obstructs one or both nasal passages.

**chordee** Ventral curvature of the penis.

**chorioamnionitis** Inflammation of the amniotic sac (fetal membranes), usually caused by bacterial or viral infections. Also called *amnionitis*.

**chorionic villus sampling (CVS)** Transcervical or transabdominal sampling of chorionic villi (projections on the outer fetal membrane) for the analysis of fetal cells.

**chronic grief** Mourning after the death of an individual that is of excessive duration and interferes with the person's ability to return to normal living.

**chronic illness or condition** A condition or illness that is long term and either is without cure or has a residual effect that limits activities of daily living.

**chronic sorrow** Recurrent feelings of grief, loss, and fear related to the child's illness and loss of the ideal, healthy child.

**chronologic age** Age in years.

**cilia** Hair-like processes on the surface of a cell. Cilia beat rhythmically to move the cell or to move fluid or other substances over the cell surface.

**circumduction** Circular movement of a limb or an eye.

**clean margins** Evidence of normal, disease-free tissue in the outermost layer of cells of a surgical sample.

**cleansing breath** A deep breath taken at the beginning and end of each labor contraction.

**climacteric** Physical and emotional changes occurring at the end of a woman's reproductive period. Also informally called *menopause*, although this term does not encompass all changes.

**closure** Reaching a decision.

**coitus** Sexual union between a male and female.

**coitus interruptus** Withdrawal of the penis from the vagina before ejaculation.

**colostrum** Breast fluid secreted during pregnancy and 7 to 10 days after childbirth.

**colposcopy** Examination of the vaginal and cervical tissue with a colposcope to magnify cells.

**comorbidity** The occurrence of two or more different disorders in the same individual; children with intellectual impairments often have coexisting psychiatric disorders.

**compensation** Maintenance of an adequate blood flow without distressing symptoms; accomplished by cardiac and circulatory adjustments, such as tachycardia, cardiac hypertrophy, and increased blood volume from sodium and water retention.

**complement** An accessory system to a humoral response that is composed of serum proteins that facilitate enzyme action and antigen death.

**complete protein food** Food containing all essential amino acids.

**compliance** Stretchability or elasticity of the lungs and thorax that allows distention without resistance during respirations.

**conceptus** Cells and membranes that result from fertilization of the ovum at any stage of prenatal development.

**condom** Latex, polyurethane, or natural membrane shield covering the penis or lining the vagina to prevent sperm from entering the cervix and to prevent infection.

**conductive hearing loss** Reversible loss caused by damage, inflammation, or obstruction to outer or middle ear; sound is prevented from progressing across middle ear.

**condyloma** A wart-like growth of the skin seen on the external genitalia, in the vagina, on the cervix, or near the anus. Condyloma may be caused by human papillomavirus (condyloma acuminatum) or by syphilis (condyloma latum).

**congenital** Present at birth.

**congenital (infantile) glaucoma** Increased intraocular fluid pressure that occurs during the first 3 years of life because of a defect in the drainage network of the eye.

**congestive heart failure** Condition resulting from failure of the heart to maintain adequate circulation; characterized by weakness, dyspnea, and edema in body parts that are lower than the heart.

**consanguinity** Blood relationship of parents.

**conservation** Ability to understand that certain properties of objects do not change simply because their order, form, or appearance has changed.

**containment** A method of increasing comfort in infants by swaddling or other methods to keep the extremities in a flexed position near the body.

**contraception** Prevention of pregnancy.

**contraction stress test (CST)** Method for evaluating fetal status during the antepartum period by observing the response of the fetal heart to intermittent stress of induced uterine contractions. Also known as *oxytocin challenge test (OCT)*.

**cooperative play** Organized play with group goals.

**coping** Efforts directed toward managing and solving various problems, events, and stressors.

**corpus luteum** Graafian follicle cells remaining after ovulation. These cells produce estrogen and progesterone.

**corrected age** Gestational age that a preterm infant would be if still *in utero* or born at full term. May also be called *developmental age.*

**couvade** Pregnancy-related rituals or a cluster of symptoms experienced by some prospective fathers during pregnancy and childbirth.

**crackles** Abnormal, discontinuous, nonmusical sounds heard on auscultation, primarily during inhalation; also called *rales.*

**craniosynostosis** Premature closure of the sutures of the infant's head.

**crepitation** A dry, crackling sound or sensation.

**crepitus** A grating sensation at a fracture site that occurs when the ends of a broken bone move against each other.

**crowning** Appearance of the fetal scalp or presenting part at the vaginal opening.

**cryotherapy** Destruction of abnormal tissue using extreme cold.

**cryptorchidism** Failure of one or both testes to descend into the scrotum.

**culture** The sum of values, beliefs, and practices of a group of people that are transmitted from one generation to the next.

**Cushing's response** Late sign of increased intracranial pressure; includes increased blood pressure, widened pulse pressure, decreased heart rate, and decreased or irregular respiratory rate.

**cystocele** Prolapse of the urinary bladder through the anterior vaginal wall.

## D

**debulking** The surgical removal of as much of a tumor as possible.

**decidua** The endometrium during pregnancy. All except the deepest layer is shed after childbirth.

**decompensation** Inability of the heart to maintain adequate circulation; may be marked by dyspnea, venous engorgement, cyanosis, and edema.

**delegated nursing interventions** Physician-prescribed nursing actions that require nursing judgment because nurses are accountable for correct implementation. *See also* independent nursing interventions.

**dental emergencies** Injuries or infections of a tooth or teeth occurring when the period of time to definitive care is critical for the survival of the tooth or to alleviate pain.

**development** Changes that occur over time in function and psychosocial and cognitive behavior.

**developmental age** Age based on functional behavior and ability to adapt to the environment; does not necessarily correspond to chronologic age.

**developmental disability** Characterized by delays and impairments of expected developmental level.

**developmental milestones** Benchmarks of development that indicate whether the infant is developing normally; not achieving milestones within a certain time frame might be a cause for concern.

**diabetes mellitus** A disorder of carbohydrate metabolism caused by a relative or complete lack of insulin secretion; characterized by glycosuria (glucose in the urine) and hyperglycemia.

**diabetic ketoacidosis** Metabolic consequence of severe insulin deficiency; marked by hyperglycemia, acidosis, and ketosis.

**diabetogenic** Refers to a condition such as pregnancy that produces the effects of diabetes mellitus.

**diaphragm** A latex dome that covers the cervix and prevents entrance of sperm; must be used with a spermicide to be effective.

**diastasis recti** Separation of the longitudinal muscles of the abdomen (rectus abdominis) during pregnancy.

**dietary reference intakes** A label for several terms that estimate nutrient needs; includes recommended dietary allowance, adequate intake,

tolerable upper intake level, and estimated average requirement.
**dilation** gradual widening of the cervix in the process of labor.
**dilation and curettage (D&C)** Stretching the cervical os to permit suctioning or scraping of the walls of the uterus. The procedure is performed in abortion, to obtain samples of uterine lining tissue for laboratory examination, and during the postpartum period to remove retained fragments of placenta.
**dilation and evacuation (D&E)** Wide cervical dilation followed by mechanical destruction and removal of fetal parts from the uterus. After complete removal of the fetus, a vacuum curet is used to remove the placenta and remaining products of conception.
**diploid** Having a pair of chromosomes (46; or 23 pairs in humans) that represents one copy of every chromosome from each parent; the number of chromosomes normally present in body cells other than gametes.
**diplopia** Double vision.
**discipline** The structure an adult sets for a child's life, designed to allow the child to interact socially in the real world in an appropriate manner; the training expected to produce a specific type or pattern of behavior.
**dislocation** Displacement of a bone from its normal articulation within a joint.
**doula** A trained support person employed to provide labor or postpartum support.
**dramatic play** Play in which children act out roles and experiences that may have happened to them, that they fear will happen to them, or that they have observed happening to someone else.
**dysfluency** Disorders in the rhythm of speech in which individuals know precisely what they wish to say but are unable to do so because of an involuntary, repetitive prolongation or cessation of sound.
**dyslipidemia** Abnormal levels of cholesterol and fat in the blood.
**dysmenorrhea** Painful menstruation; "cramps."
**dyspareunia** Difficult or painful coitus in women.
**dysphagia** Difficulty swallowing.
**dysplasia** Abnormal development of tissue.
**dyspnea** Difficulty breathing.
**dysrhythmia** Disturbance of rhythm.
**dystocia** Difficult or prolonged labor, often associated with abnormal uterine activity and cephalopelvic disproportion.
**dysuria** Painful urination, often associated with urinary tract infection.

## E

**echolalia** Stereotyped repetition of another person's words or phrases.
**eclampsia** Form of hypertension of pregnancy complicated by generalized (grand mal) seizures.
**ectopic pregnancy** Implantation of a fertilized ovum in any area other than the uterus; the most common site is the fallopian tube.
**EDD** Estimated date of delivery. May also be abbreviated EDB (estimated date of birth).
**edema** Presence of abnormally large amounts of fluid in the intercellular tissue spaces of the body.
**effacement** Cervical thinning.
**effleurage** Self-massage of the abdomen or other body part during labor contractions.
**egocentrism** Interest centered on the self rather than the needs of others.
**ejaculation** Expulsion of semen from the penis.
**embolus** A mass that may be composed of a thrombus (blood clot) or amniotic fluid released into the bloodstream to cause obstruction of pulmonary vessels.
**embryo** Developing baby from the beginning of the 3rd week through the 8th week after conception.
**embryonic period** Period of development that extends from the beginning of the 3rd week through the 8th week after conception.
**emergency** Psychologic, medical, or traumatic condition that requires immediate care or care within 1 hour to prevent further deterioration.
**empowerment** Provision of appropriate tools (education, information, support) to individuals that enable them to participate fully in decision making.
**en face** Position that allows close eye-to-eye contact between the newborn and a parent.
**encopresis** Incontinence of feces.
**endometrial hyperplasia** Excessive proliferation of normal cells of the uterine lining; may be caused by administration of estrogen during the postmenopausal period.
**endometriosis** Presence of endometrial tissue (uterine lining) outside the uterine cavity.
**endometritis** Infection of the inner lining of the uterus.
**endometrium** Lining of the uterus.
**endomyometritis** Infection of the muscle and inner lining of the uterus.
**endoparametritis** Infection of the muscle and inner lining of the uterus as well as the surrounding tissues.
**endorphins** Morphine-like substances that occur naturally in the central nervous system and modify pain sensations.
**engagement** Descent of the widest diameter of the fetal presenting part to at least a zero station (level of the ischial spines in the maternal pelvis).
**engorgement** Swelling of the breasts resulting from increased blood flow, edema, and the presence of milk.
**engrossment** Intense fascination and close face-to-face observation between father and newborn.
**enteral** By way of the digestive system (e.g., enteral feeding).
**enteral feeding** Nutrients supplied to the gastrointestinal tract orally or by feeding tube.
**entrainment** Newborn movement in rhythm with adult speech, particularly high-pitched tones, which are more easily heard.
**envenomation** Injection of venom by an animal (e.g., usually snakes, lizards, spiders, scorpions) into a human body.
**environmental injuries** Injuries occurring as a result of outside or environmental factors.
**epidemiology** The study of health, illness, and factors that determine health and illness in a selected population.
**epidural** Potential space that surrounds the spinal cord and lies outside the dura mater.
**epidural space** The area outside the dura between the dura mater and vertebral canal.
**episiotomy** Surgical incision of the perineum to enlarge the vaginal opening.
**epispadias** Abnormal placement of the urinary meatus on the dorsal side of the penis.
**erectile dysfunction** Consistent inability of a man to achieve or maintain an erection that is sufficiently rigid and sustained for vaginal intercourse.
**erythema** Redness of the skin.
**erythema toxicum** Benign rash of unknown cause in newborns, with blotchy red areas that may have white or yellow papules or vesicles in the center.
**erythroblastosis fetalis** Agglutination and hemolysis of fetal erythrocytes resulting from incompatibility between maternal and fetal blood. In most cases, the fetus is Rh-positive and the mother is Rh-negative.
**erythropoiesis** Production of erythrocytes (red blood cells [RBCs]).
**eschar** Dark plaque associated with tissue necrosis, which can form an inelastic shell over wounds.
**essential amino acids** Amino acids that cannot be synthesized by the body and must be obtained from foods.
**estimated average requirement** Amount of a nutrient estimated to meet the needs of half the healthy people in an age-group.
**estimated date of delivery (EDD)** Estimate of the date the woman will deliver. Also can be referred to as EDB, estimated date of birth.
**ethical dilemma** A situation in which no solution seems completely satisfactory.
**ethics** Rules or principles that govern right conduct and distinctions between right and wrong.
**ethnic** Pertaining to religious, racial, national, or cultural group characteristics, especially speech patterns, social customs, and physical characteristics.
**ethnicity** Condition of belonging to a particular ethnic group; also refers to ethnic pride.
**ethnocentrism** The opinion that the beliefs and customs of one's own ethnic group are superior to those of others.
**eutectic mixture of local anesthetics (EMLA)** Cream used to numb the skin at a depth of 0.5 mm; used before needle punctures.
**euthyroid** Normal thyroid function.
**exanthem** An eruption or rash on the skin.
**excoriation** Scratch or abrasion of the skin.
**exfoliation** Scaling off of dead tissue.
**extension (decerebrate) posture** Abnormal extension of the upper extremities with internal rotation of the upper arms and wrists; lower extremities will extend with some internal rotation.

**external fixation** Placement of pins, screws, or bars through bone and soft tissue to immobilize or correct a deformity.

**external rotation** Turning outward or laterally within a joint.

**externalizing disorders** Disorders with behavioral symptoms (e.g., attention, impulsivity, aggression); now included with neurodevelopmental disorders.

**extracellular fluid** Fluid found outside the cell, comprising approximately one third of the body's fluid in older children and approximately one half of the body's fluid in infants.

**extracorporeal life support** Temporary method of providing cardiovascular, pulmonary, and circulatory support for children for whom other methods of treatment are not effective.

**extramedullary** Outside the bone marrow.

**extrapyramidal motor system (tract)** Descending pathway of the motor neurons concerned with involuntary or unconscious skeletal muscle coordination and reflex control of coordination.

**extremely low-birth-weight infant** An infant weighing 1000 g (2 lb, 3 oz) or less at birth.

## F

**false labor** Braxton Hicks contractions that are mistaken for true labor.

**familial** Presence of a trait or condition in a family more often than would be expected by chance alone.

**familiarization play** Use of materials that are commonly associated with healthcare situations in creative and playful activities.

**family** A social group whose members share common goals and values and whose members are committed to each other; may or may not be biologically related.

**fantasy** Mental images formed to prepare for the birth of a child.

**fatalism** The belief that events are predestined.

**ferning (or fern test)** Microscopic appearance of amniotic fluid that resembles fern leaves when the fluid dries on a microscope slide.

**fertilization age** Prenatal age of the developing baby, calculated from the date of conception. Also called *postconceptional age.*

**fetal alcohol spectrum disorders** All disorders resulting from maternal use of alcohol during pregnancy; includes fetal alcohol syndrome.

**fetal alcohol syndrome** A group of physical, behavioral, and mental abnormalities that are the most severe effects of fetal alcohol exposure.

**fetal growth restriction** Failure of a fetus to grow as expected for gestational age.

**fetal lung fluid** Fluid that fills the fetal lungs, expanding the alveoli and promoting lung development.

**fetus** Developing baby from 9 weeks after conception until birth. In everyday practice this term is often used to describe a developing baby during pregnancy, regardless of age.

**fingertipping** First tactile (touch) experience between mother and newborn. The mother explores the infant's body, mainly with her fingertips.

**first period of reactivity** Period beginning at birth in which newborns are active and alert. It ends when the infant first falls asleep.

**fistula** Abnormal passage or communication between two organs or tissues.

**flexion (decorticate) posture** Abnormal flexion of the upper extremities and extension of the lower extremities.

**fontanel** Space at the intersection of sutures connecting fetal or infant skull bones.

**foremilk** First breast milk received in a feeding.

**fornix (pl. fornices)** Arch or pouch-like structure at the upper end of the vagina. Also called a *cul-de-sac.*

**fourth trimester** First 12 weeks after birth, a time of transition for parents and siblings.

**fremitus** A vibration perceptible on palpation or auscultation.

**frequency** Urination at short time intervals.

**functional age** The age equivalent at which the child is actually able to perform specific self-care or relational tasks; for example, the child may be 6 years old chronologically but only able to perform skills representative of children 4 years old, and thus, the child's functional age is 4 years.

**fundoplication** A 270- to 360-degree wrap of the stomach fundus around the distal esophagus to tighten the lower esophageal sphincter and prevent gastric reflux.

**fundus** Part of the uterus that is farthest from the cervix, above the openings of the fallopian tubes.

**funic souffle** Sound of blood flow through the umbilical cord, corresponds to fetal heart rate.

## G

**gamete** Reproductive cell; in the female an ovum and in the male a spermatozoon.

**gametogenesis** Creation of reproductive cells.

**gene** Segment of DNA that directs the production of a specific product needed for body structure or function.

**general anesthesia** Systemic loss of sensation with loss of consciousness.

**genetic** Pertaining to the genes or the chromosomes.

**genetic mutation** Variation (deletion, addition, or recopy of a stretch of DNA) in a gene that affects its function.

**genetic sex** Sex determined at conception by union of two X chromosomes (female) or an X and a Y chromosome (male). Also called *chromosomal sex.*

**genogram** Graphic representation of a family's medical and hereditary history and the relationships among the family members, often called a *pedigree.*

**genome** DNA encoded characteristics that may be expressed or unexpressed.

**genotype** Genetic makeup of an individual.

**germinal matrix bleeding-intraventricular hemorrhage** Bleeding around and into the ventricles of the brain.

**gestational age** Prenatal age of the developing baby (measured in weeks) calculated from the 1st day of the woman's last menstrual period. Also called *menstrual age,* approximately 2 weeks longer than the fertilization age.

**gestational surrogate** A woman who carries the embryo of an infertile couple and relinquishes the child after birth.

**gestational trophoblastic disease** Spectrum of diseases that includes both benign hydatidiform mole and gestational trophoblastic tumors, such as invasive moles and choriocarcinoma.

**gland** An organ or structure that secretes a substance or hormone to be used in another part of the body.

**glucagon** A hormone produced by the alpha cells of the pancreas; counteracts the action of insulin by converting liver stores of glycogen to blood glucose, resulting in an elevation of the blood glucose concentration.

**gluconeogenesis** Formation of glycogen by the liver from noncarbohydrate sources such as amino and fatty acids.

**glucose** The substrate of choice for cellular energy; the breakdown product of stored glycogen or dietary carbohydrate.

**glycosuria** Glucose in urine that occurs when the blood glucose level exceeds the renal threshold and glucose "spills" into the urine.

**glycosylated hemoglobin** A laboratory test used to evaluate long-term blood glucose control by measuring glycosylation (glucose attachment to a protein) of a portion of the hemoglobin molecule in red blood cells; offers a 3-month average of blood glucose control.

**gonad** Reproductive (sex) gland that produces gametes and sex hormones. The female gonads are ovaries; the male gonads are testes.

**gonadotropin-releasing hormone (GnRH)** Secretion of the anterior pituitary gland that stimulates the gonads, specifically follicle-stimulating hormone and luteinizing hormone. Chorionic gonadotropin is secreted by the placenta during pregnancy.

**Goodell's sign** Softening of the cervix during pregnancy.

**Graafian follicle** Small sac within the ovary that contains the maturing ovum.

**gradient** Difference.

**growth** Measurable physical and physiologic changes that occur over time.

**growth spurts** Brief periods of a rapid increase in growth rate.

**grunting** A sound similar to a grunting noise that can be heard with or without a stethoscope.

**gynecologic age** Number of years since menarche (first menstrual period).

## H

**hand hygiene** Cleansing of the hands with soap and water, antiseptic hand wash, alcohol-based hand rub, or surgical hand antisepsis.

**haploid** Having one copy of a chromosome from each pair (23 in humans or half the diploid number). Gametes normally have a haploid number of chromosomes.

**Hegar's sign** Softening of the lower uterine segment at 6 to 8 weeks of pregnancy.

**hematemesis** Vomiting of bright red blood or of denatured blood that looks like coffee grounds; usually represents a bleeding source proximal to the jejunum.

**hematoma** Localized collection of blood in a space or tissue.

**hematopoiesis** Production of all types of blood cells (red blood cells, white blood cells, and platelets); normally occurs in the bone marrow but may occur in extramedullary sites.

**heme iron** Iron obtained from meat, poultry, or fish sources; the form most usable by the body.

**hemolysis** Breakdown of red blood cells.

**hemosiderosis** Focal or general increase in tissue iron stores without associated tissue damage.

**hemostasis** Process of vasoconstriction and coagulation to stop bleeding.

**hepatosplenomegaly** Enlargement of the liver and spleen detected by palpation of the abdomen.

**herniation** Shift of brain tissue sideways, under the falx cerebri, or downward, causing severe neurologic dysfunction.

**heterozygous** Having two different alleles for a genetic trait.

**history** The aggregate of subjective data that describes past and present health status.

**homozygous** Having two identical alleles for a genetic trait.

**honeymoon phase** An early stage of diabetes characterized by residual endogenous insulin production that results in a lower need for exogenous insulin to maintain normal blood glucose. Also refers to the time following an incident of intimate partner violence when the batterer is contrite and remorseful.

**hormone** A chemical substance produced by one gland or tissue and transported by the blood to other tissues or organs, where it causes a specific effect.

**hormone implant** One or more small rods of progestin inserted subcutaneously to provide contraception.

**hospice care** A system of comprehensive care that provides support and assistance to patients and families affected by terminal illness; the purpose is to humanize the dying experience while providing the means for living as comfortably and as fully as possible; goals are accomplished by providing respectful, noninvasive care; pain and symptom control; and emotional, physical, psychologic, and spiritual support.

**host** The organism from which a parasite obtains its nourishment.

**hydramnios** Excessive volume of amniotic fluid (more than 2000 mL at term). Also called *polyhydramnios.*

**hydrocele** A collection of fluid around the testes.

**hydrops fetalis** Heart failure and generalized edema in the fetus secondary to severe anemia resulting from destruction of erythrocytes.

**hyperbilirubinemia** Excessive amount of bilirubin in the blood.

**hypercapnia** Excess carbon dioxide in the blood, evidenced by an elevated partial pressure of carbon dioxide ($Pco_2$).

**hyperemia** Excess blood in a part of the body.

**hyperglycemia** Blood glucose in a diabetic child above the target range; in a nondiabetic child, fasting blood glucose of 110 mg/dL or higher.

**hyperkalemia** Elevated serum potassium level above the range for age.

**hypernatremic (hypertonic) dehydration** State in which the sodium concentration is above that of normal body fluids (i.e., 150 mEq/L).

**hyperopia** Farsightedness; abnormal close vision.

**hypertonic contractions** Uterine contractions that are too long or too frequent, have too short a resting interval, or have an inadequate relaxation period to allow optimal uteroplacental exchange.

**hypertonic labor dysfunction** Ineffective labor characterized by erratic and poorly coordinated contractions. Uterine resting tone is higher than normal.

**hyphema** A hemorrhage or sanguineous exudates in the anterior chamber of the eye.

**hypoalbuminemia** Low albumin levels in the blood.

**hypoglycemia** Abnormally low blood glucose level.

**hyponatremic (hypotonic) dehydration** State in which the sodium concentration is below that of normal body fluids (i.e., 130 mEq/L).

**hypospadias** Abnormal placement of the urinary meatus on the ventral side of the penis.

**hypothalamus** Portion of the brain that secretes releasing factors to the pituitary gland for the maintenance of endocrine and metabolic activities.

**hypovolemia** Abnormally decreased volume of circulating fluid in the body.

**hypovolemic shock** Acute peripheral circulatory failure resulting from loss of circulating blood volume.

**hypoxemia** Reduced oxygenation of the blood, evident by a low partial pressure of oxygen ($Po_2$).

**hypoxia** Reduced availability of oxygen to the body tissues.

## I

**iatrogenic** An adverse condition resulting from treatment.

**identity formation** The acquisition of psychosocial, sexual, and vocational identity.

**idiopathic** For unknown reasons.

**illness trajectory** The course of a chronic illness, including the work for and effect on the lives of all those involved.

**immune (lymphoreticular) system** The body's internal defense against foreign substances, such as bacteria, viruses, parasites, and fungi.

**immunity** Resistance of the body to the effects of a harmful organism or its toxin.

**immunodeficiency** A defect in the immune system leading to increased susceptibility to multiple and repeated infections.

**immunosuppression** A weakening or cessation of the body's normal immune response.

**implanted venous access device** Surgically implanted port or reservoir in which the catheter tip is placed in the superior vena cava; used for long-term intravenous therapy.

**incompetent cervix** Inability of the cervix to remain closed long enough during pregnancy for the fetus to survive.

**incomplete protein food** Food that does not contain all the essential amino acids.

**independent nursing interventions** Nurse-prescribed actions used in both nursing diagnoses and collaboratively addressed problems. See also *delegated nursing interventions.*

**induction of labor** Artificial initiation of labor.

**infant mortality rate** Number of deaths per 1000 live births that occur within the first 12 months of life.

**infection** Condition resulting from invasion of the body by pathogenic or nonpathogenic organisms, such as bacteria, viruses, protozoa, helminths, or fungi.

**inference** The act of drawing a conclusion or making a deduction.

**infertility** Inability of a couple to conceive after 1 year of regular intercourse (two or three times weekly) without using contraception; also the involuntary inability to conceive and produce viable offspring when the couple chooses. Primary infertility occurs in a couple who have never conceived; secondary infertility occurs in a couple who have conceived at least once before.

**inflammation** A tissue response to injury or destruction of cells.

**informed consent** A requirement, both legal and ethical, that the child and the parent or guardian completely understand proposed procedures or treatments, including their benefits and risks.

**inotropic** Affects the force of muscular contractions; can cause a positive or negative effect.

**inquiry** Living with questions.

**inspection** Careful observation to identify physical findings.

**intellectual disability** Term adopted by learning specialists to describe disabilities of learning, thinking, and problem solving.

**Intellectual impairment** Replaces the term *mental retardation* as a descriptor unless specific criteria are present.

**intelligence** The innate capacity of the individual; what individuals can do relative to learning, thinking, and problem solving; results obtained on intelligence tests that measure specific skills, such as verbal, nonverbal, or mechanical abilities.

**intermittent infusion port** Intravenous catheter used to administer intermittent medications or fluids; remains clamped when not in use.

**intermittent monitoring** A variation of electronic fetal monitoring in which an initial strip is obtained on admission. If patterns are reassuring, the woman is remonitored for periods of 15 minutes at regular intervals (approximately every 30 to 60 minutes).

**internal fixation** Placement of instruments (wires, pins, rods, screws) inside the body to immobilize parts.

**internalizing disorders** Disorders of mood (depression) and anxiety.

**interstitial fluid** Extracellular fluid surrounding the cell, including lymph fluid.

**intracellular fluid** Fluid found within the cells, composing approximately two thirds of the body's fluid in older children and approximately one half of the body's fluid in infants.

**intrapartum** The time of labor and childbirth.

**intrathecal** Within the spinal column.

**intrauterine device (IUD)** A mechanical device inserted into the uterus to prevent pregnancy.

**introversion** Inward concentration on oneself and one's body.

**involution** Retrogressive changes that return the reproductive organs, particularly the uterus, to their nonpregnant size and condition.

**irreversibility** The inability to understand a process in reverse or mentally undo an action that has been performed.

**isonatremic (isotonic) dehydration** State in which the sodium concentration is practically identical to that of body fluids (i.e., between 135 and 145 mEq/L).

## J

**jaundice** Yellow discoloration of the skin and sclera caused by excessive bilirubin in the blood; also called *icterus.*

## K

**kangaroo care** Skin-to-skin contact between infants and their parents.

**karyotype** Picture of a cell's chromosomes, arranged from largest to smallest pairs.

**Kegel exercises** Alternate contracting and relaxing of the pelvic floor muscles to strengthen them.

**kernicterus** Staining of brain tissue caused by accumulation of unconjugated bilirubin in the brain. Bilirubin encephalopathy is the brain damage that results from these deposits.

**ketone, ketoacid** An acid produced in response to starvation (in the diabetic child, a result of insulin deficiency); produced from fat stores, which can be used for energy by some tissues when glucose is unavailable.

**Ketonuria** Excretion of abnormally high amounts of ketone bodies in the urine; It is a sign that diabetes mellitus is not controlled.

**ketosis** Accumulation of ketone bodies (metabolic products) in the blood; frequently associated with acidosis.

**kilocalorie** A unit of heat used to show the energy value in foods, commonly called *calorie.*

**Kussmaul respiration** Deep, rapid respiration seen with diabetic ketoacidosis in which carbon dioxide is expelled as a respiratory compensation for acidosis; also described as "air hunger."

## L

**lactation** Secretion of milk from the breasts; also describes the time when a child is breastfed.

**lactogenesis** The production of milk.

**lacto-ovovegetarian** A vegetarian whose diet includes milk products and eggs.

**lactose intolerance** Inability to digest most dairy products because of a deficiency in the enzyme lactase.

**lactovegetarian** A vegetarian whose diet includes milk products.

**lanugo** Fine, soft hair covering the fetus.

**laparoscopy** Insertion of an illuminated tube into the abdominal cavity to visualize contents, locate bleeding, and perform surgical procedures.

**laparotomy** Incision through the abdominal wall to examine the abdominal or pelvic organs.

**large-for-gestational-age infant** An infant whose size is above the 90th percentile for gestational age.

**latch-on** Attachment of the infant to the breast.

**late deceleration** Slowing of the fetal heart rate after the onset of a uterine contraction that persists after the contraction ends.

**late preterm infant** An infant born between 34 0/7 and 36 6/7 weeks of gestation.

**lavage** Wash.

**learning** Behavior changes that occur as a result of both maturation and experience with the environment.

**lecithin/sphingomyelin ratio (L/S ratio)** Ratio of two phospholipids in amniotic fluid that is used to estimate fetal lung maturity.

**let-down reflex** See *milk-ejection reflex.*

**leukocoria** Appearance of a whitish reflection or mass in the pupillary area behind the lens of the eye.

**leukocytes** White blood cells, whose chief function is to protect the body against foreign substances; includes five types: lymphocytes, monocytes, neutrophils, eosinophils, and basophils.

**libido** Sexual desire.

**lichenification** Thickening and hardening of the skin with accentuation of skin markings; often the result of chronic scratching.

**lie** Relationship of the long axis of the fetus to the long axis of the mother.

**lightening** Descent of the fetus toward the pelvic inlet before labor.

**linear salpingostomy** Incision along the length of a fallopian tube to remove an ectopic pregnancy and preserve the tube.

**lipogenic** Substances such as insulin that stimulate the production of fat.

**lochia alba** White, cream-colored, or light yellow vaginal discharge that follows lochia serosa.

**lochia rubra** Reddish or red-brown vaginal discharge that occurs immediately after childbirth; composed mostly of blood.

**lochia serosa** Pink or brown-tinged vaginal discharge that follows lochia rubra; composed largely of serous exudate, blood, and leukocytes.

**low-birth-weight infant** Infant whose weight is less than 2500 g (5 lb, 8 oz) at birth.

**lymphadenopathy** Swelling of the lymph nodes detected by palpation.

**lymphocytes** The primary white blood cells of the immune system (e.g., B lymphocytes or B cells; and T lymphocytes or T cells).

## M

**macrosomia** Unusually large fetal size; infant birth weight more than 4000 g (8 lb, 13 oz or more). Some sources define macrosomia as a birth weight of 4500 g (9 lb, 15 oz or more).

**malignant** Abnormal cells that have invasive and unregulated growth and the potential to spread to distant locations in the body; life-threatening.

**malocclusion** Misalignment of the teeth or dental arches; teeth may be crowded, crooked, or out of alignment.

**malpractice** Negligence by a professional person.

**mammogram** Study of breast tissue using very-low-dose radiography; primary tool in the diagnosis of breast cancer.

**mastitis** Infection of the breast

**mature milk** Breast milk that follows transitional milk.

**meconium aspiration syndrome** Obstruction and air trapping caused by meconium in the infant's lungs, which may cause severe respiratory distress.

**meiosis** Reduction cell division in gametes that halves the number of chromosomes in each cell.

**melasma** Brownish pigmentation of the face during pregnancy, also called *chloasma* or "*mask of pregnancy.*"

**melena** Rectal passage of black, tarry stools, indicating denatured blood from the upper gastrointestinal tract.

**menarche** Onset of menstruation.

**menometrorrhagia** Uterine bleeding that is irregular in frequency and excessive in amount.

**menopause** Permanent cessation of menstruation during the climacteric.

**metered-dose inhaler** Hand-held device that delivers "puffs" of medication for inhalation.

**methadone** A synthetic compound with opiate properties used as an oral substitute for heroin and morphine in the opiate-dependent person.

**metritis** Infection of the decidua, myometrium, and parametrial tissues of the uterus.

**metrorrhagia** Bleeding from the uterus at any time other than during the menstrual period.

**milia** White cysts, 1 mm in size, from distended sebaceous glands.

**milk-ejection reflex** Release of milk from the alveoli into the ducts. Also called the *let-down reflex.*

**mimicry** Copying the behaviors of other pregnant women or mothers as a method of "trying on" the role of advanced pregnancy or motherhood.

**mistrust** The negative resolution of the first developmental task, according to Erikson's theory; results in acute emotional tension and behavioral signs of unmet needs.

**mitosis** Cell division in body cells other than the gametes.

**mittelschmerz** Low abdominal pain that occurs at ovulation.

**molding** Shaping of fetal head during movement through the birth canal.

**Mongolian spots** Bruise-like marks that occur mostly in newborns with dark skin tones.

**monosomy** Presence of only one of a chromosome pair in every body cell.

**Monro-Kellie doctrine** Theory describing the compensatory mechanism of the cranial contents to maintain a steady volume and pressure.

**Montevideo units** A method to quantify intensity of labor contractions with internal uterine activity monitoring. The baseline intrauterine pressure for each contraction in a 10-minute period is subtracted from the peak pressure. The resulting net pressures (peak minus baseline) are added to calculate Montevideo units or MVUs.

**mood** A pervasive and sustained emotion.

**mood disorder** Recurrent disturbances or alterations in mood that inhibit functioning or cause distress.
**morbidity** Ratio of sick to well persons in a defined population.
**motor block** Loss of voluntary movement caused by regional anesthesia.
**multifetal pregnancy** A pregnancy in which the woman is carrying two or more fetuses. Also called *multiple gestation.*
**multigravida** A woman who has been pregnant more than once.
**multipara** A woman who has delivered two or more pregnancies at 20 or more weeks of gestation.
**multiple-marker screening** Analysis of maternal serum for abnormal levels of alpha-fetoprotein, human chorionic gonadotropin, and estriols that may predict chromosomal abnormalities of the fetus; often called *triple-screen* or *quad screen.* Addition of tests such as inhibin A have improved accuracy of the results, leading to alternate names for the package of tests.
**mutation** Change in a gene that usually affects its function. Mutations may be in either the gametes or somatic cells.
**myelinization** Formation of the proteolipid coating of the nerves that facilitates conduction of impulses.
**myocardial contractility** Ability of myocardial cells and tissues to shorten in response to an appropriate stimulus; force of contraction of the myocardium.
**myopia** Nearsightedness; abnormal distance vision.

## N

**nadir** Lowest point, such as the lowest pulse rate in a series.
**narcissism** Undue preoccupation with oneself.
**nasal flaring** A serious sign of air hunger demonstrated by widening of the nares to enable an infant or a young child to take in more oxygen.
**nasal polyps** Semitransparent herniations of respiratory epithelium.
**natural family planning** Method of predicting ovulation based on normal changes in a woman's body.
**necrotizing enterocolitis** Serious inflammatory condition of the intestines.
**negativism** The attitude of opposing or resisting the directions of others.
**negligence** Failure to act in the way a reasonable, prudent person of similar background would act in similar circumstances.
**neonatal abstinence syndrome** A cluster of physical signs exhibited by newborns exposed *in utero* to maternal use of substances such as heroin.
**neonatal mortality rate** Number of deaths per 1000 live births that occur before 28 days of life.
**neural tube defect (NTD)** A congenital defect in the closure of the bony encasement of the spinal cord or of the skull.
**neurons** Structural units (cells) of the nervous system that function to initiate and conduct impulses.
**neuropathic pain** Pain resulting from trauma or disease that damages the peripheral nerves or the central nervous system.
**neutral thermal environment** Environment in which body temperature is maintained without an increase in metabolic rate or oxygen use.
**neutropenia** Decrease in the number of circulating neutrophils that results in a decreased ability of the body to fight infection.
**nevus flammeus** Permanent purple birthmark; also called *port-wine stain.*
**nevus simplex (salmon patch, stork bites)** Flat, pink areas on the nape of the neck, forehead, or eyelids resulting from dilation of the capillaries.
**nevus vasculosus** Rough, red collection of capillaries with a raised surface that disappears with time. Also called *strawberry hemangioma.*
**nociceptive** Impulse from a specific body area that gives rise to the sensation of pain.
**noncompliance** Resistance of the lungs and thorax to distention with air during respirations.
**nonheme iron** Iron obtained from plants and fortified foods.
**nonnutritive sucking** Sucking during which little or no milk flow is obtained or sucking on an object such as a pacifier or finger.
**nonshivering thermogenesis** Process of heat production, without shivering, by oxidation of brown fat.
**nonstress test (NST)** A method for evaluating fetal status during the antepartum period by observing for accelerations of the fetal heart rate.
**normalization** Responses used to counteract an illness or abnormal behavior to maintain appropriate and valued social roles.
**nuchal cord** Umbilical cord around the fetal neck.
**nullipara** A woman who has never completed a pregnancy beyond 20 weeks of gestation.
**nurse anesthetist** A registered nurse who has advanced education and certification in administration of anesthetics. Also called a *certified registered nurse anesthetist (CRNA).*
**nurse practice acts** Laws that determine the scope of nursing practice in each state.
**nursing diagnosis** A clinical judgment related to individual, family, or community responses to actual or potential health problems and to normal life processes.
**nutrient density** Quantity and quality of protein, vitamins, and minerals per 100 calories in foods.
**nutrients** Foods that supply the body with elements necessary for metabolism.
**nutritive suckling or sucking** Steady, rhythmic suckling at the breast or sucking at a bottle to obtain milk.
**nystagmus** Involuntary eye movements that make the eyes appear to be darting back and forth.

## O

**object permanence** The realization that objects continue to exist even though they are out of sight.
**occult blood** Blood in such minute quantity that it can be recognized only by microscopic or chemical means.
**occult prolapse** See *prolapsed cord.*
**oligohydramnios** Abnormally small volume of amniotic fluid (less than 500 mL at term).
**oligospermia** A decreased number of sperm in semen, usually considered to be fewer than 20 million per milliliter.
**oliguria** Diminished urine output.
**ophthalmia neonatorum** Conjunctivitis noted in the first few weeks of life; usually gonococcal or chlamydial.
**opioid** Natural and synthetic agonists and antagonist with morphine-like activity.
**opportunistic infection** An infection that occurs as a result of a weakened immune system.
**oral contraceptive** Drug that inhibits ovulation; contains progestins alone or in combination with estrogen.
**orthopnea** Difficulty breathing except in an upright position.
**osmotic diuresis** Secretion and passage of large amounts of urine as a result of increased osmotic pressure that can result from hyperglycemia.
**ossification** The process of forming bone from osseous tissue or cartilage.
**osteoporosis** Increased spaces (porosity) in bone; process greatly accelerates following menopause.
**osteotomy** Surgical cutting of bone.
**ovovegetarian** A vegetarian whose diet includes eggs.
**oxytocin** Hormone produced by the posterior pituitary gland that stimulates uterine contractions and the milk-ejection reflex; also prepared synthetically.
**oxytocin challenge test (OCT)** Method for evaluating fetal status during the antepartum period by observing the response of the fetal heart to intermittent stress of induced uterine contractions. Also known as *contraction stress test (CST).*

## P

**pain** An unpleasant sensory and emotional experience associated with actual or potential tissue damage or described in terms of such damage. Pain is whatever the person experiencing the pain says it is, existing whenever the person says it does.
**pain perception (or pain threshold)** The lowest level of stimulus one perceives as painful. Pain perception is relatively constant under different conditions.
**pain tolerance** Maximum pain one is willing to endure. Pain tolerance may increase or decrease under different conditions.
**palliative care** Medical treatments or procedures that aim to promote comfort and quality of life rather than cure the underlying disease.
**palliative therapy** Medical and nursing care that either slows the progression of disease or increases the patient's comfort but is not curative.
**palpation** The use of touch to determine factors such as texture, temperature, moisture, and organ size and location.
**pancytopenia** A reduction in all types of blood cells.

**papilledema** Edema of the optic disk.

**para** Number of pregnancies that have progressed to 20 or more weeks at delivery, whether the fetus was born alive or stillborn; refers to the number of pregnancies not the number of fetuses.

**parallel play** Playing alongside but not with other children.

**parent–infant attachment** A sense of belonging to or connection between a parent and an infant.

**paresthesia** Sensation of numbness and tingling.

**passive immunity** Protection that occurs when serum containing an antibody is given or transmitted to a person who does not have that antibody.

**pathogen** A disease-producing microorganism.

**peau d'orange** Dimpled skin condition that resembles an orange; associated with lymphatic edema and often seen over the area of breast cancer.

**phenotype** Outward expression of one's genetic makeup.

**percussion** Tapping of the body to determine the density, location, and size of organs.

**percutaneous umbilical blood sampling (cordocentesis)** Procedure for obtaining fetal blood through ultrasound-guided puncture of an umbilical cord vessel to detect fetal problems such as inherited blood disorders, acidosis, or infection.

**perimenopause** Time from onset of symptoms associated with the climacteric until at least 1 year after the last menstrual period.

**periodic breathing** Cessation of breathing lasting 5 to 10 seconds followed by 10 to 15 seconds of rapid respirations without changes in color or heart rate.

**peripherally inserted central catheter (PICC)** Central line that is inserted peripherally (usually through a vein of the upper arm) into the superior vena cava.

**peristalsis** Progressive, wave-like movements caused by contraction and relaxation of the longitudinal and circular muscles of the gastrointestinal tract; propels a bolus of food or fluid forward.

**persistent pulmonary hypertension of the newborn (PPHN)** Vasoconstriction of the infant's pulmonary vessels after birth; may result in right-to-left shunting of blood flow through the ductus arteriosus, the foramen ovale, or both.

**pervasive developmental disorder** See *autism spectrum disorder.*

**petechiae** Tiny (less than 3 mm), nonblanching red spots that are the result of intradermal hemorrhage, often associated with a low platelet count.

**pharmacodynamics** Behavior of medications at the cellular level.

**pharmacokinetics** The time and movement relationships of medications.

**phenotype** Physical manifestation of DNA genetic code, such as eye color, height, and facial features.

**phimosis** Tightening of the prepuce.

**phosphatidylglycerol (PG)** A phospholipid component of surfactant; its presence in amniotic fluid indicates fetal lung maturity.

**phosphatidylinositol (PI)** A phospholipid component of surfactant that is produced and secreted in increasing amounts as the fetal lungs mature.

**physiologic anemia of pregnancy** Decrease in hemoglobin and hematocrit values caused by dilution of erythrocytes in expanded plasma volume rather than by an actual decrease in erythrocytes. Also *pseudoanemia of pregnancy.*

**physiologic anorexia** Decreased appetite because of relatively decreased caloric need.

**pica** Ingestion of nonnutritive substances, such as laundry starch, clay, or ice.

**pincer grasp** The use of index finger and thumb to grip objects.

**pituitary** An endocrine gland attached to the base of the brain that secretes numerous hormones, including thyroid-stimulating hormone, growth hormone, adrenocorticotropic hormone, antidiuretic hormone, prolactin, oxytocin, luteinizing hormone, and follicle-stimulating hormone.

**placenta** Fetal structure that provides nourishment to and removes wastes from the developing baby and secretes hormones necessary for the pregnancy to continue.

**placenta accreta** A placenta that is abnormally adherent to the uterine muscle. If the condition is more advanced, it is called *placenta increta* (the placenta extends into the uterine muscle) or *placenta percreta* (the placenta extends through the uterine muscle).

**placenta increta** A placenta that penetrates the uterine muscle.

**placenta percreta** A placenta that grows all the way through the uterine muscle.

**placenta previa** Abnormal implantation of the placenta in the lower uterus, at or near the cervical os.

**plagiocephaly** Flattening or asymmetry of the head.

**point of maximum impulse** Area of the chest in which the heart sounds are loudest when auscultated.

**polycythemia** Abnormally high number of erythrocytes.

**polydactyly** More than 10 digits on the hands or feet.

**polydipsia** Excessive thirst.

**polymerase chain reaction (PCR)** A technique to amplify a piece of DNA, generating thousands of copies of specific DNA sequences for diagnosis of infections; many hereditary characteristics can also be analyzed by the technique.

**polymorphism** Gene having two or more alternate forms (alleles), each of which occurs in more than 1% of the population.

**polyphagia** Excessive ingestion of food.

**polyploidy** Having additional full sets of chromosomes.

**polyuria** Excessive excretion of urine.

**position** Relation of a fixed reference point on the fetus to the quadrants of the maternal pelvis.

**postmaturity syndrome** Condition in which a postterm infant shows characteristics indicative of poor placental functioning before birth. Also called *dysmaturity syndrome.*

**postpartum** Refers to the first 6 weeks after childbirth.

**postpartum blues** Temporary, self-limited period of tearfulness experienced by many new mothers beginning in the 1st week after childbirth. Also called *baby blues* or *maternity blues.*

**postterm infant** An infant born after 42 weeks of gestation.

**posttraumatic stress disorder** Psychologic and cognitive disorder that results from exposure to an overwhelming traumatic event.

**precipitate birth** A birth that occurs without a trained attendant present.

**precipitate labor** An intense, unusually short labor (less than 3 hours).

**preeclampsia** A hypertensive disorder of pregnancy characterized by hypertension and proteinuria.

**pregnancy wastage** Repeated loss of pregnancies before the fetus is old enough to survive.

**pregnancy-related death ratio** Refers to the number of deaths per 100,000 women during pregnancy or within one year after pregnancy has ended.

**preload** Amount of stretch of the myocardial fibers before contraction; most easily measured by determining central venous pressure.

**premature rupture of the membranes** Spontaneous rupture of the membranes before the onset of labor. The gestation may be term, preterm, or postterm.

**preparation** Provision of information before procedures, treatments, or events; facilitates coping.

**presentation** Fetal part that first enters the pelvic inlet; also, the presenting part.

**preterm birth** A birth that occurs after the 20th week and before the start of the 38th week of gestation.

**preterm infant** An infant born before the beginning of the 38th week of gestation. Also called *premature infant.*

**preterm labor** Onset of labor after 20 weeks and before the beginning of the 38th week of gestation.

**primary sexual characteristics** Internal and external reproductive organs in males and females (i.e., uterus, fallopian tubes, ovaries, vagina, vulva, penis, testes, spermatic cord).

**primigravida** A woman who is pregnant for the first time.

**primipara** A woman who has delivered one pregnancy of at least 20 weeks.

**prodrome** The initial stage of a disease; symptoms indicating an approaching disease.

**progestin** Any natural or synthetic form of progesterone.

**projectile vomiting** Vomiting that is projected with force, perhaps 2 to 4 feet away from the mouth; may be preceded by deep gastric left to right peristaltic waves characteristic of pyloric stenosis.

**prolactin** Anterior pituitary hormone that promotes growth of breast tissue and stimulates production of milk.

**prolapsed cord** Displacement of the umbilical cord in front of or beside the fetal presenting part. An occult prolapse is one that is suspected on the basis of fetal heart rate patterns; the umbilical cord cannot be palpated or seen.
**proteinuria** Protein in the urine.
**protocol** A systematic plan of care outlining drug therapy and follow-up care based on research in cancer treatment.
**proximodistal** Progression from the center outward or from the midline to the periphery.
**pruritus** Itching.
**pseudomenstruation** Vaginal bleeding in the newborn, resulting from withdrawal of placental hormones.
**psychosis** Mental state in which a person's ability to recognize reality, communicate, and relate to others is impaired.
**ptyalism** Excess salivation.
**puberty** Period of time during which adolescents experience a growth spurt, develop secondary sexual characteristics, and achieve reproductive maturity.
**puerperal infection** A temperature of 38°C (100.4°F) or higher after the first 24 hours and occurring on at least 2 of the first 10 days following childbirth.
**puerperium** Period from the end of childbirth until involution of the reproductive organs is complete, approximately 6 weeks.
**pulmonary edema** Collection of excessive fluid in the alveoli of the lungs.
**pulmonary embolus** A potentially fatal complication that occurs when the pulmonary artery is obstructed by a blood clot that was swept into circulation from a vein or by amniotic fluid.
**pulmonary hypertension** Increased pressure in the pulmonary arteries and arterioles.
**pulmonary vascular resistance** Amount of resistance in the pulmonary vascular bed against which the right ventricle must pump to achieve blood flow to the lungs.
**pulse oximetry** Method of determining the level of blood oxygen saturation by sensors attached to the skin.
**pulse pressure** The difference between systolic and diastolic blood pressures.
**purpura** Larger (greater than 3 mm) areas of nonblanching red, blue, or purplish spots that are the result of intradermal hemorrhage (bruising), often a result of a low platelet count.
**pylorus** The distal opening of the stomach where the stomach contents pass into the duodenum; the pylorus is surrounded by muscle bands.
**pyramidal motor system (tract)** Descending pathway of the upper motor neuron concerned with voluntary movement.
**pyrogens** Substances that cause fever.
**pyrosis** Heartburn.

## Q

**quickening** The first movements of the fetus felt by the mother.

## R

**reciprocal attachment behaviors** Repertoire of infant behaviors that promotes attachment between parent and newborn.
**recommended dietary allowance (RDA)** Level of intake of a nutrient considered to meet the needs of healthy individuals.
**rectocele** Herniation (protrusion) of the rectum through the posterior vaginal wall.
**reduction** Repositioning of bone fragments into normal alignment followed by application of a device or mechanism that maintains alignment of bone until healing occurs.
**REEDA** Acronym for redness, ecchymosis, edema, discharge, and approximation. Useful for assessing wound healing or the presence of inflammation or infection.
**refeeding syndrome** A fluid and metabolic disturbance that results from introducing nutrition too rapidly to someone who has been starving; occurs most commonly in people who have lost weight rapidly.
**refractive error** Light rays passing through eye structures come into focus at an inappropriate location relative to the retina.
**regional anesthesia** Anesthesia that blocks pain impulses in a localized area without loss of consciousness.
**regression** Appearance of behavior more appropriate to an earlier stage of development; often used to cope with stress or anxiety.
**respiratory distress syndrome** Condition caused by insufficient production of surfactant in the lungs; results in atelectasis, hypoxia, and hypercapnia (increased carbon dioxide [$CO_2$]).
**respite care** The provision of temporary relief of care responsibly to people who are caring for a family member at home who might otherwise need permanent hospital or residential care.
**retention** The application of a device or mechanism that maintains alignment until healing occurs.
**reticulocyte** Immature red blood cell.
**reticuloendothelial system** The collection of cells, throughout the body, that is capable of phagocytosis.
**retinopathy of prematurity** Condition in which damage to blood vessels in the retina may cause decreased vision or blindness.
**retractions** An abnormal movement of the chest wall during inspiration that may occur intercostally and substernally.
**retrograde ejaculation** Discharge of semen into the bladder rather than from the end of the penis.
**rhonchi** Adventitious breath sounds caused by the passage of air through an airway obstructed by thick secretions; sounds usually clear with coughing.
**risk-taking behaviors** Behaviors that predispose the adolescent to physical or psychosocial harm.
**ritualism** The need to maintain sameness and reliability.
**role transition** Changing from one pattern of behavior and one image of self to another.
**ruga (pl. rugae)** Ridge or fold of tissue, as on the male's scrotum and in the female's vagina.

## S

**salpingectomy** Surgical removal of a fallopian tube.
**second period of reactivity** Period after the first sleep following birth when the newborn may have an elevated pulse and respiratory rate and excessive mucus.
**secondary glaucoma** Increased intraocular fluid pressure that occurs after 3 years of age and may be the result of disease or surgery.
**secondary sexual characteristics** Physical characteristics of males and females influenced by reproductive hormones but having no direct role in reproduction (i.e., voice, body shape, pubic hair distribution, breasts).
**self-care children** Children who care for themselves at home after school; formerly called *latch-key children*.
**self-esteem** Personal value that individuals place on themselves.
**semen** Spermatozoa with their nourishing and protective fluid, discharged at ejaculation.
**seminal fluid** Nourishes, protects, and carries sperm into the vagina until they enter the cervix.
**sensorimotor stage** Piaget's first stage of cognitive development, in which infants and young toddlers use mainly senses and movement to begin to understand and control their environment.
**sensorineural hearing loss** Result of damage or malformation of the middle ear or auditory nerve; hearing loss is usually permanent.
**sensory block** Loss of sensation caused by regional anesthesia.
**sensory information** Information gained from sight, taste, touch, smell, and hearing.
**separation anxiety** Distress and apprehension caused by being removed from parents, home, or familiar surroundings.
**seroconversion** Change in a blood test result from negative to positive, indicating the development of antibodies in response to infection or immunization.
**servocontrol** Mechanism on a radiant warmer or incubator to regulate the amount of heat produced.
**sex chromosome** X or Y chromosome. Females have two X chromosomes; males have one X and one Y chromosome.
**sexual maturity rating** Stages of sexual maturation based on pubic hair and breast development in girls and pubic hair and genital development in boys.
**shock** Inadequate tissue perfusion, usually caused by illness or injury that results in respiratory or cardiovascular compromise.
**shoulder dystocia** Delayed or difficult birth of the fetal shoulders after the head is born.
**shunt** Abnormal blood flow from one part of the circulation to another.
**situational crisis** Unanticipated event that poses a threat to an individual's psychosocial or psychologic well-being.
**small-for-gestational-age infant** An infant whose size is below the 10th percentile for gestational age.
**somatic cells** Body cells other than the gametes or germ cells.
**spermatogenesis** Formation of male gametes (sperm) in the testes.

**spinnbarkeit** Clear, slippery, stretchy quality of cervical mucus during ovulation.

**standard of care** Level of care that can be expected of a professional. This level is determined by laws, professional organizations, and healthcare agencies.

**Standard Precautions** Infection control guidelines developed by the National Center for Infectious Disease and the Hospital Control Practices Advisory Committee to prevent the spread of infectious organisms from blood, body fluids, secretions and excretions, mucous membranes, and nonintact skin.

**standardized procedures** Procedures determined by nurses, physicians, and administrators that allow nurses to perform duties, usually a part of the medical practice.

**station** Measurement of fetal descent in relation to the ischial spines of the maternal pelvis. See also *engagement.*

**stereopsis** Ability to see dimensions and perceive depth that results from convergence of visual images received by each eye.

**stomatitis** Painful inflammation of the mucous membranes lining the mouth and are often associated with oral ulcerations as a result of chemotherapy.

**strabismus** A turning inward ("crossing") or outward of the eyes caused by poor tone in the muscles that control eye movement.

**stranger anxiety** The infant's ability to distinguish between caregivers and others, to prefer parents to other caregivers, and to become distressed when separation occurs.

**stress** Any situation or condition, positive or negative, requiring adjustment on the part of the individual, family, or group.

**striae gravidarum** Irregular pink to purple streaks on the abdomen, breasts, or buttocks, resulting from tears in the connective tissue.

**stridor** A shrill, harsh sound that can be heard during inspiration, expiration, or both; produced by the flow of air through a narrowed segment of the respiratory tract.

**subarachnoid space** Space between the arachnoid mater and the pia mater that contains the cerebrospinal fluid.

**subconjunctival hemorrhages** Bleeding situated beneath the conjunctiva; in children, the most frequent cause is trauma or severe coughing or sneezing episodes (Valsalva maneuvers); also caused by infection with *Streptococcus pneumoniae* or *Haemophilus influenzae.*

**subinvolution** Delayed return of the uterus to its nonpregnant size and consistency.

**subluxation** Partial dislocation of a joint.

**submersion injury** Injury resulting from a near-drowning incident; may be immediately apparent or appear up to 48 hours after the submersion incident.

**substance abuse** Use of medications, drugs, or other substances beyond their intended or prescribed purpose. Use of substances for the purposes of intoxication, mood modification, or behavior change.

**suckling** Giving or taking nourishment from the breast. Sometimes used interchangeably with sucking, which refers to drawing into the mouth with a partial vacuum, as with a bottle or pacifier.

**suicide potential** Assessment of the individual's risk toward self-harm to end life. Includes suicidal ideation, gestures, threats, impulses, attempts, and self-termination of life.

**surfactant** A mixture of lipoproteins produced by mature fetal lungs that reduces surface tension in the alveoli, thus promoting lung expansion after birth.

**sutures** Narrow areas of flexible tissue that connect the fetal skull bones, permitting slight movement during labor.

**symbolic play** Use of games and interactions that represent an issue or a concern to be addressed.

**symbolic thought** The ability to allow a mental image (word or object) to represent something that is not present.

**syndactyly** Webbing between fingers or toes.

**systematic assessment** Organized method of collecting data.

**systemic vascular resistance** Amount of resistance in the systemic vascular bed against which the left ventricle must pump to achieve cardiac output.

## T

**tachypnea** Respiratory rate greater than 60 breaths per minute in the newborn after the first hour of life.

**taking-hold phase** Second phase of maternal adaptation, during which the mother assumes control of her own care and initiates care of the infant.

**taking-in phase** First phase of maternal adaptation, during which the mother passively accepts care and comfort and details about the newborn.

**telemetry** Wireless transmission of electronic fetal monitoring data to a bedside or central monitor unit.

**tenesmus** Ineffective, painful, or continuous urge to defecate.

**teratogen** Agent that can cause defects in a developing baby during pregnancy.

**term** The end of pregnancy. Full term is between 38 and 42 weeks of gestation.

**term birth** A birth that occurs between the 38th and 42nd weeks of gestation.

**therapeutic play** Guided play that promotes the child's psychophysiologic well-being.

**therapeutic relationship** A balance between appropriate involvement and professional separation in relation to child/family interactions.

**thermoregulation** Maintenance of body temperature.

**thrombocytopenia** A reduction in platelet count; places the individual at risk for increased bruising and bleeding.

**thrombophlebitis** Inflammation of a vein with secondary clot formation.

**thrombus** Collection of blood factors, primarily platelets and fibrin, that may cause vascular obstruction.

**time-release medication** Medication taken in a single dose but designed to dissolve slowly, releasing medication into the bloodstream over a specified period of time (usually 12 to 24 hours).

**tocolytic** A drug that inhibits uterine contractions.

**tolerable upper intake level** The highest amount of a nutrient that can be taken without probable adverse health effects by most people.

**total parenteral nutrition** Intravenous infusion of nutrients known to be needed for metabolism and growth.

**toxic shock syndrome** Rare, potentially fatal disorder caused by toxin produced by *Staphylococcus aureus*; has been associated with improper use of tampons.

**transducer** A device that translates one physical quantity into another, such as fetal heart motion into an electrical signal for rate calculation, generation of sound, or a written record.

**transductive reasoning** Reasoning from the particular to the particular rather than from the general to the particular.

**transient tachypnea of the newborn** Condition of rapid respirations caused by inadequate absorption of fetal lung fluid.

**transitional milk** The breast milk that appears between the secretion of colostrum and mature milk.

**translocation** Attachment of all or part of a chromosome to another chromosome.

**trauma score** Numeric score assessed by healthcare providers to determine the extent of trauma; usually results from adding, subtracting, dividing, or multiplying numbers representing physiologic parameters or specific types of injuries; used for field triage and serially assessed to determine whether a person's condition is improving or deteriorating; also correlated with survivability.

**traumatic brain injuries** One of the leading causes of death or permanent disability; severity of injury may range from mild to severe; can result in short- and long-term disabilities.

**triage** Sorting process used to decide the urgency of an individual's illness or injury and effectively allocate appropriate resources; purpose is to ensure that the most seriously ill or injured people receive the appropriate level of care before those with less urgent or emergent conditions.

**trimester** A division of pregnancy; one of three equal parts of approximately 13 weeks each.

**trisomy** Presence of three copies of a chromosome in each body cell.

**trophic feedings** Very small feedings designed to help the gastrointestinal tract mature. Also called *minimal enteral feedings.*

**trust** The basic emotion established during infancy as a result of satisfying interactions between child and caregiver; provides the foundation on which a healthy personality is built.

**tunneled central line** A surgically placed central line that is held in place by a Dacron polyester cuff located in a subcutaneous tunnel; most commonly placed in the external jugular vein.

## U

**ultrasound** Technique for visualizing deep structures of the body by recording the reflections (echoes) of sound waves directed into the tissue.

**urgency** Sudden urge to urinate.

**uterine atony** Decreased uterine muscle contraction; a primary cause of excessive bleeding.

**uterine inversion** Turning of the uterus inside out after the birth of the fetus.

**uterine resting tone** Degree of uterine muscle tension when the woman is not in labor or during the interval between labor contractions.

**uterine rupture** A tear in the uterus wall.

**uterine souffle** Sound of blood flow through the uterine vessels, corresponds to the maternal pulse.

**uteroplacental insufficiency** Decreased ability of the placenta to properly exchange oxygen, carbon dioxide, nutrients, and waste products between the maternal and fetal circulations.

**utilitarian theory** Ethical theory that holds that the right course of action is the one that produces the greatest good.

## V

**vacuum aspiration (vacuum curettage)** Removal of the uterine contents by applying a vacuum through a hollow curet or cannula introduced into the uterus.

**valgum** Abnormal position of a limb in which it is bent away from the midline of the body.

**validate** To make certain that the information collected during assessment is accurate.

**valvuloplasty** Mechanical procedure to open a valve.

**varum** Abnormal position of the limb in which it is bent toward the midline of the body.

**vasoconstriction** Narrowing of the lumen of blood vessels.

**vector** A carrier that transfers an infective agent from one host to another.

**vegan** A complete vegetarian who does not eat any animal products.

**vegetarian** An individual whose diet consists wholly or mostly of plant foods and who avoids animal food sources.

**vernix caseosa** Thick, white substance that protects the skin of the fetus.

**version** Turning the fetus from one presentation to another before birth, usually from breech to cephalic.

**very-low-birth-weight infant** An infant weighing 1500 g (3 lb, 5 oz) or less at birth.

**vibroacoustic stimulation** Use of sound and vibration to elicit the acceleration of the fetal heart rate.

**violence** The use of force or a destructive action that results in injury, discordance, shame, or outrage; engaging in sudden intense activity to the point of loss of control.

**virulence** Strength of effect produced by a pathogenic organism.

**visual acuity** Clarity of vision; tested through the use of vision charts, with results compared with what a person with normal vision can see at a distance of 10 or 20 feet.

## W

**wheezing** High-pitched, musical whistles that can be heard with or without a stethoscope; may be inspiratory or expiratory; caused by bronchial constriction or obstruction of the airway and commonly occurs in asthma.

**Wood light** Ultraviolet light used to help diagnose fluorescent skin lesions, including some superficial fungal infections.

## Z

**zygote** Cell formed by union of an ovum and a sperm.

# INDEX



Page numbers followed by "*f*" indicate figures, "*t*" indicate tables, and "*b*" indicate boxes.

## B

## C

## F

## G

## H

## I

## M

## N

## O

## P

## V